GERIATRIC DOSAGE HANDBOOK

Including Clinical Recommendations and Monitoring Guidelines

Todd P. Semla, PharmD, BCPS, FCCP
Judith L. Beizer, PharmD, CGP, FASCP
Martin D. Higbee, PharmD

Lexi-Comp is the official drug reference for the American Pharmacists Association

APhA

13th Edition

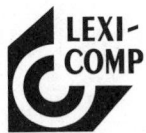

LEXI-COMP

GERIATRIC DOSAGE HANDBOOK

Including Clinical Recommendations
and Monitoring Guidelines

Todd P. Semla, BCPS, FCCP
Joseph T. Barbe, PharmD, CGP, FASCP
Martin S. Hoffman, PharmD

GERIATRIC DOSAGE HANDBOOK

Including Clinical Recommendations and Monitoring Guidelines

Todd P. Semla, PharmD, BCPS, FCCP
Clinical Pharmacy Specialist
Department of Veterans Affairs
Pharmacy Benefits Management
Associate Professor of Clinical Psychiatry
Feinberg School of Medicine
Northwestern University
Chicago, Illinois

Judith L. Beizer, PharmD, CGP, FASCP
Clinical Professor
Department of Clinical Pharmacy Practice
St John's University College of Pharmacy and Allied Health Professions
Jamaica, New York

Martin D. Higbee, PharmD
Associate Professor
Department of Pharmacy Practice and Science
The University of Arizona
Tucson, Arizona

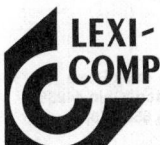

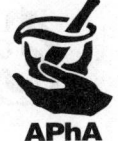

NOTICE

This data is intended to serve the user as a handy reference and not as a complete drug information resource. It does not include information on every therapeutic agent available. The publication covers over 850 commonly used drugs and is specifically designed to present important aspects of drug data in a more concise format than is typically found in medical literature or product material supplied by manufacturers.

The nature of drug information is that it is constantly evolving because of ongoing research and clinical experience and is often subject to interpretation. While great care has been taken to ensure the accuracy of the information and recommendations presented, the reader is advised that the authors, editors, reviewers, contributors, and publishers cannot be responsible for the continued currency of the information or for any errors, omissions, or the application of this information, or for any consequences arising therefrom. Therefore, the author(s) and/or the publisher shall have no liability to any person or entity with regard to claims, loss, or damage caused, or alleged to be caused, directly or indirectly, by the use of information contained herein. Because of the dynamic nature of drug information, readers are advised that decisions regarding drug therapy must be based on the independent judgment of the clinician, changing information about a drug (eg, as reflected in the literature and manufacturer's most current product information), and changing medical practices. Therefore, this data is designed to be used in conjunction with other necessary information and is not designed to be solely relied upon by any user. The user of this data hereby and forever releases the authors and publishers of this data from any and all liability of any kind that might arise out of the use of this data. The editors are not responsible for any inaccuracy of quotation or for any false or misleading implication that may arise due to the text or formulas as used or due to the quotation of revisions no longer official.

Certain of the authors, editors, and contributors have written this book in their private capacities. No official support or endorsement by any federal or state agency or pharmaceutical company is intended or inferred.

The publishers have made every effort to trace any third party copyright holders, if any, for borrowed material. If they have inadvertently overlooked any, they will be pleased to make the necessary arrangements at the first opportunity.

If you have any suggestions or questions regarding any information presented in this data, please contact our drug information pharmacists at (330) 650-6506.

This manual was produced using Lexi-Comp's Information Management System™ (LIMS) — A complete publishing service of Lexi-Comp Inc.

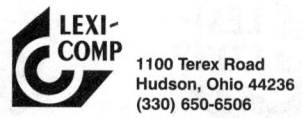

LEXI-COMP

1100 Terex Road
Hudson, Ohio 44236
(330) 650-6506

ISBN 978-1-59195-226-8

TABLE OF CONTENTS

TABLE OF CONTENTS *(Continued)*

PREFACE

The *Geriatric Dosage Handbook* is designed to be a practical and convenient guide to the dosing and usage of medications in the geriatric population. As the percentage of the population over the age of 65 increases, most healthcare professionals will be faced with the challenge of the appropriate use of medications in older adults.

Many physiologic changes occur with aging, some of which affect the pharmacokinetics and/or pharmacodynamics of medications. For the majority of drugs, exact dosing guidelines for geriatric patients have not been established and most references do not specifically address the use of medications in older adults. For practical purposes, it has been recommended to "start low, go slow." Our objective in producing this handbook is to refine this recommendation and provide the reader with specific considerations when using medications in older adults. Information has been compiled from the current literature and our clinical experiences, emphasizing choice of medication, dosing, changes in pharmacokinetics or pharmacodynamics, monitoring parameters, and adverse effects. References are listed at the end of some drug monographs to support this information. Additional clinical drug information which is relevant to the practice of geriatric pharmacotherapy is also included in each monograph and in the appendices.

With each edition, newly approved medications that would be used in the geriatric population are added. Additionally, dosage forms, indications, and adverse effects are updated, as information becomes available. The appendix information is updated to include new treatment algorithms and tables.

With this newest edition, we hope this reference continues to be a valuable and practical source of clinical drug information for healthcare professionals caring for older adults. We welcome comments to improve future editions.

ACKNOWLEDGMENTS

The *Geriatric Dosage Handbook* exists in its present form as the result of the concerted efforts of the following individuals: Robert D. Kerscher, publisher and chief executive officer of Lexi-Comp, Inc; Steven Kerscher, president and chief operating officer; Mark Bonfiglio, BS, PharmD, RPh, chief content officer; Stacy S. Robinson, editorial manager; Robin L. Farabee, project manager; David C. Marcus, chief information officer; Amy Van Orman, PharmD, pharmacotherapy specialist; Tracey J. Henterly, senior graphic designer; Alexandra Hart, composition specialist; Leslie Jo Hoppes, pharmacology database manager.

Special acknowledgment goes to all Lexi-Comp staff for their contributions to this handbook.

Special thanks goes to Chris Lomax, PharmD, director of pharmacy, Children's Hospital, Los Angeles, who played a significant role in bringing the American Pharmacists Association (APhA) and Lexi-Comp together.

Much of the material contained in this book was a result of pharmacy contributors throughout the United States and Canada. Lexi-Comp has assisted many medical institutions to develop hospital-specific formulary manuals that contain clinical drug information as well as dosing. Working with these clinical pharmacists, hospital pharmacy and therapeutics committees, and hospital drug information centers, Lexi-Comp has developed an evolutionary drug database that reflects the practice of pharmacy in these major institutions.

In addition, the authors wish to thank their families, friends, and colleagues who supported them in their efforts to complete this handbook.

EDITORIAL ADVISORY PANEL

EDITORIAL ADVISORY PANEL *(Continued)*

6

Lawrence A. Frazee, PharmD
Pharmacotherapy Specialist in Internal Medicine
Akron General Medical Center
Akron, Ohio

Matthew A. Fuller, PharmD, BCPS, BCPP, FASHP
Clinical Pharmacy Specialist, Psychiatry
Cleveland Department of Veterans Affairs Medical Center
Brecksville, Ohio
Associate Clinical Professor of Psychiatry
Clinical Instructor of Psychology
Case Western Reserve University
Cleveland, Ohio
Adjunct Associate Professor of Clinical Pharmacy
University of Toledo
Toledo, Ohio

Morton P. Goldman, PharmD
Director of Pharmacotherapy Services
The Cleveland Clinic Foundation
Cleveland, Ohio

Julie A. Golembiewski, PharmD
Clinical Associate Professor
Colleges of Pharmacy and Medicine
Clinical Pharmacist, Anesthesia/Pain
University of Illinois
Chicago, Illinois

Jeffrey P. Gonzales, PharmD, BCPS
Critical Care Clinical Pharmacy Specialist
University of Maryland Medical Center
Baltimore, Maryland

Roland Grad, MDCM, MSc, CCFP, FCFP
Department of Family Medicine
McGill University
Montreal, Quebec, Canada

Larry D. Gray, PhD, ABMM
Director of Clinical Microbiology
TriHealth
Bethesda and Good Samaritan Hospitals
Cincinnati, Ohio

Tracey Hagemann, PharmD
Associate Professor
College of Pharmacy
The University of Oklahoma
Oklahoma City, Oklahoma

Martin D. Higbee, PharmD
Associate Professor
Department of Pharmacy Practice and Science
The University of Arizona
Tucson, Arizona

Jane Hurlburt Hodding, PharmD
Director, Pharmacy
Miller Children's Hospital
Long Beach, California

Collin A. Hovinga, PharmD
Assistant Professor of Pharmacy and Pediatrics
College of Pharmacy
University of Tennessee Health Science Center
Memphis, Tennessee

EDITORIAL ADVISORY PANEL *(Continued)*

Jerrold B. Leikin, MD, FACP, FACEP, FACMT, FAACT
Director, Medical Toxicology
Evanston Northwestern Healthcare-OMEGA
Glenbrook Hospital
Glenview, Illinois
Associate Director
Toxikon Consortium at Cook County Hospital
Chicago, Illinois
Professor of Medicine
Pharmacology and Health Systems Management
Rush Medical College
Chicago, Ilinois
Professor of Medicine
Feinberg School of Medicine
Northwestern University
Chicago, Ilinois

Jeffrey D. Lewis, PharmD
Pharmacotherapy Specialist
Lexi-Comp, Inc
Hudson, Ohio

Laurie S. Mauro, BS, PharmD
Professor of Clinical Pharmacy
College of Pharmacy
Adjunct Associate Professor of Medicine
College of Medicine
The University of Toledo
Toledo, Ohio

Vincent F. Mauro, BS, PharmD, FCCP
Professor of Clinical Pharmacy
College of Pharmacy
Adjunct Professor of Medicine
College of Medicine
The University of Toledo
Toledo, Ohio

Barrie McCombs, MD, FCFP
Medical Information Service Coordinator
The Alberta Rural Physician Action Plan
Calgary, Alberta, Canada

Timothy F. Meiller, DDS, PhD
Professor
Diagnostic Sciences and Pathology
Baltimore College of Dental Surgery
Professor of Oncology
Greenebaum Cancer Center
University of Maryland Baltimore
Baltimore, Maryland

Michael A. Militello, PharmD, BCPS
Clinical Cardiology Specialist
Department of Pharmacy
The Cleveland Clinic Foundation
Cleveland, Ohio

Julie Miller, PharmD
Pharmacy Clinical Specialist, Cardiology
Columbus Children's Hospital
Columbus, Ohio

EDITORIAL ADVISORY PANEL *(Continued)*

Todd P. Semla, PharmD, BCPS, FCCP
Clinical Pharmacy Specialist
Department of Veterans Affairs
Pharmacy Benefits Management
Associate Professor of Clinical Psychiatry
Feinberg School of Medicine
Northwestern University
Chicago, Illinois

Joe Snoke, RPh
Clinical Coordinator
Department of Pharmacy
Akron General Medical Center
Akron, Ohio

Dominic A. Solimando, Jr, MA, FAPhA, FASHP, BCOP
Oncology Pharmacist
President, Oncology Pharmacy Services, Inc
Arlington, Virginia

Joni Lombardi Stahura, BS, PharmD, RPh
Pharmacotherapy Specialist
Lexi-Comp, Inc
Hudson, Ohio

Dan Streetman, PharmD, RPh
Pharmacotherapy Specialist
Lexi-Comp, Inc
Hudson, Ohio

Darcie-Ann Streetman, PharmD, RPh
Pharmacotherapy Specialist
Lexi-Comp, Inc
Hudson, Ohio

Carol K. Taketomo, PharmD
Pharmacy Manager
Children's Hospital Los Angeles
Los Angeles, California

Mary Temple, PharmD
Pediatric Clinical Research Specialist
Hillcrest Hospital
Mayfield Heights, Ohio

Elizabeth A. Tomsik, PharmD, BCPS
Pharmacotherapy Specialist
Lexi-Comp, Inc
Hudson, Ohio

Jennifer Trofe, PharmD
Clinical Transplant Pharmacist
Hospital of The University of Pennsylvania
Philadelphia, Pennsylvania

Beatrice B. Turkoski, RN, PhD
Associate Professor, Graduate Faculty
Advanced Pharmacology
College of Nursing
Kent State University
Kent, Ohio

Amy Van Orman, PharmD
Pharmacotherapy Specialist
Lexi-Comp, Inc
Hudson, Ohio

ABOUT THE AUTHORS

Todd P. Semla, MS, PharmD, BCPS, FCCP

Dr Semla received his Bachelor of Science in Pharmacy, his Master of Science in Clinical Pharmacy, and his Doctor of Pharmacy degrees from the University of Iowa. After earning his doctorate, Dr Semla was awarded the American Society of Health-System Pharmacists Fellowship in Geriatric Pharmacotherapy which he completed at the University of Iowa.

Dr Semla has more than 25 years experience in geriatric pharmacotherapy in a variety of clinical settings including ambulatory care, acute care and rehabilitation, and the nursing home. He is a Clinical Pharmacy Specialist in the Department of Veterans Affairs Pharmacy Benefits Management and an Associate Professor of Medicine and Clinical Psychiatry at the Feinberg School of Medicine, Northwestern University.

Dr Semla is the Editor for the section "Drugs and Pharmacology," for the *Journal of the American Geriatrics Society* and Chair of the Panel on Alzheimer's Disease for *The Annals of Pharmacotherapy*. He is an active member of several professional organizations, including the American College of Clinical Pharmacy (ACCP). He is currently President of the American Geriatrics Society.

Judith L. Beizer, PharmD, CGP, FASCP

Dr Beizer received her Bachelor of Science in Pharmacy from the St Louis College of Pharmacy and then earned a Doctor of Pharmacy degree from the University of Tennessee. After pursuing a residency in clinical pharmacy at the Hospital of the University of Pennsylvania, she completed a fellowship in geriatric pharmacy at Montefiore Medical Center, Bronx, NY. During her fellowship, Dr Beizer was involved in a National Institute on Aging (NIA) grant concerning medication use and pharmacist intervention in community-dwelling elderly.

Dr Beizer is a Clinical Professor in the Department of Clinical Pharmacy Practice at St John's University College of Pharmacy and Allied Health Professions. As part of her teaching responsibilities, she serves as the Clinical Pharmacist at the Center for Extended Care and Rehabilitation, a long-term care facility in Manhasset, NY. At this facility, Dr Beizer has expanded clinical pharmacy services and precepts pharmacy students. Dr Beizer speaks regularly on the topic of medication use in the elderly and has published articles and abstracts on various issues in geriatric pharmacotherapy.

Dr Beizer is a member of a number of professional organizations, including the American Society of Health-System Pharmacists (ASHP), American Society of Consultant Pharmacists (ASCP), American College of Clinical Pharmacy (ACCP), American Pharmacists Association (APhA), and the American Geriatrics Society (AGS). She currently serves as the President-Elect of ASCP. She previously served on the Board of Commissioners for the Commission for Certification in Geriatric Pharmacy. She is a past chairperson of the ASHP Special Interest Group on Geriatric Pharmacy Practice. Dr Beizer is on the Editorial Advisory Board of *The Consultant Pharmacist*.

ABOUT THE AUTHORS *(Continued)*

Martin D. Higbee, PharmD

Dr Higbee received his Bachelor of Science in Pharmacy from The University of Utah in 1973. After a year of pharmacy practice and clinical pharmacy experience at The University of Utah, he entered the Doctor of Pharmacy degree program at The University of Texas at San Antonio. After graduation in 1977, he joined the University of Utah College of Pharmacy faculty. He became involved in development of the Salt Lake Veteran Administration Medical Center's Geriatric Treatment and Evaluation Unit, and after the establishment of this unit, Dr Higbee created an ASHP accredited post-doctoral Geriatric Residency through the Veteran's Administration Medical Center and The University of Utah College of Pharmacy. Dr Higbee was also on the editorial staff for the Eli Lily - AACP Geriatric Curriculum for Pharmacists project which created a geriatric textbook and curriculum for educators.

Dr Higbee joined the faculty at The University of Arizona in 1987. As part of his teaching responsibilities, he is a Clinical Pharmacist Consultant for the Hospital-Based Primary Care Team (division of Geriatric Care Center) at the Veterans Administration Medical Center in Tucson, Arizona, where he is preceptor for doctor of pharmacy students. He is also a nursing home consultant for local nursing homes in Arizona.

Dr Higbee regularly speaks locally and nationally on geriatric drug therapy topics and has published articles, chapters, and abstracts on various geriatric research and pharmacotherapy topics. He is a member of numerous professional organizations. He is a past chairman of the ASHP Special Interest Group on Geriatric Pharmacy Practice and past member of the AACP Task Force on Aging.

DESCRIPTION OF SECTIONS AND FIELDS

The *Geriatric Dosage Handbook* is organized into four sections: Introductory information, drug information section, appendix, and pharmacologic category index.

Alphabetical Listing of Drugs

The drug information section of the handbook, wherein all drug monographs are arranged alphabetically by generic name, details information pertinent to geriatric use for each drug. U.S. brand names and synonyms are cross-referenced between monographs and marked with diamonds ◆ for easy visibility.

Individual monographs contain most or all of the following fields of information:

Generic Name	U.S. adopted name
Pronunciation Guide	Phonetic pronunciation guide
Related Information	Cross-reference to other pertinent information found elsewhere in this handbook
Medication Safety Issues	In an effort to promote the safe use of medications, this field is intended to highlight possible sources of medication errors such as look-alike/sound-alike drugs or highly concentrated formulations which require vigilance on the part of healthcare professionals. In addition, medications which have been associated with severe consequences in the event of a medication error are also identified in this field.
U.S. Brand Names	Trade names (manufacturer-specific) found in the United States. The symbol [DSC] appears after trade names that have been recently discontinued.
Canadian Brand Names	Trade name(s) found in Canada
Index Terms	Other name(s) or accepted abbreviation(s) of the generic drug
Generic Available	Indicated by a "Yes" or "No"; may include specific forms or exceptions
Pharmacologic Category	Indicates one or more systematic classifications of the drug
Use	Description of FDA-approved indications of the drug
Unlabeled / Investigational Use	Information pertaining to non-FDA-approved and investigational indications of the drug
Restrictions	The controlled substance classification from the Drug Enforcement Agency (DEA). U.S. schedules are I-V. Schedules vary by country and sometimes state (ie, Massachusetts uses I-VI)
Contraindications	Information pertaining to inappropriate use of the drug
Warnings / Precautions	Precautionary considerations, hazardous conditions related to use of the drug, and disease states or patient populations in which the drug should be cautiously used
Adverse Reactions	Side effects are grouped by percentage of incidence (if known) and/or body system; <1% effects are not listed, please consult manufacturers product labeling regarding rare serious or life threatening events; **percentages are reflective of the adult population in general, not specific for older adults**
Overdosage / Toxicology	Comments and/or considerations are offered when appropriate and include signs/symptoms of excess drug and suggested management of the patient

DESCRIPTION OF SECTIONS AND FIELDS *(Continued)*

Drug Interactions	If a drug has demonstrated involvement with cytochrome P450 enzymes, the initial line of this field will identify the drug as an inhibitor, inducer, or substrate of specific isoenzymes (ie, CYP1A2). Isoenzymes are identified as substrates (minor or major), inhibitors (weak or moderate or strong), and inducers (weak or strong). A summary of this information can also be found in a tabular format within the introductory section. The remainder of the field presents a description of the interaction between the drug listed in the monograph and other drugs or drug classes. May include possible mechanisms and effect of combined therapy. May also include a strategy to manage the patient on combined therapy (ie, quinidine).
Ethanol / Nutrition / Herb Interactions	Information regarding potential interactions with food, nutritionals, herbal products, vitamins, or ethanol
Stability	Information regarding storage of product or steps for reconstitution. Provides the time and conditions for which a solution or mixture will maintain full potency. For example, some solutions may require refrigeration after reconstitution while stored at room temperature prior to preparation. Also includes compatibility information. **Note:** Professional judgment of the individual pharmacist in application of this information is imperative. While drug products may exhibit stability over longer durations of time, it may not be appropriate to utilize the drug product due to concerns in sterility.
Mechanism of Action	How drugs work in the body to elicit a response
Pharmacodynamics	Dose-response relationships including onset of action, time of peak action, and duration of action
Pharmacokinetics	Information on drug movement through the body over time; deals with absorption, distribution, metabolism, half-life, bioavailability, protein binding, time to peak serum concentrations, and elimination/excretion of drugs; pharmacokinetic parameters help predict drug concentration and dosage requirements.
Dosage	The amount of drug to be typically given or taken during therapy; may include the following:
Geriatrics	Suggested amount of drug to be given to elderly patients; may include adjustments from adult dosing; lack of this information in the monograph may imply that the drug is not used in the elderly patient or that no specific adjustments could be identified
Geriatrics & Adults	This combined field is only used to indicate that no specific adjustments for elderly patients were identified. However, other issues should be considered (ie, renal or hepatic impairment). Also refer to Special Geriatric Considerations for additional information related to the elderly.
Adults	The recommended amount of drug to be given to adult patients
Renal Impairment	Suggested dosage adjustments or comments based on compromised renal function; may include dosing instructions for patients on dialysis
Hepatic Impairment	Suggested dosage adjustments or comments based on compromised liver function

Administration	Information regarding the recommended final concentrations, rates of administration for parenteral drugs, or other guidelines when giving the medication
Monitoring Parameters	Laboratory tests and patient physical parameters that should be monitored for safety and efficacy of drug therapy
Reference Range	Therapeutic and toxic serum concentrations listed including peak and trough levels
Test Interactions	Listing of assay interference when relevant (B = blood; S = serum; U = urine)
Patient Information	Specific information pertinent for the patient
Additional Information	Information about sodium content and/or pertinent information about specific brands
Special Geriatric Considerations	Pertinent information specific to older adults
Dosage Forms	Information with regard to form, strength, and availability of the drug. **Note:** Additional formulation information (eg, excipients, preservatives) is included when available. Please consult product labeling for further information.
Extemporaneously Prepared	Directions for preparing liquid formulations from solid drug products. May include stability information and references.
Selected References	Bibliographic information referring to specific geriatric literature findings

Appendix

The appendix offers a compilation of tables, guidelines, nomograms, and conversion information which can often be helpful when considering patient care.

Pharmacologic Category Index

This index provides a useful listing of drugs by their pharmacologic classification.

SAFE PRESCRIPTION WRITING

Health professionals and their support personnel frequently produce handwritten copies of information they see in print; therefore, such information is subjected to even greater possibilities for error or misinterpretation on the part of others. Thus, particular care must be given to how drug names and strengths are expressed when creating written health-care documents.

The following are a few examples of safe writing rules suggested by the Institute for Safe Medication Practices, Inc.*

1. There should be a space between a number and its units as it is easier to read. There should be no periods after the abbreviations mg or mL.

Correct	Incorrect
10 mg	10mg
100 mg	100mg

2. Never place a decimal and a zero after a whole number (2 mg is correct and 2.0 mg is **incorrect**). If the decimal point is not seen because it falls on a line or because individuals are working from copies where the decimal point is not seen, this causes a tenfold overdose.

3. Just the opposite is true for numbers less than one. Always place a zero before a naked decimal (0.5 mL is correct, .5 mL is **incorrect**).

4. Never abbreviate the word unit. The handwritten U or u, looks like a 0 (zero), and may cause a tenfold overdose error to be made.

5. IU is not a safe abbreviation for international units. The handwritten IU looks like IV. Write out international units or use int. units.

6. Q.D. is not a safe abbreviation for once daily, as when the Q is followed by a sloppy dot, it looks like QID which means four times daily.

7. O.D. is not a safe abbreviation for once daily, as it is properly interpreted as meaning "right eye" and has caused liquid medications such as saturated solution of potassium iodide and Lugol's solution to be administered incorrectly. There is no safe abbreviation for once daily. It must be written out in full.

8. Do not use chemical names such as 6-mercaptopurine or 6-thioguanine, as sixfold overdoses have been given when these were not recognized as chemical names. The proper names of these drugs are mercaptopurine or thioguanine.

9. Do not abbreviate drug names (5FC, 6MP, 5-ASA, MTX, HCTZ, CPZ, PBZ, etc) as they are misinterpreted and cause error.

10. Do not use the apothecary system or symbols.

11. Do not abbreviate microgram as μg; instead use mcg as there is less likelihood of misinterpretation.

12. When writing an outpatient prescription, write a complete prescription. A complete prescription can prevent the prescriber, the pharmacist, and/or the patient from making a mistake and can eliminate the need for further clarification. The legible prescriptions should contain:

    a. patient's full name

    b. for pediatric or geriatric patients: their age (or weight where applicable)

    c. drug name, dosage form and strength; if a drug is new or rarely prescribed, print this information

    d. number or amount to be dispensed

    e. complete instructions for the patient, including the purpose of the medication

    f. when there are recognized contraindications for a prescribed drug, indicate to the pharmacist that you are aware of this fact (ie, when prescribing a potassium salt for a patient receiving an ACE inhibitor, write "K serum leveling being monitored")

*From "Safe Writing" by Davis NM, PharmD and Cohen MR, MS, Lecturers and Consultants for Safe Medication Practices, 1143 Wright Drive, Huntington Valley, PA 19006. Phone: (215) 947-7566.

FDA NAME DIFFERENTIATION PROJECT THE USE OF TALL-MAN LETTERS

Confusion between similar drug names is an important cause of medication errors. For years, The Institute For Safe Medication Practices (ISMP), has urged generic manufacturers use a combination of large and small letters as well as bolding (ie, chlorpro**MAZINE** and chlorpro**PAMIDE**) to help distinguish drugs with look-alike names, especially when they share similar strengths. Recently the FDA's Division of Generic Drugs began to issue recommendation letters to manufacturers suggesting this novel way to label their products to help reduce this drug name confusion. Although this project has had marginal success, the method has successfully eliminated problems with products such as diphenhydr**A-MINE** and dimenhy**DRINATE**. Hospitals should also follow suit by making similar changes in their own labels, preprinted order forms, computer screens and printouts, and drug storage location labels.

Lexi-Comp Medical Publishing has adopted the use of these "Tall-Man" letters for the drugs suggested by the FDA.

The following is a list of product names and recommended FDA revisions:

Drug Product	Recommended Revision
acetazolamide	aceta**ZOLAMIDE**
acetohexamide	aceto**HEXAMIDE**
bupropion	bu**PROP**ion
buspirone	bus**PIR**one
chlorpromazine	chlorpro**MAZINE**
chlorpropamide	chlorpro**PAMIDE**
clomiphene	clomi**PHENE**
clomipramine	clomi**PRAMINE**
cycloserine	cyclo**SERINE**
cyclosporine	cyclo**SPORINE**
daunorubicin	**DAUNO**rubicin
dimenhydrinate	dimenhy**DRINATE**
diphenhydramine	diphenhydr**AMINE**
dobutamine	**DOBUT**amine
dopamine	**DOP**amine
doxorubicin	**DOXO**rubicin
glipizide	glipi**ZIDE**
glyburide	gly**BURIDE**
hydralazine	hydr**ALAZINE**
hydroxyzine	hydr**OXY**zine
medroxyprogesterone	medroxy**PROGESTER**one
methylprednisolone	methyl**PREDNIS**olone
methyltestosterone	methyl**TESTOSTER**one
nicardipine	ni**CARD**ipine
nifedipine	**NIFE**dipine
prednisolone	predniso**LONE**
prednisone	predni**SONE**
sulfadiazine	sulfa**DIAZINE**
sulfisoxazole	sulfi**SOXAZOLE**
tolazamide	**TOLAZ**amide
tolbutamide	**TOLBUT**amide
vinblastine	vin**BLAS**tine
vincristine	vin**CRIS**tine

Institute for Safe Medication Practices. "New Tall-Man Lettering Will Reduce Mix-Ups Due to Generic Drug Name Confusion," *ISMP Medication Safety Alert*, September 19, 2001. Available at: http://www.ismp.org.

Institute for Safe Medication Practices. "Prescription Mapping, Can Improve Efficiency While Minimizing Errors With Look-Alike Products," *ISMP Medication Safety Alert*, October 6, 1999. Available at: http://www.ismp.org.

U.S. Pharmacopeia, "USP Quality Review: Use Caution-Avoid Confusion," March 2001, No. 76. Available at: http://www.usp.org.

ALPHABETICAL LISTING OF DRUGS

♦ **A200® Lice [OTC]** *see* Permethrin *on page 1235*

Abatacept (ab a TA sept)

U.S. Brand Names Orencia®

Index Terms CTLA-4Ig

Generic Available No

Pharmacologic Category Antirheumatic, Disease Modifying

Use Treatment of rheumatoid arthritis not responsive to other disease-modifying antirheumatic drugs (DMARD); may be used as monotherapy or in combination with other DMARDs (**not** in combination with anakinra or TNF-blocking agents)

Contraindications Hypersensitivity to abatacept or any component of the formulation

Warnings/Precautions Caution should be exercised when considering the use of abatacept in patients with a history of recurrent infections, with conditions that predispose them to infections, or with chronic, latent, or localized infections. Patients who develop a new infection while undergoing treatment should be monitored closely. If a patient develops a serious infection, abatacept should be discontinued. Screen patients for latent tuberculosis infection prior to initiating abatacept; safety in tuberculosis-positive patients has not been established. Patients receiving abatacept in combination with TNF-blocking agents had higher rates of infections (including serious infections) than patients on TNF-blocking agents alone. The manufacturer does not recommend concurrent use with anakinra. Due to the affect of T-cell inhibition on host defenses, abatacept may affect immune responses against infections and malignancies; impact on the development and course of malignancies is not fully defined.

Use caution with chronic obstructive pulmonary disease (COPD), higher incidences of adverse effects (COPD exacerbation, cough, rhonchi, dyspnea) have been observed; monitor closely. May cause hypersensitivity, anaphylaxis, or anaphylactoid reactions; medications for the treatment of hypersensitivity reactions should be available for immediate use. Patients should be brought up to date with all immunizations before initiating therapy. Live vaccines should not be given concurrently; there is no data available concerning secondary transmission of live vaccines in patients receiving therapy. May contain maltose, which may result in falsely-elevated blood glucose readings on the day of infusion.

Adverse Reactions (Reflective of adult population; not specific for elderly)
Note: Percentages not always reported; COPD patients experienced a higher frequency of COPD-related adverse reactions (COPD exacerbation, cough, dyspnea, pneumonia, rhonchi)

>10%:
    Central nervous system: Headache (18%)
    Gastrointestinal: Nausea
    Respiratory: Nasopharyngitis (12%), upper respiratory tract infection
    Miscellaneous: Infection (54%)
1% to 10%:
    Cardiovascular: Hypertension (7%)
    Central nervous system: Dizziness (9%)
    Dermatologic: Rash (4%)
    Gastrointestinal: Dyspepsia (6%)
    Genitourinary: Urinary tract infection (6%)
    Neuromuscular & skeletal: Back pain (7%), limb pain (3%)
    Respiratory: Cough (8%), bronchitis, pneumonia, rhinitis, sinusitis
    Miscellaneous: Infusion-related reactions (9%), herpes simplex, influenza

Overdosage/Toxicology Doses up to 50 mg/kg have been tolerated. In the event of an overdose, monitor for signs and symptoms of adverse reactions. Treatment is symptom-directed and supportive.

Drug Interactions
    TNF-blocking agents: Concurrent use with abatacept may increase risk of infections; contraindicated.
    Vaccine (dead organism): Abatacept may decrease the effect of vaccines (dead organisms).
    Vaccines, live: Concomitant use has not be studied; currently recommended not to administer live vaccines during or for 3 months after the completion of abatacept treatment.

Ethanol/Nutrition/Herb Interactions Herb/Nutraceutical: Avoid echinacea (has immunostimulant properties; consider therapy modifications).

Stability Prior to reconstitution, store at 2°C to 8°C (36°F to 46°F); protect from light. Reconstitute each vial with 10 mL SWFI using a silicone-free disposable syringe (discard solutions accidentally reconstituted with siliconized syringe as they may develop translucent particles). Inject SWFI down the side of the vial to avoid foaming. Gently rotate or swirl vial to dissolve; do not shake. Upon dissolution, vent vial to dissipate foaming. After reconstitution, each mL will contain 25 mg abatacept. Further dilute (using a silicone-free syringe) to a final concentration of 5-10 mg/mL in 100 mL NS; gently mix.

After dilution, may be stored for up to 24 hours at room temperature or refrigerated at 2°C to 8°C (36°F to 46°F). Must be used within 24 hours of reconstitution.

Mechanism of Action Selective costimulation modulator; inhibits T-cell (T-lymphocyte) activation by binding to CD80 and CD86 on antigen presenting cells (APC), thus blocking the required CD28 interaction between APCs and T cells. Activated T lymphocytes are found in the synovium of rheumatoid arthritis patients.

Pharmacokinetics
Distribution: V_{ss}: 0.02-0.13 L/kg
Half-life elimination: 8-25 days

Dosage
Geriatrics: Refer to adult dosing. Due to potential for higher rates of infections and malignancies, use caution.

Adults: Rheumatoid arthritis: I.V.: Dosing is according to body weight. Repeat dose at 2 weeks and 4 weeks after initial dose, and every 4 weeks thereafter:
    <60 kg: 500 mg
    60-100 kg: 750 mg
    >100 kg: 1000 mg

Administration Infuse over 30 minutes. Administer through a 0.2-1.2 micron low protein-binding. filter

Monitoring Parameters Signs and symptoms of infection, signs and symptoms of infusion reaction

Test Interactions Contains maltose; may result in falsely elevated blood glucose levels with dehydrogenase pyrroloquinolinequinone or glucose-dye-oxidoreductase testing methods on the day of infusion. Glucose monitoring methods which utilize glucose dehydrogenase nicotine adenine dinucleotide (GDH-NAD), glucose oxidase, or glucose hexokinase are recommended.

Patient Information This drug can only be administered by infusion. You may be more susceptible to infections. Report signs of infection. Avoid immunizations unless approved by prescriber. May cause falsely elevated blood glucose readings on day of infusion. You may experience headache, sore throat, and nausea. Report immediately respiratory difficulty, hives, dizziness, nausea, flushing, cough, or wheezing.

Special Geriatric Considerations The number of elderly (≥65 years of age) were insufficient to draw significant clinical conclusions. The studies to date have not demonstrated any differences in safety and efficacy between young adults and elderly. However, the frequency of infections and malignancy was higher in those >65 years of age than those <65 years. Since elderly experience a higher incidence of infections and malignancies, use abatacept with caution in this population.

Dosage Forms Excipient information presented when available (limited, particularly for generics); consult specific product labeling.
Injection, powder for reconstitution [preservative free]:
    Orencia®: 250 mg [contains maltose]

Selected References
Doan T and Massarotti E, "Rheumatoid Arthritis: An Overview of New and Emerging Therapies," *J Clin Pharmacol*, 2005, 45(7):751-62.

Genovese MC, Becker JC, Schiff M, et al, "Abatacept for Rheumatoid Arthritis Refractory to Tumor Necrosis Factor Alpha Inhibition," *N Engl J Med*, 2005, 353(11):1114-23.

Kremer JM, Dougados M, Emery P, et al, "Treatment of Rheumatoid Arthritis With the Selective Costimulation Modulator Abatacept: Twelve-Month Results of a Phase IIb, Double-Blind, Randomized, Placebo-Controlled Trial," *Arthritis Rheum*, 2005, 52(8):2263-71.

Kremer JM, Genant HK, Moreland LW, et al, "Effects of Abatacept in Patients With Methotrexate-Resistant Active Rheumatoid Arthritis: A Randomized Trial," *Ann Intern Med*, 2006, 144(12):865-76.

Kremer JM, Westhovens R, Leon M, et al, "Treatment of Rheumatoid Arthritis by Selective Inhibition of T-Cell Activation With Fusion Protein CTLA4Ig," *N Engl J Med*, 2003, 349(20):1907-15.

Tay L, Leon F, Vratsanos G, et al, "Vaccination Response to Tetanus Toxoid and 23-Valent Pneumococcal Vaccines Following Administration of a Single Dose of Abatacept: A Randomized, Open-Label, Parallel Group Study in Healthy Subjects," *Arthritis Res Ther*, 2007, 9(2): R38.

Acamprosate (a kam PROE sate)

U.S. Brand Names Campral®
Canadian Brand Names Campral®
Index Terms Acamprosate Calcium; Calcium Acetylhomotaurinate
Generic Available No
(Continued)

Acamprosate *(Continued)*

Pharmacologic Category GABA Agonist/Glutamate Antagonist

Use Maintenance of alcohol abstinence

Contraindications Hypersensitivity to acamprosate or any component of the formulation; severe renal impairment (Cl$_{cr}$ <30 mL/minute)

Warnings/Precautions Should be used as part of a comprehensive program to treat alcohol dependence. Treatment should be initiated as soon as possible following the period of alcohol withdrawal, when the patient has achieved abstinence. Acamprosate does not eliminate or diminish the symptoms of alcohol withdrawal. Use caution in moderate renal impairment (Cl$_{cr}$ 30-50 mL/minute). Suicidal ideation, attempted and completed suicides have occurred in acamprosate-treated patients; monitor for depression and/or suicidal thinking. Traces of sulfites may be present in the formulation.

Adverse Reactions (Reflective of adult population; not specific for elderly)

Note: Many adverse effects associated with treatment may be related to alcohol abstinence; reported frequency range may overlap with placebo.

>10%: Gastrointestinal: Diarrhea (10% to 17%)

1% to 10%:

Cardiovascular: Syncope, palpitation, edema (peripheral)

Central nervous system: Insomnia (6% to 9%), anxiety (5% to 8%), depression (4% to 8%), dizziness (3% to 4%), pain (2% to 4%), paresthesia (2% to 3%), headache, somnolence, amnesia, tremor, chills

Dermatologic: Pruritus (3% to 4%), rash

Endocrine and metabolic: Weight gain, libido decreased

Gastrointestinal: Anorexia (2% to 5%), flatulence (1% to 3%), nausea (3% to 4%), abdominal pain, dry mouth (1% to 3%), vomiting, dyspepsia, constipation, appetite increased, taste perversion

Genitourinary: Impotence

Neuromuscular & skeletal: Weakness (5% to 7%), back pain, myalgia, arthralgia

Ocular: Abnormal vision

Respiratory: Rhinitis, dyspnea, pharyngitis, bronchitis

Miscellaneous: Diaphoresis (2% to 3%), suicide attempt

Overdosage/Toxicology Symptoms may include diarrhea and (in chronic overdose) hypocalcemia. Treatment is symptom-directed and supportive.

Drug Interactions No clinically-significant drug-to-drug interactions have been identified.

Ethanol/Nutrition/Herb Interactions

Ethanol: Abstinence is required during treatment. Ethanol does not affect the pharmacokinetics of acamprosate; however, the continued use of ethanol will decrease desired efficacy of acamprosate.

Food: Food decreases absorption of acamprosate (not clinically significant).

Stability Store at 25°C (77°F); excursions permitted to 15°C to 30°C (59°F to 86°F).

Mechanism of Action Mechanism not fully defined. Structurally similar to gamma-amino butyric acid (GABA), acamprosate appears to increase the activity of the GABA-ergic system, and decreases activity of glutamate within the CNS, including a decrease in activity at N-methyl D-aspartate (NMDA) receptors; may also affect CNS calcium channels. Restores balance to GABA and glutamate activities which appear to be disrupted in alcohol dependence. During therapeutic use, reduces alcohol intake, but does not cause a disulfiram-like reaction following alcohol ingestion.

Pharmacokinetics

Distribution: V$_d$: 1 L/kg

Protein binding: Negligible

Metabolism: Not metabolized

Bioavailability: 11%

Half-life elimination: 20-33 hours

Excretion: Urine (as unchanged drug)

Dosage

Geriatrics & Adults: Alcohol abstinence: Oral: 666 mg 3 times/day (a lower dose may be effective in some patients).

Adjustment in patients with low body weight (unlabeled): A lower dose (4 tablets/day) may be considered in patients with low body weight (eg, <60 kg).

Note: Treatment should be initiated as soon as possible following the period of alcohol withdrawal, when the patient has achieved abstinence.

Renal Impairment:

Cl$_{cr}$ 30-50 mL/minute: Initial dose should be reduced to 333 mg 3 times/day.

Cl$_{cr}$ <30 mL/minute: Contraindicated in severe renal impairment.

Administration May be administered without regard to meals.

Special Geriatric Considerations Initial studies did not include sufficient geriatric patients to be able to derive sufficient data to compare elderly to younger adults. Only 41 out of 4234 patients in clinical trials were ≥65 years of age with none ≥75 years. However, since this medication is cleared renally exclusively, caution should be used since many elderly have Cl$_{cr}$ 30-50 mL/minute where dosage reduction is required (see Dosage).

Dosage Forms Excipient information presented when available (limited, particularly for generics); consult specific product labeling.

Tablet, enteric coated, delayed release, as calcium: 333 mg [contains calcium 33 mg and sulfites]

Selected References

Brasser SM, McCaul ME, and Houtsmuller EJ, "Alcohol Effects During Acamprosate Treatment: A Dose-Response Study in Humans," *Alcohol Clin Exp Res*, 2004, 28(7):1074-83.

Graham R, Wodak AD, and Whelan G, "New Pharmacotherapies for Alcohol Dependence," *Med J Aust*, 2002, 177(2):103-7.

Overman GP, Teter CJ, and Guthrie SK, "Acamprosate For the Adjunctive Treatment of Alcohol Dependence," *Ann Pharmacother*, 2003, 37(7-8):1090-9.

♦ **Acamprosate Calcium** *see* Acamprosate *on page 23*

Acarbose (AY car bose)

Medication Safety Issues
Sound-alike/look-alike issues:
   Precose® may be confused with PreCare®

International issues:
   Precose® may be confused with Precosa® which is a brand name for *Saccharomyces boulardii* in Denmark, Finland, Norway, and Sweden

U.S. Brand Names Precose®
Canadian Brand Names Prandase®
Generic Available No
Pharmacologic Category Antidiabetic Agent, Alpha-Glucosidase Inhibitor
Use

Monotherapy, as indicated as an adjunct to diet to lower blood glucose in patients with type 2 diabetes mellitus (noninsulin dependent, NIDDM) whose hyperglycemia cannot be managed on diet alone

Combination with a sulfonylurea, metformin, or insulin in patients with type 2 diabetes mellitus (noninsulin dependent, NIDDM) when diet plus acarbose do not result in adequate glycemic control; the effect of acarbose to enhance glycemic control is additive to that of other hypoglycemic agents when used in combination

Contraindications Hypersensitivity to acarbose or any component of the formulation; patients with diabetic ketoacidosis or cirrhosis; patients with inflammatory bowel disease, colonic ulceration, partial intestinal obstruction, or in patients predisposed to intestinal obstruction; patients who have chronic intestinal diseases associated with marked disorders of digestion or absorption, and in patients who have conditions that may deteriorate as a result of increased gas formation in the intestine

Warnings/Precautions Acarbose given In combination with a sulfonylurea will cause a further lowering of blood glucose and may increase the hypoglycemic potential of the sulfonylurea. Treatment-emergent elevations of serum transaminases (AST and/or ALT) occurred in 15% of acarbose-treated patients in long-term studies. These serum transaminase elevations appear to be dose related. At doses >100 mg 3 times/day, the incidence of serum transaminase elevations greater than 3 times the upper limit of normal was 2-3 times higher in the acarbose group than in the placebo group. These elevations were asymptomatic, reversible, more common in females, and, in general, were not associated with other evidence of liver dysfunction. It may be necessary to discontinue acarbose and administer insulin if the patient is exposed to stress (ie, fever, trauma, infection, surgery).

Adverse Reactions (Reflective of adult population; not specific for elderly)
>10%:
   Gastrointestinal: Abdominal pain (21%) and diarrhea (33%) tend to return to pretreatment levels over time, and the frequency and intensity of flatulence (77%) tend to abate with time
   Hepatic: Transaminases increased

Overdosage/Toxicology An overdose of acarbose will not result in hypoglycemia. An overdose may result in transient increases in flatulence, diarrhea, and abdominal discomfort which shortly subside. However, acarbose may complicate the treatment of hypoglycemia from other causes, since it will inhibit the absorption of oral disaccharides (sucrose). Oral glucose (dextrose) should be used in mild to moderate hypoglycemia; severe hypoglycemia should be treated with I.V. glucose.

Drug Interactions
Calcium channel blocking agents: May decrease the efficacy of acarbose due to hyperglycemic effects.
Corticosteroids: May decrease the efficacy of acarbose due to hyperglycemic effects.
Digoxin: Acarbose decreases the bioavailability of digoxin, resulting in lower serum concentrations.
(Continued)

Acarbose *(Continued)*

Diuretics (including thiazides): May decrease the efficacy of acarbose due to hyperglycemic effects.

Enzyme replacement (pancrelipase, amylase): May decrease the efficacy of acarbose due to effects on carbohydrate metabolism.

Estrogens: May decrease the efficacy of acarbose due to hyperglycemic effects.

Insulin: Acarbose may increase the hypoglycemic potential of insulin. Oral glucose (dextrose) should be used in the treatment of mild-to-moderate hypoglycemia; severe hypoglycemia may require the use of either intravenous glucose infusion or glucagon injection.

Isoniazid: May decrease the efficacy of acarbose due to hyperglycemic effects.

Nicotinic acid: May decrease the efficacy of acarbose due to hyperglycemic effects.

Oral contraceptives: May decrease the efficacy of acarbose due to hyperglycemic effects.

Phenothiazines: May decrease the efficacy of acarbose due to hyperglycemic effects.

Sulfonylureas: Acarbose may increase the hypoglycemic potential of sulfonylureas. Oral glucose (dextrose) should be used in the treatment of mild-to-moderate hypoglycemia; severe hypoglycemia may require the use of either intravenous glucose infusion or glucagon injection.

Thyroid hormones: May decrease the efficacy of acarbose due to hyperglycemic effects.

Ethanol/Nutrition/Herb Interactions Ethanol: Limit ethanol.

Stability Store at <25°C (77°F); protect from moisture.

Mechanism of Action Competitive inhibitor of pancreatic α-amylase and intestinal brush border α-glucosidases, resulting in delayed hydrolysis of ingested complex carbohydrates and disaccharides and absorption of glucose; dose-dependent reduction in postprandial serum insulin and glucose peaks; inhibits the metabolism of sucrose to glucose and fructose

Pharmacokinetics

Bioavailability: Systemic: 1% to 2%

Elimination: 51% unchanged in feces; degradation by gastrointestinal enzymes and microorganisms

Dosage

Geriatrics & Adults: Type 2 diabetes: Oral:

Initial: 25 mg 3 times/day

Maintenance dose: Should be adjusted at 4- to 8-week intervals based on 1-hour postprandial glucose levels and tolerance until maintenance dose is reached; maintenance dose: 50-100 mg 3 times/day. Dosage must be individualized on the basis of effectiveness and tolerance while not exceeding the maximum recommended dose.

Maximum:

≤60 kg: 50 mg 3 times/day

>60 kg: 100 mg 3 times/day

Patients receiving sulfonylureas: Acarbose given in combination with a sulfonylurea will cause a further lowering of blood glucose and may increase the hypoglycemic potential of the sulfonylurea. If hypoglycemia occurs, appropriate adjustments in the dosage of these agents should be made.

Renal Impairment: Cl_{cr} <25 mL/minute: Peak plasma concentrations were 5 times higher and AUCs were 6 times larger than in volunteers with normal renal function; however, long-term clinical trials in patients with diabetes with significant renal dysfunction have not been conducted and treatment of these patients with acarbose is not recommended

Administration See Dosage.

Monitoring Parameters Preprandial blood glucose, glycosylated hemoglobin A_{1c}, fructosamine, serum transaminase levels (especially if ≥100 mg/day)

Patient Information Administer acarbose 3 times/day at the start (with the first bite) of each main meal. It is important to continue to adhere to dietary instructions, a regular exercise program, and regular testing of urine and/or blood glucose. The risk of hypoglycemia, its symptoms and treatment, and conditions that predispose to its development should be well understood by patients and responsible family members. A source of glucose (dextrose) should be readily available to treat symptoms of low blood glucose when taking acarbose in combination with a sulfonylurea or insulin. If side effects occur, they usually develop during the first few weeks of therapy and are mild to moderate gastrointestinal effects, such as flatulence, diarrhea, or abdominal discomfort and generally diminish in frequency and intensity with time.

Special Geriatric Considerations No specific trials in older adults have been conducted; mean age in clinical trials has been <60 years; monitor change in preprandial blood glucose concentrations to account for potential age-related changes in postprandial glucose. In clinical trials, elderly had serum concentrations 1.5 times those of younger adults. Patients with Cl_{cr} <25 mL/minute had serum concentrations

5 times those with normal renal clearance. No clinical significance can be attributed to this at this time. No adjustments in dose are recommended.

Dosage Forms Excipient information presented when available (limited, particularly for generics); consult specific product labeling.

Tablet: 25 mg, 50 mg, 100 mg

Selected References

Balfour JA and McTavish D, "Acarbose: A Reappraisal," *Drugs*, 1993, 46(6):1025-54.

Bischoff H, "Pharmacology of α-Glucosidase Inhibition," *Eur J Clin Invest*, 1994, 24(Suppl 3):3-10.

Johnston PS, Lebovitz HE, Coniff RF, et al, "Advantages of Alpha-Glucosidase Inhibition as Monotherapy in Elderly Type 2 Diabetic Patients," *J Clin Endocrinol Metab*, 1998, 83(5):1515-22.

Scheen AJ, de Magalhaes AC, Salvatore T, et al, "Reduction of the Acute Bioavailability of Metformin by the α-Glucosidase Inhibitor Acarbose in Normal Man," *Eur J Clin Invest*, 1994, 24(Suppl 3):50-4.

- ♦ **Accolate®** *see* Zafirlukast *on page 1691*
- ♦ **AccuNeb®** *see* Albuterol *on page 40*
- ♦ **Accupril®** *see* Quinapril *on page 1359*
- ♦ **Accuretic®** *see* Quinapril and Hydrochlorothiazide *on page 1362*
- ♦ **Accuzyme®** *see* Papain and Urea *on page 1201*
- ♦ **ACE** *see* Captopril *on page 226*

Acebutolol (a se BYOO toe lole)

Related Information

Beta-Blockers *on page 1751*

Medication Safety Issues

Sound-alike/look-alike issues:

Sectral® may be confused with Factrel®, Seconal®, Septra®

U.S. Brand Names Sectral®

Canadian Brand Names Apo-Acebutolol®; Gen-Acebutolol; Monitan®; Novo-Acebutolol; Nu-Acebutolol; Rhotral; Rhoxal-acebutolol; Sandoz-Acebutolol; Sectral®

Index Terms Acebutolol Hydrochloride

Generic Available Yes

Pharmacologic Category Antiarrhythmic Agent, Class II; Beta Blocker With Intrinsic Sympathomimetic Activity

Use Treatment of hypertension, ventricular arrhythmias, angina

Contraindications Hypersensitivity to beta-blocking agents; uncompensated congestive heart failure; cardiogenic shock; bradycardia or second- and third-degree heart block (except in patients with a functioning artificial pacemaker); sinus node dysfunction

Warnings/Precautions Consider pre-existing conditions such as sick sinus syndrome before initiating. Beta-blocker therapy should not be withdrawn abruptly (particularly in patients with CAD), but gradually tapered to avoid acute tachycardia, hypertension, and/or ischemia. Use with caution in diabetic patients. Beta-blockers may impair glucose tolerance, potentiate hypoglycemia, and/or mask symptoms of hypoglycemia in a diabetic patient. Use with caution in bronchospastic lung disease, hepatic impairment, myasthenia gravis, psychiatric disease (may cause CNS depression), peripheral vascular disease or renal dysfunction (especially the elderly). Beta-blockers with intrinsic sympathomimetic activity do not appear to be of benefit in CHF and should be avoided. Adequate alpha-blockade is required prior to use of any beta-blocker for patients with untreated pheochromocytoma.

Adverse Reactions (Reflective of adult population; not specific for elderly)

>10%: Central nervous system: Fatigue (11%)

1% to 10%:

Cardiovascular: Chest pain (2%), edema (2%), bradycardia, hypotension, CHF

Central nervous system: Headache (6%), dizziness (6%), insomnia (3%), depression (2%), abnormal dreams (2%), anxiety, hyperesthesia, hypoesthesia, impotence

Dermatologic: Rash (2%), pruritus

Gastrointestinal: Constipation (4%), diarrhea (4%), dyspepsia (4%), nausea (4%), flatulence (3%), vomiting, abdominal pain

Genitourinary: Micturition frequency (3%), dysuria, nocturia, impotence (2%)

Neuromuscular & skeletal: Arthralgia (2%), myalgia (2%), back pain, joint pain

Ocular: Abnormal vision (2%), conjunctivitis, dry eyes, eye pain

Respiratory: Dyspnea (4%), rhinitis (2%), cough (1%), pharyngitis, wheezing

Potential adverse effects (based on experience with other beta-blocking agents) include reversible mental depression, disorientation, catatonia, short-term memory loss, emotional lability, slightly clouded sensorium, laryngospasm, respiratory distress, allergic reactions, erythematous rash, agranulocytosis, purpura, thrombocytopenia, mesenteric artery thrombosis, ischemic colitis, alopecia, Peyronie's disease, claudication

Overdosage/Toxicology Symptoms include cardiac disturbances, CNS toxicity, bronchospasm, hypoglycemia, and hyperkalemia. The most common cardiac symptoms (Continued)

Acebutolol *(Continued)*

include hypotension and bradycardia. Atrioventricular block, intraventricular conduction disturbances, cardiogenic shock, and asystole may occur with severe overdose, especially with membrane-depressant drugs (eg, propranolol). CNS effects include convulsions, coma, and respiratory arrest is commonly seen with propranolol and other membrane-depressant and lipid-soluble drugs. Treatment is symptomatic for seizures, hypotension, hyperkalemia and hypoglycemia. Bradycardia and hypotension resistant to atropine, isoproterenol or pacing, may respond to glucagon. Wide QRS defects caused by membrane-depressant poisoning may respond to hypertonic sodium bicarbonate. Repeat-dose charcoal, hemoperfusion, or hemodialysis may be helpful.

Drug Interactions Inhibits CYP2D6 (weak)

    Alpha-blockers (prazosin, terazosin): Concurrent use of beta-blockers may increase risk of orthostasis.

    Clonidine: Hypertensive crisis after or during withdrawal of either agent.

    Drugs which slow AV conduction (digoxin): Effects may be additive with beta-blockers.

    Glucagon: Acebutolol may blunt the hyperglycemic action of glucagon.

    Insulin and oral hypoglycemics: Acebutolol masks the tachycardia from hypoglycemia.

    NSAIDs (ibuprofen, indomethacin, naproxen, piroxicam) may reduce the antihypertensive effects of beta-blockers.

    Salicylates may reduce the antihypertensive effects of beta-blockers.

    Sulfonylureas: Beta-blockers may alter response to hypoglycemic agents.

    Verapamil or diltiazem may have synergistic or additive pharmacological effects when taken concurrently with beta-blockers.

Ethanol/Nutrition/Herb Interactions

    Food: Peak serum acebutolol levels may be slightly decreased if taken with food.

    Herb/Nutraceutical: Avoid dong quai if using for hypertension (has estrogenic activity). Avoid yohimbe, ginseng (may worsen hypertension).

Stability Store at room temperature of ~25°C (77°F). Protect from light and dispense in a light-resistant, tight container.

Mechanism of Action Competitively blocks beta$_1$-adrenergic receptors with little or no effect on beta$_2$-receptors except at high doses; exhibits membrane stabilizing and intrinsic sympathomimetic activity

Pharmacokinetics

    Absorption: Oral: Well absorbed, 90%

    Protein binding: 25%

    Metabolism: Undergoes extensive first-pass

    Half-life: 3-4 hours

    Time to peak: 2-4 hours

    Elimination: Primarily excreted by bile and intestinal wall 50% to 60%; renal excretion 30% to 40%; some hepatic elimination occurs

Dosage

    Geriatrics: Oral: Initial: 200-400 mg/day; dose reduction due to age-related decrease in Cl_{cr} will be necessary; do not exceed 800 mg/day.

    Adults:

        Angina, ventricular arrhythmia: Oral: 400 mg/day in divided doses; maintenance: 600-1200 mg/day in divided doses; maximum: 1200 mg/day

        Hypertension: Oral: 400-800 mg/day (larger doses may be divided); maximum: 1200 mg/day; usual dose range (JNC 7): 200-800 mg/day in 2 divided doses

    Renal Impairment:

        Cl_{cr} 25-49 mL/minute/1.73 m^2: Reduce dose by 50%.

        Cl_{cr} <25 mL/minute/1.73 m^2: Reduce dose by 75%.

    Hepatic Impairment: Use with caution.

Administration To discontinue therapy, taper dose gradually. May be administered without regard to meals.

Monitoring Parameters Blood pressure, orthostatic hypotension, heart rate, CNS effects

Test Interactions Increased triglycerides, potassium, uric acid, cholesterol (S), glucose, thyroxine (S); decreased HDL

Patient Information Do not discontinue medication abruptly; sudden stopping of medication may precipitate or cause angina; consult pharmacist or physician before taking with other adrenergic drugs (eg, cold medications); notify physician if any of the following symptoms occur: difficult breathing, night cough, swelling of extremities, slow pulse, dizziness, lightheadedness, confusion, depression, skin rash, fever, sore throat, unusual bleeding or bruising; may produce drowsiness, dizziness, lightheadedness, blurred vision, confusion; use with caution while driving or performing tasks requiring alertness; may mask signs of hypoglycemia in diabetics; may be taken without regard to meals

Special Geriatric Considerations Since bioavailability increased in elderly about twofold, geriatric patients may require lower maintenance doses, therefore, as serum and tissue concentrations increase beta$_1$ selectivity diminishes; due to alterations in the beta-adrenergic autonomic nervous system, beta-adrenergic blockade may result in less hemodynamic response than seen in younger adults. Studies indicate that despite decreased sensitivity to the chronotropic effects of beta-blockade with age, there appears to be an increased myocardial sensitivity to the negative inotropic effect during stress (ie, exercise). Controlled trials have shown the overall response rate for propranolol to be only 20% to 50% in elderly populations. Therefore, all beta-adrenergic blocking drugs may result in a decreased response as compared to younger adults. Adjust dose for renal function.

Dosage Forms Excipient information presented when available (limited, particularly for generics); consult specific product labeling.
Capsule, as hydrochloride: 200 mg, 400 mg
  Sectral®: 200 mg, 400 mg

Selected References
Chobanian AV, Bakris GL, Black HR, et al, "The Seventh Report of the Joint National Committee on Prevention, Detection, Evaluation, and Treatment of High Blood Pressure: The JNC 7 Report," *JAMA*, 2003, 289(19):2560-71.
Kligman EW and Higbee MD, "Drug Therapy for Hypertension in the Elderly," *J Fam Pract*, 1989, 28(1):81-7.
Levison SP, "Treating Hypertension in the Elderly," *Clin Geriatr Med*, 1988, 4(1):1-12.
Vestal RE, Wood AJ, and Shand DG, "Reduced Beta-Adrenoceptor Sensitivity in the Elderly," *Clin Pharmacol Ther*, 1979, 26(2):181-6.
Yin FC, Raizes GS, Guarnieri T, et al, "Age-Associated Decrease in Ventricular Response to Haemodynamic Stress During Beta-Adrenergic Blockade," *Br Heart J*, 1978, 40(12):1349-55.

♦ **Acebutolol Hydrochloride** *see* Acebutolol *on page 27*
♦ **Aceon**® *see* Perindopril Erbumine *on page 1232*
♦ **Acephen**™ **[OTC]** *see* Acetaminophen *on page 29*
♦ **Acerola [OTC]** *see* Ascorbic Acid *on page 125*

Acetaminophen (a seet a MIN oh fen)

Medication Safety Issues
Sound-alike/look-alike issues:
  Acephen® may be confused with AcipHex®
  FeverALL® may be confused with Fiberall®
  Tylenol® may be confused with atenolol, timolol, Tuinal®, Tylox®
International issues:
  Paralen® [Czech Republic] may be confused with Aralen® which is a brand name for chloroquine in the U.S.
  Duorol® may be confused with Diuril® which is a brand name for chlorothiazide in the U.S.

Duplicate therapy issues: This product contains acetaminophen, which may be a component of combination products. Do not exceed the maximum recommended daily dose of acetaminophen.

U.S. Brand Names Acephen™ [OTC]; Apra Children's [OTC]; Aspirin Free Anacin® Maximum Strength [OTC]; Cetafen® [OTC]; Cetafen Extra® [OTC]; Comtrex® Sore Throat Maximum Strength [OTC]; FeverALL® [OTC]; Genapap™ [OTC]; Genapap™ Children [OTC]; Genapap™ Extra Strength [OTC]; Genapap™ Infant [OTC]; Genebs [OTC]; Genebs Extra Strength [OTC]; Infantaire [OTC]; Mapap [OTC]; Mapap Children's [OTC]; Mapap Extra Strength [OTC]; Mapap Infants [OTC]; Nortemp Children's [OTC]; Pain Eze [OTC]; Silapap® Children's [OTC]; Silapap® Infants [OTC]; Tycolene [OTC]; Tycolene Maximum Strength [OTC]; Tylenol® [OTC]; Tylenol® 8 Hour [OTC]; Tylenol® Arthritis Pain [OTC]; Tylenol® Children's [OTC]; Tylenol® Children's with Flavor Creator [OTC]; Tylenol® Extra Strength [OTC]; Tylenol® Infants [OTC]; Tylenol® Junior [OTC]; Valorin [OTC]; Valorin Extra [OTC]

Canadian Brand Names Abenol®; Apo-Acetaminophen®; Atasol®; Novo-Gesic; Pediatrix; Tempra®; Tylenol®

Index Terms APAP; N-Acetyl-P-Aminophenol; Paracetamol

Generic Available Yes: Excludes extended release products

Pharmacologic Category Analgesic, Miscellaneous

Use Treatment of mild to moderate pain and fever (antipyretic/analgesic); does not have antirheumatic or anti-inflammatory effects

Contraindications Hypersensitivity to acetaminophen or any component of the formulation

Warnings/Precautions Limit dose to <4 g/day. May cause severe hepatic toxicity on acute overdose; in addition, chronic daily dosing in adults has resulted in liver damage in some patients. Use with caution in patients with alcoholic liver disease; consuming ≥3 alcoholic drinks/day may increase the risk of liver damage. Use caution in patients with known G6PD deficiency.

OTC labeling: When used for self-medication, patients should be instructed to contact healthcare provider if used for fever lasting >3 days or for pain lasting >10 days in adults.
(Continued)

Acetaminophen *(Continued)*

Adverse Reactions (Reflective of adult population; not specific for elderly)
Frequency not defined.

Dermatologic: Rash

Endocrine & metabolic: May increase chloride, uric acid, glucose; may decrease sodium, bicarbonate, calcium

Hematologic: Anemia; blood dyscrasias (neutropenia, pancytopenia, leukopenia)

Hepatic: Bilirubin increased, alkaline phosphatase increased

Renal: Ammonia increased, nephrotoxicity with chronic overdose, analgesic nephropathy

Miscellaneous: Hypersensitivity reactions (rare)

Overdosage/Toxicology
Symptoms include hepatic necrosis, transient azotemia, renal tubular necrosis with acute toxicity, anemia, and GI disturbances with chronic toxicity. Acetylcysteine 140 mg/kg orally (loading) followed by 70 mg/kg every 4 hours for 17 doses. Therapy should be initiated based upon laboratory analysis suggesting high probability of hepatotoxic potential. Activated charcoal is very effective at binding acetaminophen.

Drug Interactions
Substrate (minor) of CYP1A2, 2A6, 2C9, 2D6, 2E1, 3A4; **Inhibits** CYP3A4 (weak)

Decreased effect: Barbiturates, carbamazepine, hydantoins, rifampin, sulfinpyrazone may decrease the analgesic effect of acetaminophen. Cholestyramine may decrease acetaminophen absorption (separate dosing by at least 1 hour).

Increased toxicity: Barbiturates, carbamazepine, hydantoins, isoniazid, rifampin, sulfinpyrazone may increase the hepatotoxic potential of acetaminophen. Chronic ethanol abuse increases risk for acetaminophen toxicity; effect of warfarin may be enhanced.

Ethanol/Nutrition/Herb Interactions
Ethanol: Excessive intake of ethanol may increase the risk of acetaminophen-induced hepatotoxicity. Avoid ethanol or limit to <3 drinks/day.

Food: Rate of absorption may be decreased when given with food.

Herb/Nutraceutical: St John's wort may decrease acetaminophen levels.

Stability
Do not freeze suppositories.

Mechanism of Action
Inhibits the synthesis of prostaglandins in the central nervous system and peripherally blocks pain impulse generation; produces antipyresis from inhibition of hypothalamic heat-regulating center

Pharmacokinetics
Onset of action: <1 hour

Duration: 4-6 hours

Absorption: Incomplete; varies by dosage form

Protein binding: 8% to 43% at toxic doses

Metabolism: At normal therapeutic dosages the parent compound is metabolized in the liver to sulfate and glucuronide metabolites, while a small amount is metabolized by microsomal mixed function oxidases to a highly reactive intermediate (N-acetyl-imidoquinone) which is conjugated with glutathione and inactivated; at toxic doses (as little as 4 g in a single day) glutathione can become depleted, and conjugation becomes insufficient to meet the metabolic demand causing an increase in N-acetyl-imidoquinone concentration, which is thought to cause hepatic cell necrosis

Half-life elimination: Prolonged following toxic doses: Adults: 1-3 hours (may be increased in elderly; however, this should not affect dosing)

Time to peak serum concentration: Oral: 10-60 minutes after normal doses, but may be delayed in acute overdoses

Elimination: Urine (2% to 5% unchanged; 55% as glucuronide metabolites; 30% as sulphate metabolites)

Dosage
Geriatrics & Adults: Pain or fever: Oral, rectal: 325-650 mg every 4-6 hours or 1000 mg 3-4 times/day; do **not** exceed 4 g/day.

Renal Impairment:
Cl_{cr} 10-50 mL/minute: Administer every 6 hours.

Cl_{cr} <10 mL/minute: Administer every 8 hours (metabolites accumulate).

Moderately dialyzable (20% to 50%)

Hepatic Impairment: Use with caution. Limited, low-dose therapy is usually well tolerated in hepatic disease/cirrhosis. However, cases of hepatotoxicity at daily acetaminophen dosages <4 g/day have been reported. Avoid chronic use in hepatic impairment.

Monitoring Parameters
Relief of pain or fever

Reference Range
Toxic concentration (acute ingestion) with probable hepatotoxicity: >200 mcg/mL at 4 hours after ingestion or 50 mcg/mL at 12 hours after ingestion

Test Interactions
Increased chloride, bilirubin, uric acid, glucose, ammonia (B), chloride (S), uric acid (S), alkaline phosphatase (S), chloride (S); decreased sodium, bicarbonate, calcium (S)

Patient Information Do not exceed recommended dosage; check cough and cold preparations for acetaminophen content; avoid alcohol while taking acetaminophen

Additional Information The American College of Rheumatology has recommended acetaminophen as the first-line drug in the treatment of osteoarthritis of the hip or knee.

Dosage Forms Excipient information presented when available (limited, particularly for generics); consult specific product labeling. [DSC] = Discontinued product

Caplet: 500 mg

    Cetafen Extra® Strength, Genapap™ Extra Strength, Genebs Extra Strength, Mapap Extra Strength, Tycolene Maximum Strength, Tylenol® Extra Strength: 500 mg

Caplet, extended release:

    Tylenol® 8 Hour, Tylenol® Arthritis Pain: 650 mg

Capsule: 500 mg

Elixir: 160 mg/5 mL (120 mL, 480 mL, 3780 mL)

    Apra Children's: 160 mg/5 mL (120 mL, 480 mL, 3780 mL) [alcohol free; contains benzoic acid; cherry and grape flavors]

    Mapap Children's: 160 mg/5 mL (120 mL) [alcohol free; contains benzoic acid and sodium benzoate; cherry flavor]

Gelcap:

    Mapap Extra Strength, Tylenol® Extra Strength: 500 mg

Geltab:

    Tylenol® Extra Strength: 500 mg

Geltab, extended release:

    Tylenol® 8 Hour: 650 mg [DSC]

Liquid, oral: 500 mg/15 mL (240 mL)

    Comtrex® Sore Throat Maximum Strength: 500 mg/15 mL (240 mL) [contains sodium benzoate; honey lemon flavor]

    Genapap™ Children: 160 mg/5 mL (120 mL) [contains sodium benzoate; cherry and grape flavors]

    Silapap®: 160 mg/5 mL (120 mL, 240 mL, 480 mL) [sugar free; contains sodium benzoate; cherry flavor]

    Tylenol® Extra Strength: 500 mg/15 mL (240 mL) [contains sodium benzoate; cherry flavor]

Solution, oral: 160 mg/5 mL (120 mL, 480 mL)

Solution, oral [drops]: 80 mg/0.8 mL (15 mL) [droppers are marked at 0.4 mL (40 mg) and at 0.8 mL (80 mg)]

    Genapap™ Infant: 80 mg/0.8 mL (15 mL) [fruit flavor]

    Infantaire: 80 mg/0.8mL (15 mL, 30 mL)

    Silapap® Infant's: 80 mg/0.8 mL (15 mL, 30 mL) [contains sodium benzoate; cherry flavor]

Suppository, rectal: 120 mg, 325 mg, 650 mg

    Acephen™: 120 mg, 325 mg, 650 mg

    FeverALL®: 80 mg, 120 mg, 325 mg, 650 mg

    Mapap: 125 mg, 650 mg

Suspension, oral:

    Mapap Children's: 160 mg/5 mL (120 mL) [contains sodium benzoate; cherry flavor]

    Nortemp Children's: 160 mg/5 mL (120 mL) [alcohol free; contains sodium benzoate; cotton candy flavor]

    Tylenol® Children's: 160 mg/5 mL (120 mL, 240 mL) [contains sodium benzoate; bubble gum yum, cherry blast, dye free cherry, grape splash, and very berry strawberry flavors]

    Tylenol® Children's with Flavor Creator: 160 mg/5 mL (120 mL) [contains sodium 2 mg/5 mL and sodium benzoate; cherry blast flavor; packaged with apple (4), bubblegum (8), chocolate (4), & strawberry (4) sugar free flavor packets]

Suspension, oral [drops]:

    Mapap Infants: 80 mg/0.8 mL (15 mL, 30 mL) [contains sodium benzoate; cherry flavor]

    Tylenol® Infants: 80 mg/0.8 mL (15 mL, 30 mL) [contains sodium benzoate; cherry, dye free cherry, and grape flavors]

Tablet: 325 mg, 500 mg

    Aspirin Free Anacin® Extra Strength, Genapap™ Extra Strength, Genebs Extra Strength, Mapap Extra Strength, Pain Eze, Tylenol® Extra Strength, Valorin Extra: 500 mg

    Cetafen®, Genapap™, Genebs, Mapap, Tycolene, Tylenol®, Valorin: 325 mg

Tablet, chewable: 80 mg

    Genapap™ Children: 80 mg [contains phenylalanine 6 mg/tablet; fruit and grape flavors]

    Mapap Children's: 80 mg [contains phenylalanine 3 mg/tablet; bubble gum, fruit, and grape flavors]

    Mapap Junior Strength: 160 mg [contains phenylalanine 12 mg/tablet; grape flavor]

Tablet, orally disintegrating: 80 mg, 160 mg

    Tylenol® Children's Meltaways: 80 mg [bubble gum, grape, and watermelon flavors]

    Tylenol® Junior Meltaways: 160 mg [bubble gum and grape flavors]

(Continued)

Acetaminophen *(Continued)*

Selected References

AGS Panel on Persistent Pain in Older Persons, "The Management of Persistent Pain in Older Persons," *J Am Geriatr Soc*, 2002, 50(6 Suppl):S205-24.

Hochberg MC, Altman RD, Brandt KD, et al, "Guidelines for the Medical Management of Osteoarthritis. Part I. Osteoarthritis of the Hip. American College of Rheumatology," *Arthritis Rheum*, 1995, 38(11):1535-40.

Hochberg MC, Altman RD, Brandt KD, et al, "Guidelines for the Medical Management of Osteoarthritis. Part II. Osteoarthritis of the Knee. American College of Rheumatology," *Arthritis Rheum*, 1995, 38(11):1541-6.

Acetaminophen and Codeine (a seet a MIN oh fen & KOE deen)

Related Information

Acetaminophen *on page 29*
Codeine *on page 356*

Medication Safety Issues

Sound-alike/look-alike issues:
Capital® may be confused with Capitrol®
Tylenol® may be confused with atenolol, timolol, Tuinal®, Tylox®

T3 is an error-prone abbreviation (mistaken as liothyronine)

Duplicate therapy issues: This product contains acetaminophen, which may be a component of other combination products. Do not exceed the maximum recommended daily dose of acetaminophen.

U.S. Brand Names Capital® and Codeine; Tylenol® With Codeine

Canadian Brand Names ratio-Emtec; ratio-Lenoltec; Triatec-8; Triatec-8 Strong; Triatec-30; Tylenol Elixir with Codeine; Tylenol No. 1; Tylenol No. 1 Forte; Tylenol No. 2 with Codeine; Tylenol No. 3 with Codeine; Tylenol No. 4 with Codeine

Index Terms Codeine and Acetaminophen

Generic Available Yes

Pharmacologic Category Analgesic, Opioid

Use Relief of mild to moderate pain

Restrictions C-III; C-V

Note: In countries outside of the U.S., some formulations of Tylenol® with Codeine (eg, Tylenol® No. 3) include caffeine.

Dosage

Geriatrics: Doses should be titrated to appropriate analgesic effect.
1 Tylenol® [#3] or 2 Tylenol® [#2] tablets every 4 hours; do **not** exceed 4 g/day acetaminophen.

Adults: Doses should be adjusted according to severity of pain and response of the patient. Adult doses ≥60 mg codeine fail to give commensurate relief of pain but merely prolong analgesia and are associated with an appreciably increased incidence of side effects.

Cough (Antitussive): Oral: Based on codeine (15-30 mg/dose) every 4-6 hours (maximum: 360 mg/24 hours based on codeine component)

Pain (Analgesic): Oral: Based on codeine (30-60 mg/dose) every 4-6 hours (maximum: 4000 mg/24 hours based on acetaminophen component)
1-2 tablets every 4 hours to a maximum of 12 tablets/24 hours

Renal Impairment: See individual agents.

Hepatic Impairment: Use with caution. Limited, low-dose therapy is usually well tolerated in hepatic disease/cirrhosis; however, cases of hepatotoxicity at daily acetaminophen dosages <4 g/day have been reported. Avoid chronic use in hepatic impairment.

Dosage Forms Excipient information presented when available (limited, particularly for generics); consult specific product labeling. [DSC] = Discontinued product; [CAN] = Canadian brand name

Caplet:
ratio-Lenoltec No. 1 [CAN], Tylenol No. 1 [CAN]: Acetaminophen 300 mg, codeine phosphate 8 mg, and caffeine 15 mg [not available in the U.S.]
Tylenol No. 1 Forte [CAN]: Acetaminophen 500 mg, codeine phosphate 8 mg, and caffeine 15 mg [not available in the U.S.]

Elixir, oral [C-V]: Acetaminophen 120 mg and codeine phosphate 12 mg per 5 mL (5 mL, 10 mL, 12.5 mL, 15 mL, 120 mL, 480 mL) [contains alcohol 7%]
Tylenol® with Codeine [DSC]: Acetaminophen 120 mg and codeine phosphate 12 mg per 5 mL (480 mL) [contains alcohol 7%; cherry flavor]
Tylenol Elixir with Codeine [CAN]: Acetaminophen 160 mg and codeine phosphate 8 mg per 5 mL (500 mL) [contains alcohol 7%, sucrose 31%; cherry flavor; not available in the U.S.]

Suspension, oral [C-V] (Capital® and Codeine): Acetaminophen 120 mg and codeine phosphate 12 mg per 5 mL (480 mL) [alcohol free; fruit punch flavor]

Tablet [C-III]: Acetaminophen 300 mg and codeine phosphate 15 mg; acetaminophen 300 mg and codeine phosphate 30 mg; acetaminophen 300 mg and codeine phosphate 60 mg

ratio-Emtec [CAN], Triatec-30 [CAN]: Acetaminophen 300 mg and codeine phosphate 30 mg [not available in the U.S.]

ratio-Lenoltec No. 1 [CAN]: Acetaminophen 300 mg, codeine phosphate 8 mg, and caffeine 15 mg [not available in the U.S.]

ratio-Lenoltec No. 2 [CAN], Tylenol No. 2 with Codeine [CAN]: Acetaminophen 300 mg, codeine phosphate 15 mg, and caffeine 15 mg [not available in the U.S.]

ratio-Lenoltec No. 3 [CAN], Tylenol No. 3 with Codeine [CAN]: Acetaminophen 300 mg, codeine phosphate 30 mg, and caffeine 15 mg [not available in the U.S.]

ratio-Lenoltec No. 4 [CAN], Tylenol No. 4 with Codeine [CAN]: Acetaminophen 300 mg and codeine phosphate 60 mg [not available in the U.S.]

Triatec-8 [CAN]: Acetaminophen 325 mg, codeine phosphate 8 mg, and caffeine 30 mg [not available in the U.S.]

Triatec-8 Strong [CAN]: Acetaminophen 500 mg, codeine phosphate 8 mg, and caffeine 30 mg [not available in the U.S.]

Tylenol® with Codeine No. 3: Acetaminophen 300 mg and codeine phosphate 30 mg [contains sodium metabisulfite]

Tylenol® with Codeine No. 4: Acetaminophen 300 mg and codeine phosphate 60 mg [contains sodium metabisulfite]

♦ **Acetaminophen and Hydrocodone** *see* Hydrocodone and Acetaminophen *on page 759*

♦ **Acetaminophen and Oxycodone** *see* Oxycodone and Acetaminophen *on page 1182*

♦ **Acetaminophen and Propoxyphene** *see* Propoxyphene and Acetaminophen *on page 1335*

AcetaZOLAMIDE (a set a ZOLE a mide)

Related Information
Glaucoma Drug Therapy *on page 1758*

Medication Safety Issues
Sound-alike/look-alike issues:
AcetaZOLAMIDE may be confused with acetoHEXAMIDE
Diamox® Sequels® may be confused with Diabinese®, Dobutrex®, Trimox®

U.S. Brand Names Diamox® Sequels®

Canadian Brand Names Apo-Acetazolamide®; Diamox®

Generic Available Yes: Injection, tablet

Pharmacologic Category Anticonvulsant, Miscellaneous; Carbonic Anhydrase Inhibitor; Diuretic, Carbonic Anhydrase Inhibitor; Ophthalmic Agent, Antiglaucoma

Use Treatment of glaucoma (chronic simple open-angle, secondary glaucoma, preoperatively in acute angle-closure), drug-induced edema, centrencephalic epilepsies (immediate release dosage form); prevention or amelioration of symptoms associated with acute mountain sickness; adjunctive therapy for edema due to congestive heart failure

Unlabeled/Investigational Use Urine alkalinization; respiratory stimulant in COPD

Contraindications Hypersensitivity to acetazolamide, sulfonamides, or any component of the formulation; hepatic disease or insufficiency; decreased sodium and/or potassium levels; adrenocortical insufficiency; cirrhosis; hyperchloremic acidosis; severe renal disease or dysfunction; severe pulmonary obstruction; long-term use in noncongestive angle-closure glaucoma

Warnings/Precautions Use with caution in patients with hepatic dysfunction; in cirrhosis, avoid electrolyte and acid/base imbalances that might lead to hepatic encephalopathy. Use with caution in patients with respiratory acidosis and diabetes mellitus (may change glucose control). Use with caution in the elderly; may be more sensitive to side effects. Impairment of mental alertness and/or physical coordination may occur. Chemical similarities are present among sulfonamides, sulfonylureas, carbonic anhydrase inhibitors, thiazides, and loop diuretics (except ethacrynic acid). Use in patients with sulfonamide allergy is specifically contraindicated in product labeling, however, a risk of cross-reaction exists in patients with allergy to any of these compounds; avoid use when previous reaction has been severe. Discontinue if signs of hypersensitivity are noted.

I.M. administration is painful because of the alkaline pH of the drug; use by this route is not recommended.

Adverse Reactions (Reflective of adult population; not specific for elderly)
Frequency not defined.
Cardiovascular: Flushing
Central nervous system: Ataxia, confusion, convulsions, depression, dizziness, drowsiness, excitement, fatigue, fever, headache, malaise

(Continued)

AcetaZOLAMIDE *(Continued)*

Dermatologic: Allergic skin reactions, photosensitivity, Stevens-Johnson syndrome, toxic epidermal necrolysis, urticaria

Endocrine & metabolic: Electrolyte imbalance, growth retardation (children), hyperglycemia, hypoglycemia, hypokalemia, hyponatremia, metabolic acidosis

Gastrointestinal: Appetite decreased, diarrhea, melena, nausea, taste alteration, vomiting

Genitourinary: Crystalluria, glycosuria, hematuria, polyuria, renal failure

Hematologic: Agranulocytosis, aplastic anemia, leukopenia, thrombocytopenia, thrombocytopenic purpura

Hepatic: Cholestatic jaundice, fulminant hepatic necrosis, hepatic insufficiency, liver function tests abnormal

Local: Pain at injection site

Neuromuscular & skeletal: Flaccid paralysis, paresthesia

Ocular: Myopia

Otic: Hearing disturbance, tinnitus

Miscellaneous: Anaphylaxis

Overdosage/Toxicology Symptoms include low blood sugar, tingling of lips and tongue, nausea, yawning, confusion, agitation, tachycardia, sweating, convulsions, stupor, and coma. Hypoglycemia should be managed with 50 mL I.V. dextrose 50% followed immediately with a continuous infusion of 10% dextrose in water (administer at a rate sufficient enough to approach a serum glucose level of 100 mg/dL). The use of corticosteroids to treat the hypoglycemia is controversial, however, the addition of 100 mg of hydrocortisone to the dextrose infusion may prove helpful. In certain instances, hemodialysis may be helpful.

Drug Interactions Inhibits CYP3A4 (weak)

Amphetamines: Urinary excretion of amphetamine may be decreased; magnitude and duration of effects may be enhanced.

Carbamazepine: May increase serum concentrations of carbamazepine.

Cyclosporine trough concentrations may be increased resulting in possible nephrotoxicity and neurotoxicity.

Flecainide: May decrease excretion of flecainide.

Lithium: Serum concentrations may be decreased by acetazolamide; monitor.

Memantine: May decrease excretion of memantine.

Methenamine: Urinary antiseptic effect may be prevented by acetazolamide.

Phenytoin: Serum concentrations of phenytoin may be increased; incidence of osteomalacia may be enhanced or increased in patients on chronic phenytoin therapy.

Primidone serum concentrations may be decreased; carbonic anhydrase inhibitors may enhance the adverse/toxic effects of primidone.

Quinidine: Urinary excretion of quinidine may be decreased and effects may be enhanced.

Salicylate use (high dose) may result in carbonic anhydrase inhibitor accumulation and toxicity including CNS depression and metabolic acidosis. Salicylate toxicity might also be enhanced.

Stability

Capsules, tablets: Store at controlled room temperature.

Injection: Store vial for injection (prior to reconstitution) at controlled room temperature. Reconstitute with at least 5 mL sterile water to provide a solution containing not more than 100 mg/mL. Reconstituted solution may be refrigerated (2°C to 8°C) for 1 week, however, use within 12 hours is recommended. Further dilute in D_5W or NS for I.V. infusion. Stability of IVPB solution is 5 days at room temperature (25°C) and 44 days at refrigeration (5°C).

Mechanism of Action Reversible inhibition of the enzyme carbonic anhydrase resulting in reduction of hydrogen ion secretion at renal tubule and an increased renal excretion of sodium, potassium, bicarbonate, and water to decrease production of aqueous humor; also inhibits carbonic anhydrase in central nervous system to retard abnormal and excessive discharge from CNS neurons

Pharmacodynamics

Onset of action: Lowering of intraocular pressure varies between 2 minutes with the I.V. form to 2 hours with the sustained release capsule

Peak effect:
I.V.: 15 minutes
Capsule, sustained release: 8-12 hours
Tablet: 1-4 hours

Duration:
I.V.: 4-5 hours
Capsule, sustained release: 18-24 hours
Tablet: 8-12 hours

Pharmacokinetics

Distribution: Into erythrocytes, kidneys and crosses the blood-brain barrier

Protein binding: 95% bound to serum proteins; may be lower in older adults; increased plasma concentrations secondary to decreased clearance in older persons with decreased renal function; these changes increase the risk of hyperchloremic acidosis

Half-life: 2.4-5.8 hours

Elimination: 70% to 100% of the I.V. or tablet dose is excreted unchanged in the urine within 24 hours

Dosage

Geriatrics: Oral: Initial: 250 mg once or twice daily; use lowest effective dose possible.

Adults: Note: I.M. administration is not recommended.

Glaucoma:

Chronic simple (open-angle): Oral: 250 mg 1-4 times/day or 500 mg extended release capsule twice daily

Secondary, acute (closed-angle): I.V.: 250-500 mg, may repeat in 2-4 hours to a maximum of 1 g/day

Edema: Oral, I.V.: 250-375 mg once daily

Epilepsy: Oral: 8-30 mg/kg/day in 1-4 divided doses, not to exceed 1 g/day. **Note:** Extended release capsule is not recommended for treatment of epilepsy.

Metabolic alkalosis (unlabeled use): I.V. 250 mg every 6 hours for 4 doses or 500 mg single dose; reassess need based upon acid-base status

Mountain sickness: Oral: 250 mg every 8-12 hours (or 500 mg extended release capsules every 12-24 hours). Therapy should begin 24-48 hours before and continue during ascent and for at least 48 hours after arrival at the high altitude. **Note:** In situations of rapid ascent (such as rescue or military operations), 1000 mg/day is recommended.

Urine alkalinization (unlabeled use): Oral: 5 mg/kg/dose repeated 2-3 times over 24 hours

Respiratory stimulant in COPD (unlabeled use): Oral, I.V.: 250 mg twice daily

Renal Impairment:

Cl_{cr} 10-50 mL/minute: Administer every 12 hours.

Cl_{cr} <10 mL/minute: Avoid use (ineffective).

Moderately dialyzable (20% to 50%)

Administration Reconstitute each 500 mg vial with 5 mL of sterile water for injection to yield a concentration of 100 mg/mL; may cause an alteration in taste, especially carbonated beverages; short-acting tablets may be crushed and suspended in cherry or chocolate syrup to disguise the bitter taste of the drug, do not use fruit juices, alternatively submerge tablet in 10 mL of hot water and add 10 mL honey or syrup

Monitoring Parameters Intraocular pressure, serum bicarbonate, sodium and potassium, periodic CBC with differential, blood pressure (sitting and standing)

Reference Range Total: 5-10 mcg/mL; Free (unbound) 0.25-0.5 mcg/mL

Test Interactions May cause false-positive results for urinary protein with Albustix®, Labstix®, Albutest®, Bumintest®; interferes with HPLC theophylline assay and serum uric acid levels

Patient Information Report numbness or tingling of extremities to physician; do not crush, chew, or swallow contents of long-acting capsule, but may be opened and sprinkled on soft food; ability to perform tasks requiring mental alertness and/or physical coordination may be impaired; take with food

Additional Information Drug may cause substantial increase in blood glucose in some diabetic patients; sustained release capsule is not recommended for treatment of epilepsy; the use of analgesic doses of salicylates should be avoided in patients treated with acetazolamide, especially older adults

Special Geriatric Considerations Malaise and complaints of tiredness and myalgia are signs of excessive dosing and acidosis in older adults. Orthostatic hypotension may occur; assess blood pressure.

Dosage Forms Excipient information presented when available (limited, particularly for generics); consult specific product labeling.

Capsule, extended release:

Diamox® Sequels®: 500 mg

Injection, powder for reconstitution: 500 mg

Tablet: 125 mg, 250 mg

Selected References

Chapron DJ, Gomolin IH, and Sweeney KR, "Acetazolamide Blood Concentrations are Excessive in the Elderly: Propensity for Acidosis and Relationship to Renal Function," *J Clin Pharmacol*, 1989, 29(4):348-53.

Chapron DJ, Sweeney KR, Feig PU, et al, "Influence of Advanced Age on the Disposition of Acetazolamide," *Br J Clin Pharmacol*, 1985, 19(3):363-71.

Heller I, Halevy J, Cohen S, et al, "Significant Metabolic Acidosis Induced by Acetazolamide. Not a Rare Complication," *Arch Intern Med*, 1985, 145(10):1815-7.

Reiss WG and Oles KS, "Acetazolamide in the Treatment of Seizures," *Ann Pharmacother*, 1996, 30(5):514-9.

Rousseau P and Fuentevila-Clifton A, "Acetazolamide and Salicylate Interaction in the Elderly: A Case Report," *J Am Geriatr Soc*, 1993, 41(8):868-9.

♦ **Acetoxymethylprogesterone** *see* MedroxyPROGESTERone *on page 965*

Acetylcholine (a se teel KOE leen)

Medication Safety Issues
Sound-alike/look-alike issues:
Acetylcholine may be confused with acetylcysteine
U.S. Brand Names Miochol®-E
Canadian Brand Names Miochol®-E
Index Terms Acetylcholine Chloride
Generic Available No
Pharmacologic Category Cholinergic Agonist; Ophthalmic Agent, Miotic
Use Production of complete miosis in cataract surgery, keratoplasty, iridectomy, and other anterior segment surgery where rapid miosis is required
Contraindications Hypersensitivity to acetylcholine chloride or any component of the formulation; acute iritis and acute inflammatory disease of the anterior chamber
Warnings/Precautions During cataract surgery, use only after lens is in place. Systemic effects rarely occur but can cause problems for patients with acute cardiac failure, bronchial asthma, peptic ulcer, hyperthyroidism, GI spasm, urinary tract obstruction, and Parkinson's disease; open under aseptic conditions only.
Adverse Reactions (Reflective of adult population; not specific for elderly)
Frequency not defined.
Cardiovascular: Bradycardia, flushing, hypotension
Central nervous system: Headache
Ocular: Clouding, corneal edema, decompensation
Respiratory: Dyspnea
Miscellaneous: Diaphoresis
Overdosage/Toxicology Treatment includes flushing eyes with water or normal saline and supportive measures. If accidentally ingested, induce emesis or perform gastric lavage.
Drug Interactions
Decreased effect possible with flurbiprofen and suprofen, ophthalmic.
Increased effect may be prolonged or enhanced in patients receiving tacrine.
Stability Store unopened vial at 4°C to 25°C (39°F to 77°F); prevent from freezing. Prepare solution immediately before use and discard unused portion. Acetylcholine solutions are unstable; reconstitute immediately before use.
Mechanism of Action Causes contraction of the sphincter muscles of the iris, resulting in miosis and contraction of the ciliary muscle, leading to accommodation spasm
Pharmacodynamics
Onset of miosis: In seconds
Duration: ~10-20 minutes
Dosage
Geriatrics & Adults: To produce miosis: Intraocular: 0.5-2 mL of 1% injection (5-20 mg) instilled into anterior chamber before or after securing one or more sutures
Administration Discard any solution that is not used; open under aseptic conditions only
Patient Information May sting on instillation; use caution while driving at night or performing hazardous tasks
Dosage Forms Excipient information presented when available (limited, particularly for generics); consult specific product labeling.
Powder for solution, intraocular, as chloride:
Miochol®-E: 1:100 [20 mg; packaged with diluent (2 mL)]

- **Activated Methylpolysiloxane** *see* Simethicone *on page 1467*
- **Actonel®** *see* Risedronate *on page 1413*
- **Actonel® and Calcium** *see* Risedronate and Calcium *on page 1415*
- **Actoplus Met™** *see* Pioglitazone and Metformin *on page 1269*
- **Actos®** *see* Pioglitazone *on page 1266*
- **ACT® Plus [OTC]** *see* Fluoride *on page 642*
- **ACT® x2™ [OTC]** *see* Fluoride *on page 642*
- **Acular®** *see* Ketorolac *on page 859*
- **Acular LS™** *see* Ketorolac *on page 859*
- **Acular® PF** *see* Ketorolac *on page 859*
- **ACV** *see* Acyclovir *on page 37*
- **Acycloguanosine** *see* Acyclovir *on page 37*

Acyclovir (ay SYE kloe veer)

Medication Safety Issues
Sound-alike/look-alike issues:
Zovirax® may be confused with Zostrix®, Zyvox®

International issues:
Opthavir® [Mexico] may be confused with Optivar® which is a brand name for azelastine in the U.S.
U.S. Brand Names Zovirax®
Canadian Brand Names Apo-Acyclovir®; Gen-Acyclovir; Nu-Acyclovir; ratio-Acyclovir; Zovirax®
Index Terms Aciclovir; ACV; Acycloguanosine
Generic Available Yes: Excludes cream, ointment
Pharmacologic Category Antiviral Agent
Use Treatment of initial and prophylaxis of recurrent mucosal and cutaneous herpes simplex (HSV 1 and HSV 2) infections, herpes simplex encephalitis, herpes zoster (shingles), genital herpes infection, and varicella-zoster infections in immunocompromised patients
Contraindications Hypersensitivity to acyclovir, valacyclovir, or any component of the formulation
Warnings/Precautions Use with caution in immunocompromised patients; thrombocytopenic purpura/hemolytic uremic syndrome (TTP/HUS) has been reported. Use caution in the elderly, pre-existing renal disease, or in those receiving other nephrotoxic drugs. Renal failure (sometimes fatal) has been reported. Maintain adequate hydration during oral or intravenous therapy. Use I.V. preparation with caution in patients with underlying neurologic abnormalities, serious hepatic or electrolyte abnormalities, or substantial hypoxia.

Chickenpox: Treatment should begin within 24 hours of appearance of rash

Genital herpes: Physical contact should be avoided when lesions are present; transmission may also occur in the absence of symptoms. Treatment should begin with the first signs or symptoms.

Herpes labialis: For external use only to the lips and face; do not apply to eye or inside the mouth or nose. Treatment should begin with the first signs or symptoms.

Herpes zoster: Acyclovir should be started within 72 hours of appearance of rash to be effective.
Adverse Reactions (Reflective of adult population; not specific for elderly)
Systemic: Oral:
>10%: Central nervous system: Malaise (12%)
1% to 10%:
  Central nervous system: Headache (2%)
  Gastrointestinal: Nausea (2% to 5%), vomiting (3%), diarrhea (2% to 3%)
Systemic: Parenteral:
1% to 10%:
  Dermatologic: Hives (2%), itching (2%), rash (2%)
  Gastrointestinal: Nausea/vomiting (7%)
  Hepatic: Liver function tests increased (1% to 2%)
  Local: Inflammation at injection site or phlebitis (9%)
  Renal: BUN increased (5% to 10%), creatinine increased (5% to 10%), acute renal failure
Topical:
>10%: Dermatologic: Mild pain, burning, or stinging (ointment 30%)
1% to 10%: Dermatologic: Pruritus (ointment 4%), itching
Overdosage/Toxicology Symptoms include seizures, somnolence, confusion, elevated serum creatinine, and renal failure. In the event of an overdose, sufficient
(Continued)

Acyclovir *(Continued)*

urine flow must be maintained to avoid drug precipitation within the renal tubules. Hemodialysis has resulted in up to 60% reductions in serum acyclovir levels.

Ethanol/Nutrition/Herb Interactions Food: Does not affect absorption of oral acyclovir.

Stability

Capsule, tablet: Store at controlled room temperature of 15°C to 25°C (59°F to 77°F); protect from moisture.

Cream, suspension: Store at controlled room temperature of 15°C to 25°C (59°F to 77°F).

Ointment: Store at controlled room temperature of 15°C to 25°C (59°F to 77°F) in a dry place.

Injection: Store powder at controlled room temperature of 15°C to 25°C (59°F to 77°F). Reconstitute acyclovir 500 mg with SWFI 10 mL; do not use bacteriostatic water containing benzyl alcohol or parabens. For intravenous infusion, dilute to a final concentration ≤7 mg/mL. Concentrations >10 mg/mL increase the risk of phlebitis. Reconstituted solutions remain stable for 12 hours at room temperature. Do not refrigerate reconstituted solutions as they may precipitate. Once diluted for infusion, use within 24 hours.

Mechanism of Action Acyclovir is converted to acyclovir monophosphate by virus-specific thymidine kinase then further converted to acyclovir triphosphate by other cellular enzymes. Acyclovir triphosphate inhibits DNA synthesis and viral replication by competing with deoxyguanosine triphosphate for viral DNA polymerase and being incorporated into viral DNA.

Pharmacokinetics

Absorption: Oral: 15% to 30%; food does not appear to affect absorption

Distribution: Widely throughout the body including brain, kidney, lungs, liver, spleen, muscle, uterus, vagina, and the CSF

Protein binding: <30%

Half-life (adults): Inversely affected by renal function; see table.

Creatinine Clearance (mL/min/1.73 m²)	Half-life (h)
>80	2.5
50-80	3
15-50	3.5
0-15	19.5

Time to peak serum concentration: Within 1½ to 2 hours after an oral dose, and within 1 hour following intravenous administration

Elimination: Primary route of elimination is the kidney, following a small amount of hepatic metabolism; requires dosage adjustment with renal impairment, hemodialysis removes ~60% of the dose and to a much lesser extent by peritoneal dialysis

Dosage

Geriatrics & Adults: Note: Obese patients should be dosed using ideal body weight

Genital HSV:

I.V.: Immunocompetent: Initial episode, severe: 5 mg/kg every 8 hours for 5-7 days

Oral:

Initial episode: 200 mg every 4 hours while awake (5 times/day) for 10 days (per manufacturer's labeling); 400 mg 3 times/day for 5-10 days has also been reported

Recurrence: 200 mg every 4 hours while awake (5 times/day) for 5 days (per manufacturer's labeling; begin at earliest signs of disease); 400 mg 3 times/day for 5 days has also been reported

Chronic suppression: 400 mg twice daily or 200 mg 3-5 times/day, for up to 12 months followed by re-evaluation (per manufacturer's labeling); 400-1200 mg/day in 2-3 divided doses has also been reported

Topical: Immunocompromised: Ointment: Initial episode: ½" ribbon of ointment for a 4" square surface area every 3 hours (6 times/day) for 7 days

Herpes labialis (cold sores): Topical: Apply 5 times/day for 4 days

Herpes zoster (shingles):

Oral: Immunocompetent: 800 mg every 4 hours (5 times/day) for 7-10 days

I.V.: Immunocompromised: 10 mg/kg/dose or 500 mg/m²/dose every 8 hours for 7 days

HSV encephalitis: I.V.: 10 mg/kg/dose every 8 hours for 10 days (per manufacturer's labeling); 10-15 mg/kg/dose every 8 hours for 14-21 days also reported

Mucocutaneous HSV:

I.V.: Immunocompromised: 5 mg/kg/dose every 8 hours for 7 days (per manufacturer's labeling); dosing for up to 14 days also reported

Oral: Immunocompromised (unlabeled use): 400 mg 5 times a day for 7-14 days

Topical: Ointment: Nonlife-threatening, immunocompromised: ½" ribbon of ointment for a 4" square surface area every 3 hours (6 times/day) for 7 days

Varicella-zoster (chickenpox): Begin treatment within the first 24 hours of rash onset:

Oral: >40 kg (immunocompetent): 800 mg/dose 4 times a day for 5 days

I.V.: Immunocompromised (unlabeled use): 1500 mg/m^2/day divided every 8 hours or 10 mg/kg/dose every 8 hours for 7-10 days

Prevention of HSV reactivation in HIV-positive patients, for use only when recurrences are frequent or severe (unlabeled use): Oral: 200 mg 3 times/day or 400 mg 2 times/day

Prevention of HSV reactivation in HSCT (unlabeled use): Note: Start at the beginning of conditioning therapy and continue until engraftment or until mucositis resolves (~30 days)

Oral: 200 mg 3 times/day

I.V.: 250 mg/m^2/dose every 12 hours

Bone marrow transplant recipients (unlabeled use): I.V.: Allogeneic patients who are HSV and CMV seropositive: 500 mg/m^2/dose (10 mg/kg) every 8 hours; for clinically-symptomatic CMV infection, consider replacing acyclovir with ganciclovir

Renal Impairment:

Oral:

Cl_{cr} 10-25 mL/minute/1.73 m^2: Normal dosing regimen 800 mg every 4 hours: Administer 800 mg every 8 hours

Cl_{cr} <10 mL/minute/1.73 m^2:

Normal dosing regimen 200 mg every 4 hours, 200 mg every 8 hours, or 400 mg every 12 hours: Administer 200 mg every 12 hours

Normal dosing regimen 800 mg every 4 hours: Administer 800 mg every 12 hours

I.V.:

Cl_{cr} 25-50 mL/minute/1.73 m^2: Administer recommended dose every 12 hours

Cl_{cr} 10-25 mL/minute/1.73 m^2: Administer recommended dose every 24 hours

Cl_{cr} <10 mL/minute/1.73 m^2: Administer 50% of recommended dose every 24 hours

Hemodialysis: Administer dose after dialysis

Peritoneal dialysis: No supplemental dose needed

CAVH: 3.5 mg/kg/day

CVVHD/CVVH: Adjust dose based upon Cl_{cr} 30 mL/minute

Administration

Oral: May be administered with food.

I.V.: Avoid rapid infusion; infuse over 1 hour to prevent renal damage; maintain adequate hydration of patient; check for phlebitis and rotate infusion sites

Monitoring Parameters Urinalysis, BUN, serum creatinine, liver enzymes, CBC

Reference Range

Level guidelines:

Pre: 0.1-1.6 mcg/mL

Post: 3-10 mcg/mL

Panic value: >50 mcg/mL

Infusion time: 1 hour

Patient Information Contagious only when viral shedding is occurring; avoid sexual intercourse when lesions are visible; recurrences tend to appear within 3 months of original infection; acyclovir is **not** a cure

Additional Information Injection formulations: Sodium content of 1 g: 96.6 mg (4.2 mEq)

Special Geriatric Considerations For herpes zoster, acyclovir should be started within 72 hours of the appearance of the rash to be effective. Dose adjustment may be necessary depending on creatinine clearance.

Dosage Forms Excipient information presented when available (limited, particularly for generics); consult specific product labeling. [DSC] = Discontinued product

Capsule: 200 mg

Zovirax®: 200 mg

Cream, topical:

Zovirax®: 5% (2 g, 5 g)

Injection, powder for reconstitution, as sodium: 500 mg, 1000 mg

Zovirax®: 500 mg [DSC]

Injection, solution, as sodium [preservative free]: 25 mg/mL (20 mL, 40 mL); 50 mg/mL (10 mL, 20 mL)

Ointment, topical:

Zovirax®: 5% (15 g)

Suspension, oral: 200 mg/5 mL (480 mL)

Zovirax®: 200 mg/5 mL (480 mL) [banana flavor]

Tablet: 400 mg, 800 mg

Zovirax®: 400 mg, 800 mg

(Continued)

Acyclovir *(Continued)*

Selected References

Dellamonica P, Carles M, Lokiec F, et al, "Preventing Recurrent Varicella and Herpes Zoster With Oral Acyclovir in HIV-seropositive Patients," *Clin Pharm*, 1991, 10(4):301-2.

Huff JC, Bean B, Balfour HH Jr, et al, "Therapy of Herpes Zoster With Oral Acyclovir," *Am J Med*, 1988, 85(2A):84-9.

McKendrick MW, McGill JI, White JE, et al, "Oral Acyclovir in Acute Herpes Zoster," *Br Med J (Clin Res Ed)*, 1986, 293(6561):1529-32.

Morton P and Thomson AN, "Oral Acyclovir in the Treatment of Herpes Zoster in General Practice," *N Z Med J*, 1989, 102(863):93-5.

Wood MJ, Johnson RW, McKendrick MW, et al, "A Randomized Trial of Acyclovir for 7 Days or 21 Days With and Without Prednisolone for Treatment of Acute Herpes Zoster," *N Engl J Med*, 1994, 330(13):896-900.

- **Adalat® CC** *see* NIFEdipine *on page 1119*
- **Adamantanamine Hydrochloride** *see* Amantadine *on page 68*
- **ADH** *see* Vasopressin *on page 1665*
- **Adoxa®** *see* Doxycycline *on page 479*
- **Adrenalin®** *see* Epinephrine *on page 514*
- **Adrenaline** *see* Epinephrine *on page 514*
- **Advair Diskus®** *see* Fluticasone and Salmeterol *on page 663*
- **Advair® HFA** *see* Fluticasone and Salmeterol *on page 663*
- **Advicor®** *see* Niacin and Lovastatin *on page 1111*
- **Advil® [OTC]** *see* Ibuprofen *on page 784*
- **Advil® Children's [OTC]** *see* Ibuprofen *on page 784*
- **Advil® Infants' [OTC]** *see* Ibuprofen *on page 784*
- **Advil® Junior [OTC]** *see* Ibuprofen *on page 784*
- **Advil® Migraine [OTC]** *see* Ibuprofen *on page 784*
- **AeroBid®** *see* Flunisolide *on page 637*
- **AeroBid®-M** *see* Flunisolide *on page 637*
- **Aerospan™** *see* Flunisolide *on page 637*
- **Afeditab™ CR** *see* NIFEdipine *on page 1119*
- **Afrin® Extra Moisturizing [OTC]** *see* Oxymetazoline *on page 1184*
- **Afrin® Original [OTC]** *see* Oxymetazoline *on page 1184*
- **Afrin® Severe Congestion [OTC]** *see* Oxymetazoline *on page 1184*
- **Afrin® Sinus [OTC]** *see* Oxymetazoline *on page 1184*
- **Aggrastat®** *see* Tirofiban *on page 1579*
- **Aggrenox®** *see* Aspirin and Dipyridamole *on page 131*
- **AGN 1135** *see* Rasagiline *on page 1386*
- **Ah-Chew D®** *see* Phenylephrine *on page 1247*
- **Ahist™** *see* Chlorpheniramine *on page 296*
- **A-hydroCort** *see* Hydrocortisone *on page 762*
- **AK-Con™** *see* Naphazoline *on page 1086*
- **AK-Dilate®** *see* Phenylephrine *on page 1247*
- **Akineton®** *see* Biperiden *on page 172*
- **Akne-Mycin®** *see* Erythromycin *on page 533*
- **AKTob®** *see* Tobramycin *on page 1583*
- **AK-Trol® [DSC]** *see* Neomycin, Polymyxin B, and Dexamethasone *on page 1102*
- **Akwa Tears® [OTC]** *see* Artificial Tears *on page 124*
- **Akwa Tears® Ophthalmic Ointment [OTC]** *see* Ocular Lubricant *on page 1144*
- **Alamag [OTC]** *see* Aluminum Hydroxide and Magnesium Hydroxide *on page 65*
- **Alamag Plus [OTC]** *see* Aluminum Hydroxide, Magnesium Hydroxide, and Simethicone *on page 66*
- **Alavert® [OTC]** *see* Loratadine *on page 928*
- **Alaway™ [OTC]** *see* Ketotifen *on page 863*
- **Albalon®** *see* Naphazoline *on page 1086*

Albuterol *(al BYOO ter ole)*

Related Information

Inhalant Agents *on page 1760*

Medication Safety Issues

Sound-alike/look-alike issues:

Albuterol may be confused with Albutein®, atenolol

Proventil® may be confused with Bentyl®, Prilosec® Prinivil®

Salbutamol may be confused with salmeterol

Ventolin® may be confused with phentolamine, Benylin®, Vantin®

Volmax® may be confused with Flomax®

U.S. Brand Names AccuNeb®; ProAir™ HFA; Proventil®; Proventil® HFA; Ventolin® HFA; VoSpire ER®

Canadian Brand Names Airomir; Alti-Salbutamol; Apo-Salvent®; Apo-Salvent® CFC Free; Apo-Salvent® Respirator Solution; Apo-Salvent® Sterules; Gen-Salbutamol; PMS-Salbutamol; ratio-Inspra-Sal; ratio-Salbutamol; Rhoxal-salbutamol; Salbu-2; Salbu-4; Ventolin®; Ventolin® Diskus; Ventolin® HFA; Ventolin® I.V. Infusion; Ventrodisk

Index Terms Albuterol Sulfate; Salbutamol; Salbutamol Sulphate

Generic Available Yes

Pharmacologic Category Beta$_2$-Adrenergic Agonist

Use Bronchodilator in reversible airway obstruction due to asthma or COPD

Contraindications Hypersensitivity to albuterol, adrenergic amines, or any component of the formulation

Warnings/Precautions Optimize anti-inflammatory treatment before initiating maintenance treatment with albuterol. Do not use as a component of chronic therapy without an anti-inflammatory agent. Only the mildest forms of asthma (Step 1 and/or exercise-induced) would not require concurrent use based upon asthma guidelines. Patient must be instructed to seek medical attention in cases where acute symptoms are not relieved or a previous level of response is diminished. The need to increase frequency of use may indicate deterioration of asthma, and treatment must not be delayed.

Use caution in patients with cardiovascular disease (arrhythmia or hypertension or CHF), convulsive disorders, diabetes, glaucoma, hyperthyroidism, or hypokalemia. Beta-agonists may cause elevation in blood pressure, heart rate, and result in CNS stimulation/excitation. Beta$_2$-agonists may increase risk of arrhythmia, increase serum glucose, or decrease serum potassium.

Immediate hypersensitivity reactions (urticaria, angioedema, rash, bronchospasm) have been reported. Do not exceed recommended dose; serious adverse events, including fatalities, have been associated with excessive use of inhaled sympathomimetics. Rarely, paradoxical bronchospasm may occur with use of inhaled bronchodilating agents; this should be distinguished from inadequate response. All patients should utilize a spacer device when using a metered-dose inhaler.

Because of its minimal effect on beta$_1$-receptors and its relatively long duration of action, albuterol is a rational choice in the elderly when an inhaled beta-agonist is indicated. Oral use should be avoided in the elderly due to adverse effects. Patient response may vary between inhalers that contain chlorofluorocarbons and those which are chlorofluorocarbon-free.

Adverse Reactions (Reflective of adult population; not specific for elderly) Incidence of adverse effects is dependent upon age of patient, dose, and route of administration.

Cardiovascular: Angina, atrial fibrillation, arrhythmias, chest discomfort, extrasystoles, flushing, hyper-/hypotension, palpitation, supraventricular tachycardia, tachycardia

Central nervous system: CNS stimulation, dizziness, drowsiness, headache, insomnia, irritability, lightheadedness, migraine, nervousness, nightmares, restlessness, sleeplessness, tremor

Dermatologic: Angioedema, erythema multiforme, rash, Stevens-Johnson syndrome, urticaria

Endocrine & metabolic: Hyperglycemia, hypokalemia, lactic acidosis

Gastrointestinal: Diarrhea, dry mouth, dyspepsia, gastroenteritis, nausea, unusual taste, vomiting, tooth discoloration

Genitourinary: Micturition difficulty

Local: Injection: Pain, stinging

Neuromuscular & skeletal: Muscle cramps, musculoskeletal pain, weakness

Otic: Otitis media, vertigo

Respiratory: Asthma exacerbation, bronchospasm, cough, epistaxis, laryngitis, oropharyngeal drying/irritation, oropharyngeal edema, upper respiratory inflammation, viral respiratory infection

Miscellaneous: Allergic reaction, anaphylaxis, diaphoresis, lymphadenopathy

Overdosage/Toxicology Symptoms of overdose include tachycardia, tremor, hypertension, angina, and seizures. Hypokalemia also may occur. Cardiac arrest and death may be associated with abuse of beta-agonist bronchodilators. Treatment includes immediate discontinuation and symptomatic and supportive therapies. Cautious use of beta-adrenergic blocking agents may be considered in severe cases.

Drug Interactions

Alpha-/beta blockers: May diminish the therapeutic effects of albuterol.

Atomoxetine: May enhance tachycardic effects of albuterol.

Beta-blockers (beta$_1$selective): Albuterol may diminish the bradycardic effects of beta$_1$selective beta-blockers.

Beta-blockers (nonselective): May diminish the bronchodilatory effects of albuterol; avoid concurrent use.

Betahistine: May diminish the therapeutic effect of albuterol.

(Continued)

Albuterol *(Continued)*

MAO inhibitors: May increase side effects; monitor heart rate and blood pressure.

TCAs: May increase side effects; monitor heart rate and blood pressure.

Sympathomimetics: May increase side effects of other sympathomimetics; monitor heart rate and blood pressure.

Ethanol/Nutrition/Herb Interactions

Food: Avoid or limit caffeine (may cause CNS stimulation).

Herb/Nutraceutical: Avoid ephedra, yohimbe (may cause CNS stimulation). Avoid St John's wort (may decrease the levels/effects of albuterol).

Stability

HFA aerosols: Store at 15°C to 25°C (59°F to 77°F).

Ventolin® HFA: Discard after using 200 actuations or 3 months after removal from protective pouch, whichever comes first. Store with mouthpiece down.

Infusion solution (not available in U.S.): Ventolin® I.V. : Store at 15°C to 30°C (59°F to 86°F). Protect from light. After dilution, discard after 24 hours.

Inhalation solution: AccuNeb®: Store at 2°C to 25°C (36°F to 77°F). Do not use if solution changes color or becomes cloudy. Use within 1 week of opening foil pouch.

Nebulization 0.5% solution: Store at 2°C to 30°C (36°F to 86°F). To prepare a 2.5 mg dose, dilute 0.5 mL of solution to a total of 3 mL with normal saline; also compatible with cromolyn or ipratropium nebulizer solutions.

Syrup: Store at 2°C to 30°C (36°F to 86°F).

Mechanism of Action Relaxes bronchial smooth muscle by action on beta$_2$-receptors with little effect on heart rate

Pharmacodynamics

Peak bronchodilation effect: Within 0.5-2 hours

Duration: 3-4 hours

Pharmacokinetics

Metabolism: By the liver to an inactive sulfate, with 28% appearing in the urine as unchanged drug

Half-life:

Inhaled: 3.8 hours

Oral: 3.7-5 hours

Dosage

Geriatrics:

Inhalation: Refer to adult dosing.

Bronchospasm (treatment): Oral: 2 mg 3-4 times/day; maximum: 8 mg 4 times/day

Adults:

Acute treatment of bronchospasm:

Inhalation: MDI 90 mcg/puff: 4-8 puffs every 20 minutes for up to 4 hours, then every 1-4 hours as needed

Nebulization: 2.5 mg, diluted to a total of 3 mL, 3-4 times/day over 5-15 minutes

NIH guidelines: 1.25-5 mg every 4-8 hours

Severe bronchospasm and status asthmaticus: *I.V. continuous infusion* (Ventolin® I.V. solution [not available in U.S.]): Initial: 5 mcg/minute; may increase up to 10-20 mcg/minute at 15- to 30-minute intervals if needed

Bronchospasm in ICU patients (acute):

Nebulization: 2.5-5 mg every 20 minutes for 3 doses, then 2.5-10 mg every 1-4 hours as needed, **or** 10-15 mg/hour continuously

Chronic treatment of bronchospasm:

Inhalation: MDI 90 mcg/puff: 1-2 inhalations every 4-6 hours; maximum: 12 inhalations/day

NIH guidelines: 2 puffs 3-4 times a day as needed; may double dose for mild exacerbations

Oral:

Regular release: 2-4 mg/dose 3-4 times/day; maximum dose not to exceed 32 mg/day (divided doses)

Extended release: 8 mg every 12 hours; maximum dose not to exceed 32 mg/day (divided doses). A 4 mg dose every 12 hours may be sufficient in some patients, such as adults of low body weight.

Prophylaxis of exercise-induced bronchospasm: Inhalation: MDI 90 mcg/puff: 2 puffs 5-30 minutes prior to exercise

Renal Impairment: Not removed by hemodialysis

Administration

Inhalation: MDI: Shake well before use; prime prior to first use, and whenever inhaler has not been used for >2 weeks, by releasing 4 test sprays into the air (away from face)

Oral: Volmax®: Do not crush or chew.

Monitoring Parameters Pulmonary function, blood pressure, pulse

Test Interactions Increased renin (S), increased aldosterone (S)

Patient Information Do not exceed recommended dosage; rinse mouth with water following each inhalation to help with dry throat and mouth; follow specific instructions accompanying inhaler; if more than one inhalation is necessary, wait at least 1 full minute between inhalations. May cause nervousness, restlessness, insomnia; if these effects continue after dosage reduction, notify physician; also notify physician if palpitations, tachycardia, chest pain, muscle tremors, dizziness, headache, flushing or if breathing difficulty persists.

Special Geriatric Considerations Because of its minimal effect on beta$_1$-receptors and its relatively long duration of action, albuterol is a rational choice in elderly when a beta-agonist is indicated. Elderly patients may find it beneficial to utilize a spacer device when using a metered dose inhaler. Oral use should be avoided due to adverse effects.

Dosage Forms Excipient information presented when available (limited, particularly for generics); consult specific product labeling. [CAN] = Canadian brand name
Aerosol, for oral inhalation: 90 mcg/metered inhalation (17 g) [200 metered inhalations; contains chlorofluorocarbons]
    Proventil®: 90 mcg/metered inhalation (17 g) [200 metered inhalations; contains chlorofluorocarbons]
Aerosol, for oral inhalation:
    ProAir™ HFA: 90 mcg/metered inhalation (8.5 g) [200 metered inhalations; chlorofluorocarbon free]
    Proventil® HFA: 90 mcg/metered inhalation (6.7 g) [200 metered inhalations; chlorofluorocarbon free]
    Ventolin® HFA: 90 mcg/metered inhalation (18 g) [200 metered inhalations; chlorofluorocarbon free]
Injection, solution, as sulphate:
    Ventolin® I.V. [CAN]: 1 mg/1mL (5 mL) [not available in U.S.]
Solution for nebulization: 0.042% (3 mL); 0.083% (3 mL); 0.5% (0.5 mL, 20 mL)
    AccuNeb® [preservative free]: 0.63 mg/3 mL (3 mL) [0.021%]; 1.25 mg/3 mL (3 mL) [0.042%]
    Proventil®: 0.083% (3 mL) [preservative free]; 0.5% (20 mL) [contains benzalkonium chloride]
Syrup, as sulfate: 2 mg/5 mL (480 mL)
Tablet: 2 mg, 4 mg
Tablet, extended release: 4 mg, 8 mg
    VoSpire ER®: 4 mg, 8 mg

Selected References
National Asthma Education and Prevention Program, "Expert Panel Report 2: Guidelines for the Diagnosis and Management of Asthma," Bethesda, MD, National Institutes of Health, 1997. NIH publication 97-4051.
Udezue E, D'Souza L, and Mahajan M, "Hypokalemia After Normal Doses of Nebulized Albuterol (Salbutamol)," Am J Emerg Med, 1995, 13(2):168-71.

♦ **Albuterol and Ipratropium** see Ipratropium and Albuterol on page 828
♦ **Albuterol Sulfate** see Albuterol on page 40

Alclometasone (al kloe MET a sone)

Related Information
    Corticosteroids on page 1755
Medication Safety Issues
    Sound-alike/look-alike issues:
        Aclovate® may be confused with Accolate®
U.S. Brand Names Aclovate®
Index Terms Alclometasone Dipropionate
Generic Available Yes
Pharmacologic Category Corticosteroid, Topical
Use Treatment of inflammation of corticosteroid-responsive dermatosis (low potency topical corticosteroid)
Contraindications Hypersensitivity to alclometasone or any component of the formulation; viral, fungal, or tubercular skin lesions
Warnings/Precautions Systemic absorption of topical corticosteroids may cause hypothalamic-pituitary-adrenal (HPA) axis suppression (reversible). HPA axis suppression may lead to adrenal crisis. Risk is increased when used over large surface areas, for prolonged periods, or with occlusive dressings. Adverse systemic effects including hyperglycemia, glycosuria, fluid and electrolyte changes, and HPA suppression may occur when used on large surface areas, for prolonged periods, or with an occlusive dressing. Prolonged treatment with corticosteroids has been associated with the development of Kaposi's sarcoma (case reports); if noted, discontinuation of therapy should be considered. Allergic contact dermatitis can occur, it is usually diagnosed by failure to heal rather than clinical exacerbation.
Adverse Reactions (Reflective of adult population; not specific for elderly)
Frequency not defined.
Dermatologic: Acne, allergic dermatitis, hypopigmentation, maceration of the skin, perioral dermatitis, skin atrophy, striae, miliaria, telangiectasia
(Continued)

43

Alclometasone *(Continued)*

Endocrine & metabolic: HPA suppression, Cushing's syndrome, growth retardation

Local: Burning, erythema, itching, irritation, dryness, folliculitis, hypertrichosis, papular rash

Miscellaneous: Secondary infection

Overdosage/Toxicology Symptoms include cushingoid appearance (systemic), muscle weakness (systemic), osteoporosis (systemic) all with long-term use only. When consumed in excessive quantities for prolonged periods, systemic hypercorticism and adrenal suppression may occur; in those cases, discontinuation and withdrawal of the corticosteroid should be done judiciously.

Drug Interactions No data reported

Stability Store between 2°C and 30°C (36°F and 86°F).

Mechanism of Action Stimulates the synthesis of enzymes needed to decrease inflammation, suppress mitotic activity, and cause vasoconstriction

Dosage

Geriatrics & Adults: Steroid-responsive dermatoses: Topical: Apply a thin film to the affected area 2-3 times/day. **Note:** Therapy should be discontinued when control is achieved; if no improvement is seen within 2 weeks, reassessment of diagnosis may be necessary.

Administration For external use only. Do not use on open wounds. Should not be used in the presence of open or weeping lesions. Apply sparingly to occlusive dressings.

Monitoring Parameters Relief of symptoms

Patient Information Use only as prescribed and for no longer than the period prescribed; apply sparingly in a thin film and rub in lightly; avoid contact with eyes; notify physician if condition persists or worsens

Additional Information Considered a low potency steroid; avoid use on the face

Special Geriatric Considerations Due to age-related changes in skin, limit use of topical glucocorticosteroids.

Dosage Forms Excipient information presented when available (limited, particularly for generics); consult specific product labeling.

Cream, as dipropionate: 0.05% (15 g, 45 g, 60 g)

Aclovate®: 0.05% (15 g, 45 g, 60 g)

Ointment, as dipropionate: 0.05% (15 g, 45 g, 60 g)

Aclovate®: 0.05% (15 g, 45 g, 60 g)

♦ **Alclometasone Dipropionate** *see* Alclometasone *on page 43*

♦ **Aldactazide®** *see* Hydrochlorothiazide and Spironolactone *on page 758*

♦ **Aldactone®** *see* Spironolactone *on page 1488*

♦ **Aldomet** *see* Methyldopa *on page 1012*

♦ **Aldroxicon I [OTC]** *see* Aluminum Hydroxide, Magnesium Hydroxide, and Simethicone *on page 66*

♦ **Aldroxicon II [OTC]** *see* Aluminum Hydroxide, Magnesium Hydroxide, and Simethicone *on page 66*

Alendronate *(a LEN droe nate)*

Related Information

Osteoporosis Management *on page 1779*

Medication Safety Issues

Sound-alike/look-alike issues:

Fosamax® may be confused with Flomax®

International issues:

Fosamax® may be confused with Fisamox® which is a brand name for amoxicillin in Australia

U.S. Brand Names Fosamax®

Canadian Brand Names Apo-Alendronate®; CO Alendronate; Fosamax®; Gen-Alendronate; Novo-Alendronate; PMS-Alendronate; ratio-Alendronate; Riva-Alendronate; Sandoz Alendronate

Index Terms Alendronate Sodium

Generic Available No

Pharmacologic Category Bisphosphonate Derivative

Use Treatment and prevention of osteoporosis in postmenopausal females; treatment of osteoporosis in males; treatment of Paget's disease of the bone in patients who are symptomatic, at risk for future complications, or with alkaline phosphatase ≥2 times the upper limit of normal; treatment of glucocorticoid-induced osteoporosis in males and females with low bone mineral density who are receiving a daily dosage ≥7.5 mg of prednisone (or equivalent)

Contraindications Hypersensitivity to alendronate, other bisphosphonates, or any component of the formulation; hypocalcemia; abnormalities of the esophagus which delay esophageal emptying such as stricture or achalasia; inability to stand or sit upright for at least 30 minutes; oral solution should not be used in patients at risk of aspiration

Warnings/Precautions Use caution in patients with renal impairment (not recommended for use in patients with Cl_{cr} <35 mL/minute); hypocalcemia must be corrected before therapy initiation; ensure adequate calcium and vitamin D intake. May cause irritation to upper gastrointestinal mucosa. Esophagitis, esophageal ulcers, esophageal erosions, and esophageal stricture (rare) have been reported; risk increases in patients unable to comply with dosing instructions. Use with caution in patients with dysphagia, esophageal disease, gastritis, duodenitis, or ulcers (may worsen underlying condition).

Bisphosphonate therapy has been associated with osteonecrosis, primarily of the jaw; this has been observed mostly in cancer patients, but also in patients with postmenopausal osteoporosis and other diagnoses. Dental exams and preventative dentistry should be performed prior to placing patients with risk factors on chronic bisphosphonate therapy. Invasive dental procedures should be avoided during treatment.

Infrequently, severe (and occasionally debilitating) bone, joint, and/or muscle pain have been reported during bisphosphonate treatment. The onset of pain ranged from a single day to several months. Symptoms usually resolve upon discontinuation. Some patients experienced recurrence when rechallenged with same drug or another bisphosphonate; avoid use in patients with a history of these symptoms in association with bisphosphonate therapy.

Adverse Reactions (Reflective of adult population; not specific for elderly)
Note: Incidence of adverse effects (mostly GI) increases significantly in patients treated for Paget's disease at 40 mg/day.

>10%: Endocrine & metabolic: Hypocalcemia (transient, mild, 18%); hypophosphatemia (transient, mild, 10%)

1% to 10%:
Central nervous system: Headache (up to 3%)
Gastrointestinal: Abdominal pain (1% to 7%), acid reflux (1% to 4%), dyspepsia (1% to 4%), nausea (1% to 4%), flatulence (up to 4%), diarrhea (1% to 3%), gastroesophageal reflux disease (1% to 3%), constipation (up to 3%), esophageal ulcer (up to 2%), abdominal distension (up to 1%), gastritis (up to 1%), vomiting (up to 1%), dysphagia (up to 1%), gastric ulcer (1%), melena (1%)
Neuromuscular & skeletal: Musculoskeletal pain (up to 6%), muscle cramps (up to 1%)

Overdosage/Toxicology Symptoms include hypocalcemia, hypophosphatemia, and upper GI adverse events (upset stomach, heartburn, esophagitis, gastritis or ulcer). Treat with milk or antacids to bind alendronate. Dialysis would not be beneficial. Do not induce vomiting (due to the risk of esophageal irritation); keep fully upright.

Drug Interactions
Aminoglycosides: May lower serum calcium levels with prolonged administration. Concomitant use may have an additive hypocalcemic effect.
Antacids: May decrease the absorption of bisphosphonate derivatives; should be administered at a different time of the day. Antacids containing aluminum, calcium, or magnesium are of specific concern.
Aspirin: May enhance the adverse/toxic effect of alendronate; specifically gastrointestinal adverse events.
Calcium salts: May decrease the absorption of bisphosphonate derivatives. Separate oral dosing in order to minimize risk of interaction.
Iron salts: May decrease the absorption of bisphosphonate derivatives. Only oral iron salts and oral bisphosphonates are of concern.
Magnesium salts: May decrease the absorption of bisphosphonate derivatives. Only oral magnesium salts and oral bisphosphonates are of concern.
Nonsteroidal anti-inflammatory drugs (NSAIDs): May enhance the gastrointestinal adverse/toxic effects (increased incidence of GI ulcers) of bisphosphonate derivatives.
Phosphate supplements: Bisphosphonate derivatives may enhance the hypocalcemic effect of phosphate supplements.

Ethanol/Nutrition/Herb Interactions
Ethanol: Avoid ethanol (may increase risk of osteoporosis and gastric irritation).
Food: All food and beverages interfere with absorption. Coadministration with caffeine may reduce alendronate efficacy. Coadministration with dairy products may decrease alendronate absorption. Beverages (especially orange juice and coffee) and food may reduce the absorption of alendronate as much as 60%.

Stability Store tablets and oral solution at room temperature of 15°C to 30°C (59°F to 86°F). Keep in well-closed container.

Mechanism of Action A bisphosphonate which inhibits bone resorption via actions on osteoclasts or on osteoclast precursors; decreases the rate of bone resorption, leading to an indirect increase in bone mineral density. In Paget's disease, characterized by (Continued)

Alendronate *(Continued)*

disordered resorption and formation of bone, inhibition of resorption leads to an indirect decrease in bone formation; but the newly-formed bone has a more normal architecture.

Pharmacodynamics

Onset of action: Bone mineral density increases were noted at 3 months in trials

Duration: Trials noted continuous effect for the 3 years of study with daily use; upon discontinuation of daily use, no further increases in bone mass observed. Thus, it appears daily treatment is needed to maintain effect.

Pharmacokinetics

Absorption: Oral: Male: 0.6% given in a fasting state; Female: 0.7%

Protein binding: ~78%

Metabolism: Not metabolized

Bioavailability: Fasting: 0.6%; reduced 60% with food or drink

Half-life: Terminal: Exceeds 10 years; serum concentrations cleared >95% in 6 hours

Elimination: Renal with unabsorbed drug eliminated in feces

Dosage

Geriatrics & Adults: Note: Patients treated with glucocorticoids and those with Paget's disease should receive adequate amounts of calcium and vitamin D.

Osteoporosis in postmenopausal females: Oral:

Prophylaxis: 5 mg once daily **or** 35 mg once weekly

Treatment: 10 mg once daily **or** 70 mg once weekly

Osteoporosis in males: Oral: 10 mg once daily **or** 70 mg once weekly

Osteoporosis secondary to glucocorticoids in males and females: Oral: Treatment: 5 mg once daily; a dose of 10 mg once daily should be used in postmenopausal females who are not receiving estrogen.

Paget's disease of bone in males and females: Oral: 40 mg once daily for 6 months

Retreatment: Relapses during the 12 months following therapy occurred in 9% of patients who responded to treatment. Specific retreatment data are not available. Following a 6-month post-treatment evaluation period, treatment with alendronate may be considered in patients who have relapsed based on increases in serum alkaline phosphatase, which should be measured periodically. Retreatment may also be considered in those who failed to normalize their serum alkaline phosphatase.

Renal Impairment:

Cl_{cr} 35-60 mL/minute: None necessary.

Cl_{cr} <35 mL/minute: Alendronate is not recommended due to lack of experience.

Hepatic Impairment: No adjustment necessary.

Administration Alendronate must be taken with plain water (tablets 6-8 oz; oral solution follow with 2 oz) first thing in the morning and ≥30 minutes before the first food, beverage, or other medication of the day. Do not take with mineral water or with other beverages. Patients should be instructed to stay upright (not to lie down) for at least 30 minutes **and** until after first food of the day (to reduce esophageal irritation). Patients should receive supplemental calcium and vitamin D if dietary intake is inadequate.

Monitoring Parameters Alkaline phosphatase should be periodically measured; serum calcium and phosphorus; monitor pain and fracture rate; hormonal status (male and female) prior to therapy; bone mineral density (should be done prior to initiation of therapy and after 6-12 months of combined glucocorticoid and alendronate treatment)

Reference Range Calcium (total): Adults: 9.0-11.0 mg/dL (2.05-2.54 mmol/L); may slightly decrease with aging; phosphorus: 2.5-4.5 mg/dL (0.81-1.45 mmol/L)

Test Interactions Bisphosphonates may interfere with diagnostic imaging agents such as technetium-99m-diphosphonate in bone scans.

Patient Information Take as directed, with a full glass of water first thing in the morning and at least 30 minutes before the first food or beverage of the day. Wait at least 30 minutes after taking alendronate before taking any supplement. Stay in sitting or standing position for 30 minutes following administration and until after first food of the day to reduce potential for esophageal irritation. Avoid aspirin- or aspirin-containing medications. Consult prescriber to determine necessity of lifestyle changes (decreased smoking, decreased alcohol intake) or dietary supplements of calcium and dietary vitamin D.

Additional Information Esophageal irritation and gastric pain have been reported frequently. Proper administration may prevent or decrease this common adverse effect. Patients need to take supplemental calcium while treated with alendronate appropriate for age and hormonal status; vitamin D supplements suggested if patient is deficient in this vitamin. Patients treated with 10 mg of alendronate daily had significant increases in bone mineral density. Increases were absorbed as early as 3 months and continued throughout the 3 years of study. Mean bone mineral density increases at 3 years were: spine, trochanter 8%; femoral neck 6%; total body bone mineral density 2.5%.

Special Geriatric Considerations Since many elderly patients receive diuretics, evaluation of electrolyte status (calcium, phosphate, magnesium, potassium) may need to be done periodically due to the drug class (bisphosphonate).

Dosage Forms Excipient information presented when available (limited, particularly for generics); consult specific product labeling.

Note: Strength expressed as free acid

Solution, oral, as monosodium trihydrate:

Fosamax™: 70 mg/75 mL [contains parabens; raspberry flavor]

Tablet, as sodium:

Fosamax™: 5 mg, 10 mg, 35 mg, 40 mg, 70 mg

Selected References

Chesnut CH 3rd, McClung MR, Ensrud KE, et al, "Alendronate Treatment of the Postmenopausal Osteoporotic Woman: Effect of Multiple Dosages on Bone Mass and Bone Remodeling," *Am J Med*, 1995, 99(2):144-52.

Watts NB, "Treatment of Osteoporosis With Bisphosphonates," *Rheum Dis Clin North Am*, 1994, 20(3):717-34.

♦ **Alendronate Sodium** *see* Alendronate *on page 44*
♦ **Alenic Alka [OTC]** *see* Aluminum Hydroxide and Magnesium Carbonate *on page 64*
♦ **Alenic Alka Tablet [OTC]** *see* Aluminum Hydroxide and Magnesium Trisilicate *on page 66*
♦ **Aler-Cap [OTC]** *see* DiphenhydrAMINE *on page 447*
♦ **Aler-Dryl [OTC]** *see* DiphenhydrAMINE *on page 447*
♦ **Aler-Tab [OTC]** *see* DiphenhydrAMINE *on page 447*
♦ **Aleve® [OTC]** *see* Naproxen *on page 1088*

Alfuzosin (al FYOO zoe sin)

Related Information
Pharmacotherapy of Urinary Incontinence *on page 1822*
U.S. Brand Names Uroxatral®
Canadian Brand Names Xatral
Index Terms Alfuzosin Hydrochloride
Generic Available No
Pharmacologic Category Alpha$_1$ Blocker
Use Treatment of the functional symptoms of benign prostatic hyperplasia (BPH)
Contraindications Hypersensitivity to alfuzosin or any component of the formulation; moderate or severe hepatic insufficiency (Child-Pugh class B and C); potent CYP3A4 inhibitors (ie, itraconazole, ketoconazole, ritonavir)
Warnings/Precautions Not intended for use as an antihypertensive drug. May cause significant orthostatic hypotension and syncope, especially with first dose; anticipate a similar effect if therapy is interrupted for a few days, if dosage is rapidly increased, or if another antihypertensive drug (particularly vasodilators) or a PDE5 inhibitor is introduced. Discontinue if symptoms of angina occur or worsen. Patients should be cautioned about performing hazardous tasks when starting new therapy or adjusting dosage upward. Discontinue if symptoms of angina occur or worsen. Rule out prostatic carcinoma before beginning therapy. Use caution with renal or mild hepatic impairment; not recommended in moderate to severe hepatic impairment. Intraoperative floppy iris syndrome has been observed in cataract surgery patients who were on or were previously treated with alpha$_1$-blockers. Causality has not been established and there appears to be no benefit in discontinuing alpha-blocker therapy prior to surgery.
Adverse Reactions (Reflective of adult population; not specific for elderly)
1% to 10%:
Central nervous system: Dizziness (6%), fatigue (3%), headache (3%), pain (1% to 2%)
Gastrointestinal: Abdominal pain (1% to 2%), constipation (1% to 2%), dyspepsia (1% to 2%), nausea (1% to 2%)
Genitourinary: Impotence (1% to 2%)
Respiratory: Upper respiratory tract infection (3%), bronchitis (1% to 2%), pharyngitis (1% to 2%), sinusitis (1% to 2%)
Overdosage/Toxicology Hypotension would be expected in case of overdose. Treatment is supportive.
Drug Interactions Substrate of CYP3A4 (major)
CYP3A4 inducers: CYP3A4 inducers may decrease the levels/effects of alfuzosin. Example inducers include aminoglutethimide, carbamazepine, nafcillin, nevirapine, phenobarbital, phenytoin, and rifamycins.
CYP3A4 inhibitors: May increase the levels/effects of alfuzosin. Example inhibitors include azole antifungals, clarithromycin, diclofenac, doxycycline, erythromycin, imatinib, isoniazid, nefazodone, nicardipine, propofol, protease inhibitors, quinidine, telithromycin, and verapamil. Concurrent use of itraconazole, ketoconazole, or ritonavir is contraindicated.
Ethanol/Nutrition/Herb Interactions Food: Food increases the extent of absorption.
(Continued)

Alfuzosin *(Continued)*

Stability Store at controlled room temperature of 15°C to 30°C (59°F to 86°F). Protect from light and moisture.

Mechanism of Action An antagonist of alpha₁-adrenoreceptors in the lower urinary tract. Smooth muscle tone is mediated by the sympathetic nervous stimulation of alpha₁-adrenoreceptors, which are abundant in the prostate, prostatic capsule, prostatic urethra, and bladder neck. Blockade of these adrenoreceptors can cause smooth muscles in the bladder neck and prostate to relax, resulting in an improvement in urine flow rate and a reduction in symptoms of BPH.

Pharmacokinetics

Absorption: Decreased 50% under fasting conditions

Distribution: V_d: 3.2 L/kg

Protein binding: 82% to 90%

Metabolism: Hepatic, primarily via CYP3A4; metabolism includes oxidation, O-demethylation and N-dealkylation; forms metabolites (inactive)

Bioavailability: 49% following a meal

Bioavailability and maximum serum concentrations are increased by ~50% with mild, moderate, or severe renal impairment.

Half-life: 10 hours

Time to peak, plasma: 8 hours following a meal

Elimination: Feces (69%); urine (24%)

Dosage

Geriatrics & Adults: Benign prostatic hyperplasia (BPH): Oral: 10 mg once daily

Renal Impairment: Bioavailability and maximum serum concentrations are increased by ~50% with mild, moderate, or severe renal impairment.

Note: Safety has not been evaluated in patients with creatinine clearances <30 mL/minute.

Hepatic Impairment:

Mild hepatic impairment: Use has not been studied.

Moderate or severe hepatic impairment (Child-Pugh class B and C): Clearance is decreased ¹/₃ to ¹/₄ and serum concentration is increased three- to fourfold; use is contraindicated.

Monitoring Parameters Urine flow; blood pressure

Patient Information Syncope may occur; monitor patient for dizziness and falls. Do not crush tablet.

Special Geriatric Considerations Alfuzosin is a functionally uroselective alpha-blocker, therefore, having minimal effects on the cardiovascular system. Alfuzosin has been available in Europe for many years and appears to be well tolerated in elderly. In one study, orthostatic changes were minimal and not influenced by age.

Dosage Forms Excipient information presented when available (limited, particularly for generics); consult specific product labeling.

Tablet, extended release, as hydrochloride: 10 mg

Selected References

Lee, M, "Alfuzosin Hydrochloride for the Treatment of Benign Prostatic Hyperplasia," *Am J Health Syst Pharm*, 2003, 60(14):1426-39.

van Kerrebroeck P, Jardin A, van Cangh P, et al, "Long-term Safety and Efficacy of a Once-daily Formulation of Alfuzosin 10 mg in Patients With Symptomatic Benign Prostatic Hyperplasia: Open-label Extension Study," *Eur Urol*, 2002, 41(1):54-61.

♦ **Alfuzosin Hydrochloride** *see* Alfuzosin *on page 47*

Aliskiren (a lis KYE ren)

Related Information

Angiotensin Agents *on page 1737*

Medication Safety Issues

International issues:

Aliskiren may be confused with Aliseum which is a brand name for diazepam in Italy

U.S. Brand Names Tekturna®

Index Terms Aliskiren Hemifumarate; SPP100

Generic Available No

Pharmacologic Category Renin Inhibitor

Use Treatment of hypertension, alone or in combination with other antihypertensive agents

Contraindications There are no contraindications listed in manufacturer's labeling.

Warnings/Precautions Angioedema can occur at any time during treatment (especially following first dose); it may involve head and neck (potentially affecting the airway) or the extremities. Prolonged monitoring may be required especially if tongue, glottis, or larynx are involved as they are associated with airway obstruction. Patients with a history of airway surgery may have a higher risk of airway obstruction. Discontinue immediately following any signs and symptoms of angioedema. Hyperkalemia may occur (rarely) during monotherapy; risk may increase in patients with predisposing factors (eg, renal dysfunction, diabetes mellitus or concomitant use with ACE inhibitors, potassium-sparing diuretics, potassium supplements, and/or potassium-containing salts). Symptomatic hypotension may occur (rarely) during the initiation of therapy, particularly in patients with an activated renin-angiotensin system (ie, volume or salt-depleted patients). Use with caution in patients with severe renal impairment; not studied in patients with severe renal impairment [GFR <30 mL/minute and/or S_{cr} >1.7 mg/dL (women); S_{cr} >2 mg/dL (men)], history of dialysis, nephrotic syndrome, or renovascular hypertension. Use with caution or avoid in patients with deteriorating renal function or renal artery stenosis (bilateral or unilateral).

Adverse Reactions (Reflective of adult population; not specific for elderly)
1% to 10%:
Central nervous system: Dizziness (2%)
Dermatologic: Rash (1%)
Endocrine and metabolic: Hyperkalemia (monotherapy ≤1%; concurrent with ACE inhibitor in patients with diabetes 6%)
Gastrointestinal: Diarrhea (1% to 2%)
Hematologic: Creatine kinase increased (>300%: 1%)
Renal: BUN increased (≤7%), serum creatinine increased (≤7%)
Respiratory: Cough (1%)

Overdosage/Toxicology Limited experience with overdosage. Treatment is symptom-directed and supportive.

Drug Interactions Substrate of CYP3A4 (minor)
Atorvastatin: May increase the level/effect of aliskiren; monitor blood pressure.
Furosemide: Aliskiren may decrease the level/effect of furosemide.
Ketoconazole: May increase the level/effect of aliskiren; monitor blood pressure.

Ethanol/Nutrition/Herb Interactions Food: High-fat meals decreases absorption.

Stability Store at 15°C to 30°C (59°F to 86°F). Protect from moisture.

Mechanism of Action Aliskerin is a direct renin inhibitor, resulting in blockade of the conversion of angiotensinogen to angiotensin I. Angiotensin I suppression decreases the formation of angiotensin II (Ang II), a potent blood pressure-elevating peptide (via direct vasoconstriction, aldosterone release, and sodium retention). Ang II also functions within the Renin-Angiotensin-Aldosterone System (RAAS) as a negative inhibitory feedback mediator within the renal parenchyma to suppress the further release of renin. Thus, reductions in Ang II levels suppress this feedback loop, leading to further increased plasma renin concentrations (PRC) and subsequent activity (PRA). This disinhibition effect can be potentially problematic for ACE inhibitor and ARB therapy, as increased PRA could partially overcome the pharmacologic inhibition of the RAAS. As aliskiren is a direct inhibitor of renin activity, blunting of PRA despite the increased PRC (from loss of the negative feedback) may be clinically advantageous. The effect of aliskiren on bradykinin levels is unknown.

Pharmacodynamics
Onset of action: Maximum antihypertensive effect: Within 2 weeks

Pharmacokinetics
Absorption: Poor; absorption decreased by high-fat meal
Metabolism: Extent of metabolism unknown; *in vitro* studies indicate metabolism via CYP3A4
Bioavailability: ~3%
Half-life elimination: ~24 hours (range: 16-32 hours)
Time to peak, plasma: 1-3 hours
Excretion: Urine (~25% of absorbed dose excreted unchanged in urine); feces (unchanged via biliary excretion)

Dosage
Geriatrics: Refer to adult dosing. No initial dosage adjustment required.
Adults: Hypertension: Initial: 150 mg once daily; may increase to 300 mg once daily (maximum: 300 mg/day). **Note:** Prior to initiation, correct hypovolemia and/or closely monitor volume status in patients on concurrent diuretics during treatment initiation.
Renal Impairment:
Mild-to-moderate impairment [GFR >30 mL/minute and/or S_{cr} <1.7 mg/dL (women); S_{cr} <2 mg/dL (men)]: No dose adjustment required
Severe impairment [GFR<30 mL/minute and/or S_{cr} >1.7 mg/dL (women); S_{cr} >2 mg/dL (men)]: Use caution; not studied in severe renal impairment
Hepatic Impairment: No dosage adjustment required.
Administration Administer at the same time daily; may take with or without a meal, but consistent administration with regards to meals is recommended. Avoid taking with high-fat meals.
(Continued)

Aliskiren *(Continued)*

Monitoring Parameters Serum potassium, BUN, serum creatinine

Patient Information Do not take any new prescription or over-the-counter medications or herbal products during therapy unless approved by prescriber. Take exactly as directed at same time each day; may be taken with meals. This drug does not eliminate the need for diet or exercise regimen as recommended by prescriber. May cause dizziness (use caution when driving or engaging in tasks that require alertness until response to drug is known) or hypotension (especially at beginning of therapy) (use caution when rising from lying or sitting position or climbing stairs). Report immediately any unusual swelling of eyes, face, lips, mouth, throat, or any difficulty swallowing of breathing; changes in urinary pattern; palpitations or irregular heartbeat; or any other adverse reactions.

Special Geriatric Considerations The pharmacokinetic studies in elderly (≥65 years of age) demonstrated an increased AUC; however, adjustments in starting dose are not necessary. Blood pressure response and adverse effects were similar to younger adults in studies where 19% of patients were >65 years of age.

Dosage Forms Excipient information presented when available (limited, particularly for generics); consult specific product labeling.
Tablet:
Tekturna®: 150 mg, 300 mg

Selected References
Straessen JA, Li Y, and Richart T, "Oral Renin Inhibitors," *Lancet*, 2006, 368(9545):1449-56.
Vaidyanathan S, Warren V, Yeh C, et al, "Pharmacokinetics, Safety, and Tolerability of the Oral Renin Inhibitor Aliskiren in Patients With Hepatic Impairment," *J Clin Pharmacol*, 2007, 47(2):192-200.

- ◆ **Aliskiren Hemifumarate** *see* Aliskiren *on page 48*
- ◆ **Alka-Mints® [OTC]** *see* Calcium Salts (Oral) *on page 220*
- ◆ **Alkeran®** *see* Melphalan *on page 974*
- ◆ **Allanfil 405** *see* Chlorophyllin, Papain, and Urea *on page 293*
- ◆ **Allanfil Spray** *see* Chlorophyllin, Papain, and Urea *on page 293*
- ◆ **Allanzyme** *see* Papain and Urea *on page 1201*
- ◆ **Allanzyme 650** *see* Papain and Urea *on page 1201*
- ◆ **Allegra®** *see* Fexofenadine *on page 622*
- ◆ **Aller-Chlor® [OTC]** *see* Chlorpheniramine *on page 296*
- ◆ **Allerfrim® [OTC]** *see* Triprolidine and Pseudoephedrine *on page 1638*
- ◆ **AllerMax® [OTC]** *see* DiphenhydrAMINE *on page 447*
- ◆ **Allfen-DM** *see* Guaifenesin and Dextromethorphan *on page 730*
- ◆ **Allfen Jr** *see* Guaifenesin *on page 727*
- ◆ **Alli™ [OTC]** *see* Orlistat *on page 1163*

Allopurinol *(al oh PURE i nole)*

Medication Safety Issues
Sound-alike/look-alike issues:
Allopurinol may be confused with Apresoline
Zyloprim® may be confused with Xylo-Pfan®, ZORprin®

U.S. Brand Names Aloprim™; Zyloprim®

Canadian Brand Names Alloprin®; Apo-Allopurinol®; Novo-Purol; Zyloprim®

Index Terms Allopurinol Sodium

Generic Available Yes

Pharmacologic Category Xanthine Oxidase Inhibitor

Use
Oral: Prevention of attack of gouty arthritis and nephropathy; treatment of secondary hyperuricemia which may occur during treatment of tumors or leukemia; prevention of recurrent calcium oxalate calculi

I.V.: Treatment of elevated serum and urinary uric acid levels when oral therapy is not tolerated in patients with leukemia, lymphoma, and solid tumor malignancies who are receiving cancer chemotherapy

Contraindications Hypersensitivity to allopurinol or any component of the formulation

Warnings/Precautions Do not use to treat asymptomatic hyperuricemia. Has been associated with a number of hypersensitivity reactions, including severe reactions (vasculitis and Stevens-Johnson syndrome); discontinue at first sign of rash. Reversible hepatotoxicity has been reported; use with caution in patients with pre-existing hepatic impairment. Bone marrow suppression has been reported; use caution with other drugs causing myelosuppression. Caution in renal impairment, dosage adjustments needed. Use with caution in patients taking diuretics concurrently. Risk of skin rash may be increased in patients receiving amoxicillin or ampicillin. The risk of hypersensitivity may be increased in patients receiving thiazides, and possibly ACE inhibitors. Use caution with mercaptopurine or azathioprine; dosage adjustment necessary.

Adverse Reactions (Reflective of adult population; not specific for elderly)
>1%:

Dermatologic: Rash (increased with ampicillin or amoxicillin use, 1.5% per manufacturer, >10% in some reports)

Gastrointestinal: Nausea (1.3%), vomiting (1.2%)

Renal: Renal failure/impairment (1.2%)

Overdosage/Toxicology
At high dosages, it is a theoretical possibility that oxypurinol stones could be formed but no record of such occurrence in overdose exists. Alkalinization of the urine and forced diuresis can help prevent potential xanthine stone formation.

Drug Interactions

Ampicillin, amoxicillin: Incidence of rash may be increased.

Anticoagulants: Allopurinol may prolong the half-life of anticoagulants, effect seen with dicumarol; monitor.

ACE inhibitors: Captopril may increase risk of hypersensitivity.

Azathioprine: Metabolism inhibited by allopurinol; reduce azathioprine dose by $1/3$ or $1/4$.

Chlorpropamide: Half-life of chlorpropamide may be increased.

Cyclosporine: Allopurinol may increase cyclosporine serum levels.

Mercaptopurine: Metabolism inhibited by allopurinol; reduce mercaptopurine dose by $1/3$ or $1/4$.

Thiazide diuretics: Toxicity and risk of hypersensitivity may be increased.

Theophylline: Half-life of theophylline may be increased.

Vidarabine: Neurotoxicity may be enhanced.

Ethanol/Nutrition/Herb Interactions

Ethanol: May decrease effectiveness.

Iron supplements: Hepatic iron uptake may be increased.

Vitamin C: Large amounts of vitamin C may acidify urine and increase kidney stone formation.

Stability

Powder for injection: Store at controlled room temperature of 15°C to 30°C (59°F to 86°F). Further dilution with NS or D_5W (50-100 mL) to ≤6 mg/mL is recommended. Following reconstitution, intravenous solutions should be stored at 20°C to 25°C (68°F to 77°F). Do not refrigerate reconstituted and/or diluted product. Must be administered within 10 hours of solution preparation.

Tablet: Store at controlled room temperature of 15°C to 25°C (59°F to 77°F).

Mechanism of Action
Allopurinol inhibits xanthine oxidase, the enzyme responsible for the conversion of hypoxanthine to xanthine to uric acid. Allopurinol is metabolized to oxypurinol which is also an inhibitor of xanthine oxidase; allopurinol acts on purine catabolism, reducing the production of uric acid without disrupting the biosynthesis of vital purines.

Pharmacodynamics
Decrease in serum uric acid occurs in 1-2 days with a nadir achieved in 1-3 weeks

Pharmacokinetics

Absorption: Oral: ~80% from GI tract

Protein binding: <1%

Metabolism: ~75% of the drug is metabolized to active metabolites, chiefly oxypurinol; allopurinol and oxypurinol are dialyzable

Half-life:

Parent: 1-3 hours

Oxypurinol: Normal renal function: 18-30 hours

Time to peak serum concentration: Within 2-4 hours

Dosage

Geriatrics: Oral: Initial: 100 mg/day; increase until desired uric acid level is obtained. Refer to adult dosing.

Adults: Doses >300 mg should be given in divided doses.

Gout: Oral: Mild: 200-300 mg/day; Severe: 400-600 mg/day; to reduce the possibility of acute gouty attacks, initiate dose at 100 mg/day and increase weekly to recommended dosage. Maximum daily dose: 800 mg/day.

Secondary hyperuricemia associated with chemotherapy:

Oral: 600-800 mg/day in 2-3 divided doses for prevention of acute uric acid nephropathy for 2-3 days starting 1-2 days before chemotherapy

I.V.: 200-400 mg/m^2/day (maximum: 600 mg/day)

Note: Intravenous daily dose can be given as a single infusion or in equally divided doses at 6-, 8-, or 12-hour intervals. A fluid intake sufficient to yield a daily urinary output of at least 2 L in adults and the maintenance of a neutral or, preferably, slightly alkaline urine are desirable.

Recurrent calcium oxalate stones: 200-300 mg/day in single or divided doses

Renal Impairment:

Oral:

Must be adjusted due to accumulation of allopurinol and metabolites; see table on next page.

(Continued)

Allopurinol *(Continued)*

Adult Maintenance Doses of Allopurinol[1]

Creatinine Clearance (mL/min)	Maintenance Dose of Allopurinol (mg)
140	400 daily
120	350 daily
100	300 daily
80	250 daily
60	200 daily
40	150 daily
20	100 daily
10	100 every 2 days
0	100 every 3 days

[1]This table is based on a standard maintenance dose of 300 mg of allopurinol per day for a patient with a creatinine clearance of 100 mL/min.

Hemodialysis: Administer dose after hemodialysis or administer 50% supplemental dose.

I.V.:
Cl_{cr} 10-20 mL/minute: Administer 200 mg/day.
Cl_{cr} 3-10 mL/minute: Administer 100 mg/day.
Cl_{cr} <3 mL/minute: Administer 100 mg/day at extended intervals.

Monitoring Parameters CBC, serum uric acid levels, I & O, hepatic and renal function, especially at start of therapy

Reference Range Uric acid, serum: Adults: Male: 3.4-7 mg/dL (SI: 202-416 µmol/L) or slightly more; Female: 2.4-6 mg/dL (SI: 143-357 µmol/L) or slightly more. Values >7 mg/dL (SI: 416 µmol/L) are sometimes arbitrarily regarded as hyperuricemia, but there is no sharp line between normals on the one hand, and the serum uric acid of those with clinical gout. Normal ranges cannot be adjusted for purine ingestion, but high purine diet increases uric acid. Uric acid may be increased with body size, exercise, and stress.

Patient Information Take after meals with plenty of fluid; discontinue the drug and contact physician at first sign of rash, painful urination, blood in the urine, irritation of the eyes, or swelling of the lips or mouth; may cause drowsiness

Additional Information Skin rash occurs most often in patients taking diuretics concurrently; may predispose patient to ampicillin-induced rash

Special Geriatric Considerations Adjust dose based on renal function.

Dosage Forms Excipient information presented when available (limited, particularly for generics); consult specific product labeling.
Injection, powder for reconstitution, as sodium (Aloprim™): 500 mg
Tablet (Zyloprim®): 100 mg, 300 mg

Selected References
Emmerson BT, "The Management of Gout," *N Engl J Med*, 1996, 334(7):445-51.

♦ **Allopurinol Sodium** *see* Allopurinol *on page 50*
♦ **Almacone® [OTC]** *see* Aluminum Hydroxide, Magnesium Hydroxide, and Simethicone *on page 66*
♦ **Almacone Double Strength® [OTC]** *see* Aluminum Hydroxide, Magnesium Hydroxide, and Simethicone *on page 66*
♦ **Almora® [OTC]** *see* Magnesium Salts (Various Salts) *on page 952*

Almotriptan *(al moh TRIP tan)*

Medication Safety Issues
Sound-alike/look-alike issues:
Axert™ may be confused with Antivert®
U.S. Brand Names Axert™
Canadian Brand Names Axert™
Index Terms Almotriptan Malate
Generic Available No
Pharmacologic Category Antimigraine Agent; Serotonin 5-HT$_{1B, 1D}$ Receptor Agonist
Use Acute treatment of migraine, with or without aura
Contraindications Hypersensitivity to almotriptan or any component of the formulation; use as prophylactic therapy for migraine; hemiplegic or basilar migraine; cluster headache; known or suspected ischemic heart disease (angina pectoris, MI, documented silent ischemia, coronary artery vasospasm, Prinzmetal's variant angina); peripheral vascular syndromes (including ischemic bowel disease); uncontrolled hypertension;

use within 24 hours of another 5-HT$_1$ agonist; use within 24 hours of ergotamine derivative; concurrent administration or within 2 weeks of discontinuing an MAO inhibitor (specifically MAO type A inhibitors)

Warnings/Precautions Almotriptan is indicated only in patients ≥18 years of age with a clear diagnosis of migraine headache. If a patient does not respond to the first dose, the diagnosis of migraine should be reconsidered. Do not give to patients with risk factors for CAD until a cardiovascular evaluation has been performed; if evaluation is satisfactory, the healthcare provider should administer the first dose and cardiovascular status should be periodically re-evaluated. Cardiac events (coronary artery vasospasm, transient ischemia, myocardial infarction, ventricular tachycardia/fibrillation, cardiac arrest, and death), cerebral/subarachnoid hemorrhage, stroke, peripheral vascular ischemia, and colonic ischemia have been reported with 5-HT$_1$ agonist administration. Significant elevation in blood pressure, including hypertensive crisis, has also been reported on rare occasions in patients with and without a history of hypertension. Use with caution in liver or renal dysfunction. Symptoms of agitation, confusion, hallucinations, hyper-reflexia, myoclonus, shivering, and tachycardia (serotonin syndrome) may occur with concomitant proserotonergic drugs (ie, SSRIs/SNRIs or triptans) or agents which reduce almotriptan's metabolism.

Adverse Reactions (Reflective of adult population; not specific for elderly)
1% to 10%:
Central nervous system: Headache (>1%), dizziness (>1%), somnolence (>1%)
Gastrointestinal: Nausea (1% to 2%), xerostomia (1%)
Neuromuscular & skeletal: Paresthesia (1%)

Overdosage/Toxicology Hypertension or more serious cardiovascular symptoms may occur. Clinical and electrocardiographic monitoring is needed for at least 20 hours even if the patient is asymptomatic. Treatment is symptom-directed and supportive.

Drug Interactions Substrate (minor) of CYP2D6, 3A4
Ergot-containing drugs: Prolong vasospastic reactions; do not use almotriptan or ergot-containing drugs within 24 hours of each other.
Ketoconazole: Increases almotriptan serum concentration. Monitor for increased almotriptan response.
MAO inhibitors (moclobemide [MAO type A inhibitor]): Almotriptan clearance decreased by 27%; C$_{max}$ increased by 6%. Avoid concurrent administration of MAO inhibitors or within 2 weeks of discontinuing an MAO inhibitor, specifically MAO type A inhibitors.
Selegiline: Selegiline is a selective MAO type B inhibitor; while not specifically contraindicated, combination has not been studied.
Verapamil: Increased almotriptan serum concentration by 24%. Dose adjustment not necessary.
Serotonin agonists (eg, triptans): Concurrent use of almotriptan with these agents may increase the risk of serotonin syndrome; monitor.
Serotonergic reuptake inhibitors (eg, SSRIs/SNRIs): Concurrent use of almotriptan with these agents may increase the risk of serotonin syndrome; monitor.

Stability Store at 15°C to 30°C (59°F to 86°F).

Mechanism of Action Selective agonist for serotonin (5-HT$_{1B}$, 5-HT$_{1D}$, 5-HT$_{1F}$ receptors) in cranial arteries; causes vasoconstriction and reduce sterile inflammation associated with antidromic neuronal transmission correlating with relief of migraine

Pharmacokinetics Geriatrics: Pharmacokinetic disposition is similar to that in young adults.
Absorption: Well absorbed
Distribution: V$_d$: 180-200 L
Protein binding: ~35%
Metabolism: MAO type A oxidative deamination (~27% of dose)
Bioavailability: 12.5 mg dose - 80%; 25 mg dose - 70%
Half-life: 3-4 hours
Time to peak: 1-3 hours
Elimination: Urine (40% as unchanged drug); feces (13% unchanged and metabolized)

Dosage
Geriatrics & Adults: Migraine: Oral: Initial: 6.25-12.5 mg in a single dose; if the headache returns, repeat the dose after 2 hours; no more than 2 doses in 24-hour period
Note: If the first dose is ineffective, diagnosis needs to be re-evaluated. Safety of treating more than 4 migraines/month has not been established.
Renal Impairment: Initial: 6.25 mg in a single dose; maximum daily dose: ≤12.5 mg
Hepatic Impairment: Initial: 6.25 mg in a single dose; maximum daily dose: ≤12.5 mg

Patient Information This drug is to be used to reduce your migraine, not to prevent or reduce the number of attacks. Take exactly as directed. If headache returns or is not fully resolved, the dose may be repeated after 2 hours. Do not use more than two doses in 24 hours. Do not take within 24 hours of other migraine medication without consulting prescriber. You may experience dizziness, fatigue, or drowsiness (use
(Continued)

Almotriptan *(Continued)*

caution when driving or engaging in tasks that require alertness until response to drug is known). Report immediately chest pain, palpitations, feeling of tightness or pressure in chest, jaw, or throat; acute headache or dizziness; muscle cramping, pain, or tremors; skin rash; hallucinations, anxiety, panic; or other adverse reactions.

Special Geriatric Considerations Use cautiously in elderly, particularly since many have cardiovascular disease, which would put them at risk for cardiovascular adverse effects. Safety and efficacy in elderly patients >65 years of age have not been established.

Dosage Forms Excipient information presented when available (limited, particularly for generics); consult specific product labeling.

Tablet, as malate: 6.25 mg, 12.5 mg

- ◆ **Almotriptan Malate** *see* Almotriptan *on page 52*
- ◆ **Alocril**® *see* Nedocromil *on page 1096*
- ◆ **Aloe Vesta**® **2-n-1 Antifungal [OTC]** *see* Miconazole *on page 1036*
- ◆ **Alomide**® *see* Lodoxamide *on page 924*
- ◆ **Alophen**® **[OTC]** *see* Bisacodyl *on page 173*
- ◆ **Aloprim**™ *see* Allopurinol *on page 50*
- ◆ **Alora**® *see* Estradiol *on page 549*

Alpha-Galactosidase (AL fa ga lak TOE si days)

U.S. Brand Names beano® [OTC]
Index Terms *Aspergillus niger*
Generic Available No
Pharmacologic Category Enzyme
Use Prevention of flatulence and bloating attributed to a variety of grains, cereals, nuts, and vegetables containing the sugars raffinose, stachyose, and/or verbascose
Contraindications Hypersensitivity to any component of the formulation
Warnings/Precautions Patients who are galactosemic should consult their healthcare provider prior to use. Currently, there are no FDA-approved disease-prevention or therapeutic indications for this product. Heat can inactivate; do not cook.
Stability Store at or below room temperature. Avoid heat.
Mechanism of Action Natural food enzyme that breaks down complex sugars in gassy foods, making them more digestible and less gassy.
Dosage
Geriatrics & Adults: Flatulence and bloating: Oral:
Drops: Take 5 drops per serving of problem food; adjust according to number of problem foods per meal; usual dose/meal: 10-15 drops
Tablet: One tablet per serving of problem food; adjust according to number of problem foods per meal; usual dose/meal: 2-3 tablets
Administration
Drops: Take with meal; do not cook
Tablet: Swallow, chew, or crumble. Take with meal; do not cook.
Dosage Forms Excipient information presented when available (limited, particularly for generics); consult specific product labeling.
Drops: 150 galactosidase units/5 drops
beano® Drops: 150 galactosidase units/5 drops [contains sodium 5 mg/5 drops]
Tablet: 150 galactosidase units
beano®: 150 galactosidase units/5 tablets

- ◆ **Alphagan**® **P** *see* Brimonidine *on page 183*
- ◆ **Alph-E [OTC]** *see* Vitamin E *on page 1677*
- ◆ **Alph-E-Mixed [OTC]** *see* Vitamin E *on page 1677*

Alprazolam (al PRAY zoe lam)

Related Information
Anxiolytic, Sedative / Hypnotic, and Miscellaneous Benzodiazepines *on page 1750*
Potentially Inappropriate Medications for Geriatrics *on page 1824*
Medication Safety Issues
Sound-alike/look-alike issues:
Alprazolam may be confused with alprostadil, lorazepam, triazolam
Xanax® may be confused with Lanoxin®, Tenex®, Tylox®, Xopenex®, Zantac®, Zyrtec®
U.S. Brand Names Alprazolam Intensol®; Niravam™; Xanax®; Xanax XR®
Canadian Brand Names Alti-Alprazolam; Apo-Alpraz®; Apo-Alpraz® TS; Gen-Alprazolam; Novo-Alprazol; Nu-Alprax; Xanax®; Xanax TS™
Generic Available Yes: Extended release tablet, immediate release tablet

Pharmacologic Category Benzodiazepine

Use Treatment of anxiety disorder (GAD), panic disorder (with or without agoraphobia), anxiety associated with depression; adjunct in the treatment of depression

Restrictions C-IV

Contraindications Hypersensitivity to alprazolam or any component of the formulation (cross-sensitivity with other benzodiazepines may exist); narrow-angle glaucoma; concurrent use with ketoconazole or itraconazole

Warnings/Precautions Rebound or withdrawal symptoms, including seizures, may occur 18 hours to 3 days following abrupt discontinuation or large decreases in dose (more common in patients receiving >4 mg/day or prolonged treatment). Breakthrough anxiety may occur at the end of dosing interval. Use with caution in patients receiving concurrent CYP3A4 inhibitors. Use with caution in renal impairment or predisposition to urate nephropathy. Use with caution in elderly or debilitated patients, patients with hepatic disease (including alcoholics), renal impairment, or obese patients.

Causes CNS depression (dose related) which may impair physical and mental capabilities. Patients must be cautioned about performing tasks that require mental alertness (eg, operating machinery or driving). Effects with other sedative drugs or ethanol may be potentiated. Benzodiazepines have been associated with falls and traumatic injury and should be used with extreme caution in patients who are at risk of these events (especially the elderly). Use with caution in patients with respiratory disease or impaired gag reflex.

Use caution in patients with depression, particularly if suicidal risk may be present. Episodes of mania or hypomania have occurred in depressed patients treated with alprazolam. May cause physical or psychological dependence. Acute withdrawal may be precipitated in patients after administration of flumazenil.

Benzodiazepines have been associated with anterograde amnesia. Paradoxical reactions have been reported with benzodiazepines, particularly in psychiatric patients. Does not have analgesic, antidepressant, or antipsychotic properties..

Adverse Reactions (Reflective of adult population; not specific for elderly)

>10%:
  Central nervous system: Abnormal coordination, cognitive disorder, depression, drowsiness, fatigue, irritability, lightheadedness, memory impairment, sedation, somnolence
  Gastrointestinal: Appetite increased/decreased, constipation, salivation decreased, weight gain/loss, xerostomia
  Genitourinary: Micturition difficulty
  Neuromuscular & skeletal: Dysarthria
1% to 10%:
  Cardiovascular: Hypotension
  Central nervous system: Agitation, attention disturbance, confusion, depersonalization, derealization, disorientation, disinhibition, dizziness, dream abnormalities, fear, hallucinations, hypersomnia, nightmares, seizure, talkativeness
  Dermatologic: Dermatitis, pruritus, rash
  Endocrine & metabolic: Libido decreased/increased, menstrual disorders
  Gastrointestinal: Salivation increased
  Genitourinary: Incontinence
  Hepatic: Bilirubin increased, jaundice, liver enzymes increased
  Neuromuscular & skeletal: Arthralgia, ataxia, myalgia, paresthesia
  Ocular: Diplopia
  Respiratory: Allergic rhinitis, dyspnea

Overdosage/Toxicology Symptoms include somnolence, confusion, coma, and diminished reflexes. Treatment for benzodiazepine overdose is supportive. Mechanical ventilation is rarely required. Flumazenil has been shown to selectively block the binding of benzodiazepines to CNS receptors, resulting in a reversal of benzodiazepine-induced sedation; however, its use may not alter the course of overdose.

Drug Interactions Substrate of CYP3A4 (major)
  CNS depressants: Sedative effects and/or respiratory depression may be additive with CNS depressants. Includes ethanol, barbiturates, opioid analgesics, and other sedative agents; monitor for increased effect.
  CYP3A4 inducers: CYP3A4 inducers may decrease the levels/effects of alprazolam. Example inducers include aminoglutethimide, carbamazepine, nafcillin, nevirapine, phenobarbital, phenytoin, and rifamycins.
  CYP3A4 inhibitors: May increase the levels/effects of alprazolam. Example inhibitors include azole antifungals, clarithromycin, diclofenac, doxycycline, erythromycin, imatinib, isoniazid, nefazodone, nicardipine, propofol, protease inhibitors, quinidine, telithromycin, and verapamil. Contraindicated with itraconazole and ketoconazole.
  Fluoxetine: May increase plasma concentrations/effects of alprazolam.
  Oral contraceptives: May increase serum levels/effects of alprazolam.
  Theophylline: May partially antagonize some of the effects of benzodiazepines; monitor for decreased response; may require higher doses for sedation.
  (Continued)

Alprazolam *(Continued)*

Tricyclic antidepressants: Plasma concentrations of imipramine and desipramine have been reported to be increased 31% and 20%, respectively, by concomitant administration; monitor.

Ethanol/Nutrition/Herb Interactions

Cigarette smoking: May decrease alprazolam concentrations up to 50%.

Ethanol: Avoid ethanol (may increase CNS depression).

Food: Alprazolam serum concentration is unlikely to be increased by grapefruit juice because of alprazolam's high oral bioavailability. The C_{max} of the extended release formulation is increased by 25% when a high-fat meal is given 2 hours before dosing. T_{max} is decreased 30% when food is given immediately prior to dose. T_{max} is increased by 30% when food is given ≥1 hour after dose.

Herb/Nutraceutical: St John's wort may decrease alprazolam levels. Avoid valerian, St John's wort, kava kava, gotu kola (may increase CNS depression).

Stability Orally-disintegrating tablet: Store at room temperature of 20°C to 25°C (68°F to 77°F). Protect from moisture. Seal bottle tightly and discard any cotton packaged inside bottle.

Mechanism of Action Binds to stereospecific benzodiazepine receptors on the postsynaptic GABA neuron at several sites within the central nervous system, including the limbic system, reticular formation. Enhancement of the inhibitory effect of GABA on neuronal excitability results by increased neuronal membrane permeability to chloride ions. This shift in chloride ions results in hyperpolarization (a less excitable state) and stabilization.

Pharmacodynamics Studies have shown that older adults are more sensitive to the effects of benzodiazepines as compared to younger adults.

Pharmacokinetics

Absorption: Oral: Rapidly and well absorbed

Distribution: V_d: 0.9-1.2 L/kg

Protein binding: 80%

Metabolism: Extensive in the liver; major metabolite is inactive; alphahydroxyalprazolam (active)

Half-life: 12-15 hours

Time to peak serum concentration: Within 1-2 hours

Elimination: Metabolites and parent compound in the urine; elimination is prolonged in older adult men (half-life: 19.5 hours); older adult women had no significant change in alprazolam clearance

Dosage

Geriatrics: Initial: 0.125-0.25 mg twice daily; increase by 0.125 mg/day as needed. The smallest effective dose should be used.

Immediate release: Initial 0.25 mg 2-3 times/day

Extended release: Initial: 0.5 mg once daily

Adults: Note: Treatment >4 months should be re-evaluated to determine the patient's continued need for the drug

Anxiety: Oral: *Immediate release:* Effective doses are 0.5-4 mg/day in divided doses; the manufacturer recommends starting at 0.25-0.5 mg 3 times/day; titrate dose upward; usual maximum: 4 mg/day. Patients requiring doses >4 mg/day should be increased cautiously. Periodic reassessment and consideration of dosage reduction is recommended.

Anxiety associated with depression: Oral: *Immediate release:* Average dose required: 2.5-3 mg/day in divided doses

Ethanol withdrawal (unlabeled use): Oral: *Immediate release:* Usual dose: 2-2.5 mg/day in divided doses

Panic disorder: Oral:

Immediate release: Initial: 0.5 mg 3 times/day; dose may be increased every 3-4 days in increments ≤1 mg/day. Mean effective dosage: 5-6 mg/day; many patients obtain relief at 2 mg/day, as much as 10 mg/day may be required

Extended release: 0.5-1 mg once daily; may increase dose every 3-4 days in increments ≤1 mg/day (range: 3-6 mg/day)

Switching from immediate release to extended release: Patients may be switched to extended release tablets by taking the total daily dose of the immediate release tablets and giving it once daily using the extended release preparation.

Preoperative sedation: Oral: 0.5 mg in evening at bedtime and 0.5 mg 1 hour before procedure

Dose reduction: Abrupt discontinuation should be avoided. Daily dose may be decreased by 0.5 mg every 3 days, however, some patients may require a slower reduction. If withdrawal symptoms occur, resume previous dose and discontinue on a less rapid schedule.

Renal Impairment: No guidelines for adjustment; use caution.

Hepatic Impairment: Oral: Reduce dose by 50% to 60% or avoid in cirrhosis.

Administration

Immediate release preparations: Can be administered sublingually with comparable onset and completeness of absorption.

Extended release tablet: Should be taken once daily in the morning; do not crush, break or chew.

Orally-disintegrating tablets: Using dry hands, place tablet on tongue. If using one-half of tablet, immediately discard remaining half (may not remain stable). Administration with water is not necessary.

Monitoring Parameters Respiratory and cardiovascular status, symptoms of anxiety, mental status

Patient Information Avoid alcohol and other CNS depressants; avoid activities needing good psychomotor coordination until CNS effects are known; drug may cause physical or psychological dependence; avoid abrupt discontinuation after prolonged use; do not crush, break, or chew extended release tablets

Additional Information Not intended for management of anxieties and minor distresses associated with everyday life; treatment longer than 4 months should be re-evaluated to determine the patient's need for the drug; when decreasing the dose or discontinuing alprazolam, decrease by no more than 0.5 mg every 3 days

Special Geriatric Considerations Considered to be a benzodiazepine of choice in elderly due to the short duration of action.

Dosage Forms Excipient information presented when available (limited, particularly for generics); consult specific product labeling.

Solution, oral [concentrate]:

Alprazolam Intensol®: 1 mg/mL (30 mL)

Tablet: 0.25 mg, 0.5 mg, 1 mg, 2 mg

Xanax®: 0.25 mg, 0.5 mg, 1 mg, 2 mg

Tablet, extended release: 0.5 mg, 1 mg, 2 mg, 3 mg

Xanax XR®: 0.5 mg, 1 mg, 2 mg, 3 mg

Tablet, orally disintegrating [scored]:

Niravam™: 0.25 mg, 0.5 mg, 1 mg, 2 mg [orange flavor]

Selected References

Greenblatt DJ, Divoll M, Abernethy DR, et al, "Alprazolam Kinetics in the Elderly: Relation to Antipyrine Disposition," *Arch Gen Psychiatry*, 1983, 40(3):287-90.

Reidenberg MM, Levy M, Warner H, et al, "Relationship Between Diazepam Dose, Plasma Level, Age, and Central Nervous System Depression," *Clin Pharmacol Ther*, 1978, 23(4):371-4.

♦ **Alprazolam Intensol**® *see* Alprazolam *on page 54*

Alprostadil (al PROS ta dill)

Medication Safety Issues

Sound-alike/look-alike issues:

Alprostadil may be confused with alprazolam

U.S. Brand Names Caverject®; Caverject Impulse®; Edex®; Muse®; Prostin VR Pediatric®

Canadian Brand Names Caverject®; Muse® Pellet; Prostin® VR

Index Terms PGE$_1$; Prostaglandin E$_1$

Generic Available Yes: Solution for injection

Pharmacologic Category Prostaglandin

Use

Caverject®: Treatment of erectile dysfunction of vasculogenic, psychogenic, or neurogenic etiology; adjunct in the diagnosis of erectile dysfunction

Edex®, Muse®: Treatment of erectile dysfunction of vasculogenic, psychogenic, or neurogenic etiology

Contraindications Hypersensitivity to alprostadil or any component of the formulation; when a dominant left-to-right shunt is present; respiratory distress syndrome; conditions predisposing patients to priapism (sickle cell anemia, multiple myeloma, leukemia); patients with anatomical deformation of the penis, penile implants; use in men for whom sexual activity is inadvisable or contraindicated

Warnings/Precautions When used in erectile dysfunction, priapism may occur; treat immediately to avoid penile tissue damage and permanent loss of potency; discontinue therapy if signs of penile fibrosis develop (penile angulation, cavernosal fibrosis, or Peyronie's disease). When used in erectile dysfunction (Muse®), syncope occurring within 1 hour of administration has been reported. The potential for drug-drug interactions may occur when Muse® is prescribed concomitantly with antihypertensives.

Adverse Reactions (Reflective of adult population; not specific for elderly)

Intraurethral:

>10%: Genitourinary: Penile pain, urethral burning

2% to 10%:

Central nervous system: Headache, dizziness, pain

(Continued)

Alprostadil *(Continued)*

Genitourinary: Vaginal itching (female partner), testicular pain, urethral bleeding (minor)

Intracavernosal injection:

>10%: Genitourinary: Penile pain

1% to 10%:

Cardiovascular: Hypertension

Central nervous system: Headache, dizziness

Genitourinary: Prolonged erection (>4 hours, 4%), penile fibrosis, penis disorder, penile rash, penile edema

Local: Injection site hematoma and/or bruising

Intravenous:

>10%:

Cardiovascular: Flushing

Central nervous system: Fever

Respiratory: Apnea

1% to 10%:

Cardiovascular: Bradycardia, hyper-/hypotension, tachycardia, cardiac arrest, edema

Central nervous system: Seizure, headache, dizziness

Endocrine & metabolic: Hypokalemia

Gastrointestinal: Diarrhea

Hematologic: Disseminated intravascular coagulation

Neuromuscular & skeletal: Back pain

Respiratory: Upper respiratory infection, flu syndrome, sinusitis, nasal congestion, cough

Miscellaneous: Sepsis, localized pain in structures other than the injection site

Overdosage/Toxicology Symptoms of overdose when treating patent ductus arteriosus include apnea, bradycardia, hypotension, and flushing. If hypotension or pyrexia occurs, the infusion rate should be reduced until the symptoms subside, while apnea or bradycardia requires drug discontinuation. If intracavernous overdose occurs, supervise until any systemic effects have resolved or until penile detumescence has occurred.

Drug Interactions Risk of hypotension and syncope may be increased with antihypertensives.

Ethanol/Nutrition/Herb Interactions Ethanol: Avoid concurrent use (vasodilating effect).

Stability

Caverject® Impulse™: Store at controlled room temperature of 15°C to 30°C (59°F to 86°F). Provided as a dual-chamber syringe with diluent in one chamber. To mix, hold syringe with needle pointing upward and turn plunger clockwise; turn upside down several times to mix. Device can be set to deliver specified dose, each device can be set at various increments. Following reconstitution, use within 24 hours and discard any unused solution.

Caverject® powder: The 5 mcg, 10 mcg, and 20 mcg vials should be stored at or below 25°C (77°F). The 40 mcg vial should be stored at 2°C to 8°C until dispensed. After dispensing, stable for up to 3 months at or below 25°C. Use only the supplied diluent for reconstitution (ie, bacteriostatic/sterile water with benzyl alcohol 0.945%). Following reconstitution, all strengths should be stored at or below 25°C (77°F); do not refrigerate or freeze; use within 24 hours.

Caverject® solution: Prior to dispensing, store frozen at -20°C to -10°C (-4°F to -14°F); once dispensed, may be stored frozen for up to 3 months, or under refrigeration at 2°C to 8°C (36°F to 46°F) for up to 7 days. Do not refreeze. Once removed from foil wrap, solution may be allowed to warm to room temperature prior to use. If not used immediately, solution should be discarded. Shake well prior to use.

Edex®: Store at controlled room temperature of 15°C to 30°C (59°F to 86°F); following reconstitution with NS, use immediately and discard any unused solution.

Muse®: Refrigerate at 2°C to 8°C (36°F to 46°F); may be stored at room temperature for up to 14 days.

Prostin VR Pediatric®: Refrigerate at 2°C to 8°C (36°F to 46°F); prior to infusion, dilute with D_5W or NS; use within 24 hours.

Mechanism of Action Causes vasodilation by means of direct effect on vascular and ductus arteriosus smooth muscle; relaxes trabecular smooth muscle by dilation of cavernosal arteries when injected along the penile shaft, allowing blood flow to and entrapment in the lacunar spaces of the penis (ie, corporeal veno-occlusive mechanism)

Pharmacokinetics

Distribution: Nonsignificant amounts distribute peripherally following penile injection

Protein binding, plasma: 81% to albumin

Metabolism: ~75% metabolized by oxidation in one pass through the lungs

Half-life: 5-10 minutes

Elimination: Metabolites excreted in urine (90% within 24 hours)

Dosage
  Geriatrics & Adults:
    Erectile dysfunction:
      Intracavernous (Caverject®, Edex®): Individualize dose by careful titration; doses >40 mcg (Edex®) or >60 mcg (Caverject®) are not recommended: Initial dose must be titrated in physician's office. Patient must stay in the physician's office until complete detumescence occurs; if there is no response, then the next higher dose may be given within 1 hour; if there is still no response, a 1-day interval before giving the next dose is recommended; increasing the dose or concentration in the treatment of impotence results in increasing pain and discomfort.

Vasculogenic, psychogenic, or mixed etiology: Initiate dosage titration at 2.5 mcg, increasing by 2.5 mcg to a dose of 5 mcg and then in increments of 5-10 mcg depending on the erectile response until the dose produces an erection suitable for intercourse, not lasting >1 hour; if there is absolutely no response to initial 2.5 mcg dose, the second dose may be increased to 7.5 mcg, followed by increments of 5-10 mcg

Neurogenic etiology (eg, spinal cord injury): Initiate dosage titration at 1.25 mcg, increasing to a dose of 2.5 mcg and then 5 mcg; increase further in increments 5 mcg until the dose is reached that produces an erection suitable for intercourse, not lasting >1 hour

Maintenance: Once appropriate dose has been determined, patient may self-administer injections at a frequency of no more than 3 times/week with at least 24 hours between doses

Intraurethral (Muse® Pellet):
  Initial: 125-250 mcg
  Maintenance: Administer as needed to achieve an erection; duration of action is about 30-60 minutes; use only two systems per 24-hour period

Administration Erectile dysfunction: Use a ½", 27- to 30-gauge needle; inject into the dorsolateral aspect of the proximal third of the penis, avoiding visible veins; alternate side of the penis for injections

Monitoring Parameters Degree of penile pain, length of erection, signs of infection

Patient Information Store in refrigerator; if self-injecting for the treatment of impotence, dilute with the supplied diluent and use immediately after diluting; see physician at least every 3 months to ensure proper technique and for dosage adjustment; alternate sides of the penis with each injection; do not inject more than 3 times/week, allowing at least 24 hours between each dose; dispose of the syringe, needle, and vial properly; discard single-use vials after each use; report moderate to severe penile pain or erections lasting >4 hours to a physician immediately; inform a physician as soon as possible if any new penile pain, nodules, hard tissue or signs of infection develop; the risk of transmission of blood-borne diseases is increased with use of alprostadil injections since a small amount of bleeding at the injection site is possible; do not share this medication or needles/syringes

Special Geriatric Considerations Elderly may have concomitant diseases which would contraindicate the use of alprostadil. Other forms of attaining penile tumescence are recommended.

Dosage Forms Excipient information presented when available (limited, particularly for generics); consult specific product labeling.
  Injection, powder for reconstitution:
    Caverject®: 20 mcg, 40 mcg [contains lactose; diluent contains benzyl alcohol]
    Caverject Impulse®: 10 mcg, 20 mcg [prefilled injection system; contains lactose; diluent contains benzyl alcohol]
    Edex®: 10 mcg, 20 mcg, 40 mcg [contains lactose; packaged in kits containing diluent, syringe, and alcohol swab]
  Injection, solution: 500 mcg/mL (1 mL)
    Prostin VR Pediatric®: 500 mcg/mL (1 mL) [contains dehydrated alcohol]
  Pellet, urethral (Muse®): 125 mcg (6s), 250 mcg (6s), 500 mcg (6s), 1000 mcg (6s)

Alteplase (AL te plase)

Medication Safety Issues
Sound-alike/look-alike issues:
Alteplase may be confused with Altace®
"tPA" abbreviation should not be used when writing orders for this medication; has been misread as TNKase (tenecteplase)

High alert medication: The Institute for Safe Medication Practices (ISMP) includes this medication (I.V.) among its list of drugs which have a heightened risk of causing significant patient harm when used in error.

U.S. Brand Names Activase®; Cathflo® Activase®

Canadian Brand Names Activase® rt-PA; Cathflo® Activase®

Index Terms Alteplase, Recombinant; Alteplase, Tissue Plasminogen Activator, Recombinant; tPA

Generic Available No

Pharmacologic Category Thrombolytic Agent

Use Management of acute myocardial infarction for the lysis of thrombi in coronary arteries; management of acute massive pulmonary embolism (PE) in adults

Acute myocardial infarction (AMI): Chest pain ≥20 minutes, ≤12-24 hours; S-T elevation ≥0.1 mV in at least two EKG leads

Acute pulmonary embolism (APE): Age ≤75 years: As soon as possible within 5 days of thrombotic event. Documented massive pulmonary embolism by pulmonary angiography or echocardiography or high probability lung scan with clinical shock.

Cathflo® Activase®: Restoration of central venous catheter function

Unlabeled/Investigational Use Treatment of peripheral arterial thrombotic obstruction

Contraindications Hypersensitivity to alteplase or any component of the formulation

Treatment of acute MI or PE: Active internal bleeding; history of CVA; recent intracranial or intraspinal surgery or trauma; intracranial neoplasm; arteriovenous malformation or aneurysm; known bleeding diathesis; severe uncontrolled hypertension

Treatment of acute ischemic stroke: Evidence of intracranial hemorrhage or suspicion of subarachnoid hemorrhage on pretreatment evaluation; recent (within 3 months) intracranial or intraspinal surgery; prolonged external cardiac massage; suspected aortic dissection; serious head trauma or previous stroke; history of intracranial hemorrhage; uncontrolled hypertension at time of treatment (eg, >185 mm Hg systolic or >110 mm Hg diastolic); seizure at the onset of stroke; active internal bleeding; intracranial neoplasm; arteriovenous malformation or aneurysm; known bleeding diathesis including but not limited to: current use of anticoagulants or an INR >1.7, administration of heparin within 48 hours preceding the onset of stroke and an elevated aPTT at presentation, platelet count <100,000/mm³.

Other exclusion criteria (NINDS recombinant tPA study): Stroke or serious head injury within 3 months, major surgery or serious trauma within 2 weeks, GI or urinary tract hemorrhage within 3 weeks, aggressive treatment required to lower blood pressure, glucose level <50 mg/dL or >400 mg/dL, arterial puncture at a noncompressible site or lumbar puncture within 1 week, clinical presentation suggesting post-MI pericarditis

Warnings/Precautions Concurrent heparin anticoagulation may contribute to bleeding. Monitor all potential bleeding sites. Doses >150 mg are associated with increased risk of intracranial hemorrhage. Intramuscular injections and nonessential handling of the patient should be avoided. Venipunctures should be performed carefully and only when necessary. If arterial puncture is necessary, use an upper extremity vessel that can be manually compressed. If serious bleeding occurs, the infusion of alteplase and heparin should be stopped.

For the following conditions, the risk of bleeding is higher with use of thrombolytics and should be weighed against the benefits of therapy: Recent major surgery (eg, CABG, obstetrical delivery, organ biopsy, previous puncture of noncompressible vessels), cerebrovascular disease, recent gastrointestinal or genitourinary bleeding, recent trauma, hypertension (systolic BP >175 mm Hg and/or diastolic BP >110 mm Hg), high likelihood of left heart thrombus (eg, mitral stenosis with atrial fibrillation), acute pericarditis, subacute bacterial endocarditis, hemostatic defects including ones caused by severe renal or hepatic dysfunction, significant hepatic dysfunction, diabetic hemorrhagic retinopathy or other hemorrhagic ophthalmic conditions, septic thrombophlebitis or occluded AV cannula at seriously infected site, advanced age (eg, >75 years), patients receiving oral anticoagulants, any other condition in which bleeding constitutes a significant hazard or would be particularly difficult to manage because of location.

Coronary thrombolysis may result in reperfusion arrhythmias. Treatment of patients with acute ischemic stroke more than 3 hours after symptom onset is not recommended. Treatment of patients with minor neurological deficit or with rapidly improving symptoms is not recommended. Follow standard management for MI while infusing alteplase.

Cathflo® Activase®: When used to restore catheter function, use Cathflo® cautiously in those patients with known or suspected catheter infections. Evaluate catheter for other causes of dysfunction before use. Avoid excessive pressure when instilling into catheter.

Adverse Reactions (Reflective of adult population; not specific for elderly)

As with all drugs which may affect hemostasis, bleeding is the major adverse effect associated with alteplase. Hemorrhage may occur at virtually any site. Risk is dependent on multiple variables, including the dosage administered, concurrent use of multiple agents which alter hemostasis, and patient predisposition. Rapid lysis of coronary artery thrombi by thrombolytic agents may be associated with reperfusion-related atrial and/or ventricular arrhythmia. **Note:** Lowest rate of bleeding complications expected with dose used to restore catheter function.

1% to 10%:
> Cardiovascular: Hypotension
>
> Central nervous system: Fever
>
> Dermatologic: Bruising (1%)
>
> Gastrointestinal: GI hemorrhage (5%), nausea, vomiting
>
> Genitourinary: GU hemorrhage (4%)
>
> Hematologic: Bleeding (0.5% major, 7% minor: GUSTO trial)
>
> Local: Bleeding at catheter puncture site (15.3%, accelerated administration)

Additional cardiovascular events associated **with use in MI:** AV block, cardiogenic shock, heart failure, cardiac arrest, recurrent ischemia/infarction, myocardial rupture, electromechanical dissociation, pericardial effusion, pericarditis, mitral regurgitation, cardiac tamponade, thromboembolism, pulmonary edema, asystole, ventricular tachycardia, bradycardia, ruptured intracranial AV malformation, seizure, hemorrhagic bursitis, cholesterol crystal embolization

Additional events associated **with use in pulmonary embolism:** Pulmonary re-embolization, pulmonary edema, pleural effusion, thromboembolism

Additional events associated **with use in stroke:** Cerebral edema, cerebral herniation, seizure, new ischemic stroke

Overdosage/Toxicology
Symptoms include increased incidence of intracranial bleeding.

Drug Interactions
Aminocaproic acid (antifibrinolytic agent) may decrease effectiveness.

Drugs which affect platelet function (eg, NSAIDs, dipyridamole, ticlopidine, clopidogrel, IIb/IIIa antagonists) may potentiate the risk of hemorrhage; use with caution.

Heparin and aspirin: Use with aspirin and heparin may increase the risk of bleeding. However, aspirin and heparin were used concomitantly with alteplase in many patients in myocardial infarction or pulmonary embolism trials. This combination was prohibited in the NINDS tPA stroke trial.

Nitroglycerin may increase the hepatic clearance of alteplase, potentially reducing lytic activity (limited clinical information).

Warfarin or oral anticoagulants: Risk of bleeding may be increased during concurrent therapy.

Ethanol/Nutrition/Herb Interactions
Herb/Nutraceutical: Avoid cat's claw, dong quai, evening primrose, feverfew, red clover, horse chestnut, garlic, green tea, ginseng, ginkgo (all have additional antiplatelet activity).

Stability
Activase®: The lyophilized product may be stored at room temperature (not to exceed 30°C/86°F), or under refrigeration. Once reconstituted it should be used within 8 hours. Reconstitution:

> 50 mg vial: Use accompanying diluent (50 mL sterile water for injection); do not shake. Final concentration: 1 mg/mL.

> 100 mg vial: Use transfer set with accompanying diluent (100 mL vial of sterile water for injection); no vacuum is present in 100 mg vial; final concentration: 1 mg/mL.

Cathflo® Activase®: Store lyophilized product under refrigeration. Reconstitution: Add 2.2 mL SWFI to vial; do not shake. Final concentration: 1 mg/mL. Once reconstituted, store at 2°C to 30°C (36°F to 86°F) and use within 8 hours. Do not mix other medications into infusion solution.

Mechanism of Action
Initiates local fibrinolysis by binding to fibrin in a thrombus (clot) and converts entrapped plasminogen to plasmin

Pharmacokinetics
Elimination: Cleared rapidly from circulating plasma at a rate of 550-650 mL/minute, primarily by the liver; >50% present in plasma is cleared within 5 minutes after the infusion has been terminated, and ~80% is cleared within 10 minutes
(Continued)

Alteplase *(Continued)*

Dosage

Geriatrics & Adults:

Coronary artery thrombi: I.V. Front loading dose (weight-based):

Patients >67 kg: Total dose: 100 mg over 1.5 hours; infuse 15 mg over 1-2 minutes. Infuse 50 mg over 30 minutes. Infuse remaining 35 mg of alteplase over the next hour. See "Note."

Patients ≤67 kg: Infuse 15 mg I.V. bolus over 1-2 minutes, then infuse 0.75 mg/kg (not to exceed 50 mg) over next 30 minutes, followed by 0.5 mg/kg over next 60 minutes (not to exceed 35 mg). See "Note."

Note: Concurrently, begin heparin 60 units/kg bolus (maximum: 4000 units) followed by continuous infusion of 12 units/kg/hour (maximum: 1000 units/hour) and adjust to aPTT target of 1.5-2 times the upper limit of control.

Acute pulmonary embolism: I.V.: 100 mg over 2 hours.

Acute ischemic stroke: I.V.: Doses should be given within the first 3 hours of the onset of symptoms; recommended total dose: 0.9 mg/kg (maximum dose should not exceed 90 mg) infused over 60 minutes.

Load with 0.09 mg/kg (10% of the 0.9 mg/kg dose) as an I.V. bolus over 1 minute, followed by 0.81 mg/kg (90% of the 0.9 mg/kg dose) as a continuous infusion over 60 minutes. Heparin should not be started for 24 hours or more after starting alteplase for stroke.

Central venous catheter clearance: Intracatheter (Cathflo® Activase® 1 mg/mL):

Patients <30 kg: 110% of the internal lumen volume of the catheter, not to exceed 2 mg/2 mL; retain in catheter for 0.5-2 hours; may instill a second dose if catheter remains occluded

Patients ≥30 kg: 2 mg (2 mL); retain in catheter for 0.5-2 hours; may instill a second dose if catheter remains occluded

Acute peripheral arterial occlusive disease (unlabeled use): Intra-arterial: 0.02-0.1 mg/kg/hour for up to 36 hours

Advisory Panel to the Society for Cardiovascular and Interventional Radiology on Thrombolytic Therapy recommendation: ≤2 mg/hour and subtherapeutic heparin (aPTT <1.5 times baseline)

Administration

Activase®:

Bolus dose may be prepared by one of three methods:

1) removal of 15 mL reconstituted (1 mg/mL) solution from vial

2) removal of 15 mL from a port on the infusion line after priming

3) programming an infusion pump to deliver a 15 mL bolus at the initiation of infusion

Remaining dose may be administered as follows:

50 mg vial: Either PVC bag or glass vial and infusion set

100 mg vial: Insert spike end of the infusion set through the same puncture site created by transfer device and infuse from vial

If further dilution is desired, may be diluted in equal volume of 0.9% sodium chloride or D_5W to yield a final concentration of 0.5 mg/mL AD

Cathflo® Activase®: Intracatheter: Instill dose into occluded catheter. Do not force solution into catheter. After a 30-minute dwell time, assess catheter function by attempting to aspirate blood. If catheter is functional, aspirate 4-5 mL of blood to remove Cathflo® Activase® and residual clots. Gently irrigate the catheter with NS. If catheter remains nonfunctional, let Cathflo® Activase® dwell for another 90 minutes (total dwell time: 120 minutes) and reassess function. If catheter function is not restored, a second dose may be instilled.

Reference Range

Not routinely measured; literature supports therapeutic levels of 0.52-1.8 mcg/mL

Fibrinogen: 200-400 mg/dL

Activated partial thromboplastin time (APTT): 22.5-38.7 seconds

Prothrombin time (PT): 10.9-12.2 seconds

Test Interactions
Altered results of coagulation and fibrinolytic agents

Special Geriatric Considerations
No specific changes in use in elderly patients are necessary.

Dosage Forms
Excipient information presented when available (limited, particularly for generics); consult specific product labeling.

Injection, powder for reconstitution, recombinant:

Activase®: 50 mg [29 million int. units; contains polysorbate 80; packaged with diluent]; 100 mg [58 million int. units; contains polysorbate 80; packaged with diluent and transfer device]

Cathflo® Activase®: 2 mg [contains polysorbate 80]

Selected References

Meyer BJ and Chesebro JH, "New Accelerated rt-PA Strategy Has Sufficient Advantage Over Older Streptokinase Strategies That it Should Be the Thrombolytic Strategy of Choice in Anterior and Large Infarctions," *Am J Ther*, 1995, 2(2):123-7.

Ponec D, Irwin D, Haire WD, et al, "Recombinant Tissue Plasminogen Activator (Alteplase) for Restoration of Flow in Occluded Central Venous Access Devices: A Double-Blind Placebo-Controlled Trial - The Cardiovascular Thrombolytic to Open Occluded Lines (COOL) Efficacy Trial," *J Vasc Interv Radiol*, 2001, 12(8):951-5.

"Sixth ACCP Consensus Conference on Antithrombotic Therapy," *Chest*, 2001, 119(Suppl):1S-370S.

◆ **Alteplase, Recombinant** *see* Alteplase *on page 60*

◆ **Alteplase, Tissue Plasminogen Activator, Recombinant** *see* Alteplase *on page 60*

◆ **ALternaGel®** **[OTC]** *see* Aluminum Hydroxide *on page 63*

◆ **Altoprev®** *see* Lovastatin *on page 936*

Aluminum Hydroxide (a LOO mi num hye DROKS ide)

U.S. Brand Names ALternaGel® [OTC]; Dermagran® [OTC]
Canadian Brand Names Amphojel®; Basaljel®
Generic Available Yes: Suspension
Pharmacologic Category Antacid; Antidote; Protectant, Topical
Use Treatment of hyperacidity; hyperphosphatemia; temporary protection of minor cuts, scrapes, and burns
Contraindications Hypersensitivity to aluminum salts or any component of the formulation
Warnings/Precautions Oral: Hypophosphatemia may occur with prolonged administration or large doses; aluminum intoxication and osteomalacia may occur in patients with uremia. Use with caution in patients with CHF, renal failure, edema, cirrhosis, and low sodium diets, and patients who have recently suffered gastrointestinal hemorrhage; uremic patients not receiving dialysis may develop osteomalacia and osteoporosis due to phosphate depletion.

Elderly may be predisposed to constipation and fecal impaction. Careful evaluation of possible drug interactions must be done. When used as an antacid in ulcer treatment, consider buffer capacity (mEq/mL) to calculate dose.

Topical: Not for application over deep wounds, puncture wounds, infected areas, or lacerations. When used for self medication (OTC use), consult with healthcare provider if needed for >7 days.
Adverse Reactions (Reflective of adult population; not specific for elderly)
Frequency not defined.
Gastrointestinal: Constipation, stomach cramps, fecal impaction, nausea, vomiting, discoloration of feces (white speckles)
Endocrine & metabolic: Hypophosphatemia, hypomagnesemia
Overdosage/Toxicology Aluminum antacids may cause constipation, phosphate depletion, and bezoar or fecalith formation. In patients with renal failure, aluminum may accumulate to toxic levels. Deferoxamine, traditionally used as an iron chelator, has been shown to increase urinary aluminum output. Deferoxamine chelation of aluminum has resulted in improvements of clinical symptoms and bone histology; however, remains an experimental treatment for aluminum poisoning and has a significant potential for adverse effects.
Drug Interactions
Decreased effect: Aluminum hydroxide may decrease the absorption of allopurinol, antibiotics (tetracyclines, quinolones, some cephalosporins), bisphosphonate derivatives, corticosteroids, cyclosporine, delavirdine, iron salts, imidazole antifungals, isoniazid, mycophenolate, penicillamine, phosphate supplements, phenytoin, phenothiazines, trientine.
Absorption of aluminum hydroxide may be decreased by citric acid derivatives.
Mechanism of Action Neutralizes hydrochloride in stomach to form Al $(Cl)_3$ salt $+ H_2O$
Pharmacodynamics Acid-neutralizing capacity varies from product to product. Antacids ingested in a fasting state give reduced acidity for 30 minutes; if ingested 1 hour after meals, reduced acidity may be extended for 3 hours.
Dosage
Geriatrics & Adults:
Hyperphosphatemia: Oral: Initial: 300-600 mg 3 times/day with meals
Hyperacidity: Oral: 600-1200 mg between meals and at bedtime
Skin protectant: Topical: Apply to affected area as needed; reapply at least every 12 hours
Renal Impairment: Aluminum may accumulate in renal impairment.
Administration
Oral: Dose should be followed with water.
Topical: Apply as needed to affected area; reapply at least every 12 hours
Monitoring Parameters Frequency of bowel movements, GI complaints (symptoms); phosphorous serum concentrations periodically when patient is on chronic therapy; when used as a phosphate binder, dose to achieve a serum phosphate concentration ≤4 mg/100 mL
(Continued)

Aluminum Hydroxide *(Continued)*

Reference Range Aluminum normal range (serum): 0-6 ng/mL; dialysis patients may attain up to 40 ng/mL without symptoms of toxicity; >100 ng/mL possible CNS toxicity

Test Interactions Decreased phosphorus, inorganic (S)

Patient Information Dilute dose in water or juice, shake well; chew tablets thoroughly before swallowing with water; do not take oral drugs within 1-2 hours of administration; notify physician if relief is not obtained or if there are any signs to suggest bleeding from the GI tract

Additional Information When used primarily as a phosphate binder, dose should be followed with water; when used for peptic ulcer treatment, deliver 144 mEq neutralizing capacity 1 and 3 hours after meals as needed to control symptoms; often alternated with aluminum and magnesium combinations to decrease diarrhea

Special Geriatric Considerations Elderly, due to disease and/or drug therapy, may be predisposed to constipation and fecal impaction. Careful evaluation of possible drug interactions must be done. When used as an antacid in ulcer treatment, consider buffer capacity (mEq/mL) to calculate dose. Consider renal insufficiency (<30 mL/minute) as predisposition to aluminum toxicity.

Dosage Forms Excipient information presented when available (limited, particularly for generics); consult specific product labeling.
Ointment:
Dermagran®: 0.275% (120 g)
Suspension, oral: 320 mg/5 mL (473 mL)
ALternaGel®: 600 mg/5 mL (360 mL)

Selected References
Bohannon AD and Lyles KW, "Drug-Induced Bone Disease," *Clin Geriatr Med*, 1994, 10(4):611-23.

Aluminum Hydroxide and Magnesium Carbonate
(a LOO mi num hye DROKS ide & mag NEE zhum KAR bun nate)

Related Information
Aluminum Hydroxide *on page 63*

U.S. Brand Names Acid Gone [OTC]; Acid Gone Extra Strength [OTC]; Alenic Alka [OTC]; Gaviscon® Extra Strength [OTC]; Gaviscon® Liquid [OTC]; Genaton™ [OTC]

Index Terms Magnesium Carbonate and Aluminum Hydroxide

Generic Available Yes

Pharmacologic Category Antacid

Use Temporary relief of symptoms associated with gastric acidity

Adverse Reactions (Reflective of adult population; not specific for elderly)
1% to 10%:
Endocrine & metabolic: Hypermagnesemia, aluminum intoxication (prolonged use and concomitant renal failure), hypophosphatemia
Gastrointestinal: Constipation, diarrhea
Neuromuscular & skeletal: Osteomalacia

Drug Interactions Decreased effect: Tetracyclines, digoxin, indomethacin, iron salts, isoniazid, allopurinol, benzodiazepines, corticosteroids, penicillamine, phenothiazines, ranitidine, ketoconazole, itraconazole

Dosage
Geriatrics & Adults: Dyspepsia, gastric acidity: Oral:
Liquid:
Gaviscon® Regular Strength: 15-30 mL 4 times/day after meals and at bedtime
Gaviscon® Extra Strength Relief: 15-30 mL 4 times/day after meals
Tablet (Gaviscon® Extra Strength Relief): Chew 2-4 tablets 4 times/day
Renal Impairment: Aluminum and/or magnesium may accumulate in renal impairment.

Patient Information
Liquid: Shake well. Do not use if you are on a sodium-restricted diet.
Tablet: Take tablets after meals and at bedtime, or as needed. Chew tablet, do not swallow whole. Follow tablets with $1/2$ glass of water.

Special Geriatric Considerations Elderly, due to disease or drug therapy, may be predisposed to diarrhea or constipation. Diarrhea may result in electrolyte imbalance. Decreased renal function (Cl$_{cr}$ <30 mL/minute) may result in toxicity of aluminum or magnesium. Drug interactions must be considered. If possible, administer antacid 1-2 hours apart from other drugs. When treating ulcers, consider buffer capacity (mEq/mL) to calculate dose of antacid.

Dosage Forms Excipient information presented when available (limited, particularly for generics); consult specific product labeling.
Liquid:
Acid Gone: Aluminum hydroxide 31.7 mg and magnesium carbonate 119.3 mg per 5 mL (360 mL)

Alenic Alka: Aluminum hydroxide 31.7 mg and magnesium carbonate 119.3 mg per 5 mL (355 mL) [contains magnesium 35 mg/5 mL, sodium 13 mg/5 mL, and benzyl alcohol; cool mint flavor]

Gaviscon®: Aluminum hydroxide 31.7 mg and magnesium carbonate 119.3 mg per 5 mL (355 mL) [contains sodium 0.57 mEq/5 mL and benzyl alcohol; cool mint flavor]

Gaviscon® Extra Strength: Aluminum hydroxide 84.6 mg and magnesium carbonate 79.1 mg per 5 mL (355 mL) [contains sodium 0.9 mEq/5 mL and benzyl alcohol; cool mint flavor]

Genaton™: Aluminum hydroxide 31.7 mg and magnesium carbonate 119.3 mg per 5 mL (360 mL)

Tablet, chewable:

Acid Gone Extra Strength: Aluminum hydroxide 160 mg and magnesium carbonate 105 mg

Gaviscon® Extra Strength: Aluminum hydroxide 160 mg and magnesium carbonate 105 mg [contains sodium 19 mg/tablet (1.3 mEq/tablet); cherry and original flavors]

Aluminum Hydroxide and Magnesium Hydroxide
(a LOO mi num hye DROKS ide & mag NEE zhum hye DROK side)

Related Information
Aluminum Hydroxide *on page 63*
Magnesium Hydroxide *on page 946*

Medication Safety Issues
Sound-alike/look-alike issues:
Maalox® may be confused with Maox®, Monodox®

U.S. Brand Names Alamag [OTC]; Rulox [OTC]; Rulox No. 1 [DSC]

Canadian Brand Names Diovol®; Diovol® Ex; Gelusil® Extra Strength; Mylanta™

Index Terms Magnesium Hydroxide and Aluminum Hydroxide

Generic Available Yes

Pharmacologic Category Antacid

Use Antacid; treatment of hyperphosphatemia (in renal failure), GERD, hyperacidity associated with PUD

Contraindications Known hypersensitivity to aluminum hydroxide or magnesium hydroxide

Warnings/Precautions Sodium content may be significant for patients with hypertension, renal failure, and congestive heart failure. Hypermagnesemia may result with renal insufficiency when >50 mEq of magnesium is administered daily. Patients with Cl_{cr} <30 mL/minute are at risk for hypermagnesemia. May cause aluminum intoxication, osteomalacia; use with caution in patients with GI hemorrhage.

Adverse Reactions (Reflective of adult population; not specific for elderly)
>10%: Gastrointestinal: Constipation, chalky taste, stomach cramps, fecal impaction
1% to 10%: Gastrointestinal: Nausea, vomiting, discoloration of feces (white speckles)

Drug Interactions Decreased effect: Tetracyclines, digoxin, indomethacin, iron salts, isoniazid, allopurinol, benzodiazepines, corticosteroids, penicillamine, phenothiazines, ranitidine, ketoconazole, itraconazole

Pharmacodynamics Acid-neutralizing capacity varies from product to product. Antacids ingested in a fasting state give reduced acidity for 30 minutes; if ingested 1 hour after meals, reduced acidity may be extended for 3 hours.

Dosage
Geriatrics & Adults: Dyspepsia: Oral: 5-10 mL 4-6 times/day, between meals and at bedtime; may be used every hour for severe symptoms
Renal Impairment: Aluminum and/or magnesium may accumulate in renal impairment.

Monitoring Parameters Frequency of bowel movements and GI complaints (symptoms)
Aluminum: Monitor phosphorous levels periodically when patient is on chronic therapy; when used as a phosphate binder, dose to achieve a serum phosphate concentration ≤4 mg/100 mL; observe for complaints or bone pain, malaise, and muscular weakness
Magnesium: Observe for signs of mental confusion and increased somnolence.

Reference Range
Aluminum: Normal range (serum): 0-6 ng/mL; dialysis patients may attain up to 40 ng/mL without symptoms of toxicity; >100 ng/mL possible CNS toxicity
Magnesium: Normal range (serum): 1.5-2.3 mg/dL (1.25-1.9 mEq/L); toxicity occurs with serum concentration >4 mEq/L (4.8 mg/dL)

Patient Information Chew tablets thoroughly before swallowing with water; notify physician if relief is not obtained or if signs of bleeding from GI tract occur; if prescribed dose is exceeded in order to maintain symptom-free periods, advise physician

Additional Information Sodium content varies with product; check for each product if important for patient
(Continued)

65

Aluminum Hydroxide and Magnesium Hydroxide
(Continued)

Special Geriatric Considerations Elderly, due to disease or drug therapy, may be predisposed to diarrhea or constipation. Diarrhea may result in electrolyte imbalance. Decreased renal function (Cl$_{cr}$ <30 mL/minute) may result in toxicity of aluminum or magnesium. Drug interactions must be considered. If possible, administer antacid 1-2 hours apart from other drugs. When treating ulcers, consider buffer capacity (mEq/mL) to calculate dose of antacid.

Dosage Forms Excipient information presented when available (limited, particularly for generics); consult specific product labeling. [DSC] = Discontinued product

Suspension: Aluminum hydroxide 225 mg and magnesium hydroxide 200 mg per 5 mL (360 mL)

Alamag, Rulox: Aluminum hydroxide 225 mg and magnesium hydroxide 200 mg per 5 mL (360 mL)

Tablet, chewable:

Alamag: Aluminum hydroxide 300 mg and magnesium hydroxide 150 mg

Rulox No. 1: Aluminum hydroxide 200 mg and magnesium hydroxide 200 mg [DSC]

Selected References

Bohannon AD and Lyles KW, "Drug-Induced Bone Disease," *Clin Geriatr Med*, 1994, 10(4):611-23.

Gams JG, "Clinical Significance of Magnesium: A Review," *Drug Intell Clin Pharm*, 1987, 21(3):240-6.

Peterson WL, Sturdevant RAL, Franki HD, et al, "Healing of Duodenal Ulcer With an Antacid Regimen," *N Engl J Med*, 1977, 297(7):341-5.

Aluminum Hydroxide and Magnesium Trisilicate
(a LOO mi num hye DROKS ide & mag NEE zhum trye SIL i kate)

Related Information
Aluminum Hydroxide *on page 63*

U.S. Brand Names Alenic Alka Tablet [OTC]; Gaviscon® Tablet [OTC]; Genaton Tablet [OTC]

Index Terms Magnesium Trisilicate and Aluminum Hydroxide

Generic Available Yes

Pharmacologic Category Antacid

Use Temporary relief of hyperacidity

Drug Interactions Decreased effect: Tetracyclines, digoxin, indomethacin, iron salts, isoniazid, allopurinol, benzodiazepines, corticosteroids, penicillamine, phenothiazines, ranitidine, ketoconazole, itraconazole

Dosage

Geriatrics & Adults: Dyspepsia, gastric acidity: Oral: Chew 2-4 tablets 4 times/day or as directed by healthcare provider

Renal Impairment: Aluminum and/or magnesium may accumulate in renal impairment.

Administration Tablets should be chewed and not swallowed whole.

Special Geriatric Considerations Elderly, due to disease or drug therapy, may be predisposed to diarrhea or constipation. Diarrhea may result in electrolyte imbalance. Decreased renal function (Cl$_{cr}$ <30 mL/minute) may result in toxicity of aluminum or magnesium. Drug interactions must be considered. If possible, administer antacid 1-2 hours apart from other drugs. When treating ulcers, consider buffer capacity (mEq/mL) to calculate dose of antacid.

Dosage Forms Excipient information presented when available (limited, particularly for generics); consult specific product labeling.

Tablet, chewable: Aluminum hydroxide 80 mg and magnesium trisilicate 20 mg

Alenic Alka: Aluminum hydroxide 80 mg and magnesium trisilicate 20 mg [butterscotch flavor]

Gaviscon®: Aluminum hydroxide 80 mg and magnesium trisilicate 20 mg [contains sodium 0.8 mEq/tablet; butterscotch flavor]

Genaton: Aluminum hydroxide 80 mg and magnesium trisilicate 20 mg

Aluminum Hydroxide, Magnesium Hydroxide, and Simethicone
(a LOO mi num hye DROKS ide, mag NEE zhum hye DROKS ide, & sye METH i kone)

Related Information
Aluminum Hydroxide *on page 63*
Magnesium Hydroxide *on page 946*
Simethicone *on page 1467*

Medication Safety Issues
Sound-alike/look-alike issues:
Maalox® may be confused with Maox®, Monodox®

Mylanta® may be confused with Mynatal®

Maalox® is a different formulation than Maalox® Total Stomach Relief®

U.S. Brand Names Alamag Plus [OTC]; Aldroxicon I [OTC]; Aldroxicon II [OTC]; Almacone® [OTC]; Almacone Double Strength® [OTC]; Gelusil® [OTC]; Maalox® [OTC]; Maalox® Max [OTC]; Mi-Acid [OTC]; Mi-Acid Maximum Strength [OTC]; Mintox Extra Strength [OTC]; Mintox Plus [OTC]; Mylanta® Liquid [OTC]; Mylanta® Maximum Strength Liquid [OTC]

Canadian Brand Names Diovol Plus®; Gelusil®; Mylanta® Double Strength; Mylanta® Extra Strength; Mylanta® Regular Strength

Index Terms Magnesium Hydroxide, Aluminum Hydroxide, and Simethicone; Simethicone, Aluminum Hydroxide, and Magnesium Hydroxide

Generic Available Yes

Pharmacologic Category Antacid; Antiflatulent

Use Temporary relief of hyperacidity associated with gas, hyperphosphatemia, GERD; prevention of stress ulcers

See Aluminum Hydroxide *on page 63* and Magnesium Hydroxide *on page 946* and Simethicone *on page 1467*.

Adverse Reactions (Reflective of adult population; not specific for elderly)

>10%: Gastrointestinal: Chalky taste, stomach cramps, constipation, bowel motility decreased, fecal impaction, hemorrhoids

1% to 10%: Gastrointestinal: Nausea, vomiting, discoloration of feces (white speckles)

Drug Interactions Decreased effect: Tetracyclines, digoxin, indomethacin, iron salts, isoniazid, allopurinol, benzodiazepines, corticosteroids, penicillamine, phenothiazines, ranitidine, ketoconazole, itraconazole

Dosage

Geriatrics & Adults: Dyspepsia, abdominal bloating: Oral: 10-20 mL or 2-4 tablets 4-6 times/day between meals and at bedtime; may be used every hour for severe symptoms

Renal Impairment: Aluminum and/or magnesium may accumulate in renal impairment

Administration Administer 1-2 hours apart from oral drugs

Dosage Forms Excipient information presented when available (limited, particularly for generics); consult specific product labeling.

Liquid: Aluminum hydroxide 200 mg, magnesium hydroxide 200 mg, and simethicone 20 mg per 5 mL (360 mL); aluminum hydroxide 400 mg, magnesium hydroxide 400 mg, and simethicone 40 mg per 5 mL (360 mL)

Aldroxicon I: Aluminum hydroxide 200 mg, magnesium hydroxide 200 mg, and simethicone 20 mg per 5 mL (30 mL)

Aldroxicon II: Aluminum hydroxide 400 mg, magnesium hydroxide 400 mg, and simethicone 40 mg per 5 mL (30 mL)

Almacone®: Aluminum hydroxide 200 mg, magnesium hydroxide 200 mg, and simethicone 20 mg per 5 mL (360 mL)

Almacone Double Strength®: Aluminum hydroxide 400 mg, magnesium hydroxide 400 mg, and simethicone 40 mg per 5 mL (360 mL)

Maalox®: Aluminum hydroxide 200 mg, magnesium hydroxide 200 mg, and simethicone 20 mg per 5 mL (360 mL, 770 mL) [lemon and mint flavors]

Maalox® Max: Aluminum hydroxide 400 mg, magnesium hydroxide 400 mg, and simethicone 40 mg per 5 mL (360 mL, 770 mL) [cherry, vanilla creme, and wild berry flavors]

Mi-Acid: Aluminum hydroxide 200 mg, magnesium hydroxide 200 mg, and simethicone 20 mg per 5 mL (360 mL)

Mi-Acid Maximum Strength: Aluminum hydroxide 400 mg, magnesium hydroxide 400 mg, and simethicone 40 mg per 5 mL (360 mL)

Mintox Extra Strength: Aluminum hydroxide 500 mg, magnesium hydroxide 450 mg, and simethicone 40 mg per 5 mL (360 mL) [lemon creme flavor]

Mylanta®: Aluminum hydroxide 200 mg, magnesium hydroxide 200 mg, and simethicone 20 mg per 5 mL (180 mL, 360 mL, 720 mL) [original, cherry, and mint flavors]

Mylanta® Maximum Strength: Aluminum hydroxide 400 mg, magnesium hydroxide 400 mg, and simethicone 40 mg per 5 mL (180 mL, 360 mL, 720 mL) [original, cherry, orange creme, and mint flavors]

Suspension (Alamag Plus): Aluminum hydroxide 225 mg, magnesium hydroxide 200 mg, and simethicone 25 mg per 5 mL (360 mL)

Tablet, chewable: Aluminum hydroxide 200 mg, magnesium hydroxide 200 mg, and simethicone 25 mg

Alamag Plus: Aluminum hydroxide 200 mg, magnesium hydroxide 200 mg, and simethicone 25 mg [cherry flavor]

Almacone®: Aluminum hydroxide 200 mg, magnesium hydroxide 200 mg, and simethicone 20 mg [peppermint flavor]

Gelusil®: Aluminum hydroxide 200 mg, magnesium hydroxide 200 mg, and simethicone 25 mg [peppermint flavor]

Mintox Plus: Aluminum hydroxide 200 mg, magnesium hydroxide 200 mg, and simethicone 25 mg

♦ **Aluminum Sucrose Sulfate, Basic** *see* Sucralfate *on page 1495*

Aluminum Sulfate and Calcium Acetate
(a LOO mi num SUL fate & KAL see um AS e tate)

Related Information
Calcium Acetate *on page 213*
U.S. Brand Names Domeboro® [OTC]; Gordon Boro-Packs [OTC]; Pedi-Boro® [OTC]
Index Terms Calcium Acetate and Aluminum Sulfate
Generic Available No
Pharmacologic Category Topical Skin Product
Use Astringent; wet dressing for relief of inflammatory conditions of the skin; reduction of weeping that may occur in dermatitis, such as poison ivy and insect bites
Warnings/Precautions For external use only; avoid contact with eyes. Not for OTC use >7 days.
Stability Prior to mixing, store powder or tablets at controlled room temperature, 15°C to 30°C (59°F to 86°F). Following reconstitution, unused solution may be covered and stored at room temperature for up to 7 days.

Powder, for topical solution (Domeboro®, Pedi-Boro®): 1 packet/16 ounces of water = 1:40 dilution = Modified Burow's Solution
Tablet, effervescent, for topical solution (Domeboro®): 1 tablet/12 ounces of water = 1:40 dilution = Modified Burow's Solution

Dosage
Geriatrics & Adults: Dermal inflammation, dermatitis: Topical: Soak affected area in the solution 2-4 times/day for 15-30 minutes or apply wet dressing soaked in the solution for more extended periods; rewet dressing with solution 2-4 times/day every 15-30 minutes
Administration For external use only; do not occlude dressing to prevent evaporation.
Monitoring Parameters Monitor for decreasing inflammation and swelling.
Special Geriatric Considerations No special considerations necessary
Dosage Forms Excipient information presented when available (limited, particularly for generics); consult specific product labeling.
Powder, for topical solution:
Domeboro®: Aluminum sulfate 1191 mg and calcium acetate 938 mg per packet (12s, 100s)
Gordon Boro-Packs: Aluminum sulfate 49% and calcium acetate 51% per packet (100s)
Pedi-Boro®: Aluminum sulfate 49% and calcium acetate 51% per packet (12s, 100s)

♦ **Alupent®** *see* Metaproterenol *on page 991*

Amantadine (a MAN ta deen)

Related Information
Antiparkinsonian Agents *on page 1745*
Medication Safety Issues
Sound-alike/look-alike issues:
Amantadine may be confused with ranitidine, rimantadine
Symmetrel® may be confused with Synthroid®

International issues:
Symmetrel® may be confused with Somatrel® which is a brand name for somatorelin in Denmark
U.S. Brand Names Symmetrel®
Canadian Brand Names Endantadine®; PMS-Amantadine; Symmetrel®
Index Terms Adamantanamine Hydrochloride; Amantadine Hydrochloride
Generic Available Yes
Pharmacologic Category Anti-Parkinson's Agent, Dopamine Agonist; Antiviral Agent, Adamantane
Use Symptomatic and adjunct treatment of parkinsonism; prophylaxis and treatment of influenza A viral infection; treatment of drug-induced extrapyramidal symptoms
Contraindications Hypersensitivity to amantadine, rimantadine, or any component of the formulation
Warnings/Precautions May cause CNS depression, which may impair physical or mental abilities; patients must be cautioned about performing tasks which require

mental alertness (eg, operating machinery or driving). There have been reports of suicidal ideation/attempt in patients with and without a history of psychiatric illness. Use with caution in patients with liver disease, a history of recurrent and eczematoid dermatitis, uncontrolled psychosis or severe psychoneurosis, seizures and in those receiving CNS stimulant drugs; reduce dose in renal disease; when treating Parkinson's disease, do not discontinue abruptly. In many patients, the therapeutic benefits of amantadine are limited to a few months. Elderly patients may be more susceptible to the CNS effects (using 2 divided daily doses may minimize this effect). Use with caution in patients with CHF, peripheral edema, or orthostatic hypotension. Avoid in untreated angle closure glaucoma. Due to increased resistance, in June 2006, the CDC recommended that amantadine no longer be used for the treatment or prophylaxis of influenza A in the United States until susceptibility has been re-established.

Adverse Reactions (Reflective of adult population; not specific for elderly)
1% to 10%:
Cardiovascular: Orthostatic hypotension, peripheral edema
Central nervous system: Agitation, anxiety, ataxia, confusion, delirium, depression, dizziness, dream abnormality, fatigue, hallucinations, headache, insomnia, irritability, nervousness, somnolence
Dermatologic: Livedo reticularis
Gastrointestinal: Anorexia, constipation, diarrhea, nausea, xerostomia
Respiratory: Dry nose

Overdosage/Toxicology Symptoms of overdose are generally consistent with excessive anticholinergic effects and include nausea, vomiting, slurred speech, blurred vision, lethargy, hallucinations, seizures, myoclonic jerking, and ventricular arrhythmias. Acute toxicity may be primarily due to anticholinergic effects. The minimum lethal dose may be as low as 1 g. Treatment should be supportive and directed at reducing CNS stimulation, controlling seizures, and maintaining cardiovascular function.

Drug Interactions
Anticholinergics may potentiate CNS side effects of amantadine; monitor for altered response; includes benztropine and trihexyphenidyl, as well as agents with anticholinergic activity (eg, quinidine, tricyclics, and antihistamines).
Antipsychotics (typical): May reduce the anti-Parkinsonian effects of amantadine
Triamterene: Has been reported to increase the potential for toxicity with amantadine (limited documentation); monitor response.
Vaccine: Influenza (live, attenuated): The live, attenuated form of influenza vaccine (administered intranasally) should not be administered within 2 weeks before or 48 hours after amantadine (unless medically indicated). Inactivated vaccine (trivalent) may be administered without concern to patients receiving amantadine.

Ethanol/Nutrition/Herb Interactions Ethanol: Avoid ethanol (may increase CNS adverse effects).

Stability Store at 15°C to 30°C (59°F to 86°F); protect from freezing.

Mechanism of Action As an antiviral, blocks the uncoating of influenza A virus preventing penetration of virus into host; antiparkinsonian activity may be due to its blocking the reuptake of dopamine into presynaptic neurons or by increasing dopamine release from presynaptic fibers

Pharmacodynamics Onset of action: Usually within 48 hours, antidyskinetic

Pharmacokinetics
Absorption: Well absorbed from GI tract
Distribution: Crosses the blood-brain barrier
Distribution: V_d:
Normal: 4.4 ± 0.2 L/kg
Renal failure: 5.1 ± 0.2 L/kg
Protein binding:
Normal renal function: ~67%
Hemodialysis patients: ~59%
Metabolism: Not appreciable, small amounts of an acetyl metabolite identified
Half-life:
Normal renal function: 2-7 hours
Older adult patients: 24-29 hours
Impaired renal function: 7-10 days
Hemodialysis patients: Usually within 8 days
Time to peak serum concentration: 1-4 hours
Elimination: 80% to 90% unchanged in urine by glomerular filtration and tubular secretion

Dosage
Geriatrics: Adjust dose based on renal function; some patients tolerate the drug better when it is given in 2 divided daily doses (to avoid adverse neurologic reactions).
Influenza A prophylaxis or treatment: ≤100 mg/day in patients ≥65 years
(Continued)

Amantadine *(Continued)*

Adults:

Influenza A treatment: Oral: 100 mg twice daily; initiate within 24-48 hours after onset of symptoms; discontinue as soon as possible based on clinical response (generally within 3-5 days or within 24-48 hours after symptoms disappear).

Influenza A prophylaxis: Oral: 100 mg twice daily; continue treatment throughout the peak influenza activity in the community or throughout the entire influenza season in patients who cannot be vaccinated. Development of immunity following vaccination takes ~2 weeks; amantadine therapy should be considered for high-risk patients from the time of vaccination until immunity has developed.

Drug-induced extrapyramidal symptoms: Oral: 100 mg twice daily; may increase to 300-400 mg/day, if needed

Parkinson's disease or Creutzfeldt-Jakob disease (unlabeled use): Oral: 100 mg twice daily as sole therapy; may increase to 400 mg/day if needed with close monitoring; initial dose: 100 mg/day if with other serious illness or with high doses of other anti-Parkinson drugs

Renal Impairment:

Cl_{cr} 30-50 mL/minute: Administer 200 mg on day 1, then 100 mg/day

Cl_{cr} 15-29 mL/minute: Administer 200 mg on day 1, then 100 mg on alternate days

Cl_{cr} <15 mL/minute: Administer 200 mg every 7 days

Hemodialysis: Administer 200 mg every 7 days

Peritoneal dialysis: No supplemental dose is needed

Continuous arteriovenous or venous-venous hemofiltration: No supplemental dose is needed

Monitoring Parameters Renal function, Parkinson's symptoms, mental status, influenza symptoms, blood pressure

Patient Information Do not abruptly discontinue therapy, it may precipitate a parkinsonian crisis; may impair ability to perform activities requiring mental alertness or coordination; take second dose of the day in the early afternoon to decrease the incidence of insomnia

Additional Information In many patients, the therapeutic benefits of amantadine are limited to a few months

Special Geriatric Considerations Elderly patients may be more susceptible to the CNS effects of amantadine; using 2 divided daily doses may minimize this effect. The syrup may be used to administer doses <100 mg; studies have demonstrated that young adults on 200 mg/day achieve a plasma concentration of 300 ng/mL. To achieve this concentration (for influenza prophylaxis) in elderly, studies have suggested a dose of 100 mg or 1.4 mg/kg/day.

Dosage Forms Excipient information presented when available (limited, particularly for generics); consult specific product labeling.

Capsule, as hydrochloride: 100 mg

Syrup, as hydrochloride: 50 mg/5 mL (480 mL)

Tablet, as hydrochloride: 100 mg

Symmetrel®: 100 mg

Selected References

Aoki FY and Sitar DS, "Amantadine Kinetics in Healthy Elderly Men: Implications for Influenza Prevention," *Clin Pharmacol Ther*, 1985, 37(2):137-44.

Aoki FY and Sitar DS, "Clinical Pharmacokinetics of Amantadine Hydrochloride," *Clin Pharmacokinet*, 1988, 14(1):35-51.

Centers for Disease Control, "Prevention and Control of Influenza. Recommendations of the Advisory Committee on Immunization Practices (ACIP)," *MMWR*, 2003, 52(RR-8):16-22.

Olanow CW, Watts RL, and Koller WC, "An Algorithm (Decision Tree) for the Management of Parkinson's Disease (2001): Treatment Guidelines," *Neurology*, 2001, 56(11 Suppl 5):S1-S88.

Somani SK, Degelau J, Cooper SL, et al, "Comparison of Pharmacokinetic and Safety Profiles of Amantadine 50- and 100-mg Daily Doses in Elderly Nursing Home Residents," *Pharmacotherapy*, 1991, 11(6):460-6.

Stange KC, Little DW, and Blatnik B, "Adverse Reactions to Amantadine Prophylaxis of Influenza in a Retirement Home," *J Am Geriatr Soc*, 1991, 33(7):700-5.

♦ **Amantadine Hydrochloride** *see Amantadine on page 68*

♦ **Amaryl®** *see Glimepiride on page 708*

♦ **Ambien®** *see Zolpidem on page 1709*

♦ **Ambien CR™** *see Zolpidem on page 1709*

Amcinonide *(am SIN oh nide)*

Related Information

Corticosteroids *on page 1755*

U.S. Brand Names Cyclocort® [DSC]

Canadian Brand Names Amcort®; Cyclocort®; ratio-Amcinonide; Taro-Amcinonide

Generic Available Yes

Pharmacologic Category Corticosteroid, Topical

Use Relief of inflammatory and pruritic manifestations of corticosteroid-responsive dermatoses (high potency corticosteroid)

Contraindications Hypersensitivity to amcinonide or any component of the formulation; use on the face, groin, or axilla

Warnings/Precautions Systemic absorption of topical corticosteroids may cause hypothalamic-pituitary-adrenal (HPA) axis suppression (reversible). HPA axis suppression may lead to adrenal crisis. Risk is increased when used over large surface areas, for prolonged periods, or with occlusive dressings. Adverse systemic effects including hyperglycemia, glycosuria, fluid and electrolyte changes, and HPA suppression may occur when used on large surface areas, for prolonged periods, or with an occlusive dressing. Prolonged treatment with corticosteroids has been associated with the development of Kaposi's sarcoma (case reports); if noted, discontinuation of therapy should be considered. Allergic contact dermatitis can occur, it is usually diagnosed by failure to heal rather than clinical exacerbation. Occlusive dressings should not be used in presence of infection or weeping lesions.

Adverse Reactions (Reflective of adult population; not specific for elderly)
Frequency not defined.
   Dermatologic: Acne, hypopigmentation, allergic dermatitis, maceration of the skin, skin atrophy, striae, miliaria, telangiectasia
   Endocrine & metabolic: Cushing's syndrome, growth retardation (long-term use), HPA suppression, hyperglycemia; these reactions occur more frequently with occlusive dressings
   Local: Burning, itching, irritation, dryness, folliculitis, hypertrichosis
   Miscellaneous: Secondary infection

Overdosage/Toxicology Symptoms include cushingoid appearance (systemic), muscle weakness (systemic), and osteoporosis (systemic) all with long-term use only. When consumed in excessive quantities for prolonged periods, systemic hypercorticism and adrenal suppression may occur; in those cases, discontinuation and withdrawal of the corticosteroid should be done judiciously.

Drug Interactions No data reported

Mechanism of Action Stimulates the synthesis of enzymes needed to decrease inflammation, suppress mitotic activity, and cause vasoconstriction

Pharmacokinetics
   Absorption: Adequate through intact skin; increases with skin inflammation or occlusion
   Metabolism: In the liver
   Elimination: By the kidney and in bile

Dosage
   Geriatrics & Adults: Steroid-responsive dermatoses: Topical: Apply in a thin film 2-3 times/day. Therapy should be discontinued when control is achieved; if no improvement is seen, reassessment of diagnosis may be necessary.

Monitoring Parameters Relief of symptoms

Patient Information Use only as prescribed and for no longer than the period prescribed; apply sparingly in a thin film and rub in lightly; avoid contact with eyes; notify physician if condition persists or worsens

Additional Information Considered a very high potency steroid; avoid use on the face

Special Geriatric Considerations Due to age-related changes in skin, limit use of topical glucocorticosteroids.

Dosage Forms Excipient information presented when available (limited, particularly for generics); consult specific product labeling. [DSC] = Discontinued product
   Cream: 0.1% (15 g, 30 g, 60 g) [contains benzyl alcohol]
   Lotion: 0.1% (60 mL)
      Cyclocort®: 0.1% (20 mL, 60 mL) [contains benzyl alcohol] [DSC]
   Ointment: 0.1% (30 g, 60 g) [contains benzyl alcohol]
      Cyclocort®: 0.1% (15 g, 30 g, 60 g) [contains benzyl alcohol] [DSC]

♦ **Amerge®** *see* Naratriptan *on page 1092*
♦ **A-Methapred** *see* MethylPREDNISolone *on page 1017*
♦ **Amethopterin** *see* Methotrexate *on page 1005*
♦ **Amibid DM [DSC]** *see* Guaifenesin and Dextromethorphan *on page 730*
♦ **Amigesic®** *see* Salsalate *on page 1446*

Amikacin (am i KAY sin)

Related Information
   Aminoglycoside Dosing and Monitoring *on page 1794*
   Antimicrobial Activity Against Selected Organisms *on page 1728*
   Serum Drug Concentrations Commonly Monitored Guidelines *on page 1862*
   (Continued)

Amikacin *(Continued)*

Medication Safety Issues
Sound-alike/look-alike issues:
Amikacin may be confused with Amicar®, anakinra
Amikin® may be confused with Amicar®

U.S. Brand Names Amikin®

Canadian Brand Names Amikacin Sulfate Injection, USP; Amikin®

Index Terms Amikacin Sulfate

Generic Available Yes

Pharmacologic Category Antibiotic, Aminoglycoside

Use Treatment of documented gram-negative enteric infection resistant to gentamicin and tobramycin; documented infection of mycobacterial organisms susceptible to amikacin

Contraindications Hypersensitivity to amikacin sulfate or any component of the formulation; cross-sensitivity may exist with other aminoglycosides

Warnings/Precautions [U.S. Boxed Warning]: Amikacin may cause neurotoxicity, nephrotoxicity, and/or neuromuscular blockade and respiratory paralysis; usual risk factors include pre-existing renal impairment, concomitant neuro-/nephrotoxic medications, advanced age and dehydration. Dose and/or frequency of administration must be monitored and modified in patients with renal impairment. Drug should be discontinued if signs of ototoxicity, nephrotoxicity, or hypersensitivity occur. Ototoxicity is proportional to the amount of drug given and the duration of treatment. Tinnitus or vertigo may be indications of vestibular injury and impending bilateral irreversible damage. Renal damage is usually reversible. Use with caution in patients with neuromuscular disorders, hearing loss and hypocalcemia. Prolonged use may result in fungal or bacterial superinfection, including *C. difficile*-associated diarrhea and pseudomembranous colitis. Solution contains sodium metabisulfate; use caution in patients with sulfite allergy.

Adverse Reactions (Reflective of adult population; not specific for elderly)
1% to 10%:
Central nervous system: Neurotoxicity
Otic: Ototoxicity (auditory), ototoxicity (vestibular)
Renal: Nephrotoxicity

Overdosage/Toxicology Symptoms include ototoxicity, nephrotoxicity, and neuromuscular toxicity. Treatment of choice, following a single acute overdose, appears to be the maintenance of good urine output of at least 3 mL/kg/hour. Dialysis is of questionable value in the enhancement of aminoglycoside elimination. If required, hemodialysis is preferred over peritoneal dialysis in patients with normal renal function.

Drug Interactions
Decreased effect of aminoglycoside: High concentrations of penicillins and/or cephalosporins (*in vitro* data)
Increased toxicity of aminoglycoside: Indomethacin I.V., amphotericin, loop diuretics, vancomycin, enflurane, methoxyflurane; increased effect of neuromuscular-blocking agents and polypeptide antibiotics with administration of aminoglycosides

Stability Store at controlled room temperature. Following admixture at concentrations of 0.25-5 mg/mL, amikcain is stable for 24 hours at room temperature and 2 days at refrigeration when mixed in D_5W, NS, and LR.

Mechanism of Action Inhibits protein synthesis in susceptible bacteria by binding to 30S ribosomal subunits

Pharmacokinetics
Absorption: I.M.: Aminoglycosides may be delayed in the bedridden patient
Half-life:
Adults: 2-3 hours
Anuria: 28-86 hours
Half-life and clearance are dependent on renal function primarily distributed into extracellular fluid (highly hydrophilic); penetrates the blood-brain barrier when meninges are inflamed
Time to peak serum concentration:
I.M.: Within 45-120 minutes
I.V.: Within 30 minutes
Elimination: 94% to 98% excreted unchanged in urine via glomerular filtration within 24 hours
Clearance (renal) may be reduced and half-life prolonged in geriatric patients
The pharmacokinetics of the aminoglycosides are heterogeneous in older adults; it is best to assume that clearance is reduced and half-life prolonged in older adults, while volume of distribution is usually unchanged. The establishment of each patient's pharmacokinetic parameters is important for proper dosing in order to achieve optimal therapeutic benefit and minimize the risk of toxicity.

Dosage

Geriatrics & Adults: Individualization is critical because of the low therapeutic index

Note: Use of ideal body weight (IBW) for determining the mg/kg/dose appears to be more accurate than dosing on the basis of total body weight (TBW)

In morbid obesity, dosage requirement may best be estimated using a dosing weight of IBW + 0.4 (TBW - IBW)

Initial and periodic peak and trough plasma drug levels should be determined, particularly in critically-ill patients with serious infections or in disease states known to significantly alter aminoglycoside pharmacokinetics (eg, cystic fibrosis, burns, or major surgery)

Usual dosage range: I.M., I.V.: 5-7.5 mg/kg/dose every 8 hours

Note: Some clinicians suggest a daily dose of 15-20 mg/kg for all patients with normal renal function. This dose is at least as efficacious with similar, if not less, toxicity than conventional dosing.

Indication-specific dosing:

Endophthalmitis, bacterial (unlabeled use): Intravitreal: 0.4 mg/0.1 mL NS in combination with vancomycin

Hospital-acquired pneumonia (HAP): I.V.: 20 mg/kg/day with antipseudomonal beta-lactam or carbapenem (American Thoracic Society/ATS guidelines)

Meningitis *(Pseudomonas aeruginosa):* I.V.: 5 mg/kg every 8 hours (administered with another bacteriocidal drug)

Mycobacterium fortuitum, M. chelonae, or M. abscessus: I.V.: 10-15 mg/kg daily for at least 2 weeks with high dose cefoxitin

Renal Impairment: Individualization is critical because of the low therapeutic index. Some patients may require larger or more frequent doses if serum levels document the need (ie, cystic fibrosis or febrile granulocytopenic patients).

Cl_{cr} ≥60 mL/minute: Administer every 8 hours

Cl_{cr} 40-60 mL/minute: Administer every 12 hours

Cl_{cr} 20-40 mL/minute: Administer every 24 hours

Cl_{cr} <20 mL/minute: Loading dose, then monitor levels

Dialyzable (50% to 100%)

Administer dose postdialysis or administer $^2/_3$ normal dose as a supplemental dose postdialysis and follow levels.

Peritoneal dialysis effects: Dose as for Cl_{cr} <20 mL/minute: Follow levels.

Continuous arteriovenous or venovenous hemodiafiltration effects: Dose as for Cl_{cr} 10-40 mL/minute: Follow levels.

Administration Administer I.M. injection in large muscle mass

Monitoring Parameters BUN, serum creatinine, serum peak and trough concentrations, hydration and urine output. In cases where extended treatment is warranted (>10 days), audiology testing should be considered.

Reference Range

Therapeutic:

Peak: 25-30 mcg/mL

Trough: 4-8 mcg/mL

Toxic:

Peak: >35 mcg/mL

Trough: >10 mcg/mL

Once daily or extended interval dosing: Trough: <5 mcg/mL

Test Interactions Some penicillin derivatives may accelerate the degradation of aminoglycosides *in vitro*, leading to a potential underestimation of aminoglycoside serum concentration.

Patient Information Report loss of hearing, ringing or roaring in the ears or feeling of fullness in head

Additional Information Drug should be discontinued if signs of ototoxicity, nephrotoxicity, or hypersensitivity occurs; hearing should be tested before, during, and after treatment, when indicated; sodium content of 1 g: 29.9 mg (1.3 mEq). Aminoglycoside serum concentrations measured from blood taken from silastic central catheters can sometimes give falsely high readings.

Special Geriatric Considerations The aminoglycosides are important therapeutic interventions for infections due to susceptible organisms and as empiric therapy in seriously ill patients. Their use is not without risk of toxicity, however, these risks can be minimized if initial dosing is adjusted for estimated renal function and appropriate monitoring performed. High dose, once daily aminoglycosides have been advocated as an alternative to traditional dosing regimens. Once daily or extended interval dosing is as effective and may be safer than traditional dosing. Interval must be adjusted for renal function.

Dosage Forms Excipient information presented when available (limited, particularly for generics); consult specific product labeling. [DSC] = Discontinued product

Injection, solution, as sulfate: 50 mg/mL (2 mL, 4 mL); 62.5 mg/mL (8 mL) [DSC]; 250 mg/mL (2 mL, 4 mL)

Amikin®: 50 mg/mL (2 mL); 250 mg/mL (2 mL, 4 mL) [contains metabisulfite]

(Continued)

Amikacin *(Continued)*

Selected References
Bauer LA and Blouin RA, "Influence of Age on Amikacin Pharmacokinetics in Patients Without Renal Disease. Comparison With Gentamicin and Tobramycin," *Eur J Clin Pharmacol*, 1983, 24(5):639-42.

Nicolau DP, Freeman CD, Belliveau PP, et al, "Experience With a Once-Daily Aminoglycoside Program Administered to 2184 Adult Patients," *Antimicrob Agents Chemother*, 1995, 39(3):650-5.

Preston SL and Briceland LL, "Single Daily Dosing of Aminoglycosides," *Pharmacotherapy*, 1995, 15(3):297-316.

Vanhaeverbeek M, Siska G, Douchamps J, et al, "Comparison of the Efficacy and Safety of Amikacin Once or Twice-a-Day in the Treatment of Severe Gram-Negative Infections in the Elderly," *Int J Clin Pharmacol Ther Toxicol*, 1993, 31(3):153-6.

Yasuhara H, Kobayashi S, Sakamoto K, et al, "Pharmacokinetics of Amikacin and Cephalothin in Bedridden Elderly Patients," *J Clin Pharmacol*, 1982, 22(8-9):403-9.

♦ **Amikacin Sulfate** *see* Amikacin *on page 71*

♦ **Amikin®** *see* Amikacin *on page 71*

Amiloride *(a MIL oh ride)*

Medication Safety Issues
 Sound-alike/look-alike issues:
  Amiloride may be confused with amiodarone, amlodipine, amrinone
Canadian Brand Names Apo-Amiloride®
Index Terms Amiloride Hydrochloride
Generic Available Yes
Pharmacologic Category Diuretic, Potassium-Sparing
Use Counteract potassium loss induced by other diuretics in the treatment of hypertension or edematous conditions including congestive heart failure, hepatic cirrhosis and hypoaldosteronism; usually used in conjunction with a more potent diuretic such as thiazides or loop diuretics
Unlabeled/Investigational Use Investigational: Treatment of cystic fibrosis; reduction of lithium-induced polyuria
Contraindications Hypersensitivity to amiloride or any component of the formulation; presence of elevated serum potassium levels (>5.5 mEq/L); if patient is receiving other potassium-conserving agents (eg, spironolactone, triamterene) or potassium supplementation (medicine, potassium-containing salt substitutes, potassium-rich diet); anuria; acute or chronic renal insufficiency; evidence of diabetic nephropathy. Patients with evidence of renal impairment or diabetes mellitus should not receive this medicine without close, frequent monitoring of serum electrolytes and renal function.
Warnings/Precautions [U.S. Boxed Warning]: Hyperkalemia can occur; patients at risk include those with renal impairment, diabetes, the elderly, and the severely ill. Serum potassium levels must be monitored at frequent intervals especially when dosages are changed or with any illness that may cause renal dysfunction. Excess amounts can lead to profound diuresis with fluid and electrolyte loss; close medical supervision and dose evaluation are required. Watch for and correct electrolyte disturbances; adjust dose to avoid dehydration. In cirrhosis, avoid electrolyte and acid/base imbalances that might lead to hepatic encephalopathy. Use with extreme caution in patients with diabetes mellitus; monitor closely. Discontinue amiloride 3 days prior to glucose tolerance testing. Use with caution in patients who are at risk for metabolic or respiratory acidosis (eg, cardiopulmonary disease, uncontrolled diabetes).
Adverse Reactions (Reflective of adult population; not specific for elderly)
 1% to 10%:
  Central nervous system: Headache, fatigue, dizziness
  Endocrine & metabolic: Hyperkalemia (up to 10%; risk reduced in patients receiving kaliuretic diuretics), hyperchloremic metabolic acidosis, dehydration, hyponatremia, gynecomastia
  Gastrointestinal: Nausea, diarrhea, vomiting, abdominal pain, gas pain, appetite changes, constipation
  Genitourinary: Impotence
  Neuromuscular & skeletal: Muscle cramps, weakness
  Respiratory: Cough, dyspnea
Overdosage/Toxicology Clinical signs are consistent with dehydration and electrolyte disturbance. Large amounts may result in life-threatening hyperkalemia (>6.5 mEq/L). This can be treated with I.V. glucose (dextrose 25% in water), with rapid-acting insulin, with concurrent I.V. sodium bicarbonate and, if needed, Kayexalate® oral or rectal solutions in sorbitol. Persistent hyperkalemia may require dialysis.
Drug Interactions
 Amoxicillin's absorption may be reduced; avoid concurrent use or observe for clinical response.
 ACE inhibitors or angiotensin receptor antagonists can cause hyperkalemia, especially in patients with renal impairment, potassium-rich diets, or on other drugs causing hyperkalemia; avoid concurrent use or monitor closely.

Cyclosporine or tacrolimus: Risk of hyperkalemia may be increased by concurrent therapy.

NSAIDs: May decrease the effect of diuretics.

Potassium supplements may further increase potassium retention and cause hyperkalemia; avoid concurrent use.

Quinidine and amiloride together may increase risk of malignant arrhythmias; avoid concurrent use.

Ethanol/Nutrition/Herb Interactions Food: Hyperkalemia may result if amiloride is taken with potassium-containing foods.

Mechanism of Action Interferes with potassium/sodium exchange (active transport) in the distal tubule, cortical collecting tubule, and collecting duct by inhibiting sodium, potassium-ATPase; decreases calcium excretion; increases magnesium loss

Pharmacodynamics
Onset of action: 2 hours
Duration: 24 hours

Pharmacokinetics
Absorption: Oral: ~15% to 25%
Distribution: V_d: 350-380 L
Protein binding: 23%
Metabolism: No active metabolites
Half-life: Normal renal function: 6-9 hours; End-stage renal disease: 8-144 hours
Peak serum concentration: 6-10 hours
Elimination: Unchanged equally in the urine and the feces

Dosage
Geriatrics: Oral: Initial: 5 mg once daily or every other day
Adults: Hypertension, edema (to limit potassium loss): Oral: Initial: 5-10 mg/day (up to 20 mg)
  Hypertension (JNC 7): 5-10 mg/day in 1-2 divided doses
Renal Impairment: Oral:
  Cl_{cr} 10-50 mL/minute: Administer 50% of normal dose.
  Cl_{cr} <10 mL/minute: Avoid use.

Monitoring Parameters Blood pressure (standing, sitting/supine), serum electrolytes, renal function, weight, I & O

Test Interactions Increased potassium (S)

Patient Information Take in the morning with food or milk; avoid excessive ingestion of foods high in potassium or use of salt substitutes; report any muscle cramps, weakness, nausea, or dizziness

Additional Information Medication should be discontinued if potassium serum concentration exceeds 6.5 mEq/L; combined with hydrochlorothiazide as Moduretic®; amiloride is considered an alternative to triamterene or spironolactone

Special Geriatric Considerations Use lower initial dose, and adjust dose for renal impairment.

Dosage Forms Excipient information presented when available (limited, particularly for generics); consult specific product labeling.
Tablet, as hydrochloride: 5 mg

Amiloride and Hydrochlorothiazide
(a MIL oh ride & hye droe klor oh THYE a zide)

Related Information
Amiloride *on page 74*
Hydrochlorothiazide *on page 756*
Canadian Brand Names Apo-Amilzide®; Gen-Amilazide; Moduret; Novamilor; Nu-Amilzide
Index Terms Hydrochlorothiazide and Amiloride
Generic Available Yes
Pharmacologic Category Diuretic, Combination
Use Antikaliuretic diuretic; antihypertensive
Dosage
Geriatrics: Oral: Initial: $1/2$ to 1 tablet/day
Adults: Hypertension, edema: Oral: Initial: 1 tablet/day; may be increased to 2 tablets/day if needed; usually given in a single dose
Renal Impairment: See individual agents.
Special Geriatric Considerations Potassium excretion may be decreased in the elderly, increasing the risk of hyperkalemia with potassium-sparing diuretics such as amiloride.
Dosage Forms Excipient information presented when available (limited, particularly for generics); consult specific product labeling.
Tablet: 5/50: Amiloride hydrochloride 5 mg and hydrochlorothiazide 50 mg

♦ **Amiloride Hydrochloride** *see* Amiloride *on page 74*

♦ **2-Amino-6-Trifluoromethoxy-benzothiazole** *see* Riluzole *on page 1409*
♦ **Aminobenzylpenicillin** *see* Ampicillin *on page 106*

Aminolevulinic Acid (a MEE noh lev yoo lin ik AS id)

U.S. Brand Names Levulan® Kerastick®
Canadian Brand Names Levulan®
Index Terms Aminolevulinic Acid Hydrochloride
Generic Available No
Pharmacologic Category Photosensitizing Agent, Topical; Topical Skin Product
Use Treatment of nonhyperkeratotic actinic keratoses of the face or scalp; in conjunction with blue light illumination
Contraindications Hypersensitivity to aminolevulinic acid or any component of the formulation; individuals with cutaneous photosensitivity at wavelengths of 400-450 nm; porphyria; allergy to porphyrins
Warnings/Precautions For external use only. Do not apply to eyes or mucous membranes. Treatment site will become photosensitive following application. Patients should be instructed to avoid exposure to sunlight, bright indoor lights, or tanning beds during the period prior to blue light treatment. Should be applied by a qualified health professional to avoid application to perilesional skin. Has not been tested in individuals with coagulation defects (acquired or inherited).
Adverse Reactions (Reflective of adult population; not specific for elderly)
Transient stinging, burning, itching, erythema, and edema result from the photosensitizing properties of this agent. Symptoms subside between 1 minute and 24 hours after turning off the blue light illuminator. Severe stinging or burning was reported in at least 50% of patients from at least 1 lesional site treatment.

>10%: Dermatologic: Severe stinging or burning (50%), scaling of the skin/crusted skin (64% to 71%), hyper-/hypopigmentation (22% to 36%), itching (14% to 25%), erosion (2% to 14%)
1% to 10%:
  Central nervous system: Dysesthesia (up to 2%)
  Dermatologic: Skin ulceration (2% to 4%), vesiculation (4% to 5%), pustular drug eruption (up to 4%), skin disorder (5% to 12%)
  Hematologic: Bleeding/hemorrhage (2% to 4%)
  Local: Wheal/flare (2% to 7%), local pain (1%), tenderness (1% to 2%), edema (1%), scabbing (up to 2%), ulceration (2% to 4%), excoriation (1%)
Overdosage/Toxicology Monitoring and supportive care are recommended. Patients should be advised to avoid incidental exposure to intense light sources for at least 40 hours. Consequences of exceeding the recommended topical dosage are not known.
Drug Interactions Photosensitizing agents including griseofulvin, thiazide diuretics, sulfonamides, sulfonylureas, phenothiazines, and tetracyclines theoretically may increase the photosensitizing potential of aminolevulinic acid.
Stability Store at 25°C (77°F). Prepare solution by holding applicator tube with cap pointing up. Apply finger pressure to "Position A" on cardboard sleeve to crush ampul containing solution vehicle. Apply finger pressure to "Position B" to crush ampul containing aminolevulinic acid powder. Shake gently for at least 3 minutes to dissolve; point applicator cap away from face while shaking tube. Remove cap; dab dry applicator tip on gauze pad until wet with solution. Once prepared, the topical solution should be used immediately and application must be completed within 2 hours.
Mechanism of Action Aminolevulinic acid is a metabolic precursor of protoporphyrin IX (PpIX), which is a photosensitizer. Photosensitization following application of aminolevulinic acid topical solution occurs through the metabolic conversion to PpIX. When exposed to light of appropriate wavelength and energy, accumulated PpIX produces a photodynamic reaction.
Pharmacokinetics
  Aminolevulinic acid:
    Bioavailability: Oral: 50% to 60%
    Half-life, mean: 0.7 ± 0.18 hours after oral
  PpIX:
    Peak fluorescence intensity: 11 ± 1 hour
    Half-life, mean clearance for lesions: 30 ± 10 hours
Dosage
  Geriatrics & Adults: Actinic keratoses: Topical: Apply to actinic keratoses (**not** perilesional skin) followed 14-18 hours later by blue light illumination. Application/treatment may be repeated at a treatment site after 8 weeks.
Administration Dab lesion gently with wet applicator tip. Do not apply to periorbital area, ocular tissue, or mucosal surfaces. Allow to dry then reapply to same lesion. Apply to either scalp or facial lesions, but not to both simultaneously. Follow application with blue light exposure in 14-18 hours.

Monitoring Parameters Monitor for scaling, crusting, erosion, hypo- or hyperpigmentation, pustules, and ulceration.

Patient Information Avoid exposure to sunlight, bright indoor lights, or tanning beds during the period prior to blue light treatment. Wear a wide-brimmed hat to protect from exposure. Sunscreens do not protect against photosensitization by this agent.

Additional Information To be used in conjunction with the BLU-U™ Blue Light Photodynamic Therapy Illuminator

Special Geriatric Considerations Complaints by elderly with skin lesions increase with age. Common skin lesions are actinic keratoses, squamous cell carcinoma, and basal cell carcinoma. Although other agents for treatment are commonly used for these diseases, this agent is an alternative agent.

Dosage Forms Excipient information presented when available (limited, particularly for generics); consult specific product labeling.
Powder for topical solution:
Levulan® Kerastick®: 20% (6s) [2-component system containing aminolevulinic acid hydrochloride 354 mg (powder) and diluent containing ethanol 48% (1.5 mL) packaged together in an applicator tube]

♦ **Aminolevulinic Acid Hydrochloride** *see* Aminolevulinic Acid *on page 76*

Aminophylline (am in OFF i lin)

Related Information
Serum Drug Concentrations Commonly Monitored Guidelines *on page 1862*

Medication Safety Issues
Sound-alike/look-alike issues:
Aminophylline may be confused with amitriptyline, ampicillin

Canadian Brand Names Phyllocontin®; Phyllocontin®-350

Index Terms Theophylline Ethylenediamine

Generic Available Yes

Pharmacologic Category Theophylline Derivative

Use Bronchodilator in reversible airway obstruction due to asthma or COPD; increase diaphragmatic contractility

Contraindications Hypersensitivity to theophylline, ethylenediamine, or any component of the formulation

Warnings/Precautions If a patient develops signs and symptoms of theophylline toxicity, a serum level should be measured and subsequent doses held. Due to potential saturation of theophylline clearance at serum levels within (or in some patients less than) the therapeutic range, dosage adjustment should be made in small increments (maximum: 25% reduction). Due to wide interpatient variability, theophylline serum level measurements must be used to optimize therapy and prevent serious toxicity. Use caution with peptic ulcer, hyperthyroidism, seizure disorder, hypertension, or tachyarrhythmias.

Adverse Reactions (Reflective of adult population; not specific for elderly)
Uncommon at serum theophylline concentrations ≤15 mcg/mL
1% to 10%:
Cardiovascular: Tachycardia
Central nervous system: Nervousness, restlessness
Gastrointestinal: Nausea, vomiting

Drug Interactions Substrate of CYP1A2 (major), 2E1 (minor), 3A4 (minor)
CYP1A2 inducers: May decrease the levels/effects of aminophylline. Example inducers include aminoglutethimide, carbamazepine, phenobarbital, and rifampin.
CYP1A2 inhibitors: May increase the levels/effects of aminophylline. Example inhibitors include ciprofloxacin, fluvoxamine, ketoconazole, norfloxacin, ofloxacin, and rofecoxib.

Ethanol/Nutrition/Herb Interactions Food: Food does not appreciably affect absorption. Avoid extremes of dietary protein and carbohydrate intake. Changes in diet may affect the elimination of theophylline; charcoal-broiled foods may increase elimination, reducing half-life by 50%.

Stability Do not use solutions if discolored or if crystals are present.

Mechanism of Action Causes bronchodilatation, diuresis, CNS and cardiac stimulation, and gastric acid secretion by blocking phosphodiesterase which increases tissue concentrations of cyclic adenine monophosphate (cAMP) which in turn promote catecholamine stimulation of lipolysis, glycogenolysis, and gluconeogenesis and induce release of epinephrine from adrenal medulla cells

Pharmacokinetics Aminophylline is the ethylenediamine salt of theophylline, pharmacokinetic parameters are those of theophylline.
Theophylline:
Absorption: Oral: Dosage form dependent
Distribution: 0.45 L/kg based on ideal body weight
Protein binding: 40%, primarily to albumin
(Continued)

Aminophylline *(Continued)*

Metabolism: Hepatic; extensive (85% to 90%)

Half-life: Highly variable and dependent upon age, liver function, cardiac function, lung disease, and smoking history

Time to peak, serum:
Oral: Immediate release: 1-2 hours
I.V.: Within 30 minutes

Elimination: Adults: Urine 10% unchanged

Dosage

Geriatrics & Adults:

Treatment of acute bronchospasm: I.V.:

Loading dose (in patients not currently receiving aminophylline or theophylline): 6 mg/kg (based on aminophylline) administered I.V. over 20-30 minutes; administration rate should not exceed 25 mg/minute (aminophylline)

Approximate I.V. maintenance dosages: Based upon **continuous infusions**; bolus dosing may be determined by multiplying the hourly infusion rate by 24 hours and dividing by the desired number of doses/day

Smoker: 0.8 mg/kg/hour

Nonsmoker: 0.5 mg/kg/hour

Older patients and patients with cor pulmonale: 0.3 mg/kg/hour

Patients with congestive heart failure: 0.1-0.2 mg/kg/hour

Dosage should be adjusted according to serum level measurements during the first 12- to 24-hour period.

Bronchodilator: Oral: Initial: 380 mg/day (equivalent to theophylline 300 mg/day) in divided doses every 6-8 hours; may increase dose after 3 days; maximum dose: 928 mg/day (equivalent to theophylline 800 mg/day)

Administration Dilute with I.V. fluid to a concentration of 1 mg/mL and infuse over 20-30 minutes; maximum concentration: 25 mg/mL; maximum rate of infusion: 0.36 mg/kg/minute, and no greater than 25 mg/minute. I.M. administration is not recommended. Oral and I.V. should be administered around-the-clock rather than 4 times/day, 3 times/day, etc (ie, 12-6-12-6, not 9-1-5-9) to promote less variation in peak and trough serum levels.

Monitoring Parameters Heart rate, CNS effects (insomnia, irritability); respiratory rate (COPD patients often have resting controlled respiratory rates in low 20s)

Reference Range Sample size: 0.5-1 mL serum (red top tube)

Therapeutic: 10-20 mcg/mL; Toxic: >20 mcg/mL some patients may have adequate clinical response with serum concentrations from 5-10 mcg/mL

Timing of serum samples: If toxicity is suspected, draw serum concentration any time during a continuous I.V. infusion, or 2 hours after an oral dose; if lack of therapeutic is effected, draw a trough serum concentration immediately before the next oral dose or intermittent I.V. dose

Patient Information Oral preparations should be taken with a full glass of water; avoid drinking or eating large quantities of caffeine-containing beverages or food; take at regular intervals; take sustained release tablets whole; do not chew beads; remain in bed for 15-20 minutes after inserting suppository; take with food if GI upset occurs; notify physician if nausea, vomiting, insomnia, nervousness, irritability, palpitations, seizures occur; do not change from one brand to another without consulting physician and pharmacist; do not change doses without consulting your physician

Additional Information 100 mg aminophylline = 79 mg theophylline

Older adults, the acutely ill, and patients with severe respiratory problems, pulmonary edema, or liver dysfunction are at greater risk of toxicity because of reduced drug clearance.

Special Geriatric Considerations Although there is a great intersubject variability for half-lives of methylxanthines (2-10 hours), elderly, as a group, have slower hepatic clearance. Therefore, use lower initial doses and monitor closely for response and adverse reactions. Additionally, elderly patients are at greater risk for toxicity due to concomitant disease (eg, congestive heart failure, arrhythmias), and drug use (eg, cimetidine, ciprofloxacin, etc).

Dosage Forms Excipient information presented when available (limited, particularly for generics); consult specific product labeling.

Injection, solution, as dihydrate: 25 mg/mL (10 mL, 20 mL)

Tablet, as dihydrate: 100 mg, 200 mg

Selected References

Kearney TE, Manoguerra AS, Curtis GP, et al, "Theophylline Toxicity and the Beta-Adrenergic System," *Ann Intern Med*, 1985, 102(6):766-9.

Mahler DA, Barlow PB, and Matthay RA, "Chronic Obstructive Pulmonary Disease," *Clin Geriatr Med*, 1986, 2(2):285-312.

Upton RA, "Pharmacokinetic Interactions Between Theophylline and Other Medication (Part II)," *Clin Pharmacokinet*, 1991, 20(2):135-50.

♦ **Aminosalicylate Sodium** *see* Aminosalicylic Acid *on page 79*

Aminosalicylic Acid (a mee noe sal i SIL ik AS id)

U.S. Brand Names Paser®
Index Terms Aminosalicylate Sodium; 4-Aminosalicylic Acid; Para-Aminosalicylate Sodium; PAS; Sodium PAS
Generic Available No
Pharmacologic Category Salicylate
Use Treatment of tuberculosis with combination drugs
Unlabeled/Investigational Use Treatment of Crohn's disease
Contraindications Hypersensitivity to aminosalicylic acid or any component of the formulation
Warnings/Precautions Use with caution in patients with hepatic or renal dysfunction and patients with gastric ulcer. Patients with sensitivity to tartrazine dyes, nasal polyps, and asthma may have an increased risk of salicylate sensitivity.
Adverse Reactions (Reflective of adult population; not specific for elderly) Frequency not defined.
Cardiovascular: Pericarditis, vasculitis
Central nervous system: Encephalopathy, fever
Dermatologic: Skin eruptions
Endocrine & metabolic: Goiter (with or without myxedema), hypoglycemia
Gastrointestinal: Abdominal pain, diarrhea, nausea, vomiting
Hematologic: Agranulocytosis, anemia (hemolytic), leukopenia, thrombocytopenia
Hepatic: Hepatitis, jaundice
Ocular: Optic neuritis
Respiratory: Eosinophilic pneumonia
Overdosage/Toxicology Acute overdose results in crystalluria and renal failure, nausea, and vomiting. Alkalinization of the urine with sodium bicarbonate and forced diuresis can prevent crystalluria and nephrotoxicity.
Drug Interactions
Digoxin: Serum levels may be decreased by aminosalicylic acid.
Vitamin B_{12}: Serum levels may be decreased by aminosalicylic acid.
Stability Prior to dispensing, store granules below 15°C (59°F). Once dispensed, packets may be stored at room temperature for short periods of time. Do not use if packet is swollen or if granules are dark brown or purple.
Mechanism of Action Aminosalicylic acid (PAS) is a highly-specific bacteriostatic agent active against *M. tuberculosis*. Structurally related to para-aminobenzoic acid (PABA) and its mechanism of action is thought to be similar to the sulfonamides, a competitive antagonism with PABA; disrupts plate biosynthesis in sensitive organisms.
Pharmacokinetics
Distribution: Wide with high concentrations in pleural and caseous tissue; CSF concentrations are low
Metabolism: Hepatic (>50% acetylation)
Elimination: >80% excreted in urine as metabolites or free acid
Excretion may be reduced and half-life prolonged in persons with hepatic or renal impairment
Dosage
Geriatrics & Adults:
Tuberculosis: Oral: 150 mg/kg/day in 2-3 equally divided doses
Crohn's disease (unlabeled use): 1.5 g/day
Renal Impairment:
Cl_{cr} 10-50 mL/minute: Administer 50% to 75% of dose.
Cl_{cr} <10 mL/minute: Administer 50% of dose.
Administer after hemodialysis: Administer 50% of dose.
Continuous arteriovenous hemofiltration: Dose for Cl_{cr} <10 mL/minute
Hepatic Impairment: Use with caution
Patient Information Take with food; may sprinkle on applesauce or yogurt, or swirl in tomato juice or orange juice; may discolor urine red; do not take granules when brown or purple in color; do not store in bathroom or kitchen as tablets will deteriorate in high humidity environments; notify physician of sore throat, bruising, bleeding, or skin rash
Additional Information This monograph is maintained as this drug still remains in the armamentarium for tuberculosis.
Special Geriatric Considerations Elderly may require a lower recommended dose.
Dosage Forms Excipient information presented when available (limited, particularly for generics); consult specific product labeling.
Granules, delayed release:
Paser®: 4 g/packet (30s)

♦ **4-Aminosalicylic Acid** see Aminosalicylic Acid on page 79
♦ **5-Aminosalicylic Acid** see Mesalamine on page 989
♦ **Aminoxin [OTC]** see Pyridoxine on page 1353

Amiodarone (a MEE oh da rone)

Related Information
Potentially Inappropriate Medications for Geriatrics *on page 1824*
Medication Safety Issues
Sound-alike/look-alike issues:
Amiodarone may be confused with amiloride, amrinone
Cordarone® may be confused with Cardura®, Cordran®

High alert medication: The Institute for Safe Medication Practices (ISMP) includes this medication among its list of drugs which have a heightened risk of causing significant patient harm when used in error.

U.S. Brand Names Cordarone®; Pacerone®
Canadian Brand Names Alti-Amiodarone; Amiodarone Hydrochloride for Injection®; Apo-Amiodarone®; Cordarone®; Gen-Amiodarone; Novo-Amiodarone; PMS-Amiodarone; Rhoxal-amiodarone; Sandoz-Amiodarone
Index Terms Amiodarone Hydrochloride
Generic Available Yes
Pharmacologic Category Antiarrhythmic Agent, Class III
Use Management of life-threatening recurrent ventricular fibrillation (VF) or hemodynamically-unstable ventricular tachycardia (VT) refractory to other antiarrhythmic agents or in patients intolerant of other agents used for these conditions
Unlabeled/Investigational Use
Conversion of atrial fibrillation to normal sinus rhythm; maintenance of normal sinus rhythm
Prevention of postoperative atrial fibrillation during cardiothoracic surgery
Paroxysmal supraventricular tachycardia (SVT)
Control of rapid ventricular rate due to accessory pathway conduction in pre-excited atrial arrhythmias [ACLS guidelines]
Cardiac arrest with persistent ventricular tachycardia (VT) or ventricular fibrillation (VF) if defibrillation, CPR, and vasopressor administration have failed [ACLS/PALS guidelines]
Control of hemodynamically-stable VT, polymorphic VT with a normal QT interval, or wide-complex tachycardia of uncertain origin [ACLS/PALS guidelines]
Restrictions An FDA-approved medication guide must be distributed when dispensing an outpatient prescription (new or refill) where this medication is to be used without direct supervision of a healthcare provider. Medication guides are available at http://www.fda.gov/cder/Offices/ODS/medication_guides.htm.
Contraindications Hypersensitivity to amiodarone, iodine, or any component of the formulation; severe sinus-node dysfunction; second- and third-degree heart block (except in patients with a functioning artificial pacemaker); bradycardia causing syncope (except in patients with a functioning artificial pacemaker); cardiogenic shock
Warnings/Precautions [U.S. Boxed Warning]: Only indicated for patients with life-threatening arrhythmias because of risk of toxicity. Monitor for pulmonary toxicity. Lung damage (abnormal diffusion capacity) may occur without symptoms. Pre-existing pulmonary disease does not increase risk of developing pulmonary toxicity, but if pulmonary toxicity develops then the prognosis is worse. Liver toxicity is common, but usually mild with evidence of increased liver enzymes. Severe liver toxicity can occur and has been fatal in a few cases.

Amiodarone can exacerbate the arrhythmia (including torsade de pointes), making it more difficult to tolerate or reverse. Other types of arrhythmias have occurred (eg, significant heart block, sinus bradycardia). Proarrhythmic effects may be prolonged. Use very cautiously and with close monitoring in patients with thyroid or liver disease. May cause hyper- or hypothyroidism. Hyperthyroidism may result in thyrotoxicosis and may aggravate or cause breakthrough arrhythmias. If any new signs of arrhythmia appear, hyperthyroidism should be considered. Thyroid function should be monitored prior to treatment and periodically thereafter. May cause optic neuropathy and/or optic neuritis, usually resulting in visual impairment. Corneal microdeposits occur in a majority of patients, and may cause visual disturbances in some patients (blurred vision, halos); these are not generally considered a reason to discontinue treatment. Corneal refractive laser surgery is generally contraindicated in amiodarone users. Avoid excessive exposure to sunlight; may cause photosensitivity.

[U.S. Boxed Warning]: Alternative therapies should be tried first before using amiodarone. Patients should be hospitalized when amiodarone is initiated. Due to complex pharmacokinetics, it is difficult to predict when an arrhythmia or interaction with a subsequent treatment will occur following discontinuation of amiodarone.

Amiodarone is a potent inhibitor of CYP enzymes and transport proteins (including p-glycoprotein), which may lead to increased serum concentrations/toxicity of a number of medications. Particular caution must be used when a drug with QT_c-prolonging potential relies on metabolism via these enzymes, since the effect of elevated concentrations may be additive with the effect of amiodarone. Carefully assess risk:benefit of coadministration of other drugs which may prolong QT$_c$ interval. Correct electrolyte disturbances, especially hypokalemia or hypomagnesemia, prior to use and throughout therapy.

May cause hypotension and bradycardia (infusion-rate related). Caution in surgical patients; may enhance hemodynamic effect of anesthetics; associated with increased risk of adult respiratory distress syndrome (ARDS) postoperatively.

Adverse Reactions (Reflective of adult population; not specific for elderly) In a recent meta-analysis, patients taking lower doses of amiodarone (152-330 mg daily for at least 12 months) were more likely to develop thyroid, neurologic, skin, ocular, and bradycardic abnormalities than those taking placebo (Vorperian, 1997). Pulmonary toxicity was similar in both the low dose amiodarone group and in the placebo group but there was a trend towards increased toxicity in the amiodarone group. Gastrointestinal and hepatic events were seen to a similar extent in both the low dose amiodarone group and placebo group. As the frequency of adverse events varies considerably across studies as a function of route and dose, a consolidation of adverse event rates is provided by Goldschlager, 2000.

> Cardiovascular: Hypotension (I.V. 16%, refractory in rare cases)
> Central nervous system (3% to 40%): Abnormal gait/ataxia, dizziness, fatigue, headache, malaise, impaired memory, involuntary movement, insomnia, poor coordination, peripheral neuropathy, sleep disturbances, tremor
> Dermatologic: Photosensitivity (10% to 75%)
> Endocrine & Metabolic: Hypothyroidism (1% to 22%)
> Gastrointestinal: Nausea, vomiting, anorexia, and constipation (10% to 33%)
> Hepatic: AST or ALT level >2x normal (15% to 50%)
> Ocular: Corneal microdeposits (>90%; causes visual disturbance in <10%)

> 1% to 10%:
> Cardiovascular: CHF (3%), bradycardia (3% to 5%), AV block (5%), conduction abnormalities, SA node dysfunction (1% to 3%), cardiac arrhythmia, flushing, edema. Additional effects associated with I.V. administration include asystole, cardiac arrest, electromechanical dissociation, ventricular tachycardia, and cardiogenic shock.
> Dermatologic: Slate blue skin discoloration (<10%)
> Endocrine & metabolic: Hyperthyroidism (3% to 10%; more common in iodine-deficient regions of the world), libido decreased
> Gastrointestinal: Abdominal pain, abnormal salivation, abnormal taste (oral)
> Hematologic: Coagulation abnormalities
> Hepatic: Hepatitis and cirrhosis (<3%)
> Local: Phlebitis (I.V., with concentrations >3 mg/mL)
> Ocular: Visual disturbances (2% to 9%), halo vision (<5% occurring especially at night), optic neuritis (1%)
> Respiratory: Pulmonary toxicity has been estimated to occur at a frequency between 2% and 7% of patients (some reports indicate a frequency as high as 17%). Toxicity may present as hypersensitivity pneumonitis; pulmonary fibrosis (cough, fever, malaise); pulmonary inflammation; interstitial pneumonitis; or alveolar pneumonitis. ARDS has been reported in up to 2% of patients receiving amiodarone, and postoperatively in patients receiving oral amiodarone.
> Miscellaneous: Abnormal smell (oral)

Overdosage/Toxicology Symptoms include extensions of pharmacologic effect, sinus bradycardia and/or heart block, hypotension and QT prolongation. Patients should be monitored for several days following ingestion. Intoxication with amiodarone necessitates ECG monitoring. Bradycardia may be atropine resistant. Injectable isoproterenol or a temporary pacemaker may be required. Dialysis is not beneficial.

Drug Interactions Substrate of CYP1A2 (minor), 2C8 (major at low concentrations), 2C19 (minor), 2D6 (minor), 3A4 (major); **Inhibits** CYP1A2 (weak), 2A6 (moderate), 2B6 (weak), 2C9 (moderate), 2C19 (weak), 2D6 (moderate), 3A4 (moderate)

Anesthetics (halogenated, inhaled): Amiodarone enhances the myocardial depressant and conduction effects of inhalation anesthetics; monitor.
Azole antifungals: May prolong QT$_c$, potentially leading to malignant arrhythmias; use caution.
Beta-blockers may cause excessive AV block; monitor response.
Calcium channel blockers (diltiazem, verapamil): May cause excessive AV block; monitor.
Cimetidine: May increase amiodarone blood levels.
Cholestyramine: May decrease amiodarone blood levels.
Cisapride: May prolong QT$_c$ interval potentially leading to malignant arrhythmias.
Cyclosporine: Serum levels may be increased by amiodarone; monitor.
CYP2A6 substrates: Amiodarone may increase the levels/effects of CYP2A6 substrates. Example substrates include dexmedetomidine and ifosfamide.
(Continued)

Amiodarone *(Continued)*

CYP2C8 inducers: May decrease the levels/effects of amiodarone. Example inducers include carbamazepine, phenobarbital, phenytoin, rifampin, rifapentine, and secobarbital.

CYP2C8 inhibitors: May increase the levels/effects of amiodarone. Example inhibitors include atazanavir, gemfibrozil, and ritonavir.

CYP2C9 substrates: Amiodarone may increase the levels/effects of CYP2C9 substrates. Example substrates include bosentan, dapsone, fluoxetine, glimepiride, glipizide, losartan, montelukast, nateglinide, paclitaxel, phenytoin, warfarin, and zafirlukast.

CYP2D6 substrates: Amiodarone may increase the levels/effects of CYP2D6 substrates. Example substrates include amphetamines, selected beta-blockers, dextromethorphan, fluoxetine, lidocaine, mirtazapine, nefazodone, paroxetine, risperidone, ritonavir, thioridazine, tricyclic antidepressants, and venlafaxine.

CYP2D6 prodrug substrates: Amiodarone may decrease the levels/effects of CYP2D6 prodrug substrates. Example prodrug substrates include codeine, hydrocodone, oxycodone, and tramadol.

CYP3A4 inducers: CYP3A4 inducers may decrease the levels/effects of amiodarone. Example inducers include aminoglutethimide, carbamazepine, nafcillin, nevirapine, phenobarbital, phenytoin, and rifamycins.

CYP3A4 inhibitors: May increase the levels/effects of amiodarone. Example inhibitors include azole antifungals, clarithromycin, diclofenac, doxycycline, erythromycin, imatinib, isoniazid, nefazodone, nicardipine, propofol, protease inhibitors, quinidine, telithromycin, and verapamil.

CYP3A4 substrates: Amiodarone may increase the levels/effects of CYP3A4 substrates. Example substrates include benzodiazepines, calcium channel blockers, ergot derivatives, mirtazapine, nateglinide, nefazodone, tacrolimus, and venlafaxine.

Digoxin levels may be increased by amiodarone; consider reducing digoxin dose by 50% and monitor digoxin blood levels closely.

Fentanyl: Concurrent use may lead to bradycardia, sinus arrest, and hypotension.

Flecainide blood levels may be increased; consider reducing flecainide dose by 25% to 33% with concurrent use.

Fluoroquinolones (moxifloxacin): May result in additional prolongation of the QT interval; concurrent use of sparfloxacin is contraindicated.

HMG-CoA reductase inhibitors (lovastatin, simvastatin, and others dependent on CYP3A4 metabolism): Amiodarone inhibits metabolism of lovastatin and/or simvastatin and may increase the risk of myopathy and rhabdomyolysis. Concurrent use of lovastatin or simvastatin is not recommended, but if unavoidable, dose of lovastatin should not exceed 40 mg/day. The dose of simvastatin should not exceed 20 mg/day; consider alternative HMG-CoA reductase inhibitor.

Lidocaine: Amiodarone may increase serum levels/toxicity of lidocaine. Sinus bradycardia may occur with concurrent use.

Macrolide antibiotics: May prolong QT_c, potentially leading to malignant arrhythmias. Use caution and evaluate risk:benefit.

Metoprolol blood levels may be increased; monitor response.

Phenytoin blood levels may be increased by amiodarone; amiodarone blood levels may be decreased by phenytoin.

Procainamide and NAPA plasma levels may be increased; consider reducing procainamide dosage by 25% with concurrent use.

Propranolol blood levels may be increased.

Protease inhibitors (amprenavir, indinavir, ritonavir): May increase amiodarone blood levels and toxicity; concurrent use is contraindicated.

QT_c interval prolonging agents (including but may not be limited to amitriptyline, bepridil, disopyramide, erythromycin, haloperidol, imipramine, quinidine, pimozide, procainamide, sotalol, and thioridazine): Effect/toxicity increased; use with caution.

Quinidine blood levels may be increased; monitor quinidine trough concentration.

Rifampin may decrease amiodarone blood levels.

Theophylline blood levels may be increased.

Thioridazine: Amiodarone may enhance the QTc-prolonging effect of thioridazine.

Thyroid supplements: Amiodarone may alter thyroid function; monitor closely.

Trazodone: Amiodarone may increase levels/effects of trazodone. QTC prolongation and torsade de pointes have been reported with concurrent use.

Warfarin: Hypoprothrombinemic response increased. Monitor INR closely when amiodarone is initiated or discontinued. Reduce warfarin's dose by $1/3$ to $1/2$ when amiodarone is started.

Ethanol/Nutrition/Herb Interactions

Food: Increases the rate and extent of absorption of amiodarone. Grapefruit juice increases bioavailability of oral amiodarone by 50% and decreases the conversion of amiodarone to N-DEA (active metabolite); altered effects are possible; use should be avoided during therapy.

Herb/Nutraceutical: St John's wort may decrease amiodarone levels or enhance photo-sensitization. Avoid ephedra (may worsen arrhythmia). Avoid dong quai.

Stability Store at room temperature; protect from light. When admixed in D_5W to a final concentration of 1-6 mg/mL, the solution is stable at room temperature for 24 hours in polyolefin or glass, or for 2 hours in PVC. Infusions >2 hours must be administered in glass or polyolefin bottles. Do not use evacuated glass containers; buffer may cause precipitation.

Mechanism of Action Class III antiarrhythmic agent which inhibits adrenergic stimula-tion (alpha- and beta-blocking properties), affects sodium, potassium, and calcium channels, prolongs the action potential and refractory period in myocardial tissue; decreases AV conduction and sinus node function

Pharmacodynamics

Onset of action: Oral: 2 days to 3 weeks; I.V.: May be more rapid

Duration of effects after discontinuation of therapy: 7-50 days

Pharmacokinetics

Distribution: V_d: 66 L/kg (range: 18-148 L/kg)

Protein binding: 96%

Metabolism: Hepatic via CYP2C8 and 3A4 to active N-desethylamiodarone metabolite; possible enterohepatic recirculation

Bioavailability: Oral: ~50%

Half-life elimination: Terminal: 40-55 days (range: 26-107 days)

Elimination, biphasic: 50% reduction of serum concentration in 2.5-10 days; slow terminal elimination 26-107 days; steady-state levels achieved between 130-535 days with 265 days average; <1% excreted unchanged in urine

Dosage

Geriatrics & Adults: **Note:** Lower loading and maintenance doses are preferable in women and all patients with low body weight.

Ventricular arrhythmias: Oral: 800-1600 mg/day in 1-2 doses for 1-3 weeks, then 600-800 mg/day in 1-2 doses for 1 month; maintenance: 400 mg/day; lower doses are recommended for supraventricular arrhythmias.

Breakthrough VF or VT: I.V.: 150 mg supplemental doses in 100 mL D_5W over 10 minutes

Pulseless VF or VT: I.V. push: Initial: 300 mg in 20-30 mL NS or D_5W; if VF or VT recurs, supplemental dose of 150 mg followed by infusion of 1 mg/minute for 6 hours, then 0.5 mg/minute (maximum daily dose: 2.1 g)

I.V. to oral therapy conversion: Use the following as a guide:

<1 week I.V. infusion: 800-1600 mg/day

1- to 3-week I.V. infusion: 600-800 mg/day

>3 week I.V. infusion: 400 mg

Recommendations for conversion to intravenous amiodarone after oral admin-istration: During long-term amiodarone therapy (ie, ≥4 months), the mean plasma-elimination half-life of the active metabolite of amiodarone is 61 days. Replacement therapy may not be necessary in such patients if oral therapy is discontinued for a period <2 weeks, since any changes in serum amiodarone concentrations during this period may **not** be clinically significant.

Unlabeled uses:

Atrial fibrillation prophylaxis following open heart surgery (unlabeled use): **Note:** A variety of regimens have been used in clinical trials, including oral and intravenous regimens:

Oral: Starting in postop recovery, 400 mg twice daily for up to 7 days. Alternative regimen of amiodarone: 600 mg/day for 7 days prior to surgery, followed by 200 mg/day until hospital discharge, has also been shown to decrease the risk of postoperative atrial fibrillation. Note: A variety of regimens have been used in clinical trials.

I.V.: Starting at postop recovery, 1000 mg infused over 24 hours for 2 days has been shown to reduce the risk of postoperative atrial fibrillation. **Note:** A variety of regimens have been used in clinical trials.

Atrial fibrillation pharmacologic cardioversion (ACC/AHA/ESC Practice Guidelines) (unlabeled use):

Oral: Inpatient: 1.2-1.8 g/day in divided doses until 10 g total, then 200-400 mg/day maintenance. **Note:** Other regimens have been described and may be used clinically (eg, 400 mg 3 times/day for 5-7 days, then 400 mg/day for 1 month, then 200 mg/day or 10 mg/kg/day for 14 days; followed by 300 mg/day for 4 weeks, followed by maintenance dosage of 100-200 mg/day [Roy D, 2000]).

I.V.: 5-7 mg/kg over 30-60 minutes, then 1.2-1.8 g/day continuous infusion or in divided oral doses until 10 g total. Maintenance: See oral dosing.

Recurrent atrial fibrillation (unlabeled use): No standard regimen defined; examples of regimens include: Oral: Initial: 10 mg/kg/day for 14 days; followed by 300 mg/day for 4 weeks, followed by maintenance dosage of 100-200 mg/day (Roy D, 2000). Other regimens have been described and are used clinically

(Continued)

Amiodarone *(Continued)*

(ie, 400 mg 3 times/day for 5-7 days, then 400 mg/day for 1 month, then 200 mg/day).

Stable VT or SVT (unlabeled use): I.V.: First 24 hours: 1050 mg according to following regimen

Step 1: 150 mg (100 mL) over first 10 minutes (mix 3 mL in 100 mL D_5W)

Step 2: 360 mg (200 mL) over next 6 hours (mix 18 mL in 500 mL D_5W): 1 mg/minute

Step 3: 540 mg (300 mL) over next 18 hours: 0.5 mg/minute

Note: After the first 24 hours: 0.5 mg/minute utilizing concentration of 1-6 mg/mL

Renal Impairment: Hemodialysis effects: Not removed by hemodialysis or peritoneal dialysis (0% to 5%); no supplemental doses required.

Hepatic Impairment: Dosage adjustment is probably necessary in substantial hepatic impairment. No specific guidelines available. If hepatic enzymes exceed 3 times normal or double in a patient with an elevated baseline, consider decreasing the dose or discontinuing amiodarone.

Administration

Oral: Administer consistently with regard to meals. Take in divided doses with meals if high daily dose or if GI upset occurs. If GI intolerance occurs with single-dose therapy, use twice daily dosing.

I.V.: Adjust administration rate to urgency (give more slowly when perfusing arrhythmia present). Give I.V. therapy using an infusion pump at a concentration <2 mg/mL. Slow the infusion rate if hypotension or bradycardia develops. Infusions >2 hours must be administered in glass or polyolefin bottles. **Note:** I.V. administration at lower flow rates and higher concentrations than recommended may result in leaching of plasticizers (DEHP) from intravenous tubing. DEHP may adversely affect male reproductive tract development. Alternative means of dosing and administration (1 mg/kg aliquots) may need to be considered. Use only volumetric infusion pump; use of drop counting may lead to under-dosing. Administer through I.V. line with in-line filter.

Monitoring Parameters

Blood pressure, heart rate (ECG) and rhythm throughout therapy; assess patient for signs of lethargy, edema of the hands or feet, weight loss, and pulmonary toxicity (baseline pulmonary function tests); liver function tests; monitor serum electrolytes, especially potassium and magnesium. Assess thyroid function tests before initiation of treatment and then periodically thereafter (some experts suggest every 3-6 months). If signs or symptoms of thyroid disease or arrhythmia breakthrough/exacerbation occur then immediate re-evaluation is necessary. Amiodarone partially inhibits the peripheral conversion of thyroxine (T_4) to triiodothyronine (T_3); serum T_4 and reverse triiodothyronine (rT_3) concentrations may be increased and serum T_3 may be decreased; most patients remain clinically euthyroid, however, clinical hypothyroidism or hyperthyroidism may occur.

Perform regular ophthalmic exams.

Reference Range

Therapeutic: 0.5-2.5 mg/L (SI: 1-4 µmol/L) (parent); desethyl metabolite is active and is present in equal concentration to parent drug

Patient Information

Take with food; use sunscreen or stay out of sun to prevent burns; skin discoloration is reversible; photophobia may make sunglasses necessary

Additional Information

Hospitalization required for initiation of therapy; CNS symptoms normally develop within 7 days, muscle weakness may present a great hazard for ambulation.

Special Geriatric Considerations

Information describing the clinical use and pharmacokinetics in elderly is lacking; however, elderly may be predisposed to toxicity. Half-life may be prolonged due to decreased clearance; monitor closely. It is recommended to start dosing at the lower end of dosing range.

Dosage Forms

Excipient information presented when available (limited, particularly for generics); consult specific product labeling. [DSC] = Discontinued product

Injection, solution, as hydrochloride: 50 mg/mL (3 mL, 9 mL, 18 mL) [contains benzyl alcohol and polysorbate (Tween®) 80] [DSC]

Cordarone®: 50 mg/mL (3 mL) [contains benzyl alcohol and polysorbate (Tween®) 80]

Tablet, as hydrochloride [scored]: 200 mg, 400 mg

Cordarone®: 200 mg

Pacerone®: 100 mg [not scored], 200 mg, 300 mg [DSC], 400 mg

Selected References

"2005 American Heart Association Guidelines for Cardiopulmonary Resuscitation and Emergency Cardiovascular Care," *Circulation*, 2005, 112(24 Suppl):1-211.

Fenster PE and Nolan PE, "Antiarrhythmic Drugs," *Geriatric Pharmacology*, Bressler R and Katz MD, eds, New York, NY: McGraw-Hill, 1993, 6:105-49.

Kennedy RL, Griffiths H, Gray TA, et al, "Amiodarone and the Thyroid," *Clin Chem*, 1989, 35(9):1882-7.

Martino E, Bartalena L, Bogazzi, et al, "The Effects of Amiodarone on the Thyroid," *Endocr Rev*, 2001, 22(2):240-54.

♦ **Amiodarone Hydrochloride** *see* Amiodarone *on page 80*

♦ **Amitiza**® *see* Lubiprostone *on page 942*
♦ **Amitone**® **[OTC]** *see* Calcium Salts (Oral) *on page 220*

Amitriptyline (a mee TRIP ti leen)

Related Information
Antidepressant Agents *on page 1742*
Potentially Inappropriate Medications for Geriatrics *on page 1824*
Serum Drug Concentrations Commonly Monitored Guidelines *on page 1862*

Medication Safety Issues
Sound-alike/look-alike issues:
Amitriptyline may be confused with aminophylline, imipramine, nortriptyline
Elavil® may be confused with Aldoril®, Eldepryl®, enalapril, Equanil®, Mellaril®, Oruvail®, Plavix®

Canadian Brand Names Apo-Amitriptyline®; Levate®; Novo-Triptyn; PMS-Amitriptyline

Index Terms Amitriptyline Hydrochloride; Elavil

Generic Available Yes

Pharmacologic Category Antidepressant, Tricyclic (Tertiary Amine)

Use Treatment of various forms of depression, often in conjunction with psychotherapy

Unlabeled/Investigational Use Analgesic for certain chronic and neuropathic pain; prophylaxis against migraine headaches

Restrictions An FDA-approved medication guide concerning the use of antidepressants in children, adolescents, and young adults must be distributed when dispensing an outpatient prescription (new or refill) where this medication is to be used without direct supervision of a healthcare provider. Medication guides are available at http://www.fda.gov/cder/Offices/ODS/medication_guides.htm. Dispense to parents or guardians of children and adolescents receiving this medication.

Contraindications Hypersensitivity to amitriptyline or any component of the formulation (cross-sensitivity with other tricyclics may occur); use of MAO inhibitors within past 14 days; acute recovery phase following myocardial infarction; concurrent use of cisapride

Warnings/Precautions [U.S. Boxed Warning]: Antidepressants increase the risk of suicidal thinking and behavior in children, adolescents, and young adults (18-24 years of age) with major depressive disorder (MDD) and other psychiatric disorders; consider risk prior to prescribing. Short-term studies did not show an increased risk in patients >24 years of age and showed a decreased risk in patients ≥65 years. Closely monitor for clinical worsening, suicidality, or unusual changes in behavior; the patient's family or caregiver should be instructed to closely observe the patient and communicate condition with healthcare provider. Such observation would generally include at least weekly face-to-face contact with patients or their family members or caregivers during the first 4 weeks of treatment, then every other week visits for the next 4 weeks, then at 12 weeks, and as clinically indicated beyond 12 weeks. Additional contact by telephone may be appropriate between face-to-face visits. Adults treated with antidepressants should be observed similarly for clinical worsening and suicidality, especially during the initial few months of a course of drug therapy, or at times of dose changes, either increases or decreases. A medication guide should be dispensed with each prescription.

The possibility of a suicide attempt is inherent in major depression and may persist until remission occurs. Monitor for worsening of depression or suicidality, especially during initiation of therapy (generally first 1-2 months) or with dose increases or decreases. Worsening depression and severe abrupt suicidality that are not part of the presenting symptoms may require discontinuation or modification of drug therapy. The patient's family or caregiver should be alerted to monitor patients for the emergence of suicidality and associated behaviors (such as agitation, irritability, hostility, impulsivity, and hypomania) and notify healthcare provider.

May worsen psychosis in some patients or precipitate a shift to mania or hypomania in patients with bipolar disorder. Patients presenting with depressive symptoms should be screened for bipolar disorder. Monotherapy in patients with bipolar disorder should be avoided. **Amitriptyline is not FDA approved for bipolar depression.**

The degree of sedation, anticholinergic effects, orthostasis, and conduction abnormalities are high relative to other antidepressants. Amitriptyline often causes drowsiness/sedation, resulting in impaired performance of tasks requiring alertness (eg, operating machinery or driving). Sedative effects may be additive with other CNS depressants and/or ethanol. Use with caution in patients with a history of cardiovascular disease (including previous MI, stroke, tachycardia, or conduction abnormalities). Use with caution in patients with urinary retention, benign prostatic hyperplasia, narrow-angle glaucoma, xerostomia, visual problems, constipation, or a history of bowel obstruction.

May alter glucose control - use with caution in patients with diabetes. May cause hyponatremia/SIADH. Consider discontinuing, when possible, prior to elective surgery. (Continued)

Amitriptyline *(Continued)*

Therapy should not be abruptly discontinued in patients receiving high doses for prolonged periods. May lower seizure threshold - use caution in patients with a previous seizure disorder or condition predisposing to seizures such as brain damage, alcoholism, or concurrent therapy with other drugs which lower the seizure threshold. May increase the risks associated with electroconvulsive therapy. Use with caution in hyperthyroid patients or those receiving thyroid supplementation. Use with caution in patients with hepatic or renal dysfunction and in elderly patients.

Adverse Reactions (Reflective of adult population; not specific for elderly)
Anticholinergic effects may be pronounced; moderate to marked sedation can occur (tolerance to these effects usually occurs).

Frequency not defined.

Cardiovascular: Orthostatic hypotension, tachycardia, ECG changes (nonspecific), AV conduction changes, cardiomyopathy (rare), MI, stroke, heart block, arrhythmia, syncope, hypertension, palpitation

Central nervous system: Restlessness, dizziness, insomnia, sedation, fatigue, anxiety, cognitive function (impaired), seizure, extrapyramidal symptoms, coma, hallucinations, confusion, disorientation, coordination impaired, ataxia, headache, nightmares, hyperpyrexia

Dermatologic: Allergic rash, urticaria, photosensitivity, alopecia

Endocrine & metabolic: Syndrome of inappropriate ADH secretion

Gastrointestinal: Weight gain, xerostomia, constipation, paralytic ileus, nausea, vomiting, anorexia, stomatitis, peculiar taste, diarrhea, black tongue

Genitourinary: Urinary retention

Hematologic: Bone marrow depression, purpura, eosinophilia

Neuromuscular & skeletal: Numbness, paresthesia, peripheral neuropathy, tremor, weakness

Ocular: Blurred vision, mydriasis, ocular pressure increased

Otic: Tinnitus

Miscellaneous: Diaphoresis, withdrawal reactions (nausea, headache, malaise)

Overdosage/Toxicology Symptoms include agitation, confusion, hallucinations, urinary retention, hypothermia, hypotension, ventricular tachycardia, and seizures. Following initiation of essential overdose management, toxic symptoms should be treated. Sodium bicarbonate is indicated when the QRS interval is >0.10 seconds or the QT_c is >0.42 seconds. Ventricular arrhythmias often respond to phenytoin 15-20 mg/kg with concurrent systemic alkalinization (sodium bicarbonate 0.5-2 mEq/kg I.V.). Arrhythmias unresponsive to this therapy may respond to lidocaine 1 mg/kg I.V. followed by a titrated infusion. Physostigmine (1-2 mg slow I.V.) may be indicated in reversing cardiac arrhythmias that are due to vagal blockade, or for anticholinergic effects, but should only be used as a last measure in life-threatening situations. Seizures usually respond to diazepam I.V. boluses (5-10 mg up to 30 mg). If seizures are unresponsive or recur, phenytoin or phenobarbital may be required.

Drug Interactions Substrate of CYP1A2 (minor), 2B6 (minor), 2C9 (minor), 2C19 (minor), 2D6 (major), 3A4 (minor); **Inhibits** CYP1A2 (weak), 2C9 (weak), 2C19 (weak), 2D6 (weak), 2E1 (weak)

Altretamine: Concurrent use may cause orthostatic hypertension.

Amphetamines: TCAs may enhance the effect of amphetamines; monitor for adverse CV effects.

Anticholinergics: Combined use with TCAs may produce additive anticholinergic effects.

Antihypertensives: Amitriptyline inhibits the antihypertensive response to bethanidine, clonidine, debrisoquin, guanadrel, guanethidine, guanabenz, guanfacine; monitor BP; consider alternate antihypertensive agent.

Beta-agonists: When combined with TCAs may predispose patients to cardiac arrhythmias.

Bupropion: May increase the levels of tricyclic antidepressants; based on limited information, monitor response.

Carbamazepine: Tricyclic antidepressants may increase carbamazepine levels; monitor.

Cholestyramine and colestipol: May bind TCAs and reduce their absorption; monitor for altered response.

Cisapride: May increase the risk of QT_c prolongation and/or arrhythmia; concurrent use is contraindicated.

Clonidine: Abrupt discontinuation of clonidine may cause hypertensive crisis; amitriptyline may enhance the response (also see note on antihypertensives).

CNS depressants: Sedative effects may be additive with TCAs; monitor for increased effect; includes benzodiazepines, barbiturates, antipsychotics, ethanol, and other sedative medications.

CYP2D6 inhibitors: May increase the levels/effects of amitriptyline; example inhibitors include chlorpromazine, delavirdine, fluoxetine, miconazole, paroxetine, pergolide, quinidine, quinine, ritonavir, and ropinirole.

Epinephrine (and other direct alpha-agonists): Pressor response to I.V. epinephrine, norepinephrine, and phenylephrine may be enhanced in patients receiving TCAs. (**Note:** Effect is unlikely with epinephrine or levonordefrin dosages typically administered as infiltration in combination with local anesthetics.)

Fenfluramine: May increase tricyclic antidepressant levels/effects.

Hypoglycemic agents (including insulin): TCAs may enhance the hypoglycemic effects of tolazamide, chlorpropamide, or insulin; monitor for changes in blood glucose levels; reported with chlorpropamide, tolazamide, and insulin.

Levodopa: Tricyclic antidepressants may decrease the absorption (bioavailability) of levodopa; rare hypertensive episodes have also been attributed to this combination.

Linezolid: Hyperpyrexia, hypertension, tachycardia, confusion, seizures, and **deaths have been reported** with agents which inhibit MAO (serotonin syndrome); this combination should be avoided.

Lithium: Concurrent use with a TCA may increase the risk for neurotoxicity.

MAO inhibitors: Hyperpyrexia, hypertension, tachycardia, confusion, seizures, and **deaths have been reported** (serotonin syndrome); this combination should be avoided.

Methylphenidate: Metabolism of amitriptyline may be decreased.

Phenothiazines: Serum concentrations of some TCAs may be increased; in addition, TCAs may increase concentration of phenothiazines; monitor for altered clinical response.

QT_c prolonging agents: Concurrent use of tricyclic agents with other drugs which may prolong QT_c interval may increase the risk of potentially fatal arrhythmias; includes type Ia and type III antiarrhythmics agents, selected quinolones (moxifloxacin), cisapride, and other agents.

Ritonavir: Combined use of high-dose tricyclic antidepressants with ritonavir may cause serotonin syndrome in HIV-positive patients; monitor.

Sucralfate: Absorption of tricyclic antidepressants may be reduced with coadministration.

Sympathomimetics, indirect-acting: Tricyclic antidepressants may result in a decreased sensitivity to indirect-acting sympathomimetics; includes dopamine and ephedrine; also see interaction with epinephrine (and direct-acting sympathomimetics).

Tramadol: Tramadol's risk of seizures may be increased with TCAs.

Valproic acid: May increase serum concentrations/adverse effects of some tricyclic antidepressants.

Warfarin (and other oral anticoagulants): Amitriptyline may increase the anticoagulant effect in patients stabilized on warfarin; monitor INR.

Ethanol/Nutrition/Herb Interactions

Ethanol: Avoid ethanol (may increase CNS depression).

Food: Grapefruit juice may inhibit the metabolism of some TCAs and clinical toxicity may result.

Herb/Nutraceutical: St John's wort may decrease amitriptyline levels. Avoid valerian, St John's wort, kava kava, gotu kola (may increase CNS depression).

Stability Protect injection and Elavil® 10 mg tablets from light.

Mechanism of Action Increases the synaptic concentration of serotonin and/or norepinephrine in the central nervous system by inhibition of their reuptake by the presynaptic neuronal membrane

Pharmacodynamics Onset of action:

Migraine prophylaxis: 6 weeks; higher dosage may be required in heavy smokers because of increased metabolism

Depression: 4-6 weeks; then reduce dosage to lowest effective level

Pharmacokinetics

Geriatrics: Plasma concentrations increase with age and steady-state plasma concentrations are significantly increased in older patients compared to younger patients after equal doses. Plasma concentrations do not always correlate with clinical effectiveness.

Metabolism: In the liver to nortriptyline (active), hydroxy derivatives and conjugated derivatives

Half-life: Adults: 9-25 hours (15-hour average); half-life prolonged (mean: 21.7 hours)

Time to peak serum concentration: Within 4 hours

Elimination: Renal excretion of 18% as unchanged drug; small amounts eliminated in feces by bile

Dosage

Geriatrics: Depression: Oral: Initial: 10-25 mg at bedtime; dose should be increased in 10-25 mg increments every week if tolerated; dose range: 25-150 mg/day. See Renal/Hepatic Impairment.

(Continued)

Amitriptyline *(Continued)*

Adults:
Depression: Oral: 50-150 mg/day single dose at bedtime or in divided doses; dose may be gradually increased up to 300 mg/day.

Chronic pain management (unlabeled use): Oral: Initial: 25 mg at bedtime; may increase as tolerated to 100 mg/day.

Migraine prophylaxis (unlabeled use): Oral: Initial: 10-25 mg at bedtime; usual dose: 150 mg; reported dosing ranges: 10-400 mg/day

Renal Impairment: Nondialyzable

Hepatic Impairment: Use with caution and monitor plasma levels and patient response.

Monitoring Parameters Blood pressure, pulse, EKG; target symptoms

Reference Range
Therapeutic:
Amitriptyline and nortriptyline 100-250 ng/mL (SI: 360-900 nmol/L)
Nortriptyline 50-150 ng/mL (SI: 190-570 nmol/L)
Toxic: >0.5 mcg/mL

Test Interactions May cause false-positive reaction to EMIT immunoassay for imipramine

Patient Information Avoid alcohol ingestion; do not discontinue medication abruptly; may cause urine to turn blue-green; may cause drowsiness, dry mouth, constipation, blurred vision; rise slowly to prevent dizziness

Special Geriatric Considerations Not a drug of choice for elderly. The most anticholinergic and sedating of the antidepressants; pronounced effects on the cardiovascular system (hypotension), hence, many geropsychiatrists agree it is best to avoid in elderly.

Dosage Forms Excipient information presented when available (limited, particularly for generics); consult specific product labeling.
Tablet, as hydrochloride: 10 mg, 25 mg, 50 mg, 75 mg, 100 mg, 150 mg

Selected References
Nies A, Robinson DS, Friedman MJ, et al, "Relationship Between Age and Tricyclic Antidepressant Plasma Levels," *Am J Psychiatry*, 1977, 134:790-3.

Schulz P, Turner-Tamiyasu K, Smith G, et al, "Amitriptyline Disposition in Young and Elderly Normal Men," *Clin Pharmacol Ther*, 1983, 33(3):360-6.

♦ **Amitriptyline Hydrochloride** see Amitriptyline on page 85

Amlodipine (am LOE di peen)

Related Information
Calcium Channel Blockers on page 1753

Medication Safety Issues
Sound-alike/look-alike issues:
Amlodipine may be confused with amiloride
Norvasc® may be confused with Navane®, Norvir®, Vascor®

U.S. Brand Names Norvasc®

Canadian Brand Names Norvasc®

Index Terms Amlodipine Besylate

Generic Available Yes

Pharmacologic Category Calcium Channel Blocker

Use Treatment of hypertension; treatment of symptomatic chronic stable angina, vasospastic (Prinzmetal's) angina (confirmed or suspected); prevention of hospitalization due to angina with documented CAD (limited to patients without heart failure or ejection fraction <40%)

Contraindications Hypersensitivity to amlodipine or any component of the formulation

Warnings/Precautions Increased angina and/or MI has occurred with initiation or dosage titration of calcium channel blockers. Symptomatic hypotension with or without syncope can rarely occur; blood pressure must be lowered at a rate appropriate for the patient's clinical condition. Use caution in severe aortic stenosis and/or hypertrophic cardiomyopathy. Use caution in patients with hepatic impairment. The most common side effect is peripheral edema; occurs within 2-3 weeks of starting therapy. Reflex tachycardia may occur with use. Dosage titration should occur after 7-14 days on a given dose. Initiate at a lower dose in the elderly.

Adverse Reactions (Reflective of adult population; not specific for elderly)
>10%: Cardiovascular: Peripheral edema (2% to 15% dose related)
1% to 10%:
Cardiovascular: Flushing (1% to 3%), palpitation (1% to 4%)
Central nervous system: Headache (7%; similar to placebo 8%), dizziness (1% to 3%), fatigue (4%), somnolence (1% to 2%)
Dermatologic: Rash (1% to 2%), pruritus (1% to 2%)
Endocrine & metabolic: Male sexual dysfunction (1% to 2%)

Gastrointestinal: Nausea (3%), abdominal pain (1% to 2%), dyspepsia (1% to 2%), gingival hyperplasia

Neuromuscular & skeletal: Muscle cramps (1% to 2%), weakness (1% to 2%)

Respiratory: Dyspnea (1% to 2%), pulmonary edema (15% from PRAISE trial, CHF population)

Overdosage/Toxicology Primary cardiac symptoms of calcium blocker overdose include hypotension and bradycardia. Hypotension is caused by peripheral vasodilation, myocardial depression, and bradycardia. Bradycardia results from sinus bradycardia, second- or third-degree atrioventricular block, or sinus arrest with junctional rhythm. Intraventricular conduction is usually not affected, so QRS duration is normal (verapamil prolongs the PR interval and bepridil prolongs the QT interval and may cause ventricular arrhythmias, including torsade de pointes).

Noncardiac symptoms include confusion, stupor, nausea, vomiting, metabolic acidosis, and hyperglycemia. Following initial gastric decontamination, if possible, repeated calcium administration may promptly reverse depressed cardiac contractility (but not sinus node depression or peripheral vasodilation). Glucagon, epinephrine, and inamrinone (amrinone) may treat refractory hypotension. Glucagon and epinephrine also increase the heart rate (outside the U.S., 4-aminopyridine may be available as an antidote). Dialysis and hemoperfusion are not effective in enhancing elimination, although repeat-dose activated charcoal may serve as an adjunct with sustained-release preparations.

In a few reported cases, overdose with calcium channel blockers has been associated with hypotension and bradycardia, initially refractory to atropine, but becoming more responsive to this agent when larger doses (approaching 1 g/hour for more than 24 hours) of calcium chloride were administered.

Drug Interactions Substrate of CYP3A4 (major); **Inhibits** CYP1A2 (moderate), 2A6 (weak), 2B6 (weak), 2C8 (weak), 2C9 (weak), 2D6 (weak), 3A4 (weak)

Azole antifungals may inhibit calcium channel blocker metabolism; avoid this combination. Try an antifungal like terbinafine (if appropriate) or monitor closely for altered effect of the calcium channel blocker.

Calcium may reduce the calcium channel blocker's effects, particularly hypotension.

CYP1A2 substrates: Amlodipine may increase the levels/effects of CYP1A2 substrates. Example substrates include aminophylline, fluvoxamine, mexiletine, mirtazapine, ropinirole, theophylline, and trifluoperazine.

CYP3A4 inducers: CYP3A4 inducers may decrease the levels/effects of amlodipine. Example inducers include aminoglutethimide, carbamazepine, nafcillin, nevirapine, phenobarbital, phenytoin, and rifamycins.

CYP3A4 inhibitors: May increase the levels/effects of amlodipine. Example inhibitors include azole antifungals, clarithromycin, diclofenac, doxycycline, erythromycin, imatinib, isoniazid, nefazodone, nicardipine, propofol, protease inhibitors, quinidine, telithromycin, and verapamil.

Grapefruit juice: May modestly increase amlodipine levels.

Rifampin increases the metabolism of calcium channel blockers; adjust the dose of calcium channel blocker to maintain efficacy.

Sildenafil, tadalafil, vardenafil: Blood pressure-lowering effects are additive; use caution.

Ethanol/Nutrition/Herb Interactions

Food: Grapefruit juice may modestly increase amlodipine levels.

Herb/Nutraceutical: St John's wort may decrease amlodipine levels. Avoid dong quai if using for hypertension (has estrogenic activity). Avoid ephedra, yohimbe, ginseng (may worsen hypertension). Avoid garlic (may have increased antihypertensive effects).

Stability Store at room temperature of 15°C to 30°C (59°F to 86°F).

Mechanism of Action Inhibits calcium ion from entering the "slow channels" or select voltage-sensitive areas of vascular smooth muscle and myocardium during depolarization, producing a relaxation of coronary vascular smooth muscle and coronary vasodilation; increases myocardial oxygen delivery in patients with vasospastic angina

Pharmacodynamics

Onset of action: 30-50 minutes

Peak effect: 6-12 hours

Duration: 24 hours

Pharmacokinetics

Absorption: Oral: Well absorbed; percent absorbed not determined to date

Protein binding: 93%

Metabolism: Hepatic, >90% to inactive compound

Bioavailability: 64% to 90%

Half-life: 30-50 hours

Elimination: Metabolite and parent drug excreted renally; 10% excreted unchanged in urine

(Continued)

Amlodipine *(Continued)*

Dosage
   Geriatrics: Dosing should start at the lower end of dosing range due to possible increased incidence of hepatic, renal, or cardiac impairment. Elderly patients also show decreased clearance of amlodipine.

   Hypertension: Oral: 2.5 mg once daily
   Angina: Oral: 5 mg once daily
   Adults:
      Hypertension: Oral: Initial dose: 5 mg once daily; maximum dose: 10 mg once daily. In general, titrate in 2.5 mg increments over 7-14 days. Usual dosage range (JNC 7): 2.5-10 mg once daily.
      Angina: Oral: Usual dose: 5-10 mg; lower dose suggested in elderly or hepatic impairment; most patients require 10 mg for adequate effect.
   Hepatic Impairment:
      Hypertension: Administer 2.5 mg once daily
      Angina: Administer 5 mg once daily
Administration May be taken without regard to meals.
Monitoring Parameters Heart rate, blood pressure
Patient Information Do not discontinue abruptly; report any dizziness, shortness of breath, palpitations, or edema
Additional Information The FDA's Cardiovascular and Renal Drug Advisory Committee reviewed current data regarding the risk of heart attacks in patients treated with calcium channel blockers and determined that as a class, the calcium channel antagonists are safe; however, they warned that short-acting nifedipine could increase the risk of myocardial infarction in some patients. The committee was in agreement with a statement issued September, 1995 by the National Heart Lung, and Blood Institute of the National Institute of Health, that warned that short-acting nifedipine should be used with great caution, especially at higher doses.
Special Geriatric Considerations Elderly may experience a greater hypotensive response. Constipation may be more of a problem in elderly. Calcium channel blockers are no more effective in elderly than other therapies, however, they do not cause significant CNS effects which is an advantage over some antihypertensive agents.
Dosage Forms Excipient information presented when available (limited, particularly for generics); consult specific product labeling.
   Tablet: 2.5 mg, 5 mg, 10 mg
      Norvasc®: 2.5 mg, 5 mg, 10 mg
Selected References
   Chobanian AV, Bakris GL, Black HR, et al, "The Seventh Report of the Joint National Committee on Prevention, Detection, Evaluation, and Treatment of High Blood Pressure: The JNC 7 Report," *JAMA*, 2003, 289(19):2560-71.

Amlodipine and Benazepril (am LOE di peen & ben AY ze pril)

Related Information
   Amlodipine on page 88
   Benazepril on page 155
U.S. Brand Names Lotrel®
Index Terms Benazepril Hydrochloride and Amlodipine Besylate
Generic Available Yes
Pharmacologic Category Antihypertensive Agent, Combination
Use Treatment of hypertension
Dosage
   Geriatrics: Initial dose: 2.5 mg (based on amlodipine component). Refer to adult dosing.
   Adults: Hypertension: Oral: 2.5-10 mg (amlodipine) and 10-40 mg (benazepril) once daily; maximum: Amlodipine: 10 mg/day; benazepril: 40 mg/day
   Renal Impairment: Cl_{cr} ≤30 mL/minute: Use of combination product is not recommended.
   Hepatic Impairment: Initial dose: 2.5 mg based on amlodipine component.
Special Geriatric Considerations Combination products are not recommended as first-line treatment. Only use if doses of individual agents correspond to the combination available.
Dosage Forms Excipient information presented when available (limited, particularly for generics); consult specific product labeling.
   Capsule:
      2.5/10: Amlodipine 2.5 mg and benazepril hydrochloride 10 mg
      5/10: Amlodipine 5 mg and benazepril hydrochloride 10 mg
      5/20: Amlodipine 5 mg and benazepril hydrochloride 20 mg
      10/20: Amlodipine 10 mg and benazepril hydrochloride 20 mg
      Lotrel® 2.5/10: Amlodipine 2.5 mg and benazepril hydrochloride 10 mg

Lotrel® 5/10: Amlodipine 5 mg and benazepril hydrochloride 10 mg
Lotrel® 5/20: Amlodipine 5 mg and benazepril hydrochloride 20 mg
Lotrel® 5/40: Amlodipine 5 mg and benazepril hydrochloride 40 mg
Lotrel® 10/20: Amlodipine 10 mg and benazepril hydrochloride 20 mg
Lotrel® 10/40: Amlodipine 10 mg and benazepril hydrochloride 40 mg

Amlodipine and Valsartan (am LOE di peen & val SAR tan)

Related Information
Amlodipine *on page 88*
Valsartan *on page 1657*
U.S. Brand Names Exforge®
Index Terms Amlodipine Besylate and Valsartan; Valsartan and Amlodipine
Generic Available No
Pharmacologic Category Angiotensin II Receptor Blocker Combination; Antihypertensive Agent, Combination; Calcium Channel Blocker
Use Treatment of hypertension
Dosage
Geriatrics: Refer to adult dosing. Initiate at lower end of dosing range.
Adults: Hypertension: Oral: Amlodipine 5-10 mg and valsartan 160-320 mg once daily; dose may be titrated after 3-4 weeks of therapy. Maximum recommended dose: Amlodipine 10 mg/day; valsartan 320 mg/day.
Renal Impairment:
Cl_{cr} >10 mL/minute: No dosage adjustment necessary.
Cl_{cr} ≤10 mL/minute: Use caution; not studied in severe renal impairment.
Hepatic Impairment: Use caution in hepatic impairment; amlodipine and valsartan exposure increased in presence of hepatic impairment.
Amlodipine: Lower initial doses may be required.
Valsartan: Mild-to-moderate hepatic impairment: No dosage adjustment required; however, patients with mild-to-moderate chronic disease have twice the exposure as healthy volunteers.
Special Geriatric Considerations See individual agents.
Dosage Forms Excipient information presented when available (limited, particularly for generics); consult specific product labeling.
Tablet:
Exforge®:
5/160: Amlodipine 5 mg and valsartan 160 mg
5/320 mg: Amlodipine 5 mg and valsartan 320 mg
10/160: Amlodipine 10 mg and valsartan 160 mg
10/320: Amlodipine 10 mg and valsartan 320 mg

♦ **Amlodipine Besylate** *see* Amlodipine *on page 88*
♦ **Amlodipine Besylate and Valsartan** *see* Amlodipine and Valsartan *on page 91*

Ammonium Chloride (a MOE nee um KLOR ide)

Generic Available Yes
Pharmacologic Category Electrolyte Supplement, Parenteral
Use Treatment of hypochloremic states or metabolic alkalosis
Contraindications Severe hepatic and renal dysfunction; patients with primary respiratory acidosis
Warnings/Precautions Use caution in patients with primary respiratory acidosis or pulmonary insufficiency.
Adverse Reactions (Reflective of adult population; not specific for elderly)
Frequency not defined.
Central nervous system: Headache, coma, drowsiness, EEG abnormalities, mental confusion, seizure
Dermatologic: Rash
Endocrine & metabolic: Calcium-deficient tetany, hyperchloremia, hypokalemia, metabolic acidosis, potassium and sodium may be decreased
Gastrointestinal: Abdominal pain, gastric irritation, nausea, vomiting
Hepatic: Ammonia may be increased
Local: Pain at site of injection
Neuromuscular & skeletal: Twitching
Respiratory: Hyperventilation
Overdosage/Toxicology Symptoms of overdose include abdominal pain, apnea, bradycardia, confusion, coma, diuresis, headache, hyperchloremic hypokalemic metabolic acidosis, hyperventilation, hypomagnesemia, hypovolemia, nausea, pulmonary edema, seizures, vomiting. Administer electrolytes as indicated.
Stability Prior to use, vials should be stored at controlled room temperature of 15°C to 30°C (59°F to 86°F). Solution may crystallize if exposed to low temperatures. If crystals
(Continued)

Ammonium Chloride *(Continued)*

are observed, warm vial to room temperature in a water bath prior to use. Dilute prior to use; final concentration should not exceed 1% to 2% ammonium chloride. Suggested dilution: Mix contents of 1-2 vials (100-200 mEq) in 500-1000 mL NS.

Mechanism of Action Increases acidity by increasing free hydrogen ion concentration

Pharmacokinetics
Metabolism: Hepatic; forms urea and hydrochloric acid
Elimination: Urine

Dosage
Geriatrics & Adults: Metabolic alkalosis: The following equations represent different methods of correction utilizing either the serum HCO_3^-, the serum chloride, or the base excess

Dosing of mEq NH_4Cl via the chloride-deficit method (hypochloremia):
Dose of mEq NH_4Cl = [0.2 L/kg x body weight (kg)] x [103 - observed serum chloride]; administer 50% of dose over 12 hours, then re-evaluate
Note: 0.2 L/kg is the estimated chloride volume of distribution and 103 is the average normal serum chloride concentration (mEq/L)

Dosing of mEq NH_4Cl via the bicarbonate-excess method (refractory hypochloremic metabolic alkalosis):
Dose of NH_4Cl = [0.5 L/kg x body weight (kg)] x (observed serum HCO_3^- - 24); administer 50% of dose over 12 hours, then re-evaluate
Note: 0.5 L/kg is the estimated bicarbonate volume of distribution and 24 is the average normal serum bicarbonate concentration (mEq/L)
These equations will yield different requirements of ammonium chloride

Administration Administer by slow intravenous infusion to avoid local irritation and adverse effects. Rate of infusion should not exceed 5 mL/minute in an adult.

Monitoring Parameters Serum bicarbonate; signs and symptoms of ammonia toxicity

Additional Information Do not exceed a 1% to 2% concentration of ammonium chloride or an administration rate of more than 5 mL/minute; administer over approximately 3 hours for I.V. infusion

Special Geriatric Considerations No specific data available for elderly; monitor closely with hepatic disease for signs of toxicity.

Dosage Forms Excipient information presented when available (limited, particularly for generics); consult specific product labeling.
Injection, solution: Ammonium 5 mEq/mL and chloride 5 mEq/mL (20 mL) [equivalent to ammonium chloride 267.5 mg/mL]

Selected References
Bushinsky DA and Coe FL, "Hyperkalemia During Acute Ammonium Chloride Acidosis in Man," *Nephron*, 1985, 40(1):38-40.
Martin WJ and Matzke GR, "Treating Severe Metabolic Alkalosis," *Clin Pharm*, 1982, 1(1):42-8.
Megarbane B, Bruneel F, Bedos JP, et al, "Ammonium Chloride Poisoning: A Misunderstood Cause of Metabolic Acidosis With Normal Anion Gap," *Intensive Care Med*, 2000, 26(12):1869.

♦ **Amoclan** *see* Amoxicillin and Clavulanate Potassium *on page 97*

Amoxapine (a MOKS a peen)

Related Information
Antidepressant Agents *on page 1742*

Medication Safety Issues
Sound-alike/look-alike issues:
Amoxapine may be confused with amoxicillin, Amoxil®
Asendin may be confused with aspirin

Index Terms Asendin [DSC]

Generic Available Yes

Pharmacologic Category Antidepressant, Tricyclic (Secondary Amine)

Use Treatment of neurotic and endogenous depression and mixed symptoms of anxiety and depression

Restrictions An FDA-approved medication guide concerning the use of antidepressants in children, adolescents, and young adults must be distributed when dispensing an outpatient prescription (new or refill) where this medication is to be used without direct supervision of a healthcare provider. Medication guides are available at http://www.fda.gov/cder/Offices/ODS/medication_guides.htm. Dispense to parents or guardians of children and adolescents receiving this medication.

Contraindications Hypersensitivity to amoxapine or any component of the formulation; use of MAO inhibitors within past 14 days; acute recovery phase following myocardial infarction

Warnings/Precautions Closely monitor for clinical worsening, suicidality, or unusual changes in behavior; family or caregiver should be instructed to closely observe the patient and communicate condition with healthcare provider. Such observation would generally include at least weekly face-to-face contact with patients or their family members or caregivers during the first 4 weeks of treatment, then every other week visits for the next 4 weeks, then at 12 weeks, and as clinically indicated beyond 12 weeks. Additional contact by telephone may be appropriate between face-to-face visits. Adults treated with antidepressants should be observed for clinical worsening and suicidality, especially during the initial few months of a course of drug therapy, or at times of dose changes, either increases or decreases. A medication guide should be dispensed with each prescription.

The possibility of a suicide attempt is inherent in major depression and may persist until remission occurs. Monitor for worsening of depression or suicidality, especially during initiation of therapy (generally first 1-2 months) or with dose increases or decreases. Worsening depression and severe abrupt suicidality that are not part of the presenting symptoms may require discontinuation or modification of drug therapy. Use caution in high-risk patients during initiation of therapy. Prescriptions should be written for the smallest quantity consistent with good patient care. The patient's family or caregiver should be alerted to monitor patients for the emergence of suicidality and associated behaviors such as anxiety, agitation, panic attacks, insomnia, irritability, hostility, impulsivity, akathisia, hypomania, and mania; patients should be instructed to notify their healthcare provider if any of these symptoms or worsening depression occur.

May worsen psychosis in some patients or precipitate a shift to mania or hypomania in patients with bipolar disorder. Monotherapy in patients with bipolar disorder should be avoided. Patients presenting with depressive symptoms should be screened for bipolar disorder. **Amoxapine is not FDA approved for the treatment of bipolar depression.**

May cause sedation, resulting in impaired performance of tasks requiring alertness (eg, operating machinery or driving). Sedative effects may be additive with other CNS depressants and/or ethanol. The degree of sedation is moderate relative to other antidepressants. May increase the risks associated with electroconvulsive therapy. Consider discontinuing, when possible, prior to elective surgery. Therapy should not be abruptly discontinued in patients receiving high doses for prolonged periods.

May cause extrapyramidal symptoms, including pseudoparkinsonism, acute dystonic reactions, akathisia, and tardive dyskinesia (risk of these reactions is low). May be associated with neuroleptic malignant syndrome.

May cause orthostatic hypotension (risk is moderate relative to other antidepressants) - use with caution in patients at risk of hypotension or in patients where transient hypotensive episodes would be poorly tolerated (cardiovascular disease or cerebrovascular disease). The degree of anticholinergic blockade produced by this agent is moderate relative to other cyclic antidepressants - use caution in patients with urinary retention, benign prostatic hyperplasia, narrow-angle glaucoma, xerostomia, visual problems, constipation, or history of bowel obstruction.

Use with caution in patients with a history of cardiovascular disease (including previous MI, stroke, tachycardia, or conduction abnormalities). The risk conduction abnormalities with this agent is moderate relative to other antidepressants. May lower seizure threshold - use caution in patients with a previous seizure disorder or condition predisposing to seizures such as brain damage, alcoholism, or concurrent therapy with other drugs which lower the seizure threshold. Use with caution in hyperthyroid patients or those receiving thyroid supplementation. Use with caution in patients with hepatic or renal dysfunction and in elderly patients.

Adverse Reactions (Reflective of adult population; not specific for elderly)
>10%:
    Central nervous system: Drowsiness
    Gastrointestinal: Xerostomia, constipation
1% to 10%:
    Central nervous system: Dizziness, headache, confusion, nervousness, restlessness, insomnia, ataxia, excitement, anxiety
    Dermatologic: Edema, skin rash
    Endocrine: Prolactin levels increased
    Gastrointestinal: Nausea
    Neuromuscular & skeletal: Tremor, weakness
    Ocular: Blurred vision
    Miscellaneous: Diaphoresis

Overdosage/Toxicology Symptoms include grand mal convulsions, acidosis, coma, and renal failure. Following initiation of essential overdose management, toxic symptoms should be treated. Sodium bicarbonate is indicated when the QRS interval is >0.10 seconds or the QT_c is >0.42 seconds. Ventricular arrhythmias often respond to phenytoin 15-20 mg/kg with concurrent systemic alkalinization (sodium bicarbonate 0.5-2 mEq/kg I.V.). Arrhythmias unresponsive to this therapy may respond to lidocaine 1 mg/kg I.V. followed by a titrated infusion. Physostigmine (1-2 mg slow I.V.) may be indicated in reversing cardiac arrhythmias that are due to vagal blockade, or for (Continued)

Amoxapine *(Continued)*

anticholinergic effects, but should only be used as a last measure in life-threatening situations. Seizures usually respond to diazepam I.V. boluses (5-10 mg up to 30 mg). If seizures are unresponsive or recur, phenytoin or phenobarbital may be required.

Drug Interactions Substrate of CYP2D6 (major)

Anticholinergics: Combined use with TCAs may produce additive anticholinergic effects.

Altretamine: Concurrent use may cause orthostatic hypertension.

Amphetamines: TCAs may enhance the effect of amphetamines; monitor for adverse CV effects.

Antihypertensives: Amitriptyline inhibits the antihypertensive response to bethanidine, clonidine, debrisoquin, guanadrel, guanethidine, guanabenz, guanfacine; monitor BP; consider alternate antihypertensive agent.

Beta-agonists: When combined with TCAs, may predispose patients to cardiac arrhythmias.

Bupropion: May increase the levels of tricyclic antidepressants; based on limited information; monitor response.

Carbamazepine: Tricyclic antidepressants may increase carbamazepine levels; monitor.

Cholestyramine and colestipol: May bind TCAs and reduce their absorption; monitor for altered response.

Clonidine: Abrupt discontinuation of clonidine may cause hypertensive crisis; amitriptyline may enhance the response.

CNS depressants: Sedative effects may be additive with TCAs; monitor for increased effect; includes benzodiazepines, barbiturates, antipsychotics, ethanol, and other sedative medications.

CYP2D6 inhibitors: May increase the levels/effects of amoxapine. Example inhibitors include chlorpromazine, delavirdine, fluoxetine, miconazole, paroxetine, pergolide, quinidine, quinine, ritonavir, and ropinirole.

Epinephrine (and other direct alpha-agonists): Pressor response to I.V. epinephrine, norepinephrine, and phenylephrine may be enhanced in patients receiving TCAs. (**Note:** Effect is unlikely with epinephrine or levonordefrin dosages typically administered as infiltration in combination with local anesthetics).

Fenfluramine: May increase tricyclic antidepressant levels/effects.

Hypoglycemic agents (including insulin): TCAs may enhance the hypoglycemic effects of tolazamide, chlorpropamide, or insulin; monitor for changes in blood glucose levels; reported with chlorpropamide, tolazamide, and insulin.

Levodopa: Tricyclic antidepressants may decrease the absorption (bioavailability) of levodopa; rare hypertensive episodes have also been attributed to this combination.

Linezolid: Hyperpyrexia, hypertension, tachycardia, confusion, seizures, and **deaths have been reported** with agents which inhibit MAO (serotonin syndrome); this combination should be avoided.

Lithium: Concurrent use with a TCA may increase the risk for neurotoxicity.

MAO inhibitors: Hyperpyrexia, hypertension, tachycardia, confusion, seizures, and **deaths have been reported** (serotonin syndrome); this combination should be avoided.

Methylphenidate: Metabolism of amitriptyline may be decreased.

Phenothiazines: Serum concentrations of some TCAs may be increased; in addition, TCAs may increase concentration of phenothiazines; monitor for altered clinical response.

QT_c-prolonging agents: Concurrent use of tricyclic agents with other drugs which may prolong QT_c interval may increase the risk of potentially fatal arrhythmias; includes type Ia and type III antiarrhythmics agents, selected quinolones (moxifloxacin), cisapride, and other agents.

Ritonavir: Combined use of high-dose tricyclic antidepressants with ritonavir may cause serotonin syndrome in HIV-positive patients; monitor.

Sucralfate: Absorption of tricyclic antidepressants may be reduced with coadministration.

Sympathomimetics, indirect-acting: Tricyclic antidepressants may result in a decreased sensitivity to indirect-acting sympathomimetics; includes dopamine and ephedrine; also see interaction with epinephrine (and direct-acting sympathomimetics).

Tramadol: Tramadol's risk of seizures may be increased with TCAs.

Valproic acid: May increase serum concentrations/adverse effects of some tricyclic antidepressants.

Warfarin (and other oral anticoagulants): Amitriptyline may increase the anticoagulant effect in patients stabilized on warfarin; monitor INR.

Ethanol/Nutrition/Herb Interactions

Ethanol: Avoid ethanol (may increase CNS depression).

Food: Grapefruit juice may inhibit the metabolism of some TCAs and clinical toxicity may result.

Herb/Nutraceutical: Avoid valerian, St John's wort, SAMe, kava kava.

Mechanism of Action Reduces the reuptake of serotonin and norepinephrine. The metabolite, 7-OH-amoxapine has significant dopamine receptor blocking activity similar to haloperidol.

Pharmacodynamics Antidepressant effects usually occur after 1-3 weeks; NE >5-HT

Pharmacokinetics

Absorption: Oral: Rapidly and well absorbed

Distribution: V_d: 0.9-1.2 L/kg

Protein binding: 80%

Metabolism: Extensive in the liver

Half-life: 11-16 hours

Time to peak serum concentration: Within 1-2 hours

Elimination: Excretion of metabolites and parent compound in urine

8-hydroxy metabolite is active, with a half-life: 30 hours

Dosage

Geriatrics: Oral: Initial: 25 mg at bedtime increased by 25 mg weekly for outpatients and every 3 days for inpatients if tolerated; usual dose: 50-150 mg/day, but doses up to 300 mg may be necessary. **Note:** Once symptoms are controlled, decrease gradually to lowest effective dose. See Special Geriatric Considerations.

Adults: Once symptoms are controlled, decrease gradually to lowest effective dose. Maintenance dose is usually given at bedtime to reduce daytime sedation.

Depression: Oral: Initial: 25 mg 2-3 times/day. If tolerated, dosage may be increased to 100 mg 2-3 times/day. May be given in a single bedtime dose when dosage <300 mg/day.

Maximum daily dose: 600 mg (inpatients); 400 mg (outpatients)

Monitoring Parameters Blood pressure, pulse, EKG; target symptoms

Reference Range Therapeutic: Amoxapine 20-100 ng/mL (SI: 64-319 nmol/L); 8-OH amoxapine 150-400 ng/mL (SI: 478-1275 nmol/L); both 200-500 ng/mL (SI: 637-1594 nmol/L)

Test Interactions Increased glucose, liver function tests; decreased WBC

Patient Information Dry mouth may be helped by sips of water, sugarless gum or hard candy; avoid alcohol; very important to maintain established dosage regimen; photosensitivity to sunlight can occur; rise slowly to prevent dizziness

Additional Information May take up to 2 weeks for full therapeutic effects to be apparent; maintenance dose is usually given at bedtime to reduce daytime sedation; tolerance develops in 1-3 months in some patients, close medical follow-up is essential

Special Geriatric Considerations Amoxapine is not the drug of choice in the elderly. Significant anticholinergic and orthostatic effects can occur and there is a risk for tardive dyskinesia and neuroleptic malignant syndrome.

Dosage Forms Excipient information presented when available (limited, particularly for generics); consult specific product labeling.

Tablet: 25 mg, 50 mg, 100 mg, 150 mg

Amoxicillin (a moks i SIL in)

Related Information

Antimicrobial Activity Against Selected Organisms *on page 1728*

Helicobacter pylori Treatment *on page 1759*

Prevention of Infective Endocarditis *on page 1803*

Medication Safety Issues

Sound-alike/look-alike issues:

Amoxicillin may be confused with amoxapine, Amoxil®, Atarax®

Amoxil® may be confused with amoxapine, amoxicillin

International issues:

Fisamox® [Australia] may be confused with Fosamax® which is a brand name for alendronate in the U.S.

Fisamox® [Australia] may be confused with Vigamox™ which is a brand name for moxifloxacin in the U.S.

U.S. Brand Names Amoxil®

Canadian Brand Names Apo-Amoxi®; Gen-Amoxicillin; Lin-Amox; Novamoxin®; Nu-Amoxi; PHL-Amoxicillin; PMS-Amoxicillin

Index Terms Amoxicillin Trihydrate; Amoxycillin; *p*-Hydroxyampicillin

Generic Available Yes: Excludes drops

Pharmacologic Category Antibiotic, Penicillin

Use Treatment of otitis media, sinusitis, and infections caused by susceptible organisms involving the respiratory tract, skin, and urinary tract; prophylaxis of bacterial endocarditis in patients undergoing surgical or dental procedures; as part of a multidrug regimen for *H. pylori* eradication

Unlabeled/Investigational Use Postexposure prophylaxis for anthrax exposure with documented susceptible organisms

(Continued)

Amoxicillin *(Continued)*

Contraindications Hypersensitivity to amoxicillin, penicillin, or any component of the formulation

Warnings/Precautions In patients with renal impairment, doses and/or frequency of administration should be modified in response to the degree of renal impairment. A high percentage of patients with infectious mononucleosis have developed rash during therapy with amoxicillin. Serious and occasionally severe or fatal hypersensitivity (anaphylactoid) reactions have been reported in patients on penicillin therapy, especially with a history of beta-lactam hypersensitivity, history of sensitivity to multiple allergens, or previous IgE-mediated reactions (eg, anaphylaxis, angioedema, urticaria). Use with caution in asthmatic patients. Prolonged use may result in fungal or bacterial superinfection, including *C. difficile*-associated diarrhea and pseudomembranous colitis. Chewable tablets contain phenylalanine.

Adverse Reactions (Reflective of adult population; not specific for elderly)
Frequency not defined.
Central nervous system: Hyperactivity, agitation, anxiety, insomnia, confusion, convulsions, behavioral changes, dizziness
Dermatologic: Acute exanthematous pustulosis, erythematous maculopapular rash, erythema multiforme, Stevens-Johnson syndrome, exfoliative dermatitis, toxic epidermal necrolysis, hypersensitivity vasculitis, urticaria
Gastrointestinal: Nausea, vomiting, diarrhea, hemorrhagic colitis, pseudomembranous colitis, tooth discoloration (brown, yellow, or gray; rare)
Hematologic: Anemia, hemolytic anemia, thrombocytopenia, thrombocytopenia purpura, eosinophilia, leukopenia, agranulocytosis
Hepatic: AST and ALT increased, cholestatic jaundice, hepatic cholestasis, acute cytolytic hepatitis
Renal: Crystalluria

Overdosage/Toxicology Symptoms of penicillin overdose include neuromuscular hypersensitivity (agitation, hallucinations, asterixis, encephalopathy, confusion, and seizures) and electrolyte imbalance (with potassium or sodium salts), especially in renal failure. Hemodialysis may be helpful to aid in the removal of the drug from the blood, otherwise most treatment is supportive or symptom-directed.

Drug Interactions
Allopurinol: Theoretically has an additive potential for amoxicillin rash.
Aminoglycosides: May be synergistic against selected organisms.
Fusidic acid: May decrease the therapeutic effect of penicillins; administer the penicillin at least 2 hours before fusidic acid.
Methotrexate: Penicillins may increase the exposure to methotrexate during concurrent therapy; monitor.
Oral contraceptives: Anecdotal reports suggesting decreased contraceptive efficacy with penicillins have been refuted by more rigorous scientific and clinical data.
Probenecid, disulfiram: May increase levels of penicillins (amoxicillin).
Warfarin: Effects of warfarin may be increased.

Stability Amoxil®: Oral suspension remains stable for 14 days at room temperature or if refrigerated (refrigeration preferred). Unit-dose antibiotic oral syringes are stable for 48 hours.

Mechanism of Action Inhibits bacterial cell wall synthesis by binding to one or more of the penicillin-binding proteins (PBPs) which in turn inhibits the final transpeptidation step of peptidoglycan synthesis in bacterial cell walls, thus inhibiting cell wall biosynthesis. Bacteria eventually lyse due to ongoing activity of cell wall autolytic enzymes (autolysins and murein hydrolases) while cell wall assembly is arrested.

Pharmacokinetics
Absorption: Oral: Rapid and nearly complete
Protein binding: 17% to 20%
Metabolism: Partial
Half-life (patients with Cl_{cr} <10 mL/minute): 7-21 hours
Time to peak:
Capsule: Within 2 hours
Suspension: 1 hour
Elimination: Renal excretion (80% as unchanged drug); ~30% removed by 3-hour hemodialysis

Dosage
Geriatrics & Adults:
Usual dosage range: Oral: 250-500 mg every 8 hours or 500-875 mg twice daily
Anthrax exposure (CDC guidelines): Oral: 500 mg every 8 hours
Ear, nose, throat, genitourinary tract, or skin/skin structure infections:
Mild to moderate: Oral: 500 mg every 12 hours **or** 250 mg every 8 hours
Severe: Oral: 875 mg every 12 hours **or** 500 mg every 8 hours
Endocarditis prophylaxis: Oral: 2 g 1 hour before procedure

AMOXICILLIN AND CLAVULANATE POTASSIUM

***Helicobacter pylori* eradication:** Oral: 1000 mg twice daily; requires combination therapy with at least one other antibiotic and an acid-suppressing agent (proton pump inhibitor or H₂ blocker)

Lower respiratory tract infections: Oral: 875 mg every 12 hours **or** 500 mg every 8 hours

Lyme disease: Oral: 500 mg every 6-8 hours (depending on size of patient) for 21-30 days

Renal Impairment:

The 875 mg tablet should not be used in patients with Cl_{cr} <30 mL/minute.

Cl_{cr} 10-30 mL/minute: 250-500 mg every 12 hours

Cl_{cr} <10 mL/minute: 250-500 mg every 24 hours

Moderately dialyzable (20% to 50%) by hemodialysis or peritoneal dialysis; approximately 50 mg of amoxicillin per liter of filtrate is removed by continuous arteriovenous or venovenous hemofiltration. Dose as per Cl_{cr} <10 mL/minute guidelines.

Administration Administer around-the-clock to promote less variation in peak and trough serum levels. The appropriate amount of suspension may be mixed with formula, milk, fruit juice, water, ginger ale or cold drinks; administer dose immediately after mixing.

DisperMox™: Dissolve 1 tablet in ~10 mL of water immediately before administration. Rinse container with additional water and drink entire contents to ensure that complete dose is taken. Do not chew or swallow tablet whole.

Monitoring Parameters Signs and symptoms of infection (fever, urinary frequency or pain, etc) should begin to resolve after 1-2 days

Test Interactions May interfere with urinary glucose tests using cupric sulfate (Benedict's solution, Clinitest®)

Some penicillin derivatives may accelerate the degradation of aminoglycosides *in vitro*, leading to a potential underestimation of aminoglycoside serum concentration.

Patient Information Report diarrhea promptly; entire course of medication (10-14 days) should be taken to ensure eradication of organism; should be taken in equal intervals around-the-clock to maintain adequate blood concentrations

Additional Information Food does not interfere with absorption; urticarial rash that appears after a few days of therapy may indicate hypersensitivity

Special Geriatric Considerations Resistance to amoxicillin has been a problem in patients on frequent antibiotics or in nursing homes. Alternative antibiotics may be necessary in these populations. Consider renal function.

Dosage Forms Excipient information presented when available (limited, particularly for generics); consult specific product labeling. [DSC] = Discontinued product

Capsule: 250 mg, 500 mg

Amoxil®: 500 mg

Powder for oral suspension: 125 mg/5 mL (80 mL, 100 mL, 150 mL); 200 mg/5 mL (50 mL, 75 mL, 100 mL); 250 mg/5 mL (80 mL, 100 mL, 150 mL); 400 mg/5 mL (50 mL, 75 mL, 100 mL)

Amoxil®: 200 mg/5 mL (50 mL, 75 mL, 100 mL) [contains sodium benzoate; bubble gum flavor] [DSC]; 250 mg/5 mL (100 mL, 150 mL) [contains sodium benzoate; bubble gum flavor]; 400 mg/5 mL (5 mL [DSC], 50 mL, 75 mL, 100 mL) [contains sodium benzoate; bubble gum flavor]

Powder for oral suspension [drops]:

Amoxil®: 50 mg/mL (30 mL) [contains sodium benzoate; bubble gum flavor]

Tablet: 500 mg, 875 mg

Amoxil®: 500 mg, 875 mg

Tablet, chewable: 125 mg, 200 mg, 250 mg, 400 mg

Amoxil®: 200 mg [contains phenylalanine 1.82 mg/tablet; cherry banana peppermint flavor]; 400 mg [contains phenylalanine 3.64 mg/tablet; cherry banana peppermint flavor]

Selected References

Dajani AS, Bisno AL, Chung KJ, et al, "Prevention of Bacterial Endocarditis. Recommendations by the American Heart Association," *JAMA*, 1990, 264(22):2919-22.

Hill S, Yeates M, Pathy J, et al, "A Controlled Trial of Norfloxacin and Amoxicillin in the Treatment of Uncomplicated Urinary Tract Infection in the Elderly," *J Antimicrob Chemother*, 1985, 15(4):505-6.

Amoxicillin and Clavulanate Potassium
(a moks i SIL in & klav yoo LAN ate poe TASS ee um)

Related Information

Amoxicillin *on page 95*

Antimicrobial Activity Against Selected Organisms *on page 1728*

Medication Safety Issues

Sound-alike/look-alike issues:

Augmentin® may be confused with Azulfidine®

U.S. Brand Names Amoclan; Augmentin®; Augmentin ES-600®; Augmentin XR®

Canadian Brand Names Alti-Amoxi-Clav; Apo-Amoxi-Clav®; Augmentin®; Clavulin®; Novo-Clavamoxin; ratio-Aclavulanate

(Continued)

Amoxicillin and Clavulanate Potassium *(Continued)*

Index Terms Amoxicillin and Clavulanic Acid; Clavulanic Acid and Amoxicillin

Generic Available Yes: Excludes extended release

Pharmacologic Category Antibiotic, Penicillin

Use Treatment of otitis media, sinusitis, and infections caused by susceptible organisms involving the lower respiratory tract, skin and skin structure, and urinary tract; spectrum same as amoxicillin with additional coverage of beta-lactamase producing *B. catarrhalis*, *H. influenzae*, *N. gonorrhoeae*, and *S. aureus* (not MRSA); expanded coverage of this combination makes it a useful alternative when amoxicillin resistance is present and patients cannot tolerate alternative treatments

Contraindications Hypersensitivity to amoxicillin, clavulanic acid, penicillin, or any component of the formulation; history of cholestatic jaundice or hepatic dysfunction with amoxicillin/clavulanate potassium therapy

Warnings/Precautions Hypersensitivity reactions, including anaphylaxis (some fatal), have been reported. Prolonged use may result in fungal or bacterial superinfection, including *C. difficile*-associated diarrhea and pseudomembranous colitis. In patients with renal impairment, doses and/or frequency of administration should be modified in response to the degree of renal impairment. High percentage of patients with infectious mononucleosis have developed rash during therapy. Incidence of diarrhea is higher than with amoxicillin alone. Due to differing content of clavulanic acid, not all formulations are interchangeable. Low incidence of cross-allergy with cephalosporins exists. Some products contain phenylalanine.

Adverse Reactions (Reflective of adult population; not specific for elderly)

>10%: Gastrointestinal: Diarrhea (3% to 34%; incidence varies upon dose and regimen used)

1% to 10%:

Dermatologic: Diaper rash, skin rash, urticaria

Gastrointestinal: Abdominal discomfort, loose stools, nausea, vomiting

Genitourinary: Vaginitis, vaginal mycosis

Miscellaneous: Moniliasis

Additional adverse reactions seen with **ampicillin-class antibiotics:** Agitation, agranulocytosis, alkaline phosphatase increased, anaphylaxis, anemia, angioedema, anxiety, behavioral changes, bilirubin increased, black "hairy" tongue, confusion, convulsions, crystalluria, dizziness, enterocolitis, eosinophilia, erythema multiforme, exanthematous pustulosis, exfoliative dermatitis, gastritis, glossitis, hematuria, hemolytic anemia, hemorrhagic colitis, indigestion, insomnia, hyperactivity, interstitial nephritis, leukopenia, mucocutaneous candidiasis, pruritus, pseudomembranous colitis, serum sickness-like reaction, Stevens-Johnson syndrome, stomatitis, transaminases increased, thrombocytopenia, thrombocytopenic purpura, tooth discoloration, toxic epidermal necrolysis

Overdosage/Toxicology Symptoms of overdose may include abdominal pain, diarrhea, drowsiness, rash, hyperactivity, stomach pain, and vomiting. Electrolyte imbalance may occur, especially in renal failure. Hemodialysis may be helpful to aid in removal of the drug from blood, otherwise, treatment is supportive or symptom-directed.

Drug Interactions

Allopurinol: Additive potential for amoxicillin rash.

Aminoglycosides: May be synergistic against selected organisms.

Fusidic acid: May decrease the therapeutic effect of penicillins; administer the penicillin at least 2 hours before fusidic acid.

Methotrexate: Penicillins may increase the exposure to methotrexate during concurrent therapy; monitor.

Oral contraceptives: Anecdotal reports suggesting decreased contraceptive efficacy with penicillins have been refuted by more rigorous scientific and clinical data.

Probenecid: May increase levels of penicillins (amoxicillin); concomitant use not recommended.

Warfarin: Effects of warfarin may be increased.

Stability

Powder for oral suspension: Store dry powder at room temperature of 25°C (77°F). Reconstitute powder for oral suspension with appropriate amount of water as specified on the bottle. Shake vigorously until suspended. Reconstituted oral suspension should be kept in refrigerator. Discard unused suspension after 10 days. Unit-dose antibiotic oral syringes are stable for 48 hours.

Tablet: Store at room temperature of 25°C (77°F).

Mechanism of Action Clavulanic acid binds and inhibits beta-lactamases that inactivate amoxicillin resulting in amoxicillin having an expanded spectrum of activity. Amoxicillin inhibits bacterial cell wall synthesis by binding to one or more of the penicillin-binding proteins (PBPs) which in turn inhibits the final transpeptidation step of peptidoglycan synthesis in bacterial cell walls, thus inhibiting cell wall biosynthesis. Bacteria eventually lyse due to ongoing activity of cell wall autolytic enzymes (autolysins and murein hydrolases) while cell wall assembly is arrested.

Pharmacokinetics

Absorption: Oral: Both amoxicillin and clavulanate are well absorbed

Metabolism: Clavulanic acid is metabolized in the liver

Half-life: Adults with normal renal function: Both agents are ~1 hour; amoxicillin pharmacokinetics are not affected by clavulanic acid

Time to peak: Peak levels of each appearing within 2 hours

Elimination: Amoxicillin excreted primarily unchanged in urine

Dosage

Geriatrics & Adults: Note: Dose is based on the amoxicillin component; see "Augmentin® Product-Specific Considerations" table.

Augmentin® Product-Specific Considerations

Strength	Form	Consideration
125 mg	CT, S	q8h dosing
	S	For adults having difficulty swallowing tablets, 125 mg/5 mL suspension may be substituted for 500 mg tablet.
200 mg	CT, S	q12h dosing
	CT	Contains phenylalanine
	S	For adults having difficulty swallowing tablets, 200 mg/5 mL suspension may be substituted for 875 mg tablet.
250 mg	CT, S, T	q8h dosing
	CT	Contains phenylalanine
	T	Not for use in patients <40 kg
	CT, T	Tablet and chewable tablet are not interchangeable due to differences in clavulanic acid.
	S	For adults having difficulty swallowing tablets, 250 mg/5 mL suspension may be substituted for 500 mg tablet.
400 mg	CT, S	q12h dosing
	CT	Contains phenylalanine
	S	For adults having difficulty swallowing tablets, 400 mg/5 mL suspension may be substituted for 875 mg tablet.
500 mg	T	q8h or q12h dosing
600 mg	S	q12h dosing
		Contains phenylalanine
		Not for use in adults ≥40 kg
		600 mg/5 mL suspension is not equivalent to or interchangeable with 200 mg/5 mL or 400 mg/5 mL due to differences in clavulanic acid.
875 mg	T	q12h dosing; not for use in Cl$_{cr}$ <30 mL/minute
1000 mg	XR	q12h dosing
		Not interchangeable with two 500 mg tablets
		Not for use if Cl$_{cr}$ <30 mL/minute or hemodialysis

Legend: CT = chewable tablet, S = suspension, T = tablet, XR = extended release.

Susceptible infections: Oral: 250-500 mg every 8 hours or 875 mg every 12 hours

Acute bacterial sinusitis: Oral: Extended release tablet: Two 1000 mg tablets every 12 hours for 10 days

Bite wounds (animal/human): Oral: 875 mg every 12 hours **or** 500 mg every 8 hours

Chronic obstructive pulmonary disease: Oral: 875 mg every 12 hours **or** 500 mg every 8 hours

Diabetic foot: Oral: Extended release tablet: Two 1000 mg tablets every 12 hours for 7-14 days

Diverticulitis, perirectal abscess: Oral: Extended release tablet: Two 1000 mg tablets every 12 hours for 7-10 days

Erysipelas: Oral: 875 mg every 12 hours **or** 500 mg every 8 hours

Febrile neutropenia: Oral: 875 mg every 12 hours

Pneumonia:

Aspiration: Oral: 875 mg every 12 hours

Community-acquired: Oral: Extended release tablet: Two 1000 mg tablets every 12 hours for 7-10 days

Pyelonephritis (acute, uncomplicated): Oral: 875 mg every 12 hours **or** 500 mg every 8 hours

Skin abscess: Oral: 875 mg every 12 hours

Renal Impairment

Cl$_{cr}$ <30 mL/minute: Do not use 875 mg tablet or extended release tablets.

Cl$_{cr}$ 10-30 mL/minute: 250-500 mg every 12 hours

Cl$_{cr}$ <10 mL/minute: 250-500 every 24 hours

Hemodialysis: Moderately dialyzable (20% to 50%)

(Continued)

Amoxicillin and Clavulanate Potassium *(Continued)*

250-500 mg every 24 hours; administer dose during and after dialysis. Do not use extended release tablets.

Peritoneal dialysis: Moderately dialyzable (20% to 50%)

Amoxicillin: Administer 250 mg every 12 hours

Clavulanic acid: Dose for Cl_{cr} <10 mL/minute

Continuous arteriovenous or venovenous hemofiltration effects:

Amoxicillin: ~50 mg of amoxicillin/L of filtrate is removed

Clavulanic acid: Dose for Cl_{cr} <10 mL/minute

Monitoring Parameters Assess patient at beginning and throughout therapy for infection; with prolonged therapy, monitor renal, hepatic, and hematologic function periodically; monitor for signs of anaphylaxis during first dose

Test Interactions May interfere with urinary glucose tests using cupric sulfate (Benedict's solution, Clinitest®, Fehling's solution); may inactivate aminoglycosides *in vitro*.

Some penicillin derivatives may accelerate the degradation of aminoglycosides *in vitro*, leading to a potential underestimation of aminoglycoside serum concentration.

Patient Information Report diarrhea promptly; entire course of medication (10-14 days) should be taken to ensure eradication of organism; should be taken in equal intervals around-the-clock to maintain adequate blood concentrations; females should report onset of symptoms of candidal vaginitis

Additional Information Both "250" and "500" tablets contain the same amount of clavulanic acid, thus two "250" tablets are not equivalent to one "500" tablet. Clavulanic acid inhibits beta-lactamase destruction of amoxicillin.

Special Geriatric Considerations Expanded coverage of this combination makes it a useful alternative when amoxicillin resistance is present and patients cannot tolerate alternative treatments; consider renal function. Considered one of the drugs of choice in the outpatient treatment of community-acquired pneumonia in elderly.

Dosage Forms Excipient information presented when available (limited, particularly for generics); consult specific product labeling. [DSC] = Discontinued product

Powder for oral suspension: 200: Amoxicillin 200 mg and clavulanate potassium 28.5 mg per 5 mL (50 mL, 75 mL, 100 mL) [contains phenylalanine]; 400: Amoxicillin 400 mg and clavulanate potassium 57 mg per 5 mL (50 mL, 75 mL, 100 mL) [contains phenylalanine]; 600: Amoxicillin 600 mg and clavulanic potassium 42.9 mg per 5 mL (75 mL, 125 mL, 200 mL) [contains phenylalanine]

Amoclan:

200: Amoxicillin 200 mg and clavulanate potassium 28.5 mg per 5 mL (50 mL, 75 mL, 100 mL) [contains phenylalanine 7 mg/5 mL and potassium 0.14 mEq/5 mL; fruit flavor]

400: Amoxicillin 400 mg and clavulanate potassium 57 mg per 5 mL (50 mL, 75 mL, 100 mL) [contains phenylalanine 7 mg/5 mL and potassium 0.29 mEq/5 mL; fruit flavor]

Augmentin®:

125: Amoxicillin 125 mg and clavulanate potassium 31.25 mg per 5 mL (75 mL, 100 mL, 150 mL) [contains potassium 0.16 mEq/5 mL; banana flavor]

200: Amoxicillin 200 mg and clavulanate potassium 28.5 mg per 5 mL (50 mL, 75 mL, 100 mL) [contains phenylalanine 7 mg/5 mL and potassium 0.14 mEq/5 mL; orange flavor]

250: Amoxicillin 250 mg and clavulanate potassium 62.5 mg per 5 mL (75 mL, 100 mL, 150 mL) [contains potassium 0.32 mEq/5 mL; orange flavor]

400: Amoxicillin 400 mg and clavulanate potassium 57 mg per 5 mL (50 mL, 75 mL, 100 mL) [contains phenylalanine 7 mg/5 mL and potassium 0.29 mEq/5 mL; orange flavor]

Augmentin ES-600®: Amoxicillin 600 mg and clavulanic potassium 42.9 mg per 5 mL (75 mL, 125 mL, 200 mL) [contains phenylalanine 7 mg/5 mL and potassium 0.23 mEq/5 mL; strawberry cream flavor]

Tablet: 250: Amoxicillin 250 mg and clavulanate potassium 125 mg; 500: Amoxicillin 500 mg and clavulanate potassium 125 mg; 875: Amoxicillin 875 mg and clavulanate potassium 125 mg

Augmentin®:

250: Amoxicillin 250 mg and clavulanate potassium 125 mg [contains potassium 0.63 mEq/tablet]

500: Amoxicillin 500 mg and clavulanate potassium 125 mg [contains potassium 0.63 mEq/tablet]

875: Amoxicillin 875 mg and clavulanate potassium 125 mg [contains potassium 0.63 mEq/tablet]

Tablet, chewable: 200: Amoxicillin 200 mg and clavulanate potassium 28.5 mg [contains phenylalanine]; 400: Amoxicillin 400 mg and clavulanate potassium 57 mg [contains phenylalanine]

Augmentin®:
  125: Amoxicillin 125 mg and clavulanate potassium 31.25 mg [contains potassium 0.16 mEq/tablet; lemon-lime flavor] [DSC]
  200: Amoxicillin 200 mg and clavulanate potassium 28.5 mg [contains phenylalanine 2.1 mg/tablet and potassium 0.14 mEq/tablet; cherry-banana flavor] [DSC]
  250: Amoxicillin 250 mg and clavulanate potassium 62.5 mg [contains potassium 0.32 mEq/tablet; lemon-lime flavor]
  400: Amoxicillin 400 mg and clavulanate potassium 57 mg [contains phenylalanine 4.2 mg/tablet and potassium 0.29 mEq/tablet; cherry-banana flavor] [DSC]
Tablet, extended release:
  Augmentin XR®: Amoxicillin 1000 mg and clavulanic acid 62.5 mg [contains potassium 29.3 mg (1.27 mEq) and sodium 12.6 mg (0.32 mEq) per tablet; packaged in either a 7-day or 10-day package]

Selected References
Ancill RJ, Ballard JH, and Capewell MA, "Urinary Tract Infections in Geriatric Inpatients: A Comparative Study of Amoxicillin-Clavulanic Acid and Co-trimoxazole," *Curr Ther Res*, 1987, 41(4):444-8.

Mandell LA, Bartlett JG, Dowell SF, et al, "Update of Practice Guidelines for the Management of Community-Acquired Pneumonia in Immunocompetent Adults," *Clin Infect Dis*, 2003, 37(11):1405-33.

♦ **Amoxicillin and Clavulanic Acid** *see* Amoxicillin and Clavulanate Potassium *on page 97*

♦ **Amoxicillin Trihydrate** *see* Amoxicillin *on page 95*

♦ **Amoxil®** *see* Amoxicillin *on page 95*

♦ **Amoxycillin** *see* Amoxicillin *on page 95*

♦ **Amphadase™** *see* Hyaluronidase *on page 754*

♦ **Amphocin® [DSC]** *see* Amphotericin B (Conventional) *on page 103*

♦ **Amphotec®** *see* Amphotericin B Cholesteryl Sulfate Complex *on page 101*

Amphotericin B Cholesteryl Sulfate Complex
(am foe TER i sin bee kole LES te ril SUL fate KOM plecks)

Medication Safety Issues
Safety issues:
  Lipid-based amphotericin formulations (Amphotec®) may be confused with conventional formulations (Amphocin®, Fungizone®)
  Large overdoses have occurred when conventional formulations were dispensed inadvertently for lipid-based products. Single daily doses of conventional amphotericin formulation never exceed 1.5 mg/kg.

High alert medication: The Institute for Safe Medication Practices (ISMP) includes this medication among its list of drugs which have a heightened risk of causing significant patient harm when used in error.

U.S. Brand Names Amphotec®
Canadian Brand Names Amphotec®
Index Terms ABCD; Amphotericin B Colloidal Dispersion
Generic Available No
Pharmacologic Category Antifungal Agent, Parenteral
Use Treatment of invasive aspergillosis in patients who have failed amphotericin B deoxycholate treatment, or who have renal impairment or experience unacceptable toxicity which precludes treatment with amphotericin B deoxycholate in effective doses
Contraindications Hypersensitivity to amphotericin B or any component of the formulation
Warnings/Precautions Anaphylaxis has been reported with amphotericin B-containing drugs. If severe respiratory distress occurs, the infusion should be immediately discontinued. During the initial dosing, the drug should be administered under close clinical observation. Infusion reactions, sometimes severe, usually subside with continued therapy - manage with decreased rate of infusion and pretreatment with antihistamines/corticosteroids.
Adverse Reactions (Reflective of adult population; not specific for elderly)
>10%: Central nervous system: Chills, fever
1% to 10%:
  Cardiovascular: Hypotension, tachycardia
  Central nervous system: Headache
  Dermatologic: Rash
  Endocrine & metabolic: Hypokalemia, hypomagnesemia
  Gastrointestinal: Nausea, diarrhea, abdominal pain
  Hematologic: Thrombocytopenia
  Hepatic: LFT change
  Neuromuscular & skeletal: Rigors
  Renal: Creatinine increased
  Respiratory: Dyspnea
(Continued)

Amphotericin B Cholesteryl Sulfate Complex *(Continued)*

Note: Amphotericin B colloidal dispersion has an improved therapeutic index compared to conventional amphotericin B, and has been used safely in patients with amphotericin B-related nephrotoxicity; however, continued decline of renal function has occurred in some patients.

Overdosage/Toxicology Symptoms include renal dysfunction, anemia, thrombocytopenia, granulocytopenia, fever, nausea, and vomiting. Treatment is supportive.

Drug Interactions

Increased nephrotoxicity: Aminoglycosides, cyclosporine, other nephrotoxic drugs.

Potentiation of hypokalemia: Corticosteroids, corticotropin.

Increased digitalis and neuromuscular-blocking agent toxicity due to hypokalemia.

Decreased effect: Pharmacologic antagonism may occur with azole antifungal agents (eg, miconazole, ketoconazole).

Pulmonary toxicity has occurred with concomitant administration of amphotericin B and leukocyte transfusions.

Stability

Store intact vials under refrigeration.

Reconstitute 50 mg and 100 mg vials with 10 mL and 20 mL of SWI, respectively. The reconstituted vials contain 5 mg/mL of amphotericin B. Shake the vial gently by hand until all solid particles have dissolved. After reconstitution, the solution should be refrigerated at 2°C to 8°C (36°F to 46°F) and used within 24 hours.

Further dilute amphotericin B colloidal dispersion with dextrose 5% in water. Concentrations of 0.1-2 mg/mL in dextrose 5% in water are stable for 14 days at 4°C and 23°C if protected from light, however, due to the occasional formation of subvisual particles, solutions should be used within 48 hours.

Mechanism of Action Binds to ergosterol altering cell membrane permeability in susceptible fungi and causing leakage of cell components with subsequent cell death. Proposed mechanism suggests that amphotericin causes an oxidation-dependent stimulation of macrophages (Lyman, 1992).

Pharmacokinetics

Distribution: V_d: Total amphotericin B increases with increasing doses of total amphotericin B (with 4 mg/kg/day = 4 L/kg); predominantly distributed in the liver; concentrations in kidneys and other tissues are lower than observed with conventional amphotericin B

Half-life: 28-29 hours

Plasma concentration: Total amphotericin B remains between 1-3 mcg/mL

Elimination: Clearance: 0.1 L/hour/kg (with 4 mg/kg/day)

Dosage

Geriatrics & Adults:

Note: Premedication: For patients who experience chills, fever, hypotension, nausea, or other nonanaphylactic infusion-related immediate reactions, premedicate with the following drugs 30-60 minutes prior to drug administration: A nonsteroidal (eg, ibuprofen, choline magnesium trisalicylate) with or without diphenhydramine **or** acetaminophen with diphenhydramine **or** hydrocortisone 50-100 mg. If the patient experiences rigors during the infusion, meperidine may be administered.

Usual dosage: I.V.: 3-4 mg/kg/day (infusion of 1 mg/kg/hour); maximum: 7.5 mg/kg/day

A regimen of 6 mg/kg/day has been used for treatment of life-threatening invasive mold infections in immunocompromised patients; maximum: 7.5 mg/kg/day.

Initially infuse at 1 mg/kg/hour. Rate of infusion may be increased with subsequent doses to 3 mg/kg/hour as patient tolerance allows. Treatment should continue as patient tolerance allows, until complete resolution of microbiologic and clinical evidence of fungal disease.

Monitoring Parameters Liver function tests, electrolytes, BUN, creatinine clearance, temperature, CBC, I/O, signs of hypokalemia (muscle weakness, cramping, drowsiness, EKG changes)

Special Geriatric Considerations The pharmacokinetics and dosing of amphotericin have not been studied in the elderly. It appears that use is similar to young adults. Caution should be exercised and renal function and desired effect monitored closely.

Dosage Forms Excipient information presented when available (limited, particularly for generics); consult specific product labeling.

Injection, powder for reconstitution: 50 mg, 100 mg

♦ **Amphotericin B Colloidal Dispersion** see Amphotericin B Cholesteryl Sulfate Complex on page 101

Amphotericin B (Conventional) (am foe TER i sin bee con VEN sha nal)

Medication Safety Issues
Safety issues:
Conventional amphotericin formulations (Amphocin®, Fungizone®) may be confused with lipid-based formulations (AmBisome®, Abelcet®, Amphotec®).
Large overdoses have occurred when conventional formulations were dispensed inadvertently for lipid-based products. Single daily doses of conventional amphotericin formulation never exceed 1.5 mg/kg.

High alert medication: The Institute for Safe Medication Practices (ISMP) includes this medication among its list of drugs which have a heightened risk of causing significant patient harm when used in error.

U.S. Brand Names Amphocin® [DSC]

Canadian Brand Names Fungizone®

Index Terms Amphotericin B Desoxycholate

Generic Available Yes

Pharmacologic Category Antifungal Agent, Parenteral

Use Treatment of severe systemic infections and meningitis caused by susceptible fungi; fungal peritonitis; irrigant for bladder fungal infections; and topically for cutaneous and mucocutaneous candidal infections

Contraindications Hypersensitivity to amphotericin or any component of the formulation

Warnings/Precautions Anaphylaxis has been reported with amphotericin B-containing drugs. During the initial dosing, the drug should be administered under close clinical observation. Avoid use with other nephrotoxic drugs; drug-induced renal toxicity usually improves with interrupting therapy, decreasing dosage, or increasing dosing interval. Infusion reactions are most common 1-3 hours after starting the infusion and diminish with continued therapy. Use amphotericin B with caution in patients with decreased renal function.

Adverse Reactions (Reflective of adult population; not specific for elderly)
>10%:
Central nervous system: Fever, chills, headache, malaise, generalized pain
Endocrine & metabolic: Hypokalemia, hypomagnesemia
Gastrointestinal: Anorexia
Hematologic: Anemia
Renal: Nephrotoxicity
1% to 10%:
Cardiovascular: Hypotension, hypertension, flushing
Central nervous system: Delirium, arachnoiditis, pain along lumbar nerves
Gastrointestinal: Nausea, vomiting
Genitourinary: Urinary retention
Hematologic: Leukocytosis
Local: Thrombophlebitis
Neuromuscular & skeletal: Paresthesia (especially with I.T. therapy)
Renal: Renal tubular acidosis, renal failure

Overdosage/Toxicology Symptoms include cardiac arrest, renal dysfunction, anemia, thrombocytopenia, granulocytopenia, fever, nausea, and vomiting. Treatment is supportive.

Drug Interactions
Increased nephrotoxicity: Aminoglycosides, cyclosporine, other nephrotoxic drugs.
Potentiation of hypokalemia: Corticosteroids, corticotropin.
Increased digitalis and neuromuscular-blocking agent toxicity due to hypokalemia.
Decreased effect: Pharmacologic antagonism may occur with azole antifungal agents (eg, miconazole, ketoconazole).
Pulmonary toxicity has occurred with concomitant administration of amphotericin B and leukocyte transfusions.

Stability Store intact vials under refrigeration; protect from light. Add 10 mL of SWFI (without a bacteriostatic agent) to each vial of amphotericin B. Further dilute with 250-500 mL D$_5$W; final concentration should not exceed 0.1 mg/mL (peripheral infusion) or 0.25 mg/mL (central infusion).

Reconstituted vials are stable, protected from light, for 24 hours at room temperature and 1 week when refrigerated. Parenteral admixtures are stable, protected from light, for 24 hours at room temperature and 2 days under refrigeration. Short-term exposure (<24 hours) to light during I.V. infusion does **not** appreciably affect potency.

Mechanism of Action Binds to ergosterol altering cell membrane permeability in susceptible fungi and causing leakage of cell components with subsequent cell death. Proposed mechanism suggests that amphotericin causes an oxidation-dependent stimulation of macrophages (Lyman, 1992).
(Continued)

Amphotericin B (Conventional) *(Continued)*

Pharmacokinetics

Distribution: Minimal amounts enter the aqueous humor, bile, CSF, amniotic fluid, pericardial fluid, pleural fluid and synovial fluid; poorly dialyzed

Protein binding: Plasma: 90%

Half-life:

Initial: 15-48 hours

Terminal phase: 15 days

Time to peak serum concentration: I.V.: During the first hour after a 4- to 6-hour infusion

Dosage

Geriatrics & Adults:

Note: Premedication: For patients who experience infusion-related immediate reactions, premedicate with the following drugs 30-60 minutes prior to drug administration: NSAID (with or without diphenhydramine) **or** acetaminophen with diphenhydramine **or** hydrocortisone 50-100 mg. If the patient experiences rigors during the infusion, meperidine may be administered.

Test dose: I.V.: 1 mg infused over 20-30 minutes. Many clinicians believe a test dose is unnecessary.

Systemic fungal infections: I.V.: Maintenance dose: Usual: 0.25-1.5 mg/kg/day; 1-1.5 mg/kg over 4-6 hours every other day may be given once therapy is established. Aspergillosis, mucormycosis, rhinocerebral phycomycosis often require 1-1.5 mg/kg/day; do not exceed 1.5 mg/kg/day.

Duration of therapy varies with nature of infection: Usual duration is 4-12 weeks or cumulative dose of 1-4 g.

Meningitis, coccidioidal or cryptococcal: I.T.: Initial: 25-300 mcg every 48-72 hours; increase to 500 mcg to 1 mg as tolerated; maximum total dose: 15 mg has been suggested.

Cystitis (Candidal): Bladder irrigation: Irrigate with 50 mcg/mL solution instilled periodically or continuously for 5-10 days or until cultures are clear.

Bone marrow transplantation (prophylaxis): I.V.: Low-dose amphotericin B 0.1-0.25 mg/kg/day has been administered after bone marrow transplantation to reduce the risk of invasive fungal disease.

Note: Alternative routes of administration and extemporaneous preparations have been used when standard antifungal therapy is not available (eg, inhalation, intraocular injection, subconjunctival application, intracavitary administration into various joints and the pleural space).

Renal Impairment:

If renal dysfunction is due to the drug, the daily total can be decreased by 50% or the dose can be given every other day. I.V. therapy may take several months.

Poorly dialyzed; no supplemental dose is necessary when using hemo- or peritoneal dialysis or CAVH/CAVHD.

Administration in dialysate: 1-2 mg/L of peritoneal dialysis fluid either with or without low-dose I.V. amphotericin B (a total dose of 2-10 mg/kg given over 7-14 days).

Monitoring Parameters Monitor electrolytes, BUN, serum creatinine, LFTs, CBC regularly, I & O, signs of hypokalemia (muscle weakness, cramping, drowsiness, EKG changes, etc); if BUN exceeds 40 mg/dL or the serum creatinine exceeds 3 mg/dL, discontinue the drug or reduce the dose until renal function improves

Reference Range Therapeutic: 1-2 mcg/mL (SI: 1-2.2 µmol/L)

Test Interactions Increased BUN (S), serum creatinine, alkaline phosphate, bilirubin; decreased magnesium, potassium (S)

Patient Information Amphotericin cream may slightly discolor skin and stain clothing; personal hygiene is very important to help reduce the spread and recurrence of lesions; avoid covering topical applications with occlusive bandages; most skin lesions require 1-3 weeks of therapy

Additional Information Lipid complex may be less nephrotoxic, but more expensive

Special Geriatric Considerations The pharmacokinetics and dosing of amphotericin have not been studied in elderly. It appears that use is similar to young adults; caution should be exercised and renal function and desired effect monitored closely.

Dosage Forms Excipient information presented when available (limited, particularly for generics); consult specific product labeling. [DSC] = Discontinued product

Injection, powder for reconstitution, as desoxycholate: 50 mg

Amphocin®: 50 mg [DSC]

Selected References

Gallis HA, Drew RH, and Pickard WW, "Amphotericin B: 30 Years of Clinical Experience," *Rev Infect Dis*, 1990, 12(2):308-29.

Wong-Beringer A, Beringer PM, and Rho JP, "Focus on Amphotericin B Lipid Complex," *Formulary*, 1996, 13(3):169-85.

♦ **Amphotericin B Desoxycholate** *see* Amphotericin B (Conventional) *on page 103*

Amphotericin B (Lipid Complex)
(am foe TER i sin bee LIP id KOM pleks)

Medication Safety Issues
Safety issues:
Lipid-based amphotericin formulations (Abelcet®) may be confused with conventional formulations (Amphocin®, Fungizone®)

Large overdoses have occurred when conventional formulations were dispensed inadvertently for lipid-based products. Single daily doses of conventional amphotericin formulation never exceed 1.5 mg/kg.

High alert medication: The Institute for Safe Medication Practices (ISMP) includes this medication among its list of drugs which have a heightened risk of causing significant patient harm when used in error.

U.S. Brand Names Abelcet®

Canadian Brand Names Abelcet®; Amphotec®

Index Terms ABLC

Generic Available No

Pharmacologic Category Antifungal Agent, Parenteral

Use Treatment of aspergillosis or any type of progressive fungal infection in patients who are refractory to or intolerant of conventional amphotericin B therapy

Orphan drug: Cryptococcal meningitis

Contraindications Hypersensitivity to amphotericin or any component of the formulation

Warnings/Precautions Anaphylaxis has been reported with amphotericin B-containing drugs. If severe respiratory distress occurs, the infusion should be immediately discontinued. During the initial dosing, the drug should be administered under close clinical observation. Acute reactions (including fever and chills) may occur 1-2 hours after starting an intravenous infusion. These reactions are usually more common with the first few doses and generally diminish with subsequent doses.

Adverse Reactions (Reflective of adult population; not specific for elderly) Nephrotoxicity and infusion-related hyperpyrexia, rigor, and chilling are reduced relative to amphotericin deoxycholate.

>10%:
Central nervous system: Chills, fever
Renal: Serum creatinine increased
Miscellaneous: Multiple organ failure

1% to 10%:
Cardiovascular: Hypotension, cardiac arrest
Central nervous system: Headache, pain
Dermatologic: Rash
Endocrine & metabolic: Bilirubinemia, hypokalemia, acidosis
Gastrointestinal: Nausea, vomiting, diarrhea, gastrointestinal hemorrhage, abdominal pain
Renal: Renal failure
Respiratory: Respiratory failure, dyspnea, pneumonia

Drug Interactions
Increased nephrotoxicity: Aminoglycosides, cyclosporine, other nephrotoxic drugs.
Potentiation of hypokalemia: Corticosteroids, corticotropin.
Increased digitalis and neuromuscular-blocking agent toxicity due to hypokalemia.
Decreased effect: Pharmacologic antagonism may occur with azole antifungal agents (eg, miconazole, ketoconazole).
Pulmonary toxicity has occurred with concomitant administration of amphotericin B and leukocyte transfusions.

Stability Intact vials should be stored at 2°C to 8°C (35°F to 46°F) and protected from exposure to light; do not freeze intact vials. Solutions for infusion are stable for 48 hours under refrigeration and for 6 hours at room temperature. Shake the vial gently until there is no evidence of any yellow sediment at the bottom. Dilute with D_5W to 1-2 mg/mL. Protect from light.

Do not dilute with saline solutions or mix with other drugs or electrolytes - compatibility has not been established

Do not use an in-line filter during administration.

Mechanism of Action Binds to ergosterol altering cell membrane permeability in susceptible fungi and causing leakage of cell components with subsequent cell death. Proposed mechanism suggests that amphotericin causes an oxidation-dependent stimulation of macrophages.

Dosage
Geriatrics & Adults:
Note: Premedication: For patients who experience infusion-related immediate reactions, premedicate with the following drugs 30-60 minutes prior to drug administration: A nonsteroidal anti-inflammatory agent ± diphenhydramine **or** acetaminophen
(Continued)

Amphotericin B (Lipid Complex) *(Continued)*

with diphenhydramine **or** hydrocortisone 50-100 mg. If the patient experiences rigors during the infusion, meperidine may be administered.

Usual dosage: I.V.: 2.5-5 mg/kg/day as a single infusion

Renal Impairment: The effects of renal impairment on drug pharmacokinetics or pharmacodynamics are currently unknown. The dose of amphotericin B lipid complex may be adjusted or drug administration may have to be interrupted in patients with acute kidney dysfunction to reduce the magnitude of renal impairment.

Hemodialysis: Supplemental dose is not necessary.

Peritoneal dialysis: Supplemental dose is not necessary.

Continuous arteriovenous or venovenous hemofiltration: Supplemental dose is not necessary.

Monitoring Parameters

BUN and serum creatinine concentrations should be determined every other day while therapy is increased and at least weekly thereafter; monitor input and output

Serum potassium and magnesium should be monitored closely; monitor for signs of hypokalemia (muscle weakness, cramping, drowsiness, EKG changes, etc)

Monitor electrolytes, liver function, hematocrit, CBC, blood pressure, and temperature regularly

Test Interactions Increased BUN (S), serum creatinine, alkaline phosphate, bilirubin; decreased magnesium, potassium (S)

Patient Information I.V. therapy may take several months; personal hygiene is very important to help reduce the spread and recurrence of lesions; most skin lesions require 1-3 weeks of therapy; report any hearing loss

Special Geriatric Considerations The pharmacokinetics and dosing of amphotericin have not been studied in elderly. It appears that use is similar to young adults; caution should be exercised and renal function and desired effect monitored closely.

Dosage Forms Excipient information presented when available (limited, particularly for generics); consult specific product labeling.

Injection, suspension [preservative free]: 5 mg/mL (20 mL)

Ampicillin *(am pi SIL in)*

Related Information

Antibiotic Treatment of Adults With Infective Endocarditis *on page 1797*
Antimicrobial Activity Against Selected Organisms *on page 1728*
Prevention of Infective Endocarditis *on page 1803*

Medication Safety Issues

Sound-alike/look-alike issues:

Ampicillin may be confused with aminophylline

Canadian Brand Names Apo-Ampi®; Novo-Ampicillin; Nu-Ampi

Index Terms Aminobenzylpenicillin; Ampicillin Sodium; Ampicillin Trihydrate

Generic Available Yes

Pharmacologic Category Antibiotic, Penicillin

Use Treatment of susceptible bacterial infections

Contraindications Hypersensitivity to ampicillin, any component of the formulation, or other penicillins

Warnings/Precautions Dosage adjustment may be necessary in patients with renal impairment. Serious and occasionally severe or fatal hypersensitivity (anaphylactoid) reactions have been reported in patients on penicillin therapy, especially with a history of beta-lactam hypersensitivity, history of sensitivity to multiple allergens, or previous IgE-mediated reactions (eg, anaphylaxis, angioedema, urticaria). Use with caution in asthmatic patients. High percentage of patients with infectious mononucleosis have developed rash during therapy with ampicillin. Appearance of a rash should be carefully evaluated to differentiate a nonallergic ampicillin rash from a hypersensitivity reaction. Ampicillin rash is a generalized dull red, maculopapular rash, generally appearing 3-14 days after the start of therapy. It normally begins on the trunk and spreads over most of the body. It may be most intense at pressure areas, elbows, and knees. Prolonged use may result in fungal or bacterial superinfection, including *C. difficile*-associated diarrhea and pseudomembranous colitis.

Adverse Reactions (Reflective of adult population; not specific for elderly) Frequency not defined.

Central nervous system: Fever, penicillin encephalopathy, seizure

Dermatologic: Erythema multiforme, exfoliative dermatitis, rash, urticaria

Note: Appearance of a rash should be carefully evaluated to differentiate (if possible) nonallergic ampicillin rash from hypersensitivity reaction. Incidence is higher in patients with viral infection, *Salmonella* infection, lymphocytic leukemia, or patients that have hyperuricemia.

Gastrointestinal: Black hairy tongue, diarrhea, enterocolitis, glossitis, nausea, oral candidiasis, pseudomembranous colitis, sore mouth or tongue, stomatitis, vomiting

Hematologic: Agranulocytosis, anemia, hemolytic anemia, eosinophilia, leukopenia, thrombocytopenia purpura

Hepatic: AST increased

Renal: Interstitial nephritis (rare)

Respiratory: Laryngeal stridor

Miscellaneous: Anaphylaxis, serum sickness-like reaction

Overdosage/Toxicology Symptoms of penicillin overdose include neuromuscular hypersensitivity (agitation, hallucinations, asterixis, encephalopathy, confusion, and seizures) and electrolyte imbalance (with potassium or sodium salts), especially in renal failure. Hemodialysis may be helpful to aid in the removal of the drug from the blood, otherwise most treatment is supportive or symptom-directed.

Drug Interactions

Allopurinol: Theoretically has an additive potential for ampicillin/amoxicillin rash.

Aminoglycosides: May be synergistic against selected organisms.

Fusidic acid: May decrease the therapeutic effect of penicillins; administer the penicillin at least 2 hours before fusidic acid.

Methotrexate: Penicillins may increase the exposure to methotrexate during concurrent therapy; monitor.

Oral contraceptives: Anecdotal reports suggesting decreased contraceptive efficacy with penicillins have been refuted by more rigorous scientific and clinical data.

Probenecid, disulfiram: May increase levels of penicillins (ampicillin).

Warfarin: Effects of warfarin may be increased.

Ethanol/Nutrition/Herb Interactions Food: Food decreases ampicillin absorption rate; may decrease ampicillin serum concentration.

Stability

Oral: Oral suspension is stable for 7 days at room temperature or for 14 days under refrigeration.

I.V.:

I.V. minimum volume: Concentration should not exceed 30 mg/mL due to concentration-dependent stability restrictions. Solutions for I.M. or direct I.V. should be used within 1 hour. Solutions for I.V. infusion will be inactivated by dextrose at room temperature. If dextrose-containing solutions are to be used, the resultant solution will only be stable for 2 hours versus 8 hours in the 0.9% sodium chloride injection. D_5W has limited stability.

Stability of parenteral admixture in NS at room temperature (25°C) is 8 hours.

Stability of parenteral admixture in NS at refrigeration temperature (4°C) is 2 days.

Standard diluent: 500 mg/50 mL NS; 1 g/50 mL NS; 2 g/100 mL NS

Mechanism of Action Inhibits bacterial cell wall synthesis by binding to one or more of the penicillin-binding proteins (PBPs) which in turn inhibits the final transpeptidation step of peptidoglycan synthesis in bacterial cell walls, thus inhibiting cell wall biosynthesis. Bacteria eventually lyse due to ongoing activity of cell wall autolytic enzymes (autolysins and murein hydrolases) while cell wall assembly is arrested.

Pharmacokinetics

Absorption: Oral: 50%; not affected by age

Distribution: Into bile; penetration into CSF occurs with inflamed meninges only

Protein binding: 15% to 25%

Half-life elimination:

Adults: 1-1.8 hours

Anuric/end-stage renal disease: 7-20 hours

Time to peak serum concentration: Oral: Within 1-2 hours

Elimination: ~90% of drug excreted unchanged in urine within 24 hours, ~40% is removed by hemodialysis

Clearance has been reported to be decreased and half-life prolonged in older patients

Dosage

Geriatrics: Administer usual adult dose unless renal function is markedly reduced.

Adults:

Usual dosage range:

Oral: 250-500 mg every 6 hours

I.M., I.V.: 250-500 mg every 6 hours

Actinomycosis: I.V.: 50 mg/kg/day for 4-6 weeks then oral amoxicillin

Cholangitis (acute): I.V.: 2 g every 4 hours with gentamicin

Diverticulitis: I.M., I.V.: 2 g every 6 hours with metronidazole

Endocarditis:

Infective: I.V.: 12 g/day via continuous infusion or divided every 4 hours

Prophylaxis: Dental, oral, respiratory tract, or esophageal procedures: I.M., I.V.: 2 g within 30 minutes prior to procedure in patients unable to take oral amoxicillin

Genitourinary and gastrointestinal tract (except esophageal) procedures: I.M., I.V.:

High-risk patients: 2 g within 30 minutes prior to procedure, followed by ampicillin 1 g (or amoxicillin 1g orally) 6 hours later; must be used in combination with gentamicin.

Moderate-risk patients: 2 g within 30 minutes prior to procedure

(Continued)

Ampicillin *(Continued)*

Group B strep prophylaxis (intrapartum): I.V.: 2 g initial dose, then 1 g every 4 hours until delivery

***Listeria* infections:** I.V.: 200 mg/kg/day divided every 6 hours

Sepsis/meningitis: I.M., I.V.: 150-250 mg/kg/day divided every 3-4 hours (range: 6-12 g/day)

Urinary tract infections (enterococcus suspected): I.V.: 1-2 g every 6 hours with gentamicin

Renal Impairment:

Cl_{cr} >50 mL/minute: Administer every 6 hours

Cl_{cr} 10-50 mL/minute: Administer every 6-12 hours

Cl_{cr} <10 mL/minute: Administer every 12-24 hours

Hemodialysis: Moderately dialyzable (20% to 50%); administer dose after dialysis

Peritoneal dialysis: Moderately dialyzable (20% to 50%)

Administer 250 mg every 12 hours

Continuous arteriovenous or venovenous hemofiltration effects: Dose as for Cl_{cr} 10-50 mL/minute; ~50 mg of ampicillin per liter of filtrate is removed

Administration Do not use D_5W as a diluent, D_5W has limited stability

Standard diluent: Dose/50 mL NS

Minimum volume: Concentration should not exceed 30 mg/mL; manufacturer may supply as either the anhydrous or the trihydrate form

Monitoring Parameters Signs and symptoms of infection (fever, urinary frequency or pain, etc) should begin to resolve after 1-2 days

Test Interactions May interfere with urinary glucose tests using cupric sulfate (Benedict's solution, Clinitest®)

Some penicillin derivatives may accelerate the degradation of aminoglycosides *in vitro*, leading to a potential underestimation of aminoglycoside serum concentration.

Patient Information Take on an empty stomach; complete full course of therapy; should be taken at equal intervals around-the-clock to maintain adequate blood concentrations; women should report onset of symptoms of candidal vaginitis.

Additional Information Appearance of a rash should be carefully evaluated to differentiate a nonallergic ampicillin rash from a hypersensitivity reaction; ampicillin rash is dull red, macular or maculopapular, and only mildly pruritic; normally appears on pressure areas like knees, elbows, palms, or soles, and may spread in symmetric pattern over most of the body; incidence of ampicillin rash is higher in patients with viral infections, *Salmonella* infections, lymphocytic leukemia, or patients that have hyperuricemia. Ampicillin and gentamicin should not be mixed in the same I.V. tubing or administered concurrently.

Sodium content of suspension (250 mg/5 mL, 5 mL): 10 mg (0.4 mEq)

Sodium content of 1 g: 66.7 mg (3 mEq)

Special Geriatric Considerations Adjust dose for renal function.

Dosage Forms Excipient information presented when available (limited, particularly for generics); consult specific product labeling.

Capsule: 250 mg, 500 mg

Injection, powder for reconstitution, as sodium: 125 mg, 250 mg, 500 mg, 1 g, 2 g, 10 g

Powder for oral suspension: 125 mg/5 mL (100 mL, 200 mL); 250 mg/5 mL (100 mL, 200 mL)

Selected References

Triggs EJ, Johnson JM, and Learoyd B, "Absorption and Disposition of Ampicillin in the Elderly," *Eur J Clin Pharmacol*, 1980, 18(2):195-8.

Ampicillin and Sulbactam *(am pi SIL in & SUL bak tam)*

Related Information

Ampicillin *on page 106*

Antimicrobial Activity Against Selected Organisms *on page 1728*

U.S. Brand Names Unasyn®

Canadian Brand Names Unasyn®

Index Terms Sulbactam and Ampicillin

Generic Available Yes

Pharmacologic Category Antibiotic, Penicillin

Use Treatment of susceptible bacterial infections involved with skin and skin structure, intra-abdominal infections, gynecological infections; spectrum is that of ampicillin plus organisms producing beta-lactamases such as *S. aureus*, *H. influenzae*, *E. coli*, *Klebsiella*, *Acinetobacter*, *Enterobacter*, and anaerobes

Contraindications Hypersensitivity to ampicillin, sulbactam, penicillins, or any component of the formulations

Warnings/Precautions Dosage adjustment may be necessary in patients with renal impairment. Serious and occasionally severe or fatal hypersensitivity (anaphylactoid) reactions have been reported in patients on penicillin therapy, especially with a history of beta-lactam hypersensitivity, history of sensitivity to multiple allergens, or previous IgE-mediated reactions (eg, anaphylaxis, angioedema, urticaria). Use with caution in asthmatic patients. High percentage of patients with infectious mononucleosis have developed rash during therapy with ampicillin. Appearance of a rash should be carefully evaluated to differentiate a nonallergic ampicillin rash from a hypersensitivity reaction. Prolonged use may result in fungal or bacterial superinfection, including *C. difficile*-associated diarrhea and pseudomembranous colitis.

Adverse Reactions (Reflective of adult population; not specific for elderly)
Also see Ampicillin.
>10%: Local: Pain at injection site (I.M.)
1% to 10%:
Dermatologic: Rash
Gastrointestinal: Diarrhea
Local: Pain at injection site (I.V.), thrombophlebitis
Miscellaneous: Allergic reaction (may include serum sickness, urticaria, bronchospasm, hypotension, etc)

Overdosage/Toxicology Symptoms of penicillin overdose include neuromuscular hypersensitivity (agitation, hallucinations, asterixis, encephalopathy, confusion, and seizures) and electrolyte imbalance (with potassium or sodium salts), especially in renal failure. Hemodialysis may be helpful to aid in the removal of the drug from the blood, otherwise most treatment is supportive or symptom-directed.

Drug Interactions
Allopurinol: Theoretically has an additive potential for ampicillin/amoxicillin rash.
Aminoglycosides: May be synergistic against selected organisms.
Fusidic acid: May decrease the therapeutic effect of penicillins; administer the penicillin at least 2 hours before fusidic acid.
Methotrexate: Penicillins may increase the exposure to methotrexate during concurrent therapy; monitor.
Oral contraceptives: Anecdotal reports suggesting decreased contraceptive efficacy with penicillins have been refuted by more rigorous scientific and clinical data.
Probenecid, disulfiram: May increase levels of penicillins (ampicillin).
Warfarin: Effects of warfarin may be increased.

Stability Prior to reconstitution, store at ≤30°C (86°F).

I.M. and direct I.V. administration: Use within 1 hour after preparation. Reconstitute with sterile water for injection or 0.5% or 2% lidocaine hydrochloride injection (I.M.). Sodium chloride 0.9% (NS) is the diluent of choice for I.V. piggyback use. Solutions made in NS are stable up to 72 hours when refrigerated whereas dextrose solutions (same concentration) are stable for only 4 hours.

Mechanism of Action The addition of sulbactam, a beta-lactamase inhibitor, to ampicillin extends the spectrum of ampicillin to include some beta-lactamase-producing organisms; inhibits bacterial cell wall synthesis by binding to one or more of the penicillin-binding proteins (PBPs) which in turn inhibits the final transpeptidation step of peptidoglycan synthesis in bacterial cell walls, thus inhibiting cell wall biosynthesis. Bacteria eventually lyse due to ongoing activity of cell wall autolytic enzymes (autolysins and murein hydrolases) while cell wall assembly is arrested.

Pharmacokinetics
Protein binding:
Ampicillin: 28%
Sulbactam: 38%
Half-life: Ampicillin and sulbactam are similar: 1-1.8 hours and 1-1.3 hours, respectively
Time to peak serum concentration: Immediate
Elimination: ~75% to 85% of both drugs are excreted unchanged in the urine within 8 hours following administration
Reduced clearance and prolonged half-life in older adults have been found for both compounds; age and renal function were negatively correlated with clearance

Dosage
Geriatrics & Adults: Doses expressed as ampicillin/sulbactam combination.
Susceptible infections: I.M., I.V.: 1.5-3 g every 6 hours (maximum: Unasyn® 12 g)
Amnionitis, cholangitis, diverticulitis, endometritis, endophthalmitis, epididymitis/orchitis, liver abscess, osteomyelitis (diabetic foot), peritonitis: I.V.: 3 g every 6 hours
Endocarditis: I.V.: 3 g every 6 hours with gentamicin or vancomycin for 4-6 weeks
Orbital cellulitis: I.V.: 1.5 g every 6 hours
Parapharyngeal space infections: I.V.: 3 g every 6 hours
Pasteurella multocida **(human, canine/feline bites):** I.V.: 1.5-3 g every 6 hours
Pelvic inflammatory disease: I.V.: 3 g every 6 hours with doxycycline
Peritonitis (CAPD): Intraperitoneal:
Anuric, intermittent: 3 g every 12 hours
Anuric, continuous: Loading dose: 1.5 g; maintenance dose: 150 mg
(Continued)

Ampicillin and Sulbactam *(Continued)*

Pneumonia:
Aspiration, community-acquired: I.V.: 1.5-3 g every 6 hours
Hospital-acquired: I.V.: 3 g every 6 hours
Urinary tract infections, pyelonephritis: I.V.: 3 g every 6 hours for 14 days
Renal Impairment:
Cl_{cr} 15-29 mL/minute: Administer every 12 hours
Cl_{cr} 5-14 mL/minute: Administer every 24 hours

Monitoring Parameters Signs and symptoms of infection (fever, urinary frequency or pain, etc) should begin to resolve after 1-2 days; with prolonged therapy, monitor hematologic, renal, and hepatic function

Test Interactions May interfere with urinary glucose tests using cupric sulfate (Benedict's solution, Clinitest®).

Some penicillin derivatives may accelerate the degradation of aminoglycosides *in vitro*, leading to a potential underestimation of aminoglycoside serum concentration.

Patient Information Report sore throat, fever, fatigue, or diarrhea

Additional Information Appearance of a rash should be carefully evaluated to differentiate a nonallergic ampicillin rash from a hypersensitivity reaction; ampicillin rash is dull red, macular or maculopapular, and only mildly pruritic; normally appears on pressure areas like knees, elbows, palms, or soles, and may spread in symmetric pattern over most of the body; incidence of ampicillin rash is higher in patients with viral infections, *Salmonella* infections, lymphocytic leukemia, or patients that have hyperuricemia

Special Geriatric Considerations Adjust dose for renal function.

Dosage Forms Excipient information presented when available (limited, particularly for generics); consult specific product labeling.
Injection, powder for reconstitution: 1.5 g: Ampicillin 1 g and sulbactam 0.5 g [contains sodium 115 mg (5 mEq)/1.5 g)]; 3 g: Ampicillin 2 g and sulbactam 1 g [contains sodium 115 mg (5 mEq)/1.5 g)]; 15 g: Ampicillin 10 g and sulbactam 5 g [bulk package; contains sodium 115 mg (5 mEq)/1.5 g]
Unasyn®:
1.5 g: Ampicillin 1 g and sulbactam 0.5 g [contains sodium 115 mg (5 mEq)/1.5 g)]
3 g: Ampicillin 2 g and sulbactam 1 g [contains sodium 115 mg (5 mEq)/1.5 g)]
15 g: Ampicillin 10 g and sulbactam 5 g [bulk package; contains sodium 115 mg (5 mEq)/1.5 g)]

Selected References
Meyers BR, Wilkinson P, Mendelson MH, et al, "Pharmacokinetics of Ampicillin-Sulbactam in Healthy Elderly and Young Volunteers," *Antimicrob Agents Chemother*, 1991, 35(10):2098-101.
Rho SP, Jones A, Woo M, et al, "Single Dose Pharmacokinetics of Intravenous Ampicillin plus Sulbactam in Healthy Elderly and Young Subjects," *J Antimicrob Chemother*, 1989, 24(4):573-80.

♦ **Ampicillin Sodium** *see* Ampicillin *on page 106*

♦ **Ampicillin Trihydrate** *see* Ampicillin *on page 106*

♦ **Amrinone Lactate** *see* Inamrinone *on page 797*

♦ **Anafranil®** *see* ClomiPRAMINE *on page 336*

Anakinra *(an a KIN ra)*

Medication Safety Issues
Sound-alike/look-alike issues:
Anakinra may be confused with amikacin
U.S. Brand Names Kineret®
Canadian Brand Names Kineret®
Index Terms IL-1Ra; Interleukin-1 Receptor Antagonist
Generic Available No
Pharmacologic Category Antirheumatic, Disease Modifying; Interleukin-1 Receptor Antagonist
Use Treatment of moderately- to severely-active rheumatoid arthritis in adult patients who have failed one or more disease-modifying antirheumatic drugs (DMARDs); may be used alone or in combination with DMARDs (other than tumor necrosis factor-blocking agents)
Contraindications Hypersensitivity to *E. coli*-derived proteins, anakinra, or any component of the formulation); patients with active infections (including chronic or local infection)
Warnings/Precautions Anakinra may affect defenses against infections and malignancies. Safety and efficacy in patients with immunosuppression or chronic infections have not been evaluated. Discontinue administration if patient develops a serious infection. Do not start drug administration in patients with an active infection. Patients with asthma may be at an increased risk of serious infections. Should not be used in combination with tumor necrosis factor antagonists, unless no satisfactory alternatives

exist, and then only with extreme caution. Impact on the development and course of malignancies is not fully defined. As compared to the general population, an increased risk of lymphoma has been noted in clinical trials; however, rheumatoid arthritis has been previously associated with an increased rate of lymphoma.

Use caution in patients with a history of significant hematologic abnormalities; has been associated with uncommon, but significant decreases in hematologic parameters (particularly neutrophil counts). Patients must be advised to seek medical attention if they develop signs and symptoms suggestive of blood dyscrasias. Discontinue if significant hematologic abnormalities are confirmed.

Patients should be brought up to date with all immunizations before initiating therapy. Live vaccines should not be given concurrently. Patients with a significant exposure to varicella virus should temporarily discontinue anakinra. Hypersensitivity reactions may occur. Impact on the development and course of malignancies is not fully defined. Use caution in patients with renal impairment; consider increased dosing intervals for severe renal dysfunction (Cl$_{cr}$ <30 mL/minute). Use caution in the elderly due to the potential for higher risk of infections. The packaging (needle cover) contains latex.

Adverse Reactions (Reflective of adult population; not specific for elderly)
>10%:
  Central nervous system: Headache (12%)
  Local: Injection site reaction (majority mild, typically lasting 14-28 days, characterized by erythema, ecchymosis, inflammation, and pain; up to 71%)
  Miscellaneous: Infection (39% versus 37% in placebo; serious infection 2% to 3%)
1% to 10%:
  Gastrointestinal: Nausea (8%), diarrhea (7%), abdominal pain (5%)
  Hematologic: Neutropenia (8%; grades 3/4: 0.4%)
  Respiratory: Sinusitis (7%)
  Miscellaneous: Flu-like syndrome (6%)

Overdosage/Toxicology No serious toxicities have been reported following administration of high doses of anakinra (up to 35 times the typical dosage for rheumatoid arthritis).

Drug Interactions
  Anti-TNF Agents (adalimumab, etanercept, infliximab, lenalidomide, thalidomide): May enhance the adverse/toxic effect of anakinra. An increased risk of serious infection during concomitant use has been reported with etanercept.
  Vaccine (live organism): Anakinra may increase the risk of secondary infection.

Stability Store in refrigerator at 2°C to 8°C (36°F to 46°F); do not freeze. Do not shake. Protect from light.

Mechanism of Action Antagonist of the interleukin-1 (IL-1) receptor. Endogenous IL-1 is induced by inflammatory stimuli and mediates a variety of immunological responses, including degradation of cartilage (loss of proteoglycans) and stimulation of bone resorption.

Pharmacokinetics
  Bioavailability: SubQ: 95%
  Half-life: Terminal: 4-6 hours
  Time to peak: SubQ: 3-7 hours

Dosage
  Geriatrics & Adults: Rheumatoid arthritis: SubQ: 100 mg once daily (administer at approximately the same time each day)
  Renal Impairment: Cl$_{cr}$ <30 mL/minute and/or end-stage renal disease: 100 mg every other day

Administration Rotate injection sites (thigh, abdomen, upper arm); injection should be given at least 1 inch away from previous injection site. Do not shake. Provided in single-use, preservative free syringes with 27 gauge needles; discard any unused portion.

Monitoring Parameters CBC with differential (baseline, then monthly for 3 months, then every 3 months); serum creatinine

Patient Information If self-injecting, follow instructions for injection and disposal of needles exactly. If redness, swelling, or irritation appears at the injection site, contact prescriber. Do not have any vaccinations while using this medication without consulting prescriber first. You may experience headache (use caution when driving or engaging in tasks requiring alertness until response to drug is known). If stomach pain or cramping, unusual bleeding or bruising, persistent fever, or paleness occurs, stop medication and contact prescriber **immediately**. Also, immediately report skin rash, unusual muscle or bone weakness, or signs of respiratory flu or other infection (eg, chills, fever, sore throat, easy bruising or bleeding, mouth sores, unhealed sores).

Additional Information Anakinra is produced by recombinant DNA/*E. coli* technology.

Special Geriatric Considerations Clinical trials with older adults (65% to 75%) demonstrated no clinical differences between elderly patients and younger adults in safety and efficacy. Since elderly may be more liable to infections in general, use with (Continued)

Anakinra *(Continued)*

caution. Also, since many elderly patients may have Cl$_{cr}$ <30 mL/minute, close monitoring should be followed with calculation of creatinine clearance prior to initiating therapy with anakinra.

Dosage Forms Excipient information presented when available (limited, particularly for generics); consult specific product labeling.

Injection, solution [preservative free]:

Kineret®: 100 mg/0.67 mL (1 mL) [prefilled syringe; needle cover contains latex]

Selected References

Cohen S, Hurd E, Cush J, et al, "Treatment of Rheumatoid Arthritis With Anakinra, a Recombinant Human Interleukin-1 Receptor Antagonist, in Combination With Methotrexate: Results of a Twenty-Four-Week, Multicenter, Randomized, Double-Blind, Placebo-Controlled Trial," *Arthritis Rheum*, 2002, 46(3):614-24.

Fleischmann RM, Schechtman J, Bennett R, et al, "Anakinra, a Recombinant Human Interleukin-1 Receptor Antagonist (r-metHuIL-1ra), in Patients With Rheumatoid Arthritis: A Large, International, Multicenter, Placebo-Controlled Trial," *Arthritis Rheum*, 2003, 48(4):927-34.

Fleischmann RM, Tesser J, Schiff MH, et al, Safety of Extended Treatment With Anakinra in Patients With Rheumatoid Arthritis, *Ann Rheum Dis*, 2006, 65(8):1006-12.

Genovese MC, Cohen S, Moreland L, et al, "Combination Therapy With Etanercept and Anakinra in the Treatment of Patients With Rheumatoid Arthritis Who Have Been Treated Unsuccessfully With Methotrexate," *Arthritis Rheum*, 2004, 50(5):1412-9.

♦ **Anaprox®** *see Naproxen on page 1088*
♦ **Anaprox® DS** *see Naproxen on page 1088*
♦ **Anaspaz®** *see Hyoscyamine on page 778*

Anastrozole *(an AS troe zole)*

U.S. Brand Names Arimidex®
Canadian Brand Names Arimidex®
Index Terms ICI-D1033; NSC-719344; ZD1033
Generic Available No
Pharmacologic Category Antineoplastic Agent, Aromatase Inhibitor
Use Treatment of locally-advanced or metastatic breast cancer (ER-positive or hormone receptor unknown) in postmenopausal women; treatment of advanced breast cancer in postmenopausal women with disease progression following tamoxifen therapy; adjuvant treatment of early ER-positive breast cancer in postmenopausal women

Contraindications Hypersensitivity to anastrozole or any component of the formulation

Warnings/Precautions Hazardous agent - use appropriate precautions for handling and disposal. Use with caution in patients with hyperlipidemias; total cholesterol and LDL-cholesterol increase in patients receiving anastrozole. Anastrozole may be associated with a reduction in bone mineral density.

Adverse Reactions (Reflective of adult population; not specific for elderly)

>10%:

Cardiovascular: Vasodilatation (25% to 36%), hypertension (2% to 13%)

Central nervous system: Mood disturbance (19%), fatigue (19%), pain (11% to 17%), headache (9% to 13%), depression (5% to 13%)

Dermatologic: Rash (6% to 11%)

Endocrine & metabolic: Hot flashes (12% to 36%)

Gastrointestinal: Nausea (11% to 19%), vomiting (8% to 13%)

Neuromuscular & skeletal: Weakness (16% to 19%), arthritis (17%), arthralgia (2% to 15%), back pain (10% to 12%), bone pain (6% to 11%), osteoporosis (11%)

Respiratory: Pharyngitis (6% to 14%), cough increased (8% to 11%)

1% to 10%:

Cardiovascular: Peripheral edema (5% to 10%), chest pain (5% to 7%), ischemic cardiovascular disease (4%), venous thromboembolic events (3% to 4%), ischemic cerebrovascular events (2%), angina (2%)

Central nervous system: Insomnia (2% to 10%), dizziness (6% to 8%), anxiety (2% to 6%), fever (2% to 5%), malaise (2% to 5%), confusion (2% to 5%), nervousness (2% to 5%), somnolence (2% to 5%), lethargy (1%)

Dermatologic: Alopecia (2% to 5%), pruritus (2% to 5%)

Endocrine & metabolic: Hypercholesterolemia (9%), breast pain (2% to 8%)

Gastrointestinal: Constipation (7% to 9%), abdominal pain (7% to 9%), diarrhea (8% to 9%), anorexia (5% to 7%), xerostomia (6%), dyspepsia (7%), weight gain (2% to 9%), weight loss (2% to 5%)

Genitourinary: Urinary tract infection (2% to 8%), vulvovaginitis (6%), pelvic pain (5%), vaginal bleeding (1% to 5%), vaginitis (4%), vaginal discharge (4%), vaginal hemorrhage (2% to 4%), leukorrhea (2% to 3%), vaginal dryness (2%)

Hematologic: Anemia (2% to 5%), leukopenia (2% to 5%)

Hepatic: Liver function tests increased (2% to 5%), alkaline phosphatase increased (2% to 5%), gamma GT increased (2% to 5%)

Local: Thrombophlebitis (2% to 5%)

Neuromuscular & skeletal: Fracture (2% to 10%), arthrosis (7%), paresthesia (5% to 7%), joint disorder (6%), myalgia (2% to 6%), neck pain (2% to 5%), hypertonia (3%)

Ocular: Cataracts (6%)

Respiratory: Dyspnea (8% to 10%), sinusitis (2% to 6%), bronchitis (2% to 5%), rhinitis (2% to 5%)

Miscellaneous: Lymph edema (10%), infection (2% to 9%), flu-like syndrome (2% to 7%), diaphoresis (2% to 5%), cyst (5%), tumor flare (3%)

Overdosage/Toxicology Symptoms include severe irritation to the stomach (necrosis, gastritis, ulceration and hemorrhage). There is no specific antidote. Treatment must be symptomatic. Vomiting may be induced if the patient is alert. Dialysis may be helpful because anastrozole is not highly protein bound. Treatment consists of general supportive care, including frequent monitoring of all vital signs and close observation.

Drug Interactions Inhibits CYP1A2 (weak), 2C8 (weak), 2C9 (weak), 3A4 (weak)

Estrogen derivatives (including vaginal preparations): May diminish the therapeutic effect of aromatase inhibitors; avoid concurrent use.

Tamoxifen: May decrease the serum concentration of anastrozole; avoid concurrent use.

Ethanol/Nutrition/Herb Interactions Herb/Nutraceutical: Avoid black cohosh, hops, licorice, red clover, thyme, and dong quai.

Stability Store at 20°C to 25°C (68°F to 77°F).

Mechanism of Action Potent and selective nonsteroidal aromatase inhibitor. By inhibiting aromatase, the conversion of androstenedione to estrone, and testosterone to estradiol, is prevented. Anastrozole causes an 85% decrease in estrone sulfate levels.

Pharmacodynamics

Onset of estradiol reduction: 24 hours (70% reduction; 80% after 2 weeks therapy)

Duration of estradiol reduction: 6 days

Pharmacokinetics

Absorption: Well absorbed; not affected by food

Protein binding, plasma: 40%

Metabolism: Extensively hepatic (85%) via N-dealkylation, hydroxylation, and glucuronidation; primary metabolite inactive

Half-life: 50 hours

Excretion: Feces (~75%); urine (10% as unchanged drug; 60% as metabolites)

Dosage

Geriatrics & Adults: Breast cancer: Oral (refer to individual protocols): 1 mg once daily

Renal Impairment: Dosage adjustment is not necessary.

Hepatic Impairment: Mild-to-moderate impairment: Plasma concentrations in subjects with stable hepatic cirrhosis were within the range concentrations in normal subjects across all clinical trials; therefore, no dosage adjustment required; however, patients should be monitored for side effects. Safety and efficacy in severe hepatic impairment have not been established.

Monitoring Parameters Liver function tests, total cholesterol, LDL levels

Test Interactions Lab test abnormalities: GGT, AST, ALT, alkaline phosphatase, total cholesterol, and LDL increased; threefold elevations of mean serum GGT levels have been observed among patients with liver metastases. These changes were likely related to the progression of liver metastases in these patients, although other contributing factors could not be ruled out. Mean serum total cholesterol levels increased by 0.5 mmol/L among patients.

Patient Information Take at the same time each day; may be taken with or without food

Special Geriatric Considerations No age-related changes in pharmacokinetics were noted in clinical trials.

Dosage Forms Excipient information presented when available (limited, particularly for generics); consult specific product labeling.

Tablet:

Arimidex®: 1 mg

- **Antara**™ *see* Fenofibrate *on page 604*
- **Antidiuretic Hormone** *see* Vasopressin *on page 1665*
- **Antivert®** *see* Meclizine *on page 961*
- **Anturane** *see* Sulfinpyrazone *on page 1503*
- **Anucort-HC®** *see* Hydrocortisone *on page 762*
- **Anu-Med [OTC]** *see* Phenylephrine *on page 1247*
- **Anusol-HC®** *see* Hydrocortisone *on page 762*
- **Anusol® HC-1 [OTC]** *see* Hydrocortisone *on page 762*
- **Anzemet®** *see* Dolasetron *on page 465*
- **APAP** *see* Acetaminophen *on page 29*
- **Apidra®** *see* Insulin Glulisine *on page 811*
- **Aplisol®** *see* Tuberculin Tests *on page 1643*
- **Aplonidine** *see* Apraclonidine *on page 116*
- **Apokyn®** *see* Apomorphine *on page 114*

Apomorphine (a poe MOR feen)

Related Information
Antiparkinsonian Agents *on page 1745*

U.S. Brand Names Apokyn®
Index Terms Apomorphine Hydrochloride; Apomorphine Hydrochloride Hemihydrate
Generic Available No
Pharmacologic Category Anti-Parkinson's Agent, Dopamine Agonist
Use Treatment of hypomobility, "off" episodes with Parkinson's disease
Unlabeled/Investigational Use Treatment of erectile dysfunction
Contraindications Hypersensitivity to apomorphine or any component of the formulation; concomitant use with 5HT$_3$ antagonists; intravenous administration
Warnings/Precautions May cause orthostatic hypotension, especially during dosage escalation; use extreme caution, especially in patients on antihypertensives and/or vasodilators. If patient develops clinically-significant orthostatic hypotension with test dose then apomorphine should not be used. Ergot-derived dopamine agonists have also been associated with fibrotic complications (eg, retroperitoneal fibrosis, pleural thickening, and pulmonary infiltrates). **Pretreatment with antiemetic is necessary.** Monitor patients for drowsiness. May cause hallucinations. Use caution in patients with risk factors for torsade de pointes. Use caution in cardiovascular and cerebrovascular disease. Use caution in patients with hepatic or renal dysfunction. Use with caution in patients with pre-existing dyskinesias; may be exacerbated. Dopaminergic agents have been associated with a syndrome resembling neuroleptic malignant syndrome on abrupt withdrawal or significant dosage reduction after long-term use. Retinal degeneration has been observed in animal studies when using dopamine agonists for prolonged periods. Rare cases of abuse have been reported. Contains metabisulfite.
Adverse Reactions (Reflective of adult population; not specific for elderly)
>10%:
   Cardiovascular: Chest pain/pressure or angina (15%)
   Central nervous system: Drowsiness or somnolence (35%), dizziness or orthostatic hypotension (20%)
   Gastrointestinal: Nausea and/or vomiting (30%)
   Neuromuscular & skeletal: Falls (30%), dyskinesias (24% to 35%)
   Respiratory: Yawning (40%), rhinorrhea (20%)
1% to 10%:
   Cardiovascular: Edema (10%), vasodilation (3%), hypotension (2%), syncope (2%), CHF
   Central nervous system: Hallucinations or confusion (10%), anxiety, depression, fatigue, headache, insomnia, pain
   Dermatologic: Bruising
   Endocrine & metabolic: Dehydration
   Gastrointestinal: Constipation, diarrhea
   Local: Injection site reactions
   Neuromuscular & skeletal: Arthralgias, weakness
   Miscellaneous: Diaphoresis increased
Overdosage/Toxicology An accidental overdose of 25 mg SubQ was reported resulting in nausea, loss of consciousness, bradycardia, and hypotension. Treatment should be supportive and symptomatic.
Drug Interactions Substrate (minor) of CYP1A2, 3A4, 2C19; **Inhibits** CYP1A2 (weak), 3A (weak), 2C19 (weak)

Antihypertensive medications and vasodilators: Concurrent use increased the risk of hypotension, myocardial infarction, serious falls, and bone and joint injuries. May be related to increased hypotension.

Antipsychotics (typical): May antagonize the dopaminergic action of dopamine agonist. Avoid concurrent use.

5HT$_3$ antagonists: Use with ondansetron resulted in severe hypotension and loss of consciousness. Concurrent use contraindicated.

Levodopa: Threshold levodopa concentration necessary to improve motor response was significantly reduced, leading to an increased duration of effect.

QT$_c$-prolonging agents: Doses of 6 mg or less are associated with minimal increases in QT$_c$ (mean increase of 3 msec at 20 and 90 minutes). A couple of patients exhibited large QT$_c$ increments (>60 msec from predose). Use caution with concurrent use.

Ethanol/Nutrition/Herb Interactions
Ethanol: Caution with ethanol consumption; may increase risk of hypotension.

Stability Store at 15°C to 30°C (59°F to 86°F).

Mechanism of Action Stimulates postsynaptic D2-type receptors within the caudate putamen in the brain.

Pharmacodynamics Onset: SubQ: Rapid

Pharmacokinetics
Distribution: V$_d$ (mean): 218 L
Metabolism: Not established; potential routes of metabolism include sulfation, N-demethylation, glucuronidation, and oxidation; catechol-O methyltransferase and nonenzymatic oxidation. CYP isoenzymes do not appear to play a significant role.
Half-life elimination: Terminal: 40 minutes
Time to peak, plasma: Improved motor scores: 20 minutes
Elimination: Urine 93% (as metabolites); feces 16%

Dosage
Geriatrics & Adults: Begin antiemetic therapy 3 days prior to initiation and continue for 2 months before reassessing need.
Parkinson's disease, "off" episode: SubQ: Initial test dose 2 mg, **medical supervision required; see "Note".** Subsequent dosing is based on both tolerance and response to initial test dose.
If patient tolerates test dose and responds: Starting dose: 2 mg as needed; may increase dose in 1 mg increments every few days; maximum dose: 6 mg
If patient tolerates but does not respond to 2 mg test dose: Second test dose: 4 mg
If patient tolerates and responds to 4 mg test dose: Starting dose: 3 mg, as needed for "off" episodes; may increase dose in 1 mg increments every few days; maximum dose 6 mg
If patient does not tolerate 4 mg test dose: Third test dose: 3 mg
If patient tolerates 3 mg test dose: Starting dose: 2 mg as needed for "off" episodes; may increase dose in 1 mg increments to a maximum of 3 mg
If therapy is interrupted for >1 week, restart at 2 mg and gradually titrate dose.
Note: Medical supervision is required for all test doses with standing and supine blood pressure monitoring predose and 20-, 40-, and 60 minutes postdose. If subsequent test doses are required, wait >2 hours before another test dose is given; next test dose should be timed with another "off" episode. If a single dose is ineffective for a particular "off" episode, then a second dose should not be given. The average dosing frequency was 3 times/day in the development program with limited experience in dosing >5 times/day and with total daily doses >20 mg. Apomorphine is intended to treat the "off" episodes associated with levodopa therapy of Parkinson's disease and has not been studied in levodopa-naive Parkinson's patients.
Renal Impairment:
Mild-to-moderate impairment: Reduce test dose and starting dose: 1 mg
Severe impairment: Has not been studied
Hepatic Impairment:
Mild-to-moderate impairment: Use caution
Severe impairment: Has not been studied

Administration SubQ: Initiate antiemetic 3 days before test dose of apomorphine and continue for 2 months (if patient to be treated) before reassessment. Administer in abdomen, upper arm, or upper leg; change site with each injection. 3 mL cartridges are used with a manual, reusable, multidose injector pen. Injector pen can deliver doses up to 1 mL in 0.02 mL increments. Do not give intravenously; thrombus formation or pulmonary embolism may occur.

Monitoring Parameters Each test dose: Supine and standing blood pressure predose and 20, 40, and 60 minutes postdose; drowsiness

Patient Information Patients or caregivers should be instructed to administer apomorphine as described in the Patient Instruction leaflets accompanying the product. Apomorphine is used to treat "off periods," not prevent them.

Apomorphine can cause nausea and vomiting. Patient should be on an antiemetic as prescribed by his/her physician. Avoid alcohol while on apomorphine. May cause drowsiness (do not drive until response of the drug is known). May cause dizziness (change positions slowly).
(Continued)

Apomorphine *(Continued)*

Dosage Forms Excipient information presented when available (limited, particularly for generics); consult specific product labeling.

Injection, solution, as hydrochloride:

Apokyn®: 10 mg/mL (2 mL) [ampul; contains sodium metabisulfite]; (3 mL) [multidose cartridge; contains sodium metabisulfite and benzyl alcohol]

Selected References

Olanow CW, Watts RL, and Koller WC, "An Algorithm (Decision Tree) for the Management of Parkinson's Disease (2001): Treatment Guidelines," *Neurology*, 2001, 56(11 Suppl 5):S1-S88.

♦ **Apomorphine Hydrochloride** *see* Apomorphine *on page 114*

♦ **Apomorphine Hydrochloride Hemihydrate** *see* Apomorphine *on page 114*

♦ **APPG** *see* Penicillin G Procaine *on page 1226*

♦ **Apra Children's [OTC]** *see* Acetaminophen *on page 29*

Apraclonidine *(a pra KLOE ni deen)*

Related Information

Glaucoma Drug Therapy *on page 1758*

Medication Safety Issues

Sound-alike/look-alike issues:

Iopidine® may be confused with indapamide, iodine, Lodine®

U.S. Brand Names Iopidine®

Canadian Brand Names Iopidine®

Index Terms Aplonidine; Apraclonidine Hydrochloride; p-Aminoclonidine

Generic Available No

Pharmacologic Category Alpha$_2$ Agonist, Ophthalmic

Use

0.5% solution: Short-term adjunctive therapy in patients on maximally tolerated medical therapy who require additional intraocular pressure (IOP) reduction

1% solution: Prevention and treatment of postsurgical intraocular pressure elevation

Contraindications Hypersensitivity to apraclonidine, clonidine, or any component of the formulation; use with or with 14 days of MAO inhibitors

Warnings/Precautions The IOP-lowering efficacy observed during the first month of therapy may not always reflect the long-term level of IOP reduction; routinely monitor IOP. Use with caution in patients with cardiovascular disease or a history of vasovagal reactions.

Adverse Reactions (Reflective of adult population; not specific for elderly)

Ocular:

5% to 15%: Discomfort, hyperemia, pruritus

1% to 5%: Blanching, blurred vision, conjunctivitis, discharge, dry eye, foreign body sensation, lid edema, tearing

Other body systems:

1% to 10%: Gastrointestinal: Dry mouth (10%)

<3%:

Cardiovascular: Arrhythmia, chest pain, facial edema, peripheral edema

Central nervous system: Depression, dizziness, headache, insomnia, malaise, nervousness, somnolence

Dermatologic: Contact dermatitis, dermatitis

Gastrointestinal: Constipation, nausea, taste perversion

Neuromuscular & skeletal: Abnormal coordination, myalgia, paresthesia, weakness

Respiratory: Asthma, dry nose, dyspnea, parosmia, pharyngitis, rhinitis

Drug Interactions

Antihypertensive agents: Apraclonidine may reduce pulse and blood pressure, use systemic agents with caution.

Beta-blockers: Ophthalmic agents may have additive effect on IOP; apraclonidine may reduce pulse and blood pressure, use systemic agents with caution.

CNS depressants: May have additive CNS depression.

MAO inhibitors: Concomitant use is contraindicated.

Pilocarpine: Ophthalmic use may have additive effect on IOP.

Stability Store between 2°C to 27°C (36°F to 80°F); protect from freezing and light.

Mechanism of Action Apraclonidine is a potent alpha-adrenergic agent similar to clonidine; relatively selective for alpha$_2$-receptors but does retain some binding to alpha$_1$-receptors; appears to result in reduction of aqueous humor formation; its penetration through the blood-brain barrier is more polar than clonidine which reduces its penetration through the blood-brain barrier and suggests that its pharmacological profile is characterized by peripheral rather than central effects.

Pharmacodynamics

Onset of action: 1 hour

Maximum IOP: 3-5 hours

Pharmacokinetics Half-life: 8 hours
Dosage
  Geriatrics & Adults: Postsurgical intraocular pressure elevation (prevention/treatment): Ophthalmic:
    0.5%: Instill 1-2 drops in the affected eye(s) 3 times/day
    1%: Instill 1 drop in operative eye 1 hour prior to anterior segment laser surgery, second drop in eye immediately upon completion of procedure
  Renal Impairment: Although the topical use of apraclonidine has not been studied in renal failure patients, structurally-related clonidine undergoes a significant increase in half-life in patients with severe renal impairment. Close monitoring of cardiovascular parameters in patients with impaired renal function is advised.
  Hepatic Impairment: Close monitoring of cardiovascular parameters in patients with impaired liver function is advised because the systemic dosage form of clonidine is partially metabolized in the liver.
Administration Wait 5 minutes between instillation of other ophthalmic agents to avoid washout of previous dose; after topical instillation, finger pressure should be applied to lacrimal sac to decrease drainage into the nose and throat and minimize possible systemic absorption
Monitoring Parameters Intraocular pressure, fundoscopic exam, visual field testing
Reference Range Steady-state concentration: Peak: 0.9 ng/mL; trough: 0.5 ng/mL
Patient Information May sting on instillation, do not touch dropper to eye; visual acuity may be decreased after administration; night vision may be decreased; distance vision may be altered; read package instructions for insertion
Special Geriatric Considerations Determine that the patient or caregiver can adequately administer ophthalmic medication dosage form.
Dosage Forms Excipient information presented when available (limited, particularly for generics); consult specific product labeling.
  Solution, ophthalmic:
    Iopidine®: 0.5% (5 mL, 10 mL); 1% (0.1 mL) [contains benzalkonium chloride]

♦ **Apraclonidine Hydrochloride** *see* Apraclonidine *on page 116*

Aprepitant (ap RE pi tant)

U.S. Brand Names Emend®
Index Terms L 754030; MK 869
Generic Available No
Pharmacologic Category Antiemetic; Substance P/Neurokinin 1 Receptor Antagonist
Use Prevention of acute and delayed nausea and vomiting associated with moderately- and highly-emetogenic chemotherapy in combination with a corticosteroid and 5-HT$_3$ receptor antagonist; prevention of postoperative nausea and vomiting (PONV)
Contraindications Hypersensitivity to aprepitant or any component of the formulation; use with astemizole, cisapride, pimozide, or terfenadine
Warnings/Precautions Use caution with agents primarily metabolized via CYP3A4; aprepitant is a 3A4 inhibitor. Effect on orally administered 3A4 substrates is greater than those administered intravenously. Use caution with hepatic impairment. Not intended for treatment of existing nausea and vomiting or for chronic continuous therapy.
Adverse Reactions (Reflective of adult population; not specific for elderly)
  Note: Adverse reactions reported as part of a combination chemotherapy regimen or with general anesthesia.

>10%:
  Central nervous system: Fatigue (18% to 22%)
  Gastrointestinal: Nausea (7% to 13%), constipation (9% to 12%)
  Neuromuscular & skeletal: Weakness (3% to 18%)
  Miscellaneous: Hiccups (11%)
1% to 10%:
  Cardiovascular: Hypotension (6%), bradycardia (4%)
  Central nervous system: Dizziness (>0.5% to 7%)
  Endocrine & metabolic: Dehydration (6%), hot flushing (3%)
  Gastrointestinal: Diarrhea (6% to 10%), dyspepsia (8%), abdominal pain (5%), stomatitis (5%), epigastric discomfort (4%), gastritis (4%), mucous membrane disorder (3%), throat pain (3%), vomiting (3%)
  Hematologic: Neutropenia (3% to 9%), leukopenia (9%), hemoglobin decreased (2% to 5%)
  Hepatic: ALT increased (1% to 6%), AST increased (3%)
  Renal: BUN increased (5%), proteinuria (7%), serum creatinine increased (4%)
Overdosage/Toxicology Limited data available; single doses up to 600 mg and daily doses of 375 mg for up to 42 days were well-tolerated in healthy subjects; drowsiness and headache were noted at a dose of 1440 mg. In cancer patients, a single dose of
(Continued)

Aprepitant (Continued)

375 mg followed by 250 mg on days 2 to 5 was well tolerated. In case of overdose, treatment should be symptom-directed and supportive. Not removed by hemodialysis.

Drug Interactions Substrate of CYP1A2 (minor), 2C19 (minor), 3A4 (major); **Inhibits** CYP2C9 (weak), 2C19 (weak), 3A4 (moderate); **Induces** CYP2C9 (weak), 3A4 (weak)

Antifungal agents (imidazole): May decrease the metabolism, via CYP isoenzymes, of aprepitant.

Benzodiazepines (metabolized by oxidation): Aprepitant may increase the serum concentration of benzodiazepines (metabolized by oxidation). Examples of such benzodiazepines include alprazolam, chlordiazepoxide, clonazepam, clorazepate, diazepam, estazolam, flurazepam, midazolam, quazepam, and triazolam.

Corticosteroids: Aprepitant increases the levels of systemic corticosteroids. Dexamethasone doses should be decreased by 50% (oral) when compared to dose given without aprepitant. Methylprednisolone doses should be decreased by 25% (I.V.) or by 50% (oral) when used concurrently. When using a single dose of each agent, no adjustment is required

CYP3A4 inducers: CYP3A4 inducers may decrease the levels/effects of aprepitant. Example inducers include aminoglutethimide, carbamazepine, nafcillin, nevirapine, phenobarbital, phenytoin, and rifamycins.

CYP3A4 inhibitors: May increase the levels/effects of aprepitant. Example inhibitors include azole antifungals, clarithromycin, diclofenac, doxycycline, erythromycin, imatinib, isoniazid, nefazodone, nicardipine, propofol, protease inhibitors, quinidine, telithromycin, and verapamil.

CYP3A4 substrates: Aprepitant may increase the levels/effects of CYP3A4 substrates. Example substrates include benzodiazepines, calcium channel blockers, ergot derivatives, mirtazapine, nateglinide, nefazodone, tacrolimus, and venlafaxine.

Diltiazem: May increase plasma levels of aprepitant. Aprepitant may increase diltiazem levels.

Hormone-containing contraceptives (estrogens): Aprepitant may decrease the plasma levels of ethinyl estradiol. Contraceptive efficacy may be reduced; a nonhormonal form of contraception is recommended by the manufacturer during treatment and for 1 month following the last dose.

Pimecrolimus: Aprepitant may increase the levels/effects of pimecrolimus.

Rifampin: May significantly decrease the levels/effects of aprepitant

Warfarin: Aprepitant may increase warfarin metabolism and the INR may be decreased; monitoring recommended in the 2-week period (particularly days 7-10) following start of each cycle.

Ethanol/Nutrition/Herb Interactions

Food: Aprepitant serum concentration may be increased when taken with grapefruit juice; avoid concurrent use.

Herb/Nutraceutical: St John's wort may decrease aprepitant levels.

Stability Store at controlled room temperature of 20°C to 25°C (68°F to 77°F).

Mechanism of Action Prevents acute and delayed vomiting at the substance P/neurokinin 1 (NK$_1$) receptor; augments the antiemetic activity of the 5-HT$_3$ receptor antagonist and corticosteroid activity and inhibits both acute and delayed phases of cisplatin-induced emesis.

Pharmacokinetics

Distribution: V$_d$: 70 L; crosses the blood brain barrier

Protein binding: >95%

Metabolism: Extensively hepatic

Bioavailability: 60% to 65%

Half-life: Terminal: 9-13 hours

Time to peak, plasma: 4 hours

Dosage

Geriatrics & Adults:

Prevention of chemotherapy induced nausea/vomiting: Oral: 125 mg on day 1, followed by 80 mg on days 2 and 3 in combination with a corticosteroid and 5-HT$_3$ receptor antagonist

Prevention of PONV: Oral: 40 mg within 3 hours prior to induction

Renal Impairment: No dose adjustment necessary in patients with renal disease or end-stage renal disease maintained on hemodialysis.

Hepatic Impairment:

Mild-to-moderate impairment (Child-Pugh score 5-9): No adjustment necessary.

Severe impairment (Child-Pugh score >9): No data available.

Administration Administer with or without food.

Chemotherapy induced nausea/vomiting: First dose should be given 1 hour prior to antineoplastic therapy; subsequent doses should be given in the morning.

PONV: Administer within 3 hours of induction

Patient Information May not mix well with other medicines; check medicines with prescriber. Patients taking warfarin therapy should have their clotting status monitored within a 2-week period of using aprepitant, following the initiation of therapy and each subsequent use.

Special Geriatric Considerations In two studies by the manufacturer, with a total of 544 patients, 31% were >65 years of age, while 5% were >75 years. No differences in safety and efficacy were noted between elderly subjects and younger adults. No dosing adjustment is necessary.

Dosage Forms Excipient information presented when available (limited, particularly for generics); consult specific product labeling.

Capsule:

Emend®: 40 mg, 80 mg, 125 mg

Combination package: Capsule 80 mg (2s), capsule 125 mg (1s)

Selected References

Kris MG, Hesketh PJ, Somerfield MR, et al, "American Society of Clinical Oncology Guideline for Antiemetics in Oncology: Update 2006," *J Clin Oncol*, 2006, 24(18):2932-47.

NCCN (National Comprehensive Cancer Network) "Practice Guidelines in Oncology: Antiemesis Version 2.2006." Available at http://www.nccn.org/professionals/physician_gls/PDF/antiemesis.pdf. Last accessed August 15, 2006.

♦ **Apresoline [DSC]** *see* HydrALAZINE *on page 754*
♦ **Aprodine® [OTC]** *see* Triprolidine and Pseudoephedrine *on page 1638*
♦ **Aquachloral® Supprettes®** *see* Chloral Hydrate *on page 285*
♦ **Aquanil™ HC [OTC]** *see* Hydrocortisone *on page 762*
♦ **AquaSite® [OTC]** *see* Artificial Tears *on page 124*
♦ **Aquasol E® [OTC]** *see* Vitamin E *on page 1677*
♦ **Aquavit-E [OTC]** *see* Vitamin E *on page 1677*
♦ **Aqueous Procaine Penicillin G** *see* Penicillin G Procaine *on page 1226*
♦ **Aquoral™** *see* Saliva Substitute *on page 1443*
♦ **Aranesp®** *see* Darbepoetin Alfa *on page 397*
♦ **Arava®** *see* Leflunomide *on page 879*
♦ **Aredia®** *see* Pamidronate *on page 1193*

Arformoterol (ar for MOE ter ol)

Related Information
Inhalant Agents *on page 1760*
U.S. Brand Names Brovana™
Index Terms Arformoterol Tartrate; (R,R)-Formoterol L-Tartrate
Generic Available No
Pharmacologic Category Beta$_2$-Adrenergic Agonist
Use Long-term maintenance treatment of bronchoconstriction in chronic obstructive pulmonary disease (COPD), including chronic bronchitis and emphysema
Restrictions An FDA-approved medication guide must be distributed when dispensing an outpatient prescription (new or refill) where this medication is to be used without direct supervision of a healthcare provider. Medication guides are available at http://www.fda.gov/cder/Offices/ODS/medication_guides.htm.
Contraindications Hypersensitivity to arformoterol, racemic formoterol, or any component of the formulation
Warnings/Precautions [U.S. Boxed Warning]: Long-acting beta$_2$-agonists may increase the risk of asthma-related deaths. In a large, randomized clinical trial (SMART, 2006), salmeterol was associated with a small, but statistically significant increase in asthma-related deaths (when added to usual asthma therapy); risk may be greater in African-American patients versus Caucasians. Data is not available to determine whether rate of death is increased with long-acting beta$_2$-agonists in COPD setting. Rarely, paradoxical bronchospasm may occur with use of inhaled bronchodilating agents; this should be distinguished from inadequate response. Immediate hypersensitivity reactions (urticaria, angioedema, rash, bronchospasm) have been reported. Do not exceed recommended dose; serious adverse events, including fatalities, have been associated with excessive use of inhaled sympathomimetics.

Use with caution in patients with cardiovascular disease (eg, arrhythmia, hypertension, CHF); beta-agonists may cause elevation in blood pressure, heart rate and result in CNS stimulation/excitation. Beta$_2$-agonists may also increase risk of arrhythmias and prolong QT_c interval. Arformoterol should only be used for long-term maintenance treatment and should not be used as rescue therapy in treatment of acute episodes. It should not be initiated in patients with acutely deteriorating COPD or combined with other long-acting beta$_2$-agonists. Use with caution in patients with diabetes mellitus; beta$_2$-agonists may increase serum glucose. Use caution in hepatic impairment; systemic clearance prolonged in hepatic dysfunction. Use with caution in hyperthyroidism; may stimulate thyroid activity. Use with caution in patients with hypokalemia; beta$_2$-agonists may decrease serum potassium. Use with caution in patients with seizure disorders; beta$_2$-agonists may result in CNS stimulation/excitation.
(Continued)

119

Arformoterol *(Continued)*

Tolerance/tachyplaxis to the bronchodilator effect, measured by FEV_1, has been observed in studies. Patients using inhaled, short-acting beta$_2$-agonists should be instructed to discontinue routine use of these medications prior to beginning treatment; short-acting agents should be reserved for symptomatic relief of acute symptoms. Patients must be instructed to seek medical attention in cases where acute symptoms are not relieved or a previous level of response is diminished. The need to increase frequency of use may indicate deterioration of COPD, and treatment must not be delayed.

Adverse Reactions (Reflective of adult population; not specific for elderly)
2% to 10%:
Cardiovascular: Chest pain (7%), peripheral edema (3%)
Central nervous system: Pain (8%)
Dermatologic: Rash (4%)
Gastrointestinal: Diarrhea (6%)
Neuromuscular & skeletal: Back pain (6%), leg cramps (4%)
Respiratory: Dyspnea (4%), sinusitis (5%), congestive conditions (2%)
Miscellaneous: Flu-like syndrome (3%)

Overdosage/Toxicology Symptoms of excessive beta-adrenergic stimulation include hyperglycemia, metabolic acidosis, arrhythmias, tachycardia, tremor, hypertension, angina, and seizures. Hypokalemia also may occur. Cardiac arrest and death may be associated with abuse of beta-agonist bronchodilators. Treatment should be symptom-directed and supportive. Cautious use of cardioselective beta-adrenergic blocking agents may be considered in severe cases.

Drug Interactions Substrate of CY2D6 (minor) and CYP2C19 (minor)
Alpha-/beta-blockers: May diminish the bronchodilatory effect of beta$_2$-agonists. Avoid concomitant use; if used concomitantly monitor for diminished bronchodilatory effect of beta$_2$-agonists.
Atomoxetine: May enhance the tachycardic effect of beta$_2$-agonists. Monitor for increased cardiovascular effects of beta$_2$-agonists.
Beta-blockers (beta$_1$ selective): Beta$_2$-agonists may diminish the bradycardic effect of beta-blockers (beta$_1$ selective), particularly if beta-blocker is being used at higher doses.
Beta-blockers (nonselective): May diminish the bronchodilator effect of beta$_2$ agonists. Consider avoiding concomitant use; if used concomitantly, monitor for decreased therapeutic effect.
Betahistine: May diminish the bronchodilator effect of beta$_2$-agonists; monitor.
Sympathomimetics: May enhance the adverse/toxic effect of arformoterol.

Stability Prior to dispensing, store in protective foil pouch under refrigeration at 2°C to 8°C (36°F to 46°F). Protect from light and excessive heat. After dispensing, unopened foil pouches may be stored at room temperature at 20°C to 25°C (68°F to 77°F) for up to 6 weeks. Only remove vial from foil pouch immediately before use.

Mechanism of Action Arformoterol, the (R,R)-enantiomer of the racemic formoterol, is a long-acting beta$_2$-agonist that relaxes bronchial smooth muscle by selective action on beta$_2$-receptors with little effect on cardiovascular system.

Pharmacokinetics
Onset of action: 7-20 minutes
Peak effect: 1-3 hours
Absorption: A portion of inhaled dose is absorbed into systemic circulation
Protein binding: 52% to 65%
Metabolism: Hepatic via direct glucuronidation and secondarily via O-demethylation; CYP2D6 and CYP2C19 (to a lesser extent) involved in O-demethylation
Half-life elimination: 26 hours
Time to peak: 0.5-3 hours

Dosage
Geriatrics & Adults: COPD: Nebulization: 15 mcg twice daily; maximum: 30 mcg/day
Renal Impairment: No adjustment required.
Hepatic Impairment: No dosage adjustment required, but use caution; systemic drug exposure prolonged (1.3- to 2.4-fold).

Administration Nebulization: Remove each vial from individually sealed foil pouch immediately before use. Use with standard jet nebulizer connected to an air compressor, administer with mouthpiece or face mask. Administer vial undiluted and do not mix with other medications in nebulizer.

Monitoring Parameters FEV_1, peak flow, and/or other pulmonary function tests; blood pressure, heart rate; CNS stimulation; serum glucose, serum potassium. Monitor for increased use of short-acting beta$_2$-agonist inhalers; may be marker of a deteriorating COPD condition.

Special Geriatric Considerations In clinical trials, no significant difference was seen in the AUC and C_{max} between younger and older subjects. In addition, no significant difference in clinical response was noted.

Dosage Forms Excipient information presented when available (limited, particularly for generics); consult specific product labeling.
Solution for nebulization:
Brovana™: 15 mcg/2 mL (30s)

♦ **Arformoterol Tartrate** *see Arformoterol on page 119*
♦ **8-Arginine Vasopressin** *see Vasopressin on page 1665*
♦ **Aricept®** *see Donepezil on page 467*
♦ **Aricept® ODT** *see Donepezil on page 467*
♦ **Arimidex®** *see Anastrozole on page 112*

Aripiprazole (ay ri PIP ray zole)

Related Information
Antipsychotic Agents *on page 1747*
Atypical Antipsychotics *on page 1749*
Medication Safety Issues
Sound-alike/look-alike issues:
Aripiprazole may be confused with proton pump inhibitors (eg, rabeprazole)
U.S. Brand Names Abilify®; Abilify® Discmelt™
Index Terms BMS 337039; OPC-14597
Generic Available No
Pharmacologic Category Antipsychotic Agent, Atypical
Use Treatment of schizophrenia; stabilization and maintenance therapy of bipolar disorder (with acute manic or mixed episodes); agitation associated with schizophrenia or bipolar mania
Unlabeled/Investigational Use Depression with psychotic features
Contraindications Hypersensitivity to aripiprazole or any component of the formulation
Warnings/Precautions [U.S. Boxed Warning]: Patients with dementia-related psychosis treated with atypical antipsychotics are at an increased risk of death compared to placebo. An increased incidence of cerebrovascular adverse events (including fatalities) has been reported in elderly patients with dementia-related psychosis. Risk may be increased by dehydration; use caution with concurrent diuretics. Aripiprazole is not approved for this indication.

May cause extrapyramidal symptoms, including pseudoparkinsonism, acute dystonic reactions, akathisia, and tardive dyskinesia (risk of these reactions is very low relative to typical/conventional antipsychotics, frequencies reported are similar to placebo). May be associated with neuroleptic malignant syndrome (NMS).

May be sedating, use with caution in disorders where CNS depression is a feature. May cause orthostatic hypotension (although reported rates are similar to placebo); use caution in patients at risk of this effect or those who would not tolerate transient hypotensive episodes (cerebrovascular disease, cardiovascular disease, or other medications which may predispose).

Use caution in patients with Parkinson's disease; predisposition to seizures; and severe cardiac disease. May alter cardiac conduction; life-threatening arrhythmias have occurred with therapeutic doses of antipsychotics. Esophageal dysmotility and aspiration have been associated with antipsychotic use; use caution in patients at risk of pneumonia (eg, Alzheimer's disease). May alter temperature regulation. Significant weight gain has been observed with antipsychotic therapy; incidence varies with product. Monitor waist circumference and BMI.

Atypical antipsychotics have been associated with development of hyperglycemia; in some cases, may be extreme and associated with ketoacidosis, hyperosmolar coma, or death. Reports of hyperglycemia with aripiprazole therapy have been few and specific risk associated with this agent is not known. Use caution in patients with diabetes or other disorders of glucose regulation; monitor for worsening of glucose control.

The possibility of a suicide attempt is inherent in psychotic illness or bipolar disorder; use caution in high-risk patients during initiation of therapy. Prescriptions should be written for the smallest quantity consistent with good patient care. Abilify® Discmelt™: Use caution in phenylketonuria; contains phenylalanine.
Adverse Reactions (Reflective of adult population; not specific for elderly)
Unless otherwise noted, frequency of adverse reactions is shown as reported for oral administration.
>10%:
Central nervous system: Headache (31%; injection 12%), agitation (25%), anxiety (20%), insomnia (20%), extrapyramidal symptoms (6% to 17%), somnolence (12% to 15%, dose related; injection 7%), akathisia (12% to 15%; injection 2%), light-headedness (11%)
(Continued)

Aripiprazole *(Continued)*

Gastrointestinal: Nausea (16%; injection 9%), dyspepsia (15%; injection 1%), constipation (11% to 13%), vomiting (11%; injection 3%), weight gain (8% to 30%, highest frequency in patients with BMI <23)

1% to 10%:

Cardiovascular: Edema (peripheral 2%), hypertension (2%), tachycardia, hypotension, bradycardia, chest pain

Central nervous system: Abnormal dreams, confusion, delusion, depression, fever, hallucination, hostility, mania, nervousness, paranoid reaction, schizophrenic reaction, suicidal thought

Dermatologic: Bruising, dry skin, skin ulcer

Endocrine & metabolic: Dehydration

Gastrointestinal: Salivation increased (3%), xerostomia (injection 1%), weight loss

Genitourinary: Urinary incontinence, pelvic pain

Hematologic: Anemia

Neuromuscular & skeletal: Tremor (4% to 9%), weakness (8%), myalgia (4%), neck pain, neck rigidity, muscle cramp, CPK increased, abnormal gait

Ocular: Blurred vision (3%), conjunctivitis

Respiratory: Rhinitis (4%), pharyngitis (4%), cough (3%), asthma, dyspnea, pneumonia, sinusitis

Miscellaneous: Accidental injury (5% to 6%), flu-like syndrome, diaphoresis

Overdosage/Toxicology Ingestion of 1080 mg has been reported, with full recovery. Common symptoms of overdose include somnolence, tremor, and vomiting. Treatment is supportive and symptom-directed. An ECG should be obtained and cardiac monitoring initiated if QT_c prolongation is present. Administration of 50 g activated charcoal 1 hour after a 15 mg dose reportedly decreased AUC and C_{max} values by 50%. Due to the high degree of protein binding, hemodialysis is unlikely to be effective in removing aripiprazole.

Drug Interactions Substrate (major) of CYP2D6, 3A4

Acetylcholinesterase inhibitors (central): May increase the risk of antipsychotic-related extrapyramidal symptoms; monitor.

Carbamazepine: Carbamazepine may decrease aripiprazole levels. Manufacturer recommends a doubling of the aripiprazole dose when carbamazepine is added.

CNS depressants: May increase the adverse effects/toxicity of other CNS depressants; monitor.

CYP2D6 inhibitors: May increase the levels/effects of aripiprazole. Example inhibitors include chlorpromazine, delavirdine, fluoxetine, miconazole, paroxetine, pergolide, quinidine, quinine, ritonavir, and ropinirole.

CYP3A4 inducers: CYP3A4 inducers may decrease the levels/effects of aripiprazole. Example inducers include aminoglutethimide, carbamazepine, nafcillin, nevirapine, phenobarbital, phenytoin, and rifamycins.

CYP3A4 inhibitors: May increase the levels/effects of aripiprazole. Example inhibitors include azole antifungals, clarithromycin, diclofenac, doxycycline, erythromycin, imatinib, isoniazid, nefazodone, nicardipine, propofol, protease inhibitors, quinidine, telithromycin, and verapamil.

Ketoconazole: Ketoconazole may increase aripiprazole levels. Manufacturer recommends a 50% reduction in aripiprazole dose during concurrent ketoconazole therapy.

Lithium: May increase neurotoxic effects of antipsychotics; monitor.

Quinidine: May increase the levels/effects of aripiprazole. Manufacturer recommends a 50% reduction in aripiprazole dose during concomitant therapy.

Ethanol/Nutrition/Herb Interactions

Ethanol: Avoid ethanol (may increase CNS depression).

Food: Ingestion with a high-fat meal delays time to peak plasma level.

Herb/Nutraceutical: St John's wort may decrease aripiprazole levels. Avoid kava kava, gotu kola, valerian, St John's wort (may increase CNS depression).

Stability

Injection solution: Store at 15°C to 30°C (59°F to 86°F). Protect from light.

Oral solution: Store at 15°C to 30°C (59°F to 86°F). Use within 6 months after opening.

Tablet: Store at 15°C to 30°C (59°F to 86°F).

Mechanism of Action Aripiprazole is a quinolinone antipsychotic which exhibits high affinity for D_2, D_3, $5-HT_{1A}$, and $5-HT_{2A}$ receptors; moderate affinity for D_4, $5-HT_{2C}$, $5-HT_7$, alpha$_1$ adrenergic, and H_1 receptors. It also possesses moderate affinity for the serotonin reuptake transporter; has no affinity for muscarinic (cholinergic) receptors. Aripiprazole functions as a partial agonist at the D_2 and $5-HT_{1A}$ receptors, and as an antagonist at the $5-HT_{2A}$ receptor.

Pharmacodynamics Onset: Initial: 1-3 weeks

Pharmacokinetics

Absorption: Well absorbed

Distribution: V_d: 4.9 L/kg

Protein binding: 99%, primarily to albumin

Metabolism: Hepatic, via CYP2D6, CYP3A4 (dehydro-aripiprazole metabolite has affinity for D2 receptors similar to the parent drug and represents 40% of the parent drug exposure in plasma)

Bioavailability: I.M.: 100%; Tablet: 87%

Half-life: Aripiprazole: 75 hours; CYP2D6 poor metabolizers: 146 hours; dehydro-aripiprazole: 94 hours

Time to peak, plasma: I.M.: 1-3 hours; Tablet: 3-5 hours
  With high-fat meal: Aripiprazole: Delayed by 3 hours; dehydro-aripiprazole: Delayed by 12 hours

Excretion: Feces (55%, ~18% unchanged drug); urine (25%, <1% unchanged drug)

Dosage

Geriatrics & Adults: Note: Oral solution may be substituted for the oral tablet on a mg-per-mg basis, up to 25 mg. Patients receiving 30 mg tablets should be given 25 mg oral solution. Orally disintegrating tablets (Abilify® Discmelt™) are bioequivalent to the immediate release tablets (Abilify®).

Acute agitation (schizophrenia/bipolar mania): I.M.: 9.75 mg as a single dose (range: 5.25-15 mg); repeated doses may be given at ≥2-hour intervals to a maximum of 30 mg/day. **Note:** If ongoing therapy with aripiprazole is necessary, transition to oral therapy as soon as possible.

Schizophrenia: Oral: 10-15 mg once daily; may be increased to a maximum of 30 mg once daily (efficacy at dosages above 10-15 mg has not been shown to be increased). Dosage titration should not be more frequent than every 2 weeks.

Depression (unlabeled use): 5-30 mg

Bipolar disorder (acute manic or mixed episodes):
  Stabilization: Oral: 30 mg once daily; may require a decrease to 15 mg based on tolerability (15% of patients had dose decreased); safety of doses >30 mg/day has not been evaluated
  Maintenance: Continue stabilization dose for up to 6 weeks; efficacy of continued treatment >6 weeks has not been established.

Dosage adjustment with concurrent CYP450 inducer or inhibitor therapy: Oral:
  CYP3A4 inducers (eg, carbamazepine): Aripiprazole dose should be doubled (20-30 mg/day); dose should be subsequently reduced (10-15 mg/day) if concurrent inducer agent discontinued.
  CYP3A4 inhibitors (eg, ketoconazole): Aripiprazole dose should be reduced to $\frac{1}{2}$ of the usual dose, and proportionally increased upon discontinuation of the inhibitor agent.
  CYP2D6 inhibitors (eg, fluoxetine, paroxetine): Aripiprazole dose should be reduced to $\frac{1}{2}$ of the usual dose, and proportionally increased upon discontinuation of the inhibitor agent.

Renal Impairment: No dosage adjustment required.

Hepatic Impairment: No dosage adjustment required.

Administration

Injection: For I.M. use only; do not administer SubQ or I.V.; inject slowly into deep muscle mass

Oral: May be administered with or without food. Tablet and oral solution may be interchanged on a mg-per-mg basis, up to 25 mg. Doses using 30 mg tablets should be exchanged for 25 mg oral solution. Orally disintegrating tablets (Abilify® Discmelt™) are bioequivalent to the immediate release tablets (Abilify®).

Orally-disintegrating tablet: Remove from foil blister by peeling back (do not push tablet through the foil). Place tablet in mouth immediately upon removal. Tablet dissolves rapidly in saliva and may be swallowed without liquid. If needed, can be taken with liquid. Do not split tablet.

Monitoring Parameters Vital signs; fasting lipid profile and fasting blood glucose/Hgb A_{1c} (prior to treatment, at 3 months, then annually); BMI, personal/family history of diabetes, waist circumference; blood pressure; mental status, abnormal involuntary movement scale (AIMS), extrapyramidal symptoms (EPS). Weight should be assessed prior to treatment, at 4 weeks, 8 weeks, 12 weeks, and then at quarterly intervals. Consider titrating to a different antipsychotic agent for a weight gain ≥5% of the initial weight.

Patient Information Inform prescriber of all prescriptions, OTC medications, or herbal products you are taking, and any allergies you have. Do not take any new medication during therapy without consulting prescriber. Take exactly as directed at the same time of day, without regard to meals. Do not alter dose; it may take some time to achieve desired results. Avoid alcohol. May cause headache, dizziness, lightheadedness, anxiety (use caution when driving or engaged in potentially hazardous tasks until response to drug is known), nausea or vomiting (small, frequent meals and frequent mouth care may help), orthostatic hypotension (use caution when changing position from lying or sitting to standing and when climbing stairs). Report chest pain or palpitations; persistent gastrointestinal effects; muscle or skeletal pain, weakness, cramping, or tremors; altered gait; change in vision; increased weight gain or loss; respiratory changes or flu-like symptoms.

(Continued)

Aripiprazole *(Continued)*

Special Geriatric Considerations Elderly patients have an increased risk of adverse response to side effects or adverse reactions to antipsychotics. Aripiprazole has been studied in elderly patients with psychosis associated with Alzheimer's disease. The package insert does not provide the outcomes of this study other than somnolence was more frequent with aripiprazole (8%) than placebo (1%). Clinical data have shown an increased incidence of serious cerebrovascular events in the elderly, some fatal. In light of significant risks and adverse effects in the elderly population (compared with limited data demonstrating efficacy in the treatment of dementia-related psychosis, aggression, and agitation), an extensive risk:benefit analysis should be performed prior to use. Aripiprazole's delayed onset of action and long half-life may limit its role in treating older persons with psychosis. Not approved for the treatment of patients with dementia-related psychosis.

Dosage Forms Excipient information presented when available (limited, particularly for generics); consult specific product labeling.

Injection, solution:
Abilify®: 7.5 mg/mL (1.3 mL)
Solution, oral:
Abilify®: 1 mg/mL (150 mL) [contains sucrose 400 mg/mL and fructose 200 mg/mL; orange cream flavor]
Tablet:
Abilify®: 2 mg, 5 mg, 10 mg, 15 mg, 20 mg, 30 mg
Tablet, orally disintegrating:
Abilify® Discmelt™: 10 mg [contains phenylalanine 1.12 mg; creme de vanilla flavor]; 15 mg [contains phenylalanine 1.68 mg; creme de vanilla flavor]

Selected References
Schneider LS, Tariot PN, Dagerman KS, et al, "Effectiveness of Atypical Antipsychotic Drugs in Patients With Alzheimer's Disease," *N Engl J Med*, 2006, 355(15):1525-38.

♦ **Aristospan®** *see* Triamcinolone *on page 1619*
♦ **Arixtra®** *see* Fondaparinux *on page 674*
♦ **Armour® Thyroid** *see* Thyroid *on page 1559*
♦ **Aromasin®** *see* Exemestane *on page 590*
♦ **Artane** *see* Trihexyphenidyl *on page 1631*
♦ **ArthriCare® for Women Extra Moisturizing [OTC] [DSC]** *see* Capsaicin *on page 225*
♦ **ArthriCare® for Women Multi-Action [OTC] [DSC]** *see* Capsaicin *on page 225*
♦ **ArthriCare® for Women Silky Dry [OTC] [DSC]** *see* Capsaicin *on page 225*
♦ **ArthriCare® for Women Ultra Strength [OTC] [DSC]** *see* Capsaicin *on page 225*
♦ **Arthropan®** *see* Salicylates (Various Salts) *on page 1439*
♦ **Arthrotec®** *see* Diclofenac and Misoprostol *on page 428*

Artificial Tears (ar ti FISH il tears)

Medication Safety Issues
Sound-alike/look-alike issues:
Isopto® Tears may be confused with Isoptin®
Murocel® may be confused with Murocoll-2®

U.S. Brand Names Akwa Tears® [OTC]; AquaSite® [OTC]; Bion® Tears [OTC]; HypoTears [OTC]; HypoTears PF [OTC]; Liquifilm® Tears [OTC]; Moisture® Eyes [OTC]; Moisture® Eyes PM [OTC]; Murine® Tears [OTC]; Murocel® [OTC]; Nature's Tears® [OTC]; Nu-Tears® [OTC]; Nu-Tears® II [OTC]; OcuCoat® [OTC]; OcuCoat® PF [OTC]; Puralube® Tears [OTC]; Refresh® [OTC]; Refresh Plus® [OTC]; Refresh Tears® [OTC]; Soothe® [OTC]; Systane® [OTC]; Systane® Free [OTC]; Teargen® [OTC]; Teargen® II [OTC]; Tearisol® [OTC]; Tears Again® [OTC]; Tears Naturale® [OTC]; Tears Naturale® Free [OTC]; Tears Naturale® II [OTC]; Tears Plus® [OTC]; Tears Renewed® [OTC]; Ultra Tears® [OTC]; Viva-Drops® [OTC]

Canadian Brand Names Teardrops®

Index Terms Hydroxyethylcellulose; Polyvinyl Alcohol

Generic Available Yes

Pharmacologic Category Ophthalmic Agent, Miscellaneous

Use Relief of dry eyes and eye irritation (ophthalmic)

Contraindications Hypersensitivity to any component

Warnings/Precautions Individual product formulations may include (as an active ingredient) benzalkonium chloride, polyvinyl alcohol, carboxymethylcellulose, hydroxymethylcellulose, hydroxypropyl methylcellulose, propylene glycol, dextran 70, or polysorbate 80. Refer to product labeling for specific ingredients.

Adverse Reactions (Reflective of adult population; not specific for elderly)
1% to 10%: Ocular: May cause mild stinging or temporary blurred vision

Dosage

    Geriatrics & Adults: Ocular dryness/irritation: Ophthalmic: Use as needed to relieve symptoms, 1-2 drops into eye(s) 3-4 times/day

Patient Information Wash hands thoroughly; if irritation or condition worsens or persists for longer than 3 days, discontinue use; do not touch tip of container to any surface; close immediately after use

Additional Information Not for use with soft contact lenses

Special Geriatric Considerations Assure the patient or caregiver can adequately administer ophthalmic medication.

Dosage Forms Excipient information presented when available (limited, particularly for generics); consult specific product labeling.

    Solution, ophthalmic: 15 mL and 30 mL dropper bottles

♦ **ASA** *see* Aspirin *on page 127*

♦ **5-ASA** *see* Mesalamine *on page 989*

♦ **Asacol®** *see* Mesalamine *on page 989*

♦ **Asco-Caps [OTC]** *see* Ascorbic Acid *on page 125*

♦ **Ascocid® [OTC]** *see* Ascorbic Acid *on page 125*

Ascorbic Acid (a SKOR bik AS id)

Medication Safety Issues

    International issues:

        Rubex® [Ireland] may be confused with Revex® which is a brand name for nalmefene in the U.S.

        Rubex® [Ireland]: Brand name for doxurbicin in the U.S.

U.S. Brand Names Acerola [OTC]; Asco-Caps [OTC]; Ascocid® [OTC]; Asco-Tabs [OTC]; Cecon® [OTC]; Cemill [OTC]; Cenolate®; C-Gel [OTC]; C-Gram [OTC]; Chew-C [OTC]; C-Time [OTC]; Dull-C® [OTC]; Mild-C® [OTC]; One Gram C [OTC]; Time-C [OTC]; Time-C-Bio [OTC]; Vicks® Vitamin C [OTC]; Vita-C® [OTC]

Canadian Brand Names Proflavanol C™; Revitalose C-1000®

Index Terms Vitamin C

Generic Available Yes

Pharmacologic Category Vitamin, Water Soluble

Use Prevention and treatment of scurvy; acidification of urine; dietary supplement; idiopathic methemoglobinemia

Unlabeled/Investigational Use Investigational: In large doses to decrease the severity of "colds"; dietary supplementation; a 20-year study was recently completed involving 730 individuals which indicates a possible decreased risk of death by stroke when ascorbic acid at doses ≥45 mg/day was administered

Warnings/Precautions Patients with diabetes and patients prone to recurrent renal calculi (eg, dialysis patients) should not take excessive doses for extended periods of time (some studies point to as little as 100 mg/day). Some parenteral products contain aluminum; use caution in patients with impaired renal function.

Adverse Reactions (Reflective of adult population; not specific for elderly)

    1% to 10%: Renal: Hyperoxaluria with large doses

Overdosage/Toxicology Symptoms include renal calculi, nausea, gastritis, and diarrhea. Diuresis with forced fluids may be useful following massive ingestion.

Drug Interactions

    Decreased effect:

        Aspirin (decreases ascorbate levels, increases aspirin)

        Fluphenazine (decreases fluphenazine levels)

        Warfarin (decreased effect)

    Increased effect:

        Iron (absorption enhanced)

        Oral contraceptives (increased contraceptive effect)

Stability Injectable form should be stored under refrigeration (2°C to 8°C). Protect oral dosage forms from light. Rapidly oxidized when in solution in air and alkaline media.

Mechanism of Action Not fully understood; necessary for collagen formation and tissue repair; involved in some oxidation-reduction reactions as well as other metabolic pathways, such as synthesis of carnitine, steroids, and catecholamines and conversion of folic acid to folinic acid

Pharmacokinetics

    Absorption: Oral: Readily absorbed with a wide distribution; absorption is an active process and is thought to be dose-dependent

    Metabolism: In the liver by oxidation and sulfation

    Elimination: In urine; there is an individual specific renal threshold for ascorbic acid; when blood levels are high, ascorbic acid is excreted in urine, whereas when the levels are subthreshold very little if any ascorbic acid is cleared into urine

(Continued)

Ascorbic Acid *(Continued)*

Dosage
  Geriatrics & Adults:
  Recommended daily allowance (RDA): Upper limit of intake should not exceed
    2000 mg/day
    Male: 90 mg
    Female: 75 mg;
    Adult smoker: Add an additional 35 mg/day
  Scurvy: Oral, I.M., I.V., SubQ: 100-250 mg 1-2 times/day for at least 2 weeks
  Urinary acidification: Oral, I.V.: 4-12 g/day in 3-4 divided doses
  Prevention and treatment of colds: Oral: 1-3 g/day
  Dietary supplement: Oral: 50-200 mg/day

Administration Avoid rapid I.V. injection

Monitoring Parameters Monitor for renal calculi, pH of urine (when acidifying)

Test Interactions False-positive urinary glucose with cupric sulfate reagent, false-negative urinary glucose with glucose oxidase method; false-negative stool occult blood 48-72 hours after ascorbic acid ingestion

Patient Information Do not use in large doses if diabetic or have a history of renal stones; do not exceed 3 g/day without physician's advice.

Additional Information Sodium content of 1 g of sodium ascorbate: ~5 mEq

Special Geriatric Considerations Minimum RDA for elderly is not established. Vitamin C is provided mainly in citrus fruits and tomatoes. The elderly, however, avoid citrus fruits due to cost and difficulty preparing (peeling). Daily replacement through a single multiple vitamin is recommended. Use of natural vitamin C or rose hips offers no advantages. Acidity may produce GI complaints.

Dosage Forms Excipient information presented when available (limited, particularly for generics); consult specific product labeling.
  Caplet: 1000 mg
  Caplet, timed release: 500 mg, 1000 mg
  Capsule:
    Mild-C®: 500 mg
  Capsule, softgel:
    C-Gel: 1000 mg
  Capsule, sustained release:
    C-Time: 500 mg
  Capsule, timed release: 500 mg
    Asco-Caps: 500 mg, 1000 mg [sugar free]
    Time-C®: 500 mg
  Crystals for solution, oral: 4 g/teaspoonful (170 g, 1000 g)
    Mild-C®: 3600 mg/teaspoonful [contains calcium 400 mg/teaspoonful]
    Vita-C®: 4 g/teaspoonful (100 g, 454 g)
  Injection, solution: 500 mg/mL (50 mL)
    Cenolate®: 500 mg/mL (1 mL, 2 mL) [contains sodium hydrosulfite]
  Liquid, oral: 500 mg/5 mL
  Lozenge:
    Vicks® Vitamin C: 25 mg [contains sodium 5 mg; orange flavor]
  Powder, for solution, oral:
    Ascocid®: 4000 mg/5 mL (227 g); 4300 mg/5 mL (227 g, 454 g); 5000 mg/5 mL (227
      g, 454 g)
    Dull-C®: 4 g/teaspoonful
  Solution, oral:
    Cecon®: 90 mg/mL
  Tablet: 100 mg, 250 mg, 500 mg, 1000 mg
    Asco-Tabs: 1000 mg [sugar free]
    Ascocid®: 500 mg [sugar free]
    C-Gram, One Gram C: 1000 mg
  Tablet, chewable: 250 mg, 500 mg
    Acerola: 500 mg [cherry flavor]
    Chew-C: 500 mg [orange flavor]
    Mild-C®: 250 mg
  Tablet, timed release: 500 mg, 1000 mg
    Cemill: 500 mg, 1000 mg
    Mild-C®: 1000 mg
    Time-C-Bio: 500 mg

Selected References
  Myrianthopoulos M, "Dietary Treatment of Hyperlipidemia in the Elderly," *Clin Geriatr Med*, 1987, 3(2):343-59.

Aspirin (AS pir in)

Medication Safety Issues

Sound-alike/look-alike issues:

Aspirin may be confused with Afrin®, Asendin®

Ascriptin® may be confused with Aricept®

Ecotrin® may be confused with Akineton®, Edecrin®, Epogen®

Halfprin® may be confused with Halfan®, Haltran®

ZORprin® may be confused with Zyloprim®

International issues:

Cartia® [multiple international markets] may be confused with Cartia XT™ which is a brand name for diltiazem in the U.S.

U.S. Brand Names Ascriptin® [OTC]; Ascriptin® Maximum Strength [OTC]; Aspercin [OTC]; Aspergum® [OTC]; Aspitab [OTC]; Bayer® Aspirin Extra Strength [OTC]; Bayer® Aspirin Regimen Adult Low Dose [OTC]; Bayer® Aspirin Regimen Children's [OTC]; Bayer® Aspirin Regimen Regular Strength [OTC]; Bayer® Genuine Aspirin [OTC]; Bayer® Plus Extra Strength [OTC]; Bayer® Women's Aspirin Plus Calcium [OTC]; Buffasal [OTC]; Bufferin® [OTC]; Bufferin® Extra Strength [OTC]; Buffinol [OTC]; Easprin®; Ecotrin® [OTC]; Ecotrin® Low Strength [OTC]; Ecotrin® Maximum Strength [OTC]; Genacote™ [OTC]; Halfprin® [OTC]; St. Joseph® Adult Aspirin [OTC]; ZORprin®

Canadian Brand Names Asaphen; Asaphen E.C.; Entrophen®; Novasen

Index Terms Acetylsalicylic Acid; ASA

Generic Available Yes: Excludes gum

Pharmacologic Category Salicylate

Use Treatment of mild to moderate pain, inflammation, and fever; prophylaxis of myocardial infarction, stroke and/or transient ischemic episodes; management of rheumatoid arthritis, rheumatic fever, osteoarthritis, and gout (high dose); adjunctive therapy in revascularization procedures (coronary artery bypass graft [CABG], percutaneous transluminal coronary angioplasty [PTCA], carotid endarterectomy)

Unlabeled/Investigational Use Low doses have been used in the prevention of complications associated with autoimmune disorders such as lupus

Contraindications Hypersensitivity to salicylates, other NSAIDs, or any component of the formulation; asthma; rhinitis; nasal polyps; inherited or acquired bleeding disorders (including factor VII and factor IX deficiency)

Warnings/Precautions Use with caution in patients with platelet and bleeding disorders, renal dysfunction, dehydration, erosive gastritis, or peptic ulcer disease. Heavy ethanol use (>3 drinks/day) can increase bleeding risks. Avoid use in severe renal failure or in severe hepatic failure. Discontinue use if tinnitus or impaired hearing occurs. Caution in mild-to-moderate renal failure (only at high dosages). Patients with sensitivity to tartrazine dyes, nasal polyps, and asthma may have an increased risk of salicylate sensitivity. Surgical patients should avoid ASA if possible, for 1-2 weeks prior to surgery, to reduce the risk of excessive bleeding (except in patients with cardiac stents that have not completed their full course of dual antiplatelet therapy [aspirin, clopidogrel]; patient-specific situations need to be discussed with cardiologist; AHA/ACC/SCAI/ACS/ADA Science Advisory provides recommendations).

Adverse Reactions (Reflective of adult population; not specific for elderly) As with all drugs which may affect hemostasis, bleeding is associated with aspirin. Hemorrhage may occur at virtually any site. Risk is dependent on multiple variables including dosage, concurrent use of multiple agents which alter hemostasis, and patient susceptibility. Many adverse effects of aspirin are dose related, and are rare at low dosages. Other serious reactions are idiosyncratic, related to allergy or individual sensitivity. Accurate estimation of frequencies is not possible. The reactions listed below have been reported for aspirin (frequency not defined).

Cardiovascular: Hypotension, tachycardia, dysrhythmias, edema

Central nervous system: Fatigue, insomnia, nervousness, agitation, confusion, dizziness, headache, lethargy, cerebral edema, hyperthermia, coma

Dermatologic: Rash, angioedema, urticaria

Endocrine & metabolic: Acidosis, hyperkalemia, dehydration, hypoglycemia (children), hyperglycemia, hypernatremia (buffered forms)

Gastrointestinal: Nausea, vomiting, dyspepsia, epigastric discomfort, heartburn, stomach pain, gastrointestinal ulceration (6% to 31%), gastric erosions, gastric erythema, duodenal ulcers

(Continued)

Aspirin *(Continued)*

Hematologic: Anemia, disseminated intravascular coagulation (DIC), prothrombin times prolonged, coagulopathy, thrombocytopenia, hemolytic anemia, bleeding, iron deficiency anemia

Hepatic: Hepatotoxicity, transaminases increased, hepatitis (reversible)

Neuromuscular & skeletal: Rhabdomyolysis, weakness, acetabular bone destruction (OA)

Otic: Hearing loss, tinnitus

Renal: Interstitial nephritis, papillary necrosis, proteinuria, renal impairment, renal failure (including cases caused by rhabdomyolysis), BUN increased, serum creatinine increased

Respiratory: Asthma, bronchospasm, dyspnea, laryngeal edema, hyperpnea, tachypnea, respiratory alkalosis, noncardiogenic pulmonary edema

Miscellaneous: Anaphylaxis, prolonged pregnancy and labor, stillbirths, low birth weight, peripartum bleeding, Reye's syndrome

Overdosage/Toxicology Symptoms include tinnitus, headache, dizziness, confusion, metabolic acidosis, hyperpyrexia, hypoglycemia, and coma. Treatment should also be based upon symptomatology.

Drug Interactions Substrate of CYP2C9 (minor)

ACE inhibitors: The effects of ACE inhibitors may be blunted by aspirin administration, particularly at higher dosages.

Buspirone increases aspirin's free % *in vitro*.

Carbonic anhydrase inhibitors and corticosteroids have been associated with alteration in salicylate serum concentrations.

Heparin and low molecular weight heparins: Concurrent use may increase the risk of bleeding.

Methotrexate serum levels may be increased; consider discontinuing aspirin 2-3 days before high-dose methotrexate treatment or avoid concurrent use.

NSAIDs may increase the risk of gastrointestinal adverse effects and bleeding. Serum concentrations of some NSAIDs may be decreased by aspirin. Ibuprofen, and possibly other COX-1 inhibitors, may reduce the cardioprotective effects of aspirin. Avoid giving prior to aspirin therapy or on a regular basis in patients with CAD.

Platelet inhibitors (IIb/IIIa antagonists): Risk of bleeding may be increased.

Probenecid effects may be antagonized by aspirin.

Sulfonylureas: The effects of older sulfonylurea agents (tolazamide, tolbutamide) may be potentiated due to displacement from plasma proteins. This effect does not appear to be clinically significant for newer sulfonylurea agents (glyburide, glipizide, glimepiride).

Valproic acid may be displaced from its binding sites which can result in toxicity.

Verapamil may potentiate the prolongation of bleeding time associated with aspirin.

Warfarin and oral anticoagulants may increase the risk of bleeding.

Ethanol/Nutrition/Herb Interactions

Ethanol: Avoid ethanol (may enhance gastric mucosal damage).

Food: Food may decrease the rate but not the extent of oral absorption.

Folic acid: Hyperexcretion of folate; folic acid deficiency may result, leading to macrocytic anemia.

Iron: With chronic aspirin use and at doses of 3-4 g/day, iron-deficiency anemia may result.

Sodium: Hypernatremia resulting from buffered aspirin solutions or sodium salicylate containing high sodium content. Avoid or use with caution in CHF or any condition where hypernatremia would be detrimental.

Benedictine liqueur, prunes, raisins, tea, and gherkins: Potential salicylate accumulation.

Fresh fruits containing vitamin C: Displace drug from binding sites, resulting in increased urinary excretion of aspirin.

Herb/Nutraceutical: Avoid cat's claw, dong quai, evening primrose, feverfew, garlic, ginger, ginkgo, red clover, horse chestnut, green tea, ginseng (all have additional antiplatelet activity). Limit curry powder, paprika, licorice; may cause salicylate accumulation. These foods contain 6 mg salicylate/100 g. An ordinarily American diet contains 10-200 mg/day of salicylate.

Stability Keep suppositories in refrigerator; do not freeze. Hydrolysis of aspirin occurs upon exposure to water or moist air, resulting in salicylate and acetate, which possess a vinegar-like odor. Do not use if a strong odor is present.

Mechanism of Action Inhibits prostaglandin synthesis, acts on the hypothalamus heat-regulating center to reduce fever, blocks prostaglandin synthetase action which prevents formation of the platelet-aggregating substance thromboxane A_2

Pharmacokinetics

Absorption: From the stomach and small intestine

Distribution: Readily into most body fluids and tissues; aspirin is hydrolyzed to salicylate (active) by esterases in the GI mucosa, red blood cells, synovial fluid and blood

Protein binding: Plasma protein bound (albumin) >90% at low concentrations and 76% at high concentrations (400 mcg/mL)

Metabolism: Metabolism of salicylate occurs primarily by hepatic microsomal enzymes

Half-life, aspirin: 15-20 minutes

Metabolic pathways are saturable such that salicylate half-life is dose-dependent ranging from 3 hours at lower doses (300-600 mg), 5-6 hours (after 1 g) and 15-30 hours with higher doses; in therapeutic anti-inflammatory doses, half-lives generally range from 6-12 hours

Time to peak plasma concentrations: ~1-2 hours

Dosage

Geriatrics & Adults:

Analgesic and antipyretic: Oral, rectal: 325-650 mg every 4-6 hours up to 4 g/day

Anti-inflammatory: Oral: Initial: 2.4-3.6 g/day in divided doses; usual maintenance: 3.6-5.4 g/day; monitor serum concentrations

Acute myocardial infarction: 160-325 mg/day

Myocardial infarction prophylaxis: 75-325 mg/day; use of a lower aspirin dosage has been recommended in patients receiving ACE inhibitors

CABG: 325 mg/day starting 6 hours following procedure

PTCA: Initial: 80-325 mg/day starting 2 hours before procedure; longer pretreatment durations (up to 24 hours) should be considered if lower dosages (80-100 mg) are used

Stent implantation: Oral: 325 mg 2 hours prior to implantation and 160-325 mg daily thereafter

Carotid endarterectomy: 81-325 mg/day preoperatively and daily thereafter

Acute stroke: 160-325 mg/day, initiated within 48 hours (in patients who are not candidates for thrombolytics and are not receiving systemic anticoagulation)

Stroke prevention/TIA: 30-325 mg/day (dosages up to 1300 mg/day in 2-4 divided doses have been used in clinical trials)

Renal Impairment:

Cl_{cr} <10 mL/minute: Avoid use.

Dialyzable (50% to 100%)

Hepatic Impairment: Avoid use in severe liver disease.

Administration Do not crush sustained release or enteric coated tablet. Administer with food or a full glass of water to minimize GI distress

Monitoring Parameters Serum concentrations, renal function; hearing changes or tinnitus; monitor for response (ie, pain, inflammation, range of motion, grip strength); observe for abnormal bleeding, bruising, weight gain

Reference Range

Sample size: 1.5-2 mL blood (purple top tube)

Timing of serum samples: Peak concentration usually occurs 2 hours after ingestion; the half-life increases with the dosage (eg, the half-life after 300 mg is 3 hours, and after 1 g is 5-6 hours, and after 8-10 g is 10-15 hours).

Salicylate serum concentrations correlate with the pharmacological actions and adverse effects observed. Anti-inflammatory therapeutic serum concentrations 150-300 mcg/mL. See table.

Serum Salicylate: Clinical Correlations

Serum Salicylate Concentration (mcg/mL)	Desired Effects	Adverse Effects / Intoxication
~100	Antiplatelet Antipyresis Analgesia	GI intolerance and bleeding, hypersensitivity, hemostatic defects
150-300	Anti-inflammatory	Mild salicylism
250-400	Treatment of rheumatic fever	Nausea/vomiting, hyperventilation, salicylism, flushing, sweating, thirst, headache, diarrhea, and tachycardia
>400-500		Respiratory alkalosis, hemorrhage, excitement, confusion, asterixis, pulmonary edema, convulsions, tetany, metabolic acidosis, fever, coma, cardiovascular collapse, renal and respiratory failure

Test Interactions False-negative results for glucose oxidase urinary glucose tests (Clinistix®); false-positives using the cupric sulfate method (Clinitest®); also, interferes with Gerhardt test, VMA determination; 5-HIAA, xylose tolerance test and T_3 and T_4

Patient Information Watch for bleeding gums or any signs of GI bleeding; take with food or milk to minimize GI distress, notify physician if ringing in ears or persistent GI pain occurs; do not crush or chew sustained release or enteric coated preparation; avoid other aspirin or salicylate containing products

(Continued)

Aspirin *(Continued)*

Special Geriatric Considerations Elderly are a high-risk population for adverse effects from nonsteroidal anti-inflammatory agents. As much as 60% of elderly with GI complications to NSAIDs can develop peptic ulceration and/or hemorrhage asymptomatically. The concomitant use of H_2 blockers and sucralfate is not effective as prophylaxis with the exception of NSAID-induced duodenal ulcers which may be prevented by the use of ranitidine. Misoprostol and proton pump inhibitors are the only prophylactic agents proven to help prevent the development of NSAID-induced ulcers. Also, concomitant disease and drug use contribute to the risk for GI adverse effects. Use lowest effective dose for shortest period possible. Consider renal function decline with age. Use of NSAIDs can compromise existing renal function especially when Cl_{cr} is ≤30 mL/minute. Tinnitus may be a difficult and unreliable indication of toxicity due to age-related hearing loss or eighth cranial nerve damage. CNS adverse effects such as confusion, agitation, and hallucination are generally seen in overdose or high dose situations, but elderly may demonstrate these adverse effects at lower doses than younger adults.

Dosage Forms Excipient information presented when available (limited, particularly for generics); consult specific product labeling. [DSC] = Discontinued product

Caplet:
  Bayer® Aspirin Extra Strength: 500 mg
  Bayer® Aspirin Regimen Regular Strength: 325 mg
  Bayer® Genuine Aspirin: 325 mg
  Bayer® Plus Extra Strength: 500 mg [contains calcium carbonate]
  Bayer® Women's Aspirin Plus Calcium: 81 mg [contains elemental calcium 300 mg]
Caplet, buffered:
  Ascriptin® Maximum Strength: 500 mg [contains aluminum hydroxide, calcium carbonate, and magnesium hydroxide]
Gelcap:
  Bayer® Aspirin Extra Strength: 500 mg [DSC]
Gum:
  Aspergum®: 227 mg [cherry or orange flavor]
Suppository, rectal: 300 mg, 600 mg
Tablet: 325 mg
  Aspercin, Aspirtab: 325 mg
  Bayer® Genuine Aspirin: 325 mg
Tablet, buffered: 325 mg
  Ascriptin®: 325 mg [contains aluminum hydroxide, calcium carbonate, and magnesium hydroxide]
  Buffasal: 325 mg [contains magnesium oxide]
  Bufferin®: 325 mg [contains calcium carbonate, magnesium oxide, and magnesium carbonate; contains calcium 65 mg/tablet, magnesium 50 mg/tablet]
  Bufferin® Extra Strength: 500 mg [contains calcium carbonate, magnesium oxide, and magnesium carbonate; contains calcium 90 mg/tablet, magnesium 70 mg/tablet]
  Buffinol: 325 mg [contains magnesium oxide]
Tablet, chewable: 325 mg
  Bayer® Aspirin Regimen Children's: 81 mg [cherry or orange flavor]
  St. Joseph® Adult Aspirin: 81 mg [orange flavor]
Tablet, controlled release (ZORprin®): 800 mg
Tablet, enteric coated: 81 mg, 325 mg, 500 mg, 650 mg, 975 mg
  Bayer® Aspirin Regimen Adult Low Dose, Ecotrin® Low Strength, St. Joseph Adult Aspirin: 81 mg
  Easprin®: 975 mg
  Ecotrin®, Genacote™: 325 mg
  Ecotrin® Maximum Strength: 500 mg
  Halfprin®: 81 mg, 162 mg

Selected References

Albers GW, "Atrial Fibrillation and Stroke", *Arch Intern Med*, 1994, 154(13):1443-8.

Clinch D, Banerjee AK, and Ostick G, "Absence of Abdominal Pain in Elderly Patients With Peptic Ulcer," *Age Ageing*, 1984, 13(2):120-3.

Clive DM and Stoff JS, "Renal Syndromes Associated With Nonsteroidal Anti-inflammatory Drugs," *N Engl J Med*, 1984, 310(9):563-72.

Hawkey CJ, Karrasch JA, Szczepański L, et al, "Omeprazole Compared With Misoprostol for Ulcers Associated With Nonsteroidal Anti-inflammatory Drugs," *N Engl J Med*, 1998, 338(11):727-34.

Knodel LC, "Preventing NSAID-induced Ulcers: The Role of Misoprostol," *Consult Pharm*, 1989, 4:37-41.

Schömig A, Neumann, FJ, Kastrati A, et al, "A Randomized Comparison of Antiplatelet and Anticoagulant Therapy After the Placement of Coronary-Artery Stents," *N Engl J Med*, 1996, 334(17):1084-9.

Weissmann G, "Aspirin," *Sci Am*, 1991, 264(1):84-90.

Yeomans ND, Tulassay Z, Juhasz L, et al, "A Comparison of Omeprazole With Ranitidine for Ulcers Associated With Nonsteroidal Anti-inflammatory Drugs," *N Engl J Med*, 1998, 338:719-26.

Aspirin and Dipyridamole (AS pir in & dye peer ID a mole)

Related Information
Aspirin *on page 127*
Dipyridamole *on page 454*

Medication Safety Issues
Sound-alike/look-alike issues:
Aggrenox® may be confused with Aggrastat®

U.S. Brand Names Aggrenox®

Canadian Brand Names Aggrenox®

Index Terms Aspirin and Extended-Release Dipyridamole; Dipyridamole and Aspirin

Generic Available No

Pharmacologic Category Antiplatelet Agent

Use Reduction in the risk of stroke in patients who have had transient ischemia of the brain or completed ischemic stroke due to thrombosis

Contraindications Hypersensitivity to dipyridamole, aspirin, or any component of the formulation; allergy to NSAIDs; patients with asthma, rhinitis, and nasal polyps; bleeding disorders (factor VII or IX deficiencies)

Warnings/Precautions Patients who consume ≥3 alcoholic drinks per day are at risk of bleeding. Cautious use in patients with inherited or acquired bleeding disorders including those of liver disease. Watch for signs and symptoms of GI ulcers and bleeding. Avoid use in patients with active peptic ulcer disease. Discontinue use if dizziness, tinnitus, or impaired hearing occurs. Discontinue 1-2 weeks before elective surgical procedures to avoid bleeding. Use caution in the elderly who are at high risk for adverse events. Cautious use in patients with hypotension, patients with unstable angina, recent MI, and hepatic dysfunction. Avoid in patients with severe renal failure. Dose of aspirin in this combination is inadequate to prevent MI.

Adverse Reactions (Reflective of adult population; not specific for elderly)
>10%:
Central nervous system: Headache (38%; tolerance usually develops)
Gastrointestinal: Dyspepsia, abdominal pain (18%), nausea (16%), diarrhea (13%)
1% to 10%:
Cardiovascular: Cardiac failure (2%), syncope (1%)
Central nervous system: Pain (6%), seizure (2%), fatigue (6%), malaise (2%), amnesia (2%), confusion (1%), somnolence (1%)
Dermatologic: Purpura (1%)
Gastrointestinal: Vomiting (8%), bleeding (4%), rectal bleeding (2%), hemorrhoids (1%), hemorrhage (1%), anorexia (1%)
Hematologic: Anemia (2%)
Neuromuscular & skeletal: Back pain (5%), weakness (2%), arthralgia (6%), arthritis (2%), arthrosis (1%), myalgia (1%)
Respiratory: Cough (2%), upper respiratory tract infection (1%), epistaxis (2%)

Overdosage/Toxicology Symptoms of dipyridamole overdose might predominate because of the ratio of dipyridamole to aspirin. Symptoms may include hypotension and peripheral vasodilation. Treatment would include I.V. fluids and possibly vasopressors. Careful medical management is necessary.

Drug Interactions Aspirin: **Substrate** of CYP2C9 (minor)
See individual agents.

Ethanol/Nutrition/Herb Interactions Ethanol: Avoid ethanol (due to GI irritation).

Stability Store at 25°C (77°F); excursions permitted to 15°C to 30°C (59°F to 86°F). Protect from excessive moisture.

Mechanism of Action The antithrombotic action results from additive antiplatelet effects. Dipyridamole inhibits the uptake of adenosine into platelets, endothelial cells, and erythrocytes. Aspirin inhibits platelet aggregation by irreversible inhibition of platelet cyclooxygenase and thus inhibits the generation of thromboxane A_2.

Pharmacokinetics See individual agents.

Dosage
Geriatrics & Adults: Stroke prevention: Oral: 1 capsule (200 mg dipyridamole, 25 mg aspirin) twice daily
Alternative regimen for patients with intolerable headache: 1 capsule at bedtime and low-dose aspirin in the morning. Return to usual dose (1 capsule twice daily) as soon as tolerance to headache develops (usually within a week).
Renal Impairment: Avoid use in patients with severe renal dysfunction (Cl_{cr} <10 mL/minute).
Hepatic Impairment: Avoid use in patients with severe hepatic impairment.

Administration Capsule should be swallowed whole; do not crush or chew. May be given with or without food.

Monitoring Parameters Hemoglobin, hematocrit, signs or symptoms of bleeding, signs or symptoms of stroke
(Continued)

Aspirin and Dipyridamole *(Continued)*

Patient Information Take exactly as directed (do not increase dose or frequency). Swallow capsule whole without chewing or crushing; may be taken with food to reduce GI upset. Avoid alcohol, aspirin or aspirin-containing medication and other OTC medications unless approved by prescriber. May cause dizziness, confusion, or blurred vision (avoid driving or engaging in tasks that require alertness until response to drug is known) or nausea, vomiting, anorexia (take medication with food, eating small frequent meals, and using good mouth care may help). Watch closely for signs of stroke (weakness, acute headache, numbness or loss of strength in any part of the body, disturbances in speech) and notify prescriber immediately. GI bleeding, ulceration, or perforation can occur with or without pain. Report unusual signs of bleeding or bruising, weakness, back or muscle pain, chest pain, cough, skin rash, or persistent diarrhea.

Special Geriatric Considerations Plasma concentrations were 40% higher, but specific dosage adjustments have not been recommended. Some evidence suggests that the doses of dipyridamole commonly used are ineffective for prevention of platelet aggregation, however, the addition of aspirin will add substantial efficacy. The dose of aspirin is effective for platelet inhibition, but low enough to offer a low adverse drug reaction rate.

Dosage Forms Excipient information presented when available (limited, particularly for generics); consult specific product labeling.

Capsule, variable release:
Aggrenox®: Aspirin 25 mg (immediate release) and dipyridamole 200 mg (extended release)

♦ **Aspirin and Extended-Release Dipyridamole** *see* Aspirin and Dipyridamole *on page 131*

♦ **Aspirin and Oxycodone** *see* Oxycodone and Aspirin *on page 1184*

♦ **Aspirin Free Anacin® Maximum Strength [OTC]** *see* Acetaminophen *on page 29*

♦ **Aspirtab [OTC]** *see* Aspirin *on page 127*

♦ **Asproject®** *see* Salicylates (Various Salts) *on page 1439*

♦ **Astelin®** *see* Azelastine *on page 143*

♦ **Astramorph/PF™** *see* Morphine Sulfate *on page 1065*

♦ **Atacand®** *see* Candesartan *on page 222*

♦ **Atacand HCT™** *see* Candesartan and Hydrochlorothiazide *on page 223*

Atenolol *(a TEN oh lole)*

Related Information
Beta-Blockers *on page 1751*
Medication Safety Issues
Sound-alike/look-alike issues:
Atenolol may be confused with albuterol, Altenol®, timolol, Tylenol®
Tenormin® may be confused with Imuran®, Norpramin®, thiamine, Trovan®

High alert medication: The Institute for Safe Medication Practices (ISMP) includes this medication among its list of drugs which have a heightened risk of causing significant patient harm when used in error.

International issues:
Betanol® [Bangladesh] may be confused with Patanol® which is a brand name for olopatadine in the U.S.

U.S. Brand Names Tenormin®

Canadian Brand Names Apo-Atenol®; Gen-Atenolol; Novo-Atenol; Nu-Atenol; PMS-Atenolol; RAN™-Atenolol; Rhoxal-atenolol; Riva-Atenolol; Sandoz-Atenolol; Tenolin; Tenormin®

Generic Available Yes: Tablet

Pharmacologic Category Beta Blocker, Beta₁ Selective

Use Treatment of hypertension (alone or in combination with other agents), postmyocardial infarction patients; management of angina pectoris; selective inhibitor of beta₁-adrenergic receptors

Unlabeled/Investigational Use Treatment of acute ethanol withdrawal, supraventricular and ventricular arrhythmias; migraine headache prophylaxis

Contraindications Hypersensitivity to atenolol or any component of the formulation; sinus bradycardia; sinus node dysfunction; heart block greater than first-degree (except in patients with a functioning artificial pacemaker); cardiogenic shock; uncompensated cardiac failure; pulmonary edema

Warnings/Precautions Consider pre-existing conditions such as sick sinus syndrome before initiating. Administer cautiously in compensated heart failure and monitor for a worsening of the condition (efficacy of atenolol in heart failure has not been established). Beta-blocker therapy should not be withdrawn abruptly (particularly in patients with CAD), but gradually tapered to avoid acute tachycardia, hypertension, and/or ischemia. Use caution with concurrent use of beta-blockers and either verapamil or diltiazem; bradycardia or heart block can occur. Avoid concurrent I.V. use of both agents. Beta-blockers should be avoided in patients with bronchospastic disease (asthma). Atenolol, with B_1 selectivity, has been used cautiously in bronchospastic disease with close monitoring. Use cautiously in peripheral arterial disease, especially if severe disease is present. Use cautiously in patients with diabetes - may mask hypoglycemic symptoms. Use cautiously in the renally impaired (dosage adjustment required). Use care with anesthetic agents which decrease myocardial function. Caution in myasthenia gravis or psychiatric disease (may cause CNS depression). Adequate alpha-blockade is required prior to use of any beta-blocker for patients with untreated pheochromocytoma.

Adverse Reactions (Reflective of adult population; not specific for elderly)
1% to 10%:
Cardiovascular: Persistent bradycardia, hypotension, chest pain, edema, heart failure, second- or third-degree AV block, Raynaud's phenomenon
Central nervous system: Dizziness, fatigue, insomnia, lethargy, confusion, mental impairment, depression, headache, nightmares
Gastrointestinal: Constipation, diarrhea, nausea
Genitourinary: Impotence
Miscellaneous: Cold extremities

Overdosage/Toxicology Symptoms include cardiac disturbances, CNS toxicity, bronchospasm, hypoglycemia and hyperkalemia. The most common cardiac symptoms include hypotension and bradycardia. Atrioventricular block, intraventricular conduction disturbances, cardiogenic shock, and asystole may occur with severe overdose, especially with membrane-depressant drugs (eg, propranolol). CNS effects include convulsions, coma, and respiratory arrest (commonly seen with propranolol and other membrane-depressant and lipid-soluble drugs). Treatment is symptomatic for seizures, hypotension, hyperkalemia, and hypoglycemia. Bradycardia and hypotension resistant to atropine, isoproterenol, or pacing may respond to glucagon. Wide QRS defects caused the membrane-depressant poisoning may respond to hypertonic sodium bicarbonate. Repeat-dose charcoal, hemoperfusion, or hemodialysis may be helpful in removal of only those beta-blockers with a small V_d, long half-life, or low intrinsic clearance (acebutolol, atenolol, nadolol, sotalol).

Drug Interactions
Alpha-blockers (prazosin, terazosin): Concurrent use of beta-blockers may increase risk of orthostasis.
Ampicillin, in single doses of 1 gram, decreases atenolol's pharmacologic actions.
Antacids (magnesium-aluminum, calcium antacids or salts) may reduce the bioavailability of atenolol.
Clonidine: Hypertensive crisis after or during withdrawal of either agent.
Drugs which slow AV conduction (digoxin): Effects may be additive with beta-blockers.
Glucagon: Atenolol may blunt the hyperglycemic action of glucagon.
Insulin and oral hypoglycemics: Atenolol masks the tachycardia that usually accompanies hypoglycemia.
NSAIDs (ibuprofen, indomethacin, naproxen, piroxicam) may reduce the antihypertensive effects of beta-blockers.
Salicylates may reduce the antihypertensive effects of beta-blockers.
Sulfonylureas: Beta-blockers may alter response to hypoglycemic agents.
Verapamil or diltiazem may have synergistic or additive pharmacological effects when taken concurrently with beta-blockers.

Ethanol/Nutrition/Herb Interactions
Food: Atenolol serum concentrations may be decreased if taken with food.
Herb/Nutraceutical: Avoid dong quai if using for hypertension (has estrogenic activity). Avoid ephedra, yohimbe, ginseng (may worsen hypertension). Avoid garlic (may have increased antihypertensive effect).

Stability Protect from light.

Mechanism of Action Competitively blocks response to beta-adrenergic stimulation, selectively blocks beta$_1$-receptors with little or no effect on beta$_2$-receptors except at high doses

Pharmacokinetics
Absorption: Incompletely from GI tract (50%)
Distribution: Does **not** cross the blood-brain barrier
Protein binding: Low (3% to 15%)
Half-life: 6-9 hours (longer in patients with reduced renal function; 16-27 hours with Cl_{cr} 15-35 mL/minute and >27 hours in Cl_{cr} <15 mL/minute)
Time to peak serum concentrations: Oral: Within 2-4 hours
Elimination: 40% excreted as unchanged drug in urine, 50% in feces

Dosage
Geriatrics & Adults:
Hypertension:
Oral: 25-50 mg once daily, may increase to 100 mg/day. Doses >100 mg are unlikely to produce any further benefit.
(Continued)

Atenolol *(Continued)*

I.V.: Dosages of 1.25-5 mg every 6-12 hours have been used in short-term management of patients unable to take oral enteral beta-blockers

Angina pectoris: Oral: 50 mg once daily; may increase to 100 mg/day. Some patients may require 200 mg/day.

Postmyocardial infarction:

I.V.: Early treatment: 5 mg slow I.V. over 5 minutes; may repeat in 10 minutes. If both doses are tolerated, may start oral atenolol 50 mg every 12 hours or 100 mg/day for 6-9 days postmyocardial infarction.

Oral: Follow I.V. dose with 100 mg/day or 50 mg twice daily for 6-9 days postmyocardial infarction.

Renal Impairment:

Cl_{cr} 15-35 mL/minute: Administer 50 mg/day maximum.

Cl_{cr} <15 mL/minute: Administer 50 mg every other day maximum.

Hemodialysis effects: Moderately dialyzable (20% to 50%) via hemodialysis. Administer dose postdialysis or administer 25-50 mg supplemental dose. Elimination is not enhanced with peritoneal dialysis. Supplemental dose is not necessary.

Administration Administer I.V. at 1 mg/minute; intravenous administration requires a cardiac monitor and blood pressure monitor

Monitoring Parameters Blood pressure, orthostatic hypotension, heart rate, CNS effects, EKG

Test Interactions Increased glucose; decreased HDL

Patient Information Adhere to dosage regimen; watch for postural hypotension; do not discontinue medication abruptly, sudden stopping of medication may precipitate or cause angina; consult pharmacist or physician before taking with other adrenergic drugs (eg, cold medications); notify physician if any of the following symptoms occur: difficult breathing, night cough, swelling of extremities, slow pulse, dizziness, lightheadedness, confusion, depression, skin rash, fever, sore throat, unusual bleeding or bruising; may produce drowsiness, dizziness, lightheadedness, blurred vision, confusion; use with caution while driving or performing tasks requiring alertness; may mask signs of hypoglycemia in diabetics; may be taken without regard to meals

Additional Information May potentiate hypoglycemia in a diabetic patient and mask signs and symptoms; patients who receive hemodialysis should receive 50 mg oral dose after each dialysis

Special Geriatric Considerations Due to alterations in the beta-adrenergic autonomic nervous system, beta-adrenergic blockade may result in less hemodynamic response than seen in younger adults. Studies indicate that despite decreased sensitivity to the chronotropic effects of beta-blockade with age, there appears to be an increased myocardial sensitivity to the negative inotropic effect during stress (ie, exercise). Controlled trials have shown the overall response rate for propranolol to be only 20% to 50% in the elderly. Therefore, all beta-adrenergic blocking drugs may result in a decreased response as compared to younger adults. Since many elderly have Cl_{cr} <35 mL/minute, creatinine clearance should be estimated or measured such that appropriate dose adjustment can be made.

Dosage Forms Excipient information presented when available (limited, particularly for generics); consult specific product labeling.

Injection, solution: 0.5 mg/mL (10 mL)

Tablet: 25 mg, 50 mg, 100 mg

Selected References

Aagaard GN, "Treatment of Hypertension in The Elderly," *Drug Treatment in the Elderly*, Vestal RE, ed, Boston, MA: ADIS Health Science Press, 1984, 77.

Fleisher LA, Beckman JA, Brown KA, et al, "ACC/AHA 2006 Guideline Update on Perioperative Cardiovascular Evaluation for Noncardiac Surgery: Focused Update on Perioperative Beta-Blocker Therapy. A Report of the American College of Cardiology/American Heart Association Task Force on Practice Guidelines (Writing Committee to Update the 2002 Guidelines on Perioperative Cardiovascular Evaluation for Noncardiac Surgery) Developed in Collaboration With the American Society of Echocardiography, American Society of Nuclear Cardiology, Heart Rhythm Society, Society of Cardiovascular Anesthesiologists, Society for Cardiovascular Angiography and Interventions, and Society for Vascular Medicine and Biology," *J Am Coll Cardiol*, 2006, 47(11):2343-55.

Juul AB, Wetterslev J, Gluud C, et al, "Effect of Perioperative Beta Blockade in Patients With Diabetes Undergoing Major Non-Cardiac Surgery: Randomized Placebo Controlled, Blinded Multicentre Trial. DIPOM Trial Group," *BMJ*, 2006, 332(7556):1482.

♦ **Ativan**® *see* Lorazepam *on page 929*

Atorvastatin (a TORE va sta tin)

Related Information

Hyperlipidemia Management *on page 1773*

Medication Safety Issues

Sound-alike/look-alike issues:

Lipitor® may be confused with Levatol®

U.S. Brand Names Lipitor®
Canadian Brand Names Lipitor®
Generic Available No
Pharmacologic Category Antilipemic Agent, HMG-CoA Reductase Inhibitor
Use Treatment of dyslipidemias or primary prevention of cardiovascular disease (atherosclerotic) as detailed below:

Primary prevention of cardiovascular disease (high-risk for CVD): To reduce the risk of MI or stroke in patients without evidence of heart disease who have multiple CVD risk factors or type 2 diabetes. Treatment reduces the risk for angina or revascularization procedures in patients with multiple risk factors.

Secondary prevention of cardiovascular disease: To reduce the risk of MI, stroke, revascularization procedures, and angina in patients with evidence of heart disease. To reduce the risk of hospitalization for heart failure.

Treatment of dyslipidemias: To reduce elevations in total cholesterol, LDL-C, apolipoprotein B, and triglycerides in patients with elevations of one or more components, and/or to increase HDL-C as present in Fredrickson type IIa, IIb, III, and IV hyperlipidemias; treatment of primary dysbetalipoproteinemia, homozygous familial hypercholesterolemia

Contraindications Hypersensitivity to atorvastatin or any component of the formulation; active liver disease; unexplained persistent elevations of serum transaminases

Warnings/Precautions Secondary causes of hyperlipidemia should be ruled out prior to therapy. Liver function must be monitored by periodic laboratory assessment. May cause hepatic dysfunction. Use with caution in patients who consume large amounts of ethanol or have a history of liver disease. Monitoring is recommended. Patients with a history of hemorrhagic stroke may be at increased risk for another with use.

Rhabdomyolysis with acute renal failure has occurred. Risk is dose related and is increased with concurrent use of lipid-lowering agents which may cause rhabdomyolysis (gemfibrozil, fibric acid derivatives, or niacin at doses ≥1 g/day) or during concurrent use with potent CYP3A4 inhibitors (including amiodarone, clarithromycin, cyclosporine, erythromycin, itraconazole, ketoconazole, nefazodone, grapefruit juice in large quantities, verapamil, or protease inhibitors such as indinavir, nelfinavir, or ritonavir). Monitor closely if used with other drugs associated with myopathy. Weigh the risk versus benefit when combining any of these drugs with atorvastatin. Discontinue in any patient experiencing an acute or serious condition predisposing to renal failure secondary to rhabdomyolysis. Use with caution in patients with advanced age, these patients are predisposed to myopathy.

Adverse Reactions (Reflective of adult population; not specific for elderly)
>10%: Central nervous system: Headache (3% to 17%)
2% to 10%:
  Cardiovascular: Chest pain, peripheral edema
  Central nervous system: Insomnia, dizziness
  Dermatologic: Rash (1% to 4%)
  Gastrointestinal: Abdominal pain (up to 4%), constipation (up to 3%), diarrhea (up to 4%), dyspepsia (1% to 3%), flatulence (1% to 3%), nausea
  Genitourinary: Urinary tract infection
  Hepatic: Transaminases increased (2% to 3% with 80 mg/day dosing)
  Neuromuscular & skeletal: Arthralgia (up to 5%), arthritis, back pain (up to 4%), myalgia (up to 6%), weakness (up to 4%)
  Respiratory: Sinusitis (up to 6%), pharyngitis (up to 3%), bronchitis, rhinitis
  Miscellaneous: Infection (3% to 10%), flu-like syndrome (up to 3%), allergic reaction (up to 3%)
Additional class-related events or case reports (not necessarily reported with atorvastatin therapy): Alkaline phosphatase increased, cataracts, cirrhosis, CPK increased (>10x normal), dermatomyositis, eosinophilia, erectile dysfunction, extraocular muscle movement impaired, fulminant hepatic necrosis, gynecomastia, hemolytic anemia, memory loss, ophthalmoplegia, peripheral nerve palsy, polymyalgia rheumatica, positive ANA, renal failure (secondary to rhabdomyolysis), systemic lupus erythematosus-like syndrome, thyroid dysfunction, tremor, vasculitis, vertigo

Overdosage/Toxicology Treatment is supportive.
Drug Interactions Substrate of CYP3A4 (major); **Inhibits** CYP3A4 (weak)
  Antacids: Plasma concentrations may be decreased when given with magnesium-aluminum hydroxide containing antacids (reported with atorvastatin and pravastatin). Clinical efficacy is not altered, no dosage adjustment is necessary.
  Bile acid sequestrants (cholestyramine and colestipol): Reduce absorption of several HMG-CoA reductase inhibitors; separate administration times by at least 4 hours. Cholesterol-lowering effects are additive.
  Colchicine: Concomitant therapy with an HMG-CoA reductase inhibitor may increase risk of myopathy/rhabdomyolysis; use caution.
  Cyclosporine: May increase serum concentrations of atorvastatin, increasing the risk of myopathy; monitor.
(Continued)

Atorvastatin *(Continued)*

CYP3A4 inhibitors: May increase the levels/effects of atorvastatin. Example inhibitors include azole antifungals, clarithromycin, diclofenac, doxycycline, erythromycin, imatinib, isoniazid, nefazodone, nicardipine, propofol, protease inhibitors, quinidine, telithromycin, and verapamil.

Digoxin: Plasma concentrations of digoxin may be increased by ~20%; monitor.

Diltiazem: May increase levels/effects of atorvastatin.

Fibric acid derivatives (clofibrate and fenofibrate): May increase the risk of myopathy and rhabdomyolysis.

Grapefruit juice: May inhibit metabolism of atorvastatin via CYP3A4; more likely to occur with lovastatin or simvastatin; avoid high dietary intake of grapefruit juice.

Niacin: May increase the risk of myopathy and rhabdomyolysis.

Ethanol/Nutrition/Herb Interactions

Ethanol: Avoid excessive ethanol consumption (due to potential hepatic effects).

Food: Atorvastatin serum concentrations may be increased by grapefruit juice; avoid concurrent intake of large quantities (>1 quart/day). Red yeast rice contains an estimated 2.4 mg lovastatin per 600 mg rice.

Herb/Nutraceutical: St John's wort may decrease atorvastatin levels.

Mechanism of Action Inhibitor of 3-hydroxy-3-methylglutaryl coenzyme A (HMG-CoA) reductase, the rate-limiting enzyme in cholesterol synthesis (reduces the production of mevalonic acid from HMG-CoA); this then results in a compensatory increase in the expression of LDL receptors on hepatocyte membranes and a stimulation of LDL catabolism

Pharmacodynamics Onset of action: Initial changes: 3-5 days; Maximal reduction in plasma cholesterol and triglycerides: 2 weeks

Pharmacokinetics

Absorption: Rapid

Distribution: V_d: 318 L

Protein binding: ≥98%

Metabolism: To active ortho- and parahydroxylated derivates and an inactive beta-oxidation product; undergoes enterohepatic recirculation

Half-life: Parent drug: 14 hours

Time to peak, serum: 1-2 hours

Elimination: Urine (2% as unchanged drug)

Dosage

Geriatrics & Adults:

Hyperlipidemias: Oral: Initial: 10-20 mg once daily; patients requiring >45% reduction in LDL-C may be started at 40 mg once daily; range: 10-80 mg once daily

Note: Doses should be individualized according to the baseline LDL-cholesterol levels, the recommended goal of therapy, and patient response; adjustments should be made at intervals of 2-4 weeks

Primary prevention of CVD: Oral: 10 mg once daily

Renal Impairment: No adjustment is necessary.

Hepatic Impairment: Decrease dosage with severe disease (eg, chronic alcoholic liver disease).

Administration May take with food if desired; may take without regard to time of day.

Monitoring Parameters Lipid serum concentrations after 2-4 weeks; CPK; LFT prior to initiation of therapy and at 12 weeks following initiation of therapy or following a dose increase, then periodically

Patient Information May take with meals at any time of day. Maintain adequate hydration (2-3 L/day of fluids unless instructed to restrict fluid intake). You will need laboratory evaluation during therapy. May cause headache (mild analgesic may help); diarrhea (yogurt or buttermilk may help); euphoria, giddiness, confusion (use caution when driving or engaging in tasks that require alertness until response to medication is known). Report unresolved diarrhea, excessive or acute muscle cramping or weakness, changes in mood or memory, yellowing of skin or eyes, easy bruising or bleeding, and unusual fatigue. Atorvastatin can cause severe fetal defects; do not donate blood while taking this drug or for 1 month following discontinuation.

Special Geriatric Considerations Effective and well tolerated in elderly. The definition of and, therefore, when to treat hyperlipidemia in the elderly is a controversial issue. The National Cholesterol Education Program recommends that all adults maintain a plasma cholesterol <160 mg/dL. Elderly patients with one additional risk factor, goal LDL would be <130 mg/dL. It is the authors' belief that pharmacologic treatment be reserved for those who are unable to obtain a desirable plasma cholesterol concentration by diet alone and for whom the benefits of treatment are believed to outweigh the potential adverse effects, drug interactions, and cost of treatment.

Dosage Forms Excipient information presented when available (limited, particularly for generics); consult specific product labeling.

Tablet:

Lipitor®: 10 mg, 20 mg, 40 mg, 80 mg

Selected References

Amarenco P, Bogousslavsky J, Callahan A 3rd, et al, "High-Dose Atorvastatin After Stroke or Transient Ischemic Attack. The Stroke Prevention by Aggressive Reduction in Cholesterol Levels (SPARCL) Investigators," *N Engl J Med*, 2006, 355(6):549-59.

Canadian Diabetes Association, Clinical Practice Guidelines Expert Committee, "Dyslipidemia in Adults With Diabetes," *Can J Diabetes*, 2006, 30(3):230-40.

Duell PB, Connor WE, Illingworth DR, "Rhabdomyolysis After Taking Atorvastatin With Gemfibrozil," *Am J Cardiol*, 1998, 81(3):368-9.

"Executive Summary of The Third Report of The National Cholesterol Education Program (NCEP) Expert Panel on Detection, Evaluation, And Treatment of High Blood Cholesterol In Adults (Adult Treatment Panel III)," *JAMA*, 2001, 285(19):2486-97.

Gibson DM, Bron NJ, Richens A, et al, "Effect of Age and Gender on Pharmacokinetics of Atorvastatin in Humans," *J Clin Pharmacol*, 1996, 36(3):242-6.

Smith SC Jr, Allen J, Blair SN, et al, "AHA/ACC Guidelines for Secondary Prevention for Patients With Coronary and Other Atherosclerotic Vascular Disease: 2006 Update: Endorsed by the National Heart, Lung, and Blood Institute," *J Am Coll Cardiol*, 2006, 47(10):2130-9.

Waters DD, LaRosa JC, Barter P, et al, "Effects of High-Dose Atorvastatin on Cerebrovascular Events in Patients With Stable Coronary Disease in the TNT (Treating to New Targets) Study," *J Am Coll Cardiol*, 2006, 48(9):1793-9.

◆ **Atridox**™ *see* Doxycycline Hyclate Periodontal Extended-Release Liquid *on page 483*

◆ **AtroPen**® *see* Atropine *on page 137*

Atropine (A troe peen)

Medication Safety Issues
International issues:

Genatropine® [France] may be confused with Genotropin®

U.S. Brand Names AtroPen®; Atropine-Care®; Isopto® Atropine; Sal-Tropine™

Canadian Brand Names Dioptic's Atropine Solution; Isopto® Atropine

Index Terms Atropine Sulfate

Generic Available Yes: Excludes tablet

Pharmacologic Category Anticholinergic Agent; Anticholinergic Agent, Ophthalmic; Antidote; Antispasmodic Agent, Gastrointestinal; Ophthalmic Agent, Mydriatic

Use Preoperative medication to inhibit salivation and secretions; treatment of symptomatic sinus bradycardia; antidote for organophosphate pesticide poisoning; to produce mydriasis and cycloplegia for examination of the retina and optic disc and accurate measurement of refractive errors; uveitis; AV block (nodal level); ventricular asystole; treatment of GI disorders (eg, peptic ulcer disease, irritable bowel syndrome, hypermotility of colon)

Unlabeled/Investigational Use Pulseless electric activity, asystole, neuromuscular blockade reversal

Restrictions The AtroPen® formulation is available for use primarily by the Department of Defense.

Contraindications Hypersensitivity to atropine or any component of the formulation; narrow-angle glaucoma; adhesions between the iris and lens; tachycardia; obstructive GI disease; paralytic ileus; intestinal atony of the geriatric or debilitated patient; severe ulcerative colitis; toxic megacolon complicating ulcerative colitis; hepatic disease; obstructive uropathy; renal disease; myasthenia gravis (unless used to treat side effects of acetylcholinesterase inhibitor); asthma; thyrotoxicosis; Mobitz type II block

Warnings/Precautions Use with caution in elderly patients. Low doses cause a paradoxical decrease in heart rates. Some commercial products contain sodium metabisulfite, which can cause allergic-type reactions. May accumulate with multiple inhalational administration, particularly in the elderly. Heat prostration may occur in hot weather. Use with caution in patients with autonomic neuropathy, prostatic hyperplasia, hyperthyroidism, CHF, cardiac arrhythmias, chronic lung disease, biliary tract disease; anticholinergic agents are generally not well tolerated in the elderly and their use should be avoided when possible. Atropine is rarely used except as a preoperative agent or in the acute treatment of bradyarrhythmias.

AtroPen®: There are no absolute contraindications for the use of atropine in severe organophosphate poisonings, however in mild poisonings, use caution in those patients where the use of atropine would be otherwise contraindicated. Formulation for use by trained personnel only.

Adverse Reactions (Reflective of adult population; not specific for elderly)
Severity and frequency of adverse reactions are dose related and vary greatly; listed reactions are limited to significant and/or life-threatening.

Cardiovascular: Arrhythmia, flushing, hypotension, palpitation, tachycardia

Central nervous system: Ataxia, coma, delirium, disorientation, dizziness, drowsiness, excitement, fever, hallucinations, headache, insomnia, nervousness

Dermatologic: Anhidrosis, urticaria, rash, scarlatiniform rash

Gastrointestinal: Bloating, constipation, delayed gastric emptying, loss of taste, nausea, paralytic ileus, vomiting, xerostomia, dry throat, nasal dryness

Genitourinary: Urinary hesitancy, urinary retention

Neuromuscular & skeletal: Weakness

(Continued)

Atropine *(Continued)*

Ocular: Angle-closure glaucoma, blurred vision, cycloplegia, dry eyes, mydriasis, ocular tension increased

Respiratory: Dyspnea, laryngospasm, pulmonary edema

Miscellaneous: Anaphylaxis

Overdosage/Toxicology Symptoms include dilated, unreactive pupils; blurred vision; hot, dry flushed skin; dryness of mucous membranes; difficulty in swallowing, foul breath, diminished or absent bowel sounds, urinary retention, tachycardia, hyperthermia, and hypertension, increased respiratory rate. Anticholinergic toxicity is caused by strong binding of the drug to cholinergic receptors. Anticholinesterase inhibitors reduce acetylcholinesterase, the enzyme that breaks down acetylcholine and thereby allows acetylcholine to accumulate and compete for receptor binding with the offending anticholinergic. For anticholinergic overdose with severe life-threatening symptoms, physostigmine 1-2 mg SubQ or slow I.V. may be given to reverse these effects.

Drug Interactions

Drugs with anticholinergic activity (including phenothiazines and TCAs) may increase anticholinergic effects when used concurrently.

Sympathomimetic amines may cause tachyarrhythmias; avoid concurrent use.

Stability Store injection at controlled room temperature of 15°C to 30°C (59°F to 86°F); avoid freezing. In addition, AtroPen® should be protected from light.

Mechanism of Action Blocks the action of acetylcholine at parasympathetic sites in smooth muscle, secretory glands, and the CNS; increases cardiac output, dries secretions

Pharmacokinetics

Absorption: Well absorbed from all dosage forms

Distribution: Wide throughout the body; crosses the blood-brain barrier

Metabolism: In the liver

Half-life: 2-3 hours

Elimination: Into urine of both metabolites and unchanged drug (30% to 50%)

Dosage

Geriatrics: Refer to adult dosing.

Nerve agent toxicity management (unlabeled use): See **Note**. I.M.: Elderly and frail patients:

Prehospital ("in the field"): Mild-to-moderate symptoms: 1 mg; severe symptoms: 2-4 mg

Hospital/emergency department: Mild-to-moderate symptoms: 1 mg; severe symptoms: 2 mg

Note: Pralidoxime is a component of the management of nerve agent toxicity.

Prehospital ("in the field") management: Repeat atropine I.M. (2 mg) at 5-10 minute intervals until secretions have diminished and breathing is comfortable or airway resistance has returned to near normal.

Hospital management: Repeat atropine I.M. (2 mg) at 5-10 minute intervals until secretions have diminished and breathing is comfortable or airway resistance has returned to near normal.

Adults: Doses <0.5 mg have been associated with paradoxical bradycardia.

Asystole:

I.V.: 1 mg; repeat in 3-5 minutes if asystole persists; total dose of 0.04 mg/kg.

Intratracheal: Administer 2-2.5 times the recommended I.V. dose; dilute in 10 mL NS or distilled water. **Note:** Absorption is greater with distilled water, but causes more adverse effects on PaO$_2$.

Inhibit salivation and secretions (preanesthesia):

I.M., I.V., SubQ: 0.4-0.6 mg 30-60 minutes preop and repeat every 4-6 hours as needed.

Oral: 0.4 mg; may repeat in 4 hours if necessary; 0.4 mg initial dose may be exceeded in certain cases and may repeat in 4 hours if necessary

Bradycardia: I.V.: 0.5-1 mg every 5 minutes, not to exceed a total of 3 mg or 0.04 mg/kg; may give intratracheal in 1 mg/10 mL dilution only, intratracheal dose should be 2-2.5 times the I.V. dose.

Neuromuscular blockade reversal: I.V.: 25-30 mcg/kg 30-60 seconds before neostigmine or 7-10 mcg/kg 30-60 seconds before edrophonium

Organophosphate or carbamate poisoning:

I.V.: 2 mg, followed by 2 mg every 15 minutes until adequate atropinization has occurred; initial doses of up to 6 mg may be used in life-threatening cases

I.M.: AtroPen®: Mild symptoms: Administer 2 mg as soon as exposure is known or suspected. If severe symptoms develop after first dose, 2 additional doses should be repeated in 10 minutes; do not administer more than 3 doses. Severe symptoms: Immediately administer three 2 mg doses.

Nerve agent toxicity management (unlabeled use): I.M.: See **Note**. Prehospital ("in the field") or hospital/emergency department: Mild-to-moderate symptoms: 2-4 mg; severe symptoms: 6 mg

Note: Pralidoxime is a component of the management of nerve agent toxicity; consult Pralidoxime for specific route and dose.

Prehospital ("in the field") management: Repeat atropine I.M. (2 mg) at 5-10 minute intervals until secretions have diminished and breathing is comfortable or airway resistance has returned to near normal.

Hospital management: Repeat atropine I.M. (2 mg) at 5-10 minute intervals until secretions have diminished and breathing is comfortable or airway resistance has returned to near normal.

Mydriasis, cycloplegia (preprocedure): Ophthalmic (1% solution): Instill 1-2 drops 1 hour before the procedure.

Uveitis: Ophthalmic:

1% solution: Instill 1-2 drops 4 times/day.

Ointment: Apply a small amount in the conjunctival sac up to 3 times/day. Compress the lacrimal sac by digital pressure for 1-3 minutes after instillation.

Monitoring Parameters Blood pressure, pulse, mental status, anticholinergic effects

Patient Information Maintain good oral hygiene because lack of saliva may increase chance of cavities. Observe caution while driving or performing other tasks requiring alertness; may cause drowsiness, dizziness, or blurred vision. Notify physician if skin rash, flushing or eye pain occurs, or if difficulty in urinating, constipation, or sensitivity to light becomes severe or persists.

Additional Information Because of its bothersome and potentially dangerous side effects, atropine is rarely used except as a preoperative agent or in the acute treatment of bradyarrhythmias

Special Geriatric Considerations Anticholinergic agents are generally not well tolerated in the elderly and their use should be avoided when possible. In elderly, anticholinergic agents should not be used as prophylaxis against extrapyramidal symptoms.

Dosage Forms Excipient information presented when available (limited, particularly for generics); consult specific product labeling.

Injection, solution, as sulfate: 0.05 mg/mL (5 mL); 0.1 mg/mL (5 mL, 10 mL); 0.4 mg/0.5 mL (0.5 mL); 0.4 mg/mL (0.5 mL, 1 mL, 20 mL); 1 mg/mL (1 mL)

AtroPen® [prefilled autoinjector]: 0.5 mg/0.7 mL (0.7 mL); 1 mg/0.7 mL (0.7 mL); 2 mg/0.7 mL (0.7 mL)

Ointment, ophthalmic, as sulfate: 1% (3.5 g)

Solution, ophthalmic, as sulfate: 1% (2 mL, 5 mL, 15 mL)

Atropine-Care®: 1% (2 mL) [contains benzalkonium chloride]

Isopto® Atropine: 1% (5 mL, 15 mL) [contains benzalkonium chloride]

Tablet, as sulfate (Sal-Tropine™): 0.4 mg

Selected References

Feinberg M, "The Problems of Anticholinergic Adverse Effects in Older Patients," *Drugs Aging*, 1993, 3(4):335-48.

♦ **Atropine and Diphenoxylate** *see* Diphenoxylate and Atropine *on page 450*

♦ **Atropine-Care®** *see* Atropine *on page 137*

♦ **Atropine, Hyoscyamine, Scopolamine, and Phenobarbital** *see* Hyoscyamine, Atropine, Scopolamine, and Phenobarbital *on page 780*

♦ **Atropine Sulfate** *see* Atropine *on page 137*

♦ **Atrovent®** *see* Ipratropium *on page 827*

♦ **Atrovent® HFA** *see* Ipratropium *on page 827*

♦ **Attenuvax®** *see* Measles Virus Vaccine (Live) *on page 959*

♦ **Augmentin®** *see* Amoxicillin and Clavulanate Potassium *on page 97*

♦ **Augmentin ES-600®** *see* Amoxicillin and Clavulanate Potassium *on page 97*

♦ **Augmentin XR®** *see* Amoxicillin and Clavulanate Potassium *on page 97*

Auranofin (au RANE oh fin)

Medication Safety Issues

Sound-alike/look-alike issues:

Ridaura® may be confused with Cardura®

U.S. Brand Names Ridaura®

Canadian Brand Names Ridaura®

Generic Available No

Pharmacologic Category Gold Compound

Use Management of active stage of classic or definite rheumatoid arthritis in patients that do not respond to or tolerate other agents; treatment of psoriatic arthritis; adjunctive or alternative therapy for pemphigus

Contraindications Renal disease, history of blood dyscrasias, congestive heart failure, exfoliative dermatitis, necrotizing enterocolitis, history of anaphylactic reactions

Warnings/Precautions

[U.S. Boxed Warning]: May cause significant toxicity involving dermatologic, gastrointestinal, hematologic, pulmonary, renal and hepatic systems; patient education is required. Dermatitis and lesions of the mucous membranes are common (Continued)

Auranofin (Continued)

and may be serious; pruritus may precede the early development of a skin reaction. Signs of toxicity include hematologic depression (depressed hemoglobin, leukocytes, granulocytes, or platelets); stomatitis, persistent diarrhea, enterocolitis, cholestatic jaundice; proteinuria (nephritic syndrome), and interstitial pulmonary fibrosis. Avoid use in patients with prior inflammatory bowel disease.

Concurrent use with ACE inhibitors may increase the risk of nitritoid reactions. Laboratory monitoring should be completed prior to each new prescription. Frequent monitoring of patients for signs and symptoms of toxicity will prevent serious adverse reactions.

Adverse Reactions (Reflective of adult population; not specific for elderly)
>10%:
Dermatologic: Rash (24%), pruritus (17%)
Gastrointestinal: Diarrhea/loose stools (47%), abdominal pain (14%), stomatitis (13%)
Ocular: Conjunctivitis
Renal: Proteinuria
1% to 10%:
Dermatologic: Alopecia, urticaria
Gastrointestinal: Anorexia, constipation, dyspepsia, dysgeusia, flatulence, glossitis
Hematologic: Anemia, eosinophilia, leukopenia, thrombocytopenia
Hepatic: Transaminases increased
Renal: Hematuria, proteinuria

Overdosage/Toxicology Symptoms include hematuria, proteinuria, fever, nausea, vomiting, and diarrhea. Signs of gold toxicity include decrease in hemoglobin, leukopenia, granulocytes and platelets, proteinuria, hematuria, pruritus, stomatitis or persistent diarrhea. Advise patients to report any symptoms of toxicity. Metallic taste may indicate stomatitis. For mild gold poisoning, dimercaprol 2.5 mg/kg 4 times/day for 2 days, or for more severe forms of gold intoxication, dimercaprol 3 mg/kg every 4 hours for 2 days, should be initiated. After 2 days the initial dose should be repeated twice daily on the third day and once daily thereafter for 10 days. Other chelating agents have been used with some success.

Stability Store in tight, light-resistant containers at 15°C to 30°C.

Mechanism of Action The exact mechanism of action of gold is unknown; gold is taken up by macrophages which results in inhibition of phagocytosis and lysosomal membrane stabilization; other actions observed are decreased serum rheumatoid factor and alterations in immunoglobulins. Additionally, complement activation is decreased, prostaglandin synthesis is inhibited, and lysosomal enzyme activity is decreased.

Pharmacodynamics Therapeutic response may not be seen for 3-4 months after start of therapy

Pharmacokinetics
Absorption: Oral: ~15% to 33% (25% average) of gold in a dose
Protein binding: 60%
Half-life: 21-31 days (half-life dependent upon single or multiple dosing)
Time to peak: Peak blood gold concentrations are seen within 2 hours; peak serum concentration: 1-2 hours
Elimination: 60% of absorbed gold is eliminated in urine while the remainder is eliminated in feces

Dosage
Geriatrics & Adults: Rheumatoid arthritis, psoriatic arthritis, pemphigus: Oral: Initial: 6 mg/day in 1-2 divided doses; after 3 months may be increased to 9 mg/day in 3 divided doses; if still no response after 3 months at 9 mg/day, discontinue drug

Renal Impairment:
Cl_{cr} 50-80 mL/minute: Administer 50% of dose.
Cl_{cr} <50 mL/minute: Avoid use.

Monitoring Parameters Patients should have a CBC with differential, platelet count, hemoglobin determination and urinalysis for protein, white cells, red cells and casts; at baseline and periodically during therapy (at least monthly). Skin and oral mucosa should be inspected for skin rash, bruising or oral ulceration/stomatitis. Specific questioning for symptoms such as pruritus, rash, stomatitis or metallic taste should be included. Dosing should be withheld in patients with significant gastrointestinal, renal, dermatologic, or hematologic effects (platelet count falls to <100,000/mm³, WBC <4000, granulocytes <1500/mm³

Reference Range Gold: Normal: 0-0.1 mcg/mL (SI: 0-0.0064 µmol/L); Therapeutic: 1-3 mcg/mL (SI: 0.06-0.18 µmol/L); urine <0.1 mcg/24 hours

Test Interactions May enhance the response to a tuberculin skin test

Patient Information Minimize exposure to sunlight; report any signs of toxicity to physician (ie, pruritus, rash, sore mouth, indigestion, metallic taste); joint pain may take 1-2 months to start to subside

Additional Information Metallic taste may indicate stomatitis

Special Geriatric Considerations Tolerance to gold decreases with advanced age; use cautiously only after traditional therapy and other disease modifying antirheumatic drugs (DMARDs) have been attempted.

Dosage Forms Excipient information presented when available (limited, particularly for generics); consult specific product labeling.
Capsule:
Ridaura®: 3 mg [29% gold]

Azathioprine (ay za THYE oh preen)

Medication Safety Issues
Sound-alike/look-alike issues:
Azathioprine may be confused with azatadine, azidothymidine, Azulfidine®
Imuran® may be confused with Elmiron®, Enduron®, Imdur®, Inderal®, Tenormin®

Azathioprine is metabolized to mercaptopurine; concurrent use of these commercially-available products has resulted in profound myelosuppression.

U.S. Brand Names Azasan®; Imuran®

Canadian Brand Names Alti-Azathioprine; Apo-Azathioprine®; Gen-Azathioprine; Imuran®; Novo-Azathioprine

Index Terms Azathioprine Sodium

Generic Available Yes

Pharmacologic Category Immunosuppressant Agent

Use Adjunctive therapy in prevention of rejection of kidney transplants; active rheumatoid arthritis

Unlabeled/Investigational Use Adjunct in prevention of rejection of solid organ (nonrenal) transplants; steroid-sparing agent for corticosteroid-dependent Crohn's disease (CD) and ulcerative colitis (UC); maintenance of remission in CD; fistulizing Crohn's disease

Contraindications Hypersensitivity to azathioprine or any component of the formulation

Warnings/Precautions [U.S. Boxed Warning]: Chronic immunosuppression increases the risk of neoplasia and serious infections. Azathioprine has mutagenic potential to both men and women and with possible hematologic toxicities; hematologic toxicities are dose-related and may be more severe with renal transplants undergoing rejection. Gastrointestinal toxicity may occur within the first several weeks of therapy and is reversible. Symptoms may include severe nausea, vomiting, diarrhea, rash, fever, malaise, myalgia, hypotension, and liver enzyme abnormalities. Use with caution in patients with liver disease, renal impairment; monitor hematologic function closely. Patients with genetic deficiency of thiopurine methyltransferase (TPMT) or concurrent therapy with drugs which may inhibit TPMT may be sensitive to myelosuppressive effects. Azathioprine is metabolized to mercaptopurine; concomitant use may result in profound myelosuppression and should be avoided.
(Continued)

Azathioprine *(Continued)*

Adverse Reactions (Reflective of adult population; not specific for elderly)

Frequency not defined; dependent upon dose, duration, and concomitant therapy.

Central nervous system: Chills, fever, malaise

Dermatologic: Alopecia, rash (erythematous or maculopapular)

Gastrointestinal: Diarrhea, nausea, pancreatitis, vomiting

Hematologic: Bleeding, leukopenia, macrocytic anemia, pancytopenia, thrombocytopenia

Hepatic: Hepatotoxicity, hepatic veno-occlusive disease, steatorrhea

Neuromuscular & skeletal: Arthralgia, myalgia

Respiratory: Interstitial pneumonitis

Miscellaneous: Hypersensitivity reactions (rare), infection secondary to immunosuppression, neoplasia

Overdosage/Toxicology
Symptoms include nausea, vomiting, diarrhea, and hematologic toxicity. Following initiation of essential overdose management, symptomatic and supportive treatment should be instituted. Dialysis has been reported to remove significant amounts of the drug and its metabolites, and should be considered as a treatment option in those patients who deteriorate despite established forms of therapy.

Drug Interactions
ACE inhibitors: Concomitant therapy may induce anemia and severe leukopenia.

Allopurinol: May increase serum levels of azathioprine's active metabolite (mercaptopurine). Decrease azathioprine dose to $1/3$ to $1/4$ of normal dose.

Aminosalicylates (olsalazine, mesalamine, sulfasalazine): May inhibit TPMT, increasing toxicity/myelosuppression of azathioprine. Use caution.

Mercaptopurine: Azathioprine is metabolized to mercaptopurine; concomitant use may result in profound myelosuppression and should be avoided.

Warfarin: Effect may be decreased by azathioprine.

Ethanol/Nutrition/Herb Interactions
Herb/Nutraceutical: Avoid cat's claw, echinacea (have immunostimulant properties).

Stability
Tablet: Store at room temperature of 15°C to 25°C (59°F to 77°F); protect from light.

Powder for injection: Store at room temperature of 15°C to 25°C (59°F to 77°F) and protect from light. Parenteral admixture is stable at room temperature (25°C) for 24 hours, and stable under refrigeration (4°C) for 16 days.

Mechanism of Action
Azathioprine is an imidazolyl derivative of mercaptopurine; antagonizes purine metabolism and may inhibit synthesis of DNA, RNA, and proteins; may also interfere with cellular metabolism and inhibit mitosis. The 6-thioguanine nucleotides appear to mediate the majority of azathioprine's immunosuppressive and toxic effects.

Pharmacokinetics
Protein binding: ~30%

Metabolism: Hepatic, to 6-mercaptopurine (6-MP), possibly by glutathione S-transferase (GST). Further metabolism of 6-MP (in the liver and GI tract), via three major pathways: Hypoxanthine guanine phosphoribosyltransferase (to 6-thioguanine-nucleotides, or 6-TGN), xanthine oxidase (to 6-thiouric acid), and thiopurine methyltransferase (TPMT), which forms 6-methylmercaptopurine (6-MMP).

Half-life elimination: Parent drug: 12 minutes; mercaptopurine: 0.7-3 hours; End-stage renal disease: Slightly prolonged

Time to peak, plasma: 1-2 hours (including metabolites)

Excretion: Urine (primarily as metabolites)

Dosage
Geriatrics & Adults: I.V. dose is equivalent to oral dose.

Renal transplantation: Oral, I.V.: Initial: 3-5 mg/kg/day usually given as a single daily dose, then 1-3 mg/kg/day maintenance

Rheumatoid arthritis: Oral:

Initial: 1 mg/kg/day given once daily or divided twice daily, for 6-8 weeks; increase by 0.5 mg/kg every 4 weeks until response or up to 2.5 mg/kg/day; an adequate trial should be a minimum of 12 weeks

Maintenance dose: Reduce dose by 0.5 mg/kg every 4 weeks until lowest effective dose is reached; optimum duration of therapy not specified; may be discontinued abruptly

Adjunctive management of severe recurrent aphthous stomatitis (unlabeled use): Oral: 50 mg once daily in conjunction with prednisone

Reduction of steroid use in CD or UC, maintenance of remission in CD or fistulizing disease (unlabeled uses): Oral: Initial: 50 mg daily; may increase by 25 mg/day every 1-2 weeks as tolerated to target dose of 2-3 mg/kg/day

Renal Impairment:

Cl$_{cr}$ 10-50 mL/minute: Administer 75% of normal dose.

Cl$_{cr}$ <10 mL/minute: Administer 50% of normal dose.

Hemodialysis: Dialyzable (~45% removed in 8 hours)

Administer dose posthemodialysis: CAPD effects: Unknown; CAVH effects: Unknown

Administration

I.V.: Azathioprine can be administered IVP over 5 minutes at a concentration not to exceed 10 mg/mL **or** azathioprine can be further diluted with normal saline or D_5W and administered by intermittent infusion usually over 30-60 minutes; may be extended up to 8 hours.

Oral: Administering tablets after meals or in divided doses may decrease adverse GI events.

Monitoring Parameters CBC, platelet counts, total bilirubin, liver function tests, TPMT genotyping or phenotyping

For use as immunomodulatory therapy in CD or UC, monitor CBC with differential weekly for 1 month, then biweekly for 1 month, followed by monitoring every 1-2 months throughout the course of therapy. LFT's should be assessed every 3 months.

Patient Information Response in rheumatoid arthritis may not occur for up to 3 months; do not stop taking without the physician's approval, do not have any vaccinations before checking with your physician; check with your physician if you have a persistent sore throat, unusual bleeding or bruising, fatigue, abdominal pain, pale stools, darkened urine. May cause nausea, vomiting, fever, joint pain, and diarrhea; notify physician if persistent.

Additional Information Azathioprine is an imidazolyl derivative of 6-mercaptopurine. If infection occurs, drug dosage should be reduced; NSAID therapy should be continued when beginning initial therapy with azathioprine in the treatment of rheumatoid arthritis

Special Geriatric Considerations Toxicity to immunosuppressives is increased in elderly. Start with lowest recommended adult doses. Signs of infection, such as fever and WBC rise, may not occur. Lethargy and confusion may be more prominent signs of infection. In the elderly, adjust dose to creatinine clearance.

Dosage Forms Excipient information presented when available (limited, particularly for generics); consult specific product labeling.

Injection, powder for reconstitution: 100 mg

Tablet [scored]: 50 mg

Azasan®: 75 mg, 100 mg

Imuran®: 50 mg

Selected References

Brookes MJ and Green JR, "Maintenance of Remission in Crohn's Disease: Current and Emerging Therapeutic Options," *Drugs*, 2004, 64(10):1069-89.

Hodgins C, Mosley M, and Pola-Strowd M, "Recommendations for the Diagnosis and Management of Recurrent Aphthous Stomatitis," University of Texas at Austin, School of Nursing, Family Nurse Practitioner Program, Austin; May 2003.

Hutchins LF and Lipschitz DA, "Cancer, Clinical Pharmacology, and Aging," *Clin Geriatr Med*, 1987, 3(3):483-503.

Kaplan HG, "Use of Cancer Chemotherapy in the Elderly," *Drug Treatment in the Elderly*, Vestal RE, ed, Boston, MA: ADIS Health Science Press, 1984, 338-49.

Lichtenstein GR, Abreu MT, Cohen R, et al, "American Gastroenterological Association Institute Medical Position Statement on Corticosteroids, Immunomodulators, and Infliximab in Inflammatory Bowel Disease," *Gastroenterology*, 2006, 130(3):935-9.

Matalon ST, Ornoy A, and Lishner M, et al, "Review of the \Potential Effects of Three Commonly Used Antineoplastic and Immunosuppressive Drugs (Cyclophosphamide, Azathioprine, Doxorubicin on the Embryo and Placenta)," *Reprod Toxicol*, 2004, 18(2):219-30.

Sandborn WJ, "A Review of Immune Modifier Therapy for Inflammatory Bowel Disease: Azathioprine, 6-mercaptopurine, Cyclosporine, and Methotrexate," *Am J Gastroenterol*, 1996, 91(3):423-33.

Simon L, Lipman AG, Jacox A, et al, "Guideline for the Management of Osteoarthritis, Rheumatoid Arthritis and Juvenile Chronic Arthritis Pain," 2nd ed, Glenview IL, American Pain Society, 2002.

♦ **Azathioprine Sodium** *see Azathioprine on page 141*

Azelastine (a ZEL as teen)

Medication Safety Issues

Sound-alike/look-alike issues:

Optivar® may be confused with Optiray®

International issues:

Optivar® may be confused with Opthavir® which is a brand name for acyclovir in Mexico

U.S. Brand Names Astelin®; Optivar®

Canadian Brand Names Astelin®

Index Terms Azelastine Hydrochloride

Generic Available No

Pharmacologic Category Antihistamine

Use Treatment of symptoms of seasonal allergic rhinitis (ie, rhinorrhea, sneezing, nasal pruritus) and conjunctivitis

Contraindications Hypersensitivity to azelastine or any component of the formulation (Continued)

Azelastine *(Continued)*

Warnings/Precautions

Nasal spray: May cause drowsiness in some patients; instruct patient to use caution when driving or operating machinery. Effects may be additive with CNS depressants and/or ethanol.

Ophthalmic: Solution contains benzalkonium chloride; wait at least 10 minutes after instilling solution before inserting soft contact lenses. Do not use contact lenses if eyes are red.

Adverse Reactions (Reflective of adult population; not specific for elderly)

Nasal spray:

>10%:

Central nervous system: Headache (8% to 15%), somnolence (<1% to 12%)

Gastrointestinal: Bitter taste (8% to 20%)

Respiratory: Cold symptoms/rhinitis (2% to 17%), cough (11%)

2% to 10%:

Central nervous system: Dysesthesia (8%), dizziness (2%), fatigue (2%)

Gastrointestinal: Nausea (3%), weight gain (2%), dry mouth (3%)

Ocular: Conjunctivitis (<2% to 5%)

Respiratory: Asthma (5%), nasal burning (4%), pharyngitis (4%), paroxysmal sneezing (3%), sinusitis (3%), epistaxis (2% to 3%)

<2%:

Cardiovascular: Flushing, hypertension, tachycardia

Central nervous system: Abnormal thinking, anxiety, depersonalization, depression, drowsiness, fever, hypoesthesia, malaise, nervousness, sleep disorder, vertigo

Dermatologic: Contact dermatitis, eczema, furunculosis, hair and follicle infection

Endocrine & metabolic: Amenorrhea, breast pain

Gastrointestinal: Abdominal pain, ALT increased, aphthous stomatitis, appetite increased, constipation, diarrhea, gastroenteritis, glossitis, ulcerative stomatitis, toothache, vomiting

Genitourinary: Albuminuria, hematuria, polyuria

Hepatic: Liver enzymes increased

Neuromuscular & skeletal: Back pain, extremity pain, hyperkinesia, myalgia, rheumatoid arthritis, temporomandibular dislocation

Ocular: Eye pain, watery eyes

Respiratory: Bronchitis, bronchospasm, laryngitis, nasal congestion, nocturnal dyspnea, postnasal drip, sinus hypersecretion, throat burning

Miscellaneous: Allergic reactions, viral infection

<1%, postmarketing, and/or case reports: Anaphylactoid reaction, chest pain, nasal congestion, confusion, diarrhea, dyspnea, facial edema, involuntary muscle contractions, paresthesia, parosmia, pruritus, rash, skin irritation, tolerance, urinary retention, visual abnormalities, xerophthalmia

Ophthalmic:

>10%:

Central nervous system: Headache (15%)

Ocular: Transient burning/stinging (30%)

1% to 10%:

Central nervous system: Fatigue

Gastrointestinal: Bitter taste (10%)

Ocular: Conjunctivitis, eye pain, blurred vision (temporary)

Respiratory: Asthma, dyspnea, pharyngitis

Miscellaneous: Flu-like syndrome

Overdosage/Toxicology There have been no reported overdoses with azelastine. Increased somnolence is likely to occur. Supportive measures should be employed.

Drug Interactions Substrate (minor) of CYP1A2, 2C19, 2D6, 3A4; **Inhibits** CYP2B6 (weak), 2C9 (weak), 2C19 (weak), 2D6 (weak), 3A4 (weak)

Acetylcholinesterase inhibitors (central): May diminish the therapeutic effect of anticholinergics. If the anticholinergic action is a side effect of the agent, the result may be beneficial. Anticholinergics may diminish the therapeutic effect of acetylcholinesterase inhibitors (central).

Ethanol: Azelastine may increase the CNS sedative effects of ethanol.

Anticholinergics: May enhance the adverse/toxic effect of other anticholinergics.

Antipsychotic agents (phenothiazines): Antihistamines may enhance the arrhythmogenic effect of antipsychotic agents (phenothiazines).

Cimetidine: May increase the serum levels/toxicity of azelastine.

CNS depressants: May enhance the adverse/toxic effect of other CNS depressants.

Pramlintide: May enhance the anticholinergic effect of anticholinergics. These effects are specific to the GI tract.

Ethanol/Nutrition/Herb Interactions Ethanol: Avoid ethanol (may cause increased somnolence or fatigue).

Stability
Nasal spray: Store upright at controlled room temperature of 20°C to 25°C (68°F to 77°F). Protect from freezing.
Ophthalmic solution: Store upright between 2°C to 25°C (36°F to 77°F).

Mechanism of Action Competes with histamine for H_1-receptor sites on effector cells and inhibits the release of histamine and other mediators involved in the allergic response; when used intranasally, reduces hyper-reactivity of the airways; increases the motility of bronchial epithelial cilia, improving mucociliary transport

Pharmacokinetics
Distribution: 14.5 L/kg
Protein binding: 88%, 97% for active metabolite, desmethylazelastine
Metabolism: Hepatic
Bioavailability: 40%
Half-life: Azelastine 22 hours, desmethylazelastine 54 hours
Time to peak: 2-3 hours
Elimination: 75% feces

Dosage
Geriatrics & Adults:
Seasonal allergic rhinitis: Intranasal: 1-2 sprays (137 mcg/spray) each nostril twice daily
Vasomotor rhinitis: Intranasal: 2 sprays each nostril twice daily.
Seasonal allergic conjunctivitis: Ophthalmic: Instill 1 drop into affected eye(s) twice daily

Administration Intranasal: Before initial use of the nasal spray, the delivery system should be primed with 4 sprays or until a fine mist appears. If 3 or more days have elapsed since last use, the delivery system should be reprimed with 2 sprays or until a fine mist appears.

Monitoring Parameters Relief of symptoms

Patient Information Intranasal: Avoid spraying in eyes; store bottle in upright position with pump tightly closed. Before initial use, prime the pump with 4 sprays or until a fine mist appears. If not used for 3 or more days, prime the pump with 2 sprays. Do not take other antihistamines without telling your physician.

Additional Information Absorbed systemically; will cause sedation in some patients. Although this agent is clinically effective, the side effects of sedation, bitter taste, and high cost will limit its use in many patients.

Special Geriatric Considerations Only a small number of older subjects were included in premarketing trials. In those patients, side effects were no different than in younger patients.

Dosage Forms Excipient information presented when available (limited, particularly for generics); consult specific product labeling.
Solution, intranasal, as hydrochloride [spray]:
Astelin®: 1 mg/mL(30 mL) [contains benzalkonium chloride; 137 mcg/spray; 200 metered sprays]
Solution, ophthalmic, as hydrochloride:
Optivar®: 0.05% (6 mL) [contains benzalkonium chloride]

Selected References
Dykewicz MS, Fineman S, Nicklas R, et al, "Diagnosis and Management of Rhinitis: Complete Guidelines of the Joint Task Force on Practice Parameters in Allergy, Asthma and Immunology. American Academy of Allergy, Asthma, and Immunology," *Ann Allergy Asthma Immunol*, 1998, 81(5 Pt 2):478-518.

♦ **Azelastine Hydrochloride** see Azelastine on page 143
♦ **Azilect®** see Rasagiline on page 1386

Azithromycin (az ith roe MYE sin)

Related Information
Antimicrobial Activity Against Selected Organisms on page 1728
Prevention of Infective Endocarditis on page 1803

Medication Safety Issues
Sound-alike/look-alike issues:
Azithromycin may be confused with erythromycin
Zithromax® may be confused with Zinacef®

U.S. Brand Names Azasite™; Zithromax®; Zmax™

Canadian Brand Names Apo-Azithromycin®; CO Azithromycin; Dom-Azithromycin; GMD-Azithromycin; Novo-Azithromycin; PHL-Azithromycin; PMS-Azithromycin; ratio-Azithromycin; Sandoz-Azithromycin; Zithromax®

Index Terms Azithromycin Dihydrate; Azithromycin Hydrogencitrate; Azithromycin Monohydrate; Zithromax® TRI-PAK™; Zithromax® Z-PAK®

Generic Available Yes: Injection, powder for oral suspension, tablet
(Continued)

Azithromycin *(Continued)*

Pharmacologic Category Antibiotic, Macrolide; Antibiotic, Ophthalmic

Use Treatment of acute otitis media due to *H. influenzae*, *M. catarrhalis*, or *S. pneumoniae*; pharyngitis/tonsillitis due to *S. pyogenes*; treatment of mild-to-moderate upper and lower respiratory tract infections, infections of the skin and skin structure, community-acquired pneumonia, pelvic inflammatory disease (PID), sexually-transmitted diseases (urethritis/cervicitis), pharyngitis/tonsillitis (alternative to first-line therapy), and genital ulcer disease (chancroid) due to susceptible strains of *C. trachomatis*, *M. catarrhalis*, *H. influenzae*, *S. aureus*, *S. pneumoniae*, *Mycoplasma pneumoniae*, and *C. psittaci*; acute bacterial exacerbations of chronic obstructive pulmonary disease (COPD) due to *H. influenzae*, *M. catarrhalis*, or *S. pneumoniae*; acute bacterial sinusitis

Unlabeled/Investigational Use Prevention of (or to delay onset of) or treatment of MAC in patients with advanced HIV infection; prophylaxis of bacterial endocarditis in patients who are allergic to penicillin and undergoing surgical or dental procedures; pertussis

Contraindications Hypersensitivity to azithromycin, other macrolide antibiotics, or any component of the formulation

Warnings/Precautions Use with caution in patients with pre-existing liver disease; hepatic impairment, including hepatocellular and/or cholestatic hepatitis, with or without jaundice, has been observed. Discontinue if symptoms of malaise, nausea, vomiting, abdominal colic, and fever. May mask or delay symptoms of incubating gonorrhea or syphilis, so appropriate culture and susceptibility tests should be performed prior to initiating azithromycin. Prolonged use may result in fungal or bacterial superinfection, including *C. difficile*-associated diarrhea and pseudomembranous colitis. Use caution with renal dysfunction. Prolongation of the QT_c interval has been reported with macrolide antibiotics; use caution in patients at risk of prolonged cardiac repolarization. Suspensions (immediate release and extended release) are not interchangeable.

Adverse Reactions (Reflective of adult population; not specific for elderly)

>10%: Gastrointestinal: Diarrhea (4% to 11%)

1% to 10%:

Central nervous system: Headache

Gastrointestinal: Nausea, abdominal pain, cramping, vomiting (especially with high single-dose regimens)

Ocular (with ophthalmic solution use): Eye irritation (1% to 2%)

Overdosage/Toxicology Symptoms include nausea, vomiting, diarrhea, and prostration. Treatment is supportive and symptomatic.

Drug Interactions Substrate of CYP3A4 (minor); **Inhibits** CYP3A4 (weak)

Cardiac glycosides: Macrolides may increase the serum concentrations of cardiac glycosides; monitor.

Colchicine: Macrolides may increase the adverse/toxic effects of colchicine.

Nelfinavir: May increase azithromycin serum levels; monitor for adverse effects.

Warfarin: Azithromycin and other macrolides may decrease metabolism, via CYP isoenzymes, of warfarin. Monitor for increased effects.

Ethanol/Nutrition/Herb Interactions Food: Rate and extent of GI absorption may be altered depending upon the formulation. Azithromycin suspension, not tablet form, has significantly increased absorption (46%) with food.

Stability

Injection (Zithromax®): Store intact vials of injection at room temperature. Reconstitute the 500 mg vial with 4.8 mL of sterile water for injection and shake until all of the drug is dissolved. Each mL contains 100 mg azithromycin. Reconstituted solution is stable for 24 hours when stored below 30°C (86°F). Use of a standard syringe is recommended due to the vacuum in the vial (which may draw additional solution through an automated syringe).

The initial solution should be further diluted to a concentration of 1 mg/mL (500 mL) to 2 mg/mL (250 mL) in 0.9% sodium chloride, 5% dextrose in water, or lactated Ringer's. The diluted solution is stable for 24 hours at or below room temperature (30°C or 86°F) and for 7 days if stored under refrigeration (5°C or 41°F).

Ophthalmic solution: Prior to use, store unopened under refrigeration at 2°C to 8°C (36°F to 46°F). After opening, store at 2°C to 25°C (36°F to 77°F) for ≤14 days; discard any remaining solution after 14 days.

Suspension, immediate release (Zithromax®): Store dry powder below 30°C (86°F). Following reconstitution, store at 5°C to 30°C (41°F to 86°F).

Suspension, extended release (Zmax™): Store dry powder below 30°C (86°F). Following reconstitution, store at 15°C to 30°C (59°F to 86°F); do not freeze. Should be consumed within 12 hours following reconstitution.

Tablet (Zithromax®): Store between 15°C to 30°C (59°F to 86°F).

Mechanism of Action Inhibits RNA-dependent protein synthesis at the chain elongation step; binds to the 50S ribosomal subunit resulting in blockage of transpeptidation

Pharmacokinetics

Absorption: Rapid

Distribution: Extensive tissue; distributes well into skin, lungs, sputum, tonsils, and cervix; penetration into CSF is poor; I.V.: 33.3 L/kg; Oral: 31.1 L/kg

Protein binding (concentration dependent): 7% to 51%

Metabolism: Hepatic

Bioavailability: 38%, decreased by 17% with extended release suspension; variable effect with food (increased with immediate or delayed release oral suspension, unchanged with tablet)

Half-life elimination: Terminal: Immediate release: 68-72 hours; Extended release: 59 hours

Time to peak, serum: Immediate release: 2-3 hours; Extended release: 5 hours

Excretion: Biliary (major route); urine (6%)

Dosage

Geriatrics & Adults: Note: Extended release suspension (Zmax™) is not interchangeable with immediate release formulations. Use should be limited to approved indications. All doses are expressed as immediate release azithromycin unless otherwise specified.

Bacterial conjunctivitis: Instill 1 drop into affected eye(s) twice daily (8-12 hours apart) for 2 days, then 1 drop once daily for 5 days

Bacterial sinusitis: Oral: 500 mg/day for a total of 3 days
  Extended release suspension (Zmax™): 2 g as a single dose

Cat scratch disease (unlabeled use): Oral: >45.5 kg: 500 mg as a single dose, then 250 mg once daily for 4 days

Chancroid due to *H. ducreyi:* Oral: 1 g as a single dose

Community-acquired pneumonia:
  Oral (Zmax™): 2 g as a single dose
  I.V.: 500 mg as a single dose for at least 2 days, follow I.V. therapy by the oral route with a single daily dose of 500 mg to complete a 7- to 10-day course of therapy.

Disseminated *M. avium* complex disease in patient with advanced HIV infection (unlabeled use): Oral:
  Prophylaxis: 1200 mg once weekly (may be combined with rifabutin)
  Treatment: 600 mg daily in combination with ethambutol 15 mg/kg

Endocarditis, prophylaxis (unlabeled use): Oral: 500 mg 1 hour prior to the procedure

Mild-to-moderate respiratory tract, skin, and soft tissue infections: Oral: 500 mg in a single loading dose on day 1 followed by 250 mg/day as a single dose on days 2-5
  Alternative regimen: Bacterial exacerbation of COPD: 500 mg/day for a total of 3 days

Pelvic inflammatory disease (PID): I.V.: 500 mg as a single dose for 1-2 days, follow I.V. therapy by the oral route with a single daily dose of 250 mg to complete a 7-day course of therapy.

Pertussis (CDC guidelines): Oral: 500 mg on day 1 followed by 250 mg/day on days 2-5 (maximum: 500 mg/day)

Urethritis/cervicitis: Oral:
  Due to *C. trachomatis:* 1 g as a single dose
  Due to *N. gonorrhoeae:* 2 g as a single dose

Renal Impairment: Use caution in patients with Cl_{cr} <10 mL/minute

Hepatic Impairment: Use with caution due to potential for hepatotoxicity (rare). Specific guidelines for dosing in hepatic impairment have not been established.

Administration

I.V.: Infusate concentration and rate of infusion for azithromycin for injection should be either 1 mg/mL over 3 hours or 2 mg/mL over 1 hour. Other medications should not be infused simultaneously through the same I.V. line.

Oral: Immediate release suspension and tablet may be taken without regard to food; extended release suspension should be taken on an empty stomach (at least 1 hour before or 2 hours following a meal), within 12 hours of reconstitution.

Monitoring Parameters Signs and symptoms of infection, mental status, appetite; hydration; cultures and sensitivity, if appropriate

Patient Information Complete full course of therapy; take on an empty stomach (1 hour before or 2 hours after meals); do not take with aluminum- or magnesium-containing antacids; notify physician if sore throat, unusual bleeding, or other infections occur. Take extended release oral suspension 1 hour before or 2 hours after meals; immediate release suspension may be taken with or without food; tablet form may be taken with meals to decrease GI effects.

Additional Information Capsules are no longer being produced in the United States. Zithromax® tablets and immediate release suspension may be interchanged (eg, two 250 Zithromax® tablets may be substituted for a 500 mg Zithromax® tablet or the tablets may be substituted with the immediate release suspension); however, the (Continued)

Azithromycin *(Continued)*

extended release suspension (Zmax™) is not bioequivalent with Zithromax® and therefore should not be interchanged.

Special Geriatric Considerations Dosage adjustment does not appear to be necessary in the elderly. Considered to be one of the drugs of choice in the outpatient treatment of community-acquired pneumonia in elderly.

Dosage Forms Excipient information presented when available (limited, particularly for generics); consult specific product labeling.

Note: Strength expressed as base

Injection, powder for reconstitution, as dihydrate: 500 mg
Zithromax®: 500 mg [contains sodium 114 mg (4.96 mEq) per vial]

Injection, powder for reconstitution, as hydrogencitrate: 500 mg

Injection, powder for reconstitution, as monohydrate: 500 mg

Microspheres for oral suspension, extended release, as dihydrate:
Zmax™: 2 g [single-dose bottle; contains sodium 148 mg per bottle; cherry and banana flavor]

Powder for oral suspension, as monohydrate: 100 mg/5 mL (15 mL); 200 mg/5 mL (15 mL, 22.5 mL, 30 mL)

Powder for oral suspension, immediate release, as dihydrate:
Zithromax®: 100 mg/5 mL (15 mL) [contains sodium 3.7 mg/ 5 mL; cherry creme de vanilla and banana flavor]; 200 mg/5 mL (15 mL, 22.5 mL, 30 mL) [contains sodium 7.4 mg/5 mL; cherry creme de vanilla and banana flavor]; 1 g [single-dose packet; contains sodium 37 mg per packet; cherry creme de vanilla and banana flavor]

Solution, ophthalmic:
Azasite™: 1% (2.5 mL) [contains benzalkonium chloride]

Tablet, as dihydrate:
Zithromax®: 250 mg [contains sodium 0.9 mg per tablet]; 500 mg [contains sodium 1.8 mg per tablet]; 600 mg [contains sodium 2.1 mg per tablet]
Zithromax® TRI-PAK™ [unit-dose pack]: 500 mg (3s) [contains sodium 1.8 mg per tablet]
Zithromax® Z-PAK® [unit-dose pack]: 250 mg (6s) [contains sodium 0.9 mg per tablet]

Tablet, as monohydrate: 250 mg, 500 mg, 600 mg

Selected References

American Thoracic Society, "Guidelines for the Initial Management of Adults With Community-Acquired Pneumonia: Diagnosis, Assessment of Severity, and Initial Antimicrobial Therapy," *Am Rev Respir Dis*, 1993, 148(5):1418-26.

Coates P, Daniel R, Houston AC, et al, "An Open Study to Compare the Pharmacokinetics, Safety, and Tolerability of a Multiple-Dose Regimen of Azithromycin in Young and Elderly Volunteers," *Eur J Clin Microbiol Infect Dis*, 1991, 10(10):850-2.

Peters DH, Friedel HA, and McTavish D, "Azithromycin: A Review of Its Antimicrobial Activity, Pharmacokinetic Properties and Clinical Efficacy," *Drugs*, 1992, 44(5):750-99.

Tiwari T, Murphy TV, and Moran J, "Recommended Antimicrobial Agents for the Treatment and Postexposure Prophylaxis of Pertussis: 2005 CDC Guidelines," *MMWR Recomm Rep*, 2005, 54(RR-14):1-16.

♦ **Azithromycin Dihydrate** *see* Azithromycin *on page 145*
♦ **Azithromycin Hydrogencitrate** *see* Azithromycin *on page 145*
♦ **Azithromycin Monohydrate** *see* Azithromycin *on page 145*
♦ **Azmacort®** *see* Triamcinolone *on page 1619*
♦ **AZO-Gesic®** [OTC] *see* Phenazopyridine *on page 1238*
♦ **Azopt®** *see* Brinzolamide *on page 184*
♦ **AZO-Standard®** [OTC] *see* Phenazopyridine *on page 1238*
♦ **AZO-Standard® Maximum Strength** [OTC] *see* Phenazopyridine *on page 1238*
♦ **Azthreonam** *see* Aztreonam *on page 148*

Aztreonam *(AZ tree oh nam)*

Related Information
Antimicrobial Activity Against Selected Organisms *on page 1728*

Medication Safety Issues
Sound-alike/look-alike issues:
Aztreonam may be confused with azidothymidine

U.S. Brand Names Azactam®

Canadian Brand Names Azactam®

Index Terms Azthreonam

Generic Available No

Pharmacologic Category Antibiotic, Miscellaneous

Use Treatment of patients with urinary tract infections, lower respiratory tract infections, septicemia, skin/skin structure infections, intra-abdominal infections, and gynecological infections caused by susceptible gram-negative bacilli

Contraindications Hypersensitivity to aztreonam or any component of the formulation

Warnings/Precautions Rare cross-allergenicity to penicillins and cephalosporins has been reported. Use caution in renal impairment; dosing adjustment required. Prolonged use may result in fungal or bacterial superinfection, including *C. difficile*-associated diarrhea and pseudomembranous colitis.

Adverse Reactions (Reflective of adult population; not specific for elderly)
1% to 10%:
    Dermatologic: Rash
    Gastrointestinal: Diarrhea, nausea, vomiting
    Local: Thrombophlebitis, pain at injection site

Overdosage/Toxicology Symptoms include seizures. If necessary, dialysis can reduce the drug concentration in the blood.

Drug Interactions Avoid antibiotics that induce beta-lactamase production (cefoxitin, imipenem).

Stability Prior to reconstitution, store at room temperature; avoid excessive heat. Reconstituted solutions are colorless to light yellow straw and may turn pink upon standing without affecting potency. Use reconstituted solutions and I.V. solutions (in NS and D$_5$W) within 48 hours if kept at room temperature (25°C) or 7 days under refrigeration (4°C).
    I.M.: Reconstitute with at least 3 mL SWFI, sterile bacteriostatic water for injection, NS, or bacteriostatic sodium chloride.
    I.V.:
        Bolus injection: Reconstitute with 6-10 mL SWFI.
        Infusion: Reconstitute to a final concentration ≤2%; the final concentration should not exceed 20 mg/mL. Solution for infusion may be frozen at less than -2°C (less than -4°F) for up to 3 months. Thawed solution should be used within 24 hours if thawed at room temperature or within 72 hours if thawed under refrigeration. **Do not refreeze.**

Mechanism of Action Inhibits bacterial cell wall synthesis by binding to one or more of the penicillin binding proteins (PBPs) which in turn inhibits the final transpeptidation step of peptidoglycan synthesis in bacterial cell walls, thus inhibiting cell wall biosynthesis. Bacteria eventually lyse due to ongoing activity of cell wall autolytic enzymes (autolysins and murein hydrolases) while cell wall assembly is arrested. Monobactam structure makes cross-allergenicity with beta-lactams unlikely.

Pharmacokinetics
    Absorption: I.M.: Well absorbed
    Distribution: V$_d$ (adults): 0.2 L/kg
    Protein binding: 56%
    Half-life: 1.3-2.2 hours (half-life prolonged in renal failure)
    Time to peak serum concentration: Within 60 minutes following a dose
    Elimination: 60% to 70% excreted unchanged in urine and partially excreted in feces
    In healthy older adults with normal renal function (mean Cl$_{cr}$: 99 mL/minute), there were no significant changes in pharmacokinetic parameters. However, in older adults with impaired renal function (mean Cl$_{cr}$: 24 mL/minute) serum concentrations were inversely related to Cl$_{cr}$

Dosage
    Geriatrics & Adults:
        Urinary tract infection: I.M., I.V.: 500 mg to 1 g every 8-12 hours
        Moderately severe systemic infections:
            I.M.: 1 g every 8-12 hours
            I.V.: 1-2 g every 8-12 hours
        Severe systemic or life-threatening infections (especially caused by *Pseudomonas aeruginosa*): I.V.: 2 g every 6-8 hours; maximum: 8 g/day
        Meningitis (gram-negative): I.V.: 2 g every 6-8 hours
    Renal Impairment: Adults: Following initial dose, maintenance doses should be given as follows:
        Cl$_{cr}$ 10-30 mL/minute: 50% of usual dose at the usual interval
        Cl$_{cr}$ <10 mL/minute: 25% of usual dosage at the usual interval
        Hemodialysis: Moderately dialyzable (20% to 50%); $\frac{1}{8}$ of initial dose after each hemodialysis session (given in addition to the maintenance doses)
        Peritoneal dialysis: Administer as for Cl$_{cr}$ <10 mL/minute
        Continuous arteriovenous or venovenous hemofiltration: Dose as for Cl$_{cr}$ 10-30 mL/minute

Administration I.V. route preferred for single doses >1 g or in patients with severe life-threatening infections.
    I.M.: Administer by deep injection into large muscle mass, such as upper outer quadrant of gluteus maximus or the lateral part of the thigh
    I.V.: Administer by IVP over 3-5 minutes or by intermittent infusion over 20-60 minutes at a final concentration not to exceed 20 mg/mL

Monitoring Parameters Resolution of signs and symptoms of infection, periodic liver function tests
    (Continued)

Aztreonam *(Continued)*

Test Interactions May interfere with urine glucose tests containing cupric sulfate (Benedict's solution, Clinitest®); positive Coombs' test

Additional Information Normally used with other antibiotics in life-threatening situations; member of new class of antibiotics called monobactams, with excellent gram-negative bacteria effectiveness, without ototoxicity or nephrotoxicity

Special Geriatric Considerations Adjust dose relative to renal function.

Dosage Forms Excipient information presented when available (limited, particularly for generics); consult specific product labeling.
   Infusion [premixed]: 1 g (50 mL); 2 g (50 mL)
   Injection, powder for reconstitution: 500 mg, 1 g, 2 g

Selected References
   Creasey WA, Platt TB, Frantz M, et al, "Pharmacokinetics of Aztreonam in Elderly Male Volunteers," *Br J Clin Pharmacol*, 1985, 19(2):233-7.
   Settler FR, Schramm M, Swabb EA, "Safety of Aztreonam and SQ 26,992 in Elderly Patients With Renal Insufficiency," *Rev Infect Dis*, 1985, (Suppl 4):5622.

♦ **Azulfidine®** *see* Sulfasalazine *on page 1501*

♦ **Azulfidine® EN-tabs®** *see* Sulfasalazine *on page 1501*

♦ **B2036-PEG** *see* Pegvisomant *on page 1216*

♦ **Babee® Cof Syrup [OTC]** *see* Dextromethorphan *on page 419*

♦ **Bacid® [OTC]** *see* Lactobacillus *on page 867*

Baclofen (BAK loe fen)

Medication Safety Issues
   Sound-alike/look-alike issues:
      Baclofen may be confused with Bactroban®
      Lioresal® may be confused with lisinopril, Lotensin®

   High alert medication: The Institute for Safe Medication Practices (ISMP) includes this medication among its list of drugs which have a heightened risk of causing significant patient harm when used in error.

U.S. Brand Names Lioresal®

Canadian Brand Names Apo-Baclofen®; Gen-Baclofen; Lioresal®; Liotec; Nu-Baclo; PMS-Baclofen

Generic Available Yes: Tablets only

Pharmacologic Category Skeletal Muscle Relaxant

Use Treatment of reversible spasticity associated with multiple sclerosis or spinal cord lesions
   Orphan drug: Intrathecal: Treatment of intractable spasticity caused by spinal cord injury, multiple sclerosis, and other spinal disease (spinal ischemia or tumor, transverse myelitis, cervical spondylosis, degenerative myelopathy)

Unlabeled/Investigational Use Treatment of intractable hiccups, intractable pain relief, bladder spasticity, trigeminal neuralgia, cerebral palsy, Huntington's chorea

Contraindications Hypersensitivity to baclofen or any component of the formulation

Warnings/Precautions Use with caution in patients with seizure disorder or impaired renal function. **[U.S. Boxed Warning]: Avoid abrupt withdrawal of the drug; abrupt withdrawal of intrathecal baclofen has resulted in severe sequelae (hyperpyrexia, obtundation, rebound/exaggerated spasticity, muscle rigidity, and rhabdomyolysis), leading to organ failure and some fatalities.** Risk may be higher in patients with injuries at T-6 or above, history of baclofen withdrawal, or limited ability to communicate. May cause CNS depression, which may impair physical or mental abilities; patients must be cautioned about performing tasks which require mental alertness (eg, operating machinery or driving). Elderly are more sensitive to the effects of baclofen and are more likely to experience adverse CNS effects at higher doses.

Adverse Reactions (Reflective of adult population; not specific for elderly)
   >10%:
      Central nervous system: Drowsiness, vertigo, psychiatric disturbances, insomnia, slurred speech, ataxia, hypotonia
      Neuromuscular & skeletal: Weakness
   1% to 10%:
      Cardiovascular: Hypotension
      Central nervous system: Fatigue, confusion, headache
      Dermatologic: Rash
      Gastrointestinal: Nausea, constipation
      Genitourinary: Polyuria

Overdosage/Toxicology Symptoms include vomiting, muscle hypotonia, salivation, drowsiness, coma, seizures, and respiratory depression. Atropine has been used to improve ventilation, heart rate, blood pressure, and core body temperature. Following initiation of essential overdose management, symptomatic and supportive treatment should be instituted.

For toxicity following intrathecal administration: Administer physostigmine 2 mg I.M. or I.V. (not to exceed 1 mg/minute). Consider withdrawal of 30-40 mL of CSF to reduce baclofen concentration. Abrupt withdrawal of intrathecal baclofen has resulted in severe sequelae (hyperpyrexia, obtundation, muscle rigidity, and rhabdomyolysis)

Drug Interactions
Increased effect: Opiate analgesics, benzodiazepines, hypertensive agents
Increased toxicity: CNS depressants and ethanol (sedation), tricyclic antidepressants (short-term memory loss), clindamycin (neuromuscular blockade), guanabenz (sedation), MAO inhibitors (decrease blood pressure, CNS, and respiratory effects)

Ethanol/Nutrition/Herb Interactions
Ethanol: Avoid ethanol (may increase CNS depression).
Herb/Nutraceutical: Avoid valerian, St John's wort, kava kava, gotu kola.

Mechanism of Action Inhibits the transmission of both monosynaptic and polysynaptic reflexes at the spinal cord level, possibly by hyperpolarization of primary afferent fiber terminals, with resultant relief of muscle spasticity

Pharmacodynamics
Onset of muscle relaxation effects: 3-4 days
Maximum clinical effects: Not seen for 5-10 days

Pharmacokinetics
Absorption: Oral: Rapid; absorption from the GI tract is thought to be dose dependent
Protein binding: 30%
Metabolized: Minimally in the liver
Half-life: 3.5 hours
Time to peak serum concentration: Within 2-3 hours
Elimination: 85% of oral dose excreted in urine and feces as unchanged drug

Dosage
Geriatrics: Oral (the lowest effective dose is recommended): Initial: 5 mg 2-3 times/day, increasing gradually as needed; if benefits are not seen withdraw the drug slowly.
Adults:
Spasticity:
Oral: 5 mg 3 times/day, may increase 5 mg/dose every 3 days to a maximum of 80 mg/day
Intrathecal:
Test dose: 50-100 mcg, doses >50 mcg should be given in 25 mcg increments, separated by 24 hours. A screening dose of 25 mcg may be considered in very small patients. Patients not responding to screening dose of 100 mcg should not be considered for chronic infusion/implanted pump.
Maintenance: After positive response to test dose, a maintenance intrathecal infusion can be administered via an implanted intrathecal pump. Initial dose via pump: Infusion at a 24-hourly rate dosed at twice the test dose. Avoid abrupt discontinuation.
Hiccups (unlabeled use): Oral: 10-20 mg 2-3 times/day
Renal Impairment: May be necessary to reduce dosage; no specific guidelines have been established

Monitoring Parameters Symptoms, blood pressure, mental status

Test Interactions Increased alkaline phosphatase, AST, glucose, ammonia (B); decreased bilirubin (S)

Patient Information Take this drug as prescribed. Do not discontinue without consulting prescriber (abrupt discontinuation may cause hallucinations). Do not take any prescription or OTC sleep-inducing drugs, sedatives, antispasmodics without consulting prescriber. Avoid alcohol use. You may experience transient drowsiness, lethargy, or dizziness; use caution when driving or engaging in tasks requiring alertness until response to drug is known. Frequent small meals or lozenges may reduce GI upset. Report unresolved insomnia, painful urination, change in urinary patterns, constipation, or persistent confusion.
Intrathecal: It is important not to miss scheduled appointments for refills. Contact prescriber immediately if symptoms of withdrawal occur (high fever, confusion, increased spasticity, or muscle rigidity).

Additional Information Not indicated for muscle spasm associated with rheumatic disorders; not recommended in Parkinson's disease or stroke since the efficacy has not been established

Special Geriatric Considerations The elderly are more sensitive to the effects of baclofen and are more likely to experience adverse CNS effects at higher doses. Two cases of encephalopathy were reported after inadvertent high doses (50 mg/day and 90 mg/day) were given to elderly patients.

Dosage Forms Excipient information presented when available (limited, particularly for generics); consult specific product labeling.
(Continued)

Baclofen *(Continued)*

Injection, solution, intrathecal [preservative free]:
Lioresal®: 50 mcg/mL (1 mL); 500 mcg/mL (20 mL); 2000 mcg/mL (5 mL, 20 mL)
Tablet: 10 mg, 20 mg

Selected References

Abarbanel J, Herishanu Y, Frisher S, "Encephalopathy Associated With Baclofen," *Ann Neurol,* 1985, 17(6):617-8.

Tan AK and Tan CB, "The Syndrome of Painful Legs and Moving Toes: A Case Report," *Singapore Med J,* 1996, 37(4):446-7.

- ♦ **Bactrim**™ *see* Sulfamethoxazole and Trimethoprim *on page 1498*
- ♦ **Bactrim**™ **DS** *see* Sulfamethoxazole and Trimethoprim *on page 1498*
- ♦ **Bactroban**® *see* Mupirocin *on page 1075*
- ♦ **Bactroban**® **Nasal** *see* Mupirocin *on page 1075*
- ♦ **Baking Soda** *see* Sodium Bicarbonate *on page 1474*
- ♦ **Balacet 325**™ *see* Propoxyphene and Acetaminophen *on page 1335*
- ♦ **Balsam Peru, Trypsin, and Castor Oil** *see* Trypsin, Balsam Peru, and Castor Oil *on page 1642*
- ♦ **Band-Aid**® **Hurt-Free**™ **Antiseptic Wash [OTC]** *see* Lidocaine *on page 904*
- ♦ **Banophen**® **[OTC]** *see* DiphenhydrAMINE *on page 447*
- ♦ **Banophen**® **Anti-Itch [OTC]** *see* DiphenhydrAMINE *on page 447*
- ♦ **Baridium**® **[OTC]** *see* Phenazopyridine *on page 1238*
- ♦ **Bausch & Lomb**® **Computer Eye Drops [OTC]** *see* Glycerin *on page 718*
- ♦ **Bayer**® **Aspirin Extra Strength [OTC]** *see* Aspirin *on page 127*
- ♦ **Bayer**® **Aspirin Regimen Adult Low Dose [OTC]** *see* Aspirin *on page 127*
- ♦ **Bayer**® **Aspirin Regimen Children's [OTC]** *see* Aspirin *on page 127*
- ♦ **Bayer**® **Aspirin Regimen Regular Strength [OTC]** *see* Aspirin *on page 127*
- ♦ **Bayer**® **Genuine Aspirin [OTC]** *see* Aspirin *on page 127*
- ♦ **Bayer**® **Plus Extra Strength [OTC]** *see* Aspirin *on page 127*
- ♦ **Bayer**® **Women's Aspirin Plus Calcium [OTC]** *see* Aspirin *on page 127*
- ♦ **BayGam**® **[DSC]** *see* Immune Globulin (Intramuscular) *on page 795*
- ♦ **Baza**® **Antifungal [OTC]** *see* Miconazole *on page 1036*
- ♦ **beano**® **[OTC]** *see* Alpha-Galactosidase *on page 54*

Becaplermin (be KAP ler min)

Medication Safety Issues
Sound-alike/look-alike issues:
Regranex® may be confused with Granulex®, Repronex®

U.S. Brand Names Regranex®

Canadian Brand Names Regranex®

Index Terms Recombinant Human Platelet-Derived Growth Factor B; rPDGF-BB

Generic Available No

Pharmacologic Category Growth Factor, Platelet-Derived; Topical Skin Product

Use Debridement adjunct for the treatment of diabetic ulcers that occur on the lower limbs and feet

Contraindications Hypersensitivity to becaplermin or any component of the formulation; known neoplasm(s) at the site(s) of application; active infection at ulcer site

Warnings/Precautions Concurrent use of corticosteroids, cancer chemotherapy, or other immunosuppressive agents; ulcer wounds related to arterial or venous insufficiency. Thermal, electrical, or radiation burns at wound site. Malignancy (potential for tumor proliferation, although unproven); topical absorption is minimal). Should not be used in wounds that close by primary intention. For external use only.

Stability Refrigerate at 2°C to 8°C (36°F to 46°F); do not freeze.

Mechanism of Action Recombinant B-isoform homodimer of human platelet-derived growth factor (rPDGF-BB) which enhances formation of new granulation tissue, induces fibroblast proliferation and differentiation to promote wound healing

Pharmacodynamics Onset of action: Complete healing: 15% of patients within 8 weeks, 25% at 10 weeks

Pharmacokinetics
Absorption: Minimal
Distribution: Binds to PDGF-beta receptors in normal skin and granulation tissue

Dosage
Geriatrics & Adults:
Diabetic ulcers (lower extremity): Topical: Apply appropriate amount of gel once daily with a cotton swab or similar tool, as a coating over the ulcer
Estimation of gel requirement: The amount of becaplermin to be applied will vary depending on the size of the ulcer area. To calculate the length of gel applied to

the ulcer, measure the greatest length of the ulcer by the greatest width of the ulcer in inches. Tube size will determine the formula used in the calculation. For a 15 or 7.5 g tube, multiply length x width x 0.6. For a 2 g tube, multiply length x width x 1.3.

Note: If the ulcer does not decrease in size by ~30% after 10 weeks of treatment or complete healing has not occurred in 20 weeks, continued treatment with becaplermin gel should be reassessed.

Monitoring Parameters Ulcer volume (pressure ulcers); wound area; evidence of closure; drainage (diabetic ulcers); signs/symptoms of toxicity (erythema, local infections)

Patient Information Hands should be washed thoroughly before applying. The tip of the tube should not come into contact with the ulcer or any other surface; the tube should be recapped tightly after each use. A cotton swab, tongue depressor, or other application aid should be used to apply gel.

Step-by-step instructions for application:

Squeeze the calculated length of gel on to a clean, firm, nonabsorbable surface (wax paper)

With a clean cotton swab, tongue depressor, or similar application aid, spread the measured gel over the ulcer area to obtain an even layer

Cover with a saline-moistened gauze dressing. After ~12 hours, the ulcer should be gently rinsed with saline or water to remove residual gel and covered with a saline-moistened gauze dressing (**without** gel).

Special Geriatric Considerations No specific information for use in elderly.

Dosage Forms Excipient information presented when available (limited, particularly for generics); consult specific product labeling.

Gel, topical:

Regranex®: 0.01% (2 g, 15 g)

Beclomethasone (be kloe METH a sone)

Related Information

Asthma *on page 1767*
Inhalant Agents *on page 1760*

Medication Safety Issues

Sound-alike/look-alike issues:

Vanceril® may be confused with Vancenase®

U.S. Brand Names Beconase® AQ; QVAR®

Canadian Brand Names Apo-Beclomethasone®; Gen-Beclo; Nu-Beclomethasone; Propaderm®; QVAR®; Rivanase AQ; Vanceril® AEM

Index Terms Beclomethasone Dipropionate

Generic Available No

Pharmacologic Category Corticosteroid, Inhalant (Oral); Corticosteroid, Nasal

Use

Oral inhalation: Treatment of bronchial asthma in patients who require chronic administration of corticosteroids

Nasal aerosol: Symptomatic treatment of seasonal or perennial rhinitis and nasal polyposis

Contraindications Hypersensitivity to beclomethasone or any component of the formulation; status asthmaticus

Warnings/Precautions May cause hypercorticism or suppression of hypothalamic-pituitary-adrenal (HPA) axis, particularly in patients receiving high doses for prolonged periods. HPA axis suppression may lead to adrenal crisis. Withdrawal and discontinuation of a corticosteroid should be done slowly and carefully. Particular care is required when patients are transferred from systemic corticosteroids to inhaled products due to possible adrenal insufficiency or withdrawal from steroids, including an increase in allergic symptoms. Patients receiving >20 mg per day of prednisone (or equivalent) may be most susceptible. Fatalities have occurred due to adrenal insufficiency in asthmatic patients during and after transfer from systemic corticosteroids to aerosol steroids; aerosol steroids do not provide the systemic steroid needed to treat patients having trauma, surgery, or infections.

Bronchospasm may occur with wheezing after inhalation; if this occurs stop steroid and treat with a fast-acting bronchodilator. Supplemental steroids (oral or parenteral) may be needed during stress or severe asthma attacks. Not to be used in status asthmaticus or for the relief of acute bronchospasm. Corticosteroid use may cause psychiatric disturbances, including depression, euphoria, insomnia, mood swings, and personality changes. Pre-existing psychiatric conditions may be exacerbated by corticosteroid use. Prolonged use of corticosteroids may also increase the incidence of secondary infection, mask acute infection (including fungal infections), prolong or exacerbate viral infections, or limit response to vaccines. Exposure to chickenpox should be avoided; corticosteroids should not be used to treat ocular herpes simplex. Corticosteroids (Continued)

Beclomethasone *(Continued)*

should not be used for cerebral malaria. Close observation is required in patients with latent tuberculosis and/or TB reactivity; restrict use in active TB (only in conjunction with antituberculosis treatment). Prolonged treatment with corticosteroids has been associated with the development of Kaposi's sarcoma (case reports); if noted, discontinuation of therapy should be considered.

Use with caution in patients with thyroid disease, hepatic impairment, renal impairment, cardiovascular disease, diabetes, glaucoma, cataracts, myasthenia gravis, patients at risk for osteoporosis, patients at risk for seizures, or GI diseases (diverticulitis, peptic ulcer, ulcerative colitis) due to perforation risk. Use caution following acute MI (corticosteroids have been associated with myocardial rupture). Because of the risk of adverse effects, systemic corticosteroids should be used cautiously in the elderly in the smallest possible effective dose for the shortest duration. Avoid nasal corticosteroid use in patients with recent nasal septal ulcers, nasal surgery or nasal trauma until healing has occurred.

To minimize the systemic effects of orally-inhaled and intranasal corticosteroids, each patient should be titrated to the lowest effective dose. There have been reports of systemic corticosteroid withdrawal symptoms (eg, joint/muscle pain, lassitude, depression) when withdrawing oral inhalation therapy.

Adverse Reactions (Reflective of adult population; not specific for elderly)
Frequency not defined.

Central nervous system: Agitation, depression, dizziness, dysphonia, headache, light-headedness, mental disturbances

Dermatologic: Acneiform lesions, angioedema, atrophy, bruising, pruritus, purpura, striae, rash, urticaria

Endocrine & metabolic: Cushingoid features, growth velocity reduction in children and adolescents, HPA function suppression, weight gain

Gastrointestinal: Dry/irritated nose, throat and mouth, hoarseness, localized *Candida* or *Aspergillus* infection, loss of smell, loss of taste, nausea, unpleasant smell, unpleasant taste, vomiting

Local: Nasal spray: Burning, epistaxis, localized *Candida* infection, nasal septum perforation (rare), nasal stuffiness, nosebleeds, rhinorrhea, sneezing, transient irritation, ulceration of nasal mucosa (rare)

Ocular: Cataracts, glaucoma, intraocular pressure increased

Respiratory: Cough, paradoxical bronchospasm, pharyngitis, sinusitis, wheezing

Miscellaneous: Anaphylactic/anaphylactoid reactions, death (due to adrenal insufficiency, reported during and after transfer from systemic corticosteroids to aerosol in asthmatic patients), immediate and delayed hypersensitivity reactions

Overdosage/Toxicology Symptoms include irritation and burning of the nasal mucosa, sneezing, intranasal and pharyngeal *Candida* infections, nasal ulceration, epistaxis, rhinorrhea, nasal stuffiness, and headache. When consumed in excessive quantities, systemic hypercorticism and adrenal suppression may occur; in those cases, discontinuation and withdrawal of the corticosteroid should be done judiciously.

Drug Interactions

Amphotericin: Corticosteroids may increase the hypokalemic effects of amphotericin B; monitor.

Antidiabetic agents: Corticosteroids may decrease the hypoglycemic effects of antidiabetic agents; monitor.

Diuretics, potassium-wasting (loop or thiazide): Hypokalemic effects may be increased by corticosteroids; monitor.

Fluoroquinolones: Concurrent use may increase the risk of tendinopathies (including tendonitis and rupture), particularly in elderly patients (overall incidence rare)

Stability Do not store near heat or open flame. Do not puncture canisters. Store at room temperature. Rest QVAR® on concave end of canister with actuator on top.

Mechanism of Action Controls the rate of protein synthesis; depresses the migration of polymorphonuclear leukocytes, fibroblasts; reverses capillary permeability and lysosomal stabilization at the cellular level to prevent or control inflammation

Pharmacokinetics

Absorption:

Oral: 90%

Inhalation: Readily, ~10% to 25% of an inhaled dose reaches the respiratory tract

Protein binding: 87%

Metabolism: Oral: Hepatic

Half-life: 15 hours (biphasic decay terminal decay is 15 hours, initial phase half-life: 3 hours); after inhalation, it is quickly hydrolyzed by pulmonary esterases prior to absorption

Elimination: Renal excretion with oral administration

Dosage

Geriatrics & Adults: Nasal inhalation and oral inhalation dosage forms are not to be used interchangeably.

Rhinitis, nasal polyps: Inhalation, nasal (Beconase® AQ): 1-2 inhalations each nostril twice daily; total dose 168-336 mcg/day

Asthma: Inhalation, oral (doses should be titrated to the lowest effective dose once asthma is controlled) (QVAR®):

Patients previously on bronchodilators only: Initial dose 40-80 mcg twice daily; maximum dose 320 mcg twice day

Patients previously on inhaled corticosteroids: Initial dose 40-160 mcg twice daily; maximum dose 320 mcg twice daily

NIH Asthma Guidelines (NAEPP, 2002; NIH, 1997): HFA formulation (eg, QVAR®): Administer in divided doses:

"Low" dose: 80-240 mcg/day

"Medium" dose: 240-480 mcg/day

"High" dose: >480 mcg/day

Administration Aerosol inhalation: Shake container thoroughly before using. Sit when using. Take deep breaths for 3-5 minutes, and clear nasal passages before administration (use decongestant as needed). Hold breath for 5-10 seconds after use, and wait 1-3 minutes between inhalations. Follow package insert instructions for use. Do not exceed maximum dosage. If also using inhaled bronchodilator, use before beclomethasone. Rinse mouth and throat after use to reduce aftertaste and prevent candidiasis.

Patient Information Makes many asthmatics cough; inhale drug slowly or use prescribed inhaled bronchodilator 5 minutes before beclomethasone is used; notify physician if sore throat or sore mouth occurs; do not stop abruptly. See Administration.

Additional Information Not used in status asthmaticus; shake thoroughly before using; nasal inhalation and oral inhalation dosage forms are **not** to be used interchangeably

Special Geriatric Considerations Elderly patients may have difficulty with oral metered dose inhalers and may benefit from the use of a spacer or chamber device.

Dosage Forms Excipient information presented when available (limited, particularly for generics); consult specific product labeling.

Aerosol for oral inhalation, as dipropionate:

QVAR®: 40 mcg/inhalation [100 metered actuations] (7.3 g); 80 mcg/inhalation [100 metered actuations] (7.3 g)

Suspension, intranasal, as dipropionate [aqueous spray]:

Beconase® AQ: 42 mcg/inhalation [180 metered sprays (25 g)

♦ **Beclomethasone Dipropionate** *see* Beclomethasone *on page 153*
♦ **Beconase® AQ** *see* Beclomethasone *on page 153*
♦ **Belladonna Alkaloids With Phenobarbital** *see* Hyoscyamine, Atropine, Scopolamine, and Phenobarbital *on page 780*
♦ **Benadryl® Allergy [OTC]** *see* DiphenhydrAMINE *on page 447*
♦ **Benadryl® Children's Allergy [OTC]** *see* DiphenhydrAMINE *on page 447*
♦ **Benadryl® Children's Allergy Fastmelt® [OTC]** *see* DiphenhydrAMINE *on page 447*
♦ **Benadryl® Children's Dye-Free Allergy [OTC]** *see* DiphenhydrAMINE *on page 447*
♦ **Benadryl® Injection** *see* DiphenhydrAMINE *on page 447*
♦ **Benadryl® Itch Stopping [OTC]** *see* DiphenhydrAMINE *on page 447*
♦ **Benadryl® Itch Stopping Extra Strength [OTC]** *see* DiphenhydrAMINE *on page 447*

Benazepril (ben AY ze pril)

Related Information
Angiotensin Agents *on page 1737*
Medication Safety Issues
Sound-alike/look-alike issues:
Benazepril may be confused with Benadryl®
Lotensin® may be confused with Lioresal®, lovastatin
International issues:
Lotensin® may be confused with Latensin® which is a brand name for bacillus cereus in Germany
U.S. Brand Names Lotensin®
Canadian Brand Names Apo-Benazepril®; Lotensin®
Index Terms Benazepril Hydrochloride
Generic Available Yes
Pharmacologic Category Angiotensin-Converting Enzyme (ACE) Inhibitor
Use Treatment of hypertension, either alone or in combination with other antihypertensive agents
Unlabeled/Investigational Use Treatment of left ventricular dysfunction after myocardial infarction
(Continued)

Benazepril *(Continued)*

Contraindications Hypersensitivity to benazepril or any component of the formulation; angioedema or serious hypersensitivity related to previous treatment with an ACE inhibitor; bilateral renal artery stenosis; primary hyperaldosteronism; patients with idiopathic or hereditary angioedema

Warnings/Precautions Anaphylactic reactions can occur. Angioedema can occur at any time during treatment (especially following first dose). Angioedema can occur at any time during treatment (especially following first dose). It may involve head and neck (potentially affecting the airway) or the intestine (presenting with abdominal pain). Prolonged monitoring may be required especially if tongue, glottis, or larynx are involved as they are associated with airway obstruction. Those with a history of airway surgery in this situation have a higher risk. Careful blood pressure monitoring with first dose (hypotension can occur especially in volume-depleted patients). Dosage adjustment needed in renal impairment. Use with caution in hypovolemia; collagen vascular diseases; valvular stenosis (particularly aortic stenosis); hyperkalemia; or before, during, or immediately after anesthesia. Hyperkalemia may occur. Avoid rapid dosage escalation which may lead to renal insufficiency. Rare toxicities associated with ACE inhibitors include cholestatic jaundice (which may progress to hepatic necrosis) and neutropenia/agranulocytosis with myeloid hyperplasia. Hypersensitivity reactions may be seen during hemodialysis with high-flux dialysis membranes (eg, AN69). May be associated with deterioration of renal function and/or increases in serum creatinine, particularly in patients dependent on renin-angiotensin-aldosterone system. Use with caution in unilateral renal artery stenosis and pre-existing renal insufficiency; if patient has renal impairment then a baseline WBC with differential and serum creatinine should be evaluated and monitored closely during the first 3 months of therapy.

Adverse Reactions (Reflective of adult population; not specific for elderly)
1% to 10%:
Cardiovascular: Postural dizziness (2%)
Central nervous system: Headache (6%), dizziness (4%), fatigue (3%), somnolence (2%)
Endocrine & metabolic: Hyperkalemia (1%), uric acid increased
Gastrointestinal: Nausea (2%)
Renal: Serum creatinine increased (2%), worsening of renal function may occur in patients with bilateral renal artery stenosis or hypovolemia
Respiratory: Cough (1% to 10%)
Eosinophilic pneumonitis, neutropenia, anaphylaxis, renal insufficiency, and renal failure have been reported with other ACE inhibitors. In addition, a syndrome including fever, myalgia, arthralgia, interstitial nephritis, vasculitis, rash, eosinophilia, and elevated ESR has been reported to be associated with ACE inhibitors.

Overdosage/Toxicology Mild hypotension has been the only toxic effect seen with acute overdose; bradycardia may also occur. Hyperkalemia occurs even with therapeutic doses, especially in patients with renal insufficiency and those taking NSAIDs. Following initiation of essential overdose management, toxic symptom treatment and supportive treatment should be initiated. Hypotension usually responds to I.V. fluids or Trendelenburg positioning.

Drug Interactions
Alpha₁ blockers: Hypotensive effect increased.
Aspirin: The effects of ACE inhibitors may be blunted by aspirin administration, particularly at higher dosages, and/or increase adverse renal effects.
Diuretics: Hypovolemia due to diuretics may precipitate acute hypotensive events or acute renal failure.
Gold sodium thiomalate: ACE inhibitors may enhance the adverse/toxic effects (nitritoid reaction) of gold sodium thiomalate. The reaction may include facial flushing, nausea, vomiting, hypotension, and syncope. If it is to occur, would be expected shortly after administration of gold compound in patients maintained on an ACEI.
Insulin: Risk of hypoglycemia may be increased.
Lithium: Risk of lithium toxicity may be increased; monitor lithium levels.
NSAIDs: May attenuate hypertensive efficacy; effect has been seen with captopril and may occur with other ACE inhibitors; monitor blood pressure. May increase adverse renal effects.
Potassium-sparing diuretics or potassium supplements (amiloride, potassium, spironolactone, triamterene): Increased risk of hyperkalemia.
Trimethoprim (high dose) may increase the risk of hyperkalemia.

Ethanol/Nutrition/Herb Interactions Herb/Nutraceutical: Avoid dong quai if using for hypertension (has estrogenic activity). Avoid ephedra, yohimbe, ginseng (may worsen hypertension). Avoid garlic (may have increased antihypertensive effect).

Mechanism of Action Competitive inhibition of angiotensin I being converted to angiotensin II, a potent vasoconstrictor, through the angiotensin I-converting enzyme (ACE) activity, with resultant lower levels of angiotensin II which causes an increase in plasma renin activity and a reduction in aldosterone secretion

Pharmacodynamics

Reduction in plasma angiotensin-converting enzyme activity:
  Peak effect: 1-2 hours after oral administration of 2-20 mg dose
  Duration: >90% inhibition for 24 hours has been observed after 5-20 mg oral dose
Reduction in blood pressure:
  Single oral dose: Peak effect: 2-6 hours
  With continuous therapy:
    Maximum response: 2 weeks
    Duration: 2 years

Pharmacokinetics

Absorption: Oral: Rapid, 37%; food does not alter significantly; metabolite (benazeprilat) itself unsuitable for oral administration due to poor absorption
Distribution: V_d: ~8.7 L
Protein binding: 96.7%; benazeprilat: 95.3%
Metabolism: Rapid and extensive in the liver to its active metabolite, benazeprilat, via enzymatic hydrolysis; undergoes significant first-pass metabolism and is completely eliminated from plasma in 4 hours
Half-life: Benazeprilat: Effective: 10-11 hours; Terminal: 22 hours
Time to peak: Parent drug: 0.5-1 hour
Elimination: Nonrenal clearance (ie, biliary, metabolic) appears to contribute to the elimination of benazeprilat (11% to 12%), particularly in patients with severe renal impairment; hepatic clearance is the main elimination route of unchanged benazepril
Dialyzable: ~6% of metabolite removed by 4 hours of dialysis following 10 mg of benazepril administered 2 hours prior to procedure; parent compound was not found in the dialysate

Dosage

Geriatrics: Oral: Initial: 5-10 mg/day in single or divided doses; usual range: 20-40 mg/day; adjust for renal function. Also see "Note" in adult dosing.

Adults: Hypertension: Oral: Initial: 10 mg/day in patients not receiving a diuretic; 20-40 mg/day as a single dose or 2 divided doses; the need for twice-daily dosing should be assessed by monitoring peak (2-6 hours after dosing) and trough responses.

Note: Patients taking diuretics should have them discontinued 2-3 days prior to starting benazepril. If they cannot be discontinued, then initial dose should be 5 mg; restart after blood pressure is stabilized if needed.

Renal Impairment:

Cl_{cr} <30 mL/minute: Administer 5 mg/day initially; maximum daily dose: 40 mg.
Hemodialysis: Moderately dialyzable (20% to 50%); administer dose postdialysis or administer 25% to 35% supplemental dose.
Peritoneal dialysis: Supplemental dose is not necessary.

Monitoring Parameters Serum potassium concentration, BUN, serum creatinine, renal function, WBC

Patient Information Notify physician of persistent cough; do not stop therapy except under prescriber advice; notify physician if you develop sore throat, fever, swelling of hands, feet, face, eyes, lips, and tongue; difficult breathing, irregular heartbeats, chest pains, or cough. May cause dizziness, fainting, and lightheadedness, especially in first week of therapy, sit and stand up slowly; may cause changes in taste or rash; do not add a salt substitute (potassium) without advice of physician.

Additional Information Watch for hypotensive effect within 1-3 hours of first dose or new higher dose.

Special Geriatric Considerations Due to frequent decreases in glomerular filtration (also Cl_{cr}) with aging, elderly patients may have exaggerated responses to ACE inhibitors; differences in clinical response due to hepatic changes are not observed. ACE inhibitors may be preferred agents in elderly patients with congestive heart failure and diabetes mellitus. Diabetic proteinuria is reduced and insulin sensitivity is enhanced. In general, the side effect profile is favorable in elderly and causes little or no CNS confusion; use lowest dose recommendations initially. Many elderly may be volume depleted due to diuretic use and/or blunted thirst reflex resulting in inadequate fluid intake.

Benazepril and benazeprilat are substantially excreted by the kidney. Because elderly are more likely to have decreased renal function, care should be taken in dose selection, and it may be useful to monitor renal function.

Dosage Forms Excipient information presented when available (limited, particularly for generics); consult specific product labeling.
Tablet, as hydrochloride: 5 mg, 10 mg, 20 mg, 40 mg
  Lotensin®: 5 mg, 10 mg, 20 mg, 40 mg

Extemporaneously Prepared To prepare a 2 mg/mL suspension, mix 15 benazepril 20 mg tablets in a bottle with Ora-Plus® 75 mL. Shake for 2 minutes, allow suspension to stand for ≥1 hour, then shake again for at least 1 additional minute. Add Ora-Sweet® (Continued)

Benazepril *(Continued)*

75 mL to suspension and shake to disperse. Will make 150 mL of a 2 mg/mL suspension. Store under refrigeration at 2°C to 8°C (36°F to 46°F) for up to 30 days. Shake prior to each use.

Selected References

Konstam MA, Drakup K, Baker DW, et al, "Heart Failure: Evaluation and Care of Patients With Left Ventricular Systolic Dysfunction," *Clinical Practice Guideline No 11*, Rockville, MD: Agency for Health Care Policy and Research, Public Health Service, U.S. Department of Health and Human Services, 1994.

McAreavey D and Robertson JI, "Angiotensin Converting Enzyme Inhibitors and Moderate Hypertension," *Drugs*, 1990, 40(3):326-45.

Williams JF, Bristow MR, Fowler MB, et al, "Guidelines for the Evaluation and Management of Heart Failure: Report of the American College of Cardiology/American Heart Association Task Force on Practice Guidelines (Committee on Evaluation and Management of Heart Failure)," *J Am Coll Cardiol*, 1995, 26:1376-8.

Benazepril and Hydrochlorothiazide

(ben AY ze pril & hye droe klor oh THYE a zide)

Related Information

Benazepril *on page 155*
Hydrochlorothiazide *on page 756*

U.S. Brand Names Lotensin® HCT

Index Terms Hydrochlorothiazide and Benazepril

Generic Available Yes

Pharmacologic Category Antihypertensive Agent, Combination

Use Treatment of hypertension

Dosage

Geriatrics: Dose is individualized.

Adults: Hypertension: Oral: Dose is individualized (range: benazepril: 5-20 mg; hydrochlorothiazide: 6.25-25 mg/day)

Renal Impairment: Cl_{cr} <30 mL/minute: Not recommended; loop diuretics are preferred.

Special Geriatric Considerations In clinical studies, of the total number of patients who received Lotensin® HCT in U.S., 19% were ≥65 years of age, while ~1.5% were ≥75 years. Overall differences in effectiveness or safety were not observed between these patients and younger patients, and other reported clinical experience has not identified differences in responses between elderly and younger patients, but greater sensitivity of some older individuals cannot be ruled out.

Dosage Forms Excipient information presented when available (limited, particularly for generics); consult specific product labeling.

Tablet: 5/6.25: Benazepril hydrochloride 5 mg and hydrochlorothiazide 6.25 mg; 10/12.5: Benazepril hydrochloride 10 mg and hydrochlorothiazide 12.5 mg; 20/12.5: Benazepril hydrochloride 20 mg and hydrochlorothiazide 12.5 mg; 20/25: Benazepril hydrochloride 20 mg and hydrochlorothiazide 25 mg

Lotensin® HCT 5/6.25: Benazepril hydrochloride 5 mg and hydrochlorothiazide 6.25 mg

Lotensin® HCT 10/12.5: Benazepril hydrochloride 10 mg and hydrochlorothiazide 12.5 mg

Lotensin® HCT 20/12.5: Benazepril hydrochloride 20 mg and hydrochlorothiazide 12.5 mg

Lotensin® HCT 20/25: Benazepril hydrochloride 20 mg and hydrochlorothiazide 25 mg

- ◆ **Benazepril Hydrochloride** *see* Benazepril *on page 155*
- ◆ **Benazepril Hydrochloride and Amlodipine Besylate** *see* Amlodipine and Benazepril *on page 90*
- ◆ **Benemid [DSC]** *see* Probenecid *on page 1315*
- ◆ **Benicar®** *see* Olmesartan *on page 1151*
- ◆ **Benicar HCT®** *see* Olmesartan and Hydrochlorothiazide *on page 1152*
- ◆ **Ben-Tann** *see* DiphenhydrAMINE *on page 447*
- ◆ **Bentyl®** *see* Dicyclomine *on page 430*
- ◆ **Benzathine Benzylpenicillin** *see* Penicillin G Benzathine *on page 1221*
- ◆ **Benzathine Penicillin G** *see* Penicillin G Benzathine *on page 1221*
- ◆ **Benzene Hexachloride** *see* Lindane *on page 909*
- ◆ **Benzhexol Hydrochloride** *see* Trihexyphenidyl *on page 1631*

Benzonatate (ben ZOE na tate)

U.S. Brand Names Tessalon®
Canadian Brand Names Tessalon®
Generic Available Yes

Pharmacologic Category Antitussive

Use Symptomatic relief of nonproductive cough

Contraindications Hypersensitivity to benzonatate, related compounds (such as tetracaine), or any component of the formulation

Warnings/Precautions Release of benzonatate in the mouth can cause a temporary local anesthesia of the oral mucosa; capsules should be swallowed whole

Adverse Reactions (Reflective of adult population; not specific for elderly)
1% to 10%:
Central nervous system: Sedation, headache, dizziness
Dermatologic: Rash
Gastrointestinal: GI upset
Neuromuscular & skeletal: Chest numbness
Ocular: Burning sensation in eyes
Respiratory: Nasal congestion

Overdosage/Toxicology Symptoms include restlessness, tremor, and CNS stimulation. The drug's local anesthetic activity can reduce the patient's gag reflex and, therefore, may contradict the use of ipecac following ingestion, this is especially true when the capsules are chewed. Gastric lavage may be indicated if initiated early on following an acute ingestion or in comatose patients. The remaining treatment is supportive and symptomatic.

Drug Interactions No data reported

Mechanism of Action Tetracaine congener with antitussive properties; suppresses cough by topical anesthetic action on the respiratory stretch receptors

Pharmacodynamics
Onset of action: Therapeutic: Within 15-20 minutes
Duration: 3-8 hours

Dosage
Geriatrics & Adults: Cough: Oral: 100 mg 3 times/day or every 4 hours up to 600 mg/day

Monitoring Parameters Patient's chest sounds and respiratory pattern, mental status

Patient Information Swallow capsule whole; use of hard candy may increase saliva flow to aid in protecting pharyngeal mucosa

Special Geriatric Considerations No specific geriatric information is available about benzonatate. Avoid use in patients with impaired gag reflex or who cannot swallow the capsule whole.

Dosage Forms Excipient information presented when available (limited, particularly for generics); consult specific product labeling.
Capsule, softgel: 100 mg, 200 mg
Tessalon®: 100 mg, 200 mg

Benztropine (BENZ troe peen)

Related Information
Antiparkinsonian Agents on page 1745
Medication Safety Issues
Sound-alike/look-alike issues:
Benztropine may be confused with bromocriptine
U.S. Brand Names Cogentin®
Canadian Brand Names Apo-Benztropine®
Index Terms Benztropine Mesylate
Generic Available Yes: Tablet
Pharmacologic Category Anti-Parkinson's Agent, Anticholinergic; Anticholinergic Agent
Use Adjunctive treatment of all forms of parkinsonism; treatment of drug-induced extrapyramidal effects (except tardive dyskinesia) and acute dystonic reactions
Contraindications Hypersensitivity to benztropine or any component of the formulation; pyloric or duodenal obstruction, stenosing peptic ulcers; bladder neck obstructions; achalasia; myasthenia gravis
Warnings/Precautions Use with caution in hot weather or during exercise. May cause anhidrosis and hyperthermia, which may be severe. The risk is increased in hot environments, particularly in the elderly, alcoholics, patients with CNS disease, and those with prolonged outdoor exposure.

Elderly patients frequently develop increased sensitivity and require strict dosage regulation - side effects may be more severe in elderly patients with atherosclerotic changes. Use with caution in patients with tachycardia, cardiac arrhythmias, glaucoma, hypertension, hypotension, prostatic hyperplasia (especially in the elderly), any tendency toward urinary retention, liver or kidney disorders, and obstructive disease of the GI or GU tract. When given in large doses or to susceptible patients, may cause weakness and inability to move particular muscle groups.
(Continued)

Benztropine *(Continued)*

May be associated with confusion or hallucinations (generally at higher dosages). Intensification of symptoms or toxic psychosis may occur in patients with mental disorders. May cause CNS depression, which may impair physical or mental abilities; patients must be cautioned about performing tasks which require mental alertness (eg, operating machinery or driving).

Adverse Reactions (Reflective of adult population; not specific for elderly)
Frequency not defined.
Cardiovascular: Tachycardia
Central nervous system: Confusion, disorientation, memory impairment, toxic psychosis, visual hallucinations
Dermatologic: Rash
Endocrine & metabolic: Heat stroke, hyperthermia
Gastrointestinal: Constipation, dry throat, ileus, nasal dryness, nausea, vomiting, xerostomia
Genitourinary: Urinary retention, dysuria
Ocular: Blurred vision, mydriasis
Miscellaneous: Fever

Overdosage/Toxicology Symptoms include CNS depression, confusion, nervousness, hallucinations, dizziness, blurred vision, nausea, vomiting, and hyperthermia. For anticholinergic overdose with severe life-threatening symptoms, physostigmine 1-2 mg SubQ or slow I.V., may be given to reverse these effects. Anticholinergic toxicity is caused by strong binding of the drug to cholinergic receptors. Anticholinesterase inhibitors reduce acetylcholinesterase, the enzyme that breaks down acetylcholine and thereby allows acetylcholine to accumulate and compete for receptor binding with the offending anticholinergic.

Drug Interactions Substrate of CYP2D6 (minor)
Amantadine, rimantadine: Central and/or peripheral anticholinergic syndrome can occur when administered with amantadine or rimantadine.
Anticholinergic agents: Central and/or peripheral anticholinergic syndrome can occur when administered with opioid analgesics, phenothiazines and other antipsychotics (especially with high anticholinergic activity), tricyclic antidepressants, quinidine and some other antiarrhythmics, and antihistamines.
Atenolol: Anticholinergics may increase the bioavailability of atenolol (and possibly other beta-blockers); monitor for increased effect.
Cholinergic agents: Anticholinergics may antagonize the therapeutic effect of cholinergic agents; includes tacrine and donepezil.
Digoxin: Anticholinergics may decrease gastric degradation and increase the amount of digoxin absorbed by delaying gastric emptying.
Levodopa: Anticholinergics may increase gastric degradation and decrease the amount of levodopa absorbed by delaying gastric emptying.
Neuroleptics: Anticholinergics may antagonize the therapeutic effects of neuroleptics.

Ethanol/Nutrition/Herb Interactions Ethanol: Avoid ethanol (may increase CNS depression).

Mechanism of Action Possesses both anticholinergic and antihistaminic effects. *In vitro* anticholinergic activity approximates that of atropine; *in vivo* it is only about half as active as atropine. Animal data suggest its antihistaminic activity and duration of action approach that of pyrilamine maleate. May also inhibit the reuptake and storage of dopamine, thereby prolonging the action of dopamine.

Pharmacodynamics
Onset of action:
Parenteral dose: Within 15 minutes
Oral: Within 60 minutes
Duration: Activity can last from as little as 6 hours to as long as 48 hours

Dosage
Geriatrics: Oral: Initial: 0.5 mg once or twice daily; titrate dose in 0.5 mg increments at every 5-6 days; maximum: 4 mg/day.
Adults:
Drug-induced extrapyramidal symptom: Oral, I.M., I.V.: 1-4 mg/dose 1-2 times/day
Acute dystonia: I.M., I.V.: 1-2 mg
Parkinsonism: Oral: 0.5-6 mg/day in 1-2 divided doses; if one dose is greater, give at bedtime. Titrate dose in 0.5 mg increments at 5- to 6-day intervals.

Monitoring Parameters Symptoms of EPS or Parkinson's, pulse, anticholinergic effects (ie, CNS, bowel, and bladder function)

Patient Information Take after meals or with food if GI upset occurs; do not discontinue drug abruptly; notify physician if adverse GI effects, rapid or pounding heartbeat, confusion, eye pain, rash, fever or heat intolerance occurs. Observe caution when performing hazardous tasks or those that require alertness such as driving, as may cause drowsiness. Avoid alcohol and other CNS depressants. May cause dry mouth -

adequate fluid intake or hard sugar-free candy may relieve. Difficult urination or constipation may occur - notify physician if effects persist; may increase susceptibility to heat stroke.

Additional Information No significant difference in onset of I.M. or I.V. injection, therefore, there is usually no need to use the I.V. route. Improvement is sometimes noticeable a few minutes after injection. Do not discontinue drug abruptly.

Special Geriatric Considerations Anticholinergic agents are generally not well tolerated in the elderly (often results in bowel, bladder, and CNS adverse effects) and their use should be avoided when possible. In the elderly, anticholinergic agents should not be used as prophylaxis against extrapyramidal symptoms.

Dosage Forms Excipient information presented when available (limited, particularly for generics); consult specific product labeling.

Injection, solution, as mesylate (Cogentin®): 1 mg/mL (2 mL)

Tablet, as mesylate: 0.5 mg, 1 mg, 2 mg

Selected References

Feinberg M, "The Problems of Anticholinergic Adverse Effects in Older Patients," *Drugs Aging*, 1993, 3(4):335-48.

Olanow CW, Watts RL, and Koller WC, "An Algorithm (Decision Tree) for the Management of Parkinson's Disease (2001): Treatment Guidelines," *Neurology*, 2001, 56(11 Suppl 5):S1-S88.

♦ **Benztropine Mesylate** *see* Benztropine *on page 159*

♦ **Benzylpenicillin Benzathine** *see* Penicillin G Benzathine *on page 1221*

♦ **Benzylpenicillin Potassium** *see* Penicillin G (Parenteral/Aqueous) *on page 1224*

♦ **Benzylpenicillin Sodium** *see* Penicillin G (Parenteral/Aqueous) *on page 1224*

♦ **Betagan®** *see* Levobunolol *on page 891*

♦ **Beta-HC®** *see* Hydrocortisone *on page 762*

Betamethasone (bay ta METH a sone)

Related Information
Corticosteroids *on page 1755*

Medication Safety Issues
Sound-alike/look-alike issues:
Luxiq® may be confused with Lasix®

International issues:
Beta-Val® may be confused with Betanol® which is a brand name for metipranolol in Monaco

U.S. Brand Names Beta-Val®; Celestone®; Celestone® Soluspan®; Diprolene®; Diprolene® AF; Luxiq®

Canadian Brand Names Betaderm®; Betaject™; Betnesol®; Betnovate®; Celestone® Soluspan®; Diprolene® Glycol; Diprosone®; Ectosone; Prevex® B; Taro-Sone®; Topilene®; Topisone®; Valisone® Scalp Lotion

Index Terms Betamethasone Dipropionate; Betamethasone Dipropionate, Augmented; Betamethasone Sodium Phosphate; Betamethasone Valerate; Flubenisolone

Generic Available Yes: Excludes aerosol, injection, solution

Pharmacologic Category Corticosteroid, Systemic; Corticosteroid, Topical

Use Treatment of inflammatory dermatoses such as seborrheic or atopic dermatitis, neurodermatitis, anogenital pruritus, psoriasis, inflammatory phase of xerosis, late phase of allergic dermatitis or irritant dermatitis

Contraindications Hypersensitivity to betamethasone or any component of the formulation; systemic fungal infections

Warnings/Precautions Very high potency topical products are not for treatment of rosacea, perioral dermatitis; not for use on face, groin, or axillae; not for use in a diapered area. Avoid concurrent use of other corticosteroids.

May cause hypercorticism or suppression of hypothalamic-pituitary-adrenal (HPA) axis, particularly in patients receiving high doses for prolonged periods. HPA axis suppression may lead to adrenal crisis. Withdrawal and discontinuation of a corticosteroid should be done slowly and carefully. Particular care is required when patients are transferred from systemic corticosteroids to inhaled products due to possible adrenal insufficiency or withdrawal from steroids, including an increase in allergic symptoms. Patients receiving >20 mg per day of prednisone (or equivalent) may be most susceptible. Fatalities have occurred due to adrenal insufficiency in asthmatic patients during and after transfer from systemic corticosteroids to aerosol steroids; aerosol steroids do not provide the systemic steroid needed to treat patients having trauma, surgery, or infections. In stressful situations, HPA axis-suppressed patients should receive adequate supplementation with natural glucocorticoids (hydrocortisone or cortisone) rather than betamethasone (due to lack of mineralocorticoid activity).

Acute myopathy has been reported with high dose corticosteroids, usually in patients with neuromuscular transmission disorders; may involve ocular and/or respiratory muscles; monitor creatine kinase; recovery may be delayed. Corticosteroid use may
(Continued)

Betamethasone *(Continued)*

cause psychiatric disturbances, including depression, euphoria, insomnia, mood swings, and personality changes. Pre-existing psychiatric conditions may be exacerbated by corticosteroid use. Prolonged use of corticosteroids may also increase the incidence of secondary infection, mask acute infection (including fungal infections), prolong or exacerbate viral infections, or limit response to vaccines. Exposure to chickenpox should be avoided; corticosteroids should not be used to treat ocular herpes simplex. Corticosteroids should not be used for cerebral malaria. Close observation is required in patients with latent tuberculosis and/or TB reactivity; restrict use in active TB (only in conjunction with antituberculosis treatment). Prolonged treatment with corticosteroids has been associated with the development of Kaposi's sarcoma (case reports); if noted, discontinuation of therapy should be considered.

Use with caution in patients with thyroid disease, hepatic impairment, renal impairment, cardiovascular disease, diabetes, glaucoma, cataracts, myasthenia gravis, patients at risk for osteoporosis, patients at risk for seizures, or GI diseases (diverticulitis, peptic ulcer, ulcerative colitis) due to perforation risk. Use caution following acute MI (corticosteroids have been associated with myocardial rupture). Because of the risk of adverse effects, systemic corticosteroids should be used cautiously in the elderly in the smallest possible effective dose for the shortest duration. Do not use occlusive dressings on weeping or exudative lesions and general caution with occlusive dressings should be observed; adverse effects may be increased. Discontinue if skin irritation or contact dermatitis should occur; do not use in patients with decreased skin circulation. Withdraw therapy with gradual tapering of dose.

Adverse Reactions (Reflective of adult population; not specific for elderly)
Systemic:
Cardiovascular: Congestive heart failure, edema, hyper-/hypotension
Central nervous system: Dizziness, headache, insomnia, intracranial pressure increased, lightheadedness, nervousness, pseudotumor cerebri, seizure, vertigo
Dermatologic: Ecchymoses, facial erythema, fragile skin, hirsutism, hyper-/hypopigmentation, perioral dermatitis (oral), petechiae, striae, wound healing impaired
Endocrine & metabolic: Amenorrhea, Cushing's syndrome, diabetes mellitus, growth suppression, hyperglycemia, hypokalemia, menstrual irregularities, pituitary-adrenal axis suppression, protein catabolism, sodium retention, water retention
Local: Injection site reactions (intra-articular use), sterile abscess
Neuromuscular & skeletal: Arthralgia, muscle atrophy, fractures, muscle weakness, myopathy, osteoporosis, necrosis (femoral and humeral heads)
Ocular: Cataracts, glaucoma, intraocular pressure increased
Miscellaneous: Anaphylactoid reaction, diaphoresis, hypersensitivity, secondary infection
Topical:
Dermatologic: Acneiform eruptions, allergic dermatitis, burning, dry skin, erythema, folliculitis, hypertrichosis, irritation, miliaria, pruritus, skin atrophy, striae, vesiculation
Endocrine and metabolic effects have occasionally been reported with topical use.

Overdosage/Toxicology When consumed in excessive quantities for prolonged periods, systemic hypercorticism and adrenal suppression may occur; in those cases, discontinuation and withdrawal of the corticosteroid should be done judiciously.

Drug Interactions Inhibits CYP3A4 (weak)
Aminoglutethimide: May reduce the serum levels/effects of corticosteroids; likely via induction of microsomal isoenzymes.
Amphotericin: Corticosteroids may increase the hypokalemic effects of amphotericin B; monitor.
Antacids: May decrease the absorption of corticosteroids; separate administration by 2 hours.
Anticholinesterases: Concurrent use may lead to severe weakness in patients with myasthenia gravis.
Antidiabetic agents: Corticosteroids may decrease the hypoglycemic effects of antidiabetic agents; monitor.
Aprepitant: May increase the serum levels/effects of corticosteroids; monitor.
Antifungal agents (azole): May increase the serum levels/effects of corticosteroids; monitor.
Barbiturates: May decrease the levels/effects of corticosteroids.
Bile acid sequestrants: May reduce the absorption of corticosteroids; separate administration by 2 hours.
Calcium channel blockers (nondihydropyridine): May increase the serum levels/effects of corticosteroids; monitor.
Cyclosporine: Corticosteroids may increase the serum levels/effects of cyclosporine. In addition, cyclosporine may increase levels of corticosteroids.
Diuretics, potassium-wasting (loop or thiazide): Hypokalemic effects may be increased by corticosteroids; monitor.
Estrogens: May increase the serum levels/effects of corticosteroids; monitor.

Fluoroquinolones: Concurrent use may increase the risk of tendinopathies (including tendonitis and rupture), particularly in elderly patients (overall incidence rare)

Isoniazid: Serum levels/effects may be decreased by corticosteroids.

Macrolide antibiotics: May increase the serum levels/effects of corticosteroids.

Neuromuscular-blocking agents: Concurrent use with corticosteroids may increase the risk of myopathy.

Nonsteroidal anti-inflammatory drugs (NSAIDs): Concurrent use with corticosteroids may lead to an increased incidence of gastrointestinal adverse effects; use caution.

Rifamycin derivatives: May decrease the levels/effects of corticosteroids (systemic); monitor.

Salicylates: Salicylates may increase the gastrointestinal adverse effects of corticosteroids.

Vaccine (dead organism): Corticosteroids may decrease the effect of vaccines (dead organisms). In patients receiving high doses of systemic corticosteroids for ≥14 days, wait at least 1 month between discontinuing steroid therapy and administering immunization.

Vaccine (live organism): Corticosteroids may increase the risk of vaccinal infection. The use of live vaccines is contraindicated in immunosuppressed patients.

Warfarin: Corticosteroids may increase the anticoagulant effects of warfarin; monitor INR.

Ethanol/Nutrition/Herb Interactions
Ethanol: Avoid ethanol (may enhance gastric mucosal irritation).

Food: Betamethasone interferes with calcium absorption.

Herb/Nutraceutical: Avoid cat's claw, echinacea (have immunostimulant properties).

Mechanism of Action
Controls the rate of protein synthesis; depresses the migration of polymorphonuclear leukocytes, fibroblasts; reverses capillary permeability and lysosomal stabilization at the cellular level to prevent or control inflammation

Pharmacokinetics
Protein binding: 64%

Metabolism: Extensive in the liver

Half-life: 6.5 hours

Time to peak serum concentration: I.V.: Within 10-36 minutes

Elimination: <5% of dose excreted renally as unchanged drug

Dosage
Geriatrics: Refer to adult dosing. Use the lowest effective dose.

Adults: Base dosage on severity of disease and patient response
  Inflammatory conditions:
    Oral: 2.4-4.8 mg/day in 2-4 doses; range: 0.6-7.2 mg/day
    I.M.: Betamethasone sodium phosphate and betamethasone acetate: 0.6-9 mg/day (generally, $\frac{1}{3}$ to $\frac{1}{2}$ of oral dose) divided every 12-24 hours
  Psoriasis (scalp): Topical (foam): Apply to the scalp twice daily, once in the morning and once at night.
  Rheumatoid arthritis/osteoarthritis:
    Intrabursal, intra-articular, intradermal: 0.25-2 mL
    Intralesional:
      Very large joints: 1-2 mL
      Large joints: 1 mL
      Medium joints: 0.5-1 mL
      Small joints: 0.25-0.5 mL
  Steroid-responsive dermatoses: Therapy should be discontinued when control is achieved; if no improvement is seen, reassessment of diagnosis may be necessary.
    Gel, augmented formulation: Apply once or twice daily; rub in gently. **Note:** Do not exceed 2 weeks of treatment or 50 g/week.
    Lotion: Apply a few drops twice daily
      Augmented formulation: Apply a few drops once or twice daily; rub in gently. **Note:** Do not exceed 2 weeks of treatment or 50 mL/week.
    Cream/ointment: Apply once or twice daily
      Augmented formulation: Apply once or twice daily. **Note:** Do not exceed 2 weeks of treatment or 45 g/week.

Hepatic Impairment: Adjustments may be necessary in patients with liver failure because betamethasone is extensively metabolized in the liver

Administration
Oral: Not for alternate day therapy; once daily doses should be given in the morning.

I.M.: Do **not** give injectable sodium phosphate/acetate suspension I.V.

Topical: Apply topical sparingly to areas. Not for use on broken skin or in areas of infection. Do not apply to wet skin unless directed; do not cover with occlusive dressing. Do not apply very high potency agents to face, groin, axillae, or perianal area.

  Foam: Invert can and dispense a small amount onto a saucer or other cool surface. Do not dispense directly into hands. Pick up small amounts of foam and gently

(Continued)

Betamethasone *(Continued)*

massage into affected areas until foam disappears. Repeat until entire affected scalp area is treated.

Monitoring Parameters Blood pressure, blood glucose, electrolytes

Patient Information Take with food or milk; take single daily dose in the morning; do not stop oral products abruptly; if taking oral product, carry an identification card or bracelet advising that you are on steroids; apply topical preparations in a thin layer

Additional Information

Very High Potency: Augmented betamethasone dipropionate ointment, lotion

High Potency: Augmented betamethasone dipropionate cream, betamethasone dipropionate cream and ointment

Intermediate Potency: Betamethasone dipropionate lotion, betamethasone valerate cream

Special Geriatric Considerations Because of the risk of adverse effects, systemic corticosteroids should be used cautiously in the elderly, in the smallest possible dose, and for the shortest possible time.

Dosage Forms Excipient information presented when available (limited, particularly for generics); consult specific product labeling.

Note: Potency expressed as betamethasone base.

Aerosol, topical, as valerate [foam]:

Luxiq®: 0.12% (50 g, 100 g, 150 g) [strength expressed as salt; contains ethanol 60.4%]

Cream, topical, as dipropionate: 0.05% (15 g, 45 g)

Cream, topical, as dipropionate augmented: 0.05% (15 g, 50 g)

Diprolene® AF: 0.05% (15 g, 50 g)

Cream, topical, as valerate (Beta-Val®): 0.1% (15 g, 45 g)

Beta-Val®: 0.1% (15 g, 45 g)

Gel, topical, as dipropionate augmented: 0.05% (15 g, 50 g)

Injection, suspension:

Celestone® Soluspan®: Betamethasone sodium phosphate 3 mg and betamethasone acetate 3 mg per 1 mL (5 mL) [6 mg/mL]

Lotion, topical, as dipropionate: 0.05% (60 mL)

Lotion, topical, as dipropionate augmented:

Diprolene®: 0.05% (30 mL, 60 mL)

Lotion, topical, as valerate: 0.1% (60 mL)

Beta-Val®: 0.1% (60 mL)

Ointment, topical, as dipropionate: 0.05% (15 g, 45 g)

Ointment, topical, as dipropionate augmented: 0.05% (15 g, 50 g)

Diprolene®: 0.05% (15 g, 50 g)

Ointment, topical, as valerate: 0.1% (15 g, 45 g)

Solution, as base:

Celestone®: 0.6 mg/5 mL (118 mL) [contains alcohol and sodium benzoate; cherry-orange flavor]

♦ **Betamethasone Dipropionate** *see* Betamethasone *on page 161*

♦ **Betamethasone Dipropionate, Augmented** *see* Betamethasone *on page 161*

♦ **Betamethasone Sodium Phosphate** *see* Betamethasone *on page 161*

♦ **Betamethasone Valerate** *see* Betamethasone *on page 161*

♦ **Betapace®** *see* Sotalol *on page 1485*

♦ **Betapace AF®** *see* Sotalol *on page 1485*

♦ **Betaseron®** *see* Interferon Beta-1b *on page 824*

♦ **Beta-Val®** *see* Betamethasone *on page 161*

Betaxolol *(be TAKS oh lol)*

Related Information

Beta-Blockers *on page 1751*

Glaucoma Drug Therapy *on page 1758*

Medication Safety Issues

Sound-alike/look-alike issues:

Betaxolol may be confused with bethanechol, labetalol

U.S. Brand Names Betoptic® S; Kerlone®

Canadian Brand Names Betoptic® S; Sandoz-Betaxolol

Index Terms Betaxolol Hydrochloride

Generic Available Yes: Solution, tablet

Pharmacologic Category Beta Blocker, Beta$_1$ Selective; Ophthalmic Agent, Antiglaucoma

Use Treatment of chronic open-angle glaucoma, ocular hypertension; management of hypertension

Contraindications Hypersensitivity to betaxolol or any component of the formulation; sinus bradycardia; heart block greater than first-degree (except in patients with a functioning artificial pacemaker); cardiogenic shock; uncompensated cardiac failure; pulmonary edema

Warnings/Precautions Consider pre-existing conditions (such as sick sinus syndrome) before initiating. Administer cautiously in compensated heart failure and monitor for a worsening of the condition. Beta-blocker therapy should not be withdrawn abruptly (particularly in patients with CAD), but gradually tapered to avoid acute tachycardia, hypertension, and/or ischemia. Use caution with concurrent use of beta-blockers and either verapamil or diltiazem; bradycardia or heart block can occur. Use caution in patients with PVD (can aggravate arterial insufficiency). In general, beta-blockers should be avoided in patients with bronchospastic disease. Betaxolol, with beta₁ selectivity, should be used cautiously in bronchospastic disease with close monitoring. Use cautiously in patients with diabetes because it can mask prominent hypoglycemic symptoms. May mask signs of hyperthyroidism (eg, tachycardia); use caution if hyperthyroidism is suspected, abrupt withdrawal may precipitate thyroid storm. Use with caution in patients with cerebrovascular insufficiency; hypotension and decreased heart rate may reduce cerebral blood flow. Dosage adjustment required in severe renal impairment and in patients on dialysis. Use care with anesthetic agents which decrease myocardial function. Use with caution in patients with myasthenia gravis (may potentiate myasthenia-related muscle weakness, including diplopia and ptosis) or psychiatric disease (may cause CNS depression). Adequate alpha-blockade is required prior to use of any beta-blocker for patients with untreated pheochromocytoma. Use caution with history of severe anaphylaxis to allergens; patients taking beta-blockers may become more sensitive to repeated challenges. Treatment of anaphylaxis (eg, epinephrine) in patients taking beta-blockers may be ineffective or promote undesirable effects. Should not be used alone in angle-closure glaucoma (has no effect on pupillary constriction). Ophthalmic suspension contains benzalkonium chloride which may be absorbed by contact lenses; remove contact lens prior to administration and wait 15 minutes before reinserting. Inadvertent contamination of multiple-dose ophthalmic solutions has caused bacterial keratitis.

Adverse Reactions (Reflective of adult population; not specific for elderly)
Ophthalmic:
>10%: Ocular: Short-term discomfort (25%)

Frequency not defined: Ocular: Allergic reaction, anisocoria, blurred vision, corneal punctate staining, corneal sensitivity decreased, corneal staining, crusty lashes, discharge, dry eyes, edema, erythema, foreign body sensation, inflammation, itching sensation, keratitis, ocular pain, photophobia, tearing, visual acuity decreased

Systemic:
>10%:
Central nervous system: Drowsiness, insomnia
Endocrine & metabolic: Sexual ability decreased

1% to 10%:
Cardiovascular: Bradycardia, palpitation, edema, CHF, peripheral circulation reduced
Central nervous system: Mental depression
Gastrointestinal: Diarrhea or constipation, nausea, vomiting, stomach discomfort
Respiratory: Bronchospasm
Miscellaneous: Cold extremities

Overdosage/Toxicology Symptoms of intoxication include cardiac disturbances, CNS toxicity, bronchospasm, hypoglycemia, and hyperkalemia. The most common cardiac symptoms include hypotension and bradycardia. Atrioventricular block, intraventricular conduction disturbances, cardiogenic shock, and asystole may occur with severe overdose, especially with membrane-depressant drugs (eg, propranolol). CNS effects include convulsions, coma, and respiratory arrest (commonly seen with propranolol and other membrane-depressant and lipid-soluble drugs). Treatment is symptomatic for seizures, hypotension, hyperkalemia, and hypoglycemia. Bradycardia and hypotension resistant to atropine, isoproterenol, or pacing may respond to glucagon. Wide QRS defects caused by membrane-depressant poisoning may respond to hypertonic sodium bicarbonate. Repeat-dose charcoal, hemoperfusion, or hemodialysis may be helpful in removal of only those beta-blockers with a small V_d, long half-life, or low intrinsic clearance (acebutolol, atenolol, nadolol, sotalol). Topical overdose of ophthalmic suspension may be flushed from eye(s) with warm water.

Drug Interactions Substrate (major) of CYP1A2, 2D6; **Inhibits** CYP2D6 (weak)
Acetylcholinesterase inhibitors: May enhance the bradycardic effect of beta-blockers.
Alpha-/beta-agonists (direct-acting): Beta-blockers may enhance the vasopressor effect of alpha-/beta-agonists (direct-acting).
Alpha₁-blockers: Beta-blockers may enhance the orthostatic effect of alpha₁-blockers. The risk associated with ophthalmic products is probably less than systemic products.
(Continued)

Betaxolol *(Continued)*

Alpha$_2$-agonists: Beta-blockers may enhance the rebound hypertensive effect of alpha$_2$-agonists. This effect can occur when the alpha$_2$-agonist is abruptly withdrawn.

Aminoquinolines, antimalarial (eg, hydroxychloroquine): May decrease the metabolism, via cyp isoenzymes, of beta-blockers.

Amiodarone: May enhance the bradycardic effect of beta-blockers.

Amphetamines: May diminish the antihypertensive effect of beta-blockers.

Antipsychotic agents (phenothiazines): May enhance the hypotensive effect of beta-blockers. Either group may decrease the metabolism of the other.

Barbiturates: May increase the metabolism, via cyp isoenzymes, of beta-blockers.

Beta$_2$-agonists: May diminish the bradycardic effect of beta-blockers (beta$_1$ selective).

Calcium channel blockers (nondihydropyridine): May enhance the hypotensive effect of beta-blockers; may also decrease the metabolism of beta-blockers.

Cardiac glycosides: Beta-blockers may enhance the bradycardic effect of cardiac glycosides.

CYP1A2 inducers: May decrease the levels/effects of betaxolol. Example inducers include aminoglutethimide, carbamazepine, phenobarbital, and rifampin.

CYP1A2 inhibitors: May increase the levels/effects of betaxolol. Example inhibitors include ciprofloxacin, fluvoxamine, ketoconazole, norfloxacin, ofloxacin, and rofecoxib.

CYP2D6 inhibitors: May increase the levels/effects of betaxolol. Example inhibitors include chlorpromazine, delavirdine, fluoxetine, miconazole, paroxetine, pergolide, quinidine, quinine, ritonavir, and ropinirole.

Dipyridamole: May enhance the bradycardic effect of beta-blockers.

Disopyramide: May enhance the bradycardic effect of beta-blockers.

Insulin: Beta-blockers may enhance the hypoglycemic effect of insulin.

Lidocaine: Beta-blockers may decrease the metabolism of lidocaine.

Nonsteroidal anti-inflammatory agents (NSAIDs): May diminish the antihypertensive effect of beta-blockers.

Propafenone: May decrease the metabolism, via cyp isoenzymes, of beta-blockers. Propafenone possesses some independent beta-blocking activity.

Propoxyphene: May decrease the metabolism, via cyp isoenzymes, of beta-blockers.

Quinidine: May decrease the metabolism, via cyp isoenzymes, of beta-blockers.

Rifamycin derivatives: May increase the metabolism, via cyp isoenzymes, of beta-blockers.

Selective serotonin reuptake inhibitors (SSRIs): May enhance the bradycardic effect of beta-blockers.

Sulfonylureas: Beta-blockers may enhance the hypoglycemic effect of sulfonylureas; beta-blockers appear to mask tachycardia as an initial symptom of hypoglycemia. Ophthalmic beta-blockers are probably associated with lower risk than systemic agents.

Theophylline derivatives: Beta-blockers (beta$_1$ selective) may diminish the bronchodilatory effect of theophylline derivatives. this is true at higher beta-blockers doses where cardioselectivity is lost.

Ethanol/Nutrition/Herb Interactions Herb/Nutraceutical: Avoid bayberry; blue cohosh, cayenne, ephedra, ginger, ginseng (American), gotu kola, and licorice (may worsen hypertension). Avoid black cohosh, California poppy, coleus, golden seal, hawthorn, mistletoe, periwinkle, quinine, shepherd's purse (may have increased antihypertensive effects).

Stability Avoid freezing. Store ophthalmic drops at room temperature.

Mechanism of Action Competitively blocks beta$_1$-receptors, with little or no effect on beta$_2$-receptors; ophthalmic reduces intraocular pressure by reducing the production of aqueous humor

Pharmacodynamics

Onset of action:

Ophthalmic instillation: Within 30-60 minutes with maximal effects occurring within 2 hours

Oral: Blood pressure significantly decreases within 3 hours

Duration:

Ophthalmic instillation: 12 hours or longer

Oral: 25 hours

Pharmacokinetics

Absorption: Systemically absorbed from the eye

Metabolism: To multiple metabolites

Half-life: 12-22 hours

Elimination: Renal

Dosage

Geriatrics:

Ophthalmic: Refer to adult dosing.

Hypertension: Oral: Initial: 5 mg/day

Adults:

Glaucoma: Ophthalmic:

Solution: Instill 1-2 drops into affected eye(s) twice daily.

Suspension (Betoptic®): Instill 1 drop into affected eye(s) twice daily.

Hypertension, angina: Oral: 5-10 mg/day; may increase dose to 20 mg/day after 7-14 days if desired response is not achieved

Renal Impairment: Oral: Administer 5 mg/day; can increase every 2 weeks up to a maximum of 20 mg/day.

Cl_{cr} <10 mL/minute: Administer 50% of usual dose.

Administration Ophthalmic: Shake suspension well before using. Tilt head back and instill in eye. Keep eye open and do not blink for 30 seconds. Apply gentle pressure to lacrimal sac for 1 minute. Wipe away excess from skin. Do not touch applicator to eye and do not contaminate tip of applicator.

Monitoring Parameters

Ophthalmic: Intraocular pressure

Systemic: Blood pressure, pulse

Test Interactions Oral betaxolol may interfere with glaucoma screening tests.

Patient Information May sting on instillation; do not touch dropper to eye; visual acuity may be decreased after administration; distance vision may be altered; assess patient's or caregiver's ability to administer; apply gentle pressure to lacrimal sac during and immediately following instillation (1 minute) to avoid systemic absorption; stop drug if breathing difficulty occurs

Additional Information Because of betaxolol's low lipid solubility, it is less likely to enter the CNS, decreasing the likelihood of CNS side effects

Special Geriatric Considerations Due to alterations in the beta-adrenergic autonomic nervous system, beta-adrenergic blockade may result in less hemodynamic response than seen in younger adults. Studies indicate that despite decreased sensitivity to the chronotropic effects of beta-blockade with age, there appears to be an increased myocardial sensitivity to the negative inotropic effect during stress (ie, exercise). Controlled trials have shown the overall response rate for propranolol to be only 20% to 50% in elderly populations. Therefore, all beta-adrenergic blocking drugs may result in a decreased response as compared to younger adults.

Dosage Forms Excipient information presented when available (limited, particularly for generics); consult specific product labeling. [DSC] = Discontinued product

Solution, ophthalmic: 0.5% (5 mL, 10 mL, 15 mL) [contains benzalkonium chloride]

Suspension, ophthalmic:

Betoptic® S: 0.25% (2.5 mL [DSC], 5 mL, 10 mL, 15 mL) [contains benzalkonium chloride]

Tablet, as hydrochloride: 10 mg, 20 mg

Kerlone®: 10 mg, 20 mg

Selected References

Fleisher LA, Beckman JA, Brown KA, et al, "ACC/AHA 2006 Guideline Update on Perioperative Cardiovascular Evaluation for Noncardiac Surgery: Focused Update on Perioperative Beta-Blocker Therapy. A Report of the American College of Cardiology/American Heart Association Task Force on Practice Guidelines (Writing Committee to Update the 2002 Guidelines on Perioperative Cardiovascular Evaluation for Noncardiac Surgery) Developed in Collaboration With the American Society of Echocardiography, American Society of Nuclear Cardiology, Heart Rhythm Society, Society of Cardiovascular Anesthesiologists, Society for Cardiovascular Angiography and Interventions, and Society for Vascular Medicine and Biology," *J Am Coll Cardiol*, 2006, 47(11):2343-55.

Juul AB, Wetterslev J, Gluud C, et al, "Effect of Perioperative Beta Blockade in Patients With Diabetes Undergoing Major Non-Cardiac Surgery: Randomized Placebo Controlled, Blinded Multicentre Trial. DIPOM Trial Group," *BMJ*, 2006, 332(7556):1482.

♦ **Betaxolol Hydrochloride** *see* Betaxolol *on page 164*

Bethanechol (be THAN e kole)

Medication Safety Issues

Sound-alike/look-alike issues:

Bethanechol may be confused with betaxolol

U.S. Brand Names Urecholine®

Canadian Brand Names Duvoid®; Myotonachol®; PMS-Bethanechol

Index Terms Bethanechol Chloride

Generic Available Yes

Pharmacologic Category Cholinergic Agonist

Use Treatment of nonobstructive urinary retention and retention due to neurogenic bladder

Unlabeled/Investigational Use Treatment and prevention of bladder dysfunction caused by phenothiazines; diagnosis of flaccid or atonic neurogenic bladder; treatment of gastroesophageal reflux

Contraindications Hypersensitivity to bethanechol or any component of the formulation; mechanical obstruction of the GI or GU tract or when the strength or integrity of the GI or bladder wall is in question; hyperthyroidism, peptic ulcer disease, epilepsy,

(Continued)

Bethanechol *(Continued)*

obstructive pulmonary disease, bradycardia, vasomotor instability, atrioventricular conduction defects, hypotension, or parkinsonism

Warnings/Precautions Potential for reflux infection if the sphincter fails to relax as bethanechol contracts the bladder.

Adverse Reactions (Reflective of adult population; not specific for elderly)
Frequency not defined.

Cardiovascular: Hypotension, tachycardia, flushed skin

Central nervous system: Headache, malaise

Gastrointestinal: Abdominal cramps, diarrhea, nausea, vomiting, salivation, eructation

Genitourinary: Urinary urgency

Ocular: Lacrimation, miosis

Respiratory: Asthmatic attacks, bronchial constriction

Miscellaneous: Diaphoresis

Overdosage/Toxicology Symptoms include nausea, vomiting, abdominal cramps, diarrhea, involuntary defecation, flushed skin, hypotension, and bronchospasm. Atropine is the treatment of choice for intoxications manifesting with significant muscarinic symptoms. Atropine I.V. 0.6 mg every 30-60 minutes should be repeated to control symptoms and then continued as needed for 1-2 days following the acute ingestion. Epinephrine 0.1-1 mg SubQ may be useful in reversing severe cardiovascular or pulmonary sequelae.

Drug Interactions

Decreased effect: Procainamide, quinidine.

Increased toxicity: Bethanechol and ganglionic blockers may cause a critical fall in blood pressure. Cholinergic drugs or anticholinesterase agents may have additive effects.

Stability Store at room temperature of 15°C to 30°C (59°F to 86°F).

Mechanism of Action Stimulates cholinergic receptors in the smooth muscle of the urinary bladder and gastrointestinal tract resulting in increased peristalsis, increased GI and pancreatic secretions, bladder muscle contraction, and increased ureteral peristaltic waves

Pharmacodynamics

Onset of action: Oral: 30-90 minutes

Duration: Usually 1 hour

Pharmacokinetics Absorption: Oral: Variable

Dosage

Geriatrics: Refer to adult dosing. Use the lowest effective dose.

Adults:

Urinary retention, neurogenic bladder, and/or bladder atony:

Oral: Initial: 10-50 mg 2-4 times/day (some patients may require dosages of 50-100 mg 4 times/day). To determine effective dose, may initiate at a dose of 5-10 mg, with additional doses of 5-10 mg hourly until an effective cumulative dose is reached. Cholinergic effects at higher oral dosages may be cumulative.

SubQ: Initial: 2.575 mg, may repeat in 15-30 minutes (maximum cumulative initial dose: 10.3 mg); subsequent doses may be given 3-4 times daily as needed (some patients may require more frequent dosing at 2.5- to 3-hour intervals). Chronic neurogenic atony may require doses of 7.5-10 mg every 4 hours.

Gastroesophageal reflux (unlabeled): Oral: 25 mg 4 times/day

Monitoring Parameters Urinary output, blood pressure, pulse

Test Interactions Increased lipase, amylase (S), bilirubin, aminotransferase [ALT/AST] (S)

Patient Information Oral should be taken 1 hour before meals or 2 hours after meals to avoid nausea or vomiting; may cause abdominal discomfort, salivation, sweating or flushing - notify physician if these symptoms become pronounced. Rise slowly from sitting/lying down.

Special Geriatric Considerations Urinary incontinence in elderly patients should be investigated. Bethanechol may be used for overflow incontinence (ie, dribbling) caused by an atonic or hypotonic bladder, but clinical efficacy is variable.

Dosage Forms Excipient information presented when available (limited, particularly for generics); consult specific product labeling.

Tablet, as chloride: 5 mg, 10 mg, 25 mg, 50 mg

Selected References
Romanowski GL, Shimp LA, Balson AB, et al, "Urinary Incontinence in the Elderly: Etiology and Treatment," *Drug Intell Clin Pharm*, 1988, 22(7-8):525-33.

♦ **Bethanechol Chloride** *see* Bethanechol *on page 167*

♦ **Betimol**® *see* Timolol *on page 1571*

♦ **Betoptic**® S *see* Betaxolol *on page 164*

♦ **Biaxin**® *see* Clarithromycin *on page 326*

♦ **Biaxin**® **XL** *see* Clarithromycin *on page 326*

Bicalutamide (bye ka LOO ta mide)

U.S. Brand Names Casodex®
Canadian Brand Names Casodex®; CO Bicalutamide; Novo-Bicalutamide; PMS-Bicalutamide; ratio-Bicalutamide; Sandoz-Bicalutamide
Index Terms CDX; ICI-176334; NC-722665
Generic Available No
Pharmacologic Category Antineoplastic Agent, Antiandrogen
Use In combination therapy with LHRH agonist analogues in treatment of metastatic prostate cancer
Unlabeled/Investigational Use Monotherapy for locally-advanced prostate cancer
Contraindications Hypersensitivity to bicalutamide or any component of the formulation; female patients
Warnings/Precautions Hazardous agent - use appropriate precautions for handling and disposal. Rare cases of death or hospitalization due to hepatitis have been reported postmarketing. Use with caution in moderate-to-severe hepatic dysfunction. Hepatotoxicity generally occurs within the first 3-4 months of use; patients should be monitored for signs and symptoms of liver dysfunction. Bicalutamide should be discontinued if patients have jaundice or ALT is >2 times the upper limit of normal. May cause gynecomastia, breast pain, or lead to spermatogenesis inhibition.

Adverse Reactions (Reflective of adult population; not specific for elderly) Adverse reaction percentages reported as part of combination regimen with an LHRH analogue.

>10%:
  Cardiovascular: Peripheral edema (13%)
  Central nervous system: Pain (35%)
  Endocrine & metabolic: Hot flashes (53%)
  Gastrointestinal: Constipation (22%), nausea (15%), diarrhea (12%), abdominal pain (11%)
  Genitourinary: Pelvic pain (21%), nocturia (12%), hematuria (12%)
  Hematologic: Anemia (11%)
  Neuromuscular & skeletal: Back pain (25%), weakness (22%)
  Respiratory: Dyspnea (13%)
  Miscellaneous: Infection (18%)
≥2% to 10%:
  Cardiovascular: Chest pain (8%), hypertension (8%), angina pectoris (2% to <5%), CHF (2% to <5%), edema (2% to <5%), MI (2% to <5%), coronary artery disorder (2% to <5%), syncope (2% to <5%)
  Central nervous system: Dizziness (10%), headache (7%), insomnia (7%), anxiety (5%), depression (4%), chills (2% to <5%), confusion (2% to <5%), fever (2% to <5%), nervousness (2% to <5%), somnolence (2% to <5%)
  Dermatologic: Rash (9%), alopecia (2% to <5%), dry skin (2% to <5%), pruritus (2% to <5%), skin carcinoma (2% to <5%)
  Endocrine & metabolic: Gynecomastia (9%), breast pain (6%; up to 39% as monotherapy), hyperglycemia (6%), dehydration (2% to <5%), gout (2% to <5%), hypercholesterolemia (2% to <5%), libido decreased (2% to <5%)
  Gastrointestinal: Dyspepsia (7%), weight loss (7%), anorexia (6%), flatulence (6%), vomiting (6%), weight gain (5%), dysphagia (2% to <5%), gastrointestinal carcinoma (2% to <5%), melena (2% to <5%), periodontal abscess (2% to <5%), rectal hemorrhage (2% to <5%), xerostomia (2% to <5%)
  Genitourinary: Urinary tract infection (9%), impotence (7%), polyuria (6%), urinary retention (5%), urinary impairment (5%), urinary incontinence (4%), dysuria (2% to <5%), urinary urgency (2% to <5%)
  Hepatic: LFTs increased (7%), alkaline phosphatase increased (5%)
  Neuromuscular & skeletal: Bone pain (9%), paresthesia (8%), myasthenia (7%), arthritis (5%), pathological fracture (4%), hypertonia (2% to <5%), leg cramps (2% to <5%), myalgia (2% to <5%), neck pain (2% to <5%), neuropathy (2% to <5%)
  Ocular: Cataract (2% to <5%)
  Renal: BUN increased, creatinine increased, hydronephrosis
  Respiratory: Cough (8%), pharyngitis (8%), bronchitis (6%), pneumonia (4%), rhinitis (4%), asthma (2% to <5%), epistaxis (2% to <5%), sinusitis (2% to <5%)
  Miscellaneous: Flu syndrome (7%), diaphoresis (6%), cyst (2% to <5%), hernia (2% to <5%), herpes zoster (2% to <5%), sepsis (2% to <5%)

Overdosage/Toxicology Doses up to 200 mg daily have been well tolerated in long term clinical trials. Symptoms of overdose may include hypoactivity, ataxia, anorexia, vomiting, slow respiration, and lacrimation. Vomiting may be induced if the patient is alert. Vital signs should be monitored frequently. Treatment is symptom-directed and supportive. Dialysis is of no benefit.

Stability Store at room temperature of 20°C to 25°C (68°F to 77°F).
(Continued)

Bicalutamide *(Continued)*

Mechanism of Action Pure nonsteroidal antiandrogen that binds to androgen receptors; specifically a competitive inhibitor for the binding of dihydrotestosterone and testosterone; prevents testosterone stimulation of cell growth in prostate cancer

Pharmacokinetics

Protein binding: 96%

Metabolism: Extensively hepatic; glucuronidation and oxidation of the R (active) enantiomer to inactive metabolites

Half-life: Active enantiomer ~6 days, ~10 days in severe liver disease

Time to peak, plasma: 31 hours

Excretion: Urine (36%, as inactive metabolites); feces (42%, as unchanged drug and inactive metabolites)

Dosage

Geriatrics & Adults:

Metastatic prostate cancer: Oral: 50 mg once daily (in combination with an LHRH analogue)

Locally-advanced prostate cancer (unlabeled use): Oral: 150 mg once daily (as monotherapy)

Renal Impairment: No adjustment required

Hepatic Impairment: No adjustment required for mild, moderate, or severe hepatic impairment; use caution with moderate-to-severe impairment. Discontinue if ALT >2 times ULN or patient develops jaundice.

Administration Dose should be taken at the same time each day with or without food; treatment should be started concomitantly with an LHRH analogue

Monitoring Parameters Periodically monitor CBC, ECG, echocardiograms, serum testosterone, luteinizing hormone, and prostate specific antigen. Liver function tests should be obtained at baseline and repeated regularly during the first 4 months of treatment, and periodically thereafter; monitor for signs and symptoms of liver dysfunction (discontinue if jaundice is noted or ALT is >2 times the upper limit of normal).

Patient Information Take at the same time as treatment with LHRH analog; notify the physician if any visual disturbances or yellow discoloration of the skin or eyes

Special Geriatric Considerations Renal impairment has no clinically-significant changes in elimination of the parent compound or active metabolite; therefore, no dosage adjustment is needed in the elderly. In dosage studies, no difference was found between young adults and elderly with regard to steady-state serum concentrations for bicalutamide and its active R-enantiomer metabolite.

Dosage Forms Excipient information presented when available (limited, particularly for generics); consult specific product labeling.

Tablet: 50 mg

Selected References

Cockshott ID, "Bicalutamide: Clinical Pharmacokinetics and Metabolism," *Clin Pharmacokinet*, 2004, 43(13):855-78.

Iversen P, "Bicalutamide Monotherapy for Early Stage Prostate Cancer: An Update," *J Urol*, 2003, 170(6 Pt 2 Suppl):48-52.

Iversen, P, Johansson JE, Lodding P, et al, "Bicalutamide (150 mg) Versus Placebo as Immediate Therapy Alone or as Adjuvant to Therapy With Curative Intent for Early Nonmetastatic Prostate Cancer: 5.3 Year Median Followup from the Scandinavian Prostate Cancer Group Study Number 6," *J Urol*, 2004, 172(5 Pt 1):1871-6.

Schellhammer PF, "An Evaluation of Bicalutamide in the Treatment of Prostate Cancer," *Expert Opin Pharmacother*, 2002, 3(9):1313-28.

Schellhammer PF and Davis JW, "An Evaluation of Bicalutamide in the Treatment of Prostate Cancer," *Clin Prostate Cancer*, 2004, 2(4):213-9.

Tyrell CJ, Denis L, Newling D, et al, "Casodex 10-200 mg Daily, Used as Monotherapy for the Treatment of Patients With Advanced Prostate Cancer. An Overview of the Efficacy, Tolerability and Pharmacokinetics from Three Phase II Dose-Ranging Studies. Casodex Study Group," *Eur Urol*, 1998, 33(1):39-53.

♦ **Bicillin® L-A** see Penicillin G Benzathine *on page 1221*

♦ **Bicillin® C-R** see Penicillin G Benzathine and Penicillin G Procaine *on page 1222*

♦ **Bicillin® C-R 900/300** see Penicillin G Benzathine and Penicillin G Procaine *on page 1222*

♦ **Bicitra®** see Sodium Citrate and Citric Acid *on page 1477*

♦ **Bidhist** see Brompheniramine *on page 189*

♦ **BiDil®** see Isosorbide Dinitrate and Hydralazine *on page 842*

Bimatoprost *(bi MAT oh prost)*

Related Information

Glaucoma Drug Therapy *on page 1758*

U.S. Brand Names Lumigan®

Canadian Brand Names Lumigan®

Generic Available No

Pharmacologic Category Ophthalmic Agent, Antiglaucoma; Prostaglandin, Ophthalmic

Use Reduction of intraocular pressure (IOP) in patients with open-angle glaucoma or ocular hypertension

Contraindications Hypersensitivity to bimatoprost or any component of the formulation

Warnings/Precautions May cause permanent changes in eye color (increases the amount of brown pigment in the iris), the eyelid skin, and eyelashes. In addition, may increase the length and/or number of eyelashes (may vary between eyes). Use caution in patients with intraocular inflammation, aphakic patients, pseudophakic patients with a torn posterior lens capsule, or patients with risk factors for macular edema. Contains benzalkonium chloride (may be adsorbed by contact lenses). Safety and efficacy have not been determined for use in patients with angle-closure, inflammatory, or neovascular glaucoma.

Adverse Reactions (Reflective of adult population; not specific for elderly)
>10%: Ocular (15% to 45%): Conjunctival hyperemia, growth of eyelashes, ocular pruritus
1% to 10%:
Central nervous system: Headache (1% to 5%)
Dermatologic: Hirsutism (1% to 5%)
Hepatic: Liver function tests abnormal (1% to 5%)
Neuromuscular & skeletal: Weakness (1% to 5%)
Ocular:
3% to 10%: Blepharitis, burning, cataract, dryness, eyelid redness, eyelash darkening, foreign body sensation, irritation, pain, pigmentation of periocular skin, superficial punctate keratitis, visual disturbance
1% to 3%: Allergic conjunctivitis, asthenopia, conjunctival edema, discharge, iris pigmentation increased, photophobia, tearing
Respiratory: Upper respiratory tract infection (10%)

Overdosage/Toxicology No information available. Treatment is symptom-directed and supportive.

Drug Interactions Latanoprost: Combination therapy may result in increased IOP than either agent alone.

Stability Store between 2°C to 25°C (36°F to 77°F).

Mechanism of Action As a synthetic analog of prostaglandin with ocular hypotensive activity, bimatoprost decreases intraocular pressure by increasing the outflow of aqueous humor.

Pharmacodynamics Onset of action: Reduction of IOP begins ~4 hours

Pharmacokinetics
Distribution: 0.67 L/kg
Protein binding: ~88%
Metabolism: Undergoes oxidation, N-demethylation, and glucuronidation after reaching systemic circulation; forms metabolites
Half-life: 45 minutes in systemic circulation, following I.V. administration
Time to peak: Peak plasma levels occur in 10 minutes; maximum reduction of IOP occurs in ~8-12 hours
Elimination: Urine (67%), feces (25%)

Dosage
Geriatrics & Adults: Open-angle glaucoma or ocular hypertension: Ophthalmic: Instill 1 drop into affected eye(s) once daily in the evening; do not exceed once-daily dosing (may decrease IOP-lowering effect). If used with other topical ophthalmic agents, separate administration by at least 5 minutes.

Administration May be used with other eye drops to lower intraocular pressure. If using more than one ophthalmic product, wait at least 5 minutes in between application of each medication. Remove contact lenses prior to administration and wait 15 minutes before reinserting.

Patient Information Wash hands before instilling. Sit or lie down to instill. Open eye, look at ceiling, and instill prescribed amount of solution. Apply gentle pressure to inner corner of eye. Do not let tip of applicator touch eye; do not contaminate tip of applicator (contamination may cause eye infection leading to possible eye damage or vision loss). Contact prescriber concerning continued use of drops if eye infection develops, trauma occurs to the eye, and prior to eye surgery. This product contains benzalkonium chloride which may be adsorbed by contact lenses; remove contacts prior to administration and wait 15 minutes before reinserting. May cause permanent changes in eye color (increases the amount of brown pigment in the iris), eyelid, and eyelashes. May also increase the length and/or number of eyelashes. Changes may occur slowly (months to years). May be used with other eye drops to lower intraocular pressure. If using more than one eye drop medicine, wait at least 5 minutes in between application of each medication. Notify prescriber if conjunctivitis or eyelid reactions occur with use of this product.

Additional Information The IOP-lowering effect was shown to be 7-8 mm Hg in clinical studies.

Special Geriatric Considerations Evaluate patient's ability to self-administer eye drops
(Continued)

Bimatoprost *(Continued)*

Dosage Forms Excipient information presented when available (limited, particularly for generics); consult specific product labeling.
Solution, ophthalmic:
Lumigan®: 0.03% (2.5 mL, 5 mL, 7.5 mL) [contains benzalkonium chloride]

♦ **Bion® Tears [OTC]** *see* Artificial Tears *on page 124*
♦ **Bio-Statin®** *see* Nystatin *on page 1142*

Biperiden (bye PER i den)

Medication Safety Issues
International issues:
Kinex® [Mexico] may be confused with Kionex™ which is a brand name for sodium polystyrene sulfonate in the U.S.
Kinex® [Mexico] may be confused with Tenex® which is a brand name for guanfacine in the U.S.

U.S. Brand Names Akineton®
Canadian Brand Names Akineton®
Index Terms Biperiden Hydrochloride; Biperiden Lactate
Generic Available No
Pharmacologic Category Anti-Parkinson's Agent, Anticholinergic; Anticholinergic Agent
Use Treatment of all forms of parkinsonism including drug-induced type (extrapyramidal symptoms); principally affects tremor
Contraindications Hypersensitivity to biperiden or any component of the formulation; narrow-angle glaucoma; bowel obstruction, megacolon; myasthenia gravis
Warnings/Precautions Use with caution in patients with narrow-angle glaucoma, peptic ulcer, prostatic hyperplasia, seizure disorder, cardiac arrhythmias, urinary tract obstruction, and hyperthyroidism. May be associated with confusion or hallucinations (generally at higher dosages); intensification of symptoms or toxic psychosis may occur in patients with mental disorders. May cause CNS depression, which may impair physical or mental abilities; patients must be cautioned about performing tasks which require mental alertness (eg, operating machinery or driving).
Adverse Reactions (Reflective of adult population; not specific for elderly)
Frequency not defined.
Cardiovascular: Orthostatic hypotension, bradycardia
Central nervous system: Drowsiness, euphoria, disorientation, agitation, sleep disorder (decreased REM sleep and increased REM latency)
Gastrointestinal: Constipation, xerostomia, dry throat, nasal dryness
Genitourinary: Urinary retention
Neuromuscular & skeletal: Choreic movements
Ocular: Blurred vision
Drug Interactions Inhibits CYP2D6 (weak)
Amantadine, rimantadine: Central and/or peripheral anticholinergic syndrome can occur when administered with amantadine or rimantadine.
Anticholinergic agents: Central and/or peripheral anticholinergic syndrome can occur when administered with opioid analgesics, phenothiazines and other antipsychotics (especially with high anticholinergic activity), tricyclic antidepressants, quinidine and some other antiarrhythmics, and antihistamines.
Atenolol: Anticholinergics may increase the bioavailability of atenolol (and possibly other beta-blockers); monitor for increased effect.
Cholinergic agents: Anticholinergics may antagonize the therapeutic effect of cholinergic agents; includes tacrine and donepezil.
Digoxin: Anticholinergics may decrease gastric degradation and increase the amount of digoxin absorbed by delaying gastric emptying.
Levodopa: Anticholinergics may increase gastric degradation and decrease the amount of levodopa absorbed by delaying gastric emptying.
Neuroleptics: Anticholinergics may antagonize the therapeutic effects of neuroleptics.
Ethanol/Nutrition/Herb Interactions Ethanol: Avoid ethanol (may increase sedation).
Mechanism of Action Biperiden is a weak peripheral anticholinergic agent with nicotinolytic activity. The beneficial effects in Parkinson's disease and neuroleptic-induced extrapyramidal symptoms are believed to be due to the inhibition of striatal cholinergic receptors.
Pharmacokinetics
Bioavailability: 29%
Half-life: 18.4-24.3 hours
Time to peak serum concentration: 1-1.5 hours

Dosage

Geriatrics: Initial: 2 mg 1-2 times/day

Adults:

Parkinsonism: Oral: 2 mg 3-4 times/day

Extrapyramidal symptoms: Oral: 2 mg 1-3 times/day

Monitoring Parameters Symptoms of EPS or Parkinson's, pulse, anticholinergic effects (ie, CNS, bowel, and bladder function)

Patient Information Take after meals or with food if GI upset occurs; do not discontinue drug abruptly; notify physician if adverse GI effects, rapid or pounding heartbeat, confusion, eye pain, rash, fever or heat intolerance occurs. Observe caution when performing hazardous tasks or those that require alertness such as driving, as may cause drowsiness. Avoid alcohol and other CNS depressants. May cause dry mouth - adequate fluid intake or hard sugar-free candy may relieve. Difficult urination or constipation may occur - notify physician if effects persist; may increase susceptibility to heat stroke.

Special Geriatric Considerations Anticholinergic agents are generally not well tolerated in the elderly (often results in bowel, bladder, and CNS adverse reactions) and their use should be avoided when possible; should not be used as prophylaxis against extrapyramidal symptoms.

Dosage Forms Excipient information presented when available (limited, particularly for generics); consult specific product labeling.

Tablet, as hydrochloride: 2 mg

Selected References

Feinberg M, "The Problems of Anticholinergic Adverse Effects in Older Patients," *Drugs Aging*, 1993, 3(4):335-48.

Olanow CW, Watts RL, and Koller WC, "An Algorithm (Decision Tree) for the Management of Parkinson's Disease (2001): Treatment Guidelines," *Neurology*, 2001, 56(11 Suppl 5):S1-S88.

♦ **Biperiden Hydrochloride** *see* Biperiden *on page 172*

♦ **Biperiden Lactate** *see* Biperiden *on page 172*

♦ **Bird Flu Vaccine** *see* Influenza Virus Vaccine (H5N1) *on page 807*

♦ **Bisac-Evac™ [OTC]** *see* Bisacodyl *on page 173*

Bisacodyl (bis a KOE dil)

Related Information

Potentially Inappropriate Medications for Geriatrics *on page 1824*

Treatment Options for Constipation *on page 1785*

Medication Safety Issues

Sound-alike/look-alike issues:

Doxidan® may be confused with doxepin

Modane® may be confused with Matulane®, Moban®

U.S. Brand Names Alophen® [OTC]; Bisac-Evac™ [OTC]; Bisacodyl Uniserts® [OTC] [DSC]; Bisolax™ [OTC]; Correctol® Tablets [OTC]; Dacodyl™ [OTC]; Doxidan® [OTC]; Dulcolax® [OTC]; ex-lax® Ultra [OTC]; Fematrol [OTC]; Femilax™ [OTC]; Fleet® Bisacodyl [OTC]; Fleet® Stimulant Laxative [OTC]; Veracolate [OTC]

Canadian Brand Names Apo-Bisacodyl®; Carter's Little Pills®; Dulcolax®; Gentlax®

Generic Available Yes: Excludes enema

Pharmacologic Category Laxative, Stimulant

Use Treatment of constipation; colonic evacuation prior to procedures or examination

Contraindications Hypersensitivity to bisacodyl or any component of the formulation; abdominal pain, obstruction, nausea or vomiting

Warnings/Precautions Excessive use may lead to fluid and electrolyte imbalance. Drug is habit-forming and may result in laxative dependence and loss of normal bowel function with prolonged use; rectal bleeding and failure to respond to therapy may require further evaluation; discoloration of urine may occur

Drug Interactions Decreased effect: Milk, antacids; decreased effect of warfarin

Ethanol/Nutrition/Herb Interactions Food: Milk or dairy products may disrupt enteric coating, increasing stomach irritation.

Mechanism of Action Stimulates peristalsis by directly irritating the smooth muscle of the intestine, possibly the colonic intramural plexus; alters water and electrolyte secretion producing net intestinal fluid accumulation and laxation

Pharmacodynamics Onset of action:

Oral: Within 6-10 hours

Rectal: 15-60 minutes

Pharmacokinetics

Absorption: Oral, rectal: <5% absorbed systemically

Metabolism: In the liver with conjugated metabolites

Elimination: Excreted in bile and urine

(Continued)

Bisacodyl (Continued)

Dosage

Geriatrics & Adults:

Relief of constipation:

Oral: 5-15 mg as single dose (up to 30 mg when complete evacuation of bowel is required)

Rectal: Suppository: 10 mg as single dose

Administration Administered with glass of water on empty stomach for rapid effect. Do not administer within 1 hour of milk, any dairy products, or taking an antacid, to protect the coating.

Monitoring Parameters Monitor stools daily or weekly; fluid/electrolyte status

Patient Information Swallow tablets whole, do **not** crush or chew; do not take antacid or milk within 2 hours of taking drug; patients should assure proper dietary fiber and fluid intake with adequate exercise if medically appropriate; do not use if abdominal pain, nausea, or vomiting are present; laxative use should be used for a short period of time (<1 week); prolonged use may result in abuse, dependence, as well as fluid and electrolyte loss; notify physician if bleeding occurs or if constipation is not relieved

Special Geriatric Considerations The chronic use of stimulant cathartics is inappropriate and should be avoided; although constipation is a common complaint from elderly, such complaints require evaluation; elderly are often predisposed to constipation due to disease, drugs, immobility, and a decreased fluid intake, partially because they have a blunted "thirst reflex" with aging; short-term use of stimulants is best; if prophylaxis is desired, this can be accomplished with bulk agents (psyllium), stool softeners, and hyperosmotic agents (sorbitol 70%); stool softeners are unnecessary if stools are well hydrated, soft, or "mushy".

Dosage Forms Excipient information presented when available (limited, particularly for generics); consult specific product labeling. [DSC] = Discontinued product

Solution, rectal [enema]:

Fleet® Bisacodyl: 10 mg/30 mL (37 mL)

Suppository, rectal: 10 mg

Bisac-Evac™, Bisacodyl Uniserts® [DSC], Bisolax™, Dulcolax®: 10 mg

Tablet [enteric coated]: 5 mg

Alophen®, Bisac-Evac™, Correctol®, Dacodyl™, Dulcolax®, ex-lax® Ultra, Fematrol, Femilax™, Veracolate: 5 mg

Tablet, delayed release: 5 mg

Doxidan®, Fleet® Stimulant Laxative: 5 mg

♦ **Bisacodyl Uniserts® [OTC] [DSC]** *see* Bisacodyl *on page 173*

♦ **Bismatrol** *see* Bismuth *on page 174*

♦ **Bismatrol [OTC]** *see* Bismuth *on page 174*

♦ **Bismatrol Maximum Strength [OTC]** *see* Bismuth *on page 174*

Bismuth (BIZ muth)

Related Information

Helicobacter pylori Treatment *on page 1759*

Medication Safety Issues

Sound-alike/look-alike issues:

Kaopectate® may be confused with Kayexalate®

Maalox® Total Stomach Relief® is a different formulation than Maalox®

U.S. Brand Names Bismatrol [OTC]; Bismatrol Maximum Strength [OTC]; Diotame® [OTC]; Kaopectate® [OTC]; Kaopectate® Extra Strength [OTC]; Kao-Tin [OTC]; Kapectolin [OTC]; Maalox® Total Stomach Relief® [OTC]; Peptic Relief [OTC]; Pepto-Bismol® [OTC]; Pepto-Bismol® Maximum Strength [OTC]; Pepto Relief [OTC]

Index Terms Bismatrol; Bismuth Subsalicylate; Pink Bismuth

Generic Available Yes

Pharmacologic Category Antidiarrheal

Use Symptomatic treatment of mild, nonspecific diarrhea; indigestion, nausea, control of traveler's diarrhea (enterotoxigenic *Escherichia coli*); as *H. pylori* (adjunct to reduce risk of duodenal ulcer recurrence); subgallate formulation to control fecal odors in colostomy, ileostomy, or fecal incontinence

Contraindications Do not use subsalicylate in patients with influenza or chickenpox because of risk of Reye's syndrome; hypersensitivity to salicylates or any component of the formulation; history of severe GI bleeding; history of coagulopathy

Warnings/Precautions Bismuth subsalicylate should be used with caution if patient is taking aspirin. Bismuth products may be neurotoxic with very large doses.

When used for self-medication (OTC labeling): Patients should be instructed to contact healthcare provider for diarrhea lasting >2 days, hearing loss, or ringing in the ears.

Adverse Reactions (Reflective of adult population; not specific for elderly)

Frequency not defined; subsalicylate formulation:

Central nervous system: Anxiety, confusion, headache, mental depression, slurred speech

Gastrointestinal: Discoloration of the tongue (darkening), grayish black stools, impaction may occur in infants and debilitated patients

Neuromuscular & skeletal: Muscle spasms, weakness

Ocular: Hearing loss, tinnitus

Overdosage/Toxicology

Symptoms of toxicity: **Subsalicylate**: Hyperpnea, nausea, vomiting, tinnitus, hyperpyrexia, metabolic acidoses/respiratory alkalosis, tachycardia, and confusion; seizures in severe overdose, pulmonary or cerebral edema, respiratory failure, cardiovascular collapse, coma, and death. **Note:** Each 262.4 mg tablet of bismuth subsalicylate contains an equivalent of 130 mg aspirin; 150 mg/kg of aspirin is considered to be toxic. Serious life-threatening toxicity occurs with >300 mg/kg.

Treatment: Gastrointestinal decontamination (activated charcoal for immediate release formulations (10 x dose of ASA in g), whole bowel irrigation for enteric coated tablets or when serially increasing ASA plasma levels indicate the presence of an intestinal bezoar), supportive and symptomatic treatment with emphasis on correcting fluid, electrolyte, blood glucose and acid-base disturbances; elimination is enhanced with urinary alkalinization (sodium bicarbonate infusion with potassium), multiple-dose activated charcoal, and hemodialysis.

Symptoms of toxicity: **Bismuth**: Rare with short-term administrations of bismuth salts; encephalopathy, methemoglobinemia, seizures

Treatment: Gastrointestinal decontamination; chelation with dimercaprol in doses of 3 mg/kg or penicillamine 100 mg/kg/day for 5 days can hasten recovery from bismuth-induced encephalopathy; methylene blue 1-2 mg/kg in a 1% sterile aqueous solution I.V. push over 4-6 minutes for methemoglobinemia. This may be repeated within 60 minutes if necessary, up to a total dose of 7 mg/kg. Seizures usually respond to I.V. diazepam.

Drug Interactions Tetracycline derivatives: Bismuth may decrease the absorption of tetracycline derivatives.

Mechanism of Action Bismuth subsalicylate exhibits both antisecretory and antimicrobial action. This agent may provide some anti-inflammatory action as well. The salicylate moiety provides antisecretory effect and the bismuth exhibits antimicrobial directly against bacterial and viral gastrointestinal pathogens.

Pharmacokinetics

Absorption: Minimally absorbed across the GI tract while the salt (eg, salicylate) may be readily absorbed

Metabolism: Undergoes chemical dissociation to various bismuth salts after oral administration

Dosage

Geriatrics & Adults:

Treatment of nonspecific diarrhea, control/relieve traveler's diarrhea: Oral: Subsalicylate (doses based on 262 mg/15 mL liquid or 262 mg tablets): 2 tablets or 30 mL every 30 minutes to 1 hour as needed up to 8 doses/24 hours

Helicobacter pylori eradication: Oral: Subsalicylate: 524 mg 4 times/day with meals and at bedtime; requires combination therapy

Renal Impairment: Should probably be avoided in patients with renal impairment.

Monitoring Parameters Signs/symptoms of nausea, diarrhea, tinnitus, CNS toxic effects, GI bleeding

Reference Range Mild toxicity, serum concentration ≥30 mg/dL; severe, >50 mg/dL

Test Interactions Increased uric acid, increased AST; bismuth absorbs x-rays and may interfere with diagnostic procedures of GI tract

Patient Information Chew tablet well or shake suspension well before using; may darken stools; if diarrhea persists for more than 2 days, consult a physician; tinnitus may indicate toxicity and use should be discontinued

Additional Information Pepto-Bismol® contains bismuth 58% and salicylate 42%; do not exceed 4.2 g/day dosage; bismuth is radiopaque; 2 tablets yield 204 mg salicylate; 30 mL of suspension yields 258 mg

Special Geriatric Considerations Tinnitus and CNS side effects (confusion, dizziness, high tone deafness, delirium, psychosis) may be difficult to assess in some elderly patients. Limit use of this agent in elderly.

Dosage Forms Excipient information presented when available (limited, particularly for generics); consult specific product labeling.

Caplet, as subsalicylate:

Kaopectate®: 262 mg

Pepto-Bismol®: 262 mg [sugar free; contains sodium 2 mg/caplet]

Liquid, as subsalicylate: 262 mg/15 mL (240 mL)

Bismatrol: 262 mg/15 mL (240 mL)

(Continued)

Bismuth *(Continued)*

Bismatrol Maximum Strength: 525 mg/15 mL (240 mL)

Diotame®: 262 mg/15 mL (30 mL) [sugar free]

Kaopectate®: 262 mg/15 mL (240 mL, 360 mL) [contains potassium 5 mg/15 mL, sodium 10 mg/15 mL; regular and peppermint flavors]

Kaopectate®: 262 mg/15 mL (180 mL) [contains sodium 10 mg/15 mL; cherry flavor]

Kaopectate® Extra Strength: 525 mg/15 mL (240 mL) [contains potassium 5 mg/15 mL, sodium 10 mg/15 mL; peppermint flavor]

Kao-Tin: 262 mg/15 mL (240 mL, 480 mL) [contains sodium benzoate]

Maalox® Total Stomach Relief®: 525 mg/15 mL (360 mL) [contains sodium 3.3 mg/15 mL; strawberry and peppermint flavor]

Peptic Relief: 262 mg/15 mL (240 mL) [sugar free; mint flavor]

Pepto-Bismol®: 262 mg/15 mL (120 mL, 240 mL, 360 mL, 480 mL) [sugar free; contains sodium 6 mg/15 mL and benzoic acid; cherry and wintergreen flavors]

Pepto-Bismol® Maximum Strength: 525 mg/15 mL (120 mL, 240 mL, 360 mL) [sugar free; contains sodium 6 mg/15 mL and benzoic acid; wintergreen flavor]

Suspension, as subsalicylate:

Kapectolin: 262 mg/15 mL (480 mL) [mint flavor]

Tablet, chewable, as subsalicylate: 262 mg

Bismatrol: 262 mg

Diotame®: 262 mg [sugar free]

Peptic Relief, Pepto Relief: 262 mg

Pepto-Bismol®: 262 mg [sugar free; contains sodium <1 mg; cherry and wintergreen flavors]

♦ **Bismuth Subsalicylate** *see* Bismuth *on page 174*
♦ **Bisolax™ [OTC]** *see* Bisacodyl *on page 173*

Bisoprolol (bis OH proe lol)

Related Information
Beta-Blockers *on page 1751*
Medication Safety Issues
Sound-alike/look-alike issues:
Zebeta® may be confused with DiaBeta®
U.S. Brand Names Zebeta®
Canadian Brand Names Apo-Bisoprolol®; Monocor®; Novo-Bisoprolol; Sandoz-Bisoprolol; Zebeta®
Index Terms Bisoprolol Fumarate
Generic Available Yes
Pharmacologic Category Beta Blocker, Beta$_1$ Selective
Use Treatment of hypertension, alone or in combination with other agents
Unlabeled/Investigational Use Treatment of angina pectoris, supraventricular arrhythmias, PVCs
Contraindications Hypersensitivity to bisoprolol or any component of the formulation; sinus bradycardia; heart block greater than first-degree (except in patients with a functioning artificial pacemaker); cardiogenic shock; uncompensated cardiac failure; pulmonary edema
Warnings/Precautions Consider pre-existing conditions such as sick sinus syndrome before initiating. Use with caution in patients with inadequate myocardial function, myasthenia gravis, psychiatric disease (may cause CNS depression), bronchospastic disease, undergoing anesthesia; and in those with impaired hepatic function. Beta-blocker therapy should not be withdrawn abruptly (particularly in patients with CAD), but gradually tapered to avoid acute tachycardia, hypertension, and/or ischemia. Use caution in patients with PVD (can aggravate arterial insufficiency). Use caution with concurrent use with verapamil or diltiazem; bradycardia or heart block can occur. Bisoprolol, with B$_1$selectivity, has been used cautiously in bronchospastic disease with close monitoring. Use cautiously in diabetics because it can mask prominent hypoglycemic symptoms. Use care with anesthetic agents which decrease myocardial function. Adequate alpha-blockade is required prior to use of any beta-blocker for patients with untreated pheochromocytoma.
Adverse Reactions (Reflective of adult population; not specific for elderly)
>10%:
Central nervous system: Drowsiness, insomnia
Endocrine & metabolic: Sexual ability decreased
1% to 10%:
Cardiovascular: Bradycardia, palpitation, edema, CHF, peripheral circulation reduced
Central nervous system: Mental depression
Gastrointestinal: Diarrhea, constipation, nausea, vomiting, stomach discomfort

Ocular: Mild ocular stinging and discomfort, tearing, photophobia, corneal sensitivity decreased, keratitis

Respiratory: Bronchospasm

Miscellaneous: Cold extremities

Overdosage/Toxicology Symptoms include cardiac disturbances, CNS toxicity, bronchospasm, hypoglycemia and hyperkalemia. The most common cardiac symptoms include hypotension and bradycardia. Atrioventricular block, intraventricular conduction disturbances, cardiogenic shock, and asystole may occur with severe overdose, especially with membrane-depressant drugs (eg, propranolol). CNS effects include convulsions, coma, and respiratory arrest (commonly seen with propranolol and other membrane-depressant and lipid-soluble drugs). Treatment is symptomatic for seizures, hypotension, hyperkalemia, and hypoglycemia. Bradycardia and hypotension resistant to atropine, isoproterenol, or pacing may respond to glucagon. Wide QRS defects caused by membrane-depressant poisoning may respond to hypertonic sodium bicarbonate. Repeat-dose charcoal, hemoperfusion, or hemodialysis may be helpful in removal of only those beta-blockers with a small V_d, long half-life, or low intrinsic clearance (acebutolol, atenolol, nadolol, sotalol).

Drug Interactions Substrate of CYP2D6 (minor), 3A4 (major)

Alpha-blockers (prazosin, terazosin): Concurrent use of beta-blockers may increase risk of orthostasis.

AV conduction-slowing agents (digoxin): Effects may be additive with beta-blockers.

Clonidine: Hypertensive crisis after or during withdrawal of either agent.

CYP3A4 inducers: CYP3A4 inducers may decrease the levels/effects of bisoprolol. Example inducers include aminoglutethimide, carbamazepine, nafcillin, nevirapine, phenobarbital, phenytoin, and rifamycins.

CYP3A4 inhibitors: May increase the levels/effects of bisoprolol. Example inhibitors include azole antifungals, clarithromycin, diclofenac, doxycycline, erythromycin, imatinib, isoniazid, nefazodone, nicardipine, propofol, protease inhibitors, quinidine, telithromycin, and verapamil.

Glucagon: Bisoprolol may blunt the hyperglycemic action of glucagon.

Insulin: Bisoprolol may mask tachycardia from hypoglycemia.

NSAIDs (ibuprofen, indomethacin, naproxen, piroxicam) may reduce the antihypertensive effects of beta-blockers.

Salicylates may reduce the antihypertensive effects of beta-blockers.

Sulfonylureas: Beta-blockers may alter response to hypoglycemic agents.

Ethanol/Nutrition/Herb Interactions Herb/Nutraceutical: Avoid dong quai if using for hypertension (has estrogenic activity). Avoid ephedra, yohimbe, ginseng (may worsen hypertension). Avoid garlic (may have increased antihypertensive effect).

Mechanism of Action Selective inhibitor of beta$_1$-adrenergic receptors; competitively blocks beta$_1$-receptors, with little or no effect on beta$_2$-receptors at doses <10 mg

Pharmacokinetics

Absorption: Rapid and almost complete from GI tract (≥90%)

Distribution: Wide to body tissues; highest concentrations in heart, liver, lungs, and saliva; crosses the blood-brain barrier to a limited extent

Protein binding: 26% to 33%

Metabolism: Significant first-pass metabolism; metabolized in the liver

Half-life: 9-12 hours

Time to peak serum concentration: 1.7-3 hours

Elimination: ~50% unchanged in urine, <2% excreted in feces

Dosage

Geriatrics: Oral: Initial: 2.5 mg/day; may be increased by 2.5-5 mg/day; maximum recommended dose: 20 mg/day

Adults:

Hypertension: Oral: 2.5-5 mg once daily; may be increased to 10 mg and then up to 20 mg once daily, if necessary; usual dose range (JNC 7): 2.5-10 mg once daily

CHF (unlabeled use): Initial: 1.25 mg once daily; maximum recommended dose: 10 mg once daily

Renal Impairment:

Cl_{cr} <40 mL/minute: Oral: Initial: 2.5 mg/day; increase cautiously

Not dialyzable

Monitoring Parameters Blood pressure, EKG, orthostatic hypotension, heart rate, CNS effects

Test Interactions Increased thyroxine (S), cholesterol (S), glucose, triglycerides, uric acid; decreased HDL

Patient Information Adhere to dosage regimen; watch for postural hypotension; do not discontinue medication abruptly, sudden stopping of medication may precipitate or cause angina; consult pharmacist or physician before taking with other adrenergic drugs (eg, cold medications); notify physician if any of the following symptoms occur: difficult breathing, night cough, swelling of extremities, slow pulse, dizziness, lightheadedness, confusion, depression, skin rash, fever, sore throat, unusual bleeding or (Continued)

Bisoprolol *(Continued)*

bruising; may produce drowsiness, dizziness, lightheadedness, blurred vision, confusion; use with caution while driving or performing tasks requiring alertness; may mask signs of hypoglycemia in diabetics; may be taken without regard to meals

Additional Information May potentiate hypoglycemia in a diabetic patient and mask signs and symptoms

Special Geriatric Considerations Due to alterations in the beta-adrenergic autonomic nervous system, beta-adrenergic blockade may result in less hemodynamic response than seen in younger adults. Studies indicate that despite decreased sensitivity to the chronotropic effects of beta-blockade with age, there appears to be an increased myocardial sensitivity to the negative inotropic effect during stress (ie, exercise). Controlled trials have shown the overall response rate for propranolol to be only 20% to 50% in elderly populations. Therefore, all beta-adrenergic blocking drugs may result in a decreased response as compared to younger adults.

Dosage Forms Excipient information presented when available (limited, particularly for generics); consult specific product labeling.

Tablet, as fumarate: 5 mg, 10 mg

Selected References

Aagaard GN, "Treatment of Hypertension in The Elderly," *Drug Treatment in the Elderly,* Vestal RE, ed, Boston, MA: ADIS Health Science Press, 1984, 77.

Chobanian AV, Bakris GL, Black HR, et al, "The Seventh Report of the Joint National Committee on Prevention, Detection, Evaluation, and Treatment of High Blood Pressure: The JNC 7 Report," *JAMA,* 2003, 289(19):2560-71.

Botulinum Toxin Type A (BOT yoo lin num TOKS in type aye)

U.S. Brand Names Botox®; Botox® Cosmetic
Canadian Brand Names Botox®; Botox® Cosmetic
Index Terms BTX-A
Generic Available No
Pharmacologic Category Neuromuscular Blocker Agent, Toxin; Ophthalmic Agent, Toxin

Use Treatment of strabismus and blepharospasm associated with dystonia (including benign essential blepharospasm or VII nerve disorders); cervical dystonia (spasmodic torticollis); temporary improvement in the appearance of lines/wrinkles of the face (moderate to severe glabellar lines associated with corrugator and/or procerus muscle activity) in adult patients ≤65 years of age; treatment of severe primary axillary hyperhidrosis in adults not adequately controlled with topical treatments

Unlabeled/Investigational Use Treatment of oromandibular dystonia, spasmodic dysphonia (laryngeal dystonia) and other dystonias (ie, writer's cramp, focal task-specific dystonias); migraine treatment and prophylaxis

Contraindications Hypersensitivity to albumin, botulinum toxin, or any component of the formulation; infection at the proposed injection site(s); relative contraindications include diseases of neuromuscular transmission, coagulopathy including therapeutic anticoagulation, and uncooperative patients

Warnings/Precautions Higher doses or more frequent administration may result in neutralizing antibody formation and loss of efficacy. Product contains albumin and may carry a remote risk of virus transmission. Use caution if there is inflammation, excessive weakness, or atrophy at the proposed injection site(s). Have appropriate support in case of anaphylactic reaction. Use with caution in patients with neuromuscular diseases (such as myasthenia gravis), neuropathic disorders (such as amyotrophic lateral sclerosis), or patients taking aminoglycosides or other drugs that interfere with neuromuscular transmission. Long-term effects of chronic therapy unknown.

Cervical dystonia: Dysphagia is common. It may be severe requiring alternative feeding methods. Risk factors include smaller neck muscle mass, bilateral injections into the sternocleidomastoid muscle, or injections into the levator scapulae. Dysphasia may be associated with increased risk of upper respiratory infection.

Blepharospasm: Reduced blinking from injection of the orbicularis muscle can lead to corneal exposure and ulceration.

Strabismus: Retrobulbar hemorrhages may occur from needle penetration into orbit. Spatial disorientation, double vision, or past pointing may occur if one or more extraocular muscles are paralyzed. Covering the affected eye may help. Careful testing of corneal sensation, avoidance of lower lid injections, and treatment of epithelial defects are necessary.

Primary axillary hyperhidrosis: Evaluate for secondary causes prior to treatment (eg, hyperthyroidism). Safety and efficacy for treatment of hyperhidrosis in other areas of the body have not been established.

Temporary reduction in glabellar lines: Do not use more frequently than every 3 months. Patients with marked facial asymmetry, ptosis, excessive dermatochalasis, deep dermal scarring, thick sebaceous skin, or the inability to substantially lessen glabellar lines by physically spreading them apart were excluded from clinical trials. Reduced blinking from injection of the orbicularis muscle can lead to corneal exposure and ulceration. Spatial disorientation, double vision, or past pointing may occur if one or more extraocular muscles are paralyzed.

Adverse Reactions (Reflective of adult population; not specific for elderly)
Adverse effects usually occur in 1 week and may last up to several months

>10%:
  Central nervous system: Headache (cervical dystonia up to 11%, reduction of glabellar lines up to 13%; can occur with other uses)
  Gastrointestinal: Dysphagia (cervical dystonia 19%)
  Neuromuscular & skeletal: Neck pain (cervical dystonia 11%)
  Ocular: Ptosis (blepharospasm 10% to 40%, strabismus 1% to 38%, reduction of glabellar lines 1% to 5%), vertical deviation (strabismus 17%)
  Respiratory: Upper respiratory infection (cervical dystonia 12%)
2% to 10%:
  Central nervous system: Anxiety (primary axillary hyperhydrosis), dizziness (cervical dystonia, reduction of glabellar lines), drowsiness (cervical dystonia), fever (cervical dystonia, primary axillary hyperhydrosis), speech disorder (cervical dystonia)
  Dermatologic: Nonaxillary sweating (primary axillary hyperhydrosis), pruritus (primary axillary hyperhydrosis)
  Gastrointestinal: Xerostomia (cervical dystonia), nausea (cervical dystonia, reduction of glabellar lines)
  Local: Injection site reaction
  Neuromuscular & skeletal: Back pain (cervical dystonia), facial pain (reduction of glabellar lines), hypertonia (cervical dystonia), weakness (cervical dystonia, reduction of glabellar lines)
  Ocular: Dry eyes (blepharospasm 6%), superficial punctate keratitis (blepharospasm 6%)
  Respiratory: Cough (cervical dystonia), infection (reduction of glabellar lines, primary axillary hyperhydrosis), pharyngitis (primary axillary hyperhydrosis), rhinitis (cervical dystonia)
  Miscellaneous: Flu syndrome (cervical dystonia, reduction of glabellar lines, primary axillary hyperhydrosis)

Overdosage/Toxicology Systemic weakness or muscle paralysis could occur for up to several weeks after overdose. Signs and symptoms of overdose are not apparent immediately. An antitoxin is available if there is immediate knowledge of an overdose or misinjection. Contact Allergan for additional information at (800) 433-8871 or (714) 246-5954. The antitoxin will not reverse toxin-induced muscle weakness already present.

Drug Interactions
  Aminoglycosides: May increase neuromuscular blockade.
  Neuromuscular-blocking agents: May increase neuromuscular blockade.
  Other agents which may have neuromuscular-blocking activity: Calcium channel blockers, catecholamines, chloroquine, clindamycin, colistin, corticosteroids, digitalis glycosides, diuretics, inhalation anesthetics, lidocaine, lincomycin, magnesium salts, opioids, phenytoin, phenelzine, polymyxin B, procainamide, propranolol, quinidine, and tetracyclines.

Stability Store undiluted vials under refrigeration at 2°C to 8°C for up to 24 months. Administer within 4 hours after the vial is reconstituted. Reconstitute with sterile normal saline without a preservative. Mix gently. After reconstitution, store in refrigerator (2°C to 8°C) and use within 4 hours (does not contain preservative). Do not freeze.

Botox®: Reconstitute vials with 1 mL of diluent to get 10 units per 0.1 mL; 2 mL of diluent to get 5 units per 0.1 mL; 4 mL of diluent to get 2.5 units per 0.1 mL; 8 mL of diluent to get 1.25 units per 0.1 mL.

Botox® Cosmetic: Reconstitute vials with 2.5 mL of diluent to get 4 units per 0.1 mL (20 units per 0.5 mL).

(Continued)

Botulinum Toxin Type A *(Continued)*

Mechanism of Action Botulinum A toxin is a neurotoxin produced by *Clostridium botulinum*, spore-forming anaerobic bacillus, which appears to affect only the presynaptic membrane of the neuromuscular junction in humans, where it prevents calcium-dependent release of acetylcholine and produces a state of denervation. Muscle inactivation persists until new fibrils grow from the nerve and form junction plates on new areas of the muscle-cell walls.

Pharmacodynamics

Onset of action (improvement):
Blepharospasm: ~3 days
Cervical dystonia: ~2 weeks
Strabismus: ~1-2 days
Reduction of glabellar lines (Botox® Cosmetic): 1-2 days, increasing in intensity during first week

Duration:
Blepharospasm: ~3 months
Cervical dystonia: <3 months
Strabismus: ~2-6 weeks
Primary axillary hyperhydrosis: 201 days (mean)
Reduction of glabellar lines (Botox® Cosmetic): Up to 3 months

Pharmacokinetics

Absorption: Not expected to be present in the peripheral blood at measurable levels following I.M. injection at the recommended doses.

Time to peak:
Blepharospasm: 1-2 weeks
Cervical dystonia: ~6 weeks
Strabismus: Within first week

Dosage

Geriatrics & Adults:

Cervical dystonia: I.M.: For dosing guidance, the mean dose is 236 units (25th to 75th percentile range 198-300 units) divided among the affected muscles in patients previously treated with botulinum toxin. Initial dose in previously untreated patients should be lower. Sequential dosing should be based on the patient's head and neck position, localization of pain, muscle hypertrophy, patient response, and previous adverse reactions. The total dose injected into the sternocleidomastoid muscles should be ≤100 units to decrease the occurrence of dysphagia.

Blepharospasm: I.M.: Initial dose: 1.25-2.5 units injected into the medial and lateral pretarsal orbicularis oculi of the upper and lower lid; dose may be increased up to twice the previous dose if the response from the initial dose lasted ≤2 months; maximum dose per site: 5 units; cumulative dose in a 30-day period: ≤200 units. Tolerance may occur if treatments are given more often than every 3 months, but the effect is not usually permanent.

Strabismus: I.M.:
Initial dose:
Vertical muscles and for horizontal strabismus <20 prism diopters: 1.25-2.5 units in any one muscle
Horizontal strabismus of 20-50 prism diopters: 2.5-5 units in any one muscle
Persistent VI nerve palsy >1 month: 1.5-2.5 units in the medial rectus muscle
Subsequent doses: Re-examine patients 7-14 days after each injection to assess the effect of that dose. Subsequent doses for patients experiencing incomplete paralysis of the target may be increased up to twice the previous administered dose. The maximum recommended dose as a single injection for any one muscle is 25 units. Do not administer subsequent injections until the effects of the previous dose are gone.

Primary axillary hyperhidrosis: Intradermal: 50 units/axilla. Injection area should be defined by standard staining techniques. Injections should be evenly distributed into multiple sites (10-15), administered in 0.1-0.2 mL aliquots, ~1-2 cm apart.

Reduction of glabellar lines: Adults ≤65 years: An effective dose is determined by gross observation of the patient's ability to activate the superficial muscles injected. The location, size and use of muscles may vary markedly among individuals. Inject 0.1 mL dose into each of five sites, two in each corrugator muscle and one in the procerus muscle (total dose 0.5 mL).

Renal Impairment: No adjustment is recommended.

Hepatic Impairment: No adjustment necessary.

Administration

Cervical dystonia: Use 25-, 27-, or 30-gauge needle for superficial muscles and a longer 22-gauge needle for deeper musculature; electromyography may help localize the involved muscles

Blepharospasm: Use a 27- or 30-gauge needle without electromyography guidance. Avoid injecting near the levator palpebrae superioris (may decrease ptosis); avoid medial lower lid injections (may decrease diplopia). Apply pressure at the injection site to prevent ecchymosis in the soft eyelid tissues.

Strabismus injections: Must use surgical exposure or electromyographic guidance; use the electrical activity recorded from the tip of the injections needle as a guide to placement within the target muscle. Local anesthetic and ocular decongestant should be given before injection. The volume of injection should be 0.05-0.15 mL per muscle. Many patients will require additional doses because of inadequate response to initial dose.

Primary axillary hyperhidrosis: Inject each dose intradermally to a depth of ~2mm and at a 45° angle. Do not inject directly into areas marked in ink (to avoid permanent tattoo effect). Prior to administration, injection area should be defined by standard staining techniques such as Minor's Iodine-Starch Test.

Instructions for Minor's Iodine-Starch Test: Patient should shave underarms and refrain from using deodorants or antiperspirants for 24 hours prior to test. At 30 minutes prior to test, patient should be at rest, no exercise, and not consume hot beverages. Underarm area should be dried and immediately painted with iodine solution. After area dries, lightly sprinkle with starch powder. Gently blow off excess powder. A deep blue-black color will develop over the hyperhidrotic area in ~10 minutes.

Reduction of glabellar lines (Botox® Cosmetic): Use a 30-gauge needle. Ensure injected volume/dose is accurate and where feasible keep to a minimum. Avoid injection near the levator palpebrae superioris. Medial corrugator injections should be at least 1 cm above the bony supraorbital ridge. Do not inject toxin closer than 1 cm above the central eyebrow.

Patient Information This medicine is given in a clinic or hospital setting by a prescriber. It is given as an injection. It is not a cure, but may be given on a periodic basis to help with spasms. Tell your prescriber if you have any nerve diseases or any infections where the shot might be given. Patients with blepharospasm may not have been very active. Start activity slowly and increase as you see how you feel. Call prescriber as soon as possible if you have trouble swallowing, speaking, or breathing. May have double vision or other problems where covering the eye with a patch may help.

Additional Information Units of biological activity of Botox® cannot be compared with units of any other botulinum toxin.

Special Geriatric Considerations No specific dosing adjustment recommended.

Dosage Forms Excipient information presented when available (limited, particularly for generics); consult specific product labeling.

Injection, powder for reconstitution [preservative free]: *Clostridium botulinum* toxin type A 100 units [contains human albumin]

Selected References

Borodic GE and Pearce LB, "New Concepts in Botulinum Toxin Therapy," *Drug Saf*, 1994, 11(3):145-52.

Brisinda G, Maria G, Bentivoglio AR, et al, "A Comparison of Injections of Botulinum Toxin and Topical Nitroglycerin Ointment for the Treatment of Chronic Anal Fistula," *N Engl J Med*, 1999, 341:65-9.

Bushara KO, Jones JW, and Park DM, "Localized Graying of Eyebrow Hair, A Side Effect of Botulinum Toxin Injections," *Mov Disord*, 1995, 10:382.

"Clinical Use of Botulinum Toxin," NIH Consensus Statement Online, 1990, 8(8):1-20.

Cohen S and Parkman HP, "Treatment of Achalasia - Whalebone to Botulinum Toxin," *N Engl J Med*, 1995, 332(12):815-6.

"Cosmetic Use of Botulinum Toxin," *Med Lett Drugs Ther*, 1999, 41(1057):63-4.

Ferrari AP, Jr, Siqueira ES, and Brant CQ, "Treatment of Achalasia in Chagas' Disease With Botulinum Toxin," *N Engl J Med*, 1995, 332(12):824-5.

Jankovic J and Brin MF, "Therapeutic Uses of Botulinum Toxin," *N Engl J Med*, 1991, 324(17):1186-94.

Pasricha PJ, Ravich WJ, Hendrix TR, et al, "Intrasphincteric Botulinum Toxin for the Treatment of Achalasia," *N Engl J Med*, 1995, 322(12):774-8.

Pasricha PJ, Ravich WJ, Hendrix TR, et al, "Treatment of Achalasia With Intrasphincteric Injection of Botulinum Toxin," *Ann Intern Med*, 1994, 121(8):590-1.

Repka MX, Savino PJ, and Reinecke RD, "Treatment of Acquired Nystagmus With Botulinum Neurotoxin A," *Arch Ophthalmol*, 1994, 112(10):1320-4.

Sheean GL, Murray NM, and Marsden CD, "Pain and Remote Weakness in Limbs Injected With Botulinum Toxin A for Writer's Cramp," *Lancet*, 1995, 346(8968):154-6.

Botulinum Toxin Type B (BOT yoo lin num TOKS in type bee)

U.S. Brand Names Myobloc®

Generic Available No

Pharmacologic Category Neuromuscular Blocker Agent, Toxin

Use Treatment of cervical dystonia (spasmodic torticollis)

Unlabeled/Investigational Use Treatment of cervical dystonia in patients who have developed resistance to botulinum toxin type A

Contraindications Hypersensitivity to albumin, botulinum toxin, or any component of the formulation; infection at the injection site(s); coadministration of agents known to potentiate neuromuscular blockade; relative contraindications include diseases of neuromuscular transmission, coagulopathy including therapeutic anticoagulation, and inability of patient to cooperate

(Continued)

Botulinum Toxin Type B *(Continued)*

Warnings/Precautions Higher doses or more frequent administration may result in neutralizing antibody formation and loss of efficacy. Product contains albumin and may carry a remote risk of virus transmission. Use caution if there is inflammation, excessive weakness, or atrophy at the proposed injection site(s). Concurrent use of botulinum toxin type A or within <4 months of type B is not recommended. Have appropriate support in case of anaphylactic reaction. Use with caution in patients taking aminoglycosides or other drugs that interfere with neuromuscular transmission. Long-term effects of chronic therapy unknown. Increased risk of dysphagia and respiratory complications.

Adverse Reactions (Reflective of adult population; not specific for elderly)
>10%:
- Central nervous system: Headache (10% to 16%), pain (6% to 13%; placebo 10%)
- Gastrointestinal: Dysphagia (10% to 25%), xerostomia (3% to 34%)
- Local: Injection site pain (12% to 16%)
- Neuromuscular & skeletal: Neck pain (up to 17%; placebo: 16%)
- Miscellaneous: Infection (13% to 19%; placebo: 15%)

1% to 10%:
- Cardiovascular: Chest pain, vasodilation, peripheral edema
- Central nervous system: Dizziness (3% to 6%), fever, malaise, migraine, anxiety, tremor, hyperesthesia, somnolence, confusion, vertigo
- Dermatologic: Pruritus, bruising
- Gastrointestinal: Nausea (3% to 10%; placebo: 5%), dyspepsia (up to 10%; placebo: 5%), vomiting, stomatitis, taste perversion
- Genitourinary: Urinary tract infection, cystitis, vaginal moniliasis
- Hematologic: Serum neutralizing activity
- Neuromuscular & skeletal: Torticollis (up to 8%; placebo: 7%), arthralgia (up to 7%; placebo: 5%), back pain (3% to 7%; placebo: 3%), myasthenia (3% to 6%; placebo: 3%), weakness (up to 6%; placebo: 4%), arthritis
- Ocular: Amblyopia, abnormal vision
- Otic: Otitis media, tinnitus
- Respiratory: Cough (3% to 7%; placebo: 3%), rhinitis (1% to 5%; placebo: 6%), dyspnea, pneumonia
- Miscellaneous: Flu-syndrome (6% to 9%), allergic reaction, viral infection, abscess, cyst

Overdosage/Toxicology Systemic weakness or muscle paralysis could occur for up to several weeks after overdose. Signs and symptoms of overdose are not apparent immediately. An antitoxin is available if there is immediate knowledge of an overdose or misinjection. Contact Elan Pharmaceuticals for additional information at (888) 638-7605 and your State Health Department to process a request for antitoxin through the CDC. The antitoxin will not reverse toxin-induced muscle weakness already present.

Drug Interactions
Aminoglycosides: May increase neuromuscular blockade.
Botulinum toxin type A: Potentiation of paralysis with concurrent or overlapping use; separate by ≥4 months.
Neuromuscular-blocking agents: May increase neuromuscular blockade.
Other agents which may have neuromuscular-blocking activity: Inhalation anesthetics, calcium channel blockers, catecholamines, chloroquine, clarithromycin, clindamycin, colistin, corticosteroids, digitalis glycosides, diuretics, erythromycin, inhalation anesthetics, lidocaine, lincomycin, magnesium salts, opioids, phenytoin, phenelzine, polymixin B, procainamide, propranolol, quinidine, tetracyclines, and vancomycin.

Stability Store vials under refrigeration at 2°C to 8°C (36°F to 46°F) for up to 21 months. May be diluted with normal saline; once diluted, use within 4 hours. Does not contain preservative. Single-use vial. Do not shake; do not freeze.

Mechanism of Action Botulinum B toxin is a neurotoxin produced by *Clostridium botulinum*, spore-forming anaerobic bacillus. It cleaves synaptic Vesicle Association Membrane Protein (VAMP; synaptobrevin) which is a component of the protein complex responsible for docking and fusion of the synaptic vesicle to the presynaptic membrane. By blocking neurotransmitter release, botulinum B toxin paralyzes the muscle.

Pharmacodynamics Duration: 12-16 weeks

Pharmacokinetics Absorption: Not expected to be present in the peripheral blood at measurable levels following I.M. injection at the recommended doses

Dosage
Geriatrics & Adults: Cervical dystonia: I.M.: Initial: 2500-5000 units divided among the affected muscles in patients **previously treated** with botulinum toxin; initial dose in **previously untreated** patients should be lower. Subsequent dosing should be optimized according to patient's response.

Renal Impairment: No adjustment is recommended.

Hepatic Impairment: No adjustment necessary.

Patient Information This medicine is given in a clinic or hospital setting by a prescriber. It is given as an injection. It is not a cure, but may be given on a periodic basis to help with spasms. Tell your prescriber if you have any nerve diseases or any infections where the injection might be given. Call your prescriber as soon as possible if you have trouble swallowing, speaking, breathing, or any muscle weakness.

Additional Information Units of biological activity of Myobloc® cannot be compared with units of any other botulinum toxin.

Special Geriatric Considerations No dosage adjustments required, but limited experience in patients ≥75 years of age.

Dosage Forms Excipient information presented when available (limited, particularly for generics); consult specific product labeling.

Injection, solution [preservative free]:

Myobloc®: 5000 units/mL (0.5 mL, 1 mL, 2 mL) [contains albumin 0.05%]

Selected References

Brashear A, Lew MF, Dykstra DD, et al, "Safety and Efficacy of NeuroBloc (Botulinum Toxin Type B) in Type A-Responsive Cervical Dystonia," *Neurology*, 1999, 53(7):1439-46.

Brin MF, Lew MF, Adler CH, et al, "Safety and Efficacy of NeuroBloc (Botulinum Toxin Type B) in Type A-Resistant Cervical Dystonia," *Neurology*, 1999, 53(7):1431-8.

"Clinical Use of Botulinum Toxin," NIH Consensus Statement, 1990, Nov 12-14, 8:1-20. Available at http://odp.od.nih.gov/consensus/cons/083/083_statement.htm. Accessed March 1, 2001.

♦ **Breathe Right® Saline [OTC]** *see* Sodium Chloride *on page 1475*

♦ **Brethaire [DSC]** *see* Terbutaline *on page 1533*

♦ **Brevibloc®** *see* Esmolol *on page 542*

♦ **Bricanyl [DSC]** *see* Terbutaline *on page 1533*

Brimonidine (bri MOE ni deen)

Related Information

Glaucoma Drug Therapy *on page 1758*

Medication Safety Issues

Sound-alike/look-alike issues:

Brimonidine may be confused with bromocriptine

U.S. Brand Names Alphagan® P

Canadian Brand Names Alphagan®; Apo-Brimonidine®; PMS-Brimonidine Tartrate; ratio-Brimonidine

Index Terms Brimonidine Tartrate

Generic Available Yes

Pharmacologic Category Alpha$_2$ Agonist, Ophthalmic; Ophthalmic Agent, Antiglaucoma

Use Reduction of intraocular pressure in patients with open-angle glaucoma or ocular hypertension

Contraindications Hypersensitivity to brimonidine tartrate or any component of the formulation; patients receiving MAO-inhibitor therapy

Warnings/Precautions Exercise caution in treating patients with severe cardiovascular disease. Use with caution in patients with depression, cerebral or coronary insufficiency, Raynaud's phenomenon, orthostatic hypotension, or thromboangiitis obliterans. Use with caution in patients with hepatic or renal impairment. Systemic absorption has been reported.

Products may contain benzalkonium chloride which may be absorbed by contact lenses; remove contacts prior to administration and wait 15 minutes before reinserting. The IOP-lowering efficacy observed with brimonidine tartrate during the first of month of therapy may not always reflect the long-term level of IOP reduction. Routinely monitor IOP.

Adverse Reactions (Reflective of adult population; not specific for elderly)

Actual frequency of adverse reactions may be formulation dependent; percentages reported with Alphagan® P:

>10%:

Central nervous system: Somnolence (adults 1% to 4%; children 25% to 83%)

Ocular: Allergic conjunctivitis, conjunctival hyperemia, eye pruritus

1% to 10% (unless otherwise noted 1% to 4%):

Cardiovascular: Hypertension (5% to 9%), hypotension

Central nervous system: Alertness decreased (children), dizziness, fatigue, headache, insomnia

Dermatologic: Rash

Endocrine & metabolic: Hypercholesterolemia

Gastrointestinal: Xerostomia (5% to 9%), dyspepsia

Neuromuscular & skeletal: Weakness

(Continued)

Brimonidine *(Continued)*

Ocular: Burning sensation (5% to 9%), conjunctival folliculosis (5% to 9%), ocular allergic reaction (5% to 9%), visual disturbance (5% to 9%), blepharitis, blepharo-conjunctivitis, blurred vision, cataract, conjunctival edema, conjunctival hemorrhage, conjunctivitis, dry eye, epiphora, eye discharge, eyelid disorder, eyelid edema, eyelid erythema, follicular conjunctivitis, foreign body sensation, irritation, keratitis, pain, photophobia, stinging, superficial punctate keratopathy, visual acuity worsened, visual field defect, vitreous detachment, vitreous floaters, watery eyes

Respiratory: Bronchitis, cough, dyspnea, pharyngitis, rhinitis, sinus infection, sinusitis

Miscellaneous: Allergic reaction, flu-like syndrome, infection

Overdosage/Toxicology No information is available on overdosage in humans. Treatment is symptom-directed and supportive.

Drug Interactions

Antihypertensives: Concomitant use may have additive effects

Cardiac glycosides: May increase effects

CNS depressants (eg, ethanol, barbiturates, opiates, sedatives, anesthetics): Concomitant use may have additive or potentiating effects.

MAO inhibitors: Concomitant use is contraindicated.

Pilocarpine: Additive decrease in intraocular pressure

Topical beta-blockers: Additive decreased intraocular pressure

Tricyclic antidepressants: Can affect the metabolism and uptake of circulating amines, resulting in decreased IOP-lowering effect of brimonidine.

Ethanol/Nutrition/Herb Interactions Herb/Nutraceutical: Avoid herbs with **hypertensive** properties (bayberry, blue cohosh, cayenne, ephedra, ginger, ginseng, gotu kola, licorice); may diminish antihypertensive effect. Avoid herbs with **hypotensive** properties (black cohosh, California poppy, coleus, golden seal, hawthorn, mistletoe, periwinkle, quinine, shepherd's purse); may enhance hypotensive effect.

Stability Store between 15°C to 25°C (59°F to 77°F).

Mechanism of Action Selective agonism for alpha$_2$-receptors; causes reduction of aqueous humor formation and increased uveoscleral outflow

Pharmacodynamics

Onset of action: 1-4 hours

Duration: 12 hours

Pharmacokinetics Time to peak, plasma: 0.5-2.5 hours

Dosage

Geriatrics & Adults: Glaucoma: Ophthalmic: Instill 1 drop in affected eye(s) 3 times/day (approximately every 8 hours)

Administration Remove contact lenses prior to administration; wait 15 minutes before reinserting if using products containing benzalkonium chloride. Separate administration of other ophthalmic agents by 5 minutes.

Monitoring Parameters Closely monitor patients who develop fatigue or drowsiness

Patient Information Do not touch dropper to the eyes or face.

Additional Information The use of Purite® as a preservative in Alphagan® P has lead to a reduced incidence of certain adverse effects associated with products using benzalkonium chloride as a preservative. The 0.1% and 0.15% solutions are comparable to the 0.2% solution in lowering intraocular pressure.

Special Geriatric Considerations Assess patient's ability to self-administer eye drops.

Dosage Forms Excipient information presented when available (limited, particularly for generics); consult specific product labeling.

Solution, ophthalmic, as tartrate: 0.2% (5 mL, 10 mL, 15 mL) [may contain benzalkonium chloride]

Alphagan® P: 0.1% (5 mL, 10 mL, 15 mL) [contains Purite® as preservative]; 0.15% (5 mL, 10 mL, 15 mL) [contains Purite® as preservative]

Selected References

Byles DB, Frith P, and Salmon JF, "Anterior Uveitis as a Side Effect of Topical Brimonidine," *Am J Ophthalmol*, 2000, 130(3):287-91.

♦ **Brimonidine Tartrate** *see* Brimonidine *on page 183*

Brinzolamide (brin ZOH la mide)

Related Information

Glaucoma Drug Therapy *on page 1758*

U.S. Brand Names Azopt®

Canadian Brand Names Azopt®

Generic Available No

Pharmacologic Category Carbonic Anhydrase Inhibitor; Ophthalmic Agent, Antiglaucoma

Use Reduction of intraocular pressure to treat glaucoma in patients with ocular hypertension or open-angle glaucoma

Contraindications Hypersensitivity to brinzolamide, sulfonamides, or any component of the formulation

Warnings/Precautions Although administered topically, systemic absorption occurs. Similar adverse reactions attributed to sulfonamides may occur with topical administration. Effects of prolonged use on corneal epithelial cells have not been evaluated; has not been studied in acute angle-closure glaucoma. Use caution with renal impairment (parent and metabolite may accumulate). Systemic absorption may cause serious hypersensitivity reactions to recur. Chemical similarities are present among sulfonamides, sulfonylureas, carbonic anhydrase inhibitors, thiazides, and loop diuretics (except ethacrynic acid). In patients with allergy to one of these compounds, a risk of cross-reaction exists; avoid use when previous reaction has been severe.

Adverse Reactions (Reflective of adult population; not specific for elderly)
1% to 10%:
Dermatologic: Dermatitis (1% to 5%)
Gastrointestinal: Taste disturbances (5% to 10%)
Ocular: Blurred vision (5% to 10%), blepharitis (1% to 5%), dry eye (1% to 5%), foreign body sensation (1% to 5%), eye discharge (1% to 5%), eye pain (1% to 5%), itching of eye (1% to 5%)
Respiratory: Rhinitis (1% to 5%)

Overdosage/Toxicology Theoretically, overdose could lead to electrolyte imbalance, acidosis and CNS effects; monitor serum electrolytes and blood pH. Treatment is supportive.

Drug Interactions Substrate of CYP3A4 (minor)
Carbonic anhydrase inhibitors (CAIs): Concurrent use of oral CAIs may lead to additive effects and toxicity; use is not recommended.
Salicylates: High-dose salicylates may result in toxicity from CAIs.

Stability Store at 4°C to 30°C (39°F to 86°F). Shake well before use.

Mechanism of Action Brinzolamide inhibits carbonic anhydrase, leading to decreased aqueous humor secretion. This results in a reduction of intraocular pressure.

Pharmacokinetics
Absorption: Topical: Into the systemic circulation
Distribution: Accumulates in red blood cells, binding to carbonic anhydrase (brinzolamide and metabolite)
Metabolism: To N-desmethyl brinzolamide
Elimination: Primarily in urine (unchanged drug and metabolites)

Dosage
Geriatrics & Adults: Glaucoma: Ophthalmic: Instill 1 drop in affected eye(s) 3 times/day

Administration Shake well; may be used concomitantly with other topical ophthalmic drug products to lower intraocular pressure. If more than one topical ophthalmic drug is being used, administer drugs at least 10 minutes apart.

Monitoring Parameters Intraocular pressure, ophthalmic exams

Patient Information May sting on administering instillation; shake well; teach patient or caregiver proper administration and assess ability to properly instill eye drops; do not touch dropper to eye; visual acuity may be decreased after administration; distance vision may be altered; apply gentle pressure between the eye and nose during and immediately following instillation (1 minute)

Special Geriatric Considerations The oral carbonic anhydrase inhibitors are useful for patients who have difficulty administering ophthalmic drugs, who do not achieve sufficient lowering of intraocular pressure, or who cannot tolerate other agents. Brinzolamide is a useful agent apart from those who need a carbonic anhydrase inhibitor and can administer ophthalmic drops.

Dosage Forms Excipient information presented when available (limited, particularly for generics); consult specific product labeling.
Suspension, ophthalmic: 1% (5 mL, 10 mL, 15 mL) [contains benzalkonium chloride]

Selected References
Silver LH, "Clinical Efficacy and Safety of Brinzolamide (Azopt), a New Topical Carbonic Anhydrase Inhibitor for Primary Open-Angle Glaucoma and Ocular Hypertension, Brinzolamide Primary Therapy Study Group," *Am J Ophthalmol*, 1998, 126(3):400-8.

♦ **Brioschi® [OTC]** *see* Sodium Bicarbonate *on page 1474*
♦ **BRL 43694** *see* Granisetron *on page 724*

Bromfenac (BROME fen ak)

U.S. Brand Names Xibrom™
Index Terms Bromfenac Sodium
Generic Available No
(Continued)

Bromfenac *(Continued)*

Pharmacologic Category Nonsteroidal Anti-inflammatory Drug (NSAID), Ophthalmic

Use Treatment of postoperative inflammation following cataract removal

Warnings/Precautions Use with caution in patients with previous sensitivity to acetyl-salicylic acid and phenylacetic acid derivatives, including patients who experience bronchospasm, asthma, rhinitis, or urticaria following NSAID or aspirin. May slow/delay healing or prolong bleeding time following surgery. Use caution in patients with a predisposition to bleeding (bleeding tendencies or medications which interfere with coagulation).

May cause keratitis; continued use of bromfenac in a patient with keratitis may cause severe corneal adverse reactions, potentially resulting in loss of vision. Immediately discontinue use in patients with evidence of corneal epithelial damage.

Use caution in patients with complicated ocular surgeries, corneal denervation, corneal epithelial defects, diabetes mellitus, ocular surface disease, rheumatoid arthritis, or repeat ocular surgeries (within a short timeframe); may be at risk of corneal adverse events, potentially resulting in loss of vision. Patients using ophthalmic drops should not wear soft contact lenses. Use for more than 1 day prior to surgery or for 14 days beyond surgery may increase risk and severity of corneal adverse events.

Contains sulfites, which may cause allergic reactions.

Adverse Reactions (Reflective of adult population; not specific for elderly) 2% to 7%:

Central nervous system: Headache

Ocular: Abnormal vision, abnormal sensation, conjunctival hyperemia, eye pain, iritis, pruritus

Drug Interactions

Corticosteroids, ophthalmic: Concurrent use may increase the risk of healing problems.

Latanoprost: Bromfenac may decrease the reduction in IOP produced by latanoprost; monitor.

Stability Store at 15°C to 25°C (59°F to 77°F).

Mechanism of Action Inhibits prostaglandin synthesis by decreasing the activity of the enzyme, cyclooxygenase, which results in decreased formation of prostaglandin precursors.

Pharmacokinetics

Absorption: Theoretically, systemic absorption may occur following ophthalmic use (not characterized); anticipated levels are below the limits of assay detection

Metabolism: Hepatic

Half-life elimination: 0.5-4 hours (following oral administration)

Dosage

Geriatrics & Adults: Ophthalmic: Instill 1 drop into affected eye(s) twice daily beginning 24 hours after surgery and continuing for 2 weeks postoperatively

Renal Impairment: No adjustment required.

Patient Information Do not wear contact lenses while using this medication. Report any abnormal sensation in eye, redness, severe headache, or pain.

Additional Information An oral formulation of bromfenac was previously available and was withdrawn from the market following reports of idiosyncratic hepatotoxicity.

Special Geriatric Considerations No differences in safety and efficacy noted between elderly and younger adults. No dosage adjustment necessary. Elderly may be taking other medications that will increase bleeding.

Dosage Forms Excipient information presented when available (limited, particularly for generics); consult specific product labeling.

Solution, ophthalmic:

Xibrom™: 0.09% (5 mL) [contains benzalkonium chloride and sodium sulfite]

Selected References

Fontana RJ, McCashland TM, Benner KG, et al, "Acute Liver Failure Associated With Prolonged Use of Bromfenac Leading to Liver Transplantation. The Acute Liver Failure Study Group," *Liver Transpl Surg*, 1999, 5(6):480-4.

Kashiwagi K and Tsukahara S, "Effect of Non-Steroidal Anti-Inflammatory Ophthalmic Solution on Intraocular Pressure Reduction by Latanoprost," *Br J Ophthalmol*, 2003, 87(3):297-301.

Miyake-Kashima M, Takano Y, Tanaka M, et al, "Comparison of 0.1% Bromfenac Sodium and 0.1% Pemirolast Potassium for the Treatment of Allergic Conjunctivitis," *Jpn J Ophthalmol*, 2004, 48(6):587-90.

Rabkin JM, Smith MJ, Orloff SL, et al, "Fatal Fulminant Hepatitis Associated With Bromfenac Use," *Ann Pharmacother*, 1999, 33(9):945-7.

Skjodt NM and Davies NM, "Clinical Pharmacokinetics and Pharmacodynamics of Bromfenac," *Clin Pharmacokinet*, 1999, 36(6):399-408.

♦ **Bromfenac Sodium** *see* Bromfenac *on page 185*

Bromocriptine *(broe moe KRIP teen)*

Related Information

Antiparkinsonian Agents *on page 1745*

Medication Safety Issues

Sound-alike/look-alike issues:

Bromocriptine may be confused with benztropine, brimonidine

Parlodel® may be confused with pindolol, Provera®

U.S. Brand Names Parlodel®; Parlodel® SnapTabs®

Canadian Brand Names Apo-Bromocriptine®; Parlodel®; PMS-Bromocriptine

Index Terms Bromocriptine Mesylate

Generic Available Yes

Pharmacologic Category Anti-Parkinson's Agent, Dopamine Agonist; Ergot Derivative

Use Treatment of parkinsonism in patients unresponsive or allergic to levodopa; treatment of conditions associated with hyperprolactinemia and acromegaly

Unlabeled/Investigational Use Treatment of neuroleptic malignant syndrome

Contraindications Hypersensitivity to bromocriptine, ergot alkaloids, or any component of the formulation; ergot alkaloids are contraindicated with potent inhibitors of CYP3A4 (includes protease inhibitors, azole antifungals, and some macrolide antibiotics); uncontrolled hypertension; severe ischemic heart disease or peripheral vascular disorders

Warnings/Precautions Complete evaluation of pituitary function should be completed prior to initiation of treatment. Use caution in patients with a history of peptic ulcer disease, dementia, psychosis, or cardiovascular disease (myocardial infarction, arrhythmia). Symptomatic hypotension may occur in a significant number of patients. In addition, hypertension, seizures, MI, and stroke have been rarely associated with bromocriptine therapy. Severe headache or visual changes may precede events. The onset of reactions may be immediate or delayed (often may occur in the second week of therapy). Sudden sleep onset and somnolence have been reported with use, primarily in patients with Parkinson's disease. Patients must be cautioned about performing tasks which require mental alertness.

Concurrent antihypertensives or drugs which may alter blood pressure should be used with caution. Concurrent use with levodopa has been associated with an increased risk of hallucinations. Consider dosage reduction and/or discontinuation in patients with hallucinations. Hallucinations may require weeks to months before resolution.

In the treatment of acromegaly, discontinuation is recommended if tumor expansion occurs during therapy. Digital vasospasm (cold sensitive) may occur in some patients with acromegaly; may require dosage reduction. Use of bromocriptine in patients with uncontrolled hypertension is not recommended.

Monitoring and careful evaluation of visual changes during the treatment of hyperprolactinemia is recommended to differentiate between tumor shrinkage and traction on the optic chiasm; rapidly progressing visual field loss requires neurosurgical consultation. Discontinuation of bromocriptine in patients with macroadenomas has been associated with rapid regrowth of tumor and increased prolactin serum levels. Pleural and retroperitoneal fibrosis have been reported with prolonged daily use. Cardiac valvular fibrosis has also been associated with ergot alkaloids. Safety and efficacy have not been established in patients with hepatic or renal dysfunction.

Adverse Reactions (Reflective of adult population; not specific for elderly)

Note: Frequency of adverse effects may vary by dose and/or indication.

>10%:

Central nervous system: Dizziness, headache

Gastrointestinal: Constipation, nausea

1% to 10%:

Cardiovascular: Hypotension (including postural/orthostatic), Raynaud's syndrome exacerbation, syncope

Central nervous system: Drowsiness, fatigue, lightheadedness

Gastrointestinal: Abdominal cramps, anorexia, diarrhea, dyspepsia, GI bleeding, vomiting, xerostomia

Neuromuscular & skeletal: Digital vasospasm

Respiratory: Nasal congestion

Overdosage/Toxicology Symptoms include nausea, vomiting, and hypotension. Hypotension, when unresponsive to I.V. fluids or Trendelenburg positioning, often responds to norepinephrine infusions started at 0.1-0.2 mcg/kg/minute followed by a titrated infusion.

Drug Interactions Substrate of CYP3A4 (major); **Inhibits** CYP1A2 (weak), 3A4 (weak)

Alpha agonists/sympathomimetics: May enhance the adverse/toxic effect of bromocriptine, including increased blood pressure, ventricular arrhythmias, and seizures. Monitor. **Note:** The use of epinephrine in combination local anesthetics should pose no clinical concern.

Antihypertensives: Concurrent use with bromocriptine may increase the risk of hypotension and/or orthostasis. Use caution.

(Continued)

Bromocriptine *(Continued)*

Antifungals, azole derivatives (itraconazole, ketoconazole) increase levels of ergot alkaloids by inhibiting CYP3A4 metabolism, resulting in toxicity; concomitant use is contraindicated.

Antipsychotics (atypical): May diminish the effects of bromocriptine (due to dopamine antagonism); these combinations should generally be avoided.

CYP3A4 inhibitors: May increase the levels/effects of bromocriptine. Example inhibitors include azole antifungals, clarithromycin, diclofenac, doxycycline, erythromycin, imatinib, isoniazid, nefazodone, nicardipine, propofol, protease inhibitors, quinidine, telithromycin, and verapamil.

Dopamine: Ergot derivatives may enhance the vasoconstricting effect of dopamine.

Levodopa: Concurrent use may increase the risk of hallucinations. Dosage reduction may be required.

Macrolide antibiotics: Erythromycin, clarithromycin, and telithromycin may increase levels of ergot alkaloids by inhibiting CYP3A4 metabolism, resulting in toxicity (ischemia, vasospasm); concomitant use is contraindicated.

Metoclopramide: May diminish the therapeutic effect of bromocriptine (due to dopamine antagonism).

Nitroglycerin: Ergot derivatives may decrease the vasodilatory effect of nitroglycerin.

Protease inhibitors (ritonavir, amprenavir, indinavir, nelfinavir, and saquinavir) increase blood levels of ergot alkaloids by inhibiting CYP3A4 metabolism, acute ergot toxicity has been reported; concomitant use is contraindicated.

Serotonin modulators: Concurrent use with bromocriptine may increase the risk of serotonin syndrome (includes buspirone, SSRIs, TCAs, MAO inhibitors, nefazodone, sumatriptan, and trazodone).

Sibutramine: May cause serotonin syndrome; concurrent use with ergot alkaloids is contraindicated.

Ethanol/Nutrition/Herb Interactions

Ethanol: Avoid ethanol (may increase GI side effects or ethanol intolerance).

Herb/Nutraceutical: St John's wort may decrease bromocriptine levels.

Mechanism of Action Semisynthetic ergot alkaloid derivative and a dopamine receptor agonist which activates postsynaptic dopamine receptors in the tuberoinfundibular (inhibiting pituitary prolactin secretion) and nigrostriatal pathways (enhancing coordinated motor control).

Pharmacodynamics Onset of action: Prolactin decreasing effect: 1-2 hours

Pharmacokinetics

Protein binding: 90% to 96%

Metabolism: Primarily hepatic via CYP3A; extensive first-pass biotransformation

Half-life elimination: Biphasic: Terminal: 15 hours (range 8-20 hours)

Time to peak, serum: 1-3 hours

Excretion: Feces; urine (2% to 6% as unchanged drug and metabolites)

Dosage

Geriatrics & Adults:

Parkinsonism: Oral: 1.25 mg twice daily, increased by 2.5 mg/day in 2- to 4-week intervals (usual dose range is 30-90 mg/day in 3 divided doses; maximum: 100 mg/day), though elderly patients can usually be managed on lower doses.

Neuroleptic malignant syndrome (unlabeled use): Oral: 2.5-5 mg 3 times/day

Acromegaly: Oral: Initial: 1.25-2.5 mg daily increasing by 1.25-2.5 mg daily as necessary every 3-7 days; usual dose: 20-30 mg/day (maximum: 100 mg/day)

Hyperprolactinemia: Oral: Initial: 1.25-2.5 mg/day; may be increased by 2.5 mg/day as tolerated every 2-7 days until optimal response (range: 2.5-15 mg/day)

Hepatic Impairment: No guidelines are available, however, adjustment may be necessary.

Monitoring Parameters Monitor blood pressure closely as well as hepatic, hematopoietic, and cardiovascular function

Patient Information Take with food or milk to minimize nausea; drowsiness commonly occurs upon initiation of therapy; limit use of alcohol; avoid exposure to cold; rise slowly from sitting or lying position

Additional Information Usually used with levodopa or levodopa/carbidopa to treat Parkinson's disease; when adding bromocriptine, the dose of levodopa/carbidopa can usually and should be decreased

Special Geriatric Considerations No special considerations are recommended since drug is dosed to response; however, elderly may have concomitant diseases or drug therapy which may complicate therapy.

Dosage Forms Excipient information presented when available (limited, particularly for generics); consult specific product labeling.

Capsule, as mesylate: 5 mg
   Parlodel®: 5 mg
Tablet, as mesylate: 2.5 mg
   Parlodel® SnapTabs®: 2.5 mg

Selected References

Olanow CW, Watts RL, and Koller WC, "An Algorithm (Decision Tree) for the Management of Parkinson's Disease (2001): Treatment Guidelines," *Neurology*, 2001, 56(11 Suppl 5):S1-S88.

Stern MB, "Contemporary Approaches to the Pharmacotherapeutic Management of Parkinson's Disease: An Overview," *Neurology*, 1997, 49(1 Suppl 1):S2-9.

Watts RL, "The Role of Dopamine Agonists in Early Parkinson's Disease," *Neurology*, 1997, 49(1 Suppl 1):S34-48.

♦ **Bromocriptine Mesylate** *see* Bromocriptine *on page 186*

Brompheniramine (brome fen IR a meen)

U.S. Brand Names Bidhist; BroveX™; BroveX™ CT; B-Vex; Lodrane® 12 Hour; Lodrane® 24; Lodrane® XR; LoHist-12; TanaCof-XR

Index Terms Brompheniramine Maleate; Brompheniramine Tannate

Generic Available Yes: Excludes chewable tablet

Pharmacologic Category Antihistamine

Use Symptomatic relief of perennial and seasonal allergic rhinitis, vasomotor rhinitis, and other respiratory allergies

Contraindications Hypersensitivity to brompheniramine or any component of the formulation; use with or within 14 days of MAO inhibitor therapy; narrow-angle glaucoma; urinary retention; peptic ulcer disease; during acute asthmatic attacks

Warnings/Precautions Causes sedation; caution must be used in performing tasks which require alertness (eg, operating machinery or driving). Sedative effects of CNS depressants or ethanol are potentiated. Use with caution in patients with diabetes mellitus, hyperthyroidism, increased intraocular pressure, prostatic hyperplasia, bronchial asthma, and cardiovascular disease (including hypertension and ischemic heart disease). A dose reduction in patients ≥60 years of age may be warranted due to increased adverse reactions (eg, dizziness, sedation, hypotension). Some products may contain tartrazine or phenylalanine.

Adverse Reactions (Reflective of adult population; not specific for elderly) Frequency not defined.

Cardiovascular: Angina, blood pressure increased, circulatory collapse, extrasystoles, hypotension, palpitation, tachycardia

Central nervous system: Anxiety, chills, confusion, coordination impaired, dizziness, drowsiness, euphoria, excitation, fatigue, headache, hysteria, insomnia, irritability, nervousness, neuritis, restlessness, sedation, seizure, sleepiness, stimulation, tension, vertigo

Dermatologic: Photosensitivity, rash, urticaria

Endocrine & metabolic: Early menses

Gastrointestinal: Abdominal cramps, anorexia, constipation, diarrhea, dry throat, epigastric distress, nausea, vomiting, xerostomia

Genitourinary: Dysuria, polyuria, urinary retention

Hematologic: Agranulocytosis, hemolytic anemia, hypoplastic anemia, thrombocytopenia

Neuromuscular & skeletal: Paresthesia, tremor, weakness

Ocular: Blurred vision, diplopia, mydriasis

Otic: Labyrinthitis (acute), tinnitus

Respiratory: Dry nose, nasal congestion, thickening of bronchial secretions, wheezing

Miscellaneous: Anaphylactic shock, diaphoresis

Overdosage/Toxicology Symptoms may include dizziness, sedation, hypotension, hallucinations, convulsions, and death. Treatment should be symptom-directed and supportive. Physostigmine may reverse anticholinergic symptoms.

Drug Interactions

Barbiturates (and other CNS depressants): CNS depressant effects may be increased.

MAO inhibitors: Anticholinergic effects of the antihistamine may be increased and prolonged.

Tricyclic antidepressants: Anticholinergic effects of the antihistamine may be increased and prolonged. CNS depressant effects may be increased.

Ethanol/Nutrition/Herb Interactions Ethanol: Avoid ethanol (may increase CNS depression).

Stability Store between 15°C to 30°C (59°F to 86°F).

Mechanism of Action Competes with histamine for H_1-receptor sites on effector cells

Pharmacokinetics

Metabolism: Hepatic

Excretion: Urine

Dosage

Geriatrics:

Initial (also refer to adult dosing):

B-Vex, BroveX™: 5 mL every 12 hours

BroveX™ CT, Lodrane® 12 Hour, LoHist: 1 tablet every 12 hours

Lodrane® 24: 1 capsule/24 hours

(Continued)

Brompheniramine *(Continued)*

Lodrane® XR, TanaCof-XR: 2.5 mL every 12 hours

Adults: Allergic rhinitis, allergic symptoms, vasomotor rhinitis: Oral:

B-Vex, BroveX™: 5-10 mL every 12 hours (maximum: 20 mL/day)

BroveX™ CT: 1-2 tablets every 12 hours (maximum: 4 tablets/day)

Lodrane® 12 Hour, LoHist: 1-2 tablets every 12 hours (maximum: 4 tablets/day)

Lodrane® 24: 1-2 capsules once daily

Lodrane® XR, TanaCof-XR: 5 mL every 12 hours (maximum: 10 mL/day)

Administration Extended release tablets are to be swallowed whole; do not crush or chew.

Test Interactions May interfere with skin tests using allergen extracts.

Patient Information Inform prescriber of all prescription medications, OTC medications, or herbal products you are taking. Avoid alcohol, depressants, and sleep inducing medication unless approved by prescriber. You may experience drowsiness or dizziness (use caution when driving or engaging in activities requiring alertness until response to drug is known). Report persistent sedation, confusion, or agitation; changes in urinary pattern, blurred vision, chest pain, rapid heart beat, or respiratory difficulty.

Special Geriatric Considerations Anticholinergic action may cause significant confusional symptoms, constipation, or problems voiding urine. If an antihistamine is indicated, a second generation nonsedating antihistamine would be a more appropriate choice.

Dosage Forms Excipient information presented when available (limited, particularly for generics); consult specific product labeling.

Capsule, extended release:

Lodrane® 24: 12 mg [dye free]

Suspension, as tannate:

B-Vex, BroveX™: 12 mg/5 mL (120 mL) [contains sodium benzoate and tartrazine; banana flavor]

Lodrane® XR: 8 mg/5 mL (480 mL) [alcohol free, sugar free; strawberry flavor]

TanaCof-XR: 8 mg/5 mL (480 mL) [alcohol free, sugar free; contains phenylalanine; strawberry creme flavor]

Tablet, chewable, as tannate:

BroveX™ CT: 12 mg [banana flavor]

Tablet, extended release, as maleate:

Bidhist: 6 mg

Tablet, extended release, as maleate [scored]:

Lodrane® 12 Hour, LoHist-12: 6 mg [dye free]

Tablet, timed release, as maleate: 6 mg

- ♦ **Brompheniramine Maleate** *see* Brompheniramine *on page 189*
- ♦ **Brompheniramine Tannate** *see* Brompheniramine *on page 189*
- ♦ **Broncho Saline® [OTC] [DSC]** *see* Sodium Chloride *on page 1475*
- ♦ **Brontex®** *see* Guaifenesin and Codeine *on page 729*
- ♦ **Brovana™** *see* Arformoterol *on page 119*
- ♦ **BroveX™** *see* Brompheniramine *on page 189*
- ♦ **BroveX™ CT** *see* Brompheniramine *on page 189*
- ♦ **BTX-A** *see* Botulinum Toxin Type A *on page 178*
- ♦ **B-type Natriuretic Peptide (Human)** *see* Nesiritide *on page 1106*
- ♦ **Budeprion™ SR** *see* BuPROPion *on page 198*

Budesonide *(byoo DES oh nide)*

Related Information

Asthma *on page 1767*

Inhalant Agents *on page 1760*

U.S. Brand Names Entocort® EC; Pulmicort Flexhaler®; Pulmicort Respules®; Pulmicort Turbuhaler®; Rhinocort® Aqua®

Canadian Brand Names Entocort®; Gen-Budesonide AQ; Pulmicort®; Rhinocort® Turbuhaler®

Generic Available No

Pharmacologic Category Corticosteroid, Inhalant (Oral); Corticosteroid, Nasal; Corticosteroid, Systemic

Use

Intranasal: Management of symptoms of seasonal or perennial rhinitis

Nebulization: Maintenance and prophylactic treatment of asthma

Oral capsule: Treatment of active Crohn's disease (mild to moderate) involving the ileum and/or ascending colon; maintenance of remission (for up to 3 months) of Crohn's disease (mild to moderate) involving the ileum and/or ascending colon

Oral inhalation: Maintenance and prophylactic treatment of asthma; includes patients who require corticosteroids and those who may benefit from systemic dose reduction/elimination

Contraindications Hypersensitivity to budesonide or any component of the formulation

Inhalation: Contraindicated in primary treatment of status asthmaticus, acute episodes of asthma; not for relief of acute bronchospasm

Warnings/Precautions May cause hypercorticism or suppression of hypothalamic-pituitary-adrenal (HPA) axis, particularly in patients receiving high doses for prolonged periods. HPA axis suppression may lead to adrenal crisis. Withdrawal and discontinuation of a corticosteroid should be done slowly and carefully. Particular care is required when patients are transferred from systemic corticosteroids to inhaled products due to possible adrenal insufficiency or withdrawal from steroids, including an increase in allergic symptoms. Patients receiving >20 mg per day of prednisone (or equivalent) may be most susceptible. Fatalities have occurred due to adrenal insufficiency in asthmatic patients during and after transfer from systemic corticosteroids to aerosol steroids; aerosol steroids do not provide the systemic steroid needed to treat patients having trauma, surgery, or infections. Do not use this product to transfer patients from oral corticosteroid therapy.

Bronchospasm may occur with wheezing after inhalation; if this occurs stop steroid and treat with a fast-acting bronchodilator. Supplemental steroids (oral or parenteral) may be needed during stress or severe asthma attacks. Not to be used in status asthmaticus or for the relief of acute bronchospasm. Acute myopathy has been reported with high dose corticosteroids, usually in patients with neuromuscular transmission disorders; may involve ocular and/or respiratory muscles; monitor creatine kinase; recovery may be delayed. Corticosteroid use may cause psychiatric disturbances, including depression, euphoria, insomnia, mood swings, and personality changes. Pre-existing psychiatric conditions may be exacerbated by corticosteroid use. Prolonged use of corticosteroids may also increase the incidence of secondary infection, mask acute infection (including fungal infections), prolong or exacerbate viral infections, or limit response to vaccines. Exposure to chickenpox should be avoided; corticosteroids should not be used to treat ocular herpes simplex. Corticosteroids should not be used for cerebral malaria. Close observation is required in patients with latent tuberculosis and/or TB reactivity; restrict use in active TB (only in conjunction with antituberculosis treatment). Prolonged treatment with corticosteroids has been associated with the development of Kaposi's sarcoma (case reports); if noted, discontinuation of therapy should be considered.

Use with caution in patients with thyroid disease, hepatic impairment, renal impairment, cardiovascular disease, diabetes, glaucoma, cataracts, myasthenia gravis, patients at risk for osteoporosis, patients at risk for seizures, or GI diseases (diverticulitis, peptic ulcer, ulcerative colitis) due to perforation risk. Use caution following acute MI (corticosteroids have been associated with myocardial rupture). Because of the risk of adverse effects, systemic corticosteroids should be used cautiously in the elderly in the smallest possible effective dose for the shortest duration. Avoid nasal corticosteroid use in patients with recent nasal septal ulcers, nasal surgery or nasal trauma until healing has occurred.

Adverse Reactions (Reflective of adult population; not specific for elderly)
Reaction severity varies by dose and duration; not all adverse reactions have been reported with each dosage form.

>10%:
Central nervous system: Headache (up to 21%)
Gastrointestinal: Nausea (up to 11%)
Respiratory: Respiratory infection, rhinitis
Miscellaneous: Symptoms of HPA axis suppression and/or hypercorticism may occur in >10% of patients following administration of dosage forms which result in higher systemic exposure (ie, oral capsule), but may be less frequent than rates observed with comparator drugs (prednisolone). These symptoms may be rare (<1%) following administration via methods which result in lower exposures (topical).
1% to 10%:
Cardiovascular: Chest pain, edema, flushing, hypertension, palpitation, syncope, tachycardia
Central nervous system: Dizziness, dysphonia, emotional lability, fatigue, fever, insomnia, migraine, nervousness, pain, vertigo
Dermatologic: Acne, alopecia, bruising, contact dermatitis, eczema, hirsutism, pruritus, pustular rash, rash, striae
Endocrine & metabolic: Adrenal insufficiency, hypokalemia, menstrual disorder
Gastrointestinal: Abdominal pain, anorexia, diarrhea, dry mouth, dyspepsia, flatulence, gastroenteritis, oral candidiasis, taste perversion, vomiting, weight gain
Genitourinary: Dysuria, hematuria, nocturia, pyuria
Hematologic: Cervical lymphadenopathy, leukocytosis, purpura
Hepatic: Alkaline phosphatase increased
(Continued)

Budesonide *(Continued)*

Neuromuscular & skeletal: Arthralgia, back pain, fracture, hyperkinesis, hypertonia, myalgia, neck pain, weakness, paresthesia

Ocular: Conjunctivitis, eye infection

Otic: Earache, ear infection, external ear infection

Respiratory: Bronchitis, bronchospasm, cough, epistaxis, nasal congestion, nasal irritation, pharyngitis, sinusitis, stridor

Miscellaneous: Abscess, allergic reaction, C-reactive protein increased, erythrocyte sedimentation rate increased, fat distribution (moon face, buffalo hump), flu-like syndrome, herpes simplex, infection, moniliasis, viral infection, voice alteration

Overdosage/Toxicology Symptoms of overdose with inhaled formulations include irritation and burning of the nasal mucosa, sneezing, intranasal and pharyngeal *Candida* infections, nasal ulceration, epistaxis, rhinorrhea, nasal stuffiness, and headache. When consumed in excessive quantities, systemic hypercorticism and adrenal suppression may occur; in those cases, discontinuation and withdrawal of the corticosteroid should be done judiciously. Treatment should be symptomatic and supportive.

Drug Interactions Substrate of CYP3A4 (major)

Amphotericin: Corticosteroids may increase the hypokalemic effects of amphotericin B; monitor.

Antacids: May decrease the therapeutic effect of orally-administered budesonide through adsorption; separate administration by 2 hours.

Antidiabetic agents: Corticosteroids may decrease the hypoglycemic effects of antidiabetic agents; monitor.

Antifungal agents (imidazole): May increase the serum levels/effects of corticosteroids; monitor.

Bile acid sequestrants: May decrease the therapeutic effect of orally-administered corticosteroids through adsorption; separate administration by 2 hours.

CYP3A4 inhibitors: May increase the levels/effects of budesonide. Example inhibitors include azole antifungals, clarithromycin, diclofenac, doxycycline, erythromycin, imatinib, isoniazid, nefazodone, nicardipine, propofol, protease inhibitors, quinidine, telithromycin, and verapamil.

Diuretics, potassium-wasting (loop or thiazide): Hypokalemic effects may be increased by corticosteroids; monitor.

Fluoroquinolones: Concurrent use may increase the risk of tendonopathies (including tendonitis and rupture), particularly in elderly patients (overall incidence rare)

Ethanol/Nutrition/Herb Interactions

Food: Grapefruit juice may double systemic exposure of orally-administered budesonide. Administration of capsules with a high-fat meal delays peak concentration, but does not alter the extent of absorption.

Herb/Nutraceutical: St John's wort may decrease budesonide levels.

Stability

Suspension for nebulization: Store upright at 20°C to 25°C (68°F to 77°F) and protect from light. Do not refrigerate or freeze. Once aluminum package is opened, solution should be used within 2 weeks. Continue to protect from light.

Nasal inhaler: Store with valve up at 15°C to 30°C (59°F to 86°F). Use within 6 months after opening aluminum pouch. Protect from high humidity.

Nasal spray: Store with valve up at 20°C to 25°C (68°F to 77°F) and protect from light. Do not freeze.

Oral inhaler (Pulmicort Flexhaler®): Store at 20°C to 25°C (68°F to 77°F).

Mechanism of Action Controls the rate of protein synthesis; depresses the migration of polymorphonuclear leukocytes, fibroblasts; reverses capillary permeability and lysosomal stabilization at the cellular level to prevent or control inflammation

Pharmacodynamics

Onset of action: Respules®: 2-8 days; Rhinocort® Aqua®: ~10 hours; Inhalation: 24 hours

Peak effect: Respules®: 4-6 weeks; Rhinocort® Aqua®: ~2 weeks; Inhalation: 1-2 weeks

Pharmacokinetics

Distribution: 2.2-3.9 L/kg

Protein binding: 85% to 90%

Metabolism: Hepatic

Bioavailability: Limited by high first-pass effect; Capsule: 9% to 21%; Respules®: 6%; Inhalation: 6% to 13%; Nasal: 34%

Half-life: 2-3.6 hours

Time to peak: Capsule: 0.5-10 hours (variable in Crohn's disease); Respules®: 10-30 minutes; Inhalation: 1-2 hours; Nasal: 1 hour

Elimination: Urine (60%) and feces as metabolites

Dosage

Geriatrics & Adults:

Nasal inhalation: (Rhinocort® Aqua®): 64 mcg/day as a single 32 mcg spray in each nostril. Some patients who do not achieve adequate control may benefit from increased dosage. A reduced dosage may be effective after initial control is achieved.

Maximum dose: Adults: 256 mcg/day

Oral inhalation:

Pulmicort® Turbuhaler®:

Previous therapy of bronchodilators alone: 200-400 mcg twice initially which may be increased up to 400 mcg twice daily

Previous therapy of inhaled corticosteroids: 200-400 mcg twice initially which may be increased up to 800 mcg twice daily

Previous therapy of oral corticosteroids: 400-800 mcg twice daily which may be increased up to 800 mcg twice daily

Pulmicort® Flexhaler®: Initial: 360 mcg twice daily (selected patients may be initiated at 180 mcg twice daily); maximum 720 mcg twice daily

NIH Guidelines (NIH, 1997) (give in divided doses twice daily):

"Low" dose: 200-400 mcg/day (1-2 inhalations/day)

"Medium" dose: 400-600 mcg/day (2-3 inhalations/day)

"High" dose: >600 mcg/day (>3 inhalation/day)

Oral: Crohn's disease (active): 9 mg once daily in the morning for up to 8 weeks; recurring episodes may be treated with a repeat 8-week course of treatment

Note: Patients receiving CYP3A4 inhibitors should be monitored closely for signs and symptoms of hypercorticism; dosage reduction may be required. If switching from oral prednisolone, prednisolone dosage should be tapered while budesonide (Entocort™ EC) treatment is initiated.

Maintenance of remission: Following treatment of active disease (control of symptoms with CDAI <150), treatment may be continued at a dosage of 6 mg once daily for up to 3 months. If symptom control is maintained for 3 months, tapering of the dosage to complete cessation is recommended. Continued dosing beyond 3 months has not been demonstrated to result in substantial benefit.

Hepatic Impairment: Monitor closely for signs and symptoms of hypercorticism; dosage reduction may be required.

Administration

Inhalation: Inhaler should be shaken well immediately prior to use; while activating inhaler, deep breathe for 3-5 seconds, hold breath for ~10 seconds and allow ≥1 minute between inhalations. Rinse mouth with water after use to reduce aftertaste and incidence of candidiasis.

Oral capsule: Capsule should be swallowed whole; do not crush or chew.

Monitoring Parameters Relief of symptoms

Patient Information

Oral inhalation/nebulization: Follow directions accompanying product; if you are also using an inhaled bronchodilator, wait 10 minutes before using this steroid aerosol; rinse mouth with water after treatment to decrease the risk of oral candidiasis

Nasal: For intranasal use only

Inhaler should be shaken well immediately prior to use; clear nasal passage by blowing nose prior to use; keep inhaler clean and unobstructed; wash in warm water and dry thoroughly; contact physician if symptoms are not improved by 3 weeks of treatment, if condition worsens, or if nasal irritation or burning persists

Special Geriatric Considerations Ensure that patients can correctly use nasal inhaler.

Dosage Forms Excipient information presented when available (limited, particularly for generics); consult specific product labeling. [CAN] = Canadian brand name

Capsule, enteric coated:

Entocort® EC: 3 mg

Powder for oral inhalation:

Pulmicort Flexhaler®: 90 mcg/inhalation (165 mg) [delivers ~80 mcg/inhalation; 60 actuations]

Pulmicort Flexhaler®: 180 mcg/inhalation (225 mg) [delivers ~160 mcg/inhalation; 120 actuations]

Pulmicort Turbuhaler®: 200 mcg/inhalation (104 g) [delivers ~160 mcg/inhalation; 200 metered actuations]

Pulmicort Turbuhaler® [CAN]: 100 mcg/inhalation [delivers 200 metered actuations]; 200 mcg/inhalation [delivers 200 metered actuations]; 400 mcg/inhalation [delivers 200 metered actuations] [not available in the U.S.]

Suspension, intranasal [spray]:

Rhinocort® Aqua®: 32 mcg/inhalation (8.6 g) [120 metered actuations]

Suspension for nebulization:

Pulmicort Respules®: 0.25 mg/2 mL (30s), 0.5 mg/2 mL (30s)

♦ **Buffasal [OTC]** *see* Aspirin *on page 127*
♦ **Bufferin® [OTC]** *see* Aspirin *on page 127*
♦ **Bufferin® Extra Strength [OTC]** *see* Aspirin *on page 127*
♦ **Buffinol [OTC]** *see* Aspirin *on page 127*

Bumetanide (byoo MET a nide)

Medication Safety Issues
Sound-alike/look-alike issues:
Bumetanide may be confused with Buminate®
Bumex® may be confused with Brevibloc®, Buprenex®, Permax®

U.S. Brand Names Bumex®

Canadian Brand Names Bumex®; Burinex®

Generic Available Yes

Pharmacologic Category Diuretic, Loop

Use Management of edema associated with congestive heart failure, hepatic, or renal disease (including nephrotic syndrome); used alone or in combination with antihypertensives in the treatment of hypertension

Contraindications Hypersensitivity to bumetanide, any component of the formulation, or sulfonylureas; anuria; patients with hepatic coma or in states of severe electrolyte depletion until the condition improves or is corrected

Warnings/Precautions [U.S. Boxed Warning]: Excessive amounts can lead to profound diuresis with fluid and electrolyte loss; close medical supervision and dose evaluation are required. In cirrhosis, avoid electrolyte and acid/base imbalances that might lead to hepatic encephalopathy. *In vitro* studies using pooled sera from critically-ill neonates have shown bumetanide to be a potent displacer of bilirubin. Coadministration of antihypertensives may increase the risk of hypotension.

Monitor fluid status and renal function in an attempt to prevent oliguria, azotemia, and reversible increases in BUN and creatinine; close medical supervision of aggressive diuresis required. Rapid I.V. administration, renal impairment, excessive doses, and concurrent use of other ototoxins is associated with ototoxicity. Asymptomatic hyperuricemia has been reported with use.

Chemical similarities are present among sulfonamides, sulfonylureas, carbonic anhydrase inhibitors, thiazides, and loop diuretics (except ethacrynic acid). Use in patients with sulfonylurea allergy is specifically contraindicated in product labeling, however, a risk of cross-reaction exists in patients with allergy to any of these compounds; avoid use when previous reaction has been severe. Discontinue if signs of hypersensitivity are noted.

Adverse Reactions (Reflective of adult population; not specific for elderly)
>10%:
Endocrine & metabolic: Hyperuricemia (18%), hypochloremia (15%), hypokalemia (15%)
Renal: Azotemia (11%)
1% to 10%:
Central nervous system: Dizziness (1%)
Endocrine & metabolic: Hyponatremia (9%); hyperglycemia (7%); variations in phosphorus (5%), CO_2 content (4%), bicarbonate (3%), and calcium (2%)
Neuromuscular & skeletal: Muscle cramps (1%)
Otic: Ototoxicity (1%)
Renal: Serum creatinine increased (7%)

Overdosage/Toxicology Symptoms include electrolyte depletion, and volume depletion. Treatment is primarily symptomatic and supportive.

Drug Interactions
ACE inhibitors: Hypotensive effects and/or renal effects are potentiated by hypovolemia.
Antidiabetic agents: Glucose tolerance may be decreased.
Antihypertensive agents: Hypotensive effects may be enhanced.
Cholestyramine or colestipol may reduce bioavailability of bumetanide.
Digoxin: Bumetanide-induced hypokalemia may predispose to digoxin toxicity; monitor potassium.
Indomethacin (and other NSAIDs) may reduce natriuretic and hypotensive effects of diuretics.
Lithium: Renal clearance may be reduced. Isolated reports of lithium toxicity have occurred; monitor lithium levels.
NSAIDs: Risk of renal impairment may increase when used in conjunction with diuretics.
Ototoxic drugs (aminoglycosides, cis-platinum): Concomitant use of bumetanide may increase risk of ototoxicity, especially in patients with renal dysfunction.
Peripheral adrenergic-blocking drugs or ganglionic blockers: Effects may be increased.
Salicylates (high dose) with diuretics may predispose patients to salicylate toxicity due to reduced renal excretion or alter renal function.
Thiazides: Synergistic diuretic effects occur.

Ethanol/Nutrition/Herb Interactions Herb/Nutraceutical: Avoid ephedra, yohimbe, ginseng (may worsen hypertension). Avoid dong quai if using for hypertension (has estrogenic activity). Avoid garlic (may have increased antihypertensive effect).

Stability
I.V.: Store vials at 15°C to 30°C (59°F to 86°F). Infusion solutions should be used within 24 hours after preparation. Light sensitive; discoloration may occur when exposed to light.
Tablet: Store at 15°C to 30°C (59°F to 86°F).

Mechanism of Action Inhibits reabsorption of sodium and chloride in the ascending loop of Henle and proximal renal tubule, interfering with the chloride-binding cotransport system, thus causing increased excretion of water, sodium, chloride, magnesium, phosphate, and calcium; it does not appear to act on the distal tubule

Pharmacodynamics
Onset of action:
Oral, I.M.: 30-60 minutes
I.V.: Within a few minutes
Duration: 6 hours

Pharmacokinetics
Distribution: V_d: 13-25 L/kg
Protein binding: 95%
Metabolism: Partial in the liver
Half-life: 1-1.5 hours
Elimination: Majority of unchanged drug and metabolites excreted in urine

Dosage
Geriatrics: Initial: Oral: 0.5 mg once daily, increase as necessary.
Adults:
Edema:
Oral: 0.5-2 mg/dose (maximum dose: 10 mg/day) 1-2 times/day
I.M., I.V.: 0.5-1 mg/dose; may repeat in 2-3 hours for up to 2 doses if needed (maximum dose: 10 mg/day)
Continuous I.V. infusion: Initial: 1 mg load then 0.5-2 mg/hour (ACC/AHA 2005 practice guidelines for chronic heart failure)
Hypertension: Oral: 0.5 mg daily (maximum dose: 5 mg/day)
Usual dosage range (JNC 7): 0.5-2 mg/day in 2 divided doses

Monitoring Parameters Blood pressure (standing and sitting/supine), serum electrolytes, renal function; in high doses, monitor auditory function, I & O, weight

Patient Information May be taken with food or milk; get up slowly from a lying or sitting position to minimize dizziness, lightheadedness or fainting; also use extra care when exercising, standing for long periods of time and during hot weather; take in the morning; may cause increased sensitivity to sunlight

Additional Information Can be used in furosemide-allergic patients; 1 mg = 40 mg furosemide. Administer I.V. slowly, over 1-2 minutes.

Special Geriatric Considerations Loop diuretics are potent diuretics; excess amounts can lead to profound diuresis with fluid and electrolyte loss; close medical supervision and dose evaluation is required, particularly in the elderly. Severe loss of sodium and/or increases in BUN can cause confusion; for any change in mental status in patients on bumetanide, monitor electrolytes and renal function.

Dosage Forms Excipient information presented when available (limited, particularly for generics); consult specific product labeling.
Injection, solution: 0.25 mg/mL (2 mL, 4 mL, 10 mL) [contains benzyl alcohol]
Tablet (Bumex®): 0.5 mg, 1 mg, 2 mg

♦ **Bumex**® *see* Bumetanide *on page 194*
♦ **Buprenex**® *see* Buprenorphine *on page 195*

Buprenorphine (byoo pre NOR feen)

Related Information
Narcotic / Opioid Analgesics *on page 1763*
Medication Safety Issues
Sound-alike/look-alike issues:
Buprenex® may be confused with Brevibloc®, Bumex®
U.S. Brand Names Buprenex®; Subutex®
Canadian Brand Names Buprenex®; Subutex®
Index Terms Buprenorphine Hydrochloride
Generic Available Yes: Injection
Pharmacologic Category Analgesic, Opioid
Use Management of moderate to severe pain
Unlabeled/Investigational Use Injection: Management of heroin and opioid withdrawal
Restrictions Injection: C-V/C-III; Tablet: C-III
Prescribing of tablets for opioid dependence is limited to physicians who have met the qualification criteria and have received a DEA number specific to prescribing this
(Continued)

Buprenorphine *(Continued)*

product. Tablets will be available through pharmacies and wholesalers which normally provide controlled substances.

Contraindications Hypersensitivity to buprenorphine or any component of the formulation

Warnings/Precautions An opioid-containing analgesic regimen should be tailored to each patient's needs and based upon the type of pain being treated (acute versus chronic), the route of administration, degree of tolerance for opioids (naive versus chronic user), age, weight, and medical condition. The optimal analgesic dose varies widely among patients. Doses should be titrated to pain relief/prevention.

May cause CNS depression, which may impair physical or mental abilities. Effects with other sedative drugs or ethanol may be potentiated. Elderly may be more sensitive to CNS depressant and constipating effects. May cause respiratory depression - use caution in patients with respiratory disease or pre-existing respiratory depression. Potential for drug dependency exists, abrupt cessation may precipitate withdrawal. Use caution in elderly, debilitated, depression or suicidal tendencies. Tolerance, psychological and physical dependence may occur with prolonged use. Partial antagonist activity may precipitate acute narcotic withdrawal in opioid-dependent individuals.

Use with caution in patients with hepatic, pulmonary, or renal function impairment. Also use caution in patients with head injury or increased ICP, biliary tract dysfunction, patients with history of hyperthyroidism, morbid obesity, adrenal insufficiency, prostatic hyperplasia, urinary stricture, CNS depression, toxic psychosis, pancreatitis, alcoholism, delirium tremens, or kyphoscoliosis. May cause hypotension; use with caution in patients with hypovolemia, cardiovascular disease (including acute MI), or drugs which may exaggerate hypotensive effects (including phenothiazines or general anesthetics). May obscure diagnosis or clinical course of patients with acute abdominal conditions.

Tablets, which are used for induction treatment of opioid dependence, should not be started until effects of withdrawal are evident.

Adverse Reactions (Reflective of adult population; not specific for elderly)
Injection:
>10%: Central nervous system: Sedation
1% to 10%:
    Cardiovascular: Hypotension
    Central nervous system: Respiratory depression, dizziness, headache
    Gastrointestinal: Vomiting, nausea
    Ocular: Miosis
    Otic: Vertigo
    Miscellaneous: Diaphoresis
Tablet:
>10%:
    Central nervous system: Headache (30%), pain (24%), insomnia (21% to 25%), Oralety (12%), depression (11%)
    Gastrointestinal: Nausea (10% to 14%), abdominal pain (12%), constipation (8% to 11%)
    Neuromuscular & skeletal: Back pain (14%), weakness (14%)
    Respiratory: Rhinitis (11%)
    Miscellaneous: Withdrawal syndrome (19%; placebo 37%), infection (12% to 20%), diaphoresis (12% to 13%)
1% to 10%:
    Central nervous system: Chills (6%), nervousness (6%), somnolence (5%), dizziness (4%), fever (3%)
    Gastrointestinal: Vomiting (5% to 8%), diarrhea (5%), dyspepsia (3%)
    Ocular: Lacrimation (5%)
    Respiratory: Cough (4%), pharyngitis (4%)
    Miscellaneous: Flu-like syndrome (6%)

Overdosage/Toxicology Symptoms of overdose include CNS depression, pinpoint pupils, hypotension, and bradycardia. Treatment is supportive. Naloxone may have limited effects in reversing respiratory depression; doxapram has also been used to stimulate respirations.

Drug Interactions Substrate of CYP3A4 (major); **Inhibits** CYP1A2 (weak), 2A6 (weak), 2C19 (weak), 2D6 (weak)

Cimetidine: May increase sedation from opioid analgesics; however, histamine blockers may attenuate the cardiovascular response from histamine release associated with opioid analgesics.

CNS depressants: May produce additive respiratory and CNS depression; includes benzodiazepines, barbiturates, ethanol, and other sedatives. Respiratory and CV collapse was reported in a patient who received diazepam and buprenorphine.

CYP3A4 inducers: CYP3A4 inducers may decrease the levels/effects of buprenorphine. Example inducers include aminoglutethimide, carbamazepine, nafcillin, nevirapine, phenobarbital, phenytoin, and rifamycins.

CYP3A4 inhibitors: May increase the levels/effects of buprenorphine. Example inhibitors include azole antifungals, clarithromycin, diclofenac, doxycycline, erythromycin, imatinib, isoniazid, nefazodone, nicardipine, propofol, protease inhibitors, quinidine, and verapamil.

Naltrexone: May antagonize the effect of opioid analgesics; concurrent use or use within 7-10 days of injection for pain relief is contraindicated.

Ethanol/Nutrition/Herb Interactions

Ethanol: Avoid ethanol (may increase CNS depression).

Herb/Nutraceutical: Avoid valerian, St John's wort, kava kava, gotu kola (may increase CNS depression).

Stability

Injection: Protect from excessive heat >40°C (>104°F) and light.

Tablet: Store at room temperature of 25°C (77°F).

Mechanism of Action Buprenorphine exerts its analgesic effect via high affinity binding to μ opiate receptors in the CNS; displays both agonist and antagonist activity

Pharmacodynamics Onset of analgesia: Within 10-30 minutes

Pharmacokinetics

Absorption: I.M.: 30% to 40%

Distribution: V_d: 97-187 L/kg

Protein binding: Highly protein bound

Metabolism: Mainly in the liver; undergoes extensive first-pass metabolism

Half-life: 2.2-3 hours

Elimination: 70% in feces via bile and 20% in urine as unchanged drug

Dosage

Geriatrics: Moderate to severe pain: I.M., slow I.V.: 0.15 mg every 6 hours; elderly patients are more likely to suffer from confusion and drowsiness compared to younger patients. **Long-term use is not recommended.**

Adults: Long-term use is not recommended

Note: These are guidelines and do not represent the maximum doses that may be required in all patients. Doses should be titrated to pain relief/prevention. In high-risk patients (eg, elderly, debilitated, presence of respiratory disease) and/or concurrent CNS depressant use, reduce dose by one-half. Buprenorphine has an analgesic ceiling.

Acute pain (moderate to severe):

I.M.: Initial: Opiate-naive: 0.3 mg every 6-8 hours as needed; initial dose (up to 0.3 mg) may be repeated once in 30-60 minutes after the initial dose if needed; usual dosage range: 0.15-0.6 mg every 4-8 hours as needed

Slow I.V.: Initial: Opiate-naive: 0.3 mg every 6-8 hours as needed; initial dose (up to 0.3 mg) may be repeated once in 30-60 minutes after the initial dose if needed

Heroin or opiate withdrawal (unlabeled use): I.M., slow I.V.: Variable; 0.1-0.4 mg every 6 hours

Opioid dependence: Sublingual:

Induction: Range: 12-16 mg/day (doses during an induction study used 8 mg on day 1, followed by 16 mg on day 2; induction continued over 3-4 days). Treatment should begin at least 4 hours after last use of heroin or short-acting opioid, preferably when first signs of withdrawal appear. Titrating dose to clinical effectiveness should be done as rapidly as possible to prevent undue withdrawal symptoms and patient drop-out during the induction period.

Maintenance: Target dose: 16 mg/day; range: 4-24 mg/day; patients should be switched to the buprenorphine/naloxone combination product for maintenance and unsupervised therapy

Monitoring Parameters Pain relief, respiratory and mental status, blood pressure

Patient Information May cause drowsiness and/or dizziness

Additional Information

0.3 mg = 10 mg morphine or 75 mg meperidine, has longer duration of action than either; may precipitate abstinence syndrome in narcotic-dependent patients; therefore, use buprenorphine before starting a patient on a narcotic. Long-term use is not recommended.

Prescribing of tablets for opioid dependence is limited to physicians who have met the qualification criteria and have received a DEA number specific to prescribing this product. Tablets will be available through pharmacies and wholesalers which normally provide controlled substances.

Special Geriatric Considerations One postmarketing study found that elderly patients were more likely to suffer from confusion and drowsiness after buprenorphine as compared to younger patients.

Dosage Forms Excipient information presented when available (limited, particularly for generics); consult specific product labeling.

Injection, solution: 0.3 mg/mL (1 mL) [C-III]

(Continued)

Buprenorphine *(Continued)*

Buprenex®: 0.3 mg/mL (1 mL) [C-V]
Tablet, sublingual:
Subutex®: 2 mg, 8 mg

Selected References

AGS Panel on Persistent Pain in Older Persons, "The Management of Persistent Pain in Older Persons," *J Am Geriatr Soc*, 2002, 50(6 Suppl):S205-24.

Harcus AH, Ward AE, and Smith DW, "Buprenorphine: Experience in an Elderly Population of 975 Patients During a Year's Monitored Release," *Br J Clin Pract*, 1980, 34(5):144-6.

♦ **Buprenorphine Hydrochloride** *see* Buprenorphine *on page 195*

♦ **Buproban™** *see* BuPROPion *on page 198*

BuPROPion *(byoo PROE pee on)*

Related Information
Antidepressant Agents *on page 1742*

Medication Safety Issues
Sound-alike/look-alike issues:
BuPROPion may be confused with busPIRone
Wellbutrin SR® may be confused with Wellbutrin XL™
Wellbutrin XL™ may be confused with Wellbutrin SR®
Zyban® may be confused with Zagam®

U.S. Brand Names Budeprion™ SR; Buproban™; Wellbutrin®; Wellbutrin SR®; Wellbutrin XL™; Zyban®

Canadian Brand Names Novo-Bupropion SR; Wellbutrin®; Wellbutrin XL™; Zyban®

Generic Available Yes: Excludes Wellbutrin XL™

Pharmacologic Category Antidepressant, Dopamine-Reuptake Inhibitor; Smoking Cessation Aid

Use Treatment of major depressive disorder, including seasonal affective disorder (SAD); adjunct in smoking cessation

Unlabeled/Investigational Use Attention-deficit/hyperactivity disorder (ADHD); depression associated with bipolar disorder

Restrictions An FDA-approved medication guide concerning the use of antidepressants in children, adolescents, and young adults must be distributed when dispensing an outpatient prescription (new or refill) where this medication is to be used without direct supervision of a healthcare provider. Medication guides are available at http://www.fda.gov/cder/Offices/ODS/medication_guides.htm. Dispense to parents or guardians of children and adolescents receiving this medication.

Contraindications Hypersensitivity to bupropion or any component of the formulation; seizure disorder; anorexia/bulimia; use of MAO inhibitors within 14 days; patients undergoing abrupt discontinuation of ethanol or sedatives (including benzodiazepines); patients receiving other dosage forms of bupropion

Warnings/Precautions [U.S. Boxed Warning]: Antidepressants increase the risk of suicidal thinking and behavior in children, adolescents, and young adults (18-24 years of age) with major depressive disorder (MDD) and other psychiatric disorders; consider risk prior to prescribing. Short-term studies did not show an increased risk in patients >24 years of age and showed a decreased risk in patients ≥65 years. All patients must be closely monitored for clinical worsening, suicidality, or unusual changes in behavior, especially during the initiation of therapy (generally first 1-2 months) or following an increase or decrease in dosage. The patient's family or caregiver should be instructed to closely observe the patient and communicate condition with healthcare provider. A medication guide should be dispensed with each prescription.

The possibility of a suicide attempt is inherent in major depression and may persist until remission occurs. Use caution in high-risk patients. Worsening depression and severe abrupt suicidality that are not part of the presenting symptoms may require discontinuation or modification of drug therapy. The patient's family or caregiver should be alerted to monitor patients for the emergence of suicidality and associated behaviors (such as agitation, irritability, hostility, impulsivity, and hypomania) and notify the healthcare provider.

May worsen psychosis in some patients or precipitate a shift to mania or hypomania in patients with bipolar disorder. Patients presenting with depressive symptoms should be screened for bipolar disorder. Monotherapy in patients with bipolar disorder should be avoided. **Bupropion is not FDA approved for bipolar depression.**

The risk of seizures is dose-dependent and increased in patients with a history of seizures, anorexia/bulimia, head trauma, CNS tumor, severe hepatic cirrhosis, abrupt discontinuation of sedative-hypnotics or ethanol, medications which lower seizure threshold (antipsychotics, antidepressants, theophyllines, systemic steroids), stimulants, or hypoglycemic agents. Discontinue and do not restart in patients experiencing a seizure. May cause CNS stimulation (restlessness, anxiety, insomnia) or anorexia. May increase the risks associated with electroconvulsive therapy. Consider discontinuing, when possible, prior to elective surgery. May cause weight loss; use caution in patients where weight loss is not desirable. The incidence of sexual dysfunction with bupropion is generally lower than with SSRIs.

Use caution in patients with cardiovascular disease, history of hypertension, or coronary artery disease; treatment-emergent hypertension (including some severe cases) has been reported, both with bupropion alone and in combination with nicotine transdermal systems. Use with caution in patients with hepatic or renal dysfunction and in elderly patients; reduced dose recommended. Elderly patients may be at greater risk of accumulation during chronic dosing. May cause motor or cognitive impairment in some patients; use with caution if tasks requiring alertness such as operating machinery or driving are undertaken. Arthralgia, myalgia, and fever with rash and other symptoms suggestive of delayed hypersensitivity resembling serum sickness have been reported.

Extended release tablet: Insoluble tablet shell may remain intact and be visible in the stool.

Adverse Reactions (Reflective of adult population; not specific for elderly)
Frequencies, when reported, reflect highest incidence reported with sustained release product.

>10%:
  Cardiovascular: Tachycardia (11%)
  Central nervous system: Headache (25% to 34%), insomnia (11% to 20%), dizziness (6% to 11%)
  Gastrointestinal: Xerostomia (17% to 26%), weight loss (14% to 23%), nausea (1% to 18%)
  Respiratory: Pharyngitis (3% to 13%)
1% to 10%:
  Cardiovascular: Palpitation (2% to 6%), arrhythmias (5%), chest pain (3% to 4%), hypertension (2% to 4%, may be severe), flushing (1% to 4%), hypotension (3%)
  Central nervous system: Agitation (2% to 9%), confusion (8%), anxiety (5% to 7%), hostility (6%), nervousness (3% to 5%), sleep disturbance (4%), sensory disturbance (4%), migraine (1% to 4%), abnormal dreams (3%), irritability (2% to 3%), somnolence (2% to 3%), pain (2% to 3%), memory decreased (up to 3%), fever (1% to 2%), CNS stimulation (1% to 2%), depression
  Dermatologic: Rash (1% to 5%), pruritus (2% to 4%), urticaria (1% to 2%)
  Endocrine & metabolic: Menstrual complaints (2% to 5%), hot flashes (1% to 3%), libido decreased (3%)
  Gastrointestinal: Constipation (5% to 10%), abdominal pain (2% to 9%), diarrhea (5% to 7%), flatulence (6%), anorexia (3% to 5%), appetite increased (4%), taste perversion (2% to 4%), vomiting (2% to 4%), dyspepsia (3%), dysphagia (up to 2%)
  Genitourinary: Urinary frequency (2% to 5%), urinary urgency (up to 2%), vaginal hemorrhage (up to 2%), UTI (up to 1%)
  Neuromuscular & skeletal: Tremor (3% to 6%), myalgia (2% to 6%), weakness (2% to 4%), arthralgia (1% to 4%), arthritis (2%), akathisia (2%), paresthesia (1% to 2%), twitching (1% to 2%), neck pain
  Ocular: Amblyopia (2%), blurred vision (2% to 3%)
  Otic: Tinnitus (3% to 6%), auditory disturbance (5%)
  Respiratory: Upper respiratory infection (9%), cough increased (1% to 4%), sinusitis (1% to 5%)
  Miscellaneous: Infection (8% to 9%), diaphoresis increased (5% to 6%), allergic reaction (including anaphylaxis, pruritus, urticaria)

Overdosage/Toxicology Ingestion of up to 30 g has been reported. Symptoms include labored breathing, salivation, ataxia, convulsions (~33% of all cases), sedation, coma, and respiratory depression, especially with coingestion of ethanol. Bupropion may cause sinus tachycardia and seizures. Treatment should include cardiac and EEG monitoring for the first 48 hours, but is otherwise supportive following initial decontamination with activated charcoal (lavage with massive and recent doses). Treat seizures with I.V. benzodiazepines and supportive therapies. Dialysis may be of limited value after drug absorption because of slow tissue-to-plasma diffusion.

Drug Interactions Substrate of CYP1A2 (minor), 2A6 (minor), 2B6 (major), 2C9 (minor), 2D6 (minor), 2E1 (minor), 3A4 (minor); **Inhibits** CYP2D6 (weak)

Note: Seizure threshold-lowering agents: Use with caution in individuals receiving other agents that may lower seizure threshold (antipsychotics, antidepressants, fluoroquinolones, theophylline, abrupt discontinuation of benzodiazepines, systemic steroids)

Amantadine: Concurrent use appears to result in a higher incidence of adverse effects; use caution.

CNS depressants: Concomitant use may increase adverse effects/toxicity.

(Continued)

BuPROPion *(Continued)*

CYP2B6 inducers: May decrease the levels/effects of bupropion. Example inducers include carbamazepine, nevirapine, phenobarbital, phenytoin, and rifampin.

CYP2B6 inhibitors: May increase the levels/effects of bupropion. Example inhibitors include desipramine, paroxetine, and sertraline.

Levodopa: Toxicity of bupropion is enhanced by levodopa.

MAO inhibitors: Toxicity of bupropion is enhanced by MAO inhibitors (phenelzine); concurrent use is contraindicated.

Metoprolol: Concomitant therapy may result in bradycardia; monitor.

Nicotine: Treatment-emergent hypertension may occur; monitor BP in patients treated with bupropion and nicotine patch.

Selegiline: When used in low doses (<10 mg/day), risk of interaction is theoretically lower than with nonselective MAO inhibitors.

Tricyclic antidepressants: Serum levels may be increased by bupropion; in addition, these agents lower seizure threshold (see Note).

Ethanol/Nutrition/Herb Interactions

Ethanol: Avoid ethanol (may increase CNS depression).

Herb/Nutraceutical: Avoid valerian, St John's wort, SAMe, gotu kola, kava kava (may increase CNS depression).

Stability

Store at controlled room temperature of 20°C to 25°C (68°F to 77°F).

Wellbutrin XL™: Store at 15°C to 30°C (59°F to 86°F).

Mechanism of Action Aminoketone antidepressant structurally different from all other marketed antidepressants; like other antidepressants the mechanism of bupropion's activity is not fully understood. Bupropion is a relatively weak inhibitor of the neuronal uptake of norepinephrine and dopamine, and does not inhibit monoamine oxidase or the reuptake of serotonin. Metabolite inhibits the reuptake of norepinephrine. The primary mechanism of action is thought to be dopaminergic and/or noradrenergic.

Pharmacodynamics May take up to 4 weeks or longer until full effect is seen

Pharmacokinetics

Absorption: Rapid

Distribution: V_d: 19-21 L/kg

Protein binding: 82% to 88%

Metabolism: Extensively hepatic via CYP2B6 to hydroxybupropion; non-CYP-mediated metabolism to erythrohydrobupropion and threohydrobupropion. Metabolite activity ranges from 20% to 50% potency of bupropion.

Bioavailability: 5% to 20% in animals

Half-life:

Distribution: 3-4 hours

Elimination: 21 ± 9 hours; Metabolites: Hydroxybupropion: 20 ± 5 hours; Erythrohydrobupropion: 33 ± 10 hours; Threohydrobupropion: 37 ± 13 hours (metabolite accumulation has been noted in ESRD).

Time to peak, serum: Bupropion: ~3 hours; bupropion extended release: ~5 hours

Metabolites: Hydroxybupropion, erythrohydrobupropion, threohydrobupropion: 6 hours

Elimination: Urine (87%); feces (10%)

Dosage

Geriatrics:

Depression: Oral: Initial: 37.5 mg of immediate release tablets twice daily or 100 mg/day of sustained release tablets; increase by 37.5-100 mg every 3-4 days as tolerated. **Note:** There is evidence that the elderly respond at 150 mg/day in divided doses, but some may require a higher dose.

Smoking cessation: Refer to adult dosing.

Adults:

Depression: Oral:

Immediate release: 100 mg 3 times/day; begin at 100 mg twice daily; may increase to a maximum dose of 450 mg/day.

Sustained release: Initial: 150 mg/day in the morning; may increase to 150 mg twice daily by day 4 if tolerated; target dose: 300 mg/day given as 150 mg twice daily; maximum dose: 400 mg/day given as 200 mg twice daily.

Extended release: Initial: 150 mg/day in the morning; may increase as early as day 4 of dosing to 300 mg/day; maximum dose: 450 mg/day

SAD (Wellbutrin XL™): Oral: Initial: 150 mg/day in the morning; if tolerated, may increase after 1 week to 300 mg/day

Note: Prophylactic treatment should be reserved for those patients with frequent depressive episodes and/or significant impairment. Initiate treatment in the Autumn prior to symptom onset, and discontinue in early Spring with dose tapering to 150 mg/day for 2 weeks

Smoking cessation (Zyban®): Oral: Initiate with 150 mg once daily for 3 days; increase to 150 mg twice daily; treatment should continue for 7-12 weeks.

Dosing conversion between immediate, sustained, and extended release products: Convert using same total daily dose (up to the maximum recommended dose for a given dosage form), but adjust frequency as indicated for sustained (twice daily) or extended (once daily) release products.

Renal Impairment: Per the manufacturer, the elimination of hydroxybupropion and threohydrobupropion are reduced in patients with end stage renal failure. Other research has noted a reduction in bupropion clearance (Turpeinen, 2007). Consider a reduction in frequency and/or dosage in this patient population.

Hepatic Impairment:

Mild-to-moderate hepatic impairment: Use with caution and/or reduced dose/ frequency

Severe hepatic cirrhosis: Use with extreme caution; maximum dose:

Wellbutrin®: 75 mg/day;

Wellbutrin SR®: 100 mg/day or 150 mg every other day

Wellbutrin XL™: 150 mg every other day

Zyban®: 150 mg every other day

Note: The mean AUC increased by ~1.5-fold for hydroxybupropion and ~2.5-fold for erythro/threohydrobupropion; median T_{max} was observed 19 hours later for hydroxybupropion, 31 hours later for erythro/threohydrobupropion; mean half-life for hydroxybupropion increased fivefold, and increased twofold for erythro/threo-ohydrobupropion in patients with severe hepatic cirrhosis compared to healthy volunteers.

Administration May be taken without regard to meals. Zyban® and extended release tablets should be swallowed whole; do not crush, chew, or divide. The insoluble shell of the extended-release tablet may remain intact during GI transit and is eliminated in the feces. Data from the manufacturer states that dividing Wellbutrin® SR tablets resulted in an increased rate of release at 15 minutes: "However, the divided tablet retained its sustained-release characteristics with similar increases of released bupropion at each sampling point beyond 15 minutes when compared to the intact Wellbutrin® SR tablet..." Bupropion is hygroscopic and therefore should be stored in a dry place. Splitting of large quantities in advance of administration is not advised since loss of potency may result. If necessary, splitting should be done cleanly without crushing.

Monitoring Parameters Body weight; mental status for depression, suicidal ideation (especially at the beginning of therapy or when doses are increased or decreased), anxiety, social functioning, mania, panic attacks

Patient Information Take in equally divided doses 3-4 times/day to minimize the risk of seizures; avoid alcohol; may impair driving or other motor or cognitive skills and judgment; do not discontinue without consulting prescriber.

Smoking cessation: Use as directed, do not take extra doses. Do not combine with nicotine patches unless approved by prescriber. May cause dry mouth and insomnia (these may resolve with continued use). Report any difficulty breathing, unusual cough, dizziness, or muscle tremors.

Additional Information Risk of seizures: When using immediate release tablets, seizure risk is increased at total daily dosage >450 mg, individual dosages >150 mg, or by sudden, large increments in dose. Data for the immediate-release formulation of bupropion revealed a seizure incidence of 0.4% in patients treated at doses in the 300-450 mg/day range. The estimated seizure incidence increases almost 10-fold between 450 mg and 600 mg per day. Data for the sustained release dosage form revealed a seizure incidence of 0.1% in patients treated at a dosage range of 100-300 mg/day, and increases to ~0.4% at the maximum recommended dose of 400 mg/day.

Special Geriatric Considerations Limited data available about the use of bupropion in the elderly; two studies have found it equally effective when compared to imipra-mine. Its side effect profile (minimal anticholinergic and blood pressure effects) may make it useful in persons who do not tolerate traditional cyclic antidepressants. A single and multiple dose pharmacokinetic study suggested that accumulation of bupro-pion and its metabolites may occur in the elderly.

Dosage Forms Excipient information presented when available (limited, particularly for generics); consult specific product labeling.

Tablet, as hydrochloride (Wellbutrin®): 75 mg, 100 mg

Tablet, extended release, as hydrochloride:

Budeprion™ SR: 100 mg [contains tartrazine; equivalent to Wellbutrin® SR], 150 mg [equivalent to Wellbutrin® SR]

Buproban™: 150 mg [equivalent to Zyban®]

Wellbutrin XL™: 150 mg, 300 mg

Tablet, sustained release, as hydrochloride: 100 mg, 150 mg [equivalent to Wellbutrin® SR], 150 mg [equivalent to Zyban®]

Wellbutrin® SR: 100 mg, 150 mg, 200 mg

Zyban®: 150 mg

Selected References

Branconnier RJ, Cole JO, Ghazvinian S, et al, "Clinical Pharmacology of Bupropion and Imipramine in Elderly Depressives," *J Clin Psychiatry,* 1983, 44(5 Pt 2):130-3.

Hayes PE and Kristoff CA, "Adverse Reactions to Five New Antidepressants," *Clin Pharm,* 1986, 5(6):471-80.

(Continued)

BuPROPion (Continued)

Kane JM, Cole K, Sarantakos S, et al, "Safety and Efficacy of Bupropion in Elderly Patients: Preliminary Observations," *J Clin Psychiatry*, 1983, 44(5 Pt 2):134-6.

Leverich GS, Altshuler LL, Frye MA, et al, "Risk of Switch in Mood Polarity to Hypomania or Mania in Patients with Bipolar Depression During Acute and Continuation Trials of Venlafaxine, Sertraline, and Bupropion as Adjuncts to Mood Stabilizers," *Am J Psychiatry*, 2006, 163(2):232-9.

McIntyre RS, Mancini DA, McCann S, et al, "Topiramate Versus Bupropion SR When Added to Mood Stabilizer Therapy fpr the Depressive Phase of Bipolar Disorder: A Preliminary Single-Blind Study," *Bipolar Disord*, 2002, 4(3):207-13.

Turpeinen M, Koivuviita N, Tolonen A, et al, "Effect of Renal Impairment on the Pharmacokinetics of Bupropion and Its Metabolites," *Br J Clin Pharmacol*, 2007, 28: [epub].

Wilens TE, Prince JB, Spencer T, et al, "An Open Trial of Bupropion for the Treatment of Adults with Attention-Deficit/Hyperactivity Disorder and Bipolar Disorder," *Biol Psychiatry*, 2003, 54(1):9-16.

♦ **Burnamycin [OTC]** *see* Lidocaine *on page 904*
♦ **Burn Jel [OTC]** *see* Lidocaine *on page 904*
♦ **Burn-O-Jel [OTC]** *see* Lidocaine *on page 904*
♦ **BuSpar®** *see* BusPIRone *on page 202*

BusPIRone (byoo SPYE rone)

Medication Safety Issues
Sound-alike/look-alike issues:
BusPIRone may be confused with buPROPion
U.S. Brand Names BuSpar®
Canadian Brand Names Apo-Buspirone®; BuSpar®; Buspirex; Bustab®; Gen-Buspirone; Lin-Buspirone; Novo-Buspirone; Nu-Buspirone; PMS-Buspirone
Index Terms Buspirone Hydrochloride
Generic Available Yes
Pharmacologic Category Antianxiety Agent, Miscellaneous
Use Management of anxiety
Unlabeled/Investigational Use Management of aggression in mental retardation and secondary mental disorders, major depression; potential augmenting agent for antidepressants
Contraindications Hypersensitivity to buspirone or any component of the formulation
Warnings/Precautions Use in hepatic or renal impairment is not recommended; does not prevent or treat withdrawal from benzodiazepines. Low potential for cognitive or motor impairment. Use with MAO inhibitors may result in hypertensive reactions.
Adverse Reactions (Reflective of adult population; not specific for elderly)
>10%: Central nervous system: Dizziness
1% to 10%:
Central nervous system: Drowsiness, EPS, serotonin syndrome, confusion, nervousness, lightheadedness, excitement, anger, hostility, headache
Dermatologic: Rash
Gastrointestinal: Diarrhea, nausea
Neuromuscular & skeletal: Muscle weakness, numbness, paresthesia, incoordination, tremor
Ocular: Blurred vision, tunnel vision
Miscellaneous: Diaphoresis, allergic reactions
Overdosage/Toxicology Symptoms include dizziness, drowsiness, pinpoint pupils, nausea, and vomiting. There is no known antidote for buspirone. Treatment is supportive.
Drug Interactions Substrate of CYP2D6 (minor), 3A4 (major)
Calcium channel blockers: Diltiazem and verapamil may increase serum concentrations of buspirone; consider a dihydropyridine calcium channel blocker.
CYP3A4 inducers: CYP3A4 inducers may decrease the levels/effects of buspirone. Example inducers include aminoglutethimide, carbamazepine, nafcillin, nevirapine, phenobarbital, phenytoin, and rifamycins.
CYP3A4 inhibitors: May increase the levels/effects of buspirone. Example inhibitors include azole antifungals, clarithromycin, diclofenac, doxycycline, erythromycin, imatinib, isoniazid, nefazodone, nicardipine, propofol, protease inhibitors, quinidine, telithromycin, and verapamil.
MAO inhibitors: Buspirone should not be used concurrently with an MAO inhibitor due to reports of increased blood pressure; includes classic MAO inhibitors and linezolid (due to ability to inhibit MAO).
Nefazodone: Concurrent use may increase risk of CNS adverse events. Limit buspirone initial dose (eg, 2.5 mg/day).
Selegiline: Theoretically, risk of interaction with selective MAO type B inhibitor would be less than with nonselective inhibitors; however, this combination is generally best avoided.
SSRIs: Concurrent use of buspirone with SSRIs may cause serotonin syndrome. Some SSRIs may increase buspirone serum concentrations (see CYP3A4 inhibitors).

Buspirone may increase the efficacy of fluoxetine in some patients; however, the anxiolytic activity of buspirone may be lost when combined with SSRIs (fluoxetine).

Trazodone: Concurrent use of buspirone with trazodone may cause serotonin syndrome.

Ethanol/Nutrition/Herb Interactions

Ethanol: Ethanol (may increase CNS depression).

Food: Food may decrease the absorption of buspirone, but it may also decrease the first-pass metabolism, thereby increasing the bioavailability of buspirone. Grapefruit juice may cause increased buspirone concentrations; avoid concurrent use.

Herb/Nutraceutical: St John's wort may decrease buspirone levels or increase CNS depression. Avoid valerian, gotu kola, kava kava (may increase CNS depression).

Mechanism of Action The mechanism of action of buspirone is unknown. Buspirone has a high affinity for serotonin 5-HT$_{1A}$ and 5-HT$_2$ receptors, without affecting benzodiazepine-GABA receptors. Buspirone has moderate affinity for dopamine D$_2$ receptors.

Pharmacodynamics Onset of action: Decrease in anxiety is seen after 1 week of therapy, but it may take several weeks for the full effects to be seen

Pharmacokinetics Studies in older adults found no significant changes in pharmacokinetic parameters

Protein binding: 95%

Metabolism: In the liver by oxidation and undergoes extensive first-pass metabolism

Half-life: 2-3 hours; range: 2-11 hours

Time to peak serum concentration: Within 40-60 minutes

Dosage

Geriatrics: Oral: Initial: 5 mg twice daily, increase by 5 mg/day every 2-3 days as needed up to 20-30 mg/day; maximum daily dose: 60 mg/day (see Special Geriatric Considerations).

Adults: Anxiety disorders (GAD): Oral: 15 mg/day (7.5 mg twice daily); may increase in increments of 5 mg/day every 2-4 days to a maximum of 60 mg/day. Target dose for most people is 30 mg/day (15 mg twice daily).

Renal Impairment: Use in patients with severe renal impairment cannot be recommended.

Hepatic Impairment: Buspirone is metabolized by the liver and excreted by the kidneys. Patients with impaired hepatic or renal function demonstrated increased plasma levels and a prolonged half-life of buspirone. Therefore, use in patients with severe hepatic or renal impairment cannot be recommended.

Monitoring Parameters Mental status, symptoms of anxiety

Test Interactions Increased AST, ALT, prolactin (S)

Patient Information May cause drowsiness or dizziness; take with food; report any change in senses (ie, smelling, hearing, vision); cautious use with alcohol is recommended; takes 2-3 weeks to see the full effect of this medication

Additional Information Has shown little potential for abuse; not effective when used prn; maximal effect may not be achieved until 3-4 weeks after adequate dose is achieved. Some response may be seen in 1-2 weeks after initiation of therapy. Buspirone, in the treatment of agitation, has been shown to be effective in older adults at an average daily dose of 30-35 mg; slow titration, as described in Dosage, is necessary to avoid side effects and achieve maximum tolerable doses for individual patients.

Special Geriatric Considerations Because buspirone is less sedating than other anxiolytics, it may be a useful agent in geriatric patients when an anxiolytic is indicated.

Dosage Forms Excipient information presented when available (limited, particularly for generics); consult specific product labeling.

Tablet, as hydrochloride: 5 mg, 7.5 mg, 10 mg, 15 mg, 30 mg

BuSpar®: 5 mg, 10 mg, 15 mg, 30 mg

Selected References

Gammans RE, Westrick ML, Shea JP, et al, "Pharmacokinetics of Buspirone in Elderly Subjects," *J Clin Pharmacol*, 1989, 29(1):72-8.

Kunik ME, Yudofsky SC, Silver JM, et al, "Pharmacologic Approach to Management of Agitation Associated With Dementia," *J Clin Psychiatry*, 1994, 55(Suppl 2):13-7.

Weiss KJ, "Management of Anxiety and Depression Syndromes in Elderly," *J Clin Psychiatry*, 1994, 55(Suppl 2):5-12.

♦ **Buspirone Hydrochloride** see BusPIRone on page 202

Busulfan (byoo SUL fan)

Medication Safety Issues

Sound-alike/look-alike issues:

Busulfan may be confused with Butalan®

Myleran® may be confused with Leukeran®, melphalan, Mylicon®

High alert medication: The Institute for Safe Medication Practices (ISMP) includes this medication among its list of drugs which have a heightened risk of causing significant patient harm when used in error.

(Continued)

Busulfan *(Continued)*

U.S. Brand Names Busulfex®; Myleran®
Canadian Brand Names Busulfex®; Myleran®
Index Terms NSC-750
Generic Available No
Pharmacologic Category Antineoplastic Agent, Alkylating Agent
Use Treatment of chronic myelogenous leukemia and marrow-ablative conditioning regimens prior to bone marrow transplantation
Contraindications Hypersensitivity to busulfan or any component of the formulation; failure to respond to previous courses
Warnings/Precautions Hazardous agent - use appropriate precautions for handling and disposal. **[U.S. Boxed Warning]: May induce severe bone marrow suppression.** Seizures have been reported with use; use caution in patients predisposed to seizures; initiate prophylactic anticonvulsant therapy (eg, phenytoin) prior to treatment; use caution with history of seizures or head trauma. May cause delayed pulmonary toxicity (known as "busulfan lung" - bronchopulmonary dysplasia with pulmonary fibrosis); the average onset is 4 years. Busulfan has been causally related to the development of secondary malignancies (tumors and acute leukemias). Busulfan has been associated with ovarian failure. High busulfan area under the concentration versus time curve (AUC) values (>1500 µM/minute) are associated with increased risk of hepatic veno-occlusive disease during conditioning for allogenic BMT. **[U.S. Boxed Warning]: Should be administered under the supervision of an experienced cancer chemotherapy physician.**
Adverse Reactions (Reflective of adult population; not specific for elderly)
Frequency not always defined.
Cardiovascular: Arrhythmia, atrial fibrillation, chest pain, edema, hyper-/hypotension, hypervolemia, tachycardia, tamponade (children with thalassemia: 2%), third-degree heart block, thrombosis, vasodilation, ventricular extrasystoles
Central nervous system: Anxiety, chills, depression, dizziness, fever, headache, insomnia, pain, seizure (2%)
Dermatologic: Alopecia, erythema, hyperpigmentation of skin (busulfan tan 5% to 10%), pruritus, rash, urticaria
Endocrine & metabolic: Amenorrhea, hyperglycemia, hypocalcemia, hypokalemia, hypomagnesemia
Gastrointestinal: Abdominal fullness, abdominal pain, anorexia, constipation, diarrhea, dyspepsia, hematemesis, ileus, mucositis/stomatitis, nausea, pancreatitis, vomiting, weight gain, xerostomia
Hematologic: Anemia (I.V.: 69%), bone marrow suppression, leukopenia, lymphopenia, neutropenia (I.V.: ≤100%; onset: 4 days; recovery: 9-22 days), severe pancytopenia, thrombocytopenia (I.V.: ≤98%; onset 5-6 days)
Hepatic: ALT increased, hyperbilirubinemia, veno-occlusive disease (stem cell transplantation: 8% to 12%)
Local: Injection site pain and inflammation
Neuromuscular & skeletal: Back pain, weakness
Renal: Creatinine increased
Respiratory: Cough, dyspnea, epistaxis, lung disorder, pneumonia, rhinitis
Miscellaneous: Allergic reaction, infection
Overdosage/Toxicology Symptoms include leukopenia and thrombocytopenia. Induction of vomiting or gastric lavage with charcoal is indicated for recent ingestions. The effects of dialysis are unknown. Treatment is symptom-directed and supportive.
Drug Interactions Substrate of CYP3A4 (major)
CYP3A4 inducers: CYP3A4 inducers may decrease the levels/effects of busulfan. Example inducers include aminoglutethimide, carbamazepine, nafcillin, nevirapine, phenobarbital, phenytoin, and rifamycins.
CYP3A4 inhibitors: May increase the levels/effects of busulfan. Example inhibitors include azole antifungals, clarithromycin, diclofenac, doxycycline, erythromycin, imatinib, isoniazid, nefazodone, nicardipine, propofol, protease inhibitors, quinidine, telithromycin, and verapamil.
Itraconazole: May decrease busulfan clearance and increase risk of pulmonary toxicity; monitor.
Metronidazole: May increase busulfan plasma levels.
Other cytotoxic agents: Pulmonary toxicity may be additive.
Ethanol/Nutrition/Herb Interactions
Ethanol: Avoid ethanol due to GI irritation.
Food: No clear or firm data on the effect of food on busulfan bioavailability.
Herb/Nutraceutical: St John's wort may decrease busulfan levels.
Stability
Injection: Store unopened ampuls under refrigeration at 2°C to 8°C (36°F to 46°F). Dilute (using manufacturer provided 5-micron filters) in 0.9% sodium chloride injection or dextrose 5% in water. The dilution volume should be ten times the volume of busulfan injection, ensuring that the final concentration of busulfan is 0.5 mg/mL.

This solution is stable for up to 8 hours at room temperature (25°C); the infusion must also be completed within that 8-hour timeframe. Dilution of busulfan injection in 0.9% sodium chloride is stable for up to 12 hours at refrigeration (2°C to 8°C); the infusion must be completed within that 12-hour timeframe.

Tablet: Store at room temperature at 15°C to 30°C (59°F to 86°F).

Mechanism of Action Reacts with N-7 position of guanosine and interferes with DNA replication and transcription of RNA. Busulfan has a more marked effect on myeloid cells than on lymphoid cells. The drug is also very toxic to hematopoietic stem cells. Busulfan exhibits little immunosuppressive activity. Interferes with the normal function of DNA by alkylation and cross-linking the strands of DNA.

Pharmacokinetics

Absorption: Oral: Rapidly and well absorbed

Protein binding: ~14% to 32%

Metabolism: Extensively hepatic (may increase with multiple doses); glutathione conjugation followed by oxidation

Time to peak:

I.V.: Peak plasma concentration occurs within 5 minutes

Oral: Within 4 hours

Elimination: In urine as metabolites within 24 hours

Dosage

Geriatrics: Oral (refer to individual protocols): Start with lowest recommended doses for adults.

Adults:

CML remission induction: Oral: 4-8 mg/day (may be as high as 12 mg/day); Maintenance doses: 1-4 mg/day to 2 mg/week to maintain WBC 10,000-20,000 cells/mm^3

BMT marrow-ablative conditioning regimen:

Oral: 1 mg/kg/dose (ideal body weight) every 6 hours for 16 doses

I.V.: 0.8 mg/kg (ideal body weight or actual body weight, whichever is lower) every 6 hours for 4 days (a total of 16 doses)

Polycythemia vera (unlabeled use): Oral: 2-6 mg/day

Thrombocytosis (unlabeled use): Oral: 4-6 mg/day

Administration Intravenous busulfan should be administered via a **central** venous catheter as a 2-hour infusion, every 6 hours for 4 consecutive days for a total of 16 doses; do not use polycarbonate syringes.

BMT only: Phenytoin or clonazepam should be administered prophylactically during and for at least 48 hours following completion of busulfan. Risk of seizures is increased in patients with sickle cell disease. Increased risk of VOD when busulfan AUC >3000 µmol(min)/L (mean AUC, 2012 µmol(min)/L). To facilitate ingestion of high doses, insert multiple tablets into clear gel capsules.

Monitoring Parameters CBC with differential and platelet count, hemoglobin, liver function tests (evaluate transaminases, alkaline phosphatase, and bilirubin for at least 28 days post transplant)

Patient Information Watch for signs of bleeding, bruising, coughing, difficulty breathing, fever, joint pain, or flank pain. May cause darkening of skin, dizziness, fatigue, mental confusion, nausea, vomiting, anorexia. Take medication the same time each day. Excellent oral hygiene is needed to minimize oral discomfort.

Additional Information The solvent in I.V. busulfan, DMA, may impair fertility and is associated with teratogenic effects. DMA may also be associated with hepatotoxicity, hallucinations, somnolence, lethargy, and confusion.

Special Geriatric Considerations Toxicity to immunosuppressives is increased in the elderly. Start with lowest recommended adult doses. Signs of infection, such as fever and rise in WBCs, may not occur. Lethargy and confusion may be more prominent signs of infection.

Dosage Forms Excipient information presented when available (limited, particularly for generics); consult specific product labeling.

Injection, solution:

Busulfex®: 6 mg/mL (10 mL)

Tablet:

Myleran®: 2 mg

Selected References

Heard BE and Cooke RA, "Busulphan Lung," *Thorax*, 1968, 23(2):187-93.

Hutchins LF and Lipschitz DA, "Cancer, Clinical Pharmacology, and Aging," *Clin Geriatr Med*, 1987, 3(3):483-503.

Kaplan HG, "Use of Cancer Chemotherapy in the Elderly," *Drug Treatment in the Elderly*, Vestal RE, ed, Boston, MA: ADIS Health Science Press, 1984, 338-49.

Seddon BM, Cassoni AM, Galloway MJ, et al, "Fatal Radiation Myelopathy After High-Dose Busulfan and Melphalan Chemotherapy and Radiotherapy for Ewing's Sarcoma: A Review of the Literature and Implications for Practice," *Clin Oncol (R Coll Radiol)*, 2005, 17(5):385-90.

Tosti A, Piraccini BM, Vincenzi C, et al, "Permanent Alopecia After Busulfan Chemotherapy," *Br J Dermatol*, 2005, 152(5):1056-8.

♦ **Busulfex®** *see* Busulfan *on page 203*

Butorphanol (byoo TOR fa nole)

Related Information
Narcotic / Opioid Analgesics *on page 1763*

Medication Safety Issues
Sound-alike/look-alike issues:
Stadol® may be confused with Haldol®, sotalol

U.S. Brand Names Stadol®

Canadian Brand Names Apo-Butorphanol®; PMS-Butorphanol

Index Terms Butorphanol Tartrate

Generic Available Yes

Pharmacologic Category Analgesic, Opioid

Use
Parenteral: Management of moderate to severe pain; preoperative medication; supplement to balanced anesthesia
Nasal spray: Management of moderate to severe pain, including migraine headache pain

Restrictions C-IV

Contraindications Hypersensitivity to butorphanol or any component of the formulation; avoid use in opiate-dependent patients who have not been detoxified, may precipitate opiate withdrawal

Warnings/Precautions An opioid-containing analgesic regimen should be tailored to each patient's needs and based upon the type of pain being treated (acute versus chronic), the route of administration, degree of tolerance for opioids (naive versus chronic user), age, weight, and medical condition. The optimal analgesic dose varies widely among patients. Doses should be titrated to pain relief/prevention. May cause CNS depression; use with caution in patients with head trauma, morbid obesity, thyroid dysfunction, hepatic/renal dysfunction, adrenal insufficiency, prostatic hyperplasia and/or urinary stricture, may elevate CSF pressure, may increase cardiac workload; tolerance of drug dependence may result from extended use. Use with caution in patients with biliary tract dysfunction; acute pancreatitis may cause constriction of sphincter of Oddi.

Partial antagonist activity may precipitate acute narcotic withdrawal in opioid-dependent individuals. Use with caution in patients with pre-existing respiratory compromise (hypoxia and/or hypercapnia), COPD or other obstructive pulmonary disease; critical respiratory depression may occur, even at therapeutic dosages. May cause hypotension; use with caution in patients with hypovolemia, cardiovascular disease (including acute MI), or drugs which may exaggerate hypotensive effects (including phenothiazines or general anesthetics). May obscure diagnosis or clinical course of patients with acute abdominal conditions.

Concurrent use of sumatriptan nasal spray and butorphanol nasal spray may increase risk of transient high blood pressure. Healthcare provider should be alert to problems of abuse, misuse, and diversion. Use with caution in the elderly and debilitated patients; may be more sensitive to adverse effects.

Adverse Reactions (Reflective of adult population; not specific for elderly)
>10%:
Central nervous system: Drowsiness (43%), dizziness (19%), insomnia (Stadol® NS)
Gastrointestinal: Nausea/vomiting (13%)
Respiratory: Nasal congestion (Stadol® NS)
1% to 10%:
Cardiovascular: Vasodilation, palpitation
Central nervous system: Lightheadedness, headache, lethargy, anxiety, confusion, euphoria, somnolence
Dermatologic: Pruritus
Gastrointestinal: Anorexia, constipation, xerostomia, stomach pain, unpleasant aftertaste
Neuromuscular & skeletal: Tremor, paresthesia, weakness
Ocular: Blurred vision
Otic: Ear pain, tinnitus
Respiratory: Bronchitis, cough, dyspnea, epistaxis, nasal irritation, pharyngitis, rhinitis, sinus congestion, sinusitis, upper respiratory infection
Miscellaneous: Diaphoresis increased

Overdosage/Toxicology Symptoms include respiratory depression, cardiac and CNS depression. Treatment includes airway support, establishment of an I.V. line and administration of naloxone 2 mg I.V., with repeat administration as necessary, up to a total of 10 mg.

Drug Interactions Increased toxicity: CNS depressants, phenothiazines, barbiturates, skeletal muscle relaxants, alfentanil, guanabenz, and MAO inhibitors.

Ethanol/Nutrition/Herb Interactions
Ethanol: Avoid or limit ethanol (may increase CNS depression). Watch for sedation.

Herb/Nutraceutical: Avoid valerian, St John's wort, kava kava, gotu kola (may increase CNS depression).

Stability Store at room temperature. Protect from freezing.

Mechanism of Action Mixed narcotic agonist-antagonist with central analgesic actions; binds to opiate receptors in the CNS, causing inhibition of ascending pain pathways, altering the perception of and response to pain; produces generalized CNS depression

Pharmacodynamics Peak effect:

I.M.: Within 30-60 minutes

I.V.: Within 4-5 minutes

Nasal: 1-2 hours

Pharmacokinetics Plasma concentrations after a single dose were not significantly different between older adults and young subjects.

Absorption: I.M.: Rapidly and well absorbed

Protein binding: 80%

Metabolism: In the liver

Half-life:

Geriatrics: 5.5 hours

Adults: 2.5-4 hours

Elimination: Primarily in urine

Dosage

Geriatrics:

I.M., I.V.: Initial dosage should generally be 1/2 of the recommended dose; repeated dosing must be based on initial response rather than fixed intervals, but generally should be at least 6 hours apart

Nasal spray: Initial dose should not exceed 1 mg; a second dose may be given after 90-120 minutes

Adults: Note: These are guidelines and do not represent the maximum doses that may be required in all patients. Doses should be titrated to pain relief/prevention. Butorphanol has an analgesic ceiling.

Acute pain (moderate to severe):

I.M.: Initial: 2 mg, may repeat every 3-4 hours as needed; usual range: 1-4 mg every 3-4 hours as needed

I.V.: Initial: 1 mg, may repeat every 3-4 hours as needed; usual range: 0.5-2 mg every 3-4 hours as needed

Intranasal (spray) (includes use for migraine headache pain): Initial: 1 spray (~1 mg per spray) in 1 nostril; if adequate pain relief is not achieved within 60-90 minutes, an additional 1 spray in 1 nostril may be given; may repeat initial dose sequence in 3-4 hours after the last dose as needed

Note: In some clinical trials, an initial dose of 2 mg (as 2 doses 1 hour apart or 2 mg initially - 1 spray in each nostril) has been used, followed by 1 mg in 1 hour; side effects were greater at these dosages

Migraine: Nasal spray: Refer to "moderate to severe pain" indication

Preoperative medication: I.M.: 2 mg 60-90 minutes before surgery

Supplement to balanced anesthesia: I.V.: 2 mg shortly before induction and/or an incremental dose of 0.5-1 mg (up to 0.06 mg/kg), depending on previously administered sedative, analgesic, and hypnotic medications

Renal Impairment:

I.M., I.V.: Initial dosage should generally be 1/2 of the recommended dose; repeated dosing must be based on initial response rather than fixed intervals, but generally should be at least 6 hours apart

Nasal spray: Initial dose should not exceed 1 mg; a second dose may be given after 90-120 minutes

Hepatic Impairment:

I.M., I.V.: Initial dosage should generally be 1/2 of the recommended dose; repeated dosing must be based on initial response rather than fixed intervals, but generally should be at least 6 hours apart

Nasal spray: Initial dose should not exceed 1 mg; a second dose may be given after 90-120 minutes

Administration Intranasal: Consider avoiding simultaneous intranasal migraine sprays; may want to separate by at least 30 minutes

Monitoring Parameters Pain relief, respiratory and mental status, blood pressure

Patient Information May cause drowsiness, avoid alcohol; follow instructions for use of nasal spray

Special Geriatric Considerations Adjust dose for renal function in the elderly.

Dosage Forms Excipient information presented when available (limited, particularly for generics); consult specific product labeling.

Injection, solution, as tartrate [preservative free] (Stadol®): 1 mg/mL (1 mL); 2 mg/mL (1 mL, 2 mL)

Injection, solution, as tartrate [with preservative] (Stadol®): 2 mg/mL (10 mL)

Solution, intranasal, as tartrate [spray]: 10 mg/mL (2.5 mL) [14-15 doses]

(Continued)

Butorphanol *(Continued)*

Selected References

AGS Panel on Persistent Pain in Older Persons, "The Management of Persistent Pain in Older Persons," *J Am Geriatr Soc*, 2002, 50(6 Suppl):S205-24.

Ramsey R, Higbee M, Maesner J, et al, "Influence of Age on the Pharmacokinetics of Butorphanol," *Acute Care*, 1986, 12(Suppl 1):8-16.

◆ **Butorphanol Tartrate** *see* Butorphanol *on page 206*

◆ **B-Vex** *see* Brompheniramine *on page 189*

◆ **BW-430C** *see* Lamotrigine *on page 870*

◆ **311C90** *see* Zolmitriptan *on page 1707*

◆ **Cafergot®** *see* Ergotamine and Caffeine *on page 530*

◆ **Caffeine and Ergotamine** *see* Ergotamine and Caffeine *on page 530*

◆ **Calan®** *see* Verapamil *on page 1671*

◆ **Calan® SR** *see* Verapamil *on page 1671*

◆ **Cal Carb-HD®** **[OTC]** *see* Calcium Salts (Oral) *on page 220*

◆ **Calci-Chew™** **[OTC]** *see* Calcium Salts (Oral) *on page 220*

◆ **Calciday-667®** **[OTC]** *see* Calcium Salts (Oral) *on page 220*

◆ **Calciferol™** *see* Ergocalciferol *on page 525*

◆ **Calcijex®** *see* Calcitriol *on page 210*

◆ **Calci-Mix™** **[OTC]** *see* Calcium Salts (Oral) *on page 220*

Calcipotriene *(kal si POE try een)*

U.S. Brand Names Dovonex®

Generic Available No

Pharmacologic Category Topical Skin Product; Vitamin D Analog

Use Treatment of moderate plaque psoriasis

Contraindications Hypersensitivity to calcipotriene or any component of the formulation; patients with demonstrated hypercalcemia or evidence of vitamin D toxicity; use on the face

Warnings/Precautions Use may cause irritations of lesions and surrounding uninvolved skin. If irritation develops, discontinue use. Transient, rapidly reversible elevation of serum calcium has occurred during use. If elevation in serum calcium occurs above the normal range, discontinue treatment until calcium levels are normal. For external use only; not for ophthalmic, oral, or intravaginal use. Avoid or limit excessive exposure to natural or artificial sunlight, or phototherapy.

Adverse Reactions (Reflective of adult population; not specific for elderly)
Frequency may vary with site of application.

>10%: Dermatologic: Burning, itching, rash, skin irritation, stinging, tingling

1% to 10%: Dermatologic: Dermatitis, dry skin, erythema, peeling, worsening of psoriasis

Note: Skin atrophy, hyperpigmentation, folliculitis, and hypercalcemia are potential adverse effects of calcipotriene.

Drug Interactions No data reported

Stability Store at 15° to 25°C (59° to 77°F); do not freeze. Solution should be kept away from open flame; avoid sunlight.

Mechanism of Action Synthetic vitamin D_3 analog which regulates skin cell production and proliferation

Pharmacokinetics

Absorption: ~6% when applied to psoriasis plaque

Metabolism: Within 24 hours most of the drug is converted to inactive metabolites by the liver

Dosage

Geriatrics & Adults: Psoriasis: Topical: Apply in a thin film to the affected skin twice daily and rub in gently and completely.

Monitoring Parameters Healing of lesions, serum calcium concentration

Patient Information Apply only to affected areas; do not exceed the prescribed dose; avoid contact with face or eyes; wash hands after application; report any local adverse effects

Dosage Forms Excipient information presented when available (limited, particularly for generics); consult specific product labeling. [DSC] = Discontinued product

Cream:

Dovonex®: 0.005% (60 g, 120 g)

Ointment:

Dovonex®: 0.005% (60 g, 120 g) [DSC]

Solution, topical:

Dovonex®: 0.005% (60 mL)

Calcitonin (kal si TOE nin)

Related Information
Osteoporosis Management *on page 1779*

Medication Safety Issues
Sound-alike/look-alike issues:
Calcitonin may be confused with calcitriol
Miacalcin® may be confused with Micatin®
Calcitonin nasal spray is administered as a single spray into **one** nostril daily, using alternate nostrils each day.

U.S. Brand Names Fortical®; Miacalcin®

Canadian Brand Names Apo-Calcitonin®; Calcimar®; Caltine®; Miacalcin® NS

Index Terms Calcitonin (Salmon)

Generic Available No

Pharmacologic Category Antidote; Hormone

Use Calcitonin (salmon): Treatment of Paget's disease of bone (osteitis deformans); adjunctive therapy for hypercalcemia; treatment of postmenopausal osteoporosis

Contraindications Hypersensitivity to salmon protein or gelatin diluent

Warnings/Precautions A skin test should be performed prior to initiating therapy of calcitonin salmon in patients with suspected sensitivity; have epinephrine immediately available for a possible hypersensitivity reaction. A detailed skin testing protocol is available from the manufacturers. Temporarily withdraw use of nasal spray if ulceration of nasal mucosa occurs. Patients >65 years of age may experience a higher incidence of nasal adverse events with calcitonin nasal spray.

Adverse Reactions (Reflective of adult population; not specific for elderly)
Unless otherwise noted, frequencies reported are with nasal spray.

>10%: Respiratory: Rhinitis (12%)
1% to 10%:
Cardiovascular: Flushing (nasal spray: <1%; injection: 2% to 5%), angina (1% to 3%), hypertension (1% to 3%)
Central nervous system: Depression (1% to 3%), dizziness (1% to 3%), fatigue (1% to 3%)
Dermatologic: Erythematous rash (1% to 3%)
Gastrointestinal: Abdominal pain (1% to 3%), constipation (1% to 3%), diarrhea (1% to 3%), dyspepsia (1% to 3%), nausea (injection: 10%; nasal spray: 1% to 3%)
Genitourinary: Cystitis (1% to 3%)
Local: Injection site reactions (injection: 10%)
Neuromuscular & skeletal: Back pain (5%), arthrosis (1% to 3%), myalgia (1% to 3%), paresthesia (1% to 3%)
Ocular: Conjunctivitis (1% to 3%), lacrimation abnormality (1% to 3%)
Respiratory: Bronchospasm (1% to 3%), sinusitis (1% to 3%), upper respiratory tract infection (1% to 3%)
Miscellaneous: 1% to 3%: Flu-like syndrome, infection, lymphadenopathy

Overdosage/Toxicology Symptoms of overdose include nausea, vomiting, hypocalcemia, and hypocalcemic tetany. Administer parenteral calcium for hypocalcemia and hypocalcemic tetany. Treatment is otherwise symptom-directed and supportive.

Ethanol/Nutrition/Herb Interactions Ethanol: Avoid ethanol (may increase risk of osteoporosis).

Stability
Injection: Store under refrigeration at 2°C to 8°C (36°F to 46°F); protect from freezing. NS has been recommended for the dilution to prepare a skin test in patients with suspected sensitivity.
Nasal: Store unopened bottle under refrigeration at 2°C to 8°C (36°F to 46°F); do not freeze.
Fortical®: After opening, store for up to 30 days at 20°C to 25°C (68°F to 77°F); excursions permitted to 15°C to 30°C (59°F to 86°F). Store in upright position.
Miacalcin®: After opening, store for up to 35 days at room temperature of 15°C to 30°C (59°F to 86°F). Store in upright position.

Mechanism of Action Peptide sequence similar to human calcitonin; functionally antagonizes the effects of parathyroid hormone. Directly inhibits osteoclastic bone resorption; promotes the renal excretion of calcium, phosphate, sodium, magnesium, and potassium by decreasing tubular reabsorption; increases the jejunal secretion of water, sodium, potassium, and chloride

Pharmacodynamics Hypercalcemia:
Onset of action: ~2 hours
Duration: 6-8 hours

Pharmacokinetics Hypercalcemia:
Metabolism: Rapidly by the kidneys
Half-life: SubQ: 1.2 hours
Elimination: As inactive metabolites in urine
(Continued)

Calcitonin *(Continued)*

Dosage
Geriatrics & Adults:
Paget's disease *(Miacalcin®)*: I.M., SubQ: Initial: 100 units/day; maintenance: 50 units/day or 50-100 units every 1-3 days

Hypercalcemia *(Miacalcin®)*: Initial: I.M., SubQ: 4 units/kg every 12 hours; may increase up to 8 units/kg every 12 hours to a maximum of every 6 hours

Postmenopausal osteoporosis:
Miacalcin®: I.M., SubQ: 100 units/every other day
Fortical®, Miacalcin®: Intranasal: 200 units (1 spray) in one nostril daily

Administration I.M. administration is preferred if the volume to injection exceeds 2 mL. Prior to initiating therapy, a skin test should be performed with 0.1 mL of 10 int. units of calcitonin diluted with NS and injected intradermally. Observe injection site for 15 minutes for wheal or significant erythema and have epinephrine available for a possible hypersensitivity reaction.

Nasal spray: New, unopened bottles must be stored in the refrigerator in an upright position. **Open bottles are stored at room temperature in an upright position for no more than 30 days after date opened.** Once assembled, you must activate the pump by pressing down on the arms of the pump (~6 times) until a faint spray is released. Administer spray intranasally, alternating nostrils daily.

Monitoring Parameters Serum electrolytes and calcium; alkaline phosphatase and 24-hour urine collection for hydroxyproline excretion (Paget's disease), urinalysis (urine sediment); bone mineral density

Nasal formulation: Visualization of nasal mucosa, turbinate, septum, and mucosal blood vessels

Reference Range Therapeutic: <19 pg/mL (SI: 19 ng/L) basal, depending on the assay

Patient Information Keep drug vials in refrigerator. Take at bedtime to minimize nausea and flushing (should only last about one hour). Follow instructions for administration exactly.

Special Geriatric Considerations Studies have shown calcitonin's effects on bone density and fracture rates are beneficial, particularly in women unable to tolerate estrogens. Calcium and vitamin D supplements should also be given. Calcitonin may also be effective in steroid-induced osteoporosis and other states associated with high bone turnover. Nasal spray may provide faster onset of analgesic effects than I.M.

Dosage Forms Excipient information presented when available (limited, particularly for generics); consult specific product labeling.

Injection, solution [calcitonin-salmon]:
Miacalcin®: 200 int. units/mL (2 mL)

Solution, intranasal [spray, calcitonin-salmon]:
Fortical®: 200 int. units/0.09 mL (3.7 mL) [rDNA origin; contains benzyl alcohol; delivers 30 doses, 200 units/actuation]
Miacalcin®: 200 int. units/0.09 mL (3.7 mL) [contains benzalkonium chloride; delivers 30 doses, 200 units/actuation]

Selected References
Lyritis GP, Tsakalakos N, Magiasis B, et al, "Analgesic Effect of Salmon Calcitonin in Osteoporotic Vertebral Fractures: A Double-Blind, Placebo-Controlled Clinical Study," *Calcif Tissue Int*, 1991, 49(6):369-72.

Pontiroli AE, Pajetta E, Scaglia L, et al, "Analgesic Effect of Intranasal and Intramuscular Salmon Calcitonin in Postmenopausal Osteoporosis: A Double-Blind, Double-Placebo Study," *Aging (Milane)*, 1994, 6(6):459-63.

Reginster JY, "Calcitonin for Prevention and Treatment of Osteoporosis," *Am J Med*, 1993, 95(5A):44S-47S.

Reginster JY, Deroisy R, Lecart MP, et al, "A Double-Blind, Placebo-Controlled, Dose-Finding Trial of Intermittent Nasal Salmon Calcitonin for Prevention of Postmenopausal Lumbar Spine Bone Loss," *Am J Med*, 1995, 98(5):452-8.

♦ **Calcitonin (Salmon)** *see* Calcitonin *on page 209*

Calcitriol (kal si TRYE ole)

Medication Safety Issues
Sound-alike/look-alike issues:
Calcitriol may be confused with calcifediol, Calciferol®, calcitonin
Dosage is expressed in mcg (micrograms), **not** mg (milligrams); rare cases of acute overdose have been reported

U.S. Brand Names Calcijex®; Rocaltrol®

Canadian Brand Names Calcijex®; Rocaltrol®

Index Terms 1,25 Dihydroxycholecalciferol

Generic Available Yes

Pharmacologic Category Vitamin D Analog

Use Management of hypocalcemia (in patients on chronic renal dialysis), secondary hyperparathyroidism (in moderate to severe chronic renal failure), hypocalcemia (in hypoparathyroidism and pseudohypoparathyroidism)

Unlabeled/Investigational Use Reduction in severity of psoriatic lesions in psoriatic vulgaris; treatment of vitamin D-resistant rickets

Contraindications Hypercalcemia; vitamin D toxicity; abnormal sensitivity to the effects of vitamin D

Warnings/Precautions Adequate dietary (supplemental) calcium is necessary for clinical response to vitamin D. Excessive vitamin D may cause severe hypercalcemia, hypercalciuria, and hyperphosphatemia; calcium-phosphate product (serum calcium times phosphorus) must not exceed 70 mg^2/dL^2. Other forms of vitamin D should be withheld during therapy. Immobilization may increase risk of hypercalcemia and/or hypercalciuria. Maintain adequate hydration. Use caution in patients with malabsorption syndromes (efficacy may be limited and/or response may be unpredictable). Use of calcitriol for the treatment of secondary hyperparathyroidism associated with CKD is not recommended in patients with rapidly worsening kidney function or in noncompliant patients. Increased serum phosphate levels in patients with renal failure may lead to calcification; the use of an aluminum-containing phosphate binder is recommended along with a low phosphate diet in these patients. Products may contain coconut or palm seed oil.

Adverse Reactions (Reflective of adult population; not specific for elderly)
Frequency not defined.
Cardiovascular: Cardiac arrhythmia, hypertension
Central nervous system: Apathy, headache, hypothermia, psychosis, sensory disturbances, somnolence
Dermatologic: Erythema multiforme, pruritus
Endocrine & metabolic: Dehydration, growth suppression, hypercalcemia, hypercholesterolemia, hypermagnesemia, hyperphosphatemia, libido decreased, polydipsia
Gastrointestinal: Abdominal pain, anorexia, constipation, metallic taste, nausea, pancreatitis, stomach ache, vomiting, weight loss, xerostomia
Genitourinary: Urinary tract infection
Hepatic: ALT/AST increased
Local: Injection site pain (mild)
Neuromuscular & skeletal: Bone pain, myalgia, dystrophy, soft tissue calcification, weakness
Ocular: Conjunctivitis, photophobia
Renal: Albuminuria, BUN increased, creatinine increased, hypercalciurianephrocalcinosis, nocturia, polyuria
Respiratory: Rhinorrhea
Miscellaneous: Allergic reaction

Overdosage/Toxicology Symptoms of overdose include hypercalcemia, hyperphosphatemia, and hypercalciuria. Following withdrawal of the drug, treatment consists of bedrest, liberal intake of fluids, reduced calcium intake, and cathartic administration. Severe hypercalcemia requires I.V. hydration and forced diuresis. Urine output should be monitored and maintained at >3 mL/kg/hour during the acute treatment phase. I.V. saline can quickly and significantly increase excretion of calcium into urine. Calcitonin, cholestyramine, prednisone, sodium EDTA, bisphosphonates, and mithramycin have all been used successfully to treat the more resistant cases of vitamin D-induced. Correction of hyperphosphatemia may be necessary.

Drug Interactions Induces CYP3A4 (weak)
Cholestyramine, colestipol: May decrease absorption/effect of calcitriol.
Corticosteroids: May inhibit calcium absorption, and therefore decrease the therapeutic effect of calcitriol.
Digitalis: Risk of toxicity may be increased due to hypercalcemia from calcitriol; monitor.
Magnesium-containing antacids: Toxicity may be increased by calcitriol; avoid concurrent use in patients on renal dialysis.
Phenobarbital: May decrease endogenous levels of vitamin D; higher doses of calcitriol may be needed.
Phenytoin: May decrease endogenous levels of vitamin D; higher doses of calcitriol may be needed.
Thiazide diuretics: May decrease renal calcium excretion and increase risk of hypercalcemia.

Stability Store at room temperature of 15°C to 30°C (59°F to 86°F). Protect from light.

Mechanism of Action Calcitriol is a potent active metabolite of vitamin D. Vitamin D promotes absorption of calcium in the intestines and retention at the kidneys thereby increasing calcium levels in the serum; decreases excessive serum phosphatase levels, parathyroid hormone levels, and decreases bone resorption; increases renal tubule phosphate resorption

Pharmacodynamics
Onset of action: ~2-6 hours
Duration: 3-5 days
Maximum calcemic effects: 2-4 weeks after daily administration

Pharmacokinetics
Absorption: Oral: Rapid
(Continued)

Calcitriol *(Continued)*

Protein binding: 99.9%

Metabolism: Primarily to 1,24,25-trihydroxycholecalciferol and 1,24,25-trihydroxy ergo-calciferol

Half-life: 1.5 days

Elimination: Principally in bile and feces, and 4% to 6% excreted in urine; stored primarily in liver but also in skin, fat, bone, and muscle

Dosage

Geriatrics: Refer to adult dosing. No dosage recommendations, but start at the lower end of the dosage range.

Adults:

Hypocalcemia in patients on chronic renal dialysis (manufacturer labeling):
Oral: 0.25 mcg/day or every other day (may require 0.5-1 mcg/day); increases should be made at 4- to 8-week intervals

I.V.: Initial: 1-2 mcg 3 times/week (0.02 mcg/kg) approximately every other day. Adjust dose at 2-4 week intervals; dosing range: 0.5-4 mcg 3 times/week

Hypocalcemia in hypoparathyroidism/pseudohypoparathyroidism (manufacturers labeling): Oral (evaluate dosage at 2- to 4-week intervals): Initial: 0.25 mcg/day, range: 0.5-2 mcg once daily

Secondary hyperparathyroidism associated with moderate-to-severe CKD in patients not on dialysis (manufacturer labeling): Oral: 0.25 mcg/day; may increase to 0.5 mcg/day

K/DOQI guidelines for vitamin D therapy in CKD:

CKD stage 3: Oral: 0.25 mcg/day. Treatment should only be started with serum 25(OH) D >30 ng/mL, serum iPTH >70 pg/mL, serum calcium <9.5 mg/dL and serum phosphorus <4.6 mg/dL

CKD stage 4: Oral: 0.25 mcg/day. Treatment should only be started with serum 25(OH) D >30 ng/mL, serum iPTH >110 pg/mL, serum calcium <9.5 mg/dL and serum phosphorus <4.6 mg/dL

CKD stage 5:

Peritoneal dialysis: Oral: Initial: 0.5-1 mcg 2-3 times/week or 0.25 mcg/day

Hemodialysis: **Note:** The following initial doses are based on plasma PTH and serum calcium levels for patients with serum phosphorus <5.5 mg/dL and Ca-P product <55. Adjust dose based on serum phosphate, calcium, and PTH levels. Intermittent I.V. administration may be more effective than daily oral dosing.

Plasma PTH 300-600 pg/mL and serum Ca <9.5 mg/dL: Oral, I.V.: 0.5-1.5 mcg

Plasma PTH 600-1000 pg/mL and serum Ca <9.5 mg/dL:
Oral: 1-4 mcg
I.V : 1-3 mcg

Plasma PTH >1000 pg/mL and serum Ca <10 mg/dL:
Oral: 3-7 mcg
I.V.: 3-5 mcg

Vitamin D-dependent rickets (unlabeled use): Oral: 1 mcg once daily

Monitoring Parameters Monitor renal function, serum calcium and phosphate concentrations. If patient becomes hypercalcemic on therapy, check serum calcium daily until normalized, then twice weekly on new dose. If hypercalcemia persists in predialysis patient, monitor PTH.

Reference Range Calcium (serum) 9-10 mg/dL (4.5-5 mEq/L) but do not include the I.V. dosages; phosphate 2.5-5 mg/dL

Test Interactions Increased calcium, cholesterol, creatinine, magnesium, BUN, AST, ALT; decreased alkaline phosphatase

Patient Information Do not take more than the recommended amount. While taking this medication, your physician may want you to follow a special diet or take a calcium supplement. Follow this diet closely. Avoid taking magnesium supplements or magnesium containing antacids. Early symptoms of hypercalcemia include weakness, fatigue, somnolence, headache, anorexia, dry mouth, metallic taste, nausea, vomiting, cramps, diarrhea, muscle pain, bone pain, and irritability.

Additional Information Calcitriol degrades upon prolonged exposure to light; not used as a daily supplement due to dosage forms, strengths, and cost

Special Geriatric Considerations Recommended daily allowances (RDA) have not been developed for persons >65 years of age; vitamin D, folate, and B_{12} (cyanocobalamin) have decreased absorption with age, but the clinical significance is yet unknown. Calorie requirements decrease with age and therefore, nutrient density must be increased to ensure adequate nutrient intake, including vitamins and minerals. Therefore, the use of a daily supplement with a multiple vitamin with minerals is recommended. Elderly consume less vitamin D, absorption may be decreased, and many elderly have decreased sun exposure; therefore, elderly should receive supplementation with 800 units of vitamin D (20 mcg)/day. This is a recommendation of particular need to those with high risk for osteoporosis.

Dosage Forms Excipient information presented when available (limited, particularly for generics); consult specific product labeling.
    Capsule, softgel: 0.25 mcg, 0.5 mcg
      Rocaltrol®: 0.25 mcg [contains coconut oil]; 0.5 mcg [contains coconut oil]
    Injection, solution: 1 mcg/mL (1 mL)
      Calcijex®: 1 mcg/mL (1 mL) [contains aluminum]
    Solution, oral: 1 mcg/mL (15 mL)
      Rocaltrol®: 1 mcg/mL (15 mL) [contains palm seed oil]

Selected References
Letsou AP and Price LS, "Health Aging and Nutrition: An Overview," *Clin Geriatr Med*, 1987, 3(2):253-60.
Myrianthopoulos M, "Dietary Treatment of Hyperlipidemia in the Elderly," *Clin Geriatr Med*, 1987, 3(2):343-59.
Riggs BL and Melton LJ, "The Prevention and Treatment of Osteoporosis," *N Engl J Med*, 1992, 327(9):620-7.

Calcium Acetate (KAL see um AS e tate)

Medication Safety Issues
    Sound-alike/look-alike issues:
      PhosLo® may be confused with Phos-Flur®, ProSom™

U.S. Brand Names PhosLo®

Canadian Brand Names PhosLo®

Generic Available Yes: Solution for injection

Pharmacologic Category Antidote; Calcium Salt; Phosphate Binder

Use
    Oral: Control of hyperphosphatemia in end-stage renal failure (does not promote aluminum absorption; calcium acetate binds phosphorus in the GI tract better than other calcium salts due to its lower solubility and subsequent reduction in calcium or phosphorus absorption)
    I.V.: Calcium supplementation in parenteral nutrition therapy

Contraindications Hypersensitivity to any component of the formulation; hypercalcemia, renal calculi

Warnings/Precautions Calcium absorption is impaired in achlorhydria (common in elderly - try alternate salt, administer with food); administration is followed by increased gastric acid secretion within 2 hours of administration. While hypercalcemia and hypercalciuria may result when therapeutic replacement amounts are given for prolonged periods, they are most likely to occur in hypoparathyroid patients receiving high doses of vitamin D.

Adverse Reactions (Reflective of adult population; not specific for elderly)
    Mild hypercalcemia (calcium: >10.5 mg/dL to ≤12 mg/dL) may be asymptomatic or manifest itself as constipation, anorexia, nausea, and vomiting
    More severe hypercalcemia (calcium: >12 mg/dL) is associated with confusion, delirium, stupor, and coma

Overdosage/Toxicology Acute single ingestions of calcium salts may produce mild gastrointestinal distress, but hypercalcemia or other toxic manifestations are extremely unlikely. Treatment is supportive.

Drug Interactions
    Calcium channel blockers (eg, verapamil) effects may be diminished; monitor response.
    Digitalis: Calcium acetate may potentiate digoxin toxicity.
    Levothyroxine: Calcium carbonate (and possibly other calcium salts) may decrease T_4 absorption; separate dose from levothyroxine by at least 4 hours
    Polystyrene sulfonate: Potassium-binding ability is reduced; avoid concurrent use.
    Tetracycline, atenolol (and potentially other beta-blockers), iron, quinolone antibiotics, alendronate, sodium fluoride, and zinc absorption is significantly decreased; space administration times.
    Thiazide diuretics: High doses of calcium with thiazide diuretics may result in milk-alkali syndrome and hypercalcemia; monitor response.

Mechanism of Action Combines with dietary phosphate to form insoluble calcium phosphate which is excreted in feces

Pharmacokinetics Calcium is absorbed in soluble, ionized form; solubility of calcium is increased in an acid environment (except calcium lactate); therefore, administer with meals to maximize acidity and solubility to enhance absorption
    Absorption: From the GI tract, requires vitamin D
    Elimination: Mainly in feces as unabsorbed calcium with 20% eliminated by the kidneys

Dosage
    Geriatrics & Adults:
      Dietary Reference Intake:
        Adults, Male/Female:
          19-50 years: 1000 mg/day
          ≥51 years: 1200 mg/day

      Control of hyperphosphatemia (ESRD, on dialysis): Oral: Initial: 1334 mg with each meal, can be increased gradually to bring the serum phosphate value
(Continued)

Calcium Acetate *(Continued)*

<6 mg/dL as long as hypercalcemia does not develop (usual dose: 2001-2868 mg calcium acetate with each meal); do not give additional calcium supplements

Calcium supplementation (parenteral): I.V.: Dose is dependent on the requirements of the individual patient; in central venous total parental nutrition (TPN), calcium is administered at a concentration of 5 mEq (10 mL)/L of TPN solution

Renal Impairment: Refer to adult dosing.

Administration Administer with meals.

Monitoring Parameters Serum calcium, serum phosphate; for control of hypophosphatemia, serum calcium times phosphate should not exceed 66; EKG in hyperkalemic states

Reference Range Serum calcium: 9-10.4 mg/dL; due to a poor correlation between the serum ionized calcium (free) and total serum calcium, particularly in states of low albumin or acid/base imbalances, direct measurement of ionized calcium is recommended. In low albumin states, the corrected **total** serum calcium may be estimated by this equation (assuming a normal albumin of 4 g/dL); corrected total calcium = total serum calcium + 0.8 (4 - measured serum albumin)

Patient Information Follow instructions for dosing. Take with a full glass of water or juice; take with meals; take 1-3 hours after other medications and 1-2 hours before any iron supplements. Avoid other antacids, caffeine, or other calcium supplements unless approved by healthcare provider. Report severe, unresolved nausea, vomiting, constipation, and decreased appetite; and unusual emotional lability (mood swings).

Additional Information Doses for calcium supplementation are given in elemental calcium; calcium salts vary in their amount of elemental calcium

Calcium carbonate (40% elemental calcium)
Calcium gluconate (9% elemental calcium)
Calcium lactate (13% elemental calcium)
Calcium citrate (21% elemental calcium)
Dibasic calcium phosphate (23% elemental calcium)
Calcium acetate (25% elemental calcium)
Tricalcium phosphate (39% elemental calcium)

All calcium preparations should be administered in divided doses to maximize calcium absorption; no more than 300-350 mg of elemental calcium should be given at a time. Women receiving estrogen therapy require 900-1000 mg total daily elemental calcium intake. Women not receiving estrogens require 1500 mg elemental calcium daily to maintain calcium balance.

12.7 mEq/g; 250 mg/g elemental calcium (25% elemental calcium)

Special Geriatric Considerations Constipation and gas can be significant in the elderly, but are usually mild.

Dietary Reference Intake: Adults, ≥51 years: 1200 mg/day

Dosage Forms Excipient information presented when available (limited, particularly for generics); consult specific product labeling. [DSC] = Discontinued product. **Note:** Elemental calcium listed in brackets:

Gelcap:

PhosLo®: 667 mg [169 mg]

Injection, solution: 0.5 mEq/mL (10 mL, 50 mL, 100 mL) [DSC]

♦ **Calcium Acetate and Aluminum Sulfate** *see Aluminum Sulfate and Calcium Acetate on page 68*

♦ **Calcium Acetylhomotaurinate** *see Acamprosate on page 23*

♦ **Calcium and Risedronate** *see Risedronate and Calcium on page 1415*

Calcium and Vitamin D *(KAL see um & VYE ta min dee)*

U.S. Brand Names Cal-CYUM [OTC]; Caltrate® 600+D [OTC]; Caltrate® 600+ Soy™ [OTC]; Caltrate® ColonHealth™ [OTC]; Chew-Cal [OTC]; Liqua-Cal [OTC]; Os-Cal® 500+D [OTC]; Oysco 500+D [OTC]; Oysco D [OTC]; Oyst-Cal-D [OTC]; Oyst-Cal-D 500 [OTC]

Index Terms Vitamin D and Calcium Carbonate

Generic Available Yes

Pharmacologic Category Calcium Salt; Electrolyte Supplement, Oral; Vitamin, Fat Soluble

Use Dietary supplement, antacid

Contraindications Hypersensitivity to any component of the formulation; hypophosphatemia, hypercalcemia, evidence of vitamin D toxicity; history of kidney stones

Warnings/Precautions Calcium carbonate absorption is impaired in achlorhydria Administration is followed by increased gastric acid secretion within 2 hours of administration. While hypercalcemia and hypercalciuria may result when therapeutic replacement amounts are given for prolonged periods, they are most likely to occur in hypoparathyroid patients receiving high doses of vitamin D. Use with caution in renal failure; monitoring of serum calcium may be necessary. Use with caution in patients who may be at risk of cardiac arrhythmias.

Some products may contain soy, tartrazine, or phenylalanine, or may be derived from shellfish.

Adverse Reactions (Reflective of adult population; not specific for elderly)
Frequency not defined; also see individual agents

Central nervous system: Headache

Endocrine & metabolic: Hypercalcemia, hypercalciuria

Gastrointestinal: Gastrointestinal discomfort

Drug Interactions
Calcium channel blockers (eg, verapamil) effects may be diminished; monitor response.

Digoxin: Calcium supplementation may potentiate digoxin toxicity.

Fluoroquinolones: Absorption may be significantly reduced; space administration times.

Levothyroxine: Calcium carbonate (and possibly other calcium salts) may decrease T_4 absorption; separate dose from levothyroxine by at least 4 hours.

Polystyrene sulfonate: Potassium-binding ability is reduced; avoid concurrent use.

Tetracycline, atenolol (and potentially other beta-blockers), iron, fluoroquinolone antibiotics, alendronate, sodium fluoride, and zinc absorption are significantly decreased; space administration times.

Thiazide diuretics can cause hypercalcemia (milk-alkali syndrome); monitor response.

Ethanol/Nutrition/Herb Interactions
Ethanol: Avoid ethanol (may increase risk of osteoporosis).

Food: Food may increase calcium absorption. Calcium may decrease iron absorption. Bran, foods high in oxalates, or whole grain cereals may decrease calcium absorption.

Dosage
Geriatrics & Adults: Calcium supplement, hyperphosphatemia: Oral: Refer to individual monographs for dietary reference intake.

Renal Impairment: Use caution in severe renal impairment.

Administration Administer, preferably with food, 2 hours before or after other medications.

Monitoring Parameters Monitor serum calcium (particularly if used in patients with severe renal impairment)

Patient Information Follow instructions for dosing. Take with a full glass of water or juice 1-2 hours before any iron supplements and 1-3 hours after meals or other medications. Avoid alcohol, other antacids, caffeine, or other calcium supplements, unless approved by prescriber. You may experience constipation (increased exercise, fluids, fiber, or fruit may help) or dry mouth (sucking lozenges or hard candy may help). Report severe, unresolved GI disturbances and unusual emotional liability (mood swings).

Dosage Forms Excipient information presented when available (limited, particularly for generics); consult specific product labeling.

Capsule, softgel: Calcium 500 mg and vitamin D 500 int. units; calcium 600 mg and vitamin D 100 int. units; calcium 600 mg and vitamin D 200 int. units

Liqua-Cal: Calcium 600 mg and vitamin D 200 int. units [contains beeswax, lecithin, and soybean oil]

Tablet: Calcium 250 mg and vitamin D 125 int. units; calcium 500 mg and vitamin D 125 int. units; calcium 500 mg and vitamin D 200 int. units; calcium 600 mg and vitamin D 125 int. units; calcium 600 mg and vitamin D 200 int. units

Caltrate® 600+D: Calcium 600 mg and vitamin D 200 int. units [contains soybean oil]

Caltrate® 600+ Soy™: Calcium 600 mg and vitamin D 200 int. units [contains soy isoflavones 25 mg]

Caltrate® ColonHealth™: Calcium 600 mg and vitamin D 200 int. units [contains soybean oil]

Oysco D: Calcium 250 mg and vitamin D 125 int. units

Oysco 500+D: Calcium 500 mg and vitamin D 200 int. units [contains tartrazine]

Oyst-Cal-D: Calcium 250 mg and vitamin D 125 int. units [sodium free, sugar free; contains tartrazine]

Oyst-Cal-D 500: Calcium 500 mg and vitamin D 200 int. units [sodium free, sugar free; contains tartrazine]

Tablet, chewable: Calcium 500 mg and vitamin D 100 int. units; Calcium 600 mg and vitamin D 400 int. units

Os-Cal® 500+D: Calcium 500 mg and vitamin D 400 int. units [sugar free; contains phenylalanine; light lemon flavor]

Wafer, chewable:

Cal-CYUM: Calcium 519 mg and vitamin D 150 int. units (50s) [dye free; vanilla flavor]

Chew-Cal: Calcium 333 mg and vitamin D 40 int. units (100s, 250s)

♦ **Calcium Carbonate, Magnesium Hydroxide, and Famotidine** *see* Famotidine, Calcium Carbonate, and Magnesium Hydroxide *on page 599*

Calcium Chloride (KAL see um KLOR ide)

Generic Available Yes

Pharmacologic Category Calcium Salt; Electrolyte Supplement, Parenteral

Use Cardiac resuscitation when epinephrine fails to improve myocardial contractions, cardiac disturbances of hyperkalemia, hypocalcemia; emergent treatment of hypocalcemic tetany; treatment of hypermagnesemia

Unlabeled/Investigational Use Calcium channel blocker overdose

Contraindications In ventricular fibrillation during cardiac resuscitation, hypercalcemia, and in patients with risk of digitalis toxicity, renal or cardiac disease; not recommended in treatment of asystole and electromechanical dissociation

Warnings/Precautions For I.V. use only; do not inject SubQ or I.M.; avoid too rapid I.V. administration (<1 mL/minute) and extravasation. Use with caution in patients with respiratory acidosis, renal impairment, or respiratory failure; acidifying effect of calcium chloride may potentiate acidosis. se with caution in patients with severe hyperphosphatemia. Use with caution in patients with chronic renal failure to avoid hypercalcemia; frequent monitoring of serum calcium and phosphorus is necessary. Use with caution in digitalized patients; hypercalcemia may precipitate cardiac arrhythmias. Solutions may contain aluminum; toxic levels may occur following prolonged administration in premature neonates or patients with renal impairment. Avoid metabolic acidosis (ie, administer only 2-3 days then change to another calcium salt).

Overdosage/Toxicology Symptoms include lethargy, nausea, vomiting, and coma. Following withdrawal of the drug, treatment consists of bed rest, liberal fluid intake, reduced calcium intake, and cathartic administration. Severe hypercalcemia requires I.V. hydration and forced diuresis. Urine output should be monitored and maintained at >3 mL/kg/hour. I.V. saline and natriuretic agents (eg, furosemide) can quickly and significantly increase excretion of calcium.

Drug Interactions

Calcium channel blockers (eg, verapamil) effects may be diminished; monitor response.

Levothyroxine: Calcium carbonate (and possibly other calcium salts) may decrease T_4 absorption; separate dose from levothyroxine by at least 4 hours.

Thiazide diuretics can cause hypercalcemia; monitor response.

May potentiate digoxin toxicity. High doses of calcium with thiazide diuretics may result in milk-alkali syndrome and hypercalcemia.

Stability

Do not refrigerate solutions; IVPB solutions/I.V. infusion solutions are stable for 24 hours at room temperature.

Maximum concentration in parenteral nutrition solutions: 15 mEq/L of calcium and 30 mmol/L of phosphate.

Mechanism of Action Moderates nerve and muscle performance via action potential excitation threshold regulation

Pharmacokinetics

Absorption: I.V. calcium salts are absorbed directly into the circulation

Elimination: Mainly in feces as unabsorbed calcium with 20% eliminated by the kidneys

Dosage

Geriatrics & Adults: Note: Calcium chloride has 3 times more elemental calcium than calcium gluconate. Calcium chloride is 27% elemental calcium; calcium gluconate is 9% elemental calcium. One gram of calcium chloride is equal to 270 mg of elemental calcium; one gram of calcium gluconate is equal to 90 mg of elemental calcium. Dosages are expressed in terms of the calcium chloride salt based on a solution concentration of 100 mg/mL (10%) containing 1.4 mEq (27.3 mg)/mL elemental calcium.

Cardiac arrest in the presence of hyperkalemia or hypocalcemia, magnesium toxicity: I.V.: 2-4 mg/kg, repeated every 10 minutes if necessary

Calcium channel blocker overdose (unlabeled use):

I.V.: 1 g every 15-20 minutes (total of 4 doses) **or** 1 g every 2-3 minutes until clinical effect is achieved

I.V. infusion: 0.2-0.4 mL/kg/hour

Hypocalcemia: I.V.: 500 mg to 1 g/dose repeated every 4-6 hours if needed

Hypocalcemic tetany: I.V.: 1 g over 10-30 minutes; may repeat after 6 hours

Hypocalcemia secondary to citrated blood transfusion: I.V.: 200-500 mg per 500 mL of citrated blood (infused into another vein)

Note: Routine administration of calcium, in the absence of signs/symptoms of hypocalcemia, is generally not recommended. A number of recommendations have been published seeking to address potential hypocalcemia during massive transfusion of citrated blood; however, many practitioners recommend replacement only as guided by clinical evidence of hypocalcemia and/or serial monitoring of ionized calcium.

Renal Impairment: Cl_{cr} <25 mL/minute: Dosage adjustments may be necessary depending on the serum calcium levels.

Administration For I.V. administration only; avoid extravasation. Administer slowly (0.7-1.8 mEq per minute or between 0.5 mL and 1.5 mL per minute of calcium chloride 10%); for I.V. infusion, dilute to a maximum concentration of 20 mg/mL and infuse over 1 hour or no greater than 45-90 mg/kg/hour (0.6-1.2 mEq/kg/hour); administration via a central or deep vein is preferred; do not use scalp, small hand or foot veins for I.V. administration since severe necrosis and sloughing may occur. Monitor ECG if calcium is infused faster than 2.5 mEq/minute; **stop the infusion if the patient complains of pain or discomfort.** Warm to body temperature. If used as intraventricular injection, inject into ventricular cavity - not myocardium; **do not infuse calcium chloride in the same I.V. line as phosphate-containing solutions.**

Monitoring Parameters Serum calcium and magnesium, blood pressure, heart rate, EKG, signs of extravasation and muscle weakness

Reference Range

Serum calcium: 8.4-10.2 mg/dL

Due to a poor correlation between the serum ionized calcium (free) and total serum calcium, particularly in states of low albumin or acid/base imbalances, direct measurement of ionized calcium is recommended

In low albumin states, the corrected **total** serum calcium may be estimated by this equation (assuming a normal albumin of 4 g/dL)

Corrected total calcium = total serum calcium + 0.8 (4.0 - measured serum albumin)

or

Corrected calcium = measured serum calcium - measured albumin + 4.0

Serum/plasma chloride: 95-108 mEq/L

Test Interactions Increased calcium (S); decreased magnesium

Additional Information 14 mEq/g/10 mL; 270 mg elemental calcium/g (27% elemental calcium)

Special Geriatric Considerations When using in the elderly, check albumin status and make appropriate decisions concerning reference serum concentrations. Elderly, especially the ill, often have low albumin due to malnutrition.

Dosage Forms Excipient information presented when available (limited, particularly for generics); consult specific product labeling.

Injection, solution: preservative free]: 10% (10 mL) [present as calcium chloride 100 mg (1.36 mEq)/mL; provides elemental calcium 27.2 mg/mL (1.36 mEq)/mL]

Injection, solution: 10% (10 mL) [present as calcium chloride 100 mg (1.36 mEq)/mL; provides elemental calcium 27.2 mg (1.36 mEq)/mL]

Selected References

Bilezikian JP, "Management of Acute Hypercalcemia," *N Engl J Med*, 1992, 326(18):1196-215.

Binder LS, "Acute Arthropod Envenomation: Incidence, Clinical Features, and Management," *Med Toxicol Adverse Drug Exp*, 1989, 4(3):163-73.

Chin RL, Garmel GM, and Harter PM, "Development of Ventricular Fibrillation After Intravenous Calcium Chloride Administration in a Patient With Supraventricular Tachycardia," *Ann Emerg Med*, 1995, 25(3):416-9.

DeRoos F, "Calcium Channel Blockers," Goldfrank LG, et al, ed, *Goldfrank's Toxicologic Emergencies*, 7th ed, New York, (NY):McGraw-Hill Medical Publishing, 2002, 762-74.

Howarth DM, Dawson AH, Smith AJ, et al, "Calcium Channel Blocking Drug Overdose: An Australian Series," *Hum Exp Toxicol*, 1994, 13(3):161-6.

Isbister GK, "Continuous Calcium Chloride Infusion for Massive Nifedipine Overdose," *Emerg Med J*, 2002, 19(4):355-7.

Lam YM, Tse HF, and Lau CP, "Delayed Asystolic Cardiac Arrest After Diltiazem Overdose: Resuscitation With High Dose Intravenous Calcium," *Chest*, 2001, 119(4):1280-2.

Luscher TF, Noll G, and Sturmer T, "Calcium Gluconate in Severe Verapamil Intoxication," *N Engl J Med*, 1994, 330(10):718-20.

McIvor ME, "Acute Fluoride Toxicity. Pathophysiology and Management," *Drug Saf*, 1990, 5(2):79-84.

Mokhlesi B, Leikin JB, Murray P, et al, "Adult Toxicology in Critical Care: Part II: Specific Poisonings," *Chest*, 2003, 123(3):897-922.

Pearigen PD and Benowitz NL, "Poisoning Due to Calcium Antagonists. Experience With Verapamil, Diltiazem, and Nifedipine," *Drug Saf*, 1991, 6(6):408-30.

Salhanick SD and Shannon MW, "Management of Calcium Channel Antagonist Overdose," *Drug Saf*, 2003, 26(2):65-79.

Slattery A, King WD, Nichols M, et al, "Hypercalcemia Following Damp-Rid™ Ingestion," *Clin Toxicol*, 1995, 33(5):487.

Worthley LI and Phillips PJ, "Intravenous Calcium Salts," *Lancet*, 1980, 2(8186):149.

Calcium Gluconate (KAL see um GLOO koe nate)

Medication Safety Issues

Sound-alike/look-alike issues:

Calcium gluconate may be confused with calcium glubionate

Generic Available Yes

Pharmacologic Category Calcium Salt; Electrolyte Supplement, Oral; Electrolyte Supplement, Parenteral

(Continued)

Calcium Gluconate *(Continued)*

Use Treatment and prevention of hypocalcemia; treatment of tetany, cardiac disturbances of hyperkalemia, cardiac resuscitation when epinephrine fails to improve myocardial contractions, hypocalcemia; calcium supplementation

Unlabeled/Investigational Use Hydrofluoric acid (HF) burns; calcium channel blocker overdose

Contraindications Ventricular fibrillation during cardiac resuscitation; digitalis toxicity or suspected digoxin toxicity; hypercalcemia

Warnings/Precautions Injection solution is for I.V. use only; do not inject SubQ or I.M. May produce cardiac arrest. Use caution when administering to patients with renal failure; solutions may contain aluminum; toxic levels may occur following prolonged administration in patients with renal dysfunction. Avoid too rapid I.V. administration; use with caution in digitalized patients, respiratory failure or acidosis; avoid extravasation; hypercalcemia and hypercalciuria may develop at therapeutic doses over long periods of time; hypoparathyroidism may induce hypercalcemia and hypercalciuria, especially when patients receive high doses of vitamin D; administer cautiously to a digitalized patient, may precipitate arrhythmias

Adverse Reactions (Reflective of adult population; not specific for elderly)
Frequency not defined.
I.V.:
    Cardiovascular: Arrhythmia, bradycardia, cardiac arrest, hypotension, vasodilation, and syncope may occur following rapid I.V. injection
    Central nervous system: Sense of oppression
    Gastrointestinal: Chalky taste
    Local: Abscess and necrosis following I.M. administration
    Neuromuscular & skeletal: Tingling sensation
    Miscellaneous: Heat waves
Oral: Gastrointestinal: Constipation

Overdosage/Toxicology Acute single oral ingestions of calcium salts may produce mild gastrointestinal distress, but hypercalcemia or other toxic manifestations are extremely unlikely. Symptoms of hypercalcemia include lethargy, nausea, vomiting, and coma. Treatment is supportive. Severe hypercalcemia following parenteral overdose requires I.V. hydration. Urine output should be monitored and maintained at >3 mL/kg/hour. I.V. saline and natriuretic agents (eg, furosemide) can quickly and significantly increase excretion of calcium into urine.

Drug Interactions

Bisphosphonate derivatives: Absorption may be decreased by calcium salts.

Calcium channel blockers (eg, verapamil) effects may be diminished; monitor response.

Digoxin: May potentiate digoxin toxicity.

Dobutamine: Calcium salts may diminish the therapeutic effect of dobutamine.

Levothyroxine: Calcium carbonate (and possibly other calcium salts) may decrease T_4 absorption; separate dose from levothyroxine by at least 4 hours.

Phosphate supplements: Calcium salts may decrease the absorption of phosphate supplements.

Quinolone antibiotics: Calcium salts may decrease the absorption of quinolone antibiotics with oral administration of both agents.

Thiazide diuretics: Thiazide diuretics may decrease the excretion of calcium salts. Continued concomitant use can also result in metabolic alkalosis.

Stability

Do not refrigerate solutions. IVPB solutions/I.V. infusion solutions are stable for 24 hours at room temperature.

Standard diluent: 1 g/100 mL D_5W or NS; 2 g/100 mL D_5W or NS.

Maximum concentration in parenteral nutrition solutions is variable depending upon concentration and solubility (consult detailed reference).

Mechanism of Action As dietary supplement, used to prevent or treat negative calcium balance; in osteoporosis, it helps to prevent or decrease the rate of bone loss. The calcium in calcium salts moderates nerve and muscle performance and allows normal cardiac function.

Pharmacokinetics

Absorption: Requires vitamin D; calcium is absorbed in soluble, ionized form; solubility of calcium is increased in an acid environment

Distribution: Primarily in bones and teeth

Protein binding: Primarily albumin

Excretion: Primarily feces (as unabsorbed calcium); urine (20%)

Dosage

Geriatrics & Adults:

Adequate Intake (as elemental calcium):

Adults, Male/Female:
    19-50 years: 1000 mg/day
    ≥51 years: 1200 mg/day

Dosage note: Calcium chloride has 3 times more elemental calcium than calcium gluconate. Calcium chloride is 27% elemental calcium; calcium gluconate is 9% elemental calcium. One gram of calcium chloride is equal to 270 mg of elemental calcium; 1 gram of calcium gluconate is equal to 90 mg of elemental calcium. The following dosages are expressed in terms of the calcium gluconate salt based on a solution concentration of 100 mg/mL (10%) containing 0.465 mEq (9.3 mg)/mL elemental calcium:

Hypocalcemia:

I.V.: 2-15 g/24 hours as a continuous infusion or in divided doses

Oral: 500 mg to 2 g 2-4 times/day

Hypocalcemia secondary to citrated blood infusion: I.V.: 500 mg to 1 g per 500 mL of citrated blood (infused into another vein). Single doses up to 2 g have also been recommended.

Note: Routine administration of calcium, in the absence of signs/symptoms of hypocalcemia, is generally not recommended. A number of recommendations have been published seeking to address potential hypocalcemia during massive transfusion of citrated blood; however, many practitioners recommend replacement only as guided by clinical evidence of hypocalcemia and/or serial monitoring of ionized calcium.

Hypocalcemic tetany: I.V.: 1-3 g/dose may be administered until therapeutic response occurs

Magnesium intoxication or cardiac arrest in the presence of hyperkalemia or hypocalcemia: I.V.: 500-800 mg/dose (maximum: 3 g/dose)

Maintenance electrolyte requirements for TPN: I.V.: Daily requirements: 1.7-3.4 g/1000 kcal/24 hours

Calcium channel blocker overdose (unlabeled use): I.V. infusion: 10% solution: 0.6-1.2 mL/kg/hour or I.V. 0.2-0.5 ml/kg every 15-20 minutes for 4 doses (maximum: 2-3 g/dose). In life-threatening situations, 1 g has been given every 1-10 minutes until clinical effect is achieved (case reports of resistant hypotension reported use of 12-18 g total).

Renal Impairment: Cl_{cr} <25 mL/minute: Dosage adjustments may be necessary depending on the serum calcium levels.

Administration Not for I.M. or SubQ administration. For I.V. administration only; administer slowly (~1.5 mL calcium gluconate 10% per minute) through a small needle into a large vein in order to avoid too rapid increased in serum calcium and extravasation.

Extravasation treatment example: Hyaluronidase: Add 1 mL NS to 150 unit vial to make 150 units/mL of concentration; mix 0.1 mL of above with 0.9 mL NS in 1 mL syringe to make final concentration = 15 units/mL

Monitoring Parameters EKG, plasma and urine calcium concentrations

Reference Range Mild hypercalcemia: >10.5 mg/dL; severe hypercalcemia: >12 mg/dL; serum calcium: 9-10.4 mg/dL; due to a poor correlation between the serum ionized calcium (free) and total serum calcium, particularly in states of low albumin or acid/base imbalances, direct measurement of ionized calcium is recommended. In low albumin states, the corrected **total** serum calcium may be estimated by this equation (assuming a normal albumin of 4 g/dL); corrected total calcium = total serum calcium + 0.8 (4 - measured serum albumin).

Test Interactions Increased calcium (S); decreased magnesium

Additional Information A topical 2.5% to 5% calcium gel for the treatment of hydrofluoric acid (HF) burns can be prepared by adding calcium gluconate to a surgical lubricant (water soluble such as K-Y® Jelly). Calcium chloride should not be used for this purpose. Use of injectable calcium gluconate (I.V., SubQ) has also been reported in the literature for the treatment of HF burns not amenable to topical treatment.

All calcium preparations should be administered in divided doses to maximize calcium absorption; no more than 300-350 mg of elemental calcium should be given at a time. Women receiving estrogen therapy require 900-1000 mg total daily elemental calcium intake. Women not receiving estrogens require 1500 mg elemental calcium daily to maintain calcium balance. **Note:** 1 g calcium gluconate = 90 mg elemental calcium = 4.8 mEq calcium. Doses for calcium supplementation are given in elemental calcium; calcium salts vary in their amount of elemental calcium.

Calcium carbonate (40% elemental calcium)
Calcium gluconate (9% elemental calcium)
Calcium lactate (13% elemental calcium)
Calcium citrate (21% elemental calcium)
Dibasic calcium phosphate (23% elemental calcium)
Calcium acetate (25% elemental calcium)
Tricalcium phosphate (39% elemental calcium)

Special Geriatric Considerations Constipation and gas can be significant in elderly, but are usually mild.

Dosage Forms Excipient information presented when available (limited, particularly for generics); consult specific product labeling.

(Continued)

Calcium Gluconate *(Continued)*

Injection, solution [preservative free]: 10% [100 mg/mL] (10 mL, 50 mL, 100 mL, 200 mL) [equivalent to elemental calcium 9 mg/mL; calcium 0.46 mEq/mL]

Powder: 347 mg/tablespoonful (480 g)

Tablet: 500 mg [equivalent to elemental calcium 45 mg]; 650 mg [equivalent to elemental calcium 58.5 mg]; 975 mg [equivalent to elemental calcium 87.75 mg]

Selected References

DeRoos F, "Calcium Channel Blockers," Goldfrank LG, et al, ed, *Goldfrank's Toxicologic Emergencies*, 7th ed, New York, (NY):McGraw-Hill Medical Publishing, 2002, 762-74.

Howarth DM, Dawson AH, Smith AJ, et al, "Calcium Channel Blocking Drug Overdose: An Australian Series," *Hum Exp Toxicol*, 1994, 13(3):161-6.

Isbister GK, "Continuous Calcium Chloride Infusion for Massive Nifedipine Overdose," *Emerg Med J*, 2002, 19(4):355-7.

Lam YM, Tse HF, and Lau CP, "Delayed Asystolic Cardiac Arrest After Diltiazem Overdose: Resuscitation With High Dose Intravenous Calcium," *Chest*, 2001, 119(4):1280-2.

Luscher TF, Noll G, and Sturmer T, "Calcium Gluconate in Severe Verapamil Intoxication," *N Engl J Med*, 1994, 330(10):718-20.

Millard TP, Harris AJ, and MacDonald DM, "Calcinosis Cutis Following Intravenous Infusion of Calcium Gluconate," *Br J Dermatol*, 1999, Jan;140(1):184-6.

Mokhlesi B, Leikin JB, Murray P, et al, "Adult Toxicology in Critical Care: Part II: Specific Poisonings," Chest, 2003, 123(3):897-922.

Salhanick SD and Shannon MW, "Management of Calcium Channel Antagonist Overdose," Drug Saf, 2003, 26(2):65-79.

Trujillo M, Guerrero J, Fragachan C, et al, "Pharmacologic Antidotes in Critical Care Medicine: A Practical Guide for Drug Administration, *Crit Care Med*, 1998, 26(2):377-91.

Calcium Salts (Oral) (KAL see um salts OR al)

U.S. Brand Names Alka-Mints® [OTC]; Amitone® [OTC]; Cal Carb-HD® [OTC]; Calci-Chew™ [OTC]; Calciday-667® [OTC]; Calci-Mix™ [OTC]; Cal-Plus® [OTC]; Caltrate® 600 [OTC]; Chooz® [OTC]; Citracal® [OTC]; Dicarbosil® [OTC]; Equilet® [OTC]; Florical® [OTC]; Gencalc® 600 [OTC]; Mallamint® [OTC]; Mylanta® Soothing Antacids [OTC]; Neo-Calglucon® [OTC]; Nephro-Calci® [OTC]; Os-Cal® 500 [OTC]; Oyst-Cal 500 [OTC]; Oystercal® 500; Posture® [OTC]; Rolaids® Calcium Rich [OTC]; Titralac® Plus Liquid [OTC]; Tums® [OTC]; Tums® E-X Extra Strength Tablet [OTC]; Tums® Extra Strength Liquid [OTC]; Tums® Ultra [OTC]

Generic Available Yes

Use Antacid and calcium supplement

Contraindications Hypercalcemia, renal calculi, hypophosphatemia, ventricular fibrillation. In ventricular fibrillation during cardiac resuscitation, and in patients with risk of digitalis toxicity, renal or cardiac disease

Warnings/Precautions Use caution when administering to patients with renal failure; hypercalcemia and hypercalciuria may develop at therapeutic doses over long periods of time; hypoparathyroidism may induce hypercalcemia and hypercalciuria, especially when patients receive high doses of vitamin D; administer cautiously to a digitalized patient, may precipitate arrhythmias

Drug Interactions

Calcium may antagonize the effects of verapamil; renders tetracycline antibiotics inactive (orally)

Thiazide diuretics may induce hypercalcemia

Decreased atenolol absorption

Iron salts, quinolones have decreased absorption

Stability Admixture incompatibilities: carbonates, phosphates, sulfates, tartrates

Mechanism of Action Moderates nerve and muscle performance via action potential excitation threshold regulation; may prevent negative calcium balance when used as dietary supplement as treatment or for osteoporosis; calcium carbonate is used as an antacid for acute dyspepsia

Pharmacokinetics Calcium is absorbed in soluble, ionized form; solubility of calcium is increased in an acid environment (except calcium lactate); therefore, administer with meals to maximize acidity and solubility to enhance absorption

Monitoring Parameters Plasma and urine calcium concentrations; EKG if hypercalcemic

Reference Range Mild hypercalcemia: >10.5 mg/dL; severe hypercalcemia: >12 mg/dL; serum calcium: 9-10.4 mg/dL; due to a poor correlation between the serum ionized calcium (free) and total serum calcium, particularly in states of low albumin or acid/base imbalances, direct measurement of ionized calcium is recommended. In low albumin states, the corrected **total** serum calcium may be estimated by this equation (assuming a normal albumin of 4 g/dL); corrected total calcium = total serum calcium + 0.8 (4 - measured serum albumin).

Test Interactions Increased calcium (S); decreased magnesium; decreased phosphorus

Patient Information Do not take calcium supplements within 1-2 hours of taking other medicine by mouth or eating large amounts of fiber-rich foods; do not drink large amounts of alcohol or caffeine-containing beverages or use tobacco; take with meals

Additional Information Doses for calcium supplementation are given in elemental calcium; calcium salts vary in their amount of elemental calcium

Calcium glubionate (6.5% elemental calcium)
Calcium carbonate (40% elemental calcium)
Calcium gluconate (9% elemental calcium)
Calcium lactate (13% elemental calcium)
Calcium citrate (21% elemental calcium)
Dibasic calcium phosphate (23% elemental calcium)
Calcium acetate (25% elemental calcium)
Tricalcium phosphate (39% elemental calcium)

All calcium preparations should be administered in divided doses to maximize calcium absorption; no more than 300-350 mg of elemental calcium should be given at a time. Women receiving estrogen therapy require 900-1000 mg total daily elemental calcium intake. Women not receiving estrogens require 1500 mg elemental calcium daily to maintain calcium balance.

Special Geriatric Considerations Constipation and gas can be significant in the elderly but are usually mild and may be eliminated by switching to another salt form. Calcium carbonate has been associated with the highest incidence of side effects, probably due to its high calcium content. Calcium carbonate absorption is impaired in achlorhydria. Since achlorhydria is common in the elderly, calcium carbonate may not be the ideal calcium supplement for dietary or treatment use. Administration with food helps this problem.

Dosage Forms Elemental calcium listed in brackets:
Calcium carbonate:
Capsule: 1500 mg [600 mg]
  Calci-Mix™: 1250 mg [500 mg]
  Florical®: 364 mg [145.6 mg] with sodium fluoride 8.3 mg
Liquid (Tums® Extra Strength): 1000 mg/5 mL (360 mL)
Lozenge (Mylanta® Soothing Antacids): 600 mg [240 mg]
Powder (Cal Carb-HD®): 6.5 g/packet [2.6 g]
Suspension, oral: 1250 mg/5 mL [500 mg]
Tablet: 650 mg [260 mg], 1500 mg [600 mg]
  Calciday-667®: 667 mg [267 mg]
  Os-Cal® 500, Oyst-Cal 500, Oystercal® 500: 1250 mg [500 mg]
  Cal-Plus®, Caltrate® 600, Gencalc® 600, Nephro-Calci®: 1500 mg [600 mg]
  Chewable:
    Alka-Mints®: 850 mg [340 mg]
    Amitone®: 350 mg [140 mg]
    Calci-Chew™, Os-Cal®: 750 mg [300 mg]
    Chooz®, Dicarbosil®, Equilet®, Tums®: 500 mg [200 mg]
    Mallamint®: 420 mg [168 mg]
    Rolaids® Calcium Rich: 550 mg [220 mg]
    Tums® E-X Extra Strength: 750 mg [300 mg]
    Tums® Ultra®: 1000 mg [400 mg]
    Florical®: 364 mg [145.6 mg] with sodium fluoride 8.3 mg

Calcium carbonate and simethicone (Titralac® Plus Liquid):
Liquid: Calcium carbonate 500 mg [200 mg] and simethicone 20 mg per 5 mL

Calcium citrate (Citracal®):
Tablet: 950 mg [200 mg]
Tablet, effervescent: 2376 mg [500 mg]

Calcium glubionate (Neo-Calglucon®):
Syrup: 1.8 g/5 mL [115 mg/5 mL] (480 mL)

Calcium gluconate:
Tablet: 500 mg [45 mg], 650 mg [58.5 mg], 975 mg [87.75 mg], 1 g [90 mg]

Calcium lactate:
Tablet: 325 mg [42.25 mg], 650 mg [84.5 mg]

Calcium phosphate, tribasic (Posture®):
Tablet, sugar free: 1565.2 mg [600 mg]

Selected References
Bauwens SF, Drinka PJ, and Boh LE, "Pathogenesis and Management of Primary Osteoporosis," *Clin Pharm,* 1986, 5(8):639-59.
Heaney RP, Recker RR, and Saville PD, "Menopausal Changes in Calcium Balance Performance," *J Lab Clin Med,* 1978, 92(6):953-63.
Recker RR, "Calcium Absorption and Achlorhydria," *N Engl J Med,* 1985, 313(2):70-3.
Sagraves R, "Prevention and Treatment of Osteoporosis in Women," *U.S. Pharmacist,* 1994, 19(9 Suppl):3-16.

♦ **Cal-CYUM [OTC]** *see* Calcium and Vitamin D *on page 214*

+ **Caldecort®** [OTC] *see* Hydrocortisone *on page 762*
+ **Cal-Plus®** [OTC] *see* Calcium Salts (Oral) *on page 220*
+ **Caltrate® 600** [OTC] *see* Calcium Salts (Oral) *on page 220*
+ **Caltrate® 600+D** [OTC] *see* Calcium and Vitamin D *on page 214*
+ **Caltrate® 600+ Soy™** [OTC] *see* Calcium and Vitamin D *on page 214*
+ **Caltrate® ColonHealth™** [OTC] *see* Calcium and Vitamin D *on page 214*
+ **Campral®** *see* Acamprosate *on page 23*
+ **Canasa™** *see* Mesalamine *on page 989*
+ **Cancidas®** *see* Caspofungin *on page 247*

Candesartan (kan de SAR tan)

Related Information
Angiotensin Agents *on page 1737*
U.S. Brand Names Atacand®
Canadian Brand Names Atacand®
Index Terms Candesartan Cilexetil
Generic Available No
Pharmacologic Category Angiotensin II Receptor Blocker
Use Alone or in combination with other antihypertensive agents in treating essential hypertension; treatment of heart failure (NYHA class II-IV)
Contraindications Hypersensitivity to candesartan or any component of the formulation; hypersensitivity to other A-II receptor antagonists; primary hyperaldosteronism; bilateral renal artery stenosis
Warnings/Precautions May cause hyperkalemia; avoid potassium supplementation unless specifically required by healthcare provider. Avoid use or use a smaller dose in patients who are volume depleted; correct depletion first. May be associated with deterioration of renal function and/or increases in serum creatinine, particularly in patients dependent on renin-angiotensin-aldosterone system. Use with caution in unilateral renal artery stenosis, hepatic dysfunction, pre-existing renal insufficiency, or significant aortic/mitral stenosis. Use caution when initiating in heart failure; may need to adjust dose, and/or concurrent diuretic therapy, because of candesartan-induced hypotension. Hypotension may occur during major surgery and anesthesia; use cautiously before, during, and immediately after such interventions. Although some properties may be shared between these agents, concurrent therapy with ACE inhibitor may be rational in selected patients.
Adverse Reactions (Reflective of adult population; not specific for elderly)
Cardiovascular: Angina, hypotension (CHF 19%), MI, palpitation, tachycardia
Central nervous system: Dizziness, lightheadedness, drowsiness, headache, vertigo, anxiety, depression, somnolence, fever
Dermatologic: Angioedema, rash
Endocrine & metabolic: Hyperglycemia, hyperkalemia (CHF <1% to 6%), hypertriglyceridemia, hyperuricemia
Gastrointestinal: Dyspepsia, gastroenteritis
Genitourinary: Hematuria
Neuromuscular & skeletal: Back pain, CPK increased, myalgia, paresthesia, weakness
Renal: Serum creatinine increased (up to 13% in patients with CHF with drug discontinuation required in 6%)
Respiratory: Dyspnea, epistaxis, pharyngitis, rhinitis, upper respiratory tract infection
Miscellaneous: Diaphoresis increased
Overdosage/Toxicology Symptoms include hypotension and tachycardia. Treatment is supportive.
Drug Interactions Substrate of CYP2C9 (minor); **Inhibits** CYP2C8 (weak), 2C9 (weak)
Lithium: Risk of toxicity may be increased by candesartan; monitor lithium levels.
NSAIDs: May decrease angiotensin II antagonist efficacy; effect has been seen with losartan, but may occur with other medications in this class; monitor blood pressure.
Potassium-sparing diuretics (amiloride, spironolactone, triamterene): May increase risk of hyperkalemia.
Potassium supplements: May increase the risk of hyperkalemia.
Trimethoprim (high dose): May increase the risk of hyperkalemia.
Ethanol/Nutrition/Herb Interactions
Food: Food reduces the time to maximal concentration and increases the C_{max}.
Herb/Nutraceutical: Avoid dong quai if using for hypertension (has estrogenic activity). Avoid ephedra, yohimbe, ginseng (may worsen hypertension). Avoid garlic (may have increased antihypertensive effect).
Mechanism of Action Candesartan is an angiotensin receptor antagonist. Angiotensin II acts as a vasoconstrictor. In addition to causing direct vasoconstriction, angiotensin II also stimulates the release of aldosterone. Once aldosterone is released, sodium as well as water are reabsorbed. The end result is an elevation in blood pressure.

Candesartan binds to the AT1 angiotensin II receptor. This binding prevents angiotensin II from binding to the receptor thereby blocking the vasoconstriction and the aldosterone secreting effects of angiotensin II.

Pharmacodynamics
Onset of action: 2-3 hours
Peak effect: 6-8 hours
Duration: >24 hours

Pharmacokinetics
Distribution: V_d: 0.13 L/kg
Protein binding: 99%
Metabolism: Candesartan cilexetil is metabolized to candesartan by the intestinal wall cells
Bioavailability: 15%
Half-life (dose dependent): 9 hours
Time to peak: 3-4 hours
Elimination: Total body clearance: 0.37 mL/kg/minute; renal clearance: 0.19 mL/kg/minute; 26% renal excretion (oral candesartan); 59% renal excretion after I.V. dose; biliary excretion (36% after I.V. dose) contributes to clearance
High concentrations occur in older adults compared to younger subjects; AUC may be doubled in patients with renal impairment (Cl_{cr} <30 mL/minute)

Dosage
Geriatrics: Refer to adult dosing. No initial dosage adjustment is necessary for elderly patients (although higher concentrations (C_{max}) and AUC were observed in these populations), for patients with mildly impaired renal function, or for patients with mildly impaired hepatic function.

Adults:
Hypertension: Oral: 4-32 mg once daily. Dosage must be individualized. Blood pressure response is dose related over the range of 2-32 mg. The usual recommended starting dose is 16 mg once daily when it is used as monotherapy in patients who are not volume depleted. It can be administered once or twice daily with total daily doses ranging from 8-32 mg; larger doses do not appear to have a greater effect and there is relatively little experience with such doses.

Congestive heart failure: Oral: Initial: 4 mg once daily; double the dose at 2-week intervals, as tolerated; target dose: 32 mg
Note: In selected cases, concurrent therapy with an ACE inhibitor may provide additional benefit.

Hepatic Impairment: No initial dosage adjustment required in mild hepatic impairment. Consider initiation at lower dosages in moderate hepatic impairment (AUC increased by 145%). No data available concerning dosing in severe hepatic impairment.

Administration See Dosage.

Monitoring Parameters Supine blood pressure, electrolytes, serum creatinine, BUN, urinalysis, symptomatic hypotension, and tachycardia; in CHF, serum potassium during dose escalation and periodically thereafter

Patient Information Patients may administer candesartan with other medications and food. Compliance is important for full therapeutic effect. Report episodes of hypotension (dizziness or lightheadedness); report symptoms of angioedema (swelling of the lips or tongue, or difficulty breathing) to physician.

Additional Information A potential advantage of using AIIRAs over ACE inhibitors is that they may cause less cough (71%) and may be a reasonable replacement for ACE inhibitors when cough cannot be tolerated.

Special Geriatric Considerations High concentrations occur in the elderly compared to younger subjects. AUC may be doubled in patients with renal impairment. No initial dose adjustment necessary since repeated dose did not demonstrate accumulation of drug or metabolites in elderly.

Dosage Forms Excipient information presented when available (limited, particularly for generics); consult specific product labeling.
Tablet, as cilexetil:
Atacand®: 4 mg, 8 mg, 16 mg, 32 mg

Selected References
Granger CB, McMurray JJ, Yusuf S, et al, "Effects of Candesartan in Patients With Chronic Heart Failure and Reduced Left-Ventricular Systolic Function Intolerant to Angiotensin-Converting-Enzyme Inhibitors: The CHARM-Alternative Trial," *Lancet*, 2003, 362(9386):772-6.

Candesartan and Hydrochlorothiazide
(kan de SAR tan & hye droe klor oh THYE a zide)

Related Information
Candesartan *on page 222*
Hydrochlorothiazide *on page 756*
(Continued)

Candesartan and Hydrochlorothiazide *(Continued)*

U.S. Brand Names Atacand HCT™
Canadian Brand Names Atacand® Plus
Index Terms Candesartan Cilexetil and Hydrochlorothiazide
Generic Available No
Pharmacologic Category Angiotensin II Receptor Blocker Combination; Antihypertensive Agent, Combination; Diuretic, Thiazide
Use Treatment of hypertension; combination product should not be used for initial therapy
Dosage
  Geriatrics & Adults: Hypertension, replacement therapy: Oral: Combination product can be substituted for individual agents; maximum therapeutic effect would be expected within 4 weeks

  Usual dosage range:
    Candesartan: 16-32 mg/day, given once daily or twice daily in divided doses
    Hydrochlorothiazide: 12.5-25 mg once daily
  Renal Impairment: Serum levels of candesartan are increased and the half-life of hydrochlorothiazide is prolonged in patients with renal impairment. Do not use if Cl_{cr} is <30 mL/minute.
  Hepatic Impairment: Use with caution.
Special Geriatric Considerations No initial dosage adjustment is recommended in patients with normal renal and hepatic function; some patients may have increased sensitivity.
Dosage Forms Excipient information presented when available (limited, particularly for generics); consult specific product labeling.
  Tablet:
    Atacand HCT™:
      16-12.5: Candesartan cilexetil 16 mg and hydrochlorothiazide 12.5 mg
      32-12.5: Candesartan cilexetil 32 mg and hydrochlorothiazide 12.5 mg

Capreomycin *(kap ree oh MYE sin)*

Medication Safety Issues
  Sound-alike/look-alike issues:
    Capastat® may be confused with Cepastat®
U.S. Brand Names Capastat® Sulfate
Index Terms Capreomycin Sulfate
Generic Available No
Pharmacologic Category Antibiotic, Miscellaneous; Antitubercular Agent
Use In conjunction with at least one other antituberculosis agent in the treatment of tuberculosis
Contraindications Hypersensitivity to capreomycin sulfate or any component of the formulation
Warnings/Precautions [U.S. Boxed Warnings]: Use in patients with renal insufficiency or pre-existing auditory impairment must be undertaken with great caution, and the risk of additional eighth nerve impairment or renal injury should be weighed against the benefits to be derived from therapy. Since other parenteral antituberculous agents (eg, streptomycin) also have similar and sometimes irreversible toxic effects, particularly on eighth cranial nerve and renal function, simultaneous administration of these agents with capreomycin is not recommended. Use with nonantituberculous drugs (ie, aminoglycoside antibiotics) having ototoxic or nephrotoxic potential should be undertaken only with great caution. Use caution with renal dysfunction and in the elderly. Prolonged use may result in fungal or bacterial superinfection, including *C. difficile*-associated diarrhea and pseudomembranous colitis.
Adverse Reactions (Reflective of adult population; not specific for elderly)
  >10%:
    Otic: Ototoxicity [subclinical hearing loss (11%), clinical loss (3%)], tinnitus

Renal: Nephrotoxicity (36%, increased BUN)

1% to 10%: Hematologic: Eosinophilia (dose related, mild)

Overdosage/Toxicology Symptoms include renal failure, ototoxicity, and thrombocytopenia. Treatment is supportive.

Drug Interactions

Increased effect/duration of nondepolarizing neuromuscular blocking agents

Additive toxicity (nephrotoxicity and ototoxicity, respiratory paralysis): Aminoglycosides (eg, streptomycin)

Stability Powder for injection should be stored at room temperature of 15°C to 30°C (59°F to 86°F). Dissolve powder in 2 mL of NS or SWFI; allow 2-3 minutes for dissolution. For I.V. administration, further dilute in NS 100 mL. For I.M. administration, dose <1 g may be further diluted to concentrations of 200-350 mg/mL. Following reconstitution, may store under refrigeration for up to 24 hours.

Mechanism of Action Capreomycin is a cyclic polypeptide antimicrobial. It is administered as a mixture of capreomycin IA and capreomycin IB. The mechanism of action of capreomycin is not well understood. Mycobacterial species that have become resistant to other agents are usually still sensitive to the action of capreomycin. However, significant cross-resistance with viomycin, kanamycin, and neomycin occurs.

Pharmacokinetics

Absorption: Oral: Poor absorption necessitates parenteral administration

Half-life: Dependent upon renal function and varies with creatinine clearance; 4-6 hours

Time to peak serum concentration: I.M.: 1 hour

Elimination: Essentially excreted unchanged in the urine; no significant accumulation after ≥30 day of 1 g/day dosing in patients with normal renal function

Dosage

Geriatrics: Refer to adult dosing. Use with caution due to the increased potential for pre-existing renal dysfunction or impaired hearing.

Adults: Tuberculosis: I.M., I.V.: 1 g/day (not to exceed 20 mg/kg/day) for 60-120 days, followed by 1 g 2-3 times/week

Renal Impairment: Adults:

Cl_{cr} >100 mL/minute: Administer 13-15 mg/kg every 24 hours.

Cl_{cr} 80-100 mL/minute: Administer 10-13 mg/kg every 24 hours.

Cl_{cr} 60-80 mL/minute: Administer 7-10 mg/kg every 24 hours.

Cl_{cr} 40-60 mL/minute: Administer 11-14 mg/kg every 48 hours.

Cl_{cr} 20-40 mL/minute: Administer 10-14 mg/kg every 72 hours.

Cl_{cr} <20 mL/minute: Administer 4-7 mg/kg every 72 hours.

Administration Administer by deep I.M. injection into large muscle mass

Monitoring Parameters Check hearing with audiometry and assess vestibular function regularly. Monitor BUN, creatinine, and potassium throughout the course of treatment.

Patient Information Report hearing loss to physician immediately; do not discontinue without notifying physician

Special Geriatric Considerations Has not been studied in the eldery. I.M. administration may limit use due to painful injection or lack of sites in patients with decreased muscle mass. Use with caution in patients with pre-existing hearing impairment due to potential ototoxicity.

Dosage Forms Excipient information presented when available (limited, particularly for generics); consult specific product labeling.

Injection, powder for reconstitution, as sulfate: 1 g

♦ **Capreomycin Sulfate** *see* Capreomycin *on page 224*

♦ **Capsagel® [OTC]** *see* Capsaicin *on page 225*

Capsaicin (kap SAY sin)

Medication Safety Issues

Sound-alike/look-alike issues:

Zostrix® may be confused with Zestril®, Zovirax®

U.S. Brand Names ArthriCare® for Women Extra Moisturizing [OTC] [DSC]; ArthriCare® for Women Multi-Action [OTC] [DSC]; ArthriCare® for Women Silky Dry [OTC] [DSC]; ArthriCare® for Women Ultra Strength [OTC] [DSC]; Capsagel® [OTC]; Capzasin-HP® [OTC]; Capzasin-P® [OTC]; Zostrix® [OTC]; Zostrix®-HP [OTC]

Canadian Brand Names Zostrix®; Zostrix® H.P.

Generic Available Yes: Cream

Pharmacologic Category Analgesic, Topical; Topical Skin Product

Use

Zostrix®: Temporary relief of pain (neuralgia) following herpes zoster infections

Zostrix®-HP: Relief of neuralgias such as diabetic neuropathy and postsurgical pain

Unlabeled/Investigational Use Treatment of pain associated with psoriasis, chronic neuralgias unresponsive to other forms of therapy, intractable pruritus

(Continued)

Capsaicin *(Continued)*

Contraindications Hypersensitivity to capsaicin or any component of the formulation

Warnings/Precautions Should not be applied to broken or irritated skin. Affected area should not be tightly bandaged.

Adverse Reactions (Reflective of adult population; not specific for elderly)
Frequency not defined.
Dermatologic: Itching, stinging sensation, erythema
Local: Transient burning on application which usually diminishes with repeated use
Respiratory: Cough

Drug Interactions Substrate of CYP2E1 (minor)
No drug interaction data reported

Mechanism of Action Induces release of substance P, the principal chemomediator of pain impulses from the periphery to the CNS, from peripheral sensory neurons; after repeated application, capsaicin depletes the neuron of substance P and prevents reaccumulation

Dosage

Geriatrics & Adults: Treatment of pain: Topical: Apply to affected area at least 3-4 times/day; application frequency less than 3-4 times/day prevents the total depletion, inhibition of synthesis, and transport of substance P resulting in decreased clinical efficacy and increased local discomfort

Monitoring Parameters Relief of pain

Patient Information Wash hands immediately after application; for external use only; avoid contact with eyes; do not use on broken or irritated skin; transient burning may occur upon application but should disappear after a few days; if symptoms get worse or persist longer than 28 days, or clear up and recur, discontinue use and consult physician

Additional Information If used less than 3 times/day, this product may not be effective

Special Geriatric Considerations Capsaicin products are available over-the-counter. Counsel patients about the appropriate use of these products. The American College of Rheumatology recommends capsaicin for the symptomatic treatment of osteoarthritis of the knee.

Dosage Forms Excipient information presented when available (limited, particularly for generics); consult specific product labeling. [DSC] = Discontinued product
Cream, topical: 0.025% (60 g); 0.075% (60 g)
ArthriCare® for Women Multi-Action: 0.025% (42 g) [contains menthol] [DSC]
ArthriCare® for Women Silky Dry: 0.025% (42 g) [DSC]
ArthriCare® for Women Ultra Strength: 0.075% (42 g) [contains benzalkonium chloride and menthol] [DSC]
Capzasin-P®: 0.025% (45 g)
Capzasin-HP®: 0.075% (45 g)
Zostrix®: 0.025% (60 g)
Zostrix®-HP: 0.075% (60 g)
Gel, topical:
Capsagel®: 0.025% (60 g); 0.05% (60 g); 0.075% (30 g)
Lotion, topical:
ArthriCare® for Women Extra Moisturizing: 0.025% (120 mL, 240 mL) [DSC]

Selected References
Cordell GA and Araujo OE, "Capsaicin: Identification, Nomenclature, and Pharmacotherapy," *Ann Pharmacother*, 1993, 27(3):330-6.
Hochberg MC, Altman RD, Brandt KD, et al, "Guidelines for the Medical Management of Osteoarthritis. Part II. Osteoarthritis of the Knee. American College of Rheumatology," *Arthritis Rheum*, 1995, 38(11):1541-6.

Captopril *(KAP toe pril)*

Related Information
Angiotensin Agents *on page 1737*

Medication Safety Issues
Sound-alike/look-alike issues:
Captopril may be confused with Capitrol®, carvedilol

International issues:
Acepril® [Great Britain] may be confused with Accupril® which is a brand name for quinapril in the U.S.
Acepril®: Brand name for enalapril in Hungary and Switzerland; brand name for lisinopril in Denmark

U.S. Brand Names Capoten®

Canadian Brand Names Alti-Captopril; Apo-Capto®; Capoten™; Gen-Captopril; Novo-Captopril; Nu-Capto; PMS-Captopril

Index Terms ACE

Generic Available Yes

Pharmacologic Category Angiotensin-Converting Enzyme (ACE) Inhibitor

Use Management of hypertension; treatment of systolic congestive heart failure, left ventricular dysfunction after myocardial infarction, diabetic nephropathy

Unlabeled/Investigational Use Treatment of hypertensive crisis, rheumatoid arthritis; diagnosis of anatomic renal artery stenosis, hypertension secondary to scleroderma renal crisis; diagnosis of aldosteronism, idiopathic edema, Bartter's syndrome, postmyocardial infarction for prevention of ventricular failure; increase circulation in Raynaud's phenomenon, hypertension secondary to Takayasu's disease

Contraindications Hypersensitivity to captopril or any component of the formulation; angioedema related to previous treatment with an ACE inhibitor; primary hyperaldosteronism; idiopathic or hereditary angioedema; bilateral renal artery stenosis

Warnings/Precautions Anaphylactic reactions can occur. Angioedema can occur at any time during treatment (especially following first dose). It may involve head and neck (potentially affecting the airway) or the intestine (presenting with abdominal pain). Prolonged monitoring may be required especially if tongue, glottis, or larynx are involved as they are associated with airway obstruction. Those with a history of airway surgery in this situation have a higher risk. Careful blood pressure monitoring with first dose (hypotension can occur especially in volume-depleted patients). Use with caution in collagen vascular diseases; valvular stenosis (particularly aortic stenosis); hyperkalemia; or before, during, or immediately after anesthesia. Avoid rapid dosage escalation which may lead to renal insufficiency. Hyperkalemia may rarely occur. Rare toxicities associated with ACE inhibitors include cholestatic jaundice (which may progress to hepatic necrosis) and neutropenia/agranulocytosis with myeloid hyperplasia. May be associated with deterioration of renal function and/or increases in serum creatinine, particularly in patients dependent on renin-angiotensin-aldosterone system. Use with caution in unilateral renal artery stenosis and pre-existing renal insufficiency; if patient has renal impairment then a baseline WBC with differential and serum creatinine should be evaluated and monitored closely during the first 3 months of therapy. Hypersensitivity reactions may be seen during hemodialysis with high-flux dialysis membranes (eg, AN69).

Use with caution and decrease dosage in patients with renal impairment (especially renal artery stenosis), severe CHF, or with coadministered diuretic therapy. Severe hypotension may occur in patients who are sodium and/or volume depleted; initiate lower doses and monitor closely when starting therapy in these patients. ACE inhibitors may be preferred agents in elderly patients with CHF and diabetes mellitus (diabetic proteinuria is reduced, minimal CNS effects, and enhanced insulin sensitivity); however, due to decreased renal function, tolerance must be carefully monitored.

Adverse Reactions (Reflective of adult population; not specific for elderly)
1% to 10%:
  Cardiovascular: Hypotension (1% to 3%), tachycardia (1%), chest pain (1%), palpitation (1%)
  Dermatologic: Rash (maculopapular or urticarial) (4% to 7%), pruritus (2%); in patients with rash, a positive ANA and/or eosinophilia has been noted in 7% to 10%.
  Endocrine & metabolic: Hyperkalemia (1% to 11%)
  Hematologic: Neutropenia may occur in up to 4% of patients with renal insufficiency or collagen-vascular disease.
  Renal: Proteinuria (1%), serum creatinine increased, worsening of renal function (may occur in patients with bilateral renal artery stenosis or hypovolemia)
  Respiratory: Cough (<1% to 2%)
  Miscellaneous: Hypersensitivity reactions (rash, pruritus, fever, arthralgia, and eosinophilia) have occurred in 4% to 7% of patients (depending on dose and renal function); dysgeusia - loss of taste or diminished perception (2% to 4%)
Frequency not defined:
  Cardiovascular: Angioedema, cardiac arrest, cerebrovascular insufficiency, rhythm disturbances, orthostatic hypotension, syncope, flushing, pallor, angina, MI, Raynaud's syndrome, CHF
  Central nervous system: Ataxia, confusion, depression, nervousness, somnolence
  Dermatologic: Bullous pemphigus, erythema multiforme, Stevens-Johnson syndrome, exfoliative dermatitis
  Endocrine & metabolic: Alkaline phosphatase increased, bilirubin increased, gynecomastia
  Gastrointestinal: Pancreatitis, glossitis, dyspepsia
  Genitourinary: Urinary frequency, impotence
  Hematologic: Anemia, thrombocytopenia, pancytopenia, agranulocytosis, anemia
  Hepatic: Jaundice, hepatitis, hepatic necrosis (rare), cholestasis, hyponatremia (symptomatic), transaminases increased
  Neuromuscular & skeletal: Asthenia, myalgia, myasthenia
  Ocular: Blurred vision
  Renal: Renal insufficiency, renal failure, nephrotic syndrome, polyuria, oliguria
  Respiratory: Bronchospasm, eosinophilic pneumonitis, rhinitis
  Miscellaneous: Anaphylactoid reactions
(Continued)

Captopril *(Continued)*

Overdosage/Toxicology Mild hypotension has been the only toxic effect seen with acute overdose; bradycardia may also occur. Hyperkalemia occurs even with therapeutic doses, especially in patients with renal insufficiency and those taking NSAIDs. Following initiation of essential overdose management, toxic symptom treatment and supportive treatment should be initiated. Hypotension usually responds to I.V. fluids or Trendelenburg positioning.

Drug Interactions Substrate of CYP2D6 (major)

Allopurinol: Case reports (rare) indicate a possible increased risk of Stevens-Johnson syndrome when combined with captopril.

Alpha$_1$ blockers: Hypotensive effect increased.

Aspirin: The effects of ACE inhibitors may be blunted by aspirin administration, particularly at higher dosages and/or increase adverse renal effects.

CYP2D6 inhibitors: May increase the levels/effects of captopril. Example inhibitors include chlorpromazine, delavirdine, fluoxetine, miconazole, paroxetine, pergolide, quinidine, quinine, ritonavir, and ropinirole.

Diuretics: Hypovolemia due to diuretics may precipitate acute hypotensive events or acute renal failure.

Gold sodium thiomalate: ACE inhibitors may enhance the adverse/toxic effects (nitritoid reaction) of gold sodium thiomalate. The reaction may include facial flushing, nausea, vomiting, hypotension, and syncope. If it is to occur, would be expected shortly after administration of gold compound in patients maintained on an ACEI.

Insulin: Risk of hypoglycemia may be increased.

Lithium: Risk of lithium toxicity may be increased; monitor lithium levels, especially the first 4 weeks of therapy.

Mercaptopurine: Risk of neutropenia may be increased.

NSAIDs: May attenuate hypertensive efficacy; effect has been seen with captopril and may occur with other ACE inhibitors; monitor blood pressure. May increase adverse renal effects.

Potassium-sparing diuretics (amiloride, potassium, spironolactone, triamterene): Increased risk of hyperkalemia.

Potassium supplements may increase the risk of hyperkalemia.

Trimethoprim (high dose) may increase the risk of hyperkalemia.

Ethanol/Nutrition/Herb Interactions

Food: Captopril serum concentrations may be decreased if taken with food. Long-term use of captopril may result in a zinc deficiency which can result in a decrease in taste perception.

Herb/Nutraceutical: Avoid dong quai if using for hypertension (has estrogenic activity). Avoid ephedra, yohimbe, ginseng (may worsen hypertension). Avoid garlic (may have increased antihypertensive effect).

Mechanism of Action Competitive inhibitor of angiotensin-converting enzyme (ACE); prevents conversion of angiotensin I to angiotensin II, a potent vasoconstrictor; results in lower levels of angiotensin II which causes an increase in plasma renin activity and a reduction in aldosterone secretion

Pharmacodynamics

Onset of action: Oral: Maximal decrease in blood pressure in 60-90 minutes after dose

Duration: Dose related; may require several weeks of therapy before full hypotensive effect is seen

Pharmacokinetics

Absorption: Oral: 60% to 75%

Distribution: V$_d$: 7 L/kg

Protein binding: 25% to 30%

Metabolism: 50%

Half-life:

Normal adults: Dependent upon renal and cardiac function: 1.9 hours

Impaired renal function: 3.5-32 hours

Anuria: 20-40 hours

Time to peak serum concentrations: Within 1-2 hours

Elimination: 95% excreted in urine in 24 hours; 40% to 50% excreted unchanged urine

Dosage

Geriatrics & Adults: Note: Titrate dose according to patient's response.

Acute hypertension (urgency/emergency): Oral: 12.5-25 mg, may repeat as needed (may be given sublingually, but no therapeutic advantage demonstrated)

Hypertension: Oral: Initial: 12.5-25 mg 2-3 times/day; may increase by 12.5-25 mg/dose at 1- to 2-week intervals up to 50 mg 3 times/day. Maximum: 150 mg 3 times/day. Add diuretic before further dosage increases.

Usual dose range (JNC 7): 25-100 mg/day in 2 divided doses

Congestive heart failure: Oral:

Initial: 6.25-12.5 mg 3 times/day in conjunction with cardiac glycoside and diuretic therapy. Initial dose depends upon patient's fluid/electrolyte status.

Target: 50 mg 3 times/day

Prevention of LV dysfunction following MI: Oral: Initial: 6.25 mg; followed by 12.5 mg 3 times/day; increase to 25 mg 3 times/day over the next few days; following by gradual increase to a goal of 50 mg 3 times/day (Some dosage schedules increase the dosage more aggressively to achieve goal dosage within the first few days of initiation).

Diabetic nephropathy: Oral:

25 mg 3 times/day. May be taken with other antihypertensive therapy if required to further lower blood pressure.

Renal Impairment:

Cl_{cr} 10-50 mL/minute: Administer 75% of normal dose.

Cl_{cr} <10 mL/minute: Administer 50% of normal dose.

Note: Smaller dosages given every 8-12 hours are indicated in patients with renal dysfunction. Renal function and leukocyte count should be carefully monitored during therapy.

Hemodialysis effects: Moderately dialyzable (20% to 50%); administer dose postdialysis or administer 25% to 35% supplemental dose.

Peritoneal dialysis: Supplemental dose is not necessary.

Administration Unstable in aqueous solutions; to prepare solution for oral administration, mix prior to administration and use within 10 minutes.

Monitoring Parameters Serum potassium concentrations, BUN, serum creatinine, renal function, WBC, CBC with platelets

Test Interactions Increased BUN, creatinine, potassium, positive Coombs' [direct]; decreased cholesterol (S); may cause false-positive results in urine acetone determinations using sodium nitroprusside reagent

Patient Information Administer 1 hour before meals; do not stop therapy except under prescriber advice; notify physician if you develop sore throat, fever, swelling of hands, feet, face, eyes, lips, and tongue; difficult breathing, irregular heartbeats, chest pains, or cough. May cause dizziness, fainting, and lightheadedness, especially in first week of therapy, sit and stand up slowly; may cause changes in taste or rash; do not add a salt substitute (potassium) without advice of physician.

Additional Information Watch for hypotensive effect within 1-3 hours of first dose or new higher dose. Many patients complain of transient cough during early therapy; food decreases absorption of captopril 30% to 40%; administer captopril 1 hour before meals; clinical significance not known; therefore, observe for loss of effect. Newer data demonstrate that lower doses of ACE inhibitors are effective and toxic reactions are decreased.

Special Geriatric Considerations Due to frequent decreases in glomerular filtration (also Cl_{cr}) with aging, elderly patients may have exaggerated responses to ACE inhibitors; differences in clinical response due to hepatic changes are not observed. ACE inhibitors may be preferred agents in elderly patients with congestive heart failure and diabetes mellitus. Diabetic proteinuria is reduced and insulin sensitivity is enhanced. In general, the side effect profile is favorable in the elderly and causes little or no CNS confusion; use lowest dose recommendations initially. Many elderly may be volume depleted due to diuretic use and/or blunted thirst reflex resulting in inadequate fluid intake.

Dosage Forms Excipient information presented when available (limited, particularly for generics); consult specific product labeling.

Tablet: 12.5 mg, 25 mg, 50 mg, 100 mg

Selected References

Anaizi NH and Swenson C, "Instability of Aqueous Captopril Solutions," *Am J Hosp Pharm*, 1993, 50(3):486-8.

Chobanian AV, Bakris GL, Black HR, et al, "The Seventh Report of the Joint National Committee on Prevention, Detection, Evaluation, and Treatment of High Blood Pressure: The JNC 7 Report," *JAMA*, 2003, 289(19):2560-71.

Konstam MA, Drakup K, Baker DW, et al, "Heart Failure: Evaluation and Care of Patients With Left Ventricular Systolic Dysfunction," *Clinical Practice Guideline No 11*, Rockville, MD: Agency for Health Care Policy and Research, Public Health Service, U.S. Department of Health and Human Services, 1994.

Lewis EJ, Hunsicker LG, Bain RP, et al, "The Effect of Angiotensin-Converting Enzyme Inhibition on Diabetic Nephropathy," *N Engl J Med*, 1993, 329(20):1456-62.

McAreavey D and Robertson JI, "Angiotensin Converting Enzyme Inhibitors and Moderate Hypertension," *Drugs*, 1990, 40(3):326-45.

Pereira CM and Tam YK, "Stability of Captopril in Tap Water," *Am J Hosp Pharm*, 1992, 49(3):612-5.

Taketomo CK, Chu SA, Cheng MH, et al, "Stability of Captopril in Powder Papers Under Three Storage Conditions," *Am J Hosp Pharm*, 1990, 47(8):1799-801.

Williams JF, Bristow MR, Fowler MB, et al, "Guidelines for the Evaluation and Management of Heart Failure: Report of the American College of Cardiology/American Heart Association Task Force on Practice Guidelines (Committee on Evaluation and Management of Heart Failure)," *J Am Coll Cardiol*, 1995, 26:1376-8.

Captopril and Hydrochlorothiazide

(KAP toe pril & hye droe klor oh THYE a zide)

Related Information

Captopril *on page 226*

Hydrochlorothiazide *on page 756*

(Continued)

Captopril and Hydrochlorothiazide *(Continued)*

U.S. Brand Names Capozide®
Canadian Brand Names Capozide®
Index Terms Hydrochlorothiazide and Captopril
Generic Available Yes
Pharmacologic Category Antihypertensive Agent, Combination
Use Management of hypertension and treatment of congestive heart failure
Dosage
  Geriatrics: Refer to dosing in individual monographs.
  Adults: Hypertension, CHF: May be substituted for previously titrated dosages of the individual components; alternatively, may initiate as follows: Oral:
    Initial: Single tablet (captopril 25 mg/hydrochlorothiazide 15 mg) taken once daily; daily dose of captopril should not exceed 150 mg; daily dose of hydrochlorothiazide should not exceed 50 mg
  Renal Impairment: May respond to smaller or less frequent doses.
  Special Geriatric Considerations Combination products are not recommended for first-line treatment and divided doses of diuretics may increase the incidence of nocturia in the elderly.
  Dosage Forms Excipient information presented when available (limited, particularly for generics); consult specific product labeling.
  Tablet:
    25/15: Captopril 25 mg and hydrochlorothiazide 15 mg
    25/25: Captopril 25 mg and hydrochlorothiazide 25 mg
    50/15: Captopril 50 mg and hydrochlorothiazide 15 mg
    50/25: Captopril 50 mg and hydrochlorothiazide 25 mg

♦ **Capzasin-HP® [OTC]** *see* Capsaicin *on page 225*
♦ **Capzasin-P® [OTC]** *see* Capsaicin *on page 225*
♦ **Carafate®** *see* Sucralfate *on page 1495*

Carbachol (KAR ba kole)

Related Information
  Glaucoma Drug Therapy *on page 1758*
Medication Safety Issues
  Sound-alike/look-alike issues:
    Isopto® Carbachol may be confused with Isopto® Carpine
U.S. Brand Names Isopto® Carbachol; Miostat®
Canadian Brand Names Isopto® Carbachol; Miostat®
Index Terms Carbacholine; Carbamylcholine Chloride
Generic Available No
Pharmacologic Category Cholinergic Agonist; Ophthalmic Agent, Antiglaucoma; Ophthalmic Agent, Miotic
Use Reduction of intraocular pressure in the treatment of glaucoma; production of miosis during surgery
Contraindications Hypersensitivity to carbachol or any component of the formulation; acute iritis, acute inflammatory disease of the anterior chamber
Warnings/Precautions Use with caution in patients undergoing general anesthesia and in presence of corneal abrasion. Use caution with acute cardiac failure, asthma, peptic ulcer, hyperthyroidism, gastrointestinal spasm, urinary tract obstruction, and Parkinson's disease.
Adverse Reactions (Reflective of adult population; not specific for elderly)
  Frequency not defined.
  Cardiovascular: Arrhythmia, flushing, hypotension, syncope
  Central nervous system: Headache
  Gastrointestinal: Abdominal cramps, diarrhea, epigastric distress, salivation, vomiting
  Genitourinary: Urinary bladder tightness
  Ocular: Bullous keratopathy, burning (transient), ciliary spasm, conjunctival injection, corneal clouding, irritation, postoperative iritis (following cataract extraction), retinal detachment, stinging (transient)
  Respiratory: Asthma
  Miscellaneous: Diaphoresis
Overdosage/Toxicology Symptoms include miosis, flushing, vomiting, bradycardia, bronchospasm, and involuntary urination. Atropine is the treatment of choice for intoxications manifesting with significant muscarinic symptoms. Atropine I.V. 1-2 mg every 5-60 minutes should be repeated to control symptoms and then continued as needed for 1-2 days following the acute ingestion. Epinephrine 0.1-1 mg SubQ may be useful in reversing severe cardiovascular or pulmonary sequelae.
Drug Interactions Decreased effect of carbachol possible with topical NSAIDs

Stability
Intraocular: Store at room temperature of 15°C to 30°C (59°F to 86°F).
Topical: Store at 8°C to 27°C (46°F to 80°F).
Mechanism of Action Synthetic direct-acting cholinergic agent that causes miosis by stimulating muscarinic receptors in the eye
Pharmacodynamics
Onset of miosis:
Ophthalmic: Within 10-20 minutes
Intraocular: Within 2-5 minutes
Duration:
Ophthalmic: Reductions in intraocular pressure persist for 4-8 hours
Intraocular: Lasts 24 hours
Dosage
Geriatrics & Adults:
Glaucoma: Ophthalmic: Instill 1-2 drops up to 3 times/day
Ophthalmic surgery (miosis): Intraocular: 0.5 mL instilled into anterior chamber before or after securing sutures
Administration Finger pressure should be applied on the lacrimal sac for 1-2 minutes following topical instillation; remove excess around the eye with a tissue
Patient Information May sting on instillation; may cause headache, altered distance vision, and decreased night vision; do not touch dropper to eye
Special Geriatric Considerations Assess patient's ability to self-administer.
Dosage Forms Excipient information presented when available (limited, particularly for generics); consult specific product labeling.
Solution, intraocular:
Miostat®): 0.01% (1.5 mL)
Solution, ophthalmic:
Isopto® Carbachol: 1.5% (15 mL); 3% (15 mL) [contains benzalkonium chloride]

♦ **Carbacholine** see Carbachol on page 230

Carbamazepine (kar ba MAZ e peen)

Related Information
Liquid Compatibility of Antipsychotics and Mood Stabilizers on page 1851
Serum Drug Concentrations Commonly Monitored Guidelines on page 1862
Medication Safety Issues
Sound-alike/look-alike issues:
Carbatrol® may be confused with Cartrol®
Epitol® may be confused with Epinal®
Tegretol®, Tegretol®-XR may be confused with Mebaral®, Tegrin®, Toprol-XL®, Toradol®, Trental®
U.S. Brand Names Carbatrol®; Epitol®; Equetro™; Tegretol®; Tegretol®-XR
Canadian Brand Names Apo-Carbamazepine®; Gen-Carbamazepine CR; Mapezine®; Novo-Carbamaz; Nu-Carbamazepine; PMS-Carbamazepine; Taro-Carbamazepine Chewable; Tegretol®
Index Terms CBZ; SPD417
Generic Available Yes: Excludes capsule (extended release), tablet (extended release)
Pharmacologic Category Anticonvulsant, Miscellaneous
Use
Carbatrol®, Tegretol®, Tegretol®-XR: Partial seizures with complex symptomatology (psychomotor, temporal lobe), generalized tonic-clonic seizures (grand mal), mixed seizure patterns, trigeminal neuralgia
Equetro™: Acute manic and mixed episodes associated with bipolar 1 disorder
Unlabeled/Investigational Use Treatment of bipolar disorders and other affective disorders, resistant schizophrenia, ethanol withdrawal, restless leg syndrome, psychotic behavior associated with dementia, post-traumatic stress disorders
Contraindications Hypersensitivity to carbamazepine, tricyclic antidepressants, or any component of the formulation; bone marrow depression; with or within 14 days of MAO inhibitor use
Warnings/Precautions [U.S. Boxed Warning]: Potentially fatal blood cell abnormalities have been reported. Patients with a previous history of adverse hematologic reaction to any drug may be at increased risk. Administer carbamazepine with caution to patients with history of cardiac damage, hepatic or renal disease. When used to treat bipolar disorder, the smallest effective dose is suggested to reduce the risk for overdose/suicide; high-risk patients should be monitored. Prescription should be written for the smallest quantity consistent with good patient care. Actuation of latent psychosis is possible. Potentially serious, sometimes fatal multiorgan hypersensitivity reactions have been reported with some antiepileptic drugs; monitor for signs and symptoms of possible disparate manifestations associated with lymphatic, hepatic, renal, and/or
(Continued)

Carbamazepine *(Continued)*

hematologic organ systems; gradual discontinuation and conversion to alternate therapy may be required.

Carbamazepine is not effective in absence, myoclonic, or akinetic seizures; exacerbation of certain seizure types have been seen after initiation of carbamazepine therapy in children with mixed seizure disorders. Abrupt discontinuation is not recommended in patients being treated for seizures. Dizziness or drowsiness may occur; caution should be used when performing tasks which require alertness until the effects are known. Effects with other sedative drugs or ethanol may be potentiated. Coadministration of carbamazepine and delavirdine may lead to loss of virologic response and possible resistance. Carbamazepine has mild anticholinergic activity; use with caution in patients with increased intraocular pressure, or sensitivity to anticholinergic effects. Severe dermatologic reactions, including toxic epidermal necrolysis and Stevens-Johnson syndrome, although rarely reported, have resulted in fatalities. Discontinue if there are any signs of hypersensitivity. Elderly patients may have an increased risk of SIADH-like syndrome.

Adverse Reactions (Reflective of adult population; not specific for elderly) Frequency not defined, unless otherwise specified.

Cardiovascular: Arrhythmias, AV block, bradycardia, chest pain (bipolar use), CHF, edema, hyper-/hypotension, lymphadenopathy, syncope, thromboembolism, thrombophlebitis

Central nervous system: Amnesia (bipolar use), anxiety (bipolar use), aseptic meningitis (case report), ataxia (bipolar use 15%), confusion, depression (bipolar use), dizziness (bipolar use 44%), fatigue, headache (bipolar use 22%), sedation, slurred speech, somnolence (bipolar use 32%)

Dermatologic: Alopecia, alterations in skin pigmentation, erythema multiforme, exfoliative dermatitis, photosensitivity reaction, pruritus (bipolar use 8%), purpura, rash, Stevens-Johnson syndrome, toxic epidermal necrolysis, urticaria

Endocrine & metabolic: Chills, fever, hyponatremia, syndrome of inappropriate ADH secretion (SIADH)

Gastrointestinal: Abdominal pain, anorexia, constipation, diarrhea, dyspepsia (bipolar use), gastric distress, nausea (bipolar use 29%), pancreatitis, vomiting (bipolar use 18%), xerostomia (bipolar use)

Genitourinary: Azotemia, impotence, renal failure, urinary frequency, urinary retention

Hematologic: Acute intermittent porphyria, agranulocytosis, aplastic anemia, bone marrow suppression, eosinophilia, leukocytosis, leukopenia, pancytopenia, thrombocytopenia

Hepatic: Abnormal liver function tests, hepatic failure, hepatitis, jaundice

Neuromuscular & skeletal: Back pain, pain (bipolar use 12%), peripheral neuritis, weakness

Ocular: Blurred vision, conjunctivitis, lens opacities, nystagmus

Otic: Hyperacusis, tinnitus

Miscellaneous: Diaphoresis, hypersensitivity (including multiorgan reactions, may include disorders mimicking lymphoma, eosinophilia, hepatosplenomegaly, vasculitis); infection (bipolar use 12%)

Overdosage/Toxicology Symptoms include dizziness ataxia, drowsiness, nausea, vomiting, tremor, agitation, nystagmus, urinary retention, dysrhythmias, coma, seizures, twitches, respiratory depression, and neuromuscular disturbances. Severe cardiac complications occur with very high doses. Provide general supportive care. Activated charcoal is effective at binding certain chemicals and this is especially true for carbamazepine. Other treatment is supportive/symptomatic. Treatment consists of inducing emesis or gastric lavage. ECG should also be monitored to detect cardiac dysfunction. Monitor blood pressure, body temperature, pupillary reflexes, bladder function for several days following ingestion.

Drug Interactions Substrate of CYP2C8 (minor), 3A4 (major); **Induces** CYP1A2 (strong), 2B6 (strong), 2C8 (strong), 2C9 (strong), 2C19 (strong), 3A4 (strong)

Acetaminophen: Carbamazepine may enhance hepatotoxic potential of acetaminophen; risk is greater in acetaminophen overdose.

Antimalarial drugs (chloroquine, mefloquine): Concomitant use with carbamazepine may reduce seizure control by lowering plasma levels; monitor.

Antipsychotics: Carbamazepine may decrease the serum levels/effects of antipsychotics (typical and atypical); monitor for altered response; dose adjustment may be needed.

Barbiturates: May reduce serum concentrations of carbamazepine; monitor.

Benzodiazepines: Serum concentrations and effect of benzodiazepines may be reduced by carbamazepine; monitor for decreased effect.

Calcium channel blockers: Diltiazem and verapamil may increase carbamazepine levels, due to enzyme inhibition (see below); other calcium channel blockers (felodipine) may be decreased by carbamazepine due to enzyme induction.

Chlorpromazine: **Note:** Carbamazepine suspension is incompatible with chlorpromazine solution. Schedule carbamazepine suspension at least 1-2 hours apart from other liquid medicinals.

Corticosteroids: Metabolism may be increased by carbamazepine.

Cyclosporine (and other immunosuppressants): Carbamazepine may enhance the metabolism of immunosuppressants, decreasing its clinical effect; includes both cyclosporine and tacrolimus.

CYP1A2 substrates: Carbamazepine may decrease the levels/effects of CYP1A2 substrates. Example substrates include aminophylline, estrogens, fluvoxamine, mirtazapine, ropinirole, and theophylline.

CYP2B6 substrates: Carbamazepine may decrease the levels/effects of CYP2B6 substrates. Example substrates include bupropion, efavirenz, promethazine, selegiline, and sertraline.

CYP2C8 substrates: Carbamazepine may decrease the levels/effects of CYP2C8 substrates. Example substrates include amiodarone, paclitaxel, pioglitazone, repaglinide, and rosiglitazone.

CYP2C9 substrates: Carbamazepine may decrease the levels/effects of CYP2C9 substrates. Example substrates include bosentan, celecoxib, dapsone, fluoxetine, glimepiride, glipizide, losartan, montelukast, nateglinide, paclitaxel, phenytoin, sulfonamides, trimethoprim, warfarin, and zafirlukast.

CYP2C19 substrates: Carbamazepine may decrease the levels/effects of CYP2C19 substrates. Example substrates include citalopram, diazepam, methsuximide, phenytoin, propranolol, proton pump inhibitors, sertraline, and voriconazole.

CYP3A4 inducers: CYP3A4 inducers may decrease the levels/effects of carbamazepine. Example inducers include aminoglutethimide, nafcillin, nevirapine, phenobarbital, phenytoin, and rifamycins. Carbamazepine may induce its own metabolism.

CYP3A4 inhibitors: May increase the levels/effects of carbamazepine. Example inhibitors include azole antifungals, clarithromycin, diclofenac, doxycycline, erythromycin, imatinib, isoniazid, nefazodone, nicardipine, propofol, protease inhibitors, quinidine, telithromycin, and verapamil.

CYP3A4 substrates: Carbamazepine may decrease the levels/effects of CYP3A4 substrates. Example substrates include benzodiazepines, calcium channel blockers, clarithromycin, cyclosporine, erythromycin, estrogens, mirtazapine, nateglinide, nefazodone, nevirapine, protease inhibitors, tacrolimus, and venlafaxine.

Danazol: May increase serum concentrations of carbamazepine; monitor.

Delavirdine: May lead to loss of virologic response and possible resistance.

Doxycycline: Carbamazepine may enhance the metabolism of doxycycline, decreasing its clinical effect.

Ethosuximide: Serum levels may be reduced by carbamazepine.

Felbamate: May increase carbamazepine levels and toxicity (increased epoxide metabolite concentrations); carbamazepine may decrease felbamate levels due to enzyme induction.

Immunosuppressants: Carbamazepine may enhance the metabolism of immunosuppressants, decreasing its clinical effect; includes both cyclosporine and tacrolimus.

Isoniazid: May increase the serum concentrations and toxicity of carbamazepine; in addition, carbamazepine may increase the hepatic toxicity of isoniazid (INH).

Isotretinoin: May decrease the effect of carbamazepine.

Lamotrigine: Increases the epoxide metabolite of carbamazepine resulting in toxicity; carbamazepine increases the metabolism of lamotrigine.

Lithium: Neurotoxicity may result in patients receiving concurrent carbamazepine.

Loxapine: May increase concentrations of epoxide metabolite and toxicity of carbamazepine.

Methadone: Carbamazepine may enhance the metabolism of methadone resulting in methadone withdrawal.

Methylphenidate: concurrent use of carbamazepine may reduce the therapeutic effect of methylphenidate; limited documentation; monitor for decreased effect.

Neuromuscular blocking agents, nondepolarizing: Effects may be of shorter duration when administered to patients receiving carbamazepine.

Oral contraceptives: Metabolism may be increased by carbamazepine, resulting in a loss of efficacy.

Phenytoin: Carbamazepine levels may be decreased by phenytoin. Metabolism of phenytoin may be altered by carbamazepine; phenytoin levels may be increased or decreased.

SSRIs: Metabolism may be increased by carbamazepine (due to enzyme induction).

Theophylline: Serum levels may be reduced by carbamazepine.

Thioridazine: **Note:** Carbamazepine suspension is incompatible with thioridazine liquid. Schedule carbamazepine suspension at least 1-2 hours apart from other liquid medicinals.

Thyroid: Serum levels may be reduced by carbamazepine.

Tiagabine: Carbamazepine may reduce the serum concentrations of tiagabine; monitor.

(Continued)

Carbamazepine *(Continued)*

Topiramate: Carbamazepine may reduce the serum concentrations of topiramate; monitor.

Tramadol: Tramadol's risk of seizures may be increased with TCAs (carbamazepine may be associated with similar risk due to chemical similarity to TCAs).

Trazodone: Serum concentrations may be reduced by carbamazepine; monitor.

Tricyclic antidepressants: May increase serum concentrations of carbamazepine; carbamazepine may decrease concentrations of tricyclics due to enzyme induction. The serum concentrations of clomipramine are increased by carbamazepine.

Valproic acid: Serum levels may be reduced by carbamazepine; carbamazepine levels may also be altered by valproic acid.

Warfarin: Carbamazepine may inhibit the hypoprothrombinemic effects of oral anticoagulants via increased metabolism; this combination should generally be avoided.

Zonisamide: Carbamazepine may reduce the serum concentrations of zonisamide; monitor.

Ethanol/Nutrition/Herb Interactions

Ethanol: Avoid ethanol (may increase CNS depression).

Food: Carbamazepine serum levels may be increased if taken with food. Carbamazepine serum concentration may be increased if taken with grapefruit juice; avoid concurrent use.

Herb/Nutraceutical: Avoid evening primrose (seizure threshold decreased). Avoid valerian, St John's wort, kava kava, gotu kola (may increase CNS depression).

Mechanism of Action In addition to anticonvulsant effects, carbamazepine has anticholinergic, antineuralgic, antidiuretic, muscle relaxant, antimanic, antidepressive, and antiarrhythmic properties; may depress activity in the nucleus ventralis of the thalamus or decrease synaptic transmission or decrease summation of temporal stimulation leading to neural discharge by limiting influx of sodium ions across cell membrane or other unknown mechanisms; stimulates the release of ADH and potentiates its action in promoting reabsorption of water; chemically related to tricyclic antidepressants

Pharmacokinetics

Absorption: Slow

Distribution: V_d: 0.59-2 L/kg

Protein binding: Carbamazepine: 75% to 90%; Epoxide metabolite: 50%

Metabolism: Hepatic via CYP3A4 to active epoxide metabolite; induces hepatic enzymes to increase metabolism

Bioavailability: 85%

Half-life elimination:

Carbamazepine: Initial: 18-55 hours; Multiple doses: 12-17 hours

Epoxide metabolite: Initial: 25-43 hours

Time to peak, serum: Unpredictable:

Immediate release: Suspension: 1.5 hour; tablet: 4-5 hours

Extended release: Carbatrol®, Equetro™: 12-26 hours (single dose), 4-8 hours (multiple doses); Tegretol®-XR: 3-12 hours

Excretion: Urine 72% (1% to 3% as unchanged drug); feces (28%)

Dosage

Geriatrics & Adults: Dosage must be adjusted according to patient's response and serum concentrations. Administer tablets (chewable or conventional) in 2-3 divided doses daily and suspension in 4 divided doses daily. (See Additional Information for investigational oral loading dose and rectal maintenance dose information.) Oral:

Epilepsy: Oral: Initial: 200 mg twice daily (tablets, extended release tablets, or extended release capsules) or 100 mg of suspension 4 times/day (400 mg daily); increase by up to 200 mg/day at weekly intervals using a twice daily regimen of extended release tablets or capsules, or a 3-4 times/day regimen of other formulations until optimal response and therapeutic levels are achieved; usual dose: 800-1200 mg/day

Maximum recommended dose: 1600 mg/day; however, some patients have required up to 1.6-2.4 g/day

Trigeminal or glossopharyngeal neuralgia: Oral: Initial: 100 mg twice daily with food, gradually increasing in increments of 100 mg twice daily as needed

Maintenance: Usual: 400-800 mg daily in 2 divided doses; maximum dose: 1200 mg/day

Bipolar disorder: Oral: Initial: 400 mg/day in divided doses, twice daily; may adjust by 200 mg daily increments; maximum dose: 1600 mg/day.

Note: Equetro™ is the only formulation specifically approved by the FDA for the managment of bipolar disorder.

Administration

Suspension: Must be given on a 3-4 times/day schedule versus tablets which can be given 2-4 times/day. When carbamazepine suspension has been combined with chlorpromazine or thioridazine solutions a precipitate forms which may result in loss of effect. Therefore, it is recommended that the carbamazepine suspension dosage form not be administered at the same time with other liquid medicinal agents or diluents. Since a given dose of suspension will produce higher peak levels than the same dose given as the tablet form, patients given the suspension should be started on lower doses and increased slowly to avoid unwanted side effects.

Extended release capsule (Carbatrol®, Equetro™): Consists of three different types of beads: Immediate release, extended-release, and enteric release. The bead types are combined in a ratio to allow twice daily dosing. May be opened and contents sprinkled over food such as a teaspoon of applesauce; may be administered with or without food; do not crush or chew.

Extended release tablet: Should be inspected for damage. Damaged extended release tablets (without release portal) should not be administered. Should be administered with meals; swallow whole, do not crush or chew.

Monitoring Parameters CBC with platelet count, reticulocytes, serum iron, lipid panel, liver function tests, urinalysis, BUN, serum carbamazepine levels, thyroid function tests, serum sodium; ophthalmic exams (pupillary reflexes); observe patient for excessive sedation, especially when instituting or increasing therapy

Reference Range

Timing of serum samples: Absorption is slow, peak serum concentrations occur 6-8 hours after ingestion of the first dose; the half-life ranges from 8-60 hours, therefore, steady-state is achieved in 2-5 days

Therapeutic concentration: 4-12 mcg/mL (SI: 25-51 µmol/L)

Toxic concentration: >15 mcg/mL; patients who require higher serum concentrations of 8-12 mcg/mL (SI: 34-51 µmol/L) should be observed closely. Side effects including CNS effects occur commonly at higher dosages. If other anticonvulsants are given, therapeutic range is 4-8 mcg/mL.

Test Interactions Increased BUN, AST, ALT, bilirubin, alkaline phosphatase (S); decreased calcium, T_3, T_4, sodium (S)

Patient Information Take with food, may cause drowsiness, periodic blood test monitoring required; notify physician if you observe bleeding, bruising, jaundice, abdominal pain, pale stools, mental disturbances, fever, chills, sore throat, or mouth ulcers

Additional Information Suspension dosage form must be given on a 3-4 times/day schedule versus tablets which can be given 2-4 times/day; may cause a rash, but does not necessarily mean the drug should be stopped

Special Geriatric Considerations Elderly may have increased risk of SIADH-like syndrome. Elderly are more susceptible to carbamazepine-induced confusion and agitation, AV block, and bradycardia.

Dosage Forms Excipient information presented when available (limited, particularly for generics); consult specific product labeling.

Capsule, extended release:
Carbatrol®, Equetro™: 100 mg, 200 mg, 300 mg
Suspension, oral: 100 mg/5 mL (5 mL, 10 mL, 450 mL)
Tegretol®: 100 mg/5 mL (450 mL) [citrus vanilla flavor]
Tablet: 200 mg
Epitol®, Tegretol®: 200 mg
Tablet, chewable: 100 mg
Tegretol®: 100 mg
Tablet, extended release:
Tegretol®-XR: 100 mg, 200 mg, 400 mg

Selected References

Iwahashi IS, Miyatake R, Suwaki H, et al, "The Drug-Drug Interaction Effects of Haloperidol on Plasma Carbamazepine Levels," *Clin Neuropharmacol*, 1995, 18:233-6.

Ketter TA, Kalali AH, and Weisler RH, "A 6-Month, Multicenter, Open-Label Evaluation of Beaded, Extended-Release Carbamazepine Capsule Monotherapy in Bipolar Disorder Patients With Manic or Mixed Episodes: SPD417 Study Group," *J Clin Psychiatry*, 2004, 65(5):668-73.

Weisler RH, Kalali AH, and Ketter TA, "A Multicenter, Randomized, Double-Blind, Placebo-Controlled Trial of Extended-Release Carbamazepine Capsules as Monotherapy for Bipolar Disorder Patients With Manic or Mixed Episodes: SPD417 Study Group," *J Clin Psychiatry*, 2004, 65(4):478-84.

Carbamide Peroxide (KAR ba mide per OKS ide)

U.S. Brand Names Cankaid® [OTC]; Debrox® [OTC]; Dent's Ear Wax [OTC]; E•R•O [OTC]; Gly-Oxide® [OTC]; Murine® Ear Wax Removal System [OTC]; Orajel® Perioseptic® Spot Treatment [OTC]

Index Terms Urea Peroxide

Generic Available Yes

Pharmacologic Category Anti-inflammatory, Locally Applied; Otic Agent, Cerumenolytic

Use

Oral: Relief of minor inflammation of gums, oral mucosal surfaces and lips including canker sores and dental irritation

Otic: Emulsification and dispersal of ear wax

(Continued)

Carbamide Peroxide *(Continued)*

Contraindications Hypersensitivity to carbamide peroxide or any component of the formulation; otic preparation should not be used in patients with a perforated tympanic membrane; ear drainage, ear pain or rash in the ear

Warnings/Precautions

Oral: With prolonged use of oral carbamide peroxide, there is a potential for overgrowth of opportunistic organisms, damage to periodontal tissues, and delayed wound healing; should not be used for longer than 7 days.

Otic: Do not use if ear drainage or discharge, ear pain, irritation, or rash in ear. Should not be used for longer than 4 days.

Adverse Reactions (Reflective of adult population; not specific for elderly)

Frequency not defined.

Dermatologic: Rash

Local: Irritation, redness

Miscellaneous: Superinfection

Drug Interactions No data reported

Stability Protect from excessive heat and direct sunlight.

Mechanism of Action Carbamide peroxide releases hydrogen peroxide which serves as a source of nascent oxygen upon contact with catalase; deodorant action is probably due to inhibition of odor-causing bacteria; softens impacted cerumen due to its foaming action

Dosage

Geriatrics & Adults:

Minor inflammation of gums, oral mucosal surfaces, and lips: Topical: Oral solution (should not be used for >7 days): Apply several drops undiluted on affected area 4 times/day after meals and at bedtime; expectorate after 2-3 minutes **or** place 10 drops onto tongue, mix with saliva, swish for several minutes, expectorate

Ear wax removal: Otic: Tilt head sideways and instill 5-10 drops twice daily up to 4 days, tip of applicator should not enter ear canal; keep drops in ear for several minutes by keeping head tilted and placing cotton in ear

Administration See Dosage.

Patient Information Contact physician if dizziness or otic redness, rash, irritation, tenderness, pain, drainage, or discharge develop; do not drink or rinse mouth for 5 minutes after oral use of gel

Additional Information Otic preparation should not be used for >4 days; oral preparation should not be used for longer than 7 days

Special Geriatric Considerations Avoid contact with hearing aids.

Dosage Forms Excipient information presented when available (limited, particularly for generics); consult specific product labeling.

Solution, oral: 10% (60 mL)

Cankaid®: 10% (22 mL) [in anhydrous glycerol]

Gly-Oxide®: 10% (15 mL, 60 mL) [contains glycerin]

Orajel® Perioseptic® Spot Treatment: 15% (13.3 mL) [contains anhydrous glycerin]

Solution, otic: 6.5% (15 mL)

Debrox®: 6.5% (15 mL, 30 mL) [contains propylene glycol]

Dent's Ear Wax: 6.5% (3.7 mL) [contains glycerin]

E•R•O: 6.5% (15 mL)

Murine® Ear Wax Removal System: 6.5% (15 mL) [contains alcohol 6.3% and glycerin]

♦ **Carbamylcholine Chloride** *see* Carbachol *on page 230*

♦ **Carbatrol®** *see* Carbamazepine *on page 231*

♦ **Carbaxefed RF [DSC]** *see* Carbinoxamine and Pseudoephedrine *on page 239*

Carbenicillin (kar ben i SIL in)

U.S. Brand Names Geocillin®

Index Terms Carbenicillin Indanyl Sodium; Carindacillin

Generic Available No

Pharmacologic Category Antibiotic, Penicillin

Use Treatment of serious infections caused by susceptible gram-negative aerobic bacilli or mixed aerobic-anaerobic bacterial infections and/or urinary tract infections excluding those secondary to *Klebsiella* sp and *Serratia marcescens*

Contraindications Hypersensitivity to carbenicillin, penicillins, or any component of the formulation

Warnings/Precautions Do not use in patients with severe renal impairment (Cl$_{cr}$ <10 mL/minute); dosage modification is required in patients with impaired renal and/or hepatic function. Serious and occasionally severe or fatal hypersensitivity (anaphylactoid) reactions have been reported in patients on penicillin therapy, especially with a history of beta-lactam hypersensitivity, history of sensitivity to multiple allergens, or previous IgE-mediated reactions (eg, anaphylaxis, angioedema, urticaria). Use with caution in asthmatic patients. Prolonged use may result in fungal or bacterial superinfection, including *C. difficile*-associated diarrhea and pseudomembranous colitis.

Adverse Reactions (Reflective of adult population; not specific for elderly)
>10%: Gastrointestinal: Diarrhea
1% to 10%: Gastrointestinal: Nausea, bad taste, vomiting, flatulence, glossitis

Overdosage/Toxicology Symptoms include neuromuscular hypersensitivity and convulsions. Many beta-lactam containing antibiotics have the potential to cause neuromuscular hyperirritability or convulsive seizures. Hemodialysis may be helpful to aid in the removal of the drug from the blood, otherwise, most treatment is supportive or symptom-directed.

Drug Interactions
Aminoglycosides: May be synergistic against selected organisms.
Fusidic acid: May decrease the therapeutic effect of penicillins; administer the penicillin at least 2 hours before fusidic acid.
Methotrexate: Penicillins may increase the exposure to methotrexate during concurrent therapy; monitor.
Oral contraceptives: Anecdotal reports suggesting decreased contraceptive efficacy with penicillins have been refuted by more rigorous scientific and clinical data.
Probenecid, disulfiram: May increase levels of penicillins (carbenicillin).
Tetracyclines: May decrease effectiveness of penicillins (carbenicillin).
Warfarin: Effects of warfarin may be increased.

Mechanism of Action Inhibits bacterial cell wall synthesis by binding to one or more of the penicillin-binding proteins (PBPs) which in turn inhibits the final transpeptidation step of peptidoglycan synthesis in bacterial cell walls, thus inhibiting cell wall biosynthesis. Bacteria eventually lyse due to ongoing activity of cell wall autolytic enzymes (autolysins and murein hydrolases) while cell wall assembly is arrested.

Pharmacokinetics
Absorption: Oral: 30% to 40%
Distribution: Into bile, low concentrations attained in CSF
Protein binding: 50%
Half-life: 60-90 minutes and is prolonged to 10-20 hours with renal insufficiency
Time to peak: Within 30-120 minutes; in patients with normal renal function, serum concentrations of carbenicillin following oral absorption are inadequate for the treatment of systemic infections
Elimination: ~80% to 99% of dose excreted unchanged in urine

Dosage
Geriatrics & Adults:
Prostatitis: Oral: 2 tablets every 6 hours
Urinary tract infections: Oral: 1-2 tablets every 6 hours
Renal Impairment:
Cl$_{cr}$ 10-50 mL/minute: Administer every 12-24 hours.
Cl$_{cr}$ <10 mL/minute: Administer every 24-48 hours.
Moderately dialyzable (20% to 50%)

Monitoring Parameters Signs and symptoms of infection (fever, urinary frequency, dysuria, etc)

Reference Range Therapeutic: Not established; Toxic: >250 mcg/mL (SI: >660 µmol/L)

Test Interactions May interfere with urinary glucose tests using cupric sulfate (Benedict's solution, Clinitest®); false-positive urine or serum proteins.
Some penicillin derivatives may accelerate the degradation of aminoglycosides. *In vitro*, leading to a potential underestimation of aminoglycoside serum concentration.

Patient Information Tablets have a bitter taste, can be taken with food; complete full course of treatment; notify physician of edema, difficulty breathing, bruising, or bleeding

Special Geriatric Considerations Has not been studied in the elderly. Adjust dose for renal function in the elderly.

Dosage Forms Excipient information presented when available (limited, particularly for generics); consult specific product labeling.
Tablet: 382 mg [contains sodium 23 mg/tablet]

♦ **Carbenicillin Indanyl Sodium** *see* Carbenicillin *on page 236*

Carbidopa (kar bi DOE pa)

Medication Safety Issues
International issues:
Lodosyn® may be confused with Lidosen® which is a brand name for lidocaine in Italy
U.S. Brand Names Lodosyn®
Generic Available No
(Continued)

Carbidopa (Continued)

Pharmacologic Category Anti-Parkinson's Agent, Dopamine Agonist

Use Given with levodopa in the treatment of parkinsonism to enable a lower dosage of levodopa to be used and a more rapid response to be obtained and to decrease side-effects; has no effect without levodopa.

Contraindications Hypersensitivity to carbidopa or levodopa, or any component of the formulation; use of nonselective MAO antagonists; narrow-angle glaucoma; history of melanoma or undiagnosed skin lesions

Warnings/Precautions Has no antiparkinsonian activity when administered alone. May be associated with development of movement disorders or depression with suicidal tendencies. Use caution in patients with prior mental health problems (depression, psychosis). Use caution in cardiac, pulmonary, renal, hepatic, or endocrine disease. Use caution in patients with history of arrhythmia. May cause neuroleptic malignant syndrome (NMS). Dyskinesias may occur at lower levodopa dosages than with monotherapy (levodopa dosage may need to be reduced).

Adverse Reactions (Reflective of adult population; not specific for elderly) Adverse reactions are associated with concomitant administration with levodopa

>10%: Central nervous system: Anxiety, confusion, nervousness, mental depression

1% to 10%:

Cardiovascular: Orthostatic hypotension, palpitation, cardiac arrhythmia

Central nervous system: Memory loss, insomnia, fatigue, hallucinations, ataxia, dystonic movements

Gastrointestinal: Nausea, vomiting, GI bleeding

Ocular: Blurred vision

Drug Interactions Note: Interactions apply to carbidopa/levodopa combination therapy.

Antacids: Levodopa absorption may be increased; monitor.

Anticholinergics: May reduce the efficacy of levodopa, possibly due to reduced gastrointestinal absorption (also see tricyclic antidepressants); limited evidence of clinical significance; monitor.

Antipsychotics: May inhibit the antiparkinsonian effects of levodopa via dopamine receptor blockade; use antipsychotics with low dopamine blockade (clozapine, olanzapine, quetiapine).

Benzodiazepines: May inhibit the antiparkinsonian effects of levodopa; monitor for reduced effect.

Clonidine: May reduce the efficacy of levodopa; monitor.

Dextromethorphan: Toxic reactions have occurred with dextromethorphan.

Furazolidone: May increase the effect/toxicity of levodopa; hypertensive episodes have been reported; monitor.

Iron salts: Binds levodopa and reduces its bioavailability; separate doses of iron and levodopa.

Linezolid: Due to MAO inhibition (see note on MAO inhibitors), this agent is best avoided.

MAO inhibitors: Concurrent use of levodopa with nonselective MAO inhibitors may result in hypertensive reactions via an increased storage and release of dopamine, norepinephrine, or both; use with carbidopa to minimize reactions if combination is necessary, otherwise, avoid combination.

L-methionine: May inhibit levodopa's antiparkinsonian effects; monitor for reduced effect.

Metoclopramide: May increase the absorption/effect of levodopa; hypertensive episodes have been reported. Levodopa antagonizes metoclopramide's effects on lower esophageal sphincter pressure. Avoid use of metoclopramide for reflux; monitor response to levodopa carefully if used.

Methyldopa: May potentiate the effects of levodopa; levodopa may increase the hypotensive response to methyldopa; monitor.

Papaverine: May decrease the efficacy of levodopa; includes other similar agents (ethaverine); monitor.

Penicillamine: May increase serum concentrations of levodopa; monitor for increased effect.

Phenytoin: May inhibit levodopa's antiparkinsonian effects; monitor for reduced effect.

Pyridoxine: May inhibit levodopa's antiparkinsonian effects; monitor for reduced effect.

Spiramycin: May inhibit levodopa's antiparkinsonian effects; monitor for reduced effect.

Tacrine: May inhibit the effects of levodopa via enhanced cholinergic activity; monitor for reduced effect.

Tricyclic antidepressants: May decrease the absorption (bioavailability) of levodopa; rare hypertensive episodes have been attributed to this combination.

Mechanism of Action Carbidopa is a peripheral decarboxylase inhibitor with little or no pharmacological activity when given alone in usual doses. It inhibits the peripheral decarboxylation of levodopa to dopamine; and as it does not cross the blood-brain barrier, unlike levodopa, effective brain concentrations of dopamine are produced with lower doses of levodopa. At the same time, reduced peripheral formation of dopamine reduces peripheral side-effects, notably nausea and vomiting, and cardiac arrhythmias, although the dyskinesias and adverse mental effects associated with levodopa therapy tend to develop earlier.

Dosage
    Geriatrics & Adults: Parkinson's disease (adjunct to levodopa): Oral: 70-100 mg/day; maximum daily dose: 200 mg

Additional Information Usually used in combination with levodopa (Sinemet®); plain carbidopa tablets are available from Merck & Co to physicians for use in patients requiring individual titration of carbidopa and levodopa. See Levodopa and Carbidopa on page 892.

Dosage Forms Excipient information presented when available (limited, particularly for generics); consult specific product labeling.
    Tablet: 25 mg

Selected References
    Olanow CW, Watts RL, and Koller WC, "An Algorithm (Decision Tree) for the Management of Parkinson's Disease (2001): Treatment Guidelines," *Neurology*, 2001, 56(11 Suppl 5):S1-S88.

♦ **Carbidopa and Levodopa** *see* Levodopa and Carbidopa *on page 892*

♦ **Carbidopa, Levodopa, and Entacapone** *see* Levodopa, Carbidopa, and Entacapone *on page 895*

Carbinoxamine and Pseudoephedrine
(kar bi NOKS a meen & soo doe e FED rin)

Related Information
    Pseudoephedrine *on page 1346*
U.S. Brand Names Andehist NR Drops [DSC]; Carbaxefed RF [DSC]; Carboxine-PSE [DSC]; Cordron-D NR [DSC]; Hydro-Tussin™-CBX; Palgic®-D [DSC]; Palgic®-DS [DSC]; Pediatex™-D [DSC]; Sildec [DSC]
Index Terms Pseudoephedrine and Carbinoxamine
Generic Available Yes
Pharmacologic Category Adrenergic Agonist Agent; Antihistamine, H₁ Blocker; Decongestant
Use Temporary relief of nasal congestion, runny nose, sneezing, itchy nose or throat, and itchy, watery eyes due to the common cold, hay fever, or other respiratory allergies
Contraindications Hypersensitivity to carbinoxamine, pseudoephedrine, or any component of the formulation; severe hypertension or coronary artery disease; MAO inhibitor therapy; GI or GU obstruction; peptic ulcer disease; narrow-angle glaucoma; acute asthma attack
Warnings/Precautions Use caution with hypertension, ischemic heart disease, hyperthyroidism, increased intraocular pressure, diabetes mellitus, BPH, and patients >60 years of age.
Adverse Reactions (Reflective of adult population; not specific for elderly)
    Frequency not defined.
    Cardiovascular: Arrhythmias, cardiovascular collapse, hypertension, pallor, tachycardia
    Central nervous system: Anxiety, convulsions, CNS stimulation, dizziness, excitability (children; rare), fear, hallucinations, headache, insomnia, nervousness, restlessness, sedation
    Gastrointestinal: Anorexia, diarrhea, dyspepsia, nausea, vomiting, xerostomia
    Neuromuscular skeletal: Tremors, weakness
    Ocular: Diplopia
    Renal: Dysuria, polyuria, urinary retention (with BPH)
    Respiratory: Respiratory difficulty
Overdosage/Toxicology Symptoms include dry mouth, flushed skin, dilated pupils, and CNS depression. There is no specific treatment for an antihistamine overdose, however, clinical toxicity is mostly due to anticholinergic effects. Anticholinesterase inhibitors including physostigmine, neostigmine, pyridostigmine, and edrophonium may be useful by reducing acetylcholinesterase. For anticholinergic overdose with severe life-threatening symptoms, physostigmine 1-2 mg slow I.V. may be given to reverse these effects.
Drug Interactions
    Antihypertensives: Antihypertensive effect may be decreased.
    Barbiturates (and other CNS depressants): CNS depressant effect may be increased.
    MAO inhibitors: Anticholinergic effects of the antihistamine may be increased and prolonged; sympathomimetic effect of the decongestant may be increased.
    Tricyclic antidepressants: CNS depressant effect may be increased.
Ethanol/Nutrition/Herb Interactions Ethanol: Avoid ethanol (may increase CNS depression).
Stability Store at room temperature of 15°C to 30°C (59°F to 86°F).
(Continued)

Carbinoxamine and Pseudoephedrine *(Continued)*

Mechanism of Action Carbinoxamine competes with histamine for H_1-receptor sites on effector cells in the gastrointestinal tract, blood vessels, and respiratory tract; pseudoephedrine, a sympathomimetic amine and isomer of ephedrine, acts as a decongestant in respiratory tract mucous membranes with less vasoconstrictor action than ephedrine in normotensive individuals

Dosage

Geriatrics & Adults: Nasal congestion, allergic symptoms: Oral:
Liquid (Pediatex™-D): 10 mL 4 times/day
Syrup (Hydro-Tussin™-CBX, Palgic®-DS): 10 mL 4 times/day
Tablet, timed release (Palgic®-D): 1 tablet every 12 hours

Administration

Palgic®-D: Tablets may be broken in half; do not crush or chew
Rondec-TR®: Do not crush or chew

Monitoring Parameters Monitor pulse, blood pressure; monitor for tremor, insomnia, and changes in mental function

Patient Information May cause drowsiness, impaired coordination, or judgment; may cause blurred vision; may also cause CNS excitation and difficulty sleeping

Special Geriatric Considerations Elderly are more predisposed to adverse effects of sympathomimetics since they frequently have cardiovascular diseases and diabetes mellitus, and may be on multidrug therapy. It may be advisable to treat with a short-acting immediate-release formulation before initiating sustained-release long-acting formulations. Carbinoxamine exhibits anticholinergic action which may cause constipation, urinary retention, and mental confusion in the elderly.

Dosage Forms Excipient information presented when available (limited, particularly for generics); consult specific product labeling. [DSC] = Discontinued product
Liquid:
Cordron-D NR: Carbinoxamine maleate 2 mg and pseudoephedrine hydrochloride 12.5 mg per 5 mL (480 mL) [cotton candy flavor] [DSC]
Pediatex™-D: Carbinoxamine maleate 2 mg and pseudoephedrine hydrochloride 20 mg mg per 5 mL (480 mL) [alcohol free, dye free, sugar free; cotton candy flavor] [DSC]
Solution: Carbinoxamine maleate 2 mg and pseudoephedrine hydrochloride 25 mg per 5 mL (480 mL) [DSC]
Carboxine-PSE: Carbinoxamine maleate 2 mg and pseudoephedrine hydrochloride 20 mg per 5 mL (480 mL) [peach flavor] [DSC]
Solution, oral drops:
Andehist NR: Carbinoxamine maleate 1 mg and pseudoephedrine hydrochloride 15 mg per mL (30 mL) [alcohol and sugar free; raspberry flavor] [DSC]
Carbaxefed RF: Carbinoxamine maleate 1 mg and pseudoephedrine hydrochloride 15 mg per mL (30 mL) [alcohol free; contains sodium benzoate; cherry flavor] [DSC]
Sildec: Carbinoxamine maleate 1 mg and pseudoephedrine hydrochloride 15 mg per mL (30 mL) [raspberry flavor] [DSC]
Syrup: Carbinoxamine maleate 2 mg and pseudoephedrine hydrochloride 25 mg per 5 mL (480 mL)
Hydro-Tussin™-CBX, Palgic®-DS [DSC]: Carbinoxamine maleate 2 mg and pseudo-ephedrine hydrochloride 25 mg per 5 mL (480 mL) [alcohol, dye, and sugar free; strawberry/pineapple flavor]
Tablet, timed release:
Palgic®-D: Carbinoxamine maleate 8 mg and pseudoephedrine hydrochloride 80 mg [dye free] [DSC]

♦ **Carboxine-PSE [DSC]** *see* Carbinoxamine and Pseudoephedrine *on page 239*

♦ **Cardene®** *see* NiCARdipine *on page 1113*

♦ **Cardene® I.V.** *see* NiCARdipine *on page 1113*

♦ **Cardene® SR** *see* NiCARdipine *on page 1113*

♦ **Cardizem®** *see* Diltiazem *on page 441*

♦ **Cardizem® CD** *see* Diltiazem *on page 441*

♦ **Cardizem® LA** *see* Diltiazem *on page 441*

♦ **Cardura®** *see* Doxazosin *on page 471*

♦ **Cardura® XL** *see* Doxazosin *on page 471*

♦ **Carindacillin** *see* Carbenicillin *on page 236*

♦ **Carisoprodate** *see* Carisoprodol *on page 240*

Carisoprodol *(kar eye soe PROE dole)*

Related Information

Potentially Inappropriate Medications for Geriatrics *on page 1824*
U.S. Brand Names Soma®

Canadian Brand Names Soma®

Index Terms Carisoprodate; Isobamate

Generic Available Yes

Pharmacologic Category Skeletal Muscle Relaxant

Use Relief of discomfort associated with skeletal muscle condition

Contraindications Hypersensitivity to carisoprodol, meprobamate or any component of the formulation; acute intermittent porphyria

Warnings/Precautions May cause CNS depression, which may impair physical or mental abilities. Effects with other sedative drugs or ethanol may be potentiated. Use with caution in patients with hepatic/renal dysfunction. Tolerance or drug dependence may result from extended use. Limit to 2-3 weeks; use caution in patients who may be prone to addiction. Idiosyncratic reactions and/or severe allergic reactions may occur. Idiosyncratic reactions occur following the initial dose and may include severe weakness, transient quadriplegia, euphoria, or vision loss (temporary). Has been associated (rarely) with seizures in patients with and without seizure history.

Adverse Reactions (Reflective of adult population; not specific for elderly) Frequency not defined.

Cardiovascular: Flushing of face, hypotension (postural), syncope, tachycardia, tightness in chest

Central nervous system: Agitation, allergic fever, ataxia, depression, dizziness, drowsiness, dysarthria, headache, insomnia, irritability, lightheadedness, paradoxical CNS stimulation, seizure, vertigo

Dermatologic: Angioedema, dermatitis (allergic), erythema multiforme, fixed drug reaction, pruritus, rash, urticaria

Gastrointestinal: Nausea, epigastric distress, vomiting

Hematologic: Aplastic anemia, eosinophilia, leukopenia

Neuromuscular & skeletal: Tremor

Ocular: Blurred vision, burning eyes

Respiratory: Dyspnea

Miscellaneous: Anaphylaxis, hiccups, hypersensitivity reaction, idiosyncratic reaction (symptoms may include ataxia, dysarthria, temporary vision loss, extreme weakness, agitation, euphoria, transient quadriplegia, confusion, and/or disorientation); withdrawal symptoms (abdominal cramps, headache, nausea, seizure) may occur upon abrupt discontinuation

Overdosage/Toxicology Symptoms include CNS depression, stupor, coma, shock, and respiratory depression. Treatment is supportive following attempts to enhance drug elimination. Hypotension should be treated with I.V. fluids and/or Trendelenburg positioning.

Drug Interactions Substrate of CYP2C19 (major)

CNS depressants (includes CNS depressants, benzodiazepines, and phenothiazines): Sedation may be increased; avoid concurrent use.

CYP2C19 inhibitors: May increase the levels/effects of carisoprodol. Example inhibitors include delavirdine, fluconazole, fluvoxamine, gemfibrozil, isoniazid, omeprazole, and ticlopidine.

Ethanol/Nutrition/Herb Interactions Ethanol: Avoid ethanol (may increase CNS depression).

Stability Store at 20°C to 25°C (68°F to 77°F).

Mechanism of Action Precise mechanism is not yet clear, but many effects have been ascribed to its central depressant actions

Pharmacodynamics
Onset of action: Within 30 minutes
Duration: 4-6 hours

Pharmacokinetics
Metabolism: Hepatic, via CYP2C19 to active metabolite (meprobamate)
Half-life elimination: 2.4 hours; Meprobamate: 10 hours
Excretion: Urine, as metabolite

Dosage
Geriatrics: Not recommended for use in the elderly (see Special Geriatric Considerations).

Adults: Muscle spasm (including spasm associated with acute temporomandibular joint pain): Oral: 350 mg 3-4 times/day; take last dose at bedtime

Monitoring Parameters Relief of pain and/or muscle spasm, mental status

Patient Information May cause drowsiness or dizziness; avoid alcohol and other CNS depressants; because of the risk of postural hypotension, rise slowly from sitting or lying down

Special Geriatric Considerations Avoid or use with caution in the elderly; not considered a drug of choice because of the risk of orthostatic hypotension and CNS depression; no data available on the use of skeletal muscle relaxants in the geriatric population.
(Continued)

Carisoprodol *(Continued)*

Dosage Forms Excipient information presented when available (limited, particularly for generics); consult specific product labeling.
Tablet: 350 mg
Soma®: 350 mg

♦ **Carmol® Scalp** *see* Sulfacetamide *on page 1496*
♦ **Carrington Antifungal [OTC]** *see* Miconazole *on page 1036*

Carteolol *(KAR tee oh lole)*

Related Information
Beta-Blockers *on page 1751*
Glaucoma Drug Therapy *on page 1758*
Medication Safety Issues
Sound-alike/look-alike issues:
Carteolol may be confused with carvedilol
Canadian Brand Names Ocupress® Ophthalmic
Index Terms Carteolol Hydrochloride
Generic Available Yes
Pharmacologic Category Ophthalmic Agent, Antiglaucoma
Use Treatment of chronic open-angle glaucoma and intraocular hypertension
Contraindications Hypersensitivity to carteolol or any component of the formulation; sinus bradycardia; heart block greater than first-degree (except in patients with a functioning artificial pacemaker); cardiogenic shock; bronchial asthma, bronchospasm, or COPD; uncompensated cardiac failure; pulmonary edema
Warnings/Precautions Consider pre-existing conditions such as sick sinus syndrome before initiating. Use caution in patients with PVD (can aggravate arterial insufficiency) or myasthenia gravis. In general, patients with bronchospastic disease should not receive beta-blockers; if used at all, should be used cautiously with close monitoring. Use cautiously in diabetics because it can mask prominent hypoglycemic symptoms. Systemic absorption and adverse effects may occur with ophthalmic product, including bradycardia and/or hypotension. Should not be used alone in angle-closure glaucoma (has no effect on pupillary constriction). Adequate alpha-blockade is required prior to use of any beta-blocker for patients with untreated pheochromocytoma.
Adverse Reactions (Reflective of adult population; not specific for elderly)
>10%: Ocular: Conjunctival hyperemia
1% to 10%: Ocular: Anisocoria, corneal punctate keratitis, corneal sensitivity decreased, corneal staining, eye pain, vision disturbances
Overdosage/Toxicology Symptoms include cardiac disturbances, CNS toxicity, bronchospasm, hypoglycemia, and hyperkalemia. The most common cardiac symptoms include hypotension and bradycardia. Atrioventricular block, intraventricular conduction disturbances, cardiogenic shock, and asystole may occur with severe overdose, especially with membrane-depressant drugs (eg, propranolol). CNS effects include convulsions, coma, and respiratory arrest (commonly seen with propranolol and other membrane-depressant and lipid-soluble drugs). Treatment is symptomatic for seizures, hypotension, hyperkalemia, and hypoglycemia. Bradycardia and hypotension resistant to atropine, isoproterenol, or pacing may respond to glucagon. Wide QRS defects caused by membrane-depressant poisoning may respond to hypertonic sodium bicarbonate. Repeat-dose charcoal, hemoperfusion, or hemodialysis may be helpful in removal of only those beta-blockers with a small V_d, long half-life, or low intrinsic clearance (acebutolol, atenolol, nadolol, sotalol).
Drug Interactions Substrate of CYP2D6 (minor)
Acetylcholinesterase inhibitors: May enhance the bradycardic effects of beta-blockers.
Albuterol (and other $beta_2$-agonists): Effects may be blunted by nonspecific beta-blockers.
Alpha-/beta-agonists (direct-acting): Beta-blockers may enhance the vasopressor effect of systemically active alpha- or beta-agonists.
Alpha-blockers (eg, prazosin, terazosin): Concurrent use of beta-blockers may increase risk of hypotension or orthostasis.
AV conduction-slowing drugs (eg, amiodarone, digoxin, verapamil, diltiazem): Bradycardic effects may be additive with beta-blockers.
Clonidine: Hypertensive crisis after or during withdrawal of either agent.
Glucagon: Carteolol may blunt the hyperglycemic action of glucagon.
Insulin: Carteolol may mask tachycardia from hypoglycemia.
Sulfonylureas: Beta-blockers may alter response to hypoglycemic agents.
Mechanism of Action Blocks both $beta_1$- and $beta_2$-receptors and has mild intrinsic sympathomimetic activity; reduces intraocular pressure by decreasing aqueous humor production
Pharmacodynamics Ophthalmic: 22% to 25% reduction of IOP given twice daily
Onset of action: Not known

Maximum effect: Not described
Duration: 12 hours

Pharmacokinetics
Absorption: Well absorbed, 80%
Protein binding: 25% to 30%
Bioavailability: Oral: 85%
Half-life: 6 hours
Elimination: 50% to 70% excreted unchanged in urine

Dosage
Geriatrics & Adults: Glaucoma or intraocular hypertension: Ophthalmic: Instill 1 drop in affected eye(s) twice daily

Administration Intended for twice daily dosing. Keep eye open and do not blink for 30 seconds after instillation. Wear sunglasses to avoid photophobic discomfort. Apply gentle pressure to lacrimal sac during and immediately following instillation (1 minute).

Monitoring Parameters Ophthalmic: Intraocular pressure

Patient Information Wash hands before instilling. Sit or lie down to instill. Open eye, look at ceiling, and instill prescribed amount of medication. Keep eye open and do not blink for 30 seconds after instillation. Apply gentle pressure to inner corner of eye during and immediately following installation (1 minute). Do not touch tip of applicator or let tip of applicator touch eye. Temporary stinging or burning may occur. Wear sunglasses to avoid sun sensitivity or eye discomfort. Report persistent pain, burning, vision changes, swelling, itching, or worsening of condition.

Additional Information Since bioavailability increased in older adults about twofold, geriatric patients may require lower maintenance doses, therefore, as serum and tissue concentrations increase beta$_1$ selectivity diminishes; when treating glaucoma/intraocular hypertension, if the desired IOP is not achieved, consider adding concomitant therapy with pilocarpine, dipivefrin, etc.

Special Geriatric Considerations Due to alterations in the beta-adrenergic autonomic nervous system, beta-adrenergic blockade may result in less hemodynamic response than seen in younger adults. Studies indicate that despite decreased sensitivity to the chronotropic effects of beta-blockade with age, there appears to be an increased myocardial sensitivity to the negative inotropic effect during stress (ie, exercise). Controlled trials have shown the overall response rate for propranolol to be only 20% to 50% in elderly populations. Therefore, all beta-adrenergic blocking drugs may result in a decreased response as compared to younger adults; adjust dose for renal function in the elderly.

Dosage Forms Excipient information presented when available (limited, particularly for generics); consult specific product labeling.
Solution, ophthalmic, as hydrochloride: 1% (5 mL, 10 mL, 15 mL) [contains benzalkonium chloride]

Selected References
Braunwald E, Antman EM, Beasley JW, et al, "ACC/AHA 2002 Guideline Update for the Management of Patients With Unstable Angina and Non-ST-Segment Elevation Myocardial Infarction - Summary Article: A Report of the American College of Cardiology/American Heart Association Task Force on Practice Guidelines (Committee on the Management of Patients With Unstable Angina)," J Am Coll Cardiol, 2002, 40(7):1366-74. Available at: http://www.acc.org/clinical/guidelines/unstable/incorporated/index.htm. Accessed May 20, 2003.
"Consensus Recommendations for the Management of Chronic Heart Failure. On Behalf of the Membership of the Advisory Council to Improve Outcomes Nationwide in Heart Failure," Am J Cardiol, 1999, 83(2A):1A-38A.
Gibbons RJ, Abrams J, Chatterjee K, et al, "ACC/AHA 2002 Guideline Update for the Management of Patients With Chronic Stable Angina - Summary Article: A Report of the American College of Cardiology/American Heart Association Task Force on Practice Guidelines (Committee on the Management of Patients With Chronic Stable Angina)," J Am Coll Cardiol, 2003, 41(1):159-68.
Mokhlesi B, Leikin JB, Murray P, et al, "Adult Toxicology in Critical Care: Part II: Specific Poisonings," Chest, 2003, 123(3):897-922.

♦ **Carteolol Hydrochloride** see Carteolol on page 242
♦ **Cartia XT**™ see Diltiazem on page 441

Carvedilol (KAR ve dil ole)

Related Information
Beta-Blockers on page 1751

Medication Safety Issues
Sound-alike/look-alike issues:
Carvedilol may be confused with captopril, carteolol

International issues:
Talliton® [Hungary] may be confused with Talacen® which is a brand name for pentazocine/acetaminophen combination in the U.S.

U.S. Brand Names Coreg®; Coreg CR™

Canadian Brand Names Apo-Carvedilol®; Coreg®; Novo-Carvedilol; PMS-Carvedilol; RAN™-Carvedilol; ratio-Carvedilol

(Continued)

Carvedilol *(Continued)*

Generic Available No

Pharmacologic Category Beta Blocker With Alpha-Blocking Activity

Use Mild to severe heart failure of ischemic or cardiomyopathic origin (usually in addition to standardized therapy); left ventricular dysfunction following myocardial infarction (MI); management of hypertension

Unlabeled/Investigational Use Treatment of angina pectoris

Contraindications Hypersensitivity to carvedilol or any component of the formulation; decompensated cardiac failure requiring intravenous inotropic therapy; bronchial asthma or related bronchospastic conditions; second- or third-degree AV block, sick sinus syndrome, and severe bradycardia (except in patients with a functioning artificial pacemaker); cardiogenic shock; severe hepatic impairment

Warnings/Precautions Consider pre-existing conditions such as sick sinus syndrome before initiating. Initiate cautiously and monitor for possible deterioration in patient status (including symptoms of CHF). Adjustment of other medications (ACE inhibitors and/or diuretics) may be required. In severe chronic heart failure, trial patients were excluded if they had cardiac-related rales, ascites, or a serum creatinine >2.8 mg/dL. Congestive heart failure patients may experience a worsening of renal function; risks include ischemic disease, diffuse vascular disease, underlying renal dysfunction; systolic BP <100 mm Hg. Patients should be advised to avoid driving or other hazardous tasks during initiation of therapy due to the risk of syncope. Beta-blocker therapy should not be withdrawn abruptly (particularly in patients with CAD), but gradually tapered to avoid acute tachycardia, hypertension, and/or ischemia.

Manufacturer recommends discontinuation of therapy if liver injury occurs (confirmed by laboratory testing). In general, patients with bronchospastic disease should not receive beta-blockers; if used at all, should be used cautiously with close monitoring. Use caution in patients with PVD (can aggravate arterial insufficiency). Use caution with concurrent use of verapamil or diltiazem; bradycardia or heart block can occur. Use cautiously in diabetics because it can mask prominent hypoglycemic symptoms. Use with caution in patients with myasthenia gravis or psychiatric disease (may cause CNS depression). Use with caution in patients with mild-to-moderate hepatic impairment. Adequate alpha-blockade is required prior to use of any beta-blocker for patients with untreated pheochromocytoma. Use care with anesthetic agents that decrease myocardial function.

Adverse Reactions (Reflective of adult population; not specific for elderly)
Note: Frequency ranges include data from hypertension and heart failure trials. Higher rates of adverse reactions have generally been noted in patients with CHF. However, the frequency of adverse effects associated with placebo is also increased in this population. Events occurring at a frequency > placebo in clinical trials.

>10%:
Cardiovascular: Hypotension (9% to 20%)
Central nervous system: Dizziness (2% to 32%), fatigue (4% to 24%)
Endocrine & metabolic: Hyperglycemia (5% to 12%), weight gain (10% to 12%)
Gastrointestinal: Diarrhea (1% to 12%)
Neuromuscular & skeletal: Weakness (11%)

1% to 10%:
Cardiovascular: Bradycardia (2% to 10%), syncope (3% to 8%), peripheral edema (1% to 7%), generalized edema (5% to 6%), angina (2% to 6%), dependent edema (4%), AV block (3%), hypertension (3%), postural hypotension (2%), palpitation
Central nervous system: Headache (5% to 8%), fever (3%), somnolence (2%), insomnia (1% to 2%), malaise, hypoesthesia, vertigo
Endocrine & metabolic: Alkaline phosphatase increased, gout (6%), hypercholesterolemia (4%), dehydration (2%), hyperkalemia (3%), hypervolemia (2%), hypertriglyceridemia (1%), hyperuricemia, hypoglycemia, hyponatremia
Gastrointestinal: Nausea (2% to 9%), vomiting (6%), melena, periodontitis
Genitourinary: Hematuria (3%), impotence
Hematologic: Thrombocytopenia (1% to 2%), prothrombin decreased, purpura
Hepatic: Transaminases increased
Neuromuscular & skeletal: Back pain (2% to 7%), arthralgia (6%), myalgia (3%), muscle cramps, paresthesia (1%)
Ocular: Blurred vision (3% to 5%), lacrimation
Renal: BUN increased (6%), creatinine increased (3%), renal function abnormal, albuminuria, glycosuria, kidney failure
Respiratory: Cough increased (5%), nasopharyngitis (4%), rhinitis (2%), nasal congestion (1%), sinus congestion (1%)
Miscellaneous: Injury (3% to 6%), allergy, sudden death

Overdosage/Toxicology Symptoms include cardiac disturbances, CNS toxicity, bronchospasm, hypoglycemia, and hyperkalemia. The most common cardiac symptoms include hypotension and bradycardia. Atrioventricular block, intraventricular conduction disturbances, cardiogenic shock, and asystole may occur with severe overdose, especially with membrane-depressant drugs (eg, propranolol). CNS effects include convulsions, coma, and respiratory arrest, commonly seen with propranolol and other membrane-depressant and lipid-soluble drugs. Treatment is symptomatic for seizures, hypotension, hyperkalemia, and hypoglycemia. For excessive bradycardia: consider atropine. Bradycardia and hypotension resistant to atropine, isoproterenol, or pacing may respond to glucagon. Wide QRS defects caused by membrane-depressant poisoning may respond to hypertonic sodium bicarbonate. Repeat-dose charcoal, hemoperfusion, or hemodialysis may be helpful in removal of only those beta-blockers with a small V_d, long half-life, or low intrinsic clearance (acebutolol, atenolol, nadolol, sotalol).

Drug Interactions Substrate of CYP1A2 (minor), 2C9 (major), 2D6 (major), 2E1 (minor), 3A4 (minor)

Alpha-blockers (prazosin, terazosin): Concurrent use of beta-blockers may increase risk of orthostasis.

AV conduction-slowing agents (digoxin): Effects may be additive with beta-blockers.

Beta-agonists: Beta-blockers may counteract desired effects of beta-agonists.

Calcium channel blockers (nondihydropyridine): May enhance hypotensive effects of beta-blockers.

Cimetidine: May increase carvedilol serum levels.

CYP2C9 inducers: May decrease the levels/effects of carvedilol. Example inducers include carbamazepine, phenobarbital, phenytoin, rifampin, rifapentine, and secobarbital.

CYP2C9 Inhibitors may increase the levels/effects of carvedilol. Example inhibitors include delavirdine, fluconazole, gemfibrozil, ketoconazole, nicardipine, NSAIDs, sulfonamides and tolbutamide.

CYP2D6 inhibitors: May increase the levels/effects of carvedilol. Example inhibitors include chlorpromazine, delavirdine, fluoxetine, miconazole, paroxetine, pergolide, quinidine, quinine, ritonavir, and ropinirole.

Digoxin: Carvedilol may increase the serum levels of digoxin.

Disopyramide: May exacerbate heart failure or enhance bradycardic effect of beta-blockers.

Insulin and oral hypoglycemics: Carvedilol may mask symptoms of hypoglycemia.

NSAIDs (ibuprofen, indomethacin, naproxen, piroxicam) may reduce the antihypertensive effects of beta-blockers.

Rifampin: May increase the metabolism of carvedilol.

Salicylates: May reduce the antihypertensive effects of beta-blockers.

SSRIs: May decrease the metabolism of carvedilol.

Sulfonylureas: Beta-blockers may alter response to hypoglycemic agents.

Verapamil, diltiazem: May have synergistic or additive pharmacological effects when taken concurrently with beta-blockers.

Ethanol/Nutrition/Herb Interactions

Ethanol: Coreg CR™: Avoid ethanol (including prescription and over the counter medications containing ethanol). Ethanol may affect extended release properties causing a faster release; separate by at least 2 hours.

Food: Food decreases rate but not extent of absorption. Administration with food minimizes risks of orthostatic hypotension.

Herb/Nutraceutical: Avoid dong quai if using for hypertension (has estrogenic activity). Avoid ephedra, yohimbe, ginseng (may worsen hypertension). Avoid garlic (may have increased antihypertensive effect).

Stability Store at 15°C to 30°C (59°F to 86°F).

Mechanism of Action As a racemic mixture, carvedilol has nonselective beta-adrenoreceptor and alpha-adrenergic blocking activity. No intrinsic sympathomimetic activity has been documented. Associated effects in hypertensive patients include reduction of cardiac output, exercise- or beta-agonist-induced tachycardia, reduction of reflex orthostatic tachycardia, vasodilation, decreased peripheral vascular resistance (especially in standing position), decreased renal vascular resistance, reduced plasma renin activity, and increased levels of atrial natriuretic peptide. In CHF, associated effects include decreased pulmonary capillary wedge pressure, decreased pulmonary artery pressure, decreased heart rate, decreased systemic vascular resistance, increased stroke volume index, and decreased right arterial pressure (RAP).

Pharmacodynamics Onset of action: Within 1 hour of oral administration and blood pressure lowering effect is seen within 30 minutes of ingestion

Pharmacokinetics

Absorption: Rapid

Distribution: V_d: 115 L

Protein binding: <98%, primarily to albumin

Metabolism: First-pass metabolism; extensively hepatic; primarily by aromatic ring oxidation and glucuronidation (2% excreted unchanged); three active metabolites (4-hydroxyphenyl metabolite is 13 times more potent than parent drug for (Continued)

Carvedilol *(Continued)*

beta-blockade); plasma concentrations in older adults and those with cirrhotic liver disease are 50% and 4-7 times higher, respectively

Bioavailability: Immediate release: 25% to 35%; Extended release: 85% of immediate release

Half-life: 7-10 hours; older adults have serum concentrations 50% higher than young adults

Time to peak antihypertensive effect: ~1-2 hours

Elimination: Primarily via bile into feces as metabolites

Dosage

Geriatrics & Adults: Reduce dosage if heart rate drops to <55 beats/minute.

Hypertension: Oral:

Immediate release: 6.25 mg twice daily; if tolerated, dose should be maintained for 1-2 weeks, then increased to 12.5 mg twice daily. Dosage may be increased to a maximum of 25 mg twice daily after 1-2 weeks; maximum dose: 50 mg/day.

Extended release: Initial: 20 mg once daily, if tolerated, dose should be maintained for 1-2 weeks then increased to 40 mg once daily if necessary; maximum dose: 80 mg once daily

Congestive heart failure: Oral:

Immediate release: 3.125 mg twice daily for 2 weeks; if this dose is tolerated, may increase to 6.25 mg twice daily. Double the dose every 2 weeks to the highest dose tolerated by patient. (Prior to initiating therapy, other heart failure medications should be stabilized and fluid retention minimized.)

Maximum recommended dose:

Mild-to-moderate heart failure:

<85 kg: 25 mg twice daily

>85 kg: 50 mg twice daily

Severe heart failure: 25 mg twice daily

Extended release: Initial: 10 mg once daily for 2 weeks; if the dose is tolerated, increase dose to 20 mg, 40 mg, and 80 mg over successive intervals of at least 2 weeks. Maintain on lower dose if higher dose is not tolerated.

Left ventricular dysfunction following MI: Oral: **Note:** Should be initiated only after patient is hemodynamically stable and fluid retention has been minimized.

Immediate release: Initial 3.125-6.25 mg twice daily; increase dosage incrementally (ie, from 6.25-12.5 mg twice daily) at intervals of 3-10 days, based on tolerance, to a target dose of 25 mg twice daily.

Extended release: Initial: 20 mg once daily; increase dosage incrementally at intervals of 3-10 days. Target dose: 80 mg once daily.

Angina pectoris (unlabeled use): Oral: *Immediate release:* 25-50 mg twice daily

Conversion from immediate release to extended release (Coreg CR™):

Current dose immediate release tablets 3.125 mg twice daily: Convert to extended release capsules 10 mg once daily

Current dose immediate release tablets 6.25 mg twice daily: Convert to extended release capsules 20 mg once daily

Current dose immediate release tablets 12.5 mg twice daily: Convert to extended release capsules 40 mg once daily

Current dose immediate release tablets 25 mg twice daily: Convert to extended release capsules 80 mg once daily

Renal Impairment: None necessary

Hepatic Impairment: Use is contraindicated in severe liver dysfunction.

Administration Administer with food. Extended release capsules should not be crushed or chewed. Capsules may be opened and sprinkled on applesauce for immediate use.

Monitoring Parameters Heart rate, blood pressure (base need for dosage increase on trough blood pressure measurements and for tolerance on standing systolic pressure 1 hour after dosing); renal studies, BUN, liver function; in patient with increase risk for developing renal dysfunction, monitor during dosage titration.

Patient Information Should be taken with food to minimize the risk of hypotension; do not stop or interrupt use without a physician's advice; if dizziness and fainting occur, contact physician; avoid driving or hazardous work if experiencing dizziness or fainting; patients with contact lenses may experience decreased lacrimation

Additional Information Carvedilol should not be given to patients with severe hepatic failure; addition of a diuretic or adding carvedilol to diuretic therapy can result in exaggerated hypotension. Monitor closely upon initiation. Some studies have demonstrated a reduced risk of death, hospitalization in patients with CHF treated with digoxin, diuretics, and ACEI therapy.

Special Geriatric Considerations Due to alterations in the beta-adrenergic autonomic nervous system, beta-adrenergic blockade may result in less hemodynamic response than seen in younger adults. In U.S. trials conducted by the manufacturer, hypertension patients who were elderly (>65%) had a higher incidence of dizziness

(8.8% vs 6%) than seen in younger patients. No other differences noted between young and old in these trials.

Dosage Forms Excipient information presented when available (limited, particularly for generics); consult specific product labeling.

Capsule, extended release; as phosphate:
Coreg CR™: 10 mg, 20 mg, 40 mg, 80 mg
Tablet:
Coreg®: 3.125 mg, 6.25 mg, 12.5 mg, 25 mg

Selected References

Hunt HA, Baker DW, Chin MH, et al, "ACC/AHA Guidelines for the Evaluation and Management of Chronic Heart Failure in the Adult: Executive Summary A Report of the American College of Cardiology/American Heart Association Task Force on Practice Guidelines (Committee to Revise the 1995 Guidelines for the Evaluation and Management of Heart Failure): Developed in Collaboration With the International Society for Heart and Lung Transplantation; Endorsed by the Heart Failure Society of America," *Circulation* 2001, 104(24):2996-3007.

Packer M, Bristow MR, Cohn JN, et al, "The Effect of Carvedilol on Morbidity and Mortality in Patients With Chronic Heart Failure," *N Engl J Med*, 1996, 334(21):1349-55.

Packer M, Coats AJ, Fowler MB, et al, "Effect of Carvedilol on Survival in Severe Chronic Heart Failure," *N Engl J Med*, 2001, 344(22):1651-8.

Packer M, Colucci WS, Sackner-Bernstein JD, et al, "Double-Blind, Placebo-Controlled Study of the Effects of Carvedilol in Patients With Moderate to Severe Heart Failure. The PRECISE Trial. Prospective Randomized Evaluation of Carvedilol on Symptoms and Exercise," *Circulation*, 1996, 94(11):2793-9.

♦ **Casodex®** *see* Bicalutamide *on page 169*

Caspofungin (kas poe FUN jin)

U.S. Brand Names Cancidas®
Canadian Brand Names Cancidas®
Index Terms Caspofungin Acetate
Generic Available No
Pharmacologic Category Antifungal Agent, Parenteral; Echinocandin
Use Treatment of invasive *Aspergillus* infections in patients who are refractory or intolerant of other therapy; treatment of candidemia and other *Candida* infections (intra-abdominal abscesses, esophageal, peritonitis, pleural space); empirical treatment for presumed fungal infections in febrile neutropenic patient
Contraindications Hypersensitivity to caspofungin or any component of the formulation
Warnings/Precautions Concurrent use of cyclosporine should be limited to patients for whom benefit outweighs risk, due to a high frequency of hepatic transaminase elevations observed during concurrent use. Limited data are available concerning treatment durations longer than 4 weeks.
Adverse Reactions (Reflective of adult population; not specific for elderly)
>10%:
Central nervous system: Headache (up to 11%), fever (3% to 26%), chills (up to 14%)
Endocrine & metabolic: Hypokalemia (4% to 11%)
Hematologic: Hemoglobin decreased (1% to 12%)
Hepatic: Serum alkaline phosphatase increased (3% to 11%), transaminases increased (up to 13%)
Local: Infusion site reactions (2% to 12%), phlebitis/thrombophlebitis (up to 16%)
1% to 10%:
Cardiovascular: Flushing (2% to 3%), facial edema (up to 3%), hypertension (1% to 2%), tachycardia (1% to 2%), hypotension (1%)
Central nervous system: Dizziness (2%), pain (1% to 5%), insomnia (1%)
Dermatologic: Rash (<1% to 6%), pruritus (1% to 3%), erythema (1% to 2%)
Gastrointestinal: Nausea (2% to 6%), vomiting (1% to 4%), abdominal pain (1% to 4%), diarrhea (1% to 4%), anorexia (1%)
Hematologic: Eosinophils increased (3%), neutrophils decreased (2% to 3%), WBC decreased (5% to 6%), anemia (up to 4%), platelet count decreased (2% to 3%)
Hepatic: Bilirubin increased (3%)
Local: Induration (up to 3%)
Neuromuscular & skeletal: Myalgia (up to 3%), paresthesia (1% to 3%), tremor (≤2%)
Renal: Nephrotoxicity (8%)*, proteinuria (5%), hematuria (2%), serum creatinine increased (<1% to 4%), urinary WBCs increased (up to 8%), urinary RBCs increased (1% to 4%), blood urea nitrogen increased (1%)
*Nephrotoxicity defined as serum creatinine ≥2x baseline value or ≥1 mg/dL in patients with serum creatinine above ULN range (patients with Cl_{cr} <30 mL/minute were excluded)
Miscellaneous: Flu-like syndrome (3%), diaphoresis (up to 3%)
Overdosage/Toxicology No experience with overdosage has been reported. Caspofungin is not dialyzable. Treatment is symptomatic and supportive.
(Continued)

Caspofungin (Continued)

Drug Interactions

Cyclosporine: Concurrent administration may increase caspofungin concentrations. Serum hepatic transaminases may be increased. Limit use to patients for whom benefit outweighs risk.

Rifampin: May decrease caspofungin concentrations. Caspofungin dose should be 70 mg daily during concomitant therapy.

Tacrolimus: Caspofungin may decrease blood concentrations of tacrolimus; monitor.

Stability Store vials at 2°C to 8°C (36°F to 46°F). Reconstituted solution may be stored at less than 25°C (77°F) for 1 hour prior to preparation of infusion solution. Infusion solutions may be stored at less than 25°C (77°F) and should be used within 24 hours; up to 48 hours if stored at 2°C to 8°C (36°F to 46°F).

Bring refrigerated vial to room temperature. Reconstitute vials using 0.9% sodium chloride for injection, SWFI, or bacteriostatic water for injection. Mix gently until clear solution is formed; do not use if cloudy or contains particles. Solution should be further diluted with 0.9%, 0.45%, or 0.225% sodium chloride or LR.

Mechanism of Action Inhibits synthesis of β(1,3)-D-glucan, an essential component of the cell wall of susceptible fungi. Highest activity in regions of active cell growth. Mammalian cells do not require β(1,3)-D-glucan, limiting potential toxicity.

Pharmacokinetics

Protein binding: Albumin, 97%

Metabolism: Slowly, via hydrolysis and N-acetylation as well as by spontaneous degradation, with subsequent metabolism to component amino acids

Half-life: Beta phase (distribution): 9-11 hours; terminal: 40-50 hours

Elimination: Urine (41%) and feces (35%), with only small amounts as unchanged drug (1.4% of urinary excretion) - based on 27-day radiolabel collection

Dosage

Geriatrics & Adults: Note: Duration of caspofungin treatment should be determined by patient status and clinical response. Empiric therapy should be given until neutropenia resolves. In patients with positive cultures, treatment should continue until 14 days after last positive culture. In neutropenic patients, treatment should be given at least 7 days after both signs and symptoms of infection **and** neutropenia resolve.

Empiric therapy: I.V.: Initial dose: 70 mg on day 1; subsequent dosing: 50 mg/day; may increase up to 70 mg/day if tolerated, but clinical response is inadequate.

Invasive *Aspergillus*, candidiasis: I.V.: Initial dose: 70 mg on day 1; subsequent dosing: 50 mg/day

Esophageal candidiasis: I.V.: 50 mg/day; **Note:** The majority of patients studied for this indication also had oropharyngeal involvement.

Dosage adjustment with concomitant use of an enzyme inducer:

Patients receiving rifampin: 70 mg caspofungin daily

Patients receiving carbamazepine, dexamethasone, efavirenz, nevirapine, or phenytoin (and possibly other enzyme inducers) may require an increased daily dose of caspofungin (70 mg/day).

Renal Impairment: No specific dosage adjustment is required; supplemental dose is not required following dialysis.

Hepatic Impairment:

Mild hepatic insufficiency (Child-Pugh score 5-6): No adjustment necessary.

Moderate hepatic insufficiency (Child-Pugh score 7-9): 35 mg/day; initial 70 mg loading dose should still be administered in treatment of invasive infections.

Severe hepatic insufficiency (Child-Pugh score >9): No clinical experience.

Administration Infuse slowly, over 1 hour; monitor during infusion. Isolated cases of possible histamine-related reactions have occurred during clinical trials (rash, flushing, pruritus, facial edema). Do not coadminister with other medications; do not mix with dextrose-containing solutions.

Patient Information This drug can only be administered I.V., and therapy may take several days to weeks. During infusion, report immediately any chills, chest pain, difficulty breathing, tightness in throat, or other adverse reaction. You may experience nausea or vomiting (small frequent meals, frequent mouth care, sucking lozenges, or chewing gum may help). Report any skin rash, changes in color of urine or stool, persistent GI distress, alteration in voiding or bowel patterns, pain at injection site, or other adverse reactions.

Special Geriatric Considerations The number of patients >65 years of age in clinical studies was not sufficient to establish whether a difference in response may be anticipated.

Dosage Forms Excipient information presented when available (limited, particularly for generics); consult specific product labeling.

Injection, powder for reconstitution, as acetate: 50 mg [contains sucrose 39 mg], 70 mg [contains sucrose 54 mg]

Selected References
Pappas PG, Rex JH, Sobel JD, et al, "Guidelines for Treatment of Candidiasis," *Clin Infect Dis*, 2004, 38:161-89.

♦ **Caspofungin Acetate** *see* Caspofungin *on page 247*

Castor Oil (KAS tor oyl)

Index Terms Oleum Ricini
Generic Available Yes: Oil
Pharmacologic Category Laxative, Miscellaneous
Use Preparation for rectal or bowel examination or surgery; occasionally used to relieve constipation; topical emollient and protectant
Contraindications Known hypersensitivity to castor oil; nausea, vomiting, abdominal pain, fecal impaction, GI bleeding, appendicitis, congestive heart failure, dehydration
Warnings/Precautions Castor oil induces a strong purgative action and therefore should not be used for routine treatment of constipation
Adverse Reactions (Reflective of adult population; not specific for elderly) Frequency not defined.
Cardiovascular: Hypotension
Central nervous system: Dizziness
Endocrine & metabolic: Electrolyte disturbance
Gastrointestinal: Abdominal cramps, nausea, diarrhea
Genitourinary: Pelvic congestion
Drug Interactions No data reported
Stability Protect from heat.
Mechanism of Action Acts primarily in the small intestine; hydrolyzed to ricinoleic acid which reduces net absorption of fluid and electrolytes and stimulates peristalsis
Pharmacodynamics Onset of action: Oral: 2-6 hours after dose
Dosage
Geriatrics & Adults: Bowel evacuation, constipation: Oil: Oral: 15-60 mL as a single dose
Administration Do not administer at bedtime because of rapid onset of action
Monitoring Parameters Monitor number of stools per day; consistency, fluid status, and blood pressure if fluid loss is excessive
Patient Information Laxative use should be short-term (<7 days); discontinue use when bowel regularity returns; notify physician if constipation is unrelieved, blood appears in stool, or if dizziness, muscle weakness, or cramping is experienced; take with full glass of water or juice; maintain adequate fluid intake
Special Geriatric Considerations Elderly are often predisposed to constipation due to disease, immobility, drugs, low residue diets, and a decreased fluid intake usually due to a decreased "thirst reflex" with age. Avoid stimulant cathartic use on a chronic basis if possible. Use osmotic, lubricant, stool softeners, and bulk agents as prophylaxis. Patients should be instructed for proper dietary fiber and fluid intake as well as regular exercise. Monitor closely for fluid/electrolyte imbalance, CNS signs of fluid/electrolyte loss, and hypotension. Strong and chronic purging may cause severe fluid and electrolyte loss which may affect mental function (CNS). Not a drug of first choice for constipation in the elderly.
Dosage Forms Excipient information presented when available (limited, particularly for generics); consult specific product labeling.
Oil, oral: 100% (60 mL, 120 mL, 180 mL, 480 mL, 3840 mL)

♦ **Castor Oil, Trypsin, and Balsam Peru** *see* Trypsin, Balsam Peru, and Castor Oil *on page 1642*
♦ **Cataflam®** *see* Diclofenac *on page 424*
♦ **Catapres®** *see* Clonidine *on page 342*
♦ **Catapres-TTS®** *see* Clonidine *on page 342*
♦ **Cathflo® Activase®** *see* Alteplase *on page 60*
♦ **Caverject®** *see* Alprostadil *on page 57*
♦ **Caverject Impulse®** *see* Alprostadil *on page 57*
♦ **CaviRinse™** *see* Fluoride *on page 642*
♦ **CB-1348** *see* Chlorambucil *on page 287*
♦ **CBZ** *see* Carbamazepine *on page 231*
♦ **CDX** *see* Bicalutamide *on page 169*
♦ **Cecon® [OTC]** *see* Ascorbic Acid *on page 125*
♦ **Cedax®** *see* Ceftibuten *on page 270*
♦ **CEE** *see* Estrogens (Conjugated/Equine) *on page 564*

Cefaclor (SEF a klor)

Related Information
Antimicrobial Activity Against Selected Organisms *on page 1728*

Medication Safety Issues
Sound-alike/look-alike issues:
Cefaclor may be confused with cephalexin

U.S. Brand Names Raniclor™

Canadian Brand Names Apo-Cefaclor®; Ceclor®; Novo-Cefaclor; Nu-Cefaclor; PMS-Cefaclor

Generic Available Yes: Excludes chewable tablet

Pharmacologic Category Antibiotic, Cephalosporin (Second Generation)

Use Treatment of susceptible bacterial infections including otitis media, lower respiratory tract infections, acute exacerbations of chronic bronchitis, pharyngitis and tonsillitis, urinary tract infections, skin and skin structure infections

Contraindications Hypersensitivity to cefaclor, any component of the formulation, or other cephalosporins

Warnings/Precautions Modify dosage in patients with severe renal impairment. Prolonged use may result in fungal or bacterial superinfection, including *C. difficile*-associated diarrhea and pseudomembranous colitis. Use with caution in patients with a history of penicillin allergy, especially IgE-mediated reactions (eg, anaphylaxis, urticaria). Beta-lactamase-negative, ampicillin-resistant (BLNAR) strains of *H. influenzae* should be considered resistant to cefaclor. Some products may contain phenylalanine.

Adverse Reactions (Reflective of adult population; not specific for elderly)
1% to 10%:
Dermatologic: Rash (maculopapular, erythematous, or morbilliform) (1% to 2%)
Gastrointestinal: Diarrhea (3%)
Genitourinary: Vaginitis (2%)
Hematologic: Eosinophilia (2%)
Hepatic: Transaminases increased (3%)
Miscellaneous: Moniliasis (2%)
Reactions reported with other cephalosporins: Fever, abdominal pain, superinfection, renal dysfunction, toxic nephropathy, hemorrhage, cholestasis

Overdosage/Toxicology Symptoms of overdose include diarrhea, epigastric distress, nausea, and vomiting. Many beta-lactam antibiotics have the potential to cause neuromuscular hyperirritability or seizures. Hemodialysis may be helpful to aid in removal of the drug from the blood, but is not usually indicated; otherwise, most treatment is supportive and symptom-directed.

Drug Interactions
Aminoglycosides: May be additive to nephrotoxicity.
Furosemide: May be additive to nephrotoxicity.
Probenecid: May decrease cephalosporin elimination.

Ethanol/Nutrition/Herb Interactions
Food: Cefaclor serum levels may be decreased slightly if taken with food. The bioavailability of cefaclor extended release tablets is decreased 23% and the maximum concentration is decreased 67% when taken on an empty stomach.

Stability Store at controlled room temperature. Refrigerate suspension after reconstitution. Discard after 14 days. Do not freeze.

Mechanism of Action Inhibits bacterial cell wall synthesis by binding to one or more of the penicillin-binding proteins (PBPs) which in turn inhibits the final transpeptidation step of peptidoglycan synthesis in bacterial cell walls, thus inhibiting cell wall biosynthesis. Bacteria eventually lyse due to ongoing activity of cell wall autolytic enzymes (autolysins and murein hydrolases) while cell wall assembly is arrested.

Pharmacokinetics
Absorption: Oral: Acid stable, well absorbed
Half-life: 30-60 minutes (prolonged with renal impairment)
Time to peak serum concentration: Within 30-60 minutes
Elimination: Most of a dose (80%) is excreted unchanged in urine

Dosage
Geriatrics & Adults: Treatment of infections: Oral: Dosing range: 250-500 mg every 8 hours

Renal Impairment:
Cl_{cr} 10-50 mL/minute: Administer 50% to 100% of dose
Cl_{cr} <10 mL/minute: Administer 50% of dose
Hemodialysis: Moderately dialyzable (20% to 50%)

Administration Administer around-the-clock to promote less variation in peak and trough serum levels.
Chewable tablet: Should be chewed before swallowing; should not be swallowed whole

Extended release tablet: Should not be cut, crushed, or chewed; should be administered with food

Oral suspension: Shake well before using.

Monitoring Parameters Signs and symptoms of infections, including mental status

Test Interactions Positive direct Coombs', false-positive urinary glucose test using cupric sulfate (Benedict's solution, Clinitest®, Fehling's solution), false-positive serum or urine creatinine with Jaffé reaction

Patient Information Complete full course of therapy; may take with food or milk

Special Geriatric Considerations Has not been studied in the elderly. Adjust dose for renal function in elderly. Considered to be one of the drugs of choice in the outpatient treatment of community-acquired pneumonia in elderly.

Dosage Forms Excipient information presented when available (limited, particularly for generics); consult specific product labeling.

Capsule: 250 mg, 500 mg

Powder for oral suspension: 125 mg/5 mL (75 mL, 150 mL); 250 mg/5 mL (75 mL, 150 mL); 375 mg/5 mL (50 mL, 100 mL)

Tablet, chewable:

Raniclor™: 250 mg [contains phenylalanine 5.6 mg/tablet and tartrazine; fruity flavor]; 375 mg [contains phenylalanine 8.4 mg/tablet and tartrazine; fruity flavor]

Tablet, extended release: 500 mg

Selected References

American Thoracic Society, "Guidelines for the Initial Management of Adults With Community-Acquired Pneumonia: Diagnosis, Assessment of Severity, and Initial Antimicrobial Therapy," *Am Rev Respir Dis*, 1993, 148(5):1418-26.

Cefadroxil (sef a DROKS il)

Related Information

Antimicrobial Activity Against Selected Organisms *on page 1728*

Prevention of Infective Endocarditis *on page 1803*

U.S. Brand Names Duricef®

Canadian Brand Names Apo-Cefadroxil®; Duricef®; Novo-Cefadroxil

Index Terms Cefadroxil Monohydrate

Generic Available Yes

Pharmacologic Category Antibiotic, Cephalosporin (First Generation)

Use Treatment of susceptible bacterial infections, including those caused by group A beta-hemolytic *Streptococcus*

Contraindications Hypersensitivity to cefadroxil, other cephalosporins, or any component of the formulation

Warnings/Precautions Modify dosage in patients with severe renal impairment. Use with caution in patients with a history of penicillin allergy, especially IgE-mediated reactions (eg, anaphylaxis, urticaria). Prolonged use may result in fungal or bacterial superinfection, including *C. difficile*-associated diarrhea and pseudomembranous colitis.

Adverse Reactions (Reflective of adult population; not specific for elderly)

1% to 10%: Gastrointestinal: Diarrhea

Reactions reported with other cephalosporins: Toxic epidermal necrolysis, abdominal pain, superinfection, renal dysfunction, toxic nephropathy, aplastic anemia, hemolytic anemia, hemorrhage, prothrombin time prolonged, BUN increased, creatinine increased, eosinophilia, pancytopenia, seizure

Overdosage/Toxicology After acute overdose, most agents cause only nausea, vomiting, and diarrhea, although neuromuscular hypersensitivity and seizures are possible, especially in patients with renal insufficiency. Many beta-lactam antibiotics have the potential to cause neuromuscular hyperirritability or seizures. Hemodialysis may be helpful to aid in removal of the drug from the blood, but is not usually indicated; otherwise, most treatment is supportive or symptom-directed, following GI decontamination.

Drug Interactions

Increased effect: Probenecid may decrease cephalosporin elimination.

Increased toxicity: Furosemide, aminoglycosides may be a possible additive to nephrotoxicity.

Ethanol/Nutrition/Herb Interactions Food: Concomitant administration with food or cow's milk does **not** significantly affect absorption.

Stability Refrigerate suspension after reconstitution; discard after 14 days.

Mechanism of Action Inhibits bacterial cell wall synthesis by binding to one or more of the penicillin-binding proteins (PBPs) which in turn inhibits the final transpeptidation step of peptidoglycan synthesis in bacterial cell walls, thus inhibiting cell wall biosynthesis. Bacteria eventually lyse due to ongoing activity of cell wall autolytic enzymes (autolysins and murein hydrolases) while cell wall assembly is arrested.

Pharmacokinetics

Absorption: Oral: Rapidly and well absorbed from GI tract

(Continued)

Cefadroxil *(Continued)*

Distribution: V_d: 0.31 L/kg
Protein binding: 20%
Half-life: 1-2 hours; in renal failure, the half-life increases to 20-24 hours
Time to peak serum concentration: Within 70-90 minutes
Elimination: >90% of dose excreted unchanged in urine within 8 hours
Effects of aging on the pharmacokinetics of cefadroxil are not well studied; only older patients with impaired renal function have been studied

Dosage
Geriatrics & Adults:
Susceptible infections: Oral: 1-2 g/day in 2 divided doses
Prophylaxis against bacterial endocarditis: Oral: 2 g 1 hour prior to the procedure
Renal Impairment:
Cl_{cr} 10-25 mL/minute: Administer every 24 hours.
Cl_{cr} <10 mL/minute: Administer every 36 hours.

Monitoring Parameters Signs and symptoms of infection, including mental status

Test Interactions Positive direct Coombs', false-positive urinary glucose test using cupric sulfate (Benedict's solution, Clinitest®, Fehling's solution), false-positive serum or urine creatinine with Jaffé reaction

Patient Information Complete full course of therapy; can be taken with food or milk; report persistent diarrhea to physician

Special Geriatric Considerations Adjust dose for renal function in the elderly.

Dosage Forms Excipient information presented when available (limited, particularly for generics); consult specific product labeling.
Capsule, as monohydrate: 500 mg
Powder for oral suspension, as monohydrate: 250 mg/5 mL (100 mL); 500 mg/5 mL (75 mL, 100 mL)
Duricef®: 250 mg/5 mL (50 mL, 100 mL); 500 mg/5 mL (75 mL, 100 mL) [contains sodium benzoate; orange-pineapple flavor]
Tablet, as monohydrate: 1 g

Selected References
Cutler RE, Blair AD, and Kelly MR, "Cefadroxil Kinetics in Patients With Renal Insufficiency," *Clin Pharmacol Ther*, 1979, 25(5 Pt 1):514-21.

♦ **Cefadroxil Monohydrate** *see* Cefadroxil *on page 251*

Cefazolin (sef A zoe lin)

Related Information
Antibiotic Treatment of Adults With Infective Endocarditis *on page 1797*
Antimicrobial Activity Against Selected Organisms *on page 1728*
Prevention of Infective Endocarditis *on page 1803*
Medication Safety Issues
Sound-alike/look-alike issues:
Cefazolin may be confused with cefprozil, cephalexin, cephalothin
Kefzol® may be confused with Cefzil®
Index Terms Cefazolin Sodium
Generic Available Yes
Pharmacologic Category Antibiotic, Cephalosporin (First Generation)
Use Treatment of respiratory tract, skin and skin structure, genital, urinary tract, biliary tract, bone and joint infections, and septicemia due to susceptible gram-positive cocci (except enterococcus); some gram-negative bacilli including *E. coli*, *Proteus*, and *Klebsiella* may be susceptible; perioperative prophylaxis
Unlabeled/Investigational Use Prophylaxis against bacterial endocarditis
Contraindications Hypersensitivity to cefazolin sodium, any component of the formulation, or other cephalosporins
Warnings/Precautions Modify dosage in patients with severe renal impairment. Use with caution in patients with a history of penicillin allergy, especially IgE-mediated reactions (eg, anaphylaxis, angioedema, urticaria). Prolonged use may result in fungal or bacterial superinfection, including *C. difficile*-associated diarrhea and pseudomembranous colitis. May be associated with increased INR, especially in nutritionally-deficient patients, prolonged treatment, hepatic or renal disease. Use with caution in patients with a history of seizure disorder; high levels, particularly in the presence of renal impairment, may increase risk of seizures.
Adverse Reactions (Reflective of adult population; not specific for elderly)
Frequency not defined.
Central nervous system: Fever, seizure
Dermatologic: Rash, pruritus, Stevens-Johnson syndrome
Gastrointestinal: Diarrhea, nausea, vomiting, abdominal cramps, anorexia, pseudomembranous colitis, oral candidiasis
Genitourinary: Vaginitis

Hepatic: Transaminases increased, hepatitis

Hematologic: Eosinophilia, neutropenia, leukopenia, thrombocytopenia, thrombocytosis

Local: Pain at injection site, phlebitis

Renal: BUN increased, serum creatinine increased, renal failure

Miscellaneous: Anaphylaxis

Reactions reported with other cephalosporins: Toxic epidermal necrolysis, abdominal pain, cholestasis, superinfection, toxic nephropathy, aplastic anemia, hemolytic anemia, hemorrhage, prothrombin time prolonged, pancytopenia

Overdosage/Toxicology Symptoms include neuromuscular hypersensitivity and convulsions especially with renal insufficiency. Many beta-lactam antibiotics have the potential to cause neuromuscular hyperirritability or seizures. Hemodialysis may be helpful to aid in removal of the drug from the blood; otherwise, most treatment is supportive or symptom-directed.

Drug Interactions

Aminoglycosides: Aminoglycosides increase nephrotoxic potential.

Probenecid: High-dose probenecid decreases clearance.

Warfarin: Cefazolin may increase the hypothrombinemic response to warfarin (due to alteration of GI microbial flora).

Stability Store intact vials at room temperature and protect from temperatures exceeding 40°C. Dilute large vial with 2.5 mL SWFI; 10 g vial may be diluted with 45 mL to yield 1 g/5 mL or 96 mL to yield 1 g/10 mL. May be injected or further dilution for I.V. administration in 50-100 mL compatible solution. Standard diluent is 1 g/50 mL D_5W or 2 g/50 mL D_5W.

Reconstituted solutions of cefazolin are light yellow to yellow. Protection from light is recommended for the powder and for the reconstituted solutions. Reconstituted solutions are stable for 24 hours at room temperature and for 10 days under refrigeration. Stability of parenteral admixture at room temperature (25°C) is 48 hours. Stability of parenteral admixture at refrigeration temperature (4°C) is 14 days.

DUPLEX™: Store at 20°C to 25°C (68°F to 77°F); excursions permitted to 15°C to 30°C (59°F to 86°F) prior to activation. Following activation, stable for 24 hours at room temperature and for 7 days under refrigeration.

Mechanism of Action Inhibits bacterial cell wall synthesis by binding to one or more of the penicillin-binding proteins (PBPs) which in turn inhibits the final transpeptidation step of peptidoglycan synthesis in bacterial cell walls, thus inhibiting cell wall biosynthesis. Bacteria eventually lyse due to ongoing activity of cell wall autolytic enzymes (autolysins and murein hydrolases) while cell wall assembly is arrested.

Pharmacokinetics

Distribution: V_d: No change

Protein binding: 74% to 86%

Metabolism: Hepatic metabolism is minimal

Half-life: 90-150 minutes (prolonged with renal impairment); mean half-life was twice as long, 3.5 hours, and mean total clearance was reduced by 50% in older adults compared to younger adults

CSF penetration is poor

Time to peak serum concentration:

I.M.: Within 30 minutes to 2 hours

I.V.: Within 5 minutes

Elimination: 80% to 100% excreted unchanged in urine

Dosage

Geriatrics & Adults:

Usual dosage range: I.M., I.V.: 1-2 g every 8 hours, depending on severity of infection; maximum: 12 g/day

Mild-to-moderate infections: 500 mg to 1 g every 6-8 hours

Mild infection with gram-positive cocci: 250-500 mg every 8 hours

Perioperative prophylaxis: 1 g given 30 minutes prior to surgery (repeat with 500 mg to 1 g during prolonged surgery); followed by 500 mg to 1 g every 6-9 hours for 24 hours postop

Pneumococcal pneumonia: 500 mg every 12 hours

Severe infection: 1-2 g every 6 hours

Prophylaxis against bacterial endocarditis (unlabeled use): 1 g 30 minutes before procedure

UTI (uncomplicated): 1 g every 12 hours

Renal Impairment:

Cl_{cr} 10-30 mL/minute: Administer every 12 hours.

Cl_{cr} <10 mL/minute: Administer every 24 hours.

Moderately dialyzable (20% to 50%); administer dose postdialysis or administer supplemental dose of 0.5-1 g after dialysis.

Peritoneal dialysis: Administer 0.5 g every 12 hours.

Continuous arteriovenous or venovenous hemofiltration: Dose as for Cl_{cr} 10-30 mL/minute. Removes 30 mg of cefazolin per liter of filtrate per day.

(Continued)

Cefazolin *(Continued)*

Monitoring Parameters Signs and symptoms of infection; WBC, mental status

Test Interactions Positive direct Coombs', false-positive urinary glucose test using cupric sulfate (Benedict's solution, Clinitest®, Fehling's solution), false-positive serum or urine creatinine with Jaffé reaction.

Some penicillin derivatives may accelerate the degradation of aminoglycosides *in vitro*, leading to a potential underestimation of aminoglycoside serum concentration.

Additional Information Sodium content of 1 g: 48 mg (2 mEq)

Special Geriatric Considerations Adjust dose for renal function.

Dosage Forms Excipient information presented when available (limited, particularly for generics); consult specific product labeling.
Infusion [premixed in D$_5$W]: 1 g (50 mL)
Injection, powder for reconstitution: 500 mg, 1 g, 10 g, 20 g

Selected References
Simon VC, Malerczyk V, Tenschert B, et al, "Die Geriatrische Pharmakologie von Cefazolin, Cefradin, und Sulfisomidin," *Arzneim Forsch*, 1976, 26(7):1377-82.

♦ **Cefazolin Sodium** see Cefazolin *on page 252*

Cefdinir *(SEF di ner)*

U.S. Brand Names Omnicef®
Canadian Brand Names Omnicef®
Index Terms CFDN
Generic Available No
Pharmacologic Category Antibiotic, Cephalosporin (Third Generation)

Use Treatment of community-acquired pneumonia, acute exacerbations of chronic bronchitis, acute bacterial otitis media, acute maxillary sinusitis, pharyngitis/tonsillitis, and uncomplicated skin and skin structure infections

Contraindications Hypersensitivity to cefdinir, other cephalosporins, related antibiotics, or any component of the formulation

Warnings/Precautions Administer cautiously to penicillin-sensitive patients, especially IgE-mediated reactions (eg, anaphylaxis, urticaria). Prolonged use may result in fungal or bacterial superinfection, including *C. difficile*-associated diarrhea and pseudomembranous colitis. Use caution with renal dysfunction; dose adjustment may be required.

Adverse Reactions (Reflective of adult population; not specific for elderly)
>10%: Gastrointestinal: Diarrhea (8% to 15%)
1% to 10%:
   Central nervous system: Headache (2%)
   Dermatologic: Rash (≤3%)
   Gastrointestinal: Nausea (≤3%), abdominal pain (≤1%), vomiting (≤1%)
   Genitourinary: Vaginal moniliasis (≤4%), urine leukocytes increased (2%), urine protein increased (1% to 2%), vaginitis (≤1%)
   Hematologic: Eosinophils increased (1%)
   Hepatic: Alkaline phosphatase increased (≤1%), platelets increased (1%)
   Renal: Microhematuria (1%)
   Miscellaneous: Lymphocytes increased (≤2%), GGT increased (1%), lactate dehydrogenase increased (≤1%), bicarbonate decreased (≤1%), lymphocytes decreased (≤1%), PMN changes (≤1%)
Reactions reported with other cephalosporins: Dizziness, fever, encephalopathy, asterixis, neuromuscular excitability, seizure, aplastic anemia, interstitial nephritis, toxic nephropathy, angioedema, hemorrhage, PT prolonged, and superinfection

Overdosage/Toxicology After acute overdose, most agents cause only nausea, vomiting, and diarrhea, although neuromuscular hypersensitivity and seizures are possible, especially in patients with renal insufficiency. Hemodialysis may be helpful to aid in the removal of the drug from the blood but not usually indicated, otherwise, most treatment is supportive or symptom-directed following GI decontamination.

Drug Interactions
Antacids: May reduce the rate and extent of cefdinir absorption; separate dosing by 2 hours.
Iron: May reduce the rate and extent of cefdinir absorption. Separate dosing by 2 hours.
Probenecid: May increase the effects of cefdinir by decreasing renal elimination. Peak plasma levels of cefdinir are increased by 54% and half-life is prolonged by 50%.

Stability Capsules and unmixed powder should be stored at room temperature of 25°C (77°F). Oral suspension should be mixed with 38 mL water for the 60 mL bottle and 63 mL of water for the 120 mL bottle. After mixing, the suspension can be stored at room temperature of 25°C (77°F) for 10 days.

Mechanism of Action Inhibits bacterial cell wall synthesis by binding to one or more of the penicillin-binding proteins (PBPs) which in turn inhibits the final transpeptidation

step of peptidoglycan synthesis in bacterial cell walls, thus inhibiting cell wall biosynthesis. Bacteria eventually lyse due to ongoing activity of cell wall autolytic enzymes (autolysins and murein hydrolases) while cell wall assembly is arrested.

Pharmacokinetics
Distribution: V_d: Adults: 0.06-0.64 L/kg
Protein binding: 60% to 70%
Metabolism: Minimally hepatic
Bioavailability: Capsule: 16% to 21%; suspension 25%
Half-life elimination: 100 minutes
Excretion: Primarily urine

Dosage
Geriatrics & Adults:
Acute exacerbations of chronic bronchitis, pharyngitis/tonsillitis: Oral: 300 mg twice daily for 5-10 days **or** 600 mg once daily for 10 days
Acute maxillary sinusitis: Oral: 300 mg twice daily **or** 600 mg once daily for 10 days
Community-acquired pneumonia, uncomplicated skin and skin structure infections: Oral: 300 mg twice daily for 10 days
Renal Impairment: Adults: 300 mg once daily

Monitoring Parameters Culture and sensitivity, if available; signs and symptoms of infection; mental status

Special Geriatric Considerations Cefdinir has not been studied exclusively in the elderly. Patients ≥65 years of age have been included in clinical. No information is available on their response or tolerance.

Dosage Forms Excipient information presented when available (limited, particularly for generics); consult specific product labeling.
Capsule:
Omicef®: 300 mg
Powder for oral suspension:
Omicef®: 125 mg/5 mL (60 mL, 100 mL) [contains sodium benzoate and sucrose 2.86 g/5 mL; strawberry flavor]; 250 mg/5 mL (60 mL, 100 mL) [contains sodium benzoate and sucrose 2.86 g/5 mL; strawberry flavor]

Cefditoren (sef de TOR en)

Medication Safety Issues
International issues:
Spectracef® may be confused with Spectrocef® which is a brand name for cefotaxime in Italy

U.S. Brand Names Spectracef®

Index Terms Cefditoren Pivoxil

Generic Available No

Pharmacologic Category Antibiotic, Cephalosporin

Use Treatment of acute bacterial exacerbation of chronic bronchitis (due to susceptible organisms including *Haemophilus influenzae*, *Haemophilus parainfluenzae*, *Streptococcus pneumoniae*-penicillin susceptible only, *Moraxella catarrhalis*); pharyngitis or tonsillitis (*Streptococcus pyogenes*); uncomplicated infections of skin and skin structure (*Staphylococcus aureus*-not MRSA, *Streptococcus pyogenes*)

Contraindications Hypersensitivity to cefditoren, other cephalosporins, milk protein, or any component of the formulation; carnitine deficiency

Warnings/Precautions Use with caution in patients with a history of penicillin allergy, especially IgE-mediated reactions (eg, anaphylaxis, urticaria). Prolonged use may result in fungal or bacterial superinfection, including *C. difficile*-associated diarrhea and pseudomembranous colitis. Caution in individuals with seizure disorders; high levels, particularly in the presence of renal impairment, may increase risk of seizures. Use caution in patients with renal or hepatic impairment; modify dosage in patients with severe renal impairment. Cefditoren causes renal excretion of carnitine; do not use in patients with carnitine deficiency; not for long-term therapy due to the possible development of carnitine deficiency over time. May prolong prothrombin time; use with caution in patients with a history of bleeding disorder. Cefditoren tablets contain sodium caseinate, which may cause hypersensitivity reactions in patients with milk protein hypersensitivity; this does not affect patients with lactose intolerance.

Adverse Reactions (Reflective of adult population; not specific for elderly)
>10%: Gastrointestinal: Diarrhea (11% to 15%)
1% to 10%:
Central nervous system: Headache (2% to 3%)
Endocrine & metabolic: Glucose increased (1% to 2%)
Gastrointestinal: Nausea (4% to 6%), abdominal pain (2%), dyspepsia (1% to 2%), vomiting (1%)
Genitourinary: Vaginal moniliasis (3% to 6%)
Hematologic: Hematocrit decreased (2%)
(Continued)

Cefditoren *(Continued)*

Renal: Hematuria (3%), urinary white blood cells increased (2%)

Reactions reported with other cephalosporins: Anaphylaxis, aplastic anemia, cholestasis, hemorrhage, hemolytic anemia, renal dysfunction, reversible hyperactivity, serum sickness-like reaction, toxic nephropathy

Drug Interactions

Probenecid: Serum concentration of cefditoren may be increased.

Warfarin: Prothrombin time may be prolonged by cefditoren; monitor.

Ethanol/Nutrition/Herb Interactions Food: Moderate- to high-fat meals increase bioavailability and maximum plasma concentration.

Stability Store at controlled room temperature of 15°C to 30°C (59°F to 86°F). Protect from light and moisture.

Mechanism of Action Inhibits bacterial cell wall synthesis by binding to one or more of the penicillin binding proteins (PBPs) which in turn inhibits the final transpeptidation step of peptidoglycan synthesis in bacterial cell walls, thus inhibiting cell wall biosynthesis. Bacteria eventually lyse due to ongoing activity of cell wall autolytic enzymes (autolysins and murein hydrolases) while cell wall assembly is arrested.

Pharmacokinetics

Distribution: 9.3 ± 1.6 L

Protein binding: 88% (*in vitro*), primarily to albumin

Metabolism: Cefditoren pivoxil is hydrolyzed to cefditoren (active) and pivalate

Bioavailability: ~14% to 16%, increased by moderate to high-fat meal

Half-life: 1.6 ± 0.4 hours

Time to peak: 1.5-3 hours

Elimination: Urine as cefditoren and pivaloylcarnitine

Dosage

Geriatrics & Adults:

Acute bacterial exacerbation of chronic bronchitis: Oral: 400 mg twice daily for 10 days

Community-acquired pneumonia: Oral: 400 mg twice daily for 14 days

Dental infections (unlabeled use): Oral: 400 mg twice daily for 10 days

Pharyngitis, tonsillitis, uncomplicated skin and skin structure infections: Oral: 200 mg twice daily for 10 days

Renal Impairment:

Cl_{cr} 30-49 mL/minute/1.73 m^2: Maximum dose: 200 mg twice daily

Cl_{cr} <30 mL/minute/1.73 m^2: Maximum dose: 200 mg once daily

End-stage renal disease: Appropriate dosing not established

Hepatic Impairment:

Mild-to-moderate impairment: Adjustment not required

Severe impairment (Child-Pugh class C): Specific guidelines not available

Administration Should be administered with meals.

Monitoring Parameters Assess patient at beginning and throughout therapy for infection; monitor for signs of anaphylaxis during first dose.

Test Interactions May induce a positive direct Coomb's test. May cause a false-negative ferricyanide test. Glucose oxidase or hexokinase methods recommended for blood/plasma glucose determinations. False-positive urine glucose test when using copper reduction based assays (eg, Clinitest®).

Patient Information Notify prescriber if you are allergic to any other antibiotics, if you have a carnitine deficiency, or if you have milk protein hypersensitivity. Take as directed, at regular intervals around-the-clock (with food). Complete full course of medication, even if you feel better. Do not take with antacids. Maintain adequate hydration (2-3 L/day of fluids unless instructed to restrict fluid intake). If diarrhea occurs, yogurt or buttermilk may help. May cause false-positive test with Clinitest®; use another form of testing. Report severe, unresolved diarrhea; vaginal itching or drainage; sores in mouth; blood, pus, or mucus in stool or urine; easy bleeding or bruising; unusual fever or chills, rash; or respiratory difficulty.

Special Geriatric Considerations No dose adjustment is necessary for patients with normal age-adjusted renal function.

Dosage Forms Excipient information presented when available (limited, particularly for generics); consult specific product labeling.

Tablet: Spectracef®: 200 mg [contains sodium caseinate]

♦ **Cefditoren Pivoxil** *see Cefditoren on page 255*

Cefepime *(SEF e pim)*

Related Information

Antimicrobial Activity Against Selected Organisms *on page 1728*

U.S. Brand Names Maxipime®

Canadian Brand Names Maxipime®
Index Terms Cefepime Hydrochloride
Generic Available No
Pharmacologic Category Antibiotic, Cephalosporin (Fourth Generation)
Use Treatment of uncomplicated and complicated urinary tract infections, including pyelonephritis caused by typical urinary tract pathogens; monotherapy for febrile neutropenia; uncomplicated skin and skin structure infections caused by *Streptococcus pyogenes*; moderate to severe pneumonia caused by pneumococcus, *Pseudomonas aeruginosa*, and other gram-negative organisms; complicated intra-abdominal infections (in combination with metronidazole). Also active against methicillin-susceptible staphylococci, *Enterobacter* sp, and many other gram-negative bacilli.
Contraindications Hypersensitivity to cefepime, any component of the formulation, or other cephalosporins
Warnings/Precautions Modify dosage in patients with severe renal impairment; use with caution in patients with a history of penicillin or cephalosporin allergy, especially IgE-mediated reactions (eg, anaphylaxis, urticaria). Prolonged use may result in fungal or bacterial superinfection, including *C. difficile*-associated diarrhea and pseudomembranous colitis. May be associated with increased INR, especially in nutritionally-deficient patients, prolonged treatment, hepatic or renal disease. Use with caution in patients with a history of seizure disorder; high levels, particularly in the presence of renal impairment, may increase risk of seizures.
Adverse Reactions (Reflective of adult population; not specific for elderly)
>10%: Hematologic: Positive Coombs' test without hemolysis
1% to 10%:
    Central nervous system: Fever (1%), headache (1%)
    Dermatologic: Rash, pruritus
    Gastrointestinal: Diarrhea, nausea, vomiting
    Local: Erythema at injection site, pain
    Reactions reported with other cephalosporins: Aplastic anemia, erythema multiforme, hemolytic anemia, hemorrhage, pancytopenia, PT prolonged, renal dysfunction, Stevens-Johnson syndrome, superinfection, toxic epidermal necrolysis, toxic nephropathy, vaginitis
Overdosage/Toxicology Symptoms include neuromuscular hypersensitivity and CNS toxicity (including hallucinations, confusion, seizures, and coma). Many beta-lactam antibiotics have the potential to cause neuromuscular hyperirritability or seizures. Hemodialysis may be helpful to aid in the removal of the drug from the blood, however, most often treatment is supportive and symptom-directed.
Drug Interactions
    Increased effect: High-dose probenecid decreases clearance
    Increased toxicity: Aminoglycosides increase nephrotoxic potential
Stability Stable with normal saline, D_5W, and a variety of other solutions for 24 hours at room temperature and 7 days refrigerated.
Mechanism of Action Inhibits bacterial cell wall synthesis by binding to one or more of the penicillin-binding proteins (PBPs) which in turn inhibits the final transpeptidation step of peptidoglycan synthesis in bacterial cell walls, thus inhibiting cell wall biosynthesis. Bacteria eventually lyse due to ongoing activity of cell wall autolytic enzymes (autolysis and murein hydrolases) while cell wall assembly is arrested.
Pharmacokinetics Note: A longer half-life (mean 3 hours) and reduced renal and total clearances have been reported in older adults compared to younger subjects
    Absorption: I.M.: Rapid and complete; T_{max}: 0.5-1.5 hours
    Distribution: V_d: Adults: 14-20 L; penetrates into inflammatory fluid at concentrations ~80% of serum concentrations and into bronchial mucosa at concentrations ~60% of those reached in the plasma
    Protein binding, plasma: 16% to 19%
    Metabolism: ≤15% hydrolyzed to inactive metabolites
    Half-life: 2 hours
    Elimination: ≥85% as unchanged drug in urine
Dosage
    Geriatrics & Adults:
        Brain abscess (*Pseudomonas*) and meningitis (postsurgical): I.V.: 2 g every 8 hours; if treating *Pseudomonas,* the addition of an aminoglycoside should be considered
        Hospital-acquired pneumonia (HAP): I.V.: 1-2 g every 8-12 hours (American Thoracic Society/ATS guidelines)
        Monotherapy for febrile neutropenic patients: I.V.: 2 g every 8 hours for 7 days or until neutropenia resolves
        Otitis externa (malignant) and pneumonia: I.V.: 2 g every 12 hours
        Peritonitis (spontaneous): I.V.: 2 g every 12 hours with metronidazole
        Septic lateral/cavernous sinus thrombosis: I.V.: 2 g every 8-12 hours; with metronidazole for lateral
(Continued)

Cefepime *(Continued)*

Susceptible infections: I.V.: 1-2 g every 12 hours for 7-10 days; higher doses or more frequent administration may be required in pseudomonal infections

Urinary tract infections, mild to moderate: I.M., I.V.: 500-1000 mg every 12 hours

Renal Impairment:

Adjustment of recommended maintenance schedule is required:

Normal dosing schedule: 500 mg every 12 hours

Cl_{cr} 30-60 mL/minute: 500 mg every 24 hours

Cl_{cr} 11-29 mL/minute: 500 mg every 24 hours

Cl_{cr} <11 mL/minute: 250 mg every 24 hours

Normal dosing schedule: 1 g every 12 hours

Cl_{cr} 30-60 mL/minute: 1 g every 24 hours

Cl_{cr} 11-29 mL/minute: 500 mg every 24 hours

Cl_{cr} <11 mL/minute: 250 mg every 24 hours

Normal dosing schedule: 2 g every 12 hours

Cl_{cr} 30-60 mL/minute: 2 g every 24 hours

Cl_{cr} 11-29 mL/minute: 1 g every 24 hours

Cl_{cr} <11 mL/minute: 500 mg every 24 hours

Normal dosing schedule: 2 g every 8 hours

Cl_{cr} 30-60 mL/minute: 2 g every 12 hours

Cl_{cr} 11-29 mL/minute: 2 g every 24 hours

Cl_{cr} <11 mL/minute: 1 g every 24 hours

Hemodialysis effects: Initial: 1 g (single dose) on day 1. Maintenance: 500 mg once daily (1 g once daily in febrile neutropenic patients). Dosage should be administered after dialysis on dialysis days.

Peritoneal dialysis effects: Removed to a lesser extent than hemodialysis; administer 250 mg every 48 hours.

Continuous arteriovenous hemofiltration: Dose as for Cl_{cr} >30 mL/minute.

Monitoring Parameters Obtain specimen for culture and sensitivity prior to the first dose; signs and symptoms of infection; mental status

Test Interactions Positive direct Coombs', false-positive urinary glucose test using cupric sulfate (Benedict's solution, Clinitest®, Fehling's solution), false-positive serum or urine creatinine with Jaffé reaction, false-positive urinary proteins and steroids

Patient Information Report side effects such as diarrhea, dyspepsia, headache, blurred vision, and lightheadedness to your physician

Special Geriatric Considerations Adjust dose for changes in renal function.

Dosage Forms Excipient information presented when available (limited, particularly for generics); consult specific product labeling.

Injection, powder for reconstitution, as hydrochloride: 500 mg, 1 g, 2 g

Selected References

Barbhaiya RH, Knupp CA, and Pittman KA, "Effects of Age and Gender on Pharmacokinetics of Cefepime," *J Antimicrob Chemother*, 1992, 36(6):1181-5.

Wynd MA and Paladino JA, "Cefepime: A Fourth-Generation Parenteral Cephalosporin," *Ann Pharmacother*, 1996, 30(12):1414-24.

♦ **Cefepime Hydrochloride** *see Cefepime on page 256*

Cefixime *(sef IKS eem)*

Related Information

Antimicrobial Activity Against Selected Organisms *on page 1728*

Medication Safety Issues

Sound-alike/look-alike issues:

Suprax® may be confused with Sporanox®, Surbex®

International issues:

Cefiton® [Portugal] may be confused with Cefotan® which is a brand name for cefotetan in the U.S.

Cefiton® [Portugal] may be confused with Ceftim® which is a brand name for ceftazidime in Italy

Cefiton® [Portugal] may be confused with Ceftin® which is a brand name for cefuroxime in the U.S.

Cefiton® [Portugal] may be confused with Lexotan® which is a brand name for bromazepam in multiple international markets

U.S. Brand Names Suprax®

Canadian Brand Names Suprax®

Index Terms Cefixime Trihydrate

Generic Available No

Pharmacologic Category Antibiotic, Cephalosporin (Third Generation)

Use Treatment of urinary tract infections, otitis media, respiratory infections due to susceptible organisms; documented poor compliance with other oral antimicrobials;

outpatient therapy of serious soft tissue or skeletal infections due to susceptible organisms; single dose for *N. gonorrhoeae*

Contraindications Hypersensitivity to cefixime, any component of the formulation, or other cephalosporins

Warnings/Precautions Prolonged use may result in fungal or bacterial superinfection, including *C. difficile*-associated diarrhea and pseudomembranous colitis. Modify dosage in patients with renal impairment. Use with caution in patients with a history of penicillin allergy, especially IgE-mediated reactions (eg, anaphylaxis, urticaria).

Adverse Reactions (Reflective of adult population; not specific for elderly)
>10%: Gastrointestinal: Diarrhea (16%)

2% to 10%: Gastrointestinal: Abdominal pain, nausea, dyspepsia, flatulence, loose stools

Reactions reported with other cephalosporins: Interstitial nephritis, aplastic anemia, hemolytic anemia, hemorrhage, pancytopenia, agranulocytosis, colitis, superinfection

Overdosage/Toxicology After acute overdose, most agents cause only nausea, vomiting, and diarrhea, although neuromuscular hypersensitivity and seizures are possible, especially in patients with renal insufficiency. Many beta-lactam antibiotics have the potential to cause neuromuscular hyperirritability or seizures. Hemodialysis may be helpful to aid in removal of the drug from the blood but is not usually indicated; otherwise, most treatment is supportive or symptom-directed, following GI decontamination.

Drug Interactions
Aminoglycosides: May be a possible additive to nephrotoxicity.
Carbamazepine: Cefixime may increase serum levels of carbamazepine; monitor.
Furosemide: May be a possible additive to nephrotoxicity.
Probenecid: May decrease cephalosporin elimination.
Warfarin: Cefixime may increase prothrombin time when administered with warfarin; monitor.

Ethanol/Nutrition/Herb Interactions Food: Delays cefixime absorption.

Stability After reconstitution, suspension may be stored for 14 days at room temperature or under refrigeration.

Mechanism of Action Inhibits bacterial cell wall synthesis by binding to one or more of the penicillin binding proteins (PBPs); which in turn inhibits the final transpeptidation step of peptidoglycan synthesis in bacterial cell walls, thus inhibiting cell wall biosynthesis. Bacteria eventually lyse due to ongoing activity of cell wall autolytic enzymes (autolysins and murein hydrolases) while cell wall assembly is arrested.

Pharmacokinetics
Absorption: Oral: 40% to 50%
Protein binding: 65%
Half-life:
    Normal renal function: 3-4 hours
    Renal failure: Up to 11.5 hours
Time to peak serum concentration: Within 2-6 hours
Elimination: 50% of absorbed dose is excreted as active drug in urine and 10% in bile
Decreased clearance and prolonged half-life have been reported in older adults

Dosage
Geriatrics & Adults:
    Susceptible infections: Oral: 400 mg/day divided every 12-24 hours
    ***S. pyogenes* infections:** Treat for 10 days
    Typhoid fever: Oral: 20-30 mg/kg/day in 2 divided doses for 7-14 days after I.V. therapy
    Uncomplicated cervical/urethral gonorrhea due to *N. gonorrhoeae*: Oral: 400 mg as a single dose
Renal Impairment:
    Cl_{cr} 21-60 mL/minute: Administer 75% of the standard dose.
    Cl_{cr} <20 mL/minute: Administer 50% of the standard dose.
    10% removed by hemodialysis

Monitoring Parameters With prolonged therapy, monitor renal and hepatic function periodically; signs and symptoms of infection

Test Interactions Positive direct Coombs', false-positive urinary glucose test using cupric sulfate (Benedict's solution, Clinitest®, Fehling's solution), false-positive serum or urine creatinine with Jaffé reaction

Patient Information Complete full course of therapy; can be taken with food or milk; report persistent diarrhea

Additional Information Otitis media should be treated with the suspension since it results in higher peak blood levels than the tablet

Special Geriatric Considerations Adjust dose for renal impairment.

Dosage Forms Excipient information presented when available (limited, particularly for generics); consult specific product labeling.
(Continued)

Cefixime (Continued)

Powder for oral suspension, as trihydrate:
Suprax®: 100 mg/5 mL (50 mL, 75 mL, 100 mL) [contains sodium benzoate; straw-berry flavor]; 200 mg/5 mL (50 mL, 75 mL) [contains sodium benzoate; strawberry flavor]

Selected References
Faulkner RD, Bohaycheck W, Lanc RA, et al, "Pharmacokinetics of Cefixime in Young and Elderly," *J Antimicrob Chemother*, 1988, 21(6):787-94.

♦ **Cefixime Trihydrate** see Cefixime on page 258
♦ **Cefizox®** see Ceftizoxime on page 271
♦ **Cefotan® [DSC]** see Cefotetan on page 261

Cefotaxime (sef oh TAKS eem)

Related Information
Antimicrobial Activity Against Selected Organisms on page 1728
Medication Safety Issues
Sound-alike/look-alike issues:
Cefotaxime may be confused with cefoxitin, ceftizoxime, cefuroxime

International issues:
Spectrocef® [Italy] may be confused with Spectracef® which is a brand name for cefditoren in the U.S.
U.S. Brand Names Claforan®
Canadian Brand Names Claforan®
Index Terms Cefotaxime Sodium
Generic Available Yes: Powder
Pharmacologic Category Antibiotic, Cephalosporin (Third Generation)
Use Treatment of documented or suspected infections including *N. gonorrhoeae* and meningitis due to susceptible organisms
Contraindications Hypersensitivity to cefotaxime, any component of the formulation, or other cephalosporins
Warnings/Precautions Modify dosage in patients with severe renal impairment. Prolonged use may result in superinfection. A potentially life-threatening arrhythmia has been reported in patients who received a rapid bolus injection via central line. Granulocytopenia and more rarely agranulocytosis may develop during prolonged treatment (>10 days). Minimize tissue inflammation by changing infusion sites when needed. Use with caution in patients with a history of penicillin allergy, especially IgE-mediated reactions (eg, anaphylaxis, urticaria). Prolonged use may result in fungal or bacterial superinfection, including *C. difficile*-associated diarrhea and pseudomembranous colitis.
Adverse Reactions (Reflective of adult population; not specific for elderly)
1% to 10%:
Dermatologic: Rash, pruritus
Gastrointestinal: Diarrhea, nausea, vomiting, colitis
Local: Pain at injection site
Reactions reported with other cephalosporins: Agranulocytosis, aplastic anemia, cholestasis, hemolytic anemia, hemorrhage, nephropathy, pancytopenia, renal dysfunction, seizure, superinfection.
Overdosage/Toxicology Usually well tolerated even in overdose; convulsions are possible. Many beta-lactam antibiotics have the potential to cause neuromuscular hyperirritability or seizures. Hemodialysis may be helpful to aid in removal of the drug from the blood; otherwise, most treatment is supportive or symptom-directed.
Drug Interactions
Increased effect: Probenecid may decrease cephalosporin elimination
Increased toxicity: Furosemide, aminoglycosides may be a possible additive to nephrotoxicity
Stability Reconstituted solution is stable for 12-24 hours at room temperature and 7-10 days when refrigerated and for 13 weeks when frozen. For I.V. infusion in NS or D_5W, solution is stable for 24 hours at room temperature, 5 days when refrigerated, or 13 weeks when frozen in Viaflex® plastic containers. Thawed solutions previously of frozen premixed bags are stable for 24 hours at room temperature or 10 days when refrigerated.
Mechanism of Action Inhibits bacterial cell wall synthesis by binding to one or more of the penicillin-binding proteins (PBPs) which in turn inhibits the final transpeptidation step of peptidoglycan synthesis in bacterial cell walls, thus inhibiting cell wall biosynthesis. Bacteria eventually lyse due to ongoing activity of cell wall autolytic enzymes (autolysins and murein hydrolases) while cell wall assembly is arrested.
Pharmacokinetics
Protein binding: 31% to 50%

Metabolism: Partially in the liver to active metabolite, desacetylcefotaxime

Half-life:

Cefotaxime: 1-1.5 hours (prolonged with renal and/or hepatic impairment)

Desacetylcefotaxime: 1.5-1.9 hours (prolonged with renal impairment)

Time to peak serum concentration:

I.M.: Within 30 minutes

I.V.: Within ~5 minutes

In patients 60-80 years of age, the serum half-life was prolonged, the clearance decreased, and AUC increased for cefotaxime and less so for its desacetyl metabolite. A significantly greater increase in half-life and decrease in clearance in patients >80 years of age has been reported.

Dosage

Geriatrics & Adults:

Arthritis (septic): I.V.: 1 g every 8 hours

Brain abscess and meningitis: I.V.: 2 g every 4-6 hours

C-section: 1 g as soon as the umbilical cord is clamped, then 1 g I.M., I.V. at 6- and 12-hours intervals

Epiglottitis: I.V.: 2 g every 4-8 hours

Gonorrhea: I.M.: 1 g as a single dose; disseminated 1 g every 8 hours

Life-threatening infections: I.V.: 2 g every 4 hours

Liver abscess: I.V.: 1-2 g every 6 hours

Lyme disease:

Cardiac manifestations: I.V.: 2 g every 4 hours

CNS manifestations: I.V.: 2 g every 8 hours for 14-28 days

Moderate/severe infections: I.M., I.V.: 1-2 g every 8 hours

Orbital cellulitis: I.V.: 2 g every 4 hours

Peritonitis (spontaneous): I.V.: 2 g every 8 hours, unless life-threatening then 2 g every 4 hours

Septicemia: I.V.: 2 g every 6-8 hours

Skin and soft tissue:

Mixed, necrotizing: I.V.: 2 g every 6 hours, with metronidazole or clindamycin

Bite wounds (animal): I.V.: 2 g every 6 hours

Surgical prophylaxis: I.M., I.V.: 1 g 30-90 minutes before surgery

Uncomplicated infections: I.M., I.V.: 1 g every 12 hours

Renal Impairment:

Cl_{cr} 10-50 mL/minute: Administer every 8-12 hours.

Cl_{cr} <10 mL/minute: Administer every 24 hours.

Moderately dialyzable (20% to 50%)

Continuous arteriovenous hemofiltration: 1 g every 12 hours.

Hepatic Impairment: Moderate dosage reduction is recommended in severe liver disease.

Administration Cefotaxime can be administered IVP over 3-5 minutes, or I.V. retrograde or I.V. intermittent infusion over 15-30 minutes; final concentration for I.V. administration should not exceed 100 mg/mL; I.M. dosing should be in a large muscle mass (ie, gluteus maximus)

Test Interactions Positive direct Coombs', false-positive urinary glucose test using cupric sulfate (Benedict's solution, Clinitest®, Fehling's solution), false-positive serum or urine creatinine with Jaffé reaction

Special Geriatric Considerations Adjust dose for renal impairment.

Dosage Forms Excipient information presented when available (limited, particularly for generics); consult specific product labeling.

Infusion, as sodium [premixed iso-osmotic solution]:

Claforan®: 1 g (50 mL); 2 g (50 mL) [contains sodium 50.5 mg (2.2 mEq) per cefotaxime 1 g]

Injection, powder for reconstitution, as sodium: 500 mg, 1 g, 2 g, 10 g, 20 g

Claforan®: 500 mg, 1 g, 2 g, 10 g [contains sodium 50.5 mg (2.2 mEq) per cefotaxime 1 g]

Selected References

Deeter RG, Weinstein MP, Swanson KA, et al,"Crossover Assessment of Serum Bactericidal Activity and Pharmacokinetics of Five Broad-Spectrum Cephalosporins in the Elderly," *Antimicrob Agents Chemother,* 1990, 34(6):1007-13.

Ludwig E, Székely É, Csiba A, et al,"Pharmacokinetics of Cefotaxime and Desacetylcefotaxime in Elderly Patients," *Drugs,* 1988, 35(Suppl 2):51-6.

♦ **Cefotaxime Sodium** *see* Cefotaxime *on page 260*

Cefotetan (SEF oh tee tan)

Related Information

Antimicrobial Activity Against Selected Organisms *on page 1728*

Medication Safety Issues

Sound-alike/look-alike issues:

Cefotetan may be confused with cefoxitin, Ceftin®

(Continued)

Cefotetan *(Continued)*

Cefotan® may be confused with Ceftin®

International issues:

Cefotan® may be confused with Lexotan® which is a brand name for bromazepam in multiple international markets

Cefotan® may be confused with Cefiton® which is a brand name for cefixime in Portugal

U.S. Brand Names Cefotan® [DSC]

Canadian Brand Names Cefotan®

Index Terms Cefotetan Disodium

Generic Available No

Pharmacologic Category Antibiotic, Cephalosporin (Second Generation)

Use Used predominantly for respiratory tract, skin and skin structure, bone and joint, urinary tract and gynecologic as well as septicemia; surgical prophylaxis; intra-abdominal infections and other mixed infections; active against gram-negative enteric bacilli including *E. coli*, *Klebsiella*, and *Proteus*; less active against staphylococci and streptococci than first generation cephalosporins, but active against anaerobes including *Bacteroides fragilis*

Contraindications Hypersensitivity to cefotetan, any component of the formulation, or other cephalosporins; previous cephalosporin-associated hemolytic anemia

Warnings/Precautions Modify dosage in patients with severe renal impairment. Although cefotetan contains the methyltetrazolethiol side chain, bleeding has not been a significant problem. Use with caution in patients with a history of penicillin allergy, especially IgE-mediated reactions (eg, anaphylaxis, urticaria). Cefotetan has been associated with a higher risk of hemolytic anemia relative to other cephalosporins (approximately threefold); monitor carefully during use and consider cephalosporin-associated immune anemia in patients who have received cefotetan within 2-3 weeks (either as treatment or prophylaxis). Prolonged use may result in fungal or bacterial superinfection, including *C. difficile*-associated diarrhea and pseudomembranous colitis. May be associated with increased INR, especially in nutritionally-deficient patients, prolonged treatment, hepatic or renal disease.

Adverse Reactions (Reflective of adult population; not specific for elderly)

1% to 10%:

Gastrointestinal: Diarrhea (1%)

Hepatic: Transaminases increased (1%)

Miscellaneous: Hypersensitivity reactions (1%)

Reactions reported with other cephalosporins: Seizure, Stevens-Johnson syndrome, toxic epidermal necrolysis, renal dysfunction, toxic nephropathy, cholestasis, aplastic anemia, hemolytic anemia, hemorrhage, pancytopenia, agranulocytosis, colitis, superinfection

Overdosage/Toxicology Symptoms include neuromuscular hypersensitivity and convulsions especially with renal insufficiency. Many beta-lactam antibiotics have the potential to cause neuromuscular hyperirritability or seizures. Hemodialysis may be helpful to aid in removal of the drug from the blood; otherwise, most treatment is supportive or symptom-directed.

Drug Interactions

Ethanol: Disulfiram-like reaction may occur if ethanol is consumed by a patient taking cefotetan.

Probenecid: May increase cefotetan plasma levels.

Warfarin: Cefotetan may increase risk of bleeding in patients receiving warfarin.

Ethanol/Nutrition/Herb Interactions Ethanol: Avoid ethanol (may cause a disulfiram-like reaction).

Stability Reconstituted solution is stable for 24 hours at room temperature and 96 hours when refrigerated. For I.V. infusion in NS or D_5W solution and after freezing, thawed solution is stable for 24 hours at room temperature or 96 hours when refrigerated. Frozen solution is stable for 12 weeks.

Mechanism of Action Inhibits bacterial cell wall synthesis by binding to one or more of the penicillin-binding proteins (PBPs) which in turn inhibits the final transpeptidation step of peptidoglycan synthesis in bacterial cell walls, thus inhibiting cell wall biosynthesis. Bacteria eventually lyse due to ongoing activity of cell wall autolytic enzymes (autolysins and murein hydrolases) while cell wall assembly is arrested.

Pharmacokinetics

Protein binding: 76% to 90%

Half-life: 3-5 hours

Time to peak plasma concentration: I.M.: Within 1.5-3 hours

Elimination: Primarily excreted unchanged in urine with 20% excreted in bile

Dosage
Geriatrics & Adults:
Susceptible infections: I.M., I.V.: 1-6 g/day in divided doses every 12 hours; usual dose: 1-2 g every 12 hours for 5-10 days; 1-2 g may be given every 24 hours for urinary tract infection

Orbital cellulitis, odontogenic infections: I.V.: 2 g every 12 hours

Pelvic inflammatory disease: I.V.: 2 g every 12 hours; used in combination with doxycycline

Preoperative prophylaxis: I.M., I.V.: 1-2 g 30-60 minutes prior to surgery; when used for cesarean section, dose should be given as soon as umbilical cord is clamped

Urinary tract infection: I.M., I.V.: 1-2 g may be given every 24 hours

Renal Impairment: I.M., I.V.:
Cl_{cr} 10-30 mL/minute: Administer every 24 hours
Cl_{cr} <10 mL/minute: Administer every 48 hours
Hemodialysis: Dialyzable (5% to 20%); administer $1/4$ the usual dose every 24 hours on days between dialysis; administer $1/2$ the usual dose on the day of dialysis.
Continuous arteriovenous or venovenous hemodiafiltration effects: Administer 750 mg every 12 hours

Administration I.M. doses should be given in a large muscle mass (ie, gluteus maximus)

Monitoring Parameters Signs and symptoms of infection including mental status; monitor for signs and symptoms of hemolytic anemia, including hematologic parameters where appropriate.

Test Interactions Positive direct Coombs', false-positive urinary glucose test using cupric sulfate (Benedict's solution, Clinitest®, Fehling's solution), false-positive serum or urine creatinine with Jaffé reaction

Patient Information Avoid alcoholic beverages during and for 72 hours after completion of therapy

Additional Information Sodium content of 1 g: 3.5 mEq

Special Geriatric Considerations Cefotetan has not been studied in the elderly. Adjust dose for renal function in the elderly.

Dosage Forms Excipient information presented when available (limited, particularly for generics); consult specific product labeling. [DSC] = Discontinued product
Infusion [premixed iso-osmotic solution]: 1 g (50 mL); 2 g (50 mL) [contains sodium 80 mg/g (3.5 mEq/g)] [DSC]
Injection, powder for reconstitution: 1 g, 2 g [contains sodium 80 mg/g (3.5 mEq/g)] [DSC]

♦ Cefotetan Disodium see Cefotetan on page 261

Cefoxitin (se FOKS i tin)

Related Information
Antimicrobial Activity Against Selected Organisms on page 1728

Medication Safety Issues
Sound-alike/look-alike issues:
Cefoxitin may be confused with cefotaxime, cefotetan, Cytoxan®
Mefoxin® may be confused with Lanoxin®

U.S. Brand Names Mefoxin®

Canadian Brand Names Apo-Cefoxitin®

Index Terms Cefoxitin Sodium

Generic Available Yes: Powder for injection

Pharmacologic Category Antibiotic, Cephalosporin (Second Generation)

Use Less active against staphylococci and streptococci than first generation cephalosporins, but active against anaerobes including *Bacteroides fragilis*; active against gram-negative enteric bacilli including *E. coli*, *Klebsiella*, and *Proteus*

Contraindications Hypersensitivity to cefoxitin, any component of the formulation, or other cephalosporins

Warnings/Precautions Modify dosage in patients with severe renal impairment. Prolonged use may result in superinfection. Use with caution in patients with a history of penicillin allergy, especially IgE-mediated reactions (eg, anaphylaxis, urticaria). Prolonged use may result in fungal or bacterial superinfection, including *C. difficile*-associated diarrhea and pseudomembranous colitis.

Adverse Reactions (Reflective of adult population; not specific for elderly)
1% to 10%: Gastrointestinal: Diarrhea
Reactions reported with other cephalosporins: Agranulocytosis, aplastic anemia, cholestasis, colitis, erythema multiforme, hemolytic anemia, hemorrhage, pancytopenia, renal dysfunction, serum-sickness reactions, seizure, Stevens-Johnson syndrome, superinfection, toxic nephropathy, vaginitis
(Continued)

Cefoxitin *(Continued)*

Overdosage/Toxicology Symptoms include neuromuscular hypersensitivity and convulsions especially with renal insufficiency. Many beta-lactam antibiotics have the potential to cause neuromuscular hyperirritability or seizures. Hemodialysis may be helpful to aid in removal of the drug from the blood; otherwise, most treatment is supportive or symptom-directed.

Drug Interactions

Increased effect: Probenecid may decrease cephalosporin elimination

Increased toxicity: Aminoglycosides and furosemide may increase nephrotoxic potential

Stability Reconstitute vials with SWFI, bacteriostatic water for injection, NS, or D_5W. For I.V. infusion, solutions may be further diluted in NS, $D_5^{1/4}NS$, $D_5^{1/2}NS$, D_5NS, D_5W, $D_{10}W$, LR, D_5LR, mannitol 10%, or sodium bicarbonate 5%. Reconstituted solution is stable for 6 hours at room temperature or 7 days when refrigerated; I.V. infusion in NS or D_5W solution is stable for 18 hours at room temperature or 48 hours when refrigerated. Premixed frozen solution, when thawed, is stable for 24 hours at room temperature or 21 days when refrigerated.

Mechanism of Action Inhibits bacterial cell wall synthesis by binding to one or more of the penicillin-binding proteins (PBPs) which in turn inhibits the final transpeptidation step of peptidoglycan synthesis in bacterial cell walls, thus inhibiting cell wall biosynthesis. Bacteria eventually lyse due to ongoing activity of cell wall autolytic enzymes (autolysins and murein hydrolases) while cell wall assembly is arrested.

Pharmacokinetics

Protein binding: 65% to 79%

Half-life: 45-60 minutes, increases significantly with renal insufficiency

Time to peak serum concentration:

I.M.: Within 20-30 minutes

I.V.: Within 5 minutes

Elimination: Rapidly excreted as unchanged drug (85%) in urine; poorly penetrates into CSF even with inflammation of the meninges

Compared to younger patients (<55 years), older patients (66-94 years) have been reported to have a reduced total body clearance, prolonged half-life, increased volume of distribution, and reduced protein binding

Dosage

Geriatrics & Adults:

Susceptible infections: I.M., I.V.: 1-2 g every 6-8 hours (I.M. injection is painful); up to 12 g/day

Amnionitis and endomyometritis: I.M., I.V.: 2 g every 6-8 hours

Aspiration pneumonia, empyema, orbital cellulitis, parapharyngeal space, and human bites: I.M., I.V.: 2 g every 8 hours

Liver abscess: I.V.: 1 g every 4 hours

Mycobacterium species, not MTB or MAI: I.V.: 12 g/day with amikacin

Pelvic inflammatory disease:

Inpatients: I.V.: 2 g every 6 hours **plus** doxycycline 100 mg I.V. or 100 mg orally every 12 hours until improved, followed by doxycycline 100 mg orally twice daily to complete 14 days

Outpatients: I.M.: 2 g **plus** probenecid 1 g orally as a single dose, followed by doxycycline 100 mg orally twice daily for 14 days

Perioperative prophylaxis: I.M., I.V.: 1-2 g 30-60 minutes prior to surgery followed by 1-2 g every 6-8 hours for no more than 24 hours after surgery depending on the procedure

Renal Impairment: I.M., I.V.:

Cl_{cr} 30-50 mL/minute: Administer 1-2 g every 8-12 hours

Cl_{cr} 10-29 mL/minute: Administer 1-2 g every 12-24 hours

Cl_{cr} 5-9 mL/minute: Administer 0.5-1 g every 12-24 hours

Cl_{cr} <5 mL/minute: Administer 0.5-1 g every 24-48 hours

Hemodialysis: Moderately dialyzable (20% to 50%); administer a loading dose of 1-2 g after each hemodialysis; maintenance dose as noted above based on Cl_{cr}

Continuous arteriovenous or venovenous hemodiafiltration effects: Dose as for Cl_{cr} 10-50 mL/minute

Administration I.M. dose should be administered in a large muscle mass (ie, gluteus maximus)

Monitoring Parameters Monitor renal function periodically when used in combination with other nephrotoxic drugs

Test Interactions Positive direct Coombs', false-positive urinary glucose test using cupric sulfate (Benedict's solution, Clinitest®, Fehling's solution), false-positive serum or urine creatinine with Jaffé reaction

Additional Information Sodium content of 1 g: 53 mg (2.3 mEq)

Special Geriatric Considerations Adjust dose for renal function in the elderly.

Dosage Forms Excipient information presented when available (limited, particularly for generics); consult specific product labeling.

Infusion, as sodium [premixed iso-osmotic solution]: 1 g (50 mL); 2 g (50 mL) [contains sodium 53.8 mg/g (2.3 mEq/g)]
Injection, powder for reconstitution, as sodium: 1 g, 2 g, 10 g [contains sodium 53.8 mg/g (2.3 mEq/g)]

Selected References
Garcia MJ, Garcia A, Nieto MJ, et al, "Disposition of Cefoxitin in the Elderly," *Int J Clin Pharmacol Ther Toxicol*, 1980, 18(11):503-9.

♦ **Cefoxitin Sodium** *see* Cefoxitin *on page 263*

Cefpodoxime (sef pode OKS eem)

Related Information
Antimicrobial Activity Against Selected Organisms *on page 1728*

Medication Safety Issues
Sound-alike/look-alike issues:
Vantin® may be confused with Ventolin®

U.S. Brand Names Vantin®

Canadian Brand Names Vantin®

Index Terms Cefpodoxime Proxetil

Generic Available Yes: Tablet

Pharmacologic Category Antibiotic, Cephalosporin (Third Generation)

Use Treatment of susceptible acute, community-acquired pneumonia caused by *S. pneumoniae* or nonbeta-lactamase producing *H. influenzae*; acute uncomplicated gonorrhea caused by *N. gonorrhoeae*; uncomplicated skin and skin structure infections caused by *S. aureus* or *S. pyogenes*; acute otitis media caused by *S. pneumoniae*, *H. influenzae*, or *M. catarrhalis*; pharyngitis or tonsillitis; and uncomplicated urinary tract infections caused by *E. coli*, *Klebsiella*, and *Proteus*

Contraindications Hypersensitivity to cefpodoxime, any component of the formulation, or other cephalosporins

Warnings/Precautions Modify dosage in patients with severe renal impairment. Prolonged use may result in fungal or bacterial superinfection, including *C. difficile*-associated diarrhea and pseudomembranous colitis. Use with caution in patients with a history of penicillin allergy, especially IgE-mediated reactions (eg, anaphylaxis, urticaria).

Adverse Reactions (Reflective of adult population; not specific for elderly)
>10%:
Dermatologic: Diaper rash (12%)
Gastrointestinal: Diarrhea in infants and toddlers (15%)
1% to 10%:
Central nervous system: Headache (1%)
Dermatologic: Rash (1%)
Gastrointestinal: Diarrhea (7%), nausea (4%), abdominal pain (2%), vomiting (1% to 2%)
Genitourinary: Vaginal infection (3%)
Reactions reported with other cephalosporins: Seizure, Stevens-Johnson syndrome, toxic epidermal necrolysis, erythema multiforme, urticaria, serum-sickness reactions, renal dysfunction, interstitial nephritis toxic nephropathy, cholestasis, aplastic anemia, hemolytic anemia, hemorrhage, pancytopenia, agranulocytosis, colitis, vaginitis, superinfection

Overdosage/Toxicology After acute overdose, most agents cause only nausea, vomiting, and diarrhea, although neuromuscular hypersensitivity and seizures are possible, especially in patients with renal insufficiency. Many beta-lactam antibiotics have the potential to cause neuromuscular hyperirritability or seizures. Hemodialysis may be helpful to aid in removal of the drug from the blood but not usually indicated; otherwise, most treatment is supportive or symptom-directed, following GI decontamination.

Drug Interactions
Decreased effect: Antacids and H$_2$-receptor antagonists (reduce absorption and serum concentration of cefpodoxime)
Increased effect: Probenecid may decrease cephalosporin elimination
Increased toxicity: Aminoglycosides and furosemide may increase nephrotoxic potential

Ethanol/Nutrition/Herb Interactions Food: Food delays absorption; cefpodoxime serum levels may be increased if taken with food.

Stability Shake well before using. After mixing, keep suspension in refrigerator. Discard unused portion after 14 days.

Mechanism of Action Inhibits bacterial cell wall synthesis by binding to one or more of the penicillin-binding proteins (PBPs) which in turn inhibits the final transpeptidation step of peptidoglycan synthesis in bacterial cell walls, thus inhibiting cell wall biosynthesis. Bacteria eventually lyse due to ongoing activity of cell wall autolytic enzymes (autolysins and murein hydrolases) while cell wall assembly is arrested.
(Continued)

Cefpodoxime (Continued)

Pharmacokinetics

Absorption: Oral: Rapidly and well absorbed, acid stable; enhanced in the presence of food or low gastric pH

Distribution: Good tissue penetration, including lung and tonsils; penetrates into pleural fluid

Protein binding: 18% to 23%

Metabolism: Oral: De-esterified in the GI tract to the active metabolite, cefpodoxime

Bioavailability: Oral: 50%

Half-life: 2.2 hours (prolonged with renal impairment); older adults: 3.65 hours

Peak concentrations: Within 2-3 hours

Elimination: Plasma clearance: ~200-300 mL/minute; primarily eliminated by the kidney with 80% of dose excreted unchanged in urine in 24 hours

Dosage

Geriatrics & Adults:

Acute community-acquired pneumonia and bacterial exacerbations of chronic bronchitis: Oral: 200 mg every 12 hours for 14 days and 10 days, respectively

Acute maxillary sinusitis: Oral: 200 mg every 12 hours for 10 days

Pharyngitis/tonsillitis: Oral: 100 mg every 12 hours for 5-10 days

Skin and skin structure: Oral: 400 mg every 12 hours for 7-14 days

Uncomplicated gonorrhea (male and female) and rectal gonococcal infections (female): Oral: 200 mg as a single dose

Uncomplicated urinary tract infection: Oral: 100 mg every 12 hours for 7 days

Renal Impairment:

Cl$_{cr}$ <30 mL/minute: Administer every 24 hours.

Hemodialysis: Dose 3 times/week following dialysis.

Hepatic Impairment: Dose adjustment is not necessary in patients with cirrhosis.

Monitoring Parameters Signs and symptoms of infection

Test Interactions Positive direct Coombs', false-positive urinary glucose test using cupric sulfate (Benedict's solution, Clinitest®, Fehling's solution), false-positive serum or urine creatinine with Jaffé reaction

Patient Information Take with food; chilling improves flavor (do not freeze); report persistent diarrhea; entire course of medication (10-14 days) should be taken to ensure eradication of organism; should be taken in equal intervals around-the-clock to maintain adequate blood levels; females should report symptoms of vaginitis

Additional Information Dose adjustment is not necessary in patients with cirrhosis

Special Geriatric Considerations Considered one of the drugs of choice for outpatient treatment of community-acquired pneumonia in the elderly. Adjust dosage with renal impairment.

Dosage Forms Excipient information presented when available (limited, particularly for generics); consult specific product labeling.

Granules for oral suspension: 50 mg/5 mL (50 mL, 75 mL, 100 mL); 100 mg/5 mL (50 mL, 75 mL, 100 mL) [contains sodium benzoate; lemon creme flavor]

Tablet: 100 mg, 200 mg

Selected References

American Thoracic Society, "Guidelines for the Initial Management of Adults With Community-Acquired Pneumonia: Diagnosis, Assessment of Severity, and Initial Antimicrobial Therapy," *Am Rev Respir Dis*, 1993, 148(5):1418-26.

Backhouse C, Wade A, Williamson P, et al, "Multiple Dose Pharmacokinetics of Cefpodoxime in Young Adult and Elderly Patients," *J Antimicrob Chemother*, 1990, 26(Supp E):29-34.

♦ **Cefpodoxime Proxetil** *see* Cefpodoxime *on page 265*

Cefprozil (sef PROE zil)

Related Information

Antimicrobial Activity Against Selected Organisms *on page 1728*

Medication Safety Issues

Sound-alike/look-alike issues:

Cefprozil may be confused with cefazolin, cefuroxime

Cefzil® may be confused with Cefol®, Ceftin®, Kefzol®

U.S. Brand Names Cefzil®

Canadian Brand Names Apo-Cefprozil®; Cefzil®

Generic Available Yes

Pharmacologic Category Antibiotic, Cephalosporin (Second Generation)

Use Treatment of otitis media, sinusitis, and infections caused by susceptible organisms involving the respiratory tract, skin and skin structure

Contraindications Hypersensitivity to cefprozil, any component of the formulation, or other cephalosporins

Warnings/Precautions Modify dosage in patients with severe renal impairment. Use with caution in patients with a history of penicillin allergy, especially IgE-mediated reactions (eg, anaphylaxis, urticaria). Prolonged use may result in fungal or bacterial superinfection, including *C. difficile*-associated diarrhea and pseudomembranous colitis. Some products may contain phenylalanine.

Adverse Reactions (Reflective of adult population; not specific for elderly)
1% to 10%:
Central nervous system: Dizziness (1%)
Dermatologic: Diaper rash (2%)
Gastrointestinal: Diarrhea (3%), nausea (4%), vomiting (1%), abdominal pain (1%)
Genitourinary: Vaginitis, genital pruritus (2%)
Hepatic: Transaminases increased (2%)
Miscellaneous: Superinfection
Reactions reported with other cephalosporins: Seizure, toxic epidermal necrolysis, renal dysfunction, interstitial nephritis, toxic nephropathy, aplastic anemia, hemolytic anemia, hemorrhage, pancytopenia, agranulocytosis, colitis, vaginitis, superinfection

Overdosage/Toxicology After acute overdose, most agents cause only nausea, vomiting, and diarrhea, although neuromuscular hypersensitivity and seizures are possible, especially in patients with renal insufficiency. Many beta-lactam antibiotics have the potential to cause neuromuscular hyperirritability or seizures. Hemodialysis may be helpful to aid in removal of the drug from the blood but not usually indicated; otherwise, most treatment is supportive or symptom-directed, following GI decontamination.

Drug Interactions
Increased effect: Probenecid may decrease cephalosporin elimination
Increased toxicity: Aminoglycosides and furosemide may increase nephrotoxic potential

Ethanol/Nutrition/Herb Interactions Food: Food delays cefprozil absorption.

Mechanism of Action Inhibits bacterial cell wall synthesis by binding to one or more of the penicillin-binding proteins (PBPs) which in turn inhibits the final transpeptidation step of peptidoglycan synthesis in bacterial cell walls, thus inhibiting cell wall biosynthesis. Bacteria eventually lyse due to ongoing activity of cell wall autolytic enzymes (autolysins and murein hydrolases) while cell wall assembly is arrested.

Pharmacokinetics A mixture of *cis*- (90%) and *trans*- (10%) isomers; well absorbed from the GI tract (90%); food does not delay or reduce absorption; distribution is to most body tissues including the aqueous humor, bone, soft tissues, and the CSF. Elimination is primarily renal with 60% to 70% of the drug excreted in the urine in 24 hours; hepatic dysfunction does not appear to significantly alter elimination. Significantly greater peak concentrations and area under the curve is found in patients with Cl_{cr} <30 mL/minute; also, the half-life is prolonged 1.7 vs 5.9 hours and renal clearance reduced 198 mL/minute vs 18.8 mL/minute compared to patients with normal renal function.

Dosage
Geriatrics & Adults:
  Pharyngitis/tonsillitis: Oral: 500 mg every 24 hours for 10 days
    Secondary bacterial infection of acute bronchitis or acute bacterial exacerbation of chronic bronchitis: Oral: 500 mg every 12 hours for 10 days
    Uncomplicated skin and skin structure infections: Oral: 250 mg every 12 hours, or 500 mg every 12-24 hours for 10 days
  Renal Impairment:
  Cl_{cr} <30 mL/minute: Reduce dose by 50%.
  Hemodialysis effects: 55% is removed by hemodialysis.

Monitoring Parameters Culture and sensitivity; response to treatment (fever, WBC, mental status, appetite)

Test Interactions Positive direct Coombs', false-positive urinary glucose test using cupric sulfate (Benedict's solution, Clinitest®, Fehling's solution), false-positive serum or urine creatinine with Jaffé reaction

Patient Information Complete full course of therapy; take at regular intervals; may take with food or milk; report persistent diarrhea; chilling suspension improves flavor (do not freeze)

Special Geriatric Considerations Has not been studied exclusively in the elderly. Adjust dose for estimated renal function.

Dosage Forms Excipient information presented when available (limited, particularly for generics); consult specific product labeling.
Powder for oral suspension, as anhydrous: 125 mg/5 mL (50 mL, 75 mL, 100 mL); 250 mg/5 mL (50 mL, 75 mL, 100 mL)
  Cefzil®: 125 mg/5 mL (50 mL, 75 mL, 100 mL) [contains phenylalanine 28 mg/5 mL and sodium benzoate; bubble gum flavor]; 250 mg/5 mL (50 mL, 75 mL, 100 mL) [contains phenylalanine 28 mg/5 mL and sodium benzoate; bubble gum flavor]
Tablet, as anhydrous: 250 mg, 500 mg
  Cefzil®: 250 mg, 500 mg
(Continued)

Cefprozil *(Continued)*

Selected References

Shukla UA, Pittman KA, and Barbhaiya RH, "Pharmacokinetic Interactions of Cefprozil With Food, Propantheline, Metoclopramide, and Probenecid in Healthy Volunteers," *J Clin Pharmacol*, 1992, 32(8):725-31.

Shyu WC, Pittman KA, Wilber RB, et al, "Pharmacokinetics of Cefprozil in Healthy Subjects and Patients With Hepatic Impairment," *J Clin Pharmacol*, 1991, 31(4):372-6.

Ceftazidime (SEF tay zi deem)

Related Information
Antimicrobial Activity Against Selected Organisms *on page 1728*

Medication Safety Issues
Sound-alike/look-alike issues:
Ceftazidime may be confused with ceftizoxime
Ceptaz® may be confused with Septra®
Tazicef® may be confused with Tazidime®
Tazidime® may be confused with Tazicef®

International issues:
Ceftim® [Italy] may be confused with Ceftin® which is a brand name for cefuroxime in the U.S.
Ceftim® [Italy] may be confused with Cefiton® which is a brand name for cefixime in Portugal
Ceftim® [Italy] may be confused with Ceftina® which is a brand name for cefalotin in Mexico

U.S. Brand Names Fortaz®; Tazicef®
Canadian Brand Names Fortaz®
Generic Available No
Pharmacologic Category Antibiotic, Cephalosporin (Third Generation)
Use Treatment of documented susceptible *Pseudomonas aeruginosa* infection; *Pseudomonas* infection in patient at risk of developing aminoglycoside-induced nephrotoxicity and/or ototoxicity; empiric therapy of a febrile, granulocytopenic patient
Contraindications Hypersensitivity to ceftazidime, any component of the formulation, or other cephalosporins
Warnings/Precautions Modify dosage in patients with severe renal impairment. Use with caution in patients with a history of penicillin allergy, especially IgE-mediated reactions (eg, anaphylaxis, urticaria). Prolonged use may result in fungal or bacterial superinfection, including *C. difficile*-associated diarrhea and pseudomembranous colitis. May be associated with increased INR, especially in nutritionally-deficient patients, prolonged treatment, hepatic or renal disease. Use with caution in patients with a history of seizure disorder; high levels, particularly in the presence of renal impairment, may increase risk of seizures.
Adverse Reactions (Reflective of adult population; not specific for elderly)
1% to 10%:
Gastrointestinal: Diarrhea (1%)
Local: Pain at injection site (1%)
Miscellaneous: Hypersensitivity reactions (2%)
Reactions reported with other cephalosporins: Seizure, urticaria, serum-sickness reactions, renal dysfunction, interstitial nephritis, toxic nephropathy, BUN increased, creatinine increased, cholestasis, aplastic anemia, hemolytic anemia, pancytopenia, agranulocytosis, colitis, prolonged PT, hemorrhage, superinfection
Overdosage/Toxicology Symptoms include neuromuscular hypersensitivity and convulsions, especially with renal insufficiency. Many beta-lactam antibiotics have the potential to cause neuromuscular hyperirritability or seizures. Hemodialysis may be helpful to aid in removal of the drug from the blood, otherwise, most treatment is supportive or symptom-directed.
Drug Interactions
Coumarin derivatives (eg, dicumarol, warfarin): Cephalosporins may increase the anticoagulant effect of coumarin derivatives.
Typhoid vaccine: Antibiotics may diminish the therapeutic effect of Typhoid Vaccine. Only the live attenuated Ty21a strain is affected.
Uricosuric agents (eg, probenecid, sulfinpyrazone): Uricosuric agents may decrease the excretion of cephalosporin; monitor for toxic effects.
Stability Reconstituted solution and I.V. infusion in NS or D_5W solution are stable for 24 hours at room temperature, 10 days when refrigerated, or 12 weeks when frozen. After freezing, thawed solution is stable for 24 hours at room temperature or 4 days when refrigerated; 96 hours under refrigeration, after mixing.
Mechanism of Action Inhibits bacterial cell wall synthesis by binding to one or more of the penicillin-binding proteins (PBPs) which in turn inhibits the final transpeptidation

step of peptidoglycan synthesis in bacterial cell walls, thus inhibiting cell wall biosynthesis. Bacteria eventually lyse due to ongoing activity of cell wall autolytic enzymes (autolysins and murein hydrolases) while cell wall assembly is arrested.

Pharmacokinetics

Distribution: Widely throughout the body including bone, bile, skin, CSF (diffuses into CSF with higher concentrations when the meninges are inflamed) endometrium, heart, pleural and lymphatic fluids

Protein binding: 17%, <10% protein binding in older adults; in older adults half-life increased, volume of distribution decreased, and AUC increased

Half-life: 1-2 hours (prolonged with renal impairment)

Time to peak serum concentration: I.M.: Within 60 minutes

Elimination: By glomerular filtration with 80% to 90% of the dose excreted as unchanged drug within 24 hours

Dosage

Geriatrics: I.M., I.V.: Dosage should be based on renal function with a dosing interval not more frequent then every 12 hours.

Adults:

Bacterial arthritis (gram negative bacilli): I.V.: 1-2 g every 8 hours

Bone and joint infections: I.V.: 2 g every 12 hours

Cystic fibrosis, lung infection caused by *Pseudomonas* spp: I.V.: 30-50 mg/kg every 8 hours (maximum: 6 g/day)

Endophthalmitis, bacterial (unlabeled use): Intravitreal: 2.25 mg/0.1 mL NS in combination with vancomycin

Melioidosis: I.V.: 40 mg/kg every 8 hours for 10 days, followed by oral therapy with doxycycline or TMP/SMX

Otitis externa: I.V.: 2 g every 8 hours

Peritonitis (CAPD):

Anuric, intermittent: 1000-1500 mg/day

Anuric, continuous (per liter exchange): Loading dose: 250 mg; maintenance dose: 125 mg

Pneumonia: I.V.:

Uncomplicated: 500 mg to 1 g every 8 hours

Complicated or severe: 2 g every 8 hours

Skin and soft tissue infections: I.V., I.M.: 500 mg to 1 g every 8 hours

Severe infections, including meningitis, complicated pneumonia, endophthalmitis, CNS infection, osteomyelitis, intra-abdominal and gynecological, skin and soft tissue: I.V.: 2 g every 8 hours

Urinary tract infections: I.V., I.M.:

Uncomplicated: 250 mg every 12 hours

Complicated: 500 mg every 8-12 hours

Renal Impairment:

Cl_{cr} 30-50 mL/minute: Administer every 12 hours

Cl_{cr} 10-30 mL/minute: Administer every 24 hours

Cl_{cr} <10 mL/minute: Administer every 48-72 hours

Hemodialysis: Dialyzable (50% to 100%)

Continuous arteriovenous or venovenous hemodiafiltration effects: Dose as for Cl_{cr} 30-50 mL/minute

Administration Any carbon dioxide bubbles that may be present in the withdrawn solution should be expelled prior to injection. Ceftazidime can be administered IVP over 3-5 minutes, or I.V. retrograde or I.V. intermittent infusion over 15-30 minutes; final concentration for I.V. administration should not exceed 100 mg/mL; can be reconstituted for I.M. administration with 0.5% or 1% lidocaine if volume tolerated.

Monitoring Parameters Serum creatinine with concurrent use of an aminoglycoside; a change in renal function necessitates a change in dose; signs of infection such as fever, WBC, mental status

Test Interactions Positive direct Coombs', false-positive urinary glucose test using cupric sulfate (Benedict's solution, Clinitest®, Fehling's solution), false-positive serum or urine creatinine with Jaffé reaction

Additional Information Sodium content of 1 g: 54 mg (2.3 mEq). For most older adults; weak third generation cephalosporin strongest against anaerobes and gram-positive bacteria; *Pseudomonas* sp.

Special Geriatric Considerations Changes in renal function associated with aging and corresponding alterations in pharmacokinetics result in every 12-hour dosing being an adequate dosing interval. Adjust dose based on renal function.

Dosage Forms Excipient information presented when available (limited, particularly for generics); consult specific product labeling.

Infusion [premixed iso-osmotic solution]:

Fortaz®: 1 g (50 mL) [contains sodium carbonate, sodium 54 mg (2.3 mEq)/g]; 2 g (50 mL) [contains sodium carbonate, sodium 54 mg (2.3 mEq)/g]

(Continued)

Ceftazidime (Continued)

Injection, powder for reconstitution:
Fortaz®: 500 mg, 1 g, 2 g, 6 g [contains sodium carbonate, sodium 54 mg (2.3 mEq)/g]
Tazicef®: 1 g, 2 g, 6 g [contains sodium carbonate, sodium 54 mg (2.3 mEq)/g]

Selected References

Sirgo MA and Norris S, "Ceftazidime in the Elderly: Appropriateness of Twice-Daily Dosing," *DICP Ann Pharmacother*, 1991, 25(3):284-8.

Slaker RA and Danielson B, "Neurotoxicity Associated With Ceftazidime Therapy in Geriatric Patients With Renal Dysfunction," *Pharmacotherapy*, 1991, 11(4):351-2.

Ceftibuten (sef TYE byoo ten)

Related Information
Antimicrobial Activity Against Selected Organisms *on page 1728*

Medication Safety Issues
International issues:
Cedax® may be confused with Codex which is a brand name for *Saccharomyces boulardii* in Italy

U.S. Brand Names Cedax®

Generic Available No

Pharmacologic Category Antibiotic, Cephalosporin (Third Generation)

Use Treatment of acute bacterial exacerbations of chronic bronchitis; treatment of acute bacterial otitis media due to *H. influenzae*, *Moraxella catarrhalis*, or *Streptococcus pyogenes* but not when due to *Streptococcus pneumoniae*; treatment of pharyngitis or tonsillitis due to *S. pyogenes*

Contraindications Hypersensitivity to ceftibuten, any component of the formulation, or other cephalosporins

Warnings/Precautions Modify dosage in patients with severe renal impairment. Prolonged use may result in fungal or bacterial superinfection, including *C. difficile*-associated diarrhea and pseudomembranous colitis. Use with caution in patients with a history of penicillin allergy, especially IgE-mediated reactions (eg, anaphylaxis, urticaria).

Adverse Reactions (Reflective of adult population; not specific for elderly)
1% to 10%:
Central nervous system: Headache (3%), dizziness (1%)
Gastrointestinal: Nausea (4%), diarrhea (3%), dyspepsia (2%), vomiting (1%), abdominal pain (1%)
Hematologic: Eosinophils increased (3%), hemoglobin decreased (2%), thrombocytosis
Hepatic: ALT increased (1%), bilirubin increased (1%)
Renal: BUN increased (4%)
Reactions reported with other cephalosporins: Anaphylaxis, fever, paresthesia, pruritus, Stevens-Johnson syndrome, toxic epidermal necrolysis, erythema multiforme, angioedema, pseudomembranous colitis, hemolytic anemia, candidiasis, vaginitis, encephalopathy, asterixis, neuromuscular excitability, seizure, serum-sickness reactions, renal dysfunction, interstitial nephritis, toxic nephropathy, cholestasis, aplastic anemia, hemolytic anemia, pancytopenia, agranulocytosis, colitis, prolonged PT, hemorrhage, superinfection

Overdosage/Toxicology After acute overdose, most agents cause only nausea, vomiting, and diarrhea, although neuromuscular hypersensitivity and seizures are possible, especially in patients with renal insufficiency. Many beta-lactam antibiotics have the potential to cause neuromuscular hyperirritability or seizures. Hemodialysis may be helpful to aid in removal of the drug from the blood but not usually indicated; otherwise, most treatment is supportive or symptom-directed, following GI decontamination.

Drug Interactions
Increased effect: High-dose probenecid decreases clearance
Increased toxicity: Aminoglycosides may increase nephrotoxic potential

Stability Reconstituted suspension is stable for 14 days when refrigerated.

Mechanism of Action Inhibits bacterial cell wall synthesis by binding to one or more of the penicillin-binding proteins (PBPs) which in turn inhibits the final transpeptidation step of peptidoglycan synthesis in bacterial cell walls, thus inhibiting cell wall biosynthesis. Bacteria eventually lyse due to ongoing activity of cell wall autolytic enzymes (autolysins and murein hydrolases) while cell wall assembly is arrested.

Pharmacokinetics
Absorption: T_{max}: 2-3 hours; F = 80%
Protein binding: 65% to 77%
Metabolism: 7% to 10% to weakly active olefinic isomer
Half-life: 1.5-2.5 hours
Elimination: 67% to 75% recovered unchanged in the urine after 24 hours

Dosage

Geriatrics & Adults: Susceptible infections: Oral: 400 mg once daily for 10 days; maximum: 400 mg

Renal Impairment:

Cl_{cr} 30-49 mL//minute: Administer 4.5 mg/kg or 200 mg every 24 hours.

Cl_{cr} 5-29 mL/minute: Administer 2.25 mg/kg or 100 mg every 24 hours.

Hemodialysis: Administer 400 mg or 9 mg/kg (maximum: 400 mg) after hemodialysis

Monitoring Parameters Signs and symptoms of infection including mental status

Test Interactions Positive direct Coombs', false-positive urinary glucose test using cupric sulfate (Benedict's solution, Clinitest®, Fehling's solution), false-positive serum or urine creatinine with Jaffé reaction

Patient Information Take suspension at least 2 hours before or 1 hour after meal. Complete full course of therapy; report persistent diarrhea; capsules can be taken with food

Special Geriatric Considerations Has not been studied specifically in the elderly. Adjust dose for renal function.

Dosage Forms Excipient information presented when available (limited, particularly for generics); consult specific product labeling.

Capsule:

Cedax®: 400 mg

Powder for oral suspension:

Cedax®: 90 mg/5 mL (30 mL, 60 mL, 90 mL, 120 mL) [contains sucrose 1g/5 mL and sodium benzoate; cherry flavor]

♦ **Ceftin®** *see* Cefuroxime *on page 275*

Ceftizoxime (sef ti ZOKS eem)

Related Information

Antimicrobial Activity Against Selected Organisms *on page 1728*

Medication Safety Issues

Sound-alike/look-alike issues:

Ceftizoxime may be confused with cefotaxime, ceftazidime, cefuroxime

U.S. Brand Names Cefizox®

Canadian Brand Names Cefizox®

Index Terms Ceftizoxime Sodium

Generic Available No

Pharmacologic Category Antibiotic, Cephalosporin (Third Generation)

Use Treatment of susceptible bacterial infection; mainly respiratory tract, skin and skin structure, bone and joint, urinary tract and gynecologic as well as septicemia

Contraindications Hypersensitivity to ceftizoxime, any component of the formulation, or other cephalosporins

Warnings/Precautions Modify dosage in patients with severe renal impairment. Prolonged use may result in fungal or bacterial superinfection, including *C. difficile*-associated diarrhea and pseudomembranous colitis. Use with caution in patients with a history of penicillin allergy, especially IgE-mediated reactions (eg, anaphylaxis, urticaria).

Adverse Reactions (Reflective of adult population; not specific for elderly)

1% to 10%:

Central nervous system: Fever

Dermatologic: Rash, pruritus

Hematologic: Eosinophilia, thrombocytosis

Hepatic: Alkaline phosphatase increased, transaminases increased

Local: Pain, burning at injection site

Reactions reported with other cephalosporins: Stevens-Johnson syndrome, toxic epidermal necrolysis, erythema multiforme, pseudomembranous colitis, angioedema, hemolytic anemia, candidiasis, encephalopathy, asterixis, neuromuscular excitability, seizure, serum-sickness reactions, renal dysfunction, interstitial nephritis, toxic nephropathy, cholestasis, aplastic anemia, hemolytic anemia, pancytopenia, agranulocytosis, colitis, prolonged PT, hemorrhage, superinfection

Overdosage/Toxicology Symptoms include neuromuscular hypersensitivity and convulsions especially with renal insufficiency. Many beta-lactam antibiotics have the potential to cause neuromuscular hyperirritability or seizures. Hemodialysis may be helpful to aid in removal of the drug from the blood; otherwise, most treatment is supportive or symptom-directed.

Drug Interactions

Increased effect: Probenecid may decrease cephalosporin elimination

Increased toxicity: Aminoglycosides and furosemide may increase nephrotoxic potential

Stability Reconstituted solution is stable for 24 hours at room temperature and 96 hours when refrigerated. For I.V. infusion in NS or D_5W solution is stable for 24 hours at room

(Continued)

Ceftizoxime *(Continued)*

temperature, 96 hours when refrigerated, or 12 weeks when frozen. After freezing, thawed solution is stable for 24 hours at room temperature or 10 days when refrigerated.

Mechanism of Action Inhibits bacterial cell wall synthesis by binding to one or more of the penicillin-binding proteins (PBPs) which in turn inhibits the final transpeptidation step of peptidoglycan synthesis in bacterial cell walls, thus inhibiting cell wall biosynthesis. Bacteria eventually lyse due to ongoing activity of cell wall autolytic enzymes (autolysins and murein hydrolases) while cell wall assembly is arrested.

Pharmacokinetics
Distribution: V_d: 0.35-0.5 L/kg
Protein binding: 30%
Half-life: 1.6 hours (half-life increases to 25 hours when Cl_{cr} fall <10 mL/minute)
Time to peak serum concentration: I.M.: Within 30-60 minutes
Elimination: Excreted unchanged in urine
One study has reported the pharmacokinetics of ceftizoxime in older adults. Following a single 2 g I.V. dose the mean serum half-life was 3.5 hours; mean V_{dss}: 14.2 L/1.73 m^2; mean clearance: 62.5 mL/minute/1.73 m^2

Dosage
Geriatrics & Adults: Usual dosage: I.M., I.V.: 1-2 g every 8-12 hours, up to 2 g every 4 hours or 4 g every 8 hours for life-threatening infections
Gonococcal:
Disseminated infection: I.M., I.V.: 1 g every 8 hours
Uncomplicated: I.M.: 1 g as single dose
Life-threatening infections: I.V.: 2 g every 4 hours or 4 g every 8 hours
Renal Impairment:
Cl_{cr} 50-79 mL/minute: Administer 500-1500 mg every 8 hours.
Cl_{cr} 5-49 mL/minute: Administer 250-1000 mg every 12 hours.
Cl_{cr} 0-4 mL/minute: Administer 500-1000 mg every 48 hours or 250-500 mg every 24 hours.
Moderately dialyzable (20% to 50%)
Continuous arteriovenous hemofiltration: Dose as for Cl_{cr} 10-50 mL/minute.

Administration Administer I.M. injections in a large muscle mass (ie, gluteus maximus)

Monitoring Parameters Signs and symptoms of infection including mental status

Test Interactions Positive direct Coombs', false-positive urinary glucose test using cupric sulfate (Benedict's solution, Clinitest®, Fehling's solution), false-positive serum or urine creatinine with Jaffé reaction

Additional Information Sodium content of 1 g: 60 mg (2.6 mEq)

Special Geriatric Considerations Adjust dose for renal function in the elderly.

Dosage Forms Excipient information presented when available (limited, particularly for generics); consult specific product labeling.
Infusion [premixed iso-osmotic solution]:
Cefizox®: 1 g (50 mL); 2 g (50 mL)
Injection, powder for reconstitution:
Cefizox®: 1 g, 2 g, 10 g [DSC]

Selected References
Deeter RG, Weinstein MP, Swanson KA, et al, "Crossover Assessment of Serum Bactericidal Activity and Pharmacokinetics of Five Broad-Spectrum Cephalosporins in the Elderly," *Antimicrob Agents Chemother*, 1990, 34(6):1007-13.

♦ **Ceftizoxime Sodium** *see* Ceftizoxime *on page 271*

Ceftriaxone *(sef trye AKS one)*

Related Information
Antibiotic Treatment of Adults With Infective Endocarditis *on page 1797*
Antimicrobial Activity Against Selected Organisms *on page 1728*
Medication Safety Issues
Sound-alike/look-alike issues:
Rocephin® may be confused with Roferon®
U.S. Brand Names Rocephin®
Canadian Brand Names Rocephin®
Index Terms Ceftriaxone Sodium
Generic Available Yes
Pharmacologic Category Antibiotic, Cephalosporin (Third Generation)
Use Treatment of lower respiratory tract infections, acute bacterial otitis media, skin and skin structure infections, bone and joint infections, intra-abdominal and urinary tract infections, pelvic inflammatory disease (PID), uncomplicated gonorrhea, bacterial septicemia, and meningitis; used in surgical prophylaxis

Unlabeled/Investigational Use Treatment of chancroid, epididymitis, complicated gonococcal infections; sexually-transmitted diseases (STD); periorbital or buccal cellulitis; salmonellosis or shigellosis; atypical community-acquired pneumonia; Lyme disease; used in chemoprophylaxis for high-risk contacts and persons with invasive meningococcal disease; sexual assault

Contraindications Hypersensitivity to ceftriaxone sodium, any component of the formulation, or other cephalosporins

Warnings/Precautions Modify dosage in patients with severe renal impairment. Prolonged use may result in fungal or bacterial superinfection, including *C. difficile*-associated diarrhea and pseudomembranous colitis. Use with caution in patients with a history of penicillin allergy, especially IgE-mediated reactions (eg, anaphylaxis, urticaria). Discontinue in patients with signs and symptoms of gallbladder disease. May be associated with increased INR, especially in nutritionally-deficient patients, prolonged treatment, hepatic or renal disease. Ceftriaxone may complex with calcium causing precipitation. Fatal lung and kidney damage resulting from this incompatibility has been observed in premature and term neonates. Do not reconstitute with calcium-containing solutions or co-administer with calcium-containing products, even via separate infusion lines/sites or at different times.

Adverse Reactions (Reflective of adult population; not specific for elderly)
1% to 10%:
> Dermatologic: Rash (2%)
> Gastrointestinal: Diarrhea (3%)
> Hematologic: Eosinophilia (6%), thrombocytosis (5%), leukopenia (2%)
> Hepatic: Transaminases increased (3.1% to 3.3%)
> Local: Pain, induration at injection site (I.V. 1%); warmth, tightness, induration (5% to 17%) following I.M. injection
> Renal: BUN increased (1%)

Reactions reported with other cephalosporins: Angioedema, aplastic anemia, asterixis, cholestasis, encephalopathy, erythema multiforme, hemorrhage, interstitial nephritis, neuromuscular excitability, pancytopenia, paresthesia, renal dysfunction, Stevens-Johnson syndrome, superinfection, toxic epidermal necrolysis, toxic nephropathy

Overdosage/Toxicology Symptoms include neuromuscular hypersensitivity and convulsions especially with renal insufficiency. Many beta-lactam antibiotics have the potential to cause neuromuscular hyperirritability or seizures. Hemodialysis may be helpful to aid in removal of the drug from the blood; otherwise, most treatment is supportive or symptom-directed.

Drug Interactions
> Calcium-containing solutions: Ceftriaxone may precipitate with calcium when mixed. Do not co-administer, even via separate infusion lines/sites or at different times. Do not administer calcium-containing solutions or products within 48 hours after the last dose of ceftriaxone.
> Coumarin derivative (eg, dicumarol, warfarin): Cephalosporins may increase the anticoagulant effect of coumarin derivatives.
> Uricosuric agents (eg, probenecid, sulfinpyrazone): Uricosuric agents may decrease the excretion of cephalosporin; monitor for toxic effects.

Stability
> Powder for injection: Prior to reconstitution, store at room temperature of 25°C (77°F); protect from light.
> Premixed solution (manufacturer premixed): Store at -20°C. Once thawed, solutions are stable for 3 days at room temperature of 25°C (77°F) or for 21 days refrigerated at 5°C (41°F). Do not refreeze.

Stability of reconstituted solutions:
> 10-40 mg/mL: Reconstituted in D_5W or NS: Stable for 2 days at room temperature of 25°C (77°F) or for 10 days when refrigerated at 5°C (41°F).
> 100 mg/mL:
>> Reconstituted in D_5W or NS: Stable for 2 days at room temperature of 25°C (77°F) or for 10 days when refrigerated at 5°C (41°F). Stable for 26 weeks when frozen at -20°C. Once thawed, solutions are stable for 2 days at room temperature of 25°C (77°F) or for 10 days when refrigerated at 5°C (41°F); does not apply to manufacturer's premixed bags. Do not refreeze.
>> Reconstituted in lidocaine 1% solution: Stable for 24 hours at room temperature of 25°C (77°F) or for 10 days when refrigerated at 5°C (41°F).
> 250-350 mg/mL: Reconstituted in D_5W, NS, lidocaine 1% solution, or SWFI: Stable for 24 hours at room temperature of 25°C (77°F) or for 3 days when refrigerated at 5°C (41°F).

Reconstitution:
> I.M. injection: Vials should be reconstituted with appropriate volume of diluent (including D_5W, NS, or 1% lidocaine) to make a final concentration of 250 mg/mL or 350 mg/mL.

(Continued)

Ceftriaxone *(Continued)*

Volume to add to create a **250 mg/mL** solution:
250 mg vial: 0.9 mL
500 mg vial: 1.8 mL
1 g vial: 3.6 mL
2 g vial: 7.2 mL

Volume to add to create a **350 mg/mL** solution:
500 mg vial: 1.0 mL
1 g vial: 2.1 mL
2 g vial: 4.2 mL

I.V. infusion: Infusion is prepared in two stages: Initial reconstitution of powder, followed by dilution to final infusion solution.

Vials: Reconstitute powder with appropriate I.V. diluent (including SWFI, D_5W, NS) to create an initial solution of ~100 mg/mL. Recommended volume to add:
250 mg vial: 2.4 mL
500 mg vial: 4.8 mL
1 g vial: 9.6 mL
2 g vial: 19.2 mL

Note: After reconstitution of powder, further dilution into a volume of compatible solution (eg, 50-100 mL of D_5W or NS) is recommended.

Piggyback bottle: Reconstitute powder with appropriate I.V. diluent (D_5W or NS) to create a resulting solution of ~100 mg/mL. Recommended initial volume to add:
1 g bottle:10 mL
2 g bottle: 20 mL

Note: After reconstitution, to prepare the final infusion solution, further dilution to 50 mL or 100 mL volumes with the appropriate I.V. diluent (including D_5W or NS) is recommended.

Mechanism of Action Inhibits bacterial cell wall synthesis by binding to one or more of the penicillin-binding proteins (PBPs) which in turn inhibits the final transpeptidation step of peptidoglycan synthesis in bacterial cell walls, thus inhibiting cell wall biosynthesis. Bacteria eventually lyse due to ongoing activity of cell wall autolytic enzymes (autolysins and murein hydrolases) while cell wall assembly is arrested.

Pharmacokinetics

Distribution: Widely throughout the body including gallbladder, lungs, bone, bile, CSF (diffuses into the CSF at higher concentrations when the meninges are inflamed)

Protein binding: 85% to 95%

Half-life: 5-9 hours (with normal renal and hepatic function)

Time to peak serum concentration:
I.M.: Within 1-2 hours
I.V.: Within minutes

Elimination: Excreted unchanged in urine (33% to 65%) by glomerular filtration and in feces

Studies of ceftriaxone in older adults have found a prolonged serum half-life (15 hours) and a reduced total clearance with or without a change in the volume of distribution. The change in renal clearance has been correlated to a reduction in Cl_{cr}. An increased free fraction was also found in one study suggesting a reduction in protein binding.

Dosage

Geriatrics & Adults:

Dosage range: Usual dose: 1-2 g every 12-24 hours, depending on the type and severity of infection

Arthritis (septic): I.V.: 1-2 g once daily

Brain abscess and necrotizing fasciitis: I.V.: 2 g every 12 hours

Cavernous sinus thrombosis: I.V.: 1 g every 12 hours with vancomycin or linezolid

Chancroid (unlabeled use): I.M.: 250 mg as single dose

Chemoprophylaxis for high-risk contacts and persons with invasive meningococcal disease (unlabeled use): I.M.: 250 mg in a single dose

Endocarditis, acute native valve: I.V.: 2 g once daily for 2-4 weeks

Epididymitis, acute (unlabeled use) and prostatitis: I.M.: 250 mg in a single dose with doxycycline

Gonococcal infections:

Conjunctivitis, complicated (unlabeled use): I.M., I.V.: 1 g in a single dose

Disseminated (unlabeled use): I.M., I.V.: 1 g once daily for 7 days

Endocarditis (unlabeled use): I.M., I.V.: 1-2 g every 12 hours for at least 28 days

Uncomplicated: I.M.: 125-250 mg in a single dose

Lyme disease: I.V.: 2 g once daily for 14-28 days

Mastoiditis (hospitalized): I.V.: 2 g once daily; >60 years old: 1 g once daily

Meningitis: I.V.: 2 g every 12 hours for 7-14 days (longer courses may be necessary for selected organisms

Orbital cellulitis (unlabeled use) and endophthalmitis: I.V.: 2 g once daily

PID: I.M.: 250 mg in a single dose

Pneumonia, community-acquired: I.V.: 2 g once daily; >65 years of age: 1 g once daily

Prophylaxis against infective endocarditis: I.M., I.V.: 1 g 30-60 minutes before procedure. **Note:** Intramuscular injections should be avoided in patients who are receiving anticoagulant therapy. In these circumstances, orally administered regimens should be given whenever possible. Intravenously administered antibiotics should be used for patients who are unable to tolerate or absorb oral medications.

Septic/toxic shock: I.V.: 2 g once daily; with clindamycin for toxic shock

Surgical prophylaxis: I.V.: 1 g 30 minutes to 2 hours before surgery

Syphilis: I.M., I.V.: 1 g once daily for 8-10 days

Typhoid fever: I.V.: 2-3 g once daily for 7-14 days

Renal Impairment:
No adjustment is necessary.
Not dialyzable (0% to 5%)
Administer dose postdialysis.
Peritoneal dialysis effects: Administer 750 mg every 12 hours.
Continuous arteriovenous or venovenous hemofiltration: Removes 10 mg of ceftriaxone of liter of filtrate per day.

Hepatic Impairment: No adjustment necessary.

Administration
I.M.: Inject deep I.M. into large muscle mass; a concentration of 250 mg/mL or 350 mg/mL is recommended for all vial sizes except the 250 mg size (250 mg/mL is suggested)
I.V.: Infuse intermittent infusion over 30 minutes

Monitoring Parameters Signs and symptoms of infection including mental status

Test Interactions Positive direct Coombs', false-positive urinary glucose test using cupric sulfate (Benedict's solution, Clinitest®, Fehling's solution), false-positive serum or urine creatinine with Jaffé reaction

Additional Information Sodium content of 1 g: 2.6 mEq

Special Geriatric Considerations No adjustment for changes in renal function necessary.

Dosage Forms Excipient information presented when available (limited, particularly for generics); consult specific product labeling.
Infusion [premixed in dextrose]: 1 g (50 mL); 2 g (50 mL)
Injection, powder for reconstitution: 250 mg, 500 mg, 1 g, 2 g, 10 g
Rocephin®: 250 mg, 500 mg, 1 g, 2 g, 10 g [contains sodium 83 mg (3.6 mEq) per ceftriaxone 1 g]

Selected References
Deeter RG, Weinstein MP, Swanson KA, et al, "Crossover Assessment of Serum Bactericidal Activity and Pharmacokinetics of Five Broad-Spectrum Cephalosporins in the Elderly," *Antimicrob Agents Chemother*, 1990, 34(6):1007-13.
Hayton WL and Stoeckel K, "Age-Associated Changes in Ceftriaxone Pharmacokinetics," *Clin Pharmacokinet*, 1986, 11(1):76-82.
Luderer JR, Patel IH, Durkin J, et al, "Age and Ceftriaxone Kinetics," *Clin Pharmacol Ther*, 1984, 35(1):19-25.
Richards DM, Heel RC, Brogden RN, et al, "Ceftriaxone: A Review of Its Antibacterial Activity, Pharmacological Properties and Therapeutic Use," *Drugs*, 1984, 27(6):469-527.

♦ **Ceftriaxone Sodium** *see* Ceftriaxone *on page 272*

Cefuroxime (se fyoor OKS eem)

Related Information
Antimicrobial Activity Against Selected Organisms *on page 1728*

Medication Safety Issues
Sound-alike/look-alike issues:
Cefuroxime may be confused with cefotaxime, cefprozil, ceftizoxime, deferoxamine
Ceftin® may be confused with Cefotan®, cefotetan, Cefzil®, Cipro®
Zinacef® may be confused with Zithromax®

International issues:
Ceftin® may be confused with Cefiton® which is a brand name for cefixime in Portugal
Ceftin® may be confused with Ceftina® which is a brand name for cefalotin in Mexico
Ceftin® may be confused with Ceftim® which is a brand name for ceftazidime in Italy

U.S. Brand Names Ceftin®; Zinacef®

Canadian Brand Names Apo-Cefuroxime®; Ceftin®; ratio-Cefuroxime; Zinacef®

Index Terms Cefuroxime Axetil; Cefuroxime Sodium

Generic Available Yes: Excludes powder for oral suspension

Pharmacologic Category Antibiotic, Cephalosporin (Second Generation)

Use Infections caused by staphylococci, group B streptococci, *H. influenzae* (type A and B), *E. coli*, *Enterobacter*, *Salmonella*, and *Klebsiella*; treatment of susceptible infections of the lower respiratory tract, otitis media, urinary tract, skin and soft tissue, bone and joint, sepsis, and gonorrhea
(Continued)

Cefuroxime (Continued)

Contraindications Hypersensitivity to cefuroxime, any component of the formulation, or other cephalosporins

Warnings/Precautions Modify dosage in patients with severe renal impairment. Use with caution in patients with a history of penicillin allergy, especially IgE-mediated reactions (eg, anaphylaxis, urticaria). Prolonged use may result in fungal or bacterial superinfection, including *C. difficile*-associated diarrhea and pseudomembranous colitis. May be associated with increased INR, especially in nutritionally-deficient patients, prolonged treatment, hepatic or renal disease. Tablets and oral suspension are not bioequivalent (do not substitute on a mg-per-mg basis). Some products may contain phenylalanine.

Adverse Reactions (Reflective of adult population; not specific for elderly)
1% to 10%:
Endocrine & metabolic: Alkaline phosphatase increased (2%)
Hematologic: Eosinophilia (7%), hemoglobin and hematocrit decreased (10%)
Hepatic: Transaminases increased (4%)
Local: Thrombophlebitis (2%)
Reactions reported with other cephalosporins: Agranulocytosis, aplastic anemia, asterixis, encephalopathy, hemorrhage, neuromuscular excitability, serum-sickness reactions, superinfection, toxic nephropathy

Overdosage/Toxicology After acute overdose, most agents cause only nausea, vomiting, and diarrhea, although neuromuscular hypersensitivity and seizures are possible, especially in patients with renal insufficiency. Many beta-lactam antibiotics have the potential to cause neuromuscular hyperirritability or seizures. Hemodialysis may be helpful to aid in removal of the drug from the blood but not usually indicated; otherwise, most treatment is supportive or symptom-directed, following GI decontamination.

Drug Interactions
Increased effect: High-dose probenecid decreases clearance.
Increased toxicity: Aminoglycosides increase nephrotoxic potential.

Ethanol/Nutrition/Herb Interactions Food: Bioavailability is increased with food; cefuroxime serum levels may be increased if taken with food or dairy products.

Stability Reconstituted solution is stable for 24 hours at room temperature and 48 hours when refrigerated. I.V. infusion in NS or D_5W solution is stable for 24 hours at room temperature, 7 days when refrigerated, or 26 weeks when frozen. After freezing, thawed solution is stable for 24 hours at room temperature or 21 days when refrigerated.
Oral suspension: Store in refrigerator or at room temperature. Discard after 10 days.

Mechanism of Action Inhibits bacterial cell wall synthesis by binding to one or more of the penicillin-binding proteins (PBPs) which in turn inhibits the final transpeptidation step of peptidoglycan synthesis in bacterial cell walls, thus inhibiting cell wall biosynthesis. Bacteria eventually lyse due to ongoing activity of cell wall autolytic enzymes (autolysins and murein hydrolases) while cell wall assembly is arrested.

Pharmacokinetics
Absorption: Increased when given with or shortly after food
Protein binding: 33% to 50%
Bioavailability: Oral cefuroxime axetil: 37% to 52%
Half-life (adults): 1-2 hours (prolonged in renal impairment)
The serum half-life of cefuroxime is prolonged in older adults due to decreased renal function; mean half-life: 2-4 hours
Time to peak plasma concentration:
I.M.: Within 15-60 minutes
I.V.: 2-3 minutes
Elimination: Primarily excreted 66% to 100% as unchanged drug in urine by both glomerular filtration and tubular secretion; can be removed by dialysis

Dosage
Geriatrics & Adults: Note: Cefuroxime axetil film-coated tablets and oral suspension are not bioequivalent and are not substitutable on a mg/mg basis.

Acute bacterial maxillary sinusitis: Oral: 250 mg twice daily for 10 days
Bronchitis, acute (and exacerbations of chronic bronchitis):
Oral: 250-500 mg every 12 hours for 10 days
I.V.: 500-750 mg every 8 hours (complete therapy with oral dosing)
Cellulitis:
Oral: 500 mg every 12 hours
Orbital: I.V.: 1.5 g every 8 hours
Gonorrhea:
Disseminated: I.M., I.V.: 750 mg every 8 hours
Uncomplicated:
Oral: 1 g as a single dose
I.M.: 1.5 g as single dose (administer in two different sites with probenecid)

Lyme disease (early): Oral: 500 mg twice daily for 20 days

Pharyngitis/tonsillitis and sinusitis: Oral: 250 mg twice daily for 10 days

Skin/skin structure infection, uncomplicated:
Oral: 250-500 mg every 12 hours for 10 days
I.M., I.V.: 750 mg every 8 hours

Pneumonia, uncomplicated: I.M., I.V.: 750 mg every 8 hours

Severe or complicated infections: I.M., I.V.: 1.5 g every 8 hours (up to 1.5 g every 6 hours in life-threatening infections)

Surgical prophylaxis:
I.V.: 1.5 g 30 minutes to 1 hour prior to procedure (if procedure is prolonged can give 750 mg every 8 hours I.M.)
Open heart: I.V.: 1.5 g every 12 hours to a total of 6 g

Urinary tract infection, uncomplicated:
Oral: 125-250 mg twice daily for 7-10 days
I.V., I.M.: 750 mg every 8 hours

Renal Impairment:
Cl_{cr} 10-20 mL/minute: Administer every 12 hours.
Cl_{cr} <10 mL/minute: Administer every 24 hours.
Hemodialysis: Dialyzable (25%)
Note: Cefuroxime axetil film-coated tablets and oral suspension are not bioequivalent and are not substitutable on a mg/mg basis.
Continuous arteriovenous or venovenous hemodiafiltration effects: Dose as for Cl_{cr} 10-20 mL/minute.

Administration Tablets can be crushed and given with soft foods to mask the bitter taste; I.M. doses should be given deep into a large muscle (ie, gluteus maximus)

Monitoring Parameters Observe for signs and symptoms of anaphylaxis during first dose; with prolonged therapy, monitor renal, hepatic, and hematologic function periodically; monitor prothrombin time in patients at risk of prolongation during cephalosporin therapy (nutritionally-deficient, prolonged treatment, renal or hepatic disease)

Test Interactions Positive direct Coombs', false-positive urinary glucose test with cupric sulfate (Benedict's solution, Clinitest®, Fehling's solution), false-positive serum or urine creatinine with Jaffé reaction

Patient Information Complete full course of therapy, do not skip doses; can be taken with food or milk; notify physician if severe diarrhea occurs

Additional Information Sodium content of 1 g: 54.2 mg (2.4 mEq)

Special Geriatric Considerations Adjust dose for renal function in the elderly. Considered one of the drugs of choice for outpatient treatment of community-acquired pneumonia in the elderly.

Dosage Forms Excipient information presented when available (limited, particularly for generics); consult specific product labeling.
Note: Strength expressed as base
Infusion, as sodium [premixed]: 750 mg (50 mL); 1.5 g (50 mL)
Zinacef®: 750 mg (50 mL); 1.5 g (50 mL) [contains sodium 4.8 mEq (111 mg) per 750 mg]
Injection, powder for reconstitution, as sodium: 750 mg, 1.5 g, 7.5 g
Zinacef®: 750 mg, 1.5 g, 7.5 g [contains sodium 1.8 mEq (41 mg) per 750 mg]
Powder for oral suspension, as axetil:
Ceftin®: 125 mg/5 mL (100 mL) [contains phenylalanine 11.8 mg/5 mL; tutti-frutti flavor]; 250 mg/5 mL (50 mL, 100 mL) [contains phenylalanine 25.2 mg/5 mL; tutti-frutti flavor]
Tablet, as axetil: 250 mg, 500 mg
Ceftin®: 250 mg, 500 mg

Selected References

American Thoracic Society, "Guidelines for the Initial Management of Adults With Community-Acquired Pneumonia: Diagnosis Assessment of Severity and Initial Antimicrobial Therapy," *Am Rev Respir Dis*, 1993, 148(5):1418-26.

Broekhuysen J, Deger F, Douchamps J, et al, "Pharmacokinetic Study of Cefuroxime in the Elderly," *Br J Clin Pharmacol*, 1981, 21(6):801-5.

Douglas JG, Bax RP, and Munro JF, "The Pharmacokinetics of Cefuroxime in the Elderly," *J Antimicrob Chemother*, 1980, 6(4):543-9.

♦ **Cefuroxime Axetil** *see* Cefuroxime *on page 275*

♦ **Cefuroxime Sodium** *see* Cefuroxime *on page 275*

♦ **Cefzil®** *see* Cefprozil *on page 266*

♦ **Celebrex®** *see* Celecoxib *on page 277*

Celecoxib (se le KOKS ib)

Medication Safety Issues

Sound-alike/look-alike issues:
Celebrex® may be confused with Celexa®, cerebra, Cerebyx®
(Continued)

Celecoxib *(Continued)*

U.S. Brand Names Celebrex®

Canadian Brand Names Celebrex®; GD-Celecoxib

Generic Available No

Pharmacologic Category Nonsteroidal Anti-inflammatory Drug (NSAID), COX-2 Selective

Use Relief of the signs and symptoms of osteoarthritis, ankylosing spondylitis, juvenile rheumatoid arthritis (JRA), and rheumatoid arthritis; management of acute pain; treatment of primary dysmenorrhea; decreasing intestinal polyps in familial adenomatous polyposis (FAP).

Canadian note: Celecoxib is only indicated for relief of symptoms of rheumatoid arthritis, osteoarthritis, and relief of acute pain in adults

Restrictions An FDA-approved medication guide must be distributed when dispensing an oral outpatient prescription (new or refill) where this medication is to be used without direct supervision of a healthcare provider. Medication guides are available at http://www.fda.gov/cder/Offices/ODS/medication_guides.htm.

Contraindications Hypersensitivity to celecoxib, sulfonamides, aspirin, other NSAIDs, or any component of the formulation; perioperative pain in the setting of coronary artery bypass surgery (CABG)

Warnings/Precautions [U.S. Boxed Warning]: NSAIDs are associated with an increased risk of adverse cardiovascular events, including MI, and new onset or worsening of pre-existing hypertension. Risk may be increased with duration of use or pre-existing cardiovascular risk factors or disease. Carefully evaluate individual cardiovascular risk profiles prior to prescribing. Use caution with fluid retention, CHF, cerebrovascular disease, ischemic heart disease, or hypertension.

[U.S. Boxed Warning]: Celecoxib is contraindicated for treatment of perioperative pain in the setting of coronary artery bypass surgery (CABG). Risk of MI and stroke may be increased with use following CABG surgery.

[U.S. Boxed Warning]: NSAIDs may increase risk of gastrointestinal irritation, ulceration, bleeding, and perforation. These events may occur at any time during therapy and without warning. Use caution with a history of GI disease (bleeding or ulcers), concurrent therapy with aspirin, anticoagulants and/or corticosteroids, smoking, use of alcohol, the elderly or debilitated patients.

Use the lowest effective dose for the shortest duration of time, consistent with individual patient goals, to reduce risk of cardiovascular or GI adverse events. Alternate therapies should be considered for patients at high risk.

NSAIDs may cause serious skin adverse events including exfoliative dermatitis, Stevens-Johnson syndrome (SJS), and toxic epidermal necrolysis (TEN). Anaphylactoid reactions may occur, even without prior exposure; patients with "aspirin triad" (bronchial asthma, aspirin intolerance, rhinitis) may be at increased risk. Do not use in patients who experience bronchospasm, asthma, rhinitis, or urticaria with NSAID or aspirin therapy. Use caution in other forms of asthma.

Use with caution in patients with decreased hepatic or renal function. Closely monitor patients with any abnormal LFT. Severe hepatic reactions (eg, fulminant hepatitis, liver failure) have occurred with NSAID use, rarely; discontinue if signs or symptoms of liver disease develop, or if systemic manifestations occur. Use of NSAIDs can compromise existing renal function. Renal toxicity can occur in patients with impaired renal function, dehydration, heart failure, liver dysfunction, those taking diuretics and ACE inhibitors, and the elderly. Rehydrate patient before starting therapy; monitor renal function closely. Not recommended for use in patients with advanced renal disease.

Anaphylactoid reactions may occur, even with no prior exposure to celecoxib. Use caution in patients with known or suspected deficiency of cytochrome P450 isoenzyme 2C9.

When used for the treatment of FAP, routine monitoring and care should be continued.

Adverse Reactions (Reflective of adult population; not specific for elderly)

Note: Percentages noted in adults.

>10%: Central nervous system: Headache (16%)

2% to 10%:

Cardiovascular: Peripheral edema (2%)

Central nervous system: Insomnia (2%), dizziness (2%)

Dermatologic: Skin rash (2%)

Gastrointestinal: Dyspepsia (9%), diarrhea (6%), abdominal pain (4%), nausea (4%), flatulence (2%)

Neuromuscular & skeletal: Back pain (3%)

Respiratory: Upper respiratory tract infection (8%), sinusitis (5%), pharyngitis (2%), rhinitis (2%)

Miscellaneous: Accidental injury (3%)

0.1% to 2%:

Cardiovascular: Hypertension (aggravated), chest pain, MI, palpitation, tachycardia, facial edema

Central nervous system: Migraine, vertigo, hypoesthesia, fatigue, fever, pain, hypotonia, anxiety, depression, nervousness, somnolence

Dermatologic: Alopecia, dermatitis, photosensitivity, pruritus, rash (maculopapular), rash (erythematous), dry skin, urticaria

Endocrine & metabolic: Hot flashes, diabetes mellitus, hyperglycemia, hypercholesterolemia, breast pain, dysmenorrhea, menstrual disturbances, hypokalemia

Gastrointestinal: Constipation, tenesmus, diverticulitis, eructation, esophagitis, gastroenteritis, vomiting, gastroesophageal reflux, hemorrhoids, hiatal hernia, melena, stomatitis, anorexia, appetite increased, taste disturbance, dry mouth, tooth disorder, weight gain

Genitourinary: Prostate disorder, vaginal bleeding, vaginitis, monilial vaginitis, dysuria, cystitis, urinary frequency, incontinence, urinary tract infection,

Hematologic: Anemia, thrombocytopenia, ecchymosis

Hepatic: Alkaline phosphatase increased, transaminases increased

Neuromuscular & skeletal: Leg cramps, CPK increased, neck stiffness, arthralgia, myalgia, bone disorder, fracture, synovitis, tendonitis, neuralgia, paresthesia, neuropathy, weakness

Ocular: Glaucoma, blurred vision, cataract, conjunctivitis, eye pain

Otic: Deafness, tinnitus, earache, otitis media

Renal: BUN increased, creatinine increased, albuminuria, hematuria, renal calculi

Respiratory: Bronchitis, bronchospasm, cough, dyspnea, laryngitis, pneumonia, epistaxis

Miscellaneous: Allergic reactions, diaphoresis increased, flu-like syndrome, breast cancer, herpes infection, bacterial infection, moniliasis, viral infection

Overdosage/Toxicology Doses up to 2400 mg/day for up to 10 days have been reported without serious toxicity. Symptoms may include epigastric pain, drowsiness, lethargy, nausea, and vomiting. Gastrointestinal bleeding may occur. Rare manifestations include hypertension, respiratory depression, coma, and acute renal failure. Treatment is symptomatic and supportive. Forced diuresis, hemodialysis and/or urinary alkalinization may not be useful.

Drug Interactions Substrate of CYP2C9 (major), 3A4 (minor); **Inhibits** CYP2C8 (moderate), 2D6 (weak)

ACE inhibitors: Antihypertensive effect may be diminished by celecoxib.

Aminoglycosides: Celecoxib may decrease excretion; monitor levels.

Anticoagulants: Celecoxib may enhance the anticoagulant effect of anticoagulants; monitor.

Antiplatelet agents: Celecoxib may enhance the adverse/toxic effect of antiplatelet agents. An increased risk of bleeding may occur.

Aspirin: Low-dose aspirin may be used with celecoxib, however, monitor for GI complications.

Beta-blockers: Antihypertensive effect may be diminished by celecoxib.

Bile acid sequestrants: May decrease absorption of NSAIDs.

CYP2C8 substrates: Celecoxib may increase the levels/effects of CYP2C8 substrates. Example substrates include amiodarone, paclitaxel, pioglitazone, repaglinide, and rosiglitazone.

CYP2C9 inducers: May decrease the levels/effects of celecoxib. Example inducers include carbamazepine, phenobarbital, phenytoin, rifampin, rifapentine, and secobarbital.

CYP2C9 inhibitors: May increase the levels/effects of celecoxib. Example inhibitors include delavirdine, fluconazole, gemfibrozil, ketoconazole, nicardipine, NSAIDs, pioglitazone, and sulfonamides.

Cyclosporine: NSAIDs may increase levels/nephrotoxicity of cyclosporine.

Fluconazole: Fluconazole increases celecoxib concentrations twofold. Lowest dose of celecoxib should be used.

Hydralazine: Antihypertensive effect may be diminished by celecoxib.

Lithium: Plasma levels of lithium are increased by ~17% when used with celecoxib. Monitor lithium levels closely when treatment with celecoxib is started or withdrawn.

Loop diuretics (bumetanide, furosemide, torsemide): Natriuretic effect of furosemide and other loop diuretics may be decreased by celecoxib.

Methotrexate: Severe bone marrow suppression, aplastic anemia, and GI toxicity have been reported with concomitant NSAID therapy. Selective COX-2 inhibitors appear to have a lower risk of this toxicity, however, caution is warranted.

Probenecid: Probenecid may increase the serum concentration of celecoxib; monitor.

Quinolone antibiotics: Celecoxib may enhance the neuroexcitatory and/or seizure-potentiating effect of quinolone antibiotics.

Thiazide diuretics: Natriuretic effects of thiazide diuretics may be decreased by celecoxib.

Treprostinil: Treprostinil may enhance the adverse/toxic effect of celecoxib. Bleeding may occur; monitor.

(Continued)

Celecoxib *(Continued)*

Vancomycin: Celecoxib may decrease excretion; monitor levels.

Ethanol/Nutrition/Herb Interactions

Ethanol: Avoid ethanol (increased GI irritation).

Food: Peak concentrations are delayed and AUC is increased by 10% to 20% when taken with a high-fat meal.

Herb/Nutraceutical: Avoid concomitant use with herbs possessing anticoagulation/anti-platelet properties, including alfalfa, anise, bilberry, bladderwrack, bromelain, cat's claw, celery, chamomile, coleus, cordyceps, dong quai, evening primrose oil, fenu-greek, feverfew, garlic, ginger, ginkgo biloba, ginseng, grapeseed, green tea, guggul, horse chestnut seed, horseradish, licorice, prickly ash, red clover, reishi, SAMe, sweet clover, turmeric, white willow

Stability Store at controlled room temperature of 25°C (77°F).

Mechanism of Action Inhibits prostaglandin synthesis by decreasing the activity of the enzyme, cyclooxygenase-2 (COX-2), which results in decreased formation of prosta-glandin precursors. Celecoxib does not inhibit cyclooxygenase-1 (COX-1) at thera-peutic concentrations. Celecoxib has no effect on platelets. In FAP, celecoxib reduces the number of colorectal polyps.

Pharmacokinetics

Distribution: V_d (apparent): 400 L

Protein binding: 97% prelimarily to albumin

Metabolism: Hepatic; forms inactive metabolites

Bioavailability, absolute: Has not been determined

Half-life: 11 hours

Time to peak: 3 hours

Excretion: Urine (27% as metabolites, <3% as unchanged drug); feces (57%)

Dosage

Geriatrics: Refer to adult dosing. No specific adjustment based on age is recom-mended. However, the AUC in elderly patients may be increased by 50% as compared to younger subjects. Use the lowest recommended dose in patients weighing <50 kg.

Adults: Note: Use the lowest effective dose for the shortest duration of time, consis-tent with individual patient goals.

Osteoarthritis: Oral: 200 mg/day as a single dose or in divided dose twice daily

Ankylosing spondylitis: Oral: 200 mg/day as a single dose or in divided doses twice daily; if no effect after 6 weeks, may increase to 400 mg/day. If no response following 6 weeks of treatment with 400 mg/day, consider discontinuation and alternative treatment.

Rheumatoid arthritis: Oral: 100-200 mg twice daily

Familial adenomatous polyposis: Oral: 400 mg twice daily

Acute pain or primary dysmenorrhea: Oral: Initial dose: 400 mg, followed by an additional 200 mg if needed on day 1; maintenance dose: 200 mg twice daily as needed

Renal Impairment: No specific dosage adjustment is recommended. Not recom-mended in patients with severe renal dysfunction.

Hepatic Impairment: Reduced dosage is recommended (AUC may be increased by 40% to 180%). Decrease dose by 50% in patients with moderate hepatic impairment (Child-Pugh class B). Not recommended for use with severe impairment.

Administration Lower doses (200 mg twice daily) may be taken without regard to meals. Larger doses should be taken with food to improve absorption. Capsules may be swallowed whole or the entire contents emptied onto a teaspoon of cool or room temperature applesauce. The contents of the capsules sprinkled onto applesauce may be stored under refrigeration for up to 6 hours.

Monitoring Parameters CBC; occult blood loss and periodic liver function tests; monitor response (pain, range of motion, grip strength, mobility, ADL function), inflam-mation; observe for weight gain, edema; monitor renal function (urine output, serum BUN and creatinine); observe for bleeding, bruising; evaluate gastrointestinal effects (abdominal pain, bleeding, dyspepsia); blood pressure

FAP: Continue routine endoscopic exams

Patient Information Gastrointestinal bleeding may occur as well as ulceration and perforation; pain may or may not be present. If gastric upset occurs, take with food, milk, or antacid; if gastric upset persists, contact physician.

Special Geriatric Considerations The elderly are at increased risk for adverse effects from NSAIDs. As many as 60% of elderly can develop peptic ulceration and/or hemorrhage asymptomatically. CNS adverse effects such as confusion, agitation, and hallucination are generally seen in overdose or high-dose situations; however, elderly patients may demonstrate these adverse effects at lower doses than younger adults. The elderly are also at increased risk of renal toxicity. Use the lowest recommended dose in patients weighing <50 kg.

Dosage Forms Excipient information presented when available (limited, particularly for generics); consult specific product labeling.
Capsule:
Celebrex®: 50 mg, 100 mg, 200 mg, 400 mg

Selected References
Geis GS, et al, "Efficacy and Safety of Celecoxib, A Specific COX-2 Inhibitor, in Patients With Rheumatoid Arthritis," *Arthritis Rheum*, 1998, 41(9 Suppl):S316:1699.
Karim A, et al, "Celecoxib, A Specific COX-2 Inhibitor, Lacks Significant Drug-Drug Interactions With Methotrexate or Warfarin," *Arthritis Rheum*, 1998, 41(9 Suppl):S315:1698.
Lane NE, "Pain Management in Osteoarthritis: The Role of COX-2 Inhibitors," *J Rheumatol*, 1997, 24(Suppl 49):20-4.
Lipsky PE and Isakson PC, "Outcome of Specific COX-2 Inhibition in Rheumatoid Arthritis," *J Rheumatol*, 1997, 24(Suppl 49):9-14.
Mengle-Gaw L, et al, "A Study of the Platelet Effects of SC-58635, A Novel COX-2 Selective Inhibitor," *Arthritis Rheum*, 1998, 41(9 Suppl):S93:374.
Needleman P and Isakson PC, "The Discovery and Function of COX-2," *J Rheumatol*, 1997, 24(Suppl 49):6-8.
Simon LS, et al, "Preliminary Study of the Safety and Efficacy of SC-58635, A Novel Cyclo-oxygenase 2 Inhibitor: Efficacy and Safety in Two Placebo-Controlled Trials in Osteoarthritis and Rheumatoid Arthritis, and Studies of Gastrointestinal and Platelet Effects," *Arthritis Rheum*, 1998, 41:1591-1602.

♦ **Celestone®** *see Betamethasone on page 161*
♦ **Celestone® Soluspan®** *see Betamethasone on page 161*
♦ **Celexa®** *see Citalopram on page 322*
♦ **Celontin®** *see Methsuximide on page 1011*
♦ **Cemill [OTC]** *see Ascorbic Acid on page 125*
♦ **Cenestin®** *see Estrogens (Conjugated A/Synthetic) on page 558*
♦ **Cenolate®** *see Ascorbic Acid on page 125*
♦ **Centany™** *see Mupirocin on page 1075*

Cephalexin (sef a LEKS in)

Related Information
Antimicrobial Activity Against Selected Organisms *on page 1728*
Prevention of Infective Endocarditis *on page 1803*
Medication Safety Issues
Sound-alike/look-alike issues:
Cephalexin may be confused with cefaclor, cefazolin, cephalothin, ciprofloxacin
U.S. Brand Names Keflex®
Canadian Brand Names Apo-Cephalex®; Keftab®; Novo-Lexin; Nu-Cephalex
Index Terms Cephalexin Monohydrate
Generic Available Yes
Pharmacologic Category Antibiotic, Cephalosporin (First Generation)
Use Treatment of susceptible bacterial infections including respiratory tract infections, otitis media, skin and skin structure infections, bone infections and genitourinary tract infections, including acute prostatitis; alternative therapy for acute bacterial endocarditis prophylaxis
Contraindications Hypersensitivity to cephalexin, any component of the formulation, or other cephalosporins
Warnings/Precautions Modify dosage in patients with severe renal impairment. Use with caution in patients with a history of penicillin allergy, especially IgE-mediated reactions (eg, anaphylaxis, urticaria). Prolonged use may result in fungal or bacterial superinfection, including *C. difficile*-associated diarrhea and pseudomembranous colitis. May be associated with increased INR, especially in nutritionally-deficient patients, prolonged treatment, hepatic or renal disease.
Adverse Reactions (Reflective of adult population; not specific for elderly)
Frequency not defined.
Central nervous system: Agitation, confusion, dizziness, fatigue, hallucinations, headache
Dermatologic: Angioedema, erythema multiforme (rare), rash, Stevens-Johnson syndrome (rare), toxic epidermal necrolysis (rare), urticaria
Gastrointestinal: Abdominal pain, diarrhea, dyspepsia, gastritis, nausea (rare), pseudomembranous colitis, vomiting (rare)
Genitourinary: Genital pruritus, genital moniliasis, vaginitis, vaginal discharge
Hematologic: Eosinophilia, hemolytic anemia, neutropenia, thrombocytopenia
Hepatic: AST/ALT increased, cholestatic jaundice (rare), transient hepatitis (rare)
Neuromuscular & skeletal: Arthralgia, arthritis, joint disorder
Renal: Interstitial nephritis (rare)
Miscellaneous: Allergic reactions, anaphylaxis
Overdosage/Toxicology Symptoms of overdose include epigastric distress, diarrhea, hematuria, nausea, and vomiting. Many beta-lactam containing antibiotics have the potential to cause neuromuscular hyperirritability or seizures. Hemodialysis may be helpful to aid in removal of the drug from blood; otherwise, treatment is supportive and symptom-directed.
(Continued)

Cephalexin (Continued)

Drug Interactions
Aminoglycosides: Increase nephrotoxic potential.

Probenecid: High-dose probenecid decreases clearance of cephalexin.

Typhoid vaccine: Antibiotics may diminish the efficacy of the live, attenuated Ty21a strain vaccine.

Ethanol/Nutrition/Herb Interactions Food: Peak antibiotic serum concentration is lowered and delayed, but total drug absorbed is not affected. Cephalexin serum levels may be decreased if taken with food.

Stability
Capsule: Store at 15°C to 30°C (59°F to 86°F).

Powder for oral suspension: Refrigerate suspension after reconstitution; discard after 14 days.

Tablet for oral suspension (Panixine DisperDose™): Tablet must be dissolved in ~10 mL water prior to administration, and should be used immediately after dissolving.

Mechanism of Action Inhibits bacterial cell wall synthesis by binding to one or more of the penicillin-binding proteins (PBPs) which in turn inhibits the final transpeptidation step of peptidoglycan synthesis in bacterial cell walls, thus inhibiting cell wall biosynthesis. Bacteria eventually lyse due to ongoing activity of cell wall autolytic enzymes (autolysins and murein hydrolases) while cell wall assembly is arrested.

Pharmacokinetics
Half-life: 0.5-1.2 hours (prolonged with renal impairment)

Protein binding: 6% to 15%

Time to peak serum concentration: Oral: Within 60 minutes

Elimination: 80% to 100% of dose excreted as unchanged drug in urine within 8 hours

Dosage
Geriatrics & Adults:

Dosing range: Oral: 250-1000 mg every 6 hours (maximum: 4 g/day)

Cellulitis and mastitis: Oral 500 mg every 6 hours

Furunculosis/skin abscess: Oral: 250 mg 4 times/day

Prophylaxis of bacterial endocarditis (dental, oral, respiratory tract, or esophageal procedures): Oral: 2 g 1 hour prior to procedure

Streptococcal pharyngitis, skin and skin structure infections: Oral: 500 mg every 12 hours

Uncomplicated cystitis: Oral: 500 mg every 12 hours for 7-14 days

Renal Impairment: Adults:

Cl_{cr} 10-50 mL/minute: 500 mg every 8-12 hours

Cl_{cr} <10: 250-500 mg every 12-24 hours

Hemodialysis: 250 mg every 12-24 hours; moderately dialyzable (20% to 50%); give dose after dialysis session

Administration Take without regard to food. If GI distress, take with food. Give around-the-clock to promote less variation in peak and trough serum levels.

Panixine DisperDose™: Tablets should be mixed in ~10 mL of water immediately prior to administration. Drink entire solution, then rinse glass with additional water and drink contents to ensure entire dose has been taken. Tablets should not be chewed or swallowed whole.

Monitoring Parameters Signs and symptoms of infection

Test Interactions Positive direct Coombs', false-positive urinary glucose test using cupric sulfate (Benedict's solution, Clinitest®, Fehling's solution), false-positive serum or urine creatinine with Jaffé reaction, false-positive urinary proteins and steroids

Patient Information Complete full course of therapy; may take with food or milk if GI upset occurs; notify physician if severe diarrhea occurs

Special Geriatric Considerations Adjust dose for renal function.

Dosage Forms Excipient information presented when available (limited, particularly for generics); consult specific product labeling.

Capsule: 250 mg, 500 mg

Keflex®: 250 mg, 500 mg, 750 mg

Powder for oral suspension: 125 mg/5 mL (100 mL, 200 mL); 250 mg/5 mL (100 mL, 200 mL)

Keflex®: 125 mg/5 mL (100 mL, 200 mL); 250 mg/5 mL (100 mL, 200 mL)

Tablet: 250 mg, 500 mg

♦ **Cephalexin Monohydrate** see Cephalexin on page 281

♦ **Cerebyx®** see Fosphenytoin on page 681

♦ **Cerumenex® [DSC]** see Triethanolamine Polypeptide Oleate-Condensate on page 1627

♦ **C.E.S.** see Estrogens (Conjugated/Equine) on page 564

♦ **Cetacort® [DSC]** see Hydrocortisone on page 762

♦ **Cetafen® [OTC]** see Acetaminophen on page 29

♦ **Cetafen Extra® [OTC]** see Acetaminophen on page 29

Cetirizine (se TI ra zeen)

Medication Safety Issues
Sound-alike/look-alike issues:
Zyrtec® may be confused with Serax®, Xanax®, Zantac®, Zyprexa®

U.S. Brand Names Zyrtec®
Canadian Brand Names Apo-Cetirizine®; Reactine™
Index Terms Cetirizine Hydrochloride; P-071; UCB-P071
Generic Available No
Pharmacologic Category Antihistamine
Use Treatment of perennial and seasonal allergic rhinitis and other allergic symptoms including chronic urticaria
Contraindications Hypersensitivity to cetirizine, hydroxyzine, or any component of the formulation
Warnings/Precautions Cetirizine should be used cautiously in patients with hepatic or renal dysfunction, the elderly and in nursing mothers. May cause drowsiness; use caution performing tasks which require alertness (eg, operating machinery or driving).
Adverse Reactions (Reflective of adult population; not specific for elderly)
>10%: Central nervous system: Headache (children 11% to 14%, placebo 12%), somnolence (adults 14%, children 2% to 4%)
2% to 10%:
Central nervous system: Insomnia (children 9%, adults <2%), fatigue (adults 6%), malaise (4%), dizziness (adults 2%)
Gastrointestinal: Abdominal pain (children 4% to 6%), dry mouth (adults 5%), diarrhea (children 2% to 3%), nausea (children 2% to 3%, placebo 2%), vomiting (children 2% to 3%)
Respiratory: Epistaxis (children 2% to 4%, placebo 3%), pharyngitis (children 3% to 6%, placebo 3%), bronchospasm (children 2% to 3%, placebo 2%)
Overdosage/Toxicology Symptoms of overdose may include somnolence, restlessness, or irritability. Treatment is symptomatic and supportive. Cetirizine is not removed by dialysis.
Drug Interactions Substrate of CYP3A4 (minor)
Increased toxicity: CNS depressants, anticholinergics
Ethanol/Nutrition/Herb Interactions Ethanol: Avoid ethanol (may increase CNS depression).
Stability
Syrup: Store at room temperature of 15°C to 30°C (59°F to 86°F), or under refrigeration at 2°C to 8°C (36°F to 46°F).
Tablet: Store at room temperature of 15°C to 30°C (59°F to 86°F).
Mechanism of Action Competes with histamine for H_1-receptor sites on effector cells in the gastrointestinal tract, blood vessels, and respiratory tract
Pharmacodynamics
Onset of action: Within 1 hour
Duration: 24 hours
Pharmacokinetics
Distribution: Minimal penetration into central nervous system
Protein binding: 93%
Metabolism: **Not** extensively metabolized by the liver
Half-life: 7.4-9 hours; in mild-moderate renal failure the half-life is increased to 19-21 hours
Time to peak: 0.5-1 hour; food may delay time to peak and decrease C_{max}
Elimination: 60% of dose is excreted unchanged in urine within 24 hours
Note: In older adults, there was a 50% increase in half-life and a 40% decrease in clearance, most likely due to change in renal function; not removed by hemodialysis
Dosage
Geriatrics: Oral: Initial: 5 mg once daily; may increase to 10 mg/day
Note: Manufacturer recommends 5 mg/day in patients ≥77 years of age.
Adults: Perennial or seasonal allergic rhinitis, chronic urticaria: Oral: 5-10 mg once daily, depending upon symptom severity
Renal Impairment: Adults:
Cl_{cr} 11-31 mL/minute or hemodialysis: Administer 5 mg once daily
Cl_{cr} <11 mL/minute, not on dialysis: Cetirizine use not recommended.
Hepatic Impairment: Adults: Administer 5 mg once daily
Monitoring Parameters Relief of symptoms
Patient Information May be taken at any time during the day, with or without food
Additional Information Unlike other second generation antihistamines, cetirizine has not been associated with torsade de pointes and does **not** interact with macrolide antibiotics or ketoconazole
Special Geriatric Considerations Adjust dose for renal function.
(Continued)

Cetirizine *(Continued)*

Dosage Forms Excipient information presented when available (limited, particularly for generics); consult specific product labeling.

Syrup, as hydrochloride:
Zyrtec®: 5 mg/5 mL (120 mL, 480 mL) [contains propylene glycol; banana-grape flavor]
Tablet, as hydrochloride:
Zyrtec®: 5 mg, 10 mg
Tablet, chewable, as hydrochloride:
Zyrtec®: 5 mg, 10 mg [grape flavor]

♦ **Cetirizine Hydrochloride** *see Cetirizine on page 283*

Cevimeline (se vi ME leen)

Medication Safety Issues
Sound-alike/look-alike issues:
Evoxac® may be confused with Eurax®
U.S. Brand Names Evoxac®
Canadian Brand Names Evoxac®
Index Terms Cevimeline Hydrochloride
Generic Available No
Pharmacologic Category Cholinergic Agonist
Use Treatment of symptoms of dry mouth in patients with Sjögren's syndrome
Contraindications Hypersensitivity to cevimeline or any component of the formulation; uncontrolled asthma; narrow-angle glaucoma; acute iritis; other conditions where miosis is undesirable

Warnings/Precautions May alter cardiac conduction and/or heart rate; use caution in patients with significant cardiovascular disease, including angina, myocardial infarction, or conduction disturbances. Cevimeline has the potential to increase bronchial smooth muscle tone, airway resistance, and bronchial secretions; use with caution in patients with controlled asthma, COPD, or chronic bronchitis. May cause decreased visual acuity (particularly at night and in patients with central lens changes) and impaired depth perception. Patients should be cautioned about driving at night or performing hazardous activities in reduced lighting. May cause a variety of parasympathomimetic effects, which may be particularly dangerous in elderly patients; excessive sweating may lead to dehydration in some patients.

Use with caution in patients with a history of biliary stones or nephrolithiasis; cevimeline may induce smooth muscle spasms, precipitating cholangitis, cholecystitis, biliary obstruction, renal colic, or ureteral reflux in susceptible patients. Patients with a known or suspected deficiency of CYP2D6 may be at higher risk of adverse effects.

Adverse Reactions (Reflective of adult population; not specific for elderly)
>10%:
Central nervous system: Headache (14%; placebo 20%)
Gastrointestinal: Nausea (14%), diarrhea (10%)
Respiratory: Rhinitis (11%), sinusitis (12%), upper respiratory infection (11%)
Miscellaneous: Diaphoresis increased (19%)
1% to 10%:
Cardiovascular: Peripheral edema, chest pain, edema, palpitation
Central nervous system: Dizziness (4%), fatigue (3%), pain (3%), insomnia (2%), anxiety (1%), fever, depression, migraine, hypoesthesia, vertigo
Dermatologic: Rash (4%; placebo 6%), pruritus, skin disorder, erythematous rash
Endocrine & metabolic: Hot flashes (2%)
Gastrointestinal: Dyspepsia (8%; placebo 9%), abdominal pain (8%), vomiting (5%), excessive salivation (2%), constipation, salivary gland pain, dry mouth, sialoadenitis, gastroesophageal reflux, flatulence, ulcerative stomatitis, eructation, amylase increased, anorexia, tooth disorder
Genitourinary: Urinary tract infection (6%), vaginitis, cystitis
Hematologic: Anemia
Local: Abscess
Neuromuscular & skeletal: Back pain (5%), arthralgia (4%), skeletal pain (3%), rigors (1%), hypertonia, tremor, myalgia, hyporeflexia, leg cramps
Ocular: Conjunctivitis (4%), abnormal vision, eye pain, eye abnormality, xerophthalmia
Otic: Earache, otitis media
Respiratory: Coughing (6%), bronchitis (4%), pneumonia, epistaxis
Miscellaneous: Flu-like syndrome, infection, fungal infection, allergy, hiccups
Overdosage/Toxicology Symptoms may include headache, visual disturbances, lacrimation, sweating, gastrointestinal spasm, nausea, vomiting, diarrhea, AV block, mental confusion, tremor, cardiac depression, bradycardia, tachycardia, or bronchospasm.

Atropine may be of value as an antidote, and epinephrine may be required for broncho-constriction. Additional treatment is supportive. The effect of hemodialysis is unknown.

Drug Interactions Substrate (minor) of CYP2D6, CYP3A4

Increased effect: The effects of other cholinergic agents may be increased during concurrent administration with cevimeline. Concurrent use of cevimeline and beta-blockers may increase the potential for conduction disturbances.

Decreased effect: Anticholinergic agents (atropine, TCAs, phenothiazines) may antagonize the effects of cevimeline.

Stability Store at 25°C (77°F).

Mechanism of Action Binds to muscarinic (cholinergic) receptors, causing an increase in secretion of exocrine glands (including salivary glands)

Pharmacokinetics

Distribution: V_d: 6 L/kg

Protein binding: <20%

Metabolism: Hepatic

Half-life: 5 hours

Time to peak: 1.5-2 hours

Elimination: In urine, as metabolites and unchanged drug

Dosage

Geriatrics & Adults: Xerostomia (in Sjögren's syndrome): Oral: 30 mg 3 times/day

Renal Impairment: Not studied; no specific dosage adjustment is recommended

Hepatic Impairment: Not studied; no specific dosage adjustment is recommended

Monitoring Parameters Vital signs, visual changes

Patient Information May be taken with or without food; take with food if medicine causes upset stomach. May cause decreased visual acuity (particularly at night and in patients with central lens changes) and impaired depth perception; patients should be cautioned about driving at night or performing hazardous activities in reduced lighting.

Special Geriatric Considerations No specific studies in the elderly are available. However, elderly often have cardiovascular, pulmonary, and gastrointestinal diseases which may restrict or contraindicate the use of this agent. The use of saliva substitutes should be considered initially. Although the clinical studies included elderly patients (>65 years of age), the number of elderly was insufficient to determine any significant differences between young adults and elderly.

Dosage Forms Excipient information presented when available (limited, particularly for generics); consult specific product labeling.

Capsule, as hydrochloride: 30 mg

♦ **Cevimeline Hydrochloride** see Cevimeline on page 284

♦ **CFDN** see Cefdinir on page 254

♦ **C-Gel [OTC]** see Ascorbic Acid on page 125

♦ **CGP-42446** see Zoledronic Acid on page 1704

♦ **C-Gram [OTC]** see Ascorbic Acid on page 125

♦ **CGS-20267** see Letrozole on page 882

♦ **Chantix™** see Varenicline on page 1664

♦ **Cheracol®** see Guaifenesin and Codeine on page 729

♦ **Cheracol® D [OTC]** see Guaifenesin and Dextromethorphan on page 730

♦ **Cheracol® Plus [OTC]** see Guaifenesin and Dextromethorphan on page 730

♦ **Chew-C [OTC]** see Ascorbic Acid on page 125

♦ **Chew-Cal [OTC]** see Calcium and Vitamin D on page 214

♦ **Chloral** see Chloral Hydrate on page 285

Chloral Hydrate (KLOR al HYE drate)

Medication Safety Issues

High alert medication: The Institute for Safe Medication Practices (ISMP) includes this medication among its list of drugs which have a heightened risk of causing significant patient harm when used in error.

U.S. Brand Names Aquachloral® Supprettes®; Somnote®

Canadian Brand Names PMS-Chloral Hydrate

Index Terms Chloral; Hydrated Chloral; Trichloroacetaldehyde Monohydrate

Generic Available Yes: Syrup and suppositories

Pharmacologic Category Hypnotic, Nonbenzodiazepine

Use Short-term sedative and hypnotic (<2 weeks); sedative/hypnotic for dental and diagnostic procedures; sedative prior to EEG evaluations

Restrictions C-IV

Contraindications Hypersensitivity to chloral hydrate or any component of the formulation; hepatic or renal impairment; gastritis or ulcers; severe cardiac disease

(Continued)

Chloral Hydrate *(Continued)*

Warnings/Precautions Use with caution in patients with porphyria. Trichloroethanol (TCE), a metabolite of chloral hydrate, is a carcinogen in mice; no data available in humans

Adverse Reactions (Reflective of adult population; not specific for elderly) Frequency not defined.

Central nervous system: Ataxia, disorientation, sedation, excitement (paradoxical), dizziness, fever, headache, confusion, lightheadedness, nightmares, hallucinations, drowsiness, "hangover" effect

Dermatologic: Rash, urticaria

Gastrointestinal: Gastric irritation, nausea, vomiting, diarrhea, flatulence

Hematologic: Leukopenia, eosinophilia, acute intermittent porphyria

Miscellaneous: Physical and psychological dependence may occur with prolonged use of large doses

Overdosage/Toxicology Symptoms include hypotension, respiratory depression, coma, hypothermia, cardiac arrhythmias. Treatment is supportive and symptomatic. Lidocaine or propranolol may be used for ventricular dysrhythmias, while isoproterenol or atropine may be required for torsade de pointes. Activated charcoal may prevent drug absorption.

Drug Interactions

CNS depressants: Sedative effects and/or respiratory depression with chloral hydrate may be additive with other CNS depressants; monitor for increased effect; includes ethanol, sedatives, antidepressants, opioid analgesics, and benzodiazepines.

Furosemide: Diaphoresis, flushing, and hypertension have occurred in patients who received I.V. furosemide within 24 hours after administration of chloral hydrate; consider using a benzodiazepine.

Phenytoin: Half-life may be decreased by chloral hydrate; limited documentation (small, single-dose study); monitor.

Warfarin: Effect of oral anticoagulants may be increased by chloral hydrate; monitor INR; warfarin dosage may require adjustment. Chloral hydrate's metabolite may displace warfarin from its protein binding sites resulting in an increase in the hypoprothrombinemic response to warfarin.

Ethanol/Nutrition/Herb Interactions

Ethanol: Avoid ethanol (may increase CNS depression).

Herb/Nutraceutical: Avoid valerian, St John's wort, kava kava, gotu kola (may increase CNS depression).

Stability Sensitive to light. Exposure to air causes volatilization. Store in light-resistant, airtight container.

Mechanism of Action Central nervous system depressant effects are due to its active metabolite trichloroethanol, mechanism unknown

Pharmacodynamics

Peak effect: Within 30-60 minutes

Duration: 4-8 hours

Pharmacokinetics

Absorption: Oral, rectal: Well absorbed

Protein binding: Trichloroacetic acid is highly protein bound and displaces other acidic drugs

Metabolism: Rapid to trichloroethanol; variable amounts metabolized in liver and kidney to trichloroacetic acid (inactive)

Half-life: Trichloroethanol: 8-11 hours

Elimination: Metabolites excreted in urine; small amounts excreted in feces via bile

Dosage

Geriatrics: Hypnotic: Initial: Oral: 250 mg at bedtime; adjust for renal impairment. See Special Geriatric Considerations.

Adults:

Sedation, anxiety: Oral, rectal: 250 mg 3 times/day

Hypnotic: Oral, rectal: 500-1000 mg at bedtime or 30 minutes prior to procedure, not to exceed 2 g/24 hours

Discontinuation: Withdraw gradually over 2 weeks if patient has been maintained on high doses for prolonged period of time. Do not stop drug abruptly; sudden withdrawal may result in delirium.

Renal Impairment:

Cl$_{cr}$ <50 mL/minute: Avoid use.

Hemodialysis effects: Supplemental dose is not necessary; dialyzable (50% to 100%).

Hepatic Impairment: Avoid use in patients with severe hepatic impairment.

Administration Do not crush capsule; contains drug in liquid form. Gastric irritation may be minimized by diluting dose in water or other oral liquid.

Monitoring Parameters Mental status, vital signs

Test Interactions False-positive urine glucose using Clinitest® method; may interfere with fluorometric urine catecholamine and urinary 17-hydroxycorticosteroid tests

Patient Information Take capsule with a full glass of water or fruit juice; swallow capsules whole, do not chew; avoid alcohol and other CNS depressants; avoid activities needing good psychomotor coordination until CNS effects are known; drug may cause physical or psychological dependence; avoid abrupt discontinuation after prolonged use; if taking at home prior to a diagnostic procedure, have someone else transport you

Additional Information Tolerance to hypnotic effect develops, therefore, not recommended for use >2 weeks; taper dosage to avoid withdrawal with prolonged use

Special Geriatric Considerations Chloral hydrate is considered a second- or third-line hypnotic agent in the elderly. Interpretive guidelines from the Centers for Medicare and Medicaid Services (CMS) discourage the use of chloral hydrate in residents of long-term care facilities.

Dosage Forms Excipient information presented when available (limited, particularly for generics); consult specific product labeling.

Capsule:
Somnote®: 500 mg
Suppository, rectal: 500 mg
Aquachloral® Supprettes®: 325 mg [contains tartrazine]
Syrup: 500 mg/5 mL (5 mL, 480 mL)

Chlorambucil (klor AM byoo sil)

Medication Safety Issues

Sound-alike/look-alike issues:
Chlorambucil may be confused with Chloromycetin®
Leukeran® may be confused with Alkeran®, leucovorin, Leukine®, Myleran®

High alert medication: The Institute for Safe Medication Practices (ISMP) includes this medication among its list of drugs which have a heightened risk of causing significant patient harm when used in error.

U.S. Brand Names Leukeran®

Canadian Brand Names Leukeran®

Index Terms CB-1348; Chlorambucilum; Chloraminophene; Chlorbutinum; NSC-3088; WR-139013

Generic Available No

Pharmacologic Category Antineoplastic Agent, Alkylating Agent

Use Management of chronic lymphocytic leukemia (CLL), Hodgkin's lymphoma, non-Hodgkin's lymphoma (NHL)

Unlabeled/Investigational Use Nephrotic syndrome, Waldenström's macroglobulinemia

Contraindications Hypersensitivity to chlorambucil or any component of the formulation; hypersensitivity to other alkylating agents (may have cross-hypersensitivity)

Warnings/Precautions Hazardous agent - use appropriate precautions for handling and disposal. Seizures have been observed; use with caution in patients with seizure disorder or head trauma; history of nephrotic syndrome and high pulse doses are at higher risk of seizures. **[U.S. Boxed Warning]: May cause bone marrow suppression;** reduce initial dosage if patient has received myelosuppressive or radiation therapy, or has a depressed baseline leukocyte or platelet count within the previous 4 weeks. Lymphopenia may occur. Avoid administration of live vaccines to immunocompromised patients. Rare instances of severe skin reactions (eg, erythema multiforme, Stevens-Johnson syndrome) have been reported; discontinue if a reaction occurs.

[U.S. Boxed Warning]: Affects human fertility; carcinogenic in humans and probably mutagenic and teratogenic as well; chromosomal damage has been documented. Fertility effects (reversible and irreversible sterility) include azoospermia (when administered to prepubertal and pubertal males) and amenorrhea. Secondary malignancies and acute myelocytic leukemia may be associated with chronic therapy.

Adverse Reactions (Reflective of adult population; not specific for elderly)
Frequency not always defined.

Central nervous system: Agitation (rare), ataxia (rare), confusion (rare), drug fever, focal/generalized seizure (rare), hallucinations (rare)

Dermatologic: Angioneurotic edema, erythema multiforme (rare), rash, skin hypersensitivity, Stevens-Johnson syndrome (rare), toxic epidermal necrolysis (rare), urticaria

Endocrine & metabolic: Amenorrhea, infertility, SIADH (rare)

Gastrointestinal: Diarrhea (infrequent), nausea (infrequent), oral ulceration (infrequent), vomiting (infrequent)

Genitourinary: Azoospermia, cystitis (sterile)

(Continued)

Chlorambucil *(Continued)*

Hematologic: Neutropenia (25%; dose- and duration-related; onset: 3 weeks; recovery: 10 days after last dose), bone marrow failure (irreversible), bone marrow suppression, anemia, leukemia (secondary), leukopenia, lymphopenia, pancytopenia, thrombocytopenia

Hepatic: Hepatotoxicity, jaundice

Neuromuscular & skeletal: Flaccid paresis (rare), muscular twitching (rare), myoclonia (rare), peripheral neuropathy, tremor (rare)

Respiratory: Interstitial pneumonia, pulmonary fibrosis

Miscellaneous: Allergic reactions, malignancies (secondary)

Overdosage/Toxicology Symptoms of overdose include vomiting, agitation, ataxia, coma, seizures, and pancytopenia. There are no known antidotes for chlorambucil intoxication. Treatment is symptom-directed and supportive. Monitor CBC closely; consider transfusion support. Chlorambucil is not dialyzable.

Drug Interactions Vaccines (live organism): Avoid the administration of live vaccines during chlorambucil treatment.

Stability Store in refrigerator at 2°C to 8°C (36°F to 46°F); protect from light.

Mechanism of Action Interferes with DNA replication and RNA transcription by alkylation and cross-linking the strands of DNA

Pharmacokinetics

Absorption: Rapid and complete

Protein binding (mostly albumin): ~99%

Metabolism: Hepatic; forms a major active metabolite (phenylacetic acid mustard) and inactive metabolites

Half-life elimination: ~1.5 hours; Phenylacetic acid mustard: ~1.8 hours

Time to peak plasma concentrations: Within 1 hour; Phenylacetic acid mustard: 1.2-2.6 hours

Excretion: Urine (15% to 60% primarily as inactive metabolites, <1% as unchanged drug or phenylacetic acid mustard)

Dosage

Geriatrics:

Refer to adult dosing. Begin at the lower end of dosing range(s)

Adults: Refer to individual protocols.

CLL, NHL: Oral: 0.1 mg/kg/day for 3-6 weeks **or** 0.4 mg/kg (increased by 0.1mg/kg/dose until response/toxicity observed) biweekly **or** 0.4 mg/kg (increased by 0.1mg/kg/dose until response/toxicity observed) monthly **or** 0.03-0.1 mg/kg/day continuously

Hodgkin's lymphoma: Oral: 0.2 mg/kg/day for 3-6 weeks **or** 0.4 mg/kg (increased by 0.1mg/kg/dose until response/toxicity observed) biweekly **or** 0.4 mg/kg (increased by 0.1mg/kg/dose until response/toxicity observed) monthly **or** 0.03-0.1 mg/kg/day continuously

Waldenström's macroglobulinemia (unlabeled use): Oral: 0.1 mg/kg/day (continuously) for at least 6 months **or** 0.3 mg/kg/day for 7 days every 6 weeks for at least 6 months

Administration Usually administered as a single dose; preferably on an empty stomach

Monitoring Parameters Liver function tests, CBC with differential and platelets (weekly, with WBC monitored twice weekly during the first 3-6 weeks of treatment), serum uric acid

Patient Information Any signs of infection (fever, chills, sore throat), easy bruising or bleeding, shortness of breath, black tarry stools, yellow discoloration of skin or eyes, bloody or dark urine, joint pain, swelling, or painful or burning urination should be brought to physician's attention. Nausea, vomiting or hair loss sometimes occurs. Food may delay absorption; take on empty stomach; avoid alcohol, prolonged sun exposure. May cause loss of appetite.

Additional Information Myelosuppressive effects:

WBC: Moderate

Platelets: Moderate

Onset (days): 7

Nadir (days): 10-14

Recovery (days): 28

Special Geriatric Considerations Toxicity to immunosuppressives is increased in the elderly. Start with lowest recommended adult doses. Signs of infection, such as fever and rise in WBCs, may not occur. Lethargy and confusion may be more prominent signs of infection.

Dosage Forms Excipient information presented when available (limited, particularly for generics); consult specific product labeling.

Tablet:

Leukeran®: 2 mg

Selected References

Hutchins LF and Lipschitz DA, "Cancer, Clinical Pharmacology, and Aging," *Clin Geriatr Med*, 1987, 3(3):483-503.

Kaplan HG, "Use of Cancer Chemotherapy in the Elderly," *Drug Treatment in the Elderly*, Vestal RE, ed, Boston, MA: ADIS Health Science Press, 1984, 338-49.

Kyle RA, Greipp PR, Gertz MA, et al, "Waldenström's Macroglobulinemia: A Prospective Study Comparing Daily With Intermittent Oral Chlorambucil," *Br J Haematol*, 2000, 108(4):737-42.

Wagner AM, Brunet S, Puig J, et al, "Chlorambucil-Induced Inappropriate Antidiuresis in Man with Chronic Lymphocytic Leukemia," *Ann Hemat*, 1999, 78(1):37-8.

♦ **Chlorambucilum** *see* Chlorambucil *on page 287*

♦ **Chloraminophene** *see* Chlorambucil *on page 287*

Chloramphenicol (klor am FEN i kole)

Related Information

Antimicrobial Activity Against Selected Organisms *on page 1728*

Medication Safety Issues

Sound-alike/look-alike issues:

Chloromycetin® may be confused with chlorambucil, Chlor-Trimeton®

U.S. Brand Names Chloromycetin® Sodium Succinate

Canadian Brand Names Chloromycetin®; Chloromycetin® Succinate; Diochloram®; Pentamycetin®

Generic Available Yes

Pharmacologic Category Antibiotic, Miscellaneous

Use Treatment of serious infections due to organisms resistant to other less toxic antibiotics or when its penetrability into the site of infection is clinically superior to other antibiotics to which the organism is sensitive; useful in infections caused by *Bacteroides, H. influenzae, Neisseria meningitidis, Salmonella,* and *Rickettsia*

Contraindications Hypersensitivity to chloramphenicol or any component of the formulation

Warnings/Precautions Gray syndrome characterized by circulatory collapse, cyanosis, acidosis, abdominal distention, myocardial depression, coma, and death has occurred. Use with caution in patients with impaired renal or hepatic function; reduce dose with impaired liver function. Use with care in patients with glucose 6-phosphate dehydrogenase deficiency. **[U.S. Boxed Warning]: Serious and fatal blood dyscrasias have occurred after both short-term and prolonged therapy.** Should not be used when less potentially toxic agents are effective. Prolonged use may result in fungal or bacterial superinfection, including *C. difficile*-associated diarrhea and pseudomembranous colitis.

Adverse Reactions (Reflective of adult population; not specific for elderly)
Three (3) major toxicities associated with chloramphenicol include:

Aplastic anemia, an idiosyncratic reaction which can occur with any route of administration; usually occurs 3 weeks to 12 months after initial exposure to chloramphenicol.

Bone marrow suppression is thought to be dose related with serum concentrations >25 mcg/mL and reversible once chloramphenicol is discontinued; anemia and neutropenia may occur during the first week of therapy.

Gray syndrome is characterized by circulatory collapse, cyanosis, acidosis, abdominal distention, myocardial depression, coma, and death. Reaction appears to be associated with serum levels ≥50 mcg/mL. May result from drug accumulation in patients with impaired hepatic or renal function.

Additional adverse reactions, frequency not defined:

Central nervous system: Confusion, delirium, depression, fever, headache

Dermatologic: Angioedema, rash, urticaria

Gastrointestinal: Diarrhea, enterocolitis, glossitis, nausea, stomatitis, vomiting

Hematologic: Granulocytopenia, hypoplastic anemia, pancytopenia, thrombocytopenia

Ocular: Optic neuritis

Miscellaneous: Anaphylaxis, hypersensitivity reactions

Overdosage/Toxicology Symptoms include anemia, metabolic acidosis, hypotension, and hypothermia. Treatment is supportive following GI decontamination.

Drug Interactions Inhibits CYP2C9 (weak), 3A4 (weak)

Decreased effect: Phenobarbital and rifampin may decrease concentration of chloramphenicol.

Increased toxicity: Chloramphenicol inhibits the metabolism of chlorpropamide, phenytoin, oral anticoagulants.

Ethanol/Nutrition/Herb Interactions Food: May decrease intestinal absorption of vitamin B_{12} may have increased dietary need for riboflavin, pyridoxine, and vitamin B_{12}.

Stability Store at room temperature prior to reconstitution. Reconstituted solutions remain stable for 30 days. Use only clear solutions. Frozen solutions remain stable for 6 months.

(Continued)

Chloramphenicol *(Continued)*

Mechanism of Action Reversibly binds to 50S ribosomal subunits of susceptible organisms preventing amino acids from being transferred to growing peptide chains thus inhibiting protein synthesis

Pharmacokinetics

Absorption: Oral: 75% to 100%

Chloramphenicol palmitate is hydrolyzed in the GI tract to the base; chloramphenicol sodium succinate must be hydrolyzed by esterases to active base

Protein binding: 60%

Metabolism: Extensively hepatic (90%) to inactive metabolites, principally by glucuronidation; chloramphenicol sodium succinate is hydrolyzed by esterases to active base

Half-life: 1.6-3.3 hours (increased with hepatic insufficiency)

Time to peak serum concentration: Oral: Within 0.5-3 hours

Elimination: 5% to 15% excreted as unchanged drug in urine and 4% excreted in bile

Dosage

Geriatrics & Adults: Systemic infections: I.V.: 50-100 mg/kg/day in divided doses every 6 hours; maximum daily dose: 4 g/day.

Renal Impairment: Slightly dialyzable (5% to 20%) via hemo- and peritoneal dialysis; no supplemental doses are needed in dialysis or continuous arteriovenous or venovenous hemofiltration.

Hepatic Impairment: Avoid use in severe liver impairment as increased toxicity may occur.

Administration Do not administer I.M.; can be administered IVP over at least 1 minute at a concentration of 100 mg/mL, or I.V. intermittent infusion over 15-30 minutes at a final concentration for administration of ≤20 mg/mL

Monitoring Parameters CBC with reticulocyte and platelet counts, periodic liver and renal function tests, serum drug concentration

Reference Range

Sample size: 0.5-2 mL blood (red top tube) or 0.1-1 mL serum (separated)

Therapeutic: 15-20 mcg/mL; Toxic: >40 mcg/mL

Timing of serum samples: Draw levels 0.5-1.5 hours after completion of I.V. dose

Test Interactions May cause false-positive results in urine glucose tests when using cupric sulfate (Benedict's solution, Clinitest®).

Patient Information Take on empty stomach; take with food if GI upset, at evenly spaced intervals (every 6 hours around-the-clock); notify physician if fever, sore throat, unusual bruising or bleeding, or decreased energy are experienced

Additional Information Sodium content of 1 g (injection): 51.8 mg (2.25 mEq)

Special Geriatric Considerations Chloramphenicol has not been studied in the elderly. It is not necessary to adjust the dose based upon the decrease in renal function associated with age. Chloramphenicol should be reserved for serious infections and the oral form avoided.

Dosage Forms Excipient information presented when available (limited, particularly for generics); consult specific product labeling.

Injection, powder for reconstitution: 1 g [contains sodium ~52 mg/g (2.25 mEq/g)]

Selected References

Nahata MC and Powell DA, "Bioavailability and Clearance of Chloramphenicol After Intravenous Chloramphenicol Succinate," *Clin Pharmacol Ther*, 1981, 30(3):368-72.

Yoshikawa TT, "Antimicrobial Therapy for the Elderly Patient," *J Am Geriatr Soc*, 1990, 38(12):1353-72.

♦ **Chlorbutinum** *see* Chlorambucil *on page 287*

Chlordiazepoxide *(klor dye az e POKS ide)*

Related Information

Anxiolytic, Sedative / Hypnotic, and Miscellaneous Benzodiazepines *on page 1750*

Potentially Inappropriate Medications for Geriatrics *on page 1824*

Medication Safety Issues

Sound-alike/look-alike issues:

Librium® may be confused with Librax®

U.S. Brand Names Librium®

Canadian Brand Names Apo-Chlordiazepoxide®

Index Terms Methaminodiazepoxide Hydrochloride

Generic Available Yes: Capsule

Pharmacologic Category Benzodiazepine

Use Management of anxiety, symptoms of alcohol withdrawal; preoperative sedative

Restrictions C-IV

Contraindications Hypersensitivity to chlordiazepoxide or any component of the formulation (cross-sensitivity with other benzodiazepines may also exist); narrow-angle glaucoma

Warnings/Precautions Active metabolites with extended half-lives may lead to delayed accumulation and adverse effects. Use with caution in elderly or debilitated patients, patients with hepatic disease (including alcoholics) or renal impairment, patients with respiratory disease or impaired gag reflex, patients with porphyria.

Parenteral administration should be avoided in comatose patients or shock. Adequate resuscitative equipment/personnel should be available, and appropriate monitoring should be conducted at the time of injection and for several hours following administration. The parenteral formulation should be diluted for I.M. administration with the supplied diluent only. This diluent should not be used when preparing the drug for intravenous administration.

Causes CNS depression (dose related) resulting in sedation, dizziness, confusion, or ataxia which may impair physical and mental capabilities. Patients must be cautioned about performing tasks which require mental alertness (eg, operating machinery or driving). Use with caution in patients receiving other CNS depressants or psychoactive agents (lithium, phenothiazines). Effects with other sedative drugs or ethanol may be potentiated. Benzodiazepines have been associated with falls and traumatic injury and should be used with extreme caution in patients who are at risk of these events (especially the elderly).

Use caution in patients with depression, particularly if suicidal risk may be present. Use with caution in patients with a history of drug dependence. Benzodiazepines have been associated with dependence and acute withdrawal symptoms on discontinuation or reduction in dose. Acute withdrawal, including seizures, may be precipitated in patients after administration of flumazenil to patients receiving long-term benzodiazepine therapy.

Benzodiazepines have been associated with anterograde amnesia. Paradoxical reactions, including hyperactive or aggressive behavior have been reported with benzodiazepines, particularly in psychiatric patients. Does not have analgesic, antidepressant, or antipsychotic properties.

Adverse Reactions (Reflective of adult population; not specific for elderly)
>10%:
  Central nervous system: Drowsiness, fatigue, ataxia, lightheadedness, memory impairment, dysarthria, irritability
  Dermatologic: Rash
  Endocrine & metabolic: Libido decreased, menstrual disorders
  Gastrointestinal: Xerostomia, salivation decreased, appetite increased or decreased, weight gain/loss
  Genitourinary: Micturition difficulties
1% to 10%:
  Cardiovascular: Hypotension
  Central nervous system: Confusion, dizziness, disinhibition, akathisia
  Dermatologic: Dermatitis
  Endocrine & metabolic: Libido increased
  Gastrointestinal: Salivation increased
  Genitourinary: Sexual dysfunction, incontinence
  Neuromuscular & skeletal: Rigidity, tremor, muscle cramps
  Otic: Tinnitus
  Respiratory: Nasal congestion

Overdosage/Toxicology Symptoms include hypotension, respiratory depression, coma, hypothermia, and cardiac arrhythmias. Treatment for benzodiazepine overdose is supportive. Flumazenil has been shown to selectively block the binding of benzodiazepines to CNS receptors, resulting in a reversal of benzodiazepine-induced CNS depression. Respiratory depression may not be reversed.

Drug Interactions Substrate of CYP3A4 (major)
  CNS depressants: Sedative effects and/or respiratory depression may be additive with CNS depressants; includes ethanol, barbiturates, opioid analgesics, and other sedative agents; monitor for increased effect.
  CYP3A4 inducers: CYP3A4 inducers may decrease the levels/effects of chlordiazepoxide. Example inducers include aminoglutethimide, carbamazepine, nafcillin, nevirapine, phenobarbital, phenytoin, and rifamycins.
  CYP3A4 inhibitors: May increase the levels/effects of chlordiazepoxide. Example inhibitors include azole antifungals, clarithromycin, diclofenac, doxycycline, erythromycin, imatinib, isoniazid, nefazodone, nicardipine, propofol, protease inhibitors, quinidine, telithromycin, and verapamil.
  Levodopa: Therapeutic effects may be diminished in some patients following the addition of a benzodiazepine; limited/inconsistent data.
  Oral contraceptives: May decrease the clearance of some benzodiazepines (those which undergo oxidative metabolism); monitor for increased benzodiazepine effect.
  Theophylline: May partially antagonize some of the effects of benzodiazepines; monitor for decreased response; may require higher doses for sedation.
  (Continued)

Chlordiazepoxide *(Continued)*

Ethanol/Nutrition/Herb Interactions

Ethanol: Avoid ethanol (may increase CNS depression).

Food: Serum concentrations/effects may be increased with grapefruit juice, but unlikely because of high oral bioavailability of chlordiazepoxide.

Herb/Nutraceutical: Avoid valerian, St John's wort, kava kava, gotu kola (may increase CNS depression).

Stability Injection: Prior to reconstitution, store under refrigeration and protect from light. Solution should be used immediately following reconstitution.

I.M. use: Reconstitute by adding 2 mL of provided diluent; agitate gently until dissolved. Provided diluent is **not** for I.V. use.

I.V. use: Reconstitute by adding 5 mL NS or SWFI; agitate gently until dissolved; **do not administer this dilution I.M.**

Mechanism of Action Binds to stereospecific benzodiazepine receptors on the post-synaptic GABA neuron at several sites within the central nervous system, including the limbic system, reticular formation. Enhancement of the inhibitory effect of GABA on neuronal excitability results by increased neuronal membrane permeability to chloride ions. This shift in chloride ions results in hyperpolarization (a less excitable state) and stabilization.

Pharmacodynamics Studies have shown that older adults are more sensitive to the effects of benzodiazepines as compared to younger adults

Pharmacokinetics

Absorption: I.M.: Slow and erratic

Distribution: V_d: 3.3 L/kg

Protein binding: 90% to 98%

Metabolism: Extensive in the liver to desmethyldiazepam (active and long-acting)

Half-life: 5-30 hours; increased in older adults and in severe liver disease; desmethyldiazepam has a half-life of 50-100 hours and can be prolonged in older adults

Time to peak serum concentration: Oral: Within 2 hours. I.M.: Results in lower peak plasma concentrations than oral administration.

Dosage

Geriatrics: Anxiety: Oral: 5 mg 2-4 times/day; adjust for renal impairment. Avoid use if possible. See Special Geriatric Considerations.

Adults:

Anxiety:

Oral: 15-100 mg divided 3-4 times/day

I.M., I.V.: Initial: 50-100 mg followed by 25-50 mg 3-4 times/day as needed

Preoperative anxiety: I.M.: 50-100 mg prior to surgery

Ethanol withdrawal symptoms: Oral, I.V.: 50-100 mg to start, dose may be repeated in 2-4 hours as necessary to a maximum of 300 mg/24 hours

Note: Up to 300 mg may be given I.M. or I.V. during a 6-hour period, but not more than this in any 24-hour period.

Renal Impairment:

Cl_{cr} <10 mL/minute: Administer 50% of dose.

Not dialyzable (0% to 5%)

Hepatic Impairment: Avoid use.

Administration I.V. form is a powder and should be reconstituted with 5 mL of sterile water or saline prior to administration; do not use diluent provided with ampul for I.V. administration.

Monitoring Parameters Respiratory, cardiovascular and mental status; check for orthostasis

Reference Range Therapeutic: 0.1-3 mcg/mL (SI: 0-10 μmol/L); Toxic: >23 mcg/mL (SI: >77 μmol/L)

Patient Information Avoid alcohol and other CNS depressants; may cause drowsiness; avoid activities needing good psychomotor coordination until CNS effects are known; may cause physical or psychological dependence; avoid abrupt discontinuation after prolonged use

Special Geriatric Considerations Due to its long-acting metabolite, chlordiazepoxide is not considered a drug of choice in the elderly. Long-acting benzodiazepines have been associated with falls in the elderly; interpretive guidelines from the Centers for Medicare and Medicaid Services (CMS) discourage the use of this agent in residents of long-term care facilities.

Dosage Forms Excipient information presented when available (limited, particularly for generics); consult specific product labeling.

Capsule, as hydrochloride: 5 mg, 10 mg, 25 mg

Injection, powder for reconstitution, as hydrochloride: 100 mg [diluent contains benzyl alcohol, polysorbate 80, and propylene glycol]

Selected References
Hicks R, Dysken MW, Davis JM, et al, "The Pharmacokinetics of Psychotropic Medication in the Elderly: A Review," *J Clin Psychiatry*, 1981, 42(10):374-85.
Reidenberg MM, Levy M, Warner H, et al, "Relationship Between Diazepam Dose, Plasma Level, Age, and Central Nervous System Depression," *Clin Pharmacol Ther*, 1978, 23(4):371-4.

♦ **Chlordiazepoxide and Clidinium** *see* Clidinium and Chlordiazepoxide *on page 331*

Chlordiazepoxide and Methscopolamine
(klor dye az e POKS ide & meth skoe POL a meen)

Related Information
Potentially Inappropriate Medications for Geriatrics *on page 1824*
Medication Safety Issues
Librax® formulation may be cause for confusion:
In November 2004, Valeant Pharmaceuticals licensed the Librax® trademark to Victory Pharmaceuticals. Subsequently, the product was reformulated to contain chlordiazepoxide and methscopolamine. In January 2006, Valeant Pharmaceuticals began redistributing the original formulation of Librax®, containing clidinium and chlordiazepoxide. Victory Pharmaceuticals has discontinued their product. **Note:** The formulation of Librax® distributed in Canada (Valeant Canada Ltd) always contained clidinium and chlordiazepoxide.
U.S. Brand Names Librax® *[reformulation]* [DSC]
Index Terms Methscopolamine Nitrate and Chlordiazepoxide Hydrochloride
Generic Available No
Pharmacologic Category Anticholinergic Agent; Benzodiazepine
Use Adjunctive treatment of peptic ulcer; treatment of irritable bowel syndrome, acute enterocolitis
Restrictions C-IV
Dosage
Geriatrics: Oral: Initial dose should not exceed 2 capsules/day; adjust dose as tolerated.
Adults: Peptic ulcer, irritable bowel syndrome, acute enterocolitis: Oral: 1-2 capsules 3-4 times/day; adjust dose based on individual response.
Special Geriatric Considerations Due to its long-acting metabolite, chlordiazepoxide is not considered a drug of choice in the elderly. The use of anticholinergic agents may cause problems with bladder emptying, constipation, or case confusion. This combination of benzodiazepine and anticholinergic agent may increase the risk of confusion.
Dosage Forms Excipient information presented when available (limited, particularly for generics); consult specific product labeling.
Capsule: Chlordiazepoxide hydrochloride 5 mg and methscopolamine nitrate 2.5 mg [DSC]

♦ **Chlormeprazine** *see* Prochlorperazine *on page 1320*
♦ **Chloromycetin® Sodium Succinate** *see* Chloramphenicol *on page 289*
♦ **Chlorophyllin Copper Complex Sodium, Papain, and Urea** *see* Chlorophyllin, Papain, and Urea *on page 293*

Chlorophyllin, Papain, and Urea
(KLOR oh fil in, pa PAY in, & yoor EE a)

Medication Safety Issues
Sound-alike/look-alike issues:
Ziox™ may be confused with Zyvox®
U.S. Brand Names Allanfil 405; Allanfil Spray; Panafil®; Panafil® SE; Ziox™; Ziox 405™
Index Terms Chlorophyllin Copper Complex Sodium, Papain, and Urea; Papain, Urea, and Chlorophyllin; Urea, Chlorophyllin, and Papain
Generic Available Yes: Ointment, solution
Pharmacologic Category Enzyme, Topical Debridement
Use Treatment of acute and chronic lesions, such as varicose, diabetic decubitus ulcers, burns, postoperative wounds, pilonidal cyst wounds, carbuncles, and miscellaneous traumatic or infected wounds
Dosage
Geriatrics & Adults:
Topical: Apply with each dressing change; daily or twice daily dressing changes are preferred, but may be every 2-3 days. Cover with dressing following application.
Ointment: Apply ⅛" thickness over the wound with clean applicator.
Spray: Completely cover the wound site so that the wound is not visible.
Special Geriatric Considerations Preventive skin care should be instituted in all older patients at high risk for pressure ulcers.
Dosage Forms Excipient information presented when available (limited, particularly for generics); consult specific product labeling. [DSC] = Discontinued product
(Continued)

Chlorophyllin, Papain, and Urea *(Continued)*

Emulsion [spray]:
Panafil® SE: Copper chlorophyllin complex sodium 0.5%, papain ≥521,700 USP units/g, and urea 10% (34 mL)

Ointment:
Allanfil 405, Panafil®: Chlorophyllin copper complex sodium 0.5%, papain ≥521,700 USP units/g, and urea 10% (6 g, 30 g)

Ziox™: Chlorophyllin copper complex sodium 0.5%, papain ≥521,700 units/g, and urea 10% (30 g)

Ziox 405™: Copper chlorophyllin complex sodium 0.5%, papain ≥521,700 USP units/ g, and urea 10% (30 g)

Solution [spray]:
Allanfil, Panafil® [DSC]: Copper chlorophyllin complex sodium 0.5%, papain ≥521,700 USP units/g, and urea 10% (33 mL)

Chlorothiazide (klor oh THYE a zide)

Medication Safety Issues

International issues:
Diuril® may be confused with Duorol® which is a brand name for acetaminophen in Spain

U.S. Brand Names Diuril®

Canadian Brand Names Diuril®

Generic Available Yes: Tablet

Pharmacologic Category Diuretic, Thiazide

Use Management of mild to moderate hypertension, edema associated with congestive heart failure, nephrotic syndrome in patients unable to take oral hydrochlorothiazide (when a thiazide is the diuretic of choice)

Contraindications Hypersensitivity to chlorothiazide, any component of the formulation, thiazides, or sulfonamide-derived drugs; anuria; renal decompensation

Warnings/Precautions Use with caution in severe renal disease. Electrolyte disturbances (hypokalemia, hypochloremic alkalosis, hyponatremia) can occur. Use with caution in severe hepatic dysfunction; hepatic encephalopathy can be caused by electrolyte disturbances. Gout can be precipitate in certain patients with a history of gout, a familial predisposition to gout, or chronic renal failure. Cautious use in diabetics; may see a change in glucose control. Can cause SLE exacerbation or activation. Use with caution in patients with moderate or high cholesterol concentrations. Photosensitization may occur. Correct hypokalemia before initiating therapy.

Chemical similarities are present among sulfonamides, sulfonylureas, carbonic anhydrase inhibitors, thiazides, and loop diuretics (except ethacrynic acid). Use in patients with thiazide or sulfonamide allergy is specifically contraindicated in product labeling. A risk of cross-reaction exists in patients with allergy to any of these compounds; avoid use when previous reaction has been severe. Discontinue if signs of hypersensitivity are noted.

Adverse Reactions (Reflective of adult population; not specific for elderly)

Frequency not defined.

Cardiovascular: Hypotension, orthostatic hypotension, necrotizing angiitis

Central nervous system: Dizziness, headache, restlessness, vertigo

Dermatologic: Alopecia, erythema multiforme, exfoliative dermatitis, photosensitivity, Stevens-Johnson syndrome, toxic epidermal necrolysis

Endocrine & metabolic: Cholesterol increased, hypokalemia, hypomagnesemia, triglycerides increased

Gastrointestinal: Abdominal cramping, anorexia, constipation, diarrhea, gastric irritation, nausea, pancreatitis, sialadenitis, vomiting

Genitourinary: Impotence

Hematologic: Agranulocytosis, aplastic anemia, hemolytic anemia, leukopenia, thrombocytopenia

Hepatic: Jaundice

Neuromuscular & skeletal: Muscle spasm, paresthesia, weakness

Ocular: Blurred vision, xanthopsia

Renal: Azotemia, hematuria, interstitial nephritis, renal failure, renal dysfunction

Respiratory: Pneumonitis, pulmonary edema, respiratory distress

Miscellaneous: Anaphylactic reactions, systemic lupus erythematosus

Overdosage/Toxicology Symptoms of overdose include signs and symptoms of hypovolemia, hypermotility, diuresis, lethargy, confusion, muscle weakness, and coma. Treatment is supportive.

Drug Interactions

ACE inhibitors: Increased hypotension if aggressively diuresed with a thiazide diuretic

Antidiabetic agents (insulin, oral agents): Dosage adjustment of antidiabetic agent may be needed.

Beta-blockers increase hyperglycemic effects of thiazides in type 2 diabetes mellitus (noninsulin dependent, NIDDM)

Corticosteroids: May increase electrolyte-depletion effects of chlorothiazide.

Cyclosporine and thiazides can increase the risk of gout or renal toxicity; avoid concurrent use

Digoxin toxicity can be exacerbated if a thiazide induces hypokalemia or hypomagnesemia.

Lithium toxicity can occur by reducing renal excretion of lithium; monitor lithium concentration and adjust as needed

Neuromuscular-blocking agents can prolong blockade; monitor serum potassium and neuromuscular status

NSAIDs can decrease the efficacy of thiazides reducing the diuretic and antihypertensive effects

Ethanol/Nutrition/Herb Interactions

Ethanol: May increase risk of orthostatic hypotension.

Food: Chlorothiazide serum levels may be increased if taken with food.

Herb/Nutraceutical: Avoid dong quai if using for hypertension (has estrogenic activity). Avoid dong quai, St John's wort (may also cause photosensitization). Avoid ephedra, yohimbe, ginseng (may worsen hypertension). Avoid natural licorice (due to mineralocorticoid activity). Avoid garlic (may have increased antihypertensive effect).

Stability

Powder for injection: Prior to reconstitution, store between 2°C to 25°C (36°F to 77°F). To reconstitute, add SWFI 18 mL to make 28 mg/mL. May be further diluted with dextrose or sodium chloride solutions. Reconstituted solution is stable for 24 hours at room temperature; precipitation will occur in <24 hours in pH <7.4. Single use only, discard any unused reconstituted solution.

Suspension, tablets: Store at room temperature 15°C to 30°C (59°F to 86°F); protect from freezing.

Mechanism of Action Inhibits sodium reabsorption in the distal tubules causing increased excretion of sodium and water as well as potassium and hydrogen ions, magnesium, phosphate, calcium

Pharmacodynamics

Onset of action: Oral: Diuresis: 2 hours

Duration:

Oral: 6-12 hours

I.V.: Diuretic action: ~2 hours

Pharmacokinetics

Absorption: Oral: Poor

Half-life: 1-2 hours

Time to peak serum concentration: Within 4 hours

Dosage

Geriatrics: Oral: 500 mg once daily **or** 1 g 3 times/week

Adults: Note: The manufacturer states that I.V. and oral dosing are equivalent. Some clinicians may use lower I.V. doses, however, because of chlorothiazide's poor oral absorption.

Hypertension: Oral: 500-2000 mg/day divided in 1-2 doses (manufacturer labeling); doses of 125-500 mg/day have also been recommended

Edema: Oral, I.V.: 250-1000 mg once or twice daily. Intermittent treatment (ie, therapy on alternative days) may be appropriate for some patients. Maximum daily dose: 1000 mg (ACC/AHA 2005 Heart Failure Guidelines)

Renal Impairment: Cl$_{cr}$ <10 mL/minute: Avoid use. Ineffective with low GFR (Aronoff G, 2002)

Note: ACC/AHA 2005 Heart Failure Guidelines suggest that thiazides lose their efficacy when Cl$_{cr}$ <40 mL/minute

Administration I.V. must be prepared with at least 15 mL of diluent

Monitoring Parameters Blood pressure (standing and sitting/supine), serum electrolytes, renal function, I & O, weight

Test Interactions Increased creatine phosphokinase [CPK] (S), ammonia (B), amylase (S), calcium (S), chloride (S), cholesterol (S), glucose, increased acid (S), decreased chloride (S), magnesium, potassium (S), sodium (S); may interfere with tests for parathyroid function

Patient Information Take in the morning; may cause increased sensitivity to sunlight; rise slowly from lying down or sitting

Additional Information Sodium content of 500 mg injection: 57.5 mg (2 mEq)

Special Geriatric Considerations Chlorothiazide is minimally effective in patients with a Cl$_{cr}$ <30 mL/minute. This may limit the usefulness of chlorothiazide in the elderly.

Dosage Forms Excipient information presented when available (limited, particularly for generics); consult specific product labeling.

Injection, powder for reconstitution, as sodium: 500 mg

Suspension, oral: 250 mg/5 mL (237 mL) [contains alcohol 0.5% and benzoic acid]

Tablet: 250 mg, 500 mg

♦ **Chlorphen [OTC]** *see* Chlorpheniramine *on page 296*

Chlorpheniramine (klor fen IR a meen)

Related Information
Potentially Inappropriate Medications for Geriatrics *on page 1824*
Medication Safety Issues
Sound-alike/look-alike issues:
Chlor-Trimeton® may be confused with Chloromycetin®
U.S. Brand Names Ahist™; Aller-Chlor® [OTC]; Chlorphen [OTC]; Chlor-Trimeton® [OTC]; Diabetic Tussin® Allergy Relief [OTC]; PediaTan™; QDALL® AR; Teldrin® HBP [OTC]
Canadian Brand Names Chlor-Tripolon®; Novo-Pheniram
Index Terms Chlorpheniramine Maleate; CTM
Generic Available Yes: Syrup, tablet
Pharmacologic Category Antihistamine
Use Treatment of perennial and seasonal allergic rhinitis and other allergic symptoms including urticaria
Contraindications Hypersensitivity to chlorpheniramine maleate or any component of the formulation; narrow-angle glaucoma; bladder neck obstruction; symptomatic prostate hypertrophy; during acute asthmatic attacks; stenosing peptic ulcer; pyloroduodenal obstruction.
Warnings/Precautions Antihistamines are more likely to cause dizziness, excessive sedation, syncope, toxic confusional states, and hypotension in older adults. Use with caution in patients with angle-closure glaucoma, pyloroduodenal obstruction (including stenotic peptic ulcer), urinary tract obstruction (including bladder neck obstruction and symptomatic prostatic hyperplasia), hyperthyroidism, increased intraocular pressure, and cardiovascular disease (including hypertension and tachycardia). Use with caution in patients with heart disease, hypertension, thyroid disease, and asthma.
Adverse Reactions (Reflective of adult population; not specific for elderly)
>10%:
Central nervous system: Slight to moderate drowsiness
Respiratory: Thickening of bronchial secretions
1% to 10%:
Central nervous system: Headache, excitability, fatigue, nervousness, dizziness
Gastrointestinal: Nausea, xerostomia, diarrhea, abdominal pain, appetite increase, weight gain
Genitourinary: Urinary retention
Neuromuscular & skeletal: Arthralgia, weakness
Ocular: Diplopia
Renal: Polyuria
Respiratory: Pharyngitis
Drug Interactions Substrate of CYP2D6 (minor), 3A4 (major); **Inhibits** CYP2D6 (weak)

Increased toxicity (CNS depression): CNS depressants, MAO inhibitors, tricyclic antidepressants, phenothiazines
CYP3A4 inhibitors: May increase the levels/effects of chlorpheniramine. Example inhibitors include azole antifungals, clarithromycin, diclofenac, doxycycline, erythromycin, imatinib, isoniazid, nefazodone, nicardipine, propofol, protease inhibitors, quinidine, telithromycin, and verapamil.
Ethanol/Nutrition/Herb Interactions Ethanol: Avoid ethanol (may increase CNS depression).
Stability Protect from light.
Mechanism of Action Competes with histamine for H_1-receptor sites on effector cells in the gastrointestinal tract, blood vessels, and respiratory tract
Pharmacokinetics
Protein binding: 69% to 72%
Metabolism: In the liver
Half-life: 20-24 hours; one study found no significant difference in the half-life in older adult subjects though there was wide interindividual variation
Elimination: Metabolites and parent drug (3% to 4%) excreted in urine; 35% of total within 48 hours
Dosage
Geriatrics: Allergic symptoms, rhinitis: Oral: 4 mg once or twice daily or 8 mg sustained release at bedtime. **Note:** Duration of action may be 36 hours or more when serum concentrations are low.
Adults: Allergic symptoms, allergic rhinitis: Oral: 4 mg every 4-6 hours, not to exceed 24 mg/day or sustained release 8-12 mg every 8-12 hours, not to exceed 24 mg/day
Renal Impairment: Hemodialysis: Supplemental dose is not necessary.
Administration Do not crush sustained release tablet

Monitoring Parameters Relief of symptoms

Patient Information May cause drowsiness; avoid CNS depressants and alcohol; swallow whole, do not crush or chew

Additional Information Chlorpheniramine is available in various combinations. These include acetaminophen; phenylephrine; phenylpropanolamine; pseudoephedrine; phenylephrine and phenyltoloxamine; phenylpropanolamine and acetaminophen; phenyltoloxamine, phenylpropanolamine, and phenylephrine; pseudoephedrine and iodine.

Special Geriatric Considerations Anticholinergic action may cause significant confusional symptoms, constipation, or problems voiding urine. If an antihistamine is indicated, a second generation nonsedating antihistamine would be a more appropriate choice.

Dosage Forms Excipient information presented when available (limited, particularly for generics); consult specific product labeling.

Capsule, variable release, as maleate:
QDALL® AR: Chlorpheniramine 12 mg [immediate release and sustained release]
Suspension, as tannate:
PediaTan™: 8 mg/5 mL (480 mL) [sugar free; contains sodium benzoate; bubble gum flavor]
Syrup, as maleate:
Aller-Chlor®: 2 mg/5 mL (120 mL) [contains alcohol 5%]
Diabetic Tussin® Allergy Relief: 2 mg/5 mL (120 mL) [alcohol free, dye free, sugar free]
Tablet, as maleate: 4 mg
Aller-Chlor®, Chlor-Trimeton®, Chlorphen, Teldrin® HBP: 4 mg
Tablet, extended release, as maleate:
Chlor-Trimeton®: 12 mg
Tablet, long acting, as tannate [scored]:
Ahist™: 12 mg

Selected References
Simons KJ, Martin TJ, Watson WT, et al, "Pharmacokinetics and Pharmacodynamics of Terfenadine and Chlorpheniramine in the Elderly," *J Allergy Clin Immunol*, 1990, 85(3):540-7.

♦ **Chlorpheniramine Maleate** *see* Chlorpheniramine *on page 296*

ChlorproMAZINE (klor PROE ma zeen)

Related Information
Antipsychotic Agents *on page 1747*
Liquid Compatibility of Antipsychotics and Mood Stabilizers *on page 1851*

Medication Safety Issues
Sound-alike/look-alike issues:
ChlorproMAZINE may be confused with chlorproPAMIDE, clomiPRAMINE, prochlorperazine, promethazine
Thorazine® may be confused with thiamine, thioridazine

Canadian Brand Names Largactil®; Novo-Chlorpromazine

Index Terms Chlorpromazine Hydrochloride; CPZ

Generic Available Yes

Pharmacologic Category Antipsychotic Agent, Typical, Phenothiazine

Use Treatment of schizophrenia, acute intermittent porphyria, psychoses, Tourette's syndrome, mania, behavioral problems in nonpsychotic symptoms associated with dementia (older adults), Huntington's chorea, spasmodic torticollis; control of mania, nausea and vomiting, intractable hiccups; preoperative relief of restlessness and apprehension; adjunct in the treatment of tetanus
See Special Geriatric Considerations.

Unlabeled/Investigational Use Management of psychotic disorders

Contraindications Hypersensitivity to chlorpromazine or any component of the formulation (cross-reactivity between phenothiazines may occur); severe CNS depression; coma

Warnings/Precautions Use with caution in patients with seizures, bone marrow suppression, or severe liver disease

Significant hypotension may occur, especially when the drug is administered parenterally; injection contains sulfites which may cause allergic reaction

Tardive dyskinesia: Prevalence rate may be 40% in elderly; development of the syndrome and the irreversible nature are proportional to duration and total cumulative dose over time. May be reversible if diagnosed early in therapy.

Extrapyramidal reactions are more common in elderly with up to 50% developing these reactions after 60 years of age. Drug-induced **Parkinson's syndrome** occurs often. **Akathisia** is the most common extrapyramidal symptom in elderly.

Increased confusion, memory loss, psychotic behavior, and agitation frequently occur as a consequence of anticholinergic effects

(Continued)

ChlorproMAZINE *(Continued)*

Orthostatic hypotension is due to alpha-receptor blockade, the elderly are at greater risk for orthostatic hypotension

Antipsychotic associated sedation in nonpsychotic patients is extremely unpleasant due to feelings of depersonalization, derealization, and dysphoria

Life-threatening arrhythmias have occurred at therapeutic doses of antipsychotics

Adverse Reactions (Reflective of adult population; not specific for elderly) Frequency not defined.

Cardiovascular: Postural hypotension, tachycardia, dizziness, nonspecific QT changes

Central nervous system: Drowsiness, dystonias, akathisia, pseudoparkinsonism, tardive dyskinesia, neuroleptic malignant syndrome, seizure

Dermatologic: Photosensitivity, dermatitis, skin pigmentation (slate gray)

Endocrine & metabolic: Lactation, breast engorgement, amenorrhea, gynecomastia, hyper- or hypoglycemia

Gastrointestinal: Xerostomia, constipation, nausea

Genitourinary: Urinary retention, ejaculatory disorder, impotence

Hematologic: Agranulocytosis, eosinophilia, leukopenia, hemolytic anemia, aplastic anemia, thrombocytopenic purpura

Hepatic: Jaundice

Ocular: Blurred vision, corneal and lenticular changes, epithelial keratopathy, pigmentary retinopathy

Overdosage/Toxicology Symptoms include deep sleep, coma, extrapyramidal symptoms, abnormal involuntary muscle movements, and hypotension. Following initiation of essential overdose management, toxic symptom treatment and supportive treatment should be initiated. Hypotension usually responds to I.V. fluids or Trendelenburg positioning. If unresponsive to these measures, the use of a parenteral inotrope may be required. Seizures commonly respond to diazepam (I.V. 5-10 mg bolus every 15 minutes if needed up to a total of 30 mg) or to phenytoin or phenobarbital; critical cardiac arrhythmias often respond to I.V. phenytoin (15 mg/kg up to 1 g), while other antiarrhythmics can be used. Neuroleptics often cause extrapyramidal symptoms (eg, dystonic reactions) requiring management with anticholinergic agents such as benztropine mesylate I.V. 1-2 mg may be effective. These agents are generally effective within 2-5 minutes.

Drug Interactions Substrate of CYP1A2 (minor), 2D6 (major), 3A4 (minor); **Inhibits** CYP2D6 (strong), 2E1 (weak)

Acetylcholinesterase inhibitors (central): May increase the risk of antipsychotic-related extrapyramidal symptoms; monitor.

Aluminum salts: May decrease the absorption of phenothiazines; monitor

Amphetamines: Efficacy may be diminished by antipsychotics; in addition, amphetamines may increase psychotic symptoms; avoid concurrent use

Anticholinergics: May inhibit the therapeutic response to phenothiazines and excess anticholinergic effects may occur; includes benztropine, trihexyphenidyl, biperiden, and drugs with significant anticholinergic activity (TCAs, antihistamines, disopyramide)

Antihypertensives: Concurrent use of phenothiazines with an antihypertensive may produce additive hypotensive effects (particularly orthostasis)

Bromocriptine: Phenothiazines inhibit the ability of bromocriptine to lower serum prolactin concentrations

CNS depressants: Sedative effects may be additive with phenothiazines; monitor for increased effect; includes barbiturates, benzodiazepines, opioid analgesics, ethanol and other sedative agents

CYP2D6 inhibitors: May increase the levels/effects of chlorpromazine. Example inhibitors include delavirdine, fluoxetine, miconazole, paroxetine, pergolide, quinidine, quinine, ritonavir, and ropinirole.

CYP2D6 substrates: Chlorpromazine may increase the levels/effects of CYP2D6 substrates. Example substrates include amphetamines, selected beta-blockers, dextromethorphan, fluoxetine, lidocaine, mirtazapine, nefazodone, paroxetine, risperidone, ritonavir, thioridazine, tricyclic antidepressants, and venlafaxine.

CYP2D6 prodrug substrates: Chlorpromazine may decrease the levels/effects of CYP2D6 prodrug substrates. Example prodrug substrates include codeine, hydrocodone, oxycodone, and tramadol.

Epinephrine: Chlorpromazine (and possibly other low potency antipsychotics) may diminish the pressor effects of epinephrine

Guanethidine and guanadrel: Antihypertensive effects may be inhibited by chlorpromazine

Levodopa: Chlorpromazine may inhibit the antiparkinsonian effect of levodopa; avoid this combination

Lithium: Chlorpromazine may produce neurotoxicity with lithium; this is a rare effect

Metoclopramide: May increase extrapyramidal symptoms (EPS) or risk.

Phenytoin: May reduce serum levels of phenothiazines; phenothiazines may increase phenytoin serum levels

Propranolol: Serum concentrations of phenothiazines may be increased; propranolol also increases phenothiazine concentrations

Polypeptide antibiotics: Rare cases of respiratory paralysis have been reported with concurrent use of phenothiazines

QT_c-prolonging agents: Effects on QT_c interval may be additive with phenothiazines, increasing the risk of malignant arrhythmias; includes type Ia antiarrhythmics, TCAs, and some quinolone antibiotics (moxifloxacin)

Sulfadoxine-pyrimethamine: May increase phenothiazine concentrations

Tricyclic antidepressants: Concurrent use may produce increased toxicity or altered therapeutic response

Trazodone: Phenothiazines and trazodone may produce additive hypotensive effects

Valproic acid: Serum levels may be increased by phenothiazines

Ethanol/Nutrition/Herb Interactions

Ethanol: Avoid ethanol (may increase CNS depression).

Herb/Nutraceutical: Avoid St John's wort (may decrease chlorpromazine levels, increase photosensitization, or enhance sedative effect). Avoid dong quai (may enhance photosensitization). Avoid kava kava, gotu kola, valerian (may increase CNS depression).

Stability Injection: Protect from light. A slightly yellowed solution does not indicate potency loss, but a markedly discolored solution should be discarded. Diluted injection (1 mg/mL) with NS and stored in 5 mL vials remains stable for 30 days.

Mechanism of Action Chlorpromazine is an aliphatic phenothiazine antipsychotic which blocks postsynaptic mesolimbic dopaminergic receptors in the brain; exhibits a strong alpha-adrenergic blocking effect and depresses the release of hypothalamic and hypophyseal hormones; believed to depress the reticular activating system, thus affecting basal metabolism, body temperature, wakefulness, vasomotor tone, and emesis

Pharmacokinetics

Metabolism: Extensive in the liver to active and inactive metabolites

Half-life:

Biphasic: 30 hours

Phase 1 half-life: 2 hours

Elimination: <1% excreted as unchanged drug in urine within 24 hours

Dosage

Geriatrics:

Behavioral symptoms associated with dementia (unlabeled use): Initial: 10-25 mg 1-2 times/day; increase at 4- to 7-day intervals by 10-25 mg/day. Increase dose intervals (eg, twice daily, 3 times/day) as necessary to control behavior response or side effects; maximum daily dose: 800 mg; gradual increases (titration) may prevent some side effects or decrease their severity.

Other indications: Refer to adult dosing.

Adults:

Schizophrenia/psychoses:

Oral: Range: 30-800 mg/day in 1-4 divided doses, initiate at lower doses and titrate as needed; usual dose: 200-600 mg/day; some patients may require 1-2 g/day

I.M., I.V.: Initial: 25 mg, may repeat (25-50 mg) in 1-4 hours, gradually increase to a maximum of 400 mg/dose every 4-6 hours until patient is controlled; usual dose: 300-800 mg/day

Intractable hiccups: Oral, I.M.: 25-50 mg 3-4 times/day

Nausea and vomiting:

Oral: 10-25 mg every 4-6 hours

I.M., I.V.: 25-50 mg every 4-6 hours

Renal Impairment: Not dialyzable (0% to 5%)

Hepatic Impairment: Avoid use in severe hepatic dysfunction.

Administration Note: Avoid skin contact with oral solution or injection solution; may cause contact dermatitis.

Oral: Dilute oral concentrate solution in juice before administration. Chlorpromazine concentrate is not compatible with carbamazepine suspension; schedule dosing at least 1-2 hours apart from each other.

I.V.: Direct of intermittent infusion: Infuse 1 mg or portion thereof over 1 minute.

Monitoring Parameters Monitor orthostatic blood pressures 3-5 days after initiation of therapy or a dose increase; tremors, gait changes, abnormal movement in trunk, neck, buccal area, or extremities; monitor target behaviors for which the agent is given

Reference Range Therapeutic: 30-300 ng/mL (SI: 157-942 nmol/L); Toxic: >750 ng/mL (SI: >2355 nmol/L); serum concentrations not often obtained since dose is titrated to best response, also correlation to response is controversial

Test Interactions False-positives for phenylketonuria, amylase, uroporphyrins, urobilinogen.

Patient Information Oral concentrate must be diluted in 2-4 oz of liquid (water, fruit juice, carbonated drinks, milk, or pudding); do not take antacid within 1 hour of taking (Continued)

ChlorproMAZINE *(Continued)*

drug; avoid alcohol; avoid excess sun exposure (use sun block); may cause drowsiness, rise slowly from recumbent position; use of supportive stockings may help prevent orthostatic hypotension

Special Geriatric Considerations Many elderly patients receive antipsychotic medications for inappropriate nonpsychotic behavior. Before initiating antipsychotic medication, the clinician should investigate any possible reversible cause; any stress or stress from any disease can cause acute "confusion" or worsening of baseline nonpsychotic behavior. Most commonly acute changes in behavior are due to increases in drug dose or addition of new drug to regimen; fluid electrolyte loss; infections; and changes in environment.

Any changes in disease status in any organ system can result in behavior changes.

In the treatment of agitated, demented, elderly patients, authors of meta-analysis of controlled trials of the response to the traditional antipsychotics (phenothiazines, butyrophenones) in controlling agitation have concluded that the use of neuroleptics results in a response rate of 18%. Clearly neuroleptic therapy for behavior control should be limited with frequent attempts to withdraw the agent given for behavior control.

Dosage Forms Excipient information presented when available (limited, particularly for generics); consult specific product labeling.

Injection, solution, as hydrochloride: 25 mg/mL (1 mL, 2 mL)

Tablet, as hydrochloride: 10 mg, 25 mg, 50 mg, 100 mg, 200 mg

Selected References

Peabody CA, Warner MD, Whiteford HA, et al, "Neuroleptics and the Elderly," *J Am Geriatr Soc*, 1987, 35(3):233-8.

Risse SC and Barnes R, "Pharmacologic Treatment of Agitation Associated With Dementia," *J Am Geriatr Soc*, 1986, 34(5):368-76.

Saltz BL, Woerner MG, Kane JM, et al, "Prospective Study of Tardive Dyskinesia Incidence in the Elderly," *JAMA*, 1991, 266(17):2402-6.

Seifert RD, "Therapeutic Drug Monitoring: Psychotropic Drugs," *J Pharm Pract*, 1984, 6:403-16.

♦ **Chlorpromazine Hydrochloride** *see* ChlorproMAZINE *on page 297*

ChlorproPAMIDE (klor PROE pa mide)

Related Information

Potentially Inappropriate Medications for Geriatrics *on page 1824*

Medication Safety Issues

Sound-alike/look-alike issues:

ChlorproPAMIDE may be confused with chlorproMAZINE

Diabinese® may be confused with DiaBeta®, Dialume®, Diamox®

High alert medication: The Institute for Safe Medication Practices (ISMP) includes this medication among its list of drugs which have a heightened risk of causing significant patient harm when used in error.

U.S. Brand Names Diabinese®

Canadian Brand Names Apo-Chlorpropamide®; Novo-Propamide

Generic Available Yes

Pharmacologic Category Antidiabetic Agent, Sulfonylurea

Use Adjunct to diet for the management of mild to moderately severe, stable noninsulin-dependent (type II) diabetes mellitus

Unlabeled/Investigational Use Treatment of neurogenic diabetes insipidus

Contraindications Hypersensitivity to chlorpropamide, sulfonylureas, sulfonamides, or any component of the formulation; type 1 diabetes mellitus (insulin dependent, IDDM); diabetic ketoacidosis

Warnings/Precautions All sulfonylurea drugs are capable of producing severe hypoglycemia. Hypoglycemia is more likely to occur when caloric intake is deficient, after severe or prolonged exercise, when ethanol is ingested, or when more than one glucose-lowering drug is used. It is also more likely in elderly patients, malnourished patients and in patients with impaired renal or hepatic function; use with caution.

Chemical similarities are present among sulfonamides, sulfonylureas, carbonic anhydrase inhibitors, thiazides, and loop diuretics (except ethacrynic acid). Use in patients with sulfonylurea or sulfonamide allergy is specifically contraindicated in product labeling, however, a risk of cross-reaction exists in patients with allergy to any of these compounds; avoid use when previous reaction has been severe.

Product labeling states oral hypoglycemic drugs may be associated with an increased cardiovascular mortality as compared to treatment with diet alone or diet plus insulin. Data to support this association are limited, and several studies, including a large prospective trial (UKPDS) have not supported an association.

It may be necessary to discontinue therapy and administer insulin if the patient is exposed to stress (fever, trauma, infection, surgery).

Adverse Reactions (Reflective of adult population; not specific for elderly)
Frequency not defined.

Central nervous system: Dizziness, headache

Dermatologic: Erythema multiforme, exfoliative dermatitis, maculopapular eruptions, photosensitivity, pruritus, urticaria

Endocrine & metabolic: Disulfiram-like reactions, hypoglycemia, SIADH

Gastrointestinal: Anorexia, diarrhea, hunger, nausea, proctocolitis, vomiting

Hematologic: Agranulocytosis, aplastic anemia, eosinophilia, hemolytic anemia, leukopenia, pancytopenia, porphyria cutanea tarda, thrombocytopenia

Hepatic: Cholestatic jaundice, hepatic porphyria

Drug Interactions Substrate of CYP2C9 (minor)

Allopurinol: Allopurinol may increase the serum concentration of chlorpropamide.

Beta-blockers: Beta-blockers may enhance the hypoglycemic effect of chlorpropamide and mask tachycardia as an initial symptom of hypoglycemia.

Chloramphenicol: Chloramphenicol may decrease the metabolism of chlorpropamide.

Cimetidine: Cimetidine may decrease the metabolism, via CYP isoenzymes, of chlorpropamide.

Cyclic antidepressants: Cyclic antidepressants may enhance the hypoglycemic effect of chlorpropamide.

Cyclosporine: chlorpropamide may increase the serum concentration of cyclosporine.

Fibric acid derivatives: Fibric acid derivatives may enhance the hypoglycemic effect of chlorpropamide.

Fluconazole: Fluconazole may increase the serum concentration of chlorpropamide.

Pegvisomant: Pegvisomant may enhance the hypoglycemic effect of chlorpropamide.

Rifampin: Rifampin may increase the metabolism, via CYP isoenzymes, of chlorpropamide.

Salicylates: Salicylates may enhance the hypoglycemic effect of chlorpropamide. Of concern with regular, higher doses of salicylates, not sporadic, low doses.

Sulfonamide derivatives (sulfadiazine, sulfadoxine, sulfamethoxazole, sulfisoxazole): Sulfonamide derivatives (except sulfacetamide) may enhance the hypoglycemic effect of chlorpropamide.

Ethanol/Nutrition/Herb Interactions

Ethanol: Avoid ethanol (possible disulfiram-like reaction).

Herb/Nutraceutical: Herbs with hypoglycemic properties may enhance the hypoglycemic effect of chlorpropamide. This includes alfalfa, aloe, bilberry, bitter melon, burdock, celery, damiana, fenugreek, garcinia, garlic, ginger, ginseng (American), gymnema, marshmallow, stinging nettle

Mechanism of Action Stimulates insulin release from the pancreatic beta cells; reduces glucose output from the liver; insulin sensitivity is increased at peripheral target sites

Pharmacodynamics

Onset of action: 1 hour

Peak effect: 3-6 hours

Duration of action: 24 hours

Pharmacokinetics

Absorption: Rapid

Distribution: V_d: 0.13-0.23 L/kg

Protein binding: 90%

Metabolism: Extensively hepatic (~80%), primarily via CYP2C9; forms metabolites

Half-life elimination: ~36 hours; prolonged in elderly or with renal impairment

End-stage renal disease: 50-200 hours

Time to peak, serum: 2-4 hours

Excretion: Urine

Dosage

Geriatrics: Reduce initial dose to 100-125 mg/day in older patients; subsequent dosages may be increased or decreased by 50-125 mg/day at 3- to 5-day intervals (slower upward titration may be appropriate in older patients)

Adults: Type 2 diabetes: Oral: The dosage of chlorpropamide is variable and should be individualized based upon the patient's response

Initial dose: 250 mg/day in mild-to-moderate diabetes in middle-aged, stable diabetic; 100-125 mg/day in older patients

Titration: Subsequent dosages may be increased or decreased by 50-125 mg/day at 3- to 5-day intervals

Maintenance dose: 100-250 mg/day; severe patients with diabetes may require 500 mg/day; avoid doses >750 mg/day

Renal Impairment:

Cl_{cr} <50 mL/minute: Avoid use.

Hemodialysis: Removed with hemoperfusion.

Peritoneal dialysis: Supplemental dose is not necessary.

(Continued)

ChlorproPAMIDE *(Continued)*

Hepatic Impairment: Dosage reduction is recommended. Conservative initial and maintenance doses are recommended in patients with liver impairment because chlorpropamide undergoes extensive hepatic metabolism.

Monitoring Parameters Blood glucose, Hgb A_{1c}; monitor for signs and symptoms of hypoglycemia (fatigue, sweating, numbness of extremities)

Reference Range Recommendations for glycemic control in adults with diabetes:
Hb A_{1c}: <7%
Preprandial capillary plasma glucose: 90-130 mg/dL
Peak postprandial capillary blood glucose: <180 mg/dL
Blood pressure: <130/80 mm Hg

Patient Information Avoid hypoglycemia, eat regularly, do not skip meals; carry a quick source of sugar with you

Additional Information Long half-life may complicate recovery from excess effects

Special Geriatric Considerations Because of chlorpropamide's long half-life, duration of action, drug interactions, and the increased risk for hypoglycemia, it is not considered a hypoglycemic agent of choice in the elderly. How "tightly" a geriatric patient's blood glucose should be controlled is controversial; however, a fasting blood sugar of <150 mg/dL is now an acceptable endpoint. Such a decision should be based on the patient's functional and cognitive status, how well they recognize hypoglycemic or hyperglycemic symptoms, and how to respond to them and their other disease states.

Dosage Forms Excipient information presented when available (limited, particularly for generics); consult specific product labeling.
Tablet: 100 mg, 250 mg
Diabinese®: 100 mg, 250 mg

Selected References
Arrigoni L, Fundak G, Horn J, et al, "Chlorpropamide Pharmacokinetics in Young Healthy Adults and Older Diabetic Patients," *Clin Pharm*, 1987, 6(2):162-4.
"Standards of Medical Care for Patients With Diabetes Mellitus. American Diabetes Association," *Diabetes Care*, 2007, 30(Suppl 1):4-41.
Verbalis JG, "Diabetes Insipidus," *Rev Endocr Metab Disord*, 2003, 4(2):177-85.

Chlorthalidone *(klor THAL i done)*

U.S. Brand Names Thalitone®
Canadian Brand Names Apo-Chlorthalidone®
Index Terms Hygroton
Generic Available Yes
Pharmacologic Category Diuretic, Thiazide
Use Management of mild to moderate hypertension, alone or in combination with other agents; treatment of edema associated with congestive heart failure or nephrotic syndrome

Contraindications Hypersensitivity to chlorthalidone or any component of the formulation; cross-sensitivity with other thiazides or sulfonamides; anuria; renal decompensation

Warnings/Precautions Chemical similarities are present among sulfonamides, sulfonylureas, carbonic anhydrase inhibitors, thiazides, and loop diuretics (except ethacrynic acid). Use in patients with thiazide or sulfonamide allergy is specifically contraindicated in product labeling, however, a risk of cross-reaction exists in patients with allergy to any of these compounds; avoid use when previous reaction has been severe. Use with caution in hypokalemia, renal disease, hepatic disease, gout, lupus, erythematosus, diabetes mellitus.

Adverse Reactions (Reflective of adult population; not specific for elderly)
1% to 10%:
Dermatologic: Photosensitivity
Endocrine & metabolic: Hypokalemia
Gastrointestinal: Anorexia, epigastric distress

Drug Interactions
ACE inhibitors: Increased hypotension if aggressively diuresed with a thiazide diuretic.
Beta-blockers increase hyperglycemic effects of thiazides in type 2 diabetes mellitus (noninsulin dependent, NIDDM)
Cyclosporine and thiazides can increase the risk of gout or renal toxicity; avoid concurrent use.
Digoxin toxicity can be exacerbated if a thiazide induces hypokalemia or hypomagnesemia.
Lithium toxicity can occur by reducing renal excretion of lithium; monitor lithium concentration and adjust as needed.
Neuromuscular blocking agents can prolong blockade; monitor serum potassium and neuromuscular status.

NSAIDs can decrease the efficacy of thiazides reducing the diuretic and antihypertensive effects.

Ethanol/Nutrition/Herb Interactions Herb/Nutraceutical: Avoid dong quai if using for hypertension (has estrogenic activity). Avoid dong quai, St John's Wort (may also cause photosensitization). Avoid ephedra, yohimbe, ginseng (may worsen hypertension).

Mechanism of Action Sulfonamide-derived diuretic that inhibits sodium and chloride reabsorption in the cortical-diluting segment of the ascending loop of Henle

Pharmacodynamics
Peak clinical effect: Within 2-6 hours
Duration: 24-72 hours

Pharmacokinetics
Absorption: 65%
Metabolism: In the liver
Half-life: 35-55 hours and may be prolonged with renal impairment; (anuria): 81 hours
Elimination: ~50% to 65% of dose excreted unchanged in urine

Dosage
Geriatrics: Oral: Initial: 12.5-25 mg/day or every other day; there is little advantage to using doses >25 mg/day.
Adults:
Hypertension: Oral: 25-100 mg/day or 100 mg 3 times/week; usual dosage range (JNC 7): 12.5-25 mg/day
Edema: Initial: 50-100 mg/day or 100 mg on alternate days; maximum dose: 200 mg/day
Heart failure-associated edema: 12.5-25 mg once daily; maximum daily dose: 100 mg (ACC/AHA 2005 Heart Failure Guidelines)
Renal Impairment: Cl_{cr} <10 mL/minute: Avoid use. Ineffective with low GFR (Aronoff G, 2002)
Note: ACC/AHA 2005 Heart Failure Guidelines suggest that thiazides lose their efficacy when Cl_{cr} <40 mL/minute

Monitoring Parameters Blood pressure (standing and sitting/supine), serum electrolytes, renal function, I & O, weight

Test Interactions Increased creatine phosphokinase [CPK] (S), ammonia (B), amylase (S), calcium (S), chloride (S), cholesterol (S), glucose, increased acid (S), decreased chloride (S), magnesium, potassium (S), sodium (S)

Patient Information Take in the morning; may cause increased sensitivity to sunlight; rise slowly from lying down or sitting

Special Geriatric Considerations Studies have found chlorthalidone effective in the treatment of isolated systolic hypertension in the elderly. The use of chlorthalidone as a step 1 medication reduced the incidence of stroke in the SHEP trial.

Dosage Forms Excipient information presented when available (limited, particularly for generics); consult specific product labeling.
Tablet: 25 mg, 50 mg, 100 mg
Thalitone®: 15 mg

Selected References
Hulley SB, Furberg CD, Gurland B, et al, "Systolic Hypertension in the Elderly Program (SHEP): Antihypertensive Efficacy of Chlorthalidone," *Am J Cardiol*, 1985, 56(15):913-20.
SHEP Cooperative Research Group, "Prevention of Stroke by Antihypertensive Drug Treatment in Older Persons With Isolated Systolic Hypertension," *JAMA*, 1991, 265(24):3255-64.

♦ Chlor-Trimeton® [OTC] *see* Chlorpheniramine *on page 296*

Chlorzoxazone (klor ZOKS a zone)

Related Information
Potentially Inappropriate Medications for Geriatrics *on page 1824*
Medication Safety Issues
Sound-alike/look-alike issues:
Parafon Forte® may be confused with Fam-Pren Forte
U.S. Brand Names Parafon Forte® DSC
Canadian Brand Names Parafon Forte®; Strifon Forte®
Generic Available Yes
Pharmacologic Category Skeletal Muscle Relaxant
Use Symptomatic treatment of muscle spasm and pain associated with acute musculoskeletal conditions
Contraindications Hypersensitivity to chlorzoxazone or any component of the formulation; impaired liver function
Warnings/Precautions If signs or symptoms of impaired liver dysfunction occur, discontinue drug.
Adverse Reactions (Reflective of adult population; not specific for elderly)
Frequency not defined.
(Continued)

Chlorzoxazone *(Continued)*

Central nervous system: Dizziness, drowsiness lightheadedness, paradoxical stimulation, malaise

Dermatologic: Rash, petechiae, ecchymoses (rare), angioneurotic edema

Gastrointestinal: Nausea, vomiting, stomach cramps

Genitourinary: Urine discoloration

Hepatic: Liver dysfunction

Miscellaneous: Anaphylaxis (very rare)

Overdosage/Toxicology Symptoms include nausea, vomiting, diarrhea, drowsiness, dizziness, headache, absent tendon reflexes, and hypotension. Treatment is supportive following attempts to enhance drug elimination. Hypotension should be treated with I.V. fluids and/or Trendelenburg positioning. Dialysis and hemoperfusion and osmotic diuresis have all been useful in reducing serum drug concentrations. Patients should be observed for possible relapses due to incomplete gastric emptying.

Drug Interactions Substrate of CYP1A2 (minor), 2A6 (minor), 2D6 (minor), 2E1 (major), 3A4 (minor); **Inhibits** CYP2E1 (weak), 3A4 (weak)

CNS depressants: Effects may be increased by chlorzoxazone.

CYP2E1 inhibitors: May increase the levels/effects of chlorzoxazone. Example inhibitors include disulfiram, isoniazid, and miconazole.

Disulfiram: May increase chlorzoxazone concentration; monitor.

Isoniazid: May increase chlorzoxazone concentration; monitor.

Ethanol/Nutrition/Herb Interactions Ethanol: Avoid ethanol (may increase CNS depression).

Mechanism of Action Acts on the spinal cord and subcortical levels by depressing polysynaptic reflexes

Pharmacodynamics

Onset of action: 60 minutes

Duration: 3-4 hours

Pharmacokinetics

Absorption: Oral: Readily absorbed

Metabolism: Extensive in the liver by glucuronidation

Elimination: In urine as conjugates

Dosage

Geriatrics: Oral: Initial: 250 mg 2-4 times/day; increase as necessary to 750 mg 3-4 times/day.

Adults: Muscle spasm: Oral: 250-500 mg 3-4 times/day up to 750 mg 3-4 times/day

Monitoring Parameters Liver function tests, relief of symptoms, mental status

Patient Information Avoid alcohol and CNS depressants; may cause drowsiness, dizziness, or lightheadedness; urine may turn orange or purple-red; take with food or milk

Additional Information Not useful in the chronic spasticity associated with stroke or Parkinson's disease

Special Geriatric Considerations No data available on the use of skeletal muscle relaxants in the elderly. Start dosing low and increase as necessary. The FDA recently approved a stronger warning about hepatotoxicity in the labeling of chlorzoxazone. Because it can cause unpredictable, fatal hepatic toxicity, the use of chlorzoxazone should be avoided.

Dosage Forms Excipient information presented when available (limited, particularly for generics); consult specific product labeling.

Caplet (Parafon Forte® DSC): 500 mg

Tablet: 250 mg, 500 mg

Cholecalciferol (kole e kal SI fer ole)

U.S. Brand Names Delta-D®

Canadian Brand Names D-Vi-Sol®

Index Terms D_3

Generic Available Yes

Pharmacologic Category Vitamin D Analog

Use Dietary supplement; treatment of vitamin D deficiency or prophylaxis of deficiency

Contraindications Hypercalcemia; hypersensitivity to cholecalciferol or any component of the formulation; malabsorption syndrome; evidence of vitamin D toxicity

Warnings/Precautions Administer with extreme caution in patients with impaired renal function, heart disease, renal stones, or arteriosclerosis; maintain adequate fluid intake, calcium-phosphate product must not exceed 70%; avoid hypercalcemia; must administer with supplemental calcium; use caution in patients with renal impairment and hyperparathyroidism. Use with caution in coronary artery disease and older adults.

Adverse Reactions (Reflective of adult population; not specific for elderly)

Frequency not defined.

Cardiovascular: Arrhythmia, hyper-/hypotension, cardiac arrhythmia
Central nervous system: Irritability, headache, somnolence, overt psychosis (rare)
Dermatologic: Pruritus
Endocrine & metabolic: Polydipsia
Gastrointestinal: Nausea, vomiting, anorexia, pancreatitis, metallic taste, dry mouth, constipation, weight loss
Genitourinary: Albuminuria, polyuria
Hepatic: Increased liver function test
Neuromuscular & skeletal: Bone pain, myalgia, weakness, muscle pain
Ocular: Conjunctivitis, photophobia
Renal: Azotemia, nephrocalcinosis

Drug Interactions Inhibits CYP2C9 (weak), 2C19 (weak), 2D6 (weak)
Thiazide diuretics, cholestyramine, colestipol, corticosteroids, mineral oil, orlistat, phenytoin, barbiturates, digitalis glycosides, antacids (magnesium)

Ethanol/Nutrition/Herb Interactions
Food: Olestra may impair the absorption of vitamin D.

Dosage
Geriatrics & Adults: Dietary supplement: Oral: 400-1000 units/day

Monitoring Parameters Monitor renal function, serum calcium, and phosphate concentrations; if hypercalcemia is encountered, discontinue agent until serum calcium returns to normal

Reference Range Calcium (serum) 9-10 mg/dL (4.5-5 mEq/L); phosphate 2.5-5 mg/dL

Patient Information Do not take more than the recommended amount. While taking this medication, your physician may want you to follow a special diet or take a calcium supplement. Follow this diet closely. Avoid taking magnesium supplements or magnesium-containing antacids. Early symptoms of hypercalcemia include weakness, fatigue, somnolence, headache, anorexia, dry mouth, metallic taste, nausea, vomiting, cramps, diarrhea, muscle pain, bone pain, and irritability.

Additional Information 1 mg of cholecalciferol = 40,000 units of vitamin D activity

Special Geriatric Considerations Vitamin D, folate, and B_{12} (cyanocobalamin) have decreased absorption with age (clinical significance unknown); studies in ill geriatrics demonstrated that low serum concentrations of vitamin D result in greater bone loss. Calorie requirements decrease with age and therefore, nutrient density must be increased to ensure adequate nutrient intake, including vitamins and minerals. The use of a daily supplement with a multiple vitamin with minerals is recommended because elderly consume less vitamin D, absorption may be decreased, and many have decreased sun exposure. This is a recommendation of particular need to those with high risk for osteoporosis.

Dosage Forms Excipient information presented when available (limited, particularly for generics); consult specific product labeling.
Tablet: 1000 int. units
Delta-D®: 400 int. units

Selected References
Letsou AP and Price LS, "Health Aging and Nutrition: An Overview," Clin Geriatr Med, 1987, 3(2):253-60.
Myrianthopoulos M, "Dietary Treatment of Hyperlipidemia in the Elderly," Clin Geriatr Med, 1987, 3(2):343-59.
Riggs BL and Melton LJ, "The Prevention and Treatment of Osteoporosis," N Engl J Med, 1992, 327(9):620-7.

Cholestyramine Resin (koe LES teer a meen REZ in)

Related Information
Hyperlipidemia Management on page 1773
U.S. Brand Names Prevalite®; Questran®; Questran® Light
Canadian Brand Names Novo-Cholamine; Novo-Cholamine Light; PMS-Cholestyramine; Questran®; Questran® Light Sugar Free
Generic Available Yes
Pharmacologic Category Antilipemic Agent, Bile Acid Sequestrant
Use Adjunct in the management of primary hypercholesterolemia; pruritus associated with elevated levels of bile acids; diarrhea associated with excess fecal bile acids; binding toxicologic agents; pseudomembraneous colitis
Contraindications Hypersensitivity to bile acid sequestering resins or any component of the formulation; complete biliary obstruction; bowel obstruction
Warnings/Precautions Use with caution in patients with constipation (GI dysfunction) and patients with phenylketonuria (Questran® Light contains aspartame). Overdose may result in GI obstruction. Not to be taken simultaneously with many other medicines (decreased absorption). Treat any diseases contributing to hypercholesterolemia first. May interfere with fat-soluble vitamins (A, D, E, K) and folic acid. Chronic use may be associated with bleeding problems (especially in high doses).
Adverse Reactions (Reflective of adult population; not specific for elderly)
>10%: Gastrointestinal: Constipation, heartburn, nausea, vomiting, stomach pain
1% to 10%:
Central nervous system: Headache
(Continued)

Cholestyramine Resin *(Continued)*

Gastrointestinal: Belching, bloating, diarrhea

Overdosage/Toxicology Symptoms include GI obstruction. Treatment is supportive.

Drug Interactions

Cholestyramine can reduce the absorption of numerous medications when used concurrently. Give other medications 1 hour before or 4-6 hours after giving cholestyramine. Medications which may be affected include HMG-CoA reductase inhibitors, thiazide diuretics, propranolol (and potentially other beta-blockers), corticosteroids, thyroid hormones, digoxin, valproic acid, NSAIDs, loop diuretics, sulfonylureas, troglitazone (and potentially other agents in this class).

Warfarin and other oral anticoagulants: Hypoprothrombinemic effects may be reduced by cholestyramine. Separate administration times (as detailed above) and monitor INR closely when initiating or discontinuing.

Ethanol/Nutrition/Herb Interactions

Food: Cholestyramine (especially high doses or long-term therapy) may decrease the absorption of folic acid, calcium, and iron.

Herb/Nutraceutical: Cholestyramine (especially high doses or long-term therapy) may decrease the absorption of fat-soluble vitamins (vitamins A, D, E, and K).

Stability Store powder at controlled room temperature of 15°C to 30°C (59°F to 86°F). Mix contents of 1 packet or 1 level scoop of powder with 4-6 oz of beverage. Allow to stand 1-2 minutes prior to mixing. May also be mixed with highly-fluid soups, cereals, applesauce, etc. Suspension may be used for up to 48 hours after refrigeration.

Mechanism of Action Forms a nonabsorbable complex with bile acids in the intestine, releasing chloride ions in the process; inhibits enterohepatic reuptake of intestinal bile salts and thereby increases the fecal loss of bile salt-bound low density lipoprotein cholesterol

Pharmacodynamics Peak effect: Within 21 days

Pharmacokinetics

Absorption: Not absorbed from GI tract

Elimination: In feces as an insoluble complex with bile acids

Dosage

Geriatrics & Adults: Dyslipidemia: Oral (dosages are expressed in terms of anhydrous resin): 4 g 1-2 times/day to a maximum of 16-24 g/day (and a maximum of 6 times/day)

Renal Impairment: Not removed by hemo- or peritoneal dialysis. Supplemental doses not necessary with dialysis or continuous arteriovenous or venovenous hemofiltration effects.

Monitoring Parameters Bowel function, plasma cholesterol (LDL and VLDL fractions)

Test Interactions Increased prothrombin time; decreased cholesterol (S), iron (B)

Patient Information Take before meals; mix with liquids, pulpy fruits, or soups; chew bars thoroughly and follow with fluids (at least 4 fluid oz); do not take concurrently with other medications; take other medications 1 hour before or 4-6 hours after binding resin; adhere to prescribed diet

Additional Information Overdose may result in GI obstruction; Questran® Light contains aspartame

Special Geriatric Considerations The definition of and, therefore, when to treat hyperlipidemia in the elderly is a controversial issue. The National Cholesterol Education Program recommends that all adults maintain a plasma cholesterol <160 mg/dL. Elderly with one additional risk factor, goal LDL would be <130 mg/dL. It is the authors' belief that pharmacologic treatment be reserved for those who are unable to obtain a desirable plasma cholesterol concentration by diet alone and for whom the benefits of treatment are believed to outweigh the potential adverse effects, drug interactions, and cost of treatment.

Dosage Forms Excipient information presented when available (limited, particularly for generics); consult specific product labeling.

Powder for oral suspension: 4 g of resin/5 g of powder (5 g packets, 210 g can) [contains phenylalanine 14 mg/5 g]; 4 g of resin/5.7 g of powder (5.7 g packets, 240 g can) [light formulation]; 4 g of resin/9 g of powder (9 g packets, 378 g can)

Prevalite®: 4 g of resin/5.5 g of powder (5.5 g packets, 231 g can) [contains phenylalanine 14.1 mg/5.5 g; orange flavor]

Questran®: 4 g of resin/9 g of powder (9 g packets, 378 g can)

Questran® Light: 4 g of resin/6.4 g of powder (5 g packets, 268 g can) [contains phenylalanine 28.1 mg/6.4 g]

Selected References

"Executive Summary of The Third Report of The National Cholesterol Education Program (NCEP) Expert Panel on Detection, Evaluation, and Treatment of High Blood Cholesterol in Adults (Adult Treatment Panel III)," *JAMA*, 2001, 285(19):2486-97.

Leaf DA, "Lipid Disorders: Applying New Guidelines to Your Older Patients," *Geriatrics*, 1994, 49(5):35-41.

Choline Magnesium Trisalicylate
(KOE leen mag NEE zhum trye sa LIS i late)

U.S. Brand Names Trilisate® [DSC]
Index Terms Tricosal
Generic Available Yes
Pharmacologic Category Salicylate
Use Treatment of mild to moderate pain, inflammation and fever; management of rheumatic fever, rheumatoid arthritis, osteoarthritis, gout
See Mechanism of Action.
Contraindications Hypersensitivity to salicylates, other nonacetylated salicylates, other NSAIDs, or any component of the formulation; bleeding disorders
Warnings/Precautions Salicylate salts may not inhibit platelet aggregation and, therefore, should not be substituted for aspirin in the prophylaxis of thrombosis. Use with caution in patients with impaired hepatic or renal function, dehydration, erosive gastritis, asthma, or peptic ulcer.

Elderly are a high-risk population for adverse effects from NSAIDs. As many as 60% of elderly can develop peptic ulceration and/or hemorrhage asymptomatically. Use lowest effective dose for shortest period possible. Tinnitus or impaired hearing may indicate toxicity. Tinnitus may be a difficult and unreliable indication of toxicity due to age-related hearing loss or eighth cranial nerve damage. CNS adverse effects may be observed in the elderly at lower doses than younger adults.

Adverse Reactions (Reflective of adult population; not specific for elderly)
<20%:
 Gastrointestinal: Nausea, vomiting, diarrhea, heartburn, dyspepsia, epigastric pain, constipation
 Otic: Tinnitus
<2%:
 Central nervous system: Headache, lightheadedness, dizziness, drowsiness, lethargy
 Otic: Hearing impairment
Overdosage/Toxicology Symptoms include tinnitus, vomiting, acute renal failure, hyperthermia, irritability, seizures, coma, and metabolic acidosis. For acute ingestions, determine serum salicylate levels 6 hours after ingestion. The "Done" nomogram may be helpful for estimating the severity of aspirin poisoning and directing treatment using serum salicylate levels. Treatment can also be based upon symptomatology.
Drug Interactions
 ACE inhibitors: Effects of ACE inhibitors may be decreased by concurrent therapy with NSAIDs.
 Antacids: Concomitant use may lead to decreased salicylate concentration.
 Warfarin: Concomitant use may increase the hypoprothrombinemic effect of warfarin.
Ethanol/Nutrition/Herb Interactions
 Ethanol: Avoid ethanol (may enhance gastric mucosal irritation).
 Food: May decrease the rate but not the extent of oral absorption.
 Herb/Nutraceutical: Avoid cat's claw, dong quai, evening primrose, feverfew, garlic, ginger, ginkgo, red clover, horse chestnut, green tea, ginseng (all have additional antiplatelet activity). Limit curry powder, paprika, licorice, Benedictine liqueur, prunes, raisins, tea, and gherkins; may cause salicylate accumulation. These foods contain 6 mg salicylate/100 g.
Stability Store at controlled room temperature of 15°C to 30°C (59°F to 86°F).
Mechanism of Action Inhibits prostaglandin synthesis; acts on the hypothalamus heat-regulating center to reduce fever; blocks the generation of pain impulses
Pharmacokinetics
 Absorption: From the stomach and small intestine
 Distribution: Readily into most body fluids and tissues
 Half-life: Dose-dependent ranging from 2-3 hours at low doses to 30 hours at high doses
 Time to peak plasma concentrations: Within ~2 hours
Dosage
 Geriatrics: Usual dose: 750 mg 3 times/day.
 Adults: Arthritis, pain: Oral (based on total salicylate content): 500 mg to 1.5 g 2-3 times/day **or** 3 g at bedtime; usual maintenance dose: 1-4.5 g/day
 Renal Impairment: Avoid use in severe renal impairment.
Administration Liquid may be mixed with fruit juice just before drinking. Do not administer with antacids. Take with a full glass of water and remain in an upright position for 15-30 minutes after administration.
Monitoring Parameters Serum concentrations, renal function; hearing changes or tinnitus; monitor for response (ie, pain, inflammation, range of motion, grip strength); observe for abnormal bleeding, bruising, weight gain
(Continued)

Choline Magnesium Trisalicylate *(Continued)*

Reference Range
Salicylate blood concentrations for anti-inflammatory effect: 150-300 mcg/mL (15-30 mg/dL)

Analgesia and antipyretic effect: 30-50 mcg/mL (3-5 mg/dL)

Test Interactions False-negative results for glucose oxidase urinary glucose tests (Clinistix®); false-positives using the cupric sulfate method (Clinitest®); also, interferes with Gerhardt test (urinary ketone analysis), VMA determination; 5-HIAA, xylose tolerance test, and T_3 and T_4; increased PBI

Patient Information Do not take with antacids; watch for any signs of bleeding (stool); take with food to minimize GI distress; report ringing in ears, persistent GI pain to physician or pharmacist

Additional Information Salicylate salts do not inhibit platelet aggregation and, therefore, should not be substituted for aspirin in the prophylaxis of thrombosis; use caution in patients with renal failure or reduced renal function (ie, older adults - magnesium accumulation)

Special Geriatric Considerations Elderly are a high-risk population for adverse effects from nonsteroidal anti-inflammatory agents. As much as 60% of elderly can develop peptic ulceration and/or hemorrhage asymptomatically. The concomitant use of H_2 blockers and sucralfate is not effective as prophylaxis with the exception of NSAID-induced duodenal ulcers which may be prevented by the use of ranitidine. Misoprostol and proton pump inhibitors are the only agents proven to help prevent the development of NSAID-induced ulcers. Also, concomitant disease and drug use contribute to the risk for GI adverse effects. Avoid use of multiple drugs (OTCs) which contain salicylates (eg, bismuth subsalicylate with other salicylates). Use lowest effective dose for shortest period possible. Consider renal function decline with age. Use of NSAIDs can compromise existing renal function especially when Cl_{cr} is ≤30 mL/minute. There is the consideration that the use of choline magnesium salicylate may cause less gastrointestinal and renal adverse effects than ASA or other NSAIDs in the elderly. Tinnitus may be a difficult and unreliable indication of toxicity due to age-related hearing loss or eighth cranial nerve damage. CNS adverse effects such as confusion, agitation, and hallucination are generally seen in overdose or high dose situations, but elderly may demonstrate these adverse effects at lower doses than younger adults.

Dosage Forms Excipient information presented when available (limited, particularly for generics); consult specific product labeling.

Liquid: 500 mg/5 mL (240 mL) [choline salicylate 293 mg and magnesium salicylate 362 mg per 5 mL; cherry cordial flavor]

Tablet: 500 mg [choline salicylate 293 mg and magnesium salicylate 362 mg]; 750 mg [choline salicylate 440 mg and magnesium salicylate 544 mg]; 1000 mg [choline salicylate 587 mg and magnesium salicylate 725 mg]

Selected References
Hawkey CJ, Karrasch JA, Szczepański L, et al, "Omeprazole Compared With Misoprostol for Ulcers Associated With Nonsteroidal Anti-inflammatory Drugs," *N Engl J Med*, 1998, 338(11):727-34.

Weissmann G, "Aspirin," *Sci Am*, 1991, 264(1):84-90.

Yeomans ND, Tulassay Z, Juhasz L, et al, "A Comparison of Omeprazole With Ranitidine for Ulcers Associated With Nonsteroidal Anti-inflammatory Drugs," *N Engl J Med*, 1998, 338(11):719-26.

♦ **Choline Salicylate** *see* Salicylates (Various Salts) *on page 1439*

♦ **Chooz® [OTC]** *see* Calcium Salts (Oral) *on page 220*

♦ **CI-1008** *see* Pregabalin *on page 1310*

♦ **Cialis®** *see* Tadalafil *on page 1513*

Ciclesonide *(sye KLES oh nide)*

Medication Safety Issues
International issues:

Omnaris™ is the U.S. brand name for ciclesonide **intranasal** formulation; Alvesco® is the brand name for ciclesonide **oral inhalation** formulation available in Australia, Canada, and Great Britain

U.S. Brand Names Omnaris™

Canadian Brand Names Alvesco®

Generic Available No

Pharmacologic Category Corticosteroid, Inhalant (Oral); Corticosteroid, Nasal

Use

Intranasal: Management of seasonal and perennial allergic rhinitis

Oral inhalation: Prophylactic management of bronchial asthma

Contraindications Hypersensitivity to ciclesonide or any component of the formulation

Oral inhalation (Alvesco®): Untreated fungal, bacterial, or tuberculosis infections of the respiratory tract; primary treatment of acute asthma or status asthmaticus; moderate-to-severe bronchiectasis

Warnings/Precautions May cause hypercorticism or suppression of hypothalamic-pituitary-adrenal (HPA) axis, particularly in patients receiving high doses for prolonged periods. HPA axis suppression may lead to adrenal crisis. Withdrawal and discontinuation of a corticosteroid should be done slowly and carefully. Particular care is required when patients are transferred from systemic corticosteroids to inhaled products due to possible adrenal insufficiency or withdrawal from steroids, including an increase in allergic symptoms. Patients receiving >20 mg per day of prednisone (or equivalent) may be most susceptible. Fatalities have occurred due to adrenal insufficiency in asthmatic patients during and after transfer from systemic corticosteroids to aerosol steroids; aerosol steroids do **not** provide the systemic steroid needed to treat patients having trauma, surgery, or infections.

Bronchospasm may occur with wheezing after inhalation; if this occurs stop steroid and treat with a fast-acting bronchodilator. Supplemental steroids (oral or parenteral) may be needed during stress or severe asthma attacks. Not to be used in status asthmaticus or for the relief of acute bronchospasm. Corticosteroid use may cause psychiatric disturbances, including depression, euphoria, insomnia, mood swings, and personality changes. Pre-existing psychiatric conditions may be exacerbated by corticosteroid use. Prolonged use of corticosteroids may also increase the incidence of secondary infection, mask acute infection (including fungal infections), prolong or exacerbate viral infections, or limit response to vaccines. Exposure to chickenpox should be avoided; corticosteroids should not be used to treat ocular herpes simplex. Corticosteroids should not be used for cerebral malaria. Close observation is required in patients with latent tuberculosis and/or TB reactivity; restrict use in active TB (only in conjunction with antituberculosis treatment). Prolonged treatment with corticosteroids has been associated with the development of Kaposi's sarcoma (case reports); if noted, discontinuation of therapy should be considered.

Use with caution in patients with thyroid disease, hepatic impairment, renal impairment, cardiovascular disease, diabetes, glaucoma, cataracts, myasthenia gravis, patients at risk for osteoporosis, patients at risk for seizures, or GI diseases (diverticulitis, peptic ulcer, ulcerative colitis) due to perforation risk. Use caution following acute MI (corticosteroids have been associated with myocardial rupture). Because of the risk of adverse effects, systemic corticosteroids should be used cautiously in the elderly in the smallest possible effective dose for the shortest duration. Avoid nasal corticosteroid use in patients with recent nasal septal ulcers, nasal surgery or nasal trauma until healing has occurred.

To minimize the systemic effects of orally-inhaled and intranasal corticosteroids, each patient should be titrated to the lowest effective dose.

Adverse Reactions (Reflective of adult population; not specific for elderly)
1% to 10%:
Central nervous system: Headache (6%)
Gastrointestinal: Oral candidiasis (1%)
Otic: Ear pain (2%)
Respiratory: Epistaxis (5%), nasopharyngitis (4%), paradoxical bronchospasm (2%), dysphonia (1%), hoarseness (1%), pharyngolaryngeal pain (1%), nasal discomfort

Overdosage/Toxicology No data available; acute overdose unlikely due to low systemic bioavailability. Excessive doses over prolonged periods may result in systemic hypercortisolism. In those cases, discontinuation of ciclesonide should be done slowly and treatment should be symptom-directed and supportive. In healthy subjects, doses up to 3200 mcg administered by oral inhalation were well tolerated.

Drug Interactions Substrate of CYP3A4 (major), 2D6 (minor)
Amphotericin B: Hypokalemic effects may be enhanced by corticosteroids.
Antidiabetic agents: Hypoglycemic effects may be diminished by corticosteroids.
Antifungal agents, azole (ketoconazole): May increase levels/effects of des-ciclesonide, the active metabolite of ciclesonide; monitor.
CYP3A4 inhibitors: May increase the levels/effects of ciclesonide. Example inhibitors include azole antifungals, clarithromycin, diclofenac, doxycycline, erythromycin, imatinib, isoniazid, nefazodone, nicardipine, propofol, protease inhibitors, quinidine, telithromycin, and verapamil.
Diuretics (loop, thiazide): Hypokalemic effects may be enhanced by corticosteroids.
Quinolone antibiotics: May enhance the adverse/toxic effect of corticosteroids; risk of tendon-related side effects, including tendonitis and rupture, may be enhanced.

Stability Store at 15°C to 30°C (59°F to 86°F); do not freeze. Nasal spray: Use within 4 months after opening aluminum pouch.

Mechanism of Action Ciclesonide is a nonhalogenated, glucocorticoid prodrug that is hydrolyzed to the pharmacologically active metabolite des-ciclesonide following administration. Des-ciclesonide has a high affinity for the glucocorticoid receptor and exhibits anti-inflammatory activity. The mechanism of action for corticosteroids is believed to be a combination of three important properties — anti-inflammatory activity, immunosuppressive properties, and antiproliferative actions.
(Continued)

Ciclesonide *(Continued)*

Pharmacodynamics Onset of action: Intranasal: 24-48 hours; further improvement observed over 1-2 weeks in seasonal allergic rhinitis or 5 weeks in perennial allergic rhinitis

Pharmacokinetics

Absorption: Intranasal: Minimal systemic absorption; Oral inhalation: 52% (lung deposition)

Protein binding: ≥99%

Metabolism: Ciclesonide hydrolyzed to active metabolite, des-ciclesonide via esterases in nasal mucosa and lungs; further metabolism via hepatic CYP3A4 and 2D6

Bioavailability: Intranasal <1%; oral inhalation: >50% (active metabolite)

Half-life elimination: Oral inhalation: ~5-7 hours

Time to peak: Oral inhalation: ~1 hour (active metabolite)

Excretion:

Intranasal: Feces (~66%); urine (≤20%)

Oral inhalation: Feces (78%)

Dosage

Geriatrics & Adults:

Rhinitis: Intranasal (Omnaris™): 2 sprays (50 mcg/spray) per nostril once daily; maximum: 200 mcg/day

Asthma: Oral inhalation (Alvesco®): Initial: 400 mcg once daily; maintenance: 100-800 mcg/day (1-2 puffs once or twice daily). **Note:** Titrate to the lowest effective dose once asthma stability is achieved.

Conversion from oral to inhaled steroid: Initiation of oral inhalation therapy should begin in patients who have previously been stabilized on oral corticosteroids (OCS). A gradual dose reduction of OCS should begin ~10 days after starting inhaled therapy. Decrease daily dose by 1 mg of prednisone (or equivalent of other OCS) every 7 days in closely monitored patients, and every 10 days in patients whom close monitoring is not possible. In the presence of withdrawal symptoms, resume previous OCS dose for 1 week before attempting further dose reductions.

Administration

Intranasal: Shake bottle gently before using. Prime pump prior to first use (press 8 times until fine mist appears) or if spray has not been used in 4 consecutive days (press 1 time or until a fine mist appears). Blow nose to clear nostrils. Insert applicator into nostril, keeping bottle upright, and close off the other nostril. Breathe in through nose. While inhaling, press pump to release spray. Avoid spraying directly onto the nasal septum. Nasal applicator may be removed and rinsed with warm water to clean. Discard after the "discard by" date or after labeled number of doses has been used, even if bottle is not completely empty.

Oral inhalation: Remove mouthpiece cover, place inhaler in mouth, close lips around mouthpiece, and inhale slowly and deeply. Press down on top of inhaler after slow inhalation has begun. Remove inhaler while holding breath for approximately 10 seconds. Breathe out slowly and replace mouthpiece on inhaler. Do not wash or place inhaler in water. Clean mouthpiece using a dry cloth or tissue once weekly. Discard after the "discard by" date or after labeled number of doses has been used, even if container is not completely empty.

Shaking is not necessary since drug is formulated as a solution aerosol. Prime inhaler prior to initial use or if not in use for ≥1 week by releasing 3 puffs into the air.

Monitoring Parameters Signs/symptoms of HPA axis suppression/adrenal insufficiency

Additional Information The incidence of oral candidiasis, as well as other localized oropharyngeal effects, observed with ciclesonide use has been reported to be approximately one-half of that seen with other commonly inhaled corticosteroids such as budesonide and fluticasone. Small particle size, minimal activation, and deposition in the oropharynx may explain this decreased incidence.

Special Geriatric Considerations No specific information is available for the elderly patient. Make sure the patient can correctly use the nasal inhaler.

Dosage Forms Excipient information presented when available (limited, particularly for generics); consult specific product labeling. [CAN] = Canadian brand name

Aerosol for oral inhalation:

Alvesco® [CAN]: 100 mcg/inhalation [120 metered doses]; 200 mcg/inhalation [120 metered doses] [not available in the U.S.]

Suspension, intranasal [spray]:

Omnaris™: 50 mcg/inhalation (12.5 g) [120 metered doses]

Selected References

Bateman E, Karpel J, Casale T, et al, "Ciclesonide Reduces the Need for Oral Steroid Use in Adult Patients With Severe, Persistent Asthma," *Chest*, 2006, 129(5):1176-87.

Derendorf H, "Pharmacokinetic and Pharmacodynamic Properties of Inhaled Ciclesonide," *J Clin Pharmacol*, 2007, 47(6):782-9

Nave R, Wingertzahn MA, Brookman S, et al, "Safety, Tolerability, and Exposure of Ciclesonide Nasal Spray in Healthy and Asymptomatic Subjects with Seasonal Allergic Rhinitis," *J Clin Pharmacol*, 2006, 46 (4):461-7.

Pearlman DS, Berger WE, Kerwin E, et al, "Once-Daily Ciclesonide Improves Lung Function and is Well Tolerated by Patients With Mild-to-Moderate Persistent Asthma," *J Allergy Clin Immunol*, 2005, 116(6):1206-12.

Ciclopirox (sye kloe PEER oks)

Medication Safety Issues
Sound-alike/look-alike issues:
Loprox® may be confused with Lonox®
U.S. Brand Names Loprox®; Penlac®
Canadian Brand Names Loprox®; Penlac®; Stieprox®
Index Terms Ciclopirox Olamine
Generic Available Yes: Cream, topical suspension
Pharmacologic Category Antifungal Agent, Topical
Use
Cream/lotion/suspension: Treatment of tinea pedis (athlete's foot), tinea cruris (jock itch), tinea corporis (ringworm), cutaneous candidiasis, and tinea versicolor (pityriasis)

Gel: Treatment of tinea pedis (athlete's foot), tinea corporis (ringworm); seborrheic dermatitis of the scalp

Lacquer: Topical treatment of mild-to-moderate onychomycosis of the fingernails and toenails due to *Trichophyton rubrum* (not involving the lunula) and the immediately-adjacent skin

Shampoo: Treatment of seborrheic dermatitis of the scalp
Contraindications Hypersensitivity to ciclopirox or any component of the formulation; avoid occlusive wrappings or dressings
Warnings/Precautions For external use only; avoid contact with eyes. Nail lacquer is for topical use only and has not been studied in conjunction with systemic therapy or in patients with type 1 diabetes mellitus (insulin dependent, IDDM). Use has not been evaluated in immunosuppressed or immunocompromised patients. Discontinue treatment if signs and/or symptoms of hypersensitivity are noted.
Adverse Reactions (Reflective of adult population; not specific for elderly)
Central nervous system: Headache
Dermatologic: Alopecia, dry skin, erythema, facial edema, hair discoloration (rare; shampoo formulation in light-haired individuals), nail disorder (shape or color change with lacquer), pruritus, rash
Local: Burning sensation (gel: 34%; ≤1% with other forms), irritation, redness, or pain
Drug Interactions No data reported
Stability
Cream, suspension: Store between 5°C to 25°C (41°F to 77°F).
Lacquer (solution): Store at room temperature of 15°C to 30°C (59°F to 86°F); protect from light. Flammable; keep away from heat and flame.
Gel, shampoo: Store at room temperature of 15°C to 30°C (59°F to 86°F).
Mechanism of Action Inhibiting transport of essential elements in the fungal cell disrupting the synthesis of DNA, RNA, and protein
Pharmacokinetics
Absorption: Cream, suspension: <2% through intact skin; increased with gel; <5% with lacquer
Distribution: To epidermis, corium (dermis), including hair, hair follicles, and sebaceous glands
Protein binding: 94% to 98%
Half-life elimination: Biologic: 1.7 hours (suspension); elimination: 5.5 hours (gel)
Elimination: Of the small amounts of systemically absorbed drug, the majority is excreted by the kidney (gel; 35 to 10%); small amounts excreted in feces
Dosage
Geriatrics & Adults:
Tinea pedis, tinea corporis: Topical:
Cream and suspension: Apply twice daily, gently massage into affected areas; if no improvement after 4 weeks of treatment, re-evaluate the diagnosis.
Gel: Apply twice daily, gently massage into affected areas and surrounding skin; if no improvement after 4 weeks of treatment, re-evaluate diagnosis
Tinea cruris, cutaneous candidiasis, and tinea versicolor: Topical: *Cream and suspension:* Apply twice daily, gently massage into affected areas; if no improvement after 4 weeks of treatment, re-evaluate the diagnosis.
Onychomycosis of the fingernails and toenails: Topical: *Lacquer (solution):* Apply to adjacent skin and affected nails daily (as a part of a comprehensive management program for onychomycosis). Remove with alcohol every 7 days.
(Continued)

Ciclopirox *(Continued)*

Seborrheic dermatitis of the scalp: Topical:

Gel: Apply twice daily, gently massage into affected areas and surrounding skin; if no improvement after 4 weeks of treatment, re-evaluate diagnosis.

Shampoo: Apply ~5 mL (1 teaspoonful) to wet hair; lather, and leave in place ~3 minutes; rinse. May use up to 10 mL for longer hair. Repeat twice weekly for 4 weeks; allow a minimum of 3 days between applications.

Administration Topical:

Cream, suspension: Gently massage into affected areas.

Gel: Gently massage into affected areas and adjacent skin.

Lacquer (solution): Apply evenly over nail and surrounding skin at bedtime (or allow 8 hours before washing); apply daily over previous coat for 7 days; after 7 days, may remove with alcohol and continue cycle.

Shampoo: Apply to wet hair; lather and leave in place for ~3 minutes; rinse.

Patient Information Avoid contact with eyes; if sensitivity or irritation occurs, discontinue use

Dosage Forms Excipient information presented when available (limited, particularly for generics); consult specific product labeling.

Cream, as olamine: 0.77% (15 g, 30 g, 90 g)

Loprox®: 0.77% (15 g, 30 g, 90 g)

Gel:

Loprox®: 0.77% (30 g, 45 g, 100 g)

Shampoo:

Loprox®: 1% (120 mL)

Solution, topical [nail lacquer]:

Penlac®: 8% (6.6 mL)

Suspension, topical, as olamine: 0.77% (30 mL, 60 mL)

Loprox®: 0.77% (30 mL, 60 mL)

♦ **Ciclopirox Olamine** *see* Ciclopirox *on page 311*

♦ **Cidecin** *see* Daptomycin *on page 395*

Cilostazol *(sil OH sta zol)*

Medication Safety Issues

Sound-alike/look-alike issues:

Pletal® may be confused with Plendil®

U.S. Brand Names Pletal®

Canadian Brand Names Pletal®

Index Terms OPC-13013

Generic Available Yes

Pharmacologic Category Antiplatelet Agent; Phosphodiesterase Enzyme Inhibitor

Use Symptomatic management of peripheral vascular disease, primarily intermittent claudication

Unlabeled/Investigational Use Investigational: Treatment of acute coronary syndromes and for graft patency improvement in percutaneous coronary interventions with or without stenting

Contraindications Hypersensitivity to cilostazol or any component of the formulation; heart failure (of any severity)

Warnings/Precautions Use with caution in patients receiving other platelet aggregation inhibitors or in patients with thrombocytopenia. Discontinue therapy if thrombocytopenia or leukopenia occur, progression to agranulocytosis (reversible) has been reported when cilostazol was not immediately stopped. When cilostazol and clopidogrel are used concurrently, manufacturer recommends checking bleeding times. Withhold for at least 4-6 half-lives prior to elective surgical procedures. Use with caution in patients receiving CYP3A4 inhibitors (eg, ketoconazole or erythromycin) or CYP2C19 inhibitors (eg, omeprazole). Use with caution in severe underlying heart disease. Use caution in moderate-to-severe hepatic impairment. Use cautiously in severe renal impairment (Cl_{cr} <25 mL/minute).

Adverse Reactions (Reflective of adult population; not specific for elderly)

>10%:

Central nervous system: Headache (27% to 34%)

Gastrointestinal: Abnormal stools (12% to 15%), diarrhea (12% to 19%)

Respiratory: Rhinitis (7% to 12%)

Miscellaneous: Infection (10% to 14%)

2% to 10%:

Cardiovascular: Peripheral edema (7% to 9%), palpitation (5% to 10%), tachycardia (4%)

Central nervous system: Dizziness (9% to 10%), vertigo (up to 3%)

Gastrointestinal: Dyspepsia (6%), nausea (6% to 7%), abdominal pain (4% to 5%), flatulence (2% to 3%)

Neuromuscular & skeletal: Back pain (6% to 7%), myalgia (2% to 3%)
Respiratory: Pharyngitis (7% to 10%), cough (3% to 4%)

Overdosage/Toxicology Experience with overdosage in humans is limited. Headache, diarrhea, hypotension, tachycardia and/or cardiac arrhythmias may occur. Treatment is symptomatic and supportive. Hemodialysis is unlikely to be of value. In some animal models, high-dose or long-term administration was associated with a variety of cardiovascular lesions, including endocardial hemorrhage, hemosiderin deposition and left ventricular fibrosis, coronary arteritis, and periarteritis.

Drug Interactions Substrate of CYP1A2 (minor), 2C19 (major), 2D6 (minor), 3A4 (major)

Antifungal agents (imidazole): May decrease the metabolism, via CYP isoenzymes, of cilostazol. Manufacturer recommends a reduced dose of cilostazole during concurrent therapy.

CYP2C19 inhibitors may increase the levels/effects of cilostazol. Example inhibitors include delavirdine, fluconazole, fluvoxamine, gemfibrozil, isoniazid, omeprazole, and ticlopidine.

CYP3A4 inhibitors may increase the levels/effects of cilostazol. Example inhibitors include azole antifungals, clarithromycin, diclofenac, doxycycline, erythromycin, imatinib, isoniazid, nefazodone, nicardipine, propofol, protease inhibitors, quinidine, telithromycin, and verapamil.

Drotrecogin alfa: Antiplatelet agents may enhance the adverse/toxic effect of drotrecogin alfa. Bleeding may occur.

Macrolide antibiotics: May decrease the metabolism, via CYP isoenzymes, of cilostazol. Examples include clarithromycin, erythromycin, telithromycin. The manufacturer recommends considering a reduced dose (50 mg twice daily) during coadministration of these agents.

Nonsteroidal anti-inflammatory agents: May enhance the adverse/toxic effect of antiplatelet agents. An increased risk of bleeding may occur.

Omeprazole: May enhance the adverse/toxic effect of cilostazol. The manufacturer recommends considering a reduced dose (50 mg twice daily) during coadministration of omeprazole.

Salicylates: Antiplatelet agents such as cilostazol may enhance the adverse/toxic effect of salicylates. Increased risk of bleeding may result.

Treprostinil: May enhance the adverse/toxic effect of antiplatelet agents such as cilostazol. Bleeding may occur.

Ethanol/Nutrition/Herb Interactions Food: Taking cilostazol with a high-fat meal may increase peak concentration by 90%. Avoid concurrent ingestion of grapefruit juice due to the potential to inhibit CYP3A4.

Mechanism of Action Cilostazol and its metabolites are inhibitors of phosphodiesterase III. As a result, cyclic AMP is increased leading to reversible inhibition of platelet aggregation and vasodilation. Other effects of phosphodiesterase III inhibition include increased cardiac contractility, accelerated AV nodal conduction, increased ventricular automaticity, heart rate, and coronary blood flow.

Pharmacodynamics Onset of action: 2-4 weeks; treatment for up to 12 weeks may be required before benefit is experienced

Pharmacokinetics
Protein binding: 97% to 98%
Metabolism: Hepatic; at least one metabolite has significant activity
Half-life: 11-13 hours
Elimination: In urine (74%) and feces (20%), as metabolites

Dosage
Geriatrics & Adults: Peripheral vascular disease: Oral: 100 mg twice daily taken at least 30 minutes before or 2 hours after breakfast and dinner; dosage should be reduced to 50 mg twice daily during concurrent therapy with inhibitors of CYP3A4 or CYP2C19 (see Drug Interactions).

Monitoring Parameters Monitor response (increased walking distance, increased mobility)

Patient Information It is best to take 30 minutes before or 2 hours after meal.

Special Geriatric Considerations Elderly must be evaluated for cardiac status. Since CHF is common, this disease cannot be overlooked.

Dosage Forms Excipient information presented when available (limited, particularly for generics); consult specific product labeling.
Tablet: 50 mg, 100 mg
Pletal®: 50 mg, 100 mg

♦ **Ciloxan**® *see* Ciprofloxacin *on page 317*

Cimetidine (sye MET i deen)

Related Information
Potentially Inappropriate Medications for Geriatrics *on page 1824*
(Continued)

Cimetidine *(Continued)*

Medication Safety Issues
Sound-alike/look-alike issues:
Cimetidine may be confused with simethicone

U.S. Brand Names Tagamet® [DSC]; Tagamet® HB 200 [OTC]

Canadian Brand Names Apo-Cimetidine®; Gen-Cimetidine; Novo-Cimetidine; Nu-Cimet; PMS-Cimetidine; Tagamet® HB

Generic Available Yes

Pharmacologic Category Histamine H$_2$ Antagonist

Use Short-term treatment of active duodenal ulcers, benign gastric ulcers; long-term prophylaxis of duodenal ulcer, gastric hypersecretory states, gastroesophageal reflux; prevention of upper GI bleeding in critically ill patients
Tagamet® HB [OTC]: Relief of symptoms of heartburn, acid indigestion, and sour stomach

Unlabeled/Investigational Use Part of a multidrug regimen for *H. pylori* eradication to reduce the risk of duodenal ulcer recurrence

Contraindications Hypersensitivity to cimetidine, any component of the formulation, or other H$_2$ antagonists

Warnings/Precautions Reversible confusional states, usually clearing within 3-4 days after discontinuation, have been linked to use. Increased age (>50 years) and renal or hepatic impairment are thought to be associated. Dosage should be adjusted in renal/hepatic impairment or in patients receiving drugs metabolized through the P450 system. Rapid intravenous administration has been associated with rare cases of arrhythmia and/or hypotension.

Over the counter (OTC) cimetidine should not be taken by individuals experiencing painful swallowing, vomiting with blood, or bloody or black stools; medical attention should be sought. A physician should be consulted prior to use when pain in the stomach, shoulder, arms or neck is present; if heartburn has occurred for >3 months; or if unexplained weight loss, or nausea and vomiting occur. Frequent wheezing, shortness of breath, lightheadedness, or sweating, especially with chest pain or heartburn, should also be reported. Consultation of a healthcare provider should occur by patients if also taking theophylline, phenytoin, or warfarin; if heartburn or stomach pain continues or worsens; or if use is required for >14 days. Symptoms of GI distress may be associated with a variety of conditions; symptomatic response to H$_2$ antagonists does not rule out the potential for significant pathology (eg, malignancy).

Adverse Reactions (Reflective of adult population; not specific for elderly)
1% to 10%:
Central nervous system: Headache (2% to 4%), dizziness (1%), somnolence (1%), agitation
Endocrine & metabolic: Gynecomastia (<1% to 4%)
Gastrointestinal: Diarrhea (1%)
Frequency not defined:
Cardiovascular: AV block, bradycardia, hypotension, tachycardia, vasculitis
Central nervous system: Confusion
Dermatologic: Alopecia, erythema multiforme, exfoliative dermatitis, Stevens-Johnson syndrome, toxic epidermal necrolysis, rash
Endocrine & metabolic: Edema of the breasts, sexual ability decreased
Gastrointestinal: Nausea, pancreatitis, vomiting
Hematologic: Agranulocytosis, aplastic anemia, hemolytic anemia (immune-based), neutropenia, pancytopenia, thrombocytopenia
Hepatic: AST/ALT increased, hepatic fibrosis (case report)
Neuromuscular & skeletal: Arthralgia, myalgia, polymyositis
Renal: Creatinine increased, interstitial nephritis
Miscellaneous: Anaphylaxis, pneumonia (causal relationship not established)

Overdosage/Toxicology Reported ingestions of up to 20 g have resulted in transient side effects seen with recommended doses. Reports of ingestions up to 40 g have documented severe CNS depression, including unresponsiveness. Treatment is symptom-directed and supportive. Animal data suggests that ventilation assistance and beta-blocker treatment may be effective in managing the possible respiratory depression and tachycardia, respectively.

Drug Interactions Inhibits CYP1A2 (moderate), 2C9 (weak), 2C19 (moderate), 2D6 (moderate), 2E1 (weak), 3A4 (moderate)

Note: There are many potential interactions. Listed are the most significant ones.
Alfentanil: Increased serum concentration; monitor for toxicity.
Amiodarone: Serum concentration of amiodarone is increased; avoid concurrent use.
Atazanavir: Absorption may be decreased by cimetidine; separate doses by 12 hours.
Benzodiazepines (except lorazepam, oxazepam, temazepam): Serum concentration of the benzodiazepine is increased; consider alternative H$_2$ antagonist or monitor for benzodiazepine toxicity.

Beta-blockers (except atenolol, betaxolol, bisoprolol, nadolol, penbutolol): Effects of the beta-blocker may be increased; use a renally-eliminated beta-blocker or alternative H_2 antagonist.

Calcium channel blockers (except amlodipine and nicardipine): Serum concentration of the CCB is increased; monitor for toxicity.

Carbamazepine: Plasma concentration of carbamazepine may increase transiently (1 week). Monitor for carbamazepine toxicity or use an alternative H_2 antagonist.

Carmustine: Myelotoxicity of carmustine is increased; avoid concurrent use.

Cefpodoxime, cefuroxime: Oral absorption of these agents may be reduced by increased pH; consider alternative antibiotic or separate dosing by at least 2 hours.

Cisapride: Bioavailability of cisapride is increased; avoid concurrent use.

Citalopram: Serum concentration of citalopram is increased; use an alternative H_2 antagonist or adjust citalopram dose.

Clozapine: Cimetidine may increase levels/effects; consider alternative H_2 antagonist

Cyclosporine: Serum concentration of cyclosporine may increase; monitor cyclosporine levels.

CYP1A2 substrates: Cimetidine may increase the levels/effects of CYP1A2 substrates. Example substrates include aminophylline, fluvoxamine, mexiletine, mirtazapine, ropinirole, theophylline, and trifluoperazine.

CYP2C19 substrates: Cimetidine may increase the levels/effects of CYP2C19 substrates. Example substrates include citalopram, diazepam, methsuximide, phenytoin, propranolol, and sertraline.

CYP2D6 substrates: Cimetidine may increase the levels/effects of CYP2D6 substrates. Example substrates include amphetamines, selected beta-blockers, dextromethorphan, fluoxetine, lidocaine, mirtazapine, nefazodone, paroxetine, risperidone, ritonavir, thioridazine, tricyclic antidepressants, and venlafaxine.

CYP2D6 prodrug substrates: Cimetidine may decrease the levels/effects of CYP2D6 prodrug substrates. Example prodrug substrates include codeine, hydrocodone, oxycodone, and tramadol.

CYP3A4 substrates: Cimetidine may increase the levels/effects of CYP3A4 substrates. Example substrates include benzodiazepines, calcium channel blockers, cyclosporine, mirtazapine, nateglinide, nefazodone, sildenafil (and other PDE-5 inhibitors), tacrolimus, and venlafaxine. Selected benzodiazepines (midazolam and triazolam), cisapride, ergot alkaloids, selected HMG-CoA reductase inhibitors (lovastatin and simvastatin), and pimozide are generally contraindicated with strong CYP3A4 inhibitors.

Delavirdine: Absorption of delavirdine is decreased; avoid concurrent use with H_2 antagonists.

Dofetilide: Cimetidine may increase the levels/effects of dofetilide; avoid concurrent use

Flecainide: Serum concentration of flecainide is increased, especially in patients with renal failure.

Ketoconazole, fluconazole, itraconazole (especially capsule): Decreased serum concentration; avoid concurrent use with H_2 antagonists.

Lidocaine: Serum concentration of lidocaine is increased; use alternative H_2 antagonist.

Metformin: Serum levels/effects may be increased by cimetidine; monitor for hypoglycemia.

Moricizine: Serum concentration of moricizine is increased; monitor for toxicity.

Phenytoin: Serum levels/effects may be increased by cimetidine; avoid concurrent use.

Procainamide: Cimetidine may increase levels/effects; monitor.

Propafenone: Serum concentration of propafenone is increased; monitor for toxicity.

Quinolones: Renal elimination of quinolone antibiotics may be decreased.

Selective serotonin reuptake inhibitors (eg, paroxetine, citalopram): Serum concentrations may be increased by cimetidine; monitor.

Sulfonylureas: Cimetidine may increase levels/effects; monitor for hypoglycemia

Tacrine: Plasma concentration of tacrine is increased; consider alternative H_2 antagonist.

TCAs: Serum concentration is increased; consider alternative H_2 antagonist or monitor for TCAs toxicity.

Theophylline: Serum concentration of theophylline is increased; consider alternative H_2 antagonist.

Thioridazine: Serum levels/effects may be increased by cimetidine; concurrent use contraindicated by manufacturer.

Warfarin: INR is increased; cimetidine's effect is dose related. Use an alternative H_2 antagonist if possible or monitor INR closely and adjust warfarin dose as needed.

Ethanol/Nutrition/Herb Interactions

Ethanol: Avoid ethanol (may enhance gastric mucosal irritation).

Food: Cimetidine may increase serum caffeine levels if taken with caffeine. Cimetidine peak serum levels may be decreased if taken with food.

Herb/Nutraceutical: St John's wort may decrease cimetidine levels.

(Continued)

Cimetidine *(Continued)*

Stability

Tablet: Store between 15°C and 30°C (59°F to 86°F); protect from light.

Solution for injection/infusion: Intact vials should be stored at room temperature, between 15°C and 30°C (59°F to 86°F); protect from light. May precipitate from solution upon exposure to cold, but can be redissolved by warming without degradation.

Stability at room temperature:

Prepared bags: 7 days

Premixed bags: Manufacturer expiration dating and out of overwrap stability: 15 days

Stable in parenteral nutrition solutions for up to 7 days when protected from light.

Mechanism of Action Competitive inhibition of histamine at H_2 receptors of the gastric parietal cells resulting in reduced gastric acid secretion, gastric volume and hydrogen ion concentration reduced

Pharmacodynamics 400 mg twice daily and 300 mg 4 times/day suppress nocturnal acid secretion 47% to 83% over a 6- to 8-hour interval; 800 mg at bedtime decreases acid secretion 85% over 8 hours; 1600 mg at bedtime gives 100% reduction over 8 hours

Duration: 4-8 hours

Pharmacokinetics

Absorption: Rapid

Protein binding: 13% to 25%

Bioavailability: 60% to 70%

Metabolism: Hepatic

Half-life: Adults with normal renal function: 2 hours

Time to peak serum concentrations: Oral: Within 1-2 hours

Excretion: Primarily urine (48% as unchanged drug); feces (some)

Dosage

Geriatrics & Adults:

Short-term treatment of active ulcers:

Oral: 300 mg 4 times/day or 800 mg at bedtime or 400 mg twice daily for up to 8 weeks

Note: Higher doses of 1600 mg at bedtime for 4 weeks may be beneficial for a subpopulation of patients with larger duodenal ulcers (>1 cm defined endoscopically) who are also heavy smokers (≥1 pack/day).

I.M., I.V.: 300 mg every 6 hours or 37.5 mg/hour by continuous infusion; I.V. dosage should be adjusted to maintain an intragastric pH ≥5

Prevention of upper GI bleed in critically-ill patients: 50 mg/hour by continuous infusion; I.V. dosage should be adjusted to maintain an intragastric pH ≥5

Note: Reduce dose by 50% if Cl_{cr} <30 mL/minute; treatment >7 days has not been evaluated.

Duodenal ulcer prophylaxis: Oral: 400 mg at bedtime

Gastric hypersecretory conditions: Oral, I.M., I.V.: 300-600 mg every 6 hours; dosage not to exceed 2.4 g/day

Gastroesophageal reflux disease: Oral: 400 mg 4 times/day or 800 mg twice daily for 12 weeks

Peptic ulcer disease eradication of *Helicobacter pylori* (unlabeled use): Oral: 400 mg twice daily; requires combination therapy with antibiotics

Heartburn, acid indigestion, sour stomach (OTC labeling): Oral: 200 mg up to twice daily; may take 30 minutes prior to eating foods or beverages expected to cause heartburn or indigestion

Renal Impairment:

Cl_{cr} 10-50 mL/minute: Administer 50% of normal dose

Cl_{cr} <10 mL/minute: Administer 25% of normal dose

Slightly dialyzable (5% to 20%); administer after dialysis

Hepatic Impairment: Usual dose is safe in mild liver disease but use with caution and in reduced dosage in severe liver disease. Increased risk of CNS toxicity in cirrhosis suggested by enhanced penetration of CNS.

Administration

Oral: Administer with meals so that the drug's peak effect occurs at the proper time (peak inhibition of gastric acid secretion occurs at 1 and 3 hours after dosing in fasting subjects and approximately 2 hours in nonfasting subjects; this correlates well with the time food is no longer in the stomach offering a buffering effect)

Injection: May be administered as a slow I.V. push or preferably as an I.V. intermittent or I.V. continuous infusion. Administer each 300 mg (or fraction thereof) over a minimum of 5 minutes when giving I.V. push. Give intermittent infusion over 15-30 minutes for each 300 mg dose. Intermittent infusions are administered over 15-30 minutes at a final concentration not to exceed 6 mg/mL; for patients with an active bleed, preferred method of administration is continuous infusion.

Monitoring Parameters Signs and symptoms of peptic ulcer disease, occult blood with GI bleeding, gastric pH where necessary; monitor renal function to correct dose; monitor for side effects

Reference Range Therapeutic: >1 mcg/mL (SI: 4 μmol/L); mental confusion reported with concentrations >1.25 mcg/mL

Patient Information Take with or immediately after meals; inform pharmacist and physician (nurse, practitioner) of any concomitant drug therapy; stagger doses with antacids.

Tagamet® HB [OTC]: Do not take maximum dose for more than 14 days continuously, unless directed by a physician.

Additional Information All presently available H$_2$ blockers have equivalent healing properties for both DU and GU when dose at equivalent doses; practitioners should realize that when H$_2$-blocker doses are adjusted for renal function, it is **not** a "dose reduction" that results in less than therapeutic tissue concentration. Therapeutic concentrations are maintained with doses adjusted for renal function. When prophylaxing for gastric ulcers, must use full therapeutic dose; prophylaxis for DU can be reduced as indicated.

Special Geriatric Considerations Patients diagnosed with PUD should be evaluated for *Helicobacter pylori*. H$_2$ blockers are the preferred drugs for treating PUD in elderly due to cost and ease of administration. These agents are no less or more effective than any other therapy. The preferred agents, due to favorable pharmacokinetic, side effect and drug interaction profiles are ranitidine, famotidine, and nizatidine. Due to the potential for confusion and drug interactions, cimetidine has been identified by a panel of experts as a drug to avoid in the elderly. Consider evaluating creatinine clearance before initiating H$_2$-blocker therapy.

Dosage Forms Excipient information presented when available (limited, particularly for generics); consult specific product labeling. [DSC] = Discontinued product

Infusion, as hydrochloride [premixed in NS]: 300 mg (50 mL)

Injection, solution, as hydrochloride: 150 mg/mL (2 mL, 8 mL) [8 mL size contains benzyl alcohol]

Liquid, oral, as hydrochloride: 300 mg/5 mL (240 mL, 480 mL) [contains alcohol 2.8%; mint-peach flavor]

Tablet: 200 mg [OTC], 300 mg, 400 mg, 800 mg

Tagamet®: 300 mg, 400 mg [DSC]

Tagamet® HB 200: 200 mg

Selected References

Fennerty MD and Higbee M, "Drug Therapy of Gastrointestinal Disease," *Geriatric Pharmacology*, Bressler R and Katz MD, eds, New York, NY: McGraw-Hill, 1993, 585-608.

Fick DM, Cooper JW, Wade WE, et al "Updating the Beers Criteria for Potentially Inappropriate Medication Use in Older Adults," *Intern Med*, 2003, 163(22):2716-24.

Somogyi A and Gugler R, "Clinical Pharmacokinetics of Cimetidine," *Clin Pharmacokinet*, 1983, 8(6):463-95.

Somogyi A and Muirhead M, "Pharmacokinetic Interactions of Cimetidine 1987," *Clin Pharmacokinet*, 1987, 12(5):321-66.

♦ **Cipro**® *see* Ciprofloxacin *on page 317*
♦ **Ciprodex**® *see* Ciprofloxacin and Dexamethasone *on page 322*

Ciprofloxacin (sip roe FLOKS a sin)

Related Information
Antimicrobial Activity Against Selected Organisms *on page 1728*

Medication Safety Issues
Sound-alike/look-alike issues:
Ciprofloxacin may be confused with cephalexin
Ciloxan® may be confused with cinoxacin, Cytoxan®
Cipro® may be confused with Ceftin®

U.S. Brand Names Ciloxan®; Cipro®; Cipro® XR; Proquin® XR

Canadian Brand Names Apo-Ciproflox®; Ciloxan®; Cipro®; Cipro® XL; CO Ciprofloxacin; Gen-Ciprofloxacin; Novo-Ciprofloxacin; PMS-Ciprofloxacin; RAN™-Ciprofloxacin; ratio-Ciprofloxacin; Rhoxal-ciprofloxacin; Sandoz-Ciprofloxacin; Taro-Ciprofloxacin

Index Terms Ciprofloxacin Hydrochloride

Generic Available Yes: Excludes infusion, suspension, ointment

Pharmacologic Category Antibiotic, Ophthalmic; Antibiotic, Quinolone

Use To reduce incidence or progression of disease following exposure to aerolized *Bacillus anthracis*. Ophthalmologically, for superficial ocular infections (corneal ulcers, conjunctivitis) due to susceptible strains Treatment of the following infections when caused by susceptible bacteria: Urinary tract infections; acute uncomplicated cystitis in females; chronic bacterial prostatitis; lower respiratory tract infections (including acute exacerbations of chronic bronchitis); acute sinusitis; skin and skin structure infections; bone and joint infections; complicated intra-abdominal infections (in combination with metronidazole); infectious diarrhea; typhoid fever due to *Salmonella typhi* (eradication of chronic typhoid carrier state has not been proven); uncomplicated cervical and
(Continued)

Ciprofloxacin *(Continued)*

urethra gonorrhea (due to *N. gonorrhoeae*); nosocomial pneumonia; empirical therapy for febrile neutropenic patients (in combination with piperacillin)

Note: As of April 2007, the CDC no longer recommends the use of fluoroquinolones for the treatment of gonococcal disease.

Unlabeled/Investigational Use Cutaneous/gastrointestinal/oropharyngeal anthrax (treatment); disseminated gonococcal infection; chancroid; prophylaxis to *Neisseria meningitidis* following close contact with an infected person; empirical therapy (oral) for febrile neutropenia in low-risk cancer patients

Contraindications Hypersensitivity to ciprofloxacin, any component of the formulation, or other quinolones; concurrent administration of tizanidine

Warnings/Precautions CNS stimulation may occur (tremor, restlessness, confusion, and very rarely hallucinations or seizures). Use with caution in patients with known or suspected CNS disorder. Potential for seizures, although very rare, may be increased with concomitant NSAID therapy. Use with caution in individuals at risk of seizures. Fluoroquinolones may prolong QT_c interval; avoid use in patients with a history of QT_c prolongation, uncorrected hypokalemia, hypomagnesemia, or concurrent administration of other medications known to prolong the QT interval (including Class Ia and Class III antiarrhythmics, cisapride, erythromycin, antipsychotics, and tricyclic antidepressants). Prolonged use may result in fungal or bacterial superinfection, including *C. difficile*-associated diarrhea and pseudomembranous colitis. Tendon inflammation and/or rupture have been reported with ciprofloxacin and other quinolone antibiotics. Risk may be increased with concurrent corticosteroids, particularly in the elderly. Discontinue at first sign of tendon inflammation or pain. Rare cases of peripheral neuropathy may occur.

Severe hypersensitivity reactions, including anaphylaxis, have occurred with quinolone therapy. Quinolones may exacerbate myasthenia gravis, use with caution (rare, potentially life-threatening weakness of respiratory muscles may occur). Use caution in renal impairment. Avoid excessive sunlight; may cause moderate-to-severe phototoxicity reactions.

Ciprofloxacin is a potent inhibitor of CYP1A2. Coadministration of drugs which depend on this pathway may lead to substantial increases in serum concentrations and adverse effects.

Adverse Reactions (Reflective of adult population; not specific for elderly)
1% to 10%:

> Central nervous system: Neurologic events (children 2%, includes dizziness, insomnia, nervousness, somnolence); fever (children 2%); headache (I.V. administration); restlessness (I.V. administration)
>
> Dermatologic: Rash (children 2%, adults 1%)
>
> Gastrointestinal: Nausea (children/adults 3%); diarrhea (children 5%, adults 2%); vomiting (children 5%, adults 1%); abdominal pain (children 3%, adults <1%); dyspepsia (children 3%)
>
> Hepatic: ALT/AST increased (adults 1%)
>
> Local: Injection site reactions (I.V. administration)
>
> Respiratory: Rhinitis (children 3%)

Overdosage/Toxicology Symptoms of overdose include acute renal failure and seizures. Treatment is supportive and should include adequate hydration and renal function monitoring. Magnesium or calcium containing antacids may be given to decrease absorption of oral ciprofloxacin. Only a small amount of ciprofloxacin (<10%) is removed from the body after hemodialysis or peritoneal dialysis.

Drug Interactions Inhibits CYP1A2 (strong), 3A4 (weak)

Caffeine: Ciprofloxacin may decrease the metabolism of caffeine.

Corticosteroids: Concurrent use may increase the risk of tendon rupture, particularly in elderly patients (overall incidence rare).

CYP1A2 substrates: Ciprofloxacin may increase the levels/effects of CYP1A2 substrates. Example substrates include aminophylline, fluvoxamine, mexiletine, mirtazapine, ropinirole, tizanidine, and trifluoperazine.

Foscarnet: Concomitant use with ciprofloxacin has been associated with an increased risk of seizures.

Glyburide: Quinolones may increase the effect of glyburide; monitor.

Metal cations (aluminum, calcium, iron, magnesium, and zinc) bind quinolones in the gastrointestinal tract and inhibit absorption. Concurrent administration of most antacids, oral electrolyte supplements, quinapril, sucralfate, some didanosine formulations (pediatric powder for oral suspension), and other highly-buffered oral drugs, should be avoided. Ciprofloxacin should be administered 2 hours before or 6 hours after these agents.

Methotrexate: Ciprofloxacin may decrease renal secretion of methotrexate; monitor.

NSAIDs: Risk of seizures may be increased with concomitant NSAID use. Risk is considered quite low and may only be a factor with high serum levels of either agent and/or in patients with additional predisposing factors (eg, renal dysfunction, history of seizure or other neurological disorder).

Pentoxifylline: Monitor for headache during concomitant therapy.

Phenytoin: Ciprofloxacin may decrease phenytoin levels; monitor.

Probenecid: May decrease renal secretion of quinolones.

QT_c-prolonging agents: Ciprofloxacin may enhance the QT-prolonging effects of known QT_c-prolonging agents; information based on rare case reports.

Ropivacaine: Ciprofloxacin may decrease the metabolism of ropivacaine.

Sevelamer: May decrease absorption of oral ciprofloxacin.

Theophylline: Serum levels may be increased by ciprofloxacin; in addition, CNS stimulation/seizures may occur at lower theophylline serum levels due to additive CNS effects.

Tizanidine: Ciprofloxacin may increase serum levels of tizanidine. Concurrent administration is contraindicated.

Typhoid vaccine: Antibiotics may decrease the therapeutic effect of live, attenuated Ty21a vaccine; delay vaccination for >24 hours after administration of antibacterial agents.

Warfarin: The hypoprothrombinemic effect of warfarin may be enhanced by ciprofloxacin; monitor INR.

Ethanol/Nutrition/Herb Interactions

Food: Food decreases rate, but not extent, of absorption. Ciprofloxacin serum levels may be decreased if taken with dairy products or calcium-fortified juices. Ciprofloxacin may increase serum caffeine levels if taken with caffeine.

Enteral feedings may decrease plasma concentrations of ciprofloxacin probably by >30% inhibition of absorption. Ciprofloxacin should not be administered with enteral feedings. The feeding would need to be discontinued for 1-2 hours prior to and after ciprofloxacin administration. Nasogastric administration produces a greater loss of ciprofloxacin bioavailability than does nasoduodenal administration.

Herb/Nutraceutical: Avoid dong quai, St John's wort (may also cause photosensitization).

Stability

Injection:

Premixed infusion: Store between 5°C to 25°C (41°F to 77°F); avoid freezing. Protect from light.

Vial: Store between 5°C to 30°C (41°F to 86°F); avoid freezing. Protect from light. May be diluted with NS, D_5W, SWFI, $D_{10}W$, $D_5^1/_4NS$, $D_5^1/_2NS$, LR. Diluted solutions of 0.5-2 mg/mL are stable for up to 14 days refrigerated or at room temperature.

Ophthalmic solution/ointment: Store at 36°F to 77°F (2°C to 25°C); protect from light.

Microcapsules for oral suspension: Prior to reconstitution, store below 25°C (77°F); protect from freezing. Following reconstitution, store below 30°C (86°F) for up to 14 days; protect from freezing.

Tablet:

Immediate release: Store below 30°C (86°F).

Extended release: Store at room temperature of 15°C to 30°C (59°F to 86°F).

Mechanism of Action Inhibits DNA-gyrase in susceptible organisms; inhibits relaxation of supercoiled DNA and promotes breakage of double-stranded DNA

Pharmacokinetics

Protein binding: 20% to 40%

Metabolism: Partially hepatic; forms 4 metabolites (limited activity)

Bioavailability: Oral: 50% to 85%; in older adults, the bioavailability has been reported to be increased (70% to 80%), serum half-life is prolonged (4.8-6.8 hours) secondary to reduced renal clearance

Half-life (patients with normal renal function): 3-5 hours

Time to peak serum concentration: Oral:

Immediate release tablet: 0.5-2 hours

Extended release tablet: Cipro® XR: 1-2.5 hours, Proquin® XR: 3.5-8.7 hours

Excretion: Urine (30% to 50% as unchanged drug); feces (15% to 43%)

Only small amounts of ciprofloxacin are removed by dialysis (<10%)

Dosage

Geriatrics: Refer to adult dosing. Adjust dose carefully based on renal function.

Adults: Note: Extended release tablets and immediate release formulations are not interchangeable. Unless otherwise specified, oral dosing reflects the use of immediate release formulations.

Anthrax:

Inhalational (postexposure prophylaxis):

Oral: 500 mg every 12 hours for 60 days

I.V.: 400 mg every 12 hours for 60 days

Cutaneous (treatment, CDC guidelines): Oral: Immediate release formulation: 500 mg every 12 hours for 60 days. **Note:** In the presence of systemic involvement, extensive edema, lesions on head/neck, refer to I.V. dosing for treatment of inhalational/gastrointestinal/oropharyngeal anthrax.

(Continued)

Ciprofloxacin *(Continued)*

Inhalational/gastrointestinal/oropharyngeal (treatment, CDC guidelines): I.V.: 400 mg every 12 hours. **Note:** Initial treatment should include two or more agents predicted to be effective (per CDC recommendations). Continue combined therapy for 60 days.

Bacterial conjunctivitis:
Ophthalmic solution: Instill 1-2 drops in eye(s) every 2 hours while awake for 2 days and 1-2 drops every 4 hours while awake for the next 5 days
Ophthalmic ointment: Apply a ½" ribbon into the conjunctival sac 3 times/day for the first 2 days, followed by a ½" ribbon applied twice daily for the next 5 days

Bone/joint infections:
Oral: 500-750 mg twice daily for 4-6 weeks
I.V.:
Mild/moderate: 400 mg every 12 hours for 4-6 weeks
Severe/complicated: 400 mg every 8 hours for 4-6 weeks

Chancroid (CDC guidelines): Oral: 500 mg twice daily for 3 days

Corneal ulcer: Ophthalmic solution: Instill 2 drops into affected eye every 15 minutes for the first 6 hours, then 2 drops into the affected eye every 30 minutes for the remainder of the first day. On day 2, instill 2 drops into the affected eye hourly. On days 3-14, instill 2 drops into the affected eye every 4 hours. Treatment may continue after day 14 if re-epithelialization has not occurred.

Febrile neutropenia*: I.V.: 400 mg every 8 hours for 7-14 days

Gonococcal infections:
Urethral/cervical gonococcal infections: Oral: 250-500 mg as a single dose (CDC recommends concomitant doxycycline or azithromycin due to possible coinfection with *Chlamydia*; **Note:** As of April 2007, the CDC no longer recommends the use of fluoroquinolones for the treatment of uncomplicated gonococcal disease.
Disseminated gonococcal infection (CDC guidelines): Oral: 500 mg twice daily to complete 7 days of therapy (initial treatment with ceftriaxone 1 g I.M./I.V. daily for 24-48 hours after improvement begins); **Note:** As of April 2007, the CDC no longer recommends the use of fluoroquinolones for the treatment of more serious gonococcal disease, unless no other options exist and susceptibility can be confirmed via culture.

Infectious diarrhea: Oral:
Salmonella: 500 mg twice daily for 5-7 days
Shigella: 500 mg twice daily for 3 days
Traveler's diarrhea: Mild: 750 mg for one dose; Severe: 500 mg twice daily for 3 days
Vibrio cholerae: 1 g for one dose

Intra-abdominal*:
Oral: 500 mg every 12 hours for 7-14 days
I.V.: 400 mg every 12 hours for 7-14 days

Lower respiratory tract, skin/skin structure infections:
Oral: 500-750 mg twice daily for 7-14 days
I.V.:
Mild/moderate: 400 mg every 12 hours for 7-14 days
Severe/complicated: 400 mg every 8 hours for 7-14 days

Nosocomial pneumonia: I.V.: 400 mg every 8 hours for 10-14 days

Prostatitis (chronic, bacterial): Oral: 500 mg every 12 hours for 28 days

Sinusitis (acute): Oral: 500 mg every 12 hours for 10 days

Typhoid fever: Oral: 500 mg every 12 hours for 10 days

Urinary tract infection:
Acute uncomplicated, cystitis:
Oral:
Immediate release formulation: 250 mg every 12 hours for 3 days
Extended release formulation (Cipro® XR, Proquin® XR): 500 mg every 24 hours for 3 days
I.V.: 200 mg every 12 hours for 7-14 days
Complicated (including pyelonephritis):
Oral:
Immediate release formulation: 500 mg every 12 hours for 7-14 days
Extended release formulation (Cipro® XR): 1000 mg every 24 hours for 7-14 days
I.V.: 400 mg every 12 hours for 7-14 days
*Combination therapy generally recommended.

Renal Impairment: Adults:
Cl$_{cr}$ 30-50 mL/minute: Oral: Administer 250-500 mg every 12 hours.
Cl$_{cr}$ <30 mL/minute: Acute uncomplicated pyelonephritis or complicated UTI: Oral: Extended release formulation: 500 mg every 24 hours
Cl$_{cr}$ 5-29 mL/minute:
Oral: Administer 250-500 mg every 18 hours.

I.V.: Administer 200-400 mg every 18-24 hours.

Dialysis: Only small amounts of ciprofloxacin are removed by hemo- or peritoneal dialysis (<10%); usual dose: Oral: 250-500 mg every 24 hours following dialysis.

Continuous renal replacement therapy (CRRT): I.V.:

CVVH: 200 mg every 12 hours

CVVHD or CVVHDF: 200-400 mg every 12 hours

Administration

Oral: May administer with food to minimize GI upset; avoid antacid use; maintain proper hydration and urine output. Administer immediate release ciprofloxacin and Cipro® XR at least 2 hours before or 6 hours after, and Proquin® XR at least 4 hours before or 6 hours after antacids or other products containing calcium, iron, or zinc (including dairy products or calcium-fortified juices). Separate oral administration from drugs which may impair absorption (see Drug Interactions).

Oral suspension: Should not be administered through feeding tubes (suspension is oil-based and adheres to the feeding tube). Patients should avoid chewing on the microcapsules.

Nasogastric/orogastric tube: Crush immediate-release tablet and mix with water. Flush feeding tube before and after administration. Hold tube feedings at least 1 hour before and 2 hours after administration.

Tablet, extended release: Do not crush, split, or chew. May be administered with meals containing dairy products (calcium content <800 mg), but not with dairy products alone. Proquin® XR should be administered with a main meal of the day; evening meal is preferred.

Parenteral: Administer by slow I.V. infusion over 60 minutes to reduce the risk of venous irritation (burning, pain, erythema, and swelling); final concentration for administration should not exceed 2 mg/mL

Monitoring Parameters Patients receiving concurrent ciprofloxacin and theophylline should have serum concentrations of theophylline monitored; patients receiving concurrent warfarin should have prothrombin time or INR monitored; patients receiving cyclosporine should be watched for nephrotoxicity and have their cyclosporine concentrations monitored; CBC, renal and hepatic function during prolonged therapy

Reference Range Therapeutic: 2.6-3 mcg/mL; Toxic: >5 mcg/mL

Test Interactions Some quinolones may produce a false-positive urine screening result for opiates using commercially-available immunoassay kits. This has been demonstrated most consistently with levofloxacin and ofloxacin, but other quinolones have shown cross-reactivity in certain assay kits. Confirmation of positive opiate screens by more specific methods should be considered.

Patient Information Take as directed, preferably on an empty stomach, 2 hours after meals. May be taken with food to minimize upset stomach but avoid calcium-containing foods. Extended release tablet may be taken with meals containing dairy products, but not with dairy products alone; do not crush, split, or chew extended release tablet. Swallow oral suspension, do not chew microcapsules. Take entire prescription even if feeling better. Avoid antacid use. Maintain adequate hydration (2-3 L/day of fluids unless instructed to restrict fluid intake) to avoid concentrated urine and crystal formation. You may experience nausea, vomiting, or anorexia (small frequent meals, frequent mouth care, sucking lozenges, or chewing gum may help). You may experience increased sensitivity to sunlight; use sunblock, wear protective clothing and dark glasses, or avoid direct exposure to sunlight. Report immediately any signs of skin rash, joint or back pain, or difficulty breathing. Report unusual fever or chills; vaginal itching or foul-smelling vaginal discharge; easy bruising or bleeding. Report immediately any pain, inflammation, or rupture of tendon.

Special Geriatric Considerations Ciprofloxacin should not be used as first-line therapy unless the culture and sensitivity findings show resistance to usual therapy. The interactions with caffeine and theophylline can result in serious toxicity in the elderly. Adjust dose for renal function.

Dosage Forms Excipient information presented when available (limited, particularly for generics); consult specific product labeling.

Infusion [premixed in D_5W]:

Cipro®: 200 mg (100 mL); 400 mg (200 mL) [latex free]

Injection, solution: 10 mg/mL (20 mL, 40 mL)

Cipro®: 10 mg/mL (20 mL, 40 mL)

Microcapsules for suspension, oral:

Cipro®: 250 mg/5 mL (100 mL); 500 mg/5 mL (100 mL) [strawberry flavor]

Ointment, ophthalmic, as hydrochloride:

Ciloxan®: 3.33 mg/g [0.3% base] (3.5 g)

Solution, ophthalmic, as hydrochloride: 3.5 mg/mL (2.5 mL, 5mL, 10 mL) [0.3% base]

Ciloxin®: 3.5 mg/mL (2.5 mL, 5mL, 10 mL) [0.3% base; contains benzalkonium chloride]

Tablet: 250 mg, 500 mg, 750 mg

Cipro®: 250 mg, 500 mg, 750 mg

Tablet, extended release: 500 mg, 1000 mg

(Continued)

Ciprofloxacin *(Continued)*

Cipro® XR: 500 mg [equivalent to ciprofloxacin hydrochloride 287.5 mg and ciprofloxacin base 212.6 mg]; 1000 mg [equivalent to ciprofloxacin hydrochloride 574.9 mg and ciprofloxacin base 425.2 mg]

Proquin® XR: 500 mg

Tablet, extended release [dose pack]:

Proquin® XR: 500 mg (3s)

Selected References

Bayer A, Gajewska A, Stephens M, et al, "Pharmacokinetics of Ciprofloxacin in the Elderly," *Respiration*, 1987, 51(4):292-5.

Guay DRP, Awni WM, Peterson PK, et al, "Single and Multiple Dose Pharmacokinetics of Oral Ciprofloxacin in Elderly Patients," *Int J Clin Pharmacol Ther Toxicol*, 1988, 26(6):279-84.

Ciprofloxacin and Dexamethasone
(sip roe FLOKS a sin & deks a METH a sone)

Related Information
Ciprofloxacin *on page 317*
Dexamethasone *on page 413*

U.S. Brand Names Ciprodex®

Canadian Brand Names Ciprodex®

Index Terms Ciprofloxacin Hydrochloride and Dexamethasone; Dexamethasone and Ciprofloxacin

Generic Available No

Pharmacologic Category Antibiotic/Corticosteroid, Otic

Use Treatment of acute otitis media

Dosage

Geriatrics & Adults: Acute otitis externa: Otic: Instill 4 drops into affected ear(s) twice daily for 7 days

Dosage Forms Excipient information presented when available (limited, particularly for generics); consult specific product labeling.

Suspension, otic: Ciprofloxacin 0.3% and dexamethasone 0.1% (7.5 mL) [contains benzalkonium chloride]

Ciprofloxacin and Hydrocortisone
(sip roe FLOKS a sin & hye droe KOR ti sone)

Related Information
Ciprofloxacin *on page 317*
Hydrocortisone *on page 762*

U.S. Brand Names Cipro® HC

Canadian Brand Names Cipro® HC

Index Terms Ciprofloxacin Hydrochloride and Hydrocortisone; Hydrocortisone and Ciprofloxacin

Generic Available No

Pharmacologic Category Antibiotic/Corticosteroid, Otic

Use Treatment of acute otitis externa

Dosage

Geriatrics & Adults: Otitis externa: Otic: The recommended dosage for all patients is three drops of the suspension in the affected ear twice daily for 7 days; twice-daily dosing schedule is more convenient for patients than that of existing treatments with hydrocortisone, which are typically administered three or four times a day

Dosage Forms Excipient information presented when available (limited, particularly for generics); consult specific product labeling.

Suspension, otic: Ciprofloxacin hydrochloride 0.2% and hydrocortisone 1% (10 mL) [contains benzyl alcohol]

♦ **Ciprofloxacin Hydrochloride** *see* Ciprofloxacin *on page 317*

♦ **Ciprofloxacin Hydrochloride and Dexamethasone** *see* Ciprofloxacin and Dexamethasone *on page 322*

♦ **Ciprofloxacin Hydrochloride and Hydrocortisone** *see* Ciprofloxacin and Hydrocortisone *on page 322*

♦ **Cipro® HC** *see* Ciprofloxacin and Hydrocortisone *on page 322*

♦ **Cipro® XR** *see* Ciprofloxacin *on page 317*

Citalopram *(sye TAL oh pram)*

Related Information
Antidepressant Agents *on page 1742*

Medication Safety Issues

Sound-alike/look-alike issues:

Celexa® may be confused with Celebrex®, Cerebra®, Cerebyx®, Ranexa™, Zyprexa®

U.S. Brand Names Celexa®

Canadian Brand Names Apo-Citalopram®; Celexa®; CO Citalopram; Dom-Citalopram; Gen-Citalopram; Novo-Citalopram; PHL-Citalopram; PMS-Citalopram; RAN™-Citalopram; ratio-Citalopram; Rhoxal-citalopram; Sandoz-Citalopram

Index Terms Citalopram Hydrobromide; Nitalapram

Generic Available Yes

Pharmacologic Category Antidepressant, Selective Serotonin Reuptake Inhibitor

Use Treatment of depression

Unlabeled/Investigational Use Treatment of anxiety disorders, dementia, smoking cessation, ethanol abuse, diabetic neuropathy

Restrictions An FDA-approved medication guide concerning the use of antidepressants in children, adolescents, and young adults must be distributed when dispensing an outpatient prescription (new or refill) where this medication is to be used without direct supervision of a healthcare provider. Medication guides are available at http://www.fda.gov/cder/Offices/ODS/medication_guides.htm. Dispense to parents or guardians of children and adolescents receiving this medication.

Contraindications Hypersensitivity to citalopram or any component of the formulation; hypersensitivity or other adverse sequelae during therapy with other SSRIs; concomitant use with MAO inhibitors or within 2 weeks of discontinuing MAO inhibitors.

Warnings/Precautions [U.S. Boxed Warning]: Antidepressants increase the risk of suicidal thinking and behavior in children, adolescents, and young adults (18-24 years of age) with major depressive disorder (MDD) and other psychiatric disorders; consider risk prior to prescribing. Short-term studies did not show an increased risk in patients >24 years of age and showed a decreased risk in patients ≥65 years. Closely monitor patients for clinical worsening, suicidality, or unusual changes in behavior, particularly during the initial 1-2 months of therapy or during periods of dosage adjustments (increases or decreases); the patient's family or caregiver should be instructed to closely observe the patient and communicate condition with healthcare provider. A medication guide concerning the use of antidepressants should be dispensed with each prescription.

The possibility of a suicide attempt is inherent in major depression and may persist until remission occurs. Use caution in high-risk patients. Worsening depression and severe abrupt suicidality that are not part of the presenting symptoms may require discontinuation or modification of drug therapy. The patient's family or caregiver should be alerted to monitor patients for the emergence of suicidality and associated behaviors (such as agitation, irritability, hostility, impulsivity, and hypomania) and call healthcare provider.

May worsen psychosis in some patients or precipitate a shift to mania or hypomania in patients with bipolar disorder. Patients presenting with depressive symptoms should be screened for bipolar disorder. Monotherapy in patients with bipolar disorder should be avoided. **Citalopram is not FDA approved for the treatment of bipolar depression.**

The potential for severe reaction exists when used with MAO inhibitors, SSRIs/SNRIs or triptans; serotonin syndrome (hyperthermia, muscular rigidity, mental status changes/agitation, autonomic instability) may occur. Concurrent use with MAO inhibitors is contraindicated. May increase the risks associated with electroconvulsive therapy. Has a low potential to impair cognitive or motor performance; caution operating hazardous machinery or driving.

Use with caution in patients with hepatic or renal dysfunction, in elderly patients, and concomitant CNS depressants. Use caution with concomitant use of NSAIDs, ASA, or other drugs that affect coagulation; the risk of bleeding is potentiated. May cause hyponatremia/SIADH. May cause or exacerbate sexual dysfunction. Upon discontinuation of citalopram therapy, gradually taper dose. If intolerable symptoms occur following a decrease in dosage or upon discontinuation of therapy, then resuming the previous dose with a more gradual taper should be considered.

Adverse Reactions (Reflective of adult population; not specific for elderly)

>10%:

    Central nervous system: Somnolence, insomnia

    Gastrointestinal: Nausea, xerostomia

    Miscellaneous: Diaphoresis

<10%:

    Central nervous system: Anxiety, anorexia, agitation, yawning

    Dermatologic: Rash, pruritus

    Endocrine & metabolic: Sexual dysfunction

    Gastrointestinal: Diarrhea, dyspepsia, vomiting, abdominal pain, weight gain

    Neuromuscular & skeletal: Tremor, arthralgia, myalgia

    Respiratory: Cough, rhinitis, sinusitis

(Continued)

Citalopram *(Continued)*

Overdosage/Toxicology Symptoms include dizziness, nausea, vomiting, sweating, tremor, somnolence, and sinus tachycardia. Rare symptoms have included amnesia, confusion, coma, seizures, hyperventilation, and ECG changes (including QT_c prolongation, ventricular arrhythmia, and torsade de pointes). Management is supportive.

Drug Interactions Substrate of CYP2C19 (major), 2D6 (minor), 3A4 (major); **Inhibits** CYP1A2 (weak), 2B6 (weak), 2C19 (weak), 2D6 (weak)

Aspirin: Concomitant use of citalopram and NSAIDs, aspirin, or other drugs affecting coagulation has been associated with an increased risk of bleeding; monitor.

Beta-blockers: Citalopram may increase levels of some beta-blockers (see Carvedilol and Metoprolol); monitor carefully.

Buspirone: Concurrent use of citalopram with buspirone may cause serotonin syndrome; avoid concurrent use.

Carbamazepine: May enhance the metabolism of citalopram.

Carvedilol: Serum concentrations may be increased; monitor carefully for increased carvedilol effect (hypotension and bradycardia).

Cimetidine: May inhibit the metabolism of citalopram.

CYP2C19 inducers: May decrease the levels/effects of citalopram. Example inducers include aminoglutethimide, carbamazepine, phenytoin, and rifampin.

CYP2C19 inhibitors: May increase the levels/effects of citalopram. Example inhibitors include delavirdine, fluconazole, fluvoxamine, gemfibrozil, isoniazid, omeprazole, and ticlopidine.

CYP3A4 inducers: CYP3A4 inducers may decrease the levels/effects of citalopram. Example inducers include aminoglutethimide, carbamazepine, nafcillin, nevirapine, phenobarbital, phenytoin, and rifamycins.

CYP3A4 inhibitors: May increase the levels/effects of citalopram. Example inhibitors include azole antifungals, clarithromycin, diclofenac, doxycycline, erythromycin, imatinib, isoniazid, nefazodone, nicardipine, propofol, protease inhibitors, quinidine, telithromycin, and verapamil.

Linezolid: Hyperpyrexia, hypertension, tachycardia, confusion, seizures, and **deaths have been reported** with agents which inhibit MAO (serotonin syndrome); this combination should be avoided.

MAO inhibitors: Hyperpyrexia, hypertension, tachycardia, confusion, seizures, and **deaths have been reported** with MAO inhibitors (serotonin syndrome); this combination should be avoided.

Meperidine: Combined use theoretically may increase the risk of serotonin syndrome.

Metoprolol: Citalopram may increase plasma levels of metoprolol; monitor for increased effect.

Moclobemide: Concurrent use of citalopram with moclobemide may cause serotonin syndrome; avoid concurrent use.

Nefazodone: Concurrent use of citalopram with nefazodone may cause serotonin syndrome.

NSAIDs: Concomitant use of citalopram and NSAIDs, aspirin, or other drugs affecting coagulation has been associated with an increased risk of bleeding; monitor.

Ritonavir: Combined use of citalopram with ritonavir may cause serotonin syndrome in HIV-positive patients; monitor.

Selegiline: Concurrent use with citalopram has been reported to cause serotonin syndrome; as an MAO type B inhibitor, the risk of serotonin syndrome may be less than with nonselective MAO inhibitors, and reports indicate that this combination has been well tolerated in Parkinson's patients.

Serotonin agonists (eg, triptans): Concurrent use of citalopram with these agents may increase the risk of serotonin syndrome; monitor.

Serotonergic reuptake inhibitors (eg, SSRIs/SNRIs): Concurrent use of citalopram with these agents may increase the risk of serotonin syndrome; monitor.

Sibutramine: May increase the risk of serotonin syndrome with SSRIs.

Tramadol: Concurrent use of citalopram with tramadol may cause serotonin syndrome; avoid concurrent use.

Trazodone: Concurrent use of citalopram with trazodone may cause serotonin syndrome.

Venlafaxine: Combined use with citalopram may increase the risk of serotonin syndrome.

Ethanol/Nutrition/Herb Interactions

Ethanol: Avoid ethanol (may increase CNS depression).

Herb/Nutraceutical: Avoid valerian, St John's wort, SAMe, kava kava, and gotu kola (may increase CNS depression).

Stability Store below 25°C.

Mechanism of Action A bicyclic phthalane derivative, citalopram selectively inhibits serotonin reuptake in the presynaptic neurons

Pharmacokinetics

Distribution: V_d: 12 L/kg

Protein binding, plasma: ~80%

Metabolism: Extensive in the liver to N-demethylated, N-oxide, and deaminated metabolites

Bioavailability: 80%

Half-life: 24-48 hours; average 35 hours (doubled in patients with hepatic impairment)

Time to peak serum concentration: 1-6 hours, average within 4 hours

Elimination: 10% recovered unchanged in urine; systemic clearance: 330 mL/minute (20% renal)

Clearance was decreased, while AUC and half-life were significantly increased in older adult patients and in patients with hepatic impairment. Mild to moderate renal impairment may reduce clearance of citalopram (17% reduction noted in trials). No pharmacokinetic information is available concerning patients with severe renal impairment.

Dosage

Geriatrics: Oral: Initial dose: 10-20 mg once daily. Increase dose to 40 mg/day only in nonresponders.

Adults: Depression: Oral: Initial: 20 mg/day, generally with an increase to 40 mg/day; doses of more than 40 mg are not usually necessary. Should a dose increase be necessary, it should occur in 20 mg increments at intervals of no less than 1 week. Maximum dose: 60 mg/day.

Renal Impairment: None necessary in mild-to-moderate renal impairment; best avoided in severely impaired renal function (Cl_{cr} <20 mL/minute).

Hepatic Impairment: Reduce dosage in those with hepatic impairment.

Monitoring Parameters Monitor patient periodically for symptom resolution; mental status for depression, suicidal ideation (especially at the beginning of therapy or when doses are increased or decreased), anxiety, social functioning, mania, panic attacks; akathisia

Patient Information Citalopram does not impair psychomotor performance, nevertheless, patients receiving treatment may have an impaired ability to drive or operate machinery; they should be warned of this possibility and advised to avoid these tasks if so affected

Special Geriatric Considerations In open-label and placebo-controlled studies, elderly patients with or without dementia have shown significant improvement in depressive symptoms, irritability, anxiety, behavior, and restlessness. Effects on intellectual function have not been consistent. Thus, it appears that citalopram has additional effects in stabilizing emotion. A seven- to eightfold variation in citalopram S(+) (active) and R(-) enantiomer concentrations have been reported in the elderly. The racemic citalopram concentration-to-dose ratio was 1.8 times greater in elderly patients compared to younger patients.

Clearance was decreased, while AUC and half-life were significantly increased in elderly patients and in patients with hepatic impairment. Mild to moderate renal impairment may reduce clearance of citalopram (17% reduction noted in trials). No pharmacokinetic information is available concerning patients with severe renal impairment.

Dosage Forms Excipient information presented when available (limited, particularly for generics); consult specific product labeling.

Solution, oral: 10 mg/5 mL (240 mL)

Celexa®: 10 mg/5 mL (240 mL) [alcohol free, sugar free; peppermint flavor]

Tablet: 10 mg, 20 mg, 40 mg

Celexa®: 10 mg, 20 mg, 40 mg

Selected References

Bernard L, Stern R, Lew D, et al, "Serotonin Syndrome After Concomitant Treatment With Linezolid and Citalopram," *Clin Infect Dis*, 2003, 36(9):1197.

Foglia JP, Pollock BG, Kirshner MA, et al, "Plasma Levels of Citalopram Enantiomers and Metabolites in Elderly Patients," *Psychopharmacol Bull*, 1997, 33(1):109-12.

Gottfries CG, Karlsson I, and Nyth AL, "Treatment of Depression In Elderly Patients With and Without Dementia Disorders," *Int Clin Psychopharmacol*, 1992, 6 Suppl 5:55-64.

Mahlberg R, Kunz D, Sasse J, et al, "Serotonin Syndrome With Tramadol and Citalopram," *Am J Psychiatry*, 2004, 161(6):1129.

Nyth AL, Gottfries CG, Lyby K, et al, "A Controlled Multicenter Clinical Study of Citalopram and Placebo in Elderly Depressed Patients With and Without Concomitant Dementia," *Acta Psychiatr Scand*, 1992, 86(2):138-45.

Tahir N, "Serotonin Syndrome as a Consequence of Drug-Resistant Infections: An Interaction Between Linezolid and Citalopram," *J Am Med Dir Assoc*, 2004, 5(2):111-3.

◆ **Citalopram Hydrobromide** see Citalopram on page 322

◆ **Citracal® [OTC]** see Calcium Salts (Oral) on page 220

◆ **Citrate of Magnesia** see Magnesium Citrate on page 944

Citric Acid, Sodium Citrate, and Potassium Citrate

(SIT rik AS id, SOW dee um SIT rate, & poe TASS ee um SIT rate)

U.S. Brand Names Cytra-3; Polycitra®; Polycitra®-LC

Index Terms Potassium Citrate, Citric Acid, and Sodium Citrate; Sodium Citrate, Citric Acid, and Potassium Citrate

Generic Available Yes

(Continued)

Citric Acid, Sodium Citrate, and Potassium Citrate
(Continued)

Pharmacologic Category Alkalinizing Agent, Oral

Use Conditions where long-term maintenance of an alkaline urine is desirable as in control and dissolution of uric acid and cystine calculi of the urinary tract

Contraindications Oliguria, azotemia, untreated Addison's disease

Warnings/Precautions Conversion to bicarbonate may be impaired in patients with hepatic failure, in shock, or who are severely ill.

Adverse Reactions (Reflective of adult population; not specific for elderly)
Frequency not defined.
Cardiovascular: Cardiac abnormalities
Endocrine & metabolic: Metabolic alkalosis, calcium levels, hyperkalemia, hypernatremia
Gastrointestinal: Diarrhea
Neuromuscular & skeletal: Tetany

Drug Interactions
Decreased effect/levels of lithium, chlorpropamide, salicylates due to urinary alkalinization.
Increased toxicity/levels of amphetamines, ephedrine, pseudoephedrine, flecainide, quinidine, quinine due to urinary alkalinization.

Dosage
Geriatrics & Adults: Alkalinizing agent/bicarbonate precursor/potassium supplement: Oral: 15-30 mL diluted in water after meals and at bedtime

Monitoring Parameters Blood gas (pH and bicarbonate); serum bicarbonate

Patient Information Palatability is improved by chilling solution, dilute each dose with 1-3 oz of water and follow with additional water; take after meals to prevent saline laxative effect

Dosage Forms Excipient information presented when available (limited, particularly for generics); consult specific product labeling.
Note: Equivalent to potassium 1 mEq/mL, sodium 1 mEq/mL, and bicarbonate 2 mEq/mL

Solution, oral:
Cytra-3: Citric acid 334 mg, sodium citrate 500 mg, and potassium citrate 550 mg per 5 mL (480 mL) [alcohol free, sugar free; contains sodium benzoate; raspberry flavor]
Polycitra®-LC: Citric acid 334 mg, sodium citrate 500 mg, and potassium citrate 550 mg per 5 mL (480 mL) [alcohol free, sugar free]
Syrup, oral (Polycitra®): Citric acid 334 mg, sodium citrate 500 mg, and potassium citrate 550 mg per 5 mL (480 mL) [alcohol free]

- **Citroma® [OTC]** see Magnesium Citrate on page 944
- **CL-118,532** see Triptorelin on page 1640
- **CI-719** see Gemfibrozil on page 701
- **Claforan®** see Cefotaxime on page 260
- **Clarinex®** see Desloratadine on page 409

Clarithromycin (kla RITH roe mye sin)

Related Information
Antimicrobial Activity Against Selected Organisms on page 1728
Helicobacter pylori Treatment on page 1759
Prevention of Infective Endocarditis on page 1803
Medication Safety Issues
Sound-alike/look-alike issues:
Clarithromycin may be confused with erythromycin

U.S. Brand Names Biaxin®; Biaxin® XL

Canadian Brand Names Biaxin®; Biaxin® XL; ratio-Clarithromycin

Generic Available Yes: Tablet

Pharmacologic Category Antibiotic, Macrolide

Use
Pharyngitis/tonsillitis due to susceptible *S. pyogenes*
Acute maxillary sinusitis and acute exacerbation of chronic bronchitis due to susceptible *H. influenzae*, *M. catarrhalis*, or *S. pneumoniae*
Community-acquired pneumonia due to susceptible *H. influenzae*, *H. parainfluenzae*, *Mycoplasma pneumoniae*, *S. pneumoniae*, or *Chlamydia pneumoniae* (TWAR)
Uncomplicated skin/skin structure infections due to susceptible *S. aureus*, *S. pyogenes*
Disseminated mycobacterial infections due to *M. avium* or *M. intracellulare*
Prevention of disseminated mycobacterial infections due to *M. avium* complex (MAC) disease (eg, patients with advanced HIV infection)

Duodenal ulcer disease due to *H. pylori* in regimens with other drugs including amoxicillin and lansoprazole or omeprazole, ranitidine bismuth citrate, bismuth subsalicylate, tetracycline, and/or an H_2 antagonist

Alternate antibiotic for prophylaxis of bacterial endocarditis in patients who are allergic to penicillin and undergoing surgical or dental procedures

Unlabeled/Investigational Use Pertussis (CDC guidelines); alternate antibiotic for prophylaxis of bacterial endocarditis in patients who are allergic to penicillin and undergoing surgical or dental procedures (ACC/AHA guidelines)

Contraindications Hypersensitivity to clarithromycin, erythromycin, or any macrolide antibiotic; use with ergot derivatives, pimozide, cisapride

Warnings/Precautions Dosage adjustment required with severe renal impairment; decreased dosage or prolonged dosing interval may be appropriate. Prolonged use may result in fungal or bacterial superinfection, including *C. difficile*-associated diarrhea and pseudomembranous colitis. Macrolides (including clarithromycin) have been associated with rare QT prolongation and ventricular arrhythmias, including torsade de pointes. Use caution in patients with coronary artery disease. Avoid use of extended release tablets (Biaxin® XL) in patients with known stricture/narrowing of the GI tract.

Adverse Reactions (Reflective of adult population; not specific for elderly)
1% to 10%:

Central nervous system: Headache (adults and children 2%)

Dermatologic: Rash (children 3%)

Gastrointestinal: Abnormal taste (adults 3% to 7%), diarrhea (adults 3% to 6%; children 6%), vomiting (children 6%), nausea (adults 3%), abdominal pain (adults 2%; children 3%), dyspepsia 2%

Hepatic: Prothrombin time increased (1%)

Renal: BUN increased (4%)

Overdosage/Toxicology Symptoms include nausea, vomiting, diarrhea, prostration, reversible pancreatitis, hearing loss with or without tinnitus, or vertigo. Treatment includes symptomatic and supportive care.

Drug Interactions Substrate of CYP3A4 (major); **Inhibits** CYP1A2 (weak), 3A4 (strong)

Alfentanil (and possibly other opioid analgesics): Serum levels may be increased by clarithromycin; monitor for increased effect.

Azole antifungal agents: Serum levels/effects may be increased by clarithromycin; monitor.

Benzodiazepines (those metabolized by CYP3A4, including alprazolam, midazolam, triazolam): Serum levels may be increased by clarithromycin; somnolence and confusion have been reported.

Bromocriptine: Serum levels/toxicity (eg, ergotism) may be increased by clarithromycin; monitor for increased effect.

Buspirone: Serum levels may be increased by clarithromycin; monitor.

Calcium channel blockers (felodipine, verapamil, and potentially others metabolized by CYP3A4): Serum levels may be increased by clarithromycin; monitor.

Carbamazepine: Serum levels may be increased by clarithromycin; monitor.

Cilostazol: Serum levels may be increased by clarithromycin; monitor.

Cisapride: Serum levels may be increased by clarithromycin; serious arrhythmias have occurred; concurrent use contraindicated.

Clopidogrel: Therapeutic effect may be decreased by clarithromycin; monitor.

Clozapine: Serum levels may be increased by clarithromycin; monitor.

Colchicine: Serum levels/toxicity may be increased by clarithromycin; monitor. Avoid use, if possible.

CYP3A4 inducers: CYP3A4 inducers may decrease the levels/effects of clarithromycin. Example inducers include aminoglutethimide, carbamazepine, nafcillin, nevirapine, phenobarbital, phenytoin, and rifamycins.

CYP3A4 inhibitors: May increase the levels/effects of clarithromycin. Example inhibitors include azole antifungals, diclofenac, doxycycline, erythromycin, imatinib, isoniazid, nefazodone, nicardipine, propofol, protease inhibitors, quinidine, telithromycin, and verapamil.

CYP3A4 substrates: Clarithromycin may increase the levels/effects of CYP3A4 substrates. Example substrates include benzodiazepines, calcium channel blockers, mirtazapine, nateglinide, nefazodone, tacrolimus, and venlafaxine. Selected benzodiazepines (midazolam and triazolam), cisapride, ergot alkaloids, selected HMG-CoA reductase inhibitors (lovastatin and simvastatin), and pimozide are generally contraindicated with strong CYP3A4 inhibitors.

Delavirdine: Serum levels may be increased by clarithromycin; monitor.

Digoxin: Serum levels may be increased by clarithromycin; digoxin toxicity and potentially fatal arrhythmias have been reported; monitor digoxin levels.

Disopyramide: Serum levels may be increased by clarithromycin; in addition, QT_c prolongation and risk of malignant arrhythmia may be increased; avoid combination.

Eletriptan: Serum levels/effects may be increased by clarithromycin; monitor.

Eplerenone: Serum levels/effects may be increased by clarithromycin; monitor.
(Continued)

Clarithromycin *(Continued)*

Ergot alkaloids: Concurrent use may lead to acute ergot toxicity (severe peripheral vasospasm and dysesthesia); concurrent use contraindicated.

HMG-CoA reductase inhibitors (atorvastatin, lovastatin, and simvastatin); Clarithromycin may increase serum levels of "statins" metabolized by CYP3A4, increasing the risk of myopathy/rhabdomyolysis (does not include fluvastatin, pravastatin, or rosuvastatin). Switch to pravastatin, fluvastatin, or rosuvastatin or suspend treatment during course of clarithromycin therapy.

Immunosuppressants (eg, cyclosporine, sirolimus, tacrolimus): Serum levels/effects may be increased by clarithromycin; monitor serum concentrations and for increased immune suppression.

Methylprednisolone: Serum levels may be increased by clarithromycin; monitor.

Phenytoin: Serum levels may be increased by clarithromycin; other evidence suggested phenytoin levels may be decreased in some patients; monitor.

Phosphodiesterase 5 inhibitors (eg, sildenafil, tadalafil, vardenafil): Serum levels may be increased by clarithromycin. Do not exceed single sildenafil doses of 25 mg in 48 hours, a single tadalafil dose of 10 mg in 72 hours, or a single vardenafil dose of 5 mg in 24 hours.

Pimozide: Serum levels may be increased, leading to malignant arrhythmias; concomitant use is contraindicated.

Protease inhibitors (amprenavir, nelfinavir, and ritonavir): May increase serum levels of clarithromycin.

QT_c-prolonging agents: Concomitant use may increase the risk of malignant arrhythmias.

Quinidine: Serum levels may be increased by clarithromycin; in addition, the risk of QT_c prolongation and malignant arrhythmias may be increased during concurrent use.

Quinolone antibiotics (moxifloxacin): Concurrent use may increase the risk of malignant arrhythmias.

Rifamycin derivatives (eg, rifabutin): Serum levels may be increased by clarithromycin; monitor.

Selective serotonin reuptake inhibitors (SSRIs): Serum levels/effects may be increased by clarithromycin; monitor.

Theophylline: Serum levels may be increased by clarithromycin; monitor.

Thioridazine: Risk of QT_c prolongation and malignant arrhythmias may be increased.

Valproic acid (and derivatives): Serum levels may be increased by clarithromycin; monitor.

Warfarin: Effects may be potentiated; monitor INR closely and adjust warfarin dose as needed or choose another antibiotic

Zopiclone: Serum levels may be increased by clarithromycin; monitor.

Ethanol/Nutrition/Herb Interactions

Food: Immediate release: Food delays rate, but not extent of absorption; Extended release: Food increases clarithromycin AUC by ~30% relative to fasting conditions.

Herb/Nutraceutical: St John's wort may decrease clarithromycin levels.

Stability Store tablets and granules for oral suspension at controlled room temperature. Reconstituted oral suspension should not be refrigerated because it might gel; micro-encapsulated particles of clarithromycin in suspension is stable for 14 days when stored at room temperature

Mechanism of Action Exerts its antibacterial action by binding to 50S ribosomal subunit resulting in inhibition of protein synthesis. The 14-OH metabolite of clarithromycin is twice as active as the parent compound against certain organisms.

Pharmacokinetics

Absorption: Immediate release: Rapid; food delays rate, but not extent of absorption

Distribution: Widely into most body tissues except CNS

Protein binding: 42% to 50%

Metabolism: Partially hepatic via CYP3A4; converted to 14-OH clarithromycin (active metabolite)

Bioavailability: 50%

Half-life elimination: Immediate release: Clarithromycin: 3-7 hours; 14-OH-clarithromycin: 5-9 hours

Time to peak: Immediate release: 2-3 hours

Excretion: Primarily urine (20% to 40% as unchanged drug; additional 10% to 15% as metabolite)

Clearance: Approximates normal GFR

Dosage

Geriatrics & Adults:

Usual dosage range: Oral: 250-500 mg every 12 hours **or** 1000 mg (two 500 mg extended release tablets) once daily for 7-14 days

Acute exacerbation of chronic bronchitis: Oral:

M. catarrhalis and *S. pneumoniae*: 250 mg every 12 hours for 7-14 days **or** 1000 mg (two 500 mg extended release tablets) once daily for 7 days

H. influenzae: 500 mg every 12 hours for 7-14 days or 1000 mg (two 500 mg extended release tablets) once daily for 7 days

H. parainfluenzae: 500 mg every 12 hours for 7 days or 1000 mg (two 500 mg extended release tablets) once daily for 7 days

Acute maxillary sinusitis: Oral: 500 mg every 12 hours **or** 1000 mg (two 500 mg extended release tablets) once daily for 14 days

Endocarditis, prophylaxis: Oral: 500 mg 1 hour prior to procedure

Mycobacterial infection (prevention and treatment): Oral: 500 mg twice daily (use with other antimycobacterial drugs, eg, ethambutol or rifampin)

Peptic ulcer disease: Eradication of *Helicobacter pylori*: Dual or triple combination regimens with bismuth subsalicylate, amoxicillin, an H_2-receptor antagonist, or proton-pump inhibitor: 500 mg every 8-12 hours for 10-14 days

Pertussis (unlabeled use; CDC guidelines): Oral: 500 mg twice daily for 7 days

Pharyngitis, tonsillitis: Oral: 250 mg every 12 hours for 10 days

Pneumonia: Oral:

C. pneumoniae, M. pneumoniae, and *S. pneumoniae*: 250 mg every 12 hours for 7-14 days **or** 1000 mg (two 500 mg extended release tablets) once daily for 7 days

H. influenzae: 250 mg every 12 hours for 7 days **or** 1000 mg (two 500 mg extended release tablets) once daily for 7 days

Skin and skin structure infection, uncomplicated: Oral: 250 mg every 12 hours for 7-14 days

Renal Impairment:

Cl_{cr} <30 mL/minute: Half the normal dose or double the dosing interval.

In combination with ritonavir:

Cl_{cr} 30-60 mL/minute: Reduce dose by 50%.

Cl_{cr} <30 mL/minute: Reduce dose by 75%.

Hepatic Impairment: No dosing adjustment is needed as long as renal function is normal.

Administration Clarithromycin immediate release tablets and oral solution may be given with or without meals. Give every 12 hours rather than twice daily to avoid peak and trough variation.

Biaxin® XL: Should be given with food. Do not crush or chew extended release tablet.

Patient Information Take full course of therapy; do not discontinue without consulting prescriber. Check medications with prescriber, many medicines do not mix well with clarithromycin. Maintain adequate hydration (2-3 L/day of fluids unless instructed to restrict fluid intake). You may experience nausea (small frequent meals, or sucking lozenges may help); abnormal taste (frequent mouth care or chewing gum may help); diarrhea, headache, or abdominal cramps (medication may be ordered). Report persistent fever or chills, easy bruising or bleeding, or joint pain. Report severe persistent diarrhea, skin rash, sores in mouth, foul-smelling urine, rapid heartbeat or palpitations, or difficulty breathing. May be taken with or without food; may take with milk. Extended release tablets should be taken with food. Do not crush or chew extended release tablets. Do not refrigerate oral suspension (more palatable at room temperature).

Special Geriatric Considerations Considered one of the drugs of choice in the outpatient treatment of community-acquired pneumonia in elderly. After doses of 500 mg every 12 hours for 5 days, 12 healthy elderly subjects had significantly increased C_{max} and C_{min}, elimination half-lives of clarithromycin and 14-OH clarithromycin compared to 12 healthy young subjects. These changes were attributed to a significant decrease in renal clearance; at a dose of 1000 mg twice daily, 100% of 13 elderly subjects experienced an adverse event compared to only 10% taking 500 mg twice daily.

Dosage Forms Excipient information presented when available (limited, particularly for generics); consult specific product labeling.

Granules for oral suspension:

Biaxin®: 125 mg/5 mL (50 mL, 100 mL); 250 mg/5 mL (50 mL, 100 mL) [fruit punch flavor]

Tablet: 250 mg, 500 mg

Biaxin®: 250 mg, 500 mg

Tablet, extended release: 500 mg

Biaxin® XL: 500 mg

Selected References

American Thoracic Society, "Guidelines for the Initial Management of Adults With Community-Acquired Pneumonia: Diagnosis, Assessment of Severity, and Initial Antimicrobial Therapy," *Am Rev Respir Dis*, 1993, 148(5):1418-26.

Chu SY, Wilson DS, Guay DR, et al, "Clarithromycin Pharmacokinetics in Healthy Young and Elderly Volunteers," *J Clin Pharmacol*, 1992, 32(11):1045-9.

Tiwari T, Murphy TV, and Moran J, "Recommended Antimicrobial Agents for the Treatment and Postexposure Prophylaxis of Pertussis: 2005 CDC Guidelines," *MMWR Recomm Rep*, 2005, 54(RR-14):1-16.

Wallace RJ Jr, Brown BA, and Griffith DE, "Drug Intolerance to High-Dose Clarithromycin Among Elderly Patients," *Diagn Microbiol Infect Dis*, 1993, 16(3):215-21.

◆ **Claritin® 24 Hour Allergy [OTC]** *see* Loratadine *on page 928*

♦ **Claritin® Hives Relief [OTC]** *see* Loratadine *on page 928*
♦ **Clavulanic Acid and Amoxicillin** *see* Amoxicillin and Clavulanate Potassium *on page 97*
♦ **Clear eyes® for Dry Eyes and ACR Relief [OTC]** *see* Naphazoline *on page 1086*
♦ **Clear eyes® for Dry Eyes and Redness Relief [OTC]** *see* Naphazoline *on page 1086*
♦ **Clear eyes® Redness Relief [OTC]** *see* Naphazoline *on page 1086*
♦ **Clear eyes® Seasonal Relief [OTC]** *see* Naphazoline *on page 1086*

Clemastine (KLEM as teen)

U.S. Brand Names Dayhist® Allergy [OTC]; Tavist® Allergy [OTC]
Index Terms Clemastine Fumarate
Generic Available Yes
Pharmacologic Category Antihistamine
Use Treatment of perennial and seasonal allergic rhinitis and other allergic symptoms including urticaria
Contraindications Hypersensitivity to clemastine or any component of the formulation; narrow-angle glaucoma
Warnings/Precautions Use caution with bladder neck obstruction, symptomatic prostate hypertrophy, asthmatic attacks, stenosing peptic ulcer, increased intraocular pressure, hyperthyroidism, cardiovascular disease, hypertension, and in the elderly. May cause drowsiness; use caution in performing tasks which require alertness.
Adverse Reactions (Reflective of adult population; not specific for elderly)
Frequency not defined.
Cardiovascular: Palpitation, hypotension, tachycardia
Central nervous system: Dyscoordination, sedation, somnolence slight to moderate, sleepiness, confusion, restlessness, nervousness, insomnia, irritability, fatigue, headache, dizziness increased
Dermatologic: Rash, photosensitivity
Gastrointestinal: Diarrhea, nausea, xerostomia, epigastric distress, vomiting, constipation
Genitourinary: Urinary frequency, difficult urination, urinary retention
Hematologic: Hemolytic anemia, thrombocytopenia, agranulocytosis
Ocular: Blurred vision
Otic: Tinnitus
Respiratory: Thickening of bronchial secretions
Miscellaneous: Anaphylaxis
Overdosage/Toxicology Symptoms include anemia, metabolic acidosis, hypotension, and hypothermia. There is no specific treatment for an antihistamine overdose, however, clinical toxicity is mostly due to anticholinergic effects. For anticholinergic overdose with severe life-threatening symptoms, physostigmine 1-2 mg slow I.V. may be given to reverse these effects.
Drug Interactions Inhibits CYP2D6 (weak), 3A4 (weak)
Increased toxicity (CNS depression): CNS depressants, MAO inhibitors, tricyclic antidepressants, phenothiazines
Ethanol/Nutrition/Herb Interactions Ethanol: Avoid ethanol (may increase CNS depression).
Mechanism of Action Competes with histamine for H_1-receptor sites on effector cells in the gastrointestinal tract, blood vessels, and respiratory tract
Pharmacodynamics
Peak therapeutic effect: Within 5-7 hours
Duration: 10-12 hours; some patients experience therapeutic effects for 24 hours
Pharmacokinetics
Absorption: Almost 100% from GI tract
Metabolism: In the liver
Elimination: In urine
Dosage
Geriatrics & Adults:
Rhinitis or allergic symptoms (including urticaria): Oral:
1.34 mg clemastine fumarate (1 mg base) twice daily to 2.68 mg (2 mg base) 3 times/day; do not exceed 8.04 mg/day (6 mg base)
OTC labeling: 1.34 mg clemastine fumarate (1 mg base) twice daily; do not exceed 2 mg base/24 hours
Monitoring Parameters Relief of symptoms
Patient Information May cause drowsiness; avoid CNS depressants and alcohol
Additional Information 1.34 mg of clemastine fumarate = 1 mg clemastine base. Clemastine offers no significant benefit over other antihistamines except that it may be dosed twice daily (in adults) as compared to other antihistamines with more frequent dosing.

Dosage Forms Excipient information presented when available (limited, particularly for generics); consult specific product labeling.

Syrup, as fumarate [prescription formulation]: 0.67 mg/5 mL (120 mL) [0.5 mg base/5 mL; contains alcohol 5.5%; citrus flavor]

Tablet, as fumarate: 1.34 mg [1 mg base; OTC], 2.68 mg [2 mg base; prescription formulation]

Dayhist® Allergy, Tavist® Allergy: 1.34 mg [1 mg base]

- ◆ **Clemastine Fumarate** *see* Clemastine *on page 330*
- ◆ **Cleocin®** *see* Clindamycin *on page 332*
- ◆ **Cleocin HCl®** *see* Clindamycin *on page 332*
- ◆ **Cleocin Pediatric®** *see* Clindamycin *on page 332*
- ◆ **Cleocin Phosphate®** *see* Clindamycin *on page 332*
- ◆ **Cleocin T®** *see* Clindamycin *on page 332*
- ◆ **Cleocin® Vaginal Ovule** *see* Clindamycin *on page 332*

Clidinium and Chlordiazepoxide
(kli DI nee um & klor dye az e POKS ide)

Related Information
Chlordiazepoxide *on page 290*
Potentially Inappropriate Medications for Geriatrics *on page 1824*

Medication Safety Issues
Sound-alike/look-alike issues:
Librax® may be confused with Librium®
Librax® formulation may be cause for confusion:
In November 2004, Valeant Pharmaceuticals licensed the Librax® trademark to Victory Pharmaceuticals. Subsequently, the product was reformulated to contain chlordiazepoxide and methscopolamine. In January 2006, Valeant Pharmaceuticals began redistributing the original formulation of Librax®, containing clidinium and chlordiazepoxide. Victory Pharmaceuticals has discontinued their product. **Note:** The formulation of Librax® distributed in Canada (Valeant Canada Ltd) always contained clidinium and chlordiazepoxide.

U.S. Brand Names Librax® *[original formulation]*
Canadian Brand Names Apo-Chlorax®; Librax®
Index Terms Chlordiazepoxide and Clidinium
Generic Available Yes
Pharmacologic Category Antispasmodic Agent, Gastrointestinal; Benzodiazepine
Use Adjunct treatment of peptic ulcer; treatment of irritable bowel syndrome
Contraindications Hypersensitivity to clidinium, chlordiazepoxide, or any component of the formulation; glaucoma; prostatic hyperplasia; benign bladder neck obstruction
Warnings/Precautions Causes CNS depression; patients must be cautioned about performing tasks which require mental alertness (eg, operating machinery or driving). Benzodiazepines have been associated with anterograde amnesia. Paradoxical reactions, including hyperactive or aggressive behavior have been reported with benzodiazepines, particularly in psychiatric patients. Does not have analgesic, antidepressant, or antipsychotic properties. Use caution in patients with depression, particularly if suicidal risk may be present. Use with caution in patients with a history of drug abuse or acute alcoholism; potential for drug dependency exists. Use with caution in patients receiving other CNS depressants or psychoactive agents (lithium, phenothiazines). Effects with other sedative drugs or ethanol may be potentiated. Use with caution in elderly or debilitated patients, patients with respiratory disease, impaired gag reflux, hepatic disease or renal impairment. Benzodiazepines have been associated with dependence and acute withdrawal symptoms on discontinuation or reduction in dose. Do not abruptly discontinue this medication after prolonged use; taper dose gradually.

Adverse Reactions (Reflective of adult population; not specific for elderly)
1% to 10%:
Central nervous system: Drowsiness, ataxia, confusion, anticholinergic side effects
Gastrointestinal: Dry mouth, constipation, nausea

Drug Interactions Chlordiazepoxide: **Substrate** of CYP3A4 (major)
Also see individual monograph for Chlordiazepoxide.
Additive effects may result from concomitant benzodiazepine and/or anticholinergic therapy.
CYP3A4 inducers: CYP3A4 inducers may decrease the levels/effects of chlordiazepoxide. Example inducers include aminoglutethimide, carbamazepine, nafcillin, nevirapine, phenobarbital, phenytoin, and rifamycins.
CYP3A4 inhibitors: May increase the levels/effects of chlordiazepoxide. Example inhibitors include azole antifungals, clarithromycin, diclofenac, doxycycline, erythromycin, imatinib, isoniazid, nefazodone, nicardipine, propofol, protease inhibitors, quinidine, telithromycin, and verapamil.
(Continued)

Clidinium and Chlordiazepoxide *(Continued)*

Ethanol/Nutrition/Herb Interactions Ethanol: Avoid ethanol (may increase CNS depression).

Dosage

Geriatrics & Adults: Adjunct treatment of peptic ulcer; treatment of IBS: Oral: 1-2 capsules 3-4 times/day, before meals or food and at bedtime. **Caution:** Do not abruptly discontinue after prolonged use; taper dose gradually.

Administration Should be administered before meals

Special Geriatric Considerations The use of anticholinergic agents may cause problems with bladder emptying, constipation or cause confusion. The addition of chlordiazepoxide may enhance confusion potential. Monitor closely initially.

Dosage Forms Excipient information presented when available (limited, particularly for generics); consult specific product labeling.

Capsule: Clidinium bromide 2.5 mg and chlordiazepoxide hydrochloride 5 mg

♦ **Climara**® *see* Estradiol *on page 549*
♦ **Clindagel**® *see* Clindamycin *on page 332*
♦ **ClindaMax**™ *see* Clindamycin *on page 332*

Clindamycin (klin da MYE sin)

Related Information
Antimicrobial Activity Against Selected Organisms *on page 1728*
Prevention of Infective Endocarditis *on page 1803*

Medication Safety Issues
Sound-alike/look-alike issues:
Cleocin® may be confused with bleomycin, Clinoril®, Lincocin®

U.S. Brand Names Cleocin®; Cleocin HCl®; Cleocin Pediatric®; Cleocin Phosphate®; Cleocin T®; Cleocin® Vaginal Ovule; Clindagel®; ClindaMax™; Clindesse™; Clindets® [DSC]; Evoclin™

Canadian Brand Names Alti-Clindamycin; Apo-Clindamycin®; Clindamycin Injection, USP; Clindoxyl®; Dalacin® C; Dalacin® T; Dalacin® Vaginal; Novo-Clindamycin; Riva-Clindamycin; Taro-Clindamycin

Index Terms Clindamycin Hydrochloride; Clindamycin Palmitate; Clindamycin Phosphate

Generic Available Yes: Excludes foam, granules, vaginal suppositories, vaginal cream

Pharmacologic Category Antibiotic, Lincosamide; Topical Skin Product, Acne

Use Treatment against aerobic and anaerobic streptococci (except enterococci), most staphylococci, *Bacteroides* sp and *Actinomyces*; bacterial vaginosis; prophylaxis in the prevention of bacterial endocarditis in high-risk patients undergoing surgical or dental procedures in patients allergic to penicillin; may be useful in PCP; used topically in treatment of severe acne; vaginally for *Gardnerella vaginalis* or alternate treatment for toxoplasmosis

Contraindications Hypersensitivity to clindamycin or any component of the formulation; previous pseudomembranous colitis; hepatic impairment

Warnings/Precautions Dosage adjustment may be necessary in patients with severe hepatic dysfunction. **[U.S. Boxed Warning]: Can cause severe and possibly fatal colitis.** Discontinue drug if significant diarrhea, abdominal cramps, or passage of blood and mucus occurs. Vaginal products may weaken latex or rubber condoms, or contraceptive diaphragms. Barrier contraceptives are not recommended concurrently or for 3-5 days (depending on the product) following treatment. Some dosage forms contain benzyl alcohol or tartrazine. Use caution in atopic patients.

Adverse Reactions (Reflective of adult population; not specific for elderly)
Systemic:
>10%: Gastrointestinal: Diarrhea, abdominal pain
1% to 10%:
Cardiovascular: Hypotension
Dermatologic: Urticaria, rash, Stevens-Johnson syndrome
Gastrointestinal: Pseudomembranous colitis, nausea, vomiting
Local: Thrombophlebitis, sterile abscess at I.M. injection site
Miscellaneous: Fungal overgrowth, hypersensitivity
Topical:
>10%: Dermatologic: Dryness, burning, itching, scaliness, erythema, or peeling of skin (lotion, solution); oiliness (gel, lotion)
1% to 10%: Central nervous system: Headache
Vaginal:
>10%: Genitourinary: Fungal vaginosis, vaginitis or vulvovaginal pruritus (from *Candida albicans*)
1% to 10%:
Central nervous system: Back pain, headache

Gastrointestinal: Constipation, diarrhea
Genitourinary: Urinary tract infection
Respiratory: Nasopharyngitis
Miscellaneous: Fungal infection

Overdosage/Toxicology Following GI decontamination, symptoms of overdose include diarrhea, nausea, and vomiting. Treatment is supportive.

Drug Interactions Increased duration of neuromuscular blockade from tubocurarine, pancuronium

Ethanol/Nutrition/Herb Interactions
Food: Peak concentrations may be delayed with food.
Herb/Nutraceutical: St John's wort may decrease clindamycin levels.

Stability
Capsule: Store at room temperature of 20°C to 25°C (68°F to 77°F).
Cream: Store at room temperature.
Foam: Store at room temperature of 20°C to 25°C (68°F to 77°F); avoid fire, flame, or smoking during or following application.
Gel: Store at room temperature.
Clindagel®: Do not store in direct sunlight.
I.V.: Infusion solution in NS or D_5W solution is stable for 16 days at room temperature.
Lotion: Store at room temperature of 20°C to 25°C (68°F to 77°F).
Oral solution: Do not refrigerate reconstituted oral solution (it will thicken); following reconstitution, oral solution is stable for 2 weeks at room temperature of 20°C to 25°C (68°F to 77°F).
Ovule: Store at room temperature of 15°C to 30°C (68°F to 77°F).
Pledget: Store at room temperature.
Topical solution: Store at room temperature of 20°C to 25°C (68°F to 77°F).

Mechanism of Action Reversibly binds to 50S ribosomal subunits preventing peptide bond formation thus inhibiting bacterial protein synthesis; bacteriostatic or bactericidal depending on drug concentration, infection site, and organism

Pharmacokinetics
Absorption: Topical: ~10% absorbed systemically
Distribution: No significant concentrations seen in CSF, even with inflamed meninges
Protein binding: 94%
Bioavailability: Oral: ~90%
Half-life: 1.6-5.3 hours, average: 2-3 hours
Time to peak serum concentration:
Oral: Within 60 minutes
I.M.: Within 1-3 hours
Elimination: Most of the drug is eliminated by hepatic metabolism; 10% of an oral dose is excreted in urine and 3.6% is excreted in feces as active drug and metabolites

Dosage
Geriatrics & Adults:
Usual dose:
Oral: 150-450 mg/dose every 6-8 hours; maximum dose: 1.8 g/day
I.M., I.V.: 1.2-1.8 g/day in 2-4 divided doses; maximum dose: 4.8 g/day
Pelvic inflammatory disease: *I.V.:* 900 mg every 8 hours with gentamicin 2 mg/kg, then 1.5 mg/kg every 8 hours; continue after discharge with doxycycline 100 mg twice daily to complete 14 days of total therapy
Pneumonia due to *Pneumocystis carinii* (unlabeled use):
Oral: 300-450 mg 4 times/day with primaquine
I.M., I.V.: 1200-2400 mg/day with pyrimethamine
I.V.: 600 mg 4 times/day with primaquine
Acne: *Topical:*
Gel, pledget, lotion, solution: Apply a thin film twice daily
Foam (Evoclin™): Apply once daily
Bacterial vaginosis: Intravaginal:
Suppositories: Insert one ovule (100 mg clindamycin) daily into vagina at bedtime for 3 days
Cream:
Cleocin®: One full applicator inserted intravaginally once daily before bedtime for 3 or 7 consecutive days
Clindesse™: One full applicator inserted intravaginally as a single dose at anytime during the day
Prevention of bacterial endocarditis in patients unable to take amoxicillin (unlabeled use): *Oral:* 600 mg 1 hour before procedure with no follow-up dose needed; for patients allergic to penicillin and unable to take oral medications: 600 mg I.V. within 30 minutes before procedure
Orofacial infections: 150-450 mg every 6 hours for at least 7 days; maximum dose: 1.8 g/day
Patients with prosthesis allergic to penicillin: *Oral:* 600 mg 1 hour before procedure; for patients with prosthesis allergic to penicillin and unable to take oral medication: I.V.: 600 mg 1 hour before procedure

(Continued)

Clindamycin *(Continued)*

Hepatic Impairment: Systemic use: Adjustment is recommended in patients with severe hepatic disease.

Administration Administer oral dosage form with a full glass of water to minimize esophageal ulceration. Administer around-the-clock rather than 4 times/day, 3 times/day, etc (ie, 12-6-12-6, not 9-1-5-9) to promote less variation in peak and trough serum concentrations.

Monitoring Parameters Observe for changes in bowel frequency; during prolonged therapy monitor CBC, liver and renal function tests periodically

Patient Information Report any severe diarrhea immediately and do not take antidiarrheal medication; take each oral dose with a full glass of water; finish all medication; do not skip doses; **should not engage in sexual intercourse during treatment with vaginal product**; avoid contact of topical gel/solution with eyes, abraded skin, or mucous membranes

Special Geriatric Considerations Clindamycin has not been studied in the elderly; however, since it is eliminated principally by nonrenal mechanisms, major alteration in its pharmacokinetics are not expected. Elderly patients are often at a higher risk for developing serious colitis and require close monitoring.

Dosage Forms Excipient information presented when available (limited, particularly for generics); consult specific product labeling. [DSC] = Discontinued product

Note: Strength is expressed as base

Capsule, as hydrochloride: 150 mg, 300 mg
  Cleocin HCl®: 75 mg [contains tartrazine], 150 mg [contains tartrazine], 300 mg
Cream, vaginal, as phosphate:
  Cleocin®: 2% (40 g) [contains benzyl alcohol and mineral oil; packaged with 7 disposable applicators]
  Clindesse™: 2% (5 g) [contains mineral oil; prefilled single disposable applicator]
Foam, topical, as phosphate:
  Evoclin™: 1% (50 g, 100 g) [contains ethanol 58%]
Gel, topical, as phosphate: 1% (30 g, 60 g)
  Cleocin T®: 1% (30 g, 60 g)
  Clindagel®: 1% (40 mL, 75 mL)
  ClindaMax™: 1% (30 g, 60 g)
Granules for oral solution, as palmitate:
  Cleocin Pediatric®: 75 mg/5 mL (100 mL) [cherry flavor]
Infusion, as phosphate [premixed in D₅W]:
  Cleocin Phosphate®: 300 mg (50 mL); 600 mg (50 mL); 900 mg (50 mL)
Injection, solution, as phosphate: 150 mg/mL (2 mL, 4 mL, 6 mL, 60 mL)
  Cleocin Phosphate®: 150 mg/mL (2 mL, 4 mL, 6 mL, 60 mL) [contains benzyl alcohol and disodium edetate 0.5 mg]
Lotion, as phosphate: 1% (60 mL)
  Cleocin T®, ClindaMax™: 1% (60 mL)
Pledgets, topical: 1% (60s) [contains alcohol]
  Cleocin T®: 1% (60s) [contains isopropyl alcohol 50%]
  Clindets®: 1% (69s) [contains isopropyl alcohol 52%] [DSC]
Solution, topical, as phosphate: 1% (30 mL, 60 mL)
  Cleocin T®: 1% (30 mL, 60 mL) [contains isopropyl alcohol 50%]
Suppository, vaginal, as phosphate:
  Cleocin® Vaginal Ovule: 100 mg (3s) [contains oleaginous base; single reusable applicator]

Selected References
Yoshikawa TT, "Antimicrobial Therapy for the Elderly Patient," *J Am Geriatr Soc*, 1990, 38(12):1353-72.

Clindamycin and Tretinoin *(klin da MYE sin & TRET i noyn)*

U.S. Brand Names Ziana™
Index Terms Clindamycin Phosphate and Tretinoin; Tretinoin and Clindamycin
Generic Available No
Pharmacologic Category Acne Products; Retinoic Acid Derivative; Topical Skin Product; Topical Skin Product, Acne
Use Treatment of acne vulgaris
Dosage
  Adults: Acne: Topical: Apply pea-size amount to entire face once daily at bedtime
Special Geriatric Considerations Has not been studied in elderly patients.
Dosage Forms Excipient information presented when available (limited, particularly for generics); consult specific product labeling.
  Gel, topical:
    Ziana™: Clindamycin phosphate 1.2% and tretinoin 0.025% (2 g, 30 g, 60 g)

♦ **Clindamycin Hydrochloride** *see* Clindamycin *on page 332*
♦ **Clindamycin Palmitate** *see* Clindamycin *on page 332*

◆ **Clindamycin Phosphate** see Clindamycin on page 332
◆ **Clindamycin Phosphate and Tretinoin** see Clindamycin and Tretinoin on page 334
◆ **Clindesse**™ see Clindamycin on page 332
◆ **Clindets® [DSC]** see Clindamycin on page 332
◆ **Clinoril®** see Sulindac on page 1506

Clobetasol (kloe BAY ta sol)

Related Information
Corticosteroids on page 1755
Medication Safety Issues
International issues:
Clobex® may be confused with Codex® which is a brand name for *Saccharomyces boulardii* in Italy
U.S. Brand Names Clobevate®; Clobex®; Cormax®; Olux®; Olux-E™; Temovate®; Temovate E®
Canadian Brand Names Clobex®; Dermovate®; Gen-Clobetasol; Novo-Clobetasol; Taro-Clobetasol
Index Terms Clobetasol Propionate
Generic Available Yes: Excludes foam, lotion, shampoo, spray
Pharmacologic Category Corticosteroid, Topical
Use Short-term relief (<2 weeks) of inflammatory and pruritic manifestations of corticosteroid-responsive dermatoses (super high potency topical)
Contraindications Hypersensitivity to clobetasol or any component of the formulation; viral, fungal, or tubercular skin lesions
Warnings/Precautions Systemic absorption of topical corticosteroids may cause hypothalamic-pituitary-adrenal (HPA) axis suppression (reversible). HPA axis suppression may lead to adrenal crisis. Risk is increased when used over large surface areas, for prolonged periods, or with occlusive dressings. Allergic contact dermatitis can occur, it is usually diagnosed by failure to heal rather than clinical exacerbation. Prolonged treatment with corticosteroids has been associated with the development of Kaposi's sarcoma (case reports); if noted, discontinuation of therapy should be considered. Adverse systemic effects including hyperglycemia, glycosuria, fluid and electrolyte changes, and HPA suppression may occur when used on large surface areas, for prolonged periods, or with an occlusive dressing. Do not use on the face, axillae, or groin.
Adverse Reactions (Reflective of adult population; not specific for elderly)
Frequency not defined; may depend upon formulation used, length of application, surface area covered, and the use of occlusive dressings.

Endocrine & metabolic: Adrenal suppression, Cushing's syndrome, hyperglycemia
Local: Application site: Burning, cracking/fissuring of the skin, dryness, erythema, folliculitis, irritation, numbness, pruritus, skin atrophy, stinging, telangiectasia
Renal: Glucosuria
Effects reported with other high-potency topical steroids: Acneiform eruptions, allergic contact dermatitis, hypertrichosis, hypopigmentation, maceration of the skin, miliaria, perioral dermatitis, secondary infection
Drug Interactions No data reported
Stability
Cream, emollient cream, ointment: Store at room temperature, between 15°C to 30°C (59°F to 86°F); do not refrigerate.
Foam: Store at room temperature; do not expose to temperatures >49°C (120°F). Avoid fire, flame, or smoking during and immediately following application.
Gel: Store between 2°C to 30°C (36°F to 86°F).
Lotion, shampoo, spray: Store at room temperature of 20°C to 25°C (68°F to 77°F). Spray is flammable; do not use near open flame.
Solution: Store between 4°C to 25°C (39°F to 77°F); do not use near an open flame.
Mechanism of Action Stimulates the synthesis of enzymes needed to decrease inflammation, suppress mitotic activity, and cause vasoconstriction
Pharmacokinetics
Absorption: Percutaneous absorption is variable and dependent upon many factors including vehicle used, integrity of epidermis, dose, and use of occlusive dressings
Metabolism: Hepatic
Elimination: Urine and feces
Dosage
Geriatrics & Adults: Note: Discontinue when control achieved; if improvement not seen within 2 weeks, reassessment of diagnosis may be necessary.
Oral mucosal inflammation (unlabeled use): Topical: Cream: Apply twice daily for up to 2 weeks (maximum dose: 50 g/week); discontinue application when control is achieved; if no improvement is seen, reassessment of diagnosis may be necessary
(Continued)

Clobetasol (Continued)

Steroid-responsive dermatoses: Topical:
Cream, emollient cream, gel, lotion, ointment: Apply twice daily for up to 2 weeks (maximum dose: 50 g/week)
Foam (Olux-E™): Apply to affected area twice daily for up to 2 weeks (maximum dose: 50 g/week); do not apply to face or intertriginous areas

Steroid-responsive dermatoses of the scalp: Topical: Foam (Olux®), solution: Apply to affected scalp twice daily for up to 2 weeks (maximum dose: 50 g or 50 mL/week)

Mild-to-moderate plaque-type psoriasis of nonscalp areas: Topical: Foam (Olux®): Apply to affected area twice daily for up to 2 weeks (maximum dose: 50 g/week); do not apply to face or intertriginous areas

Moderate-to-severe plaque-type psoriasis: Topical:
Emollient cream, lotion: Apply twice daily for up to 2 weeks, has been used for up to 4 weeks when application is <10% of body surface area; use with caution (maximum dose: 50 g/week)
Spray: Apply by spraying directly onto affected area twice daily; should be gently rubbed into skin. Should be used for not longer than 4 weeks; treatment beyond 2 weeks should be limited to localized lesions which have not improved sufficiently. Total dose should not exceed 50 g/week or 59 mL/week.

Scalp psoriasis: Topical: Shampoo: Apply thin film to dry scalp once daily; leave in place for 15 minutes, then add water, lather; rinse thoroughly

Administration

Cream, gel, lotion, ointment, solution: Apply the smallest amount that will cover affected area. Do not apply to face or intertriginous areas. Total dose should not exceed 50 g/week (or 50 mL/week of lotion or solution).

Foam: Turn can upside down and spray a small amount (golf ball size) of foam into the cap or another cool surface. If fingers are warm, rinse with cool water and dry prior to handling (foam will melt on contact with warm skin). Massage foam into affected area. If the can is warm or the foam is runny, run can under cold water.

Monitoring Parameters Relief of symptoms

Patient Information
Use only as prescribed and for no longer than the period prescribed; apply sparingly in a thin film and rub in lightly; avoid contact with eyes; notify physician if condition persists or worsens; do not use longer than 2 weeks

Additional Information
Considered a super high potency steroid; avoid use on face

Special Geriatric Considerations
Due to age-related changes in skin, limit use of topical glucocorticosteroids.

Dosage Forms
Excipient information presented when available (limited, particularly for generics); consult specific product labeling.
Cream, as propionate: 0.05% (15 g, 30 g, 45 g, 60 g)
Cormax®: 0.05% (30 g)
Temovate®: 0.05% (30 g, 60 g)
Cream, as propionate [in emollient base]: 0.05% (15 g, 30 g, 60 g)
Temovate E®: 0.05% (60 g)
Foam, topical, as propionate:
Olux®: 0.05% (50 g, 100 g) [contains ethanol 60%]
Olux-E™: 0.05% (50 g, 100 g)
Gel, as propionate: 0.05% (15 g, 30 g, 60 g)
Clobevate®: 0.05% (45 g)
Temovate®: 0.05% (60 g)
Lotion, as propionate:
Clobex®: 0.05% (30 mL, 59 mL)
Ointment, as propionate: 0.05% (15 g, 30 g, 45 g, 60 g)
Cormax®: 0.05% (15 g, 45 g)
Temovate®: 0.05% (15 g, 30 g)
Shampoo, as propionate:
Clobex®: 0.05% (120 mL) [contains alcohol]
Solution, topical, as propionate [for scalp application]: 0.05% (25 mL, 50 mL)
Cormax®: 0.05% (25 mL, 50 mL) [contains isopropyl alcohol 40%]
Temovate®: 0.05% (50 mL) [contains isopropyl alcohol 40%]
Solution, topical, as propionate [spray]:
Clobex®: 0.05% (60 mL, 125 mL) [contains alcohol]

◆ **Clobetasol Propionate** *see* Clobetasol *on page 335*
◆ **Clobevate®** *see* Clobetasol *on page 335*
◆ **Clobex®** *see* Clobetasol *on page 335*

ClomiPRAMINE (kloe MI pra meen)

Related Information
Antidepressant Agents *on page 1742*

Medication Safety Issues

Sound-alike/look-alike issues:

ClomiPRAMINE may be confused with chlorproMAZINE, clomiPHENE, desipramine, Norpramin®

Anafranil® may be confused with alfentanil, enalapril, nafarelin

U.S. Brand Names Anafranil®

Canadian Brand Names Anafranil®; Apo-Clomipramine®; CO Clomipramine; Gen-Clomipramine

Index Terms Clomipramine Hydrochloride

Generic Available Yes

Pharmacologic Category Antidepressant, Tricyclic (Tertiary Amine)

Use Treatment of obsessive-compulsive disorder (OCD)

Unlabeled/Investigational Use Treatment of depression, panic attacks, chronic pain

Restrictions An FDA-approved medication guide concerning the use of antidepressants in children, adolescents, and young adults must be distributed when dispensing an outpatient prescription (new or refill) where this medication is to be used without direct supervision of a healthcare provider. Medication guides are available at http://www.fda.gov/cder/Offices/ODS/medication_guides.htm. Dispense to parents or guardians of children and adolescents receiving this medication.

Contraindications Hypersensitivity to clomipramine, other tricyclic agents, or any component of the formulation; use of MAO inhibitors within 14 days; use in a patient during the acute recovery phase of MI

Warnings/Precautions [U.S. Boxed Warning]: Antidepressants increase the risk of suicidal thinking and behavior in children, adolescents, and young adults (18-24 years of age) with major depressive disorder (MDD) and other psychiatric disorders; consider risk prior to prescribing. Short-term studies did not show an increased risk in patients >24 years of age and showed a decreased risk in patients ≥65 years. Closely monitor for clinical worsening, suicidality, or unusual changes in behavior; the patient's family or caregiver should be instructed to closely observe the patient and communicate condition with healthcare provider. A medication guide should be dispensed with each prescription.

The possibility of a suicide attempt is inherent in major depression and may persist until remission occurs. Monitor for worsening of depression or suicidality, especially during initiation of therapy (generally first 1-2 months) or with dose increases or decreases. Use caution in high-risk patients. Worsening depression and severe abrupt suicidality that are not part of the presenting symptoms may require discontinuation or modification of drug therapy. The patient's family or caregiver should be alerted to monitor patients for the emergence of suicidality and associated behaviors (such as agitation, irritability, hostility, impulsivity, and hypomania) and notify the healthcare provider.

May worsen psychosis in some patients or precipitate a shift to mania or hypomania in patients with bipolar disorder. Patients presenting with depressive symptoms should be screened for bipolar disorder. Monotherapy in patients with bipolar disorder should be avoided. **Clomipramine is not FDA approved for bipolar depression.**

May cause seizures (relationship to dose and/or duration of therapy) - do not exceed maximum doses. Use caution in patients with a previous seizure disorder or condition predisposing to seizures such as brain damage, alcoholism, or concurrent therapy with other drugs which lower the seizure threshold. May increase the risks associated with electroconvulsive therapy. Has been associated with a high incidence of sexual dysfunction. Weight gain may occur.

The degree of sedation, anticholinergic effects, and conduction abnormalities are high relative to other antidepressants. Clomipramine often causes drowsiness/sedation, resulting in impaired performance of tasks requiring alertness (eg, operating machinery or driving). Sedative effects may be additive with other CNS depressants and/or ethanol. The risk of orthostasis is moderate to high relative to other antidepressants. Use with caution in patients with a history of cardiovascular disease (including previous MI, stroke, tachycardia, or conduction abnormalities). Use with caution in patients with urinary retention, benign prostatic hyperplasia, narrow-angle glaucoma, xerostomia, visual problems, constipation, or a history of bowel obstruction.

Consider discontinuing, when possible, prior to elective surgery. Therapy should not be abruptly discontinued in patients receiving high doses for prolonged periods. Use with caution in hyperthyroid patients or those receiving thyroid supplementation. Use with caution in patients with hepatic or renal dysfunction and in elderly patients.

Adverse Reactions (Reflective of adult population; not specific for elderly)

>10%:

Central nervous system: Dizziness, drowsiness, headache, insomnia, malaise, nervousness

Endocrine & metabolic: Libido changes

(Continued)

ClomiPRAMINE *(Continued)*

Gastrointestinal: Abdominal pain, anorexia, appetite increased, constipation, diarrhea, dyspepsia, nausea, weight gain, xerostomia

Genitourinary: Ejaculation failure, impotence, micturition disorder

Neuromuscular & skeletal: Fatigue, myoclonus, tremor

Ocular: Vision abnormal

Respiratory: Pharyngitis, rhinitis

Miscellaneous: Diaphoresis increased

1% to 10%:

Cardiovascular: Hypotension, palpitation, tachycardia

Central nervous system: Abnormal dreaming, agitation, anxiety, concentration impaired, confusion, coordination impaired, depersonalization, depression, emotional lability, fever, flushing, hypertonia, memory impairment, migraine, panic reaction, sleep disorder, speech disorder, twitching, yawning

Dermatologic: Dermatitis, pruritus, purpura, rash

Endocrine & metabolic: Amenorrhea, breast enlargement, breast pain, hot flashes, lactation (nonpuerperal), menstrual disorder

Gastrointestinal: Dysphagia, esophagitis, flatulence, taste disturbance, tooth disorder, vomiting

Genitourinary: Difficult urination, leukorrhea, micturition frequency, vaginitis

Neuromuscular & skeletal: Paresthesia

Ocular: Blurred vision, eye pain

Respiratory: Bronchospasm

Overdosage/Toxicology Symptoms include agitation, confusion, hallucinations, urinary retention, hypothermia, hypotension, tachycardia, ventricular tachycardia, seizures, and coma. Following initiation of essential overdose management, toxic symptoms should be treated. Sodium bicarbonate is indicated when the QRS interval is >0.10 seconds or the QT_c is >0.42 seconds. Ventricular arrhythmias and ECG abnormalities (eg, QRS widening) often respond to systemic alkalinization (sodium bicarbonate 0.5-2 mEq/kg I.V.) and/or phenytoin 15-20 mg/kg. Arrhythmias unresponsive to this therapy may respond to lidocaine 1 mg/kg I.V. followed by a titrated infusion. Physostigmine (1-2 mg slow I.V.) may be indicated in reversing life-threatening cardiac arrhythmias. Seizures usually respond to diazepam I.V. boluses (5-10 mg up to 30 mg). If seizures are unresponsive or recur, phenytoin or phenobarbital may be required.

Drug Interactions Substrate of CYP1A2 (major), 2C19 (major), 2D6 (major), 3A4 (minor); **Inhibits** CYP2D6 (moderate)

Altretamine: Concurrent use may cause orthostatic hypertension.

Amphetamines: TCAs may enhance the effect of amphetamines; monitor for adverse CV effects.

Anticholinergics: Combined use with TCAs may produce additive anticholinergic effects.

Antihypertensives: TCAs inhibit the antihypertensive response to bethanidine, clonidine, debrisoquin, guanadrel, guanethidine, guanabenz, guanfacine; monitor BP; consider alternate antihypertensive agent.

Beta-agonists: When combined with TCAs may predispose patients to cardiac arrhythmias.

Bupropion: May increase the levels of tricyclic antidepressants; based on limited information; monitor response.

Carbamazepine: Tricyclic antidepressants may increase carbamazepine levels; monitor.

Cholestyramine and colestipol: May bind TCAs and reduce their absorption; monitor for altered response.

Clonidine: Abrupt discontinuation of clonidine may cause hypertensive crisis, amitriptyline may enhance the response.

CNS depressants: Sedative effects may be additive with TCAs; monitor for increased effect; includes benzodiazepines, barbiturates, antipsychotics, ethanol, and other sedative medications.

CYP1A2 inducers: May decrease the levels/effects of clomipramine. Example inducers include aminoglutethimide, carbamazepine, phenobarbital, and rifampin.

CYP1A2 inhibitors: May increase the levels/effects of clomipramine. Example inhibitors include ciprofloxacin, fluvoxamine, ketoconazole, norfloxacin, ofloxacin, and rofecoxib.

CYP2C19 inducers: May decrease the levels/effects of clomipramine. Example inducers include aminoglutethimide, carbamazepine, phenytoin, and rifampin.

CYP2C19 inhibitors: May increase the levels/effects of clomipramine. Example inhibitors include delavirdine, fluconazole, fluvoxamine, gemfibrozil, isoniazid, omeprazole, and ticlopidine.

CYP2D6 inhibitors: May increase the levels/effects of clomipramine. Example inhibitors include chlorpromazine, delavirdine, fluoxetine, miconazole, paroxetine, pergolide, quinidine, quinine, ritonavir, and ropinirole.

CYP2D6 substrates: Clomipramine may increase the levels/effects of CYP2D6 substrates. Example substrates include amphetamines, selected beta-blockers, dextromethorphan, fluoxetine, lidocaine, mirtazapine, nefazodone, paroxetine, risperidone, ritonavir, thioridazine, tricyclic antidepressants, and venlafaxine.

CYP2D6 prodrug substrates: Clomipramine may decrease the levels/effects of CYP2D6 prodrug substrates. Example prodrug substrates include codeine, hydrocodone, oxycodone, and tramadol.

Epinephrine (and other direct alpha-agonists): Pressor response to I.V. epinephrine, norepinephrine, and phenylephrine may be enhanced in patients receiving TCAs. (**Note:** Effect is unlikely with epinephrine or levonordefrin dosages typically administered as infiltration in combination with local anesthetics.)

Fenfluramine: May increase tricyclic antidepressant levels/effects.

Hypoglycemic agents (including insulin): TCAs may enhance the hypoglycemic effects of tolazamide, chlorpropamide, or insulin; monitor for changes in blood glucose levels; reported with chlorpropamide, tolazamide, and insulin.

Levodopa: Tricyclic antidepressants may decrease the absorption (bioavailability) of levodopa; rare hypertensive episodes have also been attributed to this combination.

Linezolid: Hyperpyrexia, hypertension, tachycardia, confusion, seizures, and **deaths have been reported** with agents which inhibit MAO (serotonin syndrome); this combination should be avoided.

Lithium: Concurrent use with a TCA may increase the risk for neurotoxicity.

MAO inhibitors: Hyperpyrexia, hypertension, tachycardia, confusion, seizures, and **deaths have been reported** (serotonin syndrome); this combination should be avoided.

Methylphenidate: Metabolism of some TCAs may be decreased.

Olanzapine: When used in combination, clomipramine and olanzapine have been reported to be associated with the development of seizures; limited documentation (case report).

Phenothiazines: Serum concentrations of some TCAs may be increased; in addition, TCAs may increase concentration of phenothiazines; monitor for altered clinical response.

QT_c-prolonging agents: Concurrent use of tricyclic agents with other drugs which may prolong QT_c interval may increase the risk of potentially fatal arrhythmias; includes type Ia and type III antiarrhythmics agents, selected quinolones (moxifloxacin), cisapride, and other agents.

Ritonavir: Combined use of high-dose tricyclic antidepressants with ritonavir may cause serotonin syndrome in HIV-positive patients; monitor.

Sucralfate: Absorption of tricyclic antidepressants may be reduced with coadministration.

Sympathomimetics, indirect-acting: Tricyclic antidepressants may result in a decreased sensitivity to indirect-acting sympathomimetics; includes dopamine and ephedrine; also see interaction with epinephrine (and direct-acting sympathomimetics).

Tramadol: Tramadol's risk of seizures may be increased with TCAs.

Valproic acid: May increase serum concentrations/adverse effects of some tricyclic antidepressants.

Warfarin (and other oral anticoagulants): TCAs may increase the anticoagulant effect in patients stabilized on warfarin; monitor INR.

Ethanol/Nutrition/Herb Interactions

Ethanol: Avoid ethanol (may increase CNS depression).

Food: Serum concentrations/toxicity may be increased by grapefruit juice.

Herb/Nutraceutical: Avoid valerian, St John's wort, SAMe, kava kava.

Mechanism of Action Clomipramine appears to affect serotonin uptake while its active metabolite, desmethylclomipramine, affects norepinephrine uptake

Pharmacodynamics Onset of action: 1-3 weeks; 5-HT >NE

Pharmacokinetics

Absorption: Oral: Rapid

Metabolism: Extensive first-pass; metabolized to desmethylclomipramine (active) in the liver

Half-life: 20-30 hours

Dosage

Geriatrics & Adults: Treatment of OCD: Oral: Initial: 25 mg/day and gradually increase, as tolerated, to 100 mg/day the first 2 weeks, may then be increased to a total of 250 mg/day maximum

Monitoring Parameters Signs and symptoms of disorder, plasma concentrations, blood pressure

Reference Range Therapeutic plasma concentration: 80-100 ng/mL

Test Interactions Increased glucose

Patient Information May cause seizures; caution should be used in activities that require alertness like driving, operating machinery, or swimming; effect of drug may (Continued)

ClomiPRAMINE *(Continued)*

take several weeks to appear; avoid alcohol; do not discontinue abruptly; may cause dry mouth, constipation, blurred vision

Special Geriatric Considerations Not approved as an antidepressant, clomipramine's anticholinergic and hypotensive effects limit its use versus other preferred antidepressants. Elderly patients were found to have higher dose-normalized plasma concentrations as a result of decreased demethylation (decreased 50%) and hydroxylation (25%).

Dosage Forms Excipient information presented when available (limited, particularly for generics); consult specific product labeling.

Capsule, as hydrochloride: 25 mg, 50 mg, 75 mg
   Anafranil®: 25 mg, 50 mg, 75 mg

Selected References

Bocksberger JP, Gex-Fabry M, Gauthey L, et al, "Clomipramine Therapy in the Geriatric Hospital: Experience With Therapeutic Drug Monitoring," *Ther Drug Monit*, 1994, 16(2):113-9.

♦ **Clomipramine Hydrochloride** *see* ClomiPRAMINE *on page 336*

Clonazepam (kloe NA ze pam)

Related Information
Anxiolytic, Sedative / Hypnotic, and Miscellaneous Benzodiazepines *on page 1750*

Medication Safety Issues
Sound-alike/look-alike issues:
Clonazepam may be confused with clofazimine, clonidine, clorazepate, clozapine, lorazepam
Klonopin® may be confused with clofazimine, clonidine, clorazepate, clozapine, lorazepam

U.S. Brand Names Klonopin®

Canadian Brand Names Alti-Clonazepam; Apo-Clonazepam®; Clonapam; CO Clonazepam; Gen-Clonazepam; Klonopin®; Novo-Clonazepam; Nu-Clonazepam; PMS-Clonazepam; Rho®-Clonazepam; Rivotril®; Sandoz-Clonazepam

Generic Available Yes

Pharmacologic Category Benzodiazepine

Use Prophylaxis of absence (petit mal), petit mal variant (Lennox-Gastaut), akinetic, and myoclonic seizures

Unlabeled/Investigational Use Treatment of restless legs syndrome, neuralgia, multifocal tic disorder, parkinsonian dysarthria, bipolar disorder; adjunct therapy for schizophrenia

Restrictions C-IV

Contraindications Hypersensitivity to clonazepam or any component of the formulation (cross-sensitivity with other benzodiazepines may exist); significant liver disease; narrow-angle glaucoma

Warnings/Precautions Use with caution in elderly or debilitated patients, patients with hepatic disease (including alcoholics), or renal impairment. Use with caution in patients with respiratory disease or impaired gag reflex or ability to protect the airway from secretions (salivation may be increased). Worsening of seizures may occur when added to patients with multiple seizure types. Concurrent use with valproic acid may result in absence status. Monitoring of CBC and liver function tests has been recommended during prolonged therapy.

Causes CNS depression (dose related) resulting in sedation, dizziness, confusion, or ataxia which may impair physical and mental capabilities. Patients must be cautioned about performing tasks which require mental alertness (eg, operating machinery or driving). Use with caution in patients receiving other CNS depressants or psychoactive agents. Effects with other sedative drugs or ethanol may be potentiated. Benzodiazepines have been associated with falls and traumatic injury and should be used with extreme caution in patients who are at risk of these events (especially the elderly).

Use caution in patients with depression, particularly if suicidal risk may be present. Use with caution in patients with a history of drug dependence. Benzodiazepines have been associated with dependence and acute withdrawal symptoms, including seizures, on discontinuation or reduction in dose. Acute withdrawal, including seizures, may be precipitated in patients after administration of flumazenil to patients receiving long-term benzodiazepine therapy.

Benzodiazepines have been associated with anterograde amnesia. Paradoxical reactions, including hyperactive or aggressive behavior, have been reported with benzodiazepines, particularly in psychiatric patients. Does not have analgesic, antidepressant, or antipsychotic properties.

Adverse Reactions (Reflective of adult population; not specific for elderly)
Reactions reported in patients with seizure and/or panic disorder. Frequency not defined.

Cardiovascular: Edema (ankle or facial), palpitation

Central nervous system: Amnesia, ataxia (seizure disorder ~30%; panic disorder 5%), behavior problems (seizure disorder ~25%), coma, confusion, depression, dizziness, drowsiness (seizure disorder ~50%), emotional lability, fatigue, fever, hallucinations, headache, hypotonia, hysteria, insomnia, intellectual ability reduced, memory disturbance, nervousness; paradoxical reactions (including aggressive behavior, agitation, anxiety, excitability, hostility, irritability, nervousness, nightmares, sleep disturbance, vivid dreams); psychosis, slurred speech, somnolence (panic disorder 37%), suicidal attempt, vertigo

Dermatologic: Hair loss, hirsutism, skin rash

Endocrine & metabolic: Dysmenorrhea, libido increased/decreased

Gastrointestinal: Abdominal pain, anorexia, appetite increased/decreased, coated tongue, constipation, dehydration, diarrhea, gastritis, gum soreness, nausea, weight changes (loss/gain), xerostomia

Genitourinary: Colpitis, dysuria, ejaculation delayed, enuresis, impotence, micturition frequency, nocturia, urinary retention, urinary tract infection

Hematologic: Anemia, eosinophilia, leukopenia, thrombocytopenia

Hepatic: Alkaline phosphatase increased (transient), hepatomegaly, serum transaminases increased (transient)

Neuromuscular & skeletal: Choreiform movements, coordination abnormal, dysarthria, muscle pain, muscle weakness, myalgia, tremor

Ocular: Blurred vision, eye movements abnormal, diplopia, nystagmus

Respiratory: Chest congestion, cough, bronchitis, hypersecretions, pharyngitis, respiratory depression, respiratory tract infection, rhinitis, rhinorrhea, shortness of breath, sinusitis

Miscellaneous: Allergic reaction, aphonia, dysdiadochokinesis, encopresis, "glassy-eyed" appearance, hemiparesis, lymphadenopathy

Overdosage/Toxicology May produce somnolence, confusion, ataxia, diminished reflexes, or coma. Treatment for benzodiazepine overdose is supportive. Flumazenil has been shown to selectively block the binding of benzodiazepines to CNS receptors, resulting in a reversal of benzodiazepine-induced CNS depression, but not respiratory depression.

Drug Interactions Substrate of CYP3A4 (major)

CNS depressants: Sedative effects and/or respiratory depression may be additive with CNS depressants; includes ethanol, barbiturates, opioid analgesics, and other sedative agents; monitor for increased effect.

CYP3A4 inducers: CYP3A4 inducers may decrease the levels/effects of clonazepam. Example inducers include aminoglutethimide, carbamazepine, nafcillin, nevirapine, phenobarbital, phenytoin, and rifamycins.

CYP3A4 inhibitors: May increase the levels/effects of clonazepam. Example inhibitors include azole antifungals, clarithromycin, diclofenac, doxycycline, erythromycin, imatinib, isoniazid, nefazodone, nicardipine, propofol, protease inhibitors, quinidine, telithromycin, and verapamil.

Disulfiram: Disulfiram may inhibit the metabolism of clonazepam; monitor for increased benzodiazepine effect.

Levodopa: Therapeutic effects may be diminished in some patients following the addition of a benzodiazepine; limited/inconsistent data.

Oral contraceptives: May decrease the clearance of some benzodiazepines (those which undergo oxidative metabolism); monitor for increased benzodiazepine effect.

Theophylline: May partially antagonize some of the effects of benzodiazepines; monitor for decreased response; may require higher doses for sedation.

Valproic acid: The combined use of clonazepam and valproic acid has been associated with absence seizures.

Ethanol/Nutrition/Herb Interactions

Ethanol: Avoid ethanol (may increase CNS depression).

Food: Clonazepam serum concentration is unlikely to be increased by grapefruit juice because of clonazepam's high oral bioavailability.

Herb/Nutraceutical: St John's wort may decrease clonazepam levels. Avoid valerian, St John's wort, kava kava, gotu kola (may increase CNS depression).

Mechanism of Action The exact mechanism is unknown, but believed to be related to its ability to enhance the activity of GABA; suppresses the spike-and-wave discharge in absence seizures by depressing nerve transmission in the motor cortex

Pharmacodynamics

Onset of action: 20-60 minutes

Duration: 12 hours

Pharmacokinetics

Absorption: Oral: Well absorbed

Distribution: V_d: 1.5-4.4 L/kg

Protein binding 85%

Metabolism: Extensive

Half-life: 19-50 hours

(Continued)

Clonazepam *(Continued)*

Elimination: Metabolites excreted as glucuronide or sulfate conjugates; less than 2% excreted unchanged in urine

Dosage

Geriatrics: Refer to adult dosing. Initiate with low doses and observe closely.

Adults:

Seizure disorders: Oral:

Initial daily dose not to exceed 1.5 mg given in 3 divided doses; may increase by 0.5-1 mg every third day until seizures are controlled or adverse effects seen (maximum: 20 mg/day)

Usual maintenance dose: 0.05-0.2 mg/kg; do not exceed 20 mg/day

Panic disorder: Oral: 0.25 mg twice daily; increase in increments of 0.125-0.25 mg twice daily every 3 days; target dose: 1 mg/day (maximum: 4 mg/day)

Discontinuation of treatment: To discontinue, treatment should be withdrawn gradually. Decrease dose by 0.125 mg twice daily every 3 days until medication is completely withdrawn.

Renal Impairment: Hemodialysis: Supplemental dose is not necessary.

Administration Orally-disintegrating tablet: Open pouch and peel back foil on the blister; do not push tablet through foil. Use dry hands to remove tablet and place in mouth. May be swallowed with or without water. Use immediately after removing from package.

Monitoring Parameters Monitor blood pressure, respiratory rate, motor coordination, mental status

Reference Range

Sample size: 2 mL serum or plasma (green top tube)

Therapeutic concentrations: 20-80 ng/mL; Toxic concentration: >80 ng/mL

Timing of serum samples: Peak serum concentrations occur 1-3 hours after oral ingestion; half-life: 20-40 hours; therefore, steady-state occurs in 5-7 days

Patient Information May cause drowsiness, dizziness, confusion. Avoid alcohol; use with caution when driving or performing tasks requiring alertness

Additional Information Ethosuximide or valproic acid may be preferred for treatment of absence (petit mal) seizures; clonazepam-induced behavioral disturbances may be more frequent in mentally handicapped patients; up to 30% of patients have demonstrated a loss of anticonvulsant control within several months which requires a dosage adjustment

Special Geriatric Considerations Hepatic clearance may be decreased allowing accumulation of active drug. Also, metabolites of clonazepam are renally excreted and may accumulate in the elderly as renal function declines with age. Observe for signs of CNS and pulmonary toxicity.

Dosage Forms Excipient information presented when available (limited, particularly for generics); consult specific product labeling.

Tablet: 0.5 mg, 1 mg, 2 mg

Tablet, orally disintegrating [wafer]: 0.125 mg, 0.25 mg, 0.5 mg, 1 mg, 2 mg

Clonidine *(KLON i deen)*

Related Information

Potentially Inappropriate Medications for Geriatrics *on page 1824*

Medication Safety Issues

Sound-alike/look-alike issues:

Clonidine may be confused with Clomid®, clomiPHENE, clonazepam, clozapine, Klonopin™, quinidine

Catapres™ may be confused with Cataflam®, Cetapred®, Combipres®

Transdermal patch may contain conducting metal (eg, aluminum); remove patch prior to MRI.

U.S. Brand Names Catapres®; Catapres-TTS®; Duraclon™

Canadian Brand Names Apo-Clonidine®; Carapres®; Dixarit®; Novo-Clonidine; Nu-Clonidine

Index Terms Clonidine Hydrochloride

Generic Available Yes: Tablet

Pharmacologic Category Alpha₂-Adrenergic Agonist

Use Management of mild to moderate hypertension, alone or in combination with other antihypertensives; not recommended for first-line therapy for hypertension

Orphan drug: Duraclon™: For continuous epidural administration as adjunctive therapy with intraspinal opiates for treatment of cancer pain in patients tolerant to or unresponsive to intraspinal opiates

Unlabeled/Investigational Use Treatment of heroin or nicotine withdrawal, severe pain, vasomotor symptoms associated with menopause, ethanol dependence, glaucoma, diabetes-associated diarrhea, impulse control disorder, attention-deficit/hyperactivity disorder (ADHD), clozapine-induced sialorrhea; prophylaxis of migraines

Contraindications Hypersensitivity to clonidine hydrochloride or any component of the formulation

Warnings/Precautions Gradual withdrawal is needed (over 1 week for oral, 2-4 days with epidural) if drug needs to be stopped. Patients should be instructed about abrupt discontinuation (causes rapid increase in BP and symptoms of sympathetic overactivity). In patients on both a beta-blocker and clonidine where withdrawal of clonidine is necessary, withdraw the beta-blocker first and several days before clonidine. Then slowly decrease clonidine.

Use with caution in patients with severe coronary insufficiency; conduction disturbances; recent MI, CVA, or chronic renal insufficiency. Caution in sinus node dysfunction. Discontinue within 4 hours of surgery then restart as soon as possible after. Clonidine injection should be administered via a continuous epidural infusion device. **[U.S. Boxed Warning]: Epidural clonidine is not recommended for perioperative, obstetrical, or postpartum pain.** It is not recommended for use in patients with severe cardiovascular disease or hemodynamic instability. In all cases, the epidural may lead to cardiovascular instability (hypotension, bradycardia). Transdermal patch may contain conducting metal (eg, aluminum); remove patch prior to MRI. Due to the potential for altered electrical conductivity, remove transdermal patch before cardioversion or defibrillation. Clonidine cause significant CNS depression and xerostomia. Caution in patients with pre-existing CNS disease or depression. Elderly may be at greater risk for CNS depressive effects, favoring other agents in this population.

Adverse Reactions (Reflective of adult population; not specific for elderly)
Incidence of adverse events is not always reported.

>10%:
  Central nervous system: Drowsiness (35% oral, 12% transdermal), dizziness (16% oral, 2% transdermal)
  Dermatologic: Transient localized skin reactions characterized by pruritus, and erythema (15% to 50% transdermal)
  Gastrointestinal: Dry mouth (40% oral, 25% transdermal)
1% to 10%:
  Cardiovascular: Orthostatic hypotension (3% oral)
  Central nervous system: Headache (1% oral, 5% transdermal), sedation (3% transdermal), fatigue (6% transdermal), lethargy (3% transdermal), insomnia (2% transdermal), nervousness (3% oral, 1% transdermal), mental depression (1% oral)
  Dermatologic: Rash (1% oral), allergic contact sensitivity (5% transdermal), localized vesiculation (7%), hyperpigmentation (5% at application site), edema (3%), excoriation (3%), burning (3%), throbbing, blanching (1%), papules (1%), and generalized macular rash (1%) has occurred in patients receiving transdermal clonidine.
  Endocrine & metabolic: Sodium and water retention, sexual dysfunction (3% oral, 2% transdermal), impotence (3% oral, 2% transdermal), weakness (10% transdermal)
  Gastrointestinal: Nausea (5% oral, 1% transdermal), vomiting (5% oral), anorexia and malaise (1% oral), constipation (10% oral, 1% transdermal), dry throat (2% transdermal), taste disturbance (1% transdermal), weight gain (1% oral)
  Genitourinary: Nocturia (1% oral)
  Hepatic: Liver function test (mild abnormalities, 1% oral)
  Miscellaneous: Withdrawal syndrome (1% oral)

Overdosage/Toxicology Symptoms include bradycardia, CNS depression, hypothermia, diarrhea, respiratory depression, and apnea. Treatment is primarily supportive and symptomatic. Hypotension usually responds to I.V. fluids or Trendelenburg positioning. Naloxone may be utilized in treating CNS depression and/or apnea and should be given I.V. 0.4-2 mg, with repeated doses as needed, or as an infusion.

Drug Interactions
  Antipsychotics: Concurrent use with antipsychotics (especially low potency) or nitroprusside may produce additive hypotensive effects.
  Beta-blockers: May potentiate bradycardia in patients receiving clonidine and may increase the rebound hypertension of withdrawal; discontinue beta-blocker several days before clonidine is tapered.
  CNS depressants: Sedative effects may be additive; monitor for increased effect; includes barbiturates, benzodiazepines, opioid analgesics, ethanol, and other sedative agents.
  Cyclosporine: Clonidine may increase cyclosporine (and perhaps tacrolimus) serum concentrations; cyclosporine dosage adjustment may be needed.
  Hypoglycemic agents: Clonidine may decrease the symptoms of hypoglycemia; monitor patients receiving antidiabetic agents.
  Levodopa: Effects may be reduced by clonidine in some patients with Parkinson's disease (limited documentation); monitor.
(Continued)

Clonidine *(Continued)*

Local anesthetics: Epidural clonidine may prolong the sensory and motor blockade of local anesthetics.

Mirtazapine: Antihypertensive effects of clonidine may be antagonized by mirtazapine (hypertensive urgency has been reported following addition of mirtazapine to clonidine). In addition, mirtazapine may potentially enhance the hypertensive response associated with abrupt clonidine withdrawal. Avoid this combination; consider an alternative agent.

Narcotic analgesics: May potentiate hypotensive effects of clonidine.

Tricyclic antidepressants: Antihypertensive effects of clonidine may be antagonized by tricyclic antidepressants. In addition, tricyclic antidepressants may enhance the hypertensive response associated with abrupt clonidine withdrawal; avoid this combination; consider an alternative agent.

Verapamil: Concurrent administration may be associated with hypotension and AV block in some patients (limited documentation); monitor.

Ethanol/Nutrition/Herb Interactions

Ethanol: Avoid ethanol (may increase CNS depression).

Herb/Nutraceutical: Avoid dong quai if using for hypertension (has estrogenic activity). Avoid ephedra, yohimbe, ginseng (may worsen hypertension). Avoid valerian, St John's wort, kava kava, gotu kola (may increase CNS depression).

Mechanism of Action Stimulates alpha$_2$-adrenoceptors in the brain stem, thus activating an inhibitory neuron, resulting in reduced sympathetic outflow from the CNS, producing a decrease in peripheral resistance, renal vascular resistance, heart rate, and blood pressure; epidural clonidine may produce pain relief at spinal presynaptic and postjunctional alpha$_2$-adrenoceptors by preventing pain signal transmission; pain relief occurs only for the body regions innervated by the spinal segments where analgesic concentrations of clonidine exist

Pharmacodynamics

Onset of action: Oral: 0.5-1 hour; Transdermal: Initial application: 2-3 days

Peak effect: Within 2-4 hours

Duration: 6-10 hours

Pharmacokinetics

Distribution: V_d: 2.1 L/kg

Metabolism: Hepatic to inactive metabolites; enterohepatic recirculation

Bioavailability: Oral: 75% to 95%

Half-life:

Normal renal function: 6-20 hours

Renal impairment: 18-41 hours

Elimination: 65% excreted in urine (32% unchanged and 22% excreted in feces)

Dosage

Geriatrics: Oral: Initial: 0.1 mg once daily at bedtime, increase gradually as needed.

Adults:

Acute hypertension (urgency): Oral: Initial 0.1-0.2 mg; may be followed by additional doses of 0.1 mg every hour, if necessary, to a maximum total dose of 0.6 mg

Unlabeled route of administration: Sublingual clonidine 0.1-0.2 mg twice daily may be effective in patients unable to take oral medication

Hypertension:

Oral: Initial dose: 0.1 mg twice daily (maximum recommended dose: 2.4 mg/day); usual dose range (JNC 7): 0.1-0.8 mg/day in 2 divided doses

Transdermal: Apply once every 7 days; for initial therapy start with 0.1 mg and increase by 0.1 mg at 1- to 2-week intervals (dosages >0.6 mg do not improve efficacy); usual dose range (JNC 7): 0.1-0.3 mg once weekly

Note: If transitioning from oral to transdermal, overlap oral for 1-2 days. Transdermal route takes 2-3 days to achieve therapeutic effects.

Conversion from oral to transdermal:

Day 1: Place Catapres-TTS® 1; administer 100% of oral dose.

Day 2: Administer 50% of oral dose.

Day 3: Administer 25% of oral dose.

Day 4: Patch remains, no further oral supplement necessary.

Nicotine withdrawal symptoms: 0.1 mg twice daily to maximum of 0.4 mg/day for 3-4 weeks

Pain management: Epidural infusion: Starting dose: 30 mcg/hour; titrate as required for relief of pain or presence of side effects; minimal experience with doses >40 mcg/hour; should be considered an adjunct to intraspinal opiate therapy

Renal Impairment:

Cl_{cr} <10 mL/minute: Administer 50% to 75% of normal dose initially.

Not dialyzable (0% to 5%) via hemo- or peritoneal dialysis; supplemental dose is not necessary.

Administration Catapres-TTS® comes in 2 parts - the small patch containing the drug and an overlay to keep the patch in place for 1 week. Both parts should be used for maximum efficacy. It may be useful to note on the patch which day it should be changed.

Monitoring Parameters Blood pressure, standing and sitting/supine; mental status

Reference Range Therapeutic: 1-2 ng/mL (SI: 4.4-8.7 nmol/L)

Patient Information Do not stop drug except on instruction of physician; check daily to be sure patch present; may cause drowsiness

Special Geriatric Considerations Because of its potential CNS adverse effects, clonidine may not be considered a drug of choice in the elderly. If the decision is to use clonidine, adjust dose based on response and adverse reactions.

Dosage Forms Excipient information presented when available (limited, particularly for generics); consult specific product labeling.

Injection, epidural solution, as hydrochloride [preservative free] (Duraclon™): 100 mcg/mL (10 mL); 500 mcg/mL (10 mL)

Patch, transdermal [once-weekly patch]:
Catapres-TTS®-1: 0.1 mg/24 hours (4s)
Catapres-TTS®-2: 0.2 mg/24 hours (4s)
Catapres-TTS®-3: 0.3 mg/24 hours (4s)

Tablet, as hydrochloride (Catapres®): 0.1 mg, 0.2 mg, 0.3 mg

♦ **Clonidine Hydrochloride** see Clonidine on page 342

Clopidogrel (kloh PID oh grel)

Medication Safety Issues
Sound-alike/look-alike issues:
Plavix® may be confused with Elavil®, Paxil®

U.S. Brand Names Plavix®

Canadian Brand Names Plavix®

Index Terms Clopidogrel Bisulfate

Generic Available No

Pharmacologic Category Antiplatelet Agent

Use Reduces rate of atherothrombotic events (myocardial infarction, stroke, vascular deaths) in patients with recent MI or stroke, or established peripheral arterial disease; reduces rate of atherothrombotic events in patients with unstable angina or non-ST-segment elevation acute coronary syndromes (unstable angina and non-ST-segment elevation MI) managed medically or through PCI (with or without stent) or CABG; reduces rate of death and atherothrombotic events in patients with ST-segment elevation MI (STEMI) managed medically

Unlabeled/Investigational Use In aspirin-allergic patients, prevention of coronary artery bypass graft closure (saphenous vein)

Contraindications Hypersensitivity to clopidogrel or any component of the formulation; active pathological bleeding such as PUD or intracranial hemorrhage; coagulation disorders

Warnings/Precautions Use with caution in patients who may be at risk of increased bleeding, including patients with peptic ulcer disease, trauma, or surgery. Consider discontinuing 5 days before elective surgery (except in patients with cardiac stents that have not completed their full course of dual antiplatelet therapy; AHA/ACC/SCAI/ACS/ADA Science Advisory provides recommendations). Use caution in concurrent treatment with other antiplatelet drugs; bleeding risk is increased. Use with caution in patients with severe liver or renal disease (experience is limited). Cases of thrombotic thrombocytopenic purpura (usually occurring within the first 2 weeks of therapy) have been reported; urgent plasmapheresis is required.

Adverse Reactions (Reflective of adult population; not specific for elderly) As with all drugs which may affect hemostasis, bleeding is associated with clopidogrel. Hemorrhage may occur at virtually any site. Risk is dependent on multiple variables, including the concurrent use of multiple agents which alter hemostasis and patient susceptibility.

>10%: Gastrointestinal: The overall incidence of gastrointestinal events (including abdominal pain, vomiting, dyspepsia, gastritis and constipation) has been documented to be 27% compared to 30% in patients receiving aspirin.

3% to 10%:
Cardiovascular: Chest pain (8%), edema (4%), hypertension (4%)
Central nervous system: Headache (3% to 8%), dizziness (2% to 6%), depression (4%), fatigue (3%), general pain (6%)
Dermatologic: Rash (4%), pruritus (3%)
Endocrine & metabolic: Hypercholesterolemia (4%)
Gastrointestinal: Abdominal pain (2% to 6%), dyspepsia (2% to 5%), diarrhea (2% to 5%), nausea (3%)
Genitourinary: Urinary tract infection (3%)
Hematologic: Bleeding (major 4%; minor 5%), purpura (5%), epistaxis (3%)
Hepatic: Liver function test abnormalities (<3%; discontinued in 0.11%)

(Continued)

Clopidogrel *(Continued)*

Neuromuscular & skeletal: Arthralgia (6%), back pain (6%)

Respiratory: Dyspnea (5%), rhinitis (4%), bronchitis (4%), cough (3%), upper respiratory infection (9%)

Miscellaneous: Flu-like syndrome (8%)

1% to 3%:

Cardiovascular: Atrial fibrillation, cardiac failure, palpitation, syncope

Central nervous system: Fever, insomnia, vertigo, anxiety

Dermatologic: Eczema

Endocrine & metabolic: Gout, hyperuricemia

Gastrointestinal: Constipation, GI hemorrhage, vomiting

Genitourinary: Cystitis

Hematologic: Hematoma, anemia

Neuromuscular & skeletal: Arthritis, leg cramps, neuralgia, paresthesia, weakness

Ocular: Cataract, conjunctivitis

Overdosage/Toxicology Symptoms of acute toxicity include vomiting, prostration, difficulty breathing, and gastrointestinal hemorrhage. Only one case of overdose with clopidogrel has been reported to date; no symptoms were reported with this case and no specific treatments were required. Based on its pharmacology, platelet transfusions may be an appropriate treatment when attempting to reverse the effects of clopidogrel. After decontamination, treatment is symptomatic and supportive.

Drug Interactions Substrate (minor) of CYP1A2, 3A4; **Inhibits** CYP2C9 (weak)

Anticoagulants: May increase the risk of bleeding. Anticoagulant interacting members include antithrombin III, argatroban, bivalirudin, dalteparin, danaparoid, drotrecogin alfa, enoxaparin, fondaparinux, heparin, hirudin, lepirudin, nadroparin, tinzaparin, and warfarin. Use with heparin in acute coronary syndrome is clinically accepted.

Antiplatelet agents: May enhance the anticoagulant effect of other antiplatelet agents. Antiplatelet agent interacting members include abciximab, anagrelide, cilostazol, dipyridamole, eptifibatide, ticlopidine, and tirofiban.

Atorvastatin: Atorvastatin may attenuate the effects of clopidogrel; monitor.

Drotrecogin alfa: May increase the risk of bleeding.

Macrolide antibiotics: CYP3A4-inhibiting macrolides may attenuate the effects of clopidogrel. These include clarithromycin, erythromycin, and troleandomycin. Monitor.

NSAIDs: Concurrent use with clopidogrel may increase gastrointestinal effects, including GI blood loss. NSAID use was excluded in ACS trial (CURE).

Rifampin: Rifampin may increase the effects of clopidogrel; monitor.

Salicylates: Antiplatelet agents may enhance the adverse/toxic effect of salicylates; increased risk of bleeding may result. Though combined therapy is at times used advantageously, an increased risk of bleeding must be acknowledged and managed.

Thrombolytics: May increase the risk of bleeding.

Treprostinil: May enhance the adverse/toxic effect of antiplatelet agents. Bleeding may occur.

Ethanol/Nutrition/Herb Interactions Herb/Nutraceutical: Avoid cat's claw, dong quai, evening primrose, feverfew, garlic, ginger, ginkgo, red clover, horse chestnut, green tea, ginseng (all have additional antiplatelet activity).

Stability Store at 25°C (77°F); excursions permitted to 15°C to 3°C (59°F to 86°F).

Mechanism of Action Blocks the ADP receptors, which prevent fibrinogen binding at that site and thereby reduce the possibility of platelet adhesion and aggregation

Pharmacodynamics

Onset of action: Inhibition of platelet aggregation detected: 2 hours after 300 mg administered; after second day of treatment with 50-100 mg/day

Peak effect: 50-100 mg/day: Bleeding time: 5-6 days; Platelet function: 3-7 days

Pharmacokinetics

Absorption: Well absorbed

Metabolism: Hepatic to active metabolite

Half-life: 7-8 hours (active metabolite)

Time to peak, serum: ~1 hour

Excretion: Urine (50%); feces (46%)

Dosage

Geriatrics & Adults:

Recent MI, recent stroke, or established arterial disease: Oral: 75 mg once daily

Non-ST-segment elevation acute coronary syndrome: Initial: 300 mg loading dose, followed by 75 mg once daily (in combination with aspirin 75-325 mg once daily). **Note:** A loading dose of 600 mg has been used in some investigations; limited research exists comparing the two doses.

Note: Drug-eluting stents: Duration of clopidogrel (in combination with aspirin): Ideally 12 months following drug-eluting stent placement in patients not at high risk for bleeding; at a minimum, 1-, 3-, and 6 months for bare metal, sirolimus, and paclitaxel stents, respectively, for uninterrupted therapy.

ST-segment elevation MI: 75 mg once daily (in combination with aspirin 75-162 mg/day). CLARITY used a 300 mg loading dose of clopidogrel. The duration of therapy was <28 days (usually until hospital discharge).

Renal Impairment: No adjustment is necessary.

Hepatic Impairment: Dose adjustment may be necessary for patients with moderate-to-severe hepatic disease.

Monitoring Parameters Signs of bleeding; hemoglobin and hematocrit periodically

Patient Information May be taken with food; notify physician if bleeding or bruising occurs

Special Geriatric Considerations Because of the risk of neutropenia and its relative expense as compared with aspirin, clopidogrel should only be used in patients with a documented intolerance to aspirin. Plasma concentrations of main metabolite of clopidogrel were significantly higher in the elderly (≥75 years). This was not associated with changes in bleeding time or platelet aggregation. No dosage adjustment is recommended.

Dosage Forms Excipient information presented when available (limited, particularly for generics); consult specific product labeling.
Tablet:
Plavix®: 75 mg

Selected References
Bal dit Sollier C, Mahe I, Berge N, et al, "Reduced Thrombus Cohesion in an *ex vivo* Human Model of Arterial Thrombosis Induced by Clopidogrel Treatment: Kinetics of the Effect and Influence of Single and Double Loading-Dose Regimens," *Thromb Res*, 2003, 111(1-2):19-27.
Kastrati A, Mehilli J, Schuhlen H, et al, "A Clinical Trial of Abciximab in Elective Percutaneous Coronary Intervention After Pretreatment With Clopidogrel," *N Engl J Med*, 2004, 350(3):232-8.
Lange RA and Hillis LD, "Antiplatelet Therapy for Ischemic Heart Disease," *N Engl J Med*, 2004, 350(3):277-80.

♦ **Clopidogrel Bisulfate** *see* Clopidogrel *on page 345*

Clorazepate (klor AZ e pate)

Related Information
Anxiolytic, Sedative / Hypnotic, and Miscellaneous Benzodiazepines *on page 1750*

Medication Safety Issues
Sound-alike/look-alike issues:
Clorazepate may be confused with clofibrate, clonazepam

U.S. Brand Names Tranxene® SD™; Tranxene® SD™-Half Strength; Tranxene® T-Tab®

Canadian Brand Names Apo-Clorazepate®; Novo-Clopate

Index Terms Clorazepate Dipotassium; Tranxene T-Tab®

Generic Available Yes

Pharmacologic Category Benzodiazepine

Use Treatment of generalized anxiety and panic disorders; management of alcohol withdrawal; adjunct anticonvulsant in management of partial seizures

Restrictions C-IV

Contraindications Hypersensitivity to clorazepate or any component of the formulation (cross-sensitivity with other benzodiazepines may exist); narrow-angle glaucoma

Warnings/Precautions Not recommended for use in patients with depressive or psychotic disorders. Use with caution in elderly or debilitated patients, patients with hepatic disease (including alcoholics), or renal impairment. Active metabolites with extended half-lives may lead to delayed accumulation and adverse effects. Use with caution in patients with respiratory disease or impaired gag reflex. Avoid use in patients with sleep apnea.

Causes CNS depression (dose related) resulting in sedation, dizziness, confusion, or ataxia which may impair physical and mental capabilities. Patients must be cautioned about performing tasks which require mental alertness (eg, operating machinery or driving). Use with caution in patients receiving other CNS depressants or psychoactive agents. Effects with other sedative drugs or ethanol may be potentiated. Benzodiazepines have been associated with falls and traumatic injury and should be used with extreme caution in patients who are at risk of these events (especially the elderly).

Use caution in patients with depression, particularly if suicidal risk may be present. Use with caution in patients with a history of drug dependence. Benzodiazepines have been associated with dependence and acute withdrawal symptoms on discontinuation or reduction in dose. Acute withdrawal, including seizures, may be precipitated in patients after administration of flumazenil to patients receiving long-term benzodiazepine therapy.

Benzodiazepines have been associated with anterograde amnesia. Paradoxical reactions, including hyperactive or aggressive behavior, have been reported with benzodiazepines, particularly in psychiatric patients. Does not have analgesic, antidepressant, or antipsychotic properties.
(Continued)

Clorazepate *(Continued)*

Adverse Reactions (Reflective of adult population; not specific for elderly)
Frequency not defined.
Cardiovascular: Hypotension
Central nervous system: Drowsiness, fatigue, ataxia, lightheadedness, memory impairment, insomnia, anxiety, headache, depression, slurred speech, confusion, nervousness, dizziness, irritability
Dermatologic: Rash
Endocrine & metabolic: Libido decreased
Gastrointestinal: Xerostomia, constipation, diarrhea, nausea, salivation decreased, vomiting, appetite increased or decreased
Neuromuscular & skeletal: Dysarthria, tremor
Ocular: Blurred vision, diplopia

Overdosage/Toxicology May produce somnolence, confusion, ataxia, diminished reflexes, and coma. Treatment for benzodiazepine overdose is supportive. Mechanical ventilation is rarely required. Flumazenil has been shown to selectively block the binding of benzodiazepines to CNS receptors, resulting in a reversal of benzodiazepine-induced CNS depression, but not respiratory depression.

Drug Interactions Substrate of CYP3A4 (major)
CNS depressants: Sedative effects and/or respiratory depression may be additive with CNS depressants; includes ethanol, barbiturates, opioid analgesics, and other sedative agents; monitor for increased effect.
CYP3A4 inducers: CYP3A4 inducers may decrease the levels/effects of clorazepate. Example inducers include aminoglutethimide, carbamazepine, nafcillin, nevirapine, phenobarbital, phenytoin, and rifamycins.
CYP3A4 inhibitors: May increase the levels/effects of clorazepate. Example inhibitors include azole antifungals, clarithromycin, diclofenac, doxycycline, erythromycin, imatinib, isoniazid, nefazodone, nicardipine, propofol, protease inhibitors, quinidine, telithromycin, and verapamil.
Levodopa: Therapeutic effects may be diminished in some patients following the addition of a benzodiazepine; limited/inconsistent data.
Oral contraceptives: May decrease the clearance of some benzodiazepines (those which undergo oxidative metabolism); monitor for increased benzodiazepine effect.
Theophylline: May partially antagonize some of the effects of benzodiazepines; monitor for decreased response; may require higher doses for sedation.

Ethanol/Nutrition/Herb Interactions
Ethanol: Avoid ethanol (may increase CNS depression).
Food: Serum concentrations/toxicity may be increased by grapefruit juice.
Herb/Nutraceutical: Avoid valerian, St John's wort, kava kava, gotu kola (may increase CNS depression).

Mechanism of Action Binds to stereospecific benzodiazepine receptors on the postsynaptic GABA neuron at several sites within the central nervous system, including the limbic system, reticular formation. Enhancement of the inhibitory effect of GABA on neuronal excitability results by increased neuronal membrane permeability to chloride ions. This shift in chloride ions results in hyperpolarization (a less excitable state) and stabilization.

Pharmacodynamics Studies have shown that older adults are more sensitive to the effects of benzodiazepines as compared to younger adults.

Pharmacokinetics
Absorption: Rapidly decarboxylated to desmethyldiazepam (active) in acidic stomach prior to absorption
Metabolism: In the liver to oxazepam (active)
Half-life: Adults:
Desmethyldiazepam: 48-96 hours
Oxazepam: 6-8 hours
Time to peak serum concentration: Oral: Within 1 hour
Elimination: Metabolites excreted primarily in urine

Dosage
Geriatrics: Oral: Anxiety: 7.5 mg 1-2 times/day; use is not recommended in the elderly.
Adults:
Anxiety:
Regular release tablets (Tranxene® T-Tab®): 7.5-15 mg 2-4 times/day
Sustained release (Tranxene® SD): 11.25 or 22.5 mg once daily at bedtime
Ethanol withdrawal: Oral: Initial: 30 mg, then 15 mg 2-4 times/day on first day; maximum daily dose: 90 mg; gradually decrease dose over subsequent days.
Seizures (anticonvulsant): Oral: Initial: Up to 7.5 mg/dose 2-3 times/day; increase dose by 7.5 mg at weekly intervals; not to exceed 90 mg/day

Monitoring Parameters Respiratory, cardiovascular, and mental status
Reference Range Therapeutic: 0.12-1 mcg/mL (SI: 0.36-3.01 μmol/L)
Test Interactions Decreased hematocrit; abnormal liver and renal function tests

Patient Information Avoid alcohol and other CNS depressants; may cause drowsiness; avoid activities needing good psychomotor coordination until CNS effects are known; may cause physical or psychological dependence; avoid abrupt discontinuation after prolonged use

Additional Information Clorazepate offers no advantage over the other benzodiazepines

Special Geriatric Considerations Due to its long-acting metabolite, clorazepate is not considered a drug of choice in the elderly. Long-acting benzodiazepines have been associated with falls in the elderly. Interpretive guidelines from the Centers for Medicare and Medicaid Services (CMS) discourage the use of this agent in residents of long-term care facilities.

Dosage Forms Excipient information presented when available (limited, particularly for generics); consult specific product labeling.
Tablet, as dipotassium: 3.75 mg, 7.5 mg, 15 mg
  Tranxene® SD™: 22.5 mg [once daily]
  Tranxene® SD™-Half Strength: 11.25 mg [once daily]
  Tranxene® T-Tab®: 3.75 mg, 7.5 mg, 15 mg

♦ **Clorazepate Dipotassium** *see* Clorazepate *on page 347*

Clotrimazole (kloe TRIM a zole)

Medication Safety Issues
Sound-alike/look-alike issues:
  Clotrimazole may be confused with co-trimoxazole
  Lotrimin® may be confused with Lotrisone®, Otrivin®
  Mycelex® may be confused with Myoflex®

International issues:
  Cloderm®: Brand name for clocortolone in the United States
  Canesten® [multiple international markets] may be confused with Cenestin® which is a brand name for estrogens (conjugated a/synthetic) in the U.S.
  Canesten® [multiple international markets]: Brand name for fluconazole in Great Britain
  Mycelex® may be confused with Mucolex® which is a brand name for carbocysteine in Ireland, Portugal, and Thailand; a brand name for guaifenesin in Hong Kong

U.S. Brand Names Cruex® Cream [OTC]; Gyne-Lotrimin® 3 [OTC]; Lotrimin® AF Athlete's Foot Cream [OTC]; Lotrimin® AF Athlete's Foot Solution [OTC]; Lotrimin® AF Jock Itch Cream [OTC]; Mycelex®; Mycelex®-7 [OTC]; Mycelex® Twin Pack [OTC]

Canadian Brand Names Canesten® Topical; Canesten® Vaginal; Clotrimaderm; Trivagizole-3®

Generic Available Yes: Cream, solution, troche

Pharmacologic Category Antifungal Agent, Oral Nonabsorbed; Antifungal Agent, Topical; Antifungal Agent, Vaginal

Use Treatment of susceptible fungal infections, including oropharyngeal candidiasis, dermatophytoses, superficial mycoses, and cutaneous candidiasis, as well as vulvovaginal candidiasis; limited data suggest that the use of clotrimazole troches may be effective for prophylaxis against oropharyngeal candidiasis in neutropenic patients

Contraindications Hypersensitivity to clotrimazole or any component of the formulation

Warnings/Precautions Clotrimazole should not be used for treatment of systemic fungal infection. When using topical formulation, avoid contact with eyes.

Adverse Reactions (Reflective of adult population; not specific for elderly)
Oral:
  >10%: Hepatic: Abnormal liver function tests
  1% to 10%:
    Gastrointestinal: Nausea and vomiting may occur in patients on clotrimazole troches
    Local: Mild burning, irritation, stinging to skin or vaginal area
Vaginal:
  1% to 10%: Genitourinary: Vulvar/vaginal burning

Drug Interactions Inhibits CYP1A2 (weak), 2A6 (weak), 2B6 (weak), 2C8 (weak), 2C9 (weak), 2C19 (weak), 2D6 (weak), 2E1 (weak), 3A4 (moderate)
  CYP3A4 substrates: Clotrimazole may increase the levels/effects of CYP3A4 substrates. Example substrates include benzodiazepines, calcium channel blockers, cyclosporine, mirtazapine, nateglinide, nefazodone, sildenafil (and other PDE-5 inhibitors), tacrolimus, and venlafaxine. Selected benzodiazepines (midazolam and triazolam), cisapride, ergot alkaloids, selected HMG-CoA reductase inhibitors (lovastatin and simvastatin), and pimozide are generally contraindicated with strong CYP3A4 inhibitors.

Mechanism of Action Binds to phospholipids in the fungal cell membrane altering cell wall permeability resulting in loss of essential intracellular elements
(Continued)

Clotrimazole *(Continued)*

Pharmacokinetics

Absorption: Negligible: Through intact skin when administered topically; following oral topical administration, salivary concentrations occur within 3 hours following 30 minutes of dissolution time in the mouth; high vaginal concentrations occur following vaginal cream administration within 8-24 hours and within 1-2 days following vaginal tablet administration

Metabolism: Hepatic

Elimination: As metabolites via bile

Dosage

Geriatrics & Adults:

Oropharyngeal candidiasis: Oral:

Prophylaxis: 10 mg troche dissolved 3 times/day for the duration of chemotherapy or until steroids are reduced to maintenance levels

Treatment: 10 mg troche dissolved slowly 5 times/day for 14 consecutive days

Dermatophytosis, cutaneous candidiasis: Topical (cream, solution): Apply twice daily; if no improvement occurs after 4 weeks of therapy, re-evaluate diagnosis.

Vulvovaginal candidiasis: Intravaginal:

Cream (1%): Insert 1 applicatorful of 1% vaginal cream daily (preferably at bedtime) for 7 consecutive days.

Cream (2%): Insert 1 applicatorful of 2% vaginal cream daily (preferably at bedtime) for 3 consecutive days.

Tablet: Insert 100 mg/day for 7 days or 500 mg single dose.

Dermatologic infection (superficial): Topical (cream, solution): Apply to affected area twice daily (morning and evening) for 7 consecutive days.

Administration

Oral: Allow to dissolve slowly over 15-30 minutes.

Topical: Avoid contact with eyes. For external use only. Apply sparingly. Protect hands with latex gloves. Do not use occlusive dressings.

Monitoring Parameters Periodic liver function tests during oral therapy with clotrimazole lozenges

Patient Information

Oral: Do not swallow oral medication whole; allow to dissolve slowly in mouth. You may experience nausea or vomiting (small frequent meals, frequent mouth care, chewing gum, or sucking lozenges may help). Report signs of opportunistic infection (eg, white plaques in mouth, fever, chills, perianal itching or vaginal discharge, fatigue, unhealed wounds or sores).

Topical: Avoid contact with eyes. Wash hands before applying or wear gloves. Apply thin film of gel, lotion, or solution to affected area. May apply porous dressing. Report persistent burning, swelling, itching, worsening of condition, or lack of response to therapy.

Vaginal: Wash hands before using. Insert full applicator into vagina gently and expel cream, or insert tablet into vagina, at bedtime. Wash applicator with soap and water following use. Remain lying down for 30 minutes following administration. Avoid intercourse during therapy (sexual partner may experience penile burning or itching). Report adverse reactions (eg, vulvar itching, frequent urination, worsening of condition, or lack of response to therapy. Contact prescriber if symptoms do not improve within 3 days or you do not feel well within 7 days. Do not use tampons until therapy is complete. Contact prescriber immediately if you experience abdominal pain, fever, or foul-smelling discharge.

Special Geriatric Considerations Localized fungal infections frequently follow broad-spectrum antimicrobial therapy. Specifically, oral and vaginal infections due to *Candida.*

Dosage Forms Excipient information presented when available (limited, particularly for generics); consult specific product labeling.

Combination pack (Mycelex®-7): Vaginal tablet 100 mg (7s) and vaginal cream 1% (7 g)

Cream, topical: 1% (15 g, 30 g, 45 g)

Cruex®: 1% (15 g)

Lotrimin® AF Athlete's Foot: 1% (12 g, 24 g)

Lotrimin® AF Jock Itch: 1% (12 g)

Cream, vaginal: 2% (21 g)

Mycelex®-7: 1% (45 g)

Solution, topical: 1% (10 mL, 30 mL)

Lotrimin® AF Athlete's Foot: 1% (10 mL)

Tablet, vaginal (Gyne-Lotrimin® 3): 200 mg (3s)

Troche (Mycelex®): 10 mg

Cloxacillin (kloks a SIL in)

Related Information
Antimicrobial Activity Against Selected Organisms *on page 1728*
Canadian Brand Names Apo-Cloxi®; Novo-Cloxin; Nu-Cloxi; Riva-Cloxacillin
Index Terms Cloxacillin Sodium
Generic Available Yes
Pharmacologic Category Antibiotic, Penicillin
Use Treatment of susceptible bacterial infections, notably penicillinase-producing staphylococci (not methicillin-resistant) causing respiratory tract, skin and skin structure, bone and joint, urinary tract infections, endocarditis, septicemia, and meningitis
Restrictions Not available in U.S.
Contraindications Hypersensitivity to cloxacillin, any component of the formulation, or penicillins
Warnings/Precautions Monitor PT if patient is concurrently on warfarin. Elimination of drug is slow in renally impaired. Serious and occasionally severe or fatal hypersensitivity (anaphylactoid) reactions have been reported in patients on penicillin therapy, especially with a history of beta-lactam hypersensitivity, history of sensitivity to multiple allergens, or previous IgE-mediated reactions (eg, anaphylaxis, angioedema, urticaria). Use with caution in asthmatic patients. Prolonged use may result in fungal or bacterial superinfection, including *C. difficile*-associated diarrhea and pseudomembranous colitis.
Adverse Reactions (Reflective of adult population; not specific for elderly)
1% to 10%: Gastrointestinal: Nausea, diarrhea, abdominal pain, oral candidiasis
Overdosage/Toxicology Symptoms of penicillin overdose include neuromuscular hypersensitivity (agitation, hallucinations, asterixis, encephalopathy, confusion, and seizures) and electrolyte imbalance (with potassium or sodium salts), especially in renal failure. Hemodialysis may be helpful to aid in the removal of the drug from the blood, otherwise, most treatment is supportive or symptom-directed.
Drug Interactions
Fusidic acid: May decrease the therapeutic effect of penicillins; administer the penicillin at least 2 hours before fusidic acid.
Methotrexate: Penicillins may increase the exposure to methotrexate during concurrent therapy; monitor.
Oral contraceptives: Anecdotal reports suggesting decreased contraceptive efficacy with penicillins have been refuted by more rigorous scientific and clinical data.
Probenecid, disulfiram: May increase levels of penicillins (cloxacillin).
Warfarin: Effects of warfarin may be increased.
Stability Refrigerate oral solution after reconstitution; discard after 14 days. Stable for 3 days at room temperature.
Mechanism of Action Inhibits bacterial cell wall synthesis by binding to one or more of the penicillin-binding proteins (PBPs) which in turn inhibits the final transpeptidation step of peptidoglycan synthesis in bacterial cell walls, thus inhibiting cell wall biosynthesis. Bacteria eventually lyse due to ongoing activity of cell wall autolytic enzymes (autolysins and murein hydrolases) while cell wall assembly is arrested.
Pharmacokinetics
Absorption: Oral: ~50%
Protein binding: 90% to 98%
Metabolism: Significant in the liver to active and inactive metabolites
Half-life: 30-90 minutes (prolonged with renal impairment); reported to be longer in older adults, but is not considered clinically significant
Time to peak serum concentration: Oral: Within 0.5-2 hours
Elimination: In urine and through bile
Dosage
Geriatrics & Adults: Susceptible infections: Oral: 250-500 mg every 6 hours
Renal Impairment: Hemodialysis: Not dialyzable (0% to 5%)
Monitoring Parameters Signs and symptoms of infection; mental status, WBC; PT for patients on warfarin
Test Interactions May interfere with urinary glucose tests using cupric sulfate (Benedict's solution, Clinitest®); may inactivate aminoglycosides *in vitro*; false-positive urine and serum proteins; false-positive in uric acid, urinary steroids
Patient Information Complete full course of therapy; contact your physician or pharmacist if not improving or diarrhea develops
Special Geriatric Considerations Dosage change for renal function is not necessary.
Dosage Forms Excipient information presented when available (limited, particularly for generics); consult specific product labeling.
Capsule, as sodium: 250 mg, 500 mg
Powder for oral suspension, as sodium: 125 mg/5 mL (100 mL, 200 mL)
(Continued)

Cloxacillin *(Continued)*

Selected References
Bluhm G, Jacobson B, Julander I, et al, "Antibiotic Prophylaxis in Pacemaker Surgery - A Prospective Study," *Scand J Thorac Cardiovasc Surg,* 1984, 18(3):227-34.

♦ **Cloxacillin Sodium** *see* Cloxacillin *on page 351*

Clozapine *(KLOE za peen)*

Related Information
Antipsychotic Agents *on page 1747*
Atypical Antipsychotics *on page 1749*

Medication Safety Issues
Sound-alike/look-alike issues:
Clozapine may be confused with clofazimine, clonidine, Klonopin®
Clozaril® may be confused with Clinoril®, Colazal®

U.S. Brand Names Clozaril®; FazaClo®

Canadian Brand Names Apo-Clozapine®; Clozaril®; Gen-Clozapine

Generic Available Yes

Pharmacologic Category Antipsychotic Agent, Atypical

Use Treatment-refractory schizophrenia; to reduce risk of recurrent suicidal behavior in schizophrenia or schizoaffective disorder

Unlabeled/Investigational Use Treatment of schizoaffective disorder, bipolar disorder, severe obsessive-compulsive disorder

Restrictions Patient-specific registration is required to dispense clozapine. Monitoring systems for individual clozapine manufacturers are independent. If a patient is switched from one brand/manufacturer of clozapine to another, the patient must be entered into a new registry (must be completed by the prescriber and delivered to the dispensing pharmacy). Healthcare providers, including pharmacists dispensing clozapine, should verify the patient's hematological status and qualification to receive clozapine with all existing registries. The manufacturer of Clozaril® requests that healthcare providers submit all WBC/ANC values following discontinuation of therapy to the Clozaril National Registry for all nonrechallengable patients until WBC is ≥3500/mm³ and ANC is ≥2000/mm³.

Contraindications Hypersensitivity to clozapine or any component of the formulation; history of agranulocytosis or granulocytopenia with clozapine; uncontrolled epilepsy; severe central nervous system depression or comatose state; paralytic ileus; myeloproliferative disorders or use with other agents which have a well-known risk of agranulocytosis or bone marrow suppression

In patients with WBC ≤3500 cells/mm³ before therapy; if WBC falls to <3000 cells/mm³ during therapy the drug should be withheld until signs and symptoms of infection disappear and WBC rises to >3000 cells/mm³

Warnings/Precautions [U.S. Boxed Warning]: Patients with dementia-related psychosis treated with atypical antipsychotics are at an increased risk of death compared to placebo. An increased incidence of cerebrovascular adverse events (including fatalities) has been reported in elderly patients with dementia-related psychosis. Risk may be increased by dehydration; use caution with concurrent diuretics. Clozapine is not approved for this indication.

[U.S. Boxed Warning]: Significant risk of agranulocytosis, potentially life-threatening. Therapy should not be initiated in patients with WBC <3500 cells/mm³ or ANC <2000 cells/mm³ or history of myeloproliferative disorder. WBC testing should occur periodically on an on-going basis (see prescribing information for monitoring details) to ensure that acceptable WBC/ANC counts are maintained. Initial episodes of moderate leukopenia or granulopoietic suppression confer up to a 12-fold increased risk for subsequent episodes of agranulocytosis. WBCs must be monitored weekly for at least 4 weeks after therapy discontinuation or until WBC is ≥3500/mm³ and ANC is ≥2000/mm³. Use with caution in patients receiving other marrow suppressive agents. Eosinophilia has been reported to occur with clozapine and may require temporary or permanent interruption of therapy. Due to the significant risk of agranulocytosis, it is strongly recommended that a patient must fail at least two trials of other primary medications for the treatment of schizophrenia (of adequate dose and duration) before initiating therapy with clozapine.

Cognitive and/or motor impairment (sedation) is common with clozapine, resulting in impaired performance of tasks requiring alertness (eg, operating machinery or driving); use caution in patients receiving general anesthesia. **[U.S. Boxed Warning]: Seizures have been associated with clozapine use in a dose-dependent manner;** use with caution in patients at risk of seizures, including those with a history of seizures, head trauma, brain damage, alcoholism, or concurrent therapy with medications which may lower seizure threshold. Has been associated with benign, self-limiting fever (<100.4°F, usually within first 3 weeks). However, clozapine may also be associated with severe febrile reactions, including neuroleptic malignant syndrome (NMS). Clozapine's potential for extrapyramidal symptoms (including tardive dyskinesia) appears to be extremely low.

Deep vein thrombosis, myocarditis, pericarditis, pericardial effusion, cardiomyopathy, and CHF have also been associated with clozapine. **[U.S. Boxed Warning]: Fatalities due to myocarditis have been reported; highest risk in the first month of therapy, however, later cases also reported.** Clozapine should be discontinued in patients with confirmed cardiomyopathy unless benefit clearly outweighs risk. Rare cases of thromboembolism, including pulmonary embolism and stroke resulting in fatalities, have been associated with clozapine.

May cause anticholinergic effects; use with caution in patients with urinary retention, benign prostatic hyperplasia, narrow-angle glaucoma, xerostomia, visual problems, constipation, or history of bowel obstruction. May cause hyperglycemia; in some cases may be extreme and associated with ketoacidosis, hyperosmolar coma, or death. Use with caution in patients with diabetes or other disorders of glucose regulation; monitor for worsening of glucose control. Use with caution in patients with hepatic disease or impairment; hepatitis has been reported as a consequence of therapy.

Use caution with cardiovascular or renal disease. **[U.S. Boxed Warning]: May cause orthostatic hypotension (with or without syncope)** and tachycardia; use with caution in patients at risk of hypotension or in patients where transient hypotensive episodes would be poorly tolerated (cardiovascular disease or cerebrovascular disease). Concurrent use with benzodiazepines may increase the risk of severe cardiopulmonary reactions.

The possibility of a suicide attempt is inherent in psychotic illness or bipolar disorder; use caution in high-risk patients during initiation of therapy. Prescriptions should be written for the smallest quantity consistent with good patient care.

Medication should not be stopped abruptly; taper off over 1-2 weeks. If conditions warrant abrupt discontinuation (leukopenia, myocarditis, cardiomyopathy), monitor patient for psychosis and cholinergic rebound (headache, nausea, vomiting, diarrhea). Significant weight gain has been observed with antipsychotic therapy; incidence varies with product. Monitor waist circumference and BMI. Elderly patients are more susceptible to adverse effects (including agranulocytosis, cardiovascular, anticholinergic, and tardive dyskinesia).

Adverse Reactions (Reflective of adult population; not specific for elderly)
>10%:
Cardiovascular: Tachycardia (25%)
Central nervous system: Drowsiness (39% to 46%), dizziness (19% to 27%), insomnia (2% to 20%)
Gastrointestinal: Constipation (14% to 25%), weight gain (4% to 31%), sialorrhea (31% to 48%), nausea/vomiting (3% to 17%)
1% to 10%:
Cardiovascular: Angina (1%), ECG changes (1%), hypertension (4%), hypotension (9%), syncope (6%)
Central nervous system: Akathisia (3%), seizure (3%), headache (7%), nightmares (4%), akinesia (4%), confusion (3%), myoclonic jerks (1%), restlessness (4%), agitation (4%), lethargy (1%), ataxia (1%), slurred speech (1%), depression (1%), anxiety (1%)
Dermatologic: Rash (2%)
Gastrointestinal: Abdominal discomfort/heartburn (4% to 14%), anorexia (1%), diarrhea (2%), xerostomia (6%), throat discomfort (1%)
Genitourinary: Urinary abnormalities (eg, abnormal ejaculation, retention, urgency, incontinence; 1% to 2%)
Hematologic: Eosinophilia (1%), leukopenia, leukocytosis, agranulocytosis (1%)
Hepatic: Liver function tests abnormal (1%)
Neuromuscular & skeletal: Tremor (6%), hypokinesia (4%), rigidity (3%), hyperkinesia (1%), weakness (1%), pain (1%), spasm (1%)
Ocular: Visual disturbances (5%)
Respiratory: Dyspnea (1%), nasal congestion (1%)
Miscellaneous: Diaphoresis increased, fever, tongue numbness (1%)

Overdosage/Toxicology Symptoms include altered states of consciousness, tachycardia, hypotension, hypersalivation, and respiratory depression. Following initiation of essential overdose management, toxic symptom treatment and supportive treatment should be initiated. Hypotension usually responds to I.V. fluids or Trendelenburg positioning. If unresponsive to these measures, the use of a parenteral inotrope may be required. Seizures commonly respond to diazepam (I.V. 5-10 mg bolus every 15 minutes, if needed, up to a total of 30 mg), or to phenytoin or phenobarbital. Critical cardiac arrhythmias often respond to I.V. phenytoin (15 mg/kg up to 1 g), while other antiarrhythmics can be used. Neuroleptics often cause extrapyramidal symptoms (eg, (Continued)

Clozapine *(Continued)*

dystonic reactions) requiring management with anticholinergic agents such as benztropine mesylate I.V. 1-2 mg may be effective. These agents are generally effective within 2-5 minutes.

Drug Interactions Substrate of CYP1A2 (major), 2A6 (minor), 2C9 (minor), 2C19 (minor), 2D6 (minor), 3A4 (minor); **Inhibits** CYP1A2 (weak), 2C9 (weak), 2C19 (weak), 2D6 (moderate), 2E1 (weak), 3A4 (weak)

Acetylcholinesterase inhibitors (central): May increase the risk of antipsychotic-related extrapyramidal symptoms; monitor.

Anticholinergics: Clozapine has potent anticholinergic effects. May potentiate the effects of anticholinergic agents.

Antihypertensives: Clozapine may potentiate the hypotensive effects of antihypertensive agents.

Benzodiazepines: In combination with clozapine, may produce respiratory depression and hypotension, especially during the first few weeks of therapy; monitor for altered response.

Carbamazepine: A case of neuroleptic malignant syndrome has been reported in combination with clozapine; in addition, carbamazepine may alter clozapine levels (see enzyme inducers); monitor.

Citalopram: May increase the levels/effects of clozapine; monitor.

CNS depressants: Sedative effects may be additive with other CNS depressants; includes ethanol, barbiturates, benzodiazepines, opioid analgesics, and other sedatives.

CYP1A2 inducers: May decrease the levels/effects of clozapine. Example inducers include aminoglutethimide, carbamazepine, phenobarbital, and rifampin.

CYP1A2 inhibitors: May increase the levels/effects of clozapine. Example inhibitors include ciprofloxacin, fluvoxamine, ketoconazole, norfloxacin, ofloxacin, and rofecoxib.

CYP2D6 substrates: Clozapine may increase the levels/effects of CYP2D6 substrates. Example substrates include amphetamines, selected beta-blockers, dextromethorphan, fluoxetine, lidocaine, mirtazapine, nefazodone, paroxetine, risperidone, ritonavir, thioridazine, tricyclic antidepressants, and venlafaxine.

CYP2D6 prodrug substrates: Clozapine may decrease the levels/effects of CYP2D6 prodrug substrates. Example prodrug substrates include codeine, hydrocodone, oxycodone, and tramadol.

Epinephrine: Clozapine may reverse the pressor effect of epinephrine; use should be avoided in the treatment of drug-induced hypotension.

Metoclopramide: May increase extrapyramidal symptoms (EPS) or risk.

Omeprazole: May alter the concentrations/effects of clozapine; monitor.

Risperidone: Effects and/or toxicity may be increased when combined with clozapine; monitor.

Valproic acid: May cause reductions in clozapine concentrations; monitor for altered response.

Ethanol/Nutrition/Herb Interactions

Ethanol: Avoid ethanol (may increase CNS depression).

Herb/Nutraceutical: St John's wort may decrease clozapine levels. Avoid kava kava, gotu kola, valerian, St John's wort (may increase CNS depression).

Stability Dispensed in "clozapine patient system" packaging. Store at controlled room temperature. FazaClo™: Protect from moisture; do not remove from package until ready to use.

Mechanism of Action Clozapine (dibenzodiazepine antipsychotic) exhibits weak antagonism of D_1, D_2, D_3, and D_5 dopamine receptor subtypes, but shows high affinity for D_4; in addition, it blocks the serotonin ($5HT_2$), alpha-adrenergic, histamine H_1, and cholinergic receptors

Pharmacokinetics

Absorption: Well absorbed

Protein binding: 97% bound to serum proteins

Metabolism: Extensively hepatic; forms metabolites with limited or no activity

Bioavailability: Food does not appear to affect bioavailability

Half-life, elimination: Steady state: 12 hours (range: 4-66 hours)

Time to peak: Occurs on an average of 2.5 hours after administration (range 1-6 hours)

Elimination: ~50% of the administered dose is excreted in urine, 30% in feces

Dosage

Geriatrics: Oral: Experience in the elderly is limited; initial dose should be 25 mg/day; increase as tolerated by 25 mg/day to desired response. Maximum daily dose in the elderly should probably be 450 mg. Dose titration to 300-450 mg/day may be attained in 2 weeks if tolerated; however, elderly may require slower titration and daily increases may not be tolerated.

Adults:

Schizophrenia: Initial: 12.5 mg once or twice daily; increased, as tolerated, in increments of 25-50 mg/day to a target dose of 300-450 mg/day after 2-4 weeks; may require doses as high as 600-900 mg/day

Reduce risk of suicidal behavior: Initial: 12.5 mg once or twice daily; increased, as tolerated, in increments of 25-50 mg/day to a target dose of 300-450 mg/day after 2-4 weeks; median dose is ~300 mg/day (range: 12.5-900 mg)

Termination of therapy: If dosing is interrupted for ≥48 hours, therapy must be reinitiated at 12.5-25 mg/day; may be increased more rapidly than with initial titration, unless cardiopulmonary arrest occurred during initial titration.

In the event of planned termination of clozapine, gradual reduction in dose over a 1- to 2-week period is recommended. If conditions warrant abrupt discontinuation (leukopenia), monitor patient for psychosis and cholinergic rebound (headache, nausea, vomiting, diarrhea).

Patients discontinued on clozapine therapy due to WBC <2000/mm³ or ANC <1000/mm³ should not be restarted on clozapine.

Administration Orally-disintegrating tablet: Should be removed from foil blister by peeling apart (do not push tablet through the foil). Remove immediately prior to use. Place tablet in mouth and allow to dissolve; swallow with saliva. If dosing requires splitting tablet, throw unused portion away.

Monitoring Parameters Mental status, ECG, WBC (see below), vital signs, fasting lipid profile and fasting blood glucose/Hgb A₁c (prior to treatment, at 3 months, then annually; BMI, personal/family history of obesity; waist circumference (weight should be assessed prior to treatment, at 4 weeks, 8 weeks, 12 weeks, and then at quarterly intervals. Consider titrating to a different antipsychotic agent for a weight gain ≥5% of the initial weight); blood pressure; abnormal involuntary movement scale (AIMS); benign, self-limiting temperature elevations sometimes occur during the first 3 weeks of treatment.

WBC and ANC should be obtained at baseline and at least weekly for the first 6 months of continuous treatment. If counts remain acceptable (WBC ≥3500/mm³, ANC ≥2000/mm³) during this time period, then they may be monitored every other week for the next 6 months. If WBC/ANC continue to remain within these acceptable limits after the second 6 months of therapy, monitoring can be decreased to every 4 weeks. (**Note:** The decease in monitoring to every 4 weeks is applicable in the United States. Blood monitoring requirements related to the use of clozapine have not changed in Canada). If clozapine is discontinued, a weekly WBC should be conducted for an additional 4 weeks or until WBC is ≥3500/mm³ and ANC is ≥2000/mm³. If clozapine therapy is interrupted due to moderate leukopenia, weekly WBC/ANC monitoring is required for 12 months in patients restarted on clozapine treatment. If therapy is interrupted for reasons other than leukopenia/granulocytopenia, the 6-month time period for initiation of biweekly WBCs may need to be reset. This determination depends upon the treatment duration, the length of the break in therapy, and whether or not an abnormal blood event occurred.

Consult full prescribing information for determination of appropriate WBC/ANC monitoring interval (http://www.clozaril.com/index.jsp).

Patient Information Report any lethargy, fever, sore throat, flu-like symptoms or any other signs or symptoms of infection; may cause drowsiness, orthostatic hypotension.

Patients using clozapine should be warned of the significant risk of agranulocytosis. Therefore, weekly blood tests are imperative for the first 6 weeks, then every other week thereafter. Patients who stop taking clozapine for more than 2 days should not restart at their current dosage and contact their physician.

Patients using orally-disintegrating tablets: Patients with phenylketonuria should be aware this dosage form (FazaClo™) contains phenylalanine as a component of its flavoring, aspartame. Orally-disintegrating tablets should remain in blister pack, unopened until used. If tablets are split, unused portion should be destroyed.

Additional Information Medication should not be stopped abruptly; taper off over 1-2 weeks

Special Geriatric Considerations Not recommended for use in nonpsychotic patients (eg, dimentia-related psychotic symptoms). Studies in subjects >65 years of age have not been done. Orthostatic hypotension and sustained tachycardia have been noted in up to 25% of patients taking clozapine; therefore, elderly with cardiovascular disease may be at risk. The anticholinergic effects of clozapine may be prominent in elderly (eg, constipation, confusion, urinary retention).

Dosage Forms Excipient information presented when available (limited, particularly for generics); consult specific product labeling.

Tablet: 12.5 mg, 25 mg, 100 mg

Clozaril®: 25 mg, 100 mg

Tablet, orally disintegrating (FazaClo®): 25 mg [contains phenylalanine 1.75 mg; mint flavor], 100 mg [contains phenylalanine 6.96 mg; mint flavor]

(Continued)

Clozapine (Continued)

Selected References

American Diabetes Association; American Psychiatric Association; American Association of Clinical Endocrinologists; North American Association for the Study of Obesity, "Consensus Development Conference on Antipsychotic Drugs and Obesity and Diabetes," *Diabetes Care*, 2004, 27(2):596-601.

Aronowitz JS, Safferman AZ, Lieberman JA, "Management of Clozapine-Induced Enuresis," *Am J Psychiatry*, 1995, 152(3):472.

Campellone JV, McCluskey LF, and Greenspan D, "Fatal Outcome From Neuroleptic Malignant Syndrome Associated With Clozapine," *Neuropsychiatry, Neuropsychology, and Behavioral Neurology*, 1995, 8:70-3.

"Change in Clozapine Monitoring Requirements," *Pharm J*, 1995, 254:612.

"Clozapine and Myocarditis," *Aust Adv Drug React Bull*, 1994, 13:14-15.

Costello LE and Suppes T, "A Clinically Significant Interaction Between Clozapine and Valproate," *J Clin Psychopharmacol*, 1995, 15(2):139-41.

Cumming RG and Klineberg RJ, "Aluminum in Antacids and Cooking Pots and the Risk of Hip Fractures in Elderly People," *Age Ageing*, 1994, 23:468-72.

Drug Facts and Comparisons, New York, NY: JB Lippincott, 1990, 265E-F.

Funderberg LG, Vertrees JE, True JE, et al, "Seizure Following Addition of Erythromycin to Clozapine Treatment," *Am J Psychiatry*, 1994, 151(12):1840-1.

Gerson SL and Meltzer H, "Mechanisms of Clozapine-Induced Agranulocytosis," *Drug Saf*, 1992, 7(Suppl 1):17-25.

Ghaeli P and Dufresne RL, "Elevated Serum Triglycerides on Clozapine Resolve With Risperidone," *Pharmacotherapy*, 1995, 15:382.

Hagg S, Spigset O, and Soderstrom TG, "Association of Venous Thromboembolism and Clozapine," *Lancet*, 2000, 355(9210):1155-6.

Kane J, Honigfeld G, Singer J, et al, "Clozapine for the Treatment-Resistant Schizophrenic. A Double-Blind Comparison With Chlorpromazine," *Arch Gen Psychiatry*, 1988, 45(9):789-96.

Pacia SV and Devinsky O, "Clozapine-Related Seizures: Experience With 5629 Patients," *Neurology*, 1994, 44(12):2247-9.

Peabody CA, Warner MD, Whiteford HA, et al, "Neuroleptics and the Elderly," *J Am Geriatr Soc*, 1987, 35(3):233-8.

Radford JM, Brown TM, and Borison RL, "Unexpected Dystonia While Changing From Clozapine to Risperidone," *J Clin Psychopharmacol*, 1995, 15(3):225-6.

Risse SC and Barnes R, "Pharmacologic Treatment of Agitation Associated With Dementia," *J Am Geriatr Soc*, 1986, 34(5):368-76.

Saltz BL, Woerner MG, Kane JM, et al, "Prospective Study of Tardive Dyskinesia Incidence in the Elderly," *JAMA*, 1991, 266(17):2402-6.

Seifert RD, "Therapeutic Drug Monitoring: Psychotropic Drugs," *J Pharm Pract*, 1984, 6:403-16.

Testani M Jr, "Clozapine-Induced Orthostatic Hypotension Treated With Fludrocortisone," *J Clin Psychiatry*, 1994, 55(11):497-8.

Welber MR and Nevins S, "Clozapine Overdose, A Case Report," *J Emerg Med*, 1995, 13(2):199-202.

Wickert WA, Campbell NR, and Martin L, "Acute Severe Adverse Clozapine Reaction Resembling Systemic Lupus/Erythematosus," *Postgrad Med J*, 1994, 70(830):940-1.

Wilson WH and Claussen AM, "Seizures Associated With Clozapine Treatment in a State Hospital," *J Clin Psychiatry*, 1994, 55(5):184-8.

Wolf LR, and Otten EJ, "A Case Report of Clozapine Overdose," *Vet Hum Toxicol*, 1991, 33:370.

♦ **Clozaril®** see Clozapine on page 352

Codeine (KOE deen)

Related Information
Narcotic / Opioid Analgesics on page 1763

Medication Safety Issues
Sound-alike/look-alike issues:
Codeine may be confused with Cardene®, Cophene®, Cordran®, iodine, Lodine®

Canadian Brand Names Codeine Contin®

Index Terms Codeine Phosphate; Codeine Sulfate; Methylmorphine

Generic Available Yes

Pharmacologic Category Analgesic, Opioid; Antitussive

Use Treatment of mild to moderate pain; antitussive in lower doses

Restrictions C-II

Contraindications Hypersensitivity to codeine or any component of the formulation

Warnings/Precautions
Use with caution in patients with hypersensitivity reactions to other phenanthrene derivative opioid agonists (morphine, hydrocodone, hydromorphone, levorphanol, oxycodone, oxymorphone); respiratory diseases including asthma, emphysema, COPD, adrenal insufficiency, biliary tract impairment, CNS depression/coma, head trauma, morbid obesity, prostatic hyperplasia, urinary stricture, thyroid dysfunction, or severe liver or renal insufficiency; some preparations contain sulfites which may cause allergic reactions; tolerance or drug dependence may result from extended use. May obscure diagnosis or clinical course of patients with acute abdominal conditions. May cause CNS depression, which may impair physical or mental abilities; patients must be cautioned about performing tasks which require mental alertness (eg, operating machinery or driving). May cause hypotension; use with caution in patients with hypovolemia, cardiovascular disease (including acute MI), or drugs which may exaggerate hypotensive effects (including phenothiazines or general anesthetics).

Not recommended for use for cough control in patients with a productive cough; the elderly and debilitated patients may be particularly susceptible to adverse effects of narcotics

Not approved for I.V. administration (although this route has been used clinically). If given intravenously, must be given slowly and the patient should be lying down. Rapid intravenous administration of narcotics may increase the incidence of serious adverse effects, in part due to limited opportunity to assess response prior to administration of the full dose. Access to respiratory support should be immediately available.

Concurrent use of agonist/antagonist analgesics may precipitate withdrawal symptoms and/or reduced analgesic efficacy in patients following prolonged therapy with mu opioid agonists. Abrupt discontinuation following prolonged use may also lead to withdrawal symptoms.

Adverse Reactions (Reflective of adult population; not specific for elderly)
Frequency not defined: AST/ALT increased
>10%:
  Central nervous system: Drowsiness
  Gastrointestinal: Constipation
1% to 10%:
  Cardiovascular: Tachycardia or bradycardia, hypotension
  Central nervous system: Dizziness, lightheadedness, false feeling of well being, malaise, headache, restlessness, paradoxical CNS stimulation, confusion
  Dermatologic: Rash, urticaria
  Gastrointestinal: Xerostomia, anorexia, nausea, vomiting
  Genitourinary: Urination decreased, ureteral spasm
  Hepatic: LFTs increased
  Local: Burning at injection site
  Neuromuscular & skeletal: Weakness
  Ocular: Blurred vision
  Respiratory: Dyspnea
  Miscellaneous: Histamine release

Overdosage/Toxicology Symptoms include CNS and respiratory depression, gastrointestinal cramping, and constipation. Treatment includes naloxone 2 mg I.V., with repeat administration as necessary, up to a total of 10 mg.

Drug Interactions Substrate of CYP2D6 (major), 3A4 (minor); **Inhibits** CYP2D6 (weak)
CYP2D6 inhibitors: May decrease the effects of codeine. Example inhibitors include chlorpromazine, delavirdine, fluoxetine, miconazole, paroxetine, pergolide, quinidine, quinine, ritonavir, and ropinirole.
Decreased effect with cigarette smoking
Increased toxicity: CNS depressants, phenothiazines, TCAs, other opioid analgesics, guanabenz, MAO inhibitors, neuromuscular blockers

Ethanol/Nutrition/Herb Interactions
Ethanol: Avoid or limit ethanol (may increase CNS depression).
Herb/Nutraceutical: St John's wort may decrease codeine levels. Avoid valerian, St John's wort, kava kava, gotu kola (may increase CNS depression).

Stability Store injection between 15°C to 30°C; avoid freezing. Do not use if injection is discolored or contains a precipitate. Protect injection from light.

Mechanism of Action Binds to opiate receptors in the CNS, causing inhibition of ascending pain pathways, altering the perception of and response to pain; causes cough supression by direct central action in the medulla; produces generalized CNS depression

Pharmacodynamics
Onset of action:
  Oral: 30-60 minutes
  I.M.: 10-30 minutes
Peak action:
  Oral: 60-90 minutes
  I.M.: 30-60 minutes
Duration: 4-6 hours; may be increased in older adults; enhanced analgesia has been seen in older adult patients on therapeutic doses of narcotics

Pharmacokinetics
Absorption: Oral: Adequate
Protein binding: 7%
Metabolism: Hepatic metabolism to morphine (active)
Half-life: 2.5-3.5 hours
Elimination: 3% to 16% excreted in urine as unchanged drug, norcodeine and free and conjugated morphine

Dosage
Geriatrics & Adults: Note: These are guidelines and do not represent the maximum doses that may be required in all patients. Doses should be titrated to pain relief/prevention. Doses >1.5 mg/kg body weight are not recommended.
(Continued)

357

Codeine *(Continued)*

Pain management (analgesic):

Oral, regular release: 30 mg every 4-6 hours as needed; patients with prior opiate exposure may require higher initial doses. Usual range: 15-120 mg every 4-6 hours as needed

Oral, controlled release formulation (Codeine Contin®, not available in U.S.): 50-300 mg every 12 hours. **Note:** A patient's codeine requirement should be established using prompt release formulations; conversion to long acting products may be considered when chronic, continuous treatment is required. Higher dosages should be reserved for use only in opioid-tolerant patients.

I.M., SubQ: 30 mg every 4-6 hours as needed; patients with prior opiate exposure may require higher initial doses. Usual range: 15-120 mg every 4-6 hours as needed; more frequent dosing may be needed

Cough (antitussive): Oral (for nonproductive cough): 10-20 mg/dose every 4-6 hours as needed; maximum: 120 mg/day

Renal Impairment:

Cl_{cr} 10-50 mL/minute: Administer 75% of dose.

Cl_{cr} <10 mL/minute: Administer 50% of dose.

Hepatic Impairment: Dosing adjustment is probably necessary in hepatic insufficiency.

Monitoring Parameters Pain relief, respiratory and mental status, blood pressure

Reference Range Therapeutic: Not established; Toxic: >1.1 mcg/mL

Test Interactions Some quinolones may produce a false-positive urine screening result for opiates using commercially-available immunoassay kits. This has been demonstrated most consistently for levofloxacin and ofloxacin, but other quinolones have shown cross-reactivity in certain assay kits. Confirmation of positive opiate screens by more specific methods should be considered.

Patient Information Avoid alcohol, may cause drowsiness; may cause GI upset, can take with food

Additional Information May be habit-forming; dextromethorphan has equivalent antitussive activity but has much lower toxicity in accidental overdose

Special Geriatric Considerations The elderly may be particularly susceptible to CNS depression and confusion as well as the constipating effects of narcotics.

Dosage Forms Excipient information presented when available (limited, particularly for generics); consult specific product labeling. [CAN] = Canadian brand name

Injection, as phosphate: 15 mg/mL (2 mL); 30 mg/mL (2 mL) [contains sodium metabisulfite]

Tablet, as phosphate: 30 mg, 60 mg

Tablet, as sulfate: 15 mg, 30 mg, 60 mg

Tablet, controlled release (Codeine Contin®) [CAN]: 50 mg, 100 mg, 150 mg, 200 mg [not available in U.S.]

Selected References

AGS Panel on Persistent Pain in Older Persons, "The Management of Persistent Pain in Older Persons," *J Am Geriatr Soc*, 2002, 50(6 Suppl):S205-24.

Ferrell BA, "Pain Management in Elderly People," *J Am Geriatr Soc*, 1991, 39(1):64-73.

Kaiko RF, Wallenstein SL, Rogers AG, et al, "Narcotics in the Elderly," *Med Clin North Am*, 1982, 66(5):1079-89.

♦ **Codeine and Acetaminophen** *see* Acetaminophen and Codeine *on page 32*
♦ **Codeine and Guaifenesin** *see* Guaifenesin and Codeine *on page 729*
♦ **Codeine Phosphate** *see* Codeine *on page 356*
♦ **Codeine Sulfate** *see* Codeine *on page 356*
♦ **Cogentin®** *see* Benztropine *on page 159*
♦ **Co-Gesic®** *see* Hydrocodone and Acetaminophen *on page 759*
♦ **Cognex®** *see* Tacrine *on page 1511*
♦ **Colace® [OTC]** *see* Docusate *on page 459*
♦ **Colace® Adult/Children Suppositories [OTC]** *see* Glycerin *on page 718*
♦ **Colace® Infant/Children Suppositories [OTC]** *see* Glycerin *on page 718*
♦ **ColBenemid** *see* Colchicine and Probenecid *on page 360*

Colchicine *(KOL chi seen)*

Medication Safety Issues

High alert medication: The Institute for Safe Medication Practices (ISMP) includes this medication among its list of drugs which have a heightened risk of causing significant patient harm when used in error.

Generic Available Yes

Pharmacologic Category Colchicine

Use Treatment of acute gouty arthritis attacks; prevention of recurrences of such attacks

Unlabeled/Investigational Use Treatment of primary biliary cirrhosis; management of familial Mediterranean fever; pericarditis

Contraindications Hypersensitivity to colchicine or any component of the formulation; serious renal, gastrointestinal, hepatic, or cardiac disorders; blood dyscrasias

Warnings/Precautions Use with caution in debilitated patients or elderly patients; use caution in patients with mild-to-moderate cardiac, GI, renal, or liver disease. Severe local irritation can occur following SubQ or I.M. administration. Dosage reduction is recommended in patients who develop weakness or gastrointestinal symptoms (anorexia, diarrhea, nausea, vomiting) related to drug therapy.

Intravenous: Use only with extreme caution; potential for serious, life-threatening complications. Should not be administered to patients with renal insufficiency, hepatobiliary obstruction, patients >70 years of age, or recent oral colchicine use. Should be reserved for hospitalized patients who are under the care of a physician experienced in the use of intravenous colchicine.

Adverse Reactions (Reflective of adult population; not specific for elderly)
>10%: Gastrointestinal: Nausea, vomiting, diarrhea, abdominal pain
1% to 10%:
  Dermatologic: Alopecia
  Gastrointestinal: Anorexia

Overdosage/Toxicology Symptoms include nausea, vomiting, abdominal pain, shock, kidney damage, muscle weakness, burning in throat, watery to bloody diarrhea, hypotension, anuria, cardiovascular collapse, delirium, and convulsions. Treatment includes gastric lavage and measures to prevent shock, hemodialysis or peritoneal dialysis. Atropine and morphine may relieve abdominal pain.

Drug Interactions Substrate of CYP3A4 (major); **Induces** CYP2C8 (weak), 2C9 (weak), 2E1 (weak), 3A4 (weak)
Cyclosporine: Concurrent use with colchicine may increase toxicity of colchicine.
CYP3A4 inhibitors: May increase the levels/effects of colchicine. Example inhibitors include azole antifungals, diclofenac, doxycycline, imatinib, isoniazid, nefazodone, nicardipine, propofol, protease inhibitors, quinidine, telithromycin, and verapamil.
Macrolide antibiotics (clarithromycin, erythromycin, troleandomycin): May decrease the metabolism of colchicine resulting in severe colchicine toxicity. Avoid, if possible.
Telithromycin: May decrease the metabolism of colchicine resulting in colchicine toxicity. Avoid, if possible.
Verapamil: May increase colchicine toxicity (especially nephrotoxicity).

Ethanol/Nutrition/Herb Interactions
Ethanol: Avoid ethanol.
Food: Cyanocobalamin (vitamin B_{12}): Malabsorption of the substrate. May result in macrocytic anemia or neurologic dysfunction.
Herb/Nutraceutical: Vitamin B_{12} absorption may be decreased by colchicine.

Stability Protect tablets from light.

Mechanism of Action Decreases leukocyte motility, decreases phagocytosis in joints and lactic acid production, thereby reducing the deposition of urate crystals that perpetuates the inflammatory response

Pharmacodynamics Articular pain and swelling decrease within 12 hours; attack resolved in 1-2 days

Pharmacokinetics
Distribution: Partially deacetylated in the liver
Protein binding: 10% to 31%
Half-life: 12-30 minutes
Time to peak serum concentrations: Oral: Within 30-120 minutes then decline for 2 hours before increasing again due to enterohepatic recycling
Elimination: Primarily in feces via bile; 10% to 20% eliminated unchanged in urine

Dosage
Geriatrics: Refer to adult dosing. Reduce maintenance/prophylactic dose by 50% in individuals >70 years.
Adults:
  Familial Mediterranean fever (unlabeled use): Prophylaxis: Oral: 1-2 mg daily in divided doses (occasionally reduced to 0.6 mg/day in patients with GI intolerance)
  Gouty arthritis:
    Prophylaxis of acute attacks: Oral: 0.6 mg twice daily; initial and/or subsequent dosage may be decreased (ie, 0.6 mg once daily) in patients at risk of toxicity or in those who are intolerant (including weakness, loose stools, or diarrhea); range: 0.6 mg every other day to 0.6 mg 3 times/day
    Acute attacks:
      Oral: Initial: 0.6-1.2 mg, followed by 0.6 every 1-2 hours; some clinicians recommend a maximum of 3 doses; more aggressive approaches have recommended a maximum dose of up to 6 mg. Wait at least 3 days before initiating another course of therapy
      I.V.: Initial: 1-2 mg, then 0.5 mg every 6 hours until response, not to exceed total dose of 4 mg. If pain recurs, it may be necessary to administer additional daily
(Continued)

Colchicine *(Continued)*

doses. The amount of colchicine administered intravenously in an acute treatment period (generally ~1 week) should not exceed a total dose of 4 mg. Do not administer more colchicine by any route for at least 7 days after a full course of I.V. therapy.

Note: Many experts would avoid use because of potential for serious, life-threatening complications. Should not be administered to patients with renal insufficiency, hepatobiliary obstruction, patients >70 years of age, or recent oral colchicine use. Should be reserved for hospitalized patients who are under the care of a physician experienced in the use of intravenous colchicine.

Surgery: Gouty arthritis, prophylaxis of recurrent attacks: Oral: 0.6 mg/day or every other day; patients who are to undergo surgical procedures may receive 0.6 mg 3 times/day for 3 days before and 3 days after surgery

Primary biliary cirrhosis (unlabeled use): Oral: 0.6 mg twice daily

Pericarditis (unlabeled use): Oral: 0.6 mg twice daily

Renal Impairment:

Gouty arthritis, acute attacks: Oral: Specific dosing recommendations not available from the manufacturer:

Prophylaxis:

Cl_{cr} 35-49 mL/minute: 0.6 mg once daily

Cl_{cr} 10-34 mL/minute: 0.6 mg every 2-3 days

Cl_{cr} <10 mL/minute: Avoid chronic use of colchicine. Use in serious renal impairment is contraindicated by the manufacturer.

Treatment: Cl_{cr} <10 mL/minute: Use in serious renal impairment is contraindicated by the manufacturer. If a decision is made to use colchicine, decrease dose by 75%.

Peritoneal dialysis: Supplemental dose is not necessary

Hepatic Impairment: Avoid in hepatobiliary dysfunction and in patients with hepatic disease.

Administration

I.V.: Injection should be made over 2-5 minutes into tubing of free-flowing I.V. with compatible fluid. Do not administer I.M. or SubQ; severe local irritation can occur following SubQ or I.M. administration. Extravasation can cause tissue irritation.

Tablet: Administer orally with water and maintain adequate fluid intake.

Monitoring Parameters GI effects, symptoms

Test Interactions May cause false-positive results in urine tests for erythrocytes or hemoglobin

Patient Information Discontinue if nausea or vomiting occur; avoid alcohol; if taking for acute attack, discontinue as soon as pain resolves; do not exceed 8 mg/day orally; notify physician if sore throat, persistent abdominal pain, nausea, diarrhea, fever, bleeding, bruising, tiredness, weakness, numbness, or tingling occurs

Special Geriatric Considerations Colchicine appears to be more toxic in older adults, particularly in the presence of renal, gastrointestinal, or cardiac disease. The most predictable oral side effects are gastrointestinal (eg, vomiting, abdominal pain, and nausea). If colchicine is stopped at this point, other more severe adverse effects may be avoided, such as bone marrow suppression, peripheral neuritis, etc.

Dosage Forms Excipient information presented when available (limited, particularly for generics); consult specific product labeling.

Injection, solution: 0.5 mg/mL (2 mL)

Tablet: 0.6 mg

Selected References

Antman EM, Anbe SC, Alpert JS, et al, "ACC/AHA Guidelines for the Management of Patients With ST-Elevation Myocardial Infarction - Executive Summary: A Report of the American College of Cardiology/ American Heart Association Task Force on Practice Guidelines (Writing Committee to Revise the 1999 Guidelines for the Management of Patients With Acute Myocardial Infarction)," *Circulation*, 2004, 110:588-636. Available at: http://www.circulationaha.org/cgi/content/full/110/5/588. Last accessed October 26, 2004.

Emmerson BT, "The Management of Gout," *N Engl J Med*, 1996, 334(7):445-51.

Levy M, Spino M, and Read SE, "Colchicine: A State-of-the-Art Review," *Pharmacotherapy*, 1991, 11(3):196-211.

Colchicine and Probenecid *(KOL chi seen & proe BEN e sid)*

Related Information

Colchicine *on page 358*

Probenecid *on page 1315*

Index Terms ColBenemid; Probenecid and Colchicine

Generic Available Yes

Pharmacologic Category Anti-inflammatory Agent; Antigout Agent; Uricosuric Agent

Use Treatment of chronic gouty arthritis when complicated by frequent, recurrent acute attacks of gout

Dosage

Geriatrics & Adults: Gout: Oral: 1 tablet/day for 1 week, then 1 tablet twice daily thereafter

Renal Impairment: Probenecid may not be effective in patients with chronic renal insufficiency particularly when Cl_{cr} is ≤30 mL/minute.

Special Geriatric Considerations Refer to individual agents.

Dosage Forms Excipient information presented when available (limited, particularly for generics); consult specific product labeling.

Tablet: Colchicine 0.5 mg and probenecid 0.5 g

Colesevelam (koh le SEV a lam)

Related Information

Hyperlipidemia Management *on page 1773*

U.S. Brand Names WelChol®

Canadian Brand Names WelChol®

Generic Available No

Pharmacologic Category Antilipemic Agent, Bile Acid Sequestrant

Use Adjunctive therapy to diet and exercise in the management of elevated LDL in primary hypercholesterolemia (Fredrickson type IIa), alone or in combination with an HMG-CoA reductase inhibitor; offers a nonabsorbable alternative to systemic treatment of hypercholesterolemia

Contraindications Hypersensitivity to colesevelam or any component of the formulation; bowel obstruction

Warnings/Precautions Use caution in treating patients with serum triglyceride levels >300 mg/dL (may cause increased levels). Use caution in dysphagia, swallowing disorders, severe GI motility disorders, major GI tract surgery, and in patients susceptible to fat-soluble vitamin deficiencies. Minimal effects are seen on HDL-C and triglyceride levels. Secondary causes of hypercholesterolemia should be excluded before initiation.

Adverse Reactions (Reflective of adult population; not specific for elderly)

>10%: Gastrointestinal: Constipation (11%)

2% to 10%:

Gastrointestinal: Dyspepsia (8%)

Neuromuscular & skeletal: Weakness (4%), myalgia (2%)

Respiratory: Pharyngitis (3%)

Incidence less than or equal to placebo: Infection, headache, pain, back pain, abdominal pain, flu syndrome, flatulence, diarrhea, nausea, sinusitis, rhinitis, cough

Overdosage/Toxicology Systemic toxicity is low since the drug is not absorbed.

Drug Interactions Note: A number of medications, including digoxin, HMG-CoA reductase inhibitors (eg, atorvastatin, lovastatin, simvastatin), metoprolol, quinidine, valproic acid, verapamil, or warfarin absorption have been specifically evaluated and were not found to be significantly affected with concurrent administration.

Amiodarone: Absorption may be reduced by concurrent colesevelam. Avoid concurrent use.

Corticosteroids: Bile acid sequestrants may decrease the absorption of corticosteroids. Separating administration times by at least 1 hour before of 4 hours after dose might reduce (but not eliminate) the risk.

Diuretics: Absorption may be reduced by concurrent colesevelam. Separate administration times by at least 1 hour before or 4 hours after dose.

Ezetimibe: Absorption may be reduced by concurrent colesevelam. Separate administration times by at least 1 hour before or 4 hours after dose.

Fibric acid derivatives: Absorption may be reduced by concurrent colesevelam. Separate administration times by at least 1 hour before or 4 hours after dose.

Methotrexate: Absorption may be reduced by concurrent colesevelam. Separate administration times by at least 1 hour before or 4 hours after dose.

Niacin: Bile acid sequestrants may decrease the absorption of niacin. Separate administration times by at least 1 hour before or 4 hours after dose.

Nonsteroidal anti-inflammatory agents (NSAIDs): Absorption may be reduced by concurrent colesevelam. Separate administration times by at least 1 hour before or 4 hours after dose.

Raloxifene: Bile acid sequestrants may decrease the absorption of raloxifene. Separate administration times by at least 1 hour before or 4 hours after dose.

Tetracyclines: Absorption may be reduced by concurrent colesevelam. Separate administration times by at least 1 hour before or 4 hours after dose.

Thiazolidinediones: Absorption may be reduced by concurrent colesevelam. Monitor. Separate administration times by at least 1 hour before or 4 hours after dose.

Thyroid supplements including levothyroxine: The absorption of thyroid supplements may be reduced by colesevelam (may be noted by elevation in TSH). Separate

(Continued)

Colesevelam *(Continued)*

administration times by at least 1 hour before or 4 hours after dose, and monitor TSH levels during concurrent therapy.

Stability Store at room temperature. Protect from moisture.

Mechanism of Action Colesevelam binds bile acids including glycocholic acid in the intestine, impeding their reabsorption. Increases the fecal loss of bile salt-bound LDL-C

Pharmacokinetics

Absorption: Not significantly absorbed

Peak effect: Maximal therapeutic response seen within 2 weeks

Elimination: 0.05% was excreted in the urine after 1 month of chronic dosing

Dosage

Geriatrics & Adults:

Dyslipidemia: Oral:

Monotherapy: 3 tablets twice daily with meals or 6 tablets once daily with a meal; maximum dose: 7 tablets/day

Combination therapy with an HMG-CoA reductase inhibitor: 4-6 tablets daily; maximum dose: 6 tablets/day

Administration Administer with meal(s) and a liquid. Make sure patient understands dietary guidelines.

Monitoring Parameters Serum cholesterol, LDL, and triglyceride levels should be obtained before initiating treatment and periodically thereafter (in accordance with NCEP guidelines)

Patient Information Take once or twice daily with meals. Follow diet and exercise plan as recommended by healthcare provider.

Special Geriatric Considerations The definition of and, therefore, when to treat hyperlipidemia in elderly is a controversial issue. The National Cholesterol Education Program recommends that all adults maintain a plasma cholesterol <160 mg/dL. Elderly with one additional risk factor, goal LDL would be <130 mg/dL. It is the authors' belief that pharmacologic treatment be reserved for those who are unable to obtain a desirable plasma cholesterol concentration by diet alone and for whom the benefits of treatment are believed to outweigh the potential adverse effects, drug interactions, and cost of treatment.

Dosage Forms Excipient information presented when available (limited, particularly for generics); consult specific product labeling.

Tablet, as hydrochloride:

WelChol®: 625 mg

Selected References

Davidson MH, Dillon MA, Gordon B, et al, "Colesevelam Hydrochloride (Cholestagel): A New, Potent Bile Acid Sequestrant Associated With a Low Incidence of Gastrointestinal Side Effects," *Arch Intern Med*, 1999, 159(16):1893-900.

"Executive Summary of The Third Report of The National Cholesterol Education Program (NCEP) Expert Panel on Detection, Evaluation, And Treatment of High Blood Cholesterol In Adults (Adult Treatment Panel III)," *JAMA*, 2001, 285(19):2486-97.

♦ Colestid® *see* Colestipol *on page 362*

Colestipol *(koe LES ti pole)*

Related Information

Hyperlipidemia Management *on page 1773*

U.S. Brand Names Colestid®

Canadian Brand Names Colestid®

Index Terms Colestipol Hydrochloride

Generic Available No

Pharmacologic Category Antilipemic Agent, Bile Acid Sequestrant

Use Adjunct in the management of primary hypercholesterolemia; to relieve pruritus associated with elevated levels of bile acids, possibly used to decrease plasma half-life of digoxin as an adjunct in the treatment of toxicity

Contraindications Hypersensitivity to bile acid sequestering resins or any component of the formulation; bowel obstruction

Warnings/Precautions Not to be taken simultaneously with many other medicines (decreased absorption). Avoid in patients with high triglycerides, GI dysfunction (constipation); fecal impaction may occur; hemorrhoids may be worsened. May be associated with increased bleeding tendency as a result of hypothrombinemia secondary to vitamin K deficiency; may cause depletion of vitamins A, D, and E, and folic acid.

Adverse Reactions (Reflective of adult population; not specific for elderly)

>10%: Gastrointestinal: Constipation

1% to 10%:

Central nervous system: Headache, dizziness, anxiety, vertigo, drowsiness, fatigue

Gastrointestinal: Abdominal pain and distention, belching, flatulence, nausea, vomiting, diarrhea

Overdosage/Toxicology Symptoms include GI obstruction, nausea, and GI distress. Treatment is supportive.

Drug Interactions

Colestipol can reduce the absorption of numerous medications when used concurrently. Give other medications 1 hour before or 4 hours after giving colestipol. Medications which may be affected include HMG-CoA reductase inhibitors, thiazide diuretics, propranolol (and potentially other beta-blockers), corticosteroids, thyroid hormones, digoxin, valproic acid, NSAIDs, loop diuretics, sulfonylureas, troglitazone (and potentially other agents in this class).

Warfarin and other oral anticoagulants: Absorption is reduced by cholestyramine, may also be reduced by colestipol. Separate administration times (as detailed above) and monitor INR closely when initiating or discontinuing.

Mechanism of Action Binds with bile acids to form an insoluble complex that is eliminated in feces; it thereby increases the fecal loss of bile acid-bound low density lipoprotein cholesterol

Pharmacokinetics Absorption: Oral: Not absorbed

Dosage

Geriatrics & Adults: Dyslipidemia: Oral:

Granules: 5-30 g/day given once or in divided doses 2-4 times/day; initial dose: 5 g 1-2 times/day; increase by 5 g at 1- to 2-month intervals

Tablets: 2-16 g/day; initial dose: 2 g 1-2 times/day; increase by 2 g at 1- to 2-month intervals

Administration Dry powder should be added to at least 90 mL of liquid and stirred until completely mixed; other drugs should be administered at least 1 hour before or 4 hours after colestipol

Monitoring Parameters Serum lipid profile; plasma cholesterol (LDL and VLDL fractions); observe for gastrointestinal side effects

Test Interactions Increased prothrombin time; decreased cholesterol (S)

Patient Information Mix in liquids, cereals, soda, soup, or pulpy fruits; add at least 90 mL of liquid; do not take dry; stir well, powder will not dissolve; rinse glass with small amount of liquid to ensure full dose is taken

Special Geriatric Considerations The definition of and, therefore, when to treat hyperlipidemia in the elderly is a controversial issue. The National Cholesterol Education Program recommends that all adults maintain a plasma cholesterol <160 mg/dL. Elderly with one additional risk factor, goal LDL would be <130 mg/dL. It is the authors' belief that pharmacologic treatment be reserved for those who are unable to obtain a desirable plasma cholesterol concentration by diet alone and for whom the benefits of treatment are believed to outweigh the potential adverse effects, drug interactions, and cost of treatment.

Dosage Forms Excipient information presented when available (limited, particularly for generics); consult specific product labeling.

Granules, as hydrochloride:

5 g/7.5 g packet (30s, 90s) [unflavored]

5 g/7.5 g (300 g, 500 g) [unflavored]

5 g/7.5 g packet (60s) [contains phenylalanine 18.2 mg/7.5 g; orange flavor]

5 g/7.5 g (450 g) [contains phenylalanine 18.2 mg/7.5 g; orange flavor]

Tablet, as hydrochloride: 1 g

Selected References

"Executive Summary of The Third Report of The National Cholesterol Education Program (NCEP) Expert Panel on Detection, Evaluation, And Treatment of High Blood Cholesterol In Adults (Adult Treatment Panel III)," *JAMA*, 2001, 285(19):2486-97.

♦ **Colestipol Hydrochloride** *see* Colestipol *on page 362*
♦ **Colistin, Neomycin, Hydrocortisone, and Thonzonium** *see* Neomycin, Colistin, Hydrocortisone, and Thonzonium *on page 1101*

Collagenase (KOL la je nase)

U.S. Brand Names Santyl®

Generic Available No

Pharmacologic Category Enzyme, Topical Debridement

Use Promotes debridement of necrotic tissue in dermal ulcers and severe burns

Contraindications Hypersensitivity to collagenase or any component of the formulation

Warnings/Precautions For external use only; avoid contact with eyes; monitor debilitated patients for systemic bacterial infections because debriding enzymes may increase the risk of bacteremia

Adverse Reactions (Reflective of adult population; not specific for elderly)

Frequency not defined.

(Continued)

Collagenase *(Continued)*

Local: Irritation, pain and burning may occur at site of application

Drug Interactions Decreased effect: Enzymatic activity is inhibited by detergents, benzalkonium chloride, hexachlorophene, nitrofurazone, tincture of iodine, and heavy metal ions (silver and mercury)

Mechanism of Action Collagenase is an enzyme derived from the fermentation of *Clostridium histolyticum* and differs from other proteolytic enzymes in that its enzymatic action has a high specificity for native and denatured collagen. Collagenase will not attack collagen in healthy tissue or newly formed granulation tissue. In addition, it does not act on fat, fibrin, keratin, or muscle.

Dosage

Geriatrics & Adults: Dermal ulcers, burns: Topical: Apply once daily.

Administration Prior to application, cleanse lesion of debris and digested material. When infection is present, neomycin-bacitracin-polymyxin B may be used with collagenase. Excess ointment should be removed each time the dressing is changed. Treatment should be discontinued when debridement is complete and granulation tissue is well established.

Monitoring Parameters Healing of ulcer

Patient Information For external use only; avoid contact with eyes

Special Geriatric Considerations Preventive skin care should be instituted in all older patients at high risk for pressure ulcers. Collagenase is indicated in stage 3 and 4 pressure ulcers.

Dosage Forms Excipient information presented when available (limited, particularly for generics); consult specific product labeling.

Ointment: 250 units/g (15 g, 30 g)

Selected References

Chamberlain TM, Cali TS, Cuzzell J, et al, "Assessment and Management of Pressure Sores in Long-Term Care Facilities," *Consult Pharm*, 1992, 7(12)1328-40.

Conivaptan *(koe NYE vap tan)*

U.S. Brand Names Vaprisol®

Index Terms Conivaptan Hydrochloride; YM087

Generic Available No

Pharmacologic Category Vasopressin Antagonist

Use Treatment of euvolemic hyponatremia in hospitalized patients

Contraindications Hypersensitivity to conivaptan or any component of the formulation; use in hypovolemic hyponatremia; concurrent use with strong CYP3A4 inhibitors (eg, ketoconazole, itraconazole, ritonavir, indinavir, and clarithromycin)

Warnings/Precautions Monitor closely for rate of serum sodium increase and neurological status; overly rapid serum sodium correction (>12 mEq/L/24 hours) can lead to permanent neurological damage. Discontinue use if rate of serum sodium increase is undesirable; may reinitiate infusion (at reduced dose) if hyponatremia persists in the absence of neurological symptoms typically associated with rapid sodium rise. Discontinue if hypovolemia or hypotension occur. Safety and efficacy in heart failure patients have not been established. Use in small numbers of hypervolemic, hyponatremic heart failure patients led to increased adverse events. In other heart failure studies, conivaptan did not show significant improvements in outcomes over placebo. Use with caution in patients with hepatic and renal impairment.

Adverse Reactions (Reflective of adult population; not specific for elderly)

>10%:

Cardiovascular: Orthostatic hypotension (6% to 14%)

Central nervous system: Fever (5% to 11%)

Endocrine & metabolic: Hypokalemia (10% to 22%)
Local: Injection site reactions including pain, erythema, phlebitis, swelling (63% to 73%)
1% to 10%:
Cardiovascular: Hypertension (6% to 8%), hypotension (5% to 8%), edema (3% to 8%), phlebitis (5%), atrial fibrillation (2% to 5%), ECG abnormality (up to 5%)
Central nervous system: Headache (8% to 10%), insomnia (4% to 5%), confusion (up to 5%), pain (2%)
Dermatologic: Pruritus (1% to 5%), erythema (3%)
Endocrine & metabolic: Hyponatremia (3% to 8%), hypomagnesemia (2% to 5%), hyper-/hypoglycemia (3%)
Gastrointestinal: Constipation (6% to 8%), vomiting (5% to 7%), diarrhea (up to 7%), nausea (5%), dry mouth (4%), dehydration (2%), oral candidiasis (2%)
Genitourinary: Urinary tract infection (4% to 5%)
Hematologic: Anemia (4%)
Renal: Polyuria (5% to 6%), hematuria (2%)
Respiratory: Pneumonia (2% to 5%)
Miscellaneous: Thirst (3% to 6%)

Overdosage/Toxicology Doses of up to 120 mg/day for 2 days have been evaluated; hypotension and thirst occurred more frequently at these higher doses. Treatment should be symptom-directed and supportive.

Drug Interactions Substrate of CYP3A4 (major); **Inhibits** CYP3A4 (strong)
CYP3A4 inducers may decrease the levels/effects of conivaptan. Example inducers include aminoglutethimide, carbamazepine, nafcillin, nevirapine, phenobarbital, phenytoin, and rifamycins.
CYP3A4 inhibitors may increase the levels/effects of conivaptan. Example inhibitors include azole antifungals, clarithromycin, diclofenac, doxycycline, erythromycin, imatinib, isoniazid, nefazodone, nicardipine, propofol, protease inhibitors, quinidine, telithromycin, and verapamil. Concurrent use of strong CYP3A4 inhibitors is contraindicated.
CYP3A4 substrates: Conivaptan may increase the levels/effects of CYP3A4 substrates. Example substrates include benzodiazepines, calcium channel blockers, cyclosporine, mirtazapine, nateglinide, nefazodone, sildenafil (and other PDE-5 inhibitors), tacrolimus, and venlafaxine. Selected benzodiazepines (midazolam and triazolam), cisapride, ergot alkaloids, selected HMG-CoA reductase inhibitors (lovastatin and simvastatin), and pimozide are generally contraindicated with strong CYP3A4 inhibitors.
Digoxin: Conivaptan may increase the levels/toxicity of digoxin; monitor.
Ketoconazole: May increase the levels/effects of conivaptan; concomitant use is contraindicated.
Pimecrolimus: Conivaptan may increase levels/effects of pimecrolimus. Use cautiously especially in patients with widespread and/or erythrodermic disease.

Ethanol/Nutrition/Herb Interactions Herb/Nutraceutical: St John's wort may decrease the levels/effects of conivaptan.

Stability Store ampuls in original cardboard container at 15°C to 30°C (59°F to 86°F); protect from light. Dilute loading dose of 20 mg in 100 mL D$_5$W and continuous infusion dose of 20-40 mg in 250 mL D$_5$W. After dilution, infusion bag (final concentration of 0.08-0.2 mg/mL) is stable at room temperature for 24 hours.

Mechanism of Action Conivaptan is an arginine vasopressin (AVP) receptor antagonist with affinity for AVP receptor subtypes V$_{1A}$ and V$_2$. The antidiuretic action of AVP is mediated through activation of the V$_2$ receptor, which functions to regulate water and electrolyte balance at the level of the collecting ducts in the kidney. Serum levels of AVP are commonly elevated in euvolemic or hypervolemic hyponatremia, which results in the dilution of serum sodium and the relative hyponatremic state. Antagonism of the V$_2$ receptor by conivaptan promotes the excretion of free water (without loss of serum electrolytes) resulting in net fluid loss, increased urine output, decreased urine osmolality, and subsequent restoration of normal serum sodium levels.

Pharmacokinetics
Protein binding: 99%
Metabolism: Hepatic via CYP3A4 to four minimally-active metabolites
Half-life elimination: 6.7-8.6 hours
Excretion: Feces (83%); urine (12%, primarily as metabolites)

Dosage
Geriatrics & Adults: Euvolemic hyponatremia: I.V.:
Loading dose: 20 mg infused over 30 minutes, followed by continuous infusion of 20 mg over 24 hours
Maintenance: 20 mg/day as continuous infusion over 24 hours; may titrate to maximum of 40 mg/day if serum sodium not rising sufficiently; total duration of therapy not to exceed 4 days

Administration For intravenous use only; do not administer undiluted; infuse into large veins and change infusion site every 24 hours to minimize vascular irritation
(Continued)

Conivaptan *(Continued)*

Monitoring Parameters Rate of serum sodium increase, urine output

Special Geriatric Considerations Adverse events in elderly patients were generally similar to those seen in younger patients. In clinical studies, 52% of patients were >65 years of age and 34% were >75 years of age.

Dosage Forms Excipient information presented when available (limited, particularly for generics); consult specific product labeling.

Injection, solution:

Vaprisol®: 5 mg/mL (4 mL) [single-use ampul; contains propylene glycol and ethanol]

- ♦ **Conivaptan Hydrochloride** *see* Conivaptan *on page 364*
- ♦ **Constulose** *see* Lactulose *on page 869*
- ♦ **Contac® Cold [OTC] [DSC]** *see* Pseudoephedrine *on page 1346*
- ♦ **ControlRx®** *see* Fluoride *on page 642*
- ♦ **COPD** *see* Dyphylline and Guaifenesin *on page 496*
- ♦ **Copegus®** *see* Ribavirin *on page 1397*
- ♦ **Cordarone®** *see* Amiodarone *on page 80*
- ♦ **Cordron-D NR [DSC]** *see* Carbinoxamine and Pseudoephedrine *on page 239*
- ♦ **Coreg®** *see* Carvedilol *on page 243*
- ♦ **Coreg CR™** *see* Carvedilol *on page 243*
- ♦ **Corgard®** *see* Nadolol *on page 1079*
- ♦ **Coricidin HBP® Chest Congestion and Cough [OTC]** *see* Guaifenesin and Dextromethorphan *on page 730*
- ♦ **Cormax®** *see* Clobetasol *on page 335*
- ♦ **Correctol® Tablets [OTC]** *see* Bisacodyl *on page 173*
- ♦ **Cortaid® Intensive Therapy [OTC]** *see* Hydrocortisone *on page 762*
- ♦ **Cortaid® Maximum Strength [OTC]** *see* Hydrocortisone *on page 762*
- ♦ **Cortaid® Sensitive Skin [OTC]** *see* Hydrocortisone *on page 762*
- ♦ **Cortef®** *see* Hydrocortisone *on page 762*
- ♦ **Corticool® [OTC]** *see* Hydrocortisone *on page 762*
- ♦ **Cortifoam®** *see* Hydrocortisone *on page 762*
- ♦ **Cortisol** *see* Hydrocortisone *on page 762*

Cortisone *(KOR ti sone)*

Related Information
Corticosteroids *on page 1755*

Medication Safety Issues
Sound-alike/look-alike issues:
Cortisone may be confused with Cortizone®

Index Terms Compound E; Cortisone Acetate

Generic Available Yes

Pharmacologic Category Corticosteroid, Systemic

Use Management of adrenocortical insufficiency

Contraindications Hypersensitivity to cortisone acetate or any component of the formulation; serious infections, except septic shock or tuberculous meningitis; administration of live virus vaccines

Warnings/Precautions Use with caution in patients with thyroid disease, hepatic impairment, renal impairment, cardiovascular disease, diabetes, glaucoma, cataracts, myasthenia gravis, patients at risk for osteoporosis, patients at risk for seizures, or GI diseases (diverticulitis, peptic ulcer, ulcerative colitis) due to perforation risk. Use caution following acute MI (corticosteroids have been associated with myocardial rupture). Because of the risk of adverse effects, systemic corticosteroids should be used cautiously in the elderly in the smallest possible effective dose for the shortest duration. Withdraw therapy with gradual tapering of dose.

May cause hypercorticism or suppression of hypothalamic-pituitary-adrenal (HPA) axis, particularly in patients receiving high doses for prolonged periods. HPA axis suppression may lead to adrenal crisis. Withdrawal and discontinuation of a corticosteroid should be done slowly and carefully. Particular care is required when patients are transferred from systemic corticosteroids to inhaled products due to possible adrenal insufficiency or withdrawal from steroids, including an increase in allergic symptoms. Patients receiving >20 mg per day of prednisone (or equivalent) may be most susceptible. Fatalities have occurred due to adrenal insufficiency in asthmatic patients during and after transfer from systemic corticosteroids to aerosol steroids; aerosol steroids do not provide the systemic steroid needed to treat patients having trauma, surgery, or infections.

Acute myopathy has been reported with high dose corticosteroids, usually in patients with neuromuscular transmission disorders; may involve ocular and/or respiratory muscles; monitor creatine kinase; recovery may be delayed. Corticosteroid use may cause psychiatric disturbances, including depression, euphoria, insomnia, mood swings, and personality changes. Pre-existing psychiatric conditions may be exacerbated by corticosteroid use. Prolonged use of corticosteroids may also increase the incidence of secondary infection, mask acute infection (including fungal infections), prolong or exacerbate viral infections, or limit response to vaccines. Exposure to chickenpox should be avoided; corticosteroids should not be used to treat ocular herpes simplex. Corticosteroids should not be used for cerebral malaria. Close observation is required in patients with latent tuberculosis and/or TB reactivity; restrict use in active TB (only in conjunction with antituberculosis treatment). Prolonged treatment with corticosteroids has been associated with the development of Kaposi's sarcoma (case reports); if noted, discontinuation of therapy should be considered.

Adverse Reactions (Reflective of adult population; not specific for elderly)

>10%:
  Central nervous system: Insomnia, nervousness
  Gastrointestinal: Increased appetite, indigestion
1% to 10%:
  Dermatologic: Hirsutism
  Endocrine & metabolic: Diabetes mellitus
  Neuromuscular & skeletal: Arthralgia
  Ocular: Cataracts, glaucoma
  Respiratory: Epistaxis

Overdosage/Toxicology When consumed in excessive quantities for prolonged periods, systemic hypercorticism and adrenal suppression may occur; in those cases, discontinuation and withdrawal of the corticosteroid should be done judiciously. Cushingoid changes from continued administration of large doses results in moon face, central obesity, striae, hirsutism, acne, ecchymoses, hypertension, osteoporosis, myopathy, sexual dysfunction, diabetes, hyperlipidemia, peptic ulcer, increased susceptibility to infection, and electrolyte and fluid imbalance.

Drug Interactions

Aminoglutethimide: May reduce the serum levels/effects of corticosteroids; likely via induction of microsomal isoenzymes.

Amphotericin: Corticosteroids may increase the hypokalemic effects of amphotericin B; monitor.

Antacids: May decrease the absorption of corticosteroids; separate administration by 2 hours.

Anticholinesterases: Concurrent use may lead to severe weakness in patients with myasthenia gravis.

Antidiabetic agents: Corticosteroids may decrease the hypoglycemic effects of antidiabetic agents; monitor.

Aprepitant: May increase the serum levels/effects of corticosteroids; monitor.

Antifungal agents (azole): May increase the serum levels/effects of corticosteroids; monitor.

Barbiturates: May decrease the levels/effects of corticosteroids.

Bile acid sequestrants: May reduce the absorption of corticosteroids; separate administration by 2 hours.

Calcium channel blockers (nondihydropyridine): May increase the serum levels/effects of corticosteroids; monitor.

Cyclosporine: Corticosteroids may increase the serum levels/effects of cyclosporine. In addition, cyclosporine may increase levels of corticosteroids.

Diuretics, potassium-wasting (loop or thiazide): Hypokalemic effects may be increased by corticosteroids; monitor.

Estrogens: May increase the serum levels/effects of corticosteroids; monitor.

Fluoroquinolones: Concurrent use may increase the risk of tendinopathies (including tendonitis and rupture), particularly in elderly patients (overall incidence rare)

Isoniazid: Serum levels/effects may be decreased by corticosteroids.

Macrolide antibiotics: May increase the serum levels/effects of corticosteroids.

Neuromuscular-blocking agents: Concurrent use with corticosteroids may increase the risk of myopathy.

Nonsteroidal anti-inflammatory drugs (NSAIDs): Concurrent use with corticosteroids may lead to an increased incidence of gastrointestinal adverse effects; use caution.

Rifamycin derivatives: May decrease the levels/effects of corticosteroids (systemic); monitor.

Salicylates: Salicylates may increase the gastrointestinal adverse effects of corticosteroids.

Vaccine (dead organism): Corticosteroids may decrease the effect of vaccines (dead organisms). In patients receiving high doses of systemic corticosteroids for ≥14 days, wait at least 1 month between discontinuing steroid therapy and administering immunization.

(Continued)

Cortisone *(Continued)*

Vaccine (live organism): Corticosteroids may increase the risk of vaccinal infection. The use of live vaccines is contraindicated in immunosuppressed patients.

Warfarin: Corticosteroids may increase the anticoagulant effects of warfarin; monitor INR.

Ethanol/Nutrition/Herb Interactions Food: Limit caffeine intake.

Mechanism of Action Decreases inflammation by suppression of migration of polymorphonuclear leukocytes and reversal of increased capillary permeability

Pharmacodynamics

Peak effect:
Oral: Within 2 hours
I.M.: Within 20-48 hours
Duration: 30-36 hours

Pharmacokinetics

Absorption: Slow
Distribution: To muscles, liver, skin, intestines, and kidneys
Metabolism: In the liver to inactive metabolites
Half-life: 30 minutes; biologic half-life: 8-12 hours
Elimination: In bile and urine

Dosage

Geriatrics & Adults: If possible, administer glucocorticoids before 9 AM to minimize adrenocortical suppression; dosing depends upon the condition being treated and the response of the patient. **Note:** Supplemental doses may be warranted during times of stress in the course of withdrawing therapy.

Anti-inflammatory or immunosuppressive: Oral: 25-300 mg/day in divided doses every 12-24 hours

Physiologic replacement: Oral: 25-35 mg/day

Renal Impairment:

Hemodialysis: Supplemental dose is not necessary.
Peritoneal dialysis: Supplemental dose is not necessary.

Monitoring Parameters Blood pressure, blood glucose, electrolytes, symptoms of fluid retention

Patient Information Take with food or milk; take single daily doses in the morning; do not stop abruptly; carry an identification card or bracelet advising that you are on steroids

Additional Information Approximately 80% the potency of cortisol; the maximum activity of the adrenal cortex is between 2 AM and 8 AM and it is minimal between 4 PM and midnight; if possible, administer glucocorticoids before 9 AM to minimize adrenocortical suppression; prolonged therapy (>5 days) of pharmacologic doses of corticosteroids may lead to hypothalamic-pituitary-adrenal suppression, the degree of adrenal suppression varies with the degree and duration of glucocorticoid therapy; this must be taken into consideration when taking patients off steroids; supplemental doses may be warranted during times of stress in the course of withdrawal therapy

Special Geriatric Considerations Because of the risk of adverse effects, systemic corticosteroids should be used cautiously in the elderly, in the smallest possible dose, and for the shortest possible time.

Dosage Forms Excipient information presented when available (limited, particularly for generics); consult specific product labeling.

Tablet, as acetate: 25 mg

♦ **Crinone**® *see Progesterone on page 1325*
♦ **Crolom**® *see Cromolyn on page 369*
♦ **Cromoglycic Acid** *see Cromolyn on page 369*

Cromolyn (KROE moe lin)

Related Information
Asthma *on page 1767*
Inhalant Agents *on page 1760*
Medication Safety Issues
Sound-alike/look-alike issues:
Intal® may be confused with Endal®
NasalCrom® may be confused with Nasacort®, Nasalide®
U.S. Brand Names Crolom®; Gastrocrom®; Intal®; NasalCrom® [OTC]; Opticrom®
Canadian Brand Names Apo-Cromolyn®; Intal®; Nalcrom®; Nu-Cromolyn; Opticrom®
Index Terms Cromoglycic Acid; Cromolyn Sodium; Disodium Cromoglycate; DSCG
Generic Available Yes: Excludes aerosol, oral solution
Pharmacologic Category Mast Cell Stabilizer
Use
Inhalation: May be used as an adjunct in the prophylaxis of allergic disorders, including rhinitis, asthma; prevention of exercise-induced bronchospasm
Oral: Systemic mastocytosis
Ophthalmic: Treatment of vernal keratoconjunctivitis, vernal conjunctivitis, and vernal keratitis
Unlabeled/Investigational Use Treatment of food allergy, inflammatory bowel disease
Contraindications Hypersensitivity to cromolyn or any component of the formulation; acute asthma attacks
Warnings/Precautions Severe anaphylactic reactions may occur rarely; cromolyn is a prophylactic drug with no benefit for acute situations; caution should be used when withdrawing the drug or tapering the dose as symptoms may reoccur; use with caution in patients with a history of cardiac arrhythmias. Transient burning or stinging may occur with ophthalmic use. Dosage of oral product should be decreased with hepatic or renal dysfunction.
Adverse Reactions (Reflective of adult population; not specific for elderly)
Inhalation: >10%: Gastrointestinal: Unpleasant taste in mouth
Nasal:
>10%: Respiratory: Increase in sneezing, burning, stinging, or irritation inside of nose
1% to 10%:
Central nervous system: Headache
Gastrointestinal: Unpleasant taste
Respiratory: Hoarseness, cough, postnasal drip
<1% (Limited to important or life-threatening): Anaphylactic reactions, epistaxis
Ophthalmic: Frequency not defined:
Ocular: Conjunctival injection, dryness around the eye, edema, eye irritation, immediate hypersensitivity reactions, itchy eyes, puffy eyes, styes, rash, watery eyes
Respiratory: Dyspnea
Systemic: Frequency not defined:
Cardiovascular: Angioedema, chest pain, edema, flushing, palpitation, premature ventricular contractions, tachycardia
Central nervous system: Anxiety, behavior changes, convulsions, depression, dizziness, fatigue, hallucinations, headache, irritability, insomnia, lethargy, migraine, nervousness, hypoesthesia, postprandial lightheadedness, psychosis
Dermatologic: Erythema, photosensitivity, pruritus, purpura, rash, urticaria
Gastrointestinal: Abdominal pain, constipation, diarrhea, dyspepsia, dysphagia, esophagospasm, flatulence, glossitis, nausea, stomatitis, unpleasant taste, vomiting
Genitourinary: Dysuria, urinary frequency
Hematologic: Neutropenia, pancytopenia, polycythemia
Hepatic: Liver function test abnormal
Local: Burning
Neuromuscular & skeletal: Arthralgia, leg stiffness, leg weakness, myalgia, paresthesia
Otic: Tinnitus
Respiratory: Dyspnea, pharyngitis
Miscellaneous: Lupus erythematosus
Overdosage/Toxicology Symptoms include bronchospasm, laryngeal edema, and dysuria.
Drug Interactions Corticosteroids: Ophthalmic preparation may be used with ophthalmic corticosteroids
Stability Store at room temperature of 15°C to 30°C (59°F to 86°F); protect from light. Do not use oral solution if solution becomes discolored or forms a precipitate.
(Continued)

Cromolyn *(Continued)*

Mechanism of Action Prevents the mast cell release of histamine, leukotrienes, and slow-reacting substance of anaphylaxis by inhibiting degranulation after contact with antigens

Pharmacokinetics

Absorption:

Inhalation: ~8% reaches lungs upon inhalation; well absorbed

Oral: <1% of dose absorbed

Half-life: 80-90 minutes

Time to peak, serum: Inhalation: ~15 minutes

Elimination: Urine and feces (equal amounts as unchanged drug); exhaled gases (small amounts)

Dosage

Geriatrics & Adults:

Allergic rhinitis (treatment and prophylaxis): Nasal: Instill 1 spray in each nostril 3-4 times/day

Asthma: For chronic control of asthma, taper frequency to the lowest effective dose (ie, 4 times/day to 3 times/day to twice daily). **Note:** Not effective for immediate relief of symptoms in acute asthmatic attacks; must be used at regular intervals for 2-4 weeks to be effective.

Nebulization solution: Initial: 20 mg 4 times/day; usual dose: 20 mg 3-4 times/day

Metered spray: Initial: 2 inhalations 4 times/day; usual dose: 2-4 inhalations 3-4 times/day

Prophylaxis of bronchospasm (allergen- or exercise-induced):

Note: Administer 10-15 minutes prior to exercise or allergen exposure but no longer than 1 hour before:

Nebulization solution: Single dose of 20 mg

Metered spray: Single dose of 2 inhalations

Conjunctivitis and keratitis: Ophthalmic: 1-2 drops in each eye 4-6 times/day

Mastocytosis: Oral: 200 mg 4 times/day; given $\frac{1}{2}$ hour prior to meals and at bedtime. If control of symptoms is not seen within 2-3 weeks, dose may be increased to a maximum 40 mg/kg/day

Food allergy and inflammatory bowel disease (unlabeled use): Oral: Initial dose: 200 mg 4 times/day; may double the dose if effect is not satisfactory within 2-3 weeks; up to 400 mg 4 times/day

Renal Impairment: Specific guidelines not available; consider lower dose of oral product.

Hepatic Impairment: Specific guidelines not available; consider lower dose of oral product.

Monitoring Parameters Pulmonary function tests, spirometry

Patient Information Do not discontinue abruptly; not effective for acute relief of symptoms; must be taken on a regularly scheduled basis; store nebulizer solution away from light; follow instructions that come with the product. For ophthalmic product, put drops of suspension inside the lower eyelid; do not wear contact lenses during treatment.

Additional Information Oral administration is strictly investigational; cromolyn is a prophylactic drug with no benefit for acute situations.

Special Geriatric Considerations Elderly often have difficulty with inhaled and ophthalmic dosage forms.

Dosage Forms Excipient information presented when available (limited, particularly for generics); consult specific product labeling.

Aerosol, for oral inhalation, as sodium (Intal®): 800 mcg/inhalation (8.1 g) [112 metered inhalations; 56 doses], (14.2 g) [200 metered inhalations; 100 doses]

Solution for nebulization, as sodium (Intal®): 20 mg/2 mL (60s, 120s)

Solution, intranasal, as sodium [spray] (NasalCrom®): 40 mg/mL (13 mL, 26 mL) [5.2 mg/inhalation; contains benzalkonium chloride]

Solution, ophthalmic, as sodium (Crolom®, Opticrom®): 4% (10 mL) [contains benzalkonium chloride]

Solution, oral, as sodium (Gastrocrom®): 100 mg/5 mL (96s)

♦ **Cromolyn Sodium** *see* Cromolyn *on page 369*

Crotamiton *(kroe TAM i tonn)*

Medication Safety Issues

Sound-alike/look-alike issues:

Eurax® may be confused with Efudex®, Eulexin®, Evoxac™, Serax®, Urex®

International issues:

Eurax® may be confused with Urex® which is a brand name for furosemide in Australia

U.S. Brand Names Eurax®
Generic Available No
Pharmacologic Category Scabicidal Agent
Use Treatment of scabies and symptomatic treatment of pruritus
Contraindications Hypersensitivity to crotamiton or any component of the formulation; patients who manifest a primary irritation response to topical medications
Warnings/Precautions Avoid contact with face, eyes, mucous membranes, and urethral meatus; do not apply to acutely inflamed or raw skin; for external use only
Adverse Reactions (Reflective of adult population; not specific for elderly)
Frequency not defined. Topical:
Dermatologic: Contact dermatitis, pruritus, rash
Local: Local irritation
Miscellaneous: Allergic sensitivity reactions, warm sensation
Overdosage/Toxicology Symptoms of ingestion include burning sensation in mouth; irritation of the buccal, esophageal and gastric mucosa, nausea, vomiting, and abdominal pain. There is no specific antidote. General measures to eliminate the drug and reduce its absorption, combined with symptomatic treatment, are recommended.
Drug Interactions No data reported
Stability Store at room temperature.
Mechanism of Action Crotamiton has scabicidal activity against *Sarcoptes scabiei*; mechanism of action unknown
Dosage
Geriatrics & Adults:
Scabies: Topical: Wash thoroughly and scrub away loose scales, then towel dry; apply a thin layer and massage drug onto skin of the entire body from the neck to the toes (with special attention to skin folds, creases, and interdigital spaces). Repeat application in 24 hours. Take a cleansing bath 48 hours after the final application. Treatment may be repeated after 7-10 days if live mites are still present.
Pruritus: Topical: Massage into affected areas until medication is completely absorbed; repeat as necessary
Administration Lotion: Shake well before using; avoid contact with face, eyes, mucous membranes, and urethral meatus
Patient Information For topical use only; keep away from eyes and mucosa membranes, all contaminated clothing and bed linen should be washed to avoid reinfestation; shake lotion well
Additional Information Treatment may be repeated after 7-10 days if live mites are still present
Special Geriatric Considerations If cure is not achieved after 2 doses, use alternative therapy.
Dosage Forms Excipient information presented when available (limited, particularly for generics); consult specific product labeling.
Cream: 10% (60 g)
Lotion: 10% (60 mL, 480 mL)

Cyanocobalamin (sye an oh koe BAL a min)

U.S. Brand Names Nascobal®; Twelve Resin-K
Index Terms Vitamin B_{12}
Generic Available Yes: Excludes nasal spray
Pharmacologic Category Vitamin, Water Soluble
Use Treatment of pernicious anemia; vitamin B_{12} deficiency due to dietary deficiencies or malabsorption diseases, inadequate secretion of intrinsic factor, and inadequate utilization of B_{12} (eg, during neoplastic treatment); increased B_{12} requirements due to thyrotoxicosis, hemorrhage, malignancy, liver or kidney disease
(Continued)

Cyanocobalamin *(Continued)*

Contraindications Hypersensitivity to cyanocobalamin, cobalt, or any component of the formulation

Warnings/Precautions I.M./SubQ routes are used to treat pernicious anemia; oral and intranasal administration are not indicated until hematologic remission and no signs of nervous system involvement. Treatment of severe vitamin B_{12} megaloblastic anemia may result in thrombocytosis and severe hypokalemia, sometimes fatal, due to intracellular potassium shift upon anemia resolution. Vitamin B_{12} deficiency masks signs of polycythemia vera; use caution in other conditions where folic acid or vitamin B_{12} administration alone might mask true diagnosis, despite hematologic response. Vitamin B_{12} deficiency for >3 months results in irreversible degenerative CNS lesions; neurologic manifestations will not be prevented with folic acid unless vitamin B_{12} is also given. Spinal cord degeneration might also occur when folic acid used as a substitute for vitamin B_{12} in anemia prevention. Use caution in Leber's disease patients; B_{12} treatment may result in rapid optic atrophy. Some parenteral products contain aluminum; use caution in patients with impaired renal function. Avoid intravenous route; anaphylactic shock has occurred. Intradermal test dose of vitamin B_{12} is recommended for any patient suspected of cyanocobalamin sensitivity prior to intranasal or injectable administration.

Adverse Reactions (Reflective of adult population; not specific for elderly)
Frequency not defined.
Cardiovascular: CHF, peripheral vascular disorder, peripheral vascular thrombosis
Central nervous system: Anxiety, dizziness, headache, hypoesthesia, incoordination, pain, nervousness
Dermatologic: Itching, urticaria, exanthema (transient)
Gastrointestinal: Diarrhea, dyspepsia, glossitis, nausea, sore throat, vomiting
Hematologic: Polycythemia vera
Neuromuscular & skeletal: Abnormal gait, arthritis, back pain, myalgia, paresthesia, weakness
Respiratory: Dyspnea, pulmonary edema, rhinitis
Miscellaneous: Anaphylaxis (parenteral) and infection

Drug Interactions Chloramphenicol: Therapeutic effect of cyanocobalamin may be diminished with concurrent chloramphenicol.

Ethanol/Nutrition/Herb Interactions Ethanol: Heavy consumption >2 weeks may impair vitamin B_{12} absorption.

Stability Injection: Clear pink to red solutions are stable at room temperature. Protect from light.
Intranasal spray: Store at 15°C to 30°C (59°F to 86°F); do not freeze. Protect from light.

Mechanism of Action Coenzyme for various metabolic functions, including fat and carbohydrate metabolism and protein synthesis, used in cell replication and hematopoiesis

Pharmacokinetics
Absorption: Oral: Variable from the terminal ileum; requires the presence of calcium and gastric "intrinsic factor" to transfer the compound across the intestinal mucosa
Distribution: Principally stored in the liver and bone marrow, also stored in the kidneys and adrenals
Protein binding: Transcobalamins
Metabolism: Converted in tissues to active coenzymes, methylcobalamin and deoxyadenosylcobalamin; undergoes some enterohepatic recycling
Bioavailability: Intranasal solution: 6.1% (relative to I.M.)

Dosage
Geriatrics & Adults:
Recommended intake: 2.4 mcg/day

Vitamin B_{12} deficiency:
Intranasal: 500 mcg in one nostril once weekly
Oral: 250 mcg/day
I.M., deep SubQ: Initial: 30 mcg/day for 5-10 days; maintenance: 100-200 mcg/month
Pernicious anemia: I.M., deep SubQ (administer concomitantly with folic acid if needed, 1 mg/day for 1 month): 100 mcg/day for 6-7 days; if improvement, administer same dose on alternate days for 7 doses, then every 3-4 days for 2-3 weeks; once hematologic values have returned to normal, maintenance dosage: 100 mcg/month. **Note:** Alternative dosing of 1000 mcg/day for 5 days (followed by 500-1000 mcg/month) has been used.
Hematologic remission (without evidence of nervous system involvement):
Intranasal: 500 mcg in one nostril once weekly
Oral: 1000-2000 mcg/day
I.M., SubQ: 100-1000 mcg/month
Schilling test: I.M.: 1000 mcg

Administration

I.M./SubQ: I.M. or deep SubQ are preferred routes of administration

Intranasal: Nasal spray: Prior to initial dose, activate (prime) spray nozzle by pumping unit quickly and firmly until first appearance of spray, then prime twice more. The unit must be reprimed once immediately before each subsequent use. Administer 1 hour before or after ingestion of hot foods/liquids.

I.V.: Not recommended due to rapid elimination

Oral: Not recommended due to variable absorption; however, oral therapy of 1000-2000 mcg/day has been effective for anemia if I.M./SubQ routes refused or not tolerated.

Monitoring Parameters Vitamin B_{12}, hematocrit, reticulocyte count, folate and iron levels should be obtained prior to treatment; vitamin B_{12} and peripheral blood counts should be monitored 1 month after beginning treatment, then every 3-6 months thereafter.

Megaloblastic anemia: In addition to normal hematological parameters, serum potassium and platelet counts should be monitored during therapy

Reference Range Normal range of serum B_{12} is 150-750 pg/mL; this represents 0.1% of total body content. Metabolic requirements are 2-5 mcg/day; years of deficiency required before hematologic and neurologic signs and symptoms are seen. Occasional patients with significant neuropsychiatric abnormalities may have no hematologic abnormalities and normal serum cobalamin levels, 200 pg/mL (SI: >150 pmol/L), or more commonly between 100-200 pg/mL (SI: 75-150 pmol/L).

Test Interactions Methotrexate, pyrimethamine, and most antibiotics invalidate folic acid and vitamin B_{12} diagnostic blood assays

Patient Information Use exactly as directed. Pernicious anemia may require treatment for life. Report skin rash; swelling, pain, or redness of extremities; or acute persistent diarrhea.

Special Geriatric Considerations There exists evidence that people, particularly elderly whose serum cobalamin concentrations are <500 pg/mL, should receive replacement parenteral therapy or oral replacement (1000 mcg daily). This recommendation is based upon neuropsychiatric disorders and cardiovascular disorders associated with lower sodium cobalamin concentrations.

Dosage Forms Excipient information presented when available (limited, particularly for generics); consult specific product labeling.

Injection, solution: 1000 mcg/mL (1 mL, 10 mL, 30 mL) [may contain benzyl alcohol and/or aluminum]

Lozenge [OTC]: 100 mcg, 250 mcg, 500 mcg

Solution, intranasal [spray]:

Nascobal®: 500 mcg/0.1 mL actuation (2.3 mL) [contains benzalkonium chloride; delivers 8 doses]

Tablet [OTC]: 50 mcg, 100 mcg, 250 mcg, 500 mcg, 1000 mcg, 5000 mcg

Twelve Resin-K: 1000 mcg [may be used as oral, sublingual, or buccal]

Tablet, extended release [OTC]: 1000 mcg, 1500 mcg

Tablet, sublingual [OTC]: 2500 mcg

Selected References

Andres E, Noel E, and Goichot B, "Metformin-Associated Vitamin B_{12} Deficiency," *Arch Intern Med*, 2002, 162(19):2251-2.

"Dietary Reference Intakes for Thiamin, Riboflavin, Niacin, Vitamin B_6, Folate, Vitamin B_{12}, Pantothenic Acid, Biotin, and Choline," (Chapter 9) available at http://books.nap.edu/openbook/0309065542/html/306.html. Last accessed February 22, 2005.

Goodman M, Chen XH, and Darwish D, "Are U.S. Lower Normal B12 Limits Too Low?" *J Am Geriatr Soc*, 1996, 44(10):1274-5.

Kallstrom B and Nylof R, "Vitamin-B 12 and Folic Acid in Psychiatric Disorders," *Acta Psychiatr Scand*, 1969, 45(2):137-52.

Lane LA and Rojas-Fernandez C, "Treatment of Vitamin B_{12}-Deficiency Anemia: Oral Versus Parenteral Therapy," *Ann Pharmacother*, 2002, 36(7-8):1268-72.

Lindenbaum J, Healton EB, Savage DG, et al, "Neuropsychiatric Disorders Caused by Cobalamin Deficiency in the Absence of Anemia or Macrocytosis," *N Engl J Med*, 1988, 318(26):1720-8.

Mitsuyama Y and Kogoh H, "Serum and Cerebrospinal Fluid Vitamin B12 Levels in Demented Patients With CH3-B12 Treatment - Preliminary Study," *Jpn J Psychiatry Neurol*, 1988, 42(1):65-71.

Oh R and Brown DL, "Vitamin B_{12} Deficiency," *Am Fam Physician*, 2003, 67(5):979-86.

Olszewski AJ, Szostak WB, Bialkowska M, et al, "Reduction of Plasma Lipid and Homocysteine Levels by Pyridoxine, Folate, Cobalamin, Choline, Riboflavin, and Troxerutin in Atherosclerosis," *Atherosclerosis*, 1989, 75(1):1-6.

Regland B, Gottfries CG, and Lindstedt G, "Dementia Patients With Low Serum Cobalamin Concentration: Relationship to Atrophic Gastritis," *Aging (Milano)*, 1992, 4(1):35-41.

Schnyder G, Roffi M, Flammer Y, et al, "Effect of Homocysteine-Lowering Therapy With Folic Acid, Vitamin B12, and Vitamin B6 on Clinical Outcome After Percutaneous Coronary Intervention: The Swiss Heart Study: A Randomized Controlled Trial," *JAMA*, 2002, 288(8):973-9.

♦ **Cyanokit®** *see* Hydroxocobalamin *on page 770*

Cyclizine (SYE kli zeen)

U.S. Brand Names Marezine® [OTC]
Index Terms Cyclizine Hydrochloride; Cyclizine Lactate
Generic Available No
Pharmacologic Category Antihistamine
Use Prevention and treatment of nausea, vomiting and vertigo associated with motion sickness; control of postoperative nausea and vomiting
Contraindications Hypersensitivity to cyclizine or any component of the formulation
Warnings/Precautions Use with caution in patients with angle-closure glaucoma or prostatic hyperplasia. Older adults may be at risk for anticholinergic side effects such as glaucoma, prostate hyperplasia, constipation, gastrointestinal obstructive disease
Adverse Reactions (Reflective of adult population; not specific for elderly)
>10%:
   Central nervous system: Drowsiness
   Gastrointestinal: Xerostomia
1% to 10%:
   Central nervous system: Headache
   Dermatologic: Dermatitis
   Gastrointestinal: Nausea
   Genitourinary: Urinary retention
   Ocular: Diplopia
   Renal: Polyuria
Drug Interactions Increased effect/toxicity with CNS depressants, ethanol
Ethanol/Nutrition/Herb Interactions Ethanol: Avoid ethanol (may increase CNS depression).
Mechanism of Action Cyclizine is a piperazine derivative with properties of histamines. The precise mechanism of action in inhibiting the symptoms of motion sickness is not known. It may have effects directly on the labyrinthine apparatus and central actions on the labyrinthine apparatus and on the chemoreceptor trigger zone. Cyclizine exerts a central anticholinergic action.
Pharmacodynamics
   Onset of action: Oral: Within 30-60 minutes
   Duration: 4-6 hours
Pharmacokinetics
   Metabolism: Reportedly in the liver
   Half-life: 6 hours
   Elimination: As metabolites in urine and as unchanged drug in feces
Dosage
   Geriatrics & Adults: Emesis (prophylaxis and treatment): Oral: 50 mg taken 30 minutes before departure, may repeat in 4-6 hours if needed, up to 200 mg/day
Monitoring Parameters Monitor for CNS side effects in older adults.
Patient Information May impair ability to perform hazardous tasks; may cause drowsiness; may cause dry mouth, constipation, difficulty urinating, confusion
Special Geriatric Considerations Due to anticholinergic action, use lowest dose in divided doses to avoid side effects and their inconvenience; limit use if possible; may cause confusion or aggravate symptoms of confusion in those with dementia; constipation and difficulty voiding urine may occur
Dosage Forms Excipient information presented when available (limited, particularly for generics); consult specific product labeling.
   Tablet, as hydrochloride: 50 mg

♦ **Cyclizine Hydrochloride** see Cyclizine on page 374
♦ **Cyclizine Lactate** see Cyclizine on page 374

Cyclobenzaprine (sye kloe BEN za preen)

Related Information
   Potentially Inappropriate Medications for Geriatrics on page 1824
Medication Safety Issues
   Sound-alike/look-alike issues:
      Cyclobenzaprine may be confused with cycloSERINE, cyproheptadine
      Flexeril® may be confused with Floxin®
U.S. Brand Names Fexmid™; Flexeril®
Canadian Brand Names Apo-Cyclobenzaprine®; Flexeril®; Flexitec; Gen-Cyclobenzaprine; Novo-Cycloprine; Nu-Cyclobenzaprine
Index Terms Cyclobenzaprine Hydrochloride
Generic Available Yes

Pharmacologic Category Skeletal Muscle Relaxant

Use Treatment of muscle spasm associated with acute painful musculoskeletal conditions

Contraindications Hypersensitivity to cyclobenzaprine or any component of the formulation; do not use concomitantly or within 14 days of MAO inhibitors; hyperthyroidism; congestive heart failure, arrhythmias, heart block; acute recovery phase of MI

Warnings/Precautions Cyclobenzaprine shares the toxic potentials of the tricyclic antidepressants (including arrhythmias, tachycardia, and conduction time prolongation) and the usual precautions of tricyclic antidepressant therapy should be observed; use with caution in patients with urinary hesitancy or retention, angle-closure glaucoma or increased intraocular pressure, hepatic impairment, or in the elderly. Do not use concomitantly or within 14 days after MAO inhibitors; combination may cause hypertensive crisis, severe convulsions. Effects may be potentiated when used with other CNS depressants or ethanol.

Adverse Reactions (Reflective of adult population; not specific for elderly)

>10%:

Central nervous system: Drowsiness (29% to 39%), dizziness (1% to 11%)

Gastrointestinal: Xerostomia (21% to 32%)

1% to 10%:

Central nervous system: Fatigue (1% to 6%), confusion (1% to 3%), headache (1% to 3%), irritability (1% to 3%), mental acuity decreased (1% to 3%), nervousness (1% to 3%)

Gastrointestinal: Abdominal pain (1% to 3%), constipation (1% to 3%), diarrhea (1% to 3%), dyspepsia (1% to 3%), nausea (1% to 3%), unpleasant taste (1% to 3%)

Neuromuscular & skeletal: Weakness (1% to 3%)

Ocular: Blurred vision (1% to 3%)

Respiratory: Pharyngitis (1% to 3%), upper respiratory infection (1% to 3%)

Overdosage/Toxicology Symptoms include difficulty breathing, drowsiness, syncope, seizures, tachycardia, hallucinations, and vomiting. Following initiation of essential overdose management, toxic symptoms should be treated. Ventricular arrhythmias often respond to systemic alkalinization (sodium bicarbonate 0.5-2 mEq/kg I.V.) and/or phenytoin 15-20 mg/kg. Arrhythmias unresponsive to this therapy may respond to lidocaine 1 mg/kg I.V. followed by a titrated infusion. Physostigmine (1-2 mg I.V. slowly) may be indicated in reversing life-threatening cardiac arrhythmias. Seizures usually respond to diazepam I.V. boluses (5-10 mg up to 30 mg). If seizures are unresponsive or recur, phenytoin or phenobarbital may be required.

Drug Interactions Substrate of CYP1A2 (major), 2D6 (minor), 3A4 (minor)

Acetylcholinesterase inhibitors (central): May diminish the effects of cyclobenzaprine. Cyclobenzaprine may diminish the therapeutic effect of acetylcholinesterase inhibitors (central).

Anticholinergics: Cyclobenzaprine may enhance the adverse/toxic effect of other anticholinergics.

CNS depressants: Cyclobenzaprine may enhance adverse/toxic effects of other CNS depressants.

CYP1A2 inhibitors: May increase the levels/effects of cyclobenzaprine. Example inhibitors include amiodarone, ciprofloxacin, fluvoxamine, ketoconazole, norfloxacin, ofloxacin, and rofecoxib.

Droperidol: May have an additive effect on prolonging the QT interval; based on limited documentation; monitor.

Fluoxetine: May have an additive effect on prolonging the QT interval; based on limited documentation; monitor.

MAO inhibitors: Do not use concomitantly or within 14 days after MAO inhibitors.

Pramlintide: May enhance the anticholinergic effect of cyclobenzaprine. These effects are specific to the GI tract.

Tramadol: Cyclobenzaprine may enhance the neuroexcitatory and/or seizure-potentiating effect of tramadol.

Ethanol/Nutrition/Herb Interactions

Ethanol: Avoid ethanol (may increase CNS depression).

Herb/Nutraceutical: Avoid valerian, kava kava, gotu kola (may increase CNS depression).

Stability

Fexmid™: Store at room temperature of 20°C to 25°C (68°F to 77°F).

Flexeril®: Store at room temperature of 15°C to 30°C (59°F to 86°F).

Mechanism of Action Centrally-acting skeletal muscle relaxant pharmacologically related to tricyclic antidepressants; reduces tonic somatic motor activity influencing both alpha and gamma motor neurons

Pharmacodynamics

Onset of action: Commonly occurs within 1 hour

Duration: 12-24 hours

Pharmacokinetics

Absorption: Oral: Complete

(Continued)

Cyclobenzaprine *(Continued)*

Protein binding: 93%
Metabolism: Hepatic; may undergo enterohepatic recirculation
Bioavailability: 33% to 55%
Half-life: 18 hours (range: 8-37 hours)
Time to peak serum concentration: 3-8 hours
Elimination: Renally as inactive metabolites and in feces (via bile) as unchanged drug

Dosage

Geriatrics: 5 mg 3 times/day. Plasma concentrations and adverse effects are increased in older patients. See Special Geriatric Considerations.

Adults: Muscle spasm (including spasms associated with acute temporomandibular joint pain): Oral: Initial: 5 mg 3 times/day; may increase to 7.5-10 mg 3 times/day if needed. Do not use longer than 2-3 weeks.

Hepatic Impairment:

Mild: 5 mg 3 times/day; use with caution and titrate slowly.
Moderate to severe: Use not recommended.

Monitoring Parameters Relief of pain and muscle spasm, liver function tests, mental status

Patient Information May cause drowsiness, dizziness, or blurred vision; use caution performing activities requiring alertness; avoid alcohol and CNS depressants; may cause dry mouth

Special Geriatric Considerations High doses in the elderly caused drowsiness and dizziness; therefore, use the lowest dose possible. Because cyclobenzaprine causes anticholinergic effects, it may not be the skeletal muscle relaxant of choice in the elderly.

Dosage Forms Excipient information presented when available (limited, particularly for generics); consult specific product labeling.

Tablet, as hydrochloride: 5 mg, 10 mg
Fexmid™: 7.5 mg
Flexeril®: 5 mg, 10 mg

♦ **Cyclobenzaprine Hydrochloride** *see* Cyclobenzaprine *on page 374*
♦ **Cyclocort® [DSC]** *see* Amcinonide *on page 70*

Cyclophosphamide *(sye kloe FOS fa mide)*

Medication Safety Issues

Sound-alike/look-alike issues:

Cyclophosphamide may be confused with cycloSPORINE, ifosfamide

Cytoxan® may be confused with cefoxitin, Centoxin®, Ciloxan®, cytarabine, CytoGam®, Cytosar®, Cytosar-U®, Cytotec®

High alert medication: The Institute for Safe Medication Practices (ISMP) includes this medication among its list of drugs which have a heightened risk of causing significant patient harm when used in error.

U.S. Brand Names Cytoxan®

Canadian Brand Names Cytoxan®; Procytox®

Index Terms CPM; CTX; CYT; Neosar; NSC-26271

Generic Available Yes: Tablet

Pharmacologic Category Antineoplastic Agent, Alkylating Agent

Use Oncologic: Treatment of Hodgkin's and non-Hodgkin's lymphoma, Burkitt's lymphoma, chronic lymphocytic leukemia (CLL), chronic myelocytic leukemia (CML), acute myelocytic leukemia (AML), acute lymphocytic leukemia (ALL), mycosis fungoides, multiple myeloma, neuroblastoma, retinoblastoma, rhabdomyosarcoma, Ewing's sarcoma; treatment of breast, testicular, endometrial, ovarian, and lung cancers, and in conditioning regimens for bone marrow transplantation

Noncologic: Prophylaxis of rejection for kidney, heart, liver, and bone marrow transplants, severe rheumatoid disorders, nephrotic syndrome, Wegener's granulomatosis, idiopathic pulmonary hemosideroses, myasthenia gravis, multiple sclerosis, systemic lupus erythematosus, lupus nephritis, autoimmune hemolytic anemia, idiopathic thrombocytic purpura (ITP), macroglobulinemia, and antibody-induced pure red cell aplasia

Contraindications Hypersensitivity to cyclophosphamide or any component of the formulation

Warnings/Precautions Hazardous agent - use appropriate precautions for handling and disposal. Dosage adjustment may be needed for renal or hepatic failure. Hemorrhagic cystitis may occur; increased hydration and frequent voiding is recommended. Immunosuppression may occur; monitor for infections. May cause cardiotoxicity (CHF, usually with higher doses); may potentiate the cardiotoxicity of anthracyclines. May impair fertility; interferes with oogenesis and spermatogenesis. Secondary malignancies (usually delayed) have been reported

Adverse Reactions (Reflective of adult population; not specific for elderly)

>10%:

Dermatologic: Alopecia (40% to 60%) but hair will usually regrow although it may be a different color and/or texture. Hair loss usually begins 3-6 weeks after the start of therapy.

Endocrine & metabolic: Fertility: May cause sterility; interferes with oogenesis and spermatogenesis; may be irreversible in some patients; gonadal suppression (amenorrhea)

Gastrointestinal: Nausea and vomiting, usually beginning 6-10 hours after administration; anorexia, diarrhea, mucositis, and stomatitis are also seen

Genitourinary: Severe, potentially fatal acute hemorrhagic cystitis (7% to 40%)

Hematologic: Thrombocytopenia and anemia are less common than leukopenia

Onset: 7 days

Nadir: 10-14 days

Recovery: 21 days

1% to 10%:

Cardiovascular: Facial flushing

Central nervous system: Headache

Dermatologic: Skin rash

Renal: SIADH may occur, usually with doses >50 mg/kg (or 1 g/m^2); renal tubular necrosis, which usually resolves with discontinuation of the drug, is also reported

Respiratory: Nasal congestion occurs when I.V. doses are administered too rapidly; patients experience runny eyes, rhinorrhea, sinus congestion, and sneezing during or immediately after the infusion.

Overdosage/Toxicology Symptoms include myelosuppression, alopecia, nausea, and vomiting. Treatment is symptom-directed and supportive. Cyclophosphamide is moderately dializable (20% to 50%).

Drug Interactions Substrate of CYP2A6 (minor), 2B6 (major), 2C9 (minor), 2C19 (minor), 3A4 (major); **Inhibits** CYP3A4 (weak); **Induces** CYP2B6 (weak), 2C8 (weak), 2C9 (weak)

Allopurinol may cause increase in bone marrow depression and may result in significant elevations of cyclophosphamide cytotoxic metabolites.

Anesthetic agents: Cyclophosphamide reduces serum pseudocholinesterase concentrations and may prolong the neuromuscular blocking activity of succinylcholine; use with caution with halothane, nitrous oxide, and succinylcholine.

Cardiac glycosides: Cyclophosphamide may decrease the absorption of digoxin tablets.

CYP2B6 inducers: May increase the levels/effects of acrolein (the active metabolite of cyclophosphamide). Example inducers include carbamazepine, nevirapine, phenobarbital, phenytoin, and rifampin.

CYP2B6 inhibitors: May decrease the levels/effects of acrolein (the active metabolite of cyclophosphamide). Example inhibitors include desipramine, paroxetine, and sertraline.

CYP3A4 inducers: CYP3A4 inducers may increase the levels/effects of acrolein (the active metabolite of cyclophosphamide). Example inducers include aminoglutethimide, carbamazepine, nafcillin, nevirapine, phenobarbital, phenytoin, and rifamycins.

CYP3A4 inhibitors: May decrease the levels/effects of acrolein (the active metabolite of cyclophosphamide). Example inhibitors include azole antifungals, ciprofloxacin, clarithromycin, diclofenac, doxycycline, erythromycin, imatinib, isoniazid, nefazodone, nicardipine, propofol, protease inhibitors, quinidine, and verapamil.

Etanercept: May enhance the adverse/toxic effects of cyclophosphamide.

Mivacurium: Cyclophosphamide may increase the levels/effects of mivacurium.

Phenytoin: May decrease the levels/effects of cyclophosphamide; may increase the levels/effects of 4-hydroxycyclophosphamide.

Succinylcholine: Cyclophosphamide may increase the levels/effects of succinylcholine.

Ethanol/Nutrition/Herb Interactions Herb/Nutraceutical: Avoid black cohosh, dong quai in estrogen-dependent tumors.

Stability Store intact vials of powder at room temperature of 15°C to 30°C (59°F to 86°F). Reconstitute vials with sterile water, normal saline, or 5% dextrose to a concentration of 20 mg/mL. Reconstituted solutions are stable for 24 hours at room temperature and 6 days under refrigeration at 2°C to 8°C (36°F to 46°F). Further dilutions in D$_5$W or NS are stable for 24 hours at room temperature and 6 days at refrigeration.

Mechanism of Action Cyclophosphamide is an alkylating agent that prevents cell division by cross-linking DNA strands and decreasing DNA synthesis. It is a cell cycle phase nonspecific agent. Cyclophosphamide also possesses potent immunosuppressive activity. Cyclophosphamide is a prodrug that must be metabolized to active metabolites in the liver.

Pharmacokinetics

Absorption: Oral: Well absorbed

Distribution: V$_d$: 0.48-0.71 L/kg; crosses placenta; crosses into CSF (not in high enough concentrations to treat meningeal leukemia)

(Continued)

Cyclophosphamide *(Continued)*

Protein binding: 10% to 60%

Metabolism: Hepatic to active metabolites acrolein, 4-aldophosphamide, 4-hydroperox-ycyclophosphamide, and nor-nitrogen mustard; A large fraction of cyclophospha-mide is eliminated by hepatic metabolism.

Half-life elimination: 3-12 hours

Time to peak, serum: Oral: ~1 hour

Elimination: Urine (<30% as unchanged drug, 85% to 90% as metabolites)

Dosage

Geriatrics: Refer to individual protocols: Initial and maintenance for induction: 1-2 mg/kg/day; adjust for renal clearance.

Adults: Refer to individual protocols:

Usual dose:

Oral: 50-100 mg/m^2/day as continuous therapy or 400-1000 mg/m^2 in divided doses over 4-5 days as intermittent therapy

I.V.:

Single doses: 400-1800 mg/m^2 (30-50 mg/kg) per treatment course (1-5 days) which can be repeated at 2- to 4-week intervals

Continuous daily doses: 60-120 mg/m^2 (1-2.5 mg/kg) per day

JRA/vasculitis: I.V.: 10 mg/kg every 2 weeks

High dose BMT:

I.V.:

60 mg/kg/day for 2 days (total dose: 120 mg/kg)

50 mg/kg/day for 4 days (total dose: 200 mg/kg)

1.8 g/m^2/day for 4 days (total dose: 7.2 g/m^2)

Continuous I.V.:

1.5 g/m^2/24 hours for 96 hours (total dose: 6 g/m^2)

1875 mg/m^2/24 hours for 72 hours (total dose: 5625 mg/m^2)

Note: Duration of infusion is 1-24 hours; generally combined with other high-dose chemotherapeutic drugs, lymphocyte immune globulin, or total body irradiation (TBI).

Nephrotic syndrome: Oral: 2-3 mg/kg/day every day for up to 12 weeks when corticosteroids are unsuccessful

Renal Impairment: A large fraction of cyclophosphamide is eliminated by hepatic metabolism; some authors recommend no dose adjustment unless severe renal insufficiency (Cl$_{cr}$ <20 mL/minute).

Cl$_{cr}$ >10 mL/minute: Administer 100% of normal dose.

Cl$_{cr}$ <10 mL/minute: Administer 75% of normal dose.

Hemodialysis effects: Moderately dialyzable (20% to 50%)

Administer dose posthemodialysis

CAPD effects: Unknown

CAVH effects: Unknown

Hepatic Impairment: The pharmacokinetics of cyclophosphamide are not signifi-cantly altered in the presence of hepatic insufficiency. No dosage adjustments are recommended.

Administration May be administered I.P., intrapleurally, IVPB, or continuous I.V. infu-sion; may also be administered slow IVP in doses ≤1 g.

I.V. infusions may be administered over 1-24 hours

Doses >500 mg to approximately 2 g may be administered over 20-30 minutes

To minimize bladder toxicity, increase normal fluid intake during and for 1-2 days after cyclophosphamide dose. Most adult patients will require a fluid intake of at least 2 L/day. High-dose regimens should be accompanied by vigorous hydration with or without mesna therapy.

Oral: Tablets are not scored and should not be cut or crushed. To minimize the risk of bladder irritation, do not administer tablets at bedtime.

Monitoring Parameters Monitor WBC and platelets; observe for signs of infection, bleeding, and bladder irritation; monitor urinalysis for blood. See Additional Informa-tion.

Patient Information Drink plenty of fluids before and after doses; report any blood in the urine. May cause nausea, vomiting, and diarrhea. If these side effects persist, call physician; report any bruising, bleeding, chills, cough, shortness of breath, unusual lumps, seizures, sores in mouth, flank or joint pain.

Additional Information In patients with CYP2B6 G516T variant allele, cyclophospha-mide metabolism is markedly increased; metabolism is not influenced by CYP2C9 and CYP2C19 isotypes.

Special Geriatric Considerations Toxicity to immunosuppressives is increased in the elderly. Start with lowest recommended adult doses. Signs of infection, such as fever and WBC rise, may not occur. Lethargy and confusion may be more prominent signs of infection; adjust dose for renal function.

Dosage Forms Excipient information presented when available (limited, particularly for generics); consult specific product labeling.

Injection, powder for reconstitution:

Cytoxan®: 500 mg, 1 g, 2 g [contains mannitol 75 mg per cyclophosphamide 100 mg

Tablet: 25 mg, 50 mg

Cytoxan®: 25 mg, 50 mg

Extemporaneously Prepared A 2 mg/mL oral elixir was stable for 14 days when refrigerated when made as follows: Reconstitute a 200 mg vial with aromatic elixir, withdraw the solution, and add sufficient aromatic elixir to make a final volume of 100 mL (store in amber glass container).

Brook D, Davis RE, and Bequette RJ, "Chemical Stability of Cyclophosphamide in Aromatic Elixir U.S.P.," *Am J Health Syst Pharm*, 1973, 30:618-20.

Selected References

Bostrom BC, Weisdorf DJ, Kim TH, et al, "Bone Marrow Transplantation for Advanced Acute Leukemia: A Pilot Study of High-Energy Total Body Irradiation, Cyclophosphamide and Continuous Infusion Etoposide," *Bone Marrow Transplant*, 1990, 5(2):83-9.

deJonge ME, Huitema AD, vanDam SM, et al, "Significant Induction of Cyclophosphamide and Thiotepa Metabolism by Phenytoin," *Cancer Chemother Pharmacol*, 2005, 55(5):507-10.

Hutchins LF and Lipschitz DA, "Cancer, Clinical Pharmacology, and Aging," *Clin Geriatr Med*, 1987, 3(3):483-503.

Kaplan HG, "Use of Cancer Chemotherapy in the Elderly," *Drug Treatment in the Elderly*, Vestal RE, ed, Boston, MA: ADIS Health Science Press, 1984, 338-49.

McCune WJ, Golbus J, Zeldes W, et al, "Clinical and Immunologic Effects of Monthly Administration of Intravenous Cyclophosphamide in Severe Systemic Lupus Erythematosus," *N Engl J Med*, 1988, 318(22):1423-31.

Xie H, Griskevicius L, Stahle L, et al, "Pharmacogenetics of Cyclophosphamide in Patients With Hematologic Malignancies," *Eur J Pharm Sci*, 2006, 27(1):54-61.

CycloSERINE (sye kloe SER een)

Medication Safety Issues

Sound-alike/look-alike issues:

CycloSERINE may be confused with cyclobenzaprine, cycloSPORINE

U.S. Brand Names Seromycin®

Generic Available No

Pharmacologic Category Antibiotic, Miscellaneous; Antitubercular Agent

Use Adjunctive treatment in pulmonary or extrapulmonary tuberculosis; treatment of acute urinary tract infections caused by *E. coli* or *Enterobacter* sp when less toxic conventional therapy has failed or is contraindicated

Unlabeled/Investigational Use Treatment of Gaucher's disease

Contraindications Hypersensitivity to cycloserine or any component of the formulation

Warnings/Precautions Has been associated with CNS toxicity, including seizures, psychosis, depression, and confusion; decrease dosage or discontinue use if occurs. Use with caution in patients with epilepsy, depression, severe anxiety, psychosis, severe renal insufficiency, chronic alcoholism and patients with potential folate deficiency (malnourished, chronic anticonvulsant therapy, or elderly). Prolonged use may result in fungal or bacterial superinfection, including *C. difficile*-associated diarrhea and pseudomembranous colitis.

Adverse Reactions (Reflective of adult population; not specific for elderly)

Frequency not defined.

Cardiovascular: Cardiac arrhythmia

Central nervous system: Drowsiness, headache, dizziness, vertigo, seizure, confusion, psychosis, paresis, coma

Dermatologic: Rash

Endocrine & metabolic: Vitamin B_{12} deficiency

Hematologic: Folate deficiency

Hepatic: Liver enzymes increased

Neuromuscular & skeletal: Tremor

Overdosage/Toxicology Symptoms include confusion, agitation, CNS depression, psychosis, coma, and seizures. Decontaminate with activated charcoal. Can be hemodialyzed. Management is supportive. Administer pyridoxine 100-300 mg/day to reduce neurotoxic effects. Acute toxicity can occur with ingestions >1 g, chronic toxicity can occur with ingestions >500 mg/day.

Drug Interactions Increased toxicity: Alcohol, isoniazid, ethionamide increase toxicity of cycloserine; cycloserine inhibits the hepatic metabolism of phenytoin

Ethanol/Nutrition/Herb Interactions

Ethanol: Avoid ethanol (may increase CNS depression).

Food: May increase vitamin B_{12} and folic acid dietary requirements.

Mechanism of Action Inhibits bacterial cell wall synthesis by competing with amino acid (D-alanine) for incorporation into the bacterial cell wall; bacteriostatic or bactericidal

Pharmacokinetics

Absorption: Oral: ~70% to 90% from GI tract

(Continued)

CycloSERINE *(Continued)*

Half-life: Normal renal function: 10 hours

Time to peak serum concentration: Oral: Within 3-4 hours

Elimination: 60% to 70% of oral dose excreted unchanged in urine by glomerular filtration within 72 hours, small amounts excreted in feces, remainder is metabolized

Dosage

  Geriatrics & Adults: Note: Some of the neurotoxic effects may be relieved or prevented by the concomitant administration of pyridoxine.

    Tuberculosis: Oral: Initial: 250 mg every 12 hours for 14 days, then give 500 mg to 1 g/day in 2 divided doses for 18-24 months (maximum daily dose: 1 g)

  Renal Impairment:

    Cl_{cr} 10-50 mL/minute: Administer every 12-24 hours.

    Cl_{cr} <10 mL/minute: Administer every 24 hours.

Monitoring Parameters Check serum concentrations weekly for patients with decreased renal function, receiving >500 mg/day, or when toxicity is suspected

Reference Range Adequate CSF penetration; toxicity is greatly increased at concentrations >30 mcg/mL

Patient Information May cause drowsiness; notify physician if skin rash, mental confusion, dizziness, headache, or tremors occur

Additional Information Administer 100-300 mg/day of pyridoxine to relieve neurotoxic effects

Special Geriatric Considerations Adjust dose for renal function.

Dosage Forms Excipient information presented when available (limited, particularly for generics); consult specific product labeling.

Capsule: 250 mg

♦ **Cyclosporin A** see CycloSPORINE *on page 380*

CycloSPORINE (SYE kloe spor een)

Related Information

  Serum Drug Concentrations Commonly Monitored Guidelines *on page 1862*

Medication Safety Issues

  Sound-alike/look-alike issues:

    CycloSPORINE may be confused with cyclophosphamide, Cyklokapron®, cycloSERINE

    CycloSPORINE modified (Neoral®, Gengraf®) may be confused with cycloSPORINE non-modified (Sandimmne®)

    Gengraf® may be confused with Prograf®

    Neoral® may be confused with Neurontin®, Nizoral®

    Sandimmune® may be confused with Sandostatin®

U.S. Brand Names Gengraf®; Neoral®; Restasis®; Sandimmune®

Canadian Brand Names Neoral®; Rhoxal-cyclosporine; Sandimmune® I.V.; Sandoz-Cyclosporine

Index Terms CsA; CyA; Cyclosporin A

Generic Available Yes

Pharmacologic Category Immunosuppressant Agent

Use Prophylaxis of organ rejection in kidney, liver, and heart transplants, has been used with azathioprine and/or corticosteroids; severe, active rheumatoid arthritis (RA) not responsive to methotrexate alone; severe, recalcitrant plaque psoriasis in nonimmunocompromised adults unresponsive to or unable to tolerate other systemic therapy

  Ophthalmic emulsion (Restasis™): Increase tear production when suppressed tear production is presumed to be due to keratoconjunctivitis sicca-associated ocular inflammation (in patients not already using topical anti-inflammatory drugs or punctal plugs)

Unlabeled/Investigational Use Short-term, high-dose cyclosporine as a modulator of multidrug resistance in cancer treatment; allogenic bone marrow transplants for prevention and treatment of graft-versus-host disease; also used in some cases of severe autoimmune disease (ie, SLE, myasthenia gravis) that are resistant to corticosteroids and other therapy; focal segmental glomerulosclerosis

Contraindications Hypersensitivity to cyclosporine or any component of the formulation. Rheumatoid arthritis and psoriasis: Abnormal renal function, uncontrolled hypertension, malignancies. Concomitant treatment with PUVA or UVB therapy, methotrexate, other immunosuppressive agents, coal tar, or radiation therapy are also contraindications for use in patients with psoriasis. Ophthalmic emulsion is contraindicated in patients with active ocular infections.

Warnings/Precautions [U.S. Boxed Warning]: Renal impairment, including structural kidney damage has occurred (when used at high doses); monitor renal function closely. Use caution with other potentially nephrotoxic drugs (eg, acyclovir, aminoglycoside antibiotics, amphotericin B, ciprofloxacin). Increased risk of lymphomas and other malignancies. **[U.S. Boxed Warning]: Increased risk of infection. [U.S. Boxed Warning]: May cause hypertension.** Use caution when changing dosage forms. **[U.S. Boxed Warning]: Cyclosporine (modified) has increased bioavailability as compared to cyclosporine (non-modified) and cannot be used interchangeably without close monitoring.** Monitor cyclosporine concentrations closely following the addition, modification, or deletion of other medications; live, attenuated vaccines may be less effective; use should be avoided. Increased hepatic enzymes and bilirubin have occurred (when used at high doses); improvement usually seen with dosage reduction.

Transplant patients: To be used initially with corticosteroids. May cause significant hyperkalemia and hyperuricemia, seizures (particularly if used with high dose corticosteroids), and encephalopathy. Make dose adjustments based on cyclosporine blood concentrations. **[U.S. Boxed Warning]: Adjustment of dose should only be made under the direct supervision of an experienced physician.** Anaphylaxis has been reported with I.V. use; reserve for patients who cannot take oral form.

Psoriasis: Patients should avoid excessive sun exposure. **[U.S. Boxed Warning]: Risk of skin cancer may be increased with a history of PUVA and possibly methotrexate or other immunosuppressants, UVB, coal tar, or radiation.**

Rheumatoid arthritis: If receiving other immunosuppressive agents, radiation or UV therapy, concurrent use of cyclosporine is not recommended.

Products may contain corn oil, castor oil, ethanol, or propylene glycol; injection also contains Cremophor® EL (polyoxyethylated castor oil), which has been associated with rare anaphylactic reactions.

Adverse Reactions (Reflective of adult population; not specific for elderly)
Adverse reactions reported with systemic use, including rheumatoid arthritis, psoriasis, and transplantation (kidney, liver, and heart). Percentages noted include the highest frequency regardless of indication/dosage. Frequencies may vary for specific conditions or formulation.

>10%:
Cardiovascular: Hypertension (8% to 53%), edema (5% to 14%)
Central nervous system: Headache (2% to 25%)
Dermatologic: Hirsutism (21% to 45%), hypertrichosis (5% to 19%)
Endocrine & metabolic: Triglycerides increased (15%), female reproductive disorder (9% to 11%)
Gastrointestinal: Nausea (23%), diarrhea (3% to 13%), gum hyperplasia (2% to 16%), abdominal discomfort (<1% to 15%), dyspepsia (2% to 12%)
Neuromuscular & skeletal: Tremor (7% to 55%), paresthesia (1% to 11%), leg cramps/muscle contractions (2% to 12%)
Renal: Renal dysfunction/nephropathy (10% to 38%), creatinine increased (16% to ≥50%)
Respiratory: Upper respiratory infection (1% to 14%)
Miscellaneous: Infection (3% to 25%)

Kidney, liver, and heart transplant only (≤2% unless otherwise noted):
Cardiovascular: Flushes (<1% to 4%), MI
Central nervous system: Convulsions (1% to 5%), anxiety, confusion, fever, lethargy
Dermatologic: Acne (1% to 6%), brittle fingernails, hair breaking, pruritus
Endocrine & metabolic: Gynecomastia (<1% to 4%), hyperglycemia
Gastrointestinal: Nausea (2% to 10%), vomiting (2% to 10%), diarrhea (3% to 8%), abdominal discomfort (<1% to 7%), cramps (0% to 4%), anorexia, constipation, gastritis, mouth sores, pancreatitis, swallowing difficulty, upper GI bleed, weight loss
Hematologic: Leukopenia (<1% to 6%), anemia, thrombocytopenia
Hepatic: Hepatotoxicity (<1% to 7%)
Neuromuscular & skeletal: Paresthesia (1% to 3%), joint pain, muscle pain, tingling, weakness
Ocular: Conjunctivitis, visual disturbance
Otic: Hearing loss, tinnitus
Renal: Hematuria
Respiratory: Sinusitis (<1% to 7%)
Miscellaneous: Lymphoma (<1% to 6%), allergic reactions, hiccups, night sweats

Rheumatoid arthritis only (1% to <3% unless otherwise noted):
Cardiovascular: Hypertension (8%), edema (5%), chest pain (4%), arrhythmia (2%), abnormal heart sounds, cardiac failure, MI, peripheral ischemia
Central nervous system: Dizziness (8%), pain (6%), insomnia (4%), depression (3%), migraine (2%), anxiety, hypoesthesia, emotional lability, impaired concentration, malaise, nervousness, paranoia, somnolence, vertigo
Dermatologic: Purpura (3%), abnormal pigmentation, angioedema, cellulitis, dermatitis, dry skin, eczema, folliculitis, nail disorder, pruritus, skin disorder, urticaria
Endocrine & metabolic: Menstrual disorder (3%), breast fibroadenosis, breast pain, diabetes mellitus, goiter, hot flashes, hyperkalemia, hyperuricemia, hypoglycemia, libido increased/decreased

(Continued)

CycloSPORINE *(Continued)*

Gastrointestinal: Vomiting (9%), flatulence (5%), gingivitis (4%), gum hyperplasia (2%), constipation, dry mouth, dysphagia, enanthema, eructation, esophagitis, gastric ulcer, gastritis, gastroenteritis, gingival bleeding, glossitis, peptic ulcer, salivary gland enlargement, taste perversion, tongue disorder, tooth disorder, weight loss/gain

Genitourinary: Leukorrhea (1%), abnormal urine, micturition urgency, nocturia, polyuria, pyelonephritis, urinary incontinence, uterine hemorrhage

Hematologic: Anemia, leukopenia

Hepatic: Bilirubinemia

Neuromuscular & skeletal: Paresthesia (8%), tremor (8%), leg cramps/muscle contractions (2%), arthralgia, bone fracture, joint dislocation, myalgia, neuropathy, stiffness, synovial cyst, tendon disorder, weakness

Ocular: Abnormal vision, cataract, conjunctivitis, eye pain

Otic: Tinnitus, deafness, vestibular disorder

Renal: BUN increased, hematuria, renal abscess

Respiratory: Cough (5%), dyspnea (5%), sinusitis (4%), abnormal chest sounds, bronchospasm, epistaxis

Miscellaneous: Infection (9%), abscess, allergy, bacterial infection, carcinoma, fungal infection, herpes simplex, herpes zoster, lymphadenopathy, moniliasis, diaphoresis increased, tonsillitis, viral infection

Psoriasis only (1% to <3% unless otherwise noted):

Cardiovascular: Chest pain, flushes

Central nervous system: Psychiatric events (4% to 5%), pain (3% to 4%), dizziness, fever, insomnia, nervousness, vertigo

Dermatologic: Hypertrichosis (5% to 7%), acne, dry skin, folliculitis, keratosis, pruritus, rash, skin malignancies

Endocrine & metabolic: Hot flashes

Gastrointestinal: Nausea (5% to 6%), diarrhea (5% to 6%), gum hyperplasia (4% to 6%), abdominal discomfort (3% to 6%), dyspepsia (2% to 3%), abdominal distention, appetite increased, constipation, gingival bleeding

Genitourinary: Micturition increased

Hematologic: Bleeding disorder, clotting disorder, platelet disorder, red blood cell disorder

Hepatic: Hyperbilirubinemia

Neuromuscular & skeletal: Paresthesia (5% to 7%), arthralgia (1% to 6%)

Ocular: Abnormal vision

Respiratory: Bronchospasm (5%), cough (5%), dyspnea (5%), rhinitis (5%), respiratory infection

Miscellaneous: Flu-like syndrome (8% to 10%)

Ophthalmic emulsion (Restasis®):

>10%: Ocular: Burning (17%)

1% to 10%: Ocular: Hyperemia (conjunctival 5%), eye pain, pruritus, stinging

Overdosage/Toxicology Symptoms of overdose include hepatotoxicity, nephrotoxicity, nausea, vomiting, tremor. CNS secondary to direct action of the drug may not be reflected in serum concentrations, may be more predictable by renal magnesium loss. Forced emesis may be beneficial if done within 2 hours of ingestion of oral cyclosporine. Treatment is symptom-directed and supportive. Cyclosporine is not dialyzable.

Drug Interactions Substrate of CYP3A4 (major); **Inhibits** CYP2C9 (weak), 3A4 (moderate)

ACE inhibitors: May enhance nephrotoxic effects of cyclosporine.

Allopurinol: Increases cyclosporine concentrations by inhibiting cyclosporine metabolism.

Amiodarone: May increase cyclosporine concentrations by inhibiting cyclosporine metabolism.

Antibiotics: Concomitant use may potentiate renal dysfunction (seen with ciprofloxacin, gentamicin, tobramycin, vancomycin, trimethoprim and sulfamethoxazole); increased cyclosporine concentrations by inhibiting cyclosporine metabolism (seen with azithromycin, clarithromycin, erythromycin, and norfloxacin, quinupristin/ dalfopristin); may decrease cyclosporine concentrations by inducing cyclosporine metabolism (seen with nafcillin, and rifampin); may decrease immunosuppressant effects (seen with ciprofloxacin); CNS disturbances, seizures (seen with imipenem).

Anticonvulsants: May decrease cyclosporine concentrations by inducing cyclosporine metabolism (seen with carbamazepine, phenobarbital, and phenytoin)

Antineoplastics: Concomitant use may potentiate renal dysfunction (seen with melphalan)

Antifungals: Concomitant use may potentiate renal dysfunction (seen with amphotericin B, ketoconazole); increase cyclosporine concentrations by inhibiting cyclosporine metabolism (seen with fluconazole, itraconazole, and ketoconazole)

Bosentan: Cyclosporine may increase the serum concentration of bosentan. Bosentan may decrease the serum concentration of cyclosporine. Concurrent use is contraindicated.

Bromocriptine: Increases cyclosporine concentrations by inhibiting cyclosporine metabolism

Calcium channel blockers (diltiazem, nicardipine, verapamil): Increase cyclosporine concentrations by inhibiting cyclosporine metabolism. Nifedipine has been reported to increase the risk of gingival hyperplasia.

Colchicine: May potentiate renal dysfunction; colchicine may increase cyclosporine concentrations by inhibiting metabolism. Cyclosporine may decrease the clearance of colchicine.

Corticosteroids: Systemic corticosteroids may increase the serum concentration of cyclosporine (reported with methylprednisolone). Cyclosporine may increase the serum concentration of systemic corticosteroids. Convulsions have been reported with high-dose methylprednisolone.

CYP3A4 inducers: CYP3A4 inducers may decrease the levels/effects of cyclosporine. Example inducers include aminoglutethimide, carbamazepine, nafcillin, nevirapine, phenobarbital, phenytoin, and rifamycins.

CYP3A4 inhibitors: May increase the levels/effects of cyclosporine. Example inhibitors include azole antifungals, clarithromycin, diclofenac, doxycycline, erythromycin, imatinib, isoniazid, nefazodone, nicardipine, propofol, protease inhibitors, quinidine, telithromycin, and verapamil.

CYP3A4 substrates: Cyclosporine may increase the levels/effects of CYP3A4 substrates. Example substrates include benzodiazepines, calcium channel blockers, cyclosporine, mirtazapine, nateglinide, nefazodone, sildenafil (and other PDE-5 inhibitors), tacrolimus, and venlafaxine. Selected benzodiazepines (midazolam and triazolam), cisapride, ergot alkaloids, selected HMG-CoA reductase inhibitors (lovastatin and simvastatin), and pimozide are generally contraindicated with strong CYP3A4 inhibitors.

Danazol: Increases cyclosporine concentrations by inhibiting cyclosporine metabolism

Digoxin: Decreased clearance and decreased volume of distribution of digoxin; severe digitalis toxicity has been observed.

Fibric acid derivatives: May increase the risk of renal dysfunction and may alter cyclosporine concentrations; monitor.

H_2 blockers: Concomitant use may potentiate renal dysfunction (seen with cimetidine, ranitidine).

HMG-CoA reductase inhibitors: Cyclosporine may increase levels/effects of HMG-CoA reductase inhibitors, resulting in myalgias, rhabdomyolysis, acute renal failure; dosage adjustments of HMG-CoA reductase inhibitors are recommended.

Imatinib: May increase cyclosporine serum concentrations by inhibiting cyclosporine metabolism.

Immunosuppressives: Concomitant use may potentiate renal dysfunction (seen with tacrolimus, muromonab-CD3).

Metoclopramide: Increases cyclosporine concentrations by inhibiting cyclosporine metabolism.

Methotrexate: Cyclosporine increases plasma levels of methotrexate and decreases plasma levels of its metabolite; monitor closely for signs of toxicity.

Minoxidil: Concomitant use may lead to severe hypertrichosis.

NSAIDs: Concomitant use may potentiate renal dysfunction, especially in dehydrated patients (seen with diclofenac, naproxen, sulindac). In addition, diclofenac plasma levels are doubled when given with cyclosporine; the lowest possible dose of diclofenac should be used. Monitor serum creatinine.

Octreotide: May decrease cyclosporine concentrations by inducing cyclosporine metabolism.

Oral contraceptives (hormonal): May increase serum levels of cyclosporine; monitor for signs of toxicity.

Orlistat: May decrease absorption of cyclosporine; avoid concomitant use.

Protease inhibitors: Formal interaction studies have not been done; protease inhibitors are known to induce CYP3A4; use caution when using cyclosporine with indinavir, nelfinavir, ritonavir, or saquinavir.

Rifabutin: Formal interaction studies have not been done; rifabutin is known to increase the metabolism of medications via CYP3A4.

Sirolimus: Cyclosporine may increase serum levels/effects; monitor. Concurrent therapy may increase the risk of HUS/TTP/TMA. Administer sirolimus 4 hours after cyclosporine to minimize the increase in sirolimus blood levels.

Sulfasalazine: May decrease cyclosporine levels.

Sulfinpyrazone: May decrease cyclosporine levels by inducing cyclosporine metabolism; monitor.

Ticlopidine: May decrease cyclosporine concentrations by inducing cyclosporine metabolism.

Vaccines: Vaccination may be less effective; avoid use of live vaccines during therapy.

Voriconazole: Cyclosporine serum concentrations may be increased; monitor serum concentrations and renal function. Decrease cyclosporine dosage by 50% when initiating voriconazole.

(Continued)

CycloSPORINE *(Continued)*

Ethanol/Nutrition/Herb Interactions

Food: Grapefruit juice increases absorption; unsupervised use should be avoided.

Herb/Nutraceutical: Avoid St John's wort; as an enzyme inducer, it may increase the metabolism of and decrease plasma levels of cyclosporine; organ rejection and graft loss have been reported. Avoid cat's claw, echinacea (have immunostimulant properties).

Stability

Capsule: Store at controlled room temperature.

Injection: Store at controlled room temperature; do not refrigerate. Ampuls should be protected from light. Stability of injection of parenteral admixture at room temperature (25°C) is 6 hours in PVC; 24 hours in Excel®, PAB® containers, or glass.

Sandimmune® injection: Injection should be further diluted [1 mL (50 mg) of concentrate in 20-100 mL of D_5W or NS] for administration by intravenous infusion.

Ophthalmic emulsion: Store at 15°C to 25°C (59°F to 77°F). Vials are single-use; discard immediately following administration.

Oral solution: Store at controlled room temperature; do not refrigerate. Use within 2 months after opening; should be mixed in glass containers.

Neoral® oral solution: Orange juice, apple juice; avoid changing diluents frequently; mix thoroughly and drink at once.

Sandimmune® oral solution: Milk, chocolate milk, orange juice; avoid changing diluents frequently; mix thoroughly and drink at once.

Mechanism of Action

Inhibition of production and release of interleukin II and inhibits interleukin II-induced activation of resting T-lymphocytes.

Pharmacokinetics

Absorption:

Ophthalmic emulsion: Serum concentrations not detectable.

Oral: Incomplete and erratic

Protein binding: 90% to 98% in blood is bound to lipoproteins

Metabolism: Extensively hepatic via CYP3A4; forms at least 25 metabolites; extensive first-pass effect following oral administration

Bioavailability: Gut dysfunction, commonly seen in BMT recipients reduces oral bioavailability further

Half-life: Adults: 19-40 hours

Time to peak serum concentration: 3-4 hours

Elimination: Primarily in bile, clearance is decreased in patients with liver disease

Dosage

Geriatrics: Refer to adult dosing. **Sandimmune® and Neoral®/Genraf® are not bioequivalent and cannot be used interchangeably.**

Adults: Neoral®/Genraf® and Sandimmune® are not bioequivalent and cannot be used interchangeably.

Newly-transplanted patients: Adjunct therapy with corticosteroids is recommended. Initial dose should be given 4-12 hours prior to transplant or may be given postoperatively; adjust initial dose to achieve desired plasma concentration.

Oral: Dose is dependent upon type of transplant and formulation:

Cyclosporine (modified):

Renal: 9 ± 3 mg/kg/day, divided twice daily

Liver: 8 ± 4 mg/kg/day, divided twice daily

Heart: 7 ± 3 mg/kg/day, divided twice daily

Cyclosporine (non-modified): Initial dose: 15 mg/kg/day as a single dose (range 14-18 mg/kg); lower doses of 10-14 mg/kg/day have been used for renal transplants. Continue initial dose daily for 1-2 weeks; taper by 5% per week to a maintenance dose of 5-10 mg/kg/day; some renal transplant patients may be dosed as low as 3 mg/kg/day

Note: When using the non-modified formulation, cyclosporine levels may increase in liver transplant patients when the T-tube is closed; dose may need decreased

I.V.: Manufacturer's labeling: Cyclosporine (non-modified): Initial dose: 5-6 mg/kg/day as a single dose ($^1/_3$ the oral dose), infused over 2-6 hours; use should be limited to patients unable to take capsules or oral solution; patients should be switched to an oral dosage form as soon as possible

Note: Many transplant centers administer cyclosporine as "divided dose" infusions (in 2-3 doses/day) or as a continuous (24-hour) infusion; dosages range from 3-7.5 mg/kg/day. Specific institutional protocols should be consulted.

Note: Conversion to cyclosporine (modified) from cyclosporine (non-modified): Start with daily dose previously used and adjust to obtain preconversion cyclosporine trough concentration. Plasma concentrations should be monitored every 4-7 days and dose adjusted as necessary, until desired trough level is obtained. When transferring patients with previously poor absorption of cyclosporine (non-modified), monitor trough levels at least twice weekly (especially if initial dose exceeds 10 mg/kg/day); high plasma levels are likely to occur.

Rheumatoid arthritis: Oral: Cyclosporine (modified): Initial dose: 2.5 mg/kg/day, divided twice daily; salicylates, NSAIDs, and oral glucocorticoids may be continued (refer to Drug Interactions); dose may be increased by 0.5-0.75 mg/kg/day if insufficient response is seen after 8 weeks of treatment; additional dosage increases may be made again at 12 weeks (maximum dose: 4 mg/kg/day). Discontinue if no benefit is seen by 16 weeks of therapy.

Note: Increase the frequency of blood pressure monitoring after each alteration in dosage of cyclosporine. Cyclosporine dosage should be decreased by 25% to 50% in patients with no history of hypertension who develop sustained hypertension during therapy and, if hypertension persists, treatment with cyclosporine should be discontinued.

Psoriasis: Oral: Cyclosporine (modified): Initial dose: 2.5 mg/kg/day, divided twice daily; dose may be increased by 0.5 mg/kg/day if insufficient response is seen after 4 weeks of treatment; additional dosage increases may be made every 2 weeks if needed (maximum dose: 4 mg/kg/day). Discontinue if no benefit is seen by 6 weeks of therapy. Once patients are adequately controlled, the dose should be decreased to the lowest effective dose. Doses <2.5 mg/kg/day may be effective. Treatment longer than 1 year is not recommended.

Note: Increase the frequency of blood pressure monitoring after each alteration in dosage of cyclosporine. Cyclosporine dosage should be decreased by 25% to 50% in patients with no history of hypertension who develop sustained hypertension during therapy and, if hypertension persists, treatment with cyclosporine should be discontinued.

Focal segmental glomerulosclerosis (unlabeled use): Initial: 3 mg/kg/day divided every 12 hours

Autoimmune diseases (unlabeled use): 1-3 mg/kg/day

Keratoconjunctivitis sicca: Ophthalmic: (Restasis®): Instill 1 drop in each eye every 12 hours

Renal Impairment: For severe psoriasis:

Serum creatinine levels ≥25% above pretreatment levels: Take another sample within 2 weeks; if the level remains ≥25% above pretreatment levels, decrease dosage of cyclosporine (modified) by 25% to 50%. If two dosage adjustments do not reverse the increase in serum creatinine levels, treatment should be discontinued.

Serum creatinine levels ≥50% above pretreatment levels: Decrease cyclosporine dosage by 25% to 50%. If two dosage adjustments do not reverse the increase in serum creatinine levels, treatment should be discontinued.

Hemodialysis: Supplemental dose is not necessary.

Peritoneal dialysis: Supplemental dose is not necessary.

Hepatic Impairment: Dosage adjustment is probably necessary; monitor levels closely

Administration

Oral solution: Do not administer liquid from plastic or styrofoam cup. May dilute Neoral® oral solution with orange juice or apple juice. May dilute Sandimmune® oral solution with milk, chocolate milk, or orange juice. Avoid changing diluents frequently. Mix thoroughly and drink at once. Use syringe provided to measure dose. Mix in a glass container and rinse container with more diluent to ensure total dose is taken. Do not rinse syringe before or after use (may cause dose variation).

I.V.: The manufacturer recommends that following dilution, intravenous admixture be administered over 2-6 hours. However, many transplant centers administer as divided doses (2-3 doses/day) or as a 24-hour continuous infusion. Discard solution after 24 hours. Anaphylaxis has been reported with I.V. use; reserve for patients who cannot take oral form. Patients should be under continuous observation for at least the first 30 minutes of the infusion, and should be monitored frequently thereafter. Maintain patent airway; other supportive measures and agents for treating anaphylaxis should be present when I.V. drug is given.

Ophthalmic emulsion: Prior to use, invert vial several times to obtain a uniform emulsion. Remove contact lenses prior to instillation of drops; may be reinserted 15 minutes after administration. May be used with artificial tears; allow 15 minute interval between products.

Monitoring Parameters Cyclosporine serum concentrations, serum electrolytes, renal function, hepatic function, blood pressure, pulse

Reference Range Reference ranges are method dependent and specimen dependent; use the same analytical method consistently

Method-dependent and specimen-dependent: Trough levels should be obtained:

Oral: 12-18 hours after dose (chronic usage)

I.V.: 12 hours after dose **or** immediately prior to next dose

Therapeutic range: Not absolutely defined, dependent on organ transplanted, time after transplant, organ function and CsA toxicity:

General range of 100-400 ng/mL

Toxic level: Not well defined, nephrotoxicity may occur at any level

(Continued)

CycloSPORINE *(Continued)*

Test Interactions Specific whole blood, HPLC assay for cyclosporine may be falsely elevated if sample is drawn from the same line through which dose was administered (even if flush has been administered and/or dose was given hours before).

Patient Information Use glass container for liquid solution (do not use plastic or styrofoam cup). Diluting oral solution improves flavor. May dilute Neoral® oral solution with orange juice or apple juice. May dilute Sandimmune® oral solution with milk, chocolate milk, or orange juice. Avoid changing diluents frequently. Mix thoroughly and drink at once; rinse container to get full dose. Take at the same time each day and always take with food or always without. Do not change brands unless directed by your physician.

Ophthalmic emulsion: Prior to use, invert vial several times to obtain a uniform emulsion. Remove contact lenses prior to instillation of drops; may be reinserted 15 minutes after administration. May be used with artificial tears; allow 15-minute interval between products.

Additional Information Cyclosporine (modified): Refers to the capsule dosage formulation of cyclosporine in an aqueous dispersion (previously referred to as "microemulsion"). Cyclosporine (modified) has increased bioavailability as compared to cyclosporine (nonmodified) and cannot be used interchangeably without close monitoring.

Special Geriatric Considerations Cyclosporine has not been specifically studied in the elderly. Cyclosporine is being used in combination therapy for the treatment of severe rheumatoid arthritis.

Dosage Forms Excipient information presented when available (limited, particularly for generics); consult specific product labeling.

Capsule, soft gel, modified: 25 mg, 100 mg [contains castor oil, ethanol]
  Gengraf®: 25 mg, 100 mg [contains ethanol, castor oil, propylene glycol]
  Neoral®: 25 mg, 100 mg [contains dehydrated ethanol, corn oil, castor oil, propylene glycol]
Capsule, soft gel, non-modified (Sandimmune®): 25 mg, 100 mg [contains dehydrated ethanol, corn oil]
Emulsion, ophthalmic [preservative free, single-use vial] (Restasis®): 0.05% (0.4 mL) [contains glycerin, castor oil, polysorbate 80, carbomer 1342; 32 vials/box]
Injection, solution, non-modified (Sandimmune®): 50 mg/mL (5 mL) [contains Cremophor® EL (polyoxyethylated castor oil), ethanol]
Solution, oral, modified:
  Gengraf®: 100 mg/mL (50 mL) [contains castor oil, propylene glycol]
  Neoral®: 100 mg/mL (50 mL) [contains dehydrated ethanol, corn oil, castor oil, propylene glycol]
Solution, oral, non-modified (Sandimmune®): 100 mg/mL (50 mL) [contains olive oil, ethanol]

Selected References

Burckart GJ, Canafax DM, and Yee GC, "Cyclosporine Monitoring," *Drug Intell Clin Pharm*, 1986, 20(9):649-52.

Wells G and Tugwell P, "Cyclosporin A in Rheumatoid Arthritis: Overview of Efficacy," *Br J Rheumatol*, 1993, 32(Suppl 1):51-6.

♦ **Cymbalta®** *see* Duloxetine *on page 491*

Cyproheptadine *(si proe HEP ta deen)*

Related Information
  Potentially Inappropriate Medications for Geriatrics *on page 1824*
Medication Safety Issues
  Sound-alike/look-alike issues:
    Cyproheptadine may be confused with cyclobenzaprine
    Periactin may be confused with Perative®, Percodan®, Persantine®
Index Terms Cyproheptadine Hydrochloride; Periactin
Generic Available Yes
Pharmacologic Category Antihistamine
Use Treatment of perennial and seasonal allergic rhinitis and other allergic symptoms including urticaria
Unlabeled/Investigational Use Appetite stimulation; treatment of blepharospasm, cluster and migraine headaches, Nelson's syndrome, pruritus, schizophrenia, spinal cord damage- associated spasticity, tardive dyskinesia
Contraindications Hypersensitivity to cyproheptadine or any component of the formulation; narrow-angle glaucoma; bladder neck obstruction; acute asthmatic attack; stenosing peptic ulcer; GI tract obstruction; concurrent use of MAO inhibitors
Warnings/Precautions Do not use in symptomatic prostate hypertrophy; antihistamines are more likely to cause dizziness, excessive sedation, syncope, toxic confusion states, and hypotension in the elderly. In case reports, cyproheptadine has promoted

weight gain in anorexic adults, though it has not been specifically studied in the elderly. All cases of weight loss or decreased appetite should be adequately assessed.

Adverse Reactions (Reflective of adult population; not specific for elderly)
>10%:
  Central nervous system: Slight to moderate drowsiness
  Respiratory: Thickening of bronchial secretions
1% to 10%:
  Central nervous system: Dizziness, fatigue, headache, nervousness
  Gastrointestinal: Abdominal pain, appetitie stimulation, diarrhea, nausea, xerostomia
  Neuromuscular & skeletal: Arthralgia
  Respiratory: Pharyngitis

Overdosage/Toxicology Symptoms include CNS depression or stimulation, dry mouth, flushed skin, fixed and dilated pupils, and apnea. There is no specific treatment for an antihistamine overdose, however, clinical toxicity is mostly due to anticholinergic effects. Anticholinesterase inhibitors may be useful by reducing acetylcholinesterase. Anticholinesterase inhibitors include physostigmine, neostigmine, pyridostigmine, and edrophonium. For anticholinergic overdose with severe life-threatening symptoms, physostigmine 1-2 mg slow I.V. may be given to reverse these effects.

Drug Interactions
Cyproheptadine may potentiate the effect of CNS depressants.
MAO inhibitors may cause hallucinations when taken with cyproheptadine.

Ethanol/Nutrition/Herb Interactions Ethanol: Avoid ethanol (may increase CNS sedation).

Mechanism of Action A potent antihistamine and serotonin antagonist, competes with histamine for H_1-receptor sites on effector cells in the gastrointestinal tract, blood vessels, and respiratory tract

Pharmacokinetics
Metabolism: Almost completely
Elimination: >50% excreted in urine (primarily as metabolites) and ~25% excreted in feces

Dosage
  Geriatrics: Oral: Initial: 4 mg twice daily
  Adults:
    Appetite stimulation (including anorexia nervosa): Oral: 2 mg 4 times/day; may be increased gradually over a 3-week period to 8 mg 4 times/day
    Allergic conditions: Oral: 4-20 mg/day divided every 8 hours (not to exceed 0.5 mg/kg/day)
    Cluster headaches: Oral: 4 mg 4 times/day
    Migraine headaches: Oral: 4-8 mg 3 times/day
    Spasticity associated with spinal cord damage: Oral: 4 mg at bedtime; increase by a 4 mg dose every 3-4 days; average daily dose: 16 mg in divided doses; not to exceed 36 mg/day
  Hepatic Impairment: Dosage should be reduced in patients with significant hepatic dysfunction.

Monitoring Parameters Relief of symptoms, weight

Test Interactions Diagnostic antigen skin test results may be suppressed; false positive serum TCA screen

Patient Information May cause drowsiness; avoid CNS depressants and alcohol

Additional Information May stimulate appetite

Special Geriatric Considerations In case reports, cyproheptadine has promoted weight gain in anorexic adults, though it has not been specifically studied in the elderly. All cases of weight loss or decreased appetite should be adequately assessed. Cyproheptadine may cause less sedation than diphenhydramine or hydroxyzine and, therefore, may be useful for pruritus in elderly; however, elderly may not tolerate anticholinergic effects.

Dosage Forms Excipient information presented when available (limited, particularly for generics); consult specific product labeling.
Syrup, as hydrochloride: 2 mg/5 mL (473 mL) [contains alcohol 5%; mint flavor]
Tablet, as hydrochloride: 4 mg

DALTEPARIN

- **D₃** see Cholecalciferol *on page 304*
- **D-3-Mercaptovaline** see Penicillamine *on page 1218*
- **Dacodyl™ [OTC]** see Bisacodyl *on page 173*
- **Dalmane®** see Flurazepam *on page 653*
- **d-Alpha-Gems™ [OTC]** see Vitamin E *on page 1677*
- **d-Alpha Tocopherol** see Vitamin E *on page 1677*

Dalteparin (dal TE pa rin)

Related Information
Anticoagulants, Injectable *on page 1741*

Medication Safety Issues
High alert medication: The Institute for Safe Medication Practices (ISMP) includes this medication among its list of drugs which have a heightened risk of causing significant patient harm when used in error.

U.S. Brand Names Fragmin®
Canadian Brand Names Fragmin®
Index Terms Dalteparin Sodium; NSC-714371
Generic Available No
Pharmacologic Category Low Molecular Weight Heparin

Use Prevention of deep vein thrombosis which may lead to pulmonary embolism, in patients requiring abdominal surgery who are at risk for thromboembolism complications (eg, patients >40 years of age, obesity, patients with malignancy, history of deep vein thrombosis or pulmonary embolism, and surgical procedures requiring general anesthesia and lasting >30 minutes); prevention of DVT in patients undergoing hip-replacement surgery; patients immobile during an acute illness; acute treatment of unstable angina or non-Q-wave myocardial infarction; prevention of ischemic complications in patients on concurrent aspirin therapy; in patients with cancer, extended treatment (6 months) of acute symptomatic venous thromboembolism (DVT and/or PE) to reduce the recurrence of venous thromboembolism

Unlabeled/Investigational Use Active treatment of deep vein thrombosis (noncancer patients)

Contraindications Hypersensitivity to dalteparin or any component of the formulation; thrombocytopenia associated with a positive *in vitro* test for antiplatelet antibodies in the presence of dalteparin; hypersensitivity to heparin or pork products; patients with active major bleeding; patients with unstable angina, non-Q-wave MI, or acute venous thromboembolism undergoing regional anesthesia; not for I.M. or I.V. use

Warnings/Precautions Use with caution in patients with pre-existing thrombocytopenia, subacute bacterial endocarditis, peptic ulcer disease, pericarditis or pericardial effusion, liver or renal function impairment, recent lumbar puncture, vasculitis, concurrent use of aspirin (increased bleeding risk), previous hypersensitivity to heparin, heparin-associated thrombocytopenia. Monitor platelet count closely. Rare thrombocytopenia may occur. Consider discontinuation of dalteparin in any patient developing significant thrombocytopenia related to initiation of dalteparin. Rare cases of thrombocytopenia with thrombosis have occurred. Use caution in patients with congenital or drug-induced thrombocytopenia or platelet defects. If thromboembolism develops despite dalteparin prophylaxis, dalteparin should be discontinued and appropriate treatment should be initiated. Cancer patients with thrombocytopenia may require dose adjustments for treatment of acute venous thromboembolism.

Use with caution in patients with known hypersensitivity to methylparaben or propylparaben. Monitor patient closely for signs or symptoms of bleeding. Certain patients are at increased risk of bleeding. Risk factors include bacterial endocarditis; congenital or acquired bleeding disorders; active ulcerative or angiodysplastic GI diseases; severe uncontrolled hypertension; hemorrhagic stroke; or use shortly after brain, spinal, or ophthalmology surgery; in patient treated concomitantly with platelet inhibitors; recent GI bleeding; thrombocytopenia or platelet defects; severe liver disease; hypertensive or diabetic retinopathy; or in patients undergoing invasive procedures.

Use with caution in patients with severe renal failure (has not been studied). Rare cases of thrombocytopenia with thrombosis have occurred. Heparin can cause hyperkalemia by affecting aldosterone. Similar reactions could occur with LMWHs. Monitor for hyperkalemia. Do **not** administer intramuscularly.

[U.S. Boxed Warning]: Patients with recent or anticipated neuraxial anesthesia (epidural or spinal anesthesia) are at risk of spinal or epidural hematoma and subsequent paralysis. Consider risk versus benefit prior to neuraxial anesthesia. Risk is increased by concomitant agents which may alter hemostasis, as well as traumatic or repeated epidural or spinal puncture. Patient should be observed closely for bleeding if dalteparin is administered during or immediately following diagnostic lumbar puncture, epidural anesthesia, or spinal anesthesia.

388

Adverse Reactions (Reflective of adult population; not specific for elderly)
Note: As with all anticoagulants, bleeding is the major adverse effect of dalteparin. Hemorrhage may occur at virtually any site. Risk is dependent on multiple variables.

>10%:
  Hematologic: Bleeding (3% to 14%)
1% to 10%:
  Hematologic: Wound hematoma (up to 3%)
  Hepatic: AST >3 times upper limit of normal (5% to 9%), ALT >3 times upper limit of normal (4% to 10%)
  Local: Pain at injection site (up to 12%), injection site hematoma (up to 7%)

Overdosage/Toxicology
Symptoms of overdose include hemorrhage. Protamine sulfate has been used to reverse effects (protamine 1 mg neutralizes dalteparin 100 int. units). Monitor aPTT 2-4 hours after first infusion; consider readministration of protamine (50% of original dose). **Note:** Anti-Xa activity is never completely neutralized (maximum of 60% to 75%). Avoid overdose of protamine. Treatment is otherwise symptom-directed and supportive.

Drug Interactions
Anticoagulants: May enhance the anticoagulant effect of dalteparin.
Antiplatelet agents: May enhance the anticoagulant effect of dalteparin.
Dasatinib: May enhance the anticoagulant effect of dalteparin.
Drotrecogin alfa: Heparin (Low Molecular Weight), particularly at therapeutic doses, may enhance the adverse/toxic effect of drotrecogin alfa. Bleeding may occur.
Nonsteroidal anti-inflammatory agents: May enhance the anticoagulant effect of dalteparin.
Salicylates: May enhance the anticoagulant effect of dalteparin.
Treprostinil: May enhance the adverse/toxic effect of dalteparin. Bleeding may occur.

Ethanol/Nutrition/Herb Interactions Herb/Nutraceutical: Alfalfa, anise, bilberry, bladderwrack, bromelain, cat's claw, celery, chamomile, coleus, cordyceps, dong quai, evening primrose oil, fenugreek, feverfew, garlic, ginger, ginkgo biloba, Ginseng (american), Ginseng (panax), Ginseng (siberian), grapeseed, green tea, guggul, horse chestnut seed, horseradish, licorice, prickly ash, red clover, reishi, SAMe (s-adenosylmethionine), sweet clover, turmeric, white willow (all have additional antiplatelet/anticoagulant activity)●

Stability Store at temperatures of 20°C to 25°C (68°F to 77°F). Multidose vials may be stored for up to 2 weeks at room temperature after entering.

Mechanism of Action Low molecular weight heparin analog with a molecular weight of 4000-6000 daltons; the commercial product contains 3% to 15% heparin with a molecular weight <3000 daltons, 65% to 78% with a molecular weight of 3000-8000 daltons and 14% to 26% with a molecular weight >8000 daltons; while dalteparin has been shown to inhibit both factor Xa and factor IIa (thrombin), the antithrombotic effect of dalteparin is characterized by a higher ratio of antifactor Xa to antifactor IIa activity (ratio = 4)

Pharmacodynamics T_{max}: SubQ: 2.3-3 hours after single injection

Pharmacokinetics Geriatrics: Pharmacokinetics not shown to be significantly altered by age.
Distribution: V_d: 40-60 mL/kg
Bioavailability: SubQ: 87%
Half-life:
  Normal renal function: 1.82 hours
  Patients with chronic renal insufficiency requiring hemodialysis: 5.7 hours
Elimination: Renal; clearance: 15-25 mL/minute

Dosage
Geriatrics & Adults:
Abdominal surgery (DVT prophylaxis):
  Low-to-moderate DVT risk: SubQ: 2500 int. units 1-2 hours prior to surgery, then once daily for 5-10 days postoperatively
  High DVT risk: SubQ: 5000 int. units the evening prior to surgery and then once daily for 5-10 days postoperatively. Alternatively in patients with malignancy: 2500 int. units 1-2 hours prior to surgery, 2500 int. units 12 hours later, then 5000 int. units once daily for 5-10 days postoperatively.
Total hip surgery (DVT prophylaxis): SubQ: **Note:** Three treatment options are currently available. Dose is given for 5-10 days, although up to 14 days of treatment have been tolerated in clinical trials:
  Postoperative start:
  Initial: 2500 int. units 4-8 hours* after surgery
  Maintenance: 5000 int. units once daily; start at least 6 hours after postsurgical dose
  Preoperative (starting day of surgery):
  Initial: 2500 int. units within 2 hours before surgery
  Adjustment: 2500 int. units 4-8 hours* after surgery

(Continued)

Dalteparin *(Continued)*

Maintenance: 5000 int. units once daily; start at least 6 hours after postsurgical dose

Preoperative (starting evening prior to surgery):
Initial: 5000 int. units 10-14 hours before surgery
Adjustment: 5000 int. units 4-8 hours* after surgery
Maintenance: 5000 int. units once daily, allowing 24 hours between doses.
*Note: Dose may be delayed if hemostasis is not yet achieved.

Unstable angina or non-Q-wave myocardial infarction: SubQ: 120 int. units/kg body weight (maximum dose: 10,000 int. units) every 12 hours for 5-8 days with concurrent aspirin therapy. Discontinue dalteparin once patient is clinically stable.

Venous thromboembolism: SubQ: Cancer patients:
Initial (month 1): 200 int. units/kg (maximum dose: 18,000 int. units) once daily for 30 days
Maintenance (months 2-6): ~150 int. units/kg (maximum dose: 18,000 int. units) once daily. If platelet count between 50,000-100,000/mm^3, reduce dose by 2,500 int. units until platelet count recovers to ≥100,000/mm^3. If platelet count <50,000/mm^3, discontinue dalteparin until platelet count recover to >50,000/mm^3.

Immobility/acute illness (DVT prophylaxis): 5000 int. units once daily

Renal Impairment: In cancer patients, receiving treatment for venous thromboembolism, if Cl$_{cr}$ <30 mL/minute, manufacturer recommends monitoring anti-Xa levels to determine appropriate dose.

Administration For deep SubQ injection only. May be injected in a U-shape to the area surrounding the navel, the upper outer side of the thigh, or the upper outer quadrangle of the buttock. Apply pressure to injection site; do not massage. Use thumb and forefinger to lift a fold of skin when injecting dalteparin to the navel area or thigh. Insert needle at a 45- to 90-degree angle. The entire length of needle should be inserted. Do not expel air bubble from fixed-dose syringe prior to injection. Air bubble (and extra solution, if applicable) may be expelled from graduated syringes.

Administration once daily beginning prior to surgery and continuing 5-10 days after surgery prevents deep vein thrombosis in patients at risk for thromboembolic complications. For unstable angina or non-Q-wave myocardial infarction, dalteparin is administered every 12 hours until the patient is stable (5-8 days).

Monitoring Parameters Periodic CBC including platelet count; stool occult blood tests; monitoring of PT and PTT is not necessary. Once patient has received 3-4 doses, anti-Xa levels, drawn 4-6 hours after dalteparin administration, may be used to monitor effect in patients with severe renal dysfunction or if abnormal coagulation parameters or bleeding should occur.

Reference Range Treatment: Venous thromboembolism: Target anti-Xa range: 0.5-1.5 int. units/mL

Special Geriatric Considerations No specific recommendations are necessary for the elderly.

Dosage Forms Excipient information presented when available (limited, particularly for generics); consult specific product labeling.

Injection, solution [multidose vial]: Antifactor Xa 10,000 int. units per 1 mL (9.5 mL) [contains benzyl alcohol]; antifactor Xa 25,000 units per 1 mL (3.8 mL) [contains benzyl alcohol]

Injection, solution [preservative free; prefilled syringe]: Antifactor Xa 2500 int. units per 0.2 mL (0.2 mL); antifactor Xa 5000 int. units per 0.2 mL (0.2 mL); antifactor Xa 7500 int. units per 0.3 mL (0.3 mL); antifactor Xa 10,000 int. units per 0.4 mL (0.4 mL), antifactor Xa 12,500 int. units per 0.5 mL (0.5 mL); antifactor Xa 15,000 int. units per 0.6 mL (0.6 mL); antifactor Xa 18,000 int. units per 0.72 mL (0.72 mL)

Injection, solution [preservative free; graduated prefilled syringe]: Antifactor Xa 10,000 int. units/1 mL (1 mL)

Selected References
Simoneau G, Bergmann JF, Kher A, et al, "Pharmacokinetics of a Low Molecular Weight Heparin (Fragmin®) in Young and Elderly Subjects," *Thromb Res*, 1992, 66(5):603-7.

♦ **Dalteparin Sodium** *see* Dalteparin *on page 388*

Danaparoid (da NAP a roid)

Related Information
Anticoagulants, Injectable *on page 1741*
Canadian Brand Names Organan®
Index Terms Danaparoid Sodium
Generic Available No
Pharmacologic Category Anticoagulant
Use Prevention of postoperative deep vein thrombosis following elective hip replacement surgery

Unlabeled/Investigational Use Systemic anticoagulation for patients with heparin-induced thrombocytopenia: factor Xa inhibition is used to monitor degree of anticoagulation if necessary

Restrictions Not available in U.S.

Contraindications Hypersensitivity to danaproid or thrombocytopenia associated with a positive *in vitro* test for antiplatelet antibodies in the presence of danaproid; hypersensitivity to pork products or to sulfites (contains metabisulfite); patients with active major bleeding; severe hemorrhagic diathesis (hemophilia, idiopathic thrombocytopenic purpura); not for I.M. or I.V. use

Warnings/Precautions Do not administer intramuscularly. Danaproid shows a low cross-sensitivity with antiplatelet antibodies in individuals with type II heparin-induced thrombocytopenia. This product contains sodium sulfite which may cause allergic-type reactions, including anaphylactic symptoms and life-threatening asthmatic episodes in susceptible people; this is seen more frequently in asthmatics.

Carefully monitor patients receiving low molecular weight heparins or heparinoids. These drugs, when used concurrently with spinal or epidural anesthesia or spinal puncture, may cause bleeding or hematomas within the spinal column. Increased pressure on the spinal cord may result in permanent paralysis if not detected and treated immediately.

Use with caution in patients with known hypersensitivity to methylparaben or propylparaben. Use with caution in patients with history of heparin-induced thrombocytopenia. Monitor patient closely for signs or symptoms of bleeding. Certain patients are at increased risk of bleeding. Risk factors include bacterial endocarditis; congenital or acquired bleeding disorders; active ulcerative or angiodysplastic GI diseases; severe uncontrolled hypertension; hemorrhagic stroke; use shortly after brain, spinal, or ophthalmology surgery; patient treated concomitantly with platelet inhibitors; recent GI bleeding; thrombocytopenia or platelet defects; severe liver disease; hypertensive or diabetic retinopathy; or patients undergoing invasive procedures. Use with caution in patients with severe renal failure (has not been studied). Heparin can cause hyperkalemia by affecting aldosterone. A similar reaction could occur with danaproid. Monitor for hyperkalemia.

Note: Danaproid is **not** effectively antagonized by protamine sulfate. No other antidote is available, so extreme caution is needed in monitoring dose given and resulting Xa inhibition effect.

Adverse Reactions (Reflective of adult population; not specific for elderly) As with all anticoagulants, bleeding is the major adverse effect of danaproid. Hemorrhage may occur at virtually any site. Risk is dependent on multiple variables.

>10%:
  Central nervous system: Fever (22%)
  Gastrointestinal: Nausea (4% to 14%), constipation (4% to 11%)
1% to 10%:
  Cardiovascular: Peripheral edema (3%), edema (3%)
  Central nervous system: Insomnia (3%), headache (3%), asthenia (2%), dizziness (2%), pain (9%)
  Dermatologic: Rash (2% to 5%), pruritus (4%)
  Gastrointestinal: Vomiting (3%)
  Genitourinary: Urinary tract infection (3% to 4%), urinary retention (2%)
  Hematologic: Anemia (2%)
  Local: Injection site pain (8% to 14%), injection site hematoma (5%)
  Neuromuscular & skeletal: Joint disorder (3%)
  Miscellaneous: Infection (2%)

Overdosage/Toxicology Symptom include hemorrhage. Protamine zinc has been used to reverse effects.

Drug Interactions
  Drugs which affect platelet function (eg, aspirin, NSAIDs, dipyridamole, ticlopidine, clopidogrel) may potentiate the risk of hemorrhage.
  Thrombolytic agents increase the risk of hemorrhage.
  Warfarin (and other oral anticoagulants) may increase the risk of bleeding with danaproid.

Ethanol/Nutrition/Herb Interactions Herb/Nutraceutical: Avoid cat's claw, dong quai, evening primrose, feverfew, garlic, ginger, ginkgo, red clover, horse chestnut, green tea, and ginseng (all have additional antiplatelet activity).

Stability Store intact vials or ampuls under refrigeration.

Mechanism of Action Prevents fibrin formation in coagulation pathway via thrombin generation inhibition by anti-Xa and anti-IIa effects.

Pharmacokinetics
  Half-life, plasma: Mean terminal half-life: ~24 hours
  Elimination: Primarily by the kidneys
  (Continued)

Danaparoid *(Continued)*

Dosage
Geriatrics & Adults:

Prevention of DVT following hip replacement: SubQ: 750 anti-Xa units twice daily; beginning 1-4 hours before surgery and then not sooner than 2 hours after surgery and every 12 hours until the risk of DVT has diminished, the average duration of therapy is 7-10 days

Treatment (unlabeled uses): See table.

Adult Danaparoid Treatment Dosing Regimens (not FDA approved)

	Body Weight (kg)	I.V. Bolus aFX-aU	Long-Term Infusion aFXaU	Level of aFXaU/mL	Monitoring
Deep Vein Thrombosis OR Acute Pulmonary Embolism	<55 55-90 >90	1250 2500 3750	400 units/h over 4 h, then 300 units/h over 4 h, then 150-200 units/h maintenance dose	0.5-0.8	Days 1-3 daily, then every alternate day
Deep Vein Thrombosis OR Pulmonary Embolism >5 d old	<90 >90	1250 1250	SubQ: 3 x 750/d SubQ: 3 x 1250/d	<0.5	Not necessary
Embolectomy	<90 >90 and high risk	2500 preoperatively 2500 preoperatively	SubQ: 2 x 1250/d postoperatively 150-200 units/h I.V.; perioperative arterial irrigation, if necessary: 750 units/20 mL NaCl	<0.4 0.5 0.8	Not necessary Days 1-3 daily, then every alternate day
Peripheral Arterial Bypass		2500 preoperatively	150-200 units/h	0.5-0.8	Days 1-3 daily, then every alternate day
Cardiac Catheter	<90 >90	2500 preoperatively 3750 preoperatively			
Surgery (excluding vascular)			SubQ: 750, 1-4 h preoperatively SubQ: 750, 2-5 h postoperatively, then 2 x 750/d	<0.35	Not necessary

Renal Impairment: Adjustment may be necessary in patients with severe renal impairment. Patients with serum creatinine levels ≥2.0 mg/dL should be carefully monitored. SubQ: Hemodialysis: See table.

Hemodialysis With Danaparoid Sodium

Dialysis on alternate days:	Dosage prior to dialysis in aFXaU (dosage for body wt <55 kg):	
First dialysis	3750 (<55 kg 2500)	
Second dialysis	3750 (<55 kg 2000)	
Further dialysis:		
aFXa level before dialysis (eg, day 5)	**Bolus before next dialysis, aFXaU (eg, day 7)**	**aFXa level during dialysis**
<0.3	3000 (<55 kg 2000)	0.5-0.8
0.3-0.35	2500 (<55 kg 2000)	
0.35-0.4	2000 (<55 kg 1500)	
>0.4	No bolus; if fibrin strands occur, 1500 aFXaU I.V.	
Monitoring: 30 minutes before dialysis and after 4 hours of dialysis		
Daily Dialysis		
First dialysis	3750 (<55 kg 2500)	
Second dialysis	2500 (<55 kg 2000)	
Further dialyses	See above	
As with "dialysis on alternate days", always take the aFXa activity preceding the previous dialysis as a basis for the current dosage.		

Administration Administer SubQ, not I.M.; have patient lie down and administer by deep SubQ injection using a fine needle (25-26 gauge); rotate sites of injection

Monitoring Parameters Platelets, occult blood, and anti-Xa activity, if available; the monitoring of PT and/or PTT is not necessary; stool for occult blood; urinalysis

Special Geriatric Considerations Evaluation of elderly's creatinine serum concentrations is important before initiating therapy.

Dosage Forms Excipient information presented when available (limited, particularly for generics); consult specific product labeling. [CAN] = Canadian brand name
Injection, solution:
Orgaran® [CAN]: 750 anti-Xa units/0.6 mL (0.6 mL) [not available in the U.S.]

♦ **Danaparoid Sodium** see Danaparoid on page 390
♦ **Dantrium®** see Dantrolene on page 393

Dantrolene (DAN troe leen)

Medication Safety Issues
Sound-alike/look-alike issues:
Dantrium® may be confused with danazol, Daraprim®
U.S. Brand Names Dantrium®
Canadian Brand Names Dantrium®
Index Terms Dantrolene Sodium
Generic Available Yes: Capsule
Pharmacologic Category Skeletal Muscle Relaxant
Use Treatment of spasticity associated with spinal cord injury, stroke, cerebral palsy, or multiple sclerosis; treatment of malignant hyperthermia
Unlabeled/Investigational Use Treatment of neuroleptic malignant syndrome (NMS)
Contraindications Active hepatic disease; should not be used where spasticity is used to maintain posture or balance
Warnings/Precautions Use with caution in patients with impaired cardiac function or impaired pulmonary function. **[U.S. Boxed Warning]: Has potential for hepatotoxicity.** Overt hepatitis has been most frequently observed between the third and twelfth month of therapy. Hepatic injury appears to be greater in females and in patients >35 years of age. Idiosyncratic and hypersensitivity reactions (sometimes fatal) of the liver have also occurred.
Adverse Reactions (Reflective of adult population; not specific for elderly)
>10%:
Central nervous system: Drowsiness, dizziness, lightheadedness, fatigue
Dermatologic: Rash
Gastrointestinal: Diarrhea (mild), nausea, vomiting
Neuromuscular & skeletal: Muscle weakness
1% to 10%:
Cardiovascular: Pleural effusion with pericarditis
Central nervous system: Chills, fever, headache, insomnia, nervousness, mental depression
Gastrointestinal: Diarrhea (severe), constipation, anorexia, stomach cramps
Ocular: Blurred vision
Respiratory: Respiratory depression
Overdosage/Toxicology Symptoms include CNS depression, hypotension, nausea, and vomiting. For decontamination, lavage/activated charcoal with cathartic; do not use ipecac. Hypotension can be treated with isotonic I.V. fluids with the patient placed in the Trendelenburg position. Dopamine or norepinephrine can be given if hypotension is refractory to the above therapy.
Drug Interactions Substrate of CYP3A4 (major)
CYP3A4 inducers: CYP3A4 inducers may decrease the levels/effects of dantrolene. Example inducers include aminoglutethimide, carbamazepine, nafcillin, nevirapine, phenobarbital, phenytoin, and rifamycins.
CYP3A4 inhibitors: May increase the levels/effects of dantrolene. Example inhibitors include azole antifungals, clarithromycin, diclofenac, doxycycline, erythromycin, imatinib, isoniazid, nefazodone, nicardipine, propofol, protease inhibitors, quinidine, telithromycin, and verapamil.
Increased toxicity: Estrogens (hepatotoxicity), CNS depressants (sedation), MAO inhibitors, phenothiazines, clindamycin (increased neuromuscular blockade), verapamil (hyperkalemia and cardiac depression), warfarin, clofibrate, and tolbutamide
Ethanol/Nutrition/Herb Interactions
Ethanol: Avoid ethanol (may increase CNS depression).
Herb/Nutraceutical: Avoid valerian, St John's wort, kava kava, gotu kola (may increase CNS depression).
Stability Reconstitute vial by adding 60 mL of sterile water for injection USP (**not bacteriostatic water for injection**). Protect from light. Use within 6 hours; avoid glass bottles for I.V. infusion.
Mechanism of Action Acts directly on skeletal muscle by interfering with release of calcium ion from the sarcoplasmic reticulum; prevents or reduces the increase in myoplasmic calcium ion concentration that activates the acute catabolic processes associated with malignant hyperthermia
(Continued)

Dantrolene *(Continued)*

Pharmacokinetics
Absorption: Slow and incomplete from GI tract
Metabolism: Slowly in the liver
Half-life: 8.7 hours
Elimination: 25% in urine as metabolites and unchanged drug, and 45% to 50% in feces via bile

Dosage
Geriatrics & Adults:
Spasticity: Oral: 25 mg/day to start, increase frequency to 2-4 times/day, then increase dose by 25 mg every 4-7 days to a maximum of 100 mg 2-4 times/day or 400 mg/day
Malignant hyperthermia:
Preoperative prophylaxis:
Oral: 4-8 mg/kg/day in 4 divided doses, begin 1-2 days prior to surgery with last dose 3-4 hours prior to surgery
I.V.: 2.5 mg/kg ~1¼ hours prior to anesthesia and infused over 1 hour with additional doses as needed and individualized
Crisis: I.V.: 2.5 mg/kg; may repeat dose up to cumulative dose of 10 mg/kg; if physiologic and metabolic abnormalities reappear, repeat regimen
Postcrisis follow-up: Oral: 4-8 mg/kg/day in 4 divided doses for 1-3 days; I.V. dantrolene may be used when oral therapy is not practical; individualize dosage beginning with 1 mg/kg or more as the clinical situation dictates
Neuroleptic malignant syndrome (unlabeled use): I.V.: 1 mg/kg; may repeat dose up to maximum cumulative dose of 10 mg/kg, then switch to oral dosage

Monitoring Parameters Blood pressure, pulse, temperature, liver function tests, motor performance

Patient Information Avoid unnecessary exposure to sunlight (or use sunscreen, protective clothing); avoid CNS depressants; patients should use caution while driving or performing other tasks requiring alertness

Additional Information Avoid glass bottles for I.V. infusion; exercise caution at meals on the day of administration because difficulty swallowing and choking has been reported

Special Geriatric Considerations There is little experience with this drug in the elderly.

Dosage Forms Excipient information presented when available (limited, particularly for generics); consult specific product labeling.
Capsule, as sodium: 25 mg, 50 mg, 100 mg
Dantrium®: 25 mg, 50 mg, 100 mg
Injection, powder for reconstitution, as sodium:
Dantrium®: 20 mg [contains mannitol 3 g]

Extemporaneously Prepared A suspension can be prepared by mixing 500 mg (from capsules) with 150 mg citric acid, 10 mL distilled water, and sufficient simple syrup to bring the total volume to 100 mL (final concentration 5 mg/mL)

Selected References
Ward A, Chaffman MO, and Sorkin EM, "Dantrolene: A Review of Its Pharmacodynamic and Pharmacokinetic Properties and Therapeutic Use in Malignant Hyperthermia, the Neuroleptic Malignant Syndrome and an Update of Its Use in Muscle Spasticity," *Drugs*, 1986, 32(2):130-68.

♦ **Dantrolene Sodium** *see* Dantrolene *on page 393*
♦ **Dapcin** *see* Daptomycin *on page 395*

Dapiprazole *(DA pi pray zole)*

U.S. Brand Names Rēv-Eyes™
Index Terms Dapiprazole Hydrochloride
Generic Available No
Pharmacologic Category Alpha₁ Blocker, Ophthalmic
Use Reverse dilation due to drugs (adrenergic or parasympathomimetic) after eye exams
Contraindications Contraindicated in the presence of conditions where miosis is unacceptable, such as acute iritis and in patients with a history of hypersensitivity to any component of the formulation
Warnings/Precautions For ophthalmic use only
Adverse Reactions (Reflective of adult population; not specific for elderly)
>10%:
Central nervous system: Headache
Ocular: Conjunctival injection, burning and itching eyes, lid edema, ptosis, lid erythema, chemosis, punctate keratitis, corneal edema, photophobia
1% to 10%: Ocular: Dry eyes, blurred vision, tearing of eye
Drug Interactions No data reported

Stability After reconstitution, drops are stable at room temperature for 21 days. Store at room temperature (15°C to 30°C/59°F to 86°F).

Mechanism of Action Dapiprazole is a selective alpha-adrenergic blocking agent, exerting effects primarily on alpha$_1$-adrenoreceptors. It induces miosis via relaxation of the smooth dilator (radial) muscle of the iris, which causes pupillary constriction. It is devoid of cholinergic effects. Dapiprazole also partially reverses the cycloplegia induced with parasympatholytic agents such as tropicamide. Although the drug has no significant effect on the ciliary muscle *per se*, it may increase accommodative amplitude, therefore relieving the symptoms of paralysis of accommodation.

Dosage

Geriatrics & Adults: Reversal of dilation: Ophthalmic: Instill 2 drops followed 5 minutes later by an additional 2 drops into the conjunctiva of each eye; should not be used more frequently than once a week in the same patient

Administration Finger pressure should be applied to lacrimal sac for 1-2 minutes after instillation to decrease risk of absorption and systemic reactions; do not touch eye with dropper

Patient Information May still be sensitive to sunlight and sensitivity may return in 2 or more hours; store at room temperature

Special Geriatric Considerations No specific data in elderly.

Dosage Forms Excipient information presented when available (limited, particularly for generics); consult specific product labeling.

Powder, ophthalmic, as hydrochloride: 25 mg [contains benzalkonium chloride; 0.5% solution when mixed with supplied diluent]

♦ **Dapiprazole Hydrochloride** *see* Dapiprazole *on page 394*

Daptomycin (DAP toe mye sin)

Medication Safety Issues

Sound-alike/look-alike issues:

Daptomycin may be confused with dactinomycin

U.S. Brand Names Cubicin®

Index Terms Cidecin; Dapcin; LY146032

Generic Available No

Pharmacologic Category Antibiotic, Cyclic Lipopeptide

Use Treatment of complicated skin and skin structure infections caused by susceptible aerobic Gram-positive organisms; bacteremia, including right-sided infective endocarditis caused by MSSA or MRSA

Unlabeled/Investigational Use Treatment of severe infections caused by MRSA or VRE

Contraindications Hypersensitivity to daptomycin or any component of the formulation

Warnings/Precautions May be associated with an increased incidence of myopathy; discontinue in patients with signs and symptoms of myopathy in conjunction with an increase in CPK (>5 times ULN or 1000 units/L) or in asymptomatic patients with a CPK ≥10 times ULN. Myopathy may occur more frequently at dose and/or frequency in excess of recommended dosages. Use caution in patients receiving other drugs associated with myopathy (eg, HMG-CoA reductase inhibitors). Not indicated for the treatment of pneumonia (poor lung penetration). Use caution in renal impairment (dosage adjustment required). Symptoms suggestive of peripheral neuropathy have been observed with treatment; monitor for new-onset or worsening neuropathy. Prolonged use may result in fungal or bacterial superinfection, including *C. difficile*-associated diarrhea and pseudomembranous colitis.

Adverse Reactions (Reflective of adult population; not specific for elderly)

>10%:

Cardiovascular: Anemia (2% to 13%)

Gastrointestinal: Diarrhea (5% to 12%), vomiting (3% to 12%), constipation (6% to 11%)

1% to 10%:

Cardiovascular: Peripheral edema (7%), chest pain (7%), hypertension (1% to 6%), hypotension (2% to 5%)

Central nervous system: Insomnia (5% to 9%), headache (5% to7%), fever (2% to 7%), dizziness (2% to 6%), anxiety (5%)

Dermatologic: Rash (4% to 7%), pruritus (3% to 6%), erythema (5%)

Endocrine & metabolic: Hypokalemia (9%), hyperkalemia (5%), hyperphosphatemia (3%)

Gastrointestinal: Nausea (6% to 10%), abdominal pain (6%), dyspepsia (1% to 4%), loose stool (4%), GI hemorrhage (2%)

Genitourinary: Urinary tract infection (2% to 7%)

Hematologic: INR increased (2%), eosinophilia (2%)

Hepatic: Transaminases increased (2% to 3%), alkaline phosphatase increased (2%)

(Continued)

Daptomycin *(Continued)*

Local: Injection site reaction (3% to 6%)

Neuromuscular & skeletal: CPK increased (3% to 9%), limb pain (2% to 9%), back pain (7%), weakness (5%), arthralgia (1% to 3%)

Renal: Renal failure (2% to 3%)

Respiratory: Pharyngolaryngeal pain (8%), pleural effusion (6%), cough (3%), pneumonia (3%), dyspnea (2% to 3%)

Miscellaneous: Osteomyelitis (6%), bacteremia (5%), diaphoresis (5%), sepsis (5%), infection (fungal, 2% to 3%)

Overdosage/Toxicology Treatment is symptomatic and supportive; hemodialysis removes approximately 15% in 4 hours.

Drug Interactions No clinically-significant interactions have been identified.

Stability Store under refrigeration at 2°C to 8°C (36°F to 46°F). Reconstitute vial with 10 mL NS. Add NS to vial and rotate gently to wet powder. Allow to stand for 10 minutes, then gently swirl to obtain completely reconstituted solution. Do not shake or agitate vial vigorously. Should be further diluted following reconstitution in an appropriate volume of NS. Reconstituted solution (either in vial or in infusion bag) is stable for a cumulative time of 12 hours at room temperature and 48 hours if refrigerated (2°C to 8°C).

Mechanism of Action Daptomycin binds to components of the cell membrane of susceptible organisms and causes rapid depolarization, inhibiting intracellular synthesis of DNA, RNA, and protein. Daptomycin is bactericidal in a concentration-dependent manner.

Pharmacokinetics

Distribution: 0.09 L/kg

Protein binding: 90% to 93%; 84% to 88% in patients with Cl_{cr}<30 mL/minute

Half-life elimination: 8-9 hours (up to 28 hours in renal impairment)

Elimination: Urine (78%; primarily as unchanged drug); feces (6%)

Dosage

Geriatrics & Adults:

Skin and/or skin structure infections (complicated): I.V.: 4 mg/kg once daily for 7-14 days

Bacteremia, right-sided endocarditis caused by MSSA or MRSA: I.V.: 6 mg/kg once daily for 2-6 weeks

Renal Impairment:

Cl_{cr} <30 mL/minute:

Skin and soft tissue infections: 4 mg/kg every 48 hours

Staphylococcal bacteremia: 6 mg/kg every 48 hours

Hemodialysis (administer after hemodialysis) and/or CAPD: Dose as in Cl_{cr} <30 mL/minute

Hepatic Impairment: No adjustment required for mild-to-moderate impairment (Child-Pugh Class A or B). Not evaluated in severe hepatic impairment.

Administration Infuse over 30 minutes.

Monitoring Parameters Monitor signs and symptoms of infection. CPK should be monitored at least weekly during therapy.

Reference Range

Trough concentrations at steady-state:

4 mg/kg once daily: 5.9 ± 1.6 mcg/mL

6 mg/kg once daily: 6.7 ± 1.6 mcg/mL

Note: Trough concentrations are not predictive of efficacy/toxicity. Drug exhibits concentration-dependent bactericidal activity, so C_{max}:MIC ratios may be a more useful parameter.

Test Interactions Daptomycin may cause false prolongation of the PT and increase of INR with certain reagents. This appears to be a dose-dependent phenomenon. Therefore, it is recommended to obtain blood samples immediately prior to next daptomycin dose (eg, trough). If PT/INR elevated, clinicians should repeat PT/INR and evaluate for other causes of hypocoagulation.

Patient Information Inform prescriber of all prescriptions, OTC medications, or herbal products you are taking, and any allergies you have. This medication can only be administered via intravenous infusion. You will be monitored during and after each infusion. Report immediately any throat tightness, respiratory difficulty or chest tightness, swelling or pain at infusion site, or skin rash. Report unusual headache, insomnia, nausea or vomiting, limb or joint pain, alteration in urination patterns, itching or pain on urination, or other possible adverse reactions.

Special Geriatric Considerations The manufacturer reports that in studies of complicated skin and skin structure infections, elderly patients had a lower clinical success rate and a higher incidence of adverse effects (no quantitative data provided in product labeling). Adjust dose in renal impairment.

Dosage Forms Excipient information presented when available (limited, particularly for generics); consult specific product labeling.

Injection, powder for reconstitution:
Cubicin®: 500 mg

Selected References

Tedesco KL and Rybak MJ, "Daptomycin," *Pharmacotherapy*, 2004, 24(1):41-57.

♦ **Daranide®** *see* Dichlorphenamide *on page 423*

Darbepoetin Alfa (dar be POE e tin AL fa)

Medication Safety Issues

Sound-alike/look-alike issues:
Darbepoetin alfa may be confused with epoetin alfa

U.S. Brand Names Aranesp®

Canadian Brand Names Aranesp®

Index Terms Erythropoiesis-Stimulating Agent (ESA); Erythropoiesis-Stimulating Protein; NSC-729969

Generic Available No

Pharmacologic Category Colony Stimulating Factor; Growth Factor; Recombinant Human Erythropoietin

Use Treatment of anemia associated with chronic renal failure (CRF), including patients on dialysis (ESRD) and patients not on dialysis; anemia associated with concurrent chemotherapy for nonmyeloid malignancies

Contraindications Hypersensitivity to darbepoetin or any component of the formulation; uncontrolled hypertension

Warnings/Precautions Erythropoietic therapies may be associated with an increased risk of cardiovascular and/or neurologic events. A target hemoglobin >12 g/dL and a rapid rise in hemoglobin are associated with increased risk of cardiovascular related events. **[U.S. Boxed Warning]: Use the minimum effective dose that will gradually increase the hemoglobin level to a point sufficient to avoid red blood cell transfusion.** Avoid hemoglobin increases >1 g/dL in any 2-week period, and do not exceed a target level of 12 g/dL. Prior to and during therapy, iron stores must be evaluated. Supplemental iron is recommended if serum ferritin <100 mcg/mL or serum transferrin saturation <20%. In cancer patients, the risk of thrombotic events (eg, pulmonary emboli, thrombophlebitis, thrombosis) was increased by erythropoietic therapy. **[U.S. Boxed Warning]: A higher incidence of deep vein thrombosis was reported in patients receiving ESAs for preoperative reduction in red blood cell transfusions who were not receiving prophylactic anticoagulation.** Increased mortality was also observed in patients undergoing coronary artery bypass surgery who received ESAs; these deaths were associated with thrombotic events. Darbepoetin is **not** approved for this indication.

[U.S. Boxed Warning]: An increased risk of mortality was reported in cancer patients administered ESAs to a target hemoglobin of 12 g/dL, who were not receiving concurrent chemotherapy or radiation therapy. Darbepoetin is **not** approved for this indication. ESAs also failed to reduce the number of red blood cell transfusions in this patient population. **[U.S. Boxed Warning]: Decreased survival was reported in metastatic breast cancer patients receiving concurrent chemotherapy and ESAs to a target hemoglobin of >12g/dL.** Malignant cell lines and tumors may have surface receptors for erythropoietin; it is not known if darbepoetin stimulates these receptors. **[U.S. Boxed Warning]: There may be a potential risk of shortening time to tumor progression;** this has been reported in advanced head and neck cancer patients receiving ESAs to a target hemoglobin >12 g/dL and concurrent radiation therapy.

Use with caution in patients with hypertension or with a history of seizures; hypertensive encephalopathy and seizures have been reported. If hypertension is difficult to control, reduce or hold darbepoetin alfa. **Not** recommended for acute correction of severe anemia or as a substitute for transfusion. Consider discontinuing in patients who receive a renal transplant.

Prior to treatment, correct or exclude deficiencies of vitamin B_{12} and/or folate, as well as other factors which may impair erythropoiesis (aluminum toxicity, inflammatory conditions, infections). Poor response should prompt evaluation of these potential factors, as well as possible malignant processes, occult blood loss, hemolysis, and/or bone marrow fibrosis. Pure red cell aplasia (PRCA) with associated neutralizing antibodies to erythropoietin has been reported, predominantly in patients with CRF. Patients with loss of response to darbepoetin alfa should be evaluated. Discontinue treatment in patients with PRCA secondary to neutralizing antibodies to erythropoietin.

Due to the delayed onset of erythropoiesis, darbepoetin is of no value in the acute treatment of anemia. Safety and efficacy in patients with underlying hematologic diseases have not been established, including porphyria, thalassemia, hemolytic anemia, and sickle cell disease. Potentially serious allergic reactions have been (Continued)

397

Darbepoetin Alfa *(Continued)*

reported. The packaging of some formulations may contain latex. Do not shake solution; vigorous shaking may denature darbepoetin alfa, rendering it biologically inactive.

Adverse Reactions (Reflective of adult population; not specific for elderly)

>10%:

Cardiovascular: Hypertension (4% to 23%), hypotension (22%), edema (21%), peripheral edema (11%)

Central nervous system: Fatigue (9% to 33%), fever (4% to 19%), headache (12% to 16%), dizziness (8% to 14%)

Gastrointestinal: Diarrhea (16% to 22%), constipation (5% to 18%), vomiting (2% to 15%), nausea (14%), abdominal pain (12%)

Neuromuscular & skeletal: Myalgia (8% to 21%), arthralgia (11% to 13%)

Respiratory: Upper respiratory infection (14%), dyspnea (2% to 12%)

Miscellaneous: Infection (27%)

1% to 10%:

Cardiovascular: Arrhythmia (10%), angina/chest pain (6% to 8%), fluid overload (6%), CHF (6%), thrombosis (6%), MI (2%)

Central nervous system: Seizure (≤1%), stroke (1%), TIA (1%)

Dermatologic: Pruritus (8%), rash (7%)

Endocrine & metabolic: Dehydration (3% to 5%)

Local: Vascular access thrombosis (8%), injection site pain (7%), vascular access hemorrhage (6%), vascular access infection (6%)

Neuromuscular & skeletal: Limb pain (10%), back pain (8%), weakness (5%)

Respiratory: Cough (10%), bronchitis (6%), pneumonia (3%), pulmonary embolism (1%)

Miscellaneous: Death (7% to 10 %; similar to placebo), flu-like syndrome (6%)

Postmarketing and/or case reports: Deep vein thrombosis, pure red cell aplasia, severe anemia (with or without other cytopenias), thromboembolism, thrombophlebitis

Overdosage/Toxicology The maximum amount of darbepoetin has not been determined. However, cardiovascular and neurologic adverse events have been correlated to excessive and/or rapid rise in hemoglobin. Phlebotomy may be performed if clinically indicated.

Drug Interactions No data available

Ethanol/Nutrition/Herb Interactions Ethanol: Should be avoided due to adverse effects on erythropoiesis.

Stability Store at 2°C to 8°C (36°F to 46°F). Do not freeze or shake. Protect from light. Do not dilute or administer with other solutions.

Mechanism of Action Induces erythropoiesis by stimulating the division and differentiation of committed erythroid progenitor cells; induces the release of reticulocytes from the bone marrow into the bloodstream, where they mature to erythrocytes. There is a dose response relationship with this effect. This results in an increase in reticulocyte counts followed by a rise in hematocrit and hemoglobin levels. When administered SubQ or I.V., darbepoetin's half-life is ~3 times that of epoetin alfa concentrations.

Pharmacokinetics

Absorption: Slowly absorbed following SubQ administration

Distribution: V_d: 0.06 L/kg

Bioavailability: CRF: SubQ: Adults: ~37% (range: 30% to 50%)

Half-life elimination: CRF: Terminal: I.V.: 21 hours, SubQ: 49 hours; cancer: SubQ: 74 hours

Note: Half-life is approximately threefold longer than epoetin alfa following I.V. administration

Time to peak: SubQ: CRF: 34 hours (range: 24-72 hours); Cancer: 71-90 hours

Dosage

Geriatrics & Adults: Note: Use the minimum effective dose that will gradually increase the hemoglobin level to a point sufficient to avoid red blood cell transfusion. Hemoglobin levels should not exceed 12 g/dL and should not rise >1 g/dL per 2-week time period.

Anemia associated with CRF: I.V., SubQ: Initial: 0.45 mcg/kg once weekly; titrate to response; some patients may respond to doses given once every 2 weeks

Unlabeled dosing:

Every 2-weeks: 0.75 mcg/kg every 2 weeks (Toto, 2004)

or

Every 4-weeks: 0.75 mcg/kg every 2 weeks; once titrated, multiply dose by 2 and give every 4 weeks (Jadoul, 2004).

Dosage adjustment:

Inadequate response: Increase dose by ~25% (not more frequently than once a month) for hemoglobin increase <1 g/dL after 4 weeks

Excessive response:

Decrease dose by ~25% when hemoglobin increases >1 g/dL in any 2-week period **or** hemoglobin increases and approaches 12 g/dL in any 2-week period

Hold dose, then decrease dose by ~25% when hemoglobin increases despite previous dose decrease (hold until hemoglobin decreases)

Anemia associated with chemotherapy: SubQ: Initial: 2.25 mcg/kg once weekly; with inadequate response after 6 weeks: 4.5 mcg/kg once weekly

or

500 mcg once every 3 weeks

Unlabeled dosing:

Every 2 weeks:

Initial: 200 mcg every 2 weeks; inadequate response: 300 mcg every 2 weeks (Thames, 2003)

or

Initial: 3 mcg/kg every 2 weeks; inadequate response: 5 mcg/kg every 2 weeks (Vadhan-Raj, 2003)

or

Every 3 weeks (front load): Initial:

4.5 mcg/kg every week until desired Hgb obtained; maintenance: 4.5 mcg/kg (or titrated dose) every 3 weeks (Hesketh, 2004)

or

Initial: 325 mcg every week until desired Hgb obtained; maintenance: 325 mcg every 3 weeks (Hesketh, 2004)

Dosage adjustment: Titration may be required to limit rises of Hgb to <1 g/dL over any 2-week interval and to reach a hemoglobin concentration not to exceed 12 g/dL.

Inadequate response: Increase dose up to 4.5 mcg/kg when hemoglobin increase <1 g/dL after 6 weeks

Excessive response:

Decrease dose by ~40% when hemoglobin increases >1 g/dL in any 2-week period **or** hemoglobin exceeds 11 g/dL in any 2-week period

If hemoglobin >12 g/dL, hold until hemoglobin falls to 11 g/dL and reinitiate with a dose 40% below the previous dose.

Conversion from epoetin alfa to darbepoetin alfa: See table.

Conversion From Epoetin Alfa to Darbepoetin Alfa

Previous Dosage of Epoetin Alfa (units/week)	Adults Darbepoetin Alfa Dosage (mcg/week)	Adults Darbepoetin Alfa Dosage (mcg/every 2 weeks)
<1500	6.25	12.5
1500-2499	6.25	12.5
2500-4999	12.5	25
5000-10,999	25	50
11,000-17,999	40	80
18,000-33,999	60	120
34,000-89,999	100	200
≥90,000	200	400

Note: In patients receiving epoetin alfa 2-3 times per week, darbepoetin alfa is administered once weekly. In patients receiving epoetin alfa once weekly, darbepoetin alfa is administered once every 2 weeks.

Renal Impairment: Dosage requirements for patients with chronic renal failure who do not require dialysis may be lower than in dialysis patients. Monitor patients closely during the time period in which a dialysis regimen is initiated, dosage requirement may increase. The National Kidney Foundation 2006 guidelines recommend hemoglobin levels ≥11 g/dL; hemoglobin levels should not be maintained ≥13 g/dL. These guidelines are currently being reassessed.

Administration May be administered by SubQ or I.V. injection. The I.V. route is recommended in hemodialysis patients. Do not shake; vigorous shaking may denature darbepoetin alfa, rendering it biologically inactive. Do not dilute or administer in conjunction with other drug solutions. Discard any unused portion of the vial; do not pool unused portions. Discontinue immediately if signs/symptoms of anaphylaxis occur.

Monitoring Parameters Hemoglobin (weekly); prior to and during therapy, iron stores must be evaluated (supplemental iron is recommended in any patient with a serum ferritin <100 mcg/mL or serum transferrin saturation <20%); blood pressure (Continued)

Darbepoetin Alfa *(Continued)*

Patient Information You will require frequent blood tests to determine appropriate dosage. Do not take other medications, vitamin or iron supplements, or make significant changes in your diet without consulting prescriber. Report signs or symptoms of edema (eg, swollen extremities, difficulty breathing, rapid weight gain), onset of severe headache, acute back pain, chest pain, or muscular tremors or seizure activity. Be careful to check blood pressure regularly.

Additional Information Supplemental iron intake may be required in patients with low iron stores. Due to the delayed onset of erythropoiesis, darbepoetin is of no value in the acute treatment of anemia. Emergency/stat orders for darbepoetin are inappropriate.

Dosage Forms Excipient information presented when available (limited, particularly for generics); consult specific product labeling. [DSC] = Discontinued product

Injection, solution [preservative free; contains human albumin 2.5 mg/mL; single-dose vial]:

Aranesp®: 25 mcg/mL (1 mL); 40 mcg/mL (1 mL); 60 mcg/mL (1 mL); 100 mcg/mL (1 mL); 150 mcg/0.75 mL (0.75 mL); 200 mcg/mL (1 mL); 300 mcg/mL (1 mL); 500 mcg/mL (1 mL) [DSC]

Injection, solution [preservative free; contains human albumin 2.5 mg/mL; prefilled syringe; needle cover contains latex]:

Aranesp®: 25 mcg/0.42 mL (0.42 mL); 40 mcg/0.4 mL (0.4 mL); 60 mcg/0.3 mL (0.3 mL); 100 mcg/0.5 mL (0.5 mL); 150 mcg/0.3 mL (0.3 mL); 200 mcg/0.4 mL (0.4 mL); 300 mcg/0.6 mL (0.6 mL); 500 mcg/mL (1 mL) [DSC]

Injection, solution [preservative free; contains polysorbate 80; prefilled syringe; needle cover contains latex]:

Aranesp®: 25 mcg/0.42 mL (0.42 mL); 40 mcg/ 0.4 mL (0.4 mL); 60 mcg/0.3 mL (0.3 mL); 100 mcg/0.5 mL (0.5 mL); 150 mcg/0.3 mL (0.3 mL); 200 mcg/0.4 mL (0.4 mL); 300 mcg/0.6 mL (0.6 mL); 500 mcg/mL (1 mL)

Injection, solution [preservative free; contains polysorbate 80; single-dose vial]:

Aranesp®: 200 mcg/mL (1 mL); 300 mcg/mL (1 mL)

Selected References

Besarab A, Bolton WK, Browne JK, et al, "The Effects of Normal as Compared With Low Hematocrit Values in Patients With Cardiac Disease who are Receiving Hemodialysis and Epoetin," *N Engl J Med*, 1998, 339:584-90.

Drueke TB, Locatelli F, Clyne N, et al, "Normalization of Hemoglobin Level in Patients With Chronic Kidney Disease and Anemia," *N Engl J Med*, 2006, 355(20): 2071-84.

Egrie JC and Browne KJ, "Development and Characterization of Novel Erythropoiesis Stimulation Protein (NESP)," *Br J Cancer*, 2001, 84(Suppl 1):3-10.

Hesketh PJ, Arena F, Patel D, et al, "A randomized Controlled Trial of Darbepoetin Alfa Administered as a Fixed or Weight-Based Dose Using a Front-Loading Schedule in Patients With Anemia Who Have Nonmyeloid Malignancies," *Cancer*, 2004, 100(4):859-68.

Jadoul M, Vanrenterghem Y, Foret M, et al, "Darbepoetin Alfa Administered Once Monthly Maintains Haemoglobin Levels in Stable Dialysis Patients," *Nephrol Dial Transplant*, 2004, 19(4):898-903.

NCCN (National Comprehensive Cancer Network), "Practice Guidelines in Oncology: Cancer- and Treatment-Related Anemia Version 1.2007." Available at http://www.nccn.org/professionals/physician_gls/PDF/anemia.pdf.

Thames W, Yao B, Scheifele A, et al, "Drug Use Evaluation (DUE) of Darbepoetin Alfa in Anemic Patients Undergoing Chemotherapy Supports a Fixed Dose of 200 mcg Q2W Given Every 2 Weeks (Q2W)," Asco Annual Meeting, 2003.

Toto RD, Pichette V, Brenner R, et al, "Darbepoetin Alfa Effectively Treats Anemia in Patients With Chronic Kidney Disease With de novo Every-Other-Week Administration," *Am J Nephrol*, 2004, 24(4):453-60.

Vadhan-Raj S, Mirtsching B, Charu V, et al, "Assessment of Hematologic Effects and Fatigue in Cancer Patients With Chemotherapy-Induced Anemia Given Darbepoetin Alfa Every Two Weeks," *J Support Oncol*, 2003, 1(2):131-8.

Darifenacin (dar i FEN a sin)

Related Information
Pharmacotherapy of Urinary Incontinence *on page 1822*
U.S. Brand Names Enablex®
Canadian Brand Names Enablex®
Index Terms Darifenacin Hydrobromide; UK-88,525
Generic Available No
Pharmacologic Category Anticholinergic Agent
Use Management of symptoms of bladder overactivity (urge incontinence, urgency, and frequency)
Contraindications Hypersensitivity to darifenacin or any component of the formulation; uncontrolled narrow-angle glaucoma; urinary retention, paralytic ileus, GI or GU obstruction
Warnings/Precautions Use with caution with hepatic impairment; dosage limitation is required in moderate hepatic impairment (Child-Pugh Class B). Not recommended for use in severe hepatic impairment (Child-Pugh Class C). Use with caution in patients with clinically-significant bladder outlet obstruction or prostatic hyperplasia (nonobstructive). Use caution in patients with decreased GI motility, constipation, hiatal

hernia, reflux esophagitis, and ulcerative colitis. Use caution in patients with myasthenia gravis. In patients with controlled narrow angle glaucoma, darifenacin should be used with extreme caution and only when the potential benefit outweighs risks of treatment.

Adverse Reactions (Reflective of adult population; not specific for elderly)
>10%: Gastrointestinal: Xerostomia (19% to 35%), constipation (15% to 21%)
1% to 10%:
Cardiovascular: Hypertension, peripheral edema
Central nervous system: Headache (7%), dizziness (1% to 2%)
Dermatological: Dry skin, pruritis, rash
Gastrointestinal: Dyspepsia (3% to 8%), abdominal pain (2% to 4%), nausea (2% to 4%), diarrhea (1% to 2%), vomiting, weight gain
Genitourinary: Urinary tract infection (4% to 5%), urinary retention, urinary tract disorder, vaginitis
Neuromuscular & skeletal: Weakness (2% to 3%), arthralgia, back pain
Ocular: Dry eyes (2%), abnormal vision
Respiratory: Bronchitis, pharyngitis, rhinitis, sinusitis
Miscellaneous: Flu-like syndrome (<1% to 3%), accidental injury (<1% to 3%)

Overdosage/Toxicology Doses of up to 75 mg have been used in clinical trials, with abnormal vision as the primary adverse event. Overdose may result in severe antimuscarinic effects. Treatment should be symptom-directed and supportive. ECG monitoring is recommended.

Drug Interactions Substrate of CYP2D6 (minor), CYP3A4 (major); **Inhibits** CYP2D6 (moderate), 3A4 (weak)

Acetylcholinesterase inhibitors (central): Concomitant use with darifenacin may lead to decreased therapeutic efficacy of one or both agents; monitor.
Anticholinergic agents: Adverse anticholinergic effects may be additive with other anticholinergic agents (includes tricyclic antidepressants, antihistamines, and phenothiazines).
CYP2D6 substrates: Darifenacin may increase the levels/effects of CYP2D6 substrates. Example substrates include amphetamines, selected beta-blockers, dextromethorphan, fluoxetine, lidocaine, mirtazapine, nefazodone, paroxetine, risperidone, ritonavir, thioridazine, tricyclic antidepressants, and venlafaxine.
CYP2D6 prodrug substrates: Darifenacin may decrease the levels/effects of CYP2D6 prodrug substrates. Example prodrug substrates include codeine, hydrocodone, oxycodone, and tramadol.
CYP3A4 inducers: May decrease the levels/effects of darifenacin. Example inducers include aminoglutethimide, carbamazepine, nafcillin, nevirapine, phenobarbital, phenytoin, and rifamycins.
CYP3A4 inhibitors: May increase the levels/effects of darifenacin. Example inhibitors include azole antifungals, clarithromycin, diclofenac, doxycycline, erythromycin, imatinib, isoniazid, nefazodone, nicardipine, propofol, protease inhibitors, quinidine, telithromycin, and verapamil.
Pramlintide: Darifenacin may increase the anticholinergic effects (eg, decreased gut motility) of pramlintide.
Thioridazine: Darifenacin may result in increased levels/effects (eg, QT_c prolongation) of thioridazine; avoid concomitant use.

Stability Store at 25°C (77°F); excursions permitted to 15°C to 30°C (59°F to 86°F). Protect from light.

Mechanism of Action Selective antagonist of the M3 muscarinic (cholinergic) receptor subtype. Blockade of the receptor limits bladder contractions, reducing the symptoms of bladder irritability/overactivity (urge incontinence, urgency and frequency).

Pharmacokinetics
Distribution: V_{dss}: 163 L
Protein binding: 98%
Metabolism: Hepatic, via CYP3A4 (major) and CYP2D6 (minor)
Bioavailability: 15% to 19%
Half-life elimination: 13-19 hours
Time to peak, plasma: 7 hours
Excretion: As metabolites (inactive); urine (60%), feces (40%)

Dosage
Geriatrics & Adults:
Symptoms of bladder overactivity: Oral: Initial: 7.5 mg once daily. If response is not adequate after a minimum of 2 weeks, dosage may be increased to 15 mg once daily.
Dosage adjustment with concomitant potent CYP3A4 inhibitors: Daily dosage should not exceed 7.5 mg/day

Renal Impairment: No adjustment required.

Hepatic Impairment:
Moderate impairment (Child-Pugh Class B): Daily dosage should not exceed 7.5 mg/day

(Continued)

Darifenacin *(Continued)*

Severe impairment (Child-Pugh Class C): Has not been evaluated; use is not recommended

Administration Tablet should be swallowed whole; may be taken without regard to food.

Patient Information May cause dry mouth and constipation. Do not crush, break, or chew tablet.

Special Geriatric Considerations There is a trend for decreased clearance with age, though no change in dose is recommended. The selectivity of darifenacin for the M3 receptor on the bladder may offer an advantage (less CNS and cardiovascular effects) over other anticholinergic agents used in the treatment of overactive bladder.

Dosage Forms Excipient information presented when available (limited, particularly for generics); consult specific product labeling.

Tablet, extended release: 7.5 mg, 15 mg

Selected References

Croom KF and Keating GM, "Darifenacin in the Treatment of Overactive Bladder," *Drugs Aging*, 2004, 21(13):885-92.

♦ **Darifenacin Hydrobromide** *see* Darifenacin *on page 400*
♦ **Darvocet A500™** *see* Propoxyphene and Acetaminophen *on page 1335*
♦ **Darvocet-N® 50** *see* Propoxyphene and Acetaminophen *on page 1335*
♦ **Darvocet-N® 100** *see* Propoxyphene and Acetaminophen *on page 1335*
♦ **Darvon®** *see* Propoxyphene *on page 1333*
♦ **Darvon-N®** *see* Propoxyphene *on page 1333*
♦ **1-Day™ [OTC]** *see* Tioconazole *on page 1577*
♦ **Dayhist® Allergy [OTC]** *see* Clemastine *on page 330*
♦ **Daypro®** *see* Oxaprozin *on page 1169*
♦ **Daytrana™** *see* Methylphenidate *on page 1013*
♦ **DDAVP®** *see* Desmopressin *on page 411*
♦ **1-Deamino-8-D-Arginine Vasopressin** *see* Desmopressin *on page 411*
♦ **Debrox® [OTC]** *see* Carbamide Peroxide *on page 235*
♦ **Decavac™** *see* Diphtheria and Tetanus Toxoid *on page 451*
♦ **Declomycin®** *see* Demeclocycline *on page 404*
♦ **Deep Sea [OTC]** *see* Sodium Chloride *on page 1475*

Deferasirox *(de FER a sir ox)*

Medication Safety Issues

Sound-alike/look-alike issues:

Deferasirox may be confused with deferoxamine

U.S. Brand Names Exjade®

Canadian Brand Names Exjade®

Index Terms ICL670

Generic Available No

Pharmacologic Category Antidote; Chelating Agent

Use Treatment of chronic iron overload due to blood transfusions

Contraindications Hypersensitivity to deferasirox or any component of the formulation

Warnings/Precautions Cases of acute renal failure (some fatal) and dose-related elevations in serum creatinine have been reported. Monitor serum creatinine in patients at risk for renal complications (eg, pre-existing renal conditions, elderly, comorbid conditions, and/or with concurrent medications that may affect renal function); consider dose reduction, interruption, or discontinuation for serum creatinine elevations. Patients with baseline serum creatinine above the upper limit of normal (ULN) were excluded from clinical trials. May cause proteinuria; closely monitor. Hepatitis, elevated transaminases, and hepatic dysfunction have been reported; monitor LFTs and consider dose modifications. Use caution with hepatic impairment. May cause skin rash (dose-related); mild-to-moderate rashes may resolve without treatment interruption; for severe rash, interrupt and consider restarting at a lower dose with dose escalation and oral steroids. Hypersensitivity reactions, including severe reactions (anaphylaxis and angioedema) have been reported, usually within the first month of treatment. Auditory or ocular disturbances have been reported; monitor and consider dose reduction or treatment interruption. Cytopenias (including agranulocytosis, neutropenia, and thrombocytopenia) have been reported, predominately in patients with preexisting hematologic disorders; monitor closely; interrupt treatment for unexplained cytopenias. Do not combine with other iron chelation therapies; safety of combinations has not been established.

Adverse Reactions (Reflective of adult population; not specific for elderly)

>10%:

Central nervous system: Fever (19%), headache (16%)

Gastrointestinal: Abdominal pain (8% to 14%), diarrhea (12%), nausea (11%)
Renal: Serum creatinine increased (11% to 38%), proteinuria (19%)
Respiratory: Cough (14%), nasopharyngitis (13%), pharyngolaryngeal pain (11%)
Miscellaneous: Influenza (11%)

1% to 10%:

Central nervous system: Fatigue (6%)
Dermatologic: Rash (8% to 11%), urticaria (4%)
Gastrointestinal: Vomiting (10%)
Hepatic: ALT increased (6% to 8%), transaminitis (4%)
Neuromuscular & skeletal: Arthralgia (7%), back pain (6%)
Otic: Ear infection (5%)
Respiratory: Respiratory tract infection (10%), bronchitis (9%), pharyngitis (8%), acute tonsillitis (6%), rhinitis (6%)

Overdosage/Toxicology Overdose of 2-3 times the prescribed doses for several weeks resulted in hepatitis, which resolved upon treatment interruption. Single doses of up to 80 mg/kg have been tolerated with incidences of nausea and diarrhea. In case of overdose, induce vomiting and gastric lavage. Treatment is otherwise symptom-directed and supportive.

Drug Interactions Antacids: Aluminum-containing antacids may decrease absorption of deferasirox

Stability Store at room temperature between 15°C and 30°C (59°F and 86°F). Protect from moisture.

Mechanism of Action Selectively binds iron, forming a complex which is excreted primarily through the feces.

Pharmacokinetics

Distribution: Adults: 11.7-17.1 L
Protein binding: ~99% to serum albumin
Metabolism: Hepatic via glucuronidation by UGT1A1 and UGT1A3; minor oxidation by CYP450; undergoes enterohepatic recirculation
Bioavailability: 70%
Half-life elimination: 8-16 hours
Time to peak, plasma: 90 minutes to 4 hours
Excretion: Feces (84%), urine (6% to 8%)

Dosage

Geriatrics & Adults: Chronic iron overload due to blood transfusion: Oral:

Initial: 20 mg/kg daily (calculate dose to nearest whole tablet)
Maintenance: Adjust dose every 3-6 months based on serum ferritin levels; increase by 5-10 mg/kg/day (calculate dose to nearest whole tablet); titrate. Maximum dose: 30 mg/kg/day; consider interrupting therapy for serum ferritin <500 mcg/L. **Note:** Consider dose reduction or interruption for hearing loss or visual disturbances.

Renal Impairment: Interrupt treatment for progressive increase in serum creatinine above the age-appropriate ULN; once serum creatinine recovers to within the normal range, reinitiate treatment at a reduced dose; gradually escalate the dose if the clinical benefit outweighs potential risk.

Adults: For increase in serum creatinine >33% above the average pretreatment level at 2 consecutive levels (and cannot be attributed to other causes), reduce daily dose by 10 mg/kg

Hepatic Impairment: Consider dose adjustment or discontinuation for severe elevations in liver function tests.

Administration Do not chew or swallow whole tablets. Take at same time each day on an empty stomach, 30 minutes before food. Disperse tablets in water, orange juice, or apple juice (use 3.5 ounces for total doses <1 g; 7 ounces for doses >1 g); stir to form suspension and drink entire contents. Rinse remaining residue with more fluid; drink. Do not take simultaneously with aluminum-containing antacids.

Monitoring Parameters

CBC with differential, serum creatinine (twice prior to initiation, then monthly thereafter; monitor weekly in patients with renal risk factors or with changes in therapy; per Canadian labeling: 2 times prior to initiation, then weekly for the first month and monthly thereafter), urine protein (monthly), liver function tests (monthly), and serum ferritin (monthly); baseline and annual auditory and ophthalmic function

Additional Information Deferasirox has a low affinity for binding with zinc and copper, may cause variable decreases in the serum concentration of these trace minerals.

Special Geriatric Considerations Studies to date have not included sufficient numbers of subjects ≥65 years of age. Use caution in patients with liver dysfunction or low serum albumin. Monitor renal function. In general, this drug should be used with caution and close monitoring in elderly due to the greater incidence of decreased hepatic, renal, cardiac function, as well as concomitant disease and drug therapy.

Dosage Forms Excipient information presented when available (limited, particularly for generics); consult specific product labeling.

Tablet, for oral suspension:
Exjade®: 125 mg, 250 mg, 500 mg
(Continued)

Deferasirox *(Continued)*

Selected References
NCCN (National Comprehensive Cancer Network), "Practice Guidelines in Oncology: Myelodysplastic Syndromes Version 1.2007," available at http://www.nccn.org/professionals/physician_gls/PDF/mds.pdf

- ◆ **Dehydrobenzperidol** *see* Droperidol *on page 486*
- ◆ **Delatestryl®** *see* Testosterone *on page 1537*
- ◆ **Delestrogen®** *see* Estradiol *on page 549*
- ◆ **Delsym® [OTC]** *see* Dextromethorphan *on page 419*
- ◆ **Delta-9-tetrahydro-cannabinol** *see* Dronabinol *on page 484*
- ◆ **Delta-9 THC** *see* Dronabinol *on page 484*
- ◆ **Delta-D®** *see* Cholecalciferol *on page 304*
- ◆ **Deltacortisone** *see* PredniSONE *on page 1307*
- ◆ **Deltadehydrocortisone** *see* PredniSONE *on page 1307*
- ◆ **Deltahydrocortisone** *see* PrednisoLONE *on page 1303*
- ◆ **Demadex®** *see* Torsemide *on page 1604*

Demeclocycline *(dem e kloe SYE kleen)*

U.S. Brand Names Declomycin®
Canadian Brand Names Declomycin®
Index Terms Demeclocycline Hydrochloride; Demethylchlortetracycline
Generic Available Yes
Pharmacologic Category Antibiotic, Tetracycline Derivative
Use Treatment of susceptible bacterial infections (ie, acne, gonorrhea, pertussis, urinary tract infections) caused by both gram-negative and gram-positive organisms; used when penicillin is contraindicated
Unlabeled/Investigational Use Treatment of chronic syndrome of inappropriate secretion of antidiuretic hormone (SIADH)
Contraindications Hypersensitivity to demeclocycline, tetracyclines, or any component of the formulation; concomitant use with methoxyflurane
Warnings/Precautions Photosensitivity reactions occur frequently with this drug; avoid prolonged exposure to sunlight and do not use tanning equipment. Use caution in patients with renal or hepatic impairment (eg, elderly); dosage modification required in patients with renal impairment. May act as an antianabolic agent and increase BUN. Pseudotumor cerebri has been reported with tetracycline use (usually resolves with discontinuation). Outdated drug can cause nephropathy. Prolonged use may result in fungal or bacterial superinfection, including *C. difficile*-associated diarrhea and pseudomembranous colitis.
Adverse Reactions (Reflective of adult population; not specific for elderly)
Frequency not defined.
Cardiovascular: Pericarditis
Central nervous system: Bulging fontanels (infants), dizziness, headache, pseudotumor cerebri (adults)
Dermatologic: Angioneurotic edema, erythema multiforme, erythematous rash, maculopapular rash, photosensitivity, pigmentation of skin, Stevens-Johnson syndrome (rare), urticaria
Endocrine & metabolic: Discoloration of thyroid gland (brown/black), nephrogenic diabetes insipidus
Gastrointestinal: Anorexia, diarrhea, dysphagia, enterocolitis, esophageal ulcerations, glossitis, nausea, pancreatitis, vomiting
Genitourinary: Balanitis
Hematologic: Eosinophilia, neutropenia, hemolytic anemia, thrombocytopenia
Hepatic: Hepatitis (rare), hepatotoxicity (rare), liver enzymes increased, liver failure (rare)
Neuromuscular & skeletal: Myasthenic syndrome, polyarthralgia, tooth discoloration (children <8 years, rarely in adults)
Ocular: Visual disturbances
Otic: Tinnitus
Renal: Acute renal failure
Respiratory: Pulmonary infiltrates
Miscellaneous: Anaphylaxis, anaphylactoid purpura, lupus-like syndrome, systemic lupus erythematosus exacerbation
Overdosage/Toxicology Treatment is supportive.
Drug Interactions
Antacids: Preparations containing calcium, magnesium, aluminum bismuth, or sodium bicarbonate may decrease absorption of tetracyclines.
Bile acid sequestrants: May decrease tetracycline absorption.
Iron preparations: May decrease absorption of tetracyclines.

Methoxyflurane: Methoxyflurane anesthesia (when concurrent with tetracycline) may cause fatal nephrotoxicity; concurrent use is contraindicated.

Methotrexate: Clearance of methotrexate (high-dose therapy) may be decreased by tetracyclines.

Oral contraceptives: Anecdotal reports suggesting decreased contraceptive efficacy with tetracyclines have been refuted by more rigorous scientific and clinical data.

Penicillins: May decrease therapeutic effect of tetracyclines.

Quinapril: Magnesium-containing formulation of quinapril may decrease tetracycline absorption.

Retinoic acid derivatives: May increase adverse and toxic effects of tetracyclines, especially pseudotumor cerebri.

Warfarin: Concomitant use with tetracyclines may result in increased anticoagulation.

Zinc preparations: May decrease absorption of tetracyclines.

Ethanol/Nutrition/Herb Interactions

Food: Demeclocycline serum levels may be decreased if taken with food.

Herb/Nutraceutical: Avoid dong quai, St John's wort (may also cause photosensitization).

Stability Tetracyclines form toxic products when outdated or when exposed to light, heat, or humidity (Fanconi-like syndrome).

Mechanism of Action Inhibits protein synthesis by binding with the 30S and possibly the 50S ribosomal subunit(s) of susceptible bacteria; may also cause alterations in the cytoplasmic membrane; inhibits the action of ADH in patients with chronic SIADH

Pharmacodynamics Onset of action for diuresis in SIADH: Several days

Pharmacokinetics

Absorption: ~50% to 80% from GI tract (food and dairy products reduce absorption)

Protein binding: 41% to 50%

Metabolism: Small amounts metabolized in the liver to inactive metabolites; enterohepatically recycled

Half-life: 10-17 hours (prolonged with reduced renal function)

Time to peak serum concentration: Oral: Within 3-6 hours

Elimination: As unchanged drug (42% to 50%) in urine

Dosage

Geriatrics & Adults:

Susceptible infections: Oral: 150 mg 4 times/day or 300 mg twice daily

SIADH (unlabeled use): Oral: 900-1200 mg/day or 13-15 mg/kg/day divided every 6-8 hours initially, then decrease to 600-900 mg/day

Renal Impairment: Should be avoided in patients with renal dysfunction.

Hepatic Impairment: Should be avoided in patients with hepatic dysfunction.

Administration Administer 1 hour before or 2 hours after food or milk with plenty of fluid; avoid administration within 2-3 hours of antacids

Monitoring Parameters CBC, renal and hepatic function; PT or INR in patients taking anticoagulants

Test Interactions May interfere with tests for urinary glucose (false-negative urine glucose using Clinistix®, Tes-Tape®)

Patient Information Avoid prolonged exposure to sunlight or sunlamps; avoid taking antacids before tetracyclines

Special Geriatric Considerations Has not been studied exclusively in the elderly.

Dosage Forms Excipient information presented when available (limited, particularly for generics); consult specific product labeling.

Tablet, as hydrochloride: 150 mg, 300 mg

Selected References

Troyer AD, "Demeclocycline. Treatment for Syndrome of Inappropriate Antidiuretic Hormone Secretion," *JAMA*, 1977, 237(25):2723-6.

♦ **Depo-Provera® Contraceptive** *see* MedroxyPROGESTERone *on page 965*
♦ **depo-subQ provera 104™** *see* MedroxyPROGESTERone *on page 965*
♦ **Depo®-Testosterone** *see* Testosterone *on page 1537*
♦ **Deprenyl** *see* Selegiline *on page 1451*
♦ **DermaFungal [OTC]** *see* Miconazole *on page 1036*
♦ **Dermagran®** [OTC] *see* Aluminum Hydroxide *on page 63*
♦ **Dermagran® AF [OTC]** *see* Miconazole *on page 1036*
♦ **Dermamycin® [OTC]** *see* DiphenhydrAMINE *on page 447*
♦ **Dermarest Dricort® [OTC]** *see* Hydrocortisone *on page 762*
♦ **Derma-Smoothe/FS®** *see* Fluocinolone *on page 639*
♦ **Dermatop®** *see* Prednicarbate *on page 1302*
♦ **Dermtex® HC [OTC]** *see* Hydrocortisone *on page 762*
♦ **Desiccated Thyroid** *see* Thyroid *on page 1559*

Desipramine (des IP ra meen)

Related Information
Antidepressant Agents *on page 1742*
Pharmacotherapy of Urinary Incontinence *on page 1822*
Serum Drug Concentrations Commonly Monitored Guidelines *on page 1862*
Medication Safety Issues
Sound-alike/look-alike issues:
Desipramine may be confused with clomiPRAMINE, deserpidine, diphenhydrAMINE, disopyramide, imipramine, nortriptyline
Norpramin® may be confused with clomiPRAMINE, imipramine, Norpace®, nortriptyline, Tenormin®

International issues:
Norpramin®: Brand name for omeprazole in Spain
U.S. Brand Names Norpramin®
Canadian Brand Names Alti-Desipramine; Apo-Desipramine®; Norpramin®; Nu-Desipramine; PMS-Desipramine
Index Terms Desipramine Hydrochloride; Desmethylimipramine Hydrochloride
Generic Available Yes
Pharmacologic Category Antidepressant, Tricyclic (Secondary Amine)
Use Treatment of various forms of depression, often in conjunction with psychotherapy
Unlabeled/Investigational Use Analgesic adjunct in chronic pain; peripheral neuropathies; substance-related disorders (eg, cocaine withdrawal); attention-deficit/hyperactivity disorder (ADHD)
Restrictions An FDA-approved medication guide concerning the use of antidepressants in children, adolescents, and young adults must be distributed when dispensing an outpatient prescription (new or refill) where this medication is to be used without direct supervision of a healthcare provider. Medication guides are available at http://www.fda.gov/cder/Offices/ODS/medication_guides.htm. Dispense to parents or guardians of children and adolescents receiving this medication.
Contraindications Hypersensitivity to desipramine, drugs of similar chemical class, or any component of the formulation; use of MAO inhibitors within 14 days; use in a patient during the acute recovery phase of MI
Warnings/Precautions [U.S. Boxed Warning]: Antidepressants increase the risk of suicidal thinking and behavior in children, adolescents, and young adults (18-24 years of age) with major depressive disorder (MDD) and other psychiatric disorders; consider risk prior to prescribing. Short-term studies did not show an increased risk in patients >24 years of age and showed a decreased risk in patients ≥65 years. Closely monitor for clinical worsening, suicidality, or unusual changes in behavior; the patient's family or caregiver should be instructed to closely observe the patient and communicate condition with healthcare provider. A medication guide should be dispensed with each prescription.

The possibility of a suicide attempt is inherent in major depression and may persist until remission occurs. Monitor for worsening of depression or suicidality, especially during initiation of therapy (generally first 1-2 months) or with dose increases or decreases. Use caution in high-risk patients. Worsening depression and severe abrupt suicidality that are not part of the presenting symptoms may require discontinuation or modification of drug therapy. The patient's family or caregiver should be alerted to monitor patients for the emergence of suicidality and associated behaviors (such as agitation, irritability, hostility, impulsivity, and hypomania) and notify healthcare provider.

May worsen psychosis in some patients or precipitate a shift to mania or hypomania in patients with bipolar disorder. Patients presenting with depressive symptoms should be screened for bipolar disorder. Monotherapy in patients with bipolar disorder should be avoided. **Desipramine is not FDA approved for the treatment of bipolar depression.**

The degree of anticholinergic blockade produced by this agent is low relative to other cyclic antidepressants - however, caution should be used in patients with urinary retention, benign prostatic hyperplasia, narrow-angle glaucoma, xerostomia, visual problems, constipation, or a history of bowel obstruction. The degree of sedation and conduction disturbances with desipramine are low relative to other antidepressants. However, desipramine may cause drowsiness/sedation, resulting in impaired performance of tasks requiring alertness (eg, operating machinery or driving). Sedative effects may be additive with other CNS depressants and/or ethanol. The risk of orthostasis is moderate relative to other antidepressants. Use with caution in patients with a history of cardiovascular disease (including previous MI, stroke, tachycardia, or conduction abnormalities).

Consider discontinuing, when possible, prior to elective surgery. Therapy should not be abruptly discontinued in patients receiving high doses for prolonged periods. May lower seizure threshold - use caution in patients with a previous seizure disorder or condition predisposing to seizures such as brain damage, alcoholism, or concurrent therapy with other drugs which lower the seizure threshold. May increase the risks associated with electroconvulsive therapy. Use with caution in hyperthyroid patients or those receiving thyroid supplementation. Use with caution in patients with hepatic or renal dysfunction and in elderly patients.

Adverse Reactions (Reflective of adult population; not specific for elderly)
Frequency not defined.
Cardiovascular: Arrhythmias, edema, flushing, heart block, hyper-/hypotension, MI, palpitation, stroke, tachycardia
Central nervous system: Agitation, anxiety, ataxia, confusion, delirium, disorientation, dizziness, drowsiness, drug fever, exacerbation of psychosis, extrapyramidal symptoms, fatigue, hallucinations, headache, hypomania, incoordination, insomnia, nervousness, parkinsonian syndrome, restlessness, seizure
Dermatologic: Alopecia, itching, petechiae, photosensitivity, skin rash, urticaria
Endocrine & metabolic: Breast enlargement, galactorrhea, hyper-/hypoglycemia, impotence, libido changes, SIADH
Gastrointestinal: Abdominal cramps, anorexia, black tongue, constipation, decreased lower esophageal sphincter tone may cause GE reflux, diarrhea, heartburn, nausea, paralytic ileus, stomatitis, unpleasant taste, vomiting, weight gain/loss, xerostomia
Genitourinary: Difficult urination, polyuria, sexual dysfunction, testicular edema, urinary retention
Hematologic: Agranulocytosis, eosinophilia, purpura, thrombocytopenia
Hepatic: Cholestatic jaundice, hepatitis, liver enzymes increased
Neuromuscular & skeletal: Fine muscle tremor, numbness, paresthesia of extremities, peripheral neuropathy, tingling, weakness
Ocular: Blurred vision, disturbances of accommodation, intraocular pressure increased, mydriasis
Otic: Tinnitus
Miscellaneous: Allergic reaction, diaphoresis (excessive)

Overdosage/Toxicology Symptoms include severe hypotension, agitation, confusion, hypo-/hyperthermia, hypotension (severe), urinary retention, CNS depression, coma, cyanosis, dry mucous membranes, cardiac arrhythmias, seizures, changes in ECG (particularly in QRS axis and width), transient visual hallucinations, stupor, and muscle rigidity. Treatment is supportive and symptom-directed. Initiate gastric decontamination (emesis is contraindicated) and ECG monitoring immediately; monitor for a minimum of 6 hours. Sodium bicarbonate is indicated when the QRS interval is ≥0.10 seconds or the QT_c is >0.42 seconds. Ventricular arrhythmias and ECG changes (eg, QRS widening) often respond with concurrent systemic alkalinization (sodium bicarbonate 0.5-2 mEq/kg I.V.). Arrhythmias unresponsive to phenytoin 15-20 mg/kg (adults) may respond to lidocaine 1 mg/kg I.V. followed by a titrated infusion. Physostigmine (1-2 mg slow I.V. for adults) may be indicated in reversing life-threatening cardiac arrhythmias. Seizures usually respond to diazepam I.V. boluses (5-10 mg for adults up to 30 mg). If seizures are unresponsive or recur, phenytoin or phenobarbital may be required. Dialysis and diuresis have not been proven beneficial.

Drug Interactions Substrate of CYP1A2 (minor), 2D6 (major); **Inhibits** CYP2A6 (moderate), 2B6 (moderate), 2D6 (moderate), 2E1 (weak), 3A4 (moderate)

Alpha- and beta-agonists: When combined with TCAs, may predispose patients to cardiac arrhythmias; may also enhance vasopressor effects; consider alternate therapy.
Altretamine: Concurrent use may cause orthostatic hypertension.
Amphetamines: TCAs may enhance the effect of amphetamines; monitor for adverse CV effects.
Anticholinergics: Combined use with TCAs may produce additive anticholinergic effects.
Barbiturates: May decrease the levels/effects of TCAs; monitor.
(Continued)

Desipramine *(Continued)*

Bupropion: May increase the levels of tricyclic antidepressants; based on limited information; monitor response.

Carbamazepine: Tricyclic antidepressants may increase carbamazepine levels; monitor.

Cholestyramine and colestipol: May bind TCAs and reduce their absorption; monitor for altered response.

Clonidine: Abrupt discontinuation of clonidine may cause hypertensive crisis; amitriptyline may enhance the response.

CNS depressants: Sedative effects may be additive with TCAs; monitor for increased effect; includes benzodiazepines, barbiturates, antipsychotics, ethanol, and other sedative medications.

CYP2A6 substrates: Desipramine may increase the levels/effects of CYP2A6 substrates. Example substrates include dexmedetomidine and ifosfamide.

CYP2B6 substrates: Desipramine may increase the levels/effects of CYP2B6 substrates. Example substrates include bupropion, cyclophosphamide, irinotecan, ketamine, promethazine, propofol, and selegiline.

CYP2D6 inhibitors: May increase the levels/effects of desipramine. Example inhibitors include chlorpromazine, delavirdine, fluoxetine, miconazole, paroxetine, pergolide, quinidine, quinine, ritonavir, and ropinirole.

CYP2D6 substrates: Desipramine may increase the levels/effects of CYP2D6 substrates. Example substrates include amphetamines, selected beta-blockers, dextromethorphan, fluoxetine, lidocaine, mirtazapine, nefazodone, paroxetine, risperidone, ritonavir, thioridazine, tricyclic antidepressants, and venlafaxine. Concurrent use with thioridazine is contraindicated.

CYP2D6 prodrug substrates: Desipramine may decrease the levels/effects of CYP2D6 prodrug substrates. Example prodrug substrates include codeine, hydrocodone, oxycodone, and tramadol.

CYP3A4 substrates: Desipramine may increase the levels/effects of CYP3A4 substrates. Example substrates include benzodiazepines, calcium channel blockers, cyclosporine, mirtazapine, nateglinide, nefazodone, sildenafil (and other PDE-5 inhibitors), tacrolimus, and venlafaxine. Selected benzodiazepines (midazolam and triazolam), cisapride, ergot alkaloids, selected HMG-CoA reductase inhibitors (lovastatin and simvastatin), and pimozide are generally contraindicated with strong CYP3A4 inhibitors.

Epinephrine (and other direct alpha-agonists): Pressor response to I.V. epinephrine, norepinephrine, and phenylephrine may be enhanced in patients receiving TCAs. (**Note:** Effect is unlikely with epinephrine or levonordefrin dosages typically administered as infiltration in combination with local anesthetics.)

False neurotransmitters (eg, guanadrel, methyldopa): TCAs may diminish the antihypertensive effects of false neurotransmitters.

Fenfluramine: May increase tricyclic antidepressant levels/effects.

Hypoglycemic agents (including insulin): TCAs may enhance the hypoglycemic effects of tolazamide, chlorpropamide, or insulin; monitor for changes in blood glucose levels; reported with chlorpropamide, tolazamide, and insulin.

Levodopa: Tricyclic antidepressants may decrease the absorption (bioavailability) of levodopa; rare hypertensive episodes have also been attributed to this combination.

Linezolid: Hyperpyrexia, hypertension, tachycardia, confusion, seizures, and **deaths have been reported** with agents which inhibit MAO (serotonin syndrome); this combination should be avoided.

Lithium: Concurrent use with a TCA may increase the risk for neurotoxicity.

MAO inhibitors: Hyperpyrexia, hypertension, tachycardia, confusion, seizures, and **deaths have been reported** (serotonin syndrome); this combination should be avoided.

Methylphenidate: Metabolism of TCAs may be decreased.

Phenothiazines: Serum concentrations of some TCAs may be increased; in addition, TCAs may increase concentration of phenothiazines; monitor for altered clinical response.

Pramlintide: May increase the anticholinergic effects of TCAs.

QT_c-prolonging agents: Concurrent use of tricyclic agents with other drugs which may prolong QT_c interval may increase the risk of potentially fatal arrhythmias; includes type Ia and type III antiarrhythmics agents, selected quinolones (moxifloxacin), cisapride, and other agents.

Ritonavir: Combined use of high-dose tricyclic antidepressants with ritonavir may cause serotonin syndrome in HIV-positive patients; monitor.

Serotonin modulators, SSRIs, sibutramine: Concomitant use may increase serotonergic effects; concurrent use with sibutramine is contraindicated.

Sympathomimetics, indirect-acting: Tricyclic antidepressants may result in a decreased sensitivity to indirect-acting sympathomimetics; includes dopamine and ephedrine; also see interaction with epinephrine (and direct-acting sympathomimetics).

Terbinafine: May increase the levels/effects of TCAs; monitor.

Tramadol: Tramadol's risk of seizures may be increased with TCAs.

Valproic acid: May increase serum concentrations/adverse effects of some tricyclic antidepressants.

Warfarin (and other oral anticoagulants): TCAs may increase the anticoagulant effect in patients stabilized on warfarin; monitor INR.

Ethanol/Nutrition/Herb Interactions

Ethanol: Avoid ethanol (may increase CNS depression).

Food: Grapefruit juice may inhibit the metabolism of some TCAs and clinical toxicity may result.

Herb/Nutraceutical: Avoid valerian, St John's wort, SAMe, kava kava (may increase risk of serotonin syndrome and/or excessive sedation).

Mechanism of Action Traditionally believed to increase the synaptic concentration of norepinephrine (and to a lesser extent, serotonin) in the central nervous system by inhibition of its reuptake by the presynaptic neuronal membrane. However, additional receptor effects have been found including desensitization of adenyl cyclase, down regulation of beta-adrenergic receptors, and down regulation of serotonin receptors.

Pharmacodynamics Onset of action: 1-3 weeks; norepinephrine only

Pharmacokinetics

Absorption: Well absorbed from GI tract

Protein binding: 90%

Metabolism: Hepatic

Half-life: 12-57 hours

Plasma concentration and half-life have been found to positively correlate with age; mean half-life: >75 hours, twice that of young patients

Elimination: 70% excreted in urine

Dosage

Geriatrics: Oral: Initial: 10-25 mg/day; increase by 10-25 mg every 3 days for inpatients and every week for outpatients if tolerated; usual maintenance dose: 75-100 mg/day, but doses up to 150 mg/day may be necessary.

Adults:

Depression: Oral: Initial: 75 mg/day in divided doses; increase gradually to 150-200 mg/day in divided or single dose; maximum: 300 mg/day

Cocaine withdrawal (unlabeled use): 50-200 mg/day in divided or single dose

Renal Impairment: Hemodialysis/peritoneal dialysis effects: Supplemental dose is not necessary.

Monitoring Parameters Improvement in depressive symptoms; blood pressure, pulse

Reference Range

Therapeutic: 125-160 ng/mL

Possible toxicity: >300 ng/mL (SI: 1070 nmol/L)

Toxic: >1000 ng/mL (SI: >3750 nmol/L)

In geriatric patients the response rate is greatest with steady-state plasma concentrations >115 ng/mL

Patient Information Avoid alcohol ingestion; do not discontinue medication abruptly; may cause urine to turn blue-green; may cause drowsiness, dry mouth, blurred vision or dizziness; rise slowly to prevent dizziness

Additional Information Avoid unnecessary exposure to sunlight

Special Geriatric Considerations Preferred agent because of its milder side effect profile; patients may experience excitation or stimulation, in such cases, administer as a single morning dose or divided dose. Data from a clinical trial comparing fluoxetine to tricyclics suggest that fluoxetine is significantly less effective than nortriptyline in hospitalized elderly patients with unipolar major affective disorder, especially those with melancholia and concurrent cardiovascular disease.

Dosage Forms Excipient information presented when available (limited, particularly for generics); consult specific product labeling.

Tablet, as hydrochloride: 10 mg, 25 mg, 50 mg, 75 mg, 100 mg, 150 mg

Selected References

Nelson JC, Jatlow PI, and Mazure C, "Desipramine Plasma Levels and Response in Elderly Melancholic Patients," *J Clin Psychopharmacol*, 1985, 5(4):217-20.

Nies A, Robinson DS, Friedman MS, et al, "Relationship Between Age and Tricyclic Antidepressant Plasma Levels," *Am J Psychiatry*, 1977, 134:790-3.

Roose SP, Glassman AH, Attia E, et al, "Comparative Efficacy of Selective Serotonin Reuptake Inhibitors and Tricyclics in the Treatment of Melancholia," *Am J Psychiatry*, 1994, 151(12):1735-9.

♦ **Desipramine Hydrochloride** see Desipramine on page 406

Desloratadine (des lor AT a deen)

U.S. Brand Names Clarinex®
Canadian Brand Names Aerius®
Generic Available No
(Continued)

Desloratadine *(Continued)*

Pharmacologic Category Antihistamine, Nonsedating

Use Relief of nasal and non-nasal symptoms of seasonal allergic rhinitis (SAR) and perennial allergic rhinitis (PAR); treatment of chronic idiopathic urticaria (CIU)

Contraindications Hypersensitivity to desloratadine, loratadine, or any component of the formulation

Warnings/Precautions Dose should be adjusted in patients with liver or renal impairment. Use with caution in patients known to be slow metabolizers of desloratadine (incidence of side effects may be increased). RediTabs® contain phenylalanine.

Adverse Reactions (Reflective of adult population; not specific for elderly)
>10%: Central nervous system: Headache (14%)
1% to 10%:
   Central nervous system: Fatigue (2% to 5%), somnolence (2%), dizziness (4%)
   Endocrine & metabolic: Dysmenorrhea (2%)
   Gastrointestinal: Xerostomia (3%), nausea (5%), dyspepsia (3%)
   Neuromuscular & skeletal: Myalgia (2% to 3%)
   Respiratory: Pharyngitis (3% to 4%)

Overdosage/Toxicology Information is limited to doses studied during clinical trials (up to 45 mg/day). Symptoms included somnolence, and small increases in heart rate and QT_c interval (not clinically significant). In the event of an overdose, treatment should be symptom-directed and supportive. Desloratadine and its metabolite are not removed by hemodialysis.

Drug Interactions
   CNS depressants: May cause increased risk of sedation when combined with desloratadine; use caution.
   Erythromycin: C_{max} and AUC of desloratadine and its metabolite are increased; however, no clinically-significant changes in the safety profile of desloratadine were observed in clinical studies.
   Ketoconazole: C_{max} and AUC of desloratadine and its metabolite are increased; however, no clinically-significant changes in the safety profile of desloratadine were observed in clinical studies.

Ethanol/Nutrition/Herb Interactions
   Ethanol: Avoid ethanol (may increase risk of sedation).
   Food: Does not affect bioavailability.

Stability Syrup, tablet, orally-disintegrating tablet: Store at 25°C (77°F); excursions permitted between 15°C to 30°C (59°F to 86°F). Protect from moisture and excessive heat (85°F). Use orally-disintegrating tablet immediately after opening blister package. Syrup should be protected from light.

Mechanism of Action Desloratadine, a major metabolite of loratadine, is a long-acting tricyclic antihistamine with selective peripheral histamine H_1 receptor antagonistic activity and additional anti-inflammatory properties.

Pharmacokinetics
   Protein binding: Desloratadine: 82% to 87%; 3-hydroxydesloratadine: 85% to 89%
   Metabolism: Hepatic to active metabolite, 3-hydroxydesloratadine (specific enzymes not identified); undergoes glucuronidation. Decreased in slow metabolizers of desloratadine. Not expected to affect or be affected by medications metabolized by CYP with normal doses.
   Half-life: 27 hours
   Time to peak: 3 hours
   Elimination: Urine and feces (as metabolites)

Dosage
   Geriatrics & Adults: Seasonal or perennial allergic rhinitis, chronic idiopathic urticaria: Oral: 5 mg once daily
   Renal Impairment: 5 mg every other day
   Hepatic Impairment: 5 mg every other day

Administration May be taken with or without food. RediTabs® should be placed on the tongue; tablet will disintegrate immediately. May be taken with or without water.

Monitoring Parameters Relief of symptoms, mental status

Patient Information May be taken with or without food. Do not increase dose or take more often than recommended by prescriber. Drowsiness, tiredness, headache, or dry mouth may occur. Notify prescriber for increased heart beat, rash, itching or shortness of breath.

Dosage Forms Excipient information presented when available (limited, particularly for generics); consult specific product labeling.
   Syrup (Clarinex®): 0.5 mg/mL (120 mL, 480 mL) [bubble gum flavor]
   Tablet (Clarinex®): 5 mg
   Tablet, orally disintegrating (Clarinex® RediTabs®): 2.5 mg [contains phenylalanine 1.28 mg/tablet; tutti-frutti flavor]; 5 mg [contains phenylalanine 2.55 mg/tablet; tutti-frutti flavor]

Selected References
McClellan K and Jarvis B, "Desloratadine," *Drugs*, 2001, 61(6):789-96.

♦ **Desmethylimipramine Hydrochloride** *see* Desipramine *on page 406*

Desmopressin (des moe PRES in)

U.S. Brand Names DDAVP®; Stimate™
Canadian Brand Names Apo-Desmopressin®; DDAVP®; Minirin®; Nove-Desmopressin®; Octostim®
Index Terms 1-Deamino-8-D-Arginine Vasopressin; Desmopressin Acetate
Generic Available Yes
Pharmacologic Category Antihemophilic Agent; Hemostatic Agent; Vasopressin Analog, Synthetic
Use
Injection: Treatment of diabetes insipidus; control of bleeding in hemophilia A, and mild-to-moderate classic von Willebrand disease (type I)
Tablet, nasal solution: Treatment of diabetes insipidus; primary nocturnal enuresis
Contraindications Hypersensitivity to desmopressin or any component of the formulation; hemophilia B, severe classic von Willebrand disease (type IIB); patients with ≤5% factor VIII activity level; factor VIII antibodies; moderate to severe renal impairment (Cl$_{cr}$ <50 mL/minute)
Warnings/Precautions Fluid intake should be adjusted downward in the elderly and very young patients to decrease the possibility of water intoxication and hyponatremia. Avoid overhydration especially when drug is used for its hemostatic effect. Use may rarely lead to extreme decreases in plasma osmolality, resulting in seizures and coma. Use caution with cystic fibrosis or other conditions associated with fluid and electrolyte imbalance due to potential hyponatremia. Use caution with coronary artery insufficiency or hypertensive cardiovascular disease; may increase or decrease blood pressure leading to changes in heart rate. Consider switching from nasal to intravenous solution if changes in the nasal mucosa (scarring, edema) occur leading to unreliable absorption. Use caution in patients predisposed to thrombus formation; thrombotic events (acute cerebrovascular thrombosis, acute myocardial infarction) have occurred (rare). Injection is not for use in hemophilia B, severe classic von Willebrand disease (type IIB), or in patients with factor VIII antibodies. In general, the injection is also not recommended for use in patients with ≤5% factor VIII activity level, although it may be considered in selected patients with activity levels between 2% and 5%. Some patients may demonstrate a change in response after long-term therapy (>6 months) characterized as decreased response or a shorter duration of response.
Adverse Reactions (Reflective of adult population; not specific for elderly)
Frequency not defined (may be dose or route related).
Cardiovascular: Acute cerebrovascular thrombosis, acute MI, blood pressure increased/decreased, chest pain, edema, facial flushing, palpitation
Central nervous system: Agitation, chills, coma, dizziness, headache, insomnia, somnolence
Dermatologic: Rash
Endocrine & metabolic: Hyponatremia, water intoxication
Gastrointestinal: Abdominal cramps, dyspepsia, nausea, sore throat, vomiting
Genitourinary: Balanitis, vulval pain
Local: Injection: Burning pain, erythema, and swelling at the injection site
Ocular: Conjunctivitis, eye edema, lacrimation disorder
Respiratory: Cough, epistaxis, nasal congestion, rhinitis
Miscellaneous: Allergic reactions (rare), anaphylaxis (rare)
Overdosage/Toxicology Symptoms include drowsiness, headache, confusion, anuria, and water intoxication. In case of overdose, decrease or discontinue desmopressin.
Drug Interactions
Demeclocycline: May decrease response to endogenous antidiuretic hormone (ADH). Use caution.
Chlorpropamide: May increase response to ADH. Use caution.
Fludrocortisone: May increase response to ADH. Use caution.
Lithium: May decrease response to ADH. Use caution.
Ethanol/Nutrition/Herb Interactions Ethanol: Avoid ethanol (may decrease antidiuretic effect).
Stability
DDAVP®:
Tablet, nasal spray: Store at controlled room temperature of 20°C to 25°C (68°F to 77°F). Keep nasal spray in upright position.
Rhinal tube: Refrigerate stored at 2°C to 8°C (36°F to 46°F). May store at room temperature for up to 3 weeks.
(Continued)

Desmopressin *(Continued)*

Injection: Store refrigerated at 2°C to 8°C (36°F to 46°F). Dilute in 10-50 mL NS for I.V. infusion (50 mL for adults).

Stimate™: Store refrigerated at 2°C to 8°C (36°F to 46°F). May store at room temperature for up to 3 weeks.

Mechanism of Action Enhances reabsorption of water in the kidneys by increasing cellular permeability of the collecting ducts; possibly causes smooth muscle constriction with resultant vasoconstriction; raises plasma levels of von Willebrand factor and factor VIII

Pharmacodynamics

Intranasal administration:

Onset of increased factor VIII activity: 30 minutes (dose related)
Peak effect 1.5 hours

I.V. infusion:

Onset of increased factor VIII activity: 30 minutes (dose related)
Peak effect: 1.5-2 hours

Oral tablet:

Onset of action: ADH: ~1 hour
Peak effect: 4-7 hours

Pharmacokinetics

Intranasal administration: Bioavailability: 3.2%

I.V. infusion:

Half-life elimination: Terminal: 3 hours (up to 9 hours in renal dysfunction)
Excretion: Urine

Oral tablet:

Bioavailability: 5% compared to intranasal; 0.16% compared to I.V.
Half-life elimination: 1.5-2.5 hours

Dosage

Geriatrics & Adults:

Diabetes insipidus:

I.V., SubQ: 2-4 mcg/day (0.5-1 mL) in 2 divided doses or 1/10 of the maintenance intranasal dose

Intranasal (100 mcg/mL nasal solution): 10-40 mcg/day (0.1-0.4 mL) divided 1-3 times/day; adjust morning and evening doses separately for an adequate diurnal rhythm of water turnover. **Note:** The nasal spray pump can only deliver doses of 10 mcg (0.1 mL) or multiples of 10 mcg (0.1 mL); if doses other than this are needed, the rhinal tube delivery system is preferred.

Oral: Initial: 0.05 mg twice daily; total daily dose should be increased or decreased as needed to obtain adequate antidiuresis (range: 0.1-1.2 mg divided 2-3 times/day)

Nocturnal enuresis:

Intranasal (using 100 mcg/mL nasal solution): Initial: 20 mcg (0.2 mL) at bedtime; range: 10-40 mcg; it is recommended that $^1/_2$ of the dose be given in each nostril. For 10 mcg dose, administer in one nostril. **Note:** The nasal spray pump can only deliver doses of 10 mcg (0.1 mL) or multiples of 10 mcg (0.1 mL); if doses other than this are needed, the rhinal tube delivery system is preferred.

Oral: 0.2 mg at bedtime; dose may be titrated up to 0.6 mg to achieve desired response. Patients previously on intranasal therapy can begin oral tablets 24 hours after the last intranasal dose.

Hemophilia A and mild-to-moderate von Willebrand disease (type I):

I.V.: 0.3 mcg/kg by slow infusion, begin 30 minutes before procedure

Nasal spray: Using high concentration spray (1.5 mg/mL): <50 kg: 150 mcg (1 spray); >50 kg: 300 mcg (1 spray each nostril); repeat use is determined by the patient's clinical condition and laboratory work. If using preoperatively, administer 2 hours before surgery.

Renal Impairment: Cl_{cr} <50 mL/minute: Use is contraindicated.

Administration

I.V.: Dilute in 0.9% sodium chloride and infuse over 15-30 minutes; dose should be diluted in 50 mL NS for adults

Intranasal:

DDAVP®: Nasal pump spray: Delivers 0.1 mL (10 mcg); for other doses which are not multiples, use rhinal tube. DDAVP® Nasal spray delivers fifty 10 mcg doses. For 10 mcg dose, administer in one nostril. Any solution remaining after 50 doses should be discarded. Pump must be primed prior to first use.

DDAVP® Rhinal tube: Insert top of dropper into tube (arrow marked end) in downward position. Squeeze dropper until solution reaches desired calibration mark. Disconnect dropper. Grasp the tube ³/₄inch from the end and insert tube into nostril until the fingertips reach the nostril. Place opposite end of tube into the mouth (holding breath). Tilt head back and blow with a strong, short puff into the nostril. Reseal dropper after use.

Monitoring Parameters Blood pressure and pulse should be monitored during I.V. infusion

Diabetes insipidus: Fluid intake, urine volume, specific gravity, plasma and urine osmolality, serum electrolytes

Hemophilia: Factor VIII antigen levels, APTT

Patient Information Avoid overhydration; notify physician if headache, shortness of breath, heartburn, nausea, abdominal cramps or vulval pain occurs; follow administration guidelines for intranasal products

Additional Information Manufacturer supplies a flexible tubing for administering the nasal solution; 10 mcg of desmopressin acetate is equivalent to 40 int. units

Special Geriatric Considerations Elderly patients should be cautioned not to increase their fluid intake beyond that sufficient to satisfy their thirst in order to avoid water intoxication and hyponatremia. Under experimental conditions, elderly have been shown to have a decreased responsiveness to vasopressin with respect to its effects on water homeostasis.

Dosage Forms Excipient information presented when available (limited, particularly for generics); consult specific product labeling.

Injection, solution, as acetate (DDAVP®): 4 mcg/mL (1 mL, 10 mL)

Solution, intranasal, as acetate (DDAVP®): 100 mcg/mL (2.5 mL) [with rhinal tube]

Solution, intranasal, as acetate [spray]: 100 mcg/mL (5 mL) [delivers 10 mcg/spray]

DDAVP®: 100 mcg/mL (5 mL) [delivers 10 mcg/spray]

Stimate™: 1.5 mg/mL (2.5 mL) [delivers 150 mcg/spray]

Tablet, as acetate (DDAVP®): 0.1 mg, 0.2 mg

Selected References

Asplund R and Aberg H, "Desmopressin in Elderly Subjects With Increased Nocturnal Diuresis: A Two-Month Treatment Study," *Scand J Urol Nephrol*, 1993, 27(1):77-82.

Lindeman RD, Lee TD Jr, Yiengst MJ, et al, "Influence of Age, Renal Disease, Hypertension, Diuretics, and Calcium on the Antidiuretic Responses to Suboptimal Infusions of Vasopressin," *J Lab Clin Med*, 1966, 68(2):206-23.

Miller JH and Shock NW, "Age Differences in the Renal Tubular Response to Antidiuretic Hormone," *J Gerontol*, 1953, 8:446-50.

♦ **Desmopressin Acetate** *see* Desmopressin *on page 411*

♦ **Desoxyphenobarbital** *see* Primidone *on page 1312*

♦ **Desyrel® [DSC]** *see* Trazodone *on page 1616*

♦ **Detemir Insulin** *see* Insulin Detemir *on page 809*

♦ **Detrol®** *see* Tolterodine *on page 1597*

♦ **Detrol® LA** *see* Tolterodine *on page 1597*

Dexamethasone (deks a METH a sone)

Related Information

Corticosteroids *on page 1755*

Inhalant Agents *on page 1760*

Medication Safety Issues

Sound-alike/look-alike issues:

Dexamethasone may be confused with desoximetasone

Decadron® may be confused with Percodan®

Maxidex® may be confused with Maxzide®

U.S. Brand Names Dexamethasone Intensol™; DexPak® TaperPak®; Maxidex®

Canadian Brand Names Apo-Dexamethasone®; Dexasone®; Diodex®; Maxidex®; PMS-Dexamethasone

Index Terms Dexamethasone Sodium Phosphate

Generic Available Yes: Excludes ophthalmic suspension

Pharmacologic Category Anti-inflammatory Agent; Anti-inflammatory Agent, Ophthalmic; Antiemetic; Corticosteroid, Ophthalmic; Corticosteroid, Otic; Corticosteroid, Systemic

Use

Systemic: Primarily as an anti-inflammatory or immunosuppressant agent in the treatment of a variety of diseases including those of allergic, dermatologic, endocrine, hematologic, inflammatory, neoplastic, nervous system, renal, respiratory, rheumatic, and autoimmune origin; may be used in management of cerebral edema, septic shock, chronic swelling, as a diagnostic agent, diagnosis of Cushing's syndrome, antiemetic

Ophthalmic: Treatment of palpebral and bulbar conjunctivitis; corneal injury from chemical, radiation, thermal burns, or foreign body penetration

Otic: Treatment of inflammation of external auditory meatus; treatment of edema associated with infective otitis externa

Unlabeled/Investigational Use Dexamethasone suppression test: General indicator consistent with depression and/or suicide

(Continued)

Dexamethasone *(Continued)*

Contraindications Hypersensitivity to dexamethasone or any component of the formulation; systemic fungal infections, cerebral malaria; ophthalmic use in viral (active ocular herpes simplex), fungal, or tuberculosis diseases of the eye

Warnings/Precautions Use with caution in patients with thyroid disease, hepatic impairment, renal impairment, cardiovascular disease, diabetes, glaucoma, cataracts, myasthenia gravis, patients at risk for osteoporosis, patients at risk for seizures, or GI diseases (diverticulitis, peptic ulcer, ulcerative colitis) due to perforation risk. Use caution following acute MI (corticosteroids have been associated with myocardial rupture). Because of the risk of adverse effects, systemic corticosteroids should be used cautiously in the elderly in the smallest possible effective dose for the shortest duration. Withdraw therapy with gradual tapering of dose.

May cause hypercorticism or suppression of hypothalamic-pituitary-adrenal (HPA) axis, particularly in patients receiving high doses for prolonged periods. HPA axis suppression may lead to adrenal crisis. Withdrawal and discontinuation of a corticosteroid should be done slowly and carefully. Particular care is required when patients are transferred from systemic corticosteroids to inhaled products due to possible adrenal insufficiency or withdrawal from steroids, including an increase in allergic symptoms. Patients receiving >20 mg per day of prednisone (or equivalent) may be most susceptible. Fatalities have occurred due to adrenal insufficiency in asthmatic patients during and after transfer from systemic corticosteroids to aerosol steroids; aerosol steroids do not provide the systemic steroid needed to treat patients having trauma, surgery, or infections. Dexamethasone does not provide adequate mineralocorticoid activity in adrenal insufficiency (may be employed as a single dose while cortisol assays are performed). The lowest possible dose should be used during treatment; discontinuation and/or dose reductions should be gradual.

Acute myopathy has been reported with high dose corticosteroids, usually in patients with neuromuscular transmission disorders; may involve ocular and/or respiratory muscles; monitor creatine kinase; recovery may be delayed. Corticosteroid use may cause psychiatric disturbances, including depression, euphoria, insomnia, mood swings, and personality changes. Pre-existing psychiatric conditions may be exacerbated by corticosteroid use. Prolonged use of corticosteroids may also increase the incidence of secondary infection, mask acute infection (including fungal infections), prolong or exacerbate viral infections, or limit response to vaccines. Exposure to chickenpox should be avoided; corticosteroids should not be used to treat ocular herpes simplex. Corticosteroids should not be used for cerebral malaria. Close observation is required in patients with latent tuberculosis and/or TB reactivity; restrict use in active TB (only in conjunction with antituberculosis treatment). Prolonged treatment with corticosteroids has been associated with the development of Kaposi's sarcoma (case reports); if noted, discontinuation of therapy should be considered.

Adverse Reactions (Reflective of adult population; not specific for elderly)
Frequency not defined.

Cardiovascular: Arrhythmia, bradycardia, cardiac arrest, cardiomyopathy, CHF, circulatory collapse, edema, hypertension, myocardial rupture (post-MI), syncope, thromboembolism, vasculitis

Central nervous system: Depression, emotional instability, euphoria, headache, intracranial pressure increased, insomnia, malaise, mood swings, neuritis, personality changes, pseudotumor cerebri (usually following discontinuation), psychic disorders, seizure, vertigo

Dermatologic: Acne, allergic dermatitis, alopecia, angioedema, bruising, dry skin, erythema, fragile skin, hirsutism, hyper-/hypopigmentation, hypertrichosis, perianal pruritus (following I.V. injection), petechiae, rash, skin atrophy, skin test reaction impaired, striae, urticaria, wound healing impaired

Endocrine & metabolic: Adrenal suppression, carbohydrate tolerance decreased, Cushing's syndrome, diabetes mellitus, glucose intolerance decreased, growth suppression (children), hyperglycemia, hypokalemic alkalosis, menstrual irregularities, negative nitrogen balance, pituitary-adrenal axis suppression, protein catabolism, sodium retention

Gastrointestinal: Abdominal distention, appetite increased, gastrointestinal hemorrhage, gastrointestinal perforation, nausea, pancreatitis, peptic ulcer, ulcerative esophagitis, weight gain

Genitourinary: Altered (increased or decreased) spermatogenesis

Hepatic: Hepatomegaly, transaminases increased

Local: Postinjection flare (intra-articular use), thrombophlebitis

Neuromuscular & skeletal: Arthropathy, aseptic necrosis (femoral and humoral heads), fractures, muscle mass loss, myopathy (particularly in conjunction with neuromuscular disease or neuromuscular-blocking agents), neuropathy, osteoporosis, parasthesia, tendon rupture, vertebral compression fractures, weakness

Ocular: Cataracts, exophthalmos, glaucoma, intraocular pressure increased

Renal: Glucosuria

Respiratory: Pulmonary edema

Miscellaneous: Abnormal fat deposition, anaphylactoid reaction, anaphylaxis, avascular necrosis, diaphoresis, hiccups, hypersensitivity, impaired wound healing, infections, Kaposi's sarcoma, moon face, secondary malignancy

Overdosage/Toxicology Symptoms include moon face, central obesity, hypertension, psychosis, hallucinations, diabetes, hyperlipidemia, peptic ulcer, increased susceptibility to infection, electrolyte and fluid imbalance. When consumed in excessive quantities, systemic hypercorticism and adrenal suppression may occur; in those cases, discontinuation and withdrawal of the corticosteroid should be done judiciously.

Drug Interactions Substrate of CYP3A4 (major); **Induces** CYP2A6 (weak), 2B6 (weak), 2C8 (weak), 2C9 (weak), 3A4 (strong)

Aminoglutethimide: May reduce the serum levels/effects of dexamethasone; likely via induction of microsomal isoenzymes.

Amphotericin: Corticosteroids may increase the hypokalemic effects of amphotericin B; monitor.

Antacids: May decrease the absorption of corticosteroids; separate administration by 2 hours.

Antidiabetic agents: Corticosteroids may decrease the hypoglycemic effects of antidiabetic agents; monitor.

Anticholinesterases: Concurrent use may lead to severe weakness in patients with myasthenia gravis.

Aprepitant: May increase the serum levels/effects of corticosteroids; monitor.

Antifungal agents (azole): May increase the serum levels/effects of corticosteroids; monitor.

Barbiturates: May decrease the levels/effects of dexamethasone (systemic).

Bile acid sequestrants: May reduce the absorption of corticosteroids; separate administration by 2 hours.

Calcium channel blockers (nondihydropyridine): May increase the serum levels/effects of corticosteroids; monitor.

Cyclosporine: Corticosteroids may increase the serum levels/effects of cyclosporine. In addition, cyclosporine may increase levels of corticosteroids.

CYP3A4 Inducers may decrease the levels/effects of dexamethasone. Example inducers include aminoglutethimide, carbamazepine, nafcillin, nevirapine, phenobarbital, phenytoin, and rifamycins.

CYP3A4 Inhibitors may increase the levels/effects of dexamethasone. Example inhibitors include azole antifungals, clarithromycin, diclofenac, doxycycline, erythromycin, imatinib, isoniazid, nefazodone, nicardipine, propofol, protease inhibitors, quinidine, telithromycin, and verapamil.

CYP3A4 Substrates: Dexamethasone may decrease the levels/effects of CYP3A4 substrates. Example substrates include benzodiazepines, calcium channel blockers, clarithromycin, cyclosporine, erythromycin, estrogens, mirtazapine, nateglinide, nefazodone, nevirapine, protease inhibitors, tacrolimus, and venlafaxine.

Diuretics, potassium-wasting (loop or thiazide): Hypokalemic effects may be increased by corticosteroids; monitor.

Estrogens: May increase the serum levels/effects of corticosteroids; monitor.

Fluoroquinolones: Concurrent use may increase the risk of tendinopathies (including tendonitis and rupture), particularly in elderly patients (overall incidence rare)

Isoniazid: Serum levels/effects may be decreased by corticosteroids.

Macrolide antibiotics: May increase the serum levels/effects of dexamethasone (systemic).

Neuromuscular-blocking agents: Concurrent use with corticosteroids may increase the risk of myopathy.

Nonsteroidal anti-inflammatory drugs (NSAIDs): Concurrent use with corticosteroids may lead to an increased incidence of gastrointestinal adverse effects; use caution. NSAID (ophthalmic) may enhance the adverse/toxic effect of dexamethasone (ophthalmic).

Salicylates: Salicylates may increase the gastrointestinal adverse effects of corticosteroids.

Thalidomide: Concurrent use with corticosteroids may increase the risk of selected adverse effects (toxic epidermal necrolysis and DVT); use caution.

Vaccine (dead organism): Dexamethasone may decrease the effect of vaccines (dead organisms). In patients receiving high doses of systemic corticosteroids for ≥14 days, wait at least 1 month between discontinuing steroid therapy and administering immunization.

Vaccine (live organism): Dexamethasone may increase the risk of vaccinal infection. The use of live vaccines is contraindicated in immunosuppressed patients.

Warfarin: Corticosteroids may increase the anticoagulant effects of warfarin; monitor INR.

Ethanol/Nutrition/Herb Interactions

Ethanol: Avoid ethanol (may enhance gastric mucosal irritation).

Food: Dexamethasone interferes with calcium absorption. Limit caffeine.

Herb/Nutraceutical: Avoid cat's claw, echinacea (have immunostimulant properties).

(Continued)

Dexamethasone *(Continued)*

Stability

Injection solution: Store at room temperature; protect from light and freezing.

Stability of injection of parenteral admixture at room temperature (25°C): 24 hours

Stability of injection of parenteral admixture at refrigeration temperature (4°C): 2 days; protect from light and freezing.

Injection should be diluted in 50-100 mL NS or D_5W.

Mechanism of Action Decreases inflammation by suppression of neutrophil migration, decreased production of inflammatory mediators, and reversal of increased capillary permeability; suppresses normal immune response. Dexamethasone's mechanism of antiemetic activity is unknown.

Pharmacodynamics Duration of metabolic effects: Can last for 72 hours

Pharmacokinetics

Metabolism: In the liver

Half-life: 1.8-3.5 hours; biologic half-life: 36-54 hours

Time to peak serum concentration:

Oral: Within 1-2 hours

I.M.: Within 8 hours

Elimination: In urine and bile

Dosage

Geriatrics: Refer to adult dosing. Use cautiously in the elderly in the smallest possible dose.

Adults:

Anti-inflammatory:

Oral, I.M., I.V.: 0.75-9 mg/day in divided doses every 6-12 hours

Intra-articular, intralesional, or soft tissue: 0.4-6 mg/day

Extubation or airway edema: Oral, I.M., I.V.: 0.5-2 mg/kg/day in divided doses every 6 hours beginning 24 hours prior to extubation and continuing for 4-6 doses afterwards

Antiemetic:

Prophylaxis: Oral, I.V.: 10-20 mg 15-30 minutes before treatment on each treatment day

Continuous infusion regimen: Oral or I.V.: 10 mg every 12 hours on each treatment day

Mildly emetogenic therapy: Oral, I.M., I.V.: 4 mg every 4-6 hours

Delayed nausea/vomiting: Oral: 4-10 mg 1-2 times/day for 2-4 days **or**

8 mg every 12 hours for 2 days; then

4 mg every 12 hours for 2 days **or**

20 mg 1 hour before chemotherapy; then

10 mg 12 hours after chemotherapy; then

8 mg every 12 hours for 4 doses; then

4 mg every 12 hours for 4 doses

Ophthalmic anti-inflammatory:

Ophthalmic solution: Instill 1-2 drops into conjunctival sac every hour during the day and every other hour during the night; gradually reduce dose to every 3-4 hours, then to 3-4 times/day.

Ophthalmic suspension: Instill 1-2 drops into conjunctival sac up to 4-6 times per day; may use hourly in severe disease; taper prior to discontinuation.

Otic anti-inflammatory: Instill 3-4 drops 2-3 times a day; reduce dose gradually prior to discontinuation.

Multiple myeloma: Oral, I.V.: 40 mg/day, days 1 to 4, 9 to 12, and 17 to 20, repeated every 4 weeks (alone or as part of a regimen)

Cerebral edema: I.V. 10 mg stat, 4 mg I.M./I.V. (should be given as sodium phosphate) every 6 hours until response is maximized, then switch to oral regimen, then taper off if appropriate; dosage may be reduced after 24 days and gradually discontinued over 5-7 days

Dexamethasone suppression test (depression/suicide indicator) (unlabeled use): Oral: 1 mg at 11 PM, draw blood at 8 AM the following day for plasma cortisol determination

Cushing's syndrome, diagnostic: Oral: 1 mg at 11 PM, draw blood at 8 AM; greater accuracy for Cushing's syndrome may be achieved by the following:

Dexamethasone 0.5 mg by mouth every 6 hours for 48 hours (with 24-hour urine collection for 17-hydroxycorticosteroid excretion)

Differentiation of Cushing's syndrome due to ACTH excess from Cushing's due to other causes: Oral: Dexamethasone 2 mg every 6 hours for 48 hours (with 24-hour urine collection for 17-hydroxycorticosteroid excretion)

Multiple sclerosis (acute exacerbation): Oral: 30 mg/day for 1 week, followed by 4-12 mg/day for 1 month

Treatment of shock:

Addisonian crisis/shock (eg, adrenal insufficiency/responsive to steroid therapy): I.V.: 4-10 mg as a single dose, which may be repeated if necessary

Unresponsive shock (eg, unresponsive to steroid therapy): I.V.: 1-6 mg/kg as a single I.V. dose or up to 40 mg initially followed by repeat doses every 2-6 hours while shock persists

Physiological replacement: Oral, I.M., I.V. (should be given as sodium phosphate): 0.03-0.15 mg/kg/day **or** 0.6-0.75 mg/m^2/day in divided doses every 6-12 hours

Renal Impairment: Hemodialysis or peritoneal dialysis: Supplemental dose is not necessary.

Administration

Oral: Administer with meals to decrease GI upset.

I.V.: Administer as a 5-10 minute bolus; rapid injection is associated with a high incidence of perianal discomfort.

Ophthalmic: Remove soft contact lenses prior to using solutions containing benzalkonium chloride. Do not touch tip of container to eye.

Otic: Use ophthalmic solution for otic administration. Instill directly into aural canal or may pack canal with gauze saturated with solution. Keep wick moist and remove after 12-24 hours.

Monitoring Parameters Hemoglobin, occult blood loss, serum potassium, and glucose; intraocular pressure (with use >6 weeks)

Reference Range Dexamethasone suppression test, overnight: 8 AM cortisol <6 mcg/100 mL (dexamethasone 1 mg)

Patient Information Do not take any new medication during therapy unless approved by prescriber. Take exactly as directed, do not increase dose or discontinue abruptly without consulting prescriber.

Oral: Take with or after meals. Avoid alcohol and limit intake of caffeine or stimulants. Prescriber may recommend increased dietary vitamins, minerals, or iron. If you have diabetes, monitor glucose levels closely (antidiabetic medication may need to be adjusted). Inform prescriber if you are experiencing greater-than-normal levels of stress (medication may need adjustment). You may be more susceptible to infection (avoid crowds and persons with contagious or infective conditions and do not have any vaccinations unless approved by prescriber). Some forms of this medication may cause GI upset (small frequent meals and frequent mouth care may help). Report promptly excessive nervousness or sleep disturbances; signs of infection (eg, sore throat, unhealed injuries); excessive growth of body hair or loss of skin color; vision changes; excessive or sudden weight gain (>3 lb/week); swelling of face or extremities; respiratory difficulty; muscle weakness; tarry stool, persistent abdominal pain; worsening of condition or failure to improve.

Ophthalmic: For use in eyes only. Wash hands before using. Lie down or tilt your head back and look upward. Put drops of suspension or solution inside lower eyelid. Close eye and roll eyeball in all directions. Do not blink for 1/2 minute. Apply gentle pressure to inner corner of eye for 30 seconds. Do not use any other eye preparation for at least 10 minutes. Do not let tip of applicator touch eye; do not contaminate tip of applicator (may cause eye infection, eye damage, or vision loss). Do not share medication with anyone else. Wear sunglasses when in sunlight; you may be more sensitive to bright light. Inform prescriber if condition worsens, fails to improve, or if you experience eye pain, disturbances of vision, or other adverse eye response.

Additional Information Withdrawal/tapering of therapy: Corticosteroid tapering following short-term use is limited primarily by the need to control the underlying disease state; tapering may be accomplished over a period of days. Following longer-term use, tapering over weeks to months may be necessary to avoid signs and symptoms of adrenal insufficiency and to allow recovery of the HPA axis. Testing of HPA axis responsiveness may be of value in selected patients. Subtle deficits in HPA response may persist for months after discontinuation of therapy, and may require supplemental dosing during periods of acute illness or surgical stress.

Special Geriatric Considerations Because of the risk of adverse effects, systemic corticosteroids should be used cautiously in the elderly in the smallest possible dose, and for the shortest possible time.

Dosage Forms Excipient information presented when available (limited, particularly for generics); consult specific product labeling. [DSC] = Discontinued product

Elixir, as base: 0.5 mg/5 mL (240 mL)

Injection, solution, as sodium phosphate: 4 mg/mL (1 mL, 5 mL, 30 mL); 10 mg/mL (10 mL)

Injection, solution, as sodium phosphate [preservative free]: 10 mg/mL (1 mL)

Solution, ophthalmic, as sodium phosphate: 0.1% (5 mL)

Solution, oral: 0.5 mg/5 mL (500 mL)

Solution, oral concentrate:

Dexamethasone Intensol™: 1 mg/mL (30 mL) [contains alcohol 30%]

Suspension, ophthalmic:

Maxidex®: 0.1% (5 mL; 15 mL [DSC]) [contains benzalkonium chloride]

Tablet [scored]: 0.5 mg, 0.75 mg, 1 mg, 1.5 mg, 2 mg, 4 mg, 6 mg

DexPak® TaperPak®: 1.5 mg [51 tablets on taper dose card]

(Continued)

Dexamethasone *(Continued)*

Selected References
Kyle RA and Rajkumar SV, "Multiple Myeloma," *N Engl J Med*, 2004, 351(18): 1860-73.
Trissel LA and Zhang Y, "Compatibility and Stability of Aloxi (Palonosetron Hydrochloride) Admixed With Dexamethasone Sodium Phosphate," *Intl J Pharm Compounding*, 2004, 8(5):398-403.

♦ **Dexamethasone and Ciprofloxacin** *see* Ciprofloxacin and Dexamethasone *on page 322*

♦ **Dexamethasone and Tobramycin** *see* Tobramycin and Dexamethasone *on page 1587*

♦ **Dexamethasone Intensol™** *see* Dexamethasone *on page 413*

♦ **Dexamethasone, Neomycin, and Polymyxin B** *see* Neomycin, Polymyxin B, and Dexamethasone *on page 1102*

♦ **Dexamethasone Sodium Phosphate** *see* Dexamethasone *on page 413*

Dexchlorpheniramine (deks klor fen EER a meen)

Related Information
Potentially Inappropriate Medications for Geriatrics *on page 1824*
Index Terms Dexchlorpheniramine Maleate
Generic Available Yes
Pharmacologic Category Antihistamine
Use Treatment of perennial and seasonal allergic rhinitis and other allergic symptoms including urticaria
Contraindications Hypersensitivity to dexchlorpheniramine or any component of the formulation; narrow-angle glaucoma
Warnings/Precautions Causes sedation, caution must be used in performing tasks which require alertness (eg, operating machinery or driving). Sedative effects of CNS depressants or ethanol are potentiated. Use with caution in patients with angle-closure glaucoma, pyloroduodenal obstruction (including stenotic peptic ulcer), urinary tract obstruction (including bladder neck obstruction and symptomatic prostatic hyperplasia), hyperthyroidism, increased intraocular pressure, and cardiovascular disease (including hypertension and tachycardia). High sedative and anticholinergic properties, therefore may not be considered the antihistamine of choice for prolonged use in the elderly.
Adverse Reactions (Reflective of adult population; not specific for elderly)
>10%:
  Central nervous system: Slight to moderate drowsiness
  Respiratory: Thickening of bronchial secretions
1% to 10%:
  Central nervous system: Headache, fatigue, nervousness, dizziness
  Gastrointestinal: Appetite increase, weight gain, nausea, diarrhea, abdominal pain, xerostomia
  Neuromuscular & skeletal: Arthralgia
  Respiratory: Pharyngitis
Drug Interactions Increased effect/toxicity: CNS depressants, MAO inhibitors, TCAs, phenothiazines, guanabenz
Ethanol/Nutrition/Herb Interactions Ethanol: Avoid ethanol (may increase CNS depression).
Mechanism of Action Competes with histamine for H_1-receptor sites on effector cells in the gastrointestinal tract, blood vessels, and respiratory tract. Dexchlorpheniramine is the predominant active isomer of chlorpheniramine and is approximately twice as active as the racemic compound.
Pharmacodynamics
Peak effect: Oral: Within 3 hours
Duration: 3-6 hours
Pharmacokinetics
Absorption: Well absorbed from GI tract
Metabolism: In the liver
Elimination: In urine within 24 hours as inactive metabolites
Dosage
Geriatrics & Adults: Allergy symptoms: Oral: 2 mg every 4-6 hours or 4-6 mg timed release at bedtime or every 8-10 hours
Monitoring Parameters Monitor mental function, bowel function, and urinary retention
Patient Information May cause drowsiness, dry mouth, confusion; swallow whole, do not crush or chew sustained release product; avoid alcohol, may impair coordination and judgment
Special Geriatric Considerations Anticholinergic action may cause significant confusional symptoms, constipation, or problems voiding urine.
Dosage Forms Excipient information presented when available (limited, particularly for generics); consult specific product labeling.

Syrup, as maleate: 2 mg/5 mL (480 mL, 3840 mL) [contains alcohol 6%; orange flavor]
Tablet, sustained action, as maleate: 4 mg, 6 mg

◆ **Dexchlorpheniramine Maleate** *see* Dexchlorpheniramine *on page 418*
◆ **Dexferrum**® *see* Iron Dextran Complex *on page 832*
◆ **DexPak**® **TaperPak**® *see* Dexamethasone *on page 413*

Dextromethorphan (deks troe meth OR fan)

Medication Safety Issues
Sound-alike/look-alike issues:
Benylin® may be confused with Benadryl®, Ventolin®
Delsym® may be confused with Delfen®, Desyrel®
U.S. Brand Names Babee® Cof Syrup [OTC]; Creomulsion® Cough [OTC]; Creomul-
sion® for Children [OTC]; Creo-Terpin® [OTC]; Delsym® [OTC]; ElixSure® Cough
[OTC]; Hold® DM [OTC]; PediaCare® Children's Medicated Freezer Pops Long Acting
Cough [OTC] [DSC]; PediaCare® Infants' Long-Acting Cough [OTC]; Robitussin®
CoughGels™ [OTC]; Robitussin® Maximum Strength Cough [OTC]; Robitussin® Pedi-
atric Cough [OTC]; Scot-Tussin DM® Cough Chasers [OTC]; Silphen DM® [OTC];
Simply Cough® [OTC] [DSC]; Triaminic® Thin Strips™ Long Acting Cough [OTC];
Vicks® 44® Cough Relief [OTC]
Generic Available Yes: Excludes strip, liquid freezer pop
Pharmacologic Category Antitussive
Use Symptomatic relief of coughs caused by minor viral upper respiratory tract infections
or inhaled irritants; most effective for a chronic nonproductive cough
Unlabeled/Investigational Use *N*-methyl-D-aspartate (NMDA) antagonist in cerebral
injury
Contraindications Hypersensitivity to dextromethorphan or any component of the
formulation
Warnings/Precautions Should not be used for chronic productive coughs
Drug Interactions Substrate of CYP2B6 (minor), 2C9 (minor), 2C19 (minor), 2D6
(major), 2E1 (minor), 3A4 (minor); **Inhibits** CYP2D6 (weak)
CYP2D6 inhibitors: May increase the levels/effects of dextromethorphan. Example
inhibitors include chlorpromazine, delavirdine, fluoxetine, miconazole, paroxetine,
pergolide, quinidine, quinine, ritonavir, and ropinirole.
MAO inhibitors: Dextromethorphan may increase effect/toxicity of MAO inhibitors.
Mechanism of Action Chemical relative of morphine lacking narcotic properties
except in overdose; controls cough by depressing the medullary cough center
Pharmacodynamics
Onset of antitussive action: Within 15-30 minutes
Duration: Up to 6 hours; higher doses may have longer duration
Pharmacokinetics
Metabolism: In the liver
Elimination: Principally in urine
Dosage
Geriatrics & Adults: Cough suppressant: Oral: 10-20 mg every 4 hours or 30 mg
every 6-8 hours; extended release: 60 mg twice daily; maximum: 120 mg/day
Monitoring Parameters Cough, mental status
Patient Information May cause drowsiness; avoid CNS depressants and alcohol; do
not use for persistent or chronic cough
Additional Information Dextromethorphan is considered approximately half as potent
as codeine as an antitussive; dextromethorphan is a component in many cough and
cold preparations
Dosage Forms Excipient information presented when available (limited, particularly for
generics); consult specific product labeling. [DSC] = Discontinued product
Gelcap, as hydrobromide:
Robitussin® CoughGels™: 15 mg [contains coconut oil]
Liquid, as hydrobromide:
Creo-Terpin®: 10 mg/15 mL (120 mL) [contains alcohol 25% and tartrazine]
Simply Cough®: 5 mg/5 mL (120 mL) [contains sodium benzoate; cherry berry flavor]
[DSC]
Vicks® 44® Cough Relief: 10 mg/5 mL (120 mL) [contains alcohol, sodium 10 mg/5
mL, sodium benzoate]
Liquid, oral, as hydrobromide [freezer pops]:
PediaCare® Children's Medicated Freezer Pops Long Acting Cough: 7.5 mg/25 mL
(8s) [alcohol free; contains sodium benzoate, berry flavor also contains benzyl
alcohol; glacier grape™ and polar berry blue™ flavors] [DSC]
Liquid, oral, as hydrobromide [drops]:
PediaCare® Infants' Long-Acting Cough: 7.5 mg/0.8 mL (15 mL) [alcohol free, dye
free; contains sodium benzoate; grape flavor]
(Continued)

Dextromethorphan *(Continued)*

Lozenge, as hydrobromide:
Hold® DM: 5 mg (10s) [cherry or original flavor]
Scot-Tussin DM® Cough Chasers: 5 mg (20s)
Strips, oral, as hydrobromide:
Triaminic® Thin Strips™ Long Acting Cough: 7.5 mg [equivalent to dextromethorphan 5 mg; cherry flavor]
Suspension, extended release:
Delsym®: Dextromethorphan polistirex [equivalent to dextromethorphan hydrobromide 30 mg/5 mL] (78 mL, 148 mL) [contains sodium 6 mg/5 mL; orange flavor]
Syrup, as hydrobromide:
Babee® Cof Syrup: 7.5 mg/5 mL (120 mL) [alcohol free, dye free; cherry flavor]
Creomulsion® Cough: 20 mg/15 mL (120 mL) [alcohol free; contains sodium benzoate]
Creomulsion® for Children: 5 mg/5 mL (120 mL) [alcohol free; contains sodium benzoate; cherry flavor]
ElixSure® Cough: 7.5 mg/5 mL (120 mL) [cherry bubble gum flavor]
Robitussin® Maximum Strength Cough: 15 mg/5 mL (120 mL, 240 mL) [contains alcohol, sodium benzoate]
Robitussin® Pediatric Cough: 7.5 mg/5 mL (120 mL) [alcohol free; contains sodium benzoate; fruit punch flavor]
Silphen DM®: 10 mg/5 mL (120 mL) [strawberry flavor]

♦ **Dextromethorphan and Guaifenesin** *see* Guaifenesin and Dextromethorphan *on page 730*
♦ **Dextropropoxyphene** *see* Propoxyphene *on page 1333*
♦ **DHE** *see* Dihydroergotamine *on page 437*
♦ **D.H.E. 45®** *see* Dihydroergotamine *on page 437*
♦ **DHPG Sodium** *see* Ganciclovir *on page 697*
♦ **DHS™ Sal [OTC]** *see* Salicylic Acid *on page 1441*
♦ **DHT™ [DSC]** *see* Dihydrotachysterol *on page 439*
♦ **DHT™ Intensol™ [DSC]** *see* Dihydrotachysterol *on page 439*
♦ **Diabeta** *see* GlyBURIDE *on page 714*
♦ **DiabetAid™ Antifungal Foot Bath [OTC]** *see* Miconazole *on page 1036*
♦ **Diabetic Tussin C®** *see* Guaifenesin and Codeine *on page 729*
♦ **Diabetic Tussin® Allergy Relief [OTC]** *see* Chlorpheniramine *on page 296*
♦ **Diabetic Tussin® DM [OTC]** *see* Guaifenesin and Dextromethorphan *on page 730*
♦ **Diabetic Tussin® DM Maximum Strength [OTC]** *see* Guaifenesin and Dextromethorphan *on page 730*
♦ **Diabetic Tussin® EX [OTC]** *see* Guaifenesin *on page 727*
♦ **Diabinese®** *see* ChlorproPAMIDE *on page 300*
♦ **Diaβeta®** *see* GlyBURIDE *on page 714*
♦ **Diamode [OTC]** *see* Loperamide *on page 924*
♦ **Diamox® Sequels®** *see* AcetaZOLAMIDE *on page 33*
♦ **Diastat®** *see* Diazepam *on page 420*
♦ **Diastat® AcuDial™** *see* Diazepam *on page 420*

Diazepam *(dye AZ e pam)*

Related Information
Anxiolytic, Sedative / Hypnotic, and Miscellaneous Benzodiazepines *on page 1750*
Potentially Inappropriate Medications for Geriatrics *on page 1824*
Medication Safety Issues
Sound-alike/look-alike issues:
Diazepam may be confused with diazoxide, Ditropan®, lorazepam
Valium® may be confused with Valcyte™
U.S. Brand Names Diastat®; Diastat® AcuDial™; Diazepam Intensol®; Valium®
Canadian Brand Names Apo-Diazepam®; Diastat®; Diastat® Rectal Delivery System; Diazemuls®; Novo-Dipam; Valium®
Generic Available Yes: Injection, tablet, solution only
Pharmacologic Category Benzodiazepine
Use Management of general anxiety disorders; light anesthesia to produce amnesia, preoperative sedation; treatment of status epilepticus, convulsive disorders, ethanol withdrawal symptoms; skeletal muscle relaxant
Orphan drug: Viscous solution for rectal administration: Management of selected, refractory epilepsy patients on stable regimens of antiepileptic drugs (AEDs) requiring intermittent use of diazepam to control episodes of increased seizure activity
Unlabeled/Investigational Use Treatment of panic disorders

Restrictions C-IV

Contraindications Hypersensitivity to diazepam or any component of the formulation (cross-sensitivity with other benzodiazepines may exist); narrow-angle glaucoma

Warnings/Precautions Withdrawal has also been associated with an increase in the seizure frequency. Use with caution with drugs which may decrease diazepam metabolism. Use with caution in elderly or debilitated patients, obese patients, patients with hepatic disease (including alcoholics), or renal impairment. Active metabolites with extended half-lives may lead to delayed accumulation and adverse effects. Use with caution in patients with respiratory disease or impaired gag reflex.

Acute hypotension, muscle weakness, apnea, and cardiac arrest have occurred with parenteral administration. Acute effects may be more prevalent in patients receiving concurrent barbiturates, narcotics, or ethanol. Appropriate resuscitative equipment and qualified personnel should be available during administration and monitoring. Avoid use of the injection in patients with shock, coma, or acute ethanol intoxication. Intra-arterial injection or extravasation of the parenteral formulation should be avoided. Parenteral formulation contains propylene glycol, which has been associated with toxicity when administered in high dosages. Administration of rectal gel should only be performed by individuals trained to recognize characteristic seizure activity and monitor response.

Causes CNS depression (dose-related) resulting in sedation, dizziness, confusion, or ataxia which may impair physical and mental capabilities. Patients must be cautioned about performing tasks which require mental alertness (eg, operating machinery or driving). Use with caution in patients receiving other CNS depressants or psychoactive agents. Effects with other sedative drugs or ethanol may be potentiated. The dosage of narcotics should be reduced by approximately 1/3 when diazepam is added. Benzodiazepines have been associated with falls and traumatic injury and should be used with extreme caution in patients who are at risk of these events (especially the elderly). Use with caution in patients taking strong CYP3A4 inhibitors, moderate or strong CYP3A4 and CYP2C19 inducers and major CYP3A4 substrates.

Use with caution in patients with depression, particularly if suicidal risk may be present. Use with caution in patients with a history of drug dependence. Benzodiazepines have been associated with dependence and acute withdrawal symptoms on discontinuation or reduction in dose. Acute withdrawal, including seizures, may be precipitated in patients after administration of flumazenil to patients receiving long-term benzodiazepine therapy.

Diazepam has been associated with anterograde amnesia. Paradoxical reactions, including hyperactive or aggressive behavior, have been reported with benzodiazepines, particularly in psychiatric patients. Does not have analgesic, antidepressant, or antipsychotic properties.

Adverse Reactions (Reflective of adult population; not specific for elderly) Frequency not defined. Adverse reactions may vary by route of administration.

Cardiovascular: Hypotension, vasodilatation

Central nervous system: Agitation, amnesia, anxiety, ataxia, confusion, depression, dizziness, drowsiness, emotional lability, euphoria, fatigue, headache, incoordination, insomnia, memory impairment, paradoxical excitement or rage, seizure, slurred speech, somnolence, vertigo

Dermatologic: Rash

Endocrine & metabolic: Libido changes

Gastrointestinal: Constipation, diarrhea, nausea, salivation changes

Genitourinary: Incontinence, urinary retention

Hepatic: Jaundice

Local: Phlebitis, pain with injection

Neuromuscular & skeletal: Dysarthria, tremor, weakness

Ocular: Blurred vision, diplopia

Respiratory: Apnea, asthma, respiratory rate decreased

Overdosage/Toxicology Symptoms include somnolence, confusion, coma, hypoactive reflexes, dyspnea, hypotension, slurred speech, and impaired coordination. Treatment for benzodiazepine overdose is supportive. Rarely is mechanical ventilation required. Flumazenil has been shown to selectively block the binding of benzodiazepines to CNS receptors, resulting in a reversal of benzodiazepine-induced CNS depression, but not respiratory depression.

Drug Interactions Substrate of CYP1A2 (minor), 2B6 (minor), 2C9 (minor), 2C19 (major), 3A4 (major); **Inhibits** CYP2C19 (weak), 3A4 (weak)

Calcium channel blockers, nondihydropyridine (diltiazem, verapamil): May decrease the metabolism, via CYP isoenzymes, of diazepam.

Clozapine: Benzodiazepines may enhance the adverse/toxic effect of clozapine.

CNS depressants: Sedative effects and/or respiratory depression may be additive with CNS depressants; includes ethanol, barbiturates, opioid analgesics, and other sedative agents; monitor for increased effect.

(Continued)

Diazepam *(Continued)*

CYP2C19 inducers: May decrease the levels/effects of diazepam. Example inducers include aminoglutethimide, carbamazepine, phenytoin, and rifampin.

CYP2C19 inhibitors: May increase the levels/effects of diazepam. Example inhibitors include delavirdine, fluconazole, fluvoxamine, gemfibrozil, isoniazid, omeprazole, and ticlopidine.

CYP3A4 inducers: CYP3A4 inducers may decrease the levels/effects of diazepam. Example inducers include aminoglutethimide, carbamazepine, nafcillin, nevirapine, phenobarbital, phenytoin, and rifamycins.

CYP3A4 inhibitors: May increase the levels/effects of diazepam. Example inhibitors include azole antifungals, clarithromycin, diclofenac, doxycycline, erythromycin, imatinib, isoniazid, nefazodone, nicardipine, propofol, protease inhibitors, quinidine, telithromycin, and verapamil.

Levodopa: Therapeutic effects may be diminished in some patients following the addition of a benzodiazepine; limited/inconsistent data.

Oral contraceptives: May decrease the clearance of some benzodiazepines (those which undergo oxidative metabolism); monitor for increased benzodiazepine effect.

Theophylline: May partially antagonize some of the effects of benzodiazepines; monitor for decreased response; may require higher doses for sedation.

Ethanol/Nutrition/Herb Interactions

Ethanol: Avoid ethanol (may increase CNS depression).

Food: Diazepam serum levels may be increased if taken with food. Diazepam effect/toxicity may be increased by grapefruit juice; avoid concurrent use.

Herb/Nutraceutical: St John's wort may decrease diazepam levels. Avoid valerian, St John's wort, kava kava, gotu kola (may increase CNS depression).

Stability

Protect parenteral dosage form from light. Potency is retained for up to 3 months when kept at room temperature. Most stable at pH 4-8; hydrolysis occurs at pH <3. Per manufacturer, do not mix I.V. product with other medications.

Rectal gel: Store at 25°C (77°F); excursion permitted to 15°C to 30°C (59°F to 86°F).

Mechanism of Action

Binds to stereospecific benzodiazepine receptors on the postsynaptic GABA neuron at several sites within the central nervous system, including the limbic system, reticular formation. Enhancement of the inhibitory effect of GABA on neuronal excitability results by increased neuronal membrane permeability to chloride ions. This shift in chloride ions results in hyperpolarization (a less excitable state) and stabilization.

Pharmacodynamics

Onset of action: Almost immediate with short duration of action (20-30 minutes) when given I.V. for status epilepticus

Studies have shown that older adults are more sensitive to the effects of benzodiazepines as compared to younger adults.

Pharmacokinetics

Absorption: Oral: 85% to 100%

Distribution: V_d: Increased in older adults

Protein binding: 98%

Metabolism: In liver; active major metabolite is desmethyldiazepam

Half-life: 20-50 hours, increased half-life in older adults (~90 hours) and those with severe hepatic disorders; desmethyldiazepam has a half-life of 50-100 hours and can be prolonged in older adults; accumulation of diazepam is extensive

Dosage

Geriatrics: Oral absorption is more reliable than I.M..

Oral: Initial:

Anxiety: 1-2 mg 1-2 times/day; increase gradually as needed, rarely need to use >10 mg/day.

Skeletal muscle relaxant: 2-5 mg 2-4 times/day

Rectal gel: Due to the increased half-life in elderly and debilitated patients, consider reducing dose.

Adults: Note: Oral absorption is more reliable than I.M.

Anticonvulsant (acute treatment): Rectal gel: 0.2 mg/kg. **Note:** Dosage should be rounded upward to the next available dose, 2.5, 5, 7.5, 10, 12.5, 15, 17.5, and 20 mg/dose; dose may be repeated in 4-12 hours if needed; do not use for more than 5 episodes per month or more than one episode every 5 days.

Anxiety/sedation/skeletal muscle relaxation:

Oral: 2-10 mg 2-4 times/day

I.M., I.V.: 2-10 mg, may repeat in 3-4 hours if needed

Sedation in the ICU patient: I.V.: 0.03-0.1 mg/kg every 30 minutes to 6 hours

Status epilepticus: I.V.: 5-10 mg every 10-20 minutes, up to 30 mg in an 8-hour period; may repeat in 2-4 hours if necessary

Rapid tranquilization of agitated patient (administer every 30-60 minutes): Oral: 5-10 mg; average total dose for tranquilization: 20-60 mg

Renal Impairment: Hemodialysis effects: Not dialyzable (0% to 5%); supplemental dose is **not** necessary.

Hepatic Impairment: Reduce dose by 50% in cirrhosis and avoid in severe/acute liver disease.

Administration Intensol® should be diluted before use.

Adults: Do not exceed 5 mg/minute IVP

Rectal gel: Patient should be positioned on side (facing person responsible for monitoring), with top leg bent forward. Insert rectal tip (lubricated) into rectum and push in plunger gently over 3 seconds. Remove tip of rectal syringe after 3 additional seconds. Buttocks should be held together for 3 seconds after removal. Dispose of syringe appropriately.

Reference Range Therapeutic: Diazepam: 0.2-1.5 mcg/mL (SI: 0.7-5.3 μmol/L); N-desmethyldiazepam (nordiazepam): 0.1-0.5 mcg/mL (SI: 0.35-1.8 μmol/L)

Test Interactions False-negative urinary glucose determinations when using Clinistix® or Diastix®

Patient Information Avoid alcohol and other CNS depressants; may cause drowsiness; avoid activities needing good psychomotor coordination until CNS effects are known; may cause physical or psychological dependence; avoid abrupt discontinuation after prolonged use

Special Geriatric Considerations Due to its long-acting metabolite, diazepam is not considered a drug of choice in the elderly. Long-acting benzodiazepines have been associated with falls in the elderly. Interpretive guidelines from the Centers for Medicare and Medicaid Services (CMS) strongly discourage the use of this agent in residents of long-term care facilities.

Dosage Forms Excipient information presented when available (limited, particularly for generics); consult specific product labeling.

Gel, rectal:

Diastat®: Pediatric rectal tip [4.4 cm]: 5 mg/mL (2.5 mg, 5 mg) [contains ethyl alcohol 10%, sodium benzoate, benzyl alcohol 1.5%; twin pack]

Diastat® AcuDial™ delivery system:

10 mg: Pediatric/adult rectal tip [4.4 cm]: 5 mg/mL (delivers set doses of 5 mg, 7.5 mg, and 10 mg) [contains ethyl alcohol 10%, sodium benzoate, benzyl alcohol 1.5%; twin pack]

20 mg: Adult rectal tip [6 cm]: 5 mg/mL (delivers set doses of 10 mg, 12.5 mg, 15 mg, 17.5 mg, and 20 mg) [contains ethyl alcohol 10%, sodium benzoate, benzyl alcohol 1.5%; twin pack]

Injection, solution: 5 mg/mL (2 mL, 10 mL) [may contain benzyl alcohol, sodium benzoate, benzoic acid]

Solution, oral: 5 mg/5 mL (5 mL, 500 mL) [wintergreen-spice flavor]

Solution, oral concentrate:

Diazepam Intensol®: 5 mg/mL (30 mL)

Tablet: 2 mg, 5 mg, 10 mg

Valium®: 2 mg, 5 mg, 10 mg

Selected References

Klotz U, Avant GR, Hoyumpa A, et al, "The Effects of Age and Liver Disease on the Disposition and Elimination of Diazepam in Adult Man," *J Clin Invest*, 1975, 55(2):347-59.

Pomara N, Stanley B, Block R, et al, "Increased Sensitivity of the Elderly to the Central Depressant Effects of Diazepam," *J Clin Psychiatry*, 1985, 46(5):185-7.

Reidenberg MM, Levy M, Warner H, et al, "Relationship Between Diazepam Dose, Plasma Level, Age, and Central Nervous System Depression," *Clin Pharmacol Ther*, 1978, 23(4):371-4.

♦ **Diazepam Intensol®** *see* Diazepam *on page 420*

♦ **Dibenzyline®** *see* Phenoxybenzamine *on page 1246*

♦ **Dicarbosil® [OTC]** *see* Calcium Salts (Oral) *on page 220*

Dichlorphenamide (dye klor FEN a mide)

Medication Safety Issues

Sound-alike/look-alike issues:

Daranide® may be confused with Daraprim®

U.S. Brand Names Daranide®

Canadian Brand Names Daranide®

Index Terms Diclofenamide

Generic Available No

Pharmacologic Category Carbonic Anhydrase Inhibitor; Diuretic, Carbonic Anhydrase Inhibitor; Ophthalmic Agent, Antiglaucoma

Use Adjunct in treatment of open-angle glaucoma and perioperative treatment for angle-closure glaucoma

Contraindications Hypersensitivity to dichlorphenamide or any component of the formulation; severe pulmonary obstruction; severe renal impairment

(Continued)

Dichlorphenamide *(Continued)*

Warnings/Precautions Chemical similarities are present among sulfonamides, sulfonylureas, carbonic anhydrase inhibitors, thiazides, and loop diuretics (except ethacrynic acid). Use in patients with sulfonylurea allergy is specifically contraindicated in product labeling; however, a risk of cross-reaction exists in patients with allergy to any of these compounds; avoid use when previous reaction has been severe. Discontinue if signs of hypersensitivity are noted.

Adverse Reactions (Reflective of adult population; not specific for elderly)
>10%:
    Central nervous system: Fatigue, malaise
    Gastrointestinal: Anorexia, diarrhea, metallic taste
    Genitourinary: Polyuria
1% to 10%:
    Central nervous system: Drowsiness, mental depression
    Renal: Renal calculi

Drug Interactions Increased lithium excretion and altered excretion of other drugs by alkalinization of the urine

Dosage
Geriatrics & Adults: Glaucoma: Oral: 100-200 mg to start followed by 100 mg every 12 hours until desired response is obtained; maintenance dose: 25-50 mg 1-3 times/day

Patient Information Report numbness or tingling of extremities to physician. Ability to perform tasks requiring mental alertness and/or physical coordination may be impaired. Take with food if GI upset occurs. Notify prescriber if you experience flank pain or rash.

Special Geriatric Considerations Malaise, complaints of tiredness, and myalgia are signs of excessive dosing and acidosis in the elderly.

Dosage Forms Excipient information presented when available (limited, particularly for generics); consult specific product labeling.
Tablet: 50 mg

♦ **Dichysterol** *see* Dihydrotachysterol *on page 439*

Diclofenac *(dye KLOE fen ak)*

Medication Safety Issues
Sound-alike/look-alike issues:
    Diclofenac may be confused with Diflucan®, Duphalac®
    Cataflam® may be confused with Catapres®
    Voltaren® may be confused with tramadol, Ultram®, Verelan®

U.S. Brand Names Cataflam®; Solaraze®; Voltaren®; Voltaren Ophthalmic®; Voltaren®-XR

Canadian Brand Names Apo-Diclo®; Apo-Diclo Rapide®; Apo-Diclo SR®; Cataflam®; Novo-Difenac; Novo-Difenac K; Novo-Difenac-SR; Nu-Diclo; Nu-Diclo-SR; Pennsaid®; PMS-Diclofenac; PMS-Diclofenac SR; Riva-Diclofenac; Riva-Diclofenac-K; Voltaren®; Voltaren Ophtha®; Voltaren Rapide®

Index Terms Diclofenac Potassium; Diclofenac Sodium

Generic Available Yes; Excludes gel, ophthalmic solution

Pharmacologic Category Nonsteroidal Anti-inflammatory Drug (NSAID); Nonsteroidal Anti-inflammatory Drug (NSAID), Ophthalmic; Nonsteroidal Anti-inflammatory Drug (NSAID), Oral

Use
Immediate-release tablets: Acute treatment of mild to moderate pain; ankylosing spondylitis; acute and chronic treatment of rheumatoid arthritis, osteoarthritis
Delayed-release tablets: Acute and chronic treatment of rheumatoid arthritis, osteoarthritis, ankylosing spondylitis
Extended-release tablets: Chronic treatment of osteoarthritis, rheumatoid arthritis
Ophthalmic solution: Treatment for postoperative inflammation following cataract extraction; temporary relief of pain and photophobia in patients undergoing corneal refractive surgery
Topical gel: Treatment for actinic keratosis (AK) in conjunction with sun avoidance

Restrictions An FDA-approved medication guide must be distributed when dispensing an oral outpatient prescription (new or refill) where this medication is to be used without direct supervision of a healthcare provider. Medication guides are available at http://www.fda.gov/cder/Offices/ODS/medication_guides.htm.

Contraindications Hypersensitivity to diclofenac, aspirin, other NSAIDs, or any component of the formulation; perioperative pain in the setting of coronary artery bypass surgery (CABG)

Warnings/Precautions [U.S. Boxed Warning]: NSAIDs are associated with an increased risk of adverse cardiovascular events, including MI, stroke, and new onset or worsening of pre-existing hypertension. Risk may be increased with duration of use or pre-existing cardiovascular risk factors or disease. Carefully evaluate individual cardiovascular risk profiles prior to prescribing. Use caution with fluid retention, CHF, or hypertension. Concurrent administration of ibuprofen, and potentially other nonselective NSAIDs, may interfere with aspirin's cardioprotective effect.

Use of NSAIDs can compromise existing renal function. Renal toxicity can occur in patient with impaired renal function, dehydration, heart failure, liver dysfunction, those taking diuretics and ACEI, and the elderly. Rehydrate patient before starting therapy. Monitor renal function closely. Not recommended for use in patients with advanced renal disease.

[U.S. Boxed Warning]: NSAIDs may increase risk of gastrointestinal irritation, ulceration, bleeding, and perforation. These events may occur at any time during therapy and without warning. Use caution with a history of GI disease (bleeding or ulcers), concurrent therapy with aspirin, anticoagulants and/or corticosteroids, smoking, use of alcohol, the elderly or debilitated patients.

Use the lowest effective dose for the shortest duration of time, consistent with individual patient goals, to reduce risk of cardiovascular or GI adverse events. Alternate therapies should be considered for patients at high risk.

NSAIDs may cause serious skin adverse events including exfoliative dermatitis, Stevens-Johnson syndrome (SJS), and toxic epidermal necrolysis (TEN). Anaphylactoid reactions may occur, even without prior exposure; patients with "aspirin triad" (bronchial asthma, aspirin intolerance, rhinitis) may be at increased risk. Do not use in patients who experience bronchospasm, asthma, rhinitis, or urticaria with NSAID or aspirin therapy. Use caution in other forms of asthma.

Use with caution in patients with decreased hepatic function. Closely monitor patients with any abnormal LFT. Severe hepatic reactions (eg, fulminant hepatitis, liver failure) have occurred with NSAID use, rarely; discontinue if signs or symptoms of liver disease develop, or if systemic manifestations occur.

The elderly are at increased risk for adverse effects (especially peptic ulceration, CNS effects, renal toxicity) from NSAIDs even at low doses.

Withhold for at least 4-6 half-lives prior to surgical or dental procedures.

Topical gel should not be applied to the eyes, open wounds, infected areas, or to exfoliative dermatitis. Monitor patients for 1 year following application of ophthalmic drops for corneal refractive procedures. Patients using ophthalmic drops should not wear soft contact lenses. Ophthalmic drops may slow/delay healing or prolong bleeding time following surgery.

Adverse Reactions (Reflective of adult population; not specific for elderly)
> >10%:
> Local: Application site reactions (gel): Pruritus (31% to 52%), rash (35% to 46%), contact dermatitis (19% to 33%), dry skin (25% to 27%), pain (15% to 26%), exfoliation (6% to 24%), paresthesia (8% to 20%)
> Ocular: Ophthalmic drops (incidence may be dependent upon indication): Lacrimation (30%), keratitis (28%), elevated IOP (15%), transient burning/stinging (15%)
> 1% to 10%:
> Central nervous system: Headache (7%), dizziness (3%)
> Dermatologic: Pruritus (1% to 3%), rash (1% to 3%)
> Endocrine & metabolic: Fluid retention (1% to 3%)
> Gastrointestinal: Abdominal cramps (3% to 9%), abdominal pain (3% to 9%), constipation (3% to 9%), diarrhea (3% to 9%), flatulence (3% to 9%), indigestion (3% to 9%), nausea (3% to 9%), abdominal distention (1% to 3%), peptic ulcer/GI bleed (0.6% to 2%)
> Hepatic: ALT/AST increased (2%)
> Local: Application site reactions (gel): Edema (4%)
> Ocular: Ophthalmic drops: Abnormal vision, acute elevated IOP, blurred vision, conjunctivitis, corneal deposits, corneal edema, corneal opacity, corneal lesions, discharge, eyelid swelling, injection, iritis, irritation, itching, lacrimation disorder, ocular allergy
> Otic: Tinnitus (1% to 3%)

Overdosage/Toxicology Symptoms include acute renal failure, vomiting, drowsiness, and leukocytosis. Management of nonsteroidal anti-inflammatory drug (NSAID) intoxication is primarily supportive and symptomatic. Fluid therapy is commonly effective in managing hypotension that may occur following an acute NSAID overdose, except when due to acute blood loss.

Drug Interactions Substrate (minor) of CYP1A2, 2B6, 2C8, 2C9, 2C19, 2D6, 3A4; **Inhibits** CYP1A2 (moderate), 2C9 (weak), 2E1 (weak), 3A4 (weak)

ACE inhibitors: Antihypertensive effects may be decreased by concurrent therapy with NSAIDs; monitor blood pressure.
Angiotensin II antagonists: Antihypertensive effects may be decreased by concurrent therapy with NSAIDs; monitor blood pressure.
(Continued)

Diclofenac *(Continued)*

Anticoagulants (warfarin, heparin, LMWHs) in combination with NSAIDs can cause increased risk of bleeding.

Antiplatelet drugs (ticlopidine, clopidogrel, aspirin, abciximab, dipyridamole, eptifibatide, tirofiban) can cause an increased risk of bleeding.

Beta-blockers: NSAIDs may decrease the antihypertensive effect of beta-blockers; monitor.

Cholestyramine (and other bile acid sequestrants): May decrease the absorption of NSAIDs. Separate by at least 2 hours.

Corticosteroids may increase the risk of GI ulceration; avoid concurrent use.

Cyclosporine: NSAIDs may increase serum creatinine, potassium, blood pressure, and cyclosporine levels; monitor cyclosporine levels and renal function carefully.

CYP1A2 substrates: Diclofenac may increase the levels/effects of CYP1A2 substrates. Example substrates include aminophylline, fluvoxamine, mexiletine, mirtazapine, ropinirole, theophylline, and trifluoperazine.

Fluoroquinolone antibiotics: Risk of seizures may be increased with concomitant quinolone use. Risk is considered quite low and may only be a factor with high serum levels of either agent and/or in patients with additional predisposing factors (eg, renal dysfunction, history of seizure or other neurological disorder).

Gentamicin and amikacin serum concentrations are increased by indomethacin in premature infants. Results may apply to other aminoglycosides and NSAIDs.

Hydralazine's antihypertensive effect is decreased; avoid concurrent use.

Lithium levels can be increased; avoid concurrent use if possible or monitor lithium levels and adjust dose. Sulindac may have the least effect. When NSAID is stopped, lithium will need adjustment again.

Loop diuretics efficacy (diuretic and antihypertensive effect) is reduced. Indomethacin reduces this efficacy, however, it may be anticipated with any NSAID.

Methotrexate: Severe bone marrow suppression, aplastic anemia, and GI toxicity have been reported with concomitant NSAID therapy. Avoid use during moderate or high-dose methotrexate (increased and prolonged methotrexate levels). NSAID use during low-dose treatment of rheumatoid arthritis has not been fully evaluated; extreme caution is warranted.

Thiazides antihypertensive effects are decreased; avoid concurrent use.

Verapamil plasma concentration is decreased by diclofenac; avoid concurrent use.

Warfarin's INRs may be increased by piroxicam. Other NSAIDs may have the same effect depending on dose and duration. Monitor INR closely. Use the lowest dose of NSAIDs possible and for the briefest duration.

Ethanol/Nutrition/Herb Interactions

Ethanol: Avoid ethanol (may enhance gastric mucosal irritation).

Herb/Nutraceutical: Avoid alfalfa, anise, bilberry, bladderwrack, bromelain, cat's claw, celery, coleus, cordyceps, dong quai, evening primrose, feverfew, fenugreek, garlic, ginger, ginkgo biloba, red clover, horse chestnut, grapeseed, green tea, ginseng, guggul, horse chestnut seed, horseradish, licorice, prickly ash, red clover, reishi, SAMe, sweet clover, turmeric, white willow (all have additional antiplatelet activity).

Stability Store below 30°C (86°F). Protect from moisture; store in tight container.

Mechanism of Action Inhibits prostaglandin synthesis by decreasing the activity of the enzyme, cyclooxygenase, which results in decreased formation of prostaglandin precursors. Mechanism of action for the treatment of AK has not been established.

Pharmacokinetics

Absorption: Complete

Protein binding: 99%

Metabolism: In the liver to inactive metabolites

Half-life: 1-2 hours

Time to peak serum concentrations: Within 2-3 hours

Elimination: Primarily in urine

Dosage

Geriatrics & Adults:

Analgesia/primary dysmenorrhea: Oral: Starting dose: 50 mg 3 times/day; maximum dose: 150 mg/day

Rheumatoid arthritis: Oral: 150-200 mg/day in 2-4 divided doses (100 mg/day of sustained release product)

Osteoarthritis: Oral: 100-150 mg/day in 2-3 divided doses (100-200 mg/day of sustained release product)

Ankylosing spondylitis: Oral: 100-125 mg/day in 4-5 divided doses

Cataract surgery: Ophthalmic: Instill 1 drop into affected eye 4 times/day beginning 24 hours after cataract surgery and continuing for 2 weeks

Corneal refractive surgery: Ophthalmic: Instill 1-2 drops into affected eye within the hour prior to surgery, within 15 minutes following surgery, and then continue for 4 times/day, up to 3 days

Actinic keratosis (AK): Topical (gel): Apply gel to lesion area twice daily for 60-90 days

Renal Impairment: Not recommended in patients with advanced renal disease.

Hepatic Impairment: No adjustment necessary.

Administration

Oral: Do not crush tablets. Administer with food or milk to avoid gastric distress. Take with full glass of water to enhance absorption.

Ophthalmic: Wait at least 5 minutes before administering other types of eye drops.

Topical gel: Cover lesion with gel and smooth into skin gently. Do not cover lesion with occlusive dressings or apply sunscreens, cosmetics, or other medications to affected area.

Monitoring Parameters Monitor response (pain, range of motion, grip strength, mobility, ADL function), inflammation; observe for weight gain, edema; monitor renal function; observe for bleeding, bruising; evaluate gastrointestinal effects (abdominal pain, bleeding, dyspepsia); mental confusion, disorientation, CBC, serum, creatinine, BUN, liver function tests

Patient Information Do not crush delayed release (enteric coated) tablets. Serious gastrointestinal bleeding can occur as well as ulceration and perforation. Pain may or may not be present. Avoid aspirin and aspirin-containing products while taking this medication. If gastric upset occurs, take with food, milk, or antacid. If gastric adverse effects persist, contact physician. May cause drowsiness, dizziness, blurred vision, and confusion. Use caution when performing tasks which require alertness (eg, driving). Do not take for more than 3 days for fever or 10 days for pain without physician advice.

Topical gel: Avoid sun during therapy. Cover lesion with gel and smooth into skin gently. You may not notice complete healing until 30 days after therapy is completed. Do not cover lesion with occlusive dressings or apply sunscreens, cosmetics, or other medications to affected area.

Additional Information There are no clinical guidelines to predict which NSAID will give response in a particular patient. Trials with each must be initiated until response determined. Consider dose, patient convenience, and cost.

Special Geriatric Considerations Elderly are a high-risk population for adverse effects from nonsteroidal anti-inflammatory agents. As much as 60% of the elderly can develop peptic ulceration and/or hemorrhage asymptomatically. The concomitant use of H_2 blockers and sucralfate is not effective as prophylaxis with the exception of NSAID-induced duodenal ulcers which may be prevented by the use of ranitidine. Misoprostol and proton pump inhibitors are the only agents proven to help prevent the development of NSAID-induced ulcers. Also, concomitant disease and drug use contribute to the risk for GI adverse effects. Use lowest effective dose for shortest period possible. Consider renal function decline with age. Use of NSAIDs can compromise existing renal function especially when Cl_{cr} is $\leq$30 mL/minute. CNS adverse effects such as confusion, agitation, and hallucination are generally seen in overdose or high dose situations, but elderly may demonstrate these adverse effects at lower doses than younger adults.

Dosage Forms Excipient information presented when available (limited, particularly for generics); consult specific product labeling. [DSC] = Discontinued product

Gel, as sodium:

Solaraze®: 30 mg/g (50 g)

Solution, ophthalmic, as sodium:

Voltaren Ophthalmic®: 0.1% (2.5 mL, 5 mL)

Tablet, as potassium: 50 mg

Cataflam®: 50 mg

Tablet, delayed release, enteric coated, as sodium: 50 mg, 75 mg

Voltaren®: 25 mg [DSC], 50 mg [DSC], 75 mg

Tablet, extended release, as sodium: 100 mg

Voltaren®-XR: 100 mg

Selected References

Brooks PM and Day RO, "Nonsteroidal Anti-inflammatory Drugs - Differences and Similarities," *N Engl J Med*, 1991, 324(24):1716-25.

Clinch D, Banerjee AK, and Ostick G, "Absence of Abdominal Pain in Elderly Patients With Peptic Ulcer," *Age Ageing*, 1984, 13(2):120-3.

Clive DM and Stoff JS, "Renal Syndromes Associated With Nonsteroidal Anti-inflammatory Drugs," *N Engl J Med*, 1984, 310(9):563-72.

Graham DY, "Prevention of Gastroduodenal Injury Induced by Chronic Nonsteroidal Anti-inflammatory Drug Therapy," *Gastroenterology*, 1989, 96(2 Pt 2 Suppl):675-81.

Gurwitz JH, Avorn J, Ross-Degnan D, et al, "Nonsteroidal Anti-Inflammatory Drug-Associated Azotemia in the Very Old," *JAMA*, 1990, 264(4):471-5.

Hawkey CJ, Karrasch JA, Szczepański L, et al, "Omeprazole Compared With Misoprostol for Ulcers Associated With Nonsteroidal Anti-inflammatory Drugs," *N Engl J Med*, 1998, 338(11):727-34.

Knodel LC, "Preventing NSAID-induced Ulcers: The Role of Misoprostol," *Consult Pharm*, 1989, 4:37-41.

Pounder R, "Silent Peptic Ulceration: Deadly Silence or Golden Silence?" *Gastroenterology*, 1989, 96(2 Pt 2 Suppl):626-31.

Yeomans ND, Tulassay Z, Juhasz L, et al, "A Comparison of Omeprazole With Ranitidine for Ulcers Associated With Nonsteroidal Anti-inflammatory Drugs," *N Engl J Med*, 1998, 338(11):719-26.

Diclofenac and Misoprostol (dye KLOE fen ak & mye soe PROST ole)

Related Information
Diclofenac *on page 424*
Misoprostol *on page 1052*
U.S. Brand Names Arthrotec®
Canadian Brand Names Arthrotec®
Index Terms Misoprostol and Diclofenac
Generic Available No
Pharmacologic Category Nonsteroidal Anti-inflammatory Drug (NSAID), Oral; Prostaglandin
Use
Diclofenac: Treatment of osteoarthritis, rheumatoid arthritis
Misoprostol: Prophylaxis of NSAID-induced gastric and duodenal ulceration
Restrictions An FDA-approved medication guide must be distributed when dispensing an oral outpatient prescription (new or refill) where this medication is to be used without direct supervision of a healthcare provider. Medication guides are available at http://www.fda.gov/cder/Offices/ODS/medication_guides.htm.
Dosage
Geriatrics & Adults:
Osteoarthritis: Oral: Arthrotec® 50: 1 tablet 2-3 times/day
Rheumatoid arthritis: Oral: Arthrotec® 50: 1 tablet 3-4 times/day
Note: For both regimens, if not tolerated by patient, the dose may be reduced to 1 tablet twice daily. Arthrotec® 75 may be used in patients who cannot tolerate full daily Arthrotec® 50 regimens. Dose: 1 tablet twice daily. However, the use of these tablets may not be as effective at preventing GI ulceration.
Renal Impairment: Not recommended for use in patients with advanced renal disease. In renal insufficiency, diclofenac should be used with caution due to potential detrimental effects on renal function, and misoprostol dosage reduction may be required if adverse effects occur (misoprostol is renally eliminated).
Special Geriatric Considerations Elderly are a high-risk population for adverse effects from nonsteroidal anti-inflammatory agents. As much as 60% of the elderly can develop peptic ulceration and/or hemorrhage asymptomatically. The concomitant use of H_2 blockers and sucralfate is not effective as prophylaxis with the exception of NSAID-induced duodenal ulcers which may be prevented by the use of ranitidine. Misoprostol and proton pump inhibitors are the only agents proven to help prevent the development of NSAID-induced ulcers. Also, concomitant disease and drug use contribute to the risk for GI adverse effects. Use lowest effective dose for shortest period possible. Consider renal function decline with age. Use of NSAIDs can compromise existing renal function especially when Cl_{cr} is ≤30 mL/minute. CNS adverse effects such as confusion, agitation, and hallucination are generally seen in overdose or high dose situations, but elderly may demonstrate these adverse effects at lower doses than younger adults.
Dosage Forms Excipient information presented when available (limited, particularly for generics); consult specific product labeling.
Tablet: Diclofenac sodium 50 mg and misoprostol 200 mcg; diclofenac sodium 75 mg and misoprostol 200 mcg

♦ **Diclofenac Potassium** *see Diclofenac on page 424*
♦ **Diclofenac Sodium** *see Diclofenac on page 424*
♦ **Diclofenamide** *see Dichlorphenamide on page 423*

Dicloxacillin (dye kloks a SIL in)

Related Information
Antimicrobial Activity Against Selected Organisms *on page 1728*
Canadian Brand Names Dycill®; Pathocil®
Index Terms Dicloxacillin Sodium
Generic Available Yes
Pharmacologic Category Antibiotic, Penicillin
Use Treatment of systemic infections such as pneumonia, skin and soft tissue infections and osteomyelitis caused by penicillinase-producing staphylococci
Contraindications Hypersensitivity to dicloxacillin, penicillin, or any component of the formulation
Warnings/Precautions Monitor PT if patient concurrently on warfarin. Serious and occasionally severe or fatal hypersensitivity (anaphylactoid) reactions have been reported in patients on penicillin therapy, especially with a history of beta-lactam hypersensitivity, history of sensitivity to multiple allergens, or previous IgE-mediated reactions (eg, anaphylaxis, angioedema, urticaria). Use with caution in asthmatic

patients. Prolonged use may result in fungal or bacterial superinfection, including *C. difficile*-associated diarrhea and pseudomembranous colitis.

Adverse Reactions (Reflective of adult population; not specific for elderly)
1% to 10%: Gastrointestinal: Nausea, diarrhea, abdominal pain

Overdosage/Toxicology Symptoms of penicillin overdose include neuromuscular hypersensitivity (agitation, hallucinations, asterixis, encephalopathy, confusion, seizures) and electrolyte imbalance (with potassium or sodium salts), especially in renal failure. Hemodialysis may be helpful to aid in removal of the drug from the blood, otherwise, most treatment is supportive or symptom-directed.

Drug Interactions Induces CYP3A4 (weak)
Fusidic acid: May decrease the therapeutic effect of penicillins; administer the penicillin at least 2 hours before fusidic acid.
Methotrexate: Penicillins may increase the exposure to methotrexate during concurrent therapy; monitor.
Oral contraceptives: Anecdotal reports suggesting decreased contraceptive efficacy with penicillins have been refuted by more rigorous scientific and clinical data.
Probenecid, disulfiram: May increase levels of penicillins (dicloxacillin).
Warfarin: Concurrent use may decrease effect of warfarin.

Ethanol/Nutrition/Herb Interactions Food: Decreases drug absorption rate; decreases drug serum concentration.

Mechanism of Action Inhibits bacterial cell wall synthesis by binding to one or more of the penicillin binding proteins (PBPs) which in turn inhibits the final transpeptidation step of peptidoglycan synthesis in bacterial cell walls, thus inhibiting cell wall biosynthesis. Bacteria eventually lyse due to ongoing activity of cell wall autolytic enzymes (autolysins and murein hydrolases) while cell wall assembly is arrested.

Pharmacokinetics
Absorption: 35% to 76% from GI tract
Half-life: 0.6-0.8 hours, half-life is slightly prolonged in patients with renal impairment
Protein binding: 96%
Time to peak serum concentration: Within 0.5-2 hours
Elimination: Partially by the liver and excreted in bile, 56% to 70% is eliminated in urine as unchanged drug
The percent unbound has been reported to be increased in older adults compared to young healthy volunteers (8.8% vs 7.3%), but this is not felt to be clinically significant

Dosage
Geriatrics & Adults:
Susceptible infections: Oral: 125-500 mg every 6 hours
Erysipelas, furunculosis, mastitis, otitis externa, septic bursitis, skin abscess: Oral: 500 mg every 6 hours
Impetigo: 250 mg every 6 hours
Prosthetic joint (long-term suppression therapy): Oral: 250 mg twice daily
***Staphylococcus aureus,* methicillin susceptible infection if no I.V. access:** Oral: 500-1000 mg every 6-8 hours
Renal Impairment:
Dosage adjustment is not necessary.
Not dialyzable (0% to 5%); supplemental dose is not necessary.
Peritoneal dialysis effects: Supplemental dose is not necessary.
Continuous arteriovenous or venovenous hemofiltration: Supplemental dose is not necessary.

Administration Administer 1 hour before or 2 hours after meals; administer around-the-clock rather than 4 times/day, 3 times/day, etc (ie, 12-6-12-6, not 9-1-5-9) to promote less variation in peak and trough serum concentrations

Monitoring Parameters Signs and symptoms of infection; mental status; monitor PT or INR if patient concurrently on warfarin

Reference Range
Level guidelines: 10-25 mcg/mL
Panic value: >100 mcg/mL
Time to obtain blood for serum concentrations: 2 hours after dose

Test Interactions False-positive urine and serum proteins; false-positive in uric acid, urinary steroids; may interfere with urinary glucose tests using cupric sulfate (Benedict's solution, Clinitest®); may inactivate aminoglycosides *in vitro*

Patient Information Complete full course of therapy; report diarrhea or if symptoms not improving to physician or pharmacist

Additional Information
Sodium content of 250 mg capsule: 13 mg (0.6 mEq)
Sodium content of suspension 65 mg/5 mL: 27 mg (1.2 mEq)

Special Geriatric Considerations No dosage adjustment for renal function is necessary.

Dosage Forms Excipient information presented when available (limited, particularly for generics); consult specific product labeling.
Capsule: 250 mg, 500 mg
(Continued)

Dicloxacillin *(Continued)*

Selected References

Pacifici GM, Viani A, Taddeucci-Brunelli G, et al, "Plasma Protein Binding of Dicloxacillin: Effects of Age and Diseases," *Int J Clin Pharmacol Ther Toxicol*, 1987, 25(11):622-6.

♦ **Dicloxacillin Sodium** *see* Dicloxacillin *on page 428*

Dicyclomine *(dye SYE kloe meen)*

Related Information

Pharmacotherapy of Urinary Incontinence *on page 1822*
Potentially Inappropriate Medications for Geriatrics *on page 1824*

Medication Safety Issues

Sound-alike/look-alike issues:
Dicyclomine may be confused with diphenhydrAMINE, doxycycline, dyclonine
Bentyl® may be confused with Aventyl®, Benadryl®, Bontril®, Cantil®, Proventil®, Trental®

U.S. Brand Names Bentyl®

Canadian Brand Names Bentylol®; Formulex®; Lomine; Riva-Dicyclomine

Index Terms Dicyclomine Hydrochloride; Dicycloverine Hydrochloride

Generic Available Yes: Excludes syrup

Pharmacologic Category Anticholinergic Agent

Use Treatment of functional bowel/irritable bowel syndrome

Unlabeled/Investigational Use Treatment of urinary incontinence

Contraindications Hypersensitivity to dicyclomine or any component of the formulation; obstructive diseases of the GI tract; severe ulcerative colitis; reflux esophagitis; unstable cardiovascular status in acute hemorrhage; obstructive uropathy; narrow-angle glaucoma; myasthenia gravis

Warnings/Precautions May cause drowsiness and/or blurred vision. Use with caution in patients with hepatic or renal disease, hiatal hernia, prostatic hypertrophy (known or suspected), mild-moderate ulcerative colitis, hyperthyroidism, coronary artery disease, tachyarrhythmias, congestive heart failure, hypertension, or autonomic neuropathy. Evaluate tachycardia prior to administration. The elderly are at increased risk for anticholinergic effects, confusion, and hallucinations. Heat prostration may occur in the presence of increased environmental temperature; use caution in hot weather and/or exercise. Psychosis has been reported in patients with an extreme sensitivity to anticholinergic effects.

Adverse Reactions (Reflective of adult population; not specific for elderly) Adverse reactions are included here that have been reported for pharmacologically similar drugs with anticholinergic/antispasmodic action.

Cardiovascular: Syncope, tachycardia, palpitation
Central nervous system: Dizziness (29%), lightheadedness (11%), drowsiness (9%), tingling, headache, nervousness (6%), numbness, mental confusion and/or excitement, dyskinesia, lethargy, speech disturbance, insomnia
Dermatologic: Rash, urticaria, itching, and other dermal manifestations
Endocrine & metabolic: Suppression of lactation
Gastrointestinal: Xerostomia (33%), nausea (14%), vomiting, constipation, bloated feeling, abdominal pain, taste loss, anorexia
Genitourinary: Urinary hesitancy, urinary retention, impotence
Local: Irritation (injection), focal coagulation necrosis (injection)
Neuromuscular & skeletal: Weakness (7%)
Ocular: Blurred vision (27%), diplopia, mydriasis, cycloplegia, increased ocular tension
Respiratory: Dyspnea, apnea, asphyxia, nasal stuffiness or congestion, sneezing, throat congestion
Miscellaneous: Anaphylaxis, diaphoresis decreased, severe allergic reaction

Overdosage/Toxicology Symptoms include CNS stimulation followed by depression, confusion, delusions, nonreactive pupils, tachycardia, and hypertension. Headache, nausea, vomiting, blurred vision, dilated pupils, hot dry skin, dizziness, dryness of the mouth, and difficulty in swallowing are signs of an overdose. Anticholinergic toxicity is caused by strong binding of the drug to cholinergic receptors. For anticholinergic overdose with severe life-threatening symptoms, physostigmine 1-2 mg SubQ or slow I.V. may be given to reverse these effects.

Drug Interactions

Acetylcholinesterase inhibitors (central): Effects of dicyclomine may be diminished; in addition the effects of acetylcholinesterase inhibitors may be diminished by drugs with anticholinergic effects such as dicyclomine.
Anticholinergic agents: The anticholinergic effects of dicyclomine are additive with other anticholinergic agents, including antihistamines, amantadine, opioids, phenothiazines, and tricyclic antidepressants.
Pramlintide: Pramlintide may enhance the gastrointestinal anticholinergic effect of dicyclomine.

Ethanol/Nutrition/Herb Interactions Ethanol: Avoid ethanol (may increase CNS depression).

Stability Protect from light.

Mechanism of Action Blocks the action of acetylcholine at parasympathetic sites in smooth muscle, secretory glands and the CNS

Pharmacodynamics
Onset of action: 1-2 hours
Duration: Up to 4 hours

Pharmacokinetics
Absorption: Oral: Well absorbed
Metabolism: Extensive
Elimination: In urine with only a small amount excreted as unchanged drug

Dosage
Geriatrics: 10-20 mg 4 times/day; increasing as necessary to 160 mg/day
Adults: Gastrointestinal motility disorders/irritable bowel:
Oral: Initiate with 80 mg/day in 4 equally divided doses, then increase up to 160 mg/day
I.M. **(should not be used I.V.):** 80 mg/day in 4 divided doses (20 mg/dose)

Monitoring Parameters Pulse, anticholinergic effects, urinary output, GI symptoms

Patient Information Take 30-60 minutes before a meal; may cause drowsiness, dizziness, or blurred vision; may cause dry mouth, difficult urination, or constipation

Special Geriatric Considerations Long-term use of antispasmodics should be avoided in the elderly. The potential for a toxic reaction is greater than the potential benefit. In addition, the anticholinergic effects of dicyclomine are not well tolerated in the elderly.

Dosage Forms Excipient information presented when available (limited, particularly for generics); consult specific product labeling.
Capsule, as hydrochloride: 10 mg
Bentyl®: 10 mg
Injection, solution, as hydrochloride: 10 mg/mL (2 mL)
Bentyl®: 10 mg/mL (2 mL)
Syrup, as hydrochloride:
Bentyl®: 10 mg/5 mL (480 mL)
Tablet, as hydrochloride: 20 mg
Bentyl®: 20 mg

Selected References
Fick DM, Cooper JW, Wade WE, et al "Updating the Beers Criteria for Potentially Inappropriate Medication Use in Older Adults: Results of a U.S. Consensus Panel of Experts," *Arch Intern Med*, 2003, 163(22):2716-24.

♦ **Dicyclomine Hydrochloride** *see* Dicyclomine *on page 430*
♦ **Dicycloverine Hydrochloride** *see* Dicyclomine *on page 430*
♦ **Didronel®** *see* Etidronate Disodium *on page 585*
♦ **Difil-G** *see* Dyphylline and Guaifenesin *on page 496*
♦ **Difil®-G Forte** *see* Dyphylline and Guaifenesin *on page 496*
♦ **Diflucan®** *see* Fluconazole *on page 632*

Diflunisal (dye FLOO ni sal)

Medication Safety Issues
Sound-alike/look-alike issues:
Dolobid® may be confused with Slo-Bid®

U.S. Brand Names Dolobid® [DSC]

Canadian Brand Names Apo-Diflunisal®; Novo-Diflunisal; Nu-Diflunisal

Generic Available Yes

Pharmacologic Category Nonsteroidal Anti-inflammatory Drug (NSAID), Oral

Use Management of inflammatory disorders usually including rheumatoid arthritis and osteoarthritis; analgesic for treatment of mild to moderate pain

Restrictions An FDA-approved medication guide must be distributed when dispensing an oral outpatient prescription (new or refill) where this medication is to be used without direct supervision of a healthcare provider. Medication guides are available at http://www.fda.gov/cder/Offices/ODS/medication_guides.htm.

Contraindications Hypersensitivity to diflunisal, aspirin, other NSAIDs, or any component of the formulation; perioperative pain in the setting of coronary artery bypass surgery (CABG)

Warnings/Precautions [U.S. Boxed Warning]: NSAIDs are associated with an increased risk of adverse cardiovascular events, including MI, stroke, and new onset or worsening of pre-existing hypertension. Risk may be increased with duration of use or pre-existing cardiovascular risk factors or disease. Carefully evaluate
(Continued)

Diflunisal *(Continued)*

individual cardiovascular risk profiles prior to prescribing. Use caution with fluid retention, CHF, or hypertension. Concurrent administration of ibuprofen, and potentially other nonselective NSAIDs, may interfere with aspirin's cardioprotective effect.

[U.S. Boxed Warning]: NSAIDs may increase risk of gastrointestinal irritation, ulceration, bleeding, and perforation. Use caution with a history of GI disease (bleeding or ulcers), concurrent therapy with aspirin, anticoagulants and/or corticosteroids, smoking, use of alcohol, the elderly or debilitated patients.

Use of NSAIDs can compromise existing renal function. Diflunisal is not recommended for patients with advanced renal disease. Use with caution in patients with decreased hepatic function.

Use the lowest effective dose for the shortest duration of time, consistent with individual patient goals, to reduce risk of cardiovascular or GI adverse events.

NSAIDs may cause serious skin adverse events including exfoliative dermatitis, Stevens-Johnson syndrome (SJS), and toxic epidermal necrolysis (TEN). Do not use in patients who experience bronchospasm, asthma, rhinitis, or urticaria with NSAID or aspirin therapy. Use caution in other forms of asthma.

A hypersensitivity syndrome has been reported; monitor for constitutional symptoms and cutaneous findings; other organ dysfunction may be involved.

Diflunisal is a derivative of acetylsalicylic acid and therefore may be associated with Reye's syndrome. Withhold for at least 4-6 half-lives prior to surgical or dental procedures.

Adverse Reactions (Reflective of adult population; not specific for elderly)
1% to 10%:
Central nervous system: Headache (3% to 9%), dizziness (1% to 3%), insomnia (1% to 3%), somnolence (1% to 3%), fatigue (1% to 3%)
Dermatologic: Rash (3% to 9%)
Gastrointestinal: Nausea (3% to 9%), dyspepsia (3% to 9%), GI pain (3% to 9%), diarrhea (3% to 9%), constipation (1% to 3%), flatulence (1% to 3%), vomiting (1% to 3%), GI ulceration
Otic: Tinnitus (1% to 3%)

Overdosage/Toxicology Symptoms include drowsiness, nausea, vomiting, hyperventilation, tachycardia, tinnitus, stupor, coma, renal failure, and leukocytosis. Management of nonsteroidal anti-inflammatory drug (NSAID) intoxication is primarily supportive and symptomatic. Fluid therapy is commonly effective in managing hypotension that may occur following an acute NSAID overdose, except when due to acute blood loss.

Drug Interactions

ACE inhibitors: Antihypertensive effects may be decreased by concurrent therapy with NSAIDs; monitor blood pressure.

Aminoglycosides: NSAIDs may decrease the excretion of aminoglycosides.

Angiotensin II antagonists: Antihypertensive effects may be decreased by concurrent therapy with NSAIDs; monitor blood pressure.

Anticoagulants (warfarin, heparin, LMWHs) in combination with NSAIDs can cause increased risk of bleeding.

Antiplatelet agents (ticlopidine, clopidogrel, aspirin, abciximab, dipyridamole, eptifibatide, tirofiban) can cause an increased risk of bleeding.

Beta-blockers: NSAIDs may diminish the antihypertensive effects of beta-blockers.

Bisphosphonates: NSAIDs may increase the risk of gastrointestinal ulceration.

Cholestyramine (and other bile acid sequestrants): May decrease the absorption of NSAIDs. Separate by at least 2 hours.

Corticosteroids may increase the risk of GI ulceration; avoid concurrent use.

Cyclosporine: NSAIDs may increase serum creatinine, potassium, blood pressure, and cyclosporine levels; monitor cyclosporine levels and renal function carefully.

Fluoroquinolone antibiotics: Risk of seizures may be increased with concomitant quinolone use. Risk is considered quite low and may only be a factor with high serum levels of either agent and/or in patients with additional predisposing factors (eg, renal dysfunction, history of seizure or other neurological disorder).

Hydralazine's antihypertensive effect is decreased; avoid concurrent use.

Lithium levels can be increased; avoid concurrent use if possible or monitor lithium levels and adjust dose.

Sulindac may have the least effect. When NSAID is stopped, lithium will need adjustment again.

Loop diuretics efficacy (diuretic and antihypertensive effect) is reduced. Indomethacin reduces this efficacy, however, it may be anticipated with any NSAID.

Methotrexate: Severe bone marrow suppression, aplastic anemia, and GI toxicity have been reported with concomitant NSAID therapy. Avoid use during moderate or high-dose methotrexate (increased and prolonged methotrexate levels). NSAID use during low-dose treatment of rheumatoid arthritis has not been fully evaluated; extreme caution is warranted.

Pemetrexed: NSAIDs may decrease the excretion of pemetrexed. Patients with Cl_{cr} 45-79 mL/minute should avoid long acting NSAIDs for 5 days before and 2 days after pemetrexed treatment.

Salicylates: NSAIDs (nonselective) may diminish the cardioprotective effect of acetylated salicylates. Avoid regular use of NSAIDs if possible; consider alternatives (eg, acetaminophen). Give salicylate before NSAID; for example ibuprofen should be given 30-120 minutes after aspirin (immediate release).

Thiazides antihypertensive effects are decreased; avoid concurrent use.

Treprostinil: May enhance the risk of bleeding with concurrent use.

Vancomycin: NSAID©s may decrease the excretion of vancomycin.

Ethanol/Nutrition/Herb Interactions

Ethanol: Avoid ethanol (may enhance gastric mucosal irritation).

Herb/Nutraceutical: Avoid alfalfa, anise, bilberry, bladderwrack, bromelain, cat's claw, celery, coleus, cordyceps, dong quai, evening primrose, feverfew, fenugreek, garlic, ginger, ginkgo biloba, red clover, horse chestnut, grapeseed, green tea, ginseng, guggul, horse chestnut seed, horseradish, licorice, prickly ash, red clover, reishi, SAMe, sweet clover, turmeric, white willow (all have additional antiplatelet activity).

Mechanism of Action Inhibits prostaglandin synthesis by decreasing the activity of the enzyme, cyclooxygenase, which results in decreased formation of prostaglandin precursors

Pharmacodynamics

Onset of action: Analgesic: ~1 hour; maximal effect: 2-3 hours

Duration: 8-12 hours

Pharmacokinetics

Absorption: Well absorbed from GI tract

Protein binding: >99%

Metabolism: Extensively hepatic; metabolic pathways are saturable

Half-life: 8-12 hours, prolonged with renal impairment

Time to peak serum concentrations: Oral: Within 2-3 hours

Elimination: In urine within 72-96 hours, ~3% as unchanged drug and 90% as glucuronide conjugates

Dosage

Geriatrics & Adults:

Mild-to-moderate pain: Oral: Initial: 500-1000 mg followed by 250-500 mg every 8-12 hours; maximum daily dose: 1.5 g

Arthritis: Oral: 500-1000 mg/day in 2 divided doses; maximum daily dose: 1.5 g

Renal Impairment:

Use with caution; Cl_{cr} <50 mL/minute: Administer 50% of normal dose (Aronoff, 1998)

Hemodialysis: No supplement required

CAPD: No supplement require

CAVH: Dose for GFR 10-50

Monitoring Parameters Fecal blood loss, renal function; hearing changes or tinnitus; monitor for response (ie, pain, inflammation, range of motion, grip strength); observe for abnormal bleeding, bruising, weight gain

Test Interactions Falsely elevated increase in serum salicylate levels

Patient Information May cause GI upset, take with water, milk, or meals; do not take aspirin with diflunisal, swallow tablets whole, do not crush or chew

Additional Information Diflunisal is a salicylic acid derivative which is chemically different than aspirin and is not metabolized to salicylic acid. Diflunisal 500 mg is equal in analgesic efficacy to aspirin 650 mg, acetaminophen 650 mg, and acetaminophen 650 mg/propoxyphene napsylate 100 mg, but has a longer duration of effect (8-12 hours). Not recommended as an antipyretic. Not found to be clinically useful to treat fever; at doses of ≥2 g/day, platelets are reversibly inhibited in function. Diflunisal is uricosuric at 500-750 mg/day; causes less GI and renal toxicity than aspirin and other NSAIDs; fecal blood loss is ½ that of aspirin at 2.6 g/day.

Special Geriatric Considerations The elderly are a high-risk population for adverse effects from nonsteroidal anti-inflammatory agents. As much as 60% of elderly can develop peptic ulceration and/or hemorrhage asymptomatically. The concomitant use of H_2 blockers and sucralfate is not effective as prophylaxis with the exception of NSAID-induced duodenal ulcers which may be prevented by the use of ranitidine. Misoprostol and proton pump inhibitors are the only agents proven to help prevent the development of NSAID-induced ulcers. Also, concomitant disease and drug use contribute to the risk for GI adverse effects. Use lowest effective dose for shortest period possible. Consider renal function decline with age. Use of NSAIDs can compromise existing renal function especially when Cl_{cr} is ≤30 mL/minute. Tinnitus may be a difficult and unreliable indication of toxicity due to age-related hearing loss or eighth (Continued)

Diflunisal (Continued)

cranial nerve damage. CNS adverse effects such as confusion, agitation, and hallucination are generally seen in overdose or high dose situations, but elderly may demonstrate these adverse effects at lower doses than younger adults.

Dosage Forms Excipient information presented when available (limited, particularly for generics); consult specific product labeling. [DSC] = Discontinued product

Tablet: 500 mg

Dolobid®: 250 mg, 500 mg [DSC]

Selected References

Aronoff GR, Berns JS, Brier ME, et al. "Drug Prescribing in Renal Failure: Dosing Guidelines for Adults," 4th ed. Philadelphia, PA: American College of Physicians; 1998.

Gurwitz JH, Avorn J, Ross-Degnan D, et al, "Nonsteroidal Anti-inflammatory Drug-Associated Azotemia in the Very Old," *JAMA*, 1990, 264(4):471-5.

Hawkey CJ, Karrasch JA, Szczepański L, et al, "Omeprazole Compared With Misoprostol for Ulcers Associated With Nonsteroidal Anti-inflammatory Drugs," *N Engl J Med*, 1998, 338(11):727-34.

Hunt SA, Abraham WT, Chin MH, et al, "ACC/AHA 2005 Guideline Update for the Diagnosis and Management of Chronic Heart Failure in the Adult-Summary Article A Report of the American College of Cardiology/ American Heart Association Task Force on Practice Guidelines (Writing Committee to Update the 2001 Guidelines for the Evaluation and Management of Heart Failure)," *J Am Coll Cardiol*, 2005, 46(6):1116-43.

Yeomans ND, Tulassay Z, Juhasz L, et al, "A Comparison of Omeprazole With Ranitidine for Ulcers Associated With Nonsteroidal Anti-inflammatory Drugs," *N Engl J Med*, 1998, 338(11):719-26.

♦ **Digitek**® see Digoxin *on page 434*

Digoxin (di JOKS in)

Related Information

Potentially Inappropriate Medications for Geriatrics *on page 1824*

Serum Drug Concentrations Commonly Monitored Guidelines *on page 1862*

Medication Safety Issues

Sound-alike/look-alike issues:

Digoxin may be confused with Desoxyn®, doxepin

Lanoxin® may be confused with Lasix®, Levoxyl®, Levsinex®, Lomotil®, Lonox®, Mefoxin®, Xanax®

High alert medication: The Institute for Safe Medication Practices (ISMP) includes this medication among its list of drugs which have a heightened risk of causing significant patient harm when used in error.

International issues:

Dilacor®: Brand name for diltiazem in the U.S.; brand name for verapamil in Brazil; brand name for barnidipine in Argentina

Lanoxin® may be confused with Lemoxin® which is a brand bane for cefuroxime in Mexico

Lanoxin® may be confused with Limoxin® which is a brand name for amoxicillin in Mexico

U.S. Brand Names Digitek®; Lanoxicaps®; Lanoxin®

Canadian Brand Names Apo-Digoxin®; Digoxin CSD; Lanoxicaps®; Lanoxin®; Novo-Digoxin; Pediatric Digoxin CSD

Generic Available Yes: Excludes capsule

Pharmacologic Category Antiarrhythmic Agent, Class IV; Cardiac Glycoside

Use Treatment of congestive heart failure; slows the ventricular rate in tachyarrhythmias such as atrial fibrillation, atrial flutter, supraventricular tachycardia (paroxysmal atrial tachycardia), cardiogenic shock

Contraindications Hypersensitivity to digoxin or any component of the formulation; hypersensitivity to cardiac glycosides (another may be tried); history of toxicity; ventricular tachycardia or fibrillation; idiopathic hypertrophic subaortic stenosis; constrictive pericarditis; amyloid disease; second- or third-degree heart block (except in patients with a functioning artificial pacemaker); Wolff-Parkinson-White syndrome and atrial fibrillation concurrently

Warnings/Precautions Watch for proarrhythmic effects (especially with digoxin toxicity); monitor and adjust dose to prevent QT_c prolongation. Use with caution in patients with hypoxia, myxedema, hypothyroidism, acute myocarditis; patients with incomplete AV block (Stokes-Adams attack) may progress to complete block with digitalis drug administration; use with caution in patients with acute myocardial infarction, severe pulmonary disease, advanced heart failure, idiopathic hypertrophic subaortic stenosis, Wolff-Parkinson-White syndrome, sick-sinus syndrome (bradyarrhythmias), amyloid heart disease, and constrictive cardiomyopathies; adjust dose with renal impairment and when verapamil, quinidine or amiodarone are added to a patient on digoxin; elderly may develop exaggerated serum/tissue concentrations due to age-related alterations in clearance and pharmacodynamic differences; exercise will reduce serum concentrations of digoxin due to increased skeletal muscle uptake; recent studies indicate photopsia, chromatopsia and decreased visual acuity may occur even with therapeutic serum drug levels; reduce or hold dose 1-2 days before elective electrical cardioversion. In the Cardiac Arrhythmia Suppression Trial (CAST), recent (>6 days but <2 years ago) myocardial infarction patients with asymptomatic, nonlife-threatening ventricular arrhythmias did not benefit and may have been harmed by attempts to suppress the arrhythmia with flecainide or encainide. An increased mortality or nonfatal cardiac arrest rate (7.7%) was seen in the active treatment group compared with patients in the placebo group (3%). The applicability of the CAST results to other populations is unknown. Antiarrhythmic agents should be reserved for patients with life-threatening ventricular arrhythmias.

Adverse Reactions (Reflective of adult population; not specific for elderly)
Incidence not always reported.

Cardiovascular: Heart block; first-, second- (Wenckebach), or third-degree heart block; asystole; atrial tachycardia with block; AV dissociation; accelerated junctional rhythm; ventricular tachycardia or ventricular fibrillation; PR prolongation; ST segment depression

Central nervous system: Visual disturbances (blurred or yellow vision), headache (3%), dizziness (5%), apathy, confusion, mental disturbances (4%), anxiety, depression, delirium, hallucinations, fever

Dermatologic: Maculopapular rash (2%), erythematous, scarlatiniform, papular, vesicular or bullous rash, urticaria, pruritus, facial, angioneurotic or laryngeal edema, shedding of fingernails or toenails, alopecia

Gastrointestinal: Nausea (3%), vomiting (2%), diarrhea (3%), abdominal pain

Neuromuscular & skeletal: Weakness

Children are more likely to experience cardiac arrhythmia as a sign of excessive dosing. The most common are conduction disturbances or tachyarrhythmia (atrial tachycardia with or without block) and junctional tachycardia. Ventricular tachyarrhythmia are less common. In infants, sinus bradycardia may be a sign of digoxin toxicity. Any arrhythmia seen in a child on digoxin should be considered as digoxin toxicity. The gastrointestinal and central nervous system symptoms are not frequently seen in children.

Overdosage/Toxicology Symptoms of acute overdose include vomiting, hyperkalemia, sinus bradycardia, S-A arrest and AV block are common, ventricular tachycardia, and fibrillation. Symptoms of chronic intoxication include visual disturbances, weakness, sinus bradycardia, atrial fibrillation with slowed ventricular response, and ventricular arrhythmias. After GI decontamination, treat hyperkalemia if >5.5 mEq/L with sodium bicarbonate and glucose with insulin or Kayexalate®. Treat bradycardia or heart block with atropine or pacemaker and other arrhythmias with conventional antiarrhythmics. Use Digibind® for severe hyperkalemia, symptomatic arrhythmias unresponsive to other drugs, and for prophylactic treatment in massive overdose.

Drug Interactions Substrate of CYP3A4 (minor)

Amiloride may reduce the inotropic response to digoxin.

Amiodarone reduces renal and nonrenal clearance of digoxin and may have additive effects on heart rate. Reduce digoxin dose by 50% with start of amiodarone.

Benzodiazepines (alprazolam, diazepam) have been associated with isolated reports of digoxin toxicity.

Beta-blocking agents (propranolol) may have additive effects on heart rate.

Calcium preparations: Rare cases of acute digoxin toxicity have been associated with parenteral calcium (bolus) administration.

Carvedilol may increase digoxin blood levels in addition to potentiating its effects on heart rate.

Cholestyramine, colestipol, kaolin-pectin may reduce digoxin absorption. Separate administration.

Cyclosporine may increase digoxin levels, possibly due to reduced renal clearance.

Erythromycin, clarithromycin, and tetracyclines may increase digoxin (not capsule form) blood levels in a subset of patients.

Indomethacin has been associated with isolated reports of increased digoxin blood levels/toxicity.

Itraconazole may increase digoxin blood levels in some patients; monitor.

Levothyroxine (and other thyroid supplements) may decrease digoxin blood levels.

Metoclopramide may reduce the absorption of digoxin tablets.

Moricizine may increase the toxicity of digoxin (mechanism undefined).

Penicillamine has been associated with reductions in digoxin blood levels

Propafenone increases digoxin blood levels. Effects are highly variable; monitor closely.

Propylthiouracil (and methimazole) may increase digoxin blood levels by reducing thyroid hormone.

Quinidine increases digoxin blood levels substantially. Effect is variable (33% to 50%). Monitor digoxin blood levels/effect closely. Reduce digoxin dose by 50% with start of quinidine. Other related agents (hydroxychloroquine, quinine) should be used with caution.

Spironolactone may interfere with some digoxin assays, but may also increase blood levels directly. However, spironolactone may attenuate the inotropic effect of digoxin. Monitor effects of digoxin closely.

(Continued)

Digoxin *(Continued)*

Succinylcholine administration to patients on digoxin has been associated with an increased risk of arrhythmias.

Verapamil, diltiazem, and bepridil increased serum digoxin concentrations. Other calcium channel blocking agents do not appear to share this effect. Reduce digoxin's dose with the start of verapamil.

Drugs which cause hypokalemia (thiazide and loop diuretics, amphotericin B): Hypokalemia may potentiate digoxin toxicity.

These medications have been associated with reduced digoxin blood levels which appear to be of limited clinical significance: Aminoglutethimide, aminosalicylic acid, aluminum-containing antacids, sucralfate, sulfasalazine, neomycin, ticlopidine.

These medications have been associated with increased digoxin blood levels which appear to be of limited clinical significance: Famciclovir, flecainide, ibuprofen, fluoxetine, nefazodone, cimetidine, famotidine, ranitidine, omeprazole, trimethoprim.

Ethanol/Nutrition/Herb Interactions

Food: Digoxin peak serum levels may be decreased if taken with food. Meals containing increased fiber (bran) or foods high in pectin may decrease oral absorption of digoxin.

Herb/Nutraceutical: Avoid ephedra (risk of cardiac stimulation). Avoid natural licorice (causes sodium and water retention and increases potassium loss).

Stability Protect elixir and injection from light.

Mechanism of Action

Congestive heart failure: Inhibition of the sodium/potassium ATPase pump which acts to increase the intracellular sodium-calcium exchange to increase intracellular calcium leading to increased contractility

Supraventricular arrhythmias: Direct suppression of the AV node conduction to increase effective refractory period and decrease conduction velocity - positive inotropic effect, enhanced vagal tone, and decreased ventricular rate to fast atrial arrhythmias. Atrial fibrillation may decrease sensitivity and increase tolerance to higher serum digoxin concentrations.

Pharmacodynamics

Onset of effects:
Oral: 1-2 hours
I.V.: 5-30 minutes
Peak effect:
Oral: 2-8 hours
I.V.: 1-4 hours
Duration: 3-4 days

Pharmacokinetics

Distribution: V_d: Geriatrics: 194 L (range: 129-314 L)
Protein binding: 25%
Bioavailability: Dependent upon formulation:
Elixir: 70% to 85%
Tablets: 60% to 80% (76% in older adults)
Capsules: 90% to 100%
Half-life:
Geriatrics: 69 hours (average)
Adults: 38-48 hours
Anephric Adults: >4.5 days
Time to peak serum concentration:
Oral: 2-6 hours
I.V.: 1-5 hours
Elimination: Renal

Dosage

Geriatrics: Dose is based on lean body weight and normal renal function for age. Decrease dose in patients with decreased renal function (see Dosage: Renal Impairment).

Adults:

Note: When changing from oral (tablets or liquid) or I.M. to I.V. therapy, dosage should be reduced by 20% to 25%.

Atrial dysrhythmias (rate control), CHF:

Initial: Total digitalizing dose: Give 1/2 of the total digitalizing dose (TDD) in the initial dose, then give 1/4 of the TDD in each of two subsequent doses at 9- to 12-hour intervals. Obtain ECG 6 hours after each dose to assess potential toxicity.
Oral: 0.75-1.5 mg
I.V. or I.M.: 0.5-1 mg

Daily maintenance dose: Give once daily
Oral: 0.125-0.5 mg
I.V. or I.M.: 0.1-0.4 mg

Renal Impairment:
Cl$_{cr}$ 10-50 mL/minute: Administer 25% to 75% of dose or every 36 hours.
Cl$_{cr}$ <10 mL/minute: Administer 10% to 25% of dose or every 48 hours.
Reduce loading dose by 50% in ESRD.
Not dialyzable (0% to 5%)

Administration
I.M.: Inject no more than 2 mL per injection site. May cause intense pain.
I.V.: May be administered undiluted or diluted fourfold in D$_5$W, NS, or SWFI for direct injection. Less than fourfold dilution may lead to drug precipitation. Inject slowly over ≥5 minutes.

Monitoring Parameters Monitor apical pulse, peripheral pulse, serum concentrations, EKG in critical cases of toxicity or arrhythmias

Reference Range Therapeutic: 1-2 ng/mL (SI: 1.3-2.6 nmol/L); <0.5 ng/mL (SI: <0.6 nmol/L) probably indicates underdigitalization unless there are special circumstances; Toxic: >2 ng/mL (SI: >2.6 nmol/L)

Patient Information Do not discontinue medication without physician's advice

Additional Information The AHCPR Clinical Practice Guideline for Heart Failure recommends that digoxin should be saved for patients who do not respond to ACE inhibitors and diuretics or who present with severe dyspnea on exertion. Digoxin is useful in systolic dysfunction, but not diastolic dysfunction.

Special Geriatric Considerations Digitalis preparations (primarily digoxin) are frequently used to treat common cardiac diseases in the elderly (congestive heart failure, atrial fibrillation). Elderly are at risk for toxicity due to age-related changes; volume of distribution is diminished significantly; half-life is increased as a result of decreased total body clearance. Additionally, elderly frequently have concomitant diseases which affect the pharmacokinetics in digitalis glycosides; hypo- and hyperthyroidism and renal function decline will affect clearance of digoxin. Exercise in elderly will reduce serum concentrations of digoxin due to increased skeletal muscle uptake. Therefore, a knowledge of the physical activity of elderly helps interpret serum assays. Must be observant for noncardiac signs of toxicity in elderly such as anorexia, vision changes (blurred), confusion, and depression. Changes in dose may be necessary with declining renal function with age; monitor closely.

Dosage Forms Excipient information presented when available (limited, particularly for generics); consult specific product labeling. [CAN] = Canadian brand name
Capsule:
Lanoxicaps®: 100 mcg, 200 mcg [contains ethyl alcohol]
Injection, solution: 250 mcg/mL (1 mL, 2 mL)
Lanoxin®: 250 mcg/mL (2 mL) [contains alcohol 10% and propylene glycol 40%]
Injection, solution [pediatric]: 100 mcg/mL (1 mL)
Solution, oral: 50 mcg/mL (2.5 mL, 5 mL, 60 mL)
Tablet: 125 mcg, 250 mcg
Digitek®, Lanoxin®: 125 mcg, 250 mcg
Apo-Digoxin® [CAN]: 62.5 mcg, 125 mcg, 250 mcg

Selected References
Agency for Health Care Policy and Research, Clinical Practice Guidelines, "Heart Failure: Evaluation and Care of Patients With Left-Ventricular Systolic Dysfunction," *U.S. Department of Health and Human Services*, Pub No 94-0612, June 1994.
Nolan PE and Mooradian AD, "Digoxin," *Geriatric Pharmacology*, Bressler R and Katz MD eds, New York, NY: McGraw-Hill, 1993, 7:151-63.

Dihydroergotamine (dye hye droe er GOT a meen)

U.S. Brand Names D.H.E. 45®; Migranal®
Canadian Brand Names Migranal®
Index Terms DHE; Dihydroergotamine Mesylate
Generic Available Yes: Injection
Pharmacologic Category Antimigraine Agent; Ergot Derivative
Use Prevention or abortion of vascular headaches
Unlabeled/Investigational Use Adjunct for DVT prophylaxis for hip surgery; treatment of orthostatic hypotension, xerostomia secondary to antidepressant use, pelvic congestion with pain

Contraindications Hypersensitivity to dihydroergotamine or any component of the formulation; high-dose aspirin therapy; uncontrolled hypertension, ischemic heart disease, angina pectoris, history of MI, silent ischemia, or coronary artery vasospasm including Prinzmetal's angina; hemiplegic or basilar migraine; peripheral vascular disease; sepsis; severe hepatic or renal dysfunction; following vascular surgery; avoid use within 24 hours of sumatriptan, zolmitriptan, other serotonin agonists, or ergot-like agents; avoid during or within 2 weeks of discontinuing MAO inhibitors; ergot alkaloids are contraindicated with potent inhibitors of CYP3A4 (includes protease inhibitors, azole antifungals, and some macrolide antibiotics)

Warnings/Precautions [U.S. Boxed Warning]: Ergot alkaloids are contraindicated with potent inhibitors of CYP3A4 (includes protease inhibitors, azole antifungals,
(Continued)

Dihydroergotamine *(Continued)*

and some macrolide antibiotics); concomitant use associated with acute ergot toxicity (ergotism). Do not give to patients with risk factors for CAD until a cardiovascular evaluation has been performed; if evaluation is satisfactory, the healthcare provider should administer the first dose and cardiovascular status should be periodically evaluated. May cause vasospastic reactions; persistent vasospasm may lead to gangrene or death in patients with compromised circulation. Discontinue if signs of vasoconstriction develop. Rare reports of increased blood pressure in patients without history of hypertension. Rare reports of adverse cardiac events (acute MI, life-threatening arrhythmias, death) have been reported following use of the injection. Cerebral hemorrhage, subarachnoid hemorrhage, and stroke have also occurred following use of the injection. Not for prolonged use. Pleural and peritoneal fibrosis have been reported with prolonged daily use. Cardiac valvular fibrosis has also been associated with ergot alkaloids. Use with caution in the elderly.

Migranal® Nasal Spray: Local irritation to nose and throat (usually transient and mild-moderate in severity) can occur; long-term consequences on nasal or respiratory mucosa have not been extensively evaluated.

Adverse Reactions (Reflective of adult population; not specific for elderly)
>10%: Nasal spray: Respiratory: Rhinitis (26%)

1% to 10%: Nasal spray:
Central nervous system: Dizziness (4%), somnolence (3%)
Endocrine & metabolic: Hot flashes (1%)
Gastrointestinal: Nausea (10%), taste disturbance (8%), vomiting (4%), diarrhea (2%)
Local: Application site reaction (6%)
Neuromuscular & skeletal: Weakness (1%), stiffness (1%)
Respiratory: Pharyngitis (3%)

Overdosage/Toxicology Symptoms include peripheral ischemia, paresthesia, headache, nausea, and vomiting. Activated charcoal is effective at binding certain chemicals; this is especially true for ergot alkaloids.

Drug Interactions Substrate of CYP3A4 (major); **Inhibits** CYP3A4 (weak)

Antifungals, azole derivatives (itraconazole, ketoconazole) increase levels of ergot alkaloids by inhibiting CYP3A4 metabolism, resulting in toxicity; concomitant use is contraindicated.

Antipsychotics: May diminish the effects of dihydroergotamine (due to dopamine antagonism); these combinations should generally be avoided.

Beta-blockers: Severe peripheral vasoconstriction has been reported with concomitant use of beta-blockers and ergot derivatives. Monitor.

CYP3A4 inhibitors: May increase the levels/effects of dihydroergotamine. Example inhibitors include azole antifungals, clarithromycin, diclofenac, doxycycline, erythromycin, imatinib, isoniazid, nefazodone, nicardipine, propofol, protease inhibitors, quinidine, telithromycin, and verapamil. Ergot alkaloids are contraindicated with potent CYP3A4 inhibitors.

Heparin: When given with heparin, dihydroergotamine I.M. leads to hematoma at the injection site; combined administration not recommended.

Macrolide antibiotics: Erythromycin, clarithromycin, and troleandomycin may increase levels of ergot alkaloids by inhibiting CYP3A4 metabolism, resulting in toxicity (ischemia, vasospasm); concomitant use is contraindicated.

MAO inhibitors: The serotonergic effects of ergot derivatives may be increased by MAO inhibitors. Monitor for signs and symptoms of serotonin syndrome.

Metoclopramide: May diminish the effects of dihydroergotamine (due to dopamine antagonism); concurrent therapy should generally be avoided.

Nitroglycerin: May increase bioavailability of dihydroergotamine, decrease antianginal effects of nitrate; may need to decrease dose of dihydroergotamine. Monitor.

Protease inhibitors (ritonavir, amprenavir, atazanavir, indinavir, nelfinavir, and saquinavir) increase blood levels of ergot alkaloids by inhibiting CYP3A4 metabolism, acute ergot toxicity has been reported; concomitant use is contraindicated.

Serotonin agonists: Concurrent use with dihydroergotamine may increase the risk of serotonin syndrome (includes buspirone, SSRIs, TCAs, nefazodone, sumatriptan, and trazodone).

Sibutramine: May cause serotonin syndrome; concurrent use with ergot alkaloids is contraindicated.

Sumatriptan and other serotonin 5-HT$_1$ receptor agonists: Prolong vasospastic reactions; do not use sumatriptan or ergot-containing drugs within 24 hours of each other.

Vasoconstrictors: Concomitant use with peripheral vasoconstrictors may cause synergistic elevation of blood pressure; use is contraindicated.

Stability
Injection: Store below 25°C (77°F); do not refrigerate or freeze. Protect from heat and light.

Nasal spray: Prior to use, store below 25°C (77°F); do not refrigerate or freeze. Once spray applicator has been prepared, use within 8 hours; discard any unused solution.

Mechanism of Action Ergot alkaloid alpha-adrenergic blocker directly stimulates vascular smooth muscle to vasoconstrict peripheral and cerebral vessels; also has effects on serotonin receptors

Pharmacodynamics
Onset of action: Within 15-30 minutes
Duration: 3-4 hours

Pharmacokinetics
Distribution: V_d: 14.5 L/kg
Protein binding: 93%
Metabolism: Extensively hepatic
Half-life: 1.3-3.9 hours
Time to peak, serum: I.M.: 15-30 minutes
Elimination: Primarily feces; urine (10% mostly as metabolites)

Dosage
Geriatrics: Refer to adult dosing. Patients >65 years of age were not included in controlled clinical studies.
Adults:
Migraine, cluster headache:
I.M., SubQ: 1 mg at first sign of headache; repeat hourly to a maximum dose of 3 mg total; maximum dose: 6 mg/week
I.V.: 1 mg at first sign of headache; repeat hourly up to a maximum dose of 2 mg total; maximum dose: 6 mg/week
Intranasal: 1 spray (0.5 mg) of nasal spray should be administered into each nostril; if needed, repeat after 15 minutes, up to a total of 4 sprays. **Note:** Do not exceed 3 mg (6 sprays) in a 24-hour period and no more than 8 sprays in a week.
Renal Impairment: Contraindicated in severe renal impairment
Hepatic Impairment: Dosage reductions are probably necessary but specific guidelines are not available; contraindicated in severe hepatic dysfunction.

Administration Prior to administration of nasal spray, the nasal spray applicator must be primed (pumped 4 times); in order to let the drug be absorbed through the skin in the nose, patients should not inhale deeply through the nose while spraying or immediately after spraying; for best results, treatment should be initiated at the first symptom or sign of an attack; however, nasal spray can be used at any stage of a migraine attack

Monitoring Parameters Monitor blood pressure, heart rate, signs of tingling or numbness

Reference Range Minimum concentration for vasoconstriction is reportedly 0.06 ng/mL

Patient Information Rare feelings of numbness or tingling of fingers, toes, or face may occur; avoid using this medication if you have heart disease, hypertension, liver disease, infection, itching

Nasal spray: Follow directions for use on package insert. Prime inhaler before use. Wait 15 minutes between inhalations. Use no more than 4 inhalations (2 mg) for a single administration; do not use >3 mg (6 sprays) in a 24-hour period and no more than 8 sprays in a week.

Special Geriatric Considerations Monitor cardiac and peripheral effects closely in the elderly since they often have cardiovascular disease and peripheral vascular impairment (ie, diabetes mellitus, PVD) that will complicate therapy and monitoring for adverse effects.

Dosage Forms Excipient information presented when available (limited, particularly for generics); consult specific product labeling.
Injection, solution, as mesylate (D.H.E. 45®): 1 mg/mL (1 mL) [contains ethanol 94%]
Solution, intranasal spray, as mesylate (Migranal®): 4 mg/mL [0.5 mg/spray] (1 mL) [contains caffeine 10 mg/mL]

♦ **Dihydroergotamine Mesylate** *see* Dihydroergotamine *on page 437*
♦ **Dihydroergotoxine** *see* Ergoloid Mesylates *on page 527*
♦ **Dihydrogenated Ergot Alkaloids** *see* Ergoloid Mesylates *on page 527*
♦ **Dihydrohydroxycodeinone** *see* Oxycodone *on page 1179*
♦ **Dihydromorphinone** *see* Hydromorphone *on page 766*

Dihydrotachysterol (dye hye droe tak ISS ter ole)

U.S. Brand Names DHT™ [DSC]; DHT™ Intensol™ [DSC]; Hytakerol® [DSC]
Canadian Brand Names Hytakerol®
Index Terms Dichysterol
Generic Available No
(Continued)

Dihydrotachysterol *(Continued)*

Pharmacologic Category Vitamin D Analog

Use Treatment of hypocalcemia associated with hypoparathyroidism; prophylaxis of hypocalcemic tetany following thyroid surgery

Contraindications Hypersensitivity to dihydrotachysterol or any component of the formulation; hypercalcemia

Warnings/Precautions Must administer concomitant calcium supplementation; maintain adequate fluid intake; calcium-phosphate product (serum calcium and phosphorus) must not exceed 70; avoid hypercalcemia; may cause renal function impairment with secondary hyperparathyroidism. Use with caution in coronary artery disease, decreased renal function, renal stones, and in older adults.

Adverse Reactions (Reflective of adult population; not specific for elderly)
>10%:
Endocrine & metabolic: Hypercalcemia
Renal: Serum creatinine increased, hypercalciuria

Drug Interactions
Decreased effect/levels of vitamin D: Cholestyramine, colestipol, mineral oil; phenytoin and phenobarbital may inhibit activation may decrease effectiveness
Increased toxicity: Thiazide diuretics increase calcium

Stability Protect from light.

Mechanism of Action Synthetic analogue of vitamin D with a faster onset of action; stimulates calcium and phosphate absorption from the small intestine, promotes secretion of calcium from bone to blood; promotes renal tubule resorption of phosphate

Pharmacodynamics
Onset of action: Maximum hypercalcemic effects occur within 2-4 weeks
Duration: Can be as long as 9 weeks

Pharmacokinetics
Absorption: Well from GI tract
Elimination: In bile and feces; stored in liver, fat, skin, muscle, and bone

Dosage
Geriatrics & Adults:
Hypoparathyroidism: Oral: Initial: 0.8-2.4 mg/day for several days followed by maintenance doses of 0.2-1 mg/day
Nutritional rickets: Oral: 0.5 mg as a single dose or 13-50 mcg/day until healing occurs
Renal osteodystrophy: Oral: Maintenance: 0.25-0.6 mg/24 hours adjusted as necessary to achieve normal serum calcium levels and promote bone healing

Monitoring Parameters Monitor renal function, serum calcium and phosphate concentrations; if hypercalcemia is encountered, discontinue agent until serum calcium returns to normal

Reference Range Calcium (serum) 9-10 mg/dL (4.5-5 mEq/L); phosphate 2.5-5 mg/dL

Patient Information Do not take more than the recommended amount. While taking this medication, your physician may want you to follow a special diet or take a calcium supplement. Follow this diet closely. Avoid taking magnesium supplements or magnesium containing antacids. Early symptoms of hypercalcemia include weakness, fatigue, somnolence, headache, anorexia, dry mouth, metallic taste, nausea, vomiting, cramps, diarrhea, muscle pain, bone pain, and irritability.

Additional Information Synthetic analog of vitamin D with a faster onset of action; dose adjustment should be based on serum calcium level

Special Geriatric Considerations Recommended daily allowances (RDA) have not been developed for persons >65 years of age; vitamin D, folate, and B_{12} (cyanocobalamin) have decreased absorption with age, but the clinical significance is yet unknown. Calorie requirements decrease with age and therefore, nutrient density must be increased to ensure adequate nutrient intake, including vitamins and minerals. Therefore, the use of a daily supplement with a multiple vitamin with minerals is recommended. Elderly consume less vitamin D, absorption may be decreased, and many elderly have decreased sun exposure; therefore, elderly should receive supplementation with 800 units of vitamin D (20 mcg)/day. This is a recommendation of particular need to those with high risk for osteoporosis.

Dosage Forms Excipient information presented when available (limited, particularly for generics); consult specific product labeling. [DSC] = Discontinued product
Capsule (Hytakerol®): 0.125 mg [contains sesame oil] [DSC]
Solution, oral concentrate (DHT™ Intensol™): 0.2 mg/mL (30 mL) [contains alcohol 20%] [DSC]
Tablet (DHT™): 0.125 mg, 0.2 mg, 0.4 mg [DSC]

Selected References
Letsou AP and Price LS, "Health Aging and Nutrition: An Overview," *Clin Geriatr Med*, 1987, 3(2):253-60.
Myrianthopoulos M, "Dietary Treatment of Hyperlipidemia in the Elderly," *Clin Geriatr Med*, 1987, 3(2):343-59.
Riggs BL and Melton LJ, "The Prevention and Treatment of Osteoporosis," *N Engl J Med*, 1992, 327(9):620-7.

♦ **1,25 Dihydroxycholecalciferol** *see* Calcitriol *on page 210*

♦ **Dihydroxypropyl Theophylline** *see Dyphylline on page 496*

♦ **Diiodohydroxyquin** *see Iodoquinol on page 825*

♦ **Dilacor® XR** *See Diltiazem on page 441*

♦ **Dilantin®** *see Phenytoin on page 1250*

♦ **Dilatrate®-SR** *see Isosorbide Dinitrate on page 839*

♦ **Dilaudid®** *see Hydromorphone on page 766*

♦ **Dilaudid-HP®** *see Hydromorphone on page 766*

♦ **Dilex-G** *see Dyphylline and Guaifenesin on page 496*

♦ **Dilor-G®** *see Dyphylline and Guaifenesin on page 496*

♦ **Diltia XT®** *see Diltiazem on page 441*

Diltiazem (dil TYE a zem)

Related Information
Calcium Channel Blockers *on page 1753*

Medication Safety Issues
Sound-alike/look-alike issues:

Diltiazem may be confused with Dilantin®

Cardizem® may be confused with Cardene®, Cardene SR®, Cardizem CD®, Cardizem SR®, cardiem

Cartia XT™ may be confused with Procardia XL®

Tiazac® may be confused with Tigan®, Ziac®

Significant differences exist between oral and I.V. dosing. Use caution when converting from one route of administration to another.

International issues:

Cardizem® may be confused with Cardem® which is a brand name for celiprolol in Spain

Cartia XT™ may be confused with Cartia® which is a brand name for aspirin in multiple international markets

Dilacor®: Brand name for digoxin in Serbia, a brand name for verapamil in Brazil, and a brand name for barnidipine in Argentina

Tiazac® may be confused with Tazac® which is a brand name for nizatidine in Australia

U.S. Brand Names Cardizem®; Cardizem® CD; Cardizem® LA; Cartia XT™; Dilacor® XR; Diltia XT®; Dilt-XR; Taztia XT™; Tiazac®

Canadian Brand Names Alti-Diltiazem CD; Apo-Diltiaz®; Apo-Diltiaz CD®; Apo-Diltiaz® Injectable; Apo-Diltiaz SR®; Apo-Diltiaz TZ®; Cardizem®; Cardizem® CD; Cardizem® SR; Diltia XT®; Dilt-XR; Diltiazem Hydrochloride Injection; Gen-Diltiazem; Gen-Diltiazem CD; Med-Diltiazem; Novo-Diltiazem; Novo-Diltiazem-CD; Novo-Diltiazem HCl ER; Nu-Diltiaz; Nu-Diltiaz-CD; ratio-Diltiazem CD; Rhoxal-diltiazem CD; Rhoxal-diltiazem SR; Rhoxal-diltiazem T; Sandoz-Diltiazem CD; Sandoz-Diltiazem T; Syn-Diltiazem®; Tiazac®; Tiazac® XC

Index Terms Diltiazem Hydrochloride

Generic Available Yes: Excludes extended release tablet

Pharmacologic Category Calcium Channel Blocker

Use
Oral: Essential hypertension; chronic stable angina or angina from coronary artery spasm

Injection: Atrial fibrillation or atrial flutter; paroxysmal supraventricular tachycardia (PSVT)

Unlabeled/Investigational Use Investigational: Therapy of Duchenne muscular dystrophy

Contraindications Hypersensitivity to diltiazem or any component of the formulation; sick sinus syndrome; second- or third-degree AV block (except in patients with a functioning artificial pacemaker); hypotension (systolic <90 mm Hg); acute MI and pulmonary congestion

Warnings/Precautions Increased angina and/or MI has occurred with initiation or dosage titration of calcium channel blockers. Can cause first-degree AV block or sinus bradycardia; other conduction abnormalities are rare. The most common side effect is peripheral edema; occurs within 2-3 weeks of starting therapy. Symptomatic hypotension with or without syncope can rarely occur; blood pressure must be lowered at a rate appropriate for the patient's clinical condition. Concomitant use with beta-blockers or digoxin can result in conduction disturbances. Avoid concurrent I.V. use of diltiazem and a beta-blocker. Use caution in left ventricular dysfunction (can exacerbate condition). Use with caution with hypertrophic cardiomyopathy. Use with caution in hepatic or renal dysfunction.
(Continued)

Diltiazem *(Continued)*

Adverse Reactions (Reflective of adult population; not specific for elderly)

Note: Frequencies represent ranges for various dosage forms. Patients with impaired ventricular function and/or conduction abnormalities may have higher incidence of adverse reactions.

>10%:
  Cardiovascular: Edema (2% to 15%)
  Central nervous system: Headache (5% to 12%)

2% to 10%:
  Cardiovascular: AV block (first degree 2% to 8%), edema (lower limb 2% to 8%), pain (6%), bradycardia (2% to 6%), hypotension (<2% to 4%), vasodilation (2% to 3%), extrasystoles (2%), flushing (1% to 2%), palpitation (1% to 2%)
  Central nervous system: Dizziness (3% to 10%), nervousness (2%)
  Dermatologic: Rash (1% to 4%)
  Endocrine & metabolic: Gout (1% to 2%)
  Gastrointestinal: Dyspepsia (1% to 6%), constipation (<2% to 4%), vomiting (2%), diarrhea (1% to 2%)
  Local: Injection site reactions: Burning, itching (4%)
  Neuromuscular & skeletal: Weakness (1% to 4%), myalgia (2%)
  Respiratory: Rhinitis (<2% to 10%), pharyngitis (2% to 6%), dyspnea (1% to 6%), bronchitis (1% to 4%), sinus congestion (1% to 2%)

Overdosage/Toxicology
Primary cardiac symptoms of calcium blocker overdose include hypotension and bradycardia. Hypotension is caused by peripheral vasodilation, myocardial depression, and bradycardia. Bradycardia results from sinus bradycardia, second- or third-degree atrioventricular block, or sinus arrest with junctional rhythm. Intraventricular conduction is usually not affected, so QRS duration is normal (verapamil prolongs the PR interval and bepridil prolongs the QT interval and may cause ventricular arrhythmias, including torsade de pointes).

Noncardiac symptoms include confusion, stupor, nausea, vomiting, metabolic acidosis, and hyperglycemia. Following initial gastric decontamination, if possible, repeated calcium administration may promptly reverse depressed cardiac contractility (but not sinus node depression or peripheral vasodilation). Glucagon, epinephrine, and inamrinone (amrinone) may treat refractory hypotension. Glucagon and epinephrine also increase the heart rate (outside the U.S., 4-aminopyridine may be available as an antidote). Dialysis and hemoperfusion are not effective in enhancing elimination, although repeat-dose activated charcoal may serve as an adjunct with sustained-release preparations.

In a few reported cases, overdose with calcium channel blockers has been associated with hypotension and bradycardia, initially refractory to atropine, but becoming more responsive to this agent when larger doses (approaching 1 g/hour for more than 24 hours) of calcium chloride were administered.

Drug Interactions
Substrate of CYP2C9 (minor), 2D6 (minor), 3A4 (major); **Inhibits** CYP2C9 (weak), 2D6 (weak), 3A4 (moderate)

Alfentanil's plasma concentration is increased. Fentanyl and sufentanil may be affected similarly.

Amiodarone use may lead to bradycardia, other conduction delays, and decreased cardiac output; monitor closely if using together.

Azole antifungals may inhibit the calcium channel blocker's metabolism; avoid this combination. Try an antifungal like terbinafine (if appropriate) or monitor closely for altered effect of the calcium channel blocker.

Benzodiazepines (midazolam, triazolam) plasma concentrations are increased by diltiazem; monitor for prolonged CNS depression.

Beta-blockers may have increased pharmacodynamic interactions with diltiazem (see Warnings/Precautions).

Buspirone: Diltiazem may increase serum levels of buspirone; monitor.

Calcium may reduce the calcium channel blocker's effects, particularly hypotension.

Carbamazepine's serum concentration is increased and toxicity may result; avoid this combination.

Cimetidine reduced diltiazem's metabolism; consider an alternative H_2 antagonist.

Cyclosporine's serum concentrations are increased by diltiazem; avoid the combination. Use another calcium channel blocker or monitor cyclosporine trough levels and renal function closely.

CYP3A4 inducers: CYP3A4 inducers may decrease the levels/effects of diltiazem. Example inducers include aminoglutethimide, carbamazepine, nafcillin, nevirapine, phenobarbital, phenytoin, and rifamycins.

CYP3A4 inhibitors: May increase the levels/effects of diltiazem. Example inhibitors include azole antifungals, clarithromycin, diclofenac, doxycycline, erythromycin, imatinib, isoniazid, nefazodone, nicardipine, propofol, protease inhibitors, quinidine, telithromycin, and verapamil.

CYP3A4 substrates: Diltiazem may increase the levels/effects of CYP3A4 substrates. Example substrates include benzodiazepines, calcium channel blockers, cyclosporine, mirtazapine, nateglinide, nefazodone, sildenafil (and other PDE-5 inhibitors), tacrolimus, and venlafaxine. Selected benzodiazepines (midazolam and triazolam), cisapride, ergot alkaloids, selected HMG-CoA reductase inhibitors (lovastatin and simvastatin), and pimozide are generally contraindicated with strong CYP3A4 inhibitors.

Digoxin's serum concentration can be increased in some patients; monitor for increased effects of digoxin.

HMG-CoA reductase inhibitors (atorvastatin, lovastatin, simvastatin): Serum concentration will likely be increased; consider pravastatin/fluvastatin or a second generation dihydropyridine calcium channel blocker as an alternative.

Lithium neurotoxicity may result when diltiazem is added; monitor lithium levels.

Moricizine's serum concentration is increased; monitor clinical response closely.

Nafcillin decreases plasma concentration of diltiazem; avoid this combination.

Nitroprusside's dose required reduction in patients started on diltiazem; monitor blood pressure.

Protease inhibitor like amprenavir and ritonavir may increase diltiazem's serum concentration.

Quinidine: Diltiazem may increase serum levels of quinidine. Dosage adjustment may be required.

Rifampin increases the metabolism of calcium channel blockers; adjust the dose of the calcium channel blocker to maintain efficacy or consider an alternative to rifampin.

Sildenafil, tadalafil, vardenafil: Blood pressure-lowering effects may be additive; use caution.

Tacrolimus's serum concentrations are increased by diltiazem; avoid the combination. Use another calcium channel blocker or monitor tacrolimus trough levels and renal function closely.

Ethanol/Nutrition/Herb Interactions

Ethanol: Avoid ethanol (may increase risk of hypotension or vasodilation).

Food: Diltiazem serum levels may be elevated if taken with food. Serum concentrations were not altered by grapefruit juice in small clinical trials.

Herb/Nutraceutical: St John's wort may decrease diltiazem levels. Avoid dong quai if using for hypertension (has estrogenic activity). Avoid ephedra (may worsen arrhythmia or hypertension). Avoid yohimbe, ginseng (may worsen hypertension). Avoid garlic (may have increased antihypertensive effect).

Stability

Capsule, tablet: Store at controlled room temperature.

Solution for injection: Store in refrigerator at 2°C to 8°C (36°F to 46°F). May be stored at room temperature for up to 1 month; do not freeze. Following dilution with $D_5$1/2NS, D_5W, or NS, solution is stable for 24 hours at room temperature or under refrigeration.

Mechanism of Action Inhibits calcium ion from entering the "slow channels" or select voltage-sensitive areas of vascular smooth muscle and myocardium during depolarization, producing a relaxation of coronary vascular smooth muscle and coronary vasodilation; increases myocardial oxygen delivery in patients with vasospastic angina

Pharmacodynamics

Onset of action: Oral: Immediate release tablet: 30-60 minutes

Peak effect: 2-3 hours for plain tablets, 6-11 hours for sustained release

Pharmacokinetics

Absorption: 70% to 80%

Distribution: V_d: 3-13 L/kg; enters breast milk

Protein binding: 77% to 85%

Metabolism: Hepatic; extensive first-pass effect; following single I.V. injection, plasma concentrations of N-monodesmethyldiltiazem and desacetyldiltiazem are typically undetectable; however, these metabolites accumulate to detectable concentrations following 24-hour constant rate infusion. N-monodesmethyldiltiazem appears to have 20% of the potency of diltiazem; desacetyldiltiazem is about 50% as potent as the parent compound.

Bioavailability: Oral: ~40% to 60%

Half-life: Immediate release tablet: 3-4.5 hours, may be prolonged with renal impairment

Time to peak, serum: Immediate release tablet: 2-3 hours

Elimination: Urine and feces (primarily as metabolites)

Dosage

Geriatrics: Refer to adult dosing. **Note:** Patients ≥60 years may respond to a lower initial dose (eg, 120 mg once daily using extended release capsule)

Adults:

Angina: Oral:

Capsule, extended release (Cardizem® CD, Cartia XT™, Dilacor® XR, Diltia XT®, Tiazac®): Initial: 120-180 mg once daily (maximum dose: 480 mg/day)

(Continued)

Diltiazem *(Continued)*

Tablet, extended release (Cardizem® LA): 180 mg once daily; may increase at 7- to 14-day intervals (maximum recommended dose: 360 mg/day)

Tablet, immediate release (Cardizem®): Usual starting dose: 30 mg 4 times/day; usual range: 180-360 mg/day

Hypertension: Oral:

Capsule, extended release (Cardizem® CD, Cartia XT™, Dilacor® XR, Diltia XT®, Tiazac®): Initial: 180-240 mg once daily; dose adjustment may be made after 14 days; usual dose range (JNC 7): 180-420 mg/day; Tiazac®: usual dose range: 120-540 mg/day

Capsule, sustained release: Initial: 60-120 mg twice daily; dose adjustment may be made after 14 days; usual range: 240-360 mg/day

Tablet, extended release (Cardizem® LA): Initial: 180-240 mg once daily; dose adjustment may be made after 14 days; usual dose range (JNC 7): 120-540 mg/day

Atrial fibrillation, atrial flutter, PSVT: I.V.:

Initial bolus dose: 0.25 mg/kg actual body weight over 2 minutes (average adult dose: 20 mg)

Repeat bolus dose (may be administered after 15 minutes if the response is inadequate): 0.35 mg/kg actual body weight over 2 minutes (average adult dose: 25 mg)

Continuous infusion (requires an infusion pump; infusions >24 hours or infusion rates >15 mg/hour are not recommended): Initial infusion rate of 10 mg/hour; rate may be increased in 5 mg/hour increments up to 15 mg/hour as needed; some patients may respond to an initial rate of 5 mg/hour.

If diltiazem injection is administered by continuous infusion for >24 hours, the possibility of decreased diltiazem clearance, prolonged elimination half-life, and increased diltiazem and/or diltiazem metabolite plasma concentrations should be considered.

Conversion from I.V. diltiazem to oral diltiazem: Start oral approximately 3 hours after bolus dose.

Oral dose (mg/day) is approximately equal to [rate (mg/hour) x 3 + 3] x 10.

3 mg/hour = 120 mg/day
5 mg/hour = 180 mg/day
7 mg/hour = 240 mg/day
11 mg/hour = 360 mg/day

Renal Impairment: Use with caution as diltiazem is extensively metabolized by the liver and excreted in the kidneys and bile. Not removed by hemo- or peritoneal dialysis; supplemental dose is not necessary.

Hepatic Impairment: Use with caution as diltiazem is extensively metabolized by the liver and excreted in the kidneys and bile.

Administration

Oral: Do not crush long acting dosage forms.

Tiazac®: Capsules may be opened and sprinkled on a spoonful of applesauce. Applesauce should be swallowed without chewing, followed by drinking a glass of water.

I.V.: Bolus doses given over 2 minutes with continuous EKG and blood pressure monitoring. Continuous infusion may be via infusion pump.

Monitoring Parameters Heart rate, blood pressure, signs and symptoms of congestive heart failure

Reference Range Therapeutic: 50-200 ng/mL

Patient Information Sustained release products should be taken with food and not crushed; limit caffeine intake; avoid alcohol; notify physician if angina pain is not reduced when taking this drug, irregular heartbeat, shortness of breath, swelling, dizziness, constipation, nausea, or hypotension occur; do not stop therapy without advice of physician

Additional Information Mix injection for continuous infusion in D_5W, NS, $D_5\frac{1}{2}$ NS

The FDA's Cardiovascular and Renal Drug Advisory Committee reviewed current data regarding the risk of heart attacks in patients treated with calcium channel blockers and determined that as a class, the calcium channel antagonists are safe; however, they warned that short-acting nifedipine could increase the risk of myocardial infarction in some patients. The committee was in agreement with a statement issued September, 1995 by the National Heart Lung, and Blood Institute of the National Institute of Health, that warned that short-acting nifedipine should be used with great caution especially at higher doses.

Special Geriatric Considerations Elderly may experience a greater hypotensive response; constipation may be more of a problem in elderly; calcium channel blockers are no more effective in elderly than other therapies; however, they do not cause significant CNS effects which is an advantage over some antihypertensive agents.

Dosage Forms Excipient information presented when available (limited, particularly for generics); consult specific product labeling.

Capsule, extended release, as hydrochloride [once-daily dosing]: 120 mg, 180 mg, 240 mg, 300 mg, 360 mg, 420 mg

Cardizem® CD: 120 mg, 180 mg, 240 mg, 300 mg, 360 mg

Cartia XT™: 120 mg, 180 mg, 240 mg, 300 mg

Dilacor® XR, Dilt-XR, Diltia XT®: 120 mg, 180 mg, 240 mg

Taztia XT™: 120 mg, 180 mg, 240 mg, 300 mg, 360 mg

Tiazac®: 120 mg, 180 mg, 240 mg, 300 mg, 360 mg, 420 mg

Capsule, sustained release, as hydrochloride [twice-daily dosing]: 60 mg, 90 mg, 120 mg

Injection, solution, as hydrochloride: 5 mg/mL (5 mL, 10 mL, 25 mL)

Injection, powder for reconstitution, as hydrochloride:

Cardizem®: 25 mg

Tablet, as hydrochloride: 30 mg, 60 mg, 90 mg, 120 mg

Cardizem®: 30 mg, 60 mg, 90 mg, 120 mg

Tablet, extended release, as hydrochloride:

Cardizem® LA: 120 mg, 180 mg, 240 mg, 300 mg, 360 mg, 420 mg

Selected References

Chobanian AV, Bakris GL, Black HR, et al, "The Seventh Report of the Joint National Committee on Prevention, Detection, Evaluation, and Treatment of High Blood Pressure: The JNC 7 Report," *JAMA*, 2003, 289(19):2560-71.

♦ **Diltiazem Hydrochloride** *see* Diltiazem *on page 441*

♦ **Dilt-XR** *see* Diltiazem *on page 441*

DimenhyDRINATE (dye men HYE dri nate)

Medication Safety Issues

Sound-alike/look-alike issues:

DimenhyDRINATE may be confused with diphenhydrAMINE

U.S. Brand Names Dramamine® [OTC]; TripTone® [OTC] [DSC]

Canadian Brand Names Apo-Dimenhydrinate®; Children's Motion Sickness Liquid; Dinate®; Gravol®; Jamp® Travel Tablet; Nauseatol; Novo-Dimenate; SAB-Dimenhydrinate

Generic Available Yes

Pharmacologic Category Antihistamine

Use Treatment and prevention of nausea, vertigo, and vomiting associated with motion sickness

Dosage forms available in Canada (not available in the U.S.), including parenteral formulations and suppositories, are also approved for the treatment of postoperative nausea and vomiting and treatment of radiation sickness.

Unlabeled/Investigational Use Treatment of Meniere's disease

Contraindications Hypersensitivity to dimenhydrinate or any component

Warnings/Precautions Causes sedation, caution must be used in performing tasks which require alertness (eg, operating machinery or driving). Sedative effects of CNS depressants or ethanol are potentiated. Use with caution in patients with angle-closure glaucoma, pyloroduodenal obstruction (including stenotic peptic ulcer), urinary tract obstruction (including bladder neck obstruction and symptomatic prostatic hyperplasia), hyperthyroidism, increased intraocular pressure, and cardiovascular disease (including hypertension and tachycardia).

Note: Parenteral formulations (not available in the U.S.) intended for I.V. and I.M. use are distinct and should not be confused. The I.M. formulation can be used for I.V. administration only after dilution.

Adverse Reactions (Reflective of adult population; not specific for elderly)

>10%:

Central nervous system: Slight to moderate drowsiness

Respiratory: Thickening of bronchial secretions

1% to 10%:

Central nervous system: Headache, fatigue, nervousness, dizziness

Gastrointestinal: Abdominal pain, diarrhea, increased appetite, nausea, weight gain, xerostomia

Neuromuscular & skeletal: Arthralgia

Respiratory: Pharyngitis

Drug Interactions

Increased effect/toxicity with CNS depressants, anticholinergics, TCAs, MAO inhibitors

Increased toxicity of antibiotics, especially aminoglycosides (ototoxicity)

Ethanol/Nutrition/Herb Interactions Ethanol: Avoid ethanol (may increase CNS depression).

Mechanism of Action Competes with histamine for H_1-receptor sites on effector cells in the gastrointestinal tract, blood vessels, and respiratory tract; blocks chemoreceptor (Continued)

DimenhyDRINATE *(Continued)*

trigger zone, diminishes vestibular stimulation, and depresses labyrinthine function through its central anticholinergic activity

Pharmacodynamics
Onset of action: Oral: Within 15-30 minutes following administration
Duration: ~4-6 hours

Pharmacokinetics
Absorption: Well absorbed from GI tract
Metabolism: Extensive in the liver

Dosage
Geriatrics & Adults:
Motion sickness (prevention/treatment): Oral: 50-100 mg every 4-6 hours, not to exceed 400 mg/day
Gravol® L/A (not available in the U.S.): Oral: 75-150 mg every 8-12 hours, up to a maximum of five 75 mg caplets or three 100 mg caplets in 24 hours

Additional formulations/uses (approved in Canada) for parenteral/suppository formulations (not available in U.S.):
Postoperative nausea and vomiting: I.M., I.V., rectal: 50-100 mg administered 30-60 minutes prior to radiation therapy; may be repeated as needed up to a maximum of 400 mg in 24 hours
Radiation sickness: I.M., I.V., rectal: 50-100 mg administered 30-60 minutes prior to radiation therapy. May be repeated as needed up to a maximum of 400 mg in 24 hours

Administration I.V. injection must be diluted to 10 mL with normal saline and given at 25 mg/minute

Monitoring Parameters Monitor for anticholinergic side effects; emetic episodes and nausea

Patient Information May cause drowsiness

Special Geriatric Considerations
Monitor for anticholinergic side effects (confusion, constipation, etc); if possible, limit use to short-term therapy

Dosage Forms Excipient information presented when available (limited, particularly for generics); consult specific product labeling. [CAN] = Canadian brand name
Caplet (TripTone®): 50 mg [DSC]
Capsule, softgel (Gravol®) [CAN]: 50 mg [not available in the U.S.]
Capsule, long-acting (Gravol® L/A) [CAN]: 75 mg, 100 mg [not available in the U.S.]
Injection, solution:
Gravol® I.M. [CAN]: 50 mg/mL (1 mL, 5 mL) [not available in the U.S.]
Gravol® I.V. [CAN]: 10 mg/mL (5 mL) [not available in the U.S.]
Solution, oral (Gravol® [CAN], Children's Motion Sickness [CAN]): 3 mg/mL (75 mL) [not available in the U.S.]
Suppository, rectal (Gravol® [CAN], Sab-Dimenhydrinate [CAN]): 75 mg, 100 mg [not available in the U.S.]
Tablet:
Dinate® [CAN], Jamp® Travel Tablet [CAN], Nauseatol® [CAN]: 50 mg
Dramamine®: 50 mg
Gravol® Filmkote Jr [CAN]: 25 mg [not available in the U.S.]
Gravol® Filmkote [CAN]: 50 mg [not available in the U.S.]
Tablet, chewable:
Dramamine®: 50 mg [contains phenylalanine 1.5 mg/tablet and tartrazine; orange flavor]
Gravol® Chewable for Children [CAN]: 25 mg [not available in the U.S.]
Gravol® Chewable for Adults [CAN]: 50 mg [not available in the U.S.]

DiphenhydrAMINE (dye fen HYE dra meen)

Related Information
Potentially Inappropriate Medications for Geriatrics *on page 1824*

Medication Safety Issues
Sound-alike/look-alike issues:
DiphenhydrAMINE may be confused with desipramine, dicyclomine, dimenhyDRI-NATE
Benadryl® may be confused with benazepril, Bentyl®, Benylin®, Caladryl®

U.S. Brand Names Aler-Cap [OTC]; Aler-Dryl [OTC]; Aler-Tab [OTC]; AllerMax® [OTC]; Altaryl [OTC]; Banophen® [OTC]; Banophen® Anti-Itch [OTC]; Benadryl® Allergy [OTC]; Benadryl® Children's Allergy [OTC]; Benadryl® Children's Allergy Fastmelt® [OTC]; Benadryl® Children's Dye-Free Allergy [OTC]; Benadryl® Injection; Benadryl® Itch Stopping [OTC]; Benadryl® Itch Stopping Extra Strength [OTC]; Ben-Tann; Compoz® Nighttime Sleep Aid [OTC]; Dermamycin® [OTC]; Diphen® [OTC]; Diphen® AF [OTC]; Diphenhist [OTC]; Dytan™; Genahist® [OTC]; Hydramine® [OTC]; Nytol® Quick Caps [OTC]; Nytol® Quick Gels [OTC]; Siladryl® Allergy [OTC]; Silphen® [OTC]; Simply Sleep® [OTC]; Sleep-ettes D [OTC]; Sleepinal® [OTC]; Sominex® [OTC]; Sominex® Maximum Strength [OTC]; Triaminic® Thin Strips™ Cough and Runny Nose [OTC]; Twilite® [OTC]; Unisom® Maximum Strength SleepGels® [OTC]

Canadian Brand Names Allerdryl®; Allernix; Benadryl®; Nytol®; Nytol® Extra Strength; PMS-Diphenhydramine; Simply Sleep®

Index Terms Diphenhydramine Citrate; Diphenhydramine Hydrochloride; Diphenhydramine Tannate

Generic Available Yes: Excludes chewable tablet, gel, orally-disintegrating tablet, stick, strip

Pharmacologic Category Antihistamine

Use Symptomatic relief of allergic symptoms caused by histamine release including nasal allergies and allergic dermatosis; adjunct to epinephrine in the treatment of anaphylaxis; nighttime sleep aid; prevention or treatment of motion sickness; antitussive; management of Parkinsonian syndrome including drug-induced extrapyramidal symptoms; topically for relief of pain and itching associated with insect bites, minor cuts and burns, or rashes due to poison ivy, poison oak, and poison sumac

Contraindications Hypersensitivity to diphenhydramine or any component of the formulation; acute asthma; use as a local anesthetic (injection)

Warnings/Precautions Causes sedation, caution must be used in performing tasks which require alertness (eg, operating machinery or driving). Sedative effects of CNS depressants or ethanol are potentiated. Diphenhydramine has high sedative and anticholinergic properties, so it may not be considered the antihistamine of choice for prolonged use in the elderly. Use with caution in patients with angle-closure glaucoma, pyloroduodenal obstruction (including stenotic peptic ulcer), urinary tract obstruction (including bladder neck obstruction and symptomatic prostatic hyperplasia), asthma, hyperthyroidism, increased intraocular pressure, and cardiovascular disease (including hypertension and tachycardia). Some preparations contain soy protein; avoid use in patients with soy protein or peanut allergies.

Self-medication (OTC use): Do not use with other products containing diphenhydramine, even ones used on the skin. Topical products should not be used on large areas of the body, or on chicken pox or measles. Healthcare provider should be contacted if topical use is needed for >7 days.

Adverse Reactions (Reflective of adult population; not specific for elderly)
Frequency not defined.
Cardiovascular: Chest tightness, extrasystoles, hypotension, palpitation, tachycardia
Central nervous system: Chills, confusion, convulsion, disturbed coordination, dizziness, euphoria, excitation, fatigue, headache, insomnia, irritability, nervousness, paradoxical excitement, restlessness, sedation, sleepiness, vertigo
Dermatologic: Photosensitivity, rash, urticaria
Endocrine & metabolic: Menstrual irregularities (early menses)
Gastrointestinal: Anorexia, constipation, diarrhea, dry mucous membranes, epigastric distress, nausea, throat tightness, vomiting, xerostomia
Genitourinary: Difficult urination, urinary frequency, urinary retention
Hematologic: Agranulocytosis, hemolytic anemia, thrombocytopenia
Neuromuscular & skeletal: Neuritis, paresthesia, tremor
Ocular: Blurred vision, diplopia
Otic: Labyrinthitis (acute), tinnitus
Respiratory: Nasal stuffiness, thickening of bronchial secretions, wheezing
Miscellaneous: Anaphylactic shock, diaphoresis

Overdosage/Toxicology Symptoms include CNS stimulation or depression. There is no specific treatment for antihistamine overdose, however, clinical toxicity is mostly due to anticholinergic effects. Anticholinesterase inhibitors (eg, physostigmine, (Continued)

447

DiphenhydrAMINE *(Continued)*

neostigmine, pyridostigmine, or edrophonium) may be useful by reducing acetylcholinesterase. For anticholinergic overdose with severe life-threatening symptoms, physostigmine 1-2 mg slow I.V. may be given to reverse these effects.

Drug Interactions Inhibits CYP2D6 (moderate)

Acetylcholinesterase inhibitors (central): Acetylcholinesterase inhibitors, central (donepezil, galantamine, rivastigmine, tacrine) may diminish the therapeutic effect of anticholinergics. If the anticholinergic action is a side effect of the agent, the result may be beneficial. Anticholinergics may diminish the therapeutic effect of acetylcholinesterase inhibitors (central). Monitor for reduced therapeutic effects of either drug.

Anticholinergic agents: Diphenhydramine may enhance the adverse/toxic effect of other anticholinergics; monitor for additive effects.

Antipsychotic agents (phenothiazines): Antihistamines may enhance the arrhythmogenic effect of antipsychotic agents (phenothiazines).

Betahistine: Antihistamines may diminish the therapeutic effect of betahistine.

CNS depressants: Sedative effects may be additive with other CNS depressants; includes ethanol, benzodiazepines, barbiturates, opioid analgesics, and other sedative agents; monitor for increased effect

CYP2D6 substrates: Diphenhydramine may increase the levels/effects of CYP2D6 substrates. Example substrates include amphetamines, selected beta-blockers, dextromethorphan, fluoxetine, lidocaine, mirtazapine, nefazodone, paroxetine, risperidone, ritonavir, thioridazine, tricyclic antidepressants, and venlafaxine.

CYP2D6 prodrug substrates: Diphenhydramine may decrease the levels/effects of CYP2D6 prodrug substrates. Example prodrug substrates include codeine, hydrocodone, oxycodone, and tramadol.

Pramlintide: Pramlintide may enhance the anticholinergic GI effect of anticholinergics.

Ethanol/Nutrition/Herb Interactions

Ethanol: Avoid ethanol (may increase CNS depression).

Herb/Nutraceutical: Avoid valerian, St John's wort, kava kava, gotu kola (may increase CNS depression).

Stability Injection: Store at room temperature of 15°C to 30°C (59°F to 86°F). Protect from light and freezing

Mechanism of Action Competes with histamine for H_1-receptor sites on effector cells in the gastrointestinal tract, blood vessels, and respiratory tract; anticholinergic and sedative effects are also seen

Pharmacodynamics Duration: 4-7 hours

Pharmacokinetics

Absorption: Oral: ~65%

Distribution: V_d: 3-22 L/kg

Metabolism: Extensively hepatic n-demethylation via CYP2D6; minor demethylation via CYP1A2, 2C9 and 2C19; smaller degrees in pulmonary and renal systems; significant first-pass effect

Bioavailability: Oral: ~40% to 70%

Half-life elimination: Elderly: 13.5 hours; Adults: 2-10 hours

Time to peak serum concentration: 2-4 hours; one study showed significant increase in peak concentration in older adults

Elimination: Total body clearance is decreased in older adults

Dosage

Geriatrics: Initial: 25 mg 2-3 times/day increasing as needed

Adults: **Note:** Dosages are expressed as the hydrochloride salt.

Allergic reactions or motion sickness:

Oral: 25-50 mg every 6-8 hours

I.M., I.V.: 10-50 mg per dose; single doses up to 100 mg may be used if needed; not to exceed 400 mg/day

Antitussive: Oral: 25 mg every 4 hours; maximum 150 mg/24 hours

Nighttime sleep aid: Oral: 50 mg at bedtime

Dystonic reaction: I.M., I.V.: 50 mg in a single dose; may repeat in 20-30 minutes if necessary

Relief of pain and itching: Topical: Apply 1% or 2% to affected area up to 3-4 times/day

Administration When used to prevent motion sickness, first dose should be given 30 minutes prior to exposure. Injection solution is for I.V. or I.M. administration only; local necrosis may result with SubQ or intradermal use. For I.V. administration, inject at a rate ≤25 mg/minute.

Monitoring Parameters Relief of symptoms, mental alertness

Reference Range Therapeutic: Not established; Toxic: >0.1 mcg/mL

Test Interactions May suppress the wheal and flare reactions to skin test antigens

Patient Information May cause drowsiness; avoid CNS depressants and alcohol

Additional Information Diphenhydramine citrate 19 mg is equivalent to diphenhydramine hydrochloride 12.5 mg

Special Geriatric Considerations Diphenhydramine has high sedative and anticholinergic properties, so it may not be considered the antihistamine of choice for prolonged use in the elderly. Its use as a sleep aid is discouraged due to its anticholinergic effects; interpretive guidelines from the Centers for Medicare and Medicaid Services (CMS) discourage the use of diphenhydramine as a sedative or anxiolytic in long-term care facilities.

Dosage Forms Excipient information presented when available (limited, particularly for generics); consult specific product labeling.

Caplet, as hydrochloride: 25 mg, 50 mg

Aler-Dryl, AllerMax®, Compoz® Nighttime Sleep Aid, Sleep-ettes D, Sominex® Maximum Strength, Twilite®: 50 mg

Nytol® Quick Caps, Simply Sleep®: 25 mg

Capsule, as hydrochloride: 25 mg, 50 mg

Aler-Cap, Banophen®, Benadryl® Allergy, Diphen®, Diphenhist, Genahist®: 25 mg

Sleepinal®: 50 mg

Capsule, softgel, as hydrochloride: 50 mg

Benadryl® Dye-Free Allergy: 25 mg [dye-free]

Compoz® Nighttime Sleep Aid, Nytol® Quick Gels, Sleepinal®, Unisom® Maximum Strength SleepGels®: 50 mg

Captab, as hydrochloride:

Diphenhist®: 25 mg

Cream, as hydrochloride: 2% (30 g)

Banophen® Anti-Itch: 2% (30 g) [contains zinc acetate 0.1%]

Benadryl® Itch Stopping: 1% (30 g) [contains zinc acetate 0.1%]

Benadryl® Itch Stopping Extra Strength: 2% (30 g) [contains zinc acetate 0.1%]

Diphenhist®: 2% (30 g) [contains zinc acetate 0.1%]

Elixir, as hydrochloride:

Altaryl: 12.5 mg/5 mL (120 mL, 480 mL, 3840 mL) [cherry flavor]

Banophen®: 12.5 mg/5 mL (120 mL)

Diphen AF: 12.5 mg/5 mL (120 mL, 240 mL, 480 mL) [alcohol free; cherry flavor]

Gel, topical, as hydrochloride:

Benadryl® Itch Stopping Extra Strength: 2% (120 mL)

Injection, solution, as hydrochloride: 50 mg/mL (1 mL)

Benadryl®: 50 mg/mL (1 mL; 10 mL [DSC])

Liquid, as hydrochloride:

AllerMax®: 12.5 mg/5 mL (120 mL)

Benadryl® Allergy: 12.5 mg/5 mL (120 mL, 240 mL) [alcohol free; contains sodium benzoate; cherry flavor]

Benadryl® Children's Dye-Free Allergy: 12.5 mg/5 mL (120 mL) [alcohol free, dye free, sugar free; contains sodium benzoate; bubble gum flavor]

Genahist®: 12.5 mg/5 mL (120 mL) [alcohol free, sugar free; contains sodium benzoate; cherry flavor]

Hydramine®: 12.5 mg/5 mL (120 mL, 480 mL) [alcohol free]

Siladryl® Allergy: 12.5 mg/5 mL (120 mL, 240 mL, 480 mL) [alcohol free, sugar free; black cherry flavor]

Liquid, topical, as hydrochloride [stick]:

Benadryl® Itch Stopping Extra Strength: 2% (14 mL) [contains zinc acetate 0.1% and alcohol]

Solution, oral, as hydrochloride:

Diphenhist: 12.5 mg/5 mL (120 mL, 480 mL) [alcohol free; contains sodium benzoate]

Solution, topical, as hydrochloride [spray]:

Benadryl® Itch Stopping Extra Strength: 2% (60 mL) [contains zinc acetate 0.1% and alcohol]

Dermamycin®: 2% (60 mL) [contains menthol 1%]

Strips, oral, as hydrochloride:

Benadryl® Allergy: 25 mg (10s) [contains sodium 4 mg/strip; vanilla mint flavor]

Benadryl® Children's Allergy: 12.5 mg (10s) [vanilla mint flavor]

Triaminic® Thin Strips™ Cough and Runny Nose: 12. 5 mg (16s) [grape flavor]

Suspension, as tannate:

Ben-Tann: 25 mg/5 mL (120 ml) [contains sodium benzoate; strawberry flavor]

Dytan™: 25 mg/5 mL (120 mL) [strawberry flavor]

Syrup, as hydrochloride:

Silphen® Cough: 12.5 mg/5 mL (120 mL, 240 mL, 480 mL) [contains alcohol; 5%; strawberry flavor]

Tablet, as hydrochloride: 25 mg, 50 mg

Aler-Tab, Benadryl® Allergy, Genahist®, Sominex®: 25 mg

Tablet, chewable, as hydrochloride:

Benadryl® Children's Allergy: 12.5 mg [contains phenylalanine 4.2 mg, magnesium 15 mg, and sodium 2 mg per tablet; grape flavor]

Tablet, chewable, as tannate:

Dytan™: 25 mg [contains phenylalanine; strawberry flavor]

(Continued)

DIPHENOXYLATE AND ATROPINE

DiphenhydrAMINE (Continued)

Tablet, orally disintegrating, as citrate:
Benadryl® Children's Allergy Fastmelt®: 19 mg [equivalent to diphenhydramine hydrochloride 12.5 mg; contains phenylalanine 4.5 mg/tablet and soy protein isolate; cherry flavor]

Selected References

Akutsu T, Kobayashi K, Sakurada K, et al, "Identification of Human Cytochrome P450 Isozymes Involved in Diphenhydramine N-Demethylation," *Drug Metab Dispos*, 2007, 35(1):72-8.

Sampson HA, Munoz-Furtong A, Campbell RL, et al, "Second Symposium on the Definition and Management of Anaphylaxis: Summary Report -- Second National Institute of Allergy and Infectious Disease/Food Allergy and Anaphylaxis Network Symposium," *Ann Emerg Med*, 2006, 7(4):373-80.

Simons KJ, Watson WT, Martin TJ, et al, "Diphenhydramine: Pharmacokinetics and Pharmacodynamics in Elderly Adults, Young Adults, and Children," *J Clin Pharmacol*, 1990, 30(7):665-71.

♦ **Diphenhydramine Citrate** *see DiphenhydrAMINE on page 447*
♦ **Diphenhydramine Hydrochloride** *see DiphenhydrAMINE on page 447*
♦ **Diphenhydramine Tannate** *see DiphenhydrAMINE on page 447*

Diphenoxylate and Atropine (dye fen OKS i late & A troe peen)

Related Information
Atropine *on page 137*

Medication Safety Issues
Sound-alike/look-alike issues:
Lomotil® may be confused with Lamictal®, Lamisil®, lamotrigine, Lanoxin®, Lasix®, ludiomil
Lonox® may be confused with Lanoxin®, Loprox®

International issues:
Lomotil® may be confused with Lemesil® which is a brand name for nimesulide in Greece
Lonox® may be confused with Flomox® which is a brand of cefcapene in Japan

U.S. Brand Names Lomotil®; Lonox®
Canadian Brand Names Lomotil®
Index Terms Atropine and Diphenoxylate
Generic Available Yes
Pharmacologic Category Antidiarrheal
Use Treatment of diarrhea
Restrictions C-V
Contraindications Hypersensitivity to diphenoxylate, atropine, or any component of the formulation; obstructive jaundice; diarrhea associated with pseudomembranous enterocolitis or enterotoxin-producing bacteria
Warnings/Precautions Use in conjunction with fluid and electrolyte therapy when appropriate. In case of severe dehydration or electrolyte imbalance, withhold diphenoxylate/atropine treatment until corrective therapy has been initiated. Inhibiting peristalsis may lead to fluid retention in the intestine aggravating dehydration and electrolyte imbalance. Reduction of intestinal motility may be deleterious in diarrhea resulting from *Shigella*, *Salmonella*, toxigenic strains of *E. coli*, and pseudomembranous enterocolitis associated with broad-spectrum antibiotics; use is not recommended.

Use caution with acute ulcerative colitis, hepatic or renal dysfunction. If there is no response with 48 hours, this medication is unlikely to be effective and should be discontinued; if chronic diarrhea is not improved symptomatically within 10 days at maximum dosage, control is unlikely with further use. Physical and psychological dependence have been reported with higher than recommended dosing.

Adverse Reactions (Reflective of adult population; not specific for elderly)
Frequency not defined.
Cardiovascular: Tachycardia
Central nervous system: Confusion, depression, dizziness, drowsiness, euphoria, flushing, headache, hyperthermia, lethargy, malaise, restlessness, sedation
Dermatologic: Angioneurotic edema, dry skin, pruritus, urticaria
Gastrointestinal: Abdominal discomfort, anorexia, gum swelling, nausea, pancreatitis, paralytic ileus, toxic megacolon, vomiting, xerostomia
Genitourinary: Urinary retention
Neuromuscular & skeletal: Numbness
Miscellaneous: Anaphylaxis

Overdosage/Toxicology Symptoms of overdose include drowsiness, hypotension, blurred vision, flushing, dry mouth, and miosis. Administration of activated charcoal will reduce bioavailability of diphenoxylate. Naloxone may be used to counteract respiratory depression which may occur as late as 30 hours after ingestion. Adults may be given naloxone 0.4-2 mg I.V., with repeat administration as necessary up to a total of 10 mg; can also be used to reverse toxic effects of the opiate. For anticholinergic overdose with severe life-threatening symptoms, physostigmine 1-2 mg SubQ or I.V.

slowly, may be given to reverse these effects (adult dose). Monitor for at least 48 hours.

Drug Interactions Pramlintide: Pramlintide may enhance the anticholinergic effect of anticholinergics; additive effects on reduced GI motility may occur.

Ethanol/Nutrition/Herb Interactions Ethanol: Avoid ethanol (may increase CNS depression).

Mechanism of Action Diphenoxylate inhibits excessive GI motility and GI propulsion; commercial preparations contain a subtherapeutic amount of atropine to discourage abuse

Pharmacodynamics
Atropine: See Atropine monograph.
Diphenoxylate:
Onset of action: Antidiarrheal: 45-60 minutes
Duration: Antidiarrheal: 3-4 hours

Pharmacokinetics
Atropine: See Atropine monograph.
Diphenoxylate:
Absorption: Well absorbed
Metabolism: Extensively hepatic via ester hydrolysis to diphenoxylic acid (active)
Half-life elimination: Diphenoxylate: 2.5 hours; Diphenoxylic acid: 12-14 hours
Time to peak, serum: 2 hours
Excretion: Primarily feces (49% as unchanged drug and metabolites); urine (~14%, <1% as unchanged drug)

Dosage
Geriatrics & Adults: Diarrhea: Oral: Diphenoxylate 5 mg 4 times/day until control achieved (maximum: 20 mg/day), then reduce dose as needed; some patients may be controlled on doses of 5 mg/day

Administration If there is no response within 48 hours of continuous therapy, this medication is unlikely to be effective and should be discontinued; if chronic diarrhea is not improved symptomatically within 10 days at maximum dosage, control is unlikely with further use.

Monitoring Parameters Watch for signs of atropinism (dryness of skin and mucous membranes, tachycardia, thirst, flushing); monitor number and consistency of stools; observe for signs of toxicity, fluid and electrolyte loss, hypotension, and respiratory depression

Patient Information Do not take any new medication during therapy unless approved by prescriber. Take as directed; do not exceed recommended dosage. If no response within 48 hours, notify prescriber. Avoid alcohol or other prescriptive or OTC sedatives or depressants. May cause drowsiness, blurred vision, impaired coordination (use caution when driving or engaging in tasks that require alertness until response to drug is known); dry mouth (sucking on lozenges or chewing gum may help). Report difficulty urinating, persistent unrelieved diarrhea, respiratory difficulties, fever, or palpitations.

Additional Information If there is no response within 48 hours, the drug is unlikely to be effective and should be discontinued. If chronic diarrhea is not improved symptomatically within 10 days at maximum dosage of 20 mg/day, control is unlikely with further use. Diarrhea should also be treated with dietary measures (ie, clear liquids), and avoid milk products and high sodium foods such as bouillon and soups.

Special Geriatric Considerations Elderly are particularly sensitive to fluid and electrolyte loss. This generally results in lethargy, weakness, and confusion. Repletion and maintenance of electrolytes and water are essential in the treatment of diarrhea. Drug therapy must be limited in order to avoid toxicity with this agent.

Dosage Forms Excipient information presented when available (limited, particularly for generics); consult specific product labeling.
Solution, oral: Diphenoxylate hydrochloride 2.5 mg and atropine sulfate 0.025 mg per 5 mL (5 mL, 10 mL, 60 mL)
Lomotil®: Diphenoxylate hydrochloride 2.5 mg and atropine sulfate 0.025 mg per 5 mL (60 mL) [contains alcohol 15%; cherry flavor]
Tablet: Diphenoxylate hydrochloride 2.5 mg and atropine sulfate 0.025 mg
Lomotil®, Lonox®: Diphenoxylate hydrochloride 2.5 mg and atropine sulfate 0.025 mg

♦ **Diphenylhydantoin** see Phenytoin on page 1250

Diphtheria and Tetanus Toxoid
(dif THEER ee a & TET a nus TOKS oyd)

Related Information
Immunization Recommendations on page 1787
Tetanus Toxoid (Adsorbed) on page 1542
Tetanus Toxoid (Fluid) on page 1543
(Continued)

Diphtheria and Tetanus Toxoid *(Continued)*

U.S. Brand Names Decavac™
Canadian Brand Names Td Adsorbed
Index Terms DT; Td; Tetanus and Diphtheria Toxoid
Generic Available No
Pharmacologic Category Toxoid
Use Tetanus and diphtheria toxoids adsorbed for adult use (Td) (Decavac™): Adults: Active immunity against diphtheria and tetanus; tetanus prophylaxis in wound management

Contraindications Hypersensitivity to diphtheria, tetanus toxoid, or any component of the formulation

Warnings/Precautions Do not confuse pediatric diphtheria and tetanus (DT) with adult tetanus and diphtheria (Td). Immediate treatment for anaphylactic/anaphylactoid reaction should be available during administration. Patients with a history of severe local reaction (Arthus-type) or temperature of >39.4°C (103°F) following a previous dose should not be given further routine or emergency doses of Td more frequently than every 10 years. Continue use with caution if Guillain-Barré syndrome occurs within 6 weeks of prior tetanus toxoid. For I.M. administration, use caution with history of bleeding disorders or anticoagulant therapy. Defer administration during moderate or severe illness (with or without fever) or during outbreaks of poliomyelitis. Immune response may be decreased in immunocompromised patients.

Adverse Reactions (Reflective of adult population; not specific for elderly) All serious adverse reactions must be reported to the U.S. Department of Health and Human Services (DHHS) Vaccine Adverse Event Reporting System (VAERS) 1-800-822-7967.

>10%: Local: Injection site (adolescents and adults): Pain (81% to 85%), redness (5% to 21%), swelling (10% to 16%)

Frequency not defined; reactions reported with adult and pediatric preparations
    Cardiovascular: EEG disturbances
    Central nervous system: Brachial neuritis, Guillain-Barré syndrome, dizziness, paresthesia, seizure
    Dermatologic: Rash
    Gastrointestinal: Nausea, vomiting
    Local: Injection site: Persistent nodules; local reactions (erythema, cellulitis, swelling)
    Neuromuscular & skeletal: Arthralgia, myalgia
    Miscellaneous: Allergic/anaphylactic reactions, Arthus-type hypersensitivity reaction (severe local reaction starting 2-8 hours after injection)

Note: Other neurological conditions reported in temporal association with vaccine administration have not been demonstrated to be causally related to the vaccine. These have included demyelinating CNS diseases, mononeuropathies, and encephalopathy.

Drug Interactions
Immunosuppressant medications or therapies (antimetabolites, alkylating agents, cytotoxic drugs, corticosteroids, irradiation): The effect of the vaccine may be decreased; consider deferring vaccination for 3 months after immunosuppressant therapy is discontinued.

Stability Store at 2°C to 8°C (35°F to 46°F); do not freeze. Discard if product has been frozen.

Dosage
  Geriatrics & Adults:
    Primary immunization: I.M.: Patients previously not immunized should receive 2 primary doses of 0.5 mL each, given at an interval of 4-6 weeks; third (reinforcing) dose of 0.5 mL 6-12 months later
    Booster immunization: I.M.: 0.5 mL every 10 years. Subsequent routine doses are not recommended more often than every 10 years.
    Tetanus prophylaxis in wound management: I.M.: Use of tetanus toxoid (Td) and/or tetanus immune globulin (TIG) depends upon the number of prior tetanus toxoid doses and type of wound

Administration For I.M. administration; prior to use, shake suspension well
  Td: Administer in the deltoid muscle; do not inject in the gluteal area
  DT: Administer in the anterolateral aspect of the thigh or the deltoid muscle; do not inject in the gluteal area

For patients at risk of hemorrhage following intramuscular injection, the ACIP recommends "it should be administered intramuscularly if, in the opinion of the physician familiar with the patients bleeding risk, the vaccine can be administered with reasonable safety by this route. If the patient receives antihemophilia or other similar therapy, intramuscular vaccination can be scheduled shortly after such therapy is administered. A fine needle (23 gauge or smaller) can be used for the vaccination and firm pressure applied to the site (without rubbing) for at least 2 minutes. The patient should be instructed concerning the risk of hematoma from the injection."

Patient Information A nodule may be palpable at the injection site for a few weeks

Additional Information DT contains higher proportions of diphtheria toxoid than Td.

Special Geriatric Considerations Since protective tetanus and diphtheria antibodies decline with age, only 28% of persons >70 years of age in the U.S. are believed to be immune to tetanus, and most of the tetanus-induced deaths occur in people >60 years of age, it is advisable to offer Td, especially to elderly, concurrent with their influenza and other immunization programs if history of vaccination is unclear; boosters should be given at 10-year intervals; earlier for wounds.

Dosage Forms Excipient information presented when available (limited, particularly for generics); consult specific product labeling.

Injection, suspension, adult:

Decavac™: Diphtheria 2 Lf units and tetanus 5 Lf units per 0.5 mL (0.5 mL) [latex free prefilled syringe; contains thimerosal]

Injection, suspension, pediatric [preservative free]: Diphtheria 6.7 Lf units and tetanus 5 Lf units per 0.5 mL (0.5 mL)

Selected References

Bentley DW, "Vaccinations," *Clin Geriatr Med*, 1992, 8(4):745-60.

Centers for Disease Control, "Preventing Tetanus, Diphtheria, and Pertussis Among Adolescents: Use of Tetanus Toxoid, Reduced Diphtheria Toxoid and Acellular Pertussis Vaccines: Recommendations of the Advisory Committee on Immunization Practices (ACIP)," *MMWR*, 2006, 55(early release);1-34.

Centers for Disease Control, "Recommendations of the Advisory Committee on Immunization Practices (ACIP): General Recommendations on Immunization," *MMWR*, 2002, 51(RR-2):18.

Gardner P and Schaffner W, "Immunization of Adults," *N Engl J Med*, 1993, 328(17):1242-8.

♦ **Dipivalyl Epinephrine** *see* Dipivefrin *on page 453*

Dipivefrin (dye PI ve frin)

Related Information

Glaucoma Drug Therapy *on page 1758*

U.S. Brand Names Propine®

Canadian Brand Names Ophtho-Dipivefrin™; PMS-Dipivefrin; Propine®

Index Terms Dipivalyl Epinephrine; Dipivefrin Hydrochloride; DPE

Generic Available Yes

Pharmacologic Category Alpha/Beta Agonist; Ophthalmic Agent, Antiglaucoma; Ophthalmic Agent, Vasoconstrictor

Use Reduce elevated intraocular pressure in chronic open-angle glaucoma; also used to treat ocular hypertension, low tension, and secondary glaucomas

Contraindications Hypersensitivity to dipivefrin, any component of the formulation, or epinephrine; angle-closure glaucoma

Warnings/Precautions Use with caution in patients with vascular hypertension or cardiac disorders and in aphakic patients. Contains sulfites which cause allergic-type reactions in susceptible persons.

Adverse Reactions (Reflective of adult population; not specific for elderly)

1% to 10%:

Central nervous system: Headache

Local: Burning, stinging

Ocular: Ocular congestion, photophobia, mydriasis, blurred vision, ocular pain, bulbar conjunctival follicles, blepharoconjunctivitis, cystoid macular edema

Drug Interactions Increased or synergistic effect when used with other agents to lower intraocular pressure

Stability Avoid exposure to light and air. Discolored or darkened solutions indicate loss of potency.

Mechanism of Action Dipivefrin is a prodrug of epinephrine which is the active agent that stimulates alpha- and/or beta-adrenergic receptors increasing aqueous humor outflow

Pharmacodynamics

Ocular pressure effects: Within 30 minutes

Duration: 12 hours or longer; mydriasis may occur within 30 minutes and last for several hours

Pharmacokinetics Absorption: Rapid into the aqueous humor; converted to epinephrine

Dosage

Geriatrics & Adults: Glaucoma: Ophthalmic: Instill 1 drop every 12 hours into the eyes

Monitoring Parameters Intraocular pressure; heart rate and blood pressure

Patient Information Discolored solutions should be discarded; do not touch dropper to eye; slight amount of discomfort may follow instillation; headache or browache may occur at start of therapy; report any change in vision to physician immediately

Additional Information Contains sodium metabisulfite

Special Geriatric Considerations Use with caution in patients with heart disease. Assess patient's ability to self-administer drops.

(Continued)

Dipivefrin *(Continued)*

Dosage Forms Excipient information presented when available (limited, particularly for generics); consult specific product labeling.

Solution, ophthalmic, as hydrochloride: 0.1% (5 mL, 10 mL, 15 mL) [contains benzalkonium chloride]

Propine®: 0.1% (5 mL [DSC], 10 mL, 15 mL) [contains benzalkonium chloride]

- ◆ **Dipivefrin Hydrochloride** *see* Dipivefrin *on page 453*
- ◆ **Diprolene®** *see* Betamethasone *on page 161*
- ◆ **Diprolene® AF** *see* Betamethasone *on page 161*
- ◆ **Dipropylacetic Acid** *see* Valproic Acid and Derivatives *on page 1652*

Dipyridamole (dye peer ID a mole)

Related Information
Potentially Inappropriate Medications for Geriatrics *on page 1824*
Medication Safety Issues
Sound-alike/look-alike issues:
Dipyridamole may be confused with disopyramide
Persantine® may be confused with Periactin®, Permitil®
U.S. Brand Names Persantine®
Canadian Brand Names Apo-Dipyridamole FC®; Persantine®
Generic Available Yes
Pharmacologic Category Antiplatelet Agent; Vasodilator
Use

Oral: Used with warfarin to decrease thrombosis in patients after artificial heart valve replacement

I.V.: Diagnostic agent in CAD

Contraindications Hypersensitivity to dipyridamole or any component of the formulation

Warnings/Precautions Use with in patients with hypotension, unstable angina, and/or recent MI. Use with caution in hepatic impairment. Use caution in patients on other antiplatelet agents or anticoagulation. Severe adverse reactions have occurred rarely with I.V. administration. Use the I.V. form with caution in patients with bronchospastic disease or unstable angina. Have aminophylline ready in case of urgency or emergency with I.V. use.

Adverse Reactions (Reflective of adult population; not specific for elderly)
Oral:
>10%: Dizziness (14%)
1% to 10%:
Central nervous system: Headache (2%)
Dermatologic: Rash (2%)
Gastrointestinal: Abdominal distress (6%)
Frequency not defined: Diarrhea, vomiting, flushing, pruritus, angina pectoris, liver dysfunction
I.V.:
>10%:
Cardiovascular: Exacerbation of angina pectoris (20%)
Central nervous system: Dizziness (12%), headache (12%)
1% to 10%:
Cardiovascular: Hypotension (5%), hypertension (2%), blood pressure lability (2%), ECG abnormalities (ST-T changes, extrasystoles; 5% to 8%), pain (3%), tachycardia (3%)
Central nervous system: Flushing (3%), fatigue (1%)
Gastrointestinal: Nausea (5%)
Neuromuscular & skeletal: Paresthesia (1%)
Respiratory: Dyspnea (3%)

Overdosage/Toxicology Symptoms include hypotension and peripheral vasodilation. Dialysis is not effective. Treatment includes fluids and vasopressors although hypotension is often transient.

Drug Interactions
Adenosine: Blood levels and pharmacologic effects of adenosine are increased; consider reduced doses of adenosine.
Cholinesterase inhibitors: May counteract effect of cholinesterase inhibitor and may aggravate myasthenia gravis.
Xanthine derivatives (eg, theophylline): May reduce the pharmacologic effects of dipyridamole; hold theophylline preparations for 36-48 hours before dipyridamole facilitated stress test.

Ethanol/Nutrition/Herb Interactions Herb/Nutraceutical: Avoid cat's claw, dong quai, evening primrose, feverfew, garlic, ginger, ginkgo, red clover, horse chestnut, green tea, ginseng (all have additional antiplatelet activity).

Stability I.V.: Store between 15°C to 25°C (59°F to 77°F). Do not freeze, protect from light. Prior to administration, dilute to a ≥1:2 ratio in NS, 1/2NS, or D$_5$W. Total volume should be ~20-50 mL.

Mechanism of Action Inhibits the activity of adenosine deaminase and phosphodiesterase, which causes an accumulation of adenosine, adenine nucleotides, and cyclic AMP; these mediators then inhibit platelet aggregation and may cause vasodilation; may also stimulate release of prostacyclin or PGD$_2$; causes coronary vasodilation

Pharmacokinetics
  Absorption: Readily from GI tract
  Distribution: V$_d$: Adults: 2-3 L/kg
  Protein binding: 91% to 99%
  Metabolism: Concentrated and metabolized in the liver
  Bioavailability: Ranges from 37% to 66%
  Half-life (terminal): 10-12 hours
  Time to peak serum concentrations: Within 2-2.5 hours
  Elimination: In feces via bile as glucuronide conjugates and unchanged drug

Dosage
  Geriatrics & Adults:
    Adjunctive therapy for prophylaxis of thromboembolism with cardiac valve replacement: Oral: 75-100 mg 4 times/day
    Evaluation of coronary artery disease: I.V.: 0.14 mg/kg/minute for 4 minutes; maximum dose: 60 mg

Additional Information Dipyridamole may also be given 2 days prior to open heart surgery to prevent platelet activation by extracorporeal bypass pump; differences in bioavailability between products observed; evidence exists that doses of 400-600 mg/day have been shown to have **no effect** on platelet aggregation; this casts doubt on clinical usefulness as an antiplatelet agent

Special Geriatric Considerations Since evidence suggests that clinically used doses are ineffective for prevention of platelet aggregation, consideration for low-dose aspirin (81-325 mg/day) alone may be necessary. This will decrease cost as well as inconvenience.

Dosage Forms Excipient information presented when available (limited, particularly for generics); consult specific product labeling.
  Injection, solution: 5 mg/mL (2 mL, 10 mL)
  Tablet: 25 mg, 50 mg, 75 mg
    Persantine®: 25 mg, 50 mg, 75 mg

Selected References
Fitzgerald GA, "Dipyridamole," *N Engl J Med*, 1987, 316(20):1247-57.

♦ **Dipyridamole and Aspirin** *see* Aspirin and Dipyridamole *on page 131*
♦ **Disalicylic Acid** *see* Salsalate *on page 1446*
♦ **Disodium Cromoglycate** *see* Cromolyn *on page 369*
♦ **d-Isoephedrine Hydrochloride** *see* Pseudoephedrine *on page 1346*

Disopyramide (dye soe PEER a mide)

Related Information
  Potentially Inappropriate Medications for Geriatrics *on page 1824*
Medication Safety Issues
  Sound-alike/look-alike issues:
    Disopyramide may be confused with desipramine, dipyridamole
    Norpace® may be confused with Norpramin®
U.S. Brand Names Norpace®; Norpace® CR
Canadian Brand Names Norpace®; Rythmodan®; Rythmodan®-LA
Index Terms Disopyramide Phosphate
Generic Available Yes
Pharmacologic Category Antiarrhythmic Agent, Class Ia
Use Suppression and prevention of unifocal and multifocal premature ventricular complexes, coupled ventricular tachycardia considered to be life-threatening; also effective in the conversion of atrial fibrillation, atrial flutter, and paroxysmal atrial tachycardia to normal sinus rhythm and prevention of the recurrence of these arrhythmias after conversion by other methods
Contraindications Hypersensitivity to disopyramide or any component of the formulation; cardiogenic shock; pre-existing second- or third-degree heart block (except in patients with a functioning artificial pacemaker); congenital QT syndrome; sick sinus syndrome
Warnings/Precautions Monitor and adjust dose to prevent QT$_c$ prolongation. Avoid concurrent use with other medications that prolong QT interval or decrease myocardial (Continued)

Disopyramide *(Continued)*

contractility. Correct hypokalemia before initiating therapy; may worsen toxicity. Watch for proarrhythmic effects. **[U.S. Boxed Warning]: In the Cardiac Arrhythmia Suppression Trial (CAST), recent (>6 days but <2 years ago) myocardial infarction patients with asymptomatic, nonlife-threatening ventricular arrhythmias did not benefit and may have been harmed by attempts to suppress the arrhythmia with flecainide or encainide. An increased mortality or nonfatal cardiac arrest rate (7.7%) was seen in the active treatment group compared with patients in the placebo group (3%). The applicability of the CAST results to other populations is unknown. Antiarrhythmic agents should be reserved for patients with life-threatening ventricular arrhythmias.** May precipitate or exacerbate CHF. Due to significant anticholinergic effects, do not use in patients with urinary retention, BPH, glaucoma, or myasthenia gravis. Reduce dosage in renal or hepatic impairment. The extended release form is not recommended for Cl_{cr} <40 mL/minute. In patients with atrial fibrillation or flutter, block the AV node before initiating. Use caution in Wolff-Parkinson-White syndrome or bundle branch block. Monitor closely for hypotension during the initiation of therapy.

Adverse Reactions (Reflective of adult population; not specific for elderly)
The most common adverse effects are related to cholinergic blockade. The most serious adverse effects of disopyramide are hypotension and CHF.

>10%:
Gastrointestinal: Xerostomia (32%), constipation (11%)
Genitourinary: Urinary hesitancy (14% to 23%)

1% to 10%:
Cardiovascular: CHF, hypotension, cardiac conduction disturbance, edema, syncope, chest pain
Central nervous system: Fatigue, headache, malaise, dizziness, nervousness
Dermatologic: Rash, generalized dermatoses, pruritus
Endocrine & metabolic: Hypokalemia, elevated cholesterol, elevated triglycerides
Gastrointestinal: Dry throat, nausea, abdominal distension, flatulence, abdominal bloating, anorexia, diarrhea, vomiting, weight gain
Genitourinary: Urinary retention, urinary frequency, urinary urgency, impotence (1% to 3%)
Neuromuscular & skeletal: Muscle weakness, muscular pain
Ocular: Blurred vision, dry eyes
Respiratory: Dyspnea

Overdosage/Toxicology
Has a low toxic therapeutic ratio and may easily produce fatal intoxication (acute toxic dose: 1 g). Symptoms include sinus bradycardia, sinus node arrest or asystole; PR, QRS, or QT interval prolongation; torsade de pointes (polymorphous ventricular tachycardia) and depressed myocardial contractility; depressed myocardium, along with alpha-adrenergic or ganglionic blockade, may result in hypotension and pulmonary edema. Other effects are anticholinergic (dry mouth, dilated pupils, and delirium) as well as seizures, coma and respiratory arrest.

Treatment is primarily symptomatic and effects usually respond to conventional therapies (fluids, positioning, vasopressors, anticonvulsants, antiarrhythmics). **Note:** Do not use other type Ia or Ic antiarrhythmic agents to treat ventricular tachycardia. Sodium bicarbonate may treat wide QRS intervals or hypotension. Markedly impaired conduction or high degree AV block, unresponsive to bicarbonate, indicates consideration of a pacemaker.

Drug Interactions Substrate of CYP3A4 (major)
Beta-blockers may cause additive/excessive negative inotropic activity.
CYP3A4 inducers: CYP3A4 inducers may decrease the levels/effects of disopyramide. Example inducers include aminoglutethimide, carbamazepine, nafcillin, nevirapine, phenobarbital, phenytoin, and rifamycins.
CYP3A4 inhibitors: May increase the levels/effects of disopyramide. Example inhibitors include azole antifungals, clarithromycin, diclofenac, doxycycline, erythromycin, imatinib, isoniazid, nefazodone, nicardipine, propofol, protease inhibitors, quinidine, telithromycin, and verapamil.
Erythromycin and clarithromycin increase disopyramide blood levels; may cause QRS widening and/or QT interval prolongation.
Procainamide, quinidine, propafenone, or flecainide can cause increased/excessive negative inotropic effects or prolonged conduction.
Drugs which may prolong the QT interval (amiodarone, amitriptyline, bepridil, cisapride, disopyramide, erythromycin, haloperidol, imipramine, pimozide, quinidine, sotalol, and thioridazine) may be additive with disopyramide; use with caution.
Moxifloxacin may result in additional prolongation of the QT interval; concurrent use is contraindicated.

Ethanol/Nutrition/Herb Interactions
Ethanol: Avoid ethanol (may increase CNS depression).

Herb/Nutraceutical: St John's wort may decrease disopyramide levels. Avoid ephedra (may worsen arrhythmia).

Stability Extemporaneously prepared suspension is stable for 4 weeks refrigerated.

Mechanism of Action Class Ia antiarrhythmic: Decreases myocardial excitability and conduction velocity; reduces disparity in refractory between normal and infarcted myocardium; possesses anticholinergic, peripheral vasoconstrictive, and negative inotropic effects

Pharmacodynamics

Onset of action: 0.5-3.5 hours

Duration of effect: 1.5-8.5 hours

Pharmacokinetics

Protein binding: Concentration-dependent ranging from 20% to 60%

Metabolism: In the liver to inactive metabolites

Bioavailability: 60% to 83%

Half-life: 4-10 hours with Cl_{cr} <40 mL/minute; half-life: 8-18 hours; increased half-life with hepatic or renal disease

Time to peak concentrations: 1-2 hours

Elimination: 40% to 60% unchanged in urine and 10% to 15% in feces

Total body clearance of unbound disopyramide averages 3.2-5.4 mL/minute/kg; total disopyramide clearance range: 0.7-1.2 mL/minute/kg; the total body clearance (bound and unbound) is decreased in older adults

Dosage

Geriatrics & Adults:

Dysrhythmia: Oral:

<50 kg: 100 mg every 6 hours or 200 mg every 12 hours (controlled release)

>50 kg: 150 mg every 6 hours or 300 mg every 12 hours (controlled release); if no response, may increase to 200 mg every 6 hours; maximum dose required for patients with severe refractory ventricular tachycardia is 400 mg every 6 hours.

Hypertrophic obstructive cardiomyopathy (unlabeled use): Oral: Initial: Controlled release: 200 mg twice daily. If symptoms do not improve, increase by 100 mg/day at 2-week intervals to a maximum daily dose of 600 mg.

Renal Impairment: Oral: 100 mg (nonsustained release) given at the following intervals, based on creatinine clearance (mL/minute):

Cl_{cr} 30-40 mL/minute: Administer every 8 hours

Cl_{cr} 15-30 mL/minute: Administer every 12 hours

Cl_{cr} <15 mL/minute: Administer every 24 hours

or alter the dose as follows:

Cl_{cr} 30-<40 mL/minute: Reduce dose 50%

Cl_{cr} 15-30 mL/minute: Reduce dose 75%

Not dialyzable (0% to 5%) by hemo- or peritoneal methods; supplemental dose is not necessary.

Hepatic Impairment: Administer 100 mg every 6 hours or 200 mg every 12 hours (controlled release).

Administration Administer around-the-clock rather than 4 times/day (ie, 12-6-12-6, not 9-1-5-9) to promote less variation in peak and trough serum levels

Monitoring Parameters Congestive heart failure, hypotension and urinary retention; monitor EKG, blood pressure, pulse, and serum concentrations

Reference Range

Therapeutic:

Atrial arrhythmias: 2.8-3.2 mcg/mL (SI: 8.3-9.4 μmol/L)

Ventricular arrhythmias: 3.3-7.5 mcg/mL (SI: 9.7-22 μmol/L)

Toxic: >7 mcg/mL (SI: >20.7 μmol/L)

Patient Information May cause dry mouth, difficulty with urination, dizziness, dyspnea, blurred vision, and constipation; do not break or chew sustained release capsules

Special Geriatric Considerations Due to changes in total clearance (decreased) in the elderly, monitor closely; the anticholinergic action may be intolerable and require discontinuation; monitor for CNS anticholinergic effects (confusion, agitation, hallucinations, etc). **Note:** Dose needs to be altered with Cl_{cr} <40 mL/minute which may be found frequently in older adults.

Clinical studies of Norpace®/Norpace® CR did not include sufficient numbers of subjects ≥65 years of age to determine whether they respond differently from younger subjects. Other reported clinical experience has not identified differences in responses between elderly and younger patients. In general, dose selection for an elderly patient should be cautious, usually starting at the low end of the dosing range, reflecting the greater frequency of decreased hepatic, renal, or cardiac function, and of concomitant disease or other drug therapy.

Because of its anticholinergic activity, disopyramide phosphate should not be used in patients with glaucoma, urinary retention, or benign prostatic hyperplasia (medical conditions commonly associated with the elderly) unless adequate overriding measures are taken. In the event of increased anticholinergic side effects, plasma (Continued)

Disopyramide *(Continued)*

levels of disopyramide should be monitored and the dose of the drug adjusted accordingly. A reduction of the dose by one third, from the recommended 600 mg/day to 400 mg/day, would be reasonable, without changing the dosing interval. This drug is known to be substantially excreted by the kidney, and the risk of toxic reactions to this drug may be greater in patients with impaired renal function. Because elderly patients are more likely to have decreased renal function, care should be taken in dose selection, and it may be useful to monitor renal function.

Dosage Forms Excipient information presented when available (limited, particularly for generics); consult specific product labeling.

Capsule (Norpace®): 100 mg, 150 mg

Capsule, controlled release (Norpace® CR): 100 mg, 150 mg

Selected References

Fenster PE and Nolan PE, "Antiarrhythmic Drugs," *Geriatric Pharmacology*, Bressler R and Katz MD, eds, New York, NY: McGraw-Hill, 1993, 6:105-49.

♦ **Disopyramide Phosphate** *see Disopyramide on page 455*

♦ **Ditropan®** *see Oxybutynin on page 1177*

♦ **Ditropan® XL** *see Oxybutynin on page 1177*

♦ **Diuril®** *see Chlorothiazide on page 294*

♦ **Divalproex Sodium** *see Valproic Acid and Derivatives on page 1652*

♦ **Divigel®** *see Estradiol on page 549*

♦ **5071-1DL(6)** *see Megestrol on page 970*

♦ **dl-Alpha Tocopherol** *see Vitamin E on page 1677*

DOBUTamine *(doe BYOO ta meen)*

Medication Safety Issues

Sound-alike/look-alike issues:

DOBUTamine may be confused with DOPamine

High alert medication: The Institute for Safe Medication Practices (ISMP) includes this medication among its list of drugs which have a heightened risk of causing significant patient harm when used in error.

Canadian Brand Names Dobutamine Injection, USP; Dobutrex®

Index Terms Dobutamine Hydrochloride

Generic Available Yes

Pharmacologic Category Adrenergic Agonist Agent

Use Short-term management of patients with cardiac decompensation due to depressed contractility

Unlabeled/Investigational Use Postive inotropic agent for use in myocardial dysfunction of sepsis

Contraindications Hypersensitivity to dobutamine or sulfites (some contain sodium metabisulfate), or any component of the formulation; idiopathic hypertrophic subaortic stenosis (IHSS)

Warnings/Precautions May increase heart rate. Patients with atrial fibrillation may experience an increase in ventricular response. An increase in blood pressure is more common, but occasionally a patient may become hypotensive. May exacerbate ventricular ectopy. If needed, correct hypovolemia first to optimize hemodynamics. Ineffective therapeutically in the presence of mechanical obstruction such as severe aortic stenosis. Use caution post-MI (can increase myocardial oxygen demand). Use cautiously in the elderly starting at lower end of the dosage range. Use with extreme caution in patients taking MAO inhibitors. Dobutamine in combination with stress echo may be used diagnostically. Product may contain sodium sulfite.

Adverse Reactions (Reflective of adult population; not specific for elderly) Incidence of adverse events is not always reported.

Cardiovascular: Increased heart rate, increased blood pressure, increased ventricular ectopic activity, hypotension, premature ventricular beats (5%, dose related), anginal pain (1% to 3%), nonspecific chest pain (1% to 3%), palpitation (1% to 3%)

Central nervous system: Fever (1% to 3%), headache (1% to 3%), paresthesia

Endocrine & metabolic: Slight decrease in serum potassium

Gastrointestinal: Nausea (1% to 3%)

Hematologic: Thrombocytopenia (isolated cases)

Local: Phlebitis, local inflammatory changes and pain from infiltration, cutaneous necrosis (isolated cases)

Neuromuscular & skeletal: Mild leg cramps

Respiratory: Dyspnea (1% to 3%)

Overdosage/Toxicology Symptoms include fatigue, nervousness, tachycardia, hypertension, and arrhythmias. Reduce rate of administration or discontinue infusion until condition stabilizes.

Drug Interactions

Beta-blockers (nonselective ones) may increase hypertensive effect; avoid concurrent use.

Cocaine may cause malignant arrhythmias; avoid concurrent use.

Guanethidine can increase the pressor response; be aware of the patient's drug regimen.

MAO inhibitors potentiate hypertension and hypertensive crisis; avoid concurrent use.

Methyldopa can increase the pressor response; be aware of patient's drug regimen.

Reserpine increases the pressor response; be aware of patient's drug regimen.

TCAs increase the pressor response; be aware of patient's drug regimen.

Stability
Remix solution every 24 hours. Store reconstituted solution under refrigeration for 48 hours or 6 hours at room temperature. Pink discoloration of solution indicates slight oxidation but **no** significant loss of potency.

Stability of parenteral admixture at room temperature (25°C): 48 hours; at refrigeration (4°C): 7 days.

Standard adult diluent: 250 mg/500 mL D_5W; 500 mg/500 mL D_5W.

Mechanism of Action
Stimulates $beta_1$-adrenergic receptors, causing increased contractility and heart rate, with little effect on $beta_2$- or alpha-receptors

Pharmacodynamics
Onset of action: I.V.: 1-10 minutes following administration

Peak effect: Within 10-20 minutes

Pharmacokinetics
Metabolism: In tissues and liver to inactive metabolites

Half-life: 2 minutes

Elimination: In urine

Dosage
Geriatrics & Adults: Cardiac decompensation: I.V. infusion: 2.5-20 mcg/kg/minute; maximum: 40 mcg/kg/minute, titrate to desired response; see table.

Infusion Rates of Various Dilutions of Dobutamine

Desired Delivery Rate (mcg/kg/min)	Infusion Rate (mL/kg/min)	
	500 mcg/mL[1]	1000 mcg/mL[2]
2.5	0.005	0.0025
5.0	0.01	0.005
7.5	0.015	0.0075
10.0	0.02	0.01
12.5	0.025	0.0125
15.0	0.03	0.015

[1]500 mg per liter or 250 mg per 500 mL of diluent.

[2]1000 mg per liter or 250 mg per 250 mL of diluent.

Administration
Do not administer through same I.V. line as heparin, hydrocortisone sodium succinate, cefazolin, or penicillin; administer into large vein; use infusion device to control rate of flow

Monitoring Parameters
EKG, blood pressure, pulse, hemodynamic status

Additional Information
Most clinical experience with dobutamine is short-term (several hours)

Standard diluent: 250 mg/500 mL D_5W

Minimum volume: 500 mg/250 mL D_5W

Special Geriatric Considerations
A recent study demonstrated beneficial hemodynamic effects in elderly patients; monitor closely.

Dosage Forms
Excipient information presented when available (limited, particularly for generics); consult specific product labeling.

Infusion, as hydrochloride [premixed in dextrose]: 1 mg/mL (250 mL, 500 mL); 2 mg/mL (250 mL); 4 mg/mL (250 mL)

Injection, solution, as hydrochloride: 12.5 mg/mL (20 mL, 40 mL, 100 mL) [contains sodium bisulfite]

Selected References
Rich MN, Woods WL, Davila-Roman VG, et al, "A Randomized Comparison of Intravenous Amrinone Versus Dobutamine in Older Patients With Decompensated Congestive Heart Failure," *J Am Geriatr Soc*, 1995, 43(3):271-4.

♦ **Dobutamine Hydrochloride** *see DOBUTamine on page 458*

Docusate (DOK yoo sate)

Medication Safety Issues
Sound-alike/look-alike issues:

Docusate may be confused with Doxinate®

Colace® may be confused with Calan®

Surfak® may be confused with Surbex®

(Continued)

Docusate *(Continued)*

U.S. Brand Names Colace® [OTC]; Diocto® [OTC]; Docusoft-S™ [OTC]; DOK™ [OTC]; DOS® [OTC]; D-S-S® [OTC]; Dulcolax® Stool Softener [OTC]; Enemeez® [OTC]; Fleet® Sof-Lax® [OTC]; Genasoft® [OTC]; Phillips'® Stool Softener Laxative [OTC]; Silace [OTC]; Surfak® [OTC]

Canadian Brand Names Apo-Docusate-Sodium®; Colace®; Colax-C®; Novo-Docusate Calcium; Novo-Docusate Sodium; PMS-Docusate Calcium; PMS-Docusate Sodium; Regulex®; Selax®; Soflax™

Index Terms Dioctyl Calcium Sulfosuccinate; Dioctyl Sodium Sulfosuccinate; Docusate Calcium; Docusate Potassium; Docusate Sodium; DOSS; DSS

Generic Available Yes: Excludes gelcap

Pharmacologic Category Stool Softener

Use Stool softener in patients who should avoid straining during defecation and constipation associated with hard, dry stools; prophylaxis for straining (Valsalva) following myocardial infarction

Unlabeled/Investigational Use Ceruminolytic

Contraindications Hypersensitivity to docusate or any component of the formulation; concomitant use of mineral oil; intestinal obstruction, acute abdominal pain, nausea, or vomiting

Warnings/Precautions Prolonged, frequent or excessive use may result in dependence or electrolyte imbalance

Adverse Reactions (Reflective of adult population; not specific for elderly)
1% to 10%:
Gastrointestinal: Intestinal obstruction, diarrhea, abdominal cramping
Miscellaneous: Throat irritation

Overdosage/Toxicology Symptoms include abdominal cramps, diarrhea, fluid loss, and hypokalemia. Treatment is symptomatic.

Mechanism of Action Reduces surface tension of the oil-water interface of the stool resulting in enhanced incorporation of water and fat allowing for stool softening

Pharmacodynamics Onset of action: 12-72 hours

Dosage
Geriatrics & Adults: Note: Docusate salts are interchangeable; the amount of sodium, calcium, or potassium per dosage unit is clinically insignificant.

Stool softener:
Oral: 50-500 mg/day in 1-4 divided doses
Rectal: Add 50-100 mg of docusate liquid to enema fluid (saline or water); give as retention or flushing enema

Test Interactions Decreased potassium (S), decreased chloride (S)

Patient Information Patients should assure proper dietary fiber and fluid intake with adequate exercise if medically appropriate; do not use if abdominal pain, nausea, or vomiting are present; laxative use should be used for a short period of time (<1 week); prolonged use may result in abuse, dependence, as well as fluid and electrolyte loss; notify physician if bleeding occurs or if constipation is not relieved

Additional Information Docusate salts are interchangeable; the amount of sodium, calcium, or potassium per dosage unit is clinically insignificant; should institute nonpharmacologic therapy (ie, fluid, fiber, exercise)

Special Geriatric Considerations A safe agent to be used in the elderly. Some evidence that doses <200 mg are ineffective. Stool softeners are unnecessary if stool is well hydrated or "mushy" and soft; shown to be ineffective used long-term.

Dosage Forms Excipient information presented when available (limited, particularly for generics); consult specific product labeling.
Capsule, as calcium (Surfak®): 240 mg
Capsule, as sodium: 100 mg, 250 mg
    Colace®: 50 mg [contains sodium 3 mg], 100 mg [contains sodium 5 mg]
    Docusoft-S™: 100 mg [contains sodium 5 mg]
    DOK™, Genasoft®: 100 mg
    DOS®, D-S-S®: 100 mg, 250 mg
    Dulcolax® Stool Softener: 100 mg [contains sodium 5 mg]
    Phillips'® Stool Softener Laxative: 100 mg [contains sodium 5.2 mg]
Enema, rectal, as sodium (Enemeez®): 283 mg/5 mL 5 mL
Gelcap, as sodium (Fleet® Sof-Lax®): 100 mg
Liquid, as sodium: 150 mg/15 mL (480 mL)
    Colace®: 150 mg/15 mL (30 mL) [contains sodium 1 mg/mL]
    Diocto®: 150 mg/15 mL (480 mL) [vanilla flavor]
    Silace: 150 mg/15 mL (480 mL) [lemon-vanilla flavor]
Syrup, as sodium: 60 mg/15 mL (480 mL)
    Colace®, Diocto®: 60 mg/15 mL (480 mL) [alcohol free, sugar free; contains sodium 36 mg/5 mL]
    Silace: 20 mg/5 mL (480 mL) [peppermint flavor]

Docusate and Senna (DOK yoo sate & SEN na)

Related Information
Docusate *on page 459*
Senna *on page 1456*
Treatment Options for Constipation *on page 1785*

Medication Safety Issues
Sound-alike/look-alike issues:
Senokot® may be confused with Depakote®

U.S. Brand Names Peri-Colace® [OTC]; Senokot-S® [OTC]; SenoSol™-SS [OTC]

Index Terms Senna and Docusate; Senna-S

Generic Available Yes

Pharmacologic Category Laxative, Stimulant; Stool Softener

Use Short-term treatment of constipation

Unlabeled/Investigational Use Evacuation of the colon for bowel or rectal examinations; management/prevention of opiate-induced constipation

Contraindications Hypersensitivity to any component; intestinal obstruction; acute intestinal inflammation (eg, Crohn's disease); ulcerative colitis; appendicitis; abdominal pain of unknown origin; concurrent use of mineral oil

Warnings/Precautions Not recommended for over-the-counter (OTC) use in patients experiencing stomach pain, nausea, vomiting, or a sudden change in bowel movements which lasts >2 weeks. OTC labeling does not recommend for use longer than 1 week.

Adverse Reactions (Reflective of adult population; not specific for elderly)
Frequency not defined.
Gastrointestinal: Nausea, vomiting, diarrhea, abdominal cramps
Genitourinary: Urine discoloration (red/brown)

Mechanism of Action Docusate is a stool softener; sennosides are laxatives

Dosage
Geriatrics: Constipation: OTC ranges: Oral: Consider half the initial dose in older, debilitated patients
Adults: Constipation: OTC ranges: Oral: Initial: 2 tablets (17.2 mg sennosides plus 100 mg docusate) once daily (maximum: 4 tablets twice daily)

Administration Oral: Once-daily doses should be taken at bedtime.

Patient Information May discolor urine or feces (yellow, brown, pink, red, or violet); may cause diminished colon function with prolonged use/abuse. Bowel movements usually occur within 6-12 hours after a dose. Notify prescriber for failure to have a bowel movement after the first dose or for rectal bleeding. OTC labeling does not recommend for use longer than 1 week.

Special Geriatric Considerations The chronic use of stimulant cathartics is inappropriate and should be avoided. Although the elderly commonly complain of constipation, such complaints require evaluation; short-term use of stimulant cathartics is best. If prophylaxis is desired, then the use of bulk agents (eg, psyllium), stool softeners, and hyperosmotic agents (eg, sorbitol 70%) is preferred. Stool softeners are unnecessary if stools are well-hydrated (as in use of hyperosmotics), soft or "mushy". Patients should be instructed for proper dietary fiber and fluid intake, as well as regular exercise. Monitor closely for fluid/electrolyte imbalance, CNS signs of fluid/electrolyte loss, and hypotension.

Dosage Forms Excipient information presented when available (limited, particularly for generics); consult specific product labeling.
Tablet: Docusate sodium 50 mg and sennosides 8.6 mg
Peri-Colace®: Docusate sodium 50 mg and sennosides 8.6 mg
Senokot-S®: Docusate sodium 50 mg and sennosides 8.6 mg [sugar free; contains sodium 4 mg/tablet]
SenoSol™-SS: Docusate sodium 50 mg and sennosides 8.6 mg [contains sodium 3 mg/tablet]

♦ **Docusate Calcium** *see* Docusate *on page 459*
♦ **Docusate Potassium** *see* Docusate *on page 459*
♦ **Docusate Sodium** *see* Docusate *on page 459*
♦ **Docusoft-S™ [OTC]** *see* Docusate *on page 459*

Dofetilide (doe FET il ide)

U.S. Brand Names Tikosyn®
Canadian Brand Names Tikosyn®
Generic Available No
(Continued)

Dofetilide (Continued)

Pharmacologic Category Antiarrhythmic Agent, Class III

Use Maintenance of normal sinus rhythm in patients with atrial fibrillation/atrial flutter of ≥1-week duration who have been converted to normal sinus rhythm; conversion of atrial fibrillation and atrial flutter to normal sinus rhythm
See Additional Information.

Restrictions Tikosyn® is only available to prescribers and hospitals that have confirmed their participation in a designated Tikosyn® Education Program. The program provides comprehensive education about the importance of in-hospital treatment initiation and individualized dosing.

T.I.P.S. is the Tikosyn® In Pharmacy System designated to allow retail pharmacies to stock and dispense Tikosyn® once they have been enrolled. A participating pharmacy must confirm receipt of the T.I.P.S. program materials and educate its pharmacy staff about the procedures required to fill an outpatient prescription for Tikosyn®. The T.I.P.S. enrollment form is available at www.tikosyn.com. Tikosyn® is only available from a special mail order pharmacy, and enrolled retail pharmacies. Pharmacists must verify that the hospital/prescriber is a confirmed participant before Tikosyn® is provided. For participant verification, the pharmacist may call 1-800-788-7353 or use the web site located at www.tikosynlist.com. Further details and directions on the program are provided at www.tikosyn.com.

Dofetilide therapy must be initiated/adjusted in a hospital setting with proper monitoring under the guidance of experienced personnel.

Contraindications Hypersensitivity to dofetilide or any component of the formulation; patients with congenital or acquired long QT syndromes, do not use if a baseline QT interval or QT_c is >440 msec (500 msec in patients with ventricular conduction abnormalities); severe renal impairment (estimated Cl_{cr} <20 mL/minute); concurrent use with verapamil, cimetidine, hydrochlorothiazide (alone or in combinations), trimethoprim (alone or in combination with sulfamethoxazole), itraconazole, ketoconazole, prochlorperazine, or megestrol; baseline heart rate <50 beats/minute; other drugs that prolong QT intervals (phenothiazines, cisapride, bepridil, tricyclic antidepressants, certain oral macrolides: sparfloxacin, gatifloxacin, moxifloxacin); hypokalemia or hypomagnesemia; concurrent amiodarone

Warnings/Precautions [U.S. Boxed Warning]: Must be initiated (or reinitiated) in a setting with continuous monitoring and staff familiar with the recognition and treatment of life-threatening arrhythmias. Patients must be monitored with continuous ECG for a minimum of 3 days, or for a minimum of 12 hours after electrical or pharmacological cardioversion to normal sinus rhythm, whichever is greater. Patients should be readmitted for continuous monitoring if dosage is later increased.

Reserve for patients who are highly symptomatic with atrial fibrillation/atrial flutter; torsade de pointes significantly increases with doses >500 mcg twice daily; hold Class Ia or Class II antiarrhythmics for at least three half-lives prior to starting dofetilide; use in patients on amiodarone therapy only if serum amiodarone level is <0.3 mg/L or if amiodarone was stopped for >3 months previously; correct hypokalemia or hypomagnesemia before initiating dofetilide and maintain within normal limits during treatment. Risk of hypokalemia and/or hypomagnesemia may be increased by potassium-depleting diuretics, increasing the risk of torsade de pointes. Concurrent use with other drugs known to prolong QT_c interval is not recommended.

Patients with sick sinus syndrome or with second or third-degree heart block should not receive dofetilide unless a functional pacemaker is in place. Defibrillation threshold is reduced in patients with ventricular tachycardia or ventricular fibrillation undergoing implantation of a cardioverter-defibrillator device. Use with caution in renal impairment; not recommended in patients receiving drugs which may compete for renal secretion via cationic transport. Use with caution in patients with severe hepatic impairment.

In the Cardiac Arrhythmia Suppression Trial (CAST), recent (>6 days but <2 years ago) myocardial infarction patients with asymptomatic, nonlife-threatening ventricular arrhythmias did not benefit and may have been harmed by attempts to suppress the arrhythmia with flecainide or encainide. An increased mortality or nonfatal cardiac arrest rate (7.7%) was seen in the active treatment group compared with patients in the placebo group (3%). The applicability of the CAST results to other populations is unknown. Antiarrhythmic agents should be reserved for patients with life-threatening ventricular arrhythmias.

Adverse Reactions (Reflective of adult population; not specific for elderly)
Supraventricular arrhythmia patients (incidence > placebo)
>10%: Central nervous system: Headache (11%)
2% to 10%:
   Central nervous system: Dizziness (8%), insomnia (4%)
   Cardiovascular: Ventricular tachycardia (2.6% to 3.7%), chest pain (10%), torsade de pointes (3.3% in CHF patients and 0.9% in patients with a recent MI; up to

10.5% in patients receiving doses in excess of those recommended). Torsade de pointes occurs most frequently within the first 3 days of therapy.

Dermatologic: Rash (3%)

Gastrointestinal: Nausea (5%), diarrhea (3%), abdominal pain (3%)

Neuromuscular & skeletal: Back pain (3%)

Respiratory: Dyspnea (6%), respiratory tract infection (7%)

Miscellaneous: Flu syndrome (4%)

<2%:

Central nervous system: CVA, facial paralysis, flaccid paralysis, migraine, paralysis

Cardiovascular: AV block (0.4% to 1.5%), ventricular fibrillation (0% to 0.4%), bundle branch block, heart block, edema, heart arrest, myocardial infarct, sudden death, syncope

Dermatologic: Angioedema

Gastrointestinal: Liver damage

Neuromuscular & skeletal: Paresthesia

Respiratory: Cough

>2% (incidence ≤ placebo): Anxiety, pain, angina, atrial fibrillation, hypertension, palpitation, supraventricular tachycardia, peripheral edema, urinary tract infection, weakness, arthralgia, diaphoresis

Overdosage/Toxicology The major dose-related toxicity is torsade de pointes. Treatment should be symptomatic and supportive. Watch for excessive prolongation of the QT interval in overdose situations. Continuous cardiac monitoring is necessary. A charcoal slurry is helpful when given early (15 minutes) after the overdose. Isoproterenol infusion into anesthetized dogs with cardiac pacing has been shown to correct atrial and ventricular effective refractory periods caused by dofetilide. General treatment measures, override pacing, and magnesium therapy appear to be effective in the management of dofetilide-induced torsade de pointes.

Drug Interactions Substrate of CYP3A4 (minor)

If dofetilide needs to be discontinued to allow dosing of other potentially interacting drug(s) (see below), a washout period of at least 2 days is needed before starting the other drug(s).

Cimetidine, a cation transport system inhibitor, inhibits dofetilide's elimination and can cause a 58% increase in dofetilide's plasma levels; concomitant use is contraindicated.

Diuretics and other drugs (aminoglycosides) which deplete potassium or magnesium may increase dofetilide toxicity (torsade de pointes). Concurrent use of hydrochlorothiazide is contraindicated.

Hydrochlorothiazide: May enhance the QT_c-prolonging effect of dofetilide. May increase serum concentration of dofetilide. Concurrent use is contraindicated.

Itraconazole: May decrease the metabolism of dofetilide. Concurrent use is contraindicated.

Ketoconazole increases dofetilide's C_{max} (53% males, 97% females) and the AUC (41% males, 69% females) when used concurrently; concomitant use is contraindicated.

QT_c-prolonging agents (including bepridil, cisapride, clarithromycin, erythromycin, tricyclic antidepressants, phenothiazines, moxifloxacin): Use is contraindicated.

Renal cationic transport inhibitors (including triamterene, metformin, amiloride, prochlorperazine, megestrol) may increase dofetilide levels; coadminister with caution.

Trimethoprim (alone or in combination with sulfamethoxazole) increases dofetilide's C_{max} (103%) and AUC (93%); concomitant use is contraindicated.

Verapamil causes an increase in dofetilide's peak plasma levels by 42%. In the supraventricular arrhythmia and a higher incidence of torsade de pointes was seen in patients on verapamil; concomitant use is contraindicated.

Ethanol/Nutrition/Herb Interactions Herb/Nutraceutical: St John's wort may decrease dofetilide levels. Avoid ephedra (may worsen arrhythmia).

Mechanism of Action Vaughan Williams Class III antiarrhythmic activity. Blockade of the cardiac ion channel carrying the rapid component of the delayed rectifier potassium current. Dofetilide has no effect on sodium channels, adrenergic alpha-receptors, or adrenergic beta-receptors. It increases the monophasic action potential duration due to delayed repolarization. The increase in the QT interval is a function of prolongation of both effective and functional refractory periods in the His-Purkinje system and the ventricles. Changes in cardiac conduction velocity and sinus node function have not been observed in patients with or without structural heart disease. PR and QRS width remain the same in patients with pre-existing heart block and or sick sinus syndrome.

Pharmacokinetics

Absorption: >90%

Distribution: V_d: 3 L/kg

Protein binding: 60% to 70%

Metabolism: Dofetilide can be metabolized by CYP3A4, but has a low affinity for it. Metabolites are formed by N-dealkylation and N-oxidation.

Bioavailability: >90%

(Continued)

Dofetilide *(Continued)*

Half-life: 10 hours

Time to peak: 2-3 hours after ingested in the fasting state

Elimination: 80% excreted in the urine, of which 80% is excreted unchanged, and 20% is inactive or minimally active metabolites. Renal elimination consists of glomerular filtration and active tubular secretion via cationic transport system.

Dosage

Geriatrics: Refer to adult dosing. No specific dosage adjustments are recommended based on age; however, careful assessment of renal function is particularly important in this population. See Special Geriatric Considerations.

Adults: Note: QT_c must be determined prior to first dose

Antiarrhythmic: Oral:

Initial: 500 mcg orally twice daily. Initial dosage must be adjusted in patients with estimated Cl_{cr} <60 mL/minute. Dofetilide may be initiated at lower doses than recommended based on physician discretion.

Modification of dosage in response to initial dose: QT_c interval should be measured 2-3 hours after the initial dose. If the QT_c >15% of baseline, or if the QT_c is >500 msec (550 msec in patients with ventricular conduction abnormalities), dofetilide should be adjusted. If the starting dose is 500 mcg twice daily, then adjust to 250 mcg twice daily. If the starting dose was 250 mcg twice daily, then adjust to 125 mcg twice daily. If the starting dose was 125 mcg twice daily, then adjust to 125 mcg every day.

Continued monitoring for doses 2-5: QT_c interval must be determined 2-3 hours after each subsequent dose of dofetilide for in-hospital doses 2-5. If the measured QT_c is >500 msec (550 msec in patients with ventricular conduction abnormalities) dofetilide should be stopped.

Renal Impairment:

Cl_{cr} >60 mL/minute: Administer 500 mcg twice daily.

Cl_{cr} 40-60 mL/minute: Administer 250 mcg twice daily.

Cl_{cr} 20-39 mL/minute: Administer 125 mcg twice daily.

Cl_{cr} <20 mL/minute: Contraindicated in this group

Hepatic Impairment: No dosage adjustments required in Child-Pugh class A and B; patients with severe hepatic impairment were not studied.

Monitoring Parameters EKG monitoring with attention to QT_c and occurrence of ventricular arrhythmias, baseline serum creatinine, and changes in serum creatinine. Check serum potassium and magnesium concentrations if on medications where these electrolyte disturbances can occur, or if patient has a history of hypokalemia or hypomagnesemia.

Patient Information May be taken with or without food; take exactly the way it was prescribed; do not stop this medicine without talking with your physician. Never take an extra dose; if you miss a dose just take your scheduled dose amount at the next scheduled time. If you take more medicine than you should, call your physician immediately. If you cannot reach your physician, go to the nearest emergency room (take your medicine with you). Tell your physician about any new medicines before taking them; not all medicines mix well with this one. Call your physician immediately if you faint, become dizzy, have fast heartbeats, severe diarrhea, unusual sweating, vomiting, no appetite, or more thirst than normal. You may feel tired, weak, or have numbness, tingling, muscle cramps, constipation, vomiting, or rapid heartbeats if you have a low potassium level.

Additional Information The management of atrial fibrillation deserves careful consideration in patients with heart failure, because the loss of atrial assistance to ventricular filling may have greater negative effects on cardiac output. The choice of antiarrhythmic is important because of the risk that antiarrhythmic therapy may increase mortality in this setting.

The two DIAMOND studies were 3-year trials comparing mortality between dofetilide and placebo in patients with left ventricular dysfunction. One study included patients with moderate to severe CHF (60% of participants were NYHA class III or IV) and the other study looked at patients with a recent MI (40% had NYHA class III or IV CHF). Dofetilide was an effective therapy for atrial fibrillation in carefully selected and monitored heart failure patients. Mortality was similar between those who received placebo and dofetilide; fewer patients of dofetilide were hospitalized for heart failure. It seems prudent, therefore, to carefully select and monitor patients in this situation.

Special Geriatric Considerations No specific dosage adjustments are recommended based on age; however, evaluation for use of this drug in the elderly is imperative. A complete review of medications, to assure there is no inadvertent use of contraindicated medications and those with potential drug interactions, can be re-evaluated for continued need. Laboratory values must be assessed prior to initiating medication; careful assessment of renal function is particularly important in the elderly population.

Dosage Forms Excipient information presented when available (limited, particularly for generics); consult specific product labeling.

Capsule: 125 mcg, 250 mcg, 500 mcg

Selected References

Buxton AE, Lee KL, Fisher JD, et al, "A Randomized Study of the Prevention of Sudden Death in Patients With Coronary Artery Disease," *N Engl J Med*, 1999, 341(25):1882-90.

Choy AM, Darbar D, Dell'Orto S, et al, "Exaggerated QT Prolongation After Cardioversion of Arterial Fibrillation," *J Am Coll Cardiol*, 1999, 34(2):396-401.

Falk RH, Pollak A, Singh SN, et al, "Intravenous Dofetilide, A Class III Antiarrhythmic Agent, for the Termination of Sustained Atrial Fibrillation or Flutter. Intravenous Dofetilide Investigators," *J Am Coll Cardiol*, 1997, 29(2):385-90.

Fuster V, Rydén LE, Asinger RW, et al, "ACC/AHA/ESC Guidelines for the Management of Patients with Atrial Fibrillation: A Report of the American College of Cardiology/American Heart Association Task Force on Practice Guidelines and the European Society of Cardiology Committee for Practice Guidelines and Policy Conferences," *J Am Coll Cardiol*, 2001, 38(4):1231-66.

Norgaard BL, Wachtell K, Christensen PD, et al, "Efficacy and Safety of Intravenously Administered Dofetilide in Acute Termination of Atrial Fibrillation and Flutter: A Multicenter, Randomized, Double-Blind, Placebo-Controlled Trial. Danish Dofetilide in Atrial Fibrillation and Flutter Study Group," *Am Heart J*, 1999, 137(6):1062-9.

Prystowsky EN, Benson DW Jr, Fuster V, et al, "Management of Patients With Atrial Fibrillation: A Statement for Healthcare Professionals. From the Subcommittee on Electrocardiography and Electrophysiology, American Heart Association," *Circulation*, 1996, 93(6):1262-77.

Torp-Pederson C, Moller M, Bloch-Thomsen PE, et al, "Dofetilide in Patients with Congestive Heart Failure and Left Ventricular Dysfunction," *N Engl J Med*, 1999, 341(12):857-65.

♦ **Dofus [OTC]** *see Lactobacillus on page 867* *see Lactobacillus on page 867*

♦ **DOK™ [OTC]** *see Docusate on page 459* *see Docusate on page 459*

Dolasetron (dol A se tron)

Medication Safety Issues

Sound-alike/look-alike issues:

Anzemet® may be confused with Aldomet® and Avandamet™

Dolasetron may be confused with granisetron, ondansetron, palonosetron

U.S. Brand Names Anzemet®

Canadian Brand Names Anzemet®

Index Terms Dolasetron Mesylate; MDL 73,147EF

Generic Available No

Pharmacologic Category Antiemetic; Selective 5-HT$_3$ Receptor Antagonist

Use Prevention of nausea and vomiting associated with emetogenic cancer chemotherapy; prevention of postoperative nausea and vomiting; treatment of postoperative nausea and vomiting (injectable form only).

Note: In Canada, the use of dolasetron is contraindicated in the treatment of postoperative nausea and vomiting in adults. These are not labeled contraindications in the U.S.

Contraindications Hypersensitivity to dolasetron or any component of the formulation

Warnings/Precautions Dose-related cardiac conduction abnormalities, including PR, QT$_c$, JT prolongation and QRS widening may occur; interval prolongation usually lasts 6-8 hours, however, may last ≥24 hours and rarely lead to heart block or arrhythmia. Dolasetron should be administered with caution in patients with congenital QT syndrome or other risk factors for QT prolongation (eg, medications known to prolong QT interval, electrolyte abnormalities, and cumulative high dose anthracycline therapy). Use with caution in patients allergic to other 5-HT$_3$ receptor antagonists; cross-reactivity has been reported. **For chemotherapy, should be used on a scheduled basis, not on an "as needed" (PRN) basis,** since data support the use of this drug only in the prevention of nausea and vomiting (due to antineoplastic therapy) and not in the rescue of nausea and vomiting. Not intended for treatment of nausea and vomiting or for chronic continuous therapy.

Adverse Reactions (Reflective of adult population; not specific for elderly)

Adverse events may vary according to indication

>10%:

Central nervous system: Headache (7% to 24%)

Gastrointestinal: Diarrhea (2% to 12%)

1% to 10%:

Cardiovascular: Bradycardia (4% to 5%), hypotension (5%), hypertension (2% to 3%), tachycardia (2% to 3%)

Central nervous system: Dizziness (1% to 6%), fatigue (3% to 6%), fever (4% to 5%), pain (≤3%), chills/shivering (1% to 2%), sedation (2%)

Dermatological: Pruritus (3% to 4%)

Gastrointestinal: Dyspepsia (2% to 3%), abdominal pain (≤3%)

Hepatic: Abnormal hepatic function (4%)

Neuromuscular & skeletal: Pain (3%)

Renal: Oliguria (1% to 3%)

Overdosage/Toxicology In animal toxicity studies, doses 6.3-12.6 times the recommended human dose (based upon surface area) were lethal. Symptoms of acute (Continued)

Dolasetron *(Continued)*

poisoning included tremors, depression, and convulsions. There is no known specific antidote for dolasetron. Patients with suspected overdose should be managed with supportive therapy.

Drug Interactions Substrate (minor) of CYP2C9, 3A4; **Inhibits** CYP2D6 (weak)

Apomorphine: Due to reports of profound hypotension during concomitant therapy with ondansetron, the manufacturer of apomorphine contraindicates its use with all 5-HT$_3$ antagonists.

Ciprofloxacin: May enhance the QT$_c$-prolonging effects of dolasetron.

QT$_c$-prolonging agents: Concurrent use of dolasetron with other drugs which may prolong QT$_c$interval may increase the risk of potentially-fatal arrhythmias; includes type Ia and type III antiarrhythmic agents, selected quinolones (moxifloxacin), cisapride, palonosetron, thioridazine, and other agents.

Stability Store intact vials and tablets at room temperature; protect from light. A 20 mg/mL solution in syringes is stable for 8 months at room temperature. Dilute in 50-100 mL of a compatible solution (ie, 0.9% NS, D$_5$W, D$_5$1/2NS, D$_5$LR, LR, and 10% mannitol injection). Solutions diluted for infusion are stable at room temperature for 24 hours or under refrigeration for 48 hours.

Mechanism of Action Selective serotonin receptor (5-HT$_3$) antagonist, blocking serotonin both peripherally (primary site of action) and centrally at the chemoreceptor trigger zone

Pharmacokinetics

Absorption: Rapid and complete

Distribution: Hydrodolasetron: 5.8 L/kg

Protein binding: Hydrodolasetron: 69% to 77% (50% bound to alpha$_1$-acid glycoprotein)

Metabolism: Hepatic; reduction by carbonyl reductase to hydrodolasetron (active metabolite); further metabolized by CYP2D6, CYP3A, and flavin monooxygenase

Bioavailability: 75%

Half-life elimination: Dolasetron: 10 minutes; hydrodolasetron: Adults: 6-8 hours

Time to peak, plasma: Hydrodolasetron: I.V.: 0.6 hours; Oral: 1 hour

Excretion: Urine ~67% (53% to 61% as active metabolite hydrodolasetron); feces ~33%

Dosage

Geriatrics & Adults: Note: In Canada, the use of dolasetron is contraindicated in the treatment of postoperative nausea and vomiting in adults. These are not labeled contraindications in the U.S.

Prevention of chemotherapy-associated nausea and vomiting:

Oral:100 mg single dose 1 hour prior to chemotherapy

I.V.: 1.8 mg/kg or 100 mg 30 minutes prior to chemotherapy

Postoperative nausea and vomiting:

Prevention:

Oral: 100 mg within 2 hours before surgery (doses of 25-200 mg have been used)

I.V.: 12.5 mg ~15 minutes before stopping anesthesia

Treatment: I.V. (only): 12.5 mg as soon as needed

Additional Information A single I.V. dose of dolasetron mesylate (1.8 or 2.4 mg/kg) has comparable safety and efficacy to a single 32-mg IV dose of ondansetron in patients receiving cisplatin chemotherapy.

Special Geriatric Considerations In controlled trials, no difference in overall safety and efficacy were observed between elderly and younger adults. Pharmacokinetics are similar in younger adults and elderly. No dosage adjustment necessary.

Dosage Forms Excipient information presented when available (limited, particularly for generics); consult specific product labeling.

Injection, solution, as mesylate:

Anzemet®: 20 mg/mL (0.625 mL) [single-use Carpuject® or vial; contains mannitol 38.2 mg/mL]; 20 mg/mL (5 mL) [single-use vial; contains mannitol 38.2 mg/mL]; 20 mg/mL (25 mL) [multidose vial; contains mannitol 29 mg/mL]

Tablet, as mesylate:

Anzemet®: 50 mg, 100 mg

Extemporaneously Prepared Dolasetron injection may be diluted in apple or apple-grape juice and taken orally; this dilution is stable for 2 hours at room temperature.

♦ **Dolasetron Mesylate** *see* Dolasetron *on page 465*

♦ **Dolobid® [DSC]** *see* Diflunisal *on page 431*

♦ **Dolophine®** *see* Methadone *on page 996*

♦ **Domeboro® [OTC]** *see* Aluminum Sulfate and Calcium Acetate *on page 68*

Donepezil (doh NEP e zil)

Medication Safety Issues
Sound-alike/look-alike issues:
Aricept® may be confused with AcipHex®, Ascriptin®, and Azilect®

U.S. Brand Names Aricept®; Aricept® ODT

Canadian Brand Names Aricept®; Aricept® RDT

Index Terms E2020

Generic Available No

Pharmacologic Category Acetylcholinesterase Inhibitor (Central)

Use Treatment of mild to moderate dementia of the Alzheimer's type

Unlabeled/Investigational Use Treatment of attention-deficit/hyperactivity disorder (ADHD), behavioral syndromes in dementia

Contraindications Hypersensitivity to donepezil, piperidine derivatives, or any component of the formulation

Warnings/Precautions Cholinesterase inhibitors may have vagotonic effects which may cause bradycardia and/or heart block with or without a history of cardiac disease; syncopal episodes have been associated with donepezil. Use with caution with sick sinus syndrome or other supraventricular cardiac conduction abnormalities, with seizures, COPD, or asthma. Use with caution in patients at risk of ulcer disease (eg, previous history or NSAID use), or in patients with bladder outlet obstruction. May cause diarrhea, nausea, and/or vomiting, which may be dose-related. May exaggerate neuromuscular blockade effects of depolarizing neuromuscular-blocking agents like succinylcholine.

Adverse Reactions (Reflective of adult population; not specific for elderly)
>10%:
Central nervous system: Insomnia (5% to 14%)
Gastrointestinal: Nausea (5% to 19%), diarrhea (8% to 15%)
Miscellaneous: Accident (7% to 13%), infection (11%)
1% to 10%:
Cardiovascular: Hypertension (3%), chest pain (2%), hemorrhage (2%), syncope (2%), hypotension, atrial fibrillation, bradycardia, ECG abnormal, edema, heart failure, hot flashes, peripheral edema, vasodilation
Central nervous system: Headache (4% to 10%), pain (3% to 9%), fatigue (3% to 8%), dizziness (2% to 8%), abnormal dreams (3%), depression (2% to 3%), hostility (3%), nervousness (3%), hallucinations (3%), confusion (2%), emotional lability (2%), personality disorder (2%), fever (2%), somnolence (2%), abnormal crying, aggression, agitation, anxiety, aphasia, delusions, irritability, restlessness, seizure
Dermatologic: Bruising (4% to 5%), eczema (3%), pruritus, rash, skin ulcer, urticaria
Endocrine & metabolic: Dehydration (2%), hyperlipemia (2%), libido increased
Gastrointestinal: Anorexia (3% to 8%), vomiting (3% to 8%), weight loss (3%), abdominal pain, constipation, dyspepsia, fecal incontinence, gastroenteritis, GI bleeding, bloating, epigastric pain, toothache
Genitourinary: Urinary frequency (2%), urinary incontinence (2%), hematuria, glycosuria, nocturia, UTI
Hematologic: Anemia
Hepatic: Alkaline phosphatase increased
Neuromuscular & skeletal: Muscle cramps (3% to 8%), back pain (3%), CPK increased (3%), arthritis (2%), ataxia, bone fracture, gait abnormal, lactate dehydrogenase increased, paresthesia, tremor, weakness
Ocular: Blurred vision, cataract, eye irritation
Respiratory: Cough increased, dyspnea, bronchitis, pharyngitis, pneumonia, sore throat
Miscellaneous: Diaphoresis, fungal infection, flu symptoms, wandering

Overdosage/Toxicology Donepezil can cause cholinergic crisis characterized by severe nausea, vomiting, salivation, sweating, bradycardia, hypotension, cardiovascular collapse, and convulsions. Increased muscle weakness is a possibility and may result in death if respiratory muscles are involved. The effectiveness of dialysis is unknown.

Tertiary anticholinergics, such as atropine, may be used as an antidote. I.V. atropine sulfate titrated to effect is recommended, with an initial dose of 1-2 mg I.V., and with subsequent doses based on clinical response. Atypical blood pressure and heart rate increases have been reported with other cholinomimetics when coadministered with quaternary anticholinergics (eg, glycopyrrolate). Implement general supportive measures.

Drug Interactions Substrate (minor) of CYP2D6, 3A4
Anticholinergic agents: Effects of donepezil may be inhibited by anticholinergic agents (benztropine)
(Continued)

Donepezil *(Continued)*

Antipsychotic agents: Acetylcholinesterase inhibitors (central) may increase the risk of antipsychotic-related extrapyramidal symptoms; monitor.

Beta-blockers: Acetylcholinesterase inhibitors may enhance the bradycardic effects of beta-blockers; monitor.

Cholinergic agents: A synergistic effect may be seen with concurrent administration of succinylcholine or cholinergic agonists (bethanechol); excessive cholinergic stimulation and toxicity may occur; use caution.

Neuromuscular-blocking agents (nondepolarizing): Acetylcholinesterase inhibitors may diminish the neuromuscular-blocking effects of nondepolarizng blockers.

Ethanol/Nutrition/Herb Interactions Herb/Nutraceutical: St John's wort may decrease donepezil levels. Gingko biloba may increase adverse effects/toxicity of acetylcholinesterase inhibitors.

Stability Store at 15°C to 30°C (59°F to 86°F).

Mechanism of Action Alzheimer's disease is characterized by cholinergic deficiency in the cortex and basal forebrain, which contributes to cognitive deficits. Donepezil reversibly and noncompetitively inhibits centrally-active acetylcholinesterase, the enzyme responsible for hydrolysis of acetylcholine. This appears to result in increased concentrations of acetylcholine available for synaptic transmission in the central nervous system.

Pharmacokinetics Geriatrics: No formal pharmacokinetic studies have been done in older adults; mean donepezil plasma concentrations were no different in older Alzheimer patients as compared to younger adults.

Absorption: Well absorbed

Protein binding: 96% mainly to albumin (75%) and alpha$_1$ acid glycoprotein (21%)

Metabolism: Extensive; undergoes glucuronidation

Bioavailability: 100%

Half-life: 70 hours

Steady-state: 15 days

Time to peak plasma concentration: 3-4 hours

Excretion: Urine 57% (17% as unchanged drug); feces 15%

Dosage

Geriatrics & Adults: Alzheimer's disease: Oral: Initial: 5 mg/day at bedtime; may increase to 10 mg/day at bedtime after 4-6 weeks.

Administration Aricept® ODT: Allow tablet to dissolve completely on tongue and follow with water.

Monitoring Parameters Behavior, mood, bowel function, cognitive function, general function (eg, activities of daily living)

Patient Information May be taken with or without food; donepezil is not a cure for Alzheimer's disease, but may slow the progression of symptoms

Dosage Forms Excipient information presented when available (limited, particularly for generics); consult specific product labeling.

Tablet, as hydrochloride:

Aricept®: 5 mg, 10 mg

Tablet, orally disintegrating, as hydrochloride:

Aricept® ODT: 5 mg, 10 mg

Selected References

Rogers SL and Friedhoff LT, "The Efficacy and Safety of Donepezil in Patients With Alzheimer's Disease: Results of a U.S. Multicentre, Randomized, Double-Blind, Placebo-Controlled Trial," *Dementia*, 1996, 7(6):293-303.

♦ **Donnatal®** *see* Hyoscyamine, Atropine, Scopolamine, and Phenobarbital *on page 780*

♦ **Donnatal Extentabs®** *see* Hyoscyamine, Atropine, Scopolamine, and Phenobarbital *on page 780*

DOPamine *(DOE pa meen)*

Medication Safety Issues

Sound-alike/look-alike issues:

DOPamine may be confused with DOBUTamine, Dopram®

High alert medication: The Institute for Safe Medication Practices (ISMP) includes this medication among its list of drugs which have a heightened risk of causing significant patient harm when used in error.

Index Terms Dopamine Hydrochloride; Intropin

Generic Available Yes

Pharmacologic Category Adrenergic Agonist Agent

Use Adjunct in the treatment of shock which persists after adequate fluid volume replacement; dose related inotropic and vasopressor effects; stimulation of dopaminergic, beta- and alpha-receptors

Unlabeled/Investigational Use Treatment of symptomatic bradycardia or heart block unresponsive to atropine or pacing

Contraindications Hypersensitivity to sulfites (commercial preparation contains sodium bisulfite); pheochromocytoma; ventricular fibrillation

Warnings/Precautions Use with caution in patients with cardiovascular disease or cardiac arrhythmias or patients with occlusive vascular disease. Correct hypovolemia and electrolytes when used in hemodynamic support. May cause increases in HR and arrhythmia. Use with caution in post-MI patients. Use with extreme caution in patients taking MAO inhibitors. Avoid extravasation; infuse into a large vein if possible. Avoid infusion in leg veins. Watch I.V. site closely. **[U.S. Boxed Warning]: If extravasation occurs, infiltrate the area with diluted phentolamine (5-10 mg in 10-15 mL of saline) with a fine hypodermic needle. Phentolamine should be administered as soon as possible after extravasation is noted.** Product may contain sodium metabisulfite.

Adverse Reactions (Reflective of adult population; not specific for elderly)
Frequency not defined.
Cardiovascular: Ectopic beats, tachycardia, anginal pain, palpitation, hypotension, vasoconstriction
Central nervous system: Headache
Gastrointestinal: Nausea and vomiting
Respiratory: Dyspnea

Overdosage/Toxicology Symptoms include severe hypertension, cardiac arrhythmias, and acute renal failure. **Important:** Antidote for peripheral ischemia: To prevent sloughing and necrosis in ischemic areas, the area should be infiltrated as soon as possible with 10-15 mL of saline solution containing 5-10 mg of Regitine® (brand of phentolamine), an adrenergic blocking agent. A syringe with a fine hypodermic needle should be used, and the solution liberally infiltrated throughout the ischemic area. Sympathetic blockade with phentolamine causes immediate and conspicuous local hyperemic changes if the area is infiltrated within 12 hours. Therefore, phentolamine should be given as soon as possible after the extravasation is noted.

Drug Interactions
Beta-blockers (nonselective ones) may increase hypertensive effect; avoid concurrent use.
Cocaine may cause malignant arrhythmias; avoid concurrent use.
Guanethidine's hypotensive effects may only be partially reversed; may need to use a direct-acting sympathomimetic.
MAO inhibitors potentiate hypertension and hypertensive crisis; avoid concurrent use.
Methyldopa can increase the pressor response; be aware of patient's drug regimen.
Reserpine increases the pressor response; be aware of patient's drug regimen.
TCAs increase the pressor response; be aware of patient's drug regimen.

Stability Protect from light; solutions that are darker than slightly yellow should not be used.

Mechanism of Action Stimulates both adrenergic and dopaminergic receptors, lower doses are mainly dopaminergic stimulating and produce renal and mesenteric vasodilation, higher doses are both dopaminergic and beta$_1$-adrenergic stimulating and produce cardiac stimulation and renal vasodilation; large doses stimulate alpha-adrenergic receptors

Pharmacodynamics
Onset of action: 5 minutes upon administration
Duration: <10 minutes

Pharmacokinetics
Metabolism: In plasma, kidneys, and liver 75% to inactive metabolites by monoamine oxidase and 25% to norepinephrine (active)
Half-life: 2 minutes
Elimination: In urine; clearance is more prolonged with combined hepatic and renal dysfunction

Dosage
Geriatrics & Adults:
Hemodynamic support: I.V. infusion: 1-5 mcg/kg/minute up to 50 mcg/kg/minute, titrate to desired response; infusion may be increased by 1-4 mcg/kg/minute at 10- to 30-minute intervals until optimal response is obtained
Note: If dosages >20-30 mcg/kg/minute are needed, a more direct-acting vasopressor may be more beneficial (ie, epinephrine, norepinephrine).
Hemodynamic effects of dopamine are dose dependent:
Low-dose: 1-5 mcg/kg/minute, increased renal blood flow and urine output
Intermediate-dose: 5-15 mcg/kg/minute, increased renal blood flow, heart rate, cardiac contractility, and cardiac output
High-dose: >15 mcg/kg/minute, alpha-adrenergic effects begin to predominate, vasoconstriction, increased blood pressure

Administration Administer into large vein to prevent the possibility of extravasation; monitor continuously for free flow; use infusion device to control rate of flow; add
(Continued)

DOPamine *(Continued)*

200-400 mg to 250-500 mL of D_5W, NS, D_5NS, $D_5\frac{1}{2}NS$, D_5LR, LR, or Normosol® to dilute

Monitoring Parameters Urine output, cardiac hemodynamic status, blood pressure, EKG, pulse

Special Geriatric Considerations Has not been specifically studied in the elderly; monitor closely, especially due to increase in cardiovascular disease with age.

Dosage Forms Excipient information presented when available (limited, particularly for generics); consult specific product labeling.

Infusion, as hydrochloride [premixed in D_5W]: 0.8 mg/mL (250 mL, 500 mL); 1.6 mg/mL (250 mL, 500 mL); 3.2 mg/mL (250 mL)

Injection, solution, as hydrochloride: 40 mg/mL (5 mL, 10 mL); 80 mg/mL (5 mL); 160 mg/mL (5 mL) [contains sodium metabisulfite]

♦ **Dopamine Hydrochloride** *see* DOPamine *on page 468*
♦ **Doral**® *see* Quazepam *on page 1354*
♦ **Doryx**® *see* Doxycycline *on page 479*

Dorzolamide *(dor ZOLE a mide)*

Related Information
Glaucoma Drug Therapy *on page 1758*
U.S. Brand Names Trusopt®
Canadian Brand Names Trusopt®
Index Terms Dorzolamide Hydrochloride
Generic Available No
Pharmacologic Category Carbonic Anhydrase Inhibitor; Ophthalmic Agent, Antiglaucoma
Use Lowers intraocular pressure in patients with ocular hypertension or open-angle glaucoma
Contraindications Hypersensitivity to dorzolamide or any component of the formulation
Warnings/Precautions Although administered topically, systemic absorption occurs. Similar adverse reactions attributed to sulfonamides may occur with topical administration. Chemical similarities are present among sulfonamides, sulfonylureas, carbonic anhydrase inhibitors, thiazides, and loop diuretics (except ethacrynic acid). In patients with allergy to one of these compounds, a risk of cross-reaction exists; avoid use when previous reaction has been severe.

Because dorzolamide and its metabolite are excreted predominantly by the kidney, it is not recommended for use in patients with severe renal impairment (Cl_{cr} <30 mL/minute); use with caution in patients with hepatic impairment. Local ocular adverse effects (conjunctivitis and lid reactions) were reported with chronic administration. Many resolved with discontinuation of drug therapy. If such reactions occur, discontinue dorzolamide. Choriodal detachment has been reported after filtration procedures.

Inadvertent contamination of multiple-dose ophthalmic solutions, has caused bacterial keratitis. Contains benzalkonium chloride which may be absorbed by soft contact lenses. Dorzolamide should not be administered while wearing soft contact lenses.

Adverse Reactions (Reflective of adult population; not specific for elderly)
>10%:
Gastrointestinal: Bitter taste following administration (25%)
Ocular: Burning, stinging or discomfort immediately following administration (33%); superficial punctate keratitis (10% to 15%); signs and symptoms of ocular allergic reaction (10%)
1% to 5%: Ocular: Blurred vision, conjunctivitis, dryness, lid reactions, photophobia, tearing

Drug Interactions Substrate (minor) of CYP2C9, 3A4
Salicylates: High-dose salicylate therapy may result in carbonic anhydrase inhibitor accumulation and toxicity including CNS depression and metabolic acidosis; avoid use if possible.

Stability Store at room temperature (25°C).
Mechanism of Action Reversible inhibition of the enzyme carbonic anhydrase resulting in reduction of hydrogen ion secretion at renal tubule and an increased renal excretion of sodium, potassium, bicarbonate, and water to decrease production of aqueous humor; also inhibits carbonic anhydrase in central nervous system to retard abnormal and excessive discharge from CNS neurons

Pharmacodynamics
Onset of action: Peak effect: 2 hours
Duration: 8-12 hours

Pharmacokinetics
Absorption: Topical: Reaches systemic circulation where it accumulates in RBCs during chronic dosing as a result of binding to CA-11
Distribution: In RBCs during chronic administration
Protein binding: 33%
Metabolism: To N-desethyl metabolite (less potent than parent drug)
Half-life: Terminal RBC: 147 days; washes out of RBCs nonlinearly, resulting in a rapid decline of drug concentration initially, followed by a slower elimination phase with a half-life of about 4 months
Elimination: Urine (as unchanged drug and metabolite, N-desethyl)

Dosage
Geriatrics & Adults: Reduction of intraocular pressure: Ophthalmic: Instill 1 drop in the affected eye(s) 3 times/day

Administration See Patient Information.

Monitoring Parameters Ophthalmic exams and IOP periodically

Patient Information May sting on instillation; do not touch dropper to eye; visual acuity may be decreased after administration; distance vision may be altered; assess patient's or caregiver's ability to administer; apply gentle pressure to lacrimal sac during and immediately following instillation (1 minute) to avoid systemic absorption

Special Geriatric Considerations The oral carbonic anhydrase inhibitors are useful for patients who have difficulty administering ophthalmic drops, who do not achieve sufficient lowering of IOP, or who cannot tolerate other agents. Dorzolamide is an important addition that may be useful in the latter two groups, but with better tolerance than its oral counterpart.

Dosage Forms Excipient information presented when available (limited, particularly for generics); consult specific product labeling. [DSC] = Discontinued product
Solution, ophthalmic, as hydrochloride:
Trusopt®: 2% (5 mL [DSC]; 10 mL) [contains benzalkonium chloride]

Selected References
Biollaz J, Munafo A, Buclin T, et al, "Whole Blood Pharmacokinetics and Metabolic Affects of the Topical Carbonic Anhydrase Inhibitor Dorzolamide," *Eur J Clin Pharmacol,* 1995, 47(5):455-60.
Wilkerson M, Cyrlin M, Lippa EA, et al, "Four-Week Safety and Efficacy Study of Dorzolamide, a Novel, Active, Topical Carbonic Anhydrase Inhibitor," *Arch Ophthalmol,* 1993, 111(10):1343-50.

Dorzolamide and Timolol (dor ZOLE a mide & TYE moe lole)

Related Information
Dorzolamide *on page 470*
Timolol *on page 1571*
U.S. Brand Names Cosopt®
Canadian Brand Names Cosopt®; Preservative-Free Cosopt®
Index Terms Timolol and Dorzolamide
Generic Available No
Pharmacologic Category Beta-Adrenergic Blocker, Nonselective; Carbonic Anhydrase Inhibitor; Ophthalmic Agent, Antiglaucoma
Use Reduction of intraocular pressure in patints with ocular hypertension or open-angle glaucoma
Dosage
Geriatrics & Adults: Ocular hypertension or open-angle glaucoma: Ophthalmic: Instill 1 drop in affected eye(s) twice daily
Dosage Forms Excipient information presented when available (limited, particularly for generics); consult specific product labeling. [DSC] = Discontinued product
Solution, ophthalmic:
Cosopt®: Dorzolamide hydrochloride 2% (as base) and timolol maleate 0.5% (as base) (5 mL [DSC]; 10 mL) [contains benzalkonium chloride]

♦ **Dorzolamide Hydrochloride** *see* Dorzolamide *on page 470*
♦ **DOS® [OTC]** *see* Docusate *on page 459*
♦ **DOSS** *see* Docusate *on page 459*
♦ **Dovonex®** *see* Calcipotriene *on page 208*

Doxazosin (doks AY zoe sin)

Related Information
Pharmacotherapy of Urinary Incontinence *on page 1822*
Potentially Inappropriate Medications for Geriatrics *on page 1824*
Medication Safety Issues
Sound-alike/look-alike issues:
Doxazosin may be confused with doxapram, doxepin, DOXOrubicin
Cardura® may be confused with Cardene®, Cordarone®, Cordran®, Coumadin®, K-Dur®, Ridaura®
(Continued)

Doxazosin *(Continued)*

U.S. Brand Names Cardura®; Cardura® XL

Canadian Brand Names Alti-Doxazosin; Apo-Doxazosin®; Cardura-1™; Cardura-2™; Cardura-4™; Gen-Doxazosin; Novo-Doxazosin

Index Terms Doxazosin Mesylate

Generic Available Yes: Excludes extended release tablet

Pharmacologic Category Alpha$_1$ Blocker

Use Alpha-blocking agent for treatment of hypertension; treatment of symptoms of benign prostatic hyperplasia (BPH); can be used in combination with finasteride

Contraindications Hypersensitivity to quinazolines (prazosin, terazosin), doxazosin, or any component of the formulation

Warnings/Precautions Can cause significant orthostatic hypotension and syncope, especially with first dose; anticipate a similar effect if therapy is interrupted for a few days, if dosage is rapidly increased, or if another antihypertensive drug (particularly vasodilators) or a PDE5 inhibitor is introduced. Discontinue if symptoms of angina occur or worsen. Patients should be cautioned about performing hazardous tasks when starting new therapy or adjusting dosage upward. Prostate cancer should be ruled out before starting for BPH. Use with caution in mild to moderate hepatic impairment; not recommended in severe dysfunction. Intraoperative floppy iris syndrome has been observed in cataract surgery patients who were on or were previously treated with alpha$_1$-blockers. Causality has not been established and there appears to be no benefit in discontinuing alpha-blocker therapy prior to surgery.

The extended release formulation consists of drug within a nondeformable matrix; following drug release/absorption, the matrix/shell is expelled in the stool. The use of nondeformable products in patients with known stricture/narrowing of the GI tract has been associated with symptoms of obstruction. Use caution in patients with increased GI retention (eg, chronic constipation) as doxazosin exposure may be increased. Extended release formulation is not approved for the treatment of hypertension.

Adverse Reactions (Reflective of adult population; not specific for elderly)
Note: Type and frequency of adverse reactions reflect combined data from trials with immediate release and extended release products.

>10%: Central nervous system: Dizziness (5% to 19%), headache (5% to 14%)

1% to 10%:

Cardiovascular: Orthostatic hypotension (dose related; 0.3% up to 2%), edema (3% to 4%), hypotension (2%), palpitation (1% to 2%), chest pain (1% to 2%), arrhythmia (1%), syncope (2%), flushing (1%)

Central nervous system: Fatigue (8% to 12%), somnolence (1% to 5%), nervousness (2%), pain (2%), vertigo (2% to 4%), insomnia (1%), anxiety (1%), paresthesia (1%), movement disorder (1%), ataxia (1%), hypertonia (1%), depression (1%)

Dermatologic: Rash (1%), pruritus (1%)

Endocrine & metabolic: Sexual dysfunction (2%)

Gastrointestinal: Abdominal pain (2%), diarrhea (2%), dyspepsia (1% to 2%), nausea (1% to 3%), xerostomia (1% to 2%), constipation (1%), flatulence (1%)

Genitourinary: Urinary tract infection (1%), impotence (1%), polyuria (2%), incontinence (1%)

Neuromuscular & skeletal: Back pain (2% to 3%), weakness (1% to 7%), arthritis (1%), muscle weakness (1%), myalgia (≤1%), muscle cramps (1%)

Ocular: Abnormal vision (1% to 2%), conjunctivitis (1%)

Otic: Tinnitus (1%)

Respiratory: Respiratory tract infection (5%), rhinitis (3%), dyspnea (1% to 3%), respiratory disorder (1%), epistaxis (1%)

Miscellaneous: Diaphoresis increased (1%), flu-like syndrome (1%)

Overdosage/Toxicology Symptoms include severe hypotension, drowsiness, and tachycardia. Hypotension usually responds to I.V. fluids, Trendelenburg positioning, or a parenteral vasoconstrictor. Treatment is primarily supportive and symptomatic. Lavage, activated charcoal and fluids have shown to be effective. Dialysis not likely to benefit.

Drug Interactions

ACE inhibitors: Hypotensive effect (particularly orthostasis) may be increased.

Beta-blockers: Hypotensive effect may be increased.

Calcium channel blockers: Hypotensive effect may be increased.

Phosphodiesterase-5 (PDE5) inhibitors (eg, sildenafil, tadalafil, vardenafil): Blood pressure-lowering effects are additive. Use with caution and monitor.

Ethanol/Nutrition/Herb Interactions Herb/Nutraceutical: Avoid dong quai if using for hypertension (has estrogenic activity). Avoid ephedra, yohimbe, ginseng (may worsen hypertension). Avoid saw palmetto when used for BPH (due to limited experience with this combination). Avoid garlic (may have increased antihypertensive effect).

Mechanism of Action
Hypertension: Competitively inhibits postsynaptic alpha$_1$-adrenergic receptors which results in vasodilation of veins and arterioles and a decrease in total peripheral resistance and blood pressure; ~50% as potent on a weight by weight basis as prazosin.

BPH: Competitively inhibits postsynaptic alpha$_1$-adrenergic receptors in prostatic stromal and bladder neck tissues. This reduces the sympathetic tone-induced urethral stricture causing BPH symptoms.

Pharmacodynamics
Peak effect: Occurs 2-6 hours after a dose
Duration of effect: 24 hours

Pharmacokinetics
Increased age does not significantly affect pharmacokinetics of doxazosin. In studies of the extended-release tablets, the maximum plasma concentration was increased by 27% and the area under the curve was increased by 34% in the elderly.

Protein binding: Extended release: 98%

Metabolism: Extensively hepatic to active metabolites; primarily via CYP3A4; secondary pathways involve CYP2D6 and 2C19

Half-life elimination: 15-22 hours

Bioavailability: Extended release relative to immediate release: 54% to 59%

Time to peak, serum: Immediate release: 2-3 hours; extended release: 8-9 hours

Excretion: Feces (63% primarily as metabolites); urine (9%)

Dosage
Geriatrics: Immediate release: Oral: Initial: 0.5 mg once daily

Adults:

Hypertension: Oral: Immediate release: 1 mg once daily in morning or evening; may be increased to 2 mg once daily. Thereafter titrate upwards, if needed, over several weeks, balancing therapeutic benefit with doxazosin-induced postural hypotension. Maximum dose: 16 mg/day

BPH: Oral:

Immediate release: 1 mg once daily in morning or evening; may be increased to 2 mg once daily. Thereafter titrate upwards, if needed, over several weeks, balancing therapeutic benefit with doxazosin-induced postural hypotension. Goal: 4-8 mg/day; maximum dose: 8 mg/day

Extended release: 4 mg once daily with breakfast; titrate based on response and tolerability every 3-4 weeks to maximum recommended dose of 8 mg/day. Reinitiation of therapy: If therapy is discontinued for several days, restart at 4 mg dose and titrate as before.

Note: Conversion to extended release from immediate release: Initiate with 4 mg once daily; omit final evening dose of immediate release prior to starting morning dosing with extended release product.

Hepatic Impairment: Use with caution in mild-to-moderate hepatic dysfunction. Do not use with severe impairment.

Administration
Cardura ® XL: Tablets should be swallowed whole; do not crush, chew, or divide.

Monitoring Parameters
Blood pressure, standing and sitting/supine, urinary symptoms

Patient Information
Rise from sitting/lying carefully; may cause dizziness; take the first dose at bedtime. Do not crush or chew extended release forms, swallow whole. Tablet shell may be visible in the stool.

Additional Information
First-dose hypotension occurs less frequently with doxazosin as compared to prazosin; this may be due to its slower onset of action

Special Geriatric Considerations
Adverse reactions such as dry mouth and urinary problems can be particularly bothersome in the elderly. In studies of the extended-release tablets, the incidence of hypotension was higher in the elderly compared to younger patients.

Dosage Forms
Excipient information presented when available (limited, particularly for generics); consult specific product labeling.
Tablet: 1 mg, 2 mg, 4 mg, 8 mg
    Cardura®: 1 mg, 2 mg, 4 mg, 8 mg
Tablet, extended release:
    Cardura® XL: 4 mg, 8 mg

Selected References
McConnell JD, Roehrborn CG, Bautista OM, et al, "The Long-Term Effect of Doxazosin, Finasteride, and Combination Therapy on the Clinical Progression of Benign Prostatic Hyperplasia. Medical Therapy of Prostatic Symptoms (MTOPS) Research Group," N Engl J Med, 2003, 349(25):2387-98.

♦ Doxazosin Mesylate see Doxazosin on page 471

Doxepin (DOKS e pin)

Related Information
Antidepressant Agents on page 1742
Potentially Inappropriate Medications for Geriatrics on page 1824
(Continued)

Doxepin *(Continued)*

Medication Safety Issues

Sound-alike/look-alike issues:

Doxepin may be confused with digoxin, doxapram, doxazosin, Doxidan®, doxycycline

Sinequan® may be confused with saquinavir, Serentil®, Seroquel®, Singulair®

Zonalon® may be confused with Zone-A Forte®

International issues:

Doxal® [Finland] may be confused with Doxil® which is a brand name for doxorubicin in the U.S.

Doxal® [Finland]: Brand name for doxycycline in Austria; brand name for pyridoxine/thiamine in Brazil

U.S. Brand Names Prudoxin™; Sinequan® [DSC]; Zonalon®

Canadian Brand Names Apo-Doxepin®; Novo-Doxepin; Sinequan®; Zonalon®

Index Terms Doxepin Hydrochloride

Generic Available Yes: Capsule, solution

Pharmacologic Category Antidepressant, Tricyclic (Tertiary Amine); Topical Skin Product

Use

Oral: Treatment of various forms of depression, usually in conjunction with psychotherapy

Topical: Short-term (<8 days) management of moderate pruritus in adults with atopic dermatitis or lichen simplex chronicus

Unlabeled/Investigational Use Analgesic for certain chronic and neuropathic pain; treatment of anxiety

Restrictions An FDA-approved medication guide concerning the use of antidepressants in children, adolescents, and young adults must be distributed when dispensing an outpatient prescription (new or refill) where this medication is to be used without direct supervision of a healthcare provider. Medication guides are available at http://www.fda.gov/cder/Offices/ODS/medication_guides.htm. Dispense to parents or guardians of children and adolescents receiving this medication.

Contraindications Hypersensitivity to doxepin, drugs from similar chemical class, or any component of the formulation; narrow-angle glaucoma; urinary retention; use of MAO inhibitors within 14 days; use in a patient during acute recovery phase of MI

Warnings/Precautions [U.S. Boxed Warning]: Antidepressants increase the risk of suicidal thinking and behavior in children, adolescents, and young adults (18-24 years of age) with major depressive disorder (MDD) and other psychiatric disorders; consider risk prior to prescribing. Short-term studies did not show an increased risk in patients >24 years of age and showed a decreased risk in patients ≥65 years. Closely monitor for clinical worsening, suicidality, or unusual changes in behavior; the patient's family or caregiver should be instructed to closely observe the patient and communicate condition with healthcare provider. A medication guide should be dispensed with each prescription.

The possibility of a suicide attempt is inherent in major depression and may persist until remission occurs. Monitor for worsening of depression or suicidality, especially during initiation of therapy (generally first 1-2 months) or with dose increases or decreases. Use caution in high-risk patients. Worsening depression and severe abrupt suicidality that are not part of the presenting symptoms may require discontinuation or modification of drug therapy. The patient's family or caregiver should be alerted to monitor patients for the emergence of suicidality and associated behaviors (such as agitation, irritability, hostility, impulsivity, and hypomania) and call healthcare provider.

May worsen psychosis in some patients or precipitate a shift to mania or hypomania in patients with bipolar disorder. Patients presenting with depressive symptoms should be screened for bipolar disorder. Monotherapy in patients with bipolar disorder should be avoided. **Doxepin is not FDA approved for the treatment of bipolar depression.**

The risks of sedative and anticholinergic effects are high relative to other antidepressant agents. Doxepin frequently causes sedation, which may result in impaired performance of tasks requiring alertness (eg, operating machinery or driving). Sedative effects may be additive with other CNS depressants and/or ethanol. Also use caution in patients with benign prostatic hyperplasia, xerostomia, visual problems, constipation, or history of bowel obstruction.

May cause orthostatic hypotension or conduction disturbances (risks are moderate relative to other antidepressants). Use with caution in patients with a history of cardiovascular disease (including previous MI, stroke, tachycardia, or conduction abnormalities). Consider discontinuation, when possible, prior to elective surgery. Therapy should not be abruptly discontinued in patients receiving high doses for prolonged periods.

Use caution in patients with a previous seizure disorder or condition predisposing to seizures such as brain damage, alcoholism, or concurrent therapy with other drugs which lower the seizure threshold. Use with caution in hyperthyroid patients or those receiving thyroid supplementation. Use with caution in patients with hepatic or renal dysfunction and in elderly patients.

Cream formulation is for external use only (not for ophthalmic, vaginal, or oral use). Do not use occlusive dressings. Use for >8 days may increase risk of contact sensitization. Doxepin is significantly absorbed following topical administration; plasma levels may be similar to those achieved with oral administration.

Adverse Reactions (Reflective of adult population; not specific for elderly)
Oral: Frequency not defined.

Cardiovascular: Hyper-/hypotension, tachycardia

Central nervous system: Drowsiness, dizziness, headache, disorientation, ataxia, confusion, seizure

Dermatologic: Alopecia, photosensitivity, rash, pruritus

Endocrine & metabolic: Breast enlargement, galactorrhea, SIADH, ¡blood sugar increased/decreased, libido increased/decreased

Gastrointestinal: Xerostomia, constipation, vomiting, indigestion, anorexia, aphthous stomatitis, nausea, unpleasant taste, weight gain, diarrhea, trouble with gums, lower esophageal sphincter tone decrease may cause GE reflux

Genitourinary: Urinary retention, testicular edema

Hematologic: Agranulocytosis, leukopenia, eosinophilia, thrombocytopenia, purpura

Neuromuscular & skeletal: Weakness, tremor, numbness, paresthesia, extrapyramidal symptoms, tardive dyskinesia

Ocular: Blurred vision

Otic: Tinnitus

Miscellaneous: Diaphoresis (excessive), allergic reactions

Topical:
>10%:

   Central nervous system: Drowsiness (22%)

   Dermatologic: Stinging/burning (23%)

1% to 10%:

   Cardiovascular: Edema: (1%)

   Central nervous system: Dizziness (2%), emotional changes (2%)

   Gastrointestinal: Xerostomia (10%), taste alteration (2%)

Overdosage/Toxicology
Symptoms include confusion, hallucinations, seizures, urinary retention, hypothermia, hypotension, tachycardia, and cyanosis. Following initiation of essential overdose management, toxic symptoms should be treated. Sodium bicarbonate is indicated when the QRS interval is >0.10 seconds or the QT_c interval is >0.42 seconds. Ventricular arrhythmias often respond to systemic alkalinization with or without phenytoin 15-20 mg/kg (sodium bicarbonate 0.5-2 mEq/kg I.V.). Arrhythmias unresponsive to this therapy may respond to lidocaine 1 mg/kg I.V. followed by a titrated infusion. Physostigmine (1-2 mg slow I.V.) may be indicated in reversing life-threatening cardiac arrhythmias. Seizures usually respond to diazepam I.V. boluses (5-10 mg up to 30 mg). If seizures are unresponsive or recur, phenytoin or phenobarbital may be required.

Drug Interactions
Substrate (major) of CYP1A2, 2D6, 3A4

Altretamine: Concurrent use may cause orthostatic hypertension.

Amphetamines: TCAs may enhance the effect of amphetamines; monitor for adverse CV effects.

Anticholinergics: Combined use with TCAs may produce additive anticholinergic effects

Antihypertensives: TCAs may inhibit the antihypertensive response to bethanidine, clonidine, debrisoquin, guanadrel, guanethidine, guanabenz, guanfacine; monitor BP; consider alternate antihypertensive agent.

Beta-agonists (nonselective): When combined with TCAs may predispose patients to cardiac arrhythmias.

Bupropion: May increase the levels of tricyclic antidepressants; based on limited information; monitor response.

Carbamazepine: Tricyclic antidepressants may increase carbamazepine levels; monitor.

Cholestyramine and colestipol: May bind TCAs and reduce their absorption; monitor for altered response.

Clonidine: Abrupt discontinuation of clonidine may cause hypertensive crisis, amitriptyline may enhance the response.

CNS depressants: Sedative effects may be additive with TCAs; monitor for increased effect; includes benzodiazepines, barbiturates, antipsychotics, ethanol and other sedative medications.

CYP1A2 inducers: May decrease the levels/effects of doxepin. Example inducers include aminoglutethimide, carbamazepine, phenobarbital, and rifampin.

(Continued)

Doxepin *(Continued)*

CYP1A2 inhibitors: May increase the levels/effects of doxepin. Example inhibitors include ciprofloxacin, fluvoxamine, ketoconazole, norfloxacin, ofloxacin, and rofecoxib.

CYP2D6 inhibitors: May increase the levels/effects of doxepin. Example inhibitors include chlorpromazine, delavirdine, fluoxetine, miconazole, paroxetine, pergolide, quinidine, quinine, ritonavir, and ropinirole.

CYP3A4 inducers: CYP3A4 inducers may decrease the levels/effects of doxepin. Example inducers include aminoglutethimide, carbamazepine, nafcillin, nevirapine, phenobarbital, phenytoin, and rifamycins.

CYP3A4 inhibitors: May increase the levels/effects of doxepin. Example inhibitors include azole antifungals, clarithromycin, diclofenac, doxycycline, erythromycin, imatinib, isoniazid, nefazodone, nicardipine, propofol, protease inhibitors, quinidine, telithromycin, and verapamil.

Epinephrine (and other direct alpha-agonists): Pressor response to I.V. epinephrine, norepinephrine, and phenylephrine may be enhanced in patients receiving TCAs. (**Note:** Effect is unlikely with epinephrine or levonordefrin dosages typically administered as infiltration in combination with local anesthetics.)

Fenfluramine: May increase tricyclic antidepressant levels/effects.

Hypoglycemic agents (including insulin): TCAs may enhance the hypoglycemic effects of tolazamide, chlorpropamide, or insulin; monitor for changes in blood glucose levels; reported with chlorpropamide, tolazamide, and insulin.

Levodopa: Tricyclic antidepressants may decrease the absorption (bioavailability) of levodopa; rare hypertensive episodes have also been attributed to this combination.

Linezolid: Hyperpyrexia, hypertension, tachycardia, confusion, seizures, and **deaths have been reported** with agents which inhibit MAO (serotonin syndrome); this combination should be avoided.

Lithium: Concurrent use with a TCA may increase the risk for neurotoxicity.

MAO inhibitors: Hyperpyrexia, hypertension, tachycardia, confusion, seizures, and **deaths have been reported** (serotonin syndrome); this combination is contraindicated.

Methylphenidate: Metabolism of TCAs may be decreased.

Phenothiazines: Serum concentrations of some TCAs may be increased; in addition, TCAs may increase concentration of phenothiazines; monitor for altered clinical response.

QT_c-prolonging agents: Concurrent use of tricyclic agents with other drugs which may prolong QT_c interval may increase the risk of potentially fatal arrhythmias; includes type Ia and type III antiarrhythmics agents, selected quinolones (moxifloxacin), cisapride, and other agents.

Ritonavir: Combined use of high-dose tricyclic antidepressants with ritonavir may cause serotonin syndrome in HIV-positive patients; monitor.

Sucralfate: Absorption of tricyclic antidepressants may be reduced with coadministration.

Sympathomimetics, indirect-acting: Tricyclic antidepressants may result in a decreased sensitivity to indirect-acting sympathomimetics; includes dopamine and ephedrine; also see interaction with epinephrine (and direct-acting sympathomimetics).

Tramadol: Tramadol's risk of seizures may be increased with TCAs.

Valproic acid: May increase serum concentrations/adverse effects of some tricyclic antidepressants.

Warfarin (and other oral anticoagulants): TCAs may increase the anticoagulant effect in patients stabilized on warfarin; monitor INR.

Ethanol/Nutrition/Herb Interactions

Ethanol: Avoid ethanol (may increase CNS depression).

Food: Grapefruit juice may inhibit the metabolism of some TCAs and clinical toxicity may result.

Herb/Nutraceutical: Avoid valerian, St John's wort, SAMe, kava kava (may increase risk of serotonin syndrome and/or excessive sedation).

Stability Protect from light.

Mechanism of Action Increases the synaptic concentration of serotonin and norepinephrine in the central nervous system by inhibition of their reuptake by the presynaptic neuronal membrane

Pharmacodynamics Onset of action: Peak effect: Antidepressant: Usually >2 weeks; Anxiolytic: may occur sooner; 5-HT >NE

Pharmacokinetics

Absorption: Following topical application, plasma levels may be similar to those achieved with oral administration

Distribution: Crosses placenta; enters breast milk

Protein binding: 80% to 85%

Metabolism: Hepatic; metabolites include desmethyldoxepin (active)

Half-life: 6-8 hours

Elimination: Renal
Dosage
Geriatrics:
Depression and/or anxiety (unlabeled use): Oral: Initial: 10-25 mg at bedtime; increase by 10-25 mg every 3 days for inpatients and weekly for outpatients if tolerated. Rarely does the maximum dose required exceed 75 mg/day; a single bedtime dose is recommended.

Pruritus: Topical: Refer to adult dosing.
Adults:
Depression and/or anxiety (unlabeled use): Oral: Initial: 25-150 mg/day at bedtime or in 2-3 divided doses; may gradually increase up to 300 mg/day; single dose should not exceed 150 mg; select patients may respond to 25-50 mg/day.

Chronic urticaria, angioedema, nocturnal pruritus: Oral: 10-30 mg/day

Pruritus: Topical: Apply a thin film 4 times/day with at least 3- to 4-hour interval between applications; not recommended for use >8 days. (Oral administration of doxepin 25-50 mg has also been used, but systemic adverse effects are increased.)

Hepatic Impairment: Use a lower dose and adjust gradually.
Administration
Oral: Do not mix oral concentrate with carbonated beverages (physically incompatible).
Topical: Apply thin film to affected area; use of occlusive dressings is not recommended.

Monitoring Parameters May need to use serum concentrations to help monitor response; monitor blood pressure and pulse rate prior to and during initial therapy; monitor mental status, weight; EKG in older adults; adverse effects may be increased if topical formulation is applied to >10% of body surface area

Reference Range Proposed therapeutic concentration (doxepin plus desmethyldoxepin): 110-250 ng/mL. Toxic concentration (doxepin plus desmethyldoxepin): >500 ng/mL. Utility of serum level monitoring is controversial.

Test Interactions Increased glucose

Patient Information Avoid unnecessary exposure to sunlight; avoid alcohol ingestion; do not discontinue medication abruptly; may cause urine to turn blue-green; may cause drowsiness, dry mouth, sedation, urinary retention, blurred vision; rise slowly to prevent dizziness

Additional Information Entire daily dose may be given at bedtime; avoid unnecessary exposure to sunlight

Special Geriatric Considerations The oral form is the preferred agent when sedation is a desired property. Less potential for anticholinergic effects than amitriptyline and less orthostatic hypotension than imipramine. However, dosing should be approached cautiously, initiated at the low end of the dosage range. The pharmacokinetics of doxepin have not been studied in elderly patients. Data from a clinical trial comparing fluoxetine to tricyclics suggest that fluoxetine is significantly less effective than nortriptyline in hospitalized elderly patients with unipolar major affective disorder, especially those with melancholia and concurrent cardiovascular disease.

Dosage Forms Excipient information presented when available (limited, particularly for generics); consult specific product labeling. [DSC] = Discontinued product

Capsule, as hydrochloride: 10 mg, 25 mg, 50 mg, 75 mg, 100 mg, 150 mg
Sinequan®: 10 mg, 25 mg, 50 mg, 75 mg, 100 mg, 150 mg [DSC]
Cream, as hydrochloride:
Prudoxin™: 5% (45 g) [contains benzyl alcohol]
Zonalon®: 5% (30 g, 45 g) [contains benzyl alcohol]
Solution, oral concentrate, as hydrochloride: 10 mg/mL (120 mL)
Sinequan®: 10 mg/mL (120 mL) [DSC]

Selected References
Lakshmanan M, Mion LC, and Frengley JD, "Effective Low Dose Tricyclic Antidepressant Treatment for Depressed Geriatric Rehabilitation Patients. A Double-Blind Study," *J Am Geriatr Soc*, 1986, 34(6):421-6.
Roose SP, Glassman AH, Attia E, et al, "Comparative Efficacy of Selective Serotonin Reuptake Inhibitors and Tricyclics in the Treatment of Melancholia," *Am J Psychiatry*, 1994, 151(12):1735-9.

♦ **Doxepin Hydrochloride** see Doxepin on page 473

Doxercalciferol (doks er kal si fe FEER ole)

U.S. Brand Names Hectorol®
Canadian Brand Names Hectorol®
Index Terms 1α-Hydroxyergocalciferol
Generic Available No
Pharmacologic Category Vitamin D Analog
Use Treatment of secondary hyperparathyroidism in patients with chronic kidney disease
Contraindications Hypersensitivity to any component of the formulation; history of hypercalcemia or evidence of vitamin D toxicity
(Continued)

Doxercalciferol *(Continued)*

Warnings/Precautions Other forms of vitamin D should be discontinued when doxercalciferol is started. Overdose from vitamin D may lead to progressive hypercalcemia and needs to be avoided. Careful dosage titration and monitoring can minimize risk. Hyperphosphatemia exacerbates secondary hyperparathyroidism, diminishing the effect of doxercalciferol. Hyperphosphatemia should be corrected before initiating therapy. Use with caution in patients with hepatic impairment. Injection is intended for I.V. use only.

Adverse Reactions (Reflective of adult population; not specific for elderly)
Note: As reported in dialysis patients.
>10%:
Cardiovascular: Edema (34%)
Central nervous system: Headache (28%), malaise (28%), dizziness (12%)
Gastrointestinal: Nausea/vomiting (24%)
Respiratory: Dyspnea (12%)
1% to 10%:
Cardiovascular: Bradycardia (7%)
Central nervous system: Sleep disorder (3%)
Dermatologic: Pruritus (8%)
Gastrointestinal: Anorexia (5%), constipation (3%), dyspepsia (5%), weight gain (5%)
Neuromuscular & skeletal: Arthralgia (5%)
Miscellaneous: Abscess (3%)

Overdosage/Toxicology Doxercalciferol, in excess, can cause hypercalcemia, hypercalciuria, hyperphosphatemia, and oversuppression of PTH secretion. Following withdrawal of the drug and calcium supplements, hypercalcemia treatment consists of a low calcium diet and monitoring. Adjustments of calcium in the dialysis bath can also be made if necessary. When calcium levels normalize, doxercalciferol can be restarted. Reduce each dose by at least 2.5 mcg. Monitor serum calcium levels closely.

Signs and symptoms of early hypercalcemia include: Anorexia, bone pain, constipation, headache, metallic taste, muscle pain, nausea, somnolence, vomiting, weakness, xerostomia

Signs and symptoms of late hypercalcemia include: Albuminuria, anorexia, apathy, AST/ALT increased, BUN increased, cardiac arrhythmias, conjunctivitis (calcific), dehydration, ectopic calcification, growth arrested, hypercholesterolemia, hypertension, hyperthermia, libido decreased, nocturia, pancreatitis, photophobia, polydipsia, polyuria, pruritus, psychosis (rare), rhinorrhea, sensory disturbances, urinary tract infections, weight loss

Drug Interactions
Decreased effect: Cholestyramine, mineral oil (both reduce absorption)
Increased toxicity: Concurrent use of other vitamin D supplements, magnesium-containing antacids and supplements (hypermagnesemia)

Stability Store at controlled room temperature of 15°C to 30°C (59°F to 86°F). Protect injection from light.

Mechanism of Action Doxercalciferol is metabolized to the active form of vitamin D. The active form of vitamin D controls the intestinal absorption of dietary calcium, the tubular reabsorption of calcium by the kidneys, and in conjunction with PTH, the mobilization of calcium from the skeleton.

Pharmacokinetics
Metabolism: Hepatic
Half-life: Active metabolite: 32-37 hours; up to 96 hours

Dosage
Geriatrics & Adults: Secondary hyperparathyroidism:
Oral:
Dialysis patients: Dose should be titrated to lower iPTH to 150-300 pg/mL; dose is adjusted at 8-week intervals (maximum dose: 20 mcg 3 times/week)
Initial dose: iPTH >400 pg/mL: 10 mcg 3 times/week at dialysis
Dose titration:
iPTH level decreased by 50% and >300 pg/mL: Dose can be increased to 12.5 mcg 3 times/week for 8 more weeks; this titration process can continue at 8-week intervals; each increase should be by 2.5 mcg/dose
iPTH level 150-300 pg/mL: Maintain current dose
iPTH level <100 pg/mL: Suspend doxercalciferol for 1 week; resume at a reduced dose; decrease each dose (not weekly dose) by at least 2.5 mcg
Predialysis patients: Dose should be titrated to lower iPTH to 35-70 pg/mL with stage 3 disease or to 70-110 pg/mL with stage 4 disease: Dose may be adjusted at 2-week intervals (maximum dose: 3.5 mcg/day)
Initial dose: 1 mcg/day

Dose titration:

iPTH level >70 pg/mL with stage 3 disease or >110 pg/mL with stage 4 disease: Increase dose by 0.5 mcg every 2 weeks as necessary

iPTH level 35-70 pg/mL with stage 3 disease or 70-110 pg/mL with stage 4 disease: Maintain current dose

iPTH level is <35 pg/mL with stage 3 disease or <70 pg/mL with stage 4 disease: Suspend doxercalciferol for 1 week, then resume at a reduced dose (at least 0.5 mcg lower)

I.V.:

Dialysis patients: Dose should be titrated to lower iPTH to 150-300 pg/mL; dose is adjusted at 8-week intervals (maximum dose: 18 mcg/week)

Initial dose: iPTH level >400 pg/mL: 4 mcg 3 times/week after dialysis, administered as a bolus dose

Dose titration:

iPTH level decreased by <50% and >300 pg/mL: Dose can be increased by 1-2 mcg at 8-week intervals, as necessary

iPTH level decreased by >50% and >300 pg/mL: Maintain current dose

iPTH level 150-300 pg/mL: Maintain the current dose

iPTH level <100 pg/mL: Suspend doxercalciferol for 1 week; resume at a reduced dose (at least 1 mcg lower)

Renal Impairment: No adjustment is required.

Hepatic Impairment: Use caution in these patients; no guidelines for dosage adjustment.

Monitoring Parameters

Dialysis patients: Before initiating, check iPTH, serum calcium, and phosphorus. Check weekly thereafter until stable. Serum iPTH, calcium, phosphorus, and alkaline phosphatase should be monitored.

Predialysis patients: iPTH, serum calcium and phosphorus every 2 weeks for 3 months following initiation and dose adjustments, then monthly for 3 months, then every 3 months

Reference Range Serum calcium times phosphorus product should be <70

Patient Information Be clear on dose and directions for taking. Stop other vitamin D products. Do not miss doses. Avoid magnesium-containing antacids and supplements. Report headache, dizziness, weakness, sleepiness, severe nausea, vomiting, difficulty thinking, or concentrating to your healthcare provider. Do not take over-the-counter medicines or supplements without first consulting your healthcare provider. Follow diet and calcium supplements as directed by your healthcare provider.

Special Geriatric Considerations No special changes in dose are required. Caution should be used in the elderly using magnesium products (MOM, magnesium containing antacids, etc). These should be stopped if possible before initiating doxercalciferol.

Dosage Forms Excipient information presented when available (limited, particularly for generics); consult specific product labeling.

Capsule, softgel:

Hectorol®: 0.5 mcg, 2.5 mcg [contains coconut oil]

Injection, solution:

Hectorol®: 2 mcg/mL (2 mL) [contains disodium edetate]

♦ **Doxidan® [OTC]** *see* Bisacodyl *on page 173*

♦ **Doxy-100®** *see* Doxycycline *on page 479*

Doxycycline (doks i SYE kleen)

Medication Safety Issues

Sound-alike/look-alike issues:

Doxycycline may be confused with dicyclomine, doxepin, doxylamine

Doxy-100® may be confused with Doxil®

Monodox® may be confused with Maalox®

U.S. Brand Names Adoxa®; Doryx®; Doxy-100®; Monodox®; Oracea™; Periostat®; Vibramycin®; Vibra-Tabs®

Canadian Brand Names Apo-Doxy®; Apo-Doxy Tabs®; Doxycin; Doxytec; Novo-Doxylin; Nu-Doxycycline; Periostat®; Vibra-Tabs®

Index Terms Doxycycline Calcium; Doxycycline Hyclate; Doxycycline Monohydrate

Generic Available Yes: Excludes capsule (variable release), powder for oral solution, syrup

Pharmacologic Category Antibiotic, Tetracycline Derivative

Use Principally in the treatment of infections caused by susceptible *Rickettsia*, *Chlamydia*, and *Mycoplasma*; alternative to mefloquine for malaria prophylaxis; treatment for syphilis, uncomplicated *Neisseria gonorrhoeae*, *Listeria*, *Actinomyces israelii*, and *Clostridium* infections in penicillin-allergic patients; used for community-acquired pneumonia and other common infections due to susceptible organisms; anthrax due to (Continued)

Doxycycline *(Continued)*

Bacillus anthracis, including inhalational anthrax (postexposure); treatment of infections caused by uncommon susceptible gram-negative and gram-positive organisms including *Borrelia recurrentis, Ureaplasma urealyticum, Haemophilus ducreyi, Yersinia pestis, Francisella tularensis, Vibrio cholerae, Campylobacter fetus, Brucella* spp, *Bartonella bacilliformis*, and *Calymmatobacterium granulomatis*; treatment of inflammatory lesions associated with rosacea

Unlabeled/Investigational Use Sclerosing agent for pleural effusion injection; treatment of vancomycin-resistant enterococci (VRE)

Contraindications Hypersensitivity to doxycycline, tetracycline, or any component of the formulation; severe hepatic dysfunction

Warnings/Precautions Prolonged use may result in fungal or bacterial superinfection, including *C. difficile*-associated diarrhea and pseudomembranous colitis. Photosensitivity reaction may occur with this drug; avoid prolonged exposure to sunlight or tanning equipment. Antianabolic effects of tetracyclines can increase BUN (dose-related). Autoimmune syndromes have been reported. Hepatotoxicity rarely occurs: if symptomatic, conduct LFT and discontinue drug. Tetracyclines have been associated with pseudotumor cerebri.

Additional specific warnings: Periostat®: Effectiveness has not been established in patients with coexistent oral candidiasis; use with caution in patients with a history or predisposition to oral candidiasis. Oracea™: Should not be used for the treatment or prophylaxis of bacterial infections, since the lower dose of drug per capsule may be subefficacious and promote resistance.

Adverse Reactions (Reflective of adult population; not specific for elderly)
Frequency not defined.

Cardiovascular: Intracranial hypertension, pericarditis

Dermatologic: Angioneurotic edema, exfoliative dermatitis (rare), photosensitivity, rash, skin hyperpigmentation, urticaria

Endocrine & metabolic: Brown/black discoloration of thyroid gland (no dysfunction reported)

Gastrointestinal: Anorexia, diarrhea, dysphagia, enterocolitis, esophagitis (rare), esophageal ulcerations (rare), glossitis, inflammatory lesions in anogenital region, nausea, oral (mucosal) pigmentation, pseudomembranous colitis, tooth discoloration (children), vomiting

Hematologic: Eosinophilia, hemolytic anemia, neutropenia, thrombocytopenia

Hepatic: Hepatotoxicity

Renal: BUN increased (dose related)

Miscellaneous: Anaphylactoid purpura, anaphylaxis, bulging fontanels (infants), serum sickness, SLE exacerbation

Note: Adverse effects in clinical trials with Periostat® occurring at a frequency more than 1% greater than placebo included nausea, dyspepsia, joint pain, diarrhea, menstrual cramp, and pain.

Overdosage/Toxicology Symptoms include nausea, anorexia, and diarrhea. Following GI decontamination, care is supportive only. Fluid support may be required for hypotension.

Drug Interactions Substrate of CYP3A4 (major); **Inhibits** CYP3A4 (moderate)

Antacids (containing aluminum, calcium, or magnesium): Decreased absorption of tetracyclines

Barbiturates: May decrease the level/effect of doxycycline.

Bile acid sequestrants: May decrease the absorption of tetracycline derivatives.

Bismuth: May decrease the absorption of tetracycline derivatives.

Bismuth subsalicylate: May decrease the absorption of tetracycline derivatives.

Carbamazepine: May decrease the level/effect of doxycycline.

Coumarin derivatives: Tetracycline derivatives may enhance the anticoagulant effect of coumarin derivatives.

CYP3A4 inducers: CYP3A4 inducers may decrease the levels/effects of doxycycline. Example inducers include aminoglutethimide, carbamazepine, nafcillin, nevirapine, phenobarbital, phenytoin, and rifamycins.

CYP3A4 substrates: Doxycycline may increase the levels/effects of CYP3A4 substrates. Example substrates include benzodiazepines, calcium channel blockers, mirtazapine, nateglinide, nefazodone, tacrolimus, and venlafaxine. Selected benzodiazepines (midazolam and triazolam), cisapride, ergot alkaloids, selected HMG-CoA reductase inhibitors (lovastatin and simvastatin), and pimozide are generally contraindicated with strong CYP3A4 inhibitors.

Iron-containing products: Decreased absorption of tetracyclines.

Magnesium salts (oral): May decrease the absorption of tetracycline derivatives (oral).

Methotrexate: Tetracycline derivatives may increase the serum concentration of methotrexate.

Methoxyflurane: Concomitant use may cause fatal renal toxicity. Avoid concurrent use.

Penicillins: Tetracycline derivatives may diminish the therapeutic effect of penicillins.

Phenytoin: May decrease the level/effect of doxycycline.

Pimecrolimus: Doxycycline may decrease the metabolism, via CYP isoenzymes, of pimecrolimus.

Quinapril: May decrease the absorption of tetracycline derivatives.

Retinoic acid derivatives: Tetracycline derivatives may enhance the adverse/toxic effect of retinoic acid derivatives. The development of pseudotumor cerebri is of particular concern.

Typhoid vaccine: Antibiotics may diminish the therapeutic effect of typhoid vaccine. Only the live attenuated Ty21a strain is affected.

Ethanol/Nutrition/Herb Interactions

Ethanol: Chronic ethanol ingestion may reduce the serum concentration of doxycycline.

Food: Doxycycline serum levels may be slightly decreased if taken with food or milk. Administration with iron or calcium may decrease doxycycline absorption. May decrease absorption of calcium, iron, magnesium, zinc, and amino acids.

Herb/Nutraceutical: St John's wort may decrease doxycycline levels. Avoid dong quai, St John's wort (may also cause photosensitization).

Stability

Capsule, tablet: Store at controlled room temperature 15°C to 30°C (59°F to 86°F); protect from light

I.V. infusion: Following reconstitution with sterile water for injection, dilute to a final concentration of 0.1-1 mg/mL using a compatible solution. Solutions for I.V. infusion may be prepared using 0.9% sodium chloride, D_5W, Ringer's injection, lactated Ringer's, D_5LR. Protect from light. Stability varies based on solution.

Mechanism of Action Inhibits protein synthesis by binding with the 30S and possibly the 50S ribosomal subunit(s) of susceptible bacteria; may also cause alterations in the cytoplasmic membrane

Periostat® capsules (proposed mechanism): Has been shown to inhibit collagenase activity *in vitro*. Also has been noted to reduce elevated collagenase activity in the gingival crevicular fluid of patients with periodontal disease. Systemic levels do not reach inhibitory concentrations against bacteria.

Pharmacokinetics

Absorption: Almost completely from GI tract; can be reduced by food or milk by 20%

Protein binding: 90%

Metabolism: Not metabolized in the liver, instead partially inactivated in GI tract by chelate formation

Half-life: 12-15 hours (usually increases to 22-24 hours with multiple dosing); may be slightly increased and serum and tissue concentrations have been reported to be higher in older adults

Time to peak serum concentration: Within 1.5-4 hours

Elimination: Urine (23%), feces (30%)

Dosage

Geriatrics & Adults:

Usual dosage range: Oral, I.V.: 100-200 mg/day in 1-2 divided doses

Anthrax:

Inhalational (postexposure prophylaxis): Oral, I.V. (use oral route when possible): 100 mg every 12 hours for 60 days (*MMWR*, 2001, 50:889-93); **Note:** Preliminary recommendation, FDA review and update is anticipated.

Cutaneous (treatment): Oral: 100 mg every 12 hours for 60 days. **Note:** In the presence of systemic involvement, extensive edema, lesions on head/neck, refer to I.V. dosing for treatment of inhalational/gastrointestinal/oropharyngeal anthrax

Inhalational/gastrointestinal/oropharyngeal (treatment): I.V.: Initial: 100 mg every 12 hours; switch to oral therapy when clinically appropriate; some recommend initial loading dose of 200 mg, followed by 100 mg every 8-12 hours (*JAMA*, 1997, 278:399-411).

Note: Initial treatment should include two or more agents predicted to be effective (per CDC recommendations). Agents suggested for use in conjunction with doxycycline or ciprofloxacin include rifampin, vancomycin, imipenem, penicillin, ampicillin, chloramphenicol, clindamycin, and clarithromycin. May switch to oral antimicrobial therapy when clinically appropriate. Continue combined therapy for 60 days.

Brucellosis: Oral: 100 mg twice daily for 6 weeks with rifampin or streptomycin

Chlamydial infections, uncomplicated: Oral: 100 mg twice daily for ≥7 days

Community-acquired pneumonia, bronchitis: Oral, I.V.: 100 mg twice daily

Endometritis, salpingitis, parametritis, or peritonitis: I.V.: 100 mg twice daily with cefoxitin 2 g every 6 hours for 4 days and for ≥48 hours after patient improves; then continue with oral therapy 100 mg twice daily to complete a 10- to 14-day course of therapy

Gonococcal infection, acute (PID) in combination with another antibiotic: I.V.: 100 mg every 12 hours until improved, followed by 100 mg orally twice daily to complete 14 days

(Continued)

Doxycycline *(Continued)*

Lyme disease, Q fever, or Tularemia: Oral: 100 mg twice daily for 14-21 days

Malaria prophylaxis: 100 mg/day. Start 1-2 days prior to travel to endemic area; continue daily during travel and for 4 weeks after leaving endemic area

Nongonococcal urethritis: Oral: 100 mg twice daily for 7 days

Periodontitis: Oral (Periostat®): 20 mg twice daily as an adjunct following scaling and root planing; may be administered for up to 9 months. Safety beyond 12 months of treatment and efficacy beyond 9 months of treatment have not been established.

Rickettsial disease or ehrlichiosis: Oral, I.V.: 100 mg twice daily for 7-14 days

Rosacea: (Oracea™): Oral: 40 mg once daily in the morning

Sclerosing agent for pleural effusion injection (unlabeled use): Irrigation: 500 mg as a single dose in 30-50 mL of NS or SWI

Syphilis:

Early syphilis: Oral, I.V.: 200 mg/day in divided doses for 14 days

Late syphilis: Oral, I.V.: 200 mg/day in divided doses for 28 days

Yersinia pestis (plague): Oral: 100 mg twice daily for 7 days

Vibrio cholerae: Oral: 300 mg as a single dose

Renal Impairment: No adjustment necessary.

Not dialyzable; 0% to 5% by hemo- and peritoneal methods or by continuous arterio-venous or venovenous hemofiltration; supplemental dose is not necessary.

Administration

Oral: May give with meals to decrease GI upset. Capsule and tablet: Administer with at least 8 ounces of water and have patient sit up for at least 30 minutes after taking to reduce the risk of esophageal irritation and ulceration.

Oracea™: Take on an empty stomach 1 hour before or 2 hours after meals.

Doryx®: May be administered by carefully breaking up the tablet and sprinkling tablet contents on a spoonful of applesauce. The delayed release pellets must not be crushed or damaged when breaking up tablet. Should be administered immediately after preparation and without chewing.

I.V.: Infuse I.V. doxycycline over 1-4 hours; avoid extravasation

Monitoring Parameters Signs and symptoms of infection including mental status; blood glucose in diabetics

Test Interactions False elevations of urine catecholamine levels; false-negative urine glucose using Clinistix®, Tes-Tape®

Patient Information Avoid unnecessary exposure to sunlight; do not take with antacids, iron products, or dairy products; complete full course of therapy

Special Geriatric Considerations Dose adjustment for renal function is not necessary.

Dosage Forms Excipient information presented when available (limited, particularly for generics); consult specific product labeling. [DSC] = Discontinued product

Note: Strength expressed as base.

Capsule, as hyclate: 50 mg, 100 mg

Vibramycin®: 100 mg

Capsule, as monohydrate: 50 mg, 100 mg

Monodox®: 50 mg, 100 mg

Capsule, variable release:

Oracea™: 40 mg [30 mg (immediate-release) and 10 mg (delayed-release)]

Injection, powder for reconstitution, as hyclate: 100 mg

Doxy-100®: 100 mg

Powder for oral suspension, as monohydrate:

Vibramycin®: 25 mg/5 mL (60 mL) [raspberry flavor]

Syrup, as calcium:

Vibramycin®: 50 mg/5 mL (480 mL) [contains sodium metabisulfite; raspberry-apple flavor]

Tablet, as hyclate: 20 mg, 100 mg

Periostat®: 20 mg

Vibra-Tabs®: 100 mg

Tablet, as monohydrate: 50 mg, 75 mg, 100 mg, 150 mg

Adoxa®: 50 mg, 75 mg, 100 mg

Adoxa® Pak™ 1/75 [unit-dose pack]: 75 mg (31s)

Adoxa® Pak™ 1/100 [unit-dose pack]: 100 mg (31s)

Adoxa® Pak™ 1/150 [unit-dose pack]: 150 mg (30s)

Adoxa® Pak™ 2/100 [unit-dose pack]: 100 mg (60s)

Tablet, delayed-release coated pellets, as hyclate:

Doryx®: 75 mg [contains sodium 4.5 mg (0.196 mEq)], 100 mg [contains sodium 6 mg (0.261 mEq)]

Selected References

Böcker R, Mühlberg W, Platt D, et al, "Serum Level, Half-Life and Apparent Volume of Distribution of Doxycycline in Geriatric Patients," *Eur J Clin Pharmacol*, 1986, 30(1):105-8.

Centers for Disease Control and Prevention, "1998 Guidelines for Treatment of Sexually Transmitted Diseases," *MMWR*, 1998, 47(RR-1):1-111.

Centers for Disease Control and Prevention, "Update: Investigation of Anthrax Associated With Intentional Exposure and Interim Public Health Guidelines, October 2001," *MMWR*, 2001, 50(41):889-93. Accessed October 19, 2001, at http://www.cdc.gov/mmwr/preview/mmwrhtml/mm5041a1.htm.

Ljungberg B and Nilsson-Ehle I, "Pharmacokinetics of Antimicrobial Agents in the Elderly," *Rev Infect Dis*, 1987, 9(2):250-64.

♦ **Doxycycline Calcium** *see* Doxycycline *on page 479*
♦ **Doxycycline Hyclate** *see* Doxycycline *on page 479*

Doxycycline Hyclate Periodontal Extended-Release Liquid
(doks i SYE kleen HI klayt per ee oh DON tal ik STEN did ri LES LIK wid)

U.S. Brand Names Atridox™
Canadian Brand Names Atridox™
Generic Available No
Pharmacologic Category Antibiotic, Tetracycline Derivative
Use Dental: Treatment of periodontitis associated with presence of *Actinobacillus actino-mycetemcomitans* (AA); Atridox™ gel is indicated for the treatment of adult periodontitis for a gain in clinical attachment, reduction in probing depth, and reduction in bleeding on probing
Warnings/Precautions Prolonged use may result in fungal or bacterial superinfection, including *C. difficile*-associated diarrhea and pseudomembranous colitis. Photosensitivity reaction may occur with this drug; avoid prolonged exposure to sunlight or tanning equipment

Additional specific warnings for doxycycline gel (Atridox™) for subgingival application: This product has not been evaluated or tested in immunocompromised patients, in patients with oral candidiasis, or in conditions characterized by severe periodontal defects with little remaining periodontium. May result in overgrowth of nonsusceptible organisms, including fungi. Effects of treatment >6 months have not been evaluated. Has not been evaluated for use in regeneration of alveolar bone
Adverse Reactions (Reflective of adult population; not specific for elderly)
>10%: Discoloration of teeth in children
Doxycycline periodontal gel (Atridox™): The adverse effects reported in clinical trials were similar in incidence between doxycycline-containing product and vehicle alone. In addition, these effects were comparable to standard therapies including scaling and root planning or oral hygiene. Events associated with application reported with an incidence >1% included: gum discomfort (18%), toothache (14%), periodontal abscess (10%), tooth sensitivity (8%), broken tooth (5%), tooth mobility (2%), endodontic abscess (2%) and jaw pain (1%). Systemic adverse events included headache (27%), muscle aches (7%), diarrhea (3%), upset stomach (4%), and nausea (2%). Although there is no known relationship between doxycycline and hypertension, unspecified essential hypertension was noted in 1.6% of the doxycycline gel group, as compared to 0.2% in the vehicle group. Allergic reactions to the vehicle were also reported in two patients.
Drug Interactions Iron and bismuth subsalicylate may decrease doxycycline bioavailability; barbiturates, phenytoin, and carbamazepine decrease doxycycline's half-life; increased effect of warfarin. Concurrent use of tetracycline and Penthrane® has been reported to result in fatal renal toxicity.
Stability Dental gel: Store at 2°C to 8°C (36°F to 46°F). After mixing, coupled syringes may be stored for a maximum of 3 days at room temperature.
Mechanism of Action Inhibits protein synthesis by binding with the 30S and possibly the 50S ribosomal subunit(s) of susceptible bacteria; may also cause alterations in the cytoplasmic membrane

Doxycycline inhibits collagenase *in vitro* and has been shown to inhibit collagenase in the gingival crevicular fluid in adults with periodontitis
Pharmacokinetics Systemic absorption from dental subgingival gel may occur, but is limited by the slow rate of dissolution from this formulation over 7 days.
Dosage
  Geriatrics & Adults:
    Periodontitis: Subgingival application: Dose depends on size, shape and number of pockets treated. Contains 50 mg doxycycline per 500 mg of formulation in each final blended syringe product. Application may be repeated four months after initial treatment.

    Atridox™ subgingival controlled-release product: The delivery system consists of 2 separate syringes in a single pouch. Syringe A contains 450 mg of a bioabsorbable polymer gel; syringe B contains doxycycline hyclate 50 mg. To prepare for instillation, couple syringe A to syringe B. Inject contents of syringe A (purple stripe) into syringe B, then push contents back into syringe A. Repeat this mixing cycle at a rate of one cycle per second for 100 cycles. If syringes are stored prior to use (a maximum of 3 days), repeat mixing cycle 10 times before use. After appropriate mixing, contents should be in syringe A. Holding syringes vertically, with syringe A at
(Continued)

Doxycycline Hyclate Periodontal Extended-Release Liquid
(Continued)

the bottom, pull back on the syringe A plunger, allowing contents to flow down barrel for several seconds. Uncouple syringes and attach enclosed blunt cannula to syringe A. Local anesthesia is not required for placement. Cannula tip may be bent to resemble periodontal probe and used to explore pocket. Express product from syringe until pocket is filled. To separate tip from formulation, turn tip towards the tooth and press against tooth surface to achieve separation. An appropriate dental instrument may be used to pack gel into the pocket. Pockets may be covered with either Coe-Pak™ or Octyldent™ dental adhesive.

Administration Atridox™ subgingival controlled-release product: The delivery system consists of 2 separate syringes in a single pouch. Syringe A contains 450 mg of a bioabsorbable polymer gel; syringe B contains doxycycline hyclate 50 mg. To prepare for instillation, couple syringe A to syringe B. Inject contents of syringe A (purple stripe) into syringe B, then push contents back into syringe A. Repeat this mixing cycle at a rate of one cycle per second for 100 cycles. If syringes are stored prior to use (a maximum of 3 days), repeat mixing cycle 10 times before use. After appropriate mixing, contents should be in syringe A. Holding syringes vertically, with syringe A at the bottom, pull back on the syringe A plunger, allowing contents to flow down barrel for several seconds. Uncouple syringes and attach enclosed blunt cannula to syringe A. Local anesthesia is not required for placement. Cannula tip may be bent to resemble periodontal probe and used to explore pocket. Express product from syringe until pocket is filled. To separate tip from formulation, turn tip towards the tooth and press against tooth surface to achieve separation. An appropriate dental instrument may be used to pack gel into the pocket. Pockets may be covered with either Coe-Pak™ or Octyldent™ dental adhesive.

Patient Information Avoid excessive sunlight or artificial ultraviolet light while receiving doxycycline. After application of dental gel, toothbrushing and flossing should be avoided on any treated areas for 7 days.

Dosage Forms Excipient information presented when available (limited, particularly for generics); consult specific product labeling.

Gel, subgingival: 50 mg in each 500 mg of blended formulation [2-syringe system includes doxycycline syringe (50 mg) and delivery system syringe (450 mg) with a blunt cannula]

♦ **Doxycycline Monohydrate** see Doxycycline on page 479

♦ **DPA** see Valproic Acid and Derivatives on page 1652

♦ **DPE** see Dipivefrin on page 453

♦ **D-Penicillamine** see Penicillamine on page 1218

♦ **DPH** see Phenytoin on page 1250

♦ **Dramamine® [OTC]** see DimenhyDRINATE on page 445

♦ **Dramamine® Less Drowsy Formula [OTC]** see Meclizine on page 961

♦ **Drisdol®** see Ergocalciferol on page 525

♦ **Dristan™ 12-Hour [OTC]** see Oxymetazoline on page 1184

Dronabinol (droe NAB i nol)

Medication Safety Issues
Sound-alike/look-alike issues:
Dronabinol may be confused with droperidol

U.S. Brand Names Marinol®

Canadian Brand Names Marinol®

Index Terms Delta-9-tetrahydro-cannabinol; Delta-9 THC; Tetrahydrocannabinol; THC

Generic Available No

Pharmacologic Category Antiemetic; Appetite Stimulant

Use Chemotherapy-associated nausea and vomiting refractory to other antiemetic(s); AIDS-related anorexia

Unlabeled/Investigational Use
Cancer-related anorexia

Restrictions C-III

Contraindications Hypersensitivity to dronabinol, cannabinoids, sesame oil, or any component of the formulation, or marijuana; should be avoided in patients with a history of schizophrenia

Warnings/Precautions Use with caution in patients with hepatic disease or seizure disorders. Reduce dosage in patients with severe hepatic impairment. May cause additive CNS effects with sedatives, hypnotics or other psychoactive agents; patients must be cautioned about performing tasks which require mental alertness (eg, operating machinery or driving).

May have potential for abuse; drug is psychoactive substance in marijuana; use caution in patients with a history of substance abuse or potential. May cause withdrawal symptoms upon abrupt discontinuation. Use with caution in patients with mania, depression, or schizophrenia; careful psychiatric monitoring is recommended. Use caution in elderly; they are more sensitive to adverse effects.

Adverse Reactions (Reflective of adult population; not specific for elderly)
>10%:
Central nervous system: Drowsiness (48%), sedation (53%), confusion (30%), dizziness (21%), detachment, anxiety, difficulty concentrating, mood change
Gastrointestinal: Appetite increased (when used as an antiemetic), xerostomia (38% to 50%)
1% to 10%:
Cardiovascular: Orthostatic hypotension, tachycardia
Central nervous system: Ataxia (4%), depression (7%), headache, vertigo, hallucinations (5%), memory lapse (4%)
Neuromuscular & skeletal: Paresthesia, weakness

Overdosage/Toxicology Symptoms may include tachycardia, hyper- or hypotension, behavioral disturbances, lethargy, panic reactions, seizures or motor incoordination. Benzodiazepines may be helpful for agitative behavior; Trendelenburg position and hydration may be helpful for hypotensive effects. For other manifestations, treatment should be symptom-directed and supportive.

Drug Interactions
CNS depressants: Sedative effects may be additive with CNS depressants; includes barbiturates, opioid analgesics, and other sedative agents; monitor for increased effect.
Phenothiazines (prochlorperazine): Combinations may result in additive or synergistic effects (as antiemetics), but sedation must be monitored.

Ethanol/Nutrition/Herb Interactions
Ethanol: Avoid ethanol (may increase CNS depression).
Food: Administration with high-lipid meals may increase absorption.
Herb/Nutraceutical: St John's wort may decrease dronabinol levels.

Stability Store under refrigeration (or in a cool environment) between 8°C and 15°C (46°F and 59°F). Protect from freezing.

Mechanism of Action Unknown, may inhibit endorphins in the brain's emetic center, suppress prostaglandin synthesis, and/or inhibit medullary activity through an unspecified cortical action. Some pharmacologic effects appear to involve sympathimometic activity; tachyphylaxis to some effect (eg, tachycardia) may occur, but appetite-stimulating effects do not appear to wane over time. Antiemetic activity may be due to effect on cannabinoid receptors (CB1) within the central nervous system.

Pharmacokinetics
Onset of action: Within 1 hour
Peak effect: 2-4 hours
Duration: 24 hours (appetite stimulation)
Absorption: Oral: 90% to 95%; 10% to 20% of dose gets into systemic circulation
Distribution: V_d: 10 L/kg; dronabinol is highly lipophilic and distributes to adipose tissue
Protein binding: 97% to 99%
Metabolism: Hepatic to at least 50 metabolites, some of which are active; 11-hydroxy-delta-9-tetrahydrocannabinol (11-OH-THC) is the major metabolite; extensive first-pass effect
Half-life elimination: Dronabinol: 25-36 hours (terminal); Dronabinol metabolites: 44-59 hours
Time to peak, serum: 0.5-4 hours
Excretion: Feces (50% as unconjugated metabolites, 5% as unchanged drug); urine (10% to 15% as acid metabolites and conjugates)

Dosage
Geriatrics & Adults:
Antiemetic: Oral: 5 mg/m² 1-3 hours before chemotherapy, then give 5 mg/m²/dose every 2-4 hours after chemotherapy for a total of 4-6 doses/day; dose may be increased up to a maximum of 15 mg/m²/dose if needed (dosage may be increased by 2.5 mg/m² increments).
Appetite stimulant (AIDS-related): Oral: Initial: 2.5 mg twice daily (before lunch and dinner); titrate up to a maximum of 20 mg/day.
Hepatic Impairment: Usual dose should be reduced in patients with severe liver failure.

Monitoring Parameters CNS effects, heart rate, blood pressure, behavioral profile
Reference Range Antinauseant effects: 5-10 ng/mL
Test Interactions Decreased FSH, LH, and testosterone
Patient Information Do not take any new medication during therapy unless approved by prescriber (especially barbiturates and benzodiazepines). Take exactly as directed; do not increase dose or take more often than prescribed. Avoid alcohol. May cause
(Continued)

Dronabinol *(Continued)*

psychotic reaction, impaired coordination or judgment, faintness, dizziness, or drowsiness (do not drive or engage in activities that require alertness and coordination until response to drug is known); or clumsiness, unsteadiness, or muscular weakness (change position slowly and use caution when climbing stairs). Report excessive or persistent CNS changes (euphoria, anxiety, depression, memory lapse, bizarre thought patterns, excitability, inability to control thoughts or behavior, fainting); respiratory difficulties; rapid heartbeat; or other adverse reactions.

Special Geriatric Considerations Elderly patients may be more sensitive to the CNS effects and postural hypotensive effects of dronabinol. Titrate the dose slowly and monitor for adverse effects.

Dosage Forms Excipient information presented when available (limited, particularly for generics); consult specific product labeling.

Capsule, gelatin:

Marinol®: 2.5 mg, 5 mg, 10 mg [contains sesame oil]

Droperidol (droe PER i dole)

Medication Safety Issues

Sound-alike/look-alike issues:

Droperidol may be confused with dronabinol

Inapsine® may be confused with Nebcin®

U.S. Brand Names Inapsine®

Canadian Brand Names Droperidol Injection, USP

Index Terms Dehydrobenzperidol

Generic Available Yes

Pharmacologic Category Antiemetic; Antipsychotic Agent, Typical

Use Antiemetic in surgical and diagnostic procedures; preoperative medication in patients when other treatments are ineffective or inappropriate

Contraindications Hypersensitivity to droperidol or any component of the formulation; known or suspected QT prolongation, including congenital long QT syndrome (prolonged QT_c is defined as >440 msec in males or >450 msec in females)

Warnings/Precautions May alter cardiac conduction. **[U.S. Boxed Warning]: Cases of QT prolongation and torsade de pointes, including some fatal cases, have been reported.** Use extreme caution in patients with bradycardia (<50 bpm), cardiac disease, concurrent MAO inhibitor therapy, Class I and Class III antiarrhythmics or other drugs known to prolong QT interval, and electrolyte disturbances (hypokalemia or hypomagnesemia), including concomitant drugs which may alter electrolytes (diuretics).

Use with caution in patients with seizures or severe liver disease. May be sedating, use with caution in disorders where CNS depression is a feature. Caution in patients with hemodynamic instability, predisposition to seizures, subcortical brain damage, pheochromocytoma or renal disease. Esophageal dysmotility and aspiration have been associated with antipsychotic use - use with caution in patients at risk of pneumonia (ie, Alzheimer's disease). Caution in breast cancer or other prolactin-dependent tumors (may elevate prolactin levels). May alter temperature regulation or mask toxicity of other drugs due to antiemetic effects. May cause orthostatic hypotension - use with caution in patients at risk of this effect or those who would tolerate transient hypotensive episodes (cerebrovascular disease, cardiovascular disease, or other medications which may predispose). Significant hypotension may occur; injection contains benzyl alcohol; injection also contains sulfites which may cause allergic reaction.

May cause anticholinergic effects (confusion, agitation, constipation, xerostomia, blurred vision, urinary retention). Therefore, they should be used with caution in patients with decreased gastrointestinal motility, urinary retention, BPH, xerostomia, or visual problems. Conditions which also may be exacerbated by cholinergic blockade include narrow-angle glaucoma (screening is recommended) and worsening of myasthenia gravis. Relative to other neuroleptics, droperidol has a low potency of cholinergic blockade.

May cause extrapyramidal symptoms, including pseudoparkinsonism, acute dystonic reactions, akathisia, and tardive dyskinesia (risk of these reactions is high relative to other neuroleptics). May be associated with neuroleptic malignant syndrome (NMS) or pigmentary retinopathy. May mask toxicity of other drugs or conditions (eg, intestinal obstruction, Reye's syndrome, brain tumor) due to antiemetic effects. Use with caution in the elderly; reduce initial dose.

Adverse Reactions (Reflective of adult population; not specific for elderly)

>10%:

Cardiovascular: QT_c prolongation (dose dependent)

Central nervous system: Restlessness, anxiety, extrapyramidal symptoms, dystonic reactions, pseudoparkinsonian signs and symptoms, tardive dyskinesia, seizure, altered central temperature regulation, sedation, drowsiness

Endocrine & metabolic: Swelling of breasts

Gastrointestinal: Weight gain, constipation

1% to 10%:

Cardiovascular: Hypotension (especially orthostatic), tachycardia, abnormal T waves with prolonged ventricular repolarization, hypertension

Central nervous system: Hallucinations, persistent tardive dyskinesia, akathisia

Gastrointestinal: Nausea, vomiting

Genitourinary: Dysuria

Overdosage/Toxicology Symptoms include hypotension, tachycardia, hallucinations, and extrapyramidal symptoms. Prolonged QT interval, seizures, and arrhythmias have been reported. Following initiation of essential overdose management, toxic symptom and supportive treatment should be initiated. Hypotension usually responds to I.V. fluids or Trendelenburg positioning. If unresponsive to these measures, the use of a parenteral inotrope may be required (eg, norepinephrine 0.1-0.2 mcg/kg/minute titrated to response). Seizures commonly respond to diazepam (I.V. 5-10 mg bolus every 15 minutes, if needed, up to a total of 30 mg) or to phenytoin or phenobarbital. Arrhythmia management is per ACLS protocols (**Note:** Potential for QT prolongation and/or torsade de pointes). Neuroleptics often cause extrapyramidal symptoms (eg, dystonic reactions) requiring management with diphenhydramine 1-2 mg/kg, up to a maximum of 50 mg I.M. or slow I.V. push, followed by a maintenance dose for 48-72 hours. When these reactions are unresponsive to diphenhydramine, anticholinergic agents such as benztropine mesylate I.V. 1-2 mg may be effective. These agents are generally effective within 2-5 minutes.

Drug Interactions

Acetylcholinesterase inhibitors (central): May increase the risk of antipsychotic-related extrapyramidal symptoms; monitor.

CNS depressants: Sedative effects may be additive with other CNS depressants; monitor for increased effect; includes benzodiazepines, barbiturates, antipsychotics, ethanol, opiates, and other sedative medications

Cyclobenzaprine: Droperidol and cyclobenzaprine may have an additive effect on prolonging the QT interval; based on limited documentation; monitor

Inhalation anesthetics: Droperidol in combination with certain forms of induction anesthesia may produce peripheral vasodilatation and hypotension

Metoclopramide: May increase extrapyramidal symptoms (EPS) or risk.

Potassium- or magnesium-depleting agents: May increase the risk of serious arrhythmias with droperidol; includes many diuretics, aminoglycosides, cyclosporine, supra-physiologic doses of corticosteroids with mineralocorticoid effects, laxatives, and amphotericin B; monitor serum potassium and magnesium levels closely.

Propofol: An increased incidence of postoperative nausea and vomiting have been reported following coadministration

QT_c-prolonging agents: May result in additive effects on cardiac conduction, potentially resulting in malignant or lethal arrhythmias; concurrent use is contraindicated. Includes cisapride, Class I and Class III antiarrhythmics (amiodarone, dofetilide, procainamide, quinidine, sotalol), pimozide, some quinolone antibiotics (moxiflox-acin), tricyclic antidepressants, and some phenothiazines (mesoridazine, thiorida-zine).

Stability Droperidol ampuls/vials should be stored at room temperature and protected from light. Solutions diluted in NS or D_5W are stable at room temperature for up to 7 days.

Mechanism of Action Droperidol is a butyrophenone antipsychotic; antiemetic effect is a result of blockade of dopamine stimulation of the chemoreceptor trigger zone. Other effects include alpha-adrenergic blockade, peripheral vascular dilation, and reduction of the pressor effect of epinephrine resulting in hypotension and decreased peripheral vascular resistance; may also reduce pulmonary artery pressure

Pharmacodynamics

Onset of action: I.M., I.V.: 3-10 minutes

Peak effect: Parenteral: Within 30 minutes

Duration: 2-4 hours (may extend to 12 hours)

Pharmacokinetics

Metabolism: In the liver

Half-life: 2.3 hours

Elimination: In urine (75%) and feces (22%); ~1% excreted in urine unchanged

Dosage

Geriatrics & Adults: Titrate carefully to desired effect: Nausea and vomiting: I.M., I.V.: Initial: 2.5 mg; additional doses of 1.25 mg may be administered to achieve desired effect; administer additional doses with caution

Administration Administer I.M. or I.V.; according to the manufacturer, I.V. push administration should be slow (generally regarded as 2-5 minutes); however, many clinicians administer I.V. doses rapidly (over 30-60 seconds) in an effort to reduce the incidence (Continued)

Droperidol *(Continued)*

of EPS. The effect, if any, of rapid administration on QT prolongation is unclear. For I.V. infusion, dilute in 50-100 mL NS or D_5W; ECG monitoring for 2-3 hours after administration is recommended regardless of rate of infusion.

Monitoring Parameters To identify QT prolongation, a 12-lead EKG prior to use is recommended (use is contraindicated); continued EKG monitoring for 2-3 hours following administration is recommended. Monitor blood pressure, respiratory rate; observe for dystonias, extrapyramidal side effects, and temperature changes

Additional Information Has good antiemetic effect as well as sedative and antianxiety effects

Special Geriatric Considerations Many elderly patients receive antipsychotic medications for inappropriate nonpsychotic behavior although the use of droperidol is seldom used for this indication. Since elderly frequently have cardiac disease which may result in QT prolongation, evaluation should be made prior to considering use of this agent.

Dosage Forms Excipient information presented when available (limited, particularly for generics); consult specific product labeling.
Injection, solution: 2.5 mg/mL (1 mL, 2 mL)

Selected References
Peabody CA, Warner MD, Whiteford HA, et al, "Neuroleptics and the Elderly," *J Am Geriatr Soc*, 1987, 35(3):233-8.

Risse SC and Barnes R, "Pharmacologic Treatment of Agitation Associated With Dementia," *J Am Geriatr Soc*, 1986, 34(5):368-76.

Saltz BL, Woerner MG, Kane JM, et al, "Prospective Study of Tardive Dyskinesia Incidence in the Elderly," *JAMA*, 1991, 266(17):2402-6.

Seifert RD, "Therapeutic Drug Monitoring: Psychotropic Drugs," *J Pharm Pract*, 1984, 6:403-16.

Drospirenone and Estradiol (droh SPYE re none & es tra DYE ole)

U.S. Brand Names Angeliq®
Canadian Brand Names Angeliq®
Index Terms E2 and DRSP; Estradiol and Drospirenone
Generic Available No
Pharmacologic Category Estrogen and Progestin Combination
Use Treatment of moderate-to-severe vasomotor symptoms associated with menopause; treatment of vulvar and vaginal atrophy associated with menopause
Contraindications Hypersensitivity to drospirenone, estradiol, or any component of the formulation; undiagnosed abnormal vaginal bleeding; history of or current thrombophlebitis or venous thromboembolic disorders (including DVT, PE); active or recent (within 1 year) arterial thromboembolic disease (eg, stroke, MI); carcinoma of the breast; estrogen-dependent tumor; hepatic or renal dysfunction or disease; adrenal insufficiency

Warnings/Precautions Drospirenone has antimineralocorticoid activity that may lead to hyperkalemia in patients with renal insufficiency, hepatic dysfunction, or adrenal insufficiency. Use caution with medications that may increase serum potassium.

Cardiovascular-related considerations: Estrogens with or without progestin should not be used to prevent coronary heart disease. Use caution with cardiovascular disease or dysfunction. May increase the risks of hypertension, myocardial infarction (MI), stroke, pulmonary emboli (PE), and deep vein thrombosis; incidence of these effects was shown to be significantly increased in postmenopausal women using conjugated equine estrogens (CEE) in combination with medroxyprogesterone acetate (MPA). Nonfatal MI, PE, and thrombophlebitis have also been reported in males taking high doses of CEE (eg, for prostate cancer). Estrogen compounds are generally associated with lipid effects such as increased HDL-cholesterol and decreased LDL-cholesterol. Triglycerides may also be increased; use with caution in patients with familial defects of lipoprotein metabolism. Whenever possible, estrogens should be discontinued at least 4 weeks prior to and for 2 weeks following elective surgery associated with an increased risk of thromboembolism or during periods of prolonged immobilization.

Neurological considerations: The risk of dementia may be increased in postmenopausal women; increased incidence was observed in women ≥65 years of age taking CEE alone or in combination with MPA.

Cancer-related considerations: Unopposed estrogens may increase the risk of endometrial carcinoma in postmenopausal women. Estrogens may exacerbate endometriosis. Malignant transformation of residual endometrial implants has been reported posthysterectomy with estrogen only therapy. Estrogens may increase the risk of breast cancer. An increased risk of invasive breast cancer was observed in postmenopausal women using CEE in combination with MPA; a smaller increase in risk was seen with estrogen therapy alone in observational studies. An increase in abnormal mammograms has also been reported with estrogen and progestin therapy. Estrogen use may lead to severe hypercalcemia in patients with breast cancer and bone metastases; discontinue estrogen if hypercalcemia occurs.

Estrogens may cause retinal vascular thrombosis; discontinue permanently if papilledema or retinal vascular lesions are observed on examination. Use with caution in patients with diseases which may be exacerbated by fluid retention, including asthma, epilepsy, migraine, diabetes, or renal dysfunction. Use with caution in patients with a history of severe hypocalcemia, SLE, hepatic hemangiomas, porphyria, endometriosis, and gallbladder disease. Use caution with history of cholestatic jaundice associated with past estrogen use or pregnancy.

Before prescribing estrogen therapy to postmenopausal women, the risks and benefits must be weighed for each patient. Women should be informed of these risks and benefits, as well as possible effects of progestin when added to estrogen therapy. Estrogens with or without progestin should be used for shortest duration possible consistent with treatment goals. Conduct periodic risk:benefit assessments. When used solely for the treatment of vulvar and vaginal atrophy, topical vaginal products should be considered. Not for use prior to menopause.

Adverse Reactions (Reflective of adult population; not specific for elderly)
>10%:
  Endocrine & metabolic: Breast pain (19%)
  Gastrointestinal: Abdominal pain (11%)
  Respiratory: Upper respiratory tract infection (19%)
1% to 10%:
  Cardiovascular: Peripheral edema (2%)
  Central nervous system: Headache (10%), pain (8%)
  Gastrointestinal: Abdomen enlarged (7%)
  Genitourinary: Vaginal hemorrhage (9%), endometrial disorder (2%), leukorrhea (1%)
  Neuromuscular & skeletal: Back pain (7%)
  Respiratory: Flu-like syndrome (7%), sinusitis (5%)
Additional adverse effects reported with estrogens and/or progestins: Abdominal cramps, acne, abnormal uterine bleeding, aggravation of porphyria, amenorrhea, anaphylactoid reactions, anaphylaxis, antifactor Xa decreased, antithrombin III decreased, appetite changes, bloating, breast enlargement, breast tenderness, cerebral embolism, cerebral thrombosis, chloasma, cholestatic jaundice, cholecystitis, cholelithiasis, chorea, contact lens intolerance, corneal curvature steepening, cystitis-like syndrome, decreased carbohydrate tolerance, depression, dementia, dizziness, dysmenorrhea; factors VII, VIII, IX, X, XII, VII-X complex, and II-VII-X complex increased; endometrial hyperplasia, erythema multiforme, erythema nodosum, galactorrhea, hemorrhagic eruption, fatigue, fibrinogen increased, impaired glucose tolerance, HDL-cholesterol increased, hirsutism, hypertension, gallbladder disease, insomnia, LDL-cholesterol decreased, libido changes, melasma, migraine, mood disturbances, nausea, nervousness, optic neuritis, pancreatitis, platelet aggregability and platelet count increased, premenstrual-like syndrome, PT and PTT accelerated, pulmonary embolism, pyrexia, retinal thrombosis, scalp hair loss, somnolence, stroke, thrombophlebitis, thyroid-binding globulin increased, total thyroid hormone (T_4) increased, triglycerides increased, urticaria, uterine leiomyomata size increased, vaginal candidiasis, vomiting, weight gain/loss

Overdosage/Toxicology
Overdose may cause nausea; withdrawal bleeding may occur in females. Monitor potassium and sodium serum concentrations. Treatment should be symptom directed and supportive.

Drug Interactions
  Drospirenone: **Substrate** of CYP3A4 (minor); **Inhibits** CYP1A2 (weak), 2C9 (weak), 2C19 (weak), 3A4 (weak)
  Estradiol: **Substrate** of CYP1A2 (major), 2A6 (minor), 2B6 (minor), 2C9 (minor), 2C19 (minor), 2D6 (minor), 2E1 (minor), 3A4 (major); **Inhibits** CYP1A2 (weak), 2C8 (weak); **Induces** CYP3A4 (weak)

  See Estradiol monograph for related drug interactions. The following interaction information is for drospirenone.
  ACE inhibitors: Potential for hyperkalemia with concomitant use; monitor serum potassium during first cycle.
  Aldosterone antagonists: Potential for hyperkalemia with concomitant use; monitor serum potassium during first cycle.
  Aminoglutethimide: May increase CYP metabolism of progestins.
  Angiotensin II receptor antagonists: Potential for hyperkalemia with concomitant use; monitor serum potassium during first cycle.
  Anticoagulants: Oral contraceptives may increase or decrease the effects of coumarin derivatives.
  Anticonvulsants (carbamazepine, felbamate, phenobarbital, phenytoin, topiramate): Increase the metabolism of ethinyl estradiol and/or some progestins, leading to possible decrease in contraceptive effectiveness.
(Continued)

Drospirenone and Estradiol *(Continued)*

Heparin: Potential for hyperkalemia with concomitant use; monitor serum potassium during first cycle.

NSAIDs: Potential for hyperkalemia with concomitant use when taken daily, long term; monitor serum potassium during first cycle.

Phenylbutazone: May decrease contraceptive effectiveness and increase menstrual irregularities.

Potassium-sparing diuretics: Potential for hyperkalemia with concomitant use; monitor serum potassium during first cycle.

Ethanol/Nutrition/Herb Interactions Ethanol: Avoid ethanol (routine use increases estrogen level and risk of breast cancer). Ethanol may also increase the risk of osteoporosis.

Stability Store at controlled room temperature of 15°C to 30°C (59°F to 86°F).

Mechanism of Action

Drospirenone is a synthetic progestin and spironolactone analog with antimineralocorticoid and antiandrogenic activity. Counteracts estrogen effects causing endometrial thinning.

Estrogens are responsible for the development and maintenance of the female reproductive system and secondary sexual characteristics. Estradiol is the principal intracellular human estrogen and is more potent than estrone and estriol at the receptor level; it is the primary estrogen secreted prior to menopause. Following menopause, estrone and estrone sulfate are more highly produced. Estrogens modulate the pituitary secretion of gonadotropins, luteinizing hormone, and follicle-stimulating hormone through a negative feedback system; estrogen replacement reduces elevated levels of these hormones in postmenopausal women.

Pharmacokinetics

Distribution: Drospirenone: 4.2 L/kg

Protein binding:

Drospirenone: 97%; does not bind to sex hormone binding globulin or corticosteroid binding globulin

Estradiol: 37% bound to sex hormone binding globulin; 61% bound to albumin

Metabolism: Hepatic

Drospirenone forms two metabolites (inactive)

Estradiol: Converted to estrone and estriol; also undergoes enterohepatic recirculation; estrone sulfite is the main metabolite in postmenopausal women

Bioavailability: Drospirenone: 76% to 85%

Time to peak, plasma: Drospirenone: 1 hour; Estradiol: 6-8 hours

Dosage

Geriatrics & Adults:

Moderate-to-severe vasomotor symptoms associated with menopause: Oral: One tablet daily; re-evaluate patients at 3- and 6-month intervals to determine if treatment is still necessary.

Atrophic vaginitis in females with an intact uterus: Oral: One tablet daily; re-evaluate patients at 3- and 6-month intervals to determine if treatment is still necessary.

Note: The lowest dose of estrogen/progestin that will control symptoms should be used; medication should be discontinued as soon as possible.

Renal Impairment: Use in contraindicated.

Hepatic Impairment: Use in contraindicated.

Monitoring Parameters Yearly physical examination that includes blood pressure and Papanicolaou smear, breast exam, mammogram. Monitor for signs of endometrial cancer. Adequate diagnostic measures, including endometrial sampling, if indicated, should be performed to rule out malignancy in all cases of undiagnosed abnormal vaginal bleeding. Monitor for loss of vision, sudden onset of proptosis, diplopia, migraine; signs and symptoms of thromboembolic disorders; glycemic control in diabetics; lipid profiles in patients being treated for hyperlipidemias; thyroid function in patients on thyroid hormone replacement therapy.

Menopausal symptoms: Assess need for therapy at 3- to 6-month intervals.

Test Interactions Pathologist should be advised of estrogen/progesterone therapy when specimens are submitted. Reduced response to metyrapone test.

Patient Information Avoid alcohol. Maintain adequate hydration (2-3 L/day) unless instructed to restrict intake by prescriber. If diabetic, monitor blood glucose levels closely. May impair glucose tolerance. You may experience headache, pain in your breast, irregular vaginal bleeding or spotting, abdominal cramps, bloated sensation, nausea and vomiting, or hair loss. Report lumps in the breast, unusual vaginal bleeding, dizziness or faintness (use caution when driving or engaging in activities requiring alertness until response to drug is known), changes in speech, severe headaches, chest pain, shortness of breath, pain or swelling in legs, changes in vision, upper respiratory infection, or severe vomiting.

Special Geriatric Considerations Before prescribing estrogen therapy to postmenopausal women, the risks and benefits must be weighed for each patient. Women should be informed of these risks and benefits, as well as possible side effects and the return of menstrual bleeding (when cycled with a progestin), and be involved in the decision to prescribe. A higher incidence of stroke and invasive breast cancer was observed in women >75 years in a WHI substudy. Oral therapy may be more convenient for vaginal atrophy and urinary incontinence.

Dosage Forms Excipient information presented when available (limited, particularly for generics); consult specific product labeling.

Tablet: Drospirenone 0.5 mg and estradiol 1 mg

Selected References

Rossouw JE, Anderson GL, Prentice RL, et al, "Risks and Benefits of Estrogen Plus Progestin in Healthy Postmenopausal Women: Principle Results From the Women's Health Initiative Randomized Controlled Trial," *JAMA*, 2002, 288(3):321-33.

Shumaker SA, Legault C, Rapp SR, et al, "WHIMS Investigators. Estrogen Plus Progestin and the Incidence of Dementia and Mild Cognitive Impairment in Postmenopausal Women: The Women's Health Initiative Memory Study: A Randomized Controlled Trial," *JAMA*, 2003, 289(20):2651-62.

U.S. Food and Drug Administration, Department of Health and Human Services, "FDA Approves New Labels for Estrogen and Estrogen With Progestin Therapies for Postmenopausal Women Following Review of Women's Health Initiative Data," January 8, 2003. Available at: http://www.fda.gov/medwatch/SAFETY/2003/safety03.htm#prempr.

U.S. Food and Drug Administration, Department of Health and Human Services, "WHIMS Study on Estrogen/Progestin," May 27, 2003. Available at: http://www.fda.gov/ bs/topics/ANSWERS/2003/ANS01226.html.

Wassertheil-Smoller S, Hendrix S, Limacher M, et al, "Effect of Estrogen Plus Progestin on Stroke in Postmenopausal Women: The Women's Health Initiative: A Randomized Trial," *JAMA*, 2003, 289:2673-84.

♦ **Droxia®** *see* Hydroxyurea *on page 774*

♦ **Dr. Scholl's® Callus Remover [OTC]** *see* Salicylic Acid *on page 1441*

♦ **Dr. Scholl's® Clear Away [OTC]** *see* Salicylic Acid *on page 1441*

♦ **Dry Eyes® Ophthalmic Ointment [OTC]** *see* Ocular Lubricant *on page 1144*

♦ **DSCG** *see* Cromolyn *on page 369*

♦ **D-Ser(Bu^t)^6,Azgly^{10}-LHRH** *see* Goserelin *on page 722*

♦ **DSS** *see* Docusate *on page 459*

♦ **D-S-S® [OTC]** *see* Docusate *on page 459*

♦ **DT** *see* Diphtheria and Tetanus Toxoid *on page 451*

♦ **D-Trp(6)-LHRH** *see* Triptorelin *on page 1640*

♦ **Duetact™** *see* Pioglitazone and Glimepiride *on page 1268*

♦ **Dulcolax® [OTC]** *see* Bisacodyl *on page 173*

♦ **Dulcolax® Stool Softener [OTC]** *see* Docusate *on page 459*

♦ **Dull-C® [OTC]** *see* Ascorbic Acid *on page 125*

Duloxetine (doo LOX e teen)

Related Information
Antidepressant Agents *on page 1742*

Medication Safety Issues
Sound-alike/look-alike issues:
Duloxetine may be confused with fluoxetine.

U.S. Brand Names Cymbalta®

Index Terms Duloxetine Hydrochloride; LY248686; (+)-(S)-N-Methyl-γ-(1-naphthyloxy)-2-thiophenepropylamine Hydrochloride

Generic Available No

Pharmacologic Category Antidepressant, Serotonin/Norepinephrine Reuptake Inhibitor

Use Treatment of major depressive disorder (MDD); management of pain associated with diabetic neuropathy; treatment of generalized anxiety disorder (GAD)

Unlabeled/Investigational Use Treatment of stress incontinence; management of chronic pain syndromes; management of fibromyalgia

Restrictions An FDA-approved medication guide concerning the use of antidepressants in children, adolescents, and young adults must be distributed when dispensing an outpatient prescription (new or refill) where this medication is to be used without direct supervision of a healthcare provider. Medication guides are available at http://www.fda.gov/cder/Offices/ODS/medication_guides.htm. Dispense to parents or guardians of children and adolescents receiving this medication.

Contraindications Hypersensitivity to duloxetine or any component of the formulation; concomitant use or within 2 weeks of MAO inhibitors; uncontrolled narrow angle glaucoma

Warnings/Precautions [U.S. Boxed Warning]: Antidepressants increase the risk of suicidal thinking and behavior in children, adolescents, and young adults (18-24 years of age) with major depressive disorder (MDD) and other psychiatric disorders; consider risk prior to prescribing. Short-term studies did not show an increased risk in patients >24 years of age and showed a decreased risk in patients ≥65 years. Closely monitor for clinical worsening, suicidality, or unusual changes in
(Continued)

Duloxetine *(Continued)*

behavior; the patient's family or caregiver should be instructed to closely observe the patient and communicate condition with healthcare provider.

The possibility of a suicide attempt is inherent in major depression and may persist until remission occurs. Patients treated with antidepressants should be observed for clinical worsening and suicidality, especially during the initial (generally first 1-2 months) few months of a course of drug therapy, or at times of dose changes, either increases or decreases. Use caution in high-risk patients. Worsening depression and severe abrupt suicidality that are not part of the presenting symptoms may require discontinuation or modification of drug therapy. The patient's family or caregiver should be alerted to monitor patients for the emergence of suicidality and associated behaviors (such as agitation, irritability, hostility, impulsivity, and hypomania) and call healthcare provider.

May worsen psychosis in some patients or precipitate a shift to mania or hypomania in patients with bipolar disorder. Patients presenting with depressive symptoms should be screened for bipolar disorder. Monotherapy in patients with bipolar disorder should be avoided. **Duloxetine is not FDA approved for the treatment of bipolar depression.**

Duloxetine may cause increased urinary resistance; advise patient to report symptoms of urinary hesitation/difficulty. Has a low potential to impair cognitive or motor performance. Use caution with a previous seizure disorder or condition predisposing to seizures such as brain damage or alcoholism. May cause hepatotoxicity; avoid use in patients with substantial alcohol intake, evidence of chronic liver disease, or hepatic impairment. Use with caution in patients with controlled narrow angle glaucoma. May cause or exacerbate sexual dysfunction. Use caution with renal impairment or with concomitant CNS depressants.

A potential exists for severe reactions when used with MAO inhibitors, SSRIs/SNRIs or triptans; serotonin syndrome (hyperthermia, muscular rigidity, mental status changes/ agitation, autonomic instability) may occur. Use caution during concurrent therapy with other drugs which lower the seizure threshold.

To discontinue therapy with duloxetine, gradually taper dose. If intolerable symptoms occur following a decrease in dosage or upon discontinuation of therapy, then resuming the previous dose with a more gradual taper should be considered. May increase the risks associated with electroconvulsive therapy. Consider discontinuing, when possible, prior to elective surgery.

Adverse Reactions (Reflective of adult population; not specific for elderly)

>10%:

Central nervous system: Somnolence (7% to 15%), dizziness (1% to 14%), headache (13%), insomnia (8% to 11%)

Gastrointestinal: Nausea (4% to 22%), xerostomia (5% to 15%), diarrhea (8% to 13%), constipation (5% to 11%)

1% to 10%:

Cardiovascular: Palpitation (1%)

Central nervous system: Fatigue (2% to 10%), anxiety (3%), fever (1% to 2%), hypoesthesia (1%), irritability (1%), lethargy (1%), nervousness (1%), nightmares (1%), restlessness (1%), sleep disorder (1%), vertigo (1%), yawning (1%)

Dermatologic: Hyperhidrosis (6%), pruritus (1%), rash (1%)

Endocrine & metabolic: Libido decreased (3% to 6%), orgasm abnormality (3% to 4%), hot flushes (2%), anorgasmia (1%), hypoglycemia (1%)

Gastrointestinal: Appetite decreased (3% to 8%), vomiting (1% to 6%), dyspepsia (4%), loose stools (2% to 3%), weight loss (1% to 2%), gastritis (1%)

Genitourinary: Erectile dysfunction (1% to 4%), ejaculation delayed (3%), ejaculatory dysfunction (3%), pollakiuria (1% to 3%), dysuria (1%), urinary symptoms (hesitancy, obstructive symptoms)

Hepatic: Transaminases increased: Occasionally associated with hyperbilirubinemia and/or increased alkaline phosphatase (1%)

Neuromuscular & skeletal: Muscle cramp (4% to 5%), weakness (2% to 4%), myalgia (1% to 3%), tremor (1% to 3%), muscle tightness (1%), muscle twitching (1%), rigors (1%)

Ocular: Blurred vision (4%)

Respiratory: Nasopharyngitis (7% to 9%), cough (3% to 6%), pharyngolaryngeal pain (1% to 3%)

Miscellaneous: Diaphoresis increased (6%), night sweats (1%)

Drug Interactions Substrate (major) of CYP1A2, 2D6; **inhibits** CYP2D6 (moderate)

Buspirone: Concurrent use of duloxetine with buspirone may cause serotonin syndrome; avoid concurrent use.

CYP1A2 inducers: May decrease the levels/effects of duloxetine. Example inducers include aminoglutethimide, carbamazepine, phenobarbital, and rifampin.

CYP1A2 inhibitors: May increase the levels/effects of duloxetine. Example inhibitors include ciprofloxacin, fluvoxamine, ketoconazole, norfloxacin, ofloxacin, and rofecoxib.

CYP2D6 inhibitors: May increase the levels/effects of duloxetine. Example inhibitors include chlorpromazine, delavirdine, fluoxetine, miconazole, paroxetine, pergolide, quinidine, quinine, ritonavir, and ropinirole.

Desipramine: Duloxetine may increase desipramine levels.

Linezolid: Hyperpyrexia, hypertension, tachycardia, confusion, seizures, and deaths have been reported with agents which inhibit MAO (serotonin syndrome); this combination should be avoided.

MAO inhibitors: Hyperpyrexia, hypertension, tachycardia, confusion, seizures, and deaths have been reported with MAO inhibitors (serotonin syndrome); this combination is contraindicated. Wait 5 days after discontinuation of duloxetine before initiating therapy with a MAO inhibitor.

Meperidine: Combined use theoretically may increase the risk of serotonin syndrome.

Moclobemide: Concurrent use of duloxetine with moclobemide may cause serotonin syndrome; avoid concurrent use.

Nefazodone: Concurrent use of duloxetine with nefazodone may cause serotonin syndrome.

Selegiline: Concurrent use with SSRIs has been reported to cause serotonin syndrome; as an MAO type B inhibitor, the risk of serotonin syndrome may be less than with nonselective MAO inhibitors, and reports indicate that this combination has been well tolerated in Parkinson's patients.

Serotonin agonists (eg, triptans): Concurrent use of duloxetine with these agents may increase the risk of serotonin syndrome; monitor.

Serotonergic reuptake inhibitors (eg, SSRIs/SNRIs): Concurrent use of duloxetine with these agents may increase the risk of serotonin syndrome; monitor.

Sibutramine: May increase the risk of serotonin syndrome with SNRIs.

Thioridazine: Duloxetine may increase serum concentrations of thioridazine, which has been associated with the development of malignant ventricular arrhythmias; use caution

Tramadol: Concurrent use of duloxetine with tramadol may cause serotonin syndrome; avoid concurrent use.

Trazodone: Concurrent use of duloxetine with trazodone may cause serotonin syndrome.

Tricyclic antidepressants: Serum levels/effects may be increased by duloxetine; use caution

Venlafaxine: Combined use with duloxetine may increase the risk of serotonin syndrome.

Ethanol/Nutrition/Herb Interactions

Ethanol: Avoid ethanol (may increase CNS depression and/or hepatotoxic potential of duloxetine).

Herb/Nutraceutical: Avoid valerian, St John's wort, SAMe, kava kava, and gotu kola (may increase CNS depression).

Stability Store at 25°C (77°F); excursions permitted to 15°C to 30°C (59°F to 86°F)

Mechanism of Action Duloxetine is a potent inhibitor of neuronal serotonin and norepinephrine reuptake and a weak inhibitor of dopamine reuptake. Duloxetine has no significant activity for muscarinic cholinergic, H_1-histaminergic, or alpha$_2$-adrenergic receptors. Duloxetine does not possess MAO-inhibitory activity.

Pharmacokinetics

Absorption: Well absorbed, 2-hour delay in absorption after ingestion

Distribution: 1640 L

Protein binding: >90%

Metabolism: Hepatic, via CYP1A2 and CYP2D6; forms multiple metabolites (inactive)

Half-life elimination: 12 hours (range 8-17 hours)

Time to peak: 6 hours

Elimination: As metabolites; urine (70%), feces (20%)

Dosage

Geriatrics:

MDD: Oral: Manufacturer does not recommend specific dosage adjustment. Conservatively, may initiate at a dose of 20 mg 1-2 times/day; increase to 40-60 mg/day as a single daily dose or in divided doses

Other indications: Refer to adult dosing.

Adults:

MDD: Oral: Initial: 40-60 mg/day; dose may be divided (ie, 20 or 30 mg twice daily) or given as a single daily dose of 60 mg; maximum dose: 60 mg/day

Diabetic neuropathy: Oral: 60 mg once daily; lower initial doses may be considered in patients where tolerability is a concern and/or renal impairment is present

GAD: Oral: Initial: 30-60 mg/day as a single daily dose; patients initiated at 30 mg/day should be titrated to 60 mg/day after 1 week; maximum dose: 120 mg/day.

Note: Doses >60 mg/day have not been demonstrated to be more effective than 60 mg/day.

(Continued)

Duloxetine *(Continued)*

Chronic pain syndromes (unlabeled use): Oral: 60 mg once daily
Fibromyalgia (unlabeled use): Oral: 60 mg twice daily
Stress incontinence (unlabeled use): Oral: 40 mg twice daily
Renal Impairment: Not recommended for use in Cl_{cr} <30 mL/minute or ESRD. In mild-moderate impairment, lower initial doses may be considered with titration guided by response and tolerability.

Hepatic Impairment: Not recommended for use in hepatic impairment.

Special Geriatric Considerations In an 8-week study of elderly patients with a history of recurrent major depressive disorder, improvements in verbal learning and memory, and depression response and remission rates were significantly greater in subjects randomized to duloxetine 60 mg per day compared to placebo. Duloxetine was well tolerated. No dose adjustment is necessary for age alone; adjust dose for renal function in the elderly. Higher doses are generally required for treatment of general anxiety disorder, neuropathic pain and stress urinary incontinence (unlabeled use).

Dosage Forms Excipient information presented when available (limited, particularly for generics); consult specific product labeling.
Capsule, enteric coated pellets:
Cymbalta®: 20 mg, 30 mg, 60 mg

Selected References

Arnold LM, Lu Y, Crofford LJ, et al, "A Double-Blind, Multicenter Trial Comparing Duloxetine With Placebo in the Treatment of Fibromyalgia Patients With or Without Major Depressive Disorder," *Arthritis Rheum*, 2004, 50(9):2974-84.

Dmochowski RR, Miklos JR, Norton PA, et al, "Duloxetine Versus Placebo for the Treatment of North American Women With Stress Urinary Incontinence," *J Urol*, 2003, 170(4 Pt 1):1259-63.

Fava M, Mallinckrodt CH, Detke MJ, et al, "The Effect of Duloxetine on Painful Physical Symptoms in Depressed Patients: Do Improvements in These Symptoms Result in Higher Remission Rates?", *J Clin Psychiatry*, 2004, 65(4):521-30.

Goldstein DJ, Lu Y, Detke MJ, et al, "Duloxetine in the Treatment of Depression: A Double-Blind Placebo-Controlled Comparison With Paroxetine," *J Clin Psychopharmacol*, 2004, 24(4):389-99.

Millard RJ, Moore K, Rencken R, et al, "Duloxetine vs Placebo in the Treatment of Stress Urinary Incontinence: A Four-Continent Randomized Clinical Trial," *BJU Int*, 2004, 93(3):311-8.

Raskin J, Wiltse CG, Siegal A, et al, "Efficacy of Duloxetine on Cognition, Depression, and Pain in Elderly Patients With Major Depressive Disorder: An 8-Week, Double-Blind, Placebo-Controlled Trial," *Am J Psychiatry*, 2007, 164(6):900-9.

van Kerrebroeck P, Abrams P, Lange R, et al, "Duloxetine Versus Placebo in the Treatment of European and Canadian Women With Stress Urinary Incontinence," *BJOG*, 2004, 111(3):249-57.

♦ **Duloxetine Hydrochloride** *see* Duloxetine *on page 491*

♦ **DuoFilm® [OTC]** *see* Salicylic Acid *on page 1441*

♦ **DuoNeb™** *see* Ipratropium and Albuterol *on page 828*

♦ **DuoPlant® [DSC] [OTC]** *see* Salicylic Acid *on page 1441*

♦ **DuP 753** *see* Losartan *on page 932*

♦ **Duraclon™** *see* Clonidine *on page 342*

♦ **Duragesic®** *see* Fentanyl *on page 609*

♦ **Duramist® Plus [OTC]** *see* Oxymetazoline *on page 1184*

♦ **Duramorph®** *see* Morphine Sulfate *on page 1065*

♦ **Duratears® Naturale® Ophthalmic Ointment [OTC]** *see* Ocular Lubricant *on page 1144*

♦ **Duration® [OTC]** *see* Oxymetazoline *on page 1184*

♦ **Duratuss® DM** *see* Guaifenesin and Dextromethorphan *on page 730*

♦ **Duricef®** *see* Cefadroxil *on page 251*

Dutasteride *(doo TAS teer ide)*

U.S. Brand Names Avodart™
Canadian Brand Names Avodart™
Generic Available No
Pharmacologic Category 5 Alpha-Reductase Inhibitor
Use Treatment of symptomatic benign prostatic hyperplasia (BPH)
Unlabeled/Investigational Use Treatment of male patterned baldness
Contraindications Hypersensitivity to dutasteride, other 5α-reductase inhibitors (eg, finasteride), or any component of the formulation; not indicated for use in women
Warnings/Precautions Hazardous agent - use appropriate precautions for handling and disposal. Pregnant women or women trying to conceive should not handle the product. Urological diseases including cancer should be ruled out before initiating. Men should not donate blood until ≥6 months after last dose. Use caution in hepatic impairment and with concurrent use of potent, chronic CYP3A4 inhibitors. Reduces prostate specific antigen (PSA); re-establish a new baseline after 3-6 months of use.

Adverse Reactions (Reflective of adult population; not specific for elderly)

>10%: Endocrine & metabolic: Serum testosterone increased, thyroid-stimulating hormone increased

1% to 10%: Endocrine & metabolic: Impotence (1% to 5%), libido decreased (1% to 3%), ejaculation disorders (1%), gynecomastia (including breast tenderness, breast enlargement) (1%)

Note: Frequency of adverse events (except gynecomastia) tends to decrease with continued use (>6 months).

Overdosage/Toxicology Treatment is symptom-directed and supportive.

Drug Interactions Substrate of CYP3A4 (minor)

Calcium channel blockers, nondihydropyridine (diltiazem, verapamil): Increase in dutasteride levels with concurrent use

Ethanol/Nutrition/Herb Interactions

Ethanol: No effect or interaction noted.

Food: Maximum serum concentrations reduced by 10% to 15% when taken with food; not clinically significant.

Herb/Nutraceutical: St John's wort may decrease dutasteride levels. Avoid saw palmetto (concurrent use has not been adequately studied).

Stability Store at 25°C (77°F); excursions permitted to 15°C to 30°C (59°F to 86°F).

Mechanism of Action Dutasteride is a 4-azo analog of testosterone and is a competitive, selective inhibitor of both reproductive tissues (type 2) and skin and hepatic (type 1) 5α-reductase. This results in inhibition of the conversion of testosterone to dihydrotestosterone and markedly suppresses serum dihydrotestosterone levels.

Pharmacokinetics

Absorption: Via skin when handling capsules

Distribution: ~12% of serum concentrations partitioned into semen

Protein binding: 99% to albumin; ~97% to α_1-acid glycoprotein; >96% to semen protein

Metabolism: Hepatic; forms metabolites: 6-hydroxydutasteride has activity similar to parent compound, 4′-hydroxydutasteride and 1,2-dihydrodutasteride are much less potent than parent *in vitro*

Bioavailability: 60% (range: 40% to 94%)

Half-life: Terminal: ~5 weeks

Time to peak: 2-3 hours

Elimination: Feces (40% as metabolites, 5% as unchanged drug); urine (<1% as unchanged drug); 55% of dose unaccounted for

Dosage

Geriatrics & Adults: Male: Benign prostatic hyperplasia: Oral: 0.5 mg once daily

Renal Impairment: No adjustment is required.

Hepatic Impairment: Use caution; no specific adjustments recommended.

Administration May be administered with or without food. Capsule should be swallowed whole. Healthcare professionals who are pregnant (or may become pregnant) should **not handle** the product.

Monitoring Parameters Objective and subjective signs of relief of benign prostatic hyperplasia, including improvement in urinary flow, reduction in symptoms of urgency, and relief of difficulty in micturition.

Test Interactions PSA levels decrease in treated patients. After 6 months of therapy, PSA levels stabilize to a new baseline that is ~50% of pretreatment values. If following serial PSAs in a patient, re-establish a new baseline after 3-6 months of use. If interpreting an isolated PSA value in a patient treated for 6 months, then double the PSA value for comparison.

Patient Information Results of therapy may take several months. Take with or without food. Report any increase in urinary volume or voiding patterns that occur and decreased libido or impotence during therapy. Do not donate blood for at least 6 months after the last dose. See Warnings/Precautions.

Dosage Forms Excipient information presented when available (limited, particularly for generics); consult specific product labeling.

Capsule, softgel: 0.5 mg

Dyphylline (DYE fi lin)

Medication Safety Issues
International issues:
Dilor® [Canada] may be confused with Dilar® which is a brand name for paramethasone in France and Mexico

U.S. Brand Names Dylix; Lufyllin®

Canadian Brand Names Dilor®; Lufyllin®

Index Terms Dihydroxypropyl Theophylline

Generic Available Yes: Elixir

Pharmacologic Category Theophylline Derivative

Use Bronchodilator in reversible airway obstruction due to asthma, chronic bronchitis, or emphysema

Contraindications Hypersensitivity to dyphylline, xanthine compounds, or any component of the formulation; status asthmaticus

Warnings/Precautions Excessive doses may increase risk of adverse reactions. Use caution with severe cardiac disease, acute myocardial injury, hypertension, CHF, hyperthyroidism, or peptic ulcer disease. Use caution with renal dysfunction; dose adjustment may be required. Xanthine derivatives, including theophylline, are not indicated for the management of status asthmaticus.

Adverse Reactions (Reflective of adult population; not specific for elderly)
Uncommon at serum theophylline concentrations ≤20 mcg/mL
1% to 10%:
Cardiovascular: Tachycardia
Central nervous system: Nervousness, restlessness
Gastrointestinal: Nausea, vomiting

Drug Interactions
Adenosine: Theophylline derivatives may diminish the therapeutic effect of adenosine. Monitor for decreased therapeutic effects of adenosine.
Benzodiazepines: Theophylline derivatives may diminish the therapeutic effect of benzodiazepines. Monitor for decreased therapeutic effects of benzodiazepines.
Beta-blockers (nonselective): May diminish the bronchodilatory effect of theophylline derivatives. If dyphylline is being as a bronchodilator, consider avoiding the use of nonselective beta-blockers.
Probenecid: Probenecid may decrease the excretion of dyphylline.

Stability Store at controlled room temperature.

Mechanism of Action Causes bronchodilatation, through phosphodiesterase inhibition which increases concentrations of cyclic adenine monophosphate (cAMP) and produces relaxation of bronchial smooth muscle.

Dosage
Geriatrics & Adults: Bronchoconstriction (asthma, COPD): Oral: Up to 15 mg/kg 4 times/day, individualize dosage
Renal Impairment:
Cl_{cr} 50-80 mL/minute: Administer 75% of normal dose.
Cl_{cr} 10-50 mL/minute: Administer 50% of normal dose.
Cl_{cr} <10 mL/minute: Administer 25% of normal dose.

Dosage Forms Excipient information presented when available (limited, particularly for generics); consult specific product labeling.
Elixir:
Dylix: 100 mg/15 mL (473 mL) [contains alcohol 20%]
Tablet:
Lufyllin®: 200 mg, 400 mg

Dyphylline and Guaifenesin (DYE fi lin & gwye FEN e sin)

U.S. Brand Names COPD; Difil-G; Difil®-G Forte; Dilex-G; Dilor-G®; Lufyllin®-GG

Index Terms Guaifenesin and Dyphylline

Generic Available Yes: Excludes syrup

Pharmacologic Category Expectorant; Theophylline Derivative

Use Treatment of bronchial asthma and reversible bronchospasm associated with chronic bronchitis and emphysema

Contraindications Hypersensitivity to dyphylline, guaifenesin, or any component of the formulation

Warnings/Precautions Use with caution in patients with severe cardiac disease, acute myocardial injury, hypertension, hyperthyroidism, severe renal impairment, or peptic ulcer. Xanthine derivatives, including theophylline, are not indicated for the management of status asthmaticus.

Adverse Reactions (Reflective of adult population; not specific for elderly)
Frequency not defined. Also see individual agents.

Cardiovascular: Circulatory failure, extrasystoles, flushing, hypotension, palpitation, tachycardia, ventricular arrhythmias

Central nervous system: Agitation, dizziness, drowsiness, headache, hyperexcitability, insomnia, irritability, restlessness, seizure (generalized tonic-clonic)

Endocrine & metabolic: Hyperglycemia, SIADH, uric acid serum concentration decreased

Gastrointestinal: Diarrhea, epigastric pain, hematemesis, nausea, vomiting

Neuromuscular: Muscle twitching

Renal: Albuminuria, diuresis, hematuria

Respiratory: Tachypnea

Drug Interactions

Adenosine: Theophylline derivatives may diminish the therapeutic effect of adenosine. Monitor for decreased therapeutic effects of adenosine.

Benzodiazepines: Theophylline derivatives may diminish the therapeutic effect of benzodiazepines. Monitor for decreased therapeutic effects of benzodiazepines.

Beta-blockers (nonselective): May diminish the bronchodilatory effect of theophylline derivatives. If dyphylline is being used as a bronchodilator, consider avoiding the use of nonselective beta-blockers.

Probenecid: May increase the levels/effect of dyphylline. Dyphylline plasma half-life has been shown to be increased due to competition for tubular secretion.

Stability Store at room temperature.

Mechanism of Action

Dyphylline primarily causes bronchodilation by competitively inhibiting phosphodiesterases resulting in the increase of cyclic AMP and the relaxation of bronchial smooth muscles.

Guaifenesin is thought to act as an expectorant by irritating the gastric mucosa and stimulating respiratory tract secretions, thereby increasing respiratory fluid volumes and decreasing phlegm viscosity.

Pharmacokinetics See individual agents.

Dosage

Geriatrics & Adults: Asthma/bronchospasm: Oral:

Elixir: Lufyllin®-GG: 30 mL 4 times/day

Syrup:

Dilex-G: 5-10 mL 4 times/day

Difil®-G Forte: 5-10 mL 3 or 4 times/day; may double or triple (in severe cases) according to patient response

Tablet: Difil-G, Dilex-G, Lufyllin®-GG: One tablet 3 or 4 times/day

Renal Impairment: Dosage reduction should be considered in severe renal impairment. Half-life of dyphylline is significantly prolonged in anuria.

Administration Administer after meals to decrease stomach irritation.

Test Interactions Guaifenesin: Possible color interference with determination of 5-HIAA and VMA; discontinue for 48 hours prior to test.

Patient Information

Do not take any new medication during therapy without consulting prescriber. Take as prescribed; do not exceed prescribed dose or frequency. Maintain adequate hydration (2-3 L/day of fluids) unless instructed to restrict fluid intake. Avoid dietary stimulants (eg, caffeine, tea, colas, or chocolate; may increase adverse side effects). If diabetic, monitor blood sugars closely. Can cause elevated blood sugars. You may experience hyperexcitability, restlessness, insomnia, headache, nausea (small frequent meals, frequent mouth care, chewing gum, or sucking lozenges may help), vomiting, or diarrhea. Report respiratory difficulty, rapid or erratic heart beat, seizures, emotional lability or agitation, muscle tremors, cramping, or persistent abdominal pain.

Special Geriatric Considerations There is a lack of significant studies to document the efficacy of guaifenesin. Best to encourage adequate hydration to enhance response to guaifenesin since elderly have a blunted thirst reflex. Elderly are at greater risk for toxicity due to concomitant disease (eg, CHF, arrhythmias); therefore, start at lowest recommended doses.

Dosage Forms Excipient information presented when available (limited, particularly for generics); consult specific product labeling.

Elixir: Dyphylline 100 mg and guaifenesin 100 mg per 15 mL (480 mL)

Lufyllin®-GG: Dyphylline 100 mg and guaifenesin 100 mg per 15 mL (480 mL) [contains alcohol 17%; wine-like flavor]

Liquid: Dyphylline 100 mg and guaifenesin 100 mg per 5 mL (480 mL)

Difil®-G Forte: Dyphylline 100 mg and guaifenesin 100 mg per 5 mL (240 mL) [menthol flavor]

Syrup:

Dilex-G: Dyphylline 100 mg and guaifenesin 200 mg per 5 mL (480 mL) [alcohol free, dye free, and sugar free]

Tablet: Dyphylline 200 mg and guaifenesin 200 mg

COPD, Lufyllin®-GG: Dyphylline 200 mg and guaifenesin 200 mg

Difil-G: Dyphylline 200 mg and guaifenesin 300 mg

Dilex-G: Dyphylline 200 mg and guaifenesin 400 mg

(Continued)

◆ **Dyrenium**® *see* Triamterene *on page 1624*

◆ **Dytan**™ *see* DiphenhydrAMINE *on page 447*

◆ **E2 and DRSP** *see* Drospirenone and Estradiol *on page 488*

◆ **E2020** *see* Donepezil *on page 467*

◆ **EarSol**® **HC** *see* Hydrocortisone *on page 762*

◆ **Easprin**® *see* Aspirin *on page 127*

Echothiophate Iodide (ek oh THYE oh fate EYE oh dide)

Related Information
Glaucoma Drug Therapy *on page 1758*

U.S. Brand Names Phospholine Iodide®

Index Terms Ecostigmine Iodide

Generic Available No

Pharmacologic Category Acetylcholinesterase Inhibitor; Ophthalmic Agent, Antiglaucoma; Ophthalmic Agent, Miotic

Use Reversal of toxic CNS effects caused by anticholinergic drugs; miotic in treatment of open-angle glaucoma; may be useful in specific case of narrow-angle glaucoma; accommodative esotropia

Contraindications Hypersensitivity to echothiophate or any component of the formulation; most cases of angle-closure glaucoma; active uveal inflammation or any inflammatory disease of the iris or ciliary body, glaucoma associated with iridocyclitis

Warnings/Precautions If general anesthesia required, use succinylcholine with great caution due to potential for respiratory or cardiovascular collapse. Use caution in patients on concomitant anticholinesterase agents; warn patients of possible additive effects if chronically exposed to organophosphate/carbamate pesticides/insecticides. Baseline measurement of anterior chamber angle recommended; routine lens examinations (for opacities) should be conducted. Do not use for tonometric glaucoma, or with active or history of uveitis, or retinal detachment. Discontinue if cardiac irregularities or symptoms of excess cholinergic activity (eg, salivation, sweating, urinary incontinence). Not generally recommended for use in patients with any of the following: Vagotonia, asthma GI disturbances, PUD, bradycardia or hypotension, recent MI, epilepsy, parkinsonism. Use cautiously prior to ophthalmic surgery due to risk of blood in the anterior chamber. May depress plasma and erythrocyte cholinesterase levels after a few weeks of therapy. Tolerance may develop after prolonged use; a rest period restores response to the drug.

Adverse Reactions (Reflective of adult population; not specific for elderly)
Frequency not defined.
Cardiovascular: Bradycardia, cardiac irregularities, flushing, hypotension
Gastrointestinal: Diarrhea, nausea, vomiting
Neurologic & skeletal: Muscle weakness
Ocular: Blurred vision, browache, burning eyes, ciliary redness, conjunctival redness/thickening, intraocular pressure increases (paradoxical), iris cysts, lacrimation, lid muscle twitching, miosis, myopia, latent iritis or uveitis activation, lens opacities, retinal detachment, stinging
Respiratory: Dyspnea
Miscellaneous: Diaphoresis, nasolacrimal canal obstruction

Drug Interactions Succinylcholine: May increase or prolong the effects of succinylcholine; use cautiously and monitor closely, possibly reducing dose of succinylcholine

Stability Store undiluted vials at room temperature of 2°C to 8°C (36°F to 46°F). Reconstituted solutions remain stable for 30 days at room temperature or 6 months when refrigerated.

Mechanism of Action Long-acting inhibition of cholinesterase enhances activity of endogenous acetylcholine. Reduced degradation of acetylcholine leads to continuous stimulation of the ciliary muscle producing miosis; other effects include potentiation of accommodation and facilitation of aqueous humor outflow, with attendant reduction in intraocular pressure.

Pharmacodynamics
Onset of action: Following ophthalmic instillation, miosis occurs within 10-30 minutes and a decrease in intraocular pressure (IOP) occurs within 4-8 hours
Duration: Miosis and IOP reduction can persist for 1-4 weeks

Dosage
Geriatrics & Adults: Open-angle or secondary glaucoma: Ophthalmic:
Initial: Instill 1 drop (0.03%) twice daily into eyes with 1 dose just prior to bedtime
Maintenance: Some patients have been treated with 1 dose daily or every other day
Conversion from other ophthalmic agents: If IOP control was unsatisfactory, patients may be expected to require higher doses of echothiophate (eg, ≥0.06%); however,

patients should be initially started on the 0.03% strength for a short period to better tolerance.

Monitoring Parameters Intraocular pressure

Patient Information Be sure of solution expiration date; local irritation and headache may occur; notify physician if abdominal cramps, diarrhea, or salivation occurs; use caution if driving at night or performing hazardous tasks; do not touch dropper to eye; report any change in vision to physician

Special Geriatric Considerations Assess patient's ability to self-administer eye drops.

Dosage Forms Excipient information presented when available (limited, particularly for generics); consult specific product labeling.

Powder for reconstitution, ophthalmic: 6.25 mg [0.125%]
   Phospholine Iodide®: 6.25 mg [0.125%] (5 mL) [packaged with sterile diluent containing mannitol]

Edrophonium (ed roe FOE nee um)

U.S. Brand Names Enlon®; Reversol®
Canadian Brand Names Enlon®; Tensilon®
Index Terms Edrophonium Chloride
Generic Available No
Pharmacologic Category Antidote; Cholinergic Agonist; Diagnostic Agent
Use Diagnosis of myasthenia gravis; differentiation of cholinergic crises from myasthenia crises; reversal of nondepolarizing neuromuscular blockers; treatment of paroxysmal atrial tachycardia; adjunct in treating respiratory depression by curare overdosage; **not** indicated for maintenance therapy due to its short duration of action
Contraindications Hypersensitivity to edrophonium, sulfites, or any component of the formulation; GI or GU obstruction
Warnings/Precautions Use with caution in patients with bronchial asthma and those receiving a cardiac glycoside; atropine sulfate should always be readily available as an antagonist. Overdosage can cause cholinergic crisis which may be fatal. I.V. atropine should be readily available for treatment of cholinergic reactions. Use with caution in patients with cardiac arrhythmias (eg, bradyarrhythmias). Avoid use in myasthenia gravis; may exacerbate muscular weakness. Products may contain sodium sulfite.
Adverse Reactions (Reflective of adult population; not specific for elderly) Frequency not defined.
   Cardiovascular: Arrhythmias (especially bradycardia), AV block, cardiac arrest, decreased carbon monoxide, flushing, hypotension, nodal rhythm, nonspecific ECG changes, syncope, tachycardia
   Central nervous system: Convulsions, dizziness, drowsiness, dysarthria, dysphonia, headache, loss of consciousness
   Dermatologic: Skin rash, thrombophlebitis (I.V.), urticaria
   Gastrointestinal: Diarrhea, dysphagia, flatulence, hyperperistalsis, nausea, salivation, stomach cramps, vomiting
   Genitourinary: Urinary urgency
   Neuromuscular & skeletal: Arthralgias, fasciculations, muscle cramps, spasms, weakness
   Ocular: Lacrimation, small pupils
   Respiratory: Bronchiolar constriction, bronchospasm, dyspnea, bronchial secretions increased, laryngospasm, respiratory arrest, respiratory depression, respiratory muscle paralysis
   Miscellaneous: Allergic reactions, anaphylaxis, diaphoresis increased
Overdosage/Toxicology Symptoms of overdose include muscle weakness, nausea, vomiting, miosis, bronchospasm, and respiratory paralysis. Maintain an adequate airway. For muscarinic symptoms, the antidote is atropine 0.4-0.5 mg I.V. repeated every 3-10 minutes (initial doses as high as 1.2 mg have been administered). Skeletal muscle effects of edrophonium are not alleviated by atropine.
Drug Interactions
   Decreased effect: Atropine, nondepolarizing muscle relaxants, procainamide, quinidine
   Increased effect: Succinylcholine, digoxin, I.V. acetazolamide, neostigmine, physostigmine
   (Continued)

Edrophonium *(Continued)*

Mechanism of Action Inhibits destruction of acetylcholine by acetylcholinesterase. This facilitates transmission of impulses across myoneural junction and results in increased cholinergic responses such as miosis, increased tonus of intestinal and skeletal muscles, bronchial and ureteral constriction, bradycardia, and increased salivary and sweat gland secretions.

Pharmacodynamics

I.M.:

    Onset of effect: Within 2-10 minutes

    Duration: 5-30 minutes

I.V.:

    Onset of effect: Within 30-60 seconds

    Duration: 10 minutes

Pharmacokinetics

Distribution: V_d: 1.1 L/kg

Half-life: 1.8 hours

Dosage

Geriatrics & Adults: Usually administered I.V.; however, if not possible, I.M. or SubQ may be used.

    Diagnosis of Myasthenia gravis:

      I.V.: 2 mg test dose administered over 15-30 seconds; 8 mg given 45 seconds later if no response is seen. Test dose may be repeated after 30 minutes.

      I.M.: Initial: 10 mg; if no cholinergic reaction occurs, give 2 mg 30 minutes later to rule out false-negative reaction.

    Titration of oral anticholinesterase therapy: 1-2 mg given 1 hour after oral dose of anticholinesterase; if strength improves, an increase in neostigmine or pyridostigmine dose is indicated.

    Differentiation of cholinergic from myasthenic crisis: I.V.: 1 mg; may repeat after 1 minute. **Note:** Intubation and controlled ventilation may be required if patient has cholinergic crisis.

    Reversal of nondepolarizing neuromuscular blocking agents (neostigmine with atropine usually preferred): I.V.: 10 mg over 30-45 seconds; may repeat every 5-10 minutes up to 40 mg.

    Termination of paroxysmal atrial tachycardia: I.V. rapid injection: 5-10 mg

Renal Impairment: Dose may need to be reduced in patients with chronic renal failure.

Administration Edrophonium is administered by direct I.V. injection; see Dosage

Monitoring Parameters Monitor blood pressure, pulse, respiratory rate; monitor for muscle strength, fasciculations, and side effects. See Adverse Reactions.

Test Interactions Increased aminotransferase [ALT/AST] (S), amylase (S)

Additional Information In the diagnosis of myasthenia gravis, all anticholinesterase medications should be discontinued for at least 8 hours before administering neostigmine; monitor for signs of cholinergic crisis

Special Geriatric Considerations Many elderly will have diseases which may influence the use of edrophonium. Also, many elderly will need doses reduced 50% due to creatinine clearances in the 10-50 mL/minute range (common in the aged). Side effects or concomitant disease may warrant use of pyridostigmine.

Dosage Forms Excipient information presented when available (limited, particularly for generics); consult specific product labeling.

Injection, solution, as chloride:

    Enlon®: 10 mg/mL (15 mL) [contains sodium sulfite]

    Reversol®: 10 mg/mL (10 mL) [contains sodium sulfite]

Selected References

Rossen RN, Krikorian J, and Hancock EW, "Ventricular Asystole After Edrophonium Chloride Administration," *JAMA*, 1976, 235(10):1041-2.

Youngberg JA, "Cardiac Arrest Following Treatment of Paroxysmal Atrial Tachycardia With Edrophonium," *Anesthesiology*, 1979, 50(3):234-5.

◆ **Edrophonium Chloride** *see* Edrophonium *on page 499*

◆ **E.E.S.**® *see* Erythromycin *on page 533*

◆ **Effexor**® *see* Venlafaxine *on page 1667*

◆ **Effexor**® **XR** *see* Venlafaxine *on page 1667*

◆ **E-Gems**® **[OTC]** *see* Vitamin E *on page 1677*

◆ **E-Gems Elite**® **[OTC]** *see* Vitamin E *on page 1677*

◆ **E-Gems Plus**® **[OTC]** *see* Vitamin E *on page 1677*

◆ **EHDP** *see* Etidronate Disodium *on page 585*

◆ **Elavil** *see* Amitriptyline *on page 85*

◆ **Eldepryl**® *see* Selegiline *on page 1451*

◆ **Electrolyte Lavage Solution** *see* Polyethylene Glycol-Electrolyte Solution and Bisacodyl *on page 1284*

◆ **Elestat**™ *see* Epinastine *on page 513*
◆ **Elestrin**™ *see* Estradiol *on page 549*

Eletriptan (el e TRIP tan)

U.S. Brand Names Relpax®
Canadian Brand Names Relpax®
Index Terms Eletriptan Hydrobromide
Generic Available No
Pharmacologic Category Antimigraine Agent; Serotonin 5-HT$_{1B, 1D}$ Receptor Agonist
Use Treatment of acute treatment of migraine, with or without aura
Contraindications Hypersensitivity to eletriptan or any component of the formulation; ischemic heart disease or signs or symptoms of ischemic heart disease (including Prinzmetal's angina, angina pectoris, MI, silent myocardial ischemia); cerebrovascular syndromes (including strokes, transient ischemic attacks); peripheral vascular syndromes (including ischemic bowel disease); uncontrolled hypertension; use within 24 hours of ergotamine derivatives; use within 24 hours of another 5-HT$_1$ agonist; use within 72 hours of potent CYP3A4 inhibitors; management of hemiplegic or basilar migraine; prophylactic treatment of migraine; severe hepatic impairment
Warnings/Precautions Eletriptan is indicated only in patients with a clear diagnosis of migraine headache. If a patient does not respond to the first dose, the diagnosis of migraine should be reconsidered. Do not give to patients with risk factors for CAD until a cardiovascular evaluation has been performed; if evaluation is satisfactory, the healthcare provider should administer the first dose and cardiovascular status should be periodically evaluated. Cardiac events (coronary artery vasospasm, transient ischemia, MI, ventricular tachycardia/fibrillation, cardiac arrest, and death), cerebral/subarachnoid hemorrhage, stroke, peripheral vascular ischemia, and colonic ischemia have been reported with 5-HT$_1$ agonist administration. Significant elevation in blood pressure, including hypertensive crisis, has also been reported on rare occasions in patients with and without a history of hypertension. Use with caution with mild to moderate hepatic impairment. Symptoms of agitation, confusion, hallucinations, hyper-reflexia, myoclonus, shivering, and tachycardia (serotonin syndrome) may occur with concomitant proserotonergic drugs (ie, SSRIs/SNRIs or triptans) or agents which reduce eletriptan's metabolism. Concurrent use of serotonin precursors (eg, trypto-phan) is not recommended.
Adverse Reactions (Reflective of adult population; not specific for elderly)
1% to 10%:
Cardiovascular: Chest pain/tightness (1% to 4%; placebo 1%), palpitation
Central nervous system: Dizziness (3% to 7%; placebo 3%), somnolence (3% to 7%; placebo 4%), headache (3% to 4%; placebo 3%), chills, pain, vertigo
Gastrointestinal: Nausea (4% to 8%; placebo 5%), xerostomia (2% to 4%, placebo 2%), dysphagia (1% to 2%), abdominal pain/discomfort (1% to 2%; placebo 1%), dyspepsia (1% to 2%; placebo 1%)
Neuromuscular & skeletal: Weakness (4% to 10%), paresthesia (3% to 4%), back pain, hypertonia, hypoesthesia
Respiratory: Pharyngitis
Miscellaneous: Diaphoresis
Overdosage/Toxicology Hypertension or more serious cardiovascular symptoms may occur. Clinical and electrocardiographic monitoring needed for at least 20 hours even if patient is asymptomatic. Treatment is symptom-directed and supportive.
Drug Interactions Substrate of CYP3A4 (major)
CYP3A4 inhibitors: May increase the levels/effects of eletriptan. Example inhibitors include azole antifungals, clarithromycin, diclofenac, doxycycline, erythromycin, imatinib, isoniazid, nefazodone, nicardipine, propofol, protease inhibitors, quinidine, telithromycin, and verapamil.
Ergot-containing drugs: Prolong vasospastic reactions; do not use eletriptan or ergot-containing drugs within 24 hours of each other.
Serotonergic reuptake inhibitors (eg, SSRIs/SNRIs): Concurrent use of eletriptan with these agents may increase the risk of serotonin syndrome; monitor.
Serotonin agonists (eg, triptans): Concurrent use of eletriptan with these agents may increase the risk of serotonin syndrome; monitor.
Ethanol/Nutrition/Herb Interactions Food: High-fat meal increases bioavailability.
Stability Store at 25°C (77°F); excursions permitted to 15°C to 30°C (59°F to 86°F).
Mechanism of Action Selective agonist for serotonin (5-HT$_{1B}$, 5-HT$_{1D}$, 5-HT$_{1F}$ receptors) in cranial arteries; causes vasoconstriction and reduce sterile inflammation associated with antidromic neuronal transmission correlating with relief of migraine
Pharmacokinetics
Absorption: Well absorbed
Distribution: V$_d$: 138 L
Protein binding: ~85%
Metabolism: Hepatic
(Continued)

Eletriptan *(Continued)*

Bioavailability: ~50%, increased with high-fat meal
Half-life: 4 hours (Geriatric: 4.4-5.7 hours); Metabolite: ~13 hours
Time to peak, plasma: 1.5-2 hours

Dosage

Geriatrics & Adults: Acute migraine: Oral: 20-40 mg; if the headache improves but returns, dose may be repeated after 2 hours have elapsed since first dose; maximum 80 mg/day

Note: If the first dose is ineffective, diagnosis needs to be re-evaluated. Safety of treating >3 headaches/month has not been established.

Renal Impairment: No dosing adjustment needed; monitor for increased blood pressure.

Hepatic Impairment:
Mild-to-moderate impairment: No adjustment necessary.
Severe impairment: Use is contraindicated.

Patient Information Inform prescriber of all prescriptions, OTC medications, or herbal products you are taking, and any allergies you have. This drug is to be used to reduce your migraine, not to prevent or reduce the number of attacks. Follow exact instructions for use. Do not use more than two doses in 24 hours and do not take within 24 hours of any other migraine medication without consulting prescriber. May cause dizziness, fatigue, or drowsiness (use caution when driving or engaging in tasks requiring alertness until response to drug is known). Report immediately any chest pain, palpitations, or throbbing; feelings of tightness or pressure in jaw or throat; acute headache or dizziness; muscle cramping, pain, or tremors; skin rash; hallucinations, anxiety, panic; or other adverse reactions.

Special Geriatric Considerations Since elderly often have cardiovascular disease, careful evaluation of the use of 5-HT agonists is needed to avoid complications with the use of these agents. Safety and efficacy in elderly >65 years of age have not been established, however, pharmacokinetic disposition is similar to that in younger adults. Use lowest recommended doses initially.

Dosage Forms Excipient information presented when available (limited, particularly for generics); consult specific product labeling.
Tablet, as hydrobromide: 20 mg, 40 mg [as base]

♦ **Eletriptan Hydrobromide** *see* Eletriptan *on page 501*
♦ **Eligard®** *see* Leuprolide *on page 883*
♦ **Elimite®** *see* Permethrin *on page 1235*
♦ **Elixophyllin®** *see* Theophylline *on page 1548*
♦ **ElixSure® Cough [OTC]** *see* Dextromethorphan *on page 419*
♦ **ElixSure™ IB [OTC]** *see* Ibuprofen *on page 784*
♦ **Elocon®** *see* Mometasone *on page 1059*
♦ **Emadine®** *see* Emedastine *on page 502*

Emedastine *(em e DAS teen)*

U.S. Brand Names Emadine®
Index Terms Emedastine Difumarate
Pharmacologic Category Antihistamine, H$_1$ Blocker, Ophthalmic
Use Treatment of allergic conjunctivitis
Contraindications Hypersensitivity to emedastine or any component of the formulation
Warnings/Precautions Emadine® is for topical ophthalmic use only, **not** for injection. Soft contact lenses should not be worn during treatment if eyes are red; if there is no redness, wait 10 minutes following emedastine instillation before inserting contact lenses.

Adverse Reactions (Reflective of adult population; not specific for elderly)
>10%: Central nervous system: Headache (11%)
1% to 10%:
Cardiovascular: Hyperemia
Central nervous system: Abnormal dreams
Dermatologic: Dermatitis, keratitis, pruritus
Gastrointestinal: Taste (unpleasant)
Neuromuscular & skeletal: Weakness
Ocular: Blurred vision, corneal infiltrates, corneal staining, dry eyes, transient burning or stinging
Respiratory: Rhinitis, sinusitis
Miscellaneous: Tearing

Drug Interactions No data reported.
Stability Store at 4°C to 30°C (39°F to 86°F). Solution should not be used if it becomes discolored.

Mechanism of Action Selective histamine H_1-receptor antagonist for topical ophthalmic use

Pharmacokinetics
Absorption: Ocular: Minimal
Half-life: Oral: Plasma: 3-4 hours

Dosage
Geriatrics & Adults: Allergic conjunctivitis: Ophthalmic: Instill 1 drop in affected eye up to 4 times/day

Patient Information Do not wear soft contact lenses during treatment if eyes are red; if eyes are not red, wait 10 minutes after instilling emedastine before inserting contact lenses. This medication may cause drowsiness in some patients. Take care to not touch dropper tip to eyelids or area surrounding the eye. Do not use if solution has become discolored.

Dosage Forms Excipient information presented when available (limited, particularly for generics); consult specific product labeling.
Solution, ophthalmic, as difumarate: 0.05% (5 mL) [contains benzalkonium chloride]

◆ **Emedastine Difumarate** see Emedastine on page 502
◆ **Emend®** see Aprepitant on page 117
◆ **Emsam®** see Selegiline on page 1451
◆ **ENA 713** see Rivastigmine on page 1421
◆ **Enablex®** see Darifenacin on page 400

Enalapril (e NAL a pril)

Related Information
Angiotensin Agents on page 1737

Medication Safety Issues
Sound-alike/look-alike issues:
Enalapril may be confused with Anafranil®, Elavil®, Eldepryl®, nafarelin, ramipril

Significant differences exist between oral and I.V. dosing. Use caution when converting from one route of administration to another.

International issues:
Acepril® [Hungary, Switzerland] may be confused with Accupril® which is a brand name for quinapril in the U.S.
Acepril®: Brand name for lisinopril in Denmark; brand name for captopril in Great Britain
Nacor® [Spain] may be confused with Niacor® which is a brand name for niacin in the U.S.

U.S. Brand Names Vasotec®
Canadian Brand Names Vasotec®
Index Terms Enalaprilat; Enalapril Maleate
Generic Available Yes
Pharmacologic Category Angiotensin-Converting Enzyme (ACE) Inhibitor
Use Management of mild to severe hypertension; treatment of systolic congestive heart failure, asymptomatic left ventricular dysfunction after myocardial infarction, diabetic nephropathy

Unlabeled/Investigational Use
Unlabeled: Hypertensive crisis, diabetic nephropathy, rheumatoid arthritis, diagnosis of anatomic renal artery stenosis, hypertension secondary to scleroderma renal crisis, diagnosis of aldosteronism, idiopathic edema, Bartter's syndrome, postmyocardial infarction for prevention of ventricular failure
Investigational: Acute pulmonary edema

Contraindications Hypersensitivity to enalapril or enalaprilat; angioedema related to previous treatment with an ACE inhibitor; patients with idiopathic or hereditary angioedema; bilateral renal artery stenosis; primary hyperaldosteronism

Warnings/Precautions Anaphylactic reactions can occur. Angioedema can occur at any time during treatment (especially following first dose). It may involve head and neck (potentially affecting the airway) or the intestine (presenting with abdominal pain). Prolonged monitoring may be required especially if tongue, glottis, or larynx are involved as they are associated with airway obstruction. Those with a history of airway surgery in this situation have a higher risk. Careful blood pressure monitoring with first dose (hypotension can occur especially in volume-depleted patients). Dosage adjustment needed in renal impairment. Use with caution in hypovolemia; collagen vascular diseases; valvular stenosis (particularly aortic stenosis); hyperkalemia; or before, during, or immediately after anesthesia. Avoid rapid dosage escalation which may lead to renal insufficiency.
(Continued)

Enalapril *(Continued)*

Rare toxicities associated with ACE inhibitors include cholestatic jaundice (which may progress to hepatic necrosis) and neutropenia/agranulocytosis with myeloid hyperplasia. Hyperkalemia may rarely occur. May be associated with deterioration of renal function and/or increases in serum creatinine, particularly in patients dependent on renin-angiotensin-aldosterone system. Use with caution in unilateral renal artery stenosis and pre-existing renal insufficiency; if patient has renal impairment then a baseline WBC with differential and serum creatinine should be evaluated and monitored closely during the first 3 months of therapy. Hypersensitivity reactions may be seen during hemodialysis with high-flux dialysis membranes (eg, AN69).

Adverse Reactions (Reflective of adult population; not specific for elderly)
Note: Frequency ranges include data from hypertension and heart failure trials. Higher rates of adverse reactions have generally been noted in patients with CHF. However, the frequency of adverse effects associated with placebo is also increased in this population.

1% to 10%:
Cardiovascular: Hypotension (0.9% to 7%), chest pain (2%), syncope (0.5% to 2%), orthostasis (2%), orthostatic hypotension (2%)
Central nervous system: Headache (2% to 5%), dizziness (4% to 8%), fatigue (2% to 3%)
Dermatologic: Rash (2%)
Gastrointestinal: Abnormal taste, abdominal pain, vomiting, nausea, diarrhea, anorexia, constipation
Neuromuscular & skeletal: Weakness
Renal: Serum creatinine increased (0.2% to 20%), worsening of renal function (in patients with bilateral renal artery stenosis or hypovolemia)
Respiratory (1% to 2%): Bronchitis, cough, dyspnea

Overdosage/Toxicology Mild hypotension has been the only toxic effect seen with acute overdose. Bradycardia may also occur. Hyperkalemia occurs even with therapeutic doses, especially in patients with renal insufficiency, and those taking NSAIDs. Following initiation of essential overdose management, toxic symptom and supportive treatment should be initiated. Hypotension usually responds to I.V. fluids or Trendelenburg positioning.

Drug Interactions Substrate of CYP3A4 (major)
Alpha$_1$ blockers: Hypotensive effect increased.
Aspirin: The effects of ACE inhibitors may be blunted by aspirin administration, particularly at higher dosages and/or increase adverse renal effects.
CYP3A4 inducers: CYP3A4 inducers may decrease the levels/effects of enalapril. Example inducers include aminoglutethimide, carbamazepine, nafcillin, nevirapine, phenobarbital, phenytoin, and rifampicins.
Diuretics: Hypovolemia due to diuretics may precipitate acute hypotensive events or acute renal failure.
Insulin: Risk of hypoglycemia may be increased.
Lithium: Risk of lithium toxicity may be increased; monitor lithium levels, especially in the first 4 weeks of therapy.
Mercaptopurine: Risk of neutropenia may be increased.
NSAIDs: May attenuate hypertensive efficacy; effect has been seen with captopril and may occur with other ACE inhibitors; monitor blood pressure. May increase risk of renal adverse effects.
Potassium-sparing diuretics (amiloride, spironolactone, triamterene): Increased risk of hyperkalemia.
Potassium supplements may increase the risk of hyperkalemia.
Trimethoprim (high dose) may increase the risk of hyperkalemia.

Ethanol/Nutrition/Herb Interactions Herb/Nutraceutical: St John's wort may decrease enalapril levels. Avoid dong quai if using for hypertension (has estrogenic activity). Avoid ephedra, yohimbe, ginseng (may worsen hypertension). Avoid natural licorice (causes sodium and water retention and increases potassium loss). Avoid garlic (may have increased antihypertensive effect).

Stability Enalaprilat: Clear, colorless solution which should be stored at <30°C. I.V. is 24 hours at room temperature in D$_5$W or NS.

Mechanism of Action Competitive inhibitor of angiotensin-converting enzyme (ACE); prevents conversion of angiotensin I to angiotensin II, a potent vasoconstrictor; results in lower levels of angiotensin II which causes an increase in plasma renin activity and a reduction in aldosterone secretion

Pharmacodynamics
Onset of action: Oral: ~1 hour following administration
Peak effect: 4-8 hours
Duration: 12-24 hours

Pharmacokinetics
Absorption: Oral: 55% to 75% (enalapril)

Protein binding: 50% to 60%

Enalapril is a prodrug and undergoes biotransformation to enalaprilat in the liver

Half-life:

Healthy: 2 hours

Enalapril half-life (CHF): 3.4-5.8 hours

Enalaprilat half-life: 11 hours

Time to peak serum concentrations:

Enalapril: Within 0.5-1.5 hours

Enalaprilat (active): Within 3-4.5 hours

Elimination: Principally in urine (60% to 80%) with some fecal excretion

Dosage

Geriatrics & Adults: Use lower listed initial dose in patients with hyponatremia, hypovolemia, severe congestive heart failure, decreased renal function, or in those receiving diuretics.

Asymptomatic left ventricular dysfunction: Oral: 2.5 mg twice daily, titrated as tolerated to 20 mg/day

Hypertension:

Oral: 2.5-5 mg/day then increase as required, usually at 1- to 2-week intervals; usual dose range (JNC 7): 2.5-40 mg/day in 1-2 divided doses. **Note:** Initiate with 2.5 mg if patient is taking a diuretic which cannot be discontinued. May add a diuretic if blood pressure cannot be controlled with enalapril alone.

I.V. (Enalaprilat): 1.25 mg/dose, given over 5 minutes every 6 hours; doses as high as 5 mg/dose every 6 hours have been tolerated for up to 36 hours. **Note:** If patients are concomitantly receiving diuretic therapy, begin with 0.625 mg I.V. over 5 minutes; if the effect is not adequate after 1 hour, repeat the dose and administer 1.25 mg at 6-hour intervals thereafter; if adequate, administer 0.625 mg I.V. every 6 hours.

Heart failure:

Oral: Initial: 2.5 mg once or twice daily (usual range: 5-40 mg/day in 2 divided doses). Titrate slowly at 1- to 2-week intervals. Target dose: 10-20 mg twice daily (ACC/AHA 2005 Heart Failure Guidelines)

I.V.: Avoid I.V. administration in patients with unstable heart failure or those suffering acute myocardial infarction.

Conversion from I.V. to oral therapy if not concurrently on diuretics: 5 mg once daily; subsequent titration as needed; if concurrently receiving diuretics and responding to 0.625 mg I.V. every 6 hours, initiate with 2.5 mg/day.

Renal Impairment:

Oral: Enalapril: Hypertension:

Cl_{cr} 30-80 mL/minute: Administer 5 mg/day titrated upwards to maximum of 40 mg.

Cl_{cr} <30 mL/minute: Administer 2.5 mg day titrated upward until blood pressure is controlled up to a maximum of 40 mg.

For heart failure patients with sodium <130 mEq/L or serum creatinine >1.6 mg/dL, initiate dosage with 2.5 mg/day, increasing to twice daily as needed; increase further in increments of 2.5 mg/dose at >4-day intervals to a maximum daily dose of 40 mg.

I.V.: Enalaprilat:

Cl_{cr} >30 mL/minute: Initiate with 1.25 mg every 6 hours and increase dose based on response.

Cl_{cr} <30 mL/minute: Initiate with 0.625 mg every 6 hours and increase dose based on response.

Moderately dialyzable (20% to 50%)

Administer dose postdialysis (eg, 0.625 mg I.V. every 6 hours) or administer 20% to 25% supplemental dose following dialysis; Clearance: 62 mL/minute

Peritoneal dialysis effects: Supplemental dose is not necessary, although some removal of drug occurs.

Hepatic Impairment: Hydrolysis of enalapril to enalaprilat may be delayed and/or impaired in patients with severe hepatic impairment, but the pharmacodynamic effects of the drug do not appear to be significantly altered. No dosage adjustment is necessary.

Administration Administer direct IVP over at least 5 minutes or dilute up to 50 mL and infuse; discontinue diuretic, if possible, for 2-3 days before beginning enalapril therapy

Monitoring Parameters Blood pressure, serum potassium concentrations, BUN, serum creatinine, renal function, and WBC

Test Interactions Positive Coombs' [direct]; may cause false-positive results in urine acetone determinations using sodium nitroprusside reagent

Patient Information Do not stop therapy except under prescriber's advice; notify physician if you develop sore throat, fever, swelling of hands, feet, face, eyes, lips, and tongue; difficulty breathing, irregular heartbeats, chest pains, or cough. May cause dizziness, fainting, and lightheadedness, especially in first week of therapy, sit and stand up slowly; may cause changes in taste or rash; do not add a salt substitute (potassium) without advice of physician.

(Continued)

Enalapril *(Continued)*

Additional Information Severe hypotension may occur in patients who are sodium and/or volume depleted; initiate lower doses and watch for hypotensive effect within 1-3 hours of first dose or new higher dose.

Special Geriatric Considerations Due to frequent decreases in glomerular filtration (also creatinine clearance) with aging, elderly patients may have exaggerated responses to ACE inhibitors; differences in clinical response due to hepatic changes are not observed. ACE inhibitors may be preferred agents in elderly patients with congestive heart failure and diabetes mellitus. Diabetic proteinuria is reduced and insulin sensitivity is enhanced. In general, the side effect profile is favorable in the elderly and causes little or no CNS confusion; use lowest dose recommendations initially; adjust dose for renal function in the elderly. Many elderly may be volume depleted due to diuretic use and/or blunted thirst reflex resulting in inadequate fluid intake.

Dosage Forms Excipient information presented when available (limited, particularly for generics); consult specific product labeling.

Injection, solution, as enalaprilat: 1.25 mg/mL (1 mL, 2 mL) [contains benzyl alcohol]

Tablet, as maleate (Vasotec®): 2.5 mg, 5 mg, 10 mg, 20 mg

Extemporaneously Prepared An enalapril oral suspension (1 mg/mL) has been made using 20 mg tablets and mL Bicitra®. Add 50 mL Bicitra® to a polyethylene terephthalate (PET) bottle containing ten 20 mg tablets and shake for at least 2 minutes. Let concentrate stand for 60 minutes. Following the 60-minute hold time, shake the concentration for an additional minute. Add 150 mL Bicitra® to the concentrate and shake the suspension to disperse the ingredients. The suspension should refrigerated at 2°C to 8°C (36°F to 46°F); it can be stored for up to 30 days. Shake suspension well before use.

Package labeling, Merck & Co, Inc, issued October 2000.

Selected References

Chobanian AV, Bakris GL, Black HR, et al, "The Seventh Report of the Joint National Committee on Prevention, Detection, Evaluation, and Treatment of High Blood Pressure: The JNC 7 Report," *JAMA*, 2003, 289(19):2560-71.

Konstam MA, Drakup K, Baker DW, et al, "Heart Failure: Evaluation and Care of Patients With Left Ventricular Systolic Dysfunction," *Clinical Practice Guideline No 11*, Rockville, MD: Agency for Health Care Policy and Research, Public Health Service, U.S. Department of Health and Human Services, 1994.

McAreavey D and Robertson JI, "Angiotensin Converting Enzyme Inhibitors and Moderate Hypertension," *Drugs*, 1990, 40(3):326-45.

Williams JF, Bristow MR, Fowler MB, et al, "Guidelines for the Evaluation and Management of Heart Failure: Report of the American College of Cardiology/American Heart Association Task Force on Practice Guidelines (Committee on Evaluation and Management of Heart Failure)," *J Am Coll Cardiol*, 1995, 26:1376-8.

Enalapril and Felodipine (e NAL a pril & fe LOE di peen)

Related Information
Enalapril *on page 503*
Felodipine *on page 602*

U.S. Brand Names Lexxel®

Canadian Brand Names Lexxel®

Index Terms Felodipine and Enalapril

Generic Available No

Pharmacologic Category Antihypertensive Agent, Combination

Use Treatment of hypertension (**not** initial treatment); replacement therapy in patients receiving separate dosage forms (for patient convenience); when monotherapy with one component fails to achieve desired antihypertensive effect, or when dose-limiting adverse effects limit upward titration of monotherapy

Dosage

Geriatrics: Recommended initial dose of felodipine is 2.5 mg daily. Titration of individual components is preferred.

Adults: Hypertension: Oral: Enalapril 5-20 mg and felodipine 2.5-10 mg once daily

Renal Impairment: Cl_{cr} <30 mL/minute: Recommended initial dose of enalapril is 2.5 mg/day. Titration of individual components is preferred.

Hepatic Impairment: Recommended initial dose of felodipine is 2.5 mg daily. Titration of individual components is preferred.

Dosage Forms Excipient information presented when available (limited, particularly for generics); consult specific product labeling.

Tablet, extended release:
Enalapril maleate 5 mg and felodipine 2.5 mg
Enalapril maleate 5 mg and felodipine 5 mg

Enalapril and Hydrochlorothiazide
(e NAL a pril & hye droe klor oh THYE a zide)

Related Information
Enalapril *on page 503*
Hydrochlorothiazide *on page 756*
U.S. Brand Names Vaseretic®
Canadian Brand Names Vaseretic®
Index Terms Hydrochlorothiazide and Enalapril
Generic Available Yes
Pharmacologic Category Antihypertensive Agent, Combination
Use Treatment of hypertension
Dosage
Geriatrics: Refer to dosing in individual monographs; adjust for renal impairment.
Adults: Hypertension: Oral: Enalapril 5-10 mg and hydrochlorothiazide 12.5-25 mg once daily (maximum: 20 mg/day [enalapril]; 50 mg/day [hydrochlorothiazide])
Renal Impairment:
Cl_{cr} >30 mL/minute: Administer usual dose.
Severe renal failure: Avoid; loop diuretics are recommended.
Dosage Forms Excipient information presented when available (limited, particularly for generics); consult specific product labeling.
Tablet:
5-12.5: Enalapril maleate 5 mg and hydrochlorothiazide 12.5 mg
10-25: Enalapril maleate 10 mg and hydrochlorothiazide 25 mg

♦ **Enalaprilat** *see* Enalapril *on page 503*
♦ **Enalapril Maleate** *see* Enalapril *on page 503*
♦ **Enbrel®** *see* Etanercept *on page 577*
♦ **Encort™** *see* Hydrocortisone *on page 762*
♦ **Endocet®** *see* Oxycodone and Acetaminophen *on page 1182*
♦ **Endodan®** *see* Oxycodone and Aspirin *on page 1184*
♦ **Endometrin®** *see* Progesterone *on page 1325*
♦ **Enemeez® [OTC]** *see* Docusate *on page 459*
♦ **Engerix-B®** *see* Hepatitis B Vaccine *on page 750*
♦ **Engerix-B® and Havrix®** *see* Hepatitis A Inactivated and Hepatitis B (Recombinant) Vaccine *on page 744*
♦ **Enhanced-potency Inactivated Poliovirus Vaccine** *see* Poliovirus Vaccine (Inactivated) *on page 1280*
♦ **Enjuvia™** *see* Estrogens (Conjugated B/Synthetic) *on page 561*
♦ **Enlon®** *see* Edrophonium *on page 499*

Enoxaparin (ee noks a PA rin)

Related Information
Anticoagulants, Injectable *on page 1741*
Medication Safety Issues
Sound-alike/look-alike issues:
Lovenox® may be confused with Lotronex®, Protonix®

High alert medication: The Institute for Safe Medication Practices (ISMP) includes this medication among its list of drugs which have a heightened risk of causing significant patient harm when used in error.

International issues:
Lovenox® may be confused with Lotanax® which is a brand name for terfenadine in the Czech Republic
U.S. Brand Names Lovenox®
Canadian Brand Names Enoxaparin Injection; Lovenox®; Lovenox® HP
Index Terms Enoxaparin Sodium
Generic Available No
Pharmacologic Category Low Molecular Weight Heparin
Use
Acute coronary syndromes: Unstable angina (UA), non-ST-segment elevation (NSTEMI), and ST-segment elevation myocardial infarction (STEMI)
DVT prophylaxis: Following hip or knee replacement surgery, abdominal surgery, or in medical patients with severely-restricted mobility during acute illness in patients at risk of thromboembolic complications
DVT treatment (acute): Inpatient treatment (patients with and without pulmonary embolism) and outpatient treatment (patients without pulmonary embolism)
(Continued)

Enoxaparin *(Continued)*

Note: High-risk patients include those with one or more of the following risk factors: >40 years of age, obesity, general anesthesia lasting >30 minutes, malignancy, history of deep vein thrombosis or pulmonary embolism

Contraindications Hypersensitivity to enoxaparin, heparin, or any component of the formulation; thrombocytopenia associated with a positive *in vitro* test for antiplatelet antibodies in the presence of enoxaparin; hypersensitivity to pork products; active major bleeding; not for I.M. use

Warnings/Precautions

[U.S. Boxed Warning]: Patients with recent or anticipated neuraxial anesthesia (epidural or spinal anesthesia) are at risk of spinal or epidural hematoma and subsequent paralysis. Consider risk versus benefit prior to neuraxial anesthesia; risk is increased by concomitant agents which may alter hemostasis, as well as traumatic or repeated epidural or spinal puncture. Patient should be observed closely for bleeding if enoxaparin is administered during or immediately following diagnostic lumbar puncture, epidural anesthesia, or spinal anesthesia.

Do not administer intramuscularly. Not recommended for thromboprophylaxis in patients with prosthetic heart valves. Not to be used interchangeably (unit for unit) with heparin or any other low molecular weight heparins. Use caution in patients with history of heparin-induced thrombocytopenia. Monitor patient closely for signs or symptoms of bleeding. Certain patients are at increased risk of bleeding. Risk factors include bacterial endocarditis; congenital or acquired bleeding disorders; active ulcerative or angiodysplastic GI diseases; severe uncontrolled hypertension; hemorrhagic stroke; use shortly after brain, spinal, or ophthalmology surgery; patients treated concomitantly with platelet inhibitors; recent GI bleeding; thrombocytopenia or platelet defects; severe liver disease; hypertensive or diabetic retinopathy; or in patients undergoing invasive procedures. Monitor platelet count closely. Rare cases of thrombocytopenia have occurred. Manufacturer recommends discontinuation of therapy if platelets are <100,000/mm^3. Rare cases of thrombocytopenia with thrombosis has occurred. Use caution in patients with congenital or drug-induced thrombocytopenia or platelet defects. Risk of bleeding may be increased in women <45 kg and in men <57 kg. Use caution in patients with renal failure; dosage adjustment needed if Cl_{cr} <30 mL/minute. Use with caution in the elderly (delayed elimination may occur); dosage alteration/adjustment may be required (eg, omission of I.V. bolus in acute STEMI in patients ≥75 years of age). Heparin can cause hyperkalemia by affecting aldosterone. Similar reactions could occur with LMWHs. Monitor for hyperkalemia. Multiple-dose vials contain benzyl alcohol.

Adverse Reactions (Reflective of adult population; not specific for elderly)

As with all anticoagulants, bleeding is the major adverse effect of enoxaparin. Hemorrhage may occur at virtually any site. Risk is dependent on multiple variables. At the recommended doses, single injections of enoxaparin do not significantly influence platelet aggregation or affect global clotting time (ie, PT or aPTT).

1% to 10%:

Central nervous system: Fever (5% to 8%), confusion, pain

Dermatologic: Erythema, bruising

Gastrointestinal: Nausea (3%), diarrhea

Hematologic: Hemorrhage (major, <1% to 4%; includes cases of intracranial, retroperitoneal, or intraocular hemorrhage; incidence varies with indication/population), thrombocytopenia (moderate 1%; severe 0.1% - see note below), hypochromic anemia (2%)

Hepatic: ALT/AST increased

Local: Injection site hematoma (9%), local reactions (irritation, pain, ecchymosis, erythema)

Note: Thrombocytopenia with thrombosis: Cases of heparin-induced thrombocytopenia (some complicated by organ infarction, limb ischemia, or death) have been reported.

Overdosage/Toxicology Symptoms of overdose include hemorrhage. Protamine sulfate has been used to reverse effects (protamine 1 mg neutralizes enoxaparin 1 mg). Monitor aPTT 2-4 hours after first infusion; consider readministration of protamine (50% of original dose). Note: anti-Xa activity is never completely neutralized (maximum of 60% to 75%). Avoid overdose of protamine.

Drug Interactions

Drugs which affect platelet function (eg, aspirin, NSAIDs, dipyridamole, ticlopidine, clopidogrel) may potentiate the risk of hemorrhage.

Thrombolytic agents increase the risk of hemorrhage.

Warfarin: Risk of bleeding may be increased during concurrent therapy. Enoxaparin is commonly continued during the initiation of warfarin therapy to assure anticoagulation and to protect against possible transient hypercoagulability.

Ethanol/Nutrition/Herb Interactions Herb/Nutraceutical: Avoid cat's claw, dong quai, evening primrose, feverfew, garlic, ginger, ginkgo, red clover, horse chestnut, green tea, ginseng (all have additional antiplatelet activity).

Stability Store at 15°C to 25°C (59°F to 77°F); do not freeze.

Mechanism of Action Standard heparin consists of components with molecular weights ranging from 4000-30,000 daltons with a mean of 16,000 daltons. Heparin acts as an anticoagulant by enhancing the inhibition rate of clotting proteases by anti-thrombin III impairing normal hemostasis and inhibition of factor Xa. Low molecular weight heparins have a small effect on the activated partial thromboplastin time and strongly inhibit factor Xa. Enoxaparin is derived from porcine heparin that undergoes benzylation followed by alkaline depolymerization. The average molecular weight of enoxaparin is 4500 daltons which is distributed as (≤20%) 2000 daltons (≥68%) 2000-8000 daltons, and (≤15%) >8000 daltons. Enoxaparin has a higher ratio of antifactor Xa to antifactor IIa activity than unfractionated heparin.

Pharmacodynamics
Peak effect: 3 hours
Duration: 275 minutes

Pharmacokinetics
Half-life: 275 minutes
Elimination: In the kidney

Dosage
  Geriatrics: SubQ: Refer to adult dosing. Increased incidence of bleeding with doses of 1.5 mg/kg/day or 1 mg/kg every 12 hours; injection-associated bleeding and serious adverse reactions are also increased in the elderly. Careful attention should be paid to elderly patients, particularly those <45 kg. **Note:** Dosage alteration/adjustment may be required.

  Adults:
    DVT prophylaxis: SubQ:
      Hip replacement surgery:
        Twice-daily dosing: 30 mg twice daily, with initial dose within 12-24 hours after surgery, and every 12 hours until risk of DVT has diminished or the patient is adequately anticoagulated on warfarin.
        Once-daily dosing: 40 mg once daily, with initial dose within 9-15 hours before surgery, and daily until risk of DVT has diminished or the patient is adequately anticoagulated on warfarin.
      Knee replacement surgery: 30 mg twice daily, with initial dose within 12-24 hours after surgery, and every 12 hours until risk of DVT has diminished (usually 7-10 days).
      Abdominal surgery: 40 mg once daily, with initial dose given 2 hours prior to surgery; continue until risk of DVT has diminished (usual 7-10 days).
      Medical patients with severely-restricted mobility during acute illness: 40 mg once daily; continue until risk of DVT has diminished
    DVT treatment (acute): SubQ: **Note:** Start warfarin within 72 hours and continue enoxaparin until INR is between 2.0 and 3.0 (usually 7 days).
      Inpatient treatment (with or without pulmonary embolism): 1 mg/kg/dose every 12 hours or 1.5 mg/kg once daily.
      Outpatient treatment (without pulmonary embolism): 1 mg/kg/dose every 12 hours.
    ST-segment elevation MI (STEMI):
      Patients <75 years of age: Initial: 30 mg I.V. single bolus plus 1 mg/kg (maximum 100 mg for the first 2 doses only) SubQ every 12 hours. The first SubQ dose should be administered with the I.V. bolus. Maintenance: After first 2 doses, administer 1 mg/kg SubQ every 12 hours.
      Patients ≥75 years of age: Initial: SubQ: 0.75 mg/kg every 12 hours (**Note:** No I.V. bolus is administered in this population); a maximum dose of 75 mg is recommended for the first 2 doses. Maintenance: After first 2 doses, administer 0.75 mg/kg SubQ every 12 hours
    Additional notes on STEMI treatment: Therapy was continued for 8 days or until hospital discharge; optimal duration not defined. Unless contraindicated, all patients received aspirin (75-325 mg daily) in clinical trials. In patients with STEMI receiving thrombolytics, initiate enoxaparin dosing between 15 minutes before and 30 minutes after fibrinolytic therapy. In patients undergoing PCI, if balloon inflation occurs <8 hours after the last SubQ enoxaparin dose, no additional dosing is needed. If balloon inflation occurs ≥8 hours after last SubQ enoxaparin dose, a single I.V. dose of 0.3 mg/kg should be administered.
    Unstable angina or non-ST-segment MI (NSTEMI): 1 mg/kg every 12 hours in conjunction with oral aspirin therapy (100-325 mg once daily); continue until clinical stabilization (a minimum of at least 2 days)

  Renal Impairment:
    Cl_cr ≥30 mL/minute: No specific adjustment recommended (per manufacturer); monitor closely for bleeding.
(Continued)

Enoxaparin *(Continued)*

Cl$_{cr}$ <30 mL/minute:

DVT prophylaxis in abdominal surgery, hip replacement, knee replacement, or in medical patients during acute illness: SubQ: 30 mg once daily

DVT treatment (inpatient or outpatient treatment in conjunction with warfarin): SubQ: 1 mg/kg once daily

STEMI: Initial: I.V.: 30 mg as a single dose in patients <75 years of age; omit I.V. bolus in patients ≥75 years of age. The first dose of the SubQ maintenance regimen is administered at the same time as the I.V. bolus. Maintenance: SubQ: 1 mg/kg every 24 hours in all patients

Unstable angina, NSTEMI: SubQ: 1 mg/kg once daily

Dialysis: Enoxaparin has not been FDA approved for use in dialysis patients. It's elimination is primarily via the renal route. Serious bleeding complications have been reported with use in patients who are dialysis dependent or have severe renal failure. LMWH administration at fixed doses without monitoring has greater unpredictable anticoagulant effects in patients with chronic kidney disease. If used, dosages should be reduced and anti-Xa activity frequently monitored, as accumulation may occur with repeated doses. Many clinicians would not use enoxaparin in this population especially without timely anti-Xa activity assay results.

Hemodialysis: Supplemental dose is not necessary.

Peritoneal dialysis: Significant drug removal is unlikely based on physiochemical characteristics.

Administration Should be administered by deep SubQ injection to the left or right anterolateral and left or right posterolateral abdominal wall. A single dose may be administered I.V. as part of treatment for ST-segment elevation myocardial infarction (STEMI) to patients <75 years of age; no I.V. bolus is given to patients ≥75 years of age. To avoid loss of drug from the 30 mg and 40 mg syringes, do not expel the air bubble from the syringe prior to injection. In order to minimize bruising, do not rub injection site. An automatic injector (Lovenox EasyInjector™) is available with the 30 mg and 40 mg syringes to aid the patient with self-injections. **Note:** Enoxaparin is available in 100 mg/mL and 150 mg/mL concentrations.

Monitoring Parameters Periodic CBC including platelets, occult blood, and anti-Xa activity, if available

Special Geriatric Considerations No specific dosage adjustment recommendations for most indications, however, total clearance is lower and elimination is delayed in patients with renal failure. Adjustment may be necessary if renal impairment is present. In the treatment of STEMI, a lower dosage (0.75 mg/kg every 12 hours) and omission of the I.V. bolus, are recommended in patients ≥75 years of age.

Over 2800 patients, ≥65 years of age, have received enoxaparin sodium in pivotal clinical trials. The efficacy of enoxaparin injection in elderly (≥65 years) was similar to that seen in younger patients (<65 years). The incidence of bleeding complications was similar between elderly and younger patients when 30 mg every 12 hours or 40 mg once daily doses of enoxaparin injection was administered at doses of 1.5 mg/kg/day or 1 mg/kg every 12 hours. The risk of enoxaparin injection associated bleeding increased with age. Serious adverse events increased with age for patients receiving enoxaparin injections. Other clinical experience (including postmarketing surveillance and literature reports) has not revealed additional differences in the safety of enoxaparin injection between elderly and younger patients. Careful attention to dosing intervals and concomitant medications (especially antiplatelet medications) is advised. Monitoring of elderly patients with low body weight (<45 kg) and those predisposed to decreased renal function should be considered.

Dosage Forms Excipient information presented when available (limited, particularly for generics); consult specific product labeling.

Injection, solution, as sodium [graduated prefilled syringe; preservative free]:

Lovenox®: 60 mg/0.6 mL (0.6 mL); 80 mg/0.8 mL (0.8 mL); 100 mg/mL (1 mL); 120 mg/0.8 mL (0.8 mL); 150 mg/mL (1 mL)

Injection, solution, as sodium [multidose vial]:

Lovenox®: 100 mg/mL (3 mL) [contains benzyl alcohol]

Injection, solution, as sodium [prefilled syringe; preservative free]:

Lovenox®: 30 mg/0.3 mL (0.3 mL); 40 mg/0.4 mL (0.4 mL)

Selected References

Levine M, Gent M, Hirsh J, et al, "A Comparison of Low-Molecular-Weight Heparin Administered Primarily at Home With Unfractionated Heparin Administered in the Hospital for Proximal Deep Vein Thrombosis," *N Engl J Med,* 1996, 334(11):677-81.

Simonneau G, Charbonnier B, Decousus H, et al, "Subcutaneous Low-Molecular-Weight Heparin Compared With Continuous Intravenous Unfractionated Heparin in the Treatment of Proximal Deep Vein Thrombosis," *Arch Intern Med,* 1993, 153(13):1541-6.

♦ **Enoxaparin Sodium** *see* Enoxaparin *on page 507*

Entacapone (en TA ka pone)

Related Information
Antiparkinsonian Agents *on page 1745*
U.S. Brand Names Comtan®
Canadian Brand Names Comtan®
Generic Available No
Pharmacologic Category Anti-Parkinson's Agent, COMT Inhibitor
Use Adjunct to levodopa/carbidopa therapy in patients with idiopathic Parkinson's disease who experience "wearing-off" symptoms at the end of a dosing interval
Contraindications Hypersensitivity to entacapone or any of component of the formulation
Warnings/Precautions Patient should not be treated concomitantly with entacapone and a nonselective MAO inhibitor. Orthostatic hypotension may be increased in patients on dopaminergic therapy in Parkinson's disease.
Adverse Reactions (Reflective of adult population; not specific for elderly)
>10%:
Gastrointestinal: Nausea (14%)
Neuromuscular & skeletal: Dyskinesia (25%), placebo (15%)
1% to 10%:
Cardiovascular: Orthostatic hypotension (4%), syncope (1%)
Central nervous system: Dizziness (8%), fatigue (6%), hallucinations (4%), anxiety (2%), somnolence (2%), agitation (1%)
Dermatologic: Purpura (2%)
Gastrointestinal: Diarrhea (10%), abdominal pain (8%), constipation (6%), vomiting (4%), dry mouth (3%), dyspepsia (2%), flatulence (2%), gastritis (1%), taste perversion (1%)
Genitourinary: Brown-orange urine discoloration (10%)
Neuromuscular & skeletal: Hyperkinesia (10%), hypokinesia (9%), back pain (4%), weakness (2%)
Respiratory: Dyspnea (3%)
Miscellaneous: Diaphoresis increased (2%), bacterial infection (1%)
Overdosage/Toxicology There have been no reported cases of intentional or accidental overdose with this drug. COMT inhibition by entacapone treatment is dose dependent.
Drug Interactions Inhibits CYP1A2 (weak), 2A6 (weak), 2C9 (weak), 2C19 (weak), 2D6 (weak), 2E1 (weak), 3A4 (weak)

COMT substrates (eg, apomorphine, bitolterol, dobutamine, dopamine, epinephrine, norepinephrine, isoproterenol, isoetharine, and methyldopa): Entacapone may decrease the metabolism and increase the side effects of these agents.
CNS depressants: Effects on mental status may be additive with other CNS depressants; includes barbiturates, benzodiazepines, TCAs, antipsychotics, ethanol, opioid analgesics, and other sedative-hypnotics.
MAO inhibitors: Concurrent use of nonselective MAO inhibitors with entacapone may increase the risk of cardiovascular side effects; selective MAO inhibitors (eg, selegiline) appear to pose limited risk.
Ethanol/Nutrition/Herb Interactions Ethanol: Avoid ethanol (may increase CNS adverse effects).
Mechanism of Action Entacapone is a reversible and selective inhibitor of catechol-O-methyltransferase (COMT). When entacapone is taken with levodopa, the pharmacokinetics are altered, resulting in more sustained levodopa serum levels compared to levodopa taken alone. The resulting levels of levodopa provide for increased concentrations available for absorption across the blood-brain barrier, thereby providing for increased CNS levels of dopamine, the active metabolite of levodopa.
Pharmacodynamics A 200 mg dose will inhibit erythrocyte COMT by 65% with return to baseline within 8 hours.
Pharmacokinetics No age-related changes in pharmacokinetics were seen.
Absorption: Rapid; food does not affect absorption
Protein binding: 98% mainly to albumin
Metabolism: >99%; the main pathway is isomerization to the cis-isomer, followed by glucuronidation. The glucuronide conjugate is inactive.
Bioavailability: 35%
Half-life: 2.4 hours
Time to peak: 1 hour
Elimination: 0.2% of a dose is found unchanged in the urine
Dosage
Geriatrics & Adults: Parkinson's disease: Oral: 200 mg with each dose of levodopa/carbidopa, up to a maximum of 8 times/day (maximum daily dose: 1600 mg/day). To optimize therapy, the dosage of levodopa may need reduced or the dosing interval may need extended. Patients taking levodopa ≥800 mg/day or who had
(Continued)

Entacapone *(Continued)*

moderate-to-severe dyskinesias prior to therapy required an average decrease of 25% in the daily levodopa dose.

Renal Impairment: No adjustment is required; dialysis patients were not studied.

Hepatic Impairment: Dosage adjustment in chronic therapy with standard treatment has not been studied.

Administration Always given with a dose of levodopa/carbidopa. Entacapone has no anti-Parkinson activity of its own.

Monitoring Parameters Symptoms of Parkinson's, blood pressure

Patient Information Take only as prescribed; can be taken with or without food. Possible nausea, hallucinations, and change in color of urine (not clinically relevant) may occur. Do not drive a car or operate other complex machinery until there is sufficient experience with entacapone. Do not withdraw medication unless advised by healthcare professional.

Additional Information No increase in LFTs has been noted; therefore, does not require LFT monitoring. Because of this, entacapone may be preferred over the other COMT inhibitor, tolcapone, in patients with "wearing off". Entacapone has not been studied in patients with stable Parkinson's disease.

Special Geriatric Considerations No difference in adverse effects was noted in the elderly. Monitor levodopa dose.

Dosage Forms Excipient information presented when available (limited, particularly for generics); consult specific product labeling.

Tablet: 200 mg

Selected References

Holm KJ and Spencer CM, "Entacapone. A Review of Its Use in Parkinson's Disease," *Drugs*, 1999, 58(1):159-77.

Olanow CW, Watts RL, and Koller WC, "An Algorithm (Decision Tree) for the Management of Parkinson's Disease (2001): Treatment Guidelines," *Neurology*, 2001, 56(11 Suppl 5):S1-S88.

Pahwa R, Factor SA, Lyons KE, et al, "Practice Parameter: Treatment of Parkinson Disease With Motor Fluctuations and Dyskinesia (An Evidence-Based Review): Report of the Quality Standards Subcommittee of the American Academy of Neurology," *Neurology*, 2006, 66(7):983-95.

♦ **Entacapone, Carbidopa, and Levodopa** *see* Levodopa, Carbidopa, and Entacapone *on page 895*

♦ **Entertainer's Secret® [OTC]** *see* Saliva Substitute *on page 1443*

♦ **Entocort® EC** *see* Budesonide *on page 190*

♦ **Entsol® [OTC]** *see* Sodium Chloride *on page 1475*

♦ **Enulose** *see* Lactulose *on page 869*

Ephedrine *(e FED rin)*

Medication Safety Issues

Sound-alike/look-alike issues:

Ephedrine may be confused with Epifrin®, epinephrine

U.S. Brand Names Pretz-D® [OTC]

Index Terms Ephedrine Sulfate

Generic Available Yes

Pharmacologic Category Alpha/Beta Agonist

Use Treatment of bronchial asthma, nasal congestion (intranasal topical), acute bronchospasm

Contraindications Hypersensitivity to ephedrine or any component of the formulation; cardiac arrhythmias; angle-closure glaucoma; concurrent use of other sympathomimetic agents

Warnings/Precautions Blood volume depletion should be corrected before injectable ephedrine therapy is instituted; use caution in patients with unstable vasomotor symptoms, diabetes, hyperthyroidism, prostatic hyperplasia, a history of seizures or those on other sympathomimetic agents; also use caution in the elderly and those patients with cardiovascular disorders such as coronary artery disease, arrhythmias, and hypertension. Ephedrine may cause hypertension. Long-term use may cause anxiety and symptoms of paranoid schizophrenia. Avoid as a bronchodilator; generally not used as a bronchodilator since new beta$_2$-agents are less toxic. Use with caution in the elderly, since it crosses the blood-brain barrier and may cause confusion. Use with extreme caution in patients taking MAO inhibitors.

Adverse Reactions (Reflective of adult population; not specific for elderly) Frequency not defined.

Cardiovascular: Arrhythmias, chest pain, elevation or depression of blood pressure, hypertension, palpitation, tachycardia, unusual pallor

Central nervous system: Agitation, anxiety, apprehension, CNS stimulating effects, dizziness, excitation, fear, headache hyperactivity, insomnia, irritability, nervousness, restlessness, tension

Gastrointestinal: Anorexia, GI upset, nausea, vomiting, xerostomia

Genitourinary: Painful urination

Neuromuscular & skeletal: Trembling, tremor (more common in the elderly), weakness

Respiratory: Dyspnea

Miscellaneous: Diaphoresis increased

Overdosage/Toxicology Symptoms include dysrhythmias, CNS excitation, respiratory depression, vomiting, and convulsions. There is no specific antidote for ephedrine intoxication and the bulk of the treatment is supportive. Hyperactivity and agitation usually respond to reduced sensory input; however, with extreme agitation, haloperidol (2-5 mg I.M. for adults) may be required. Hyperthermia is best treated with external cooling measures; or when severe or unresponsive, muscle paralysis with pancuronium may be needed. Hypertension is usually transient and generally does not require treatment unless severe. For diastolic blood pressures >110 mm Hg, a nitroprusside infusion should be initiated. Seizures usually respond to diazepam I.V. and/or phenytoin maintenance regimens.

Drug Interactions

Alpha- and beta-adrenergic-blocking agents decrease ephedrine vasopressor effects. Cardiac glycosides or general anesthetics may increase cardiac stimulation.

MAO inhibitors or atropine may increase blood pressure

Sympathomimetic agents: Additive cardiostimulation with other sympathomimetic agents.

Theophylline may lead to cardiostimulation.

Ethanol/Nutrition/Herb Interactions Herb/Nutraceutical: Avoid ephedra, yohimbe (may cause CNS stimulation).

Stability Protect all dosage forms from light.

Mechanism of Action Releases tissue stores of epinephrine and thereby produces an alpha- and beta-adrenergic stimulation; longer-acting and less potent than epinephrine

Pharmacodynamics

Onset of bronchodilation: Oral: 15-60 minutes

Duration: 3-6 hours

Pharmacokinetics

Metabolism: Little hepatic metabolism

Half-life: 3-6 hours

Elimination: 60% to 77% of dose excreted as unchanged drug in urine within 24 hours; renal excretion is dependent on urine pH; decreased excretion with alkaline urine

Dosage

Geriatrics & Adults:

Asthma, nasal congestion, acute bronchospasm, idiopathic orthostatic hypotension, hypotension induced by anesthesia:

Oral: 25-50 mg every 3-4 hours as needed

I.M., SubQ: 25-50 mg, parenteral adult dose should not exceed 150 mg in 24 hours

I.M.: 25 mg

I.V.: 5-25 mg/dose slow I.V. push repeated after 5-10 minutes as needed, then every 3-4 hours not to exceed 150 mg/24 hours

Nasal congestion: Nasal spray: 2-3 sprays into each nostril, not more frequently than every 4 hours

Monitoring Parameters Blood pressure, pulse, mental status

Test Interactions Can cause a false-positive amphetamine EMIT assay

Patient Information May cause wakefulness or nervousness; available over-the-counter, but older adult patients should consult physician before using

Additional Information Ephedrine is generally not used as a bronchodilator since newer beta$_2$-specific agents are less toxic

Special Geriatric Considerations Avoid as a bronchodilator. Use caution since it crosses the blood-brain barrier and may cause confusion.

Dosage Forms Excipient information presented when available (limited, particularly for generics); consult specific product labeling.

Capsule, as sulfate: 25 mg

Injection, solution, as sulfate: 50 mg/mL (1 mL, 10 mL)

Solution, intranasal spray, as sulfate (Pretz-D®): 0.25% (50 mL)

♦ **Ephedrine Sulfate** *see* Ephedrine *on page 512*

Epinastine (ep i NAS teen)

U.S. Brand Names Elestat™

Index Terms Epinastine Hydrochloride

Generic Available No

Pharmacologic Category Antihistamine, H$_1$ Blocker, Ophthalmic

Use Treatment of allergic conjunctivitis

Contraindications Hypersensitivity to epinastine or any component of the formulation *(Continued)*

Epinastine *(Continued)*

Warnings/Precautions Contains benzalkonium chloride; contact lenses should be removed prior to use. Not for the treatment of contact lens irritation.

Adverse Reactions (Reflective of adult population; not specific for elderly)
1% to 10%:
Central nervous system: Headache (1% to 3%)
Ocular: Burning sensation, folliculosis, hyperemia, pruritus
Respiratory: Cough (1% to 3%), pharyngitis (1% to 3%), rhinitis (1% to 3%), sinusitis (1% to 3%)
Miscellaneous: Infection (10%; defined as cold symptoms and upper respiratory infection)

Stability Store at controlled room temperature of 15°C to 25°C (59°F to 77°F). Keep tightly closed.

Mechanism of Action Selective H_1-receptor antagonist; inhibits release of histamine from the mast cell

Pharmacokinetics
Onset: 3-5 minutes
Duration: 8 hours
Absorption: Low systemic absorption following topical application
Distribution: Does not cross blood-brain barrier
Protein binding: 64%
Metabolism: <10% metabolized
Half-life elimination: 12 hours

Dosage
Geriatrics & Adults: Allergic conjunctivitis: Ophthalmic: Instill 1 drop into each eye twice daily. Continue throughout period of exposure, even in the absence of symptoms.

Administration For ophthalmic use only; avoid touching tip of applicator to eye or other surfaces. Contact lenses should be removed prior to application, may be reinserted after 10 minutes. Do not wear contact lenses if eyes are red.

Special Geriatric Considerations No difference in safety and efficacy was observed between elderly and younger patients.

Dosage Forms Excipient information presented when available (limited, particularly for generics); consult specific product labeling.
Solution, ophthalmic, as hydrochloride: 0.05% (5 mL) [contains benzalkonium chloride]

♦ **Epinastine Hydrochloride** *see* Epinastine *on page 513*

Epinephrine (ep i NEF rin)

Related Information
Glaucoma Drug Therapy *on page 1758*
Inhalant Agents *on page 1760*
Medication Safety Issues
Sound-alike/look-alike issues:
Epinephrine may be confused with ephedrine
Epifrin® may be confused with ephedrine, EpiPen®
EpiPen® may be confused with Epifrin®

High alert medication: The Institute for Safe Medication Practices (ISMP) includes this medication among its list of drugs which have a heightened risk of causing significant patient harm when used in error.

Medication errors have occurred due to confusion with epinephrine products expressed as ratio strengths (eg, 1:1000 vs 1:10,000).
Epinephrine 1:1000 = 1 mg/mL and is most commonly used SubQ.
Epinephrine 1:10,000 = 0.1 mg/mL and is used I.V.

International issues:
EpiPen® may be confused with Epigen® which is a brand name for glycyrrhizinic acid in Mexico
EpiPen® may be confused with Epopen® which is a brand name for epoetin alfa in Spain

U.S. Brand Names Adrenalin®; EpiPen®; EpiPen® Jr; Primatene® Mist [OTC]; Raphon [OTC]; S2® [OTC]; Twinject™

Canadian Brand Names Adrenalin®; EpiPen®; EpiPen® Jr; Twinject™

Index Terms Adrenaline; Epinephrine Bitartrate; Epinephrine Hydrochloride; Racepinephrine

Generic Available Yes: Solution for injection

Pharmacologic Category Alpha/Beta Agonist; Antidote

Use Treatment of bronchospasms, bronchial asthma, nasal congestion, viral croup, anaphylactic reactions, cardiac arrest; added to local anesthetics to decrease systemic absorption of local anesthetics and increase duration of action; decrease superficial hemorrhage

Unlabeled/Investigational Use ACLS guidelines: Ventricular fibrillation (VF) or pulseless ventricular tachycardia (VT) unresponsive to initial defibrillatory shocks; pulseless electrical activity, asystole, hypotension unresponsive to volume resuscitation; symptomatic bradycardia or hypotension unresponsive to atropine or pacing; inotropic support

Contraindications Hypersensitivity to epinephrine or any component of the formulation; cardiac arrhythmias; angle-closure glaucoma

Warnings/Precautions Use with caution in elderly patients, patients with diabetes mellitus, cardiovascular diseases (angina, tachycardia, myocardial infarction), thyroid disease, cerebrovascular disease, Parkinson's or taking MAO inhibitors; some products contain sulfites as preservatives. Rapid I.V. infusion may cause death from cerebrovascular hemorrhage or cardiac arrhythmias. Oral inhalation of epinephrine is **not** the preferred route of administration. Avoid topical application where reduced perfusion could lead to ischemic tissue damage (eg, penis, ears, digits).

Adverse Reactions (Reflective of adult population; not specific for elderly) Frequency not defined.

Cardiovascular: Angina, cardiac arrhythmia, chest pain, flushing, hypertension, increased myocardial oxygen consumption, pallor, palpitation, sudden death, tachycardia (parenteral), vasoconstriction, ventricular ectopy

Central nervous system: Anxiety, dizziness, headache, insomnia, lightheadedness, nervousness, restlessness

Gastrointestinal: Dry throat, nausea, vomiting, xerostomia

Genitourinary: Acute urinary retention in patients with bladder outflow obstruction

Neuromuscular & skeletal: Trembling, weakness

Ocular: Allergic lid reaction, burning, eye pain, ocular irritation, precipitation of or exacerbation of narrow-angle glaucoma, transient stinging

Renal: Decreased renal and splanchnic blood flow

Respiratory: Dyspnea, wheezing

Miscellaneous: Diaphoresis increased

Overdosage/Toxicology Symptoms of overdose include arrhythmias, unusually large pupils, pulmonary edema, renal failure, metabolic acidosis; and hypertension, which may result in subarachnoid hemorrhage and hemiplegia. There is no specific antidote for epinephrine intoxication and the bulk of treatment is supportive. Hyperactivity and agitation usually respond to reduced sensory input; however, with extreme agitation, haloperidol (2-5 mg I.M.) may be required. Hyperthermia is best treated with external cooling measures; or when severe or unresponsive, muscle paralysis with pancuronium may be needed. Hypertension is usually transient and generally does not require treatment unless severe. For diastolic blood pressures >110 mm Hg, a nitroprusside infusion should be initiated. Seizures usually respond to diazepam I.V. and/or phenytoin maintenance regimens.

Drug Interactions Increased toxicity: Increased cardiac irritability if administered concurrently with halogenated inhalational anesthetics, beta-blocking agents, alpha-blocking agents

Ethanol/Nutrition/Herb Interactions Herb/Nutraceutical: Avoid ephedra, yohimbe (may cause CNS stimulation).

Stability

Epinephrine is sensitive to light and air; protection from light is recommended. Oxidation turns drug pink, then a brown color. **Solutions should not be used if they are discolored or contain a precipitate.**

Adrenalin®: Store between 15°C to 25°C (59°F to 77°F); do not freeze. Protect from light. The 1:1000 solution should be discarded 30 days after initial use.

Raphon: Store between 2°C to 25°C (36°F to 77°F). Refrigerate after opening.

Twinject™: Store between 20°C to 25°C (68°F to 77°F); do not freeze or refrigerate. Protect from light.

Stability of injection of parenteral admixture at room temperature (25°C) or refrigeration (4°C) is 24 hours.

Standard I.V. diluent: 1 mg/250 mL NS.

Preparation of adult I.V. infusion: Dilute 1 mg in 250 mL of D_5W or NS (4 mcg/mL). Administer at an initial rate of 1 mcg/minute and increase to desired effects. At 20 mcg/minute pure alpha effects occur.

S2®: Dilution not required when administered via hand-nebulizer; dilute with NS 3-5 mL if using jet nebulizer

Mechanism of Action Stimulates alpha-, beta$_1$-, and beta$_2$-adrenergic receptors resulting in relaxation of smooth muscle of the bronchial tree, cardiac stimulation, and dilation of skeletal muscle vasculature; small doses can cause vasodilation via beta$_2$-vascular receptors; large doses may produce constriction of skeletal and vascular smooth muscle

Pharmacodynamics

Onset of action:

SubQ: Bronchodilation occurs within 3-5 minutes following administration

(Continued)

Epinephrine *(Continued)*

Inhalation: Within 1 minute

Following conjunctival instillation, intraocular pressures fall within 1 hour with a maximal response occurring within 4-8 hours

Duration: Ocular effects persist for 12-24 hours; decreased beta-receptor responsiveness has been seen in older adults

Pharmacokinetics

Absorption: Oral: Degraded in the GI tract and, therefore, is not useful

Metabolism: Following administration, drug is taken up into the adrenergic neuron and metabolized by monoamine oxidase and catechol-o-methyltransferase, circulating drug is metabolized in the liver

Elimination: Inactive metabolites (metanephrine and the sulfate and hydroxy derivatives of mandelic acid) and a small amount of unchanged drug is excreted in urine

Dosage

Geriatrics & Adults:

Asystole/pulseless arrest, bradycardia, VT/VF:

I.V., I.O.: 1 mg every 3-5 minutes; if this approach fails, higher doses of epinephrine (up to 0.2 mg/kg) may be indicated for treatment of specific problems (eg, beta-blocker or calcium channel blocker overdose)

Intratracheal: Administer 2-2.5 mg for VF or pulseless VT if I.V./I.O. access is delayed or cannot be established; dilute in 5-10 mL NS or distilled water. **Note:** Absorption is greater with distilled water, but causes more adverse effects on PaO_2.

Bradycardia (symptomatic) or hypotension (not responsive to atropine or pacing): *I.V. infusion:* 2-10 mcg/minute; titrate to desired effect

Bronchodilator:

SubQ: 0.3-0.5 mg **(1:1000)** every 20 minutes for 3 doses

Nebulization: 1-3 inhalations up to every 3 hours using solution prepared with 10 drops of the **1:100** product

S2® (racepinephrine, OTC labeling): 0.5 mL (~10 drops). Dose may be repeated not more frequently than very 3-4 hours if needed. Solution should be diluted if using jet nebulizer.

Inhalation: Primatene® Mist (OTC labeling): One inhalation, wait at least 1 minute; if relieved, may use once more. Do not use again for at least 3 hours.

Decongestant: *Intranasal:* Apply 1:1000 locally as drops or spray or with sterile swab

Hypersensitivity reaction:

SubQ, I.M.: 0.3-0.5 mg (1:1000) every 15-20 minutes if condition requires (I.M route is preferred)

I.V.: 0.1 mg (1:10,000) over 5 minutes. May infuse at 1-4 mcg/minute to prevent the need to repeat injections frequently.

Self-administration following severe allergic reactions (eg, insect stings, food): **Note:** The World Health Organization (WHO) and Anaphylaxis Canada recommend the availability of one dose for every 10 to 20 minutes of travel time to a medical emergency facility. More than 2 doses should only be administered under direct medical supervision.

Twinject™: SubQ, I.M.: 0.3 mg

Epipen®: I.M.: 0.3 mg

Administration Central line administration only. I.V. infusions require an infusion pump. Epinephrine solutions for injection can be administered SubQ, I.M., I.V., I.O.; I.M. administration into the buttocks should be avoided.

Inhalation: S2®: Administer over ~15 minutes; must be diluted if using jet nebulizer

Intratracheal: Dilute in NS or distilled water. Absorption is greater with distilled water, but causes more adverse effects on PaO_2. Pass catheter beyond tip of tracheal tube, stop compressions, spray drug quickly down tube. Follow immediately with several quick insufflations and continue chest compressions.

Extravasation management: Use phentolamine as antidote. Mix 5 mg with 9 mL of NS. Inject a small amount of this dilution into extravasated area. Blanching should reverse immediately. Monitor site. If blanching should recur, additional injections of phentolamine may be needed.

Monitoring Parameters Pulmonary function, heart rate, blood pressure, site of infusion for blanching, extravasation; cardiac monitor and blood pressure monitor required. If using to treat hypotension, assess intravascular volume and support as needed.

Reference Range Therapeutic: 31-95 pg/mL (SI: 170-520 pmol/L)

Test Interactions Increased bilirubin (S), catecholamines (U), glucose, uric acid (S)

Patient Information After instilling, apply pressure on the side of the nose near the eye to minimize systemic absorption; stinging may occur upon instillation; headache or aching in the brow area may occur

Additional Information Oral inhalation of epinephrine is **not** the preferred route of administration. Patients should be cautioned to avoid the use of over-the-counter epinephrine inhalation products (eg, Primatene® Mist [OTC]); beta$_2$-adrenergic agents for inhalation are preferred.

Special Geriatric Considerations The use of epinephrine in the treatment of acute exacerbations of asthma was studied in the elderly. A dose of 0.3 mg SubQ every 20 minutes for three doses was well tolerated in elderly patients with no history of angina or recent myocardial infarction. There was no significant difference in the incidence of ventricular arrhythmias in elderly versus younger adults.

Dosage Forms Excipient information presented when available (limited, particularly for generics); consult specific product labeling.

Aerosol for oral inhalation:
Primatene® Mist: 0.22 mg/inhalation (15 mL, 22.5 mL) [contains CFCs]

Injection, solution [prefilled auto injector]:
EpiPen®: 0.3 mg/0.3 mL [1:1000] (2 mL) [contains sodium metabisulfite; available as single unit or in double-unit pack with training unit]
EpiPen® Jr: 0.15 mg/0.3 mL [1:2000] (2 mL) [contains sodium metabisulfite; available as single unit or in double-unit pack with training unit]
Twinject™: 0.15 mg/0.15 mL [1:1000] (1.1 mL) [contains sodium bisulfite; two 0.15 mg doses per injector]; 0.3 mg/0.3 mL [1:1000] (1.1 mL) [contains sodium bisulfite; two 0.3 mg doses per injector]

Injection, solution, as hydrochloride: 0.1 mg/mL [1:10,000] (10 mL); 1 mg/mL [1:1000] (1 mL) [products may contain sodium metabisulfite]
Adrenalin®: 1 mg/mL [1:1000] (1 mL, 30 mL) [contains sodium bisulfite]

Solution for oral inhalation, as hydrochloride:
Adrenalin®: 1% [10 mg/mL, 1:100] (7.5 mL) [contains sodium bisulfite]

Solution for oral inhalation [racepinephrine]:
S2®: 2.25% (0.5 mL, 15 mL) [as d-epinephrine 1.125% and l-epinephrine 1.125%; contains metabisulfites]

Solution, topical [racepinephrine]:
Raphon: 2.25% (15 mL) [as d-epinephrine 1.125% and l-epinephrine 1.125%; contains metabisulfites]

Selected References
"2005 American Heart Association Guidelines for Cardiopulmonary Resuscitation and Emergency Cardiovascular Care," *Circulation*, 2005, 112(24 Suppl): 1-211.
Cydulka R, Davison R, Grammer L, et al, "The Use of Epinephrine in the Treatment of Older Adult Asthmatics," *Ann Emerg Med*, 1988, 17(4):322-6.
National Asthma Education and Prevention Program, "Expert Panel Report 2: Guidelines for the Diagnosis and Management of Asthma," Bethesda, MD, National Institutes of Health, 1997. NIH publication 97-4051.

◆ **Epinephrine Bitartrate** *see* Epinephrine *on page 514*
◆ **Epinephrine Hydrochloride** *see* Epinephrine *on page 514*
◆ **EpiPen®** *see* Epinephrine *on page 514*
◆ **EpiPen® Jr** *see* Epinephrine *on page 514*
◆ **Epitol®** *see* Carbamazepine *on page 231*

Eplerenone (e PLER en one)

Medication Safety Issues
Sound-alike/look-alike issues:
Inspra™ may be confused with Spiriva®

U.S. Brand Names Inspra™

Generic Available No

Pharmacologic Category Diuretic, Potassium-Sparing; Selective Aldosterone Blocker

Use Treatment of hypertension, alone or in combination with other antihypertensive agents; treatment of CHF following acute MI

Contraindications Hypersensitivity to eplerenone or any component of the formulation; serum potassium >5.5 mEq/L; Cl$_{cr}$ ≤30 mL/minute; concomitant use of strong CYP3A4 inhibitors (see Drug Interactions for details).

The following additional contraindications apply to patients with hypertension: Type 2 diabetes mellitus (noninsulin dependent, NIDDM) with microalbuminuria; serum creatinine >2.0 mg/dL in males or >1.8 mg/dL in females; Cl$_{cr}$ <50 mL/minute; concomitant use with potassium supplements or potassium-sparing diuretics

Warnings/Precautions Dosage adjustment needed for patients on moderate CYP3A4 inhibitors (see drug interactions for details). Monitor closely for hyperkalemia; increases in serum potassium were dose related during clinical trials and rates of hyperkalemia also increased with declining renal function. Safety and efficacy have not been established in patients with severe hepatic impairment. Use with caution in CHF patients post-MI with diabetes.

Adverse Reactions (Reflective of adult population; not specific for elderly)
>10%: Endocrine & metabolic: Hypertriglyceridemia (1% to 15%, dose related)
1% to 10%:
Central nervous system: Dizziness (3%), fatigue (2%)
(Continued)

Eplerenone *(Continued)*

Endocrine & metabolic: Breast pain (males <1% to 1%), serum creatinine increased (6% in CHF), gynecomastia (males <1% to 1%), hyponatremia (2%, dose related), hypercholesterolemia (<1% to 1%); hyperkalemia (mild-to-moderate hypertension <1%; left ventricular dysfunction ~6% had serum potassium ≥6 mEq/L)

Gastrointestinal: Diarrhea (2%), abdominal pain (1%)

Genitourinary: Abnormal vaginal bleeding (<1% to 2%)

Renal: Albuminuria (1%)

Respiratory: Cough (2%)

Miscellaneous: Flu-like syndrome (2%)

Overdosage/Toxicology Cases of human overdose have not been reported; hypotension or hyperkalemia would be expected. Treatment should be symptom-directed and supportive. Eplerenone is not removed by hemodialysis; binds extensively to charcoal.

Drug Interactions Substrate of CYP3A4 (major)

ACE inhibitors: Concomitant use increases serum potassium, use of ACE inhibitors and another mineralocorticoid receptor blocker has led to clinically relevant hyperkalemia. Use with caution; monitoring of potassium levels recommended.

Angiotensin II receptor antagonists: Concomitant use increases serum potassium, use of angiotensin II receptor antagonists and another mineralocorticoid receptor blocker has led to clinically relevant hyperkalemia. Use with caution; monitoring of potassium levels recommended.

CYP3A4 inducers: CYP3A4 inducers may decrease the levels/effects of eplerenone. Example inducers include aminoglutethimide, carbamazepine, nafcillin, nevirapine, phenobarbital, phenytoin, and rifamycins.

CYP3A4 inhibitors: May increase the levels/effects of eplerenone. Example inhibitors include azole antifungals, ciprofloxacin, clarithromycin, diclofenac, doxycycline, erythromycin, imatinib, isoniazid, nefazodone, nicardipine, propofol, protease inhibitors, quinidine, and verapamil.

Lithium: Interaction studies have not been conducted, however, monitoring of lithium levels is recommended.

NSAIDs: Interaction studies have not been conducted, however, NSAIDs may decrease the antihypertensive effects and cause hyperkalemia in patients with impaired renal function. Blood pressure should be monitored closely.

Potassium-sparing diuretics (amiloride, spironolactone, triamterene): Increase risk of hyperkalemia; concurrent use is contraindicated.

Potassium supplements: Increase risk of hyperkalemia; concurrent use is contraindicated.

Ethanol/Nutrition/Herb Interactions

Food: Grapefruit juice increases eplerenone AUC ~25%.

Herb/Nutraceutical: St John's wort decreases eplerenone AUC ~30%.

Stability Store at controlled room temperature of 25°C (77°F).

Mechanism of Action Aldosterone increases blood pressure primarily by inducing sodium reabsorption. Eplerenone reduces blood pressure by blocking aldosterone binding at mineralocorticoid receptors found in the kidney, heart, blood vessels and brain.

Pharmacokinetics

Distribution: V_d: 43-90 L

Protein binding: ~50%; primarily to alpha$_1$-acid glycoproteins

Metabolism: Primarily; metabolites inactive

Half-life: 4-6 hours

Time to peak, plasma: 1.5 hours; may take up to 4 weeks for full therapeutic effect

Elimination: Urine (67%; <5% as unchanged drug), feces (32%)

Dosage

Geriatrics: See Special Geriatric Considerations.

Adults:

Hypertension: Oral: Initial: 50 mg once daily; may increase to 50 mg twice daily if response is not adequate; may take up to 4 weeks for full therapeutic response. Doses >100 mg/day are associated with increased risk of hyperkalemia and no greater therapeutic effect.

Dose modification during concurrent use with moderate CYP3A4 inhibitors: Initial: 25 mg once daily

Congestive heart failure (post-MI): Oral: Initial: 25 mg once daily; dosage goal: titrate to 50 mg once daily within 4 weeks, as tolerated

Dosage adjustment per serum potassium concentrations for CHF:

Serum level <5.0 mEq/L:

Increase dose from 25 mg every other day to 25 mg daily **or**

Increase dose from 25 mg daily to 50 mg daily

5.0-5.4 mEq/L: No adjustment needed

5.5-5.9 mEq/L:

Decrease dose from 50 mg daily to 25 mg daily **or**

Decrease dose from 25 mg daily to 25 mg every other day **or**

Decrease does from 25 mg every other day to withhold medication
Potassium level ≥6.0 mEq/L: Withhold medication until potassium <5.5 mEq/L, then restart at 25 mg every other day

Renal Impairment:
Patients with hypertension with Cl$_{cr}$ <50 mL/minute or serum creatinine >2.0 mg/dL in males or >1.8 mg/dL in females: Use is contraindicated; risk of hyperkalemia increases with declining renal function.
Patients with CHF post-MI: Use with caution.

Hepatic Impairment: No dosage adjustment needed for mild-to-moderate impairment. Safety and efficacy not established for severe impairment.

Administration May be administered with or without food.

Monitoring Parameters Blood pressure; serum potassium (levels monitored every 2 weeks for the first 1-2 months, then monthly in clinical trials); renal function

Patient Information Inform prescriber of all prescriptions, OTC medications, or herbal products you are taking, and any allergies you have. Do not take anything new during treatment without consulting prescriber. Do not use potassium supplement or salt substitutes without consulting prescriber. Take exactly as directed and do not discontinue without consulting prescriber. This drug does not eliminate need for diet or exercise regimen as recommended by prescriber. May cause dizziness or lightheadedness (use caution when driving or engaging in tasks that require alertness until response to drug is known); or diarrhea (boiled milk, buttermilk, or yogurt may help). Report chest pain, palpitations, or irregular heartbeat; unrelenting headache; persistent fatigue or flu-like symptoms; or other persistent adverse reactions.

Special Geriatric Considerations Since this medication is contraindicated in patients with a Cl$_{cr}$ <50 mL/minute, it will have limited use in the elderly. Due to physiologic changes, elderly may be at increased risk of hyperkalemia when using this medication.

Dosage Forms Excipient information presented when available (limited, particularly for generics); consult specific product labeling.
Tablet: 25 mg, 50 mg

♦ **EPO** *see* Epoetin Alfa *on page 519*

Epoetin Alfa (e POE e tin AL fa)

Medication Safety Issues
Sound-alike/look-alike issues:
Epoetin alfa may be confused with darbepoetin alfa

International issues:
Epopen® [Spain] may be confused with EpiPen® which is a brand name for epinephrine in the U.S.

U.S. Brand Names Epogen®; Procrit®

Canadian Brand Names Eprex®

Index Terms EPO; Erythropoiesis-Stimulating Agent (ESA); Erythropoietin; NSC-724223; rHuEPO-α

Generic Available No

Pharmacologic Category Colony Stimulating Factor

Use Treatment of anemia related to HIV (zidovudine) therapy, chronic renal failure, antineoplastic therapy (for nonmyeloid malignancies); reduction of allogeneic blood transfusion for elective, noncardiac, nonvascular surgery

Unlabeled/Investigational Use Treatment of anemia associated with rheumatic disease; hypogenerative anemia of Rh hemolytic disease; sickle cell anemia; acute renal failure; Gaucher's disease; Castleman's disease; paroxysmal nocturnal hemoglobinuria; anemia of critical illness (limited documentation)

Contraindications Hypersensitivity to albumin (human) or mammalian cell-derived products; uncontrolled hypertension

Warnings/Precautions Erythropoietic therapies may be associated with an increased risk of cardiovascular and/or neurologic events. A target hemoglobin >12 g/dL and a rapid rise in hemoglobin are associated with increased risk of cardiovascular related events. **[U.S. Boxed Warning]: Use the minimum effective dose that will gradually increase the hemoglobin level to a point sufficient to avoid red blood cell transfusion.** Avoid hemoglobin increases >1 g/dL in any 2-week period, and do not exceed a target level of 12 g/dL. Prior to and during therapy, iron stores must be evaluated. Supplemental iron is recommended if serum ferritin <100 mcg/mL or serum transferrin saturation <20%. In cancer patients, the risk of thrombotic events (eg, pulmonary emboli, thrombophlebitis, thrombosis) was increased by erythropoietic therapy. **[U.S. Boxed Warning]: A higher incidence of deep vein thrombosis was reported in patients receiving ESAs for preoperative reduction in red blood cell transfusions who were not receiving prophylactic anticoagulation.** Antithrombotic prophylaxis is recommended when ESAs are used in surgical patients to reduce red blood cell transfusions. Increased mortality was also observed in patients undergoing coronary
(Continued)

Epoetin Alfa *(Continued)*

artery bypass surgery who received ESAs; these deaths were associated with thrombotic events. Epoetin is **not** approved for reduction of red blood cell transfusion in patients undergoing cardiac or vascular surgery.

[U.S. Boxed Warning]: An increased risk of mortality was reported in cancer patients administered ESAs to a target hemoglobin of 12 g/dL, who were not receiving concurrent chemotherapy or radiation therapy. Epoetin is **not** approved for this indication. ESAs also failed to reduce the number of red blood cell transfusions in this patient population. **[U.S. Boxed Warning]: Decreased survival was reported in metastatic breast cancer patients receiving concurrent chemotherapy and ESAs to a target hemoglobin of >12 g/dL.** Malignant cell lines and tumors may have surface receptors for erythropoietin; it is not known if epoetin stimulates these receptors. **[U.S. Boxed Warning]: There may be a potential risk of shortening time to tumor progression;** this has been reported in advanced head and neck cancer patients receiving ESAs to a target hemoglobin >12 g/dL and concurrent radiation therapy.

Use with caution in patients with hypertension or with a history of seizures; hypertensive encephalopathy and seizures have been reported. If hypertension is difficult to control, reduce or hold epoetin alfa. **Not** recommended for acute correction of severe anemia or as a substitute for transfusion.

Prior to treatment, correct or exclude deficiencies of vitamin B_{12} and/or folate, as well as other factors which may impair erythropoiesis (aluminum toxicity, inflammatory conditions, infections). Poor response should prompt evaluation of these potential factors, as well as possible malignant processes, occult blood loss, hemolysis, and/or bone marrow fibrosis. Pure red cell aplasia (PRCA) with associated neutralizing antibodies to erythropoietin has been reported, predominantly in patients with CRF. Patients with loss of response to epoetin alfa should be evaluated. Discontinue treatment in patients with PRCA secondary to neutralizing antibodies to epoetin.

Due to the delayed onset of erythropoiesis, epoetin is of no value in the acute treatment of anemia. Safety and efficacy in patients with underlying hematologic diseases have not been established, including porphyria, thalassemia, hemolytic anemia, and sickle cell disease. Potentially serious allergic reactions have been reported. Use caution with porphyria, exacerbation of porphyria has been reported (rarely) in patients with chronic renal failure.

Adverse Reactions (Reflective of adult population; not specific for elderly)
>10%:
- Cardiovascular: Hypertension (5% to 24%), thrombotic/vascular events (coronary artery bypass graft surgery: 23%), edema (6% to 17%), deep vein thrombosis (3% to 11%)
- Central nervous system: Fever (29% to 51%), dizziness (<7% to 21%), insomnia (13% to 21%), headache (10% to 19%)
- Dermatologic: Pruritus (14% to 22%), skin pain (4% to 18%), rash (≤16%)
- Gastrointestinal: Nausea (11% to 58%), constipation (42% to 53%), vomiting (8% to 29%), diarrhea (9% to 21%), dyspepsia (7% to 11%)
- Genitourinary: Urinary tract infection (3% to 12%)
- Local: Injection site reaction (<10% to 29%)
- Neuromuscular & skeletal: Arthralgia (11%), paresthesia (11%)
- Respiratory: Cough (18%), congestion (15%), dyspnea (13% to 14%), upper respiratory infection (11%)

1% to 10%:
- Central nervous system: Seizure (1% to 3%)
- Local: Clotted vascular access (7%)

Overdosage/Toxicology Symptoms of overdose include erythrocytosis and polycythemia. A rapid or excessive rise in hemoglobin may be associated with an increased risk for cardiovascular and/or thrombotic events. Phlebotomy may be indicated for polycythemia; treatment is otherwise symptom-directed and supportive.

Stability
Vials should be stored at 2°C to 8°C (36°F to 46°F); **do not freeze or shake**.

Single-dose 1 mL vial contains no preservative: Use one dose per vial. Do not re-enter vial; discard unused portions.
Single-dose vials (except 40,000 units/mL vial) are stable for 2 weeks at room temperature. Single-dose 40,000 units/mL vial is stable for 1 week at room temperature.

Multidose 1 mL or 2 mL vial contains preservative. Store at 2°C to 8°C after initial entry and between doses. Discard 21 days after initial entry.
Multidose vials (with preservative) are stable for 1 week at room temperature.
Prefilled syringes containing the 20,000 units/mL formulation with preservative are stable for 6 weeks refrigerated (2°C to 8°C).
Dilutions of 1:10 and 1:20 (1 part epoetin:19 parts sodium chloride) are stable for 18 hours at room temperature.

Prior to SubQ administration, preservative free solutions may be mixed with bacteriostatic NS containing benzyl alcohol 0.9% in a 1:1 ratio. Dilutions of 1:10 in $D_{10}W$ with human albumin 0.05% or 0.1% are stable for 24 hours.

Mechanism of Action Induces erythropoiesis by stimulating the division and differentiation of committed erythroid progenitor cells; induces the release of reticulocytes from the bone marrow into the bloodstream, where they mature to erythrocytes. There is a dose response relationship with this effect. This results in an increase in reticulocyte counts followed by a rise in hematocrit and hemoglobin levels.

Pharmacodynamics

Onset on action: Increase in reticulocyte count in 10 days, with an increase in RBC count, hemoglobin, and hematocrit within 2-6 weeks

Peak effect: 2-3 weeks

Pharmacokinetics

Distribution: V_d: 9 L; rapid in the plasma compartment; majority of drug is taken up by the liver, kidneys, and bone marrow

Metabolism: Some metabolic degradation does occur

Bioavailability: SubQ: ~21% to 31%; intraperitoneal epoetin in a few patients demonstrated a bioavailability of only 3%

Half-life elimination: Cancer: SubQ: 16-67 hours; Chronic renal failure: 4-13 hours

Time to peak, serum: Chronic renal failure: 5-24 hours

Elimination: Small amounts recovered in the urine; majority hepatically eliminated; 10% excreted unchanged in the urine of normal volunteers

Dosage

Geriatrics & Adults: Individuals with anemia due to iron deficiency, sickle cell disease, autoimmune hemolytic anemia, and bleeding, generally have appropriate endogenous EPO levels to drive erythropoiesis and would not ordinarily be candidates for EPO therapy.

Note: Use the minimum effective dose that will gradually increase the hemoglobin level to a point sufficient to avoid red blood cell transfusion. Hemoglobin levels should not exceed 12 g/dL and should not rise >1 g/dL per 2-week time period.

Chronic renal failure patients: I.V., SubQ: Initial dose: 50-100 units/kg 3 times/week. **Note:** Target hemoglobin levels should not exceed 12 g/dL.

Titration: Reduce dose by 25% when hemoglobin approaches 12 g/dL **or** hemoglobin increases 1 g/dL in any 2-week period. Increase dose by 25% if hemoglobin does not increase by 2 g/dL after 8 weeks of therapy (with adequate iron stores, may increase dose by 25% if hemoglobin increase <1 g/dL over 4 weeks) and hemoglobin is below suggested target range. Do not increase dose more frequently than at 4-week intervals.

Maintenance dose: Individualize to target range; limit additional dosage increases to every 4 weeks (or longer)

Dialysis patients: Median dose: 75 units/kg 3 times/week

Nondialysis patients: Median dose: 75-150 units/kg/week

Zidovudine-treated, HIV-infected patients (with serum erythropoietin levels ≤500 and zidovudine doses ≤4200 mg; patient with erythropoietin levels >500 mU/mL is unlikely to respond): I.V., SubQ: 100 units/kg 3 times/week for 8 weeks. **Note:** Target hemoglobin levels should not exceed 12 g/dL.

Increase dose by 50-100 units/kg 3 times/week if response is not satisfactory in terms of reducing transfusion requirements or increasing hemoglobin after 8 weeks of therapy. Evaluate response every 4-8 weeks thereafter and adjust the dose accordingly by 50-100 units/kg increments 3 times/week. If patient has not responded satisfactorily to a 300 unit/kg dose 3 times/week, a response to higher doses is unlikely. Withhold dose if hemoglobin exceeds 12 g/dL and resume treatment at a 25% dose reduction when hemoglobin drops below 11 g/dL.

Cancer patients on chemotherapy: Treatment of patients with erythropoietin levels >200 mU/mL is **not recommended. Note:** Target hemoglobin levels should not exceed 12 g/dL. SubQ:

150 units/kg 3 times/week or 40,000 units once weekly; commonly used doses range from 10,000 units 3 times/week to 40,000-60,000 units once weekly.

Dose adjustment: If response is not satisfactory after a sufficient period of evaluation (8 weeks of 3 times/week and 4 weeks of once-weekly therapy), the dose may be increased every 4 weeks (or longer) up to 300 units/kg 3 times/week, **or** when dosed weekly, increased all at once to 60,000 units weekly. If patient does not respond, a response to higher doses is unlikely. Stop dose if hemoglobin exceeds 12 g/dL and resume treatment at a 25% dose reduction when hemoglobin drops below 11 g/dL; reduce dose by 25% if hemoglobin increases by 1 g/dL in any 2-week period, or if hemoglobin approaches 12 g/dL.

Surgery patients: Prior to initiating treatment, obtain a hemoglobin to establish that is >10 mg/dL or ≤13 mg/dL: SubQ: Initial dose: 300 units/kg/day for 10 days before surgery, on the day of surgery, and for 4 days after surgery

(Continued)

Epoetin Alfa *(Continued)*

Alternative dose: 600 units/kg in once weekly doses (21, 14, and 7 days before surgery) plus a fourth dose on the day of surgery

Anemia of critical illness (unlabeled use): SubQ: 40,000 units once weekly

Renal Impairment: The National Kidney Foundation 2006 guidelines recommend hemoglobin levels ≥11 g/dL; hemoglobin levels should not be maintained ≥13 g/dL. These guidelines are currently being reassessed.

Hemodialysis: Supplemental dose is not necessary.

Peritoneal dialysis: Supplemental dose is not necessary.

Administration SubQ, I.M. (I.V. not recommended unless on hemodialysis; I.V. administration may require up to 40% more drug as SubQ/I.M. administration to achieve the same therapeutic result)

Patients with CRF on dialysis: I.V. route preferred; may be administered I.V. bolus into the venous line after dialysis.

Patients with CRF not on dialysis: May be administered I.V. or SubQ

Monitoring Parameters

Careful monitoring of blood pressure is indicated; problems with hypertension have been noted in renal failure patients treated with rHuEPO-α. Other patients are less likely to develop this complication.

Follow serum ferritin and serum transferrin saturation monthly

Hematocrit should be determined twice weekly until stabilization within the target range (30% to 33%), and twice weekly at least 2-6 weeks after a dose increase

Baseline and follow-up of blood urea nitrogen (BUN), uric acid, serum creatinine, phosphorous, and potassium

Reference Range Hematocrit: 30% to 33%

Patient Information Frequent blood tests are needed to determine the correct dose; notify physician if any severe headache develops

Additional Information Due to the delayed onset of erythropoiesis (7-10 days to ↑ reticulocyte count; 2-6 weeks to ↑ hemoglobin), erythropoietin is of no value in the acute treatment of anemia. Emergency/stat orders for erythropoietin are inappropriate.

Factors Limiting Response to Epoetin Alfa

Factor	Mechanism
Iron deficiency	Limits hemoglobin synthesis
Blood loss/hemolysis	Counteracts epoetin alfa-stimulated erythropoiesis
Infection/inflammation	Inhibits iron transfer from storage to bone marrow
	Suppresses erythropoiesis through activated macrophages
Aluminum overload	Inhibits iron incorporation into heme protein
Bone marrow replacement Hyperparathyroidism Metastatic, neoplastic	Limits bone marrow volume
Folic acid/vitamin B_{12} deficiency	Limits hemoglobin synthesis
Patient compliance	Self-administered epoetin alfa or iron therapy

Professional Services:
Amgen (Epogen®): 1-800-772-6436
Ortho Biotech (Procrit®): 1-800-325-7504
Reimbursement Assistance:
Amgen: 1-800-272-9376
Ortho Biotech: 1-800-553-3851

Special Geriatric Considerations There is limited information about the use of epoetin alfa in the elderly. Endogenous erythropoietin secretion has been reported to be decreased in elderly with normocytic or iron deficiency anemias or those with a serum hemoglobin concentration <12 g/dL; one study did not find such a relationship in the elderly with chronic anemia. A blunted erythropoietin response to anemia has been reported in patients with cancer, rheumatoid arthritis, and AIDS.

Dosage Forms Excipient information presented when available (limited, particularly for generics); consult specific product labeling.

Injection, solution [preservative free]:
Epogen®, Procrit®: 2000 units/mL (1 mL); 3000 units/mL (1 mL); 4000 units/mL (1 mL); 10,000 units/mL (1 mL); 40,000 units/mL (1 mL) [contains human albumin]

Injection, solution [with preservative]:
Epogen®, Procrit®: 10,000 units/mL (2 mL); 20,000 units/mL (1 mL) [contains human albumin and benzyl alcohol]

Selected References

Carpenter MA, Kendall RG, O'Brien AE, et al, "Reduced Erythropoietin Response to Anaemia in Elderly Patients With Normocytic Anaemia," *Eur J Haematol*, 1992, 49(3):119-21.

Drueke TB, Locatelli F, Clyne N, et al, "Normalization of Hemoglobin Level in Patients With Chronic Kidney Disease and Anemia," *N Engl J Med*, 2006, 355(20): 2071-84.

Erslev AJ, "Erythropoietin," *N Engl J Med*, 1991, 324(19):1339-44.

Goodnough LT, Price TH, Parvin CA, "The Endogenous Erythropoietin Response and the Erythropoietic Response to Blood Loss Anemia: The Effects of Age and Gender," *J Lab Clin Med*, 1995, 126(1):57-64.

Joosten E, Van Hove L, Lesaffre E, et al, "Serum Erythropoietin Levels in Elderly Inpatients With Anemia of Chronic Disorders and Iron Deficiency Anemia," *J Am Geriatr Soc*, 1993, 41(12):1301-4.

Kario K, Matsuo T, and Nakao K, "Serum Erythropoietin Levels in the Elderly," *Gerontology*, 1991, 37(6):345-8.

Nafziger J, Pailla K, Luciani L, et al, "Decreased Erythropoietin Responsiveness to Iron Deficiency Anemia in the Elderly," *Am J Hematol*, 1993, 43(3):172-6.

National Kidney Foundation, "KDOQI Clinical Practice Guidelines and Clinical Practice Recommentaions for Anemia in Chronic Kidney Disease," *Am J Kidney Dis*, 2006, 47(5 Suppl 3):1-145. Available at http://www.kidney.org/professionals/KDOQI/guidelines_anemia/cpr31.htm. Accessed March 12, 2007.

Powers JS, Krantz SB, Collins JC, et al, "Erythropoietin Response to Anemia as a Function of Age," *J Am Geriatr Soc*, 1991, 39(1):30-2.

Singh AJ, Szczech L, Tang Kl, et al, "Correction of Anemia With Epoetin Alfa in Chronic Kidney Disease," *N Engl J Med*, 2006, 355(20):2085-98.

♦ **Epogen®** see Epoetin Alfa *on page 519*

Eprosartan (ep roe SAR tan)

Related Information
Angiotensin Agents *on page 1737*
U.S. Brand Names Teveten®
Canadian Brand Names Teveten®
Generic Available No
Pharmacologic Category Angiotensin II Receptor Blocker
Use Treatment of hypertension, alone or in combination with other antihypertensive agents
Contraindications Hypersensitivity to eprosartan or any component of the formulation; sensitivity to other A-II receptor antagonists; bilateral renal artery stenosis; primary hyperaldosteronism
Warnings/Precautions May cause hyperkalemia; avoid potassium supplementation unless specifically required by healthcare provider. Avoid use or use a smaller dose in patients who are volume depleted; correct depletion first. May be associated with deterioration of renal function and/or increases in serum creatinine, particularly in patients dependent on renin-angiotensin-aldosterone system. Use with caution in unilateral renal artery stenosis and pre-existing renal insufficiency; significant aortic/mitral stenosis.
Adverse Reactions (Reflective of adult population; not specific for elderly)
1% to 10%:
Central nervous system: Fatigue (2%), depression (1%)
Endocrine & metabolic: Hypertriglyceridemia (1%)
Gastrointestinal: Abdominal pain (2%)
Genitourinary: Urinary tract infection (1%)
Respiratory: Upper respiratory tract infection (8%), rhinitis (4%), pharyngitis (4%), cough (4%)
Miscellaneous: Viral infection (2%), injury (2%)
Overdosage/Toxicology The most likely manifestations of overdose would be hypotension and tachycardia. Initiate supportive care for symptomatic hypotension.
Drug Interactions Inhibits CYP2C9 (weak)
Lithium: Risk of toxicity may be increased by eprosartan; monitor lithium levels.
NSAIDs: May decrease angiotensin II antagonist efficacy; effect has been seen with losartan, but may occur with other medications in this class; monitor blood pressure
Potassium-sparing diuretics (amiloride, potassium, spironolactone, triamterene): Increased risk of hyperkalemia.
Potassium supplements may increase the risk of hyperkalemia.
Trimethoprim (high dose) may increase the risk of hyperkalemia.
Ethanol/Nutrition/Herb Interactions Herb/Nutraceutical: Avoid dong quai if using for hypertension (has estrogenic activity). Avoid ephedra, yohimbe, ginseng (may worsen hypertension). Avoid garlic (may have increased antihypertensive effect).
Mechanism of Action Angiotensin II is formed from angiotensin I in a reaction catalyzed by angiotensin-converting enzyme (ACE, kininase II). Angiotensin II is the principal pressor agent of the renin-angiotensin system, with effects that include vasoconstriction, stimulation of synthesis and release of aldosterone, cardiac stimulation, and renal reabsorption of sodium. Eprosartan blocks the vasoconstrictor and aldosterone-secreting effects of angiotensin II by selectively blocking the binding of angiotensin II to the AT1 receptor in many tissues, such as vascular smooth muscle and the adrenal gland. Its action is therefore independent of the pathways for angiotensin II synthesis. Blockade of the renin-angiotensin system with ACE inhibitors, which inhibit the biosynthesis of angiotensin II from angiotensin I, is widely used in the treatment of hypertension. ACE inhibitors also inhibit the degradation of bradykinin, a reaction also catalyzed by ACE. Because eprosartan does not inhibit ACE (kininase II), (Continued)

Eprosartan *(Continued)*

it does not affect the response to bradykinin. Whether this difference has clinical relevance is not yet known. Eprosartan does not bind to or block other hormone receptors or ion channels known to be important in cardiovascular regulation.

Pharmacodynamics Peak effect: 1-2 hours after oral dose (fasting state)

Pharmacokinetics

Distribution: V_d: 308 L

Protein binding: 98%

Metabolism: No active metabolites; glucuronidation

Bioavailability: 13%

Half-life (terminal): 5-9 hours

Elimination: 90% excreted in the feces via the biliary route; 7% excreted in the urine (80% unchanged)

Dosage

Geriatrics & Adults: Hypertension: Oral: Dosage must be individualized. Can administer once or twice daily with total daily doses of 400-800 mg. Usual starting dose is 600 mg once daily as monotherapy in patients who are euvolemic. Limited clinical experience with doses >800 mg.

Renal Impairment: No starting dosage adjustment is necessary; however, carefully monitor the patient.

Hepatic Impairment: No starting dosage adjustment is necessary; however, carefully monitor the patient.

Monitoring Parameters Supine blood pressure, electrolytes, serum creatinine, BUN, urinalysis, symptomatic hypotension, tachycardia

Patient Information Take with or without food. Take with food if medicine causes stomach upset. Take at a similar time every day. Follow diet given by healthcare provider. Check blood pressure regularly.

Additional Information The angiotensin II receptor antagonists appear to have similar indications as the ACE inhibitors. While these drugs have been shown to be effective in treating hypertension, their efficacy in heart failure is being vigorously evaluated. The angiotensin II antagonists are especially useful in providing an alternative therapy in those patients who have intractable cough in response to ACE inhibitor therapy. Similar to ACE inhibitors, pre-existing volume depletion caused by diuretic therapy may potentiate hypotension in response to angiotensin II antagonists.

Because of the lack of effect on the response to bradykinin, angiotensin-receptor blockers are less likely to be associated with nonrenin-angiotensin effects such as cough and angioedema. Because of a different site of action in comparison to ACE inhibitors, the angiotensin II antagonists do not cause increases in levels of bradykinin. These different sites of action have lead to the supposition that the ACE inhibitors and the angiotensin II antagonists may be used in combination for enhanced response. This possibility is currently being evaluated.

Special Geriatric Considerations No specific dose adjustments are necessary in the elderly due to the drug's major route of elimination. However, since many elderly may be volume depleted due to their "blunted thirst reflex" and use of diuretics, care and monitoring of blood pressure and volume status are necessary upon initiation.

Dosage Forms Excipient information presented when available (limited, particularly for generics); consult specific product labeling.

Tablet: 400 mg, 600 mg

Eprosartan and Hydrochlorothiazide

(ep roe SAR tan & hye droe klor oh THYE a zide)

Related Information

Eprosartan *on page 523*

Hydrochlorothiazide *on page 756*

U.S. Brand Names Teveten® HCT

Canadian Brand Names Teveten® HCT; Teveten® Plus

Index Terms Eprosartan Mesylate and Hydrochlorothiazide; Hydrochlorothiazide and Eprosartan

Generic Available No

Pharmacologic Category Angiotensin II Receptor Blocker Combination; Antihypertensive Agent, Combination; Diuretic, Thiazide

Use Treatment of hypertension (not indicated for initial treatment)

Dosage

Geriatrics & Adults: Hypertension: Oral: Dose is individualized (combination substituted for individual components)

Usual recommended dose: Eprosartan 600 mg/hydrochlorothiazide 12.5 mg once daily (maximum dose: Eprosartan 600 mg/hydrochlorothiazide 25 mg once daily)

Renal Impairment: Initial dose adjustments not recommended by manufacturer; carefully monitor patient. Hydrochlorothiazide is ineffective in patients with Cl$_{cr}$ <30 mL/minute.

Hepatic Impairment: Initial dose adjustments not recommended by manufacturer; carefully monitor patient.

Dosage Forms Excipient information presented when available (limited, particularly for generics); consult specific product labeling.
Tablet:
600 mg/12.5 mg: Eprosartan 600 mg and hydrochlorothiazide 12.5 mg
600 mg/25 mg: Eprosartan 600 mg and hydrochlorothiazide 25 mg

♦ **Eprosartan Mesylate and Hydrochlorothiazide** see Eprosartan and Hydrochlorothiazide on page 524

♦ **Epsom Salt [OTC]** see Magnesium Salts (Various Salts) on page 952

♦ **Equalactin® [OTC]** see Polycarbophil on page 1282

♦ **Equalizer Gas Relief [OTC]** see Simethicone on page 1467

♦ **Equanil** see Meprobamate on page 984

♦ **Equetro™** see Carbamazepine on page 231

♦ **Equilet® [OTC]** see Calcium Salts (Oral) on page 220

Ergocalciferol (er goe kal SIF e role)

Medication Safety Issues
Sound-alike/look-alike issues:
Calciferol™ may be confused with calcitriol
Drisdol® may be confused with Drysol™

U.S. Brand Names Calciferol™; Drisdol®
Canadian Brand Names Drisdol®; Ostoforte®
Index Terms Activated Ergosterol; Viosterol; Vitamin D$_2$
Generic Available Yes: Tablet
Pharmacologic Category Vitamin D Analog
Use Treatment of refractory rickets, hypophosphatemia, hypoparathyroidism
Unlabeled/Investigational Use Prevention and treatment of vitamin D deficiency in patients with chronic kidney disease (CKD)
Contraindications Hypersensitivity to ergocalciferol or any component of the formulation; hypercalcemia; malabsorption syndrome; hypervitaminosis D or abnormal sensitivity to the toxic effects of vitamin D
Warnings/Precautions Adequate calcium supplementation is required; calcium and phosphorous levels must be monitored during therapy. The range between therapeutic and toxic doses is narrow in vitamin D-resistant rickets. Adjust dose based on clinical response to avoid toxicity. Use caution with cardiovascular disease or renal dysfunction. Products may contain tartrazine, which may cause allergic reactions in certain individuals.
Adverse Reactions (Reflective of adult population; not specific for elderly)
Frequency not defined.
Cardiovascular: Hypertension, vascular calcification
Central nervous system: Mental retardation
Endocrine & metabolic: Acidosis, growth suppression (children), hyperphosphatemia, polydypsia
Gastrointestinal: Anorexia, constipation, nausea, weight loss
Hematologic: Anemia
Neuromuscular & skeletal: Aches, osteoporosis (adults), stiffness, weakness
Renal: Azotemia (reversible), hypercalciuria, nephrocalcinosis, nocturia, polyuria, renal dysfunction
Miscellaneous: Dwarfism (children); soft tissue calcification (blood vessels, heart, lungs, renal tubules)
Overdosage/Toxicology Effects of overdose may persist for >2 months. Symptoms of chronic overdose include hypercalcemia, weakness, fatigue, lethargy, and anorexia. Following withdrawal of the drug and oral decontamination, treatment consists of bedrest, liberal fluid intake, reduced calcium intake, and cathartic administration. Severe hypercalcemia requires I.V. hydration and forced diuresis with I.V. furosemide. Urine output should be monitored and maintained at >3 mL/kg/hour. I.V. saline can quickly and significantly increase excretion of calcium into urine. Calcitonin and bisphosphonates have all been used successfully to treat the more resistant cases of vitamin D-induced hypercalcemia.
Drug Interactions
Mineral oil: Absorption of ergocalciferol may be decreased.
Thiazide diuretics: Concomitant use may cause hypercalcemia.
Stability Store at room temperature of 15°C to 30°C (59°F to 86°F). Protect from light.
(Continued)

Ergocalciferol *(Continued)*

Mechanism of Action Stimulates calcium and phosphate absorption from the small intestine, promotes secretion of calcium from bone to blood; promotes renal tubule phosphate resorption

Pharmacodynamics Peak effect: Within a month following daily doses

Pharmacokinetics

Absorption: Readily from GI tract; absorption requires intestinal levels of bile

Inactive until hydroxylated in the liver and the kidney to calcifediol and then to calcitriol (most active form)

Dosage

Geriatrics: Refer to adult dosing (see Special Geriatric Considerations and Additional Information).

Adequate intake (each 1 mcg = 40 int. units): >70 years: Oral: 15 mcg/day (600 int. units/day)

Adults: Note: 1 mcg = 40 int. units

Adequate intake: Oral:

18-50 years: 5 mcg/day (200 int. units/day)

51-70 years: 10 mcg/day (400 int. units/day)

Elderly >70 years: 15 mcg/day (600 int. units/day)

Dietary supplementation: Oral: 10 mcg/day (400 int. units/day)

Vitamin D deficiency/insufficiency in patients with CKD stages 3-4 (K/DOQI guidelines). **Note:** Dose is based on 25-hydroxyvitamin D serum level [25(OH) D]: Oral (treatment duration should be a total of 6 months):

Serum 25(OH)D <5 ng/mL:

50,000 int. units/week for 12 weeks, then 50,000 int. units/month

Serum 25(OH)D 5-15 ng/mL:

50,000 int. units/week for 4 weeks, then 50,000 int. units/month

Serum 25(OH)D 16-30 ng/mL:

50,000 int. units/month

Hypoparathyroidism: Oral: 625 mcg to 5 mg/day (25,000-200,000 int. units) and calcium supplements

Nutritional rickets and osteomalacia: Oral:

Adults with normal absorption: 25-125 mcg/day (1000-5000 int. units)

Adults with malabsorption: 250-7500 mcg (10,000-300,000 int. units)

Vitamin D-*dependent* rickets: Oral: 250 mcg to 1.5 mg/day (10,000-60,000 int. units)

Vitamin D-*resistant* rickets: Oral: 12,000-500,000 int. units/day

Familial hypophosphatemia: Oral: 10,000-60,000 int. units plus phosphate supplements

Administration Parenteral injection for I.M. use only

Monitoring Parameters Serum calcium, creatinine, BUN, and phosphorus every 1-2 weeks; x-ray bones monthly until stabilized; signs and symptoms of vitamin D intoxication

Vitamin D deficiency/insufficiency in patients with CKD stages 3-4: Measure serum 25(OH)D levels after 3 months of treatment in children or after 6 months in adults. Discontinue ergocalciferol (or any vitamin D supplements) if the corrected total serum calcium level is >10.2 mg/dL.

Reference Range

Serum calcium times phosphorus should not exceed 70 mg^2/dL^2 to avoid ectopic calcification

Vitamin D insufficiency: Serum 25(OH)D <27-32 ng/mL

CKD K/DOQI guidelines definition of stages; chronic disease is kidney damage or GFR <60 mL/minute/1.73 m^2 for ≥3 months:

Stage 2: GFR 60-89 mL/minute/1.73 m^2 (kidney damage with mild decrease GFR)

Stage 3: GFR 30-59 mL/minute/1.73 m^2 (moderate decrease GFR)

Stage 4: GFR 15-29 mL/minute/1.73 m^2 (severe decrease GFR)

Stage 5: GFR <15 mL/minute/1.73 m^2 or dialysis (kidney failure)

Patient Information Early symptoms of hypercalcemia include weakness, fatigue, somnolence, headache, anorexia, dry mouth, metallic taste, nausea, vomiting, cramps, diarrhea, muscle pain, bone pain, and irritability; do not take more than the recommended amount. While taking this medication, your physician may want you to follow a special diet or take a calcium supplement. Follow this diet closely. Avoid taking magnesium supplements or magnesium containing antacids.

Additional Information 1.25 mg ergocalciferol provides 50,000 units of vitamin D activity

Special Geriatric Considerations Vitamin D, folate, and B$_{12}$ (cyanocobalamin) have decreased absorption with age (clinical significance unknown); studies in ill geriatrics demonstrated that low serum concentrations of vitamin D result in greater bone loss. Calorie requirements decrease with age and therefore, nutrient density must be increased to ensure adequate nutrient intake, including vitamins and minerals. The use of a daily supplement with a multiple vitamin with minerals is recommended because elderly consume less vitamin D, absorption may be decreased, and many have decreased sun exposure. This is a recommendation of particular need to those with high risk for osteoporosis.

Dosage Forms Excipient information presented when available (limited, particularly for generics); consult specific product labeling.

Capsule:

Drisdol®: 50,000 int. units [1.25 mg; contains tartrazine and soybean oil]

Liquid, oral [drops]:

Calciferol™, Drisdol®: 8000 int. units/mL (60 mL) [200 mcg/mL; OTC]

Tablet: 400 int. units [10 mcg; OTC]

Selected References

"K/DOQI Clinical Practice Guidelines for Bone Metabolism and Disease in Chronic Kidney Disease. Guideline 7. Prevention and Treatment of Vitamin D Insufficiency and Vitamin D Deficiency in CKD Patients," *Am J Kidney Dis*, 2003, 42(4 Suppl 3):84-89.

Letsou AP and Price LS, "Health Aging and Nutrition: An Overview," *Clin Geriatr Med*, 1987, 3(2):253-60.

Myrianthopoulos M, "Dietary Treatment of Hyperlipidemia in the Elderly," *Clin Geriatr Med*, 1987, 3(2):343-59.

Riggs BL and Melton LJ, "The Prevention and Treatment of Osteoporosis," *N Engl J Med*, 1992, 327(9):620-7.

Thomas MK, Lloyd-Jones, DM, Thadhani RI, et al, "Hypovitaminosis D in Medical Inpatients," *N Engl J Med*, 1998, 338(12):777-83.

Ergoloid Mesylates (ER goe loid MES i lates)

Related Information

Potentially Inappropriate Medications for Geriatrics *on page 1824*

Canadian Brand Names Hydergine®

Index Terms Dihydroergotoxine; Dihydrogenated Ergot Alkaloids; Hydergine [DSC]

Generic Available Yes

Pharmacologic Category Ergot Derivative

Use Treatment of age-related declines in mental capacity related to primary progressive dementia, Alzheimer's dementia, senile onset, and multi-infarct dementia

Contraindications Hypersensitivity to ergot or any component of the formulation; acute or chronic psychosis; ergot alkaloids are contraindicated with potent inhibitors of CYP3A4 (includes protease inhibitors, azole antifungals, and some macrolide antibiotics)

Warnings/Precautions Pleural and peritoneal fibrosis have been reported with prolonged daily use. Cardiac valvular fibrosis has also been associated with ergot alkaloids. Concomitant use with potent inhibitors of CYP3A4 (includes protease inhibitors, azole antifungals, and some macrolide antibiotics) and ergot alkaloids has been associated with acute ergot toxicity (ergotism); certain ergot alkaloids (eg, ergotamine and dihydroergotamine) are contraindicated by the manufacturer. Use with caution in the elderly.

Adverse Reactions (Reflective of adult population; not specific for elderly) Adverse effects are minimal; most common include transient nausea, gastrointestinal disturbances and sublingual irritation with SL tablets; other common side effects include:

Cardiovascular: Orthostatic hypotension, bradycardia

Dermatologic: Skin rash, flushing

Ocular: Blurred vision

Respiratory: Nasal congestion

Drug Interactions Substrate of CYP3A4 (major)

Antipsychotics: May diminish the effects of ergoloid mesylates (due to dopamine antagonism); these combinations should generally be avoided.

Beta-blockers: Severe peripheral vasoconstriction has been reported with concomitant use of beta-blockers and ergot derivatives; monitor.

CYP3A4 inhibitors: May increase the levels/effects of ergoloid mesylates. Example inhibitors include azole antifungals, clarithromycin, diclofenac, doxycycline, erythromycin, imatinib, isoniazid, nefazodone, nicardipine, propofol, protease inhibitors, quinidine, telithromycin, and verapamil. Certain ergot alkaloids are contraindicated with potent CYP3A4 inhibitors.

MAO inhibitors: The serotonergic effects of ergot derivatives may be increased by MAO inhibitors. Monitor for signs and symptoms of serotonin syndrome.

Metoclopramide: May diminish the effects of ergoloid mesylates (due to dopamine antagonism); concurrent therapy should generally be avoided.

Serotonin agonists: Concurrent use with ergoloid mesylates may increase the risk of serotonin syndrome (includes buspirone, SSRIs, TCAs, nefazodone, sumatriptan, and trazodone).

Sibutramine: May cause serotonin syndrome; concurrent use with certain ergot alkaloids is contraindicated.

Sumatriptan and other serotonin 5-HT$_1$ receptor agonists: Prolong vasospastic reactions; do not use sumatriptan or ergot-containing drugs within 24 hours of each other.

(Continued)

Ergoloid Mesylates (Continued)

Vasoconstrictors: Concomitant use with peripheral vasoconstrictors may cause synergistic elevation of blood pressure; use is contraindicated with many ergot derivatives.

Mechanism of Action Ergoloid mesylates do not have the vasoconstrictor effects of the natural ergot alkaloids; exact mechanism in dementia is unknown; originally classed as peripheral and cerebral vasodilator, now considered a "metabolic enhancer"; there is no specific evidence which clearly establishes the mechanism by which ergoloid mesylate preparations produce mental effects, nor is there conclusive evidence that the drug particularly affects cerebral arteriosclerosis or cerebrovascular insufficiency

Pharmacokinetics
Absorption: Rapid yet incomplete
Metabolism: Significant first-pass metabolism
Half-life: 3.5 hours
Time to peak serum concentration: Within 1 hour

Dosage
Geriatrics & Adults: Primary progressive dementia, Alzheimer's dementia: Oral: 1 mg 3 times/day up to 4.5-12 mg/day; up to 6 months of therapy may be necessary

Monitoring Parameters Blood pressure, heart rate, mental status

Patient Information Do not chew or crush sublingual tablets, allow to dissolve under tongue

Special Geriatric Considerations Ergoloid mesylates have no role in the treatment of dementia. Many clinicians regard it as no better than placebo and most patients do not experience significant benefits. Improvement in social function has been shown in some studies, but no consistent improvement in memory or cognitive function was reported.

Dosage Forms Excipient information presented when available (limited, particularly for generics); consult specific product labeling.
Tablet: 1 mg
Tablet, sublingual: 1 mg

♦ **Ergomar**® see Ergotamine on page 528

Ergotamine (er GOT a meen)

U.S. Brand Names Ergomar®
Index Terms Ergotamine Tartrate
Generic Available No
Pharmacologic Category Antimigraine Agent; Ergot Derivative
Use Treatment or prevention of vascular headaches, such as migraine, migraine variants, or so-called "histaminic cephalalgia"
Contraindications Hypersensitivity to ergotamine or any component of the formulation; peripheral vascular disease; hepatic or renal disease; coronary artery disease; hypertension; sepsis; ergot alkaloids are contraindicated with potent inhibitors of CYP3A4 (includes protease inhibitors, azole antifungals, and some macrolide antibiotics)
Warnings/Precautions Ergot alkaloids have been associated with fibrotic valve thickening (eg, aortic, mitral, tricuspid); usually associated with long-term, chronic use; vasospasm or vasoconstriction can occur; ergot alkaloid use may result in ergotism (intense vasoconstriction) resulting in peripheral vascular ischemia and possible gangrene; rare cases of pleural and/or retroperitoneal fibrosis have been reported with prolonged daily use. Discontinuation after extended use may result in withdrawal symptoms (eg, rebound headache). Use with caution in the elderly.

[U.S. Boxed Warning]: Ergot alkaloids are contraindicated with potent inhibitors of CYP3A4 (includes protease inhibitors, azole antifungals, and some macrolide antibiotics); concomitant use associated with acute ergot toxicity (ergotism).

Adverse Reactions (Reflective of adult population; not specific for elderly)
Frequency not defined.
Cardiovascular: Absence of pulse, bradycardia, cardiac valvular fibrosis, cyanosis, edema, ECG changes, gangrene, hypertension, ischemia, precordial distress and pain, tachycardia, vasospasm
Central nervous system: Vertigo
Dermatologic: Itching
Gastrointestinal: Nausea, vomiting
Genitourinary: Retroperitoneal fibrosis
Neuromuscular & skeletal: Muscle pain, numbness, paresthesia, weakness
Respiratory: Pleuropulmonary fibrosis
Miscellaneous: Cold extremities

Overdosage/Toxicology Symptoms include vasospastic effects, nausea, vomiting, lassitude, impaired mental function, hypotension, hypertension, unconsciousness, seizures, shock, and death. Treatment includes general supportive therapy, gastric lavage, or induction of emesis, and saline cathartic, Keep extremities warm. Activated charcoal is effective at binding certain chemicals, this is especially true for ergot alkaloids. Treatment is symptomatic, with heparin and vasodilators (nitroprusside). Use vasodilators with caution to avoid exaggerating any pre-existing hypotension.

Drug Interactions Substrate of CYP3A4 (major); Inhibits CYP3A4 (weak)

Antifungals, azole derivatives (itraconazole, ketoconazole) increase levels of ergot alkaloids by inhibiting CYP3A4 metabolism, resulting in toxicity; concomitant use is contraindicated.

Antipsychotics: May diminish the effects of ergotamine (due to dopamine antagonism); these combinations should generally be avoided.

Beta-blockers: Severe peripheral vasoconstriction has been reported with concomitant use of beta-blockers and ergot derivatives; monitor.

CYP3A4 inhibitors: May increase the levels/effects of ergotamine. Example inhibitors include azole antifungals, clarithromycin, diclofenac, doxycycline, erythromycin, imatinib, isoniazid, nefazodone, nicardipine, propofol, protease inhibitors, quinidine, telithromycin, and verapamil. Ergot alkaloids are contraindicated with potent CYP3A4 inhibitors.

Macrolide antibiotics: Erythromycin, clarithromycin, and troleandomycin may increase levels of ergot alkaloids by inhibiting CYP3A4 metabolism, resulting in toxicity (ischemia, vasospasm); concomitant use is contraindicated.

MAO inhibitors: The serotonergic effects of ergot derivatives may be increased by MAO inhibitors. Monitor for signs and symptoms of serotonin syndrome.

Metoclopramide: May diminish the effects of ergotamine (due to dopamine antagonism); concurrent therapy should generally be avoided.

Protease inhibitors (ritonavir, amprenavir, atazanavir, indinavir, nelfinavir, and saquinavir) increase blood levels of ergot alkaloids by inhibiting CYP3A4 metabolism, acute ergot toxicity has been reported; concomitant use is contraindicated.

Sibutramine: May cause serotonin syndrome; concurrent use with ergot alkaloids is contraindicated.

Serotonin agonists: Concurrent use with ergotamine may increase the risk of serotonin syndrome (includes buspirone, SSRIs, TCAs, nefazodone, sumatriptan, and trazodone).

Sumatriptan and other serotonin 5-HT$_1$ receptor agonists: Prolong vasospastic reactions; do not use sumatriptan or ergot-containing drugs within 24 hours of each other.

Vasoconstrictors: Concomitant use of some ergot derivatives and peripheral vasoconstrictors may cause synergistic elevation of blood pressure; use is contraindicated.

Ethanol/Nutrition/Herb Interactions Food: Avoid tea, cola, and coffee (caffeine may increase GI absorption of ergotamine). Grapefruit juice may cause increased blood levels of ergotamine, leading to increased toxicity.

Stability Store sublingual tablet at room temperature. Protect from light and heat.

Mechanism of Action Has partial agonist and/or antagonist activity against tryptaminergic, dopaminergic and alpha-adrenergic receptors depending upon their site; is a highly active uterine stimulant; it causes constriction of peripheral and cranial blood vessels and produces depression of central vasomotor centers

Pharmacokinetics

Absorption: Ergotamine: Oral: Erratic; enhanced by caffeine coadministration

Metabolism: Extensively hepatic

Time to peak, serum: Ergotamine: 0.5-3 hours

Half-life: 2 hours

Elimination: Feces (90% as metabolites)

Dosage

Geriatrics: See Special Geriatric Considerations.

Adults: Migraine: Sublingual: One tablet under tongue at first sign, then 1 tablet every 30 minutes if needed; maximum dose: 3 tablets/24 hours, 5 tablets/week

Administration Do not crush sublingual drug product.

Monitoring Parameters Relief of symptoms, blood pressure, pulse, peripheral circulation

Patient Information Inform prescriber of all prescriptions, OTC medications, or herbal products you are taking, and any allergies you have. Do not take any new medication during therapy without consulting prescriber. Take this drug as directed; do not increase dose or use more often than prescribed. If relief is not obtained, contact your prescriber. Avoid products that contain caffeine (eg, tea, coffee, colas, cocoa); caffeine increases GI absorption of ergotamines. May cause drowsiness (avoid activities requiring alertness until effects of medication are known); mild nausea or vomiting (consult prescriber for approved antiemetic); or mild weakness or numbness of extremities (avoid activities that may have a potential for injury). Inspect your extremities for coldness, numbness, or injury. Report immediately any extreme numbness, pain, tingling or weakness in extremities (toes, fingers); severe unresolved nausea or vomiting; or respiratory difficulty or irregular heartbeat.
(Continued)

Ergotamine *(Continued)*

Special Geriatric Considerations Not recommended for use in the elderly. May be harmful due to reduction in cerebral blood flow. May precipitate angina, myocardial infarction, or aggravate intermittent claudication.

Dosage Forms Excipient information presented when available (limited, particularly for generics); consult specific product labeling.

Tablet, sublingual: Ergotamine tartrate 2 mg

Ergotamine and Caffeine (er GOT a meen & KAF een)

Related Information

Ergotamine *on page 528*

Medication Safety Issues

Sound-alike/look-alike issues:

Cafergot® may be confused with Carafate®

U.S. Brand Names Cafergot®; Migergot

Canadian Brand Names Cafergor®

Index Terms Caffeine and Ergotamine; Ergotamine Tartrate and Caffeine

Generic Available Yes

Pharmacologic Category Antimigraine Agent; Ergot Derivative; Stimulant

Use Abort or prevent vascular headaches, such as migraine, migraine variants, or so-called "histaminic cephalalgia"

Contraindications Hypersensitivity to ergotamine, caffeine, or any component of the formulation; peripheral vascular disease; hepatic or renal disease; coronary artery disease; hypertension; sepsis; ergot alkaloids are contraindicated with strong inhibitors of CYP3A4 (includes protease inhibitors, azole antifungals, and some macrolide antibiotics)

Warnings/Precautions Ergot alkaloids have been associated with fibrotic valve thickening (eg, aortic, mitral, tricuspid); usually associated with long-term, chronic use; vasospasm or vasoconstriction can occur; ergot alkaloid use may result in ergotism (intense vasoconstriction) resulting in peripheral vascular ischemia and possible gangrene; rare cases of pleural and/or retroperitoneal fibrosis have been reported with prolonged daily use. Discontinuation after extended use may result in withdrawal symptoms (eg, rebound headache). Use with caution in the elderly.

[U.S. Boxed Warning]: Ergot alkaloids are contraindicated with potent inhibitors of CYP3A4 (includes protease inhibitors, azole antifungals, and some macrolide antibiotics); concomitant use associated with acute ergot toxicity (ergotism).

Adverse Reactions (Reflective of adult population; not specific for elderly)

Frequency not defined.

Cardiovascular: Absence of pulse, bradycardia, cardiac valvular fibrosis, cyanosis, edema, ECG changes, gangrene, hypertension, ischemia, precordial distress and pain, tachycardia, vasospasm

Central nervous system: Vertigo

Dermatologic: Itching

Gastrointestinal: Anal or rectal ulcer (with overuse of suppository), nausea, vomiting

Genitourinary: Retroperitoneal fibrosis

Neuromuscular & skeletal: Muscle pain, numbness, paresthesia, weakness

Respiratory: Pleuropulmonary fibrosis

Miscellaneous: Cold extremities

Overdosage/Toxicology Symptoms include vasospastic effects, nausea, vomiting, lassitude, impaired mental function, hypotension, hypertension, unconsciousness, seizures, shock, and death. Treatment includes general supportive therapy, gastric lavage, or induction of emesis, and saline cathartic, Keep extremities warm. Activated charcoal is effective at binding certain chemicals, this is especially true for ergot alkaloids. Treatment is symptomatic, with heparin and vasodilators (nitroprusside). Use vasodilators with caution to avoid exaggerating any pre-existing hypotension.

Drug Interactions

Ergotamine: **Substrate** of CYP3A4 (major); **Inhibits** CYP3A4 (weak)

Caffeine: **Substrate** of CYP1A2 (major), 2C9 (minor), 2D6 (minor), 2E1 (minor), 3A4 (minor); **Inhibits** CYP1A2 (weak), 3A4 (moderate)

See Ergotamine monograph for related interactions.

CYP1A2 inhibitors: May increase the levels/effects of caffeine. Example inhibitors include amiodarone, fluvoxamine, ketoconazole, and rofecoxib.

CYP3A4 substrates: Caffeine may increase the levels/effects of CYP3A4 substrates. Example substrates include benzodiazepines, calcium channel blockers, cyclosporine, mirtazapine, nateglinide, nefazodone, sildenafil (and other PDE-5 inhibitors), tacrolimus, and venlafaxine. Selected benzodiazepines (midazolam and triazolam), cisapride, ergot alkaloids, selected HMG-CoA reductase inhibitors (lovastatin and simvastatin), and pimozide are generally contraindicated with strong CYP3A4 inhibitors.

Quinolone antibiotics (specifically ciprofloxacin, norfloxacin, ofloxacin): Caffeine levels may be increased by quinolone antibiotics.

Ethanol/Nutrition/Herb Interactions Food: Avoid tea, cola, and coffee (caffeine may increase GI absorption of ergotamine). Grapefruit juice may cause increased blood levels of ergotamine, leading to increased toxicity.

Stability

Suppositories: Store below 25°C (77°F) in sealed foil. Protect from moisture.

Tablet: Store at room temperature 15°C to 30°C (59°F to 86°F).

Mechanism of Action Has partial agonist and/or antagonist activity against tryptaminergic, dopaminergic and alpha-adrenergic receptors depending upon their site; is a highly active uterine stimulant; it causes constriction of peripheral and cranial blood vessels and produces depression of central vasomotor centers

Pharmacokinetics

Absorption: Ergotamine: Oral, rectal: Erratic; enhanced by caffeine coadministration

Metabolism: Extensively hepatic

Time to peak, serum: Ergotamine: 0.5-3 hours

Half-life elimination: 2 hours

Elimination: Feces (90% as metabolites)

Dosage

Adults: Migraine:

Oral: Two tablets at onset of attack; then 1 tablet every 30 minutes as needed; maximum: 6 tablets per attack; do not exceed 10 tablets/week.

Rectal: One suppository rectally at first sign of an attack; follow with second dose after 1 hour, if needed; maximum: 2 per attack; do not exceed 5/week.

Monitoring Parameters Relief of symptoms, blood pressure, pulse, peripheral circulation

Patient Information Inform prescriber of all prescriptions, OTC medications, or herbal products you are taking, and any allergies you have. Do not take any new medication during therapy without consulting prescriber. Take this drug as directed; do not increase dose or use more often than prescribed. If relief is not obtained, contact your prescriber. Avoid products that contain caffeine (eg, tea, coffee, colas, cocoa); caffeine increases GI absorption of ergotamines. May cause drowsiness (avoid activities requiring alertness until effects of medication are known); mild nausea or vomiting (consult prescriber for approved antiemetic); or mild weakness or numbness of extremities (avoid activities that may have a potential for injury). Inspect your extremities for coldness, numbness, or injury. Report immediately any extreme numbness, pain, tingling or weakness in extremities (toes, fingers); severe unresolved nausea or vomiting; or respiratory difficulty or irregular heartbeat.

Special Geriatric Considerations Not recommended for use in the elderly. May be harmful due to reduction in cerebral blood flow. May precipitate angina, myocardial infarction, or aggravate intermittent claudication.

Dosage Forms Excipient information presented when available (limited, particularly for generics); consult specific product labeling.

Suppository, rectal:

Migergot: Ergotamine tartrate 2 mg and caffeine 100 mg (12s)

Tablet: Ergotamine tartrate 1 mg and caffeine 100 mg

Cafergot®: Ergotamine tartrate 1 mg and caffeine 100 mg

♦ **Ergotamine Tartrate** see Ergotamine on page 528

♦ **Ergotamine Tartrate and Caffeine** see Ergotamine and Caffeine on page 530

Ertapenem (er ta PEN em)

Medication Safety Issues

Sound-alike/look-alike issues:

Invanz® may be confused with Avinza™

U.S. Brand Names Invanz®

Canadian Brand Names Invanz®

Index Terms Ertapenem Sodium; L-749,345; MK0826

Generic Available No

Pharmacologic Category Antibiotic, Carbapenem

Use Treatment of the following moderate-severe infections: Complicated intra-abdominal infections, complicated skin and skin structure infections (including diabetic foot infections without osteomyelitis), complicated UTI (including pyelonephritis), acute pelvic infections, and community-acquired pneumonia. Prophylaxis of surgical site infection following elective colorectal surgery. Antibacterial coverage includes aerobic gram-positive organisms, aerobic gram-negative organisms, anaerobic organisms.

Note: Methicillin-resistant *Staphylococcus*, *Enterococcus* spp, penicillin-resistant strains of *Streptococcus pneumoniae*, beta-lactamase-positive strains of *Haemophilus influenzae* are **resistant** to ertapenem, as are most *Pseudomonas aeruginosa*. (Continued)

Ertapenem *(Continued)*

Contraindications Hypersensitivity to ertapenem, other carbapenems, or any other component of the formulation; anaphylactic reactions to beta-lactam antibiotics. If using intramuscularly, known hypersensitivity to local anesthetics of the amide type (lidocaine as the diluent).

Warnings/Precautions Use caution with renal impairment. Dosage adjustment required in patients with moderate-to-severe renal dysfunction; elderly patients often require lower doses (based upon renal function). Prolonged use may result in fungal or bacterial superinfection, including *C. difficile*-associated diarrhea and pseudomembranous colitis. Has been associated with CNS adverse effects, including confusional states and seizures; use caution with CNS disorders (eg, brain lesions, history of seizures, or renal impairment). Serious hypersensitivity reactions, including anaphylaxis, have been reported (some without a history of previous allergic reactions to beta-lactams). Doses for I.M. administration are mixed with lidocaine; consult Lidocaine *on page 904* information for associated Warnings/Precautions.

Adverse Reactions (Reflective of adult population; not specific for elderly)
Note: Percentages reported in adults.
1% to 10%:
    Cardiovascular: Swelling/edema (3%), chest pain (1% to 2%), hypertension (1% to 2%), hypotension (1% to 2%), tachycardia (1% to 2%)
    Central nervous system: Headache (6% to 7%), altered mental status (ie, agitation, confusion, disorientation, decreased mental acuity, changed mental status, somnolence, stupor) (3% to 5%), fever (2% to 5%), insomnia (3%), dizziness (2%), fatigue (1%), anxiety (1%)
    Dermatologic: Rash (2% to 3%), pruritus (1% to 2%), erythema (1% to 2%), wound complication (3%)
    Gastrointestinal: Diarrhea (9% to 10%), nausea (6% to 9%), abdominal pain (4%), vomiting (4%), constipation (3% to 4%), acid regurgitation (1% to 2%), dyspepsia (1%), oral candidiasis (≤1%)
    Genitourinary: Vaginitis (1% to 3%), dysuria (1%), proteinuria
    Hematologic: Platelet count increased (3% to 7%), leukopenia (1% to 2%), neutrophils decreased (1% to 2%), prothrombin time increased (1% to 2%)
    Hepatic: Hepatic enzyme increased (5% to 9%), alkaline phosphatase increase (3% to 7%)
    Local: Infused vein complications (5% to 7%), phlebitis/thrombophlebitis (2%), extravasation (1% to 2%)
    Neuromuscular & skeletal: Leg pain (≤1%), weakness (1%)
    Respiratory: Atelectasis (3%), dyspnea (1% to 3%), cough (1% to 2%), pharyngitis (1%), rales/rhonchi (1%), respiratory distress (≤1%)

Overdosage/Toxicology Treatment is symptom-directed and supportive. Ertapenem is removed by hemodialysis (plasma clearance increased by 30% following 4-hour session).

Drug Interactions Typhoid vaccine: Antibiotics may decrease effectiveness of the Ty21a live, attenuated typhoid vaccine; delay vaccination for >24 hours after administration of antibiotic.
    Uricosuric agents (eg, probenecid): Serum concentrations of ertapenem may be increased; use caution.
    Valproic acid: Ertapenem may decrease valproic acid serum concentrations to subtherapeutic levels; monitor.

Stability Before reconstitution store at ≤25°C (77°F).
    I.M.: Reconstitute 1 g vial with 3.2 mL of 1% lidocaine HCl injection (without epinephrine). Shake well. Use within 1 hour after preparation.
    I.V.: Reconstitute 1 g vial with 10 mL of water for injection, 0.9% sodium chloride injection, or bacteriostatic water for injection. Shake well. For adults, transfer dose to 50 mL of 0.9% sodium chloride injection. Reconstituted I.V. solution may be stored at room temperature and must be used within 6 hours **or** refrigerated, stored for up to 24 hours and used within 4 hours after removal from refrigerator. Do not freeze.

Mechanism of Action Inhibits bacterial cell wall synthesis by binding to one or more of the penicillin binding proteins; which in turn inhibits the final transpeptidation step of peptidoglycan synthesis in bacterial cell walls, thus inhibiting cell wall biosynthesis. Bacteria eventually lyse due to ongoing activity of cell wall autolytic enzymes (autolysins and murein hydrolases) while cell wall assembly is arrested.

Pharmacokinetics
    Absorption: I.M.: Almost complete
    Distribution: V_{dss}: 0.12 L/kg
    Protein binding: Concentration-dependent; 85% at 300 mcg/mL, 95% at <100 mcg/mL
    Metabolism: Hydrolysis to inactive metabolite
    Bioavailability: I.M.: ~90%
    Half-life: 4 hours
    Time to peak: I.M.: ~2.3 hours
    Elimination: Urine (80%) as unchanged drug and metabolite; feces (10%)

Dosage

Geriatrics & Adults: Note: I.V. therapy may be administered for up to 14 days; I.M. for up to 7 days

Community-acquired pneumonia and complicated urinary tract infections (including pyelonephritis): I.M., I.V.: 1 g/day; duration of total antibiotic treatment: 10-14 days (**Note:** Duration includes possible switch to appropriate oral therapy after at least 3 days of parenteral treatment, once clinical improvement demonstrated.)

Intra-abdominal infection: I.M., I.V.: 1 g/day for 5-14 days

Pelvic infections (acute): I.M., I.V.: 1 g/day for 3-10 days

Prophylaxis of surgical site following colorectal surgery: 1 g given 1 hour preoperatively

Skin and skin structure infections (including diabetic foot infections): I.M., I.V.: 1 g/day for 7-14 days

Renal Impairment:

Adults: Cl_{cr} ≤30 mL/minute/1.73 m^2 and ESRD: 500 mg/day

Hemodialysis: When the daily dose is given within 6 hours prior to hemodialysis, a supplementary dose of 150 mg is required following hemodialysis.

Hepatic Impairment: Adjustments cannot be recommended (lack of experience and research in this patient population).

Administration

I.M.: Avoid injection into a blood vessel. Make sure patient does not have an allergy to lidocaine or another anesthetic of the amide type. Administer by deep I.M. injection into a large muscle mass (eg, gluteal muscle or lateral part of the thigh). Do not administer I.M. preparation or drug reconstituted for I.M. administration intravenously.

I.V.: Infuse over 30 minutes

Monitoring Parameters Periodic renal, hepatic, and hematopoietic assessment during prolonged therapy; neurological assessment

Patient Information Report warmth, swelling, irritation at infusion or injection site. Maintain adequate hydration (2-3 L/day of fluids unless instructed to restrict fluid intake) and nutrition. Report unresolved nausea or vomiting (small, frequent meals may help). Report feelings of excessive dizziness, palpitations, visual disturbances, headache, diarrhea, and CNS changes. Report chills, or unusual discharge, or foul-smelling urine.

Special Geriatric Considerations According to the package insert, the total and unbound AUCs were increased 37% and 67%, respectively, in healthy men and women ≥65 years of age compared to younger adults. No dose adjustment is required for patients with normal age-adjusted renal function.

Dosage Forms Excipient information presented when available (limited, particularly for generics); consult specific product labeling.

Injection, powder for reconstitution: 1 g [contains sodium 137 mg/g (~6 mEq/g)]

Selected References

Invanz™ [package insert]. Whitehouse Station, NJ: Merck & Company, Inc, 2001. Available at: http://www.merck.com/product/usa/pi_circulars/i/invanz_pi.pdf. Accessed March 11, 2002.

♦ **Ertapenem Sodium** *see* Ertapenem *on page 531*

♦ **Eryc® [DSC]** *see* Erythromycin *on page 533*

♦ **Eryderm®** *see* Erythromycin *on page 533*

♦ **Erygel®** *see* Erythromycin *on page 533*

♦ **EryPed®** *see* Erythromycin *on page 533*

♦ **Ery-Tab®** *see* Erythromycin *on page 533*

♦ **Erythrocin®** *see* Erythromycin *on page 533*

Erythromycin (er ith roe MYE sin)

Related Information

Antimicrobial Activity Against Selected Organisms *on page 1728*

Medication Safety Issues

Sound-alike/look-alike issues:

Erythromycin may be confused with azithromycin, clarithromycin, Ethmozine®

Akne-Mycin® may be confused with AK-Mycin®

E.E.S.® may be confused with DES®

Eryc® may be confused with Emcyt®, Ery-Tab®

Ery-Tab® may be confused with Eryc®

Erythrocin® may be confused with Ethmozine®

U.S. Brand Names Akne-Mycin®; E.E.S.®; Eryc® [DSC]; Eryderm®; Erygel®; EryPed®; Ery-Tab®; Erythrocin®; PCE®; Romycin®

Canadian Brand Names Apo-Erythro Base®; Apo-Erythro E-C®; Apo-Erythro-ES®; Apo-Erythro-S®; Diomycin®; EES®; Erybid™; Eryc®; Novo-Rythro Estolate; (Continued)

Erythromycin *(Continued)*

Novo-Rythro Ethylsuccinate; Nu-Erythromycin-S; PCE®; PMS-Erythromycin; Sans Acne®

Index Terms Erythromycin Base; Erythromycin Ethylsuccinate; Erythromycin Lactobionate; Erythromycin Stearate

Generic Available Yes: Capsule, gel, ophthalmic ointment, topical solution, suspension (as ethylsuccinate), swab, tablet (as base, ethylsuccinate, and stearate)

Pharmacologic Category Acne Products; Antibiotic, Macrolide; Antibiotic, Ophthalmic; Antibiotic, Topical; Topical Skin Product; Topical Skin Product, Acne

Use

Systemic: Treatment of susceptible bacterial infections including *S. pyogenes*, some *S. pneumoniae*, some *S. aureus*, *M. pneumoniae*, *Legionella pneumophila*, diphtheria, pertussis, *Chlamydia*, erythrasma, *N. gonorrhoeae*, *E. histolytica*, syphilis and nongonococcal urethritis, and *Campylobacter* gastroenteritis; used in conjunction with neomycin for decontaminating the bowel

Ophthalmic: Treatment of superficial eye infections involving the conjunctiva or cornea; neonatal ophthalmia

Topical: Treatment of acne vulgaris

Unlabeled/Investigational Use Systemic: Treatment of gastroparesis, chancroid; preoperative gut sterilization

Contraindications Hypersensitivity to erythromycin or any component of the formulation

Systemic: Concomitant use with pimozide or cisapride

Warnings/Precautions Systemic: Use caution with hepatic impairment with or without jaundice has occurred, it may be accompanied by malaise, nausea, vomiting, abdominal colic, and fever; discontinue use if these occur. Use caution with other medication relying on CYP3A4 metabolism; high potential for drug interactions exists. Prolonged use may result in fungal or bacterial superinfection, including *C. difficile*-associated diarrhea and pseudomembranous colitis. Macrolides have been associated with rare QT_c prolongation and ventricular arrhythmias, including torsade de pointes. Use caution in elderly patients, as risk of adverse events may be increased. Use caution in myasthenia gravis patients; erythromycin may aggravate muscular weakness.

Adverse Reactions (Reflective of adult population; not specific for elderly) Frequency not defined. Incidence may vary with formulation.

Systemic:

Cardiovascular: QT_c prolongation, torsade de pointes, ventricular arrhythmia, ventricular tachycardia

Central nervous system: Seizure

Dermatitis: Pruritus, rash

Gastrointestinal: Abdominal pain, anorexia, diarrhea, infantile hypertrophic pyloric stenosis, nausea, oral candidiasis, pancreatitis, pseudomembranous colitis, vomiting

Hepatic: Cholestatic jaundice (most common with estolate), hepatitis, liver function tests abnormal

Local: Phlebitis at the injection site, thrombophlebitis

Neuromuscular & skeletal: Weakness

Otic: Hearing loss

Miscellaneous: Allergic reactions, anaphylaxis, hypersensitivity reactions, urticaria

Topical: 1% to 10%: Dermatologic: Erythema, desquamation, dryness, pruritus

Overdosage/Toxicology Symptoms include nausea, vomiting, and diarrhea. Treatment is symptom-directed and supportive. Erythromycin is not dialyzable.

Drug Interactions Substrate of CYP2B6 (minor), 3A4 (major); **Inhibits** CYP1A2 (weak), 3A4 (moderate)

Alfentanil (and possibly other opioid analgesics): Serum levels may be increased by erythromycin; monitor for increased effect.

Antifungal agents (imidazole): Reciprocal inhibition of metabolism may lead to increased levels/effects of both azole antifungal and erythromycin; monitor.

Antipsychotic agents (particularly mesoridazine and thioridazine): Risk of QT_c prolongation and malignant arrhythmias may be increased.

Benzodiazepines (those metabolized by CYP3A4, including alprazolam and triazolam): Serum levels may be increased by erythromycin; somnolence and confusion have been reported.

Bromocriptine: Serum levels may be increased by erythromycin; monitor for increased effect (eg, ergotism).

Buspirone: Serum levels may be increased by erythromycin; monitor.

Calcium channel blockers (felodipine, verapamil, and potentially others metabolized by CYP3A4): Serum levels may be increased by erythromycin; monitor.

Carbamazepine: Serum levels may be increased by erythromycin; monitor.

Cilostazol: Serum levels may be increased by erythromycin.

Cisapride: Serum levels may be increased by erythromycin; serious arrhythmias have occurred; concurrent use contraindicated.

Clindamycin (and lincomycin): Use with erythromycin may result in pharmacologic antagonism; manufacturer recommends avoiding this combination.

Clopidogrel: Erythromycin may decrease the anticoagulant effects of clopidogrel; monitor.

Clozapine: Serum levels may be increased by erythromycin; monitor.

Colchicine: serum levels/toxicity may be increased by erythromycin; monitor. Avoid use, if possible.

Corticosteroids: Erythromycin may increase the levels/effects of systemic steroids; monitor for increased effects.

Cyclosporine: Serum levels may be increased by erythromycin; monitor serum levels.

CYP3A4 inducers: CYP3A4 inducers may decrease the levels/effects of erythromycin. Example inducers include aminoglutethimide, carbamazepine, nafcillin, nevirapine, phenobarbital, phenytoin, and rifamycins.

CYP3A4 inhibitors: May increase the levels/effects of erythromycin. Example inhibitors include azole antifungals, clarithromycin, diclofenac, doxycycline, imatinib, isoniazid, nefazodone, nicardipine, propofol, protease inhibitors, quinidine, telithromycin, and verapamil.

CYP3A4 substrates: Erythromycin may increase the levels/effects of CYP3A4 substrates. Example substrates include benzodiazepines, calcium channel blockers, cyclosporine, mirtazapine, nateglinide, nefazodone, sildenafil (and other PDE-5 inhibitors), tacrolimus, and venlafaxine. Selected benzodiazepines (midazolam and triazolam), cisapride, ergot alkaloids, selected HMG-CoA reductase inhibitors (lovastatin and simvastatin), and pimozide are generally contraindicated with strong CYP3A4 inhibitors.

Delavirdine: Serum levels of erythromycin may be increased; also, serum levels of delavirdine may increased by erythromycin (low risk); monitor.

Digoxin: Serum levels may be increased by erythromycin; monitor digoxin levels.

Disopyramide: Serum levels may be increased by erythromycin; in addition, QT_c prolongation and risk of malignant arrhythmia may be increased; avoid combination.

Eletriptan: Serum levels/effects may be increased by erythromycin; monitor.

Eplerenone: Serum levels/effects may be increased by erythromycin; monitor.

Ergot alkaloids: Concurrent use may lead to acute ergot toxicity (severe peripheral vasospasm and dysesthesia).

HMG-CoA reductase inhibitors (atorvastatin, lovastatin, and simvastatin); Erythromycin may increase serum levels of "statins" metabolized by CYP3A4, increasing the risk of myopathy/rhabdomyolysis (does not include fluvastatin, pravastatin, and rosuvastatin). Switch to pravastatin/fluvastatin/rosuvastatin or suspend treatment during course of erythromycin therapy.

Immunosuppressants (eg, cyclosporine, tacrolimus, sirolimus): Serum levels/effects may be increased by erythromycin; monitor.

Phenytoin: Serum levels may be increased by erythromycin; other evidence suggested phenytoin levels may be decreased in some patients; monitor.

Phosphodiesterase-5 inhibitors (eg, sildenafil, tadalafil, vardenafil): Serum concentration may be substantially increased by erythromycin. Do not exceed single sildenafil doses of 25 mg in 48 hours, a single tadalafil dose of 10 mg in 72 hours, or a single vardenafil dose of 2.5 mg in 24 hours.

Pimozide: Serum levels may be increased, leading to malignant arrhythmias; concomitant use is contraindicated.

QT_c-prolonging agents: Concomitant use may increase the risk of malignant arrhythmias.

Quinidine: Serum levels may be increased by erythromycin; in addition, the risk of QT_c prolongation and malignant arrhythmias may be increased during concurrent use.

Repaglinide: Serum levels/effects may be increased by erythromycin; monitor.

Rifamycin derivatives (eg, rifabutin, rifampin): Serum levels may be increased by erythromycin; monitor.

SSRIs: Macrolides may increase the levels/effects; monitor.

Theophylline: Serum levels may be increased by erythromycin; monitor.

Thioridazine: Risk of QT_c prolongation may be increased; concomitant use not recommended.

Valproic acid (and derivatives): Serum levels may be increased by erythromycin; monitor.

Vinblastine (and vincristine): Serum levels may be increased by erythromycin.

Warfarin: Effects may be potentiated; monitor INR closely and adjust warfarin dose as needed or choose another antibiotic.

Zafirlukast: Serum levels may be decreased by erythromycin; monitor.

Zopiclone: Serum levels may be increased by erythromycin; monitor.

Ethanol/Nutrition/Herb Interactions

Ethanol: Avoid ethanol (may decrease absorption of erythromycin or enhance ethanol effects).

(Continued)

Erythromycin *(Continued)*

Food: Erythromycin serum levels may be altered if taken with food (formulation-dependent).

Herb/Nutraceutical: St John's wort may decrease erythromycin levels.

Stability

Injection:

Store unreconstituted vials at 15°C to 30°C (59°F to 86°F). Erythromycin lactobionate should be reconstituted with sterile water for injection without preservatives to avoid gel formation. The reconstituted solution is stable for 2 weeks when refrigerated or for 8 hours at room temperature.

Erythromycin I.V. infusion solution is stable at pH 6-8. Stability of lactobionate is pH dependent. I.V. form has the longest stability in 0.9% sodium chloride (NS) and should be prepared in this base solution whenever possible. Do not use D₅W as a diluent unless sodium bicarbonate is added to solution. If I.V. must be prepared in D₅W, 0.5 mL of the 8.4% sodium bicarbonate solution should be added per each 100 mL of D₅W.

Stability of parenteral admixture at room temperature (25°C) and at refrigeration temperature (4°C) is 24 hours.

Standard diluent: 500 mg/250 mL D₅W/NS; 750 mg/250 mL D₅W/NS; 1 g/250 mL D₅W/NS.

Oral suspension:

Granules: Prior to mixing, store at <30°C (<86°F). After mixing, store under refrigeration and use within 10 days.

Powder: Refrigerate to preserve taste. Erythromycin ethylsuccinate may be stored at room temperature if used within 14 days. EryPed® drops should be used within 35 days following reconstitution. May store at room temperature or under refrigeration.

Tablet and capsule formulations: Store at <30°C (<86°F).

Topical and ophthalmic formulations: Store at room temperature.

Mechanism of Action Inhibits RNA-dependent protein synthesis at the chain elongation step; binds to the 50S ribosomal subunit resulting in blockage of transpeptidation

Pharmacokinetics

Absorption: Oral: Variable but better with salt forms than with base form; 18% to 45%; ethylsuccinate may be better absorbed with food

Distribution: Crosses placenta; enters breast milk

Relative diffusion from blood into CSF: Minimal even with inflammation

CSF:blood level ratio: Normal meninges: 2% to 13%; Inflamed meninges: 7% to 25%

Protein binding: 73% to 81%

Metabolism: Demethylation primarily via hepatic CYP3A4

Half-life: Peak: 1.5-2 hours; End-stage renal disease: 5-6 hours

Time to peak, serum: Base: 4 hours; Ethylsuccinate: 0.5-2.5 hours; delayed with food due to differences in absorption

Elimination: Primarily feces; urine (2% to 15% as unchanged drug)

Dosage

Geriatrics & Adults: Note: Due to differences in absorption, 400 mg erythromycin ethylsuccinate produces the same serum levels as 250 mg erythromycin base or stearate.

Usual dosage range:

Ophthalmic: Instill ½" (1.25 cm) 2-6 times/day depending on the severity of the infection

Topical: Apply over the affected area twice daily after the skin has been thoroughly washed and patted dry

Oral:

Base: 250-500 mg every 6-12 hours

Ethylsuccinate: 400-800 mg every 6-12 hours

I.V.: Lactobionate: 15-20 mg/kg/day divided every 6 hours or 500 mg to 1 g every 6 hours, or given as a continuous infusion over 24 hours (maximum: 4 g/24 hours)

Indication-specific dosing:

Bartonella sp infections (bacillary angiomatosis [BA], peliosis hepatis [PH]) (unlabeled use): Oral: 500 mg (base) 4 times/day for 3 months (BA) or 4 months (PH)

Chancroid (unlabeled use): Oral: 500 mg (base) 3 times/day for 7 days; Note: Not a preferred agent; isolates with intermediate resistance have been documented

Gastrointestinal prokinetic (unlabeled use): I.V.: 200 mg initially followed by 250 mg (base) orally 3 times/day 30 minutes before meals. Lower dosages have been used in some trials.

Granuloma inguinale *(K. granulomatis)* (unlabeled use): Oral: 500 mg (base) 4 times/day for 21 days

Legionnaires' disease: Oral: 1.6-4 g (ethylsuccinate)/day or 1-4 g (base)/day in divided doses for 21 days. **Note:** No longer preferred therapy and only used in nonhospitalized patients.

Lymphogranuloma venereum: Oral: 500 mg (base) 4 times/day for 21 days

Nongonococcal urethritis (including coinfection with *C. trachomatis*): Oral: 500 mg (base) 4 times/day for 7 days or 800 mg (ethylsuccinate) 4 times/day for 7 days. **Note:** May use 250 mg (base) or 400 mg (ethylsuccinate) 4 times/day for 14 days if gastrointestinal intolerance.

Pelvic inflammatory disease: I.V.: 500 mg every 6 hours for 3 days, followed by 1000 mg (base)/day orally in 2-4 divided doses for 7 days. **Note:** Not recommended therapy per current treatment guidelines.

Pertussis: Oral: 500 mg (base) every 6 hours for 14 days

Preop bowel preparation (unlabeled use): Oral: 1 g erythromycin base at 1, 2, and 11 PM on the day before surgery combined with mechanical cleansing of the large intestine and oral neomycin

Syphilis, primary: Oral: 48-64 g (ethylsuccinate) or 30-40 g (base) in divided doses over 10-15 days. **Note:** Not recommended therapy per current treatment guidelines.

Renal Impairment: Slightly dialyzable (5% to 20%); supplemental dose is not necessary in hemo- or peritoneal dialysis or in continuous arteriovenous or venovenous hemofiltration.

Administration

Oral: Do not crush enteric coated drug product. GI upset, including diarrhea, is common. May be administered with food to decrease GI upset. Do not give with milk or acidic beverages.

I.V.: Infuse 1 g over 20-60 minutes. I.V. infusion may be very irritating to the vein. If phlebitis/pain occurs with used dilution, consider diluting further (eg, 1:5) if fluid status of the patient will tolerate, or consider administering in larger available vein. The addition of lidocaine or bicarbonate does not decrease the irritation of erythromycin infusions.

Ophthalmic: Avoid contact of tip of ophthalmic ointment tube with affected eye

Monitoring Parameters Signs and symptoms of infection

Test Interactions False-positive urinary catecholamines

Patient Information Complete full course of therapy, do not skip doses; refrigerate after reconstitution; chewable tablets should not be swallowed whole; notify physician or pharmacist if GI side effects are intolerable, diarrhea develops, or symptoms are not improving

Additional Information

Erythromycin base: E-Mycin®, Eryc®, Ery-Tab®, PCE®, Ilotycin®, Robimycin®

Erythromycin estolate: Ilosone®

Erythromycin ethylsuccinate: E.E.S.®, E-Mycin® E, EryPed®, Wyamycin® E

Erythromycin glucceptate: Ilotycin® Gluceptate

Erythromycin lactobionate: Erythrocin® Lactobionate-IV

Erythromycin stearate: Eramycin®, Erypar®, Erythrocin®, Ethril®, Wintrocin®, Wyamycin® S Due to differences in absorption, 400 mg erythromycin ethylsuccinate produces the same serum levels as 250 mg erythromycin base, stearate, or estolate. Do not use D_5W as a diluent unless sodium bicarbonate is added to solution; infuse over 20-60 minutes.

Sodium content of oral suspension (ethylsuccinate) 200 mg/5 mL: 29 mg (1.3 mEq)

Sodium content of base Filmtab® 250 mg: 70 mg (3 mEq)

Special Geriatric Considerations Dose does not need to be adjusted unless there is severe renal or hepatic impairment. Elderly may be at an increased risk for torsade de pointes, ototoxicity (particularly when dose is ≥4 g/day in conjunction with renal or hepatic impairment).

Dosage Forms Excipient information presented when available (limited, particularly for generics); consult specific product labeling. [DSC] = Discontinued product; [CAN] = Canadian brand name

Note: Strength expressed as base

Capsule, delayed release, enteric-coated pellets, as base: 250 mg
Eryc®: 250 mg [DSC]

Gel, topical: 2% (30 g, 60 g)
Erygel®: 2% (30 g, 60 g) [contains alcohol 92%]

Granules for oral suspension, as ethylsuccinate:
E.E.S.®: 200 mg/5 mL (100 mL, 200 mL) [contains sodium 25.9 mg (1.1 mEq)/5 mL; cherry flavor]

Injection, powder for reconstitution, as lactobionate:
Erythrocin®: 500 mg, 1 g

Ointment, ophthalmic: 0.5% [5 mg/g] (1 g, 3.5 g)
Romycin®: 0.5% [5 mg/g] (3.5 g)

Ointment, topical:
Akne-Mycin®: 2% (25 g)

(Continued)

Erythromycin *(Continued)*

Powder for oral suspension, as ethylsuccinate:
EryPed®: 200 mg/5 mL (100 mL, 200 mL) [contains sodium 117.5 mg (5.1 mEq)/5 mL; fruit flavor]; 400 mg/5 mL (100 mL, 200 mL) [contains sodium 117.5 mg (5.1 mEq)/5 mL; banana flavor]

Powder for oral suspension, as ethylsuccinate [drops]:
EryPed®: 100 mg/2.5 mL (50 mL) [contains sodium 58.8 mg (2.6 mEq)/dropperful; fruit flavor]

Solution, topical: 2% (60 mL)
Eryderm®: 2% (60 mL) [contain alcohol]
Sans acne [CAN]: 2% (60 mL) [contains ethyl alcohol 44%; not available in U.S.]

Suspension, oral, as ethylsuccinate: 200 mg/5 mL (480 mL); 400 mg/5 mL (480 mL)
E.E.S.®: 200 mg/5 mL (100 mL, 480 mL) [fruit flavor]; 400 mg/5 mL (100 mL, 480 mL) [orange flavor]

Tablet, as base: 250 mg, 500 mg
Tablet, as base [polymer-coated particles]:
PCE®: 333 mg, 500 mg

Tablet, as ethylsuccinate: 400 mg
E.E.S.®: 400 mg

Tablet, as stearate: 250 mg, 500 mg
Erythrocin®: 250 mg, 500 mg

Tablet, delayed release, enteric coated, as base:
Ery-Tab®: 250 mg, 333 mg, 500 mg

Selected References

Tiwari T, Murphy TV, and Moran J, "Recommended Antimicrobial Agents for the Treatment and Postexposure Prophylaxis of Pertussis: 2005 CDC Guidelines," *MMWR Recomm Rep*, 2005, 54(RR-14):1-16.
Yoshikawa TT, "Antimicrobial Therapy for the Elderly Patient," *J Am Geriatr Soc*, 1990, 38(12):1353-72.

Erythromycin and Sulfisoxazole

(er ith roe MYE sin & sul fi SOKS a zole)

Related Information

Erythromycin *on page 533*
SulfiSOXAZOLE *on page 1504*

Medication Safety Issues

Sound-alike/look-alike issues:
Pediazole® may be confused with Pediapred®

U.S. Brand Names Pediazole® [DSC]

Canadian Brand Names Pediazole®

Index Terms Sulfisoxazole and Erythromycin

Generic Available Yes

Pharmacologic Category Antibiotic, Macrolide; Antibiotic, Macrolide Combination; Antibiotic, Sulfonamide Derivative

Use Treatment of susceptible bacterial infections of the upper and lower respiratory tract; and other infections in patients allergic to penicillin

Contraindications Hypersensitivity to erythromycin, sulfonamides, or any component of the formulation; hepatic dysfunction; porphyria; concurrent use with pimozide, astemizole, or cisapride

Warnings/Precautions Use with caution in patients with impaired renal or hepatic function, myasthenia gravis, G6PD deficiency (hemolysis may occur). Macrolides have been associated with rare QT_c prolongation and ventricular arrhythmias, including torsade de pointes; use with caution in patients at risk of prolonged cardiac repolarization. Chemical similarities are present among sulfonamides, sulfonylureas, carbonic anhydrase inhibitors, thiazides, and loop diuretics (except ethacrynic acid). In patients with allergy to one of these compounds, a risk of cross-reaction exists; avoid use when previous reaction has been severe. Prolonged use may result in fungal or bacterial superinfection, including *C. difficile*-associated diarrhea and pseudomembranous colitis.

Adverse Reactions (Reflective of adult population; not specific for elderly)
Frequency not defined.
Cardiovascular: Ventricular arrhythmia,
Central nervous system: Headache, fever
Dermatologic: Rash, Stevens-Johnson syndrome, toxic epidermal necrolysis
Gastrointestinal: Abdominal pain, cramping, nausea, vomiting, oral candidiasis, hypertrophic pyloric stenosis, diarrhea, pseudomembranous colitis
Hematologic: Agranulocytosis, aplastic anemia, eosinophilia
Hepatic: Hepatic necrosis, cholestatic jaundice
Local: Phlebitis at the injection site, thrombophlebitis
Renal: Toxic nephrosis, crystalluria
Miscellaneous: Hypersensitivity reactions

Overdosage/Toxicology Symptoms include nausea, vomiting, diarrhea, prostration, reversible pancreatitis, and hearing loss with or without tinnitus or vertigo. Treatment consists of general and supportive care only. Keep well hydrated.

Drug Interactions

Erythromycin: **Substrate** of CYP2B6 (minor), 3A4 (major); **Inhibits** CYP1A2 (weak), 3A4 (moderate)

Sulfisoxazole: **Substrate** of CYP2C8/9 (major); **Inhibits** CYP2C8/9 (strong)

Also see individual agents.

Increased effect/toxicity/levels with erythromycin/sulfisoxazole on alfentanil, bromocriptine, carbamazepine, cyclosporine, digoxin, disopyramide, theophylline, triazolam, lovastatin/simvastatin, ergots, methylprednisolone, cisapride, pimozide, felodipine, phenytoin, barbiturate anesthetics, methotrexate, sulfonylureas, uricosuric agents, and warfarin; may inhibit metabolism of protease inhibitors.

Increased toxicity of sulfonamides occurs with concurrent diuretics, indomethacin, methenamine, probenecid, and salicylates.

Stability Reconstituted suspension is stable for 14 days when refrigerated.

Mechanism of Action Erythromycin inhibits bacterial protein synthesis; sulfisoxazole competitively inhibits bacterial synthesis of folic acid from para-aminobenzoic acid

Pharmacokinetics

Erythromycin ethylsuccinate:

Absorption: Well from the GI tract

Protein binding: 75% to 90%

Metabolism: In the liver

Half-life: 1-1.5 hours

Elimination: Unchanged drug excreted and concentrated in bile

Sulfisoxazole acetyl:

Hydrolyzed in GI tract to sulfisoxazole which is readily absorbed

Protein binding: 85%

Half-life: 6 hours, prolonged in renal impairment

Elimination: 50% excreted in urine as unchanged drug

Dosage

Geriatrics: Not recommended for use in the elderly.

Adults: Susceptible infections: Oral (dosage recommendation is based on the product's erythromycin content): 400 mg erythromycin and 1200 mg sulfisoxazole every 6 hours

Renal Impairment: Sulfisoxazole must be adjusted in renal impairment.

Cl_{cr} 10-50 mL/minute: Administer every 8-12 hours.

Cl_{cr} <10 mL/minute: Administer every 12-24 hours.

Monitoring Parameters CBC and periodic liver function test

Test Interactions False-positive urinary protein

Patient Information Maintain adequate fluid intake; avoid prolonged exposure to sunlight; discontinue if rash appears

Dosage Forms Excipient information presented when available (limited, particularly for generics); consult specific product labeling. [DSC] = Discontinued product

Powder for oral suspension: Erythromycin ethylsuccinate 200 mg and sulfisoxazole acetyl 600 mg per 5 mL (100 mL, 200 mL)

Pediazole®: Erythromycin ethylsuccinate 200 mg and sulfisoxazole acetyl 600 mg per 5 mL (100 mL, 150 mL, 200 mL) [strawberry-banana flavor] [DSC]

♦ **Erythromycin Base** *see* Erythromycin *on page 533*

♦ **Erythromycin Ethylsuccinate** *see* Erythromycin *on page 533*

♦ **Erythromycin Lactobionate** *see* Erythromycin *on page 533*

♦ **Erythromycin Stearate** *see* Erythromycin *on page 533*

♦ **Erythropoiesis-Stimulating Agent (ESA)** *see* Darbepoetin Alfa *on page 397*

♦ **Erythropoiesis-Stimulating Agent (ESA)** *see* Epoetin Alfa *on page 519*

♦ **Erythropoiesis-Stimulating Protein** *see* Darbepoetin Alfa *on page 397*

♦ **Erythropoietin** *see* Epoetin Alfa *on page 519*

Escitalopram (es sye TAL oh pram)

Related Information

Antidepressant Agents *on page 1742*

U.S. Brand Names Lexapro®

Canadian Brand Names Cipralex®

Index Terms Escitalopram Oxalate; Lu-26-054; S-Citalopram

Generic Available No

Pharmacologic Category Antidepressant, Selective Serotonin Reuptake Inhibitor

Use Treatment of major depressive disorder; generalized anxiety disorders (GAD)

Unlabeled/Investigational Use Treatment of anxiety disorders

(Continued)

Escitalopram *(Continued)*

Restrictions An FDA-approved medication guide concerning the use of antidepressants in children, adolescents, and young adults must be distributed when dispensing an outpatient prescription (new or refill) where this medication is to be used without direct supervision of a healthcare provider. Medication guides are available at http://www.fda.gov/cder/Offices/ODS/medication_guides.htm. Dispense to parents or guardians of children and adolescents receiving this medication.

Contraindications Hypersensitivity to escitalopram, citalopram, or any component of the formulation; concomitant use or within 2 weeks of MAO inhibitors

Warnings/Precautions [U.S. Boxed Warning]: Antidepressants increase the risk of suicidal thinking and behavior in children, adolescents, and young adults (18-24 years of age) with major depressive disorder (MDD) and other psychiatric disorders; consider risk prior to prescribing. Short-term studies did not show an increased risk in patients >24 years of age and showed a decreased risk in patients ≥65 years. Closely monitor patients for clinical worsening, suicidality, or unusual changes in behavior, particularly during the initial 1-2 months of therapy or during periods of dosage adjustments (increases or decreases); the patient's family or caregiver should be instructed to closely observe the patient and communicate condition with healthcare provider. A medication guide concerning the use of antidepressants should be dispensed with each prescription.

The possibility of a suicide attempt is inherent in major depression and may persist until remission occurs. Use caution in high-risk patients. Worsening depression and severe abrupt suicidality that are not part of the presenting symptoms may require discontinuation or modification of drug therapy. The patient's family or caregiver should be alerted to monitor patients for the emergence of suicidality and associated behaviors (such as agitation, irritability, hostility, impulsivity, and hypomania) and call healthcare provider.

May worsen psychosis in some patients or precipitate a shift to mania or hypomania in patients with bipolar disorder. Patients presenting with depressive symptoms should be screened for bipolar disorder. Monotherapy in patients with bipolar disorder should be avoided. Escitalopram is not FDA approved for the treatment of bipolar depression.

The potential for a severe reaction exists when used with MAO inhibitors, SSRIs/SNRIs or triptans; serotonin syndrome (hyperthermia, muscular rigidity, mental status changes/agitation, autonomic instability) may occur. Concurrent use with MAO inhibitors is contraindicated. May increase the risks associated with electroconvulsive therapy. Has a low potential to impair cognitive or motor performance; caution operating hazardous machinery or driving.

Use caution with a previous seizure disorder or condition predisposing to seizures such as brain damage, alcoholism, or concurrent therapy with other drugs which lower the seizure threshold. May cause hyponatremia/SIADH. May cause or exacerbate sexual dysfunction. Use caution with renal or liver impairment; concomitant CNS depressants. Use caution with concomitant use of NSAIDs, ASA, or other drugs that affect coagulation; the risk of bleeding is potentiated.

Upon discontinuation of escitalopram therapy, gradually taper dose. If intolerable symptoms occur following a decrease in dosage or upon discontinuation of therapy, then resuming the previous dose with a more gradual taper should be considered.

Adverse Reactions (Reflective of adult population; not specific for elderly)
>10%:
  Central nervous system: Headache (24%), somnolence (6% to 13%), insomnia (9% to 12%)
  Gastrointestinal: Nausea (15%)
  Genitourinary: Ejaculation disorder (9% to 14%)
1% to 10%:
  Cardiovascular: Chest pain, hypertension, palpitation
  Central nervous system: Dizziness (5%), fatigue (5% to 8%), dreaming abnormal, concentration impaired, fever, irritability, lethargy, lightheadedness, migraine, vertigo, yawning
  Dermatologic: Rash
  Endocrine & metabolic: Libido decreased (3% to 7%), anorgasmia (2% to 6%), hot flashes, menstrual cramps, menstrual disorder
  Gastrointestinal: Diarrhea (8%), xerostomia (6% to 9%), appetite decreased (3%), constipation (3% to 5%), indigestion (3%), abdominal pain (2%), abdominal cramps, appetite increased, flatulence, gastroenteritis, gastroesophageal reflux, heartburn, toothache, vomiting, weight gain/loss
  Genitourinary: Impotence (3%), urinary tract infection, urinary frequency
  Neuromuscular & skeletal: Arthralgia, limb pain, muscle cramp, myalgia, neck/shoulder pain, paresthesia, tremor
  Ocular: Blurred vision
  Otic: Earache, tinnitus

Respiratory: Rhinitis (5%), sinusitis (3%), bronchitis, cough, nasal or sinus congestion, sinus headache

Miscellaneous: Diaphoresis (4% to 5%), flu-like syndrome (5%), allergy

Overdosage/Toxicology Treatment should be symptom-directed and supportive.

Drug Interactions Substrate (major) of CYP2C19, 3A4; **Inhibits** CYP2D6 (weak)

Aspirin: Concomitant use of escitalopram and NSAIDs, aspirin, or other drugs affecting coagulation has been associated with an increased risk of bleeding; monitor.

Buspirone: Concurrent use of citalopram with buspirone may cause serotonin syndrome; avoid concurrent use.

Cimetidine: May inhibit the metabolism of citalopram.

CYP2C19 inducers: May decrease the levels/effects of escitalopram. Example inducers include aminoglutethimide, carbamazepine, phenytoin, and rifampin.

CYP2C19 inhibitors: May increase the levels/effects of escitalopram. Example inhibitors include delavirdine, fluconazole, fluvoxamine, gemfibrozil, isoniazid, omeprazole, and ticlopidine.

CYP3A4 inducers: CYP3A4 inducers may decrease the levels/effects of escitalopram. Example inducers include aminoglutethimide, carbamazepine, nafcillin, nevirapine, phenobarbital, phenytoin, and rifamycins.

CYP3A4 inhibitors: May increase the levels/effects of escitalopram. Example inhibitors include azole antifungals, clarithromycin, diclofenac, doxycycline, erythromycin, imatinib, isoniazid, nefazodone, nicardipine, propofol, protease inhibitors, quinidine, telithromycin, and verapamil.

Desipramine: Escitalopram may increase desipramine levels.

Linezolid: Hyperpyrexia, hypertension, tachycardia, confusion, seizures, and deaths have been reported with agents which inhibit MAO (serotonin syndrome); this combination should be avoided.

MAO inhibitors: Hyperpyrexia, hypertension, tachycardia, confusion, seizures, and deaths have been reported with MAO inhibitors (serotonin syndrome); this combination should be avoided.

Meperidine: Combined use theoretically may increase the risk of serotonin syndrome.

Metoprolol: Escitalopram may increase plasma levels of metoprolol; monitor for increased effect.

Moclobemide: Concurrent use of citalopram with moclobemide may cause serotonin syndrome; avoid concurrent use.

Nefazodone: Concurrent use of citalopram with nefazodone may cause serotonin syndrome.

NSAIDs: Concomitant use of escitalopram and NSAIDs, aspirin, or other drugs affecting coagulation has been associated with an increased risk of bleeding; monitor.

Selegiline: Concurrent use with citalopram has been reported to cause serotonin syndrome; as an MAO type B inhibitor, the risk of serotonin syndrome may be less than with nonselective MAO inhibitors, and reports indicate that this combination has been well tolerated in Parkinson's patients.

SSRIs: Concurrent use with other reuptake inhibitors may increase the risk of serotonin syndrome.

Serotonin agonists (eg, triptans): Concurrent use of escitalopram with these agents may increase the risk of serotonin syndrome; monitor.

Serotonergic reuptake inhibitors (eg, SSRIs/SNRIs): Concurrent use of escitalopram with these agents may increase the risk of serotonin syndrome; monitor.

Sibutramine: May increase the risk of serotonin syndrome with SSRIs.

Tramadol: Concurrent use of citalopram with tramadol may cause serotonin syndrome; avoid concurrent use.

Trazodone: Concurrent use of citalopram with trazodone may cause serotonin syndrome.

Venlafaxine: Combined use with citalopram may increase the risk of serotonin syndrome.

Warfarin: Use with caution; may increase risk of bleeding.

Ethanol/Nutrition/Herb Interactions

Ethanol: Avoid ethanol (may increase CNS depression).

Herb/Nutraceutical: Avoid valerian, St John's wort, SAMe, kava kava, and gotu kola (may increase CNS depression).

Stability Store at 25°C (77°F).

Mechanism of Action Escitalopram is the S-enantiomer of the racemic derivative citalopram, which selectively inhibits the reuptake of serotonin with little to no effect on norepinephrine or dopamine reuptake. It has no or very low affinity for 5-HT$_{1-7}$, alpha- and beta-adrenergic, D$_{1-5}$, H$_{1-3}$, M$_{1-5}$, and benzodiazepine receptors. Escitalopram does not bind or has low affinity for Na$^+$, K$^+$, Cl$^-$, and Ca^{++} ion channels.

Pharmacodynamics Onset of action: 1-2 weeks

Pharmacokinetics

Onset: 1-2 weeks

Distribution: V$_d$: 12 L/kg

Protein binding: 56% to plasma proteins

(Continued)

Escitalopram *(Continued)*

Metabolism: Hepatic via CYP2D6, 2C19, and 3A4 to an active metabolite, S-desmethylcitalopram (S-DCT); S-DCT is metabolized to S-didesmethylcitalopram (active) via CYP2D6

Bioavailability: ~80%

Half-life: Escitalopram: 27-32 hours; S-desmethylcitalopram: 59 hours

Time to peak: Escitalopram: 5 ± 1.5 hours; S-desmethylcitalopram: 14 hours

Elimination: Urine (Escitalopram: 8%; S-DCT: 10%)

Clearance: Total body: 37-40 L/hour; Renal: Escitalopram: 2.7 L/hour; S-desmethylcitalopram: 6.9 L/hour

Dosage

Geriatrics: Depression: Oral: 5-10 mg/day; doses may be increased by 5-10 mg/day after at least 1 week.

Adults: Depression, GAD: Oral: Initial: 10 mg/day; dose may be increased to 20 mg/day after at least 1 week

Renal Impairment:

Mild-to-moderate impairment: No dosage adjustment needed.

Severe impairment: Cl_{cr} <20 mL/minute: Use caution.

Hepatic Impairment: 10 mg/day

Administration Administer once daily (morning or evening), with or without food.

Monitoring Parameters Depression, suicidal ideation, anxiety, social functioning

Patient Information The full effects of this medication may take up to 3 weeks to occur. Take as directed; do not alter dose or frequency without consulting prescriber. May be taken with or without food. Avoid alcohol, caffeine, and CNS stimulants. You may experience sexual dysfunction (reversible). May cause dizziness, anxiety, or blurred vision (rise slowly from sitting or lying position and use caution when driving or engaging in tasks requiring alertness until response to drug is known); nausea or dry mouth (frequent small meals, frequent mouth care, chewing gum, or sucking lozenges may help). Report confusion or impaired concentration, severe headache, palpitations, rash, insomnia or nightmares, changes in personality, muscle weakness or tremors, altered gait pattern, signs and symptoms of respiratory infection, or excessive perspiration.

Additional Information The tablet and oral solution dosage forms are bioequivalent. Clinically, escitalopram 20 mg is equipotent to citalopram 40 mg. Do not coadminister with citalopram.

Special Geriatric Considerations Bioavailability and half-life are increased by 50% in the elderly.

Dosage Forms Excipient information presented when available (limited, particularly for generics); consult specific product labeling.

Solution, oral: 1 mg/mL (240 mL) [peppermint flavor]

Tablet: 5 mg, 10 mg, 20 mg

Note: Cipralex® [CAN] is available only in 10 mg and 20 mg strengths.

Selected References

Bernard L, Stern R, Lew D, et al, "Serotonin Syndrome After Concomitant Treatment With Linezolid and Citalopram," *Clin Infect Dis*, 2003, 36(9):1197.

Mahlberg R, Kunz D, Sasse J, et al, "Serotonin Syndrome With Tramadol and Citalopram," *Am J Psychiatry*, 2004, 161(6):1129.

Montgomery SA, Loft H, Sanchez C, et al, "Escitalopram (S-Enantiomer of Citalopram): Clinical Efficacy and Onset of Action Predicted From a Rat Model," *Pharmacol Toxicol*, 2001, 88(5):282-6.

Tahir N, "Serotonin Syndrome as a Consequence of Drug-Resistant Infections: An Interaction Between Linezolid and Citalopram," *J Am Med Dir Assoc*, 2004, 5(2):111-3.

von Moltke LL, Greenblatt DJ, Giancarlo GM, et al, "Escitalopram (S-Citalopram) and its Metabolites *In Vitro*: Cytochromes Mediating Biotransformation, Inhibitory Effects, and Comparison to R-Citalopram," *Drug Metab Dispos*, 2001, 29(8):1102-9.

♦ **Escitalopram Oxalate** *see* Escitalopram *on page 539*

♦ **Esclim**® *see* Estradiol *on page 549*

♦ **Eserine Salicylate** *see* Physostigmine *on page 1256*

♦ **Eskalith**® **[DSC]** *see* Lithium *on page 920*

♦ **Eskalith CR**® **[DSC]** *see* Lithium *on page 920*

Esmolol *(ES moe lol)*

Related Information

Beta-Blockers *on page 1751*

Medication Safety Issues

Sound-alike/look-alike issues:

Esmolol may be confused with Osmitrol®

Brevibloc® may be confused with bretylium, Brevital®, Bumex®, Buprenex®

High alert medication: The Institute for Safe Medication Practices (ISMP) includes this medication among its list of drugs which have a heightened risk of causing significant patient harm when used in error.

ESMOLOL

U.S. Brand Names Brevibloc®
Canadian Brand Names Brevibloc®
Index Terms Esmolol Hydrochloride
Generic Available Yes: Excludes infusion
Pharmacologic Category Antiarrhythmic Agent, Class II; Beta Blocker, Beta$_1$ Selective

Use Treatment of supraventricular tachycardia and atrial fibrillation/flutter (primarily to control ventricular rate), tachycardia and/or hypertension (especially intraoperative or postoperative)

Unlabeled/Investigational Use In children, for SVT and postoperative hypertension

Contraindications Hypersensitivity to esmolol or any component of the formulation; sinus bradycardia; heart block greater than first degree (except in patients with a functioning artificial pacemaker); cardiogenic shock; bronchial asthma; uncompensated cardiac failure; hypotension

Warnings/Precautions Consider pre-existing conditions such as sick sinus syndrome before initiating. Hypotension is common; patients need close blood pressure monitoring. Administer cautiously in compensated heart failure and monitor for a worsening of the condition. Use caution in patients with PVD (can aggravate arterial insufficiency). Use caution with concurrent use of beta-blockers and either verapamil or diltiazem; bradycardia or heart block can occur. Avoid concurrent I.V. use of both agents. Use beta-blockers cautiously in patients with bronchospastic disease; monitor pulmonary status closely. Use cautiously in diabetics because it can mask prominent hypoglycemic symptoms. Use with caution in patients with myasthenia gravis and psychiatric disease (may cause CNS depression). Use caution in patients with renal dysfunction (active metabolite retained). Adequate alpha-blockade is required prior to use of any beta-blocker for patients with untreated pheochromocytoma. Beta-blocker therapy should not be withdrawn abruptly (particularly in patients with CAD), but gradually tapered to avoid acute tachycardia, hypertension, and/or ischemia. Do not use in the treatment of hypertension associated with vasoconstriction related to hypothermia. Concentrations >10 mcg/mL or infusion into small veins or through a butterfly catheter should be avoided (can cause thrombophlebitis). Extravasation can lead to skin necrosis and sloughing.

Adverse Reactions (Reflective of adult population; not specific for elderly)
>10%:
Cardiovascular: Asymptomatic hypotension (dose related: 25% to 38%), symptomatic hypotension (dose related: 12%)
Miscellaneous: Diaphoresis (10%)
1% to 10%:
Cardiovascular: Peripheral ischemia (1%)
Central nervous system: Dizziness (3%), somnolence (3%), confusion (2%), headache (2%), agitation (2%), fatigue (1%)
Gastrointestinal: Nausea (7%), vomiting (1%)
Local: Pain on injection (8%), infusion site reaction

Overdosage/Toxicology Symptoms of overdose include hypotension, bradycardia, bronchospasm, congestive heart failure, and heart block. Initially, a decrease/discontinuation of the esmolol infusion and administration of fluids may be the best treatment for hypotension. Sympathomimetics (eg, epinephrine or dopamine), glucagon, or an anticholinergic or a pacemaker can be used to treat the toxic bradycardia, asystole, and/or hypotension. Bradycardia and hypotension resistant to atropine, isoproterenol, or pacing may respond to glucagon. Wide QRS defects caused by membrane-depressant poisoning may respond to hypertonic sodium bicarbonate. Repeat-dose charcoal, hemoperfusion, or hemodialysis may be helpful in removal of only those beta-blockers with a small V_d, long half-life, or low intrinsic clearance (acebutolol, atenolol, nadolol, sotalol).

Drug Interactions
Acetylcholinesterase Inhibitors: May enhance the bradycardic effect of beta-blockers.
Alpha-/beta-agonists (direct acting): Beta-blockers may enhance the vasopressor effect of alpha-/beta-agonists (direct-acting). Epinephrine used as a local anesthetic for dental procedures will not likely cause clinically-relevant problems.
Alpha$_1$-blockers: Beta-blockers may enhance the orthostatic effect of alpha$_1$ blockers. The risk associated with ophthalmic products is probably less than systemic products.
Alpha$_2$ agonists: Beta-blockers may enhance the rebound hypertensive effect of alpha$_2$ agonists. This effect can occur when the alpha$_2$ agonist is abruptly withdrawn.
Amiodarone: May enhance the bradycardic effect of beta-blockers. Possibly to the point of cardiac arrest. Consider therapy modification.
Beta$_2$-agonists: May diminish the bradycardic effect of beta-blockers (beta$_1$ selective); of concern with high doses of some beta-blockers.
Calcium channel blockers (nondihydropyridine): May enhance the hypotensive effect of beta-blockers. Bradycardia and signs of heart failure have also been reported.
(Continued)

543

Esmolol (Continued)

Cardiac glycosides: Beta-blockers may enhance the bradycardic effect of cardiac glycosides.

Disopyramide; May enhance the bradycardic effect of beta-blockers. Use caution if coadministering disopyramide and a beta-blocker (especially if both are I.V.).

Insulin preparations: Beta-blockers may enhance the hypoglycemic effect of insulin preparations.

NSAIDs: May diminish the antihypertensive effect of beta-blockers.

Sulfonylureas: Beta-blockers may enhance the hypoglycemic effect of sulfonylureas. Cardioselective beta-blockers (eg, esmolol) may be safer than nonselective beta-blockers. All beta-blockers appear to mask tachycardia as an initial symptom of hypoglycemia.

Stability Clear, colorless to light yellow solution which should be stored at 15°C to 30°C (59°F to 85°F); do not freeze. Protect from excessive heat.

Stability of parenteral admixture at room temperature (25°C) is 24 hours.

Mechanism of Action Class II antiarrhythmic: Competitively blocks response to $beta_1$-adrenergic stimulation with little or no effect of $beta_2$-receptors except at high doses, no intrinsic sympathomimetic activity, no membrane stabilizing activity

Pharmacodynamics

Onset of action: Beta blockade occurs within 2-10 minutes following initiation of I.V. administration (onset of effects is quickest when loading doses are administered)

Duration of hemodynamic effects: 10-30 minutes; prolonged following higher cumulative doses, extended duration of use

Pharmacokinetics

Protein binding: 55%

Metabolism: By esterase in cytosol or red blood cells

Half-life: 9 minutes

Elimination: ~69% of dose excreted in urine as metabolites and 2% as unchanged drug

Dosage

Geriatrics & Adults: Infusion requires an infusion pump (must be adjusted to individual response and tolerance):

Intraoperative tachycardia and/or hypertension (immediate control): I.V.: Initial bolus: 80 mg (~1 mg/kg) over 30 seconds, followed by a 150 mcg/kg/minute infusion, if necessary. Adjust infusion rate as needed to maintain desired heart rate and/or blood pressure, up to 300 mcg/kg/minute.

For control of postoperative hypertension, as many as one-third of patients may require higher doses (250-300 mcg/kg/minute) to control blood pressure; the safety of doses >300 mcg/kg/minute has not been studied.

Supraventricular tachycardia or gradual control of postoperative tachycardia/ hypertension: I.V.: Loading dose: 500 mcg/kg over 1 minute; follow with a 50 mcg/kg/minute infusion for 4 minutes; response to this initial infusion rate may be a rough indication of the responsiveness of the ventricular rate.

Infusion may be continued at 50 mcg/kg/minute or, if the response is inadequate, titrated upward in 50 mcg/kg/minute increments (increased no more frequently than every 4 minutes) to a maximum of 200 mcg/kg/minute.

Note: To achieve more rapid response, following the initial loading dose and 50 mcg/kg/minute infusion, rebolus with a second 500 mcg/kg loading dose over 1 minute, and increase the maintenance infusion to 100 mcg/kg/minute for 4 minutes. If necessary, a third (and final) 500 mcg/kg loading dose may be administered, prior to increasing to an infusion rate of 150 mcg/kg/minute. After 4 minutes of the 150 mcg/kg/minute infusion, the infusion rate may be increased to a maximum rate of 200 mcg/kg/minute (without a bolus dose).

Supraventricular tachycardias (SVT); usual dose range: Usual dosage range: 50-200 mcg/kg/minute with average dose of 100 mcg/kg/minute.

Guidelines for transfer to oral therapy (beta-blocker, calcium channel blocker): Infusion should be reduced by 50% 30 minutes following the first dose of the alternative agent

Manufacturer suggests following the second dose of the alternative drug, patient's response should be monitored and if control is adequate for the first hours, esmolol may be discontinued.

Renal Impairment: Not removed by hemo- or peritoneal dialysis. Supplemental dose is not necessary.

Administration Infusions must be administered with an infusion pump. The concentrate (250 mg/mL ampul) is **not** for direct I.V. injection, but rather must first be diluted to a final concentration of 10 mg/mL (ie, 2.5 g in 250 mL or 5 g in 500 mL). Concentrations >10 mg/mL or infusion into small veins or through a butterfly catheter should be avoided (can cause thrombophlebitis). Decrease or discontinue infusion if hypotension or congestive heart failure occur. Medication port of premixed bags should be used to withdraw only the initial bolus, if necessary (not to be used for withdrawal of additional bolus doses).

Monitoring Parameters Blood pressure, apical and peripheral pulse, EKG

Test Interactions Increases cholesterol (S), glucose

Special Geriatric Considerations Due to alterations in the beta-adrenergic auto-nomic nervous system, beta-adrenergic blockade may result in less hemodynamic response than seen in younger adults. Studies indicate that despite decreased sensi-tivity to the chronotropic effects of beta-blockade with age, there appears to be an increased myocardial sensitivity to the negative inotropic effect during stress (ie, exer-cise). Controlled trials have shown the overall response rate for propranolol to be only 20% to 50% in elderly populations. Therefore, all beta-adrenergic blocking drugs may result in a decreased response as compared to younger adults.

Dosage Forms Excipient information presented when available (limited, particularly for generics); consult specific product labeling.

Infusion [premixed in sodium chloride; preservative free]:

Brevibloc®: 2000 mg (100 mL) [20 mg/mL; double strength]; 2500 mg (250 mL) [10 mg/mL]

Injection, solution, as hydrochloride: 10 mg/mL (10 mL) [premixed in sodium chloride]

Brevibloc®: 10 mg/mL (10 mL) [alcohol free; premixed in sodium chloride]; 20 mg/mL (5 mL, 100 mL) [alcohol free; double strength; premixed in sodium chloride]; 250 mg/mL (10 mL) [contains alcohol 25%, propylene glycol 25%; concentrate]

Selected References

Vincent RN, Click LA, Williams HM, et al, "Esmolol As an Adjunct in the Treatment of Systemic Hypertension After Operative Repair of Coarctation of the Aorta," *Am J Cardiol*, 1990, 65(13):941-3.

♦ **Esmolol Hydrochloride** *see* Esmolol *on page 542*

Esomeprazole (es oh ME pray zol)

Related Information

Helicobacter pylori Treatment *on page 1759*

U.S. Brand Names Nexium®

Canadian Brand Names Nexium®

Index Terms Esomeprazole Magnesium; Esomeprazole Sodium

Generic Available No

Pharmacologic Category Proton Pump Inhibitor; Substituted Benzimidazole

Use

Oral: Short-term (4-8 weeks) treatment of erosive esophagitis; maintaining symptom resolution and healing of erosive esophagitis; treatment of symptomatic gastroe-sophageal reflux disease (GERD); as part of a multidrug regimen for *Helicobacter pylori* eradication in patients with duodenal ulcer disease (active or history of within the past 5 years); prevention of gastric ulcers in patients at risk (age ≥60 years and/ or history of gastric ulcer) associated with continuous NSAID therapy; long-term treatment of pathological hypersecretory conditions

I.V.: Short-term (≤10 weeks) treatment of gastroesophageal reflux disease (GERD) when oral therapy is not possible or appropriate

Contraindications Hypersensitivity to esomeprazole, lansoprazole, omeprazole, rabeprazole, or any component of the formulation

Warnings/Precautions Relief of symptoms does not preclude the presence of a gastric malignancy. Atrophic gastritis (by biopsy) has been noted with long-term omeprazole therapy; this may also occur with esomeprazole. No reports of enterochro-maffin-like (ECL) cell carcinoids, dysplasia, or neoplasia have occurred. Severe liver dysfunction may require dosage reductions. Safety and efficacy of I.V. therapy >10 days have not been established; transition from I.V. to oral therapy as soon possible.

Adverse Reactions (Reflective of adult population; not specific for elderly) Unless otherwise specified, percentages represent adverse reactions identified in clin-ical trials evaluating the intravenous formulation.

>10%: Central nervous system: Headache (I.V. 11%; oral 5% to 6%)

1% to 10%:

Central nervous system: Dizziness (3%)

Dermatologic: Pruritus (≤1%)

Gastrointestinal: Flatulence (10%), nausea (I.V. 6%; oral 2%), abdominal pain (I.V. 6%; oral 3% to 4%), diarrhea (4%), xerostomia (I.V. 4%; oral ≥1%), dyspepsia (<1% to 6%), constipation (3%)

Local: Injection site reaction (2%)

Respiratory: Sinusitis (I.V. 2%; oral <1%), respiratory infection (1%)

Overdosage/Toxicology Doses up to 2400 mg have been reported. Symptoms of overdose may include confusion, drowsiness, blurred vision, tachycardia, nausea, sweating, headache or dry mouth. Treatment is symptom-directed and supportive; not dialyzable.

Drug Interactions Substrate of CYP2C19 (major), 3A4 (major); **Inhibits** CYP2C19 (moderate)

(Continued)

Esomeprazole *(Continued)*

Antifungal agents (imidazole): Proton pump inhibitors may decrease the absorption of itraconazole and ketoconazole.

Benzodiazepines metabolized by oxidation (eg, diazepam, midazolam, triazolam): Esomeprazole and omeprazole may increase levels of benzodiazepines metabolized by oxidation.

CYP2C19 inducers: May decrease the levels/effects of esomeprazole. Example inducers include aminoglutethimide, carbamazepine, phenytoin, and rifampin.

CYP2C19 substrates: Esomeprazole may increase the levels/effects of CYP2C19 substrates. Example substrates include citalopram, diazepam, methsuximide, phenytoin, propranolol, and sertraline.

Dasatinib: Esomeprazole may decrease the absorption of dasatinib.

HMG-CoA reductase inhibitors: Esomeprazole may increase the levels/effects; monitor.

Iron salts: Esomeprazole may decrease the absorption of orally-administered iron salts.

Methotrexate: Proton pump inhibitors may decrease the excretion of methotrexate; monitor for increased methotrexate toxic effects. Lower antirheumatic doses likely to carry less of a risk compared with higher antineoplastic doses.

Protease inhibitors: Proton pump inhibitors may decrease absorption of some protease inhibitors (atazanavir and indinavir).

Ethanol/Nutrition/Herb Interactions Food: Absorption is decreased by 43% to 53% when taken with food.

Stability

Capsule, granules: Store at 15°C to 30°C (59°F to 86°F). Keep container tightly closed.

Powder for injection: Store at 15°C to 30°C (59°F to 86°F). Protect from light.

For I.V. injection: Reconstitute powder with 5 mL NS.

For I.V. infusion: Initially reconstitute powder with 5 mL of NS, LR, or D_5W, then further dilute to a final volume of 50 mL.

Following reconstitution, solution for injection prepared in NS, and solution for infusion prepared in NS or LR should be used within 12 hours. Following reconstitution, solution for infusion prepared in D_5W should be used within 6 hours. Refrigeration is not required following reconstitution.

Mechanism of Action Proton pump inhibitor suppresses gastric acid secretion by inhibition of the H^+/K^+-ATPase in the gastric parietal cell

Pharmacokinetics

Distribution: V_{dss}: 16 L

Protein binding: 97%

Metabolism: Hepatic to hydroxy, desmethyl, and sulfone metabolites (all inactive)

Bioavailability: 90% with repeated dosing

Half-life: 1-1.5 hours

Time to peak: 1.5 hours

Excretion: Urine (80%, primarily as inactive metabolites; <1% as active drug); feces (20%)

Dosage

Geriatrics: Refer to adult dosing. No dosage adjustment needed.

Adults:

Healing of erosive esophagitis: Oral: Initial: 20-40 mg once daily for 4-8 weeks; if incomplete healing, may continue for an additional 4-8 weeks; maintenance: 20 mg once daily

Maintenance of healing of erosive esophagitis: Oral: 20 mg once daily; clinical trials evaluated therapy for ≤6 months

Symptomatic gastroesophageal reflux: Oral: 20 mg once daily for 4 weeks; may consider an additional 4 weeks of treatment if symptoms do not resolve

Treatment of GERD (short-term): I.V.: 20 mg or 40 mg once daily for ≤10 days; change to oral therapy as soon as appropriate

Peptic ulcer disease: Eradication of *Helicobacter pylori*: Oral: 40 mg once daily for 10 days; requires combination therapy

Prevention of NSAID-induced gastric ulcers: 20-40 mg once daily for up to 6 months

Pathological hypersecretory conditions (Zollinger-Ellison syndrome): 40 mg twice daily; adjust regimen to individual patient needs; doses up to 240 mg/day have been administered

Renal Impairment: No adjustment is necessary.

Hepatic Impairment:

Mild-to-moderate hepatic impairment (Child-Pugh Class A or B): No dosage adjustment needed.

Severe hepatic impairment (Child-Pugh Class C): Dose should not exceed 20 mg/day.

Administration

Oral:

Capsule: Should be swallowed whole and taken at least 1 hour before eating (best if taken before breakfast). Capsule can be opened and contents mixed with 1 tablespoon of applesauce. Swallow immediately; mixture should not be chewed or warmed. For patients with difficulty swallowing, use of granules may be easiest.

Granules: Empty into container with 1 tablespoon of water and stir; leave 2-3 minutes to thicken. Stir and drink within 30 minutes. If any medicine remains after drinking, add more water, stir and drink immediately.

I.V.: May be administered by injection (≥3 minutes) or infusion (10-30 minutes). Flush line prior to and after administration with NS, LR, or D_5W.

Nasogastric tube:

Capsule: Open capsule and place intact granules into a 60 mL syringe; mix with 50 mL of water. Replace plunger and shake vigorously for 15 seconds. Ensure that no granules remain in syringe tip. Do not administer if pellets dissolve or disintegrate. Use immediately after preparation. After administration, flush nasogastric tube with additional water.

Granules: Delayed release oral suspension granules can also be given by nasogastric or gastric tube. Add 15 mL of water to a syringe, add granules from packet. Shake the syringe, leave 2-3 minutes to thicken. Shake the syringe and administer through nasogastric or gastric tube (French size 6 or greater) within 30 minutes. Refill the syringe with 15 mL of water, shake and flush nasogastric/gastric tube.

Monitoring Parameters Susceptibility testing recommended in patients who fail *H. pylori* eradication regimen (esomeprazole, clarithromycin, and amoxicillin)

Patient Information Take as directed, 1 hour before eating at same time each day. Swallow capsule whole; do not crush or chew. If you cannot swallow capsule whole, open capsule, mix contents with 1 tablespoon of applesauce, and swallow immediately; do not chew mixture. Do not store for future use. You may experience headache; constipation (increased exercise, fluids, fruit, or fiber may help); diarrhea (boiled milk, yogurt, or buttermilk may help); or abdominal pain (should diminish with use). Report persistent headache, diarrhea, constipation, abdominal pain, changes in urination or pain on urination, chest pain or palpitations, changes in respiratory status, CNS changes, persistent muscular aches or pain, ringing in ears or visual changes, or other adverse reactions.

Additional Information Esomeprazole is the S-isomer of omeprazole.

Special Geriatric Considerations Dose adjustment is not necessary

Dosage Forms Excipient information presented when available (limited, particularly for generics); consult specific product labeling.

Note: Strength expressed as base

Capsule, delayed release, as magnesium:

Nexium®: 20 mg, 40 mg

Granules, for oral suspension, delayed release, as magnesium:

Nexium®: 20 mg, 40 mg

Injection, powder for reconstitution, as sodium:

Nexium®: 20 mg, 40 mg [contains edetate sodium]

♦ **Esomeprazole Magnesium** *see* Esomeprazole *on page 545*

♦ **Esomeprazole Sodium** *see* Esomeprazole *on page 545*

Estazolam (es TA zoe lam)

Related Information

Anxiolytic, Sedative / Hypnotic, and Miscellaneous Benzodiazepines *on page 1750*

Medication Safety Issues

Sound-alike/look-alike issues:

ProSom® may be confused with PhosLo®, Proscar®, Pro-Sof® Plus, Prozac®, Psorcon®

U.S. Brand Names ProSom® [DSC]

Generic Available Yes

Pharmacologic Category Benzodiazepine

Use Short-term management of insomnia

Restrictions C-IV

Contraindications Hypersensitivity to estazolam or any component of the formulation (cross-sensitivity with other benzodiazepines may exist)

Note: Manufacturer states concurrent therapy with itraconazole or ketoconazole is contraindicated.

Warnings/Precautions As a hypnotic, should be used only after evaluation of potential causes of sleep disturbance. Failure of sleep disturbance to resolve after 7-10 days may indicate psychiatric or medical illness. Use is not recommended in patients with depressive disorders or psychoses. Avoid use in patients with sleep apnea. Postmarketing studies have indicated that the use of hypnotic/sedative agents for
(Continued)

Estazolam *(Continued)*

sleep has been associated with hypersensitivity reactions including anaphylaxis as well as angioedema. An increased risk for hazardous sleep-related activities such as sleep-driving; cooking and eating food, and making phone calls while asleep have also been noted. Use with caution in patients receiving concurrent CYP3A4 inhibitors, particularly when these agents are added to therapy. Use with caution in elderly or debilitated patients, patients with hepatic disease (including alcoholics), renal impairment, respiratory disease, impaired gag reflex, or obese patients. Rebound or withdrawal symptoms may occur following abrupt discontinuation or large decreases in dose. Use caution when reducing dose or withdrawing therapy; decrease slowly and monitor for withdrawal symptoms.

Causes CNS depression (dose related) which may impair physical and mental capabilities. Use with caution in patients receiving other CNS depressants or psychoactive agents. Benzodiazepines have been associated with falls and traumatic injury and should be used with extreme caution in patients who are at risk of these events (especially the elderly). May cause physical or psychological dependence - use with caution in patients with a history of drug dependence.

Benzodiazepines have been associated with anterograde amnesia. Paradoxical reactions, including hyperactive or aggressive behavior, have been reported with benzodiazepines, particularly in psychiatric patients. Does not have analgesic, antidepressant, or antipsychotic properties.

Adverse Reactions (Reflective of adult population; not specific for elderly)

>10%:
  Central nervous system: Somnolence
  Neuromuscular & skeletal: Weakness

1% to 10%:
  Cardiovascular: Flushing, palpitation
  Central nervous system: Anxiety, confusion, dizziness, hypokinesia, abnormal coordination, hangover effect, agitation, amnesia, apathy, emotional lability, euphoria, hostility, seizure, sleep disorder, stupor, twitch
  Dermatologic: Dermatitis, pruritus, rash, urticaria
  Gastrointestinal: Xerostomia, constipation, appetite increased/decreased, flatulence, gastritis, perverse taste
  Genitourinary: Frequent urination, menstrual cramps, urinary hesitancy, urinary frequency, vaginal discharge/itching
  Neuromuscular & skeletal: Paresthesia
  Ocular: Photophobia, eye pain, eye swelling
  Respiratory: Cough, dyspnea, asthma, rhinitis, sinusitis
  Miscellaneous: Diaphoresis

Drug Interactions Substrate of CYP3A4 (minor)
  CNS depressants: Sedative effects and/or respiratory depression may be additive with CNS depressants; includes ethanol, barbiturates, opioid analgesics, and other sedative agents; monitor for increased effect.
  Itraconazole, ketoconazole: Concurrent use is contraindicated (per manufacturer); however, estazolam is a minor CYP3A4 substrate and an effect has not been documented in clinical studies.
  Levodopa: Therapeutic effects may be diminished in some patients following the addition of a benzodiazepine; limited/inconsistent data.
  Oral contraceptives: May decrease the clearance of some benzodiazepines (those which undergo oxidative metabolism); monitor for increased benzodiazepine effect.
  Theophylline: May partially antagonize some of the effects of benzodiazepines; monitor for decreased response; may require higher doses for sedation.

Ethanol/Nutrition/Herb Interactions
  Ethanol: Avoid ethanol (may increase CNS depression).
  Food: Serum levels and/or toxicity may be increased by grapefruit juice.

Mechanism of Action Binds to stereospecific benzodiazepine receptors on the postsynaptic GABA neuron at several sites within the central nervous system, including the limbic system, reticular formation. Enhancement of the inhibitory effect of GABA on neuronal excitability results by increased neuronal membrane permeability to chloride ions. This shift in chloride ions results in hyperpolarization (a less excitable state) and stabilization.

Pharmacodynamics Studies have shown that older adults are more sensitive to the effects of benzodiazepines as compared to younger adults

Pharmacokinetics
  Metabolism: Rapid and extensive in the liver to inactive metabolites
  Half-life: 10-24 hours (no significant changes in older adults)
  Time to peak serum concentration: 0.5-1.6 hours
  Elimination: <5% excreted unchanged in urine

Dosage
Geriatrics: Start at doses of 0.5 mg in small elderly patients.
Adults: Insomnia: Oral: 1 mg at bedtime, some patients may require 2 mg; start at doses of 0.5 mg in debilitated patients.
Hepatic Impairment: Adjustment may be necessary.
Monitoring Parameters Respiratory, cardiovascular, and mental status
Patient Information Avoid alcohol and other CNS depressants; may cause drowsiness; avoid activities needing good psychomotor coordination until CNS effects are known; may cause physical or psychological dependence; avoid abrupt discontinuation after prolonged use
Special Geriatric Considerations There has been little experience with this drug in the elderly, but because of its lack of active metabolites, estazolam would be a reasonable choice for elderly patients when a benzodiazepine hypnotic is indicated.
Dosage Forms Excipient information presented when available (limited, particularly for generics); consult specific product labeling. [DSC] = Discontinued product
Tablet: 1 mg, 2 mg
ProSom®: 1 mg, 2 mg [DSC]

♦ **Ester-E™ [OTC]** *see* Vitamin E *on page 1677*
♦ **Esterified Estrogens** *see* Estrogens (Esterified) *on page 572*
♦ **Estrace®** *see* Estradiol *on page 549*
♦ **Estraderm®** *see* Estradiol *on page 549*

Estradiol (es tra DYE ole)

Related Information
Osteoporosis Management *on page 1779*
Medication Safety Issues
Sound-alike/look-alike issues:
Alora® may be confused with Aldara™
Elestrin™ may be confused with alosetron
Estraderm® may be confused with Testoderm®

International issues:
Vivelle®: Brand name for ethinyl estradiol and norgestimate in Austria
Estring® may be confused with Estrena® [Finland]
Estrena® [Finland] may be confused with estrone in the U.S.

Transdermal patch may contain conducting metal (eg, aluminum); remove patch prior to MRI.
U.S. Brand Names Alora®; Climara®; Delestrogen®; Depo®-Estradiol; Divigel®; Elestrin™; Esclim®; Estrace®; Estraderm®; Estrasorb™; Estring®; EstroGel®; Femring®; Femtrace®; Gynodiol®; Menostar™; Vagifem®; Vivelle®; Vivelle-Dot®
Canadian Brand Names Climara®; Depo®-Estradiol; Estrace®; Estraderm®; Estradot®; Estring®; EstroGel®; Menostar™; Oesclim®; Sandoz-Estradiol Derm 50; Sandoz-Estradiol Derm 75; Sandoz-Estradiol Derm 100; Vagifem®
Index Terms Estradiol Acetate; Estradiol Cypionate; Estradiol Hemihydrate; Estradiol Transdermal; Estradiol Valerate
Generic Available Yes: Oral tablet, patch
Pharmacologic Category Estrogen Derivative
Use Treatment of atrophic vaginitis, urinary incontinence secondary to estrogen deficiency, atrophic dystrophy of vulva, menopausal symptoms, female hypogonadism, oophorectomy, ovariectomy, primary ovarian failure, inoperable breast cancer, inoperable prostatic cancer, mild to severe vasomotor symptoms associated with menopause, prevention of osteoporosis
Contraindications Hypersensitivity to estradiol or any component of the formulation; undiagnosed abnormal vaginal bleeding; history of or current thrombophlebitis or venous thromboembolic disorders (including DVT, PE); active or recent (within 1 year) arterial thromboembolic disease (eg, stroke, MI); carcinoma of the breast, except in appropriately selected patients being treated for metastatic disease; estrogen-dependent tumor; porphyria
Warnings/Precautions
Cardiovascular-related considerations: **[U.S. Boxed Warning]: Estrogens with or without progestin should not be used to prevent coronary heart disease.** Use caution with cardiovascular disease or dysfunction. May increase the risks of hypertension, myocardial infarction (MI), stroke, pulmonary emboli (PE), and deep vein thrombosis; incidence of these effects was shown to be significantly increased in postmenopausal women using conjugated equine estrogens (CEE) in combination with medroxyprogesterone acetate (MPA). Nonfatal MI, PE, and thrombophlebitis have also been reported in males taking high doses of CEE (eg, for prostate cancer). Estrogen compounds are generally associated with lipid effects such as increased HDL-cholesterol and decreased LDL-cholesterol. Triglycerides may also be increased; (Continued)

Estradiol *(Continued)*

use with caution in patients with familial defects of lipoprotein metabolism. Whenever possible, estrogens should be discontinued at least 4 weeks prior to and for 2 weeks following elective surgery associated with an increased risk of thromboembolism or during periods of prolonged immobilization.

Neurological considerations: **[U.S. Boxed Warning]: The risk of dementia may be increased in postmenopausal women;** increased incidence was observed in women ≥65 years of age taking CEE alone or in combination with MPA.

Cancer-related considerations: **[U.S. Boxed Warning]: Unopposed estrogens may increase the risk of endometrial carcinoma in postmenopausal women with an intact uterus.** Estrogens may exacerbate endometriosis. Malignant transformation of residual endometrial implants has been reported posthysterectomy with estrogen only therapy. Consider adding a progestin in women with residual endometriosis posthysterectomy. Estrogens may increase the risk of breast cancer. An increased risk of invasive breast cancer was observed in postmenopausal women using CEE in combination with MPA; a smaller increase in risk was seen with estrogen therapy alone in observational studies. An increase in abnormal mammograms has also been reported with estrogen and progestin therapy. Estrogen use may lead to severe hypercalcemia in patients with breast cancer and bone metastases; discontinue estrogen if hypercalcemia occurs.

Estrogens may cause retinal vascular thrombosis; discontinue permanently if papilledema or retinal vascular lesions are observed on examination. Use with caution in patients with diseases which may be exacerbated by fluid retention, including asthma, epilepsy, migraine, diabetes or renal dysfunction. Use with caution in patients with a history of severe hypocalcemia, SLE, hepatic hemangiomas, porphyria (use is contraindicated with certain products), endometriosis, and gallbladder disease. Use caution with history of cholestatic jaundice associated with past estrogen use or pregnancy.

Before prescribing estrogen therapy to postmenopausal women, the risks and benefits must be weighed for each patient. Women should be informed of these risks and benefits, as well as possible effects of progestin when added to estrogen therapy. Estrogens with or without progestin should be used for shortest duration possible consistent with treatment goals. Conduct periodic risk:benefit assessments.

When used solely for prevention of osteoporosis in women at significant risk, nonestrogen treatment options should be considered. When used solely for the treatment of vulvar and vaginal atrophy, topical vaginal products should be considered. Use caution applying topical products to severely atrophic vaginal mucosa. Absorption of the topical emulsion (Estrasorb™) and topical gel (Elestrin™) is increased by application of sunscreen; do not apply sunscreen within close proximity of estradiol. Application of Divigel® or EstroGel® with sunscreen has not been evaluated. Transdermal patch may contain conducting metal (eg, aluminum); remove patch prior to MRI. Use of the vaginal ring may not be appropriate in women with narrow vagina, vaginal stenosis, vaginal infections, cervical prolapse, rectoceles, cystoceles, or other conditions which may increase the risk of vaginal irritation, ulceration, or increase the risk of expulsion.

Adverse Reactions (Reflective of adult population; not specific for elderly)
Frequency not defined. Some adverse reactions observed with estrogen and/or progestin combination therapy.

Cardiovascular: DVT, edema, hypertension, MI, stroke, venous thromboembolism

Central nervous system: Anxiety, dementia, dizziness, epilepsy exacerbation, headache, irritability, mental depression, migraine, mood disturbances, nervousness

Dermatologic: Angioedema, chloasma, erythema multiforme, erythema nodosum, hemorrhagic eruption, hirsutism, loss of scalp hair, melasma, rash, pruritus, urticaria

Endocrine & metabolic: Breast cancer, breast enlargement, breast pain, breast tenderness, fibrocystic breast changes, HDL-cholesterol increased, galactorrhea, glucose intolerance, hypocalcemia, LDL-cholesterol decreased, libido changes, nipple pain, serum triglycerides/phospholipids increased, thyroid-binding globulin increased, total thyroid hormone (T_4) increased, vaginal discharge, vaginitis

Gastrointestinal: Abdominal cramps, abdominal distension, abdominal pain, bloating, cholecystitis, cholelithiasis, diarrhea, flatulence, gallbladder disease, nausea, pancreatitis, vomiting, weight gain/loss

Genitourinary: Alterations in frequency and flow of menses, cervical secretion changes, dysmenorrhea, endometrial cancer, endometrial hyperplasia, metrorrhagia, ovarian cancer, Pap smear suspicious, urinary tract infection, uterine leiomyomata size increased, uterine pain, vaginal candidiasis

Vaginal: Trauma from applicator insertion may occur in women with severely atrophic vaginal mucosa

Hematologic: Aggravation of porphyria, antithrombin III and antifactor Xa decreased, fibrinogen levels increased, platelet aggregability increased, platelet count increased, prothrombin increased; factors VII, VIII, IX, X increased

Hepatic: Cholestatic jaundice, hepatic hemangioma enlargement

Local: Thrombophlebitis
  Gel: Application site reaction
  Transdermal patches: Burning, erythema, irritation
Neuromuscular & skeletal: Arthralgia, back pain, chorea, leg cramps, muscle cramps
Ocular: Contact lens intolerance, corneal curvature steepening, retinal vascular thrombosis
Respiratory: Asthma exacerbation, pulmonary thromboembolism
Miscellaneous: Anaphylactoid/anaphylactic reactions

Overdosage/Toxicology Symptoms include fluid retention, jaundice, thrombophlebitis, nausea, and vomiting. Toxicity is unlikely following single exposures of excessive doses. Treatment following emesis and charcoal administration should be supportive and symptomatic.

Drug Interactions Substrate of CYP1A2 (major), 2A6 (minor), 2B6 (minor), 2C9 (minor), 2C19 (minor), 2D6 (minor), 2E1 (minor), 3A4 (major); **Inhibits** CYP1A2 (weak), 2C8 (weak); **Induces** CYP3A4 (weak)

Anticoagulants: Increase potential for thromboembolic events.
Corticosteroids: Estrogens may enhance the effects of hydrocortisone and prednisone.
Cyclosporine: Estrogen derivatives may enhance the hepatotoxic effect of cyclosporine. Estrogen derivatives may increase the serum concentration of cyclosporine.
CYP1A2 inducers: May decrease the levels/effects of estradiol. Example inducers include aminoglutethimide, carbamazepine, phenobarbital, and rifampin.
CYP3A4 inducers: CYP3A4 inducers may decrease the levels/effects of estradiol. Example inducers include aminoglutethimide, carbamazepine, nafcillin, nevirapine, phenobarbital, phenytoin, and rifamycins.
Thyroid products: Estrogen derivatives may diminish the therapeutic effect of thyroid products; monitor.

Ethanol/Nutrition/Herb Interactions
Ethanol: Avoid ethanol (routine use increases estrogen level and risk of breast cancer). Ethanol may also increase the risk of osteoporosis.
Food: Folic acid absorption may be decreased
Herb/Nutraceutical: St John's wort may decrease levels. Herbs with estrogenic properties may enhance the adverse/toxic effect of estrogen derivatives; examples include alfalfa, black cohosh, bloodroot, hops, kudzu, licorice, red clover, saw palmetto, soybean, thyme, wild yam, yucca.

Mechanism of Action Estrogens are responsible for the development and maintenance of the female reproductive system and secondary sexual characteristics. Estradiol is the principle intracellular human estrogen and is more potent than estrone and estriol at the receptor level; it is the primary estrogen secreted prior to menopause. Following menopause, estrone and estrone sulfate are more highly produced. Estrogens modulate the pituitary secretion of gonadotropins, luteinizing hormone, and follicle-stimulating hormone through a negative feedback system; estrogen replacement reduces elevated levels of these hormones in postmenopausal women.

Pharmacokinetics
Absorption: Readily through skin and GI tract
Protein binding: 80%
Half-life: 50-60 minutes
Elimination: Principally degraded in the liver and excreted in urine as conjugates; small amounts excreted in feces via bile, reabsorbed from the GI tract and enterohepatically recycled

Dosage
  Geriatrics & Adults: All dosage needs to be adjusted based upon the patient's response:
    Atrophic vaginitis, vulvar/vaginal atrophy:
      Intravaginal:
        Vaginal cream: Atrophic vaginitis, kraurosis vulvae: Insert 2-4 g/day for 2 weeks then gradually reduce to $^1/_2$ the initial dose for 2 weeks followed by a maintenance dose of 1 g 1-3 times/week
        Vaginal ring:
          Postmenopausal vaginal atrophy, urogenital symptoms (Estring®): 2 mg intravaginally; following insertion, ring should remain in place for 90 days
          Vulvar/vaginal atrophy (Femring®): 0.05 mg intravaginally; following insertion, ring should remain in place for 3 months; dose may be increased to 0.1 mg if needed
        Vaginal tablets (Vagifem®); Atrophic vaginitis: Initial: Insert 1 tablet once daily for 2 weeks; maintenance: Insert 1 tablet twice weekly. Attempts to discontinue or taper medication should be made at 3- to 6-month intervals
      Topical gel: Vulvar/vaginal atrophy:
        Elestrin™: 0.87 g/day applied at the same time each day
        EstroGel®: 1.25 g/day applied at the same time each day
      Transdermal: Refer to product-specific dosing (below)
(Continued)

Estradiol *(Continued)*

Breast cancer (females; inoperable, progressing): Oral: 10 mg 3 times/day for at least 3 months

Hypogonadism:
Oral: 1-2 mg/day in a cyclic regimen for 3 weeks on drug, then 1 week off drug
I.M.: Cypionate: 1.5-2 mg monthly; Valerate: 10-20 mg every 4 weeks
Transdermal: Refer to product-specific dosing (below)

Osteoporosis prevention (females):
Oral: 0.5 mg/day in a cyclic regimen (3 weeks on and 1 week off of drug)
Transdermal: Refer to product-specific dosing (below)

Prostate cancer:
I.M. (valerate): ≥30 mg or more every 1-2 weeks
Oral (androgen-dependent, inoperable, progressing): 10 mg 3 times/day for at least 3 months

Vasomotor symptoms (moderate to severe) associated with menopause:
Oral (in addition to I.M. dosing): 1-2 mg daily, adjusted as necessary to limit symptoms. Administrations should be cyclic (3 weeks on, 1 week off). Patients should be re-evaluated at 3-6 month intervals to determine if treatment is still necessary
I.M.: Cypionate: 1-5 mg every 3-4 weeks; Valerate: 10-20 mg every 4 weeks
Topical emulsion: 3.84 g applied once daily in the morning
Topical gel:
Divigel®: 0.25 g per day; adjust dose based on patient response. Dosing range: 0.25-1 g/day
Elestrin™: 0.87 g/day applied at the same time each day
EstroGel®: 1.25 g/day applied at the same time each day
Vaginal ring (Femring®): 0.05 mg intravaginally; following insertion, ring should remain in place for 3 months; dose may be increased to 0.1 mg if needed
Transdermal: See product-specific dosing (below)

Transdermal product-specific dosing:
Note: Indicated dose may be used continuously in patients without an intact uterus. May be given continuously or cyclically (3 weeks on, 1 week off) in patients with an intact uterus **(exception - Menostar™, see specific dosing instructions).** When changing patients from oral to transdermal therapy, start transdermal patch 1 week after discontinuing oral hormone (may begin sooner if symptoms reappear within 1 week):
Transdermal once-weekly patch:
Moderate-to-severe vasomotor symptoms associated with menopause (Climara®): Apply 0.025 mg/day patch once weekly. Adjust dose as necessary to control symptoms. Patients should be re-evaluated at 3- to 6-month intervals to determine if treatment is still necessary.
Prevention of osteoporosis in postmenopausal women:
Climara®: Apply patch once weekly; minimum effective dose 0.025 mg/day; adjust dosage based on response to therapy as indicated by biological markers and bone mineral density.
Menostar™: Apply patch once weekly. In women with a uterus, also administer a progestin for 14 days every 6-12 months.
Transdermal twice-weekly patch (Alora®, Esclim®, Estraderm®, Vivelle®):
Moderate to severe vasomotor symptoms associated with menopause, vulvar/vaginal atrophy, female hypogonadism: Titrate to lowest dose possible to control symptoms, adjusting initial dose after the first month of therapy; re-evaluate therapy at 3- to 6-month intervals to taper or discontinue medication:
Alora®, Esclim®, Estraderm®, Vivelle-Dot®: Apply 0.05 mg patch twice weekly
Vivelle®: Apply 0.0375 mg patch twice weekly
Prevention of osteoporosis in postmenopausal women:
Alora®, Vivelle®, Vivelle-Dot®: Apply 0.025 mg patch twice weekly, increase dose as necessary
Estraderm®: Apply 0.05 mg patch twice weekly

Administration

Injection formulation: Intramuscular use only

Emulsion: Apply to clean, dry skin while in a sitting position. Contents of two pouches (total 3.48 g) are to be applied individually, once daily in the morning. Apply contents of first pouch to left thigh; massage into skin of left thigh and calf until thoroughly absorbed (~3 minutes). Apply excess from both hands to the buttocks. Apply contents of second pouch to the right thigh; massage into skin of right thigh and calf until thoroughly absorbed (~3 minutes). Apply excess from both hands to buttocks. Wash hands with soap and water. Allow skin to dry before covering legs with clothing. Do not apply to other areas of body. Do not apply to red or irritated skin.

Gel: Apply to clean, dry, unbroken skin at the same time each day. Allow to dry for 5 minutes prior to dressing. Gel is flammable; avoid fire or flame until dry. After application, wash hands with soap and water. Prior to the first use, pump must be primed. Do not apply gel to breast.

Elestrin™: Apply to upper arm and shoulder area using two fingers to spread gel. Apply after bath or shower; allow at least 2 hours between applying gel and going swimming. Wait at least 25 minutes before applying sunscreen to application area. Do not apply sunscreen to application area for ≥7 days (may increase absorption of gel).

EstroGel®: Apply gel to the arm, from the wrist to the shoulder. Spread gel as thinly as possible over one arm.

Transdermal patch: Aerosol topical corticosteroids applied under the patch may reduce allergic reactions. Do not apply transdermal system to breasts, but place on trunk of body (preferably abdomen). Rotate application sites.

Vaginal ring: Exact positioning is not critical for efficacy, however, patient should not feel anything once inserted. In case of discomfort, ring should be pushed further into vagina. If ring is expelled prior to 90 days, it may be rinsed off and reinserted.

Monitoring Parameters Yearly physical examination that includes blood pressure and Papanicolaou smear, breast exam, mammogram. Monitor for signs of endometrial cancer in female patients with uterus. Adequate diagnostic measures, including endometrial sampling, if indicated, should be performed to rule out malignancy in all cases of undiagnosed abnormal vaginal bleeding. Monitor for loss of vision, sudden onset of proptosis, diplopia, migraine; signs and symptoms of thromboembolic disorders; glycemic control in diabetics; lipid profiles in patients being treated for hyperlipidemias; thyroid function in patients on thyroid hormone replacement therapy.

When using Menostar™ in a woman with a uterus, endometrial sampling is recommended at yearly intervals or when clinically indicated.

Menopausal symptoms: Assess need for therapy at 3- to 6-month intervals

Prevention of osteoporosis: Bone density measurement

Reference Range Male: 10-50 pg/mL (SI: 37-184 pmol/L); postmenopausal female: 0-30 pg/mL (SI: 0-110 pmol/L)

Test Interactions Pathologist should be advised of estrogen/progesterone therapy when specimens are submitted. Reduced response to metyrapone test.

Patient Information Women should inform their physicians if signs or symptoms of any of the following occur: thromboembolic or thrombotic disorders including sudden severe headache or vomiting, disturbance of vision or speech, loss of vision, numbness or weakness in an extremity, sharp or crushing chest pain, calf pain, shortness of breath, severe abdominal pain or mass, mental depression or unusual bleeding. Women should perform regular self exams on breasts. Notify physician if area under dermal patch becomes irritated or a rash develops.

Transdermal patch: Apply to clean dry skin. Do not apply transdermal patch to breasts. Apply to trunk of body (preferably abdomen). Rotate application sites. Aerosol topical corticosteroids may reduce allergic skin reaction; report persistent skin reaction.

Intravaginal cream: Insert high in vagina. Wash hands and applicator before and after use.

Topical emulsion: Contents of two pouches are applied one at time to each thigh and rubbed into thigh and calf. Excess on hands should be applied to buttocks. Wash hands with soap and water after application. Allow skin to dry before covering legs with clothes. Do not apply sunscreen soon after or before applying emulsion. Do not apply to red or irritated skin.

Topical gel: Apply dose to one arm at the same time each day. Allow to dry for 5 minutes prior to dressing. Wash hands with soap and water after application. Do not apply to red or irritated skin. Do not apply to breast.

Special Geriatric Considerations Before prescribing estrogen therapy to postmenopausal women, the risks and benefits must be weighed for each patient. Data in women ≥80 years are minimal and it is unclear if the reduced risk is applicable to women in this age group. Women should be informed of these risks and benefits, as well as possible side effects and the return of menstrual bleeding (when cycled with a progestin), and be involved in the decision to prescribe. Oral therapy may be more convenient for vaginal atrophy and urinary incontinence.

Dosage Forms Excipient information presented when available (limited, particularly for generics); consult specific product labeling.

Cream, vaginal:

Estrace®: 0.1 mg/g (12 g) [refill]; 0.1 mg/g (42.5 g) [packaged with applicator]

Emulsion, topical, as hemihydrate:

Estrasorb™: 2.5 mg/g (56s) [each pouch contains 4.35 mg estradiol hemihydrate; contents of two pouches delivers estradiol 0.05 mg/day]

Gel, topical:

Divigel®: 0.1% (0.25 g) [foil packet; delivers estradiol 0.25 mg/packet]; (0.5 g) [foil packet; delivers 0.5 mg estradiol/packet]; (1 g) [foil packet; delivers estradiol 1 mg/packet]

Elestrin™: 0.06% (144 g) [pump; delivers estradiol 0.52 mg/0.87 g; 100 actuations]

(Continued)

Estradiol *(Continued)*

EstroGel®: 0.06% (93 g) [pump; delivers estradiol 0.75 mg/1.25 g; 64 actuations]

Injection, oil, as cypionate:

Depo®-Estradiol: 5 mg/mL (5 mL) [contains chlorobutanol; in cottonseed oil]

Injection, oil, as valerate:

Delestrogen®:

10 mg/mL (5 mL) [contains chlorobutanol; in sesame oil]

20 mg/mL (5 mL) [contains benzyl alcohol; in castor oil]

40 mg/mL (5 mL) [contains benzyl alcohol; in castor oil]

Ring, vaginal, as base:

Estring®: 2 mg [total estradiol 2 mg; releases 7.5 mcg/day over 90 days] (1s)

Ring, vaginal, as acetate:

Femring®: 0.05 mg [total estradiol 12.4 mg; releases 0.05 mg/day over 3 months] (1s); 0.1 mg [total estradiol 24.8 mg; releases 0.1 mg/day over 3 months] (1s)

Tablet, oral, as acetate:

Femtrace®: 0.45 mg, 0.9 mg, 1.8 mg

Tablet, oral, micronized: 0.5 mg, 1 mg, 2 mg

Estrace®: 0.5 mg, 1 mg, 2 mg [2 mg tablets contain tartrazine]

Gynodiol®: 0.5 mg, 1 mg, 1.5 mg, 2 mg

Tablet, vaginal, as base:

Vagifem®: 25 mcg [contains lactose]

Transdermal system: 0.025 mg/24 hours [once-weekly patch] (4s); 0.0375 mg/24 hours (4s) [once-weekly patch]; 0.05 mg/24 hours (4s) [once-weekly patch]; 0.06 mg/24 hours (4s) [once-weekly patch]; 0.075 mg/24 hours [once-weekly patch]; 0.1 mg/24 hours (4s) [once-weekly patch]

Alora® [twice-weekly patch]:

0.025 mg/24 hours [9 cm^2, total estradiol 0.77 mg] (8s)

0.05 mg/24 hours [18 cm^2, total estradiol 1.5 mg] (8s, 24s)

0.075 mg/24 hours [27 cm^2, total estradiol 2.3 mg] (8s)

0.1 mg/24 hours [36 cm^2, total estradiol 3.1 mg] (8s)

Climara® [once-weekly patch]:

0.025 mg/24 hours [6.5 cm^2, total estradiol 2.04 mg] (4s)

0.0375 mg/24 hours [9.375 cm^2, total estradiol 2.85 mg] (4s)

0.05 mg/24 hours [12.5 cm^2, total estradiol 3.8 mg] (4s)

0.06 mg/24 hours [15 cm^2, total estradiol 4.55 mg] (4s)

0.075 mg/24 hours [18.75 cm^2, total estradiol 5.7 mg] (4s)

0.1 mg/24 hours [25 cm^2, total estradiol 7.6 mg] (4s)

Esclim® [twice-weekly patch]:

0.025 mg/day [11 cm^2, total estradiol 5 mg] (8s)

0.0375 mg/day [16.5 cm^2, total estradiol 7.5 mg] (8s)

0.05 mg/day [22 cm^2, total estradiol 10 mg] (8s)

0.075 mg/day [33 cm^2, total estradiol 15 mg] (8s)

0.1 mg/day [44 cm^2, total estradiol 20 mg] (8s)

Estraderm® [twice-weekly patch]:

0.05 mg/24 hours [10 cm^2, total estradiol 4 mg] (8s)

0.1 mg/24 hours [20 cm^2, total estradiol 8 mg] (8s)

Menostar™ [once-weekly patch]: 0.014 mg/24 hours [3.25 cm^2, total estradiol 1 mg] (4s)

Vivelle® [twice-weekly patch]:

0.05 mg/24 hours [14.5 cm^2, total estradiol 4.33 mg] (8s)

0.1 mg/24 hours [29 cm^2, total estradiol 8.66 mg] (8s)

Vivelle-Dot® [twice-weekly patch]:

0.025 mg/day [2.5 cm^2, total estradiol 0.39 mg] (8s)

0.0375 mg/day [3.75 cm^2, total estradiol 0.585 mg] (8s)

0.05 mg/day [5 cm^2, total estradiol 0.78 mg] (8s)

0.075 mg/day [7.5 cm^2, total estradiol 1.17 mg] (8s)

0.1 mg/day [10 cm^2, total estradiol 1.56 mg] (8s)

Selected References

American College of Physicians, "Guidelines for Counseling Postmenopausal Women About Preventive Hormone Therapy," *Ann Intern Med*, 1992, 117(12):1038-41.

Belchetz PE, "Hormonal Treatment for Postmenopausal Women," *N Engl J Med*, 1994, 330(15):1062-71.

♦ **Estradiol Acetate** *see* Estradiol *on page 549*

♦ **Estradiol and Drospirenone** *see* Drospirenone and Estradiol *on page 488*

♦ **Estradiol and NGM** *see* Estradiol and Norgestimate *on page 554*

Estradiol and Norgestimate (es tra DYE ole & nor JES ti mate)

Related Information

Estradiol *on page 549*

U.S. Brand Names Prefest™

Index Terms Estradiol and NGM; Norgestimate and Estradiol; Ortho Prefest

Generic Available No

Pharmacologic Category Estrogen and Progestin Combination

Use Women with an intact uterus: Treatment of moderate to severe vasomotor symptoms associated with menopause, atrophic vaginitis; prevention of osteoporosis

Contraindications Hypersensitivity to estradiol, norgestimate, or any component of the formulation; undiagnosed abnormal vaginal bleeding; history of or current thrombophlebitis or thromboembolic disorders; carcinoma of the breast; estrogen-dependent tumor

Warnings/Precautions

Cardiovascular-related considerations: Estrogens with or without progestin should not be used to prevent coronary heart disease. Use caution with cardiovascular disease or dysfunction. May increase the risks of hypertension, myocardial infarction (MI), stroke, pulmonary emboli (PE), and deep vein thrombosis; incidence of these effects was shown to be significantly increased in postmenopausal women using conjugated equine estrogens (CEE) in combination with medroxyprogesterone acetate (MPA). Nonfatal MI, PE, and thrombophlebitis have also been reported in males taking high doses of CEE (eg, for prostate cancer). Estrogen compounds are generally associated with lipid effects such as increased HDL-cholesterol and decreased LDL-cholesterol. Triglycerides may also be increased; use with caution in patients with familial defects of lipoprotein metabolism. Whenever possible, combination hormonal contraceptives should be discontinued at least 4 weeks prior to and for 2 weeks following elective surgery associated with an increased risk of thromboembolism or during periods of prolonged immobilization.

Neurological considerations: The risk of dementia may be increased in postmenopausal women; increased incidence was observed in women ≥65 years of age taking CEE alone or in combination with MPA.

Cancer-related considerations: Unopposed estrogens may increase the risk of endometrial carcinoma in postmenopausal women. Estrogens may exacerbate endometriosis. Malignant transformation of residual endometrial implants has been reported posthysterectomy with estrogen only therapy. Estrogens may increase the risk of breast cancer. An increased risk of invasive breast cancer was observed in postmenopausal women using CEE in combination with MPA; a smaller increase in risk was seen with estrogen therapy alone in observational studies. An increase in abnormal mammograms has also been reported with estrogen and progestin therapy. Estrogen use may lead to severe hypercalcemia in patients with breast cancer and bone metastases; discontinue estrogen if hypercalcemia occurs.

Estrogens may cause retinal vascular thrombosis; discontinue permanently if papilledema or retinal vascular lesions are observed on examination. Use with caution in patients with diseases which may be exacerbated by fluid retention, including asthma, epilepsy, migraine, diabetes or renal dysfunction. Use with caution in patients with a history of severe hypocalcemia, SLE, hepatic hemangiomas, porphyria, endometriosis, and gallbladder disease. Use caution with history of cholestatic jaundice associated with past estrogen use or pregnancy. Not for use prior to menopause.

Before prescribing estrogen therapy to postmenopausal women, the risks and benefits must be weighed for each patient. Women should be informed of these risks and benefits, as well as possible effects of progestin when added to estrogen therapy. Estrogens with or without progestin should be used for shortest duration possible consistent with treatment goals. Conduct periodic risk:benefit assessments.

When used solely for prevention of osteoporosis in women at significant risk, nonestrogen treatment options should be considered. When used solely for the treatment of vulvar and vaginal atrophy, topical vaginal products should be considered.

Adverse Reactions (Reflective of adult population; not specific for elderly)

>10%:

Central nervous system: Headache (23%)

Endocrine & metabolic: Breast pain (16%)

Gastrointestinal: Abdominal pain (12%)

Neuromuscular & skeletal: Back pain (12%)

Respiratory: Upper respiratory tract infection (21%)

Miscellaneous: Flu-like syndrome (11%)

1% to 10%:

Central nervous system: Fatigue (6%), pain (6%), depression (5%), dizziness (5%)

Endocrine & metabolic: Vaginal bleeding (9%), dysmenorrhea (8%), vaginitis (7%)

Gastrointestinal: Nausea (6%), flatulence (5%)

Neuromuscular & skeletal: Arthralgia (9%), myalgia (5%)

Respiratory: Sinusitis (8%), pharyngitis (7%), cough (5%)

Miscellaneous: Viral infection (6%)

(Continued)

Estradiol and Norgestimate *(Continued)*

Additional adverse effects associated with **estrogens and progestins**; frequency not defined:

Cardiovascular: Edema, hypertension, MI, stroke, venous thrombosis

Central nervous system: Anxiety, epilepsy exacerbation, insomnia, irritability, migraine, mood disturbances, nervousness, pyrexia, somnolence

Dermatologic: Acne, chloasma, erythema multiforme, erythema nodosum, hemorrhagic eruptions, hirsutism, itching, melasma, pruritus, rash, scalp hair loss, urticaria

Endocrine & metabolic: Amenorrhea, breast cancer, breast discharge, breast enlargement, Breast tenderness, carbohydrate tolerance decreased, endometrial cancer, endometrial hyperplasia, fibrocystic breast changes, galactorrhea, hypocalcemia, libido changes, ovarian cancer, triglycerides increased

Gastrointestinal: Abdominal cramps, appetite changes, bloating, gallbladder disease, pancreatitis, vomiting, weight gain/loss

Genitourinary: Abnormal withdrawal bleeding/flow, breakthrough bleeding, cervical secretion changes, cystitis syndrome, uterine leiomyomata size increased, vaginal candidiasis, vaginal bleeding/spotting

Hematologic: Anemia, porphyria

Hepatic: Cholestatic jaundice

Local: Thrombophlebitis

Neuromuscular & skeletal: Chorea

Ocular: Contact lens intolerance, corneal curvature steepening, neuro-ocular lesions

Respiratory: Asthma exacerbation, pulmonary embolism

Miscellaneous: Anaphylaxis

Drug Interactions

Estradiol: **Substrate** of CYP1A2 (major), 2A6 (minor), 2B6 (minor), 2C9 (minor), 2C19 (minor), 2D6 (minor), 2E1 (minor), 3A4 (major); **Inhibits** CYP1A2 (weak), 2C8 (weak); **Induces** CYP3A4 (weak)

Acetaminophen: May increase plasma concentration of synthetic estrogens, possibly by inhibiting conjugation. Estrogen/progestin combinations may also decrease the plasma concentration of acetaminophen.

Aminoglutethimide: May increase CYP metabolism of progestins leading to possible decrease in serum concentration.

Anticoagulants: Estrogen/progestin combinations may increase or decrease the effects of coumarin derivatives; may also increase risk of thromboembolic disorders.

Anticonvulsants (carbamazepine, felbamate, phenobarbital, phenytoin, topiramate): Increase the metabolism of ethinyl estradiol and/or some progestins, leading to possible decrease in serum concentration.

Ascorbic acid: Doses of ascorbic acid (vitamin C) 1 g/day have been reported to increase plasma concentration of synthetic estrogens by ~47%, possibly by inhibiting conjugation; clinical implications are unclear.

Atorvastatin: Atorvastatin increases the AUC for norethindrone and ethinyl estradiol.

Benzodiazepines: Estrogen/progestin combinations may decrease the clearance of some benzodiazepines (alprazolam, chlordiazepoxide, diazepam) and increase the clearance of others (lorazepam, oxazepam, temazepam).

Clofibric acid: Estrogen/progestin combinations may increase the clearance of clofibric acid.

Cyclosporine: Estrogen/progestin combinations may inhibit the metabolism of cyclosporine, leading to increased plasma concentrations; monitor cyclosporine levels.

Griseofulvin: Griseofulvin may induce the metabolism of estrogen/progestin combinations.

Morphine: Estrogen/progestin combinations may increase the clearance of morphine.

Non-nucleoside reverse transcriptase inhibitors (NNRTIs): Nevirapine may decrease plasma levels of estrogen/progestin combinations.

Prednisolone: Ethinyl estradiol may inhibit the metabolism of prednisolone, leading to increased plasma concentrations.

Protease inhibitors: Amprenavir, lopinavir, nelfinavir, and ritonavir have been shown to decrease plasma levels of estrogen/progestin combinations. Indinavir has been shown to increase plasma levels of estrogen/progestin combinations.

Rifampin: Rifampin increases the metabolism of ethinyl estradiol and some progestins (norethindrone) leading to decreased serum concentrations.

Salicylic acid: Estrogen/progestin combinations may increase the clearance of salicylic acid.

Selegiline: Estrogen/progestin combinations may increase the serum concentration of selegiline.

Theophylline: Ethinyl estradiol may inhibit the metabolism of theophylline, leading to increased plasma concentrations.

Tricyclic antidepressants (amitriptyline, imipramine, nortriptyline): Metabolism may be inhibited by estrogen/progestin combinations, increasing plasma levels of antidepressant; use caution.

Ethanol/Nutrition/Herb Interactions

Ethanol: Avoid ethanol (routine use increases estrogen level and risk of breast cancer). Ethanol may also increase the risk of osteoporosis.

Food: CNS effects of caffeine may be enhanced if combination estrogen/progestins are used concurrently with caffeine. Grapefruit juice increases ethinyl estradiol concentrations and would be expected to increase progesterone serum levels as well; clinical implications are unclear.

Herb/Nutraceutical: St John's wort may decrease the plasma levels of combination estrogen/progestin combinations by inducing hepatic enzymes. Avoid dong quai and black cohosh (have estrogen activity). Avoid saw palmetto, red clover, ginseng.

Stability Store at 25°C (77°F).

Mechanism of Action Estrogens are responsible for the development and maintenance of the female reproductive system and secondary sexual characteristics. Estradiol is the principle intracellular human estrogen and is more potent than estrone and estriol at the receptor level; it is the primary estrogen secreted prior to menopause. Following menopause, estrone and estrone sulfate are more highly produced. Estrogens modulate the pituitary secretion of gonadotropins, luteinizing hormone, and follicle-stimulating hormone through a negative feedback system; estrogen replacement reduces elevated levels of these hormones in postmenopausal women.

Progestins inhibit gonadotropin production which then prevents follicular maturation and ovulation. In women with adequate estrogen, progestins transform a proliferative endometrium into a secretory endometrium; when administered with estradiol, reduces the incidence of endometrial hyperplasia and risk of adenocarcinoma.

Pharmacokinetics

Protein binding:

Estradiol: Albumin and sex hormone binding globulin

17-deacetylnorgestimate: 99%

Metabolism:

Estradiol: Metabolized in the liver; converted to estrone and estriol; also undergoes enterohepatic recirculation

Norgestimate: Undergoes first-pass metabolism in the gut/liver; forms 17-deacetylnorgestimate (major active metabolite) and other metabolites

Half-life:

Estradiol: 16 hours

17-deacetylnorgestimate: 37 hours

Elimination:

Estradiol, estrone, estriol, and metabolites: Urine

Norgestimate metabolites: Urine and feces

Dosage

Geriatrics & Adults: Females with an intact uterus:

Treatment of menopausal symptoms, atrophic vaginitis, prevention of osteoporosis: Oral: Treatment is cyclical and consists of the following: One tablet of estradiol 1 mg (pink tablet) once daily for 3 days, followed by 1 tablet of estradiol 1 mg and norgestimate 0.09 mg (white tablet) once daily for 3 days; repeat sequence continuously. **Note:** This dose may not be the lowest effective combination for these indications. In case of a missed tablet, restart therapy with next available tablet in sequence (taking only 1 tablet each day).

Administration In case of a missed tablet, restart therapy with next available tablet in sequence (taking only 1 tablet each day).

Monitoring Parameters Yearly physical examination that includes blood pressure and Papanicolaou smear, breast exam, mammogram. Monitor for signs of endometrial cancer. Adequate diagnostic measures, including endometrial sampling, if indicated, should be performed to rule out malignancy in all cases of undiagnosed abnormal vaginal bleeding. Monitor for loss of vision, sudden onset of proptosis, diplopia, migraine; signs and symptoms of thromboembolic disorders; glycemic control in diabetics; lipid profiles in patients being treated for hyperlipidemias; thyroid function in patients on thyroid hormone replacement therapy.

Menopausal symptoms: Assess need for therapy at 3- to 6-month intervals

Prevention of osteoporosis: Bone density measurement

Test Interactions Pathologist should be advised of estrogen/progesterone therapy when specimens are submitted. Reduced response to metyrapone test.

Patient Information Take this medication as prescribed; maintain schedule. Avoid alcohol. Annual gynecologic and breast exams are important. You may experience nausea or vomiting (small frequent meals may help); abdominal pain, difficult/painful menstrual cycles; dizziness or mental depression; rash, headache, breast pain, or increased/decreased libido. Report significant swelling of extremities; sudden acute pain in legs or calves, chest or abdomen; shortness of breath; severe headache or vomiting; sudden blindness; weakness or numbness of arm or leg; unusual vaginal bleeding; yellowing of skin or eyes; or unusual bruising or bleeding. You may become (Continued)

Estradiol and Norgestimate *(Continued)*

intolerant to wearing contact lenses, notify prescriber if this occurs. If taking for prevention of osteoporosis, ask prescriber about calcium and vitamin D intake, and weight-bearing exercises.

Special Geriatric Considerations See Estradiol monograph *on page 549.*

Dosage Forms Excipient information presented when available (limited, particularly for generics); consult specific product labeling.

Tablet: Estradiol 1 mg [15 pink tablets] and estradiol 1 mg and norgestimate 0.09 mg [15 white tablets] (supplied in blister card of 30)

- ♦ **Estradiol Cypionate** *see Estradiol on page 549*
- ♦ **Estradiol Hemihydrate** *see Estradiol on page 549*
- ♦ **Estradiol Transdermal** *see Estradiol on page 549*
- ♦ **Estradiol Valerate** *see Estradiol on page 549*
- ♦ **Estrasorb™** *see Estradiol on page 549*
- ♦ **Estring®** *see Estradiol on page 549*
- ♦ **EstroGel®** *see Estradiol on page 549*
- ♦ **Estrogenic Substances, Conjugated** *see Estrogens (Conjugated/Equine) on page 564*

Estrogens (Conjugated A/Synthetic)
(ES troe jenz, KON joo gate ed, aye, sin THET ik)

Related Information
Osteoporosis Management *on page 1779*
Pharmacotherapy of Urinary Incontinence *on page 1822*

Medication Safety Issues
Sound-alike/look-alike issues:
Cenestin® may be confused with Senexon®

International issues:
Cenestin® may be confused with Canesten® which is a brand name for clotrimazole in multiple international markets and a brand name for fluconazole in Great Britain

U.S. Brand Names Cenestin®

Canadian Brand Names Cenestin

Generic Available No

Pharmacologic Category Estrogen Derivative

Use Treatment of moderate to severe vasomotor symptoms of menopause

Contraindications Hypersensitivity to estrogens or any component of the formulation; undiagnosed abnormal vaginal bleeding; history of or current thrombophlebitis or thromboembolic disorders; liver disease; carcinoma of the breast; estrogen dependent tumor

Warnings/Precautions

Cardiovascular-related considerations: **[U.S. Boxed Warning]: Estrogens with or without progestin should not be used to prevent coronary heart disease.** Use caution with cardiovascular disease or dysfunction. May increase the risks of hypertension, myocardial infarction (MI), stroke, pulmonary emboli (PE), and deep vein thrombosis; incidence of these effects was shown to be significantly increased in postmenopausal women using conjugated equine estrogens (CEE) in combination with medroxyprogesterone acetate (MPA). Nonfatal MI, PE, and thrombophlebitis have also been reported in males taking high doses of CEE (eg, for prostate cancer). Estrogen compounds are generally associated with lipid effects such as increased HDL-cholesterol and decreased LDL-cholesterol. Triglycerides may also be increased; use with caution in patients with familial defects of lipoprotein metabolism. Whenever possible, estrogens should be discontinued at least 4 weeks prior to and for 2 weeks following elective surgery associated with an increased risk of thromboembolism or during periods of prolonged immobilization.

Neurological considerations: **[U.S. Boxed Warning]: The risk of dementia may be increased in postmenopausal women;** increased incidence was observed in women ≥65 years of age taking CEE alone or in combination with MPA.

Cancer-related considerations: **[U.S. Boxed Warning]: Unopposed estrogens may increase the risk of endometrial carcinoma in postmenopausal women.** Estrogens may exacerbate endometriosis. Malignant transformation of residual endometrial implants has been reported posthysterectomy with estrogen only therapy. Consider adding a progestin in women with residual endometriosis posthysterectomy. Estrogens may increase the risk of breast cancer. An increased risk of invasive breast cancer was observed in postmenopausal women using CEE in combination with MPA; a smaller increase in risk was seen with estrogen therapy alone in observational studies. An increase in abnormal mammograms has also been reported with estrogen and progestin therapy. Estrogen use may lead to severe hypercalcemia in patients with breast cancer and bone metastases; discontinue estrogen if hypercalcemia occurs.

Estrogens may cause retinal vascular thrombosis; discontinue permanently if papilledema or retinal vascular lesions are observed on examination. Use with caution in patients with diseases which may be exacerbated by fluid retention, including asthma, epilepsy, migraine, diabetes or renal dysfunction. Use with caution in patients with a history of severe hypocalcemia, SLE, hepatic hemangiomas, porphyria, endometriosis, and gallbladder disease. Use caution with history of cholestatic jaundice associated with past estrogen use or pregnancy.

Before prescribing estrogen therapy to postmenopausal women, the risks and benefits must be weighed for each patient. Women should be informed of these risks and benefits, as well as possible effects of progestin when added to estrogen therapy. Estrogens with or without progestin should be used for shortest duration possible consistent with treatment goals. Conduct periodic risk:benefit assessments.

When used solely for prevention of osteoporosis in women at significant risk, nonestrogen treatment options should be considered. When used solely for the treatment of vulvar and vaginal atrophy, topical vaginal products should be considered.

Adverse Reactions (Reflective of adult population; not specific for elderly)
>10%:
  Central nervous system: Headache (11% to 68%), dizziness (11%), pain (11%)
  Endocrine & metabolic: Breast pain (29%), endometrial thickening (19%), metrorrhagia (14%)
  Gastrointestinal: Abdominal pain (9% to 28%), nausea (9% to 18%)
  Neuromuscular & skeletal: Paresthesia (8% to 33%), back pain (14%)
  Respiratory: Upper respiratory tract infection (13%)
  Miscellaneous: Infection (2% to 14%)
1% to 10%:
  Central nervous system: Anxiety (6%), fever (1%)
  Gastrointestinal: Dyspepsia (10%), vomiting (7%), constipation (6%), diarrhea (6%), weight gain (6%)
  Genitourinary: Vaginitis (8%)
  Neuromuscular & skeletal: Leg cramps (10%), hypertonia (6%)
  Respiratory: Rhinitis (6% to 8%), cough (6%)

In addition, the following have been reported with estrogen and/or progestin therapy:
  Cardiovascular: Edema, hypertension, MI, stroke, venous thromboembolism
  Central nervous system: Epilepsy exacerbation, irritability, mental depression, migraine, mood disturbances, nervousness
  Dermatologic: Angioedema, chloasma, erythema multiforme, erythema nodosum, hemorrhagic eruption, hirsutism, melasma, pruritus, rash, scalp hair loss, urticaria
  Endocrine & metabolic: Breast cancer, breast enlargement, breast tenderness, glucose tolerance impaired, HDL-cholesterol increased, hyper-/hypocalcemia, LDL-cholesterol decreased, libido changes, serum triglycerides/phospholipids increased, thyroid-binding globulin increased, total thyroid hormone (T_4) increased
  Gastrointestinal: Abdominal cramps, bloating, cholecystitis, cholelithiasis, gallbladder disease, pancreatitis, weight gain/loss
  Genitourinary: Alterations in frequency and flow of menses, cervical secretion changes, endometrial cancer, endometrial hyperplasia, uterine leiomyomata size increased, vaginal candidiasis
  Hematologic: Aggravation of porphyria, antithrombin III and antifactor Xa decreased, fibrinogen levels increased, platelet aggregability and platelet count increased; prothrombin and factors VII, VIII, IX, X increased
  Hepatic: Cholestatic jaundice, hepatic hemangiomas enlarged
  Neuromuscular & skeletal: Arthralgias, chorea, leg cramps
  Local: Thrombophlebitis
  Ocular: Contact lens intolerance, retinal vascular thrombosis, corneal curvature steepening
  Respiratory: Asthma exacerbation, pulmonary thromboembolism
  Miscellaneous: Anaphylactoid/anaphylactic reactions, carbohydrate intolerance

Overdosage/Toxicology Symptoms of overdose include nausea and vomiting; withdrawal bleeding may occur in females. Toxicity is unlikely following single exposures of excessive doses, any treatment following emesis and charcoal administration should be supportive and symptomatic.

Drug Interactions Based on estradiol and estrone: **Substrate** of CYP1A2 (major), 2A6 (minor), 2B6 (minor), 2C9 (minor), 2C19 (minor), 2D6 (minor), 2E1 (minor), 3A4 (major); **Inhibits** CYP1A2 (weak); **Induces** CYP3A4 (weak)
  Anticoagulants: Increase potential for thromboembolic events.
  Corticosteroids: Estrogens may enhance the effects of hydrocortisone and prednisone.
  Cyclosporine: Estrogen derivatives may enhance the hepatotoxic effect of cyclosporine. Estrogen derivatives may increase the serum concentration of cyclosporine.
  (Continued)

Estrogens (Conjugated A/Synthetic) *(Continued)*

CYP1A2 inducers: May decrease the levels/effects of estrogens. Example inducers include aminoglutethimide, carbamazepine, phenobarbital, and rifampin.

CYP3A4 inducers: CYP3A4 inducers may decrease the levels/effects of estrogens. Example inducers include aminoglutethimide, carbamazepine, nafcillin, nevirapine, phenobarbital, phenytoin, and rifamycins.

Thyroid products: Estrogen derivatives may diminish the therapeutic effect of thyroid products; monitor.

Ethanol/Nutrition/Herb Interactions

Ethanol: Avoid ethanol (routine use increases estrogen level and risk of breast cancer).

Food: Grapefruit juice may increase estrogen levels, leading to increased adverse effects.

Herb/Nutraceutical: St John's wort may decrease levels. Herbs with estrogenic properties may enhance the adverse/toxic effect of estrogen derivatives; examples include alfalfa, black cohosh, bloodroot, hops, kudzu, licorice, red clover, saw palmetto, soybean, thyme, wild yam, yucca.

Stability Store at room temperature of 25°C (77°F).

Mechanism of Action Conjugated A/synthetic estrogens contain a mixture of 9 synthetic estrogen substances, including sodium estrone sulfate, sodium equilin sulfate, sodium 17 alpha-dihydroequilin, sodium 17 alpha-estradiol and sodium 17 beta-dihydroequilin. Estrogens are responsible for the development and maintenance of the female reproductive system and secondary sexual characteristics. Estradiol is the principle intracellular human estrogen and is more potent than estrone and estriol at the receptor level; it is the primary estrogen secreted prior to menopause. Following menopause, estrone and estrone sulfate are more highly produced. Estrogens modulate the pituitary secretion of gonadotropins, luteinizing hormone, and follicle-stimulating hormone through a negative feedback system; estrogen replacement reduces elevated levels of these hormones in postmenopausal women.

Pharmacokinetics

Absorption: Well absorbed over a period of several hours

Protein-binding: Sex hormone-binding globulin (SHBG) and albumin

Metabolism: Hepatic via CYP3A4; estradiol is converted to estrone and estriol; also undergoes enterohepatic recirculation; estrone sulfate is the main metabolite in postmenopausal women

Excretion: Urine (primarily estriol, also as estradiol, estrone, and conjugates)

Dosage

Geriatrics: Refer to adult dosing. A higher incidence of stroke and invasive breast cancer were observed in women >75 years in a WHI substudy using conjugated equine estrogen.

Adults: The lowest dose that will control symptoms should be used. Medication should be discontinued as soon as possible.

Menopause, moderate-to-severe vasomotor symptoms: Oral: 0.45 mg/day; may be titrated up to 1.25 mg/day; attempts to discontinue medication should be made at 3- to 6-month intervals

Vulvar and vaginal atrophy: Oral: 0.3 mg/day

Monitoring Parameters Yearly physical examination that includes blood pressure and Papanicolaou smear, breast exam, mammogram. Monitor for signs of endometrial cancer in female patients with uterus. Adequate diagnostic measures, including endometrial sampling, if indicated, should be performed to rule out malignancy in all cases of undiagnosed abnormal vaginal bleeding. Monitor for loss of vision, sudden onset of proptosis, diplopia, migraine; signs and symptoms of thromboembolic disorders; glycemic control in diabetics; lipid profiles in patients being treated for hyperlipidemias; thyroid function in patients on thyroid hormone replacement therapy.

Menopausal symptoms: Assess need for therapy at 3- to 6-month intervals

Test Interactions Pathologist should be advised of estrogen/progesterone therapy when specimens are submitted. Reduced response to metyrapone test observed with conjugated estrogens (equine).

Patient Information Follow prescribed schedule and dose. Periodic gynecologic exam and breast exams are important with long-term use. Consult prescriber for specific dietary recommendations. You may experience nausea or vomiting (small frequent meals may help); dizziness or mental depression (use caution when driving); photosensitivity (use sunscreen, wear protective clothing and eyewear, and avoid direct sunlight); rash, loss of scalp hair (reversible); enlargement/tenderness of breasts; increased (female) libido; or headache (use of mild analgesic may help). Report swelling of extremities or unusual weight gain; chest pain or palpitations; sudden acute pain, warmth, or weakness in legs or calves; shortness of breath; severe headache or vomiting; or unusual vaginal bleeding.

Additional Information Not biologically equivalent to conjugated estrogens from equine source. Contains 9 unique estrogenic compounds (equine source contains at least 10 active estrogenic compounds).

Special Geriatric Considerations Before prescribing estrogen therapy to postmeno-pausal women, the risks and benefits must be weighed for each patient. Women should be informed of these risks and benefits, as well as possible side effects and the return of menstrual bleeding (when cycled with a progestin), and be involved in the decision to prescribe. A higher incidence of stroke and invasive breast cancer were observed in women >75 years in a WHI substudy using conjugated equine estrogen. Oral therapy may be more convenient for vaginal atrophy and urinary incontinence.

Dosage Forms Excipient information presented when available (limited, particularly for generics); consult specific product labeling.

Tablet: 0.3 mg, 0.45 mg, 0.625 mg, 0.9 mg, 1.25 mg

Selected References

American College of Physicians, "Guidelines for Counseling Postmenopausal Women About Preventive Hormone Therapy," *Ann Intern Med*, 1992, 117(12):1038-41.

Belcheze PE, "Hormonal Treatment of Postmenopausal Women," *N Engl J Med*, 1994, 330(15):1062-71.

The Writing Group for the PEPI Trial, "Effects of Estrogen or Estrogen/Progestin Regimens on Heart Disease Risk Factors in Postmenopausal Women," *JAMA*, 1995, 273(3):199-208.

U.S. Food and Drug Administration, Department of Health and Human Services, "FDA Approves New Labels for Estrogen and Estrogen with Progestin Therapies for Postmenopausal Women Following Review of Women's Health Initiative Data," January 8, 2003, viewable at http://www.fda.gov/medwatch/SAFETY/2003/safety03.htm#prempr, last accessed January 9, 2003.

"Writing Group for the Women's Health Initiative Investigators. Risks and Benefits of Estrogen Plus Progestin in Healthy Postmenopausal Women: Principle Results From the Women's Health Initiative Randomized Controlled Trial," *JAMA*, 2002, 288:321-33.

Estrogens (Conjugated B/Synthetic)

(ES troe jenz, KON joo gate ed, bee, sin THET ik)

U.S. Brand Names Enjuvia™

Generic Available No

Pharmacologic Category Estrogen Derivative

Use Treatment of moderate-to-severe vasomotor symptoms of menopause

Contraindications Hypersensitivity to estrogens or any component of the formulation; undiagnosed abnormal vaginal bleeding; history of or current thrombophlebitis or venous thromboembolic disorders (including DVT, PE); active or recent (within 1 year) arterial thromboembolic disease (eg, stroke, MI); carcinoma of the breast; estrogen-dependent tumor; hepatic dysfunction or disease

Warnings/Precautions

Cardiovascular-related considerations: **[U.S. Boxed Warning]: Estrogens with or without progestin should not be used to prevent coronary heart disease.** Use caution with cardiovascular disease or dysfunction. May increase the risks of hypertension, myocardial infarction (MI), stroke, pulmonary emboli (PE), and deep vein thrombosis; incidence of these effects was shown to be significantly increased in postmenopausal women using conjugated equine estrogens (CEE) in combination with medroxyprogesterone acetate (MPA). Nonfatal MI, PE, and thrombophlebitis have also been reported in males taking high doses of CEE (eg, for prostate cancer). Estrogen compounds are generally associated with lipid effects such as increased HDL-cholesterol and decreased LDL-cholesterol. Triglycerides may also be increased; use with caution in patients with familial defects of lipoprotein metabolism. Whenever possible, estrogens should be discontinued at least 4 weeks prior to and for 2 weeks following elective surgery associated with an increased risk of thromboembolism or during periods of prolonged immobilization.

Neurological considerations: **[U.S. Boxed Warning]: The risk of dementia may be increased in postmenopausal women;** increased incidence was observed in women ≥65 years of age taking CEE alone or in combination with MPA.

Cancer-related considerations: **[U.S. Boxed Warning]: Unopposed estrogens may increase the risk of endometrial carcinoma in postmenopausal women.** Estrogens may exacerbate endometriosis. Malignant transformation of residual endometrial implants has been reported posthysterectomy with estrogen only therapy. Consider adding a progestin in women with residual endometriosis posthysterectomy. Estrogens may increase the risk of breast cancer. An increased risk of invasive breast cancer was observed in postmenopausal women using CEE in combination with MPA; a smaller increase in risk was seen with estrogen therapy alone in observational studies. An increase in abnormal mammograms has also been reported with estrogen and progestin therapy. Estrogen use may lead to severe hypercalcemia in patients with breast cancer and bone metastases; discontinue estrogen if hypercalcemia occurs.

Estrogens may cause retinal vascular thrombosis; discontinue permanently if papilledema or retinal vascular lesions are observed on examination. Use with caution in patients with diseases which may be exacerbated by fluid retention, including asthma, epilepsy, migraine, diabetes or renal dysfunction. Use with caution in patients with a history of severe hypocalcemia, SLE, hepatic hemangiomas, porphyria, endometriosis, and gallbladder disease. Use caution with history of cholestatic jaundice associated with past estrogen use or pregnancy.

(Continued)

Estrogens (Conjugated B/Synthetic) *(Continued)*

Before prescribing estrogen therapy to postmenopausal women, the risks and benefits must be weighed for each patient. Women should be informed of these risks and benefits, as well as possible effects of progestin when added to estrogen therapy. Estrogens with or without progestin should be used for shortest duration possible consistent with treatment goals. Conduct periodic risk:benefit assessments. When used solely for the treatment of vaginal dryness and pain with intercourse, or vulvar and vaginal atrophy, topical vaginal products should be considered.

Adverse Reactions (Reflective of adult population; not specific for elderly)
>10%:
    Central nervous system: Headache (15% to 25%), pain (10% to 19%)
    Endocrine & metabolic: Breast pain (up to 14%)
    Gastrointestinal: Abdominal pain (4% to 15%), nausea (7% to 12%)
1% to 10%:
    Central nervous system: Dizziness (1% to 7%)
    Endocrine & metabolic: Dysmenorrhea (1% to 8%)
    Gastrointestinal: Flatulence (4% to 7%)
    Genitourinary: Vaginitis (2% to 7%)
    Neuromuscular & skeletal: Paresthesia (up to 6%)
    Respiratory: Bronchitis (up to 7%), rhinitis (4% to 7%), sinusitis (3% to 7%)
    Miscellaneous: Flu-like syndrome (4% to 7%)
In addition, the following have been reported with estrogen and/or progestin therapy:
    Cardiovascular: Edema, hypertension, MI, stroke, venous thromboembolism
    Central nervous system: Epilepsy exacerbation, irritability, mental depression, migraine, mood disturbances, nervousness
    Dermatologic: Angioedema, chloasma, erythema multiforme, erythema nodosum, hemorrhagic eruption, hirsutism, loss of scalp hair, melasma, pruritus, rash, urticaria
    Endocrine & metabolic: Breast cancer, breast enlargement, breast tenderness, HDL-cholesterol increased, hyper-/hypocalcemia, impaired glucose tolerance, LDL-cholesterol decreased, libido (changes in), serum triglycerides/phospholipids increased, thyroid-binding globulin increased, total thyroid hormone (T_4) increased
    Gastrointestinal: Abdominal cramps, bloating, cholecystitis, cholelithiasis, gallbladder disease, pancreatitis, weight gain/loss
    Genitourinary: Alterations in frequency and flow of menses, changes in cervical secretions, endometrial cancer, endometrial hyperplasia, increased size of uterine leiomyomata, vaginal candidiasis
    Hematologic: Aggravation of porphyria; antithrombin III and antifactor Xa decreased; fibrinogen levels increased; platelet aggregability and platelet count increased; prothrombin and factors VII, VIII, IX, X increased
    Hepatic: Cholestatic jaundice, hepatic hemangiomas enlarged
    Local: Thrombophlebitis
    Neuromuscular & skeletal: Arthralgias, chorea, leg cramps
    Ocular: Contact lens intolerance, corneal curvature steepening, retinal vascular thrombosis
    Respiratory: Asthma exacerbation, pulmonary thromboembolism
    Miscellaneous: Anaphylactoid/anaphylactic reactions, carbohydrate intolerance

Overdosage/Toxicology Symptoms include nausea and vomiting; withdrawal bleeding may occur in females. Toxicity is unlikely following single exposures of excessive doses, any treatment following emesis and charcoal administration should be supportive and symptomatic.

Drug Interactions Based on estradiol and estrone: **Substrate** of CYP1A2 (major), 2A6 (minor), 2B6 (minor), 2C9 (minor), 2C19 (minor), 2D6 (minor), 2E1 (minor), 3A4 (major); **Inhibits** CYP1A2 (weak); **Induces** CYP3A4 (weak)
Anticoagulants: Increase potential for thromboembolic events.
Corticosteroids: Estrogens may enhance the levels/effects of systemic corticosteroids.
Cyclosporine: Estrogen derivatives may enhance the hepatotoxic effect of cyclosporine. Estrogen derivatives may increase the serum concentration of cyclosporine.
CYP1A2 inducers: May decrease the levels/effects of estrogens. Example inducers include aminoglutethimide, carbamazepine, phenobarbital, and rifampin.
CYP3A4 inducers: CYP3A4 inducers may decrease the levels/effects of estrogens. Example inducers include aminoglutethimide, carbamazepine, nafcillin, nevirapine, phenobarbital, phenytoin, and rifamycins.
Thyroid products: Estrogen derivatives may diminish the therapeutic effect of thyroid products; monitor.

Ethanol/Nutrition/Herb Interactions
Ethanol: Avoid ethanol (routine use increases estrogen level and risk of breast cancer).
Food: Grapefruit juice may increase estrogen levels, leading to increased adverse effects.
Herb/Nutraceutical: St John's wort may decrease levels. Herbs with estrogenic properties may enhance the adverse/toxic effect of estrogen derivatives; examples include

alfalfa, black cohosh, bloodroot, hops, kudzu, licorice, red clover, saw palmetto, soybean, thyme, wild yam, and yucca.

Stability Store at room temperature of 25°C (77°F).

Mechanism of Action Conjugated B/synthetic estrogens contain a mixture of 10 synthetic estrogen substances, including sodium estrone sulfate, sodium equilin sulfate, sodium 17-alpha-dihydroequilin, sodium 17-alpha-estradiol, and sodium 17-beta-dihydroequilin. Estrogens are responsible for the development and maintenance of the female reproductive system and secondary sexual characteristics. Estradiol is the principle intracellular human estrogen and is more potent than estrone and estriol at the receptor level; it is the primary estrogen secreted prior to menopause. Following menopause, estrone and estrone sulfate are more highly produced. Estrogens modulate the pituitary secretion of gonadotropins, luteinizing hormone, and follicle-stimulating hormone through a negative feedback system; estrogen replacement reduces elevated levels of these hormones in postmenopausal women.

Pharmacokinetics

Absorption: Well absorbed over a period of several hours

Protein-binding: Sex hormone-binding globulin (SHBG) and albumin

Metabolism: Hepatic via CYP3A4; estradiol is converted to estrone and estriol; also undergoes enterohepatic recirculation; estrone sulfate is the main metabolite in postmenopausal women

Excretion: Urine (primarily estriol, also as estradiol, estrone, and conjugates)

Dosage

Geriatrics: Refer to adult dosing. A higher incidence of stroke and invasive breast cancer were observed in women >75 years in a WHI substudy using conjugated equine estrogen.

Adults: The lowest dose that will control symptoms should be used. Medication should be discontinued as soon as possible.

Menopause, moderate-to-severe vasomotor symptoms: Oral: 0.3 mg/day; may be titrated up to 1.25 mg/day. Attempts to discontinue medication should be made at 3- to 6-month intervals.

Vaginal dryness/vulvar and vaginal atrophy associated with menopause: Oral: 0.3 mg/day. Attempts to discontinue medication should be made at 3- to 6-month intervals.

Monitoring Parameters Yearly physical examination that may include blood pressure and Papanicolaou smear, breast exam, mammogram. Monitor for signs of endometrial cancer in female patients with uterus. Adequate diagnostic measures, including endometrial sampling, if indicated, should be performed to rule out malignancy in all cases of undiagnosed abnormal vaginal bleeding. Monitor for loss of vision, sudden onset of proptosis, diplopia, migraine; signs and symptoms of thromboembolic disorders; glycemic control in diabetics; lipid profiles in patients being treated for hyperlipidemias; thyroid function in patients on thyroid hormone replacement therapy.

Test Interactions Pathologist should be advised of estrogen/progesterone therapy when specimens are submitted. Reduced response to metyrapone test observed with conjugated estrogens (equine).

Patient Information Do not take any new medication during therapy without consulting prescriber. Take exactly as directed and maintain prescribed cycles or term as prescribed. Routine use of alcohol may increase estrogen level and risk of breast cancer. Annual gynecologic and regular self-breast exams are important. If you have diabetes, monitor glucose levels closely (may impair glucose tolerance). You may experience nausea, vomiting or abdominal pain (small, frequent meals may help); dizziness or mental depression (use caution when driving); rash; hair loss; headache; or breast pain, increased/decreased libido, enlargement/tenderness of breasts, or difficult/painful menstrual cycles. Report significant swelling of extremities; sudden acute pain in legs or calves, chest, or abdomen; shortness of breath; severe headache or vomiting; sudden blindness; weakness or numbness of arm or leg; unusual vaginal bleeding; yellowing of skin or eyes; unusual bruising or bleeding; or other persistent adverse reactions. You may become intolerant to wearing contact lenses, notify prescriber if this occurs. Not for use in premenopausal women.

Additional Information Not biologically equivalent to conjugated estrogens from equine source. Contains 10 unique estrogenic compounds (equine source contains at least 10 active estrogenic compounds).

Special Geriatric Considerations Enjuvia™ has not been studied in an elderly population. Before prescribing estrogen therapy to postmenopausal women, the risks and benefits must be weighed for each patient. Women should be informed of these risks and benefits, as well as possible side effects and the return of menstrual bleeding (when cycled with a progestin), and be involved in the decision to prescribe. A higher incidence of stroke and invasive breast cancer was observed in women >75 years of age in a WHI substudy. Oral therapy may be more convenient for vaginal atrophy and urinary incontinence.

Dosage Forms Excipient information presented when available (limited, particularly for generics); consult specific product labeling.

(Continued)

Estrogens (Conjugated B/Synthetic) *(Continued)*

Tablet:

Enjuvia™: 0.3 mg, 0.45 mg, 0.625 mg, 1.25 mg

Selected References

Grodstein F, Stampfer MJ, Colditz GA, et al, "Postmenopausal Hormone Therapy and Mortality," *N Engl J Med*, 1997, 336(25):1769-75.

Hulley S, Grady D, Bush T, et al, "Randomized Trial of Estrogen Plus Progestin for Secondary Prevention of Coronary Heart Disease in Postmenopausal Women. Heart and Estrogen/Progestin Replacement Study (HERS) Research Group," *JAMA*, 1998, 280(7):605-13.

Shumaker S, Legault C, Thal L, et al, "Estrogen Plus Progestin and the Incidence of Dementia and Mild Cognitive Impairment in Postmenopausal Women: The Women's Health Initiative Memory Study: A Randomized Controlled Trial," *JAMA*, 2003, 289:2651-62.

U.S. Food and Drug Administration, Department of Health and Human Services, "FDA Approves New Labels for Estrogen and Estrogen With Progestin Therapies for Postmenopausal Women Following Review of Women's Health Initiative Data," January 8, 2003. Available at: http://www.fda.gov/medwatch/SAFETY/2003/safety03.htm#prempr. Accessed January 9, 2003.

"Writing Group for the Women's Health Initiative Investigators. Risks and Benefits of Estrogen Plus Progestin in Healthy Postmenopausal Women: Principle Results From the Women's Health Initiative Randomized Controlled Trial," *JAMA*, 2002, 288:321-33.

Estrogens (Conjugated/Equine)

(ES troe jenz KON joo gate ed, EE kwine)

Related Information

Osteoporosis Management *on page 1779*

Pharmacotherapy of Urinary Incontinence *on page 1822*

Medication Safety Issues

Sound-alike/look-alike issues:

Premarin® may be confused with Primaxin®, Provera®, Remeron®

U.S. Brand Names Premarin®

Canadian Brand Names C.E.S.®; Premarin®

Index Terms CEE; C.E.S.; Estrogenic Substances, Conjugated

Generic Available No

Pharmacologic Category Estrogen Derivative

Use Treatment of atrophic vaginitis, atrophic dystrophy of vulva, urinary incontinence secondary to estrogen deficiency, hypogonadism, primary ovarian failure, vasomotor symptoms of menopause, prostatic carcinoma, inoperable breast cancer; prevention of osteoporosis

Unlabeled/Investigational Use Treatment of uremic bleeding

Contraindications Hypersensitivity to estrogens or any component of the formulation; undiagnosed abnormal vaginal bleeding; history of or current thrombophlebitis or thromboembolic disorders; carcinoma of the breast (except in appropriately selected patients being treated for metastatic disease); estrogen-dependent tumor

Warnings/Precautions

Cardiovascular-related considerations: **[U.S. Boxed Warning]: Estrogens with or without progestin should not be used to prevent coronary heart disease.** Use caution with cardiovascular disease or dysfunction. May increase the risks of hypertension, myocardial infarction (MI), stroke, pulmonary emboli (PE), and deep vein thrombosis; incidence of these effects was shown to be significantly increased in postmenopausal women using conjugated equine estrogens (CEE) in combination with medroxyprogesterone acetate (MPA). Nonfatal MI, PE, and thrombophlebitis have also been reported in males taking high doses of CEE (eg, for prostate cancer). Estrogen compounds are generally associated with lipid effects such as increased HDL-cholesterol and decreased LDL-cholesterol. Triglycerides may also be increased; use with caution in patients with familial defects of lipoprotein metabolism. Whenever possible, estrogens should be discontinued at least 4 weeks prior to and for 2 weeks following elective surgery associated with an increased risk of thromboembolism or during periods of prolonged immobilization.

Neurological considerations: **[U.S. Boxed Warning]: The risk of dementia may be increased in postmenopausal women;** increased incidence was observed in women ≥65 years of age taking CEE alone or in combination with MPA.

Cancer-related considerations: **[U.S. Boxed Warning]: Unopposed estrogens may increase the risk of endometrial carcinoma in postmenopausal women.** Estrogens may exacerbate endometriosis. Malignant transformation of residual endometrial implants has been reported posthysterectomy with estrogen only therapy. Consider adding a progestin in women with residual endometriosis posthysterectomy. Estrogens may increase the risk of breast cancer. An increased risk of invasive breast cancer was observed in postmenopausal women using CEE in combination with MPA; a smaller increase in risk was seen with estrogen therapy alone in observational studies. An increase in abnormal mammograms has also been reported with estrogen and progestin therapy. Estrogen use may lead to severe hypercalcemia in patients with breast cancer and bone metastases; discontinue estrogen if hypercalcemia occurs.

Estrogens may cause retinal vascular thrombosis; discontinue permanently if papille-dema or retinal vascular lesions are observed on examination. Use with caution in patients with diseases which may be exacerbated by fluid retention, including asthma, epilepsy, migraine, diabetes or renal dysfunction. Use with caution in patients with a history of severe hypocalcemia, SLE, hepatic hemangiomas, porphyria, endometriosis, and gallbladder disease. Use caution with history of cholestatic jaundice associated with past estrogen use or pregnancy.

Before prescribing estrogen therapy to postmenopausal women, the risks and benefits must be weighed for each patient. Women should be informed of these risks and benefits, as well as possible effects of progestin when added to estrogen therapy. Estrogens with or without progestin should be used for shortest duration possible consistent with treatment goals. Conduct periodic risk:benefit assessments.

When used solely for prevention of osteoporosis in women at significant risk, nones-trogen treatment options should be considered. When used solely for the treatment of vulvar and vaginal atrophy, topical vaginal products should be considered. Use caution applying topical products to severely atrophic vaginal mucosa.

Adverse Reactions (Reflective of adult population; not specific for elderly)

Note: Percentages reported in postmenopausal women.

>10%:

Central nervous system: Headache (26% to 32%; placebo 28%)

Endocrine & metabolic: Breast pain (7% to 12%; placebo 9%)

Gastrointestinal: Abdominal pain (15% to 17%)

Genitourinary: Vaginal hemorrhage (2% to 14%)

Neuromuscular & skeletal: Back pain (13% to 14%)

1% to 10%:

Central nervous system: Nervousness (2% to 5%)

Endocrine & metabolic: Leukorrhea (4% to 7%)

Gastrointestinal: Flatulence (6% to 7%)

Genitourinary: Vaginitis (5% to 7%), vaginal moniliasis (5% to 6%)

Neuromuscular & skeletal: Weakness (7% to 8%), leg cramps (3% to 7%)

In addition, the following have been reported with estrogen and/or progestin therapy:

Cardiovascular: Edema, hypertension, MI, stroke, venous thromboembolism

Central nervous system: Dizziness, epilepsy exacerbation, headache, irritability, mental depression, migraine, mood disturbances, nervousness

Dermatologic: Angioedema, chloasma, erythema multiforme, erythema nodosum, hemorrhagic eruption, hirsutism, loss of scalp hair, melasma, pruritus, rash, urticaria

Endocrine & metabolic: Breast cancer, breast enlargement, breast tenderness, libido (changes in), increased thyroid-binding globulin, increased total thyroid hormone (T_4), increased serum triglycerides/phospholipids, increased HDL-cholesterol, decreased LDL-cholesterol, impaired glucose tolerance, hypercalcemia, hypocalcemia

Gastrointestinal: Abdominal cramps, bloating, cholecystitis, cholelithiasis, gallbladder disease, nausea, pancreatitis, vomiting, weight gain/loss

Genitourinary: Alterations in frequency and flow of menses, changes in cervical secretions, endometrial cancer, endometrial hyperplasia, increased size of uterine leiomyomata, vaginal candidiasis

Hematologic: Aggravation of porphyria, decreased antithrombin III and antifactor Xa, increased levels of fibrinogen, increased platelet aggregability and platelet count; increased prothrombin and factors VII, VIII, IX, X

Hepatic: Cholestatic jaundice, hepatic hemangiomas enlarged

Neuromuscular & skeletal: Arthralgias, chorea, leg cramps

Local: Thrombophlebitis

Ocular: Contact lens intolerance, corneal curvature steepening, retinal vascular thrombosis

Respiratory: Asthma exacerbation, pulmonary thromboembolism

Miscellaneous: Anaphylactoid/anaphylactic reactions, carbohydrate intolerance

Overdosage/Toxicology Toxicity is unlikely following single exposures of excessive doses. Effects noted after large doses include headache, nausea, and vomiting. Bleeding may occur in females. Treatment following emesis and charcoal administration should be supportive and symptomatic.

Drug Interactions

Based on estradiol and estrone: **Substrate** of CYP1A2 (major), 2A6 (minor), 2B6 (minor), 2C9 (minor), 2C19 (minor), 2D6 (minor), 2E1 (minor), 3A4 (major); **Inhibits** CYP1A2 (weak), 2C8 (weak); **Induces** CYP3A4 (weak)

Anticoagulants: Increase potential for thromboembolic events

Cyclosporine: Estrogen derivatives may enhance the hepatotoxic effect of cyclosporine. Estrogen derivatives may increase the serum concentration of cyclosporine.

CYP1A2 inducers: May decrease the levels/effects of estrogens. Example inducers include aminoglutethimide, carbamazepine, phenobarbital, and rifampin.

(Continued)

Estrogens (Conjugated/Equine) *(Continued)*

CYP3A4 inducers: CYP3A4 inducers may decrease the levels/effects of estrogens. Example inducers include aminoglutethimide, carbamazepine, nafcillin, nevirapine, phenobarbital, phenytoin, and rifamycins.

Thyroid products: Estrogen derivatives may diminish the therapeutic effect of thyroid products; monitor.

Ethanol/Nutrition/Herb Interactions

Ethanol: Avoid ethanol (routine use increases estrogen level and risk of breast cancer). Ethanol may also increase the risk of osteoporosis.

Food: Folic acid absorption may be decreased.

Herb/Nutraceutical: St John's wort may decrease levels. Herbs with estrogenic properties may enhance the adverse/toxic effect of estrogen derivatives; examples include alfalfa, black cohosh, bloodroot, hops, kudzu, licorice, red clover, saw palmetto, soybean, thyme, wild yam, yucca.

Stability

Injection: Refrigerate at 2°C to 8°C (36°F to 46°F) prior to reconstitution. Reconstitute using provided diluent; do not shake violently. Following reconstitution, solution may be stored under refrigeration for up to 60 days. Do not use if darkening or precipitation occurs.

Tablets, vaginal cream: Store at room temperature (25°C).

Mechanism of Action

Conjugated estrogens contain a mixture of estrone sulfate, equilin sulfate, 17 alpha-dihydroequilin, 17 alpha-estradiol and 17 beta-dihydroequilin. Estrogens are responsible for the development and maintenance of the female reproductive system and secondary sexual characteristics. Estradiol is the principle intracellular human estrogen and is more potent than estrone and estriol at the receptor level; it is the primary estrogen secreted prior to menopause. Following menopause, estrone and estrone sulfate are more highly produced. Estrogens modulate the pituitary secretion of gonadotropins, luteinizing hormone, and follicle-stimulating hormone through a negative feedback system; estrogen replacement reduces elevated levels of these hormones in postmenopausal women.

Pharmacokinetics

Absorption: Readily from GI tract

Metabolism: To inactive compounds occurs in the liver

Elimination: In bile and urine

Dosage

Geriatrics: Refer to adult dosing. A higher incidence of stroke and breast cancer was observed in women >75 years in a WHI substudy.

Adults:

Breast cancer palliation, metastatic disease in selected patients (male and female): Oral: 10 mg 3 times/day for at least 3 months

Uremic bleeding (unlabeled use): I.V.: 0.6 mg/kg/day for 5 days

Androgen-dependent prostate cancer palliation (males): Oral: 1.25-2.5 mg 3 times/day

Prevention of postmenopausal osteoporosis: Oral: Initial: 0.3 mg/day, cyclically* or daily, depending on medical assessment of patient. Dose may be adjusted based on bone mineral density and clinical response. The lowest effective dose should be used.

Menopause (moderate to severe vasomotor symptoms): Oral: Initial: 0.3 mg/day. May be given cyclically* or daily, depending on medical assessment of patient. The lowest dose that will control symptoms should be used. Medication should be discontinued as soon as possible.

Vulvar and vaginal atrophy: Oral: Initial: 0.3 mg/day. The lowest dose that will control symptoms should be used. May be given cyclically* or daily, depending on medical assessment of patient. Medication should be discontinued as soon as possible.

Vaginal cream: Intravaginal: 1/2 to 2 g/day given cyclically*

Female hypogonadism: Oral: 0.3-0.625 mg/day given cyclically*; dose may be titrated in 6- to 12-month intervals; progestin treatment should be added to maintain bone mineral density once skeletal maturity is achieved.

Female castration, primary ovarian failure: Oral: 1.25 mg/day given cyclically*; adjust according to severity of symptoms and patient response. For maintenance, adjust to the lowest effective dose.

Abnormal uterine bleeding:

Acute/heavy bleeding:

Oral (unlabeled route): 1.25 mg, may repeat every 4 hours for 24 hours, followed by 1.25 mg once daily for 7-10 days

I.M., I.V.: 25 mg, may repeat in 6-12 hours if needed

Note: Treatment should be followed by a low-dose oral contraceptive; medroxyprogesterone acetate along with or following estrogen therapy can also be given

Nonacute/lesser bleeding: Oral (unlabeled route): 1.25 mg once daily for 7-10 days

*Cyclic administration: Either 3 weeks on, 1 week off **or** 25 days on, 5 days off
Hepatic Impairment:
Mild to moderate liver impairment: Dosage reduction of estrogens is recommended.
Severe liver impairment: **Not recommended.**

Monitoring Parameters Yearly physical examination that includes blood pressure and Papanicolaou smear, breast exam, mammogram as appropriate. Monitor for signs of endometrial cancer in female patients with uterus; rule out malignancy if unexplained vaginal bleeding occurs

Reference Range Male: 15-40 mcg/24 hours (SI: 52-139 μmol/day); Female, postmenopausal: <20 mcg/24 hours (SI: 69 μmol/day) (values at Mayo Medical Laboratories)

Test Interactions Pathologist should be advised of estrogen/progesterone therapy when specimens are submitted. Reduced response to metyrapone test.

Patient Information It is important to maintain schedule. Estrogens have been shown to increase the risk of endometrial cancer. Annual gynecologic and breast exams are important. You may experience nausea or vomiting (small frequent meals may help); abdominal pain; dizziness or mental depression; headaches; rash; breast pain; or increased/decreased libido. Report significant swelling of extremities, sudden acute pain in legs or calves, chest or abdomen; shortness of breath; severe headache or vomiting; weakness or numbness of arms or legs; or unusual vaginal bleeding. You may become intolerant to wearing contact lenses, notify healthcare provider if this occurs. If taking for prevention of osteoporosis, ask healthcare provider about calcium and vitamin D intake, and weight-bearing exercises.

Additional Information May 28, 2003 (Updated from January, 2003 and July, 2002): Updated Risk/Benefit Labeling Based on Women's Health Initiative Study: Conjugated estrogens are currently indicated for the treatment of menopausal symptoms and prevention of osteoporosis. Use of conjugated estrogens for the prevention of other chronic diseases, as well as their potential negative effects on women's health, has been debated. Data published from the Women's Health Initiative (WHI) has provided some additional insight on this controversial topic.[1] Based on preliminary data from this trial, the Premarin® product labeling has been updated to strengthen the warnings section and to clarify the FDA-approved indications.

In the WHI, one arm of the study compared postmenopausal women with an intact uterus using conjugated equine estrogen 0.625 mg in combination with medroxyprogesterone acetate 2.5 mg daily, versus placebo. The primary outcome was to see the effect on coronary heart disease (CHD). This arm of the study was stopped early when it was observed that the incidence of CHD, breast cancer, ischemic stroke[2], and venous thromboembolism was increased in the treatment group.

Based on the preliminary findings, a new boxed warning has been placed on the Premarin®, Prempro™, and Premphase® product labeling. The warning emphasizes that these products should not be used for the prevention of cardiovascular disease and includes information from the WHI. Two of the approved indications have also been updated to clarify their use. When used solely for the treatment of moderate to severe symptoms of vulvar and vaginal atrophy associated with menopause, topical vaginal products should be considered. When used solely for the prevention of postmenopausal osteoporosis, nonestrogen products should be considered and estrogen products should only be used in women with significant risk, when the benefits of use outweigh the possible risks of the medication.

Additional data from a WHI substudy have recently been published[3]. The Women's Health Initiative Memory Study (WHIMS) evaluated a subset of WHI participants between the ages of 65-79 years of age to see if hormone replacement therapy reduces the risk of dementia, including Alzheimer's disease, in women. The estrogen/progesterone arm of this substudy was terminated early when this arm of the WHI study was halted. Researchers have found that conjugated equine estrogen plus progesterone may increase an older woman's risk of dementia and that this combination does not protect against mild cognitive impairment. Effects when using other forms or routes of estrogen are not known. Estrogens have never been approved for the prevention of cognitive disorders, including dementia. The use of conjugated equine estrogens and progestin to prevent dementia or preserve memory is not recommended.

Data collection from the WHI is still underway and additional or adjusted information from the completed study may be forthcoming. It should be noted that these results (increased incidence of CHD, breast cancer, ischemic stroke, venous thromboembolism, or increased dementia) have not been seen in another arm of the WHI study, testing conjugated equine estrogen alone in women without an intact uterus. This arm of the study has not been stopped and is expected to complete the planned 8 years of data collection. Meanwhile, the FDA advises that estrogen- and progestin-containing products be used at the lowest appropriate dose and for the shortest duration possible (Continued)

Estrogens (Conjugated/Equine) *(Continued)*

in carefully selected patients. Refer to the following FDA website for further information and links to revised product labeling:

http://www.fda.gov/medwatch/SAFETY/2003/safety03.htm#prempr, last accessed January 9, 2003.

http://www.fda.gov/bbs/topics/ANSWERS/2003/ANS01226.html, last accessed May 28, 2003.

[1]"Writing Group for the Women's Health Initiative Investigators. Risks and Benefits of Estrogen Plus Progestin in Healthy Postmenopausal Women: Principle Results From the Women's Health Initiative Randomized Controlled Trial," *JAMA*, 2002, 288:321-33.

[2]Wassertheil-Smoller S, Hendrix S, Limacher M, et al, "Effect of Estrogen Plus Progestin on Stroke in Postmenopausal Women: The Women's Health Initiative: A Randomized Trial," *JAMA*, 2003, 289:2673-84.

[3]Shumaker S, Legault C, Thal L, et al, "Estrogen Plus Progestin and the Incidence of Dementia and Mild Cognitive Impairment in Postmenopausal Women: The Women's Health Initiative Memory Study: A Randomized Controlled Trial," *JAMA*, 2003, 289:2651-62.

Special Geriatric Considerations Before prescribing estrogen therapy to postmenopausal women, the risks and benefits must be weighed for each patient. Women should be informed of these risks and benefits, as well as possible side effects and the return of menstrual bleeding (when cycled with a progestin), and be involved in the decision to prescribe. A higher incidence of stroke and invasive breast cancer was observed in women >75 years in a WHI substudy. Oral therapy may be more convenient for vaginal atrophy and urinary incontinence.

Dosage Forms Excipient information presented when available (limited, particularly for generics); consult specific product labeling.

Cream, vaginal: 0.625 mg/g (42.5 g)

Injection, powder for reconstitution: 25 mg [contains lactose 200 mg; diluent contains benzyl alcohol]

Tablet: 0.3 mg, 0.45 mg, 0.625 mg, 0.9 mg, 1.25 mg

Selected References

American College of Physicians, "Guidelines for Counseling Postmenopausal Women About Preventive Hormone Therapy," *Ann Intern Med*, 1992, 117(12):1038-41.

Belchetz PE, "Hormonal Treatment of Postmenopausal Women," *N Engl J Med*, 1994, 330(15):1062-71.

U.S. Food and Drug Administration, Department of Health and Human Services, "FDA Approves New Labels for Estrogen and Estrogen with Progestin Therapies for Postmenopausal Women Following Review of Women's Health Initiative Data," January 8, 2003, viewable at http://www.fda.gov/medwatch/SAFETY/2003/safety03.htm#prempr, last accessed January 9, 2003.

"Writing Group for the Women's Health Initiative Investigators. Risks and Benefits of Estrogen Plus Progestin in Healthy Postmenopausal Women: Principle Results From the Women's Health Initiative Randomized Controlled Trial," *JAMA*, 2002, 288:321-33.

Estrogens (Conjugated/Equine) and Medroxyprogesterone

(ES troe jenz KON joo gate ed/EE kwine & me DROKS ee proe JES te rone)

Related Information

Estrogens (Conjugated/Equine) *on page 564*

MedroxyPROGESTERone *on page 965*

Medication Safety Issues

Sound-alike/look-alike issues:

Premphase® may be confused with Prempro™

Prempro™ may be confused with Premphase®

U.S. Brand Names Premphase®; Prempro™

Canadian Brand Names Premphase®; Premplus®; Prempro™

Index Terms Medroxyprogesterone and Estrogens (Conjugated); MPA and Estrogens (Conjugated)

Generic Available No

Pharmacologic Category Estrogen and Progestin Combination

Use Women with an intact uterus: Treatment of moderate to severe vasomotor symptoms associated with the menopause, atrophic vaginitis, primary ovarian failure, osteoporosis prophylactic

Contraindications Hypersensitivity to conjugated estrogens, medroxyprogesterone (MPA), or any component of the formulation; undiagnosed abnormal vaginal bleeding; history of or current thrombophlebitis or thromboembolic disorders; carcinoma of the breast; estrogen-dependent tumor; hepatic dysfunction or disease

Warnings/Precautions

Cardiovascular-related considerations: **[U.S. Boxed Warning]: Estrogens with or without progestin should not be used to prevent coronary heart disease.** Use caution with cardiovascular disease or dysfunction. May increase the risks of hypertension, myocardial infarction (MI), stroke, pulmonary emboli (PE), and deep vein thrombosis; incidence of these effects was shown to be significantly increased in postmenopausal women using conjugated equine estrogens (CEE) in combination with medroxyprogesterone acetate (MPA). Nonfatal MI, PE, and thrombophlebitis have also been reported in males taking high doses of CEE (eg, for prostate cancer). Estrogen compounds are generally associated with lipid effects such as increased HDL-cholesterol and decreased LDL-cholesterol. Triglycerides may also be increased; use with caution in patients with familial defects of lipoprotein metabolism. Whenever possible, estrogens should be discontinued at least 4 weeks prior to and for 2 weeks following elective surgery associated with an increased risk of thromboembolism or during periods of prolonged immobilization.

Neurological considerations: **[U.S. Boxed Warning]: The risk of dementia may be increased in postmenopausal women;** increased incidence was observed in women ≥65 years of age taking CEE alone or in combination with MPA.

Cancer-related considerations: Unopposed estrogens may increase the risk of endometrial carcinoma in postmenopausal women. Estrogens may exacerbate endometriosis. Malignant transformation of residual endometrial implants has been reported posthysterectomy with estrogen only therapy. Estrogens may increase the risk of breast cancer. An increased risk of invasive breast cancer was observed in postmenopausal women using CEE in combination with MPA; a smaller increase in risk was seen with estrogen therapy alone in observational studies. An increase in abnormal mammograms has also been reported with estrogen and progestin therapy. Estrogen use may lead to severe hypercalcemia in patients with breast cancer and bone metastases; discontinue estrogen if hypercalcemia occurs.

Estrogens may cause retinal vascular thrombosis; discontinue permanently if papilledema or retinal vascular lesions are observed on examination. Use with caution in patients with diseases which may be exacerbated by fluid retention, including asthma, epilepsy, migraine, diabetes, or renal dysfunction. Use with caution in patients with a history of severe hypocalcemia, SLE, hepatic hemangiomas, porphyria, endometriosis, and gallbladder disease. Use caution with history of cholestatic jaundice associated with past estrogen use or pregnancy.

Before prescribing estrogen therapy to postmenopausal women, the risks and benefits must be weighed for each patient. Women should be informed of these risks and benefits, as well as possible effects of progestin when added to estrogen therapy. Estrogens with or without progestin should be used for shortest duration possible consistent with treatment goals. Conduct periodic risk:benefit assessments.

When used solely for prevention of osteoporosis in women at significant risk, nonestrogen treatment options should be considered. When used solely for the treatment of vulvar and vaginal atrophy, topical vaginal products should be considered.

Adverse Reactions (Reflective of adult population; not specific for elderly)
>10%:
    Central nervous system: Headache (28% to 37%), pain (11% to 13%), depression (6% to 11%)
    Endocrine & metabolic: Breast pain (32% to 38%), dysmenorrhea (8% to 13%)
    Gastrointestinal: Abdominal pain (16% to 23%), nausea (9% to 11%)
    Neuromuscular & skeletal: Back pain (13% to 16%)
    Respiratory: Pharyngitis (11% to 13%)
    Miscellaneous: Infection (16% to 18%), flu-like syndrome (10% to 13%)
1% to 10%:
    Cardiovascular: Peripheral edema (3% to 4%)
    Central nervous system: Dizziness (3% to 5%)
    Dermatologic: Pruritus (5% to 10%), rash (4% to 6%)
    Endocrine & metabolic: Leukorrhea (5% to 9%)
    Gastrointestinal: Flatulence (8% to 9%), diarrhea (5% to 6%), dyspepsia (5% to 6%)
    Genitourinary: Vaginitis (5% to 7%), cervical changes (4% to 5%), vaginal hemorrhage (1% to 3%)
    Neuromuscular & skeletal: Weakness (6% to 10%), arthralgia (7% to 9%), leg cramps (3% to 5%), hypertonia (3% to 4%)
    Respiratory: Sinusitis (7% to 8%), rhinitis (6% to 8%)
Additional adverse effects reported with conjugated estrogens and/or progestins: Abdominal cramps, acne, abnormal uterine bleeding, aggravation of porphyria, amenorrhea, anaphylactoid reactions, anaphylaxis, antifactor Xa decreased, antithrombin III decreased, appetite changes, bloating, breast enlargement, breast tenderness, cerebral embolism, cerebral thrombosis, chloasma, cholestatic jaundice, cholecystitis, cholelithiasis, chorea, contact lens intolerance, cystitis-like syndrome, decreased carbohydrate tolerance, dizziness; factors VII, VIII, IX, X, XII, VII-X complex, and II-VII-X complex increased; endometrial hyperplasia, erythema multiforme, erythema nodosum, galactorrhea, hemorrhagic eruption, fatigue, fibrinogen increased, impaired glucose tolerance, HDL-cholesterol increased, hirsutism, hypertension, increase in size of uterine leiomyomata, gallbladder disease, insomnia, LDL-cholesterol decreased, libido changes, loss of scalp hair, melasma, migraine, nervousness, optic neuritis, pancreatitis, platelet aggregability and platelet count
(Continued)

Estrogens (Conjugated/Equine) and Medroxyprogesterone
(Continued)

increased, premenstrual like syndrome, PT and PTT accelerated, pulmonary embolism, pyrexia, retinal thrombosis, somnolence, steepening of corneal curvature, thrombophlebitis, thyroid-binding globulin increased, total thyroid hormone (T_4) increased, triglycerides increased, urticaria, vaginal candidiasis, vomiting, weight gain/loss

Drug Interactions

Based on estradiol and estrone: **Substrate** of CYP1A2 (major), 2A6 (minor), 2B6 (minor), 2C9 (minor), 2C19 (minor), 2D6 (minor), 2E1 (minor), 3A4 (major); **Inhibits** CYP1A2 (weak), 2C8 (weak); **Induces** CYP3A4 (weak)

Medroxyprogesterone: **Substrate** of CYP3A4 (major); **Induces** CYP3A4 (weak)

See individual agents.

Ethanol/Nutrition/Herb Interactions

Ethanol: Avoid ethanol (routine use increases estrogen level and risk of breast cancer). Ethanol may also increase the risk of osteoporosis.

Food: Folic acid absorption may be decreased.

Herb/Nutraceutical: St John's wort may decrease levels. Avoid black cohosh, dong quai (has estrogenic activity). Avoid red clover, saw palmetto, ginseng (due to potential hormonal effects).

Stability Store at room temperature 20°C to 25°C (68°F to 77°F).

Mechanism of Action

Conjugated estrogens contain a mixture of estrone sulfate, equilin sulfate, 17 alpha-dihydroequilin, 17 alpha-estradiol, and 17 beta-dihydroequilin. Estrogens are responsible for the development and maintenance of the female reproductive system and secondary sexual characteristics. Estradiol is the principle intracellular human estrogen and is more potent than estrone and estriol at the receptor level; it is the primary estrogen secreted prior to menopause. Following menopause, estrone and estrone sulfate are more highly produced. Estrogens modulate the pituitary secretion of gonadotropins, luteinizing hormone, and follicle-stimulating hormone through a negative feedback system; estrogen replacement reduces elevated levels of these hormones in postmenopausal women.

MPA inhibits gonadotropin production which then prevents follicular maturation and ovulation. In women with adequate estrogen, MPA transforms a proliferative endometrium into a secretory endometrium; when administered with conjugated estrogens, reduces the incidence of endometrial hyperplasia and risk of adenocarcinoma.

Pharmacokinetics

Absorption: Well absorbed

Protein binding:

Conjugated estrogens: Albumin

Unconjugated estrogens: Albumin and sex-hormone-binding globulin (SHBG)

MPA: Plasma proteins (90%), but not SHBG

Metabolism:

Conjugated estrogens and MPA are both metabolized in the liver

MPA is hydroxylated and conjugated

Half-life: Conjugated estrogens: 10-24 hours; MPA: 38-46 hours

Time to peak: Conjugated estrogens: 4-10 hours; MPA: 2-4 hours

Elimination:

Conjugated estrogens: Urine, bile

MPA: Urine as glucuronide conjugates (major) and sulfates (minor)

Dosage

Geriatrics: Refer to adult dosing. A higher incidence of stroke and breast cancer was observed in women >75 years in a WHI substudy.

Adults:

Treatment of moderate-to-severe vasomotor symptoms associated with menopause or treatment of atrophic vaginitis in females with an intact uterus: (**Note:** The lowest dose that will control symptoms should be used; medication should be discontinued as soon as possible): Oral:

Premphase®: One maroon conjugated estrogen 0.625 mg tablet daily on days 1 through 14 and one light blue conjugated estrogen 0.625 mg/MPA 5 mg tablet daily on days 15 through 28; re-evaluate patients at 3- and 6-month intervals to determine if treatment is still necessary; monitor patients for signs of endometrial cancer; rule out malignancy if unexplained vaginal bleeding occurs

Prempro™: One conjugated estrogen 0.3 mg/MPA 1.5 mg tablet daily; re-evaluate at 3-and 6-month intervals to determine if therapy is still needed; dose may be increased to a maximum of one conjugated estrogen 0.625 mg/MPA 5 mg tablet daily in patients with bleeding or spotting, once malignancy has been ruled out

Osteoporosis prophylaxis in females with an intact uterus: Oral:

Premphase®: One maroon conjugated estrogen 0.625 tablet daily on days 1 through 14 and one light blue conjugated estrogen 0.625 mg/MPA 5 mg tablet daily on days 15 through 28; monitor patients for signs of endometrial cancer; rule out malignancy if unexplained vaginal bleeding occurs

Prempro™: One conjugated estrogen 0.3 mg/MPA 1.5 mg tablet daily; dose may be increased to one conjugated estrogen 0.625 mg/MPA 5 mg tablet daily; in patients with bleeding or spotting, once malignancy has been ruled out

Monitoring Parameters Yearly physical examination that includes blood pressure and Papanicolaou smear, breast exam, mammogram. Monitor for signs of endometrial cancer. Adequate diagnostic measures, including endometrial sampling, if indicated, should be performed to rule out malignancy in all cases of undiagnosed abnormal vaginal bleeding. Monitor for loss of vision, sudden onset of proptosis, diplopia, migraine; signs and symptoms of thromboembolic disorders; glycemic control in diabetics; lipid profiles in patients being treated for hyperlipidemias; thyroid function in patients on thyroid hormone replacement therapy.

Menopausal symptoms: Assess need for therapy at 3- to 6-month intervals

Prevention of osteoporosis: Bone density measurement

Test Interactions Pathologist should be advised of estrogen/progesterone therapy when specimens are submitted. Reduced response to metyrapone test.

Patient Information Take this as prescribed; maintain schedule. Annual gynecologic and breast exams are important. You may experience nausea or vomiting (small frequent meals may help); abdominal pain, dizziness or mental depression; rash, headache, breast pain, or increased/decreased libido. Report significant swelling of extremities; sudden acute pain in legs or calves, chest or abdomen; shortness of breath; severe headache or vomiting; sudden blindness; weakness or numbness of arm or leg; unusual vaginal bleeding; yellowing of skin or eyes; or unusual bruising or bleeding. You may become intolerant to wearing contact lenses, notify healthcare provider if this occurs. If taking for prevention of osteoporosis, ask healthcare provider about calcium and vitamin D intake, and weight-bearing exercises.

Additional Information The use of estrogens for the prevention of other chronic diseases, as well as their potential negative effects on women's health, has been debated. Data published from the Women's Health Initiative (WHI) has provided some additional insight on this controversial topic.

In the WHI, one arm of the study compared postmenopausal women with an intact uterus using conjugated equine estrogen 0.625 mg in combination with medroxyprogesterone acetate 2.5 mg daily, versus placebo. The primary outcome was to see the effect on coronary heart disease (CHD). This arm of the study was stopped early (2002) when it was observed that the incidence of CHD, breast cancer, stroke, and venous thromboembolism was increased in the treatment group.

Based on the preliminary findings, a black warning was placed on the Premarin®, Prempro™, and Premphase® product labeling. The warning emphasizes that these products should not be used for the prevention of cardiovascular disease. Two of the approved indications were also been updated to clarify their use: Topical vaginal products should be considered if used solely for the treatment of moderate to severe symptoms of vulvar and vaginal atrophy associated with menopause; nonestrogen products should be considered for the prevention of osteoporoses and estrogen products should only be used in women with significant risk. These products should be used at the lowest dose for the shortest duration with careful monitoring. The FDA recommended that similar changes be made to the labeling of other estrogen products used in postmenopausal women.

Data collection from the WHI is still underway and additional or adjusted information from the completed study may be forthcoming. It should be noted that these results have not been seen in another arm of the WHI study, testing conjugated equine estrogen alone in women without an intact uterus. This arm of the study has not been stopped and is expected to complete the planned 8 years of data collection.

Special Geriatric Considerations Before prescribing estrogen therapy to postmenopausal women, the risks and benefits must be weighed for each patient. Women should be informed of these risks and benefits, as well as possible side effects and the return of menstrual bleeding (when cycled with a progestin), and be involved in the decision to prescribe. A higher incidence of stroke and invasive breast cancer was observed in women >75 years in a WHI substudy. Oral therapy may be more convenient for vaginal atrophy and urinary incontinence.

Dosage Forms Excipient information presented when available (limited, particularly for generics); consult specific product labeling.

Tablet:

Premphase® [therapy pack contains 2 separate tablet formulations]: Conjugated estrogens 0.625 mg [14 maroon tablets] and conjugated estrogen 0.625 mg/medroxyprogesterone acetate 5 mg [14 light blue tablets] (28s)

Prempro™:

0.3/1.5: Conjugated estrogens 0.3 mg and medroxyprogesterone acetate 1.5 mg (28s)

(Continued)

Estrogens (Conjugated/Equine) and Medroxyprogesterone
(Continued)

0.45/1.5: Conjugated estrogens 0.45 mg and medroxyprogesterone acetate 1.5 mg (28s)

0.625/2.5: Conjugated estrogens 0.625 mg and medroxyprogesterone acetate 2.5 mg (28s)

0.625/5: Conjugated estrogens 0.625 mg and medroxyprogesterone acetate 5 mg (28s)

Selected References

U.S. Food and Drug Administration, Department of Health and Human Services, "FDA Approves New Labels for Estrogen and Estrogen with Progestin Therapies for Postmenopausal Women Following Review of Women's Health Initiative Data," January 8, 2003, viewable at http://www.fda.gov/medwatch/SAFETY/2003/safety03.htm#prempr, last accessed January 9, 2003.

"Writing Group for the Women's Health Initiative Investigators. Risks and Benefits of Estrogen Plus Progestin in Healthy Postmenopausal Women: Principle Results From the Women's Health Initiative Randomized Controlled Trial," *JAMA*, 2002, 288:321-33.

Estrogens (Esterified) (ES troe jenz, es TER i fied)

Related Information
Osteoporosis Management *on page 1779*

Medication Safety Issues
Sound-alike/look-alike issues:
Estratab® may be confused with Estratest®, Estratest® H.S.

U.S. Brand Names Menest®

Canadian Brand Names Estratab®; Menest®

Index Terms Esterified Estrogens

Generic Available No

Pharmacologic Category Estrogen Derivative

Use Treatment of moderate to severe vasomotor symptoms associated with menopause, vulvar and vaginal atrophy, hypoestrogenism (due to hypogonadism, castration, or primary ovarian failure), prostatic cancer (palliation), breast cancer (palliation); osteoporosis prophylaxis (in women at significant risk only)

Contraindications Hypersensitivity to estrogens or any component of the formulation; undiagnosed abnormal vaginal bleeding; history of or current thrombophlebitis or thromboembolic disorders; carcinoma of the breast, except in appropriately selected patients being treated for metastatic disease; estrogen-dependent tumor

Warnings/Precautions

Cardiovascular-related considerations: **[U.S. Boxed Warning]: Estrogens with or without progestin should not be used to prevent coronary heart disease.** Use caution with cardiovascular disease or dysfunction. May increase the risks of hypertension, myocardial infarction (MI), stroke, pulmonary emboli (PE), and deep vein thrombosis; incidence of these effects was shown to be significantly increased in postmenopausal women using conjugated equine estrogens (CEE) in combination with medroxyprogesterone acetate (MPA). Nonfatal MI, PE, and thrombophlebitis have also been reported in males taking high doses of CEE (eg, for prostate cancer). Estrogen compounds are generally associated with lipid effects such as increased HDL-cholesterol and decreased LDL-cholesterol. Triglycerides may also be increased; use with caution in patients with familial defects of lipoprotein metabolism. Whenever possible, estrogens should be discontinued at least 4 weeks prior to and for 2 weeks following elective surgery associated with an increased risk of thromboembolism or during periods of prolonged immobilization.

Neurological considerations: **[U.S. Boxed Warning]: The risk of dementia may be increased in postmenopausal women;** increased incidence was observed in women ≥65 years of age taking CEE alone or in combination with MPA.

Cancer-related considerations: **[U.S. Boxed Warning]: Unopposed estrogens may increase the risk of endometrial carcinoma in postmenopausal women.** Estrogens may exacerbate endometriosis. Malignant transformation of residual endometrial implants has been reported post-hysterectomy with estrogen only therapy. Consider adding a progestin in women with residual endometriosis post-hysterectomy. Estrogens may increase the risk of breast cancer. An increased risk of invasive breast cancer was observed in postmenopausal women using CEE in combination with MPA; a smaller increase in risk was seen with estrogen therapy alone in observational studies. An increase in abnormal mammograms has also been reported with estrogen and progestin therapy. Estrogen use may lead to severe hypercalcemia in patients with breast cancer and bone metastases; discontinue estrogen if hypercalcemia occurs.

Estrogens may cause retinal vascular thrombosis; discontinue permanently if papilledema or retinal vascular lesions are observed on examination. Use with caution in patients with diseases which may be exacerbated by fluid retention, including asthma, epilepsy, migraine, diabetes or renal dysfunction. Use with caution in patients with a history of severe hypocalcemia, SLE, hepatic hemangiomas, porphyria, endometriosis, and gallbladder disease. Use caution with history of cholestatic jaundice associated with past estrogen use or pregnancy.

Before prescribing estrogen therapy to postmenopausal women, the risks and benefits must be weighed for each patient. Women should be informed of these risks and benefits, as well as possible effects of progestin when added to estrogen therapy. Estrogens with or without progestin should be used for shortest duration possible consistent with treatment goals. Conduct periodic risk:benefit assessments.

When used solely for prevention of osteoporosis in women at significant risk, nonestrogen treatment options should be considered. When used solely for the treatment of vulvar and vaginal atrophy, topical vaginal products should be considered.

Adverse Reactions (Reflective of adult population; not specific for elderly)
Frequency not defined.

Cardiovascular: Edema, hypertension, venous thromboembolism

Central nervous system: Dizziness, headache, mental depression, migraine

Dermatologic: Chloasma, erythema multiforme, erythema nodosum, hemorrhagic eruption, hirsutism, loss of scalp hair, melasma

Endocrine & metabolic: Breast enlargement, breast tenderness, libido (changes in), increased thyroid-binding globulin, increased total thyroid hormone (T_4), increased serum triglycerides/phospholipids, increased HDL-cholesterol, decreased LDL-cholesterol, impaired glucose tolerance, hypercalcemia

Gastrointestinal: Abdominal cramps, bloating, cholecystitis, cholelithiasis, gallbladder disease, nausea, pancreatitis, vomiting, weight gain/loss

Genitourinary: Alterations in frequency and flow of menses, changes in cervical secretions, endometrial cancer, increased size of uterine leiomyomata, vaginal candidiasis

Hematologic: Aggravation of porphyria, decreased antithrombin III and antifactor Xa, increased levels of fibrinogen, increased platelet aggregability and platelet count; increased prothrombin and factors VII, VIII, IX, X

Hepatic: Cholestatic jaundice

Neuromuscular & skeletal: Chorea

Ocular: Ocular: Contact lens intolerance, corneal curvature steepening

Respiratory: Pulmonary thromboembolism

Miscellaneous: Carbohydrate intolerance

Overdosage/Toxicology Toxicity is unlikely following single exposures of excessive doses. Effects noted after large doses include headache, nausea, and vomiting. Bleeding may occur in females. Treatment following emesis and charcoal administration should be supportive and symptomatic.

Drug Interactions Based on estrone: **Substrate** of CYP1A2 (major), 2B6 (minor), 2C9 (minor), 2E1 (minor), 3A4 (major)

Anticoagulants: Increases potential for thromboembolic events with anticoagulants

Corticosteroids: Estrogens may enhance the effects of hydrocortisone and prednisone.

Cyclosporine: Estrogen derivatives may enhance the hepatotoxic effect of cyclosporine. Estrogen derivatives may increase the serum concentration of cyclosporine.

CYP1A2 inducers: May decrease the levels/effects of estrogens. Example inducers include aminoglutethimide, carbamazepine, phenobarbital, and rifampin.

CYP3A4 inducers: CYP3A4 inducers may decrease the levels/effects of estrogens. Example inducers include aminoglutethimide, carbamazepine, nafcillin, nevirapine, phenobarbital, phenytoin, and rifamycins.

Thyroid products: Estrogen derivatives may diminish the therapeutic effect of thyroid products; monitor.

Ethanol/Nutrition/Herb Interactions

Ethanol: Avoid ethanol (routine use increases estrogen level and risk of breast cancer). Ethanol may also increase the risk of osteoporosis.

Food: Folic acid absorption may be decreased.

Herb/Nutraceutical: St John's wort may decrease levels. Herbs with estrogenic properties may enhance the adverse/toxic effect of estrogen derivatives; examples include alfalfa, black cohosh, bloodroot, hops, kudzu, licorice, red clover, saw palmetto, soybean, thyme, wild yam, yucca.

Stability Store below 30°C (86°F). Protect from moisture.

Mechanism of Action Esterified estrogens contain a mixture of estrogenic substances; the principle component is estrone. Preparations contain 75% to 85% sodium estrone sulfate and 6% to 15% sodium equilin sulfate such that the total is not <90%. Estrogens are responsible for the development and maintenance of the female reproductive system and secondary sexual characteristics. Estradiol is the principle intracellular human estrogen and is more potent than estrone and estriol at the receptor level; it is the primary estrogen secreted prior to menopause. In males and following menopause in females, estrone and estrone sulfate are more highly produced. Estrogens modulate the pituitary secretion of gonadotropins, luteinizing hormone, and follicle-stimulating hormone through a negative feedback system; estrogen replacement reduces elevated levels of these hormones.

(Continued)

Estrogens (Esterified) *(Continued)*

Pharmacokinetics
Absorption: Readily absorbed from GI tract
Metabolism: Rapidly in the liver to less active metabolites
Elimination: In urine as unchanged compound and metabolites

Dosage
Geriatrics: Refer to adult dosing. A higher incidence of stroke and invasive breast cancer were observed in women >75 years in a WHI substudy using conjugated equine estrogen.

Adults:

Prostate cancer (palliation): Oral: 1.25-2.5 mg 3 times/day

Female hypogonadism: Oral: 2.5-7.5 mg of estrogen daily for 20 days followed by a 10-day rest period. Administer cyclically (3 weeks on and 1 week off). If bleeding does not occur by the end of the 10-day period, repeat the same dosing schedule; the number of courses dependent upon the responsiveness of the endometrium. If bleeding occurs before the end of the 10-day period, begin an estrogen-progestin cyclic regimen of 2.5-7.5 mg esterified estrogens daily for 20 days. During the last 5 days of estrogen therapy, give an oral progestin. If bleeding occurs before regimen is concluded, discontinue therapy and resume on the fifth day of bleeding.

Menopause, moderate to severe vasomotor symptoms: Oral: 1.25 mg/day administered cyclically (3 weeks on and 1 week off). If patient has not menstruated within the last 2 months or more, cyclic administration is started arbitrary. If the patient is menstruating, cyclical administration is started on day 5 of the bleeding. For short-term use only and should be discontinued as soon as possible. Re-evaluate at 3- to 6-month intervals for tapering or discontinuation of therapy.

Atopic vaginitis and kraurosis vulvae: Oral: 0.3 to ≥1.25 mg/day, depending on the tissue response of the individual patient. Administer cyclically. For short-term use only and should be discontinued as soon as possible. Re-evaluate at 3- to 6-month intervals for tapering or discontinuation of therapy.

Breast cancer (palliation): Oral: 10 mg 3 times/day for at least 3 months

Osteoporosis in postmenopausal women: Oral: Initial: 0.3 mg/day and increase to a maximum daily dose of 1.25 mg/day; initiate therapy as soon as possible after menopause; cyclically or daily, depending on medical assessment of patient. Monitor patients with an intact uterus for signs of endometrial cancer; rule out malignancy if unexplained vaginal bleeding occurs

Female castration and primary ovarian failure: Oral: 1.25 mg/day, cyclically. Adjust dosage upward or downward, according to the severity of symptoms and patient response. For maintenance, adjust dosage to lowest level that will provide effective control.

Hepatic Impairment:
Mild to moderate liver impairment: Dosage reduction of estrogens is recommended.
Severe liver impairment: **Not recommended**.

Monitoring Parameters Yearly physical examination that includes blood pressure and Papanicolaou smear, breast exam, mammogram. Monitor for signs of endometrial cancer in female patients with uterus. Adequate diagnostic measures, including endometrial sampling, if indicated, should be performed to rule out malignancy in all cases of undiagnosed abnormal vaginal bleeding. Monitor for loss of vision, sudden onset of proptosis, diplopia, migraine; signs and symptoms of thromboembolic disorders; glycemic control in diabetics; lipid profiles in patients being treated for hyperlipidemias; thyroid function in patients on thyroid hormone replacement therapy.

Menopausal symptoms: Assess need for therapy at 3- to 6-month intervals
Prevention of osteoporosis: Bone density measurement

Test Interactions Pathologist should be advised of estrogen/progesterone therapy when specimens are submitted. Reduced response to metyrapone test.

Patient Information It is important to maintain schedule. Estrogens have been shown to increase the risk of endometrial cancer. Annual gynecologic and breast exams are important. You may experience nausea or vomiting (small frequent meals may help); abdominal pain; dizziness or mental depression; headaches; rash; breast pain; or increased/decreased libido. Report significant swelling of extremities, sudden acute pain in legs or calves, chest or abdomen; shortness of breath; severe headache or vomiting; weakness or numbness of arms or legs; or unusual vaginal bleeding. You may become intolerant to wearing contact lenses, notify healthcare provider if this occurs. If taking for prevention of osteoporosis, ask healthcare provider about calcium and vitamin D intake, and weight-bearing exercises.

Additional Information Esterified estrogens are a combination of the sodium salts of the sulfate esters of estrogenic substances; the principal component is estrone, with preparations containing 75% to 85% sodium estrone sulfate and 6% to 15% sodium equilin sulfate such that the total is not <90%.

The use of estrogens for the prevention of other chronic diseases, as well as their potential negative effects on women's health, has been debated. Data published from the Women's Health Initiative (WHI) has provided some additional insight on this controversial topic.

In the WHI, one arm of the study compared postmenopausal women with an intact uterus using conjugated equine estrogen 0.625 mg in combination with medroxypro-gesterone acetate 2.5 mg daily, versus placebo. The primary outcome was to see the effect on coronary heart disease (CHD). This arm of the study was stopped early (2002) when it was observed that the incidence of CHD, breast cancer, stroke, and venous thromboembolism was increased in the treatment group.

Based on the preliminary findings, a boxed warning was placed on the Premarin®, Prempro™, and Premphase® product labeling. The warning emphasizes that these products should not be used for the prevention of cardiovascular disease. Two of the approved indications were also been updated to clarify their use: Topical vaginal products should be considered if used solely for the treatment of moderate to severe symptoms of vulvar and vaginal atrophy associated with menopause; nonestrogen products should be considered for the prevention of osteoporoses and estrogen products should only be used in women with significant risk. These products should be used at the lowest dose for the shortest duration with careful monitoring. The FDA recommended that similar changes be made to the labeling of other estrogen products used in postmenopausal women.

Data collection from the WHI is still underway and additional or adjusted information from the completed study may be forthcoming. It should be noted that these results have not been seen in another arm of the WHI study, testing conjugated equine estrogen alone in women without an intact uterus. This arm of the study has not been stopped and is expected to complete the planned 8 years of data collection.

Special Geriatric Considerations Before prescribing estrogen therapy to postmeno-pausal women, the risks and benefits must be weighed for each patient. Women should be informed of these risks and benefits, as well as possible side effects and the return of menstrual bleeding (when cycled with a progestin), and be involved in the decision to prescribe. A higher incidence of stroke and invasive breast cancer were observed in women >75 years in a WHI substudy using conjugated equine estrogen. Oral therapy may be more convenient for vaginal atrophy and urinary incontinence.

Dosage Forms Tablet: 0.3 mg, 0.625 mg, 1.25 mg, 2.5 mg

Selected References

American College of Physicians, "Guidelines for Counseling Postmenopausal Women About Preventive Hormone Therapy," *Ann Intern Med*, 1992, 117(12):1038-41.

Belchetz PE, "Hormonal Treatment of Postmenopausal Women," *N Engl J Med*, 1994, 330 (15): 1062-71.

The Writing Group for the PEPI Trial, "Effects of Estrogen or Estrogen/Progestin Regimens on Heart Disease Risk Factors in Postmenopausal Women," *JAMA*, 1995, 273(3):199-208.

U.S. Food and Drug Administration, Department of Health and Human Services, "FDA Approves New Labels for Estrogen and Estrogen with Progestin Therapies for Postmenopausal Women Following Review of Women's Health Initiative Data," January 8, 2003, viewable at http://www.fda.gov/medwatch/SAFETY/2003/safety03.htm#prempr, last accessed January 9, 2003.

"Writing Group for the Women's Health Initiative Investigators. Risks and Benefits of Estrogen Plus Progestin in Healthy Postmenopausal Women: Principle Results From the Women's Health Initiative Randomized Controlled Trial," *JAMA*, 2002, 288:321-33.

Eszopiclone (es zoe PIK lone)

Medication Safety Issues
Sound-alike/look-alike issues:
Lunesta™ may be confused with Neulasta®

U.S. Brand Names Lunesta™

Generic Available No

Pharmacologic Category Hypnotic, Nonbenzodiazepine

Use Treatment of insomnia

Restrictions C-IV

Contraindications Hypersensitivity to eszopiclone or any component of the formulation

Warnings/Precautions Symptomatic treatment of insomnia should be initiated only after careful evaluation of potential causes of sleep disturbance. Tolerance did not develop over 6 months of use. Use with caution in patients with depression or a history of drug dependence. Abrupt discontinuance may lead to withdrawal symptoms. Use with caution in patients receiving other CNS depressants or psychoactive medications. Hypnotics/sedatives have been associated with abnormal thinking and behavior changes including decreased inhibition, aggression, bizarre behavior, agitation, halluci-nations, and depersonalization. These changes may occur unpredictably and may indicate previously unrecognized psychiatric disorders; evaluate appropriately. Amnesia may occur. May impair physical and mental capabilities. Postmarketing studies have indicated that the use of hypnotic/sedative agents for sleep has been associated with hypersensitivity reactions including anaphylaxis as well as angioe-dema. An increased risk for hazardous sleep-related activities such as sleep-driving; cooking and eating food, and making phone calls while asleep have also been noted. Use caution in patients with respiratory compromise, hepatic dysfunction, elderly or
(Continued)

Eszopiclone *(Continued)*

those taking strong CYP3A4 inhibitors. Because of the rapid onset of action, administer immediately prior to bedtime or after the patient has gone to bed and is having difficulty falling asleep.

Adverse Reactions (Reflective of adult population; not specific for elderly)
>10%:

Central nervous system: Headache (15% to 21%)

Gastrointestinal: Unpleasant taste (8% to 34%)

1% to 10%:

Cardiovascular: Chest pain, peripheral edema

Central nervous system: Somnolence (8% to 10%), dizziness (5% to 7%), hallucinations (1% to 3%), anxiety (1% to 3%), nervousness (up to 5%), confusion (up to 3%), depression (1% to 4%), abnormal dreams (1% to 3%), migraine

Dermatologic: Rash (3% to 4%), pruritus (1% to 4%)

Endocrine & metabolic: Libido decreased (up to 3%), dysmenorrhea (up to 3%), gynecomastia (males up to 3%)

Gastrointestinal: Xerostomia (3% to 7%), dyspepsia (5% to 6%), nausea (5%), diarrhea (2% to 4%), vomiting (up to 3%)

Genitourinary: Urinary tract infection (up to 3%)

Neuromuscular & skeletal: Neuralgia (up to 3%)

Miscellaneous: Infection (5% to 10%), viral infection (3%)

Overdosage/Toxicology Overdose symptoms range from somnolence to coma. Treatment is symptom-directed and supportive. Flumazenil may be useful.

Drug Interactions Substrate of CYP2E1 (minor), 3A4 (major)

CYP3A4 inducers: May decrease the levels/effects of eszopiclone. Example inducers include aminoglutethimide, carbamazepine, nafcillin, nevirapine, phenobarbital, phenytoin, and rifamycins.

CYP3A4 inhibitors: May increase the levels/effects of eszopiclone. Example inhibitors include azole antifungals, clarithromycin, diclofenac, doxycycline, erythromycin, imatinib, isoniazid, nefazodone, nicardipine, propofol, protease inhibitors, quinidine, telithromycin, and verapamil.

Ketoconazole: May increase serum concentration of eszopiclone.

Olanzapine: Concurrent use may lead to decreased psychomotor function.

Ethanol/Nutrition/Herb Interactions

Ethanol: Use caution with concurrent use. Effects are additive and may decrease psychomotor function.

Food: Onset of action may be reduced if taken with or immediately after a heavy meal.

Herb/Nutraceutical: Avoid valerian, St John's wort, kava kava, gotu kola (may increase CNS depression).

Stability Store at 15°C to 30°C (59°F to 86°F).

Mechanism of Action May interact with GABA-receptor complexes at binding domains located close to or allosterically coupled to benzodiazepine receptors.

Pharmacokinetics

Absorption: Rapid; high-fat/heavy meal may delay absorption

Protein binding: 52% to 59%

Metabolism: Hepatic via oxidation and demethylation (CYP2E1, 3A4); 2 primary metabolites; one with activity less than parent.

Half-life elimination: 6 hours; Elderly (≥65 years): ~9 hours

Time to peak, plasma: 1 hour

Excretion: Urine (75%, primarily as metabolites; <10% as parent drug)

Dosage

Geriatrics:

Difficulty **falling** asleep: Initial: 1 mg before bedtime; maximum dose: 2 mg.

Difficulty **staying** asleep: 2 mg before bedtime.

Adults:

Insomnia: Oral: Initial: 2 mg before bedtime (maximum dose: 3 mg)

Concurrent use with strong CYP3A4 inhibitor: 1 mg before bedtime; if needed, dose may be increased to 2 mg

Renal Impairment: No adjustment required.

Hepatic Impairment:

Mild-to-moderate: Use with caution; dosage adjustment unnecessary

Severe: Maximum dose: 2 mg

Administration Because of the rapid onset of action, eszopiclone should be administered immediately prior to bedtime or after the patient has gone to bed and is having difficulty falling asleep. Do not take with, or immediately following, a high-fat meal; do not crush or break tablet.

Patient Information Avoid alcohol and other CNS depressants while taking this medication. Only take this medication if you are able to get 8 or more hours of sleep before you must wake up. Take immediately before going to bed. For best results, avoid taking it with or immediately after a high-fat, heavy meal. Do not crush, break, or chew tablet.

Special Geriatric Considerations In subjects >65 years of age, the AUC was increased by 41%. The manufacturer reports that in studies, the pattern of adverse reactions in elderly subjects was not different from that seen in younger adults.

Dosage Forms Excipient information presented when available (limited, particularly for generics); consult specific product labeling.

Tablet: 1 mg, 2 mg, 3 mg

Etanercept (et a NER sept)

U.S. Brand Names Enbrel®
Canadian Brand Names Enbrel®
Generic Available No
Pharmacologic Category Antirheumatic, Disease Modifying; Tumor Necrosis Factor (TNF) Blocking Agent
Use Treatment of moderately- to severely-active rheumatoid arthritis (RA); moderately- to severely-active polyarticular juvenile rheumatoid arthritis (JRA) in patients with inadequate response to at least one disease-modifying antirheumatic drug; psoriatic arthritis; active ankylosing spondylitis (AS); moderate-to-severe chronic plaque psoriasis
Unlabeled/Investigational Use Treatment of Crohn's disease
Contraindications Hypersensitivity to etanercept or any component of the formulation; patients with sepsis (mortality may be increased); active infections (including chronic or local infection)
Warnings/Precautions Serious and potentially fatal rare infections, including reactivation of hepatitis or cases of tuberculosis have been reported. Discontinue administration if patient develops a serious infection. Caution should be exercised when considering the use in patients with chronic infection, history of recurrent infection, or predisposition to infection (such as poorly-controlled diabetes). Do not give to patients with an active chronic or localized infection. Patients who develop a new infection while undergoing treatment should be monitored closely. If a patient develops a serious infection, therapy should be discontinued. Patients should be brought up to date with all immunizations before initiating therapy. Live vaccines should not be given concurrently. Patients with a significant exposure to varicella virus should temporarily discontinue etanercept. Treatment with varicella zoster immune globulin should be considered.

Impact on the development and course of malignancies is not fully defined. As compared to the general population, an increased risk of lymphoma has been noted in clinical trials; however, rheumatoid arthritis has been previously associated with an increased rate of lymphoma. Etanercept is not recommended for use in patients with Wegener's granulomatosis who are receiving immunosuppressive therapy. Treatment may result in the formation of autoimmune antibodies; cases of autoimmune disease have not been described. Non-neutralizing antibodies to etanercept may also be formed. Rarely, a reversible lupus-like syndrome has occurred.

Use caution in patients with pre-existing or recent-onset demyelinating CNS disorders; cases of optic neuritis, demyelinating disease and/or seizures have been reported. Use caution in patients with CHF; has been associated with worsening and new-onset CHF. Use caution in patients with a history of significant hematologic abnormalities; has been associated with pancytopenia and aplastic anemia (rare). Discontinue if significant hematologic abnormalities are confirmed.

Should not be used in combination with anakinra, unless no satisfactory alternatives exist, and then only with extreme caution. Some dosage forms may contain dry natural rubber (latex).
Adverse Reactions (Reflective of adult population; not specific for elderly)
>10%:
    Central nervous system: Headache (17%)
    Local: Injection site reaction (14% to 37%; erythema, itching, pain or swelling)
    Respiratory: Respiratory tract infection (upper, 20% to 29%), rhinitis (12%)
    Miscellaneous: Infection (35%), positive ANA (11%), positive antidouble-stranded DNA antibodies (15% by RIA, 3% by *Crithidia luciliae* assay)
≥3% to 10%:
    Central nervous system: Dizziness (7%)
    Dermatologic: Rash (5%)
    Gastrointestinal: Abdominal pain (5%), dyspepsia (4%), nausea (9%), vomiting (3%)
    Neuromuscular & skeletal: Weakness (5%)
    Respiratory: Pharyngitis (7%), respiratory disorder (5%), sinusitis (3%), cough (6%)
    Pediatric patients (JRA): The percentages of patients reporting abdominal pain (17%) and vomiting (13%) were higher than in adult RA. Two patients developed varicella infection associated with aseptic meningitis which resolved without complications
(Continued)

Etanercept *(Continued)*

(see Warnings/Precautions). Other severe reactions included gastroenteritis, depression, cutaneous ulcer, esophagitis/gastritis, group A streptococcal septic shock, and wound infections.

Overdosage/Toxicology No dose-limiting toxicities have been observed during clinical trials. Single I.V. doses up to 60 mg/m^2 have been administered to healthy volunteers in an endotoxemia study, without evidence of dose-limiting toxicities.

Drug Interactions

Abatacept: Concurrent use may increase the risk of infection; avoid concurrent use.

Anakinra: An increased rate of serious infections has been noted with concurrent therapy, without additional improvement in American College of Rheumatology (ACR) response criteria; concurrent use is not recommended.

Cyclophosphamide: May increase the risk of noncutaneous solid malignancy when used with etanercept. Concurrent therapy is not recommended.

Vaccines (killed organism or component): Etanercept may decrease the effect of vaccines; monitor.

Vaccines (live organism): Etanercept increase the risk of vaccinal infection; avoid concurrent use.

Ethanol/Nutrition/Herb Interactions Herb/Nutraceutical: Echinacea may decrease the therapeutic effects of etanercept (avoid concurrent use).

Stability Store prefilled syringes at 2°C to 8°C (36°F to 46°F); protect from light; do not freeze or shake. Powder for reconstitution must be refrigerated at 2°C to 8°C (36°F to 46°F). Do not freeze. Reconstitute lyophilized powder aseptically with 1 mL sterile bacteriostatic water for injection, USP (supplied); swirl gently, do not shake. Do not filter reconstituted solution during preparation or administration. Reconstituted vials of etanercept should be administered as soon as possible after reconstitution. If not administered immediately after reconstitution, etanercept may be stored in the vial at 2°C to 8°C (36°F to 46°F) for up to 14 days.

Mechanism of Action Etanercept is a recombinant DNA-derived protein composed of tumor necrosis factor receptor (TNFR) linked to the Fc portion of human IgG1. Etanercept binds tumor necrosis factor (TNF) and blocks its interaction with cell surface receptors. TNF plays an important role in the inflammatory processes and the resulting joint pathology of rheumatoid arthritis (RA), polyarticular-course juvenile arthritis (JRA), ankylosing spondylitis (AS), and plaque psoriasis.

Pharmacokinetics

Onset of action: ~2-3 weeks; RA: 1-2 weeks

Half-life elimination: RA: SubQ: 72-132 hours

Time to peak: RA: SubQ: 35-103 hours

Excretion: Clearance: 89 mL/hour (52 mL/hour/m^2)

Dosage

Geriatrics: SubQ: Refer to adult dosing. Although greater sensitivity of some elderly patients cannot be ruled out, no overall differences in safety or effectiveness were observed.

Adults:

Rheumatoid arthritis, psoriatic arthritis, ankylosing spondylitis: SubQ:

Once-weekly dosing: 50 mg once weekly

Twice-weekly dosing: 25 mg given twice weekly (individual doses should be separated by 72-96 hours)

Plaque psoriasis:

Initial: 50 mg twice weekly, 3-4 days apart (starting doses of 25 or 50 mg once weekly have also been used successfully); maintain initial dose for 3 months

Maintenance dose: 50 mg weekly

Administration Follow package instructions carefully for reconstitution. **Note:** The needle cover of the diluent syringe may contain dry natural rubber (latex) which should not be handled by persons sensitive to this substance. Injection sites should be rotated. New injections should be given at least one inch from an old site and never into areas where the skin is tender, bruised, red, or hard.

Monitoring Parameters Monitor for response (inflammation, pain, grip strength), mobility; ADLs; observe for infections, allergic reactions. See Warnings/Precautions and Adverse Reactions. Monitor injection site for signs of reaction (swelling, pain, itching).

Patient Information If self-injecting, follow instructions for injection and disposal of needles exactly. If redness, swelling, or irritation appears at the injection site, contact prescriber. Do not have any vaccinations while using this medication without consulting prescriber first. You may experience headache or dizziness (use caution when driving or engaging in tasks requiring alertness until response to drug is known). If stomach pain or cramping, unusual bleeding or bruising, persistent fever, paleness, blood in vomitus, stool, or urine occurs, stop taking medication and contact prescriber **immediately**. Also immediately report skin rash, unusual muscle or bone weakness, or signs of respiratory flu or other infection (eg, chills, fever, sore throat, easy bruising or bleeding, mouth sores, unhealed sores).

Special Geriatric Considerations Clinical trials including those ≥65 years of age with rheumatoid arthritis have not demonstrated any differences in safety and efficacy between elderly and younger adults to date. Since elderly have a higher incidence of infections in general, caution should be used.

Dosage Forms Excipient information presented when available (limited, particularly for generics); consult specific product labeling.

Injection, powder for reconstitution:

Enbrel®: 25 mg [contains sucrose; diluent contains benzyl alcohol]

Injection, solution:

Enbrel®: 50 mg/mL (0.51 mL, 0.98 mL) [contains sucrose; packaging may contain dry natural rubber (latex)]

Selected References

Breedveld F, "New Tumor Necrosis Factor-Alpha Biologic Therapies for Rheumatoid Arthritis," *Eur Cytokine Netw*, 1998, 9(3):233-8.

Data on file, Immunex Corporation.

Feldmann M, Brennan FM, and Maini RN, "Role of Cytokines in Rheumatoid Arthritis," *Annu Rev Immunol*, 1996, 14:397-440.

Felson DT, Anderson JJ, Boers M, et al, "American College of Rheumatology. Preliminary Definition of Improvement in Rheumatoid Arthritis," *Arthritis Rheum*, 1995, 38(6):727-35.

Fisher CJ Jr, Agosti JM, Opal SM, et al, "Treatment of Septic Shock With the Tumor Necrosis Factor Receptor:Fc Fusion Protein. The Soluble TNF Receptor Sepsis Study Group," *N Engl J Med*, 1996, 334(26):1697-702.

Giannini EH, Ruperto N, Ravelli A, et al, "Preliminary Definition of Improvement in Juvenile Arthritis," *Arthritis Rheum*, 1997, 40(7):1202-9.

Mease PJ, Goffe BS, Metz J, et al, "Etanercept in the Treatment of Psoriatic Arthritis and Psoriasis: A Randomised Trial," *Lancet*, 2000, 356(9227):385-90.

Moreland LW, Baumgartner SW, Schiff MH, et al, "Treatment of Rheumatoid Arthritis With a Recombinant Human Tumor Necrosis Factor Receptor (p75)-Fc Fusion Protein," *N Engl J Med*, 1997, 337(3):141-7.

"New Drugs for Rheumatoid Arthritis," *Med Lett Drugs Ther*, 1998, 40(1040):110-2.

Ramey DR, Fries JF, and Singh G, "The Health Assessment Questionnaire 1995 - Status and Review," Spilker B, ed, *Quality of Life and Pharmacoeconomics in Clinical Trials*, 2nd ed, Philadelphia, PA: Lippincott-Raven, 1996.

Saxne T, Palladino MA Jr, Heinegard D, et al, "Detection of Tumor Necrosis Factor Alpha But Not Tumor Necrosis Factor Beta in Rheumatoid Arthritis Synovial Fluid and Serum," *Arthritis Rheum*, 1988, 31(8):1041-5.

Smith CA, Farrah T, and Goodwin RG, "The TNF Receptor Superfamily of Cellular and Viral Proteins: Activation, Costimulation, and Death," *Cell*, 1994, 76(6):959-62.

Weinblatt ME, Kremer JM, Bankhurst AD, et al, "A Trial of Etanercept, A Recombinant Tumor Necrosis Factor Receptor:Fc Fusion Protein, in Patients With Rheumatoid Arthritis Receiving Methotrexate," *N Engl J Med*, 1999, 340(4):253-9.

Wooley PH, Dutcher J, Widmer MB, et al, "Influence of a Recombinant Human Soluble Tumor Necrosis Factor Receptor FC Fusion Protein on Type II Collagen-Induced Arthritis in Mice," *J Immunol*, 1993, 151(11):6602-7.

van Oosten BW, Barkhof F, Truyen L, et al, "Increased MRI Activity and Immune Activation in Two Multiple Sclerosis Patients Treated With the Monoclonal Anti-tumor Necrosis Factor Antibody cA2," *Neurology*, 1996, 47(6):1531-4.

♦ **Ethacrynate Sodium** *see* Ethacrynic Acid *on page 579*

Ethacrynic Acid (eth a KRIN ik AS id)

Related Information

Potentially Inappropriate Medications for Geriatrics *on page 1824*

Medication Safety Issues

Sound-alike/look-alike issues:

Edecrin® may be confused with Eulexin®, Ecotrin®

U.S. Brand Names Edecrin®

Canadian Brand Names Edecrin®

Index Terms Ethacrynate Sodium

Generic Available No

Pharmacologic Category Diuretic, Loop

Use Management of edema associated with congestive heart failure, hepatic cirrhosis, or renal disease; short-term management of ascites due to malignancy, idiopathic edema, and lymphedema

Contraindications Hypersensitivity to ethacrynic acid or any component of the formulation; anuria; history of severe watery diarrhea caused by this product

Warnings/Precautions Loop diuretics are potent diuretics; excess amounts can lead to profound diuresis with fluid and electrolyte loss; close medical supervision and dose evaluation are required. Watch for and correct electrolyte disturbances; adjust dose to avoid dehydration. In cirrhosis, avoid electrolyte and acid/base imbalances that might lead to hepatic encephalopathy. Monitor fluid status and renal function in an attempt to prevent oliguria, azotemia, and reversible increases in BUN and creatinine; close medical supervision of aggressive diuresis required. Rapid I.V. administration, renal impairment, excessive doses, and concurrent use of other ototoxins is associated with ototoxicity; has been associated with a higher incidence of ototoxicity than other loop diuretics. Hypersensitivity reactions can rarely occur; however, ethacrynic acid has no

(Continued)

Ethacrynic Acid *(Continued)*

cross-reactivity to sulfonamides or sulfonylureas. Coadministration of antihypertensives may increase the risk of hypotension.

Adverse Reactions (Reflective of adult population; not specific for elderly)
Frequency not defined.

Central nervous system: Headache, fatigue, apprehension, confusion, fever, chills, encephalopathy (patients with pre-existing liver disease); vertigo

Dermatologic: Skin rash, Henoch-Schönlein purpura (in patient with rheumatic heart disease)

Endocrine & metabolic: Hyponatremia, hyperglycemia, variations in phosphorus, CO_2 content, bicarbonate, and calcium; reversible hyperuricemia, gout, hyperglycemia, hypoglycemia (occurred in two uremic patients who received doses above those recommended)

Gastrointestinal: Anorexia, malaise, abdominal discomfort or pain, dysphagia, nausea, vomiting, diarrhea, gastrointestinal bleeding, acute pancreatitis (rare)

Genitourinary: Hematuria

Hepatic: Jaundice, abnormal liver function tests

Hematology: Agranulocytosis, severe neutropenia, thrombocytopenia

Local: Thrombophlebitis (with intravenous use), local irritation and pain,

Ocular: Blurred vision

Otic: Tinnitus, temporary or permanent deafness

Renal: Serum creatinine increased

Overdosage/Toxicology Symptoms include electrolyte depletion, volume depletion, dehydration, and circulatory collapse. Following GI decontamination, treatment is supportive. Hypotension responds to fluids and Trendelenburg positioning.

Drug Interactions

ACE inhibitors: Hypotensive effects and/or renal effects are potentiated by hypovolemia.

Antidiabetic agents: Glucose tolerance may be decreased.

Antihypertensive agents: Hypotensive effects may be enhanced.

Cephaloridine or cephalexin: Nephrotoxicity may occur.

Cholestyramine or colestipol may reduce bioavailability of ethacrynic acid.

Clofibrate: Protein binding may be altered in hypoalbuminemic patients receiving ethacrynic acid, potentially increasing toxicity.

Digoxin: Ethacrynic acid-induced hypokalemia may predispose to digoxin toxicity; monitor potassium.

Indomethacin (and other NSAIDs) may reduce natriuretic and hypotensive effects of diuretics.

Lithium: Renal clearance may be reduced. Isolated reports of lithium toxicity have occurred; monitor lithium levels.

NSAIDs: Risk of renal impairment may increase when used in conjunction with diuretics.

Ototoxic drugs (aminoglycosides, cis-platinum): Concomitant use of ethacrynic acid may increase risk of ototoxicity, especially in patients with renal dysfunction.

Peripheral adrenergic-blocking drugs or ganglionic blockers: Effects may be increased.

Salicylates (high-dose) with diuretics may predispose patients to salicylate toxicity due to reduced renal excretion or alter renal function.

Thiazides: Synergistic diuretic effects occur.

Mechanism of Action Inhibits reabsorption of sodium and chloride in the ascending loop of Henle and distal renal tubule, interfering with the chloride-binding cotransport system, thus causing increased excretion of water, sodium, chloride, magnesium, and calcium

Pharmacodynamics

Onset of action:

Oral: Following administration diuretic effects occur within 30 minutes and peak in 2 hours

I.V.: Diuresis occurs in 5 minutes and peaks in 30 minutes

Duration:

Oral: 12 hours

I.V.: 2 hours

Pharmacokinetics

Absorption: Oral: Rapid

Metabolism: In the liver to active cysteine conjugate

Elimination: In bile and urine

Dosage

Geriatrics: Oral: Initial: 25-50 mg/day

Adults: I.V. formulation should be diluted in D_5W or NS (1 mg/mL) and infused over several minutes.

Edema:

Oral: 50-100 mg/day in 1-2 divided doses; may increase in increments of 25-50 mg at intervals of several days to a maximum of 400 mg/24 hours.

I.V.: 0.5-1 mg/kg/dose (maximum: 100 mg/dose); repeat doses not routinely recommended; however, if indicated, repeat doses every 8-12 hours.

Renal Impairment:

Cl$_{cr}$ <10 mL/minute: Avoid use.

Not removed by hemo- or peritoneal dialysis; supplemental dose is not necessary.

Administration Injection should **not** be given SubQ or I.M. due to local pain and irritation; single I.V. doses should not exceed 100 mg; use a new injection site if a second dose is needed, to avoid possible thrombophlebitis

Monitoring Parameters Blood pressure (standing, sitting, and supine), serum electrolytes, renal function, auditory function, weight, I & O

Patient Information May be taken with food or milk; get up slowly from a lying or sitting position to minimize dizziness, lightheadedness, or fainting; also use extra care when exercising, standing for long periods of time and during hot weather; take in the morning; take the last dose of multiple doses before 6 PM unless instructed otherwise

Additional Information Injection form may be given orally while hospitalized. Ethacrynic acid should be reserved for patients who are either allergic or resistant to furosemide, bumetanide, or torsemide.

Special Geriatric Considerations Ethacrynic acid is rarely used because of its increased incidence of ototoxicity as compared to the other loop diuretics.

Dosage Forms Excipient information presented when available (limited, particularly for generics); consult specific product labeling.

Injection, powder for reconstitution, as ethacrynate sodium: 50 mg

Tablet: 25 mg

Ethambutol (e THAM byoo tole)

Medication Safety Issues

Sound-alike/look-alike issues:

Myambutol® may be confused with Nembutal®

U.S. Brand Names Myambutol®

Canadian Brand Names Etibi®

Index Terms Ethambutol Hydrochloride

Generic Available Yes

Pharmacologic Category Antitubercular Agent

Use Treatment of tuberculosis and other mycobacterial diseases in conjunction with other antituberculosis agents

Contraindications Hypersensitivity to ethambutol or any component of the formulation; optic neuritis; use in unconscious patients or any other patient who may be unable to discern and report visual changes

Warnings/Precautions May cause optic neuritis, resulting in decreased visual acuity or other vision changes. Discontinue promptly in patients with changes in vision, color blindness, or visual defects (effects normally reversible, but reversal may require up to a year). Dosage modification is required in patients with renal insufficiency. Hepatic toxicity has been reported, possibly due to concurrent therapy.

Adverse Reactions (Reflective of adult population; not specific for elderly)

Frequency not defined.

Cardiovascular: Myocarditis, pericarditis

Central nervous system: Headache, confusion, disorientation, malaise, mental confusion, fever, dizziness, hallucinations

Dermatologic: Rash, pruritus, dermatitis, exfoliative dermatitis

Endocrine & metabolic: Acute gout or hyperuricemia

Gastrointestinal: Abdominal pain, anorexia, nausea, vomiting

Hematologic: Leukopenia, thrombocytopenia, eosinophilia, neutropenia, lymphadenopathy

Hepatic: Abnormal LFTs, hepatotoxicity (possibly related to concurrent therapy), hepatitis

Neuromuscular & skeletal: Peripheral neuritis, arthralgia

Ocular: Optic neuritis; symptoms may include decreased acuity, scotoma, color blindness, or visual defects (usually reversible with discontinuation, irreversible blindness has been described)

Renal: Nephritis

Respiratory: Infiltrates (with or without eosinophilia), pneumonitis

Miscellaneous: Anaphylaxis, anaphylactoid reaction; hypersensitivity syndrome (rash, eosinophilia, and organ-specific inflammation)

Overdosage/Toxicology Symptoms include decreased visual acuity, anorexia, joint pain, and numbness of the extremities. Following GI decontamination, treatment is supportive.

(Continued)

Ethambutol *(Continued)*

Drug Interactions Decreased absorption with aluminum hydroxide. Avoid concurrent administration of aluminum-containing antacids for at least 4 hours following ethambutol.

Stability Store at controlled room temperature of 20°C to 25°C (68°F to 77°F).

Mechanism of Action Suppresses mycobacteria multiplication by interfering with RNA synthesis

Pharmacokinetics

Absorption: Oral: ~80%

Distribution: Well throughout the body with high concentrations in kidneys, lungs, saliva and red blood cells

Protein binding: 20% to 30%

Metabolism: 20% by the liver to inactive metabolite

Half-life: 2.5-3.6 hours (up to 7 hours or longer with renal impairment)

Time to peak serum concentration: 2-4 hours

Elimination: ~50% in urine and 20% excreted in feces as unchanged drug

Dosage

Geriatrics & Adults:

Treatment of tuberculosis (suggested doses by lean body weight):

Daily therapy: 15-25 mg/kg

40-55 kg: 800 mg

56-75 kg: 1200 mg

76-90 kg: 1600 mg (maximum dose regardless of weight)

Twice weekly directly observed therapy (DOT): 50 mg/kg

40-55 kg: 2000 mg

56-75 kg: 2800 mg

76-90 kg: 4000 mg (maximum dose regardless of weight)

Three times/week DOT: 25-30 mg/kg (maximum: 2.5 g)

40-55 kg: 1200 mg

56-75 kg: 2000 mg

76-90 kg: 2400 mg (maximum dose regardless of weight)

Note: Used as part of a multidrug regimen. Treatment regimens consist of an initial 2 month phase, followed by a continuation phase of 4 or 7 additional months; frequency of dosing may differ depending on phase of therapy.

Disseminated *Mycobacterium avium* complex (MAC) in patients with advanced HIV infection: 15 mg/kg ethambutol in combination with azithromycin 600 mg daily

Renal Impairment:

Cl_{cr} 10-50 mL/minute: Administer every 24-36 hours.

Cl_{cr} <10 mL/minute: Administer every 48 hours.

Slightly dialyzable (5% to 20%); administer dose postdialysis.

Peritoneal dialysis: Dose as for Cl_{cr} <10 mL/minute.

Continuous arteriovenous or venovenous hemofiltration: Administer every 24-36 hours.

Monitoring Parameters Baseline and periodic (monthly) visual testing (each eye individually, as well as both eyes tested together) in patients receiving >15 mg/kg/day; baseline and periodic renal, hepatic, and hematopoietic tests

Patient Information Report any vision, visual, or color changes to physician; may cause stomach upset, take with food

Special Geriatric Considerations Since most elderly patients acquired their tuberculosis before current antituberculin regimens were available, ethambutol is only indicated when patients are from areas where drug resistant *M. tuberculosis* is endemic, in HIV-infected elderly patients, and when drug resistant *M. tuberculosis* is suspected (see dose adjustments for renal impairment).

Dosage Forms Excipient information presented when available (limited, particularly for generics); consult specific product labeling.

Tablet, as hydrochloride: 100 mg, 400 mg

Selected References

American Thoracic Society, "Targeted Tuberculin Testing and Treatment of Latent Tuberculosis Infection," *MMWR*, 2000, 49(RR-6):1-51.

Blumberg HM, Burman WJ, Chaisson RE, et al, "American Thoracic Society/Centers for Disease Control and Prevention/Infectious Diseases Society of America: Treatment of Tuberculosis," *Am J Respir Crit Care Med*, 2003, 167(4):603-62.

Centers for Disease Control and Prevention (CDC) and American Thoracic Society, "Update: Adverse Event Data and Revised American Thoracic Society/CDC Recommendations Against the Use of Rifampin and Pyrazinamide for Treatment of Latent Tuberculosis Infection - United States, 2003," *MMWR*, 2003, 52(31):735-9. Available at http://www.cdc.gov/mmwr/preview/mmwrhtml/mm5231a4.htm. Last accessed February 16, 2005.

"Treatment of Latent Tuberculosis Infection (LTBI), Last Updated: April 8, 2004," available at http://www.cdc.gov/nchstp/tb/pubs/tbfactsheets/250110.htm. Last accessed February 16, 2005.

Yoshikawa TT, "Tuberculosis in Aging Adults," *J Am Geriatr Soc*, 1992, 40(2):178-87.

♦ **Ethambutol Hydrochloride** *see* Ethambutol *on page 581*

◆ EtheDent™ *see* Fluoride *on page 642*
◆ Ethezyme™ *see* Papain and Urea *on page 1201*
◆ Ethezyme™ 830 *see* Papain and Urea *on page 1201*

Ethionamide (e thye on AM ide)

U.S. Brand Names Trecator®
Canadian Brand Names Trecator®
Generic Available No
Pharmacologic Category Antitubercular Agent
Use In conjunction with other antituberculosis agents in the treatment of tuberculosis and other mycobacterial diseases
Contraindications Hypersensitivity to ethionamide or any component of the formulation; severe hepatic impairment
Warnings/Precautions Use with caution in patients with diabetes mellitus; use with caution in patients receiving cycloserine or isoniazid. Use caution when switching patients from the sugar-coated tablet formulation (Trecator®-SC) to film-coated tablet (Trecator®); the dosage may need retitrated in order to avoid intolerance.
Adverse Reactions (Reflective of adult population; not specific for elderly) Frequency not defined.
Cardiovascular: Postural hypotension
Central nervous system: Depression, dizziness, drowsiness, headache, psychiatric disturbances, restlessness, seizure
Dermatologic: Acne, alopecia, photosensitivity, purpura, rash
Endocrine & metabolic: Gynecomastia, hypoglycemia, hypothyroidism or goiter, pellagra-like syndrome
Gastrointestinal: Abdominal pain, anorexia, diarrhea, excessive salivation, metallic taste, nausea, stomatitis, vomiting, weight loss
Genitourinary: Impotence
Hematologic: Thrombocytopenia
Hepatic: Hepatitis, jaundice, liver function tests increased
Neuromuscular & skeletal: Peripheral neuritis, weakness (common)
Ocular: Blurred vision, diplopia, optic neuritis
Respiratory: Olfactory disturbances
Miscellaneous: Hypersensitivity reaction
Overdosage/Toxicology Symptoms include peripheral neuropathy, anorexia, and joint pain. Following GI decontamination, treatment is supportive. Pyridoxine may be given to prevent peripheral neuropathy.
Ethanol/Nutrition/Herb Interactions
Ethanol: Avoid excessive ethanol ingestion; psychotic reaction may occur.
Mechanism of Action Inhibits peptide synthesis
Pharmacokinetics
Absorption: Rapid, complete
Distribution: V_d: 93.5 L
Protein binding: ~30%
Metabolism: Extensively hepatic to active and inactive metabolites
Bioavailability: 80%
Half-life elimination: 2-3 hours
Time to peak, serum: 1 hour
Excretion: Urine (<1% as unchanged drug; as active and inactive metabolites)
Dosage
Geriatrics & Adults: Tuberculosis: Oral: 15-20 mg/kg/day; initiate dose at 250 mg/day for 1-2 days, then increase to 250 mg twice daily for 1-2 days, with gradual increases to highest tolerated dose; average adult dose: 750 mg/day (maximum: 1 g/day in 3-4 divided doses)
Renal Impairment: Cl_{cr} <30 mL/minute: 250-500 mg/day
Administration Neurotoxic effects may be relieved by the administration of pyridoxine (6-100 mg daily, lower doses are more common). May be taken with or without meals. Gastrointestinal adverse effects may be decreased by administration at bedtime, decreased dose, or giving antiemetics.
Monitoring Parameters Initial and periodic serum ALT and AST; ophthalmic exams; thyroid function
Patient Information Take with meals, may cause upset stomach and loss of appetite, metallic taste or salivation
Special Geriatric Considerations Since many elderly have Cl_{cr} <50 mL/minute, adjust dose for renal function.
Dosage Forms Excipient information presented when available (limited, particularly for generics); consult specific product labeling.
Tablet: 250 mg
(Continued)

Ethionamide *(Continued)*

Selected References
Centers for Disease Control and Prevention, "Treatment of Tuberculosis. American Thoracic Society, CDC, and Infectious Diseases Society of America," *MMWR*, 2003, 52(RR11);26, 64.

♦ **Ethmozine®** *see Moricizine on page 1063*

Ethosuximide *(eth oh SUKS i mide)*

Related Information
Serum Drug Concentrations Commonly Monitored Guidelines *on page 1862*

Medication Safety Issues
Sound-alike/look-alike issues:
Ethosuximide may be confused with methsuximide
Zarontin® may be confused with Xalatan®, Zantac®, Zaroxolyn®

U.S. Brand Names Zarontin®

Canadian Brand Names Zarontin®

Generic Available Yes

Pharmacologic Category Anticonvulsant, Succinimide

Use Management of absence (petit mal) seizures, myoclonic seizures, and akinetic epilepsy; considered to be drug of choice for simple absence seizures

Contraindications Hypersensitivity to succinimides or any component of the formulation

Warnings/Precautions Succinimides have been associated with severe blood dyscrasias and cases of systemic lupus erythematosus. Abrupt withdrawal of the drug may precipitate absence status; ethosuximide may increase tonic-clonic seizures in patients with mixed seizure disorders. Consider evaluation of blood counts in patients with signs/symptoms of infection. Effects with other sedative drugs or ethanol may be potentiated.

Adverse Reactions (Reflective of adult population; not specific for elderly)
Frequency not defined.
Central nervous system: Aggressiveness, ataxia, disturbance in sleep, dizziness, drowsiness, euphoria, fatigue, headache, hyperactivity, inability to concentrate, irritability, lethargy, mental depression (with cases of overt suicidal intentions), night terrors, paranoid psychosis
Dermatologic: Hirsutism, pruritus, rash, Stevens-Johnson syndrome, urticaria
Endocrine & metabolic: Libido increased
Gastrointestinal: Abdominal pain, anorexia, cramps, diarrhea, epigastric pain, gastric upset, gum hypertrophy, nausea, tongue swelling, vomiting, weight loss
Genitourinary: Hematuria (microscopic), vaginal bleeding
Hematologic: Agranulocytosis, eosinophilia, leukopenia, pancytopenia
Ocular: Myopia
Miscellaneous: Hiccups, systemic lupus erythematosus

Drug Interactions Substrate of CYP3A4 (major)
CNS depressants: Ethosuximide may enhance the adverse/toxic effect of other CNS depressants.
CYP3A4 inducers: May decrease the level/effect of ethosuximide. Example inducers include aminoglutethimide, carbamazepine, nafcillin, nevirapine, phenobarbital, phenytoin, and rifamycins.
CYP3A4 inhibitors: May increase the levels/effects of ethosuximide. Example inhibitors include azole antifungals, clarithromycin, diclofenac, doxycycline, erythromycin, imatinib, isoniazid, nefazodone, nicardipine, propofol, protease inhibitors, quinidine, telithromycin, and verapamil.
Isoniazid: May increase levels/effects of ethosuximide.
Phenytoin: May decrease levels/effects of ethosuximide.

Ethanol/Nutrition/Herb Interactions
Ethanol: Avoid ethanol (may increase CNS depression).
Herb/Nutraceutical: St John's wort may decrease ethosuximide levels.

Mechanism of Action Increases the seizure threshold and suppresses paroxysmal spike-and-wave pattern in absence seizures; depresses nerve transmission in the motor cortex

Pharmacokinetics
Absorption: Well absorbed from GI tract
Distribution: Adults: V_d: 0.62-0.72 L/kg
Metabolism: ~80% in the liver to three inactive metabolites
Half-life: 50-60 hours
Time to peak serum concentration:
Capsule: Within 3-7 hours
Syrup: <2-4 hours
Elimination: Slowly excreted in urine as metabolites (50%) and as unchanged drug (10% to 20%); small amounts excreted in feces

Dosage

Geriatrics & Adults: Management of absence (petit mal) seizures: Oral: Initial: 500 mg/day; increase by 250 mg as needed every 4-7 days up to 1.5 g/day in divided doses

Renal Impairment: Use with caution.

Hepatic Impairment: Use with caution.

Administration Administer with food or milk to avoid GI upset

Monitoring Parameters CBC, platelets, liver enzymes, trough ethosuximide serum concentration

Reference Range Therapeutic: 40-100 mcg/mL (SI: 280-710 µmol/L); Toxic: >150 mcg/mL (SI: >1062 µmol/L)

Patient Information Take with food; do not discontinue abruptly; may cause drowsiness and impair judgment; patient should have a "Medic Alert" identification; call physician if experiencing rash, fever, sore throat, bleeding, dizziness, blurred vision

Additional Information Considered to be drug of choice for simple absence seizures

Special Geriatric Considerations No specific studies with the use of this medication in the elderly. Consider renal function and proceed slowly with dosing increases; monitor closely.

Dosage Forms Excipient information presented when available (limited, particularly for generics); consult specific product labeling.

Capsule: 250 mg
Zarontin®: 250 mg
Syrup: 250 mg/5 mL (473 mL)
Zarontin®: 250 mg/5 mL [contains sodium benzoate; raspberry flavor]

- ♦ **ETH-Oxydose**™ *see* Oxycodone *on page 1179*
- ♦ **Ethoxynaphthamido Penicillin Sodium** *see* Nafcillin *on page 1081*
- ♦ **Ethyl Esters of Omega-3 Fatty Acids** *see* Omega-3-Acid Ethyl Esters *on page 1155*

Etidronate Disodium (e ti DROE nate dye SOW dee um)

Medication Safety Issues
Sound-alike/look-alike issues:
Etidronate may be confused with etidocaine, etomidate, etretinate

U.S. Brand Names Didronel®

Canadian Brand Names Didronel®; Gen-Etidronate

Index Terms EHDP; Sodium Etidronate

Generic Available No

Pharmacologic Category Bisphosphonate Derivative

Use Symptomatic treatment of Paget's disease; prevention and treatment of heterotopic ossification due to spinal cord injury or after total hip replacement

Unlabeled/Investigational Use Postmenopausal osteoporosis

Contraindications Hypersensitivity to bisphosphonates or any component of the formulation; overt osteomalacia

Warnings/Precautions Ensure adequate calcium and vitamin D intake. Etidronate may retard mineralization of bone; treatment may need delayed or interrupted until callus is present. Use caution in patients with renal impairment. Use caution with enterocolitis; diarrhea has been reported at high doses and therapy may need to be withheld.

Bisphosphonate therapy has been associated with osteonecrosis, primarily of the jaw; this has been observed mostly in cancer patients, but also in patients with postmenopausal osteoporosis and other diagnoses. Dental exams and preventative dentistry should be performed prior to placing patients with risk factors on chronic bisphosphonate therapy. Invasive dental procedures should be avoided during treatment. Esophagitis, esophageal ulcers, esophageal erosions, and esophageal stricture (rare) have been reported with oral bisphosphonates; use with caution in patients with dysphagia, esophageal disease, gastritis, duodenitis, or ulcers (may worsen underlying condition).

Infrequently, severe (and occasionally debilitating) bone, joint, and/or muscle pain have been reported during bisphosphonate treatment. The onset of pain ranged from a single day to several months. Symptoms usually resolve upon discontinuation. Some patients experienced recurrence when rechallenged with same drug or another bisphosphonate; avoid use in patients with a history of these symptoms in association with bisphosphonate therapy.

Adverse Reactions (Reflective of adult population; not specific for elderly)
Frequency not defined.
Gastrointestinal: Diarrhea, nausea
Neuromuscular & skeletal: Bone pain

Overdosage/Toxicology Hypocalcemia, vomiting, paresthesia, diarrhea, and hematologic abnormalities may be expected following acute overdose. Nephrotic syndrome
(Continued)

Etidronate Disodium *(Continued)*

and fracture may be observed with chronic overdose. Intravenous calcium may be used to treat hypocalcemia.

Drug Interactions

Aminoglycosides: May lower serum calcium levels with prolonged administration. Concomitant use may have an additive hypocalcemic effect.

Antacids: May decrease the absorption of bisphosphonate derivatives; should be administered at a different time of the day. Antacids containing aluminum, calcium, or magnesium are of specific concern.

Calcium salts: May decrease the absorption of bisphosphonate derivatives. Separate oral dosing in order to minimize risk of interaction.

Iron salts: May decrease the absorption of bisphosphonate derivatives. Only oral iron salts and oral bisphosphonates are of concern.

Magnesium salts: May decrease the absorption of bisphosphonate derivatives. Only oral magnesium salts and oral bisphosphonates are of concern.

Nonsteroidal anti-inflammatory drugs (NSAIDs): May enhance the gastrointestinal adverse/toxic effects (increased incidence of GI ulcers) of bisphosphonate derivatives.

Phosphate supplements: Bisphosphonate derivatives may enhance the hypocalcemic effect of phosphate supplements.

Ethanol/Nutrition/Herb Interactions Food: Food decreases the absorption and bioavailability of the drug.

Stability Store at controlled room temperature of 15°C to 30°C (59°F to 86°F).

Mechanism of Action Decreases bone resorption by inhibiting osteocystic osteolysis; decreases mineral release and matrix or collagen breakdown in bone

Pharmacodynamics

Onset of action: Within 1-3 months of therapy

Duration: 12 months without continuous therapy

Pharmacokinetics

Absorption: ~3%

Half-life: 1-6 hours

Metabolism: Not metabolized

Elimination: Excreted as unchanged drug primarily in urine with unabsorbed oral drug being eliminated in feces

Dosage

Geriatrics & Adults:

Paget's disease: Oral:

Initial: 5-10 mg/kg/day (not to exceed 6 months) or 11-20 mg/kg/day (not to exceed 3 months). Doses >20 mg/kg/day are **not** recommended.

Retreatment: Initiate only after etidronate-free period ≥90 days. Monitor patients every 3-6 months. Retreatment regimens are the same as for initial treatment.

Heterotopic ossification: Oral:

Caused by spinal cord injury: 20 mg/kg/day for 2 weeks, then 10 mg/kg/day for 10 weeks; total treatment period: 12 weeks

Complicating total hip replacement: 20 mg/kg/day for 1 month preoperatively then 20 mg/kg/day for 3 months postoperatively; total treatment period is 4 months

Postmenopausal osteoporosis (unlabeled use)**:** Oral: 400 mg/day orally for 2 weeks followed by a 13-week period with no etidronate, then repeat cycle; maintain adequate calcium and vitamin D intake during entire 15-week treatment cycle

Renal Impairment: Use with caution; specific guidelines are not available, however consider dose reduction.

Administration Administer tablet should be administered on an empty stomach 2 hours before food.

Monitoring Parameters Serum calcium, phosphorous, potassium

Reference Range Calcium (total): Adults: 9.0-11.0 mg/dL (2.05-2.54 mmol/L), may slightly decrease with aging; phosphorus: 2.5-4.5 mg/dL (0.81-1.45 mmol/L)

Test Interactions Bisphosphonates may interfere with diagnostic imaging agents such as technetium-99m-diphosphonate in bone scans.

Patient Information Maintain adequate intake of calcium and vitamin D; take medicine on an empty stomach; do not take with calcium, separate by 2 hours

Special Geriatric Considerations Monitor serum electrolytes periodically since the elderly are often receiving diuretics which can result in decreases in serum calcium, potassium, and magnesium

Dosage Forms Excipient information presented when available (limited, particularly for generics); consult specific product labeling.

Tablet: 200 mg, 400 mg

Selected References

Storm T, Thamsborg G, Steiniche T, et al, "Effect of Intermittent Cyclical Etidronate Therapy on Bone Mass and Fracture Rate in Women With Postmenopausal Osteoporosis," *N Engl J Med*, 1990, 322(18):1265-71.

Watts NB, Harris ST, Genant HK, et al, "Intermittent Cyclical Etidronate Treatment of Postmenopausal Osteoporosis," *N Engl J Med*, 1990, 323(2):73-9.

Etodolac (ee toe DOE lak)

Medication Safety Issues
Sound-alike/look-alike issues:
Lodine® may be confused with codeine, iodine, Iopidine®, Lopid®
U.S. Brand Names Lodine® [DSC]; Lodine® XL [DSC]
Canadian Brand Names Apo-Etodolac®; Lodine®; Utradol™
Index Terms Etodolic Acid
Generic Available Yes
Pharmacologic Category Nonsteroidal Anti-inflammatory Drug (NSAID), Oral
Use Acute and long-term use in the management of signs and symptoms of osteoarthritis and management of pain
Unlabeled/Investigational Use Treatment of rheumatoid arthritis
Restrictions An FDA-approved medication guide must be distributed when dispensing an oral outpatient prescription (new or refill) where this medication is to be used without direct supervision of a healthcare provider. Medication guides are available at http://www.fda.gov/cder/Offices/ODS/medication_guides.htm.
Contraindications Hypersensitivity to etodolac, aspirin, other NSAIDs, or any component of the formulation; perioperative pain in the setting of coronary artery bypass surgery (CABG)
Warnings/Precautions [U.S. Boxed Warning]: NSAIDs are associated with an increased risk of adverse cardiovascular events, including MI, stroke, and new onset or worsening of pre-existing hypertension. Risk may be increased with duration of use or pre-existing cardiovascular risk factors or disease. Carefully evaluate individual cardiovascular risk profiles prior to prescribing. Use caution with fluid retention, CHF, or hypertension. Concurrent administration of ibuprofen, and potentially other nonselective NSAIDs, may interfere with aspirin's cardioprotective effect.

[U.S. Boxed Warning]: NSAIDs may increase risk of gastrointestinal irritation, ulceration, bleeding, and perforation. These events may occur at any time during therapy and without warning. Use caution with a history of GI disease (bleeding or ulcers), concurrent therapy with aspirin, anticoagulants and/or corticosteroids, smoking, use of alcohol, the elderly or debilitated patients.

Use of NSAIDs can compromise existing renal function. Renal toxicity can occur in patient with impaired renal function, dehydration, heart failure, liver dysfunction, those taking diuretics and ACE inhibitors and the elderly. Rehydrate patient before starting therapy. Monitor renal function closely. Etodolac is not recommended for patients with advanced renal disease.

Use the lowest effective dose for the shortest duration of time, consistent with individual patient goals, to reduce risk of cardiovascular or GI adverse events. Alternate therapies should be considered for patients at high risk.

NSAIDs may cause serious skin adverse events including exfoliative dermatitis, Stevens-Johnson syndrome (SJS), and toxic epidermal necrolysis (TEN). Anaphylactoid reactions may occur, even without prior exposure; patients with "aspirin triad" (bronchial asthma, aspirin intolerance, rhinitis) may be at increased risk. Do not use in patients who experience bronchospasm, asthma, rhinitis, or urticaria with NSAID or aspirin therapy. Use caution in other forms of asthma.

Use with caution in patients with decreased hepatic function. Closely monitor patients with any abnormal LFT. Severe hepatic reactions (eg, fulminant hepatitis, liver failure) have occurred with NSAID use, rarely; discontinue if signs or symptoms of liver disease develop, or if systemic manifestations occur. The elderly are at increased risk for adverse effects (especially peptic ulceration, CNS effects, renal toxicity) from NSAIDs even at low doses.

Withhold for at least 4-6 half-lives prior to surgical or dental procedures.

Use of extended release product consisting of a nondeformable matrix should be avoided in patients with stricture/narrowing of the GI tract; symptoms of obstruction have been associated with nondeformable products.
Adverse Reactions (Reflective of adult population; not specific for elderly)
1% to 10%:
Central nervous system: Dizziness (3% to 9 %), chills/fever (1% to 3%), depression (1% to 3%), nervousness (1% to 3%)
Dermatologic: Rash (1% to 3%), pruritus (1% to 3%)
Gastrointestinal: Abdominal cramps (3% to 9%), nausea (3% to 9%), vomiting (1% to 3%), dyspepsia (10%), diarrhea (3% to 9%), constipation (1% to 3%), flatulence (3% to 9%), melena (1% to 3%), gastritis (1% to 3%)
Genitourinary: Dysuria (1% to 3%)
Neuromuscular & skeletal: Weakness (3% to 9%)
Ocular: Blurred vision (1% to 3%)
Otic: Tinnitus (1% to 3%)
(Continued)

Etodolac *(Continued)*

Renal: Polyuria (1% to 3%)

Overdosage/Toxicology Symptoms include acute renal failure, vomiting, drowsiness, and leukocytosis. Management of nonsteroidal anti-inflammatory drug (NSAID) intoxication is primarily supportive and symptomatic. Fluid therapy is commonly effective in managing hypotension that may occur following an acute NSAID overdose, except when due to acute blood loss.

Drug Interactions

ACE inhibitors: Antihypertensive effects may be decreased by concurrent therapy with NSAIDs; monitor blood pressure.

Aminoglycosides: NSAIDs may decrease the excretion of aminoglycosides.

Angiotensin II antagonists: Antihypertensive effects may be decreased by concurrent therapy with NSAIDs; monitor blood pressure.

Anticoagulants (warfarin, heparin, LMWHs) in combination with NSAIDs can cause increased risk of bleeding.

Antiplatelet agents (ticlopidine, clopidogrel, aspirin, abciximab, dipyridamole, eptifibatide, tirofiban) can cause an increased risk of bleeding.

Beta-blockers: NSAIDs may diminish the antihypertensive effects of beta-blockers.

Bisphosphonates: NSAIDs may increase the risk of gastrointestinal ulceration.

Cholestyramine and colestipol reduce the bioavailability of some NSAIDs; separate administration times.

Corticosteroids may increase the risk of GI ulceration; avoid concurrent use.

Cyclosporine: NSAIDs may increase serum creatinine, potassium, blood pressure, and cyclosporine levels; monitor cyclosporine levels and renal function carefully.

Fluoroquinolone antibiotics: Risk of seizures may be increased with concomitant quinolone use. Risk is considered quite low and may only be a factor with high serum levels of either agent and/or in patients with additional predisposing factors (eg, renal dysfunction, history of seizure or other neurological disorder).

Hydralazine's antihypertensive effect is decreased; avoid concurrent use.

Lithium levels can be increased; avoid concurrent use if possible or monitor lithium levels and adjust dose. Sulindac may have the least effect. When NSAID is stopped, lithium will need adjustment again.

Loop diuretics efficacy (diuretic and antihypertensive effect) is reduced. Indomethacin reduces this efficacy, however, it may be anticipated with any NSAID.

Methotrexate: Severe bone marrow suppression, aplastic anemia, and GI toxicity have been reported with concomitant NSAID therapy. Avoid use during moderate or high-dose methotrexate (increased and prolonged methotrexate levels). NSAID use during low-dose treatment of rheumatoid arthritis has not been fully evaluated; extreme caution is warranted.

Pemetrexed: NSAIDs may decrease the excretion of pemetrexed. Patients with Cl_{cr} 45-79 mL/minute should avoid short acting NSAIDs for 2 days before and 2 days after pemetrexed treatment.

Salicylates: NSAIDs (nonselective) may diminish the cardioprotective effect of acetylated salicylates. Avoid regular use of NSAIDs if possible; consider alternatives (eg, acetaminophen). Give salicylate before NSAID; for example ibuprofen should be given 30-120 minutes after aspirin (immediate release).

Thiazides antihypertensive effects are decreased; avoid concurrent use.

Treprostinil: May enhance the risk of bleeding with concurrent use.

Vancomycin: NSAIDs may decrease the excretion of vancomycin. Avoid concurrent use.

Verapamil plasma concentration is decreased by some NSAIDs; avoid concurrent use.

Ethanol/Nutrition/Herb Interactions

Ethanol: Avoid ethanol (may enhance gastric mucosal irritation).

Food: Etodolac peak serum levels may be decreased if taken with food.

Herb/Nutraceutical: Avoid alfalfa, anise, bilberry, bladderwrack, bromelain, cat's claw, celery, coleus, cordyceps, dong quai, evening primrose, feverfew, fenugreek, garlic, ginger, ginkgo biloba, red clover, horse chestnut, grapeseed, green tea, ginseng, guggul, horse chestnut seed, horseradish, licorice, prickly ash, red clover, reishi, SAMe, sweet clover, turmeric, white willow (all have additional antiplatelet activity)

Stability Store at 20°C to 25°C (68°F to 77°F). Protect from moisture.

Mechanism of Action Inhibits prostaglandin synthesis by decreasing the activity of the enzyme, cyclooxygenase, which results in decreased formation of prostaglandin precursors

Pharmacodynamics

Onset of analgesic action: Within 30 minutes to 1 hour

Duration: 4-12 hours

Pharmacokinetics

Absorption: Oral: Well absorbed

Distribution: V_d: 0.4 L/kg

Protein binding: Highly protein-bound

Half-life elimination: Terminal: Adults: 5-8 hours

Time to peak serum concentration: Within 1-2 hours

Dosage

Geriatrics & Adults: Note: For chronic conditions, response is usually observed within 2 weeks.

Acute pain: Oral: 200-400 mg every 6-8 hours, as needed, not to exceed total daily doses of 1000 mg

Rheumatoid arthritis, osteoarthritis: Oral: 400 mg 2 times/day **or** 300 mg 2-3 times/day **or** 500 mg 2 times/day (doses >1000 mg/day have not been evaluated)
Lodine® XL: 400-1000 mg once daily

Renal Impairment:

Mild to moderate: No adjustment required

Severe: Use not recommended; use with caution

Hemodialysis: Not removed

Hepatic Impairment: No adjustment required.

Monitoring Parameters Monitor CBC, liver enzymes; monitor BUN/serum creatinine in patients receiving diuretics; monitor response (pain, range of motion, grip strength, mobility, ADL function), inflammation; observe for weight gain, edema; monitor renal function; observe for bleeding, bruising; evaluate gastrointestinal effects (abdominal pain, bleeding, dyspepsia); mental confusion, disorientation

Test Interactions False-positive for urinary bilirubin and ketone

Patient Information Take with food, milk, or water; report any signs of blood in stool; serious gastrointestinal bleeding can occur as well as ulceration and perforation. Pain may or may not be present. Avoid aspirin and aspirin-containing products while taking this medication. If gastric upset occurs, take with food, milk, or antacid. If gastric adverse effects persist, contact physician. May cause drowsiness, dizziness, blurred vision, and confusion. Use caution when performing tasks which require alertness (eg, driving). Do not take for more than 3 days for fever or 10 days for pain without physician's advice.

Additional Information Single dose of 76-100 mg is comparable to the analgesic effect of aspirin 650 mg; there are no clinical guidelines to predict which NSAID will give response in a particular patient. Trials with each must be initiated until response determined. Consider dose, patient convenience, and cost.

Special Geriatric Considerations The elderly are a high-risk population for adverse effects from nonsteroidal anti-inflammatory agents. As much as 60% of older adults who experience GI side effects can develop peptic ulceration and/or hemorrhage asymptomatically. The concomitant use of H_2 blockers and sucralfate is not effective as prophylaxis with the exception of NSAID-induced duodenal ulcers which may be prevented by the use of ranitidine. Misoprostol and proton pump inhibitors are the only agents proven to help prevent the development of NSAID-induced ulcers. Also, concomitant disease and drug use contribute to the risk for GI adverse effects. Use lowest effective dose for shortest period possible. Consider renal function decline with age. Use of NSAIDs can compromise existing renal function especially when Cl_{cr} is ≤30 mL/minute.

Tinnitus may be a difficult and unreliable indication of toxicity due to age-related hearing loss or eighth cranial nerve damage. CNS adverse effects such as confusion, agitation, and hallucination are generally seen in overdose or high dose situations, but older adults may demonstrate these adverse effects at lower doses than younger adults. In patients ≥65 years, no substantial differences in the pharmacokinetics or side-effects profile were seen compared with the general population. Studies with etodolac in elderly demonstrated no difference in safety or efficacy compared to younger adults. No dosing adjustment necessary in elderly.

Dosage Forms Excipient information presented when available (limited, particularly for generics); consult specific product labeling. [DSC] = Discontinued product

Capsule: 200 mg, 300 mg

Lodine®: 200 mg, 300 mg [DSC]

Tablet: 400 mg, 500 mg

Tablet, extended release (Lodine® XL): 400 mg, 500 mg [DSC]

Selected References

Brooks PM and Day RO, "Nonsteroidal Anti-inflammatory Drugs - Differences and Similarities," *N Engl J Med*, 1991, 324(24):1716-25.

Clinch D, Banerjee AK, and Ostick G, "Absence of Abdominal Pain in Elderly Patients With Peptic Ulcer," *Age Ageing*, 1984, 13(2):120-3.

Clive DM and Stoff JS, "Renal Syndromes Associated With Nonsteroidal Anti-inflammatory Drugs," *N Engl J Med*, 1984, 310(9):563-72.

Graham DY, "Prevention of Gastroduodenal Injury Induced by Chronic Nonsteroidal Anti-inflammatory Drug Therapy," *Gastroenterology*, 1989, 96(2 Pt 2 Suppl):675-81.

Gurwitz JH, Avorn J, Ross-Degnan D, et al, "Nonsteroidal Anti-inflammatory Drug-Associated Azotemia in the Very Old," *JAMA*, 1990, 264(4):471-5.

Hawkey CJ, Karrasch JA, Szczepański L, et al, "Omeprazole Compared With Misoprostol for Ulcers Associated With Nonsteroidal Anti-inflammatory Drugs," *N Engl J Med*, 1998, 338(11):727-34.

Knodel LC, "Preventing NSAID-induced Ulcers: The Role of Misoprostol," *Consult Pharm*, 1989, 4:37-41.

Pounder R, "Silent Peptic Ulceration: Deadly Silence or Golden Silence?" *Gastroenterology*, 1989, 96(2 Pt 2 Suppl):626-31.

(Continued)

Etodolac *(Continued)*

Yeomans ND, Tulassay Z, Juhasz L, et al, "A Comparison of Omeprazole With Ranitidine for Ulcers Associated With Nonsteroidal Anti-inflammatory Drugs," *N Engl J Med*, 1998, 338(11):719-26.

- ◆ **Etodolic Acid** *see Etodolac on page 587*
- ◆ **Eulexin®** *see Flutamide on page 658*
- ◆ **Eurax®** *see Crotamiton on page 370*
- ◆ **Evac-U-Gen [OTC]** *see Senna on page 1456*
- ◆ **Evista®** *see Raloxifene on page 1374*
- ◆ **Evoclin™** *see Clindamycin on page 332*
- ◆ **Evoxac®** *see Cevimeline on page 284*
- ◆ **Exelon®** *see Rivastigmine on page 1421*

Exemestane *(ex e MES tane)*

Medication Safety Issues
Sound-alike/look-alike issues:
Exemestane may be confused with estramustine.

U.S. Brand Names Aromasin®

Canadian Brand Names Aromasin®

Generic Available No

Pharmacologic Category Antineoplastic Agent, Aromatase Inactivator

Use Treatment of advanced breast cancer in postmenopausal women whose disease has progressed following tamoxifen therapy; adjuvant treatment of postmenopausal estrogen receptor-positive early breast cancer following 2-3 years of tamoxifen (for a total of 5 years of adjuvant therapy)

Contraindications Hypersensitivity to exemestane or any component of the formulation

Warnings/Precautions Hazardous agent - use appropriate precautions for handling and disposal. Exemestane should not be administered concurrently with estrogen-containing drugs; not recommended for use in premenopausal women.

Adverse Reactions (Reflective of adult population; not specific for elderly)
>10%:
Cardiovascular: Hypertension (5% to 15%)
Central nervous system: Fatigue (8% to 22%), insomnia (11% to 14%), pain (13%), headache (7% to 13%), depression (6% to 13%)
Dermatological: Hyperhidrosis (4% to 18%), alopecia (15%)
Endocrine & metabolic: Hot flashes (13% to 21%)
Gastrointestinal: Nausea (9% to 18%), abdominal pain (6% to 11%)
Hepatic: Alkaline phosphatase increased (14% to 15%)
Neuromuscular & skeletal: Arthralgia (15% to 29%)
1% to 10%:
Cardiovascular: Edema (6% to 7%); cardiac ischemic events (2%: MI, angina, myocardial ischemia); chest pain
Central nervous system: Dizziness (8% to 10%), anxiety (4% to 10%), fever (5%), confusion, hypoesthesia
Dermatologic: Dermatitis (8%), itching, rash
Endocrine & metabolic: Weight gain (8%)
Gastrointestinal: Diarrhea (4% to 10%), vomiting (7%), anorexia (6%), constipation (5%), appetite increased (3%), dyspepsia
Genitourinary: Urinary tract infection
Hepatic: Bilirubin increased (5% to 7%)
Neuromuscular & skeletal: Back pain (9%), limb pain (9%), osteoarthritis (6%), weakness (6%), osteoporosis (5%), pathological fracture (4%), paresthesia (3%), carpal tunnel syndrome (2%), cramps (2%)
Ocular: Visual disturbances (5%)
Renal: Creatinine increased (6%)
Respiratory: Dyspnea (10%), cough (6%), bronchitis, pharyngitis, rhinitis, sinusitis, upper respiratory infection
Miscellaneous: Influenza-like symptoms (6%), diaphoresis (6%), lymphedema, infection

A dose-dependent decrease in sex hormone-binding globulin has been observed with daily doses of 25 mg or more. Serum luteinizing hormone and follicle-stimulating hormone levels have increased with this medicine.

Overdosage/Toxicology In case of overdose, treatment should be symptom-directed and supportive.

Drug Interactions Substrate of CYP3A4 (major)
CYP3A4 inducers: May decrease the levels/effects of exemestane. Example inducers include aminoglutethimide, carbamazepine, efavirenz, fosphenytoin, nafcillin,

nevirapine, oxcarbazepine, pentobarbital, phenobarbital, phenytoin, primidone, rifabutin, rifampin, and rifapentine. Dosage adjustment required with potent inducers.
Rifampin: May decrease exemestane levels; consider therapy modification.

Ethanol/Nutrition/Herb Interactions
Food: Plasma levels increased by 40% when exemestane was taken with a fatty meal.
Herb/Nutraceutical: St John's wort may decrease exemestane levels. Avoid black cohosh, dong quai in estrogen-dependent tumors.

Stability Store at 25°C (77°F)

Mechanism of Action Exemestane is an irreversible, steroidal aromatase inactivator. It prevents conversion of androgens to estrogens by tying up the enzyme aromatase. In breast cancers where growth is estrogen-dependent, this medicine will lower circulating estrogens.

Pharmacokinetics
Absorption: Rapidly absorbed; mean AUC: 75.4 ng•h/mL
Distribution: Extensive
Protein binding: 90%
Metabolism: Extensively metabolized; oxidation of the methylene group, reduction of the 17-keto group with formation of many secondary metabolites which are inactive or inhibit aromatase with decreased potency compared to the parent drug
Half-life: 24 hours
Time to peak: T_{max} (women with breast cancer): 1.2 hours
Elimination: <1% of parent drug excreted in urine; 42% of metabolites excreted in urine; 42% excreted in feces

Dosage
Geriatrics & Adults: Breast cancer: Oral: 25 mg once daily
Dosage adjustment with CYP3A4 inducers: 50 mg once daily when used with potent inducers (eg, rifampin, phenytoin)
Renal Impairment: Safety of chronic dosing in renal impairment has not been established.
Hepatic Impairment: Safety of chronic dosing in hepatic impairment has not been established.

Administration Administer after a meal.

Patient Information Take after a meal; use caution if you have uncontrolled high blood pressure. Avoid driving or doing other tasks or hobbies that require alertness until you know how this medicine affects you. Take at a similar time every day.

Additional Information The safety of chronic dosing in patients with moderate or severe hepatic or renal impairment has not been studied.

Special Geriatric Considerations In pharmacokinetic trials, no significant changes were seen in women <68 years of age.

Dosage Forms Excipient information presented when available (limited, particularly for generics); consult specific product labeling.
Tablet: 25 mg

Selected References
Morandi P, Rouzier R, Altundag K, et al, "The Role of Aromatase Inhibitors in the Adjuvant Treatment of Breast Carcinoma: The M. D. Anderson Cancer Center Evidence-Based Approach," *Cancer*, 2004, 101(7):1482-9.
Winer EP, Hudis C, Burstein HJ, et al, "American Society of Clinical Oncology Technology Assessment on the Use of Aromatase Inhibitors as Adjuvant Therapy for Postmenopausal Women With Hormone Receptor-Positive Breast Cancer: Status Report 2004," *J Clin Oncol*, 2005, 23(3):619-29.

♦ **Exforge**® *see* Amlodipine and Valsartan *on page 91*
♦ **Exjade**® *see* Deferasirox *on page 402*
♦ **ex-lax**® [OTC] *see* Senna *on page 1456*
♦ **ex-lax**® **Maximum Strength** [OTC] *see* Senna *on page 1456*
♦ **ex-lax**® **Ultra** [OTC] *see* Bisacodyl *on page 173*
♦ **Extina**® *see* Ketoconazole *on page 853*
♦ **Extra Strength Doan's**® [OTC] *see* Salicylates (Various Salts) *on page 1439*
♦ **Exubera**® *see* Insulin Inhalation *on page 811*
♦ **EYE001** *see* Pegaptanib *on page 1211*
♦ **Eye-Sine**™ [OTC] *see* Tetrahydrozoline *on page 1547*

Ezetimibe (ez ET i mibe)

Related Information
Hyperlipidemia Management *on page 1773*
Medication Safety Issues
Sound-alike/look-alike issues:
Zetia™ may be confused with Zestril®
U.S. Brand Names Zetia™
Canadian Brand Names Ezetrol®
Generic Available No
(Continued)

Ezetimibe *(Continued)*

Pharmacologic Category Antilipemic Agent, 2-Azetidinone

Use Use in combination with dietary therapy for the treatment of primary hypercholesterolemia (as monotherapy or in combination with HMG-CoA reductase inhibitors); homozygous sitosterolemia; homozygous familial hypercholesterolemia (in combination with atorvastatin or simvastatin); mixed hyperlipidemia (in combination with fenofibrate)

Contraindications Hypersensitivity to ezetimibe or any component of the formulation

Warnings/Precautions Secondary causes of hyperlipidemia should be ruled out prior to therapy. Use caution with renal or mild hepatic impairment; not recommended for use with moderate or severe hepatic impairment. Use of ezetimibe and fenofibrate (160 mg daily) may increase rate of cholecystectomy.

Adverse Reactions (Reflective of adult population; not specific for elderly) 1% to 10%:
Cardiovascular: Chest pain (3%), dizziness (3%), fatigue (2%)
Central nervous system: Headache (8%)
Gastrointestinal: Diarrhea (3% to 4%), abdominal pain (3%)
Neuromuscular & skeletal: Arthralgia (4%)
Respiratory: Sinusitis (4% to 5%), pharyngitis (2% to 3%, placebo 2%)

Overdosage/Toxicology Doses of up to 50 mg/day were well-tolerated. Treatment should be symptom-directed and supportive.

Drug Interactions
Bile acid sequestrants (cholestyramine): May decrease ezetimibe bioavailability; administer ≥2 hours before or ≥4 hours after bile acid sequestrants
Cyclosporine: Ezetimibe serum levels may be increased. Ezetimibe may also increase serum levels of cyclosporine. Monitor.
Fibric acid derivatives: May increase serum concentrations of ezetimibe.

Ethanol/Nutrition/Herb Interactions Food: Ezetimibe did not cause meaningful reductions in fat-soluble vitamin concentrations during a 2-week clinical trial. Effects of long-term therapy have not been evaluated.

Stability Store at controlled room temperature of 15°C to 30°C (59°F to 86°F). Protect from moisture.

Mechanism of Action Inhibits absorption of cholesterol at the brush border of the small intestine via the sterol transporter, Niemann-Pick C1-Like1 (NPC1L1). This leads to a decreased delivery of cholesterol to the liver, reduction of hepatic cholesterol stores and an increased clearance of cholesterol from the blood; decreases total C, LDL-cholesterol (LDL-C), ApoB, and triglycerides (TG) while increasing HDL-cholesterol (HDL-C).

Pharmacokinetics
Protein binding: >90% to plasma proteins
Metabolism: Undergoes conjugation in the small intestine and liver; forms metabolite (active); may undergo enterohepatic recycling
Bioavailability: Variable
Half-life: 22 hours (ezetimibe and metabolite)
Time to peak, plasma: 4-12 hours
Excretion: Feces (78%, 69% as ezetimibe); urine (11%, 9% as metabolite)

Dosage
Geriatrics & Adults:
Hyperlipidemias: Oral: 10 mg/day
Sitosterolemia: Oral: 10 mg/day
Renal Impairment: Bioavailability increased with severe impairment; no dosing adjustment recommended.
Hepatic Impairment: Bioavailability increased with hepatic impairment
Mild impairment (Child-Pugh score 5-6): No dosing adjustment necessary.
Moderate to severe impairment (Child-Pugh score 7-15): Use of ezetimibe not recommended.

Administration May be administered without regard to meals. May be taken at the same time as HMG-CoA reductase inhibitors. Administer ≥2 hours before or ≥4 hours after bile acid sequestrants.

Monitoring Parameters Total cholesterol profile prior to therapy, and when clinically indicated and/or periodically thereafter. When used in combination with fenofibrate, monitor LFTs and signs and symptoms of cholelithiasis.

Patient Information Inform prescriber of all prescriptions, OTC medications, or herbal products you are taking, and any allergies you have. Do not take any new medication during therapy without consulting prescriber. Take at the same time of day, without regard for meals. Take 2 hours before or 4 hours after bile acid binding agents (ie, Questran®). This medication does not replace the need for dietary and exercise recommendations of prescriber. May cause headache, dizziness, or fatigue (use caution when driving or engaged in potentially hazardous tasks until response to drug is known); diarrhea (boiled milk, buttermilk, or yogurt may help); abdominal pain. Report any severe or persistent side effects (eg, chest pain; muscle, skeletal, or joint pain; increased perspiration).

Additional Information When studied in combination with fenofibrate for mixed hyperlipidemia, the dose of fenofibrate was 160 mg daily.

Dosage Forms Excipient information presented when available (limited, particularly for generics); consult specific product labeling.

Tablet: 10 mg [capsule shaped]

Selected References

Gustavson LE, Schweitzer SM, Burt DA, et al, "Evaluation of the Potential for Pharmacokinetic Interaction Between Fenofibrate and Ezetimibe: A Phase I, Open-Label, Multiple-Dose, Three-Period Crossover Study in Healthy Subjects," *Clin Ther*, 2006, 28 (3):373-87.

Mauro VF and Tuckerman CE, "Ezetimibe for Management of Hypercholesterolemia," *Ann Pharmacother*, 2003, 37(6):839-48.

"Three New Drugs for Hyperlipidemia," *Med Lett Drugs Ther*, 2003, 45(1151):17-9.

von Bergmann K, Salen G, Lutjohann D, et al, "Ezetimibe Effectively Reduces Serum Plant Sterols in Patients With Sitosterolemia (abstract). 73rd European Atherosclerosis Society Congress, 2002. Available at: www.kenes.com/73eas/program/abstracts/405.doc. Accessed July 7, 2003.

Ezetimibe and Simvastatin (ez ET i mibe & SIM va stat in)

Medication Safety Issues

Sound-alike/look-alike issues:

Vytorin® may be confused with Vyvanse™

U.S. Brand Names Vytorin®

Generic Available No

Pharmacologic Category Antilipemic Agent, 2-Azetidinone; Antilipemic Agent, HMG-CoA Reductase Inhibitor

Use Used in combination with dietary modification for the treatment of primary hypercholesterolemia and homozygous familial hypercholesterolemia

Contraindications Hypersensitivity to ezetimibe, simvastatin, or any component of the formulation; acute liver disease; unexplained persistent elevations of serum transaminases

Warnings/Precautions Secondary causes of hyperlipidemia should be ruled out prior to therapy. Liver function must be monitored by laboratory assessment. Rhabdomyolysis with acute renal failure has occurred with simvastatin. Risk is dose-related and is increased with concurrent use of lipid-lowering agents which may cause rhabdomyolysis (gemfibrozil, fibric acid derivatives, or niacin at doses ≥1 g/day) or during concurrent use with danazol or potent CYP3A4 inhibitors (including amiodarone, clarithromycin, cyclosporine, erythromycin, itraconazole, ketoconazole, nefazodone, grapefruit juice in large quantities, telithromycin, verapamil, or protease inhibitors). Avoid use with clarithromycin, erythromycin, fibrates, itraconazole, ketoconazole, nefazodone, protease inhibitors, telithromycin, or other drugs associated with myopathy. Weigh the risk versus benefit when combining any of these drugs with a simvastatin-containing product. Do not initiate simvastatin-containing treatment in a patient with pre-existing therapy of cyclosporine or danazol, unless the patient has previously demonstrated tolerance to ≥5 mg/day simvastatin.

Use caution with renal or mild hepatic impairment; not recommended for use with moderate or severe hepatic impairment. Temporarily discontinue in any patient experiencing an acute or serious condition predisposing to renal failure secondary to rhabdomyolysis. Stop a few days prior to elective major surgery. Use with caution in patients who consume large amounts of ethanol or have a history of liver disease.

Adverse Reactions (Reflective of adult population; not specific for elderly)

Percentages below refer to combination Vytorin®. Also see individual agents.

1% to 10%:

Central nervous system: Headache (7%)

Neuromuscular & skeletal: Myalgia (4%), pain in extremity (2%)

Respiratory: Upper respiratory infection (4%)

Miscellaneous: Influenza (3%)

Overdosage/Toxicology See individual agents.

Drug Interactions Simvastatin: **Substrate** of CYP3A4 (major); **Inhibits** CYP2C8 (weak), 2C9 (weak), 2D6 (weak)

Amiodarone: May increase the levels/effects of simvastatin; do not exceed ezetimibe 10 mg/simvastatin 20 mg once daily.

Antifungal agents (imidazole): May increase the levels/effects of simvastatin. Avoid using Vytorin® with itraconazole or ketoconazole (manufacturer's recommendation).

Bile acid seqestrants: May decrease the absorption of ezetimibe. Consider administering Vytorin® at least 2 hours before or at least 4 hours after the bile acid sequestrant.

Bosentan: May decrease levels/effects of HMG-CoA reductase inhibitors.

Colchicine: Concomitant therapy with an HMG-CoA reductase inhibitor may increase risk of myopathy/rhabdomyolysis; use caution

(Continued)

Ezetimibe and Simvastatin *(Continued)*

Cyclosporine: May increase the serum concentration of ezetimibe. Ezetimibe may increase the serum concentration of cyclosporine. Concurrent use may increase the risk of myopathy and rhabdomyolysis. Do not exceed ezetimibe 10 mg/simvastatin 10 mg once daily.

CYP3A4 inhibitors: May increase the levels/effects of simvastatin. Example inhibitors include azole antifungals, clarithromycin, diclofenac, doxycycline, erythromycin, imatinib, isoniazid, nefazodone, nicardipine, propofol, protease inhibitors, quinidine, telithromycin, and verapamil. Manufacturer recommends avoiding concurrent use with clarithromycin, erythromycin, itraconazole, ketoconazole, nefazodone, protease inhibitors, telithromycin.

Danazol: May increase risk of myopathy and rhabdomyolysis; do not exceed ezetimibe 10 mg/simvastatin 10 mg once daily.

Diclofenac: May increase the levels/effects of simvastatin.

Fibric acid derivatives: May enhance the myopathic (rhabdomyolysis) effect of HMG-CoA reductase inhibitors. The manufacturer does not recommend concurrent use, but suggests that if gemfibrozil is used, doses should not exceed ezetimibe 10 mg and simvastatin 10 mg once daily.

Imatinib: May increase the levels/effects of simvastatin.

Macrolide antibiotics: May increase the levels/effects of HMG-CoA reductase inhibitors. Avoid Vytorin® with clarithromycin, erythromycin, or telithromycin (manufacturer's recommendation).

Nefazodone: May increase levels/effects of HMG-CoA reductase inhibitors. Avoid concurrent use with Vytorin® (manufacturer's recommendation).

Phenytoin: May decrease the levels/effects of HMG-CoA reductase inhibitors.

Protease inhibitors: May increase the levels/effects of HMG-CoA reductase inhibitors. Avoid concurrent use with Vytorin® (manufacturer's recommendation).

Proton pump inhibitors: May increase the serum concentration of HMG-CoA reductase inhibitors.

Ranolazine: May increase the serum concentration of simvastatin.

Rifamycin derivatives: May decrease the levels/effects of HMG-CoA reductase inhibitors.

Sildenafil: May increase the levels/effects of HMG-CoA reductase inhibitors.

Verapamil: May increase the levels/effects of HMG-CoA reductase inhibitors. Do not exceed ezetimibe 10 mg/simvastatin 20 mg once daily.

Warfarin: Simvastatin may increase levels/effects of warfarin; monitor INR closely when simvastatin is initiated or discontinued.

Ethanol/Nutrition/Herb Interactions

Ethanol: Avoid excessive ethanol consumption (due to potential hepatic effects).

Food: Simvastatin serum concentration may be increased when taken with grapefruit juice; avoid concurrent intake of large quantities (>1 quart/day). Red yeast rice contains an estimated 2.4 mg lovastatin per 600 mg rice. Ezetimibe did not cause meaningful reductions in fat-soluble vitamin concentrations during a 2-week clinical trial. Effects of long-term therapy have not been evaluated.

Herb/Nutraceutical: St John's wort may decrease simvastatin levels.

Stability Store at 20°C to 25°C (68°F to 77°F).

Mechanism of Action

Ezetimibe: Inhibits absorption of cholesterol at the brush border of the small intestine, leading to a decreased delivery of cholesterol to the liver. Ezetimibe inhibits the enzyme Niemann-Pick C1-Like1 (NPC1L1), a sterol transporter.

Simvastatin: A methylated derivative of lovastatin that acts by competitively inhibiting 3-hydroxy-3-methylglutaryl-coenzyme A (HMG-CoA) reductase, the enzyme that catalyzes the rate-limiting step in cholesterol biosynthesis.

Pharmacokinetics See individual agents.

Bioavailability: Vytorin™ is equivalent to coadministered ezetimibe and simvastatin.

Dosage

Geriatrics & Adults:

Homozygous familial hypercholesterolemia: Ezetimibe 10 mg and simvastatin 40 mg once daily or ezetimibe 10 mg and simvastatin 80 mg once daily in the evening. Dosing range: Ezetimibe 10 mg and simvastatin 10-80 mg once daily.

Hyperlipidemias: Oral: Initial: Ezetimibe 10 mg and simvastatin 20 mg once daily in the evening; those patients requiring less aggressive LDL-C reductions can start with ezetimibe 10 mg and simvastatin 10 mg once daily

Patients who require less aggressive reduction in LDL-C: Initial: Ezetimibe 10 mg and simvastatin 10 mg once daily

Patients who require >55% reduction in LDL-C: Initial: Ezetimibe 10 mg and simvastatin 40 mg once daily

Dosage adjustment with concomitant medications: Oral:

Amiodarone or verapamil: Dose should not exceed ezetimibe 10 mg and simvastatin 20 mg once daily.

Danazol or cyclosporine: Patient must first demonstrate tolerance to simvastatin ≥5 mg once daily. Dose should not exceed ezetimibe 10 mg and simvastatin 10 mg once daily.

Gemfibrozil: Although concurrent use is not recommended by manufacturer, dose should not exceed ezetimibe 10 mg and simvastatin 10 mg once daily.

Renal Impairment: Dosage adjustment unnecessary in mild to moderate renal dysfunction. In severe dysfunction, start only if patient tolerates 5 mg daily of simvastatin; monitor closely.

Hepatic Impairment: Dosage adjustment unnecessary in mild hepatic dysfunction.

Monitoring Parameters Creatine phosphokinase levels due to possibility of myopathy; serum cholesterol (total and fractionated)

Obtain liver function tests prior to initiation, dosage increase, and thereafter when clinically indicated. Patients titrated to the simvastatin 80 mg dose should be tested prior to initiation and 3 months after initiating the 80 mg dose. Thereafter, periodic monitoring (ie, semiannually) is recommended for the first year of treatment. Patients with elevated transaminase levels should have a second (confirmatory) test and frequent monitoring until values normalize. Discontinue if increase in ALT/AST is persistently >3 times ULN.

Special Geriatric Considerations Clinical studies of Vytorin® included a total of 792 patients >65 years of age with 176 of these patients ≥75 years. The safety in this group was similar to the younger patients. No adjustment of dose is necessary for initiation of treatment in the elderly.

Dosage Forms Excipient information presented when available (limited, particularly for generics); consult specific product labeling.

Tablet:
10/10: Ezetimibe 10 mg and simvastatin 10 mg
10/20: Ezetimibe 10 mg and simvastatin 20 mg
10/40: Ezetimibe 10 mg and simvastatin 40 mg
10/80: Ezetimibe 10 mg and simvastatin 80 mg

◆ **E•R•O [OTC]** *see* Carbamide Peroxide *on page 235*
◆ **F₃T** *see* Trifluridine *on page 1630*
◆ **Factive®** *see* Gemifloxacin *on page 702*

Famciclovir (fam SYE kloe veer)

U.S. Brand Names Famvir®
Canadian Brand Names Apo-Famciclovir; Famvir®; PMS-Famciclovir
Generic Available No
Pharmacologic Category Antiviral Agent
Use Treatment of acute herpes zoster (shingles); treatment and suppression of recurrent episodes of genital herpes in immunocompetent patients; treatment of herpes labialis (cold sores) in immunocompetent patients; treatment of recurrent mucocutaneous/genital herpes simplex in HIV-infected patients
Contraindications Hypersensitivity to famciclovir or any component of the formulation
Warnings/Precautions Has not been studied in immunocompromised patients or patients with ophthalmic, disseminated zoster, or with initial episode of genital herpes. Dosage adjustment is required in patients with renal insufficiency. Tablets contain lactose; do not use with galactose intolerance, severe lactase deficiency, or glucose-galactose malabsorption syndromes.
Adverse Reactions (Reflective of adult population; not specific for elderly)
Note: Frequencies vary with dose and duration. Single-dose treatment (herpes labialis) was associated only with headache (10%), diarrhea (2%), fatigue (1%), and dysmenorrhea (1%).

>10%:
Central nervous system: Headache (17% to 39%)
Gastrointestinal: Nausea (7% to 13%)
1% to 10%:
Central nervous system: Fatigue (4% to 6%), migraine (1% to 3%)
Dermatologic: Pruritus (1% to 4%), rash (<1% to 3%)
Endocrine and metabolic: Dysmenorrhea (up to 8%)
Gastrointestinal: Diarrhea (5% to 9%), flatulence (2% to 5%), vomiting (1% to 5%), abdominal pain (1% to 8%)
Hematologic: Neutropenia (3%), leukopenia (1%)
Hepatic: Transaminases increased (2% to 3%), bilirubin increased (2%)
Neuromuscular & skeletal: Paresthesia (1% to 3%)
Overdosage/Toxicology Supportive and symptomatic care is recommended. Hemodialysis may enhance elimination of penciclovir.
(Continued)

Famciclovir *(Continued)*

Ethanol/Nutrition/Herb Interactions Food: Rate of absorption and/or conversion to penciclovir and peak concentration are reduced with food, but bioavailability is not affected.

Stability Store at controlled room temperature.

Mechanism of Action Famciclovir undergoes rapid biotransformation to the active compound, penciclovir, which is phosphorylated by viral thymidine kinase in HSV-1, HSV-2, and VZV-infected cells to a monophosphate form; this is then converted to penciclovir triphosphate and competes with deoxyguanosine triphosphate to inhibit HSV-2 polymerase (eg, herpes viral DNA synthesis/replication is selectively inhibited)

Pharmacokinetics

Absorption: Food decreases maximum peak concentration and delays time to peak; AUC remains the same

Distribution: V_{dss}: 0.91-1.25 L/kg

Protein binding: ≤20%

Metabolism: Rapidly deacetylated and oxidized to penciclovir; not via CYP

Bioavailability: 69% to 85%

Half-life elimination: Penciclovir: 2-3 hours (10, 20, and 7 hours in HSV-1, HSV-2, and VZV-infected cells, respectively); prolonged with renal impairment

Time to peak: 0.9 hours; C_{max} and T_{max} are decreased and prolonged with noncompensated hepatic impairment

Excretion: Urine (73% primarily as penciclovir); feces (27%)

Dosage

Geriatrics & Adults:

Acute herpes zoster: Oral: 500 mg every 8 hours for 7 days (**Note:** Initiate therapy within 72 hours of rash onset.)

Recurrent genital herpes simplex in immunocompetent patients: Oral:

Initial: 1000 mg twice daily for 1 day (**Note:** initiate therapy within 6 hours of symptoms/lesions.)

Suppressive therapy: 250 mg twice daily for up to 1 year

Recurrent herpes labialis (cold sores): Oral: 1500 mg as a single dose; initiate therapy at first sign or symptom such as tingling, burning, or itching (initiated within 1 hour in clinical studies)

Recurrent mucocutaneous/genital herpes simplex in HIV patients: Oral: 500 mg twice daily for 7 days

Renal Impairment:

Herpes zoster:

Cl_{cr} 40-59 mL/minute: Administer 500 mg every 12 hours

Cl_{cr} 20-39 mL/minute: Administer 500 mg every 24 hours

Cl_{cr} <20 mL/minute: Administer 250 mg every 24 hours

Hemodialysis: Administer 250 mg after each dialysis session.

Recurrent genital herpes: Treatment (single day regimen):

Cl_{cr} 40-59 mL/minute: Administer 500 mg every 12 hours for 1 day

Cl_{cr} 20-39 mL/minute: Administer 500 mg as a single dose

Cl_{cr} <20 mL/minute: Administer 250 mg as a single dose

Hemodialysis: Administer 250 mg as a single dose after dialysis session.

Recurrent genital herpes: Suppression:

Cl_{cr} 20-39 mL/minute: Administer 125 mg every 12 hours

Cl_{cr} <20 mL/minute: Administer 125 mg every 24 hours

Hemodialysis: Administer 125 mg after each dialysis session.

Recurrent herpes labialis: Treatment (single dose regimen):

Cl_{cr} 40-59 mL/minute: Administer 750 mg as a single dose

Cl_{cr} 20-39 mL/minute: Administer 500 mg as a single dose

Cl_{cr} <20 mL/minute: Administer 250 mg as a single dose

Hemodialysis: Administer 250 mg as a single dose after dialysis session.

Recurrent orolabial or genital herpes in HIV-infected patients:

Cl_{cr} 20-39 mL/minute: Administer 500 mg every 12 hours

Cl_{cr} <20 mL/minute: Administer 250 mg every 24 hours

Hemodialysis: Administer 250 mg after each dialysis session.

Monitoring Parameters BUN, serum creatinine

Patient Information Patient may take medication without regard to meals; contagious only when viral shedding is occurring; avoid sexual intercourse when lesions are visible; begin medication at first sign or symptom of genital herpes or at diagnosis of herpes zoster

Additional Information Most effective for herpes zoster if therapy is initiated within 48 hours of initial lesion. Resistance may occur by alteration of thymidine kinase, resulting in loss of or reduced penciclovir phosphorylation (cross-resistance occurs between acyclovir and famciclovir). When treatment for herpes labialis is initiated within 1 hour of symptom onset, healing time is reduced by ~2 days.

Special Geriatric Considerations For herpes zoster (shingles) infections, famciclovir should be started within 72 hours of the appearance of the rash to be effective.

Famciclovir has been shown to accelerate healing, reduce the duration of viral shedding, and resolve posthepatic neuralgia faster than placebo. Comparison trials to acyclovir or valacyclovir are not available. Adjust dose for estimated renal function.

Dosage Forms Excipient information presented when available (limited, particularly for generics); consult specific product labeling.

Tablet: 125 mg, 250 mg, 500 mg [contains lactose]

Selected References

Pue MA and Benet LZ, "Pharmacokinetics of Famciclovir in Man," *Antivir Chem Chemother*, 1993, 4(Suppl 1):47-55.

Spruance SL, Bodsworth N, Resnick H, et al, "Single-Dose, Patient-Initiated Famciclovir: A Randomized, Double-Blind, Placebo-Controlled Trial for Episodic Treatment of Herpes Labialis," *J Am Acad Dermatol*, 2006, 55(1):47-53.

Tyring S, Barbarash RA, Nahlik JE, et al, "Famciclovir for the Treatment of Acute Herpes Zoster: Effects on Acute Disease and Postherpetic Neuralgia," *Ann Intern Med*, 1995, 123(2):89-96.

Famotidine (fa MOE ti deen)

U.S. Brand Names Pepcid®; Pepcid® AC [OTC]

Canadian Brand Names Apo-Famotidine®; Apo-Famotidine® Injectable; Famotidine Omega; Gen-Famotidine; Novo-Famotidine; Nu-Famotidine; Pepcid®; Pepcid® AC; Pepcid® I.V.; ratio-Famotidine; Riva-Famotidine; Ulcidine

Generic Available Yes: Injection, tablet

Pharmacologic Category Histamine H_2 Antagonist

Use Therapy and treatment of duodenal ulcer, gastric ulcer, control gastric pH in critically-ill patients, symptomatic relief in gastritis, gastroesophageal reflux, active benign ulcer, and pathological hypersecretory conditions

OTC labeling: Relief of heartburn, acid indigestion, and sour stomach

Unlabeled/Investigational Use Part of a multidrug regimen for *H. pylori* eradication to reduce the risk of duodenal ulcer recurrence

Contraindications Hypersensitivity to famotidine, other H_2 antagonists, or any component of the formulation

Warnings/Precautions Modify dose in patients with renal impairment. Relief of symptoms does not preclude the presence of a gastric malignancy. Reversible confusional states, usually clearing within 3-4 days after discontinuation, have been linked to use. Increased age (>50 years) and renal or hepatic impairment are thought to be associated. Chewable tablets contain phenylalanine; multidose vials contain benzyl alcohol.

OTC labeling: When used for self-medication, patients should be instructed not to use if they have difficulty swallowing, vomiting with blood, or bloody or black stools. Not for use with other acid reducers.

Adverse Reactions (Reflective of adult population; not specific for elderly)

1% to 10%:

Central nervous system: Dizziness (1%), headache (5%)

Gastrointestinal: Constipation (1%), diarrhea (2%)

Overdosage/Toxicology Symptoms include hypotension, tachycardia, vomiting, and drowsiness. Treatment is symptomatic and supportive.

Drug Interactions

Antifungal agents, azole: Histamine H_2 antagonists may decrease the absorption of azole antifungals; monitor.

Cefpodoxime: Histamine H_2 antagonists may decrease the absorption of cefpodoxime; separate oral doses by at least 2 hours. Risk: Moderate.

Cefuroxime: Histamine H_2 antagonists may decrease the absorption of cefuroxime; separate oral doses by at least 2 hours. Risk: Moderate.

Cyclosporine: Histamine H_2 antagonists may increase the serum concentration of cyclosporine; monitor.

Delavirdine: Delavirdine's absorption is decreased; avoid concurrent use with H_2 antagonists.

Ethanol/Nutrition/Herb Interactions

Ethanol: Avoid ethanol (may cause gastric mucosal irritation).

Food: Famotidine bioavailability may be increased if taken with food.

Stability

Oral:

Powder for oral suspension: Prior to mixing, dry powder should be stored at room temperature of 25°C (77°F). Reconstituted oral suspension is stable for 30 days at room temperature; do not freeze.

Tablet: Store at 20°C (77°F); excursions permitted between 15°C to 30°C (59°F to 86°F). Protect from moisture.

I.V.:

Solution for injection: Prior to use, store at 2°C to 8°C (36°F to 46°F). If solution freezes, allow to solubilize at room temperature.

(Continued)

Famotidine *(Continued)*

I.V. push: Dilute famotidine with NS (or another compatible solution) to a total of 5-10 mL (some centers also administer undiluted). Following reconstitution, solutions for I.V. push should be used immediately, or may be stored in refrigerator and used within 48 hours.

Infusion: Dilute with D_5W 100 mL or another compatible solution. Following reconstitution, solutions for infusion are stable for 7 days at room temperature.

Solution for injection, premixed bags: Store at room temperature of 25°C (77°F). Avoid excessive heat.

Mechanism of Action Competitive inhibition of histamine at H_2 receptors of the gastric parietal cells, which inhibits gastric acid secretion

Pharmacodynamics

Onset of action: GI: Oral: Within 1-3 hours

Peak effect: Oral: Within 1-3 hours after doses

Duration: 10-12 hours

Duodenal ulcer healing rates at 40 mg/day: 4 weeks: 67% to 77%: 8 weeks: 82% to 95% in young adults

Pharmacokinetics

Protein binding: 15% to 20%

Metabolism: 30% to 35%

Bioavailability: Oral: 40% to 50%

Half-life elimination:

Injection, oral suspension, tablet: 2.5-3.5 hours; prolonged with renal impairment; Oliguria: 20 hours

Orally-disintegrating tablet: 2.5-5 hours

Elimination: Excreted as unchanged drug in urine 25% to 30% oral and 65% to 70% I.V.; excreted in bile and feces

Dosage

Geriatrics & Adults:

Duodenal ulcer: Oral: Acute therapy: 40 mg/day at bedtime for 4-8 weeks; maintenance therapy: 20 mg/day at bedtime

Gastric ulcer: Oral: Acute therapy: 40 mg/day at bedtime

Hypersecretory conditions: Oral: Initial: 20 mg every 6 hours, may increase in increments up to 160 mg every 6 hours

GERD: Oral: 20 mg twice daily for 6 weeks

Esophagitis and accompanying symptoms due to GERD: Oral: 20 mg or 40 mg twice daily for up to 12 weeks

Peptic ulcer disease: Eradication of *Helicobacter pylori* (unlabeled use): Oral: 40 mg once daily; requires combination therapy with antibiotics

Patients unable to take oral medication: I.V.: 20 mg every 12 hours

Heartburn, indigestion, sour stomach: OTC labeling: Oral: 10-20 mg every 12 hours; dose may be taken 15-60 minutes before eating foods known to cause heartburn

Renal Impairment: Cl_{cr} <50 mL/minute: Manufacturer recommendation: Administer 50% of dose **or** increase the dosing interval to every 36-48 hours (to limit potential CNS adverse effects).

Administration

I.V. push: Inject over at least 2 minutes

Solution for infusion: Administer over 15-30 minutes

Monitoring Parameters Signs and symptoms of peptic ulcer disease, occult blood with GI bleeding, gastric pH where necessary; monitor renal function to correct dose; monitor for side effects

Patient Information Take with or immediately after meals; inform pharmacist and physician (nurse, practitioner) of any concomitant drug therapy; stagger doses with antacids

Orally-disintegrating tablet: Do not break tablet.

OTC use: Do not take maximum dose for more than 14 days continuously unless directed by physician

Additional Information The expensive parenteral route should only be used when a patient is unable to take oral medication

Special Geriatric Considerations H_2 blockers are the preferred drugs for treating PUD in the elderly due to cost and ease of administration. They are no less or more effective than any other therapy. Famotidine is one of the preferred agents (due to side effects, drug interaction profile, and pharmacokinetics). Treatment for PUD in the elderly is recommended for 12 weeks since their lesions are typically larger; therefore, take longer to heal. Always adjust dose based upon creatinine clearance, since slight accumulation may result in CNS side effects, mainly confusion.

Dosage Forms Excipient information presented when available (limited, particularly for generics); consult specific product labeling. [DSC] = Discontinued product

Gelcap:
Pepcid® AC: 10 mg [DSC]
Infusion [premixed in NS]: 20 mg (50 mL)
Pepcid®: 20 mg (50 mL)
Injection, solution: 10 mg/mL (4 mL, 20 mL)
Pepcid®: 10 mg/mL (20 mL) [contains benzyl alcohol]
Injection, solution [preservative free]: 10 mg/mL (2 mL)
Pepcid®: 10 mg/mL (2 mL)
Powder for oral suspension:
Pepcid®: 40 mg/5 mL (50 mL) [contains sodium benzoate; cherry-banana-mint flavor]
Tablet: 10 mg [OTC], 20 mg, 40 mg
Pepcid®: 20 mg, 40 mg
Pepcid® AC: 10 mg, 20 mg
Tablet, chewable:
Pepcid® AC: 10 mg [contains phenylalanine 1.4 mg/tablet; mint flavor]

Selected References
Fennerty MD and Higbee M, "Drug Therapy of Gastrointestinal Disease," *Geriatric Pharmacology*, Bressler R and Katz MD, eds, New York, NY: McGraw-Hill, 1993, 585-608.

Famotidine, Calcium Carbonate, and Magnesium Hydroxide
(fa MOE ti deen, KAL see um KAR bun ate, & mag NEE zhum hye DROKS ide)

Related Information
Famotidine *on page 597*
Magnesium Hydroxide *on page 946*
U.S. Brand Names Pepcid® Complete [OTC]
Canadian Brand Names Pepcid® Complete [OTC]
Index Terms Calcium Carbonate, Magnesium Hydroxide, and Famotidine; Magnesium Hydroxide, Famotidine, and Calcium Carbonate
Generic Available No
Pharmacologic Category Antacid; Histamine H_2 Antagonist
Use Relief of heartburn due to acid indigestion
Contraindications Hypersensitivity to famotidine or other H_2 antagonists, calcium carbonate, magnesium hydroxide, or any component of the formulation. See individual agents for additional information.
Warnings/Precautions See individual agents.
Adverse Reactions (Reflective of adult population; not specific for elderly) See individual agents.
Drug Interactions See individual agents.
Stability Store at 25°C to 30°C (77°F to 86°F). Protect from moisture.
Mechanism of Action
Famotidine: H_2 antagonist
Calcium carbonate: Antacid
Magnesium hydroxide: Antacid
Dosage
Geriatrics & Adults: Relief of heartburn due to acid indigestion: Oral: Pepcid® Complete: 1 tablet as needed; no more than 2 tablets in 24 hours; do **not** swallow whole, chew tablet completely before swallowing; do not use for longer than 14 days (see Additional Information for dosing ranges for individual ingredients)
Patient Information Do **not** swallow tablet whole; chew completely before swallowing. Contact prescriber if your symptoms last for more than 14 days. Should not be used in combination with other products for acid indigestion (prescription or over the counter). Certain foods are more likely to cause acid indigestion in some patients, including foods that are rich, spicy, fatty, or fried; chocolate; caffeine; alcohol; some fruits or vegetables. Avoid meals close to bedtime, eat slowly and avoid big meals to help decrease symptoms. Avoid smoking.
Additional Information Presented in dosage field is the specific OTC labeling for the indicated product. Dosing ranges of the individual ingredients include:

Adults:
Famotidine: Duodenal/gastric ulcer: 40 mg/day at bedtime
Calcium carbonate: Antacid: ≤3 g/day of elemental calcium
Magnesium hydroxide: Antacid: Approximately ≤5 g/day of magnesium hydroxide
Healthcare providers should also refer to the individual monographs for more specific information.
Special Geriatric Considerations Use with caution in the elderly with reduced renal function (Cl_{cr} <30 mL/minute), since accumulation of magnesium and famotidine may occur and potentiate side effects
Dosage Forms Excipient information presented when available (limited, particularly for generics); consult specific product labeling.
(Continued)

Famotidine, Calcium Carbonate, and Magnesium Hydroxide *(Continued)*

Tablet, chewable: Famotidine 10 mg, calcium carbonate 800 mg, and magnesium hydroxide 165 mg [berry blend and mint flavors]

◆ **Famvir**® *see Famciclovir on page 595*
◆ **Fareston**® *see Toremifene on page 1602*
◆ **Faslodex**® *see Fulvestrant on page 688*
◆ **FazaClo**® *see Clozapine on page 352*
◆ **5-FC** *see Flucytosine on page 634*
◆ **FC1157a** *see Toremifene on page 1602*

Felbamate (FEL ba mate)

U.S. Brand Names Felbatol®
Generic Available No
Pharmacologic Category Anticonvulsant, Miscellaneous
Use Not as a first-line antiepileptic treatment; only in those patients who respond inadequately to alternative treatments and whose epilepsy is so severe that a substantial risk of aplastic anemia and/or liver failure is deemed acceptable in light of the benefits conferred by its use. Patient must be fully advised of risk and provide signed written informed consent. Felbamate can be used as either monotherapy or adjunctive therapy in the treatment of partial seizures (with and without generalization) and in adults with epilepsy.
Restrictions A patient "informed consent" form should be completed and signed by the patient and physician. Copies are available from Wallace Pharmaceuticals by calling 609-655-6147.
Contraindications Hypersensitivity to felbamate or any component of the formulation; use with caution in those patients who have demonstrated hypersensitivity reactions to other carbamates
Warnings/Precautions Use with caution in patients allergic to other carbamates (eg, meprobamate); antiepileptic drugs should not be suddenly discontinued because of the possibility of increasing seizure frequency. **[U.S. Boxed Warning]: Ten cases of aplastic anemia reported in the U.S. after 2 1/2 to 6 months of therapy.** Carter Wallace and the FDA recommended the use of this agent be suspended unless withdrawal of the product would place a patient at greater risk as compared to the frequently fatal form of anemia. **[U.S. Boxed Warning]: Felbamate has also been associated with rare cases of hepatic failure (estimated >6 cases per 75,000 patients per year).** Do not initiate treatment in patients with pre-existing hepatic dysfunction. Use caution in renal impairment (dose adjustment recommended). "Informed consent" (concerning hematological/hepatic risks) should be documented prior to initiation of therapy. Effects with other sedative drugs or ethanol may be potentiated.
Adverse Reactions (Reflective of adult population; not specific for elderly)
>10%:
  Central nervous system: Somnolence, headache, fatigue, dizziness
  Gastrointestinal: Nausea, anorexia, vomiting, constipation
1% to 10%:
  Cardiovascular: Chest pain, palpitation, tachycardia
  Central nervous system: Depression or behavior changes, nervousness, anxiety, ataxia, stupor, malaise, agitation, psychological disturbances, aggressive reaction
  Dermatologic: Skin rash, acne, pruritus
  Gastrointestinal: Xerostomia, diarrhea, abdominal pain, weight gain, taste perversion
  Neuromuscular & skeletal: Tremor, abnormal gait, paresthesia, myalgia
  Ocular: Diplopia, abnormal vision
  Respiratory: Sinusitis, pharyngitis
  Miscellaneous: ALT increased
Overdosage/Toxicology Symptoms include sedation, gastrointestinal upset, and tachycardia. Provide general supportive care.
Drug Interactions Substrate of CYP2E1 (minor), 3A4 (major); **Inhibits** CYP2C19 (weak); **Induces** CYP3A4 (weak)
  Carbamazepine: Felbamate may decrease carbamazepine levels and increase levels of the active metabolite of carbamazepine (10,11-epoxide) resulting in carbamazepine toxicity; monitor for signs of carbamazepine toxicity (dizziness, ataxia, nystagmus, drowsiness)
  CYP3A4 inducers: CYP3A4 inducers may decrease the levels/effects of felbamate. Example inducers include aminoglutethimide, carbamazepine, nafcillin, nevirapine, phenobarbital, phenytoin, and rifamycins.
  CYP3A4 inhibitors: May increase the levels/effects of felbamate. Example inhibitors include azole antifungals, clarithromycin, diclofenac, doxycycline, erythromycin,

imatinib, isoniazid, nefazodone, nicardipine, propofol, protease inhibitors, quinidine, telithromycin, and verapamil.

Gabapentin: May increase serum concentrations of felbamate; monitor for increased effect

Oral contraceptives: Serum levels have been noted to decrease modestly in some patients receiving felbamate; clinical significance in terms of contraceptive failure has not been established

Phenytoin: Felbamate may increase serum concentrations, consider decreasing phenytoin dosage by 25%

Phenobarbital: Felbamate may increase serum concentrations, consider decreasing phenobarbital dosage by 25%

Valproic acid: Felbamate may increase serum concentrations; a decrease in valproic acid dosage may be necessary; monitor for valproic acid toxicity (confusion, irritability, restlessness)

Ethanol/Nutrition/Herb Interactions

Ethanol: Avoid ethanol (may increase CNS depression).

Food: Food does not affect absorption.

Herb/Nutraceutical: Avoid evening primrose (seizure threshold decreased).

Stability Store medication in tightly closed container at room temperature away from excessive heat.

Mechanism of Action Mechanism of action is unknown but has properties in common with other marketed anticonvulsants; has weak inhibitory effects on GABA-receptor binding, benzodiazepine receptor binding, and is devoid of activity at the MK-801 receptor binding site of the NMDA receptor-ionophore complex.

Pharmacokinetics Geriatrics: Reduced clearance and prolonged half-life have been reported in persons 66-78 years of age, compared to persons 18-45 years of age.

Absorption: Rapid and almost complete; food has no effect upon the tablet's absorption

Distribution: V_d: 0.7-1 L/kg

Protein binding: 22% to 25%, primarily to albumin

Half-life: 20-23 hours (average); prolonged in renal dysfunction

Time to peak, serum: ~3 hours

Elimination: Urine (40% to 50% as unchanged drug, 40% as inactive metabolites)

Dosage

Geriatrics & Adults:

Anticonvulsant, monotherapy: Oral:

Initial: 1200 mg/day in divided doses 3 or 4 times/day; titrate previously untreated patients under close clinical supervision, increasing the dosage in 600 mg increments every 2 weeks to 2400 mg/day based on clinical response and thereafter to 3600 mg/day as clinically indicated

Conversion to monotherapy: Initiate at 1200 mg/day in divided doses 3 or 4 times/day, reduce the dosage of the concomitant anticonvulsant(s) by 20% to 33% at the initiation of felbamate therapy; at week 2, increase the felbamate dosage to 2400 mg/day while reducing the dosage of the other anticonvulsant(s) up to an additional 33% of their original dose; at week 3, increase the felbamate dosage up to 3600 mg/day and continue to reduce the dosage of the other anticonvulsant(s) as clinically indicated

Renal Impairment: Use caution; reduce initial and maintenance doses by 50% (half-life prolonged by 9-15 hours)

Monitoring Parameters Monitor serum concentrations of concomitant anticonvulsant therapy

Reference Range Not necessary to routinely monitor serum drug concentrations, since dose should be titrated to clinical response

Patient Information Shake oral suspension well before using

Additional Information Monotherapy has not been associated with gingival hyperplasia, impaired concentration, weight gain, or abnormal thinking

Special Geriatric Considerations Clinical studies have not included large numbers of patients >65 years of age. Due to decreased hepatic and renal function, dosing should start at the lower end of the dosage range.

Dosage Forms Excipient information presented when available (limited, particularly for generics); consult specific product labeling. [DSC] = Discontinued product

Suspension, oral:

Felbatol®: 600 mg/5 mL (240 mL, 960 mL)

Tablet:

Felbatol®: 400 mg; 600 mg [DSC]

Selected References

Richens A, Banfield CR, Salfi M, et al, "Single and Multiple Dose Pharmacokinetics of Felbamate in the Elderly," *Br J Clin Pharmacol*, 1997, 44(2):129-34.

♦ **Felbatol®** *see* Felbamate *on page 600*

♦ **Feldene®** *see* Piroxicam *on page 1276*

Felodipine (fe LOE di peen)

Related Information
Calcium Channel Blockers *on page 1753*
Medication Safety Issues
Sound-alike/look-alike issues:
Plendil® may be confused with Isordil®, pindolol, Pletal®, Prilosec®, Prinivil®
U.S. Brand Names Plendil®
Canadian Brand Names Plendil®; Renedil®
Generic Available Yes
Pharmacologic Category Calcium Channel Blocker
Use Treatment of hypertension
Contraindications Hypersensitivity to felodipine, any component of the formulation, or other calcium channel blocker
Warnings/Precautions Increased angina and/or MI has occurred with initiation or dosage titration of calcium channel blockers. Use caution in patients with heart failure and/or hypertrophic cardiomyopathy. Elderly patients and patients with hepatic impairment should start off with a lower dose. Peripheral edema is the most common side effect (occurs within 2-3 weeks of starting therapy). May cause reflex tachycardia. Symptomatic hypotension with or without syncope can rarely occur; blood pressure must be lowered at a rate appropriate for the patient's clinical condition. Use caution in hepatic impairment. Dosage titration should occur after 14 days on a given dose.
Adverse Reactions (Reflective of adult population; not specific for elderly)
>10%: Central nervous system: Headache (11% to 15%)
2% to 10%: Cardiovascular: Peripheral edema (2% to 17%), tachycardia (0.4% to 2.5%), flushing (4% to 7%)
Overdosage/Toxicology Primary cardiac symptoms of calcium blocker overdose include hypotension and bradycardia. Hypotension is caused by peripheral vasodilation, myocardial depression, and bradycardia. Bradycardia results from sinus bradycardia, second- or third-degree atrioventricular block, or sinus arrest with junctional rhythm. Intraventricular conduction is usually not affected so QRS duration is normal (verapamil prolongs the PR interval and bepridil prolongs the QT interval and may cause ventricular arrhythmias, including torsade de pointes).

Noncardiac symptoms include confusion, stupor, nausea, vomiting, metabolic acidosis and hyperglycemia. Following gastric decontamination, if possible, repeated calcium administration may promptly reverse depressed cardiac contractility (but not sinus node depression or peripheral vasodilation). Glucagon, epinephrine, and inamrinone (amrinone) may treat refractory hypotension. Glucagon and epinephrine also increase the heart rate (outside the U.S., 4-aminopyridine may be available as an antidote). Dialysis and hemoperfusion are not effective in enhancing elimination, although repeat-dose activated charcoal may serve as an adjunct with sustained-release preparations.

In a few reported cases, overdose with calcium channel blockers has been associated with hypotension and bradycardia, initially refractory to atropine, but becoming more responsive to this agent when larger doses (approaching 1 g/hour for more than 24 hours) of calcium chloride were administered.
Drug Interactions Substrate of CYP3A4 (major); **Inhibits** CYP2C8 (moderate), 2C9 (weak), 2D6 (weak), 3A4 (weak)
Azole antifungals may inhibit calcium channel blocker's metabolism; avoid this combination. Try an antifungal like terbinafine (if appropriate) or monitor closely for altered effect of the calcium channel blocker.
Beta-blockers may have increased pharmacokinetic or pharmacodynamic interactions with felodipine.
Calcium may reduce the calcium channel blocker's effects, particularly hypotension.
Carbamazepine significantly reduces felodipine's bioavailability; avoid this combination.
Cimetidine may inhibit felodipine metabolism (AUC increased by 50%); use caution and monitor for potential hypotension.
Cyclosporine increases felodipine's serum concentration; avoid the combination or reduce dose of felodipine and monitor blood pressure.
CYP2C8 Substrates: Felodipine may increase the levels/effects of CYP2C8 substrates. Example substrates include amiodarone, paclitaxel, pioglitazone, repaglinide, and rosiglitazone.
CYP3A4 inducers: CYP3A4 inducers may decrease the levels/effects of felodipine. Example inducers include aminoglutethimide, carbamazepine, nafcillin, nevirapine, phenobarbital, phenytoin, and rifamycins.
CYP3A4 inhibitors: May increase the levels/effects of felodipine. Example inhibitors include azole antifungals, clarithromycin, diclofenac, doxycycline, erythromycin, imatinib, isoniazid, nefazodone, nicardipine, propofol, protease inhibitors, quinidine, telithromycin, and verapamil.

Erythromycin decreases felodipine's metabolism; coadministration results in a twofold increase in the AUC and half-life of felodipine; monitor for hypotension.

Nafcillin decreases plasma concentration of felodipine; avoid this combination.

Rifampin increases the metabolism of the calcium channel blocker; adjust the dose of the calcium channel blocker to maintain efficacy.

Sildenafil, tadalafil, vardenafil: Blood pressure-lowering effects may be additive; use caution.

Tacrolimus: Felodipine may increase tacrolimus serum levels; monitor.

Ethanol/Nutrition/Herb Interactions

Ethanol: Increases felodipine's absorption; watch for a greater hypotensive effect.

Food: Increased therapeutic and vasodilator side effects, including severe hypotension and myocardial ischemia, may occur if felodipine is taken with grapefruit juice; avoid concurrent use. High-fat/carbohydrate meals will increase C_{max} by 60%; grapefruit juice will increase C_{max} by twofold.

Herb/Nutraceutical: St John's wort may decrease felodipine levels. Avoid dong quai if using for hypertension (has estrogenic activity). Avoid ephedra, yohimbe, ginseng (may worsen hypertension). Avoid garlic (may have increased antihypertensive effect).

Mechanism of Action Inhibits calcium ions from entering the "slow channels" or select voltage-sensitive areas of vascular smooth muscle and myocardium during depolarization, producing a relaxation of coronary vascular smooth muscle and coronary vasodilation; increases myocardial oxygen delivery in patients with vasospastic angina

Pharmacodynamics Onset of action: 2-5 hours

Pharmacokinetics

Absorption: 98% to 100%

Protein bound: 99%

Metabolism: Hepatic

Bioavailability: Due to first-pass elimination, absolute bioavailability is ~20%

Time to peak serum concentrations: Oral: 2-5 hours

Dosage

Geriatrics: Oral: Initial 2.5 mg/day

Adults: Hypertension: Oral: 2.5-10 mg once daily; increase by 5 mg at 2-week intervals, as needed, to a maximum of 20 mg/day; usual dose range (JNC 7): 2.5-20 mg once daily.

Hepatic Impairment: Initial: 2.5 mg/day; monitor blood pressure

Administration Do not crush or chew extended release tablets; swallow whole.

Monitoring Parameters Heart rate, blood pressure

Reference Range None described

Patient Information Do not crush or chew tablets; do not discontinue abruptly; report any dizziness, shortness of breath, palpitations, or edema

Additional Information

The FDA's Cardiovascular and Renal Drug Advisory Committee reviewed current data regarding the risk of heart attacks in patients treated with calcium channel blockers and determined that as a class, the calcium channel antagonists are safe; however, they warned that short-acting nifedipine could increase the risk of myocardial infarction in some patients. The committee was in agreement with a statement issued September, 1995 by the National Heart Lung, and Blood Institute of the National Institute of Health, that warned that short-acting nifedipine should be used with great caution especially at higher doses.

Special Geriatric Considerations Elderly may experience a greater hypotensive response. Constipation may be more of a problem in the elderly. Calcium channel blockers are no more effective in the elderly than other therapies; however, they do not cause significant CNS effects which is an advantage over some antihypertensive agents.

Dosage Forms Excipient information presented when available (limited, particularly for generics); consult specific product labeling.

Tablet, extended release: 2.5 mg, 5 mg, 10 mg

Plendil®: 2.5 mg, 5 mg, 10 mg

Selected References

Chobanian AV, Bakris GL, Black HR, et al, "The Seventh Report of the Joint National Committee on Prevention, Detection, Evaluation, and Treatment of High Blood Pressure: The JNC 7 Report," *JAMA*, 2003, 289(19):2560-71.

♦ **Felodipine and Enalapril** *see* Enalapril and Felodipine *on page 506*

♦ **Femara®** *see* Letrozole *on page 882*

♦ **Fematrol [OTC]** *see* Bisacodyl *on page 173*

♦ **Femilax™ [OTC]** *see* Bisacodyl *on page 173*

♦ **Femiron® [OTC]** *see* Ferrous Fumarate *on page 618*

♦ **Femring®** *see* Estradiol *on page 549*

♦ **Femtrace®** *see* Estradiol *on page 549*

Fenofibrate (fen oh FYE brate)

Related Information
Hyperlipidemia Management *on page 1773*

U.S. Brand Names Antara™; Lipofen™; Lofibra™; TriCor®; Triglide™

Canadian Brand Names Apo-Fenofibrate®; Apo-Feno-Micro™; Dom-Fenofibrate Supra; Gen-Fenofibrate Micro; Lipidil EZ®; Lipidil Micro®; Lipidil Supra®; Novo-Fenofibrate; Novo-Fenofibrate-S; Nu-Fenofibrate; PHL-Fenofibrate Supra; PMS-Fenofibrate Micro; PMS-Fenofibrate Supra; ratio-Fenofibrate MC; Sandoz Fenofibrate S; TriCor®

Index Terms Procetofene; Proctofene

Generic Available Yes: Micronized capsule and tablet

Pharmacologic Category Antilipemic Agent, Fibric Acid

Use Adjunct to dietary therapy for the treatment of adults with very high elevations of serum triglyceride levels (types IV and V hyperlipidemia) who are at risk of pancreatitis and who do not respond adequately to a determined dietary effort; adjunct to dietary therapy for the reduction of low density lipoprotein cholesterol (LDL-C), total cholesterol (total-C), triglycerides, and apolipoprotein B (apo B) in adult patients with primary hypercholesterolemia or mixed dyslipidemia (Fredrickson types IIa and IIb)

Contraindications Hypersensitivity to fenofibrate or any component of the formulation; hepatic or severe renal dysfunction including primary biliary cirrhosis and unexplained persistent liver function abnormalities; pre-existing gallbladder disease

Warnings/Precautions Hepatic transaminases can become significantly elevated (dose-related); hepatocellular, chronic active, and cholestatic hepatitis have been reported. Regular monitoring of liver function tests is required. May cause cholelithiasis. Use caution with warfarin; adjustments in warfarin therapy may be required. Use caution with HMG-CoA reductase inhibitors (may lead to myopathy, rhabdomyolysis). Therapy should be withdrawn if an adequate response is not obtained after 2 months of therapy at the maximal daily dose. May cause mild to moderate decreases in hemoglobin, hematocrit and WBC upon initiation of therapy which usually stabilizes with long-term therapy. Rare hypersensitivity reactions may occur. Dose adjustment is required for renal impairment and elderly patients.

Adverse Reactions (Reflective of adult population; not specific for elderly)
>10%: Hepatic: ALT/AST increased (3% to 13%)

1% to 10%:
   Gastrointestinal: Abdominal pain (5%), constipation (2%)
   Neuromuscular & skeletal: Back pain (3%)
   Respiratory: Respiratory disorder (6%), rhinitis (2%)

Frequency not defined:
   Cardiovascular: Angina pectoris, arrhythmia, atrial fibrillation, cardiovascular disorder, chest pain, coronary artery disorder, edema, electrocardiogram abnormality, extrasystoles, hyper-/hypotension, MI, palpitation, peripheral edema, peripheral vascular disorder, phlebitis, tachycardia, varicose veins, vasodilatation
   Central nervous system: Anxiety, depression, dizziness, fever, headache, insomnia, malaise, nervousness, neuralgia, pain, somnolence, vertigo
   Dermatologic: Acne, alopecia, bruising, contact dermatitis, eczema, fungal dermatitis, maculopapular rash, nail disorder, photosensitivity reaction, pruritus, skin ulcer, Stevens-Johnson syndrome, toxic epidermal necrolysis, urticaria
   Endocrine & metabolic: Diabetes mellitus, gout, gynecomastia, hypoglycemia, hyperuricemia, libido decreased
   Gastrointestinal: Anorexia, appetite increased, colitis, diarrhea, dry mouth, duodenal ulcer, dyspepsia, eructation, esophagitis, flatulence, gastroenteritis, gastritis, gastrointestinal disorder, nausea, peptic ulcer, rectal disorder, rectal hemorrhage, tooth disorder, vomiting, weight gain/loss
   Genitourinary: Cystitis, dysuria, prostatic disorder, libido decreased, pregnancy (unintended), urinary frequency, urolithiasis, vaginal moniliasis
   Hematologic: Agranulocytosis, anemia, eosinophilia, leukopenia, lymphadenopathy, thrombocytopenia
   Hepatic: Cholelithiasis, cholecystitis, creatine phosphokinase increased, fatty liver deposits, liver function tests abnormal
   Neuromuscular & skeletal: Arthralgia, arthritis, arthrosis, bursitis, hypertonia, joint disorder, leg cramps, muscle pain, myalgia, myasthenia, myopathy, myositis, paresthesia, rhabdomyolysis, tenderness, tenosynovitis, weakness
   Ocular: Abnormal vision, amblyopia, cataract, conjunctivitis, eye disorder, refraction disorder
   Otic: Ear pain, otitis media
   Renal: Creatinine increased, kidney function abnormality
   Respiratory: Asthma, bronchitis, cough increased, dyspnea, laryngitis, pharyngitis, pneumonia, sinusitis

Miscellaneous: Allergic reaction, cyst, diaphoresis, hernia, herpes simplex, herpes zoster, hypersensitivity reaction, infection

Overdosage/Toxicology Symptoms include nausea, vomiting, diarrhea, and GI distress. Treatment is supportive. Hemodialysis has no effect on removal of fenofibric acid from the plasma.

Drug Interactions Substrate of CYP3A4 (minor); **Inhibits** CYP2A6 (weak), 2C8 (moderate), 2C9 (moderate), 2C19 (weak)

Bile acid sequestrants: May decrease absorption of fenofibrate; administer fenofibrate at least 1 hour before or 4-6 hours after a bile acid binding resin.

CYP2C8 substrates: Fenofibrate may increase the levels/effects of CYP2C8 substrates. Example substrates include amiodarone, paclitaxel, pioglitazone, repaglinide, and rosiglitazone.

CYP2C9 substrates: Fenofibrate may increase the levels/effects of CYP2C9 substrates. Example substrates include bosentan, dapsone, fluoxetine, glimepiride, glipizide, losartan, montelukast, nateglinide, paclitaxel, phenytoin, warfarin, and zafirlukast.

Ezetimibe: Fibric acid derivatives may increase serum concentrations of ezetimibe.

HMG-CoA reductase inhibitors (atorvastatin, fluvastatin, lovastatin, pravastatin, rosuvastatin, simvastatin): May increase the risk of myopathy and rhabdomyolysis. The manufacturer warns against concomitant use. However, combination therapy with statins has been used in some patients with resistant hyperlipidemias (with great caution). Current labeling of statins allows concurrent therapy, however, maximum statin dosages may be reasonably avoided.

Sulfonylureas: Fibric acid derivatives may enhance the hypoglycemic effects of sulfonylureas.

Warfarin: Increased anticoagulant response; monitor INRs closely when fenofibrate is initiated or discontinued.

Stability Store at 15°C to 30°C (59°F to 86°F). Protect from moisture.

Mechanism of Action Fenofibric acid is believed to increase VLDL catabolism by enhancing the synthesis of lipoprotein lipase; as a result of a decrease in VLDL levels, total plasma triglycerides are reduced by 30% to 60%; modest increase in HDL occurs in some hypertriglyceridemic patients

Pharmacokinetics

Absorption: Increased when taken with meals

Distribution: Widely to most tissues except brain or eye; concentrates in liver, kidneys, and gut

Protein binding: >99%

Metabolism: Tissue and plasma via esterases to active form, fenofibric acid; undergoes inactivation by glucuronidation hepatically or renally

Half-life elimination: 20-23 hours

Time to peak: 4-8 hours

Elimination: Urine (60% as metabolites); feces (25%); hemodialysis has no effect on removal of fenofibric acid from the plasma

Dosage

Geriatrics: Oral: Initial:
Antara™: 43 mg/day
Lipofen™: 50 mg/day
Lofibra™: 67 mg/day
TriCor®: 48 mg/day
Triglide™: 50 mg/day

Adults:

Hypertriglyceridemia: Oral: Initial:
Antara™: 43-130 mg/day
Lipofen™: 50-150 mg/day; maximum dose: 150 mg/day
Lofibra™: 67 mg/day with meals, up to 200 mg/day
TriCor®: 48 mg/day, up to 145 mg/day
Triglide™: 50-160 mg/day

Hypercholesterolemia or mixed hyperlipidemia: Oral:
Antara™: 130 mg/day
Lipofen™: 150 mg/day
Lofibra™: 200 mg/day with meals
TriCor®: 145 mg/day
Triglide™: 160 mg/day

Renal Impairment: Monitor renal function and lipid panel before adjusting. Decrease dose or increase dosing interval for patients with renal failure: Initial:
Antara™: 43 mg/day
Lipofen™: 50 mg/day
Lofibra™: 67 mg/day
TriCor®: 48 mg/day
Triglide™: 50 mg/day

Administration 6-8 weeks of therapy is required to determine efficacy.
(Continued)

Fenofibrate *(Continued)*

Lofibra™: Administer with meals.

Antara™, Lipofen™, TriCor®, Triglide™: May be administered with or without food.

Monitoring Parameters Periodic blood counts during first year of therapy. Total cholesterol, LDL-C, triglycerides, and HDL-C should be measured periodically; If only marginal changes are noted in 6-8 weeks, the drug should be discontinued. Monitor LFTs regularly and discontinue therapy if levels remain >3 times normal limits.

Patient Information Take with food. Do not change dosage without consulting prescriber. Maintain diet and exercise program as prescribed. You may experience mild GI disturbances (eg, gas, diarrhea, constipation, nausea); inform prescriber if these are severe. Report skin rash or irritation, insomnia, unusual muscle pain or tremors, or persistent dizziness.

Special Geriatric Considerations The definition of and, therefore, when to treat hyperlipidemia in 89 is a controversial issue. The National Cholesterol Education Program recommends that all adults maintain a plasma cholesterol <160 mg/dL. Older adults with one additional risk factor, goal LDL would be <130 mg/dL. It is the authors' belief that pharmacologic treatment be reserved for those who are unable to obtain a desirable plasma cholesterol concentration by diet alone and for whom the benefits of treatment are believed to outweigh the potential adverse effects, drug interactions, and cost of treatment.

Dosage Forms Excipient information presented when available (limited, particularly for generics); consult specific product labeling. [DSC] = Discontinued product

Capsule:

Lipofen™: 50 mg, 100 mg, 150 mg

Capsule [micronized]: 67 mg, 134 mg, 200 mg

Antara™: 43 mg, 87 mg [DSC], 130 mg

Lofibra™: 67 mg, 134 mg, 200 mg

Tablet: 54 mg, 160 mg

TriCor®: 48 mg, 145 mg

Triglide™: 50 mg, 160 mg

Fenoprofen *(fen oh PROE fen)*

Medication Safety Issues

Sound-alike/look-alike issues:

Fenoprofen may be confused with flurbiprofen

Nalfon® may be confused with Naldecon®

U.S. Brand Names Nalfon®

Canadian Brand Names Nalfon®

Index Terms Fenoprofen Calcium

Generic Available Yes: Tablet

Pharmacologic Category Nonsteroidal Anti-inflammatory Drug (NSAID), Oral

Use Symptomatic treatment of acute and chronic rheumatoid arthritis and osteoarthritis; relief of mild to moderate pain, sunburn; prophylaxis of migraine headache

Restrictions An FDA-approved medication guide must be distributed when dispensing an oral outpatient prescription (new or refill) where this medication is to be used without direct supervision of a healthcare provider. Medication guides are available at http://www.fda.gov/cder/Offices/ODS/medication_guides.htm.

Contraindications Hypersensitivity to fenoprofen, aspirin, or other NSAIDs, or any component of the formulation; perioperative pain in the setting of coronary artery bypass surgery (CABG); significant renal dysfunction

Warnings/Precautions [U.S. Boxed Warning]: NSAIDs are associated with an increased risk of adverse cardiovascular events, including MI, stroke, and new onset or worsening of pre-existing hypertension. Risk may be increased with duration of use or pre-existing cardiovascular risk factors or disease. Carefully evaluate individual cardiovascular risk profiles prior to prescribing. Use caution with fluid retention, CHF, or hypertension. Concurrent administration of ibuprofen, and potentially other nonselective NSAIDs, may interfere with aspirin's cardioprotective effect.

Use of NSAIDs can compromise existing renal function. Renal toxicity can occur in patient with impaired renal function, dehydration, heart failure, liver dysfunction, those taking diuretics and ACEI, and the elderly. Rehydrate patient before starting therapy. Monitor renal function closely. Not recommended for use in patients with advanced renal disease.

[U.S. Boxed Warning]: NSAIDs may increase risk of gastrointestinal irritation, ulceration, bleeding, and perforation. These events may occur at any time during therapy and without warning. Use caution with a history of GI disease (bleeding or ulcers), concurrent therapy with aspirin, anticoagulants and/or corticosteroids, smoking, use of alcohol, the elderly or debilitated patients.

Use the lowest effective dose for the shortest duration of time, consistent with individual patient goals, to reduce risk of cardiovascular or GI adverse events. Alternate therapies should be considered for patients at high risk.

NSAIDs may cause serious skin adverse events including exfoliative dermatitis, Stevens-Johnson syndrome (SJS), and toxic epidermal necrolysis (TEN). Anaphylactoid reactions may occur, even without prior exposure; patients with "aspirin triad" (bronchial asthma, aspirin intolerance, rhinitis) may be at increased risk. Do not use in patients who experience bronchospasm, asthma, rhinitis, or urticaria with NSAID or aspirin therapy. Use caution in other forms of asthma.

Use with caution in patients with decreased hepatic function. Closely monitor patients with any abnormal LFT. Severe hepatic reactions (eg, fulminant hepatitis, liver failure) have occurred with NSAID use, rarely; discontinue if signs or symptoms of liver disease develop, or if systemic manifestations occur.

The elderly are at increased risk for adverse effects (especially peptic ulceration, CNS effects, renal toxicity) from NSAIDs even at low doses.

Withhold for at least 4-6 half-lives prior to surgical or dental procedures.

Adverse Reactions (Reflective of adult population; not specific for elderly)
>10%:
    Central nervous system: Dizziness (7% to 15%), somnolence (9% to 15%)
    Gastrointestinal: Abdominal cramps (2% to 4%), heartburn, indigestion, nausea (8% to 14%), dyspepsia (10% to 14%), flatulence (14%), anorexia (14%), constipation (7% to 14%), occult blood in stool (14%), vomiting (3% to 14%), diarrhea (2% to 14%)
1% to 10%:
    Central nervous system: Headache (9%)
    Dermatologic: Itching
    Endocrine & metabolic: Fluid retention

Overdosage/Toxicology Symptoms include acute renal failure, vomiting, drowsiness, and leukocytosis. Management of nonsteroidal anti-inflammatory drug (NSAID) intoxication is primarily supportive and symptomatic. Fluid therapy is commonly effective in managing hypotension that may occur following an acute NSAID overdose, except when due to acute blood loss.

Drug Interactions
    ACE inhibitors: Antihypertensive effects may be decreased by concurrent therapy with NSAIDs; monitor blood pressure.
    Angiotensin II antagonists: Antihypertensive effects may be decreased by concurrent therapy with NSAIDs; monitor blood pressure.
    Anticoagulants (warfarin, heparin, LMWHs) in combination with NSAIDs can cause increased risk of bleeding.
    Antiplatelet drugs (ticlopidine, clopidogrel, aspirin, abciximab, dipyridamole, eptifibatide, tirofiban) can cause an increased risk of bleeding.
    Beta-blockers: NSAIDs may decrease the antihypertensive effect of beta-blockers. Monitor.
    Cholestyramine (and other bile acid sequestrants): May decrease the absorption of NSAIDs. Separate by at least 2 hours.
    Corticosteroids may increase the risk of GI ulceration; avoid concurrent use.
    Cyclosporine: NSAIDs may increase serum creatinine, potassium, blood pressure, and cyclosporine levels; monitor cyclosporine levels and renal function carefully.
    Fluoroquinolone antibiotics: Risk of seizures may be increased with concomitant quinolone use. Risk is considered quite low and may only be a factor with high serum levels of either agent and/or in patients with additional predisposing factors (eg, renal dysfunction, history of seizure or other neurological disorder).
    Gentamicin and amikacin serum concentrations are increased by indomethacin in premature infants. Results may apply to other aminoglycosides and NSAIDs.
    Hydralazine's antihypertensive effect is decreased; avoid concurrent use.
    Lithium levels can be increased; avoid concurrent use if possible or monitor lithium levels and adjust dose. Sulindac may have the least effect. When NSAID is stopped, lithium will need adjustment again.
    Loop diuretics efficacy (diuretic and antihypertensive effect) is reduced. Indomethacin reduces this efficacy, however, it may be anticipated with any NSAID.
    Methotrexate: Severe bone marrow suppression, aplastic anemia, and GI toxicity have been reported with concomitant NSAID therapy. Avoid use during moderate or high-dose methotrexate (increased and prolonged methotrexate levels). NSAID use during low-dose treatment of rheumatoid arthritis has not been fully evaluated; extreme caution is warranted.
    Salicylates: NSAIDs (nonselective) may diminish the cardioprotective effect of acetylated salicylates. Avoid regular use of NSAIDs if possible; consider alternatives (eg, acetaminophen). Give salicylate before NSAID; for example ibuprofen should be given 30-120 minutes after aspirin.
(Continued)

Fenoprofen *(Continued)*

Thiazide efficacy (diuretic and antihypertensive effect) may be reduced. Indomethacin may reduce this efficacy and it may be anticipated with any NSAID.

Verapamil plasma concentration is decreased by diclofenac; avoid concurrent use.

Warfarin's INRs may be increased by piroxicam. Other NSAIDs may have the same effect depending on dose and duration. Monitor INR closely. Use the lowest dose of NSAIDs possible and for the briefest duration.

Ethanol/Nutrition/Herb Interactions

Ethanol: Avoid ethanol (may enhance gastric mucosal irritation).

Food: Fenoprofen peak serum levels may be decreased if taken with food.

Herb/Nutraceutical: Avoid alfalfa, anise, bilberry, bladderwrack, bromelain, cat's claw, celery, coleus, cordyceps, dong quai, evening primrose, feverfew, fenugreek, garlic, ginger, ginkgo biloba, red clover, horse chestnut, grapeseed, green tea, ginseng, guggul, horse chestnut seed, horseradish, licorice, prickly ash, red clover, reishi, SAMe, sweet clover, turmeric, white willow (all have additional antiplatelet activity).

Mechanism of Action Inhibits prostaglandin synthesis by decreasing the activity of the enzyme, cyclooxygenase, which results in decreased formation of prostaglandin precursors

Pharmacodynamics

Onset of anti-inflammatory action: 2 days

Maximum response: 2-3 weeks

Pharmacokinetics

Absorption: Rapid (to 80%) from upper GI tract

Protein binding: 99%

Metabolism: Extensive in the liver

Half-life: 2.5-3 hours

Time to peak serum concentration: Within 1-2 hours

Elimination: In urine 2% to 5% as unchanged drug; small amounts appear in feces

Dosage

Geriatrics & Adults:

Rheumatoid arthritis and osteoarthritis: Oral: 300-600 mg 3-4 times/day up to 3.2 g/day

Mild to moderate pain: Oral: 200 mg every 4-6 hours as needed

Renal Impairment: Not recommended in patients with advanced renal disease.

Monitoring Parameters Monitor response (pain, range of motion, grip strength, mobility, ADL function), inflammation; observe for weight gain, edema; monitor renal function; observe for bleeding, bruising; evaluate gastrointestinal effects (abdominal pain, bleeding, dyspepsia); mental confusion, disorientation, CBC, serum, creatinine, BUN, liver function tests

Reference Range Therapeutic: 20-65 mcg/mL (SI: 82-268 μmol/L)

Test Interactions Increased chloride (S), increased sodium (S)

Patient Information Serious gastrointestinal bleeding can occur as well as ulceration and perforation. Pain may or may not be present. Avoid aspirin and aspirin-containing products while taking this medication. If gastric upset occurs, take with food, milk, or antacid. If gastric adverse effects persist, contact physician. May cause drowsiness, dizziness, blurred vision, and confusion. Use caution when performing tasks which require alertness (eg, driving). Do not take for more than 3 days for fever or 10 days for pain without physician advice.

Additional Information There are no clinical guidelines to predict which NSAID will give response in a particular patient. Trials with each must be initiated until response determined. Consider dose, patient convenience, and cost.

Special Geriatric Considerations Elderly are a high-risk population for adverse effects from NSAIDs. As much as 60% of elderly can develop peptic ulceration and/or hemorrhage asymptomatically. The concomitant use of H_2 blockers and sucralfate is not effective as prophylaxis with the exception of NSAID-induced duodenal ulcers which may be prevented by the use of ranitidine. Misoprostol and proton pump inhibitors are the only agents proven to help prevent the development of NSAID-induced ulcers. Also, concomitant disease and drug use contribute to the risk for GI adverse effects. Use lowest effective dose for shortest period possible. Consider renal function decline with age. Use of NSAIDs can compromise existing renal function especially when Cl_{cr} is ≤30 mL/minute. Tinnitus may be a difficult and unreliable indication of toxicity due to age-related hearing loss or eighth cranial nerve damage. CNS adverse effects such as confusion, agitation, and hallucination are generally seen in overdose or high-dose situations, but elderly may demonstrate these adverse effects at lower doses than younger adults.

Dosage Forms Excipient information presented when available (limited, particularly for generics); consult specific product labeling.

Capsule, as calcium (Nalfon®): 200 mg, 300 mg

Tablet, as calcium: 600 mg

Selected References

Brooks PM and Day RO, "Nonsteroidal Anti-inflammatory Drugs - Differences and Similarities," *N Engl J Med*, 1991, 324(24):1716-25.

Clinch D, Banerjee AK, and Ostick G, "Absence of Abdominal Pain in Elderly Patients With Peptic Ulcer," *Age Ageing*, 1984, 13(2):120-3.

Clive DM and Stoff JS, "Renal Syndromes Associated With Nonsteroidal Anti-inflammatory Drugs," *N Engl J Med*, 1984, 310(9):563-72.

Graham DY, "Prevention of Gastroduodenal Injury Induced by Chronic Nonsteroidal Anti-inflammatory Drug Therapy," *Gastroenterology*, 1989, 96(2 Pt 2 Suppl):675-81.

Gurwitz JH, Avorn J, Ross-Degnan D, et al, "Nonsteroidal Anti-inflammatory Drug-Associated Azotemia in the Very Old," *JAMA*, 1990, 264(4):471-5.

Hawkey CJ, Karrasch JA, Szczepañski L, et al, "Omeprazole Compared With Misoprostol for Ulcers Associated With Nonsteroidal Anti-inflammatory Drugs," *N Engl J Med*, 1998, 338(11):727-34.

Knodel LC, "Preventing NSAID-induced Ulcers: The Role of Misoprostol," *Consult Pharm*, 1989, 4:37-41.

Pounder R, "Silent Peptic Ulceration: Deadly Silence or Golden Silence?" *Gastroenterology*, 1989, 96(2 Pt 2 Suppl):626-31.

Yeomans ND, Tulassay Z, Juhasz L, et al, "A Comparison of Omeprazole With Ranitidine for Ulcers Associated With Nonsteroidal Anti-inflammatory Drugs," *N Engl J Med*, 1998, 338(11):719-26.

♦ **Fenoprofen Calcium** *see Fenoprofen on page 606*

Fentanyl (FEN ta nil)

Related Information
Narcotic / Opioid Analgesics *on page 1763*

Medication Safety Issues
Sound-alike/look-alike issues:
Fentanyl may be confused with alfentanil, sufentanil

Dosing of transdermal fentanyl patches may be confusing. Transdermal fentanyl patches should always be prescribed in mcg/hour, not size.

High alert medication: The Institute for Safe Medication Practices (ISMP) includes this medication among its list of drugs which have a heightened risk of causing significant patient harm when used in error.

New patch dosage form of Duragesic®-12 actually delivers 12.5 mcg/hour of fentanyl. Use caution, as orders may be written as "Duragesic 12.5" which can be erroneously interpreted as a 125 mcg dose.

Iontophoretic transdermal system (Ionsys™) may contain conducting metal (eg, aluminum); remove patch prior to MRI. Transdermal patch (eg, Duragesic®) does not contain any metal-based compounds; however, the printed ink used to indicate strength on the outer surface of the patch does contain titanium dioxide, but the amount is minimal.

U.S. Brand Names Actiq®; Duragesic®; Fentora™; Ionsys™; Sublimaze®

Canadian Brand Names Actiq®; Duragesic®; Fentanyl Citrate Injection, USP

Index Terms Fentanyl Citrate; Fentanyl Hydrochloride; OTFC (Oral Transmucosal Fentanyl Citrate)

Generic Available Yes: Excludes buccal tablet and iontophoretic transdermal system

Pharmacologic Category Analgesic, Opioid; General Anesthetic

Use
Injection: Sedation, relief of pain, preoperative medication, adjunct to general or regional anesthesia
Iontophoretic transdermal system (Ionsys™): Short-term in-hospital management of acute postoperative pain
Transdermal patch (eg, Duragesic®): Management of moderate-to-severe chronic pain
Transmucosal lozenge (eg, Actiq®), buccal tablet (Fentora™): Management of breakthrough cancer pain

Restrictions C-II
An FDA-approved medication guide for buccal tablet (Fentora™) and transmucosal lozenge (eg, Actiq®) must be distributed when dispensing an outpatient prescription (new or refill) where this medication is to be used without direct supervision of a healthcare provider. Medication guides are available at http://www.fda.gov/cder/Offices/ODS/medication_guides.htm.

Contraindications Hypersensitivity to fentanyl or any component of the formulation; increased intracranial pressure; severe respiratory disease or depression including acute asthma (unless patient is mechanically ventilated); paralytic ileus; severe liver or renal insufficiency

Iontophoretic transdermal system (Ionsys™): Hypersensitivity to fentanyl, cetylpyridinium chloride (eg, Cepacol®) or any component of Ionsys™ system

Transmucosal buccal tablets (Fentora™), lozenges (eg, Actiq®), and/or transdermal patches (eg, Duragesic®) are recommended for use only in patients who are opioid-tolerant. Patients are considered opioid-tolerant if they are taking at least 60 mg morphine/day, 30 mg oral oxycodone/day, 8 mg oral hydromorphone/day, 25 mcg (Continued)

Fentanyl *(Continued)*

transdermal fentanyl/hour, or an equivalent dose of another opioid for ≥1 week. Transmucosal buccal tablets (Fentora™), lozenges (eg, Actiq®), and transdermal patches (eg, Duragesic®) are not for use in acute pain, mild pain, intermittent pain, or postoperative pain management.

Warnings/Precautions An opioid-containing analgesic regimen should be tailored to each patient's needs and based upon the type of pain being treated (acute versus chronic), the route of administration, degree of tolerance for opioids (naive versus chronic user), age, weight, and medical condition. The optimal analgesic dose varies widely among patients. Doses should be titrated to pain relief/prevention. When using with other CNS depressants, reduce dose of one or both agents. Fentanyl shares the toxic potentials of opiate agonists, and precautions of opiate agonist therapy should be observed; use with caution in patients with bradycardia; rapid I.V. infusion may result in skeletal muscle and chest wall rigidity leading to respiratory distress and/or apnea, bronchoconstriction, laryngospasm; inject slowly over 3-5 minutes. Tolerance or drug dependence may result from extended use. Use caution in patients with a history of drug dependence or abuse. The elderly may be particularly susceptible to the CNS depressant and constipating effects of narcotics. Use extreme caution in patients with COPD or other chronic respiratory conditions. Use caution with head injuries, morbid obesity, or hepatic dysfunction. **[U.S. Boxed Warning]: Use with strong or moderate CYP3A4 inhibitors may result in increased effects and potential respiratory depression.** Concurrent use of agonist/antagonist analgesics may precipitate withdrawal symptoms and/or reduced analgesic efficacy in patients following prolonged therapy with mu opioid agonists. Abrupt discontinuation following prolonged use may also lead to withdrawal symptoms. Opioid-nontolerant patients should not receive some formulations/strengths of fentanyl, including buccal tablets (Fentora™), lozenges (Actiq®), or transdermal patches.

Transmucosal: Lozenge (eg, Actiq®), buccal tablet (Fentora™): **[U.S. Boxed Warning]: Do not substitute Fentora™ on a mcg-per-mcg basis when converting from transmucosal lozenge to buccal tablet. Buccal tablet has higher bioavailability. [U.S. Boxed Warning]: Should be used only for the care of opioid-tolerant cancer patients.** Not approved for use in management of acute or postoperative pain. **[U.S. Boxed Warning]: Buccal tablet and lozenge contain an amount of medication that can be fatal to children.** Keep all units out of the reach of children and discard any open units properly.

Transdermal patches (eg, Duragesic®): **[U.S. Boxed Warning]: Serious or life-threatening hypoventilation may occur, even in opioid-tolerant patients.** Serum fentanyl concentrations may increase approximately one-third for patients with a body temperature of 40°C secondary to a temperature-dependent increase in fentanyl release from the patch and increased skin permeability. Avoid exposure of application site to direct external heat sources. Patients who experience adverse reactions should be monitored for at least 24 hours after removal of the patch. Transdermal patch does not contain any metal-based compounds; the printed ink used to indicate strength on the outer surface of the patch does contain titanium dioxide but the amount is minimal; adverse events have not been reported while wearing during an MRI.

Iontophoretic transdermal system (Ionsys™): **[U.S. Boxed Warning]: Should only be used for the treatment of hospitalized patients. To avoid overdose, the patient should be the only one to activate the system. Unintended exposure to fentanyl hydrogel could lead to absorption of fatal dose; hydrogel should not come in contact with fingers or mouth.** Should be used only in patients who are able to understand and follow instructions to operate the system. Use caution in patients who have high frequency hearing impairment. Remove prior to MRI procedure, cardioversion, or defibrillation. May interfere with radiographic image or CAT scan. Patients on chronic opioids or with a history of opioid abuse may require higher analgesic doses than Ionsys™ is able to provide. Prior to patient's hospital discharge, the system must be removed and disposed of. **[U.S. Boxed Warning]: A significant amount of fentanyl remains in the iontophoretic transdermal system and requires proper removal and disposal to avoid misuse, abuse, or diversion.**

Adverse Reactions (Reflective of adult population; not specific for elderly)

>10%:
  Cardiovascular: Hypotension, bradycardia
  Central nervous system: CNS depression, confusion, drowsiness, sedation
  Gastrointestinal: Nausea, vomiting, constipation, xerostomia
  Local: Application-site reaction (iontophoretic system 14%)
  Neuromuscular & skeletal: Chest wall rigidity (high dose I.V.), weakness
  Ocular: Miosis
  Respiratory: Respiratory depression
  Miscellaneous: Diaphoresis

1% to 10%:
  Cardiovascular: Cardiac arrhythmia, edema, orthostatic hypotension, hypertension, syncope, tachycardia
  Central nervous system: Abnormal dreams, abnormal thinking, agitation, amnesia, anxiety, dizziness, euphoria, fatigue, fever, hallucinations, headache, insomnia, nervousness, paranoid reaction
  Dermatologic: Erythema, papules, pruritus (iontophoretic system 6%), rash
  Gastrointestinal: Abdominal pain, anorexia, biliary tract spasm, diarrhea, dyspepsia, flatulence, ileus
  Genitourinary: Urinary retention (iontophoretic transdermal system 3%)
  Hematologic: Anemia
  Local: Application site reactions (buccal tablet)
  Neuromuscular & skeletal: Abnormal coordination, abnormal gait, back pain, paresthesia, rigors, tremor
  Respiratory: Apnea, bronchitis, dyspnea, hemoptysis, hypoxia, pharyngitis, rhinitis, sinusitis, upper respiratory infection
  Miscellaneous: Hiccups, flu-like syndrome, speech disorder

Overdosage/Toxicology Symptoms of overdose include CNS depression, respiratory depression, and miosis; muscle and chest wall rigidity (may require nondepolarizing skeletal muscle relaxant). Treatment is symptom-directed and supportive. If overdose from transdermal patch (eg, Duragesic®), remove system from patient's skin. Naloxone, 2 mg I.V. with repeat administration as necessary up to a total of 10 mg, can also be used to reverse toxic effects of the opiate. Use of an opioid antagonist can precipitate withdrawal in opioid-tolerant patients. Patients who experience adverse reactions during use of transdermal patch (eg, Duragesic®) should be monitored for at least 24 hours after removal of the patch.

Drug Interactions Substrate of CYP3A4 (major); **Inhibits** CYP3A4 (weak)
  Ammonium chloride: May increase the excretion of analgesics (opioid).
  Antipsychotic agents (phenothiazines): May enhance the hypotensive effect of analgesics (opioid).
  CNS depressants: Increased sedation with fentanyl; monitor closely.
  CYP3A4 inhibitors: May increase the levels/effects of fentanyl. Potentially fatal respiratory depression may occur when a potent inhibitor is used in a patient receiving chronic fentanyl (eg, transdermal patch). Example inhibitors include azole antifungals, clarithromycin, diclofenac, doxycycline, erythromycin, imatinib, isoniazid, nefazodone, nicardipine, propofol, protease inhibitors, quinidine, telithromycin, and verapamil.
  MAO inhibitors: Not recommended to use Actiq® within 14 days. Severe and unpredictable potentiation by MAO inhibitors has been reported with opioid analgesics.
  Pegvisomant: Analgesics (opioid) may diminish the therapeutic effect of pegvisomant.
  Protease inhibitors: May decrease the metabolism, via CYP isoenzymes, of fentanyl.
  Rifamycin derivatives: May decrease the serum concentration of fentanyl.
  Selective serotonin reuptake inhibitors (SSRIs): Analgesics (opioid) may enhance the serotonergic effect of SSRIs. This may cause serotonin syndrome.
  Sibutramine: Fentanyl may enhance the serotonergic effect of sibutramine.

Ethanol/Nutrition/Herb Interactions
  Ethanol: Avoid ethanol (may increase CNS depression).
  Food: Glucose may cause hyperglycemia.
  Herb/Nutraceutical: St John's wort may decrease fentanyl levels. Avoid valerian, St John's wort, kava kava, gotu kola (may increase CNS depression).

Stability
  Injection formulation: Store at controlled room temperature of 15°C to 25°C (59°F to 86°F). Protect from light.
  Iontophoretic transdermal system: Store at 15°C to 30°C (59°F to 86°F).
  Transdermal patch: Do not store above 25°C (77°F).
  Transmucosal (buccal tablets, lozenges): Store at controlled room temperature of 15°C to 30°C (59°F to 86°F). Protect from freezing and moisture.

Mechanism of Action Binds with stereospecific receptors at many sites within the CNS, increases pain threshold, alters pain reception, inhibits ascending pain pathways

Pharmacodynamics
  Onset of action: Analgesic: I.M.: 7-15 minutes; I.V.: Almost immediate; Transmucosal: 5-15 minutes
  Peak effect: Transmucosal: Analgesic: 15-30 minutes
  Duration: I.M.: 1-2 hours; I.V.: 0.5-1 hour; Transmucosal: Related to blood level; respiratory depressant effect may last longer than analgesic effect

Pharmacokinetics
  Absorption:
    Transmucosal, buccal tablet: Rapid, ~50% from the buccal mucosa; remaining 50% swallowed with saliva and slowly absorbed from GI tract.
    Transmucosal, lozenge: Rapid, ~25% from the buccal mucosa; 75% swallowed with saliva and slowly absorbed from GI tract
(Continued)

Fentanyl *(Continued)*

Iontophoretic transdermal system (Ionsys™): Fentanyl levels continue to rise for 5 minutes after the completion of each 10-minute dose

Distribution: Highly lipophilic, redistributes into muscle and fat

Protein binding: 80% to 85%

Metabolism: Hepatic, primarily via CYP3A4

Bioavailability: Total (transmucosal and GI absorption): Buccal: 65% (range: 45% to 85%); Lozenge: 47% (range: 37% to 57%)

Half-life elimination:

I.V.: 2-4 hours

Iontophoretic transdermal system (Ionsys™): 11 hours

Transdermal patch: 17 hours (half-life is influenced by absorption rate)

Transmucosal: Lozenge: 7 hours; Buccal tablet: 100-200 mcg: 3-4 hours, 400-800 mcg: 11-12 hours

Time to peak: Buccal tablet: 46 minutes; Lozenge: ~91 minutes; Transdermal patch: 24-72 hours

Excretion: Urine (primarily as metabolites, <7% to 10% as unchanged drug)

Dosage

Geriatrics: Elderly have been found to be twice as sensitive as younger patients to the effects of fentanyl. A wide range of doses may be used. When choosing a dose, take into consideration the following patient factors: age, weight, physical status, underlying disease states, other drugs used, type of anesthesia used, and the surgical procedure to be performed.

Transmucosal lozenge (eg, Actiq®): Dose should be reduced to 2.5-5 mcg/kg. Suck on lozenge vigorously approximately 20-40 minutes before the start of procedure.

Adults: Note: These are guidelines and do not represent the maximum doses that may be required in all patients. Doses should be titrated to pain relief/prevention. Monitor vital signs routinely. Single I.M. doses have a duration of 1-2 hours, single I.V. doses last 0.5-1 hour.

Sedation for minor procedures/analgesia: I.V.: 25-50 mcg; may repeat every 3-5 minutes to desired effect or adverse event; maximum dose of 500 mcg/4 hours; higher doses are used for major procedures

Surgery:

Premedication: I.M., slow I.V.: 25-100 mcg/dose 30-60 minutes prior to surgery

Adjunct to regional anesthesia: Slow I.V.: 25-100 mcg/dose over 1-2 minutes. **Note:** An I.V. should be in place with regional anesthesia so the I.M. route is rarely used but still maintained as an option in the package labeling.

Adjunct to general anesthesia: Slow I.V.:

Low dose: 0.5-2 mcg/kg/dose depending on the indication. For example, 0.5 mcg/kg will provide analgesia or reduce the amount of propofol needed for laryngeal mask airway insertion with minimal respiratory depression. However, to blunt the hemodynamic response to intubation 2 mcg/kg is often necessary.

Moderate dose: Initial: 2-15 mcg/kg/dose; maintenance (bolus or infusion): 1-2 mcg/kg/hour. Discontinuing fentanyl infusion 30-60 minutes prior to the end of surgery will usually allow adequate ventilation upon emergence from anesthesia. For "fast-tracking" and early extubation following major surgery, total fentanyl doses are limited to 10-15 mcg/kg.

High dose: **Note:** High-dose (20-50 mcg/kg/dose) fentanyl is rarely used, but is still maintained in the package labeling.

Acute pain management:

Severe: I.M, I.V.: 50-100 mcg/dose every 1-2 hours as needed; patients with prior opiate exposure may tolerate higher initial doses

Patient-controlled analgesia (PCA): I.V.: Usual concentration: 10 mcg/mL

Demand dose: Usual: 10 mcg; range: 10-50 mcg

Lockout interval: 5-8 minutes

Mechanically-ventilated patients (based on 70 kg patient): Slow I.V.: 0.35-1.5 mcg/kg every 30-60 minutes as needed; infusion: 0.7-10 mcg/kg/hour

Iontophoretic transdermal: 40 mcg per activation on-demand (maximum: 6 doses/hour). **Note:** Patient's pain should be controlled prior to initiating system. Instruct patient how to operate system. Only the patient should initiate system. Each system operates for 24 hours or until 80 doses have been administered, whichever comes first.

Breakthrough cancer pain: For patients who are tolerant to and currently receiving opioid therapy for persistent cancer pain; dosing should be individually titrated to provide adequate analgesia with minimal side effects. Dose titration should be done if patient requires more than 1 dose/breakthrough pain episode for several consecutive episodes. Patients experiencing >4 breakthrough pain episodes/day should have the dose of their long-term opioid re-evaluated.

Lozenge: Initial dose: 200 mcg; the second dose may be started 15 minutes after completion of the first dose. Consumption should be limited to ≤4 units/day.

Buccal tablet (Fentora™): Initial dose: 100 mcg; a second 100 mcg dose, if needed, may be started 30 minutes after the start of the first dose.

Dose titration, if required, should be done using multiples of the 100 mcg tablets. Patient can take two 100 mcg tablets (one on each side of mouth). If that dose is not successful, can use four 100 mcg tablets (two on each side of mouth). If titration requires >400 mcg/dose, then use 200 mcg tablets.

Conversion from lozenge to buccal tablet (Fentora™):

Lozenge dose 200-400 mcg, then buccal tablet 100 mcg

Lozenge dose 600-800 mcg, then buccal tablet 200 mcg

Lozenge dose 1200 mcg, then buccal tablet 400 mcg

Note: Four 100 mcg buccal tablets deliver approximately 12% and 13% higher values of C_{max} and AUC, respectively, compared to one 400 mcg buccal tablet. To prevent confusion, patient should only have one strength available at a time. Using more than four buccal tablets at a time has not been studied.

Chronic pain management: Opioid-tolerant patients: Transdermal patch (eg, Duragesic®):

Initial: To convert patients from oral or parenteral opioids to transdermal formulation, a 24-hour analgesic requirement should be calculated (based on prior opiate use). Using the tables, the appropriate initial dose can be determined. The initial fentanyl dosage may be approximated from the 24-hour morphine dosage and titrated to minimize adverse effects and provide analgesia. With the initial application, the absorption of transdermal fentanyl requires several hours to reach plateau; therefore transdermal fentanyl is inappropriate for management of acute pain. Change patch every 72 hours.

Conversion from continuous infusion of fentanyl: In patients who have adequate pain relief with a fentanyl infusion, fentanyl may be converted to transdermal dosing at a rate equivalent to the intravenous rate. A two-step taper of the infusion to be completed over 12 hours has been recommended (Kornick, 2001) after the patch is applied. The infusion is decreased to 50% of the original rate six hours after the application of the first patch, and subsequently discontinued twelve hours after application.

Titration: Short-acting agents may be required until analgesic efficacy is established and/or as supplements for "breakthrough" pain. The amount of supplemental doses should be closely monitored. Appropriate dosage increases may be based on daily supplemental dosage using the ratio of 45 mg/24 hours of oral morphine to a 12.5 mcg/hour increase in fentanyl dosage.

Frequency of adjustment: The dosage should not be titrated more frequently than every 3 days after the initial dose or every 6 days thereafter. Patients should wear a consistent fentanyl dosage through two applications (6 days) before dosage increase based on supplemental opiate dosages can be estimated.

Frequency of application: The majority of patients may be controlled on every 72-hour administration; however, a small number of patients require every 48-hour administration.

Dose conversion guidelines for transdermal fentanyl[1] (see tables below and on next pages).

Hepatic Impairment: Fentanyl kinetics may be altered in hepatic disease.

Recommended Initial Duragesic® Dose Based Upon Daily Oral Morphine Dose[1]

Oral 24-Hour Morphine (mg/d)	Duragesic® Dose (mcg/h)
60-134	25
135-224	50
225-314	75
315-404	100
405-494	125
495-584	150
585-674	175
675-764	200
765-854	225
855-944	250
945-1034	275
1035-1124	300

[1]The table should NOT be used to convert from transdermal fentanyl to other opioid analgesics. Rather, following removal of the patch, titrate the dose of the new opioid until adequate analgesia is achieved.

(Continued)

Fentanyl *(Continued)*

Opioid Analgesics Initial Oral Dosing Commonly Used for Severe Pain

Drug	Equianalgesic Dose (mg) Oral[1]	Equianalgesic Dose (mg) Parenteral[2]	Initial Oral Dose Adults (mg)
Buprenorphine	—	0.4	—
Butorphanol	—	2	—
Hydromorphone	7.5	1.5	4-8
Levorphanol	4 (acute) 1 (chronic)	2 (acute) 1 (chronic)	2-4
Meperidine	300	75	Not Recommended
Methadone	10	5	0.2
Morphine	30	10	15-30
Nalbuphine	—	10	—
Pentazocine	50	30	—
Oxycodone	20	—	10-20
Oxymorphone	1	—	—

From "Principles of Analgesic Use in the Treatment of Acute Pain and Cancer Pain," *Am Pain Soc*, Fifth Ed.

[1]Elderly: Starting dose should be lower for this population group

[2]Standard parenteral doses for acute pain in adults; can be used to doses for I.V. infusions and repeated small I.V. boluses. Single I.V. boluses, use half the I.M. dose.

Administration

I.V.: Muscular rigidity may occur with rapid I.V. administration.

Transdermal patch (eg, Duragesic®): Apply to nonirritated and nonirradiated skin, such as chest, back, flank, or upper arm. Do not shave skin; hair at application site should be clipped. Prior to application, clean site with clear water and allow to dry completely. Do not use damaged or cut patches; a rapid release of fentanyl and increased systemic absorption may occur. Firmly press in place and hold for 30 seconds. Change patch every 72 hours. Do **not** use soap, alcohol, or other solvents to remove transdermal gel if it accidentally touches skin; use copious amounts of water. Avoid exposing application site to external heat sources (eg, heating pad, electric blanket, heat lamp, hot tub).

Iontophoretic transdermal system: System should be tested and applied by healthcare professional. The sticker on the back of the pouch is intended for use by the registered nurse. The sticker should be removed and applied to the Ionsys™ system with a date and time of application so that subsequent healthcare providers will know when the system expires (24 hours after application). Apply to intact, nonirritated, nonirradiated skin on chest or upper outer arm. Do not apply to scarred, burned, or tattooed areas. Any excessive hair at application site should be clipped; do not shave. Remove clear, plastic release liner before placement on skin. Avoid pulling on red tab. To administer a dose, the patient must press the button twice firmly within 3 seconds. An audible tone (beep) indicates the start of the delivery of the dose; red light remains on throughout the 10-minute dosing period. Each system operates for 24 hours or until 80 doses have been used (whichever comes first). Rotate skin site if another system is required after the first one is finished. Do not touch sticky side of system or the gels. If the hydrogel (where fentanyl is housed) becomes separated from the delivery system during removal, use gloves or tweezers to remove the hydrogel from skin. Do not use soap, alcohol, or other solvents to remove the hydrogel as they can increase absorption of fentanyl. Once a system has been removed, the same system can not be reapplied. Contains metal; remove prior to MRi procedure, cardioversion, or defibrillation.

Lozenge: Foil overwrap should be removed just prior to administration. Place the unit in mouth and allow it to dissolve. Do not chew. Lozenge may be moved from one side of the mouth to the other. The unit should be consumed over a period of 15 minutes. Handle should be removed after it is consumed or if patient has achieved an adequate response and/or shows signs of respiratory depression.

Buccal tablet: Patient should not open blister until ready to administer. The blister backing should be peeled back to expose the tablet; tablet should not be pushed out through the blister. Immediately use tablet once removed from blister. Place entire tablet in the buccal cavity (above a rear molar, between the upper cheek and gum). Tablet should not be broken, sucked, chewed, or swallowed. Should dissolve in about 14-25 minutes when left between the cheek and the gum. If remnants remain they may be swallowed with water.

Dosing Conversion Guidelines[1,2]

Current Analgesic	Daily Dosage (mg/day)			
Morphine (I.M./I.V.)	10-22	23-37	38-52	53-67
Oxycodone (oral)	30-67	67.5-112	112.5-157	157.5-202
Oxycodone (I.M./I.V.)	15-33	33.1-56	56.1-78	78.1-101
Codeine (oral)	150-447	448-747	748-1047	1048-1347
Hydromorphone (oral)	8-17	17.1-28	28.1-39	39.1-51
Hydromorphone (I.V.)	1.5-3.4	3.5-5.6	5.7-7.9	8-10
Meperidine (I.M.)	75-165	166-278	279-390	391-503
Methadone (oral)	20-44	45-74	75-104	105-134
Methadone (I.M.)	10-22	23-37	38-52	53-67
Fentanyl transdermal recommended dose (mcg/h)	**25 mcg/h**	**50 mcg/h**	**75 mcg/h**	**100 mcg/h**

[1]The table should NOT be used to convert from transdermal fentanyl (eg, Duragesic®) to other opioid analgesics. Rather, following removal of the patch, titrate the dose of the new opioid until adequate analgesia is achieved.

[2]Duragesic® product insert, Janssen Pharmaceutica, Feb 2005.

Monitoring Parameters Respiratory and cardiovascular status, blood pressure, heart rate; signs of misuse, abuse, or addiction

Transdermal: Monitor for 24 hours after application of first dose

Patient Information Transdermal system: Apply to intact skin on the upper torso; clip hair at application site (do not shave) before applying system. If cleansing skin before application, use clear water and allow skin to dry completely before applying system; firmly press in place and hold for 30 seconds, change patch every 72 hours; dispose of system by folding it (medication side in) and flushing down the toilet; may cause dizziness or drowsiness, avoid alcohol, and CNS depressants.

Additional Information Fentanyl is 50-100 times as potent as morphine; morphine 10 mg I.M. is equivalent to fentanyl 0.1-0.2 mg I.M.; fentanyl has less hypotensive effects than morphine due to lack of histamine release. However, fentanyl may cause rigidity with high doses. If the patient has required high-dose analgesia or has used for a prolonged period (~7 days), taper dose to prevent withdrawal; monitor for signs and symptoms of withdrawal.

Iontophoretic transdermal system: Pharmacist should test before dispensing for patient. Without opening pouch, pharmacist should locate button side, find button and firmly press and release button twice within 3 seconds. Listen for a single audible tone (beep) confirming that the system is functional. The pharmacist should sign the front of the pouch after performing the functionality test.

Four minutes after the functional test, the system will beep for 15 seconds indicating that it is not in contact with skin. Open by cutting on dotted line of pouch, remove and discard plastic liner covering adhesive. Do not pull on red tab while removing. Press system firmly in place with sticky side down, on skin for at least 15 seconds. Make sure all sides of outer edge stick to skin. May tape sides down if they loosen; don't tape over button or red light. To determine the number of doses delivered, the red light will flash between doses in one second pulses to indicate the approximate number of doses that have been administered up to the present time. Each flash indicates up to 5 doses have been administered: One flash 1-5 doses; two flashes 6-10 doses; three flashes 11-15 doses; four flashes 16-20 doses, continuing up to 16 flashes (76-80 doses).

To dispose of system, wear gloves and pull the red tab to separate the bottom from the top. Fold the bottom in half with the sticky side facing in and flush down the toilet (needs to be witnessed by second healthcare provider). Dispose of top section according to hospital procedures for batteries.

Transmucosal (oral lozenge): Disposal of lozenge units: After consumption of a complete unit, the handle may be disposed of in a trash container that is out of the reach of children. For a partially-consumed unit, or a unit that still has any drug matrix remaining on the handle, the handle should be placed under hot running tap water until (Continued)

Fentanyl *(Continued)*

the drug matrix has dissolved. Special child-resistant containers are available to temporarily store partially consumed units that cannot be disposed of immediately.

Transdermal patch (Duragesic®): Upon removal of the patch, ~17 hours are required before serum concentrations fall to 50% of their original values. Opioid withdrawal symptoms are possible. Gradual downward titration (potentially by the sequential use of lower-dose patches) is recommended. Keep transdermal patch (both used and unused) out of the reach of children. Do **not** use soap, alcohol, or other solvents to remove transdermal gel if it accidentally touches skin as they may increase transdermal absorption, use copious amounts of water. Avoid exposure of direct external heat sources (eg, heating pads, electric blankets, heat lamps, saunas, hot tubs, heated water beds) to application site.

Special Geriatric Considerations The elderly may be particularly susceptible to the CNS depressant and constipating effects of narcotics; therefore, use with caution. For Ionsys™, age does not significantly affect the extent of drug absorption. Before using Ionsys™ in elderly patients, assess cognitive function and ability to operate the dosage system. The effect of age on the pharmacokinetics of Fentora™ (oral transmucosal buccal tablets) has not been studied.

Dosage Forms Excipient information presented when available (limited, particularly for generics); consult specific product labeling.

Note: Strengths expressed as base.

Infusion, as citrate [premixed in NS]: 0.05 mg (10 mL); 1 mg (100 mL); 1.25 mg (250 mL); 2 mg (100 mL); 2.5 mg (250 mL)

Injection, solution, as citrate [preservative free]: 0.05 mg/mL (2 mL, 5 mL, 10 mL, 20 mL, 30 mL, 50 mL)

Sublimaze®: 0.05 mg/mL (2 mL, 5 mL, 10 mL, 20 mL)

Lozenge, oral, as citrate [transmucosal]: 200 mcg, 400 mcg, 600 mcg, 800 mcg, 1200 mcg, 1600 mcg

Actiq®: 200 mcg, 400 mcg, 600 mcg, 800 mcg, 1200 mcg, 1600 mcg [mounted on a plastic radiopaque handle; contains sugar 2 g/unit; raspberry flavor]

Tablet, for buccal application, as citrate:

Fentora™: 100 mcg, 200 mcg, 300 mcg, 400 mcg, 600 mcg, 800 mcg

Transdermal system, topical, as base: 12 (5s) [delivers 12.5 mcg/hour; 3.13 cm^2]; 12 (5s) [delivers 12.5 mcg/hour; 5 cm^2]; 25 (5s) [delivers 25 mcg/hour; 10 cm^2]; 25 (5s) [delivers 25 mcg/hour; 6.25 cm^2]; 50 (5s) [delivers 50 mcg/hour; 12.5 cm^2]; 50 (5s) [delivers 50 mcg/hour; 20 cm^2]; 75 (5s) [delivers 75 mcg/hour; 18.75 cm^2]; 75 (5s) [delivers 75 mcg/hour; 30 cm^2]; 100 (5s) [delivers 100 mcg/hour; 25 cm^2]; 100 (5s) [delivers 100 mcg/hour; 40 cm^2]

Duragesic®: 12 [delivers 12.5 mcg/hour; 5 cm^2; contains alcohol 0.1 mL/10 cm^2] (5s); 25 [delivers 25 mcg/hour; 10 cm^2; contains alcohol 0.1 mL/10 cm^2] (5s); 50 [delivers 50 mcg/hour; 20 cm^2; contains alcohol 0.1 mL/10 cm^2] (5s); 75 [delivers 75 mcg/hour; 30 cm^2; contains alcohol 0.1 mL/10 cm^2]; 100 [delivers 100 mcg/hour; 40 cm^2; contains alcohol 0.1 mL/10 cm^2] (5s)

Transdermal iontophoretic system, topical, as hydrochloride:

Ionsys™: Fentanyl 40 mcg/dose [80 doses/patch; contains 3-volt lithium battery]

Selected References

AGS Panel on Persistent Pain in Older Persons, "The Management of Persistent Pain in Older Persons," *J Am Geriatr Soc*, 2002, 50(6 Suppl):S205-24.

Ferric Gluconate *(FER ik GLOO koe nate)*

Medication Safety Issues

Sound-alike/look-alike issues:

Ferrlecit® may be confused with Ferralet®

U.S. Brand Names Ferrlecit®

Canadian Brand Names Ferrlecit®

Index Terms Sodium Ferric Gluconate

Generic Available No

Pharmacologic Category Iron Salt

Use Repletion of total body iron content in patients with iron deficiency anemia who are undergoing hemodialysis in conjunction with erythropoietin therapy

Contraindications Hypersensitivity to ferric gluconate or any component of the formulation; use in any anemia not caused by iron deficiency; iron overload

Warnings/Precautions Potentially serious hypersensitivity reactions may occur. Fatal immediate hypersensitivity reactions have occurred with other iron carbohydrate complexes. Avoid rapid administration. Flushing and transient hypotension may occur. May augment hemodialysis-induced hypotension. Use with caution in elderly patients. Use only in patients with documented iron deficiency; caution with hemoglobinopathies or other refractory anemias.

Adverse Reactions (Reflective of adult population; not specific for elderly)

Cardiovascular: Angina, bradycardia, chest pain, edema, hyper-/hypotension, hypervolemia, MI, pulmonary edema, syncope, tachycardia, thrombosis, vasodilation

Central nervous system: Agitation, chills, dizziness, fatigue, fever, headache, insomnia, malaise, pain, somnolence

Dermatologic: Pruritus, rash

Endocrine & metabolic: Hyper-/hypokalemia, hypoglycemia

Gastrointestinal: Abdominal pain, anorexia, diarrhea, dyspepsia, epigastric pain, eructation, flatulence, melena, nausea, vomiting

Genitourinary: Urinary tract infection

Hematologic: Abnormal erythrocytes, leukocytosis, lymphadenopathy

Local: Injection site reactions, injection site pain

Neuromuscular & skeletal: Arthralgia, back pain, cramps, groin pain, leg cramps, myalgia, paresthesia, rigors, weakness

Ocular: Blurred vision, conjunctivitis

Respiratory: Cough, dyspnea, pneumonia, rhinitis, upper respiratory infection

Miscellaneous: Carcinoma, diaphoresis increased, flu-like syndrome, hypersensitivity reactions, infection, sepsis

Overdosage/Toxicology Serum iron levels >300 mcg/dL may indicate iron poisoning. Initially, symptoms include abdominal pain, diarrhea, and/or vomiting and may progress to pallor, cyanosis, lassitude, drowsiness, acidosis and cardiovascular collapse. Treatment is generally symptom-directed and supportive.

Drug Interactions Iron preparations, oral: Ferric gluconate injection may reduce the absorption of oral iron preparations

Stability Store at 20°C to 25°C (68°F to 77°F). Do not freeze. For I.V. infusion, dilute 10 mL ferric gluconate in 0.9% sodium chloride (100 mL NS); use immediately after dilution.

Mechanism of Action Supplies a source to elemental iron necessary to the function of hemoglobin, myoglobin and specific enzyme systems; allows transport of oxygen via hemoglobin

Pharmacokinetics Pharmacokinetic studies have not been conducted. The total body iron content normally ranges from 2-4 g of elemental iron.

Dosage

Geriatrics & Adults: Repletion of iron in hemodialysis patients: I.V.: 125 mg elemental iron per 10 mL (either by I.V. infusion or slow I.V. injection). Most patients will require a cumulative dose of 1 g elemental iron over approximately 8 sequential dialysis treatments to achieve a favorable response.

Note: A test dose of 2 mL diluted in NS 50 mL administered over 60 minutes was previously recommended (not in current manufacturer labeling). Doses >125 mg are associated with increased adverse events.

Administration I.V.: Monitor patient for hypotension or hypersensitivity reactions during infusion.

Adults: May be diluted prior to administration; avoid rapid administration. Infusion rate should not exceed 2.1 mg/minute. If administered undiluted, infuse slowly at a rate of up to 12.5 mg/minute.

Monitoring Parameters Hemoglobin and hematocrit, serum ferritin, iron saturation; vital signs

NKF K/DOQI guidelines recommend that iron status should be monitored monthly during initiation through the percent transferrin saturation (TSAT) and serum ferritin.

Reference Range CKD patients should have sufficient iron to achieve and maintain hemoglobin of 11-12 g/dL. To achieve and maintain this target Hgb, sufficient iron should be administered to maintain a TSAT of 20%, and a serum ferritin level >100 ng/mL (nondialysis chronic kidney disease and peritoneal dialysis chronic kidney disease) or serum ferritin level >200 ng/mL (hemodialysis chronic kidney disease).

Test Interactions Serum or transferrin bound iron levels may be falsely elevated if assessed within 24 hours of ferric gluconate administration. Serum ferritin levels may be falsely elevated for 5 days after ferric gluconate administration.

Special Geriatric Considerations Studies in the elderly have not been done, nor were there sufficient numbers of the elderly in premarketing studies to identify any
(Continued)

Ferric Gluconate *(Continued)*

differences in the elderly using this drug. Monitor dose closely so as to avoid iron overload.

Dosage Forms Excipient information presented when available (limited, particularly for generics); consult specific product labeling.

Injection, solution:

Ferrlecit®: Elemental iron 12.5 mg/mL (5 mL) [contains benzyl alcohol and sucrose 20%]

Selected References

National Kidney Foundation, "KDOQI Clinical Practice Guidelines and Clinical Practice Recommentaions for Anemia in Chronic Kidney Disease." Available at www.kidney.org/professionals/KDOQI/guidelines_anemia/cpr32.htm. Last accessed November 20, 2006.

♦ **Ferrlecit®** *see* Ferric Gluconate *on page 616*
♦ **Ferro-Sequels® [OTC]** *see* Ferrous Fumarate *on page 618*

Ferrous Fumarate (FER us FYOO ma rate)

Medication Safety Issues

Sound-alike/look-alike issues:

Feostat® may be confused with Feosol®

U.S. Brand Names Femiron® [OTC]; Feostat® [OTC] [DSC]; Ferretts [OTC]; Ferro-Sequels® [OTC]; Hemocyte® [OTC]; Ircon® [OTC]; Nephro-Fer® [OTC]

Canadian Brand Names Palafer®

Index Terms Iron Fumarate

Generic Available Yes: Tablet

Pharmacologic Category Iron Salt

Use Prevention and treatment of iron deficiency anemias

Contraindications Hypersensitivity to iron salts or any component of the formulation; hemochromatosis, hemolytic anemia

Warnings/Precautions Avoid in patients with peptic ulcer, enteritis, or ulcerative colitis. Administration of iron for >6 months should be avoided except in patients with continuous bleeding or menorrhagia. Anemia in the elderly is often caused by "anemia of chronic disease" or associated with inflammation rather than blood loss. Iron stores are usually normal or increased, with a serum ferritin >50 ng/mL and a decreased total iron binding capacity. Hence, the "anemia of chronic disease" is not secondary to iron deficiency but the inability of the reticuloendothelial system to reclaim available iron stores. Avoid in patients receiving frequent blood transfusions. **[U.S. Boxed Warning]: Severe iron toxicity may occur in overdose, particularly when ingested by children; iron is a leading cause of fatal poisoning in children; store out of children's reach and in child-resistant containers.**

Adverse Reactions (Reflective of adult population; not specific for elderly)

>10%: Gastrointestinal: Stomach cramping, constipation, nausea, vomiting, dark stools

1% to 10%:

Gastrointestinal: Heartburn, diarrhea, staining of teeth

Genitourinary: Discoloration of urine

Overdosage/Toxicology Symptoms include acute GI irritation, erosion of GI mucosa, hepatic and renal impairment, coma, hematemesis, lethargy, and acidosis. Due to severe toxicity, serum iron ≥300 mcg/mL requires treatment. Following treatment for fluid losses, metabolic acidosis, and shock, a severe iron overdose may be treated with deferoxamine. Deferoxamine may be administered I.V. (80 mg/kg over 24 hours) or I.M. (40-90 mg/kg every 8 hours). The usual toxic dose of elemental iron is ≥35 mg/kg.

Drug Interactions

Antacids and H$_2$ blockers (cimetidine): Concurrent administration may decrease iron absorption.

Chloramphenicol: Response to iron therapy may be delayed.

Levodopa, methyldopa, penicillamine: Iron may decrease absorption when given at the same time.

Quinolones: Absorption may be decreased due to formation of a ferric ion-quinolone complex

Tetracyclines: Absorption of oral preparation of iron and tetracyclines are decreased when both of these drugs are given together

Vitamin C: Concurrent administration of ≥200 mg vitamin C per 30 mg elemental iron increases absorption of oral iron.

Ethanol/Nutrition/Herb Interactions Food: Cereals, dietary fiber, tea, coffee, eggs, and milk may decrease absorption.

Stability Iron is a leading cause of fatal poisoning in children. Store out of children's reach and in child-resistant containers.

Mechanism of Action Replaces iron found in hemoglobin, myoglobin, and enzymes; allows the transportation of oxygen via hemoglobin

Pharmacodynamics
Onset of action: Hematologic response to oral iron in red blood cells form and color changes occur within 3-10 days
Peak action: Within 5-10 days, and hemoglobin values increase within 2-4 weeks

Pharmacokinetics
Absorption: Iron is absorbed in the duodenum and upper jejunum; in persons with normal iron stores 10% of an oral dose is absorbed, this is increased to 20% to 30% in persons with inadequate iron stores. Food and achlorhydria will decrease absorption; aging has not been shown to affect absorption, but the percent uptake by red cells decreases from 91.2% in healthy young adults to 60% in healthy older adults.
Elimination: Iron is largely bound to serum transferrin and excreted in the urine, sweat, sloughing of intestinal mucosa, and by menstrual bleeding. sloughing of intestinal mucosa, and by menstrual bleeding.

Dosage
Geriatrics: 200 mg 3-4 times/day
Adults: (Dose expressed in terms of elemental iron):
　Treatment of iron deficiency: Oral: 60-100 mg twice daily up to 60 mg 2 times/day
　Prophylaxis of iron deficiency: Oral: 60-100 mg/day
　　Note: To avoid GI upset, start with a single daily dose and increase by 1 tablet/day each week or as tolerated until desired daily dose is achieved

Administration Administer 2 hours prior to or 4 hours after antacids

Monitoring Parameters Hemoglobin, hematocrit, ferritin, reticulocyte count

Reference Range Therapeutic: Male: 75-175 mcg/dL (SI: 13.4-31.3 µmol/L); Female: 65-165 mcg/dL (SI: 11.6-29.5 µmol/L); ranges may vary by laboratory

Patient Information May color stool black, take between meals for maximum absorption; may take with food if GI upset occurs, do not take with milk or antacids

Additional Information The elemental iron content in ferrous fumarate is 33% (ie, 200 mg ferrous fumarate is equivalent to 66 mg ferrous iron). Administration of iron for longer than 6 months should be avoided except in patients with continuous bleeding or menorrhagia.

Special Geriatric Considerations Anemia in the elderly is often caused by "anemia of chronic disease", a result of aging changes in the bone marrow, or associated with inflammation rather than blood loss. Iron stores are usually normal or increased, with a serum ferritin >50 ng/mL and a decreased total iron binding capacity. Hence, the anemia is not secondary to iron deficiency but the inability of the reticuloendothelial system to use available iron stores. Timed release iron preparations should be avoided due to their erratic absorption. Products combined with a laxative or stool softener should not be used unless the need for the combination is demonstrated.

Dosage Forms Excipient information presented when available (limited, particularly for generics); consult specific product labeling. [DSC] = Discontinued product
　Tablet: 324 mg [elemental iron 106 mg]
　　Femiron®: 63 mg [elemental iron 20 mg]
　　Ferretts: 325 mg [elemental iron 106 mg]
　　Hemocyte®: 324 mg [elemental iron 106 mg]
　　Ircon®: 200 mg [elemental iron 66 mg]
　　Nephro-Fer®: 350 mg [elemental iron 115 mg; contains tartrazine]
　Tablet, chewable (Feostat®): 100 mg [elemental iron 33 mg; chocolate flavor] [DSC]
　Tablet, timed release (Ferro-Sequels®): 150 mg [elemental iron 50 mg; contains docusate sodium and sodium benzoate]

Selected References
Lipschitz DA, "The Anemia of Chronic Disease," *J Am Geriatr Soc*, 1990, 38(11):1258-64.
Marx JJ, "Normal Iron Absorption and Decreased Red Cell Iron Uptake in the Aged," *Blood*, 1979, 53(2):204-11.

Ferrous Gluconate (FER us GLOO koe nate)

U.S. Brand Names Fergon® [OTC]
Canadian Brand Names Apo-Ferrous Gluconate®; Novo-Ferrogluc
Index Terms Iron Gluconate
Generic Available Yes
Pharmacologic Category Iron Salt
Use Prevention and treatment of iron deficiency anemias
Contraindications Hypersensitivity to iron salts or any component of the formulation; hemochromatosis, hemolytic anemia
Warnings/Precautions Avoid in patients with peptic ulcer, enteritis, or ulcerative colitis. Administration of iron for >6 months should be avoided except in patients with continuous bleeding or menorrhagia. Anemia in the elderly is often caused by "anemia of chronic disease" or associated with inflammation rather than blood loss. Iron stores are usually normal or increased, with a serum ferritin >50 ng/mL and a decreased total iron binding capacity. Hence, the "anemia of chronic disease" is not secondary to iron deficiency but the inability of the reticuloendothelial system to reclaim available iron
(Continued)

Ferrous Gluconate *(Continued)*

stores. Avoid in patients receiving frequent blood transfusions. **[U.S. Boxed Warning]: Severe iron toxicity may occur in overdose, particularly when ingested by children; iron is a leading cause of fatal poisoning in children; store out of children's reach and in child-resistant containers.**

Adverse Reactions (Reflective of adult population; not specific for elderly)

>10%: Gastrointestinal: Stomach cramping, constipation, nausea, vomiting, dark stools

1% to 10%:

Gastrointestinal: Heartburn, diarrhea, staining of teeth

Genitourinary: Discoloration of urine

Overdosage/Toxicology Symptoms include acute GI irritation, erosion of GI mucosa, hepatic and renal impairment, coma, hematemesis, lethargy, and acidosis. Due to severe toxicity, serum iron ≥300 mcg/mL requires treatment. Following treatment for fluid losses, metabolic acidosis, and shock, a severe iron overdose may be treated with deferoxamine. Deferoxamine may be administered I.V. (80 mg/kg over 24 hours) or I.M. (40-90 mg/kg every 8 hours). The usual toxic dose of elemental iron is ≥35 mg/kg.

Drug Interactions

Antacids and H_2 blockers (cimetidine): Concurrent administration may decrease iron absorption.

Chloramphenicol: Response to iron therapy may be delayed.

Levodopa, methyldopa, penicillamine: Iron may decrease absorption when given at the same time.

Quinolones: Absorption may be decreased due to formation of a ferric ion-quinolone complex

Tetracyclines: Absorption of oral preparation of iron and tetracyclines are decreased when both of these drugs are given together

Vitamin C: Concurrent administration of ≥200 mg vitamin C per 30 mg elemental iron increases absorption of oral iron.

Ethanol/Nutrition/Herb Interactions Food: Cereals, dietary fiber, tea, coffee, eggs, and milk may decrease absorption.

Stability Iron is a leading cause of fatal poisoning in children. Store out of children's reach and in child-resistant containers.

Mechanism of Action Replaces iron found in hemoglobin, myoglobin, and enzymes; allows the transportation of oxygen via hemoglobin

Pharmacodynamics

Onset of action: Hematologic response to either oral or parenteral iron salts is essentially the same; red blood cell form and color changes within 3-10 days

Peak effect: Within 5-10 days, and hemoglobin values increase within 2-4 weeks

Pharmacokinetics

Absorption: Iron is absorbed in the duodenum and upper jejunum; in persons with normal iron stores 10% of an oral dose is absorbed, this is increased to 20% to 30% in persons with inadequate iron stores. Food and achlorhydria will decrease absorption; aging has not been shown to affect absorption, but the percent uptake by red cells decreases from 91.2% in healthy young adults to 60% in healthy older adults.

Elimination: Iron is largely bound to serum transferrin and excreted in the urine, sweat, sloughing of intestinal mucosa, and by menstrual bleeding

Dosage

Geriatrics & Adults: (Dose expressed in terms of elemental iron):

Treatment of iron deficiency anemia: Oral: 60 mg twice daily up to 60 mg 4 times/day

Prophylaxis of iron deficiency: Oral: 60 mg/day

Administration Administer 2 hours before or 4 hours after antacids

Monitoring Parameters Hemoglobin, hematocrit, ferritin, reticulocyte count

Reference Range Therapeutic: Male: 75-175 mcg/dL (SI: 13.4-31.3 µmol/L); Female: 65-165 mcg/dL (SI: 11.6-29.5 µmol/L); ranges may vary by laboratory

Test Interactions False-positive for blood in stool by the guaiac test

Patient Information May color the stool black; take between meals for maximum absorption; may take with food if GI upset occurs; do **not** take with milk or antacid

Additional Information Gluconate contains 12% elemental iron (ie, 300 mg ferrous gluconate is equivalent to 34 mg ferrous iron); administration of iron for longer than 6 months should be avoided except in patients with continued bleeding or menorrhagia

Special Geriatric Considerations Anemia in the elderly is often caused by "anemia of chronic disease", a result of aging changes in the bone marrow, or associated with inflammation rather than blood loss. Iron stores are usually normal or increased, with a serum ferritin >50 ng/mL and a decreased total iron binding capacity. Hence, the anemia is not secondary to iron deficiency but the inability of the reticuloendothelial system to use available iron stores. Timed release iron preparations should be avoided due to their erratic absorption. Products combined with a laxative or stool softener should not be used unless the need for the combination is demonstrated.

Dosage Forms Excipient information presented when available (limited, particularly for generics); consult specific product labeling.

Tablet: 246 mg [elemental iron 28 mg]; 300 mg [elemental iron 34 mg]; 325 mg [elemental iron 36 mg]

Fergon®: 240 mg [elemental iron 27 mg]

Selected References

Lipschitz DA, "The Anemia of Chronic Disease," *J Am Geriatr Soc*, 1990, 38(11):1258-64.

Marx JJ, "Normal Iron Absorption and Decreased Red Cell Iron Uptake in the Aged," *Blood*, 1979, 53(2):204-11.

Ferrous Sulfate (FER us SUL fate)

Related Information

Potentially Inappropriate Medications for Geriatrics *on page 1824*

Medication Safety Issues

Sound-alike/look-alike issues:

Feosol® may be confused with Feostat®, Fer-In-Sol®

Fer-In-Sol® may be confused with Feosol®

Slow FE® may be confused with Slow-K®

U.S. Brand Names Feosol® [OTC]; Feratab® [OTC]; Fer-Gen-Sol [OTC]; Fer-In-Sol® [OTC]; Fer-Iron® [OTC]; Slow FE® [OTC]

Canadian Brand Names Apo-Ferrous Sulfate®; Fer-In-Sol®; Ferodan™

Index Terms FeSO$_4$; Iron Sulfate

Generic Available Yes

Pharmacologic Category Iron Salt

Use Prevention and treatment of iron deficiency anemias

Contraindications Hypersensitivity to iron salts or any component of the formulation; hemochromatosis, hemolytic anemia

Warnings/Precautions Avoid in patients with peptic ulcer, enteritis, or ulcerative colitis. Administration of iron for >6 months should be avoided except in patients with continuous bleeding or menorrhagia. Anemia in the elderly is often caused by "anemia of chronic disease" or associated with inflammation rather than blood loss. Iron stores are usually normal or increased, with a serum ferritin >50 ng/mL and a decreased total iron binding capacity. Hence, the "anemia of chronic disease" is not secondary to iron deficiency but the inability of the reticuloendothelial system to reclaim available iron stores. Avoid in patients receiving frequent blood transfusions. **[U.S. Boxed Warning]: Severe iron toxicity may occur in overdose, particularly when ingested by children; iron is a leading cause of fatal poisoning in children; store out of children's reach and in child-resistant containers.**

Adverse Reactions (Reflective of adult population; not specific for elderly)

>10%: Gastrointestinal: GI irritation, epigastric pain, nausea, dark stools, vomiting, stomach cramping, constipation

1% to 10%:

Gastrointestinal: Heartburn, diarrhea

Genitourinary: Discoloration of urine

Miscellaneous: Liquid preparations may temporarily stain the teeth

Overdosage/Toxicology Symptoms include acute GI irritation, erosion of GI mucosa, hepatic and renal impairment, coma, hematemesis, lethargy, and acidosis. Due to severe toxicity, serum iron ≥300 mcg/mL requires treatment. Following treatment for fluid losses, metabolic acidosis, and shock, a severe iron overdose may be treated with deferoxamine. Deferoxamine may be administered I.V. (80 mg/kg over 24 hours) or I.M. (40-90 mg/kg every 8 hours). The usual toxic dose of elemental iron is ≥35 mg/kg.

Drug Interactions

Antacids and H$_2$ blockers (cimetidine): Concurrent administration may decrease iron absorption.

Chloramphenicol: Response to iron therapy may be delayed.

Levodopa, methyldopa, penicillamine: Iron may decrease absorption when given at the same time.

Quinolones: Absorption may be decreased due to formation of a ferric ion-quinolone complex

Tetracyclines: Absorption of oral preparation of iron and tetracyclines are decreased when both of these drugs are given together

Vitamin C: Concurrent administration of ≥200 mg vitamin C per 30 mg elemental iron increases absorption of oral iron.

Ethanol/Nutrition/Herb Interactions Food: Cereals, dietary fiber, tea, coffee, eggs, and milk may decrease absorption.

Stability Iron is a leading cause of fatal poisoning in children. Store out of children's reach and in child-resistant containers.

Mechanism of Action Replaces iron, found in hemoglobin, myoglobin, and other enzymes; allows the transportation of oxygen via hemoglobin

(Continued)

Ferrous Sulfate *(Continued)*

Pharmacodynamics

Onset of action: Hematologic response to either oral or parenteral iron salts is essentially the same; red blood cell form and color changes within 3-10 days

Peak effect: Reticulocytosis occurs in 5-10 days, and hemoglobin values increase within 2-4 weeks

Pharmacokinetics

Absorption: Iron is absorbed in the duodenum and upper jejunum; in persons with normal serum iron stores, 10% of an oral dose is absorbed; this is increased to 20% to 30% in persons with inadequate iron stores. Food and achlorhydria will decrease absorption; aging has not been shown to affect absorption, but the percent uptake by red cells decreases from 91.2% in healthy young adults to 60% in healthy older adults.

Elimination: Iron is largely bound to serum transferrin and excreted in the urine, sweat, sloughing of the intestinal mucosa, and by menstrual bleeding

Dosage

Geriatrics & Adults: Dose expressed in terms of ferrous sulfate:

Treatment of iron deficiency anemia: Oral: 300 mg twice daily up to 300 mg 4 times/day or 250 mg (extended release) 1-2 times/day

Prophylaxis of iron deficiency: Oral: 300 mg/day

Administration Administer 2 hours prior to or 4 hours after antacids

Monitoring Parameters Hemoglobin, hematocrit, ferritin, reticulocyte count

Reference Range Therapeutic: Male: 75-175 mcg/dL (SI: 13.4-31.3 μmol/L); Female: 65-165 mcg/dL (SI: 11.6-29.5 μmol/L); values may vary by laboratory

Test Interactions False-positive for blood in stool by the guaiac test

Patient Information May color stool black, take between meals for maximum absorption; may take with food if GI upset occurs, do not take with milk or antacids

Additional Information The elemental iron content of ferrous sulfate is 20% (ie, 300 mg ferrous sulfate is equivalent to 60 mg ferrous iron). Administration of iron for longer than 6 months should be avoided except in patients with continued bleeding, or menorrhagia.

Special Geriatric Considerations Anemia in the elderly is often caused by "anemia of chronic disease", a result of aging changes in the bone marrow, or associated with inflammation rather than blood loss. Iron stores are usually normal or increased, with a serum ferritin >50 ng/mL and a decreased total iron binding capacity. Hence, the anemia is not secondary to iron deficiency but the inability of the reticuloendothelial system to use available iron stores. Timed release iron preparations should be avoided due to their erratic absorption. Products combined with a laxative or stool softener should not be used unless the need for the combination is demonstrated.

Dosage Forms Excipient information presented when available (limited, particularly for generics); consult specific product labeling.

Elixir: 220 mg/5 mL (480 mL) [elemental iron 44 mg/5 mL; contains alcohol]

Liquid, oral drops: 75 mg/0.6 mL (50 mL) [elemental iron 15 mg/0.6 mL]

Fer-Gen-Sol: 75 mg/0.6 mL (50 mL) [elemental iron 15 mg/0.6 mL]

Fer-In-Sol®: 75 mg/0.6 mL (50 mL) [elemental iron 15 mg/0.6 mL; contains alcohol 0.2% and sodium bisulfite]

Fer-Iron®: 75 mg/0.6 mL (50 mL) [elemental iron 15 mg/0.6 mL]

Tablet: 324 mg [elemental iron 65 mg]; 325 mg [elemental iron 65 mg]

Feratab®: 300 mg [elemental iron 60 mg]

Tablet, exsiccated (Feosol®): 200 mg [elemental iron 65 mg]

Tablet, exsiccated, timed release (Slow FE®): 160 mg [elemental iron 50 mg]

Selected References

Lipschitz DA, "The Anemia of Chronic Disease," *J Am Geriatr Soc*, 1990, 38(11):1258-64.

Marx JJ, "Normal Iron Absorption and Decreased Red Cell Iron Uptake in the Aged," *Blood*, 1979, 53(2):204-11.

♦ **FeSO₄** see Ferrous Sulfate *on page 621*

♦ **FeverALL® [OTC]** see Acetaminophen *on page 29*

♦ **Fexmid™** see Cyclobenzaprine *on page 374*

Fexofenadine *(feks oh FEN a deen)*

Medication Safety Issues

Sound-alike/look-alike issues:

Allegra® may be confused with Viagra®

International issues:

Allegra® may be confused with Allegro® which is a brand name for frovatriptan in Germany; a brand name for fluticasone in Israel

U.S. Brand Names Allegra®
Canadian Brand Names Allegra®
Index Terms Fexofenadine Hydrochloride
Generic Available Yes: Excludes suspension
Pharmacologic Category Antihistamine, Nonsedating
Use Relief of symptoms associated with seasonal allergic rhinitis; treatment of chronic idiopathic urticaria
Contraindications Hypersensitivity to fexofenadine or any component of the formulation
Warnings/Precautions See Drug Interactions.
Adverse Reactions (Reflective of adult population; not specific for elderly)
>10%:
  Central nervous system: Headache (5% to 11%)
  Gastrointestinal: Vomiting (children 6 months to 5 years): 4% to 12%
1% to 10%:
  Central nervous system: Somnolence (1% to 3%), dizziness (2%), drowsiness (2%), pain (2%), fatigue (1%)
  Endocrine & metabolic: Dysmenorrhea (2%)
  Gastrointestinal: Dyspepsia (1% to 5%), diarrhea (3% to 4%), nausea (2%)
  Neuromuscular & skeletal: Myalgia (3%), back pain (2% to 3%)
  Otic: Otitis media (2%)
  Respiratory: Upper respiratory tract infection (4%), cough (2% to 4%), nasopharyngitis (2%)
  Miscellaneous: Viral infection (3%)
Overdosage/Toxicology Symptoms may include: dizziness, drowsiness, and xerostomia. Not effectively removed by hemodialysis. Doses up to 690 mg twice daily were administered for 1 month without significant adverse effects. Treatment is symptom-directed and supportive.
Drug Interactions Substrate of CYP3A4 (minor); **Inhibits** CYP2D6 (weak)
  Acetylcholinesterase inhibitors (central): May diminish the adverse effects of fexofenadine. Fexofenadine may diminish the therapeutic effect of acetylcholinesterase inhibitors (central).
  Anticholinergics: Fexofenadine may enhance the adverse/toxic effect of other anticholinergics.
  Betahistine: Fexofenadine may diminish the therapeutic effect of betahistine.
  CNS depressants: Fexofenadine may worsen the adverse/toxic effect of other CNS depressants.
  Pramlintide: May enhance the anticholinergic effect of fexofenadine. These effects are specific to the GI tract.
  Rifampin: May decrease the serum concentration of fexofenadine.
  Verapamil: May increase the bioavailability of fexofenadine.
Ethanol/Nutrition/Herb Interactions
  Ethanol: Avoid ethanol (although limited with fexofenadine, may increase risk of sedation).
  Food: Fruit juice (apple, grapefruit, orange) may decrease bioavailability of fexofenadine by ~36%.
  Herb/Nutraceutical: St John's wort may decrease fexofenadine levels.
Stability Store at controlled room temperature of 20°C to 25°C (68°F to 77°F). Protect from excessive moisture.
Mechanism of Action Fexofenadine is an active metabolite of terfenadine and like terfenadine it competes with histamine for H_1-receptor sites on effector cells in the gastrointestinal tract, blood vessels and respiratory tract; it appears that fexofenadine does not cross the blood brain barrier to any appreciable degree, resulting in a reduced potential for sedation
Pharmacokinetics
  Absorption: Rapid
  Protein binding: 60% to 70% bound to albumin and alpha$_1$-acid glycoprotein
  Metabolism: Minimal (~5%)
  Half-life, mean: 14.4 hours
  Pharmacokinetics in renal impairment:
    Cl_{cr} 41-80 mL/minute:
      Peak concentration: 87% higher
      Half-life: 59% longer
    Cl_{cr} 11-40 mL/minute:
      Peak concentration: 111% higher
      Half-life: 72% longer
  Time to peak plasma concentration: 2.6 hours; peak plasma fexofenadine concentrations were 99% higher in older adult patients as compared to younger volunteers; no unusual adverse effects were seen with these elevated concentrations
  Elimination: 80% in feces; 11% in urine
(Continued)

Fexofenadine *(Continued)*

Dosage

Geriatrics: Chronic idiopathic urticaria, seasonal allergic rhinitis: Starting dose: 60 mg once daily; adjust for renal impairment.

Adults:

Allergic rhinitis, idiopathic urticaria: Oral: 60 mg twice daily **or** 180 mg once daily

Renal Impairment: Cl_{cr} <80 mL/minute: Initial: 60 mg once daily

Not effectively removed by hemodialysis

Administration Administer with water only; do not administer with fruit juices. Shake suspension well before use.

Monitoring Parameters Symptoms of allergic rhinitis

Patient Information Do not exceed recommended dose

Special Geriatric Considerations Plasma levels in the elderly are generally higher than those observed in other age groups. Once daily dosing is recommended when starting therapy in elderly patients or patients with decreased renal function.

Dosage Forms Excipient information presented when available (limited, particularly for generics); consult specific product labeling.

Suspension:

Allegra®: 6 mg/mL (30 mL, 300 mL) [raspberry cream]

Tablet, as hydrochloride: 30 mg, 60 mg, 180 mg

Allegra®: 30 mg, 60 mg, 180 mg

♦ **Fexofenadine Hydrochloride** *see Fexofenadine on page 622*

♦ **Fiberall®** *see Psyllium on page 1347*

♦ **FiberCon® [OTC]** *see Polycarbophil on page 1282*

♦ **Fiber-Lax® [OTC]** *see Polycarbophil on page 1282*

♦ **Fiber-Tabs™ [OTC]** *see Polycarbophil on page 1282*

♦ **Fibro-XL [OTC]** *see Psyllium on page 1347*

♦ **Fibro-Lax [OTC]** *see Psyllium on page 1347*

Filgrastim *(fil GRA stim)*

Medication Safety Issues

Sound-alike/look-alike issues:

Neupogen® may be confused with Epogen®, Neumega®, Neupro®, Nutramigen®

U.S. Brand Names Neupogen®

Canadian Brand Names Neupogen®

Index Terms G-CSF; Granulocyte Colony Stimulating Factor; NSC-614629

Generic Available No

Pharmacologic Category Colony Stimulating Factor

Use Decreases the period of neutropenia and the associated risk of infection in patients with nonmyeloid malignancies receiving myelosuppressive chemotherapeutic regimens associated with a significant incidence of severe neutropenia with fever; it has also been used in AIDS patients on zidovudine and in patients with noncancer chemotherapy-induced neutropenia

Unlabeled/Investigational Use Treatment of anemia in myelodysplastic syndrome; treatment of drug-induced (nonchemotherapy) agranulocytosis in the elderly

Contraindications Hypersensitivity to filgrastim, *E. coli*-derived proteins, or any component of the formulation

Warnings/Precautions Do not use filgrastim in the period 24 hours before to 24 hours after administration of cytotoxic chemotherapy because of the potential sensitivity of rapidly dividing myeloid cells to cytotoxic chemotherapy. May potentially act as a growth factor for any tumor type, particularly myeloid malignancies; precaution should be exercised in the usage of filgrastim in any malignancy with myeloid characteristics. Safety and efficacy have not been established with patients receiving radiation therapy, or with chemotherapy associated with delayed myelosuppression (eg, nitrosoureas, mitomycin C).

Allergic-type reactions (rash, urticaria, wheezing, dyspnea, tachycardia and/or hypotension) have occurred with first or later doses. Reactions tended to occur more frequently with intravenous administration and within 30 minutes of administration. Rare cases of splenic rupture or adult respiratory distress syndrome have been reported in association with filgrastim; patients must be instructed to report left upper quadrant pain or shoulder tip pain or respiratory distress. Use caution in patients with sickle cell diseases; sickle cell crises have been reported following filgrastim therapy. Cytogenetic abnormalities, transformation to AML and MDS have been observed in patients treated with filgrastim for congenital neutropenia; a longer duration of treatment and poorer ANC response appear to increase the risk. The packaging of some forms may contain latex.

Adverse Reactions (Reflective of adult population; not specific for elderly)

>10%:

Central nervous system: Fever (12%)

Dermatologic: Petechiae (17%), rash (12%)

Gastrointestinal: Splenomegaly (severe chronic neutropenia: 30%; rare in other patients)

Hepatic: Alkaline phosphatase increased (21%)

Neuromuscular & skeletal: Bone pain (22% to 33%), commonly in the lower back, posterior iliac crest, and sternum

Respiratory: Epistaxis (9% to 15%)

1% to 10%:

Cardiovascular: Hyper-/hypotension (4%), S-T segment depression (3%), myocardial infarction/arrhythmias (3%)

Central nervous system: Headache (7%)

Gastrointestinal: Nausea (10%), vomiting (7%), peritonitis (2%)

Hematologic: Leukocytosis (2%)

Miscellaneous: Transfusion reaction (10%)

Overdosage/Toxicology No clinical adverse effects have been seen with high doses producing ANC >10,000/mm^3. Filgrastim discontinuation should result in a 50% decrease in circulating neutrophils within 1-2 days and a return to pretreatment levels in 1-7 days.

Stability Intact vials and prefilled syringes should be stored under refrigeration at 2°C to 8°C (36°F to 46°F) and protected from direct sunlight. Filgrastim should be protected from freezing and temperatures >30°C to avoid aggregation. If inadvertently frozen, thaw in a refrigerator and use within 24 hours; do not use if frozen >24 hours or frozen more than once. Do not shake.

Filgrastim vials and prefilled syringes are stable for 24 hours at 9°C to 30°C (47°F to 86°F).

Undiluted filgrastim is stable for 24 hours at 15°C to 30°C (59°F to 86°F) and for up to 14 days at 2°C to 8°C (36°F to 46°F) (data on file, Amgen Medical Information) in BD tuberculin syringes; however, sterility has only been assessed and maintained for up to 7 days when prepared under strict aseptic conditions (Singh, 1994; Jacobson, 1996). The manufacturer recommends using syringes within 24 hours due to the potential for bacterial contamination.

Do not dilute with saline at any time; product may precipitate. Filgrastim may be diluted with D$_5$W or with D$_5$W with albumin for I.V. infusion administration (5-15 mcg/mL; minimum concentration is 5 mcg/mL). This diluted solution is stable for 7 days at 2°C to 8°C (36°F to 46°F), however, should be used within 24 hours due to the possibility for bacterial contamination. Dilution to <5 mcg/mL is not recommended. Concentrations 5-15 mcg/mL require addition of albumin (final concentration of 2 mg/mL) to prevent absorption to plastics.

Mechanism of Action Stimulates the production, maturation, and activation of neutrophils; filgrastim activates neutrophils to increase both their migration and cytotoxicity.

Pharmacodynamics

Onset of action: Rapid elevation in neutrophil counts within the first 24 hours, reaching a plateau in 3-5 days

Duration: ANC decreases by 50% within 2 days after discontinuing G-CSF white counts return to the normal range in 4-7 days

Pharmacokinetics

Absorption: SubQ: 100%; peak plasma concentrations can be maintained for up to 12 hours

Distribution: V$_d$: 150 mL/kg; no evidence of drug accumulation over a 11- to 20-day period

Metabolism: Systemic

Bioavailability: Oral: Not bioavailable

Half-life: 1.8-3.5 hours

Time to peak, serum: SubQ: 2-8 hours

Dosage

Geriatrics: Refer to adult dosing.

Drug-induced agranulocytosis (nonchemotherapy) in the elderly (unlabeled use): SubQ: 300 mcg daily until ANC >1500/mm^3

Adults: Refer to individual protocols.

Note: Dosing should be based on actual body weight (even in morbidly obese patients). Rounding doses to the nearest vial size often enhances patient convenience and reduces costs without compromising clinical response.

Chemotherapy-induced neutropenia I.V., SubQ: 5 mcg/kg/day; doses may be increased by 5 mcg/kg according to the duration and severity of the neutropenia; continue for up to 14 days or until the ANC reaches 10,000/mm^3

(Continued)

Filgrastim *(Continued)*

Bone marrow transplantation: I.V., SubQ: 10 mcg/kg/day; adjust the dose according to the duration and severity of neutropenia; recommended steps based on neutrophil response:

When ANC >1000/mm^3 for 3 consecutive days: Reduce filgrastim dose to 5 mcg/kg/day.

If ANC remains >1000/mm^3 for 3 more consecutive days: Discontinue filgrastim.

If ANC decreases to <1000/mm^3: Resume at 5 mcg/kg/day.

If ANC decreases <1000/mm^3 during the 5 mcg/kg/day dose: Increase filgrastim to 10 mcg/kg/day and follow the above steps.

Peripheral blood progenitor cell (PBPC) collection: SubQ: 10 mcg/kg daily in donors, usually for 6-7 days. Begin at least 4 days before the first leukopheresis and continue until the last leukopheresis; consider dose adjustment for WBC >100,000/mm^3

Severe chronic neutropenia: SubQ:

Congenital: 6 mcg/kg twice daily; adjust the dose based on ANC and clinical response

Idiopathic/cyclic: 5 mcg/kg/day; adjust the dose based on ANC and clinical response

Anemia in myelodysplastic syndrome (unlabeled use - in combination with epoetin): SubQ: 0.3-3 mcg/kg daily **or** 30-150 mcg daily **or** 1-2 mcg/kg 2-3 times weekly

Administration May be administered undiluted by SubQ injection. May also be administered by I.V. bolus over 15-30 minutes in D$_5$W, or by continuous SubQ or I.V. infusion. Do not administer earlier than 24 hours after or in the 24 hours prior to cytotoxic chemotherapy.

Monitoring Parameters CBC with differential prior to treatment and twice weekly during filgrastim treatment for chemotherapy-induced neutropenia (3 times a week following marrow transplantation). For severe chronic neutropenia, monitor CBC twice weekly during the first month of therapy and for 2 weeks following dose adjustments; monthly thereafter.

Reference Range No clinical benefit seen with ANC >10,000/mm^3

Test Interactions May interfere with bone imaging studies; increased hematopoietic activity of the bone marrow may appear as transient positive bone imaging changes

Patient Information Possible bone pain

Additional Information

Reimbursement Hotline: 1-800-272-9376

Professional Services [Amgen]: 1-800-77-AMGEN

Special Geriatric Considerations No specific data available for the elderly.

Dosage Forms Excipient information presented when available (limited, particularly for generics); consult specific product labeling.

Injection, solution [preservative free]:

Neupogen®: 300 mcg/mL (1 mL, 1.6 mL) [vial; contains sodium 0.035 mg/mL and sorbitol]

Injection, solution [preservative free]:

Neupogen®: 600 mcg/mL (0.5 mL, 0.8 mL) [prefilled Singleject® syringe; contains sodium 0.035 mg/mL and sorbitol; needle cover contains latex]

Selected References

Andres E, Kurtz JE, Martin-Hunyadi C, et al, "Nonchemotherapy Drug-Induced Agranulocytosis in Elderly Patients: The Effects of Granulocyte Colony-Stimulating Factor," *Am J Med*, 2002, 112(6):460-4.

Rosenberg PS, Alter BP, Bolyard AA, et al, "The Incidence of Leukemia and Mortality From Sepsis in Patients With Severe Congenital Neutropenia Receiving Long-Term G-CSF Therapy," *Blood*, 2006, 107(12): 4628-35.

Finasteride (fi NAS teer ide)

Medication Safety Issues

Sound-alike/look-alike issues:

Proscar® may be confused with ProSom®, Prozac®, Psorcon®

High alert medication: The Institute for Safe Medication Practices (ISMP) includes this medication among its list of drugs which have a heightened risk of causing significant patient harm when used in error.

U.S. Brand Names Propecia®; Proscar®

Canadian Brand Names Propecia®; Proscar®

Generic Available Yes

Pharmacologic Category 5 Alpha-Reductase Inhibitor

Use

Propecia®: Treatment of male pattern hair loss in **men only**

Proscar®: Treatment of symptomatic benign prostatic hyperplasia (BPH); can be used in combination with an alpha blocker, doxazosin

Unlabeled/Investigational Use Adjuvant monotherapy after radical prostatectomy in the treatment of prostatic cancer; treatment of female hirsutism

Contraindications Hypersensitivity to finasteride or any component of the formulation

Warnings/Precautions Hazardous agent - use appropriate precautions for handling and disposal. Other urological diseases including cancer should be ruled out before initiating. A minimum of 6 months of treatment may be necessary to determine whether an individual will respond to finasteride. Reduces prostate specific antigen (PSA) by 50%; in patients treated for ≥6 months the PSA should be doubled when comparing to normal ranges in untreated patients. Use with caution in those patients with hepatic dysfunction. Carefully monitor patients with a large residual urinary volume or severely diminished urinary flow for obstructive uropathy. These patients may not be candidates for finasteride therapy.

Adverse Reactions (Reflective of adult population; not specific for elderly)
Note: "Combination therapy" refers to finasteride and doxazosin.
>10%:
Endocrine & metabolic: Impotence (19%; combination therapy 23%), libido decreased (10%; combination therapy 12%)
Genitourinary: Neuromuscular & skeletal: Weakness (5%; combination therapy 17%)
1% to 10%:
Cardiovascular: Postural hypotension (9%; combination therapy 18%), edema (1%, combination therapy 3%)
Central nervous system: Dizziness (7%; combination therapy 23%), somnolence (2%; combination therapy 3%)
Genitourinary: Ejaculation disturbances (7%; combination therapy 14%), decreased volume of ejaculate
Endocrine & metabolic: Gynecomastia (2%)
Respiratory: Dyspnea (1%; combination therapy 2%), rhinitis (1%; combination therapy 2%)

Drug Interactions Substrate of CYP3A4 (minor)

Ethanol/Nutrition/Herb Interactions
Herb/Nutraceutical: St John's wort may decrease finasteride levels. Avoid saw palmetto (concurrent use has not been adequately studied).

Stability Store below 30°C (86°F). Protect from light.

Mechanism of Action Finasteride is a competitive inhibitor of both tissue and hepatic 5-alpha reductase. This results in inhibition of the conversion of testosterone to dihydrotestosterone and markedly suppresses serum dihydrotestosterone levels

Pharmacodynamics
Onset of clinical effect: Within 12 weeks to 6 months of ongoing therapy
Duration:
After a single oral dose as small as 0.5 mg: 65% depression of plasma dihydrotestosterone levels persists 5-7 days
After 6 months of treatment with 5 mg/day: Circulating dihydrotestosterone levels are reduced to castration levels without significant effects on circulating testosterone; levels return to normal within 14 days of discontinuation of treatment

Pharmacokinetics
Absorption: Oral: Extent of absorption may be reduced if administered with food
Distribution: V_{dss}: 76 L
Protein binding: 90%
Metabolism: Hepatic via CYP3A4; two active metabolites (<20% activity of finasteride)
Bioavailability: Mean: 63%
Half-life elimination, serum: Elderly: 8 hours; Adults: 6 hours (3-16)
Elimination: Excreted as metabolites in urine and feces; elimination rate is decreased in older adults, but no dosage adjustment is needed

Dosage
Geriatrics & Adults:
Benign prostatic hyperplasia (Proscar®): Oral: 5 mg/day as a single dose; clinical responses occur within 12 weeks to 6 months of initiation of therapy; long-term administration is recommended for maximal response
Male pattern baldness (Propecia®): Oral: 1 mg daily
Female hirsutism (unlabeled use): Oral: 5 mg/day
Renal Impairment: No adjustment is necessary.
Hepatic Impairment: Use with caution in patients with liver function abnormalities because finasteride is metabolized extensively in the liver

Administration Women of childbearing age should not touch or handle broken tablets.

Monitoring Parameters Objective and subjective signs of relief of benign prostatic hyperplasia, including improvement in urinary flow, reduction in symptoms of urgency, and relief of difficulty in micturition

Patient Information Inform prescriber of all prescriptions, OTC medications, or herbal products you are taking, and any allergies you have. Do not take any new medication during therapy unless approved by prescriber. Results of therapy may take several months. Take with or without meals. May cause decreased libido or impotence during
(Continued)

Finasteride *(Continued)*

therapy. Report any increase in urinary volume or voiding patterns occurs. Report changes in breast condition (pain, lumps, or nipple discharge) in male and female patients.

Additional Information Finasteride may be useful in men with moderately sympto-matic BPH who either refuse prostatectomy or are poor surgical candidates. Risk:benefit ratio and cost must be explained to the patient. Currently, there is no way to predict which men will respond to finasteride. A recent study found finasteride to be no more effective than placebo in men with BPH. When added to terazosin (an alpha antagonist), the combination was no more effective than terazosin alone.

Propecia®: Daily use for 3 or more months is necessary before benefit is observed. Withdrawal of treatment leads to reversal of effect within 12 months.

Special Geriatric Considerations Clearance of finasteride is decreased in the elderly, but no dosage reductions are necessary.

Dosage Forms Excipient information presented when available (limited, particularly for generics); consult specific product labeling.

Tablet: 5 mg
Propecia®: 1 mg
Proscar®: 5 mg

Selected References

Lepor H, Williford WO, Barry MJ, et al, "The Efficacy of Terazosin, Finasteride, or Both in Benign Prostatic Hyperplasia," *N Engl J Med*, 1996, 335(8):533-9.

McConnell JD, Roehrborn CG, Bautista OM, et al, "The Long-Term Effect of Doxazosin, Finasteride, and Combination Therapy on the Clinical Progression of Benign Prostatic Hyperplasia. Medical Therapy of Prostatic Symptoms (MTOPS) Research Group," *N Engl J Med*, 2003, 349(25):2387-98.

Thompson IM, Goodman PJ, Tangen CM, et al, "The Influence of Finasteride on the Development of Prostate Cancer," *N Engl J Med*, 2003, Jul 349(3):215-24.

- ◆ **First® Testosterone** *see* Testosterone *on page 1537*
- ◆ **First® Testosterone MC** *see* Testosterone *on page 1537*
- ◆ **Fisalamine** *see* Mesalamine *on page 989*
- ◆ **Fish Oil** *see* Omega-3-Acid Ethyl Esters *on page 1155*
- ◆ **Flagyl®** *see* Metronidazole *on page 1031*
- ◆ **Flagyl ER®** *see* Metronidazole *on page 1031*

Flavoxate (fla VOKS ate)

Medication Safety Issues

Sound-alike/look-alike issues:

Flavoxate may be confused with fluvoxamine
Urispas® may be confused with Urised®

U.S. Brand Names Urispas®

Canadian Brand Names Apo-Flavoxate®; Urispas®

Index Terms Flavoxate Hydrochloride

Generic Available Yes

Pharmacologic Category Antispasmodic Agent, Urinary

Use Antispasmodic to provide symptomatic relief of dysuria, nocturia, suprapubic pain, urgency, and incontinence due to detrusor instability and hyper-reflexia in older adults with cystitis, urethritis, urethrocystitis, urethrotrigonitis, and prostatitis

Contraindications Hypersensitivity to flavoxate; pyloric or duodenal obstruction; GI hemorrhage; GI obstruction; ileus; achalasia; obstructive uropathies of lower urinary tract (BPH)

Warnings/Precautions May cause drowsiness, vertigo, and ocular disturbances; administer cautiously in patients with suspected glaucoma.

Adverse Reactions (Reflective of adult population; not specific for elderly)

Frequency not defined.

Cardiovascular: Tachycardia, palpitation

Central nervous system: Drowsiness, confusion (especially in the elderly), nervous-ness, fatigue, vertigo, headache, hyperpyrexia

Dermatologic: Rash. urticaria

Gastrointestinal: Constipation, nausea, vomiting, xerostomia, dry throat

Genitourinary: Dysuria

Hematologic: Leukopenia

Ocular: Increased intraocular pressure, blurred vision

Drug Interactions No data reported

Ethanol/Nutrition/Herb Interactions Ethanol: Avoid ethanol (may increase CNS depression).

Mechanism of Action Synthetic antispasmotic with similar actions to that of propan-theline; it exerts a direct relaxant effect on smooth muscles via phosphodiesterase inhibition, providing relief to a variety of smooth muscle spasms; it is especially useful for the treatment of bladder spasticity, whereby it produces an increase in urinary capacity

Pharmacodynamics Onset of action: 55-60 minutes

Pharmacokinetics
Metabolism: To methyl- flavone carboxylic acid active
Elimination: 10% to 30% in urine within 6 hours

Dosage
Geriatrics & Adults: Urinary spasms: Oral: 100-200 mg 3-4 times/day; reduce the dose when symptoms improve.

Monitoring Parameters Monitor incontinence episodes; postvoid residual (PVR); monitor for anticholinergic side effects

Patient Information May cause drowsiness, dizziness, or visual disturbances; use with caution if performing tasks requiring coordination or mental alertness; avoid other substances that may cause similar effects (eg, alcohol)

Special Geriatric Considerations Caution should be used in the elderly due to anticholinergic activity (eg, confusion, constipation, blurred vision, and tachycardia).

Dosage Forms Excipient information presented when available (limited, particularly for generics); consult specific product labeling.
Tablet, as hydrochloride: 100 mg

♦ **Flavoxate Hydrochloride** *see Flavoxate on page 628*

Flecainide (fle KAY nide)

Medication Safety Issues
Sound-alike/look-alike issues:
Flecainide may be confused with fluconazole
Tambocor™ may be confused with tamoxifen

U.S. Brand Names Tambocor™

Canadian Brand Names Apo-Flecainide®; Tambocor™

Index Terms Flecainide Acetate

Generic Available Yes

Pharmacologic Category Antiarrhythmic Agent, Class Ic

Use Prevention and suppression of documented life-threatening ventricular arrhythmias (ie, sustained ventricular tachycardia); control of symptomatic, disabling supraventricular tachycardias in patients without structural heart disease

Contraindications Hypersensitivity to flecainide or any component of the formulation; pre-existing second- or third-degree AV block or with right bundle branch block when associated with a left hemiblock (bifascicular block) (except in patients with a functioning artificial pacemaker); cardiogenic shock; coronary artery disease (based on CAST study results); concurrent use of ritonavir or amprenavir

Warnings/Precautions [U.S. Boxed Warning]: In the Cardiac Arrhythmia Suppression Trial (CAST), recent (>6 days but <2 years ago) myocardial infarction patients with asymptomatic, nonlife-threatening ventricular arrhythmias did not benefit and may have been harmed by attempts to suppress the arrhythmia with flecainide or encainide. An increased mortality or nonfatal cardiac arrest rate (7.7%) was seen in the active treatment group compared with patients in the placebo group (3%). The applicability of the CAST results to other populations is unknown. The risks of class 1C agents and the lack of improved survival make use in patients without life-threatening arrhythmias generally unacceptable. **[U.S. Boxed Warning]: Watch for proarrhythmic effects;** monitor and adjust dose to prevent QT_c prolongation. Not recommended for patients with chronic atrial fibrillation. **[U.S. Boxed Warning]: When treating atrial flutter, 1:1 atrioventricular conduction may occur; pre-emptive negative chronotropic therapy (eg, digoxin, beta-blockers) may lower the risk.** Pre-existing hypokalemia or hyperkalemia should be corrected before initiation (can alter drug's effect). A worsening or new arrhythmia may occur (proarrhythmic effect). Use caution in heart failure (may precipitate or exacerbate CHF). Dose-related increases in PR, QRS, and QT intervals occur. Use with caution in sick sinus syndrome or with permanent pacemakers or temporary pacing wires (can increase endocardial pacing thresholds). Cautious use in significant hepatic impairment.

Adverse Reactions (Reflective of adult population; not specific for elderly)
>10%:
Central nervous system: Dizziness (19% to 30%)
Ocular: Visual disturbances (16%)
Respiratory: Dyspnea (~10%)
1% to 10%:
Cardiovascular: Palpitation (6%), chest pain (5%), edema (3.5%), tachycardia (1% to 3%), proarrhythmic (4% to 12%), sinus node dysfunction (1.2%)
Central nervous system: Headache (4% to 10%), fatigue (8%), nervousness (5%) additional symptoms occurring at a frequency between 1% and 3%: fever,
(Continued)

Flecainide *(Continued)*

malaise, hypoesthesia, paresis, ataxia, vertigo, syncope, somnolence, tinnitus, anxiety, insomnia, depression

Dermatologic: Rash (1% to 3%)

Gastrointestinal: Nausea (9%), constipation (1%), abdominal pain (3%), anorexia (1% to 3%), diarrhea (0.7% to 3%)

Neuromuscular & skeletal: Tremor (5%), weakness (5%), paresthesia (1%)

Ocular: Diplopia (1% to 3%), blurred vision

Overdosage/Toxicology Has a narrow therapeutic index; severe toxicity may occur slightly above the therapeutic range, especially if combined with other antiarrhythmic drugs. An acute single ingestion of twice the daily therapeutic dose is life-threatening. Symptoms include increased PR, QRS, and QT intervals; amplitude of the T wave, AV block, bradycardia, hypotension, ventricular arrhythmias (monomorphic or polymorphic ventricular tachycardia); and asystole. Other symptoms include dizziness, blurred vision, headache, and GI upset. Treatment is supportive, using conventional treatment (fluids, positioning, anticonvulsants, antiarrhythmics). **Note:** Type Ia antiarrhythmic agents should not be used to treat cardiotoxicity caused by type Ic antiarrhythmics. Sodium bicarbonate may reverse QRS prolongation, bradycardia, and hypotension. Ventricular pacing may be needed. Hemodialysis is only of possible benefit for tocainide or flecainide overdose in patients with renal failure.

Drug Interactions Substrate of CYP1A2 (minor), 2D6 (major); **Inhibits** CYP2D6 (weak)

Amiodarone increases in flecainide plasma levels; consider reducing flecainide dose by 25% to 33% with concurrent use.

Amprenavir and ritonavir may increase cardiotoxicity of flecainide (decrease metabolism).

Cimetidine may decrease flecainide's metabolism; monitor cardiac status or use an alternative H_2 antagonist.

CYP2D6 inhibitors: May increase the levels/effects of flecainide. Example inhibitors include chlorpromazine, delavirdine, fluoxetine, miconazole, paroxetine, pergolide, quinidine, quinine, ritonavir, and ropinirole.

Digoxin's serum concentration may increase slightly.

Propranolol (and possibly other beta-blockers) increases flecainide blood levels, and propranolol blood levels are increased with concurrent use; monitor for excessive negative inotropic effects.

Quinidine may decrease flecainide's metabolism; monitor cardiac status.

Urinary alkalinizers (antacids, sodium bicarbonate, acetazolamide) may increase flecainide blood levels.

Ethanol/Nutrition/Herb Interactions Food: Clearance may be decreased in patients following strict vegetarian diets due to urinary pH ≥8.

Mechanism of Action Class Ic antiarrhythmic; slows conduction in cardiac tissue by altering transport of ions across cell membranes; causes slight prolongation of refractory periods; decreases the rate of rise of the action potential without affecting its duration; increases electrical stimulation threshold of ventricle, His-Purkinje system; possesses local anesthetic and moderate negative inotropic effects

Pharmacokinetics

Absorption: Oral: Rapid

Distribution: V_d: Adults: 5-13.4 L/kg

Protein binding: 40% to 50% (alpha$_1$ glycoprotein)

Metabolism: In the liver

Bioavailability: 85% to 90%

Half-life: Adults: 7-22 hours (average: 14 hours); increased half-life with congestive heart failure or renal dysfunction

Time to peak serum concentrations: Within 1.5-3 hours

Elimination: 80% to 90% in urine as unchanged drug and metabolites (10% to 50%)

Dosage

Geriatrics & Adults:

Life-threatening ventricular arrhythmias: Oral:

Initial: 100 mg every 12 hours; increase by 50-100 mg/day (given in 2 doses/day) every 4 days; maximum: 400 mg/day

For patients receiving 400 mg/day who are not controlled and have trough concentrations <0.6 mcg/mL, dosage may be increased to 600 mg/day.

Prevention of paroxysmal supraventricular arrhythmias: Oral: (**Note:** In patients with disabling symptoms but no structural heart disease): Initial: 50 mg every 12 hours; increase by 50 mg twice daily at 4-day intervals; maximum: 300 mg/day

Paroxysmal atrial fibrillation: Outpatient: "Pill-in-the-pocket" dose (unlabeled dose): Oral: 200 mg (weight <70 kg), 300 mg (weight ≥70 kg). May not repeat in ≤24 hours. **Note:** An initial inpatient conversion trial should have been successful before sending patient home on this approach. Patient must be taking an AV nodal-blocking agent (eg, beta-blocker, nondihydropyridine calcium channel blocker) prior to initiation of antiarrhythmic.

Renal Impairment: GFR ≤50 mL/minute: Decrease dose by 50%; dose increases should be made cautiously at intervals >4 days and serum levels monitored frequently.

Hemodialysis: No supplemental dose recommended.

Peritoneal dialysis: No supplemental dose recommended.

Hepatic Impairment: Monitoring of plasma levels is recommended because half-life is significantly increased. When transferring from another antiarrhythmic agent, allow for 2-4 half-lives of the agent to pass before initiating flecainide therapy.

Administration Administer around-the-clock to promote less variation in peak and trough serum levels

Monitoring Parameters EKG, blood pressure, pulse, periodic serum concentrations, especially in patients with renal or hepatic impairment

Reference Range Therapeutic: 0.2-1 mcg/mL (SI: 0.4-2 μmol/L)

Patient Information Take exactly as directed, around-the-clock. Do not discontinue without consulting prescriber. You will require frequent monitoring while taking this medication. You may experience lightheadedness, nervousness, dizziness, visual disturbances (use caution when driving or engaging in tasks requiring alertness until response to drug is known); or nausea, vomiting, or loss of appetite (small frequent meals may help). Report palpitations, chest pain, excessively slow or rapid heartbeat; acute nervousness, headache, or fatigue; unusual weight gain; unusual cough; respiratory difficulty; swelling of hands or ankles; or muscle tremor, numbness, or weakness.

Special Geriatric Considerations Decreased clearance and, therefore, prolonged half-life is possible; however, studies have shown no difference in response to usual doses in the elderly despite slight decrease in clearance; calculate or measure GFR since elderly patients may have GFR ≤50 mL/minute.

Dosage Forms Excipient information presented when available (limited, particularly for generics); consult specific product labeling.

Tablet, as acetate: 50 mg, 100 mg, 150 mg

Selected References

Fenster PE and Nolan PE, "Antiarrhythmic Drugs," *Geriatric Pharmacology*, Bressler R and Katz MD, eds, New York, NY: McGraw-Hill, 1993, 6:105-49.

Fuster V, Ryden LE, Cannom DS, et al, "ACC/AHA/ESC 2006 Guidelines for the Management of Patients With Atrial Fibrillation-Executrive Summary. A Report of the American College of Cardiology/American Heart Association Task Force on Practice Guidelines and the European Society of Cardiology Committee for Practice Guidelines (Writing Committee to Revise the 2001 Guidelines for the Management of Patients With Atrial Fibrillation). Developed in Collaboration With the European Heart Rhythm Association and the Heart Rhythm Society," *J Am Coll Cardiol*, 2006, 48(4):854-906.

♦ **Flecainide Acetate** *see* Flecainide *on page 629*

♦ **Fleet® Accu-Prep® [OTC]** *see* Sodium Phosphates *on page 1478*

♦ **Fleet® Babylax® [OTC]** *see* Glycerin *on page 718*

♦ **Fleet® Bisacodyl [OTC]** *see* Bisacodyl *on page 173*

♦ **Fleet® Enema [OTC]** *see* Sodium Phosphates *on page 1478*

♦ **Fleet® Glycerin Suppositories [OTC]** *see* Glycerin *on page 718*

♦ **Fleet® Glycerin Suppositories Maximum Strength [OTC]** *see* Glycerin *on page 718*

♦ **Fleet® Liquid Glycerin Suppositories [OTC]** *see* Glycerin *on page 718*

♦ **Fleet® Mineral Oil Enema [OTC]** *see* Mineral Oil *on page 1045*

♦ **Fleet® Phospho-Soda® [OTC]** *see* Sodium Phosphates *on page 1478*

♦ **Fleet® Sof-Lax® [OTC]** *see* Docusate *on page 459*

♦ **Fleet® Stimulant Laxative [OTC]** *see* Bisacodyl *on page 173*

♦ **Fletcher's® [OTC]** *see* Senna *on page 1456*

♦ **Flexeril®** *see* Cyclobenzaprine *on page 374*

♦ **Flomax®** *see* Tamsulosin *on page 1518*

♦ **Flonase®** *see* Fluticasone *on page 659*

♦ **Flora-Q™ [OTC]** *see* Lactobacillus *on page 867*

♦ **Florastor® [OTC]** *see* Saccharomyces boulardii *on page 1438*

♦ **Florastor® Kids [OTC]** *see* Saccharomyces boulardii *on page 1438*

♦ **Florical® [OTC]** *see* Calcium Salts (Oral) *on page 220*

♦ **Florinef® [DSC]** *see* Fludrocortisone *on page 635*

♦ **Flovent® HFA** *see* Fluticasone *on page 659*

♦ **Floxin®** *see* Ofloxacin *on page 1144*

♦ **Floxin Otic Singles** *see* Ofloxacin *on page 1144*

♦ **Fluarix®** *see* Influenza Virus Vaccine *on page 803*

♦ **Flubenisolone** *see* Betamethasone *on page 161*

Fluconazole (floo KOE na zole)

Medication Safety Issues
Sound-alike/look-alike issues:
Fluconazole may be confused with flecainide
Diflucan® may be confused with diclofenac, Diprivan®, disulfiram

International issues:
Canesten® [Great Britain]: Brand name for clotrimazole in multiple international markets

U.S. Brand Names Diflucan®

Canadian Brand Names Apo-Fluconazole®; Diflucan®; Fluconazole Injection; Fluconazole Omega; Gen-Fluconazole; GMD-Fluconazole; Novo-Fluconazole; Riva-Fluconazole

Generic Available Yes

Pharmacologic Category Antifungal Agent, Oral; Antifungal Agent, Parenteral

Use Treatment of susceptible fungal infections (including oropharyngeal and esophageal candidiasis), systemic candidal infections (including urinary tract infection, peritonitis, and pneumonia), cryptococcal meningitis

Contraindications Hypersensitivity to fluconazole, other azoles, or any component of the formulation; concomitant administration with cisapride or astemizole

Warnings/Precautions Should be used with caution in patients with renal and hepatic dysfunction or previous hepatotoxicity from other azole derivatives. Patients who develop abnormal liver function tests during fluconazole therapy should be monitored closely and discontinued if symptoms consistent with liver disease develop. Rare exfoliative skin disorders have been observed; monitor closely if rash develops. The manufacturer reports rare cases of QT_c prolongation and TdP associated with fluconazole use and advises caution in patients with concomitant medications or conditions which are arrhythmogenic. However, given the limited number of cases and the presence of multiple confounding variables, the likelihood that fluconazole causes conduction abnormalities appears remote.

Adverse Reactions (Reflective of adult population; not specific for elderly)
Frequency not always defined.
Cardiovascular: Angioedema, pallor, QT prolongation (rare, case reports), torsade de pointes (rare, case reports)
Central nervous system: Headache (2% to 13%), seizure, dizziness
Dermatologic: Rash (2%), alopecia, toxic epidermal necrolysis, Stevens-Johnson syndrome
Endocrine & metabolic: Hypercholesterolemia, hypertriglyceridemia, hypokalemia
Gastrointestinal: Nausea (4% to 7%), vomiting (2%), abdominal pain (2% to 6%), diarrhea (2% to 3%), taste perversion, dyspepsia
Hematologic: Agranulocytosis, leukopenia, neutropenia, thrombocytopenia
Hepatic: Hepatic failure (rare), hepatitis, cholestasis, jaundice, increased ALT/AST, increased alkaline phosphatase
Respiratory: Dyspnea
Miscellaneous: Anaphylactic reactions (rare)

Overdosage/Toxicology Symptoms include decreased lacrimation, salivation, respiration, GI motility, urinary incontinence, and cyanosis. Treatment includes supportive measures. A 3-hour hemodialysis will remove 50% of the drug.

Drug Interactions Inhibits CYP1A2 (weak), 2C9 (strong), 2C19 (strong), 3A4 (moderate)

Benzodiazepines (metabolized by oxidation, eg, alprazolam, triazolam, midazolam, diazepam) serum concentrations are increased by fluconazole which may cause increased CNS sedation. Consider a benzodiazepine not metabolized by CYP3A4 or another antifungal.
Caffeine's metabolism is decreased; monitor for tachycardia, nervousness, and anxiety.
Calcium channel blockers may have increased serum concentrations; consider another agent instead of a calcium channel blocker, another antifungal, or reduce the dose of the calcium channel blocker. Monitor blood pressure.
Cisapride's serum concentration is increased which may lead to malignant arrhythmias; concurrent use is contraindicated.
Cyclosporine's serum concentration is increased; monitor cyclosporine's serum concentration and renal function.
CYP2C9 Substrates: Fluconazole may increase the levels/effects of CYP2C9 substrates. Example substrates include bosentan, dapsone, fluoxetine, glimepiride, glipizide, losartan, montelukast, nateglinide, paclitaxel, phenytoin, warfarin, and zafirlukast.
CYP2C19 substrates: Fluconazole may increase the levels/effects of CYP2C19 substrates. Example substrates include citalopram, diazepam, methsuximide, phenytoin, propranolol, and sertraline.

CYP3A4 substrates: Fluconazole may increase the levels/effects of CYP3A4 substrates. Example substrates include benzodiazepines, calcium channel blockers, cyclosporine, mirtazapine, nateglinide, nefazodone, sildenafil (and other PDE-5 inhibitors), tacrolimus, and venlafaxine. Selected benzodiazepines (midazolam and triazolam), cisapride, ergot alkaloids, selected HMG-CoA reductase inhibitors (lovastatin and simvastatin), and pimozide are generally contraindicated with strong CYP3A4 inhibitors.

HMG-CoA reductase inhibitors (except pravastatin and fluvastatin) have increased serum concentrations; switch to pravastatin/fluvastatin or monitor for development of myopathy.

Losartan's active metabolite is reduced in concentration; consider another antihypertensive agent unaffected by the azole antifungals, another antifungal, or monitor blood pressure closely.

Phenytoin's serum concentration is increased; monitor phenytoin levels and adjust dose as needed.

Rifampin decreases fluconazole's serum concentration; monitor infection status.

Tacrolimus's serum concentration is increased; monitor tacrolimus's serum concentration and renal function.

Warfarin's effects are increased; monitor INR and adjust warfarin's dose as needed.

Stability

Powder for oral suspension: Store dry powder at ≤30°C (86°F). Following reconstitution, store at 5°C to 30°C (41°F to 86°F). Discard unused portion after 2 weeks. Do not freeze.

Injection: Store injection in glass at 5°C to 30°C (41°F to 86°F). Store injection in Viaflex® at 5°C to 25°C (41°F to 77°F). Do not freeze. Do not unwrap unit until ready for use.

Mechanism of Action Interferes with cytochrome P450 activity, decreasing ergosterol synthesis (principal sterol in fungal cell membrane) and inhibiting cell membrane formation

Pharmacokinetics

Protein binding, plasma: 11% to 12%

Metabolism: Hepatic

Bioavailability: Oral: >90%

Half-life: Normal renal function: 25-30 hours

Time to peak: Oral: Within 2-4 hours

Elimination: 80% of dose excreted unchanged in urine

Dosage

Geriatrics & Adults: The daily dose of fluconazole is the same for both oral and I.V. administration

Usual dosage range: 200-800 mg daily; duration and dosage depends on severity of infection

Indication-specific dosing:

Candidiasis:

Candidemia (neutropenic and non-neutropenic): 400-800 mg/day for 14 days after last positive blood culture and resolution of signs/symptoms

Chronic, disseminated: 400-800 mg/day for 3-6 months

Oropharyngeal (long-term suppression): 200 mg/day; chronic therapy is recommended in immunocompromised patients with history of oropharyngeal candidiasis (OPC)

Osteomyelitis: 400-800 mg/day for 6-12 months

Esophageal: 200 mg on day 1, then 100-200 mg/day for 2-3 weeks after clinical improvement

Prophylaxis in bone marrow transplant: 400 mg/day; begin 3 days before onset of neutropenia and continue for 7 days after neutrophils >1000 cells/mm³

Urinary: 200 mg/day for 1-2 weeks

Vaginal: 150 mg as a single dose

Coccidiomycosis (unlabeled use, IDSA guideline): 400 mg/day; doses of 800-1000 mg/day have been used for meningeal disease; usual duration of therapy ranges from 3-6 months for primary uncomplicated infections and up to 1 year for pulmonary (chronic and diffuse) infection

Endocarditis, prosthetic valve, early (unlabeled use, IDSA guideline): 400-800 mg/day for 6 weeks after valve replacement; long-term suppression in absence of valve replacement: 200-400 mg/day

Endophthalmitis: 400-800 mg/day for 6-12 weeks after surgical intervention.

Meningitis, cryptococcal: Amphotericin 0.7-1 mg/kg +/- 5-FC for 2 weeks then fluconazole 400 mg/day for at least 10 weeks (consider life-long in HIV-positive); maintenance (HIV-positive): 200-400 mg/day life-long

Pneumonia, cryptococcal (mild-to-moderate) (unlabeled use, IDSA guideline): 200-400 mg/day for 6-12 months (consider life-long in HIV-positive patients)

(Continued)

Fluconazole *(Continued)*

Renal Impairment:
No adjustment for vaginal candidiasis single-dose therapy

For multiple dosing, administer usual load then adjust daily doses as follows:

Cl_{cr} ≤50 mL/minute (no dialysis): Administer 50% of recommended dose or administer every 48 hours.

Hemodialysis: 50% is removed by hemodialysis; administer 100% of daily dose (according to indication) after each dialysis treatment.

Continuous arteriovenous or venovenous hemofiltration: Dose as for Cl_{cr} 10-50 mL/minute.

Administration Parenteral fluconazole must be administered by I.V. infusion over ~1-2 hours; do not exceed 200 mg/hour when giving I.V. infusion

Monitoring Parameters AST, ALT, and alkaline phosphatase, potassium

Patient Information Take with or without food. Complete full course of therapy; contact physician or pharmacist if side effects develop

Additional Information An expensive oral alternative to I.V. amphotericin B infusions; in some clinical studies it has been as effective as amphotericin B, but is less likely to cause serious adverse reactions

Special Geriatric Considerations Has not been specifically studied in the elderly.

Dosage Forms Excipient information presented when available (limited, particularly for generics); consult specific product labeling.

Infusion [premixed in sodium chloride or dextrose]: 200 mg (100 mL); 400 mg (200 mL)
Diflucan® [premixed in sodium chloride or dextrose]: 200 mg (100 mL); 400 mg (200 mL)

Powder for oral suspension: 10 mg/mL (35 mL); 40 mg/mL (35 mL)
Diflucan®: 10 mg/mL (35 mL); 40 mg/mL (35 mL) [contains sodium benzoate; orange flavor]

Tablet: 50 mg, 100 mg, 150 mg, 200 mg
Diflucan®: 50 mg, 100 mg, 150 mg, 200 mg

Selected References

Grant SM and Clissold SP, "Fluconazole: A Review of Its Pharmacodynamic and Pharmacokinetic Properties and Therapeutic Potential in Superficial and Systemic Mycoses," *Drugs*, 1990, 39(6):877-916.

Pappas PG, Rex JH, Sobel JD, et al, "Guidelines for Treatment of Candidiasis. Infectious Diseases Society of America," *Clin Infect Dis*, 2004, 38(2):161-89.

Flucytosine *(floo SYE toe seen)*

Medication Safety Issues
Sound-alike/look-alike issues:

Flucytosine may be confused with fluorouracil

Ancobon® may be confused with Oncovin®

High alert medication: The Institute for Safe Medication Practices (ISMP) includes this medication among its list of drugs which have a heightened risk of causing significant patient harm when used in error.

U.S. Brand Names Ancobon®

Canadian Brand Names Ancobon®

Index Terms 5-FC; 5-Fluorocytosine; 5-Flurocytosine

Generic Available No

Pharmacologic Category Antifungal Agent, Oral

Use Adjunctive treatment of systemic fungal infections (eg, septicemia, endocarditis, UTI, meningitis, or pulmonary) caused by susceptible strains of *Candida* or *Cryptococcus*

Contraindications Hypersensitivity to flucytosine or any component of the formulation

Warnings/Precautions [U.S. Boxed Warning]: Use with extreme caution in patients with renal dysfunction; dosage adjustment required. Avoid use as monotherapy; resistance rapidly develops. Use with caution in patients with bone marrow depression; patients with hematologic disease or who have been treated with radiation or drugs that suppress the bone marrow may be at greatest risk. Bone marrow toxicity can be irreversible. **[U.S. Boxed Warning]: Closely monitor hematologic, renal, and hepatic status.** Hepatotoxicity and bone marrow toxicity appear to be dose related; monitor levels closely and adjust dose accordingly.

Adverse Reactions (Reflective of adult population; not specific for elderly)
Frequency not defined.

Cardiovascular: Cardiac arrest, myocardial toxicity, ventricular dysfunction, chest pain

Central nervous system: Ataxia, confusion, dizziness, drowsiness, fatigue, hallucinations, headache, parkinsonism, psychosis, pyrexia, sedation, seizure, vertigo

Dermatologic: Rash, photosensitivity, pruritus, toxic epidermal necrolysis, urticaria

Endocrine & metabolic: Hypoglycemia, hypokalemia

Gastrointestinal: Abdominal pain, diarrhea, dry mouth, duodenal ulcer, hemorrhage, loss of appetite, nausea, ulcerative colitis, vomiting

Hematologic: Agranulocytosis, anemia, aplastic anemia, eosinophilia, leukopenia, pancytopenia, thrombocytopenia

Hepatic: Acute hepatic injury, bilirubin increased, hepatic dysfunction, jaundice, liver enzymes increased

Neuromuscular & skeletal: Paresthesia, peripheral neuropathy, weakness

Otic: Hearing loss

Renal: Azotemia, BUN increased, crystalluria, renal failure, serum creatinine increased

Respiratory: Dyspnea, respiratory arrest

Miscellaneous: Allergic reaction

Overdosage/Toxicology Symptoms include nausea, vomiting, diarrhea, hepatitis, and bone marrow suppression. Monitor hematologic, renal, and hepatic parameters frequently. Treatment is symptom-directed and supportive. Removed by hemodialysis.

Drug Interactions Cytarabine: May decrease levels/effects of flucytosine; monitor.

Ethanol/Nutrition/Herb Interactions Food: Food decreases the rate, but not the extent of absorption.

Stability Store at room temperature of 15°C to 30°C (59°F to 86°F); protect from light.

Mechanism of Action Penetrates fungal cells and is converted to fluorouracil which competes with uracil interfering with fungal RNA and protein synthesis

Pharmacokinetics
Absorption: 76% to 89%
Protein binding: 3% to 4%
Metabolism: Minimal
Half-life: 3-8 hours (may be as long as 200 hours in anuria)
Time to peak, serum: ~1-2 hours
Elimination: 75% to 90% excreted unchanged in urine by glomerular filtration

Dosage
Geriatrics & Adults:
  Endocarditis: Oral: 0.7-1 mg/kg/day (with amphotericin B) for at least 6 weeks after valve replacement
  Meningoencephalitis, cryptococcal: Induction: Oral: 25 mg/kg/day (with amphotericin B) every 6 hours for 2 weeks; if clinical improvement, may discontinue both amphotericin and flucytosine and follow with an extended course of fluconazole (400 mg/day); alternatively, may continue flucytosine for 6-10 weeks (with amphotericin B) without conversion to fluconazole treatment

Renal Impairment: Use lower initial dose:
  Cl_{cr} 20-40 mL/minute: Administer 37.5 mg/kg every 12 hours
  Cl_{cr} 10-20 mL/minute: Administer 37.5 mg/kg every 24 hours
  Cl_{cr} <10 mL/minute: Administer 37.5 mg/kg every 24-48 hours, but monitor drug concentrations frequently
  Hemodialysis: Dialyzable (50% to 100%); administer dose posthemodialysis
  Peritoneal dialysis: Adults: Administer 0.5-1 g every 24 hours
  Continuous arteriovenous or venovenous hemodiafiltration effects: Change dosing frequency to every 12-24 hours (monitor serum concentrations and adjust)

Monitoring Parameters
Pretreatment: Electrolytes (especially potassium), CBC with differential, BUN, renal function, blood culture
During treatment: CBC with differential, and LFTs (eg, alkaline phosphatase, AST/ALT) frequently, serum flucytosine concentration, renal function

Reference Range Therapeutic: 25-100 mcg/mL (SI: 195-775 µmol/L)

Test Interactions Flucytosine causes markedly false elevations in serum creatinine values when the Ektachem® analyzer is used. The Jaffé reaction is recommended for determining serum creatinine.

Patient Information Take capsules a few at a time with food over a 15-minute period

Special Geriatric Considerations Adjust for renal function.

Dosage Forms Excipient information presented when available (limited, particularly for generics); consult specific product labeling.
Capsule: 250 mg, 500 mg

Fludrocortisone (floo droe KOR ti sone)

Related Information
Corticosteroids on page 1755
Medication Safety Issues
Sound-alike/look-alike issues:
Florinef® may be confused with Fiorinal®
U.S. Brand Names Florinef® [DSC]
Canadian Brand Names Florinef®
Index Terms 9α-Fluorohydrocortisone Acetate; Fludrocortisone Acetate; Fluohydrisone Acetate; Fluohydrocortisone Acetate
Generic Available Yes
(Continued)

Fludrocortisone *(Continued)*

Pharmacologic Category Corticosteroid, Systemic

Use Treatment of Addison's disease; partial replacement therapy for adrenal insufficiency and for treatment of salt-losing forms of congenital adrenogenital syndrome

Contraindications Hypersensitivity to fludrocortisone or any component of the formulation; systemic fungal infections

Warnings/Precautions May cause hypercorticism or suppression of hypothalamic-pituitary-adrenal (HPA) axis, particularly in patients receiving high doses for prolonged periods. HPA axis suppression may lead to adrenal crisis. Withdrawal and discontinuation of a corticosteroid should be done slowly and carefully. Fludrocortisone is primarily a mineralocorticoid agonist, but may also inhibit the HPA axis. May increase risk of infection and/or limit response to vaccinations; close observation is required in patients with latent tuberculosis and/or TB reactivity. Restrict use in active TB (only in conjunction with antituberculosis treatment). Use with caution in patients with sodium retention and potassium loss, hepatic impairment, myocardial infarction, osteoporosis, and/or renal impairment. Use with caution in the elderly. Withdraw therapy with gradual tapering of dose.

Adverse Reactions (Reflective of adult population; not specific for elderly)
Frequency not defined.

Cardiovascular: Hypertension, edema, CHF

Central nervous system: Convulsions, headache, dizziness

Dermatologic: Acne, rash, bruising

Endocrine & metabolic: Hypokalemic alkalosis, suppression of growth, hyperglycemia, HPA suppression

Gastrointestinal: Peptic ulcer

Neuromuscular & skeletal: Muscle weakness

Ocular: Cataracts

Miscellaneous: Diaphoresis, anaphylaxis (generalized)

Overdosage/Toxicology Symptoms include hypertension, edema, hypokalemia, and excessive weight gain. When consumed in excessive quantities, systemic hypercorticism and adrenal suppression may occur; in those cases, discontinuation and withdrawal of the corticosteroid should be done judiciously.

Drug Interactions

Aminoglutethimide: May reduce the serum levels/effects of corticosteroids; likely via induction of microsomal isoenzymes.

Amphotericin: Corticosteroids may increase the hypokalemic effects of amphotericin B; monitor.

Antacids: May decrease the absorption of corticosteroids; separate administration by 2 hours.

Anticholinesterases: Concurrent use may lead to severe weakness in patients with myasthenia gravis.

Antidiabetic agents: Corticosteroids may decrease the hypoglycemic effects of antidiabetic agents; monitor.

Aprepitant: May increase the serum levels/effects of corticosteroids; monitor.

Antifungal agents (azole): May increase the serum levels/effects of corticosteroids; monitor.

Barbiturates: May decrease the levels/effects of fludrocortisone; monitor.

Bile acid sequestrants: May reduce the absorption of corticosteroids; separate administration by 2 hours.

Calcium channel blockers (nondihydropyridine): May increase the serum levels/effects of corticosteroids; monitor.

Cyclosporine: Corticosteroids may increase the serum levels/effects of cyclosporine. In addition, cyclosporine may increase levels of corticosteroids.

Diuretics, potassium-wasting (loop or thiazide): Hypokalemic effects may be increased by corticosteroids; monitor.

Estrogens: May increase the serum levels/effects of corticosteroids; monitor.

Fluoroquinolones: Concurrent use may increase the risk of tendinopathies (including tendonitis and rupture), particularly in elderly patients (overall incidence rare)

Isoniazid: Serum levels/effects may be decreased by corticosteroids.

Macrolide antibiotics: May increase the serum levels/effects of fludrocortisone.

Neuromuscular-blocking agents: Concurrent use with corticosteroids may increase the risk of myopathy.

Nonsteroidal anti-inflammatory drugs (NSAIDs): Concurrent use with corticosteroids may lead to an increased incidence of gastrointestinal adverse effects; use caution.

Rifamycin derivatives: May decrease the levels/effects of corticosteroids (systemic); monitor.

Salicylates: Salicylates may increase the gastrointestinal adverse effects of corticosteroids.

Vaccine (dead organism): Corticosteroids may decrease the effect of vaccines (dead organisms). In patients receiving high doses of systemic corticosteroids for ≥14 days, wait at least 1 month between discontinuing steroid therapy and administering immunization.

Vaccine (live organism): Corticosteroids may increase the risk of vaccinal infection. The use of live vaccines is contraindicated in immunosuppressed patients.

Warfarin: Corticosteroids may increase the anticoagulant effects of warfarin; monitor INR.

Mechanism of Action Promotes increased reabsorption of sodium and loss of potassium from renal distal tubules

Pharmacodynamics Duration: 1-2 days

Pharmacokinetics
Absorption: Rapid and completely from GI tract
Protein binding: 42%
Metabolism: In the liver
Half-life: 30-35 minutes; biological: 18-36 hours
Time to peak serum concentration: 1-7 hours

Dosage
Geriatrics & Adults: Mineralocorticoid deficiency: Oral: 0.05-0.2 mg/day with ranges of 0.1 mg 3 times/week to 0.2 mg/day

Monitoring Parameters Blood pressure, standing and sitting/lying down, signs of edema, electrolytes

Patient Information Notify physician if dizziness, severe or continuing headaches, swelling of feet or lower legs, or unusual weight gain occur

Additional Information Very potent mineralocorticoid with high glucocorticoid activity

Special Geriatric Considerations The most common use of fludrocortisone in the elderly is orthostatic hypotension that is unresponsive to more conservative measures. Attempt nonpharmacologic measures (hydration, support stockings etc) before starting drug therapy.

Dosage Forms Excipient information presented when available (limited, particularly for generics); consult specific product labeling. [DSC] = Discontinued product
Tablet, as acetate: 0.1 mg
Florinef®: 0.1 mg [DSC]

♦ **Fludrocortisone Acetate** see Fludrocortisone on page 635
♦ **FluLaval**™ see Influenza Virus Vaccine on page 803
♦ **Flumadine**® see Rimantadine on page 1411
♦ **fluMist**® see Influenza Virus Vaccine on page 803

Flunisolide (floo NISS oh lide)

Related Information
Asthma on page 1767
Inhalant Agents on page 1760

Medication Safety Issues
Sound-alike/look-alike issues:
Flunisolide may be confused with Flumadine®, fluocinonide
Nasarel® may be confused with Nizoral®

U.S. Brand Names AeroBid®; AeroBid®-M; Aerospan™; Nasarel®

Canadian Brand Names Alti-Flunisolide; Apo-Flunisolide®; Nasalide®; PMS-Flunisolide; Rhinalar®

Generic Available Yes: Nasal spray

Pharmacologic Category Corticosteroid, Inhalant (Oral); Corticosteroid, Nasal

Use Treatment of steroid-dependent asthma, seasonal or perennial rhinitis (intranasal product)

Contraindications Hypersensitivity to flunisolide or any component of the formulation; acute status asthmaticus; viral, tuberculosis, fungal, or bacterial respiratory infections; infections of the nasal mucosa

Warnings/Precautions May cause hypercorticism or suppression of hypothalamic-pituitary-adrenal (HPA) axis, particularly in patients receiving high doses for prolonged periods. HPA axis suppression may lead to adrenal crisis. Withdrawal and discontinuation of a corticosteroid should be done slowly and carefully. Particular care is required when patients are transferred from systemic corticosteroids to inhaled products due to possible adrenal insufficiency or withdrawal from steroids, including an increase in allergic symptoms. Patients receiving >20 mg per day of prednisone (or equivalent) may be most susceptible. Fatalities have occurred due to adrenal insufficiency in asthmatic patients during and after transfer from systemic corticosteroids to aerosol steroids; aerosol steroids do **not** provide the systemic steroid needed to treat patients having trauma, surgery, or infections. Do not use this product to transfer patients from oral corticosteroid therapy.

Bronchospasm may occur with wheezing after inhalation; if this occurs stop steroid and treat with a fast-acting bronchodilator. Supplemental steroids (oral or parenteral) may (Continued)

Flunisolide *(Continued)*

be needed during stress or severe asthma attacks. Not to be used in status asthmaticus or for the relief of acute bronchospasm. Corticosteroid use may cause psychiatric disturbances, including depression, euphoria, insomnia, mood swings, and personality changes. Pre-existing psychiatric conditions may be exacerbated by corticosteroid use. Prolonged use of corticosteroids may also increase the incidence of secondary infection, mask acute infection (including fungal infections), prolong or exacerbate viral infections, or limit response to vaccines. Exposure to chickenpox should be avoided; corticosteroids should not be used to treat ocular herpes simplex. Corticosteroids should not be used for cerebral malaria. Close observation is required in patients with latent tuberculosis and/or TB reactivity; restrict use in active TB (only in conjunction with antituberculosis treatment). Prolonged treatment with corticosteroids has been associated with the development of Kaposi's sarcoma (case reports); if noted, discontinuation of therapy should be considered.

Use with caution in patients with thyroid disease, hepatic impairment, renal impairment, cardiovascular disease, diabetes, glaucoma, cataracts, myasthenia gravis, patients at risk for osteoporosis, patients at risk for seizures, or GI diseases (diverticulitis, peptic ulcer, ulcerative colitis) due to perforation risk. Use caution following acute MI (corticosteroids have been associated with myocardial rupture). Because of the risk of adverse effects, systemic corticosteroids should be used cautiously in the elderly in the smallest possible effective dose for the shortest duration. Avoid nasal corticosteroid use in patients with recent nasal septal ulcers, nasal surgery or nasal trauma until healing has occurred.

To minimize the systemic effects of orally-inhaled and intranasal corticosteroids, each patient should be titrated to the lowest effective dose. There have been reports of systemic corticosteroid withdrawal symptoms (eg, joint/muscle pain, lassitude, depression) when withdrawing oral inhalation therapy.

Adverse Reactions (Reflective of adult population; not specific for elderly)
>10%:
    Central nervous system: Headache (intranasal <5%; oral 9% to 25%)
    Gastrointestinal: Aftertaste (10% to 17%)
    Respiratory: Nasal burning (intranasal 45%), pharyngitis (14% to 20%), rhinitis (<15%), nasal irritation (>1% to 13%)
1% to 10%:
    Cardiovascular: Chest pain (1% to 3%), edema (1% to 3%), chest tightness, hypertension, palpitation, tachycardia
    Central nervous system: Fever (1% to 9%), dizziness (1% to 3%), insomnia (1% to 3%), migraine (1% to 3%), chills, malaise, irritability, shakiness, anxiety, depression, faintness, fatigue, moodiness, vertigo
    Dermatologic: Erythema multiform (1% to 3%), acne, eczema, pruritus, urticaria
    Endocrine & metabolic: Dysmenorrhea (1% to 3%)
    Gastrointestinal: Dyspepsia (2% to 4%), abdominal pain (1% to 3%), diarrhea (1% to 10%), gastroenteritis (1% to 3%), nausea (Aerospan™: 1% to 3%), oral candidiasis (1% to 3%), taste perversion (1% to 3%), abdominal fullness, constipation, gas, heartburn, sore throat, dry throat, mouth discomfort, throat irritation
    Genitourinary: Vaginitis (1% to 3%), urinary tract infection (1% to 4%)
    Neuromuscular & skeletal: Myalgia (1% to 3%), neck pain (1% to 3%), numbness, weakness
    Ocular: Conjunctivitis (1% to 3%), blurred vision
    Renal: Laryngitis (1% to 3%)
    Respiratory: Sinusitis (<9%), epistaxia (<3%), bronchospasm, cough increased, dyspnea, hoarseness, nasal ulcer, sneezing, wheezing
    Miscellaneous: Allergy (4% to 5%), infection (3% to 9%), loss of smell, voice alteration (1% to 3%), flu-like syndrome, diaphoresis
<1%: Adrenal suppression

Overdosage/Toxicology When consumed in excessive quantities, systemic hypercorticism and adrenal suppression may occur; in those cases, discontinuation and withdrawal of the corticosteroid should be done judiciously.

Drug Interactions Substrate of CYP3A4 (major)
    Amphotericin: Corticosteroids may increase the hypokalemic effects of amphotericin B; monitor.
    Antidiabetic agents: Corticosteroids may decrease the hypoglycemic effects of antidiabetic agents; monitor.
    CYP3A4 inhibitors: May increase the levels/effects of flunisolide. Example inhibitors include azole antifungals, clarithromycin, diclofenac, doxycycline, erythromycin, imatinib, isoniazid, nefazodone, nicardipine, propofol, protease inhibitors, quinidine, telithromycin, and verapamil.
    Diuretics, potassium-wasting (loop or thiazide): Hypokalemic effects may be increased by corticosteroids; monitor.

Antifungal agents (azole): May increase the serum levels/effects of corticosteroids; monitor.

Fluoroquinolones: Concurrent use may increase the risk of tendinopathies (including tendonitis and rupture), particularly in elderly patients (overall incidence rare)

Stability
Aerospan™: Store at 15°C to 30°C (59°F to 86°F). Do not store near heat or flame. Protect from freezing and sunlight.

AeroBid®: Store below 49°C (below 120°F).

Mechanism of Action Decreases inflammation by suppression of migration of poly-morphonuclear leukocytes and reversal of increased capillary permeability; does not depress hypothalamus

Pharmacokinetics
Absorption: Nasal inhalation: ~50%

Metabolism: Rapid in the liver to active metabolites

Half-life: 1.8 hours

Elimination: Equally excreted in urine and feces

Dosage
Geriatrics & Adults: Note: AeroBid® and Aerospan™ are not interchangeable; dosing changes when switching from one to another.

Asthma: Oral Inhalation:

AeroBid®: 2 inhalations twice daily (morning and evening); up to 8 inhalations/day maximum

Aerospan™: 2 inhalations twice daily; up to 8 inhalations/day

Seasonal allergic rhinitis: Intranasal: 2 sprays each nostril twice daily (morning and evening); may increase to 2 sprays 3 times daily; maximum dose: 8 sprays/day in each nostril (400 mcg/day)

Administration Inhalation: Shake well before using. Rinse mouth following use of oral inhalers.

Aerospan™: Has a self-contained spacer; do not use with another spacer. Prime inhaler prior to first use. Begin inhalation immediately prior to actuation; a delay may reduce dose by ≥75%.

Monitoring Parameters Relief of symptoms

Patient Information Follow instructions that accompany the product; do not exceed recommended dosage; do not confuse or interchange oral and nasal inhalers

Additional Information Aerospan™ and AeroBid® doses are not interchangeable because of differences in delivery characteristics.

Special Geriatric Considerations Many elderly patients have difficulty using metered dose inhalers, which can limit their effectiveness. Assess technique in all older patients. A spacer device may be beneficial for the oral inhaler. Aerospan™ has its own spacer device attached to the unit and may be easier to use for elderly patients.

Dosage Forms Excipient information presented when available (limited, particularly for generics); consult specific product labeling.

Aerosol for oral inhalation:

AeroBid®: 250 mcg/actuation (7 g) [100 metered inhalations; contains CFCs]

AeroBid®-M: 250 mcg/actuation (7 g) [100 metered inhalations; contains CFCs; menthol flavor]

Aerospan™: 80 mcg/actuation (5.1 g) [60 metered inhalations; CFC free]; 80 mcg/actuation (8.9 g) [120 metered inhalations; CFC free]

Solution, intranasal [spray]: 29 mcg/actuation (25 mL) [200 sprays]

Nasarel®: 29 mcg/actuation (25 mL) [200 sprays; contains benzalkonium chloride]

Fluocinolone (floo oh SIN oh lone)

Related Information
Corticosteroids on page 1755

Medication Safety Issues
Sound-alike/look-alike issues:
Fluocinolone may be confused with fluocinonide

U.S. Brand Names Capex™; Derma-Smoothe/FS®; Retisert™; Synalar®

Canadian Brand Names Capex™; Derma-Smoothe/FS®; Synalar®

Index Terms Fluocinolone Acetonide

Generic Available Yes: Excludes ocular implant, oil, shampoo

Pharmacologic Category Corticosteroid, Ophthalmic; Corticosteroid, Topical

Use Relief of the inflammatory and pruritic manifestations of corticosteroid-responsive dermatoses

Ocular implant (Retisert™): Treatment of chronic, noninfectious uveitis affecting the posterior segment of the eye.

Contraindications Hypersensitivity to fluocinolone or any component of the formulation; TB of skin, herpes (including varicella)

(Continued)

Fluocinolone *(Continued)*

Ocular implant: Additional contraindications include ocular infections of viral or fungal origin

Warnings/Precautions Adverse systemic effects may occur when used on large areas of the body, denuded areas, for prolonged periods of time, with an occlusive dressing. Derma-Smoothe/FS® contains peanut oil; use caution in peanut-sensitive patients.

Ocular implant: May cause transient decrease in visual acuity of 1-4 weeks duration; caution with use in glaucoma patients; routine monitoring of IOP recommended. May require IOP-lowering treatments within 2 years postimplantation. Prolonged use of ocular corticosteroids may increase risk of secondary infection, cataract formation, optic nerve damage, and/or glaucoma. Recommend unilateral implantation only to minimize risk of postoperative infections developing in both eyes.

Adverse Reactions (Reflective of adult population; not specific for elderly)

Topical: Frequency not defined.

Dermatologic: Acneiform eruptions, allergic contact dermatitis, burning, dryness, folliculitis, irritation, itching, hypertrichosis, hypopigmentation, miliaria, perioral dermatitis, skin atrophy, striae

Endocrine & metabolic: Cushing's syndrome, HPA axis suppression

Miscellaneous: Secondary infection

Ocular implant:

>50%: Ocular: Cataract, intraocular pressure increased, eye pain; procedural complications (eg, cataract fragments, implant migration, wound complications)

10% to 35%:

Central nervous system: Dizziness (5% to 15%), headache (31%), pain (5% to 15%), pyrexia (5% to 15%)

Dermatologic: Rash (5% to 15%)

Gastrointestinal (5% to 15%): Nausea, vomiting

Neuromuscular & skeletal (5% to 15%): Arthralgia, back pain, limb pain

Ocular: Blurred vision, conjunctival hemorrhage, conjunctival hyperemia, dry eye, eye irritation/inflammation, eyelid edema, glaucoma, hypotony, maculopathy, pruritus, ptosis, tearing, visual acuity decrease, vitreous floaters, vitreous hemorrhage

Respiratory (5% to 15%): Cough, influenza, nasopharyngitis, sinusitis, upper respiratory infection

5% to 9%: Ocular: Blepharitis, choroidal detachment, conjunctival edema/chemosis, corneal edema, eye discharge, eye swelling, macular edema, photophobia, photopsia, retinal hemorrhage, visual disturbance, vitreous opacitites

Frequency not specified: Miscellaneous: Secondary infection (bacterial, viral, or fungal)

Overdosage/Toxicology Topically-applied products may be absorbed in sufficient amounts to produce systemic effects, particularly if applied to a large surface area or to inflamed/damaged skin. Systemic hypercorticism and adrenal suppression may occur; in those cases, discontinuation and withdrawal of the corticosteroid should be done judiciously.

Drug Interactions No data reported

Stability

Topical: Store at controlled room temperature in tightly-closed container.

Capex™: Prior to dispensing, the contents of the capsule should be emptied into the liquid shampoo; shake well; discard after 3 months

Ocular implant (Retisert™): Store in original container at 15°C to 25°C (59°F to 77°F); protect from freezing

Mechanism of Action A synthetic corticosteroid which differs structurally from triamcinolone acetonide in the presence of an additional fluorine atom in the 6-alpha position on the steroid nucleus. The mechanism of action for all topical corticosteroids is not well defined, however, is believed to be a combination of anti-inflammatory, antipruritic, and vasoconstrictive properties.

Pharmacokinetics

Absorption:

Topical: Dependent on strength of preparation, amount applied, nature of skin at application site, vehicle, and use of occlusive dressing; increased in areas of skin damage, inflammation, or occlusion

Ocular implant: Systemic absorption is negligible

Duration: Ocular implant: Releases fluocinolone acetonide at a rate of 0.6 mcg/day, decreasing over 30 days to a steady-state release rate of 0.3-0.4 mcg/day for 30 months

Distribution:

Topical: Throughout local skin; absorbed drug is distributed rapidly into muscle, liver, skin, intestines, and kidneys

Ocular implant: Aqueous and vitreous humor

Metabolism: Primarily in skin; small amount absorbed into systemic circulation is primarily hepatic to inactive compounds

Excretion: Urine (primarily as glucuronide and sulfate, also as unconjugated products); feces (small amounts)

Dosage
Geriatrics & Adults:
Corticosteroid-responsive dermatoses: Topical: Cream, ointment, solution: Apply a thin layer to affected area 2-4 times/day; may use occlusive dressings to manage psoriasis or recalcitrant conditions

Atopic dermatitis (Derma-Smoothe/FS®): Topical: Apply thin film to affected area 3 times/day

Scalp psoriasis (Derma-Smoothe/FS®): Topical: Massage thoroughly into wet or dampened hair/scalp; cover with shower cap. Leave on overnight (or for at least 4 hours). Remove by washing hair with shampoo and rinsing thoroughly.

Seborrheic dermatitis of the scalp (Capex™): Topical: Apply no more than 1 ounce to scalp once daily; work into lather and allow to remain on scalp for ~5 minutes. Remove from hair and scalp by rinsing thoroughly with water.

Chronic uveitis: Ocular implant: One silicone-encased tablet (0.59 mg) surgically implanted into the posterior segment of the eye is designed to release 0.6 mcg/day, decreasing over 30 days to a steady-state release rate of 0.3-0.4 mcg/day for 30 months. Recurrence of uveitis denotes depletion of tablet, requiring reimplantation.

Administration
Topical, cream/ointment: Apply thin film to affected area; avoid eyes.
Ocular implant: Handle only by suture tab to avoid damaging the tablet integrity and adversely affecting release characteristics. Maintain strict adherence to aseptic handling of product; do not resterilize.

Monitoring Parameters Relief of symptoms

Patient Information Use only as prescribed and for no longer than the period prescribed; apply sparingly in a thin film and rub in lightly; avoid contact with eyes; notify physician if condition persists or worsens

Additional Information Considered a moderate-potency steroid; avoid prolonged use on the face, may cause atrophic changes

Special Geriatric Considerations Due to age-related changes in skin, limit use of topical glucocorticosteroids.

Dosage Forms Excipient information presented when available (limited, particularly for generics); consult specific product labeling.
Cream, as acetonide: 0.01% (15 g, 60 g); 0.025% (15 g, 60 g)
Synalar®: 0.025% (15 g, 60 g)
Oil, as acetonide:
Derma-Smoothe/FS® [eczema oil]: 0.01% (120 mL) [contains peanut oil]
Derma-Smoothe/FS® [scalp oil]: 0.01% (120 mL) [contains peanut oil; packaged with shower caps]
Ointment, as acetonide (Synalar®): 0.025% (15 g, 60 g)
Shampoo, as acetonide (Capex™): 0.01% (120 mL)
Solution, as acetonide: 0.01% (60 mL)
Synalar®: 0.01% (20 mL, 60 mL)
Tablet, ocular implant, as acetonide (Retisert™): 0.59 mg [enclosed in silicone elastomer]

♦ **Fluocinolone Acetonide** see Fluocinolone on page 639

Fluocinonide (floo oh SIN oh nide)

Related Information
Corticosteroids on page 1755
Medication Safety Issues
Sound-alike/look-alike issues:
Fluocinonide may be confused with flunisolide, fluocinolone
Lidex® may be confused with Lasix®, Videx®, Wydase®
U.S. Brand Names Lidex®; Lidex-E®; Vanos™
Canadian Brand Names Lidemol®; Lidex®; Lyderm®; Tiamol®; Topsyn®
Generic Available Yes
Pharmacologic Category Corticosteroid, Topical
Use Anti-inflammatory, antipruritic; treatment of plaque-type psoriasis (up to 10% of body surface area) [high-potency topical corticosteroid]
Contraindications Hypersensitivity to fluocinonide or any component of the formulation; viral, fungal, or tubercular skin lesions, herpes simplex
Warnings/Precautions Systemic absorption of topical corticosteroids may cause hypothalamic-pituitary-adrenal (HPA) axis suppression (reversible). HPA axis suppression may lead to adrenal crisis. Risk is increased when used over large surface areas, for prolonged periods, or with occlusive dressings. Allergic contact dermatitis can occur, it is usually diagnosed by failure to heal rather than clinical exacerbation. (Continued)

Fluocinonide *(Continued)*

Prolonged treatment with corticosteroids has been associated with the development of Kaposi's sarcoma (case reports); if noted, discontinuation of therapy should be considered. Adverse systemic effects including hyperglycemia, glycosuria, fluid and electrolyte changes, and HPA suppression may occur when used on large surface areas, for prolonged periods, or with an occlusive dressing. Lower-strength cream (0.05%) may be used cautiously on face or opposing skin surfaces that may rub or touch (eg, skin folds of the groin, axilla, and breasts); higher-strength (0.1%) should not be used on the face, groin, or axillae. Use of the 0.1% cream for >2 weeks is not recommended.

Adverse Reactions (Reflective of adult population; not specific for elderly) Frequency not defined.

Cardiovascular: Intracranial hypertension

Dermatologic: Acne, allergic dermatitis, contact dermatitis, dry skin, folliculitis, hypertrichosis, hypopigmentation, maceration of the skin, miliaria, perioral dermatitis, pruritus, skin atrophy, striae, telangiectasia

Endocrine & metabolic: Cushing's syndrome, growth retardation, HPA suppression, hyperglycemia

Local: Burning, irritation

Renal: Glycosuria

Miscellaneous: Secondary infection

Drug Interactions No data reported. Concomitant use with other corticosteroids (by any route) may increase the risk of HPA axis suppression.

Mechanism of Action Fluorinated topical corticosteroid considered to be of high potency. The mechanism of action for all topical corticosteroids is not well defined, however, is felt to be a combination of three important properties: anti-inflammatory activity, immunosuppressive properties, and antiproliferative actions.

Dosage

Geriatrics & Adults:

Pruritus and inflammation: Topical (0.5% cream): Apply thin layer to affected area 2-4 times/day depending on the severity of the condition. Therapy should be discontinued when control is achieved; if no improvement is seen, reassessment of diagnosis may be necessary.

Plaque-type psoriasis (Vanos™): Topical (0.1% cream): Apply a thin layer once or twice daily to affected areas (limited to <10% of body surface area). **Note:** Not recommended for use >2 consecutive weeks or >60 g/week total exposure. Discontinue when control is achieved.

Monitoring Parameters Relief of symptoms

Patient Information Use only as prescribed and for no longer than the period prescribed; apply sparingly in a thin film and rub in lightly; avoid contact with eyes; notify physician if condition persists or worsens

Additional Information Considered a high potency steroid; avoid prolonged use on the face; may cause atrophic changes

Special Geriatric Considerations Due to age-related changes in skin, limit use of topical glucocorticosteroids.

Dosage Forms Excipient information presented when available (limited, particularly for generics); consult specific product labeling.

Cream, anhydrous, emollient (Lidex®): 0.05% (15 g, 30 g, 60 g)

Cream, aqueous, emollient (Lidex-E®): 0.05% (15 g, 30 g, 60 g)

Cream (Vanos™): 0.1% (30 g, 60 g)

Gel (Lidex®): 0.05% (15 g, 30 g, 60 g)

Ointment (Lidex®): 0.05% (15 g, 30 g, 60 g)

Solution (Lidex®): 0.05% (60 mL) [contains alcohol 35%]

♦ **Fluohydrisone Acetate** *see* Fludrocortisone *on page 635*
♦ **Fluohydrocortisone Acetate** *see* Fludrocortisone *on page 635*
♦ **Fluor-A-Day** *see* Fluoride *on page 642*

Fluoride *(FLOR ide)*

Medication Safety Issues

Sound-alike/look-alike issues:

Luride® may be confused with Lortab®

Phos-Flur® may be confused with PhosLo®

Thera-Flur-N® may be confused with Thera-Flu®

International issues:

Fluorex® [France] may be confused with Flarex® which is a brand name for fluorometholone in the U.S.

U.S. Brand Names ACT® [OTC]; ACT® Plus [OTC]; ACT® x2™ [OTC]; CaviRinse™; ControlRx™; Denta 5000 Plus; DentaGel; EtheDent™; Fluor-A-Day; Fluorigard® [OTC]; Fluorinse®; Flura-Drops®; Gel-Kam® [OTC]; Gel-Kam® Rinse; Just for Kids™ [OTC];

Lozi-Flur™; Luride®; Luride® Lozi-Tab®; NeutraCare®; NeutraGard® [OTC]; Neutra-Gard® Advanced; NeutraGard® Plus; Omnii Gel™ [OTC]; Pediaflor® [DSC]; Peri-oMed™; Pharmaflur®; Pharmaflur® 1.1; Phos-Flur®; Phos-Flur® Rinse [OTC]; PreviDent®; PreviDent® 5000 Plus™; StanGard®; StanGard® Perio; Stop®; Thera-Flur-N®

Canadian Brand Names Fluor-A-Day

Index Terms Acidulated Phosphate Fluoride; Sodium Fluoride; Stannous Fluoride

Generic Available Yes: Excludes lozenge, gel drops

Pharmacologic Category Nutritional Supplement

Use Prevention of dental caries

Contraindications Hypersensitivity to fluoride, tartrazine, or any component of the formulation; when fluoride content of drinking water exceeds 0.7 ppm; low sodium or sodium-free diets

Warnings/Precautions Prolonged ingestion with excessive doses may result in dental fluorosis and osseous changes; do **not** exceed recommended dosage. Some products contain tartrazine.

Overdosage/Toxicology Symptoms include hypersalivation, salty or soapy taste, epigastric pain, nausea, vomiting, diarrhea, rash, muscle weakness, tremor, seizures, cardiac failure, respiratory arrest, shock, and death. The fatal dose not known. Treatment consists of gastric lavage with $CaCl_2$ or $Ca(OH)_2$ solution. Administer a large quantity of milk at frequent intervals. $Al(OH)_3$ may also bind the fluoride ion.

Drug Interactions Decreased effect/absorption with magnesium-, aluminum-, and calcium-containing products.

Stability Store in tight plastic containers (not glass).

Mechanism of Action Promotes remineralization of decalcified enamel; inhibits the cariogenic microbial process in dental plaque; increases tooth resistance to acid dissolution

Pharmacokinetics

Absorption: In the GI tract, lungs and skin; 50% of fluoride is deposited in teeth and bone after ingestion; topical application works superficially on enamel and plaque

Elimination: In urine and feces

Dosage

Geriatrics & Adults: Prevention of dental caries: Oral:

Dental rinse or gel: 10 mL rinse or apply to teeth and spit daily after brushing

Product-specific dosing:

PreviDent® rinse: Once weekly, rinse 10 mL vigorously around and between teeth for 1 minute, then spit; this should be done preferably at bedtime, after thoroughly brushing teeth; for maximum benefit, do not eat, drink, or rinse mouth for at least 30 minutes after treatment; do not swallow

Fluorinse®: Once weekly, vigorously swish 5-10 mL in mouth for 1 minute, then spit

Patient Information Take with food (but not milk) to eliminate GI upset; with dental rinse or dental gel do **not** swallow, do **not** eat or drink for 30 minutes after use; notify physician of GI or lower extremity complaints

Additional Information 2.2 mg of sodium fluoride is equivalent to 1 mg of fluoride ion

Special Geriatric Considerations Postmenopausal women taking high doses of sodium fluoride have increased their bone density in the lumbar spine by 35% with a smaller increase in the femoral neck. In spite of these increases, the overall rate of vertebral fracture did not decline significantly while the rate of hip fracture increased. The results of a randomized, placebo-controlled trial using an investigational slow-release fluoride formulation at a lower dose (50 mg/day) are encouraging. Patients who received fluoride for 1 year or more had a lower vertebral fracture rate and substantial increase in L2-L4 bone mass and femoral neck bone density compared to placebo. Both groups took calcium. At the present time, restricted to investigational protocols.

Dosage Forms Excipient information presented when available (limited, particularly for generics); consult specific product labeling. [DSC] = Discontinued product

Cream, oral, as sodium [toothpaste]: 1.1% (51 g) [fluoride 2.5 mg/dose]

Denta 5000 Plus: 1.1% (51g) [fluoride 2.5 mg/dose; spearmint flavor]

EtheDent™: 1.1% (51g) [fluoride 2.5 mg/dose]

Gel-drops, as sodium fluoride (Thera-Flur-N®): 1.1% (24 mL) [fluoride 0.5%; neutral pH; no artificial color or flavor]

Gel, topical, as acidulated phosphate fluoride (Phos-Flur®): 1.1% (60 g) [fluoride 0.5%; cherry and mint flavors]

Gel, topical, as sodium fluoride: 1.1% (56 g) [fluoride 2 mg/dose]

DentaGel, EtheDent™: 1.1% (56 g) [fluoride 2 mg/dose; fresh mint flavor]

NeutraCare®: 1.1% (60 g) [neutral pH; grape and mint flavors]

NeutraGard® Advanced: 1.1% (60 g) [cinnamon and mint flavors]

PreviDent®: 1.1% (60 g) [fluoride 2 mg/dose; berry, cherry, and mint flavors]

Gel, topical, as stannous fluoride:

Gel-Kam®: 0.4% (129 g) [bubble gum, cinnamon, fruit/berry, and mint flavors]

(Continued)

Fluoride *(Continued)*

Just for Kids™: 0.4% (122 g) [bubble gum, fruit punch, and grapey grape flavors]

Omnii Gel™: 0.4% (122 g) [cinnamon, grape, natural, mint, and raspberry flavors]

StanGard®: 0.4% (122 g) [bubble gum, cherry, mint, and raspberry flavors]

Stop®: 0.4% (120 g) [bubble gum, cinnamon, grape, and mint flavors]

Lozenge, as sodium (Lozi-Flur™): 2.21 mg [fluoride 1 mg; cherry flavor]

Paste, oral, as sodium [toothpaste] (ControlRx®): 1.1% (56 g) [vanilla mint flavor]

Solution, oral drops, as sodium: 1.1 mg/mL (50 mL) [fluoride 0.5 mg/mL]

Flura-Drops®: 0.55 mg/drop (24 mL) [fluoride 0.25 mg/drop; dye free, sugar free]

Luride®: 1.1 mg/mL (50 mL) [fluoride 0.5 mg/mL; sugar free]

Pediaflor®: 1.1 mg/mL (50 mL) [fluoride 0.5 mg/mL; contains alcohol <0.5%; sugar free; cherry flavor] [DSC]

Solution, oral rinse, as sodium:

ACT®: 0.05% (530 mL) [fluoride 0.02%; bubble gum, cinnamon (contains tartrazine), and mint flavors]

ACT® Plus: 0.05% (530 mL) [fluoride 0.02%; alcohol free; icy cool mint flavor]

ACT® x2™: 0.5% (530 mL) [fluoride 0.02%; contains alcohol 11%; icy cool mint and spearmint flavors]

CaviRinse™: 0.2% (240 mL) [mint flavor]

Fluorigard®: 0.05% (480 mL) [alcohol free, sugar free; contains sodium benzoate and tartrazine; mint flavor]

Fluorinse®: 0.2% (480 mL) [alcohol free; cinnamon and mint flavors]

NeutraGard®: 0.05% (480 mL) [neutral pH; mint and tropical blast flavors]

NeutraGard® Plus: 0.2% (480 mL) [neutral pH; mint and tropical blast flavors]

Phos-Flur®: 0.44% (500 mL) [bubble gum, cherry, grape, and mint flavors]

PreviDent®: 0.2% (250 mL) [contains alcohol; mint flavor]

Solution, oral rinse concentrate, as stannous fluoride:

Gel-Kam®: 0.63% (300 mL) [fluoride 0.1%/dose; cinnamon and mint flavors]

PerioMed™: 0.63% (284 mL) [fluoride 7 mg/30 mL; alcohol free; cinnamon, mint and tropical fruit flavors]

StanGard® Perio: 0.63% (284 mL) [mint flavor]

Tablet, chewable, as sodium: 0.5 mg [fluoride 0.25 mg]; 1.1 mg [fluoride 0.5 mg]; 2.2 mg [fluoride 1 mg]

EtheDent™:

0.55 mg [fluoride 0.25 mg; sugar free; contains aspartame; vanilla flavor]

1.1 mg [fluoride 0.5 mg; sugar free; contains aspartame; grape flavor]

2.2 mg [fluoride 1 mg; sugar free; contains aspartame; cherry flavor]

Fluor-A-Day:

0.56 mg [fluoride 0.25 mg; raspberry flavor]

1.1 mg [fluoride 0.5 mg; raspberry flavor]

2.21 mg [fluoride 1 mg; raspberry flavor]

Luride® Lozi-Tab®:

0.55 mg [fluoride 0.25 mg; sugar free; vanilla flavor]

1.1 mg [fluoride 0.5 mg; sugar free; grape flavor]

2.2 mg [fluoride 1 mg; sugar free; cherry flavor]

Pharmaflur®: 2.2 mg [fluoride 1 mg; dye free, sugar free; cherry flavor]

Pharmaflur® 1.1: 1.1 mg [fluoride 0.5 mg; dye free, sugar free; grape flavor]

Selected References

Pak CYS, Sakhaee K, Adams-Huet B, et al, "Treatment of Postmenopausal Osteoporosis With Slow-Release Sodium Fluoride: Final Report of a Randomized Controlled Trial," *Ann Intern Med*, 1995, 123(6):401-8.

Riggs BL, Hodgson SF, O'Fallon WM, et al, "Effect of Fluoride Treatment on the Fracture Rate in Postmenopausal Women With Osteoporosis," *N Engl J Med*, 1990, 322(12):802-9.

- ◆ **Fluorigard® [OTC]** *see* Fluoride *on page 642*
- ◆ **Fluorinse®** *see* Fluoride *on page 642*
- ◆ **5-Fluorocytosine** *see* Flucytosine *on page 634*
- ◆ **9α-Fluorohydrocortisone Acetate** *see* Fludrocortisone *on page 635*

Fluoxetine *(floo OKS e teen)*

Related Information

Antidepressant Agents *on page 1742*

Potentially Inappropriate Medications for Geriatrics *on page 1824*

Medication Safety Issues

Sound-alike/look-alike issues:

Fluoxetine may be confused with duloxetine, fluvastatin, fluvoxamine

Prozac® may be confused with Prilosec®, Proscar®, ProSom®, ProStep®

Sarafem® may be confused with Serophene®

International issues:

Fluoxin® [Czech Republic and Romania] may be confused with Floxin® which is a brand name for ofloxacin in the U.S.

Prozac® may be confused with Prazac® a brand of prazosin in Denmark
Reneuron® [Spain] may be confused with Remeron® a brand of mirtazapine in the U.S.

U.S. Brand Names Prozac®; Prozac® Weekly™; Sarafem®

Canadian Brand Names Alti-Fluoxetine; Apo-Fluoxetine®; BCI-Fluoxetine; CO Fluoxetine; FXT; Gen-Fluoxetine; Novo-Fluoxetine; Nu-Fluoxetine; PMS-Fluoxetine; Prozac®; Rhoxal-fluoxetine; Sandoz-Fluoxetine

Index Terms Fluoxetine Hydrochloride

Generic Available Yes: Excludes delayed release capsule

Pharmacologic Category Antidepressant, Selective Serotonin Reuptake Inhibitor

Use Treatment of major depression, geriatric depression, binge-eating and vomiting in patients with moderate-to-severe bulimia nervosa, obsessive-compulsive disorder (OCD)

Unlabeled/Investigational Use Treatment of selective mutism

Restrictions An FDA-approved medication guide concerning the use of antidepressants in children, adolescents, and young adults must be distributed when dispensing an outpatient prescription (new or refill) where this medication is to be used without direct supervision of a healthcare provider. Medication guides are available at http://www.fda.gov/cder/Offices/ODS/medication_guides.htm. Dispense to parents or guardians of children and adolescents receiving this medication.

Contraindications Hypersensitivity to fluoxetine or any component of the formulation; patients receiving MAO inhibitors, thioridazine, or mesoridazine currently or within prior 14 days; MAO inhibitor, thioridazine, or mesoridazine should not be initiated until 5 weeks after the discontinuation of fluoxetine

Warnings/Precautions [U.S. Boxed Warning]: Antidepressants increase the risk of suicidal thinking and behavior in children, adolescents, and young adults (18-24 years of age) with major depressive disorder (MDD) and other psychiatric disorders; consider risk prior to prescribing. Short-term studies did not show an increased risk in patients >24 years of age and showed a decreased risk in patients ≥65 years. Closely monitor patients for clinical worsening, suicidality, or unusual changes in behavior, particularly during the initial 1-2 months of therapy or during periods of dosage adjustments (increases or decreases); the patient's family or caregiver should be instructed to closely observe the patient and communicate condition with healthcare provider. A medication guide concerning the use of antidepressants should be dispensed with each prescription.

The possibility of a suicide attempt is inherent in major depression and may persist until remission occurs. Use caution in high-risk patients. Worsening depression and severe abrupt suicidality that are not part of the presenting symptoms may require discontinuation or modification of drug therapy. The patient's family or caregiver should be alerted to monitor patients for the emergence of suicidality and associated behaviors (such as agitation, irritability, hostility, impulsivity, and hypomania) and call healthcare provider.

May worsen psychosis in some patients or precipitate a shift to mania or hypomania in patients with bipolar disorder. Patients presenting with depressive symptoms should be screened for bipolar disorder. Monotherapy in patients with bipolar disorder should be avoided. **Fluoxetine is not FDA approved for the treatment of bipolar depression.** May cause insomnia, anxiety, nervousness, or anorexia. Use with caution in patients where weight loss is undesirable. May impair cognitive or motor performance; caution operating hazardous machinery or driving.

The potential for severe reactions exists when used with MAO inhibitors, SSRIs/SNRIs or triptans; serotonin syndrome (hyperthermia, muscular rigidity, mental status changes/agitation, autonomic instability) may occur. Concurrent use with MAO inhibitors is contraindicated. Fluoxetine may elevate plasma levels of thioridazine and increase the risk of QT$_c$ interval prolongation. This may lead to serious ventricular arrhythmias, such as torsade de pointes-type arrhythmias, and sudden death. Fluoxetine use has been associated with occurrences of significant rash and allergic events, including vasculitis, lupus-like syndrome, laryngospasm, anaphylactoid reactions, and pulmonary inflammatory disease. Discontinue if underlying cause of rash cannot be identified.

Use caution in patients with a previous seizure disorder or condition predisposing to seizures such as brain damage, alcoholism, or concurrent therapy with other drugs which lower the seizure threshold. Use with caution in patients with hepatic or renal dysfunction and in elderly patients. May cause hyponatremia/SIADH. May increase the risks associated with electroconvulsive treatment. Use with caution in patients at risk of bleeding or receiving concurrent anticoagulant therapy - may cause impairment in platelet function. Use caution with history of MI or unstable heart disease; use in these patients is limited. May alter glycemic control in patients with diabetes. Due to the long half-life of fluoxetine and its metabolites, the effects and interactions noted may persist for prolonged periods following discontinuation. May cause or exacerbate sexual dysfunction. Discontinuation symptoms (eg, dysphoric mood, irritability, agitation, (Continued)

Fluoxetine *(Continued)*

confusion, anxiety, insomnia, hypomania) may occur upon abrupt discontinuation. Taper dose when discontinuing therapy.

Adverse Reactions (Reflective of adult population; not specific for elderly) Percentages listed for adverse effects as reported in placebo-controlled trials and were generally similar in adults and children; actual frequency may be dependent upon diagnosis and in some cases the range presented may be lower than or equal to placebo for a particular disorder.

>10%:

Central nervous system: Insomnia (10% to 33%), headache (21%), anxiety (6% to 15%), nervousness (8% to 14%), somnolence (5% to 17%)

Endocrine & metabolic: Libido decreased (1% to 11%)

Gastrointestinal: Nausea (12% to 29%), diarrhea (8% to 18%), anorexia (4% to 11%), xerostomia (4% to 12%)

Neuromuscular & skeletal: Weakness (7% to 21%), tremor (3% to 13%)

Respiratory: Pharyngitis (3% to 11%), yawn (<1% to 11%)

1% to 10%:

Cardiovascular: Vasodilation (1% to 5%), fever (2%), chest pain, hemorrhage, hypertension, palpitation

Central nervous system: Dizziness (9%), dream abnormality (1% to 5%), thinking abnormality (2%), agitation, amnesia, chills, confusion, emotional lability, sleep disorder

Dermatologic: Rash (2% to 6%), pruritus (4%)

Endocrine & metabolic: Ejaculation abnormal (<1% to 7%), impotence (<1% to 7%)

Gastrointestinal: Dyspepsia (6% to 10%), constipation (5%), flatulence (3%), vomiting (3%), weight loss (2%), appetite increased, taste perversion, weight gain

Genitourinary: Urinary frequency

Ocular: Vision abnormal (2%)

Otic: Ear pain, tinnitus

Respiratory: Sinusitis (1% to 6%)

Miscellaneous: Flu-like syndrome (3% to 10%), diaphoresis (2% to 8%)

Overdosage/Toxicology Among 633 adult patients who overdosed on fluoxetine alone, 34 resulted in a fatal outcome. Symptoms include ataxia, sedation, coma, and ECG abnormalities (QT prolongation, torsade de pointes). Respiratory depression may occur, especially with coingestion of alcohol or other drugs. Seizures rarely occur. Treatment is supportive.

Drug Interactions Substrate of CYP1A2 (minor), 2B6 (minor), 2C9 (major), 2C19 (minor), 2D6 (major), 2E1 (minor), 3A4 (minor); **Inhibits** CYP1A2 (moderate), 2B6 (weak), 2C9 (weak), 2C19 (moderate), 2D6 (strong), 3A4 (weak)

Amphetamines: SSRIs may increase the sensitivity to amphetamines, and amphetamines may increase the risk of serotonin syndrome.

Benzodiazepines: Fluoxetine may inhibit the metabolism of alprazolam and diazepam resulting in elevated serum levels; monitor for increased sedation and psychomotor impairment.

Beta-blockers: Fluoxetine may inhibit the metabolism of metoprolol and propranolol resulting in cardiac toxicity; monitor for bradycardia, hypotension, and heart failure if combination is used; not established for all beta-blockers (unlikely with atenolol or nadolol due to renal elimination).

Buspirone: Fluoxetine inhibits the reuptake of serotonin; combined use with a serotonin agonist (buspirone) may cause serotonin syndrome.

Carbamazepine: Fluoxetine may inhibit the metabolism of carbamazepine resulting in increased carbamazepine levels and toxicity; monitor for altered carbamazepine response.

Carvedilol: Serum concentrations may be increased; monitor carefully for increased carvedilol effect (hypotension and bradycardia).

Clozapine: Fluoxetine may increase serum levels of clozapine; levels may increase by 76%; monitor for increased effect/toxicity.

Cyclosporine: Fluoxetine may increase serum levels of cyclosporine (and possibly tacrolimus); monitor.

CYP1A2 substrates: Fluoxetine may increase the levels/effects of CYP1A2 substrates. Example substrates include aminophylline, fluvoxamine, mexiletine, mirtazapine, ropinirole, theophylline, and trifluoperazine.

CYP2C9 inducers: May decrease the levels/effects of fluoxetine. Example inducers include carbamazepine, phenobarbital, phenytoin, rifampin, rifapentine, and secobarbital.

CYP2C9 inhibitors: May increase the levels/effects of fluoxetine. Example inhibitors include delavirdine, fluconazole, gemfibrozil, ketoconazole, nicardipine, NSAIDs, sulfonamides, and tolbutamide.

CYP2C19 substrates: Fluoxetine may increase the levels/effects of CYP2C19 substrates. Example substrates include citalopram, diazepam, methsuximide, phenytoin, propranolol, and sertraline.

CYP2D6 inhibitors: May increase the levels/effects of fluoxetine. Example inhibitors include chlorpromazine, delavirdine, miconazole, paroxetine, pergolide, quinidine, quinine, ritonavir, and ropinirole.

CYP2D6 substrates: Fluoxetine may increase the levels/effects of CYP2D6 substrates. Example substrates include amphetamines, selected beta-blockers, dextromethorphan, lidocaine, mirtazapine, nefazodone, paroxetine, risperidone, ritonavir, thioridazine, tricyclic antidepressants, and venlafaxine.

CYP2D6 prodrug substrates: Fluoxetine may decrease the levels/effects of CYP2D6 prodrug substrates. Example prodrug substrates include codeine, hydrocodone, oxycodone, and tramadol.

Cyproheptadine: May inhibit the effects of serotonin reuptake inhibitors (fluoxetine); monitor for altered antidepressant response; cyproheptadine acts as a serotonin agonist.

Dextromethorphan: Fluoxetine inhibits the metabolism of dextromethorphan; visual hallucinations occurred in a patient receiving this combination; monitor for serotonin syndrome.

Digoxin: Fluoxetine may increase serum levels of digoxin; monitor.

Haloperidol: Fluoxetine may inhibit the metabolism of haloperidol and cause extrapyramidal symptoms (EPS); monitor patients for EPS if combination is utilized.

HMG-CoA reductase inhibitors: Fluoxetine may inhibit the metabolism of lovastatin and simvastatin resulting in myositis and rhabdomyolysis; these combinations are best avoided.

Lithium: Reports of both increased and decreased lithium levels when used concomitantly with fluoxetine. Patients receiving fluoxetine and lithium have developed neurotoxicity. If combination is used; monitor lithium levels and for neurotoxicity.

Loop diuretics: Fluoxetine may cause hyponatremia; additive hyponatremic effects may be seen with combined use of a loop diuretic (bumetanide, furosemide, torsemide); monitor for hyponatremia.

MAO inhibitors: Combined use of fluoxetine with nonselective MAOIs (ie, isocarboxazid, phenelzine) is contraindicated; fatal reactions have been reported; wait 5 weeks after stopping fluoxetine before starting an MAO inhibitor and 2 weeks after stopping an MAO inhibitor before starting fluoxetine.

Meperidine: Combined use with fluoxetine theoretically may increase the risk of serotonin syndrome.

Nefazodone: May increase the risk of serotonin syndrome with SSRIs; monitor.

NSAIDs: Concomitant use of fluoxetine and NSAIDs, aspirin, or other drugs affecting coagulation has been associated with an increased risk of bleeding; monitor.

Phenytoin: Fluoxetine inhibits the metabolism of phenytoin and may result in phenytoin toxicity; monitor for phenytoin toxicity (ataxia, confusion, dizziness, nystagmus, involuntary muscle movement).

Pimozide: Due to potential QT_c interval prolongation, concomitant use is contraindicated.

Propafenone: Serum concentrations and/or toxicity may be increased by fluoxetine; avoid concurrent administration.

Ritonavir: Combined use of fluoxetine with ritonavir may cause serotonin syndrome in HIV-positive patients; monitor.

Selegiline: Fluoxetine has been reported to cause mania or hypertension when combined with selegiline; this combination is best avoided. Concurrent use with SSRIs has also been reported to cause serotonin syndrome. As a MAO type B inhibitor, the risk of serotonin syndrome may be less than with nonselective MAO inhibitors.

Sibutramine: May increase the risk of serotonin syndrome with SSRIs; avoid coadministration.

Serotonin agonists (eg, triptans): Concurrent use of fluoxetine with these agents may increase the risk of serotonin syndrome; monitor.

Serotonergic reuptake inhibitors (eg, SSRIs/SNRIs): Concurrent use of fluoxetine with these agents may increase the risk of serotonin syndrome; monitor.

Sympathomimetics: May increase the risk of serotonin syndrome with SSRIs.

Thioridazine: Fluoxetine may inhibit the metabolism of thioridazine, resulting in increased plasma levels and increasing the risk of QT_c interval prolongation. This may lead to serious ventricular arrhythmias, such as torsade de pointes-type arrhythmias and sudden death. Do not use together. Wait at least 5 weeks after discontinuing fluoxetine prior to starting thioridazine.

Tramadol: Fluoxetine combined with tramadol (serotonergic effects) may cause serotonin syndrome; monitor.

Trazodone: Fluoxetine may inhibit the metabolism of trazodone resulting in increased toxicity; monitor.

Tricyclic antidepressants: Fluoxetine inhibits the metabolism of tricyclic antidepressants (amitriptyline, desipramine, imipramine, nortriptyline) resulting is elevated serum levels; if combination is warranted, a low dose of TCA (10-25 mg/day) should be utilized.

(Continued)

Fluoxetine *(Continued)*

Tryptophan: Fluoxetine inhibits the reuptake of serotonin; combination with tryptophan, a serotonin precursor, may cause agitation and restlessness; this combination is best avoided.

Valproic acid: Fluoxetine may increase serum levels of valproic acid; monitor.

Venlafaxine: Fluoxetine may increase the risk of serotonin syndrome.

Warfarin: Fluoxetine may alter the hypoprothrombinemic response to warfarin; monitor.

Ethanol/Nutrition/Herb Interactions

Ethanol: Avoid ethanol (may increase CNS depression). Depressed patients should avoid/limit intake.

Herb/Nutraceutical: Avoid valerian, St John's wort, kava kava, gotu kola (may increase CNS depression).

Stability All dosage forms should be stored at controlled room temperature of 15°C to 30°C (50°F to 86°F). Oral liquid should be dispensed in a light-resistant container.

Mechanism of Action Inhibits CNS neuron serotonin reuptake; minimal or no effect on reuptake of norepinephrine or dopamine; does not significantly bind to alpha-adrenergic, histamine, or cholinergic receptors

Pharmacodynamics Peak antidepressant effects: Usually occur after more than 4 weeks; due to long half-life, resolution of adverse reactions after discontinuation may be slow

Pharmacokinetics

Absorption: Oral: well absorbed; delayed 1-2 hours with weekly formulation

Protein binding: 95%

Metabolism: Hepatic, to norfluoxetine (active; equal to fluoxetine)

Half-life:

Parent drug: 1-3 days (acute), 4-6 days (chronic), 7.6 days (cirrhosis)

Metabolite (norfluoxetine): 9.3 days (range: 4-16 days), 12 days (cirrhosis)

Due to long half-life, resolution of adverse reactions after discontinuation may be slow

Time to peak: 6-8 hours

Elimination: In urine as fluoxetine (2.5% to 5%) and norfluoxetine (10%)

Note: Weekly formulation results in greater fluctuations between peak and trough concentrations of fluoxetine and norfluoxetine compared to once-daily dosing (24% daily/164% weekly; 17% daily/43% weekly, respectively). Trough concentrations are 76% lower for fluoxetine and 47% lower for norfluoxetine than the concentrations maintained by 20 mg once-daily dosing. Steady-state fluoxetine concentrations are ~50% lower following the once-weekly regimen compared to 20 mg once daily. Average steady-state concentrations of once-daily dosing in adults: fluoxetine 91-302 ng/mL; norfluoxetine 72-258 ng/mL

Dosage

Geriatrics: Oral: Some patients may require an initial dose of 10 mg/day with dosage increases of 10 mg and 20 mg every several weeks as tolerated; should not be taken at night unless patient experiences sedation.

Adults:

Depression, OCD, bulimia: 20 mg/day in the morning; may increase after several weeks by 20 mg/day increments; maximum: 80 mg/day; doses >20 mg may be given once daily or divided twice daily. **Note:** Lower doses of 5-10 mg/day have been used for initial treatment.

Usual dosage range:

Depression: 20-40 mg/day; patients maintained on Prozac® 20 mg/day may be changed to Prozac® Weekly™ 90 mg/week, starting dose 7 days after the last 20 mg/day dose

Obsessive compulsive disorder (OCD): 40-80 mg/day

Bulimia nervosa: 60-80 mg/day

Panic disorder: Initial: 10 mg/day; after 1 week, increase to 20 mg/day; may increase after several weeks; doses >60 mg/day have not been evaluated

Renal Impairment:

Single dose studies: Pharmacokinetics of fluoxetine and norfluoxetine were similar among subjects with all levels of impaired renal function, including anephric patients on chronic hemodialysis.

Chronic administration: Additional accumulation of fluoxetine or norfluoxetine may occur in patients with severely impaired renal function.

Not removed by hemodialysis; use of lower dose or less frequent dosing is not usually necessary.

Hepatic Impairment: Elimination half-life of fluoxetine is prolonged in patients with hepatic impairment. A lower dose or less frequent dosing of fluoxetine should be used in these patients.

Cirrhosis patient: Administer a lower dose or less frequent dosing interval.

Compensated cirrhosis without ascites: Administer 50% of normal dose.

Monitoring Parameters Signs and symptoms of depression, anxiety, sleep, appetite, and weight; signs of EPS in patients taking haloperidol

Reference Range Therapeutic: Fluoxetine 100-800 ng/mL (SI: 289-2314 nmol/L); norfluoxetine 100-600 ng/mL (SI: 289-1735 nmol/L); not well correlated

Patient Information Use sugarless hard candy for dry mouth; avoid alcoholic beverages, may cause drowsiness or insomnia, improvement may take several weeks; rise slowly to prevent dizziness

Special Geriatric Considerations Fluoxetine's favorable side effect profile makes it a useful alternative to the traditional tricyclic antidepressants. Its potential stimulating and anorexic effects may be bothersome to some patients and has not been shown to be superior in efficacy to the traditional tricyclic antidepressants or other SSRIs. The long half-life in the elderly makes it less attractive compared to other SSRIs. Data from a clinical trial comparing fluoxetine to tricyclics suggest that fluoxetine is significantly less effective than nortriptyline in hospitalized elderly patients with unipolar major affective disorder, especially those with melancholia and concurrent cardiovascular diseases. As with other SSRIs, fluoxetine has been associated with hyponatremia in elderly patients.

Dosage Forms Excipient information presented when available (limited, particularly for generics); consult specific product labeling. [DSC] = Discontinued product

Capsule, as hydrochloride: 10 mg, 20 mg, 40 mg

Prozac®: 10 mg, 20 mg, 40 mg

Sarafem®: 10 mg, 20 mg

Capsule, delayed release, as hydrochloride (Prozac® Weekly™): 90 mg

Solution, oral, as hydrochloride (Prozac®): 20 mg/5 mL (120 mL) [contains alcohol 0.23% and benzoic acid; mint flavor]

Tablet, as hydrochloride: 10 mg, 20 mg

Prozac® [scored]: 10 mg [DSC]

Extemporaneously Prepared A 20 mg capsule may be mixed with 4 oz of water, apple juice, or Gatorade® to provide a solution that is stable for 14 days under refrigeration

Selected References

Beasley CM, Bosomworth JC, and Wernicke JF, "Fluoxetine: Relationships Among Dose, Response, Adverse Events, and Plasma Concentrations in the Treatment of Depression," *Psychopharmacol Bull*, 1990, 26(1):18-24.

Feighner JP and Cohn JB, "Double-Blind Comparative Trials of Fluoxetine and Doxepin in Geriatric Patients With Major Depressive Disorder," *J Clin Psychiatry*, 1985, 46(3 Pt 2):20-5.

Harvey AT and Preskorn SH, "Fluoxetine Pharmacokinetics and Effect on CYP2C19 in Young and Elderly Volunteers," *J Clin Psychopharmacol*, 2001, 21(2):161-6.

Lemberger L, Bergstrom RF, Wolen RL, et al, "Fluoxetine: Clinical Pharmacology and Physiologic Disposition," *J Clin Psychiatry*, 1985, 46(3 Pt 2):14-9.

Roose SP, Glassman AH, Attia E, et al, "Comparative Efficacy of Selective Serotonin Reuptake Inhibitors and Tricyclics in the Treatment of Melancholia," *Am J Psychiatry*, 1994, 151(12):1735-9.

Schone W and Ludwig M, "A Double-Blind Study of Paroxetine Compared With Fluoxetine in Geriatric Patients With Major Depression," *J Clin Psychopharmacol*, 1993, 13(6 Suppl 2):34S-9S.

♦ **Fluoxetine Hydrochloride** *see* Fluoxetine *on page 644*

Fluphenazine (floo FEN a zeen)

Related Information

Antipsychotic Agents *on page 1747*

Liquid Compatibility of Antipsychotics and Mood Stabilizers *on page 1851*

Medication Safety Issues

Sound-alike/look-alike issues:

Prolixin® may be confused with Proloprim®

International issues:

Prolixin® may be confused with Prolixan® which is a brand name for azapropazone in multiple international markets

U.S. Brand Names Prolixin® [DSC]; Prolixin Decanoate®

Canadian Brand Names Apo-Fluphenazine®; Apo-Fluphenazine Decanoate®; Modecate®; Modecate® Concentrate; PMS-Fluphenazine Decanoate

Index Terms Fluphenazine Decanoate

Generic Available Yes: Injection, tablet

Pharmacologic Category Antipsychotic Agent, Typical, Phenothiazine

Use Management of manifestations of psychotic disorders, depressive neurosis; treatment of alcohol withdrawal, nausea and vomiting, nonpsychotic symptoms associated with dementia in older adults, Tourette's syndrome, Huntington's chorea, spiromatic torticollis, Reye's syndrome

See Special Geriatric Considerations.

Contraindications Hypersensitivity to fluphenazine or any component of the formulation (cross-reactivity between phenothiazines may occur); severe CNS depression; coma; subcortical brain damage; blood dyscrasias; hepatic disease

(Continued)

Fluphenazine *(Continued)*

Warnings/Precautions May be sedating; use with caution in disorders where CNS depression is a feature. Use with caution in Parkinson's disease. Caution in patients with hemodynamic instability; predisposition to seizures; or severe cardiac, renal, or respiratory disease. Esophageal dysmotility and aspiration have been associated with antipsychotic use - use with caution in patients at risk of pneumonia (ie, Alzheimer's disease). Caution in breast cancer or other prolactin-dependent tumors (may elevate prolactin levels). May alter temperature regulation or mask toxicity of other drugs due to antiemetic effects. May alter cardiac conduction; life-threatening arrhythmias have occurred with therapeutic doses of phenothiazines. Hypotension may occur, particularly with I.M. administration. May cause orthostatic hypotension - use with caution in patients at risk of this effect or those who would tolerate transient hypotensive episodes (cerebrovascular disease, cardiovascular disease, or other medications which may predispose). Adverse effects of depot injections may be prolonged. Check blood counts periodically and discontinue at first signs of blood dyscrasias; use is contraindicated in patients with bone marrow suppression.

Phenothiazines may cause anticholinergic effects (confusion, agitation, constipation, xerostomia, blurred vision, urinary retention); therefore, they should be used with caution in patients with decreased gastrointestinal motility, urinary retention, BPH, xerostomia, or visual problems. Conditions which also may be exacerbated by cholinergic blockade include narrow-angle glaucoma (screening is recommended) and worsening of myasthenia gravis. Relative to other antipsychotics, fluphenazine has a low potency of cholinergic blockade.

May cause extrapyramidal reactions, including pseudoparkinsonism, acute dystonic reactions, akathisia, and tardive dyskinesia (risk of these reactions is high relative to other antipsychotics). Use caution in the elderly. May be associated with neuroleptic malignant syndrome (NMS) or pigmentary retinopathy.

Adverse Reactions (Reflective of adult population; not specific for elderly)
Frequency not defined.

Cardiovascular: Hyper-/hypotension, tachycardia, fluctuations in blood pressure, arrhythmia, edema

Central nervous system: Parkinsonian symptoms, akathisia, dystonias, tardive dyskinesia, dizziness, hyper-reflexia, headache, cerebral edema, drowsiness, lethargy, restlessness, excitement, bizarre dreams, EEG changes, depression, seizure, NMS, altered central temperature regulation

Dermatologic: Dermatitis, eczema, erythema, itching, photosensitivity, rash, seborrhea, skin pigmentation, urticaria

Endocrine & metabolic: Menstrual cycle changes, breast pain, amenorrhea, galactorrhea, gynecomastia, libido changes, prolactin increased, SIADH

Gastrointestinal: Weight gain, appetite loss, salivation, xerostomia, constipation, paralytic ileus, laryngeal edema

Genitourinary: Ejaculatory disturbances, impotence, polyuria, bladder paralysis, enuresis

Hematologic: Agranulocytosis, leukopenia, thrombocytopenia, nonthrombocytopenic purpura, eosinophilia, pancytopenia

Hepatic: Cholestatic jaundice, hepatotoxicity

Neuromuscular & skeletal: Trembling of fingers, SLE, facial hemispasm

Ocular: Pigmentary retinopathy, cornea and lens changes, blurred vision, glaucoma

Respiratory: Nasal congestion, asthma

Overdosage/Toxicology Symptoms include deep sleep, hypotension, hypertension, dystonia, seizures, extrapyramidal symptoms, and respiratory failure. Following initiation of essential overdose management, toxic symptom and supportive treatment should be initiated. Hypotension usually responds to I.V. fluids or Trendelenburg positioning. If unresponsive to these measures, the use of a parenteral inotrope may be required. Seizures commonly respond to diazepam (I.V. 5-10 mg bolus every 15 minutes, if needed, up to a total of 30 mg) or to phenytoin or phenobarbital. Cardiac arrhythmias often respond to I.V. lidocaine while other antiarrhythmics can be used. Neuroleptics often cause extrapyramidal symptoms (eg, dystonic reactions) requiring management with anticholinergic agents such as benztropine mesylate I.V. 1-2 mg may be effective. These agents are generally effective within 2-5 minutes.

Drug Interactions Substrate of CYP2D6 (major); **Inhibits** CYP1A2 (weak), 2C9 (weak), 2D6 (weak), 2E1 (weak)

Acetylcholinesterase inhibitors (central): May increase the risk of antipsychotic-related extrapyramidal symptoms; monitor.

Aluminum salts: May decrease the absorption of phenothiazines; monitor.

Amphetamines: Efficacy may be diminished by antipsychotics; in addition, amphetamines may increase psychotic symptoms; avoid concurrent use.

Anticholinergics: May inhibit the therapeutic response to phenothiazines and excess anticholinergic effects may occur; includes benztropine, trihexyphenidyl, biperiden, and drugs with significant anticholinergic activity (TCAs, antihistamines, disopyramide).

Antihypertensives: Concurrent use of phenothiazines with an antihypertensive may produce additive hypotensive effects (particularly orthostasis).

Bromocriptine: Phenothiazines inhibit the ability of bromocriptine to lower serum prolactin concentrations.

CNS depressants: Sedative effects may be additive with phenothiazines; monitor for increased effect; includes barbiturates, benzodiazepines, opioid analgesics, ethanol, and other sedative agents.

CYP2D6 inhibitors: May increase the levels/effects of fluphenazine. Example inhibitors include chlorpromazine, delavirdine, fluoxetine, miconazole, paroxetine, pergolide, quinidine, quinine, ritonavir, and ropinirole.

Epinephrine: Chlorpromazine (and possibly other low potency antipsychotics) may diminish the pressor effects of epinephrine.

Guanethidine and guanadrel: Antihypertensive effects may be inhibited by phenothiazines.

Levodopa: Phenothiazines may inhibit the antiparkinsonian effect of levodopa; avoid this combination.

Lithium: Phenothiazines may produce neurotoxicity with lithium; this is a rare effect.

Metoclopramide: May increase extrapyramidal symptoms (EPS) or risk.

Phenytoin: May reduce serum levels of phenothiazines; phenothiazines may increase phenytoin serum levels.

Propranolol: Serum concentrations of phenothiazines may be increased; propranolol also increases phenothiazine concentrations.

Polypeptide antibiotics: Rare cases of respiratory paralysis have been reported with concurrent use of phenothiazines.

QT_c-prolonging agents: Effects on QT_c interval may be additive with phenothiazines, increasing the risk of malignant arrhythmias; includes type Ia antiarrhythmics, TCAs, and some quinolone antibiotics (moxifloxacin).

Sulfadoxine-pyrimethamine: May increase phenothiazine concentrations

Tricyclic antidepressants: Concurrent use may produce increased toxicity or altered therapeutic response.

Trazodone: Phenothiazines and trazodone may produce additive hypotensive effects.

Valproic acid: Serum levels may be increased by phenothiazines.

Ethanol/Nutrition/Herb Interactions

Ethanol: Avoid ethanol (may increase CNS depression).

Herb/Nutraceutical: Avoid dong quai, St John's wort (may also cause photosensitization). Avoid kava kava, gotu kola, valerian, St John's wort (may increase CNS depression).

Stability Avoid freezing. Protect all dosage forms from light. Clear or slightly yellow solutions may be used. Should be dispensed in amber or opaque vials/bottles. Solutions may be diluted or mixed with fruit juices or other liquids, but must be administered immediately after mixing. Do not prepare bulk dilutions or store bulk dilutions.

Mechanism of Action Fluphenazine is a piperazine phenothiazine antipsychotic which blocks postsynaptic mesolimbic dopaminergic D_1 and D_2 receptors in the brain; depresses the release of hypothalamic and hypophyseal hormones; believed to depress the reticular activating system, thus affecting basal metabolism, body temperature, wakefulness, vasomotor tone, and emesis

Pharmacodynamics

Onset of action: I.M., SubQ: 24-72 hours

Peak effect: 48-96 hours; derivative dependent; the hydrochloride salt acts quickly and persists briefly, while the decanoate lasts the longest and requires more time for onset

Following hydrochloride derivative administration, the onset of activity occurs within 1 hour yet persists for only 6-8 hours

Pharmacokinetics

Absorption: Oral: May be affected by the inherent anticholinergic action on the gastrointestinal tissue causing variable absorption. Absorption from tablets is erratic with less variation seen with solutions. These agents are widely distributed in tissues with CNS concentrations exceeding that of plasma due to their lipophilic characteristics.

Protein binding: Antipsychotic agents are bound 90% to 99% to plasma or proteins; highly bound to brain and lung tissue and other tissues with a high blood perfusion

Metabolism: Hepatic

Half-life (derivative dependent):
Enanthate: 84-96 hours
Hydrochloride: 33 hours
Decanoate: 163-232 hours

Time to peak serum concentrations: 2-4 hours

Elimination: Excretion occurs through hepatic metabolism (oxidation) where numerous active metabolites are produced; active metabolites excreted in urine; elimination half-lives of antipsychotics ranges from 20-40 hours which may be extended in older adults due to decline in oxidative hepatic reactions (phase I) with age.

(Continued)

Fluphenazine *(Continued)*

The biologic effect of a single dose persists for 24 hours. When the patient has accommodated to initial side effects (sedation), once daily dosing is possible due to the long half-life of antipsychotics.

Steady-state plasma concentrations are achieved in 4-7 days; therefore, if possible, do not make dose adjustments more than once in a 7-day period.

Due to the long half-lives of antipsychotics, as needed (prn) use is ineffective since repeated doses are necessary to achieve therapeutic tissue concentrations in the CNS.

Dosage

Geriatrics: Nonpsychotic patient, dementia behavior (unlabeled use): Oral: 1-2.5 mg/day; increase dose at 4- to 7-day intervals by 1-2.5 mg/day. Increase dosing intervals (bid, tid) as necessary to control response or side effects. Maximum daily dose: 20 mg; gradual increases (titration) may prevent some side effects or decrease their severity.

Adults:

Psychosis:

Oral: 0.5-10 mg/day in divided doses at 6- to 8-hour intervals; some patients may require up to 40 mg/day

I.M.: 2.5-10 mg/day in divided doses at 6- to 8-hour intervals (parenteral dose is ⅓ to ½ the oral dose for the hydrochloride salts)

Long-acting maintenance injections (Depot):

I.M. (decanoate): 12.5-37.5 mg every 2 weeks

Conversion from hydrochloride to decanoate I.M.: 0.5 mL (12.5 mg) decanoate every 3 weeks is approximately equivalent to 10 mg hydrochloride/day

Renal Impairment: Use with caution; not dialyzable (0% to 5%).

Hepatic Impairment: Use with caution.

Administration Avoid contact of oral solution or injection with skin (contact dermatitis). Oral liquid should be diluted in the following **only**: Water, saline, homogenized milk, carbonated orange beverages, pineapple, apricot, prune, orange, tomato, and grapefruit juices. Do **not** dilute in beverages containing caffeine, tannics, or pectinate. Watch for hypotension when administering I.M.

Monitoring Parameters Monitor orthostatic blood pressures 3-5 days after initiation of therapy or a dose increase; tremors, gait changes, abnormal movement in trunk, neck, buccal area, or extremities; monitor target behaviors for which the agent is given

Reference Range Therapeutic: 0.13-2.8 ng/mL; correlation of serum concentrations and efficacy is controversial; most often dosed to best response

Patient Information Oral concentrate must be diluted in 2-4 oz of liquid (water, fruit juice, carbonated drinks, milk, or pudding); do not take antacid within 1 hour of taking drug; avoid alcohol; avoid excess sun exposure (use sun block); may cause drowsiness, rise slowly from recumbent position; use of supportive stockings may help prevent orthostatic hypotension

Additional Information Oral liquid to be diluted in the following **only**: water, saline, 7-UP, homogenized milk, carbonated orange beverages, pineapple, apricot, prune, orange, V-8 juice, tomato, and grapefruit juices; do not mix with beverages containing caffeine, tannins, or pectin (ie, coffee, tea, apple juice)

Special Geriatric Considerations Any changes in disease status in any organ system can result in behavior changes.

Many elderly patients receive antipsychotic medications for inappropriate nonpsychotic behavior. Before initiating antipsychotic medication, the clinician should investigate any possible reversible cause; any stress or stress from any disease can cause acute "confusion" or worsening of baseline nonpsychotic behavior. Most commonly, acute changes in behavior are due to increases in drug dose or addition of a new drug to regimen, fluid electrolyte loss, infections, and changes in environment.

In the treatment of agitated, demented, and elderly patients, authors of meta-analysis of controlled trials of the response to the traditional antipsychotics (phenothiazines, butyrophenones) in controlling agitation have concluded that the use of neuroleptics results in a response rate of 18%. Clearly, neuroleptic therapy for behavior control should be limited with frequent attempts to withdraw the agent given for behavior control.

Dosage Forms Excipient information presented when available (limited, particularly for generics); consult specific product labeling. [DSC] = Discontinued product

Elixir, as hydrochloride (Prolixin®): 2.5 mg/5 mL (60 mL) [contains alcohol 14% and sodium benzoate] [DSC]

Injection, oil, as decanoate: 25 mg/mL (5 mL) [may contain benzyl alcohol, sesame oil]
Prolixin Decanoate®: 25 mg/mL (5 mL) [contains benzyl alcohol, sesame oil]

Injection, solution, as hydrochloride (Prolixin® [DSC]): 2.5 mg/mL (10 mL)

Solution, oral concentrate, as hydrochloride (Prolixin®): 5 mg/mL (120 mL) [contains alcohol 14%] [DSC]

Tablet, as hydrochloride: 1 mg, 2.5 mg, 5 mg, 10 mg

Prolixin®: 1 mg, 2.5 mg, 5 mg [contains tartrazine], 10 mg [DSC]

Selected References

Peabody CA, Warner MD, Whiteford HA, et al, "Neuroleptics and the Elderly," *J Am Geriatr Soc*, 1987, 35(3):233-8.

Risse SC and Barnes R, "Pharmacologic Treatment of Agitation Associated With Dementia," *J Am Geriatr Soc*, 1986, 34(5):368-76.

Saltz BL, Woerner MG, Kane JM, et al, "Prospective Study of Tardive Dyskinesia Incidence in the Elderly," *JAMA*, 1991, 266(17):2402-6.

Seifert RD, "Therapeutic Drug Monitoring: Psychotropic Drugs," *J Pharm Pract*, 1984, 6:403-16.

♦ **Fluphenazine Decanoate** *see* Fluphenazine *on page 649*

♦ **Flura-Drops®** *see* Fluoride *on page 642*

Flurazepam (flure AZ e pam)

Related Information

Anxiolytic, Sedative / Hypnotic, and Miscellaneous Benzodiazepines *on page 1750*
Potentially Inappropriate Medications for Geriatrics *on page 1824*

Medication Safety Issues

Sound-alike/look-alike issues:
Flurazepam may be confused with temazepam
Dalmane® may be confused with Demulen®, Dialume®

U.S. Brand Names Dalmane®

Canadian Brand Names Apo-Flurazepam®; Dalmane®; Som Pam

Index Terms Flurazepam Hydrochloride

Generic Available Yes

Pharmacologic Category Hypnotic, Benzodiazepine

Use Short-term treatment of insomnia

Restrictions C-IV

Contraindications Hypersensitivity to flurazepam or any component of the formulation (cross-sensitivity with other benzodiazepines may exist); narrow-angle glaucoma

Warnings/Precautions Use with caution in elderly or debilitated patients, patients with hepatic disease (including alcoholics), or renal impairment. Use with caution in patients with respiratory disease or impaired gag reflex. Avoid use in patients with sleep apnea.

Causes CNS depression (dose related); patients must be cautioned about performing tasks which require mental alertness (eg, operating machinery or driving). Use with caution in patients receiving other CNS depressants or psychoactive agents. Benzodiazepines have been associated with falls and traumatic injury and should be used with extreme caution in patients who are at risk of these events (especially the elderly).

Use caution in patients with depression, particularly if suicidal risk may be present. Use with caution in patients with a history of drug dependence. Benzodiazepines have been associated with dependence and acute withdrawal symptoms on discontinuation or reduction in dose (may occur after as little as 10 days of use).

As a hypnotic, should be used only after evaluation of potential causes of sleep disturbance. Failure of sleep disturbance to resolve after 7-10 days may indicate psychiatric or medical illness. A worsening of insomnia or the emergence of new abnormalities of thought or behavior may represent unrecognized psychiatric or medical illness and requires immediate and careful evaluation. Postmarketing studies have indicated that the use of hypnotic/sedative agents for sleep has been associated with hypersensitivity reactions including anaphylaxis as well as angioedema. An increased risk for hazardous sleep-related activities such as sleep-driving; cooking and eating food, and making phone calls while asleep have also been noted.

Benzodiazepines have been associated with anterograde amnesia. Paradoxical reactions have been reported, particularly in psychiatric patients. Does not have analgesic, antidepressant, or antipsychotic properties.

Adverse Reactions (Reflective of adult population; not specific for elderly)

Frequency not defined.

Cardiovascular: Chest pain, flushing, hypotension, palpitation

Central nervous system: Apprehension, ataxia, confusion, depression, dizziness, drowsiness, euphoria, faintness, falling, hallucinations, hangover effect, headache, irritability, lightheadedness, memory impairment, nervousness, paradoxical reactions, restlessness, slurred speech, staggering, talkativeness

Dermatologic: Pruritus, rash

Gastrointestinal: Appetite increased/decreased, bitter taste, constipation, diarrhea, GI pain, heartburn, nausea, salivation increased/excessive, upset stomach, vomiting, weight gain/loss, xerostomia

Hematologic: Granulocytopenia, leukopenia

Hepatic: Alkaline phosphatase increased, ALT/AST increased, cholestatic jaundice, total bilirubin increased

Neuromuscular & skeletal: Body/joint pain, dysarthria, reflex slowing, weakness

Ocular: Blurred vision, burning eyes, difficulty focusing

(Continued)

Flurazepam *(Continued)*

Respiratory: Apnea, dyspnea

Miscellaneous: Diaphoresis, drug dependence

Postmarketing and/or case reports: Anaphylaxis, angioedema, complex sleep-related behavior (sleep-driving, cooking or eating food, making phone calls)

Overdosage/Toxicology Symptoms include respiratory depression, hypoactive reflexes, unsteady gait, and hypotension. Treatment for benzodiazepine overdose is supportive. Rarely is mechanical ventilation required. Flumazenil has been shown to selectively block the binding of benzodiazepines to CNS receptors, resulting in a reversal of benzodiazepine-induced CNS depression.

Drug Interactions Substrate of CYP3A4 (major); **Inhibits** CYP2E1 (weak)

CNS depressants: Sedative effects and/or respiratory depression may be additive with CNS depressants; includes ethanol, barbiturates, opioid analgesics, and other sedative agents; monitor for increased effect.

CYP3A4 inducers: CYP3A4 inducers may decrease the levels/effects of flurazepam. Example inducers include aminoglutethimide, carbamazepine, nafcillin, nevirapine, phenobarbital, phenytoin, and rifamycins.

CYP3A4 inhibitors: May increase the levels/effects of flurazepam. Example inhibitors include azole antifungals, clarithromycin, diclofenac, doxycycline, erythromycin, imatinib, isoniazid, nefazodone, nicardipine, propofol, protease inhibitors, quinidine, telithromycin, and verapamil.

Levodopa: Therapeutic effects may be diminished in some patients following the addition of a benzodiazepine; limited/inconsistent data.

Oral contraceptives: May decrease the clearance of some benzodiazepines (those which undergo oxidative metabolism); monitor for increased benzodiazepine effect.

Theophylline: May partially antagonize some of the effects of benzodiazepines; monitor for decreased response; may require higher doses for sedation.

Ethanol/Nutrition/Herb Interactions

Ethanol: Avoid ethanol (may increase CNS depression).

Food: Serum levels and response to flurazepam may be increased by grapefruit juice, but unlikely because of flurazepam's high oral bioavailability.

Herb/Nutraceutical: Avoid valerian, St John's wort, kava kava, gotu kola (may increase CNS depression).

Stability Store at 15°C to 30°C (59°F to 86°F).

Mechanism of Action Binds to stereospecific benzodiazepine receptors on the postsynaptic GABA neuron at several sites within the central nervous system, including the limbic system, reticular formation. Enhancement of the inhibitory effect of GABA on neuronal excitability results by increased neuronal membrane permeability to chloride ions. This shift in chloride ions results in hyperpolarization (a less excitable state) and stabilization.

Pharmacodynamics Geriatrics: Because of a long-acting metabolite, residual, daytime sedation or "hangover effect" may occur, particularly in older adults. Studies have shown that older adults are more sensitive to the effects of benzodiazepines as compared to younger adults.

Onset of hypnotic effects: 15-20 minutes

Peak effect: 3-6 hours

Duration: 7-8 hours

Pharmacokinetics

Metabolism: Hepatic to N-desalkylflurazepam (active)

Half-life: Desalkylflurazepam:

Adults: Single dose: 74-90 hours; Multiple doses: 111-113 hours

Geriatrics (61-85 years): Single dose: 120-160 hours; Multiple doses: 126-158 hours

Elimination: Prolonged in older adults; accumulation of the parent drug and its metabolite occurs.

Dosage

Geriatrics: Oral: 15 mg at bedtime. Avoid use if possible.

Adults: Insomnia (short-term treatment): Oral: 15-30 mg at bedtime

Monitoring Parameters Respiratory, cardiovascular, and mental status

Reference Range Therapeutic: 0-4 ng/mL (SI: 0-9 nmol/L); metabolite N-desalkylflurazepam: 20-110 ng/mL (SI: 43-240 nmol/L); Toxic: >0.12 mcg/mL

Patient Information Avoid alcohol and other CNS depressants, may cause drowsiness or "hangover" effect; avoid activities needing good psychomotor coordination until CNS effects are known; may cause physical or psychological dependence; avoid abrupt discontinuation after prolonged use

Special Geriatric Considerations Due to its long-acting metabolite, flurazepam is not considered a drug of choice in the elderly. Long-acting benzodiazepines have been associated with falls in the elderly. Interpretive guidelines from the Centers for Medicare and Medicaid Services (CMS) discourage the use of this agent in residents of long-term care facilities.

Dosage Forms Excipient information presented when available (limited, particularly for generics); consult specific product labeling.

Capsule, as hydrochloride: 15 mg, 30 mg

Dalmane®: 15 mg, 30 mg

Selected References

Maletta G, Mattox KM, and Dysken M, "Guidelines for Prescribing Psychoactive Drugs in the Elderly: Part 1," *Geriatrics*, 1991, 46(9):40-7.

Reidenberg MM, Levy M, Warner H, et al, "Relationship Between Diazepam Dose, Plasma Level, Age, and Central Nervous System Depression," *Clin Pharmacol Ther*, 1978, 23(4):371-4.

♦ **Flurazepam Hydrochloride** see Flurazepam on page 653

Flurbiprofen (flure BI proe fen)

Medication Safety Issues

Sound-alike/look-alike issues:

Flurbiprofen may be confused with fenoprofen

Ansaid® may be confused with Asacol®, Axid®

Ocufen® may be confused with Ocuflox®, Ocupress®

U.S. Brand Names Ansaid® [DSC]; Ocufen®

Canadian Brand Names Alti-Flurbiprofen; Ansaid®; Apo-Flurbiprofen®; Froben®; Froben-SR®; Novo-Flurprofen; Nu-Flurprofen; Ocufen®

Index Terms Flurbiprofen Sodium

Generic Available Yes

Pharmacologic Category Nonsteroidal Anti-inflammatory Drug (NSAID), Ophthalmic; Nonsteroidal Anti-inflammatory Drug (NSAID), Oral

Use Acute or long-term treatment of signs and symptoms of rheumatoid arthritis and osteoarthritis; inhibition of intraoperative miosis; topical treatment of cystoid macular edema; postcataract surgery inflammation and uveitis syndromes

Restrictions An FDA-approved medication guide must be distributed when dispensing an oral outpatient prescription (new or refill) where this medication is to be used without direct supervision of a healthcare provider. Medication guides are available at http://www.fda.gov/cder/Offices/ODS/medication_guides.htm.

Contraindications Hypersensitivity to flurbiprofen, aspirin, other NSAIDs, or any component of the formulation; perioperative pain in the setting of coronary artery bypass surgery (CABG); dendritic keratitis

Warnings/Precautions [U.S. Boxed Warning]: NSAIDs are associated with an increased risk of adverse cardiovascular events, including MI, stroke, and new onset or worsening of pre-existing hypertension. Risk may be increased with duration of use or pre-existing cardiovascular risk factors or disease. Carefully evaluate individual cardiovascular risk profiles prior to prescribing. Use caution with fluid retention, CHF, or hypertension. Concurrent administration of ibuprofen, and potentially other nonselective NSAIDs, may interfere with aspirin's cardioprotective effect.

Use of NSAIDs can compromise existing renal function. Renal toxicity can occur in patient with impaired renal function, dehydration, heart failure, liver dysfunction, those taking diuretics and ACEIs, and the elderly. Rehydrate patient before starting therapy. Monitor renal function closely. Not recommended for use in patients with advanced renal disease.

[U.S. Boxed Warning]: NSAIDs may increase risk of gastrointestinal irritation, ulceration, bleeding, and perforation. These events may occur at any time during therapy and without warning. Use caution in patients with a history of GI disease (bleeding or ulcers), concurrent therapy with aspirin, anticoagulants and/or corticosteroids, smoking, use of alcohol, the elderly, or debilitated patients.

Use the lowest effective dose for the shortest duration of time, consistent with individual patient goals, to reduce risk of cardiovascular or GI adverse events. Alternate therapies should be considered for patients at high risk.

NSAIDs may cause serious skin adverse events including exfoliative dermatitis, Stevens-Johnson syndrome (SJS), and toxic epidermal necrolysis (TEN). Anaphylactoid reactions may occur, even without prior exposure; patients with "aspirin triad" (bronchial asthma, aspirin intolerance, rhinitis) may be at increased risk. Do not use in patients who experience bronchospasm, asthma, rhinitis, or urticaria with NSAID or aspirin therapy. Use caution in other forms of asthma.

Use with caution in patients with decreased hepatic function. Closely monitor patients with any abnormal LFT. Severe hepatic reactions (eg, fulminant hepatitis, liver failure) have occurred with NSAID use, rarely; discontinue if signs or symptoms of liver disease develop, or if systemic manifestations occur.

The elderly are at increased risk for adverse effects (especially peptic ulceration, CNS effects, renal toxicity) from NSAIDs even at low doses.

Withhold for at least 4-6 half-lives prior to surgical or dental procedures.

(Continued)

Flurbiprofen *(Continued)*

Adverse Reactions (Reflective of adult population; not specific for elderly)

Ophthalmic: Frequency not defined: Ocular: Slowing of corneal wound healing, mild ocular stinging, itching and burning, ocular irritation, fibrosis, miosis, mydriasis, bleeding tendency increased

Oral:

>1%:

Cardiovascular: Edema

Central nervous system: Amnesia, anxiety, depression, dizziness, headache, insomnia, malaise, nervousness, somnolence, vertigo

Dermatologic: Rash

Gastrointestinal: Abdominal pain, constipation, diarrhea, dyspepsia, flatulence, GI bleeding, nausea, vomiting, weight changes

Hepatic: Liver enzymes increased

Neuromuscular & skeletal: Reflexes increased, tremor, weakness

Ocular: Vision changes

Otic: Tinnitus

Respiratory: Rhinitis

Overdosage/Toxicology Symptoms include apnea, metabolic acidosis, coma, nystagmus, leukocytosis, and renal failure. Management of nonsteroidal anti-inflammatory drug (NSAID) intoxication is primarily supportive and symptomatic. Fluid therapy is commonly effective in managing hypotension that may occur following an acute NSAID overdose, except when due to acute blood loss. Seizures tend to be very short-lived and often do not require drug treatment, although recurrent seizures should be treated with I.V. diazepam. Since many of NSAIDs undergo enterohepatic cycling, multiple doses of charcoal may be needed to reduce the potential for delayed toxicities.

Drug Interactions Substrate of CYP2C9 (minor); **Inhibits** CYP2C9 (strong)

ACE inhibitors: Antihypertensive effects may be decreased by concurrent therapy with NSAIDs; monitor blood pressure.

Angiotensin II antagonists: Antihypertensive effects may be decreased by concurrent therapy with NSAIDs; monitor blood pressure.

Anticoagulants (warfarin, heparin, LMWHs) in combination with NSAIDs can cause increased risk of bleeding.

Antiplatelet drugs (ticlopidine, clopidogrel, aspirin, abciximab, dipyridamole, eptifibatide, tirofiban) can cause an increased risk of bleeding.

Beta-blockers: NSAIDs may decrease the antihypertensive effect of beta-blockers; monitor.

Cholestyramine (and other bile acid sequestrants): May decrease the absorption of NSAIDs; separate by at least 2 hours.

Corticosteroids may increase the risk of GI ulceration; avoid concurrent use.

Cyclosporine: NSAIDs may increase serum creatinine, potassium, blood pressure, and cyclosporine levels; monitor cyclosporine levels and renal function carefully.

CYP2C9 substrates: Flurbiprofen may increase the levels/effects of CYP2C9 substrates. Example substrates include bosentan, dapsone, fluoxetine, glimepiride, glipizide, losartan, montelukast, nateglinide, paclitaxel, phenytoin, warfarin, and zafirlukast.

Gentamicin and amikacin serum concentrations are increased by indomethacin in premature infants. Results may apply to other aminoglycosides and NSAIDs.

Fluoroquinolone antibiotics: Risk of seizures may be increased with concomitant quinolone use. Risk is considered quite low and may only be a factor with high serum levels of either agent and/or in patients with additional predisposing factors (eg, renal dysfunction, history of seizure or other neurological disorder).

Hydralazine's antihypertensive effect is decreased; avoid concurrent use.

Lithium levels can be increased; avoid concurrent use if possible or monitor lithium levels and adjust dose. Sulindac may have the least effect. When NSAID is stopped, lithium will need adjustment again.

Loop diuretics efficacy (diuretic and antihypertensive effect) is reduced. Indomethacin reduces this efficacy, however, it may be anticipated with any NSAID.

Methotrexate: Severe bone marrow suppression, aplastic anemia, and GI toxicity have been reported with concomitant NSAID therapy. Avoid use during moderate or high-dose methotrexate (increased and prolonged methotrexate levels). NSAID use during low-dose treatment of rheumatoid arthritis has not been fully evaluated; extreme caution is warranted.

Salicylates: NSAIDs (nonselective) may diminish the cardioprotective effect of acetylated salicylates. Avoid regular use of NSAIDs, if possible; consider alternatives (eg, acetaminophen). Give salicylate before NSAID; for example ibuprofen should be given 30-120 minutes after aspirin (immediate release).

Thiazides antihypertensive effects are decreased; avoid concurrent use.

Verapamil plasma concentration is decreased by some NSAIDs; avoid concurrent use.

Warfarin's INRs may be increased by piroxicam. Other NSAIDs may have the same effect depending on dose and duration. Monitor INR closely. Use the lowest dose of NSAIDs possible and for the briefest duration.

Ethanol/Nutrition/Herb Interactions

Ethanol: Avoid ethanol (may enhance gastric mucosal irritation).

Food: Food may decrease the rate but not the extent of absorption.

Herb/Nutraceutical: Avoid alfalfa, anise, bilberry, bladderwrack, bromelain, cat's claw, celery, coleus, cordyceps, dong quai, evening primrose, feverfew, fenugreek, garlic, ginger, ginkgo biloba, red clover, horse chestnut, grapeseed, green tea, ginseng, guggul, horse chestnut seed, horseradish, licorice, prickly ash, red clover, reishi, SAMe, sweet clover, turmeric, white willow (all have additional antiplatelet activity).

Mechanism of Action Inhibits prostaglandin synthesis by decreasing the activity of the enzyme, cyclooxygenase, which results in decreased formation of prostaglandin precursors

Pharmacodynamics Onset of action: Within 1-2 hours

Pharmacokinetics

Absorption: Oral: Rapid

Protein binding: 99%

Metabolism: Metabolized in the liver

Half-life: 5-6 hours

Time to peak serum concentration: Within 1-2 hours

Elimination: Excreted by kidneys primarily as glucuronides and sulfates

Dosage

Geriatrics & Adults:

Rheumatoid arthritis and osteoarthritis: Oral: 200-300 mg/day in 2, 3, or 4 divided doses; do not administer more than 100 mg for any single dose; maximum: 300 mg/day

Management of postoperative dental pain: 100 mg every 12 hours

Ophthalmic anti-inflammatory/surgical aid: Ophthalmic: Instill 1 drop every 30 minutes, beginning 2 hours prior to surgery (total of 4 drops in each affected eye)

Renal Impairment: Not recommended in patients with advanced renal disease.

Administration Tablet: Take with a full glass of water.

Monitoring Parameters Monitor response (pain, range of motion, grip strength, mobility, ADL function), inflammation; observe for weight gain, edema; monitor renal function; observe for bleeding, bruising; evaluate gastrointestinal effects (abdominal pain, bleeding, dyspepsia); mental confusion, disorientation, CBC, serum creatinine, BUN, liver function tests

Patient Information Serious gastrointestinal bleeding can occur as well as ulceration and perforation. Pain may or may not be present. Avoid aspirin and aspirin-containing products while taking this medication. If gastric upset occurs, take with food, milk, or antacid. If gastric adverse effects persist, contact physician. May cause drowsiness, dizziness, blurred vision, and confusion. Use caution when performing tasks which require alertness (eg, driving). Do not take for more than 3 days for fever and 10 days for pain without physician's advice.

Ophthalmic: May sting on instillation; do not touch dropper to eye; visual acuity may be decreased after administration; assess patient's or caregiver's ability to administer

Additional Information There are no clinical guidelines to predict which NSAID will give response in a particular patient. Trials with each must be initiated until response is determined. Consider dose, patient convenience, and cost.

Special Geriatric Considerations Elderly are a high-risk population for adverse effects from NSAIDs. As much as 60% of the elderly can develop peptic ulceration and/ or hemorrhage asymptomatically. The concomitant use of H_2 blockers, omeprazole, and sucralfate is not effective as prophylaxis with the exception of NSAID-induced duodenal ulcers which may be prevented by the use of ranitidine. Misoprostol and proton pump inhibitors are the only agents proven to help prevent the development of NSAID-induced ulcers. Also, concomitant disease and drug use contribute to the risk for GI adverse effects. Use lowest effective dose for shortest period possible. Consider renal function decline with age. Use of NSAIDs can compromise existing renal function, especially when Cl_{cr} is ≤30 mL/minute. Tinnitus may be a difficult and unreliable indication of toxicity due to age-related hearing loss or eighth cranial nerve damage. CNS adverse effects, such as confusion, agitation, and hallucinations, are generally seen in overdose or high-dose situations, but elderly may demonstrate these adverse effects at lower doses than younger adults.

Dosage Forms Excipient information presented when available (limited, particularly for generics); consult specific product labeling. [DSC] = Discontinued product

Solution, ophthalmic, as sodium (Ocufen®): 0.03% (2.5 mL) [contains thimerosal]

Tablet: 50 mg, 100 mg

Ansaid®: 50 mg, 100 mg [DSC]

Selected References

Brooks PM and Day RO, "Nonsteroidal Anti-inflammatory Drugs - Differences and Similarities," *N Engl J Med*, 1991, 324(24):1716-25.

(Continued)

Flurbiprofen *(Continued)*

Clinch D, Banerjee AK, and Ostick G, "Absence of Abdominal Pain in Elderly Patients With Peptic Ulcer," *Age Ageing*, 1984, 13(2):120-3.

Clive DM and Stoff JS, "Renal Syndromes Associated With Nonsteroidal Anti-inflammatory Drugs," *N Engl J Med*, 1984, 310(9):563-72.

Graham DY, "Prevention of Gastroduodenal Injury Induced by Chronic Nonsteroidal Anti-inflammatory Drug Therapy," *Gastroenterology*, 1989, 96(2 Pt 2 Suppl):675-81.

Hawkey CJ, Karrasch JA, Szczepański L, et al, "Omeprazole Compared With Misoprostol for Ulcers Associated With Nonsteroidal Anti-inflammatory Drugs," *N Engl J Med*, 1998, 338(11):727-34.

Knodel LC, "Preventing NSAID-induced Ulcers: The Role of Misoprostol," *Consult Pharm*, 1989, 4:37-41.

Pounder R, "Silent Peptic Ulceration: Deadly Silence or Golden Silence?" *Gastroenterology*, 1989, 96(2 Pt 2 Suppl):626-31.

Yeomans ND, Tulassay Z, Juhasz L, et al, "A Comparison of Omeprazole With Ranitidine for Ulcers Associated With Nonsteroidal Anti-inflammatory Drugs," *N Engl J Med*, 1998, 338(11):719-26.

♦ **Flurbiprofen Sodium** *see* Flurbiprofen *on page 655*

♦ **5-Flurocytosine** *see* Flucytosine *on page 634*

Flutamide (FLOO ta mide)

Medication Safety Issues
Sound-alike/look-alike issues:
Flutamide may be confused with Flumadine®, thalidomide
Eulexin® may be confused with Edecrin®, Eurax®

U.S. Brand Names Eulexin®

Canadian Brand Names Apo-Flutamide®; Euflex®; Eulexin®; Novo-Flutamide

Index Terms Niftolid; NSC-147834; 4′-Nitro-3′-Trifluoromethylisobutyrantide; SCH 13521

Generic Available Yes

Pharmacologic Category Antineoplastic Agent, Antiandrogen

Use Treatment of metastatic prostatic carcinoma in combination therapy with LHRH agonist analogues

Unlabeled/Investigational Use Treatment of female hirsutism

Contraindications Hypersensitivity to flutamide or any component of the formulation; severe hepatic impairment

Warnings/Precautions Hazardous agent - use appropriate precautions for handling and disposal. **[U.S. Boxed Warning]: Hospitalization and, rarely, death due to liver failure have been reported in patients taking flutamide.** Elevated serum transaminase levels, jaundice, hepatic encephalopathy, and acute hepatic failure have been reported. Product labeling states flutamide is not for use in women, particularly for nonlife-threatening conditions. In some patients, the toxicity reverses after discontinuation of therapy. About 50% of the cases occur within the first 3 months of treatment. Serum transaminase levels should be measured prior to starting treatment, monthly for 4 months, and periodically thereafter. Liver function tests should be obtained at the first suggestion of liver dysfunction (nausea, vomiting, abdominal pain, fatigue, anorexia, "flu-like" symptoms, hyperbilirubinuria, jaundice, or right upper quadrant tenderness). Flutamide should be immediately discontinued any time a patient has jaundice, and/or an ALT level greater than twice the upper limit of normal. Flutamide should not be used in patients whose ALT values are greater than twice the upper limit of normal.

Patients with glucose-6 phosphate dehydrogenase deficiency or hemoglobin M disease or smokers are at risk of toxicities associated with aniline exposure, including methemoglobinemia, hemolytic anemia, and cholestatic jaundice. Monitor methemoglobin levels.

Adverse Reactions (Reflective of adult population; not specific for elderly)
>10%:
Endocrine & metabolic: Gynecomastia, hot flashes, breast tenderness, galactorrhea (9% to 42%), impotence, libido decreased, tumor flare
Gastrointestinal: Nausea, vomiting (11% to 12%)
Hepatic: AST and LDH levels increased, transient, mild
1% to 10%:
Cardiovascular: Hypertension (1%), edema
Central nervous system: Drowsiness, confusion, depression, anxiety, nervousness, headache, dizziness, insomnia
Dermatologic: Pruritus, ecchymosis, photosensitivity
Gastrointestinal: Anorexia, appetite increased, constipation, indigestion, upset stomach (4% to 6%); diarrhea
Hematologic: Anemia (6%), leukopenia (3%), thrombocytopenia (1%)
Neuromuscular & skeletal: Weakness (1%)
Miscellaneous: Herpes zoster

Overdosage/Toxicology Symptoms include hypoactivity, ataxia, anorexia, vomiting, slow respirations, and lacrimation. Induce vomiting. Management is supportive. There is no benefit from dialysis.

Drug Interactions Substrate (major) of CYP1A2, 3A4; **Inhibits** CYP1A2 (weak)

CYP1A2 inducers: May decrease the levels/effects of flutamide. Example inducers include aminoglutethimide, carbamazepine, phenobarbital, and rifampin.

CYP1A2 inhibitors: May increase the levels/effects of flutamide. Example inhibitors include ciprofloxacin, fluvoxamine, ketoconazole, lomefloxacin, ofloxacin, and rofecoxib.

CYP3A4 inducers: CYP3A4 inducers may decrease the levels/effects of flutamide. Example inducers include aminoglutethimide, carbamazepine, nafcillin, nevirapine, phenobarbital, phenytoin, and rifamycins.

CYP3A4 inhibitors: May increase the levels/effects of flutamide. Example inhibitors include azole antifungals, clarithromycin, diclofenac, doxycycline, erythromycin, imatinib, isoniazid, nefazodone, nicardipine, propofol, protease inhibitors, quinidine, telithromycin, and verapamil.

Warfarin: Warfarin effects may be increased.

Ethanol/Nutrition/Herb Interactions

Food: No effect on bioavailability of flutamide.

Herb/Nutraceutical: St John's wort may decrease flutamide levels.

Stability Store at room temperature.

Mechanism of Action Nonsteroidal antiandrogen that inhibits androgen uptake or inhibits binding of androgen in target tissues

Pharmacokinetics

Absorption: Oral: Rapid and complete

Protein binding: Parent drug: 94% to 96%; 2-hydroxyflutamide: 92% to 94%

Metabolism: Extensively hepatic to more than 10 metabolites, primarily 2-hydroxyflutamide (active)

Half-life: 5-6 hours (2-hydroxyflutamide)

Elimination: Primarily urine (as metabolites)

Dosage

Geriatrics & Adults: Refer to individual protocols.

Prostate carcinoma: Oral: 250 mg 3 times/day; alternatively, once-daily doses of 0.5-1.5 g have been used (unlabeled dosing)

Female hirsutism (unlabeled use): Oral: 250 mg daily

Administration Usually administered orally in 3 divided doses; contents of capsule may be opened and mixed with applesauce, pudding, or other soft foods; mixing with a beverage is not recommended

Monitoring Parameters Serum transaminase levels should be measured prior to starting treatment and should be repeated monthly for the first 4 months of therapy, and periodically thereafter. LFTs should be checked at the first sign or symptom of liver dysfunction (eg, nausea, vomiting, abdominal pain, fatigue, anorexia, flu-like symptoms, hyperbilirubinuria, jaundice, or right upper quadrant tenderness). Other parameters include tumor reduction, testosterone/estrogen, and phosphatase serum concentrations.

Patient Information Do not discontinue therapy without physician's advice

Special Geriatric Considerations A study has shown that the addition of flutamide to leuprolide therapy in patients with advanced prostatic cancer increased median actuarial survival time to 34.9 months versus 27.9 months with leuprolide alone. No specific dose alterations are necessary in the elderly.

Dosage Forms Excipient information presented when available (limited, particularly for generics); consult specific product labeling.

Capsule: 125 mg

Selected References

Crawford ED, Eisenberger MA, McLeod DG, et al, "A Controlled Trial of Leuprolide With and Without Flutamide in Prostatic Carcinoma," *N Engl J Med*, 1989, 321(7):419-24.

Fluticasone (floo TIK a sone)

Related Information

Asthma *on page 1767*
Corticosteroids *on page 1755*
Inhalant Agents *on page 1760*

Medication Safety Issues

Sound-alike/look-alike issues:

Cutivate® may be confused with Ultravate®

International issues:

Allegro® [Israel] may be confused with Allegra® which is a brand name for fexofenadine in the U.S.

Allegro®: Brand name for frovatriptan in Germany

Flovent® may be confused with Flogen® which is a brand name for naproxen in Mexico

(Continued)

Fluticasone *(Continued)*

U.S. Brand Names Cutivate®; Flonase®; Flovent® HFA; Veramyst™

Canadian Brand Names Cutivate™; Flonase®; Flovent® Diskus®; Flovent® HFA

Index Terms Fluticasone Furoate; Fluticasone Propionate

Generic Available Yes: Cream, nasal spray, ointment

Pharmacologic Category Corticosteroid, Inhalant (Oral); Corticosteroid, Nasal; Corticosteroid, Topical; Corticosteroid, Topical (Medium Potency)

Use

Oral inhalation: Maintenance treatment of asthma as prophylactic therapy; also indicated for patients requiring oral corticosteroid therapy for asthma to assist in total discontinuation or reduction of total oral dose

Intranasal:

Flonase®: Management of seasonal and perennial allergic rhinitis and nonallergic rhinitis

Veramyst™: Management of seasonal and perennial allergic rhinitis

Topical: Relief of inflammation and pruritus associated with corticosteroid-responsive dermatoses; atopic dermatitis

Contraindications Hypersensitivity to fluticasone or any component of the formulation; primary treatment of status asthmaticus or acute bronchospasm

Topical: Do not use if infection is present at treatment site, in the presence of skin atrophy, or for the treatment of rosacea or perioral dermatitis

Warnings/Precautions May cause hypercorticism or suppression of hypothalamic-pituitary-adrenal (HPA) axis, particularly in patients receiving high doses for prolonged periods. HPA axis suppression may lead to adrenal crisis. Withdrawal and discontinuation of a corticosteroid should be done slowly and carefully. Particular care is required when patients are transferred from systemic corticosteroids to inhaled products due to possible adrenal insufficiency or withdrawal from steroids, including an increase in allergic symptoms. Patients receiving >20 mg per day of prednisone (or equivalent) may be most susceptible. Concurrent use of ritonavir (and potentially other strong inhibitors of CYP3A4) may increase fluticasone levels and effects on HPA suppression. Fatalities have occurred due to adrenal insufficiency in asthmatic patients during and after transfer from systemic corticosteroids to aerosol steroids; aerosol steroids do **not** provide the systemic steroid needed to treat patients having trauma, surgery, or infections.

Bronchospasm may occur with wheezing after inhalation; if this occurs, stop steroid and treat with a fast-acting bronchodilator. Supplemental steroids (oral or parenteral) may be needed during stress or severe asthma attacks. Corticosteroid use may cause psychiatric disturbances, including depression, euphoria, insomnia, mood swings, and personality changes. Pre-existing psychiatric conditions may be exacerbated by corticosteroid use. Prolonged use of corticosteroids may also increase the incidence of secondary infection, mask acute infection (including fungal infections), prolong or exacerbate viral infections, or limit response to vaccines. Exposure to chickenpox should be avoided; corticosteroids should not be used to treat ocular herpes simplex. Corticosteroids should not be used for cerebral malaria. Close observation is required in patients with latent tuberculosis and/or TB reactivity; restrict use in active TB (only in conjunction with antituberculosis treatment). Rare cases of vasculitis (Churg-Strauss syndrome) or other eosinophilic conditions can occur. Prolonged treatment with corticosteroids has been associated with the development of Kaposi's sarcoma (case reports); if noted, discontinuation of therapy should be considered.

Use with caution in patients with thyroid disease, hepatic impairment, renal impairment, cardiovascular disease, diabetes, glaucoma, cataracts, myasthenia gravis, patients at risk for osteoporosis, patients at risk for seizures, or GI diseases (diverticulitis, peptic ulcer, ulcerative colitis) due to perforation risk. Use caution following acute MI (corticosteroids have been associated with myocardial rupture). Because of the risk of adverse effects, systemic corticosteroids should be used cautiously in the elderly in the smallest possible effective dose for the shortest duration. Avoid nasal corticosteroid use in patients with recent nasal septal ulcers, nasal surgery, or nasal trauma until healing has occurred.

Inhalation: Not to be used in status asthmaticus or for the relief of acute bronchospasm. Flovent® Diskus® [CAN] contains lactose; very rare anaphylactic reactions have been reported in patients with severe milk protein allergy. There have been reports of systemic corticosteroid withdrawal symptoms (eg, joint/muscle pain, lassitude, depression) when withdrawing oral inhalation therapy.

Topical: May also cause suppression of HPA axis, especially when used on large areas of the body, denuded areas, for prolonged periods of time, or with an occlusive dressing.

Adverse Reactions (Reflective of adult population; not specific for elderly)
Oral inhalation:
>10%:
Central nervous system: Headache (5% to 11%)
Respiratory: Upper respiratory tract infection (16% to 18%)
3% to 10%:
Respiratory: Throat irritation (8% to 10%), sinusitis/sinus infection (4% to 7%), cough (4% to 6%), bronchitis (2% to 6%), hoarseness/dysphonia (2% to 6%), upper respiratory tract inflammation (2% to 5%)
Miscellaneous: Candidiasis (2% to 5%)
1% to 3%:
Cardiovascular: Chest symptoms
Central nervous system: Dizziness, fever, migraine, pain
Gastrointestinal: Diarrhea, dyspepsia, gastrointestinal infection (viral), gastrointestinal discomfort/pain, hyposalivation
Genitourinary: Urinary tract infection
Neuromuscular & skeletal: Musculoskeletal pain, muscle pain, muscle stiffness/tightness/rigidity
Respiratory: Rhinitis, pharyngitis/throat infection, rhinorrhea/postnasal drip, nasal sinus disorder, laryngitis
Miscellaneous: Viral infection, injuries (including muscle, soft tissue)

Nasal inhalation (includes reactions from Flonase® and Veramyst™ trials):
>10%: Central nervous system: Headache (7% to 16%)
1% to 10%:
Central nervous system: Dizziness (1% to 3%), fever (1% to 5%)
Gastrointestinal: Nausea/vomiting (3% to 5%), abdominal pain (1% to 3%), diarrhea (1% to 3%)
Neuromuscular & skeletal: Back pain (1%)
Respiratory: Pharyngitis (6% to 8%), epistaxis (4% to 7%), asthma symptoms (3% to 7%), cough (3% to 4%), pharyngolaryngeal pain (2% to 4%), blood in nasal mucous (1% to 3%), bronchitis (1% to 3%), runny nose (1% to 3%), nasal ulcer (1%)
Miscellaneous: Aches and pains (1% to 3%), flu-like syndrome (1% to 3%)

Topical: 1% to 10%:
Dermatologic: Dry skin (7%), skin burning/stinging (2% to 5%), pruritus (3%), skin irritation (3%), viral skin infection (1% to 3%), exacerbation of eczema (2%)
Neuromuscular & skeletal: Numbness of fingers (1%)

Reported with other topical corticosteroids (in decreasing order of occurrence): Irritation, folliculitis, acneiform eruptions, hypopigmentation, perioral dermatitis, allergic contact dermatitis, secondary infection, skin atrophy, striae, miliaria, pustular psoriasis from chronic plaque psoriasis

Overdosage/Toxicology When consumed in excessive quantities, systemic hypercorticism and adrenal suppression may occur; in those cases, discontinuation and withdrawal of the corticosteroid should be done judiciously.

Drug Interactions Substrate of CYP3A4 (major)
Antifungal agents, azole (eg, ketoconazole): May increase the serum levels/effects of corticosteroids; monitor for signs and symptoms of adrenal suppression.
CYP3A4 inhibitors: May increase the levels/effects of fluticasone. Example inhibitors include azole antifungals, clarithromycin, diclofenac, doxycycline, erythromycin, imatinib, isoniazid, nefazodone, nicardipine, propofol, protease inhibitors, quinidine, telithromycin, and verapamil.
Fluoroquinolones: Concurrent use may increase the risk of tendinopathies (including tendonitis and rupture), particularly in elderly patients (overall incidence rare)
Protease inhibitors: May increase the levels/effects of fluticasone; avoid concurrent use with ritonavir.

Ethanol/Nutrition/Herb Interactions Herb/Nutraceutical: In theory, St John's wort may decrease serum levels of fluticasone by inducing CYP3A4 isoenzymes.

Stability
Nasal spray:
Flonase®: Store between 4°C to 30°C (39°F to 86°F).
Veramyst™: Store between 15°C to 30°C (59°F to 86°F); do not refrigerate or freeze. Store in upright position with cap on.
Oral inhalation: Flovent®, Flovent® HFA: Store at 15°C to 30°C (59°F to 86°F). Store with mouthpiece down.
Powder for oral inhalation: Flovent® Diskus® [CAN]: Store between 2°C to 30°C in a dry place away from direct frost, heat, or sunlight. Do not store in a damp environment (eg, bathroom).
Topical, cream: Store at 15°C to 30°C (59°F to 86°F).
Cutivate® lotion: Store at 15°C to 30°C (59°F to 86°F); do not refrigerate.
Cutivate® cream, ointment: Store at 2°C to 30°C (36°F to 86°F).
(Continued)

Fluticasone *(Continued)*

Mechanism of Action Fluticasone belongs to a new group of corticosteroids which utilizes a fluorocarbothioate ester linkage at the 17 carbon position; extremely potent vasoconstrictive and anti-inflammatory activity; has a weak HPA inhibitory potency when applied topically, which gives the drug a high therapeutic index. The effectiveness of inhaled fluticasone is due to its direct local effect. The mechanism of action for all topical corticosteroids is believed to be a combination of three important properties: anti-inflammatory activity, immunosuppressive properties, and antiproliferative actions.

Pharmacodynamics

Onset of action: Intranasal: Maximal benefit may take several days

Flovent® HFA: Maximal benefit may take 1-2 weeks or longer

Pharmacokinetics

Absorption:

Topical cream: 5% (increased with inflammation)

Oral inhalation: Absorbed systemically (DISKUS®: ~18%) primarily via lungs, minimal GI absorption (<1%) due to presystemic metabolism

Distribution: 4.2 L/kg

Protein binding: 91%

Metabolism: Hepatic via CYP3A4 to 17β-carboxylic acid (negligible activity)

Bioavailability: Nasal: ≤2%; Oral inhalation: (~18% to 21%)

Excretion: Feces (as parent drug and metabolites); urine (<5% as metabolites)

Dosage

Geriatrics & Adults:

Asthma: Inhalation, oral: **Note:** Titrate to the lowest effective dose once asthma stability is achieved

Flovent® HFA: Manufacturers labeling: Dosing based on previous therapy

Bronchodilator alone: Recommended starting dose: 88 mcg twice daily; highest recommended dose: 440 mcg twice daily

Inhaled corticosteroids: Recommended starting dose: 88-220 mcg twice daily; highest recommended dose: 440 mcg twice daily; a higher starting dose may be considered in patients previously requiring higher doses of inhaled corticosteroids

Oral corticosteroids:

Recommended starting dose:

Flovent® HFA: 440 mcg twice daily

Highest recommended dose: 880 mcg twice daily; starting dose is patient dependent. In patients on chronic oral corticosteroids therapy, reduce prednisone dose no faster than 2.5-5 mg/day on a weekly basis; begin taper after 1 week of fluticasone therapy.

NIH Asthma Guidelines (administer in divided doses twice daily).

"Low" dose: 88-264 mcg/day

"Medium" dose: 264-660 mcg/day

"High" dose: >660 mcg/day

Flovent® Diskus® [CAN]:

Mild asthma: 100-250 mcg twice daily

Moderate asthma: 250-500 mcg twice daily

Severe asthma: 500 mcg twice daily; may increase to 1000 mcg twice daily in very severe patients requiring high doses of corticosteroids

Corticosteroid-responsive dermatoses: Topical: Cream, lotion, ointment: Apply sparingly to affected area twice daily. If no improvement is seen within 2 weeks, reassessment of diagnosis may be necessary.

Atopic dermatitis: Topical: Cream, lotion: Apply sparingly to affected area once or twice daily. If no improvement is seen within 2 weeks, reassessment of diagnosis may be necessary.

Rhinitis: Intranasal:

Flonase® (fluticasone propionate): Initial: 2 sprays (50 mcg/spray) per nostril once daily; may also be divided into 100 mcg twice a day. After the first few days, dosage may be reduced to 1 spray per nostril once daily for maintenance therapy.

Veramyst™ (fluticasone furoate): Initial: 2 sprays (27.5 mcg/spray) per nostril once daily (110 mcg/day). Once symptoms are controlled, may reduce dosage to 1 spray per nostril once daily (55 mcg/day) for maintenance therapy.

Hepatic Impairment: Fluticasone is primarily cleared in the liver. Fluticasone plasma levels may be increased in patients with hepatic impairment, use with caution; monitor.

Administration

Aerosol inhalation: Flovent® HFA: Shake container thoroughly before using. Take 3-5 deep breaths. Use inhaler on inspiration. Allow 1 full minute between inhalations. Rinse mouth with water after use to reduce aftertaste and incidence of candidiasis. Inhaler must be primed before first use, when not used for 7 days, or if dropped. To prime the first time, release 4 sprays into air; shake well before each spray and spray away from face. If dropped or not used for 7 days, prime by releasing a single test spray. Discard after 120 actuations; do not use "float" test to determine contents.

Nasal spray: Administer at regular intervals. Shake bottle gently before using. Blow nose to clear nostrils. Insert applicator into nostril, keeping bottle upright, and close off the other nostril. Breathe in through nose. While inhaling, press pump to release spray. Discard after labeled number of doses has been used, even if bottle is not completely empty.

Flonase®: Prime pump (press 6 times until fine spray appears) prior to first use or if spray unused for ≥7 days. Once weekly, nasal applicator may be removed and rinsed with warm water to clean.

Veramyst™: Prime pump (press 6 times until fine spray appears) prior to first use, if spray unused for ≥30 days, or if cap left off bottle for ≥5 days. After each use, nozzle should be wiped with a clean, dry tissue. Once weekly, inside of cap should be cleaned with a clean, dry tissue.

Powder for oral inhalation: Flovent® Diskus® [CAN]: Do not use with a spacer device. Do not exhale into Diskus®. Do not wash or take apart. Use in horizontal position.

Topical cream, lotion, ointment: Apply sparingly in a thin film. Rub in lightly. Unless otherwise directed by healthcare professional, do not use with occlusive dressing; do not use on skin covered by diapers or plastic pants.

Monitoring Parameters Relief of symptoms; FEV_1, peak flow, and/or other pulmonary function tests; asthma symptoms

Patient Information Use only as prescribed, and for no longer than the period prescribed; apply thin film of cream lotion, or ointment, rub in lightly, avoid contact with eyes; notify physician if condition being treated persists or worsens; for intranasal and oral inhalers, follow the instructions accompanying the medication; do not confuse or interchange intranasal and oral inhalers

Additional Information In the United States, dosage for the metered dose inhaler (Flovent®, Flovent® HFA) is expressed as the amount of drug which leaves the actuater and is delivered to the patient. This differs from other countries, which express the dosage as the amount of drug which leaves the valve.

Special Geriatric Considerations No specific geriatric information is available. No differences in safety have been observed in the elderly when compared to younger patients. Based on current data, no dosage adjustment is needed based on age.

Dosage Forms Excipient information presented when available (limited, particularly for generics); consult specific product labeling. [CAN] = Canadian brand name

Aerosol for oral inhalation, as propionate [CFC free]:
Flovent® HFA: 44 mcg/inhalation (10.6 g) [120 metered doses]
Flovent® HFA: 110 mcg/inhalation (12 g) [120 metered doses]
Flovent® HFA: 220 mcg/inhalation (12 g) [120 metered doses]

Cream, as propionate: 0.05% (15 g, 30 g, 60 g)
Cutivate®: 0.05% (30 g, 60 g)

Lotion, as propionate:
Cutivate®: 0.05% (60 mL)

Ointment, as propionate: 0.005% (15 g, 30 g, 60 g)
Cutivate®: 0.005% (30 g, 60 g)

Powder for oral inhalation, as propionate [prefilled blister pack]:
Flovent® Diskus® [CAN]: 50 mcg (28s, 60s) [contains lactose] [not available in the U.S.]
Flovent® Diskus® [CAN]: 100 mcg (28s, 60s) [contains lactose] [not available in the U.S.]
Flovent® Diskus® [CAN]: 250 mcg (28s, 60s) [contains lactose] [not available in the U.S.]
Flovent® Diskus® [CAN]: 500 mcg (28s, 60s) [contains lactose] [not available in the U.S.]

Suspension, intranasal, as furoate [spray]:
Veramyst™: 27.5 mcg/inhalation (10 g) [120 metered actuations; contains benzalkonium chloride]

Suspension, intranasal, as propionate [spray]: 50 mcg/inhalation (16 g) [120 metered actuations]
Flonase®: 50 mcg/inhalation (16 g) [120 metered actuations]

Fluticasone and Salmeterol (floo TIK a sone & sal ME te role)

Related Information
Fluticasone on page 659
Salmeterol on page 1444

Medication Safety Issues
Sound-alike/look-alike issues:
Advair may be confused with Advicor®

(Continued)

Fluticasone and Salmeterol *(Continued)*

U.S. Brand Names Advair Diskus®; Advair® HFA

Canadian Brand Names Advair Diskus®

Index Terms Fluticasone Propionate and Salmeterol Xinafoate; Salmeterol and Fluticasone

Generic Available No

Pharmacologic Category Beta$_2$-Adrenergic Agonist; Corticosteroid, Inhalant (Oral)

Use Maintenance treatment of asthma; **not** for use for relief of acute bronchospasm; maintenance treatment of COPD associated with chronic bronchitis

Restrictions An FDA-approved medication guide must be distributed when dispensing an outpatient prescription (new or refill) where this medication is to be used without direct supervision of a healthcare provider. Medication guides are available at http://www.fda.gov/cder/Offices/ODS/medication_guides.htm.

Contraindications Hypersensitivity to fluticasone, salmeterol, or any component of the formulation; status asthmaticus; acute episodes of asthma

Warnings/Precautions

Asthma treatment: Long-acting beta$_2$ agonists may increase the risk of asthma-related deaths. In a large, randomized clinical trial (SMART, 2006), salmeterol was associated with an increase in asthma-related deaths (when added to usual asthma therapy); risk may be greater in African-American patients versus Caucasians. Should only be used as adjuvant therapy in patients not adequately controlled on inhaled corticosteroids or whose disease requires two maintenance therapies. Salmeterol is not meant to relieve acute asthmatic symptoms, should not be initiated in patients with significantly worsening or acutely deteriorating asthma, and is not a substitute for inhaled or oral corticosteroids. Short-acting beta$_2$ agonist should be used for acute symptoms and symptoms occurring between treatments. Corticosteroids should not be stopped or reduced when salmeterol is initiated. During the initiation of salmeterol watch for signs of worsening asthma. Patients must be instructed to seek medical attention in cases where acute symptoms are not relieved or a previous level of response is diminished. The need to increase frequency of use may indicate deterioration of asthma, and treatment must not be delayed.

Concurrent diseases: Use caution in patients with cardiovascular disease (eg, arrhythmia, hypertension, or CHF); seizure disorders, diabetes, ocular disease, thyroid disease, osteoporosis, gastrointestinal disease, hepatic impairment, renal impairment, myasthenia gravis, osteoporosis, or hypokalemia. Beta-agonists may cause elevation in blood pressure, heart rate, CNS stimulation/excitation, increase risk of arrhythmia, increase serum glucose, decrease serum potassium.

Adverse events: Salmeterol should not be used more than twice daily; do not exceed recommended dose. Do not use with other long-acting beta$_2$ agonists; serious adverse events, have been associated with excessive use of inhaled sympathomimetics. There have been reports of laryngeal spasm, irritation, and swelling (stridor, choking) with use. Rarely, paradoxical bronchospasm may occur with use of inhaled bronchodilating agents; this should be distinguished from inadequate response. Powder for oral inhalation contains lactose; very rare anaphylactic reactions have been reported in patients with severe milk protein allergy. Immediate hypersensitivity reactions (urticaria, angioedema, rash, bronchospasm) have been reported. Rare cases of vasculitis (Churg-Strauss syndrome) have been reported with fluticasone use. Glaucoma, increased intraocular pressure, and cataracts have occurred with fluticasone inhalation; consider routine eye exams in chronic users. Local yeast infections (eg, oral pharyngeal candidiasis) may occur. Corticosteroid use may cause psychiatric manifestations, including depression, euphoria, insomnia, mood swings, and personality changes. Pre-existing psychiatric conditions may be exacerbated by corticosteroid use.

Adrenal suppression: Fluticasone may cause hypercorticism or suppression of hypothalamic-pituitary-adrenal (HPA) axis, particularly in patients receiving high doses for prolonged periods. Withdrawal and discontinuation of a corticosteroid should be done slowly and carefully. Particular care is required when patients are transferred from systemic corticosteroids to inhaled products. Patients receiving >20 mg per day of prednisone (or equivalent) may be most susceptible. Concurrent use of ritonavir (and potentially other strong inhibitors of CYP3A4) may increase fluticasone levels and effects on HPA suppression. Fatalities have occurred due to adrenal insufficiency in asthmatic patients during and after transfer from systemic corticosteroids to aerosol steroids; aerosol steroids do not provide the systemic steroid needed to treat patients having trauma, surgery, or infections. Do not use this product to transfer patients from oral corticosteroid therapy.

Immune system: Prolonged use of corticosteroids may also increase the incidence of secondary infection, mask acute infection (including fungal infections), prolong or exacerbate viral infections, or limit response to vaccines. Exposure to chickenpox should be avoided; corticosteroids should not be used to treat ocular herpes simplex. Corticosteroids should not be used for cerebral malaria. Close observation is required in patients with latent tuberculosis and/or TB reactivity; restrict use in active TB (only in conjunction with antituberculosis treatment).

There have been reports of systemic corticosteroid withdrawal symptoms (eg, joint/ muscle pain, lassitude, depression) when withdrawing oral inhalation therapy.

Adverse Reactions (Reflective of adult population; not specific for elderly)
Percentages reported in patients with asthma; also see individual agents:
>10%:
Central nervous system: Headache (12% to 21%)
Respiratory: Upper respiratory tract infection (16% to 27%), pharyngitis (9% to 13%)
>3% to 10%:
Central nervous system: Dizziness (1% to 4%)
Gastrointestinal: Nausea/vomiting (4% to 6%), diarrhea (2% to 4%), pain/discomfort (1% to 4%), oral candidiasis (1% to 4%)
Neuromuscular & skeletal: Musculoskeletal pain (2% to 7%)
Respiratory: Bronchitis (2% to 8%), upper respiratory tract inflammation (4% to 7%), cough (3% to 6%), sinusitis (4% to 5%), hoarseness/dysphonia (1% to 5%), viral respiratory tract infection (4%), epistaxis (1% to 4%)
1% to 3%:
Cardiovascular: Arrhythmia, chest symptoms, fluid retention, MI, palpitation, syncope, tachycardia
Central nervous system: Compressed nerve syndromes, hypnagogic effects, migraine, pain, sleep disorders, tremor
Dermatologic: Dermatitis, dermatosis, eczema, hives, skin flakiness, urticaria, viral skin infection
Endocrine & metabolic: Hypothyroidism
Gastrointestinal: Appendicitis, constipation, dental discomfort/pain, gastrointestinal infection, gastrointestinal signs and symptoms (nonspecified), hemorrhoids, oral discomfort/pain, oral erythema/rash, oral ulcerations, unusual taste, viral GI infection (0% to 3%), weight gain
Genitourinary: Urinary tract infection
Hematologic: Contusions/hematomas, lymphatic signs and symptoms (nonspecified)
Hepatic: Abnormal liver function tests
Neuromuscular & skeletal: Arthralgia, articular rheumatism, bone/cartilage disorders, bone pain, cramps, fractures, muscle injuries, muscle spasm, muscle stiffness, tightness/rigidity
Ocular: Conjunctivitis, edema, eye redness, keratitis, xerophthalmia
Otic: Ear signs and symptoms (nonspecified)
Respiratory: Blood in nasal mucosa, congestion, ear/nose/throat infection, laryngitis, lower respiratory tract infection, lower respiratory signs and symptoms (nonspecified), nasal irritation, nasal signs and symptoms (nonspecified), nasal sinus disorders, pneumonia, rhinitis, rhinorrhea/postnasal drip, sneezing, wheezing
Miscellaneous: Allergies/allergic reactions, bacterial infection, burns, candidiasis (0% to 3%), diaphoresis, sweat/sebum disorders, viral infection, wounds and lacerations

Overdosage/Toxicology Symptoms of overdose include tachycardia, tremor, hypertension, angina, and seizures. Hypokalemia also may occur. Cardiac arrest and death may be associated with abuse of beta-agonist bronchodilators. Treatment includes immediate discontinuation and symptomatic and supportive therapies. Cautious use of beta-adrenergic blocking agents may be considered in severe cases.

Drug Interactions Fluticasone: **Substrate** of CYP3A4 (major); Salmeterol: **Substrate** of CYP3A4 (major)
Antifungal agents (imidazole): May decrease the metabolism, via CYP isoenzymes, of corticosteroids (orally inhaled).
Atomoxetine: May enhance the tachycardia effect of beta$_2$-agonists.
Beta$_2$-agonists: May diminish the bradycardia effect of beta-blockers (beta$_1$ selective).
Beta-blockers (nonselective): May diminish the bronchodilator effect of beta$_2$-agonists.
Protease inhibitors: May decrease the metabolism, via CYP isoenzymes, of corticosteroids (orally inhaled). Examples include amprenavir, atazanavir, fosamprenavir, indinavir, lopinavir, nelfinavir, ritonavir, and saquinavir; **exception** is tipranavir.
Sympathomimetics: May enhance the adverse/toxic effect of salmeterol.

Stability
Advair Diskus®: Store at 20°C to 25°C (68°F to 77°F). Store in a dry place out of direct heat or sunlight. Diskus® device should be discarded 1 month after removal from foil pouch, or when dosing indicator reads "zero," whichever comes first. Device is not reusable.
Advair® HFA: Store at 15°C to 30°C (59°F to 86°F). Store with mouthpiece down. Discard after 120 inhalations. Device is not reusable.

Mechanism of Action Combination of fluticasone (corticosteroid) and salmeterol (long-acting beta$_2$-agonist) designed to improve pulmonary function and control over what is produced by either agent when used alone. Because fluticasone and salmeterol act locally in the lung, plasma levels do not predict therapeutic effect.
(Continued)

Fluticasone and Salmeterol *(Continued)*

Fluticasone: The mechanism of action for all topical corticosteroids is believed to be a combination of three important properties: Anti-inflammatory activity, immunosuppressive properties, and antiproliferative actions. Fluticasone has extremely potent vasoconstrictive and anti-inflammatory activity.

Salmeterol: Relaxes bronchial smooth muscle by selective action on beta$_2$-receptors with little effect on heart rate

Pharmacokinetics See individual agents.

Duration: 12 hours

Dosage

Geriatrics & Adults: Do not use to transfer patients from systemic corticosteroid therapy.

COPD: Oral Inhalation: Advair Diskus®: Fluticasone 250 mcg/salmeterol 50 mcg twice daily, 12 hours apart. **Note:** This is the maximum dose.

Asthma (maintenance): Oral inhalation:

Advair Diskus®: One inhalation twice daily, morning and evening, 12 hours apart

Maximum dose: Fluticasone 500 mcg/salmeterol 50 mcg per inhalation

Advair® HFA: Two inhalations twice daily, morning and evening, 12 hours apart

Maximum dose: Fluticasone 230 mcg/salmeterol 21 mcg per inhalation

Note: Initial dose prescribed should be based upon previous dose of inhaled-steroid asthma therapy. Dose should be increased after 2 weeks if adequate response is not achieved. Patients should be titrated to lowest effective dose once stable. Each suggestion below specifies the product strength to use; remember to **use 1 inhalation for Diskus® and 2 inhalations for HFA.**

Patients not currently on inhaled corticosteroids:

Advair Diskus®: Fluticasone 100 mcg/salmeterol 50 mcg **or** fluticasone 250 mcg/salmeterol 50 mcg

Advair® HFA: Fluticasone 45 mcg/salmeterol 21 mcg **or** fluticasone 115 mcg/salmeterol 21 mcg

Patients currently using inhaled beclomethasone dipropionate:

≤160 mcg/day: Advair Diskus®: Fluticasone 100 mcg/salmeterol 50 mcg **or** Advair® HFA: Fluticasone 45 mcg/salmeterol 21 mcg

320 mcg/day: Advair Diskus®:Fluticasone 250 mcg/salmeterol 50 mcg **or** Advair® HFA: Fluticasone 115 mcg/salmeterol 21 mcg

640 mcg/day: Advair Diskus®: Fluticasone 500 mcg/salmeterol 50 mcg **or** Advair® HFA: Fluticasone 230 mcg/salmeterol 21 mcg

Patients currently using inhaled budesonide:

≤400 mcg/day: Advair Diskus®: Fluticasone 100 mcg/salmeterol 50 mcg **or** Advair® HFA: Fluticasone 45 mcg/salmeterol 21 mcg

800-1200 mcg/day: Advair Diskus®: Fluticasone 250 mcg/salmeterol 50 mcg **or** Advair® HFA: Fluticasone 115 mcg/salmeterol 21mcg

1600 mcg/day: Advair Diskus®: Fluticasone 500 mcg/salmeterol 50 mcg **or** Advair® HFA: Fluticasone 230 mcg/salmeterol 21 mcg

Patients currently using inhaled flunisolide CFC aerosol:

≤1000 mcg/day: Advair Diskus®: Fluticasone 100 mcg/salmeterol 50 mcg **or** Advair® HFA: Fluticasone 45 mcg/salmeterol 21 mcg

1250-2000 mcg/day: Advair Diskus®: Fluticasone 250 mcg/salmeterol 50 mcg **or** Advair® HFA: Fluticasone 115 mcg/salmeterol 21 mcg

Patients currently using inhaled fluticasone HFA aerosol:

≤176 mcg/day: Advair Diskus®: Fluticasone 100 mcg/salmeterol 50 mcg **or** Advair® HFA: Fluticasone 45 mcg/salmeterol 21 mcg

440 mcg/day: Advair Diskus®: Fluticasone 250 mcg/salmeterol 50 mcg **or** Advair® HFA: Fluticasone 115 mcg/salmeterol 21 mcg

660-880 mcg/day: Advair Diskus®: Fluticasone 500 mcg/salmeterol 50 mcg **or** Advair® HFA: Fluticasone 230 mcg/salmeterol 21 mcg

Patients currently using inhaled fluticasone propionate powder:

≤200 mcg/day: Advair Diskus®: Fluticasone 100 mcg/salmeterol 50 mcg **or** Advair® HFA: Fluticasone 45 mcg/salmeterol 21 mcg

500 mcg/day: Advair Diskus®: Fluticasone 250 mcg/salmeterol 50 mcg **or** Advair® HFA: Fluticasone 115 mcg/salmeterol 21 mcg

1000 mcg/day: Advair Diskus®: Fluticasone 500 mcg/salmeterol 50 mcg **or** Advair® HFA: Fluticasone 230 mcg/salmeterol 21 mcg

Patients currently using inhaled mometasone furoate powder:

220 mcg/day: Advair Diskus®: Fluticasone 100 mcg/salmeterol 50 mcg **or** Advair® HFA: Fluticasone 45 mcg/salmeterol 21 mcg

440 mcg/day: Advair Diskus®: Fluticasone 250 mcg/salmeterol 50 mcg **or** Advair® HFA: Fluticasone 115 mcg/salmeterol 21 mcg

880 mcg/day: Advair Diskus®: Fluticasone 500 mcg/salmeterol 50 mcg **or** Advair® HFA: Fluticasone 230 mcg/salmeterol 21 mcg

Patients currently using inhaled triamcinolone acetonide:
≤1000 mcg/day: Advair Diskus®: Fluticasone 100 mcg/salmeterol 50 mcg **or** Advair® HFA: Fluticasone 45 mcg/salmeterol 21 mcg
1100-1600 mcg/day: Advair Diskus®: Fluticasone 250 mcg/salmeterol 50 mcg **or** Advair® HFA: Fluticasone 115 mcg/salmeterol 21 mcg

Hepatic Impairment: Systemic absorption is poor from inhalation therapy; therefore, no dosage adjustment recommended. Manufacturer suggests close monitoring of patients with hepatic impairment.

Administration Advair® HFA: Shake well for 5 seconds before each spray; prime with 4 test sprays (into air and away from face) before using for the first time. If canister is dropped or not used for >4 weeks, prime with 2 sprays. Patient must keep track of the number of uses. Throw away canister after 120 inhalations. Do not spray in eyes. Rinse mouth with water after use to reduce risk of oral candidiasis.

Patient Information Use at regular intervals, as directed; do not overuse. Do not use for acute attacks. It may take ≥1 week to see full benefits from treatment. You may experience nervousness, dizziness, or fatigue (use caution when driving or engaging in tasks requiring alertness until response to drug is known); or dry mouth, stomach upset (frequent small meals, frequent mouth care, chewing gum, or sucking hard candy may help). Report unresolved GI upset; dizziness or fatigue; vision changes; chest pain, rapid heartbeat, or palpitations; insomnia; nervousness or hyperactivity; muscle cramping, tremors, or pain; unusual cough or spasm; or rash (hypersensitivity). Notify health care provider immediately if there is an increased need for short-acting beta₂ agonists, a decrease in peak flow, or general worsening of condition. May be more susceptible to infection; avoid exposure to chickenpox and measles unless immunity has been established.

Special Geriatric Considerations No differences in safety or effectiveness have been seen in studies of patients ≥65 years of age. However, increased sensitivity may be seen in the elderly. Use with caution in patients with concomitant cardiovascular disease.

Dosage Forms Excipient information presented when available (limited, particularly for generics); consult specific product labeling.
Aerosol, for oral inhalation:
Advair® HFA:
45/21: Fluticasone propionate 45 mcg and salmeterol xinafoate 30.45 mcg (12 g) [120 metered inhalations]
115/21: Fluticasone propionate 115 mcg and salmeterol xinafoate 30.45 mcg (12 g) [120 metered inhalations]
230/21: Fluticasone propionate 230 mcg and salmeterol xinafoate 30.45 mcg (12 g) [120 metered inhalations]
Powder, for oral inhalation:
Advair Diskus®:
100/50: Fluticasone propionate 100 mcg and salmeterol xinafoate 50 mcg (28s, 60s) [contains lactose; chlorofluorocarbon free]
250/50: Fluticasone propionate 250 mcg and salmeterol xinafoate 50 mcg (28s, 60s) [contains lactose; chlorofluorocarbon free]
500/50: Fluticasone propionate 500 mcg and salmeterol xinafoate 50 mcg (28s, 60s) [contains lactose; chlorofluorocarbon free]

Selected References
Nelson HS, Weiss ST, Bleecker ER, et al, "The Salmeterol Multicenter Asthma Research Trial: A Comparison of Usual Pharmacotherapy for Asthma or Usual Pharmacotherapy Plus Salmeterol," *Chest*, 2006, 129(1):15-26.

♦ **Fluticasone Furoate** *see Fluticasone on page 659*
♦ **Fluticasone Propionate** *see Fluticasone on page 659*
♦ **Fluticasone Propionate and Salmeterol Xinafoate** *see Fluticasone and Salmeterol on page 663*

Fluvastatin (FLOO va sta tin)

Related Information
Hyperlipidemia Management *on page 1773*
Medication Safety Issues
Sound-alike/look-alike issues:
Fluvastatin may be confused with fluoxetine
U.S. Brand Names Lescol®; Lescol® XL
Canadian Brand Names Lescol®; Lescol® XL
Generic Available No
Pharmacologic Category Antilipemic Agent, HMG-CoA Reductase Inhibitor
Use Adjunct to dietary therapy to decrease elevated serum total and LDL cholesterol concentrations in primary hypercholesterolemia; mixed dyslipidemia to lower triglycerides and apolipoprotein B (APOB)
(Continued)

Fluvastatin *(Continued)*

Contraindications Hypersensitivity to fluvastatin or any component of the formulation; active liver disease; unexplained persistent elevations of serum transaminases

Warnings/Precautions Secondary causes of hyperlipidemia should be ruled out prior to therapy. Liver function must be monitored by periodic laboratory assessment. Rhabdomyolysis with acute renal failure has occurred with fluvastatin and other HMG-CoA reductase inhibitors. Risk may be increased with concurrent use of other drugs which may cause rhabdomyolysis (including gemfibrozil, fibric acid derivatives, or niacin at doses ≥1 g/day). Monitor closely if used with other drugs associated with myopathy (eg, colchicine). Temporarily discontinue in any patient experiencing markedly elevated CPK levels, myopathy, or an acute/serious condition predisposing to renal failure secondary to rhabdomyolysis. Use with caution in patients with advanced age; these patients are predisposed to myopathy. Use caution in patients with previous liver disease or heavy ethanol use. Use caution in patients with concurrent medications or conditions which reduce steroidogenesis.

Adverse Reactions (Reflective of adult population; not specific for elderly)
As reported with fluvastatin capsules; in general, adverse reactions reported with fluvastatin extended release tablet were similar, but the incidence was less.

1% to 10%:
  Central nervous system: Headache (9%), fatigue (3%), insomnia (3%)
  Gastrointestinal: Dyspepsia (8%), diarrhea (5%), abdominal pain (5%), nausea (3%)
  Genitourinary: Urinary tract infection (2%)
  Neuromuscular & skeletal: Myalgia (5%)
  Respiratory: Sinusitis (3%), bronchitis (2%)

Overdosage/Toxicology GI complaints and elevated ALT (SGOT) and AST (SGPT) have been reported following large doses of the extended release tablets. In case of overdose, supportive measures should be instituted, as required. Dialyzability is not known.

Drug Interactions Substrate of CYP2C9 (major), 2C8 (minor), 2D6 (minor), 3A4 (minor); **Inhibits** CYP1A2 (weak), 2C8 (weak), 2C9 (moderate); 2D6 (weak), 3A4 (weak)

Cholestyramine: Cholestyramine may decrease the absorption of fluvastatin. Separate administration times by at least 4 hours. Cholestyramine may increase the therapeutic effects of fluvastatin.

Colchicine: Concomitant therapy with an HMG-CoA reductase inhibitor may increase risk of myopathy/rhabdomyolysis; use caution.

CYP2C9 inhibitors: May increase the levels/effects of fluvastatin. Example inhibitors include delavirdine, fluconazole, gemfibrozil, ketoconazole, nicardipine, NSAIDs, sulfonamides, and tolbutamide.

CYP2C9 substrates: Fluvastatin may increase levels/effects of CYP2C9 substrates. Example substrates include bosentan, dapsone, fluoxetine, glimepiride, glipizide, losartan, montelukast, nateglinide, paclitaxel, phenytoin, warfarin, and zafirlukast.

Fibric acid derivatives: May increase the risk of myopathy and rhabdomyolysis.

Fluconazole: May increase the levels/effects of fluvastatin; monitor.

Glyburide: C_{max} and AUC of both fluvastatin and glyburide may increase; half-life of glyburide may also increase; monitor

Omeprazole: Omeprazole may increase serum concentrations of fluvastatin.

Phenytoin: C_{max} and AUC of both phenytoin and fluvastatin may be increased when given together; monitor phenytoin when fluvastatin is initiated, modified, or discontinued.

Rifamycin derivatives: May decrease serum concentrations of fluvastatin.

Warfarin: Fluvastatin may increase hypoprothrombinemic effects of warfarin; monitor INR closely when fluvastatin is initiated, modified, or discontinued.

Ethanol/Nutrition/Herb Interactions

Ethanol: Avoid excessive ethanol consumption (due to potential hepatic effects).

Food: Reduces rate but not the extent of absorption. Red yeast rice contains an estimated 2.4 mg lovastatin per 600 mg rice.

Stability Store at 15°C to 30°C (59°F to 86°F). Protect from light.

Mechanism of Action Acts by competitively inhibiting 3-hydroxyl-3-methylglutaryl-coenzyme A (HMG-CoA) reductase, the enzyme that catalyzes the reduction of HMG-CoA to mevalonate; this is an early rate-limiting step in cholesterol biosynthesis. HDL is increased while total, LDL, and VLDL cholesterols; apolipoprotein B; and plasma triglycerides are decreased.

Pharmacodynamics Onset: Peak effect: Maximal LDL-C reductions achieved within 4 weeks

Pharmacokinetics
  Distribution: V_d: 0.35 L/kg
  Protein binding: >98%

Metabolism: To inactive and active metabolites (oxidative metabolism via CYP2C9 [75%], 2C8 [~5%], and 3A4 [~20%] isoenzymes); active forms do not circulate systemically; extensive (saturable) first-pass hepatic extraction

Bioavailability: Absolute: Capsule: 24%; Extended release tablet: 29%

Half-life elimination: Capsule: <3 hours; Extended release tablet: 9 hours

Elimination: Feces (90%): urine (5%)

Dosage
Geriatrics & Adults:
Dyslipidemia (also delay in progression of CAD): Oral:

Patients requiring ≥25% decrease in LDL-C: 40 mg capsule once daily in the evening, 80 mg extended release tablet once daily (anytime), or 40 mg capsule twice daily

Patients requiring <25% decrease in LDL-C: Initial: 20 mg capsule once daily in the evening; may increase based on tolerability and response to a maximum recommended dose of 80 mg/day, given in 2 divided doses (immediate release capsule) or as a single daily dose (extended release tablet)

Renal Impairment: Less than 6% is excreted renally. No dosage adjustment needed with mild-to-moderate renal impairment; use with caution in severe impairment.

Hepatic Impairment: Levels may accumulate in patients with liver disease (increased AUC and C_{max}). Use caution with severe hepatic impairment or heavy ethanol ingestion. Contraindicated in active liver disease or unexplained transaminase elevations. Decrease dose and monitor effects carefully in patients with hepatic insufficiency.

Administration Patient should be placed on a standard cholesterol-lowering diet before and during treatment; fluvastatin may be taken without regard to meals; adjust dosage as needed in response to periodic lipid determinations during the first 4 weeks after a dosage change; lipid-lowering effects are additive when fluvastatin is combined with a bile-acid binding resin or niacin, however, it must be administered at least 2 hours following these drugs. Do not break, chew, or crush extended release tablets; do not open capsules.

Monitoring Parameters Obtain baseline LFTs and total cholesterol profile; repeat tests at 12 weeks after initiation of therapy or elevation in dose, and periodically thereafter. Monitor LDL-C at intervals no less than 4 weeks.

Patient Information Follow diet and exercise regimen as prescribed. Have periodic ophthalmic exam to check for cataract development. Avoid prolonged exposure to the sun and other ultraviolet light. Report unexplained muscle pain or weakness, especially if accompanied by fever or malaise. Fluvastatin may cause severe fetal defects; do not donate blood while taking this drug or for 1 month following discontinuation.

Special Geriatric Considerations The definition of and, therefore, when to treat hyperlipidemia in the elderly is a controversial issue. The National Cholesterol Education Program recommends that all adults maintain a plasma cholesterol <160 mg/dL. In elderly patients with one additional risk factor, goal LDL would decrease to <130 mg/dL. Pharmacologic treatment should be reserved for those who are unable to obtain a desirable plasma cholesterol concentration by diet alone and for whom the benefits of treatment are believed to outweigh the potential adverse effects, drug interactions, and cost of treatment.

Dosage Forms Excipient information presented when available (limited, particularly for generics); consult specific product labeling.

Capsule (Lescol®): 20 mg, 40 mg

Tablet, extended release (Lescol® XL): 80 mg

Selected References
"Executive Summary of The Third Report of The National Cholesterol Education Program (NCEP) Expert Panel on Detection, Evaluation, And Treatment of High Blood Cholesterol In Adults (Adult Treatment Panel III)," *JAMA*, 2001, 285(19):2486-97.

♦ **Fluvirin®** *see* Influenza Virus Vaccine *on page 803*

Fluvoxamine (floo VOKS a meen)

Related Information
Antidepressant Agents *on page 1742*

Medication Safety Issues
Sound-alike/look-alike issues:
Fluvoxamine may be confused with flavoxate, fluoxetine
Luvox may be confused with Lasix®, Levoxyl®

Canadian Brand Names Alti-Fluvoxamine; Apo-Fluvoxamine®; Luvox®; Novo-Fluvoxamine; Nu-Fluvoxamine; PMS-Fluvoxamine; Rhoxal-fluvoxamine; Sandoz-Fluvoxamine

Index Terms Luvox

Generic Available Yes

Pharmacologic Category Antidepressant, Selective Serotonin Reuptake Inhibitor

Use Treatment of obsessive-compulsive disorder (OCD)
(Continued)

Fluvoxamine *(Continued)*

Unlabeled/Investigational Use Treatment of major depression, panic disorder

Restrictions An FDA-approved medication guide concerning the use of antidepressants in children, adolescents, and young adults must be distributed when dispensing an outpatient prescription (new or refill) where this medication is to be used without direct supervision of a healthcare provider. Medication guides are available at http://www.fda.gov/cder/Offices/ODS/medication_guides.htm. Dispense to parents or guardians of children and adolescents receiving this medication.

Contraindications Hypersensitivity to fluvoxamine or any component of the formulation; concurrent use with alosetron, pimozide, thioridazine, tizanidine, mesoridazine, or cisapride; use of MAO inhibitors within 14 days

Warnings/Precautions [U.S. Boxed Warning]: Antidepressants increase the risk of suicidal thinking and behavior in children, adolescents, and young adults (18-24 years of age) with major depressive disorder (MDD) and other psychiatric disorders; consider risk prior to prescribing. Short-term studies did not show an increased risk in patients >24 years of age and showed a decreased risk in patients ≥65 years. Closely monitor patients for clinical worsening, suicidality, or unusual changes in behavior, particularly during the initial 1-2 months of therapy or during periods of dosage adjustments (increases or decreases); the patient's family or caregiver should be instructed to closely observe the patient and communicate condition with healthcare provider. A medication guide concerning the use of antidepressants should be dispensed with each prescription.

The possibility of a suicide attempt is inherent in major depression and may persist until remission occurs. Use caution in high-risk patients. Worsening depression and severe abrupt suicidality that are not part of the presenting symptoms may require discontinuation or modification of drug therapy. The patient's family or caregiver should be alerted to monitor patients for the emergence of suicidality and associated behaviors (such as agitation, irritability, hostility, impulsivity, and hypomania) and call healthcare provider.

May worsen psychosis in some patients or precipitate a shift to mania or hypomania in patients with bipolar disorder. Patients presenting with depressive symptoms should be screened for bipolar disorder. Monotherapy in patients with bipolar disorder should be avoided. **Fluvoxamine is not FDA approved for the treatment of bipolar depression.**

The potential for severe reaction exits when used with MAO inhibitors, SSRIs/SNRIs, or triptans; serotonin syndrome (hyperthermia, muscular rigidity, mental status changes/agitation, autonomic instability) may occur. Concurrent use with MAO inhibitors is contraindicated. Fluvoxamine has a low potential to impair cognitive or motor performance; caution operating hazardous machinery or driving. Use caution in patients with a previous seizure disorder or condition predisposing to seizures such as brain damage, alcoholism, or concurrent therapy with other drugs which lower the seizure threshold.

May increase the risks associated with electroconvulsive therapy. Use with caution in patients with hepatic or renal dysfunction and in elderly patients. May cause hyponatremia/SIADH. Use with caution in patients with renal insufficiency or other concurrent illness (cardiovascular disease). Use with caution in patients at risk of bleeding or receiving concurrent anticoagulant therapy, although not consistently noted, fluvoxamine may cause impairment in platelet function. May cause or exacerbate sexual dysfunction.

Adverse Reactions (Reflective of adult population; not specific for elderly)

>10%:

Central nervous system: Headache (22%), somnolence (22%), insomnia (21%), nervousness (12%), dizziness (11%)

Gastrointestinal: Nausea (40%), diarrhea (11%), xerostomia (14%)

Neuromuscular & skeletal: Weakness (14%)

1% to 10%:

Cardiovascular: Palpitation

Central nervous system: Somnolence, mania, hypomania, vertigo, abnormal thinking, agitation, anxiety, malaise, amnesia, yawning, hypertonia, CNS stimulation, depression

Endocrine & metabolic: Libido decreased

Gastrointestinal: Abdominal pain, vomiting, dyspepsia, constipation, abnormal taste, anorexia, flatulence, weight gain

Genitourinary: Ejaculation delayed, impotence, anorgasmia, urinary frequency, urinary retention

Neuromuscular & skeletal: Tremors

Ocular: Blurred vision

Respiratory: Dyspnea

Miscellaneous: Diaphoresis

Overdosage/Toxicology Symptoms include nausea, vomiting, somnolence, hypotension, hypokalemia, tachycardia, respiratory distress, and coma. Other symptoms reported in overdose (single- or multiple-drug ingestion) include bradycardia, ECG abnormalities, seizures, tremor, diarrhea, and increased reflexes. A specific antidote does not exist. Treatment is supportive. Although vomiting has not been extensive in overdose to date, patients should be monitored for fluid and electrolyte loss, and appropriate replacement therapy instituted when necessary.

Drug Interactions Substrate (major) of CYP1A2, 2D6; **Inhibits** CYP1A2 (strong), 2B6 (weak), 2C9 (weak), 2C19 (strong), 2D6 (weak), 3A4 (weak)

Alosetron: Serum concentrations may be increased by fluvoxamine; concurrent use is not recommended.

Amphetamines: SSRIs may increase the sensitivity to amphetamines, and amphetamines may increase the risk of serotonin syndrome.

Benzodiazepines: Fluvoxamine may inhibit the metabolism of alprazolam, diazepam, and triazolam resulting in elevated serum levels; monitor for increased sedation and psychomotor impairment.

Beta-blockers: Fluvoxamine may inhibit the metabolism of metoprolol and propranolol resulting in cardiac toxicity; monitor for bradycardia, hypotension, and heart failure if combination is used. Not established for all beta-blockers (unlikely with atenolol or nadolol due to renal elimination).

Buspirone: Fluvoxamine inhibits the reuptake of serotonin; combined use with a serotonin agonist (buspirone) may cause serotonin syndrome. Fluvoxamine may also increase serum concentrations of buspirone.

Carbamazepine: Fluvoxamine may inhibit the metabolism of carbamazepine resulting in increased carbamazepine levels and toxicity; monitor for altered carbamazepine response.

Carvedilol: Serum concentrations may be increased; monitor carefully for increased carvedilol effect (hypotension and bradycardia).

Cisapride: Concurrent use is contraindicated.

Clozapine: Fluvoxamine inhibits the metabolism of clozapine; adjust clozapine dosage downward or use an alternative SSRI.

CYP1A2 inducers: May decrease the levels/effects of fluvoxamine. Example inducers include aminoglutethimide, carbamazepine, phenobarbital, and rifampin.

CYP1A2 inhibitors: May increase the levels/effects of fluvoxamine. Example inhibitors include ciprofloxacin, ketoconazole, norfloxacin, ofloxacin, and rofecoxib.

CYP1A2 substrates: Fluvoxamine may increase the levels/effects of CYP1A2 substrates. Example substrates include aminophylline, mexiletine, mirtazapine, ropinirole, theophylline, and trifluoperazine.

CYP2C19 substrates: Fluvoxamine may increase the levels/effects of CYP2C19 substrates. Example substrates include citalopram, diazepam, methsuximide, phenytoin, propranolol, and sertraline.

CYP2D6 inhibitors: May increase the levels/effects of fluvoxamine. Example inhibitors include chlorpromazine, delavirdine, fluoxetine, miconazole, paroxetine, pergolide, quinidine, quinine, ritonavir, and ropinirole.

Cyproheptadine: May inhibit the effects of serotonin reuptake inhibitors (fluvoxamine); monitor for altered antidepressant response. Cyproheptadine acts as a serotonin agonist.

Dextromethorphan: Fluvoxamine inhibits the metabolism of dextromethorphan; visual hallucinations occurred in a patient receiving this combination; monitor for serotonin syndrome.

Haloperidol: Fluvoxamine may inhibit the metabolism of haloperidol and cause extrapyramidal symptoms (EPS); monitor patients for EPS if combination is utilized.

HMG-CoA reductase inhibitors: Fluvoxamine may inhibit the metabolism of lovastatin and simvastatin resulting in myositis and rhabdomyolysis; these combinations are best avoided.

Lithium: Patients receiving SSRIs and lithium have developed neurotoxicity; if combination is used, monitor for neurotoxicity.

Loop diuretics: Fluvoxamine may cause hyponatremia; additive hyponatremic effects may be seen with combined use of a loop diuretic (bumetanide, furosemide, torsemide); monitor for hyponatremia.

MAO inhibitors: Fluvoxamine should not be used with nonselective MAO inhibitors (isocarboxazid, phenelzine); fatal reactions have been reported. This combination should be avoided.

Meperidine: Combined use with fluvoxamine, theoretically, may increase the risk of serotonin syndrome.

Methadone: Fluvoxamine may increase serum concentrations of methadone; monitor for increased effect.

Mexiletine: Clearance of mexiletine was reduced by 38% following coadministration with fluvoxamine. If used concurrently, mexiletine levels should be monitored.

Nefazodone: May increase the risk of serotonin syndrome with SSRIs.

NSAIDs: Concomitant use of fluvoxamine and NSAIDs, aspirin, or other drugs affecting coagulation has been associated with an increased risk of bleeding; monitor.

(Continued)

Fluvoxamine *(Continued)*

Pimozide: Concurrent use is contraindicated.

Phenothiazines: Fluvoxamine may inhibit metabolism of phenothiazines; **concurrent use of agents associated with QT prolongation (thioridazine, mesoridazine) is contraindicated**.

Phenytoin: Fluvoxamine inhibits the metabolism of phenytoin and may result in phenytoin toxicity; monitor for phenytoin toxicity (ataxia, confusion, dizziness, nystagmus, involuntary muscle movement).

Propafenone: Serum concentrations and/or toxicity may be increased by fluoxetine; avoid concurrent administration.

Quinidine: Serum concentrations may be increased with fluvoxamine; avoid concurrent use.

Ritonavir: Combined use of fluvoxamine with ritonavir may cause serotonin syndrome in HIV-positive patients; monitor.

Selegiline: SSRIs have been reported to cause mania or hypertension when combined with selegiline; this combination is best avoided. In addition, use with some SSRIs has been reported to cause serotonin syndrome. As an MAO type B inhibitor, the risk of serotonin syndrome may be less than with nonselective MAO inhibitors.

Serotonin agonists (eg, triptans): Concurrent use of fluvoxamine with these agents may increase the risk of serotonin syndrome; monitor.

Serotonergic reuptake inhibitors (eg, SSRIs/SNRIs): Concurrent use of fluvoxamine with these agents may increase the risk of serotonin syndrome; monitor.

Sibutramine: May increase the risk of serotonin syndrome with SSRIs.

Sympathomimetics: May increase the risk of serotonin syndrome with SSRIs.

Tacrine: Fluvoxamine inhibits the metabolism of tacrine; use alternative SSRI.

Tacrolimus: Fluvoxamine may inhibit the metabolism of tacrolimus; monitor for adverse effects; consider an alternative SSRI.

Theophylline: Fluvoxamine inhibits the metabolism of theophylline; monitor for theophylline toxicity or use alternative SSRI.

Tizanidine: Serum concentrations may be increased by fluvoxamine; concurrent use is not recommended.

Tramadol: Fluvoxamine combined with tramadol (serotonergic effects) may cause serotonin syndrome; monitor.

Trazodone: Fluvoxamine may inhibit the metabolism of trazodone resulting in increased toxicity; monitor.

Tricyclic antidepressants Fluvoxamine inhibits the metabolism of tricyclic antidepressants (amitriptyline, desipramine, imipramine, nortriptyline) resulting is elevated serum levels; if combination is warranted, a low dose of TCA (10-25 mg/day) should be utilized.

Tryptophan: Fluvoxamine inhibits the reuptake of serotonin; combination with tryptophan, a serotonin precursor, may cause agitation and restlessness. This combination is best avoided.

Venlafaxine: Combined use with fluvoxamine may increase the risk of serotonin syndrome.

Warfarin: Fluvoxamine may alter the hypoprothrombinemic response to warfarin; monitor.

Ethanol/Nutrition/Herb Interactions

Ethanol: Avoid ethanol. Depressed patients should avoid/limit intake.

Food: The bioavailability of melatonin has been reported to be increased by fluvoxamine.

Herb/Nutraceutical: Avoid valerian, St John's wort, SAMe, kava kava (may increase risk of serotonin syndrome and/or excessive sedation).

Stability Protect from high humidity and store at controlled room temperature 15°C to 30°C (59°F to 86°F). Dispense in tight containers.

Mechanism of Action Inhibits CNS neuron serotonin uptake; minimal or no effect on reuptake of norepinephrine or dopamine; does not significantly bind to alpha-adrenergic, histamine or cholinergic receptors

Pharmacodynamics Maximum effect: Requires at least 4-6 weeks of treatment

Pharmacokinetics Geriatrics: The pharmacokinetics of fluvoxamine do not appear to be affected by age.

Absorption: Oral: Readily complete in the fasting and nonfasting state

Distribution: V_d: >5-20 L/kg

Protein binding: 77%

Metabolism: Via oxidative pathways to 14 inactive compounds which are renally eliminated. See Drug Interactions.

Bioavailability, systemic: 53%

Half-life: 16 hours after multiple dosing

Peak plasma concentration: Within 2-8 hours after a single dose

Time to steady-state: ~10 days

Elimination: ~3% recovered unchanged in the urine

Dosage

Geriatrics: Reduce dose; titrate slowly. See Special Geriatric Considerations.

Adults: Obsessive-compulsive disorder: Oral: Initial: 50 mg at bedtime; adjust in 50 mg increments in 4- to 7-day intervals; usual dose range: 100-300 mg/day; divide total daily dose into 2 doses. Administer larger portion at bedtime.

Note: When total daily dose exceeds 50 mg, the dose should be given in 2 divided doses.

Hepatic Impairment: Reduce dose; titrate slowly.

Monitoring Parameters Signs and symptoms of depression, anxiety, weight gain or loss, nutritional intake, sleep

Reference Range A therapeutic range has not been established.

Patient Information Avoid alcoholic beverages; its favorable side effect profile makes it a useful alternative to the traditional agents; use sugarless hard candy for dry mouth; avoid alcoholic beverages, may cause drowsiness; improvement may take several weeks; rise slowly to prevent dizziness. As with all psychoactive drugs, fluvoxamine may impair judgment, thinking, or motor skills, so use caution when operating hazardous machinery, including automobiles, especially early on into therapy. Inform your physician of any concurrent medications you may be taking or antidepressants you have been taking. Avoid abrupt discontinuation.

Additional Information Abrupt withdrawal may result in CNS side effects (agitation, GI symptoms, "feelings of electrical shock").

Special Geriatric Considerations Given fluvoxamine's approved indication (OCD), the number of drug interactions, and the limited information available on its use in the elderly, it may be best to select a different agent when treating depression.

Dosage Forms Excipient information presented when available (limited, particularly for generics); consult specific product labeling.

Tablet, as maleate: 25 mg, 50 mg, 100 mg

Selected References

de Vries MH, Raghoebar M, Mathlener IS, et al, "Single and Multiple Oral Dose Fluvoxamine Kinetics in Young and Elderly Subjects," *Ther Drug Monit*, 1992, 14(6):493-8.

Grimsley SR and Jann MW, "Paroxetine, Sertraline, and Fluvoxamine: New Selective Serotonin Reuptake Inhibitors," *Clin Pharm*, 1992, 11(11):930-57.

Roose SP, Glassman AH, Attia E, et al, "Comparative Efficacy of Selective Serotonin Reuptake Inhibitors and Tricyclics in the Treatment of Melancholia," *Am J Psychiatry*, 1994, 151(12):1735-9.

♦ **Fluzone**® *see* Influenza Virus Vaccine *on page 803*

♦ **Folacin** *see* Folic Acid *on page 673*

♦ **Folate** *see* Folic Acid *on page 673*

Folic Acid (FOE lik AS id)

Medication Safety Issues

Sound-alike/look-alike issues:

Folic acid may be confused with folinic acid

Canadian Brand Names Apo-Folic®

Index Terms Folacin; Folate; Pteroylglutamic Acid

Generic Available Yes

Pharmacologic Category Vitamin, Water Soluble

Use Treatment of megaloblastic and macrocytic anemias due to folate deficiency

Contraindications Hypersensitivity to folic acid or any component of the formulation

Warnings/Precautions Not appropriate for monotherapy with pernicious, aplastic, or normocytic anemias when anemia is present with vitamin B_{12} deficiency. Doses >0.1 mg/day may obscure pernicious anemia with continuing irreversible nerve damage progression. Resistance to treatment may occur with depressed hematopoiesis, alcoholism, and deficiencies of other vitamins. Injection contains benzyl alcohol (1.5%) as preservative.

Adverse Reactions (Reflective of adult population; not specific for elderly)

Frequency not defined.

Allergic reaction, bronchospasm, flushing (slight), malaise (general), pruritus, rash

Drug Interactions

Phenytoin: Folic acid may decrease phenytoin concentrations.

Raltitrexed: Folic acid may diminish the therapeutic effect of raltitrexed.

Stability Do not use with oxidizing and reducing agents or heavy metal ions.

Mechanism of Action Folic acid is necessary for formation of a number of coenzymes in many metabolic systems, particularly for purine and pyrimidine synthesis; required for nucleoprotein synthesis and maintenance in erythropoiesis; stimulates WBC and platelet production in folate deficiency anemia

Pharmacodynamics Peak effect: Oral: Within 30-60 minutes

Pharmacokinetics Absorption: In the proximal part of the small intestine

(Continued)

Folic Acid *(Continued)*

Dosage

Geriatrics: Refer to adult dosing. Vitamin B_{12} deficiency must be ruled out before initiating folate therapy due to frequency of combined nutritional deficiencies: RDA requirements (1999): 400 mcg/day (0.4 mg) minimum.

Adults:

Anemia: Oral, I.M., I.V., SubQ: 0.4 mg/day

RDA: Expressed as dietary folate equivalents: 400 mcg/day

Administration Oral preferred, but may also be administered by deep I.M., SubQ, or I.V. injection; a diluted solution for oral or for parenteral administration may be prepared by diluting 1 mL of folic acid injection (5 mg/mL), with 49 mL sterile water for injection; resulting solution is 0.1 mg folic acid per 1 mL

Monitoring Parameters Reticulocyte count within 5-10 days of initiation of therapy; hematocrit, hemoglobin, RBC count at monthly intervals; diarrheal episodes should stop in 2-3 days of therapy; monitor seizure activity, serum phenytoin concentration should be monitored more often

Reference Range Therapeutic: 0.005-0.015 mcg/mL

Test Interactions Falsely low serum concentrations may occur with the *Lactobacillus casei* assay method in patients on anti-infectives (eg, tetracycline)

Patient Information Take folic acid replacement only under recommendation of physician

Additional Information The RDA for folic acid is presented as dietary folate equivalents (DFE). DFE adjusts for the difference in bioavailability of folic acid from food as compared to dietary supplements.

Special Geriatric Considerations Elderly frequently have combined nutritional deficiencies. Must rule out vitamin B_{12} deficiency before initiating folate therapy. Elderly, due to decreased nutrient intake, may benefit from daily intake of a multiple vitamin with minerals.

Dosage Forms Excipient information presented when available (limited, particularly for generics); consult specific product labeling.

Injection, solution, as sodium folate: 5 mg/mL (10 mL) [contains benzyl alcohol]

Tablet: 0.4 mg, 0.8 mg, 1 mg

Selected References

"Dietary Reference Intakes for Thiamin, Riboflavin, Niacin, Vitamin B6, Folate, Vitamin B12, Pantothenic Acid, Biotin and Choline. Standing Committee on the Scientific Evaluation of Dietary Reference Intakes, Food and Nutrition Board, Institute of Medicine," National Academy of Sciences, Washington, DC: National Academy Press, 1999. Available at: http://www.nap.edu.

Liem A, Reynierse-Buitenwerf GH, Zwinderman AH, et al, "Secondary Prevention With Folic Acid: Effects on Clinical Outcomes," *J Am Coll Cardiol*, 2003, 41(12):2105-13.

Olszewski AJ, Szostak WB, Bialkowska M, et al, "Reduction of Plasma Lipid and Homocysteine Levels by Pyridoxine, Folate, Cobalamin, Choline, Riboflavin, and Troxerutin in Atherosclerosis," *Atherosclerosis*, 1989, 75(1):1-6.

Schnyder G, Roffi M, Flammer Y, et al, "Effect of Homocysteine-Lowering Therapy With Folic Acid, Vitamin B12, and Vitamin B6 on Clinical Outcome After Percutaneous Coronary Intervention: The Swiss Heart Study: A Randomized Controlled Trial," *JAMA*, 2002, 288(8):973-9.

Fondaparinux *(fon da PARE i nuks)*

Related Information

Anticoagulants, Injectable *on page 1741*

Medication Safety Issues

High alert medication: The Institute for Safe Medication Practices (ISMP) includes this medication among its list of drugs which have a heightened risk of causing significant patient harm when used in error.

U.S. Brand Names Arixtra®

Canadian Brand Names Arixtra®

Index Terms Fondaparinux Sodium

Generic Available No

Pharmacologic Category Factor Xa Inhibitor

Use Prophylaxis of deep vein thrombosis (DVT) in patients undergoing surgery for hip replacement, knee replacement, hip fracture (including extended prophylaxis following hip fracture surgery), or abdominal surgery (in patients at risk for thromboembolic complications); treatment of acute pulmonary embolism (PE); treatment of acute DVT without PE

Note: Additional Canadian approvals (not approved in U.S.): Unstable angina or non-ST segment elevation myocardial infarction (UA/NSTEMI) for the prevention of death and subsequent MI; ST segment elevation MI (STEMI) for the prevention of death and myocardial reinfarction

Unlabeled/Investigational Use Treatment of DVT

Contraindications Hypersensitivity to fondaparinux or any component of the formulation; severe renal impairment (Cl_{cr} <30 mL/minute); body weight <50 kg (prophylaxis);

active major bleeding; bacterial endocarditis; thrombocytopenia associated with a positive *in vitro* test for antiplatelet antibody in the presence of fondaparinux

Warnings/Precautions [U.S. Boxed Warning]: Patients with recent or anticipated neuraxial anesthesia (epidural or spinal anesthesia) are at risk of spinal or epidural hematoma and subsequent paralysis. Not to be used interchangeably (unit-for-unit) with heparin, low molecular weight heparins (LMWHs), or heparinoids. Use caution in patients with moderate renal dysfunction (Cl$_{cr}$ 30-50 mL/minute). Discontinue if severe dysfunction or labile function develops.

Use caution in congenital or acquired bleeding disorders; active ulcerative or angiodysplastic gastrointestinal disease; hemorrhagic stroke; shortly after brain, spinal, or ophthalmologic surgery; or in patients taking platelet inhibitors. Risk of major bleeding may be increased if initial dose is administered earlier then recommended (initiation recommended at 6-8 hours following surgery). Discontinue agents that may enhance the risk of hemorrhage if possible. If thrombocytopenia occurs discontinue fondaparinux. Use caution in the elderly, patients with a history of heparin-induced thrombocytopenia, patients with a bleeding diathesis, uncontrolled hypertension, recent gastrointestinal ulceration, diabetic retinopathy, and hemorrhage. Use caution in patients <50 kg who are being treated for DVT/PE.

Canadian labeling warnings/precautions: The administration of fondaparinux is not recommended prior to and during primary percutaneous coronary intervention (PCI) for reperfusion in STEMI patients, due to an increased risk for guiding catheter thrombosis. UA/NSTEMI and STEMI patients undergoing any PCI should not receive fondaparinux as a sole anticoagulant agent. Use of an antithrombin regimen (eg, unfractionated heparin) is recommended as adjunctive therapy to PCI. Following sheath removal, fondaparinux therapy should not resume for at least 2 hours in UA/NSTEMI patients and 3 hours in STEMI patients. Use caution in UA/NSTEMI/STEMI patients <50 kg. Avoid administration 24 hours before and 48 hours after coronary artery bypass graft (CABG) surgery.

Adverse Reactions (Reflective of adult population; not specific for elderly)
As with all anticoagulants, bleeding is the major adverse effect. Hemorrhage may occur at any site. Risk appears increased by a number of factors including renal dysfunction, age (>75 years), and weight (<50 kg).

>10%:
  Central nervous system: Fever (4% to 14%)
  Gastrointestinal: Nausea (11%)
  Hematologic: Anemia (20%)

1% to 10%:
  Cardiovascular: Edema (9%), hypotension (4%), thrombosis PCI catheter (without heparin 1%)
  Central nervous system: Insomnia (5%), dizziness (4%), headache (2% to 5%), confusion (3%), pain (2%)
  Dermatologic: Rash (8%), purpura (4%), bullous eruption (3%)
  Endocrine & metabolic: Hypokalemia (1% to 4%)
  Gastrointestinal: Constipation (5% to 9%), nausea (3%), vomiting (6%), diarrhea (3%), dyspepsia (2%)
  Genitourinary: Urinary tract infection (4%), urinary retention (3%)
  Hematologic: Moderate thrombocytopenia (50,000-100,000/mm^3: 3%), major bleeding (1% to 3%), minor bleeding (2% to 4%), hematoma (3%); risk of major bleeding increased as high as 5% in patients receiving initial dose <6 hours following surgery
  Hepatic: AST increased (2%), ALT increased (3%)
  Local: Injection site reaction (bleeding, rash, pruritus)
  Miscellaneous: Wound drainage increased (5%)

Overdosage/Toxicology Treatment is symptom-directed and supportive. Hemodialysis may increase clearance by 20%.

Drug Interactions
  Anticoagulants: May enhance the effects of other anticoagulants.
  Antiplatelet agents (including abciximab, anagrelide, cilostazol, clopidogrel, dipyridamole, eptifibatide, ticlopidine, tirofiban): May enhance the anticoagulant effect of fondaparinux.
  Drotrecogin alfa: May enhance the bleeding potential with drotrecogin alfa.
  NSAIDs: May enhance the anticoagulant effect of fondaparinux.
  Salicylates: May enhance the anticoagulant effect of fondaparinux.
  Thrombolytic agents: Increase the risk of hemorrhage.

Ethanol/Nutrition/Herb Interactions Herb/Nutraceutical: Avoid alfalfa, anise, bilberry, bladderwrack, bromelain, cat's claw, celery, coleus, cordyceps, dong quai, evening primrose oil, fenugreek, feverfew, garlic, ginger, ginkgo biloba, ginseng (American/Panax/Siberian), grapeseed, green tea, guggul, horse chestnut seed, horseradish, licorice, prickly ash, red clover, reishi, sweet clover, turmeric, white willow (all possess anticoagulant or antiplatelet activity and as such, may enhance the anticoagulant effects of fondaparinux).
(Continued)

Fondaparinux *(Continued)*

Stability Store at 15°C to 30°C (59°F to 86°F).

Canadian labeling: For I.V. administration: May mix with 25 mL or 50 mL NS; manufacturer recommends immediate use once diluted in NS, but is stable for up to 24 hours at 15°C to 30°C (59°F to 86°F).

Mechanism of Action Fondaparinux is a synthetic pentasaccharide that causes an antithrombin III-mediated selective inhibition of factor Xa. Neutralization of factor Xa interrupts the blood coagulation cascade and inhibits thrombin formation and thrombus development.

Pharmacokinetics

Absorption: SubQ: Rapid and complete

Distribution: V_d: 7-11 L; mainly in blood

Protein binding: ≥94% (to antithrombin III)

Bioavailability: SubQ: 100%

Half-life: 17-21 hours; increases with decreasing renal function

Time to peak: SubQ: 2-3 hours

Excretion: Urine (as unchanged drug); decreased clearance in patients <50 kg

Dosage

Geriatrics & Adults:

DVT prophylaxis: SubQ: Adults ≥50 kg: 2.5 mg once daily.

DVT prophylaxis with history of HIT (unlabeled use): 2.5 mg once daily.

Note: Initiate dose after hemostasis has been established, 6-8 hours postoperatively.

Usual duration: 5-9 days (up to 10 days following abdominal surgery or up to 11 days following hip replacement or knee replacement).

Extended prophylaxis is recommended following hip fracture surgery (has been tolerated for up to 32 days).

Acute DVT/PE treatment: SubQ: **Note:** Concomitant treatment with warfarin sodium should be initiated as soon as possible, usually within 72 hours:

<50 kg: 5 mg once daily

50-100 kg: 7.5 mg once daily

>100 kg: 10 mg once daily

Usual duration: 5-9 days (has been administered up to 26 days)

Canadian labeling only: Adults:

UA/NSTEMI: SubQ: 2.5 mg once daily; initiate as soon as possible after diagnosis; treat for up to 8 days or until hospital discharge.

STEMI: I.V.: 2.5 mg once; subsequent doses SubQ: 2.5 mg once daily; treat for up to 8 days or until hospital discharge

Renal Impairment:

Cl_{cr} 30-50 mL/minute: Use caution

Cl_{cr} <30 mL/minute: Contraindicated

Administration Do not administer I.M.; for SubQ administration only. Do not mix with other injections or infusions. Do not expel air bubble from syringe before injection. Administer according to recommended regimen; early initiation (before 6 hours after surgery) has been associated with increased bleeding.

Canadian labeling only: STEMI patients: I.V. push or mixed in 25-50 mL of NS and infused over 1-2 minutes. Flush tubing with NS after infusion to ensure complete administration of fondaparinux. Infusion bag should not be mixed with other agents.

Monitoring Parameters Periodic monitoring of CBC, serum creatinine, occult blood testing of stools is recommended. Antifactor Xa activity of fondaparinux can be measured by the assay if fondaparinux is used as the calibrator. PT and aPTT are insensitive measures of fondaparinux activity.

Test Interactions International standards of heparin or LMWH are not the appropriate calibrators for antifactor Xa activity of fondaparinux.

Patient Information This drug can only be administered by injection. You may have a tendency to bleed easily while taking this drug; brush your teeth with a soft brush, floss with waxed floss, use an electric razor, and avoid scissors or sharp knives and potentially harmful activities. Report unusual bleeding or bruising (bleeding gums, nosebleed, blood in urine, dark stool), any falls or accidents, new joint pain or swelling, dizziness, severe headache, shortness of breath, weakness, and fainting or passing out.

Special Geriatric Considerations Patients studied for DVT prophylaxis following elective knee or hip fracture surgery averaged 67.5 and 77 years of age, respectively. Use with caution in patients with estimated or actual creatinine clearance between 30-50 mL/minute. Contraindicated in patients with Cl_{cr} <30 mL/minute.

Dosage Forms Excipient information presented when available (limited, particularly for generics); consult specific product labeling.

Injection, solution, as sodium [preservative free]: 2.5 mg/0.5 mL (0.5 mL); 5 mg/0.4 mL (0.4 mL); 7.5 mg/0.6 mL (0.6 mL); 10 mg/0.8 mL (0.8 mL) [prefilled syringe]

Selected References

Bauer KA, Eriksson BI, Lassen MR, et al, "Fondaparinux Compared With Enoxaparin for the Prevention of Venous Thromboembolism After Elective Major Knee Surgery," *N Engl J Med*, 2001, 345(18):1305-10.

Bauer KA, "Fondaparinux Sodium: A Selective Inhibitor of Factor Xa," *Am J Health Syst Pharm*, 2001, 58(Suppl 2): S14-S17.

Eriksson BI, Bauer KA, Lassen MR, et al, "Fondaparinux Compared With Enoxaparin for the Prevention of Venous Thromboembolism After Hip-Fracture Surgery," *N Engl J Med*, 2001, 345(18):1298-1304.

♦ **Fondaparinux Sodium** *see* Fondaparinux *on page 674*

♦ **Foradil® Aerolizer™** *see* Formoterol *on page 677*

Formoterol (for MOH te rol)

Related Information
Inhalant Agents *on page 1760*

Medication Safety Issues
Sound-alike/look-alike issues:
Foradil® may be confused with Toradol®
Foradil® capsules for inhalation are for administration via Aerolizer™ inhaler and are not for oral use.

International issues:
Foradil® may be confused with Theradol® which is a brand name for tramadol in the Netherlands.

U.S. Brand Names Foradil® Aerolizer™

Canadian Brand Names Foradil®; Oxeze® Turbuhaler®

Index Terms Formoterol Fumarate

Generic Available No

Pharmacologic Category Beta$_2$-Adrenergic Agonist

Use Maintenance treatment of asthma and prevention of bronchospasm in patients with reversible obstructive airway disease, including patients with symptoms of nocturnal asthma, who require regular treatment with inhaled, short-acting beta$_2$ agonists; maintenance treatment of bronchoconstriction in patients with chronic obstructive pulmonary disease (COPD); prevention of exercise-induced bronchospasm

Restrictions An FDA-approved medication guide must be distributed when dispensing an outpatient prescription (new or refill) where this medication is to be used without direct supervision of a healthcare provider. Medication guides are available at http://www.fda.gov/cder/Offices/ODS/medication_guides.htm.

Contraindications Hypersensitivity to adrenergic amines, formoterol, or any component of the formulation; need for acute bronchodilation

Warnings/Precautions [U.S. Boxed Warning]: Long-acting beta$_2$-agonists may increase the risk of asthma-related deaths. Formoterol should only be used as adjuvant therapy in patients not adequately controlled on other asthma medications (eg, low-to-medium dose inhaled corticosteroids) or whose disease warrants initiation of two maintenance therapies. Optimize anti-inflammatory treatment before initiating maintenance treatment with formoterol. Do not use as a component of chronic therapy without an anti-inflammatory agent. Corticosteroids should not be stopped or reduced at formoterol initiation. Patients using inhaled, short-acting beta$_2$-agonists should be instructed to discontinue routine use of these medications prior to beginning treatment; short-acting agents should be reserved for symptomatic relief of acute symptoms. Patient must be instructed to seek medical attention in cases where acute symptoms are not relieved by a rapid-onset beta-agonist or when a previous level of response is diminished. Treatment must not be delayed. Rarely, paradoxical bronchospasm may occur with use of inhaled bronchodilating agents; this should be distinguished from inadequate response.

Acute episodes should be treated with a rapid-onset beta$_2$-agonist. The approved U.S. labeling states that formoterol is not meant to relieve acute asthmatic symptoms; although, a formulation of formoterol (Oxeze®) is approved for acute treatment outside the U.S. (eg, Canada).

Immediate hypersensitivity reactions (urticaria, angioedema, rash, bronchospasm) have been reported. Do not exceed recommended dose; serious adverse events (including serious asthma exacerbations and fatalities) have been associated with excessive use of inhaled sympathomimetics. Beta$_2$-agonists may increase risk of arrhythmias, decrease serum potassium, prolong QT$_c$ interval, or increase serum glucose. These effects may be exacerbated in hypoxemia. Use caution in patients with cardiovascular disease (arrhythmia or hypertension or CHF), seizures, diabetes, glaucoma, hyperthyroidism, or hypokalemia. Beta-agonists may cause elevation in blood pressure and heart rate, and result in CNS stimulation/excitation. Powder for oral inhalation contains lactose; very rare anaphylactic reactions have been reported in patients with severe milk protein allergy.

Adverse Reactions (Reflective of adult population; not specific for elderly)
>10%: Miscellaneous: Viral infection (17%)
(Continued)

Formoterol *(Continued)*

1% to 10%:
Cardiovascular: Chest pain (2%)
Central nervous system: Anxiety (2%), dizziness (2%), fever (2%), insomnia (2%), dysphonia (1%)
Dermatologic: Rash (1%)
Gastrointestinal: Abdominal pain, dyspepsia, gastroenteritis, nausea, xerostomia (1%)
Respiratory: Asthma exacerbation (age 5-12 years: 5% to 6%; age >12 years: <4%), bronchitis (5%), infection (3% to 7%), pharyngitis (4%), sinusitis (3%), dyspnea (2%), tonsillitis (1%)

Overdosage/Toxicology Symptoms of overdose include tachycardia, tremor, hypertension, angina, and seizures. Hypokalemia also may occur. Cardiac arrest and death may be associated with abuse of beta-agonist bronchodilators. Treatment includes immediate discontinuation and symptomatic and supportive therapies. Cautious use of beta-adrenergic blocking agents may be considered in severe cases.

Drug Interactions Substrate (minor) of CYP2A6, 2C9, 2C19, 2D6
Atomoxetine: May enhance the tachycardic effect of beta$_2$-agonists.
Beta$_2$-agonists: May diminish the bradycardic effect of beta-blockers (beta$_1$ selective).
Beta-blockers (nonselective): May diminish the bronchodilatory effect of beta$_2$-agonists.
Sympathomimetics: May enhance the adverse/toxic effect of formoterol.

Stability Prior to dispensing, store in refrigerator at 2°C to 8°C (36°F to 46°F). After dispensing, store at room temperature at 20°C to 25°C (68°F to 77°F). Protect from heat and moisture. Capsules should always be stored in the blister and only removed immediately before use. Always check expiration date. Use within 4 months of purchase date or product expiration date, whichever comes first.

Mechanism of Action Relaxes bronchial smooth muscle by selective action on beta$_2$ receptors with little effect on heart rate. Formoterol has a long-acting effect.

Pharmacodynamics
Onset: Within 3 minutes
Peak effect: 80% of peak effect within 15 minutes
Duration: Improvement in FEV$_1$ observed for 12 hours in most patients

Pharmacokinetics
Absorption: Rapidly absorbed into plasma following oral inhalation
Protein binding: 61% to 64% *in vitro* at higher concentrations than achieved with usual dosing
Metabolism: Hepatic via direct glucuronidation and O-demethylation
Half-life: ~10-14 hours
Time to peak: Maximum improvement in FEV$_1$ in 1-3 hours
Elimination: 10% excreted in the urine as unchanged drug; 15% to 18% excreted as direct glucuronide metabolites

Dosage
Geriatrics & Adults:
Asthma (maintenance): Inhalation: 12 mcg capsule every 12 hours
Oxeze® (CAN): **Note:** Not labeled for use in the U.S.: Inhalation: 6 mcg or 12 mcg every 12 hours. Maximum dose: Adults: 48 mcg/day
Exercise-induced bronchospasm: Inhalation: 12 mcg capsule at least 15 minutes before exercise on an "as needed" basis; additional doses should not be used for another 12 hours. **Note:** If already using for asthma maintenance then should not use additional doses for exercise-induced bronchospasm.
Oxeze® (CAN): **Note:** Not labeled for use in the U.S.: Adults: Inhalation: 6 mcg or 12 mcg at least 15 minutes before exercise.
COPD (maintenance): Inhalation: 12 mcg capsule every 12 hours
Acute ("on demand") relief of bronchoconstriction: *Indication for Oxeze® approved in Canada:* 6 mcg or 12 mcg as a single dose (maximum dose: 72 mcg in any 24-hour period). The prolonged use of high dosages (48 mcg/day for ≥3 consecutive days) may be a sign of suboptimal control, and should prompt the re-evaluation of therapy.
Renal Impairment: Not studied

Administration Remove capsule from foil blister **immediately** before use. Place capsule in the capsule-chamber in the base of the Aerolizer™ Inhaler. Must only use the Aerolizer™ Inhaler. Press both buttons **once only** and then release. Keep inhaler in a level, horizontal position. Exhale fully. Do not exhale into inhaler. Tilt head slightly back and inhale (rapidly, steadily, and deeply). Hold breath as long as possible. If any powder remains in capsule, exhale and inhale again. Repeat until capsule is empty. Throw away empty capsule; do not leave in inhaler. Do not use a spacer with the Aerolizer™ Inhaler. Always keep capsules and inhaler dry.

Monitoring Parameters Peak flow meter

Patient Information Do not swallow capsules; this medication can only be used in the Aerolizer™ Inhaler. Use exactly as directed and do not use more often than recommended. Store capsules in blister and do not remove from blister until ready for treatment. Maintain adequate hydration (2-3 L/day) unless instructed to restrict fluids. It is recommended that you wear identification (Med-Alert bracelet) if you have an asthmatic condition. You may experience nervousness, dizziness, or insomnia (use caution when driving or engaging in hazardous activities until response to medication is known); dry mouth, nausea, or GI discomfort (small frequent meals, good mouth care, sucking lozenges, or chewing gum may help); difficulty voiding (always void before treatment). Report any unresolved GI upset, nervousness or dizziness, muscle cramping, chest pain or palpitations, skin rash, signs of infection, unusual cough, or worsening of condition.

Special Geriatric Considerations Elderly patients should be specifically counseled about the proper use of this inhaler and spacing of doses.

Dosage Forms Excipient information presented when available (limited, particularly for generics); consult specific product labeling. [CAN] = Canadian brand name
  Powder for oral inhalation, as fumarate:
    Foradil® Aerolizer™ [capsule]: 12 mcg (12s, 60s) [contains lactose 25 mg]
    Oxeze® Turbuhaler® [CAN]: 6 mcg/inhalation [delivers 60 metered doses; contains lactose 600 mcg/dose]; 12 mcg/inhalation [delivers 60 metered doses; contains lactose 600 mcg/dose] [not available in the U.S.]

Selected References
Cazzola M, Centanni S, Regorda C, et al, "Onset of Action of Single Doses of Formoterol Administered Via Turbuhaler in Patients With Stable COPD," *Pulm Pharmacol Ther*, 2001, 14(1):41-5.
Cazzola M and Donner CF, "Long-acting Beta2 Agonists in the Management of Stable Chronic Obstructive Pulmonary Disease," *Drugs*, 2000, 60:307-20.

♦ **Formoterol Fumarate** *see* Formoterol *on page 677*
♦ **Formulation R™ [OTC]** *see* Phenylephrine *on page 1247*
♦ **Fortamet®** *see* Metformin *on page 993*
♦ **Fortaz®** *see* Ceftazidime *on page 268*
♦ **Forteo™** *see* Teriparatide *on page 1535*
♦ **Fortical®** *see* Calcitonin *on page 209*
♦ **Fosamax®** *see* Alendronate *on page 44*

Fosinopril (foe SIN oh pril)

Related Information
Angiotensin Agents *on page 1737*
Medication Safety Issues
  Sound-alike/look-alike issues:
    Fosinopril may be confused with lisinopril
    Monopril® may be confused with Accupril®, minoxidil, moexipril, Monoket®, Monurol™, ramipril
U.S. Brand Names Monopril®
Canadian Brand Names Apo-Fosinopril®; Monopril®; Novo-Fosinopril; ratio-Fosinopril; Riva-Fosinopril
Index Terms Fosinopril Sodium
Generic Available Yes
Pharmacologic Category Angiotensin-Converting Enzyme (ACE) Inhibitor
Use Treatment of hypertension, either alone or in combination with other antihypertensive agents; management of systolic congestive heart failure
Contraindications Hypersensitivity to fosinopril or any component of the formulation; angioedema related to previous treatment with an ACE inhibitor; idiopathic or hereditary angioedema; bilateral renal artery stenosis; primary hyperaldosteronism
Warnings/Precautions Anaphylactic reactions can occur. Angioedema can occur at any time during treatment (especially following first dose). It may involve head and neck (potentially affecting the airway) or the intestine (presenting with abdominal pain). Prolonged monitoring may be required, especially if tongue, glottis, or larynx are involved as they are associated with airway obstruction. Those with a history of airway surgery in this situation have a higher risk. Careful blood pressure monitoring (hypotension can occur especially in volume-depleted patients). Dosage adjustment needed in severe renal impairment (Cl_{cr} <10 mL/minute). Use with caution in hypovolemia; collagen vascular diseases; valvular stenosis (particularly aortic stenosis); hyperkalemia; or before, during, or immediately after anesthesia. Avoid rapid dosage escalation which may lead to renal insufficiency. Rare toxicities associated with ACE inhibitors include cholestatic jaundice (which may progress to hepatic necrosis) and neutropenia/agranulocytosis with myeloid hyperplasia. Hyperkalemia may rarely occur. May be associated with deterioration of renal function and/or increases in serum creatinine, particularly in patients dependent on renin-angiotensin-aldosterone system. Use with caution in unilateral renal artery stenosis and pre-existing renal insufficiency; (Continued)

Fosinopril *(Continued)*

if patient has renal impairment, then a baseline WBC with differential and serum creatinine should be evaluated and monitored closely during the first 3 months of therapy. Hypersensitivity reactions may be seen during hemodialysis with high-flux dialysis membranes (eg, AN69).

Adverse Reactions (Reflective of adult population; not specific for elderly)
Note: Frequency ranges include data from hypertension and heart failure trials. Higher rates of adverse reactions have generally been noted in patients with CHF. However, the frequency of adverse effects associated with placebo is also increased in this population.

>10%: Central nervous system: Dizziness (2% to 12%)
1% to 10%:
  Cardiovascular: Orthostatic hypotension (1% to 2%), palpitation (1%)
  Central nervous system: Dizziness (1% to 2%; up to 12% in CHF patients), headache (3%), fatigue (1% to 2%)
  Endocrine & metabolic: Hyperkalemia (2.6%)
  Gastrointestinal: Diarrhea (2%), nausea/vomiting (1.2% to 2.2%)
  Hepatic: Transaminases increased
  Neuromuscular & skeletal: Musculoskeletal pain (<1% to 3%), noncardiac chest pain (<1% to 2%), weakness (<1% to 2%)
  Renal: Serum creatinine increased, renal function worsening (in patients with bilateral renal artery stenosis or hypovolemia)
  Respiratory: Cough (2% to 10%)
  Miscellaneous: Upper respiratory infection (2%)
>1% but ≤ frequency in patients receiving placebo: Sexual dysfunction, fever, flu-like syndrome, dyspnea, rash, headache, insomnia
Other events reported with ACE inhibitors: Neutropenia, agranulocytosis, eosinophilic pneumonitis, cardiac arrest, pancytopenia, hemolytic anemia, anemia, aplastic anemia, thrombocytopenia, acute renal failure, hepatic failure, jaundice, symptomatic hyponatremia, bullous pemphigus, exfoliative dermatitis, Stevens-Johnson syndrome. In addition, a syndrome which may include fever, myalgia, arthralgia, interstitial nephritis, vasculitis, rash, eosinophilia and positive ANA, and elevated ESR has been reported for other ACE inhibitors.

Overdosage/Toxicology Mild hypotension has been the only toxic effect seen with acute overdose. Bradycardia may also occur; hyperkalemia occurs even with therapeutic doses, especially in patients with renal insufficiency and those taking NSAIDs. Following initiation of essential overdose management, toxic symptom and supportive treatment should be initiated. Hypotension usually responds to I.V. fluids or Trendelenburg positioning.

Drug Interactions
Alpha₁-blockers: Hypotensive effect increased.
Antacids (aluminum hydroxide, magnesium hydroxide and simethicone): Absorption of fosinopril impaired; separate dose by 2 hours.
Aspirin: The effects of ACE inhibitors may be blunted by aspirin administration, particularly at higher dosages and/or increase adverse renal effects.
Diuretics: Hypovolemia due to diuretics may precipitate acute hypotensive events or acute renal failure.
Gold sodium thiomalate: ACE inhibitors may enhance the adverse/toxic effects (nitritoid reaction) of gold sodium thiomalate. The reaction may include facial flushing, nausea, vomiting, hypotension, and syncope. If it is to occur, would be expected shortly after administration of gold compound in patients maintained on an ACEI.
Insulin: Risk of hypoglycemia may be increased.
Lithium: Risk of lithium toxicity may be increased; monitor lithium levels, especially the first 4 weeks of therapy.
Mercaptopurine: Risk of neutropenia may be increased.
NSAIDs: May attenuate hypertensive efficacy; effect has been seen with captopril and may occur with other ACE inhibitors; monitor blood pressure. May increase risk of adverse renal effects.
Potassium-sparing diuretics (amiloride, spironolactone, triamterene): Increased risk of hyperkalemia.
Potassium supplements: May increase the risk of hyperkalemia.
Trimethoprim (high dose): May increase the risk of hyperkalemia.

Ethanol/Nutrition/Herb Interactions Herb/Nutraceutical: Avoid dong quai if using for hypertension (has estrogenic activity). Avoid ephedra, garlic, yohimbe, ginseng (may worsen hypertension).

Stability Store at 25°C (77°F); excursions permitted to 15°C to 30°C (59°F to 86°F). Protect from moisture by keeping bottle tightly closed.

Mechanism of Action Competitive inhibitor of angiotensin-converting enzyme (ACE); prevents conversion of angiotensin I to angiotensin II, a potent vasoconstrictor; results in lower levels of angiotensin II which causes an increase in plasma renin activity and a reduction in aldosterone secretion; a CNS mechanism may also be involved in hypotensive effect as angiotensin II increases adrenergic outflow from CNS; vasoactive kallikreins may be decreased in conversion to active hormones by ACE inhibitors, thus reducing blood pressure

Pharmacodynamics Duration of effect: ~12-24 hours

Pharmacokinetics
Absorbed: 36%
Metabolism: Fosinopril is a prodrug and is hydrolyzed to its active metabolite fosinoprilat by intestinal wall and hepatic esterases
Half-life, serum (fosinoprilat): Effective: 12 hours
Time to peak serum concentration: ~3 hours
Elimination: In the urine and bile as fosinoprilat and it conjugates in roughly equal proportions (45% to 50%)

Dosage
Geriatrics & Adults:
Hypertension: Oral: Initial: 10 mg/day; increase to a maximum dose of 80 mg/day. Most patients are maintained on 20-40 mg/day. May need to divide the dose into two if trough effect is inadequate. Discontinue the diuretic, if possible 2-3 days before initiation of therapy. Resume diuretic therapy carefully, if needed.
Heart failure: Oral: Initial: 10 mg/day (5 mg if renal dysfunction present) and increase, as needed, to a maximum of 40 mg once daily over several weeks. Usual dose: 20-40 mg/day. If hypotension, orthostasis, or azotemia occurs during titration, consider decreasing concomitant diuretic dose, if any.
Renal Impairment: None needed since hepatobiliary elimination compensates adequately diminished renal elimination.
Hemodialysis: Moderately dialyzable (20% to 50%)
Hepatic Impairment: Decrease dose and monitor effects

Monitoring Parameters Serum potassium concentration, BUN, serum creatinine, renal function, WBC

Test Interactions Positive Coombs' [direct]; may cause false-positive results in urine acetone determinations using sodium nitroprusside reagent

Patient Information Notify physician if vomiting, diarrhea, excessive perspiration, or dehydration should occur; also if swelling of face, lips, tongue, or difficulty in breathing occurs or if persistent cough develops; may be taken with meals; do not stop therapy or add a potassium salt replacement without physician's advice

Additional Information Watch for hypotensive effect within 1-3 hours of first dose or new higher dose. Some patients may have a decreased hypotensive effect between 12-16 hours; consider dividing total daily dose into 2 doses 12 hours apart; if patient is receiving a diuretic, a potential for first-dose hypotension is increased; to decrease this potential, stop diuretic for 2-3 days prior to initiating fosinopril if possible; continue diuretic if needed to control blood pressure

Special Geriatric Considerations Due to frequent decreases in glomerular filtration (also creatinine clearance) with aging, elderly patients may have exaggerated responses to ACE inhibitors. Differences in clinical response due to hepatic changes are not observed. ACE inhibitors may be preferred agents in elderly patients with congestive heart failure and diabetes mellitus. Diabetic proteinuria is reduced and insulin sensitivity is enhanced. In general, the side effect profile is favorable in the elderly and causes little or no CNS confusion; use lowest dose recommendations initially. Many elderly may be volume depleted due to diuretic use and/or blunted thirst reflex resulting in inadequate fluid intake.

Dosage Forms Excipient information presented when available (limited, particularly for generics); consult specific product labeling.
Tablet, as sodium: 10 mg, 20 mg, 40 mg
Monopril®: 10 mg, 20 mg, 40 mg

Selected References
Konstam MA, Drakup K, Baker DW, et al, "Heart Failure: Evaluation and Care of Patients With Left Ventricular Systolic Dysfunction," *Clinical Practice Guideline No 11*, Rockville, MD: Agency for Health Care Policy and Research, Public Health Service, U.S. Department of Health and Human Services, 1994.
McAreavey D and Robertson JI, "Angiotensin Converting Enzyme Inhibitors and Moderate Hypertension," *Drugs*, 1990, 40(3):326-45.
Williams JF, Bristow MR, Fowler MB, et al, "Guidelines for the Evaluation and Management of Heart Failure: Report of the American College of Cardiology/American Heart Association Task Force on Practice Guidelines (Committee on Evaluation and Management of Heart Failure)," *J Am Coll Cardiol*, 1995, 26:1376-8.

♦ **Fosinopril Sodium** see Fosinopril on page 679

Fosphenytoin (FOS fen i toyn)

Medication Safety Issues
Sound-alike/look-alike issues:
Cerebyx® may be confused with Celebrex®, Celexa™, Cerezyme®
(Continued)

Fosphenytoin *(Continued)*

U.S. Brand Names Cerebyx®
Canadian Brand Names Cerebyx®
Index Terms Fosphenytoin Sodium
Generic Available No
Pharmacologic Category Anticonvulsant, Hydantoin

Use Short-term parenteral administration when other means of phenytoin administration are unavailable, inappropriate or deemed less advantageous; the safety and effectiveness of fosphenytoin in this use has not been systematically evaluated for more than 5 days; may be used for the control of generalized convulsive status epilepticus and prevention and treatment of seizures occurring during neurosurgery

Contraindications Hypersensitivity to phenytoin, other hydantoins, or any component of the formulation; patients with sinus bradycardia, sinoatrial block, second- and third-degree AV block, or Adams-Stokes syndrome; occurrence of rash during treatment (should not be resumed if rash is exfoliative, purpuric, or bullous)

Warnings/Precautions Doses of fosphenytoin are expressed as their phenytoin sodium equivalent (PE). Antiepileptic drugs should not be abruptly discontinued. Hypotension may occur, especially after I.V. administration at high doses and high rates of administration. Administration of phenytoin has been associated with atrial and ventricular conduction depression and ventricular fibrillation. Careful cardiac monitoring is needed when administering I.V. loading doses of fosphenytoin. Acute hepatotoxicity associated with a hypersensitivity syndrome characterized by fever, skin eruptions, and lymphadenopathy has been reported to occur within the first 2 months of treatment. Discontinue if skin rash or lymphadenopathy occurs. A spectrum of hematologic effects have been reported with use (eg, neutropenia, leukopenia, thrombocytopenia, pancytopenia, and anemias). Use with caution in patients with hypotension, severe myocardial insufficiency, diabetes mellitus, porphyria, hypoalbuminemia, hypothyroidism, fever, or hepatic or renal dysfunction. Effects with other sedative drugs or ethanol may be potentiated.

Adverse Reactions (Reflective of adult population; not specific for elderly)
The more important adverse clinical events caused by the I.V. use of fosphenytoin or phenytoin are cardiovascular collapse and/or central nervous system depression. Hypotension can occur when either drug is administered rapidly by the I.V. route. Do not exceed a rate of 150 mg phenytoin equivalent/minute when administering fosphenytoin.

The adverse clinical events most commonly observed with the use of fosphenytoin in clinical trials were nystagmus, dizziness, pruritus, paresthesia, headache, somnolence, and ataxia. Paresthesia and pruritus were seen more often following fosphenytoin (versus phenytoin) administration and occurred more often with I.V. fosphenytoin than with I.M. administration. These events were dose and rate related (doses ≥15 mg/kg at a rate of 150 mg/minute). These sensations, generally described as itching, burning, or tingling are usually not at the infusion site. The location of the discomfort varied with the groin mentioned most frequently. The paresthesia and pruritus were transient events that occurred within several minutes of the start of infusion and generally resolved within 10 minutes after completion of infusion.

Transient pruritus, tinnitus, nystagmus, somnolence, and ataxia occurred 2-3 times more often at doses ≥15 mg/kg and rates ≥150 mg/minute.

I.V. administration (maximum dose/rate):
>10%:
  Central nervous system: Nystagmus, dizziness, somnolence, ataxia
  Dermatologic: Pruritus
1% to 10%:
  Cardiovascular: Hypotension, vasodilation, tachycardia
  Central nervous system: Stupor, incoordination, paresthesia, extrapyramidal syndrome, tremor, agitation, hypoesthesia, dysarthria, vertigo, brain edema, headache
  Gastrointestinal: Nausea, tongue disorder, dry mouth, vomiting
  Neuromuscular & skeletal: Pelvic pain, muscle weakness, back pain
  Ocular: Diplopia, amblyopia
  Otic: Tinnitus, deafness
  Miscellaneous: Taste perversion
I.M. administration (substitute for oral phenytoin):
1% to 10%:
  Central nervous system: Nystagmus, tremor, ataxia, headache, incoordination, somnolence, dizziness, paresthesia, reflexes decreased
  Dermatologic: Pruritus
  Gastrointestinal: Nausea, vomiting
  Hematologic/lymphatic: Ecchymosis
  Neuromuscular & skeletal: Muscle weakness

Overdosage/Toxicology Signs and symptoms include unsteady gait, tremors, hyperglycemia, chorea (extrapyramidal), gingival hyperplasia, gynecomastia, myoglobinuria, nephrotic syndrome, slurred speech, mydriasis, myoclonus, confusion, encephalopathy, hyperthermia, drowsiness, nausea, hypothermia, fever, hypotension, respiratory depression, hyper-reflexia, coma, systemic lupus erythematosus (SLE), ophthalmoplegia; as well as, leukopenia, neutropenia, agranulocytosis, and granulocytopenia. Treatment for hypotension is supportive. Treat with I.V. fluids and Trendelenburg positioning. Seizures may be controlled with lorazepam or diazepam 5-10 mg; intravenous albumin (25 g every 6 hours) has been used to increase the bound fraction of drug. Multiple dosing of activated charcoal may be effective. Peritoneal dialysis, diuresis, hemodialysis, hemoperfusion, and plasmapheresis are of little value.

Drug Interactions As phenytoin: **Substrate** of CYP2C9 (major), 2C19 (major), 3A4 (minor); **Induces** CYP2B6 (strong), 2C8 (strong), 2C9 (strong), 2C19 (strong), 3A4 (strong)

Acetaminophen: Phenytoin may enhance the hepatotoxic potential of acetaminophen overdoses.

Acetazolamide: Concurrent use with phenytoin may result in an increased risk of osteomalacia.

Acyclovir: May decrease phenytoin serum levels; limited documentation; monitor.

Allopurinol: May increase phenytoin serum concentrations; monitor.

Antiarrhythmics: Phenytoin may increase the metabolism of antiarrhythmics, decreasing their clinical effect; includes disopyramide, propafenone, and quinidine. Amiodarone also may increase phenytoin concentrations (see CYP inhibitors).

Anticonvulsants: Phenytoin may increase the metabolism of anticonvulsants; includes barbiturates, carbamazepine, ethosuximide, felbamate, lamotrigine, tiagabine, topiramate, and zonisamide; does not appear to affect gabapentin or levetiracetam. Felbamate and gabapentin may increase phenytoin levels; monitor

Antineoplastics: Several chemotherapeutic agents have been associated with a decrease in serum phenytoin levels; includes cisplatin, bleomycin, carmustine, methotrexate, and vinblastine; monitor phenytoin serum levels. Limited evidence also suggest that enzyme-inducing anticonvulsant therapy may reduce the effectiveness of some chemotherapy regimens (specifically in ALL). Teniposide and methotrexate may be cleared more rapidly in these patients.

Antipsychotics: Phenytoin may enhance the metabolism (decrease the efficacy) of antipsychotics; monitor for altered response. Dose adjustment may be needed. Also see note on clozapine.

Benzodiazepines: Phenytoin may decrease the serum concentrations of some benzodiazepines; monitor for decreased benzodiazepine effect.

Beta-blockers: Metabolism of beta-blockers may be increased and clinical effect decreased; atenolol and nadolol are unlikely to interact given their renal elimination.

Calcium channel blockers: Phenytoin may enhance the metabolism of calcium channel blockers, decreasing their clinical effect. Calcium channel blockers (diltiazem, nifedipine) have been reported to increase phenytoin levels (case report); monitor.

Capecitabine: May increase the serum concentrations of phenytoin; monitor.

Chloramphenicol: Phenytoin may increase the metabolism of chloramphenicol and chloramphenicol may inhibit phenytoin metabolism; monitor for altered response.

Cimetidine: May increase the serum concentrations of phenytoin; monitor.

Ciprofloxacin: Case reports indicate ciprofloxacin may increase or decrease serum phenytoin concentrations; monitor.

Clozapine: May decrease phenytoin serum concentrations; monitor.

CNS depressants: Sedative effects may be additive with other CNS depressants; monitor for increased effect; includes ethanol, barbiturates, sedatives, antidepressants, opioid analgesics, and benzodiazepines.

Corticosteroids: Phenytoin may increase the metabolism of corticosteroids, decreasing their clinical effect. Also see dexamethasone.

Cyclosporine and tacrolimus: Levels may be decreased by phenytoin; monitor.

CYP2B6 substrates: Phenytoin may decrease the levels/effects of CYP2B6 substrates. Example substrates include bupropion, efavirenz, promethazine, selegiline, and sertraline.

CYP2C9 inducers: May decrease the levels/effects of phenytoin. Example inducers include carbamazepine, phenobarbital, rifampin, rifapentine, and secobarbital.

CYP2C9 inhibitors: May increase the levels/effects of phenytoin. Example inhibitors include delavirdine, fluconazole, gemfibrozil, ketoconazole, nicardipine, NSAIDs, sulfonamides, and tolbutamide.

CYP2C8 substrates: Phenytoin may decrease the levels/effects of CYP2C8 substrates. Example substrates include amiodarone, paclitaxel, pioglitazone, repaglinide, and rosiglitazone.

CYP2C9 substrates: Phenytoin may decrease the levels/effects of CYP2C9 substrates. Example substrates include bosentan, celecoxib, dapsone, fluoxetine, glimepiride, glipizide, losartan, montelukast, nateglinide, paclitaxel, sulfonamides, trimethoprim, warfarin, and zafirlukast.

(Continued)

Fosphenytoin (Continued)

CYP2C19 inducers: May decrease the levels/effects of phenytoin. Example inducers include aminoglutethimide, carbamazepine, phenytoin, and rifampin.

CYP2C19 inhibitors: May increase the levels/effects of phenytoin. Example inhibitors include delavirdine, fluconazole, fluvoxamine, gemfibrozil, isoniazid, omeprazole, and ticlopidine.

CYP2C19 substrates: Phenytoin may decrease the levels/effects of CYP2C19 substrates. Example substrates include citalopram, diazepam, methsuximide, phenytoin, propranolol, proton pump inhibitors, sertraline, and voriconazole.

CYP3A4 substrates: Phenytoin may decrease the levels/effects of CYP3A4 substrates. Example substrates include benzodiazepines, calcium channel blockers, clarithromycin, cyclosporine, erythromycin, estrogens, mirtazapine, nateglinide, nefazodone, nevirapine, protease inhibitors, tacrolimus, and venlafaxine.

Dexamethasone: May decrease serum phenytoin due to increased metabolism; monitor.

Digoxin: Effects and/or levels of digitalis glycosides may be decreased by phenytoin.

Disulfiram: May increase serum phenytoin concentrations; monitor.

Dopamine: Phenytoin (I.V.) may increase the effect of dopamine (enhanced hypotension).

Doxycycline: Phenytoin may enhance the metabolism of doxycycline, decreasing its clinical effect; higher dosages may be required.

Estrogens: Phenytoin may increase the metabolism of estrogens, decreasing their clinical effect; monitor.

Folic acid: Replacement of folic acid has been reported to increase the metabolism of phenytoin, decreasing its serum concentrations and/or increasing seizures.

HMG-CoA reductase inhibitors: Phenytoin may increase the metabolism of these agents, reducing their clinical effect; monitor.

Itraconazole: Phenytoin may decrease the effect of itraconazole.

Levodopa: Phenytoin may inhibit the anti-Parkinson effect of levodopa.

Lithium: Concurrent use of phenytoin and lithium has resulted in lithium intoxication.

Methadone: Phenytoin may enhance the metabolism of methadone resulting in methadone withdrawal.

Methylphenidate: May increase serum phenytoin concentrations; monitor.

Metronidazole: May increase the serum concentrations of phenytoin; monitor.

Neuromuscular-blocking agents: Duration of effect may be decreased by phenytoin.

Omeprazole: May increase serum phenytoin concentrations; monitor.

Oral contraceptives: Phenytoin may enhance the metabolism of oral contraceptives, decreasing their clinical effect; an alternative method of contraception should be considered.

Primidone: Phenytoin enhances the conversion of primidone to phenobarbital resulting in elevated phenobarbital serum concentrations.

Quetiapine: Serum concentrations may be substantially reduced by phenytoin, potentially resulting in a loss of efficacy; limited documentation; monitor.

SSRIs: May increase phenytoin serum concentrations; fluoxetine and fluvoxamine are known to inhibit metabolism via CYP enzymes. Sertraline and paroxetine have also been shown to increase concentrations in some patients; monitor.

Theophylline: Phenytoin may increase metabolism of theophylline derivatives and decrease their clinical effect. Theophylline may also increase phenytoin concentrations.

Thyroid hormones (including levothyroxine): Phenytoin may alter the metabolism of thyroid hormones, reducing its effect. There is limited documentation of this interaction, but monitoring should be considered.

Ticlopidine: May increase serum phenytoin concentrations and/or toxicity; monitor.

Tricyclic antidepressants: Phenytoin may increase metabolism of tricyclic antidepressants and decrease their clinical effect; sedative effects may be additive. Tricyclics may also increase phenytoin concentrations.

Topiramate: Phenytoin may decrease serum levels of topiramate; topiramate may increase the effect of phenytoin.

Trazodone: Serum levels of phenytoin may be increased; limited documentation; monitor.

Trimethoprim: May increase serum phenytoin concentrations; monitor.

Valproic acid (and sulfisoxazole): May displace phenytoin from binding sites; valproic acid may increase, decrease, or have no effect on phenytoin serum concentrations.

Vigabatrin: May reduce phenytoin serum concentrations; monitor.

Warfarin: Phenytoin transiently increased the hypothrombinemia response to warfarin initially; this is followed by an inhibition of the hypoprothrombinemic response.

Ethanol/Nutrition/Herb Interactions

Ethanol:
Acute use: Avoid or limit ethanol (inhibits metabolism of phenytoin); watch for sedation.
Chronic use: Avoid or limit ethanol (stimulates metabolism of phenytoin).

Stability Refrigerate at 2°C to 8°C (36°F to 46°F). Do not store at room temperature for more than 48 hours. Do not use vials that develop particulate matter. Must be diluted to concentrations of 1.5-25 mg PE/mL, in normal saline or D_5W, for I.V. infusion.

Mechanism of Action Diphosphate ester salt of phenytoin which acts as a water soluble prodrug of phenytoin; after administration, plasma esterases convert fosphenytoin to phosphate, formaldehyde, and phenytoin as the active moiety; phenytoin works by stabilizing neuronal membranes and decreasing seizure activity by increasing efflux or decreasing influx of sodium ions across cell membranes in the motor cortex during generation of nerve impulses

Pharmacokinetics Also refer to Phenytoin monograph for additional information.

Protein binding: Fosphenytoin: 95% to 99% to albumin; can displace phenytoin and increase free fraction (up to 30% unbound) during the period required for conversion of fosphenytoin to phenytoin

Metabolism: Fosphenytoin is rapidly converted via hydrolysis to phenytoin; phenytoin is metabolized in the liver and forms metabolites

Bioavailability: I.M.: Fosphenytoin: 100%

Half-life elimination:

Fosphenytoin: 15 minutes

Phenytoin: Variable (mean: 12-29 hours); kinetics of phenytoin are saturable

Time to peak: Conversion to phenytoin: Following I.V. administration (maximum rate of administration): 15 minutes; following I.M. administration, peak phenytoin levels are reached in 3 hours

Elimination: Phenytoin: Urine (as inactive metabolites)

Dosage

Geriatrics: Phenytoin clearance is decreased in geriatric patients; lower doses may be required. In addition, older adults may have lower serum albumin which may increase the free fraction and, therefore, pharmacologic response. Refer to adult dosing.

Adults:

The dose, concentration in solutions, and infusion rates for fosphenytoin are expressed as phenytoin sodium equivalents (PE); fosphenytoin should always be prescribed and dispensed in phenytoin sodium equivalents (PE)

Status epilepticus: I.V.: Loading dose: 15-20 mg PE/kg I.V. administered at 100-150 mg PE/minute

Nonemergent loading and maintenance dosing: I.V. or I.M.:

Loading dose: 10-20 mg PE/kg I.V. or I.M. (maximum I.V. rate: 150 mg PE/minute)

Initial daily maintenance dose: 4-6 mg PE/kg/day I.V. or I.M.

Substitution for oral phenytoin therapy: I.M. or I.V.: May be substituted for oral phenytoin sodium at the same total daily dose; however, Dilantin® capsules are ~90% bioavailable by the oral route; phenytoin, supplied as fosphenytoin, is 100% bioavailable by both the I.M. and I.V. routes; for this reason, plasma phenytoin concentrations may increase when I.M. or I.V. fosphenytoin is substituted for oral phenytoin sodium therapy; in clinical trials, I.M. fosphenytoin was administered as a single daily dose utilizing either 1 or 2 injection sites; some patients may require more frequent dosing

Renal Impairment: Free phenytoin levels should be monitored closely in patients with renal disease or in those with hypoalbuminemia; furthermore, fosphenytoin clearance to phenytoin may be increased without a similar increase in phenytoin clearance in these patients leading to increase frequency and severity of adverse events.

Hepatic Impairment: Phenytoin clearance may be substantially reduced in cirrhosis and plasma level monitoring with dose adjustment advisable. Free phenytoin levels should be monitored closely in patients with hepatic disease or in those with hypoalbuminemia; furthermore, fosphenytoin clearance to phenytoin may be increased without a similar increase in phenytoin clearance in these patients leading to increased frequency and severity of adverse events.

Administration Since there is no precipitation problem with fosphenytoin, no I.V. filter is required; I.V. administration rate should not exceed 150 mg/minute

Monitoring Parameters Blood pressure, EKG, respiratory rate for 10-20 minutes after completion of administration; plasma concentration monitoring, CBC, liver function tests; monitor gait, CNS effects, speech, free fraction measurements

Reference Range

Therapeutic: 10-20 mcg/mL (SI: 40-79 µmol/L); toxicity is measured clinically, and some patients require serum concentrations outside the suggested therapeutic range

Toxic: 30-50 mcg/mL (SI: 120-200 µmol/L)

Lethal: >100 mcg/mL (SI: >400 µmol/L)

Manifestations of toxicity:

Nystagmus: 20 mcg/mL (SI: 79 µmol/L)

Ataxia: 30 mcg/mL (SI: 118.9 µmol/L)

(Continued)

Fosphenytoin (Continued)

Decreased mental status: 40 mcg/mL (SI: 159 µmol/L)

Coma: 50 mcg/mL (SI: 200 µmol/L)

Peak serum phenytoin concentration after a 375 mg I.M. fosphenytoin dose in healthy males: 5.7 mcg/mL

Peak serum fosphenytoin concentrations and phenytoin concentrations after a 1.2 g infusion (I.V.) in healthy subjects over 30 minutes were 129 mcg/mL and 17.2 mcg/mL respectively

Do not obtain serum for analysis 8-12 hours after administration; spurious elevations will be seen due to slow distribution of phenytoin

Test Interactions Increased glucose, alkaline phosphatase (S); decreased thyroxine (S), calcium (S); serum sodium increased in overdose setting

Additional Information 1.5 mg fosphenytoin is approximately equivalent to 1 mg phenytoin; equimolar fosphenytoin dose is 375 mg (75 mg/mL solution) to phenytoin 250 mg (50 mg/mL); 0.0037 mmol phosphate/mg PE fosphenytoin

Water solubility: 142 mg/mL at pH of 9

Antiarrhythmic effects may be similar to phenytoin; parenteral product contains no propylene sterol; this should allow for rapid intravenous bolus dosing without cardiovascular complications; formaldehyde production is not expected to be clinically consequential (about 200 mg) if used for one week

Special Geriatric Considerations No significant changes in fosphenytoin pharmacokinetics with age have been noted. Phenytoin clearance is decreased in the elderly and lower doses may be needed. Elderly may have reduced hepatic clearance due to age decline in Phase I metabolism. Elderly may have low albumin which will increase free fraction and, therefore, pharmacologic response. Monitor closely in those who are hypoalbuminemic. Free fraction measurements advised, also elderly may display a higher incidence of adverse effects (cardiovascular) when using the I.V. loading regimen; therefore, it is recommended to decrease loading I.V. dose to 25 mg/minute.

Dosage Forms Excipient information presented when available (limited, particularly for generics); consult specific product labeling.

Injection, solution, as sodium: 75 mg/mL [equivalent to phenytoin sodium 50 mg/mL] (2 mL, 10 mL)

Selected References

Bebin M and Bleck TP, "New Anticonvulsant Drugs. Focus on Flunarizine, Fosphenytoin, Midazolam, and Stiripentol," Drugs, 1994, 48(2):153-71.

Jamerson BD, Dukes GE, Brouwer KL, et al, "Venous Irritation Related to Intravenous Administration of Phenytoin Versus Fosphenytoin," Pharmacotherapy, 1994, 14(1):47-52.

Leppik IE, Boucher R, Wilder BJ, et al, "Phenytoin Prodrug: Preclinical and Clinical Studies," Epilepsia, 1989, 30(Suppl 2):S22-6.

♦ **Fosphenytoin Sodium** see Fosphenytoin on page 681

♦ **Fosrenol™** see Lanthanum on page 877

♦ **Fragmin®** see Dalteparin on page 388

♦ **Freezone® [OTC]** see Salicylic Acid on page 1441

♦ **Frova®** see Frovatriptan on page 686

Frovatriptan (froe va TRIP tan)

Medication Safety Issues

International issues:

Allegro® [Germany] may be confused with Allegra® which is a brand name for fexofenadine in the U.S.

Allegro®: Brand name for fluticasone in Israel

U.S. Brand Names Frova®

Index Terms Frovatriptan Succinate

Generic Available No

Pharmacologic Category Antimigraine Agent; Serotonin 5-HT$_{1B, 1D}$ Receptor Agonist

Use Acute treatment of migraine with or without aura in adults

Contraindications Hypersensitivity to frovatriptan or any component of the formulation; patients with ischemic heart disease or signs or symptoms of ischemic heart disease (including Prinzmetal's angina, angina pectoris, myocardial infarction, silent myocardial ischemia); cerebrovascular syndromes (including strokes, transient ischemic attacks); peripheral vascular syndromes (including ischemic bowel disease); uncontrolled hypertension; use within 24 hours of ergotamine derivatives; use within 24 hours of another 5-HT$_1$ agonist; management of hemiplegic or basilar migraine; prophylactic treatment of migraine; severe hepatic impairment

Warnings/Precautions Not intended for migraine prophylaxis, or treatment of cluster headaches, hemiplegic or basilar migraines. Cardiac events (coronary artery vasospasm, transient ischemia, MI, ventricular tachycardia/fibrillation, cardiac arrest, and death), cerebral/subarachnoid hemorrhage, stroke, peripheral vascular ischemia, and colonic ischemia have been reported with 5-HT$_1$ agonist administration. May cause vasospastic reactions resulting in colonic, peripheral, or coronary ischemia. Do not give to patients with risk factors for CAD until a cardiovascular evaluation has been performed; if evaluation is satisfactory, the healthcare provider should administer the first dose and cardiovascular status should be periodically evaluated. Significant elevation in blood pressure, including hypertensive crisis, has also been reported on rare occasions in patients using other 5-HT$_{1D}$ agonists with and without a history of hypertension. Symptoms of agitation, confusion, hallucinations, hyper-reflexia, myoclonus, shivering, and tachycardia (serotonin syndrome) may occur with concomitant proserotonergic drugs (ie, SSRIs/SNRIs or triptans) or agents which reduce frovatriptan's metabolism.

Adverse Reactions (Reflective of adult population; not specific for elderly)
1% to 10%:
Cardiovascular: Chest pain (2%), flushing (4%), palpitation (1%)
Central nervous system: Dizziness (8%), fatigue (5%), headache (4%), hot or cold sensation (3%), anxiety (1%), dysesthesia (1%), hypoesthesia (1%), insomnia (1%), pain (1%)
Gastrointestinal: Hyposalivation (3%), dyspepsia (2%), abdominal pain (1%), diarrhea (1%), vomiting (1%)
Neuromuscular & skeletal: Paresthesia (4%), skeletal pain (3%)
Ocular: Visual abnormalities (1%)
Otic: Tinnitus (1%)
Respiratory: Rhinitis (1%), sinusitis (1%)
Miscellaneous: Diaphoresis (1%)

Overdosage/Toxicology Single oral doses up to 100 mg have been reported without adverse effects. Treatment should be supportive and symptomatic. Monitor for at least 48 hours or until signs and symptoms subside. It is not known if hemodialysis or peritoneal dialysis is effective.

Drug Interactions Substrate of CYP1A2 (minor)
Ergot derivatives: Ergot derivatives may cause prolonged vasospastic reactions, creating additive toxicity with frovatriptan. Do not use within 24 hours of each other.
Estrogens (oral contraceptives): Estradiol may increase serum concentrations of frovatriptan.
Propranolol: Propranolol may increase serum concentrations of frovatriptan.
Serotonergic reuptake inhibitors (eg, SSRIs/SNRIs): Concurrent use of frovatriptan with these agents may increase the risk of serotonin syndrome; monitor.
Serotonin agonists (eg, triptans): Concurrent use of frovatriptan with these agents may increase the risk of serotonin syndrome; monitor.

Ethanol/Nutrition/Herb Interactions Food: Food does not affect frovatriptan bioavailability.

Stability Store at room temperature of 25°C (77°F). Protect from moisture and light.

Mechanism of Action Selective agonist for serotonin (5-HT$_{1B}$ and 5-HT$_{1D}$ receptor) in cranial arteries to cause vasoconstriction and reduces sterile inflammation associated with antidromic neuronal transmission correlating with relief of migraine.

Pharmacokinetics
Distribution: 4.2 L/kg (males); 3.0 L/kg (females)
Protein binding: 15%
Metabolism: Primarily hepatic; forms metabolites
Bioavailability: 20% to 30%
Half-life: 26 hours
Time to peak: 2-4 hours
Elimination: Urine (32%), feces (62%)

Dosage
Geriatrics & Adults: Migraine: Oral: 2.5 mg; if headache recurs, a second dose may be given if first dose provided some relief and at least 2 hours have elapsed since the first dose (maximum daily dose: 7.5 mg)
Renal Impairment: No adjustment necessary.
Hepatic Impairment: No adjustment necessary in mild-to-moderate hepatic impairment; use with caution in severe impairment

Administration Administer with fluids.

Patient Information Take at first sign of migraine attack. This drug is to be used to relieve your migraine, not to prevent or reduce number of attacks. If headache returns or is not fully resolved after first dose, the dose may be repeated after 2 hours. **Do not exceed 7.5 mg (3 tablets) in 24 hours.** Take tablet whole with fluids. **Do not take within 24 hours of any other migraine medication without first consulting prescriber.** You may experience some dizziness (use caution); hot flashes (cool room may help); nausea or vomiting (frequent small meals, frequent mouth care, sucking lozenges or chewing gum may help); or excess sweating (will resolve). Report chest tightness or pain; excessive drowsiness; acute abdominal pain; skin rash or burning sensation; muscle weakness, soreness, or numbness; or respiratory difficulty.

Additional Information Blocks 5-HT$_{1B}$ and 5-HT$_{1D}$ receptors. Relieves symptoms of migraine by blocking vasoconstrictive and other effects of serotonin.
(Continued)

Frovatriptan *(Continued)*

Special Geriatric Considerations Since elderly often have cardiovascular disease, careful evaluation of the use of 5-HT agonists is needed to avoid complications with the use of these agents. The pharmacokinetic disposition of these agents is similar to that seen in younger adults.

Dosage Forms Excipient information presented when available (limited, particularly for generics); consult specific product labeling.

Tablet, as base: 2.5 mg

♦ **Frovatriptan Succinate** *see* Frovatriptan *on page 686*

♦ **Frusemide** *see* Furosemide *on page 690*

Fulvestrant *(fool VES trant)*

U.S. Brand Names Faslodex®

Index Terms ICI-182,780; Zeneca 182,780; ZM-182,780

Generic Available No

Pharmacologic Category Antineoplastic Agent, Estrogen Receptor Antagonist

Use Treatment of hormone receptor positive metastatic breast cancer in postmenopausal women with disease progression following antiestrogen therapy

Unlabeled/Investigational Use Treatment of endometriosis, uterine bleeding

Contraindications Hypersensitivity to fulvestrant or any component of the formulation; contraindications to I.M. injections (bleeding diatheses, thrombocytopenia, or therapeutic anticoagulation)

Warnings/Precautions Hazardous agent - use appropriate precautions for handling and disposal. Use caution in hepatic impairment.

Adverse Reactions (Reflective of adult population; not specific for elderly)

>10%:

Cardiovascular: Vasodilation (18%)

Central nervous system: Pain (19%), headache (15%)

Endocrine & metabolic: Hot flushes (19% to 24%)

Gastrointestinal: Nausea (26%), vomiting (13%), constipation (13%), diarrhea (12%), abdominal pain (12%)

Local: Injection site reaction (11%)

Neuromuscular & skeletal: Weakness (23%), bone pain (16%), back pain (14%)

Respiratory: Pharyngitis (16%), dyspnea (15%)

1% to 10%:

Cardiovascular: Edema (9%), chest pain (7%)

Central nervous system: Dizziness (7%), insomnia (7%), paresthesia (6%), fever (6%), depression (6%), anxiety (5%)

Dermatologic: Rash (7%)

Gastrointestinal: Anorexia (9%), weight gain (1% to 2%)

Genitourinary: Pelvic pain (10%), urinary tract infection (6%), vaginitis (2% to 3%)

Hematologic: Anemia (5%)

Neuromuscular and skeletal: Arthritis (3%)

Respiratory: Cough (10%)

Miscellaneous: Diaphoresis increased (5%)

Overdosage/Toxicology No specific experience in overdose. Treatment is supportive.

Drug Interactions Substrate of CYP3A4 (minor)

Stability Store under refrigeration at 2°C to 8°C (36°F to 46°F).

Mechanism of Action Steroidal compound which competitively binds to estrogen receptors on tumors and other tissue targets, producing a nuclear complex that decreases DNA synthesis and inhibits estrogen effects. Fulvestrant has no estrogen-receptor agonist activity. Causes down-regulation of estrogen receptors and inhibits tumor growth.

Pharmacodynamics Duration: I.M.: Plasma levels maintained for at least 1 month

Pharmacokinetics

Distribution: V_d: 3-5 L/kg

Protein binding: 99%

Metabolism: Hepatic via multiple pathways

Bioavailability: Oral: Poor

Half-life: ~40 days

Time to peak plasma concentration: I.M.: 7-9 days

Elimination: Feces (>90%); urine (<1%)

Dosage

Geriatrics & Adults: Metastatic breast cancer (postmenopausal women): I.M.: 250 mg at 1-month intervals

Renal Impairment: No dosage adjustment required.

Hepatic Impairment: Use in moderate-to-severe hepatic impairment has not been evaluated; use caution

Administration I.M. injection into a relatively large muscle (ie, buttock); do not administer I.V., SubQ, or intra-arterially. May be administered as a single 5 mL injection or two concurrent 2.5 mL injections.

Patient Information Take as directed. You may experience an initial "flare" of disease (increased bone pain and hot flashes) which will subside with continued use. You may experience nausea, vomiting, or loss of appetite (frequent mouth care, frequent small meals, chewing gum, or sucking lozenges may help); dizziness (use caution when driving, climbing stairs, or engaging in tasks requiring alertness until response to drug is known). Report chest pain, palpitations, or swollen extremities; vaginal bleeding; chest pain, unusual coughing, or difficulty breathing.

Dosage Forms Excipient information presented when available (limited, particularly for generics); consult specific product labeling.

Injection, solution: 50 mg/mL (2.5 mL, 5 mL) [prefilled syringe; contains alcohol, benzyl alcohol, benzyl stearate, castor oil]

- ♦ **Fungi-Guard [OTC]** *see* Tolnaftate *on page 1596*
- ♦ **Fung-O® [OTC]** *see* Salicylic Acid *on page 1441*
- ♦ **Fungoid® Tincture [OTC]** *see* Miconazole *on page 1036*
- ♦ **Furadantin®** *see* Nitrofurantoin *on page 1128*

Furazolidone (fyoor a ZOE li done)

Canadian Brand Names Furoxone®
Index Terms Furoxone
Generic Available No
Pharmacologic Category Antiprotozoal
Use Treatment of bacterial or protozoal diarrhea and enteritis caused by susceptible organisms: *Giardia lamblia* and *Vibrio cholerae*
Restrictions Not available in U.S.
Contraindications Hypersensitivity to furazolidone or any component of the formulation; concurrent use of ethanol; foods high in tyramine content
Warnings/Precautions Use caution in patients with G6PD deficiency when administering large doses for prolonged periods. Furazolidone inhibits monoamine oxidase.
Adverse Reactions (Reflective of adult population; not specific for elderly)
>10%: Genitourinary: Discoloration of urine (dark yellow to brown)
1% to 10%:
Central nervous system: Headache
Gastrointestinal: Abdominal pain, diarrhea, nausea, vomiting
Overdosage/Toxicology Symptoms include nausea, vomiting, and serotonin crisis. Treatment is supportive care only. Serotonin crisis may require dantrolene/bromocriptine.
Drug Interactions
Increases toxicity of sympathomimetic amines, tricyclic antidepressants, MAO inhibitors, meperidine, anorexiants, dextromethorphan, fluoxetine, paroxetine, sertraline, and trazodone.
Increased effect/toxicity of levodopa.
Disulfiram-like reaction with ethanol.
Ethanol/Nutrition/Herb Interactions
Ethanol: Avoid ethanol (a disulfiram-like reaction may occur).
Food: Concurrent ingestion of foods rich in tyramine may cause sudden and severe high blood pressure (hypertensive crisis). Avoid tyramine-containing foods with MAOIs. Food's freshness is also an important concern; improperly stored or spoiled food can create an environment where tyramine concentrations may increase.
Herb/Nutraceuticals: Avoid supplements containing caffeine, tyrosine, tryptophan, or phenylalanine. Ingestion of large quantities may increase the risk of severe side effects (eg, hypertensive reactions, serotonin syndrome).
Mechanism of Action Inhibits several vital enzymatic reactions causing antibacterial and antiprotozoal action
Pharmacokinetics
Absorption: Oral: Poor
Elimination: 33% of oral dose excreted in urine as active drug and metabolites
Dosage
Geriatrics & Adults: Diarrhea/enteritis: Oral: 100 mg 4 times/day; not more than 8.8 mg/kg/day; treatment duration: 7 days
Test Interactions False-positive results for urine glucose with Clinitest®
Patient Information May discolor urine to a brown tint; avoid drinking alcohol with or within 4 days of taking furazolidone or eating tyramine-containing foods; avoid medications containing sympathomimetics (cold and allergy medications, etc); if result not achieved at the end of treatment contact physician
Dosage Forms Excipient information presented when available (limited, particularly for generics); consult specific product labeling. [CAN] = Canadian brand name
(Continued)

Furazolidone *(Continued)*

Liquid:
    Furoxone® [CAN]: 50 mg/15 mL [not available in the U.S.]
Tablet:
    Furoxone® [CAN]: 100 mg [not available in the U.S.]

◆ **Furazosin** *see Prazosin on page 1301*

Furosemide *(fyoor OH se mide)*

Medication Safety Issues
Sound-alike/look-alike issues:
    Furosemide may be confused with torsemide
    Lasix® may be confused with Esidrix®, Lanoxin®, Lidex®, Lomotil®, Luvox®, Luxiq®

International issues:
    Urex® [Australia] may be confused with Eurax® which is a brand name for crotamiton in the U.S.
    Urex® [Australia]: Brand name for methenamine in the U.S.

U.S. Brand Names Lasix®
Canadian Brand Names Apo-Furosemide®; Furosemide Injection, USP; Furosemide Special; Lasix®; Lasix® Special; Novo-Semide
Index Terms Frusemide
Generic Available Yes
Pharmacologic Category Diuretic, Loop
Use Management of edema associated with congestive heart failure and hepatic or renal disease; used alone or in combination with antihypertensives in treatment of hypertension
Contraindications Hypersensitivity to furosemide, any component, or sulfonylureas; anuria; patients with hepatic coma or in states of severe electrolyte depletion until the condition improves or is corrected
Warnings/Precautions Loop diuretics are potent diuretics; excess amounts can lead to profound diuresis with fluid and electrolyte loss; close medical supervision and dose evaluation are required. Watch for and correct electrolyte disturbances; adjust dose to avoid dehydration. In cirrhosis, avoid electrolyte and acid/base imbalances that might lead to hepatic encephalopathy. Coadministration of antihypertensives may increase the risk of hypotension.

Monitor fluid status and renal function in an attempt to prevent oliguria, azotemia, and reversible increases in BUN and creatinine; close medical supervision of aggressive diuresis is required. Rapid I.V. administration, renal impairment, excessive doses, and concurrent use of other ototoxins is associated with ototoxicity. Asymptomatic hyperuricemia has been reported with use.

Chemical similarities are present among sulfonamides, sulfonylureas, carbonic anhydrase inhibitors, thiazides, and loop diuretics (except ethacrynic acid). Use in patients with sulfonylurea allergy is specifically contraindicated in product labeling, however, a risk of cross-reaction exists in patients with allergy to any of these compounds; avoid use when previous reaction has been severe. Discontinue if signs of hypersensitivity are noted.

Adverse Reactions (Reflective of adult population; not specific for elderly)
Frequency not defined.
    Cardiovascular: Acute hypotension, chronic aortitis, necrotizing angiitis, orthostatic hypotension, thrombophlebitis, sudden death from cardiac arrest (with I.V. or I.M. administration)
    Central nervous system: Blurred vision, dizziness, fever, headache, lightheadedness, restlessness, vertigo, xanthopsia
    Dermatologic: Cutaneous vasculitis, erythema multiforme, exfoliative dermatitis, photosensitivity, pruritus, purpura, rash, urticaria
    Endocrine & metabolic: Gout, hyperglycemia, hyperuricemia, hypocalcemia, hypochloremia, hypokalemia, hypomagnesemia, hyponatremia, metabolic alkalosis
    Gastrointestinal: Anorexia, constipation, cramping, diarrhea, intrahepatic cholestatic jaundice, ischemia hepatitis, nausea, oral and gastric irritation, pancreatitis, vomiting
    Genitourinary: Urinary bladder spasm, urinary frequency
    Hematological: Agranulocytosis (rare), anemia, aplastic anemia (rare), hemolytic anemia, leukopenia, purpura, thrombocytopenia
    Neuromuscular & skeletal: Muscle spasm, paresthesia, weakness
    Otic: Hearing impairment (reversible or permanent with rapid I.V. or I.M. administration), reversible deafness (with rapid I.V. or I.M. administration), tinnitus
    Renal: Allergic interstitial nephritis, fall in glomerular filtration rate and renal blood flow (due to overdiuresis), glycosuria, transient rise in BUN, vasculitis
    Miscellaneous: Anaphylaxis (rare), exacerbate or activate systemic lupus erythematosus

Overdosage/Toxicology Symptoms include electrolyte imbalance, volume depletion, hypotension, dehydration, hypokalemia and hypochloremic alkalosis. Following GI decontamination, treatment is supportive. Hypotension responds to fluids and Trendelenburg position.

Drug Interactions

ACE inhibitors: Hypotensive effects and/or renal effects are potentiated by hypovolemia.

Antidiabetic agents: Glucose tolerance may be decreased.

Antihypertensive agents: Hypotensive effects may be enhanced.

Cephaloridine or cephalexin: Nephrotoxicity may occur.

Cholestyramine or colestipol may reduce bioavailability of furosemide.

Digoxin: Furosemide-induced hypokalemia may predispose to digoxin toxicity. Monitor potassium.

Fibric acid derivatives: Blood levels of furosemide and fibric acid derivatives (ie, clofibrate and fenofibrate) may be increased during concurrent dosing (particularly in hypoalbuminemia). Limited documentation; monitor for increased effect/toxicity.

Indomethacin (and other NSAIDs) may reduce natriuretic and hypotensive effects of furosemide.

Lithium: Renal clearance may be reduced. Isolated reports of lithium toxicity have occurred; monitor lithium levels.

Metformin may decrease furosemide concentrations.

Metformin blood levels may be increased by furosemide.

NSAIDs: Risk of renal impairment may increase when used in conjunction with furosemide.

Ototoxic drugs (aminoglycosides, cis-platinum): Concomitant use of furosemide may increase risk of ototoxicity, especially in patients with renal dysfunction.

Peripheral adrenergic-blocking drugs or ganglionic blockers: Effects may be increased.

Phenobarbital or phenytoin may reduce diuretic response to furosemide.

Salicylates (high dose) with furosemide may predispose patients to salicylate toxicity due to reduced renal excretion or alter renal function.

Succinylcholine: Action may be potentiated by furosemide.

Sucralfate may limit absorption of furosemide, effects may be significantly decreased; separate oral administration by 2 hours.

Thiazides: Synergistic diuretic effects occur.

Tubocurarine: The skeletal muscle-relaxing effect may be attenuated by furosemide.

Ethanol/Nutrition/Herb Interactions

Food: Furosemide serum levels may be decreased if taken with food.

Herb/Nutraceutical: Avoid dong quai if using for hypertension (has estrogenic activity). Avoid ephedra, yohimbe, and ginseng (may worsen hypertension). Limit intake of natural licorice. Avoid garlic (may have increased antihypertensive effect).

Stability Furosemide injection should be stored at controlled room temperature and protected from light. Exposure to light may cause discoloration; do not use furosemide solutions if they have a yellow color. Furosemide solutions are unstable in acidic media, but very stable in basic media Refrigeration may result in precipitation or crystallization, however, resolubilization at room temperature or warming may be performed without affecting the drug's stability.

I.V. infusion solution mixed in NS or D_5W solution is stable for 24 hours at room temperature. May also be diluted for infusion 1-2 mg/mL (maximum: 10 mg/mL) over 10-15 minutes (following infusion rate parameters).

Mechanism of Action Inhibits reabsorption of sodium and chloride in the ascending loop of Henle and distal renal tubule, interfering with the chloride-binding cotransport system, thus causing increased excretion of water, sodium, chloride, magnesium, and calcium

Pharmacodynamics

Oral:

Onset of action: Diuresis begins within 30-60 minutes

Peak effect: Within 1-2 hours

Duration: 6-8 hours

I.V.:

Onset of action: Diuresis starts in 5 minutes

Peak effect: Reduced and delayed in older adults as compared to younger adults

Duration: 2 hours

Pharmacokinetics

Absorption: Oral: 60% to 67%

Protein binding: >90%

Elimination: In older adults, total clearance is decreased and dependent on renal function

(Continued)

Furosemide (Continued)

Dosage

Geriatrics: Oral, I.M., I.V.: Initial: 20 mg/day; increase slowly to desired response.

Adults:

Edema, CHF, or hypertension (diuresis):

Oral: 20-80 mg/dose initially increased in increments of 20-40 mg/dose at intervals of 6-8 hours; usual maintenance dose interval is twice daily or every day

Usual dosage range for hypertension (JNC 7): 20-80 mg/day in 2 divided doses

I.M., I.V.: 20-40 mg/dose, may be repeated in 1-2 hours as needed and increased by 20 mg/dose with each succeeding dose up to 1000 mg/day; usual dosing interval: 6-12 hours. **Note:** ACC/AHA 2005 guidelines for chronic congestive heart failure recommend a maximum single dose of 160-200 mg.

Continuous I.V. infusion: Initial I.V. bolus dose 20-40 mg, followed by continuous I.V. infusion doses of 10-40 mg/hour. If urine output is <1 mL/kg/hour, double as necessary to a maximum of 80-160 mg/hour. The risk associated with higher infusion rates (80-160 mg/hour) must be weighed against alternative strategies. **Note:** ACC/AHA 2005 guidelines for chronic congestive heart failure recommend 40 mg I.V. load, then 10-40 mg/hour infusion.

Refractory heart failure: Oral, I.V.: Doses up to 8 g/day have been used.

Renal Impairment:

Acute renal failure: Doses up to 1-3 g/day may be necessary to initiate desired response; avoid use in oliguric states.

Not removed by hemo- or peritoneal dialysis; supplemental dose is not necessary.

Hepatic Impairment: Diminished natriuretic effect with increased sensitivity to hypokalemia and volume depletion in cirrhosis. Monitor effects, particularly with high doses.

Administration Replace parenteral therapy with oral therapy as soon as possible. I.V. injections should be given slowly. In adults, undiluted direct I.V. injections may be administered at a rate of 40 mg over 1-2 minutes; maximum rate of adminstration for IVPB or continuous infusion: 4 mg/minute.

Monitoring Parameters Blood pressure both standing and sitting/supine, serum electrolytes, renal function, I & O, weight; in high doses monitor auditory function

Reference Range Therapeutic: 1-2 mcg/mL (SI: 3-6 μmol/L)

Patient Information May be taken with food or milk; get up slowly from a lying or sitting position to minimize dizziness, lightheadedness or fainting; also use extra care when exercising, standing for long periods of time and during hot weather; take in the morning; may cause increased sensitivity to sunlight

Additional Information Injection contains 0.162 mEq of sodium per mL; do not use solutions that are yellow in color

Standard diluent: Dose/50 mL D_5W

Minimum volume: 50 mL D_5W

Special Geriatric Considerations Loop diuretics are potent diuretics; excess amounts can lead to profound diuresis with fluid and electrolyte loss; close medical supervision and dose evaluation is required, particularly in the elderly. Severe loss of sodium and/or increase in BUN can cause confusion. For any change in mental status in patients on furosemide, monitor electrolytes and renal function.

Dosage Forms Excipient information presented when available (limited, particularly for generics); consult specific product labeling.

Injection, solution: 10 mg/mL (2 mL, 4 mL, 8 mL, 10 mL)

Solution, oral: 10 mg/mL (60 mL, 120 mL) [orange flavor]; 40 mg/5 mL (5 mL, 500 mL) [pineapple-peach flavor]

Tablet (Lasix®): 20 mg, 40 mg, 80 mg

Selected References

Chaudhry AY, Bing RF, Castleden CM, et al, "The Effect of Aging on the Response to Frusemide in Normal Subjects," *Eur J Clin Pharmacol*, 1984, 27(3):303-6.

Mühlberg W, "Pharmacokinetics of Diuretics in Geriatric Patients," *Arch Gerontol Geriatr*, 1989, 9(3):283-90.

Murray MD, Haag, KM, Black PK, et al, "Variable Furosemide Absorption and Poor Predictability of Response in Elderly Patients," *Pharmacotherapy*, 1997, 17(1):98-106.

♦ **Furoxone** *see* Furazolidone *on page 689*

Gabapentin (GA ba pen tin)

Related Information

Serum Drug Concentrations Commonly Monitored Guidelines *on page 1862*

Medication Safety Issues

Sound-alike/look-alike issues:

Neurontin® may be confused with Neoral®, Noroxin®

U.S. Brand Names Neurontin®

Canadian Brand Names Apo-Gabapentin®; BCI-Gabapentin; Gen-Gabapentin; Neurontin®; Novo-Gabapentin; Nu-Gabapentin; PMS-Gabapentin

Generic Available Yes: Capsule, tablet

Pharmacologic Category Anticonvulsant, Miscellaneous

Use Adjunct for treatment of partial seizures with and without secondary generalized seizures in patients with epilepsy

Unlabeled/Investigational Use Social phobia; chronic pain

Contraindications Hypersensitivity to gabapentin or any component of the formulation

Warnings/Precautions Avoid abrupt withdrawal, may precipitate seizures; use cautiously in patients with severe renal dysfunction; male rat studies demonstrated an association with pancreatic adenocarcinoma (clinical implication unknown). May cause CNS depression, which may impair physical or mental abilities. Patients must be cautioned about performing tasks which require mental alertness (eg, operating machinery or driving). Effects with other sedative drugs or ethanol may be potentiated.

Adverse Reactions (Reflective of adult population; not specific for elderly)
>10%:
   Central nervous system: Somnolence (20%), dizziness (17% to 28%), ataxia (13%), fatigue (11%)
   Miscellaneous: Viral infection
1% to 10%:
   Cardiovascular: Peripheral edema (2% to 8%), vasodilatation (1%)
   Central nervous system: Fever, hostility, emotional lability, fatigue, headache (3%), ataxia (3%), abnormal thinking (2% to 3%), amnesia (2%), depression (2%), dysarthria (2%), nervousness (2%), abnormal coordination (1% to 2%), twitching (1%), hyperesthesia (1%)
   Dermatologic: Pruritus (1%), rash (1%)
   Endocrine & metabolic: Hyperglycemia (1%)
   Gastrointestinal: Diarrhea (6%), Nausea/vomiting (3% to 4%), abdominal pain (3%), weight gain (2% to 3%), dyspepsia (2%), flatulence (2%), dry throat (2%), xerostomia (2% to 5%), constipation (2% to 4%), dental abnormalities (2%), appetite stimulation (1%)
   Genitourinary: Impotence (2%)
   Hematologic: Leukopenia (1%), decreased WBC (1%)
   Neuromuscular & skeletal: Tremor (7%), weakness (6%), hyperkinesia, abnormal gait (2%), back pain (2%), myalgia (2%), fracture (1%)
   Ocular: Nystagmus (8%), diplopia (1% to 6%), blurred vision (3% to 4%), conjunctivitis (1%)
   Otic: Otitis media (1%)
   Respiratory: Rhinitis (4%), bronchitis, respiratory infection, pharyngitis (1% to 3%), cough (2%)
   Miscellaneous: Infection (5%)

Overdosage/Toxicology Acute oral overdoses up to 49 g have been reported; double vision, slurred speech, drowsiness, lethargy, and diarrhea were observed. Patients recovered with supportive care. Decontaminate using lavage/activated charcoal with cathartic. Multiple dosing of activated charcoal may be useful. Hemodialysis may be useful.

Drug Interactions CNS depressants: Sedative effects may be additive with CNS depressants; includes ethanol, barbiturates, opioid analgesics, and other sedative agents. Monitor for increased effect.

Ethanol/Nutrition/Herb Interactions
   Ethanol: Avoid ethanol (may increase CNS depression).
   Food: Does not change rate or extent of absorption.
   Herb/Nutraceutical: Avoid evening primrose (seizure threshold decreased). Avoid valerian, St John's wort, kava kava, gotu kola (may increase CNS depression).

Stability Store at 25°C (77°F); excursions permitted to 15°C to 30°C (59°F to 86°F).

Mechanism of Action Gabapentin is structurally related to GABA. However, it does not bind to $GABA_A$ or $GABA_B$ receptors, and it does not appear to influence synthesis or uptake of GABA. High affinity gabapentin binding sites have been located throughout the brain; these sites correspond to the presence of voltage-gated calcium channels specifically possessing the alpha-2-delta-1 subunit. This channel appears to be located presynaptically, and may modulate the release of excitatory neurotransmitters which participate in epileptogenesis and nociception.

Pharmacokinetics
   Absorption: 50% to 60% from proximal small bowel by L-amino transport system
   Distribution: V_d: 0.6-0.8 L/kg
   Protein binding: <3%
   Bioavailability: Inversely proportional to dose due to saturable absorption:
      900 mg/day: 60%
      1200 mg/day: 47%
      2400 mg/day: 34%
(Continued)

Gabapentin *(Continued)*

3600 mg/day: 33%

4800 mg/day: 27%

Half-life elimination: 5-7 hours; anuria 132 hours; during dialysis 3.8 hours

Excretion: Proportional to renal function; urine (as unchanged drug)

Dosage

Geriatrics: Studies in elderly patients have shown a decrease in clearance as age increases. This is most likely due to age-related decreases in renal function; dose reductions may be needed.

Adults:

Anticonvulsant: Oral:

Initial: 300 mg 3 times/day, if necessary the dose may be increased up to 1800 mg/day

Maintenance: 900-1800 mg/day administered in 3 divided doses; doses of up to 2400 mg/day have been tolerated in long-term clinical studies; up to 3600 mg/day has been tolerated in short-term studies

Note: If gabapentin is discontinued or if another anticonvulsant is added to therapy, it should be done slowly over a minimum of 1 week.

Chronic pain (unlabeled use): Oral: 300-1800 mg/day given in 3 divided doses has been the most common dosage range

Postoperative pain (unlabeled use): 300-1200 mg 1-2 hours before surgery

Postherpetic neuralgia: Day 1: 300 mg, Day 2: 300 mg twice daily, Day 3: 300 mg 3 times/day; dose may be titrated as needed for pain relief (range: 1800-3600 mg/day, daily doses >1800 mg do not generally show greater benefit)

Renal Impairment: Adults: See table.

Hemodialysis: Dialyzable

Gabapentin Dosing Adjustments in Renal Impairment

Creatinine Clearance (mL/min)	Daily Dose Range
≥60	300-1200 mg tid
>30-59	200-700 mg bid
>15-29	200-700 mg daily
15[1]	100-300 mg daily
Hemodialysis[2]	125-350 mg

[1]Cl_{cr}<15 mL/minute: Reduce daily dose in proportion to creatinine clearance.

[2]Single supplemental dose administered after each 4 hours of hemodialysis

Administration Administer first dose on first day at bedtime to avoid somnolence and dizziness. Dosage must be adjusted for renal function; when given 3 times daily, the maximum time between doses should not exceed 12 hours.

Reference Range Minimum effective serum concentration may be 2 mcg/mL; **routine monitoring of drug levels is not required even with concomitant drug therapy**

Test Interactions False positives have been reported with the Ames N-Multistix SG® dipstick test for urine protein

Patient Information Take only as prescribed; may cause dizziness, somnolence, and other symptoms and signs of CNS depression; do not operate machinery or drive a car until you have experience with the drug; may be administered without regard to meals

Special Geriatric Considerations Studies in the elderly have shown a decrease in clearance as age increases. This is most likely due to age-related decreases in renal function; calculations of Cl_{cr} recommended since dose reductions may be needed.

Dosage Forms Excipient information presented when available (limited, particularly for generics); consult specific product labeling.

Capsule: 100 mg, 300 mg, 400 mg

Neurontin®: 100 mg, 300 mg, 400 mg

Solution, oral:

Neurontin®: 250 mg/5 mL (480 mL) [cool strawberry anise flavor]

Tablet: 100 mg, 300 mg, 400 mg, 600 mg, 800 mg

Neurontin®: 600 mg, 800 mg

Selected References

Adler CH, "Treatment of Restless Legs Syndrome With Gabapentin," *Clin Neuropharmacol*, 1997, 20(2):148-51.

Backonja M, Beydoun A, Edwards KR, et al, "Gabapentin for the Symptomatic Treatment of Painful Neuropathy in Patients With Diabetes Mellitus: A Randomized Controlled Trial," *JAMA*, 1998, 280(21):1831-6.

Bennett J, Goldman WT, and Suppes T, "Gabapentin for Treatment of Bipolar and Schizoaffective Disorders," *J Clin Psychopharmacol*, 1997, 17:141-1.

McElroy SL, Soutullo CA, Keck PE Jr, et al, "A Pilot Trial of Adjunctive Gabapentin in the Treatment of Bipolar Disorder," *Ann Clin Psychiatry*, 1997, 9(2):99-103.

Pande AC, Crockatt JG, Janney CA, et al, "Gabapentin in Bipolar Disorder: A Placebo-Controlled Trial of Adjunctive Therapy. Gabapentin Bipolar Disorder Study Group," *Bipolar Disord*, 2000, 2(3):249-55.

Regan WM and Gordon SM, "Gabapentin for Behavioral Agitation in Alzheimer's Disease," *J Clin Psychopharmacol*, 1997, 17:59-60.

Rosenberg JM, Harrell C, Ristic H, et al, "The Effect of Gabapentin on Neuropathic Pain," *Clin J Pain*, 1997, 13(3):251-5.

Rosner H, Rubin L, and Kestenbaum A, "Gabapentin Adjunctive Therapy in Neuropathic Pain States," *Clin J Pain*, 1996, 12(1):56-8.

Rowbotham M, Harden N, Stacey B, et al, "Gabapentin for the Treatment of Postherpetic Neuralgia: A Randomized Controlled Trial," *JAMA*, 1998, 280(21):1837-42.

Ryback R and Ryback L, "Gabapentin for Behavioral Dyscontrol," *Am J Psychiatry*, 1995, 152(9):1399.

Schaffer CB and Schaffer LC, "Gabapentin in the Treatment of Bipolar Disorder," *Am J Psychiatry*, 1997, 154(2):291-2.

Stanton SP, Keck PE Jr, and McElroy SL, "Treatment of Acute Mania With Gabapentin," *Am J Psychiatry*, 1997, 154(2):287.

♦ **Gabitril**® see Tiagabine on page 1561

Galantamine (ga LAN ta meen)

Medication Safety Issues
Sound-alike/look-alike issues:

Razedyne™ may be confused with Rozerem™

Reminyl® may be confused with Amaryl®

Due to patient safety concerns regarding prescribing and dispensing errors between Reminyl® and Amaryl®, Reminyl® (galantamine) is being renamed to Razadyne™ (immediate-release) and Razadyne™ ER (extended-release). The brand name Reminyl® was discontinued with the July, 2005 distribution of Razadyne™.

U.S. Brand Names Razadyne™; Razadyne™ ER; Reminyl® [DSC]

Canadian Brand Names Reminyl®; Reminyl® ER

Index Terms Galantamine Hydrobromide

Generic Available No

Pharmacologic Category Acetylcholinesterase Inhibitor (Central)

Use Treatment of mild to moderate dementia of Alzheimer's disease

Contraindications Hypersensitivity to galantamine or any component of the formulation; severe liver dysfunction (Child-Pugh score 10-15); severe renal dysfunction (Cl_{cr} <9 mL/minute)

Warnings/Precautions Use caution in patients with supraventricular conduction delays (without a functional pacemaker in place) or patients taking medicines that slow conduction through SA or AV node. Use caution in peptic ulcer disease (or in patients at risk); seizure disorder; asthma; COPD; mild-to-moderate liver dysfunction; moderate renal dysfunction. May cause bladder outflow obstruction. May exaggerate neuromuscular blockade effects of succinylcholine and like agents. May cause nausea, vomiting, diarrhea, weight los and anorexia.

Adverse Reactions (Reflective of adult population; not specific for elderly)

>10%: Gastrointestinal: Nausea (6% to 24%), vomiting (4% to 13%), diarrhea (6% to 12%)

1% to 10%:

Cardiovascular: Bradycardia (2% to 3%), syncope (0.4% to 2.2%: dose related), chest pain (≥1%)

Central nervous system: Dizziness (9%), headache (8%), depression (7%), fatigue (5%), insomnia (5%), somnolence (4%)

Gastrointestinal: Anorexia (7% to 9%), weight loss (5% to 7%), abdominal pain (5%), dyspepsia (5%), flatulence (≥1%)

Genitourinary: Urinary tract infection (8%), hematuria (<1% to 3%), incontinence (≥1%)

Hematologic: Anemia (3%)

Neuromuscular & skeletal: Tremor (3%)

Respiratory: Rhinitis (4%)

Overdosage/Toxicology Symptoms of overdose may include bradycardia, collapse, convulsions, defecation, gastrointestinal cramping, hypotension, lacrimation, muscle fasciculations, muscle weakness, QT prolongation, respiratory depression, salivation, severe nausea, sweating, torsade de pointes, urination, ventricular tachycardia, vomiting. Treatment is symptom-directed and supportive. Atropine may be used as an antidote; initial dose 0.5-1 mg I.V. and titrate to effect. An atypical response in blood pressure and heart rate has been reported. Effects of hemodialysis are unknown.

Drug Interactions Substrate (minor) of CYP2D6, 3A4

Amiodarone: Concurrent use may lead to bradycardia

Anticholinergic agents (eg, atropine, benztropine, tolterodine): Galantamine may antagonize anticholinergic actions

Antipsychotic agents: Acetylcholinesterase inhibitors (central) may increase the risk of antipsychotic-related extrapyramidal symptoms; monitor.

Beta-blockers without ISA activity: Concurrent use may lead to bradycardia

Cholinergic agonists: May have synergistic effects

Digoxin: Concurrent use may lead to AV block

Diltiazem: Concurrent use may lead to bradycardia

NSAIDs: Concurrent use may increase risk of gastrointestinal ulcer because of increased gastric acid secretion.

(Continued)

Galantamine *(Continued)*

Succinylcholine: Concurrent use may lead to enhanced neuromuscular blockade
Verapamil: Concurrent use may lead to bradycardia

Ethanol/Nutrition/Herb Interactions

Ethanol: Avoid ethanol (may increase CNS adverse events).
Herb/Nutraceutical: St John's wort may decrease galantamine serum levels; avoid concurrent use.

Stability Store at 15°C to 30°C (59°F to 86°F). Do not freeze oral solution; protect from light.

Mechanism of Action Centrally-acting cholinesterase inhibitor (competitive and reversible). It elevates acetylcholine in cerebral cortex by slowing the degradation of acetylcholine. Modulates nicotinic acetylcholine receptor to increase acetylcholine from surviving presynaptic nerve terminals. May increase glutamate and serotonin levels.

Pharmacodynamics Duration: Maximum inhibition of erythrocyte acetylcholinesterase ~40% at 1 hour post 10 mg oral dose; levels return to baseline at 30 hour

Pharmacokinetics

Absorption: Rapidly and completely absorbed
Distribution: V_d 1.8-2.6 L/kg
Protein binding: 18%
Metabolism: Hepatic; linear, metabolized to epigalanthaminone and galanthaminone both of which have acetylcholinesterase inhibitory activity 130 times less than galantamine
Bioavailability: 90%
Half-life: 7 hours
Time to peak: Immediate release: 1 hour (2.5 hours with food); extended release: 4.5-5 hours
Elimination: 95% urine, 5% feces; 20% to 32% excreted as unchanged galantamine

Dosage

Geriatrics & Adults:

Alzheimer's dementia (mild-to-moderate): Oral:

Immediate release tablet or solution: Mild-to-moderate dementia of Alzheimer's: Initial: 4 mg twice a day for 4 weeks; if tolerated, increase to 8 mg twice daily for ≥4 weeks; if tolerated, increase to 12 mg twice daily
Range: 16-24 mg/day in 2 divided doses

Extended-release capsule: Initial: 8 mg once daily for 4 weeks; if tolerated, increase to 16 mg once daily for ≥4 weeks; if tolerated, increase to 24 mg once daily
Range: 16-24 mg once daily

Note: Oral solution and tablet should be taken with breakfast and dinner; capsule should be taken with breakfast. If therapy is interrupted for ≥3 days, restart at the lowest dose and increase to current dose.

Conversion to galantamine from other cholinesterase inhibitors: Patients experiencing poor tolerability with donepezil or rivastigmine should wait until side effects subside or allow a 7-day washout period prior to beginning galantamine. Patients not experiencing side effects with donepezil or rivastigmine may begin galantamine therapy the day immediately following discontinuation of previous therapy (Morris, 2001).

Renal Impairment:

Moderate renal impairment: Maximum dose: 16 mg/day.
Severe renal dysfunction (Cl_{cr} <9 mL/minute): Use is not recommended

Hepatic Impairment:

Moderate liver dysfunction (Child-Pugh score 7-9): Maximum dose: 16 mg/day
Severe liver dysfunction (Child-Pugh score 10-15): Use is not recommended

Administration Administer oral solution or tablet with breakfast and dinner; administer extended release capsule with breakfast. If therapy is interrupted for ≥3 days, restart at the lowest dose and increase to current dose. If using oral solution, mix dose with 3-4 ounces of any nonalcoholic beverage; mix well and drink immediately.

Patient Information This medication will not cure Alzheimer's disease, but may help reduce symptoms. Use exactly as directed; do not increase dose or discontinue without consulting prescriber. Maintain adequate hydration (2-3 L/day) unless instructed to restrict fluids. May cause dizziness, sedation, hypotension, or tremor (use caution when driving or engaging in hazardous tasks, rise slowly from sitting or lying position, and use caution when climbing stairs until response to drug is known); diarrhea (boiled milk, yogurt, or buttermilk may help); or nausea or vomiting (frequent small meals, good mouth care, sucking lozenges, or chewing gum may help). Report persistent gastrointestinal disturbances; significantly increased salivation, sweating, or tearing; excessive fatigue, insomnia, dizziness, or depression; increased muscle, joint, or body pain or spasms; vision changes; respiratory changes, wheezing, or signs of dyspnea; chest pain or palpitations; or other adverse reactions.

Special Geriatric Considerations No dosage adjustment needed.

Dosage Forms Excipient information presented when available (limited, particularly for generics); consult specific product labeling.

Capsule, extended release, as hydrobromide (Razadyne™ ER): 8 mg, 16 mg, 24 mg [contains gelatin]

Solution, oral, as hydrobromide (Razadyne™): 4 mg/mL (100 mL) [with calibrated pipette]

Tablet, as hydrobromide (Razadyne™): 4 mg, 8 mg, 12 mg

Selected References

Morris JC, Farlow MR, Ferris SH, et al, "Therapeutic Continuity in Alzheimer's Disease: Switching Patients to Galantamine. Panel Discussion: Recommendations for Prescribers," *Clin Ther*, 2001, 23 (Suppl A):31-9.

Raskind MA, Peskind ER, Wessel T, et al, "Galantamine in AD: A 6-month Randomized, Placebo-controlled Trial With a 6-month Extension. The Galantamine USA-1 Study Group," *Neurology*, 2000, 54(12):2261-8.

Tariot PN, Solomon PR, Morris JC, et al, "A 5-month, Randomized, Placebo-controlled Trial of Galantamine in AD. The Galantamine USA-10 Study Group," *Neurology*, 2000, 54(12):2269-76.

♦ **Galantamine Hydrobromide** *see* Galantamine *on page 695*

♦ **Gamma Benzene Hexachloride** *see* Lindane *on page 909*

♦ **Gamma E-Gems® [OTC]** *see* Vitamin E *on page 1677*

♦ **Gamma-E Plus [OTC]** *see* Vitamin E *on page 1677*

♦ **Gamma Globulin** *see* Immune Globulin (Intramuscular) *on page 795*

♦ **GammaSTAN™ S/D** *see* Immune Globulin (Intramuscular) *on page 795*

Ganciclovir (gan SYE kloe veer)

Medication Safety Issues

Sound-alike/look-alike issues:

Cytovene® may be confused with Cytosar®, Cytosar-U®

U.S. Brand Names Cytovene®; Vitrasert®

Canadian Brand Names Cytovene®; Vitrasert®

Index Terms DHPG Sodium; GCV Sodium; Nordeoxyguanosine

Generic Available Yes: Capsule

Pharmacologic Category Antiviral Agent

Use CMV retinitis treatment of immunocompromised individuals, including patients with acquired immunodeficiency syndrome; treatment of CMV pneumonia in marrow transplant recipients, promising results have been achieved in AIDS patients and organ transplant recipients with CMV colitis, pneumonitis, and multiorgan involvement; attenuation of CMV infection in transplant patients

Contraindications Hypersensitivity to ganciclovir, acyclovir, or any component of the formulation; absolute neutrophil count <500/mm^3; platelet count <25,000/mm^3

Warnings/Precautions Hazardous agent - use appropriate precautions for handling and disposal. **[U.S. Boxed Warning]: Granulocytopenia (neutropenia), anemia, and thrombocytopenia may occur.** Dosage adjustment or interruption of ganciclovir therapy may be necessary in patients with neutropenia and/or thrombocytopenia and patients with impaired renal function. **[U.S. Boxed Warning]: Animal studies have demonstrated carcinogenic and teratogenic effects, and inhibition of spermatogenesis;** contraceptive precautions for female and male patients need to be followed during and for at least 90 days after therapy with the drug; take care to administer only into veins with good blood flow. **[U.S. Boxed Warning]: Indicated only for treatment of CMV retinitis in the immunocompromised patient and CMV prevention in transplant patients at risk.**

Adverse Reactions (Reflective of adult population; not specific for elderly)

>10%:

Central nervous system: Fever (38% to 48%)

Dermatologic: Rash (15% oral, 10% I.V.)

Gastrointestinal: Abdominal pain (17% to 19%), diarrhea (40%), nausea (25%), anorexia (15%), vomiting (13%)

Hematologic: Anemia (20% to 25%), leukopenia (30% to 40%)

1% to 10%:

Central nervous system: Confusion, neuropathy (8% to 9%), headache (4%)

Dermatologic: Pruritus (5%)

Hematologic: Thrombocytopenia (6%), neutropenia with ANC <500/mm^3 (5% oral, 14% I.V.)

Neuromuscular & skeletal: Paresthesia (6% to 10%), weakness (6%)

Ocular: Retinal detachment (8% oral, 11% I.V.; relationship to ganciclovir not established)

Miscellaneous: Sepsis (4% oral, 15% I.V.)

Overdosage/Toxicology Symptoms include neutropenia, vomiting, hypersalivation, bloody diarrhea, cytopenia, and testicular atrophy. Treatment is supportive. Hemodialysis removes 50% of drug. Hydration may be of some benefit.

Drug Interactions

Decreased effect: Didanosine: A decrease in steady-state ganciclovir AUC may occur (Continued)

Ganciclovir *(Continued)*

Increased toxicity:

Immunosuppressive agents may increase cytotoxicity of ganciclovir

Imipenem/cilastatin may increase seizure potential

Zidovudine: Oral ganciclovir increased the AUC of zidovudine, although zidovudine decreases steady state levels of ganciclovir. Since both drugs have the potential to cause neutropenia and anemia, some patients may not tolerate concomitant therapy with these drugs at full dosage.

Probenecid: The renal clearance of ganciclovir is decreased in the presence of probenecid

Didanosine levels are increased with concurrent ganciclovir

Other nephrotoxic drugs (eg, amphotericin and cyclosporine) may have additive nephrotoxicity with ganciclovir

Stability Intact vials should be stored at room temperature and protected from temperatures >40°C Reconstitute powder with unpreserved sterile water **not** bacteriostatic water because parabens may cause precipitation; dilute in 250-1000 mL D_5W or NS to a concentration ≤10 mg/mL for infusion.

Reconstituted solution is stable for 12 hours at room temperature, however, conflicting data indicates that reconstituted solution is stable for 60 days under refrigeration (4°C). Stability of parenteral admixture at room temperature (25°C) and at refrigeration temperature (4°C) is 5 days.

Mechanism of Action Ganciclovir is phosphorylated to a substrate which competitively inhibits the binding of deoxyguanosine triphosphate to DNA polymerase resulting in inhibition of viral DNA synthesis

Pharmacokinetics

Protein binding: 1% to 2%

Half-life: 1.7-5.8 hours; increases with impaired renal function

Elimination: Majority (94% to 99%) is excreted as unchanged drug in urine

Dosage

Geriatrics & Adults: Dosing is based on total body weight.

CMV retinitis:

I.V. (slow infusion):

Induction therapy: 5 mg/kg/dose every 12 hours for 14-21 days followed by maintenance therapy

Maintenance therapy: 5 mg/kg/day as a single daily dose for 7 days/week or 6 mg/kg/day for 5 days/week

Oral: 1000 mg 3 times/day with food **or** 500 mg 6 times/day with food

Ocular implant: Intravitreally: One implant for 5- to 8-month period; following depletion of ganciclovir, as evidenced by progression of retinitis, implant may be removed and replaced

Prevention of CMV disease in patients with advanced HIV infection and normal renal function: Oral: 1000 mg 3 times/day with food

Prevention of CMV disease in transplant patients: Same initial and maintenance dose as CMV retinitis except duration of initial course is 7-14 days, duration of maintenance therapy is dependent on clinical condition and degree of immunosuppression

Renal Impairment:

I.V. (Induction):

Cl_{cr} 50-69 mL/minute: Administer 2.5 mg/kg/dose every 12 hours.

Cl_{cr} 25-49 mL/minute: Administer 2.5 mg/kg/dose every 24 hours.

Cl_{cr} 10-24 mL/minute: Administer 1.25 mg/kg/dose every 24 hours.

Cl_{cr} <10 mL/minute: Administer 1.25 mg/kg/dose 3 times/week following hemodialysis.

I.V. (Maintenance):

Cl_{cr} 50-69 mL/minute: Administer 2.5 mg/kg/dose every 24 hours.

Cl_{cr} 25-49 mL/minute: Administer 1.25 mg/kg/dose every 24 hours.

Cl_{cr} 10-24 mL/minute: Administer 0.625 mg/kg/dose every 24 hours

Cl_{cr} <10 mL/minute: Administer 0.625 mg/kg/dose 3 times/week following hemodialysis.

Oral:

Cl_{cr} 50-69 mL/minute: Administer 1500 mg/day or 500 mg 3 times/day.

Cl_{cr} 25-49 mL/minute: Administer 1000 mg/day or 500 mg twice daily.

Cl_{cr} 10-24 mL/minute: Administer 500 mg/day.

Cl_{cr} <10 mL/minute: Administer 500 mg 3 times/week following hemodialysis.

Hemodialysis effects: Dialyzable (50%) following hemodialysis; administer dose postdialysis. During peritoneal dialysis, dose as for Cl_{cr} <10 mL/minute. During continuous arteriovenous or venovenous hemofiltration, administer 2.5 mg/kg/dose every 24 hours.

Administration The same precautions utilized with antineoplastic agents should be followed with ganciclovir administration. Ganciclovir should not be administered by I.M., SubQ, or rapid IVP administration; administer by slow I.V. infusion over at least

1 hour at a final concentration for administration not to exceed 10 mg/mL. Oral ganciclovir should be administered with food.

Monitoring Parameters CBC with differential and platelet count, serum creatinine, ophthalmologic exams

Patient Information Ganciclovir is not a cure for CMV retinitis; regular ophthalmologic examinations should be done; close monitoring of blood counts should be done while on therapy and dosage adjustments may need to be made

Additional Information Sodium content of 500 mg vial: 46 mg

Special Geriatric Considerations Adjust dose based upon renal function.

Dosage Forms Excipient information presented when available (limited, particularly for generics); consult specific product labeling. [DSC] = Discontinued product

Capsule: 250 mg, 500 mg
  Cytovene®: 250 mg, 500 mg [DSC]
Implant, intravitreal (Vitrasert®): 4.5 mg [released gradually over 5-8 months]
Injection, powder for reconstitution, as sodium (Cytovene®): 500 mg

♦ **Ganidin NR** see Guaifenesin on page 727
♦ **Gani-Tuss DM NR** see Guaifenesin and Dextromethorphan on page 730
♦ **Gani-Tuss® NR** see Guaifenesin and Codeine on page 729
♦ **Gantrisin®** see SulfiSOXAZOLE on page 1504
♦ **GAR-936** see Tigecycline on page 1568
♦ **Gas-X® [OTC]** see Simethicone on page 1467
♦ **Gas-X® Extra Strength [OTC]** see Simethicone on page 1467
♦ **Gas-X® Maximum Strength [OTC]** see Simethicone on page 1467
♦ **GasAid [OTC]** see Simethicone on page 1467
♦ **Gastrocrom®** see Cromolyn on page 369

Gatifloxacin (gat i FLOKS a sin)

Related Information
Antimicrobial Activity Against Selected Organisms on page 1728
U.S. Brand Names Zymar®
Canadian Brand Names Zymar®
Generic Available No
Pharmacologic Category Antibiotic, Ophthalmic; Antibiotic, Quinolone
Use
Oral: Treatment of the following infections when caused by susceptible bacteria: Acute bacterial exacerbation of chronic bronchitis due to *S. pneumoniae, H. influenzae, H. parainfluenzae, M. catarrhalis,* or *S. aureus*; acute sinusitis due to *S. pneumoniae, H. influenzae*; community-acquired pneumonia including pneumonia caused by multidrug-resistant *S. pneumoniae* (MDRSP); community acquired pneumonia due to *S. pneumoniae, H. influenzae, H. parainfluenzae, M. catarrhalis, S. aureus, M. pneumoniae, C. pneumoniae,* or *L. pneumophilia*; uncomplicated urinary tract infections (cystitis) due to *E. coli, K. pneumoniae,* or *P. mirabilis*; complicated urinary tract infections due to *E. coli, K. pneumoniae,* or *P. mirabilis*; pyelonephritis due to *E. coli*; uncomplicated urethral and cervical gonorrhea; acute, uncomplicated rectal infections in women due to *N. gonorrhoeae*; bacterial conjunctivitis
Ophthalmic: Bacterial conjunctivitis

Contraindications Hypersensitivity to gatifloxacin, other quinolone antibiotics, or any component of the formulation

Warnings/Precautions Use with caution in patients with significant bradycardia or acute myocardial ischemia. May prolong QT interval (concentration related). Use caution in patients with known prolongation of QT interval, uncorrected hypokalemia, or concurrent administration of other medications known to prolong the QT interval (including Class Ia and Class III antiarrhythmics, cisapride, erythromycin, antipsychotics, and tricyclic antidepressants). May cause increased CNS stimulation, increased intracranial pressure, convulsions, or psychosis. Use with caution in individuals at risk for seizures. Potential for seizures, although very rare, may be increased with concomitant NSAID therapy. Discontinue in patients who experience significant CNS adverse effects. Use caution in renal dysfunction (dosage adjustment required) and in severe hepatic insufficiency (no data available). Serious disruptions in glucose regulation (including hyperglycemia and severe hypoglycemia) may occur, usually (but not always) in patients with diabetes. Other risk factors for glucose dysregulation include advanced age, renal insufficiency, and use of concurrent medications which alter glucose utilization. Hypoglycemia may be more prevalent in the initial 3 days of therapy while a greater risk of hyperglycemia may be present after the initial 3 days (particularly days 4-10). Monitor closely and discontinue if hyper- or hypoglycemia occur. Tendon inflammation and/or rupture has been reported with this and other (Continued)

Gatifloxacin *(Continued)*

quinolone antibiotics. Discontinue at first signs or symptoms of tendon or pain. Quinolones may exacerbate myasthenia gravis. May cause peripheral neuropathy (rare); discontinue if symptoms of sensory or sensorimotor neuropathy occur.

Severe hypersensitivity reactions, including anaphylaxis, have occurred with quinolone therapy. Prolonged use may result in fungal or bacterial superinfection, including *C. difficile*-associated diarrhea and pseudomembranous colitis. Avoid excessive sunlight; other quinolones have been associated with moderate-to-severe phototoxicity reactions. Do not inject ophthalmic solution subconjunctivally or introduce directly into the anterior chamber of the eye.

Adverse Reactions (Reflective of adult population; not specific for elderly)
5% to 10%: Ocular: Conjunctival irritation, keratitis, lacrimation increased, papillary conjunctivitis
1% to 4%:
Central nervous system: Headache
Gastrointestinal: Taste disturbance
Ocular: Chemosis, conjunctival hemorrhage, discharge, dry eye, edema, irritation, pain, visual acuity decreased

Overdosage/Toxicology Potential symptoms of overdose include CNS excitation, seizures, QT prolongation, and arrhythmias (including torsade de pointes). Monitor by continuous ECG in the event of an overdose. Management is supportive and symptomatic. The drug is not removed by dialysis.

Stability Store between 15°C to 25°C (59°F to 77°F); do not freeze.

Mechanism of Action Gatifloxacin is a DNA gyrase inhibitor, and also inhibits topoisomerase IV. DNA gyrase (topoisomerase II) is an essential bacterial enzyme that maintains the superhelical structure of DNA. DNA gyrase is required for DNA replication and transcription, DNA repair, recombination, and transposition; inhibition is bactericidal.

Pharmacokinetics
Absorption: Well absorbed after oral administration
Distribution: V_d: 1.5-2.0 L/kg; concentrates in alveolar macrophages and lung parenchyma
Protein binding: 20%
Metabolism: Only 1% metabolized. No interaction with hepatic microsomal enzymes.
Bioavailability: 96%
Half-life: 7.1-13.9 hours (up to 30-40 hours in ESRD or CAPD)
Time to peak: Oral: 1 hour
Elimination: In urine, as unchanged drug (5% in feces)

Dosage
Geriatrics & Adults:
Bacterial conjunctivitis: Ophthalmic:
Days 1 and 2: Instill 1 drop into affected eye(s) every 2 hours while awake (maximum: 8 times/day)
Days 3-7: Instill 1 drop into affected eye(s) up to 4 times/day while awake

Administration Concentrated injection (10 mg/mL) must be diluted to 2 mg/mL prior to administration. No further dilution is required for premixed 100 mL and 200 mL solutions. Suspension may be administered through a gastric feeding tube.

Monitoring Parameters WBC, signs of infection, mental status

Patient Information May be taken with or without food. Drink plenty of fluids. Avoid exposure to direct sunlight during therapy and for several days following. Do not take antacids within 4 hours before or 2 hours after dosing. Contact your physician immediately if signs of allergy occur or if signs of tendon inflammation or pain occur. Do not discontinue therapy until your course has been completed. Take a missed dose as soon as possible, unless it is almost time for your next dose.

Additional Information Gatifloxacin causes a dose-dependent QT prolongation. Coadministration of gatifloxacin with other drugs that also prolong the QT interval or induce bradycardia (eg, beta-blockers, amiodarone) should be avoided. Careful consideration should be given in the use of gatifloxacin in patients with cardiovascular disease, particularly in those with conduction abnormalities.

Special Geriatric Considerations No dosage adjustment is required based on age, however, assessment of renal function is particularly important in this population.

Dosage Forms Excipient information presented when available (limited, particularly for generics); consult specific product labeling.
Solution, ophthalmic:
Zymar®: 0.3% (5 mL) [contains benzalkonium chloride]

♦ **Gaviscon® Extra Strength [OTC]** *see* Aluminum Hydroxide and Magnesium Carbonate *on page 64*

♦ **Gaviscon® Liquid [OTC]** *see* Aluminum Hydroxide and Magnesium Carbonate *on page 64*

♦ **Gaviscon® Tablet [OTC]** *see* Aluminum Hydroxide and Magnesium Trisilicate *on page 66*

- ◆ **G-CSF** see Filgrastim on page 624
- ◆ **G-CSF (PEG Conjugate)** see Pegfilgrastim on page 1212
- ◆ **GCV Sodium** see Ganciclovir on page 697
- ◆ **GD-Sildenafil** see Sildenafil on page 1463
- ◆ **Gel-Kam® [OTC]** see Fluoride on page 642
- ◆ **Gel-Kam® Rinse** see Fluoride on page 642
- ◆ **Gelusil® [OTC]** see Aluminum Hydroxide, Magnesium Hydroxide, and Simethicone on page 66

Gemfibrozil (jem FI broe zil)

Related Information
Hyperlipidemia Management on page 1773
Medication Safety Issues
Sound-alike/look-alike issues:
Lopid® may be confused with Levbid®, Lodine®, Lorabid®, Slo-bid™
U.S. Brand Names Lopid®
Canadian Brand Names Apo-Gemfibrozil®; Gen-Gemfibrozil; GMD-Gemfibrozil; Lopid®; Novo-Gemfibrozil; Nu-Gemfibrozil; PMS-Gemfibrozil
Index Terms CI-719
Generic Available Yes
Pharmacologic Category Antilipemic Agent, Fibric Acid
Use Hypertriglyceridemia in types IV and V hyperlipidemia for patients who are at greater risk for pancreatitis and who have not responded to dietary intervention; reduction of coronary heart disease in type IIb patients who have low HDL cholesterol, increased LDL cholesterol, and decreased triglycerides
Contraindications Hypersensitivity to gemfibrozil or any component of the formulation; significant hepatic or renal dysfunction; primary biliary cirrhosis; pre-existing gallbladder disease
Warnings/Precautions Abnormal elevation of AST, ALT, LDH, bilirubin, and alkaline phosphatase has occurred; if no appreciable triglyceride or cholesterol lowering effect occurs after 3 months, the drug should be discontinued; not useful for type I hyperlipidemia; myositis may be more common in patients with poor renal function
Adverse Reactions (Reflective of adult population; not specific for elderly)
>10%: Gastrointestinal: Dyspepsia (20%)
1% to 10%:
Central nervous system: Fatigue (4%), vertigo (2%), headache (1%)
Dermatologic: Eczema (2%), rash (2%)
Gastrointestinal: Abdominal pain (10%), diarrhea (7%), nausea/vomiting (3%), constipation (1%)

Reports where causal relationship has not been established: Weight loss, extrasystoles, pancreatitis, hepatoma, colitis, confusion, seizure, syncope, retinal edema, decreased fertility (male), renal dysfunction, positive ANA, drug-induced lupus-like syndrome, thrombocytopenia, anaphylaxis, vasculitis, alopecia, photosensitivity
Overdosage/Toxicology Symptoms include abdominal pain, diarrhea, nausea, and vomiting. Following GI decontamination, treatment is supportive.
Drug Interactions **Substrate** of CYP3A4 (minor); **Inhibits** CYP1A2 (moderate), 2C8 (strong), 2C9 (strong), 2C19 (strong)
Bexarotene's serum concentration is significantly increased; avoid concurrent use.
Chlorpropamide: May increase risk of hypoglycemia.
Cyclosporine's blood levels may be reduced; monitor cyclosporine levels and renal function.
CYP1A2 substrates: Gemfibrozil may increase the levels/effects of CYP1A2 substrates. Example substrates include aminophylline, fluvoxamine, mexiletine, mirtazapine, ropinirole, theophylline, and trifluoperazine.
CYP2C8 substrates: Gemfibrozil may increase the levels/effects of CYP2C8 substrates. Example substrates include amiodarone, paclitaxel, pioglitazone, repaglinide, and rosiglitazone.
CYP2C9 substrates: Gemfibrozil may increase the levels/effects of CYP2C9 substrates. Example substrates include bosentan, dapsone, fluoxetine, glimepiride, glipizide, losartan, montelukast, nateglinide, paclitaxel, phenytoin, warfarin, and zafirlukast.
CYP2C19 substrates: Gemfibrozil may increase the levels/effects of CYP2C19 substrates. Example substrates include citalopram, diazepam, methsuximide, phenytoin, propranolol, and sertraline.
Furosemide: Increased blood levels of both in hypoalbuminemia.
Glyburide (and possibly other sulfonylureas): The hypoglycemic effects may be increased.
HMG-CoA reductase inhibitors (atorvastatin, fluvastatin, lovastatin, pravastatin, simvastatin) may increase the risk of myopathy and rhabdomyolysis. The manufacturer
(Continued)

Gemfibrozil *(Continued)*

warns against the concurrent use of lovastatin (if unavoidable, limit lovastatin to <20 mg/day). Combination therapy with statins has been used in some patients with resistant hyperlipidemias (with great caution).

Repaglinide: Gemfibrozil may increase the serum concentration of repaglinide (prolonged, severe hypoglycemia has been reported). The addition of itraconazole may augment the effects of gemfibrozil on repaglinide. Consider alternative therapy.

Rifampin: Decreased gemfibrozil blood levels.

Warfarin: Hypoprothrombinemic response increased; monitor INRs closely when gemfibrozil is initiated or discontinued.

Ethanol/Nutrition/Herb Interactions Ethanol: Avoid ethanol to decrease triglycerides.

Mechanism of Action The exact mechanism of action of gemfibrozil is unknown, however, several theories exist regarding the VLDL effect; it can inhibit lipolysis and decrease subsequent hepatic fatty acid uptake as well as inhibit hepatic secretion of VLDL; together these actions decrease serum VLDL levels; increases HDL-cholesterol; the mechanism behind HDL elevation is currently unknown

Pharmacokinetics

Absorption: Oral: Well absorbed

Protein binding: 99%; a portion of the drug undergoes enterohepatic recycling

Metabolism: In the liver by oxidation to 2 inactive metabolites

Half-life: 1.4 hours

Time to peak serum concentration: Within 1-2 hours

Elimination: In urine (70%) primarily as glucuronide conjugate; some enterohepatic recycling

Dosage

Geriatrics & Adults: Hyperlipidemia/hypertriglyceridemia: Oral: 1200 mg/day in 2 divided doses, 30 minutes before breakfast and dinner

Renal Impairment: Hemodialysis effects: Not removed by hemodialysis; supplemental dose is not necessary.

Monitoring Parameters Fractionated cholesterol and triglycerides; CBC; liver function tests; blood glucose, especially in diabetics

Patient Information May cause dizziness or blurred vision, medication may cause abdominal or epigastric pain, diarrhea, nausea, or vomiting; notify physician if these become pronounced; take before meals

Additional Information If no appreciable triglyceride or cholesterol lowering effect occurs after 3 months, the drug should be discontinued

Special Geriatric Considerations Gemfibrozil is the drug of choice for the treatment of hypertriglyceridemia and hypoalphaproteinemia in the elderly; it is usually well tolerated; myositis may be more common in patients with poor renal function. The definition of and, therefore, when to treat hyperlipidemia in the elderly is a controversial issue. The National Cholesterol Education Program recommends that all adults maintain a plasma cholesterol <160 mg/dL. Older adults with one additional risk factor, goal LDL would be <130 mg/dL. It is the authors' belief that pharmacologic treatment be reserved for those who are unable to obtain a desirable plasma cholesterol concentration by diet alone and for whom the benefits of treatment are believed to outweigh the potential adverse effects, drug interactions, and cost of treatment.

Dosage Forms Excipient information presented when available (limited, particularly for generics); consult specific product labeling.

Tablet: 600 mg

Selected References

Duell PB, Connor WE, Illingworth DR, "Rhabdomyolysis After Taking Atorvastatin With Gemfibrozil," *Am J Cardiol*, 1998, 81(3):368-9.

"Executive Summary of The Third Report of The National Cholesterol Education Program (NCEP) Expert Panel on Detection, Evaluation, And Treatment of High Blood Cholesterol In Adults (Adult Treatment Panel III)," *JAMA*, 2001, 285(19):2486-97.

Gemifloxacin *(je mi FLOKS a sin)*

U.S. Brand Names Factive®

Canadian Brand Names Factive®

Index Terms DW286; Gemifloxacin Mesylate; LA 20304a; SB-265805

Generic Available No

Pharmacologic Category Antibiotic, Quinolone

Use Treatment of acute exacerbation of chronic bronchitis and community-acquired pneumonia, including pneumonia caused by multidrug-resistant strains of *S. pneumoniae* (MDRSP)

Unlabeled/Investigational Use Acute sinusitis

Contraindications Hypersensitivity to gemifloxacin, other fluoroquinolones, or any component of the formulation

Warnings/Precautions Fluoroquinolones may prolong QT_c interval; avoid use of gemifloxacin in patients with a history of QT_c prolongation, uncorrected hypokalemia, hypomagnesemia, or concurrent administration of other medications known to prolong the QT interval (including Class Ia and Class III antiarrhythmics, cisapride, erythromycin, antipsychotics, and tricyclic antidepressants). Use with caution in patients with significant bradycardia or acute myocardial ischemia. Use with caution in individuals at risk of seizures (CNS disorders or concurrent therapy with medications which may lower seizure threshold). Potential for seizures, although very rare, may be increased with concomitant NSAID therapy. Discontinue in patients who experience significant CNS adverse effects (dizziness, hallucinations, suicidal ideation or actions). Use caution in renal dysfunction; dosage adjustment required for Cl_{cr} ≤40 mL/minute.

Severe hypersensitivity reactions, including anaphylaxis, have occurred with quinolone therapy. If an allergic reaction occurs (itching, urticaria, dyspnea or facial edema, loss of consciousness, tingling, cardiovascular collapse), discontinue drug immediately. May cause mild-to-moderate maculopapular rash, usually 8-10 days after treatment initiation; risk factors may include age <40 years, female gender (including postmenopausal women on HRT), and treatment duration >7 days; discontinue therapy if rash develops. Avoid excessive sunlight; may rarely cause moderate-to-severe phototoxicity reaction similar to ciprofloxacin. Prolonged use may result in fungal or bacterial superinfection, including *C. difficile*-associated diarrhea and pseudomembranous colitis. Tendon inflammation and/or rupture has been reported with other quinolone antibiotics; risk may increase with concurrent corticosteroids, particularly in the elderly. Discontinue at first sign of tendon inflammation or pain. Peripheral neuropathy has been linked to the use of quinolones; these cases were rare.

Adverse Reactions (Reflective of adult population; not specific for elderly)
1% to 10%:
  Central nervous system: Headache (1%), dizziness (1%)
  Dermatologic: Rash (3%)
  Gastrointestinal: Diarrhea (4%), nausea (3%), abdominal pain (1%), vomiting (1%)
  Hepatic: Transaminases increased (1% to 2%)
Important adverse effects reported with other agents in this drug class include (not reported for gemifloxacin): Allergic reactions, CNS stimulation, hepatitis, jaundice, peripheral neuropathy, pneumonitis (eosinophilic), seizure; sensorimotor-axonal neuropathy (paresthesia, hypoesthesias, dysesthesias, weakness); severe dermatologic reactions (toxic epidermal necrolysis, Stevens-Johnson syndrome); tendon rupture, torsade de pointes, vasculitis

Overdosage/Toxicology Based on animal data, acute toxicity may manifest as ataxia, lethargy, tremor and/or seizures. Treatment is symptom-directed and supportive; 20% to 30% removed by hemodialysis.

Drug Interactions
  Corticosteroids: Concurrent use may increase the risk of tendon rupture, particularly in elderly patients (overall incidence rare).
  Glyburide: Quinolones may increase the effect of glyburide; monitor.
  Metal cations (aluminum, iron, magnesium, and zinc) bind quinolones in the gastrointestinal tract and inhibit absorption. Concurrent administration of most antacids (not calcium carbonate), oral electrolyte supplements, quinapril, sucralfate, some didanosine formulations (pediatric powder for oral suspension), and other highly-buffered oral drugs, should be avoided. Gemifloxacin should be administered 2 hours before or 3 hours after these agents.
  NSAIDs: Risk of seizures may be increased with concomitant NSAID use. Risk is considered quite low and may only be a factor with high serum levels of either agent and/or in patients with additional predisposing factors (eg, renal dysfunction, history of seizure or other neurological disorder)
  Probenecid: May decrease renal secretion of quinolones.
  QT_c-prolonging agents: Effects may be additive with gemifloxacin. Avoid concurrent use with Class Ia and Class III antiarrhythmics, erythromycin, cisapride, antipsychotics, and cyclic antidepressants.
  Typhoid vaccine: Antibiotics may decrease the therapeutic effect of live, attenuated Ty21a vaccine; delay vaccination for >24 hours after administration of antibacterial agents.
  Warfarin: The hypoprothrombinemic effect of warfarin may be enhanced by some quinolone antibiotics; monitor INR.

Ethanol/Nutrition/Herb Interactions Herb/Nutraceutical: Avoid dong quai, St John's wort (may also cause photosensitization).

Stability Store at 15°C to 30°C (59°F to 86°F). Protect from light.

Mechanism of Action Gemifloxacin is a DNA gyrase inhibitor and also inhibits topoisomerase IV. DNA gyrase (topoisomerase IV) is an essential bacterial enzyme that maintains the superhelical structure of DNA. DNA gyrase is required for DNA replication and transcription, DNA repair, recombination, and transposition; bactericidal

Pharmacokinetics
  Absorption: Well absorbed from the GI tract
  (Continued)

Gemifloxacin *(Continued)*

Distribution: V_{dss}: 4.2 L/kg
Bioavailability: 71%
Metabolism: Hepatic (minor); forms metabolites (CYP isoenzymes are not involved)
Time to peak, plasma: 0.5-2 hours
Protein binding: 60% to 70%
Half-life: 7 hours (range 4-12 hours)
Excretion: Feces (61%); urine (36%)

Dosage

Geriatrics & Adults:

Susceptible infections: Oral: 320 mg once daily

Acute exacerbations of chronic bronchitis: Oral: 320 mg once daily for 5 days

Community-acquired pneumonia (mild to moderate): Oral: 320 mg once daily for 5 or 7 days (decision to use 5- or 7-day regimen should be guided by initial sputum culture; 7 days are recommended for MDRSP, *Klebsiella*, or *M. catarrhalis* infection)

Sinusitis (unlabeled use): Oral: 320 mg once daily for 10 days

Renal Impairment: Cl_{cr} ≤40 mL/minute (or patients on hemodialysis/CAPD): 160 mg once daily (administer dose following hemodialysis)

Hepatic Impairment: No adjustment required.

Administration Gemifloxacin should be taken 3 hours before or 2 hours after supplements (including multivitamins) containing iron, zinc, or magnesium.

Monitoring Parameters WBC, signs/symptoms of infection, renal function

Patient Information Do not take any new medication during therapy without consulting prescriber. Take exactly as directed (with or without food). Should be taken at least 3 hours before or 2 hours after antacids or other drug products containing iron, aluminum, magnesium, or zinc (including multivitamins). Take entire prescription, even if feeling better. Unless instructed to restrict fluid intake, maintain adequate hydration (2-3 L/day of fluids) to avoid concentrated urine and crystal formation. May cause headache or dizziness (use caution when driving or engaging in hazardous tasks until response to drug is known); nausea, vomiting, or abdominal discomfort (small, frequent meals, frequent mouth care, chewing gum, or sucking lozenges may help); diarrhea (consult prescriber if persistent). If signs of inflammation or tendon pain occur, discontinue use immediately and report to prescriber. Discontinue use immediately and report to prescriber if you experience signs of allergic reaction (eg, itching, rash, respiratory difficulty, facial edema, or difficulty swallowing), chest pain, or palpitations. Report CNS changes (eg, hallucinations, suicidal ideation, seizures) or signs of opportunistic infection (unusual fever or chills; vaginal itching or foul-smelling vaginal discharge; easy bruising or bleeding; tendon or muscle pain).

Special Geriatric Considerations The risk of torsade de pointes and tendon inflammation and/or rupture associated with the concomitant use of corticosteroids and quinolones is increased in the elderly population.

Dosage Forms Excipient information presented when available (limited, particularly for generics); consult specific product labeling.
Tablet:
Factive®: 320 mg

- ♦ **Gemifloxacin Mesylate** *see* Gemifloxacin *on page 702*
- ♦ **Genac®** **[OTC]** *see* Triprolidine and Pseudoephedrine *on page 1638*
- ♦ **Genacote™** **[OTC]** *see* Aspirin *on page 127*
- ♦ **Genahist®** **[OTC]** *see* DiphenhydrAMINE *on page 447*
- ♦ **Genapap™** **[OTC]** *see* Acetaminophen *on page 29*
- ♦ **Genapap™ Children [OTC]** *see* Acetaminophen *on page 29*
- ♦ **Genapap™ Extra Strength [OTC]** *see* Acetaminophen *on page 29*
- ♦ **Genapap™ Infant [OTC]** *see* Acetaminophen *on page 29*
- ♦ **Genaphed®** **[OTC]** *see* Pseudoephedrine *on page 1346*
- ♦ **Genasal [OTC]** *see* Oxymetazoline *on page 1184*
- ♦ **Genasoft®** **[OTC]** *see* Docusate *on page 459*
- ♦ **Genasyme®** **[OTC]** *see* Simethicone *on page 1467*
- ♦ **Genaton™** **[OTC]** *see* Aluminum Hydroxide and Magnesium Carbonate *on page 64*
- ♦ **Genaton Tablet [OTC]** *see* Aluminum Hydroxide and Magnesium Trisilicate *on page 66*
- ♦ **Genatuss DM®** **[OTC]** *see* Guaifenesin and Dextromethorphan *on page 730*
- ♦ **Gencalc®** **600 [OTC]** *see* Calcium Salts (Oral) *on page 220*
- ♦ **Genebs [OTC]** *see* Acetaminophen *on page 29*
- ♦ **Genebs Extra Strength [OTC]** *see* Acetaminophen *on page 29*
- ♦ **Generlac** *see* Lactulose *on page 869*
- ♦ **Geneye®** **[OTC]** *see* Tetrahydrozoline *on page 1547*
- ♦ **Genfiber®** **[OTC]** *see* Psyllium *on page 1347*

Gentamicin (jen ta MYE sin)

Related Information
Aminoglycoside Dosing and Monitoring *on page 1794*
Antibiotic Treatment of Adults With Infective Endocarditis *on page 1797*
Antimicrobial Activity Against Selected Organisms *on page 1728*
Prevention of Infective Endocarditis *on page 1803*
Serum Drug Concentrations Commonly Monitored Guidelines *on page 1862*

Medication Safety Issues
Sound-alike/look-alike issues:
Gentamicin may be confused with kanamycin
Garamycin® may be confused with kanamycin, Terramycin®

U.S. Brand Names Genoptic® [DSC]; Gentak®

Canadian Brand Names Alcomicin®; Diogent®; Garamycin®; Gentamicin Injection, USP; SAB-Gentamicin

Index Terms Gentamicin Sulfate

Generic Available Yes

Pharmacologic Category Antibiotic, Aminoglycoside; Antibiotic, Ophthalmic; Antibiotic, Topical

Use Treatment of susceptible bacterial infections, normally gram-negative organisms including *Pseudomonas, Proteus, Serratia*, treatment of bone infections, CNS infections, respiratory tract infections, skin and soft tissue infections, as well as abdominal and urinary tract infections, endocarditis, and septicemia

Contraindications Hypersensitivity to gentamicin or other aminoglycosides

Warnings/Precautions [U.S. Boxed Warning]: Aminoglycosides may cause neurotoxicity and/or nephrotoxicity; usual risk factors include pre-existing renal impairment, concomitant neuro-/nephrotoxic medications, advanced age and dehydration. Ototoxicity may be directly proportional to the amount of drug given and the duration of treatment; tinnitus or vertigo are indications of vestibular injury and impending hearing loss; renal damage is usually reversible. May cause neuromuscular blockade and respiratory paralysis; especially when given soon after anesthesia or muscle relaxants.

Not intended for long-term therapy due to toxic hazards associated with extended administration; use caution in pre-existing renal insufficiency, vestibular or cochlear impairment, myasthenia gravis, hypocalcemia, conditions which depress neuromuscular transmission. Dosage modification required in patients with impaired renal function. Prolonged use may result in fungal or bacterial superinfection, including *C. difficile*-associated diarrhea and pseudomembranous colitis.

Adverse Reactions (Reflective of adult population; not specific for elderly)
>10%:
Central nervous system: Neurotoxicity (vertigo, ataxia)
Neuromuscular & skeletal: Gait instability
Otic: Ototoxicity (auditory), ototoxicity (vestibular)
Renal: Nephrotoxicity, decreased creatinine clearance
1% to 10%:
Cardiovascular: Edema
Dermatologic: Skin itching, reddening of skin, rash

Overdosage/Toxicology Symptoms include ototoxicity, nephrotoxicity, and neuromuscular toxicity. Serum level monitoring is recommended. The treatment of choice, following a single acute overdose, appears to be the maintenance of urine output of at least 3 mL/kg/hour. Dialysis is of questionable value in enhancing aminoglycoside elimination. If required, hemodialysis is preferred over peritoneal dialysis in patients with normal renal function. Careful hydration may be all that is required to promote diuresis and therefore enhance the drug's elimination. Chelation with penicillins is experimental.

Drug Interactions
Increased toxicity:
Aminoglycosides may potentiate the effects of neuromuscular-blocking agents.
Penicillins, cephalosporins, amphotericin B, loop diuretics may increase nephrotoxic potential
Decreased effect: Gentamicin's efficacy reduced when given concurrently with carbenicillin, ticarcillin, or piperacillin to patients with severe renal impairment (inactivation). Separate administration.

(Continued)

Gentamicin *(Continued)*

Stability

Gentamicin is a colorless to slightly yellow solution which should be stored between 2°C to 30°C, but refrigeration is not recommended.

I.V. infusion solutions mixed in NS or D_5W solution are stable for 24 hours at room temperature and refrigeration.

Premixed bag: Manufacturer expiration date.

Out of overwrap stability: 30 days.

Mechanism of Action
Interferes with bacterial protein synthesis by binding to 30S and 50S ribosomal subunits resulting in a defective bacterial cell membrane

Pharmacokinetics

Distribution: V_d: Increased by edema, ascites, fluid overload; decreased in patients with dehydration

Adults: 0.2-0.3 L/kg

Protein binding: <30%

Half-life: Adults: 1.5-3 hours; with anuria: 36-70 hours

Time to peak serum concentration:

I.M.: Within 30-90 minutes

I.V.: 30 minutes after a 30-minute I.V. infusion

Elimination: Clearance is directly related to renal function, eliminated almost completely by glomerular filtration of unchanged drug with excretion into the urine

The pharmacokinetics of the aminoglycosides are heterogeneous in older adults; it is best to assume that clearance is reduced and half-life prolonged in older adults, while volume of distribution is usually unchanged. The establishment of each patient's pharmacokinetic parameters is important for proper dosing in order to achieve optimal therapeutic benefit and minimize the risk of toxicity.

Dosage

Geriatrics & Adults: Individualization is **critical** because of the low therapeutic index.

Use of ideal body weight (IBW) for determining the mg/kg/dose appears to be more accurate than dosing on the basis of total body weight (TBW). In morbid obesity, dosage requirement may best be estimated using a dosing weight of IBW + 0.4 (TBW - IBW).

Initial and periodic plasma drug levels (eg, peak and trough with conventional dosing) should be determined, particularly in critically-ill patients with serious infections or in disease states known to significantly alter aminoglycoside pharmacokinetics (eg, cystic fibrosis, burns, or major surgery).

Usual dosage ranges:

I.M., I.V.:

Conventional: 1-2.5 mg/kg/dose every 8-12 hours; to ensure adequate peak concentrations early in therapy, higher initial dosage may be considered in selected patients when extracellular water is increased (edema, septic shock, postsurgical, or trauma)

Once daily: 4-7 mg/kg/dose once daily; some clinicians recommend this approach for all patients with normal renal function; this dose is at least as efficacious with similar, if not less, toxicity than conventional dosing

Intrathecal: 4-8 mg/day

Ophthalmic:

Ointment: Instill 1/2" (1.25 cm) 2-3 times/day to every 3-4 hours

Solution: Instill 1-2 drops every 2-4 hours, up to 2 drops every hour for severe infections

Topical: Apply 3-4 times/day to affected area

Indication-specific dosing: I.M., I.V.:

Brucellosis: 240 mg (I.M.) daily or 5 mg/kg (I.V.) daily for 7 days; either regimen recommended in combination with doxycycline

Cholangitis: 4-6 mg/kg once daily with ampicillin

Diverticulitis (complicated): 1.5-2 mg/kg every 8 hours (with ampicillin and metronidazole)

Endocarditis prophylaxis: Dental, oral, upper respiratory procedures, GI/GU procedures: 1.5 mg/kg with ampicillin (50 mg/kg) 30 minutes prior to procedure

Endocarditis or synergy (for Gram-positive infections): 1 mg/kg every 8 hours (with ampicillin)

Meningitis *(Enterococcus* sp or *Pseudomonas aeruginosa):* I.V.: Loading dose 2 mg/kg, then 1.7 mg/kg/dose every 8 hours (administered with another bacteriocidal drug)

Pelvic inflammatory disease: Loading dose: 2 mg/kg, then 1.5 mg/kg every 8 hours

Alternate therapy: 4.5 mg/kg once daily

Plague *(Yersinia pestis):* Treatment: 5 mg/kg/day, followed by postexposure prophylaxis with doxycycline

Pneumonia, hospital- or ventilator-associated: 7 mg/kg/day (with antipseudomonal beta-lactam or carbapenem)

Tularemia: 5 mg/kg/day divided every 8 hours for 1-2 weeks

Urinary tract infection: 1.5 mg/kg/dose every 8 hours

Renal Impairment:

Conventional dosing:

Cl_{cr} ≥60 mL/minute: Administer every 8 hours

Cl_{cr} 40-60 mL/minute: Administer every 12 hours

Cl_{cr} 20-40 mL/minute: Administer every 24 hours

Cl_{cr} <20 mL/minute: Loading dose, then monitor levels

High-dose therapy: Interval may be extended (eg, every 48 hours) in patients with moderate renal impairment (Cl_{cr} 30-59 mL/minute) and/or adjusted based on serum level determinations.

Hemodialysis: Dialyzable; removal by hemodialysis: 30% removal of aminoglycosides occurs during 4 hours of HD; administer dose after dialysis and follow levels

Removal by continuous ambulatory peritoneal dialysis (CAPD):

Administration via CAPD fluid:

Gram-negative infection: 4-8 mg/L (4-8 mcg/mL) of CAPD fluid

Gram-positive infection (eg, synergy): 3-4 mg/L (3-4 mcg/mL) of CAPD fluid

Administration via I.V., I.M. route during CAPD: Dose as for Cl_{cr} <10 mL/minute and follow levels

Removal via continuous arteriovenous or venovenous hemofiltration: Dose as for Cl_{cr} 10-40 mL/minute and follow levels

Hepatic Impairment: Monitor plasma concentrations.

Monitoring Parameters Urinalysis, urine output, BUN, serum creatinine; hearing should be tested before, during, and after treatment; particularly in those at risk for ototoxicity or who will be receiving prolonged therapy (>2 weeks). Obtain peak levels 30 minutes after the end of a 30-minute infusion; trough levels are drawn within 30 minutes before the next dose.

Reference Range

Therapeutic:

Peak: 4-8 mcg/mL (SI: 8-17 μmol/L)

Trough: <2 mcg/mL (SI: 4 μmol/L) (peak depends in part on the minimal inhibitory concentration of drug against organism being treated)

Once daily or extended interval: Trough: <0.5 mcg/mL

Toxic:

Peak: >12 mcg/mL (SI: >21 μmol/L)

Trough: >2 mcg/mL (SI: >8.4 μmol/L)

Test Interactions

Some penicillin derivatives may accelerate the degradation of aminoglycosides *in vitro*, leading to a potential underestimation of aminoglycoside serum concentration.

Patient Information Report any dizziness or sensations of ringing or fullness in ears; do not touch ophthalmics to eye; use no other eye drops within 5-10 minutes of instilling ophthalmic

Special Geriatric Considerations The aminoglycosides are important therapeutic interventions for infections due to susceptible organisms and as empiric therapy in seriously ill patients. Their use is not without risk of toxicity, however, these risks can be minimized if initial dosing is adjusted for estimated renal function and appropriate monitoring performed. High dose, once daily aminoglycosides have been advocated as an alternative to traditional dosing regimens. Once daily or extended interval dosing is as effective and may be safer than traditional dosing. The interval must be adjusted for renal function.

Dosage Forms Excipient information presented when available (limited, particularly for generics); consult specific product labeling. [DSC] = Discontinued product

Cream, topical, as sulfate: 0.1% (15 g, 30 g)

Infusion, as sulfate [premixed in NS]: 40 mg (50 mL); 60 mg (50 mL, 100 mL); 70 mg (50 mL); 80 mg (50 mL, 100 mL); 90 mg (100 mL); 100 mg (50 mL, 100 mL); 120 mg (100 mL)

Injection, solution, as sulfate [ADD-Vantage® vial]: 10 mg/mL (6 mL, 8 mL, 10 mL)

Injection, solution, as sulfate: 40 mg/mL (2 mL, 20 mL) [may contain sodium metabisulfite]

Injection, solution, pediatric, as sulfate: 10 mg/mL (2 mL) [may contain sodium metabisulfite]

Injection, solution, pediatric, as sulfate [preservative free]: 10 mg/mL (2 mL)

Ointment, ophthalmic, as sulfate (Gentak®): 0.3% [3 mg/g] (3.5 g)

Ointment, topical, as sulfate: 0.1% (15 g, 30 g)

Solution, ophthalmic, as sulfate: 0.3% (5 mL, 15 mL) [contains benzalkonium chloride]

Genoptic®: 0.3% (1 mL) [contains benzalkonium chloride] [DSC]

Gentak®: 0.3% (5 mL; 15 mL [DSC]) [contains benzalkonium chloride]

Selected References

Matzke GR, Jameson JJ, and Halstenson CE, "Gentamicin Disposition in Young and Elderly Patients With Various Degrees of Renal Function," *J Clin Pharmacol*, 1987, 27(3):216-20.

(Continued)

Gentamicin *(Continued)*

Nicolau DP, Freeman CD, Belliveau PP, et al, "Experience With a Once-Daily Aminoglycoside Program Administered to 2184 Adult Patients," *Antimicrob Agents Chemother*, 1995, 39(3):650-5.

Preston SL and Briceland LL, "Single Daily Dosing of Aminoglycosides," *Pharmacotherapy*, 1995, 15(3):297-316.

Zaske DE, Irvine P, Strand LM, et al, "Wide Interpatient Variations in Gentamicin Dose Requirements for Geriatric Patients," *JAMA*, 1982, 248(23):3122-6.

♦ **Gentamicin and Prednisolone** *see* Prednisolone and Gentamicin *on page 1306*
♦ **Gentamicin Sulfate** *see* Gentamicin *on page 705*
♦ **Geocillin**® *see* Carbenicillin *on page 236*
♦ **Geodon**® *see* Ziprasidone *on page 1701*
♦ **German Measles Vaccine** *see* Rubella Virus Vaccine (Live) *on page 1436*
♦ **GF196960** *see* Tadalafil *on page 1513*
♦ **GG** *see* Guaifenesin *on page 727*
♦ **Gladase**® *see* Papain and Urea *on page 1201*
♦ **Glargine Insulin** *see* Insulin Glargine *on page 810*
♦ **Glibenclamide** *see* GlyBURIDE *on page 714*

Glimepiride *(GLYE me pye ride)*

Medication Safety Issues
Sound-alike/look-alike issues:
Glimepiride may be confused with glipiZIDE
Amaryl® may be confused with Altace®, Amerge®, Reminyl®

High alert medication: The Institute for Safe Medication Practices (ISMP) includes this medication among its list of drugs which have a heightened risk of causing significant patient harm when used in error.

U.S. Brand Names Amaryl®

Canadian Brand Names Amaryl®; CO Glimepiride; Novo-Glimepiride; ratio-Glimepiride; Rhoxal-glimepiride; Sandoz-Glimepiride

Generic Available Yes

Pharmacologic Category Antidiabetic Agent, Sulfonylurea

Use Management of type 2 diabetes mellitus (noninsulin dependent, NIDDM) as an adjunct to diet and exercise to lower blood glucose; may be used in combination with metformin or insulin in patients whose hyperglycemia cannot be controlled by diet and exercise in conjunction with a single oral hypoglycemic agent

Contraindications Hypersensitivity to glimepiride, any component of the formulation, or sulfonamides; diabetic ketoacidosis (with or without coma)

Warnings/Precautions All sulfonylurea drugs are capable of producing severe hypoglycemia. Hypoglycemia is more likely to occur when caloric intake is deficient, after severe or prolonged exercise, when ethanol is ingested, or when more than one glucose-lowering drug is used. It is also more likely in elderly patients, malnourished patients and in patients with impaired renal or hepatic function; use with caution.

Chemical similarities are present among sulfonamides, sulfonylureas, carbonic anhydrase inhibitors, thiazides, and loop diuretics (except ethacrynic acid). Use in patients with sulfonamide allergy is specifically contraindicated in product labeling, however, a risk of cross-reaction exists in patients with allergy to any of these compounds; avoid use when previous reaction has been severe.

Product labeling states oral hypoglycemic drugs may be associated with an increased cardiovascular mortality as compared to treatment with diet alone or diet plus insulin. Data to support this association are limited, and several studies, including a large prospective trial (UKPDS) have not supported an association.

It may be necessary to discontinue therapy and administer insulin if the patient is exposed to stress (fever, trauma, infection, surgery).

Adverse Reactions (Reflective of adult population; not specific for elderly)
1% to 10%:
Central nervous system: Dizziness (2%), headache (2%)
Endocrine & metabolic: Hypoglycemia (1% to 2%)
Gastrointestinal: Nausea (1%)
Neuromuscular & skeletal: Weakness (2%)

Overdosage/Toxicology Symptoms include low blood sugar, tingling of lips and tongue, nausea, yawning, confusion, agitation, tachycardia, sweating, convulsions, stupor, and coma. Intoxications with sulfonylureas can cause hypoglycemia and are best managed with glucose administration (orally for milder hypoglycemia or by injection in more severe forms). Patients should be monitored for a minimum of 24-48 hours after ingestion.

Drug Interactions Substrate of CYP2C9 (major)
Beta-blockers: Beta-blockers may enhance the effects of sulfonylureas.

Chloramphenicol: Chloramphenicol may increase the effects of sulfonylureas.

Cimetidine: Cimetidine may increase the effects of glimepiride.

Cyclosporine: Sulfonylureas may increase the levels of cyclosporine.

CYP2C9 inducers: May decrease the levels/effects of glimepiride. Example inducers include carbamazepine, phenobarbital, phenytoin, rifampin, rifapentine, and secobarbital.

CYP2C9 inhibitors: May increase the levels/effects of glimepiride. Example inhibitors include delavirdine, fluconazole, gemfibrozil, ketoconazole, nicardipine, NSAIDs, sulfonamides, and tolbutamide.

Ethanol: Sulfonylureas may induce a disulfiram-like reaction.

Fibric acid derivatives: May increase the hypoglycemic effects of sulfonylureas; monitor.

Fluconazole: Fluconazole may increase the levels of sulfonylureas.

Hyperglycemia-producing agents: Certain drugs tend to produce hyperglycemia and may lead to loss of control. These drugs include the thiazides and other diuretics, corticosteroids, phenothiazines, thyroid products, estrogens, oral contraceptives, phenytoin, nicotinic acid, sympathomimetics, and isoniazid.

Pegvisomant: Pegvisomant may increase the effects of sulfonylureas.

Rifampin: Rifampin may decrease the effects of sulfonylureas.

Salicylates: Salicylates may increase the effects of sulfonylureas.

Sulfonamides: Sulfonamides may increase the effects of sulfonylureas.

Tricyclic antidepressants: TCAs may increase the effects of sulfonylureas.

Ethanol/Nutrition/Herb Interactions

Ethanol: Caution with ethanol (may cause hypoglycemia).

Herb/Nutraceutical: Caution with chromium, garlic, gymnema (may cause hypoglycemia).

Mechanism of Action Stimulates insulin release from the pancreatic beta cells; reduces glucose output from the liver; insulin sensitivity is increased at peripheral target sites

Pharmacodynamics

Onset of action: Peak effect: Blood glucose reductions: 2-3 hours

Duration: 24 hours

Pharmacokinetics

Absorption: 100%; delayed when given with food

Distribution: V_d: 8.8 L

Protein binding: >99.5%

Metabolism: Hepatic oxidation via CYP2C9 to M1 metabolite (~33% activity of parent compound); further oxidative metabolism to inactive M2 metabolite

Half-life elimination: 5-9 hours

Time to peak, plasma: 2-3 hours

Excretion: Urine (60%, 80% to 90% M1 and M2); feces (40%, 70% M1 and M2)

Dosage

Geriatrics: Initial: 1 mg/day; dose titration and maintenance dosing should be conservative to avoid hypoglycemia

Adults:

Type 2 diabetes: Oral:

Initial: 1-2 mg once daily, administered with breakfast or the first main meal

Adjustment: Allow several days between dose titrations: usual maintenance dose: 1-4 mg once daily; after a dose of 2 mg once daily, increase in increments of 2 mg at 1- to 2-week intervals based upon the patient's blood glucose response to a maximum of 8 mg once daily. If inadequate response to maximal dose, combination therapy with metformin may be considered.

Combination with insulin therapy:

Note: Fasting glucose level for instituting combination therapy is in the range of >150 mg/dL in plasma or serum depending on the patient)

Initial: 8 mg once daily with the first main meal

Adjustment: After starting with low-dose insulin, upward adjustments of insulin can be done approximately weekly as guided by frequent measurements of fasting blood glucose. Once stable, combination-therapy patients should monitor their capillary blood glucose on an ongoing basis, preferably daily.

Conversion from therapy with long half-life agents: Observe patient carefully for 1-2 weeks when converting from a longer half-life agent (eg, chlorpropamide) to glimepiride due to overlapping hypoglycemic effects.

Renal Impairment: Cl_{cr} <22 mL/minute: Initial starting dose should be 1 mg and dosage increments should be based on fasting blood glucose levels.

Administration Administer once daily with breakfast or first main meal of the day. Patients who are NPO may need to have their dose held to avoid hypoglycemia.

Monitoring Parameters Fasting blood glucose, hemoglobin A_{1c}, fructosamine

Reference Range Fasting blood glucose: Geriatrics: 100-150 mg/dL; Adults: 80-140 mg/dL

(Continued)

Glimepiride *(Continued)*

Patient Information Take with breakfast or first main meal; seek counseling by someone experienced in diabetes education about the signs and symptoms of hyper- and hypoglycemia, exercise, and diet; blood glucose monitoring, and other related topics; eat regularly, do not skip meals; carry quick source of sugar; wear medical alert bracelet

Special Geriatric Considerations Rapid and prolonged hypoglycemia (>12 hours) despite hypertonic glucose injections have been reported with glimepiride. Age, hepatic impairment, and renal impairment are independent risk factors for hypoglycemia; dosage titration should be made at weekly intervals. How "tightly" a geriatric patient's blood glucose should be controlled is controversial; however, a fasting blood sugar of <150 mg/dL is now an acceptable endpoint. Such a decision should be based on the patient's functional and cognitive status, how well they recognize hypoglycemic or hyperglycemic symptoms, and how to respond to them and their other disease states.

Dosage Forms Excipient information presented when available (limited, particularly for generics); consult specific product labeling.

Tablet: 1 mg, 2 mg, 4 mg

Amaryl®: 1 mg, 2 mg, 4 mg

♦ **Glimepiride and Pioglitazone** *see* Pioglitazone and Glimepiride *on page 1268*

♦ **Glimepiride and Pioglitazone Hydrochloride** *see* Pioglitazone and Glimepiride *on page 1268*

♦ **Glimepiride and Rosiglitazone Maleate** *see* Rosiglitazone and Glimepiride *on page 1430*

GlipiZIDE (GLIP i zide)

Medication Safety Issues

Sound-alike/look-alike issues:

GlipiZIDE may be confused with glimepiride, glyBURIDE

Glucotrol® may be confused with Glucophage®, Glucotrol® XL, glyBURIDE

Glucotrol® XL may be confused with Glucotrol®

High alert medication: The Institute for Safe Medication Practices (ISMP) includes this medication among its list of drugs which have a heightened risk of causing significant patient harm when used in error.

U.S. Brand Names Glucotrol®; Glucotrol® XL

Index Terms Glydiazinamide

Generic Available Yes

Pharmacologic Category Antidiabetic Agent, Sulfonylurea

Use Management of noninsulin-dependent diabetes mellitus (type II)

Contraindications Hypersensitivity to glipizide or any component of the formulation; other sulfonamides; type 1 diabetes mellitus (insulin dependent, IDDM); diabetic keto-acidosis

Warnings/Precautions All sulfonylurea drugs are capable of producing severe hypoglycemia. Hypoglycemia is more likely to occur when caloric intake is deficient, after severe or prolonged exercise, when ethanol is ingested, or when more than one glucose-lowering drug is used. It is also more likely in elderly patients, malnourished patients and in patients with impaired renal or hepatic function; use with caution.

Chemical similarities are present among sulfonamides, sulfonylureas, carbonic anhydrase inhibitors, thiazides, and loop diuretics (except ethacrynic acid). Use in patients with sulfonamide allergy is specifically contraindicated in product labeling, however, a risk of cross-reaction exists in patients with allergy to any of these compounds; avoid use when previous reaction has been severe.

Product labeling states oral hypoglycemic drugs may be associated with an increased cardiovascular mortality as compared to treatment with diet alone or diet plus insulin. Data to support this association are limited, and several studies, including a large prospective trial (UKPDS) have not supported an association.

Use with caution in patients with severe hepatic disease. It may be necessary to discontinue therapy and administer insulin if the patient is exposed to stress (fever, trauma, infection, surgery).

Avoid use of extended release tablets (Glucotrol® XL) in patients with known stricture/narrowing of the GI tract.

Adverse Reactions (Reflective of adult population; not specific for elderly)

Frequency not defined.

Cardiovascular: Edema, syncope

Central nervous system: Anxiety, depression, dizziness, drowsiness, headache, hypoesthesia, insomnia, nervousness, pain

Dermatologic: Eczema, erythema, maculopapular eruptions, morbilliform eruptions, photosensitivity, pruritus, rash, urticaria

Endocrine & metabolic: Disulfiram-like reaction, hypoglycemia, hyponatremia, SIADH (rare)

Gastrointestinal: Anorexia, constipation, diarrhea, epigatsric fullness, flatulence, gastralgia, hearburn, nausea, vomiting

Hematologic: Agranulocytopenia, aplastic anemia, blood dyscrasias, hemolytic anemia, leukopenia, pancytopenia, porphyria cutanea tarda, thrombocytopenia

Hepatic: Cholestatic jaundice, hepatic porphyria

Neuromuscular & skeletal: Arthralgia, leg cramps, myalgia, paresthesia, tremor

Ocular: Blurred vision

Renal: Diuretic effect (minor)

Respiratory: Rhinitis

Miscellaneous: Diaphoresis

Overdosage/Toxicology Symptoms include low blood sugar, tingling of lips and tongue, nausea, yawning, confusion, agitation, tachycardia, sweating, convulsions, stupor, and coma. Intoxications with sulfonylureas can cause hypoglycemia and are best managed with glucose administration (orally for milder hypoglycemia or by injection in more severe forms).

Drug Interactions Substrate of 2C9 (major)

Beta-blockers decrease hypoglycemic effect, mask most hypoglycemic symptoms, decrease glycogenolysis; avoid use in patients with diabetes with frequent hypoglycemic episodes.

Chloramphenicol: Chloramphenicol may decrease the metabolism of glipizide.

Cimetidine: Cimetidine may decrease the metabolism, via CYP isoenzymes, of glipizide.

Cyclic antidepressants: Cyclic antidepressants may enhance the hypoglycemic effect of glipizide.

Cyclosporine serum concentration is increased; monitor cyclosporine levels and renal function.

CYP2C9 inducers: May decrease the levels/effects of glipizide. Example inducers include carbamazepine, phenobarbital, phenytoin, rifampin, rifapentine, and secobarbital.

CYP2C9 inhibitors: May increase the levels/effects of glipizide. Example inhibitors include delavirdine, fluconazole, gemfibrozil, ketoconazole, nicardipine, NSAIDs, pioglitazone, and sulfonamides.

Fibric acid derivatives: Fibric acid derivatives may enhance the hypoglycemic effect of glipizide.

Fluconazole: Fluconazole may increase the serum concentration of glipizide.

Pegvisomant: Pegvisomant may enhance the hypoglycemic effect of glipizide.

Salicylates: Salicylates may enhance the hypoglycemic effect of glipizide. Of concern with regular, higher doses of salicylates, not sporadic, low doses.

Sulfonamide derivatives (sulfadiazine, sulfadoxine, sulfamethoxazole, sulfisoxazole): Sulfonamide derivatives (except sulfacetamide) may enhance the hypoglycemic effect of glipizide.

Ethanol/Nutrition/Herb Interactions

Ethanol: Caution with ethanol (may cause hypoglycemia or rare disulfiram reaction).

Food: A delayed release of insulin may occur if glipizide is taken with food. Immediate release tablets should be administered 30 minutes before meals to avoid erratic absorption.

Herb/Nutraceutical: Herbs with hypoglycemic properties may enhance the hypoglycemic effect of glipizide. This includes alfalfa, aloe, bilberry, bitter melon, burdock, celery, damiana, fenugreek, garcinia, garlic, ginger, ginseng (American), gymnema, marshmallow, stinging nettle

Mechanism of Action Stimulates insulin release from the pancreatic beta cells; reduces glucose output from the liver; insulin sensitivity is increased at peripheral target sites

Pharmacodynamics

Duration: 12-24 hours

Pharmacokinetics

Absorption: Rapid and complete; delayed with food

Distribution: 10-11 L

Protein binding: 98% to 99%; primarily to albumin

Bioavailability: 90% to 100%

Metabolism: Hepatic via CYP2C9; forms metabolites (inactive)

Half-life elimination: 2-5 hours

Time to peak: 1-3 hours; extended release tablets: 6-12 hours

Excretion: Urine (60% to 80%, 91% to 97% as metabolites); feces (11%)

(Continued)

GlipiZIDE *(Continued)*

Dosage

Geriatrics: Initial: 2.5 mg/day; increase by 2.5-5 mg/day at 1- to 2-week intervals.

Adults:

Type 2 diabetes: Oral (allow several days between dose titrations): Initial: 5 mg/day; adjust dosage at 2.5-5 mg daily increments as determined by blood glucose response at intervals of several days.

Immediate release tablet: Maximum recommended once-daily dose: 15 mg; maximum recommended total daily dose: 40 mg. Doses >15 mg/day should be administered in divided doses.

Extended release tablet (Glucotrol® XL): Maximum recommended dose: 20 mg

When transferring from insulin to glipizide:

Current insulin requirement ≤20 units: Discontinue insulin and initiate glipizide at usual dose

Current insulin requirement >20 units: Decrease insulin by 50% and initiate glipizide at usual dose; gradually decrease insulin dose based on patient response. Several days should elapse between dosage changes.

Renal Impairment: Cl_{cr} <10 mL/minute: Some investigators recommend not using.

Hepatic Impairment: Initial dosage should be 2.5 mg/day.

Administration Administer immediate release tablets 30 minutes before a meal to achieve greatest reduction in postprandial hyperglycemia. Extended release tablets should be given with breakfast. Patients who are NPO may need to have their dose held to avoid hypoglycemia.

Monitoring Parameters Signs and symptoms of hypoglycemia (fatigue, excessive hunger, profuse sweating, numbness of extremities), blood glucose, hemoglobin A_{1c}

Reference Range Recommendations for glycemic control in adults with diabetes:

Hb A_{1c}: <7%

Preprandial capillary plasma glucose: 90-130 mg/dL

Peak postprandial capillary blood glucose: <180 mg/dL

Blood pressure: <130/80 mm Hg

Patient Information Patients must be counseled by someone experienced in diabetes education about the signs and symptoms of hyper- and hypoglycemia, exercise and diet, blood glucose monitoring, and other related topics; eat regularly, do not skip meals; carry quick source of sugar; medical alert bracelet

Special Geriatric Considerations Glipizide is a useful agent since there are few drug to drug interactions and elimination of the active drug is not dependent upon renal function. How "tightly" a geriatric patient's blood glucose should be controlled is controversial; however, a fasting blood sugar <150 mg/dL is now an acceptable endpoint. Such a decision should be based on the patient's functional and cognitive status, how well they recognize hypoglycemic or hyperglycemic symptoms, and how to respond to them and their other disease states.

Dosage Forms Excipient information presented when available (limited, particularly for generics); consult specific product labeling.

Tablet: 5 mg, 10 mg

Glucotrol®: 5 mg, 10 mg

Tablet, extended release: 2.5 mg, 5 mg, 10 mg

Glucotrol® XL: 2.5 mg, 5 mg, 10 mg

Selected References

Brodows RG, "Benefits and Risks With Glyburide and Glipizide in Elderly NIDDM Patients," *Diabetes Care*, 1992, 15(1):75-80.

Kradjan WA, Kobayashi KA, Bauer LA, et al, "Glipizide Pharmacokinetics: Effects of Age, Diabetes, and Multiple Dosing," *J Clin Pharmacol*, 1989, 29(12):1121-7.

Kradjan WA, Takeuchi KY, Opheim KE, et al, "Pharmacokinetics and Pharmacodynamics of Glipizide After Once-Daily and Divided Doses," *Pharmacotherapy*, 1995, 15(4):465-71.

Rosenstock J, Corrao PJ, Goldberg RB, et al, "Diabetes Control in the Elderly: A Randomized, Comparative Study of Glyburide Versus Glipizide in Noninsulin Dependent Diabetes Mellitus," *Clin Ther*, 1993, 15(6):1031-40.

"Standards of Medical Care for Patients With Diabetes Mellitus. American Diabetes Association," *Diabetes Care*, 2007, 30(Suppl 1):4-41.

Glipizide and Metformin (GLIP i zide & met FOR min)

Related Information

GlipiZIDE *on page 710*

Metformin *on page 993*

Medication Safety Issues

High alert medication: The Institute for Safe Medication Practices (ISMP) includes this medication among its list of drugs which have a heightened risk of causing significant patient harm when used in error.

U.S. Brand Names Metaglip™

Index Terms Glipizide and Metformin Hydrochloride; Metformin and Glipizide

Generic Available Yes

Pharmacologic Category Antidiabetic Agent, Biguanide; Antidiabetic Agent, Sulfonylurea

Use Initial therapy for management of type 2 diabetes mellitus (noninsulin dependent, NIDDM) when hyperglycemia cannot be managed with diet and exercise alone; second-line therapy for management of type 2 diabetes (NIDDM) when hyperglycemia cannot be managed with a sulfonylurea or metformin along with diet and exercise

Dosage

Geriatrics: Conservative doses are recommended in the elderly due to potentially decreased renal function; **do not titrate to maximum dose**; should not be used in patients ≥80 years unless renal function is verified as normal

Adults:

Type 2 diabetes, first-line therapy: Oral: Initial: Glipizide 2.5 mg/metformin 250 mg once daily with a meal. Dose adjustment: Increase dose by 1 tablet/day every 2 weeks, up to a maximum of glipizide 10 mg/metformin 1000 mg daily

Patients with fasting plasma glucose (FPG) 280-320 mg/dL: Oral: Consider glipizide 2.5 mg/metformin 500 mg twice daily. Dose adjustment: Increase dose by 1 tablet/day every 2 weeks, up to a maximum of glipizide 10 mg/metformin 2000 mg daily in divided doses

Type 2 diabetes, second-line therapy: Oral: Glipizide 2.5 mg/metformin 500 mg **or** glipizide 5 mg/metformin 500 mg twice daily with morning and evening meals; starting dose should not exceed current daily dose of glipizide (or sulfonylurea equivalent) or metformin. Dose adjustment: Titrate dose in increments of no more than glipizide 5 mg/metformin 500 mg, up to a maximum dose of glipizide 20 mg/metformin 2000 mg daily.

Renal Impairment: Risk of lactic acidosis increases with degree of renal impairment; contraindicated in renal disease or renal dysfunction (see Contraindications).

Hepatic Impairment: Use should be avoided; liver disease is a risk factor for the development of lactic acidosis during metformin therapy.

Dosage Forms Excipient information presented when available (limited, particularly for generics); consult specific product labeling.

Tablet: 2.5/250: Glipizide 2.5 mg and metformin hydrochloride 250 mg; 2.5/500: Glipizide 2.5 mg and metformin hydrochloride 500 mg; 5/500: Glipizide 5 mg and metformin hydrochloride 500 mg

Metaglip™ 2.5/250: Glipizide 2.5 mg and metformin hydrochloride 250 mg
Metaglip™ 2.5/500: Glipizide 2.5 mg and metformin hydrochloride 500 mg
Metaglip™ 5/500: Glipizide 5 mg and metformin hydrochloride 500 mg

♦ **Glipizide and Metformin Hydrochloride** *see* Glipizide and Metformin *on page 712*
♦ **GlucaGen**® *see* Glucagon *on page 713*
♦ **GlucaGen**® **Diagnostic Kit** *see* Glucagon *on page 713*
♦ **GlucaGen**® **HypoKit**™ *see* Glucagon *on page 713*

Glucagon (GLOO ka gon)

Medication Safety Issues

Sound-alike/look-alike issues:

Glucagon may be confused with Glaucon®

U.S. Brand Names GlucaGen®; GlucaGen® Diagnostic Kit; GlucaGen® HypoKit™; Glucagon Diagnostic Kit [DSC]; Glucagon Emergency Kit

Index Terms Glucagon Hydrochloride

Generic Available No

Pharmacologic Category Antidote; Diagnostic Agent

Use Management of hypoglycemia; diagnostic aid in radiologic examinations to temporarily inhibit GI tract movement

Unlabeled/Investigational Use Used with some success as a cardiac stimulant in management of severe cases of beta-adrenergic blocking agent overdosage; treatment of myocardial depression due to calcium channel blocker overdose

Contraindications Hypersensitivity to glucagon or any component of the formulation; insulinoma; pheochromocytoma

Warnings/Precautions Use caution with prolonged fasting, starvation, adrenal insufficiency or chronic hypoglycemia; levels of glucose stores in liver may be decreased. Following response to therapy, oral carbohydrates should be administered to prevent hypoglycemia. Monitor blood glucose levels closely.

Adverse Reactions (Reflective of adult population; not specific for elderly)

Frequency not defined.

Cardiovascular: Hypotension (up to 2 hours after GI procedures), hypertension, tachycardia

Gastrointestinal: Nausea, vomiting (high incidence with rapid administration of high doses)

Miscellaneous: Hypersensitivity reactions, anaphylaxis

(Continued)

Glucagon (Continued)

Overdosage/Toxicology Symptoms include hypokalemia, nausea and vomiting, inhibition of GI tract motility, decreased blood pressure, tachycardia

Drug Interactions Oral anticoagulant: Hypoprothrombinemic effects may be increased possibly with bleeding; effect seen with glucagon doses of 50 mg administered over 1-2 days

Ethanol/Nutrition/Herb Interactions Glucagon depletes glycogen stores.

Stability Prior to reconstitution, store at controlled room temperature of 20°C to 25°C (69°F to 77°F); do not freeze. Reconstitute powder for injection by adding 1 mL of sterile diluent to a vial containing 1 unit of the drug, to provide solutions containing 1 mg of glucagon/mL. Gently roll vial to dissolve. If dose to be administered is <2 mg of the drug, then use only the diluent provided by the manufacturer. If >2 mg, use sterile water for injection. Use immediately after reconstitution. May be kept at 5°C for up to 48 hours if necessary.

Mechanism of Action Stimulates adenylate cyclase to produce increased cyclic AMP, which promotes hepatic glycogenolysis and gluconeogenesis, causing a raise in blood glucose levels

Pharmacokinetics
Metabolism: In the liver with some inactivation occurring in the kidneys and plasma
Half-life, plasma: 3-10 minutes

Dosage
Geriatrics & Adults:
Hypoglycemia or insulin shock therapy: I.M., I.V., SubQ: 1 mg; may repeat in 20 minutes as needed
Note: If patient fails to respond to glucagon, I.V. dextrose must be given.
Beta-blocker overdose, calcium channel blocker overdose (unlabeled use): I.V.: 5-10 mg over 1 minutes followed by an infusion of 1-10 mg/hour. The following has also been reported for beta-blocker overdose: 3-10 mg or initially 0.5-5 mg bolus followed by continuous infusion 1-5 mg/hour
Diagnostic aid: I.M., I.V.: 0.25-2 mg 10 minutes prior to procedure

Administration I.V.: Bolus may be associated with nausea and vomiting. Continuous infusions may be used in beta-blocker overdose/toxicity.

Monitoring Parameters Blood pressure, blood glucose, heart rate

Patient Information Instruct a close associate on how to prepare and administer as a treatment for insulin shock

Additional Information 1 unit = 1 mg

Special Geriatric Considerations No specific recommendations needed.

Dosage Forms Excipient information presented when available (limited, particularly for generics); consult specific product labeling.
Injection, powder for reconstitution, as hydrochloride:
GlucaGen®: 1 mg [equivalent to 1 unit; contains lactose 107 mg]
GlucaGen® Diagnostic Kit: 1 mg [equivalent to 1 unit; contains lactose 107 mg; packaged with sterile water]
GlucaGen® HypoKit™: 1 mg [equivalent to 1 unit; contains lactose 107 mg; packaged with prefilled syringe containing sterile water]
Glucagon®: 1 mg [equivalent to 1 unit; contains lactose 49 mg]
Glucagon Diagnostic Kit, Glucagon Emergency Kit: 1 mg [equivalent to 1 unit; contains lactose 49 mg; packaged with diluent syringe containing glycerin 12 mg/mL and water for injection]

♦ **Glucagon Diagnostic Kit [DSC]** see Glucagon on page 713
♦ **Glucagon Emergency Kit** see Glucagon on page 713
♦ **Glucagon Hydrochloride** see Glucagon on page 713
♦ **Glucophage®** see Metformin on page 993
♦ **Glucophage® XR** see Metformin on page 993
♦ **Glucotrol®** see GlipiZIDE on page 710
♦ **Glucotrol® XL** see GlipiZIDE on page 710
♦ **Glucovance®** see Glyburide and Metformin on page 717
♦ **Glulisine Insulin** see Insulin Glulisine on page 811
♦ **Glumetza™** see Metformin on page 993
♦ **Glybenclamide** see GlyBURIDE on page 714
♦ **Glybenzcyclamide** see GlyBURIDE on page 714

GlyBURIDE (GLYE byoor ide)

Medication Safety Issues
Sound-alike/look-alike issues:
GlyBURIDE may be confused with glipiZIDE, Glucotrol®
Diaβeta® may be confused with Diabinese®, Zebeta®

Micronase® may be confused with microK®, miconazole, Micronor®, Microzide™

High alert medication: The Institute for Safe Medication Practices (ISMP) includes this medication among its list of drugs which have a heightened risk of causing significant patient harm when used in error.

U.S. Brand Names Diaβeta®; Glynase® PresTab®; Micronase®

Canadian Brand Names Albert® Glyburide; Apo-Glyburide®; Diaβeta®; Euglucon®; Gen-Glybe; Novo-Glyburide; Nu-Glyburide; PMS-Glyburide; ratio-Glyburide; Sandoz-Glyburide

Index Terms Diabeta; Glibenclamide; Glybenclamide; Glybenzcyclamide

Generic Available Yes

Pharmacologic Category Antidiabetic Agent, Sulfonylurea

Use Management of noninsulin-dependent diabetes mellitus (type II)

Contraindications Hypersensitivity to glyburide, any component of the formulation, or other sulfonamides; type 1 diabetes mellitus (insulin dependent, IDDM), diabetic keto-acidosis; concurrent use with bosentan

Warnings/Precautions All sulfonylurea drugs are capable of producing severe hypo-glycemia. Hypoglycemia is more likely to occur when caloric intake is deficient, after severe or prolonged exercise, when ethanol is ingested, or when more than one glucose-lowering drug is used. It is also more likely in elderly patients, malnourished patients and in patients with impaired renal or hepatic function; use with caution.

Elderly: Rapid and prolonged hypoglycemia (>12 hours) despite hypertonic glucose injections have been reported; age and hepatic and renal impairment are independent risk factors for hypoglycemia; dosage titration should be made at weekly intervals.

Chemical similarities are present among sulfonamides, sulfonylureas, carbonic anhy-drase inhibitors, thiazides, and loop diuretics (except ethacrynic acid). Use in patients with sulfonamide allergy is specifically contraindicated in product labeling, however, a risk of cross-reaction exists in patients with allergy to any of these compounds; avoid use when previous reaction has been severe.

Product labeling states oral hypoglycemic drugs may be associated with an increased cardiovascular mortality as compared to treatment with diet alone or diet plus insulin. Data to support this association are limited, and several studies, including a large prospective trial (UKPDS) have not supported an association.

It may be necessary to discontinue therapy and administer insulin if the patient is exposed to stress (fever, trauma, infection, surgery).

Adverse Reactions (Reflective of adult population; not specific for elderly)
Frequency not defined.
Cardiovascular: Vasculitis
Central nervous system: Headache, dizziness
Dermatologic: Erythema, maculopapular eruptions, morbilliform eruptions, pruritus, purpura, rash, urticaria, photosensitivity reaction
Endocrine & metabolic: Disulfiram-like reaction, hypoglycemia, hyponatremia (SIADH reported with other sulfonylureas)
Gastrointestinal: Nausea, epigastric fullness, heartburn, constipation, diarrhea, anorexia
Genitourinary: Nocturia
Hematologic: Leukopenia, thrombocytopenia, hemolytic anemia, agranulocytosis, aplastic anemia, pancytopenia, porphyria cutanea tarda
Hepatic: Cholestatic jaundice, hepatitis, transaminase increased
Neuromuscular & skeletal: Arthralgia, myalgia, paresthesia
Ocular: Blurred vision
Renal: Diuretic effect (minor)
Miscellaneous: Allergic reaction

Overdosage/Toxicology Symptoms include severe hypoglycemia, seizures, cerebral damage, tingling of lips and tongue, nausea, yawning, confusion, agitation, tachy-cardia, sweating, convulsions, stupor, and coma. Intoxications with sulfonylureas can cause hypoglycemia and are best managed with glucose administration (orally for milder hypoglycemia or by injection in more severe forms).

Drug Interactions Inhibits CYP2C8 (weak), 3A4 (weak)
Beta-blockers: Beta-blockers may enhance the hypoglycemic effect of glyburide and mask tachycardia as an initial symptom of hypoglycemia.
Bosentan: Glyburide may enhance the hepatotoxic effect and increase the metabolism of bosentan. Bosentan may increase the metabolism of glyburide. Concomitant use is contraindicated
Chloramphenicol: Chloramphenicol may decrease the metabolism of glyburide.
Cimetidine: Cimetidine may decrease the metabolism, via CYP isoenzymes, of glybu-ride.
Cyclic antidepressants: Cyclic antidepressants may enhance the hypoglycemic effect of glyburide.
Cyclosporine: Glyburide may increase the serum concentration of cyclosporine.
(Continued)

GlyBURIDE *(Continued)*

Fibric acid derivatives: Fibric acid derivatives may enhance the hypoglycemic effect of glyburide.

Fluconazole: Fluconazole may increase the serum concentration of glyburide.

Pegvisomant: Pegvisomant may enhance the hypoglycemic effect of glyburide.

Quinolone antibiotics: Quinolone antibiotics may enhance the hypoglycemic effect of glyburide.

Rifampin: Rifampin may increase the metabolism, via CYP isoenzymes, of glyburide.

Salicylates: Salicylates may enhance the hypoglycemic effect of glyburide. Of concern with regular, higher doses of salicylates, not sporadic, low doses.

Sulfonamide derivatives (sulfadiazine, sulfadoxine, sulfamethoxazole, sulfisoxazole): Sulfonamide derivatives (except sulfacetamide) may enhance the hypoglycemic effect of glyburide.

Ethanol/Nutrition/Herb Interactions

Ethanol: Caution with ethanol (may cause hypoglycemia).

Herb/Nutraceutical: Herbs with hypoglycemic properties may enhance the hypoglycemic effect of glyburide. This includes alfalfa, aloe, bilberry, bitter melon, burdock, celery, damiana, fenugreek, garcinia, garlic, ginger, ginseng (American), gymnema, marshmallow, stinging nettle

Mechanism of Action Stimulates insulin release from the pancreatic beta cells; reduces glucose output from the liver; insulin sensitivity is increased at peripheral target sites

Pharmacodynamics

Onset of action: Serum insulin levels begin to increase 15-60 minutes after a single dose

Duration: ≤24 hours

Pharmacokinetics

Absorption: Significant within 1 hour

Distribution: 9-10 L

Protein binding, plasma: >99% primarily to albumin

Metabolism: Hepatic; forms metabolites (weakly active)

Half-life elimination: Diabeta®, Micronase®: 10 hours; Glynase® PresTab®: ~4 hours; may be prolonged with renal or hepatic impairment

Time to peak, serum: Adults: 2-4 hours

Excretion: Feces (50%) and urine (50%) as metabolites

Dosage

Geriatrics: Regular tablets (Diaβeta®, Micronase®): Oral: Initial: 1.25-2.5 mg/day, increase by 1.25-2.5 mg/day every 1-3 weeks. Refer to adult dosing.

Adults:

Type 2 diabetes: Oral:

Note: Regular tablets cannot be used interchangeably with micronized tablet formulations

Regular tablets (Diaβeta®, Micronase®):

Initial: 2.5-5 mg/day, administered with breakfast or the first main meal of the day. In patients who are more sensitive to hypoglycemic drugs, start at 1.25 mg/day.

Adjustment: Increase in increments of no more than 2.5 mg/day at weekly intervals based on the patient's blood glucose response

Maintenance: 1.25-20 mg/day given as single or divided doses; maximum: 20 mg/day

Micronized tablets (Glynase® PresTab®):

Initial: 1.5-3 mg/day, administered with breakfast or the first main meal of the day in patients who are more sensitive to hypoglycemic drugs, start at 0.75 mg/day. Increase in increments of no more than 1.5 mg/day in weekly intervals based on the patient's blood glucose response.

Maintenance: 0.75-12 mg/day given as a single dose or in divided doses. Some patients (especially those receiving >6 mg/day) may have a more satisfactory response with twice-daily dosing. Maximum: 12 mg/day

Renal Impairment: Cl_{cr} <50 mL/minute: Not recommended

Hepatic Impairment: Use conservative initial and maintenance doses and avoid use in severe disease.

Monitoring Parameters Fasting blood glucose, hemoglobin A_{1c}, fructosamine

Reference Range Recommendations for glycemic control in adults with diabetes:

Hb A_{1c}: <7%

Preprandial capillary plasma glucose: 90-130 mg/dL

Peak postprandial capillary blood glucose: <180 mg/dL

Blood pressure: <130/80 mm Hg

Patient Information Patients must be counseled by someone experienced in diabetes education about the signs and symptoms of hyper- and hypoglycemia, exercise and diet, blood glucose monitoring, and other related topics; eat regularly, do not skip meals; carry quick source of sugar; medical alert bracelet

Special Geriatric Considerations Rapid and prolonged hypoglycemia (>12 hours) despite hypertonic glucose injections has been reported; age, hepatic, and renal impairment are independent risk factors for hypoglycemia; dosage titration should be made at weekly intervals. How "tightly" a geriatric patient's blood glucose should be controlled is controversial; however, a fasting blood sugar <150 mg/dL is now an acceptable endpoint. Such a decision should be based on the patient's functional and cognitive status, how well they recognize hypoglycemic or hyperglycemic symptoms, and how to respond to them and their other disease states. Use with caution in the elderly with renal insufficiency.

Dosage Forms Excipient information presented when available (limited, particularly for generics); consult specific product labeling.
Tablet: 1.25 mg, 2.5 mg, 5 mg
DiaβBeta®, Micronase®: 1.25 mg, 2.5 mg, 5 mg
Tablet, micronized: 1.5 mg, 3 mg, 6 mg
Glynase® PresTab®: 3 mg, 6 mg

Selected References
Brodows RG, "Benefits and Risks With Glyburide and Glipizide in Elderly NIDDM Patients," *Diabetes Care*, 1992, 15(1):75-80.

Rosenstock J, Corrao PJ, Goldberg RB, et al, "Diabetes Control in the Elderly: A Randomized, Comparative Study of Glyburide Versus Glipizide in Non-insulin-Dependent Diabetes Mellitus," *Clin Ther*, 1993, 15(6):1031-40.

Sonnenblick M and Shilo S, "Glibenclamide Induced Prolonged Hypoglycaemia," *Age Ageing*, 1986, 15(3):185-9.

"Standards of Medical Care for Patients With Diabetes Mellitus. American Diabetes Association," *Diabetes Care*, 2007, 30(Suppl 1):4-41.

Glyburide and Metformin (GLYE byoor ide & met FOR min)

Related Information
GlyBURIDE *on page 714*
Metformin *on page 993*

Medication Safety Issues
Sound-alike/look-alike issues:
Glucovance may be confused with Vyvanse™

High alert medication: The Institute for Safe Medication Practices (ISMP) includes this medication among its list of drugs which have a heightened risk of causing significant patient harm when used in error.

U.S. Brand Names Glucovance®

Index Terms Glyburide and Metformin Hydrochloride; Metformin and Glyburide

Generic Available Yes

Pharmacologic Category Antidiabetic Agent, Biguanide; Antidiabetic Agent, Sulfonylurea

Use Initial treatment as an adjunct to diet and exercise in patients with type 2 diabetes whose diabetes is not adequately controlled by diet and exercise. Second-line therapy when diet and exercise and a sulfonylurea or metformin do not result in adequate glycemic control in patients with type 2 diabetes.

Dosage
Geriatrics: Refer to adult dosing. Adjust carefully to renal function. Should not be used in patients ≥80 years of age unless renal function is verified as normal.

Adults: Note: Dose must be individualized. All doses should be taken with a meal. Twice daily dosage should be taken with the morning and evening meals. Dosages expressed as glyburide/metformin components.

Type 2 diabetes: Oral:
No prior treatment with sulfonylurea or metformin: Initial: 1.25 mg/250 mg once daily with a meal; patients with Hb A$_{1c}$ >9% or fasting plasma glucose (FPG) >200 mg/dL may start with 1.25 mg/250 mg twice daily. Adjustment: Dosage may be increased in increments of 1.25 mg/250 mg, at intervals of not less than 2 weeks; maximum daily dose: 10 mg/2000 mg (limited experience with higher doses)

Previously treated with a sulfonylurea or metformin alone: Initial: 2.5 mg/500 mg or 5 mg/500 mg twice daily; increase in increments no greater than 5 mg/500 mg; maximum daily dose: 20 mg/2000 mg

Note: When switching patients previously on a sulfonylurea and metformin together, do not exceed the daily dose of glyburide (or glyburide equivalent) or metformin.

Combination with thiazolidinedione: May be combined with a thiazolidinedione in patients with an inadequate response to glyburide/metformin therapy, however the risk of hypoglycemia may be increased.

Special Geriatric Considerations Conservative doses are recommended in the elderly due to potentially decreased renal function. **Do not titrate to maximum dose.** Should not be used in patients ≥80 years of age unless renal function is verified as normal.
(Continued)

Glyburide and Metformin *(Continued)*

Dosage Forms Excipient information presented when available (limited, particularly for generics); consult specific product labeling.
Tablet:
1.25 mg/250 mg: Glyburide 1.25 mg and metformin hydrochloride 250 mg
2.5 mg/500 mg: Glyburide 2.5 mg and metformin hydrochloride 500 mg
5 mg/500 mg: Glyburide 5 mg and metformin hydrochloride 500 mg

♦ **Glyburide and Metformin Hydrochloride** *see* Glyburide and Metformin *on page 717*

Glycerin (GLIS er in)

U.S. Brand Names Bausch & Lomb® Computer Eye Drops [OTC]; Colace® Adult/Children Suppositories [OTC]; Colace® Infant/Children Suppositories [OTC]; Fleet® Babylax® [OTC]; Fleet® Glycerin Suppositories [OTC]; Fleet® Glycerin Suppositories Maximum Strength [OTC]; Fleet® Liquid Glycerin Suppositories [OTC]; Osmoglyn® [DSC]; Sani-Supp® [OTC]
Index Terms Glycerol
Generic Available Yes: Suppositories
Pharmacologic Category Laxative, Osmotic; Ophthalmic Agent, Miscellaneous
Use Treatment of constipation; reduction of intraocular pressure, corneal edema; has been administered orally to reduce intracranial pressure acutely
Contraindications Known hypersensitivity to glycerin, anuria, acute pulmonary edema, severe dehydration
Warnings/Precautions Use oral glycerin with caution in patients with cardiac, renal, or hepatic disease and in diabetics
Adverse Reactions (Reflective of adult population; not specific for elderly)
Frequency not defined.
Cardiovascular: Arrhythmias
Central nervous system: Headache, confusion, dizziness, hyperosmolar nonketotic coma
Endocrine: Polydipsia, hyperglycemia, dehydration
Gastrointestinal: Nausea, vomiting, tenesmus, rectal irritation, cramping pain, diarrhea, dry mouth
Stability
Refrigerate suppositories; avoid freezing. Protect from heat.
Ophthalmic: Store at room temperature. Keep bottle tightly closed. Discard 6 months after dropper is first placed in the solution.
Mechanism of Action Osmotic dehydrating agent which increases osmotic pressure; draws fluid into colon and thus stimulates evacuation
Pharmacodynamics
Onset of action:
For glycerin suppository: 15-30 minutes
In decreasing IOP: Within 10-30 minutes
Peak effect: Following oral absorption, within 60-90 minutes
Duration: 4-8 hours; increased intracranial pressure decreases within 10-60 minutes following an oral dose with a duration of action around 2-3 hours
Pharmacokinetics
Absorbed:
Oral: Well absorbed
Rectal: Poor
Metabolism: Primarily in the liver with 20% metabolized in the kidney
Half-life: 30-45 minutes
Elimination: Only a small percentage of drug is excreted unchanged in urine
Dosage
Geriatrics & Adults:
Constipation: Rectal: 1 adult suppository 1-2 times/day as needed or 5-15 mL as an enema
Reduction of intracranial pressure: Oral: 1.5 g/kg/day divided every 4 hours; 1 g/kg/dose every 6 hours has also been used
Reduction of corneal edema: Ophthalmic solution: Instill 1-2 drops in eye(s) prior to examination OR for lubricant effect, instill 1-2 drops in eye(s) every 3-4 hours
Reduction of intraocular pressure: Oral: 1-1.8 g/kg 1-1½ hours preoperatively; additional doses may be administered at 5-hour intervals
Administration Apply topical anesthetic before instilling ophthalmic drops
Patient Information Do not use if experiencing abdominal pain, nausea, or vomiting
Additional Information Suppository needs to melt to provide laxative effect
Special Geriatric Considerations The primary use of glycerin in the elderly is as a laxative, although it is not recommended as a first-line treatment

Dosage Forms Excipient information presented when available (limited, particularly for generics); consult specific product labeling. [DSC] = Discontinued product

Solution, ophthalmic, sterile (Bausch & Lomb® Computer Eye Drops): 1% (15 mL) [contains benzalkonium chloride]

Solution, oral (Osmoglyn®): 50% (220 mL) [lime flavor] [DSC]

Solution, rectal:
Fleet® Babylax®: 2.3 g/2.3 mL (4 mL) [6 units per box]
Fleet® Liquid Glycerin Suppositories: 5.6 g/5.5 mL (7.5 mL) [4 units per box]

Suppository, rectal: 82.5% (12s, 25s) [pediatric size]; 82.5% (12s, 24s, 25s, 50s, 100s) [adult size]
Colace® Adult/Children: 2.1 g (12s, 24s, 48s, 100s)
Colace® Infant/Children: 1.2 g (12s, 24s)
Fleet® Glycerin Suppositories: 1 g (12s) [pediatric size]; 2g (12s, 24s, 50s) [adult size]
Fleet® Glycerin Suppositories Maximum Strength: 3g (18s) [adult size]
Sani-Supp®: 82.5% (10s, 25s) [pediatric size]; 82.5% (10s, 25s, 50s) [adult size]

Selected References

Heinemeyer G, "Clinical Pharmacokinetic Considerations in the Treatment of Increased Intracranial Pressure," *Clin Pharmacokinet*, 1987, 13(1):1-25.

Rottenberg DA, Hurwitz BJ, and Posner JB, "The Effect of Oral Glycerol on Intraventricular Pressure in Man," *Neurology*, 1977, 27(7):600-8.

♦ **Glycerol** *see* Glycerin *on page 718*

♦ **Glycerol Guaiacolate** *see* Guaifenesin *on page 727*

♦ **Glyceryl Trinitrate** *see* Nitroglycerin *on page 1129*

♦ **GlycoLax®** *see* Polyethylene Glycol 3350 *on page 1283*

Glycopyrrolate (glye koe PYE roe late)

U.S. Brand Names Robinul®; Robinul® Forte
Canadian Brand Names Glycopyrrolate Injection, USP
Index Terms Glycopyrronium Bromide
Generic Available Yes
Pharmacologic Category Anticholinergic Agent

Use Adjunct in treatment of peptic ulcer disease; preoperative inhibition of salivation and excessive secretions of the respiratory tract; reversal of neuromuscular blockade; control of upper airway secretions

Contraindications Hypersensitivity to glycopyrrolate or any component of the formulation; severe ulcerative colitis, toxic megacolon complicating ulcerative colitis, paralytic ileus, obstructive disease of GI tract, intestinal atony in the elderly or debilitated patient; unstable cardiovascular status in acute hemorrhage; narrow-angle glaucoma; acute hemorrhage; tachycardia; obstructive uropathy; myasthenia gravis

Warnings/Precautions Use caution in elderly, patients with autonomic neuropathy, hepatic or renal disease, ulcerative colitis may predispose megacolon, hyperthyroidism, CAD, CHF, arrhythmias, tachycardia, BPH, or hiatal hernia with reflux. Use of anticholinergics in gastric ulcer treatment may cause a delay in gastric emptying due to antral statis. May cause drowsiness, eye sensitivity to light, or blurred vision; caution should be used when performing tasks which require mental alertness, such as driving. The risk of heat stroke with this medication may be increased during exercise or hot weather. Patients with Down syndrome may be hypersensitive to antimuscarine effects.

Adverse Reactions (Reflective of adult population; not specific for elderly)
Frequency not defined. **Note:** Includes adverse effects which may occur as an extension of the pharmacologic action of anticholinergics (including glycopyrrolate) and adverse effects reported postmarketing with glycopyrrolate.

Cardiovascular: Arrhythmias, cardiac arrest, heart block, hyper-/hypotension, malignant hyperthermia, palpitation, QT_c interval prolongation, tachycardia

Central nervous system: Confusion, dizziness, drowsiness, excitement, headache, insomnia, nervousness, seizure

Dermatologic: Dry skin, pruritus, sensitivity to light increased

Endocrine & metabolic: Lactation suppression

Gastrointestinal: Bloated feeling, constipation, loss of taste, nausea, vomiting, xerostomia

Genitourinary: Impotence, urinary hesitancy, urinary retention

Local: Irritation at injection site

Neuromuscular & skeletal: Weakness

Ocular: Blurred vision, cycloplegia, mydriasis, ocular tension increased, photophobia, sensitivity to light increased

Respiratory: Respiratory depression

Miscellaneous: Anaphylactoid reactions, diaphoresis decreased, hypersensitivity reactions

(Continued)

Glycopyrrolate *(Continued)*

Overdosage/Toxicology

Symptoms of overdose include blurred vision, urinary retention, tachycardia, and absent bowel sounds. For peripheral adverse effects, a quaternary ammonium anticholinesterase, such as neostigmine methylsulfate, may be given I.V. in increments of 0.25 mg in adults; may repeat every 5-10 minutes (up to a maximum of 2.5 mg) based upon decrease in heart rate and return of bowel sounds. For overdose exhibiting CNS symptoms (eg, excitement, restlessness, convulsions, psychotic behavior), physostigmine 0.5-2 mg I.V. slowly, may be given and repeated as necessary, up to 5 mg. Artificial respiration should be given to individuals experiencing a neuromuscular or curare-like effect which could lead to muscular weakness or possible paralysis. Additional care should be symptomatic and supportive.

Drug Interactions

Anticholinergic agents: Effects of other anticholinergic agents or medications with anticholinergic activity may be increased by glycopyrrolate.

Potassium chloride: Severity of potassium chloride-induced gastrointestinal lesions (when potassium is given in a wax matrix formulation, eg, Klor-Con®) may be increased by glycopyrrolate.

Pramlinitide: May enhance the anticholinergic effects of anticholinergics. These effects are specific to the GI tract.

Stability Store at 20°C to 25°C (68°F to 77°F).

Mechanism of Action Blocks the action of acetylcholine at parasympathetic sites in smooth muscle, secretory glands, and the CNS

Pharmacodynamics

Onset of action: Oral: 50 minutes; I.M.: 15-30 minutes; I.V.: ~1 minute

Peak effect: Oral: ~1 hour; I.M.: 30-45 minutes

Duration: Vagal effect: 2-3 hours; Inhibition of salivation: Up to 7 hours; Anticholinergic: Oral: 8-12 hours

Pharmacokinetics

Absorption: Oral: Poor and erratic

Distribution: V_d: 0.2-0.62 L/kg

Metabolism: Hepatic (minimal)

Bioavailability: ~10%

Half-life elimination: Adults: ~30-75 minutes

Excretion: Urine (as unchanged drug, I.M.: 80%, I.V.: 85%); bile (as unchanged drug)

Dosage

Geriatrics & Adults:

Reduction of secretions: I.M.:

Preoperative: I.M.: 4 mcg/kg 30-60 minutes before procedure

Intraoperative: I.V.: 0.1 mg repeated as needed at 2- to 3-minute intervals

Reversal of neuromuscular blockade: I.V.: 0.2 mg for each 1 mg of neostigmine or 5 mg of pyridostigmine administered or 5-15 mcg/kg glycopyrrolate with 25-70 mcg/kg of neostigmine or 0.1-0.3 mg/kg of pyridostigmine (agents usually administered simultaneously, but glycopyrrolate may be administered first if bradycardia is present)

Peptic ulcer:

Oral: 1-2 mg 2-3 times/day

I.M., I.V.: 0.1-0.2 mg 3-4 times/day

Administration For I.V. administration, glycopyrrolate may also be administered via the tubing of a running I.V. infusion of a compatible solution; may be administered in the same syringe with neostigmine or pyridostigmine.

Monitoring Parameters Pulse, anticholinergic effects; bowel sounds

Patient Information Take as directed before meals. Maintain good oral hygiene habits, because lack of saliva may increase chance of cavities. Observe caution while driving or performing other tasks requiring alertness, as may cause drowsiness, dizziness, or blurred vision. Notify physician if skin rash, flushing or eye pain occurs; or if difficulty in urinating, constipation or sensitivity to light becomes severe or persists.

Additional Information Because of its bothersome and potentially dangerous side effects, glycopyrrolate is rarely used for the treatment of peptic ulcer disease

Special Geriatric Considerations Anticholinergic agents are generally not well tolerated in the elderly and their use should be avoided when possible.

Dosage Forms Excipient information presented when available (limited, particularly for generics); consult specific product labeling. [DSC] = Discontinued product

Injection, solution: 0.2 mg/mL (1 mL, 2 mL, 5 mL, 20 mL)

Robinul®: 0.2 mg/mL (1 mL, 2 mL, 5 mL; 20 mL [DSC]) [contains benzyl alcohol]

Tablet: 1 mg, 2 mg

Robinul®: 1 mg

Robinul® Forte: 2 mg

Selected References

Friedl KE, Hannan CJ, Mader TH, et al, "Effect of Eye Color on Heart Rate Response to Intramuscular Administration of Atropine," *J Auton Nerv Syst*, 1988, 24(1-2):51-6.

- **Glycopyrronium Bromide** *see* Glycopyrrolate *on page 719*
- **Glydiazinamide** *see* GlipiZIDE *on page 710*
- **Glynase® PresTab®** *see* GlyBURIDE *on page 714*
- **Gly-Oxide® [OTC]** *see* Carbamide Peroxide *on page 235*
- **Glyset®** *see* Miglitol *on page 1044*
- **Gold Bond® Antifungal [OTC] [DSC]** *see* Tolnaftate *on page 1596*

Gold Sodium Thiomalate (gold SOW dee um thye oh MAL ate)

U.S. Brand Names Myochrysine®
Canadian Brand Names Myochrysine®
Index Terms Sodium Aurothiomalate
Generic Available No
Pharmacologic Category Gold Compound
Use Adjunctive treatment in adult active rheumatoid arthritis; alternative or adjunct in treatment of pemphigus; for psoriatic patients who do not respond to NSAIDs
Contraindications Hypersensitivity to gold compounds or any component of the formulation; systemic lupus erythematosus; history of blood dyscrasias; congestive heart failure, exfoliative dermatitis, colitis
Warnings/Precautions Frequent monitoring of patients for signs and symptoms of toxicity will prevent/limit serious adverse reactions. Must not be administered by I.V. injection. In patients with hematologic abnormalities (blood dyscrasias, hemorrhagic diathesis), renal impairment, hepatic impairment, SLE or dermatitis: Consider alternative therapy (these conditions may be considered relative contraindications); may increase risk and/or symptoms of gold toxicity may be more difficult to detect.

[U.S. Boxed Warning]: May cause significant toxicity involving dermatologic, gastrointestinal, hematologic, pulmonary, renal and hepatic systems; patient education is required. Dermatitis and lesions of the mucous membranes are common and may be serious; pruritus may precede the early development of a skin reaction. Signs of toxicity include hematologic depression (depressed hemoglobin, leukocytes, granulocytes, or platelets); stomatitis, persistent diarrhea, enterocolitis, cholestatic jaundice; proteinuria (nephritic syndrome), and interstitial pulmonary fibrosis. Use caution in patients with CHF, hypertension, or cerebrovascular disease. Avoid use in patients with prior inflammatory bowel disease.

In general, NSAIDS and corticosteroids may be discontinued after initiation of therapy (corticosteroid tapering may be required). Concurrent ACE inhibitors may be associated with a higher risk of nitritoid reactions.
Adverse Reactions (Reflective of adult population; not specific for elderly)
Frequency not defined.
Dermatologic: Alopecia, angioedema, pruritus, rash, urticaria
Gastrointestinal: Stomatitis, gingivitis, glossitis, dysphagia, taste disturbance (metallic), nausea, GI hemorrhage, diarrhea, enterocolitis (ulcerative)
Hematologic: Agranulocytosis, aplastic anemia, eosinophilia, leukopenia, thrombocytopenia
Hepatic: Cholestasis, hepatitis, hepatotoxicity, jaundice
Neuromuscular & skeletal: Peripheral neuropathy
Ocular: Conjunctivitis
Respiratory: Gold bronchitis, interstitial pneumonitis
Renal: Hematuria, proteinuria
Miscellaneous: Anaphylactoid reaction, anaphylaxis, nitritoid reaction
Overdosage/Toxicology Symptoms include hematuria, proteinuria, fever, nausea, vomiting, and diarrhea. For mild gold poisoning, dimercaprol 2.5 mg/kg 4 times/day for 2 days, or for more severe forms of gold intoxication, dimercaprol 3-5 mg/kg every 4 hours for 2 days should be initiated. Then after 2 days, the initial dose should be repeated twice daily on the third day, and once daily thereafter for 10 days. Other chelating agents have been used with some success.
Drug Interactions ACE inhibitors: May enhance the adverse/toxic effects (nitritoid reaction) of gold sodium thiomalate. The reaction may include facial flushing, nausea, vomiting, hypotension, and syncope. If it is to occur, would be expected shortly after administration of gold compound in patients maintained on an ACEI.
Stability Should not be used if solution is darker than pale yellow.
Mechanism of Action Unknown, may decrease prostaglandin synthesis or may alter cellular mechanisms by inhibiting sulfhydryl systems
Pharmacodynamics Gold injections may result in decreased morning stiffness in 1-2 months; significant benefit may not be noted for 3-6 months
Pharmacokinetics
Protein binding: 95% to 99%
Half-life: 3-27 days (single dose); 14-40 days (third dose); up to 168 days (11th dose)
Time to peak serum concentrations: I.M.: Within 2-6 hours
(Continued)

Gold Sodium Thiomalate *(Continued)*

Elimination: Majority (60% to 90%) is excreted in urine with smaller amounts (10% to 40%) excreted in feces (via bile)

Dosage

Geriatrics & Adults: Rheumatoid arthritis: I.M.: 10 mg first week; 25 mg second week; then 25-50 mg/week until 1 g cumulative dose has been given; if improvement occurs without adverse reactions, administer 25-50 mg every 2-3 weeks for 2-20 weeks, then every 3-4 weeks indefinitely

Renal Impairment:

Cl_{cr} 50-80 mL/minute: Administer 50% of normal dose.

Cl_{cr} <50 mL/minute: Avoid use.

Administration Deep I.M. injection into the upper outer quadrant of the gluteal region addition of 0.1 mL of 1% lidocaine to each injection may reduce the discomfort associated with I.M. administration

Monitoring Parameters Patients should have a CBC with differential, platelet count, hemoglobin determination and urinalysis for protein, white cells, red cells and casts; at baseline and prior to each injection. Skin and oral mucosa should be inspected for skin rash, bruising or oral ulceration/stomatitis. Specific questioning for symptoms such as pruritus, rash, stomatitis or metallic taste should be included. Dosing should be withheld in patients with significant gastrointestinal, renal, dermatologic, or hematologic effects (platelet count falls to <100,000/mm³, WBC <4000, granulocytes <1500/mm³

Reference Range Gold: Normal: 0-0.1 mcg/mL (SI: 0-0.0064 μmol/L); Therapeutic: 1-3 mcg/mL (SI: 0.06-0.18 μmol/L); urine <0.1 mcg/24 hours

Patient Information Minimize exposure to sunlight; report any signs of toxicity to physician (ie, pruritus, rash, sore mouth, indigestion, metallic taste); joint pain may take 1-2 months to start to subside

Special Geriatric Considerations Tolerance to gold decreases with advanced age; use cautiously only after traditional therapy and other disease-modifying antirheumatic drugs (DMARDs) have been attempted. Since elderly frequently have Cl_{cr} <50 mL/minute, it is advisable to measure or calculate creatinine clearance before use.

Dosage Forms Excipient information presented when available (limited, particularly for generics); consult specific product labeling.

Injection, solution:

Myochrysine®: 50 mg/mL (1 mL, 10 mL)

♦ **Gordofilm® [OTC]** *see* Salicylic Acid *on page 1441*

♦ **Gordon Boro-Packs [OTC]** *see* Aluminum Sulfate and Calcium Acetate *on page 68*

Goserelin (GOE se rel in)

U.S. Brand Names Zoladex®

Canadian Brand Names Zoladex®; Zoladex® LA

Index Terms D-Ser(But)⁶,Azgly¹⁰-LHRH; Goserelin Acetate; ICI-118630; NSC-606864

Generic Available No

Pharmacologic Category Gonadotropin Releasing Hormone Agonist

Use Palliative treatment of advanced breast cancer and carcinoma of the prostate; treatment of endometriosis, including pain relief and reduction of endometriotic lesions; endometrial thinning agent as part of treatment for dysfunctional uterine bleeding

Contraindications Hypersensitivity to goserelin or any component of the formulation

Warnings/Precautions Hazardous agent - use appropriate precautions for handling and disposal. Transient worsening of signs and symptoms (tumor flare) may develop during the first few weeks of treatment. Urinary tract obstruction or spinal cord compression have been reported when used for prostate cancer; closely observe patients for weakness, paresthesias, and urinary tract obstruction in first few weeks of therapy. Decreased bone density has been reported in women and may be irreversible; use caution if other risk factors are present; evaluate and institute preventative treatment if necessary. Rare cases of pituitary apoplexy (frequently secondary to pituitary adenoma) have been observed with leuprolide administration (onset from 1 hour to usually <2 weeks); may present as sudden headache, vomiting, visual or mental status changes, and infrequently cardiovascular collapse; immediate medical attention required.

Adverse Reactions (Reflective of adult population; not specific for elderly)

Percentages reported in males with prostatic carcinoma and females with endometriosis using the 1-month implant:

>10%:

Central nervous system: Headache (female 75%, male 1% to 5%), emotional lability (female 60%), depression (female 54%, male 1% to 5%), pain (female 17%, male 8%), insomnia (female 11%, male 5%)

Endocrine & metabolic: Hot flashes (female 96%, male 62%), sexual dysfunction (21%), erections decreased (18%), libido decreased (female 61%), breast enlargement (female 18%)

Genitourinary: Lower urinary symptoms (male 13%), vaginitis (75%), dyspareunia (female 14%)

Miscellaneous: Diaphoresis (female 45%, male 6%); infection (female 13%)

1% to 10%:

Cardiovascular: CHF (male 5%), arrhythmia, cerebrovascular accident, hypertension, MI, peripheral vascular disorder, chest pain, palpitation, tachycardia, edema

Central nervous system: Lethargy (male 8%), dizziness (female 6%, male 5%), abnormal thinking, anxiety, chills, fever, malaise, migraine, somnolence

Dermatologic: Rash (female >1%, male 6%), alopecia, bruising, dry skin, skin discoloration

Endocrine & metabolic: Breast pain (female 7%), breast swelling/tenderness (male 1% to 5%), dysmenorrhea, gout, hyperglycemia

Gastrointestinal: Anorexia (female >1%, male 5%), nausea (male 5%), constipation, diarrhea, flatulence, dyspepsia, ulcer, vomiting, weight increased, xerostomia

Genitourinary: Renal insufficiency, urinary frequency, urinary obstruction, urinary tract infection, vaginal hemorrhage

Hematologic: Anemia, hemorrhage

Neuromuscular & skeletal: Arthralgia, bone mineral density decreased (female; ~4% decrease in 6 months), joint disorder, paresthesia

Ocular: Amblyopia, dry eyes

Respiratory: Upper respiratory tract infection (male 7%), COPD (male 5%), pharyngitis (female 5%), bronchitis, cough, epistaxis, rhinitis, sinusitis

Miscellaneous: Allergic reaction

Overdosage/Toxicology Treatment is symptomatic.

Stability Zoladex® should be stored at room temperature not to exceed 25°C or 77°F. Protect from light; should be dispensed in a lightproof bag.

Mechanism of Action Goserelin is a synthetic analog of luteinizing-hormone-releasing hormone (LHRH). Following an initial increase in luteinizing hormone (LH) and follicle stimulating hormone (FSH), chronic administration of goserelin results in a sustained suppression of pituitary gonadotropins. Serum testosterone falls to levels comparable to surgical castration. The exact mechanism of this effect is unknown, but may be related to changes in the control of LH or down-regulation of LH receptors.

Pharmacokinetics Data reported using the 1-month implant:

Absorption: SubQ: Rapid and can be detected in serum in 10 minutes

Distribution: V_d: Male: 44.1 L; Female: 20.3 L

Time to peak, serum: SubQ: Male: 12-15 days, Female: 8-22 days

Half-life: SubQ: Male: ~4 hours, Female: ~2 hours; Renal impairment: Male: 12 hours

Elimination: Urine (90%)

Dosage

Geriatrics & Adults:

Prostate cancer: SubQ:

Monthly implant: 3.6 mg injected into upper abdomen every 28 days

3-month implant: 10.8 mg injected into the upper abdominal wall every 12 weeks

Breast cancer, endometriosis, endometrial thinning: SubQ: Monthly implant: 3.6 mg injected into upper abdomen every 28 days

Note: For breast cancer, treatment may continue indefinitely; for endometriosis, it is recommended that duration of treatment not exceed 6 months. Only 1-2 doses are recommended for endometrial thinning.

Administration Subcutaneous implant: Insert the hypodermic needle into the subcutaneous fat. Do not try to aspirate with the goserelin syringe. If the needle is in a large vessel, blood will immediately appear in the syringe chamber. Change the direction of the needle so it parallels the abdominal wall. Push the needle in until the barrel hub touches the patient's skin. Fully depress the plunger to discharge. Withdraw needle and bandage the site. Confirm discharge by ensuring tip of the plunger is visible within the tip of the needle.

Test Interactions Serum alkaline phosphatase, serum acid phosphatase, serum testosterone, serum LH and FSH, serum estradiol

Patient Information This drug must be implanted under the skin of your abdomen every 28 days; it is important to maintain appointment schedule. You may experience systemic hot flashes (cool clothes and temperatures may help), headache (analgesic may help), constipation (increased bulk and water in diet or stool softener may help), sexual dysfunction (decreased libido, decreased erection). Symptoms may worsen temporarily during first weeks of therapy. Report unusual nausea or vomiting, any chest pain, respiratory difficulty, unresolved dizziness, or constipation. Females must use reliable contraception during therapy.

Additional Information Emetic potential: Low (10% to 30%)

(Continued)

Goserelin *(Continued)*

Special Geriatric Considerations No dosage adjustments are needed in the elderly. Monitoring for bone density changes, serum lipid and serum calcium changes is recommended.

Dosage Forms Excipient information presented when available (limited, particularly for generics); consult specific product labeling.

Injection, solution, 1-month implant [disposable syringe; single-dose]: 3.6 mg [with 16-gauge hypodermic needle]

Injection, solution, 3-month implant [disposable syringe; single-dose]: 10.8 mg [with 14-gauge hypodermic needle]

Selected References

Ahmann FR, Citrin DL, deHaan HA, et al, "Zoladex: A Sustained-Release, Monthly Luteinizing Hormone-Releasing Hormone Analog for the Treatment of Advanced Prostate Cancer," *J Clin Oncol*, 1987, 5(6):912-7.

Brogden RN and Faulds D, "Goserelin. A Review of Its Pharmacodynamic and Pharmacokinetic Properties and Therapeutic Efficacy in Prostate Cancer," *Drugs Aging*, 1995, 6(4);324-43.

Goldspiel BR and Kohler DR, "Goserelin Acetate Implant: A Depot Luteinizing Hormone-Releasing Hormone Analog for Advanced Prostate Cancer," *DICP*, 1991, 25(7-8):796-804.

Peeling WB, "Phase III Studies to Compare Goserelin (Zoladex) With Orchiectomy and With Diethylstilbestrol in Treatment of Prostatic Carcinoma," *Urol*, 1989, 33(5 Suppl):45-52.

Robertson JF, Nicholson RI, Walker KJ, et al, "Zoladex in Advanced Breast Cancer," *Horm Res*, 1989, 32 (Suppl 1):206-8.

♦ **Goserelin Acetate** *see* Goserelin *on page 722*

♦ **GP 47680** *see* Oxcarbazepine *on page 1174*

♦ **GR38032R** *see* Ondansetron *on page 1160*

♦ **Gramicidin, Neomycin, and Polymyxin B** *see* Neomycin, Polymyxin B, and Gramicidin *on page 1103*

Granisetron *(gra NI se tron)*

Medication Safety Issues

Sound-alike/look-alike issues:

Granisetron may be confused with dolasetron, ondansetron, palonosetron

U.S. Brand Names Kytril®

Canadian Brand Names Kytril®

Index Terms BRL 43694

Generic Available No

Pharmacologic Category Antiemetic; Selective 5-HT$_3$ Receptor Antagonist

Use Prophylaxis of chemotherapy-related emesis; prophylaxis of nausea and vomiting associated with radiation therapy, including total body irradiation and fractionated abdominal radiation; prophylaxis of postoperative nausea and vomiting (PONV)

Generally **not** recommended for treatment of existing chemotherapy-induced emesis (CIE) or for prophylaxis of nausea from agents with a low emetogenic potential

Contraindications Previous hypersensitivity to granisetron, other 5-HT$_3$ receptor antagonists, or any component of the formulation

Warnings/Precautions For chemotherapy-related emesis, **granisetron should be used on a scheduled basis, not on an "as needed" (PRN) basis**, since data support the use of this drug in the prevention of nausea and vomiting and not in the rescue of nausea and vomiting. Granisetron should be used only in the first 24-48 hours of receiving chemotherapy or radiation. Data do not support any increased efficacy of granisetron in delayed nausea and vomiting.

Use with caution in patients allergic to other 5-HT$_3$ receptor antagonists; cross-reactivity has been reported. Routine prophylaxis for PONV is not recommended in patients where there is little expectation of nausea and vomiting postoperatively. In patients where nausea and vomiting must be avoided postoperatively, administer to all patients even when expected incidence of nausea and vomiting is low. Use caution following abdominal surgery or in chemotherapy-induced nausea and vomiting; may mask progressive ileus or gastric distention.

Adverse Reactions (Reflective of adult population; not specific for elderly)

>10%:

Central nervous system: Headache (9% to 21%)

Gastrointestinal: Constipation (3% to 18%)

Neuromuscular & skeletal: Weakness (5% to 18%)

1% to 10%:

Cardiovascular: Hypertension (1% to 2%)

Central nervous system: Pain (10%), fever (3% to 9%), dizziness (4% to 5%), insomnia (<2% to 5%), somnolence (1% to 4%), anxiety (2%), agitation (<2%), CNS stimulation (<2%)

Dermatologic: Rash (1%)

Gastrointestinal: Diarrhea (3% to 9%), abdominal pain (4% to 6%), dyspepsia (3% to 6%), taste perversion (2%)

Hepatic: Liver enzymes increased (5% to 6%)
Renal: Oliguria (2%)
Respiratory: Cough (2%)
Miscellaneous: Infection (3%)

Overdosage/Toxicology Treatment should be symptomatic and supportive.

Drug Interactions Substrate of CYP3A4 (minor)

Apomorphine: Due to reports of profound hypotension during concomitant therapy with other 5-HT3 antagonists, the manufacturer of apomorphine contraindicates its use with granisetron.

Ethanol/Nutrition/Herb Interactions Herb/Nutraceutical: St John's wort may decrease granisetron levels.

Stability

I.V.: Store at 15°C to 30°C (59°F to 86°F). Stable when mixed in NS or D_5W for 7 days under refrigeration and for 3 days at room temperature. Protect from light. Do not freeze vials.

Oral: Store tablet or oral solution at 15°C to 30°C (59°F to 86°F). Protect from light.

Mechanism of Action Selective 5-HT$_3$-receptor antagonist, blocking serotonin, both peripherally on vagal nerve terminals and centrally in the chemoreceptor trigger zone

Pharmacodynamics

Onset of action: Commonly controls emesis within 1-3 minutes of administration
Duration: Effects generally last no more than 24 hours maximum

Pharmacokinetics

Distribution: V_d: 2-4 L/kg; widely throughout body
Protein binding: 65%
Metabolism: Hepatic via N-demethylation, oxidation, and conjugation; some metabolites may have 5-HT$_3$ antagonist activity
Half-life: Cancer patients: 10-12 hours; Healthy volunteers: 4-5 hours; PONV: 9 hours
Elimination: Urine (12% as unchanged drug, 49% as metabolites); feces (34% as metabolites)

Dosage

Geriatrics & Adults:

Prophylaxis of chemotherapy-related emesis:

Oral: 2 mg once daily up to 1 hour before chemotherapy or 1 mg twice daily; the first 1 mg dose should be given up to 1 hour before chemotherapy.

I.V.:

Within U.S.: 10 mcg/kg/dose (maximum: 1 mg/dose) given 30 minutes prior to chemotherapy; for some drugs (eg, carboplatin, cyclophosphamide) with a later onset of emetic action, 10 mcg/kg every 12 hours may be necessary.

Outside U.S.: 40 mcg/kg/dose (or 3 mg/dose); maximum: 9 mg/24 hours

Breakthrough: Granisetron has not been shown to be effective in terminating nausea or vomiting once it occurs and should not be used for this purpose.

Prophylaxis of radiation therapy-associated emesis: Oral: 2 mg once daily given 1 hour before radiation therapy.

Postoperative nausea and vomiting (PONV): I.V.:

Prevention: 1 mg given undiluted over 30 seconds; administer before induction of anesthesia or immediately before reversal of anesthesia

Treatment: 1 mg given undiluted over 30 seconds

Renal Impairment: No dosage adjustment required.

Hepatic Impairment: Kinetic studies in patients with hepatic impairment showed that total clearance was approximately halved; however, standard doses were very well tolerated, and dose adjustments are not necessary.

Administration

Oral: Doses should be given up to 1 hour prior to initiation of chemotherapy/radiation
I.V.: Administer as rapid (30 second) I.V. push or a short (5-10 minutes) infusion

For prevention of PONV, administer before induction of anesthesia or before reversal of anesthesia.

For PONV, administer undiluted over 30 seconds.

Monitoring Parameters Monitor for control of nausea and vomiting

Special Geriatric Considerations Clinical trials with patients older than 65 years of age are limited; however, the data indicates that safety and efficacy are similar to that observed in younger adults. No adjustment in dose necessary for elderly.

Dosage Forms Excipient information presented when available (limited, particularly for generics); consult specific product labeling.

Injection, solution: 1 mg/mL (1 mL, 4 mL) [contains benzyl alcohol]
Injection, solution [preservative free]: 0.1 mg/mL (1 mL)
Solution, oral: 2 mg/10 mL (30 mL) [contains sodium benzoate; orange flavor]
Tablet: 1 mg

Extemporaneously Prepared A 0.2 mg/mL oral suspension may be prepared by crushing twelve (12) 1 mg tablets and mixing with 30 mL water and enough cherry syrup to provide a final volume of 60 mL; this preparation is stable for 14 days at room temperature or when refrigerated

(Continued)

Granisetron *(Continued)*

Quercia RA, Zhang JH, Fan C, et al, "Stability of Granisetron (Kytril®) in an Extemporaneously Prepared Oral Liquid," *International Pharmaceutical Abstracts*, 1996, May 15, Vol 33.

♦ **Granulex®** *see* Trypsin, Balsam Peru, and Castor Oil *on page 1642*
♦ **Granulocyte Colony Stimulating Factor** *see* Filgrastim *on page 624*
♦ **Granulocyte Colony Stimulating Factor (PEG Conjugate)** *see* Pegfilgrastim *on page 1212*
♦ **Grifulvin® V** *see* Griseofulvin *on page 726*

Griseofulvin *(gri see oh FUL vin)*

Medication Safety Issues
Sound-alike/look-alike issues:
Fulvicin® may be confused with Furacin®
U.S. Brand Names Grifulvin® V; Gris-PEG®
Index Terms Griseofulvin Microsize; Griseofulvin Ultramicrosize
Generic Available Yes: Suspension, ultramicrosized product
Pharmacologic Category Antifungal Agent, Oral
Use Treatment of susceptible tinea infections of the skin, hair, and nails
Contraindications Hypersensitivity to griseofulvin or any component of the formulation; severe liver disease; porphyria (interferes with porphyrin metabolism)
Warnings/Precautions During long-term therapy, periodic assessment of hepatic, renal, and hematopoietic functions should be performed; avoid exposure to intense sunlight to prevent photosensitivity reactions; hypersensitivity cross reaction between penicillins and griseofulvin is possible
Adverse Reactions (Reflective of adult population; not specific for elderly)
Frequency not defined.
Central nervous system: Dizziness, fatigue, headache, insomnia, mental confusion
Dermatologic: Angioneurotic edema (rare), erythema multiforme-like drug reaction, photosensitivity, rash (most common), urticaria (most common),
Gastrointestinal: Nausea, vomiting, epigastric distress, diarrhea, GI bleeding
Genitourinary: Menstrual irregularities (rare)
Hematologic: Granulocytopenia, leukopenia
Hepatic: Hepatotoxicity
Neuromuscular & skeletal: Paresthesia (rare)
Renal: Nephrosis, proteinuria
Miscellaneous: Drug-induced lupus-like syndrome (rare), oral thrush
Overdosage/Toxicology Symptoms include lethargy, vertigo, blurred vision, nausea, vomiting, and diarrhea. Following GI decontamination, treatment is symptom-directed and supportive.
Drug Interactions Induces CYP1A2 (weak), 2C8 (weak), 2C9 (weak), 3A4 (weak)
Barbiturates: May decrease levels/effects of griseofulvin.
Cyclosporine: Levels/effects may be decreased by griseofulvin.
Estrogen and hormonal contraceptives: Effectiveness may be decreased by griseofulvin.
Warfarin: Levels/effects may be decreased by griseofulvin.
Ethanol/Nutrition/Herb Interactions
Ethanol: Avoid ethanol (may increase CNS depression). Concomitant use with ethanol will cause "disulfiram"-type reaction consisting of tachycardia, flushing, headache, nausea, and in some patients, vomiting and chest and/or abdominal pain.
Food: Griseofulvin concentrations may be increased if taken with food, especially with high-fat meals.
Mechanism of Action Inhibits fungal cell mitosis at metaphase; binds to human keratin making it resistant to fungal invasion
Pharmacokinetics
Absorption: Ultramicrosize griseofulvin is almost complete; absorption of microsize griseofulvin is variable (25% to 70% of an oral dose); absorption is enhanced by ingestion of a fatty meal
Distribution: Deposited in varying concentrations in the keratin layer of the skin, hair, and nails; only a very small fraction is distributed in the body fluids and tissues
Metabolism: Extensive in the liver
Half-life: 9-22 hours
Time to peak serum concentration: ~4 hours
Elimination: <1% excreted unchanged in urine; also excreted in feces and perspiration
Dosage
Geriatrics & Adults:
Tinea infections: Oral:
Microsize: 500-1000 mg/day in single or divided doses

Ultramicrosize: 375 mg/day in single or divided doses; doses up to 750 mg/day have been used for infections more difficult to eradicate such as tinea unguium and tinea pedis.

Note: Duration of therapy depends on the site of infection:
Tinea corporis: 2-4 weeks
Tinea capitis: 4-6 weeks or longer (up to 8-12 weeks)
Tinea pedis: 4-8 weeks
Tinea unguium: 4-6 months

Administration Oral: Administer with a fatty meal (peanuts or ice cream) to increase absorption, or with food or milk to avoid GI upset
Gris-PEG® tablets: May be swallowed whole or crushed and sprinkled onto 1 tablespoonful of applesauce and swallowed immediately without chewing.

Monitoring Parameters Periodic renal, hepatic, and hematopoietic function tests

Test Interactions False-positive urinary VMA levels

Patient Information Avoid exposure to sunlight, take with fatty meal; if patient gets headache, it usually goes away with continued therapy; may cause dizziness, drowsiness, and impair judgment

Additional Information
Microsize: Fulvicin-U/F®, Grifulvin® V, Grisactin®
Ultramicrosize: Fulvicin® P/G, Grisactin® Ultra, Gris-PEG®; GI absorption of ultramicrosize is ~1.5 times that of microsize

Special Geriatric Considerations No specific changes in dosing are needed.

Dosage Forms Excipient information presented when available (limited, particularly for generics); consult specific product labeling.
Suspension, oral, microsize: 125 mg/5mL (120 mL)
Grifulvin® V: 125 mg/5 mL (120 mL) [contains alcohol 0.2%]
Tablet, microsize:
Grifulvin® V: 500 mg
Tablet, ultramicrosize:
Gris-PEG®: 125 mg, 250 mg

♦ **Griseofulvin Microsize** *see* Griseofulvin *on page 726*
♦ **Griseofulvin Ultramicrosize** *see* Griseofulvin *on page 726*
♦ **Gris-PEG®** *see* Griseofulvin *on page 726*
♦ **Guaicon DM [OTC]** *see* Guaifenesin and Dextromethorphan *on page 730*
♦ **Guaicon DMS [OTC]** *see* Guaifenesin and Dextromethorphan *on page 730*

Guaifenesin (gwye FEN e sin)

Medication Safety Issues
Sound-alike/look-alike issues:
Guaifenesin may be confused with guanfacine
Mucinex® may be confused with Mucomyst®
Naldecon® may be confused with Nalfon®

International issues:
Mucolex® [Hong Kong] may be confused with Mycelex® which is a brand name for clotrimazole in the U.S.

U.S. Brand Names Allfen Jr; Diabetic Tussin® EX [OTC]; Ganidin NR; Guiatuss™ [OTC]; Mucinex® [OTC]; Mucinex®, Children's [OTC]; Mucinex®, Children's Mini-Melts™ [OTC]; Mucinex®, Junior Mini-Melts™ [OTC]; Mucinex® Maximum Strength [OTC]; Organidin® NR; Phanasin® [OTC]; Phanasin® Diabetic Choice [OTC]; Robitussin® [OTC]; Scot-Tussin® Expectorant [OTC]; Siltussin DAS [OTC]; Siltussin SA [OTC]; Vicks® Casero™ Chest Congestion Relief [OTC]; XPECT™ [OTC]

Canadian Brand Names Balminil Expectorant; Benylin® E Extra Strength; Koffex Expectorant; Robitussin®

Index Terms GG; Glycerol Guaiacolate

Generic Available Yes: Excludes extended release and granules

Pharmacologic Category Expectorant

Use Symptomatic relief of respiratory conditions characterized by a dry, nonproductive cough and in the presence of mucous in the respiratory tract

Contraindications Hypersensitivity to guaifenesin or any component of the formulation

Warnings/Precautions Not for persistent cough such as occurs with smoking, asthma, chronic bronchitis, or emphysema or cough accompanied by excessive secretions. When used for self-medication (OTC), contact healthcare provider if needed for >7 days or for a cough with a fever, rash, or persistent headache.

Adverse Reactions (Reflective of adult population; not specific for elderly)
Frequency not defined.
Central nervous system: Dizziness, drowsiness, headache
Dermatologic: Rash
Endocrine & metabolic: Uric acid levels decreased
(Continued)

Guaifenesin *(Continued)*

Gastrointestinal: Nausea, vomiting, stomach pain

Postmarketing and/or case reports: Kidney stone formation (with consumption of large quantities)

Overdosage/Toxicology Symptoms include vomiting, lethargy, coma, and respiratory depression. Treatment is supportive.

Mechanism of Action Thought to act as an expectorant by irritating the gastric mucosa and stimulating respiratory tract secretions, thereby increasing respiratory fluid volumes and decreasing mucous viscosity

Pharmacokinetics

Absorption: Well absorbed from the GI tract

Metabolism: Undergoes hepatic metabolism (60%)

Elimination: Renal excretion of changed and unchanged drug

Dosage

Geriatrics & Adults:

Cough (expectorant): Oral: 200-400 mg every 4 hours to a maximum of 2.4 g/day

Extended release tablet: 600-1200 mg every 12 hours, not to exceed 2.4 g/day

Monitoring Parameters Cough, sputum consistency and volume

Test Interactions Possible color interference with determination of 5-HIAA and VMA; discontinue for 48 hours prior to test

Patient Information Take with a large quantity of fluid to ensure proper action; if cough persists for more than 1 week, is recumbent, or is accompanied by fever, rash or persistent headache, physician should be consulted

Additional Information Should not be used for persistent or chronic cough such as that occurring with smoking, asthma, chronic bronchitis, or emphysema or for cough associated with excessive phlegm; there is lack of convincing studies to document the efficacy of guaifenesin. Guaifenesin is available in various combinations: With pseudo-ephedrine; dextromethorphan; pseudoephedrine and dextromethorphan; codeine; pseudoephedrine and codeine; phenylephrine; hydrocodone; pseudoephedrine and hydrocodone; theophylline.

Dosage Forms Excipient information presented when available (limited, particularly for generics); consult specific product labeling.

Granules, oral:

Mucinex® Children's Mini-Melts™: 50 mg/packet (12s) [contains phenylalanine 0.6 mg/packet and magnesium 6 mg/packet; grape flavor]

Mucinex® Junior Mini-Melts™: 100 mg/packet (12s) [contains phenylalanine 1 mg/packet and magnesium 10 mg/packet; bubble gum flavor]

Liquid: 100 mg/5 mL (120 mL, 480 mL)

Diabetic Tussin EX®: 100 mg/5 mL (120 mL) [alcohol free, sugar free, dye free; contains phenylalanine 8.4 mg/5 mL]

Ganidin NR: 100 mg/5 mL (480 mL) [raspberry flavor]

Mucinex® Children's: 100 mg/5 mL (120 mL) [alcohol free; grape flavor]

Organidin® NR: 100 mg/5 mL (480 mL) [contains sodium benzoate; raspberry flavor]

Siltussin DAS: 100 mg/5 mL (120 mL) [alcohol free, dye free, sugar free; strawberry flavor]

Syrup: 100 mg/5 mL (120 mL, 480 mL)

Guiatuss™: 100 mg/5 mL (120 mL, 480 mL) [alcohol free; fruit-mint flavor]

Phanasin®: 100 mg/5 mL (120 mL, 240 mL) [alcohol free, sugar free; mint flavor]

Phanasin® Diabetic Choice: 100 mg/5 mL (120 mL) [alcohol free, sugar free; mint flavor]

Robitussin®: 100 mg/5 mL (5 mL, 10 mL, 15 mL, 30 mL, 120 mL, 240 mL, 480 mL) [alcohol free; contains sodium benzoate]

Scot-Tussin® Expectorant: 100 mg/5 mL (120 mL) [alcohol free, dye free, sugar free; contains benzoic acid; grape flavor]

Siltussin SA: 100 mg/5 mL (120 mL, 240 mL, 480 mL) [alcohol free, sugar free; strawberry flavor]

Vicks® Casero™ Chest Congestion Relief: 100 mg/6.25 mL (120 mL, 240 mL) [contains phenylalanine 5.5 mg/12.5 mL, sodium 32 mg/12.5 mL, and sodium benzoate; honey menthol flavor]

Tablet: 200 mg

Allfen Jr: 400 mg [dye free]

Organidin® NR: 200 mg

XPECT™: 400 mg

Tablet, extended release:

Mucinex®: 600 mg

Mucinex® Maximum Strength: 1200 mg

♦ **Guaifenesin AC** *see* Guaifenesin and Codeine *on page 729*

Guaifenesin and Codeine (gwye FEN e sin & KOE deen)

Related Information
Codeine *on page 356*
Guaifenesin *on page 727*

U.S. Brand Names Brontex®; Cheracol®; Diabetic Tussin C®; Gani-Tuss® NR; Guaifenesin AC; Guaituss AC; Kolephrin® #1; Mytussin® AC; Robafen® AC; Romilar® AC; Tussi-Organidin® NR; Tussi-Organidin® S-NR

Index Terms Codeine and Guaifenesin

Generic Available Yes

Pharmacologic Category Antitussive; Cough Preparation; Expectorant

Use Temporary control of cough due to minor throat and bronchial irritation

Restrictions C-V

Contraindications Hypersensitivity to guaifenesin, codeine, or any component of the formulation; asthma

Warnings/Precautions Use with caution in patients with hypersensitivity reactions to other phenanthrene derivative opioid agonists (morphine, hydrocodone, hydromorphone, levorphanol, oxycodone, oxymorphone). Use caution with respiratory diseases (including emphysema, COPD, decreased respiratory reserve), CNS depression, acute alcoholism, acute abdominal conditions, fever, hypothyroidism, Addison's disease, ulcerative colitis, prostatic hyperplasia, recent GI or urinary tract surgery, seizure disorders, head injury or increased intracranial pressure, or severe liver or renal insufficiency; tolerance or drug dependence may result from extended use.

The elderly may be particularly susceptible to the CNS depressant and confusion, as well as constipating effects of narcotics. Causes sedation; caution must be used in performing tasks which require alertness (eg, operating machinery or driving). Dose should not be increased if cough does not respond; reevaluate within 5 days for possible underlying pathology.

Adverse Reactions (Reflective of adult population; not specific for elderly)
Frequency not defined; also see individual agents.
Cardiovascular: Bradycardia, circulatory depression, flushing, orthostatic hypotension, palpitation, syncope, tachycardia
Central nervous system: Convulsions, CNS depression, disorientation, dizziness, dysphoria, euphoria, faintness, hallucinations (transient), headache, lightheadedness, sedation
Dermatologic: Angioneurotic edema, pruritus, urticaria
Gastrointestinal: Biliary tract spasm, colonic motility increase (with chronic ulcerative colitis), constipation, nausea, stomach pain, toxic dilation (with acute ulcerative colitis), vomiting
Genitourinary: Oliguria, urinary retention
Neuromuscular & skeletal: Weakness
Ocular: Visual disturbances
Respiratory: Laryngeal edema, respiratory depression
Miscellaneous: Anaphylaxis, diaphoresis

Drug Interactions See individual agents.

Ethanol/Nutrition/Herb Interactions Ethanol: Avoid or limit ethanol (may increase CNS depression). Watch for sedation.

Mechanism of Action
Guaifenesin may act as an expectorant by irritating the gastric mucosa and stimulating respiratory tract secretions, thereby increasing respiratory fluid volumes and decreasing phlegm viscosity
Codeine is an antitussive that controls cough by depressing the medullary cough center

Dosage
Geriatrics & Adults: Cough (antitussive/expectorant): Oral:
Brontex® tablets: 1 tablet every 4 hours; maximum 6 tablets/24 hours
Diabetic Tussin C®, Kolephrin® #1, Romilar® AC, Tussi-Organidin® NR liquid: 10 mL every 4 hours; maximum 60 mL/24 hours
Note: Also refer to specific product labeling.

Monitoring Parameters Cough, sputum consistency and volume, mental status, respiratory status

Patient Information Take with a large quantity of fluid to ensure proper action. May cause drowsiness; avoid CNS depressants and alcohol; do not use for chronic or persistent coughs

Special Geriatric Considerations Elderly may be more sensitive to the CNS depressant effects of codeine; monitor closely for excessive sedation.

Dosage Forms Excipient information presented when available (limited, particularly for generics); consult specific product labeling.
(Continued)

Guaifenesin and Codeine *(Continued)*

Liquid:

Brontex®: Guaifenesin 75 mg and codeine phosphate 2.5 mg per 5 mL (480 mL) [alcohol free; strawberry mint flavor]

Diabetic Tussin C®: Guaifenesin 200 mg and codeine phosphate 10 mg per 5 mL (480 mL) [contains phenylalanine 0.03 mcg/5 mL; cherry vanilla flavor]

Gani-Tuss® NR: Guaifenesin 100 mg and codeine phosphate 10 mg per 5 mL (480 mL) [raspberry flavor]

Guiatuss AC: Guaifenesin 100 mg and codeine phosphate 10 mg per 5 mL (120 mL, 480 mL) [alcohol free, sugar free; raspberry flavor]

Kolephrin® #1: Guaifenesin 100 mg and codeine phosphate 10 mg per 5 mL (120 mL) [contains sodium 1.1 mg/5 mL and sodium benzoate]

Tussi-Organidin® NR: Guaifenesin 300 mg and codeine phosphate 10 mg per 5 mL (480 mL) [alcohol free, sugar free; contains sodium benzoate; raspberry flavor]

Tussi-Organidin® S-NR: Guaifenesin 300 mg and codeine phosphate 10 mg per 5 mL (120 mL) [alcohol free, sugar free; contains sodium benzoate; raspberry flavor]

Syrup:

Cheracol®: Guaifenesin 100 mg and codeine phosphate 10 mg per 5 mL (120 mL) [contains alcohol 4.75% and benzoic acid]

Guaituss AC: Guaifenesin 100 mg and codeine phosphate 10 mg per 5 mL (120 mL, 480 mL) [contains alcohol; sugar free; fruit-mint flavor]

Mytussin® AC: Guaifenesin 100 mg and codeine phosphate 10 mg per 5 mL (120 mL, 480 mL) [contains alcohol; sugar free; fruit flavor]

Robafen® AC: Guaifenesin 100 mg and codeine phosphate 10 mg per 5 mL (120 mL, 480 mL)

Romilar® AC: Guaifenesin 100 mg and codeine phosphate 10 mg per 5 mL (480 mL) [alcohol free, sugar free, dye free; contains benzoic acid and phenylalanine; grape flavor]

Tablet: Guaifenesin 300 mg and codeine phosphate 10 mg

Brontex®: Guaifenesin 300 mg and codeine phosphate 10 mg

Guaifenesin and Dextromethorphan

(gwye FEN e sin & deks troe meth OR fan)

Related Information

Dextromethorphan *on page 419*

Guaifenesin *on page 727*

Medication Safety Issues

Sound-alike/look-alike issues:

Benylin® may be confused with Benadryl®, Ventolin®

U.S. Brand Names Allfen-DM; Altarussin DM [OTC]; Amibid DM [DSC]; Cheracol® D [OTC]; Cheracol® Plus [OTC]; Coricidin HBP® Chest Congestion and Cough [OTC]; Diabetic Tussin® DM [OTC]; Diabetic Tussin® DM Maximum Strength [OTC]; Duratuss® DM; Gani-Tuss DM NR; Genatuss DM® [OTC]; Guaicon DM [OTC]; Guaicon DMS [OTC]; Guaifenex® DM; Guia-D; Guiatuss-DM® [OTC]; Hydro-Tussin™ DM; Kolephrin® GG/DM [OTC]; Mintab DM; Mucinex® Children's Cough [OTC]; Mucinex® DM [OTC]; Mucinex® DM Maximum Strength [OTC]; Phanatuss® DM [OTC]; Phlemex; Respa-DM®; Robafen DM [OTC]; Robafen DM Clear [OTC]; Robitussin® Cough and Congestion [OTC]; Robitussin® DM [OTC]; Robitussin® DM Infant [OTC]; Robitussin® Sugar Free Cough [OTC]; Safe Tussin® [OTC]; Scot-Tussin® Senior [OTC]; Silexin [OTC]; Siltussin DM [OTC]; Siltussin DM DAS [OTC]; Simuc-DM; Su-Tuss DM; Touro® DM; Tussi-Organidin® DM NR; Tussi-Organidin® DM-S NR; Vicks® 44E [OTC]; Vicks® Pediatric Formula 44E [OTC]; Z-Cof LA™

Canadian Brand Names Balminil DM E; Benylin® DM-E; Koffex DM-Expectorant; Robitussin® DM

Index Terms Dextromethorphan and Guaifenesin

Generic Available Yes

Pharmacologic Category Antitussive; Cough Preparation; Expectorant

Use Temporary control of cough due to minor throat and bronchial irritation

Contraindications Hypersensitivity to guaifenesin, dextromethorphan, or any component of the formulation; use with or within 14 days of MAO inhibitor therapy

Warnings/Precautions Should not be used for persistent or chronic cough such as that occurring with smoking, asthma, chronic bronchitis, or emphysema or for cough associated with excessive phlegm. Use caution in patients who are sedated, debilitated or confined to a supine position. When used for self-medication (OTC), contact healthcare provider if needed for >7 days or for a cough with a fever, rash, or persistent headache.

Adverse Reactions (Reflective of adult population; not specific for elderly)

See individual agents.

Drug Interactions Dextromethorphan: **Substrate** of CYP2B6 (minor), 2C9 (minor), 2C19 (minor), 2D6 (major), 2E1 (minor), 3A4 (minor); **Inhibits** CYP2D6 (weak) Also see individual agents.

Stability Store at room temperature.

Mechanism of Action

Guaifenesin is thought to act as an expectorant by irritating the gastric mucosa and stimulating respiratory tract secretions, thereby increasing respiratory fluid volumes and decreasing phlegm viscosity

Dextromethorphan is a chemical relative of morphine lacking narcotic properties except in overdose; controls cough by depressing the medullary cough center

Dosage

Geriatrics & Adults: Cough (antitussive/expectorant): Oral:

General dosing guidelines: Guaifenesin 200-400 mg and dextromethorphan 10-20 mg every 4 hours (maximum dose: Guaifenesin 2400 mg and dextromethorphan 120 mg per day)

Product-specific labeling:

Guaifenex® DM, Mucinex® DM, Touro® DM: 1-2 tablets every 12 hours (maximum: 4 tablets/24 hours)

Robitussin® DM, Robitussin® Sugar Free Cough: 10 mL every 4 hours (maximum: 6 doses/24 hours)

Vicks® 44E: 15 mL every 4 hours (maximum: 6 doses/24 hours)

Vicks® Pediatric Formula 44E: 30 mL every 4 hours (maximum: 6 doses/24 hours)

Z-Cof LA™: 1 tablet every 12 hours

Administration Take with water. Do not crush or chew extended release or long acting formulations.

Monitoring Parameters Cough, sputum consistency and volume, mental status

Patient Information Take with a large quantity of fluid to ensure proper action; if cough persists for more than 1 week, is recumbent, or is accompanied by fever, rash or persistent headache, physician should be consulted; may cause drowsiness; avoid CNS depressants and alcohol

Additional Information Should not be used for persistent or chronic cough such as that occurring with smoking, asthma, chronic bronchitis, or emphysema or for cough associated with excessive phlegm

Dosage Forms Excipient information presented when available (limited, particularly for generics); consult specific product labeling. [DSC] = Discontinued product

Capsule, softgel:

Coricidin HBP® Chest Congestion and Cough: Guaifenesin 200 mg and dextromethorphan hydrobromide 10 mg

Elixir:

Duratuss DM®: Guaifenesin 225 mg and dextromethorphan hydrobromide 25 mg per 5 mL (480 mL) [contains sodium benzoate; grape flavor]

Simuc-DM: Guaifenesin 225 mg and dextromethorphan hydrobromide 25 mg per 5 mL (480 mL) [grape flavor]

Su-Tuss DM: Guaifenesin 200 mg and dextromethorphan hydrobromide 20 mg per 5 mL (480 mL) [fruit flavor]

Liquid: Guaifenesin 100 mg and dextromethorphan hydrobromide 10 mg per 5 mL (480 mL)

Diabetic Tussin® DM: Guaifenesin 100 mg and dextromethorphan hydrobromide 10 mg per 5 mL (120 mL) [alcohol free, sugar free, dye free; contains phenylalanine 8.4 mg/5 mL]

Diabetic Tussin® DM Maximum Strength: Guaifenesin 200 mg and dextromethorphan hydrobromide 10 mg per 5 mL (120 mL) [alcohol free, sugar free, dye free; contains phenylalanine 8.4 mg/5 mL]

Gani-Tuss® DM NR: Guaifenesin 100 mg and dextromethorphan hydrobromide 10 mg per 5 mL (480 mL) [raspberry flavor]

Hydro-Tussin™ DM: Guaifenesin 200 mg and dextromethorphan hydrobromide 20 mg per 5 mL (480 mL) [alcohol free, sugar free; contains sodium benzoate]

Kolephrin® GG/DM: Guaifenesin 150 mg and dextromethorphan hydrobromide 10 mg per 5 mL (120 mL) [alcohol free; cherry flavor]

Mucinex® Children's Cough: Guaifenesin 100 mg and dextromethorphan hydrobromide 5 mg per 5 mL (120 mL) [contains sodium 3 mg/5 mL; cherry flavor]

Safe Tussin®: Guaifenesin 100 mg and dextromethorphan hydrobromide 15 mg per 5 mL (120 mL) [alcohol free, sodium free, sugar free, dye free; mint flavor]

Scot-Tussin® Senior: Guaifenesin 200 mg and dextromethorphan hydrobromide 15 mg per 5 mL (120 mL) [alcohol free, sodium free, sugar free]

Tussi-Organidin® DM NR: Guaifenesin 300 mg and dextromethorphan hydrobromide 10 mg per 5 mL (480 mL) [alcohol free, sugar free; contains sodium benzoate; grape flavor]

Tussi-Organidin® DM-S NR: Guaifenesin 300 mg and dextromethorphan hydrobromide 10 mg per 5 mL (120 mL) [alcohol free, sugar free; contains sodium benzoate; grape flavor]

(Continued)

Guaifenesin and Dextromethorphan *(Continued)*

Vicks® 44E: Guaifenesin 200 mg and dextromethorphan hydrobromide 20 mg per 15 mL (120 mL, 235 mL) [contains sodium 31 mg/15 mL, alcohol, sodium benzoate]

Vicks® Pediatric Formula 44E: Guaifenesin 100 mg and dextromethorphan hydrobromide 10 mg per 15 mL (120 mL) [alcohol free; contains sodium 30 mg/15 mL, sodium benzoate; cherry flavor]

Liquid, oral [drops]:

Robitussin® DM Infant: Guaifenesin 100 mg and dextromethorphan hydrobromide 5 mg per 2.5 mL (30 mL) [alcohol free; contains sodium benzoate; fruit punch flavor]

Syrup: Guaifenesin 100 mg and dextromethorphan hydrobromide 10 mg per 5 mL (120 mL, 480 mL)

Altarussin DM: Guaifenesin 100 mg and dextromethorphan hydrobromide 10 mg per 5 mL (120 mL, 240 mL, 480 mL, 3840 mL)

Cheracol® D: Guaifenesin 100 mg and dextromethorphan hydrobromide 10 mg per 5 mL (120 mL, 180 mL) [contains alcohol 4.75%, benzoic acid]

Cheracol® Plus: Guaifenesin 100 mg and dextromethorphan hydrobromide 10 mg per 5 mL (120 mL) [contains alcohol 4.75%, benzoic acid]

Genatuss DM®: Guaifenesin 100 mg and dextromethorphan hydrobromide 10 mg per 5 mL (120 mL)

Guiatuss® DM: Guaifenesin 100 mg and dextromethorphan hydrobromide 10 mg per 5 mL (120 mL, 480 mL, 3840 mL) [alcohol free; contains sodium benzoate]

Guaicon DM®: Guaifenesin 100 mg and dextromethorphan hydrobromide 10 mg per 5 mL (10 mL) [alcohol free]

Guaicon DMS®: Guaifenesin 100 mg and dextromethorphan hydrobromide 10 mg per 5 mL (10 mL) [alcohol free, sugar free]

Mintab DM: Guaifenesin 200 mg and dextromethorphan hydrobromide 10 mg per 5 mL (480 mL) [alcohol free, dye free; cherry vanilla flavor]

Phanatuss® DM: Guaifenesin 100 mg and dextromethorphan hydrobromide 10 mg per 5 mL (120 mL) [alcohol free, sugar free]

Robafen® DM: Guaifenesin 100 mg and dextromethorphan hydrobromide 10 mg per 5 mL (120 mL, 240 mL, 480 mL) [cherry flavor]

Robafen® DM Clear: Guaifenesin 100 mg and dextromethorphan hydrobromide 10 mg per 5 mL (120 mL)

Robitussin® Cough and Congestion: Guaifenesin 100 mg and dextromethorphan hydrobromide 10 mg per 5 mL (120 mL) [alcohol free; contains sodium benzoate]

Robitussin®-DM: Guaifenesin 100 mg and dextromethorphan hydrobromide 10 mg per 5 mL (5 mL, 120 mL, 340 mL, 360 mL) [alcohol free; contains sodium benzoate]

Robitussin® Sugar Free Cough: Guaifenesin 100 mg and dextromethorphan hydrobromide 10 mg per 5 mL (120 mL) [alcohol free, sugar free; contains sodium benzoate]

Silexin: Guaifenesin 100 mg and dextromethorphan hydrobromide 10 mg per 5 mL (45 mL) [alcohol free, sugar free)]

Siltussin DM: Guaifenesin 100 mg and dextromethorphan hydrobromide 10 mg per 5 mL (120 mL, 240 mL, 480 mL) [strawberry flavor]

Siltussin DM DAS: Guaifenesin 100 mg and dextromethorphan hydrobromide 10 mg per 5 mL (120 mL) [alcohol free, dye free, sugar free; strawberry flavor]

Tablet: Guaifenesin 1000 mg and dextromethorphan hydrobromide 60 mg; guaifenesin 1200 mg and dextromethorphan hydrobromide 60 mg

Silexin: Guaifenesin 100 mg and dextromethorphan hydrobromide 10 mg

Tablet, extended release:

Amibid DM [DSC], Guaifenex® DM, Mucinex® DM, Respa-DM®: Guaifenesin 600 mg and dextromethorphan hydrobromide 30 mg

Mucophen® DM: Guaifenesin 1000 mg and dextromethorphan hydrobromide 60 mg

Mucinex® DM Maximum Strength: Guaifenesin 1200 mg and dextromethorphan hydrobromide 60 mg

Phlemex: Guaifenesin 1200 mg and dextromethorphan hydrobromide 20 mg

Touro® DM: Guaifenesin 575 mg and dextromethorphan hydrobromide 30 mg

Tablet, long-acting: Guaifenesin 1000 mg and dextromethorphan hydrobromide 60 mg

Z-Cof LA [scored]: Guaifenesin 650 mg and dextromethorphan hydrobromide 30 mg

Tablet, sustained release:

Allfen-DM: Guaifenesin 1000 mg and dextromethorphan hydrobromide 55 mg

Relacon LAX: Guaifenesin 835 mg and dextromethorphan hydrobromide 30 mg

Tussi-Bid®: Guaifenesin 1200 mg and dextromethorphan hydrobromide 60 mg

Tablet, timed release [scored]: Guaifenesin 1200 mg and dextromethorphan hydrobromide 60 mg

Guia-D: Guaifenesin 1000 mg and dextromethorphan hydrobromide 60 mg [dye free]

- ♦ **Guaifenesin and Dyphylline** *see* Dyphylline and Guaifenesin *on page 496*
- ♦ **Guaifenex® DM** *see* Guaifenesin and Dextromethorphan *on page 730*
- ♦ **Guaituss AC** *see* Guaifenesin and Codeine *on page 729*

Guanabenz (GWAHN a benz)

Medication Safety Issues
Sound-alike/look-alike issues:
Guanabenz may be confused with guanadrel, guanfacine
Canadian Brand Names Wytensin®
Index Terms Guanabenz Acetate
Generic Available Yes
Pharmacologic Category Alpha$_2$-Adrenergic Agonist
Use Management of hypertension
Contraindications Hypersensitivity to guanabenz or any component of the formulation
Warnings/Precautions May cause significant orthostasis. Do not abruptly discontinue this medication; use with caution in patients with severe coronary insufficiency, recent myocardial infarction, severe renal or hepatic impairment
Adverse Reactions (Reflective of adult population; not specific for elderly)
Higher rates with larger doses
>5% (at doses of 16 mg/day):
Cardiovascular: Orthostasis
Central nervous system: Drowsiness or sedation (39%), dizziness (12% to 17%), headache (5%)
Gastrointestinal: Xerostomia (28% to 38%)
Neuromuscular & skeletal: Weakness (~10%)
≤3% (may be similar to placebo):
Cardiovascular: Arrhythmias, chest pain, edema, palpitation
Central nervous system: Anxiety, ataxia, depression, sleep disturbances
Dermatologic: Pruritus, rash
Endocrine & metabolic: Disturbances of sexual function, gynecomastia, decreased sexual function
Gastrointestinal: Constipation, diarrhea, nausea, vomiting
Genitourinary: Polyuria
Neuromuscular & skeletal: Myalgia
Ocular: Blurring of vision
Respiratory: Dyspnea, nasal congestion
Miscellaneous: Taste disorders
Drug Interactions Substrate of CYP1A2 (major)
CYP1A2 inducers: May decrease the levels/effects of guanabenz. Example inducers include aminoglutethimide, carbamazepine, phenobarbital, and rifampin.
CYP1A2 inhibitors: May increase the levels/effects of guanabenz. Example inhibitors include ciprofloxacin, fluvoxamine, ketoconazole, norfloxacin, ofloxacin, and rofecoxib.
Hypoglycemic symptoms may be reduced. Educate patient about decreased signs and symptoms of hypoglycemia or avoid use in patients with frequent episodes of hypoglycemia.
Nitroprusside and guanabenz have additive hypotensive effects.
Noncardioselective beta-blockers (nadolol, propranolol, timolol) may exacerbate rebound hypertension when guanabenz is withdrawn. The beta-blocker should be withdrawn first. The gradual withdrawal of guanabenz or a cardioselective beta-blocker could be substituted.
TCAs decrease the hypotensive effect of guanabenz.
Stability Protect from light.
Mechanism of Action Stimulates alpha$_2$-adrenoreceptors in the brain stem, thus activating an inhibitory neuron, resulting in reduced sympathetic outflow, producing a decrease in vasomotor tone and heart rate
Dosage
Geriatrics: Initial: 4 mg once daily, increase every 1-2 weeks
Adults: Hypertension: Oral: Initial: 4 mg twice daily; increase in increments of 4-8 mg/day every 1-2 weeks to a maximum of 32 mg twice daily.
Hepatic Impairment: Dosage adjustment is probably necessary; however, no specific guidelines are available.
Patient Information May cause drowsiness; rise from sitting/lying position carefully, may cause dizziness; do not discontinue without notifying physician
Special Geriatric Considerations Because of its CNS adverse effects, guanabenz is not considered a drug of choice for the treatment of hypertension in the elderly.
Dosage Forms Excipient information presented when available (limited, particularly for generics); consult specific product labeling.
Tablet: 4 mg, 8 mg
Selected References
Chobanian AV, Bakris GL, Black HR, et al, "The Seventh Report of the Joint National Committee on Prevention, Detection, Evaluation, and Treatment of High Blood Pressure: The JNC 7 Report," *JAMA*, 2003, 289(19):2560-71.

♦ **Guanabenz Acetate** *see* Guanabenz *on page 733*

Guanfacine (GWAHN fa seen)

Medication Safety Issues
Sound-alike/look-alike issues:
Guanfacine may be confused with guaifenesin, guanabenz, guanidine
Tenex® may be confused with Entex®, Ten-K®, Xanax®

International issues:
Tenex® may be confused with Kinex® which is a brand name for biperiden in Mexico
U.S. Brand Names Tenex®
Canadian Brand Names Tenex®
Index Terms Guanfacine Hydrochloride
Generic Available Yes
Pharmacologic Category Alpha$_2$-Adrenergic Agonist
Use Management of hypertension
Unlabeled/Investigational Use ADHD, tic disorder, aggression
Contraindications Hypersensitivity to guanfacine or any component of the formulation
Warnings/Precautions Use caution with severe coronary insufficiency, recent MI, cerebrovascular disease, or chronic renal or hepatic disease. Abrupt discontinuation can result in nervousness, anxiety and rarely, rebound hypertension (occurs 2-4 days after withdrawal). Avoid use in CNS disease, elderly, or with other CNS depressants (can cause sedation and drowsiness alone). Caution in diabetes; may mask signs of hypoglycemia. May cause orthostasis.
Adverse Reactions (Reflective of adult population; not specific for elderly)
>10%:
Central nervous system: Somnolence (5% to 40%), headache (3% to 13%), dizziness (2% to 15%)
Gastrointestinal: Xerostomia (10% to 54%), constipation (2% to 15%)
1% to 10%:
Central nervous system: Fatigue (2% to 10%)
Endocrine & metabolic: Impotence (up to 7%)
Drug Interactions
Nitroprusside and guanfacine have additive hypotensive effects.
Noncardioselective beta-blockers (nadolol, propranolol, timolol) may exacerbate rebound hypertension when guanfacine is withdrawn. The beta-blocker should be withdrawn first. The gradual withdrawal of guanfacine or a cardioselective beta-blocker could be substituted.
TCAs decrease the hypotensive effect of guanfacine.
Mechanism of Action Stimulates alpha$_2$-adrenoreceptors in the brain stem, thus activating an inhibitory neuron, resulting in reduced sympathetic outflow, producing a decrease in vasomotor tone and heart rate
Dosage
Geriatrics & Adults:
Hypertension: Oral: 1 mg usually at bedtime, may increase if needed at 3- to 4-week intervals; usual dose range (JNC 7): 0.5-2 mg once daily
ADHD, tic disorder, aggression (unlabeled uses): Oral: Initial: 0.5 mg at bedtime; increase as tolerated (every 3-14 days) to usual dose range (1.5-3 mg/day) given in 3 divided doses (maximum: 4 mg/day)
Patient Information May cause drowsiness, dizziness; do not discontinue this medication without consulting your physician; take at bedtime
Special Geriatric Considerations Because of adverse effects such as CNS depression, dry mouth, and constipation, guanfacine may not be considered a drug of choice in the elderly.
Dosage Forms Excipient information presented when available (limited, particularly for generics); consult specific product labeling.
Tablet: 1 mg, 2 mg
Tenex®: 1 mg, 2 mg
Selected References
Chobanian AV, Bakris GL, Black HR, et al, "The Seventh Report of the Joint National Committee on Prevention, Detection, Evaluation, and Treatment of High Blood Pressure: The JNC 7 Report," *JAMA*, 2003, 289(19):2560-71.

♦ **Guanfacine Hydrochloride** *see* Guanfacine *on page 734*
♦ **Guia-D** *see* Guaifenesin and Dextromethorphan *on page 730*
♦ **Guiatuss™ [OTC]** *see* Guaifenesin *on page 727*
♦ **Guiatuss-DM® [OTC]** *see* Guaifenesin and Dextromethorphan *on page 730*
♦ **Gyne-Lotrimin® 3 [OTC]** *see* Clotrimazole *on page 349*
♦ **Gynodiol®** *see* Estradiol *on page 549*
♦ **H5N1 Influenza Vaccine** *see* Influenza Virus Vaccine (H5N1) *on page 807*

♦ **Habitrol** *see* Nicotine *on page 1116*

Halcinonide (hal SIN oh nide)

Related Information
   Corticosteroids *on page 1755*
Medication Safety Issues
   Sound-alike/look-alike issues:
      Halcinonide may be confused with Halcion®
      Halog® may be confused with Haldol®, Mycolog®
U.S. Brand Names Halog®
Canadian Brand Names Halog®
Generic Available No
Pharmacologic Category Corticosteroid, Topical
Use Relief of the inflammatory and pruritic manifestations of corticosteroid-responsive dermatoses (very high potency topical corticosteroid)
Contraindications Hypersensitivity to halcinonide or any component of the formulation; viral, fungal, or tubercular skin lesions
Warnings/Precautions Systemic absorption of topical corticosteroids may cause hypothalamic-pituitary-adrenal (HPA) axis suppression (reversible). HPA axis suppression may lead to adrenal crisis. Risk is increased when used over large surface areas, for prolonged periods, or with occlusive dressings. Allergic contact dermatitis can occur, it is usually diagnosed by failure to heal rather than clinical exacerbation. Prolonged treatment with corticosteroids has been associated with the development of Kaposi's sarcoma (case reports); if noted, discontinuation of therapy should be considered. Adverse systemic effects including hyperglycemia, glycosuria, fluid and electrolyte changes, and HPA suppression may occur when used on large surface areas, for prolonged periods, or with an occlusive dressing.
Adverse Reactions (Reflective of adult population; not specific for elderly) Frequency not defined: Itching; dry skin; folliculitis; hypertrichosis; acneiform eruptions; hypopigmentation; perioral dermatitis; allergic contact dermatitis; skin maceration; skin atrophy; striae; local burning, irritation, miliaria; secondary infection
Drug Interactions No data reported
Mechanism of Action Decreases inflammation by suppression of migration of polymorphonuclear leukocytes and reversal of increased capillary permeability
Pharmacokinetics Absorption: Percutaneous absorption varies by location of topical application and the use of occlusive dressings
Dosage
   Geriatrics & Adults: Steroid-responsive dermatoses: Topical: Apply sparingly 1-3 times/day, occlusive dressing may be used for severe or resistant dermatoses; a thin film is effective; do not overuse. Therapy should be discontinued when control is achieved; if no improvement is seen, reassessment of diagnosis may be necessary.
Monitoring Parameters Relief of symptoms
Patient Information Use only as prescribed and for no longer than the period prescribed; apply sparingly in a thin film and rub in lightly; avoid contact with eyes; notify physician if condition persists or worsens
Additional Information Considered a very high potency steroid; avoid use on face
Special Geriatric Considerations Due to age-related changes in skin, limit use of topical glucocorticosteroids.
Dosage Forms Excipient information presented when available (limited, particularly for generics); consult specific product labeling. [DSC] = Discontinued product
   Cream (Halog®): 0.1% (15 g, 30 g, 60 g, 240 g) [DSC]
   Ointment (Halog®): 0.1% (15 g, 30 g, 60 g, 240 g) [DSC]
   Solution, topical (Halog®): 0.1% (20 mL, 60 mL)

♦ **Halcion® [DSC]** *see* Triazolam *on page 1625*
♦ **Haldol®** *see* Haloperidol *on page 736*
♦ **Haldol® Decanoate** *see* Haloperidol *on page 736*
♦ **Haley's M-O** *see* Magnesium Hydroxide and Mineral Oil *on page 948*
♦ **HalfLytely® and Bisacodyl** *see* Polyethylene Glycol-Electrolyte Solution and Bisacodyl *on page 1284*
♦ **Halfprin® [OTC]** *see* Aspirin *on page 127*

Halobetasol (hal oh BAY ta sol)

Related Information
   Corticosteroids *on page 1755*
Medication Safety Issues
   Sound-alike/look-alike issues:
      Ultravate® may be confused with Cutivate®
(Continued)

Halobetasol *(Continued)*

U.S. Brand Names Ultravate®

Canadian Brand Names Ultravate®

Index Terms Halobetasol Propionate

Generic Available Yes

Pharmacologic Category Corticosteroid, Topical

Use Short-term relief (<2 weeks) of inflammatory and pruritic manifestations of cortico-steroid-response dermatoses [super high potency topical corticosteroid]

Contraindications Hypersensitivity to halobetasol or any component of the formulation; viral, fungal, or tubercular skin lesions

Warnings/Precautions Systemic absorption of topical corticosteroids may cause hypothalamic-pituitary-adrenal (HPA) axis suppression (reversible). HPA axis suppression may lead to adrenal crisis. Risk is increased when used over large surface areas, for prolonged periods, or with occlusive dressings. Allergic contact dermatitis can occur, it is usually diagnosed by failure to heal rather than clinical exacerbation. Prolonged treatment with corticosteroids has been associated with the development of Kaposi's sarcoma (case reports); if noted, discontinuation of therapy should be considered. Adverse systemic effects including hyperglycemia, glycosuria, fluid and electrolyte changes, and HPA suppression may occur when used on large surface areas, for prolonged periods, or with an occlusive dressing. Not for ophthalmic use. Topical halobetasol should not be used for the treatment of rosacea or perioral dermatitis. Not recommended for application to the face, groin, or axillae.

Adverse Reactions (Reflective of adult population; not specific for elderly) 1% to 4%: Dermatologic: Burning, itching, stinging

Overdosage/Toxicology When applied in excessive quantities, systemic hypercorti-cism and adrenal suppression may occur; HPA axis suppression was observed in psoriasis patients using 7 g/day for 1 week; discontinuation of the corticosteroid should be done judiciously

Drug Interactions No data reported

Mechanism of Action Corticosteroids inhibit the initial manifestations of the inflammatory process (ie, capillary dilation and edema, fibrin deposition, and migration and diapedesis of leukocytes into the inflamed site) as well as later sequelae (angiogenesis, fibroblast proliferation)

Pharmacokinetics

Absorption: Percutaneous absorption varies by location of topical application; ~6% of a topically applied dose of ointment enters circulation within 96 hours

Metabolism: Primarily hepatic

Elimination: Urine

Dosage

Geriatrics & Adults: Steroid-responsive dermatoses: Topical: Apply sparingly to skin twice daily, rub in gently and completely; treatment should not exceed 2 consecutive weeks and total dosage should not exceed 50 g/week. Therapy should be discontinued when control is achieved; if no improvement is seen, reassessment of diagnosis may be necessary.

Monitoring Parameters Relief of symptoms

Patient Information Use only as prescribed and for no longer than the period prescribed; apply sparingly in a thin film and rub in lightly; avoid contact with eyes; notify physician if condition persists or worsens; do not use longer than 2 weeks

Additional Information Considered a super high potency steroid; avoid use on face

Special Geriatric Considerations Due to age-related changes in skin, limit use of topical glucocorticosteroids.

Dosage Forms Excipient information presented when available (limited, particularly for generics); consult specific product labeling.

Cream, as propionate: 0.05% (15 g, 50 g)

Ointment, as propionate: 0.05% (15 g, 50 g)

♦ **Halobetasol Propionate** *see Halobetasol on page 735*

♦ **Halog®** *see Halcinonide on page 735*

Haloperidol *(ha loe PER i dole)*

Related Information

Antipsychotic Agents *on page 1747*

Liquid Compatibility of Antipsychotics and Mood Stabilizers *on page 1851*

Medication Safety Issues

Sound-alike/look-alike issues:

Haloperidol may be confused Halotestin®

Haldol® may be confused with Halcion®, Halenol®, Halog®, Halotestin®, Stadol®

U.S. Brand Names Haldol®; Haldol® Decanoate

Canadian Brand Names Apo-Haloperidol®; Apo-Haloperidol LA®; Haloperidol Injection, USP; Haloperidol-LA; Haloperidol-LA Omega; Haloperidol Long Acting; Novo-Peridol; Peridol; PMS-Haloperidol LA

Index Terms Haloperidol Decanoate; Haloperidol Lactate

Generic Available Yes

Pharmacologic Category Antipsychotic Agent, Typical

Use Management of psychotic disorders, nonpsychotic symptoms associated with dementia in older adults, Tourette's syndrome, Huntington's chorea
See Special Geriatric Considerations.

Unlabeled/Investigational Use Treatment of psychosis; may be used for the emergency sedation of severely-agitated or delirious patients; adjunctive treatment of ethanol dependence; antiemetic

Contraindications Hypersensitivity to haloperidol or any component of the formulation; Parkinson's disease; severe CNS depression; bone marrow suppression; severe cardiac or hepatic disease; coma

Warnings/Precautions Hypotension may occur, particularly with parenteral administration. Although the short-acting form is used clinically, the I.V. use of the injection is not an FDA-approved route of administration; the decanoate form should never be administered intravenously. Avoid in thyrotoxicosis. May be sedating, use with caution in disorders where CNS depression is a feature. Caution in patients with hemodynamic instability, predisposition to seizures, subcortical brain damage, renal or respiratory disease. Esophageal dysmotility and aspiration have been associated with antipsychotic use - use with caution in patients at risk of pneumonia (eg, Alzheimer's disease). Caution in breast cancer or other prolactin-dependent tumors (may elevate prolactin levels). May alter temperature regulation or mask toxicity of other drugs due to antiemetic effects. May alter cardiac conduction - life-threatening arrhythmias have occurred with therapeutic doses of antipsychotics. Avoid use in patients with underlying QT prolongation, in those taking medicines that prolong the QT interval, or cause polymorphic ventricular tachycardia. Even when used at recommended doses, cardiac arrhythmias have occurred. Monitor ECG closely for dose-related QT effects. Adverse effects of decanoate may be prolonged. May cause orthostatic hypotension; use with caution in patients at risk of this effect or those who would tolerate transient hypotensive episodes (cerebrovascular disease, cardiovascular disease, or other medications which may predispose). Some tablets contain tartrazine.

May cause anticholinergic effects (confusion, agitation, constipation, xerostomia, blurred vision, urinary retention). Therefore, they should be used with caution in patients with decreased gastrointestinal motility, urinary retention, BPH, xerostomia, or visual problems. Conditions which also may be exacerbated by cholinergic blockade include narrow-angle glaucoma (screening is recommended) and worsening of myasthenia gravis. Relative to other neuroleptics, haloperidol has a low potency of cholinergic blockade.

May cause extrapyramidal reactions, including pseudoparkinsonism, acute dystonic reactions, akathisia, and tardive dyskinesia (risk of these reactions is high relative to other neuroleptics). May be associated with neuroleptic malignant syndrome (NMS) or pigmentary retinopathy.

Adverse Reactions (Reflective of adult population; not specific for elderly)
Frequency not defined.
Cardiovascular: Abnormal T waves with prolonged ventricular repolarization, arrhythmia, hyper-/hypotension, tachycardia, torsade de pointes
Central nervous system: Agitation, akathisia, altered central temperature regulation, anxiety, confusion, depression, drowsiness, dystonic reactions, euphoria, extrapyramidal reactions, headache, insomnia, lethargy, neuroleptic malignant syndrome (NMS), pseudoparkinsonian signs and symptoms, restlessness, seizure, tardive dyskinesia, tardive dystonia, vertigo
Dermatologic: Alopecia, contact dermatitis, hyperpigmentation, photosensitivity (rare), pruritus, rash
Endocrine & metabolic: Amenorrhea, breast engorgement, galactorrhea, gynecomastia, hyper-/hypoglycemia, hyponatremia, lactation, mastalgia, menstrual irregularities, sexual dysfunction
Gastrointestinal: Anorexia, constipation, diarrhea, dyspepsia, hypersalivation, nausea, vomiting, xerostomia
Genitourinary: Priapism, urinary retention
Hematologic: Cholestatic jaundice, obstructive jaundice
Ocular: Blurred vision
Respiratory: Bronchospasm, laryngospasm
Miscellaneous: Diaphoresis, heat stroke

Overdosage/Toxicology Symptoms include deep sleep, dystonia, agitation, dysrhythmias, and extrapyramidal symptoms. Following initiation of essential overdose management, toxic symptom treatment and supportive treatment should be initiated. Critical cardiac arrhythmias often respond to I.V. lidocaine, while other antiarrhythmics
(Continued)

Haloperidol *(Continued)*

can be used. Neuroleptics often cause extrapyramidal symptoms (eg, dystonic reactions) requiring management with anticholinergic agents such as benztropine mesylate I.V. 1-2 mg (adult). These agents are generally effective within 2-5 minutes.

Drug Interactions Substrate of CYP1A2 (minor), 2D6 (major), 3A4 (major); **Inhibits** CYP2D6 (moderate), 3A4 (moderate)

Acetylcholinesterase inhibitors (central): May increase the risk of antipsychotic-related extrapyramidal symptoms; monitor.

Anticholinergics: May inhibit the therapeutic response to haloperidol and excess anticholinergic effects may occur; tardive dyskinesias have also been reported; includes benztropine and trihexyphenidyl

Antihypertensives: Concurrent use of haloperidol with an antihypertensive may produce additive hypotensive effects (particularly orthostasis)

Bromocriptine: Antipsychotics inhibit the ability of bromocriptine to lower serum prolactin concentrations

Chloroquine: Serum concentrations of haloperidol may be increased by chloroquine

CNS depressants: Sedative effects may be additive; monitor for increased effect; includes barbiturates, benzodiazepines, opioid analgesics, ethanol and other sedative agents

CYP2D6 inhibitors: May increase the levels/effects of haloperidol. Example inhibitors include chlorpromazine, delavirdine, fluoxetine, miconazole, paroxetine, pergolide, quinidine, quinine, ritonavir, and ropinirole.

CYP2D6 substrates: Haloperidol may increase the levels/effects of CYP2D6 substrates. Example substrates include amphetamines, selected beta-blockers, dextromethorphan, fluoxetine, lidocaine, mirtazapine, nefazodone, paroxetine, risperidone, ritonavir, thioridazine, tricyclic antidepressants, and venlafaxine.

CYP2D6 prodrug substrates: Haloperidol may decrease the levels/effects of CYP2D6 prodrug substrates. Example prodrug substrates include codeine, hydrocodone, oxycodone, and tramadol.

CYP3A4 inducers: CYP3A4 inducers may decrease the levels/effects of haloperidol. Example inducers include aminoglutethimide, carbamazepine, nafcillin, nevirapine, phenobarbital, phenytoin, and rifamycins.

CYP3A4 inhibitors: May increase the levels/effects of haloperidol. Example inhibitors include azole antifungals, clarithromycin, diclofenac, doxycycline, erythromycin, imatinib, isoniazid, nefazodone, nicardipine, propofol, protease inhibitors, quinidine, telithromycin, and verapamil.

CYP3A4 substrates: Haloperidol may increase the levels/effects of CYP3A4 substrates. Example substrates include benzodiazepines, calcium channel blockers, cyclosporine, mirtazapine, nateglinide, nefazodone, sildenafil (and other PDE-5 inhibitors), tacrolimus, and venlafaxine. Selected benzodiazepines (midazolam and triazolam), cisapride, ergot alkaloids, selected HMG-CoA reductase inhibitors (lovastatin and simvastatin), and pimozide are generally contraindicated with strong CYP3A4 inhibitors.

Indomethacin: Haloperidol in combination with indomethacin may result in drowsiness, tiredness, and confusion; monitor for adverse effects

Inhalation anesthetics: Haloperidol in combination with certain forms of induction anesthesia may produce peripheral vasodilitation and hypotension

Levodopa: Haloperidol may inhibit the antiparkinsonian effect of levodopa; avoid this combination

Lithium: Haloperidol may produce neurotoxicity with lithium; this is a rare effect

Methyldopa: Effect of haloperidol may be altered; enhanced effects, as well as reduced efficacy have been reported

Metoclopramide: May increase extrapyramidal symptoms (EPS) or risk.

Nefazodone: Haloperidol and nefazodone may produce additive CNS toxicity, including sedation

Propranolol: Serum concentrations of haloperidol may be increased

Quinidine: May increase haloperidol concentrations; monitor for EPS and/or QT_c prolongation

SSRIs: Fluoxetine, fluvoxamine, and paroxetine may inhibit the metabolism of haloperidol resulting in EPS; monitor for EPS

Sulfadoxine-pyrimethamine: May increase fluphenazine concentrations

Tricyclic antidepressants: Concurrent use may produce increased toxicity or altered therapeutic response

Trazodone: Haloperidol and trazodone may produce additive hypotensive effects

Ethanol/Nutrition/Herb Interactions

Ethanol: Avoid ethanol (may increase CNS depression).

Herb/Nutraceutical: Avoid valerian, St John's wort, kava kava, gotu kola (may increase CNS depression).

Stability

Protect oral dosage forms from light.

Haloperidol lactate injection should be stored at controlled room temperature; do not freeze or expose to temperatures >40°C. Protect from light; exposure to light may cause discoloration and the development of a grayish-red precipitate over several weeks.

Haloperidol lactate may be administered IVPB or I.V. infusion in D_5W solutions. NS solutions should not be used due to reports of decreased stability and incompatibility. Standardized dose: 0.5-100 mg/50-100 mL D_5W.

Stability of standardized solutions is 38 days at room temperature (24°C).

Mechanism of Action Haloperidol is a butyrophenone antipsychotic which blocks postsynaptic mesolimbic dopaminergic D_1 and D_2 receptors in the brain; depresses the release of hypothalamic and hypophyseal hormones; believed to depress the reticular activating system thus affecting basal metabolism, body temperature, wakefulness, vasomotor tone, and emesis

Pharmacodynamics
Onset of action: Sedation: I.M., I.V.: 30-60 minutes
Duration: Decanoate: 2-4 weeks

Pharmacokinetics
Distribution: V_d: 8-18 L/kg
Protein binding: 90%
Metabolism: Hepatic to inactive compounds
Bioavailability: Oral: 60%
Half-life elimination: 18 hours; Decanoate: ~1 day
Time to peak, serum: Oral: 2-6 hours; I.M.: 20 minutes; Decanoate: 7 days
Excretion: Urine (33% to 40% as metabolites) within 5 days; feces (15%)
Clearance: 550 ± 133 mL/minute

Dosage
Geriatrics: Nonpsychotic patient, dementia behavior (unlabeled use): Initial: Oral: 0.25-0.5 mg 1-2 times/day; increase dose at 4- to 7-day intervals by 0.25-0.5 mg/day. Increase dosing intervals (twice daily, 3 times/day, etc) as necessary to control response or side effects.

Adults:
Psychosis:
Oral: 0.5-5 mg 2-3 times/day; usual maximum: 30 mg/day
I.M. (as lactate): 2-5 mg every 4-8 hours as needed
I.M. (as decanoate): Initial: 10-20 times the daily oral dose administered at 4-week intervals. Maintenance dose: 10-15 times initial oral dose; used to stabilize psychiatric symptoms

Delirium in the intensive care unit (unlabeled use, unlabeled route):
I.V.: 2-10 mg; may repeat bolus doses every 20-30 minutes until calm achieved then administer 25% of the maximum dose every 6 hours; monitor ECG and QT_c interval
Intermittent I.V.: 0.03-0.15 mg/kg every 30 minutes to 6 hours
Oral: Agitation: 5-10 mg
Continuous I.V. infusion (100 mg/100 mL D_5W): Rates of 3-25 mg/hour have been used

Rapid tranquilization of severely-agitated patient (unlabeled use; administer every 30-60 minutes):
Oral: 5-10 mg
I.M. (as lactate): 5 mg
Average total dose (oral or I.M.) for tranquilization: 10-20 mg

Renal Impairment: Hemodialysis/peritoneal dialysis: Supplemental dose is not necessary.

Administration The decanoate injectable formulation should be administered I.M. only, **do not administer decanoate I.V.** Dilute the oral concentrate with water or juice before administration. Avoid skin contact with oral suspension or solution; may cause contact dermatitis.

Monitoring Parameters Orthostatic blood pressures; tremors, gait changes, abnormal movement in trunk, neck, buccal area, or extremities; monitor target behaviors for which the agent is given

Reference Range Therapeutic: 5-20 ng/mL (SI: 10-30 nmol/L) (psychotic disorders - less for Tourette's and mania); Toxic: >42 mcg/mL (SI: >84 nmol/L). Therapeutic levels are controversial; dosed by response most commonly.

Patient Information Oral concentrate must be diluted in 2-4 oz of liquid (water, fruit juice, carbonated drinks, milk, or pudding); do not take antacid within 1 hour of taking drug; avoid alcohol; avoid excess sun exposure (use sun block); may cause drowsiness, rise slowly from recumbent position; use of supportive stockings may help prevent orthostatic hypotension

Special Geriatric Considerations Many elderly patients receive antipsychotic medications for inappropriate nonpsychotic behavior. Before initiating antipsychotic medication, the clinician should investigate any possible reversible cause; any stress or stress from any disease can cause acute "confusion" or worsening of baseline nonpsychotic (Continued)

Haloperidol *(Continued)*

behavior. Most commonly acute changes in behavior are due to increases in drug dose or addition of new drug to regimen; fluid electrolyte loss; infections; and changes in environment.

Any changes in disease status in any organ system can result in behavior changes.

In the treatment of agitated, demented, elderly patients, authors of meta-analysis of controlled trials of the response to the traditional antipsychotics (phenothiazines, butyrophenones) in controlling agitation have concluded that the use of neuroleptics results in a response rate of 18%. Clearly neuroleptic therapy for behavior control should be limited with frequent attempts to withdraw the agent given for behavior control.

Clinical studies of haloperidol did not include sufficient numbers of subjects ≥65 years of age to determine whether they respond differently from younger subjects. Other reported clinical experience has not consistently identified differences between the elderly and younger patients. However, the prevalence of tardive dyskinesia appears to be highest among the elderly, especially elderly women. Also, the pharmacokinetics of haloperidol in geriatric patients generally warrants the use of lower doses.

Dosage Forms Excipient information presented when available (limited, particularly for generics); consult specific product labeling. [DSC] = Discontinued product
Note: Strength expressed as base.
Injection, oil, as decanoate: 50 mg/mL (1 mL, 5 mL); 100 mg/mL (1 mL, 5 mL)
Haldol® Decanoate: 50 mg/mL (1 mL; 5 mL [DSC]); 100 mg/mL (1 mL; 5 mL [DSC]) [contains benzyl alcohol, sesame oil]
Injection, solution, as lactate: 5 mg/mL (1 mL, 10 mL)
Haldol®: 5 mg/mL (1 mL)
Solution, oral concentrate, as lactate: 2 mg/mL (15 mL, 120 mL)
Tablet: 0.5 mg, 1 mg, 2 mg, 5 mg, 10 mg, 20 mg

Selected References
Peabody CA, Warner MD, Whiteford HA, et al, "Neuroleptics and the Elderly," *J Am Geriatr Soc*, 1987, 35(3):233-8.
Risse SC and Barnes R, "Pharmacologic Treatment of Agitation Associated With Dementia," *J Am Geriatr Soc*, 1986, 34(5):368-76.
Saltz BL, Woerner MG, Kane JM, et al, "Prospective Study of Tardive Dyskinesia Incidence in the Elderly," *JAMA*, 1991, 266(17):2402-6.
Seifert RD, "Therapeutic Drug Monitoring: Psychotropic Drugs," *J Pharm Pract*, 1984, 6:403-16.

♦ **Haloperidol Decanoate** *see* Haloperidol *on page 736*
♦ **Haloperidol Lactate** *see* Haloperidol *on page 736*
♦ **Havrix®** *see* Hepatitis A Vaccine *on page 746*
♦ **Havrix® and Engerix-B®** *see* Hepatitis A Inactivated and Hepatitis B (Recombinant) Vaccine *on page 744*
♦ **HBIG** *see* Hepatitis B Immune Globulin *on page 748*
♦ **hBNP** *see* Nesiritide *on page 1106*
♦ **HCTZ (error-prone abbreviation)** *see* Hydrochlorothiazide *on page 756*
♦ **HDCV** *see* Rabies Virus Vaccine *on page 1372*
♦ **Heavy Mineral Oil** *see* Mineral Oil *on page 1045*
♦ **Hectorol®** *see* Doxercalciferol *on page 477*
♦ **Hemocyte® [OTC]** *see* Ferrous Fumarate *on page 618*
♦ **Hemorrhoidal HC** *see* Hydrocortisone *on page 762*
♦ **Hemril®-30** *see* Hydrocortisone *on page 762*
♦ **HepaGam B™** *see* Hepatitis B Immune Globulin *on page 748*

Heparin *(HEP a rin)*

Related Information
Anticoagulants, Injectable *on page 1741*
Anticoagulant Therapy Guidelines *on page 1813*
Medication Safety Issues
Sound-alike/look-alike issues:
Heparin may be confused with Hespan®

High alert medication: The Institute for Safe Medication Practices (ISMP) includes this medication among its list of drugs which have a heightened risk of causing significant patient harm when used in error.

Heparin sodium injection 10,000 units/mL and Hep-Lock U/P 10 units/mL have been confused with each other. Fatal medication errors have occurred between the two whose labels are both blue. **Never rely on color as a sole indicator to differentiate product identity.**

Heparin lock flush solution is intended only to maintain patency of I.V. devices and is **not** to be used for anticoagulant therapy.

Note: The 100 unit/mL concentration should not be used in neonates or infants <10 kg. The 10 unit/mL concentration may cause systemic anticoagulation in infants <1 kg who receive frequent flushes.

U.S. Brand Names HepFlush®-10; Hep-Lock®; Hep-Lock U/P
Canadian Brand Names Hepalean®; Hepalean® Leo; Hepalean®-LOK
Index Terms Heparin Calcium; Heparin Lock Flush; Heparin Sodium
Generic Available Yes
Pharmacologic Category Anticoagulant
Use Prophylaxis and treatment of thromboembolic disorders
Unlabeled/Investigational Use Acute MI — combination regimen of heparin (unlabeled dose), tenecteplase (half dose), and abciximab (full dose)
Contraindications Hypersensitivity to heparin or any component of the formulation; severe thrombocytopenia; uncontrolled active bleeding except when due to DIC; suspected intracranial hemorrhage; not for I.M. use; not for use when appropriate monitoring parameters cannot be obtained
Warnings/Precautions Use cautiously in patients with a documented hypersensitivity reaction and only in life-threatening situations. Hemorrhage is the most common complication. Monitor for signs and symptoms of bleeding. Certain patients are at increased risk of bleeding. Risk factors include bacterial endocarditis; congenital or acquired bleeding disorders; active ulcerative or angiodysplastic GI diseases; severe uncontrolled hypertension; hemorrhagic stroke; or use shortly after brain, spinal, or ophthalmology surgery; patient treated concomitantly with platelet inhibitors; conditions associated with increased bleeding tendencies (hemophilia, vascular purpura); recent GI bleeding; thrombocytopenia or platelet defects; severe liver disease; hypertensive or diabetic retinopathy; or in patients undergoing invasive procedures. A higher incidence of bleeding has been reported in patients >60 years of age, particularly women. They are also more sensitive to the dose. Discontinue heparin if hemorrhage occurs; severe hemorrhage or overdosage may require protamine.

May cause thrombocytopenia; monitor platelet count closely. Patients who develop thrombocytopenia on heparin may be at risk of developing a new thrombus (heparin-induced thrombocytopenia and thrombosis [HITT]). Discontinue therapy and consider alternatives if platelets are <100,000/mm^3 and/or thrombosis develops. HIT or HITT can occur up to several weeks after discontinuation of heparin. Hypersensitivity reactions can occur. Osteoporosis can occur following long-term use (>6 months). Monitor for hyperkalemia. Patients >60 years of age may require lower doses of heparin.

Some preparations contain sulfite which may cause allergic reactions.

Heparin resistance may occur in patients with fever, thrombosis, thrombophlebitis, infections with thromboing tendencies, MI, cancer, and in postsurgical patients.

Adverse Reactions (Reflective of adult population; not specific for elderly)
Cardiovascular: Chest pain, hemorrhagic shock, thrombosis, vasospasm (possibly related to thrombosis)
Central nervous system: Fever, headache, chills
Dermatologic: Unexplained bruising, urticaria, alopecia, dysesthesia pedis, purpura, eczema, cutaneous necrosis (following deep SubQ injection), erythematous plaques (case reports)
Endocrine & metabolic: Hyperkalemia (supression of aldosterone), rebound hyperlipidemia on discontinuation
Gastrointestinal: Nausea, vomiting, constipation, hematemesis
Genitourinary: Frequent or persistent erection
Hematologic: Hemorrhage, blood in urine, bleeding from gums, epistaxis, adrenal hemorrhage, ovarian hemorrhage, retroperitoneal hemorrhage, thrombocytopenia (see note)
Hepatic: Elevated liver enzymes (AST/ALT)
Local: Irritation, ulceration, cutaneous necrosis have been rarely reported with deep SubQ injections, I.M. injection (not recommended) is associated with a high incidence of these effects
Neuromuscular & skeletal: Peripheral neuropathy, osteoporosis (chronic therapy effect)
Ocular: Conjunctivitis (allergic reaction)
Respiratory: Hemoptysis, pulmonary hemorrhage, asthma, rhinitis, bronchospasm (case reports)
Miscellaneous: Allergic reactions, anaphylactoid reactions

Note: Thrombocytopenia has been reported to occur at an incidence between 0% and 30%. It is often of no clinical significance. However, immunologically mediated heparin-induced thrombocytopenia has been estimated to occur in 1% to 2% of patients, and is marked by a progressive fall in platelet counts and, in some cases, thromboembolic complications (skin necrosis, pulmonary embolism, gangrene of the extremities, stroke or MI). For recommendations regarding platelet monitoring during
(Continued)

Heparin *(Continued)*

heparin therapy, consult "Seventh ACCP Consensus Conference on Antithrombotic and Thrombolytic Therapy."

Overdosage/Toxicology The primary symptom of overdose is bleeding. The antidote is protamine: 1 mg per 100 units of heparin. Discontinue all heparin if evidence of progressive immune thrombocytopenia occurs.

Drug Interactions

Cephalosporins which contain the MTT side chain may increase the risk of hemorrhage.

Drugs which affect platelet function (eg, aspirin, NSAIDs, dipyridamole, ticlopidine, clopidogrel, IIb/IIIa antagonists) may potentiate the risk of hemorrhage.

Nitroglycerin (I.V.) may decrease heparin's anticoagulant effect. This interaction has not been validated in some studies, and may only occur at high nitroglycerin dosages.

Penicillins (parenteral) may prolong bleeding time via inhibition of platelet aggregation, potentially increasing the risk of hemorrhage.

Thrombolytic agents increase the risk of hemorrhage.

Warfarin: Risk of bleeding may be increased during concurrent therapy. Heparin is commonly continued during the initiation of warfarin therapy to assure anticoagulation and to protect against possible transient hypercoagulability.

Other drugs reported to increase heparin's anticoagulant effect include antihistamines, tetracycline, quinine, nicotine, and cardiac glycosides (digoxin).

Ethanol/Nutrition/Herb Interactions

Food: When taking for >6 months, may interfere with calcium absorption.

Herb/Nutraceutical: Avoid cat's claw, dong quai, evening primrose, feverfew, red clover, horse chestnut, garlic, green tea, ginseng, ginkgo (all have additional antiplatelet activity).

Stability

Heparin solutions are colorless to slightly yellow; minor color variations do not affect therapeutic efficacy.

Heparin should be stored at controlled room temperature. Protect from freezing and temperatures >40°C.

Stability at room temperature and refrigeration:

Prepared bag: 24 hours.

Premixed bag: After seal is broken 4 days.

Out of overwrap stability: 30 days.

Standard diluent: 25,000 units/500 mL D_5W (premixed).

Minimum volume: 250 mL D_5W.

Mechanism of Action Potentiates the action of antithrombin III and thereby inactivates thrombin (as well as activated coagulation factors IX, X, XI, XII, and plasmin) and prevents the conversion of fibrinogen to fibrin; heparin also stimulates release of lipoprotein lipase (lipoprotein lipase hydrolyzes triglycerides to glycerol and free fatty acids)

Pharmacodynamics

Onset of action:

SubQ: Anticoagulation occurs within 20-30 minutes

I.V.: Immediate

Duration: Dose-dependent

Pharmacokinetics

Absorption: Oral, rectal, SubQ, I.M.: Erratic

Metabolism: Believed to be partially metabolized in the reticuloendothelial system

Half-life: Mean: 90 minutes with range: 30 minutes to 3 hours (half-life affected by obesity, renal function, hepatic function, malignancy, presence of pulmonary embolism, and infections), half-life is dose-dependent

Elimination: Hepatic metabolism is followed by renal excretion, small amount excreted unchanged in urine

Dosage

Geriatrics: Patients >60 years of age may have higher serum levels and clinical response (longer aPTTs) as compared to younger patients receiving similar dosages. Lower dosages may be required.

Adults:

DVT Prophylaxis (low-dose heparin): SubQ: 5000 units every 8-12 hours

Systemic anticoagulation: I.V. infusion (weight-based dosing per institutional nomogram recommended):

Acute coronary syndromes or MI: Fibrinolytic therapy: I.V. infusion:

Full-dose alteplase, reteplase, or tenecteplase with dosing as follows: Concurrent bolus of 60 units/kg (maximum: 4000 units), then 12 units/kg/hour (maximum: 1000 units/hour) as continuous infusion. Check aPTT every 4-6 hours; adjust to target of 1.5-2 times the upper limit of control (50-70 seconds in clinical trials); usual range 10-30 units/kg/hour. Duration of heparin therapy depends on concurrent therapy and the specific patient risks for systemic or venous thromboembolism.

Combination regimen (unlabeled): Half-dose tenecteplase (15-25 mg based on weight) and abciximab 0.25 mg/kg bolus then 0.125 mcg/kg/minute (maximum 10 mcg/minute) for 12 hours with heparin dosing as follows: Concurrent bolus of 40 units/kg (maximum 3000 units), then 7 units/kg/hour (maximum: 800 units/hour) as continuous infusion. Adjust to a aPTT target of 50-70 seconds.

Streptokinase: Heparin use optional depending on concurrent therapy and specific patient risks for systemic or venous thromboembolism (anterior MI, CHF, previous embolus, atrial fibrillation, LV thrombus): If heparin is administered, start when aPTT <2 times the upper limit of control; do not use a bolus, but initiate infusion adjusted to a target aPTT of 1.5-2 times the upper limit of control (50-70 seconds in clinical trials). If heparin is not administered by infusion, 7500-12,500 units SubQ every 12 hours (when aPTT <2 times the upper limit of control) is recommended.

Percutaneous coronary intervention: Heparin bolus and infusion may be administered to an activated clotting time (ACT) of 300-350 seconds if no concurrent GPIIb/IIIa receptor antagonist is administered or 200-250 seconds if a GPIIb/IIIa receptor antagonist is administered.

Unstable angina (high-risk and some intermediate-risk patients): Initial bolus of 60-70 units/kg (maximum: 5000 units), followed by an initial infusion of 12-15 units/kg/hour (maximum: 1000 units/hour). The American College of Chest Physicians consensus conference has recommended dosage adjustments to correspond to a therapeutic range equivalent to heparin levels of 0.3-0.7 units/mL by antifactor Xa determinations.

Venous thromboembolism :
DVT/PE: I.V. push: 80 units/kg followed by continuous infusion of 18 units/kg/hour
DVT: SubQ: 17,500 units every 12 hours

Intermittent I.V. Anticoagulation: Intermittent I.V.: Initial: 10,000 units, then 50-70 units/kg (5000-10,000 units) every 4-6 hours

Maintenance of line patency (line flushing): When using daily flushes of heparin to maintain patency of single and double lumen central catheters, 100 units/mL is commonly used in adults. Capped PVC catheters and peripheral heparin locks require flushing more frequently (eg, every 6-8 hours). Volume of heparin flush is usually similar to volume of catheter (or slightly greater). Additional flushes should be given when stagnant blood is observed in catheter, after catheter is used for drug or blood administration, and after blood withdrawal from catheter.

Parenteral nutrition: Addition of heparin (0.5-3 unit/mL) to peripheral and central parenteral nutrition has not been shown to decrease catheter-related thrombosis. Arterial lines are heparinized with a final concentration of 1 unit/mL.

Administration Do not administer I.M. due to pain, irritation, and hematoma formation

Monitoring Parameters PTT, platelets, hemoglobin, hematocrit, and signs of bleeding

Reference Range Therapeutic: 0.3-0.5 units/mL

Test Interactions Increased thyroxine (S) (competitive protein binding methods); increased PT

Aprotinin significantly increases aPTT and celite Activated Clotting Time (ACT) which may not reflect the actual degree of anticoagulation by heparin. Kaolin-based ACTs are not affected by aprotinin to the same degree as celite ACTs. While institutional protocols may vary, a minimal celite ACT of 750 seconds or kaolin-ACT of 480 seconds is recommended in the presence of aprotinin. Consult the manufacturer's information on specific ACT test interpretation in the presence of aprotinin.

Additional Information Heparin does not possess fibrinolytic activity and, therefore, cannot lyse established thrombi; discontinue heparin if hemorrhage occurs; severe hemorrhage or overdosage may require protamine; monitor platelet counts, signs of bleeding, PTT.

When using daily flushes of heparin to maintain patency of single and double lumen central catheters. Capped PVC catheters and peripheral heparin locks require flushing more frequently (eg, every 6-8 hours). Volume of heparin flush is usually similar to volume of catheter (or slightly greater) or may be standardized according to specific hospital's policy (eg, 2-5 mL/flush). Dose of heparin flush used should not approach therapeutic per kg dose. Additional flushes should be given when stagnant blood is observed in catheter, after catheter is used for drug or blood administration, and after blood withdrawal from catheter.

Heparin 1 unit/mL (final concentration) may be added to TPN solutions, both central and peripheral. (Addition of heparin to peripheral TPN has been shown to increase duration of line patency.)

Arterial lines are heparinized with a final concentration of 1 unit/mL.

Special Geriatric Considerations In the clinical setting, age has not been shown to be a reliable predictor of a patient's anticoagulant response to heparin. However, it is common for the elderly to have a "standard" response for the first 24-48 hours after a
(Continued)

Heparin *(Continued)*

loading dose (5000 units) and a maintenance infusion of 800-1000 units/hour. After this period, they then have an exaggerated response (ie, elevated PTT), requiring a lower infusion rate. Hence, monitor closely during this period of therapy. Elderly women are more likely to have bleeding complications and osteoporosis may be a problem when used >3 months or total daily dose exceeds 30,000 units.

Dosage Forms Excipient information presented when available (limited, particularly for generics); consult specific product labeling.

Infusion, as sodium [premixed in NaCl 0.45%; porcine intestinal mucosa source]: 12,500 units (250 mL); 25,000 units (250 mL, 500 mL)

Infusion, as sodium [preservative free; premixed in D$_5$W; porcine intestinal mucosa source]: 10,000 units (100 mL) [contains sodium metabisulfite]; 12,500 units (250 mL) [contains sodium metabisulfite]; 20,000 units (500 mL) [contains sodium metabisulfite]; 25,000 units (250 mL, 500 mL) [contains sodium metabisulfite]

Infusion, as sodium [preservative free; premixed in NaCl 0.9%; porcine intestinal mucosa source]: 1000 units (500 mL); 2000 units (1000 mL)

Injection, solution, as sodium [lock flush preparation; porcine intestinal mucosa source; multidose vial]: 10 units/mL (1 mL, 10 mL, 30 mL) [contains parabens]; 100 units/mL (1 mL, 5 mL) [contains parabens]

Injection, solution, as sodium [lock flush preparation; porcine intestinal mucosa source; multidose vial]: 10 units/mL (10 mL, 30 mL); 100 units/mL (10 mL, 30 mL) [contains benzyl alcohol]

Hep-Lock®: 10 units/mL (1 mL, 2 mL, 10 mL, 30 mL); 100 units/mL (1 mL, 2 mL, 10 mL, 30 mL) [contains benzyl alcohol]

Injection, solution, as sodium [lock flush preparation; porcine intestinal mucosa source; prefilled syringe]: 10 units/mL (1 mL, 2 mL, 3 mL, 5 mL); 100 units/mL (1 mL, 2 mL, 3 mL, 5 mL) [contains benzyl alcohol]

Injection, solution, as sodium [preservative free; lock flush preparation; porcine intestinal mucosa source; prefilled syringe]: 100 units/mL (5 mL)

Injection, solution, as sodium [preservative free; lock flush preparation; porcine intestinal mucosa source; vial]:

HepFlush®-10: 10 units/mL (10 mL)

Hep-Lock U/P: 10 units/mL (1 mL); 100 units/mL (1 mL)

Injection, solution, as sodium [porcine intestinal mucosa source; multidose vial]: 1000 units/mL (1 mL, 10 mL, 30 mL) [contains benzyl alcohol]; 1000 units/mL (1 mL, 10 mL, 30 mL) [contains methylparabens]; 5000 units/mL (1 mL, 10 mL) [contains benzyl alcohol]; 5000 units/mL (1 mL) [contains methylparabens]; 10,000 units/mL (1 mL, 4 mL) [contains benzyl alcohol]; 10,000 units/mL (1 mL, 5 mL) [contains methylparabens]; 20,000 units/mL (1 mL) [contains methylparabens]

Injection, solution, as sodium [porcine intestinal mucosa source; prefilled syringe]: 5000 units/mL (1 mL) [contains benzyl alcohol]

Injection, solution, as sodium [preservative free; porcine intestinal mucosa source; prefilled syringe]: 10,000 units/mL (0.5 mL)

Injection, solution, as sodium [preservative free; porcine intestinal mucosa source; vial]: 1000 units/mL (2 mL); 2000 units/mL (5 mL); 2500 units/mL (10 mL)

Selected References

Bohannon AD and Lyles KW, "Drug-Induced Bone Disease," *Clin Geriatr Med*, 1994, 10(4):611-23.

Bull BS, Korpman RA, Huse WM, et al, "Heparin Therapy During Extracorporeal Circulation. I. Problems Inherent in Existing Heparin Protocols," *J Thorac Cardiovasc Surg*, 1975, 69(5):674-84.

Jick H, Slone D, Borda IT, et al, "Efficacy and Toxicity of Heparin in Relation to Age and Sex," *N Engl J Med*, 1968, 279(6):284-6.

♦ **Heparin Calcium** *see* Heparin *on page 740*
♦ **Heparin Lock Flush** *see* Heparin *on page 740*
♦ **Heparin Sodium** *see* Heparin *on page 740*

Hepatitis A Inactivated and Hepatitis B (Recombinant) Vaccine
(hep a TYE tis aye in ak ti VAY ted & hep a TYE tis bee ree KOM be nant vak SEEN)

Related Information
Hepatitis A Vaccine *on page 746*
Hepatitis B Vaccine *on page 750*
U.S. Brand Names Twinrix®
Canadian Brand Names Twinrix®
Index Terms Engerix-B® and Havrix®; Havrix® and Engerix-B®; Hepatitis B (Recombinant) and Hepatitis A Inactivated Vaccine
Generic Available No

Pharmacologic Category Vaccine

Use Active immunization against disease caused by hepatitis A virus and hepatitis B virus (all known subtypes) in populations desiring protection against or at high risk of exposure to these viruses.

Populations include travelers to areas of intermediate/high endemicity for **both** HAV and HBV; those at increased risk of HBV infection due to behavioral or occupational factors; patients with chronic liver disease; laboratory workers who handle live HAV and HBV; healthcare workers, police, and other personnel who render first-aid or medical assistance; workers who come in contact with sewage; employees of day care centers and correctional facilities; patients/staff of hemodialysis units; male homosexuals; patients frequently receiving blood products; military personnel; users of injectable illicit drugs; close household contacts of patients with hepatitis A and hepatitis B infection; residents of drug and alcohol treatment centers

Contraindications Hypersensitivity to hepatitis A vaccine or hepatitis B vaccine, or any component of the formulation

Warnings/Precautions Use caution in patients on anticoagulants, with thrombocytopenia, or bleeding disorders (bleeding may occur following intramuscular injection). Treatment for anaphylactic reactions should be immediately available. Postpone vaccination in moderate to severe acute illness (minor illness is not a contraindication). May not prevent infection if adequate antibody titers are not achieved (including immunosuppressed patients, patients on immunosuppressant therapy). Contains yeast and aluminum, and trace amounts of neomycin and thimerosal; packaging may contain latex. Also see individual agents.

Adverse Reactions (Reflective of adult population; not specific for elderly)
All serious adverse reactions must be reported to the U.S. Department of Health and Human Services (DHHS) Vaccine Adverse Event Reporting System (VAERS) 1-800-822-7967.

Incidence of adverse effects of the combination product were similar to those occurring after administration of hepatitis A vaccine and hepatitis B vaccine alone. (Incidence reported is not versus placebo.)

>10%:
  Central nervous system: Headache (13% to 22%), fatigue (11% to 14%)
  Local: Injection site reaction: Soreness (37% to 41%), redness (8% to 11%)

1% to 10%:
  Central nervous system: Fever (2% to 4%)
  Gastrointestinal: Diarrhea (4% to 6%), nausea (2% to 4%), vomiting (≤1%)
  Local: Injection site reaction: Swelling (4% to 6%), induration
  Respiratory: Upper respiratory tract infection

Drug Interactions Immunosuppressant agents: May decrease immune response to vaccine

Stability Store in refrigerator at 2°C to 8°C (36°F to 46°F); do not freeze (discard if frozen).

Mechanism of Action
Hepatitis A vaccine, an inactivated virus vaccine, offers active immunization against hepatitis A virus infection at an effective immune response rate in up to 99% of subjects.

Recombinant hepatitis B vaccine is a noninfectious subunit viral vaccine. The vaccine is derived from hepatitis B surface antigen (HB$_s$Ag) produced through recombinant DNA techniques from yeast cells. The portion of the hepatitis B gene which codes for HB$_s$Ag is cloned into yeast which is then cultured to produce hepatitis B vaccine.

In immunocompetent people, Twinrix® provides active immunization against hepatitis A virus infection (at an effective immune response rate >99% of subjects) and against hepatitis B virus infection (at an effective immune response rate of 93% to 97%) 30 days after completion of the 3-dose series. This is comparable to using hepatitis A vaccine and hepatitis B vaccine concomitantly.

Pharmacodynamics
Onset of action: Seroconversion for antibodies against HAV and HBV were detected one month after completion of the 3-dose series.
Duration: Patients remained seropositive for at least 4 years during the clinical studies.

Dosage
Geriatrics & Adults: Primary immunization: I.M.: Three doses (1 mL each) given on a 0-, 1-, and 6-month schedule
  Alternative regimen: Accelerated regimen (1 mL doses at day 0, 7, and 21-30, followed by a booster at 12 months) has demonstrated similar safety, tolerability, and immunogenicity to the standard regimen.

Administration I.M.: Shake well prior to use. Do not dilute prior to administration. Administer in the deltoid region; do not administer in the gluteal region (may give suboptimal response). Do not administer at the same site, or using the same syringe, as additional vaccines or immunoglobulins.

(Continued)

Hepatitis A Inactivated and Hepatitis B (Recombinant) Vaccine *(Continued)*

For patients at risk of hemorrhage following intramuscular injection, the ACIP recommends "it should be administered intramuscularly if, in the opinion of the physician familiar with the patients bleeding risk, the vaccine can be administered with reasonable safety by this route. If the patient receives antihemophilia or other similar therapy, intramuscular vaccination can be scheduled shortly after such therapy is administered. A fine needle (23 gauge or smaller) can be used for the vaccination and firm pressure applied to the site (without rubbing) for at least 2 minutes. The patient should be instructed concerning the risk of hematoma from the injection."

Patient Information Must complete full course of injections for adequate immunization. Notify prescriber of any reactions following prior vaccines. May cause soreness, redness, or swelling at the injection site. Other side effects may be headache, tiredness, diarrhea, nausea, vomiting, or fever. Notify prescriber if these are severe or last longer than 48 hours.

Additional Information Federal law requires that the date of administration, the vaccine manufacturer, lot number of vaccine, and the administering person's name, title, and address be entered into the patient's permanent medical record.

Special Geriatric Considerations No adjustment for age is necessary. Some studies with HBV demonstrate a lower antibody titer in the elderly as compared to younger adults.

Dosage Forms Excipient information presented when available (limited, particularly for generics); consult specific product labeling.

Injection, suspension:

Twinrix®: Inactivated hepatitis A virus 720 ELISA units and hepatitis B surface antigen 20 mcg per mL (1 mL) [contains aluminum, yeast, and trace amounts of neomycin and thimerosal; rubber plunger and tip cap in prefilled syringe contain latex]

Selected References

Centers for Disease Control, "Recommendations of the Advisory Committee on Immunization Practices (ACIP): General Recommendations on Immunization," *MMWR*, 1994, 43(RR-1):23.

Hepatitis A Vaccine (hep a TYE tis aye vak SEEN)

Related Information

Immunization Recommendations *on page 1787*

U.S. Brand Names Havrix®; VAQTA®

Canadian Brand Names Avaxim®; Avaxim®-Pediatric; Havrix®; VAQTA®

Generic Available No

Pharmacologic Category Vaccine

Use

Active immunization against disease caused by hepatitis A virus in populations desiring protection against or at high risk of exposure

Populations at high risk of exposure to hepatitis A virus may include children and adolescents in selected states and regions, travelers to developing countries, household and sexual contacts of persons infected with hepatitis A, child day care employees, patients with chronic liver disease, illicit drug users, male homosexuals, institutional workers (eg, institutions for the mentally and physically handicapped persons, prisons), and healthcare workers who may be exposed to hepatitis A virus (eg, laboratory employees)

Contraindications Hypersensitivity to hepatitis A vaccine or any component of the formulation

Warnings/Precautions Use caution in patients on anticoagulants, with thrombocytopenia, or bleeding disorders (bleeding may occur following intramuscular injection). Treatment for anaphylactic reactions should be immediately available. Postpone vaccination with acute infection or febrile illness. May not prevent infection if adequate antibody titers are not achieved (including immunosuppressed patients, patients on immunosuppressant therapy). Packaging may contain natural latex rubber..

Adverse Reactions (Reflective of adult population; not specific for elderly)

All serious adverse reactions must be reported to the U.S. Department of Health and Human Services (DHHS) Vaccine Adverse Event Reporting System (VAERS) 1-800-822-7967.

Frequency dependent upon age, product used, and concomitant vaccine administration. In general, injection site reactions were less common in younger children.

>10%:

Central nervous system: Irritability (11% to 36%), drowsiness (15% to 17%), headache (≤1% to 16%), fever ≥100.4°F (9% to 11%)

Gastrointestinal: Anorexia (1% to 19%)

Local: Injection site: Pain, soreness, tenderness (3% to 56%), erythema (1% to 22%), warmth (<1% to 17%), swelling (1% to 14%)

1% to 10%:

Central nervous system: Fever ≥102°F (3% to 4%)

Dermatologic: Rash (≤1% to 5%)

Endocrine & metabolic: Menstrual disorder (1%)

Gastrointestinal: Diarrhea (<1% to 6%), vomiting (<1% to 4%), nausea (2%), abdominal pain (<1% to 2%), anorexia (1%)

Local: Injection site bruising (1% to 2%)

Neuromuscular & skeletal: Weakness/fatigue (4%), myalgia (<1% to 2%), arm pain (1%), back pain (1%), stiffness (1%)

Ocular: Conjunctivitis (1%)

Otic: Otitis media (8%), otitis (2%)

Respiratory: Upper respiratory tract infection (<1% to 10%), rhinorrhea (6%), cough (1% to 5%), pharyngitis (<1% to 3%), respiratory congestion (2%), nasal congestion (1%), laryngotracheobronchitis (1%)

Miscellaneous: Crying (2%), viral exanthema (1%)

Drug Interactions

Immune globulin: May be administered concomitantly (using separate sites and syringes)

Vaccines: May be administered concomitantly with cholera, diphtheria, MMR II, Japanese encephalitis, poliovirus, rabies, tetanus, typhoid or yellow fever vaccines using separate sites and syringes. May be administered simultaneously with hepatitis B vaccine.

Stability Store under refrigeration at 2°C to 8°C (36°F to 46°F); do not freeze.

Mechanism of Action As an inactivated virus vaccine, hepatitis A vaccine offers active immunization against hepatitis A virus infection at an effective immune response rate in up to 99% of subjects

Pharmacodynamics

Onset of action (protection): 4 weeks after a single dose

Duration: Neutralizing antibodies have persisted for up to 8 years; based on kinetic models, antibodies may be present >20 years

Dosage

Geriatrics & Adults: Immunization: I.M.: **Note:** Primary immunization should be given at least 2 weeks prior to expected exposure:

Havrix®:

1440 ELISA units (1 mL) with a booster dose of 1440 ELISA units given 6-12 months following primary immunization

VAQTA®:

50 units (1 mL) with 50 units (1 mL) booster dose of 50 units to be given 6-18 months after primary immunization (6-12 months if initial dose was with Havrix®)

Administration Shake vial or syringe well before withdrawing or injecting; discard if suspension does not appear as an opaque, uniform suspension. For patients at risk of hemorrhage following intramuscular injection, the ACIP recommends "it should be administered intramuscularly if, in the opinion of the physician familiar with the patients bleeding risk, the vaccine can be administered with reasonable safety by this route. If the patient receives antihemophilia or other similar therapy, intramuscular vaccination can be scheduled shortly after such therapy is administered. A fine needle (23 gauge or smaller) can be used for the vaccination and firm pressure applied to the site (without rubbing) for at least 2 minutes. The patient should be instructed concerning the risk of hematoma from the injection."

Monitoring Parameters Liver function tests

Reference Range Seroconversion for Havrix®: Antibody >20 mIU/mL

Patient Information Report any serious side effects such as seizures, dizziness, hives, rash, or swelling to your physician.

Additional Information Some investigators suggest simultaneous or sequential administration of inactivated hepatitis A vaccine and immune globulin for postexposure protection, especially for travelers requiring rapid immunization, although a slight decrease in vaccine immunogenicity may be observed with this technique. If concomitant administration with other vaccines or IgG is anticipated, administer at different sites or injections with separate syringes.

Federal law requires that the date of administration, the vaccine manufacturer, lot number of vaccine, and the administering person's name, title, and address be entered into the patient's permanent medical record.

Special Geriatric Considerations There is no specific data to suggest dosing is different than it is for younger adults.

Dosage Forms Excipient information presented when available (limited, particularly for generics); consult specific product labeling.

Injection, suspension [adult formulation; preservative free]:

Havrix®: Viral antigen 1440 ELISA units/mL (1 mL) [contains trace amounts of neomycin; syringe plunger contains latex rubber; available in prefilled syringe or single-dose vial]

(Continued)

Hepatitis A Vaccine *(Continued)*

VAQTA®: HAV antigen 50 units/mL (1 mL) [vial stopper and syringe plunger contain latex rubber; available in prefilled syringe or single-dose vial]

Injection, suspension [pediatric formulation; preservative free]:

Havrix®: Viral antigen 720 ELISA units/0.5 mL (0.5 mL) [contains trace amounts of neomycin; syringe plunger contains latex rubber; available in prefilled syringe or single-dose vial]

Injection, suspension [pediatric/adolescent formulation; preservative free]:

VAQTA®: HAV antigen 25 units/0.5 mL (0.5 mL) [vial stopper and syringe plunger contain latex rubber; available in prefilled syringe or single-dose vial]

Selected References

Bancroft WH, "Hepatitis A Vaccine," *N Engl J Med*, 1992, 327(7):453-7.

Centers for Disease Control and Prevention, "Prevention of Hepatitis A Through Active or Passive Immunization: Recommendations of the Advisory Committee on Immunization Practices (ACIP)," *MMWR Recomm Rep*, 1999, 48(RR-12):1-37.

Centers for Disease Control, "Recommendations of the Advisory Committee on Immunization Practices (ACIP): General Recommendations on Immunization," *MMWR*, 1994, 43(RR-1):23.

Koff RS, "Hepatitis A," *Lancet*, 1998, 351(9116):1643-9.

Lemon SM, "Inactivated Hepatitis A Vaccines," *JAMA*, 1994, 271(17):1363-4.

Niu MT, Salive M, Krueger C, et al, "Two-Year Review of Hepatitis A Vaccine Safety: Data From the Vaccine Adverse Event Reporting System (VAERS)," *Clin Infect Dis*, 1998, 26(6):1475-6.

Hepatitis B Immune Globulin (hep a TYE tis bee i MYUN GLOB yoo lin)

Related Information
Immunization Recommendations *on page 1787*

U.S. Brand Names HepaGam B™; HyperHEP B™ S/D; Nabi-HB®

Canadian Brand Names HepaGam B™; HyperHep B®

Index Terms HBIG

Generic Available No

Pharmacologic Category Immune Globulin

Use
Passive prophylactic immunity to hepatitis B following: Acute exposure to blood containing hepatitis B surface antigen (HBsAg); perinatal exposure of infants born to HBsAg-positive mothers; sexual exposure to HBsAg-positive persons; household exposure to persons with acute HBV infection

Prevention of hepatitis B virus recurrence after liver transplantation in HBsAg-positive transplant patients

Note: Hepatitis B immune globulin is not indicated for treatment of active hepatitis B infection and is ineffective in the treatment of chronic active hepatitis B infection.

Contraindications Hypersensitivity to hepatitis B immune globulin or any component of the formulation; severe allergy to gamma globulin or anti-immunoglobulin therapies

Warnings/Precautions Hypersensitivity and anaphylactic reactions can occur; immediate treatment (including epinephrine 1:1000) should be available. Use with caution in patients with previous systemic hypersensitivity to human immunoglobulins. Use with caution in patients with thrombocytopenia or coagulation disorders; I.M. injections may be contraindicated. Use with caution in patients with IgA deficiency. Product of human plasma; may potentially contain infectious agents which could transmit disease. Screening of donors, as well as testing and/or inactivation or removal of certain viruses, reduces the risk. Infections thought to be transmitted by this product should be reported to the manufacturer. Some products may contain maltose, which may result in falsely-elevated blood glucose readings.

Adverse Reactions (Reflective of adult population; not specific for elderly)
Reported with postexposure prophylaxis; frequency not defined. Adverse events reported in liver transplant patients included tremor and hypotension, were associated with a single infusion during the first week of treatment, and did not recur with additional infusions.

Central nervous system: Fainting, headache, lightheadedness, malaise

Dermatologic: Angioedema, bruising, urticaria

Gastrointestinal: Nausea, vomiting

Hematologic: WBC decreased

Hepatic: Alkaline phosphatase increased, AST increased

Local: Ache, erythema, pain, and/or tenderness at injection site

Neuromuscular & skeletal: Arthralgia, joint stiffness, myalgia

Renal: Creatinine increased

Respiratory: Cold symptoms

Miscellaneous: Anaphylaxis, flu-like syndrome

Drug Interactions Live virus vaccines: Interferes with immune response of live virus vaccines; defer live virus vaccine for about 3 months after immune globulin

Note: HBIG may be administered at the same time (but at a different site) or up to 1 month preceding hepatitis B vaccination without impairing the active immune response

Stability Refrigerate at 2°C to 8°C (36°F to 46°F); do not freeze. Use within 6 hours of entering vial. Do not shake vial; avoid foaming.

Mechanism of Action Hepatitis B immune globulin (HBIG) is a nonpyrogenic sterile solution containing immunoglobulin G (IgG) specific to hepatitis B surface antigen (HB$_s$Ag). HBIG differs from immune globulin in the amount of anti-HB$_s$. Immune globulin is prepared from plasma that is not preselected for anti-HB$_s$ content. HBIG is prepared from plasma preselected for high titer anti-HB$_s$. In the U.S., HBIG has an anti-HB$_s$ high titer >1:100,000 by IRA.

Pharmacodynamics Duration of action: Postexposure prophylaxis: 3-6 months

Pharmacokinetics
> Absorption: I.M.: Slow
> Half-life: 17-25 days
> Distribution: V$_d$: 7-15 L
> Time to peak, serum: I.M.: 2-10 days

Dosage
> **Geriatrics & Adults:**
> > **Postexposure prophylaxis:** I.M.: 0.06 mL/kg as soon as possible after exposure (ie, within 24 hours of needlestick, ocular, or mucosal exposure or within 14 days of sexual exposure); usual dose: 3-5 mL; repeat at 28-30 days after exposure in nonresponders to hepatitis B vaccine or in patients who refuse vaccination
> > **Note:** HBIG may be administered at the same time (but at a different site) or up to 1 month preceding hepatitis B vaccination without impairing the active immune response
> >
> > **Prevention of hepatitis B virus recurrence after liver transplantation (HepaGam B™):** I.V.: 20,000 int. units/dose according to the following schedule:
> > Anhepatic phase (Initial dose): One dose given with the liver transplant
> > Week 1 postop: One dose daily for 7 days (days 1-7)
> > Weeks 2-12 postop: One dose every 2 weeks starting day 14
> > Month 4 onward: One dose monthly starting on month 4
> > Dose adjustment: Adjust dose to reach anti-HBs levels of 500 int. units/L within the first week after transplantation. In patients with surgical bleeding, abdominal fluid drainage >500 mL or those undergoing plasmapheresis, administer 10,000 int. units/dose every 6 hours until target anti-HBs levels are reached.

Administration
> I.M.: Postexposure prophylaxis: I.M. injection only in anterolateral aspect of upper thigh and deltoid muscle of upper arm; to prevent injury from injection, care should be taken when giving to patients with thrombocytopenia or bleeding disorders
> I.V.:
> > HepaGam B™: Liver transplant: Administer at 2 mL/minute. Decrease infusion to ≤1 mL/minute for patient discomfort or infusion-related adverse events. Actual volume of infusion is dependant upon potency labeled on each individual vial.
> > Nabi-HB®: Although not an FDA-approved for this purpose, Nabi-HB® has been administered intravenously in hepatitis B-positive liver transplant patients.

Monitoring Parameters Liver transplant: Serum HBsAg; infusion-related adverse events

Test Interactions
> Glucose testing: HepaGam B™ contains maltose. Falsely-elevated blood glucose levels may occur when glucose monitoring devices and test strips utilizing the glucose dehydrogenase pyrroloquinolinequinone (GDH-PQQ) based methods are used.
> Serological testing: Antibodies transferred following administration of immune globulins may provide misleading positive test results (eg, Coombs' test)

Patient Information Be aware of adverse effects

Additional Information Hepatitis B immune globulin is not indicated for treatment of active hepatitis B infections and is ineffective in the treatment of chronic active hepatitis B infection. Administration of HBIG preceding or concomitantly with hepatitis B vaccine does not interfere with the immune response to vaccine; the two together provide more rapid protective antibodies to hepatitis B than when vaccine is used alone; rapid levels may be necessary in certain settings. Has been administered intravenously in hepatitis B-positive liver transplant patients.

Special Geriatric Considerations No data available to suggest different dosing in the elderly than in younger adults.

Dosage Forms Excipient information presented when available (limited, particularly for generics); consult specific product labeling.
> **Note:** Potency expressed in international units (as compared to the WHO standard) is noted by individual lot on the vial label.
> Injection, solution [preservative free]:
> > HyperHEP B™ S/D: 15% to 18% (0.5 mL, 1 mL, 5 mL)
> > Nabi-HB®: 5% (1 mL, 5 mL) [>312 int. units/mL; contains polysorbate 80]
> > HepaGam B™: 5% (1 mL, 5 mL) [>312 int. units/mL; contains maltose and polysorbate 80]

(Continued)

749

Hepatitis B Immune Globulin *(Continued)*
Selected References
Dickson RC, Terrault NA, Ishitani M, et al, "Protective Antibody Levels and Dose Requirements for IV 5% Nabi Hepatitis B Immune Globulin Combined With Lamivudine in Liver Transplantation for Hepatitis B-Induced End Stage Liver Disease," *Liver Transpl*, 2006, 12(1):124-33.

Mast EE, Weinbaum CM, Fiore AE, et al, "A Comprehensive Immunization Strategy to Eliminate Transmission of Hepatitis B Virus Infection in the United States: Recommendations of the Advisory Committee on Immunization Practices (ACIP) Part II: Immunization of Adults," *MMWR Recomm Rep*, 2006, 55(RR-16):1-33.

Tung BY and Kowdley KV, "Hepatitis B and Liver Transplantation," *Clin Infect Dis*, 2005, 41(10):1461-6.

♦ **Hepatitis B Inactivated Virus Vaccine (recombinant DNA)** *see* Hepatitis B Vaccine *on page 750*

♦ **Hepatitis B (Recombinant) and Hepatitis A Inactivated Vaccine** *see* Hepatitis A Inactivated and Hepatitis B (Recombinant) Vaccine *on page 744*

Hepatitis B Vaccine *(hep a TYE tis bee vak SEEN)*

Related Information
Immunization Recommendations *on page 1787*
Medication Safety Issues
Sound-alike/look-alike issues:
Recombivax HB® may be confused with Comvax®
U.S. Brand Names Engerix-B®; Recombivax HB®
Canadian Brand Names Engerix-B®; Recombivax HB®
Index Terms Hepatitis B Inactivated Virus Vaccine (recombinant DNA)
Generic Available No
Pharmacologic Category Vaccine
Use Immunization against infection caused by all known subtypes of hepatitis B virus (HBV), in individuals seeking protection from HBV infection and/or in the following individuals considered at high risk of potential exposure to hepatitis B virus or HB$_s$Ag-positive materials:

Workplace Exposure:
- Healthcare workers[1] (including students, custodial staff, lab personnel, etc)
- Police and fire personnel
- Military personnel
- Morticians and embalmers
- Clients/staff of institutions for the developmentally disabled

Lifestyle Factors:
- Homosexual men
- Heterosexually-active persons with multiple partners in a 6-month period or those with recently acquired sexually-transmitted disease
- Intravenous drug users

Specific Patient Groups:
- Those on hemodialysis[2], receiving transfusions[3], or in hematology/oncology units
- Adolescents
- Infants born of HBsAG-positive mothers
- Individuals with chronic liver disease
- Individual with HIV infection

Others:
- Prison inmates and staff of correctional facilities
- Household and sexual contacts of HBV carriers
- Residents, immigrants, adoptees, and refugees from areas with endemic HBV infection (eg, Alaskan Eskimos, Pacific Islanders, Indochinese, and Haitian descent)
- International travelers to areas of endemic HBV
- Children born after 11/21/1991

[1]The risk of hepatitis B virus (HBV) infection for healthcare workers varies both between hospitals and within hospitals. Hepatitis B vaccination is recommended for all healthcare workers with blood exposure.

[2]Hemodialysis patients often respond poorly to hepatitis B vaccination; higher vaccine doses or increased number of doses are required. A special formulation of one vaccine is now available for such persons (Recombivax HB®, 40 mcg/mL). The anti-HB$_s$(antibody to hepatitis B surface antigen) response of such persons should be tested after they are vaccinated, and those who have not responded should be revaccinated with 1-3 additional doses. Patients with chronic renal disease should be vaccinated as early as possible, ideally before they require hemodialysis. In addition, their anti-HB$_s$ levels should be monitored at 6- to 12-month intervals to assess the need for revaccination.

[3]Patients with hemophilia should be immunized subcutaneously, not intramuscularly.

Contraindications Hypersensitivity to yeast, hepatitis B vaccine, or any component of the formulation

Warnings/Precautions Immediate treatment for anaphylactic/anaphylactoid reaction should be available during vaccine use. Consider delaying vaccination during acute, moderate-to-severe febrile illness. Use caution with decreased cardiopulmonary function Unrecognized hepatitis B infection may be present, immunization may not prevent infection in these patients Patients >65 years may have lower response rates. Consider delaying vaccination for ≥3 months after receiving immunosuppressive therapy. Use caution in multiple sclerosis patients; rare exacerbations of symptoms have been observed. Some dosage forms contain dry natural latex rubber.

Adverse Reactions (Reflective of adult population; not specific for elderly)
All serious adverse reactions must be reported to the U.S. Department of Health and Human Services (DHHS) Vaccine Adverse Event Reporting System (VAERS) 1-800-822-7967.

Frequency not defined. The most common adverse effects reported with both products included injection site reactions (>10%).

Cardiovascular: Flushing, hypotension

Central nervous system: Agitation, chills, dizziness, fatigue, fever (≥37.5°C / 100°F), headache, insomnia, irritability, lightheadedness, malaise, somnolence, vertigo

Dermatologic: Angioedema, petechiae, pruritus, rash, urticaria

Gastrointestinal: Abdominal pain, appetite decreased, constipation, cramps, diarrhea, dyspepsia, nausea, vomiting

Genitourinary: Dysuria

Local: Injection site reactions: Ecchymosis, erythema, induration, pain, nodule formation, soreness, swelling, tenderness, warmth

Neuromuscular & skeletal: Achiness, arthralgia, back pain, myalgia, neck pain, neck stiffness, paresthesia, shoulder pain, tingling, weakness

Otic: Earache

Respiratory: Cough, pharyngitis, rhinitis, upper respiratory tract infection

Miscellaneous: Diaphoresis, lymphadenopathy, flu-like syndrome

Drug Interactions

Immunosuppressant medications: The effect of the vaccine may be decreased; consider deferring vaccination for at least 3 months after immunosuppressant therapy is discontinued.

Vaccines: DTaP, *Haemophilus* b conjugate vaccine (PedvaxHIB®), MMR, and OPV vaccines may be administered together (using separate sites and syringes).

Stability Refrigerate at 2°C to 8°C (36°F to 46°F); do not freeze.

Mechanism of Action Recombinant hepatitis B vaccine is a noninfectious subunit viral vaccine, which confers active immunity via formation of antihepatitis B antibodies. The vaccine is derived from hepatitis B surface antigen (HB$_s$Ag) produced through recombinant DNA techniques from yeast cells. The portion of the hepatitis B gene which codes for HB$_s$Ag is cloned into yeast which is then cultured to produce hepatitis B vaccine.

Pharmacokinetics Duration of action: Following a 3-dose series in children, up to 50% of patients will have low or undetectable anti-HB antibody 5-15 years postvaccination. However, anamnestic increases in anti-HB have been shown up to 23 years later suggesting a lifelong immune memory response.

Routine Immunization Regimen of Three I.M. Hepatitis B Vaccine Doses

Age	Initial		1 mo		2 mo	6 mo[1]	
	Recom-bivax HB® (mL)	Enger-ix-B® (mL)	Recom-bivax HB® (mL)	Enger-ix-B® (mL)	Enger-ix-B® (mL)	Recom-bivax HB® (mL)	Enger-ix-B® (mL)
Birth[2] to 19 y	0.5[3]	0.5[4]	0.5[3]	0.5[4]	--	0.5[3]	0.5[4]
≥20 y[5]	1[6]	1[7]	1[6]	1[7]	--	1[6]	1[7]
Dialysis or immunocompromised patients[8]	1[9]	2[10]	1[9]	2[10]	2[10]	1[9]	2[10]

[1]Final dose in series should not be administered before age of 24 weeks
[2]Infants born of HB$_s$Ag **negative** mothers.
[3]5 mcg/0.5 mL pediatric/adolescent formulation
[4]10 mcg/0.5 mL formulation
[5]Alternately, doses may be administered at 0, 1, and 4 months **or** at 0, 2, and 4 months
[6]10 mcg/mL adult formulation
[7]20 mcg/mL formulation
[8]Revaccinate if anti-HB$_s$ <10 mIU/mL ≥1-2 months after third dose.
[9]40 mcg/mL dialysis formulation
[10]Two 1 mL doses given at different sites using the 20 mcg/mL formulation

(Continued)

Hepatitis B Vaccine *(Continued)*

Dosage

Geriatrics & Adults:

Immunization regimen:

Note: Regimen consists of 3 doses (0, 1, and 6 months): First dose given on the elected date, second dose given 1 month later, third dose given 6 months after the first dose; see table on previous page.

*Alternative dosing schedule for **Recombivax HB®**:* Adults ≥20 years: Doses may be administered at 0, 1, and 4 months **or** at 0, 2, and 4 months

*Alternative dosing schedules for **Engerix-B®**:* Adults ≥20 years:

Doses may be administered at 0, 1, and 4 months **or** at 0, 2, and 4 months

High-risk adults (20 mcg/mL formulation): 1 mL at 0, 1, 2, and 12 months. If booster dose is needed, revaccinate with 1 mL.

Administration It is possible to interchange the vaccines for completion of a series or for booster doses; the antibody produced in response to each type of vaccine is comparable, however, the quantity of the vaccine will vary

I.M. injection only; in adults, the deltoid muscle is the preferred site. Not for gluteal administration. Shake well prior to withdrawal and use.

For patients at risk of hemorrhage following intramuscular injection, hepatitis B vaccine may be administered subcutaneously although lower titers and/or increased incidence of local reactions may result. The ACIP recommends "it should be administered intramuscularly if, in the opinion of the physician familiar with the patients bleeding risk, the vaccine can be administered with reasonable safety by this route. If the patient receives antihemophilia or other similar therapy, intramuscular vaccination can be scheduled shortly after such therapy is administered. A fine needle (23 gauge or smaller) can be used for the vaccination and firm pressure applied to the site (without rubbing) for at least 2 minutes. The patient should be instructed concerning the risk of hematoma from the injection."

Federal law requires that the date of administration, the vaccine manufacturer, lot number of vaccine, and the administering person's name, title, and address be entered into the patient's permanent medical record.

Monitoring Parameters Measure serum antibody titers

Reference Range Maintain >10 mIU/mL

Patient Information Report any rash, edema, hives, changes in heartbeat, dizziness, or cough to your physician.

Additional Information Recombivax HB® is a recombinant vaccine derived from HB_sAg produced in yeast cells. Inactivated virus vaccine.

Federal law requires that the date of administration, the vaccine manufacturer, lot number of vaccine, and the administering person's name, title, and address be entered into the patient's permanent medical record.

Special Geriatric Considerations No dose adjustments required based on age. Some studies demonstrate a lower antibody titer in the elderly as compared to young adults.

Dosage Forms Excipient information presented when available (limited, particularly for generics); consult specific product labeling.

Injection, suspension [preservative free] [recombinant DNA]:

Engerix-B®:

Adult: Hepatitis B surface antigen 20 mcg/mL (1 mL) [contains trace amounts of thimerosal; some dosage forms contain dry natural latex rubber]

Pediatric/adolescent: Hepatitis B surface antigen 10 mcg/0.5 mL (0.5 mL) [contains trace amounts of thimerosal; some dosage forms contain dry natural latex rubber]

Recombivax HB®:

Adult: Hepatitis B surface antigen 10 mcg/mL (1 mL, 3 mL)

Dialysis: Hepatitis B surface antigen 40 mcg/mL (1 mL)

Pediatric/adolescent: Hepatitis B surface antigen 5 mcg/0.5 mL (0.5 mL)

Selected References

Centers for Disease Control and Prevention, "A Comprehensive Immunization Strategy to Eliminate Transmission of Hepatitis B Virus Infection in the United States: Recommendations of the Advisory Committee on Immunization Practices (ACIP) Part I: Immunization of Infants, Children, and Adolescents," *MMWR Recomm Rep*, 2005, 54(RR16):1-23.

Centers for Disease Control and Prevention, "A Comprehensive Immunization Strategy to Eliminate Transmission of Hepatitis B Virus Infection in the United States: Recommendations of the Advisory Committee on Immunization Practices (ACIP) Part II: Immunization of Adults," *MMWR Recomm Rep*, 2006, 54(RR16):1-25.

Centers for Disease Control, "Hepatitis B Virus: A Comprehensive Strategy for Eliminating Transmission in the United States Through Universal Childhood Vaccination: Recommendations of the Immunization Practices Advisory Committee (ACIP)," *MMWR Recomm Rep*, 1991, 40(RR-13):23.

Centers for Disease Control, "Recommendations of the Advisory Committee on Immunization Practices (ACIP): General Recommendations on Immunization," *MMWR Recomm Rep*, 2006, 55(RR-15):1-48.

Gardner P and Schaffner W, "Immunization of Adults," *N Engl J Med*, 1993, 328(17):1252-8.

◆ **HepFlush®-10** *see* Heparin *on page 740*
◆ **Hep-Lock®** *see* Heparin *on page 740*
◆ **Hep-Lock U/P** *see* Heparin *on page 740*
◆ **Hexachlorocyclohexane** *see* Lindane *on page 909*
◆ **Hexamethylenetetramine** *see* Methenamine *on page 1001*
◆ **High Gamma Vitamin E Complete™ [OTC]** *see* Vitamin E *on page 1677*
◆ **Hiprex®** *see* Methenamine *on page 1001*
◆ **Hi-Vegi-Lip [OTC]** *see* Pancreatin *on page 1195*
◆ **HMR 3647** *see* Telithromycin *on page 1523*
◆ **Hold® DM [OTC]** *see* Dextromethorphan *on page 419*

Homatropine (hoe MA troe peen)

U.S. Brand Names Isopto® Homatropine
Index Terms Homatropine Hydrobromide
Generic Available No
Pharmacologic Category Anticholinergic Agent, Ophthalmic; Ophthalmic Agent, Mydriatic
Use Producing cycloplegia and mydriasis for refraction; treatment of acute inflammatory conditions of the uveal tract
Contraindications Hypersensitivity to the drug or any component of the formulation; narrow-angle glaucoma, acute hemorrhage
Warnings/Precautions Use with caution in patients with hypertension, cardiac disease, or increased intraocular pressure; use with caution in obstructive uropathy, paralytic ileus, ulcerative colitis, unstable cardiovascular status in acute hemorrhage
Adverse Reactions (Reflective of adult population; not specific for elderly)
>10%: Ocular: Blurred vision, photophobia
1% to 10%:
    Local: Stinging, local irritation
    Ocular: Increased intraocular pressure
    Respiratory: Congestion
Overdosage/Toxicology Symptoms include blurred vision, urinary retention, and tachycardia. Anticholinergic toxicity is caused by strong binding of the drug to cholinergic receptors. For anticholinergic overdose with severe life-threatening symptoms, physostigmine 1-2 mg SubQ or slow I.V. may be given to reverse these effects.
Stability Protect from light.
Mechanism of Action Blocks response of iris sphincter muscle and the accommodative muscle of the ciliary body to cholinergic stimulation resulting in dilation and loss of accommodation
Pharmacodynamics
Onset of action: Following ophthalmic instillation, accommodation and pupil effects occur within 30-90 minutes
Duration: Mydriasis persists for 6-24 hours or more and cycloplegia lasts for 10-48 hours
Dosage
Geriatrics & Adults:
    Mydriasis and cycloplegia for refraction: Ophthalmic: Instill 1-2 drops of 2% solution or 1 drop of 5% solution before the procedure; repeat at 5- to 10-minute intervals as needed; maximum of 3 doses for refraction
    Uveitis: Ophthalmic: Instill 1-2 drops of 2% or 5% 2-3 times/day up to every 3-4 hours as needed
Administration Finger pressure should be applied to lacrimal sac for 1-2 minutes after instillation to decrease risk of absorption and systemic reactions
Patient Information If irritation persists or increases, discontinue use; may cause blurred vision and sensitivity to bright light
Dosage Forms Excipient information presented when available (limited, particularly for generics); consult specific product labeling.
    Solution, ophthalmic, as hydrobromide: 2% (5 mL); 5% (5 mL, 15 mL) [contains benzalkonium chloride]
Selected References
Barker DB and Solomon DA, "The Potential for Mental Status Changes Associated With Systemic Absorption of Anticholinergic Ophthalmic Medications: Concerns in the Elderly," *DICP Ann Pharmacother*, 1990, 24(9):847-50.

◆ **Homatropine Hydrobromide** *see* Homatropine *on page 753*
◆ **HTF919** *see* Tegaserod *on page 1520*
◆ **Humalog®** *see* Insulin Lispro *on page 812*
◆ **Humalog® Mix 50/50™** *see* Insulin Lispro Protamine and Insulin Lispro *on page 813*
◆ **Humalog® Mix 75/25™** *see* Insulin Lispro Protamine and Insulin Lispro *on page 813*

- ◆ **Human Diploid Cell Cultures Rabies Vaccine** *see* Rabies Virus Vaccine *on page 1372*
- ◆ **Humulin® 50/50** *see* Insulin NPH and Insulin Regular *on page 814*
- ◆ **Humulin® 70/30** *see* Insulin NPH and Insulin Regular *on page 814*
- ◆ **Humulin® N** *see* Insulin NPH *on page 813*
- ◆ **Humulin® R** *see* Insulin Regular *on page 815*
- ◆ **Humulin® R (Concentrated) U-500** *see* Insulin Regular *on page 815*

Hyaluronidase (hye al yoor ON i dase)

Medication Safety Issues
Sound-alike/look-alike issues:
Wydase may be confused with Lidex®, Wyamine®
U.S. Brand Names Amphadase™; Hydase™; Hylenex™; Vitrase®
Generic Available No
Pharmacologic Category Enzyme
Use Increase the dispersion and absorption of other drugs; increase rate of absorption of parenteral fluids given by hypodermoclysis; adjunct in subcutaneous urography for improving resorption of radiopaque agents
Unlabeled/Investigational Use Management of drug extravasations
Dosage
Geriatrics: Refer to adult dosing. Adjust dose carefully to individual patient.
Adults: Note: A preliminary skin test for hypersensitivity can be performed. ACTH, antihistamines, corticosteroids, estrogens, and salicylates, when used in large doses, may cause tissues to be partly resistant to hyaluronidase. May require larger doses of hyaluronidase for the same effect.
Skin test: Intradermal: 0.02 mL (3 units) of a 150 units/mL solution. Positive reaction consists of a wheal with pseudopods appearing within 5 minutes and persisting for 20-30 minutes with localized itching.
Hypodermoclysis: SubQ: 15 units is added to each 100 mL of I.V. fluid to be administered; 150 units facilitates absorption of >1000 mL of solution; rate and volume of a single clysis should not exceed those used for infusion of I.V. fluids
Urography: SubQ: 75 units over each scapula followed by injection of contrast medium at the same site; patient should be in the prone position.
Extravasation (unlabeled use): SubQ: Inject 1 mL of a 150 unit/mL solution (as 5-10 injections of 0.1-0.2 mL) into affected area; doses of 15-250 units have been reported. **Note:** Do not use for extravasation of pressor agents (eg, dopamine, norepinephrine).
Special Geriatric Considerations The most common use of hyaluronidase in the elderly is in hypodermoclysis. Hypodermoclysis is very useful in dehydrated patients in whom oral intake is minimal and I.V. access is a problem.
Dosage Forms Excipient information presented when available (limited, particularly for generics); consult specific product labeling.
Injection, powder for reconstitution:
Vitrase®: 6200 units [ovine derived; contains lactose]
Injection, solution:
Amphadase™: 150 units/mL (1 mL) [bovine derived; contains edetate disodium 1 mg, thimerosal ≤0.1 mg]
Injection, solution [preservative free]:
Hydase™: 150 units/mL (2 mL) [bovine derived; contains edetate disodium 1 mg]
Hylenex™: 150 units/mL (1 mL, 2 mL) [recombinant; contains human albumin and edetate disodium]
Vitrase®: 200 units/mL (2 mL) [ovine derived; contains lactose]

- ◆ **hycet™** *see* Hydrocodone and Acetaminophen *on page 759*
- ◆ **Hydase™** *see* Hyaluronidase *on page 754*
- ◆ **Hydergine [DSC]** *see* Ergoloid Mesylates *on page 527*

HydrALAZINE (hye DRAL a zeen)

Medication Safety Issues
Sound-alike/look-alike issues:
HydrALAZINE may be confused with hydrOXYzine
Canadian Brand Names Apo-Hydralazine®; Apresoline®; Novo-Hylazin; Nu-Hydral
Index Terms Apresoline [DSC]; Hydralazine Hydrochloride
Generic Available Yes
Pharmacologic Category Vasodilator
Use Management of moderate to severe hypertension, congestive heart failure
Contraindications Hypersensitivity to hydralazine or any component of the formulation; mitral valve rheumatic heart disease

Warnings/Precautions May cause a drug-induced lupus-like syndrome (more likely on larger doses, longer duration). Discontinue hydralazine in patients who develop SLE-like syndrome or positive ANA. Use with caution in patients with severe renal disease or cerebral vascular accidents or with known or suspected coronary artery disease; monitor blood pressure closely with I.V. use. Slow acetylators, patients with decreased renal function, and patients receiving >200 mg/day (chronically) are at higher risk for SLE. Titrate dosage to patient's response. Usually administered with diuretic and a beta-blocker to counteract side effects of sodium and water retention and reflex tachycardia.

Adjust dose in severe renal dysfunction. Use with caution in CAD (increase in tachycardia may increase myocardial oxygen demand). Use with caution in pulmonary hypertension (may cause hypotension). Patients may be poorly compliant because of frequent dosing. Hydralazine-induced fluid and sodium retention may require addition or increased dosage of a diuretics.

Adverse Reactions (Reflective of adult population; not specific for elderly)
Frequency not defined.
Cardiovascular: Tachycardia, angina pectoris, orthostatic hypotension (rare), dizziness (rare), paradoxical hypertension, peripheral edema, vascular collapse (rare), flushing
Central nervous system: Increased intracranial pressure (I.V., in patient with pre-existing increased intracranial pressure), fever (rare), chills (rare), anxiety*, disorientation*, depression*, coma*
Dermatologic: Rash (rare), urticaria (rare), pruritus (rare)
Gastrointestinal: Anorexia, nausea, vomiting, diarrhea, constipation, adynamic ileus
Genitourinary: Difficulty in micturition, impotence
Hematologic: Hemolytic anemia (rare), eosinophilia (rare), decreased hemoglobin concentration (rare), reduced erythrocyte count (rare), leukopenia (rare), agranulocytosis (rare), thrombocytopenia (rare)
Neuromuscular & skeletal: Rheumatoid arthritis, muscle cramps, weakness, tremor, peripheral neuritis (rare)
Ocular: Lacrimation, conjunctivitis
Respiratory: Nasal congestion, dyspnea
Miscellaneous: Drug-induced lupus-like syndrome (dose related; fever, arthralgia, splenomegaly, lymphadenopathy, asthenia, myalgia, malaise, pleuritic chest pain, edema, positive ANA, positive LE cells, maculopapular facial rash, positive direct Coombs' test, pericarditis, pericardial tamponade), diaphoresis
*Seen in uremic patients and severe hypertension where rapidly escalating doses may have caused hypotension leading to these effects.

Overdosage/Toxicology Symptoms include hypotension, tachycardia, and shock. Hypotension usually responds to I.V. fluids, Trendelenburg positioning, or vasoconstrictors. Treatment is primarily supportive and symptomatic.

Drug Interactions Inhibits CYP3A4 (weak)
Beta-blockers (metoprolol, propranolol) serum concentrations and pharmacologic effects may be increased. Monitor cardiovascular status.
Propranolol increases hydralazine's serum concentrations. Acebutolol, atenolol, and nadolol (low hepatic clearance or no first-pass metabolism) are unlikely to be affected.
NSAIDs may decrease the hemodynamic effects of hydralazine; avoid use if possible or closely monitor cardiovascular status.

Ethanol/Nutrition/Herb Interactions
Ethanol: Avoid ethanol (may increase CNS depression).
Food: Food enhances bioavailability of hydralazine.
Herb/Nutraceutical: Avoid dong quai if using for hypertension (has estrogenic activity). Avoid ephedra, yohimbe, ginseng (may worsen hypertension). Avoid garlic (may have increased antihypertensive effect).

Stability Intact ampuls/vials of hydralazine should not be stored under refrigeration because of possible precipitation or crystallization. Hydralazine should be diluted in NS for IVPB administration due to decreased stability in D_5W. Stability of IVPB solution in NS is 4 days at room temperature.

Mechanism of Action Direct vasodilation of arterioles (with little effect on veins) with decreased systemic resistance

Pharmacodynamics
Onset of action:
Oral: 20-30 minutes
I.V.: 5-20 minutes
Duration: **Note:** May vary depending on acetylator status of patient.
Oral: Up to 8 hours
I.V.: 1-4 hours

Pharmacokinetics
Metabolism: Oral: Large first-pass effect
Bioavailability: 30% to 50%; enhanced by the concurrent ingestion of food
(Continued)

HydrALAZINE *(Continued)*

Dosage

Geriatrics: Oral: Initial: 10 mg 2-3 times/day; increase by 10-25 mg/day every 2-5 days.

Adults:

Hypertension: Oral:

Initial: 10 mg 4 times/day; increase by 10-25 mg/dose every 2-5 days (maximum: 300 mg/day); usual dose range (JNC 7): 25-100 mg/day in 2 divided doses

Acute hypertension: I.M., I.V.: Initial: 10-20 mg/dose every 4-6 hours as needed, may increase to 40 mg/dose; change to oral therapy as soon as possible.

Congestive heart failure: Oral:

Initial dose: 10-25 mg 3-4 times/day

Adjustment: Dosage must be adjusted based on individual response

Target dose: 225-300 mg/day in divided doses; use in combination with isosorbide dinitrate

Renal Impairment:

Cl_{cr} 10-50 mL/minute: Administer every 8 hours.

Cl_{cr} <10 mL/minute: Administer every 8-16 hours in fast acetylators and every 12-24 hours in slow acetylators.

Hemodialysis effects: Supplemental dose is not necessary.

Peritoneal dialysis effects: Supplemental dose is not necessary.

Monitoring Parameters Blood pressure, standing and sitting/supine

Patient Information Report flu-like symptoms; rise from sitting/lying carefully, may cause dizziness; take with meals

Additional Information Has also been used to treat primary pulmonary hypertension. Slow acetylators, patients with decreased renal function and patients receiving >200 mg/day (chronically) are at higher risk for SLE. Titrate dosage to patient's response. Usually administered with diuretic and a beta-blocker to counteract side effects of sodium and water retention and reflex tachycardia although the beta-blocker may not be necessary in older adults. For the treatment of CHF where hydralazine is used in place of an ACE inhibitor, it is necessary to use a combination of hydralazine and isosorbide. See Isosorbide Dinitrate *on page 839*.

Dosage Forms Excipient information presented when available (limited, particularly for generics); consult specific product labeling.

Injection, solution, as hydrochloride: 20 mg/mL (1 mL)

Tablet, as hydrochloride: 10 mg, 25 mg, 50 mg, 100 mg

Selected References

Birkenhager WH, "Choosing the Optimum Therapy for Older Hypertensive Patients," *Drugs Aging*, 1991, 1(1):36-47.

Sproat TT and Lopez LM, "Hypertension," *Therapeutics in the Elderly*, 2nd ed, Delauente JC, Stewart RB, eds, Cincinnati, OH: Harvey Whitney Books, 1995, 228-46.

♦ **Hydralazine and Isosorbide Dinitrate** *see* Isosorbide Dinitrate and Hydralazine *on page 842*

♦ **Hydralazine Hydrochloride** *see* HydrALAZINE *on page 754*

♦ **Hydramine® [OTC]** *see* DiphenhydrAMINE *on page 447*

♦ **Hydrated Chloral** *see* Chloral Hydrate *on page 285*

♦ **Hydrea®** *see* Hydroxyurea *on page 774*

♦ **Hydrisalic™ [OTC]** *see* Salicylic Acid *on page 1441*

Hydrochlorothiazide *(hye droe klor oh THYE a zide)*

Medication Safety Issues

Sound-alike/look-alike issues:

Hydrochlorothiazide may be confused with hydrocortisone, hydroflumethiazide

Esidrix may be confused with Lasix®

HCTZ is an error-prone abbreviation (mistaken as hydrocortisone)

Microzide™ may be confused with Micronase®

International issues:

Microzide™ may be confused with Nitrobide® which is a brand name for isosorbide dinitrate in Japan

Microzide™ may be confused with Mikrozid® which is a brand name for ethanol/propanol combination in Great Britain

U.S. Brand Names Microzide™

Canadian Brand Names Apo-Hydro®; Novo-Hydrazide; PMS-Hydrochlorothiazide

Index Terms HCTZ (error-prone abbreviation)

Generic Available Yes

Pharmacologic Category Diuretic, Thiazide

Use Management of mild to moderate hypertension; treatment of edema in congestive heart failure and nephrotic syndrome

Unlabeled/Investigational Use Treatment of lithium-induced diabetes insipidus

Contraindications Hypersensitivity to hydrochlorothiazide or any component of the formulation, thiazides, or sulfonamide-derived drugs; anuria; renal decompensation

Warnings/Precautions Avoid in severe renal disease (ineffective). Electrolyte disturbances (hypokalemia, hypochloremic alkalosis, hyponatremia) can occur. Use with caution in severe hepatic dysfunction; hepatic encephalopathy can be caused by electrolyte disturbances. Gout can be precipitate in certain patients with a history of gout, a familial predisposition to gout, or chronic renal failure. Cautious use in prediabetics and diabetics; may see a change in glucose control. Can cause SLE exacerbation or activation. Use with caution in patients with moderate or high cholesterol concentrations. Photosensitization may occur. Correct hypokalemia before initiating therapy.

Chemical similarities are present among sulfonamides, sulfonylureas, carbonic anhydrase inhibitors, thiazides, and loop diuretics (except ethacrynic acid). Use in patients with sulfonamide allergy is specifically contraindicated in product labeling, however, a risk of cross-reaction exists in patients with allergy to any of these compounds; avoid use when previous reaction has been severe. Discontinue if signs of hypersensitivity are noted.

Adverse Reactions (Reflective of adult population; not specific for elderly)
1% to 10%:
Cardiovascular: Orthostatic hypotension, hypotension
Dermatologic; Photosensitivity
Endocrine & metabolic: Hypokalemia
Gastrointestinal: Anorexia, epigastric distress

Overdosage/Toxicology Symptoms include hypermotility, diuresis, lethargy, confusion, and muscle weakness. Following GI decontamination, therapy is supportive with I.V. fluids, electrolytes, and I.V. pressors if needed.

Drug Interactions
ACE inhibitors: Increased hypotension if aggressively diuresed with a thiazide diuretic.
Beta-blockers increase hyperglycemic effects in type 2 diabetes mellitus (noninsulin dependent, NIDDM)
Cholestyramine: Hydrochlorothiazide absorption may be decreased.
Colestipol: Hydrochlorothiazide absorption may be decreased.
Cyclosporine and thiazides can increase the risk of gout or renal toxicity; avoid concurrent use.
Digoxin toxicity can be exacerbated if a thiazide induces hypokalemia or hypomagnesemia.
Lithium toxicity can occur by reducing renal excretion of lithium; monitor lithium concentration and adjust as needed.
Neuromuscular blocking agents can prolong blockade; monitor serum potassium and neuromuscular status.
NSAIDs can decrease the efficacy of thiazides reducing the diuretic and antihypertensive effects.

Ethanol/Nutrition/Herb Interactions
Food: Hydrochlorothiazide peak serum levels may be decreased if taken with food. This product may deplete potassium, sodium, and magnesium.
Herb/Nutraceutical: Avoid dong quai if using for hypertension (has estrogenic activity). Dong quai may also cause photosensitization. Avoid ephedra, ginseng, yohimbe (may worsen hypertension). Avoid garlic (may have increased antihypertensive effect).

Mechanism of Action Inhibits sodium reabsorption in the distal tubules causing increased excretion of sodium and water as well as potassium and hydrogen ions

Pharmacodynamics
Onset of diuretic action: Oral: Within 2 hours
Peak effect: 4 hours; diuresis can continue for 6-12 hours
Duration: 6-12 hours

Pharmacokinetics Absorption: Oral: ~60% to 80%

Dosage
Geriatrics: Oral: 12.5-25 mg once daily; minimal increase in response and more electrolyte disturbances are seen with doses >50 mg/day (see Special Geriatric Considerations).
Adults:
Edema (diuresis): Oral: 25-100 mg/day in 1-2 doses; maximum: 200 mg/day
Hypertension: Oral: 12.5-50 mg/day; minimal increase in response and more electrolyte disturbances are seen with doses >50 mg/day
Renal Impairment: Cl_{cr} <10 mL/minute: Avoid use. Usually ineffective with GFR <30 mL/minute. Effective at lower GFR in combination with a loop diuretic.

Monitoring Parameters Blood pressure (both standing and sitting/supine), serum electrolytes, renal function, weight, I & O

Test Interactions Increased creatine phosphokinase [CPK] (S), ammonia (B), amylase (S), calcium (S), chloride (S), cholesterol (S), glucose, increased acid (S), decreased
(Continued)

Hydrochlorothiazide *(Continued)*

chloride (S), magnesium, potassium (S), sodium (S); Tyramine and phentolamine tests, histamine tests for pheochromocytoma

Patient Information May be taken with food or milk; take early in day to avoid nocturia; take the last dose of multiple doses no later than 6 PM unless instructed otherwise. A few people who take this medication become more sensitive to sunlight and may experience skin rash, redness, itching or severe sunburn, especially if sun block SPF ≥15 is not used on exposed skin areas.

Additional Information Effect of drug may be decreased when used every day

Special Geriatric Considerations Hydrochlorothiazide is not effective in patients with a Cl_{cr} <30 mL/minute, therefore, it may not be a useful agent in many elderly patients.

Dosage Forms Excipient information presented when available (limited, particularly for generics); consult specific product labeling.

Capsule: 12.5 mg

Microzide™: 12.5 mg

Tablet: 25 mg, 50 mg

♦ **Hydrochlorothiazide and Amiloride** *see* Amiloride and Hydrochlorothiazide *on page 75*

♦ **Hydrochlorothiazide and Benazepril** *see* Benazepril and Hydrochlorothiazide *on page 158*

♦ **Hydrochlorothiazide and Captopril** *see* Captopril and Hydrochlorothiazide *on page 229*

♦ **Hydrochlorothiazide and Enalapril** *see* Enalapril and Hydrochlorothiazide *on page 507*

♦ **Hydrochlorothiazide and Eprosartan** *see* Eprosartan and Hydrochlorothiazide *on page 524*

♦ **Hydrochlorothiazide and Irbesartan** *see* Irbesartan and Hydrochlorothiazide *on page 831*

♦ **Hydrochlorothiazide and Lisinopril** *see* Lisinopril and Hydrochlorothiazide *on page 920*

♦ **Hydrochlorothiazide and Losartan** *see* Losartan and Hydrochlorothiazide *on page 934*

♦ **Hydrochlorothiazide and Metoprolol** *see* Metoprolol and Hydrochlorothiazide *on page 1030*

♦ **Hydrochlorothiazide and Metoprolol Tartrate** *see* Metoprolol and Hydrochlorothiazide *on page 1030*

♦ **Hydrochlorothiazide and Olmesartan Medoxomil** *see* Olmesartan and Hydrochlorothiazide *on page 1152*

♦ **Hydrochlorothiazide and Propranolol** *see* Propranolol and Hydrochlorothiazide *on page 1340*

♦ **Hydrochlorothiazide and Quinapril** *see* Quinapril and Hydrochlorothiazide *on page 1362*

♦ **Hydrochlorothiazide and Ramipril** *see* Ramipril and Hydrochlorothiazide *on page 1380*

Hydrochlorothiazide and Spironolactone

(hye droe klor oh THYE a zide & speer on oh LAK tone)

Related Information

Hydrochlorothiazide *on page 756*
Spironolactone *on page 1488*

Medication Safety Issues

Sound-alike/look-alike issues:

Aldactazide® may be confused with Aldactone®

U.S. Brand Names Aldactazide®

Canadian Brand Names Aldactazide 25®; Aldactazide 50®; Novo-Spirozine

Index Terms Spironolactone and Hydrochlorothiazide

Generic Available Yes

Pharmacologic Category Antihypertensive Agent, Combination

Use Management of mild to moderate hypertension; treatment of edema in congestive heart failure and nephrotic syndrome, cirrhosis of the liver accompanied by edema or ascites

Refer to individual agents.

Dosage

Geriatrics: Oral: Initial: 1 tablet/day; increase as necessary.

Adults: Hypertension, edema: Oral: Hydrochlorothiazide 12.5-50 mg/day and spironolactone 12.5-50 mg/day; manufacturer labeling states hydrochlorothiazide maximum 200 mg/day, however, usual dose in JNC-7 is 12.5-50 mg/day

Renal Impairment: Efficacy of hydrochlorothiazide is limited in patients with Cl_cr <30 mL/minute.

Special Geriatric Considerations The efficacy of hydrochlorothiazide is limited in patients with a Cl_cr <30 mL/minute; monitor serum potassium.

Dosage Forms Excipient information presented when available (limited, particularly for generics); consult specific product labeling.

Tablet: Hydrochlorothiazide 25 mg and spironolactone 25 mg
Aldactazide®:
25/25: Hydrochlorothiazide 25 mg and spironolactone 25 mg
50/50: Hydrochlorothiazide 50 mg and spironolactone 50 mg

♦ **Hydrochlorothiazide and Telmisartan** see Telmisartan and Hydrochlorothiazide on page 1527

Hydrochlorothiazide and Triamterene
(hye droe klor oh THYE a zide & trye AM ter een)

Related Information
Hydrochlorothiazide on page 756
Triamterene on page 1624
Medication Safety Issues
Sound-alike/look-alike issues:
Dyazide® may be confused with diazoxide, Dynacin®
Maxzide® may be confused with Maxidex®
U.S. Brand Names Dyazide®; Maxzide®; Maxzide®-25
Canadian Brand Names Apo-Triazide®; Novo-Triamzide; Nu-Triazide; Penta-Triamterene HCTZ; Riva-Zide
Index Terms Triamterene and Hydrochlorothiazide
Generic Available Yes
Pharmacologic Category Antihypertensive Agent, Combination; Diuretic, Potassium-Sparing; Diuretic, Thiazide
Use Management of mild to moderate hypertension; treatment of edema in congestive heart failure and nephrotic syndrome
Refer to individual agents.
Dosage
Geriatrics & Adults: Hypertension, edema: Oral:
Triamterene 37.5 mg and hydrochlorothiazide 25 mg: 1-2 tablets/capsules once daily
Triamterene 75 mg and hydrochlorothiazide 50 mg: ½-1 tablet daily
Special Geriatric Considerations The efficacy of hydrochlorothiazide is limited in patients with a Cl_cr <30 mL/minute; monitor serum potassium.
Dosage Forms Excipient information presented when available (limited, particularly for generics); consult specific product labeling.
Capsule (Dyazide®): Hydrochlorothiazide 25 mg and triamterene 37.5 mg
Tablet:
Maxzide®: Hydrochlorothiazide 50 mg and triamterene 75 mg
Maxzide®-25: Hydrochlorothiazide 25 mg and triamterene 37.5 mg

♦ **Hydrochlorothiazide and Valsartan** see Valsartan and Hydrochlorothiazide on page 1659
♦ **Hydrocil® Instant [OTC]** see Psyllium on page 1347

Hydrocodone and Acetaminophen
(hye droe KOE done & a seet a MIN oh fen)

Related Information
Acetaminophen on page 29
Narcotic / Opioid Analgesics on page 1763
Medication Safety Issues
Sound-alike/look-alike issues:
Lorcet® may be confused with Fioricet®
Lortab® may be confused with Cortef®, Lorabid®, Luride®
Vicodin® may be confused with Hycodan®, Hycomine®, Indocin®, Uridon®
Zydone® may be confused with Vytone®

Duplicate therapy issues: This product contains acetaminophen, which may be a component of other combination products. Do not exceed the maximum recommended daily dose of acetaminophen.
U.S. Brand Names Anexsia®; Co-Gesic®; hycet™; Lorcet® 10/650; Lorcet® Plus; Lortab®; Margesic® H; Maxidone™; Norco®; Stagesic®; Vicodin®; Vicodin® ES; Vicodin® HP; Xodol® 5/300; Xodol® 7.5/300; Xodol® 10/300; Zydone®
Index Terms Acetaminophen and Hydrocodone
Generic Available Yes
(Continued)

Hydrocodone and Acetaminophen *(Continued)*

Pharmacologic Category Analgesic Combination (Opioid)

Use Relief of moderate to severe pain

Restrictions C-III

Contraindications Hypersensitivity to hydrocodone, acetaminophen, or any component of the formulation; CNS depression; severe respiratory depression

Warnings/Precautions Use with caution in patients with hypersensitivity reactions to other phenanthrene derivative opioid agonists (morphine, hydromorphone, levorphanol, oxycodone, oxymorphone); tolerance or drug dependence may result from extended use. Concurrent use of agonist/antagonist analgesics may precipitate withdrawal symptoms and/or reduced analgesic efficacy in patients following prolonged therapy with mu opioid agonists. Abrupt discontinuation following prolonged use may also lead to withdrawal symptoms.

Respiratory depressant effects may be increased with head injuries. Use caution with acute abdominal conditions; clinical course may be obscured. Use caution with adrenal insufficiency, biliary tract impairment, morbidly obese patients, toxic psychosis, thyroid dysfunction, prostatic hyperplasia, hepatic or renal disease, and in the debilitated or elderly. Causes sedation; caution must be used in performing tasks which require alertness (eg, operating machinery or driving). Effects may be potentiated when used with other sedative drugs or ethanol. May cause hypotension.

Limit acetaminophen to <4 g/day. May cause severe hepatic toxicity in acute overdose; in addition, chronic daily dosing in adults has resulted in liver damage in some patients. Use with caution in patients with alcoholic liver disease; consuming ≥3 alcoholic drinks/day may increase the risk of liver damage. Use caution in patients with known G6PD deficiency.

Adverse Reactions (Reflective of adult population; not specific for elderly)
Frequency not defined.

Cardiovascular: Bradycardia, cardiac arrest, circulatory collapse, coma, hypotension

Central nervous system: anxiety, dizziness, drowsiness, dysphoria, euphoria, fear, lethargy, lightheadedness, malaise, mental clouding, mental impairment, mood changes, physiological dependence, sedation, somnolence, stupor

Dermatologic: Pruritus, rash

Endocrine & metabolic: Hypoglycemic coma

Gastrointestinal: Abdominal pain, constipation, gastric distress, heartburn, nausea, peptic ulcer, vomiting, xerostomia

Genitourinary: Ureteral spasm, urinary retention, vesical sphincter spasm

Hematologic: Agranulocytosis, bleeding time prolonged, hemolytic anemia, iron deficiency anemia, occult blood loss, thrombocytopenia

Hepatic: Hepatic necrosis, hepatitis

Neuromuscular & skeletal: Skeletal muscle rigidity

Otic: Hearing impairment or loss (chronic overdose)

Renal: Renal toxicity, renal tubular necrosis

Respiratory: Acute airway obstruction, apnea, dyspnea, respiratory depression (dose related)

Miscellaneous: Allergic reactions, clamminess, diaphoresis

Overdosage/Toxicology Symptoms include hepatic necrosis, blood dyscrasias, and respiratory depression. Treatment consists of acetylcysteine 140 mg/kg orally (loading), followed by 70 mg/kg every 4 hours for 17 doses. Therapy should be initiated based upon laboratory analysis suggesting a high probability of hepatotoxic potential. Naloxone (2 mg I.V.) can also be used to reverse toxic effects of the opiate. Activated charcoal is effective at binding certain chemicals, and this is especially true for acetaminophen.

Drug Interactions

Hydrocodone: **Substrate** (minor) of CYP2D6, 3A

Acetaminophen: **Substrate** (minor) of CYP1A2, 2A6, 2C9, 2D6, 2E1, 3A4; **Inhibits** CYP3A4 (weak)

Acetaminophen component: Refer to Acetaminophen monograph.

Hydrocodone component:

CNS depressants (including antianxiety agents, antihistamines, antipsychotics, narcotics): CNS depression is additive; dose adjustment may be needed

MAO inhibitors: May see increased effects of MAO inhibitor and hydrocodone.

Tricyclic antidepressants (TCAs): May see increased effects of TCA and hydrocodone.

Ethanol/Nutrition/Herb Interactions

Ethanol: Avoid ethanol (may increase CNS depression); consuming ≥3 alcoholic drinks/day may increase the risk of liver damage

Herb/Nutraceutical: Avoid valerian, St John's wort, SAMe, kava kava (may increase risk of excessive sedation).

Mechanism of Action Hydrocodone, as with other narcotic (opiate) analgesics, blocks pain perception in the cerebral cortex by binding to specific receptor molecules (opiate receptors) within the neuronal membranes of synapses. This binding results in a decreased synaptic chemical transmission throughout the CNS thus inhibiting the flow of pain sensations into the higher centers. Mu and kappa are the two subtypes of the opiate receptor which hydrocodone binds to cause analgesia.

Acetaminophen inhibits the synthesis of prostaglandins in the CNS and peripherally blocks pain impulse generation; produces antipyresis from inhibition of hypothalamic heat-regulating center.

Pharmacodynamics
Onset of action: Oral: Narcotic analgesia occurs within 10-20 minutes following administration
Duration: 3-6 hours; enhanced analgesia has been seen in older adult patients on therapeutic doses of narcotics; duration of action may be increased in older adults

Pharmacokinetics
Metabolism: In the liver
Half-life: 3.8 hours
Elimination: In urine

Dosage
Geriatrics: Doses should be titrated to appropriate analgesic effect; 2.5-5 mg of the hydrocodone component every 4-6 hours. Do not exceed 4 g/day of acetaminophen.
Adults:
Pain management (analgesic): Oral (doses should be titrated to appropriate analgesic effect): Average starting dose in opioid naive patients: Hydrocodone 5-10 mg 4 times/day; the dosage of acetaminophen should be limited to ≤4 g/day (and possibly less in patients with hepatic impairment or ethanol use).
Dosage ranges (based on specific product labeling): Hydrocodone 2.5-10 mg every 4-6 hours; maximum: 60 mg hydrocodone/day (maximum dose of hydrocodone may be limited by the acetaminophen content of specific product)
Hepatic Impairment: Use with caution. Limited, low-dose therapy usually well tolerated in hepatic disease/cirrhosis; however, cases of hepatotoxicity at daily acetaminophen dosages <4 g/day have been reported. Avoid chronic use in hepatic impairment.

Monitoring Parameters Pain relief, respiratory and mental status, blood pressure

Patient Information May cause drowsiness; avoid alcoholic beverages; do not exceed recommended dose

Special Geriatric Considerations Elderly may be particularly susceptible to the CNS depressant action (sedation, confusion) and constipating effects of narcotics. If 1 tablet/dose is used, it may be useful to add an additional 325 mg of acetaminophen to maximize analgesic effect.

Dosage Forms Excipient information presented when available (limited, particularly for generics); consult specific product labeling. [DSC] = Discontinued product
Capsule:
Margesic® H, Stagesic®: Hydrocodone bitartrate 5 mg and acetaminophen 500 mg
Elixir: Hydrocodone bitartrate 7.5 mg and acetaminophen 500 mg per 15 mL (480 mL)
Lortab®: Hydrocodone bitartrate 7.5 mg and acetaminophen 500 mg per 15 mL (480 mL) [contains alcohol 7%; tropical fruit punch flavor]
Solution, oral:
hycet™: Hydrocodone bitartrate 7.5 mg and acetaminophen 325 mg per 15 mL (480 mL) [contains alcohol 7%; tropical fruit punch flavor]
Tablet:
Hydrocodone bitartrate 2.5 mg and acetaminophen 500 mg
Hydrocodone bitartrate 5 mg and acetaminophen 325 mg
Hydrocodone bitartrate 5 mg and acetaminophen 500 mg
Hydrocodone bitartrate 7.5 mg and acetaminophen 325 mg
Hydrocodone bitartrate 7.5 mg and acetaminophen 500 mg
Hydrocodone bitartrate 7.5 mg and acetaminophen 650 mg
Hydrocodone bitartrate 7.5 mg and acetaminophen 750 mg
Hydrocodone bitartrate 10 mg and acetaminophen 325 mg
Hydrocodone bitartrate 10 mg and acetaminophen 500 mg
Hydrocodone bitartrate 10 mg and acetaminophen 650 mg
Hydrocodone bitartrate 10 mg and acetaminophen 660 mg
Hydrocodone bitartrate 10 mg and acetaminophen 750 mg
Anexsia®:
5/325: Hydrocodone bitartrate 5 mg and acetaminophen 325 mg
7.5/325: Hydrocodone bitartrate 7.5 mg and acetaminophen 325 mg
Co-Gesic® 5/500: Hydrocodone bitartrate 5 mg and acetaminophen 500 mg
Lorcet® 10/650: Hydrocodone bitartrate 10 mg and acetaminophen 650 mg
Lorcet® Plus: Hydrocodone bitartrate 7.5 mg and acetaminophen 650 mg
Lortab®:
5/500: Hydrocodone bitartrate 5 mg and acetaminophen 500 mg
7.5/500: Hydrocodone bitartrate 7.5 mg and acetaminophen 500 mg
10/500: Hydrocodone bitartrate 10 mg and acetaminophen 500 mg
(Continued)

Hydrocodone and Acetaminophen *(Continued)*

Maxidone™: Hydrocodone bitartrate 10 mg and acetaminophen 750 mg
Norco®:
    Hydrocodone bitartrate 5 mg and acetaminophen 325 mg
    Hydrocodone bitartrate 7.5 mg and acetaminophen 325 mg
    Hydrocodone bitartrate 10 mg and acetaminophen 325 mg
Vicodin®: Hydrocodone bitartrate 5 mg and acetaminophen 500 mg
Vicodin® ES: Hydrocodone bitartrate 7.5 mg and acetaminophen 750 mg
Vicodin® HP: Hydrocodone bitartrate 10 mg and acetaminophen 660 mg
Xodol®:
    10/300: Hydrocodone bitartrate 10 mg and acetaminophen 300 mg
    5/300: Hydrocodone bitartrate 5 mg and acetaminophen 300 mg
    7/300: Hydrocodone bitartrate 7 mg and acetaminophen 300 mg
Zydone®:
    Hydrocodone bitartrate 5 mg and acetaminophen 400 mg
    Hydrocodone bitartrate 7.5 mg and acetaminophen 400 mg
    Hydrocodone bitartrate 10 mg and acetaminophen 400 mg

Selected References
Carpenter RL, "Optimizing Postoperative Pain Management," *Am Fam Physician*, 1997, 56(3):835-44, 847-50. Available at http://www.aafp.org/afp/970901ap/painmgmt.html. Accessed May 4, 2004.
"Principles of Analgesic Use in the Treatment of Acute Pain and Cancer Pain," 5th ed, Glenview, IL: American Pain Society, 2003.

Hydrocortisone *(hye droe KOR ti sone)*

Related Information
Corticosteroids *on page 1755*

Medication Safety Issues
Sound-alike/look-alike issues:
Hydrocortisone may be confused with hydrocodone, hydroxychloroquine, hydrochlorothiazide
Anusol® may be confused with Anusol-HC®, Aplisol®, Aquasol®
Anusol-HC® may be confused with Anusol®
Cortef® may be confused with Lortab®
Cortizone® may be confused with cortisone
HCT (occasional abbreviation for hydrocortisone) is an error-prone abbreviation (mistaken as hydrochlorothiazide)
Hytone® may be confused with Vytone®
Proctocort® may be confused with ProctoCream®
ProctoCream® may be confused with Proctocort®

International issues:
Hytone® may be confused with Hysone® [Australia]
Nutracort® may be confused with Nitrocor® which is a brand name of nitroglycerin in Chile and Italy

U.S. Brand Names Anucort-HC®; Anusol-HC®; Anusol® HC-1 [OTC]; Aquanil™ HC [OTC]; Beta-HC®; Caldecort® [OTC]; Cetacort® [DSC]; Colocort®; Cortaid® Intensive Therapy [OTC]; Cortaid® Maximum Strength [OTC]; Cortaid® Sensitive Skin [OTC]; Cortef®; Corticool® [OTC]; Cortifoam®; Cortizone®-10 Maximum Strength [OTC]; Cortizone®-10 Plus Maximum Strength [OTC]; Cortizone®-10 Quick Shot [OTC]; Dermarest Dricort® [OTC]; Dermtex® HC [OTC]; EarSol® HC; Encort™; Hemril®-30; HydroZone Plus [OTC]; Hytone®; IvySoothe® [OTC]; Locoid®; Locoid Lipocream®; Nupercainal® Hydrocortisone Cream [OTC]; Nutracort®; Pandel®; Post Peel Healing Balm [OTC]; Preparation H® Hydrocortisone [OTC]; Proctocort®; ProctoCream® HC; Procto-Kit™; Procto-Pak™; Proctosert; Proctosol-HC®; Proctozone-HC™; Sarnol®-HC [OTC]; Solu-Cortef®; Summer's Eve® SpecialCare™ Medicated Anti-Itch Cream [OTC] [DSC]; Texacort®; Tucks® Anti-Itch [OTC]; Westcort®

Canadian Brand Names Aquacort®; Cortamed®; Cortef®; Cortenema®; Cortifoam™; Emo-Cort®; Hycort™; Hyderm; HydroVal®; Locoid®; Prevex® HC; Sarna® HC; Solu-Cortef®; Westcort®

Index Terms A-hydroCort; Compound F; Cortisol; Hemorrhoidal HC; Hydrocortisone Acetate; Hydrocortisone Butyrate; Hydrocortisone Probutate; Hydrocortisone Sodium Succinate; Hydrocortisone Valerate

Generic Available Yes: Excludes acetate foam, butyrate cream and ointment, gel as base, otic drops as base, probutate cream, sodium succinate injection

Pharmacologic Category Corticosteroid, Rectal; Corticosteroid, Systemic; Corticosteroid, Topical

Use Management of adrenocortical insufficiency; relief of inflammation of corticosteroid-responsive dermatoses (low and medium potency topical corticosteroid); adjunctive treatment of ulcerative colitis

Contraindications Hypersensitivity to hydrocortisone or any component of the formulation; serious infections, except septic shock or tuberculous meningitis; viral, fungal, or tubercular skin lesions

Warnings/Precautions Use with caution in patients with thyroid disease, hepatic impairment, renal impairment, cardiovascular disease, diabetes, glaucoma, cataracts, myasthenia gravis, patients at risk for osteoporosis, patients at risk for seizures, or GI diseases (diverticulitis, peptic ulcer, ulcerative colitis) due to perforation risk. Use caution following acute MI (corticosteroids have been associated with myocardial rupture). Because of the risk of adverse effects, systemic corticosteroids should be used cautiously in the elderly in the smallest possible effective dose for the shortest duration. Withdraw therapy with gradual tapering of dose.

May cause hypercorticism or suppression of hypothalamic-pituitary-adrenal (HPA) axis, particularly in patients receiving high doses for prolonged periods. HPA axis suppression may lead to adrenal crisis. Withdrawal and discontinuation of a corticosteroid should be done slowly and carefully. Particular care is required when patients are transferred from systemic corticosteroids to inhaled products due to possible adrenal insufficiency or withdrawal from steroids, including an increase in allergic symptoms. Patients receiving >20 mg per day of prednisone (or equivalent) may be most susceptible. Fatalities have occurred due to adrenal insufficiency in asthmatic patients during and after transfer from systemic corticosteroids to aerosol steroids; aerosol steroids do not provide the systemic steroid needed to treat patients having trauma, surgery, or infections. Avoid use of topical preparations with occlusive dressings or on weeping or exudative lesions.

Acute myopathy has been reported with high dose corticosteroids, usually in patients with neuromuscular transmission disorders; may involve ocular and/or respiratory muscles; monitor creatine kinase; recovery may be delayed. Corticosteroid use may cause psychiatric disturbances, including depression, euphoria, insomnia, mood swings, and personality changes. Pre-existing psychiatric conditions may be exacerbated by corticosteroid use. Prolonged use of corticosteroids may also increase the incidence of secondary infection, mask acute infection (including fungal infections), prolong or exacerbate viral infections, or limit response to vaccines. Exposure to chickenpox should be avoided; corticosteroids should not be used to treat ocular herpes simplex. Corticosteroids should not be used for cerebral malaria. Close observation is required in patients with latent tuberculosis and/or TB reactivity; restrict use in active TB (only in conjunction with antituberculosis treatment). Prolonged treatment with corticosteroids has been associated with the development of Kaposi's sarcoma (case reports); if noted, discontinuation of therapy should be considered.

Adverse Reactions (Reflective of adult population; not specific for elderly)
Systemic:
>10%:
Central nervous system: Insomnia, nervousness
Gastrointestinal: Increased appetite, indigestion
1% to 10%:
Dermatologic: Hirsutism
Endocrine & metabolic: Diabetes mellitus
Neuromuscular & skeletal: Arthralgia
Ocular: Cataracts
Respiratory: Epistaxis

Topical:
>10%: Dermatologic: Eczema (12.5%)
1% to 10%: Dermatologic: Pruritus (6%), stinging (2%), dry skin (2%)

Overdosage/Toxicology Symptoms include cushingoid appearance (systemic), muscle weakness (systemic), and osteoporosis (systemic) - all with long-term use only. When consumed in excessive quantities for prolonged periods, systemic hypercorticism and adrenal suppression may occur. In those cases, discontinuation and withdrawal of the corticosteroid should be done judiciously.

Drug Interactions Substrate of CYP3A4 (minor); **Induces** CYP3A4 (weak)

Aminoglutethimide: May reduce the serum levels/effects of corticosteroids; likely via induction of microsomal isoenzymes.
Amphotericin: Corticosteroids may increase the hypokalemic effects of amphotericin B; monitor.
Antacids: May decrease the absorption of corticosteroids; separate administration by 2 hours.
Anticholinesterases: Concurrent use may lead to severe weakness in patients with myasthenia gravis.
Antidiabetic agents: Corticosteroids may decrease the hypoglycemic effects of antidiabetic agents; monitor.
Aprepitant: May increase the serum levels/effects of corticosteroids; monitor.
Antifungal agents (azole): May increase the serum levels/effects of corticosteroids; monitor.
(Continued)

Hydrocortisone *(Continued)*

Barbiturates: May decrease the levels/effects of corticosteroids.

Bile acid sequestrants: May reduce the absorption of corticosteroids; separate administration by 2 hours.

Calcium channel blockers (nondihydropyridine): May increase the serum levels/effects of corticosteroids; monitor.

Cyclosporine: Corticosteroids may increase the serum levels/effects of cyclosporine. In addition, cyclosporine may increase levels of corticosteroids.

Diuretics, potassium-wasting (loop or thiazide): Hypokalemic effects may be increased by corticosteroids; monitor.

Estrogens: May increase the serum levels/effects of corticosteroids; monitor.

Fluoroquinolones: Concurrent use may increase the risk of tendinopathies (including tendonitis and rupture), particularly in elderly patients (overall incidence rare)

Isoniazid: Serum levels/effects may be decreased by corticosteroids.

Macrolide antibiotics: May increase the serum levels/effects of corticosteroids.

Neuromuscular-blocking agents: Concurrent use with corticosteroids may increase the risk of myopathy.

Nonsteroidal anti-inflammatory drugs (NSAIDs): Concurrent use with corticosteroids may lead to an increased incidence of gastrointestinal adverse effects; use caution.

Rifamycin derivatives: May decrease the levels/effects of corticosteroids (systemic); monitor.

Salicylates: Salicylates may increase the gastrointestinal adverse effects of corticosteroids.

Vaccine (dead organism): Corticosteroids may decrease the effect of vaccines (dead organisms). In patients receiving high doses of systemic corticosteroids for ≥14 days, wait at least 1 month between discontinuing steroid therapy and administering immunization.

Vaccine (live organism): Corticosteroids may increase the risk of vaccinal infection. The use of live vaccines is contraindicated in immunosuppressed patients.

Warfarin: Corticosteroids may increase the anticoagulant effects of warfarin; monitor INR.

Ethanol/Nutrition/Herb Interactions

Ethanol: Avoid ethanol (may enhance gastric mucosal irritation).

Food: Hydrocortisone interferes with calcium absorption.

Herb/Nutraceutical: St John's wort may decrease hydrocortisone levels. Avoid cat's claw, echinacea (have immunostimulant properties).

Stability Store at controlled room temperature 20°C to 25°C (59°F to 86°F). Hydrocortisone sodium phosphate and hydrocortisone sodium succinate are clear, light yellow solutions which are heat labile.

Sodium succinate: Reconstitute 100 mg vials with bacteriostatic water (not >2 mL). Act-O-Vial (self-contained powder for injection plus diluent) may be reconstituted by pressing the activator to force diluent into the powder compartment. Following gentle agitation, solution may be withdrawn via syringe through a needle inserted into the center of the stopper. May be administered (I.V. or I.M.) without further dilution. After initial reconstitution, hydrocortisone sodium succinate solutions are stable for 3 days at room temperature or under refrigeration when protected from light. Stability of parenteral admixture (Solu-Cortef®) at room temperature (25°C) and at refrigeration temperature (4°C) is concentration-dependent:

Stability of concentration 1 mg/mL: 24 hours.

Stability of concentration 2 mg/mL to 60 mg/mL: At least 4 hours.

Solutions for I.V. infusion: Reconstituted solutions may be added to an appropriate volume of compatible solution for infusion. Concentration should generally not exceed 1 mg/mL. However, in cases where administration of a small volume of fluid is desirable, 100-3000 mg may be added to 50 mL of D_5W or NS (stability limited to 4 hours).

Mechanism of Action Decreases inflammation by suppression of migration of polymorphonuclear leukocytes and reversal of increased capillary permeability

Pharmacokinetics

Absorption: Rapid by all routes, except rectally

Metabolism: In the liver and excreted renally, mainly as 17-hydroxysteroids and 17-ketosteroids

Half-life: Biologic: 8-12 hours

Dosage

Geriatrics & Adults: Dose should be based on severity of disease and patient response.

Acute adrenal insufficiency: I.M., I.V.: Succinate: 100 mg I.V. bolus, then 300 mg/day in divided doses every 8 hours or as a continuous infusion for 48 hours. Once patient is stable change to oral, 50 mg every 8 hours for 6 doses, then taper to 30-50 mg/day in divided doses.

Chronic adrenal corticoid insufficiency/physiologic replacement: Oral: 20-30 mg/day

Anti-inflammatory or immunosuppressive: Oral, I.M., I.V.: Succinate: 15-240 mg every 12 hours

Congenital adrenal hyperplasia: Oral: Initial: 10-20 mg/m^2/day in 3 divided doses; a variety of dosing schedules have been used. **Note:** Inconsistencies have occurred with liquid formulations; tablets may provide more reliable levels. Doses must be individualized by monitoring growth, bone age, and hormonal levels. Mineralocorticoid and sodium supplementation may be required based upon electrolyte regulation and plasma renin activity.

Shock: I.M., I.V.: Succinate: 500 mg to 2 g every 2-6 hours

Status asthmaticus: I.V.: Succinate: 1-2 mg/kg/dose every 6 hours for 24 hours, then maintenance of 0.5-1 mg/kg every 6 hours

Stress dosing (surgery) in patients known to be adrenally-suppressed or on chronic systemic steroids: I.V.:

Minor stress (ie, inguinal herniorrhaphy): 25 mg/day for 1 day

Moderate stress (ie, joint replacement, cholecystectomy): 50-75 mg/day (25 mg every 8-12 hours) for 1-2 days

Major stress (pancreatoduodenectomy, esophagogastrectomy, cardiac surgery): 100-150 mg/day (50 mg every 8-12 hours) for 2-3 days

Rheumatic diseases:

Intralesional, intra-articular, soft tissue injection: Acetate:
Large joints: 25 mg (up to 37.5 mg)
Small joints: 10-25 mg
Tendon sheaths: 5-12.5 mg
Soft tissue infiltration: 25-50 mg (up to 75 mg)
Bursae: 25-37.5 mg
Ganglia: 12.5-25 mg

Dermatosis: Topical: Apply to affected area 2-4 times/day.

Ulcerative colitis: Rectal: 10-100 mg 1-2 times/day for 2-3 weeks

Monitoring Parameters Blood pressure, blood glucose, electrolytes, weight, symptoms of fluid retention

Reference Range Therapeutic: AM: 5-25 mcg/dL (SI: 138-690 nmol/L); PM: 2-9 mcg/dL (SI: 55-248 nmol/L) depending on test, assay

Patient Information Notify surgeon or dentist before surgical repair; may cause GI upset; take with food or milk; notify physician if any sign of infection occurs; avoid abrupt withdrawal when on long-term oral therapy; carry an identification card or bracelet advising that you are on steroids; do not use topical products on broken skin

Additional Information Hydrocortisone base topical cream, lotion, and ointments in concentrations of 0.25%, 0.5%, and 1% may be OTC or prescription depending on the product labeling.

Special Geriatric Considerations Because of the risk of adverse effects, systemic corticosteroids should be used cautiously in the elderly, in the smallest possible dose, and for the shortest possible time.

Dosage Forms Excipient information presented when available (limited, particularly for generics); consult specific product labeling. [DSC] = Discontinued product

Aerosol, rectal, as acetate (Cortifoam®): 10% (15 g) [90 mg/applicator]

Cream, rectal, as acetate (Nupercainal® Hydrocortisone Cream): 1% (30 g) [strength expressed as base]

Cream, rectal, as base:
Cortizone®-10: 1% (30 g) [contains aloe]
Preparation H® Hydrocortisone: 1% (27 g)

Cream, topical, as acetate: 0.5% (9 g, 30 g, 60 g) [available with aloe]; 1% (30 g, 454 g) [available with aloe]

Cream, topical, as base: 0.5% (30 g); 1% (1.5 g, 30 g, 114 g, 454 g); 2.5% (20 g, 30 g, 454 g)
Anusol-HC®: 2.5% (30 g) [contains benzyl alcohol]
Caldecort®: 1% (30 g) [contains aloe vera gel]
Cortaid® Intensive Therapy: 1% (60 g)
Cortaid® Maximum Strength: 1% (15 g, 30 g, 40 g, 60 g) [contains aloe vera gel and benzyl alcohol]
Cortaid® Sensitive Skin: 0.5% (15 g) [contains aloe vera gel]
Cortizone®-10 Maximum Strength: 1% (15 g, 30 g, 60 g) [contains aloe]
Cortizone®-10 Plus Maximum Strength: 1% (30 g, 60 g) [contains vitamins A, D, E and aloe]
Dermarest® Dricort®: 1% (15 g, 30 g)
HydroZone Plus, Proctocort®, Procto-Pak™: 1% (30 g)
Hytone®: 2.5% (30 g, 60 g)
IvySoothe®: 1% (30 g) [contains aloe]
Post Peel Healing Balm: 1% (23 g)
ProctoCream® HC: 2.5% (30 g) [contains benzyl alcohol]
Procto-Kit™: 1% (30 g) [packaged with applicator tips and finger cots]; 2.5% (30 g) [packaged with applicator tips and finger cots]
Proctosol-HC®, Proctozone-HC™: 2.5% (30 g)

(Continued)

Hydrocortisone *(Continued)*

Summer's Eve® SpecialCare™ Medicated Anti-Itch Cream: 1% (30 g) [DSC]
Cream, topical, as butyrate (Locoid®, Locoid Lipocream®): 0.1% (15 g, 45 g)
Cream, topical, as probutate (Pandel®): 0.1% (15 g, 45 g, 80 g)
Cream, topical, as valerate (Westcort®): 0.2% (15 g, 45 g, 60 g)
Gel, topical, as base (Corticool®): 1% (45 g)
Injection, powder for reconstitution, as sodium succinate:
A-Hydrocort: 100 mg
Solu-Cortef®: 100 mg, 250 mg, 500 mg, 1 g [diluent contains benzyl alcohol; strength expressed as base]
Lotion, topical, as base: 1% (120 mL); 2.5% (60 mL)
Aquanil™ HC: 1% (120 mL)
Beta-HC®, Cetacort® [DSC], Sarnol®-HC: 1% (60 mL)
HydroZone Plus: 1% (120 mL)
Hytone®: 2.5% (60 mL)
Nutracort®: 1% (60 mL, 120 mL); 2.5% (60 mL, 120 mL)
Ointment, topical, as acetate: 1% (30 g) [strength expressed as base; available with aloe]
Anusol® HC-1: 1% (21 g) [strength expressed as base]
Cortaid® Maximum Strength: 1% (15 g, 30 g) [strength expressed as base]
Ointment, topical, as base: 0.5% (30 g); 1% (30 g, 454 g); 2.5% (20 g, 30 g, 454 g)
Cortizone®-10 Maximum Strength: 1% (30 g, 60 g)
Hytone®: 2.5% (30 g) [DSC]
Ointment, topical, as butyrate (Locoid®): 0.1% (15 g, 45 g)
Ointment, topical, as valerate (Westcort®): 0.2% (15 g, 45 g, 60 g)
Solution, otic, as base (EarSol® HC): 1% (30 mL) [contains alcohol 44%, benzyl benzoate, yerba santa]
Solution, topical, as base (Texacort®): 2.5% (30 mL) [contains alcohol]
Solution, topical, as butyrate (Locoid®): 0.1% (20 mL, 60 mL) [contains alcohol 50%]
Solution, topical spray, as base:
Cortaid® Intensive Therapy: 1% (60 mL) [contains alcohol]
Cortizone®-10 Quick Shot: 1% (44 mL) [contains benzyl alcohol]
Dermtex® HC: 1% (52 mL) [contains menthol 1%]
Suppository, rectal, as acetate: 25 mg (12s, 24s, 100s)
Anucort-HC®, Tucks® Anti-Itch: 25 mg (12s, 24s, 100s) [strength expressed as base; Anucort-HC® *renamed* Tucks® Anti-Itch]
Anusol-HC®, Proctosol-HC®: 25 mg (12s, 24s)
Encort™, Proctocort®: 30 mg (12s)
Hemril®-30, Proctosert: 30 mg (12s, 24s)
Suspension, rectal, as base: 100 mg/60 mL (7s)
Colocort®: 100 mg/60 mL (1s, 7s)
Tablet, as base: 20 mg
Cortef®: 5 mg, 10 mg, 20 mg

◆ **Hydrocortisone Acetate** *see* Hydrocortisone *on page 762*
◆ **Hydrocortisone and Ciprofloxacin** *see* Ciprofloxacin and Hydrocortisone *on page 322*
◆ **Hydrocortisone Butyrate** *see* Hydrocortisone *on page 762*
◆ **Hydrocortisone, Neomycin, Colistin, and Thonzonium** *see* Neomycin, Colistin, Hydrocortisone, and Thonzonium *on page 1101*
◆ **Hydrocortisone Probutate** *see* Hydrocortisone *on page 762*
◆ **Hydrocortisone Sodium Succinate** *see* Hydrocortisone *on page 762*
◆ **Hydrocortisone Valerate** *see* Hydrocortisone *on page 762*

Hydromorphone *(hye droe MOR fone)*

Related Information
Narcotic / Opioid Analgesics *on page 1763*
Medication Safety Issues
Sound-alike/look-alike issues:
Dilaudid® may be confused with Demerol®, Dilantin®
Hydromorphone may be confused with morphine; significant overdoses have occurred when hydromorphone products have been inadvertently administered instead of morphine sulfate. Commercially available prefilled syringes of both products looks similar and are often stored in close proximity to each other. **Note:** Hydromorphone 1 mg oral is approximately equal to morphine 4 mg oral; hydromorphone 1 mg I.V. is approximately equal to morphine 5 mg I.V.

Dilaudid®, Dilaudid-HP®: Extreme caution should be taken to avoid confusing the highly-concentrated (Dilaudid-HP®) injection with the less-concentrated (Dilaudid®) injectable product.

Significant differences exist between oral and I.V. dosing. Use caution when converting from one route of administration to another.

U.S. Brand Names Dilaudid®; Dilaudid-HP®

Canadian Brand Names Dilaudid®; Dilaudid-HP®; Dilaudid-HP-Plus®; Dilaudid® Sterile Powder; Dilaudid-XP®; Hydromorph Contin®; Hydromorph-IR®; Hydromorphone HP; Hydromorphone HP® 10; Hydromorphone HP® 20; Hydromorphone HP® 50; Hydromorphone HP® Forte; Hydromorphone Hydrochloride Injection, USP; PMS-Hydromorphone

Index Terms Dihydromorphinone; Hydromorphone Hydrochloride

Generic Available Yes: Excludes capsule, liquid, powder for injection

Pharmacologic Category Analgesic, Opioid

Use Management of moderate to severe pain

Restrictions C-II

Contraindications Hypersensitivity to hydromorphone, any component of the formulation, or other phenanthrene derivative; increased intracranial pressure; acute or severe asthma, severe respiratory depression (in absence of resuscitative equipment or ventilatory support); severe CNS depression

Warnings/Precautions Use with caution in patients with hypersensitivity reactions to other phenanthrene derivative opioid agonists (codeine, hydrocodone, levorphanol, oxycodone, oxymorphone). Hydromorphone shares toxic potential of opiate agonists, including CNS depression and respiratory depression. Precautions associated with opiate agonist therapy should be observed. May cause CNS depression, which may impair physical or mental abilities; patients must be cautioned about performing tasks which require mental alertness (eg, operating machinery or driving). Myoclonus and seizures have been reported with high doses. Critical respiratory depression may occur, even at therapeutic dosages, particularly in elderly or debilitated patients or in patients with pre-existing respiratory compromise (hypoxia and/or hypercapnia). Use caution in COPD or other obstructive pulmonary disease. Use with caution in patients with hypersensitivity to other phenanthrene opiates, kyphoscoliosis, biliary tract disease, acute pancreatitis, morbid obesity, adrenocortical insufficiency, hypothyroidism, acute alcoholism, toxic psychoses, prostatic hyperplasia and/or urinary stricture, or severe liver or renal failure. Use extreme caution in patients with head injury, intracranial lesions, or elevated intracranial pressure; exaggerated elevation of ICP may occur (in addition, hydromorphone may complicate neurologic evaluation due to pupillary dilation and CNS depressant effects). Use with caution in patients with depleted blood volume or drugs which may exaggerate hypotensive effects (including phenothiazines or general anesthetics). May obscure diagnosis or clinical course of patients with acute abdominal conditions.

[U.S. Boxed Warning]: Hydromorphone has a high potential for abuse. Those at risk for opioid abuse include patients with a history of substance abuse or mental illness. Tolerance or drug dependence may result from extended use; however, concerns for abuse should not prevent effective management of pain. In general, abrupt discontinuation of therapy in dependent patients should be avoided.

An opioid-containing analgesic regimen should be tailored to each patient's needs and based upon the type of pain being treated (acute versus chronic), the route of administration, degree of tolerance for opioids (naive versus chronic user), age, weight, and medical condition. The optimal analgesic dose varies widely among patients. Doses should be titrated to pain relief/prevention. I.M. use may result in variable absorption and a lag time to peak effect.

Dosage form specific warnings:

    [U.S. Boxed Warning]: Dilaudid-HP®: Extreme caution should be taken to avoid confusing the highly-concentrated (Dilaudid-HP®) injection with the less-concentrated (Dilaudid®) injectable product. Dilaudid-HP® should only be used in patients who are opioid-tolerant.

    Controlled release: Capsules should only be used when continuous analgesia is required over an extended period of time. Controlled release products are not to be used on an "as needed" (PRN) basis.

    Some dosage forms contain trace amounts of sodium metabisulfite which may cause allergic reactions in susceptible individuals.

Adverse Reactions (Reflective of adult population; not specific for elderly) Frequency not defined.

Cardiovascular: Bradycardia, flushing of face, hyper-/hypotension, palpitation, peripheral vasodilation, syncope, tachycardia

Central nervous system: Agitation, chills, CNS depression, dizziness, drowsiness, dysphoria, euphoria, fatigue, hallucinations, headache, increased intracranial pressure, insomnia, lightheadedness, mental depression, nervousness, restlessness, sedation, seizure

Dermatologic: Pruritus, rash, urticaria

Endocrine & metabolic: Antidiuretic hormone release

(Continued)

Hydromorphone *(Continued)*

Gastrointestinal: Anorexia, biliary tract spasm, constipation, diarrhea, nausea, paralytic ileus, stomach cramps, taste perversion, vomiting, xerostomia

Genitourinary: Ureteral spasm, urinary retention, urinary tract spasm, urination decreased

Hepatic: AST/ALT increased, LFTs increased

Local: Pain at injection site (I.M.), wheal/flare over vein (I.V.)

Neuromuscular & skeletal: Myoclonus, paresthesia, trembling, tremor, weakness

Ocular: Blurred vision, diplopia, miosis, nystagmus

Respiratory: Apnea, bronchospasm, dyspnea, laryngospasm, respiratory depression

Miscellaneous: Diaphoresis, histamine release, physical and psychological dependence

Overdosage/Toxicology Symptoms of overdose include CNS depression, bradycardia, hypotension, respiratory depression, miosis, apnea, pulmonary edema, and convulsions. Along with supportive measures, naloxone, 2 mg I.V. with repeat administration as necessary up to a total of 10 mg, can also be used to reverse toxic effects of the opiate. Longer observation times may be required with overdose of longer duration products. Activated charcoal or gut decontamination may be used with oral overdose.

Drug Interactions

Ammonium chloride: May decrease the levels/effects of hydromorphone.

CNS depressants: Effects with hydromorphone may be additive.

General anesthetics: May enhance the hypotensive and CNS depressant effects of hydromorphone.

Pegvisomant: Analgesics (narcotic) may diminish the therapeutic effect of pegvisomant; increased pegvisomant doses may be needed.

Phenothiazines: May enhance the hypotensive and CNS depressant effects of hydromorphone.

Selective serotonin reuptake inhibitors (SSRIs): Serotonergic effects may be additive, leading to serotonin syndrome.

Ethanol/Nutrition/Herb Interactions

Ethanol: Avoid ethanol (may increase CNS depression).

Herb/Nutraceutical: Avoid valerian, St John's wort, kava kava, gotu kola (may increase CNS depression).

Stability Store injection and oral dosage forms at 15°C to 30°C (59°F to 86°F). Protect tablets from light. A slightly yellowish discoloration has not been associated with a loss of potency.

Mechanism of Action Binds to opiate receptors in the CNS, causing inhibition of ascending pain pathways, altering the perception of and response to pain; causes cough supression by direct central action in the medulla; produces generalized CNS depression

Pharmacodynamics

Onset of action: Analgesic: Immediate release formulations:

Oral: 15-30 minutes

Peak effect: Oral: 30-60 minutes

Duration: Immediate release formulations: 4-5 hours

Pharmacokinetics

Absorption: I.M.: Variable and delayed

Distribution: V_d: 4 L/kg

Protein binding: ~8% to 19%

Metabolism: Hepatic via glucuronidation; to inactive metabolites

Bioavailability: 62%

Half-life elimination: Immediate release formulations: 1-3 hours

Excretion: Urine (primarily as glucuronide conjugates)

Dosage

Geriatrics: Doses should be titrated to appropriate analgesic effects. When changing routes of administration, note that oral doses are less than half as effective as parenteral doses (may be only 20% as effective).

Pain: Oral: 1-2 mg every 4-6 hours

Antitussive: Refer to adult dosing.

Adults:

Antitussive (unlabeled use): Oral: 1 mg every 3-4 hours as needed

Acute pain (moderate to severe): Note: These are guidelines and do not represent the maximum doses that may be required in all patients. Doses should be titrated to pain relief/prevention. Doses should be titrated to appropriate analgesic effects; when changing routes of administration, note that oral doses are <50% as effective as parenteral doses (may be only one-fifth as effective).

Oral:

Initial: Opiate-naive: 2-4 mg every 3-6 hours as needed; elderly/debilitated patients may require lower doses; patients with prior opiate exposure may require higher initial doses

Usual dosage range: 2-8 mg every 3-4 hours as needed

I.V.: Initial: Opiate-naive: 0.2-0.6 mg every 2-3 hours as needed; patients with prior opiate exposure may tolerate higher initial doses

Note: More frequent dosing may be needed.

Mechanically-ventilated patients (based on 70 kg patient): 0.7-2 mg every 1-2 hours as needed; infusion (based on 70 kg patient): 0.5-1 mg/hour

Patient-controlled analgesia (PCA): (Opiate-naive: Consider lower end of dosing range)

Usual concentration: 0.2 mg/mL

Demand dose: Usual: 0.1-0.2 mg; range: 0.05-0.5 mg

Lockout interval: 5-15 minutes

4-hour limit: 4-6 mg

Epidural:

Bolus dose: 1-1.5 mg

Infusion concentration: 0.05-0.075 mg/mL

Infusion rate: 0.04-0.4 mg/hour

Demand dose: 0.15 mg

Lockout interval: 30 minutes

I.M., SubQ: **Note:** I.M. use may result in variable absorption and a lag time to peak effect.

Initial: Opiate-naive: 0.8-1 mg every 4-6 hours as needed; patients with prior opiate exposure may require higher initial doses

Usual dosage range: 1-2 mg every 3-6 hours as needed

Rectal: 3 mg every 4-8 hours as needed

Chronic pain: Note: Patients taking opioids chronically may become tolerant and require doses higher than the usual dosage range to maintain the desired effect. Tolerance can be managed by appropriate dose titration. There is no optimal or maximal dose for hydromorphone in chronic pain. The appropriate dose is one that relieves pain throughout its dosing interval without causing unmanageable side effects.

Controlled release formulation (Hydromorph Contin®, not available in U.S.): Oral: 3-30 mg every 12 hours. **Note:** A patient's hydromorphone requirement should be established using prompt release formulations; conversion to long acting products may be considered when chronic, continuous treatment is required. Higher dosages should be reserved for use only in opioid-tolerant patients.

Hepatic Impairment: Dose adjustment should be considered.

Administration

Parenteral: May be given SubQ or I.M.; vial stopper contains latex

I.V.: For IVP, must be given slowly over 2-3 minutes (rapid IVP has been associated with an increase in side effects, especially respiratory depression and hypotension)

Oral: Hydromorph Contin®: Capsule should be swallowed whole; do not crush or chew; contents may be sprinkled on soft food and swallowed

Monitoring Parameters Pain relief, respiratory and mental status, blood pressure

Test Interactions Some quinolones may produce a false-positive urine screening result for opiates using commercially-available immunoassay kits. This has been demonstrated most consistently for levofloxacin and ofloxacin, but other quinolones have shown cross-reactivity in certain assay kits. Confirmation of positive opiate screens by more specific methods should be considered.

Patient Information May cause drowsiness; avoid the use of alcohol and other CNS depressants

Additional Information Equianalgesic doses: Morphine 10 mg I.M. = hydromorphone 1.5 mg I.M.

Special Geriatric Considerations Elderly may be particularly susceptible to the CNS depressant and constipating effects of narcotics.

Dosage Forms Excipient information presented when available (limited, particularly for generics); consult specific product labeling. [CAN] = Canadian brand name

Capsule, controlled release:

Hydromorph Contin® [CAN]: 3 mg, 6 mg, 12 mg, 18 mg, 24 mg, 30 mg [not available in U.S.]

Injection, powder for reconstitution, as hydrochloride:

Dilaudid-HP®: 250 mg [may contain trace amounts of sodium bisulfite]

Injection, solution, as hydrochloride: 1 mg/mL (1 mL); 2 mg/mL (1 mL, 20 mL); 4 mg/mL (1 mL); 10 mg/mL (1 mL, 5 mL, 10 mL)

Dilaudid®: 1 mg/mL (1 mL); 2 mg/mL (1 mL, 20 mL) [20 mL size contains edetate sodium; vial stopper contains latex]; 4 mg/mL (1 mL)

Dilaudid-HP®: 10 mg/mL (1 mL, 5 mL, 50 mL) [50 mL packaging contains latex]

Liquid, oral, as hydrochloride:

Dilaudid®: 1 mg/mL (480 mL) [may contain trace amounts of sodium bisulfite]

Suppository, rectal, as hydrochloride: 3 mg

Dilaudid®: 3 mg (6s)

Tablet, as hydrochloride: 2 mg, 4 mg, 8 mg

(Continued)

Hydromorphone (Continued)

Dilaudid®: 2 mg, 4 mg, 8 mg (8 mg tablets may contain trace amounts of sodium bisulfite)

Selected References

AGS Panel on Persistent Pain in Older Persons, "The Management of Persistent Pain in Older Persons," *J Am Geriatr Soc*, 2002, 50(6 Suppl):S205-24.

Ferrell BA, "Pain Management in Elderly People," *J Am Geriatr Soc*, 1991, 39(1):64-73.

Kaiko RF, Wallenstein SL, Rogers AG, et al, "Narcotics in the Elderly," *Med Clin North Am*, 1982, 66(5):1079-89.

Mokhlesi B, Leikin JB, Murray P, et al, "Adult Toxicology in Critical Care: Part II: Specific Poisonings," *Chest*, 2003, 123(3):897-922.

♦ **Hydromorphone Hydrochloride** *see* Hydromorphone *on page 766*

♦ **Hydro-Tussin™-CBX** *see* Carbinoxamine and Pseudoephedrine *on page 239*

♦ **Hydro-Tussin™ DM** *see* Guaifenesin and Dextromethorphan *on page 730*

Hydroxocobalamin (hye droks oh koe BAL a min)

U.S. Brand Names Cyanokit®

Index Terms Vitamin B_{12a}

Generic Available Yes: Excludes powder for injection

Pharmacologic Category Antidote; Vitamin, Water Soluble

Use Treatment of pernicious anemia, vitamin B_{12} deficiency due to dietary deficiencies or malabsorption diseases, inadequate secretion of intrinsic factor, and inadequate utilization of B_{12} (eg, during neoplastic treatment); diagnostic agent for Schilling test

Cyanokit®: Treatment of cyanide poisoning (known or suspected)

Unlabeled/Investigational Use Treatment of neuropathies, multiple sclerosis

Contraindications Hypersensitivity to hydroxocobalamin, cyanocobalamin, cobalt, or any component of the formulation

Warnings/Precautions

Solution for I.M. injection: Treatment of severe vitamin B_{12} megaloblastic anemia may result in thrombocytosis and severe hypokalemia, sometimes fatal, due to intracellular potassium shift upon anemia resolution. Use caution in folic acid deficient megaloblastic anemia; administration of vitamin B_{12} alone is not a substitute for folic acid and might mask true diagnosis. Vitamin B_{12} deficiency masks signs of polycythemia vera; vitamin B_{12} administration may unmask this condition. Neurologic manifestations of vitamin B_{12} deficiency will not be prevented with folic acid unless vitamin B_{12} is also given; spinal cord degeneration might also occur when folic acid is used as a substitute for vitamin B_{12} in anemia prevention. Blunted therapeutic response to vitamin B_{12} may occur in certain conditions (eg, infection, uremia, concurrent iron or folic acid deficiency) or in patients on medications with bone marrow suppressant properties (eg, chloramphenicol). Approved for use as I.M. injection only.

Cyanokit®: Use caution or consider alternatives in patients with known allergic reactions, including anaphylaxis, to hydroxocobalamin or cyanocobalamin. Increased blood pressure (≥180 mm Hg diastolic or ≥110 mm Hg diastolic) is associated with infusion; elevations usually noted at beginning of infusion, peak toward the end of infusion and return to baseline within 4 hours of infusion. Collection of pretreatment blood cyanide concentrations does not preclude administration and should not delay administration in the emergency management of highly suspected or confirmed cyanide toxicity. Pretreatment levels may be useful as post infusion levels may be inaccurate. Treatment of cyanide poisoning should include decontamination and supportive therapy. Photosensitivity is a potential concern; avoid direct sunlight while skin remains discolored.

Adverse Reactions (Reflective of adult population; not specific for elderly)

I.M. injection: Frequency not defined:

Dermatologic: Exanthema (transient), itching

Gastrointestinal: Diarrhea (mild, transient)

Local: Injection site pain

Miscellaneous: Anaphylaxis

I.V. infusion (Cyanokit®):

>10%:

Cardiovascular: Blood pressure increased (18% to 28%; systolic ≥180 mm Hg or diastolic ≥110 mm Hg)

Central nervous system: Headache (6% to 33%)

Dermatologic: Erythema (94% to 100%; may last up to 2 weeks), rash (predominantly acneiform; 20% to 44%; can appear 7-28 days after administration and usually resolves within a few weeks)

Gastrointestinal: Nausea (6% to 11%)

Genitourinary: Chromaturia (100%; may last up to 5 weeks after administration)

Hematologic: Lymphocytes decreased (8% to 17%)

Local: Infusion site reaction (6% to 39%)

Frequency not defined:

Cardiovascular: Chest discomfort, heart rate increased/decreased, hot flashes, peripheral edema

Central nervous system: Dizziness, memory impairment, restlessness

Dermatologic: Pruritus, urticaria

Gastrointestinal: Abdominal discomfort, diarrhea, dyspepsia, dysphagia, hematochezia, vomiting

Ocular: Irritation, redness, swelling

Respiratory: Dry throat, dyspnea, throat tightness

Miscellaneous: Allergic reaction (including anaphylaxis)

Drug Interactions No data reported

Stability

Solution for I.M. injection: Store at 20°C to 25°C (68°F to 77°F). Protect from light.

I.V. infusion (Cyanokit®): Prior to reconstitution, store at 15°C to 30°C (59°F to 86°F). Temperature variation exposure allowed for transport of lyophilized form:

Usual transport: ≤15 days at 5°C to 40°C (41°F to 104°F)

Desert transport: ≤4 days at 5°C to 60°C (41°F to 140°F)

Freezing/defrosting cycles: ≤15 days at -20°C to 40°C (-4°F to 104°F)

Reconstitute each 2.5 g vial with 100 mL of NS using provided sterile transfer spike. If NS unavailable, may use LR or D_5W. Invert or rock each vial for at least 30 seconds prior to infusion; do not shake. Do not use if solution is **not** dark red. Following reconstitution, store up to 6 hours at ≤40°C (104°F); do not freeze. Discard any remaining solution after 6 hours.

Mechanism of Action Hydroxocobalamin (vitamin B_{12a}) is a precursor to cyanocobalamin (vitamin B_{12}). Cyanocobalamin acts as a coenzyme for various metabolic functions, including fat and carbohydrate metabolism and protein synthesis, used in cell replication and hematopoiesis. In the presence of cyanide, each hydroxocobalamin molecule can bind one cyanide ion by displacing it for the hydroxo ligand linked to the trivalent cobalt ion, forming cyanocobalamin.

Pharmacokinetics Following I.V. administration of Cyanokit®:

Protein binding: Significant; forms various cobalamin-(III) complexes

Half-life elimination: 26-31 hours

Excretion: Urine (50% to 60% within initial 72 hours)

Dosage

Geriatrics & Adults:

Vitamin B_{12} deficiency: I.M.: 30 mcg/day for 5-10 days, followed by 100-200 mcg/month

Note: Larger doses may be required in critically-ill patients or if patient has neurologic disease, an infectious disease, or hyperthyroidism.

Schilling test: I.M.: 1000 mcg

Cyanide toxicity (Cyanokit®): I.V.: Initial: 5 g as single infusion; may repeat a second 5 g dose depending on severity of poisoning and clinical response. Maximum cumulative dose: 10 g. **Note:** If suspected, antidotal therapy must be given immediately.

Administration

Solution for I.M. injection: Administer 1000 mcg/mL solution I.M. only

Cyanokit®: Administer by I.V. infusion over 15 minutes; if repeat dose needed, administer second dose over 15 minutes to 2 hours

Monitoring Parameters Vitamin B_{12}, hematocrit, hemoglobin, reticulocyte count, red blood cell counts, folate and iron levels should be obtained prior to treatment and periodically during treatment.

Cyanide toxicity: Blood pressure and heart rate during and after infusion, serum lactate levels, venous-arterial PO_2 gradient.

Megaloblastic anemia: In addition to normal hematological parameters, serum potassium and platelet counts should be monitored during therapy, particularly in the first 48 hours of treatment.

Reference Range Blood cyanide levels may be used for diagnosis confirmation; however, reliable levels require prompt testing and proper storage conditions.

Tachycardia/flushing: 0.5-1 mg/L

Obtundation: 1-2.5 mg/L

Coma: 2.5-3 mg/L

Death: >3 mg/L

Test Interactions The following values may be affected, *in vitro*, following hydroxocobalamin 5 g dose. Interference following hydroxocobalamin 10 g dose can be expected to last up to an additional 24 hours. **Note:** Extent and duration of interference dependant on analyzer used and patient variability.

Falsely elevated:

Basophils, hemoglobin, MCH, and MCHC [duration: 12-16 hours]

Albumin, alkaline phosphatase, cholesterol, creatinine, glucose, total protein, and triglycerides [duration: 24 hours]

Bilirubin [duration: up to 4 days]

(Continued)

Hydroxocobalamin *(Continued)*

Urinalysis: Glucose, protein, erythrocytes, leukocytes, ketones, bilirubin, urobilinogen, nitrite [duration: 2-8 days]

Falsely decreased: ALT and amylase [duration: 24 hours]

Unpredictable:

AST, CK, CKMB, LDH, phosphate, and uric acid [duration: 24 hours]

PT (quick or INR) and aPTT [duration: 24-48 hours]

Urine pH [duration: 2-8 days]

May also interfere with colorimetric tests

Patient Information Therapy is required throughout life; do not take folic acid instead of B_{12} to prevent anemia

Additional Information Expert advice from a regional poison control center for appropriate use may be obtained (1-800-222-1222). Cyanide is a clear colorless gas or liquid with a faint bitter almond odor. Cyanide reacts with trivalent ions in cytochrome oxidase in the mitochondria leading to histotoxic hypoxia and lactic acidosis. Signs and symptoms of cyanide toxicity include headache, altered mental status, dyspnea, mydriasis, chest tightness, nausea, vomiting, tachycardia/hypertension (initially), bradycardia/hypotension (later), seizures, cardiovascular collapse, or coma.

Special Geriatric Considerations Evidence exists that people, particularly elderly, whose serum cobalamin concentrations are <500 pg/mL, should receive replacement parenteral therapy. This recommendation is based upon neuropsychiatric disorders and cardiovascular disorders associated with lower sodium cobalamin concentrations.

Dosage Forms Excipient information presented when available (limited, particularly for generics); consult specific product labeling.

Injection, solution: 1000 mcg/mL (30 mL)

Injection, powder for reconstitution:

Cyanokit®: 2.5 g (2 vials) [provided in a kit which also contains one I.V. infusion set]

Selected References

Cottrell JE, Casthely P, Brodie JD, et al, "Prevention of Nitroprusside-Induced Cyanide Toxicity With Hydroxocobalamin," *N Engl J Med*, 1978, 298(15):809-11.

Curry SC, Connor DA, and Raschke RA, "Effect of the Cyanide Antidote Hydroxocobalamin on Commonly Ordered Serum Chemistry Studies," *Ann Emerg Med*, 1994, 24(1):65-7.

Holland MA and Kozlowski LM, "Clinical Features and Management of Cyanide Poisoning," *Clin Pharm*, 1986, 5(9):737-41.

Kayser SR and Kurisu S, "Hydroxocobalamin in Nitroprusside Induced Cyanide Toxicity," *Drug Intell Clin Pharm*, 1986, 20:365-6.

Lindenbaum J, Healton EB, Savage DG, et al, "Neuropsychiatric Disorders Caused by Cobalamin Deficiency in the Absence of Anemia or Macrocytosis," *N Engl J Med*, 1988, 318(26):1720-8.

Olszewski AJ, Szostak WB, Bialkowska M, et al, "Reduction of Plasma Lipid and Homocysteine Levels by Pyridoxine, Folate, Cobalamin, Choline, Riboflavin, and Troxerutin in Atherosclerosis," *Atherosclerosis*, 1989, 75(1):1-6.

Regland B, Gottfries CG, and Lindstedt G, "Dementia Patients With Low Serum Cobalamin Concentration: Relationship to Atrophic Gastritis," *Aging (Milano)*, 1992, 4(1):35-41.

Sauer SW and Keim ME, "Hydroxocobalamin: Improved Public Health Readiness for Cyanide Disasters," *Ann Emerg Med*, 2001, 37(6):635-41.

♦ **Hydroxycarbamide** *see* Hydroxyurea *on page 774*

Hydroxychloroquine *(hye droks ee KLOR oh kwin)*

Medication Safety Issues

Sound-alike/look-alike issues:

Hydroxychloroquine may be confused with hydrocortisone

Plaquenil® may be confused with Platinol®

U.S. Brand Names Plaquenil®

Canadian Brand Names Apo-Hydroxyquine®; Gen-Hydroxychloroquine; Plaquenil®

Index Terms Hydroxychloroquine Sulfate

Generic Available Yes

Pharmacologic Category Aminoquinoline (Antimalarial)

Use Suppression and treatment of acute attacks of malaria; treatment of systemic lupus erythematosus, rheumatoid arthritis

Unlabeled/Investigational Use Treatment of porphyria cutanea tarda, polymorphous light eruptions

Contraindications Hypersensitivity to hydroxychloroquine, 4-aminoquinoline derivatives, or any component of the formulation; retinal or visual field changes attributable to 4-aminoquinolines

Warnings/Precautions Use with caution in patients with hepatic disease, G6PD deficiency, psoriasis, and porphyria; perform baseline and periodic (6 months) ophthalmologic examinations; test periodically for muscle weakness. **[U.S. Boxed Warning]: Should be prescribed by physicians familiar with its use.**

Adverse Reactions (Reflective of adult population; not specific for elderly)

Frequency not defined.

Cardiovascular: Cardiomyopathy (rare, relationship to hydroxychloroquine unclear)

Central nervous system: Irritability, nervousness, emotional changes, nightmares, psychosis, headache, dizziness, vertigo, seizure, ataxia, lassitude

Dermatologic: Bleaching of hair, alopecia, pigmentation changes (skin and mucosal; black-blue color), rash (urticarial, morbilliform, lichenoid, maculopapular, purpuric, erythema annulare centrifugum, Stevens-Johnson syndrome, acute generalized exanthematous pustulosis, and exfoliative dermatitis)

Endocrine & metabolic: Weight loss

Gastrointestinal: Anorexia, nausea, vomiting, diarrhea, abdominal cramping

Hematologic: Aplastic anemia, agranulocytosis, leukopenia, thrombocytopenia, hemolysis (in patients with glucose-6-phosphate deficiency)

Hepatic: Abnormal liver function/hepatic failure (isolated cases)

Neuromuscular & skeletal: Myopathy, palsy, or neuromyopathy leading to progressive weakness and atrophy of proximal muscle groups (may be associated with mild sensory changes, loss of deep tendon reflexes, and abnormal nerve conduction)

Ocular: Disturbance in accommodation, keratopathy, corneal changes/deposits (visual disturbances, blurred vision, photophobia - reversible on discontinuation), macular edema, atrophy, abnormal pigmentation, retinopathy (early changes reversible - may progress despite discontinuation if advanced), optic disc pallor/atrophy, attenuation of retinal arterioles, pigmentary retinopathy, scotoma, decreased visual acuity, nystagmus

Otic: Tinnitus, deafness

Miscellaneous: Exacerbation of porphyria and nonlight sensitive psoriasis

Overdosage/Toxicology Symptoms include headache, drowsiness, visual changes, cardiovascular collapse, and seizures, followed by respiratory and cardiac arrest. Treatment is symptomatic. Activated charcoal will bind the drug following GI decontamination. Urinary alkalinization will enhance renal elimination.

Drug Interactions

Chloroquine and other 4-aminoquinolones may be decreased due to GI binding with kaolin or magnesium trisilicate

Increased effect: Cimetidine increases levels of chloroquine and probably other 4-aminoquinolones

Ethanol/Nutrition/Herb Interactions Ethanol: Avoid ethanol (due to GI irritation).

Mechanism of Action Interferes with digestive vacuole function within sensitive malarial parasites by increasing the pH and interfering with lysosomal degradation of hemoglobin; inhibits locomotion of neutrophils and chemotaxis of eosinophils; impairs complement-dependent antigen-antibody reactions

Pharmacokinetics

Absorption: Oral: Complete

Protein binding: 55%

Metabolism: In the liver

Elimination: Metabolites and unchanged drug slowly excreted in urine, may be enhanced by urinary acidification

Dosage

Geriatrics & Adults:

Note: Hydroxychloroquine sulfate 200 mg is equivalent to 155 mg hydroxychloroquine base and 250 mg chloroquine phosphate.

Chemoprophylaxis of malaria: 310 mg base weekly on same day each week; begin 2 weeks before exposure. Continue for 4-6 weeks after leaving endemic area; if suppressive therapy is not begun prior to the exposure, double the initial dose and give in 2 doses, 6 hours apart.

Malaria, acute attack: 620 mg first dose day 1; 310 mg in 6 hours day 1; 310 mg in 1 dose day 2; and 310 mg in 1 dose on day 3

Rheumatoid arthritis: 310-465 mg/day to start taken with food or milk; increase dose until optimum response level is reached; usually after 4-12 weeks dose should be reduced by $1/2$ and a maintenance dose of 155-310 mg/day given

Lupus erythematosus: 310 mg every day or twice daily for several weeks depending on response; 155-310 mg/day for prolonged maintenance therapy

Hepatic Impairment: Use with caution; dosage adjustment may be necessary.

Monitoring Parameters Ophthalmologic exam, CBC

Patient Information Take with food or milk; complete full course of therapy; wear sunglasses in bright sunlight; notify physician if blurring or other vision changes, ringing in the ears, or hearing loss occurs; may cause nausea, vomiting, diarrhea, loss of appetite, stomach pain, and muscle weakness; should this remain for a prolonged period, report to your physician

Additional Information If long-term use of drug is contemplated, it is recommended to have a complete eye examination performed prior to therapy and at periodic intervals (eg, 6 months)

Special Geriatric Considerations No specific recommendations for dosing.

Dosage Forms Excipient information presented when available (limited, particularly for generics); consult specific product labeling.

Tablet, as sulfate: 200 mg [equivalent to 155 mg base]

♦ **Hydroxychloroquine Sulfate** *see* Hydroxychloroquine *on page 772*

♦ **1α-Hydroxyergocalciferol** *see* Doxercalciferol *on page 477*

♦ **Hydroxyethylcellulose** *see* Artificial Tears *on page 124*

♦ **9-hydroxy-risperidone** *see* Paliperidone *on page 1190*

Hydroxyurea (hye droks ee yoor EE a)

Medication Safety Issues
Sound-alike/look-alike issues:
Hydroxyurea may be confused with hydrOXYzine

High alert medication: The Institute for Safe Medication Practices (ISMP) includes this medication among its list of drugs which have a heightened risk of causing significant patient harm when used in error.

International issues:
Hydrea® may be confused with Hydra® which is a brand name for isoniazid in Japan

U.S. Brand Names Droxia®; Hydrea®; Mylocel™

Canadian Brand Names Apo-Hydroxyurea®; Gen-Hydroxyurea; Hydrea®

Index Terms Hydroxycarbamide

Generic Available Yes: Capsule

Pharmacologic Category Antineoplastic Agent, Antimetabolite

Use Treatment of melanoma, refractory chronic myelocytic leukemia (CML), relapsed and refractory metastatic ovarian cancer; radiosensitizing agent in the treatment of squamous cell head and neck cancer (excluding lip cancer); adjunct in the management of sickle cell patients who have had at least three painful crises in the previous 12 months (to reduce frequency of these crises and the need for blood transfusions)

Unlabeled/Investigational Use Treatment of HIV; treatment of psoriasis, treatment of hematologic conditions such as essential thrombocythemia, polycythemia vera, hypereosinophilia, and hyperleukocytosis due to acute leukemia; treatment of uterine, cervix and nonsmall cell lung cancers; radiosensitizing agent in the treatment of primary brain tumors; has shown activity against renal cell cancer and prostate cancer

Contraindications Hypersensitivity to hydroxyurea or any component of the formulation; severe anemia; severe bone marrow suppression; WBC <2500/mm³ or platelet count <100,000/mm³

Warnings/Precautions Hazardous agent - use appropriate precautions for handling and disposal. Patients with a history of prior cytotoxic chemotherapy and radiation therapy are more likely to experience bone marrow depression. Patients with a history of radiation therapy are also at risk for exacerbation of post irradiation erythema. Megaloblastic erythropoiesis may be seen early in hydroxyurea treatment; plasma iron clearance may be delayed and the rate of utilization of iron by erythrocytes may be delayed. HIV-infected patients treated with hydroxyurea and antiretroviral agents (including didanosine) are at higher risk for potentially fatal pancreatitis, hepatotoxicity, hepatic failure, and severe peripheral neuropathy. **[U.S. Boxed Warning]: Hydroxyurea is mutagenic and clastogenic. Treatment of myeloproliferative disorders (polycythemia vera and thrombocythemia) with long-term hydroxyurea is associated with secondary leukemia**; it is unknown if this is drug-related or disease-related. Cutaneous vasculitic toxicities (vasculitic ulceration and gangrene) have been reported with hydroxyurea treatment, most often in patients with a history of or receiving concurrent interferon therapy; discontinue hydroxyurea and consider alternate cytoreductive therapy if cutaneous vasculitic toxicity develops. Use caution with renal dysfunction; may require dose reductions. **[U.S. Boxed Warning]: Should be administered under the supervision of a physician experienced in cancer chemotherapy or in the treatment of sickle cell anemia.**

Adverse Reactions (Reflective of adult population; not specific for elderly)
Frequency not defined.
Cardiovascular: Edema
Central nervous system: Chills, disorientation, dizziness, drowsiness (dose-related), fever, hallucinations, headache, malaise, seizure
Dermatologic: Alopecia (rare), cutaneous vasculitic toxicities, dermatomyositis-like skin changes, dry skin, facial erythema, gangrene, hyperpigmentation, maculopapular rash, nail atrophy, nail pigmentation, peripheral erythema, scaling, skin atrophy, skin cancer, skin ulcer, vasculitis ulcerations, violet papules
Endocrine & metabolic: Hyperuricemia
Gastrointestinal: Anorexia, constipation, diarrhea, gastrointestinal irritation and mucositis, (potentiated with radiation therapy), nausea, pancreatitis, stomatitis, vomiting
Genitourinary: Dysuria (rare)
Hematologic: Myelosuppression (primarily leukopenia; onset: 24-48 hours; nadir: 10 days; recovery: 7 days after stopping drug; reversal of WBC count occurs rapidly but the platelet count may take 7-10 days to recover); thrombocytopenia and anemia,

megaloblastic erythropoiesis, macrocytosis, hemolysis, serum iron decreased, persistent cytopenias, secondary leukemias (long-term use)

Hepatic: Hepatic enzymes increased, hepatotoxicity

Neuromuscular & skeletal: Peripheral neuropathy, weakness

Renal: BUN increased, creatinine increased

Respiratory: Acute diffuse pulmonary infiltrates (rare), dyspnea, pulmonary fibrosis (rare)

Overdosage/Toxicology Symptoms include myelosuppression, facial swelling, hallucinations, and disorientation. Treatment is supportive.

Drug Interactions

Didanosine: Hydroxyurea may increase risk of didanosine-induced pancreatitis, hepatotoxicity, or neuropathy; concomitant use is not recommended

Stability Store at room temperature between 15°C and 30°C (59°F and 86°F).

Mechanism of Action Thought to interfere (unsubstantiated hypothesis) with synthesis of DNA, during the S phase of cell division, without interfering with RNA synthesis; inhibits ribonucleoside diphosphate reductase, preventing conversion of ribonucleotides to deoxyribonucleotides; cell-cycle specific for the S phase and may hold other cells in the G_1 phase of the cell cycle. In sickle cell anemia, hydroxyurea increases red blood cell (RBC) hemoglobin F levels, RBC water content, deformability of sickled cells, and alters adhesion of RBCs to endothelium.

Pharmacokinetics

Absorption: Readily from the GI tract ($\geq$80%)

Distribution: Readily crosses blood-brain barrier; distributes into intestine, brain, lung, kidney tissues, effusions and ascites

Metabolism: 60% via hepatic and GI tract

Half-life: 3-4 hours

Time to peak: 1-4 hours

Elimination: Renal excretion of urea (metabolite) and respiratory excretion of CO_2 (metabolic end product); 50% of the drug is excreted unchanged in urine

Dosage

Geriatrics & Adults: Refer to individual protocols.

Note: Dose should always be titrated to patient response and WBC counts; usual oral doses range from 10-30 mg/kg/day or 500-3000 mg/day; if WBC count falls to <2500 cells/mm^3, or the platelet count to <100,000/mm^3, therapy should be stopped for at least 3 days and resumed when values rise toward normal.

Solid tumors: Oral:

Intermittent therapy: 80 mg/kg as a single dose every third day

Continuous therapy: 20-30 mg/kg/day given as a single dose/day

Concomitant therapy with irradiation: 80 mg/kg as a single dose every third day starting at least 7 days before initiation of irradiation

Resistant chronic myelocytic leukemia: Oral: Continuous therapy: 20-30 mg/kg once daily

HIV (unlabeled use; in combination with antiretroviral agents): 1000-1500 mg daily in single or divided doses

Psoriasis: 1000-1500 mg daily in single or divided doses

Sickle cell anemia (moderate/severe disease): Initial: 15 mg/kg/day, increased by 5 mg/kg every 12 weeks if blood counts are in an acceptable range until the maximum tolerated dose of 35 mg/kg/day is achieved or the dose that does not produce toxic effects

Renal Impairment:

Sickle cell anemia: Cl_{cr} <60 mL/minute or ESRD: Reduce initial dose to 7.5 mg/kg; titrate to response/avoidance of toxicity (refer to usual dosing).

Other indications:

Cl_{cr} 10-50 mL/minute: Administer 50% of normal dose.

Cl_{cr} <10 mL/minute: Administer 20% of normal dose.

Hemodialysis: Administer dose after dialysis on dialysis days; supplemental dose is not necessary. Hydroxyurea is a low molecular weight compound with high aqueous solubility that may be freely dialyzable, however, clinical studies confirming this hypothesis have not been performed.

CAPD effects: Unknown

CAVH effects: Dose for GFR 10-50 mL/minute.

Administration Capsules may be opened and emptied into water (will not dissolve completely); observe proper handling procedures

Monitoring Parameters CBC with differential and platelets, renal function and liver function tests, serum uric acid

Sickle cell disease: Monitor for toxicity every 2 weeks. If toxicity occurs, stop treatment until the bone marrow recovers; restart at 2.5 mg/kg/day less than the dose at which toxicity occurs. If no toxicity occurs over the next 12 weeks, then the subsequent dose should be increased by 2.5 mg/kg/day. Reduced dosage of hydroxyurea alternating with erythropoietin may decrease myelotoxicity and increase levels of fetal hemoglobin in patients who have not been helped by hydroxyurea alone.

(Continued)

Hydroxyurea (Continued)

Acceptable range: Neutrophils ≥2500 cells/mm³, platelets ≥95,000/mm³, hemoglobin >5.3 g/dL, and reticulocytes ≥95,000/mm³ if the hemoglobin concentration is <9 g/dL

Toxic range: Neutrophils <2000 cells/mm³, platelets <80,000/mm³, hemoglobin <4.5 g/dL, and reticulocytes <80,000/mm³ if the hemoglobin concentration is <9 g/dL

Patient Information Do not take any new medication during therapy unless approved by prescriber. Take capsules exactly as directed by prescriber (dosage and timing will be specific to purpose of therapy). Contents of capsule may be emptied into a glass of water and taken immediately. You will require frequent monitoring and blood tests while taking this medication to assess effectiveness and monitor adverse reactions. You will be susceptible to infection (avoid crowds and exposure to infection and do not have any vaccinations without consulting prescriber). May cause nausea, vomiting, or loss of appetite (small frequent meals, frequent mouth care, sucking lozenges, or chewing gum may help); constipation (increased exercise, fluid, fruit, or fiber may help); diarrhea (buttermilk, boiled milk, or yogurt may help); or mouth sores (frequent mouth care will help). Report persistent vomiting, diarrhea, constipation, stomach pain, or mouth sores; skin rash, redness, irritation, or sores; painful or difficult urination; anemia (unusual fatigue, lethargy), CNS changes (increased confusion, depression, hallucinations, or seizures); opportunistic infection (persistent fever or chills, white plaques in mouth, vaginal discharge, or unhealed sores); unusual lassitude, muscle tremors or weakness; easy bruising/bleeding; or blood in vomitus, stool, or urine. **Note:** People taking hydroxyurea should not be exposed to it. If powder from capsule is spilled, wipe up with damp, disposable towel immediately, and discard the towel in a closed container, such as a plastic bag. Wash hands thoroughly.

Additional Information Although I.V. use is reported, no parenteral product is commercially available in the U.S.

If WBC decreases to <2500/mm³ or platelet count to <100,000/mm³, interrupt therapy until values rise significantly toward normal. Treat anemia with whole blood replacement; do not interrupt therapy. Adequate trial period to determine the antineoplastic effectiveness is 6 weeks. Almost all patients receiving hydroxyurea in clinical trials needed to have their medication stopped for a time to allow their low blood count to return to acceptable levels.

Special Geriatric Considerations Elderly may be more sensitive to the effects of this drug and may require a lower dosage regimen; advance dose slowly and adjust dose for renal function with careful monitoring.

Dosage Forms Excipient information presented when available (limited, particularly for generics); consult specific product labeling.

Capsule: 500 mg

Droxia®: 200 mg, 300 mg, 400 mg

Hydrea®: 500 mg

Tablet:

Mylocel™: 1000 mg

Selected References

Aronoff GR, Berns JS, Brier ME, et al, "Drug Prescribing in Renal Failure: Dosing Guidelines for Adults," 4th ed. Philadelphia, PA: American College of Physicians; 1999, p. 74.

Bauman JL, Shulruff S, Hasegawa GR, et al, "Fever Caused by Hydroxyurea," *Arch Intern Med*, 1981, 141(2):260-1.

Bennett WM, Aronoff GR, Morrison G, et al, "Drug Prescribing in Renal Failure: Dosing Guidelines for Adults," *Am J Kidney Dis*, 1983, 3(3):155-93.

Charache S, "Mechanism of Action of Hydroxyurea in the Management of Sickle Cell Anemia in Adults," *Semin Hematol*, 1997, 34(3 Suppl 3):15-21.

Charache S, Terrin ML, Moore RD, et al, "Effect of Hydroxyurea on the Frequency of Painful Crises in Sickle Cell Anemia," *N Engl J Med*, 1995, 332(20):1317-22.

Cortelazzo S, Finazzi G, Ruggeri M, et al, "Hydroxyurea for Patients With Essential Thrombocythemia and a High Risk of Thrombosis," *N Engl J Med*, 1995, 332(17):1132-6.

Donehower RC, "An Overview of the Clinical Experience With Hydroxyurea," *Semin Oncol*, 1992, 19(3 Suppl 9):11-9.

Howard LW and Kennedy LD, "Hydroxyurea in the Treatment of Sickle-Cell Anemia," *Ann Pharmacother*, 1997, 31(11):1393-6.

Kennedy BJ, "The Evolution of Hydroxyurea Therapy in Chronic Myelogenous Leukemia," *Semin Oncol*, 1992, 19(3 Suppl 9):21-6.

Longhurst HJ and Pinching AJ, "Drug Points: Pancreatitis Associated With Hydroxyurea in Combination With Didanosine," *BMJ*, 2001, 322(7278):81.

Lossos IS and Matzner Y, "Hydroxyurea-Induced Fever: Case Report and Review of the Literature," *Ann Pharmacother*, 1995, 29(2):132-3. *Blood*, 1998, 91(12):4472-9.

Marwick CM, "Trial Halted as Sickle Cell Treatment Proves Itself," *JAMA*, 1995, 273:(8)611.

Montaner JS, Zala C, Conway B, et al, "A Pilot Study of Hydroxyurea Among Patients With Advanced Human Immunodeficiency Virus (HIV) Disease Receiving Chronic Didanosine Therapy: Canadian HIV Trials Network Protocol 080," *J Infect Dis*, 1997, 175(4):801-6.

Renfro L, Kamino H, Raphael B, et al, "Ulcerative Lichen Planus-Like Dermatitis Associated With Hydroxyurea," *J Am Acad Dermatol*, 1991, 24(1):143-5.

Rodgers GP, Dover GJ, Noguchi CT, et al, "Hematologic Responses of Patients With Sickle Cell Disease to Treatment With Hydroxyurea," *N Engl J Med*, 1990, 322(15):1037-45.

Rodgers GP, "Recent Approaches to the Treatment of Sickle Cell Anemia," *JAMA*, 1991, 265(16):2097-101.

Yarboro JW, "Mechanism of Action of Hydroxyurea," *Semin Oncol*, 1992, 19(3 Suppl 9):1-10.

HydrOXYzine (hye DROKS i zeen)

Related Information
Potentially Inappropriate Medications for Geriatrics *on page 1824*

Medication Safety Issues
Sound-alike/look-alike issues:
HydrOXYzine may be confused with hydrALAZINE, hydroxyurea
Atarax® may be confused with amoxicillin, Ativan®
Vistaril® may be confused with Restoril®, Versed, Zestril®

International issues:
Vistaril® may be confused with Vastarel® which is a brand name for trimetazidine in multiple international markets

U.S. Brand Names Vistaril®

Canadian Brand Names Apo-Hydroxyzine®; Atarax®; Hydroxyzine Hydrochloride Injection, USP; Novo-Hydroxyzin; PMS-Hydroxyzine; Vistaril®

Index Terms Hydroxyzine Hydrochloride; Hydroxyzine Pamoate

Generic Available Yes

Pharmacologic Category Antiemetic; Antihistamine

Use Treatment of anxiety; preoperative sedation; antipruritic

Unlabeled/Investigational Use Antiemetic; treatment of ethanol withdrawal symptoms

Contraindications Hypersensitivity to hydroxyzine or any component of the formulation; SubQ, intra-arterial, or I.V. administration of injection

Warnings/Precautions Causes sedation, caution must be used in performing tasks which require alertness (eg, operating machinery or driving). Sedative effects of CNS depressants or ethanol are potentiated. SubQ, I.V., and intra-arterial administration are contraindicated since tissue damage, intravascular hemolysis, thrombosis, and digital gangrene can occur. Use with caution with narrow-angle glaucoma, prostatic hyperplasia, bladder neck obstruction, asthma, or COPD.

Anticholinergic effects are not well tolerated in the elderly. Hydroxyzine may be useful as a short-term antipruritic, but it is not recommended for use as a sedative or anxiolytic in the elderly.

Adverse Reactions (Reflective of adult population; not specific for elderly)
Frequency not defined.
Central nervous system: Dizziness, drowsiness, fatigue, hallucination, headache, nervousness, seizure
Dermatologic: Pruritus, rash, urticaria
Gastrointestinal: Xerostomia
Neuromuscular & skeletal: Involuntary movements, paresthesia, tremor
Ocular: Blurred vision
Respiratory: Thickening of bronchial secretions
Miscellaneous: Allergic reaction

Overdosage/Toxicology Symptoms include seizures, sedation, and hypotension. There is no specific treatment for antihistamine overdose, however, clinical toxicity is mostly due to anticholinergic effects. Anticholinesterase inhibitors may be useful by reducing acetylcholinesterase. For anticholinergic overdose with severe life-threatening symptoms, physostigmine 1-2 mg slow I.V. may be given to reverse these effects.

Drug Interactions Inhibits CYP2D6 (weak)
Acetylcholinesterase Inhibitors (Central): May diminish the anticholinergic of hydroxyzine. If the anticholinergic effect is a side effect of the agent, as is the case with hydroxyzine, the result may be beneficial.
Anticholinergic agents: Central and/or peripheral anticholinergic syndrome can occur when administered with opioid analgesics, phenothiazines and other antipsychotics (especially with high anticholinergic activity), tricyclic antidepressants, quinidine and some other antiarrhythmics, and antihistamines
CNS depressants: Sedative effects of hydroxyzine may be additive with CNS depressants; includes ethanol, benzodiazepines, barbiturates, opioid analgesics, and other sedative agents; monitor for increased effect
Pramlintide: May enhance the GI-related anticholinergic effect of hydroxyzine.

Ethanol/Nutrition/Herb Interactions
Ethanol: Avoid ethanol (may increase CNS depression).
Herb/Nutraceutical: Avoid valerian, St John's wort, kava kava, gotu kola (may increase CNS depression).

Stability Injection: Store at 15°C to 30°C. Protect from light.

Mechanism of Action Competes with histamine for H_1-receptor sites on effector cells in the gastrointestinal tract, blood vessels, and respiratory tract. Possesses skeletal muscle relaxing, bronchodilator, antihistamine, antiemetic, and analgesic properties.

Pharmacodynamics Onset of action: Within 15-30 minutes
(Continued)

HydrOXYzine (Continued)

Pharmacokinetics
Absorption: Oral: Rapid
Distribution: V_d: Increased in older adults
Metabolism: Forms metabolites
Half-life: 3-7 hours; increased in older adults
Time to peak serum concentration: Within 2 hours and lingers for 4-6 hours
Excretion: Urine

Dosage
Geriatrics: Management of pruritus: 10 mg 3-4 times/day; increase to 25 mg 3-4 times/day if necessary.

Adults:
Antiemetic (unlabeled use): I.M.: 25-100 mg/dose every 4-6 hours as needed
Anxiety: Oral, I.M.: 50-100 mg 4 times/day
Preoperative sedation:
Oral: 50-100 mg
I.M.: 25-100 mg
Pruritus: Oral, I.M.: 25 mg 3-4 times/day

Hepatic Impairment: Change dosing interval to every 24 hours in patients with primary biliary cirrhosis.

Administration
Do not administer SubQ or intra-arterially. Administer I.M. deep in large muscle. With I.V. administration, extravasation can result in sterile abscess and marked tissue induration.

Monitoring Parameters
Relief of symptoms, mental status, blood pressure

Patient Information
Will cause drowsiness, avoid alcohol and other CNS depressants, avoid driving and other hazardous tasks until the CNS effects are known

Additional Information
Hydroxyzine hydrochloride: Atarax®, Vistaril® injection
Hydroxyzine pamoate: Vistaril® capsule and suspension

Special Geriatric Considerations
Anticholinergic effects are not well tolerated in the elderly and frequently result in bowel, bladder, and mental status changes (ie, constipation, confusion, and urinary retention). Hydroxyzine may be useful as a short-term antipruritic, but it is not recommended for use as a sedative or anxiolytic in the elderly.

Dosage Forms
Excipient information presented when available (limited, particularly for generics); consult specific product labeling. [DSC] = Discontinued product
Capsule, as pamoate: 25 mg, 50 mg, 100 mg
Vistaril®: 25 mg, 50 mg
Injection, solution, as hydrochloride: 25 mg/mL (1 mL); 50 mg/mL (1 mL, 2 mL, 10 mL)
Suspension, oral, as pamoate:
Vistaril®: 25 mg/5 mL (120 mL, 480 mL) [lemon flavor] [DSC]
Syrup, as hydrochloride: 10 mg/5 mL (120 mL, 480 mL)
Tablet, as hydrochloride: 10 mg, 25 mg, 50 mg

Selected References
Simons KJ, Watson WT, Chen XY, et al, "Pharmacokinetic and Pharmacodynamic Studies of the H₁-Receptor Antagonist Hydroxyzine in the Elderly," Clin Pharmacol Ther, 1989, 45(1):9-14.

Hyoscyamine (hye oh SYE a meen)

Related Information
Potentially Inappropriate Medications for Geriatrics on page 1824

Medication Safety Issues
Sound-alike/look-alike issues:
Anaspaz® may be confused with Anaprox®, Antispas®
Levbid® may be confused with Lithobid®, Lopid®, Lorabid®
Levsinex® may be confused with Lanoxin®

U.S. Brand Names Anaspaz®; Cystospaz®; Cystospaz-M® [DSC]; Hyosine; Levbid®; Levsin®; Levsinex®; Levsin/SL®; NuLev™; Spacol [DSC]; Spacol T/S [DSC]; Symax SL; Symax SR
Canadian Brand Names Cystospaz®; Levsin®
Index Terms Hyoscyamine Sulfate; l-Hyoscyamine Sulfate
Generic Available Yes

Pharmacologic Category Anticholinergic Agent
Use
  Oral: Adjunctive therapy for peptic ulcers, irritable bowel, neurogenic bladder/bowel; treatment of GI tract disorders caused by spasm; reduction of rigidity, tremors, sialorrhea, and hyperhidrosis associated with parkinsonism; drying agent in acute rhinitis

  Injection: Preoperative antimuscarinic to reduce secretions and block cardiac vagal inhibitory reflexes; improvement of radiologic visibility of the kidneys; symptomatic relief of biliary and renal colic; reduction of GI motility to facilitate diagnostic procedures (ie, endoscopy, hypotonic duodenography); reduction of pain and hypersecretion in pancreatitis, certain cases of partial heart block associated with vagal activity; reversal of neuromuscular blockade

Contraindications Hypersensitivity to belladonna alkaloids or any component of the formulation; glaucoma; obstructive uropathy; myasthenia gravis; obstructive GI tract disease, paralytic ileus, intestinal atony of geriatric or debilitated patients, severe ulcerative colitis, toxic megacolon complicating ulcerative colitis; unstable cardiovascular status in acute hemorrhage, myocardial ischemia

Warnings/Precautions Heat prostration may occur in hot weather. Diarrhea may be a sign of incomplete intestinal obstruction, treatment should be discontinued if this occurs. May produce side effects as seen with other anticholinergic medications including drowsiness, dizziness, blurred vision, or psychosis. The elderly may be more susceptible to these effects. Use with caution in patients with autonomic neuropathy, coronary heart disease, CHF, cardiac arrhythmias, prostatic hyperplasia, hyperthyroidism, hypertension, chronic lung disease, renal disease, and hiatal hernia associated with reflux esophagitis. Use with caution in the elderly, may precipitate undiagnosed glaucoma and/or severely impair memory function (especially in those patients with previous memory problems).

NuLev™: Contains phenylalanine

Adverse Reactions (Reflective of adult population; not specific for elderly)
Frequency not defined.
  Cardiovascular: Palpitation, tachycardia
  Central nervous system: Ataxia, dizziness, drowsiness, headache, insomnia, mental confusion/excitement, nervousness, speech disorder
  Dermatologic: Urticaria
  Endocrine & metabolic: Lactation suppression
  Gastrointestinal: Bloating, constipation, dry mouth, loss of taste, nausea, vomiting
  Genitourinary: Impotence, urinary hesitancy, urinary retention
  Neuromuscular & skeletal: Weakness
  Ocular: Blurred vision, cycloplegia, increased ocular tension, mydriasis
  Miscellaneous: Allergic reactions, sweating decreased

Overdosage/Toxicology Symptoms include dilated, unreactive pupils; blurred vision; hot, dry, flushed skin; dry mucous membranes; difficulty swallowing, foul breath, diminished or absent bowel sounds, urinary retention, tachycardia, hyperthermia, hypertension, and increased respiratory rate. Anticholinergic toxicity is caused by strong binding of the drug to cholinergic receptors. Anticholinesterase inhibitors reduce acetylcholinesterase, the enzyme that breaks down acetylcholine and thereby allows acetylcholine to accumulate and compete for receptor binding with the offending anticholinergic. For anticholinergic overdose with severe life-threatening symptoms, physostigmine 1-2 mg SubQ or slow I.V. may be given to reverse these effects.

Drug Interactions
  Amantadine: Additive adverse effects may occur due to cholinergic blockade.
  Antacids: Antacids may decrease absorption of hyoscyamine; administer hyoscyamine before meals and give antacids after meals.
  Antihistamines: Additive adverse effects may occur with some antihistamines due to cholinergic blockade.
  Antimuscarinics: Additive adverse effects may occur due to cholinergic blockade.
  Haloperidol: Additive adverse effects may occur due to cholinergic blockade.
  MAO inhibitors: Additive adverse effects may occur due to cholinergic blockade.
  Phenothiazines: Additive adverse effects may occur due to cholinergic blockade.
  Tricyclic antidepressants: Additive adverse effects may occur due to cholinergic blockade.

Stability Store at controlled room temperature. Protect NuLev™ from moisture.

Mechanism of Action Blocks the action of acetylcholine at parasympathetic sites in smooth muscle, secretory glands and the CNS; increases cardiac output, dries secretions, antagonizes histamine and serotonin

Pharmacodynamics
  Onset of action: Within 2-3 minutes
  Duration: 4-6 hours

Pharmacokinetics
  Absorption: Well absorbed
  Protein binding: 50%
  (Continued)

Hyoscyamine *(Continued)*

Metabolism: In the liver
Half-life: 2-3.5 hours
    Capsule, extended release: 6 hours
    Tablet, extended release: 7.47 hours
Elimination: In urine

Dosage
Geriatrics & Adults:
Gastrointestinal spasms:
Oral or S.L.: 0.125-0.25 mg every 4 hours or as needed (before meals or food); maximum: 1.5 mg/24 hours
    Product-specific dosing: Cystospaz®: 0.15-0.3 mg up to 4 times/day
Oral, timed release: 0.375-0.75 mg every 12 hours; maximum: 1.5 mg/24 hours
I.M., I.V., SubQ: 0.25-0.5 mg; may repeat as needed up to 4 times/day, at 4-hour intervals
Diagnostic procedures: I.V.: 0.25-0.5 mg given 5-10 minutes prior to procedure
Preanesthesia: I.V.: 5 mcg/kg given 30-60 minutes prior to induction of anesthesia or at the time preoperative narcotics or sedatives are administered
To reduce drug-induced bradycardia during surgery: I.V.: 0.125 mg; repeat as needed
Reverse neuromuscular blockade: I.V.: 0.2 mg for every 1 mg neostigmine (or the physostigmine/pyridostigmine equivalent)

Monitoring Parameters Pulse, anticholinergic effects, urine output, GI symptoms

Patient Information Take as directed before meals; do not increase dose and do not discontinue without consulting prescriber. Do not crush or chew extended release forms. Void before taking medication. You may experience dizziness or blurred vision (use caution when driving or engaging in tasks that require alertness until response to drug is known); dry mouth (sucking on lozenges may help); photosensitivity (wear dark glasses in bright sunlight); or impotence (temporary). Report chest pain or palpitations, or excessive and persistent anticholinergic effects (blurred vision, headache, flushing, tachycardia, nervousness, constipation, dizziness, insomnia, mental confusion or excitement, hyperthermia, dry mouth, altered taste perception, dysphagia, palpitations, bradycardia, urinary hesitancy or retention, impotence, decreased sweating).
Sublingual tablets: Place tablet under tongue and allow to dissolve.
Levbid® and Levsinex® may not completely disintegrate and may be excreted.
NuLev™ Orally disintegrating tablet: Tablet is placed on tongue and allowed to disintegrate before swallowing; may take with or without water.

Special Geriatric Considerations Avoid long-term use; the potential for toxic reactions is higher than the potential benefit; elderly are particularly prone to CNS side effects of anticholinergics (eg, confusion, delirium, hallucinations). Side effects often occur before clinical response is obtained.

Dosage Forms Excipient information presented when available (limited, particularly for generics); consult specific product labeling. [DSC] = Discontinued product
Capsule, timed release, as sulfate (Cystospaz-M® [DSC], Levsinex®): 0.375 mg
Elixir, as sulfate: 0.125 mg/5 mL (480 mL)
    Hyosine: 0.125 mg/5 mL (480 mL) [contains alcohol 20% and sodium benzoate; orange flavor]
    Levsin®: 0.125 mg/5 mL (480 mL) [contains alcohol 20%; orange flavor]
Injection, solution, as sulfate (Levsin®): 0.5 mg/mL (1 mL)
Liquid, as sulfate (Spacol [DSC]): 0.125 mg/5 mL (120 mL) [sugar free, alcohol free, simethicone based, bubble gum flavor]
Solution, oral drops, as sulfate: 0.125 mg/mL (15 mL)
    Hyosine: 0.125 mg/mL (15 mL) [contains alcohol 5% and sodium benzoate; orange flavor]
    Levsin®: 0.125 mg/mL (15 mL) [contains alcohol 5%; orange flavor]
Tablet (Cystospaz®): 0.15 mg
Tablet, as sulfate (Anaspaz®, Levsin®, Spacol [DSC]): 0.125 mg
Tablet, extended release, as sulfate (Levbid®, Symax SR, Spacol T/S [DSC]): 0.375 mg
Tablet, orally disintegrating, as sulfate (NuLev™): 0.125 mg [contains phenylalanine 1.7 mg/tablet, mint flavor]
Tablet, sublingual, as sulfate: 0.125 mg
    Levsin/SL®: 0.125 mg [peppermint flavor]
    Symax SL: 0.125 mg

Hyoscyamine, Atropine, Scopolamine, and Phenobarbital
(hye oh SYE a meen, A troe peen, skoe POL a meen, & fee noe BAR bi tal)

Related Information
Atropine *on page 137*
Hyoscyamine *on page 778*

Phenobarbital *on page 1243*
Scopolamine Derivatives *on page 1448*

Medication Safety Issues
Sound-alike/look-alike issues:
Donnatal® may be confused with Donnagel®

U.S. Brand Names Donnatal®; Donnatal Extentabs®

Index Terms Atropine, Hyoscyamine, Scopolamine, and Phenobarbital; Belladonna Alkaloids With Phenobarbital; Phenobarbital, Hyoscyamine, Atropine, and Scopolamine; Scopolamine, Hyoscyamine, Atropine, and Phenobarbital

Generic Available Yes: Tablet

Pharmacologic Category Anticholinergic Agent; Antispasmodic Agent, Gastrointestinal

Use Adjunct in treatment of irritable bowel syndrome, acute enterocolitis, duodenal ulcer

Contraindications Hypersensitivity to hyoscyamine, atropine, scopolamine, phenobarbital, or any component of the formulation; narrow-angle glaucoma; tachycardia; GI and GU obstruction; myasthenia gravis; paralytic ileus; intestinal atony; unstable cardiovascular status in acute hemorrhage; severe ulcerative colitis; hiatal hernia associated with reflux esophagitis; acute intermittent porphyria

Warnings/Precautions Use with caution in patients with hepatic or renal disease, hyperthyroidism, cardiovascular disease, CHF, hypertension, autonomic neuropathy. Use caution with diarrhea; may be an early symptom of incomplete intestinal obstruction. May causes sedation or blurred vision, caution must be used in performing tasks which require alertness (eg, operating machinery or driving). Due to the phenobarbital component, a potential for drug dependency exists, abrupt cessation may precipitate withdrawal, including status epilepticus in epileptic patients. Use caution in the elderly, may be more sensitive to adverse reactions.

Adverse Reactions (Reflective of adult population; not specific for elderly)
Frequency not defined.
Cardiovascular: Palpitation, tachycardia
Central nervous system: Dizziness, drowsiness, headache, insomnia, nervousness
Dermatologic: Urticaria
Gastrointestinal: Bloating, constipation, nausea, taste loss, vomiting, xerostomia
Genitourinary: Impotence, urinary hesitancy, urinary retention
Neuromuscular & skeletal: Musculoskeletal pain, weakness
Ocular: Blurred vision, cycloplegia, mydriasis, ocular tension increased
Miscellaneous: Allergic reaction (may be severe), anaphylaxis, lactation suppressed, diaphoresis decreased

Overdosage/Toxicology Symptoms include unsteady gait, slurred speech, confusion, hypotension, respiratory collapse, dilated unreactive pupils, hot or flushed skin, diminished bowel sounds, and urinary retention. Anticholinergic toxicity is caused by strong binding of the drug to cholinergic receptors. Anticholinesterase inhibitors reduce acetylcholinesterase, the enzyme that breaks down acetylcholine and thereby allows acetylcholine to accumulate and compete for receptor binding with the offending anticholinergic. For anticholinergic overdose with severe life-threatening symptoms, physostigmine 1-2 mg SubQ or slow I.V. may be given to reverse these effects.

Drug Interactions Phenobarbital: **Substrate** (minor) of CYP2C8/9, 2C19, 2E1; **Induces** CYP1A2 (strong), 2A6 (strong), 2B6 (strong), 2C8/9 (strong), 3A4 (strong)
Increased toxicity: CNS depressants, coumarin anticoagulants, amantadine, antihistamine, phenothiazines, antidiarrheal suspensions, corticosteroids, digitalis, griseofulvin, tetracyclines, anticonvulsants, MAO inhibitors, tricyclic antidepressants
CYP1A2 substrates: Phenobarbital may decrease the levels/effects of CYP1A2 substrates. Example substrates include aminophylline, estrogens, fluvoxamine, mirtazapine, ropinirole, and theophylline.
CYP2A6 substrates: Phenobarbital may decrease the levels/effects of CYP2A6 substrates. Example substrates include ifosfamide and rifampin.
CYP2B6 substrates: Phenobarbital may decrease the levels/effects of CYP2B6 substrates. Example substrates include bupropion, efavirenz, promethazine, selegiline, and sertraline.
CYP2C8/9 substrates: Phenobarbital may decrease the levels/effects of CYP2C8/9 substrates. Example substrates include amiodarone, fluoxetine, glimepiride, glipizide, losartan, nateglinide, phenytoin, pioglitazone, rosiglitazone, sertraline, sulfonamides, warfarin, and zafirlukast.
CYP3A4 substrates: Phenobarbital may decrease the levels/effects of CYP3A4 substrates. Example substrates include benzodiazepines, calcium channel blockers, clarithromycin, cyclosporine, erythromycin, estrogens, mirtazapine, nateglinide, nefazodone, nevirapine, protease inhibitors, tacrolimus, and venlafaxine

Mechanism of Action A fixed combination of belladonna alkaloids and phenobarbital which provides anticholinergic/antispasmodic action and mild sedation.

Pharmacokinetics Absorption: Well absorbed from GI tract
(Continued)

Hyoscyamine, Atropine, Scopolamine, and Phenobarbital
(Continued)

Dosage

Geriatrics & Adults: Spasmolytic: Oral:

Donnatal®: 1-2 tablets or 5-10 mL of elixir 3-4 times/day

Donnatal Extentabs®: 1 tablet every 12 hours; may increase to 1 tablet every 8 hours if needed

Patient Information Maintain good oral hygiene habits, because lack of saliva may increase chance of cavities. Observe caution while driving or performing other tasks requiring alertness, as may cause drowsiness, dizziness, or blurred vision. Notify physician if skin rash, flushing or eye pain occurs; or if difficulty in urinating, constipation or sensitivity to light becomes severe or persists. Do not attempt tasks requiring mental alertness or physical coordination until you know the effects of the drug. Swallow extended release tablet whole, do not crush or chew.

Special Geriatric Considerations Because of the anticholinergic effects of this product, it is not recommended for use in the elderly.

Dosage Forms Excipient information presented when available (limited, particularly for generics); consult specific product labeling.

Elixir:

Donnatal®: Hyoscyamine sulfate 0.1037 mg, atropine sulfate 0.0194 mg, scopolamine hydrobromide 0.0065 mg, and phenobarbital 16.2 mg per 5 mL (120 mL, 480 mL) [contains alcohol 95%; grape flavor]

Tablet: Hyoscyamine sulfate 0.1037 mg, atropine sulfate 0.0194 mg, scopolamine hydrobromide 0.0065 mg, and phenobarbital 16.2 mg

Donnatal®: Hyoscyamine sulfate 0.1037 mg, atropine sulfate 0.0194 mg, scopolamine hydrobromide 0.0065 mg, and phenobarbital 16.2 mg

Tablet, extended release:

Donnatal Extentabs®: Hyoscyamine sulfate 0.3111 mg, atropine sulfate 0.0582 mg, scopolamine hydrobromide 0.0195 mg, and phenobarbital 48.6 mg

♦ **Hyoscyamine Sulfate** *see* Hyoscyamine *on page 778*

♦ **Hyosine** *see* Hyoscyamine *on page 778*

♦ **HyperHEP B™ S/D** *see* Hepatitis B Immune Globulin *on page 748*

♦ **HyperRAB™ S/D** *see* Rabies Immune Globulin (Human) *on page 1371*

♦ **HyperTET™ S/D** *see* Tetanus Immune Globulin (Human) *on page 1541*

♦ **HypoTears [OTC]** *see* Artificial Tears *on page 124*

♦ **HypoTears® Ophthalmic Ointment [OTC]** *see* Ocular Lubricant *on page 1144*

♦ **HypoTears PF [OTC]** *see* Artificial Tears *on page 124*

♦ **Hytakerol® [DSC]** *see* Dihydrotachysterol *on page 439*

♦ **Hytone®** *see* Hydrocortisone *on page 762*

♦ **Hytrin® [DSC]** *see* Terazosin *on page 1530*

♦ **Hyzaar®** *see* Losartan and Hydrochlorothiazide *on page 934*

Ibandronate (eye BAN droh nate)

Related Information

Osteoporosis Management *on page 1779*

U.S. Brand Names Boniva®

Canadian Brand Names Bondronat®

Index Terms Ibandronate Sodium; Ibandronic Acid; NSC-722623

Generic Available No

Pharmacologic Category Bisphosphonate Derivative

Use Treatment and prevention of osteoporosis in postmenopausal females

Unlabeled/Investigational Use Hypercalcemia of malignancy; corticosteroid-induced osteoporosis; Paget's disease; reduce bone pain and skeletal complications from metastatic bone disease

Contraindications Hypersensitivity to ibandronate, other bisphosphonates, or any component of the formulation; hypocalcemia; oral tablets are also contraindicated in patients unable to stand or sit upright for at least 60 minutes

Warnings/Precautions Hypocalcemia must be corrected before therapy initiation. Ensure adequate calcium and vitamin D intake. Bisphosphonate therapy has been associated with osteonecrosis, primarily of the jaw; this has been observed mostly in cancer patients, but also in patients with postmenopausal osteoporosis and other diagnoses. Dental exams and preventative dentistry should be performed prior to placing patients with risk factors on chronic bisphosphonate therapy. Invasive dental procedures should be avoided during treatment.

Infrequently, severe (and occasionally debilitating) bone, joint, and/or muscle pain have been reported during bisphosphonate treatment. The onset of pain ranged from a single day to several months. Symptoms usually resolve upon discontinuation. Some patients experienced recurrence when rechallenged with same drug or another bisphosphonate; avoid use in patients with a history of these symptoms in association with bisphosphonate therapy.

Oral bisphosphonates may cause dysphagia, esophagitis, esophageal or gastric ulcer; risk may increase in patients unable to comply with dosing instructions. Intravenous bisphosphonates may cause transient decreases in serum calcium and have also been associated with renal toxicity.

Use not recommended with severe renal impairment (Cl_{cr} <30 mL/minute or serum creatinine >2.3 mg/dL).

Adverse Reactions (Reflective of adult population; not specific for elderly)
Percentages vary based on frequency of administration (daily vs monthly). Unless specified, percentages are reported with oral use.
>10%:
  Gastrointestinal: Dyspepsia (6% to 12%)
  Neuromuscular & skeletal: Back pain (4% to 14%)
1% to 10%:
  Central nervous system: Headache (3% to 7%), dizziness (1% to 4%), insomnia (1% to 2%)
  Dermatologic: Rash (1% to 2%)
  Endocrine & metabolic: Hypercholesterolemia (5%)
  Gastrointestinal: Abdominal pain (5% to 8%), diarrhea (4% to 7%), nausea (5%), tooth disorder (4%), vomiting (3%), constipation (3% to 4%)
  Genitourinary: Urinary tract infection (2% to 6%)
  Hepatic: Alkaline phosphatase decreased (frequency not defined)
  Local: Injection site reaction (<2%)
  Neuromuscular & skeletal: Pain in extremity (8%), myalgia (1% to 6%), joint disorder (4%), weakness (4%), muscle cramp (2%)
  Respiratory: Bronchitis (3% to 10%), pneumonia (6%), pharyngitis/nasopharyngitis (3% to 4%), upper respiratory infection (2%)
  Miscellaneous: Acute phase reaction (I.V. 10%; oral 4%), allergic reaction (3%), flu-like syndrome (1% to 3%)

Overdosage/Toxicology Dyspepsia, esophagitis, gastritis, ulcer, hypocalcemia, hypophosphatemia, hypomagnesemia, or upset stomach may be seen with overdose. Milk or antacids may be used to bind ibandronate. Patient should remain fully upright, and vomiting should not be induced to avoid esophageal irritation. Following overdose with I.V. formulation, dialysis may be of benefit if administered within 2 hours of overdose.

Drug Interactions
  Aminoglycosides: May lower serum calcium levels with prolonged administration. Concomitant use may have an additive hypocalcemic effect.
  Antacids: May decrease the absorption of bisphosphonate derivatives; should be administered at a different time of the day. Antacids containing aluminum, calcium, or magnesium are of specific concern.
  Calcium salts: May decrease the absorption of ibandronate. Separate oral dosing in order to minimize risk of interaction.
  Iron salts: May decrease the absorption of bisphosphonate derivatives. Only oral iron salts and oral bisphosphonates are of concern.
  Magnesium salts: May decrease the absorption of bisphosphonate derivatives. Only oral magnesium salts and oral bisphosphonates are of concern.
  Nonsteroidal anti-inflammatory drugs (NSAIDs): May enhance the gastrointestinal adverse/toxic effects (increased incidence of GI ulcers) of bisphosphonate derivatives.
  Phosphate supplements: Bisphosphonate derivatives may enhance the hypocalcemic effect of phosphate supplements.

Ethanol/Nutrition/Herb Interactions
  Ethanol: Avoid ethanol (may increase risk of osteoporosis).
  Food: May reduce absorption; mean oral bioavailability is decreased up to 90% when given with food.

Stability Store at controlled room temperature of 15°C to 30°C (59°F to 86°F).

Mechanism of Action A bisphosphonate which inhibits bone resorption via actions on osteoclasts or on osteoclast precursors; decreases the rate of bone resorption, leading to an indirect increase in bone mineral density.

Pharmacokinetics
  Distribution: Terminal V_d: 90 L; 40% to 50% of circulating ibandronate binds to bone
  Protein binding: 85% to 99%
  Bioavailability: Oral: Reduced by 90% following standard breakfast
  Half-life elimination:
    Oral: 150 mg dose: Terminal: 37-157 hours
    I.V.: Terminal: ~5-25 hours
  Time to peak, plasma: Oral: 0.5-2 hours
(Continued)

Ibandronate *(Continued)*

Excretion: Urine (50% to 60% of absorbed dose, excreted as unchanged drug); feces (unabsorbed drug)

Dosage

Geriatrics & Adults:

Treatment of postmenopausal osteoporosis:
Oral: 2.5 mg/day or 150 mg once a month
I.V.: 3 mg every 3 months

Prevention of postmenopausal osteoporosis: Oral: 2.5 mg/day; 150 mg once a month may be considered

Hypercalcemia of malignancy (unlabeled use): I.V.: 2-4 mg over 2 hours

Metastatic bone disease (unlabeled use):
Oral: 50 mg once daily
I.V.: 6 mg over 1 hour every 3-4 weeks

Renal Impairment:

Mild or moderate impairment: Dosing adjustment not needed.

Severe impairment (Cl_{cr} <30 mL/minute): Use not recommended.

Dosage adjustment in renal impairment for oncologic uses (unlabeled): Severe impairment (Cl_{cr} <30 mL/minute):
Oral: 50 mg once weekly
I.V.: 2 mg over 1 hour every 3-4 weeks

Hepatic Impairment: Dosing adjustment not needed.

Administration

Oral: Should be administered 60 minutes before the first food or drink of the day (other than water). Ibandronate should be taken in an upright position with a full glass (6-8 oz) of plain water and the patient should avoid lying down for 60 minutes to minimize the possibility of GI side effects. Mineral water with a high calcium content should be avoided. The tablet should be swallowed whole; do not chew or suck.

Once-monthly dosing: The 150 mg tablet should be taken on the same date each month. In case of a missed dose, do not take two 150 mg tablets within the same week. If the next scheduled dose is 1-7 days away, wait until the next scheduled dose to take the tablet. If the next scheduled dose is >7 days away, take the dose the morning it is remembered, and then resume taking the once-monthly dose on the originally scheduled day.

I.V.: Administer as a 15-30 second bolus. Do not mix with calcium-containing solutions or other drugs. For osteoporosis, do not administer more frequently than every 3 months. Infuse over 1 hour for metastatic bone disease and over 2 hours for hypercalcemia of malignancy.

Monitoring Parameters Bone mineral density; serum creatinine prior to each I.V. dose

Test Interactions Bisphosphonates may interfere with diagnostic imaging agents such as technetium-99m-diphosphonate in bone scans.

Special Geriatric Considerations Studies with elderly found no difference between younger adults and the elderly. No special dosage changes are necessary.

Dosage Forms Excipient information presented when available (limited, particularly for generics); consult specific product labeling.

Injection, solution: 1 mg/mL (3 mL) [prefilled syringe]

Tablet: 2.5 mg [once-daily formulation]; 150 mg [once-monthly formulation]

Selected References

Barrett J, Worth E, Bauss F, et al, "Ibandronate: A Clinical Pharmacological and Pharmacokinetic Update," *J Clin Pharmacol*, 2004, 44(9):951-65.

McCormack PL and Plosker GL, "Ibandronic Acid: A Review of Its Use in the Treatment of Bone Metastases of Breast Cancer," *Drugs*, 2006, 66(5):711-28.

Ruggiero SL, Mehrotra B, Rosenberg TJ, et al, "Osteonecrosis of the Jaws Associated With the Use of Bisphosphonates: A Review of 63 Cases," *J Oral Maxillofac Surg*, 2004, 62(5):527-34.

Tripathy D, Body JJ, and Bergstrom B, "Review of Ibandronate in the Treatment of Metastatic Bone Disease: Experience From Phase III Trials," *Clin Ther*, 2004, 26(12):1947-59.

Von Moos R, "Bisphosphonate Treatment Recommendations for Oncologists," *Oncologist*, 2005, 10(Suppl 1):19-24.

♦ **Ibandronate Sodium** *see* Ibandronate *on page 782*

♦ **Ibandronic Acid** *see* Ibandronate *on page 782*

♦ **Ibidomide Hydrochloride** *see* Labetalol *on page 864*

♦ **Ibu-200 [OTC]** *see* Ibuprofen *on page 784*

Ibuprofen *(eye byoo PROE fen)*

Medication Safety Issues

Sound-alike/look-alike issues:

Haltran® may be confused with Halfprin®

U.S. Brand Names Advil® [OTC]; Advil® Children's [OTC]; Advil® Infants' [OTC]; Advil® Junior [OTC]; Advil® Migraine [OTC]; ElixSure™ IB [OTC]; Genpril® [OTC]; Ibu-200 [OTC]; I-Prin [OTC]; Midol® Cramp and Body Aches [OTC]; Motrin®; Motrin® Children's

[OTC]; Motrin® IB [OTC]; Motrin® Infants' [OTC]; Motrin® Junior Strength [OTC]; Proprinal [OTC]; Ultraprin [OTC]

Canadian Brand Names Advil®; Apo-Ibuprofen®; Motrin® (Children's); Motrin® IB; Novo-Profen; Nu-Ibuprofen

Index Terms *p*-Isobutylhydratropic Acid

Generic Available Yes: Caplet, suspension, tablet

Pharmacologic Category Nonsteroidal Anti-inflammatory Drug (NSAID), Oral

Use Treatment of inflammatory diseases and rheumatoid disorders including rheumatoid arthritis; temporary relief of mild to moderate pain, fever, gout, osteoarthritis, sunburn, ankylosing spondylitis, acute migraine headache

Unlabeled/Investigational Use Treatment of cystic fibrosis

Restrictions An FDA-approved medication guide must be distributed when dispensing an oral outpatient prescription (new or refill) where this medication is to be used without direct supervision of a healthcare provider. Medication guides are available at http://www.fda.gov/cder/Offices/ODS/medication_guides.htm.

Contraindications Hypersensitivity to ibuprofen, aspirin, other NSAIDs, or any component of the formulation; perioperative pain in the setting of coronary artery bypass surgery (CABG)

Warnings/Precautions [U.S. Boxed Warning]: NSAIDs are associated with an increased risk of adverse cardiovascular events, including MI, stroke, and new onset or worsening of pre-existing hypertension. Risk may be increased with duration of use or pre-existing cardiovascular risk factors or disease. Carefully evaluate individual cardiovascular risk profiles prior to prescribing. Use caution with fluid retention, CHF or hypertension. Concurrent administration of ibuprofen, and potentially other nonselective NSAIDs, may interfere with aspirin's cardioprotective effect.

Use of NSAIDs can compromise existing renal function. Renal toxicity can occur in patient with impaired renal function, dehydration, heart failure, liver dysfunction, those taking diuretics and ACEI and the elderly. Rehydrate patient before starting therapy. Monitor renal function closely. Ibuprofen is not recommended for patients with advanced renal disease.

NSAIDs may increase risk of gastrointestinal irritation, ulceration, bleeding, and perforation. These events may occur at any time during therapy and without warning. Use caution with a history of GI disease (bleeding or ulcers), concurrent therapy with aspirin, anticoagulants and/or corticosteroids, smoking, use of alcohol, the elderly or debilitated patients.

Use the lowest effective dose for the shortest duration of time, consistent with individual patient goals, to reduce risk of cardiovascular or GI adverse events. Alternate therapies should be considered for patients at high risk.

NSAIDs may cause serious skin adverse events including exfoliative dermatitis, Stevens-Johnson syndrome (SJS) and toxic epidermal necrolysis (TEN). Anaphylactoid reactions may occur, even without prior exposure; patients with "aspirin triad" (bronchial asthma, aspirin intolerance, rhinitis) may be at increased risk. Do not use in patients who experience bronchospasm, asthma, rhinitis, or urticaria with NSAID or aspirin therapy. Use caution in other forms of asthma.

Use with caution in patients with decreased hepatic function. Closely monitor patients with any abnormal LFT. Severe hepatic reactions (eg, fulminant hepatitis, liver failure) have occurred with NSAID use, rarely; discontinue if signs or symptoms of liver disease develop, or if systemic manifestations occur.

The elderly are at increased risk for adverse effects (especially peptic ulceration, CNS effects, renal toxicity) from NSAIDs even at low doses.

Withhold for at least 4-6 half-lives prior to surgical or dental procedures.

Injection: Hold second or third doses if urinary output is <0.6 mL/kg/hour. May alter signs of infection. May inhibit platelet aggregation; monitor for signs of bleeding. May displace bilirubin; use caution when total bilirubin is elevated. A second course of treatment, alternative pharmacologic therapy or surgery may be needed if the ductus arteriosus fails to close or reopens following the initial course of therapy.

OTC labeling: Prior to self-medication, patients should contact healthcare provider if they have had recurring stomach pain or upset, ulcers, bleeding problems, high blood pressure, heart or kidney disease, other serious medical problems, are currently taking a diuretic, or are ≥60 years of age. Recommended dosages should not be exceeded, due to an increased risk of GI bleeding. Consuming ≥3 alcoholic beverages/day or taking longer than recommended may increase the risk of GI bleeding.

Adverse Reactions (Reflective of adult population; not specific for elderly)
Oral:
1% to 10%:
  Cardiovascular: Edema (1% to 3%)
  Central nervous system: Dizziness (3% to 9%), headache (1% to 3%), nervousness (1% to 3%)
(Continued)

Ibuprofen *(Continued)*

Dermatologic: Itching (1% to 3%), rash (3% to 9%)

Endocrine & metabolic: Fluid retention (1% to 3%)

Gastrointestinal: Dyspepsia (1% to 3%), vomiting (1% to 3%), abdominal pain/cramps/distress (1% to 3%), heartburn (3% to 9%), nausea (3% to 9%), diarrhea (1% to 3%), constipation (1% to 3%), flatulence (1% to 3%), epigastric pain (3% to 9%), appetite decreased (1% to 3%)

Otic: Tinnitus (3% to 9%)

Injection:

>10%:

Cardiovascular: Intraventricular hemorrhage (29%; grade 3/4: 15%)

Dermatologic: Skin irritation (16%)

Endocrine & metabolic: Hypocalcemia (12%), hypoglycemia (12%)

Gastrointestinal: GI disorders, non NEC (22%)

Hematologic: Anemia (32%)

Respiratory: Apnea (28%), respiratory infection (19%)

Miscellaneous: Sepsis (43%)

1% to 10%:

Cardiovascular: Edema (4%)

Endocrine & metabolic: Adrenal insufficiency (7%), hypernatremia (7%)

Genitourinary: Urinary tract infection (9%)

Renal: Urea increased (7%), renal impairment (6%), creatinine increased (3%), urine output decreased (3%; small decrease reported on days 2-6 with compensatory increase in output on day 9)

Respiratory: Respiratory failure (10%), atelectasis (4%)

Frequency not defined: Abdominal distension, cardiac failure, cholestasis, convulsions, feeding problems, gastritis, GI reflux, hyperglycemia, hypotension, ileus, infection, inguinal hernia, injection-site reaction, jaundice, neutropenia, tachycardia, thrombocytopenia

Overdosage/Toxicology Symptoms include apnea, metabolic acidosis, coma, and nystagmus; leukocytosis, renal failure. Management of nonsteroidal anti-inflammatory drug (NSAID) intoxication is primarily supportive and symptomatic. Fluid therapy is commonly effective in managing hypotension that may occur following an acute NSAID overdose, except when due to acute blood loss. Seizures tend to be very short-lived and often do not require drug treatment, although recurrent seizures should be treated with I.V. diazepam. Since many of NSAIDs undergo enterohepatic cycling, multiple doses of charcoal may be needed to reduce the potential for delayed toxicities.

Drug Interactions Substrate (minor) of CYP2C9, 2C19; **Inhibits** CYP2C9 (strong)

ACE inhibitors: Antihypertensive effects may be decreased by concurrent therapy with NSAIDs; monitor blood pressure.

Aminoglycosides: NSAIDs may decrease the excretion of aminoglycosides.

Angiotensin II antagonists: Antihypertensive effects may be decreased by concurrent therapy with NSAIDs; monitor blood pressure.

Anticoagulants (warfarin, heparin, LMWHs) in combination with NSAIDs can cause increased risk of bleeding.

Antiplatelet drugs (ticlopidine, clopidogrel, aspirin, abciximab, dipyridamole, eptifibatide, tirofiban) can cause an increased risk of bleeding.

Aspirin: Ibuprofen and other COX-1 inhibitors may reduce the cardioprotective effects of aspirin. Avoid giving prior to aspirin therapy or on a regular basis in patients with CAD.

Beta-blockers: NSAIDs may decrease the antihypertensive effect of beta-blockers. Monitor.

Bisphosphonate derivatives: NSAIDs may enhance the adverse/toxic effect of bisphosphonate derivatives. An increased incidence of gastrointestinal ulceration is of concern.

Cholestyramine (and other bile acid sequestrants): May decrease the absorption of NSAIDs. Separate by at least 2 hours.

Corticosteroids: May increase the risk of GI ulceration; avoid concurrent use

Cyclosporine: NSAIDs may increase serum creatinine, potassium, blood pressure, and cyclosporine levels; monitor cyclosporine levels and renal function carefully.

CYP2C9 Substrates: Ibuprofen may increase the levels/effects of CYP2C9 substrates. Example substrates include bosentan, dapsone, fluoxetine, glimepiride, glipizide, losartan, montelukast, nateglinide, paclitaxel, phenytoin, warfarin, and zafirlukast.

Hydralazine's antihypertensive effect is decreased; avoid concurrent use

Lithium levels can be increased; avoid concurrent use if possible or monitor lithium levels and adjust dose. Sulindac may have the least effect. When NSAID is stopped, lithium will need adjustment again.

Loop diuretics efficacy (diuretic and antihypertensive effect) is reduced. Indomethacin reduces this efficacy, however, it may be anticipated with any NSAID.

Methotrexate: Severe bone marrow suppression, aplastic anemia, and GI toxicity have been reported with concomitant NSAID therapy. Avoid use during moderate or high-dose methotrexate (increased and prolonged methotrexate levels). NSAID use during low-dose treatment of rheumatoid arthritis has not been fully evaluated; extreme caution is warranted.

Pemetrexed: NSAIDs may decrease the excretion of pemetrexed.

Probenecid: Probenecid may increase the serum concentration of NSAIDs.

Vancomycin: NSAIDs may decrease the excretion of vancomycin.

Warfarin's INRs may be increased by piroxicam. Other NSAIDs may have the same effect depending on dose and duration. Monitor INR closely. Use the lowest dose of NSAIDs possible and for the briefest duration. May alter the anticoagulant effects of warfarin; concurrent use with other antiplatelet agents or anticoagulants may increase risk of bleeding.

Ethanol/Nutrition/Herb Interactions

Ethanol: Avoid ethanol (may enhance gastric mucosal irritation).

Food: Ibuprofen peak serum levels may be decreased if taken with food.

Herb/Nutraceutical: Avoid alfalfa, anise, bilberry, bladderwrack, bromelain, cat's claw, celery, coleus, cordyceps, dong quai, evening primrose, feverfew, fenugreek, garlic, ginger, ginkgo biloba, red clover, horse chestnut, grapeseed, green tea, ginseng, guggul, horse chestnut seed, horseradish, licorice, prickly ash, red clover, reishi, SAMe, sweet clover, turmeric, white willow (all have additional antiplatelet activity).

Stability

Suspension: Store at room temperature of 15°C to 30°C (59°F to 86°F).

Tablet: Store at room temperature of 20°C to 25°C (68°F to 77°F).

Mechanism of Action Inhibits prostaglandin synthesis by decreasing the activity of the enzyme, cyclooxygenase, which results in decreased formation of prostaglandin precursors

Pharmacodynamics

Onset of action: Analgesic: 30-60 minutes; Anti-inflammatory: ≤7 days

Peak effect: 1-2 weeks

Duration: 4-6 hours

Pharmacokinetics

Absorption: Oral: Rapid (85%)

Protein binding: 90% to 99%

Metabolism: Hepatic via oxidation

Half-life elimination: Adults: 2-4 hours; End-stage renal disease: Unchanged

Time to peak: ~1-2 hours

Excretion: Urine (1% as free drug); some feces

Dosage

Geriatrics & Adults:

Inflammatory disease: Oral: 400-800 mg/dose 3-4 times/day (maximum: 3.2 g/day)

Analgesia/pain/fever/dysmenorrhea: Oral: 200-400 mg/dose every 4-6 hours (maximum daily dose: 1.2 g, unless directed by physician)

OTC labeling (analgesic, antipyretic): Oral: 200 mg every 4-6 hours as needed (maximum: 1200 mg/24 hours)

Hepatic Impairment: Avoid use in severe hepatic impairment.

Administration Administer with food

Monitoring Parameters Monitor response (pain, range of motion, grip strength, mobility, ADL function), inflammation; observe for weight gain, edema; monitor renal function; observe for bleeding, bruising; evaluate gastrointestinal effects (abdominal pain, bleeding, dyspepsia); mental confusion, disorientation, CBC, serum, creatinine, BUN, liver function tests

Reference Range Plasma concentrations >200 mcg/mL may be associated with severe toxicity

Patient Information Serious gastrointestinal bleeding can occur as well as ulceration and perforation. Pain may or may not be present. Avoid aspirin and aspirin-containing products while taking this medication. If gastric upset occurs, take with food, milk, or antacid. If gastric adverse effects persist, contact physician. May cause drowsiness, dizziness, blurred vision, and confusion. Use caution when performing tasks which require alertness (eg, driving). Do not take for more than 3 days for fever or 10 days for pain without physician's advice.

Additional Information There are no clinical guidelines to predict which NSAID will give response in a particular patient. Trials with each must be initiated until response determined. Consider dose, patient convenience, and cost.

Special Geriatric Considerations Elderly are a high-risk population for adverse effects from NSAIDs. As much as 60% of elderly can develop peptic ulceration and/or hemorrhage asymptomatically. The concomitant use of H_2 blockers and sucralfate is not effective as prophylaxis with the exception of NSAID-induced duodenal ulcers which may be prevented by the use of ranitidine. Misoprostol and proton pump inhibitors are the only agents proven to help prevent the development of NSAID-induced ulcers. Also, concomitant disease and drug use contribute to the risk for GI adverse effects. Use lowest effective dose for shortest period possible. Consider renal function decline with age. Use of NSAIDs can compromise existing renal function especially (Continued)

Ibuprofen *(Continued)*

when Cl$_{cr}$ is ≤30 mL/minute. Tinnitus may be a difficult and unreliable indication of toxicity due to age-related hearing loss or eighth cranial nerve damage. CNS adverse effects such as confusion, agitation, and hallucination are generally seen in overdose or high dose situations, but the elderly may demonstrate these adverse effects at lower doses than younger adults.

Dosage Forms

Caplet: 200 mg [OTC]
  Advil®: 200 mg [contains sodium benzoate]
  Ibu-200, Motrin® IB: 200 mg
  Motrin® Junior Strength: 100 mg
Capsule, liqui-gel:
  Advil®: 200 mg
  Advil® Migraine: 200 mg [solubilized ibuprofen; contains potassium 20 mg]
Gelcap:
  Advil®: 200 mg [contains coconut oil]
Suspension, oral: 100 mg/5 mL (5 mL, 120 mL, 480 mL)
  Advil® Children's: 100 mg/5 mL (60 mL, 120 mL) [contains sodium benzoate; blue raspberry, fruit, and grape flavors]
  ElixSure™ IB: 100 mg/5 mL (120 mL) [berry flavor]
  Motrin® Children's: 100 mg/5 mL (60 mL, 120 mL) [contains sodium benzoate; berry, dye free berry, bubble gum, and grape flavors]
Suspension, oral drops: 40 mg/mL (15 mL)
  Advil' Infants': 40 mg/mL (15 mL) [contains sodium benzoate; fruit and grape flavors]
  Motrin® Infants': 40 mg/mL (15 mL, 30 mL) [contains sodium benzoate; berry and dye-free berry flavors]
Tablet: 200 mg [OTC], 400 mg, 600 mg, 800 mg
  Advil®: 200 mg [contains sodium benzoate]
  Advil® Junior: 100 mg [contains sodium benzoate; coated tablets]
  Genpril®, I-Prin, Midol® Cramp and Body Aches, Motrin® IB, Proprinal, Ultraprin: 200 mg
  Motrin®: 400 mg, 600 mg, 800 mg
Tablet, chewable:
  Advil® Children's: 50 mg [contains phenylalanine 2.1 mg; grape flavors]
  Advil® Junior: 100 mg [contains phenylalanine 4.2 mg; grape flavors]
  Motrin® Children's: 50 mg [contains phenylalanine 1.4 mg; grape and orange flavor]
  Motrin® Junior Strength: 100 mg [contains phenylalanine 2.1 mg; grape and orange flavors]

Selected References
Brooks PM and Day RO, "Nonsteroidal Anti-inflammatory Drugs - Differences and Similarities," *N Engl J Med*, 1991, 324(24):1716-25.

Clinch D, Banerjee AK, and Ostick G, "Absence of Abdominal Pain in Elderly Patients With Peptic Ulcer," *Age Ageing*, 1984, 13(2):120-3.

Clive DM and Stoff JS, "Renal Syndromes Associated With Nonsteroidal Anti-inflammatory Drugs," *N Engl J Med*, 1984, 310(9):563-72.

Graham DY, "Prevention of Gastroduodenal Injury Induced by Chronic Nonsteroidal Anti-inflammatory Drug Therapy," *Gastroenterology*, 1989, 96(2 Pt 2 Suppl):675-81.

Gurwitz JH, Avorn J, Ross-Degnan D, et al, "Nonsteroidal Anti-Inflammatory Drug-Associated Azotemia in the Very Old," *JAMA*, 1990, 264(4):471-5.

Hawkey CJ, Karrasch JA, Szczepański L, et al, "Omeprazole Compared With Misoprostol for Ulcers Associated With Nonsteroidal Anti-inflammatory Drugs," *N Engl J Med*, 1998, 338(11):727-34.

Knodel LC, "Preventing NSAID-induced Ulcers: The Role of Misoprostol," *Consult Pharm*, 1989, 4:37-41.

Pounder R, "Silent Peptic Ulceration: Deadly Silence or Golden Silence?" *Gastroenterology*, 1989, 96:(2 Pt 2 Suppl)626-31.

Yeomans ND, Tulassay Z, Juhasz L, et al, "A Comparison of Omeprazole With Ranitidine for Ulcers Associated With Nonsteroidal Anti-inflammatory Drugs," *N Engl J Med*, 1998, 338(11):719-26.

Imipenem and Cilastatin (i mi PEN em & sye la STAT in)

Related Information
Antimicrobial Activity Against Selected Organisms *on page 1728*

Medication Safety Issues
Sound-alike/look-alike issues:
Primaxin® may be confused with Premarin®, Primacor®

U.S. Brand Names Primaxin®

Canadian Brand Names Primaxin®; Primaxin® I.V.

Index Terms Imipemide

Generic Available No

Pharmacologic Category Antibiotic, Carbapenem

Use Treatment of lower respiratory tract, urinary tract, intra-abdominal, gynecologic, bone and joint, skin and skin structure, and polymicrobic infections as well as bacterial septicemia and endocarditis. Antibacterial activity includes resistant gram-negative bacilli (*Pseudomonas aeruginosa* and *Enterobacter* sp), gram-positive bacteria (methicillin-sensitive *Staphylococcus aureus* and *Streptococcus* sp) and anaerobes.

Contraindications Hypersensitivity to imipenem/cilastatin or any component of the formulation; consult information on Lidocaine for contraindications associated with I.M. dosing

Warnings/Precautions Dosage adjustment required in patients with impaired renal function; elderly patients often require lower doses (adjust carefully to renal function). Prolonged use may result in fungal or bacterial superinfection, including *C. difficile*-associated diarrhea and pseudomembranous colitis. Has been associated with CNS adverse effects, including confusional states and seizures (myoclonic); use with caution in patients with a history of seizures or hypersensitivity to beta-lactams (including penicillins and cephalosporins); patients with impaired renal function are at increased risk of seizures if not properly dose adjusted. Serious hypersensitivity reactions, including anaphylaxis, have been reported (some without a history of previous allergic reactions to beta-lactams). Doses for I.M. administration are mixed with lidocaine; consult information on lidocaine for associated warnings/precautions. Two different imipenem/cilastatin products are available; due to differences in formulation, the I.V. and I.M. preparations **cannot** be interchanged.

Adverse Reactions (Reflective of adult population; not specific for elderly)
Adverse reactions reported with use for both I.V. and I.M. formulations in adults, except where noted.

1% to 10%:
Cardiovascular: Tachycardia (infants 2%; adults <1%)
Central nervous system: Seizure (infants 6%; adults <1%)
Dermatologic: Rash (≤1%, children 2%)
Gastrointestinal: Nausea (1% to 2%), diarrhea (children 3% to 4%; adults 1% to 2%), vomiting (≤2%)
Genitourinary: Oliguria/anuria (infants 2%; adults <1%)
Local: Phlebitis/thrombophlebitis (3%), pain at I.M. injection site (1.2%)

Overdosage/Toxicology Symptoms include neuromuscular hypersensitivity and seizures. Hemodialysis may be helpful to aid in removal of the drug from the blood, otherwise most treatment is supportive or symptom-directed.

Drug Interactions
Cyclosporine: May increase neurotoxicity of imipenem; conversely, imipenem may increase the serum levels/effects of cyclosporine; monitor.
Ganciclovir: May increase the risk of seizures; concomitant use not recommended.
Typhoid vaccine: Concomitant antibiotics may decrease the effectiveness of live, attenuated Ty21a typhoid vaccine; delay vaccination for >24 hours after administration of antibiotic.
Uricosuric agents: May increase the levels/effects imipenem; monitor.
Valproic acid: Imipenem may decrease valproic acid concentrations to subtherapeutic levels; monitor.

Stability Imipenem/cilastatin powder for injection should be stored at <25°C (77°F).
I.M.: Prepare 500 mg vial with 2 mL 1% lidocaine (do not use lidocaine with epinephrine). The I.V. formulation does not form a stable suspension in lidocaine and cannot be used to prepare an I.M dose. The I.M. suspension should be used within 1 hour of reconstitution.
I.V.: Prior to use, dilute dose into 100-250 mL of an appropriate solution. Imipenem is inactivated at acidic or alkaline pH. Final concentration should not exceed 5 mg/mL. The I.M. formulation is not buffered and cannot be used to prepare I.V. solutions. Reconstituted I.V. solutions are stable for 4 hours at room temperature and 24 hours when refrigerated. Do not freeze.

Mechanism of Action Inhibits bacterial cell wall synthesis by binding to one or more of the penicillin binding proteins (PBPs); which in turn inhibits the final transpeptidation
(Continued)

Imipenem and Cilastatin *(Continued)*

step of peptidoglycan synthesis in bacterial cell walls, thus inhibiting cell wall biosynthesis. Bacteria eventually lyse due to ongoing activity of cell wall autolytic enzymes (autolysins and murein hydrolases) while cell wall assembly is arrested. Cilastatin prevents renal metabolism of imipenem by competitive inhibition of dehydropeptidase along the brush border of the renal tubules.

Pharmacokinetics

Absorption: I.M.: Imipenem: 60% to 75%; cilastatin: 95% to 100%

Protein binding: Imipenem: 20%; cilastatin: 40%

Metabolism:
  Imipenem: Metabolized in the kidney by dehydropeptidase
  Cilastatin: Partially metabolized in the kidneys

Half-life elimination: I.V.: Both drugs: 60 minutes; prolonged with renal impairment;
  I.M.: Imipenem: 2-3 hours

Time to peak: I.M.: 3.5 hours

Elimination: When imipenem is given with cilastatin, urinary excretion of unchanged
  imipenem increases to 70%

Cilastatin: 70% to 80% of a dose is excreted unchanged in the urine

Half-life and V_d (L/kg) have been reported to be increased and decreased, respectively,
  in the older adult compared to younger adults

Dosage

Geriatrics & Adults: Doses based on **imipenem** content. **Note:** I.M. administration is not intended for severe or life-threatening infections (eg, septicemia, endocarditis, shock), UTI, bone/joint or polymicrobic infections. For adults weighing <70 kg, refer to Dosage: Renal Impairment:

Burkholderia mallei (melioidosis) (unlabeled use): I.V.: 20 mg/kg (up to 1 g) every
  6-8 hours for 10 days

Intra-abdominal infections:
  I.V.: Mild infection: 250-500 mg every 6 hours; severe: 500 mg every 6 hours
  I.M.: Mild-to-moderate infection: 750 mg every 12 hours

Liver abscess (unlabeled use): I.V.: 500 mg every 6 hours for 2-3 weeks, then
  appropriate oral therapy for a total of 4-6 weeks

Lower respiratory tract, skin/skin structure, gynecologic infections: I.M.: Mild/
  moderate: 500-750 mg every 12 hours

Moderate infections:
  I.M.: 750 mg every 12 hours
  I.V.:
    Fully-susceptible organisms: 500 mg every 6-8 hours
    Moderately-susceptible organisms: 500 mg every 6 hours or 1 g every 8 hours

Neutropenic fever (unlabeled use): I.V.: 500 mg every 6 hours

Pseudomonas infections: I.V.: 500 mg every 6 hours; **Note:** Higher doses may be
  required based on organism sensitivity.

Severe infections: I.V.: **Note:** I.M. administration is not intended for severe or
  life-threatening infections (eg, septicemia, endocarditis, shock):
    Fully-susceptible organisms: 500 mg every 6 hours
    Moderately-susceptible organisms: 1 g every 6-8 hours
    Maximum daily dose should not exceed 50 mg/kg or 4 g/day, whichever is lower

Urinary tract infection, uncomplicated: I.V.: 250 mg every 6 hours

Urinary tract infection, complicated: I.V.: 500 mg every 6 hours

Mild infections: Note: Rarely a suitable option in mild infections; normally reserved
  for moderate-severe cases:
    I.M.: 500 mg every 12 hours
    I.V.:
      Fully-susceptible organisms: 250 mg every 6 hours
      Moderately-susceptible organisms: 500 mg every 6 hours

Renal Impairment: I.V.: **Note:** Adjustments have not been established for I.M.
  dosing:
  Patients with a Cl_{cr} ≤5 mL/minute/1.73 m^2 should not receive imipenem/cilastatin
    unless hemodialysis is instituted within 48 hours.
  Patients weighing <30 kg with impaired renal function should not receive imipenem/
    cilastatin.
  Hemodialysis: Use the dosing recommendation for patients with a Cl_{cr} 6-20 mL/
    minute; administer dose after dialysis session and every 12 hours thereafter
  Peritoneal dialysis: Dose as for Cl_{cr} <10 mL/minute.
  Continuous arteriovenous or venovenous hemofiltration: Dose as for Cl_{cr} 20-30 mL/
    minute; monitor for seizure activity. Imipenem is well removed by CAVH but
    cilastatin is not; removes 20 mg of imipenem per liter of filtrate per day.

  See table on next page.

Administration Do not interchange I.M. and I.V. products
  I.M.: Prepare 500 mg vial with 2 mL 1% lidocaine; prepare 750 mg vial with 3 mL 1%
    lidocaine **(do not use lidocaine with epinephrine)**. Administer by deep injection

into a large muscle (gluteal or lateral thigh). Aspiration is necessary to avoid inadvertent injection into a blood vessel.

I.V.: Not for direct infusion; vial contents must be transferred to 100 mL of infusion solution; final concentration should not exceed 5 mg/mL; infuse each 250-500 mg dose over 20-30 minutes; infuse each 1 g dose over 40-60 minutes; watch for convulsions. If nausea and/or vomiting occur during administration, decrease the rate of I.V. infusion; do not mix with or physically add to other antibiotics; however, may administer concomitantly

Imipenem and Cilastatin Dosage in Renal Impairment

Reduced I.V. Dosage Regimen Based on Creatinine Clearance (mL/minute/1.73 m^2) and/or Body Weight <70 kg				
Body Weight (kg)				
≥70	60	50	40	30
Total daily dose for normal renal function: 1 g/day				
Cl$_{cr}$ ≥71	250 mg q6h	250 mg q8h	125 mg q6h	125 mg q6h	125 mg q8h
Cl$_{cr}$ 41-70	250 mg q8h	125 mg q6h	125 mg q6h	125 mg q8h	125 mg q8h
Cl$_{cr}$ 21-40	250 mg q12h	250 mg q12h	125 mg q8h	125 mg q12h	125 mg q12h
Cl$_{cr}$ 6-20	250 mg q12h	250 mg q12h	125 mg q12h	125 mg q12h	125 mg q12h
Total daily dose for normal renal function: 1.5 g/day				
Cl$_{cr}$ ≥71	500 mg q8h	250 mg q6h	250 mg q6h	250 mg q8h	125 mg q6h
Cl$_{cr}$ 41-70	250 mg q6h	250 mg q8h	250 mg q8h	125 mg q6h	125 mg q8h
Cl$_{cr}$ 21-40	250 mg q8h	250 mg q8h	250 mg q12h	125 mg q8h	125 mg q8h
Cl$_{cr}$ 6-20	250 mg q12h	250 mg q12h	250 mg q12h	125 mg q12h	125 mg q12h
Total daily dose for normal renal function: 2 g/day				
Cl$_{cr}$ ≥71	500 mg q6h	500 mg q8h	250 mg q6h	250 mg q8h	250 mg q8h
Cl$_{cr}$ 41-70	500 mg q8h	250 mg q6h	250 mg q6h	250 mg q8h	125 mg q6h
Cl$_{cr}$ 21-40	250 mg q6h	250 mg q8h	250 mg q8h	250 mg q8h	125 mg q8h
Cl$_{cr}$ 6-20	250 mg q12h	250 mg q12h	250 mg q12h	250 mg q12h	125 mg q12h
Total daily dose for normal renal function: 3 g/day				
Cl$_{cr}$ ≥71	1000 mg q8h	750 mg q8h	500 mg q6h	500 mg q8h	250 mg q6h
Cl$_{cr}$ 41-70	500 mg q6h	500 mg q8h	500 mg q8h	250 mg q6h	250 mg q8h
Cl$_{cr}$ 21-40	500 mg q8h	500 mg q8h	250 mg q6h	250 mg q8h	250 mg q8h
Cl$_{cr}$ 6-20	500 mg q12h	500 mg q12h	250 mg q8h	250 mg q12h	250 mg q12h
Total daily dose for normal renal function: 4 g/day				
Cl$_{cr}$ ≥71	1000 mg q6h	1000 mg q8h	750 mg q8h	500 mg q6h	500 mg q8h
Cl$_{cr}$ 41-70	750 mg q8h	750 mg q8h	500 mg q6h	500 mg q8h	250 mg q6h
Cl$_{cr}$ 21-40	500 mg q6h	500 mg q8h	500 mg q8h	250 mg q6h	250 mg q8h
Cl$_{cr}$ 6-20	500 mg q12h	500 mg q12h	500 mg q12h	250 mg q12h	250 mg q12h

Monitoring Parameters Signs and symptoms of infection; mental status, WBC, periodic renal, hepatic, and hematologic function tests

Test Interactions Interferes with urinary glucose determination using Clinitest®

Additional Information Sodium content of 1 g: 3.2 mEq

Special Geriatric Considerations Imipenem/cilastatin's role is limited to the treatment of infections caused by susceptible multiresistant organism(s) and in patients whose bacterial infection(s) have failed to respond to other appropriate antimicrobials; many of the seizures attributed to imipenem/cilastatin were in elderly patients; dose must be adjusted for creatinine clearance and body weight.

Dosage Forms Excipient information presented when available (limited, particularly for generics); consult specific product labeling.
(Continued)

Imipenem and Cilastatin *(Continued)*

Injection, powder for reconstitution [I.M.]:

Primaxin®: Imipenem 500 mg and cilastatin 500 mg [contains sodium 32 mg (1.4 mEq)]

Injection, powder for reconstitution [I.V.]:

Primaxin®: Imipenem 250 mg and cilastatin 250 mg [contains sodium 18.8 mg (0.8 mEq)]; imipenem 500 mg and cilastatin 500 mg [contains sodium 37.5 mg (1.6 mEq)]

Selected References

Finch RG, Craddock C, Kelly J, et al, "Pharmacokinetic Studies of Imipenem/Cilastatin in Elderly Patients," *J Antimicrob Chemother*, 1986, 18(Suppl E):103-7.

Toon S, Hopkins KJ, Garstang FM, et al, "Pharmacokinetics of Imipenem and Cilastatin After Their Simultaneous Administration to the Elderly," *Br J Clin Pharmacol*, 1987, 23(2):143-9.

Yoshikawa TT, "Antimicrobial Therapy for the Elderly Patient," *J Am Geriatr Soc*, 1990, 38(12):1353-72.

Imipramine *(im IP ra meen)*

Related Information

Antidepressant Agents *on page 1742*

Pharmacotherapy of Urinary Incontinence *on page 1822*

Serum Drug Concentrations Commonly Monitored Guidelines *on page 1862*

Medication Safety Issues

Sound-alike/look-alike issues:

Imipramine may be confused with amitriptyline, desipramine, Norpramin®

U.S. Brand Names Tofranil®; Tofranil-PM®

Canadian Brand Names Apo-Imipramine®; Novo-Pramine; Tofranil®

Index Terms Imipramine Hydrochloride; Imipramine Pamoate

Generic Available Yes

Pharmacologic Category Antidepressant, Tricyclic (Tertiary Amine)

Use Treatment of various forms of depression, often in conjunction with psychotherapy

Unlabeled/Investigational Use Analgesic for certain chronic and neuropathic pain; treatment of panic disorder, attention-deficit/hyperactivity disorder (ADHD)

Restrictions An FDA-approved medication guide concerning the use of antidepressants in children, adolescents, and young adults must be distributed when dispensing an outpatient prescription (new or refill) where this medication is to be used without direct supervision of a healthcare provider. Medication guides are available at http://www.fda.gov/cder/Offices/ODS/medication_guides.htm. Dispense to parents or guardians of children and adolescents receiving this medication.

Contraindications Hypersensitivity to imipramine (cross-reactivity with other dibenzodiazepines may occur) or any component of the formulation; concurrent use of MAO inhibitors (within 14 days); in a patient during acute recovery phase of MI

Warnings/Precautions [U.S. Boxed Warning]: Antidepressants increase the risk of suicidal thinking and behavior in children, adolescents, and young adults (18-24 years of age) with major depressive disorder (MDD) and other psychiatric disorders; consider risk prior to prescribing. Short-term studies did not show an increased risk in patients >24 years of age and showed a decreased risk in patients ≥65 years. Closely monitor for clinical worsening, suicidality, or unusual changes in behavior; the patient's family or caregiver should be instructed to closely observe the patient and communicate condition with healthcare provider. A medication guide should be dispensed with each prescription.

The possibility of a suicide attempt is inherent in major depression and may persist until remission occurs. Monitor for worsening of depression or suicidality, especially during initiation of therapy (generally first 1-2 months) or with dose increases or decreases. Use caution in high-risk patients. Worsening depression and severe abrupt suicidality that are not part of the presenting symptoms may require discontinuation or modification of drug therapy. The patient's family or caregiver should be alerted to monitor patients for the emergence of suicidality and associated behaviors (such as agitation, irritability, hostility, impulsivity, and hypomania) and notify healthcare provider.

May worsen psychosis in some patients or precipitate a shift to mania or hypomania in patients with bipolar disorder. Patients presenting with depressive symptoms should be screened for bipolar disorder. Monotherapy in patients with bipolar disorder should be avoided. **Imipramine is not FDA approved for the treatment of bipolar depression.**

The degree of sedation, anticholinergic effects, orthostasis, and conduction abnormalities are high relative to other antidepressants. Imipramine often causes drowsiness/sedation, resulting in impaired performance of tasks requiring alertness (eg, operating machinery or driving). Sedative effects may be additive with other CNS depressants and/or ethanol. Use with caution in patients with a history of cardiovascular disease (including previous MI, stroke, tachycardia, or conduction abnormalities). Use with caution in patients with urinary retention, benign prostatic hyperplasia, narrow-angle glaucoma, xerostomia, visual problems, constipation, or a history of bowel obstruction.

Consider discontinuing, when possible, prior to elective surgery. Therapy should not be abruptly discontinued in patients receiving high doses for prolonged periods. May lower seizure threshold - use caution in patients with a previous seizure disorder or condition predisposing to seizures such as brain damage, alcoholism, or concurrent therapy with other drugs which lower the seizure threshold. May increase the risks associated with electroconvulsive therapy. Use with caution in hyperthyroid patients or those receiving thyroid supplementation. Use with caution in patients with hepatic or renal dysfunction and in elderly patients. Has been associated with photosensitization.

Adverse Reactions (Reflective of adult population; not specific for elderly)
Frequency not defined.

Cardiovascular: Orthostatic hypotension, arrhythmia, tachycardia, hypertension, palpitation, MI, heart block, ECG changes, CHF, stroke

Central nervous system: Dizziness, drowsiness, headache, agitation, insomnia, nightmares, hypomania, psychosis, fatigue, confusion, hallucinations, disorientation, delusions, anxiety, restlessness, seizure

Endocrine & metabolic: Gynecomastia, breast enlargement, galactorrhea, increase or decrease in libido, increase or decrease in blood sugar, SIADH

Gastrointestinal: Nausea, unpleasant taste, weight gain, xerostomia, constipation, ileus, stomatitis, abdominal cramps, vomiting, anorexia, epigastric disorders, diarrhea, black tongue, weight loss

Genitourinary: Urinary retention, impotence

Neuromuscular & skeletal: Weakness, numbness, tingling, paresthesia, incoordination, ataxia, tremor, peripheral neuropathy, extrapyramidal symptoms

Ocular: Blurred vision, disturbances of accommodation, mydriasis

Otic: Tinnitus

Miscellaneous: Diaphoresis

Overdosage/Toxicology Symptoms include confusion, hallucinations, constipation, cyanosis, tachycardia, urinary retention, ventricular tachycardia, and seizures. Following initiation of essential overdose management, toxic symptoms should be treated. Sodium bicarbonate is indicated when the QRS interval is >0.10 seconds or the QT_c interval is >0.42 seconds. Ventricular arrhythmias often respond to concurrent systemic alkalinization (sodium bicarbonate 0.5-2 mEq/kg I.V.). Arrhythmias unresponsive to this therapy may respond to lidocaine 1 mg/kg I.V., followed by a titrated infusion. Physostigmine (1-2 mg slow I.V.) may be indicated in reversing life-threatening cardiac arrhythmias. Seizures usually respond to diazepam I.V. boluses (5-10 mg up to 30 mg). If seizures are unresponsive or recur, phenytoin or phenobarbital may be required.

Drug Interactions Substrate of CYP1A2 (minor), 2B6 (minor), 2C19 (major), 2D6 (major), 3A4 (minor); **Inhibits** CYP1A2 (weak), 2C19 (weak), 2D6 (moderate), 2E1 (weak)

Altretamine: Concurrent use may cause orthostatic hypertension

Amphetamines: TCAs may enhance the effect of amphetamines; monitor for adverse CV effects

Anticholinergics: Combined use with TCAs may produce additive anticholinergic effects

Antihypertensives: TCAs may inhibit the antihypertensive response to bethanidine, clonidine, debrisoquin, guanadrel, guanethidine, guanabenz, guanfacine; monitor BP; consider alternate antihypertensive agent

Beta-agonists: When combined with TCAs may predispose patients to cardiac arrhythmias

Bupropion: May increase the levels of tricyclic antidepressants; based on limited information; monitor response

Carbamazepine: Tricyclic antidepressants may increase carbamazepine levels; monitor

Cholestyramine and colestipol: May bind TCAs and reduce their absorption; monitor for altered response

Clonidine: Abrupt discontinuation of clonidine may cause hypertensive crisis, amitriptyline may enhance the response

CNS depressants: Amitriptyline may be additive with or may potentiate sedation; sedative effects may be additive with TCAs; monitor for increased effect; includes benzodiazepines, barbiturates, antipsychotics, ethanol, and other sedative medications

CYP2C19 inducers: May decrease the levels/effects of imipramine. Example inducers include aminoglutethimide, carbamazepine, phenytoin, and rifampin.

CYP2C19 inhibitors: May increase the levels/effects of imipramine. Example inhibitors include delavirdine, fluconazole, fluvoxamine, gemfibrozil, isoniazid, omeprazole, and ticlopidine.

CYP2D6 inhibitors: May increase the levels/effects of imipramine. Example inhibitors include chlorpromazine, delavirdine, fluoxetine, miconazole, paroxetine, pergolide, quinidine, quinine, ritonavir, and ropinirole.

(Continued)

Imipramine *(Continued)*

Epinephrine (and other direct alpha-agonists): The pressor response to I.V. epinephrine, norepinephrine, and phenylephrine may be enhanced in patients receiving TCAs; this combination is best avoided

Fenfluramine: May increase tricyclic antidepressant levels/effects

Hypoglycemic agents (including insulin): TCAs may enhance the hypoglycemic effects of tolazamide, chlorpropamide, or insulin; monitor for changes in blood glucose levels; reported with chlorpropamide, tolazamide, and insulin

Levodopa: Tricyclic antidepressants may decrease the absorption (bioavailability) of levodopa; rare hypertensive episodes have also been attributed to this combination

Linezolid: Hyperpyrexia, hypertension, tachycardia, confusion, seizures, and **deaths have been reported** with agents which inhibit MAO (serotonin syndrome); this combination should be avoided

Lithium: Concurrent use with a TCA may increase the risk for neurotoxicity

MAO inhibitors: Hyperpyrexia, hypertension, tachycardia, confusion, seizures, and **deaths have been reported** (serotonin syndrome); this combination should be avoided

Methylphenidate: Metabolism of TCAs may be decreased

Phenothiazines: Serum concentrations of some TCAs may be increased; in addition, TCAs may increase concentration of phenothiazines; monitor for altered clinical response

QT_c-prolonging agents: Concurrent use of tricyclic agents with other drugs which may prolong QT_c interval may increase the risk of potentially fatal arrhythmias; includes type Ia and type III antiarrhythmics agents, selected quinolones (moxifloxacin), cisapride, and other agents

Ritonavir: Combined use of high-dose tricyclic antidepressants with ritonavir may cause serotonin syndrome in HIV-positive patients; monitor

Sucralfate: Absorption of tricyclic antidepressants may be reduced with coadministration

Sympathomimetics, indirect-acting: Tricyclic antidepressants may result in a decreased sensitivity to indirect-acting sympathomimetics; includes dopamine and ephedrine; also see interaction with epinephrine (and direct-acting sympathomimetics)

Tramadol: Tramadol's risk of seizures may be increased with TCAs

Valproic acid: May increase serum concentrations/adverse effects of some tricyclic antidepressants

Warfarin (and other oral anticoagulants): TCAs may increase the anticoagulant effect in patients stabilized on warfarin; monitor INR

Ethanol/Nutrition/Herb Interactions

Ethanol: Avoid ethanol (may increase CNS depression).

Food: Grapefruit juice may inhibit the metabolism of some TCAs and clinical toxicity may result.

Herb/Nutraceutical: St John's wort may decrease imipramine levels. Avoid valerian, St John's wort, SAMe, kava kava (may increase risk of serotonin syndrome and/or excessive sedation).

Mechanism of Action Traditionally believed to increase the synaptic concentration of serotonin and/or norepinephrine in the central nervous system by inhibition of their reuptake by the presynaptic neuronal membrane. However, additional receptor effects have been found including desensitization of adenyl cyclase, down regulation of beta-adrenergic receptors, and down regulation of serotonin receptors.

Pharmacodynamics Onset of action: Peak antidepressant effect: Usually after ≥2 weeks

Pharmacokinetics

Absorption: Well absorbed

Distribution: Crosses placenta

Metabolism: Hepatic to desipramine (active) and other metabolites; significant first-pass effect

Half-life: 6-18 hours

Elimination: Urine (as metabolites)

Dosage

Geriatrics:

Antidepressant: Initial: 10-25 mg at bedtime; increase by 10-25 mg every 3 days for inpatients and weekly for outpatients if tolerated. Average daily dose to achieve a therapeutic concentration: 100 mg/day; range: 50-150 mg/day.

Urinary incontinence (urge or mixed type): 10-50 mg at bedtime or twice daily

Adults: Antidepressant:

Oral: Initial: 25 mg 3-4 times/day; increase dose gradually, total dose may be given at bedtime; maximum: 300 mg/day.

Note: Maximum antidepressant effect may not be seen for 2 or more weeks after initiation of therapy.

Monitoring Parameters Improvement of depressive symptoms; blood pressure, pulse; may need to use serum concentrations to help monitor response

Reference Range Therapeutic: Imipramine and desipramine: 150-250 ng/mL (SI: 530-890 nmol/L); desipramine: 150-300 ng/mL (SI: 560-1125 nmol/L); Toxic: >500 ng/mL (SI: 446-893 nmol/L); utility of serum level monitoring controversial

Patient Information May require 2-4 weeks to achieve desired effect; avoid alcohol ingestion; do not discontinue medication abruptly; may cause urine to turn blue-green; may cause drowsiness, constipation, blurred vision; use water or hard candy for dry mouth; rise slowly to avoid dizziness

Special Geriatric Considerations Orthostatic hypotension is a concern with this agent, especially in patients taking other medications that may affect blood pressure. May precipitate arrhythmias in predisposed patients; may aggravate seizures. A less anticholinergic antidepressant may be a better choice. Data from a clinical trial comparing fluoxetine to tricyclics suggests that fluoxetine is significantly less effective than nortriptyline in hospitalized elderly patients with unipolar major affective disorder, especially those with melancholia and concurrent cardiovascular diseases.

Dosage Forms Excipient information presented when available (limited, particularly for generics); consult specific product labeling.

Capsule, as pamoate: 75 mg, 100 mg, 125 mg, 150 mg

　Tofranil-PM®: 75 mg, 100 mg, 125 mg, 150 mg

Tablet, as hydrochloride: 10 mg, 25 mg, 50 mg

　Tofranil®: 10 mg, 25 mg, 50 mg

Selected References

Nies A, Robinson DS, Friedman MS, et al, "Relationship Between Age and Tricyclic Antidepressant Plasma Levels," *Am J Psychiatry*, 1977, 134:790-3.

Roose SP, Glassman AH, Attia E, et al, "Comparative Efficacy of Selective Serotonin Reuptake Inhibitors and Tricyclics in the Treatment of Melancholia," *Am J Psychiatry*, 1994, 151(12):1735-9.

♦ **Imipramine Hydrochloride** *see* Imipramine *on page 792*

♦ **Imipramine Pamoate** *see* Imipramine *on page 792*

♦ **Imitrex®** *see* Sumatriptan *on page 1508*

Immune Globulin (Intramuscular)
(i MYUN GLOB yoo lin, IN tra MUS kyoo ler)

Related Information

Immunization Recommendations *on page 1787*

U.S. Brand Names BayGam® [DSC]; GammaSTAN™ S/D

Canadian Brand Names BayGam®

Index Terms Gamma Globulin; IG; IGIM; Immune Serum Globulin; ISG

Generic Available No

Pharmacologic Category Immune Globulin

Use Treatment of immunodeficiency syndrome, idiopathic thrombocytopenia purpura, B-cell chronic lymphocytic leukemia, Kawasaki syndrome; prophylaxis against hepatitis A, measles, varicella, and possibly rubella and immunoglobulin deficiency

Contraindications Hypersensitivity to immune globulin, thimerosal, or any component of the formulation; IgA deficiency; I.M. injections in patients with thrombocytopenia or coagulation disorders

Warnings/Precautions Hypersensitivity and anaphylactic reactions can occur; immediate treatment (including epinephrine 1:1000) should be available. Product of human plasma; may potentially contain infectious agents which could transmit disease. Screening of donors, as well as testing and/or inactivation or removal of certain viruses, reduces the risk. Infections thought to be transmitted by this product should be reported to the manufacturer. Skin testing should not be performed as local irritation can occur and be misinterpreted as a positive reaction. Not for I.V. administration.

Adverse Reactions (Reflective of adult population; not specific for elderly)

Frequency not defined.

Cardiovascular: Flushing, angioedema

Central nervous system: Chills, lethargy, fever

Dermatologic: Urticaria, erythema

Gastrointestinal: Nausea, vomiting

Local: Pain, tenderness, muscle stiffness at I.M. site

Neuromuscular & skeletal: Myalgia

Miscellaneous: Hypersensitivity reactions

Drug Interactions

Hepatitis A vaccine: IG and hepatitis A vaccine may be administered simultaneously, given at separate injection sites.

Live virus, vaccines: Do not administer MMR within 3 months after administration of IGIM; do not administer varicella vaccine within 5 months. If IG is given <2 weeks after MMR vaccine or <3 weeks after varicella vaccine, revaccination is required.

Stability Store under refrigeration at 2°C to 8°C (36°F to 46°F).

(Continued)

Immune Globulin (Intramuscular) *(Continued)*

Mechanism of Action Provides passive immunity by increasing the antibody titer and antigen-antibody reaction potential

Pharmacodynamics Duration of immune effects: Usually 3-4 weeks

Pharmacokinetics
Half-life: 21-23 days
Time to peak:
I.M.: Peak antibody serum concentration occur within 2-5 days
I.V.: Provides immediate antibody levels

Dosage
Geriatrics & Adults:
Hepatitis A: I.M.:
Pre-exposure prophylaxis upon travel into endemic areas (hepatitis A vaccine preferred):
0.02 mL/kg for anticipated risk of exposure <3 months
0.06 mL/kg for anticipated risk of exposure ≥3 months
Repeat approximate dose every 5 months if exposure continues
Postexposure prophylaxis: 0.02 mL/kg given within 14 days of exposure. IG is not needed if at least 1 dose of hepatitis A vaccine was given at ≥1 month before exposure
Measles: I.M.:
Prophylaxis, immunocompetent: 0.25 mL/kg/dose (maximum dose: 15 mL) given within 6 days of exposure followed by live attenuated measles vaccine in 5-6 months when indicated
Prophylaxis, immunocompromised: 0.5 mL/kg (maximum dose: 15 mL) immediately following exposure
Varicella: I.M.: Prophylaxis: 0.6-1.2 mL/kg (varicella zoster immune globulin preferred) within 72 hours of exposure
IgG deficiency: I.M.: 0.66 mL/kg/dose every 3-4 weeks. A double dose may be given at onset of therapy; some patients may require more frequent injections.

Administration Intramuscular injection only

Monitoring Parameters I.V. may cause hypotension; monitor for anaphylaxis, platelet counts, serum IgG concentration

Reference Range Serum IgG: 300 mg/dL

Test Interactions Skin tests should **not** be done

Additional Information Epidemiologic and laboratory data indicate that current IMIG products do not have a discernible risk of transmitting HIV.

Special Geriatric Considerations No special recommendations are made for the elderly, doses are same as recommended for younger adults.

Dosage Forms Excipient information presented when available (limited, particularly for generics); consult specific product labeling.
Injection, solution [preservative free]:
BayGam® [DSC], GammaSTAN™ S/D: 15% to 18% (2 mL, 10 mL)

Immune Globulin (Subcutaneous)
(i MYUN GLOB yoo lin sub kyoo TAY nee us)

U.S. Brand Names Vivaglobin®

Index Terms Immune Globulin Subcutaneous (Human); SCIG

Generic Available No

Pharmacologic Category Immune Globulin

Use Treatment of primary immune deficiency (PID)

Dosage
Geriatrics & Adults: Note: Consider premedicating with acetaminophen and diphenhydramine.
Primary immune deficiency: SubQ infusion: 100-200 mg/kg weekly (maximum rate: 20 mL/hour; doses >15 mL should be divided between sites); adjust the dose over time to achieve desired clinical response or target IgG levels
Conversion from I.V. to SubQ: Multiply previous I.V. dose by 1.37, then divide into a weekly regimen by dividing by the previous I.V. dosing interval (eg, if the dosing interval was every 3 weeks, divide by 3); adjust the dose over time to achieve desired clinical response or target IgG levels. SubQ infusion administration should begin 1 week after the last I.V. dose.

Special Geriatric Considerations No clinical data specific to elderly at this time. Use caution and monitor closely.

Dosage Forms Excipient information presented when available (limited, particularly for generics); consult specific product labeling.
Injection, solution [preservative free]: IgG 160 mg/mL (3 mL, 10 mL, 20 mL)

♦ **Immune Globulin Subcutaneous (Human)** *see Immune Globulin (Subcutaneous) on page 796*

♦ **Immune Serum Globulin** *see Immune Globulin (Intramuscular) on page 795*

♦ **Imodium® A-D [OTC]** *see Loperamide on page 924*

♦ **Imodium® Advanced** *see Loperamide and Simethicone on page 926*

♦ **Imogam® Rabies-HT** *see Rabies Immune Globulin (Human) on page 1371*

♦ **Imovax® Rabies** *see Rabies Virus Vaccine on page 1372*

♦ **Imuran®** *see Azathioprine on page 141*

Inamrinone (eye NAM ri none)

Medication Safety Issues
Sound-alike/look-alike issues:
  Amrinone may be confused with amiloride, amiodarone
Index Terms Amrinone Lactate
Generic Available Yes
Pharmacologic Category Phosphodiesterase Enzyme Inhibitor
Use Treatment of low cardiac output states (eg, sepsis, congestive heart failure); adjunctive therapy of pulmonary hypertension
Contraindications Hypersensitivity to inamrinone, any component of the formulation, or bisulfites (contains sodium metabisulfite); patients with severe aortic or pulmonic valvular disease
Warnings/Precautions Due to a slight effect on AV conduction, may increase ventricular response rate in atrial fibrillation/atrial flutter; prior treatment with digoxin is recommended. Monitor liver function. Discontinue therapy if alteration in LFTs and clinical symptoms of hepatotoxicity occur. Observe for arrhythmias in this very high-risk patient population. Not recommended in acute MI treatment. Monitor fluid status closely; patients may require adjustment of diuretic and electrolyte replacement therapy. Can cause thrombocytopenia (dose dependent). Correct hypokalemia before initiating therapy. Increase risk of hospitalization and death with long-term therapy.
Adverse Reactions (Reflective of adult population; not specific for elderly)
1% to 10%:
  Cardiovascular: Arrhythmias (3%, especially in high-risk patients), hypotension (1% to 2%), (may be infusion rate-related)
  Gastrointestinal: Nausea (1% to 2%)
  Hematologic: Thrombocytopenia (may be dose related)
Drug Interactions
Furosemide: A precipitate forms on admixture with inamrinone.
Diuretics may cause significant hypovolemia and decrease filling pressure.
Digitalis: Inotropic effects are additive.
Stability May be administered undiluted for I.V. bolus doses. For continuous infusion, dilute with 0.45% or 0.9% sodium chloride to final concentration of 1-3 mg/mL. Use within 24 hours. Do not directly dilute with dextrose-containing solutions, chemical interaction occurs. May be administered I.V. into running dextrose infusions. Furosemide forms a precipitate when injected in I.V. lines containing inamrinone.
Mechanism of Action Inhibits myocardial cyclic adenosine monophosphate (cAMP) phosphodiesterase activity and increases cellular levels of cAMP resulting in a positive inotropic effect and increased cardiac output; also possesses systemic and pulmonary vasodilator effects resulting in pre- and afterload reduction; slightly increases atrioventricular conduction
Pharmacodynamics
Onset of action: I.V.: Following administration, hemodynamic actions occur within 2-5 minutes
Peak effect: Within 10 minutes
Duration: Dose dependent with low doses lasting ~30 minutes and higher doses lasting ~2 hours
Pharmacokinetics
Distribution: V_d: 1.2 L/kg
Protein binding: 10% to 49%
Metabolism: In the liver
Half-life:
  Normal adult volunteers: 3.6 hours
  Congestive heart failure: 5.8 hours, range: 3-15 hours
Elimination: Excreted (60% to 90% as metabolites) in urine within 24 hours; 10% to 40% excreted unchanged in urine
Dosage
Geriatrics & Adults: Dosage is based on clinical response (**Note:** Dose should not exceed 10 mg/kg/24 hours).

  Heart failure: 0.75 mg/kg I.V. bolus over 2-3 minutes followed by maintenance infusion of 5-10 mcg/kg/minute; I.V. bolus may need to be repeated in 30 minutes.
(Continued)

Inamrinone *(Continued)*

Renal Impairment: Cl_{cr} <10 mL/minute: Administer 50% to 75% of dose.

Administration May be administered undiluted for I.V. bolus doses. For continuous infusion: Dilute with 0.45% or 0.9% sodium chloride to final concentration of 1-3 mg/mL use within 24 hours.

Monitoring Parameters Thrombocytopenia, hepatotoxicity, GI effects, blood pressure and heart rate every 5 minutes during infusion, CVP, PCWP, respiratory rate; monitor renal function and fluid/electrolyte status (particularly potassium)

Reference Range 0.5-7 mcg/mL

Patient Information Change position slowly because of postural hypotension

Additional Information Normally prescribed for patients who have not responded well to therapy with digitalis, diuretics, and vasodilators; dosage is based on clinical response

Special Geriatric Considerations While inamrinone is not specifically arrhythmogenic, the elderly may be at high risk for ventricular and particularly atrial arrhythmias due to high incidence of arrhythmias in this population. Also, the elderly are often hypovolemic due to dehydration; therefore, monitor fluid status carefully (CVP line) in order to have effective falling pressure for maximal response. Found to be as effective as dobutamine in the elderly with heart failure in one study despite the decline in beta-adrenergic response with age.

Dosage Forms Excipient information presented when available (limited, particularly for generics); consult specific product labeling.

Injection, solution, as lactate: 5 mg/mL (20 mL) [contains sodium metabisulfite]

Selected References
Rich MW, Woods WL, Davila-Roman VG, et al, "A Randomized Comparison of Intravenous Amrinone Versus Dobutamine in Older Patients With Decompensated Congestive Heart Failure," *J Am Geriatr Soc,* 1995, 43(3):271-4.

♦ **Inapsine®** *see Droperidol on page 486*

Indapamide *(in DAP a mide)*

Medication Safety Issues

Sound-alike/look-alike issues:
   Indapamide may be confused with Iopidine®

International issues:
   Pretanix® [Hungary] may be confused with Protonix® which is a brand name for pantoprazole in the U.S.

U.S. Brand Names Lozol® [DSC]

Canadian Brand Names Apo-Indapamide®; Gen-Indapamide; Lozide®; Lozol®; Novo-Indapamide; Nu-Indapamide; PMS-Indapamide

Generic Available Yes

Pharmacologic Category Diuretic, Thiazide-Related

Use Management of mild to moderate hypertension; treatment of edema in congestive heart failure and nephrotic syndrome

Contraindications Hypersensitivity to indapamide or any component of the formulation, thiazides, or sulfonamide-derived drugs; anuria; renal decompensation

Warnings/Precautions Use with caution in severe renal disease. Electrolyte disturbances (hypokalemia, hypochloremic alkalosis, hyponatremia) can occur. Use with caution in severe hepatic dysfunction; hepatic encephalopathy can be caused by electrolyte disturbances. Gout can be precipitate in certain patients with a history of gout, a familial predisposition to gout, or chronic renal failure. Cautious use in prediabetics or diabetics; may see a change in glucose control. I.V. use is generally not recommended (but is available). Can cause SLE exacerbation or activation. Use with caution in patients with moderate or high cholesterol concentrations. Photosensitization may occur. Correct hypokalemia before initiating therapy.

Chemical similarities are present among sulfonamides, sulfonylureas, carbonic anhydrase inhibitors, thiazides, and loop diuretics (except ethacrynic acid). Use in patients with thiazide or sulfonamide allergy is specifically contraindicated in product labeling, however, a risk of cross-reaction exists in patients with allergy to any of these compounds; avoid use when previous reaction has been severe. Discontinue if signs of hypersensitivity are noted.

Adverse Reactions (Reflective of adult population; not specific for elderly)
1% to 10%:
   Cardiovascular: Orthostatic hypotension, palpitation (<5%), flushing
   Central nervous system: Dizziness (<5%), lightheadedness (<5%), vertigo (<5%), headache (≥5%), restlessness (<5%), drowsiness (<5%), fatigue, lethargy, malaise, lassitude, anxiety, agitation, depression, nervousness (≥5%)
   Dermatologic: Rash (<5%), pruritus (<5%), hives (<5%)
   Endocrine & metabolic: Hyperglycemia (<5%), hyperuricemia (<5%)

Gastrointestinal: Anorexia, gastric irritation, nausea, vomiting, abdominal pain, cramping, bloating, diarrhea, constipation, dry mouth, weight loss

Genitourinary: Nocturia, frequent urination, polyuria, impotence (<5%), reduced libido (<5%), glycosuria (<5%)

Neuromuscular & skeletal: Muscle cramps, spasm, weakness (≥5%)

Ocular: Blurred vision (<5%)

Renal: Necrotizing angiitis, vasculitis, cutaneous vasculitis (<5%)

Respiratory: Rhinorrhea (<5%)

Overdosage/Toxicology Symptoms include lethargy, diuresis, hypermotility, confusion, and muscle weakness. Following GI decontamination, therapy is supportive with I.V. fluids, electrolytes, and I.V. pressors if needed.

Drug Interactions

ACE inhibitors: Increased hypotension if aggressively diuresed with a thiazide diuretic.

Beta-blockers increase hyperglycemic effects in type 2 diabetes mellitus (noninsulin dependent, NIDDM)

Cyclosporine and thiazides can increase the risk of gout or renal toxicity; avoid concurrent use.

Digoxin toxicity can be exacerbated if a thiazide induces hypokalemia or hypomagnesemia.

Lithium toxicity can occur by reducing renal excretion of lithium; monitor lithium concentration and adjust as needed.

Neuromuscular blocking agents can prolong blockade; monitor serum potassium and neuromuscular status.

NSAIDs can decrease the efficacy of thiazides reducing the diuretic and antihypertensive effects.

Ethanol/Nutrition/Herb Interactions Herb/Nutraceutical: Avoid dong quai if using for hypertension (has estrogenic activity). Avoid ephedra, yohimbe, ginseng (may worsen hypertension). Avoid garlic (may have increased antihypertensive effect).

Mechanism of Action Diuretic effect is localized at the proximal segment of the distal tubule of the nephron; it does not appear to have significant effect on glomerular filtration rate nor renal blood flow; like other diuretics, it enhances sodium, chloride, and water excretion by interfering with the transport of sodium ions across the renal tubular epithelium

Pharmacokinetics

Absorption: Oral: Completely from GI tract

Protein binding: 71% to 79%

Metabolism: Extensive in the liver

Half-life: 14-18 hours

Time to peak serum concentration: 2-2.5 hours

Elimination: ~60% of dose excreted in urine within 48 hours, about 16% to 23% excreted via bile into feces

Dosage

Geriatrics & Adults:

Edema (diuretic): Oral: 2.5-5 mg/day. **Note:** There is little therapeutic benefit to increasing the dose >5 mg/day; there is, however, an increased risk of electrolyte disturbances.

Hypertension: Oral: 1.25 mg in the morning, may increase to 5 mg/day by increments of 1.25-2.5 mg; consider adding another antihypertensive and decreasing the dose if response is not adequate.

Monitoring Parameters Blood pressure (both standing and sitting/supine), serum electrolytes, renal function, weight, I & O

Patient Information Take early in the day to avoid nocturia. May cause photosensitivity; use a sun block with an SPF of 15 or more.

Additional Information Indapamide offers no specific advantage over thiazides except it is effective in patients with impaired renal function (Cl$_{cr}$ <30 mL/minute).

Special Geriatric Considerations Thiazide diuretics lose efficacy when Cl$_{cr}$ is <30-35 mL/minute. Many elderly may have Cl$_{cr}$ below this limit. Calculate Cl$_{cr}$ for elderly before initiating therapy. Indapamide has the advantage over thiazide diuretics in that it is effective when Cl$_{cr}$ is <30 mL/minute.

Dosage Forms Excipient information presented when available (limited, particularly for generics); consult specific product labeling.

Tablet: 1.25 mg, 2.5 mg

Lozol®: 1.25 mg [DSC]

♦ **Inderal®** see Propranolol on page 1336

♦ **Inderal® LA** see Propranolol on page 1336

♦ **Inderide®** see Propranolol and Hydrochlorothiazide on page 1340

♦ **Indocin®** see Indomethacin on page 800

♦ **Indocin® I.V.** see Indomethacin on page 800

♦ **Indometacin** see Indomethacin on page 800

Indomethacin (in doe METH a sin)

Related Information
Potentially Inappropriate Medications for Geriatrics *on page 1824*

Medication Safety Issues
Sound-alike/look-alike issues:
Indocin® may be confused with Imodium®, Lincocin®, Minocin®, Vicodin®

International issues:
Flexin® [Great Britain] may be confused with Floxin® which is a brand name for ofloxacin in the U.S.
Flexin® [Great Britain]: Brand name for orphenadrine in Israel

U.S. Brand Names Indocin®; Indocin® I.V.

Canadian Brand Names Apo-Indomethacin®; Indocid® P.D.A.; Indocin®; Indo-Lemmon; Indotec; Novo-Methacin; Nu-Indo; Rhodacine®

Index Terms Indometacin; Indomethacin Sodium Trihydrate

Generic Available Yes: Capsule

Pharmacologic Category Nonsteroidal Anti-inflammatory Drug (NSAID), Oral; Nonsteroidal Anti-inflammatory Drug (NSAID), Parenteral

Use Acute gouty arthritis, acute bursitis/tendonitis, moderate to severe osteoarthritis, rheumatoid arthritis, ankylosing spondylitis

Restrictions An FDA-approved medication guide must be distributed when dispensing an oral outpatient prescription (new or refill) where this medication is to be used without direct supervision of a healthcare provider. Medication guides are available at http://www.fda.gov/cder/Offices/ODS/medication_guides.htm.

Contraindications Hypersensitivity to indomethacin, aspirin, other NSAIDs, or any component of the formulation; perioperative pain in the setting of coronary artery bypass surgery (CABG)

Warnings/Precautions [U.S. Boxed Warning]: NSAIDs are associated with an increased risk of adverse cardiovascular events, including MI, stroke, and new onset or worsening of pre-existing hypertension. Risk may be increased with duration of use or pre-existing cardiovascular risk factors or disease. Use caution with fluid retention, CHF or hypertension. Concurrent administration of ibuprofen, and potentially other nonselective NSAIDs, may interfere with aspirin's cardioprotective effect.

Use of NSAIDs can compromise existing renal function. Indomethacin is not recommended for patients with advanced renal disease. Use with caution in patients with decreased hepatic function.

[U.S. Boxed Warning]: NSAIDs may increase risk of gastrointestinal irritation, ulceration, bleeding, and perforation. Use caution with a history of GI disease (bleeding or ulcers), concurrent therapy with aspirin, anticoagulants and/or corticosteroids, smoking, use of alcohol, the elderly or debilitated patients.

Use the lowest effective dose for the shortest duration of time, consistent with individual patient goals, to reduce risk of cardiovascular or GI adverse events.

NSAIDs may cause serious skin adverse events including exfoliative dermatitis, Stevens-Johnson syndrome (SJS) and toxic epidermal necrolysis (TEN). Do not use in patients who experience bronchospasm, asthma, rhinitis, or urticaria with NSAID or aspirin therapy. Use caution in other forms of asthma.

The elderly are at increased risk for adverse effects (especially peptic ulceration, CNS effects, renal toxicity) from NSAIDs even at low doses. Prolonged use may cause corneal deposits and retinal disturbances; discontinue if visual changes are observed. Use caution with depression, epilepsy or Parkinson's disease.

Withhold for at least 4-6 half-lives prior to surgical or dental procedures.

Adverse Reactions (Reflective of adult population; not specific for elderly)
>10%: Central nervous system: Headache (12%)
1% to 10%:
Central nervous system: Dizziness (3% to 9%), fatigue (<3%), vertigo (<3%), depression (<3%), malaise (<3%), somnolence (<3%)
Gastrointestinal: Nausea (3% to 9%), epigastric pain (3% to 9%), abdominal pain/cramps/distress (<3%), heartburn (3% to 9%), indigestion (3% to 9%), constipation (<3%), diarrhea (<3%), dyspepsia (3% to 9%), vomiting
Otic: Tinnitus (<3%)

Overdosage/Toxicology Symptoms include drowsiness, lethargy, nausea, vomiting, seizures, paresthesias, headache, dizziness, GI bleeding, cerebral edema, tinnitus, leukocytosis, and renal failure. Management of nonsteroidal anti-inflammatory drug (NSAID) intoxication is symptom-directed and supportive. Fluid therapy is commonly effective in managing hypotension that may occur following an acute NSAID overdose, except when due to acute blood loss. Seizures tend to be very short-lived and often do not require drug treatment, although recurrent seizures should be treated with I.V. diazepam.

Drug Interactions Substrate (minor) of CYP2C9, 2C19; **Inhibits** CYP2C9 (strong), 2C19 (weak)

ACE inhibitors: Antihypertensive effects may be decreased by concurrent therapy with NSAIDs; monitor blood pressure.

Aminoglycosides: NSAIDs may decrease the excretion of aminoglycosides.

Anticoagulants (warfarin, heparin, LMWHs) in combination with NSAIDs can cause increased risk of bleeding.

Antiplatelet drugs (ticlopidine, clopidogrel, aspirin, abciximab, dipyridamole, eptifibatide, tirofiban) can cause an increased risk of bleeding.

Beta-blockers: NSAIDs may diminish the antihypertensive effects of beta-blockers.

Bisphosphonates: NSAIDs may increase the risk of gastrointestinal ulceration.

Cholestyramine (and other bile acid sequestrants): May decrease the absorption of NSAIDs. Separate by at least 2 hours.

Cyclosporine: NSAIDs may increase serum creatinine, potassium, blood pressure, and cyclosporine levels; monitor cyclosporine levels and renal function carefully.

CYP2C9 Substrates: Indomethacin may increase the levels/effects of CYP2C9 substrates. Example substrates include bosentan, dapsone, fluoxetine, glimepiride, glipizide, losartan, montelukast, nateglinide, paclitaxel, phenytoin, warfarin, and zafirlukast.

Fluoroquinolone antibiotics: Risk of seizures may be increased with concomitant quinolone use. Risk is considered quite low and may only be a factor with high serum levels of either agent and/or in patients with additional predisposing factors (eg, renal dysfunction, history of seizure or other neurological disorder).

Hydralazine's antihypertensive effect may be decreased; avoid concurrent use.

Lithium: Levels can be increased; avoid concurrent use if possible or monitor lithium levels and adjust dose. Sulindac may have the least effect. When NSAID is stopped, lithium dose will need adjustment; use levels to titrate.

Loop diuretics: Diuretic and antihypertensive efficacy is reduced. This effect may be anticipated with any NSAID.

Methotrexate: Severe bone marrow suppression, aplastic anemia, and GI toxicity have been reported with concomitant NSAID therapy. Avoid use during moderate or high-dose methotrexate (increased and prolonged methotrexate levels). NSAID use during low-dose treatment of rheumatoid arthritis has not been fully evaluated; extreme caution is warranted.

Pemetrexed: NSAIDs may decrease the excretion of pemetrexed. Patients with Cl_{cr} 45-79 mL/minute should avoid short acting NSAIDs for 2 days before and 2 days after pemetrexed treatment.

Probenecid: Probenecid may increase the serum concentration of NSAIDs.

Salicylates: NSAIDs (nonselective) may diminish the cardioprotective effect of acetylated salicylates. Avoid regular use of NSAIDs if possible; consider alternatives (eg, acetaminophen). Give salicylate before NSAID; for example ibuprofen should be given 30-120 minutes after aspirin (immediate release)..

Tiludronate: Indomethacin may increase serum concentration of tiludronate.

Treprostinil: May enhance the risk of bleeding with concurrent use.

Triamterene: Indomethacin may enhance the nephrotoxic effect of triamterene; avoid concomitant use.

Vancomycin: NSAIDs may decrease the excretion of vancomycin.

Ethanol/Nutrition/Herb Interactions

Ethanol: Avoid ethanol (may enhance gastric mucosal irritation).

Food: Food may decrease the rate but not the extent of absorption. Indomethacin peak serum levels may be delayed if taken with food.

Herb/Nutraceutical: Avoid alfalfa, anise, bilberry, bladderwrack, bromelain, cat's claw, celery, coleus, cordyceps, dong quai, evening primrose, feverfew, fenugreek, garlic, ginger, ginkgo biloba, ginseng, grapeseed, green tea, guggul, horse chestnut seed, horseradish, licorice, prickly ash, red clover, reishi, SAMe, sweet clover, turmeric, white willow (all have additional antiplatelet activity).

Stability I.V.: Store below 30°C (86°F). Protect from light. Not stable in alkaline solution. Reconstitute with 1-2 mL preservative free NS or SWFI just prior to administration. Discard any unused portion. Do not use preservative-containing diluents for reconstitution.

Mechanism of Action Inhibits prostaglandin synthesis by decreasing the activity of the enzyme, cyclooxygenase, which results in decreased formation of prostaglandin precursors

Pharmacodynamics

Onset of action: Within 30 minutes

Duration: 4-6 hours

Onset of anti-inflammatory action: Within 7 days

Peak effect: 1-2 weeks

Pharmacokinetics

Absorption: Promptly and extensively

(Continued)

Indomethacin *(Continued)*

Distribution: V_d: 0.34-1.57 L/kg; crosses blood brain barrier

Protein binding: 99%

Metabolism: In the liver with significant enterohepatic recycling

Half-life: 4-6 hours

Bioavailability: 100%

Time to peak: Oral: 2 hours

Excretion: Urine (60%, primarily as glucuronide conjugates); feces (33%, primarily as metabolites)

Dosage

Geriatrics: Refer to adult dosing. Use lowest recommended dose and frequency in elderly to initiate therapy for indications listed in adult dosing.

Adults:

Inflammatory/rheumatoid disorders (use lowest effective dose): Oral: 25-50 mg/dose 2-3 times/day; maximum dose: 200 mg/day. In patients with arthritis and persistent night pain and/or morning stiffness may give the larger portion (up to 100 mg) of the total daily dose at bedtime.

Bursitis/tendonitis: Oral: Initial dose: 75-150 mg/day in 3-4 divided doses; usual treatment is 7-14 days

Acute gouty arthritis: Oral: 50 mg 3 times daily until pain is tolerable then reduce dose; usual treatment <3-5 days

Renal Impairment: Not recommended with advanced renal disease.

Administration

Oral: Administer with food, milk, or antacids to decrease GI adverse effects.

I.V.: Administer over 20-30 minutes. Reconstitute I.V. formulation just prior to administration; discard any unused portion; avoid I.V. bolus administration or infusion via an umbilical catheter into vessels near the superior mesenteric artery as these may cause vasoconstriction and can compromise blood flow to the intestines. Do not administer intra-arterially.

Monitoring Parameters Monitor response (pain, range of motion, grip strength, mobility, ADL function), inflammation; observe for weight gain, edema; monitor renal function (serum creatinine, BUN); observe for bleeding, bruising; evaluate gastrointestinal effects (abdominal pain, bleeding, dyspepsia); mental confusion, disorientation, CBC, liver function tests; ophthalmologic exams with prolonged therapy

Test Interactions False-negative dexamethasone suppression test

Patient Information Extended release capsules must be swallowed intact. Serious gastrointestinal bleeding can occur as well as ulceration and perforation. Pain may or may not be present. Avoid aspirin and aspirin-containing products while taking this medication. If gastric upset occurs, take with food, milk, or antacid. If gastric adverse effects persist, contact physician. May cause drowsiness, dizziness, blurred vision, and confusion. Use caution when performing tasks which require alertness (eg, driving). Do not take for more than 3 days for fever or 10 days for pain without physician advice.

Additional Information There are no clinical guidelines to predict which NSAID will give response in a particular patient; trials with each must be initiated until response determined; consider dose, patient convenience, and cost

Special Geriatric Considerations Elderly are a high-risk population for adverse effects from NSAIDs. As much as 60% of elderly can develop peptic ulceration and/or hemorrhage asymptomatically. The concomitant use of H_2 blockers and sucralfate is not effective as prophylaxis with the exception of NSAID-induced duodenal ulcers which may be prevented by the use of ranitidine. Misoprostol and proton pump inhibitors are the only agents proven to help prevent the development of NSAID-induced ulcers. Also, concomitant disease and drug use contribute to the risk for GI adverse effects. Use lowest effective dose for shortest period possible. Consider renal function decline with age. Use of NSAIDs can compromise existing renal function especially when Cl_{cr} is ≤30 mL/minute. Tinnitus may be a difficult and unreliable indication of toxicity due to age-related hearing loss or eighth cranial nerve damage. CNS adverse effects such as confusion, agitation, and hallucination are generally seen in overdose or high dose situations, but the elderly may demonstrate these adverse effects at lower doses than younger adults. Indomethacin frequently causes confusion at recommended doses in the elderly.

Dosage Forms Excipient information presented when available (limited, particularly for generics); consult specific product labeling.

Capsule: 25 mg, 50 mg

Injection, powder for reconstitution:

Indocin® I.V.: 1 mg

Suspension, oral:

Indocin®: 25 mg/5 mL (237 mL) [contains alcohol 1%; pineapple-coconut-mint flavor]

Selected References

Brooks PM and Day RO, "Nonsteroidal Anti-inflammatory Drugs - Differences and Similarities," *N Engl J Med*, 1991, 324(24):1716-25.

Clinch D, Banerjee AK, and Ostick G, "Absence of Abdominal Pain in Elderly Patients With Peptic Ulcer," *Age Ageing*, 1984, 13(2):120-3.

Clive DM and Stoff JS, "Renal Syndromes Associated With Nonsteroidal Anti-inflammatory Drugs," *N Engl J Med*, 1984, 310(9):563-72.

Graham DY, "Prevention of Gastroduodenal Injury Induced by Chronic Nonsteroidal Anti-inflammatory Drug Therapy," *Gastroenterology*, 1989, 96(2 Pt 2 Suppl):675-81.

Gurwitz JH, Avorn J, Ross-Degnan D, et al, "Nonsteroidal Anti-Inflammatory Drug-Associated Azotemia in the Very Old," *JAMA*, 1990, 264(4):471-5.

Hawkey CJ, Karrasch JA, Szczepañski L, et al, "Omeprazole Compared With Misoprostol for Ulcers Associated With Nonsteroidal Anti-inflammatory Drugs," *N Engl J Med*, 1998, 338(11):727-34.

Hunt SA, Abraham WT, Chin MH , et al, "ACC/AHA 2005 Guideline Update for the Diagnosis and Management of Chronic Heart Failure in the Adult: A Report of the American College of Cardiology/American Heart Association Task Force on Practice Guidelines (Writing Committee to Update the 2001 Guidelines for the Evaluation and Management of Heart Failure)," available at: http://www.acc.org/clinical/guidelines/failure//index.pdf

Knodel LC, "Preventing NSAID-induced Ulcers: The Role of Misoprostol," *Consult Pharm*, 1989, 4:37-41.

Pounder R, "Silent Peptic Ulceration: Deadly Silence or Golden Silence?" *Gastroenterology*, 1989, 96(2 Pt 2 Suppl):626-31.

Yeomans ND, Tulassay Z, Juhasz L, et al, "A Comparison of Omeprazole With Ranitidine for Ulcers Associated With Nonsteroidal Anti-inflammatory Drugs," *N Engl J Med*, 1998, 338(11):719-26.

♦ **Indomethacin Sodium Trihydrate** *see* Indomethacin *on page 800*

♦ **Infantaire [OTC]** *see* Acetaminophen *on page 29*

♦ **Infantaire Gas Drops [OTC]** *see* Simethicone *on page 1467*

♦ **INFeD®** *see* Iron Dextran Complex *on page 832*

Influenza Virus Vaccine (in floo EN za VYE rus vak SEEN)

Related Information
Immunization Recommendations *on page 1787*

Medication Safety Issues
Sound-alike/look-alike issues:

Fluarix® may be confused with Flarex®

Influenza virus vaccine may be confused with tetanus toxoid and tuberculin products. Medication errors have occurred when tuberculin skin tests (PPD) have been inadvertently administered instead of tetanus toxoid products and influenza virus vaccine. These products are refrigerated and often stored in close proximity to each other.

Influenza virus vaccine (human strain) may be confused with the avian strain (H5N1) of influenza virus vaccine

U.S. Brand Names Fluarix®; FluLaval™; fluMist®; Fluvirin®; Fluzone®

Canadian Brand Names Fluviral S/F®; Vaxigrip®

Index Terms Influenza Virus Vaccine (Purified Surface Antigen); Influenza Virus Vaccine (Split-Virus); Influenza Virus Vaccine (Trivalent, Live); Live Attenuated Influenza Vaccine (LAIV); Trivalent Inactivated Influenza Vaccine (TIV)

Generic Available No

Pharmacologic Category Vaccine

Use Provide active immunity to influenza virus strains contained in the vaccine

Advisory Committee on Immunization Practices (ACIP) target groups for vaccination:
- Persons ≥50 years of age
- Residents of nursing homes and other chronic-care facilities that house persons of any age with chronic medical conditions
- Adults and children with chronic disorders of the pulmonary or cardiovascular systems, including asthma
- Adults and children who have required regular medical follow-up or hospitalization during the preceding year because of chronic metabolic diseases (including diabetes mellitus), renal dysfunction, hemoglobinopathies, or immunosuppression (including immunosuppression caused by medications or HIV)
- Adults and children with conditions which may compromise respiratory function, the handling of respiratory secretions, or that can increase the risk of aspiration (eg, cognitive dysfunction, spinal; cord injuries, seizure disorders, other neuromuscular disorders)
- Children and adolescents (6 months to 18 years of age) who are receiving long-term aspirin therapy and therefore, may be at risk for developing Reye's syndrome after influenza
- Women who will be pregnant during the influenza season
- Children 6-59 months of age

The ACIP also recommends vaccination for close contacts of children 0-59 months of age, healthy persons who may transmit influenza to those at risk, all healthcare workers, and all persons (including school-aged children) who want to decrease their risk of influenza infection or transmitting influenza to others.

Contraindications Hypersensitivity to influenza virus vaccine, or any component of the formulation; presence of acute respiratory disease or other active infections or
(Continued)

INFLUENZA VIRUS VACCINE

Influenza Virus Vaccine *(Continued)*

illnesses; delay immunization in a patient with an active neurological disorder (immunization should be delayed)

Nasal spray: Patients at increased risk for influenza-related complications (see Use); history of Guillain-Barré syndrome; history of asthma or reactive airway disease; underlying medical conditions such as diabetes, renal dysfunction, cardiovascular disease, hemoglobinopathies; immunosuppressed or concomitant immunosuppressant therapy

Warnings/Precautions Antigenic response may not be as great as expected in patients requiring immunosuppressive drug therapy or HIV-infected persons with CD4 cells <100/mm^3 and with viral copies of HIV type 1 >30,000/mL. Some products contain thimerosal, latex, or are manufactured with egg protein, chicken protein, and/or gentamicin; hypersensitivity reactions may occur. Due to potential for febrile reactions, risks and benefits must carefully be considered in patients with history of febrile convulsions. Influenza vaccines from previous seasons must not be used. Inactivated vaccine is preferred over live virus vaccine for household members, healthcare workers and others coming in close contact with severely-immunosuppressed persons requiring care in a protected environment. Treatment for anaphylactic reactions (including epinephrine) should be readily available.

Injection (inactivated, split virus, TIV): For I.M. use only; use caution with thrombocytopenia or any coagulation disorder. Use with caution in patients with history of Guillain-Barré (GBS); patients with history of GBS have a greater likelihood of developing GBS than those without. May consider avoiding vaccination in patients with a history of GBS and who are at low risk for severe influenza complications, and in patients known to have experienced GBS within 6 weeks following previous vaccination (consider influenza antiviral chemoprophylaxis in these patients). Immunization should be delayed during moderate-to-severe febrile illness; minor illnesses with or without fever generally do not preclude use of vaccine.

Nasal spray (live, attenuated virus): For intranasal use only. **Avoid contact with severely immunocompromised individuals for at least 7 days following vaccination.** Safety and efficacy for use in adults ≥50 years of age have not been established. Defer immunization if nasal congestion is present which may impede delivery of vaccine.

Adverse Reactions (Reflective of adult population; not specific for elderly) All serious adverse reactions must be reported to the U.S. Department of Health and Human Services (DHHS) Vaccine Adverse Event Reporting System (VAERS) 1-800-822-7967.

Injection:

Frequency not defined.

Central nervous system: Chills; fever and malaise (may start within 6-12 hours and last 1-2 days; incidence equal to placebo in adults; occurs more frequently than placebo in children); Guillain-Barré syndrome (GBS)

Dermatologic: Angioedema, rash, urticaria

Local: Tenderness, redness, or induration at the site of injection (10% to 64%; may last up to 2 days); injection site pain

Neuromuscular & skeletal: Myalgia (may start within 6-12 hours and last 1-2 days; incidence equal to placebo in adults; occurs more frequently than placebo in children)

Miscellaneous: Allergic or anaphylactoid reactions (most likely to residual egg protein; includes allergic asthma, angioedema, hives, systemic anaphylaxis)

Postmarketing and/or case reports: Seizure (rare; majority associated with fever)

Nasal spray: Frequency of events reported within 10 days

>10%:

Central nervous system: Headache (children 18% after first dose, < placebo after second dose; adults 40%) irritability (children 10% to 18%)

Neuromuscular & skeletal: Tiredness/weakness (adults 26%), muscle aches (children 5% to 6%; adults 17%)

Respiratory: Cough (children 26% to 38%; adults 14%), nasal congestion/ runny nose (children 46% to 48%; adults 9% to 45%), sore throat (children < placebo; adults 28%)

Miscellaneous: Activity decreased (children 14% after first dose, < placebo after second dose)

1% to 10%:

Central nervous system: Chills

Gastrointestinal: Abdominal pain, diarrhea, vomiting

Otic: Otitis media

Respiratory: Rhinitis, sinusitis

Drug Interactions

Aspirin: Concomitant use of aspirin and the nasal spray formulation may increase the risk of Reye syndrome in patients 5-17 years due to the presence of wild-type influenza in the preparation; concomitant use in this age group is contraindicated.

Immune globulins: Efficacy of influenza (live) vaccines may be diminished. Live virus vaccinations should be withheld for as long as 6 months.

Immunosuppressive agents: Decreased effect of vaccine may occur.

Influenza antiviral agents (amantadine, oseltamivir, ribavirin, rimantadine, zanamivir): Safety and efficacy for use with influenza virus vaccine nasal spray have not been established. Do not administer nasal spray until 48 hours after stopping antiviral; do not administer antiviral for 2 weeks after receiving influenza virus vaccine nasal spray.

Tuberculin test: Live virus vaccines may diminish the diagnostic effect of tuberculin tests.

Vaccines: Some manufacturers and clinicians recommend that the flu vaccine not be administered concomitantly with DTP due to the potential for increased febrile reactions (specifically whole-cell pertussis) and that one should wait at least 3 days. However, ACIP recommends that children at high risk for influenza may get the vaccine concomitantly with DTP. Safety and efficacy of nasal spray with other vaccines have not been established; do not give within 1 month of other live virus vaccines or within 2 weeks of inactivated or subunit vaccines.

Stability

Injection: Store between 2°C to 8°C (36°F to 46°F). Potency is destroyed by freezing; do not use if product has been frozen.

Fluarix®: Protect from light.

FluLaval™: Discard 28 days after initial entry. Protect from light.

Nasal spray: Store in a freezer at or below -15°C (5°F). May thaw in refrigerator and store at 2°C to 8°C (36°F to 46°F) ≤60 hours. Do not refreeze after thawing.

Mechanism of Action Promotes immunity to influenza virus by inducing specific antibody production. Each year the formulation is standardized according to the U.S. Public Health Service. Preparations from previous seasons must not be used.

Pharmacodynamics

Onset: Protective antibody levels achieved ~2 weeks after vaccination

Duration: Protective antibody titers persist approximately ≥6 months. Elderly: Protective antibody titers may fall ≤4 months after vaccination.

Dosage

Geriatrics & Adults: Optimal time to receive vaccine is October-November, prior to exposure to influenza; however, vaccination can continue into December and throughout the influenza season as long as vaccine is available.

Immunization:

Fluarix®, FluLaval™: I.M.: 0.5 mL/dose (1 dose per season)

Fluzone®, Fluvirin®: I.M.: 0.5 mL/dose (1 dose per season)

FluMist®: Intranasal: Adults ≤49 years: 0.5 mL/dose (1 dose per season)

Administration

Injection: For I.M. administration only. Inspect for particulate matter and discoloration prior to administration. Adults should be vaccinated in the deltoid muscle using a ≥1 inch needle length. Suspensions should be shaken well prior to use. **Note:** For patients at risk of hemorrhage following intramuscular injection, the ACIP recommends "it should be administered intramuscularly if, in the opinion of the physician familiar with the patients bleeding risk, the vaccine can be administered with reasonable safety by this route. If the patient receives antihemophilia or other similar therapy, intramuscular vaccination can be scheduled shortly after such therapy is administered. A fine needle (23 gauge or smaller) can be used for the vaccination and firm pressure applied to the site (without rubbing) for at least 2 minutes. The patient should be instructed concerning the risk of hematoma from the injection."

Intranasal: Must be thawed prior to administration. May thaw in refrigerator and store at 2°C to 8°C (36°F to 46°F) ≤60 hours. May also be thawed by holding sprayer in the palm of the hand and supporting the plunger rod with thumb; use immediately. Half the dose (0.25 mL) is administered to each nostril; patient should be in upright position. A dose divider clip is provided. Severely-immunocompromised persons should not administer the live vaccine. If recipient sneezes following administration, the dose should not be repeated.

Reference Range Less than a fourfold increase in titer; >1:10 IgG and IgM

Patient Information Be aware of possible adverse effects

Additional Information Pharmacies will stock the formulations(s) standardized according to the USPHS requirements for the season. Influenza vaccines from previous seasons must not be used. Federal law requires that the date of administration, the vaccine manufacturer, lot number of vaccine, and the administering person's name, title, and address be entered into the patient's permanent medical record.

The optimal time to receive vaccine is October-November, prior to exposure to influenza; however, vaccination can continue into December and later as long as vaccine is (Continued)

Influenza Virus Vaccine *(Continued)*

available. To avoid missed opportunities for vaccination, patients at risk for complications can be offered the vaccine during routine healthcare visits as early as September if vaccine is available. Avoid vaccination before October in older persons in nursing homes or similar housing facilities because antibody levels can decline more rapidly following vaccination.

Priority groups for vaccination with inactivated influenza vaccine during periods of vaccine shortage:

Tier 1A:

Persons ≥65 years with comorbid conditions

Residents of long-term-care facilities

Tier 1B:

Persons 2-64 years with comorbid conditions

Persons ≥65 years without comorbid conditions

Children 6-23 months

Pregnant women

Tier 1C:

Healthcare personnel

Household contacts and out-of-home caregivers of children <6 months

Tier 2:

Household contacts of children and adults at increased risk of influenza associated complications

Healthy persons 50-64 years

Tier 3:

Persons 2-49 years without high-risk conditions

Further information available at http://www.cdc.gov/mmwr/preview/mmwrhtml/ mm5430a4.htm

Federal law requires that the date of administration, the vaccine manufacturer, lot number of vaccine, and the administering person's name, title, and address be entered into the patient's permanent medical record.

Special Geriatric Considerations Limited data on the elderly exists due to ethical considerations precluding use of placebo and differences in studies and vaccines; 80% develop a 1:40 HA titer, 70% are completely protected, 90% protected from death. Amantadine may be used to prophylax against influenza type A in the following situations:

High-risk institutionalized patients, both vaccinated and unvaccinated

Epidemic environment

Supplement vaccine in those who may have inadequate response (immunosuppressed)

Those who refuse vaccine

Those hypersensitive to vaccine or its components

Amantadine dose must be adjusted for renal failure. Administer for 2 weeks in vaccinated patients and 6-12 weeks in unvaccinated patients.

Dosage Forms Excipient information presented when available (limited, particularly for generics); consult specific product labeling.

Injection, solution, purified split-virus [preservative free]:

Fluvirin®: (0.5 mL) [TIV; contains thimerosal (trace amounts); manufactured using chicken eggs, neomycin, and polymyxin]

Injection, suspension, purified split-virus:

FluLaval™: (5 mL) [TIV; latex-free; contains thimerosal; produced in chick embryo cell culture]

Fluzone®: (5 mL) [TIV; latex free; contains thimerosal; produced in chick embryo cell culture]

Injection, suspension, purified split-virus [preservative free]:

Fluarix®: (0.5 mL) [TIV; syringe cap and rubber plunger contain natural latex rubber; produced in chick embryo cell culture; may contain residual amounts of thimerosal, hydrocortisone, gentamicin, and ovalbumin]

Fluzone®: (0.25 mL) [TIV; latex free; produced in chick embryo cell culture]; (0.5 mL) [TIV; latex free; produced in chick embryo cell culture]

Solution, intranasal [preservative free; trivalent; live virus; spray]:

fluMist®: (0.5 mL) [LAIV; manufactured using eggs and gentamicin]

Selected References

Bentley DW, "Vaccinations," *Clin Geriatr Med*, 1992, 8(4):745-60.

Centers for Disease Control, "Prevention and Control of Influenza. Recommendations of the Advisory Committee on Immunization Practices (ACIP)," *MMWR Recomm Rep*, 2007, 56 (early release):1-54. Available at http://www.cdc.gov/mmwr/preview/mmwrhtml/rr56e629a1.htm

Centers for Disease Control, "Recommendations of the Advisory Committee on Immunization Practices (ACIP): General Recommendations on Immunization," *MMWR*, 1994, 43(RR-1):23.

Gardner P and Schaffner W, "Immunization of Adults," *N Engl J Med*, 1993, 328(17):1252-8.

"Influenza Vaccine 2006-2007," *Med Lett Drugs Ther*, 2006, 48(1245):81-3.

INFLUENZA VIRUS VACCINE (H5N1)

Influenza Virus Vaccine (H5N1) (in floo EN za VYE rus vak SEEN H5N1)

Related Information
Immunization Recommendations *on page 1787*

Medication Safety Issues
Sound-alike/look-alike issues:
Influenza virus vaccine (H5N1) may be confused with the nonavian strain of influenza virus vaccine

Index Terms Avian Influenza Virus Vaccine; Bird Flu Vaccine; H5N1 Influenza Vaccine; Influenza Virus Vaccine (Monovalent)

Generic Available No

Pharmacologic Category Vaccine

Use Active immunization of adults at increased risk of exposure to the H5N1 viral subtype of influenza

Restrictions Commercial distribution is not planned. The vaccine will be included as part of the U.S. Strategic National Stockpile. It will be distributed by public health officials if needed.

Contraindications Manufacturer states no contraindications

Warnings/Precautions Immediate treatment (including epinephrine 1:1000) for anaphylactoid and/or hypersensitivity reactions should be available during vaccine use. Use with caution in patients with a history of Guillain-Barré syndrome (GBS); these patients may have a greater likelihood of developing GBS. If recent occurrence of GBS (≤6 weeks), decision to administer vaccine should entail careful consideration of risk:benefit. Use with caution in severely immunocompromised patients (eg, patients receiving chemo/radiation therapy or other immunosuppressive therapy [including high-dose corticosteroids]); may have a reduced response to vaccination. Safety and efficacy in patients >64 years of age have not been established.

Adverse Reactions (Reflective of adult population; not specific for elderly)
All serious adverse reactions must be reported to the U.S. Department of Health and Human Services (DHHS) Vaccine Adverse Event Reporting System (VAERS) 1-800-822-7967.
>10%:
Central nervous system: Headache (3% to 36%), malaise (22%)
Local: Pain (74%), tenderness (70%), erythema/redness (20%), induration/swelling (15%)
Neuromuscular & skeletal: Myalgia (16%)
1% to 10%:
Central nervous system: Fever (up to 7%)
Gastrointestinal: Nausea (10%), diarrhea (6%)
Respiratory: Nasopharyngitis (2%), upper respiratory infection (2%), nasal congestion (1%)
Additional reactions observed with other influenza vaccine formulations: Allergic reaction, anaphylaxis, angioedema, asthma, encephalopathy, facial paralysis, hives, GBS, neuropathy, optic neuritis, vasculitis

Drug Interactions Immunosuppressive agents: Decreased protective effect of vaccine may occur.

Stability Store between 2°C to 8°C (36°F to 46°F). Potency is destroyed by freezing; do not use if product has been frozen. Protect from light.

Mechanism of Action A monovalent, split virus (inactivated) preparation of the H5N1 avian strain of influenza virus (A/Vietnam/1203/2004) which promotes active immunity to avian influenza.

Pharmacokinetics Onset of action: Four-fold increase in antibody titers occurred in up to 58% of patients 28 days after second dose.

Dosage
Adults: Immunization: Adults 18-64 years: I.M.: 1 mL, followed by second 1 mL dose given 28 days later (acceptable range: 21-35 days)

Administration For I.M. administration only. Inspect for particulate matter and discoloration prior to administration. Vaccinate in the deltoid muscle using a ≥1 inch needle length. Suspension should be shaken well prior to use. **Note:** For patients at risk of hemorrhage following intramuscular injection, the ACIP recommends "it should be administered intramuscularly if, in the opinion of the physician familiar with the patients bleeding risk, the vaccine can be administered with reasonable safety by this route. If the patient receives antihemophilia or other similar therapy, intramuscular vaccination can be scheduled shortly after such therapy is administered. A fine needle (23 gauge or smaller) can be used for the vaccination and firm pressure applied to the site (without rubbing) for at least 2 minutes. The patient should be instructed concerning the risk of hematoma from the injection."

Patient Information
Notify prescriber immediately of any acute reaction to vaccination (eg, difficulty breathing, chest pain, acute headache, rash, difficulty swallowing). May cause mild
(Continued)

807

Influenza Virus Vaccine (H5N1) *(Continued)*

headache, fever, muscle pain, or some redness, pain, or swelling at injection site; consult prescriber if excessive or persisting.

Additional Information Federal law requires that the date of administration, the vaccine manufacturer, lot number of vaccine, and the administering person's name, title, and address be entered into the patient's permanent medical record.

The 2-dose regimen prompted antibody response consistent with a protective titer in up to 58% of patients. However, there are no clinical data evaluating whether vaccination protects patients against development of infection. Therefore, protection against a pandemic avian flu strain cannot be assured.

Special Geriatric Considerations No clinical studies in elderly have been done to date. Differences in immune response may be different than the titer response seen in younger adults.

Dosage Forms Injection, suspension [monovalent]: Hemagglutinin (H5N1 strain) 90 mcg/1 mL (5 mL) [contains thimerosal, and chicken, porcine, and egg proteins]

Selected References
Centers for Disease Control, "General Recommendations on Immunization. Recommendations of the Advisory Committee on Immunization Practices (ACIP)," *MMWR Recomm Rep*, 2006, 55(RR-15):1-48.
Treanor JJ, Campbell JD, Zangwill KM, et al, "Safety and Immunogenicity of an Inactivated Subvirion Influenza A (H5N1) Vaccine," *N Engl J Med*, 2006, 354(13):1343-51.

Insulin Aspart *(IN soo lin AS part)*

Related Information
Insulin Regular *on page 815*
Medication Safety Issues
Sound-alike/look-alike issues:
NovoLog® may be confused with Novolin®
NovoLog® Mix 70/30 may be confused with NovoLog®

High alert medication: The Institute for Safe Medication Practices (ISMP) includes this medication among its list of drugs which have a heightened risk of causing significant patient harm when used in error. *Due to the number of insulin preparations, it is essential to identify/clarify the type of insulin to be used.*

U.S. Brand Names NovoLog®
Canadian Brand Names NovoRapid®
Index Terms Aspart Insulin
Generic Available No
Pharmacologic Category Antidiabetic Agent, Insulin
Use Treatment of type 1 diabetes mellitus (insulin dependent, IDDM); type 2 diabetes mellitus (noninsulin dependent, NIDDM) to control hyperglycemia
Dosage
Geriatrics & Adults: Refer to Insulin Regular *on page 815*. Insulin aspart is a rapid-acting insulin analog which is normally administered as a premeal component of the insulin regimen. It is normally used along with a long-acting (basal) form of insulin.
SubQ: When used in a meal-related treatment regimen, 50% to 70% of total daily insulin requirement may be provided by insulin aspart and the remainder provided by an intermediate or long-acting insulin. Due to rapid onset and short duration, some patients may require more basal insulin to prevent premeal hypoglycemia when using insulin aspart as opposed to regular insulin.
SubQ infusion pump: ~50% of total dose given as meal related bolus and ~50% of total dose given as basal infusion; adjust dose as necessary
Renal Impairment: Insulin requirements are reduced due to changes in insulin clearance or metabolism. Close monitoring of blood glucose and adjustment of therapy is required in renal impairment.

Special Geriatric Considerations How "tightly" a geriatric patient's blood glucose should be controlled is controversial; however, a fasting blood sugar <150 mg/dL is now an acceptable endpoint. Such a decision should be based on the patient's functional and cognitive status, how well he/she recognizes hypoglycemic or hyperglycemic symptoms, and how to respond to them and any other disease states. Patients who are unable to accurately draw up their dose will need assistance such as prefilled syringes. Initial doses may require considerations for renal function in the elderly with dosing adjusted subsequently based on blood glucose monitoring.

Dosage Forms Excipient information presented when available (limited, particularly for generics); consult specific product labeling.

Injection, solution:

NovoLog®: 100 units/mL (3 mL) [FlexPen® prefilled syringe or PenFill® prefilled cartridge]; (10 mL) [vial]

♦ **Insulin Aspart and Insulin Aspart Protamine** *see* Insulin Aspart Protamine and Insulin Aspart *on page 809*

Insulin Aspart Protamine and Insulin Aspart
(IN soo lin AS part PROE ta meen & IN soo lin AS part)

Related Information
Insulin Regular *on page 815*

Medication Safety Issues

Sound-alike/look-alike issues:

NovoLog® Mix 70/30 may be confused with Novolin® 70/30

High alert medication: The Institute for Safe Medication Practices (ISMP) includes this medication among its list of drugs which have a heightened risk of causing significant patient harm when used in error. *Due to the number of insulin preparations, it is essential to identify/clarify the type of insulin to be used.*

U.S. Brand Names NovoLog® Mix 70/30

Canadian Brand Names NovoMix® 30

Index Terms Insulin Aspart and Insulin Aspart Protamine

Generic Available No

Pharmacologic Category Antidiabetic Agent, Insulin

Use Treatment of type 1 diabetes mellitus (insulin dependent, IDDM); type 2 diabetes mellitus (noninsulin dependent, NIDDM) to control hyperglycemia

Dosage

Geriatrics & Adults: Refer to Insulin Regular *on page 815*. Fixed ratio insulins (such as insulin aspart protamine and insulin aspart combination) are normally administered in 2 daily doses.

Renal Impairment: Insulin requirements are reduced due to changes in insulin clearance or metabolism.

Special Geriatric Considerations How "tightly" a geriatric patient's blood glucose should be controlled is controversial; however, a fasting blood sugar <150 mg/dL is now an acceptable endpoint. Such a decision should be based on the patient's functional and cognitive status, how well he/she recognizes hypoglycemic or hyperglycemic symptoms, and how to respond to them and any other disease states. Patients who are unable to accurately draw up their dose will need assistance such as prefilled syringes. Initial doses may require considerations for renal function in the elderly with dosing adjusted subsequently based on blood glucose monitoring.

Dosage Forms Excipient information presented when available (limited, particularly for generics); consult specific product labeling.

Injection, suspension:

NovoLog® Mix 70/30: Insulin aspart protamine suspension 70% [intermediate acting] and insulin aspart solution 30% [rapid acting]: 100 units/mL (3 mL) [PenFill® prefilled cartridge or FlexPen® prefilled syringe]; (10 mL) [vial]

Insulin Detemir (IN soo lin DE te mir)

Related Information
Insulin Regular *on page 815*

Medication Safety Issues

High alert medication: The Institute for Safe Medication Practices (ISMP) includes this medication among its list of drugs which have a heightened risk of causing significant patient harm when used in error. *Due to the number of insulin preparations, it is essential to identify/clarify the type of insulin to be used.*

Note: Insulin detemir is a clear solution, but it is NOT intended for I.V. or I.M. administration.

(Continued)

Insulin Detemir *(Continued)*

U.S. Brand Names Levemir®
Canadian Brand Names Levemir®
Index Terms Detemir Insulin
Generic Available No
Pharmacologic Category Antidiabetic Agent, Insulin
Use Treatment of type 1 diabetes mellitus (insulin dependent, IDDM); type 2 diabetes mellitus (noninsulin dependent, NIDDM) to control hyperglycemia
Dosage
  Geriatrics & Adults: Also refer to Insulin Regular *on page 815.*
    Note: Duration is dose-dependent. Dosage must be carefully titrated (adjustment of dose and timing. Adjustment of concomitant antidiabetic treatment (short-acting insulins or oral antidiabetic agents) may be required.
    Type 1 or type 2 diabetes:
      Basal insulin or basal-bolus: May be substituted on a unit-per-unit basis. Adjust dose to achieve glycemic targets.
      Insulin-naive patients (type 2 diabetes only): 0.1-0.2 units/kg once daily in the evening or 10 units once or twice daily. Adjust dose to achieve glycemic targets. Note: Canadian labeling recommends 10 units once daily (twice daily dosing is not included).
  Renal Impairment: Insulin requirements are reduced due to changes in insulin clearance or metabolism.
  Special Geriatric Considerations How "tightly" a geriatric patient's blood glucose should be controlled is controversial; however, a fasting blood sugar <150 mg/dL is now an acceptable endpoint. Such a decision should be based on the patient's functional and cognitive status, how well he/she recognizes hypoglycemic or hyperglycemic symptoms, and how to respond to them and any other disease states. Patients who are unable to accurately draw up their dose will need assistance such as prefilled syringes. Initial doses may require considerations for renal function in the elderly with dosing adjusted subsequently based on blood glucose monitoring.
  Dosage Forms Excipient information presented when available (limited, particularly for generics); consult specific product labeling.
    Injection, solution: Levemir®: 100 units/mL (3 mL) [FlexPen® prefilled syringe]; (10 mL) [vial]

Insulin Glargine *(IN soo lin GLAR jeen)*

Related Information
  Insulin Regular *on page 815*
Medication Safety Issues
  Sound-alike/look-alike issues:
    Lantus® may be confused with Lente®
    Lente® may be confused with Lantus®
  High alert medication: The Institute for Safe Medication Practices (ISMP) includes this medication among its list of drugs which have a heightened risk of causing significant patient harm when used in error. *Due to the number of insulin preparations, it is essential to identify/clarify the type of insulin to be used.*
U.S. Brand Names Lantus®
Canadian Brand Names Lantus®; Lantus® OptiSet®
Index Terms Glargine Insulin
Generic Available No
Pharmacologic Category Antidiabetic Agent, Insulin
Use Treatment of type 1 diabetes mellitus (insulin dependent, IDDM); type 2 diabetes mellitus (noninsulin dependent, NIDDM) requiring basal (long-acting) insulin to control hyperglycemia
Dosage
  Geriatrics & Adults: SubQ
    Type 1 diabetes: Refer to Insulin Regular *on page 815.*
    Type 2 diabetes:
      Patient not already on insulin: 10 units once daily, adjusted according to patient response (range in clinical study: 2-100 units/day)
      Patient already receiving insulin: In clinical studies, when changing to insulin glargine from once-daily NPH or Ultralente® insulin, the initial dose was not changed; when changing from twice-daily NPH to once-daily insulin glargine, the total daily dose was reduced by 20% and adjusted according to patient response
  Renal Impairment: Insulin requirements are reduced due to changes in insulin clearance or metabolism.
  Dosage Forms Excipient information presented when available (limited, particularly for generics); consult specific product labeling.
    Injection, solution: Lantus®: 100 units/mL (3 mL) [cartridge]; (10 mL) [vial]

Insulin Glulisine (IN soo lin gloo LIS een)

Related Information
Insulin Regular *on page 815*

Medication Safety Issues
High alert medication: The Institute for Safe Medication Practices (ISMP) includes this medication among its list of drugs which have a heightened risk of causing significant patient harm when used in error. *Due to the number of insulin preparations, it is essential to identify/clarify the type of insulin to be used.*

U.S. Brand Names Apidra®

Canadian Brand Names Apidra®

Index Terms Glulisine Insulin

Generic Available No

Pharmacologic Category Antidiabetic Agent, Insulin

Use Treatment of type 1 diabetes mellitus (insulin dependent, IDDM); type 2 diabetes mellitus (noninsulin dependent, NIDDM) to control hyperglycemia

Dosage
Geriatrics & Adults: Refer to Insulin Regular *on page 815*. Insulin glulisine is a rapid-acting insulin analog which is normally administered as a premeal component of the insulin regimen. It is normally used along with a long-acting (basal) form of insulin.

SubQ: When used in a meal-related treatment regimen, 50% to 70% of total daily insulin requirement may be provided by insulin glulisine (in divided doses) and the remainder provided by an intermediate or long-acting insulin. Insulin glulisine may also be administered by external subcutaneous infusion pumps.

I.V.: Under close medical supervision, insulin glulisine may be administered by infusion.

Renal Impairment: Insulin requirements are reduced due to changes in insulin clearance or metabolism. Close monitoring of blood glucose and adjustment of therapy is required in renal impairment.

Special Geriatric Considerations How "tightly" a geriatric patient's blood glucose should be controlled is controversial; however, a fasting blood sugar <150 mg/dL is now an acceptable endpoint. Such a decision should be based on the patient's functional and cognitive status, how well he/she recognizes hypoglycemic or hyperglycemic symptoms, and how to respond to them and any other disease states. Patients who are unable to accurately draw up their dose will need assistance such as prefilled syringes. Initial doses may require considerations for renal function in the elderly with dosing adjusted subsequently based on blood glucose monitoring.

Dosage Forms Excipient information presented when available (limited, particularly for generics); consult specific product labeling.
Injection, solution:
Apidra®: 100 units/mL (3 mL [cartridge], 10 mL [vial])

Insulin Inhalation (IN soo lin in ha LAY shun)

Related Information
Insulin Regular *on page 815*

Medication Safety Issues
High alert medication: The Institute for Safe Medication Practices (ISMP) includes this medication among its list of drugs which have a heightened risk of causing significant patient harm when used in error. *Due to the number of insulin preparations, it is essential to identify/clarify the type of insulin to be used. The inhalation form of insulin is expressed in milligrams rather than units, potentially leading to confusion. Absolute conversion between doses of inhalation and injection insulin is not possible.*

U.S. Brand Names Exubera®

Canadian Brand Names Exubera®

Index Terms Inhaled Insulin

Pharmacologic Category Antidiabetic Agent, Insulin

Use Treatment of type 1 diabetes mellitus (insulin dependent, IDDM); type 2 diabetes mellitus (noninsulin dependent, NIDDM)

Restrictions An FDA-approved medication guide must be distributed when dispensing an outpatient prescription (new or refill) where this medication is to be used without direct supervision of a healthcare provider. Medication guides are available at http://www.fda.gov/cder/Offices/ODS/medication_guides.htm.
(Continued)

Insulin Inhalation *(Continued)*

Dosage

Geriatrics & Adults: Diabetes mellitus (type 1 or 2): Inhalation:

Initial: 0.05 mg/kg (rounded down to nearest whole milligram) 3 times/daily administered within 10 minutes of a meal

Adjustment: Dosage may be increased or decreased based on serum glucose monitoring, meal size, nutrient composition, time of day, and exercise patterns.

Note: A 1 mg blister is approximately equivalent to 3 units of regular insulin, while a 3 mg blister is approximately equivalent to 8 units of regular insulin administered subcutaneously. Patients should combine 1 mg and 3 mg blisters so that the fewest blisters are required to achieve the prescribed dose. Consecutive inhalation of three 1 mg blisters results in significantly higher insulin levels as compared to inhalation of a single 3 mg blister (do not substitute). In a patient stabilized on a dosage which uses 3 mg blisters, if 3 mg blister is temporarily unavailable, inhalation of two 1 mg blisters may be substituted.

Renal Impairment: Insulin requirements are reduced due to changes in insulin clearance or metabolism.

Special Geriatric Considerations How "tightly" a geriatric patient's blood glucose should be controlled is controversial; however, a fasting blood sugar <150 mg/dL is now an acceptable endpoint. Such a decision should be based on the patient's functional and cognitive status, how well he/she recognizes hypoglycemic or hyperglycemic symptoms, and how to respond to them and any other disease states. Patients who are unable to accurately draw up their dose will need assistance, such as prefilled syringes. Initial doses may require considerations for renal function in the elderly with dosing adjusted subsequently based on blood glucose monitoring.

The manufacturer reports that 266 patients with diabetes ≥65 years of age, including 30 subjects ≥75 years were included in the Phase 2/3 clinical trials. Clinical response, measured as a change in hemoglobin A_{1c}, and the rate of hypoglycemia did not differ from younger patients with diabetes.

Prior to being prescribed inhaled insulin, elderly patients with type 2 diabetes must demonstrate the ability to prepare and administer their dose.

Dosage Forms Excipient information presented when available (limited, particularly for generics); consult specific product labeling.

Combination package:

Exubera® Kit [packaged with inhaler, chamber and release unit]:

Powder for oral inhalation [prefilled blister pack]: 1 mg/blister (180s)

Powder for oral inhalation [prefilled blister pack]: 3 mg/blister (90s)

Exubera® Combination Pack 15 [packaged with 2 release units]:

Powder for oral inhalation [prefilled blister pack]: 1 mg/blister (180s)

Powder for oral inhalation [prefilled blister pack]: 3 mg/blister (90s)

Exubera® Combination Pack 12 [packaged with 2 release units]:

Powder for oral inhalation [prefilled blister pack]: 1 mg/blister (90s)

Powder for oral inhalation [prefilled blister pack]: 3 mg/blister (90s)

Insulin Lispro *(IN soo lin LYE sproe)*

Related Information

Insulin Regular *on page 815*

Medication Safety Issues

Sound-alike/look-alike issues:

Humalog® may be confused with Humulin®, Humira®

High alert medication: The Institute for Safe Medication Practices (ISMP) includes this medication among its list of drugs which have a heightened risk of causing significant patient harm when used in error. *Due to the number of insulin preparations, it is essential to identify/clarify the type of insulin to be used.*

U.S. Brand Names Humalog®

Canadian Brand Names Humalog®

Index Terms Lispro Insulin

Generic Available No

Pharmacologic Category Antidiabetic Agent, Insulin

Use Treatment of type 1 diabetes mellitus (insulin dependent, IDDM); type 2 diabetes mellitus (noninsulin dependent, NIDDM) to control hyperglycemia

Note: In type 1 diabetes mellitus (insulin dependent, IDDM), insulin lispro (Humalog®) should be used in combination with a long-acting insulin. However, in type 2 diabetes mellitus (noninsulin dependent, NIDDM), insulin lispro (Humalog®) may be used without a long-acting insulin when used in combination with a sulfonylurea.

Dosage

Geriatrics & Adults: Refer to Insulin Regular *on page 815*. Insulin lispro is equipotent to insulin regular, but has a more rapid onset.

Renal Impairment: Insulin requirements are reduced due to changes in insulin clearance or metabolism. Close monitoring of blood glucose and adjustment of therapy is required in renal impairment.

Special Geriatric Considerations How "tightly" a geriatric patient's blood glucose should be controlled is controversial; however, a fasting blood sugar <150 mg/dL is now an acceptable endpoint. Such a decision should be based on the patient's functional and cognitive status, how well he/she recognizes hypoglycemic or hyperglycemic symptoms, and how to respond to them and any other disease states. Patients who are unable to accurately draw up their dose will need assistance such as prefilled syringes. Initial doses may require considerations for renal function in the elderly with dosing adjusted subsequently based on blood glucose monitoring.

Dosage Forms Excipient information presented when available (limited, particularly for generics); consult specific product labeling.

Injection, solution:

Humalog®: 100 units/mL (3 mL) [prefilled cartridge or prefilled disposable pen]; (10 mL) [vial]

♦ **Insulin Lispro and Insulin Lispro Protamine** *see* Insulin Lispro Protamine and Insulin Lispro *on page 813*

Insulin Lispro Protamine and Insulin Lispro
(IN soo lin LYE sproe PROE ta meen & IN soo lin LYE sproe)

Related Information
Insulin Regular *on page 815*

Medication Safety Issues
Sound-alike/look-alike issues:

Humalog® Mix 75/25™ may be confused with Humulin® 70/30.

High alert medication: The Institute for Safe Medication Practices (ISMP) includes this medication among its list of drugs which have a heightened risk of causing significant patient harm when used in error. ***Due to the number of insulin preparations, it is essential to identify/clarify the type of insulin to be used.***

U.S. Brand Names Humalog® Mix 50/50™; Humalog® Mix 75/25™

Canadian Brand Names Humalog® Mix 25

Index Terms Insulin Lispro and Insulin Lispro Protamine

Generic Available No

Pharmacologic Category Antidiabetic Agent, Insulin

Use Treatment of type 1 diabetes mellitus (insulin dependent, IDDM); type 2 diabetes mellitus (noninsulin dependent, NIDDM) to control hyperglycemia

Dosage

Geriatrics & Adults: Refer to Insulin Regular *on page 815*. Fixed ratio insulins (such as insulin lispro protamine and insulin lispro) are normally administered in 2 daily doses.

Renal Impairment: Insulin requirements are reduced due to changes in insulin clearance or metabolism.

Dosage Forms Excipient information presented when available (limited, particularly for generics); consult specific product labeling.

Injection, suspension:

Humalog® Mix 50/50™: Insulin lispro protamine suspension 50% [intermediate acting] and insulin lispro solution 50% [rapid acting]: 100 units/mL (3 mL) [disposable pen]

Humalog® Mix 75/25™: Insulin lispro protamine suspension 75% [intermediate acting] and insulin lispro solution 25% [rapid acting]: 100 units/mL (3 mL) [disposable pen]; (10 mL) [vial]

Insulin NPH (IN soo lin N P H)

Related Information
Insulin Regular *on page 815*

Medication Safety Issues
Sound-alike/look-alike issues:

Humulin® may be confused with Humalog®, Humira®

Novolin® may be confused with NovoLog®

High alert medication: The Institute for Safe Medication Practices (ISMP) includes this medication among its list of drugs which have a heightened risk of causing significant patient harm when used in error. ***Due to the number of insulin preparations, it is essential to identify/clarify the type of insulin to be used.***

(Continued)

Insulin NPH *(Continued)*

U.S. Brand Names Humulin® N; Novolin® N

Canadian Brand Names Humulin® N; Novolin® ge NPH

Index Terms Isophane Insulin; NPH Insulin

Generic Available No

Pharmacologic Category Antidiabetic Agent, Insulin

Use Treatment of type 1 diabetes mellitus (insulin dependent, IDDM); type 2 diabetes mellitus (noninsulin dependent, NIDDM) to control hyperglycemia

Dosage

Geriatrics & Adults: Refer to Insulin Regular *on page 815*. Insulin NPH is usually administered 1-2 times daily.

Renal Impairment: Insulin requirements are reduced due to changes in insulin clearance or metabolism.

Special Geriatric Considerations How "tightly" a geriatric patient's blood glucose should be controlled is controversial; however, a fasting blood sugar <150 mg/dL is now an acceptable endpoint. Such a decision should be based on the patient's functional and cognitive status, how well he/she recognizes hypoglycemic or hyperglycemic symptoms, and how to respond to them and any other disease states. Patients who are unable to accurately draw up their dose will need assistance such as prefilled syringes. Initial doses may require considerations for renal function in the elderly with dosing adjusted subsequently based on blood glucose monitoring.

Dosage Forms Excipient information presented when available (limited, particularly for generics); consult specific product labeling. [CAN] = Canadian brand name

Injection, suspension:

Humulin® N: 100 units/mL (3 mL) [disposable pen]; (10 mL) [vial]

Novolin® ge NPH [CAN]: 100 units/mL (3 mL) [NovolinSet® prefilled syringe or PenFill® prefilled cartridge]; 10 mL [vial]

Novolin® N: 100 units/mL (3 mL) [InnoLet® prefilled syringe or PenFill® prefilled cartridge]; (10 mL) [vial]

Insulin NPH and Insulin Regular
(IN soo lin N P H & IN soo lin REG yoo ler)

Related Information

Insulin Regular *on page 815*

Medication Safety Issues

Sound-alike/look-alike issues:

Humulin® 70/30 may be confused with Humalog® Mix 75/25

Novolin® 70/30 may be confused with NovoLog® Mix 70/30

High alert medication: The Institute for Safe Medication Practices (ISMP) includes this medication among its list of drugs which have a heightened risk of causing significant patient harm when used in error. *Due to the number of insulin preparations, it is essential to identify/clarify the type of insulin to be used.*

U.S. Brand Names Humulin® 50/50; Humulin® 70/30; Novolin® 70/30

Canadian Brand Names Humulin® 20/80; Humulin® 70/30; Novolin® ge 10/90; Novolin® ge 20/80; Novolin® ge 30/70; Novolin® ge 40/60; Novolin® ge 50/50

Index Terms Insulin Regular and Insulin NPH; Isophane Insulin and Regular Insulin; NPH Insulin and Regular Insulin

Generic Available No

Pharmacologic Category Antidiabetic Agent, Insulin

Use Treatment of type 1 diabetes mellitus (insulin dependent, IDDM); type 2 diabetes mellitus (noninsulin dependent, NIDDM) to control hyperglycemia

Dosage

Geriatrics & Adults:

Refer to Insulin Regular *on page 815*. Fixed ratio insulins are normally administered in 1-2 daily doses.

Dosage Forms Excipient information presented when available (limited, particularly for generics); consult specific product labeling.

Injection, suspension:

Humulin® 50/50: Insulin NPH suspension 50% [intermediate acting] and insulin regular solution 50% [short acting]: 100 units/mL (10 mL) [vial]

Humulin® 70/30: Insulin NPH suspension 70% [intermediate acting] and insulin regular solution 30% [short acting]: 100 units/mL (3 mL) [disposable pen]; (10 mL) [vial]

Novolin® 70/30: Insulin NPH suspension 70% [intermediate acting] and insulin regular solution 30% [short acting]: 100 units/mL (3 mL) [InnoLet® prefilled syringe or PenFill® prefilled cartridge]; (10 mL) [vial]

Additional formulations available in Canada: Injection, suspension:

Humulin® 20/80: Insulin regular solution 20% [short acting] and insulin NPH suspension 80% [intermediate acting]: 100 units/mL (3 mL) [PenFill® prefilled cartridge]

Novolin® ge 10/90: Insulin regular solution 10% [short acting] and insulin NPH suspension 90% [intermediate acting]: 100 units/mL (3 mL) [PenFill® prefilled cartridge]

Novolin® ge 20/80: Insulin regular solution 20% [short acting] and insulin NPH suspension 80% [intermediate acting]: 100 units/mL (3 mL) [PenFill® prefilled cartridge]

Novolin® ge 30/70: Insulin regular solution 30% [short acting] and insulin NPH suspension 70% [intermediate acting]: 100 units/mL (3 mL) [prefilled syringe or PenFill® prefilled cartridge]; (10 mL) [vial]

Novolin® ge 40/60: Insulin regular solution 40% [short acting] and insulin NPH suspension 60% [intermediate acting]: 100 units/mL (3 mL) [PenFill® prefilled cartridge]

Novolin® ge 50/50: Insulin regular solution 50% [short acting] and insulin NPH suspension 50% [intermediate acting]: 100 units/mL (3 mL) [PenFill® prefilled cartridge]

Insulin Regular (IN soo lin REG yoo ler)

Related Information
Insulin Aspart *on page 808*
Insulin Aspart Protamine and Insulin Aspart *on page 809*
Insulin Detemir *on page 809*
Insulin Glargine *on page 810*
Insulin Glulisine *on page 811*
Insulin Inhalation *on page 811*
Insulin Lispro *on page 812*
Insulin Lispro Protamine and Insulin Lispro *on page 813*
Insulin NPH *on page 813*
Insulin NPH and Insulin Regular *on page 814*

Medication Safety Issues
Sound-alike/look-alike issues:
Humulin® may be confused with Humalog®, Humira®
Novolin® may be confused with NovoLog®

High alert medication: The Institute for Safe Medication Practices (ISMP) includes this medication among its list of drugs which have a heightened risk of causing significant patient harm when used in error. *Due to the number of insulin preparations, it is essential to identify/clarify the type of insulin to be used.*

Concentrated solutions (eg, U-500) should not be available in patient care areas.

U.S. Brand Names Humulin® R; Humulin® R (Concentrated) U-500; Novolin® R

Canadian Brand Names Humulin® R; Novolin® ge Toronto

Index Terms Regular Insulin

Generic Available No

Pharmacologic Category Antidiabetic Agent, Insulin; Antidote

Use Treatment of type 1 diabetes mellitus (insulin dependent, IDDM); type 2 diabetes mellitus (noninsulin dependent, NIDDM) unresponsive to treatment with diet and/or oral hypoglycemics; to control hyperglycemia; adjunct to parenteral nutrition; diabetic ketoacidosis (DKA)

Unlabeled/Investigational Use Hyperkalemia (regular insulin only; use with glucose to shift potassium into cells to lower serum potassium levels)

Contraindications Hypersensitivity to any component of the formulation

Warnings/Precautions Hypoglycemia is the most common adverse effect of insulin. The timing of hypoglycemia differs among various insulin formulations. Hypoglycemia may result from increased work or exercise without eating; use of long-acting insulin preparations (insulin glargine, Ultralente®, insulin U) may delay recovery from hypoglycemia. Insulin requirements may be altered during illness, emotional disturbances or other stresses. Use with caution in renal or hepatic impairment.

Human insulin differs from animal-source insulin. Any change of insulin should be made cautiously; changing manufacturers, type, and/or method of manufacture may result in the need for a change of dosage.

Regular insulin is the only insulin to be used intravenously. Insulin aspart may also be administered I.V. in selected clinical situations to control hyperglycemia; close medical supervision is required.

The general objective of insulin replacement therapy is to approximate the physiologic pattern of insulin secretion. This requires a basal level of insulin throughout the day, supplemented by additional insulin at mealtimes. Since combinations of agents are frequently used, dosage adjustment must address the individual component of the (Continued)

Insulin Regular *(Continued)*

insulin regimen which most directly influences the blood glucose value in question, based on the known onset and duration of the insulin component. The frequency of doses and monitoring must be individualized in consideration of the patient's ability to manage therapy. Diabetic education and nutritional counseling are essential to maximize the effectiveness of therapy.

In type 1 diabetes mellitus (insulin dependent, IDDM), insulin lispro (Humalog®) and insulin glulisine (Apidra™) should be used in combination with a long-acting insulin. However, in type 2 diabetes mellitus (noninsulin dependent, NIDDM), insulin lispro (Humalog®) may be used without a long-acting insulin when used in combination with a sulfonylurea.

Adverse Reactions (Reflective of adult population; not specific for elderly)
Frequency not defined.

Cardiovascular: Palpitation, pallor, tachycardia

Central nervous system: Fatigue, headache, hypothermia, loss of consciousness, mental confusion

Dermatologic: Urticaria, redness

Endocrine & metabolic: Hypoglycemia

Gastrointestinal: Hunger, nausea, numbness of mouth

Local: Atrophy or hypertrophy of SubQ fat tissue; edema, itching, pain or warmth at injection site; stinging

Neuromuscular & skeletal: Muscle weakness, paresthesia, tremor

Ocular: Transient presbyopia or blurred vision

Miscellaneous: Anaphylaxis, diaphoresis, local allergy, systemic allergic symptoms

Overdosage/Toxicology Symptoms of overdose include tachycardia, anxiety, hunger, tremor, pallor, headache, motor dysfunction, speech disturbances, sweating, palpitations, coma, and death. Antidote is glucose (15-20 g) and glucagon, if necessary. Retest plasma glucose ~15 minutes after administration of glucose; additional treatment may be needed.

Drug Interactions Induces CYP1A2 (weak)

Drugs which **DECREASE** hypoglycemic effect of insulin:

Contraceptives (oral), corticosteroids, dextrothyroxine, diltiazem, dobutamine, epinephrine, niacin, smoking, thiazide diuretics, thyroid hormone

Drugs which **INCREASE** hypoglycemic effect of insulin:

Alcohol, alpha-blockers, anabolic steroids, beta-blockers (see "Note", clofibrate, guanethidine, MAO inhibitors, pentamidine, phenylbutazone, salicylates, sulfinpyrazone, tetracyclines. **Note:** Nonselective beta-blockers may delay recovery from hypoglycemic episodes and mask signs/symptoms of hypoglycemia. Cardioselective agents may be alternatives.

Insulin increases the risk of hypoglycemia associated with oral hypoglycemic agents (including sulfonylureas, metformin, pioglitazone, rosiglitazone, and troglitazone).

Ethanol/Nutrition/Herb Interactions

Ethanol: Caution with ethanol (may increase hypoglycemia).

Food: Insulin shifts potassium from extracellular to intracellular space. Decreases potassium serum concentration.

Herb/Nutraceutical: Use caution with chromium, garlic, gymnema (may increase hypoglycemia).

Stability Insulin, regular (Humulin® R, Novolin® R): Store unopened containers in refrigerator at 2°C to 8°C (36°F to 46°F); do not freeze. Vial in use may be stored under refrigeration or at room temperature; store below 30°C (86°F) away from direct heat or light. Regular insulin should only be used if clear.

Note: Standard diluent for regular insulin: 100 units/100 mL NS; all bags should be prepared fresh; tubing should be flushed 30 minutes prior to administration to allow adsorption as time permits. Can be given as a more diluted solution (eg, 100 units/250 mL 0.45% NS).

Mechanism of Action Insulin acts via specific membrane-bound receptors on target tissues to regulate metabolism of carbohydrate, protein, and fats. Insulin facilitates entry of glucose into muscle, adipose, and other tissues via hexose transporters, including GLUT4. Insulin stimulates the cellular uptake of amino acids and increases cellular permeability to several ions, including potassium, magnesium, and phosphate. By activating sodium-potassium ATPases, insulin promotes the intracellular movement of potassium.

Target organs for insulin include the liver, skeletal muscle, and adipose tissue. Within the liver, insulin stimulates hepatic glycogen synthesis through the activation of the enzymes hexokinase, phosphofructokinase, and glycogen synthase as well as the inhibition of glucose-6 phosphatase. Insulin promotes hepatic synthesis of fatty acids, which are released into the circulation as lipoproteins. Skeletal muscle effects of insulin include increased protein synthesis and increased glycogen synthesis. Within adipose tissue, insulin stimulates the processing of circulating lipoproteins to provide free fatty acids, facilitating triglyceride synthesis and storage by adipocytes. Insulin also directly inhibits the hydrolysis of triglycerides.

Normally secreted by the pancreas, insulin products are manufactured for pharmacologic use through recombinant DNA technology using either *E. coli* or *Saccharomyces cerevisiae*. Insulins are categorized based on promptness and duration of effect, including rapid-, short-, intermediate-, and long-acting insulins.

Pharmacodynamics
Onset of action: 0.5 hours
Duration of action: 6-8 hours (may increase with dose)

Pharmacokinetics
Time to peak: 2-4 hours
Excretion: Urine

Dosage
Geriatrics & Adults: SubQ (regular insulin may also be administered I.V.): The number and size of daily doses, time of administration, and diet and exercise require continuous medical supervision. In addition, specific formulations may require distinct administration procedures (see Administration).

Type 1 Diabetes Mellitus: Note: Multiple daily doses guided by blood glucose monitoring are the standard of diabetes care. Combinations of insulin are commonly used.

Initial dose: 0.2-0.6 unit/kg/day in divided doses. Conservative initial doses of 0.2-0.4 units/kg/day are often recommended to avoid the potential for hypoglycemia.

Division of daily insulin requirement: Generally, 50% to 75% of the daily insulin dose is given as an intermediate- or long-acting form of insulin (in 1-2 daily injections). The remaining portion of the 24-hour insulin requirement is divided and administered as a rapid-acting or short-acting form of insulin. These may be given with meals (before or at the time of meals depending on the form of insulin) or at the same time as injections of intermediate forms (some premixed combinations are intended for this purpose).

Adjustment of dose: Dosage must be titrated to achieve glucose control and avoid hypoglycemia. Adjust dose to maintain premeal and bedtime glucose of 80-140 mg/dL. Since combinations of agents are frequently used, dosage adjustment must address the individual component of the insulin regimen which most directly influences the blood glucose value in question, based on the known onset and duration of the insulin component. Also see Additional Information.

Usual maintenance range: 0.5-1.2 units/kg/day in divided doses. An estimate of anticipated needs may be based on body weight and/or activity factors as follows:
Nonobese: 0.4-0.6 units/kg/day
Obese: 0.8-1.2 units/kg/day
Renal failure: Due to alterations in pharmacokinetics of insulin, may require <0.2 units/kg/day

Type 2 Diabetes Mellitus:
Augmentation therapy: Dosage must be carefully adjusted.
Insulins other than glargine: Initial dosage of 0.15-0.2 units/kg/day have been recommended
Insulin glargine: Initial dose: 10 units/day
Note: Administered when residual beta-cell function is present, as a supplemental agent when oral hypoglycemics have not achieved goal glucose control. Twice daily NPH, or an evening dose of NPH, lente, or glargine insulin may be added to oral therapy with metformin or a sulfonylurea. Augmentation to control postprandial glucose may be accomplished with regular, glulisine, aspart, or lispro insulin.

Monotherapy: Initial dose: Highly variable: See Augmentation therapy dosing.
Note: An empirically-defined scheme for dosage estimation based on fasting plasma glucose and degree of obesity has been published with recommended doses ranging from 6-77 units/day (Holman, 1995). In the setting of glucose toxicity (loss of beta-cell sensitivity to glucose concentrations), insulin therapy may be used for short-term management to restore sensitivity of beta-cells; in these cases, the dose may need to be rapidly reduced/withdrawn when sensitivity is re-established.

Hyperkalemia (unlabeled use): I.V.: Administer dextrose at 0.5-1 mL/kg and regular insulin 1 unit for every 4-5 g dextrose given

Diabetic ketoacidosis:
I.V.: Regular insulin 0.15 units/kg initially followed by an infusion of 0.1 units/kg/hour
SubQ, I.M.: Regular insulin 0.4 units/kg given half as I.V. bolus and half as SubQ or I.M., followed by 0.1 units/kg/hour SubQ or I.M.
(Continued)

Insulin Regular *(Continued)*

If serum glucose does not fall by 50-70 mg/dL in the first hour, double insulin dose hourly until glucose falls at an hourly rate of 50-70 mg/dL. Decrease dose to 0.05-0.1 units/kg/hour once serum glucose reaches 250 mg/dL.

Note: Newly-diagnosed patients with IDDM presenting in DKA and patients with blood sugars <800 mg/dL may be relatively "sensitive" to insulin and should receive loading and initial maintenance doses ~50% of those indicated.

Infusion should continue until reversal of acid-base derangement/ketonemia. Serum glucose is not a direct indicator of these abnormalities, and may decrease more rapidly than correction of the range of metabolic abnormalities.

Renal Impairment: Insulin requirements are reduced due to changes in insulin clearance or metabolism. Close monitoring of blood glucose and adjustment of therapy is required in renal impairment.

Cl_{cr} 10-50 mL/minute: Administer 75% of normal dose.

Cl_{cr} <10 mL/minute: Administer 25% to 50% of normal dose and monitor glucose closely.

Hemodialysis: Because of a large molecular weight (6000 daltons), insulin is not significantly removed by either peritoneal or hemodialysis.

Supplemental dose is not necessary.

Peritoneal dialysis: Supplemental dose is not necessary.

Continuous arteriovenous or venovenous hemofiltration effects: Supplemental dose is not necessary.

Administration

SubQ administration: Cold injections should be avoided. SubQ administration is usually made into the thighs, arms, buttocks, or abdomen, with sites rotated. When mixing regular insulin with other preparations of insulin, regular insulin should be drawn into syringe first. Except for rapid-acting, short-acting, or insulin glargine, gently roll vial or pen in the palms of the hands to resuspend before using. When rapid-acting insulin is mixed with an intermediate or long-acting insulin, it should be administered within 15 minutes before a meal.

Human regular insulin: Should be administered within 30-60 minutes before a meal; may be administered by SubQ, I.M., or I.V. routes

I.V. administration (requires use of an infusion pump): **Only regular insulin** may be administered I.V.

I.V. infusions: To minimize adsorption problems to I.V. solution bag:

If new tubing is **not** needed: Wait a minimum of 30 minutes between the preparation of the solution and the initiation of the infusion

If new tubing is needed: After receiving the insulin drip solution, the administration set should be attached to the I.V. container and the line should be flushed with the insulin solution. The nurse should then wait 30 minutes, then flush the line again with the insulin solution prior to initiating the infusion

If insulin is required prior to the availability of the insulin drip, regular insulin should be administered by I.V. push injection

Because of adsorption, the actual amount of insulin being administered could be substantially less than the apparent amount. Therefore, adjustment of the insulin drip rate should be based on effect and not solely on the apparent insulin dose. Furthermore, the apparent dose should not be used as the basis for determining the subsequent insulin dose upon discontinuing the insulin drip. Dose requires continuous medical supervision.

Monitoring Parameters Urine sugar and acetone, serum glucose, electrolytes, Hb A_{1c}, lipid profile

DKA: Arterial blood gases, CBC with differential, urinalysis, serum glucose (baseline and every hour until reaches 250 mg/dL), BUN, creatinine, electrolytes, anion gap

Reference Range

Therapeutic, serum insulin (fasting): 5-20 µIU/mL (SI: 35-145 pmol/L)

Glucose, fasting:

Newborns: 60-110 mg/dL

Adults: 60-110 mg/dL

Elderly: 100-180 mg/dL

Recommendations for glycemic control, adults with type 1 diabetes:

Hb A_{1c}: <7%

Preprandial capillary plasma glucose: 90-130 mg/dL

Peak postprandial capillary blood glucose: <180 mg/dL

Blood pressure: <130/80 mm Hg

Criteria for diagnosis of DKA:

Serum glucose: >250 mg/dL

Arterial pH: <7.3

Bicarbonate: <15 mEq/L

Moderate ketonuria or ketonemia

Patient Information Do not take any new medication during therapy unless approved by prescriber. This medication is used to control diabetes; it is not a cure. It is imperative to follow other components of prescribed treatment (eg, diet and exercise regimen). Take exactly as directed. Do not change dose or discontinue unless advised by prescriber. With insulin aspart (NovoLog®), you must start eating within 5-10 minutes after injection. Insulin glulisine (Apidra™) should be administered within 15 minutes before or within 20 minutes after start of meal. If you experience hypoglycemic reaction, contact prescriber immediately. Always carry quick source of sugar with you. Monitor glucose levels as directed by prescriber. Report adverse side effects, including chest pain or palpitations; persistent fatigue, confusion, headache; skin rash or redness; numbness of mouth, lips, or tongue; muscle weakness or tremors; vision changes; respiratory difficulty; or nausea, vomiting, or flu-like symptoms.

Additional Information

Split-mixed or basal-bolus regimens: Combination regimens which exploit differences in the onset and duration of different insulin products are commonly used to approximate physiologic secretion. In split-mixed regimens, an intermediate-acting insulin (such as NPH insulin) is administered once or twice daily and supplemented by short-acting (regular) or rapid-acting (lispro, aspart, or glulisine) insulin. Blood glucose measurements are completed several times daily. Dosages are adjusted emphasizing the individual component of the regimen which most directly influences the blood sugar in question (either the intermediate-acting component or the shorter-acting component). Fixed-ratio formulations (eg, 70/30 mix) may be used as twice daily injections in this scenario; however, the ability to titrate the dosage of an individual component is limited. A example of a "split-mixed" regimen would be 21 units of NPH plus 9 units of regular in the morning and an evening meal dose consisting of 14 units of NPH plus 6 units of regular insulin.

Basal-bolus regimens are designed to more closely mimic physiologic secretion. These employ a long-acting insulin (eg, glargine) to simulate basal insulin secretion. The basal component is frequently administered at bedtime or in the early morning. This is supplemented by multiple daily injections of very rapid-acting products (lispro or aspart) immediately prior to a meal, which provides insulin at the time when nutrients are absorbed. An example of basal-bolus regimen would be 30 units of glargine at bedtime and 12 units of lispro insulin prior to each meal.

Estimation of the effect per unit: A "Rule of 1500" has been frequently used as a means to estimate the change in blood sugar relative to each unit of insulin administered. In fact, the recommended values used in these calculations may vary from 1500-2200 (a value of at least 1800 is recommended for lispro). The higher values lead to more conservative estimates of the effect per unit of insulin, and therefore lead to more cautious adjustments. The effect per unit of insulin is approximated by dividing the selected numerical value (eg, 1500-2200) by the number of units/day received by the patient. This may be used as a crude approximation of the patient's insulin sensitivity as adjustments to individual components of the regimen are made. Each additional unit of insulin added to the corresponding insulin dose may be expected to lower the blood glucose by this amount.

To illustrate, in the "basal-bolus" regimen example presented above, the rule of 1800 would indicate an expected change of 27 mg/dL per unit of lispro insulin (the total daily insulin dose is 66 units; using the formula: 1800/66 = 27). A patient may be instructed to add additional insulin if the preprandial glucose is >125 mg/dL. For a prelunch glucose of 195 mg/dL, this would mean the patient would administer the scheduled 12 units of lispro along with an additional "correctional" 3 units for a total of 15 units prior to the meal. If correctional doses are required on a consistent basis, an adjustment of the patients diet and/or scheduled insulin dose may be necessary.

Special Geriatric Considerations How "tightly" a geriatric patient's blood glucose should be controlled is controversial; however, a fasting blood sugar <150 mg/dL is now an acceptable endpoint. Such a decision should be based on the patient's functional and cognitive status, how well he/she recognizes hypoglycemic or hyperglycemic symptoms, and how to respond to them and any other disease states. Patients who are unable to accurately draw up their dose will need assistance such as prefilled syringes. Initial doses may require considerations for renal function in the elderly with dosing adjusted subsequently based on blood glucose monitoring.

Dosage Forms Excipient information presented when available (limited, particularly for generics); consult specific product labeling.

Injection, solution:

Humulin® R: 100 units/mL (10 mL) [vial]

Novolin® R: 100 units/mL (3 mL) [InnoLet® prefilled syringe or PenFill® prefilled cartridge]; (10 mL) [vial]

Injection, solution [concentrate]:

Humulin® R U-500: 500 units/mL (20 mL vial)

Selected References

American Diabetes Association, "Standards of Medical Care in Diabetes," *Diabetes Care*, 2007, 30(Suppl 1):4-41.

Antman EM, Anbe SC, Alpert JS, et al, "ACC/AHA Guidelines for the Management of Patients With ST-Elevation Myocardial Infarction - Executive Summary: A Report of the American College of Cardiology/

(Continued)

Insulin Regular *(Continued)*

American Heart Association Task Force on Practice Guidelines (Writing Committee to Revise the 1999 Guidelines for the Management of Patients With Acute Myocardial Infarction)," Circulation, 2004, 110:588-636. Available at: http://www.circulationaha.org/cgi/content/full/110/5/588. Last accessed October 26, 2004.

Brown G and Dodek P, "Intravenous Insulin Nomogram Improves Blood Glucose Control in the Critically Ill," *Crit Care Med*, 2001, 29(9):1714-9.

Brown AF, Mangione CM, Saliba D, et al, "Guidelines for Improving the Care of the Older Person With Diabetes Mellitus," *J Am Geriatr Soc*, 2003, 51(5 Suppl Guidelines):S265-80.

Dailey G, "New Strategies for Basal Insulin Treatment in Type 2 Diabetes Mellitus, *Clin Ther*, 2004, 26(6):889-901.

Holman RR and Turner RC, "Insulin Therapy in Type II Diabetes," *Diabetes Res Clin Pract*, 1995, (28 Suppl):179-84.

Hopkins DF, Cotton SJ, and Williams G, "Effective Treatment of Insulin-Induced Edema Using Ephedrine," *Diabetes Care*, 1993, 16(7):1026-8.

Joint Commission on Accreditation of Healthcare Organizations, "2005 National Patient Safety Goals," available at http://www.jcaho.org/accredited+organizations/patient+safety/05_npsg_guidelines.

Kitabchi AE, Umpierrez GE, Murphy MB, et al, "Hyperglycemic Crises in Diabetes," *Diabetes Care*, 2004, 27(Suppl 1): 94-102.

Lazar HL, Philippides G, Fitzgerald C, et al, "Glucose-Insulin-Potassium Solutions Enhance Recovery After Urgent Coronary Artery Bypass Grafting," *J Thorac Cardiovasc Surg*, 1997, 113(2):354-60.

Levine DF and Bulstrode C, "Managing Suicidal Insulin Overdose," *Br Med J (Clin Res Ed)*, 1982, 285(6346):974-5.

Malmberg K, "Prospective Randomised Study of Intensive Insulin Treatment on Long Term Survival After Acute Myocardial Infarction in Patients With Diabetes Mellitus. DIGAMI (Diabetes Mellitus, Insulin Glucose Infusion in Acute Myocardial Infarction) Study Group," *BMJ*, 1997, 314(7093):1512-5.

Mokhlesi B, Leikin JB, Murray P, et al, "Adult Toxicology in Critical Care: Part II: Specific Poisonings," *Chest*, 2003, 123(3):897-922.

Morley JE and Perry HM 3d, "The Management of Diabetes Mellitus in Older Individuals," *Drugs*, 1991, 41(4):548-65.

Mueller-Schoop J, "Accidental Intravenous Self-Injection With Insulin Pen," *Lancet*, 1993, 341(8849):894.

Nathan DM, "Insulin Treatment in the Elderly Diabetic Patient," *Clin Geriatr Med*, 1990, 6(4):923-31.

Oiknine R, Bernbaum M, and Mooradian AD, "A Critical Appraisal of the Role of Insulin Analogues in the Management of Diabetes Mellitus," *Drugs*, 2005, 65(3):325-40.

"Proceedings of the American College of Endocrinology Task Force on Inpatient Diabetes and Metabolic Control Consensus Conference, Washington, DC, USA, December 2003," *Endocr Pract*, 2004, (10 Suppl 2):3-108.

Roberge RJ, Martin TG, and Delbridge TR, "Intentional Massive Insulin Overdose: Recognition and Management," *Ann Emerg Med*, 1993, 22(2):228-34.

Van den Berghe G, Wouters P, Weekers F, et al, "Intensive Insulin Therapy in the Critically Ill Patients," *N Engl J Med*, 2001, 345(19):1359-67.

♦ **Insulin Regular and Insulin NPH** *see* Insulin NPH and Insulin Regular *on page 814*

♦ **Intal®** *see* Cromolyn *on page 369*

♦ **Interferon Alfa-2b (PEG Conjugate)** *see* Peginterferon Alfa-2b *on page 1213*

Interferon Alfa-2a *(in ter FEER on AL fa too aye)*

Medication Safety Issues
Sound-alike/look-alike issues:
Interferon alfa-2a may be confused with interferon alfa-2b, interferon alfa-n3, pegylated interferon alfa-2b
Roferon-A® may be confused with Rocephin®

International issues:
Interferon alfa-2a may be confused with interferon alpha multi-subtype which is available in international markets

U.S. Brand Names Roferon®-A

Canadian Brand Names Roferon®-A

Index Terms IFLrA; Interferon Alpha-2a; NSC-367982; rIFN-A

Generic Available No

Pharmacologic Category Interferon

Use
Patients >18 years of age: Treatment of hairy cell leukemia, chronic hepatitis C
Treatment of Philadelphia chromosome-positive (Ph+) chronic myelogenous leukemia (CML) in chronic phase, within 1 year of diagnosis

Unlabeled/Investigational Use Adjuvant therapy for malignant melanoma; treatment of AIDS-related Kaposi's sarcoma, carcinoid tumors; bladder, cervical, and ovarian cancers; hemangioma; chronic hepatitis D; low-grade non-Hodgkin's lymphoma; multiple myeloma; renal cell carcinoma; basal and squamous cell skin cancer; cutaneous T-cell lymphoma

Restrictions An FDA-approved medication guide must be distributed when dispensing an outpatient prescription (new or refill) where this medication is to be used without direct supervision of a healthcare provider. Medication guides are available at http://www.fda.gov/cder/Offices/ODS/medication_guides.htm.

Contraindications Hypersensitivity to alfa interferon, benzyl alcohol, or any component of the formulation; autoimmune hepatitis; visceral AIDS-related Kaposi's sarcoma associated with rapidly-progressing or life-threatening disease; hepatic decompensation (Child-Pugh Class B or C)

Warnings/Precautions Hazardous agent - use appropriate precautions for handling and disposal.

[U.S. Boxed Warning]: May cause or aggravate fatal or life-threatening autoimmune disorders, neuropsychiatric symptoms (including depression and/or suicidal thoughts/behaviors), ischemic and/or infectious disorders; discontinue treatment for persistent severe or worsening symptoms.

Neuropsychiatric disorders: May cause severe psychiatric adverse events (eg, depression, psychosis, mania, suicidal behavior/ideation) in patients with and without previous psychiatric symptoms; use with extreme caution in patients with a history of depression. Careful neuropsychiatric monitoring is required during therapy. Patients developing severe depression may require discontinuation of treatment. Although dose reduction or discontinuation may resolve symptoms, depression may persist; suicides have been reported after therapy has been discontinued. Use with caution in patients with seizure disorders, brain metastases, or compromised CNS function. Higher doses in the elderly or in malignancies other than hairy cell leukemia may result in severe obtundation.

Hepatic disease: Transient liver abnormalities may occur when treating chronic hepatitis C with interferon alfa-2a; increased ascites, hepatic failure, and death may occur with poorly-compensated liver disease.

Bone marrow suppression: Causes bone marrow suppression, including potentially severe cytopenias, and very rarely, aplastic anemia. Use caution in patients with pre-existing myelosuppression and/or with concomitant medications which cause myelosuppression.

Cardiovascular disease: Use caution and monitor closely in patients with history of cardiovascular disease; acute toxicities may exacerbate pre-existing cardiac conditions. MI has been observed (rarely) in patients receiving interferon alfa-2a; cardiomyopathy has been reported (rarely) in patients receiving interferon alfa.

Gastrointestinal disorders: Pancreatitis (occasionally fatal) has been observed; hypertriglyceridemia increases the risk for pancreatitis; consider discontinuing treatment in patients with pancreatitis. Hypertriglyceridemia has been reported; consider discontinuing with persistent elevations, particularly if combined with symptoms of pancreatitis. Gastrointestinal hemorrhage, ulcerative and hemorrhagic/ischemic colitis have been observed with interferon alfa treatment; may be severe and/or life-threatening; discontinue if symptoms (eg, abdominal pain, bloody diarrhea, and/or fever) develop.

Pulmonary disease: Dyspnea, pulmonary infiltrates, pneumonia, bronchiolitis obliterans, interstitial pneumonia, and sarcoidosis, resulting in potential fatal respiratory failure may occur with interferon alfa treatment. Discontinue with unexplained pulmonary infiltrates or evidence of impaired pulmonary function. Use caution in patients with a history of pulmonary disease.

Endocrine disorders: Thyroid disorders (hyper- or hypothyroidism) have been reported; use caution in patients with pre-existing thyroid disease. Hyperglycemia has been reported; use caution in patients with diabetes mellitus, may require adjustments in medications.

Autoimmune disorders: Avoid use in patients with history of autoimmune disorders. Development or exacerbation of autoimmune disorders (thrombocytopenic purpura, vasculitis, Raynaud's disease, rheumatoid arthritis, interstitial nephritis, thyroiditis, lupus erythematosus, and rhabdomyolysis) has been associated with interferon alfa. Monitor closely and consider discontinuing if autoimmune disease develops.

Ophthalmic disorders: Decreased/loss of vision, retinopathy (including macular edema), retinal artery or vein thrombosis, retinal hemorrhages, cotton wool spots, optic neuritis and papilledema have occurred in patients receiving interferon alfa. Use caution in patients with pre-existing ophthalmic disorders; monitor closely and discontinue with new or worsening ophthalmic symptoms.

Infections: Commonly associated with flu-like symptoms, including fever; rule out other causes/infection with persistent or high fever. Serious and severe infections (bacterial, viral and fungal) have been reported in with treatment; evaluate and treat promptly; consider discontinuing interferon.

Renal disorders: Renal toxicities, some requiring dialysis, have been reported with interferon alfa (alone or in combination with interleukin-2). Use caution in patients with renal impairment (Cl_{cr} <50 mL/minute); monitor closely for signs/symptoms of toxicity.

Acute hypersensitivity reactions have been reported. **Due to differences in dosage, patients should not change brands of interferons without the concurrence of their healthcare provider.**

(Continued)

Interferon Alfa-2a *(Continued)*

Adverse Reactions (Reflective of adult population; not specific for elderly)

Note: A flu-like syndrome (fever, chills, tachycardia, malaise, myalgia, arthralgia, headache) occurs within 1-2 hours of administration; may last up to 24 hours and may be dose-limiting.

>10%:

Cardiovascular: Chest pain (<4% to 11%), edema (1% to 11%), hypertension (11%)

Central nervous system: Fever (28% to 92%), fatigue (58% to 88%), headache (44% to 64%), chills (23% to 64%), depression (16% to 28%), pain (24%), dizziness (11% to 21%), mental status decreased (10% to 16%), irritability (15%), insomnia (14%), sleep disturbances (10% to 11%)

Dermatologic: Rash (8% to 44%), alopecia (17% to 19%), pruritus (7% to 13%), dry skin (7% to 17%)

Endocrine & metabolic: Hypocalcemia (28%), hypophosphatemia (22%)

Gastrointestinal: Anorexia (14% to 48%), nausea (33% to 39%), vomiting (33% to 39%), diarrhea (20% to 37%), weight loss (33%), throat irritation (21%), abdominal pain (12%)

Hematologic (often due to underlying disease): Myelosuppression (onset: 7-10 days; nadir 14 days [may be delayed 20-40 days in hairy cell leukemia], recovery: 21 days), neutropenia (≤68%; dose dependant); thrombocytopenia (5% to 62%), leukopenia (2% to 45%), anemia (≤31%)

Hepatic: Alkaline phosphatase increased (≤50%), transaminases increased (≤50%)

Local: Injection site reaction (29%)

Neuromuscular & skeletal: Weakness (6% to 88%) myalgia (51% to 71%), arthralgia (47% to 51%), bone pain (25% to 47%), joint pain (25%), back pain (16%), numbness (12%), paresthesia (7% to 12%)

Respiratory: Cough (1% to 19%), rhinorrhea/rhinitis (3% to 12%), dyspnea (1% to 12%), pneumonia (11%), sinusitis (11%)

Miscellaneous: Flu-like syndrome (16% to 33%), diaphoresis (1% to 22%)

1% to 10%:

Cardiovascular: Dysrhythmia (7%), hypotension (<5%), syncope (<5%), murmur (<5%), thrombophlebitis (<5%), palpitations (<3%), vasculitis (<3%), arrhythmia (1%)

Central nervous system: Confusion (<4% to 7%), anxiety (5% to 6%), lethargy (1% to 6%), nervousness (<5%), vertigo (<5%), concentration impaired (4%), memory loss (<4%), seizure (<4%), behavior disturbances (3%), malaise (1%)

Dermatologic: Bruising (<4%), skin lesions (1% to 3%)

Endocrine & metabolic: Hyperphosphatemia (9%), diabetes (<5%), hyper-/hypothyroidism (<5%), hypertriglyceridemia (<4%), libido changes (<4%), sexual dysfunction (1% to 3%), menstrual irregularity (2%)

Gastrointestinal: Colitis (<5%), gastrointestinal hemorrhage (<5%), pancreatitis (<5%), flatulence (3%), taste change (3% to <4%), stomatitis (1% to <5%), constipation (<3%), digestion impaired (2%), gingival bleeding (≤2%)

Genitourinary: Impotence (<4%), urinary tract infection (1% to 3%)

Hematologic: Coagulopathy (<4%), hemolytic anemia (<3%), hematoma (1%)

Hepatic: Liver pain (3%)

Neuromuscular & skeletal: Involuntary movements (7%), arthritis (≤5%), polyarthritis (5%), gait disturbance (<5%), leg cramps (3%), muscle cramps (1% to 3%)

Ocular: Visual disturbance (6%), conjunctivitis (4%), eye pain (1% to 3%)

Otic: Hearing alteration (<4%)

Renal: Proteinuria (≤10%)

Respiratory: Oropharynx dryness/inflammation (6%), pneumonitis (<5%), epistaxis (≤4%), bronchospasm (<4%), chest congestion (<3%)

Miscellaneous: Herpes virus reactivation (1% to 3%), lupus erythematosus syndrome (<3%)

Overdosage/Toxicology Symptoms include CNS depression, obtundation, flu-like symptoms, and myelosuppression. Treatment is symptom-directed and supportive.

Drug Interactions Inhibits CYP1A2 (weak)

Ribavirin: Concurrent therapy may increase the risk of hemolytic anemia.

Theophylline derivatives: Interferon alfa may increase the levels/effects of theophylline; monitor.

Zidovudine: Interferons may decrease the metabolism of zidovudine; the neutropenic effects of zidovudine and interferon may be synergistic; monitor.

Stability Refrigerate (2°C to 8°C/36°F to 46°F); do not freeze. Protect from light. Do not shake.

Mechanism of Action Following activation, multiple effects can be detected including induction of gene transcription. Inhibits cellular growth, alters the state of cellular differentiation, interferes with oncogene expression, alters cell surface antigen expression, increases phagocytic activity of macrophages, and augments cytotoxicity of lymphocytes for target cells

Pharmacokinetics

Distribution: The V_d of interferon is 31 L; but has been noted to be much greater (370-720 L) in leukemia patients receiving continuous infusion IFN; IFN does not penetrate the CSF

Metabolism: Alfa interferons are filtered through the glomeruli; majority of dose thought to be metabolized by proteolytic degradation during tubular reabsorption

Bioavailability:

I.M.: 83%

SubQ: 90%

Half-life: Elimination: 4-8 hours (mean: 5 hours)

Time to peak serum concentration: I.M., SubQ: ~4-7 hours

Dosage

Geriatrics & Adults: Refer to individual protocols.

Hairy cell leukemia: SubQ: 3 million units/day for 16-24 weeks, then 3 million units 3 times/week for up to 6-24 months

Ph+ chronic myelogenous leukemia (CML): SubQ: 9 million units/day, continue treatment until disease progression **or** 3 million units/day for 3 days, followed by 6 million units/day for 3 days, followed by 9 million units daily until disease progression

AIDS-related Kaposi's sarcoma (unlabeled use): SubQ, I.M.: 36 million units/day for 10-12 weeks, then 36 million units 3 times/week; to minimize adverse reactions, can use escalating dose (3-, 9-, then 18 million units each day for 3 days, then 36 million units daily thereafter)

Chronic hepatitis C: SubQ: 3 million units 3 times/week for 12 months **or** 6 million units 3 times/week for 12 weeks followed by 3 million units 3 times/week for 36 weeks

Renal Impairment: Not removed by hemodialysis

Administration

SubQ: For SubQ administration, rotate SubQ injection site.

I.M.: May also be administered I.M. (unlabeled route).

Monitoring Parameters CBC with differential and platelets, liver function, electrolytes, triglycerides. Baseline chest x-ray and ECG. Baseline ophthalmologic exam should be performed in all patients, with periodic reassessment in patients with impairment. Patients with thyroid dysfunction should be monitored by TSH levels at baseline and every 3 months during therapy.

Chronic hepatitis C: Monitor ALT (at baseline, after 2 weeks, and monthly thereafter) and HCV-RNA (particularly in first 3 months of therapy)

CML/hairy cell leukemia: Hematologic monitoring should be performed monthly

Reference Range Peak serum concentration following an I.V. dose of 36 million units: 10,400-17,470 pg/mL

Patient Information Use as directed; do not change dosage or schedule of administration without consulting prescriber. Maintain adequate hydration (2-3 L/day of fluids unless instructed to restrict fluid intake). You may experience flu-like syndrome (acetaminophen may help); this syndrome subsides after several weeks of continuous dosing, but usually recurs during each cycle of intermittent therapy. You may also experience nausea, vomiting, dry mouth, or metallic taste (frequent small meals, frequent mouth care, sucking lozenges, or chewing gum may help); drowsiness, dizziness, agitation, abnormal thinking (use caution when driving or engaging in tasks requiring alertness until response to drug is known). Inform prescriber **immediately** if you feel depressed or have any thoughts of suicide. Report unusual bruising or bleeding; persistent abdominal disturbances; unusual fatigue; muscle pain or tremors; chest pain or palpitation; swelling of extremities or unusual weight gain; difficulty breathing; pain, swelling, or redness at injection site; or other unusual symptoms.

Additional Information Indications and dosage regimens are specific for a particular brand of interferon; other brands of interferon (ie, Intron® A) have different indications and dosage guidelines; do not change brands of interferon as changes in dosage may result; a flu-like syndrome (fever, chills) occurs in the majority of patients 2-6 hours after a dose; pretreatment with nonsteroidal anti-inflammatory drug (NSAID) or acetaminophen can decrease fever and its severity and alleviate headache

Special Geriatric Considerations No specific data is available for the elderly; however, pay close attention to Warnings/Precautions since the elderly often have reduced Cl_{cr} (<50 mL/minute), diabetes, and hyper-/hypothyroidism.

Dosage Forms Excipient information presented when available (limited, particularly for generics); consult specific product labeling.

Injection, solution:

Roferon®-A: 3 million units/0.5 mL (0.5 mL) [contains benzyl alcohol and polysorbate 80]; 6 million units/0.5 mL (0.5 mL) [contains benzyl alcohol and polysorbate 80]; 9 million units/0.5 mL (0.5 mL) [contains benzyl alcohol and polysorbate 80]

♦ **Interferon Alpha-2a** see Interferon Alfa-2a on page 820

Interferon Beta-1b (in ter FEER on BAY ta won bee)

U.S. Brand Names Betaseron®
Canadian Brand Names Betaseron®
Index Terms rIFN beta-1b
Generic Available No
Pharmacologic Category Interferon
Use Treatment of relapsing forms of multiple sclerosis (MS); treatment of first clinical episode with MRI features consistent with MS
Restrictions An FDA-approved medication guide must be distributed when dispensing an outpatient prescription (new or refill) where this medication is to be used without direct supervision of a healthcare provider. Medication guide is available at http://www.berlex.com/html/products/pi/Betaseron_Medication_Guide.pdf.
Contraindications Hypersensitivity to *E. coli*-derived products, natural or recombinant interferon beta, albumin human or any other component of the formulation
Warnings/Precautions Anaphylaxis has been reported rarely with use. Associated with a high incidence of flu-like adverse effects. Hepatotoxicity has been reported with beta interferons, including rare reports of hepatitis (autoimmune) and hepatic failure requiring transplant. Interferons have been associated with severe psychiatric adverse events (psychosis, mania, depression, suicidal behavior/ideation) in patients with and without previous psychiatric symptoms, avoid use in severe psychiatric disorders and use caution in patients with a history of depression; patients exhibiting symptoms of depression should be closely monitored and discontinuation of therapy should be considered. Use caution in patients with pre-existing cardiovascular disease, pulmonary disease, seizure disorders, renal impairment or hepatic impairment. Use caution in myelosuppression. Severe injection site reactions (necrosis) may occur, which may or may not heal with continued therapy; patient and/or caregiver competency in injection technique should be confirmed and periodically re-evaluated. Contains albumin, which may carry a remote risk of transmitting viral diseases.
Adverse Reactions (Reflective of adult population; not specific for elderly)
Note: Flu-like syndrome (including at least two of the following - headache, fever, chills, malaise, diaphoresis, and myalgia) are reported in the majority of patients (60%) and decrease over time (average duration ~1 week).

>10%:
  Cardiovascular: Peripheral edema (15%), chest pain (11%)
  Central nervous system: Headache (57%), fever (36%), pain (51%), chills (25%), dizziness (24%), insomnia (24%)
  Dermatologic: Rash (24%), skin disorder (12%)
  Endocrine & metabolic: Metrorrhagia (11%)
  Gastrointestinal: Nausea (27%), diarrhea (19%), abdominal pain (19%), constipation (20%), dyspepsia (14%)
  Genitourinary: Urinary urgency (13%)
  Hematologic: Lymphopenia (88%), neutropenia (14%), leukopenia (14%)
  Local: Injection site reaction (85%), inflammation (53%), pain (18%)
  Neuromuscular & skeletal: Weakness (61%), myalgia (27%), hypertonia (50%), myasthenia (46%), arthralgia (31%), incoordination (21%)
  Miscellaneous: Flu-like syndrome (decreases over treatment course; 60%)
1% to 10%:
  Cardiovascular: Palpitation (4%), vasodilation (8%), hypertension (7%), tachycardia (4%), peripheral vascular disorder (6%)
  Central nervous system: Anxiety (10%), malaise (8%), nervousness (7%)
  Dermatologic: Alopecia (4%)
  Endocrine & metabolic: Menorrhagia (8%), dysmenorrhea (7%)
  Gastrointestinal: Weight gain (7%)
  Genitourinary: Impotence (9%), pelvic pain (6%), cystitis (8%), urinary frequency (7%), prostatic disorder (3%)
  Hematologic: Lymphadenopathy (8%)
  Hepatic: ALT increased >5x baseline (10%), AST increased >5x baseline (3%)
  Local: Injection site necrosis (4% to 5%), edema (3%), mass (2%)
  Neuromuscular & skeletal: Leg cramps (4%)
  Respiratory: Dyspnea (7%)
  Miscellaneous: Diaphoresis (8%), hypersensitivity (3%)
Overdosage/Toxicology Symptoms include CNS depression, obtundation, flu-like symptoms, and myelosuppression. Treatment is supportive.
Drug Interactions
  Theophylline: Interferons may decrease the metabolism of theophylline derivatives.
Stability Store at room temperature of 25°C (77°F); excursions permitted to 15°C to 30°C (59°F to 86°F). To reconstitute solution, inject 1.2 mL of diluent (provided); gently swirl to dissolve, do not shake. Reconstituted solution provides 0.25 mg/mL (8 million

units). If not used immediately following reconstitution, refrigerate solution at 2°C to 8°C (36°F to 46°F) and use within 3 hours; do not freeze or shake solution.

Mechanism of Action Interferon beta-1b differs from naturally occurring human protein by a single amino acid substitution and the lack of carbohydrate side chains; mechanism in the treatment of MS is unknown; however, immunomodulatory effects attributed to interferon beta-1b include enhancement of suppressor T cell activity, reduction of proinflammatory cytokines, down-regulation of antigen presentation, and reduced trafficking of lymphocytes into the central nervous system. Improves MRI lesions, decreases relapse rate, and disease severity in patients with secondary progressive MS.

Pharmacokinetics Limited data due to small doses used
Time to peak serum concentration: 1-8 hours
Bioavailability: 50%
Half-life: 8 minutes to 4.3 hours

Dosage
Geriatrics & Adults: **Note:** Gradual dose-titration, analgesics, and/or antipyretics may help decrease flu-like symptoms on treatment days.
Multiple sclerosis (relapsing): SubQ: Initial: 0.0625 mg (2 million units; 0.25 mL) every other day; gradually increase dose by 0.0625 every 2 weeks
Target dose: 0.25 mg (8 million units; 1 mL) every other day

Administration Withdraw dose of reconstituted solution from the vial into a sterile syringe fitted with a 27-gauge needle and inject the solution subcutaneously; sites for self-injection include outer surface of the arms, abdomen, hips, and thighs. Rotate SubQ injection site. Patient should be well hydrated.

Monitoring Parameters Complete blood chemistries (including platelet count) and liver function tests are recommended at 1, 3, and 6 months following initiation of therapy and periodically thereafter. Thyroid function should be assessed every 6 months in patients with history of thyroid dysfunction.

Patient Information Patients must be instructed in aseptic technique when injecting themselves, proper disposal of needles and syringes; injection site may develop a reaction, but this does not dictate the stopping of therapy; flu-like symptoms may occur but the use of aspirin or acetaminophen will relieve the symptoms; warn about depression, feelings of suicide, and photosensitivity; report changes in mental state to physician; use sun block to prevent photosensitivity reactions

Inform healthcare provider **immediately** if you feel depressed or have any thoughts of suicide. Report any broken skin, or black-blue discoloration around the injection site. Report unusual bruising or bleeding; persistent abdominal disturbances; unusual fatigue; muscle pain or tremors; chest pain or palpitations, swelling of extremities; visual disturbances; pain, swelling, or redness at injection site; or other unusual symptoms.

Additional Information American Academy of Neurology and MS Council guidelines suggest that, based upon published data, 6 million units of Avonex® (interferon beta-1a) (30 mcg) is equivalent to approximately 7-9 million units of Betaseron® (220-280 mcg).

Special Geriatric Considerations No specific recommendations necessary for use in the elderly. Monitor for CNS adverse effects which may be significant in the elderly.

Dosage Forms Excipient information presented when available (limited, particularly for generics); consult specific product labeling.
Injection, powder for reconstitution [preservative free]:
Betaseron®: 0.3 mg [9.6 million units] [contains albumin; packaged with prefilled syringe containing diluent]

Selected References
Sheremata WA, Taylor JR, and Elgart GW, "Severe Necrotizing Cutaneous Lesions Complicating Treatment With Interferon Beta-1b," *N Engl J Med*, 1995, 332(23):1584.

♦ **Interleukin-1 Receptor Antagonist** *see* Anakinra *on page 110*
♦ **Intropin** *see* DOPamine *on page 468*
♦ **Invanz®** *see* Ertapenem *on page 531*
♦ **Invega™** *see* Paliperidone *on page 1190*

Iodoquinol (eye oh doe KWIN ole)

U.S. Brand Names Yodoxin®
Canadian Brand Names Diodoquin®
Index Terms Diiodohydroxyquin
Generic Available No
Pharmacologic Category Amebicide
Use Treatment of acute and chronic intestinal amebiasis; asymptomatic cyst passers; *Blastocystis hominis* infections
Contraindications Hypersensitivity to iodine or iodoquinol or any component of the formulation; hepatic damage; pre-existing optic neuropathy
(Continued)

Iodoquinol *(Continued)*

Warnings/Precautions Optic neuritis, optic atrophy, and peripheral neuropathy have occurred following prolonged use; avoid long-term therapy

Adverse Reactions (Reflective of adult population; not specific for elderly)
Frequency not defined.
Central nervous system: Fever, chills, agitation, retrograde amnesia, headache
Dermatologic: Rash, urticaria, pruritus
Endocrine & metabolic: Thyroid gland enlargement
Gastrointestinal: Diarrhea, nausea, vomiting, stomach pain, abdominal cramps
Neuromuscular & skeletal: Peripheral neuropathy, weakness
Ocular: Optic neuritis, optic atrophy, visual impairment
Miscellaneous: Itching of rectal area

Overdosage/Toxicology Chronic overdose can result in vomiting, diarrhea, abdominal pain, metallic taste, paresthesias, paraplegia, and loss of vision. Can lead to destruction of the long fibers of the spinal cord and optic nerve. Acute overdose symptoms includes delirium, stupor, coma, and amnesia. Following GI decontamination, treatment is symptomatic.

Drug Interactions No data reported

Mechanism of Action Contact amebicide that works in the lumen of the intestine by an unknown mechanism

Pharmacokinetics
Absorption: Oral: Poor and irregular
Metabolism: In the liver
Elimination: High percentage of dose excreted in feces

Dosage
Geriatrics: This agent is no longer a drug of choice; use only if other therapy is contraindicated or has failed. Due to optic nerve damage, use cautiously in the elderly.
Adults: Treatment of susceptible infections: Oral: 650 mg 3 times/day after meals for 20 days; not to exceed 2 g/day

Administration Tablets may be crushed and mixed with applesauce or chocolate syrup

Test Interactions May increase protein-bound serum iodine concentrations reflecting a decrease in ^{131}I uptake; false-positive ferric chloride test for phenylketonuria

Patient Information Complete full course of therapy; may cause nausea, vomiting, or diarrhea

Special Geriatric Considerations No special considerations for the elderly, however, this agent is no longer a drug of choice. Use only if other therapy is contraindicated or has failed. Due to optic nerve damage, use cautiously in the elderly.

Dosage Forms Excipient information presented when available (limited, particularly for generics); consult specific product labeling.
Tablet: 210 mg, 650 mg

♦ **Ionil® [OTC]** *see* Salicylic Acid *on page 1441*

♦ **Ionil® Plus [OTC]** *see* Salicylic Acid *on page 1441*

♦ **Ionsys™** *see* Fentanyl *on page 609*

♦ **Iopidine®** *see* Apraclonidine *on page 116*

Ipecac Syrup *(IP e kak SIR up)*

Index Terms Syrup of Ipecac
Generic Available Yes
Pharmacologic Category Antidote
Use Treatment of acute oral drug overdosage and in certain poisonings
Contraindications Hypersensitivity to ipecac or any component of the formulation; do not use in unconscious patients; patients with no gag reflex; following ingestion of strong bases, acids, or volatile oils; when seizures are likely
Warnings/Precautions Do not confuse ipecac syrup with ipecac fluid extract, which is 14 times more potent; use with caution in patients with cardiovascular disease and bulimics; may not be effective in antiemetic overdose
Adverse Reactions (Reflective of adult population; not specific for elderly)
Frequency not defined.
Cardiovascular: Cardiotoxicity
Central nervous system: Lethargy
Gastrointestinal: Protracted vomiting, diarrhea
Neuromuscular & skeletal: Myopathy
Overdosage/Toxicology Ipecac syrup contains cardiotoxin. Symptoms include tachycardia, CHF, atrial fibrillation, depressed myocardial contractility, myocarditis, diarrhea, persistent vomiting, and hypotension. Treatment consists of activated charcoal and gastric lavage.

Drug Interactions
Decreased effect: Activated charcoal, milk, carbonated beverages
Increased toxicity: Phenothiazines (chlorpromazine has been associated with serious dystonic reactions)
Ethanol/Nutrition/Herb Interactions Food: Milk, carbonated beverages may decrease effectiveness.
Mechanism of Action Irritates the gastric mucosa and stimulates the medullary chemoreceptor trigger zone to induce vomiting
Pharmacodynamics
Onset of emesis: Within 15-30 minutes
Duration: 20-25 minutes; can last longer, 60 minutes in some cases
Dosage
Geriatrics & Adults: Emetic: Oral: 15-30 mL followed by 200-300 mL of water; repeat dose one time if vomiting does not occur within 20 minutes.
Administration Do **not** administer to unconscious patients; patients should be kept active and moving following administration of ipecac; if vomiting does not occur after second dose, gastric lavage may be considered to remove ingested substance
Patient Information Call the Poison Center before administering. Patients should be kept active and moving following administration of ipecac; follow dose with 8 oz of water following initial episode; if vomiting, no food or liquids should be ingested for 1 hour.
Dosage Forms Excipient information presented when available (limited, particularly for generics); consult specific product labeling.
Syrup: 70 mg/mL (30 mL) [contains alcohol]

◆ **IPOL**® *see* Poliovirus Vaccine (Inactivated) *on page 1280*

Ipratropium (i pra TROE pee um)

Related Information
Inhalant Agents *on page 1760*
Medication Safety Issues
Sound-alike/look-alike issues:
Atrovent® may be confused with Alupent®
U.S. Brand Names Atrovent®; Atrovent® HFA
Canadian Brand Names Alti-Ipratropium; Apo-Ipravent®; Atrovent®; Atrovent® HFA; Gen-Ipratropium; Novo-Ipramide; Nu-Ipratropium; PMS-Ipratropium
Index Terms Ipratropium Bromide
Generic Available Yes: Excludes solution for oral inhalation, aerosol for oral inhalation
Pharmacologic Category Anticholinergic Agent
Use Anticholinergic bronchodilator for prevention of bronchospasm associated with COPD, bronchitis, and emphysema; symptomatic relief of perennial rhinitis (0.03%), common cold (0.06%) [nasal spray]
Contraindications Hypersensitivity to atropine, its derivatives, or any component of the formulation
Warnings/Precautions Not indicated for the initial treatment of acute episodes of bronchospasm; use with caution in patients with myasthenia gravis, narrow-angle glaucoma, benign prostatic hyperplasia (BPH), or bladder neck obstruction
Adverse Reactions (Reflective of adult population; not specific for elderly)
Inhalation aerosol and inhalation solution:
>10%: Bronchitis (10% to 23%), upper respiratory tract infection (13%)
1% to 10%:
Cardiovascular: Palpitation
Central nervous system: Dizziness (2% to 3%)
Dermatologic: Rash (1%)
Gastrointestinal: Nausea, xerostomia, stomach upset, dry mucous membranes
Renal: Urinary tract infection
Respiratory: Nasal congestion, dyspnea (10%), sputum increased (1%), bronchospasm (2%), pharyngitis (3%), rhinitis (2%), sinusitis (5%)
Miscellaneous: Flu-like syndrome

Nasal spray: Respiratory: Epistaxis (8%), nasal dryness (5%), nausea (2%)
Overdosage/Toxicology Symptoms include dry mouth, drying of respiratory secretions, cough, nausea, GI distress, blurred vision or impaired visual accommodation, headache, and nervousness. Acute overdose by inhalation is unlikely since it is so poorly absorbed. However, if poisoning occurs, it can be treated like any other anticholinergic toxicity. An anticholinergic overdose with severe life-threatening symptoms may be treated with physostigmine 1-2 mg SubQ or slow I.V.
Drug Interactions Anticholinergics: Concurrent use with ipratropium may increase risk of adverse events.
Stability Store at 15°C to 30°C (59°F to 86°F). Do not store near heat or open flame.
(Continued)

Ipratropium *(Continued)*

Mechanism of Action Blocks the action of acetylcholine at parasympathetic sites in bronchial smooth muscle causing bronchodilation

Pharmacodynamics

Onset of action: Bronchodilation begins 1-3 minutes after administration with a maximal effect occurring within 1.5-2 hours

Duration: ≤4 hours

Pharmacokinetics

Absorption: Inhalation: Not readily absorbed into the systemic circulation from the surface of the lung or from GI tract

Distribution: 15% of dose reaches the lower airways

Dosage

Geriatrics & Adults:

Bronchospasm:

Nebulization: 500 mcg (one unit-dose vial) 3-4 times/day with doses 6-8 hours apart

Metered-dose inhaler: 2 inhalations 4 times/day, up to 12 inhalations/24 hours

Colds (symptomatic relief of rhinorrhea): Safety and efficacy of use beyond 4 days not established: Nasal spray (0.06%): 2 sprays in each nostril 3-4 times/day

Allergic/nonallergic rhinitis: Nasal spray (0.03%): 2 sprays in each nostril 2-3 times/day

Administration

Atrovent®: Shake inhaler before each use; rinsing mouth after each use decreases dry mouth side effect

Atrovent® HFA: Prime inhaler by releasing 2 test sprays into the air. If the inhaler has not been used for >3 days, reprime.

Monitoring Parameters Pulmonary function tests

Patient Information Temporary blurred vision may occur if sprayed into eyes. Follow instructions for use accompanying the product. Close eyes when administering ipratropium; wait at least one full minute between inhalations. Nasal spray: Initial pump priming requires 7 actuations. Do not interchange oral and nasal products.

Additional Information Some COPD patients may require higher doses (3-8 inhalations/dose); ipratropium solution may be mixed with albuterol solution if used within 1 hour

Special Geriatric Considerations The elderly may find it difficult to use the metered dose inhaler. A spacer device may be useful. Ipratropium has not been specifically studied in the elderly, but it is poorly absorbed from the airways and appears to be safe in this population.

Dosage Forms Excipient information presented when available (limited, particularly for generics); consult specific product labeling.

Aerosol for oral inhalation, as bromide:

Atrovent® HFA: 17 mcg/actuation (12.9 g)

Solution for nebulization, as bromide: 0.02% (2.5 mL)

Solution, intranasal, as bromide [spray]:

Atrovent®: 0.03% (30 mL); 0.06% (15 mL)

Selected References

Hughes DT, "The Use of Anticholinergic Drugs in Nocturnal Asthma," *Postgrad Med J*, 1987, 63(Suppl 1):47-51.

"Strategies in Preserving Lung Health and Preventing COPD and Associated Diseases. The National Lung Health Education Program (NLHEP)," *Chest*, 1998, 113(2 Suppl):123-63S.

Ipratropium and Albuterol (i pra TROE pee um & al BYOO ter ole)

Related Information

Albuterol *on page 40*

Ipratropium *on page 827*

Medication Safety Issues

Sound-alike/look-alike issues:

Combivent® may be confused with Combivir®

International issues:

DuoNeb™ may be confused with DuoTrav™ which is a brand name for travoprost/timolol combination product in Canada

U.S. Brand Names Combivent®; DuoNeb™

Canadian Brand Names CO Ipra-Sal; Combivent®; Gen-Combo Sterinebs

Index Terms Albuterol and Ipratropium; Salbutamol and Ipratropium

Generic Available Yes: Solution for nebulization

Pharmacologic Category Bronchodilator

Use Treatment of chronic obstructive pulmonary disease (COPD) in those patients that are currently on a regular bronchodilator who continue to have bronchospasms and require a second bronchodilator

Contraindications Hypersensitivity to atropine or its derivatives, albuterol or its adrenergic amines, any component of the formulation

Warnings/Precautions

Based on **ipratropium** component: Not indicated for the initial treatment of acute episodes of bronchospasm; use with caution in patients with narrow-angle glaucoma, prostatic hyperplasia, or bladder neck obstruction; ipratropium has not been specifically studied in the elderly, but it is poorly absorbed from the airways and appears to be safe in this population.

Based on **albuterol** component: Use with caution in patients with hyperthyroidism, diabetes mellitus, or sensitivity to sympathomimetic amines; cardiovascular disorders including coronary insufficiency or hypertension; excessive use may result in tolerance. Because of its minimal effect on beta$_1$-receptors and its relatively long duration of action, albuterol is a rational choice in the elderly when a beta agonist is indicated. All patients should utilize a spacer device when using a metered dose inhaler. Oral use should be avoided in the elderly due to adverse effects.

Adverse Reactions (Reflective of adult population; not specific for elderly)

Based on **ipratropium** component: **Note:** Ipratropium is poorly absorbed from the lung, so systemic effects are rare.

Inhalation aerosol and inhalation solution:

<10%: Respiratory: Upper respiratory infection (13%), bronchitis (15%)

1% to 10%:
Cardiovascular: Palpitation (2%)
Central nervous system: Nervousness (3%), dizziness (2%), fatigue, headache (6%), pain (4%)
Dermatologic: Rash (1%)
Gastrointestinal: Nausea, xerostomia, stomach upset, dry mucous membranes
Respiratory: Nasal congestion, dyspnea (10%), increased sputum (1%), bronchospasm (2%), pharyngitis (3%), rhinitis (2%), sinusitis (5%)
Miscellaneous: Influenza-like symptoms

Based on **albuterol** component:

>10%:
Cardiovascular: Tachycardia, palpitation, pounding heartbeat
Gastrointestinal: GI upset, nausea

1% to 10%:
Cardiovascular: Flushing of face, hypertension or hypotension
Central nervous system: Nervousness, CNS stimulation, hyperactivity, insomnia, dizziness, lightheadedness, drowsiness, headache
Gastrointestinal: Xerostomia, heartburn, vomiting, unusual taste
Genitourinary: Dysuria
Neuromuscular & skeletal: Muscle cramping, tremor, weakness
Respiratory: Coughing
Miscellaneous: Diaphoresis (increased)

Drug Interactions Albuterol: **Substrate** of CYP3A4 (major)
Also see individual agents.

Stability DuoNeb™: Store at 2°C to 25°C (36°F to 77°F). Protect from light.
Combivent®: Store at 15°C to 30°C (59°F to 86°F). Avoid excessive humidity.

Mechanism of Action See individual agents.

Dosage

Geriatrics & Adults:

COPD:

Inhalation: 2 metered-dose inhalations 4 times/day; may receive additional doses as necessary, but total number of doses in 24 hours should not exceed 12 inhalations.

Inhalation via nebulization: Initial: 3 mL every 6 hours (maximum: 3 mL every 4 hours)

Administration Nebulization: Administer via jet nebulizer to an air compressor with an adequate air flow, equipped with a mouthpiece or face mask

Patient Information Inhalers should be primed (test sprayed) three times before use and when not used for more than 24 hours.

Dosage Forms Excipient information presented when available (limited, particularly for generics); consult specific product labeling.

Aerosol for oral inhalation:
Combivent®: Ipratropium bromide 18 mcg and albuterol sulfate 103 mcg per actuation [200 doses] (14.7 g) [contains soya lecithin]

Solution for nebulization: Ipratropium bromide 0.5 mg [0.017%] and albuterol base 2.5 mg [0.083%] per 3 mL vial (30s, 60s)
DuoNeb™: Ipratropium bromide 0.5 mg [0.017%] and albuterol base 2.5 mg [0.083%] per 3 mL vial (30s, 60s)

♦ **Ipratropium Bromide** *see* Ipratropium *on page 827*
♦ **I-Prin [OTC]** *see* Ibuprofen *on page 784*

♦ **Iproveratril Hydrochloride** see Verapamil on page 1671
♦ **IPV** see Poliovirus Vaccine (Inactivated) on page 1280
♦ **Iquix®** see Levofloxacin on page 896

Irbesartan (ir be SAR tan)

Related Information
Angiotensin Agents on page 1737

Medication Safety Issues
Sound-alike/look-alike issues:
Avapro® may be confused with Anaprox®

U.S. Brand Names Avapro®

Canadian Brand Names Avapro®

Generic Available No

Pharmacologic Category Angiotensin II Receptor Blocker

Use Treatment of hypertension alone or in combination with other antihypertensives

Contraindications Hypersensitivity to irbesartan or any component of the formulation; hypersensitivity to other A-II receptor antagonists; primary hyperaldosteronism; bilateral renal artery stenosis

Warnings/Precautions May cause hyperkalemia; avoid potassium supplementation unless specifically required by healthcare provider. May be associated with deterioration of renal function and/or increases in serum creatinine, particularly in patients dependent on renin-angiotensin-aldosterone system. Avoid use or use a much smaller dose in patients who are intravascularly volume-depleted; use caution in patients with unilateral or bilateral renal artery stenosis to avoid a decrease in renal function; AUCs of irbesartan (not the active metabolite) are about 50% greater in patients with Cl_{cr} <30 mL/minute and are doubled in hemodialysis patients.

Adverse Reactions (Reflective of adult population; not specific for elderly)
Unless otherwise indicated, percentage of incidence is reported for patients with hypertension.
>10%: Endocrine & metabolic: Hyperkalemia (19%, diabetic nephropathy; rarely seen in HTN)
1% to 10%:
Cardiovascular: Orthostatic hypotension (5%, diabetic nephropathy)
Central nervous system: Fatigue (4%), dizziness (10%, diabetic nephropathy)
Gastrointestinal: Diarrhea (3%), dyspepsia (2%)
Respiratory: Upper respiratory infection (9%), cough (2.8% versus 2.7% in placebo)
>1% but frequency ≤ placebo: Abdominal pain, anxiety, chest pain, edema, headache, influenza, musculoskeletal pain, nausea, nervousness, pharyngitis, rash, rhinitis, sinus abnormality, syncope, tachycardia, urinary tract infection, vertigo, vomiting

Overdosage/Toxicology The most likely overdose manifestations would be hypotension and tachycardia. Bradycardia could occur from parasympathetic (vagal) stimulation. If symptomatic hypotension should occur, institute supportive treatment. Not removed by hemodialysis.

Drug Interactions Substrate of CYP2C9 (minor); Inhibits CYP2C8 (moderate), 2C9 (moderate), 2D6 (weak), 3A4 (weak)
CYP2C8 Substrates: Irbesartan may increase the levels/effects of CYP2C8 substrates. Example substrates include amiodarone, paclitaxel, pioglitazone, repaglinide, and rosiglitazone.
CYP2C9 Substrates: Irbesartan may increase the levels/effects of CYP2C9 substrates. Example substrates include bosentan, dapsone, fluoxetine, glimepiride, glipizide, losartan, montelukast, nateglinide, paclitaxel, phenytoin, warfarin, and zafirlukast.
Lithium: Risk of toxicity may be increased by irbesartan; monitor lithium levels.
NSAIDs: May decrease angiotensin II antagonist efficacy; effect has been seen with losartan, but may occur with other medications in this class; monitor blood pressure
Potassium-sparing diuretics (amiloride, potassium, spironolactone, triamterene): Increased risk of hyperkalemia.
Potassium supplements may increase the risk of hyperkalemia.
Trimethoprim (high dose) may increase the risk of hyperkalemia.

Ethanol/Nutrition/Herb Interactions Herb/Nutraceutical: Avoid dong quai if using for hypertension (has estrogenic activity). Avoid ephedra, yohimbe, ginseng (may worsen hypertension). Avoid garlic (may have increased antihypertensive effect).

Stability Store at room temperature of 15°C to 30°C (59°F to 86°F).

Mechanism of Action Irbesartan is an angiotensin receptor antagonist. Angiotensin II acts as a vasoconstrictor. In addition to causing direct vasoconstriction, angiotensin II also stimulates the release of aldosterone. Once aldosterone is released, sodium as well as water are reabsorbed. The end result is an elevation in blood pressure. Irbesartan binds to the AT1 angiotensin II receptor. This binding prevents angiotensin II from binding to the receptor thereby blocking the vasoconstriction and the aldosterone secreting effects of angiotensin II.

Pharmacokinetics
Distribution: 53-93 L
Protein binding: 90%
Metabolism: Metabolized in the liver; <20% metabolites
Bioavailability: 60% to 80%
Half-life: 11-15 hours
Time to peak concentration: 1.5-2 hours
Elimination: Urine unchanged ~20%; recovered in feces ~80%

Dosage
Geriatrics & Adults:
Hypertension: Oral: 150 mg once daily; patients may be titrated to 300 mg once daily. **Note:** Starting dose in volume-depleted patients should be 75 mg.
Nephropathy in patients with type 2 diabetes and hypertension: Oral: Target dose: 300 mg once daily
Renal Impairment: No dosage adjustment necessary with mild to severe impairment unless the patient is also volume depleted.

Monitoring Parameters Baseline and periodic electrolyte panels, renal and liver function tests, urinalysis; symptoms of hypotension or hypersensitivity; monitor blood pressure and pulse

Patient Information Do not stop taking this medication unless instructed by a physician; take a missed dose as soon as possible unless it is almost time for your next dose; call your physician immediately if you have symptoms of allergy or develop side effects including headache and dizziness

Additional Information Addition of a diuretic gives an additive effect. For patients who have an adequate response to 300 mg, no gain in antihypertensive effect can be seen by increasing dose beyond 300 mg/day. Consider adding a diuretic or other antihypertensive.

Special Geriatric Considerations No dosage adjustment is necessary when initiating angiotensin II receptor antagonists in the elderly. In clinical studies, no differences between younger adults and the elderly were demonstrated. Many elderly may be volume depleted due to diuretic use and/or blunted thirst reflex resulting in inadequate fluid intake.

Dosage Forms Excipient information presented when available (limited, particularly for generics); consult specific product labeling.
Tablet: 75 mg, 150 mg, 300 mg

Selected References
Munger MA and Furniss SM, "Angiotensin II Receptor Blockers: Novel Therapy for Heart Failure?" *Pharmacotherapy*, 1996, 16(2 Pt 2):59S-68S.

Irbesartan and Hydrochlorothiazide
(ir be SAR tan & hye droe klor oh THYE a zide)

Related Information
Hydrochlorothiazide *on page 756*
Irbesartan *on page 830*

Medication Safety Issues
Sound-alike/look-alike issues:
Avalide® may be confused with Avandia®

U.S. Brand Names Avalide®

Canadian Brand Names Avalide®

Index Terms Avapro® HCT; Hydrochlorothiazide and Irbesartan

Generic Available No

Pharmacologic Category Angiotensin II Receptor Blocker Combination; Antihypertensive Agent, Combination; Diuretic, Thiazide

Use Treatment of hypertension

Dosage
Geriatrics & Adults: Hypertension: Oral: Dose must be individualized. A patient who is not controlled with either agent alone may be switched to the combination product. Mean effect increases with the dose of each component. The lowest dosage available is irbesartan 150 mg/hydrochlorothiazide 12.5 mg. Dose increases should be made not more frequently than every 2-4 weeks.

Canadian dosing (not approved in U.S.): Severe hypertension: Oral: Initial: Combination product irbesartan 150 mg/hydrochlorothiazide 12.5 mg once daily. Titrate dose after 2-4 weeks, if needed, to a maximum dose of irbesartan 300 mg/hydrochlorothiazide 25 mg once daily.

Dosage Forms Excipient information presented when available (limited, particularly for generics); consult specific product labeling.
Tablet:
Irbesartan 150 mg and hydrochlorothiazide 12.5 mg
Irbesartan 300 mg and hydrochlorothiazide 12.5 mg
Irbesartan 300 mg and hydrochlorothiazide 25 mg
(Continued)

IRON DEXTRAN COMPLEX

♦ Ircon® [OTC] *see* Ferrous Fumarate *on page 618*

Iron Dextran Complex (EYE ern DEKS tran KOM pleks)

Medication Safety Issues
Sound-alike/look-alike issues:
Dexferrum® may be confused with Desferal®

U.S. Brand Names Dexferrum®; INFeD®

Canadian Brand Names Dexiron™; Infufer®

Generic Available No

Pharmacologic Category Iron Salt

Use Treatment of microcytic hypochromic anemia resulting from iron deficiency in whom oral administration is infeasible or ineffective

Contraindications Hypersensitivity to iron dextran or any component of the formulation; all anemias that are not involved with iron deficiency; hemochromatosis; hemolytic anemia

Warnings/Precautions Use with caution in patients with history of asthma, hepatic impairment, rheumatoid arthritis. **[U.S. Boxed Warning]: Deaths associated with parenteral administration following anaphylactic-type reactions have been reported.** Use only in patients where the iron deficient state is not amenable to oral iron therapy. A test dose of 0.5 mL I.V. or I.M. should be given to observe for adverse reactions. Anemia in the elderly is often caused by "anemia of chronic disease" or associated with inflammation rather than blood loss. Iron stores are usually normal or increased, with a serum ferritin >50 ng/mL and a decreased total iron binding capacity. I.V. administration of iron dextran is often preferred over I.M. in the elderly secondary to a decreased muscle mass and the need for daily injections.

Adverse Reactions (Reflective of adult population; not specific for elderly)
>10%:
Cardiovascular: Flushing
Central nervous system: Dizziness, fever, headache, pain
Gastrointestinal: Nausea, vomiting, metallic taste
Local: Staining of skin at the site of I.M. injection
Miscellaneous: Diaphoresis
1% to 10%:
Cardiovascular: Hypotension (1% to 2%)
Dermatologic: Urticaria (1% to 2%), phlebitis (1% to 2%)
Gastrointestinal: Diarrhea
Genitourinary: Discoloration of urine
Note: Diaphoresis, urticaria, arthralgia, fever, chills, dizziness, headache, and nausea may be delayed 24-48 hours after I.V. administration or 3-4 days after I.M. administration.
Anaphylactoid reactions: Respiratory difficulties and cardiovascular collapse have been reported and occur most frequently within the first several minutes of administration.

Overdosage/Toxicology Symptoms include erosion of GI mucosa, pulmonary edema, hyperthermia, convulsions, tachycardia, hepatic and renal impairment, coma, hematemesis, lethargy, tachycardia, and acidosis. Serum iron >300 mcg/mL requires overdose treatment, due to severe toxicity. Although rare, if a severe iron overdose (when the serum iron concentration exceeds the total iron-binding capacity) occurs, it may be treated with deferoxamine. Deferoxamine may be administered I.V. (80 mg/kg over 24 hours) or I.M. (40-90 mg/kg every 8 hours).

Drug Interactions Decreased effect with chloramphenicol

Ethanol/Nutrition/Herb Interactions Food: Iron bioavailability may be decreased if taken with dairy products.

Stability Store at room temperature. Stability of parenteral admixture is 3 months refrigerated. Solutions for infusion should be diluted in 250-1000 mL NS.

Mechanism of Action The released iron, from the plasma, eventually replenishes the depleted iron stores in the bone marrow where it is incorporated into hemoglobin

Pharmacokinetics
Absorption: I.M.: Prompt, 50% to 90% absorbed, balance slowly absorbed over months
Elimination: By reticuloendothelial system and excreted in urine and feces (via bile)

Dosage
Geriatrics & Adults:
Note: A 0.5 mL test dose should be given prior to starting iron dextran therapy.
Iron-deficiency anemia: I.M., I.V.:
Dose (mL) = 0.0442 (desired Hgb - observed Hgb) x LBW + (0.26 x LBW)
Desired hemoglobin: Usually 14.8 g/dL
LBW = Lean body weight in kg

Iron replacement therapy for blood loss: I.M., I.V.: Replacement iron (mg) = blood loss (mL) x Hct

Maximum daily dosage:
Manufacturer's labeling: **Note:** Replacement of larger estimated iron deficits may be achieved by serial administration of smaller incremental dosages. Daily dosages should be limited to: Adults >50 kg: 100 mg iron (2 mL)

Total dose infusion (unlabeled): The entire dose (estimated iron deficit) may be diluted and administered as a one-time I.V. infusion.

Administration Note: Test dose: A test dose should be given on the first day of therapy; patient should be observed for 1 hour for hypersensitivity reaction, then the remaining dose (dose minus test dose) should be given. Epinephrine should be available.

I.M.: Use Z-track technique (displacement of the skin laterally prior to injection); injection should be deep into the upper outer quadrant of buttock; subsequent injections should be given into alternate buttock

I.V.: Test dose should be given gradually over at least 5 minutes. Subsequent dose(s) may be administered by I.V. bolus at rate of ≤50 mg/minute or diluted in 250-1000 mL NS and infused over 1-6 hours (initial 25 mL should be given slowly and patient should be observed for allergic reactions); avoid dilutions with dextrose (increased incidence of local pain and phlebitis)

Monitoring Parameters Hemoglobin, hematocrit, ferritin, reticulocyte count

Reference Range Therapeutic: Male: 75-175 mcg/dL (SI: 13.4-31.3 µmol/L); Female: 65-165 mcg/dL (SI: 11.6-29.5 µmol/L); ranges may vary by laboratory

Test Interactions May cause falsely elevated values of serum bilirubin and falsely decreased values of serum calcium

Patient Information Report any unusual systemic or local reactions to your physician; pain on administration .

Additional Information Avoid iron injection if oral intake is feasible; a test dose of 0.5 mL I.V. or I.M. should be given to observe for adverse reactions

Special Geriatric Considerations Anemia in the elderly is most often caused by "anemia of chronic disease", a result of aging effect in bone marrow, or associated with inflammation rather than blood loss. Iron stores are usually normal or increased, with a serum ferritin >50 ng/mL and a decreased total iron binding capacity. Hence, the anemia is not secondary to iron deficiency but the inability of the reticuloendothelial system to use available iron stores. I.V. administration of iron dextran is often preferred over I.M. in the elderly secondary to a decreased muscle mass and the need for daily injections.

Dosage Forms Excipient information presented when available (limited, particularly for generics); consult specific product labeling.
Note: Strength expressed as elemental iron
Injection, solution:
Dexferrum®: 50 mg/mL (1 mL, 2 mL)
INFeD®: 50 mg/mL (2 mL)

Selected References
Lipschitz DA, "The Anemia of Chronic Disease," *J Am Geriatr Soc*, 1990, 38(11):1258-64.

♦ **Iron Fumarate** *see* Ferrous Fumarate *on page 618*
♦ **Iron Gluconate** *see* Ferrous Gluconate *on page 619*
♦ **Iron Sulfate** *see* Ferrous Sulfate *on page 621*
♦ **ISD** *see* Isosorbide Dinitrate *on page 839*
♦ **ISDN** *see* Isosorbide Dinitrate *on page 839*
♦ **ISG** *see* Immune Globulin (Intramuscular) *on page 795*
♦ **ISMN** *see* Isosorbide Mononitrate *on page 842*
♦ **Ismo®** *see* Isosorbide Mononitrate *on page 842*
♦ **Isobamate** *see* Carisoprodol *on page 240*

Isocarboxazid (eye soe kar BOKS a zid)

Related Information
Antidepressant Agents *on page 1742*
U.S. Brand Names Marplan®
Generic Available No
Pharmacologic Category Antidepressant, Monoamine Oxidase Inhibitor
Use Symptomatic treatment of atypical, nonendogenous or neurotic depression
Restrictions An FDA-approved medication guide concerning the use of antidepressants in children, adolescents, and young adults must be distributed when dispensing an outpatient prescription (new or refill) where this medication is to be used without direct supervision of a healthcare provider. Medication guides are available at http://www.fda.gov/cder/Offices/ODS/medication_guides.htm. Dispense to parents or guardians of children and adolescents receiving this medication.
(Continued)

Isocarboxazid *(Continued)*

Contraindications Hypersensitivity to isocarboxazid or any component of the formulation; uncontrolled hypertension; pheochromocytoma; hepatic or renal disease; cerebrovascular defect; cardiovascular disease (CHF); concurrent use of sympathomimetics (and related compounds), CNS depressants, ethanol, meperidine, bupropion, buspirone, guanethidine, and serotonergic drugs (including SSRIs) - do not use within 5 weeks of fluoxetine discontinuation or 2 weeks of other antidepressant discontinuation; general anesthesia, local vasoconstrictors; spinal anesthesia (hypotension may be exaggerated). Foods which are high in tyramine, tryptophan, or dopamine, chocolate, or caffeine.

Warnings/Precautions [U.S. Boxed Warning]: Antidepressants increase the risk of suicidal thinking and behavior in children, adolescents, and young adults (18-24 years of age) with major depressive disorder (MDD) and other psychiatric disorders; consider risk prior to prescribing. Short-term studies did not show an increased risk in patients >24 years of age and showed a decreased risk in patients ≥65 years. Closely monitor for clinical worsening, suicidality, or unusual changes in behavior; the patient's family or caregiver should be instructed to closely observe the patient and communicate condition with healthcare provider. A medication guide should be dispensed with each prescription.

The possibility of a suicide attempt is inherent in major depression and may persist until remission occurs. Monitor for worsening of depression or suicidality, especially during initiation of therapy (generally first 1-2 months) or with dose increases or decreases. Use caution in high-risk patients. Worsening depression and severe abrupt suicidality that are not part of the presenting symptoms may require discontinuation or modification of drug therapy. The patient's family or caregiver should be alerted to monitor patients for the emergence of suicidality and associated behaviors (such as agitation, irritability, hostility, impulsivity, and hypomania) and notify healthcare provider.

May worsen psychosis in some patients or precipitate a shift to mania or hypomania in patients with bipolar disorder. Patients presenting with depressive symptoms should be screened for bipolar disorder. Monotherapy in patients with bipolar disorder should be avoided. Isocarboxazid is not FDA approved for the treatment of bipolar depression.

Use with caution in patients who are hyperactive, hyperexcitable, or who have glaucoma, hyperthyroidism, or diabetes; avoid use of meperidine within 2 weeks of isocarboxazid use. Toxic reactions have occurred with dextromethorphan. Hypertensive crisis may occur with foods/supplements high in tyramine, tryptophan, phenylalanine, or tyrosine content. Should not be used in combination with other antidepressants. Hypotensive effects of antihypertensives (beta-blockers, thiazides) may be exaggerated. May cause orthostatic hypotension (especially at dosages >30 mg/day) - use with caution in patients with hypotension or patients who would not tolerate transient hypotensive episodes - effects may be additive when used with other agents known to cause orthostasis (phenothiazines).

Discontinue at least 48 hours prior to myelography. May increase the risks associated with electroconvulsive therapy. Consider discontinuing, when possible, prior to elective surgery. Use with caution in patients receiving disulfiram. Use with caution in patients with renal impairment.

Adverse Reactions (Reflective of adult population; not specific for elderly)
>10%:
  Cardiovascular: Orthostatic hypotension
  Central nervous system: Drowsiness
  Endocrine & metabolic: Decreased sexual ability
  Neuromuscular & skeletal: Weakness, trembling
  Ocular: Blurred vision
1% to 10%:
  Cardiovascular: Tachycardia, peripheral edema
  Central nervous system: Nervousness, chills
  Dermatologic: Xerostomia
  Gastrointestinal: Diarrhea, anorexia, constipation, xerostomia

Drug Interactions
  Amphetamines: MAO inhibitors in combination with amphetamines may result in severe hypertensive reaction; these combinations are best avoided.
  Anorexiants: Concurrent use of anorexiants may result in serotonin syndrome; these combinations are best avoided; includes dexfenfluramine, fenfluramine, or sibutramine.
  Barbiturates: MAO inhibitors may inhibit the metabolism of barbiturates and prolong their effect.
  CNS stimulants: MAO inhibitors in combination with stimulants (methylphenidate) may result in severe hypertensive reaction; these combinations are best avoided
  Dextromethorphan: Concurrent use of MAO inhibitors may result in serotonin syndrome; these combinations are best avoided.

Disulfiram: MAO inhibitors may produce delirium in patients receiving disulfiram; monitor.

Guanadrel and guanethidine: MAO inhibitors inhibit the antihypertensive response to guanadrel or guanethidine; use an alternative antihypertensive agent.

Hypoglycemic agents: MAO inhibitors may produce hypoglycemia in patients with diabetes; monitor.

Levodopa: MAO inhibitors in combination with levodopa may result in hypertensive reactions; monitor.

Lithium: MAO inhibitors in combination with lithium have resulted in malignant hyperpyrexia; this combination is best avoided.

Meperidine: May cause serotonin syndrome when combined with an MAO inhibitor; avoid this combination.

Nefazodone: Concurrent use of MAO inhibitors may result in serotonin syndrome; these combinations are best avoided.

Norepinephrine: MAO inhibitors may increase the pressor response of norepinephrine (effect is generally small); monitor.

Reserpine: MAO inhibitors in combination with reserpine may result in hypertensive reactions; monitor.

Serotonin agonists: Theoretically, may increase the risk of serotonin syndrome; includes sumatriptan, naratriptan, rizatriptan, and zolmitriptan.

SSRIs: May cause serotonin syndrome when combined with an MAO inhibitor; avoid this combination.

Succinylcholine: MAO inhibitors may prolong the muscle relaxation produced by succinylcholine via decreased plasma pseudocholinesterase.

Sympathomimetics (indirect-acting): MAO inhibitors in combination with sympathomimetics such as dopamine, metaraminol, phenylephrine, and decongestants (pseudoephedrine) may result in severe hypertensive reaction; these combinations are best avoided.

Tramadol: May increase the risk of seizures and serotonin syndrome in patients receiving an MAO inhibitor.

Trazodone: Concurrent use of MAO inhibitors may result in serotonin syndrome; these combinations are best avoided.

Tricyclic antidepressants: May cause serotonin syndrome when combined with an MAO inhibitor; avoid this combination.

Venlafaxine: Concurrent use of MAO inhibitors may result in serotonin syndrome; these combinations are best avoided.

Ethanol/Nutrition/Herb Interactions

Ethanol: Avoid ethanol (based on CNS depressant effects and potential tyramine content)

Food: Concurrent ingestion of foods rich in tyramine may cause sudden and severe high blood pressure (hypertensive crisis). Avoid tyramine-containing foods with MAOIs. Food's freshness is also an important concern; improperly stored or spoiled food can create an environment where tyramine concentrations may increase.

Herb/Nutraceuticals: Avoid supplements containing caffeine, tyrosine, tryptophan or phenylalanine. Ingestion of large quantities may increase the risk of severe side effects (eg, hypertensive reactions, serotonin syndrome).

Mechanism of Action Thought to act by increasing endogenous concentrations of epinephrine, norepinephrine, dopamine, and serotonin through inhibition of the enzyme (monoamine oxidase) responsible for the breakdown of these neurotransmitters

Pharmacokinetics

Absorption: Oral: Well absorbed; undergoes acetylation in the liver; older patients have been reported to have higher blood concentrations than younger adults after 2 weeks of continuous treatment

Elimination: In urine primarily as metabolites and unchanged drug

Dosage

Geriatrics & Adults: Depression: Oral: 10 mg 2-3 times/day; reduce to 10-20 mg/day in divided doses when condition improves

Monitoring Parameters Blood pressure, especially at therapy onset or if other CNS drugs or cardiovascular drugs are added

Reference Range Inhibition of platelet monoamine oxidase (≥80%) correlates with clinical response

Patient Information Avoid tyramine-containing foods and drinks; see Warnings/Precautions.

Additional Information Isocarboxazid was reintroduced to the market in January 1999.

Special Geriatric Considerations The MAO inhibitors are effective and generally well tolerated by elderly patients. It is their potential interactions with tyramine-containing foods and other drugs and their effects on blood pressure that have limited their use. The MAO inhibitors are usually reserved for patients who do not tolerate or respond to the traditional "cyclic" or "second generation" antidepressants. The brain activity of monoamine oxidase increases with age and even more so in (Continued)

Isocarboxazid (Continued)

patients with Alzheimer's disease. Therefore, the MAO inhibitor may have an increased role in patients with Alzheimer's disease who are depressed. Information on the use of isocarboxazid in the elderly is limited.

Dosage Forms Excipient information presented when available (limited, particularly for generics); consult specific product labeling.
Tablet: 10 mg

♦ **Isochron**™ *see* Isosorbide Dinitrate *on page 839*

Isoniazid (eye soe NYE a zid)

Medication Safety Issues
International issues:
Hydra® [Japan] may be confused with Hydrea®
U.S. Brand Names Nydrazid® [DSC]
Canadian Brand Names Isotamine®; PMS-Isoniazid
Index Terms INH; Isonicotinic Acid Hydrazide
Generic Available Yes
Pharmacologic Category Antitubercular Agent
Use Treatment of susceptible tuberculosis infections; treatment of latent tuberculosis infection (LTBI)
Contraindications Hypersensitivity to isoniazid or any component of the formulation; acute liver disease; previous history of hepatic damage during isoniazid therapy
Warnings/Precautions Use with caution in patients with renal impairment and chronic liver disease. **[U.S. Boxed Warning]: Severe and sometimes fatal hepatitis may occur or develop even after many months of treatment.** Patients must report any prodromal symptoms of hepatitis, such as fatigue, weakness, malaise, anorexia, nausea, or vomiting. Periodic ophthalmic examinations are recommended even when usual symptoms do not occur; pyridoxine (10-50 mg/day) is recommended in individuals likely to develop peripheral neuropathies.
Adverse Reactions (Reflective of adult population; not specific for elderly)
Frequency not defined.
Cardiovascular: Hypertension, palpitation, tachycardia, vasculitis
Central nervous system: Dizziness, encephalopathy, memory impairment, slurred speech, lethargy, fever, depression, psychosis, seizure
Dermatologic: Rash (morbilliform, maculopapular, pruritic, or exfoliative), flushing
Endocrine & metabolic: Hyperglycemia, metabolic acidosis, gynecomastia, pellagra, pyridoxine deficiency
Gastrointestinal: Anorexia, nausea, vomiting, stomach pain
Hematologic: Agranulocytosis, anemia (sideroblastic, hemolytic, or aplastic), thrombocytopenia, eosinophilia, lymphadenopathy
Hepatic: LFTs mildly increased (10% to 20%); hyperbilirubinemia, jaundice, hepatitis (may involve progressive liver damage; risk increases with age; 2.3% in patients >50 years)
Neuromuscular & skeletal: Weakness, peripheral neuropathy (dose-related incidence, 10% to 20% incidence with 10 mg/kg/day), hyper-reflexia, arthralgia, lupus-like syndrome
Ocular: Blurred vision, loss of vision, optic neuritis and atrophy
Overdosage/Toxicology Symptoms include nausea, vomiting, slurred speech, dizziness, blurred vision, hallucinations, stupor, coma, and intractable seizures. The onset of metabolic acidosis is 30 minutes to 3 hours. Because of severe morbidity and high mortality rates associated with isoniazid overdose, patients who are asymptomatic after an overdose should be monitored for 4-6 hours. Pyridoxine has been shown to be effective in the treatment of intoxication, especially when seizures occur. Pyridoxine I.V. is administered on a milligram to milligram dose. If the amount of isoniazid ingested is unknown, 5 g of pyridoxine should be given over 3-5 minutes and may be followed by an additional 5 g in 30 minutes. Treatment is supportive. Airway protection and ventilation may be required, with diazepam for seizures, and sodium bicarbonate for acidosis. Forced diuresis and hemodialysis can result in more rapid removal.
Drug Interactions Substrate of CYP2E1 (major); **Inhibits** CYP1A2 (weak), 2A6 (moderate), 2C9 (weak), 2C19 (strong), 2D6 (moderate), 2E1 (moderate), 3A4 (strong); **Induces** CYP2E1 (after discontinuation) (weak)
Acetaminophen: Isoniazid may enhance the adverse/toxic effect of acetaminophen.
Antacids: Antacids may decrease the absorption of isoniazid.
Benzodiazepines (metabolized by oxidation): Isoniazid may decrease the metabolism, via CYP isoenzymes, of benzodiazepines (metabolized by oxidation).
Carbamazepine: Isoniazid may decrease the metabolism of carbamazepine.
Cycloserine: Cycloserine may enhance the CNS depressant effect of isoniazid.
CYP2A6 substrates: Isoniazid may increase the levels/effects of CYP2A6 substrates. Example substrates include dexmedetomidine and ifosfamide.

CYP2C19 substrates: Isoniazid may increase the levels/effects of CYP2C19 substrates. Example substrates include citalopram, diazepam, methsuximide, phenytoin, propranolol, and sertraline.

CYP2D6 substrates: Isoniazid may increase the levels/effects of CYP2D6 substrates. Example substrates include amphetamines, selected beta-blockers, dextromethorphan, fluoxetine, lidocaine, mirtazapine, nefazodone, paroxetine, risperidone, ritonavir, thioridazine, tricyclic antidepressants, and venlafaxine.

CYP2D6 prodrug substrates: Isoniazid may decrease the levels/effects of CYP2D6 prodrug substrates. Example prodrug substrates include codeine, hydrocodone, oxycodone, and tramadol.

CYP2E1 substrates: Isoniazid may increase the levels/effects of CYP2E1 substrates. Example substrates include inhalational anesthetics, theophylline, and trimethadione.

CYP3A4 substrates: Isoniazid may increase the levels/effects of CYP3A4 substrates. Example substrates include benzodiazepines, calcium channel blockers, mirtazapine, nateglinide, nefazodone, tacrolimus, and venlafaxine. Selected benzodiazepines (midazolam and triazolam), cisapride, ergot alkaloids, selected HMG-CoA reductase inhibitors (lovastatin and simvastatin), and pimozide are generally contraindicated with strong CYP3A4 inhibitors.

Disulfiram: Isoniazid may enhance the adverse/toxic effect of disulfiram.

Phenytoin: Isoniazid may decrease the metabolism, via CYP isoenzymes, of phenytoin.

Theophylline: Isoniazid may decrease the metabolism, via CYP isoenzymes, of theophylline derivatives.

Valproic Acid: Isoniazid may increase the serum concentration of valproic acid.

Ethanol/Nutrition/Herb Interactions

Ethanol: Avoid ethanol (increases the risk of hepatitis).

Food: Isoniazid serum levels may be decreased if taken with food. Has some ability to inhibit tyramine metabolism; several case reports of mild reactions (flushing, palpitations) after ingestion of cheese with or without wine. Isoniazid decreases folic acid absorption. Isoniazid alters pyridoxine metabolism.

Stability Protect oral dosage forms from light.

Mechanism of Action Unknown, but may include the inhibition of myocolic acid synthesis resulting in disruption of the bacterial cell wall

Pharmacokinetics

Absorption: Oral, I.M.: Rapid and complete

Distribution: Into all body tissues and fluids including the CSF

Protein binding: 10% to 15%

Metabolism: By the liver with decay rate determined genetically by acetylation phenotype

Half-life:

Fast acetylators: 30-100 minutes

Slow acetylators: 2-5 hours; half-life may be prolonged in patients with impaired hepatic function or severe renal impairment

Time to peak serum concentration: Oral: Within 1-2 hours; rate of absorption can be slowed when administered with food

Elimination: In urine (75% to 95%), feces, and saliva

Dosage

Geriatrics & Adults: Recommendations often change due to resistant strains and newly-developed information; consult *MMWR* for current CDC recommendations. Intramuscular is available in patients who are unable to either take or absorb oral therapy.

Treatment of latent tuberculosis infection (LTBI): 300 mg/day or 900 mg twice weekly for 6-9 months in patients who do not have HIV infection (9 months is optimal, 6 months may be considered to reduce costs of therapy) and 9 months in patients who have HIV infection. Extend to 12 months of therapy if interruptions in treatment occur.

Treatment of active TB infection (drug susceptible):

Daily therapy: 5 mg/kg/day given daily (usual dose: 300 mg/day); 10 mg/kg/day in 1-2 divided doses in patients with disseminated disease

Twice weekly directly observed therapy (DOT): 15 mg/kg (maximum: 900 mg); 3 times/week therapy: 15 mg/kg (maximum: 900 mg)

Note: Treatment may be defined by the number of doses administered (eg, "six-month" therapy involves 192 doses of INH and rifampin, and 56 doses of pyrazinamide. Six months is the shortest interval of time over which these doses may be administered, assuming no interruption of therapy.

Note: Concomitant administration of 6-50 mg/day pyridoxine is recommended in malnourished patients or those prone to neuropathy (eg, alcoholics, patients with diabetes)

Renal Impairment:

Cl_{cr} <10 mL/minute: Administer 50% of normal dose

Hemodialysis: Dialyzable (50% to 100%)

Administer dose postdialysis

(Continued)

Isoniazid *(Continued)*

Peritoneal dialysis, continuous arteriovenous or venovenous hemofiltration: Dose for Cl$_{cr}$ <10 mL/minute

Hepatic Impairment: Dose should be reduced in severe hepatic disease.

Monitoring Parameters Periodic liver function tests; sputum cultures monthly (until 2 consecutive negative cultures reported); monitoring for prodromal signs of hepatitis

Reference Range Therapeutic: 1-7 mcg/mL (SI: 7-51 µmol/L); Toxic: 20-710 mcg/mL (SI: 146-5176 µmol/L)

Test Interactions False-positive urinary glucose with Clinitest®

Patient Information Report any prodromal symptoms of hepatitis (fatigue, weakness, nausea, vomiting, dark urine, or yellowing of eyes) or any burning, tingling, or numbness in the extremities

Additional Information Pyridoxine should be given concomitantly in persons with conditions in which neuropathy is common (eg, diabetes, alcoholism, malnutrition)

Special Geriatric Considerations Age has not been shown to affect the pharmacokinetics of INH since acetylation phenotype determines clearance and half-life, acetylation rate does not change significantly with age. Most strains of *M. tuberculosis* found the elderly should be susceptible to INH since most acquired their initial infection prior to INH's introduction.

Dosage Forms Excipient information presented when available (limited, particularly for generics); consult specific product labeling. [DSC] = Discontinued product

Injection, solution (Nydrazid®): 100 mg/mL (10 mL) [DSC]

Syrup: 50 mg/5 mL (473 mL) [orange flavor]

Tablet: 100 mg, 300 mg

Selected References

American Thoracic Society, "Targeted Tuberculin Testing and Treatment of Latent Tuberculosis Infection," *MMWR*, 2000, 49(RR-6):1-51.

Bass JB Jr, Farer LS, Hopewell PC, et al, "Treatment of Tuberculosis and Tuberculosis Infection in Adults and Children," *Am J Respir Crit Care Med*, 1994, 149(5):1359-74.

Blumberg HM, Burman WJ, Chaisson RE, et al, "American Thoracic Society/Centers for Disease Control and Prevention/Infectious Diseases Society of America: Treatment of Tuberculosis," *Am J Respir Crit Care Med*, 2003, 167(4):603-62.

Centers for Disease Control and Prevention (CDC) and American Thoracic Society, "Update: Adverse Event Data and Revised American Thoracic Society/CDC Recommendations Against the Use of Rifampin and Pyrazinamide for Treatment of Latent Tuberculosis Infection - United States, 2003," *MMWR*, 2003, 52(31):735-9. Available at http://www.cdc.gov/mmwr/preview/mmwrhtml/mm5231a4.htm. Last accessed February 16, 2005.

Kergueris MF, Bourin M, and Larousse C, "Pharmacokinetics of Isoniazid: Influence of Age," *Eur J Clin Pharmacol*, 1986, 30(3):335-40.

"Treatment of Latent Tuberculosis Infection (LTBI), Last Updated: April 8, 2004," available at http://www.cdc.gov/nchstp/tb/pubs/tbfactsheets/250110.htm. Last accessed February 16, 2005.

Van Scoy RE and Wilkowske CJ, "Antituberculous Agents: Isoniazid, Rifampin, Streptomycin, Ethambutol, and Pyrazinamide," *Mayo Clin Proc*, 1983, 58(4):233-40.

Yoshikawa TT, "Tuberculosis in Aging Adults," *J Am Geriatr Soc*, 1992, 40(2):178-87.

♦ **Isonicotinic Acid Hydrazide** *see* Isoniazid *on page 836*

♦ **Isonipecaine Hydrochloride** *see* Meperidine *on page 980*

♦ **Isophane Insulin** *see* Insulin NPH *on page 813*

♦ **Isophane Insulin and Regular Insulin** *see* Insulin NPH and Insulin Regular *on page 814*

Isoproterenol *(eye soe proe TER e nole)*

Medication Safety Issues

Sound-alike/look-alike issues:

Isuprel® may be confused with Disophrol®, Ismelin®, Isordil®

U.S. Brand Names Isuprel®

Index Terms Isoproterenol Hydrochloride

Generic Available Yes

Pharmacologic Category Beta$_1$- & Beta$_2$-Adrenergic Agonist Agent

Use Treatment of asthma or COPD (reversible airway obstruction), AV nodal block, hemodynamically compromised bradyarrhythmias or atropine-resistant bradyarrhythmias; temporary use in third degree AV block until pacemaker insertion, low cardiac output, vasoconstrictive shock states

Unlabeled/Investigational Use Temporizing measure before transvenous pacing for torsade de pointes; diagnostic aid (vasovagal syncope)

Contraindications Hypersensitivity to sulfites or isoproterenol, any component of the formulation, or other sympathomimetic amines; angina, pre-existing cardiac arrhythmias (ventricular); tachycardia or AV block caused by cardiac glycoside intoxication

Warnings/Precautions Use with extreme caution; not currently a treatment of choice; use with caution in elderly patients, diabetics, renal or cardiovascular disease, seizure disorder, or hyperthyroidism; excessive or prolonged use may result in decreased effectiveness.

Adverse Reactions (Reflective of adult population; not specific for elderly)
Frequency not defined.
Cardiovascular: Premature ventricular beats, bradycardia, hyper-/hypotension, chest pain, palpitation, tachycardia, ventricular arrhythmia, MI size increased
Central nervous system: Headache, nervousness or restlessness
Endocrine & metabolic: Serum glucose increased, serum potassium decreased, hypokalemia
Gastrointestinal: Nausea, vomiting
Respiratory: Dyspnea

Overdosage/Toxicology Symptoms of overdose include tachycardia, tremor, hypertension or hypotension, angina, and seizures. Hypokalemia also may occur. Cardiac arrest and death may be associated with abuse of beta-agonist bronchodilators. Treatment includes immediate discontinuation and symptomatic and supportive therapies. Cautious use of beta-adrenergic blocking agents may be considered in severe cases.

Drug Interactions Increased toxicity: Sympathomimetic agents may cause headaches and elevate blood pressure; general anesthetics may cause arrhythmias

Ethanol/Nutrition/Herb Interactions Herb/Nutraceutical: Avoid ephedra, yohimbe (may cause CNS stimulation).

Stability Isoproterenol solution should be stored at room temperature. It should not be used if a color or precipitate is present. Exposure to air, light, or increased temperature may cause a pink to brownish pink color to develop. Stability of parenteral admixture at room temperature (25°C) or at refrigeration (4°C) is 24 hours.
Standard diluent: 2 mg/500 mL D_5W; 4 mg/500 mL D_5W.
Minimum volume: 1 mg/100 mL D_5W.

Mechanism of Action Stimulates beta$_1$- and beta$_2$-receptors resulting in relaxation of bronchial, GI, and uterine smooth muscle, increased heart rate and contractility, vasodilation of peripheral vasculature

Pharmacokinetics
Metabolism: By conjugation in many tissues including the liver and lungs
Half-life: 2.5-5 minutes
Time to peak serum concentration: Oral: Within 1-2 hours
Elimination: In urine principally as sulfate conjugates

Dosage
Geriatrics & Adults: Cardiac arrhythmias: I.V.: Initial: 2 mcg/minute; titrate to patient response (2-10 mcg/minute)

Administration I.V. infusion administration requires the use of an infusion pump. To prepare for infusion: 1 mg isoproterenol to 500 mL D_5W, final concentration 2 mcg/mL

Monitoring Parameters Pulmonary function, blood pressure, pulse

Patient Information You may experience nervousness, dizziness, or fatigue (use caution when driving or engaging in tasks requiring alertness until response to drug is known); or dry mouth, nausea, or vomiting (frequent small meals may reduce the incidence of nausea or vomiting). Report chest pain, rapid heartbeat or palpitations, unresolved/persistent GI upset, dizziness, fatigue, trembling, increased anxiety, sleeplessness, or difficulty breathing.

Additional Information Isoproterenol is not a drug of first choice in the chronic treatment of asthma because of its beta$_1$ effects.

Dosage Forms Excipient information presented when available (limited, particularly for generics); consult specific product labeling.
Injection, solution, as hydrochloride: 0.02 mg/mL (10 mL); 0.2 mg/mL (1:5000) (1 mL, 5 mL) [contains sodium metabisulfite]

♦ **Isoproterenol Hydrochloride** *see* Isoproterenol *on page 838*
♦ **Isoptin® SR** *see* Verapamil *on page 1671*
♦ **Isopto® Atropine** *see* Atropine *on page 137*
♦ **Isopto® Carbachol** *see* Carbachol *on page 230*
♦ **Isopto® Carpine** *see* Pilocarpine *on page 1259*
♦ **Isopto® Homatropine** *see* Homatropine *on page 753*
♦ **Isopto® Hyoscine** *see* Scopolamine Derivatives *on page 1448*
♦ **Isordil®** *see* Isosorbide Dinitrate *on page 839*

Isosorbide Dinitrate (eye soe SOR bide dye NYE trate)

Medication Safety Issues
Sound-alike/look-alike issues:
Isordil® may be confused with Inderal®, Isuprel®

International issues:
Nitrobide® [Japan] may be confused with Microzide™ which is a brand name for hydrochlorothiazide in the U.S.

(Continued)

Isosorbide Dinitrate *(Continued)*

U.S. Brand Names Dilatrate®-SR; Isochron™; Isordil®

Canadian Brand Names Apo-ISDN®; Cedocard®-SR; Coronex®; Novo-Sorbide; PMS-Isosorbide

Index Terms ISD; ISDN

Generic Available Yes: Tablet, sublingual tablet

Pharmacologic Category Vasodilator

Use Prevention and treatment of angina pectoris; treatment of congestive heart failure; relief of pain, dysphagia, and spasm in esophageal spasm with GE reflux

Unlabeled/Investigational Use Esophageal spastic disorders

Contraindications Hypersensitivity to isosorbide dinitrate or any component of the formulation; hypersensitivity to organic nitrates; concurrent use with sildenafil; angle-closure glaucoma (intraocular pressure may be increased); head trauma or cerebral hemorrhage (increase intracranial pressure); severe anemia

Warnings/Precautions Use with caution in patients with increased intracranial pressure, hypotension, hypovolemia, glaucoma; sustained release products may be absorbed erratically in patients with GI hypermotility or malabsorption syndrome; do not crush or chew sublingual dosage form; abrupt withdrawal may result in angina; tolerance may develop (adjust dose or change agent). Nitrates may aggravate angina caused by hypertrophic cardiomyopathy. Avoid concurrent use with PDE-5 inhibitors (eg, sildenafil, tadalafil, vardenafil).

Adverse Reactions (Reflective of adult population; not specific for elderly) Frequency not defined.

Cardiovascular: Hypotension (infrequent), postural hypotension, crescendo angina (uncommon), rebound hypertension (uncommon), pallor, cardiovascular collapse, tachycardia, shock, flushing, peripheral edema

Central nervous system: Headache (most common), lightheadedness (related to blood pressure changes), syncope (uncommon), dizziness, restlessness

Gastrointestinal: Nausea, vomiting, bowel incontinence, xerostomia

Genitourinary: Urinary incontinence

Hematologic: Methemoglobinemia (rare, overdose)

Neuromuscular & skeletal: Weakness

Ocular: Blurred vision

Miscellaneous: Cold sweat

The incidence of hypotension and adverse cardiovascular events may be increased when used in combination with sildenafil (Viagra®).

Overdosage/Toxicology The most common symptoms of overdose include hypotension, throbbing headache, tachycardia, and flushing. Methemoglobinemia may occur with massive doses. Hypotension may aggravate symptoms of cardiac ischemia or cerebrovascular disease, and may even cause seizures (rare). Treatment consists of recumbent positioning and administration of fluids. Alpha-adrenergic vasopressors may be required. Treat methemoglobinemia with oxygen and methylene blue at a dose of 1-2 mg/kg slow I.V.

Drug Interactions Substrate of CYP3A4 (major)

CYP3A4 inducers: CYP3A4 inducers may decrease the levels/effects of isosorbide dinitrate. Example inducers include aminoglutethimide, carbamazepine, nafcillin, nevirapine, phenobarbital, phenytoin, and rifamycins.

CYP3A4 inhibitors: May increase the levels/effects of isosorbide dinitrate. Example inhibitors include azole antifungals, clarithromycin, diclofenac, doxycycline, erythromycin, imatinib, isoniazid, nefazodone, nicardipine, propofol, protease inhibitors, quinidine, telithromycin, and verapamil.

Sildenafil, tadalafil, vardenafil: Significant reduction of systolic and diastolic blood pressure with concurrent use (contraindicated). Do not administer sildenafil, tadalafil, or vardenafil within 24 hours of a nitrate preparation.

Ethanol/Nutrition/Herb Interactions Ethanol: Caution with ethanol (may increase risk of hypotension).

Mechanism of Action Stimulation of intracellular cyclic-GMP results in vascular smooth muscle relaxation of both arterial and venous vasculature. Increased venous pooling decreases left ventricular pressure (preload) and arterial dilatation decreases arterial resistance (afterload). Therefore, this reduces cardiac oxygen demand by decreasing left ventricular pressure and systemic vascular resistance by dilating arteries. Additionally, coronary artery dilation improves collateral flow to ischemic regions; esophageal smooth muscle is relaxed via the same mechanism.

Pharmacodynamics

Onset of action: Sublingual tablet: 2-10 minutes; Chewable tablet: 3 minutes; Oral tablet: 45-60 minutes

Duration: Sublingual tablet: 1-2 hours; Chewable tablet: 0.5-2 hours; Oral tablet: 4-6 hours

Pharmacokinetics

Metabolism: Extensive in the liver to conjugated metabolites, including isosorbide 5-mononitrate (active) and 2-mononitrate (active); oral first pass bioavailability: ~50%

Half-life:

Parent: 1-4 hours

5-mononitrate: 4 hours

Elimination: In urine and feces

Dosage

Geriatrics: Elderly patients should be given lowest recommended adult daily doses initially and titrate upward.

Adults:

Angina:

Oral: 5-40 mg 4 times/day or 40 mg every 8-12 hours in sustained released dosage form

Sublingual: 2.5-5 mg every 5-10 minutes for maximum of 3 doses in 15-30 minutes; may also use prophylactically 15 minutes prior to activities which may provoke an attack

Congestive heart failure:

Initial dose: 20 mg 3-4 times/day

Target dose: 120-160 mg/day in divided doses; use in combination with hydralazine

Esophageal spastic disorders (unlabeled use):

Oral: 5-10 mg before meals

Sublingual: 2.5 mg after meals

Note: Tolerance to nitrate effects develops with chronic exposure. Dose escalation does not overcome this effect. Tolerance can only be overcome by short periods of nitrate absence from the body. Short periods (10-12 hours) of nitrate withdrawal help minimize tolerance. General recommendations are to take the last dose of short-acting agents no later than 7 PM; administer 2-3 times/day rather than 4 times/day. Sustained release preparations could be administered at times to allow a 15- to 17-hour interval between first and last daily dose. Example: Administer sustained release at 8 AM and 2 PM for a twice daily regimen.

Renal Impairment: Hemodialysis: During hemodialysis, administer dose postdialysis or administer supplemental 10-20 mg dose. During peritoneal dialysis, supplemental dose is not necessary.

Administration Do not administer around-the-clock; the first dose of nitrates should be administered in a physician's office to observe for maximal cardiovascular dynamic effects and adverse effects (orthostatic blood pressure drop, headache); when immediate release products are prescribed twice daily - recommend 7 AM and noon; for 3 times/day dosing - recommend 7 AM, noon, and 5 PM; when sustained-release products are indicated, suggest once a day in morning or via twice daily dosing at 8 AM and 2 PM

Monitoring Parameters Monitor number of anginal episodes, orthostatic blood pressures; a decrease of 15 mm Hg pressure systolic and/or 10 mm Hg diastolic or an increase in heart rate of 10 beats/minute from baseline (no drug) indicates approximate maximal cardiodynamic effects to nitrates and end point for dosing

Test Interactions Decreased cholesterol (S)

Patient Information Dispense drug in easy-to-open container; do not chew or crush sublingual or sustained-release dosage form; do not change brands without consulting your pharmacist or physician; patient should be instructed to take sublingual and chewable tablets while sitting down; any angina that persists for more than 20 minutes should be evaluated by a physician immediately

Additional Information For the treatment of CHF where isosorbide dinitrate is used in place of an ACE inhibitor, it is necessary to use a combination of isosorbide and hydralazine.

Special Geriatric Considerations The first dose of nitrates (sublingual, chewable, oral) should be taken in a physician's office to observe for maximal cardiovascular dynamic effects and adverse effects (eg, orthostatic blood pressure drop, headache). The use of nitrates for angina may occasionally promote reflux esophagitis. This may require dose adjustments or changing therapeutic agents to correct this adverse effect.

Dosage Forms Excipient information presented when available (limited, particularly for generics); consult specific product labeling. [DSC] = Discontinued product

Capsule, sustained release (Dilatrate®-SR): 40 mg

Tablet: 5 mg, 10 mg, 20 mg, 30 mg

Isordil®: 5 mg, 10 mg [DSC], 20 mg [DSC], 30 mg [DSC], 40 mg

Tablet, extended release (Isochron™): 40 mg

Tablet, sublingual: 2.5 mg, 5 mg

Isordil®: 2.5 mg, 5 mg, 10 mg [DSC]

Selected References

Flaherty JT, "Hemodynamic Attenuation and the Nitrate-Free Interval: Alternative Dosing Strategies for Transdermal Nitroglycerin," *Am J Cardiol,* 1985, 56(17):321-71.

(Continued)

Isosorbide Dinitrate *(Continued)*

Gibbons RJ, Abrams J, Chatterjee K, et al, "ACC/AHA 2002 Guideline Update for the Management of Patients With Chronic Stable Angina - Summary Article: A Report of the American College of Cardiology/American Heart Association Task Force on Practice Guidelines (Committee on the Management of Patients With Chronic Stable Angina)," *J Am Coll Cardiol*, 2003, 41(1):159-68. Available at: http://http://www.acc.org/clinical/guidelines/stable/stable_clean.pdf. Accessed May 5, 2004.

Parker JO, "Eccentric Dosing With Isosorbide-5-Mononitrate in Angina Pectoris," *Am J Cardiol*, 1993, 72(12):871-6.

Parker JO, Fanell B, Lahey KA, et al, "Effect of Intervals Between Doses on the Development or Tolerance to Isosorbide Dinitrate," *N Engl J Med*, 1987, 316(23):1440-4.

Isosorbide Dinitrate and Hydralazine
(eye soe SOR bide dye NYE trate & hye DRAL a zeen)

U.S. Brand Names BiDil®
Index Terms Hydralazine and Isosorbide Dinitrate
Generic Available No
Pharmacologic Category Vasodilator
Use Treatment of heart failure, adjunct to standard therapy, in African-Americans
Dosage

Geriatrics & Adults: Heart failure: Oral: Initial: 1 tablet 3 times/day; titrate to a maximum dose of 2 tablets 3 times/day; see individual agents for CHF target doses

Dosage adjustment for toxicity: If patient experiences persistent headache, adjust dosing to twice daily.

Special Geriatric Considerations The pharmacokinetics of hydralazine and isosorbide alone or in combination have not been studied. As with all antihypertensives and nitrate products, caution should be used on initiation of therapy, as hypotension may be encountered. Since many elderly are volume depleted, secondary to their blunted thirst reflex and/or use of diuretics, doses used initially should be at lowest recommended dose. The use of nitrates may occasionally promote reflux esophagitis. Monitor for these effects at start of therapy.

Dosage Forms Excipient information presented when available (limited, particularly for generics); consult specific product labeling.

Tablet: Isosorbide dinitrate 20 mg and hydralazine 37.5 mg

Isosorbide Mononitrate (eye soe SOR bide mon oh NYE trate)

Medication Safety Issues
Sound-alike/look-alike issues:
Imdur® may be confused with Imuran®, Inderal LA®, K-Dur®
Monoket® may be confused with Monopril®

International issues:
Nitrex® [Italy] may be confused with Imitrex® which is a brand name for sumatriptan in the U.S.

U.S. Brand Names Imdur®; Ismo®; Monoket®
Canadian Brand Names Apo-ISMN; Imdur®
Index Terms ISMN
Generic Available Yes
Pharmacologic Category Vasodilator
Use Long-acting metabolite of the vasodilator isosorbide dinitrate used for the prophylactic treatment of angina pectoris
Contraindications Hypersensitivity to isosorbide or any component of the formulation; hypersensitivity to organic nitrates; concurrent use with sildenafil; angle-closure glaucoma (intraocular pressure may be increased); head trauma or cerebral hemorrhage (increase intracranial pressure); severe anemia
Warnings/Precautions Postural hypotension, transient episodes of weakness, dizziness, or syncope may occur even with small doses; ethanol accentuates these effects; tolerance and cross-tolerance to nitrate antianginal and hemodynamic effects may occur during prolonged isosorbide mononitrate therapy; (minimized by using the smallest effective dose, by alternating coronary vasodilators or offering drug-free intervals of as little as 12 hours). Excessive doses may result in severe headache, blurred vision, or xerostomia; increased anginal symptoms may be a result of dosage increases. Nitrates may aggravate angina caused by hypertrophic cardiomyopathy. Avoid concurrent use with PDE-5 inhibitors (eg, sildenafil, tadalafil, vardenafil).
Adverse Reactions (Reflective of adult population; not specific for elderly)
>10%: Central nervous system: Headache (19% to 38%)
1% to 10%:
Central nervous system: Dizziness (3% to 5%)
Gastrointestinal: Nausea/vomiting (2% to 4%)

The incidence of hypotension and adverse cardiovascular events may be increased when used in combination with sildenafil (Viagra®).

Overdosage/Toxicology The most common symptoms of overdose include hypotension, throbbing headache, tachycardia, and flushing. Methemoglobinemia may occur with massive doses. Hypotension may aggravate symptoms of cardiac ischemia or cerebrovascular disease and may even cause seizures (rare). Treatment consists of placing patient in recumbent position and administering fluids; alpha-adrenergic vasopressors may be required; treat methemoglobinemia with oxygen and methylene blue at a dose of 1-2 mg/kg I.V. slowly.

Drug Interactions Substrate of CYP3A4 (major)

CYP3A4 inducers: CYP3A4 inducers may decrease the levels/effects of isosorbide mononitrate. Example inducers include aminoglutethimide, carbamazepine, nafcillin, nevirapine, phenobarbital, phenytoin, and rifamycins.

CYP3A4 inhibitors: May increase the levels/effects of isosorbide mononitrate. Example inhibitors include azole antifungals, clarithromycin, diclofenac, doxycycline, erythromycin, imatinib, isoniazid, nefazodone, nicardipine, propofol, protease inhibitors, quinidine, telithromycin, and verapamil.

Sildenafil, tadalafil, vardenafil: Significant reduction of systolic and diastolic blood pressure with concurrent use (contraindicated). Do not administer sildenafil, tadalafil, or vardenafil within 24 hours of a nitrate preparation.

Ethanol/Nutrition/Herb Interactions Ethanol: Caution with ethanol (may increase risk of hypotension).

Stability Tablets should be stored in a tight container at room temperature of 15°C to 30°C (59°F to 86°F).

Mechanism of Action Prevailing mechanism of action for nitroglycerin (and other nitrates) is systemic venodilation, decreasing preload as measured by pulmonary capillary wedge pressure and left ventricular end diastolic volume and pressure; the average reduction in left ventricular end diastolic volume is 25% at rest, with a corresponding increase in ejection fractions of 50% to 60%. This effect improves congestive symptoms in heart failure and improves the myocardial perfusion gradient in patients with coronary artery disease.

Pharmacokinetics

Absorption: Oral: Nearly complete and low intersubject variability in its pharmacokinetic parameters and plasma concentrations

Metabolism: Metabolite of isosorbide dinitrate

Half-life: Mononitrate: ~4 hours (8 times that of dinitrate)

Dosage

Geriatrics: Start with lowest recommended adult dose.

Adults:

Angina: Oral:

Regular tablet: 5-20 mg twice daily with the two doses given 7 hours apart (eg, 8 AM and 3 PM) to decrease tolerance development; then titrate to 10 mg twice daily in first 2-3 days.

Extended release tablet: Initial: 30-60 mg given in morning as a single dose; titrate upward as needed, giving at least 3 days between increases; maximum daily single dose: 240 mg

Note: Tolerance to nitrate effects develops with chronic exposure. Dose escalation does not overcome this effect. Tolerance can only be overcome by short periods of nitrate absence from the body. Short periods (10-12 hours) of nitrate withdrawal help minimize tolerance. Recommended dosage regimens incorporate this interval. General recommendations are to take the last dose of short-acting agents no later than 7 PM; administer 2 times/day rather than 4 times/day. Administer sustained release tablet once daily in the morning.

Renal Impairment: Not necessary for elderly or patients with altered renal or hepatic function. Tolerance to nitrate effects develops with chronic exposure.

Administration Do not administer around-the-clock; Monoket® and Ismo® should be scheduled twice daily with doses 7 hours apart (8 AM and 3 PM); Imdur® may be administered once daily. Extended release tablets should not be chewed or crushed. Should be swallowed with a half-glassful of fluid.

Monitoring Parameters Monitor number of anginal episodes, orthostatic blood pressures; a decrease of 15 mm Hg pressure systolic and/or 10 mm Hg diastolic or an increase in heart rate of 10 beats/minute from baseline (no drug) indicates approximate maximal cardiodynamic effects to nitrates and end point for dosing

Patient Information Dispense drug in easy-to-open container; do not change brands without consulting pharmacist or physician; keep tablets or capsules tightly closed in original container; extended release tablets should not be chewed or crushed and should be swallowed together with a half-glassful of fluid; the antianginal efficacy of tablets (Ismo®, Monoket®) can be maintained by carefully following the prescribed schedule of dosing (2 doses taken 7 hours apart); the sustained-release tablet (Imdur®) should be given once daily; headaches are sometimes a marker of the activity of the (Continued)

Isosorbide Mononitrate *(Continued)*

drug; any angina that persists for more than 20 minutes should be evaluated by a physician immediately

Special Geriatric Considerations The first dose of nitrates (sublingual, chewable, oral) should be taken in a physician's office to observe for maximal cardiovascular dynamic effects and adverse effects (eg, orthostatic blood pressure drop, headache). The use of nitrates for angina may occasionally promote reflux esophagitis. This may require dose adjustments or changing therapeutic agents to correct this adverse effect.

Dosage Forms Excipient information presented when available (limited, particularly for generics); consult specific product labeling.

Tablet: 10 mg, 20 mg
    Ismo®: 20 mg
    Monoket®: 10 mg, 20 mg
Tablet, extended release: 30 mg, 60 mg, 120 mg
    Imdur®: 30 mg, 60 mg, 120 mg

Selected References

Flaherty JT, "Hemodynamic Attenuation and the Nitrate Dose-Free Interval: Alternative Dosing Strategies for Transdermal Nitroglycerin," *Am J Cardiol*, 1985, 56(17):321-71.

Gibbons RJ, Abrams J, Chatterjee K, et al, "ACC/AHA 2002 Guideline Update for the Management of Patients With Chronic Stable Angina - Summary Article: A Report of the American College of Cardiology/American Heart Association Task Force on Practice Guidelines (Committee on the Management of Patients With Chronic Stable Angina)," *J Am Coll Cardiol*, 2003, 41(1):159-68. Available at: http://http://www.acc.org/clinical/guidelines/stable/stable_clean.pdf. Accessed May 5, 2004.

Parker JO, "Eccentric Dosing With Isosorbide-5-Mononitrate in Angina Pectoris," *Am J Cardiol*, 1993, 72(12):871-6.

Parker JO, Fanell B, Lahey KA, et al, "Effect of Intervals Between Doses on the Development to Tolerance to Isosorbide Dinitrate," *N Engl J Med*, 1987, 316(23):1440-4.

Isoxsuprine *(eye SOKS syoo preen)*

Related Information
Potentially Inappropriate Medications for Geriatrics *on page 1824*

Medication Safety Issues
Sound-alike/look-alike issues:
    Vasodilan® may be confused with Vasocidin®

U.S. Brand Names Vasodilan® [DSC]

Index Terms Isoxsuprine Hydrochloride

Generic Available Yes

Pharmacologic Category Vasodilator

Use Considered "possibly effective" for treatment of peripheral vascular diseases, such as arteriosclerosis obliterans and Raynaud's disease

Contraindications Hypersensitivity to isoxsuprine or any component of the formulation; presence of arterial bleeding

Warnings/Precautions May cause hypotension in older adults.

Adverse Reactions (Reflective of adult population; not specific for elderly)
Frequency not defined.
Cardiovascular: Hypotension, chest pain, tachycardia
Central nervous system: Dizziness
Dermatologic: Rash
Gastrointestinal: Nausea, vomiting
Neuromuscular & skeletal: Weakness

Drug Interactions May enhance effects of other vasodilators/hypotensive agents; use with caution in elderly

Mechanism of Action In studies on normal human subjects, isoxsuprine increases muscle blood flow, but skin blood flow is usually unaffected. Rather than increasing muscle blood flow by beta-receptor stimulation, isoxsuprine probably has a direct action on vascular smooth muscle. The generally accepted mechanism of action of isoxsuprine on the uterus is beta-adrenergic stimulation. Isoxsuprine was shown to inhibit prostaglandin synthetase at high serum concentrations, with low concentrations there was an increase in the P-G synthesis.

Pharmacokinetics
Absorption: Nearly completely
Metabolism: Partially conjugated in the liver
Serum half-life: 1.25 hours mean
Time to peak serum concentration: Oral, I.M.: Within 1 hour
Elimination: Primarily in urine

Dosage
Geriatrics & Adults: Peripheral vascular disease: Oral: 10-20 mg 3-4 times/day; start with lower dose in elderly due to potential hypotension

Monitoring Parameters Monitor orthostatic blood pressure

Patient Information May cause skin rash; discontinue use if rash occurs; arise slowly from prolonged sitting or lying

Special Geriatric Considerations Vasodilators have been used to treat dementia upon the premise that dementia is secondary to a cerebral blood flow insufficiency. The hypothesis is that if blood flow could be increased, cognitive function would be increased. This hypothesis is no longer valid. The use of vasodilators for cognitive dysfunction is not recommended or proven by appropriate scientific study.

Dosage Forms Excipient information presented when available (limited, particularly for generics); consult specific product labeling.

Tablet, as hydrochloride: 10 mg, 20 mg

Selected References

Erwin WG, "Senile Dementia of the Alzheimer Type," *Clin Pharm*, 1984, 3(4):497-504.

Higbee MD, "Noncholinergic Approaches to Treating Senile Dementia of the Alzheimer's Type," *Consult Pharm*, 1992, 7(6):635-41.

Waters C, "Cognitive Enhancing Agents: Current Status in the Treatment of Alzheimer's Disease," *Can J Neurol Sci*, 1988, 15(3):249-56.

Yesavage JA, Tinklenberg JR, Hollister LE, et al, "Vasodilators in Senile Dementias: A Review of the Literature," *Arch Gen Psychiatry*, 1979, 36:220-3.

♦ **Isoxsuprine Hydrochloride** *see* Isoxsuprine *on page 844*

Isradipine (iz RA di peen)

Related Information
Calcium Channel Blockers *on page 1753*

Medication Safety Issues
Sound-alike/look-alike issues:
DynaCirc® may be confused with Dynabac®, Dynacin®

U.S. Brand Names DynaCirc® [DSC]; DynaCirc® CR

Canadian Brand Names DynaCirc®

Generic Available Yes: Capsule

Pharmacologic Category Calcium Channel Blocker

Use Management of hypertension, alone or concurrently with thiazide-type diuretics

Contraindications Hypersensitivity to isradipine or any component of the formulation; hypotension (<90 mm Hg systolic)

Warnings/Precautions Increased angina and/or MI has occurred with initiation or dosage titration of calcium channel blockers. The most common side effect is peripheral edema; occurs within 2-3 weeks of starting therapy. Reflex tachycardia may occur with use. Symptomatic hypotension with or without syncope can rarely occur; blood pressure must be lowered at a rate appropriate for the patient's clinical condition. Use cautiously in CHF, hypertrophic cardiomyopathy (IHSS), and in hepatic dysfunction. Use controlled release tablets with caution in patients with severe GI narrowing. Adjust doses at 2- to 4-week intervals.

Adverse Reactions (Reflective of adult population; not specific for elderly)
Percentages reported with capsule formulation.
>10%: Central nervous system: Headache (dose related 2% to 22%)
1% to 10%:
Cardiovascular: Edema (dose related 1% to 9%), palpitation (dose related 1% to 5%), flushing (dose related 1% to 5%), tachycardia (1% to 3%), chest pain (2% to 3%)
Central nervous system: Dizziness (2% to 8%), fatigue (dose related 1% to 9%)
Dermatologic: Rash (2%)
Gastrointestinal: Nausea (1% to 5%), abdominal discomfort (≤3%), vomiting (≤1%), diarrhea (≤3%)
Neuromuscular & skeletal: Weakness (≤1%)
Renal: Urinary frequency (1% to 3%)
Respiratory: Dyspnea (1% to 3%)

Overdosage/Toxicology Primary cardiac symptoms of calcium blocker overdose include hypotension and bradycardia. Hypotension is caused by peripheral vasodilation, myocardial depression, and bradycardia. Bradycardia results from sinus bradycardia, second- or third-degree atrioventricular block, or sinus arrest with junctional rhythm. Intraventricular conduction is usually not affected so the QRS duration is normal (verapamil prolongs the PR interval and bepridil prolongs the QT interval and may cause ventricular arrhythmias, including torsade de pointes).

Noncardiac symptoms include confusion, stupor, nausea, vomiting, metabolic acidosis and hyperglycemia. Following initial gastric decontamination, if possible, repeated calcium administration may promptly reverse depressed cardiac contractility (but not sinus node depression or peripheral vasodilation). Glucagon, epinephrine, and inamrinone (amrinone) may treat refractory hypotension. Glucagon and epinephrine also increase the heart rate (outside the U.S., 4-aminopyridine may be available as an antidote). Dialysis and hemoperfusion are not effective in enhancing elimination, although repeat-dose activated charcoal may serve as an adjunct with sustained-release preparations.

(Continued)

Isradipine *(Continued)*

In a few reported cases, overdose with calcium channel blockers has been associated with hypotension and bradycardia, initially refractory to atropine, but becoming more responsive to this agent when larger doses (approaching 1 g/hour for more than 24 hours) of calcium chloride were administered.

Drug Interactions Substrate of CYP3A4 (major); **Inhibits** CYP3A4 (weak)

Alpha$_1$-blockers: Alpha$_1$-blockers may enhance the hypotensive effect of isradipine.

Azole antifungals may inhibit the calcium channel blocker's metabolism; avoid this combination. Try an antifungal like terbinafine (if appropriate) or monitor closely for altered effect of the calcium channel blocker.

Beta-blockers may have increased pharmacokinetic or pharmacodynamic interactions with isradipine.

Calcium may reduce the effect of calcium channel blockers, particularly hypotension.

Cimetidine: Cimetidine may decrease the metabolism, via CYP isoenzymes, of israpidine.

Cyclosporine: Cyclosporine may decrease the metabolism, via CYP isoenzymes, of isradipine. Cyclosporine dosage adjustments might be needed.

CYP3A4 inducers: CYP3A4 inducers may decrease the levels/effects of isradipine. Example inducers include aminoglutethimide, carbamazepine, nafcillin, nevirapine, phenobarbital, phenytoin, and rifamycins.

CYP3A4 inhibitors: May increase the levels/effects of isradipine. Example inhibitors include azole antifungals, clarithromycin, diclofenac, doxycycline, erythromycin, imatinib, isoniazid, nefazodone, nicardipine, propofol, protease inhibitors, quinidine, telithromycin, and verapamil.

Magnesium salts: Calcium channel blockers may enhance the adverse/toxic effect of magnesium salts. Monitor for hypotension in patients receiving calcium channel blockers with elevated serum magnesium concentrations.

QT$_c$-prolonging agents: Isradipine may enhance the adverse/toxic effect of other QT$_c$-prolonging agents.

Rifampin increases the metabolism of the calcium channel blocker; adjust the dose of the calcium channel blocker to maintain efficacy.

Sildenafil, tadalafil, vardenafil: Blood pressure-lowering effects may be additive; use caution.

Thioridazine: Isradipine may enhance the QT$_c$-prolonging effect of thioridazine.

Ethanol/Nutrition/Herb Interactions

Food: Administration with food delays absorption, but does not affect availability

Herb/Nutraceutical: St John's wort may decrease isradipine levels. Avoid dong quai if using for hypertension. Avoid bayberry, blue cohosh, cayenne, ephedra, ginger, ginseng (American), gotu kola, licorice (may worsen hypertension) Avoid garlic (may have increased antihypertensive effect).

Mechanism of Action Inhibits calcium ion from entering the "slow channels" or select voltage-sensitive areas of vascular smooth muscle and myocardium during depolarization, producing a relaxation of coronary vascular smooth muscle and coronary vasodilation; increases myocardial oxygen delivery in patients with vasospastic angina

Pharmacodynamics

Onset of action: 2 hours

Peak effect: 2-4 weeks

Pharmacokinetics

Absorption: Oral: 90% to 95%

Protein binding: 95%

Metabolism: In the liver

Bioavailability: Absolute due to first-pass elimination 15% to 24%

Half-life: 8 hours

Time to peak serum concentration: 1-1.5 hours

Elimination: Renal excretion by metabolites (cyclic lactone and monoacids)

Dosage

Geriatrics:

Capsule: Refer to adult dosing.

Controlled release tablet: Initial dose: 5 mg once daily

Adults: Hypertension: Oral:

Capsule: 2.5 mg twice daily; antihypertensive response occurs in 2-3 hours; maximal response in 2-4 weeks; increase dose at 2- to 4-week intervals at 2.5-5 mg increments; usual dose range (JNC 7): 2.5-10 mg/day in 2 divided doses. **Note:** Most patients show no improvement with doses >10 mg/day except adverse reaction rate increases; therefore, maximal dose in older adults should be 10 mg/day.

Controlled release tablet: 5 mg once daily; antihypertensive response occurs in 2 hours. Adjust dose in increments of 5 mg at 2-4 week intervals. Maximum dose 20 mg/day; adverse events are increased at doses >10 mg/day.

Renal Impairment:

Cl$_{cr}$ 30-80 mL/minute: Bioavailability increased by 45%

Cl$_{cr}$ <10 mL/minute on hemodialysis: Bioavailability decreased by 20% to 50%

Capsule: Refer to adult dosing.
Controlled release tablet: Initial dose: 5 mg once daily

Hepatic Impairment:
Peak serum concentrations are increased by 32% and bioavailability is increased by 52%.

Capsule: Refer to adult dosing.
Controlled release tablet: Initial dose: 5 mg once daily

Administration Controlled release tablets should be swallowed whole; do not divide or chew

Monitoring Parameters Heart rate, blood pressure, signs and symptoms of congestive heart failure

Patient Information Notify physician if you experience irregular heartbeat, shortness of breath, swelling, constipation, nausea, hypotension, or dizziness; do not stop or interrupt therapy without physician advice

Additional Information Only approved indication is hypertension, but may be used for congestive heart failure; similar to nifedipine in actions, except for fewer side effects

The FDA's Cardiovascular and Renal Drug Advisory Committee reviewed current data regarding the risk of heart attacks in patients treated with calcium channel blockers and determined that as a class, the calcium channel antagonists are safe; however, they warned that short-acting nifedipine could increase the risk of myocardial infarction in some patients. The committee was in agreement with a statement issued September, 1995 by the National Heart Lung, and Blood Institute of the National Institute of Health, that warned that short-acting nifedipine should be used with great caution especially at higher doses.

Special Geriatric Considerations Elderly may experience a greater hypotensive response. Constipation may be more of a problem in the elderly. Calcium channel blockers are no more effective in the elderly than other therapies; however, they do not cause significant CNS effects which is an advantage over some antihypertensive agents.

Dosage Forms Excipient information presented when available (limited, particularly for generics); consult specific product labeling.
Capsule: 2.5 mg, 5 mg
    DynaCirc®: 2.5 mg [DSC], 5 mg [DSC]
Tablet, controlled release:
    DynaCirc® CR: 5 mg, 10 mg

Selected References
Chobanian AV, Bakris GL, Black HR, et al, "The Seventh Report of the Joint National Committee on Prevention, Detection, Evaluation, and Treatment of High Blood Pressure: The JNC 7 Report," *JAMA*, 2003, 289(19):2560-71.

♦ **Istalol**™ *see* Timolol *on page 1571*
♦ **Isuprel**® *see* Isoproterenol *on page 838*

Itraconazole (i tra KOE na zole)

Medication Safety Issues
Sound-alike/look-alike issues:
    Sporanox® may be confused with Suprax®
U.S. Brand Names Sporanox®
Canadian Brand Names Sporanox®
Generic Available No
Pharmacologic Category Antifungal Agent, Oral
Use Treatment of susceptible fungal infections in immunocompromised and immunocompetent patients including blastomycosis and histoplasmosis; indicated for aspergillosis, and onychomycosis of the toenail; treatment of onychomycosis of the fingernail without concomitant toenail infection via a pulse-type dosing regimen; has activity against *Aspergillus*, *Candida*, *Coccidioides*, *Cryptococcus*, *Sporothrix*, tinea unguium

Oral: Useful in superficial mycoses including dermatophytoses (eg, tinea capitis), pityriasis versicolor, seboppsoriasis, vaginal and chronic mucocutaneous candidiases; systemic mycoses including candidiasis, meningeal and disseminated cryptococcal infections, paracoccidioidomycosis, coccidioidomycoses; miscellaneous mycoses such as sporotrichosis, chromomycosis, leishmaniasis, fungal keratitis, alternariosis, zygomycosis
Oral solution: Treatment of oral and esophageal candidiasis
Intravenous solution: Indicated in the treatment of blastomycosis, histoplasmosis (nonmeningeal), and aspergillosis (in patients intolerant or refractory to amphotericin B therapy)

Contraindications Hypersensitivity to itraconazole, any component of the formulation, or to other azoles; concurrent administration with astemizole, cisapride, dofetilide, (Continued)

Itraconazole *(Continued)*

ergot derivatives, lovastatin, midazolam, pimozide, quinidine, simvastatin, or triazolam; treatment of onychomycosis in patients with evidence of left ventricular dysfunction, CHF, or a history of CHF

Warnings/Precautions Discontinue if signs or symptoms of CHF or neuropathy occur during treatment. **[U.S. Boxed Warning]: Rare cases of serious cardiovascular adverse events (including death), ventricular tachycardia, and torsade de pointes have been observed due to increased cisapride, pimozide, quinidine, dofetilide or levomethadyl concentrations induced by itraconazole; concurrent use contraindicated. Use with caution in patients with left ventricular dysfunction or a history of CHF; not recommended for treatment of onychomycosis in these patients.** Not recommended for use in patients with active liver disease, elevated liver enzymes, or prior hepatotoxic reactions to other drugs. Itraconazole has been associated with rare cases of serious hepatotoxicity (including fatal cases and cases within the first week of treatment); treatment should be discontinued in patients who develop clinical symptoms of liver dysfunction or abnormal liver function tests during itraconazole therapy except in cases where expected benefit exceeds risk. Large differences in itraconazole pharmacokinetic parameters have been observed in cystic fibrosis patients receiving the solution; if a patient with cystic fibrosis does not respond to therapy, alternate therapies should be considered. Due to differences in bioavailability, oral capsules and oral solution **cannot be used interchangeably.** Intravenous formulation should be used with caution in renal impairment; consider conversion to oral therapy if renal dysfunction/toxicity is noted. Initiation of treatment with oral solution is not recommended in patients at immediate risk for systemic candidiasis (eg, patients with severe neutropenia).

Adverse Reactions (Reflective of adult population; not specific for elderly)
Listed incidences are for higher doses appropriate for systemic fungal infection.

>10%: Gastrointestinal: Nausea (11%)

1% to 10%:

Cardiovascular: Edema (4%), hypertension (3%)

Central nervous system: Headache (4%), fatigue (2% to 3%), malaise (1%), fever (3%), dizziness (2%)

Dermatologic: Rash (9%), pruritus (3%)

Endocrine & metabolic: Decreased libido (1%), hypertriglyceridemia, hypokalemia (2%)

Gastrointestinal: Abdominal pain (2%), anorexia (1%), vomiting (5%), diarrhea (3%)

Hepatic: Abnormal LFTs (3%), hepatitis

Renal: Albuminuria (1%)

Overdosage/Toxicology Overdoses are well tolerated. Following decontamination, if possible, supportive measures only are required. Dialysis is not effective.

Drug Interactions Substrate of CYP3A4 (major); **Inhibits** CYP3A4 (strong)

Antacids: May decrease serum concentration of itraconazole. Administer antacids 1 hour before or 2 hours after itraconazole capsules.

Alfentanil: Serum concentrations may be increased; monitor.

Anticonvulsants: Itraconazole may increase the serum concentration of carbamazepine; carbamazepine, phenobarbital, and phenytoin may decrease the serum concentration of itraconazole.

Benzodiazepines: Alprazolam, diazepam, temazepam, triazolam, and midazolam serum concentrations may be increased; consider a benzodiazepine not metabolized by CYP3A4 (such as lorazepam) or another antifungal that is metabolized by CYP3A4

Buspirone: Serum concentrations may be increased; monitor for sedation

Busulfan: Serum concentrations may be increased; avoid concurrent use

Calcium channel blockers: Serum concentrations may be increased (applies to those agents metabolized by CYP3A4, including felodipine, nifedipine, and verapamil); consider another agent instead of a calcium channel blocker, another antifungal, or reduce the dose of the calcium channel blocker; monitor blood pressure

Cisapride; Serum concentration is increased which may lead to malignant arrhythmias; concurrent use is contraindicated

Corticosteroids: Serum levels/effects of the corticosteroid may be increased; use caution.

CYP3A4 inducers: CYP3A4 inducers may decrease the levels/effects of itraconazole. Example inducers include aminoglutethimide, carbamazepine, nafcillin, nevirapine, phenobarbital, phenytoin, and rifamycins.

CYP3A4 substrates: Itraconazole may increase the levels/effects of CYP3A4 substrates. Example substrates include benzodiazepines, calcium channel blockers, mirtazapine, nateglinide, nefazodone, tacrolimus, and venlafaxine. Selected benzodiazepines (midazolam and triazolam), cisapride, ergot alkaloids, selected HMG-CoA reductase inhibitors (lovastatin and simvastatin), and pimozide are generally contraindicated with strong CYP3A4 inhibitors.

Didanosine: May decrease absorption of itraconazole (due to buffering capacity of oral solution); applies only to oral solution formulation of didanosine

Digoxin: Serum concentrations may be increased; monitor.

Disopyramide: Serum levels/effects (including QT_c prolongation) may be increased; use caution.

Docetaxel: Serum concentrations may be increased; avoid concurrent use

Dofetilide: Serum levels/toxicity may be increased; concurrent use is contraindicated.

Eletriptan: Serum level/toxicity of eletriptan may be increased; use caution.

Ergot alkaloids: Toxicity (vasospasm, ischemia) may be significantly increased by itraconazole; concurrent use is contraindicated.

Erythromycin (and clarithromycin): May increase serum concentrations of itraconazole.

H_2 blockers: May decrease itraconazole absorption. Itraconazole depends on gastric acidity for absorption. Avoid concurrent use.

HMG-CoA reductase inhibitors (except pravastatin and fluvastatin): Serum concentrations may be increased. The risk of myopathy/rhabdomyolysis may be increased. Switch to pravastatin/fluvastatin or suspend treatment during course of itraconazole therapy.

Hypoglycemic agents, oral: Serum concentrations may be increased; monitor.

Immunosuppressants: Cyclosporine, sirolimus, and tacrolimus: Serum concentrations may be increased; monitor serum concentrations and renal function.

Levomethadyl: Serum levels/effects may be increased by itraconazole, potentially resulting in malignant arrhythmia; concurrent use is contraindicated.

Nevirapine: May decrease serum concentrations of itraconazole; monitor

Oral contraceptives: Efficacy may be reduced by itraconazole (limited data); use barrier birth control method during concurrent use

Pimozide: Serum levels/toxicity may be increased; concurrent use is contraindicated.

Protease inhibitors: May increase serum concentrations of itraconazole. Includes amprenavir, indinavir, nelfinavir, ritonavir, and saquinavir; monitor. Serum concentrations of indinavir, ritonavir, or saquinavir may be increased by itraconazole.

Proton pump inhibitors: May decrease itraconazole absorption. Itraconazole depends on gastric acidity for absorption. Avoid concurrent use (includes omeprazole, lansoprazole).

Quinidine: Serum levels may be increased. Concurrent use is contraindicated.

Rifabutin: Serum concentrations may be increased; monitor.

Sildenafil: Serum concentrations may be increased by itraconazole; consider dosage reduction. A maximum sildenafil dose of 25 mg in 48 hours is recommended with other strong CYP3A4 inhibitors.

Tadalafil: Serum concentrations may be increased by itraconazole. A maximum tadalafil dose of 10 mg in 72 hours is recommended with strong CYP3A4 inhibitors.

Vardenafil: Serum concentrations may be increased by itraconazole. If itraconazole dose is 200 mg/day, limit vardenafil dose to a maximum of 5 mg/24 hours. If itraconazole dose is 400 mg/day, limit vardenafil dose to a maximum of 2.5 mg/24 hours.

Warfarin: Anticoagulant effects may be increased; monitor INR and adjust warfarin's dose as needed

Vinca alkaloids: Serum concentrations may be increased.

Zolpidem: Serum levels may be increased; monitor

Ethanol/Nutrition/Herb Interactions

Food:

Capsules: Enhanced by food and possibly by gastric acidity. cola drinks have been shown to increase the absorption of the capsules in patients with achlorhydria or those taking H_2-receptor antagonists or other gastric acid suppressors. Avoid grapefruit juice.

Solution: Decreased by food, time to peak concentration prolonged by food.

Herb/Nutraceutical: St John's wort may decrease itraconazole levels.

Stability

Capsule: Store at room temperature, 15°C to 25°C (59°F to 77°F). Protect from light and moisture.

Oral solution: Store at ≤25°C (77°F); do not freeze.

Solution for injection: Store at ≤25°C (77°F); do not freeze. Protect from light. Dilute with 0.9% sodium chloride. Stable for 48 hours at room temperature or under refrigeration. A precise mixing ratio is required to maintain stability (3.33:1) and avoid precipitate formation. Add 25 mL (1 ampul) to 50 mL 0.9% sodium chloride. Mix and withdraw 15 mL of solution before infusing.

Mechanism of Action Interferes with cytochrome P450 activity, decreasing ergosterol synthesis (principal sterol in fungal cell membrane) and inhibiting cell membrane formation

Pharmacokinetics

Absorption: Requires gastric acidity; capsule better absorbed with food, solution better absorbed on empty stomach; hypochlorhydria has been reported in HIV-infected patients; therefore, oral absorption in these patients may be decreased

(Continued)

849

Itraconazole *(Continued)*

Distribution: V_d (average): 796 ± 185 L or 10 L/kg; highly lipophilic and tissue concentrations are higher than plasma concentrations. The highest concentrations: adipose, omentum, endometrium, cervical and vaginal mucus, and skin/nails. Aqueous fluids (eg, CSF and urine) contain negligible amounts.

Protein binding, plasma: 99.9%; metabolite hydroxy-itraconazole: 99.5%

Metabolism: Extensively hepatic via CYP3A4 into >30 metabolites including hydroxy-itraconazole (major metabolite); appears to have *in vitro* antifungal activity. Main metabolic pathway is oxidation; may undergo saturation metabolism with multiple dosing.

Bioavailability: Variable, ~55% (oral solution) in 1 small study; **Note:** Oral solution has a higher degree of bioavailability (149% ± 68%) relative to oral capsules; should not be interchanged

Half-life: Oral: After single 200 mg dose: 21 ± 5 hours; 64 hours at steady-state; I.V.: steady-state: 35 hours; steady-state concentrations are achieved in 13 days with multiple administration of itraconazole 100-400 mg/day.

Elimination: Feces (~3% to 18%); urine (~0.03% as parent drug, 40% as metabolites)

Dosage

Geriatrics & Adults:

Aspergillosis:
Oral: 200-400 mg/day
I.V.: 200 mg twice daily for 4 doses, followed by 200 mg daily

Blastomycosis/histoplasmosis:
Oral: 200 mg once daily, if no obvious improvement or there is evidence of progressive fungal disease, increase the dose in 100 mg increments to a maximum of 400 mg/day. Doses >200 mg/day are given in 2 divided doses. Length of therapy varies from 1 day to >6 months depending on the condition and mycological response.
I.V.: 200 mg twice daily for 4 doses, followed by 200 mg daily

Brain abscess: Cerebral phaeohyphomycosis (dematiaceous): Oral: 200 mg twice daily for at least 6 months with amphotericin

Candidiasis:
Oropharyngeal: Oral (solution): 200 mg once daily for 1-2 weeks; in patients unresponsive or refractory to fluconazole: 100 mg twice daily (clinical response expected in 1-2 weeks)
Esophageal: Oral (solution): 100-200 mg once daily for a minimum of 3 weeks; continue dosing for 2 weeks after resolution of symptoms

Coccidioides: Oral: 200 mg twice daily

Infections, Life-threatening:
Oral: Loading dose: 200 mg 3 times/day (600 mg/day) should be given for the first 3 days of therapy.
I.V.: 200 mg twice daily for 4 doses, followed by 200 mg/day

Meningitis: Oral:
Coccidioides: 400-800 mg/day
Cryptococcal: HIV positive (unlabeled use): Induction: 400 mg/day for 10-12 weeks; maintenance: 200 mg twice daily lifelong

Onychomycosis: Oral: 200 mg once daily for 12 consecutive weeks

Pneumonia:
Coccidioides: Mild to moderate: Oral, I.V.: 200 mg twice daily
Cryptococcal: Mild to moderate (unlabeled use): 200-400 mg/day for 6-12 months (lifelong for HIV positive)

Prototothecal infection: 200 mg once daily for 2 months

Sporotrichosis: Oral:
Lymphocutaneous: 100-200 mg/day for 3-6 months
Osteoarticular and pulmonary: 200 mg twice daily for 1-2 years (may use amphotericin B initially for stabilization)

Renal Impairment: Not necessary. Itraconazole injection is not recommended in patients with a creatinine clearance <30 mL/minute; hydroxypropyl-β-cyclodextrin (the excipient) is eliminated primarily by the kidneys.

Not dialyzable

Hepatic Impairment: May be necessary, but specific guidelines are not available. Risk-to-benefit evaluation should be undertaken in patients who develop liver function abnormalities during treatment.

Administration

Oral: Doses >200 mg/day are administered in 2 divided doses; do not administer with antacids.

I.V.: Using a flow control device, infuse 60 mL of the dilute solution (3.33 mg/mL = 200 mg itraconazole, pH ~4.8) intravenously over 60 minutes, using an extension line and the infusion set provided. After administration, flush the infusion set with 15-20 mL of 0.9% sodium chloride over 30 seconds to 15 minutes, via the two-way stopcock. Do not use bacteriostatic sodium chloride injection, USP. The compatibility of

Sporanox® injection with flush solutions other than 0.9% sodium chloride (normal saline) is not known. Discard the entire infusion line.

Monitoring Parameters Signs and symptoms of infection, baseline LFTs, recheck LFTs if therapy is to go beyond 2 weeks (see Drug Interactions)

Patient Information Take with food; do not take with antacids

Special Geriatric Considerations No specific data for the elderly.

Dosage Forms Excipient information presented when available (limited, particularly for generics); consult specific product labeling.

Capsule: 100 mg

Injection, solution: 10 mg/mL (25 mL) [packaged in a kit containing sodium chloride 0.9% (50 mL); filtered infusion set (1)]

Solution, oral: 100 mg/10 mL (150 mL) [cherry flavor]

- ◆ **IvySoothe® [OTC]** *see* Hydrocortisone *on page 762*
- ◆ **Jantoven™** *see* Warfarin *on page 1682*
- ◆ **Janumet™** *see* Sitagliptin and Metformin *on page 1472*
- ◆ **Januvia™** *see* Sitagliptin *on page 1470*
- ◆ **Just for Kids™ [OTC]** *see* Fluoride *on page 642*
- ◆ **Kadian®** *see* Morphine Sulfate *on page 1065*
- ◆ **Kala® [OTC]** *see* Lactobacillus *on page 867*

Kanamycin (kan a MYE sin)

Medication Safety Issues
Sound-alike/look-alike issues:
Kanamycin may be confused with Garamycin®, gentamicin

U.S. Brand Names Kantrex®

Canadian Brand Names Kantrex®

Index Terms Kanamycin Sulfate

Generic Available No

Pharmacologic Category Antibiotic, Aminoglycoside

Use Treatment of susceptible bacterial infection including gram-negative aerobes, gram-positive *Bacillus* as well as some mycobacteria

Oral: Preoperative bowel preparation in the prophylaxis of infections and adjunctive treatment of hepatic coma (oral kanamycin is not indicated in the treatment of systemic infections)

Parenteral: Rarely used in antibiotic irrigations during surgery

Contraindications Hypersensitivity to kanamycin, any component of the formulation, or other aminoglycosides

Warnings/Precautions [U.S. Boxed Warning]: Aminoglycosides may cause neurotoxicity and/or nephrotoxicity; usual risk factors include pre-existing renal impairment, concomitant neuro-/nephrotoxic medications, advanced age, and dehydration. Ototoxicity may be directly proportional to the amount of drug given and the duration of treatment. Tinnitus or vertigo are indications of vestibular injury and impending hearing loss. Renal damage is usually reversible. May cause neuromuscular blockade and respiratory paralysis; especially when given soon after anesthesia or muscle relaxants.

Not intended for long-term therapy due to toxic hazards associated with extended administration. Use caution in pre-existing renal insufficiency, vestibular or cochlear impairment, myasthenia gravis, hypocalcemia, and conditions which depress neuromuscular transmission. Dosage modification required in patients with impaired renal function. Prolonged use may result in fungal or bacterial superinfection, including *C. difficile*-associated diarrhea and pseudomembranous colitis.

Adverse Reactions (Reflective of adult population; not specific for elderly)
Frequency not defined.
Cardiovascular: Edema
Central nervous system: Neurotoxicity, drowsiness, headache, pseudomotor cerebri
Dermatologic: Skin itching, redness, rash, photosensitivity, erythema
Gastrointestinal: Nausea, vomiting, diarrhea, malabsorption syndrome (with prolonged and high-dose therapy of hepatic coma), anorexia, weight loss, salivation increased, enterocolitis
Hematologic: Granulocytopenia, agranulocytosis, thrombocytopenia
Local: Burning, stinging
Neuromuscular & skeletal: Weakness, tremor, muscle cramps
Otic: Ototoxicity (auditory), ototoxicity (vestibular)
Renal: Nephrotoxicity
Respiratory: Dyspnea

Overdosage/Toxicology Symptoms of overdose include ototoxicity, nephrotoxicity, and neuromuscular toxicity. The treatment of choice following a single acute overdose
(Continued)

Kanamycin *(Continued)*

appears to be the maintenance of good urine output of at least 3 mL/kg/hour. Hemodialysis or peritoneal dialysis may enhance kanamycin elimination.

Drug Interactions

Amphotericin B: Concomitant use may lead to nephrotoxicity (reported with gentamicin).

Bisphosphonate derivatives: Concomitant use may lead to hypocalcemia (reported with amikacin and clodronate).

Cisplatin: Concomitant use may lead to increased nephrotoxicity.

Loop diuretics: May increase risk of ototoxicity (reported with ethacrynic acid) and nephrotoxicity.

Neuromuscular-blocking agents: Increase risk of neuromuscular blockade

Stability Store vial at controlled room temperature. Darkening of vials does not indicate loss of potency.

I.V.: Must be further diluted prior to I.V. infusion. For adults, dilute 500 mg in 100-200 mL of appropriate solution or 1 g in 200-400 mL.

Intraperitoneal: Dilute dose in 20 mL sterile distilled water.

Aerosol: Dilute 250 mg in 3 mL normal saline.

Mechanism of Action Interferes with protein synthesis in bacterial cell by binding to ribosomal subunit

Pharmacokinetics

Distribution: V_d: 0.19 L/kg

Half-life: 2-4 hours, increases in anuria to 80 hours

Geriatrics: Mean half-life has been reported to be longer, 2.5 hours in 50-70 years of age and 4.7 hours in 70-90 years of age; the plasma half-life and V_d have also been reported to be increased in older bedridden patients.

Time to peak serum concentration: I.M.: Within 1-2 hours

Elimination: Entirely in the kidney, principally by glomerular filtration

Dosage

Geriatrics: I.M., I.V.: Initial dose should be 5-7.5 mg/kg based on ideal body weight (except in obese patients); maintenance dose and interval should be adjusted for estimated renal function; dosing interval in most older patients is every 12-24 hours (see Dosage: Renal Impairment).

Adults: Note: Dosing should be based on ideal body weight

Susceptible systemic infections: I.M., I.V.: 5-7.5 mg/kg/dose in divided doses every 8-12 hours (<15 mg/kg/day)

Following surgical contamination, peritonitis: Intraperitoneal: 500 mg

Irrigating solution: 0.25%; maximum 1.5 g/day (via all administration routes)

Aerosol: 250 mg 2-4 times/day

Renal Impairment:

Cl_{cr} 50-80 mL/minute: Administer 60% to 90% of dose or administer every 8-12 hours.

Cl_{cr} 10-50 mL/minute: Administer 30% to 70% of dose or administer every 12 hours.

Cl_{cr} <10 mL/minute: Administer 20% to 30% of dose or administer every 24-48 hours.

Administration Dilute to 100-200 mL and infuse over 30 minutes; I.M. doses should be given in a large muscle mass (ie, gluteus maximus)

Monitoring Parameters Serum creatinine and BUN every 2-3 days; peak and trough concentrations; hearing

Reference Range

Therapeutic:

Peak: 25-35 mcg/mL (SI: 52-72 µmol/L)

Trough: 4-8 mcg/mL (SI: 8-16 µmol/L)

Toxic:

Peak: >35 mcg/mL (SI: >72 µmol/L)

Trough: >10 mcg/mL (SI: >21 µmol/L)

Test Interactions Some penicillin derivatives may accelerate the degradation of aminoglycosides *in vitro*, leading to a potential underestimation of aminoglycoside serum concentration.

Additional Information Aminoglycoside levels in blood taken from silastic central catheters can sometime give falsely high readings.

Special Geriatric Considerations This is not a drug of choice since elderly may have increased adverse effects (renal).

Dosage Forms Excipient information presented when available (limited, particularly for generics); consult specific product labeling.

Injection, solution, as sulfate: 1 g/3 mL (3 mL) [contains sodium bisulfate]

Selected References

Kristensen M, Molholm HJ, Kampmann J, et al, "Letter: Drug Elimination and Renal Function," *J Clin Pharmacol*, 1974, 14(5-6):307-8.

Yasuhara H, Kobayashi S, Sakamoto K, et al, "Pharmacokinetics of Amikacin and Cephalothin in Bedridden Elderly Patients," *J Clin Pharmacol*, 1982, 22(8-9):403-9.

♦ **Kanamycin Sulfate** *see* Kanamycin *on page 851*

- **Kantrex®** *see* Kanamycin *on page 851*
- **Kaon-Cl-10®** *see* Potassium Chloride *on page 1288*
- **Kaon-Cl® 20** *see* Potassium Chloride *on page 1288*
- **Kao-Paverin® [OTC]** *see* Loperamide *on page 924*
- **Kaopectate® [OTC]** *see* Bismuth *on page 174*
- **Kaopectate® Extra Strength [OTC]** *see* Bismuth *on page 174*
- **Kao-Tin [OTC]** *see* Bismuth *on page 174*
- **Kapectolin [OTC]** *see* Bismuth *on page 174*
- **Kay Ciel®** *see* Potassium Chloride *on page 1288*
- **Kayexalate®** *see* Sodium Polystyrene Sulfonate *on page 1481*
- **KCl** *see* Potassium Chloride *on page 1288*
- **K-Dur® 10** *see* Potassium Chloride *on page 1288*
- **K-Dur® 20** *see* Potassium Chloride *on page 1288*
- **Keflex®** *see* Cephalexin *on page 281*
- **Kemadrin®** *see* Procyclidine *on page 1323*
- **Kenalog®** *see* Triamcinolone *on page 1619*
- **Kenalog-10®** *see* Triamcinolone *on page 1619*
- **Kenalog-40®** *see* Triamcinolone *on page 1619*
- **Keoxifene Hydrochloride** *see* Raloxifene *on page 1374*
- **Keppra®** *see* Levetiracetam *on page 889*
- **Keralyt® [OTC]** *see* Salicylic Acid *on page 1441*
- **Kerlone®** *see* Betaxolol *on page 164*
- **Ketek®** *see* Telithromycin *on page 1523*

Ketoconazole (kee toe KOE na zole)

Medication Safety Issues
Sound-alike/look-alike issues:
Nizoral® may be confused with Nasarel®, Neoral®, Nitrol®

U.S. Brand Names Extina®; Kuric™; Nizoral®; Nizoral® A-D [OTC]; Xolegel™

Canadian Brand Names Apo-Ketoconazole®; Ketoderm®; Novo-Ketoconazole; Xolegel™

Generic Available Yes: Cream, shampoo, tablet

Pharmacologic Category Antifungal Agent, Oral; Antifungal Agent, Topical

Use

Systemic: Treatment of susceptible fungal infections, including candidiasis, oral thrush, blastomycosis, histoplasmosis, paracoccidioidomycosis, coccidioidomycosis, chromomycosis, candiduria, chronic mucocutaneous candidiasis, as well as certain recalcitrant cutaneous dermatophytoses

Topical: Treatment of tinea corporis, tinea cruris, tinea versicolor, cutaneous candidiasis, seborrheic dermatitis

Unlabeled/Investigational Use Treatment of prostate cancer (androgen synthesis inhibitor)

Contraindications Hypersensitivity to ketoconazole or any component of the formulation; CNS fungal infections (due to poor CNS penetration); coadministration with ergot derivatives, astemizole, or cisapride is contraindicated due to risk of potentially fatal cardiac arrhythmias

Warnings/Precautions [U.S. Boxed Warning]: Ketoconazole has been associated with hepatotoxicity, including some fatalities; use with caution in patients with impaired hepatic function and perform periodic liver function tests. **[U.S. Boxed Warning]: Concomitant use with cisapride is contraindicated due to the occurrence of ventricular arrhythmias.** High doses of ketoconazole may depress adrenocortical function.

Topical: Formulations may contain sulfites. Avoid exposure of gel to open flames during or immediately after application.

Adverse Reactions (Reflective of adult population; not specific for elderly)
Oral: 1% to 10%:
Dermatologic: Pruritus (2%)
Gastrointestinal: Nausea/vomiting (3% to 10%), abdominal pain (1%)
Topical cream/gel: Pruritus, severe irritation, stinging (~5%)
Topical foam: Application site burning (10%), application site reaction (6%), contact sensitization, dryness, erythema, pruritus, rash
Shampoo: Abnormal hair texture, hair loss increase, itching, mild dryness of skin, oiliness/dryness of hair, scalp pustules

Overdosage/Toxicology Symptoms include dizziness, headache, nausea, vomiting, and diarrhea. Overdoses are well tolerated. Treatment includes supportive measures and gastric decontamination.
(Continued)

Ketoconazole *(Continued)*

Drug Interactions Substrate of CYP3A4 (major); **Inhibits** CYP1A2 (strong), 2A6 (moderate), 2B6 (weak), 2C8 (weak), 2C9 (strong), 2C19 (moderate), 2D6 (moderate), 3A4 (strong)

Benzodiazepines: Alprazolam, diazepam, temazepam, triazolam, and midazolam serum concentrations may be increased; consider a benzodiazepine not metabolized by CYP3A4 (such as lorazepam) or another antifungal that is metabolized by CYP3A4. Concurrent use is contraindicated.

Buspirone: Serum concentrations may be increased; monitor for sedation.

Busulfan: Serum concentrations may be increased; avoid concurrent use.

Calcium channel blockers: Serum concentrations may be increased (applies to those agents metabolized by CYP3A4, including felodipine, nifedipine, and verapamil); consider another agent instead of a calcium channel blocker, another antifungal, or reduce the dose of the calcium channel blocker. Monitor blood pressure.

Cisapride: Serum concentration is increased which may lead to malignant arrhythmias; concurrent use is contraindicated.

CYP1A2 substrates: Ketoconazole may increase the levels/effects of CYP1A2 substrates. Example substrates include aminophylline, fluvoxamine, mexiletine, mirtazapine, ropinirole, theophylline, and trifluoperazine.

CYP2A6 substrates: Ketoconazole may increase the levels/effects of CYP2A6 substrates. Example substrates include dexmedetomidine and ifosfamide.

CYP2C9 substrates: Ketoconazole may increase the levels/effects of CYP2C9 substrates. Example substrates include bosentan, dapsone, fluoxetine, glimepiride, glipizide, losartan, montelukast, nateglinide, paclitaxel, phenytoin, warfarin, and zafirlukast.

CYP2C19 substrates: Ketoconazole may increase the levels/effects of CYP2C19 substrates. Example substrates include citalopram, diazepam, methsuximide, phenytoin, propranolol, and sertraline.

CYP2D6 substrates: Ketoconazole may increase the levels/effects of CYP2D6 substrates. Example substrates include amphetamines, selected beta-blockers, dextromethorphan, fluoxetine, lidocaine, mirtazapine, nefazodone, paroxetine, risperidone, ritonavir, thioridazine, tricyclic antidepressants, and venlafaxine.

CYP2D6 prodrug substrates: Ketoconazole may decrease the levels/effects of CYP2D6 prodrug substrates. Example prodrug substrates include codeine, hydrocodone, oxycodone, and tramadol.

CYP3A4 inducers: CYP3A4 inducers may decrease the levels/effects of ketoconazole. Example inducers include aminoglutethimide, carbamazepine, nafcillin, nevirapine, phenobarbital, phenytoin, and rifamycins.

CYP3A4 substrates: Ketoconazole may increase the levels/effects of CYP3A4 substrates. Example substrates include benzodiazepines, calcium channel blockers, mirtazapine, nateglinide, nefazodone, tacrolimus, and venlafaxine. Selected benzodiazepines (midazolam and triazolam), cisapride, ergot alkaloids, selected HMG-CoA reductase inhibitors (lovastatin and simvastatin), and pimozide are generally contraindicated with strong CYP3A4 inhibitors.

Didanosine: May decrease absorption of ketoconazole (due to buffering capacity of oral solution); applies only to oral solution formulation of didanosine.

Docetaxel: Serum concentrations may be increased; avoid concurrent use.

Erythromycin (and clarithromycin): May increase serum concentrations of ketoconazole.

H_2 blockers: May decrease ketoconazole absorption. Ketoconazole depends on gastric acidity for absorption. Avoid concurrent use.

HMG-CoA reductase inhibitors (except pravastatin and fluvastatin): Serum concentrations may be increased. The risk of myopathy/rhabdomyolysis may be increased. Switch to pravastatin/fluvastatin or suspend treatment during course of ketoconazole therapy.

Immunosuppressants: Cyclosporine, sirolimus, and tacrolimus: Serum concentrations may be increased; monitor serum concentrations and renal function.

Methylprednisolone: Serum concentrations may be increased; monitor.

Nevirapine: May decrease serum concentrations of ketoconazole; monitor.

Oral contraceptives: Efficacy may be reduced by ketoconazole (limited data); use barrier birth control method during concurrent use.

Phenytoin: Serum concentrations may be increased; monitor phenytoin levels and adjust dose as needed.

Protease inhibitors: May increase serum concentrations of ketoconazole. Includes amprenavir, indinavir, nelfinavir, ritonavir, and saquinavir; monitor.

Proton pump inhibitors: May decrease ketoconazole absorption. Ketoconazole depends on gastric acidity for absorption. Avoid concurrent use (includes omeprazole, lansoprazole).

Quinidine: Serum levels may be increased; monitor.

Rifampin: Rifampin decreases ketoconazole's serum concentration to levels which are no longer effective; avoid concurrent use.

Sildenafil: Serum concentrations may be increased by ketoconazole; consider dosage reduction. A maximum sildenafil dose of 25 mg in 48 hours is recommended with other strong CYP3A4 inhibitors.

Tadalafil: Serum concentrations may be increased by ketoconazole. A maximum tadalafil dose of 10 mg in 72 hours is recommended with strong CYP3A4 inhibitors.

Vardenafil: Serum concentrations may be increased by ketoconazole. If ketoconazole dose is 200 mg/day, limit vardenafil to a maximum of 5 mg/24 hours. If ketoconazole dose is 400 mg/day, limit vardenafil dose to a maximum of 2.5 mg/24 hours.

Warfarin: Anticoagulant effects may be increased; monitor INR and adjust warfarin's dose as needed.

Vinca alkaloids: Serum concentrations may be increased.

Zolpidem: Serum levels may be increased; monitor.

Ethanol/Nutrition/Herb Interactions

Food: Ketoconazole peak serum levels may be prolonged if taken with food.

Herb/Nutraceutical: St John's wort may decrease ketoconazole levels.

Stability

Cream: Store at <25°C (<77°F).

Foam: Store at 20°C to 25°C (68°F to 77°F). Do not refrigerate. Do not store in direct sunlight. Contents are flammable.

Gel: Store at 15°C to 30°C (59°F to 86°F).

Shampoo: Store between 2°C to 30°C (35°F to 86°F); protect from freezing. Protect from light.

Tablet: Store at 15°C to 25°C (59°F to 77°F).

Mechanism of Action Alters the permeability of the cell wall by blocking fungal cytochrome P450; inhibits biosynthesis of triglycerides and phospholipids by fungi; inhibits several fungal enzymes that results in a build-up of toxic concentrations of hydrogen peroxide; also inhibits androgen synthesis

Pharmacokinetics

Absorption: Oral: Rapid (~75%)

Distribution: Minimal into the CNS

Protein binding: 93% to 96%

Metabolism: Partially in the liver by enzymes to inactive compounds

Bioavailability: Decreases as pH of the gastric contents increase

Half-life, biphasic:

Initial: 2 hours

Terminal: 8 hours

Time to peak serum concentration: Within 1-2 hours

Elimination: Primarily in feces (57%) with smaller amounts excreted in urine (13%)

Dosage

Geriatrics & Adults:

Fungal infections:

Oral: 200-400 mg/day as a single daily dose

Topical: Tinea infections: Cream: Rub gently into the affected area once daily. Duration of treatment: Tinea corporis, cruris: 2 weeks; tinea pedis: 6 weeks

Shampoo: Tinea versicolor: Apply twice weekly for 4 weeks with at least 3 days between each shampoo

Seborrheic dermatitis: *Topical:*

Cream: Rub gently into the affected area twice daily for 4 weeks or until clinical response is noted.

Foam: Apply to affected area twice daily for 4 weeks

Gel: Rub gently into the affected area once daily for 2 weeks.

Shampoo: Apply twice weekly for 4 weeks with at least 3 days between each shampoo

Prostate cancer (unlabeled use): Oral: Adults: 400 mg 3 times/day

Renal Impairment: Not dialyzable (0% to 5%)

Hepatic Impairment: Dose reductions should be considered in patients with severe liver disease.

Administration Administer oral tablets 2 hours prior to antacids to prevent decreased absorption due to the high pH of gastric contents. Cream, gel, and shampoo are for external use only.

Monitoring Parameters Signs and symptoms of infection, baseline LFTs; recheck if therapy is to go beyond 2 weeks; serum concentration and subjective response (see Drug Interactions)

Reference Range Therapeutic: Peak: 1-4 mg/L; Trough: ≤1 mg/L

Patient Information Cream is for topical application to the skin only; avoid contact with the eye; avoid taking antacids or H₂ antagonists at the same time as ketoconazole; may cause headache, dizziness or drowsiness, observe caution when driving or operating machinery; notify physician of GI side effects or if dark urine or pale stools occur

Special Geriatric Considerations No specific recommendations.

Dosage Forms Excipient information presented when available (limited, particularly for generics); consult specific product labeling.

(Continued)

Ketoconazole *(Continued)*

Aerosol, topical [foam]:
Extina®: 2% (10 g, 50 g, 100 g)
Cream, topical: 2% (15 g, 30 g, 60 g)
Kuric™: 2%: (25 g, 75 g)
Gel, topical:
Xolegel™: 2% (15 g) [contains dehydrated alcohol 34%]
Shampoo, topical: 1% (120 mL), 2% (120 mL)
Nizoral® : 2% (120 mL)
Nizoral® A-D: 1% (120 mL, 210 mL)
Tablet: 200 mg
Nizoral®: 200 mg

Ketoprofen (kee toe PROE fen)

Medication Safety Issues

Sound-alike/look-alike issues:
Oruvail® may be confused with Clinoril®, Elavil®

U.S. Brand Names Orudis® KT [OTC] [DSC]

Canadian Brand Names Apo-Keto®; Apo-Keto-E®; Apo-Keto SR®; Novo-Keto; Novo-Keto-EC; Nu-Ketoprofen; Nu-Ketoprofen-E; Oruvail®; Rhodis™; Rhodis-EC™; Rhodis SR™

Generic Available Yes: Capsule

Pharmacologic Category Nonsteroidal Anti-inflammatory Drug (NSAID), Oral

Use Acute or long-term treatment of rheumatoid arthritis and osteoarthritis; relief of mild to moderate pain, sunburn; migraine headache prophylaxis

Restrictions An FDA-approved medication guide must be distributed when dispensing an oral outpatient prescription (new or refill) where this medication is to be used without direct supervision of a healthcare provider. Medication guides are available at http://www.fda.gov/cder/Offices/ODS/medication_guides.htm.

Contraindications Hypersensitivity to ketoprofen, aspirin, other NSAIDs, or any component of the formulation; perioperative pain in the setting of coronary artery bypass surgery (CABG)

Warnings/Precautions [U.S. Boxed Warning]: NSAIDs are associated with an increased risk of adverse cardiovascular events, including MI, stroke, and new onset or worsening of pre-existing hypertension. Risk may be increased with duration of use or pre-existing cardiovascular risk factors or disease. Carefully evaluate individual cardiovascular risk profiles prior to prescribing. Use caution with fluid retention, CHF, or hypertension. Concurrent administration of ibuprofen, and potentially other nonselective NSAIDs, may interfere with aspirin's cardioprotective effect.

Use of NSAIDs can compromise existing renal function. Ketoprofen is not recommended for patients with advanced renal disease. **[U.S. Boxed Warning]: NSAIDs may increase risk of gastrointestinal irritation, ulceration, bleeding, and perforation.** Use with caution in patients with decreased hepatic function.

Use the lowest effective dose for the shortest duration of time, consistent with individual patient goals, to reduce risk of cardiovascular or GI adverse events. Alternate therapies should be considered for patients at high risk.

NSAIDs may cause serious skin adverse events including exfoliative dermatitis, Stevens-Johnson syndrome (SJS), and toxic epidermal necrolysis (TEN). Do not use in patients who experience bronchospasm, asthma, rhinitis, or urticaria with NSAID or aspirin therapy. Use caution in other forms of asthma.

The elderly are at increased risk for adverse effects (especially peptic ulceration, CNS effects, renal toxicity) from NSAIDs, even at low doses.

Withhold for at least 4-6 half-lives prior to surgical or dental procedures.

Adverse Reactions (Reflective of adult population; not specific for elderly
>10%: Gastrointestinal: Dyspepsia (11%)
1% to 10%:
Central nervous system: Headache (3% to 9%), depression, dizziness (>1%), dreams, insomnia, malaise, nervousness, somnolence
Dermatologic: Rash
Gastrointestinal: Abdominal pain (3% to 9%), constipation (3% to 9%), diarrhea (3% to 9%), flatulence (3% to 9%), nausea (3% to 9%), anorexia (>1%), stomatitis (>1%), vomiting (>1%)
Genitourinary: Urinary tract infection (>1%)
Ocular: Visual disturbances
Otic: Tinnitus
Renal: Renal dysfunction (3% to 9%)

Overdosage/Toxicology Common symptoms of acute NSAID overdose include lethargy, drowsiness, nausea, vomiting and epigastric pain. Respiratory depression, coma, convulsions, GI bleeding, or acute renal failure are rare. Management of NSAID intoxication is supportive and symptomatic; multiple dosing of activated charcoal may be effective.

Drug Interactions Inhibits CYP2C9 (weak)

ACE inhibitors: Antihypertensive effects may be decreased by concurrent therapy with NSAIDs; monitor blood pressure.

Aminoglycosides: NSAIDs may decrease the excretion of aminoglycosides.

Angiotensin II antagonists: Antihypertensive effects may be decreased by concurrent therapy with NSAIDs; monitor blood pressure.

Anticoagulants (warfarin, heparin, LMWHs): In combination with NSAIDs can cause increased risk of bleeding.

Antiplatelet agents (ticlopidine, clopidogrel, aspirin, abciximab, dipyridamole, eptifibatide, tirofiban): In combination with NSAIDs can cause an increased risk of bleeding.

Beta-blockers: NSAIDs may decrease the antihypertensive effect of beta-blockers; monitor.

Bisphosphonates: NSAIDs may increase the risk of gastrointestinal ulceration.

Cholestyramine (and other bile acid sequestrants): May decrease the absorption of NSAIDs; separate by at least 2 hours.

Corticosteroids: May increase the risk of GI ulceration; avoid concurrent use.

Cyclosporine: NSAIDs may increase serum creatinine, potassium, blood pressure, and cyclosporine levels; monitor cyclosporine levels and renal function carefully.

Fluoroquinolone antibiotics: Risk of seizures may be increased with concomitant quinolone use. Risk is considered quite low and may only be a factor with high serum levels of either agent and/or in patients with additional predisposing factors (eg, renal dysfunction, history of seizure, or other neurological disorder).

Hydralazine: Antihypertensive effect is decreased; avoid concurrent use.

Lithium: Lithium levels can be increased; avoid concurrent use if possible or monitor lithium levels and adjust dose. Sulindac may have the least effect. When NSAID is stopped, lithium will need adjustment again.

Loop diuretics: Antihypertensive and diuretic effects may be diminished. Indomethacin reduces this efficacy, however, it may be anticipated with any NSAID.

Methotrexate: Severe bone marrow suppression, aplastic anemia, and GI toxicity have been reported with concomitant NSAID therapy. Avoid use during moderate or high-dose methotrexate (increased and prolonged methotrexate levels). NSAID use during low-dose treatment of rheumatoid arthritis has not been fully evaluated; extreme caution is warranted.

Pemetrexed: NSAIDs may decrease the excretion of pemetrexed. Patients with Cl_{cr} 45-79 mL/minute should avoid long-acting NSAIDs for 5 days before and 2 days after pemetrexed treatment.

Probenecid: May increase the serum concentration of ketoprofen.

Salicylates: NSAIDs (nonselective) may diminish the cardioprotective effect of acetylated salicylates. Avoid regular use of NSAIDs if possible; consider alternatives (eg, acetaminophen). Give salicylate before NSAID; for example ibuprofen should be given 30-120 minutes after aspirin (immediate release).

Thiazides: Antihypertensive effects may be decreased; avoid concurrent use.

Treprostinil: May enhance the risk of bleeding with concurrent use.

Vancomycin: NSAIDs may decrease the excretion of vancomycin.

Ethanol/Nutrition/Herb Interactions

Ethanol: Avoid ethanol (due to GI irritation).

Food: Food slows rate of absorption resulting in delayed and reduced peak serum concentrations.

Herb/Nutraceutical: Avoid alfalfa, anise, bilberry, bladderwrack, bromelain, cat's claw, celery, coleus, cordyceps, dong quai, evening primrose, feverfew, fenugreek, garlic, ginger, ginkgo biloba, red clover, horse chestnut, grapeseed, green tea, ginseng, guggul, horse chestnut seed, horseradish, licorice, prickly ash, red clover, reishi, SAMe, sweet clover, turmeric, and white willow (all have additional antiplatelet activity).

Mechanism of Action Inhibits prostaglandin synthesis by decreasing the activity of the enzyme, cyclooxygenase, which results in decreased formation of prostaglandin precursors

Pharmacokinetics

Absorption: Almost complete

Protein binding: >99%, primarily albumin

Metabolism: Hepatic via glucuronidation; metabolite can be converted back to parent compound; may have enterohepatic recirculation

Half-life elimination:

Capsule: 2-4 hours; moderate-severe renal impairment: 5-9 hours

Capsule, extended release: ~3-7.5 hours

Time to peak, serum: Capsule: 0.5-2 hours; Capsule, extended release: 6-7 hours

Elimination: Urine (~80%, primarily as glucuronide conjugates)

(Continued)

Ketoprofen *(Continued)*

Dosage

Geriatrics: Initial: 25-50 mg 3-4 times/day; increase up to 150-300 mg/day (maximum daily dose: 300 mg)

Adults:

Rheumatoid arthritis or osteoarthritis: Oral:

Capsule: 50-75 mg 3-4 times/day up to a maximum of 300 mg/day

Capsule, extended release: 200 mg once daily

Note: Lower doses may be used in small patients or in the elderly, or debilitated.

Mild-to-moderate pain: Oral: Capsule: 25-50 mg every 6-8 hours up to a maximum of 300 mg/day

OTC labeling: 12.5 mg every 4-6 hours, up to a maximum of 6 tablets/24 hours

Renal Impairment: In general, NSAIDs are not recommended for use in patients with advanced renal disease, but the manufacturer of ketoprofen does provide some guidelines for adjustment in renal dysfunction:

Mild impairment: Maximum dose: 150 mg/day

Severe impairment: Cl_{cr} <25 mL/minute: Maximum dose: 100 mg/day

Hepatic Impairment: Hepatic impairment and serum albumin <3.5 g/dL: Maximum dose: 100 mg/day

Administration May take with food to reduce GI upset. Do not crush or break extended release capsules.

Monitoring Parameters Monitor response (pain, range of motion, grip strength, mobility, ADL function), inflammation; observe for weight gain, edema; monitor renal function; observe for bleeding, bruising; evaluate gastrointestinal effects (abdominal pain, bleeding, dyspepsia); mental confusion, disorientation, CBC, serum, creatinine, BUN, liver function tests

Patient Information Serious gastrointestinal bleeding can occur as well as ulceration and perforation. Pain may or may not be present. Avoid aspirin and aspirin-containing products while taking this medication. If gastric upset occurs, take with food, milk, or antacid. If gastric adverse effects persist, contact physician. May cause drowsiness, dizziness, blurred vision, and confusion. Use caution when performing tasks which require alertness (eg, driving). Do not take for more than 3 days for fever or 10 days for pain without physician advice.

Additional Information Dose must be lowest recommended in renal insufficiency. There are no clinical guidelines to predict which NSAID will give response in a particular patient. Trials with each must be initiated until response determined. Consider dose, patient convenience, and cost.

Special Geriatric Considerations Elderly are a high-risk population for adverse effects from NSAIDs. As much as 60% of the elderly can develop peptic ulceration and/or hemorrhage asymptomatically. The concomitant use of H_2 blockers and sucralfate is not effective as prophylaxis with the exception of NSAID-induced duodenal ulcers which may be prevented by the use of ranitidine. Misoprostol and proton pump inhibitors are the only agents proven to help prevent the development of NSAID-induced ulcers. Also, concomitant disease and drug use contribute to the risk for GI adverse effects. Use lowest effective dose for shortest period possible. Consider renal function decline with age. Use of NSAIDs can compromise existing renal function especially when Cl_{cr} is ≤30 mL/minute. Tinnitus may be a difficult and unreliable indication of toxicity due to age-related hearing loss and eighth cranial nerve damage. CNS adverse effects such as confusion, agitation, and hallucination are generally seen in overdose or high dose situations, but elderly may demonstrate these adverse effects at lower doses than younger adults.

Dosage Forms Excipient information presented when available (limited, particularly for generics); consult specific product labeling. [DSC] = Discontinued product

Capsule: 50 mg, 75 mg

Capsule, extended release: 200 mg

Tablet (Orudis® KT): 12.5 mg [contains tartrazine and sodium benzoate] [DSC]

Selected References

Brooks PM and Day RO, "Nonsteroidal Anti-inflammatory Drugs - Differences and Similarities," *N Engl J Med,* 1991, 324(24):1716-25.

Clinch D, Banerjee AK, and Ostick G, "Absence of Abdominal Pain in Elderly Patients With Peptic Ulcer," *Age Ageing,* 1984, 13(2):120-3.

Clive DM and Stoff JS, "Renal Syndromes Associated With Nonsteroidal Anti-inflammatory Drugs," *N Engl J Med,* 1984, 310(9):563-72.

Graham DY, "Prevention of Gastroduodenal Injury Induced by Chronic Nonsteroidal Anti-inflammatory Drug Therapy," *Gastroenterology,* 1989, 96(2 Pt 2 Suppl):675-81.

Gurwitz JH, Avorn J, Ross-Degnan D, et al, "Nonsteroidal Anti-Inflammatory Drug-Associated Azotemia in the Very Old," *JAMA,* 1990, 264(4):471-5.

Hawkey CJ, Karrasch JA, Szczepañski L, et al, "Omeprazole Compared With Misoprostol for Ulcers Associated With Nonsteroidal Anti-inflammatory Drugs," *N Engl J Med,* 1998, 338(11):727-34.

Knodel LC, "Preventing NSAID-induced Ulcers: The Role of Misoprostol," *Consult Pharm,* 1989, 4:37-41.

Pounder R, "Silent Peptic Ulceration: Deadly Silence or Golden Silence?" *Gastroenterology,* 1989, 96(2 Pt 2 Suppl):626-31.

Yeomans ND, Tulassay Z, Juhasz L, et al, "A Comparison of Omeprazole With Ranitidine for Ulcers Associated With Nonsteroidal Anti-inflammatory Drugs," *N Engl J Med,* 1998, 338(11):719-26.

Ketorolac (KEE toe role ak)

Related Information
Potentially Inappropriate Medications for Geriatrics *on page 1824*

Medication Safety Issues
Sound-alike/look-alike issues:
Acular® may be confused with Acthar®, Ocular®
Toradol® may be confused with Foradil®, Inderal®, Tegretol®, Torecan®, tramadol

International issues:
Toradol® may be confused with Theradol® which is a brand name for tramadol in the Netherlands

U.S. Brand Names Acular®; Acular LS™; Acular® PF; Toradol®

Canadian Brand Names Acular®; Acular LS™; Apo-Ketorolac®; Apo-Ketorolac Inject-able®; Ketorolac Tromethamine Injection, USP; Novo-Ketorolac; ratio-Ketorolac; Toradol®; Toradol® IM

Index Terms Ketorolac Tromethamine

Generic Available Yes: Injection, tablet

Pharmacologic Category Nonsteroidal Anti-inflammatory Drug (NSAID), Ophthalmic; Nonsteroidal Anti-inflammatory Drug (NSAID), Oral; Nonsteroidal Anti-inflammatory Drug (NSAID), Parenteral

Use
Oral, injection: Short-term (≤5 days) management of moderately-severe acute pain requiring analgesia at the opioid level
Ophthalmic: Temporary relief of ocular itching due to seasonal allergic conjunctivitis; postoperative inflammation following cataract extraction; reduction of ocular pain and photophobia following incisional refractive surgery

Restrictions An FDA-approved medication guide must be distributed when dispensing an oral outpatient prescription (new or refill) where this medication is to be used without direct supervision of a healthcare provider. Medication guides are available at http://www.fda.gov/cder/Offices/ODS/medication_guides.htm.

Contraindications Hypersensitivity to ketorolac, aspirin, other NSAIDs, or any component of the formulation; active or history of peptic ulcer disease; recent or history of GI bleeding or perforation; patients with advanced renal disease or risk of renal failure; prophylaxis before major surgery; suspected or confirmed cerebrovascular bleeding; hemorrhagic diathesis or high risk of bleeding; concurrent ASA or other NSAIDs; concomitant probenecid or pentoxifylline; epidural or intrathecal administration; perioperative pain in the setting of coronary artery bypass surgery (CABG)

Warnings/Precautions
Systemic: Treatment should be started with I.V./I.M. administration then changed to oral only as a continuation of treatment. Total therapy is not to exceed 5 days. Should not be used for minor or chronic pain.

May prolong bleeding time; do not use when hemostasis is critical. Patients should be euvolemic prior to treatment. Low doses of narcotics may be needed for breakthrough pain.

[U.S. Boxed Warning]: NSAIDs are associated with an increased risk of adverse cardiovascular events, including MI, stroke, and new onset or worsening of pre-existing hypertension. Risk may be increased with duration of use or pre-existing cardiovascular risk factors or disease. Carefully evaluate individual cardiovascular risk profiles prior to prescribing. Use caution with fluid retention, CHF or hypertension. Concurrent administration of ibuprofen, and potentially other nonselective NSAIDs, may interfere with aspirin's cardioprotective effect.

Use of NSAIDs can compromise existing renal function. Renal toxicity can occur in patient with impaired renal function, dehydration, heart failure, liver dysfunction, those taking diuretics and ACEI, and the elderly. Rehydrate patient before starting therapy. Monitor renal function closely. Ketorolac is not recommended for patients with advanced renal disease.

[U.S. Boxed Warning]: NSAIDs may increase risk of gastrointestinal irritation, ulceration, bleeding, and perforation. These events may occur at any time during therapy and without warning. Use caution with a history of GI disease (bleeding or ulcers), concurrent therapy with aspirin, anticoagulants and/or corticosteroids, smoking, use of alcohol, the elderly, or debilitated patients.

Use the lowest effective dose for the shortest duration of time, consistent with individual patient goals, to reduce risk of cardiovascular or GI adverse events. Alternate therapies should be considered for patients at high risk.

NSAIDs may cause serious skin adverse events including exfoliative dermatitis, Stevens-Johnson syndrome (SJS), and toxic epidermal necrolysis (TEN). Anaphylactoid reactions may occur, even without prior exposure; patients with "aspirin triad" (bronchial asthma, aspirin intolerance, rhinitis) may be at increased risk. Do not use in (Continued)

Ketorolac *(Continued)*

patients who experience bronchospasm, asthma, rhinitis, or urticaria with NSAID or aspirin therapy. Use caution in other forms of asthma.

Use with caution in patients with decreased hepatic function. Closely monitor patients with any abnormal LFT. Severe hepatic reactions (eg, fulminant hepatitis, liver failure) have occurred with NSAID use, rarely; discontinue if signs or symptoms of liver disease develop, or if systemic manifestations occur.

The elderly are at increased risk for adverse effects (especially peptic ulceration, CNS effects, renal toxicity) from NSAIDs, even at low doses. Patients with low body weight (<50 kg) or moderate elevation of serum creatinine require adjusted doses to limit risk of bleeding.

Withhold for at least 4-6 half-lives prior to surgical or dental procedures.

Ophthalmic: May increase bleeding time associated with ocular surgery. Use with caution in patients with known bleeding tendencies or those receiving anticoagulants. Healing time may be slowed or delayed. Corneal thinning, erosion, or ulceration have been reported with topical NSAIDs; discontinue if corneal epithelial breakdown occurs. Use caution with complicated ocular surgery, corneal denervation, corneal epithelial defects, diabetes, rheumatoid arthritis, ocular surface disease, or ocular surgeries repeated within short periods of time; risk of corneal epithelial breakdown may be increased. Use for >24 hours prior to or for >14 days following surgery also increases risk of corneal adverse effects. Do not administer while wearing soft contact lenses.

Adverse Reactions (Reflective of adult population; not specific for elderly)
Systemic (frequencies noted for parenteral administration):
>10%:
Central nervous system: Headache (17%)
Gastrointestinal: Gastrointestinal pain (13%), dyspepsia (12%), nausea (12%)
>1% to 10%:
Cardiovascular: Edema (4%), hypertension
Central nervous system: Dizziness (7%), drowsiness (6%)
Dermatologic: Pruritus, purpura, rash
Gastrointestinal: Diarrhea (7%), constipation, flatulence, gastrointestinal fullness, vomiting, stomatitis
Local: Injection site pain (2%)
Miscellaneous: Diaphoresis

Ophthalmic solution:
>10%: Ocular: Transient burning/stinging (Acular®: 40%; Acular® PF: 20%)
>1% to 10%:
Central nervous system: Headache
Ocular: Conjunctival hyperemia, corneal infiltrates, iritis, ocular edema, ocular inflammation, ocular irritation, ocular pain, superficial keratitis, superficial ocular infection
Miscellaneous: Allergic reactions

Overdosage/Toxicology Symptoms include abdominal pain, peptic ulcers, and metabolic acidosis. Management of nonsteroidal anti-inflammatory (NSAID) intoxication is supportive and symptomatic. Dialysis is not effective.

Drug Interactions
ACE inhibitors: Antihypertensive effects may be decreased by concurrent therapy with NSAIDs; monitor blood pressure.
Angiotensin II antagonists: Antihypertensive effects may be decreased by concurrent therapy with NSAIDs; monitor blood pressure.
Anticoagulants: Increased risk of bleeding complications with concomitant use; monitor closely.
Antiepileptic drugs (carbamazepine, phenytoin): Sporadic cases of seizures have been reported with concomitant use.
Beta-blockers: NSAIDs may decrease the antihypertensive effect of beta-blockers; monitor.
Cholestyramine (and other bile acid sequestrants): May decrease the absorption of NSAIDs; separate by at least 2 hours.
Diuretics: May see decreased effect of diuretics.
Fluoroquinolone antibiotics: Risk of seizures may be increased with concomitant quinolone use. Risk is considered quite low and may only be a factor with high serum levels of either agent and/or in patients with additional predisposing factors (eg, renal dysfunction, history of seizure or other neurological disorder).
Hydralazine's antihypertensive effect may be reduced; monitor.
Lithium: May increase lithium levels; monitor.
Methotrexate: Severe bone marrow suppression, aplastic anemia, and GI toxicity have been reported with concomitant NSAID therapy. Avoid use during moderate or high-dose methotrexate (increased and prolonged methotrexate levels). NSAID use during low-dose treatment of rheumatoid arthritis has not been fully evaluated; extreme caution is warranted.

Nondepolarizing muscle relaxants: Concomitant use has resulted in apnea.

NSAIDs, salicylates: Concomitant use increases NSAID-induced adverse effects; contraindicated.

Pentoxifylline: Concomitant use may increase risk of bleeding; contraindicated.

Probenecid: Probenecid significantly decreases ketorolac clearance, increases keto-rolac plasma levels, and doubles the half-life of ketorolac; concomitant use is contra-indicated.

Psychoactive drugs (alprazolam, fluoxetine, thiothixene): Hallucinations have been reported with concomitant use.

Salicylates: NSAIDs (nonselective) may diminish the cardioprotective effect of acety-lated salicylates. Avoid regular use of NSAIDs, if possible; consider alternatives (eg, acetaminophen). Give salicylate before NSAID; for example, ibuprofen should be given 30-120 minutes after aspirin (immediate release).

Ethanol/Nutrition/Herb Interactions

Ethanol: Avoid ethanol (may enhance gastric mucosal irritation).

Food: Oral: High-fat meals may delay time to peak (by ~1 hour) and decrease peak concentrations.

Herb/Nutraceuticals: Avoid alfalfa, anise, bilberry, bladderwrack, bromelain, cat's claw, celery, coleus, cordyceps, dong quai, evening primrose, feverfew, fenugreek, garlic, ginger, ginkgo biloba, red clover, horse chestnut, grapeseed, green tea, ginseng, guggul, horse chestnut seed, horseradish, licorice, prickly ash, red clover, reishi, SAMe, sweet clover, turmeric, and white willow (all have additional antiplatelet activity).

Stability

Injection: Store at controlled room temperature. Protect from light. Injection is clear and has a slight yellow color. Precipitation may occur at relatively low pH values.

Ophthalmic solution: Store at controlled room temperature. Protect from light.

Tablet: Store at 15°C to 30°C (59°F to 86°F).

Mechanism of Action Inhibits prostaglandin synthesis by decreasing the activity of the enzyme, cyclooxygenase, which results in decreased formation of prostaglandin precursors

Pharmacodynamics

Onset of action: I.M.: Within 10 minutes

Peak effect: Within 75-150 minutes

Duration: 6-8 hours

Pharmacokinetics

Absorption: Oral: Well absorbed

Protein binding: 99%

Metabolism: In the liver

Half-life elimination: 2-6 hours; prolonged 30% to 50% in elderly; up to 19 hours in renal impairment

Time to peak serum concentration: Within 30-60 minutes

Excretion: Urine (92%, 61% as unchanged drug)

Dosage

Geriatrics: Dosage adjustments in elderly (>65 years), renal insufficiency, or low body weight (<50 kg): **Note:** These groups have an increased incidence of GI bleeding, ulceration, and perforation. The maximum combined duration of treatment (for parenteral and oral) is 5 days.

I.M.: 30 mg as a single dose or 15 mg every 6 hours (maximum daily dose: 60 mg)

I.V.: 15 mg as a single dose or 15 mg every 6 hours (maximum daily dose: 60 mg)

Oral: 10 mg, followed by 10 mg every 4-6 hours; do not exceed 40 mg/day; oral dosing is intended to be a continuation of I.M. or I.V. therapy only

Adults:

Pain management (acute; moderately-severe):

Note: The maximum combined duration of treatment (for parenteral and oral) is 5 days; do not increase dose or frequency; supplement with low dose opioids if needed for breakthrough pain. For patients <50 kg and/or ≥65 years of age, see Geriatric dosing.

I.M.: 60 mg as a single dose or 30 mg every 6 hours (maximum daily dose: 120 mg)

I.V.: 30 mg as a single dose or 30 mg every 6 hours (maximum daily dose: 120 mg)

Oral: 20 mg, followed by 10 mg every 4-6 hours; do not exceed 40 mg/day; oral dosing is intended to be a continuation of I.M. or I.V. therapy only

Ophthalmic uses:

Seasonal allergic conjunctivitis (relief of ocular itching) (Acular®): Ophthalmic: Instill 1 drop (0.25 mg) 4 times/day for seasonal allergic conjunctivitis

Inflammation following cataract extraction (Acular®): Ophthalmic: Instill 1 drop (0.25 mg) to affected eye(s) 4 times/day beginning 24 hours after surgery; continue for 2 weeks

(Continued)

Ketorolac *(Continued)*

Pain and photophobia following incisional refractive surgery (Acular® PF): Ophthalmic: Instill 1 drop (0.25 mg) 4 times/day to affected eye for up to 3 days

Pain following corneal refractive surgery (Acular LS™): Ophthalmic: Instill 1 drop 4 times/day as needed to affected eye for up to 4 days

Renal Impairment: Contraindicated in patients with advanced renal impairment. Patients with moderately-elevated serum creatinine should use half the recommended dose, not to exceed 60 mg/day I.M./I.V.

Hepatic Impairment: Use with caution, may cause elevation of liver enzymes

Administration

Oral: May take with food to reduce GI upset

I.M.: Administer slowly and deeply into the muscle. Analgesia begins in 30 minutes and maximum effect within 2 hours

I.V.: Administer I.V. bolus over a minimum of 15 seconds; onset within 30 minutes; peak analgesia within 2 hours

Ophthalmic solution: Contact lenses should be removed before instillation.

Monitoring Parameters Monitor response (pain, range of motion, grip strength, mobility, ADL function), inflammation; observe for weight gain, edema; monitor renal function (creatinine, BUN); observe for bleeding, bruising; evaluate gastrointestinal effects (abdominal pain, bleeding, dyspepsia); mental confusion, disorientation, CBC, serum, liver function tests

Reference Range Serum concentration: Therapeutic: 0.3-5 mcg/mL; Toxic: >5 mcg/mL

Test Interactions Increased chloride (S), sodium (S), bleeding time

Patient Information

Serious gastrointestinal bleeding can occur as well as ulceration and perforation. Pain may or may not be present. If gastric upset occurs, take with food, milk, or antacid. If gastric adverse effects persist, contact physician. May cause drowsiness, dizziness, blurred vision, and confusion. Use caution when performing tasks which require alertness (eg, driving). Do not take for more than 3 days for fever or 5 days for pain without physician's advice.

If self-administered, use exactly as directed (do not increase dose or frequency); adverse reactions can occur with overuse. While using this medication, do not use alcohol, other prescription or OTC medications including aspirin, aspirin-containing medications, or other NSAIDs without consulting healthcare provider. Maintain adequate hydration (2-3 L/day of fluids unless instructed to restrict fluid intake). You may experience nausea, vomiting, gastric discomfort (frequent mouth care, small frequent meals, chewing gum, or sucking lozenges may help). GI bleeding, ulceration, or perforation can occur with or without pain. Stop taking medication and report ringing in ears; persistent cramping or pain in stomach; unresolved nausea or vomiting; difficulty breathing or shortness of breath; unusual bruising or bleeding (mouth, urine, stool); skin rash; unusual swelling of extremities; chest pain; or palpitations.

Ophthalmic: Instill drops as often as recommended. Wash hands before instilling. Sit or lie down to instill. Open eye, look at ceiling, and instill prescribed amount of solution. Close eye and roll eye in all directions, and apply gentle pressure to inner corner of eye for 1-2 minutes after instillation. Do not let tip of applicator touch eye or contaminate tip of applicator. Temporary stinging or blurred vision may occur. Do not wear soft contact lenses. Report persistent pain, burning, double vision, swelling, itching, worsening of condition.

Additional Information First parenteral NSAID for analgesia; 30 mg provides the analgesia comparable to 12 mg of morphine or 100 mg of meperidine; pain relief usually begins within 10 minutes; there are no clinical guidelines to predict which NSAID will give response in a particular patient. Trials with each must be initiated until response determined. Consider dose, patient convenience, and cost.

Special Geriatric Considerations Ketorolac is cleared more slowly in the elderly. It is recommended to use lower doses in the elderly. Elderly are a high-risk population for adverse effects from NSAIDs. As much as 60% of elderly can develop peptic ulceration and/or hemorrhage asymptomatically. The concomitant use of H_2 blockers and sucralfate is not effective as prophylaxis with the exception of NSAID-induced duodenal ulcers which may be prevented by the use of ranitidine. Misoprostol and proton pump inhibitors are the only agents proven to help prevent the development of NSAID-induced ulcers. Also, concomitant disease and drug use contribute to the risk for GI adverse effects. Use lowest effective dose for shortest period possible. Consider renal function decline with age. Use of NSAIDs can compromise existing renal function especially when Cl_{cr} is ≤30 mL/minute or weight <50 kg. Tinnitus may be a difficult and unreliable indication of toxicity due to age-related hearing loss or eighth cranial nerve damage. CNS adverse effects such as confusion, agitation, and hallucination are generally seen in overdose or high dose situations, but elderly may demonstrate these adverse effects at lower doses than younger adults.

Dosage Forms Excipient information presented when available (limited, particularly for generics); consult specific product labeling. [DSC] = Discontinued product

Injection, solution, as tromethamine: 15 mg/mL (1 mL); 30 mg/mL (1 mL, 2 mL, 10 mL) [contains alcohol]

Solution, ophthalmic, as tromethamine:
Acular®: 0.5% (3 mL, 5 mL, 10 mL) [contains benzalkonium chloride]
Acular LS™: 0.4% (5 mL) [contains benzalkonium chloride]
Acular® P.F. [preservative free]: 0.5% (0.4 mL)
Tablet, as tromethamine: 10 mg
Toradol®: 10 mg [DSC]

Selected References

Brooks PM and Day RO, "Nonsteroidal Anti-inflammatory Drugs - Differences and Similarities," *N Engl J Med*, 1991, 324(24):1716-25.

Clinch D, Banerjee AK, and Ostick G, "Absence of Abdominal Pain in Elderly Patients With Peptic Ulcer," *Age Ageing*, 1984, 13(2):120-3.

Clive DM and Stoff JS, "Renal Syndromes Associated With Nonsteroidal Anti-inflammatory Drugs," *N Engl J Med*, 1984, 310(9):563-72.

Graham DY, "Prevention of Gastroduodenal Injury Induced by Chronic Nonsteroidal Anti-inflammatory Drug Therapy," *Gastroenterology*, 1989, 96(2 Pt 2 Suppl):675-81.

Hawkey CJ, Karrasch JA, Szczepański L, et al, "Omeprazole Compared With Misoprostol for Ulcers Associated With Nonsteroidal Anti-inflammatory Drugs," *N Engl J Med*, 1998, 338(11):727-34.

Jallad NS, Garg DC, Martinez JJ, et al, "Pharmacokinetics of Single-Dose Oral and Intramuscular Ketorolac Tromethamine in the Young and Elderly," *J Clin Pharmacol*, 1990, 30(1):76-81.

Knodel LC, "Preventing NSAID-induced Ulcers: The Role of Misoprostol," *Consult Pharm*, 1989, 4:37-41.

Obase Y, Matsuse H, Shimoda T, et al, "Pathogenesis and Management of Aspirin-Intolerant Asthma," *Treat Respir Med*, 2005, 4(5):325-36.

Pounder R, "Silent Peptic Ulceration: Deadly Silence or Golden Silence?" *Gastroenterology*, 1989, 96(2 Pt 2 Suppl):626-31.

Yeomans ND, Tulassay Z, Juhasz L, et al, "A Comparison of Omeprazole With Ranitidine for Ulcers Associated With Nonsteroidal Anti-inflammatory Drugs," *N Engl J Med*, 1998, 338(11):719-26.

♦ **Ketorolac Tromethamine** *see Ketorolac on page 859*

Ketotifen (kee toe TYE fen)

U.S. Brand Names Alaway™ [OTC]; Zaditor® [OTC]
Canadian Brand Names Apo-Ketotifen®; Novo-Ketotifen; Zaditen®; Zaditor®
Index Terms Ketotifen Fumarate
Generic Available Yes
Pharmacologic Category Antihistamine, H₁ Blocker, Ophthalmic
Use Temporary prevention of eye itching due to allergic conjunctivitis
Contraindications Hypersensitivity to ketotifen or any component of the formulation (the preservative is benzalkonium chloride)
Warnings/Precautions For topical ophthalmic use only. Not to treat contact lens-related irritation. After ketotifen use, soft contact lens wearers should wait at least 10 minutes before putting their lenses in. Do not wear contact lenses if eyes are red. Do not contaminate dropper tip or solution when placing drops in eyes.
Adverse Reactions (Reflective of adult population; not specific for elderly)
1% to 10%:
Ocular: Allergic reactions, burning or stinging, conjunctivitis, discharge, dry eyes, eye pain, eyelid disorder, itching, keratitis, lacrimation disorder, mydriasis, photophobia, rash
Respiratory: Pharyngitis
Miscellaneous: Flu syndrome
Overdosage/Toxicology No serious signs or symptoms have been seen after ingestion up to 20 mg.
Stability Stable at room temperature.
Mechanism of Action Relatively selective, noncompetitive H₁-receptor antagonist and mast cell stabilizer, inhibiting the release of mediators from cells involved in hypersensitivity reactions
Pharmacodynamics
Onset of action: Within minutes
Duration: 8-12 hours
Dosage
Geriatrics & Adults: Allergic conjunctivitis: Ophthalmic: Instill 1 drop into the affected eye(s) twice daily, every 8-12 hours
Patient Information For topical ophthalmic use only. Not to be used to treat contact lens-related irritation. After ketotifen's use, soft contact lens wearers should wait at least 10 minutes before putting their contact lenses in. Do not wear contact lenses if eyes are red. Do not contaminate dropper tip or solution when placing drops in eyes. Store at room temperature
Special Geriatric Considerations Instruct the patient on proper instillation of ophthalmic solution.
Dosage Forms Excipient information presented when available (limited, particularly for generics); consult specific product labeling.
Solution, ophthalmic [drops]: 0.025% (5 mL)
(Continued)

Ketotifen *(Continued)*

Alaway™: 0.025% (10 mL) [contains benzalkonium chloride]
Zaditor®: 0.025% (5 mL) [contains benzalkonium chloride]

Labetalol *(la BET a lole)*

Related Information
Beta-Blockers *on page 1751*
Medication Safety Issues
Sound-alike/look-alike issues:
Labetalol may be confused with betaxolol, Hexadrol®, lamotrigine
Trandate® may be confused with tramadol, Trendar®, Trental®, Tridrate®

High alert medication: The Institute for Safe Medication Practices (ISMP) includes this medication among its list of drugs which have a heightened risk of causing significant patient harm when used in error.

Significant differences exist between oral and I.V. dosing. Use caution when converting from one route of administration to another.
U.S. Brand Names Trandate®
Canadian Brand Names Apo-Labetalol®; Labetalol Hydrochloride Injection, USP; Normodyne®; Trandate®
Index Terms Ibidomide Hydrochloride; Labetalol Hydrochloride
Generic Available Yes

Pharmacologic Category Beta Blocker With Alpha-Blocking Activity

Use Treatment of mild to severe hypertension; I.V. for hypertensive emergencies

Contraindications Hypersensitivity to labetalol or any component of the formulation; sinus bradycardia; heart block greater than first degree (except in patients with a functioning artificial pacemaker); cardiogenic shock; bronchial asthma; uncompensated cardiac failure

Warnings/Precautions Consider pre-existing conditions such as sick sinus syndrome before initiating. Paradoxical increase in blood pressure has been reported with treatment of pheochromocytoma or clonidine withdrawal syndrome; orthostatic hypotension may occur with I.V. administration; patient should remain supine during and for up to 3 hours after I.V. administration; use with caution in impaired hepatic function (discontinue if signs of liver dysfunction occur); may mask the signs and symptoms of hypoglycemia; a lower hemodynamic response rate and higher incidence of toxicity may be observed with administration to elderly patients.

Use only with extreme caution in compensated heart failure and monitor for a worsening of the condition. Beta-blocker therapy should not be withdrawn abruptly (particularly in patients with CAD), but gradually tapered to avoid acute tachycardia, hypertension, and/or ischemia. Use caution with concurrent use of beta-blockers and either verapamil or diltiazem; bradycardia or heart block can occur. Patients with bronchospastic disease should not receive beta-blockers. Labetalol may be used with caution in patients with nonallergic bronchospasm (chronic bronchitis, emphysema). Use cautiously in diabetics because it can mask prominent hypoglycemic symptoms. Use with caution in patients with myasthenia gravis, psychiatric disease (may cause CNS depression), or peripheral vascular disease. Adequate alpha-blockade is required prior to use of any beta-blocker for patients with untreated pheochromocytoma. Use with caution in patients receiving anesthetic agents which decrease myocardial function.

Adverse Reactions (Reflective of adult population; not specific for elderly)
>10%:
    Central nervous system: Dizziness (1% to 16%)
    Gastrointestinal: Nausea (0% to 19%)
1% to 10%:
    Cardiovascular: Edema (0% to 2%), hypotension (1% to 5%); with I.V. use, hypotension may occur in up to 58%
    Central nervous system: Fatigue (1% to 10%), headache (2%), vertigo (2%)
    Dermatologic: Rash (1%), scalp tingling (1% to 5%)
    Gastrointestinal: Vomiting (<1% to 3%), dyspepsia (1% to 4%)
    Genitourinary: Ejaculatory failure (0% to 5%), impotence (1% to 4%)
    Hepatic: Transaminases increased (4%)
    Neuromuscular & skeletal: Paresthesia (1% to 5%), weakness (1%)
    Respiratory: Nasal congestion (1% to 6%), dyspnea (2%)
    Miscellaneous: Taste disorder (1%), abnormal vision (1%)
Other adverse reactions noted with beta-adrenergic blocking agents include mental depression, catatonia, disorientation, short-term memory loss, emotional lability, clouded sensorium, intensification of pre-existing AV block, laryngospasm, respiratory distress, agranulocytosis, thrombocytopenic purpura, nonthrombocytopenic purpura, mesenteric artery thrombosis, and ischemic colitis.

Overdosage/Toxicology Symptoms of intoxication include cardiac disturbances, CNS toxicity, bronchospasm, hypoglycemia and hyperkalemia. The most common cardiac symptoms include hypotension and bradycardia. Atrioventricular block, intraventricular conduction disturbances, cardiogenic shock, and asystole may occur with severe overdose, especially with membrane-depressant drugs (eg, propranolol). CNS effects include convulsions, coma, and respiratory arrest, commonly seen with propranolol and other membrane-depressant and lipid-soluble drugs. Treatment is symptomatic for seizures, hypotension, hyperkalemia and hypoglycemia. Bradycardia and hypotension resistant to atropine, isoproterenol or pacing may respond to glucagon. Wide QRS defects caused by membrane-depressant poisoning may respond to hypertonic sodium bicarbonate. Repeat-dose charcoal, hemoperfusion, or hemodialysis may be helpful in removal of only those beta-blockers with a small V_d, long half-life, or low intrinsic clearance (acebutolol, atenolol, nadolol, sotalol).

Drug Interactions Substrate of CYP2D6 (major); **Inhibits** CYP2D6 (weak)
    Alpha-blockers (prazosin, terazosin): Concurrent use of beta-blockers may increase risk of orthostasis.
    Cimetidine increases the bioavailability of labetalol.
    CYP2D6 inhibitors: May increase the levels/effects of labetalol. Example inhibitors include chlorpromazine, delavirdine, fluoxetine, miconazole, paroxetine, pergolide, quinidine, quinine, ritonavir, and ropinirole.
    Halothane, isoflurane, enflurane (possibly other inhalational anesthetics): Excessive hypotension may occur.
    NSAIDs may reduce antihypertensive efficacy of labetalol.
    Salicylates may reduce the antihypertensive effects of beta-blockers.
    (Continued)

Labetalol *(Continued)*

Sulfonylureas: Effects may be decreased by beta-blockers.

Verapamil or diltiazem may have synergistic or additive pharmacological effects when taken concurrently with beta-blockers; avoid concurrent I.V. use.

Ethanol/Nutrition/Herb Interactions

Food: Labetalol serum concentrations may be increased if taken with food.

Herb/Nutraceutical: Avoid dong quai if using for hypertension (has estrogenic activity). Avoid ephedra, yohimbe, ginseng (may worsen hypertension). Avoid natural licorice (causes sodium and water retention and increases potassium loss). Avoid garlic (may have increased antihypertensive effect).

Stability

Labetalol should be stored at room temperature or under refrigeration and should be protected from light and freezing. The solution is clear to slightly yellow.

Stability of parenteral admixture at room temperature (25°C) and refrigeration temperature (4°C): 3 days.

Standard diluent: 500 mg/250 mL D_5W.

Minimum volume: 250 mL D_5W.

Mechanism of Action Blocks alpha-, beta$_1$-, and beta$_2$-adrenergic receptor sites; elevated renins are reduced. The ratios of alpha- to beta-blockade differ depending on the route of administration: 1:3 (oral) and 1:7 (I.V.).

Pharmacodynamics

Onset of action:

Oral: 20 minutes to 2 hours; maximum: 1-4 hours

I.V.: 2-5 minutes; maximum: 5-15 minutes

Duration:

Oral: 8-24 hours (dose-dependent)

I.V.: 2-4 hours

Pharmacokinetics

Distribution: V_d: Adults: 3-16 L/kg, mean: 9.4 L/kg; moderately lipid soluble, therefore, it can enter the CNS

Protein binding: 50%

Metabolism: Extensive first-pass effect; metabolized in liver primarily via glucuronide conjugation

Bioavailability: Oral: 25%; increased bioavailability with liver disease, in older adults, and with concurrent cimetidine

Half-life: 6-8 hours

Elimination: In older adults, total body clearance of labetalol is decreased; <5% excreted in urine unchanged

Dosage

Geriatrics: Oral: Initial: 100 mg 1-2 times/day increasing as needed

Adults:

Hypertension: Oral: Initial: 100 mg twice daily, may increase as needed every 2-3 days by 100 mg until desired response is obtained; usual dose: 200-400 mg twice daily; not to exceed 2.4 g/day

Usual dose range (JNC 7): 200-800 mg/day in 2 divided doses

Acute hypertension (hypertensive urgency/emergency):

I.V. bolus: 20 mg IVP over 2 minutes, may give 40-80 mg at 10-minute intervals, up to 300 mg total dose

I.V. infusion (acute loading): Initial: 2 mg/minute; titrate to response up to 300 mg total dose. Administration requires the use of an infusion pump.

Note: Although loading infusions are well described in the product labeling, the labeling is silent in specific clinical situations, such as in the patient who has an initial response to labetalol infusions but cannot be converted to an oral route for subsequent dosing. There is limited documentation of prolonged continuous infusions. In rare clinical situations, higher dosages (up to 6 mg/minute) have been used in the critical care setting (eg, aortic dissection). At the other extreme, continuous infusions at relatively low doses (2-6 mg/hour - note difference in units) have been used in some settings (following loading infusion in patients who are unable to be converted to oral regimens or in some cases as a continuation of outpatient oral regimens). These prolonged infusions should not be confused with loading infusions. Because of wide variation in the use of infusions, an awareness of institutional policies and practices is extremely important. Careful clarification of orders and specific infusion rates/units is required to avoid confusion. Due to the prolonged duration of action, careful monitoring should be extended for the duration of the infusion and for several hours after the infusion. Excessive administration may result in prolonged hypotension and/or bradycardia.

Renal Impairment: Not removed by hemo- or peritoneal dialysis; supplemental dose is not necessary.

Hepatic Impairment: Dosage reduction may be necessary.

Administration Bolus administered over 2 minutes. Loading infusions (2 mg/minute) require close monitoring of heart rate and blood pressure and are usually terminated after response or cumulative dose of 300 mg. There is limited documentation of prolonged continuous infusions. In clinical experience, prolonged continuous infusions have been used. In rare clinical situations, higher dosages (up to 6 mg/minute) have been used in the critical care setting (eg, aortic dissection). At the other extreme, continuous infusions at relatively low doses (2-6 mg/hour: note difference in units) have been used in some settings (following loading infusion in patients who are unable to be converted to oral regimens or in some cases as a continuation of outpatient oral regimens). These prolonged infusions should not be confused with loading infusions. Because of wide variation in the use of infusions, an awareness of institutional policies and practices is extremely important. Careful clarification of orders and specific infusion rates/units is required to avoid confusion. Due to the prolonged duration of action, careful monitoring should be extended for the duration of the infusion and for several hours after the infusion. Excessive administration may result in prolonged hypotension and/or bradycardia.

Monitoring Parameters Blood pressure, standing and sitting/supine, pulse, mental status; if used in a diabetic patient, monitor glucose carefully; if used in patients with COPD, monitor pulmonary function

Test Interactions False-positive urine catecholamines, VMA if measured by fluorometric or photometric methods; use HPLC or specific catecholamine radioenzymatic technique

Patient Information Do not take any new medication during therapy unless approved by prescriber. Take as directed, with meals. Do not skip dose or discontinue without consulting prescriber. This medication does not replace other antihypertensive interventions; follow prescriber's instructions for diet and lifestyle changes. If you have diabetes, monitor serum glucose closely and notify prescriber of changes (this medication can alter glycemic response). You may experience drowsiness, dizziness, or impaired judgment (use caution when driving or engaging in tasks that require alertness until response to drug is known); postural hypotension (use caution when rising from sitting or lying position or when climbing stairs); dry mouth, nausea, or loss of appetite (frequent mouth care or sucking lozenges may help); or sexual dysfunction (reversible, may resolve with continued use). Report altered CNS status (eg, fatigue, depression, numbness or tingling of fingers, toes, or skin); palpitations or slowed heartbeat; respiratory difficulty; edema or cold extremities; or other persistent side effects.

Special Geriatric Considerations Due to alterations in the beta-adrenergic autonomic nervous system, beta-adrenergic blockade may result in less hemodynamic response than seen in younger adults. Studies indicate that despite decreased sensitivity to the chronotropic effects of beta-blockade with age, there appears to be an increased myocardial sensitivity to the negative inotropic effect during stress (ie, exercise). Controlled trials have shown the overall response rate for propranolol to be only 20% to 50% in elderly populations. Therefore, all beta-adrenergic blocking drugs may result in a decreased response as compared to younger adults.

Dosage Forms Excipient information presented when available (limited, particularly for generics); consult specific product labeling.

Injection, solution, as hydrochloride: 5 mg/mL (4 mL, 20 mL, 40 mL)
    Trandate®: 5 mg/mL (20 mL, 40 mL)
Tablet, as hydrochloride: 100 mg, 200 mg, 300 mg
    Trandate®: 100 mg, 200 mg [contains sodium benzoate], 300 mg

♦ **Labetalol Hydrochloride** see Labetalol on page 864
♦ **Lacri-Lube® NP Ophthalmic Ointment [OTC]** see Ocular Lubricant on page 1144
♦ **Lacri-Lube® S.O.P. Ophthalmic Ointment [OTC]** see Ocular Lubricant on page 1144
♦ **Lactinex™ [OTC]** see Lactobacillus on page 867

Lactobacillus (lak toe ba SIL us)

U.S. Brand Names Bacid® [OTC]; Culturelle® [OTC]; Dofus [OTC]; Flora-Q™ [OTC]; Kala® [OTC]; Lactinex™ [OTC]; Lacto-Bifidus [OTC]; Lacto-Key [OTC]; Lacto-Pectin [OTC]; Lacto-TriBlend [OTC]; Megadophilus® [OTC]; MoreDophilus® [OTC]; Superdophilus® [OTC]

Canadian Brand Names Bacid®; Fermalac

Index Terms Lactobacillus acidophilus; Lactobacillus bifidus; Lactobacillus bulgaricus; Lactobacillus casei; Lactobacillus paracasei; Lactobacillus reuteri; Lactobacillus rhamnosus GG

Generic Available Yes

Pharmacologic Category Dietary Supplement; Probiotic

Use Promote normal bacterial flora of the intestinal tract
(Continued)

Lactobacillus (Continued)

Contraindications Hypersensitivity to any component of the formulation

Warnings/Precautions Lactobacillus species have been studied for various gastrointestinal disorders including diarrhea, inflammatory bowel disease, gastrointestinal infection. Effectiveness may be dependent upon actual species used; studies are ongoing. Currently, there are no FDA-approved disease-prevention or therapeutic indications for these products.

Adverse Reactions (Reflective of adult population; not specific for elderly)
Gastrointestinal: Flatulence

Drug Interactions No data reported

Stability
Bacid®: Store at room temperature.
Flora-Q™: Store at or below room temperature; do not store in bathroom.
Kala®, MoreDophilus®: Refrigeration recommended after opening.
Lactinex™, Dofus: Store in refrigerator.

Mechanism of Action Helps re-establish normal intestinal flora; suppresses the growth of potentially pathogenic microorganisms by producing lactic acid which favors the establishment of an aciduric flora.

Pharmacokinetics
Absorption: Oral: None
Distribution: Locally, primarily colon
Excretion: feces

Dosage
Geriatrics & Adults: Dietary supplement: Oral: Dosing varies by manufacturer; consult product labeling

Bacid®: 2 caplets/day
Culturelle®: 1 capsule daily; may increase to twice daily
Flora-Q™: 1 capsule/day
Lacto-Key 100 or 600: 1-2 capsules/day
Lactinex™: 1 packet or 4 tablets 3-4 times/day

Administration
Culturelle®: Capsules may be opened and mixed in a cool beverage or sprinkled onto baby food or applesauce.
Flora-Q™: May be taken with or without food.
Lactinex™: Granules may be added to or administered with cereal, food, or milk.
Megadophilus®, Superdophilus®: Administer on an empty stomach; powder should be mixed in unchilled water.

Monitoring Parameters Monitor for decrease in frequency of stool and increased mass of stool

Patient Information Granules may be added to or taken with cereal, food, milk, fruit juice, or water. You may experience increased flatus while taking this medication. Discontinue and notify prescriber if a high fever develops. Refrigerate Lactinex™ and Bacid®.

Additional Information Pro-Bionate®, Superdophilus® and Lactinex®, mixed L. acidophilus and L. bulgaricus, More-Dophilus® can be stored at room temperature

Special Geriatric Considerations No specific recommendations due to age; keep in mind that elderly suffer significantly with fluid and electrolyte loss (lethargy, confusion, etc) and diarrhea should be aggressively treated

Dosage Forms Excipient information presented when available (limited, particularly for generics); consult specific product labeling.
Capsule:
Culturelle®: L. rhamnosus GG 10 billion colony-forming units [contains casein and whey]
Dofus: L. acidophilus and L. bifidus 10:1 ratio [beet root powder base]
Flora-Q™: L. acidophilus and L. paracasei ≥8 billion colony-forming units [also contains Bifidobacterium and S. thermophilus]
Lacto-Key:
100: L. acidophilus 1 billion colony-forming units [milk, soy, and yeast free; rice derived]
600: L. acidophilus 6 billion colony-forming units [milk, soy, and yeast free; rice derived]
Lacto-Bifidus:
100: L. bifidus 1 billion colony-forming units [milk, soy, and yeast free; rice derived]
600: L. bifidus 6 billion colony-forming units [milk, soy, and yeast free; rice derived]
Lacto-Pectin: L. acidophilus and L. casei ≥5 billion colony-forming units [also contains Bifidobacterium lactis and citrus pectin cellulose complex]
Lacto-TriBlend:
100: L. acidophilus, L. bifidus, and L. bulgaricus 1 billion colony-forming units [milk, soy and yeast free; rice derived]

600: *L. acidophilus*, *L. bifidus*, and *L. bulgaricus* 6 billion colony-forming units [milk, soy and yeast free; rice derived]

Megadophilus®, Superdophilus®: *L. acidophilus* 2 billion units [available in dairy based or dairy free formulations]

Capsule, softgel: *L. acidophilus* 100 active units

Caplet (Bacid®): *L. acidophilus* *80%* and *L. bulgaricus* 10% [also contains *Bifidobacterium biffidum* 5% and *S. thermophilus* 5%]

Granules (Lactinex™): *L. acidophilus* and *L. bulgaricus* 100 million live cells per 1 g packet (12s) [contains whey, evaporated milk, soy peptone, lactose, and beef extract]

Powder:

Lacto-TriBlend: *L. acidophilus*, *L. bifidus*, and *L. bulgaricus* 10 billion colony-forming units per ¹/₄ teaspoon (60 g) [milk, soy, and yeast free; rice derived]

Megadophilus®, Superdophilus®: *L. acidophilus* 2 billion units per half-teaspoon (49 g, 70 g, 84 g, 126 g) [available in dairy based or dairy free (garbanzo bean) formulations]

MoreDophilus®: *L. acidophilus* 12.4 billion units per teaspoon (30 g, 120 g) [dairy free, yeast free; soy and carrot derived]

Tablet:

Kala®: *L. acidophilus* 200 million units [dairy free, yeast free; soy based]

Lactinex™: *L. acidophilus* and *L. bulgaricus* 1 million live cells [contains whey, evaporated milk, soy peptone, lactose, and beef extract; contains sodium 5.6 mg/4 tablets]

Tablet, chewable: *L. reuteri* 100 million organisms

Wafer: *L. acidophilus* 90 mg and *L. bifidus* 25 mg (100s) [provides 1 billion organisms/ wafer at time of manufacture; milk free]

♦ **Lactobacillus acidophilus** *see Lactobacillus on page 867*
♦ **Lactobacillus bifidus** *see Lactobacillus on page 867*
♦ **Lactobacillus bulgaricus** *see Lactobacillus on page 867*
♦ **Lactobacillus casei** *see Lactobacillus on page 867*
♦ **Lactobacillus paracasei** *see Lactobacillus on page 867*
♦ **Lactobacillus reuteri** *see Lactobacillus on page 867*
♦ **Lactobacillus rhamnosus** **GG** *see Lactobacillus on page 867*
♦ **Lacto-Bifidus [OTC]** *see Lactobacillus on page 867*
♦ **Lacto-Key [OTC]** *see Lactobacillus on page 867*
♦ **Lacto-Pectin [OTC]** *see Lactobacillus on page 867*
♦ **Lacto-TriBlend [OTC]** *see Lactobacillus on page 867*

Lactulose (LAK tyoo lose)

Related Information
Treatment Options for Constipation *on page 1785*

Medication Safety Issues
Sound-alike/look-alike issues:
Lactulose may be confused with lactose

U.S. Brand Names Constulose; Enulose; Generlac; Kristalose®

Canadian Brand Names Acilac; Apo-Lactulose®; Laxilose; PMS-Lactulose

Generic Available Yes

Pharmacologic Category Ammonium Detoxicant; Laxative, Osmotic

Use Adjunct in the prevention and treatment of portal-systemic encephalopathy; treatment of chronic constipation

Contraindications Hypersensitivity to lactulose or any component of the formulation; galactosemia (or patients requiring a low galactose diet)

Warnings/Precautions Use with caution in patients with diabetes mellitus; solution contains galactose and lactose; monitor periodically for electrolyte imbalance when lactulose is used >6 months or in patients predisposed to electrolyte abnormalities (eg, elderly); patients receiving lactulose and an oral anti-infective agent should be monitored for possible inadequate response to lactulose

Adverse Reactions (Reflective of adult population; not specific for elderly)
Frequency not defined: Gastrointestinal: Flatulence, diarrhea (excessive dose), abdominal discomfort, nausea, vomiting, cramping

Overdosage/Toxicology Symptoms include diarrhea, abdominal pain, hypochloremic alkalosis, dehydration, hypotension, and hypokalemia. Treatment is supportive.

Drug Interactions Decreased effect: Oral neomycin, laxatives, antacids

Stability Keep solution at room temperature to reduce viscosity. Discard solution if cloudy or very dark.

Mechanism of Action The bacterial degradation of lactulose resulting in an acidic pH inhibits the diffusion of NH_3 into the blood by causing the conversion of NH_3 to NH_4+; also enhances the diffusion of NH_3 from the blood into the gut where conversion to

(Continued)

Lactulose *(Continued)*

NH_4+ occurs; produces an osmotic effect in the colon with resultant distention promoting peristalsis

Pharmacokinetics

Absorption: Oral: Not absorbed appreciably, this is desirable since the intended site of action is within the colon; requires colonic flora for primary drug activation

Metabolism: By colonic flora to lactic acid and acetic acid

Elimination: Primarily in feces and urine (~3%)

Dosage

Geriatrics & Adults:

Note: Diarrhea may indicate overdosage and responds to dose reduction.

Acute portal-systemic encephalopathy (PSE):

Oral: 20-30 g (30-45 mL) every 1-2 hours to induce rapid laxation; adjust dosage daily to produce 2-3 soft stools; doses of 30-45 mL may be given hourly to cause rapid laxation, then reduce to recommended dose; usual daily dose: 60-100 g (90-150 mL) daily

Rectal: 200 g (300 mL) diluted with 700 mL of H_2O or NS; administer rectally via rectal balloon catheter and retain 30-60 minutes every 4-6 hours.

Constipation: Oral: 10-20 g/day (15-30 mL/day) increased to 60 mL/day in 1-2 divided doses if necessary

Administration Dilute lactulose in water, usually 60-120 mL, prior to administering through a gastric or feeding tube.

Monitoring Parameters Monitor for number of stools per day, dehydration, hypotension; measure serum electrolytes with long-term use; monitor serum ammonia concentrations when treating hepatic encephalopathy

Patient Information Lactulose can be taken "as is" or diluted with water, fruit juice or milk, or taken in a food; laxative results may not occur for 24-48 hours; take with a full glass of water

Additional Information Diarrhea indicates overdosage and responds to dose reduction

Special Geriatric Considerations Elderly are more likely to show CNS signs of dehydration and electrolyte loss than younger adults. Therefore, monitor closely for fluid and electrolyte loss with chronic use. Sorbitol is equally effective as a laxative and less expensive. However, sorbitol **cannot be substituted** in the treatment of hepatic encephalopathy.

Dosage Forms Excipient information presented when available (limited, particularly for generics); consult specific product labeling.

Crystals for solution, oral:

Kristalose®: 10 g/packet (30s), 20 g/packet (30s)

Syrup: 10 g/15 mL (15 mL, 30 mL, 237 mL, 473 mL, 946 mL, 1890 mL)

Constulose: 10 g/15 mL (240 mL, 960 mL)

Enulose: 10 g/15 mL (480 mL)

Generlac: 10 g/15 mL (480 mL, 1920 mL)

Selected References

Lederle FA, Busch DL, Mattox KM, et al, "Cost-Effective Treatment of Constipation in the Elderly: A Randomized Double-Blind Comparison of Sorbitol and Lactulose," *Am J Med*, 1990, 89(5):597-601.

♦ **Lamictal®** *see* Lamotrigine *on page 870*
♦ **Lamisil®** *see* Terbinafine *on page 1531*
♦ **Lamisil® AT™ [OTC]** *see* Terbinafine *on page 1531*

Lamotrigine *(la MOE tri jeen)*

Medication Safety Issues

Sound-alike/look-alike issues:

Lamotrigine may be confused with labetalol, Lamisil®, lamivudine, Lomotil®, ludiomil

Lamictal® may be confused with Lamisil®, Lomotil®, ludiomil

U.S. Brand Names Lamictal®

Canadian Brand Names Apo-Lamotrigine®; Gen-Lamotrigine; Lamictal®; Novo-Lamotrigine; PMS-Lamotrigine; ratio-Lamotrigine

Index Terms BW-430C; LTG

Generic Available Yes: Chewable tablet

Pharmacologic Category Anticonvulsant, Miscellaneous

Use Adjunctive therapy in the treatment of generalized seizures of Lennox-Gastaut syndrome, primary generalized tonic-clonic seizures, and partial seizures; conversion to monotherapy in adults with partial seizures who are receiving treatment with valproic acid or a single enzyme-inducing antiepileptic drug (specifically carbamazepine, phenytoin, phenobarbital or primidone); maintenance treatment of bipolar I disorder

Contraindications Hypersensitivity to lamotrigine or any component of the formulation

Warnings/Precautions [U.S. Boxed Warning]: Severe and potentially life-threatening skin rashes requiring hospitalization have been reported; risk may be increased by coadministration with valproic acid, higher than recommended starting doses, and rapid dose titration. The majority of cases occur in the first 8 weeks; however, isolated cases may occur after prolonged treatment. Discontinue at first sign of rash unless rash is clearly not drug related. Acute multiorgan failure has also been reported. A spectrum of hematologic effects have been reported with use (eg, neutropenia, leukopenia, thrombocytopenia, pancytopenia, and anemias); patients with a previous history of adverse hematologic reaction to any drug may be at increased risk. Early detection of hematologic change is important; advise patients of early signs and symptoms including fever, sore throat, mouth ulcers, infections, easy bruising, petechial or purpuric hemorrhage. May be associated with hypersensitivity syndrome. Use caution in patients with impaired renal, hepatic, or cardiac function. Avoid abrupt cessation, taper over at least 2 weeks if possible. May cause CNS depression, which may impair physical or mental abilities. Patients must be cautioned about performing tasks which require mental alertness (eg, operating machinery or driving). Effects with other sedative drugs or ethanol may be potentiated. Binds to melanin and may accumulate in the eye and other melanin-rich tissues; the clinical significance of this is not known. Safety and efficacy have not been established for use as initial monotherapy, conversion to monotherapy from antiepileptic drugs (AED) other than carbamazepine, phenytoin, phenobarbital, primidone or valproic acid or conversion to monotherapy from two or more AEDs. Patients treated for bipolar disorder should be monitored closely for clinical worsening or suicidality; prescriptions should be written for the smallest quantity consistent with good patient care. Hormonal contraceptives may cause a decrease in lamotrigine levels requiring dose adjustment.

Adverse Reactions (Reflective of adult population; not specific for elderly)
Percentages reported in adults on monotherapy for epilepsy or bipolar disorder.

>10%: Gastrointestinal: Nausea (7% to 14%)

1% to 10%:

Cardiovascular: Chest pain (5%), peripheral edema (2% to 5%), edema (1% to 5%)

Central nervous system: Somnolence (9%), fatigue (8%), dizziness (7%), anxiety (5%), insomnia (5% to 10%), pain (5%), ataxia (2% to 5%), irritability (2% to 5%), suicidal ideation (2% to 5%), agitation (1% to 5%), amnesia (1% to 5%), depression (1% to 5%), dream abnormality (1% to 5%), emotional lability (1% to 5%), fever (1% to 5%), hypoesthesia (1% to 5%), migraine (1% to 5%), thought abnormality (1% to 5%), confusion (1%)

Dermatologic: Rash (nonserious: 7%), dermatitis (2% to 5%), dry skin (2% to 5%)

Endocrine & metabolic: Dysmenorrhea (5%), libido increased (2% to 5%)

Gastrointestinal: Vomiting (5% to 9%), dyspepsia (7%), abdominal pain (6%), xerostomia (2% to 6%), constipation (5%), weight loss (5%), anorexia (2% to 5%), peptic ulcer (2% to 5%), rectal hemorrhage (2% to 5%), flatulence (1% to 5%), weight gain (1% to 5%)

Genitourinary: Urinary frequency (1% to 5%)

Neuromuscular & skeletal: Back pain (8%), coordination abnormal (7%), weakness (2% to 5%), arthralgia (1% to 5%), myalgia (1% to 5%), neck pain (1% to 5%), paresthesia (1%)

Ocular: Nystagmus (2% to 5%), vision abnormal (2% to 5%), amblyopia (1%)

Respiratory: Rhinitis (7%), cough (5%), pharyngitis (5%), bronchitis (2% to 5%), dyspnea (2% to 5%), epistaxis (2% to 5%), sinusitis (1% to 5%)

Miscellaneous: Infection (5%), diaphoresis (2% to 5%), reflexes increased/decreased (2% to 5%), dyspraxia (1% to 5%)

Overdosage/Toxicology Most common symptoms reported following lamotrigine overdose include ataxia, drowsiness, lethargy, nausea and vomiting. Coma, respiratory depression, and seizures have also been reported. Symptoms such as hypokalemia, hypertonia, motor weakness, nystagmus, QRS prolongation, tremor, and xerostomia have been noted in case reports. Treatment should be symptom directed and supportive and may include activated charcoal. Effectiveness of hemodialysis is uncertain; ~20% removed during 4-hour dialysis session.

Drug Interactions

Carbamazepine: Lamotrigine may increase the epoxide metabolite of carbamazepine resulting in toxicity. Carbamazepine may decrease plasma levels of lamotrigine. Dosage adjustments may be needed when adding or withdrawing agents; monitor.

CNS depressants: Lamotrigine may enhance the adverse/toxic effect of other CNS depressants.

Oral contraceptives (estrogens): Oral contraceptives may decrease the serum concentration of lamotrigine; monitor. Dosage adjustment of lamotrigine may be required when starting/stopping oral contraceptives. Lamotrigine levels may increase (~twofold) during the inactive (pill-free) week of oral combination hormonal contraceptives; dose dependent adverse effects may be observed

Phenytoin: May decrease plasma levels of lamotrigine. Dosage adjustments may be needed when adding or withdrawing agents; monitor.

(Continued)

Lamotrigine *(Continued)*

Phenobarbital (barbiturates, primidone): May increase the metabolism of lamotrigine. Dosage adjustment may be needed when adding or withdrawing agent; monitor.

Rifampin: May reduce serum concentrations and effects of lamotrigine.

Valproic acid: Inhibits the clearance of lamotrigine, dosage adjustment required when adding or withdrawing valproic acid. Inhibition appears maximal at valproic acid 250-500 mg/day. The incidence of serious rash may be increased by valproic acid.

Ethanol/Nutrition/Herb Interactions

Ethanol: Avoid ethanol (may increase CNS depression).

Food: Has no effect on absorption.

Herb/Nutraceutical: Avoid evening primrose (seizure threshold decreased).

Stability Store at 25°C (77°F); excursions are permitted to 15°C to 30°C (59°F to 86°F). Protect from light.

Mechanism of Action A triazine derivative which inhibits release of glutamate (an excitatory amino acid) and inhibits voltage-sensitive sodium channels, which stabilizes neuronal membranes. Lamotrigine has weak inhibitory effect on the 5-HT$_3$ receptor; *in vitro* inhibits dihydrofolate reductase.

Pharmacokinetics

Absorption: Rapid and complete

Distribution: V_d: ~1 L/kg

Protein binding: 55%

Metabolism: Hepatic and renal; metabolized by glucuronic acid conjugation to inactive metabolites

Bioavailability: 98%

Half-life elimination: Adults: 25-33 hours

Concomitant valproic acid therapy: 59-70 hours

Concomitant phenytoin or carbamazepine therapy: 13-14 hours

Chronic renal failure: 43 hours

Hemodialysis: 13 hours during dialysis; 57 hours between dialysis

Hepatic impairment: 26-148 hours

Time to peak, plasma: 1-5 hours

Excretion: Urine (94%, ~90% as glucuronide conjugates and ~10% unchanged); feces (2%)

Dosage

Geriatrics & Adults: Note: Only whole tablets should be used for dosing, round calculated dose down to the nearest whole tablet. Enzyme-inducing regimens specifically refer to those containing carbamazepine, phenytoin, phenobarbital, or primidone. Oral:

Lennox-Gastaut (adjunctive), primary generalized tonic-clonic seizures (adjunctive) or partial seizures (adjunctive): Initial: 25 mg/day for weeks 1 and 2, then increase to 50 mg/day for weeks 3 and 4; maintenance: titrate dose to effect; after week 4 increase daily dose every 1-2 weeks by 50 mg/day; usual maintenance: 225-375 mg/day in 2 divided doses.

Adjustment for AED regimens **containing** valproic acid (see "Note"): Initial: 25 mg every other day for weeks 1 and 2, then increase to 25 mg every day for weeks 3 and 4. Maintenance: Titrate dose to effect; after week 4 increase daily dose every 1-2 weeks by 25-50 mg/day; usual maintenance: 100-400 mg/day in 1 or 2 divided doses.

Note: For patients taking lamotrigine with valproic acid alone, the usual maintenance dose is 100-200 mg/day.

Adjustment for **enzyme-inducing** AED regimens **without** valproic acid: Initial: 50 mg/day for weeks 1 and 2, then increase to 100 mg/day in 2 divided doses for weeks 3 and 4. Maintenance: Titrate dose to effects; after week 4 increase daily dose every 1-2 weeks by 100 mg/day; usual maintenance: 300-500 mg/day in 2 divided doses. Doses as high as 700 mg/day have been used, though additional benefit has not been established.

Conversion to monotherapy with lamotrigine:

Conversion from adjunctive therapy with valproic acid: Initiate and titrate as per recommendations to a lamotrigine dose of 200 mg/day. Then taper valproic acid dose in decrements of not >500 mg/day at intervals of 1 week (or longer) to a valproic acid dosage of 500 mg/day; this dosage should be maintained for 1 week. The lamotrigine dosage should then be increased to 300 mg/day while valproic acid is decreased to 250 mg/day; this dosage should be maintained for 1 week. Valproic acid may then be discontinued, while the lamotrigine dose is increased by 100 mg/day at weekly intervals to achieve a lamotrigine maintenance dose of 500 mg/day.

Conversion from adjunctive therapy with carbamazepine, phenytoin, phenobarbital, or primidone: Initiate and titrate as per recommendations to a lamotrigine dose of 500 mg/day. Concomitant enzyme-inducing AED should then be withdrawn by 20% decrements each week over a 4-week period. Patients should be monitored for rash.

Conversion from adjunctive therapy with AED other than carbamazepine, phenytoin, phenobarbital, primidone or valproic acid: No specific guidelines available.

Bipolar disorder: Initial: 25 mg/day for weeks 1 and 2, then increase to 50 mg/day for weeks 3 and 4, then increase to 100 mg/day for week 5; Maintenance: Increase dose to 200 mg/day beginning week 6.

Adjustment for regimens **containing** valproic acid: Initial: 25 mg every other day for weeks 1 and 2, then increase to 25 mg every day for weeks 3 and 4, then increase to 50 mg/day for week 5. Maintenance: 100 mg/day beginning week 6.

Adjustment for **enzyme-inducing** regimens **without** valproic acid: Initial: 50 mg/day for weeks 1 and 2, then increase to 100 mg/day in divided doses for weeks 3 and 4, then increase to 200 mg/day in divided doses for week 5, then increase to 300 mg/day in divided dose for week 6. Maintenance: 400 mg/day in divided doses beginning week 7.

Adjustment following discontinuation of psychotropic medication:

Discontinuing valproic acid with current dose of lamotrigine 100 mg/day: 150 mg/day for week 1, then increase to 200 mg/day beginning week 2.

Discontinuing carbamazepine, phenytoin, phenobarbital, primidone, or rifampin with current dose of lamotrigine 400 mg/day: 400 mg/day for week 1, then decrease to 300 mg/day for week 2, then decrease to 200 mg/day beginning week 3.

Discontinuing therapy: Decrease dose by ~50% per week, over at least 2 weeks unless safety concerns require a more rapid withdrawal. Discontinuing carbamazepine, phenytoin, phenobarbital, or primidone should prolong the half-life of lamotrigine; discontinuing valproic acid should shorten the half-life of lamotrigine

Restarting therapy after discontinuation: If lamotrigine has been withheld for >5 half-lives, consider restarting according to initial dosing recommendations.

Dosage adjustment with combination hormonal contraceptives: Follow initial dosing guidelines, maintenance dose should be adjusted as follows: Patients taking carbamazepine, phenytoin, phenobarbital, primidone or rifampin: No dosing adjustment required

Patients **not** taking carbamazepine, phenytoin, phenobarbital, primidone or rifampin: Maintenance dose may need increased by twofold over target dose. If already taking a stable dose of lamotrigine and starting contraceptive, maintenance dose may need increased by twofold. Dose increases should start when contraceptive is started and titrated to clinical response increasing no more rapidly than 50-100 mg/day every week. Gradual increases of lamotrigine plasma levels may occur during the inactive "pill-free" week and will be greater when dose increases are made the week before. If increased adverse events consistently occur during "pill-free" week, overall dose adjustments may be required. When discontinuing combination hormonal contraceptive, dose of lamotrigine may need decreased by as much as 50%; do not decrease by more than 25% of total daily dose over a 2-week period unless clinical response or plasma levels indicate otherwise. Dose adjustments during "pill-free" week are not recommended.

Renal Impairment: Decreased dosage may be effective in patients with significant renal impairment; use with caution.

Hepatic Impairment:

Moderate-to-severe impairment without ascites: Decrease initial, escalation, and maintenance doses by ~25%

Moderate-to-severe impairment with ascites: Decrease initial, escalation, and maintenance doses by ~50%

Administration Doses should be rounded down to the nearest whole tablet. Dispersible tablets may be chewed, dispersed in water or diluted fruit juice, or swallowed whole. To disperse tablets, add to a small amount of liquid (just enough to cover tablet); let sit ~1 minute until dispersed; swirl solution and consume immediately. Do not administer partial amounts of liquid. If tablets are chewed, a small amount of water or diluted fruit juice should be used to aid in swallowing.

Monitoring Parameters Monitor for therapeutic response and for adverse reactions; no established therapeutic serum concentrations

Reference Range A therapeutic serum concentration range has not been established for lamotrigine. Dosing should be based on therapeutic response. Lamotrigine plasma concentrations of 0.25-29.1 mcg/mL have been reported in the literature.

Patient Information Take exactly as directed; do not increase dose or frequency or discontinue without consulting prescriber. Only whole tablets should be used for dosing, rounded down to the nearest whole tablet. When having the prescription refilled, contact the prescriber if the medicine looks different or the label name has changed. While using this medication, do not use alcohol and other prescription or OTC medications (especially pain medications, sedatives, antihistamines, or hypnotics) without consulting prescriber. Maintain adequate hydration (2-3 L/day of (Continued)

Lamotrigine *(Continued)*

fluids) unless advised by prescriber to restrict fluids. You may experience drowsiness, dizziness, or blurred vision (use caution when driving or engaging in tasks requiring alertness until response to drug is known); or nausea, vomiting, loss of appetite, heartburn, or dry mouth (small, frequent meals, frequent mouth care, chewing gum, or sucking lozenges may help). Wear identification of epileptic status and medications. Report CNS changes, mentation changes, or changes in cognition; persistent GI symptoms (cramping, constipation, vomiting, anorexia); skin rash; swelling of face, lips, or tongue; easy bruising or bleeding (mouth, urine, stool); vision changes; worsening of seizure activity, or loss of seizure control.

Special Geriatric Considerations No pharmacokinetic differences noted between young adults and the elderly. Use with caution in the elderly with significant renal decline.

Dosage Forms Excipient information presented when available (limited, particularly for generics); consult specific product labeling.

Tablet:
   Lamictal®: 25 mg, 100 mg, 150 mg, 200 mg
Tablet, combination package [each unit-dose starter kit contains]:
   Lamictal® (blue kit; for patients taking valproic acid):
      Tablet: Lamotrigine 25 mg (35s)
   Lamictal® (green kit; for patients taking carbamazepine, phenytoin, phenobarbital, primidone, or rifampin and **not** taking valproic acid):
      Tablet: Lamotrigine 25 mg (84s)
      Tablet: Lamotrigine 100 mg (14s)
   Lamictal® (orange kit; for patients **not** taking carbamazepine, phenytoin, phenobarbital, primidone, or valproic acid):
      Tablet: Lamotrigine 25 mg (42s)
      Tablet: Lamotrigine 100 mg (7s)
Tablet, dispersible/chewable: 5 mg, 25 mg
   Lamictal®: 2 mg, 5 mg, 25 mg [black currant flavor]

Extemporaneously Prepared A 1 mg/mL oral suspension may be compounded as follows: Crush one 100 mg tablet and reduce to a fine powder. Add small amount of Ora-Sweet® or Ora-Plus® and mix to uniform paste. Transfer to graduate and qs to 100 mL. Shake well before using and refrigerate. Suspension is stable for 91 days.

   Nahata M, Morosco R, Hipple T. "Stability of Lamotrigine in Two Extemporaneously Prepared Oral Suspensions at 4 and 25°C," *Am J Health Syst Pharm*, 1999, 56:240-2.

Selected References

Battino D, Estienne M, and Avanzini G, "Clinical Pharmacokinetics of Antiepileptic Drugs in Paediatric Patients: Part II. Phenytoin, Carbamazepine, Sulthiame, Lamotrigine, Vigabatrin, Oxcarbazepine, and Felbamate," *Clin Pharmacokinet*, 1995, 29(5):341-69.

Brodie MJ, "Lamotrigine," *Lancet*, 1992, 339(8806):1397-400.

Burstein AH, "Lamotrigine," *Pharmacotherapy*, 1995, 15(2):129-43.

Calabrese JR, Suppes T, Bowden CL, et al, "Double-Blind, Placebo-Controlled, Prophylaxis Study of Lamotrigine in Rapid-Cycling Bipolar Disorder," *J Clin Psychiatry*, 2000, 61:841-50.

de Haan GJ, Edelbroek P, Segers J, et al, "Gestation-Induced Changes in Lamotrigine Pharmacokinetics: A monotherapy Study," *Neurology*, 2004, 63(3):571-3.

Fitton A, and Goa KL, "Lamotrigine: An Update of its Pharmacology and Therapeutic Use in Epilepsy," *Drugs*, 1995, 50(4):691-713.

Garnett WR and Pellock JM, "Focus on Lamotrigine: A New Antiepileptic Drug for Patients With Partial Seizures," *Hosp Formul*, 1994, 29:806-12.

Gilman JT, "Lamotrigine: An Antiepileptic Agent for the Treatment of Partial Seizures," *Ann Pharmacother*, 1995, 29(2):144-51.

Goa KL, Ross SR, and Chrisp P, "Lamotrigine: A Review of Its Pharmacological Properties and Clinical Efficacy in Epilepsy," *Drugs*, 1993, 46(1):152-76.

Harchelroad F, Lang D, and Valeriano J, "Lamotrigine Overdose," *Vet Hum Toxicol*, 1994, 36:372.

Lofton AL and Klein-Schwartz W, "Evaluation of Lamotrigine Toxicity Reported to Poison Control Centers," *Ann Pharmacother*, 2004, 38(11):1811-5

Messenheimer JA, "Lamotrigine," *Epilepsia*, 1995, 36(Suppl 2):S87-94.

Myllynen PK, Pienimaki PK, and Vahakangas KH, "Transplacental Passage of Lamotrigine in a Human Placental Perfusion System *in vitro* and in Maternal and Cord Blood *in vivo*," *Eur J Clin Pharmacol*, 2003, 58(10):677-82.

Schirop Th, Lufft H, Winkler M, et al, "Bronchial Mucosa Reaction in Lyell-Stevens-Johnson Syndrome Following Lamotrigine," *Intensivmedizin und Notfallmedizin*, 1994, 31:343.

♦ **Lanoxicaps®** *see* Digoxin *on page 434*
♦ **Lanoxin®** *see* Digoxin *on page 434*

Lansoprazole *(lan SOE pra zole)*

Related Information
   Helicobacter pylori Treatment *on page 1759*
Medication Safety Issues
   Sound-alike/look-alike issues:
      Prevacid® may be confused with Pravachol®, Prevpac®, Prilosec®, Prinivil®

U.S. Brand Names Prevacid®; Prevacid® SoluTab™
Canadian Brand Names Prevacid®
Generic Available No
Pharmacologic Category Proton Pump Inhibitor; Substituted Benzimidazole
Use

Oral: Short-term treatment of active duodenal ulcers; maintenance treatment of healed duodenal ulcers; as part of a multidrug regimen for *H. pylori* eradication to reduce the risk of duodenal ulcer recurrence; short-term treatment of active benign gastric ulcer; treatment of NSAID-associated gastric ulcer; to reduce the risk of NSAID-associated gastric ulcer in patients with a history of gastric ulcer who require an NSAID; short-term treatment of symptomatic GERD; short-term treatment for all grades of erosive esophagitis; to maintain healing of erosive esophagitis; long-term treatment of pathological hypersecretory conditions, including Zollinger-Ellison syndrome

I.V.: Short-term treatment (≤7 days) of erosive esophagitis in adults unable to take oral medications

Contraindications Hypersensitivity to lansoprazole, substituted benzimidazoles (ie, esomeprazole, omeprazole, pantoprazole, rabeprazole), or any component of the formulation

Warnings/Precautions Relief of symptoms does not preclude the presence of a gastric malignancy. Atrophic gastritis (by biopsy) has been noted with long-term omeprazole therapy; this may also occur with lansoprazole. No reports of enterochromaffin-like (ECL) cell carcinoids, dysplasia, or neoplasia have occurred. Severe liver dysfunction may require dosage reductions.

Adverse Reactions (Reflective of adult population; not specific for elderly)
1% to 10%:

Central nervous system: Headache (children 1-11 years 3%, 12-17 years 7%)

Gastrointestinal: Abdominal pain (children 12-17 years 5%; adults 2%), constipation (children 1-11 years 5%; adults 1%), diarrhea (60 mg/day 7%), nausea (children 12-17 years 3%; adults 1%)

Local: Injection site reaction (1%)

Overdosage/Toxicology No toxicity has been observed in animal studies. There is limited human overdose experience. Treatment is symptomatic and supportive. Lansoprazole is not removed by hemodialysis.

Drug Interactions Substrate of CYP2C9 (minor), 2C19 (major), 3A4 (major); **Inhibits** CYP2C9 (weak), 2C19 (moderate), 2D6 (weak), 3A4 (weak); **Induces** CYP1A2 (weak)

Antifungal agents (imidazoles): Proton pump inhibitors may decrease the absorption of itraconazole and ketoconazole.

CYP2C19 inducers: May decrease the levels/effects of lansoprazole. Example inducers include aminoglutethimide, carbamazepine, fosphenytoin, phenytoin, and rifampin.

CYP2C19 substrates: Lansoprazole may increase the levels/effects of CYP2C19 substrates. Example substrates include citalopram, diazepam, methsuximide, phenytoin, propranolol, and sertraline.

CYP3A4 inducers: CYP3A4 inducers may decrease the levels/effects of lansoprazole. Example inducers include aminoglutethimide, carbamazepine, nafcillin, nevirapine, phenobarbital, phenytoin, and rifamycins.

HMG-CoA reductase inhibitors: Proton pump inhibitors may increase the serum concentration of HMG-CoA reductase inhibitors.

Imatinib: Lansoprazole may worsen the dermatologic adverse effect of imatinib.

Iron salts (oral): Lansoprazole may decrease the absorption of oral iron salts.

Methotrexate: Proton pump inhibitors may decrease the excretion of methotrexate. Antirheumatic doses of methotrexate probably hold minimal risk.

Protease inhibitors: Proton pump inhibitors may decrease absorption of some protease inhibitors (atazanavir and indinavir). The manufacturer of atazanavir recommends avoiding concurrent use with a proton pump inhibitor.

Ethanol/Nutrition/Herb Interactions

Ethanol: Avoid ethanol (may cause gastric mucosal irritation).

Food: Lansoprazole serum concentrations may be decreased if taken with food.

Herb/Nutraceutical: Avoid St John's wort (may decrease the levels/effect of lansoprazole).

Stability Store at 15°C to 30°C (59°F to 86°F). Protect from light and moisture.

Oral suspension: Empty packet into container with 2 tablespoons of water. Do **not** mix with other liquids or food. Stir well and drink immediately.

Powder for injection: Reconstitute with sterile water 5 mL; mix gently until dissolved. Prior to administration, further dilute with 50 mL of NS, LR, or D_5W. After reconstitution, the solution may be stored for up to 1 hour at room temperature prior to final dilution. Following final dilution, solutions mixed with NS or LR are stable at room temperature for 24 hours; solutions mixed with D_5W are stable for 8-12 hours.

Mechanism of Action Decreases acid secretion in gastric parietal cells through inhibition of (H+, K+)-ATPase enzyme system, blocking the final step in gastric acid production.

(Continued)

Lansoprazole *(Continued)*

Pharmacodynamics Duration: >24 hours

Pharmacokinetics The clearance of lansoprazole is decreased in older adults, however, the half-life is only increased by 50% to 100%. This still results in a short half-life and no accumulation is seen in older adults.

Absorption: Rapid

Distribution: V_d: 14-18 L

Protein binding: 97%

Metabolism: Hepatic via CYP2C19 and 3A4, and in parietal cells to two active metabolites that are not present in systemic circulation

Bioavailability: 80% (decreased by 50% if given 30 minutes after food)

Half-life elimination: 1-2 hours; Elderly: 2-3 hours; Hepatic impairment: ≤7 hours

Peak plasma levels: 1.7 hours

Elimination: 33% in urine; 67% in feces

Dosage

Geriatrics & Adults:

Symptomatic GERD: Oral: Short-term treatment: 15 mg once daily for up to 8 weeks

Erosive esophagitis:

Oral: Short-term treatment: 30 mg once daily for up to 8 weeks; continued treatment for an additional 8 weeks may be considered for recurrence or for patients who do not heal after the first 8 weeks of therapy; maintenance therapy: 15 mg once daily

I.V.: 30 mg once daily for up to 7 days; patients should be switched to an oral formulation as soon as they can take oral medications.

Hypersecretory conditions: Oral: Initial: 60 mg once daily; adjust dose based upon patient response and to reduce acid secretion to <10 mEq/hour (5 mEq/hour in patients with prior gastric surgery); doses of 90 mg twice daily have been used; administer doses >120 mg/day in divided doses

Duodenal ulcer: Oral: Short-term treatment: 15 mg once daily for 4 weeks; maintenance therapy: 15 mg once daily

Peptic ulcer disease: Eradication of *Helicobacter pylori:* Currently accepted recommendations (may differ from product labeling): Oral: Dose varies with regimen: 30 mg once daily or 60 mg/day in 2 divided doses; requires combination therapy with antibiotics

Gastric ulcer: Oral: Short-term treatment: 30 mg once daily for up to 8 weeks

NSAID-associated gastric ulcer (healing): Oral: 30 mg once daily for 8 weeks; controlled studies did not extend past 8 weeks

NSAID-associated gastric ulcer (to reduce risk): Oral: 15 mg once daily for up to 12 weeks; controlled studies did not extend past 12 weeks

Prevention of rebleeding in peptic ulcer bleed (unlabeled use): I.V.: 60 mg, followed by 6 mg/hour infusion for 72 hours

Renal Impairment: No adjustment is necessary.

Hepatic Impairment: May require a dose reduction.

Administration

Oral: Administer before food; best if taken before breakfast. The intact granules should not be chewed or crushed; however, in addition to oral suspension, several options are available for those patients unable to swallow capsules:

Capsules may be opened and the intact granules sprinkled on 1 tablespoon of applesauce, Ensure® pudding, cottage cheese, yogurt, or strained pears. The granules should then be swallowed immediately.

Capsules may be opened and emptied into ~60 mL orange juice, apple juice, or tomato juice; mix and swallow immediately. Rinse the glass with additional juice and swallow to assure complete delivery of the dose.

Capsule granules may be mixed with apple, cranberry, grape, orange, pineapple, prune, tomato and V-8® juice and stored for up to 30 minutes.

Delayed release oral suspension granules should be mixed with 2 tablespoonfuls (30 mL) of water; no other liquid should be used. Stir well and drink immediately. Should not be administered through enteral administration tubes.

Orally-disintegrating tablets: Should not be swallowed whole or chewed. Place tablet on tongue; allow to dissolve (with or without water) until particles can be swallowed. Orally-disintegrating tablets may also be administered via an oral syringe: Place the 15 mg tablet in an oral syringe and draw up ~4 mL water, or place the 30 mg tablet in an oral syringe and draw up ~10 mL water. After tablet has dispersed, administer within 15 minutes. Refill the syringe with water (2 mL for the 15 mg tablet; 4 mL for the 30 mg tablet), shake gently, then administer any remaining contents.

I.V.: Administer over 30 minutes. A 1.2 micron in-line filter is required (provided by manufacturer). Before and after administration, flush I.V. line with NS, LR, or D_5W. Do not administer with other medications.

Nasogastric tube administration:

Capsule: Capsule can be opened, the granules mixed (not crushed) with 40 mL of apple juice and then injected through the NG tube into the stomach, then flush tube with additional apple juice.

Orally-disintegrating tablet: Nasogastric tube ≥8 French: Place a 15 mg tablet in a syringe and draw up ~4 mL water, or place the 30 mg tablet in a syringe and draw up ~10 mL water. After tablet has dispersed, administer within 15 minutes. Refill the syringe with ~5 mL water, shake gently, and then flush the nasogastric tube.

Monitoring Parameters Symptoms of peptic ulcer disease, occult blood; use of gastroscopy is preferred

Patient Information Take before eating; capsules should not be crushed or chewed; swallow capsules whole

Special Geriatric Considerations The clearance of lansoprazole is decreased in the elderly; however, the half-life is only increased by 50% to 100%, resulting in a short half-life and no accumulation in the elderly. No dosage adjustment is required with normal hepatic function. The rate of healing and side effects are similar to younger adults.

Dosage Forms Excipient information presented when available (limited, particularly for generics); consult specific product labeling.

Capsule, delayed release:
    Prevacid®: 15 mg, 30 mg
Granules, for oral suspension, delayed release:
    Prevacid®: 15 mg/packet (30s), 30 mg/packet (30s) [strawberry flavor]
Injection, powder for reconstitution:
    Prevacid®: 30 mg [contains mannitol 60 mg]
Tablet, orally disintegrating:
    Prevacid® SoluTab™: 15 mg [contains phenylalanine 2.5 mg; strawberry flavor]; 30 mg [contains phenylalanine 5.1 mg; strawberry flavor]

Selected References

Cockayne SE, Glet RJ, Gawkrodger DJ, et al, "Severe Erythrodermic Reactions to the Proton Pump Inhibitors Omeprazole and Lansoprazole," Br J Dermatol, 1999, 141(1):173-5.

DeVault KR and Castell DO, "Practice Guidelines. Updated Guidelines for the Diagnosis and Treatment of Gastroesophageal Reflux Disease", Am J Gastroenterol, 2005,100(1):190-200.

Natsch S, Vinks MH, Voogt AK, et al, "Anaphylactic Reactions to Proton-Pump Inhibitors," Ann Pharmacother, 2000, 34(4):474-6.

Lanthanum (LAN tha num)

U.S. Brand Names Fosrenol™
Index Terms Lanthanum Carbonate
Generic Available No
Pharmacologic Category Phosphate Binder
Use Reduction of serum phosphate in patients with end-stage renal disease (ESRD)
Contraindications Hypersensitivity to lanthanum or any component of the formulation
Warnings/Precautions Use caution with active peptic ulcer, ulcerative colitis, Crohn's disease, or bowel obstruction. Abdominal x-rays may have a radiopaque appearance.

Adverse Reactions (Reflective of adult population; not specific for elderly)
Reported in short-term (4-6 weeks) trials at frequency > placebo:
>10%:
    Gastrointestinal: Nausea (11%), vomiting (9%), diarrhea (13%), abdominal pain (5%)
    Miscellaneous: Dialysis graft occlusion (8%)
1% to 10%: Endocrine & metabolic: Hypercalcemia was reported in longer-term trials at frequencies ≤4% (less frequently than with alternate therapy)

Note: Additional adverse effects noted in longer-term trials at rates higher than alternate therapy included headache, dialysis graft occlusion, and vomiting.

Drug Interactions Lanthanum may bind to some drugs in the gastrointestinal tract and decrease their absorption. It is recommended that compounds known to interact with antacids, especially those with significant clinical consequences (eg, antiarrhythmic and antiseizure medications), not be administered within 2 hours of the administration of lanthanum.

Stability Store at 15°C to 30°C (59°F to 86°F). Protect from moisture.

Mechanism of Action Disassociates in the upper gastrointestinal tract to lanthanum ions (La^{3+}) which bind to dietary phosphate resulting in insoluble lanthanum phosphate complexes and a net decrease in serum phosphate and calcium levels.

Pharmacokinetics
Absorption: <0.1%
Protein binding: 99%
Metabolism: Not metabolized
Half-life elimination: Plasma: 53 hours; Bone: 2-3.6 years
Excretion: Feces primarily; urine <0.1%
(Continued)

Lanthanum *(Continued)*

Dosage

Geriatrics & Adults: Initial: Oral: 750-1500 mg/day divided and taken with meals; typical increases of 750 mg/day every 2-3 weeks are suggested as needed to bring the serum phosphate level <6 mg/dL. Usual dosage range: 1500-3000 mg; doses of up to 3750 mg have been used.

Administration Administer with or immediately after meals; tablet should be chewed prior to swallowing; do not swallow whole

Monitoring Parameters Calcium and phosphate levels

Test Interactions Abdominal x-rays may have a radiopaque appearance.

Patient Information Inform prescriber of all prescription medications, OTC medications, or herbal products you are taking. Chew tablets prior to swallowing. Maintain adequate hydration (2-3 L/day unless instructed to restrict intake by prescriber). You may experience dizziness or lightheadedness, (use caution when climbing stairs or changing position), headache, nausea, vomiting, diarrhea, abdominal pain, and constipation (increasing exercise, fluids, fruit/fiber may help). Report persistent dizziness, headache, nausea, vomiting, and diarrhea.

Special Geriatric Considerations In initial studies, no overall clinical differences were noted in those >65 years old compared to younger adults.

Dosage Forms Excipient information presented when available (limited, particularly for generics); consult specific product labeling.
Tablet, chewable: 250 mg, 500 mg, 750 mg, 1000 mg

Selected References
Behets GJ, Verberckmoes SC, D'Haese PC, et al, "Lanthanum Carbonate: A New Phosphate Binder," *Curr Opin Nephrol Hypertens*, 2004, 13:403-9.

♦ **Lanthanum Carbonate** *see* Lanthanum *on page 877*

♦ **Lantus®** *see* Insulin Glargine *on page 810*

♦ **Lapase** *see* Pancreatin *on page 1195*

♦ **Lasix®** *see* Furosemide *on page 690*

Latanoprost *(la TA noe prost)*

Related Information
Glaucoma Drug Therapy *on page 1758*
Medication Safety Issues
Sound-alike/look-alike issues:
Xalatan® may be confused with Travatan®, Zarontin®
U.S. Brand Names Xalatan®
Canadian Brand Names Xalatan®
Generic Available No
Pharmacologic Category Ophthalmic Agent, Antiglaucoma; Prostaglandin, Ophthalmic
Use Reduction of elevated intraocular pressure in patients with open-angle glaucoma and ocular hypertension
Contraindications Hypersensitivity to latanoprost or any component of the formulation
Warnings/Precautions May permanently change/increase brown pigmentation of the iris, the eyelid skin, and eyelashes. In addition, may increase the length and/or number of eyelashes (may vary between eyes); changes occur slowly and may not be noticeable for months or years. Long-term consequences and potential injury to eye are not known. Use with caution in patients with intraocular inflammation, aphakic patients, pseudophakic patients with a torn posterior lens capsule, or patients with risk factors for macular edema. Safety and efficacy have not been determined for use in patients with angle-closure-, inflammatory-, or neovascular glaucoma.

There have been reports of bacterial keratitis associated with the use of multiple-dose containers of topical ophthalmic products. Contains benzalkonium chloride which may be adsorbed by contact lenses; remove contacts prior to administration and wait 15 minutes before reinserting. Use with caution in patients with intraocular inflammation, aphakic patients, pseudophakic patients with a torn posterior lens capsule, or patients with risk factors for macular edema. Safety and efficacy have not been determined for use in patients with angle-closure-, inflammatory-, or neovascular glaucoma.

Adverse Reactions (Reflective of adult population; not specific for elderly)
>10%: Ocular: Blurred vision, burning and stinging, conjunctival hyperemia, foreign body sensation, itching, increased pigmentation of the iris, and punctate epithelial keratopathy
1% to 10%:
Cardiovascular: Chest pain, angina pectoris
Dermatologic: Rash, allergic skin reaction
Neuromuscular & skeletal: Myalgia, arthralgia, back pain

Ocular: Dry eye, excessive tearing, eye pain, lid crusting, lid edema, lid erythema, lid discomfort/pain, photophobia

Respiratory: Upper respiratory tract infection, cold, flu

Drug Interactions

May be used concomitantly with other topical ophthalmic drugs if administration is separated by at least 5 minutes.

Bimatoprost: Combination therapy may result in higher IOP than either agent alone.

Thimerosal-containing eye drops: Precipitation occurs when eye drops containing thimerosal are mixed with latanoprost. If such drugs are used, administer with an interval of at least 5 minutes between applications.

Stability Store intact bottles under refrigeration (2°C to 8°C/36°F to 46°F). Protect from light. Once opened, the container may be stored at room temperature up to 25°C (77°F) for 6 weeks.

Mechanism of Action Latanoprost is a prostaglandin F_2-alpha analog believed to reduce intraocular pressure by increasing the outflow of the aqueous humor

Pharmacodynamics

Onset of effect: 3-4 hours

Maximum effect: 8-12 hours

Pharmacokinetics

Absorption: Through the cornea where the isopropyl ester prodrug is hydrolyzed by esterases to the biologically active acid. Peak concentration in the aqueous humor is reached in 2 hours after topical administration.

Distribution: V_d: 0.16 L/kg

Half-life: 17 minutes (prodrug ester)

Metabolism: Primarily metabolized by the liver via fatty acid beta-oxidation

Elimination: After hepatic metabolism, the metabolites are mainly eliminated via the kidneys

Dosage

Geriatrics & Adults: Glaucoma: Ophthalmic: 1 drop (1.5 mcg) in the affected eye(s) once daily in the evening; do not exceed the once daily dosage because it has been shown that more frequent administration may decrease the IOP lowering effect

Note: A medication delivery device (Xal-Ease™) is available for use with Xalatan®.

Administration If more than one topical ophthalmic drug is being used, administer the drugs at least 5 minutes apart

Monitoring Parameters Intraocular pressure, funduscopic exam, visual field testing

Patient Information There is a possibility of iris color change because of an increase of the brown pigment and resultant cosmetically different eye coloration that may occur. Iris pigmentation changes may be more noticeable in patients with green-brown, blue/gray-brown, or yellow-brown irises. Latanoprost contains benzalkonium chloride, which may be absorbed by contact lenses. Remove contact lenses prior to administration of the solution. Lenses may be reinserted 15 minutes following latanoprost administration. Do not touch the tip of the dropper to eye or any other surface. If any ocular reactions occur, such as conjunctivitis or lid reactions, immediately report to eye specialist. If more than one topical ophthalmic drug is being used, administer the drugs at least 5 minutes apart.

Special Geriatric Considerations Evaluate patient's ability to self-administer eye drops

Dosage Forms Excipient information presented when available (limited, particularly for generics); consult specific product labeling.

Solution, ophthalmic: 0.005% (2.5 mL) [contains benzalkonium chloride]

Selected References

Patel SS and Spencer CM, "Latanoprost: A Review of Its Pharmacological Properties, Clinical Efficacy and Tolerability in the Management of Primary Open-Angle Glaucoma and Ocular Hypertension," *Drugs Aging*, 1996, 9(5):363-78.

♦ *l*-Bunolol Hydrochloride *see* Levobunolol *on page 891*

♦ **L-Deoxythymidine** *see* Telbivudine *on page 1522*

♦ **L-Deprenyl** *see* Selegiline *on page 1451*

Leflunomide (le FLOO noh mide)

U.S. Brand Names Arava®

Canadian Brand Names Apo-Leflunomide®; Arava®; Novo-Leflunomide

Generic Available Yes

Pharmacologic Category Antirheumatic, Disease Modifying

Use Treatment of active rheumatoid arthritis to reduce signs and symptoms and to retard structural damage as evidenced by x-ray erosions and joint space narrowing

Contraindications Hypersensitivity to leflunomide or any component of the formulation

Warnings/Precautions Leflunomide has been associated with rare reports of hepatotoxicity, hepatic failure, and death. Multiple risk factors for hepatotoxicity including hepatic disease (including seropositive hepatitis B or C patients) and/or concurrent

(Continued)

Leflunomide *(Continued)*

exposure to other hepatotoxins may increase the risk of hepatotoxicity. Most severe cases occur within 6 months of initiation. Monitoring of hepatic function is required.

Not recommended for patients with severe immune deficiency, bone marrow dysplasia, or uncontrolled infection. Has been associated with rare pancytopenia, agranulocytosis, and thrombocytopenia, particularly when given in combination with methotrexate or other immunosuppressive agents. Monitoring of hematologic function is required. Use with caution in patients with a prior history of significant hematologic abnormalities. Discontinue if evidence of bone marrow suppression or severe dermatologic reaction occurs, and begin procedure to accelerate elimination (cholestyramine or activated charcoal, see Overdosage/Toxicology). Interstitial lung disease has been associated (rarely) with leflunomide use. Discontinue in patients who develop new onset or worsening of pulmonary symptoms; accelerated elimination procedures should be considered if interstitial lung disease occurs; fatal outcomes have been reported. Consider interruption of therapy and accelerated elimination in patients who develop serious infections while receiving leflunomide. The use of live vaccines is not recommended.

Caution in renal impairment. Leflunomide will increase uric acid excretion. Immunosuppression may increase the risk of lymphoproliferative disorders or other malignancies.

Adverse Reactions (Reflective of adult population; not specific for elderly)

>10%:

Gastrointestinal: Diarrhea (17%)

Respiratory: Respiratory tract infection (15%)

1% to 10%:

Cardiovascular: Hypertension (10%), chest pain (2%), palpitation, tachycardia, vasculitis, vasodilation, varicose vein, edema (peripheral)

Central nervous system: Headache (7%), dizziness (4%), pain (2%), fever, malaise, migraine, anxiety, depression, insomnia, sleep disorder

Dermatologic: Alopecia (10%), rash (10%), pruritus (4%), dry skin (2%), eczema (2%), acne, dermatitis, hair discoloration, hematoma, nail disorder, subcutaneous nodule, skin disorder/discoloration, skin ulcer, bruising

Endocrine & metabolic: Hypokalemia (1%), diabetes mellitus, hyperglycemia, hyperlipidemia, hyperthyroidism, menstrual disorder

Gastrointestinal: Nausea (9%), abdominal pain (5%), dyspepsia (5%), weight loss (4%), anorexia (3%), gastroenteritis (3%), stomatitis (3%), vomiting (3%), cholelithiasis, colitis, constipation, esophagitis, flatulence, gastritis, gingivitis, melena, candidiasis (oral), enlarged salivary gland, tooth disorder, xerostomia, taste disturbance

Genitourinary: Urinary tract infection (5%), albuminuria, cystitis, dysuria, hematuria, vaginal candidiasis, prostate disorder, urinary frequency

Hematologic: Anemia

Hepatic: Abnormal LFTs (5%)

Neuromuscular & skeletal: Back pain (5%), joint disorder (4%), weakness (3%), tenosynovitis (3%), synovitis (2%), arthralgia (1%), paresthesia (2%), muscle cramps (1%), neck pain, pelvic pain, increased CPK, arthrosis, bursitis, myalgia, bone necrosis, bone pain, tendon rupture, neuralgia, neuritis

Ocular: Blurred vision, cataract, conjunctivitis, eye disorder

Respiratory: Bronchitis (7%), cough (3%), pharyngitis (3%), pneumonia (2%), rhinitis (2%), sinusitis (2%), asthma, dyspnea, epistaxis

Miscellaneous: Infection (4%), accidental injury (5%), allergic reactions (2%), diaphoresis, herpes infection

Overdosage/Toxicology

There is no human experience with overdose. Leflunomide is not dialyzable. Cholestyramine and/or activated charcoal enhance elimination of leflunomide's active metabolite (M1). In cases of significant overdose or toxicity, cholestyramine 8 g every 8 hours for 1-3 days or activated charcoal 50 g every 6 hours for 24 hours may be administered to enhance elimination. Plasma levels are reduced by ~40% in 24 hours and 49% to 65% after 48 hours of cholestyramine dosing. Activated charcoal reduces plasma levels by 37% after 24 hours and 48% after 48 hours of continuous dosing. Activated charcoal without sorbitol should be used.

Drug Interactions

Inhibits CYP2C9 (weak)

Bile acid sequestrants (cholestyramine): May interfere with enterohepatic recycling of leflunomide. This is used emergently to remove drug from the circulation, but may decrease levels inadvertently if used concomitantly.

Hepatotoxic agents: Leflunomide may increase the risk of hepatotoxicity when combined with drugs which may cause hepatic injury; use caution.

Methotrexate: Concomitant treatment with leflunomide may increase the risk of hepatotoxicity or hematologic toxicity; monitor.

Rifampin: May increase the serum concentration of leflunomide's active metabolite; use caution.

Warfarin: Leflunomide may increase the effects of warfarin; monitor.

Ethanol/Nutrition/Herb Interactions Food: No interactions with food have been noted.

Stability Store at 25°C (77°F). Protect from light.

Mechanism of Action Inhibits pyrimidine synthesis, resulting in antiproliferative and anti-inflammatory effects. For CMV, may interfere with virion assembly.

Pharmacokinetics

Distribution: V_d: 0.13 L/kg

Metabolism: Hepatic, to A77 1726 (MI) which accounts for nearly all pharmacologic activity; further metabolism to multiple inactive metabolites

Bioavailability: 80%

Half-life: Mean 14-15 days; enterohepatic recycling appears to contribute to the long half-life of this agent, since activated charcoal and cholestyramine substantially reduce plasma half-life

Time to peak: 6-12 hours

Elimination: Urine 43%; Feces 48%

Dosage

Geriatrics & Adults:

Rheumatoid arthritis: Oral: Initial: 100 mg/day for 3 days, followed by 20 mg/day; dosage may be decreased to 10 mg/day in patients who have difficulty tolerating the 20 mg dose. Due to the long half-life of the active metabolite, plasma levels may require a prolonged period to decline after dosage reduction.

CMV (unlabeled): Some authors recommend 200 mg daily for 7 days, followed by 40-60 mg/day targeting blood levels of 100 mcg/mL. Others have utilized the standard arthritis dosing.

Renal Impairment: No specific dosage adjustment is recommended. There is no clinical experience in the use of leflunomide in patients with renal impairment. The free fraction of MI is doubled in dialysis patients. Patients should be monitored closely for adverse effects requiring dosage adjustment.

Hepatic Impairment: No specific dosage adjustment is recommended. Since the liver is involved in metabolic activation and subsequent metabolism/elimination of leflunomide, patients with hepatic impairment should be monitored closely for adverse effects requiring dosage adjustment.

Dosing adjustment in hepatic toxicity: Guidelines for dosage adjustment or discontinuation based on the severity and persistence of ALT elevation secondary to leflunomide have been developed. If ALT elevations >2 times but ≤3 times ULN are noted, reduce dose to 10 mg/day, and monitor closely. If elevations persist or if elevations >3 times ULN are observed, discontinue leflunomide and initiate protocol to accelerate elimination. Cholestyramine (8 g 3 times/day for 1-3 days) or activated charcoal (50 g every 6 hours for 24 hours) may be administered to decrease leflunomide concentrations rapidly. If elevations >3 times ULN persist additional cholestyramine and/or activated charcoal may be required.

Monitoring Parameters A complete blood count (WBC, hemoglobin, hematocrit, and platelet count), serum phosphate, as well as serum transaminase determinations should be monitored at baseline and monthly during the initial 6 months of treatment; if stable, monitoring frequency may be decreased to every 6-8 weeks thereafter (continue monthly when used in combination with other immunosuppressive agents). In addition, monitor for signs/symptoms of severe infection, abnormalities in hepatic function tests, or symptoms of hepatotoxicity. If coadministered with methotrexate, monthly transaminase and serum albumin levels are recommended.

Patient Information Take as directed; do not increase dose without consulting prescriber. Maintain adequate hydration (2-3 L/day of fluids) unless instructed to restrict fluid intake. Store medication away from light. You may experience diarrhea (buttermilk, boiled milk, or yogurt may help); nausea, vomiting, loss of appetite, and flatulence (small frequent meals, frequent mouth care, chewing gum, or sucking lozenges may help); or dizziness (use caution when driving or engaging in tasks requiring alertness until response to drug is known). If you have diabetes, monitor blood sugars closely; this medication may alter glucose levels. If you experience symptoms such as nausea, vomiting, stomach pain or swelling, jaundice, dark urine, or unusual tiredness, report these to your prescriber **immediately**. Report chest pain, palpitations, rapid heartbeat, or swelling of extremities; persistent GI problems; skin rash, mucous membrane lesions, redness, irritation, acne, ulcers; frequent, painful, or difficult urination, or genital itching or irritation; depression, acute headache, anxiety, or difficulty sleeping; muscle tremors, cramping or weakness, back pain, or altered gait; cough, cold symptoms, wheezing, or respiratory difficulty; easy bruising/bleeding; blood in vomitus, stool, urine; or other unusual effects related to this medication.

Special Geriatric Considerations No dosage reduction necessary based on age alone; monitor in renal and hepatic impairment.

Dosage Forms Excipient information presented when available (limited, particularly for generics); consult specific product labeling.

Tablet (Arava®): 10 mg, 20 mg

(Continued)

Leflunomide *(Continued)*

Selected References

Fox RI, "Mechanism of Action of Leflunomide in Rheumatoid Arthritis," *J Rheumatol*, 1998, 53:20-6.

"New Drugs for Rheumatoid Arthritis," *Med Lett Drugs Ther*, 1998, 40(1040):110-2.

Popovic M, Stefanovic D, Pejnovic N, et al, "Comparative Study of the Clinical Efficacy of Four DMARDs (Leflunomide, Methotrexate, Cyclosporine, and Levamisole) in Patients With Rheumatoid Arthritis," *Transplant Proc*, 1998, 30(8):4135-6.

Rozman B, "Clinical Experience With Leflunomide in Rheumatoid Arthritis. Leflunomide Investigators' Group," *J Rheumatol Suppl*, 1998, 53:27-32.

Smolen JS, Kalden JR, Scott DL, et al, "Efficacy and Safety of Leflunomide Compared With Placebo and Sulfasalazine in Active Rheumatoid Arthritis: A Double-Blind, Ramdomised, Multicentre Trial. European Leflunomide Study Group," *Lancet*, 1999, 353(9149):259-66.

♦ **Lescol®** *see* Fluvastatin *on page 667*

♦ **Lescol® XL** *see* Fluvastatin *on page 667*

Letrozole (LET roe zole)

Medication Safety Issues

Sound-alike/look-alike issues:

Femara® may be confused with femhrt®

U.S. Brand Names Femara®

Canadian Brand Names Femara®

Index Terms CGS-20267; NSC-719345

Generic Available No

Pharmacologic Category Antineoplastic Agent, Aromatase Inhibitor

Use Adjuvant treatment of postmenopausal hormone receptor positive early breast cancer; treatment of postmenopausal hormone receptor positive or hormone receptor unknown, locally-advanced, or metastatic breast cancer

Contraindications Hypersensitivity to letrozole or any component of the formulation; women of premenopausal endocrine status

Warnings/Precautions Hazardous agent - use appropriate precautions for handling and disposal. Use caution with hepatic impairment; dose adjustment may be required. Increases in transaminases ≥5 times the upper limit of normal and in bilirubin ≥1.5 times the upper limit of normal were most often, but not always, associated with metastatic liver disease. May cause dizziness, fatigue, and somnolence; patients should be cautioned before performing tasks which require mental alertness (eg, operating machinery or driving). May increase total serum cholesterol. May cause decreases in bone mineral density.

Adverse Reactions (Reflective of adult population; not specific for elderly)

>10%:

Cardiovascular: Edema (7% to 18%)

Central nervous system: Headache (4% to 20%), dizziness (2% to 14%), fatigue (6% to 13%)

Endocrine & metabolic: Hot flashes (5% to 50%), hypercholesterolemia (3% to 16%)

Gastrointestinal: Nausea (9% to 17%), constipation (2% to 11%), weight gain (2% to 11%),

Neuromuscular & skeletal: Weakness (4% to 34%), bone pain (22%), arthralgia (8% to 22%), arthritis (7% to 21%), back pain (5% to 18%)

Respiratory: Dyspnea (6% to 18%), cough (5% to 13%)

Miscellaneous: Diaphoresis (<5% to 24%), night sweats (14%)

2% to 10%:

Cardiovascular: Chest pain (3% to 8%), hypertension (5% to 8%), peripheral edema (5%)

Central nervous system: Insomnia (6% to 7%), pain (5%), somnolence (2% to 3%), depression (<5%), anxiety (<5%), vertigo (<5%)

Dermatologic: Rash (4% to 5%), alopecia (<5%), pruritus (1% to 2%)

Endocrine & metabolic: Breast pain (7%), hypercalcemia (<5%)

Gastrointestinal: Diarrhea (5% to 8%), vomiting (3% to 7%), weight loss (7%), abdominal pain (5% to 6%), anorexia (3% to 5%), dyspepsia (3% to 4%)

Genitourinary: Urinary tract infection (6%), vaginal bleeding (5%), vaginal dryness (5%), vaginal hemorrhage (5%), vaginal irritation (4%)

Hepatic: Transaminases increased (<1% to 3%)

Neuromuscular & skeletal: Limb pain (10%), myalgia (6% to 7%), bone fractures (<5% to 6%), bone mineral density decreased/osteoporosis (2% to 7%)

Renal: Renal disorder (5%)

Respiratory: Pleural effusion (<5%)

Miscellaneous: Infection (7%), flu (6%), viral infection (5% to 6%)

Overdosage/Toxicology Firm recommendations for treatment are not possible; emesis could be induced if the patient is alert. In general, treatment is symptom-directed and supportive. Frequent monitoring of vital signs is appropriate.

Drug Interactions Substrate (minor) of CYP2A6, 3A4; **Inhibits** CYP2A6 (strong), 2C19 (weak)

CYP2A6 substrates: Letrozole may increase the levels/effects of CYP2A6 substrates. Example substrates include dexmedetomidine and ifosfamide.

Tamoxifen: May decrease serum concentrations of letrozole.

Stability Store at 15°C to 30°C (59°F to 86°F).

Mechanism of Action Nonsteroidal competitive inhibitor of the aromatase enzyme system which binds to the heme group of aromatase, a cytochrome P450 enzyme which catalyzes conversion of androgens to estrogens (specifically, androstenedione to estrone and testosterone to estradiol). This leads to inhibition of the enzyme and a significant reduction in plasma estrogen levels. Does not affect synthesis of adrenal or thyroid hormones, aldosterone, or androgens.

Pharmacokinetics

Absorption: Rapid and well absorbed; not affected by food

Distribution: V_d: ~1.9 L/kg

Protein binding, plasma: Weakly bound

Metabolism: Hepatic via CYP3A4 and 2A6 to an inactive carbinol metabolite

Half-life: Terminal elimination: ~2 days

Time to steady state plasma concentrations: 2-6 weeks

Elimination: Urine (90%; 6% as unchanged drug, 75% as glucuronide carbinol metabolite, 9% as unidentified metabolites)

Dosage

Geriatrics & Adults: Refer to individual protocols.

Breast cancer: Female: Oral: 2.5 mg once daily

Renal Impairment: No dosage adjustment is required in patients with renal impairment if Cl_{cr} is ≥10 mL/minute.

Hepatic Impairment:

Mild-to-moderate impairment (Child-Pugh class A and B): No adjustment recommended

Severe impairment (Child-Pugh class C): 2.5 mg every other day

Monitoring Parameters Monitor periodically during therapy: Complete blood counts; thyroid function tests; serum electrolytes, cholesterol, transaminases, and creatinine; blood pressure; bone density

Patient Information May experience nausea, vomiting, hot flashes, or loss of appetite; musculoskeletal pain or headache; sleepiness, fatigue, or dizziness (use caution when driving, climbing stairs, or engaging in tasks that require alertness until response to drug is known); constipation; diarrhea; or loss of hair. Report chest pain, pressure, palpitations, or swollen extremities; weakness, severe headache, numbness, or loss of strength in any part of the body; difficulty speaking; vaginal bleeding; unusual signs of bleeding or bruising; difficulty breathing; severe nausea, or muscle pain; or skin rash. For use in postmenopausal women only.

Special Geriatric Considerations No dosage adjustment recommended.

Dosage Forms Excipient information presented when available (limited, particularly for generics); consult specific product labeling.

Tablet: 2.5 mg

Femara®: 2.5 mg

Selected References

Coates AS, Keshaviah A, Thurlimann B, et al, "Five Years of Letrozole Compared With Tamoxifen as Initial Adjuvant Therapy for Postmenopausal Women With Endocrine-Responsive Early Breast Cancer: Update of Study BIG 1-98," *J Clin Oncol*, 2007, 25(5):486-92.

Smith IE and Dowsett M, "Aromatase Inhibitors in Breast Cancer," *N Engl J Med*, 2003, 348(24):2431-42.

Winer EP, Hudis C, Burstein HJ, et al, "American Society of Clinical Oncology Technology Assessment on the Use of Aromatase Inhibitors as Adjuvant Therapy for Postmenopausal Women With Hormone Receptor-Positive Breast Cancer: Status Report 2004," *J Clin Oncol*, 2005, 23(3):619-29.

♦ **Leukeran**® *see* Chlorambucil *on page 287*

Leuprolide (loo PROE lide)

Medication Safety Issues

Sound-alike/look-alike issues:

Lupron® may be confused with Nuprin®

Lupron Depot®-3 Month may be confused with Lupron Depot-Ped®

U.S. Brand Names Eligard®; Lupron®; Lupron Depot®; Lupron Depot-Ped®; Viadur®

Canadian Brand Names Eligard®; Lupron®; Lupron® Depot®; Viadur®

Index Terms Abbott-43818; Leuprolide Acetate; Leuprorelin Acetate; NSC-377526; TAP-144

Generic Available Yes: Injection (solution)

Pharmacologic Category Antineoplastic Agent, Gonadotropin-Releasing Hormone Agonist; Gonadotropin Releasing Hormone Agonist

(Continued)

Leuprolide *(Continued)*

Use Palliative treatment of advanced prostate carcinoma (alternative when orchiectomy or estrogen administration are not indicated or are unacceptable to the patient); combination therapy with flutamide for treating metastatic prostatic carcinoma; treatment of endometriosis as initial treatment and/or treatment of recurrent symptoms; uterine leiomyomata (fibroids)

Unlabeled/Investigational Use Treatment of prostatic hyperplasia; breast, ovarian, and endometrial cancer

Contraindications Hypersensitivity to leuprolide, GnRH, GnRH-agonist analogs, or any component of the formulation; spinal cord compression (orchiectomy suggested); undiagnosed abnormal vaginal bleeding

Warnings/Precautions Hazardous agent - use appropriate precautions for handling and disposal. Transient increases in testosterone serum levels occur at the start of treatment. Tumor flare, bone pain, neuropathy, urinary tract obstruction, and spinal cord compression have been reported when used for prostate cancer; closely observe patients for weakness, paresthesias, hematuria, and urinary tract obstruction in first few weeks of therapy. Observe patients with metastatic vertebral lesions or urinary obstruction closely. Exacerbation of endometriosis or uterine leiomyomata may occur initially. Decreased bone density has been reported when used for ≥6 months. Use caution in patients with a history of psychiatric illness; alteration in mood, memory impairment, and depression have been associated with use. Rare cases of pituitary apoplexy (frequently secondary to pituitary adenoma) have been observed with leuprolide administration (onset from 1 hour to usually <2 weeks); may present as sudden headache, vomiting, visual or mental status changes, and infrequently cardiovascular collapse; immediate medical attention required.

Adverse Reactions (Reflective of adult population; not specific for elderly)

Note: For prostate cancer treatment, an initial rise in serum testosterone concentrations may cause "tumor flare" or worsening of symptoms, including bone pain, neuropathy, hematuria, or ureteral or bladder outlet obstruction during the first 2 weeks. Similarly, an initial increase in estradiol levels, with a temporary worsening of symptoms, may occur in women treated with leuprolide.

Delayed release formulations:

10%:

Cardiovascular: Edema (≤14%)

Central nervous system: Headache (≤65%), pain (<2% to 33%), depression (≤31%), insomnia (≤31%), fatigue (≤17%), dizziness/vertigo (≤16%)

Dermatologic: Skin reaction (≤12%)

Endocrine & metabolic: Hot flashes (47% to 98%), testicular atrophy (≤20%), hyperlipidemia (≤12%), libido decreased (≤11%)

Gastrointestinal: Nausea/vomiting (≤25%), weight gain/loss (≤13%)

Genitourinary: Vaginitis (11% to 28%), urinary disorder (13% to 15%)

Local: Implant site bruising (35%), injection site reaction (≤16%)

Neuromuscular & skeletal: Joint disorder (≤12%), weakness (≤12%)

Miscellaneous: Flu-like syndrome (≤12%)

1% to 10% (limited to important or life-threatening):

Cardiovascular: Angina (<5%), arrhythmia (<5%), atrial fibrillation (<5%), bradycardia (<5%), CHF (<5%), deep thrombophlebitis (<5%), hyper-/hypotension (<5%), palpitation (<5%), syncope (<5%), tachycardia (<5%)

Central nervous system: Nervousness (≤8%), anxiety (≤6%), confusion (<5%), delusions (<5%), dementia (<5%), fever (<5%), seizure (<5%)

Dermatologic: Acne (≤10%), alopecia (≤5%), bruising (≤5%), cellulitis (<5%), pruritus (≤3%), hirsutism (<2%), rash (<2%)

Endocrine & metabolic: Dehydration (≤8%), gynecomastia (≤7%), breast tenderness/pain (≤6%), bicarbonate decreased (≥5%), hyper-/hypocholesterolemia (≥5%), hyperglycemia (≥5%), hyperphosphatemia (≥5%), hyperuricemia (≥5%), hypoalbuminemia (≥5%), hypoproteinemia (≥5%), lactation (<5%), testicular pain (≤4%), menstrual disorder (≤2%)

Gastrointestinal: Dysphagia (<5%), gastrointestinal hemorrhage (<5%), intestinal obstruction (<5%), ulcer (<5%), gastroenteritis/colitis (≤3%), diarrhea (≤2%), constipation (≤2%)

Genitourinary: Prostatic acid phosphatase increased/decreased (≥5%), urine specific gravity increased/decreased (≥5%), impotence (≤5%), balanitis (<5%), incontinence (<5%), penile/testis disorder (<5%), urinary tract infection (<5%), nocturia (≤4%), urinary frequency (4%), dysuria (<2%), urinary retention (<2%), urinary urgency (<2%)

Hematologic: Eosinophilia (≥5%), leukopenia (≥5%), platelets increased (≥5%), anemia

Hepatic: Liver function tests abnormal (≥5%), partial thromboplastin time increased (≥5%), prothrombin time increased (≥5%), hepatomegaly (<5%)

Local: Implant site reaction (persistent or delayed: 9% to 10%), implant site burning (6%)

Neuromuscular & skeletal: Myalgia (≤8%), paresthesia (≤8%), neuropathy (<5%), paralysis (<5%), pathologic fracture (<5%), bone pain (<2%)

Renal: BUN increased (≥5%), creatinine increased (≥5%)

Respiratory: Emphysema (<5%), epistaxis (<5%), hemoptysis (<5%), pleural effusion (<5%), pulmonary edema (<5%), dyspnea (≤2%)

Miscellaneous: Diaphoresis (≤5%), allergic reaction (<5%), infection (5%), lymphadenopathy (<5%)

Immediate release formulation:

>10%:

Cardiovascular: ECG changes/ischemia (19%), peripheral edema (12%)

Central nervous system: Pain (13%)

Endocrine & metabolic: Hot flashes (55%)

1% to 10% (limited to important or life-threatening):

Cardiovascular: Hypertension (8%), murmur (3%), thrombosis/phlebitis (2%), CHF (1%), angina, arrhythmia, MI, syncope

Central nervous system: Headache (7%), insomnia (7%), dizziness/lightheadedness (5%), anxiety, depression, fatigue, fever, nervousness

Dermatologic: Dermatitis (5%), alopecia, bruising, itching, lesions, pigmentation

Endocrine & metabolic: Gynecomastia/breast tenderness/pain (7%), testicular size decreased (7%), diabetes, hypercalcemia, hypoglycemia, libido decreased, thyroid enlarged

Gastrointestinal: Constipation (7%), anorexia (6%), nausea/vomiting (5%), diarrhea, dysphagia, gastrointestinal bleeding, peptic ulcer, rectal polyps

Genitourinary: Urinary frequency/urgency (6%), impotence (4%), urinary tract infection (3%), bladder spasm, dysuria, incontinence, testicular pain, urinary obstruction

Hematologic: Anemia (5%)

Local: Injection site reaction

Neuromuscular & skeletal: Weakness (10%), bone pain (5%), peripheral neuropathy

Ocular: Blurred vision

Renal: Hematuria (6%), BUN increased, creatinine increased

Respiratory: Dyspnea (2%), cough, pneumonia, pulmonary embolus, pulmonary fibrosis

Miscellaneous: Infection, inflammation

Overdosage/Toxicology Treatment is symptom-directed and supportive.

Stability

Lupron®: Store unopened vials of injection in refrigerator. Vial in use can be kept at room temperature ≤30°C (86°F) for several months with minimal loss of potency. Protect from light and store vial in carton until use. Do not freeze.

Eligard®: Store at 2°C to 8°C (36°F to 46°C). Allow to reach room temperature prior to using. Once mixed, must be administered within 30 minutes. Eligard® is packaged in two syringes; one contains the Atrigel® polymer system and the second contains leuprolide acetate powder. Follow package instructions for mixing.

Lupron Depot® may be stored at room temperature of 15°C to 30°C (59°F to 86°F). Upon reconstitution, the suspension does not contain a preservative and should be used immediately. Reconstitute only with diluent provided.

Viadur® may be stored at room temperature of 15°C to 30°C (59°F and 86°F).

Mechanism of Action Leuprolide, is an agonist of luteinizing hormone-releasing hormone (LHRH). Acting as a potent inhibitor of gonadotropin secretion; continuous daily administration results in suppression of ovarian and testicular steroidogenesis due to decreased levels of LH and FSH with subsequent decrease in testosterone (male) and estrogen (female) levels. Leuprolide may also have a direct inhibitory effect on the testes, and act by a different mechanism not directly related to reduction in serum testosterone.

Pharmacodynamics Onset of action: Following transient increase, testosterone suppression occurs in ~2-4 weeks of continued therapy

Pharmacokinetics Serum testosterone concentrations first increase within 3 days of therapy, then decrease after 2-4 weeks with continued therapy; requires parenteral administration since it is rapidly destroyed within the GI tract

Distribution: Males: V_d: 27 L

Protein binding: 43% to 49%

Metabolism: Major metabolite, pentapeptide (M-1)

Bioavailability: Not bioavailable if given orally; bioavailability of SubQ and I.V. doses is comparable

Half-life: 3-4.25 hours

Elimination: Urine (<5% as parent and major metabolite)

(Continued)

Leuprolide *(Continued)*

Dosage

Geriatrics & Adults:

Advanced prostatic carcinoma:

SubQ:

Eligard®: 7.5 mg monthly **or** 22.5 mg every 3 months **or** 30 mg every 4 months **or** 45 mg every 6 months

Lupron®: 1 mg/day

Viadur®: 65 mg implanted subcutaneously every 12 months

I.M.:

Lupron Depot®: 7.5 mg/dose given monthly (every 28-33 days) **or**

Lupron Depot®-3: 22.5 mg every 3 months **or**

Lupron Depot®-4: 30 mg every 4 months

Breast cancer, premenopausal ovarian ablation (unlabeled use): I.M.:

Lupron Depot®: 3.75 mg every 28 days **or**

Lupron Depot®-3: 11.25 mg every 3 months

Endometriosis: I.M.: Initial therapy may be with leuprolide alone or in combination with norethindrone; if retreatment for an additional 6 months is necessary, norethindrone should be used. Retreatment is not recommended for longer than one additional 6-month course.

Lupron Depot®: 3.75 mg/month for up to 6 months **or**

Lupron Depot®-3: 11.25 mg every 3 months for up to 2 doses (6 months total duration of treatment)

Uterine leiomyomata (fibroids): I.M. (in combination with iron):

Lupron Depot®: 3.75 mg/month for up to 3 months **or**

Lupron Depot®-3: 11.25 mg as a single injection

Administration

Eligard™: Packaged in two syringes; one contains the Atrigel® polymer system, and the second contains leuprolide acetate powder; follow instructions for mixing. Must be administered within 30 minutes of mixing.

Lupron Depot®: Do not use needles smaller than 22 gauge; reconstitute only with diluent provided.

Viadur® implant: Requires surgical implantation and removal at 12-month intervals

Monitoring Parameters Monitor for paresthesia and urinary tract obstruction during first weeks of therapy. Monitor for adverse reactions. Teach patient/caregiver appropriate administration procedures.

Test Interactions Interferes with pituitary gonadotropic and gonadal function tests during and up to 3 months after monthly administration of leuprolide therapy. Viadur®: Efficacy and stability of product not affected by MRI or radiographic exposure, although device will be visualized during these diagnostic procedures.

Patient Information Use as directed. Do not discontinue abruptly; consult prescriber. You may experience disease flare (increased bone pain) and urinary retention during early treatment (usually resolves), dizziness, headache, lethargy, or faintness (use caution when driving or engaging in tasks that require alertness until response to drug is known), nausea or vomiting (small frequent meals or analgesics may help), hot flashes - flushing or redness (cold clothes and cool environment may help). Report irregular or rapid heartbeat, unresolved nausea or vomiting, numbness of extremities, breast swelling or pain, difficulty breathing, or infection at injection sites. May cause depression; report changes in mood or memory immediately.

Additional Information

Eligard® Atrigel®: A nongelatin-based, biodegradable, polymer matrix

Viadur®: Leuprolide acetate implant containing 72 mg of leuprolide acetate, equivalent to 65 mg leuprolide free base. One Viadur® implant delivers 120 mcg of leuprolide/day over 12 months.

Guidelines from the American Society of Clinical Oncology (ASCO) for hormonal management of advanced prostate cancer which is androgen-sensitive (Loblaw, 2007) recommend either orchiectomy or luteinizing hormone-releasing hormone (LHRH) agonists as initial treatment for androgen deprivation.

Special Geriatric Considerations Leuprolide has the advantage of not increasing risk of atherosclerotic vascular disease, causing swelling of breasts, fluid retention, and thromboembolism as compared to estrogen therapy.

Dosage Forms Excipient information presented when available (limited, particularly for generics); consult specific product labeling.

Implant (Viadur®): 65 mg [released over 12 months; packaged with administration kit]

Injection, solution, as acetate (Lupron®): 5 mg/mL (2.8 mL) [contains benzyl alcohol; packaged with syringes and alcohol swabs]

Injection, powder for reconstitution, as acetate [depot formulation; prefilled syringe]:

Eligard®:

7.5 mg [released over 1 month]

22.5 mg [released over 3 months]

30 mg [released over 4 months]

45 mg [released over 6 months]
Lupron Depot®: 3.75 mg, 7.5 mg [released over 1 month; contains polysorbate 80]
Lupron Depot®-3 Month: 11.25 mg, 22.5 mg [released over 3 months; contains polysorbate 80]
Lupron Depot®-4 Month: 30 mg [released over 4 months; contains polysorbate 80]
Lupron Depot-Ped®: 7.5 mg, 11.25 mg, 15 mg [released over 1 month; contains polysorbate 80]

Selected References

Adjuvant Breast Cancer Trials Collaborative Group, "Ovarian Ablation or Suppression in Premenopausal Early Breast Cancer: Results From the International Adjuvant Breast Cancer Ovarian Ablation or Suppression Randomized Trial," *J Natl Cancer Inst*, 2007, 99(7):516-25.

Boccardo F, Rubagotti A, Amoroso D, et al, "Endocrinological and Clinical Evaluation of Two Depot Formulations of Leuprolide Acetate in Pre- and Perimenopausal Breast Cancer Patients," *Cancer Chemother Pharmacol*, 1999, 43(6):461-6.

♦ **Leuprolide Acetate** see Leuprolide on page 883
♦ **Leuprorelin Acetate** see Leuprolide on page 883

Levalbuterol (leve al BYOO ter ole)

Related Information
Inhalant Agents on page 1760
Medication Safety Issues
Sound-alike/look-alike issues:
Xopenex® may be confused with Xanax®
U.S. Brand Names Xopenex®; Xopenex HFA™
Canadian Brand Names Xopenex®
Index Terms Levalbuterol Hydrochloride; Levalbuterol Tartrate; R-albuterol
Generic Available No
Pharmacologic Category Beta$_2$-Adrenergic Agonist
Use Treatment or prevention of bronchospasm in adults with reversible obstructive airway disease
Contraindications Hypersensitivity to levalbuterol, albuterol, or any component of the formulation
Warnings/Precautions Optimize anti-inflammatory treatment before initiating maintenance treatment with levalbuterol. Do not use as a component of chronic therapy without an anti-inflammatory agent. Only the mildest form of asthma (Step 1 and/or exercise-induced) would not require concurrent use based upon asthma guidelines. Patient must be instructed to seek medical attention in cases where acute symptoms are not relieved or a previous level of response is diminished. The need to increase frequency of use may indicate deterioration of asthma, and treatment must not be delayed.

Use caution in patients with cardiovascular disease (arrhythmia or hypertension or CHF), convulsive disorders, diabetes, glaucoma, hyperthyroidism, or hypokalemia. Beta-agonists may cause elevation in blood pressure, heart rate, and result in CNS stimulation/excitation. Beta$_2$-agonists may increase risk of arrhythmia, increase serum glucose, or decrease serum potassium.

Immediate hypersensitivity reactions (urticaria, angioedema, rash, bronchospasm) have been reported. Do not exceed recommended dose; serious adverse events including fatalities, have been associated with excessive use of inhaled sympathomimetics. Rarely, paradoxical bronchospasm may occur with use of inhaled bronchodilating agents; this should be distinguished from inadequate response.

Adverse Reactions (Reflective of adult population; not specific for elderly)
>10%:
Endocrine & metabolic: Serum glucose increased, serum potassium decreased
Respiratory: Viral infection (7% to 12%), rhinitis (3% to 11%)
>2% to 10%:
Central nervous system: Nervousness (3% to 10%), tremor (≤7%), anxiety (≤3%), dizziness (1% to 3%), migraine (≤3%), pain (1% to 3%)
Cardiovascular: Tachycardia (~3%)
Gastrointestinal: Dyspepsia (1% to 3%)
Neuromuscular & skeletal: Leg cramps (≤3%)
Respiratory: Asthma (9%), pharyngitis (8%), cough (1% to 4%), nasal edema (1% to 3%), sinusitis (1% to 4%)
Miscellaneous: Flu-like syndrome (1% to 4%), accidental injury (≤3%)
Overdosage/Toxicology Symptoms of overdose include tachycardia, tremor, hypertension, angina, and seizures. Hypokalemia also may occur. Cardiac arrest and death may be associated with abuse of beta-agonist bronchodilators. Treatment includes immediate discontinuation and symptomatic and supportive therapies. Cautious use of beta-adrenergic blocking agents may be considered in severe cases.
(Continued)

Levalbuterol *(Continued)*

Drug Interactions

Anesthetics (inhaled): Cardiac effects of levalbuterol may be potentiated; use with caution.

Beta-blockers (particularly nonselective agents): May block the effect of levalbuterol and also produce severe bronchospasm.

Diuretics (nonpotassium-sparing): ECG changes and/or hypokalemia may result from concomitant use; use caution.

Digoxin: Plasma levels of digoxin may be decreased by 16% to 22%; monitor.

MAO inhibitors: Cardiac effects of levalbuterol may be potentiated; use with extreme caution or within 2 weeks of discontinuing MAO inhibitor.

Sympathomimetics (including amphetamine, dobutamine): Cardiac effects of levalbuterol may be potentiated; use with caution.

Tricyclic antidepressants (TCAs): Cardiac effects of levalbuterol may be potentiated; use with extreme caution or within 2 weeks of discontinuing TCAs

Stability

Aerosol: Store at room temperature of 20°C to 25°C (68°F to 77°F); protect from freezing and direct sunlight. Store with mouthpiece up. Discard after 200 actuations.

Solution for nebulization: Store in protective foil pouch at room temperature of 20°C to 25°C (68°F to 77°F). Protect from light and excessive heat. Vials should be used within 2 weeks after opening protective pouch. Use within 1 week and protect from light if removed from pouch. Vials of concentrated solution should be used immediately after removing from protective pouch. Concentrated solution should be diluted with 2.5 mL NS prior to use.

Mechanism of Action Relaxes bronchial smooth muscle by action on beta$_2$-receptors with little effect on heart rate

Pharmacodynamics

Onset of action:

Aerosol: 5.5-10.2 minutes

Peak effect: ~77 minutes

Nebulization: 10-17 minutes (measured as a 15% increase in FEV$_1$)

Peak effect: 1.5 hours

Duration:

Aerosol: 3-4 hours (up to 6 hours in some patients)

Nebulization: 5-6 hours (up to 8 hours in some patients)

Pharmacokinetics

Absorption: A portion of inhaled dose is absorbed to systemic circulation

Half-life elimination: 3.3-4.0 hours

Time to peak serum concentration:

Aerosol: 0.5 hours

Nebulization: 0.2 hours

Dosage

Geriatrics: Only a small number of patients have been studied. Although greater sensitivity of some elderly patients cannot be ruled out, no overall differences in safety or effectiveness were observed. An initial dose of 0.63 mg should be used in all patients >65 years of age.

Adults: Bronchospasm:

Metered-dose inhalation: Aerosol: 1-2 puffs every 4-6 hours

Nebulization: 0.63 mg 3 times/day at intervals of 6-8 hours; dosage may be increased to 1.25 mg 3 times/day with close monitoring for adverse effects. Most patients gain optimal benefit from regular use

Administration Inhalation:

Aerosol: Shake well before use; prime with 4 test sprays prior to first use or if inhaler has not been use of more than 3 days. Clean actuator (mouthpiece) weekly.

Solution for nebulization: Safety and efficacy were established when administered with the following nebulizers: PARI LC Jet™, PARI LC Plus™, as well as the following compressors: PARI Master®, Dura-Neb® 2000, and Dura-Neb® 3000. Concentrated solution should be diluted prior to use.

Monitoring Parameters Pulmonary function, heart rate, blood pressure, CNS status, arterial blood gases (if condition warrants). In selected patients: Serum, glucose, and potassium

Patient Information If a previously effective regimen fails to provide expected relief, medical advice should be sought immediately. Only available via nebulization.

Additional Information Slightly smaller increase in heart rate and slightly lower incidence of nervousness were seen with levalbuterol compared to albuterol.

Special Geriatric Considerations For aerosol formulation, start with low end of dosage range. Refer to dosing information for nebulization dosing specifics.

Dosage Forms Excipient information presented when available (limited, particularly for generics); consult specific product labeling.

Note: Strength expressed as base.

Aerosol, oral, as tartrate:
Xopenex HFA™: 45 mcg/actuation (15 g) [200 doses; chlorofluorocarbon free]
Solution for nebulization, as hydrochloride:
Xopenex®: 0.31 mg/3 mL (24s); 0.63 mg/3 mL (24s); 1.25 mg/3 mL (24s)
Solution for nebulization, concentrate, as hydrochloride:
Xopenex®: 1.25 mg/0.5 mL (30s)

♦ **Levalbuterol Hydrochloride** *see* Levalbuterol *on page 887*
♦ **Levalbuterol Tartrate** *see* Levalbuterol *on page 887*
♦ **Levaquin®** *see* Levofloxacin *on page 896*
♦ **Levatol®** *see* Penbutolol *on page 1217*
♦ **Levbid®** *see* Hyoscyamine *on page 778*
♦ **Levemir®** *see* Insulin Detemir *on page 809*

Levetiracetam (lee va tye RA se tam)

Medication Safety Issues
Sound-alike/look-alike issues:
Potential for dispensing errors between Keppra® and Kaletra® (lopinavir/ritonavir)
U.S. Brand Names Keppra®
Canadian Brand Names CO Levetiracetam; Keppra®
Generic Available No
Pharmacologic Category Anticonvulsant, Miscellaneous
Use Adjunctive therapy in the treatment of partial onset, myoclonic, and/or primary generalized tonic-clonic seizures
Unlabeled/Investigational Use Bipolar disorder
Contraindications Hypersensitivity to levetiracetam or any component of the formulation
Warnings/Precautions Psychotic symptoms (psychosis, hallucinations) and behavioral symptoms (including aggression, anger, anxiety, depersonalization, depression, personality disorder) may occur. Dose reduction may be required. Levetiracetam should be withdrawn gradually to minimize the potential of increased seizure frequency. Use caution with renal impairment; dosage adjustment may be necessary. Weakness, dizziness, and somnolence occur mostly during the first month of therapy.
Adverse Reactions (Reflective of adult population; not specific for elderly)
>10%:
Central nervous system: Behavioral symptoms (agitation, aggression, anger, anxiety, apathy, depersonalization, depression, emotional lability, hostility, hyperkinesias, irritability, nervousness, neurosis and personality disorder: adults 5% to 13%; children 5% to 38%), somnolence (12% to 23%), headache (14%), hostility (2% to 12%)
Gastrointestinal: Vomiting (15%), anorexia (3% to 13%)
Neuromuscular & skeletal: Weakness (9% to 15%)
Respiratory: Pharyngitis (6% to 14%), rhinitis (4% to 13%), cough (2% to 11%)
Miscellaneous: Accidental injury (17%), infection (2% to 13%)
1% to 10%:
Cardiovascular: Facial edema (2%)
Central nervous system: Fatigue (10%), nervousness (4% to 10%), dizziness (7% to 9%), personality disorder (8%), pain (6% to 7%), agitation (6%), irritability (6%), emotional lability (2% to 6%), mood swings (5%), depression (3% to 5%), vertigo (3% to 5%), ataxia (3%), amnesia (2%), anxiety (2%), confusion (2%)
Dermatologic: Bruising (4%), pruritus (2%), rash (2%), skin discoloration (2%)
Endocrine & metabolic: Dehydration (2%)
Gastrointestinal: Diarrhea (8%), gastroenteritis (4%), constipation (3%)
Genitourinary: Urine abnormality (2%)
Hematologic: Leukocytes decreased (2% to 3%)
Neuromuscular & skeletal: Neck pain (2% to 8%), paresthesia (2%), reflexes increased (2%)
Ocular: Conjunctivitis (3%), diplopia (2%), amblyopia (2%)
Otic: Ear pain (2%)
Renal: Albuminuria (4%)
Respiratory: Influenza (5%), asthma (2%), sinusitis (2%)
Miscellaneous: Flu-like syndrome (3%), viral infection (2%)
Overdosage/Toxicology Symptoms may include aggression, agitation, ataxia, coma, decreased consciousness, drowsiness, respiratory depression and somnolence. Monitor vital signs. Treatment is symptomatic and supportive. Hemodialysis may be effective (estimated clearance of ~50% in 4 hours).
Drug Interactions CNS depressants: May enhance the adverse/toxic effect of levetiracetam.
Ethanol/Nutrition/Herb Interactions
Ethanol: Avoid ethanol (may increase CNS depression).
(Continued)

Levetiracetam *(Continued)*

Food: Food may delay, but does not affect the extent of absorption.

Stability

Oral solution, tablet: Store at 15°C to 30°C (59°F to 86°F).

Injection solution: Store at 15°C to 30°C (59°F to 86°F). Must dilute dose in 100 mL of NS, LR, or D_5W. Admixed solution is stable for 24 hours in PVC bags kept at room temperature.

Mechanism of Action The precise mechanism by which levetiracetam exerts its antiepileptic effect is unknown. However, several studies have suggested the mechanism may involve one or more of the following central pharmacologic effects: inhibition of voltage-dependent N-type calcium channels; facilitation of GABA-ergic inhibitory transmission through displacement of negative modulators; reduction of delayed rectifier potassium current; and/or binding to synaptic proteins which modulate neurotransmitter release.

Pharmacokinetics

Absorption: Oral: Rapid and complete

Protein binding: <10%

Metabolism: Not extensive; primarily by enzymatic hydrolysis; forms metabolites (inactive)

Bioavailability: 100%

Half-life elimination: 6-8 hours

Time to peak, plasma: Oral: 1 hour

Excretion: Urine (66% as unchanged drug)

Dosage

Geriatrics & Adults:

Myoclonic seizures: Oral: Initial: 500 mg twice daily; may increase every 2 weeks by 500 mg/dose to the recommended dose of 1500 mg twice daily. Efficacy of doses >3000 mg/day has not been established.

Partial onset seizures:

Oral: Initial: 500 mg twice daily; may increase every 2 weeks by 500 mg/dose to a maximum of 1500 mg twice daily. Doses >3000 mg/day have been used in trials; however, there is no evidence of increased benefit.

I.V.: Initial: 500 mg twice daily; may increase every 2 weeks by 500 mg/dose to a maximum of 1500 mg twice daily. Doses >3000 mg/day have been used in trials; however, there is no evidence of increased benefit.

Note: When switching from oral to I.V. formulations, the total daily dose should be the same.

Tonic-clonic seizures: Oral: Initial: 500 mg twice daily; may increase every 2 weeks by 500 mg/dose to the recommended dose of 1500 mg twice daily. Efficacy of doses >3000 mg/day has not been established.

Bipolar disorder (unlabeled use): Oral: Initial: 500 mg twice daily; if tolerated, increase to 500 mg twice daily; dose may be increased every 3 days until target dose of 3000 mg/day is reached; maximum: 4000 mg/day

Renal Impairment: Adults:

Cl_{cr} >80 mL/minute: 500-1500 mg every 12 hours

Cl_{cr} 50-80 mL/minute: 500-1000 mg every 12 hours

Cl_{cr} 30-50 mL/minute: 250-750 mg every 12 hours

Cl_{cr} <30 mL/minute: 250-500 mg every 12 hours

End-stage renal disease patients using dialysis: 500-1000 mg every 24 hours; a supplemental dose of 250-500 mg following dialysis is recommended

Hepatic Impairment: No adjustment required

Administration

I.V.: Infuse over 15 minutes

Oral solution: Should be administered with a calibrated measuring device (not a household teaspoon or tablespoon)

Tablet: Only administer as whole tablet.

Patient Information Be advised that levetiracetam may cause dizziness and somnolence and accordingly, you should not drive or operate machinery or engage in other hazardous activities until sufficient experience has been gained on levetiracetam to gauge whether it adversely affects your performance of these activities

Special Geriatric Considerations In a study of 16 older adults (61-88 years of age) receiving levetiracetam daily and with creatinine clearances ranging from 30-74 mL/minute, a decrease in creatinine clearance (38%) and a 2.5 hour longer half-life were recorded in the elderly compared to younger adults. The authors concluded that the difference was due to renal function. Other studies show no overall difference in safety and efficacy, although larger numbers in studies are needed to verify efficacy. When using the drug in elderly, it is essential to base the dose on estimated creatinine clearance and adjust appropriately.

Dosage Forms Excipient information presented when available (limited, particularly for generics); consult specific product labeling.

Injection, solution:
Keppra®: 100 mg/mL (5 mL)
Solution, oral:
Keppra®: 100 mg/mL (480 mL) [dye free; grape flavor]
Tablet:
Keppra®: 250 mg, 500 mg, 750 mg, 1000 mg

Selected References

Hovinga CA, "Levetiracetam: A Novel Antiepileptic Drug," *Pharmacotherapy*, 2001, 21(11):1375-88.

Sankar R and Holmes GL, "Mechanisms of Action for the Commonly Used Antiepileptic Drugs: Relevance to Antiepileptic Drug-Associated Neurobehavioral Adverse Effects," *J Child Neurol*, 2004, 19(Suppl 1):6-14.

Roberts GM, Majoie HJ, Leenen LA, et al, "Ketter's Hypothesis of the Mood Effects of Antiepileptic Drugs Coupled to the Mechanism of Action of Topiramate and Levetiracetam," *Epilepsy Behav*, 2005, 6(3):366-72.

Welty TE, Gidal BE, Ficker DM, et al, "Levetiracetam: A Different Approach to the Pharmacotherapy of Epilepsy," *Ann Pharmacother*, 2002, 36(2):296-304.

♦ **Levitra®** *see* Vardenafil *on page 1662*

Levobunolol (lee voe BYOO noe lole)

Related Information
Glaucoma Drug Therapy *on page 1758*

Medication Safety Issues
Sound-alike/look-alike issues:
Levobunolol may be confused with levocabastine
Betagan® may be confused with Betadine®

International issues:
Betagan® may be confused with Betagon® which is a brand name for mepindolol in Italy

U.S. Brand Names Betagan®

Canadian Brand Names Apo-Levobunolol®; Betagan®; Novo-Levobunolol; Optho-Bunolol®; PMS-Levobunolol; Sandoz-Levobunolol

Index Terms *l*-Bunolol Hydrochloride; Levobunolol Hydrochloride

Generic Available Yes

Pharmacologic Category Beta-Adrenergic Blocker, Nonselective; Ophthalmic Agent, Antiglaucoma

Use Reduction in intraocular pressure in chronic open-angle glaucoma or ocular hypertension

Contraindications Hypersensitivity to levobunolol or any component of the formulation; bronchial asthma, severe COPD, sinus bradycardia, second- or third-degree AV block, cardiac failure, cardiogenic shock

Warnings/Precautions Consider pre-existing conditions such as sick sinus syndrome before initiating. Use with caution in patients with CHF, diabetes mellitus, bronchospastic disease, myasthenia gravis, peripheral vascular disease, psychiatric disease, hyperthyroidism; contains metabisulfite. Because systemic absorption does occur with ophthalmic administration, the elderly with other disease states or syndromes that may be affected by a beta-blocker (CHF, COPD, etc) should be monitored closely. Product contains benzalkonium chloride which may be absorbed by soft contact lenses; do not administer while wearing soft contact lenses. Ophthalmic solutions contain metabisulfite.

Adverse Reactions (Reflective of adult population; not specific for elderly)
>10%: Ocular: Stinging/burning eyes
1% to 10%:
Cardiovascular: Bradycardia, arrhythmia, hypotension
Central nervous system: Dizziness, headache
Dermatologic: Alopecia, erythema
Local: Stinging, burning
Ocular: Blepharoconjunctivitis, conjunctivitis
Respiratory: Bronchospasm

Drug Interactions Increased toxicity:
Systemic beta-adrenergic blocking agents
Ophthalmic epinephrine (increased blood pressure/loss of IOP effect)
Quinidine (sinus bradycardia)
Verapamil (bradycardia and asystole have been reported)

Mechanism of Action A nonselective beta-adrenergic blocking agent that lowers intraocular pressure by reducing aqueous humor production and possibly increases the outflow of aqueous humor

Pharmacodynamics
Onset of action: Following ophthalmic instillation decreases in intraocular pressure (IOP) can be noted within 1 hour
Peak effect: Within 2-6 hours; reductions in IOP can last from 1-7 days
(Continued)

Levobunolol *(Continued)*

Dosage

Geriatrics & Adults: Glaucoma: Ophthalmic: Instill 1 drop in the affected eye(s) 1-2 times/day

Administration Apply finger pressure over nasolacrimal duct to decrease systemic absorption.

Monitoring Parameters Intraocular pressure, heart rate, funduscopic exam, visual field testing

Patient Information May sting on instillation, do not touch dropper to eye; visual acuity may be decreased after administration; night vision may be decreased; distance vision may be altered; apply finger pressure between the bridge of the nose and corner of the eye to decrease systemic absorption; assess patient's or caregiver's ability to administer

Additional Information Contains metabisulfite

Special Geriatric Considerations Because systemic absorption does occur with ophthalmic administration, the elderly with other disease states or syndromes that may be affected by a beta-blocker (CHF, COPD, etc) should be monitored closely

Dosage Forms Excipient information presented when available (limited, particularly for generics); consult specific product labeling.

Solution, ophthalmic, as hydrochloride: 0.25% (5 mL, 10 mL); 0.5% (5 mL, 10 mL, 15 mL) [contains benzalkonium chloride and sodium metabisulfite]

Betagan®: 0.25% (5 mL, 10 mL); 0.5% (2 mL, 5 mL, 10 mL, 15 mL) [contains benzalkonium chloride and sodium metabisulfite]

♦ **Levobunolol Hydrochloride** *see* Levobunolol *on page 891*

Levodopa and Carbidopa (lee voe DOE pa & kar bi DOE pa)

Related Information

Antiparkinsonian Agents *on page 1745*

Carbidopa *on page 237*

U.S. Brand Names Parcopa™; Sinemet®; Sinemet® CR

Canadian Brand Names Apo-Levocarb®; Apo-Levocarb® CR; Endo®-Levodopa/Carbidopa; Novo-Levocarbidopa; Nu-Levocarb; Sinemet®; Sinemet® CR

Index Terms Carbidopa and Levodopa

Generic Available Yes: Excludes orally-disintegrating tablet

Pharmacologic Category Anti-Parkinson's Agent, Dopamine Agonist

Use Treatment of idiopathic Parkinson's disease, postencephalitic parkinsonism, symptomatic parkinsonism

Unlabeled/Investigational Use Treatment of restless leg syndrome

Contraindications Hypersensitivity to levodopa, carbidopa, or any component of the formulation; narrow-angle glaucoma; use of MAO inhibitors within prior 14 days (however, may be administered concomitantly with the manufacturer's recommended dose of an MAO inhibitor with selectivity for MAO type B); history of melanoma or undiagnosed skin lesions

Warnings/Precautions Use with caution in patients with history of cardiovascular disease (including myocardial infarction and arrhythmias); pulmonary diseases such as asthma, psychosis, wide-angle glaucoma, peptic ulcer disease; as well as in renal, hepatic, or endocrine disease. Sudden discontinuation of levodopa may cause a worsening of Parkinson's disease. Elderly may be more sensitive to CNS effects of levodopa. May cause or exacerbate dyskinesias. Patients have reported falling asleep while engaging in activities of daily living; this has been reported to occur without significant warning signs. May cause orthostatic hypotension; Parkinson's disease patients appear to have an impaired capacity to respond to a postural challenge; use with caution in patients at risk of hypotension (such as those receiving antihypertensive drugs) or where transient hypotensive episodes would be poorly tolerated (cardiovascular disease or cerebrovascular disease). Observe patients closely for development of depression with concomitant suicidal tendencies. Dopaminergic agents have been associated with a syndrome resembling neuroleptic malignant syndrome on abrupt withdrawal or significant dosage reduction after long-term use. Protein in the diet should be distributed throughout the day to avoid fluctuations in levodopa absorption.

Adverse Reactions (Reflective of adult population; not specific for elderly)

Frequency not defined.

Cardiovascular: Orthostatic hypotension, arrhythmia, chest pain, hypertension, syncope, palpitation, phlebitis

Central nervous system: Dizziness, anxiety, confusion, nightmares, headache, hallucinations, on-off phenomenon, decreased mental acuity, memory impairment, disorientation, delusions, euphoria, agitation, somnolence, insomnia, gait abnormalities, nervousness, ataxia, EPS, falling, psychosis, peripheral neuropathy, seizure (causal relationship not established)

Dermatologic: Rash, alopecia, malignant melanoma, hypersensitivity (angioedema, urticaria, pruritus, bullous lesions, Henoch-Schönlein purpura)

Endocrine & metabolic: Increased libido

Gastrointestinal: Anorexia, nausea, vomiting, constipation, GI bleeding, duodenal ulcer, diarrhea, dyspepsia, taste alterations, sialorrhea, heartburn

Genitourinary: Discoloration of urine, urinary frequency

Hematologic: Hemolytic anemia, agranulocytosis, thrombocytopenia, leukopenia; decreased hemoglobin and hematocrit; abnormalities in AST and ALT, LDH, bilirubin, BUN, Coombs' test

Neuromuscular & skeletal: Choreiform and involuntary movements, paresthesia, bone pain, shoulder pain, muscle cramps, weakness

Ocular: Blepharospasm, oculogyric crises (may be associated with acute dystonic reactions)

Renal: Difficult urination

Respiratory: Dyspnea, cough

Miscellaneous: Hiccups, discoloration of sweat, diaphoresis (increased)

Overdosage/Toxicology Symptoms include palpitations, arrhythmias, spasms, and hypotension. May cause hypertension or hypotension. Treatment is supportive. Initiate gastric lavage, administer I.V. fluids judiciously and monitor ECG. Use fluids judiciously to maintain pressures. May precipitate a variety of arrhythmias.

Drug Interactions

Antacids: Levodopa absorption may be increased; monitor

Anticholinergics: May reduce the efficacy of levodopa, possibly due to reduced gastrointestinal absorption (also see tricyclic antidepressants); limited evidence of clinical significance; monitor

Antipsychotics: May inhibit the antiparkinsonian effects of levodopa via dopamine receptor blockade; use antipsychotics with low dopamine blockade (clozapine, olanzapine, quetiapine)

Benzodiazepines: May inhibit the antiparkinsonian effects of levodopa; monitor for reduced effect

Clonidine: May reduce the efficacy of levodopa; monitor

Dextromethorphan: Toxic reactions have occurred with dextromethorphan

Furazolidone: May increase the effect/toxicity of levodopa; hypertensive episodes have been reported; monitor

Iron salts: Binds levodopa and reduces its bioavailability; separate doses of iron and levodopa

Linezolid: Due to MAO inhibition (see note on MAO inhibitors), this agent is best avoided

MAO inhibitors: Concurrent use of levodopa with nonselective MAO inhibitors may result in hypertensive reactions via an increased storage and release of dopamine, norepinephrine, or both; use with carbidopa to minimize reactions if combination is necessary, otherwise avoid combination.

L-methionine: May inhibit levodopa's antiparkinsonian effects; monitor for reduced effect

Metoclopramide: May increase the absorption/effect of levodopa; hypertensive episodes have been reported. Levodopa antagonizes metoclopramide's effects on lower esophageal sphincter pressure. Avoid use of metoclopramide for reflux, monitor response to levodopa carefully if used.

Methyldopa: May potentiate the effects of levodopa; levodopa may increase the hypotensive response to methyldopa; monitor

Papaverine: May decrease the efficacy of levodopa; includes other similar agents (ethaverine); monitor

Penicillamine: May increase serum concentrations of levodopa; monitor for increased effect

Phenytoin: May inhibit levodopa's antiparkinsonian effects; monitor for reduced effect

Pyridoxine: May inhibit levodopa's antiparkinsonian effects; monitor for reduced effect (pyridoxine in doses >10-25 mg for levodopa alone, higher doses >200 mg/day may be a problem for levodopa/carbidopa)

Spiramycin: May inhibit levodopa's antiparkinsonian effects; monitor for reduced effect

Tacrine: May inhibit the effects of levodopa via enhanced cholinergic activity; monitor for reduced effect

Tricyclic antidepressants: May decrease the absorption (bioavailability) of levodopa; rare hypertensive episodes have also been attributed to this combination

Ethanol/Nutrition/Herb Interactions

Ethanol: Avoid ethanol (due to CNS depression).

Food: Avoid high protein diets and high intakes of vitamin B_6.

Herb/Nutraceutical: Avoid kava kava (may decrease effects). Pyridoxine in doses >10-25 mg (for levodopa alone) or higher doses >200 mg/day (for levodopa/carbidopa) may decrease efficacy.

Stability Store at 20°C to 25°C (68°F to 77°F); excursions permitted between 15°C to 30°C (59°F to 86°F). Protect from light and moisture.

(Continued)

Levodopa and Carbidopa *(Continued)*

Mechanism of Action Parkinson's symptoms are due to a lack of striatal dopamine; levodopa circulates in the plasma to the blood-brain-barrier (BBB), where it crosses, to be converted by striatal enzymes to dopamine; carbidopa inhibits the peripheral plasma breakdown of levodopa by inhibiting its decarboxylation, and thereby increases available levodopa at the BBB

Pharmacodynamics Peak effect: Oral: Within 1-2 hours after administration; may take 2-3 weeks to see the full therapeutic effect

Pharmacokinetics

Carbidopa:

Absorption: Oral: 40% to 70%

Protein binding: 36%

Half-life: 1-2 hours

Elimination: Excreted unchanged

Levodopa:

Absorption: May be decreased if given with a high protein meal

Half-life: 1.2-2.3 hours

Elimination: Primarily in urine (80%) as dopamine, norepinephrine, and homovanillic acid

Dosage

Geriatrics: Initial dose: 25/100 twice daily, increase as necessary. Sinemet® CR may be used as initial therapy.

Adults:

Parkinson's disease: Oral: Initial:

Immediate release tablet:

Initial: Carbidopa 25 mg/levodopa 100 mg 3 times/day

Dosage adjustment: Alternate tablet strengths may be substituted according to individual carbidopa/levodopa requirements. Increase by 1 tablet every other day as necessary, except when using the carbidopa 25 mg/levodopa 250 mg tablets where increases should be made using $1/2$-1 tablet every 1-2 days. Use of more than 1 dosage strength or dosing 4 times/day may be required (maximum: 8 tablets of any strength/day or 200 mg of carbidopa and 2000 mg of levodopa)

Sustained release tablet:

Initial: Carbidopa 50 mg/levodopa 200 mg 2 times/day, at intervals not <6 hours

Dosage adjustment: May adjust every 3 days; intervals should be between 4-8 hours during the waking day (maximum: 8 tablets/day)

Restless leg syndrome (unlabeled use): Oral: Carbidopa 25 mg/levodopa 100 mg given 30-60 minutes before bedtime; may repeat dose once

Administration Space doses evenly over the waking hours. Give with meals to decrease GI upset. Sustained release product should not be crushed. Orally-disintegrating tablets do not require water; the tablet should disintegrate on the tongue's surface before swallowing.

Monitoring Parameters Blood pressure, standing and sitting/supine; symptoms of parkinsonism, dyskinesias, mental status

Test Interactions False-positive reaction for urinary glucose with Clinitest®; false-negative reaction using Clinistix®; false-positive urine ketones with Acetest®, Ketostix®, Labstix®

Patient Information Take on an empty stomach if possible; if GI distress occurs, take with meals; rise carefully from lying or sitting position; do not crush or chew sustained release product

Additional Information 50-100 mg/day of carbidopa is needed to block the peripheral conversion of levodopa to dopamine. "On-off" (a clinical syndrome characterized by sudden periods of drug activity/inactivity), can be managed by giving smaller, more frequent doses of Sinemet® or adding a dopamine agonist or selegiline; when adding a new agent, doses of Sinemet® can usually be decreased. Protein in the diet should be distributed throughout the day to avoid fluctuations in levodopa absorption. Levodopa is the drug of choice when rigidity is the predominant presenting symptom.

Conversion from immediate release carbidopa/levodopa (Sinemet® or Parcopa™) to Sinemet® CR (50/200):

Sinemet® or Parcopa™ [total daily dose of levodopa]/Sinemet® CR:

Sinemet® or Parcopa™ (levodopa 300-400 mg/day): Sinemet® CR (50/200) 1 tablet twice daily

Sinemet® or Parcopa™ (levodopa 500-600 mg/day): Sinemet® CR (50/200) 1 $1/2$ tablets twice daily or 1 tablet 3 times/day

Sinemet® or Parcopa™ (levodopa 700-800 mg/day): Sinemet® CR (50/200) 4 tablets in 3 or more divided doses

Sinemet® or Parcopa™ (levodopa 900-1000 mg/day): Sinemet® CR (50/200) 5 tablets in 3 or more divided doses

Intervals between doses of Sinemet® CR should be 4-8 hours while awake; when divided doses are not equal, smaller doses should be given toward the end of the day,

Special Geriatric Considerations The elderly may be more sensitive to the CNS effects of levodopa.

Dosage Forms Excipient information presented when available (limited, particularly for generics); consult specific product labeling.

Tablet immediate release (Sinemet®):
10/100: Carbidopa 10 mg and levodopa 100 mg
25/100: Carbidopa 25 mg and levodopa 100 mg
25/250: Carbidopa 25 mg and levodopa 250 mg

Tablet, immediate release, orally disintegrating (Parcopa™):
10/100: Carbidopa 10 mg and levodopa 100 mg [contains phenylalanine 3.4 mg/ tablet; mint flavor]
25/100: Carbidopa 25 mg and levodopa 100 mg [contains phenylalanine 3.4 mg/ tablet; mint flavor]
25/250: Carbidopa 25 mg and levodopa 250 mg [contains phenylalanine 8.4 mg/ tablet; mint flavor]

Tablet, sustained release (Sinemet® CR):
Carbidopa 25 mg and levodopa 100 mg
Carbidopa 50 mg and levodopa 200 mg

Selected References

Olanow CW, Watts RL, and Koller WC, "An Algorithm (Decision Tree) for the Management of Parkinson's Disease (2001): Treatment Guidelines," *Neurology*, 2001, 56(11 Suppl 5):S1-S88.

Restless Leg Syndrome Foundation, Inc, *2001 Medical Bulletin*, revised April 2001. Available at: http://www.rls.org/frames/home_frame.htm. Accessed May 1, 2002.

Stern MB, "Contemporary Approaches to the Pharmacotherapeutic Management of Parkinson's Disease: An Overview," *Neurology*, 1997, 49(1 Suppl 1):S2-9.

Walker SW, Fina A, and Kryger MH, "L-Dopa/Carbidopa for Nocturnal Movement Disorders in Uremia," *Sleep*, 1996, 19(3):214-8.

Levodopa, Carbidopa, and Entacapone
(lee voe DOE pa, kar bi DOE pa, & en TA ka pone)

Related Information
Carbidopa *on page 237*
Entacapone *on page 511*

U.S. Brand Names Stalevo™

Index Terms Carbidopa, Levodopa, and Entacapone; Entacapone, Carbidopa, and Levodopa

Generic Available No

Pharmacologic Category Anti-Parkinson's Agent, COMT Inhibitor; Anti-Parkinson's Agent, Dopamine Agonist

Use Treatment of idiopathic Parkinson's disease

Dosage

Geriatrics & Adults:

Note: All strengths of Stalevo™ contain a carbidopa/levodopa ratio of 1:4 plus entacapone 200 mg.

Parkinson's disease: Oral: Dose should be individualized based on therapeutic response; doses may be adjusted by changing strength or adjusting interval. Fractionated doses are not recommended and only 1 tablet should be given at each dosing interval; maximum dose: 8 tablets/day (equivalent to entacapone 1600 mg/day)

Patients previously treated with carbidopa/levodopa immediate release tablets (ratio of 1:4):

With current entacapone therapy: May switch directly to corresponding strength of combination tablet. No data available on transferring patients from controlled release preparations or products with a 1:10 ratio of carbidopa/levodopa.

Without entacapone therapy:
If current levodopa dose is >600 mg/day: Levodopa dose reduction may be required when adding entacapone to therapy; therefore, titrate dose using individual products first (carbidopa/levodopa immediate release with a ratio of 1:4 plus entacapone 200 mg); then transfer to combination product once stabilized.

If current levodopa dose is <600 mg without dyskinesias: May transfer to corresponding dose of combination product; monitor, dose reduction of levodopa may be required.

Renal Impairment: Use caution with severe renal impairment; specific dosing recommendations not available.

Hepatic Impairment: Use with caution; specific dosing recommendations not available.

(Continued)

Levodopa, Carbidopa, and Entacapone *(Continued)*

Dosage Forms Excipient information presented when available (limited, particularly for generics); consult specific product labeling.
Tablet:
50: Carbidopa 12.5 mg, levodopa 50 mg, and entacapone 200 mg
100: Carbidopa 25 mg, levodopa 100 mg, and entacapone 200 mg
150: Carbidopa 37.5 mg, levodopa 150 mg, and entacapone 200 mg

♦ **Levo-Dromoran®** *see* Levorphanol *on page 899*

Levofloxacin (lee voe FLOKS a sin)

Related Information
Antimicrobial Activity Against Selected Organisms *on page 1728*
U.S. Brand Names Iquix®; Levaquin®; Quixin™
Canadian Brand Names Levaquin®; Novo-Levofloxacin
Generic Available No
Pharmacologic Category Antibiotic, Quinolone
Use

Systemic: Treatment of mild, moderate, or severe infections caused by susceptible organisms. Includes the treatment of community-acquired pneumonia, including multidrug resistant strains of *S. pneumoniae* (MDRSP); nosocomial pneumonia; chronic bronchitis (acute bacterial exacerbation); acute bacterial sinusitis; urinary tract infection (uncomplicated or complicated), including acute pyelonephritis caused by *E. coli*; prostatitis (chronic bacterial); skin or skin structure infections (uncomplicated or complicated); prevention of inhalational anthrax (postexposure)

Ophthalmic: Treatment of bacterial conjunctivitis caused by susceptible organisms (Quixin™ 0.5% ophthalmic solution); treatment of corneal ulcer caused by susceptible organisms (Iquix® 1.5% ophthalmic solution)

Contraindications Hypersensitivity to levofloxacin, any component of the formulation, or other quinolones

Warnings/Precautions

Systemic: CNS stimulation may occur (tremor, restlessness, confusion, and very rarely hallucinations or seizures). Potential for seizures, although very rare, may be increased with concomitant NSAID therapy. Use with caution in individuals at risk of seizures, with known or suspected CNS disorders or renal dysfunction; use caution to avoid possible photosensitivity reactions during and for several days following fluoroquinolone therapy

Rare cases of torsade de pointes have been reported in patients receiving levofloxacin. Use caution in patients with known prolongation of QT interval, bradycardia, hypokalemia, hypomagnesemia, or in those receiving concurrent therapy with Class Ia or Class III antiarrhythmics.

Severe hypersensitivity reactions, including anaphylaxis, have occurred with quinolone therapy. If an allergic reaction occurs (itching, urticaria, dyspnea or facial edema, loss of consciousness, tingling, cardiovascular collapse), discontinue drug immediately. Prolonged use may result in fungal or bacterial superinfection, including *C. difficile*-associated diarrhea and pseudomembranous colitis. Tendon inflammation and/or rupture has been reported; risk may be increased with concurrent corticosteroids, particularly in the elderly. Discontinue at first sign of tendon inflammation or pain. Peripheral neuropathies have been linked to levofloxacin use; discontinue if numbness, tingling, or weakness develops. Quinolones may exacerbate myasthenia gravis.

Ophthalmic solution: For topical use only. Do not inject subconjunctivally or introduce into anterior chamber of the eye. Contact lenses should not be worn during treatment for bacterial conjunctivitis. **Note:** Indications for ophthalmic solutions are product concentration-specific and should not be used interchangeably.

Adverse Reactions (Reflective of adult population; not specific for elderly)
1% to 10%:
Cardiovascular: Chest pain (1%)
Central nervous system: Headache (6%), insomnia (5%), dizziness (2%), fatigue (1%), pain (1%), fever
Dermatologic: Pruritus (1%), rash (1%)
Gastrointestinal: Nausea (7%), diarrhea (5%), abdominal pain (3%), constipation (3%), dyspepsia (2%), vomiting (2%), flatulence (1%)
Genitourinary: Vaginitis (1%)
Hematologic: Lymphopenia (2%)
Ocular (with ophthalmic solution use): Decreased vision (transient), foreign body sensation, transient ocular burning, ocular pain or discomfort, photophobia
Respiratory: Pharyngitis (4%), dyspnea (1%), rhinitis (1%), sinusitis (1%)

Overdosage/Toxicology Symptoms include acute renal failure and seizures. Treatment should include GI decontamination and supportive care. Not removed by peritoneal or hemodialysis.

Drug Interactions

Corticosteroids: Concurrent use may increase the risk of tendon rupture, particularly in elderly patients (overall incidence rare).

Glyburide: Quinolones may increase the effect of glyburide; monitor

Metal cations (aluminum, calcium, iron, magnesium, and zinc) bind quinolones in the gastrointestinal tract and inhibit absorption. Concurrent administration of most antacids, oral electrolyte supplements, quinapril, sucralfate, some didanosine formulations (pediatric powder for oral suspension), and other highly-buffered oral drugs, should be avoided. Levofloxacin should be administered 2 hours before or 2 hours after these agents.

NSAIDs: Risk of seizures may be increased with concomitant NSAID use. Risk is considered quite low and may only be a factor with high serum levels of either agent and/or in patients with additional predisposing factors (eg, renal dysfunction, history of seizure or other neurological disorder)

Probenecid: May decrease renal secretion of levofloxacin.

QT_c-prolonging agents: Effects may be additive with levofloxacin. Avoid concurrent use with Class Ia and Class III antiarrhythmics, erythromycin, cisapride, antipsychotics, and cyclic antidepressants.

Typhoid vaccine: Antibiotics may decrease the therapeutic effect of live, attenuated Ty21a vaccine; delay vaccination for >24 hours after administration of antibacterial agents.

Warfarin: The hypoprothrombinemic effect of warfarin may be enhanced by some quinolone antibiotics; monitor INR.

Stability

Solution for injection:

Vial: Store at room temperature. Protect from light. When diluted to 5 mg/mL in a compatible I.V. fluid, solution is stable for 72 hours when stored at room temperature; stable for 14 days when stored under refrigeration. When frozen, stable for 6 months; do not refreeze. Do not thaw in microwave or by bath immersion.

Premixed: Store at ≤25°C (77°F); do not freeze. Brief exposure to 40°C (104°F) does not affect product. Protect from light.

Tablet, oral solution: Store at 25°C (77°F); excursions permitted to 15°C to 25°C (59°F to 77°F).

Ophthalmic solution: Store at 15°C to 25°C (59°F to 77°F).

Mechanism of Action As the S (-) enantiomer of the fluoroquinolone, ofloxacin, levofloxacin, inhibits DNA-gyrase in susceptible organisms thereby inhibits relaxation of supercoiled DNA and promotes breakage of DNA strands. DNA gyrase (topoisomerase II), is an essential bacterial enzyme that maintains the superhelical structure of DNA and is required for DNA replication and transcription, DNA repair, recombination, and transposition.

Pharmacokinetics

Absorption: Well absorbed

Distribution: V_d: 1.25 L/kg; CSF concentrations ~15% of serum concentrations; high concentrations are achieved in prostate and gynecological tissues, sinus, breast milk, and saliva

Protein binding: 50%

Metabolism: Minimally hepatic

Bioavailability: 100%

Half-life: 6 hours

Time to peak, serum: 1 hour

Elimination: Primarily urine (as unchanged drug)

Dosage

Geriatrics & Adults: Note: Sequential therapy (intravenous to oral) may be instituted based on prescriber's discretion.

Anthrax (inhalational): 500 mg every 24 hours for 60 days, beginning as soon as possible after exposure

Chronic bronchitis (acute bacterial exacerbation): Oral, I.V.: 500 mg every 24 hours for at least 7 days

Conjunctivitis (0.5% ophthalmic solution): Ophthalmic:

Treatment day 1 and day 2: Instill 1-2 drops into affected eye(s) every 2 hours while awake, up to 8 times/day

Treatment day 3 through day 7: Instill 1-2 drops into affected eye(s) every 4 hours while awake, up to 4 times/day

Corneal ulceration (1.5% ophthalmic solution): Ophthalmic: Treatment day 1 through day 3: Instill 1-2 drops into affected eye(s) every 30 minutes to 2 hours while awake and 4-6 hours after retiring.

Diverticulitis, peritonitis (unlabeled use): Oral, I.V.: 750 mg every 24 hours for 7-10 days; use adjunctive metronidazole therapy

(Continued)

Levofloxacin *(Continued)*

Dysenteric enterocolitis, *Shigella spp.* (unlabeled use): Oral, I.V.: 500 mg every 24 hours for 3-5 days

Epididymitis, nongonococcal (unlabeled use): 500 mg once daily for 10 days

Gonococcal infection (unlabeled use): Oral, I.V.:

Cervicitis, urethritis: 250 mg for one dose with azithromycin or doxycycline; **Note:** As of April 2007, the CDC no longer recommends the use of fluoroquinolones for the treatment of uncomplicated gonococcal disease.

Disseminated infection: 250 mg I.V. once daily; 24 hours after symptoms improve may change to 500 mg orally every 24 hours to complete total therapy of 7 days; **Note:** As of April 2007, the CDC no longer recommends the use of fluoroquinolones for the treatment of more serious gonococcal disease, unless no other options exist and susceptibility can be confirmed via culture.

Pelvic inflammatory disease (unlabeled use): 500 mg once daily for 14 days with or without adjunctive metronidazole; **Note:** The CDC recommends use only if standard cephalosporin therapy is not feasible and community prevalence of quinolone-resistant gonococcal organisms is low. Culture sensitivity must be confirmed.

Pneumonia: Oral, I.V.:

Community-acquired: 500 mg every 24 hours for 7-14 days or 750 mg every 24 hours for 5 days (efficacy of 5-day regimen for MDRSP not established)

Nosocomial: 750 mg every 24 hours for 7-14 days

Prostatitis (chronic bacterial): Oral, I.V.: 500 mg every 24 hours for 28 days

Sinusitis (acute bacterial): Oral, I.V.: 500 mg every 24 hours for 10-14 days or 750 mg every 24 hours for 5 days

Skin and skin structure infections: Oral, I.V.:

Uncomplicated: 500 mg every 24 hours for 7-10 days

Complicated: 750 mg every 24 hours for 7-14 days

Traveler's diarrhea (unlabeled use): Oral, I.V.: 500 mg for one dose

Urinary tract infections: Oral, I.V.:

Uncomplicated: 250 mg once daily for 3 days

Complicated, including acute pyelonephritis: 250 mg every 24 hours for 10 days

Renal Impairment:

Chronic bronchitis, acute bacterial sinusitis, uncomplicated skin infection, community-acquired pneumonia, chronic bacterial prostatitis, or inhalational anthrax: Initial: 500 mg, then as follows:

Cl_{cr} 20-49 mL/minute: 250 mg every 24 hours

Cl_{cr} 10-19 mL/minute: 250 mg every 48 hours

Hemodialysis/CAPD: 250 mg every 48 hours

Uncomplicated UTI: No dosage adjustment required

Complicated UTI, acute pyelonephritis: Cl_{cr} 10-19 mL/minute: 250 mg every 48 hours

Complicated skin infection, acute bacterial sinusitis, community-acquired pneumonia, or nosocomial pneumonia: Initial: 750 mg, then as follows:

Cl_{cr} 20-49 mL/minute: 750 mg every 48 hours

Cl_{cr} 10-19 mL/minute: 500 mg every 48 hours

Hemodialysis/CAPD: 500 mg every 48 hours

Administration

Oral: Tablets may be administered without regard to meals. Oral solution should be administered 1 hour before or 2 hours after meals.

I.V.: Infuse 250-500 mg I.V. solution over 60 minutes; infuse 750 mg I.V. solution over 90 minutes. Too rapid of infusion can lead to hypotension. Avoid administration through an intravenous line with a solution containing multivalent cations (eg, magnesium, calcium).

Monitoring Parameters Evaluation of organ system functions (renal, hepatic, ophthalmologic, and hematopoietic) is recommended periodically during therapy; the possibility of crystalluria should be assessed; WBC and signs of infection

Test Interactions Some quinolones may produce a false-positive urine screening result for opiates using commercially-available immunoassay kits. This has been demonstrated most consistently for levofloxacin and ofloxacin, but other quinolones have shown cross-reactivity in certain assay kits. Confirmation of positive opiate screens by more specific methods should be considered.

Patient Information

Oral: Take per recommended schedule, preferably on an empty stomach (1 hour before or 2 hours after meals). Maintain adequate hydration (2-3 L/day of fluids unless instructed to restrict fluid intake). Take complete prescription; do not skip doses. Do not take with antacids; separate by 2 hours. Insomnia may occur; take early in the day to lessen sleep disturbances. You may experience dizziness, lightheadedness, or confusion; use caution when driving or engaging in tasks that require alertness until response to drug is known. Small frequent meals and frequent mouth care may reduce nausea or vomiting. You may experience photosensitivity; use sunscreen, wear protective clothing and eyewear, and avoid direct sunlight. Report palpitations or chest pain, persistent diarrhea, GI disturbances or abdominal pain, muscle tremor or pain, yellowing of eyes or skin, easy bruising or bleeding, unusual fatigue, fever, chills, signs of infection, or worsening of condition. Report immediately any rash, itching, unusual CNS changes, or any facial swelling. Report immediately any pain, inflammation, or rupture of tendon.

Ophthalmic: Wash hands before instilling solution. Sit or lie down to instill. Open eye, look at ceiling, and instill prescribed amount of solution. Close eye and roll eye in all directions, and apply gentle pressure to inner corner of eye. Do not let tip of applicator touch eye or contaminate tip of applicator. Temporary stinging or blurred vision may occur. Report persistent pain, burning, vision disturbances, swelling, itching, or worsening of condition. Discontinue medication and contact prescriber immediately if you develop a rash or allergic reaction. Do not wear contact lenses.

Special Geriatric Considerations The risk of torsade de pointes and tendon inflammation and/or rupture associated with the concomitant use of corticosteroids and quinolones is increased in the elderly population. Adjust dose for renal function.

Dosage Forms Excipient information presented when available (limited, particularly for generics); consult specific product labeling.

Infusion [premixed in D$_5$W] (Levaquin®): 250 mg (50 mL); 500 mg (100 mL); 750 mg (150 mL)

Injection, solution [preservative free] (Levaquin®): 25 mg/mL (20 mL, 30 mL)

Solution, ophthalmic:

Iquix®: 1.5% (5 mL)

Quixin™: 0.5% (5 mL) [contains benzalkonium chloride]

Solution, oral (Levaquin®): 25 mg/mL (480 mL) [contains benzyl alcohol]

Tablet (Levaquin®): 250 mg, 500 mg, 750 mg

Levaquin® Leva-Pak: 750 mg (5s)

Selected References

Nicolle LN, Bradley S, Colgan R et al, "Infectious Disease Society of America Guidelines for the Diagnosis and Treatment of Asymptomatic Bacteriuria in Adults," *Clinical Infectious Diseases*, 2005, 40:643-54.

Levorphanol (lee VOR fa nole)

Related Information
Narcotic / Opioid Analgesics *on page 1763*
U.S. Brand Names Levo-Dromoran®
Index Terms Levorphanol Tartrate; Levorphan Tartrate
Generic Available Yes: Tablet
Pharmacologic Category Analgesic, Opioid
Use Relief of moderate to severe pain; preoperative sedation (parenteral); adjunct to nitrous oxide/oxygen anesthesia
Restrictions C-II
Contraindications Hypersensitivity to levorphanol or any component of the formulation
Warnings/Precautions An opioid-containing analgesic regimen should be tailored to each patient's needs and based upon the type of pain being treated (acute versus chronic), the route of administration, degree of tolerance for opioids (naive versus chronic user), age, weight, and medical condition. The optimal analgesic dose varies widely among patients. Doses should be titrated to pain relief/prevention.

May cause CNS depression, which may impair physical or mental abilities; patients must be cautioned about performing tasks which require mental alertness (eg, operating machinery or driving). Effects may be potentiated when used with other sedative drugs or ethanol. Use with caution in patients with hypersensitivity reactions to other phenanthrene derivative opioid agonists (morphine, hydrocodone, hydromorphone, oxycodone, oxymorphone); respiratory diseases including asthma, emphysema, COPD, hypothyroidism, head trauma, morbid obesity, adrenal insufficiency, prostatic hyperplasia/urinary stricture, or severe liver or renal insufficiency; some preparations contain sulfites which may cause allergic reactions; tolerance or dependence may result from extended use. Use with caution in patients with biliary tract dysfunction; acute pancreatitis may cause constriction of sphincter of Oddi. May cause hypotension; use with caution in patients with depleted blood volume or drugs which may exaggerate hypotensive effects (including phenothiazines or general anesthetics). May obscure diagnosis or clinical course of patients with acute abdominal conditions. Concurrent use of agonist/antagonist analgesics may precipitate withdrawal symptoms and/or reduced analgesic efficacy in patients following prolonged therapy with mu opioid agonists. Abrupt discontinuation following prolonged use may also lead to withdrawal symptoms. Elderly and debilitated patients may be particularly susceptible to the adverse of narcotics.

Adverse Reactions (Reflective of adult population; not specific for elderly)
Frequency not defined.
Cardiovascular: Palpitation, hypotension, bradycardia, peripheral vasodilation, cardiac arrest, shock, tachycardia
(Continued)

Levorphanol *(Continued)*

Central nervous system: CNS depression, fatigue, drowsiness, dizziness, nervousness, headache, restlessness, anorexia, malaise, confusion, coma, convulsion, insomnia, amnesia, mental depression, hallucinations, paradoxical CNS stimulation, intracranial pressure (increased)

Dermatologic: Pruritus, urticaria, rash

Endocrine & metabolic: Antidiuretic hormone release

Gastrointestinal: Nausea, vomiting, dyspepsia, stomach cramps, xerostomia, constipation, abdominal pain, dry mouth, biliary tract spasm, paralytic ileus

Genitourinary: Decreased urination, urinary tract spasm, urinary retention

Local: Pain at injection site

Neuromuscular & skeletal: Weakness

Ocular: Miosis, diplopia

Respiratory: Respiratory depression, apnea, hypoventilation, cyanosis

Miscellaneous: Histamine release, physical and psychological dependence

Overdosage/Toxicology Symptoms include CNS depression, respiratory depression, miosis, apnea, pulmonary edema, and convulsions. Treatment includes naloxone 2 mg I.V., with repeat administration as necessary, up to a total of 10 mg.

Drug Interactions Increased toxicity: CNS depressants increase CNS depression

Ethanol/Nutrition/Herb Interactions

Ethanol: Avoid or limit ethanol (may increase CNS depression). Watch for sedation.

Herb/Nutraceutical: Avoid valerian, St John's wort, kava kava, gotu kola (may increase CNS depression).

Stability Store at room temperature; do not freeze.

Mechanism of Action Levorphanol tartrate is a synthetic opioid agonist that is classified as a morphinan derivative. Opioids interact with stereospecific opioid receptors in various parts of the central nervous system and other tissues. Analgesic potency parallels the affinity for these binding sites. These drugs do not alter the threshold or responsiveness to pain, but the perception of pain.

Pharmacodynamics

Onset of action: Oral: 10-60 minutes

Duration: 6-8 hours; enhanced analgesia has been seen in older adult patients on therapeutic dose of narcotics; duration of action may be increased in older adults

Pharmacokinetics

Metabolism: In the liver

Half-life: 11 hours

Elimination: In urine as glucuronide

Dosage

Geriatrics & Adults: Note: These are guidelines and do not represent the maximum doses that may be required in all patients. Doses should be titrated to pain relief/prevention.

Acute pain (moderate to severe):

Oral: Initial: Opiate-naive: 2 mg every 6-8 hours as needed; patients with prior opiate exposure may require higher initial doses; usual dosage range: 2-4 mg every 6-8 hours as needed

I.M., SubQ: Initial: Opiate-naive: 1 mg every 6-8 hours as needed; patients with prior opiate exposure may require higher initial doses; usual dosage range: 1-2 mg every 6-8 hours as needed

I.V. (slow): Initial: Opiate-naive: Up to 1 mg/dose every 3-6 hours as needed; patients with prior opiate exposure may require higher initial doses

Chronic pain: Patients taking opioids chronically may become tolerant and require doses higher than the usual dosage range to maintain the desired effect. Tolerance can be managed by appropriate dose titration. **There is no optimal or maximal dose for levorphanol in chronic pain. The appropriate dose is one that relieves pain throughout its dosing interval without causing unmanageable side effects.**

Premedication: I.M., SubQ: 1-2 mg/dose 60-90 minutes prior to surgery; older or debilitated patients usually require less drug

Hepatic Impairment: Reduce dose in patients with liver disease.

Monitoring Parameters Pain relief, respiratory and mental status, blood pressure

Patient Information May cause drowsiness; avoid alcoholic beverages

Additional Information 2 mg levorphanol I.M. produces analgesia comparable to that produced by 10 mg of morphine I.M.

Special Geriatric Considerations The elderly may be particularly susceptible to the CNS depressant and constipating effects of narcotics.

Dosage Forms Excipient information presented when available (limited, particularly for generics); consult specific product labeling.

Injection, solution, as tartrate: 2 mg/mL (1 mL, 10 mL)

Tablet, as tartrate: 2 mg

Selected References
AGS Panel on Persistent Pain in Older Persons, "The Management of Persistent Pain in Older Persons," *J Am Geriatr Soc*, 2002, 50(6 Suppl):S205-24.

♦ **Levorphanol Tartrate** *see* Levorphanol *on page 899*
♦ **Levorphan Tartrate** *see* Levorphanol *on page 899*
♦ **Levothroid®** *see* Levothyroxine *on page 901*

Levothyroxine (lee voe thye ROKS een)

Medication Safety Issues
Sound-alike/look-alike issues:
  Levothyroxine may be confused with liothyronine
  Levoxyl® may be confused with Lanoxin®, Luvox®
  Synthroid® may be confused with Symmetrel®

To avoid errors due to misinterpretation of a decimal point, always express dosage in mcg (**not** mg).

Significant differences exist between oral and I.V. dosing. Use caution when converting from one route of administration to another.

U.S. Brand Names Levothroid®; Levoxyl®; Synthroid®; Unithroid®

Canadian Brand Names Eltroxin®; Gen-Levothyroxine; Levothyroxine Sodium; Synthroid®

Index Terms Levothyroxine Sodium; *L*-Thyroxine Sodium; T_4

Generic Available Yes

Pharmacologic Category Thyroid Product

Use Replacement or supplemental therapy in hypothyroidism; pituitary TSH suppression

Contraindications Hypersensitivity to levothyroxine sodium or any component of the formulation; recent MI or thyrotoxicosis; uncorrected adrenal insufficiency

Warnings/Precautions [U.S. Boxed Warning]: Ineffective and potentially toxic for weight reduction. High doses may produce serious or even life-threatening toxic effects particularly when used with some anorectic drugs. Use with caution and reduce dosage in patients with angina pectoris or other cardiovascular disease; use cautiously in elderly since they may be more likely to have compromised cardiovascular functions. Patients with adrenal insufficiency, myxedema, diabetes mellitus and insipidus may have symptoms exaggerated or aggravated. Chronic hypothyroidism predisposes patients to coronary artery disease. Levoxyl® may rapidly swell and disintegrate causing choking or gagging (should be administered with a full glass of water); use caution in patients with dysphagia or other swallowing disorders.

Adverse Reactions (Reflective of adult population; not specific for elderly)
Frequency not defined.
  Cardiovascular: Angina, arrhythmia, blood pressure increased, cardiac arrest, flushing, heart failure, MI, palpitation, pulse increased, tachycardia
  Central nervous system: Anxiety, emotional lability, fatigue, fever, headache, hyperactivity, insomnia, irritability, nervousness, pseudotumor cerebri (children), seizure (rare)
  Dermatologic: Alopecia
  Endocrine & metabolic: Fertility impaired, menstrual irregularities
  Gastrointestinal: Abdominal cramps, appetite increased, diarrhea, vomiting, weight loss
  Hepatic: Liver function tests increased
  Neuromuscular & skeletal: Bone mineral density decreased, muscle weakness, tremor, slipped capital femoral epiphysis (children)
  Respiratory: Dyspnea
  Miscellaneous: Diaphoresis, heat intolerance, hypersensitivity (to inactive ingredients, symptoms include urticaria, pruritus, rash, flushing, angioedema, GI symptoms, fever, arthralgia, serum sickness, wheezing)
  Levoxyl®: Choking, dysphagia, gagging

Overdosage/Toxicology Chronic overdose is treated by withdrawal of the drug. Massive overdose may require beta-blockers for increased sympathomimetic activity. Chronic overdose may cause hyperthyroidism, weight loss, nervousness, sweating, tachycardia, insomnia, heat intolerance, menstrual irregularities, palpitations, psychosis, and fever. Acute overdose may cause fever, hypoglycemia, CHF, and unrecognized adrenal insufficiency. Reduce the dose or temporarily discontinue therapy. The hypothalamic-pituitary-thyroid axis will return to normal in 6-8 weeks. Serum T_4 levels do not correlate well with toxicity. In massive acute ingestion, reduce GI absorption and administer general supportive care. Treat congestive heart failure with digitalis glycosides. Excessive adrenergic activity (tachycardia) requires propranolol 1-3 mg I.V. over 10 minutes or 80-160 mg orally/day. Fever may be treated with acetaminophen.

Drug Interactions Also refer to Additional Information.
(Continued)

Levothyroxine *(Continued)*

Aluminum- and magnesium-containing antacids, calcium carbonate, simethicone, or sucralfate: May decrease T_4 absorption; separate dose from levothyroxine by at least 4 hours.

Antidiabetic agents (biguanides, meglitinides, sulfonylureas, thiazolidinediones, insulin): Changes in thyroid function may alter requirements of antidiabetic agent. Monitor closely at initiation of therapy, or when dose is changed or discontinued.

Cholestyramine and colestipol: Decrease T_4 absorption; separate dose from levothyroxine by at least 2 hours.

Digoxin: Digoxin levels may be reduced in hyperthyroidism; therapeutic effect may be reduced. Impact of thyroid replacement should be monitored.

Estrogens: May decrease serum free thyroxine concentrations.

Imatinib: May decrease the effects of thyroid replacement therapy; monitor.

Iron: Decreases T_4 absorption; separate dose from levothyroxine by at least 4 hours.

Kayexalate®: Decreases T_4 absorption; separate dose from levothyroxine by at least 4 hours.

Ketamine: May cause marked hypertension and tachycardia; monitor.

Theophylline, caffeine: Decreased theophylline clearance in hypothyroid patients; monitor during thyroid replacement.

Tricyclic and tetracyclic antidepressants: Therapeutic and toxic effects of levothyroxine and the antidepressant are increased.

Warfarin (and other oral anticoagulants): The hypoprothrombinemic response to warfarin may be altered by a change in thyroid function or replacement. Replacement may dramatically increase response to warfarin. However, initiation of warfarin in a patient stabilized on a dose of levothyroxine does not appear to require a significantly different approach.

Ethanol/Nutrition/Herb Interactions Food: Taking levothyroxine with enteral nutrition may cause reduced bioavailability and may lower serum thyroxine levels leading to signs or symptoms of hypothyroidism. Limit intake of goitrogenic foods (eg, asparagus, cabbage, peas, turnip greens, broccoli, spinach, Brussels sprouts, lettuce, soybeans). Soybean flour, cottonseed meal, walnuts, and dietary fiber may decrease absorption of levothyroxine from the GI tract.

Stability

Tablet: Store at room temperature of 15°C to 30°C (59°F to 86°F). Protect from light and moisture.

Injection: Store at room temperature of 15°C to 30°C (59°F to 86°F). Dilute vials for injection with 5 mL normal saline and shake well. Reconstituted solutions should be used immediately and any unused portions discarded.

Mechanism of Action Exact mechanism of action is unknown; however, it is believed the thyroid hormone exerts its many metabolic effects through control of DNA transcription and protein synthesis; involved in normal metabolism, growth, and development; promotes gluconeogenesis, increases utilization and mobilization of glycogen stores, and stimulates protein synthesis, increases basal metabolic rate

Pharmacodynamics Onset of action:

Oral: Therapeutic effects require 3-5 days

I.V.: Within 6-8 hours, with maximum effect within 24 hours; 4-6 weeks may be required to see maximal effect for each dose

Pharmacokinetics

Absorption: Oral: Erratic, 48% to 79%; T_3 is 95% absorbed

Distribution: 80% of T_3 is derived from monodeiodination of T_4 in the periphery (liver, kidneys, other tissues)

Half-life: 6-7 days for T_4 and 1-2 days for T_3

Time to peak serum concentrations: Within 2-4 hours

Elimination: As conjugated forms in feces, bile

Dosage

Geriatrics: Doses should be adjusted based on clinical response and laboratory parameters.

Hypothyroidism:

Oral:

>50 years without cardiac disease **or** <50 years with cardiac disease: Initial: 25-50 mcg/day; adjust dose at 6- to 8-week intervals as needed

>50 years with cardiac disease: Initial: 12.5-25 mcg/day; adjust dose by 12.5-25 mcg increments at 4- to 6-week intervals. (**Note:** Many clinicians prefer to adjust at 6- to 8-week intervals.)

Note: Elderly patients may require <1 mcg/kg/day

I.M., I.V.: 50% of the oral dose

Myxedema coma: I.V.: Refer to adult dosing; lower doses may be needed

Adults: Doses should be adjusted based on clinical response and laboratory parameters.

Hypothyroidism:

Oral: 1.7 mcg/kg/day in otherwise healthy adults <50 years old and older adults who have been recently treated for hyperthyroidism or who have been hypothyroid for only a few months. Titrate dosage every 6 weeks. Average starting dose ~100 mcg; usual doses are ≤200 mcg/day; doses ≥300 mcg/day are rare (consider poor compliance, malabsorption, and/or drug interactions). **Note:** For patients >50 years or patients with cardiac disease, refer to geriatric dosing.

I.M., I.V.: 50% of the oral dose

Severe hypothyroidism: Oral: Initial: 12.5-25 mcg/day; adjust dose by 25 mcg/day every 2-4 weeks as appropriate

Subclinical hypothyroidism (if treated): Oral: 1 mcg/kg/day

TSH suppression: Oral:

Well-differentiated thyroid cancer: Highly individualized; Doses >2 mcg/kg/day may be needed to suppress TSH to <0.1 mU/L.

Benign nodules and nontoxic multinodular goiter: Goal TSH suppression: 0.1-0.3 mU/L

Myxedema coma or stupor: I.V.: 200-500 mcg, then 100-300 mcg the next day if necessary; smaller doses should be considered in patients with cardiovascular disease

Administration

Oral: Administer in the morning on an empty stomach, at least 30 minutes before food. Tablets may be crushed and suspended in 1-2 teaspoonfuls of water; suspension should be used immediately.

Parenteral: Dilute vial with 5 mL normal saline; use immediately after reconstitution; should not be admixed with other solutions

Monitoring Parameters Thyroid function test (serum thyroxine, thyrotropin concentrations), resin triiodothyronine uptake (RT_3U), free thyroxine index (FTI), T_4, TSH, heart rate, blood pressure, clinical signs of hypo- and hyperthyroidism. TSH is the most reliable guide for evaluating adequacy of thyroid replacement dosage. TSH may be elevated during the first few months of thyroid replacement despite being clinically euthyroid. In cases where T_4 remains low and TSH is within normal limits, an evaluation of "free" (unbound) T_4 is needed to evaluate further dosage increase.

Reference Range

TSH: 0.4-10 (for those ≥80 years) mIU/L

T_4: 4-12 mcg/dL (SI: 51-154 nmol/L)

T_3 (RIA) (total T_3): 80-230 ng/dL (SI: 1.2-3.5 nmol/L)

T_4 free (Free T_4): 0.7-1.8 ng/dL (SI: 9-23 pmol/L)

Test Interactions Many drugs may have effects on thyroid function tests (see Additional Information). Infectious hepatitis and acute intermittent porphyria may increase TBG concentrations; nephrosis, severe hypoproteinemia, severe liver disease, and acromegaly may decrease TBG concentrations.

Patient Information Do not change brands without physician's knowledge; report immediately to physician any chest pain, increased pulse, palpitations, heat intolerance, excessive sweating; do not stop use without physician's advice; replacement therapy will be for life; take as a single dose before breakfast

Additional Information Levothroid® tablets contain lactose; use caution when interchanging brands, they may not be equally effective.

Equivalent doses: Thyroid USP 60 mg ~ levothyroxine 0.05-0.06 mg ~ liothyronine 0.015-0.0375 mg

50-60 mg thyroid ~ 50-60 mcg levothyroxine and 12.5-15 mcg liothyronine Liotrix®

Note: Several medications have effects on thyroid production or conversion. The impact in thyroid replacement has not been specifically evaluated, but patient response should be monitored:

Methimazole: Decreases thyroid hormone secretion, while propylthiouracil decrease thyroid hormone secretion and decreases conversion of T_4 to T_3.

Beta-adrenergic antagonists: Decrease conversion of T_4 to T_3 (dose related, propranolol ≥160 mg/day); patients may be clinically euthyroid.

Iodide, iodine-containing radiographic contrast agents may decrease thyroid hormone secretion; may also increase thyroid hormone secretion, especially in patients with Graves' disease.

Other agents reported to impact on thyroid production/conversion include aminoglutethimide, amiodarone, chloral hydrate, diazepam, ethionamide, interferon-alpha, interleukin-2, lithium, lovastatin (case report), glucocorticoids (dose-related), 6-mercaptopurine, sulfonamides, thiazide diuretics, and tolbutamide.

In addition, a number of medications have been noted to cause transient depression in TSH secretion, which may complicate interpretation of monitoring tests for levothyroxine, including corticosteroids, octreotide, and dopamine. Metoclopramide may increase TSH secretion.

Special Geriatric Considerations Elderly do not have a change in serum thyroxine associated with aging; however, plasma T_3 concentrations are decreased 25% to 40% in the elderly. There is not a compensatory rise in thyrotropin suggesting that lower T_3 (Continued)

Levothyroxine *(Continued)*

is not reacted upon as a deficiency by the pituitary. This indicates a slightly lower than normal dosage of thyroid hormone replacement is usually sufficient in elderly patients than in younger adult patients. TSH must be monitored since insufficient thyroid replacement (elevated TSH) is a risk for coronary artery disease and excessive replacement (low TSH) may cause signs of hyperthyroidism and excessive bone loss. Some clinicians suggest levothyroxine is the drug of choice for replacement therapy.

Dosage Forms Excipient information presented when available (limited, particularly for generics); consult specific product labeling.

Injection, powder for reconstitution, as sodium: 0.2 mg, 0.5 mg

Tablet, as sodium: 25 mcg, 50 mcg, 75 mcg, 88 mcg, 100 mcg, 112 mcg, 125 mcg, 137 mcg, 150 mcg, 175 mcg, 200 mcg, 300 mcg

Levothroid®: 25 mcg, 50 mcg, 75 mcg, 88 mcg, 100 mcg, 112 mcg, 125 mcg, 150 mcg, 175 mcg, 200 mcg, 300 mcg

Levoxyl®: 25 mcg, 50 mcg, 75 mcg, 88 mcg, 100 mcg, 112 mcg, 125 mcg, 137 mcg, 150 mcg, 175 mcg, 200 mcg; 300 mcg [DSC]

Synthroid®: 25 mcg, 50 mcg, 75 mcg, 88 mcg, 100 mcg, 112 mcg, 125 mcg, 137 mcg, 150 mcg, 175 mcg, 200 mcg, 300 mcg

Unithroid®: 25 mcg, 50 mcg, 75 mcg, 88 mcg, 100 mcg, 112 mcg, 125 mcg, 150 mcg, 175 mcg, 200 mcg, 300 mcg

Selected References

de Groot JW, Zonnenberg BA, Plukker JT, et al, "Imatinib Induces Hypothyroidism in Patients Receiving Levothyroxine," *Clin Pharmacol Ther*, 2005, 78(4):433-8.

Helfand M and Crapo LM, "Monitoring Therapy in Patients Taking Levothyroxine," *Ann Intern Med*, 1990, 113(6):450-4.

Johnson DG and Campbell S, "Hormonal and Metabolic Agents," *Geriatric Pharmacology*, Bressler R and Katz MD, eds, New York, NY: McGraw-Hill, 1993, 427-50.

Sanders LR, "Pituitary, Thyroid, Adrenal and Parathyroid Diseases in the Elderly," *Geriatric Medicine*, 1990, 475-87.

Sawin CT, Geller A, Hershman JM, et al, "The Aging Thyroid. The Use of Thyroid Hormone in Older Persons," *JAMA*, 1989, 261(18):2653-5.

Watts NB, "Use of a Sensitive Thyrotropin Assay for Monitoring Treatment With Levothyroxine," *Arch Intern Med*, 1989, 149(2):309-12.

www.synthroid.com, Drug Interactions Chart, August 17, 2000.

Lidocaine *(LYE doe kane)*

Related Information

Serum Drug Concentrations Commonly Monitored Guidelines *on page 1862*

Medication Safety Issues

High alert medication: The Institute for Safe Medication Practices (ISMP) includes this medication (I.V. formulation) among its list of drugs which have a heightened risk of causing significant patient harm when used in error.

Transdermal patch may contain conducting metal (eg, aluminum); remove patch prior to MRI.

International issues:

Lidpen® may be confused with Linoten® which is a brand name for pamidronate in Spain

U.S. Brand Names Anestacon®; Band-Aid® Hurt-Free™ Antiseptic Wash [OTC]; Burnamycin [OTC]; Burn Jel [OTC]; Burn-O-Jel [OTC]; LidaMantle®; Lidoderm®; L-M-X™ 4 [OTC]; L-M-X™ 5 [OTC]; LTA® 360; Premjact® [OTC]; Solarcaine® Aloe Extra Burn Relief [OTC]; Topicaine® [OTC]; Xylocaine®; Xylocaine® MPF; Xylocaine® Viscous; Zilactin-L® [OTC]

Canadian Brand Names Betacaine®; Lidodan™; Lidoderm®; Xylocaine®; Xylocard®; Zilactin®

Index Terms Lidocaine Hydrochloride; Lignocaine Hydrochloride

Generic Available Yes: Cream, infusion, injection, jelly, lotion, ointment, solution

Pharmacologic Category Analgesic, Topical; Antiarrhythmic Agent, Class Ib; Local Anesthetic

Use Local anesthetic and acute treatment of ventricular arrhythmias from myocardial infarction, or cardiac manipulation

Rectal: Temporary relief of pain and itching due to anorectal disorders

Topical: Local anesthetic for use in laser, cosmetic, and outpatient surgeries; minor burns, cuts, and abrasions of the skin

Lidoderm® Patch: Relief of allodynia (painful hypersensitivity) and chronic pain in postherpetic neuralgia

Unlabeled/Investigational Use ACLS guidelines (not considered drug of choice): Stable monomorphic VT (preserved ventricular function), polymorphic VT (preserved ventricular function), drug-induced monomorphic VT

Contraindications Hypersensitivity to lidocaine or any component of the formulation; hypersensitivity to another local anesthetic of the amide type; Adam-Stokes syndrome; severe degrees of SA, AV, or intraventricular heart block (except in patients with a functioning artificial pacemaker); premixed injection may contain corn-derived dextrose and its use is contraindicated in patients with allergy to corn-related products

Warnings/Precautions

Intravenous: Constant ECG monitoring is necessary during I.V. administration. Use cautiously in hepatic impairment, any degree of heart block, Wolff-Parkinson-White syndrome, CHF, marked hypoxia, severe respiratory depression, hypovolemia, history of malignant hyperthermia, or shock. Increased ventricular rate may be seen when administered to a patient with atrial fibrillation. Correct electrolyte disturbances, especially hypokalemia or hypomagnesemia, prior to use and throughout therapy. Correct any underlying causes of ventricular arrhythmias. Monitor closely for signs and symptoms of CNS toxicity. The elderly may be prone to increased CNS and cardiovascular side effects. Reduce dose in hepatic dysfunction and CHF.

Injectable anesthetic: Follow appropriate administration techniques so as not to administer any intravascularly. Solutions containing antimicrobial preservatives should not be used for epidural or spinal anesthesia. Some solutions contain a bisulfite; avoid in patients who are allergic to bisulfite. Resuscitative equipment, medicine and oxygen should be available in case of emergency. Use products containing epinephrine cautiously in patients with significant vascular disease, compromised blood flow, or during or following general anesthesia (increased risk of arrhythmias). Adjust the dose for the elderly, acutely ill, and debilitated patients.

Topical: Do not leave on large body areas for >2 hours. Potentially life threatening side effects (eg, irregular heart beat, seizures, coma, respiratory depression, death) have occurred when used prior to cosmetic procedures. Observe young children closely to prevent accidental ingestion. Not for use ophthalmic use or for use on mucous membranes.

Adverse Reactions (Reflective of adult population; not specific for elderly)
Effects vary with route of administration. Many effects are dose related.
Frequency not defined.

Cardiovascular: Arrhythmia, bradycardia, arterial spasms, cardiovascular collapse, defibrillator threshold increased, edema, flushing, heart block, hypotension, sinus node supression, vascular insufficiency (periarticular injections)

Central nervous system: Agitation, anxiety, apprehension, coma, confusion, disorientation, dizziness, drowsiness, euphoria, hallucinations, headache, hyperesthesia, hypoesthesia, lethargy, lightheadedness, nervousness, psychosis, seizure, slurred speech, somnolence, unconsciousness

Dermatologic: Angioedema, bruising (transdermal system), contact dermatitis, depigmentation (transdermal system), edema of the skin, itching, petechia (transdermal system), pruritus, rash, urticaria

Gastrointestinal: Metallic taste, nausea, vomiting

Local: Irritation (transdermal system), thrombophlebitis

Neuromuscular & skeletal: Pain exacerbation (transdermal system), paresthesia, transient radicular pain (subarachnoid administration; up to 1.9%), tremor, twitching, weakness

Ocular: Diplopia, visual changes

Otic: Tinnitus

Respiratory: Bronchospasm, dyspnea, respiratory depression or arrest

Miscellaneous: Allergic reactions, anaphylactoid reaction, sensitivity to temperature extremes

Following spinal anesthesia positional headache (3%), shivering (2%) nausea, peripheral nerve symptoms, respiratory inadequacy and double vision (<1%), hypotension, cauda equina syndrome

(Continued)

Lidocaine *(Continued)*

Overdosage/Toxicology Has a narrow therapeutic index and severe toxicity may occur slightly above the therapeutic range, especially with other antiarrhythmic drugs. Symptoms include sedation, confusion, coma, seizures, respiratory arrest and cardiac toxicity (sinus arrest, AV block, asystole, and hypotension). The QRS and QT intervals are usually normal, although they may be prolonged after massive overdose. Other effects include dizziness, paresthesias, tremor, ataxia, and GI disturbance. Treatment is supportive, using conventional therapies (fluids, positioning, vasopressors, antiarrhythmics, anticonvulsants). Sodium bicarbonate may reverse QRS prolongation, bradyarrhythmias and hypotension. Enhanced elimination with dialysis, hemoperfusion or repeat charcoal is not effective.

Drug Interactions Substrate of CYP1A2 (minor), 2A6 (minor), 2B6 (minor), 2C9 (minor), 2D6 (major), 3A4 (major); **Inhibits** CYP1A2 (strong), 2D6 (moderate), 3A4 (moderate)

Cimetidine increases lidocaine blood levels; monitor levels or use an alternative H_2 antagonist.

CYP1A2 substrates: Lidocaine may increase the levels/effects of CYP1A2 substrates. Example substrates include aminophylline, fluvoxamine, mexiletine, mirtazapine, ropinirole, theophylline, and trifluoperazine.

CYP2D6 inhibitors: May increase the levels/effects of lidocaine. Example inhibitors include chlorpromazine, delavirdine, fluoxetine, miconazole, paroxetine, pergolide, quinidine, quinine, ritonavir, and ropinirole.

CYP2D6 substrates: Lidocaine may increase the levels/effects of CYP2D6 substrates. Example substrates include amphetamines, selected beta-blockers, dextromethorphan, fluoxetine, mirtazapine, nefazodone, paroxetine, risperidone, ritonavir, thioridazine, tricyclic antidepressants, and venlafaxine.

CYP2D6 prodrug substrates: Lidocaine may decrease the levels/effects of CYP2D6 prodrug substrates. Example prodrug substrates include codeine, hydrocodone, oxycodone, and tramadol.

CYP3A4 inducers: CYP3A4 inducers may decrease the levels/effects of lidocaine. Example inducers include aminoglutethimide, carbamazepine, nafcillin, nevirapine, phenobarbital, phenytoin, and rifamycins.

CYP3A4 inhibitors: May increase the levels/effects of lidocaine. Example inhibitors include amiodarone (doses >400 mg/day), azole antifungals, clarithromycin, diclofenac, doxycycline, erythromycin, imatinib, isoniazid, nefazodone, nicardipine, propofol, protease inhibitors, quinidine, telithromycin, and verapamil.

CYP3A4 substrates: Lidocaine may increase the levels/effects of CYP3A4 substrates. Example substrates include benzodiazepines, calcium channel blockers, cyclosporine, mirtazapine, nateglinide, nefazodone, sildenafil (and other PDE-5 inhibitors), tacrolimus, and venlafaxine. Selected benzodiazepines (midazolam and triazolam), cisapride, ergot alkaloids, selected HMG-CoA reductase inhibitors (lovastatin and simvastatin), and pimozide are generally contraindicated with strong CYP3A4 inhibitors.

Propranolol: Increases lidocaine blood levels.

Protease inhibitors (eg, amprenavir, ritonavir): May increase lidocaine blood levels.

Ethanol/Nutrition/Herb Interactions Herb/Nutraceutical: St John's wort may decrease lidocaine levels; avoid concurrent use.

Stability Lidocaine injection is stable at room temperature. Stability of parenteral admixture at room temperature (25°C) is the expiration date on premixed bag; out of overwrap stability is 30 days.

Standard diluent: 2 g/250 mL D_5W.

Mechanism of Action Class Ib antiarrhythmic; suppresses automaticity of conduction tissue, by increasing electrical stimulation threshold of ventricle, His-Purkinje system, and spontaneous depolarization of the ventricles during diastole by a direct action on the tissues; blocks both the initiation and conduction of nerve impulses by decreasing the neuronal membrane's permeability to sodium ions, which results in inhibition of depolarization with resultant blockade of conduction

Pharmacodynamics

Onset of action (single bolus dose): 45-90 seconds

Duration: 10-20 minutes

Pharmacokinetics

Distribution: V_d alterable by many patient factors, decreased in congestive heart failure and liver disease

Protein binding: 60% to 80%; binds to alpha$_1$-acid glycoprotein

Metabolism: 90% metabolized in liver; active metabolites monoethylglycinexylidide (MEGX) and glycinexylidide (GX) can accumulate and may cause CNS toxicity

Half-life: Biphasic:

Alpha: 7-30 minutes

Beta: Terminal: Adults: 1.5-2 hours

Dosage
Geriatrics & Adults:
Antiarrhythmic:

I.V.: 1-1.5 mg/kg bolus over 2-3 minutes; may repeat doses of 0.5-0.75 mg/kg in 5-10 minutes up to a total of 3 mg/kg; continuous infusion: 1-4 mg/minute

Ventricular fibrillation or pulseless ventricular tachycardia (after defibrillation, CPR, and vasopressor administration): I.V.: Initial: 1-1.5 mg/kg. Refractory ventricular tachycardia or ventricular fibrillation, a repeat 0.5-0.75 mg/kg bolus may be given every 5-10 minutes after initial dose for a maximum of 3 doses. Total dose should not exceed 3 mg/kg. Follow with continuous infusion (1-4 mg/minute) after return of perfusion. Reappearance of arrhythmia during constant infusion: 0.5 mg/kg bolus and reassessment of infusion.

E.T. (loading dose only): 2-2.5 times the I.V. dose

Note: Decrease dose in patients with CHF, shock, or hepatic disease.

Anesthetic, topical:
Cream:

LidaMantle®: Skin irritation: Apply to affected area 2-3 times/day as needed

L-M-X™ 4: Apply ¼ inch thick layer to intact skin. Leave on until adequate anesthetic effect is obtained. Remove cream and cleanse area before beginning procedure.

L-M-X™ 5: Relief of anorectal pain and itching: Rectal: Apply topically to clean, dry area **or** using applicator, insert rectally, up to 6 times/day

Gel, ointment, solution: Apply to affected area ≤3 times/day as needed (maximum dose: 4.5 mg/kg, not to exceed 300 mg)

Jelly: Maximum dose: 30 mL (600 mg) in any 12-hour period:

Anesthesia of male urethra: 5-30 mL (100-600 mg)

Anesthesia of female urethra: 3-5 mL (60-100 mg)

Lubrication of endotracheal tube: Apply a moderate amount to external surface only

Liquid: Cold sores and fever blisters: Apply to affected area every 6 hours as needed

Patch: Postherpetic neuralgia: Apply patch to most painful area. Up to 3 patches may be applied in a single application. Patch may remain in place for up to 12 hours in any 24-hour period.

Anesthetic, local injectable: Varies with procedure, degree of anesthesia needed, vascularity of tissue, duration of anesthesia required, and physical condition of patient; maximum: 4.5 mg/kg/dose; do not repeat within 2 hours.

Renal Impairment: Not dialyzable (0% to 5%) by hemo- or peritoneal dialysis; supplemental dose is not necessary.

Hepatic Impairment: Reduce dose in acute hepatitis and decompensated cirrhosis by 50%.

Administration

Intratracheal: Dilute in NS or distilled water. Absorption is greater with distilled water, but causes more adverse effects on PaO_2. Pass catheter beyond tip of tracheal tube, stop compressions, spray drug quickly down tube. Follow immediately with several quick insufflations and continue chest compressions.

I.V.: Use microdrip (60 gtt/mL) or infusion pump to administer an accurate dose; local thrombophlebitis may occur in patients receiving prolonged I.V. infusions

Infusion rates: 2 g/250 mL D_5W (infusion pump should be used):

1 mg/minute: 7.5 mL/hour

2 mg/minute: 15 mL/hour

3 mg/minute: 22.5 mL/hour

4 mg/minute: 30 mL/hour

Buffered lidocaine for injectable local anesthetic: Add 2 mL of sodium bicarbonate 8.4% to 18 mL of lidocaine 1%

Topical:

Gel (Topicaine®): Avoid mucous membranes; remove prior to laser treatment.

Patch: May be cut to appropriate size; remove immediately if burning sensation occurs; wash hands after application

Monitoring Parameters EKG, blood pressure, pulse, paresthesias

Reference Range Therapeutic: 1.5-4.0 mcg/mL (SI: 6.4-17.1 µmol/L), up to 6.0 mcg/mL (SI: 25.6 µmol/L) if necessary; Toxic: >8 mcg/mL (SI: >34.2 µmol/L)

Special Geriatric Considerations Due to decreases in Phase I metabolism and possibly decrease in splanchnic perfusion with age, there may be a decreased clearance or increased half-life in the elderly and increased risk for CNS side effects and cardiac effects.

Dosage Forms Excipient information presented when available (limited, particularly for generics); consult specific product labeling. [DSC] = Discontinued product

Cream, rectal (L-M-X™ 5): 5% (15 g) [contains benzyl alcohol; packaged with applicator]; (30 g) [contains benzyl alcohol]

(Continued)

Lidocaine *(Continued)*

Cream, topical (L-M-X™ 4): 4% (5 g) [contains benzyl alcohol; packaged with Tegaderm™ dressing]; (15 g, 30 g) [contains benzyl alcohol]

Cream, topical, as hydrochloride: 3% (30 g)

LidaMantle®: 3% (30 g, 85 g)

Gel, topical:

Burn-O-Jel: 0.5% (90 g)

Topicaine®: 4% (10 g, 30 g, 113 g) [contains alcohol 35%, benzyl alcohol, aloe vera, and jojoba]

Gel, topical, as hydrochloride:

Burn Jel: 2% (3.5 g, 120 g)

Solarcaine® Aloe Extra Burn Relief: 0.5% (113 g, 226 g) [contains aloe vera gel and tartrazine]

Infusion, as hydrochloride [premixed in D_5W]: 0.4% [4 mg/mL] (250 mL, 500 mL); 0.8% [8 mg/mL] (250 mL, 500 mL)

Injection, solution, as hydrochloride: 0.5% [5 mg/mL] (50 mL); 1% [10 mg/mL] (2 mL, 10 mL, 20 mL, 30 mL, 50 mL); 2% [20 mg/mL] (2 mL, 5 mL, 20 mL, 50 mL)

Xylocaine®: 0.5% [5 mg/mL] (50 mL); 1% [10 mg/mL] (10 mL, 20 mL, 50 mL); 2% [20 mg/mL] (1.8 mL, 10 mL, 20 mL, 50 mL)

Injection, solution, as hydrochloride [preservative free]: 0.5% [5 mg/mL] (50 mL); 1% [10 mg/mL] (2 mL, 5 mL, 30 mL); 1.5% [15 mg/mL] (20 mL); 2% [20 mg/mL] (2 mL, 5 mL, 10 mL); 4% [40 mg/mL] (5 mL)

Xylocaine®: 10% [100 mg/mL] (5 mL) [for ventricular arrhythmias]

Xylocaine® MPF: 0.5% [5 mg/mL] (50 mL); 1% [10 mg/mL] (2 mL, 5 mL, 10 mL, 30 mL); 1.5% [15 mg/mL] (10 mL, 20 mL); 2% [20 mg/mL] (2 mL, 5 mL, 10 mL); 4% [40 mg/mL] (5 mL)

Injection, solution, as hydrochloride [premixed in $D_{7.5}W$, preservative free]: 5% (2 mL)

Xylocaine® MPF: 1.5% (2 mL) [DSC]

Jelly, topical, as hydrochloride: 2% (5 mL, 30 mL)

Anestacon®: 2% (15 mL) [contains benzalkonium chloride]

Xylocaine®: 2% (5 mL, 30 mL)

Liquid, topical (Zilactin®-L): 2.5% (7.5 mL)

Lotion, topical, as hydrochloride (LidaMantle®): 3% (177 mL)

Ointment, topical: 5% (37 g, 50 g)

Solution, topical, as hydrochloride: 4% [40 mg/mL] (50 mL)

Band-Aid® Hurt-Free™ Antiseptic Wash: 2% (180 mL)

LTA® 360: 4% [40 mg/mL] (4 mL) [packaged with cannula for laryngotracheal administration]

Xylocaine®: 4% [40 mg/mL] (50 mL)

Solution, viscous, as hydrochloride: 2% [20 mg/mL] (20 mL, 100 mL)

Xylocaine® Viscous: 2% [20 mg/mL] (100 mL, 450 mL)

Spray, topical:

Burnamycin: 0.5% (60 mL) [contains aloe vera gel and menthol]

Premjact®: 9.6% (13 mL)

Solarcaine® Aloe Extra Burn Relief: 0.5% (127 g) [contains aloe vera]

Transdermal system, topical (Lidoderm®): 5% (30s)

Lidocaine and Tetracaine (LYE doe kane & TET ra kane)

U.S. Brand Names Synera™

Index Terms Tetracaine and Lidocaine

Generic Available No

Pharmacologic Category Analgesic, Topical; Local Anesthetic

Use Topical anesthetic for use on normal intact skin for minor procedures (eg, I.V. cannulation or venipuncture) and superficial dermatologic procedures

Dosage

Geriatrics & Adults: Note: Adults can use another patch at a new location to facilitate venous access after a failed attempt; remove previous patch.

Venipuncture or intravenous cannulation: Transdermal patch: Prior to procedure, apply to intact skin for 20-30 minutes.

Superficial dermatological procedures: Transdermal patch: Prior to procedure, apply to intact skin for 30 minutes.

Hepatic Impairment:

Use caution in patients with severe hepatic dysfunction.

Special Geriatric Considerations

The manufacturer reports that in clinical studies there were no significant differences in safety between geriatric adjustments and younger subjects.

Dosage Forms Excipient information presented when available (limited, particularly for generics); consult specific product labeling.

Transdermal system:

Synera™: Lidocaine 70 mg and tetracaine 70 mg (10s) [contains heating component; each patch is 50 cm²]

♦ **Lidocaine Hydrochloride** *see Lidocaine on page 904*

♦ **Lidoderm®** *see Lidocaine on page 904*

♦ **Lignocaine Hydrochloride** *see Lidocaine on page 904*

Lindane (LIN dane)

Canadian Brand Names Hexit™; PMS-Lindane

Index Terms Benzene Hexachloride; Gamma Benzene Hexachloride; Hexachlorocyclohexane

Generic Available Yes

Pharmacologic Category Antiparasitic Agent, Topical; Pediculocide; Scabicidal Agent

Use Treatment of scabies and pediculosis

Restrictions An FDA-approved medication guide must be distributed when dispensing an outpatient prescription (new or refill) where this medication is to be used without direct supervision of a healthcare provider. Medication guides are available at http://www.fda.gov/cder/Offices/ODS/medication_guides.htm.

Contraindications Hypersensitivity to lindane or any component of the formulation; uncontrolled seizure disorders; crusted (Norwegian) scabies, acutely-inflamed skin or raw, weeping surfaces or other skin conditions which may increase systemic absorption

Warnings/Precautions [U.S. Boxed Warning]: Not considered a drug of first choice; use only in patients who have failed first-line treatments, or in patients who cannot tolerate these agents. Because of the potential for systemic absorption and CNS side effects, lindane should be used with caution; consider permethrin or crotamiton agent first. Oil-based hair dressing may increase toxic potential.

[U.S. Boxed Warning]: May be associated with severe neurologic toxicities (contraindicated in uncontrolled seizure disorders). Seizures and death have been reported with use; use with caution in patients <50 kg or patients with a history of seizures; use caution with conditions which may increase risk of seizures or medications which decrease seizure threshold; use caution with hepatic impairment; avoid contact with face, eyes, mucous membranes, and urethral meatus.

[U.S. Boxed Warning]: A lindane medication use guide must be given to all patients along with instructions for proper use. Patients should be informed that itching may occur following successful killing of lice and re-treatment may not be indicated. Should be used as a part of an overall lice management program

Adverse Reactions (Reflective of adult population; not specific for elderly) Frequency not defined (includes postmarketing and/or case reports).

Cardiovascular: Cardiac arrhythmia

Central nervous system: Ataxia, dizziness, headache, restlessness, seizure, pain

Dermatologic: Alopecia, contact dermatitis, skin and adipose tissue may act as repositories, eczematous eruptions, pruritus, urticaria

Gastrointestinal: Nausea, vomiting

Hematologic: Aplastic anemia

Hepatic: Hepatitis

Local: Burning and stinging

Neuromuscular & skeletal: Paresthesia

Renal: Hematuria

Respiratory: Pulmonary edema

Overdosage/Toxicology Symptoms include vomiting, restlessness, ataxia, seizures, arrhythmias, pulmonary edema, hematuria, and hepatitis. The drug is absorbed through skin, mucous membranes, and the GI tract. When used excessively for prolonged periods or when accidental ingestion has occurred, the drug has occasionally caused serious CNS, hepatic, and renal toxicity. If ingested, perform gastric lavage and general supportive measures. Diazepam 0.01 mg/kg can be used to control seizures.

Drug Interactions Increased toxicity: Drugs which lower seizure threshold

Mechanism of Action Directly absorbed by parasites and ova through the exoskeleton; stimulates the nervous system resulting in seizures and death of parasitic arthropods

Pharmacokinetics

Absorption: Up to 13% systemically; stored in body fat

Metabolism: By the liver

Elimination: In urine and feces

(Continued)

Lindane *(Continued)*

Dosage

Geriatrics & Adults:

Scabies: Topical: Apply a thin layer of lotion and massage it on skin from the neck to the toes; after 8-12 hours, bathe and remove the drug

Head lice, crab lice: Topical: Apply shampoo to dry hair and massage into hair for 4 minutes; add small quantities of water to hair until lather forms, then rinse hair thoroughly and comb with a fine tooth comb to remove nits. Amount of shampoo needed is based on length and density of hair; most patients will require 30 mL (maximum: 60 mL).

Administration For topical use only; never administer orally. Caregivers should apply with gloves (avoid natural latex, may be permeable to lindane). Rinse off with warm (not hot) water.

Lotion: Apply to dry, cool skin; do not apply to face or eyes. Wait at least 1 hour after bathing or showering (wet or warm skin increases absorption). Skin should be clean and free of any other lotions, creams, or oil prior to lindane application.

Shampoo: Apply to clean, dry hair. Wait at least 1 hour after washing hair before applying lindane shampoo. Hair should be washed with a shampoo not containing a conditioner; hair and skin of head and neck should be free of any lotions, oils, or creams prior to lindane application.

Patient Information For topical use only; do not apply to face; avoid getting in eyes, do not bathe prior to application

Special Geriatric Considerations Because of the potential for systemic absorption and CNS side effects, lindane should be used with caution. Not considered a drug of first choice; consider permethrin or crotamiton agent first.

Dosage Forms Excipient information presented when available (limited, particularly for generics); consult specific product labeling.

Lotion, topical: 1% (60 mL)

Shampoo, topical: 1% (60 mL) [contains alcohol 0.5%]

Linezolid *(li NE zoh lid)*

Related Information

Antimicrobial Activity Against Selected Organisms *on page 1728*

Medication Safety Issues

Sound-alike/look-alike issues:

Zyvox® may be confused with Vioxx®, Ziox™, Zosyn®, Zovirax®

U.S. Brand Names Zyvox®

Canadian Brand Names Zyvoxam®

Generic Available No

Pharmacologic Category Antibiotic, Oxazolidinone

Use Treatment of vancomycin-resistant *Enterococcus faecium* (VRE) infections, nosocomial pneumonia caused by *Staphylococcus aureus* including MRSA or *Streptococcus pneumoniae* (including multidrug-resistant strains [MDRSP]), complicated and uncomplicated skin and skin structure infections (including diabetic foot infections without concomitant osteomyelitis), and community-acquired pneumonia caused by susceptible gram-positive organisms

Contraindications Hypersensitivity to linezolid or any other component of the formulation

Warnings/Precautions Myelosuppression has been reported and may be dependent on duration of therapy (generally >2 weeks of treatment); use with caution in patients with pre-existing myelosuppression, in patients receiving other drugs which may cause bone marrow suppression, or in chronic infection (previous or concurrent antibiotic therapy). Weekly CBC monitoring is recommended. Discontinue linezolid in patients developing myelosuppression (or in whom myelosuppression worsens during treatment).

Lactic acidosis has been reported with use. Linezolid exhibits mild MAO inhibitor properties and has the potential to have the same interactions as other MAO inhibitors; use with caution in uncontrolled hypertension, pheochromocytoma, carcinoid syndrome, or untreated hyperthyroidism; avoid use with serotonergic agents such as TCAs, venlafaxine, trazodone, sibutramine, meperidine, dextromethorphan, and SSRIs; concomitant use has been associated with the development of serotonin syndrome. Unnecessary use may lead to the development of resistance to linezolid; consider alternatives before initiating outpatient treatment.

Peripheral and optic neuropathy (with vision loss) has been reported and may occur primarily with extended courses of therapy >28 days; any symptoms of visual change or impairment warrant immediate ophthalmic evaluation and possible discontinuation of therapy. Seizures have been reported; use with caution in patients with a history of seizures. Prolonged use may result in fungal or bacterial superinfection, including *C. difficile*-associated diarrhea and pseudomembranous colitis.

Adverse Reactions (Reflective of adult population; not specific for elderly)
Percentages as reported in adults; frequency similar in pediatric patients
>10%:
  Central nervous system: Headache (<1% to 11%)
  Gastrointestinal: Diarrhea (3% to 11%)
1% to 10%:
  Central nervous system: Insomnia (3%), dizziness (0.4% to 2%), fever (2%)
  Dermatologic: Rash (2%)
  Gastrointestinal: Nausea (3% to 10%), vomiting (1% to 4%), pancreatic enzymes increased (<1% to 4%), constipation (2%), taste alteration (1% to 2%), tongue discoloration (0.2% to 1%), oral moniliasis (0.4% to 1%), pancreatitis
  Genitourinary: Vaginal moniliasis (1% to 2%)
  Hematologic: Thrombocytopenia (0.3% to 10%), hemoglobin decreased (0.9% to 7%), anemia, leukopenia, neutropenia; **Note:** Myelosuppression (including anemia, leukopenia, pancytopenia, and thrombocytopenia; may be more common in patients receiving linezolid for >2 weeks)
  Hepatic: Abnormal LFTs (0.4% to 1%)
  Renal: BUN increased (<1% to 2%)
  Miscellaneous: Fungal infection (0.1% to 2%), lactate dehydrogenase increased (<1% to 2%)

Overdosage/Toxicology Treatment is supportive. Hemodialysis may improve elimination (30% of a dose is removed during a 3-hour hemodialysis session).

Drug Interactions
Adrenergic agents (eg, phenylpropanolamine, pseudoephedrine, sympathomimetic agents, vasopressor or dopaminergic agents) may cause hypertension.
Myelosuppressive medications: Concurrent use may increase risk of myelosuppression with linezolid.
Serotonergic agents (eg, TCAs, venlafaxine, trazodone, sibutramine, meperidine, dextromethorphan, and SSRIs) may cause a serotonin syndrome (eg, hyperpyrexia, cognitive dysfunction) when used concomitantly.
Tramadol: Concurrent use may increase risk of seizures.

Ethanol/Nutrition/Herb Interactions
Ethanol: Avoid ethanol (based on CNS depressant effects and potential tyramine content)
Food: Concurrent ingestion of foods rich in tyramine may cause sudden and severe high blood pressure (hypertensive crisis). Avoid tyramine-containing foods with MAOIs. Food's freshness is also an important concern; improperly stored or spoiled food can create an environment where tyramine concentrations may increase.
Herb/Nutraceutical: Avoid supplements containing caffeine, tyrosine, tryptophan or phenylalanine. Ingestion of large quantities may increase the risk of severe side effects (eg, hypertensive reactions, serotonin syndrome).

Stability
Infusion: Store at 25°C (77°F). Protect from light. Keep infusion bags in overwrap until ready for use. Protect infusion bags from freezing.
Oral suspension: Following reconstitution, store at room temperature. Use reconstituted suspension within 21 days.

Mechanism of Action Inhibits bacterial protein synthesis by binding to bacterial 23S ribosomal RNA of the 50S subunit. This prevents the formation of a functional 70S initiation complex that is essential for the bacterial translation process. Linezolid is bacteriostatic against enterococci and staphylococci and bactericidal against most strains of streptococci.

Pharmacokinetics
Absorption: Rapid and extensive
Distribution: Steady state V_d 40-50 L
Protein binding: 31%
Metabolism: Hepatic by oxidation of the morpholine ring which results in 2 inactive metabolites (aminoethoxyacetic acid, hydroxyethyl glycine); does not involve cytochrome P450 isoenzymes.
Bioavailability: 100%
Half-life: 4-5 hours
Time to peak: Oral: 1-2 hours
Elimination: Urine (30% as parent drug, 50% as metabolites); feces (9% as metabolites)
  Nonrenal clearance: 65%

Dosage
Geriatrics & Adults:
  VRE infections: Oral, I.V.: 600 mg every 12 hours for 14-28 days
  Nosocomial pneumonia, complicated skin and skin structure infections, community-acquired pneumonia including concurrent bacteremia: Oral, I.V.: 600 mg every 12 hours for 10-14 days
(Continued)

Linezolid *(Continued)*

Uncomplicated skin and skin structure infections: Oral: 400 mg every 12 hours for 10-14 days

Note: 400 mg dose is recommended in the product labeling; however, 600 mg dose is commonly employed clinically

Renal Impairment: No adjustment is recommended. The two primary metabolites may accumulate in patients with renal impairment but the clinical significance is unknown. Weigh the risk of accumulation of metabolites versus the benefit of therapy. Monitor for hematopoietic (eg, anemia, leukopenia, thrombocytopenia) and neuropathic (eg, peripheral neuropathy) adverse events when administering for extended periods. Both linezolid and the two metabolites are eliminated by dialysis. Linezolid should be given after hemodialysis.

Continuous venovenous hemofiltration, continuous venovenous hemodialysis, and continuous venovenous hemodiafiltration: No adjustment needed.

Hepatic Impairment: No dosage adjustment required for mild to moderate hepatic insufficiency (Child-Pugh class A or B). Use in severe hepatic insufficiency has not been adequately evaluated.

Administration

I.V.: Administer intravenous infusion over 30-120 minutes. Do not mix or infuse with other medications. When the same intravenous line is used for sequential infusion of other medications, flush line with D_5W, NS, or LR before and after infusing linezolid. The yellow color of the injection may intensify over time without affecting potency.

Oral suspension: Invert gently to mix prior to administration, do not shake.

Monitoring Parameters Weekly CBC and platelet counts, particularly in patients at increased risk of bleeding; with pre-existing myelosuppression or thrombocytopenia; on concomitant medications that decrease platelet count/function or cause bone marrow suppression; who require >2 weeks of therapy; or with chronic infection, who have received previous or concomitant antibiotic therapy; visual function with extended therapy (≥3 months) or in patients with new onset visual symptoms, regardless of therapy length

Patient Information Take with food if medicine causes stomach upset. Tell your healthcare provider if you have hypertension or are taking any cold remedy or decongestant. Limit quantities of tyramine-containing foods. Gently mix suspension. Store at room temperature.

Special Geriatric Considerations According to the manufacturer the pharmacokinetics of linezolid are not significantly altered in persons ≥65 years of age.

Dosage Forms Excipient information presented when available (limited, particularly for generics); consult specific product labeling. [CAN] = Canadian brand name

Infusion [premixed]:

Zyvox®: 200 mg (100 mL) [contains sodium 1.7 mEq]

Zyvox® [CAN]: 600 mg (300 mL) [contains sodium 5 mEq] [not available in the U.S.]

Powder for oral suspension:

Zyvox®: 20 mg/mL (150 mL) [contains phenylalanine 20 mg/5 mL, sodium benzoate, and sodium 0.4 mEq/5 mL; orange flavor]

Tablet:

Zyvox®: 600 mg [contains sodium 0.1 mEq/tablet]

Selected References

Bain KT and Wittbrodt ET, "Linezolid for the Treatment of Resistant Gram-Positive Cocci," *Ann Pharmacother*, 2001, 35(5):566-75.

Perry CM and Jarvis B, "Linezolid: A Review of Its Use in the Management of Serious Gram-Positive Infections," *Drugs*, 2001, 61(4):525-51.

♦ **Lioresal**® *see* Baclofen *on page 150*

Liothyronine (lye oh THYE roe neen)

Medication Safety Issues

Sound-alike/look-alike issues:

Liothyronine may be confused with levothyroxine

T3 is an error-prone abbreviation (mistaken as acetaminophen and codeine [ie, Tylenol® #3])

U.S. Brand Names Cytomel®; Triostat®

Canadian Brand Names Cytomel®

Index Terms Liothyronine Sodium; Sodium *L*-Triiodothyronine; T_3 Sodium (error-prone abbreviation)

Generic Available No

Pharmacologic Category Thyroid Product

Use

Oral: Replacement or supplemental therapy in hypothyroidism; management of nontoxic goiter; a diagnostic aid

I.V.: Treatment of myxedema coma/precoma

Contraindications Hypersensitivity to liothyronine sodium or any component of the formulation; undocumented or uncorrected adrenal insufficiency; recent myocardial infarction or thyrotoxicosis; artificial rewarming (injection)

Warnings/Precautions [U.S. Boxed Warning]: Ineffective and potentially toxic for weight reduction. High doses may produce serious or even life-threatening toxic effects particularly when used with some anorectic drugs. Use with extreme caution in patients with angina pectoris or other cardiovascular disease (including hypertension) or coronary artery disease; use with caution in elderly patients since they may be more likely to have compromised cardiovascular function. Patients with adrenal insufficiency, myxedema, diabetes mellitus and insipidus may have symptoms exaggerated or aggravated; thyroid replacement requires periodic assessment of thyroid status. Chronic hypothyroidism predisposes patients to coronary artery disease.

Adverse Reactions (Reflective of adult population; not specific for elderly)
1% to 10%: Cardiovascular: Arrhythmia (6%), tachycardia (3%), cardiopulmonary arrest (2%), hypotension (2%), MI (2%)

Drug Interactions
Aluminum- and magnesium-containing antacids, calcium carbonate, simethicone, or sucralfate: May decrease T_4 absorption; separate dose from thyroid hormones by at least 4 hours.

Antidiabetic agents (biguanides, meglitinides, sulfonylureas, thiazolidinediones, insulin): Changes in thyroid function may alter requirements of antidiabetic agent. Monitor closely at initiation of therapy, or when dose is changed or discontinued.

Cholestyramine and colestipol: Decrease T_4 absorption; separate dose from thyroid hormones by at least 2 hours.

Digoxin: Digoxin levels may be reduced in hyperthyroidism; therapeutic effect may be reduced. Impact of thyroid replacement should be monitored.

Estrogens: May decrease serum free-thyroxine concentrations.

Iron: Decreases T_4 absorption; separate dose from thyroid hormones by at least 4 hours

Kayexalate®: Decreases T_4 absorption; separate dose from thyroid hormones by at least 4 hours

Ketamine: May cause marked hypertension and tachycardia; monitor

Theophylline, caffeine: Decreased theophylline clearance in hypothyroid patients; monitor during thyroid replacement.

Tricyclic and tetracyclic antidepressants: Therapeutic and toxic effects of thyroid hormones and the antidepressant are increased.

Warfarin (and other oral anticoagulants): The hypoprothrombinemic response to warfarin may be altered by a change in thyroid function or replacement. Replacement may dramatically increase response to warfarin. However, initiation of warfarin in a patient stabilized on a dose of thyroid hormones does not appear to require a significantly different approach.

Stability Vials must be stored under refrigeration at 2°C to 8°C (36°F to 46°F). Store tablets at 15°C to 30°C (59°F to 86°F).

Mechanism of Action Exact mechanism of action is unknown; however, it is believed the thyroid hormone exerts its many metabolic effects through control of DNA transcription and protein synthesis; involved in normal metabolism, growth, and development; promotes gluconeogenesis, increases utilization and mobilization of glycogen stores, and stimulates protein synthesis, increases basal metabolic rate

Pharmacodynamics
Onset of action: 2-4 hours
Peak response: 2-3 days

Pharmacokinetics
Absorption: Oral: Well absorbed (95% in 4 hours)
Half-life: 2.5 days
Elimination: Urine

Dosage
Geriatrics: Oral: 5 mcg/day; increase by 5 mcg/day every 2 weeks
Adults:
Hypothyroidism: Oral: 25 mcg/day increase by 12.5-25 mcg/day every 1-2 weeks to a maximum of 100 mcg/day
Patients with cardiovascular disease: Refer to geriatric dosing.
Suppression test: (T_3): Oral: 75-100 mcg/day for 7 days; use lowest dose for elderly
Myxedema: Oral: Initial: 5 mcg/day; increase in increments of 5-10 mcg/day every 1-2 weeks. When 25 mcg/day is reached, dosage may be increased at intervals of 5-25 mcg/day every 1-2 weeks. Usual maintenance dose: 50-100 mcg/day.
Myxedema coma: I.V.: 25-50 mcg
Patients with known or suspected cardiovascular disease: 10-20 mcg
Note: Normally, at least 4 hours should be allowed between doses to adequately assess therapeutic response and no more than 12 hours should elapse between doses to avoid fluctuations in hormone levels. Oral therapy should be resumed as soon as the clinical situation has been stabilized and the patient is able to
(Continued)

Liothyronine *(Continued)*

take oral medication. If levothyroxine rather than liothyronine sodium is used in initiating oral therapy, the prescriber should bear in mind that there is a delay of several days in the onset of levothyroxine activity and that I.V. therapy should be discontinued gradually.

Simple (nontoxic) goiter: Oral: Initial: 5 mcg/day; increase by 5-10 mcg every 1-2 weeks; after 25 mcg/day is reached, may increase dose by 12.5-25 mcg. Usual maintenance dose: 75 mcg/day.

Administration I.V.: For I.V. use only; **do not administer I.M. or SubQ**

Administer doses at least 4 hours, and no more than 12 hours, apart

Resume oral therapy as soon as the clinical situation has been stabilized and the patient is able to take oral medication

When switching to tablets, discontinue the injectable, initiate oral therapy at a low dosage and increase gradually according to response

If **levothyroxine** is used for oral therapy, there is a delay of several days in the onset of activity; therefore, discontinue I.V. therapy gradually

Monitoring Parameters T_3, TSH, heart rate, blood pressure, renal function, clinical signs of hypo- and hyperthyroidism; TSH is the most reliable guide for evaluating adequacy of thyroid replacement dosage. TSH may be elevated during the first few months of thyroid replacement despite patients being clinically euthyroid. In cases where T_4 remains low and TSH is within normal limits, an evaluation of "free" (unbound) T_4 is needed to evaluate further increase in dosage.

Reference Range Free T_3, serum: 250-390 pg/dL; TSH: 0.4 and up to 10 ($\geq$80 years) mIU/L

Patient Information Take as directed; do not discontinue without consulting prescriber. Do not change diet without consulting prescriber. Limit intake of goitrogenic foods (asparagus, cabbage, peas, turnip greens, broccoli, spinach, Brussels sprouts, lettuce, soybeans). Report chest pain, increased heartbeat, palpitations, excessive weight gain or loss, change in level of energy (increased or decreased), excessive sweating, or intolerance to heat.

Additional Information

Equivalent doses: Thyroid USP 60 mg $\sim$ levothyroxine 0.05-0.06 mg $\sim$ liothyronine 0.015-0.0375 mg

50-60 mg thyroid $\sim$ 50-60 mcg levothyroxine and 12.5-15 mcg liothyronine

A synthetic form of *L*-Triiodothyronine (T_3) can be used in patients allergic to products derived from pork or beef.

Note: Several medications have effects on thyroid production or conversion. The impact in thyroid replacement has not been specifically evaluated, but patient response should be monitored:

Methimazole: Decreases thyroid hormone secretion, while propylthiouracil decrease thyroid hormone secretion and decreases conversion of T_4 to T_3.

Beta-adrenergic antagonists: Decrease conversion of T_4 to T_3 (dose related, propranolol $\geq$160 mg/day); patients may be clinically euthyroid.

Iodide, iodine-containing radiographic contrast agents may decrease thyroid hormone secretion; may also increase thyroid hormone secretion, especially in patients with Graves' disease.

Other agents reported to impact on thyroid production/conversion include aminoglutethimide, amiodarone, chloral hydrate, diazepam, ethionamide, interferon-alpha, interleukin-2, lithium, lovastatin (case report), glucocorticoids (dose-related), 6-mercaptopurine, sulfonamides, thiazide diuretics, and tolbutamide.

In addition, a number of medications have been noted to cause transient depression in TSH secretion, which may complicate interpretation of monitoring tests for thyroid hormones, including corticosteroids, octreotide, and dopamine. Metoclopramide may increase TSH secretion.

Special Geriatric Considerations Elderly do not have a change in serum thyroxine associated with aging; however, plasma T_3 concentrations are decreased 25% to 40% in the elderly. There is not a compensatory rise in thyrotropin suggesting that lower T_3 is not reacted upon as a deficiency by the pituitary. This indicates a slightly lower than normal dosage of thyroid hormone replacement is usually sufficient in elderly patients than in younger adult patients. TSH must be monitored since insufficient thyroid replacement (elevated TSH) is a risk for coronary artery disease and excessive replacement (low TSH) may cause signs of hyperthyroidism and excessive bone loss.

Dosage Forms Excipient information presented when available (limited, particularly for generics); consult specific product labeling.

Injection, solution, as sodium (Triostat®): 10 mcg/mL (1 mL) [contains alcohol 6.8%]

Tablet, as sodium (Cytomel®): 5 mcg, 25 mcg, 50 mcg

Selected References

Helfand M and Crapo LM, "Monitoring Therapy in Patients Taking Levothyroxine," *Ann Intern Med*, 1990, 113(6):450-4.

Johnson DG and Campbell S, "Hormonal and Metabolic Agents," *Geriatric Pharmacology*, Bressler R and Katz MD, eds, New York, NY: McGraw-Hill, 1993, 427-50.

Sanders LR, "Pituitary, Thyroid, Adrenal and Parathyroid Diseases in the Elderly," *Geriatric Medicine*, 1990, 475-87.

Sawin CT, Geller A, Hershman JM, et al, "The Aging Thyroid. The Use of Thyroid Hormone in Older Persons," *JAMA*, 1989, 261(18):2653-5.

Watts NB, "Use of a Sensitive Thyrotropin Assay for Monitoring Treatment With Levothyroxine," *Arch Intern Med*, 1989, 149(2):309-12.

♦ **Liothyronine Sodium** *see* Liothyronine *on page 912*

Liotrix (LYE oh triks)

Medication Safety Issues
Sound-alike/look-alike issues:
Liotrix may be confused with Klotrix®
Thyrolar® may be confused with Theolair™, Thyrogen®, Thytropar®

U.S. Brand Names Thyrolar®

Canadian Brand Names Thyrolar®

Index Terms T_3/T_4 Liotrix

Generic Available No

Pharmacologic Category Thyroid Product

Use Replacement or supplemental therapy in hypothyroidism and thyroid cancer

Contraindications Hypersensitivity to liotrix or any component of the formulation; recent myocardial infarction or thyrotoxicosis, uncomplicated by hypothyroidism; uncorrected adrenal insufficiency, hypersensitivity to active or extraneous constituents

Warnings/Precautions [U.S. Boxed Warning]: Ineffective and potentially toxic for weight reduction; high doses may produce serious or even life-threatening toxic effects particularly when used with some anorectic drugs. Use with caution and reduce dosage in patients with angina pectoris or other cardiovascular disease; chronic hypothyroidism predisposes patients to coronary artery disease, elderly since they may be more likely to have compromised cardiovascular function. Use with caution in patients with adrenal insufficiency, diabetes mellitus or insipidus, and myxedema; symptoms may be exaggerated or aggravated.

Adverse Reactions (Reflective of adult population; not specific for elderly)
Frequency not defined.
Cardiovascular: Cardiac arrhythmia, chest pain, palpitation, tachycardia
Central nervous system: Ataxia, fever, headache, insomnia, nervousness
Dermatologic: Alopecia
Endocrine & metabolic: Changes in menstrual cycle, increased appetite, weight loss
Gastrointestinal: Abdominal cramps, constipation, diarrhea, vomiting
Neuromuscular & skeletal: Hand tremor, myalgia, tremor
Respiratory: Dyspnea
Miscellaneous: Allergic skin reactions (rare), diaphoresis

Drug Interactions
Aluminum- and magnesium-containing antacids, calcium carbonate, simethicone, or sucralfate: May decrease T_4 absorption; separate dose from thyroid hormones by at least 4 hours.

Antidiabetic agents (biguanides, meglitinides, sulfonylureas, thiazolidinediones, insulin): Changes in thyroid function may alter requirements of antidiabetic agent. Monitor closely at initiation of therapy, or when dose is changed or discontinued.

Cholestyramine and colestipol: Decrease T_4 absorption; separate dose from thyroid hormones by at least 4 hours.

Digoxin: Digoxin levels may be reduced in hyperthyroidism; therapeutic effect may be reduced. Impact of thyroid replacement should be monitored.

Iron: Decreases T_4 absorption; separate dose from thyroid hormones by at least 4 hours

Kayexalate®: Decreases T_4 absorption; separate dose from thyroid hormones by at least 4 hours

Ketamine: May cause marked hypertension and tachycardia; monitor

Ritonavir: May alter response to thyroid hormones (limited documentation/case report); monitor

Somatrem, somatropin: Excessive thyroid hormone levels lead to accelerated epiphyseal closure; inadequate replacement interferes with growth response to growth hormone. Effect of thyroid replacement not specifically evaluated; use caution.

SSRI antidepressants: May need to increase dose of thyroid hormones when SSRI is added to a previously stabilized patient.

Sympathomimetics: Effects of sympathomimetic agent or thyroid hormones may be increased. Risk of coronary insufficiency is increased in patients with coronary artery disease when these agents are used together.

Theophylline, caffeine: Decreased theophylline clearance in hypothyroid patients; monitor during thyroid replacement.

Tricyclic and tetracyclic antidepressants: Therapeutic and toxic effects of thyroid hormones and the antidepressant are increased.

(Continued)

Liotrix *(Continued)*

Warfarin (and other oral anticoagulants): The hypoprothrombinemic response to warfarin may be altered by a change in thyroid function or replacement. Replacement may dramatically increase response to warfarin. However, initiation of warfarin in a patient stabilized on a dose of thyroid hormones does not appear to require a significantly different approach.

Note: Several medications have effects on thyroid production or conversion. The impact in thyroid replacement has not been specifically evaluated, but patient response should be monitored:

Methimazole: Decreases thyroid hormone secretion, while propylthiouracil decrease thyroid hormone secretion and decreases conversion of T_4 to T_3.

Beta-adrenergic antagonists: Decrease conversion of T_4 to T_3 (dose related, propranolol ≥160 mg/day); patients may be clinically euthyroid.

Iodide, iodine-containing radiographic contrast agents may decrease thyroid hormone secretion; may also increase thyroid hormone secretion, especially in patients with Graves' disease.

Other agents reported to impact on thyroid production/conversion include aminoglutethimide, amiodarone, chloral hydrate, diazepam, ethionamide, interferon-alpha, interleukin-2, lithium, lovastatin (case report), glucocorticoids (dose-related), mercaptopurine, sulfonamides, thiazide diuretics, and tolbutamide.

In addition, a number of medications have been noted to cause transient depression in TSH secretion, which may complicate interpretation of monitoring tests for thyroid hormones, including corticosteroids, octreotide, and dopamine. Metoclopramide may increase TSH secretion.

Stability Store at 2°C to 8°C (36°F to 46°F). Protect from light.

Mechanism of Action The primary active compound is T_3 (triiodothyronine), which may be converted from T_4 (thyroxine) and then circulates throughout the body to influence growth and maturation of various tissues. Liotrix is uniform mixture of synthetic T_4 and T_3 in 4:1 ratio; exact mechanism of action is unknown; however, it is believed the thyroid hormone exerts its many metabolic effects through control of DNA transcription and protein synthesis; involved in normal metabolism, growth, and development; promotes gluconeogenesis, increases utilization and mobilization of glycogen stores and stimulates protein synthesis, increases basal metabolic rate

Pharmacokinetics

Absorption: 50% to 95% from GI tract

Metabolism: Partially in liver, kidneys, and intestines

Half-life: 6-7 days

Time to peak: 12-48 hours

Elimination: In feces and bile as conjugated metabolites

Dosage

Geriatrics: Initial: 15 mg, adjust dose at 2- to 4-week intervals by increments of 15 mg

Adults: Hypothyroidism (dose of thyroid equivalent): Oral: 30 mg/day (15 mg/day if cardiovascular impairment), increasing by increments of 15 mg/day at 2- to 3-week intervals to a maximum of 180 mg/day (usual maintenance dose: 60-120 mg/day)

Monitoring Parameters T_4, TSH, heart rate, blood pressure, clinical signs of hypo- and hyperthyroidism; TSH is the most reliable guide for evaluating adequacy of thyroid replacement dosage. TSH may be elevated during the first few months of thyroid replacement despite patients being clinically euthyroid. In cases where T_4 remains low and TSH is within normal limits, an evaluation of "free" (unbound) T_4 is needed to evaluate further increase in dosage. See Special Geriatric Considerations.

Reference Range

TSH: 0.4-10 (for those ≥80 years) mIU/L

T_4: 4-12 mcg/dL (SI: 51-154 nmol/L)

T_3 (RIA) (total T_3): 80-230 ng/dL (SI: 1.2-3.5 nmol/L)

T_4 free (Free T_4): 0.7-1.8 ng/dL (SI: 9-23 pmol/L)

Test Interactions Many drugs may have effects on thyroid function tests; para-aminosalicylic acid, aminoglutethimide, amiodarone, barbiturates, carbamazepine, chloral hydrate, clofibrate, colestipol, corticosteroids, danazol, diazepam, estrogens, ethionamide, fluorouracil, I.V. heparin, insulin, lithium, methadone, methimazole, mitotane, nitroprusside, oxyphenbutazone, phenylbutazone, PTU, perphenazine, phenytoin, propranolol, salicylates, sulfonylureas, and thiazides

Patient Information Do not change brands without physician's knowledge; report immediately to physician any chest pain, increased pulse, palpitations, heat intolerances, excessive sweating; do not stop use without physician's advice; replacement therapy will be for life; take as a single dose before breakfast

Additional Information Since T_3 is produced by monodeiodination of T_4 in peripheral tissues (80%) and since older adults have decreased T_3 (25% to 40%), little advantage to this product exists and cost is not justified; no advantage over synthetic levothyroxine sodium; 1 grain (60 mg) liotrix is equivalent to 0.05-0.06 mg levothyroxine; 60 mg thyroid USP and thyroglobulin; and 45 mg of Thyroid Strong®

Special Geriatric Considerations Elderly do not have a change in serum thyroxine associated with aging; however, plasma T_3 concentrations are decreased 25% to 40% in older adults. There is not a compensatory rise in thyrotropin suggesting that lower T_3 is not reacted upon as a deficiency by the pituitary. This indicates a slightly lower than normal dosage of thyroid hormone replacement is usually sufficient in older patients than in younger adult patients. TSH must be monitored since insufficient thyroid replacement (elevated TSH) is a risk for coronary artery disease and excessive replacement (low TSH) may cause signs of hyperthyroidism and excessive bone loss.

Dosage Forms Excipient information presented when available (limited, particularly for generics); consult specific product labeling.

Tablet:

$1/4$ [levothyroxine sodium 12.5 mcg and liothyronine sodium 3.1 mcg]

$1/2$ [levothyroxine sodium 25 mcg and liothyronine sodium 6.25 mcg]

1 [levothyroxine sodium 50 mcg and liothyronine sodium 12.5 mcg]

2 [levothyroxine sodium 100 mcg and liothyronine sodium 25 mcg]

3 [levothyroxine sodium 150 mcg and liothyronine sodium 37.5 mcg]

Selected References

Helfand M and Crapo LM, "Monitoring Therapy in Patients Taking Levothyroxine," *Ann Intern Med*, 1990, 113(6):450-4.

Johnson DG and Campbell S, "Hormonal and Metabolic Agents," *Geriatric Pharmacology*, Bressler R and Katz MD, eds, New York, NY: McGraw-Hill, 1993, 427-50.

Sanders LR, "Pituitary, Thyroid, Adrenal and Parathyroid Diseases in the Elderly," *Geriatric Medicine*, 1990, 475-87.

Sawin CT, Geller A, Hershman JM, et al, "The Aging Thyroid. The Use of Thyroid Hormone in Older Persons," *JAMA*, 1989, 261(18):2653-5.

Watts NB, "Use of a Sensitive Thyrotropin Assay for Monitoring Treatment With Levothyroxine," *Arch Intern Med*, 1989, 149(2):309-12.

♦ **Lipancreatin** *see* Pancrelipase *on page 1196*

♦ **Lipitor**® *see* Atorvastatin *on page 134*

♦ **Lipofen**™ *see* Fenofibrate *on page 604*

♦ **Lipram 4500** *see* Pancrelipase *on page 1196*

♦ **Lipram-CR** *see* Pancrelipase *on page 1196*

♦ **Lipram-PN** *see* Pancrelipase *on page 1196*

♦ **Lipram-UL** *see* Pancrelipase *on page 1196*

♦ **Liqua-Cal [OTC]** *see* Calcium and Vitamin D *on page 214*

♦ **Liquid Paraffin** *see* Mineral Oil *on page 1045*

♦ **Liquifilm**® **Tears [OTC]** *see* Artificial Tears *on page 124*

Lisinopril (lyse IN oh pril)

Related Information

Angiotensin Agents *on page 1737*

Medication Safety Issues

Sound-alike/look-alike issues:

Lisinopril may be confused with fosinopril, Lioresal®, Risperdal®

Prinivil® may be confused with Plendil®, Pravachol®, Prevacid®, Prilosec®, Proventil®

Zestril® may be confused with Desyrel®, Restoril®, Vistaril®, Zetia™, Zostrix®

International issues:

Acepril® [Denmark] may be confused with Accupril® which is a brand name for quinapril in the U.S.

Acepril®: Brand name for enalapril in Hungary and Switzerland; brand name for captopril in Great Britain

Carace® [Ireland; Great Britain] may be confused with Carac™ which is a brand name for fluorouracil in the U.S.

Zetril® may be confused with Nostril® which is a brand name for chlorhexidine/cetrimonium in France

U.S. Brand Names Prinivil®; Zestril®

Canadian Brand Names Apo-Lisinopril®; Prinivil®; Zestril®

Generic Available Yes

Pharmacologic Category Angiotensin-Converting Enzyme (ACE) Inhibitor

Use Treatment of hypertension (alone or in combination with other antihypertensive agents), acute myocardial infarction (hemodynamically stable) within 24 hours of onset; adjunctive therapy in treatment of systolic congestive heart failure

Contraindications Hypersensitivity to lisinopril or any component of the formulation; angioedema related to previous treatment with an ACE inhibitor; bilateral renal artery stenosis; primary hyperaldosteronism

Warnings/Precautions Anaphylactic reactions can occur. Angioedema can occur at any time during treatment (especially following first dose). It may involve head and neck (potentially affecting the airway) or the intestine (presenting with abdominal pain). Prolonged monitoring may be required especially if tongue, glottis, or larynx are involved as they are associated with airway obstruction. Those with a history of airway (Continued)

Lisinopril *(Continued)*

surgery in this situation have a higher risk. Careful blood pressure monitoring with first dose (hypotension can occur especially in volume-depleted patients).

Dosage adjustment needed in renal impairment. Use with caution in hypovolemia; collagen vascular diseases; valvular stenosis (particularly aortic stenosis); or before, during, or immediately after anesthesia. Hyperkalemia may occur; risk factors include renal dysfunction, diabetes mellitus, concomitant use of potassium-sparing diuretics, potassium supplements and/or potassium containing salts. Use cautiously, if at all, with these agents and monitor potassium closely. Avoid rapid dosage escalation, which may lead to renal insufficiency. Rare toxicities associated with ACE inhibitors include cholestatic jaundice (which may progress to hepatic necrosis) and neutropenia/agranulocytosis with myeloid hyperplasia. May be associated with deterioration of renal function and/or increases in serum creatinine, particularly in patients dependent on renin-angiotensin-aldosterone system. Use with caution in unilateral renal artery stenosis and pre-existing renal insufficiency; if patient has renal impairment then a baseline WBC with differential and serum creatinine should be evaluated and monitored closely during the first 3 months of therapy. Hypersensitivity reactions may be seen during hemodialysis with high-flux dialysis membranes (eg, AN69).

Adverse Reactions (Reflective of adult population; not specific for elderly)
Note: Frequency ranges include data from hypertension and heart failure trials. Higher rates of adverse reactions have generally been noted in patients with CHF. However, the frequency of adverse effects associated with placebo is also increased in this population.

1% to 10%:
    Cardiovascular: Orthostatic effects (1%), hypotension (1% to 4%)
    Central nervous system: Headache (4% to 6%), dizziness (5% to 12%), fatigue (3%)
    Dermatologic: Rash (1% to 2%)
    Endocrine & metabolic: Hyperkalemia (2% to 5%)
    Gastrointestinal: Diarrhea (3% to 4%), nausea (2%), vomiting (1%), abdominal pain (2%)
    Genitourinary: Impotence (1%)
    Hematologic: Decreased hemoglobin (small)
    Neuromuscular & skeletal: Chest pain (3%), weakness (1%)
    Renal: BUN increased (2%); deterioration in renal function (in patients with bilateral renal artery stenosis or hypovolemia); serum creatinine increased (often transient)
    Respiratory: Cough (4% to 9%), upper respiratory infection (1% to 2%)

Overdosage/Toxicology Mild hypotension has been the only toxic effect seen with acute overdose; bradycardia may also occur. Hyperkalemia occurs even with therapeutic doses, especially in patients with renal insufficiency and those taking NSAIDs. Following initiation of essential overdose management, toxic symptom and supportive treatment should be initiated. Hypotension usually responds to I.V. fluids or Trendelenburg positioning.

Drug Interactions
    Allopurinol: Case reports (rare) indicate a possible increased risk of hypersensitivity reactions when combined with lisinopril.
    Antacids: May decrease the serum concentration of ACE inhibitors.
    Aprotinin: May diminish the antihypertensive effect of ACE inhibitors during infusion.
    Azathioprine: ACE inhibitors may enhance the neutropenic effect of azathioprine.
    Cyclosporine: ACE inhibitors may enhance the nephrotoxic effect of cyclosporine.
    Eplerenone: May increase the risk of hyperkalemia.
    Ferric gluconate: ACE inhibitors may enhance the adverse/toxic effect of ferric gluconate.
    Gold sodium thiomalate: ACE inhibitors may enhance the adverse/toxic effects (nitritoid reaction) of gold sodium thiomalate. The reaction may include facial flushing, nausea, vomiting, hypotension, and syncope. If it is to occur, would be expected shortly after administration of gold compound in patients maintained on an ACEI.
    Insulin: Risk of hypoglycemia may be increased.
    Lithium: ACE inhibitors may increase the serum concentration of lithium. Monitor lithium levels, especially the first 4 weeks of therapy.
    Loop diuretics: Hypovolemia due to diuretics may precipitate acute hypotensive events or acute renal failure.
    Mercaptopurine: Risk of neutropenia may be increased.
    NSAIDs: May attenuate hypertensive efficacy; effect has been seen with captopril and may occur with other ACE inhibitors; monitor blood pressure. May increase adverse renal effects.
    Potassium-sparing diuretics (eg, amiloride, spironolactone, triamterene): May increase the risk of hyperkalemia.
    Salicylates: May diminish the effects of ACE inhibitors and/or increase renal toxicity, particularly when used at higher doses.

Thiazide diuretics: May enhance the hypotensive effect and/or the nephrotoxic effect of ACE inhibitors.

Trimethoprim: May increase the risk of hyperkalemia.

Ethanol/Nutrition/Herb Interactions

Food: Potassium-containing salt substitutes may increase risk of hyperkalemia.

Herb/Nutraceutical: Avoid dong quai if using for hypertension (has estrogenic activity). Avoid ephedra, yohimbe, ginseng (may worsen hypertension). Avoid garlic (may have increased antihypertensive effect).

Mechanism of Action Competitive inhibitor of angiotensin-converting enzyme (ACE); prevents conversion of angiotensin I to angiotensin II, a potent vasoconstrictor; results in lower levels of angiotensin II which causes an increase in plasma renin activity and a reduction in aldosterone secretion; a CNS mechanism may also be involved in hypotensive effect as angiotensin II increases adrenergic outflow from CNS; vasoactive kallikreins may be decreased in conversion to active hormones by ACE inhibitors, thus reducing blood pressure

Pharmacodynamics Oral:

Onset of action: Within 1 hour

Peak effect: Within 6 hours

Duration: 24 hours

Pharmacokinetics

Absorption: Oral: Well absorbed

Protein binding: 25%

Half-life: 11-12 hours

Time to peak concentration: 6-7 hours; unaffected by food

Elimination: Almost entirely in urine as unchanged drug (100%)

Dosage

Geriatrics: Oral:

Initial: 2.5-5 mg/day; increase doses 2.5-5 mg/day at 1- to 2-week intervals; maximum daily dose: 40 mg

Patients taking diuretics should have them discontinued 2-3 days prior to initiating lisinopril if possible. Restart diuretic after blood pressure is stable if needed. In patients with hyponatremia (<130 mEq/L), start dose at 2.5 mg/day (see Dosage: Renal Impairment).

Adults:

Hypertension: Oral: Usual dosage range (JNC 7): 10-40 mg/day

Not maintained on diuretic: Initial: 10 mg/day

Maintained on diuretic: Initial: 5 mg/day

Note: Antihypertensive effect may diminish toward the end of the dosing interval especially with doses of 10 mg/day. An increased dose may aid in extending the duration of antihypertensive effect. Doses up to 80 mg/day have been used, but do not appear to give greater effect (Zesteril® Product Information, 12/04).

Patients taking diuretics should have them discontinued 2-3 days prior to initiating lisinopril if possible. Restart diuretic after blood pressure is stable if needed. If diuretic cannot be discontinued prior to therapy, begin with 5 mg with close supervision until stable blood pressure. In patients with hyponatremia (<130 mEq/L), start dose at 2.5 mg/day.

Congestive heart failure: Oral: Initial: 2.5-5 mg once daily; then increase by no more than 10 mg increments at intervals no less than 2 weeks to a maximum daily dose of 40 mg. Usual maintenance: 5-40 mg/day as a single dose. Target dose: 20-40 mg once daily (ACC/AHA 2005 Heart Failure Guidelines)

Note: If patient has hyponatremia (serum sodium <130 meq/L) or renal impairment (Cl_{cr} <30 mL/minute or creatinine >3 mg/dL), then initial dose should be 2.5 mg/day

Acute myocardial infarction (within 24 hours in hemodynamically stable patients): Oral: 5 mg immediately, then 5 mg at 24 hours, 10 mg at 48 hours, and 10 mg every day thereafter for 6 weeks. Patients should continue to receive standard treatments such as thrombolytics, aspirin, and beta-blockers.

Renal Impairment: Adults: Initial doses should be modified and upward titration should be cautious, based on response (maximum: 40 mg/day)

Cl_{cr} >30 mL/minute: Initial: 10 mg/day

Cl_{cr} 10-30 mL/minute: Initial: 5 mg/day

Hemodialysis: Initial: 2.5 mg/day; dialyzable (50%)

Administration Watch for hypotensive effects within 1-3 hours of first dose or new higher dose.

Monitoring Parameters Serum potassium concentration, BUN, serum creatinine, WBC

Test Interactions May cause false-positive results in urine acetone determinations using sodium nitroprusside reagent; increased potassium (S); increased serum creatinine/BUN

Patient Information Do not stop therapy except under prescriber advice; notify physician if you develop sore throat, fever, swelling of hands, feet, face, eyes, lips, and *(Continued)*

Lisinopril *(Continued)*

tongue; difficult breathing, irregular heartbeats, chest pains, or cough. May cause dizziness, fainting, and lightheadedness, especially in first week of therapy, sit and stand up slowly; may cause changes in taste or rash; do not add a salt substitute (potassium) without advice of physician.

Special Geriatric Considerations Due to frequent decreases in glomerular filtration (also creatinine clearance) with aging, elderly patients may have exaggerated responses to ACE inhibitors. Differences in clinical response due to hepatic changes are not observed. ACE inhibitors may be preferred agents in elderly patients with congestive heart failure and diabetes mellitus. Diabetic proteinuria is reduced and insulin sensitivity is enhanced. In general, the side effect profile is favorable in the elderly and causes little or no CNS confusion. Use lowest dose recommendations initially. Many elderly may be volume depleted due to diuretic use and/or blunted thirst reflex resulting in inadequate fluid intake.

Dosage Forms Excipient information presented when available (limited, particularly for generics); consult specific product labeling. [DSC] = Discontinued product

Tablet: 2.5 mg, 5 mg, 10 mg, 20 mg, 30 mg, 40 mg

   Prinivil®: 5 mg, 10 mg, 20 mg, 30 mg; 40 mg [DSC]

   Zestril®: 2.5 mg, 5 mg, 10 mg, 20 mg, 30 mg, 40 mg

Selected References

Konstam MA, Drakup K, Baker DW, et al, "Heart Failure: Evaluation and Care of Patients With Left Ventricular Systolic Dysfunction," *Clinical Practice Guideline No 11*, Rockville, MD: Agency for Health Care Policy and Research, Public Health Service, U.S. Department of Health and Human Services, 1994.

McAreavey D and Robertson JI, "Angiotensin Converting Enzyme Inhibitors and Moderate Hypertension," *Drugs*, 1990, 40(3):326-45.

Williams JF, Bristow MR, Fowler MB, et al, "Guidelines for the Evaluation and Management of Heart Failure: Report of the American College of Cardiology/American Heart Association Task Force on Practice Guidelines (Committee on Evaluation and Management of Heart Failure)," *J Am Coll Cardiol*, 1995, 26(5):1376-8.

Lisinopril and Hydrochlorothiazide
(lyse IN oh pril & hye droe klor oh THYE a zide)

Related Information

Hydrochlorothiazide *on page 756*
Lisinopril *on page 917*

U.S. Brand Names Prinzide®; Zestoretic®

Canadian Brand Names Prinzide®; Zestoretic®

Index Terms Hydrochlorothiazide and Lisinopril

Generic Available Yes

Pharmacologic Category Antihypertensive Agent, Combination

Use Treatment of hypertension

Dosage

Geriatrics & Adults: Hypertension: Oral: Initial: Lisinopril 10 mg/hydrochlorothiazide 12.5 mg or lisinopril 20 mg/hydrochlorothiazide 12.5 mg with further increases of either or both components could depend on clinical response. Doses >80 mg/day lisinopril or >50 mg/day hydrochlorothiazide are not recommended.

Renal Impairment: Dosage adjustments should be made with caution. Usual regimens of therapy need not be adjusted as long as patient's Cl$_{cr}$ >30 mL/minute. In patients with more severe renal impairment, loop diuretics are preferred.

Dosage Forms Excipient information presented when available (limited, particularly for generics); consult specific product labeling. [DSC] = Discontinued product

Tablet: 10/12.5: Lisinopril 10 mg and hydrochlorothiazide 12.5 mg; 20/12.5: Lisinopril 20 mg and hydrochlorothiazide 12.5 mg; 20/25: Lisinopril 20 mg and hydrochlorothiazide 25 mg

   Prinzide®:

   10/12.5: Lisinopril 10 mg and hydrochlorothiazide 12.5 mg

   20/12.5: Lisinopril 20 mg and hydrochlorothiazide 12.5 mg [DSC]

   20/25: Lisinopril 20 mg and hydrochlorothiazide 25 mg

   Zestoretic®:

   10/12.5: Lisinopril 10 mg and hydrochlorothiazide 12.5 mg

   20/12.5: Lisinopril 20 mg and hydrochlorothiazide 12.5 mg

   20/25: Lisinopril 20 mg and hydrochlorothiazide 25 mg

♦ **Lispro Insulin** *see* Insulin Lispro *on page 812*

Lithium (LITH ee um)

Related Information

Liquid Compatibility of Antipsychotics and Mood Stabilizers *on page 1851*
Serum Drug Concentrations Commonly Monitored Guidelines *on page 1862*

Medication Safety Issues

Sound-alike/look-alike issues:

Eskalith® may be confused with Estratest®

Lithobid® may be confused with Levbid®, Lithostat®

Do not confuse **mEq** (milliequivalent) with **mg** (milligram). **Note:** 8 mEq lithium carbonate equals 300 mg lithium carbonate. Dosage should be written in **mg** (milligrams) to avoid confusion. Check prescriptions for unusually high volumes of the syrup for dosing errors.

U.S. Brand Names Eskalith® [DSC]; Eskalith CR® [DSC]; Lithobid®

Canadian Brand Names Apo-Lithium® Carbonate; Apo-Lithium® Carbonate SR; Carbolith™; Duralith®; Lithane™; PMS-Lithium Carbonate; PMS-Lithium Citrate

Index Terms Lithium Carbonate; Lithium Citrate

Generic Available Yes

Pharmacologic Category Lithium

Use Management of bipolar disorders; treatment of mania in individuals with bipolar disorder (maintenance treatment prevents or diminishes intensity of subsequent episodes)

Unlabeled/Investigational Use Potential augmenting agent for antidepressants; treatment of aggression, post-traumatic stress disorder

Contraindications Hypersensitivity to lithium or any component of the formulation; avoid use in patients with severe cardiovascular or renal disease, or with severe debilitation, dehydration, or sodium depletion

Warnings/Precautions [U.S. Boxed Warning]: Lithium toxicity is closely related to serum levels and can occur at therapeutic doses; serum lithium determinations are required to monitor therapy. Use with caution in patients with thyroid disease, mild-moderate renal impairment, or mild-moderate cardiovascular disease. Use caution in patients receiving medications which alter sodium excretion (eg, diuretics, ACE inhibitors, NSAIDs), or in patients with significant fluid loss (protracted sweating, diarrhea, or prolonged fever); temporary reduction or cessation of therapy may be warranted. Some elderly patients may be extremely sensitive to the effects of lithium, see Dosage and Reference Range. Chronic therapy results in diminished renal concentrating ability (nephrogenic DI); this is usually reversible when lithium is discontinued. Changes in renal function should be monitored, and re-evaluation of treatment may be necessary. Use caution in patients at risk of suicide (suicidal thoughts or behavior).

Use with caution in patients receiving neuroleptic medications - a syndrome resembling NMS has been associated with concurrent therapy. Lithium may impair the patient's alertness, affecting the ability to operate machinery or driving a vehicle. Neuromuscular-blocking agents should be administered with caution; the response may be prolonged.

Higher serum concentrations may be required and tolerated during an acute manic phase; however, the tolerance decreases when symptoms subside. Normal fluid and salt intake must be maintained during therapy.

Adverse Reactions (Reflective of adult population; not specific for elderly)

Frequency not defined.

Cardiovascular: Cardiac arrhythmia, hypotension, sinus node dysfunction, flattened or inverted T waves (reversible), edema, bradycardia, syncope

Central nervous system: Dizziness, vertigo, slurred speech, blackout spells, seizure, sedation, restlessness, confusion, psychomotor retardation, stupor, coma, dystonia, fatigue, lethargy, headache, pseudotumor cerebri, slowed intellectual functioning, tics

Dermatologic: Dry or thinning of hair, folliculitis, alopecia, exacerbation of psoriasis, rash

Endocrine & metabolic: Euthyroid goiter and/or hypothyroidism, hyperthyroidism, hyperglycemia, diabetes insipidus

Gastrointestinal: Polydipsia, anorexia, nausea, vomiting, diarrhea, xerostomia, metallic taste, weight gain, salivary gland swelling, excessive salivation

Genitourinary: Incontinence, polyuria, glycosuria, oliguria, albuminuria

Hematologic: Leukocytosis

Neuromuscular & skeletal: Tremor, muscle hyperirritability, ataxia, choreoathetoid movements, hyperactive deep tendon reflexes, myasthenia gravis (rare)

Ocular: Nystagmus, blurred vision, transient scotoma

Miscellaneous: Coldness and painful discoloration of fingers and toes

Overdosage/Toxicology Symptoms include sedation, confusion, tremors, joint pain, visual changes, seizures, and coma. There is no specific antidote for lithium poisoning. For acute ingestion, following initiation of essential overdose management, discontinue lithium and remove any unabsorbed lithium via gastric lavage (activated charcoal is ineffective as it does not bind lithium). Correct fluid and electrolyte imbalances, provide supportive care. In severe cases, patient should be dialyzed. Hemodialysis is preferred (and more effective) than peritoneal dialysis. The goal is to decrease serum lithium

(Continued)

Lithium *(Continued)*

level to <1 mEq/L on a serum sample drawn 6-8 hours after completion of dialysis. Agents that increase the excretion of lithium are of questionable value.

Drug Interactions

ACE inhibitors: May increase the risk of lithium toxicity via sodium depletion; monitor

Angiotensin receptor antagonists (losartan): May reduce the renal clearance of lithium; monitor

Caffeine (xanthine derivatives): May lower lithium serum concentrations by increasing urinary lithium excretion; monitor.

Carbamazepine: Concurrent use of lithium with carbamazepine may increase the risk for neurotoxicity; monitor

Carbonic anhydrase inhibitors: May decrease lithium levels; includes acetazolamide; monitor

Calcium channel blockers (diltiazem and verapamil): May increase the risk for neurotoxicity (ataxia, tremors, nausea, vomiting, diarrhea, and/or tinnitus); monitor; does not appear to involve dihydropyridine class

Chlorpromazine: May lower serum concentrations of both drugs; monitor

COX-2 inhibitors (celecoxib): May increase lithium plasma concentrations (similar to NSAIDs); monitor.

Haloperidol: May increase the risk for neurotoxicity and encephalopathy; a rare encephalopathic syndrome resulting in irreversible brain damage and possible recovery in a few patients (causal relationship not established); monitor

Iodine salts: May enhance the hypothyroid effects of lithium; monitor

Loop diuretics: May decrease the renal excretion of lithium, leading to toxicity; monitor

MAO inhibitors: Should generally be avoided due to use reports of fatal malignant hyperpyrexia when combined with lithium

Methyldopa: May increase the risk for neurotoxicity; monitor

Metronidazole: May increase lithium toxicity (rare); monitor

Neuromuscular-blocking agents: Lithium may potentiate the response to neuromuscular blockade, resulting in prolonged blockade and possible delayed recovery

NSAIDs: Renal lithium excretion may be decreased leading to increased serum lithium concentrations; sulindac and aspirin may be the exceptions; monitor

Phenothiazines: May increase the risk for neurotoxicity; monitor

Phenytoin: May enhance lithium toxicity; monitor

Selegiline: Risk of severe reactions when combined with MAO inhibitors may be decreased when administered with selective MAO type B inhibitor, particularly at selegiline doses <10 mg/day; however, theoretical risk is still present

SSRIs: May increase the risk for neurotoxicity; monitor; effect noted with fluoxetine, fluvoxamine

Sibutramine: Combined use of lithium with sibutramine may increase the risk of serotonin syndrome; this combination is best avoided

Sodium-containing products: Bicarbonate and/or high sodium intake may reduce serum lithium concentrations via enhanced excretion; monitor. **Note:** Reabsorption of lithium in the proximal convoluted tubule occurs against electrical and concentration gradients that do not distinguish between lithium and sodium. Therefore, lithium clearance may increase or decrease 30% to 50% with sodium load or depletion, respectively. Sodium depletion usually has the greater effect.

Sympathomimetics: Lithium may blunt the pressor response to sympathomimetics (epinephrine, phenylephrine, norepinephrine)

Tetracyclines: May increase lithium levels; monitor

Theophylline: May increase real clearance of lithium, resulting in a decrease in serum lithium concentrations; monitor

Thiazide diuretics: May increase serum lithium concentration via sodium depletion and decreased lithium clearance; a lithium dose reduction of 50% is commonly recommended

Tricyclic antidepressants: May increase the risk for neurotoxicity; monitor

Urea: May lower lithium serum concentrations by increasing urinary lithium excretion; monitor.

Ethanol/Nutrition/Herb Interactions Food: Lithium serum concentrations may be increased if taken with food. Limit caffeine.

Mechanism of Action Alters cation transport across cell membrane in nerve and muscle cells and influences reuptake of serotonin and/or norepinephrine; second messenger systems involving the phosphatidylinositol cycle are inhibited; postsynaptic D2 receptor supersensitivity is inhibited

Pharmacokinetics

Absorption: Rapid and complete

Distribution: V_d: Initial: 0.3-0.4 L/kg; V_{dss}: 0.7-1 L/kg

Metabolism: Not metabolized

Half-life: 18-24 hours; can increase to more than 36 hours in older adults or with renal impairment

Time to peak, serum: Nonsustained release: ~0.5-2 hours

Elimination: Urine (90% to 98% as unchanged drug); sweat (4% to 5%); feces (1%)

Dosage

Geriatrics: Bipolar disorders: Oral: Initial: 300 mg twice daily; increase weekly in increments of 300 mg/day, monitoring levels; rarely need to go >900-1200 mg/day.

Adults:

Bipolar disorders: Oral: 900-2400 mg/day in 3-4 divided doses or 900-1800 mg/day in two divided doses of sustained release

Note: Monitor serum concentrations and clinical response (efficacy and toxicity) to determine proper dose

Renal Impairment:

Cl_{cr} 10-50 mL/minute: Administer 50% to 75% of normal dose.

Cl_{cr} <10 mL/minute: Administer 25% to 50% of normal dose.

Dialyzable (50% to 100%); 4-7 times more efficient than peritoneal dialysis

Administration Administer with meals to decrease GI upset. Slow release tablets must be swallowed whole; do not crush or chew.

Monitoring Parameters Serum lithium every 4-5 days during initial therapy; draw lithium serum concentrations 12 hours postdose; renal, thyroid, and cardiovascular function; fluid status; serum electrolytes; CBC with differential, urinalysis; monitor for signs of toxicity

Reference Range Levels should be obtained twice weekly until both patient's clinical status and levels are stable, then levels may be obtained every 1-3 months.

Timing of serum samples: Draw trough just before next dose (8-12 hours after previous dose).

Therapeutic levels:

Acute mania: 0.6-1.2 mEq/L (SI: 0.6-1.2 mmol/L)

Protection against future episodes in most patients with bipolar disorder: 0.8-1 mEq/L (SI: 0.8-1.0 mmol/L); a higher rate of relapse is described in subjects who are maintained at <0.4 mEq/L (SI: 0.4 mmol/L)

Older adults can usually be maintained at lower end of therapeutic range (0.6-0.8 mEq/L)

Toxic concentration: >1.5 mEq/L (SI: >2 mmol/L)

Adverse effect levels:

GI complaints/tremor: 1.5-2 mEq/L

Confusion/somnolence: 2-2.5 mEq/L

Seizures/death: >2.5 mEq/L

Patient Information Avoid tasks requiring psychomotor coordination until the CNS effects are known, blood level monitoring is required to determine the proper dose; maintain a steady salt and fluid intake especially during the summer months; do not crush or chew slow or extended release dosage form, swallow whole

Additional Information Lithium levels should be obtained 12 hours after the last dose of the day; 5 mL of lithium citrate syrup contains 8 mEq of lithium and is approximately equivalent to 300 mg of lithium carbonate

Lithium citrate: Cibalith-S®

Lithium carbonate: Eskalith®, Lithane®, Lithobid®, Lithonate®, Lithotabs®

Special Geriatric Considerations Some elderly patients may be extremely sensitive to the effects of lithium. Initial doses need to be adjusted for renal function in the elderly; thereafter, adjust doses based upon serum concentrations and response.

Dosage Forms Excipient information presented when available (limited, particularly for generics); consult specific product labeling. [DSC] = Discontinued product

Capsule, as carbonate: 150 mg, 300 mg, 600 mg

Eskalith®: 300 mg [contains benzyl alcohol] [DSC]

Solution, as citrate: 300 mg/5 mL (5 mL, 500 mL) [equivalent to amount of lithium in lithium carbonate]

Syrup, as citrate: 300 mg/5 mL (480 mL) [equivalent to amount of lithium in lithium carbonate]

Tablet, as carbonate: 300 mg

Tablet, controlled release, as carbonate: 450 mg

Eskalith CR®: 450 mg [DSC]

Tablet, slow release, as carbonate: 300 mg

Lithobid®: 300 mg

Selected References

Foster JF, Gershell WJ, and Goldfarb AI, "Lithium Treatment in the Elderly. I. Clinical Usage," *J Gerontol,* 1977, 32(3):299-302.

Hicks R, Dysken MW, Davis JM, et al, "The Pharmacokinetics of Psychotropic Medication in the Elderly: A Review," *J Clin Psychiatry,* 1981, 42(10):374-85.

Ward ME, Musa MN, Bailey L, "Clinical Pharmacokinetics of Lithium," *J Clin Pharmacol,* 1994, 34(4):280-5.

- **Locoid Lipocream®** *see* Hydrocortisone *on page 762*
- **Lodine® [DSC]** *see* Etodolac *on page 587*
- **Lodine® XL [DSC]** *see* Etodolac *on page 587*
- **Lodosyn®** *see* Carbidopa *on page 237*

Lodoxamide (loe DOKS a mide)

Medication Safety Issues
International issues:
Thilomide® [Turkey] may be confused with Thalomid® which is a brand name for thalidomide in the U.S.
U.S. Brand Names Alomide®
Canadian Brand Names Alomide®
Index Terms Lodoxamide Tromethamine
Generic Available No
Pharmacologic Category Mast Cell Stabilizer
Use Treatment of vernal keratoconjunctivitis, vernal conjunctivitis, and vernal keratitis
Contraindications Hypersensitivity to lodoxamide tromethamine or any component of the formulation
Warnings/Precautions Not for injection; not for use in patients wearing soft contact lenses during treatment
Adverse Reactions (Reflective of adult population; not specific for elderly)
>10%: Local: Transient burning, stinging, discomfort
1% to 10%:
Central nervous system: Headache
Ocular: Blurred vision, corneal erosion/ulcer, eye pain, corneal abrasion, blepharitis
Drug Interactions No data reported
Mechanism of Action Mast cell stabilizer that inhibits the *in vivo* type I immediate hypersensitivity reaction to increase cutaneous vascular permeability associated with IgE and antigen-mediated reactions
Pharmacokinetics Absorption: Topical: Very small and undetectable
Dosage
Geriatrics & Adults: Vernal conjunctivitis, keratitis: Ophthalmic: Instill 1-2 drops in eye(s) 4 times/day for up to 3 months
Patient Information May sting or burn upon instillation; do not touch dropper to the eye
Special Geriatric Considerations Assure the patient or caregiver can adequately administer ophthalmic medication.
Dosage Forms Excipient information presented when available (limited, particularly for generics); consult specific product labeling.
Solution, ophthalmic: 0.1% (10 mL) [contains benzalkonium chloride]

- **Lodoxamide Tromethamine** *see* Lodoxamide *on page 924*
- **Lodrane® 12 Hour** *see* Brompheniramine *on page 189*
- **Lodrane® 24** *see* Brompheniramine *on page 189*
- **Lodrane® XR** *see* Brompheniramine *on page 189*
- **Lofibra™** *see* Fenofibrate *on page 604*
- **LoHist-12** *see* Brompheniramine *on page 189*
- **Lomotil®** *see* Diphenoxylate and Atropine *on page 450*
- **Lonox®** *see* Diphenoxylate and Atropine *on page 450*

Loperamide (loe PER a mide)

Medication Safety Issues
Sound-alike/look-alike issues:
Imodium® A-D may be confused with Indocin®, Ionamin®
U.S. Brand Names Diamode [OTC]; Imodium® A-D [OTC]; Kao-Paverin® [OTC]; K-Pek II [OTC]
Canadian Brand Names Apo-Loperamide®; Diarr-Eze; Imodium®; Loperacap; Novo-Loperamide; PMS-Loperamine; Rho®-Loperamine; Riva-Loperamine
Index Terms Loperamide Hydrochloride
Generic Available Yes
Pharmacologic Category Antidiarrheal
Use Treatment of chronic diarrhea associated with inflammatory bowel disease; acute nonspecific diarrhea; increased volume of ileostomy discharge
OTC labeling: Control of symptoms of diarrhea, including Traveler's diarrhea
Unlabeled/Investigational Use Cancer treatment-induced diarrhea (eg, irinotecan induced); chronic diarrhea caused by bowel resection
Contraindications Hypersensitivity to loperamide or any component of the formulation; abdominal pain without diarrhea

Avoid use as primary therapy in acute dysentery, acute ulcerative colitis, bacterial enterocolitis, pseudomembranous colitis

Warnings/Precautions Rare cases of anaphylaxis and anaphylactic shock have been reported. Should not be used if diarrhea is accompanied by high fever or blood in stool. Concurrent fluid and electrolyte replacement is often necessary in all age groups depending upon severity of diarrhea. Should not be used when inhibition of peristalsis is undesirable or dangerous. Discontinue if constipation, abdominal pain, or ileus develop. Use caution in treatment of AIDS patients; stop therapy at the sign of abdominal distention. Cases of toxic megacolon have occurred in this population. Loperamide is a symptom-directed treatment; if an underlying diagnosis is made, other disease-specific treatment may be indicated. Use caution in patients with hepatic impairment because of reduced first-pass metabolism; monitor for signs of CNS toxicity.

OTC labeling: If diarrhea lasts longer than 2 days, patient should stop taking loperamide and consult healthcare provider.

Adverse Reactions (Reflective of adult population; not specific for elderly)
1% to 10%:
Central nervous system: Dizziness (1%)
Gastrointestinal: Constipation (2% to 5%), abdominal cramping (<1% to 3%), nausea (<1% to 3%)
Postmarketing and/or case reports: Abdominal distention, abdominal pain, allergic reactions, anaphylactic shock, anaphylactoid reactions, angioedema, bullous eruption (rare), drowsiness, dry mouth, dyspepsia, erythema multiforme (rare), fatigue, flatulence, paralytic ileus, megacolon, pruritus, rash, Stevens-Johnson syndrome, toxic epidermal necrolysis, toxic megacolon, urinary retention, urticaria, vomiting

Overdosage/Toxicology Symptoms of overdose include CNS depression, urinary retention, and paralytic ileus. Treatment of overdose includes gastric lavage followed by 100 g activated charcoal through a nasogastric tube. Naloxone can be given as an antidote. The prolonged action of loperamide may necessitate naloxone's repeated administration and close patient monitoring for recurrent CNS depression.

Drug Interactions Substrate (minor) of CYP2B6
P-glycoprotein inhibitors: May increase CNS depressant effects of loperamide. Examples of inhibitors include cyclosporine, ketoconazole, quinidine, quinine, and ritonavir. Monitor.
Saquinavir: Loperamide may decrease levels/effects of saquinavir.

Stability Store at 15°C to 25°C (59°F to 77°F).

Mechanism of Action Acts directly on circular and longitudinal intestinal muscles, through the opioid receptor, to inhibit peristalsis and prolong transit time; reduces fecal volume, increases viscosity, and diminishes fluid and electrolyte loss; demonstrates antisecretory activity. Loperamide increases tone on the anal sphincter

Pharmacokinetics
Absorption: Poor
Distribution: Poor penetration into brain
Metabolism: Hepatic via oxidative N-demethylation
Half-life elimination: 7-14 hours
Time to peak, plasma: Liquid: 2.5 hours; Capsule: 5 hours
Excretion: Urine and feces (1% as metabolites, 30% to 40% as unchanged drug)

Dosage
Geriatrics & Adults:
Acute diarrhea: Oral: Initial: 4 mg, followed by 2 mg after each loose stool, up to 16 mg/day
Chronic diarrhea: Oral: Initial: Follow acute diarrhea; maintenance dose should be slowly titrated downward to minimum required to control symptoms (typically, 4-8 mg/day in divided doses)
Traveler's diarrhea: Oral: Initial: 4 mg after first loose stool, followed by 2 mg after each subsequent stool (maximum dose: 8 mg/day)
Irinotecan-induced diarrhea (unlabeled use): Oral: 4 mg after first loose or frequent bowel movement, then 2 mg every 2 hours until 12 hours have passed without a bowel movement. If diarrhea recurs, then repeat administration
Hepatic Impairment: No specific guidelines available.

Monitoring Parameters Monitor stool frequency and consistency; observe for toxicity with use more than 48 hours

Patient Information Do not take more than 8 capsules/80 mL in 24 hours; may cause drowsiness; use caution when driving; may cause dry mouth; notify physician if diarrhea persists or abdominal distention occurs; if diarrhea does not subside in 2-3 days, consult physician when buying without physician's advice.

Additional Information Therapy for chronic diarrhea should not exceed 10 days; if diarrhea persists longer than 48 hours for acute diarrhea, etiology should be examined

Special Geriatric Considerations Elderly are particularly sensitive to fluid and electrolyte loss. This generally results in lethargy, weakness, and confusion. Repletion and (Continued)

Loperamide *(Continued)*

maintenance of electrolytes and water are essential in the treatment of diarrhea. Drug therapy must be limited in order to avoid toxicity with this agent.

Dosage Forms Excipient information presented when available (limited, particularly for generics); consult specific product labeling.

Caplet, as hydrochloride: 2 mg
    Diamode, Imodium® A-D, Kao-Paverin®: 2 mg
Capsule, as hydrochloride: 2 mg
Liquid, oral, as hydrochloride: 1 mg/5 mL (5 mL, 10 mL, 120 mL)
    Imodium® A-D: 1 mg/5 mL (60 mL, 120 mL) [contains alcohol, sodium benzoate, benzoic acid; cherry mint flavor]
    Imodium® A-D [new formulation]: 1 mg/7.5 mL (60 mL, 120 mL, 360 mL) [contains sodium 10 mg/30 mL, sodium benzoate; creamy mint flavor]
Tablet, as hydrochloride: 2 mg
    K-Pek II: 2 mg

Selected References

Benson AB 3rd, Ajani JA, Catalano RB, et al, "Recommended Guidelines for the Treatment of Cancer Treatment-Induced Diarrhea," *J Clin Oncol*, 2004, 22(14):2918-26.

Ericsson CD, "Nonantimicrobial Agents in the Prevention and Treatment of Traveler's Diarrhea," *Clin Infect Dis*, 2005, 41(Suppl 8):557-63.

Rothenberg ML, Eckardt JR, Kuhn JG, et al, "Phase II Trial of Irinotecan in Patients With Progressive or Rapidly Recurrent Colorectal Cancer," *J Clin Oncol*, 1996, 14(4):1128-35.

Loperamide and Simethicone *(loe PER a mide & sye METH i kone)*

U.S. Brand Names Imodium® Advanced
Index Terms Simethicone and Loperamide Hydrochloride
Generic Available No
Pharmacologic Category Antidiarrheal; Antiflatulent
Use Control of symptoms of diarrhea and gas (bloating, pressure, and cramps)
Dosage
  Geriatrics & Adults: Acute diarrhea: Oral: 1 caplet or tablet after first loose stool, followed by 1 caplet or tablet with each subsequent loose stool (maximum: 4 caplets or tablets/24 hours)
Special Geriatric Considerations
Elderly are particularly sensitive to fluid and electrolyte loss. This generally results in lethargy, weakness, and confusion. Repletion and maintenance of electrolytes and water are essential in the treatment of diarrhea. Drug therapy must be limited in order to avoid toxicity with this agent. Before treating excess gas or pain due to gas accumulation, a thorough evaluation must be made to determine cause since many bowel diseases may present with flatulence and bloating.

Dosage Forms Excipient information presented when available (limited, particularly for generics); consult specific product labeling.

Caplet: Loperamide hydrochloride 2 mg and simethicone 125 mg
Tablet, chewable: Loperamide hydrochloride 2 mg and simethicone 125 mg [mint flavor]

♦ **Loperamide Hydrochloride** *see* Loperamide *on page 924*
♦ **Lopid®** *see* Gemfibrozil *on page 701*
♦ **Lopressor®** *see* Metoprolol *on page 1027*
♦ **Lopressor HCT®** *see* Metoprolol and Hydrochlorothiazide *on page 1030*
♦ **Loprox®** *see* Ciclopirox *on page 311*
♦ **Lorabid® [DSC]** *see* Loracarbef *on page 926*

Loracarbef *(lor a KAR bef)*

Related Information
  Antimicrobial Activity Against Selected Organisms *on page 1728*
Medication Safety Issues
  Sound-alike/look-alike issues:
    Lorabid® may be confused with Levbid®, Lopid®, Lortab®, Slo-bid™
U.S. Brand Names Lorabid® [DSC]
Canadian Brand Names Lorabid®
Generic Available No
Pharmacologic Category Antibiotic, Carbacephem
Use Treatment of infections caused by susceptible organisms involving the upper and lower respiratory tract, uncomplicated skin and skin structure, and urinary tract (including uncomplicated pyelonephritis)
Contraindications Hypersensitivity to loracarbef, any component of the formulation, or cephalosporins

Warnings/Precautions Modify dosage in patients with severe renal impairment. Prolonged use may result in fungal or bacterial superinfection, including *C. difficile*-associated diarrhea and pseudomembranous colitis. Use with caution in patients with a previous history of hypersensitivity to other beta-lactam antibiotics (eg, penicillins, cephalosporins).

Adverse Reactions (Reflective of adult population; not specific for elderly)
1% to 10%:
Central nervous system: Headache (1% to 3%), somnolence (<1% to 2%)
Dermatologic: Rash (1% to 3%)
Gastrointestinal: Diarrhea (4% to 6%), nausea (2% to 3%), vomiting (1% to 3%), anorexia (<1% to 2%), abdominal pain (1%)
Genitourinary: Vaginitis (1%), vaginal moniliasis (1%)
Respiratory: Rhinitis (2% to 6%)
Miscellaneous: Hypersensitivity reactions (1%; eg, urticaria, pruritus, erythema multiforme)

Other adverse reactions observed with beta-lactam antibiotics: Agranulocytosis, allergic reactions, aplastic anemia, hemolytic anemia, hemorrhage, interstitial nephritis, LDH increased, neutropenia, pancytopenia, positive direct Coombs' test, pseudomembranous colitis, seizure (with high doses and renal dysfunction), toxic epidermal necrolysis

Overdosage/Toxicology Symptoms include nausea and vomiting, abdominal discomfort and diarrhea. Treatment is symptom-directed and supportive.

Drug Interactions Probenecid: May decrease cephalosporin elimination.

Ethanol/Nutrition/Herb Interactions Food: Administration with food decreases and delays the peak plasma concentration.

Stability
Capsule: Store at 15°C to 30°C (59°F to 86°F).
Suspension: Prior to reconstitution, store at 15°C to 30°C (59°F to 86°F). After reconstitution, suspension may be kept at room temperature for 14 days.

Mechanism of Action Inhibits bacterial cell wall synthesis by binding to one or more of the penicillin binding proteins (PBPs); inhibits the final transpeptidation step of peptidoglycan synthesis in bacterial cell walls, thus inhibiting cell wall biosynthesis. It is thought that beta-lactam antibiotics inactivate transpeptidase via acylation of the enzyme with cleavage of the CO-N bond of the beta-lactam ring. Upon exposure to beta-lactam antibiotics, bacteria eventually lyse due to ongoing activity of cell wall autolytic enzymes (autolysins and murein hydrolases) while cell wall assembly is arrested.

Pharmacokinetics
Absorption: Oral: Rapid
Half-life, elimination: ~1 hour
Bioavailability: ~90%; decreased by food
Protein binding: ~25%
Time to peak serum concentration: Oral: Within 1 hour
Elimination: Plasma clearance: ~200-300 mL/minute

Dosage
Geriatrics & Adults:
Bronchitis: Oral: 200-400 mg every 12 hours for 7 days
Pharyngitis/tonsillitis: Oral: 200 mg every 12 hours for 10 days
Pneumonia: Oral: 400 mg every 12 hours for 14 days
Sinusitis: Oral: 400 mg every 12 hours for 10 days
Skin and soft tissue, uncomplicated: Oral: 200 mg every 12 hours for 7 days
Urinary tract infections, uncomplicated: Oral: 200 mg once daily for 7 days
Pyelonephritis, uncomplicated: Oral: 400 mg every 12 hours for 14 days
Renal Impairment:
Cl_{cr} ≥50 mL/minute: Administer usual dose.
Cl_{cr} 10-49 mL/minute: Administer 50% of usual dose at usual interval or usual dose given half as often.
Cl_{cr} <10 mL/minute: Administer usual dose every 3-5 days.
Hemodialysis: Doses should be administered after dialysis sessions.

Administration Take on an empty stomach

Monitoring Parameters Signs and symptoms of infection, WBC, mental status

Patient Information Take on an empty stomach at least 1 hour before or 2 hours after meals; complete full course of therapy.

Special Geriatric Considerations Half-life is slightly prolonged with age, presumably due to the reduced creatinine clearance related to aging. Adjust dose for renal function.

Dosage Forms Excipient information presented when available (limited, particularly for generics); consult specific product labeling. [DSC] = Discontinued product
Capsule:
Lorabid®: 200 mg, 400 mg [DSC]
(Continued)

Loracarbef *(Continued)*

Powder for oral suspension:
Lorabid®: 100 mg/5 mL (100 mL); 200 mg/5 mL (100 mL) [strawberry bubble gum flavor] [DSC]

Selected References
DeSante KA and Zeckel ML, "Pharmacokinetic Profile of Loracarbef," *Am J Med*, 1992, 92(6A):16S-9S.

Loratadine *(lor AT a deen)*

Medication Safety Issues
Sound-alike/look-alike issues:
Dimetapp® may be confused with Dermatop®, Dimetabs®, Dimetane®

U.S. Brand Names Alavert® [OTC]; Claritin® 24 Hour Allergy [OTC]; Claritin® Hives Relief [OTC]; Tavist® ND [OTC]; Triaminic® Allerchews™ [OTC]

Canadian Brand Names Apo-Loratadine®; Claritin®; Claritin® Kids

Generic Available Yes

Pharmacologic Category Antihistamine, Nonsedating

Use Relief of nasal and non-nasal symptoms of seasonal allergic rhinitis

Contraindications Hypersensitivity to loratadine or any component of the formulation

Warnings/Precautions Use with caution and modify dose in patients with liver or renal impairment

Adverse Reactions (Reflective of adult population; not specific for elderly)

Adults:
Central nervous system: Headache (12%), somnolence (8%), fatigue (4%)
Gastrointestinal: Xerostomia (3%)

Children:
Central nervous system: Nervousness (4% ages 6-12 years), fatigue (3% ages 6-12 years, 2% to 3% ages 2-5 years), malaise (2% ages 6-12 years)
Dermatologic: Rash (2% to 3% ages 2-5 years)
Gastrointestinal: Abdominal pain (2% ages 6-12 years), stomatitis (2% to 3% ages 2-5 years)
Neuromuscular & skeletal: Hyperkinesia (3% ages 6-12 years)
Ocular: Conjunctivitis (2% ages 6-12 years)
Respiratory: Wheezing (4% ages 6-12 years), dysphonia (2% ages 6-12 years), upper respiratory infection (2% ages 6-12 years), epistaxis (2% to 3% ages 2-5 years), pharyngitis (2% to 3% ages 2-5 years)
Miscellaneous: Flu-like syndrome (2% to 3% ages 2-5 years), viral infection (2% to 3% ages 2-5 years)

Overdosage/Toxicology Symptoms include somnolence, tachycardia, and headache. No specific antidote is available. Treatment is symptomatic and supportive. Loratadine is not eliminated by dialysis.

Drug Interactions Substrate (minor) of CYP2D6, 3A4; **Inhibits** CYP2C8 (weak), 2C19 (moderate), 2D6 (weak)
CYP2C19 substrates: Loratadine may increase the levels/effects of CYP2C19 substrates. Example substrates include citalopram, diazepam, methsuximide, phenytoin, propranolol, and sertraline.
Protease inhibitors (amprenavir, ritonavir, nelfinavir) may increase the serum levels of loratadine
Increased toxicity: Other antihistamines

Ethanol/Nutrition/Herb Interactions
Ethanol: Avoid ethanol (although sedation is limited with loratadine, may increase risk of CNS depression).
Food: Increases bioavailability and delays peak.
Herb/Nutraceutical: St John's wort may decrease loratadine levels.

Stability Store at 2°C to 25°C (36°F to 77°F).
Rapidly-disintegrating tablets: Use within 6 months of opening foil pouch, and immediately after opening individual tablet blister. Store in a dry place.

Mechanism of Action Long-acting tricyclic antihistamine with selective peripheral histamine H_1-receptor antagonistic properties

Pharmacokinetics
Absorption: Rapid
Metabolism: Extensive to an active metabolite
Half-life:
Geriatrics: 18.2 hours (6.7-37 hours)
Adults: 12-15 hours
Elimination: In one study, the AUC and peak plasma levels of both loratadine and its active metabolite were approximately 50% higher in older adult patients as compared to younger adults

Dosage

Geriatrics & Adults: Seasonal allergic rhinitis, chronic idiopathic urticaria: Oral: 10 mg/day

Renal Impairment:

Cl_{cr} ≤30 mL/minute: 10 mg every other day

Hepatic Impairment:

Elimination half-life increases with severity of disease.

Adults: 10 mg every other day

Monitoring Parameters Relief of symptoms, mental status

Patient Information Drink plenty of water; may cause dry mouth, sedation, drowsiness, and can impair judgment and coordination

Special Geriatric Considerations Loratadine is a nonsedating antihistamines; because of its low incidence of side effects, it seems to be a good choice in the elderly. However, there is a wide variation in loratadine half-life reported in the elderly and this should be kept in mind when initiating dosing. Because of its new OTC status, patients should be advised of appropriate use.

Dosage Forms Excipient information presented when available (limited, particularly for generics); consult specific product labeling.

Syrup: 1 mg/mL (120 mL)

Claritin®: 1 mg/mL (120 mL) [contains sodium benzoate; fruit flavor]; (60 mL, 120 mL) [alcohol free, dye free, sugar free; contains sodium 6 mg/5 mL and sodium benzoate; grape flavor]

Tablet: 10 mg

Alavert®, Claritin®, Claritin® Hives Relief, Claritin® 24 Hour Allergy, Tavist® ND: 10 mg

Tablet, rapidly disintegrating: 10 mg

Alavert®: 10 mg [contains phenylalanine 8.4 mg/tablet; mint and citrus burst flavors]

Claritin® RediTabs®: 10 mg [mint flavor]

Triaminic® Allerchews™: 10 mg

Lorazepam (lor A ze pam)

Related Information

Anxiolytic, Sedative / Hypnotic, and Miscellaneous Benzodiazepines *on page 1750*
Potentially Inappropriate Medications for Geriatrics *on page 1824*

Medication Safety Issues

Sound-alike/look-alike issues:

Lorazepam may be confused with alprazolam, clonazepam, diazepam, temazepam

Ativan® may be confused with Atarax®, Atgam®, Avitene®

Injection dosage form contains propylene glycol. Monitor for toxicity when administering continuous lorazepam infusions.

U.S. Brand Names Ativan®; Lorazepam Intensol®

Canadian Brand Names Apo-Lorazepam®; Ativan®; Lorazepam Injection, USP; Novo-Lorazepam; Nu-Loraz; PMS-Lorazepam; Riva-Lorazepam

Generic Available Yes

Pharmacologic Category Benzodiazepine

Use

Oral: Management of anxiety disorders or short-term (≤4 months) relief of the symptoms of anxiety or anxiety associated with depressive symptoms

I.V.: Status epilepticus, preanesthesia for desired amnesia

Unlabeled/Investigational Use Ethanol detoxification; treatment of insomnia, psychogenic catatonia, partial complex seizures, agitation (I.V.)

Restrictions C-IV

Contraindications Hypersensitivity to lorazepam or any component of the formulation (cross-sensitivity with other benzodiazepines may exist); acute narrow-angle glaucoma; sleep apnea (parenteral); intra-arterial injection of parenteral formulation; severe respiratory insufficiency (except during mechanical ventilation)

Warnings/Precautions Use with caution in elderly or debilitated patients, patients with hepatic disease (including alcoholics) or renal impairment. Use with caution in patients with respiratory disease (COPD or sleep apnea) or limited pulmonary reserve, or impaired gag reflex. Initial doses in elderly or debilitated patients should be at the lower end of the dosing range. May worsen hepatic encephalopathy.

Causes CNS depression (dose-related) resulting in sedation, dizziness, confusion, or ataxia which may impair physical and mental capabilities. Patients must be cautioned about performing tasks which require mental alertness (eg, operating machinery or driving). Use with caution in patients receiving other CNS depressants or psychoactive agents. Effects with other sedative drugs or ethanol may be potentiated. Benzodiazepines have been associated with falls and traumatic injury and should be used with extreme caution in patients who are at risk of these events (especially the elderly). (Continued)

Lorazepam *(Continued)*

Lorazepam may cause anterograde amnesia. Paradoxical reactions, including hyperactive or aggressive behavior have been reported with benzodiazepines, particularly in psychiatric patients. Does not have analgesic, antidepressant, or antipsychotic properties.

Use caution in patients with depression, particularly if suicidal risk may be present. Pre-existing depression may worsen or emerge during therapy. Not recommended for use in primary depressive or psychotic disorders. Use with caution in patients with a history of drug dependence, alcoholism, or significant personality disorders. Benzodiazepines have been associated with dependence and acute withdrawal symptoms on discontinuation or reduction in dose. Acute withdrawal, including seizures, may be precipitated after administration of flumazenil to patients receiving long-term benzodiazepine therapy.

As a hypnotic agent, should be used only after evaluation of potential causes of sleep disturbance. Failure of sleep disturbance to resolve after 7-10 days may indicate psychiatric or medical illness. A worsening of insomnia or the emergence of new abnormalities of thought or behavior may represent unrecognized psychiatric or medical illness and requires immediate and careful evaluation.

The parenteral formulation of lorazepam contains polyethylene glycol and propylene glycol which have resulted in toxicity during high dose and/or longer term infusions.

Adverse Reactions (Reflective of adult population; not specific for elderly)
>10%:
    Central nervous system: Sedation
    Respiratory: Respiratory depression
1% to 10%:
    Cardiovascular: Hypotension
    Central nervous system: Confusion, dizziness, akathisia, ataxia, headache, depression, disorientation, amnesia
    Dermatologic: Dermatitis, rash
    Gastrointestinal: Weight gain/loss, nausea, changes in appetite
    Neuromuscular & skeletal: Weakness
    Ocular: Visual disturbances
    Respiratory: Nasal congestion, hyperventilation, apnea

Overdosage/Toxicology Symptoms include confusion, coma, hypoactive reflexes, dyspnea, and labored breathing. **Note:** Prolonged infusions have been associated with toxicity from propylene glycol and/or polyethylene glycol. Treatment for benzodiazepine overdose is supportive. Rarely is mechanical ventilation required. Flumazenil has been shown to selectively block the binding of benzodiazepines to CNS receptors, resulting in a reversal of benzodiazepine-induced CNS depression, but not respiratory depression. Treatment requires blood pressure and respiratory support until drug effects subside.

Drug Interactions
    Clozapine: Benzodiazepines may enhance the adverse/toxic effect of clozapine (sedation, hypersalivation, hypotension, ataxia, delirium, and respiratory distress reported).
    CNS depressants: Sedative effects and/or respiratory depression may be additive with CNS depressants; includes ethanol, barbiturates, opioid analgesics, and other sedative agents; monitor for increased effect
    Loxapine: There are rare reports of significant respiratory depression, stupor, and/or hypotension with concomitant use of loxapine and lorazepam; use caution if concomitant administration of loxapine and CNS drugs is required
    Probenecid: May increase the levels/effects of lorazepam; adjust lorazepam dose (decrease by 50%).
    Theophylline: May partially antagonize some of the effects of benzodiazepines; monitor for decreased response; may require higher doses for sedation
    Valproic acid derivatives: May increase the levels/effects of lorazepam; adjust lorazepam dose (decrease by 50%).

Ethanol/Nutrition/Herb Interactions
    Ethanol: Avoid or limit ethanol (may increase CNS depression).
    Herb/Nutraceutical: Avoid valerian, St John's wort, kava kava, gotu kola (may increase CNS depression).

Stability
    I.V.: Intact vials should be refrigerated. Protect from light. Do not use discolored or precipitate-containing solutions. May be stored at room temperature for up to 60 days. Parenteral admixture is stable at room temperature (25°C) for 24 hours. Dilute I.V. dose with equal volume of compatible diluent (D_5W, NS, SWI).
    Infusion: Use 2 mg/mL injectable vial to prepare; there may be deceased stability when using 4 mg/mL vial. Dilute ≤1 mg/mL and mix in glass bottle. Precipitation may develop. Can also be administered undiluted via infusion.
    Tablet: Store at room temperature.

Mechanism of Action Binds to stereospecific benzodiazepine receptors on the post-synaptic GABA neuron at several sites within the central nervous system, including the limbic system, reticular formation. Enhancement of the inhibitory effect of GABA on neuronal excitability results by increased neuronal membrane permeability to chloride ions. This shift in chloride ions results in hyperpolarization (a less excitable state) and stabilization.

Pharmacodynamics

Onset of action: I.M.: Hypnosis occurs in ~20-30 minutes

Duration: 6-8 hours

Studies have shown that older adults are more sensitive to the effects of benzodiazepines as compared to younger adults.

Pharmacokinetics

Absorption: Oral, I.M.: Promptly absorbed

Protein binding: 85%; free fraction may be significantly higher in older adults

Metabolism: In the liver to inactive compounds with urinary excretion and minimal fecal clearance; metabolism is not significantly affected in older adults

Bioavailability: Oral: 90%

Half-life: 10-16 hours; one study found the half-life in older adults to be 15.9 hours as compared to 14.1 hours in younger adults

Time to peak: Oral: 2 hours

Dosage

Geriatrics: Anxiety and sedation: Oral, I.V.: 0.5-4 mg/day; refer to adult dosing for other indications. Dose selection should generally be on the low end of the dosage range (ie, initial dose not to exceed 2 mg)

Adults:

Antiemetic: Oral, I.V. (**Note:** May be administered sublingually; not a labeled route): 0.5-2 mg every 4-6 hours as needed

Anxiety and sedation: Oral: 1-10 mg/day in 2-3 divided doses; usual dose: 2-6 mg/day in divided doses; initial dose should not exceed 2 mg in debilitated patients

Insomnia: Oral: 2-4 mg at bedtime

Preoperative:

I.M.: 0.05 mg/kg administered 2 hours before surgery; maximum: 4 mg/dose

I.V.: 0.044 mg/kg 15-20 minutes before surgery; usual maximum: 2 mg/dose

Operative amnesia: I.V.: Up to 0.05 mg/kg; maximum: 4 mg/dose

Status epilepticus: I.V.: 4 mg/dose given slowly over 2-5 minutes; may repeat in 10-15 minutes; usual maximum dose: 8 mg

Rapid tranquilization of agitated patient (administer every 30-60 minutes):

Oral: 1-2 mg

I.M.: 0.5-1 mg

Average total dose for tranquilization: 4-8 mg

Agitation in the ICU patient (unlabeled):

I.V.: 0.02-0.06 mg/kg every 2-6 hours

I.V. infusion: 0.01-0.1 mg/kg/hour

Concurrent use of probenecid or valproic acid: Reduce lorazepam dose by 50%

Renal Impairment: I.V.: Risk of propylene glycol toxicity. Monitor closely if using for prolonged periods or at high doses.

Hepatic Impairment: Use cautiously.

Administration See Warnings/Precautions.

Monitoring Parameters Respiratory, cardiovascular and mental status, symptoms of anxiety

Reference Range Therapeutic: 50-240 ng/mL (SI: 156-746 nmol/L)

Patient Information Avoid alcohol and other CNS depressants; may cause drowsiness; avoid activities needing good psychomotor coordination until CNS effects are known; may cause physical or psychological dependence; avoid abrupt discontinuation after prolonged use

Additional Information I.M. lorazepam is rapidly and completely absorbed and, therefore, may be more predictable as compared to I.M. chlordiazepoxide or diazepam

Special Geriatric Considerations Because lorazepam is relatively short-acting with an inactive metabolite, it is a preferred agent to use in elderly patients when a benzodiazepine is indicated.

Dosage Forms Excipient information presented when available (limited, particularly for generics); consult specific product labeling.

Injection, solution: 2 mg/mL (1 mL, 10 mL); 4 mg/mL (1 mL, 10 mL)

Ativan®: 2 mg/mL (1 mL, 10 mL); 4 mg/mL (1 mL, 10 mL) [contains benzyl alcohol, polyethylene glycol, and propylene glycol]

Solution, oral concentrate:

Lorazepam Intensol®: 2 mg/mL (30 mL) [alcohol free, dye free]

Tablet: 0.5 mg, 1 mg, 2 mg

Ativan®: 0.5 mg, 1 mg, 2 mg

(Continued)

Lorazepam *(Continued)*

Selected References

Divoll M and Greenblatt DJ, "Effect of Age and Sex on Lorazepam Protein Binding," *J Pharm Pharmacol*, 1982, 34(2):122-3.

Greenblatt DJ, Allen MD, Locniskar A, et al, "Lorazepam Kinetics in the Elderly," *Clin Pharmacol Ther*, 1979, 26(1):103-13.

◆ **Lorazepam Intensol**® *see* Lorazepam *on page 929*

◆ **Lorcet**® **10/650** *see* Hydrocodone and Acetaminophen *on page 759*

◆ **Lorcet**® **Plus** *see* Hydrocodone and Acetaminophen *on page 759*

◆ **Lortab**® *see* Hydrocodone and Acetaminophen *on page 759*

Losartan *(loe SAR tan)*

Related Information

Angiotensin Agents *on page 1737*

Medication Safety Issues

Sound-alike/look-alike issues:

Losartan may be confused with valsartan

Cozaar® may be confused with Hyzaar®, Zocor®

U.S. Brand Names Cozaar®

Canadian Brand Names Cozaar®

Index Terms DuP 753; Losartan Potassium; MK594

Generic Available No

Pharmacologic Category Angiotensin II Receptor Blocker

Use Treatment of hypertension, alone or in combination with other hypertensive medications

Contraindications Hypersensitivity to losartan or any component of the formulation; hypersensitivity to other A-II receptor antagonists; primary hyperaldosteronism; bilateral renal artery stenosis

Warnings/Precautions Avoid use or use a much smaller dose in patients who are volume-depleted; correct depletion first. Use with caution in patients with pre-existing renal insufficiency or significant aortic/mitral stenosis. May cause hyperkalemia; avoid potassium supplementation unless specifically required by healthcare provider. May be associated with deterioration of renal function and/or increases in serum creatinine, particularly in patients dependent on renin-angiotensin-aldosterone system. Use caution in patients with unilateral or bilateral renal artery stenosis to avoid a decrease in renal function. AUCs of losartan (not the active metabolite) are about 50% greater in patients with Cl$_{cr}$ <30 mL/minute and are doubled in hemodialysis patients. When used to reduce the risk of stroke in patients with HTN and LVH, may not be effective in African-American population. Use caution with hepatic dysfunction, dose adjustment may be needed.

Adverse Reactions (Reflective of adult population; not specific for elderly)

>10%:

Cardiovascular: Chest pain (12% diabetic nephropathy)

Central nervous system: Fatigue (14% diabetic nephropathy)

Endocrine: Hypoglycemia (14% diabetic nephropathy)

Gastrointestinal: Diarrhea (2% hypertension to 15% diabetic nephropathy)

Genitourinary: Urinary tract infection (13% diabetic nephropathy)

Hematologic: Anemia (14% diabetic nephropathy)

Neuromuscular & skeletal: Weakness (14% diabetic nephropathy), back pain (2% hypertension to 12% diabetic nephropathy)

Respiratory: Cough (≤3% to 11%; similar to placebo; incidence higher in patients with previous cough related to ACE inhibitor therapy)

1% to 10%:

Cardiovascular: Hypotension (7% diabetic nephropathy), orthostatic hypotension (4% hypertension to 4% diabetic nephropathy), first-dose hypotension (dose related: <1% with 50 mg, 2% with 100 mg)

Central nervous system: Dizziness (4%), hypoesthesia (5% diabetic nephropathy), fever (4% diabetic nephropathy), insomnia (1%)

Dermatology: Cellulitis (7% diabetic nephropathy)

Endocrine: Hyperkalemia (<1% hypertension to 7% diabetic nephropathy)

Gastrointestinal: Gastritis (5% diabetic nephropathy), weight gain (4% diabetic nephropathy), dyspepsia (1% to 4%), abdominal pain (2%), nausea (2%)

Neuromuscular & skeletal: Muscular weakness (7% diabetic nephropathy), knee pain (5% diabetic nephropathy), leg pain (1% to 5%), muscle cramps (1%), myalgia (1%)

Respiratory: Bronchitis (10% diabetic nephropathy), upper respiratory infection (8%), nasal congestion (2%), sinusitis (1% hypertension to 6% diabetic nephropathy)

Miscellaneous: Infection (5% diabetic nephropathy), flu-like syndrome (10% diabetic nephropathy)

Overdosage/Toxicology Symptoms including hypotension and tachycardia may occur with very significant overdoses. Treatment should be supportive. Not removed via hemodialysis.

Drug Interactions Substrate (major) of CYP2C9, 3A4; **Inhibits** CYP1A2 (weak), 2C8 (moderate), 2C9 (moderate), 2C19 (weak), 3A4 (weak)

CYP2C9 inducers: May decrease the levels/effects of losartan. Example inducers include carbamazepine, phenobarbital, phenytoin, rifampin, rifapentine, and seco-barbital.

CYP2C8 Substrates: Losartan may increase the levels/effects of CYP2C8 substrates. Example substrates include amiodarone, paclitaxel, pioglitazone, repaglinide, and rosiglitazone.

CYP2C9 Substrates: Losartan may increase the levels/effects of CYP2C9 substrates. Example substrates include bosentan, dapsone, fluoxetine, glimepiride, glipizide, montelukast, nateglinide, paclitaxel, phenytoin, warfarin, and zafirlukast.

CYP3A4 inducers: CYP3A4 inducers may decrease the levels/effects of losartan. Example inducers include aminoglutethimide, carbamazepine, nafcillin, nevirapine, phenobarbital, phenytoin, and rifamycins.

Fluconazole: Increases plasma levels of losartan via 2C8/9 inhibition (decreases the plasma levels of the active metabolite). Monitor for increased losartan efficacy.

Lithium: Risk of toxicity may be increased by losartan; monitor lithium levels.

NSAIDs: May decrease angiotensin II antagonist efficacy; effect has been seen with losartan, but may occur with other medications in this class; monitor blood pressure

Potassium-sparing diuretics (amiloride, potassium, spironolactone, triamterene): Increased risk of hyperkalemia.

Potassium supplements may increase the risk of hyperkalemia.

Rifampin may reduce antihypertensive efficacy of losartan.

Trimethoprim (high dose) may increase the risk of hyperkalemia.

Ethanol/Nutrition/Herb Interactions Herb/Nutraceutical: St John's wort may decrease levels. Avoid dong quai if using for hypertension (has estrogenic activity). Avoid ephedra, yohimbe, ginseng (may worsen hypertension). Avoid garlic (may have increased antihypertensive effect).

Stability Store at 15°C to 30°C (59°F to 86°F). Protect from light.

Mechanism of Action As a selective and competitive, nonpeptide angiotensin II receptor antagonist, losartan blocks the vasoconstrictor and aldosterone-secreting effects of angiotensin II; losartan interacts reversibly at the AT1 and AT2 receptors of many tissues and has slow dissociation kinetics; its affinity for the AT1 receptor is 1000 times greater than the AT2 receptor. Angiotensin II receptor antagonists may induce a more complete inhibition of the renin-angiotensin system than ACE inhibitors, they do not affect the response to bradykinin, and are less likely to be associated with nonrenin-angiotensin effects (eg, cough and angioedema). Losartan increases urinary flow rate and in addition to being natriuretic and kaliuretic, increases excretion of chloride, magnesium, uric acid, calcium, and phosphate.

Pharmacodynamics Losartan inhibits pressor effect 85% at peak serum concentrations and maintains a 25% to 40% reduction for 24 hours.

Pharmacokinetics

Absorption: Well absorbed from gastrointestinal tract

Distribution: V_d: Losartan: 34 L; active metabolite: 12 L

Metabolism: Significant first-pass metabolism; the carboxylic acid metabolite is active (14%)

Bioavailability: 33%

Half-life: Losartan: 2 hours; active metabolite: 6-9 hours

Protein binding: Losartan and its active metabolite are highly bound to albumin; (free fractions 1.3% and 0.2% respectively).

Time to peak serum concentration: 1 hour for losartan; 3-4 hours for active metabolite

Elimination: ~35% of losartan and its metabolites eliminated renally with the remainder excreted in the feces; biliary excretion contributes significantly to elimination. Serum concentrations of losartan are not affected by mild renal impairment (Cl_{cr} as low as 31 mL/minute). Creatinine clearances <30 mL/minute are 50% higher than patients with normal renal function. Plasma concentrations of the active metabolite are not changed with renal impairment.

Dosage

Geriatrics & Adults:

Hypertension: Oral: Initial: 25-50 mg once daily; can be administered once or twice daily with total daily doses ranging from 25-100 mg

Usual initial doses in patients receiving diuretics or those with intravascular volume depletion: 25 mg

Nephropathy in patients with type 2 diabetes and hypertension: Oral: Initial: 50 mg once daily; can be increased to 100 mg once daily based on blood pressure response

Stroke reduction (HTN with LVH): Oral: 50 mg once daily (maximum daily dose: 100 mg); may be used in combination with a thiazide diuretic

(Continued)

Losartan (Continued)

Renal Impairment: Adults: No adjustment necessary.

Hepatic Impairment: Reduce the initial dose to 25 mg/day; divide dosage intervals into two.

Administration May be administered with or without food.

Monitoring Parameters Monitor blood pressure and pulse; no clinically important changes seen with laboratory electrolytes, glucose, uric acid, triglycerides, or cholesterol

Patient Information Patients may administer losartan with other medications and food. Compliance is important for full therapeutic effect. Report episodes of hypotension (dizziness or lightheadedness); report symptoms of angioedema (swelling of the lips or tongue, or difficulty breathing) to physician.

Additional Information It is not uncommon to find hyperuricemia associated with hypertension. In those patients, losartan may offer an advantage due to its uricosuric action and may be of benefit in patients who have hyperuricemia and hypertension. Available in combination with hydrochlorothiazide as Hyzaar®.

Special Geriatric Considerations Serum concentrations of losartan and its metabolites are not significantly different and no initial dose adjustment is necessary even in low creatinine clearance states (<30 mL/minute). Many elderly may be volume depleted due to diuretic use and/or blunted thirst reflex resulting in inadequate fluid intake.

Dosage Forms Excipient information presented when available (limited, particularly for generics); consult specific product labeling.

Tablet, as potassium: 25 mg, 50 mg, 100 mg

Extemporaneously Prepared To prepare losartan suspension, combine 10 mL of purified water and ten (10) losartan 50 mg tablets in an 8 ounce bottle. Shake well for ≥2 minutes. Allow concentrate to stand for 1 hour then shake for 1 minute. Separately, prepare 190 mL of a 50/50 mixture of Ora-Plus™ and Ora-Sweet SF™. Add to tablet and water mixture; shake for 1 minute. Resulting 200 mL suspension will contain losartan 2.5 mg/mL. Store under refrigeration for up to 4 weeks; shake well before use.

Selected References

Chobanian AV, Bakris GL, Black HR, et al, "The Seventh Report of the Joint National Committee on Prevention, Detection, Evaluation, and Treatment of High Blood Pressure: The JNC 7 Report," *JAMA*, 2003, 289(19):2560-71.

Cohn JN and Tognoni G, "Valsartan Heart Failure Trial Investigators. A Randomized Trial of the Angiotensin-Receptor Blocker Valsartan in Chronic Heart Failure," *N Engl J Med*, 2001, 345(23):1667-75.

Conlin P, Moore T, Swartz S, et al, "Effect of Indomethacin on Blood Pressure Lowering by Captopril and Losartan in Hypertensive Patients," *Hypertension*, 2000, 36(3):461-5.

"Consensus Recommendations for the Management of Chronic Heart Failure. On Behalf of the Membership of the Advisory Council to Improve Outcomes Nationwide in Heart Failure," *Am J Cardiol*, 1999, 83(2A):1A-38A.

Dahlof B, Devereux RB, Kjeldsen SE, et al, "Cardiovascular Morbidity and Mortality in the Losartan Intervention For Endpoint Reduction in Hypertension Study (LIFE): A Randomised Trial Against Atenolol," *Lancet*, 2002, 359(9311):995-1003.

Dickstein K, Kjekshus J, et al, "Effects of Losartan and Captopril on Mortality and Morbidity in High-Risk Patients After Acute Myocardial Infarction: The OPTIMAAL Randomised Trial. Optimal Trial in Myocardial Infarction with Angiotensin II Antagonist Losartan," *Lancet*, 2002, 360(9335):752-60.

Epstein BJ and Gums JG, "Angiotensin Receptor Blockers Versus ACE Inhibitors: Prevention of Death and Myocardial Infarction in High-Risk Populations," *Ann Pharmacother*, 2005, 39(3):470-80.

Granger CB, McMurray JJ, Yusuf S, et al, "Effects of Candesartan in Patients With Chronic Heart Failure and Reduced Left-Ventricular Systolic Function Intolerant to Angiotensin-Converting-Enzyme Inhibitors: The CHARM-Alternative Trial," *Lancet*, 2003, 362(9386):772-6.

Hunt SA, Baker DW, Chin MH, et al, "ACC/AHA Guidelines for the Evaluation and Management of Chronic Heart Failure in the Adult: A Report of the American College of Cardiology/American Heart Association Task Force on Practice Guidelines (Committee to Revise the 1995 Guidelines for the Evaluation and Management of Heart Failure). 2001. American College of Cardiology Web site. Available at: http://www.acc.org/clinical/guidelines/failure/hf_index.htm. Accessed June 9, 2003.

"K/DOQI Clinical Practice Guidelines for Chronic Kidney Disease: Evaluation, Classification, and Stratification. Kidney Disease Outcome Quality Initiative," *Am J Kidney Dis*, 2002, 39(2 Suppl 2):1-246. Available at: http://www.kidney.org/professionals/doqi/kdoqi/toc.htm. Accessed August 1, 2003.

McMurray JJ, Ostergren J, Swedberg K, et al, "Effects of Candesartan in Patients With Chronic Heart Failure and Reduced Left-Ventricular Systolic Function Taking Angiotensin-Converting-Enzyme Inhibitors: The CHARM-Added Trial," *Lancet*, 2003, 362(9386):767-71.

Pfeffer MA, McMurray JJ, Velazquez EJ, et al, "Valsartan, Captopril, or Both in Myocardial Infarction Complicated by Heart Failure, Left Ventricular Dysfunction, or Both," *N Engl J Med*, 2004, 350(2):203.

Pitt B, Poole-Wilson PA, Segal R, et al, "Effect of Losartan Compared With Captopril on Mortality in Patients With Symptomatic Heart Failure: Randomised Trial - The Losartan Heart Failure Survival Study ELITE II," *Lancet*, 2000, 355(9215):1582-7.

Losartan and Hydrochlorothiazide
(loe SAR tan & hye droe klor oh THYE a zide)

Related Information

Hydrochlorothiazide *on page 756*
Losartan *on page 932*

Medication Safety Issues
Sound-alike/look-alike issues:
Hyzaar® may be confused with Cozaar®
U.S. Brand Names Hyzaar®
Canadian Brand Names Hyzaar®; Hyzaar® DS
Index Terms Hydrochlorothiazide and Losartan
Generic Available No
Pharmacologic Category Angiotensin II Receptor Blocker Combination; Antihypertensive Agent, Combination; Diuretic, Thiazide
Use Treatment of hypertension; stroke risk reduction in patients with HTN and left ventricular hypertrophy (LVH)
Dosage
Geriatrics: Refer to dosing in individual monographs.
Adults: Hypertension (dosage must be individualized): Oral: 1 tablet/day
Renal Impairment: Cl$_{cr}$ ≤30 mL/minute: Use of combination formulation is not recommended.
Hepatic Impairment: Use is not recommended.
Dosage Forms Excipient information presented when available (limited, particularly for generics); consult specific product labeling.
Tablet:
Hyzaar® 50-12.5: Losartan potassium 50 mg and hydrochlorothiazide 12.5 mg
Hyzaar® 100-12.5: Losartan potassium 100 mg and hydrochlorothiazide 12.5 mg
Hyzaar® 100-25: Losartan potassium 100 mg and hydrochlorothiazide 25 mg

♦ **Losartan Potassium** see Losartan on page 932
♦ **Lotemax®** see Loteprednol on page 935
♦ **Lotensin®** see Benazepril on page 155
♦ **Lotensin® HCT** see Benazepril and Hydrochlorothiazide on page 158

Loteprednol (loe te PRED nol)

Medication Safety Issues
International issues:
Lotemax® may be confused with Lotanax® which is a brand name for terfenadine in the Czech Republic
U.S. Brand Names Alrex®; Lotemax®
Canadian Brand Names Alrex®; Lotemax®
Index Terms Loteprednol Etabonate
Generic Available No
Pharmacologic Category Corticosteroid, Ophthalmic
Use
0.2% suspension (Alrex®): Temporary relief of signs and symptoms of seasonal allergic conjunctivitis
0.5% suspension (Lotemax®): Treatment of inflammatory conditions (steroid-responsive inflammatory conditions of the palpebral and bulbar conjunctiva, cornea, and anterior segment of the globe, such as allergic conjunctivitis, acne rosacea, superficial punctate keratitis, herpes zoster keratitis, iritis, cyclitis, selected infective conjunctivitis when the inherent hazard of steroid use is accepted to obtain an advisable diminution in edema and inflammation); treatment of postoperative inflammation following ocular surgery
Contraindications Hypersensitivity to loteprednol, other corticosteroids, and any component of the formulation; viral diseases of the cornea and conjunctiva; mycobacterial infection of the eye; fungal diseases of ocular structures
Warnings/Precautions For ophthalmic use only; patients should be re-evaluated if symptoms fail to improve after 2 days. Intraocular pressure should be monitored if this product is used >10 days. Prolonged use may result in glaucoma and injury to the optic nerve. Visual defects in acuity and field of vision may occur. Posterior subcapsular cataracts may form after long-term use. Use with caution in presence of glaucoma (steroids increase intraocular pressure). Perforation may occur with topical steroids in diseases which thin the cornea or sclera. Steroids may mask infection or enhance existing infection. Steroid use may delay healing after cataract surgery.
Adverse Reactions (Reflective of adult population; not specific for elderly)
>10%:
Central nervous system: Headache
Respiratory: Rhinitis, pharyngitis
1% to 10%: Ocular: Abnormal vision/blurring, burning on instillation, chemosis, dry eyes, itching, injection, conjunctivitis/irritation, corneal abnormalities, eyelid erythema, papillae uveitis
Mechanism of Action Corticosteroids inhibit the inflammatory response including edema, capillary dilation, leukocyte migration, and scar formation. Loteprednol is highly
(Continued)

Loteprednol *(Continued)*

lipid soluble and penetrates cells readily to induce the production of lipocortins. These proteins modulate the activity of prostaglandins and leukotrienes.

Pharmacokinetics Plasma levels following intraocular administration were not detectable

Dosage

Geriatrics & Adults:

Seasonal allergic conjunctivitis: Ophthalmic: 0.2% suspension (Alrex®): Instill 1 drop into affected eye(s) 4 times/day.

Inflammatory conditions: Ophthalmic: 0.5% suspension (Lotemax®): Apply 1-2 drops into the conjunctival sac of the affected eye(s) 4 times/day. During the initial treatment within the first week, the dosing may be increased up to 1 drop every hour. Advise patients not to discontinue therapy prematurely. If signs and symptoms fail to improve after 2 days, re-evaluate the patient.

Postoperative inflammation: Ophthalmic: 0.5% suspension (Lotemax®): Apply 1-2 drops into the conjunctival sac of the operated eye(s) 4 times/day beginning 24 hours after surgery and continuing throughout the first 2 weeks of the postoperative period.

Administration Shake well before using.

Monitoring Parameters Intraocular pressure (if >10 days)

Special Geriatric Considerations Assess patient's ability to administer eye drops.

Dosage Forms Excipient information presented when available (limited, particularly for generics); consult specific product labeling.

Suspension, ophthalmic, as etabonate:

Alrex®: 0.2% (5 mL, 10 mL) [contains benzalkonium chloride]

Lotemax®: 0.5% (2.5 mL, 5 mL, 10 mL, 15 mL) [contains benzalkonium chloride]

Loteprednol and Tobramycin (loe te PRED nol & toe bra MYE sin)

U.S. Brand Names Zylet™

Index Terms Loteprednol Etabonate and Tobramycin; Tobramycin and Loteprednol Etabonate

Generic Available No

Pharmacologic Category Antibiotic/Corticosteroid, Ophthalmic

Use Treatment of steroid-responsive ocular inflammatory conditions where either a superficial bacterial ocular infection or the risk of a superficial bacterial ocular infection exists

Dosage

Geriatrics & Adults: Ophthalmic: Instill 1-2 drops into the affected eye(s) every 4-6 hours; may increase frequency during the first 24-48 hours to every 1-2 hours. Interval should increase as signs and symptoms improve. Further evaluation should occur for use of greater than 20 mL.

Special Geriatric Considerations Assess patient's ability to correctly self-administer eye drops.

Dosage Forms Excipient information presented when available (limited, particularly for generics); consult specific product labeling.

Suspension, ophthalmic: Loteprednol 0.5% and tobramycin 0.3% (2.5 mL, 5 mL, 10 mL) [contains benzalkonium chloride]

♦ **Loteprednol Etabonate** *see* Loteprednol *on page 935*
♦ **Loteprednol Etabonate and Tobramycin** *see* Loteprednol and Tobramycin *on page 936*
♦ **Lotrel®** *see* Amlodipine and Benazepril *on page 90*
♦ **Lotrimin® AF Athlete's Foot Cream [OTC]** *see* Clotrimazole *on page 349*
♦ **Lotrimin® AF Athlete's Foot Solution [OTC]** *see* Clotrimazole *on page 349*
♦ **Lotrimin® AF Jock Itch Cream [OTC]** *see* Clotrimazole *on page 349*
♦ **Lotrimin® AF Jock Itch Powder Spray [OTC]** *see* Miconazole *on page 1036*
♦ **Lotrimin® AF Powder/Spray [OTC]** *see* Miconazole *on page 1036*

Lovastatin (LOE va sta tin)

Related Information

Hyperlipidemia Management *on page 1773*

Medication Safety Issues

Sound-alike/look-alike issues:

Lovastatin may be confused with Leustatin®, Livostin®, Lotensin®

Mevacor® may be confused with Mivacron®

International issues:

Lovacol® [Chile and Finland] may be confused with Levatol® which is a brand name for penbutolol in the U.S.

Lovastin® [Poland] may be confused with Livostin® which is a brand name for levocabastine in the U.S.

U.S. Brand Names Altoprev®; Mevacor®

Canadian Brand Names Apo-Lovastatin®; CO Lovastatin; Gen-Lovastatin; Mevacor®; Novo-Lovastatin; Nu-Lovastatin; PMS-Lovastatin; RAN™-Lovastatin; ratio-Lovastatin; Riva-Lovastatin; Sandoz-Lovastatin

Index Terms Mevinolin; Monacolin K

Generic Available Yes: Immediate release tablet

Pharmacologic Category Antilipemic Agent, HMG-CoA Reductase Inhibitor

Use Adjunct to dietary therapy to decrease elevated serum total and LDL cholesterol concentrations in primary hypercholesterolemia; lower the risk of first heart attack, unstable angina, and in coronary revascularization procedures in persons whose total cholesterol levels are average but whose HDL levels are below average

Contraindications Hypersensitivity to lovastatin or any component of the formulation; active liver disease; unexplained persistent elevations of serum transaminases

Warnings/Precautions Secondary causes of hyperlipidemia should be ruled out prior to therapy. Liver function must be monitored by periodic laboratory assessment. Rhabdomyolysis with or without acute renal failure has occurred. Risk is dose-related and is increased with concurrent use of lipid-lowering agents which may cause rhabdomyolysis (gemfibrozil, fibric acid derivatives, or niacin at doses ≥1 g/day) or during concurrent use with potent CYP3A4 inhibitors. Avoid concurrent use of azole antifungals, macrolide antibiotics, and protease inhibitors. Use caution/limit dose with amiodarone, cyclosporine, danazol, gemfibrozil (or other fibrates), lipid-lowering doses of niacin, or verapamil. Monitor closely if used with other drugs associated with myopathy (eg, colchicine). Patients should be instructed to report unexplained muscle pain or weakness; lovastatin should be discontinued if myopathy is suspected/confirmed. Temporarily discontinue in any patient experiencing an acute or serious condition predisposing to renal failure secondary to rhabdomyolysis. Use with caution in patients with advanced age, these patients are predisposed to myopathy. Use with caution in patients who consume large amounts of ethanol or have a history of liver disease.

Adverse Reactions (Reflective of adult population; not specific for elderly)

Percentages as reported with immediate release tablets; similar adverse reactions seen with extended release tablets.

>10%: Neuromuscular & skeletal: Increased CPK (>2x normal) (11%)

1% to 10%:

Central nervous system: Headache (2% to 3%), dizziness (0.5% to 1%)

Dermatologic: Rash (0.8% to 1%)

Gastrointestinal: Abdominal pain (2% to 3%), constipation (2% to 4%), diarrhea (2% to 3%), dyspepsia (1% to 2%), flatulence (4% to 5%), nausea (2% to 3%)

Neuromuscular & skeletal: Myalgia (2% to 3%), weakness (1% to 2%), muscle cramps (0.6% to 1%)

Ocular: Blurred vision (0.8% to 1%)

Overdosage/Toxicology Few adverse events have been reported. Treatment is symptomatic.

Drug Interactions **Substrate** of CYP3A4 (major); **Inhibits** CYP2C9 (weak), 2D6 (weak), 3A4 (weak)

Amiodarone: Inhibits metabolism of lovastatin and may increase lovastatin-induced myopathy and rhabdomyolysis. Concurrent use is not recommended, but if unavoidable, dose of lovastatin should be limited.

Antacids: Plasma concentrations may be decreased when given with magnesium-aluminum hydroxide containing antacids (reported with atorvastatin and pravastatin). Clinical efficacy is not altered, no dosage adjustment is necessary

Azole antifungals: May decrease the metabolism, via CYP isoenzymes, of HMG-CoA reductase inhibitors and may increase risk of lovastatin-induced myopathy and rhabdomyolysis. Avoid concurrent use.

Cholestyramine reduces absorption of several HMG-CoA reductase inhibitors. Separate administration times by at least 4 hours.

Cholestyramine and colestipol (bile acid sequestrants): Cholesterol-lowering effects are additive.

Clofibrate and fenofibrate may increase the risk of myopathy and rhabdomyolysis; limit dose of lovastatin

Colchicine: Concomitant therapy with an HMG-CoA reductase inhibitor may increase risk of myopathy/rhabdomyolysis; use caution.

Cyclosporine: Concurrent use may increase risk of myopathy; limit dose of lovastatin

CYP3A4 inhibitors: May increase the levels/effects of lovastatin. Example inhibitors include azole antifungals, clarithromycin, diclofenac, doxycycline, erythromycin, imatinib, isoniazid, nefazodone, nicardipine, propofol, protease inhibitors, quinidine, telithromycin, and verapamil. Avoid concurrrent use.

(Continued)

Lovastatin *(Continued)*

Danazol: Concurrent use may increase risk of myopathy; limit dose of lovastatin.

Diltiazem: May increase levels/effects of lovavastatin.

Gemfibrozil: Increased risk of myopathy and rhabdomyolysis; limit dose of lovastatin

Grapefruit juice may inhibit metabolism of lovastatin via CYP3A4; avoid high dietary intakes of grapefruit juice.

Isradipine may decrease lovastatin blood levels.

Macrolide antibiotics: May decrease the metabolism, via CYP isoenzymes, of HMG-CoA reductase inhibitors and may increase risk of lovastatin-induced myopathy and rhabdomyolysis. Avoid concurrent use.

Nefazodone: May decrease the metabolism, via CYP isoenzymes, of HMG-CoA reductase inhibitors and may increase risk of lovastatin-induced myopathy and rhabdomyolysis. Avoid concurrent use.

Niacin (at higher dosages ≥1 g/day) may increase risk of myopathy and rhabdomyolysis; limit dose of lovastatin

Protease inhibitors: Concurrent use increases the risk of myopathy and rhabdomyolysis; concurrent use should be avoided.

Verapamil: Inhibits metabolism of lovastatin and may increase lovastatin-induced myopathy and rhabdomyolysis. Concurrent use is not recommended, but if unavoidable, dose of lovastatin should be limited.

Warfarin effect (hypoprothrombinemic response) may be increased; monitor INR closely when lovastatin is initiated or discontinued.

Ethanol/Nutrition/Herb Interactions

Ethanol: Avoid excessive ethanol consumption (due to potential hepatic effects).

Food: Food **decreases** the bioavailability of lovastatin extended release tablets and **increases** the bioavailability of lovastatin immediate release tablets. Lovastatin serum concentrations may be increased if taken with grapefruit juice; avoid concurrent intake of large quantities (>1 quart/day). Red yeast rice contains an estimated 2.4 mg lovastatin per 600 mg rice.

Herb/Nutraceutical: St John's wort may decrease lovastatin levels.

Stability

Tablet, immediate release: Store between 5°C to 30°C (41°F to 86°F). Protect from light

Tablet, extended release: Store between 20°C to 25°C (68°F to 77°F). Avoid excessive heat and humidity.

Mechanism of Action Lovastatin acts by competitively inhibiting 3-hydroxyl-3-methylglutaryl-coenzyme A (HMG-CoA) reductase, the enzyme that catalyzes the rate-limiting step in cholesterol biosynthesis

Pharmacodynamics Onset of action: LDL-cholesterol reduction: 3 days

Pharmacokinetics

Absorption: 30%; increased with extended release tablets when taken in the fasting state

Protein binding: 95%

Metabolism: Hepatic; extensive first-pass effect; hydrolyzed to B-hydroxy acid (active)

Bioavailability: Increased with extended release tablets

Half-life: 1.1-1.7 hours

Time to peak, serum: 2-4 hours

Elimination: Feces (~80% to 85%); urine (10%)

Dosage

Geriatrics & Adults:

Dyslipidemia and primary prevention of CAD: Oral: Initial: 20 mg with evening meal, then adjust at 4-week intervals; maximum: 80 mg/day immediate release tablet **or** 60 mg/day extended release tablet.

Dosage modification/limits based on concurrent therapy:

Cyclosporine and other immunosuppressant drugs: Initial dose: 10 mg/day with a maximum recommended dose of 20 mg/day

Concurrent therapy with fibrates, danazol, and/or lipid-lowering doses of niacin (>1 g/day): Maximum recommended dose: 20 mg/day. Concurrent use with fibrates should be avoided unless risk to benefit favors use.

Concurrent therapy with amiodarone or verapamil: Maximum recommended dose: 40 mg/day of regular release or 20 mg/day with extended release.

Dosage adjustment in renal impairment: Cl$_{cr}$ <30 mL/minute: Use doses >20 mg/day with caution.

Renal Impairment: Cl$_{cr}$ <30 mL/minute: Use with caution and carefully consider doses >20 mg/day.

Administration Administer immediate release tablets with meals. Administer extended-release tablet at bedtime; do not crush or chew.

Monitoring Parameters Obtain baseline LFTs and total cholesterol profile. LFTs should also be assessed prior to upwards dosage adjustment to ≥40 mg daily or when otherwise indicated clinically. Enzyme levels should be followed periodically thereafter as clinically warranted.

Test Interactions Altered thyroid function tests

Patient Information Promptly report any unexplained muscle pain, tenderness or weakness, especially if accompanied by malaise or fever. Follow prescribed diet; take with meals.

Additional Information Before initiation of therapy, patients should be placed on a standard cholesterol-lowering diet for 6 weeks and the diet should be continued during drug therapy. For explicit guidelines on the risk factors for CHD and when to treat high blood cholesterol (see Selected References)

Special Geriatric Considerations The definition of and, therefore, when to treat hyperlipidemia in the elderly is a controversial issue. The National Cholesterol Education Program recommends that all adults maintain a plasma cholesterol <160 mg/dL. Elderly with one additional risk factor, goal LDL would be <130 mg/dL. It is the authors' belief that pharmacologic treatment be reserved for those who are unable to obtain a desirable plasma cholesterol concentration by diet alone and for whom the benefits of treatment are believed to outweigh the potential adverse effects, drug interactions, and cost of treatment.

Dosage Forms Excipient information presented when available (limited, particularly for generics); consult specific product labeling.
Tablet: 10 mg, 20 mg, 40 mg
  Mevacor®: 20 mg, 40 mg
Tablet, extended release:
  Altoprev®: 20 mg, 40 mg, 60 mg

Selected References
"Executive Summary of The Third Report of The National Cholesterol Education Program (NCEP) Expert Panel on Detection, Evaluation, And Treatment of High Blood Cholesterol In Adults (Adult Treatment Panel III)," *JAMA*, 2001, 285(19):2486-97.

♦ **Lovastatin and Niacin** *see* Niacin and Lovastatin *on page 1111*
♦ **Lovenox®** *see* Enoxaparin *on page 507*

Loxapine (LOKS a peen)

Related Information
  Antipsychotic Agents *on page 1747*
  Liquid Compatibility of Antipsychotics and Mood Stabilizers *on page 1851*

Medication Safety Issues
  Sound-alike/look-alike issues:
    Loxitane® may be confused with Soriatane®

  International issues:
    Loxitane® may be confused with Lexotan® which is a brand name for bromazepam in multiple international markets

U.S. Brand Names Loxitane®

Canadian Brand Names Apo-Loxapine®; Loxapac® IM; Nu-Loxapine; PMS-Loxapine

Index Terms Loxapine Succinate; Oxilapine Succinate

Generic Available Yes

Pharmacologic Category Antipsychotic Agent, Typical

Use Management of psychotic disorders, nonpsychotic symptoms associated with dementia in older adults, Tourette's syndrome, Huntington's chorea

Contraindications Hypersensitivity to loxapine or any component of the formulation; severe CNS depression; coma

Warnings/Precautions Watch for hypotension when administering I.M.; should not be given I.V. Moderately sedating, use with caution in disorders where CNS depression is a feature. Use with caution in Parkinson's disease. Caution in patients with hemodynamic instability; bone marrow suppression; predisposition to seizures; subcortical brain damage; severe cardiac, hepatic, renal or respiratory disease. Esophageal dysmotility and aspiration have been associated with antipsychotic use - use with caution in patients at risk of pneumonia (ie, Alzheimer's disease). Caution in breast cancer or other prolactin-dependent tumors (may elevate prolactin levels). May alter temperature regulation or mask toxicity of other drugs due to antiemetic effects. May alter cardiac conduction; life-threatening arrhythmias have occurred with therapeutic doses of phenothiazines. May cause orthostatic hypotension - use with caution in patients at risk of this effect or those who would tolerate transient hypotensive episodes (cerebrovascular disease, cardiovascular disease, or other medications which may predispose).

Phenothiazines may cause anticholinergic effects (confusion, agitation, constipation, xerostomia, blurred vision, urinary retention); therefore, they should be used with caution in patients with decreased gastrointestinal motility, urinary retention, BPH, xerostomia, or visual problems. Conditions which also may be exacerbated by cholinergic blockade include narrow-angle glaucoma (screening is recommended) and worsening of myasthenia gravis. Relative to other antipsychotics, loxapine has a low potency of cholinergic blockade.
(Continued)

Loxapine *(Continued)*

May cause extrapyramidal reactions, including pseudoparkinsonism, acute dystonic reactions, akathisia, and tardive dyskinesia (risk of these reactions is moderate-high relative to other neuroleptics). May be associated with neuroleptic malignant syndrome (NMS) or pigmentary retinopathy.

Adverse Reactions (Reflective of adult population; not specific for elderly)
Frequency not defined.

Cardiovascular: Abnormal T waves with prolonged ventricular repolarization, arrhythmia, hyper-/hypotension, orthostatic hypotension, tachycardia, syncope

Central nervous system: Agitation, altered central temperature regulation, ataxia, confusion, dizziness, drowsiness, extrapyramidal reactions (akathisia, akinesia, dystonia, pseudoparkinsonism, tardive dyskinesia), faintness, headache, insomnia, lightheadedness, neuroleptic malignant syndrome (NMS), seizure, slurred speech, tension

Dermatologic: Alopecia, dermatitis, photosensitivity, pruritus, rash, seborrhea

Endocrine & metabolic: Amenorrhea, enlargement of breasts, galactorrhea, gynecomastia, menstrual irregularity

Gastrointestinal: Adynamic ileus, constipation, nausea, polydipsia, vomiting, weight gain/loss, xerostomia

Genitourinary: Sexual dysfunction, urinary retention

Hematologic: Agranulocytosis, leukopenia, thrombocytopenia

Neuromuscular & skeletal: Weakness

Ocular: Blurred vision

Respiratory: Nasal congestion

Overdosage/Toxicology Symptoms include deep sleep, dystonia, agitation, dysrhythmias, extrapyramidal symptoms, hypotension, and seizures. Following initiation of essential overdose management, toxic symptom and supportive treatment should be initiated. Hypotension usually responds to I.V. fluids or Trendelenburg positioning. If unresponsive to these measures, the use of a parenteral inotrope may be required (eg, norepinephrine 0.1-0.2 mcg/kg/minute titrated to response). Seizures commonly respond to diazepam (I.V. 5-10 mg bolus every 15 minutes, if needed, up to a total of 30 mg) or to phenytoin or phenobarbital. Critical cardiac arrhythmias often respond to I.V. phenytoin (15 mg/kg up to 1 g), while other antiarrhythmics can be used. Neuroleptics often cause extrapyramidal symptoms (eg, dystonic reactions) requiring management with diphenhydramine 1-2 mg/kg, up to a maximum of 50 mg I.M. or slow I.V. push, followed by a maintenance dose for 48-72 hours. When these reactions are unresponsive to diphenhydramine, anticholinergic agents such as benztropine mesylate I.V. 1-2 mg may be effective. These agents are generally effective within 2-5 minutes.

Drug Interactions

Acetylcholinesterase inhibitors (central): May increase the risk of antipsychotic-related extrapyramidal symptoms; monitor.

Aluminum salts: May decrease the absorption of antipsychotics; monitor

Amphetamines: Efficacy may be diminished by antipsychotics; in addition, amphetamines may increase psychotic symptoms; avoid concurrent use

Anticholinergics: May inhibit the therapeutic response to antipsychotics and excess anticholinergic effects may occur; includes benztropine, trihexyphenidyl, biperiden, and drugs with significant anticholinergic activity (TCAs, antihistamines, disopyramide)

Antihypertensives: Concurrent use of antipsychotics with an antihypertensive may produce additive hypotensive effects (particularly orthostasis)

Bromocriptine: Antipsychotics inhibit the ability of bromocriptine to lower serum prolactin concentrations

CNS depressants: Sedative effects may be additive with antipsychotics; monitor for increased effect; includes barbiturates, benzodiazepines, opioid analgesics, ethanol, and other sedative agents

Epinephrine: Chlorpromazine (and possibly other low potency antipsychotics) may diminish the pressor effects of epinephrine

Guanethidine and guanadrel: Antihypertensive effects may be inhibited by antipsychotics

Levodopa: Antipsychotics may inhibit the antiparkinsonian effect of levodopa; avoid this combination

Lithium: Antipsychotics may produce neurotoxicity with lithium; this is a rare effect

Metoclopramide: May increase extrapyramidal symptoms (EPS) or risk.

Phenytoin: May reduce serum levels of antipsychotics; antipsychotics may increase phenytoin serum levels

Propranolol: Serum concentrations of antipsychotics may be increased; propranolol also increases antipsychotic concentrations

QT_c-prolonging agents: Effects on QT_c interval may be additive with antipsychotics, increasing the risk of malignant arrhythmias. Other QT_c-prolonging agents include type Ia antiarrhythmics, TCAs, and some quinolone antibiotics (moxifloxacin). Concomitant use with thioridazine is contraindicated.

Sulfadoxine-pyrimethamine: May increase antipsychotic concentrations

Tricyclic antidepressants: Concurrent use may produce increased toxicity or altered therapeutic response

Trazodone: Antipsychotics and trazodone may produce additive hypotensive effects

Valproic acid: Serum levels may be increased by antipsychotics

Ethanol/Nutrition/Herb Interactions

Ethanol: Avoid ethanol (may increase CNS depression).

Herb/Nutraceutical: Avoid kava kava, gotu kola, valerian, St John's wort (may increase CNS depression).

Stability Protect from light. Dispense in amber or opaque vials.

Mechanism of Action Loxapine is a dibenzoxazepine antipsychotic which blocks postsynaptic mesolimbic D_1 and D_2 receptors in the brain, and also possesses serotonin 5-HT$_2$ blocking activity

Pharmacodynamics

Onset of action: Oral: Within 20-30 minutes

Peak effect: 90-180 minutes

Duration: ~12 hours

Pharmacokinetics

Metabolism: Liver metabolism to glucuronide conjugates

Half-life: Biphasic:

Initial: 5 hours

Terminal: 12-19 hours

Elimination: In urine, and to a smaller degree, the feces within 24 hours

Dosage

Geriatrics: Oral: 20-60 mg/day

Adults:

Psychosis: Oral: 10 mg twice daily, increase dose until psychotic symptoms are controlled; usual dose range: 20-100 mg/day in divided doses 2-4 times/day; dosages >250 mg/day are not recommended.

Administration Dilute the oral concentrate with water or juice before administration; avoid skin contact with solution; may cause contact dermatitis.

Monitoring Parameters Monitor orthostatic blood pressures 3-5 days after initiation of therapy or a dose increase; tremors, gait changes, abnormal movement in trunk, neck, buccal area, or extremities; monitor target behaviors for which the agent is given

Test Interactions False-positives for phenylketonuria, amylase, uroporphyrins, urobilinogen

Patient Information Oral concentrate must be diluted in 2-4 oz of liquid (water, fruit juice, carbonated drinks, milk, or pudding); do not take antacid within 1 hour of taking drug; avoid alcohol; avoid excess sun exposure (use sun block); may cause drowsiness, rise slowly from recumbent position; use of supportive stockings may help prevent orthostatic hypotension

Special Geriatric Considerations Many elderly patients receive antipsychotic medications for inappropriate nonpsychotic behavior. Before initiating antipsychotic medication, the clinician should investigate any possible reversible cause; any stress or stress from any disease can cause acute "confusion" or worsening of baseline nonpsychotic behavior. Most commonly acute changes in behavior are due to increases in drug dose or addition of new drug to regimen; fluid electrolyte loss; infections; and changes in environment.

Any changes in disease status in any organ system can result in behavior changes.

In the treatment of agitated, demented, elderly patients, authors of meta-analysis of controlled trials of the response to the traditional antipsychotics (phenothiazines, butyrophenones) in controlling agitation have concluded that the use of neuroleptics results in a response rate of 18%. Clearly neuroleptic therapy for behavior control should be limited with frequent attempts to withdraw the agent given for behavior control.

Dosage Forms Excipient information presented when available (limited, particularly for generics); consult specific product labeling.

Capsule, as succinate: 5 mg, 10 mg, 25 mg, 50 mg

Selected References

Peabody CA, Warner MD, Whiteford HA, et al, "Neuroleptics and the Elderly," *J Am Geriatr Soc*, 1987, 35(3):233-8.

Risse SC and Barnes R, "Pharmacologic Treatment of Agitation Associated With Dementia," *J Am Geriatr Soc*, 1986, 34(5):368-76.

Saltz BL, Woerner MG, Kane JM, et al, "Prospective Study of Tardive Dyskinesia Incidence in the Elderly," *JAMA*, 1991, 266(17):2402-6.

Seifert RD, "Therapeutic Drug Monitoring: Psychotropic Drugs," *J Pharm Pract*, 1984, 6:403-16.

♦ **Loxapine Succinate** *see* Loxapine *on page 939*

♦ **Loxitane**® *see* Loxapine *on page 939*

♦ **Lozi-Flur**™ *see* Fluoride *on page 642*

♦ **Lozol**® **[DSC]** *see* Indapamide *on page 798*

+ **L-PAM** *see* Melphalan *on page 974*
+ **L-Sarcolysin** *see* Melphalan *on page 974*
+ **LTA® 360** *see* Lidocaine *on page 904*
+ **LTG** *see* Lamotrigine *on page 870*
+ **Lu-26-054** *see* Escitalopram *on page 539*

Lubiprostone (loo bi PROS tone)

U.S. Brand Names Amitiza®
Index Terms RU 0211; SPI 0211
Generic Available No
Pharmacologic Category Chloride Channel Activator; Gastrointestinal Agent, Miscellaneous
Use Treatment of chronic idiopathic constipation
Contraindications Hypersensitivity to lubiprostone or any component of the formulation; history of bowel obstruction
Warnings/Precautions Symptoms of mechanical gastrointestinal obstruction should be evaluated before prescribing this medicine. Avoid use in patients with severe diarrhea. May consider reducing dose if nausea is severe. Safety and efficacy have not been established in renal or hepatic dysfunction.
Adverse Reactions (Reflective of adult population; not specific for elderly)
>10%:
    Central nervous system: Headache (11%)
    Gastrointestinal: Nausea (29%; severe: 3%; dose related), diarrhea (12%; severe 3%)
1% to 10%:
    Cardiovascular: Edema (3%), chest discomfort/pain (2%), hypertension (1%)
    Central nervous system: Dizziness (3%), fatigue (2%), fever (1%), depression (1%), insomnia (1%)
    Gastrointestinal: Abdominal pain (8%), abdominal distention (6%), flatulence (6%), vomiting (3%), loose stools (3%), dyspepsia (2%), gastroesophageal reflux disease (2%), xerostomia (1%), weight gain (1%)
    Neuromuscular & skeletal: Arthralgia (3%), back pain (2%)
    Renal: Urinary tract infection (4%)
    Respiratory: Sinusitis (5%), upper respiratory tract infection (4%), nasopharyngitis (3%), bronchitis (2%), dyspnea (2%), cough (2%)
Overdosage/Toxicology Symptoms may include nausea, vomiting, diarrhea, dizziness, loose/watery stools, headache, flushing, dyspnea, abdominal pain/discomfort, syncope, xerostomia, and chest discomfort.
Stability Store at room temperature of 15°C to 30°C (59°F to 86°F).
Mechanism of Action Bicyclic fatty acid that acts locally at the apical portion of the intestine as a chloride channel activator, increasing intestinal water secretion and intestinal motility. Does not alter serum sodium or potassium concentrations.
Pharmacokinetics
    Absorption: Systemic: Parent drug: Poor (below levels of detection); Active metabolite (M3): Low
    Distribution: Gastrointestinal tissue
    Metabolism: Within stomach and jejunum by carbonyl reductase to M3 (active metabolite) and others
    Half-life elimination: M3: 0.9-1.4 hours
    Bioavailability: Minimal
    Excretion: M3: Feces (trace amounts)
Dosage
    Geriatrics & Adults: Idiopathic constipation: Oral: 24 mcg twice daily
    Renal Impairment: Has not been studied.
    Hepatic Impairment: Has not been studied.
Administration Administer with food.
Special Geriatric Considerations No studies have been done in elderly populations to date. Data in subpopulation analysis demonstrate lubiprostone is safe and well tolerated in all sexes, races, and age groups.
Dosage Forms Excipient information presented when available (limited, particularly for generics); consult specific product labeling.
    Capsule:
        Amitiza®: 24 mcg
Selected References
Amitiza™ (lubiprostone) package insert, Bethesda, MD, Sucampo Pharmaceuticals, Inc, 2006.
"Lubiprostone: RU 0211, SPI 0211," *Drugs R D* 2005, 6(4):245-8.
Winpenny JP, "Lubiprostone," *IDrugs*, 2005, 8(5):416-22.

+ **LubriTears® Ophthalmic Ointment [OTC]** *see* Ocular Lubricant *on page 1144*
+ **Lucentis®** *see* Ranibizumab *on page 1380*

- **Ludiomil** *see* Maprotiline *on page 954*
- **Lufyllin®** *see* Dyphylline *on page 496*
- **Lufyllin®-GG** *see* Dyphylline and Guaifenesin *on page 496*
- **Lugol's Solution** *see* Potassium Iodide and Iodine *on page 1291*
- **Lumigan®** *see* Bimatoprost *on page 170*
- **Luminal® Sodium** *see* Phenobarbital *on page 1243*
- **Lunesta™** *see* Eszopiclone *on page 575*
- **LupiCare™ II Psoriasis [OTC]** *see* Salicylic Acid *on page 1441*
- **LupiCare™ Dandruff [OTC]** *see* Salicylic Acid *on page 1441*
- **LupiCare™ Psoriasis [OTC]** *see* Salicylic Acid *on page 1441*
- **Lupron®** *see* Leuprolide *on page 883*
- **Lupron Depot®** *see* Leuprolide *on page 883*
- **Lupron Depot-Ped®** *see* Leuprolide *on page 883*
- **Luride®** *see* Fluoride *on page 642*
- **Luride® Lozi-Tab®** *see* Fluoride *on page 642*
- **LuSonal™** *see* Phenylephrine *on page 1247*
- **Luvox** *see* Fluvoxamine *on page 669*
- **Luxiq®** *see* Betamethasone *on page 161*
- **LY146032** *see* Daptomycin *on page 395*
- **LY170053** *see* Olanzapine *on page 1148*
- **LY248686** *see* Duloxetine *on page 491*
- **Lyrica®** *see* Pregabalin *on page 1310*
- **M-M-R® II** *see* Measles, Mumps, and Rubella Vaccines (Combined) *on page 957*
- **Maalox® [OTC]** *see* Aluminum Hydroxide, Magnesium Hydroxide, and Simethicone *on page 66*
- **Maalox® Max [OTC]** *see* Aluminum Hydroxide, Magnesium Hydroxide, and Simethicone *on page 66*
- **Maalox® Total Stomach Relief® [OTC]** *see* Bismuth *on page 174*
- **Macrobid®** *see* Nitrofurantoin *on page 1128*
- **Macrodantin®** *see* Nitrofurantoin *on page 1128*
- **Macugen®** *see* Pegaptanib *on page 1211*

Magaldrate and Simethicone (MAG al drate & sye METH i kone)

Related Information
Simethicone *on page 1467*

Medication Safety Issues
Sound-alike/look-alike issues:
Riopan Plus® may be confused with Repan®

U.S. Brand Names
Riopan Plus® [OTC] [DSC]; Riopan Plus® Double Strength [OTC] [DSC]

Index Terms
Simethicone and Magaldrate

Generic Available
Yes

Pharmacologic Category
Antacid; Antiflatulent

Use
Relief of hyperacidity associated with peptic ulcer, gastritis, peptic esophagitis, and hiatal hernia, which are accompanied by symptoms of gas
Refer to individual agents.

Contraindications
Based on **magaldrate** component: Hypersensitivity to magaldrate or any component of the formulation; patients with colostomy or an ileostomy; appendicitis; ulcerative colitis; diverticulitis
Based on **simethicone** component: Hypersensitivity to simethicone or any component of the formulation

Adverse Reactions (Reflective of adult population; not specific for elderly)
Frequency not defined.
Based on **magaldrate** component:
Central nervous system: Encephalopathy
Gastrointestinal: Constipation, chalky taste, stomach cramps, fecal impaction, diarrhea, nausea, vomiting, discoloration of feces (white speckles), rebound hyperacidity
Endocrine & metabolic: Hypophosphatemia, hypermagnesemia, milk-alkali syndrome
Neuromuscular & metabolic: Osteomalacia
Miscellaneous: Aluminum intoxication
Based on **simethicone** component: No data reported

Drug Interactions
See individual agents.
(Continued)

943

Magaldrate and Simethicone *(Continued)*

Dosage

Geriatrics & Adults: Hyperacidity/gas: Oral: 5-10 mL (540-1080 mg magaldrate) between meals and at bedtime

Additional Information Magaldrate is not a mixture of aluminum and magnesium, but a chemical complex (chemical entity). It contains 29% to 40% magnesium oxide and 18% to 26% aluminum oxide.

Dosage Forms Excipient information presented when available (limited, particularly for generics); consult specific product labeling. [DSC] = Discontinued product

Suspension, oral: Magaldrate 540 mg and simethicone 20 mg per 5 mL (360 mL)

Riopan Plus®: Magaldrate 540 mg and simethicone 20 mg per 5 mL (360 mL) [DSC]

Riopan Plus® Double Strength: Magaldrate 1080 mg and simethicone 40 mg per 5 mL (360 mL) [DSC]

- ♦ **Magan®** *see* Salicylates (Various Salts) *on page 1439*
- ♦ **Mag-Caps [OTC]** *see* Magnesium Oxide *on page 951*
- ♦ **MagGel™ [OTC]** *see* Magnesium Oxide *on page 951*
- ♦ **Maginex™ [OTC]** *see* Magnesium L-aspartate Hydrochloride *on page 948*
- ♦ **Maginex™ DS [OTC]** *see* Magnesium L-aspartate Hydrochloride *on page 948*
- ♦ **Magnacet™** *see* Oxycodone and Acetaminophen *on page 1182*
- ♦ **Magnesia Magma** *see* Magnesium Hydroxide *on page 946*
- ♦ **Magnesium L-lactate Dihydrate** *see* Magnesium L-lactate *on page 950*
- ♦ **Magnesium Carbonate and Aluminum Hydroxide** *see* Aluminum Hydroxide and Magnesium Carbonate *on page 64*

Magnesium Citrate *(mag NEE zhum SIT rate)*

U.S. Brand Names Citroma® [OTC]

Canadian Brand Names Citro-Mag®

Index Terms Citrate of Magnesia

Generic Available Yes

Pharmacologic Category Laxative, Saline; Magnesium Salt

Use Evacuation of bowel prior to certain surgical and diagnostic procedures or overdose situations

Contraindications Renal failure, appendicitis, abdominal pain, intestinal impaction, obstruction or perforation, diabetes mellitus, complications in gastrointestinal tract, patients with colostomy or ileostomy, ulcerative colitis or diverticulitis

Warnings/Precautions Use with caution in patients with impaired renal function, especially if Cl_{cr} <30 mL/minute (accumulation of magnesium which may lead to magnesium intoxication). Use caution in patients receiving a cardiac glycoside; may increase the AV-blocking effects. Use with caution in patients with lithium administration; use with caution with neuromuscular-blocking agents, and CNS depressants.

Adverse Reactions (Reflective of adult population; not specific for elderly)

1% to 10%:

Cardiovascular: Hypotension

Endocrine & metabolic: Hypermagnesemia

Gastrointestinal: Abdominal cramps, diarrhea, gas formation

Respiratory: Respiratory depression

Overdosage/Toxicology

Due to diarrhea, serious potentially life-threatening electrolyte disturbances may occur with long-term use or overdose; hypermagnesemia may occur, as well as, CNS depression, confusion, hypotension, muscle weakness, and blockage of peripheral neuromuscular transmission.

Serum level >4 mEq/L (4.8 mg/dL): Deep tendon reflexes may be depressed

Serum level ≥10 mEq/L (12 mg/dL): Deep tendon reflexes may disappear, respiratory paralysis may occur, heart block may occur

I.V. calcium (5-10 mEq) will reverse respiratory depression or heart block. In extreme cases, peritoneal dialysis or hemodialysis may be required.

Serum level >12 mEq/L may be fatal, serum level ≥10 mEq/L may cause complete heart block

Mechanism of Action Promotes bowel evacuation by causing osmotic retention of fluid which distends the colon with increased peristaltic activity

Pharmacodynamics Onset of cathartic action: Oral: Within 1-2 hours

Pharmacokinetics

Absorption: Oral: 15% to 30%

Elimination: Renal

Dosage

Geriatrics & Adults: Cathartic: Oral: Adults: $^1/_2$ to 1 full bottle (120-300 mL)

Renal Impairment: Patients in severe renal failure should not receive magnesium due to toxicity from accumulation. Patients with a Cl_{cr} <25 mL/minute should be monitored by serum magnesium levels.

Monitoring Parameters See Overdosage/Toxicology.

Reference Range Adults: 2.2-2.8 mg/dL ~1.8-2.3 mEq/L

Test Interactions Increased magnesium; decreased protein, decreased calcium (S), decreased potassium (S)

Patient Information Take with a glass of water, fruit juice, or citrus flavored carbonated beverage; report severe abdominal pain to physician

Additional Information To increase palatability, manufacturer suggests chilling the solution prior to administration. See Overdosage/Toxicology.

3.85-4.71 mEq of magnesium/5 mL

Special Geriatric Considerations Elderly, due to disease or drug therapy, may be predisposed to diarrhea. Diarrhea may result in electrolyte imbalance. Decreased renal function (Cl_{cr} <30 mL/minute) may result in toxicity; monitor for toxicity and Cl_{cr} <30 mL/minute.

Dosage Forms Excipient information presented when available (limited, particularly for generics); consult specific product labeling.

Solution, oral: 290 mg/5 mL (300 mL) [cherry and lemon flavors]

Citroma®: 290 mg/5 mL (300 mL) [contains magnesium 48 mg and potassium 13 mg per 5 mL; cherry and lemon flavors]; (300 mL) [contains magnesium 48 mg and sodium 7.5 mg per 5 mL; grape and lemony flavors]

Tablet: 100 mg [as elemental magnesium]

Selected References

Chernow B, Smith J, Rainey TG, et al, "Hypomagnesemia: Implications for the Critical Care Specialist," *Crit Care Med*, 1982, 10(3):193-6.

Gams JG, "Clinical Significance of Magnesium: A Review," *Drug Intell Clin Pharm*, 1987, 21(3):240-6.

♦ **Magnesium Gluceptate** *see* Magnesium Glucoheptonate *on page 945*

Magnesium Glucoheptonate (mag NEE zhum gloo koh HEP toh nate)

Canadian Brand Names Magnelium®; Magnolex®; Magnorol® Sirop; ratio-Magnesium

Index Terms Magnesium Gluceptate

Generic Available Yes

Pharmacologic Category Magnesium Salt

Use Treatment and prevention of hypomagnesemia

Restrictions Not available in U.S.

Contraindications Heart block, serious renal impairment, myocardial damage, hepatitis, Addison's disease

Warnings/Precautions Use with caution in patients with impaired renal function (accumulation of magnesium which may lead to magnesium intoxication). Use caution in patients receiving a cardiac glycoside; may increase the AV-blocking effects. Use with extreme caution in patients with myasthenia gravis or other neuromuscular disease.

Adverse Reactions (Reflective of adult population; not specific for elderly)

Adverse effects on neuromuscular function may occur at lower levels in patients with neuromuscular disease (eg, myasthenia gravis).

Serum magnesium levels >3 mg/dL:

Central nervous system: Depressed CNS

Gastrointestinal: Diarrhea

Neuromuscular & skeletal: Blocked peripheral neuromuscular transmission leading to anticonvulsant effects

Serum magnesium levels >5 mg/dL:

Cardiovascular: Flushing

Central nervous system: Somnolence

Serum magnesium levels >12.5 mg/dL:

Cardiovascular: Complete heart block, cardiac conduction affected

Respiratory: Respiratory paralysis

Overdosage/Toxicology

Symptoms of overdose usually present with serum level >4 mEq/L

Serum magnesium >4: Deep tendon reflexes may be depressed

Serum magnesium ≥10: Deep tendon reflexes may disappear, respiratory paralysis may occur, heart block may occur

Serum level >12 mEq/L may be fatal, serum level ≥10 mEq/L may cause complete heart block

I.V. calcium (5-10 mEq) 1-2 g calcium gluconate will reverse respiratory depression or heart block; in extreme cases, peritoneal dialysis or hemodialysis may be required

(Continued)

Magnesium Glucoheptonate *(Continued)*

Drug Interactions
Increased effect: Nifedipine decreased blood pressure and increased neuromuscular blockade
Increased toxicity: Aminoglycosides increased neuromuscular blockade; CNS depressants increased CNS depression; neuromuscular antagonists, betamethasone (pulmonary edema), ritodrine increased cardiotoxicity

Mechanism of Action When taken orally, magnesium promotes bowel evacuation by causing osmotic retention of fluid which distends the colon with increased peristaltic activity; parenterally, magnesium decreases acetylcholine in motor nerve terminals and acts on myocardium by slowing rate of S-A node impulse formation and prolonging conduction time.

Pharmacokinetics Excretion: Urine (as magnesium)

Dosage
Geriatrics & Adults: The recommended dietary allowance (RDA) of magnesium is 4.5 mg/kg which is a total daily allowance of 350-400 mg for adult men and 280-300 mg for adult women. Average daily intakes of dietary magnesium have declined in recent years due to processing of food. The latest estimate of the average American dietary intake was 349 mg/day. Dose represented as magnesium sulfate unless stated otherwise.

Note: Serum magnesium is poor reflection of repletional status as the majority of magnesium is intracellular; serum levels may be transiently normal for a few hours after a dose is given, therefore, aim for consistently high normal serum levels in patients with normal renal function for most efficient repletion
Hypomagnesemia: Oral: 100-600 mg (5-30 mg elemental magnesium) 1-2 times/day with food.
Maintenance electrolyte requirements:
Daily requirements: 0.2-0.5 mEq/kg/24 hours or 3-10 mEq/1000 kcal/24 hours
Maximum: 8-16 mEq/24 hours
Dosing adjustment/comments in renal impairment: Cl_{cr} <25 mL/minute: Do not administer or monitor serum magnesium levels carefully.

Monitoring Parameters Serum magnesium levels should be monitored to avoid overdose; monitor for diarrhea

Reference Range Serum magnesium: 1.5-2.5 mg/dL; slightly different ranges are reported by different laboratories

Test Interactions Increased magnesium; decreased protein, calcium (S), decreased potassium (S)

Patient Information Take in divided doses. Report diarrhea (>5 stools/day) or changes in mental function to prescriber.

Special Geriatric Considerations
Elderly, due to disease or drug therapy, may be predisposed to diarrhea. Diarrhea may result in electrolyte imbalance. Decreased renal function (Cl_{cr} <30 mL/minute) may result in toxicity; monitor for toxicity and Cl_{cr} <30 mL/minute.

Dosage Forms Excipient information presented when available (limited, particularly for generics); consult specific product labeling.
Capsule:
Magnelium®, Magnorol®: 20 mg [contains 20 mg elemental magnesium]
Magnolex®: 300 mg [contains 15 mg elemental magnesium]
Solution, oral (ratio-Magnesium): 100 mg/mL (500 mL, 2000 mL) [contains 5 mg/mL elemental magnesium]
Syrup (Magnorol® Sirop): 90 mg/mL (400 mL) [contains 4.5 mg/mL elemental magnesium]

Selected References
Bashuk RG and Krendel DA, "Myasthenia Gravis Presenting as Weakness After Magnesium Administration," *Muscle Nerve*, 1990, 13(8):708-12.
Bohman VR and Cotton DB, "Supralethal Magnesemia With Patient Survival," *Obstet Gynecol*, 1990, 76(5 Pt 2):984-6.
Gams JG, "Clinical Significance of Magnesium: A Review," *Drug Intell Clin Pharm*, 1987, 21(3):240-6.
Kaeser HE, "Drug-Induced Myasthenia Gravis," *Acta Neurol Scand Suppl*, 1984, 100:39-47.
Nichols B, "Minerals," *Pediatrics*, Norwalk, CT: Appleton & Lange, 1987, 176-7.

Magnesium Hydroxide (mag NEE zhum hye DROKS ide)

U.S. Brand Names Phillips'® Chews [OTC]; Phillips'® Milk of Magnesia [OTC]
Index Terms Magnesia Magma; Milk of Magnesia; MOM
Generic Available Yes: Liquid
Pharmacologic Category Antacid; Laxative; Magnesium Salt
Use Short-term treatment of occasional constipation and symptoms of hyperacidity
Contraindications Hypersensitivity to any component of the formulation; patients with colostomy or an ileostomy, intestinal obstruction, fecal impaction, renal failure, appendicitis

Warnings/Precautions Use with caution in patients with severe renal impairment (especially when doses are >50 mEq magnesium/day); hypermagnesemia and toxicity may occur due to decreased renal clearance of absorbed magnesium. Decreased renal function (Cl$_{cr}$ <30 mL/minute) may result in toxicity; monitor for toxicity.

For self-medication (OTC use): Patients should notify healthcare provider of any sudden change in bowel habits which last >14 days, stomach pain, nausea, or vomiting or if use is needed for >1 week.

Overdosage/Toxicology Magnesium antacids are also laxatives and may cause diarrhea and hypokalemia. In patients with renal failure, magnesium may accumulate to toxic levels. I.V. calcium (5-10 mEq) will reverse respiratory depression or heart block. In extreme cases, peritoneal dialysis or hemodialysis may be required.

Mechanism of Action Promotes bowel evacuation by causing osmotic retention of fluid which distends the colon with increased peristaltic activity; reacts with hydrochloric acid in stomach to form magnesium chloride

Pharmacodynamics Onset of laxative action: Within 4-8 hours

Pharmacokinetics

Absorption: Absorbed magnesium ions (up to 30%)

Elimination: Usually by kidneys, unabsorbed drug is excreted in feces

Dosage

Geriatrics & Adults:

Antacid: OTC labeling: Oral:

Liquid: Magnesium hydroxide 400 mg/5 mL: 5-15 mL as needed up to 4 times/day

Tablet: Magnesium hydroxide 311 mg/tablet: 2-4 tablets every 4 hours up to 4 times/day

Dietary supplement: OTC labeling (Phillips'® Chews): Oral: Magnesium 500 mg: 2-4 tablets/day once daily at bedtime or in divided doses

Laxative: OTC labeling: Oral:

Liquid:

Magnesium hydroxide 400 mg/5 mL: 30-60 mL/day once daily at bedtime or in divided doses

Magnesium hydroxide 800 mg/5 mL: 15-30 mL/day once daily at bedtime or in divided doses

Tablet: Magnesium hydroxide 311 mg/tablet: 8 tablets/day once daily at bedtime or in divided doses

Renal Impairment: Patients in severe renal failure should not receive magnesium due to toxicity from accumulation. Patients with a Cl$_{cr}$ <30 mL/minute should be monitored by serum magnesium levels.

Administration Liquid doses may be diluted with a small amount of water prior to administration. All doses should be followed by 8 ounces of water.

Monitoring Parameters See Overdosage/Toxicology.

Reference Range Adults: 2.2-2.8 mg/dL ~1.8-2.3 mEq/L

Test Interactions Increased magnesium; decreased protein, calcium (S), decreased potassium (S)

Patient Information Dilute dose in water or juice, shake well; chew tablets well

Additional Information 1.05 g magnesium = ~87 mEq magnesium/30 mL

Special Geriatric Considerations Elderly, due to disease or drug therapy, may be predisposed to diarrhea. Diarrhea may result in electrolyte imbalance. Decreased renal function (Cl$_{cr}$ <30 mL/minute) may result in toxicity; monitor for toxicity.

Dosage Forms Excipient information presented when available (limited, particularly for generics); consult specific product labeling.

Liquid, oral: 400 mg/5 mL (360 mL, 480 mL, 960 mL, 3780 mL)

Phillips'® Milk of Magnesia: 400 mg/5 mL (120 mL, 360 mL, 780 mL) [contains magnesium 167 mg/5 mL, cherry flavor also contains sodium 2 mg/5 mL; original, cherry, and mint flavors]

Liquid, oral concentrate: 800 mg/5 mL (100 mL, 400 mL)

Phillips'® Milk of Magnesia [concentrate]: 800 mg/5 mL (240 mL) [strawberry flavor]

Tablet, chewable:

Phillips'® Chews: Magnesium 500 mg [contains sodium 10 mg/tablet, coconut oil and soybean oil; chocolate flavor]

Phillips'® Milk of Magnesia: 311 mg [contains magnesium 130 mg/tablet; mint flavor]

Selected References

Chernow B, Smith J, Rainey TG, et al, "Hypomagnesemia: Implications for the Critical Care Specialist," *Crit Care Med*, 1982, 10(3):193-6.

Gams JG, "Clinical Significance of Magnesium: A Review," *Drug Intell Clin Pharm*, 1987, 21(3):240-6.

♦ **Magnesium Hydroxide, Aluminum Hydroxide, and Simethicone** *see* Aluminum Hydroxide, Magnesium Hydroxide, and Simethicone *on page 66*

♦ **Magnesium Hydroxide and Aluminum Hydroxide** *see* Aluminum Hydroxide and Magnesium Hydroxide *on page 65*

Magnesium Hydroxide and Mineral Oil
(mag NEE zhum hye DROKS ide & MIN er al oyl)

Related Information
Magnesium Hydroxide *on page 946*
Mineral Oil *on page 1045*
U.S. Brand Names Phillips'® M-O [OTC]
Index Terms Haley's M-O; MOM/Mineral Oil Emulsion
Generic Available No
Pharmacologic Category Laxative
Use Short-term treatment of occasional constipation
Contraindications Patients with colostomy or an ileostomy, intestinal obstruction, fecal impaction, renal failure, appendicitis; heart block, myocardial damage, serious renal impairment, hepatitis, and Addison's disease
Warnings/Precautions Use magnesium with caution in patients with severe renal impairment (especially when doses are >50 mEq magnesium/day); hypermagnesemia and toxicity may occur due to decreased renal clearance of absorbed magnesium. Decreased renal function (Cl_{cr} <30 mL/minute) may result in toxicity; monitor for toxicity.

For self-medication (OTC use): Patients should notify healthcare provider of any sudden change in bowel habits which last >14 days, stomach pain, nausea, vomiting, or if use is needed for >1 week. Not for OTC use in bedridden patients or patients with dysphagia. Avoid concomitant use with stool softener laxatives.
Pharmacodynamics Onset of action: 4-8 hours
Pharmacokinetics
Absorption: Absorbed magnesium ions (up to 30%)
Elimination: Usually by kidneys, unabsorbed drug is excreted in feces
Dosage
Geriatrics & Adults: Laxative: OTC labeling: Oral: 45-60 mL at bedtime
Renal Impairment: Patients in severe renal failure should not receive magnesium due to toxicity from accumulation. Patients with a Cl_{cr} <30 mL/minute should be monitored by serum magnesium levels.
Administration Shake well; administer with full glass of water
Reference Range Adults: 2.2-2.8 mg/dL ~1.8-2.3 mEq/L
Patient Information Shake well; take with full glass of water; report persistent diarrhea or abdominal pains with incidence of blood in stool or vomit
Special Geriatric Considerations The use of mineral oil products may be hazardous in the elderly with conditions predisposing them to aspiration. Elderly, due to disease or drug therapy, may be predisposed to diarrhea. Diarrhea may result in electrolyte imbalance. Decreased renal function (Cl_{cr} <30 mL/minute) may result in toxicity from magnesium absorption; monitor for toxicity.
Dosage Forms Excipient information presented when available (limited, particularly for generics); consult specific product labeling.
Suspension, oral:
Phillips'® M-O: Magnesium hydroxide 300 mg and mineral oil 1.25 mL per 5 mL (360 mL, 780 mL) [contains magnesium 125 mg and sodium 1.5 mg per 5 mL mint flavors]
Selected References

Chernow B, Smith J, Rainey TG, et al, "Hypomagnesemia: Implications for the Critical Care Specialist," *Crit Care Med*, 1982, 10(3):193-6.
Gams JG, "Clinical Significance of Magnesium: A Review," *Drug Intell Clin Pharm*, 1987, 21(3):240-6.

♦ **Magnesium Hydroxide, Famotidine, and Calcium Carbonate** *see* Famotidine, Calcium Carbonate, and Magnesium Hydroxide *on page 599*

Magnesium L-aspartate Hydrochloride
(mag NEE zhum el as PAR tate hye droe KLOR ide)

U.S. Brand Names Maginex™ [OTC]; Maginex™ DS [OTC]
Index Terms MAH
Generic Available No
Pharmacologic Category Electrolyte Supplement, Oral; Magnesium Salt
Use Dietary supplement
Contraindications Hypersensitivity to any component of the formulation
Warnings/Precautions Use magnesium with caution in patients with impaired renal function, hepatitis or Addison's disease (accumulation of magnesium may lead to magnesium intoxication). Use with extreme caution in patients with myasthenia gravis or other neuromuscular disease.
Adverse Reactions (Reflective of adult population; not specific for elderly)
Frequency not defined: Gastrointestinal: Diarrhea (excessive oral doses)

Overdosage/Toxicology Serious, potentially life-threatening electrolyte disturbances may occur with long-term use or overdosage due to diarrhea; hypermagnesemia may occur.

Symptoms of overdose usually present with magnesium serum level >4 mEq/L

Serum magnesium >4 mEq/L: Deep tendon reflexes may be depressed; drowsiness, flushing, headache, lethargy, or nausea may be present

Serum magnesium 6-10 mEq/L: Deep tendon reflexes may disappear; respiratory paralysis may occur; bradycardia, ECG changes, hypocalcemia, hypotension, or somnolence may be present

Serum level 10 mEq/L may be fatal; muscle or respiratory paralysis may be present, complete heart block or cardiac arrest may occur

Drug Interactions

Bisphosphonate derivatives: Oral magnesium salts may decrease the absorption of bisphosphonate derivatives.

Calcium channel blockers: Calcium channel blockers may enhance the adverse/toxic effect of magnesium salts. Magnesium salts may enhance the hypotensive effect of calcium channel blockers.

Mycophenolate: Oral magnesium salts may decrease the absorption of mycophenolate.

Neuromuscular-blocking agents: Magnesium salts may enhance the neuromuscular-blocking effect of neuromuscular-blocking agents. Only of concern in patients with increased serum magnesium concentrations.

Phosphate supplements: Oral magnesium salts may decrease the absorption of phosphate supplements.

Quinolone antibiotics: Magnesium salts may decrease the absorption of quinolone antibiotics. Of concern only with oral administration of both agents.

Tetracyclines: Magnesium salts may decrease the absorption of tetracycline antibiotics. Of concern only with oral administration of both agents.

Mechanism of Action Magnesium is important as a cofactor in many enzymatic reactions in the body involving protein synthesis and carbohydrate metabolism (at least 300 enzymatic reactions require magnesium). Actions on lipoprotein lipase have been found to be important in reducing serum cholesterol and on sodium/potassium ATPase in promoting polarization (eg, neuromuscular functioning).

Pharmacokinetics

Absorption: Oral: Inversely proportional to amount ingested; 40% to 60% under controlled dietary conditions; 15% to 36% at higher doses. Absorption of the Maginex™ formulation may be increased compared to other magnesium salts.

Distribution: Bone (50% to 60%); extracellular fluid (1% to 2%)

Protein binding: 30%, to albumin

Excretion: Urine (as magnesium)

Dosage

Geriatrics & Adults:

RDA (elemental magnesium):

19-30 years:

Female: 310 mg/day

Male: 400 mg/day

≥31 years:

Female: 320 mg/day

Male: 420 mg/day

Dietary supplement: Oral: Magnesium-L-aspartate 1230 mg (magnesium 122 mg) up to 3 times/day

Renal Impairment: Cl_{cr} <30 mL/minute: Use with caution; monitor for hypermagnesemia

Administration

Granules: Mix each packet in 4 ounces of water or juice prior to administration

Tablet, enteric coated: Do not crush or chew

Reference Range Serum magnesium: 1.5-2.5 mg/dL; slightly different ranges are reported by different laboratories

Patient Information Not for use in patients with kidney/renal disease.

Special Geriatric Considerations Elderly, due to disease or drug therapy, may be predisposed to diarrhea. Diarrhea may result in electrolyte imbalance. Decreased renal function (Cl_{cr} <30 mL/minute) may result in toxicity; monitor for toxicity. Monitor for signs of confusion or worsening signs of dementia.

Dosage Forms Excipient information presented when available (limited, particularly for generics); consult specific product labeling.

Granules:

Maginex™ DS: 1230 mg [magnesium 10 mEq; equivalent to magnesium 122 mg; lemon flavor]

Tablet [enteric coated]:

Maginex™: 615 mg [magnesium 5 mEq; equivalent to magnesium 61 mg]

(Continued)

Magnesium L-aspartate Hydrochloride *(Continued)*

Selected References

Bashuk RG and Krendel DA, "Myasthenia Gravis Presenting as Weakness After Magnesium Administration," *Muscle Nerve*, 1990, 13(8):708-12.

"Dietary Reference Intakes for Calcium, Phosphorus, Magnesium, Vitamin D, and Fluoride. Standing Committee on the Scientific Evaluation of Dietary Reference Intakes, Food and Nutrition Board, Institute of Medicine," National Academy of Sciences, Washington, DC: National Academy Press, 1997. Available at: http://www.nap.edu.

Gams JG, "Clinical Significance of Magnesium: A Review," *Drug Intell Clin Pharm*, 1987, 21(3):240-6.

Magnesium L-lactate (mag NEE zhum el LAK tate)

U.S. Brand Names Mag-Tab® SR
Index Terms Magnesium L-lactate Dihydrate
Generic Available No
Pharmacologic Category Electrolyte Supplement; Magnesium Salt
Use Dietary supplement
Contraindications Hypersensitivity to any component of the formulation
Warnings/Precautions Use magnesium with caution in patients with impaired renal function, hepatitis, or Addison's disease. Use with extreme caution in patients with myasthenia gravis or other neuromuscular disease.
Adverse Reactions (Reflective of adult population; not specific for elderly)
Frequency not defined: Gastrointestinal: Diarrhea
Overdosage/Toxicology Serious, potentially life-threatening electrolyte disturbances may occur with high dose or long-term use, especially in patients with significant renal dysfunction or failure. Hypermagnesemia may cause CNS depression, confusion, hypotension, muscle weakness, blockage of peripheral neuromuscular transmission may occur.

Symptoms of overdose usually present with serum magnesium level >4 mEq/L

Serum magnesium >4 mEq/L: Deep tendon reflexes may be depressed; drowsiness, flushing, headache, lethargy, or nausea may be present

Serum magnesium 6-10 mEq/L: Deep tendon reflexes may disappear; respiratory paralysis may occur; bradycardia, ECG changes, hypocalcemia, hypotension, or somnolence may be present

Serum magnesium 10 mEq/L may be fatal; muscle or respiratory paralysis may be present, complete heart block or cardiac arrest may occur

Drug Interactions

Aminoglycosides: Magnesium salts may enhance the neuromuscular-blocking effect of aminoglycosides. Primarily of concern in patients with elevated serum magnesium concentrations.

Bisphosphonate derivatives: Oral magnesium salts may decrease the absorption of bisphosphonate derivatives.

Calcium channel blockers: May enhance the adverse/toxic effect of magnesium salts. Magnesium salts may enhance the hypotensive effect of calcium channel blockers.

Mycophenolate: Oral magnesium salts may decrease the absorption of mycophenolate.

Neuromuscular-blocking agents: Magnesium salts may enhance the neuromuscular-blocking effect of neuromuscular-blocking agents. Only of concern in patients with increased serum magnesium concentrations.

Phosphate supplements: Oral magnesium salts may decrease the absorption of phosphate supplements.

Quinolone antibiotics: Magnesium salts may decrease the absorption of quinolone antibiotics. Of concern only with oral administration of both agents.

Tetracyclines: Magnesium salts may decrease the absorption of tetracycline antibiotics. Of concern only with oral administration of both agents.

Mechanism of Action Magnesium is important as a cofactor in many enzymatic reactions in the body involving protein synthesis and carbohydrate metabolism (at least 300 enzymatic reactions require magnesium). Actions on lipoprotein lipase have been found to be important in reducing serum cholesterol and on sodium/potassium ATPase in promoting polarization (eg, neuromuscular functioning).

Pharmacokinetics

Absorption: Oral: Inversely proportional to amount ingested; 40% to 60% under controlled dietary conditions; 15% to 36% at higher doses; majority occurs in jejunum and ileum.

Distribution: Bone (50% to 60%); extracellular fluid (1% to 2%)

Protein binding: 30%, to albumin

Bioavailability: 41%

Excretion: Urine (as magnesium)

Dosage

Geriatrics & Adults:

Dietary supplement: Oral:1-2 caplets every 12 hours

RDA (elemental magnesium):
19-30 years:
  Female: 310 mg/day
  Male: 400 mg/day
≥31 years:
  Female: 320 mg/day
  Male: 420 mg/day

Renal Impairment: Cl_{cr} <30 mL/minute: Use with caution; monitor for hypermagnesemia

Administration Should be administered with food.

Reference Range Serum magnesium: 1.5-2.5 mg/dL; slightly different ranges are reported by different laboratories

Special Geriatric Considerations Elderly, due to disease or drug therapy, may be predisposed to diarrhea. Diarrhea may result in electrolyte imbalance. Decreased renal function (Cl_{cr} <30 mL/minute) may result in toxicity; monitor for toxicity and Cl_{cr} <30 mL/minute.

Dosage Forms Excipient information presented when available (limited, particularly for generics); consult specific product labeling.
Caplet, sustained-release:
  Mag-Tab® SR: Elemental magnesium 84 mg (7 mEq)

Magnesium Oxide (mag NEE zhum OKS ide)

U.S. Brand Names Mag-Caps [OTC]; MagGel™ [OTC]; Mag-Ox® 400 [OTC]; Uro-Mag® [OTC]

Generic Available Yes

Pharmacologic Category Electrolyte Supplement, Oral; Magnesium Salt

Use Electrolyte replacement

Contraindications Hypersensitivity to any component of the formulation

Warnings/Precautions Use magnesium with caution in patients with impaired renal function, hepatitis, or Addison's disease (accumulation of magnesium may lead to magnesium intoxication). Use with extreme caution in patients with myasthenia gravis or other neuromuscular disease.

Adverse Reactions (Reflective of adult population; not specific for elderly)
Frequency not defined: Gastrointestinal: Diarrhea (excessive oral doses)

Overdosage/Toxicology Serious, potentially life-threatening electrolyte disturbances may occur with long-term use or overdosage due to diarrhea; hypermagnesemia may occur.
Symptoms of overdose usually present with magnesium serum level >4 mEq/L
  Serum magnesium >4 mEq/L: Deep tendon reflexes may be depressed; drowsiness, flushing, headache, lethargy, or nausea may be present
  Serum magnesium 6-10 mEq/L: Deep tendon reflexes may disappear; respiratory paralysis may occur; bradycardia, ECG changes, hypocalcemia, hypotension, or somnolence may be present
  Serum level 10 mEq/L may be fatal; muscle or respiratory paralysis may be present, complete heart block or cardiac arrest may occur

Drug Interactions
Bisphosphonate derivatives: Oral magnesium salts may decrease the absorption of bisphosphonate derivatives.
Calcium channel blockers: Calcium channel blockers may enhance the adverse/toxic effect of magnesium salts. Magnesium salts may enhance the hypotensive effect of calcium channel blockers.
Mycophenolate: Oral magnesium salts may decrease the absorption of mycophenolate.
Neuromuscular-blocking agents: Magnesium salts may enhance the neuromuscular-blocking effect of neuromuscular-blocking agents. Only of concern in patients with increased serum magnesium concentrations.
Phosphate supplements: Oral magnesium salts may decrease the absorption of phosphate supplements.
Quinolone antibiotics: Magnesium salts may decrease the absorption of quinolone antibiotics. Of concern only with oral administration of both agents.
Tetracyclines: Magnesium salts may decrease the absorption of tetracycline antibiotics. Of concern only with oral administration of both agents.

Mechanism of Action Magnesium is important as a cofactor in many enzymatic reactions in the body involving protein synthesis and carbohydrate metabolism (at least 300 enzymatic reactions require magnesium). Actions on lipoprotein lipase have been found to be important in reducing serum cholesterol and on sodium/potassium ATPase in promoting polarization (eg, neuromuscular functioning).

Pharmacokinetics
Absorption: Oral: Inversely proportional to amount ingested; 40% to 60% under controlled dietary conditions; 15% to 36% at higher doses
(Continued)

Magnesium Oxide *(Continued)*

Distribution: Bone (50% to 60%); extracellular fluid (1% to 2%)
Protein binding: 30%, to albumin
Excretion: Urine (as magnesium)

Dosage
Geriatrics & Adults:
RDA (elemental magnesium): Oral:
19-30 years:
Female: 310 mg/day
Male: 400 mg/day
≥31 years:
Female: 320 mg/day
Male: 420 mg/day

Dietary supplement: Oral:
Mag-Ox 400®: 2 tablets daily with food
Mag-Caps, Uro-Mag®: 4-5 capsules daily with food
Renal Impairment: Cl_{cr} <30 mL/minute: Use with caution; monitor for hypermagnesemia

Reference Range Serum magnesium: 1.5-2.5 mg/dL; slightly different ranges are reported by different laboratories

Special Geriatric Considerations Elderly, due to disease or drug therapy, may be predisposed to diarrhea. Diarrhea may result in electrolyte imbalance. Decreased renal function (Cl_{cr} <30 mL/minute) may result in toxicity; monitor for toxicity.

Dosage Forms Excipient information presented when available (limited, particularly for generics); consult specific product labeling.
Caplet: 250 mg
Capsule:
Mag-Caps: Elemental magnesium 85 mg
Uro-Mag®: 140 mg [magnesium 7 mEq; equivalent to elemental magnesium 84.5 mg]
Capsule, softgel:
MagGel™: 600 mg [magnesium 28.64 mEq; equivalent to elemental magnesium 348 mg]
Tablet: 400 mg [magnesium 20 mEq; equivalent to elemental magnesium 242 mg], 500 mg
Mag-Ox® 400: 400 mg [magnesium 20 mEq; equivalent to elemental magnesium 242 mg]

Selected References
Chernow B, Smith J, Rainey TG, et al, "Hypomagnesemia: Implications for the Critical Care Specialist," *Crit Care Med*, 1982, 10(3):193-6.
Gams JG, "Clinical Significance of Magnesium: A Review," *Drug Intell Clin Pharm*, 1987, 21(3):240-6.

♦ **Magnesium Salicylate** *see* Salicylates (Various Salts) *on page 1439*

Magnesium Salts (Various Salts) (mag NEE zhum salts)

U.S. Brand Names Almora® [OTC]; Epsom Salt [OTC]; Magonate® [OTC]; Mg-plus® [OTC]; Slow-Mag® [OTC]
Generic Available Yes
Use Treatment and prevention of hypomagnesemia; short-term treatment of constipation
Restrictions See Warnings/Precautions and Contraindications.
Contraindications Heart block, myocardial damage, serious renal impairment, hepatitis and Addison's disease
Warnings/Precautions Use with caution in patients with impaired renal function, especially when Cl_{cr} <30 mL/minute (accumulation of magnesium which may lead to magnesium intoxication); monitor serum magnesium concentration and renal function when magnesium sulfate is administered parenterally; use with caution in digitalized patients (may alter cardiac conduction leading to heart block); use with caution with neuromuscular blocking agents, lithium administration
Drug Interactions
Magnesium compounds decrease the pharmacologic effect of benzodiazepines, chloroquine, glucocorticosteroids, digoxin, H_2 antagonists, hydantoins, iron compounds, nitrofurantoin, penicillamine, phenothiazines, tetracyclines, ticlopidine
Magnesium compounds increase the pharmacologic effect of dicumarol, quinidine, sulfonylureas
Stability Refrigeration of intact ampuls may result in precipitation or crystallization; stability of parenteral admixture at room temperature (25°C): 60 days
Mechanism of Action Promotes bowel evacuation by causing osmotic retention of fluid which distends the colon with increased peristaltic activity when taken orally; parenterally, decreases acetylcholine in motor nerve terminals and acts on myocardium by slowing rate of S-A node impulse formation and prolonging conduction time

Pharmacodynamics
  Onset of action:
    Oral: Within 1-2 hours
    I.M.: Within 60 minutes
    I.V.: Immediately
  Duration:
    I.M.: 3-4 hours
    I.V.: 30 minutes
Pharmacokinetics
  Absorption: Absorbed magnesium is rapidly eliminated by the kidneys. See Special Geriatric Considerations.
  Elimination: Primarily excreted in feces
Reference Range Adults: 2.2-2.8 mg/dL ~1.8-2.3 mEq/L
Test Interactions Increased magnesium; decreased protein, calcium (S), decreased potassium (S)
Patient Information Take in divided doses; report diarrhea (>5 stools/day) or changes in mental function to physician, nurse, or pharmacist
Additional Information 1 g magnesium = 8.3 mEq (41.1 mmol); see individual agents for magnesium content per dose
Special Geriatric Considerations Elderly, due to disease or drug therapy, may be predisposed to diarrhea. Diarrhea may result in electrolyte imbalance. Decreased renal function (Cl$_{cr}$ <30 mL/minute) may result in toxicity; monitor for toxicity.
Dosage Forms
  Granules, as sulfate: ~40 mEq magnesium/5 g (240 g)
  Injection, as sulfate: 10% = 0.8 mEq/mL (2 mL, 10 mL, 20 mL, 30 mL, 50 mL); 20% = 1.97 mEq/mL (2 mL, 10 mL, 20 mL, 30 mL, 50 mL); 50% = 4 mEq/mL (2 mL, 10 mL, 20 mL, 50 mL)
  Liquid, as sulfate: 54 mg/5 mL; gluconate: 54 mg/5 mL (gluconate has 27 mg magnesium)
  Tablet, as various salts: 140 mg, 400 mg, 500 mg
Selected References
  Chernow B, Smith J, Rainey TG, et al, "Hypomagnesemia: Implications for the Critical Care Specialist," *Crit Care Med*, 1982, 10(3):193-6.
  Gams JG, "Clinical Significance of Magnesium: A Review," *Drug Intell Clin Pharm*, 1987, 21(3):240-6.

♦ **Magnesium Trisilicate and Aluminum Hydroxide** *see* Aluminum Hydroxide and Magnesium Trisilicate *on page 66*
♦ **Magonate® [OTC]** *see* Magnesium Salts (Various Salts) *on page 952*
♦ **Mag-Ox® 400 [OTC]** *see* Magnesium Oxide *on page 951*
♦ **Mag-Tab® SR** *see* Magnesium L-lactate *on page 950*
♦ **MAH** *see* Magnesium L-aspartate Hydrochloride *on page 948*
♦ **Maldemar™** *see* Scopolamine Derivatives *on page 1448*
♦ **Mallamint® [OTC]** *see* Calcium Salts (Oral) *on page 220*

Maltodextrin (mal toe DEK strin)

U.S. Brand Names Multidex® [OTC]; OraRinse™ [OTC]
Generic Available No
Pharmacologic Category Anti-inflammatory, Locally Applied
Use
  Oral: Management and relief of pain due to oral lesions (including mucositis/stomatitis), oral ulcers, or irritation; treatment of aphthous ulcers
  Topical: Treatment of infected or noninfected wounds
Contraindications Hypersensitivity to maltodextrin or any component of the formulation
Warnings/Precautions Oral: Avoid eating or drinking for 1 hour; products are not harmful if accidentally swallowed; notify healthcare provider if improvement is not seen within 7 days
Stability OraRinse™: Fill bottle with water to first arrow; shake vigorously until suspended; continue to fill to second arrow; shake well
Mechanism of Action Forms a protective barrier over wound providing an environment which promotes tissue growth.
Dosage
  Geriatrics & Adults:
    Management of pain due to oral lesions: Oral: OraRinse™: 1 tablespoonful, swish or gargle for ~1 minute, 4 times/day or more if needed
    Wound dressing: Topical: Multidex®: After debridement and irrigation of wound, apply and cover with a nonadherent, nonocclusive dressing. May be applied to moist or dry, infected or noninfected wounds.
Dosage Forms Excipient information presented when available (limited, particularly for generics); consult specific product labeling.
  (Continued)

Maltodextrin *(Continued)*

Gel, topical dressing:
   Multidex®: (4 mL, 7 mL, 14 mL, 85 mL)
Powder, for oral suspension:
   OraRinse™: (19 g) [contains phenylalanine; also contains aloe vera, fructose, and sodium benzoate; vanilla flavor]
Powder, topical dressing:
   Multidex®: (6 g, 12 g, 25 g, 45 g)

♦ **Mandelamine®** *see* Methenamine *on page 1001*
♦ **Mantoux** *see* Tuberculin Tests *on page 1643*
♦ **Mapap [OTC]** *see* Acetaminophen *on page 29*
♦ **Mapap Children's [OTC]** *see* Acetaminophen *on page 29*
♦ **Mapap Extra Strength [OTC]** *see* Acetaminophen *on page 29*
♦ **Mapap Infants [OTC]** *see* Acetaminophen *on page 29*

Maprotiline *(ma PROE ti leen)*

Related Information
   Antidepressant Agents *on page 1742*
Medication Safety Issues
   Sound-alike/look-alike issues:
      Ludiomil may be confused with Lamictal®, lamotrigine, Lomotil®
Canadian Brand Names Novo-Maprotiline
Index Terms Ludiomil; Maprotiline Hydrochloride
Generic Available Yes
Pharmacologic Category Antidepressant, Tetracyclic
Use Treatment of depression and anxiety associated with depression
Unlabeled/Investigational Use Treatment of bulimia, duodenal ulcers, enuresis, urinary symptoms of multiple sclerosis, pain, panic attacks, tension headache, cocaine withdrawal
Restrictions An FDA-approved medication guide concerning the use of antidepressants in children, adolescents, and young adults must be distributed when dispensing an outpatient prescription (new or refill) where this medication is to be used without direct supervision of a healthcare provider. Medication guides are available at http://www.fda.gov/cder/Offices/ODS/medication_guides.htm. Dispense to parents or guardians of children and adolescents receiving this medication.
Contraindications Hypersensitivity to maprotiline or any component of the formulation; use of MAO inhibitors within 14 days; use in a patient during the acute recovery phase of MI
Warnings/Precautions [U.S. Boxed Warning]: Antidepressants increase the risk of suicidal thinking and behavior in children, adolescents, and young adults (18-24 years of age) with major depressive disorder (MDD) and other psychiatric disorders; consider risk prior to prescribing. Short-term studies did not show an increased risk in patients >24 years of age and showed a decreased risk in patients ≥65 years. Closely monitor for clinical worsening, suicidality, or unusual changes in behavior; the patient's family or caregiver should be instructed to closely observe the patient and communicate condition with healthcare provider. A medication guide should be dispensed with each prescription.

The possibility of a suicide attempt is inherent in major depression and may persist until remission occurs. Monitor for worsening of depression or suicidality, especially during initiation of therapy (generally first 1-2 months) or with dose increases or decreases. Use caution in high-risk patients. Worsening depression and severe abrupt suicidality that are not part of the presenting symptoms may require discontinuation or modification of drug therapy. The patient's family or caregiver should be alerted to monitor patients for the emergence of suicidality and associated behaviors (such as agitation, irritability, hostility, impulsivity, and hypomania) and call healthcare provider.

May worsen psychosis in some patients or precipitate a shift to mania or hypomania in patients with bipolar disorder. Patients presenting with depressive symptoms should be screened for bipolar disorder. Monotherapy in patients with bipolar disorder should be avoided. **Maprotiline is not FDA approved for the treatment of bipolar depression.**

Maprotiline has a high risk of sedation relative to other antidepressants. Sedation is common, and may result in impaired performance of tasks requiring alertness (eg, operating machinery or driving). Sedative effects may be additive with other CNS depressants and/or ethanol.

The risk of orthostatic hypotension and/or cardiac conduction abnormalities is moderate relative to other antidepressants. Use with caution in patients with a history of cardiovascular disease (including previous MI, stroke, tachycardia, or conduction abnormalities). The degree of anticholinergic blockade produced by this agent is moderate relative to other cyclic antidepressants, however, caution should still be used in patients with urinary retention, benign prostatic hyperplasia, narrow-angle glaucoma, xerostomia, visual problems, constipation, or history of bowel obstruction.

Consider discontinuing, when possible, prior to elective surgery. Therapy should not be abruptly discontinued in patients receiving high doses for prolonged periods. Use caution in patients with a previous seizure disorder or condition predisposing to seizures such as brain damage, alcoholism, or concurrent therapy with other drugs which lower the seizure threshold. May increase the risks associated with electroconvulsive therapy. Use with caution in hyperthyroid patients or those receiving thyroid supplementation. Use with caution in patients with hepatic or renal dysfunction and in elderly patients.

Adverse Reactions (Reflective of adult population; not specific for elderly)
>10%:
  Central nervous system: Drowsiness
  Gastrointestinal: Xerostomia
1% to 10%:
  Central nervous system: Insomnia, nervousness, anxiety, agitation, dizziness, fatigue, headache
  Gastrointestinal: Constipation, nausea
  Neuromuscular & skeletal: Tremor, weakness
  Ocular: Blurred vision

Drug Interactions Substrate of CYP2D6 (major)
  Altretamine: Concurrent use may cause orthostatic hypertension
  Amphetamines: Cyclic antidepressants may enhance the effect of amphetamines; monitor for adverse CV effects
  Anticholinergics: Combined use with cyclic antidepressants may produce additive anticholinergic effects
  Antihypertensives: Cyclic antidepressants may inhibit the antihypertensive response to bethanidine, clonidine, debrisoquin, guanadrel, guanethidine, guanabenz, guanfacine; monitor BP; consider alternate antihypertensive agent
  Beta-agonists: When combined with cyclic antidepressants may predispose patients to cardiac arrhythmias
  Bupropion: May increase the levels of cyclic antidepressants; based on limited information; monitor response
  Carbamazepine: Cyclic antidepressants may increase carbamazepine levels; monitor
  Cholestyramine and colestipol: May bind cyclic antidepressants and reduce their absorption; monitor for altered response
  Clonidine: Abrupt discontinuation of clonidine may cause hypertensive crisis, cyclic antidepressants may enhance the response
  CNS depressants: Sedative effects may be additive with cyclic antidepressants; monitor for increased effect; includes benzodiazepines, barbiturates, antipsychotics, ethanol and other sedative medications
  CYP2D6 inhibitors: May increase the levels/effects of maprotiline. Example inhibitors include chlorpromazine, delavirdine, fluoxetine, miconazole, paroxetine, pergolide, quinidine, quinine, ritonavir, and ropinirole.
  Epinephrine (and other direct alpha-agonists): The pressor response to I.V. epinephrine, norepinephrine, and phenylephrine may be enhanced in patients receiving cyclic antidepressants; this combination is best avoided
  Fenfluramine: May increase cyclic antidepressant levels/effects
  Hypoglycemic agents (including insulin): Hypoglycemic effects may be enhanced, profound hypoglycemia has been reported; monitor for changes in blood glucose levels; reported with chlorpropamide, tolazamide, and insulin
  Levodopa: Cyclic antidepressants may decrease the absorption (bioavailability) of levodopa; rare hypertensive episodes have also been attributed to this combination
  Linezolid: Hyperpyrexia, hypertension, tachycardia, confusion, seizures, and **deaths have been reported** with agents which inhibit MAO (serotonin syndrome); this combination should be avoided
  Lithium: Concurrent use with a cyclic antidepressant may increase the risk for neurotoxicity
  MAO inhibitors: Hyperpyrexia, hypertension, tachycardia, confusion, seizures, and **deaths have been reported** (serotonin syndrome); this combination should be avoided
  Methylphenidate: Metabolism of maprotiline may be decreased
  Phenothiazines: Serum concentrations of some TCAs may be increased; in addition, TCAs may increase concentration of phenothiazines; monitor for altered clinical response
  QT_c-prolonging agents: Concurrent use of cyclic agents with other drugs which may prolong QT_c interval may increase the risk of potentially fatal arrhythmias; includes type Ia and type III antiarrhythmics agents, selected quinolones (moxifloxacin), cisapride, and other agents
  Sucralfate: Absorption of cyclic antidepressants may be reduced with coadministration. (Continued)

Maprotiline *(Continued)*

Sympathomimetics, indirect-acting: Cyclic antidepressants may result in a decreased sensitivity to indirect-acting sympathomimetics; includes dopamine and ephedrine; also see interaction with epinephrine (and direct-acting sympathomimetics)

Tramadol: Tramadol's risk of seizures may be increased with TCAs

Valproic acid: May increase serum concentrations/adverse effects of some cyclic antidepressants

Warfarin (and other oral anticoagulants): Cyclic antidepressants may increase the anticoagulant effect in patients stabilized on warfarin; monitor INR

Ethanol/Nutrition/Herb Interactions Ethanol: Avoid ethanol (may increase CNS depression).

Mechanism of Action Traditionally believed to increase the synaptic concentration of norepinephrine in the central nervous system by inhibition of their reuptake by the presynaptic neuronal membrane. However, additional receptor effects have been found including desensitization of adenyl cyclase, down regulation of beta-adrenergic receptors, and down regulation of serotonin receptors.

Pharmacodynamics Onset of therapeutic effects: May take 1-3 weeks before effects are seen; norepinephrine only

Pharmacokinetics

Absorption: Oral: Slow

Protein binding: 88%

Metabolism: In the liver to active and inactive compounds

Half-life: 21-25 hours

Time to peak serum concentration: Within 12 hours

Elimination: In urine (70%) and feces (30%)

Geriatrics: After a single 125 mg oral dose in 5 subjects between 75-83 years of age 50% of the dose was absorbed, the average time to peak was 7 hours, and the average elimination half-life was 31.5 hours

Dosage

Geriatrics: Initial: 25 mg at bedtime, increase by 25 mg every 3 days for inpatients and weekly for outpatients if tolerated. Usual maintenance dose: 50-75 mg/day, higher doses may be necessary in nonresponders.

Adults: Depression/anxiety: Oral: 75 mg/day to start, increase by 25 mg every 2 weeks up to 150-225 mg/day; given in 3 divided doses or in a single daily dose

Monitoring Parameters Sleep, appetite, mood, somatic complaints, mental status, weight, blood pressure and heart rate, urine flow/output

Reference Range Therapeutic: 200-600 ng/mL (SI: 721-2163 nmol/L); not well established

Patient Information Do not drink alcoholic beverages, may cause drowsiness, dry mouth, constipation, blurred vision; rise slowly to avoid dizziness

Special Geriatric Considerations Use with caution due to sedation and anticholinergic effects (eg, confusion, constipation, difficulty urinating, dry mouth).

Dosage Forms Excipient information presented when available (limited, particularly for generics); consult specific product labeling.

Tablet, as hydrochloride: 25 mg, 50 mg, 75 mg

Selected References

Hrdina PD, Rovei V, Henry JF, et al, "Comparison of Single-Dose Pharmacokinetics of Imipramine and Maprotiline in the Elderly," *Psychopharmacology*, 1980, 70(1):29-34.

Measles, Mumps, and Rubella Vaccines (Combined)
(MEE zels, mumpz & roo BEL a vak SEENS, kom BINED)

Related Information
Immunization Recommendations *on page 1787*
Measles Virus Vaccine (Live) *on page 959*
Mumps Virus Vaccine (Live/Attenuated) *on page 1073*
Rubella Virus Vaccine (Live) *on page 1436*
U.S. Brand Names M-M-R® II
Canadian Brand Names M-M-R® II; Priorix™
Index Terms MMR; Mumps, Measles and Rubella Vaccines, Combined; Rubella, Measles and Mumps Vaccines, Combined
Generic Available No
Pharmacologic Category Vaccine, Live Virus
Use Measles, mumps, and rubella prophylaxis in adults born after 1956 with no evidence of immunity to measles or mumps
Contraindications Hypersensitivity to measles, mumps, and rubella vaccine or any component of the formulation; hypersensitivity to neomycin or gelatin; current febrile respiratory illness or other febrile infection; patients receiving immunosuppressive therapy; primary and acquired immunodeficiency states; blood dyscrasias, cancers affecting the bone marrow or lymphatic systems
Warnings/Precautions Use caution with history of cerebral injury, seizures, or other conditions where stress due to fever should be avoided. Immediate treatment for anaphylactic/anaphylactoid reaction should be available during vaccine use. Use extreme caution in patients with immediate-type hypersensitivity reactions to eggs. Use caution in patients with thrombocytopenia and those who develop thrombocytopenia after first dose; thrombocytopenia may worsen. Consider delaying vaccination during acute moderate or severe febrile illness; patients with minor illnesses with or without fever (diarrhea, mild upper respiratory tract infection, otitis media) may receive vaccine. Use is contraindicated in severely immunocompromised patients. However, leukemia patients who are in remission and who have not received chemotherapy for at least 3 months may be vaccinated; patients with HIV infection, who are asymptomatic and not severely immunosuppressed may be vaccinated. Therapy to treat tuberculosis should be started prior to administering vaccine to patients with untreated, active tuberculosis. Exposure to measles is not a contraindication to vaccine; use within 72 hours of exposure may provide some protection. Recent administration of immune globulins, blood or blood products may interfere with immune response. Acceptable evidence of immunity is recommended for students entering institutions of higher learning, healthcare workers at time of employment, and for travelers to endemic areas.
Adverse Reactions (Reflective of adult population; not specific for elderly)
All serious adverse reactions must be reported to the U.S. Department of Health and Human Services (DHHS) Vaccine Adverse Event Reporting System (VAERS) 1-800-822-7967.
Frequency not defined:
Cardiovascular: Syncope, vasculitis
Central nervous system: Ataxia, dizziness, febrile convulsions, fever, encephalitis, encephalopathy, Guillain-Barré syndrome, headache, irritability, malaise, measles inclusion body encephalitis, polyneuritis, polyneuropathy, seizure, subacute sclerosing panencephalitis,
Dermatologic: Angioneurotic edema, erythema multiforme, purpura, rash, Stevens-Johnson syndrome, urticaria
Endocrine & metabolic: Diabetes mellitus, parotitis
Gastrointestinal: Diarrhea, nausea, pancreatitis, sore throat, vomiting
Genitourinary: Orchitis
Hematologic: Leukocytosis, thrombocytopenia
Local: Injection site reactions which include burning, induration, redness, stinging, swelling, tenderness, wheal and flare, vesiculation
Neuromuscular & skeletal: Arthralgia/arthritis (variable; highest rates in women, 12% to 26% versus children, up to 3%), myalgia, paresthesia
Ocular: Ocular palsies
Otic: Otitis media
Renal: Conjunctivitis, retinitis, optic neuritis, papillitis, retrobulbar neuritis
Respiratory: Bronchospasm, cough, pneumonitis, rhinitis
Miscellaneous: Anaphylactoid reactions, anaphylaxis, atypical measles, panniculitis, regional lymphadenopathy
Drug Interactions
Corticosteroids: In patients receiving high doses of systemic corticosteroids for ≥14 days, wait at least 1 month between discontinuing steroid therapy and administering immunization.
Immune globulin, whole blood, plasma: May diminish the therapeutic effect of live vaccines. Live virus vaccination should be withheld for ~3-11 months following
(Continued)

Measles, Mumps, and Rubella Vaccines (Combined)
(Continued)

immune globulin administration; length of time depends on dose of IgG given. Live virus vaccine administered during the days prior to immune globulin administration may require repeat vaccination.

Immunosuppressants medications: Immunosuppressants may enhance the adverse/toxic effect of live vaccines; vaccinial infections may develop.

Vaccines: Using separate sites and syringes, MMR may be administered concurrently with DTaP, *Haemophilus* b conjugate vaccine, or varicella virus vaccine. Unless otherwise specified, MMR should be given 1 month before or 1 month after live virus vaccines.

Stability Prior to reconstitution, store the powder at 2°C to 8°C (36°F to 46°F) or colder (freezing does not affect potency). Protect from light. Diluent may be stored with powder or at room temperature. Use entire contents of the provided diluent to reconstitute vaccine. Gently agitate to mix thoroughly. Discard if powder does not dissolve. Use as soon as possible following reconstitution (may be stored at 2°C to 8°C/36°F to 46°F; protect from light); discard if not used within 8 hours.

Mechanism of Action As a live, attenuated vaccine, MMR vaccine offers active immunity to disease caused by the measles, mumps, and rubella viruses.

Dosage

Adults: Immunization: *Born ≥1957 without evidence of immunity* (also see Additional Information): SubQ: 1 or 2 doses (0.5 mL/dose); minimum interval between doses is 28 days

Routine vaccination of healthcare workers:

Born ≥1957 without evidence of immunity: SubQ: 2 doses of a live mumps virus vaccine; minimum interval between doses is 28 days

Born <1957 without evidence of immunity: SubQ: 1 dose of a live mumps virus vaccine.

Mumps outbreak:

Healthcare workers born <1957 without other evidence of immunity: SubQ: Consider 2 doses of a live mumps virus vaccine; minimum interval between doses is 28 days

Low-risk adults: SubQ: A second dose of a live mumps virus vaccine should be considered in adults who previously received 1 dose; minimum interval between doses is 28 days

Administration Administer SubQ with a 25-gauge ⅝" needle in outer aspect of the upper arm. **Not for I.V. administration.** Federal law requires that the date of administration, the vaccine manufacturer, lot number of vaccine, and the administering person's name, title and address be entered into the patient's permanent medical record.

Monitoring Parameters Monitor site of injection and for systemic side effects.

Test Interactions Temporary suppression of TB skin test reactivity with onset approximately 3 days after administration

Patient Information Report any serious side effects to your physician such as seizures or sore throat.

Additional Information Live, attenuated vaccine. Federal law requires that the date of administration, the vaccine manufacturer, lot number of vaccine, and the administering person's name, title and address be entered into the patient's permanent medical record

Adults born before 1957 are generally considered to be immune to measles and mumps; all born in or after 1957 without documentation of live vaccine on or after first birthday, physician-diagnosed measles or mumps, or laboratory evidence of immunity should be vaccine with two doses separated by no less than 1 month; for those previously vaccinated with one dose of measles vaccine, revaccination is indicated healthcare workers at time of employment, and for travelers to endemic areas. Guidelines for rubella vaccination are the same with the exception of birth year; all adults should be vaccinated against rubella. Booster doses of mumps and rubella are not necessary.

Measles vaccine:

A rash may occur from 1-2 weeks after receiving the measles vaccine

A fever ≥103°F after receiving the first measles vaccine; fever occurs less often after a second injection.

Mumps vaccine: A little swelling of the glands in the cheeks and under the jaw that lasts for a few days; this could happen from 1-2 weeks after the mumps vaccine; happens rarely

Rubella vaccine: Swelling of the lymph glands in the neck or a rash that lasts 1-2 days

Mild pain or stiffness in the joints that may last up to 3 days; happens in 25 out of 100 adults who are vaccinated. Women have this side effect more than men in up to 40 women out of every 100. Rarely, pain or stiffness can last for months or longer.

Painful swelling of the joints (arthritis) happens in 10 out of 100 adults which usually lasts a few days to a week. Rarely, this swelling has been reported to last longer. Pain or numbness, or "pins and needles" feeling in the hands and feet that lasts for a short time; happens rarely

Special Geriatric Considerations Most adults and elderly are immune to measles (rubeola) and it is not necessary to vaccinate. If no history of measles exposure or patient is from an isolated community where measles is not endemic, vaccination may be required. Testing may be indicated; may need to test for rubella. Vaccinate those traveling into endemic areas with no evidence of immunity. No dose restriction necessary.

Dosage Forms Excipient information presented when available (limited, particularly for generics); consult specific product labeling.
Injection, powder for reconstitution [preservative free]:
M-M-R® II: Measles virus 1000 TCID$_{50}$, mumps virus 20,000 TCID$_{50}$, and , rubella virus 1000 TCID$_{50}$ [contains neomycin 25 mcg, gelatin, human albumin, and bovine serum; produced in chick embryo cell culture]

Selected References

Centers for Disease Control and Prevention (CDC), "Notice to Readers: Updated Recommendations of the Advisory Committee on Immunization Practices (ACIP) for the Control and Elimination of Mumps," *MMWR Recomm Rep*, 2006, 55(early release):1-2. Available at http://www.cdc.gov/mmwr/pdf/wk/mm55e601.pdf
Centers for Disease Control, "Recommendations of the Advisory Committee on Immunization Practices (ACIP): General Recommendations on Immunization," *MMWR Recomm Rep*, 1994, 43(RR-1):23.
Plichta AM, "Immunization: Protecting Older Patients From Infectious Disease," *Geriatrics*, 1996, 51(9):47-52.
Watson JC, Hadler SC, Dykewicz CA, et al, "Measles, Mumps, and Rubella — Vaccine Use and Strategies for Elimination of Measles, Rubella, and Congenital Rubella Syndrome and Control of Mumps: Recommendations of the Advisory Committee on Immunization Practices (ACIP)," *MMWR Recomm Rep*, 1998, 47(RR-8):1-57.

Measles Virus Vaccine (Live) (MEE zels VYE rus vak SEEN, live)

Related Information
Immunization Recommendations *on page 1787*
Medication Safety Issues
Sound-alike/look-alike issues:
Attenuvax® may be confused with Meruvax®
U.S. Brand Names Attenuvax®
Index Terms More Attenuated Enders Strain; Rubeola Vaccine
Generic Available No
Pharmacologic Category Vaccine, Live Virus
Use Active immunization against measles (rubeola)
Note: Trivalent measles - mumps - rubella (MMR) is the vaccine of choice if recipients are likely to be susceptible to rubella and/or mumps as well as to measles.
Contraindications Hypersensitivity to measles vaccine or any component of the formulation; current febrile illness; patients receiving immunosuppressive therapy (not including steroid replacement); primary and acquired immunodeficiency states; blood dyscrasias, cancers affecting the bone marrow or lymphatic systems
Warnings/Precautions Use caution with history of cerebral injury, seizures, or other conditions where stress due to fever should be avoided. Immediate treatment for anaphylactic/anaphylactoid reaction should be available during vaccine use. Vaccine is produced in chick embryo cell culture; use extreme caution in patients with immediate-type hypersensitivity reactions to eggs. Vaccine also contains albumin, neomycin, and gelatin. A history of contact dermatitis to neomycin is not a contraindication to use, however, do not use with previous anaphylactic reaction to neomycin. Use caution in patients with thrombocytopenia and those who develop thrombocytopenia after first dose; thrombocytopenia may worsen. The manufacturer contraindicates use with febrile infections; however, the ACIP notes that patients with minor illnesses with or without fever (diarrhea, mild upper respiratory tract infection, otitis media) may receive vaccines.

Use is contraindicated in severely immunocompromised patients. However, leukemia patients who are in remission and who have not received chemotherapy for at least 3 months may be vaccinated; patients with HIV infection, who are asymptomatic and not severely immunosuppressed may be vaccinated. Therapy to treat tuberculosis should be started prior to administering vaccine to patients with untreated, active tuberculosis. Exposure to measles is not a contraindication to vaccine; use within 72 hours of exposure may provide some protection. Recent administration of immune globulins, blood, or blood products may interfere with immune response. Acceptable evidence of immunity is recommended for students entering institutions of higher learning, healthcare workers at time of employment, and for travelers to endemic areas.

Adverse Reactions (Reflective of adult population; not specific for elderly)
All serious adverse reactions must be reported to the U.S. Department of Health and Human Services (DHHS) Vaccine Adverse Event Reporting System (VAERS) 1-800-822-7967.
(Continued)

Measles Virus Vaccine (Live) *(Continued)*

Frequency not defined.

Cardiovascular: Peripheral edema, syncope, vasculitis

Central nervous system: Ataxia, dizziness, encephalitis, encephalopathy, febrile seizure, fever, Guillain-Barré syndrome, headache, irritability, malaise, seizure

Dermatologic: Angioneurotic edema, erythema multiforme, panniculitis, purpura, rash, Stevens-Johnson syndrome, urticaria

Gastrointestinal: Diarrhea, nausea, vomiting

Hematologic: Leukocytosis, thrombocytopenia

Local: Injection site reactions: Burning, redness, stinging, swelling, vesiculation, wheal and flare

Neuromuscular & skeletal: Arthralgia, myalgia

Ocular: Conjunctivitis, ocular palsies, optic neuritis, papillitis, retinitis, retrobulbar neuritis

Otic: Nerve deafness, otitis media

Respiratory: Bronchial spasm, cough, pneumonitis, rhinitis

Miscellaneous: Anaphylaxis/anaphylactoid reactions, atypical measles, facial edema, lymphadenopathy, measles inclusion body encephalitis, subacute sclerosing pancephalitis

Drug Interactions

Corticosteroids: In patients receiving high doses of systemic corticosteroids for ≥14 days, wait at least 1 month between discontinuing steroid therapy and administering immunization.

Immune globulin, whole blood, plasma: Do not administer together; immune response may be compromised. Defer vaccine administration for ≥3 months.

Immunosuppressant medications: Immunosuppressants may enhance the adverse/toxic effect of live vaccines; vaccinial infections may develop.

Vaccines: Using separate sites and syringes, may be administered concurrently with *Haemophilus* b conjugate vaccine or varicella virus vaccine. Unless otherwise specified, should be given 1 month before or 1 month after live virus vaccines.

Stability During shipment, store at ≤10°C (50°F). Prior to and following reconstitution, refrigerate at 2°C to 8°C (36°F to 46°F). Protect from light at all times. Following reconstitution, use within 8 hours.

Mechanism of Action Promotes active immunity to measles virus by inducing specific measles IgG and IgM antibodies. Measles antibodies develop in ~95% of children vaccinated at 12 months of age and in 98% of children vaccinated at 15 months of age. Life-long immunity is induced in most persons completing vaccination schedule.

Dosage

Geriatrics & Adults: Immunization: SubQ: 0.5 mL in outer aspect of the upper arm. **Note:** Trivalent measles - mumps - rubella (MMR) vaccine should be used unless contraindicated in adults.

Adults born in or after 1957 without documentation of live vaccine on or after first birthday, without physician-diagnosed measles, or without laboratory evidence of immunity should be vaccinated, ideally with 2 doses of vaccine separated by no less than 1 month. For those previously vaccinated with 1 dose of measles vaccine, revaccination is recommended for students entering colleges and other institutions of higher education, for healthcare workers at the time of employment, and for international travelers who visit endemic areas. Persons vaccinated between 1963 and 1967 with a killed measles vaccine, followed by live vaccine within 3 months, or with a vaccine of unknown type should be revaccinated with live measles virus vaccine.

Administration Vaccine should not be administered I.V.; SubQ injection preferred with a 25-gauge ⁵⁄₈" needle.

Monitoring Parameters Monitor for side effects

Test Interactions May temporarily depress tuberculin skin test sensitivity; tuberculin test may be given simultaneously on the same day as vaccine or ≥4 weeks later.

Additional Information Federal law requires that the date of administration, the vaccine manufacturer, lot number of vaccine, and the administering person's name, title, and address be entered into the patient's permanent medical record.

Acceptable presumptive evidence of immunity includes one of the following:

1. Documentation of adequate vaccination. Adequate vaccination is defined as 1 dose of a live mumps virus vaccine for preschool children and adults not at high risk; 2 doses of a live mumps virus vaccine for school-aged children and high-risk adults. Healthcare workers, international travelers, and students in institutions of higher learning are considered high-risk adults.
2. Laboratory evidence of immunity
3. Birth prior to 1957
4. Documentation of physician-diagnosed disease

Special Geriatric Considerations Generally not recommended for adults since most have become immune; if from an isolated community where measles is not endemic, may require vaccination; no dose reduction is necessary

Dosage Forms Excipient information presented when available (limited, particularly for generics); consult specific product labeling.

Injection, powder for reconstitution [preservative free]:

Attenuvax®: ≥1000 $TCID_{50}$/0.5 mL (0.5 mL) [contains human albumin, bovine serum, neomycin, gelatin, neomycin, sorbitol, and sucrose; produced in chick embryo cell culture]

Selected References

Centers for Disease Control and Prevention, "Measles, Mumps, and Rubella — Vaccine Use and Strategies for Elimination of Measles, Rubella, and Congenital Rubella Syndrome and Control of Mumps: Recommendations of the Advisory Committee on Immunization Practices (ACIP)," *MMWR Recomm Rep*, 1998, 47(RR-8):1-57.

Centers for Disease Control and Prevention, "Notice to Readers: Revised ACIP Recommendation for Avoiding Pregnancy After Receiving a Rubella-Containing Vaccine," *MMWR Morb Mortal Wkly Rep*, 2001, 50(49):1117.

Centers for Disease Control, "Recommendations of the Advisory Committee on Immunization Practices (ACIP): General Recommendations on Immunization," *MMWR Recomm Rep*, 2006, 55(RR-15):1-48.

Gardner P and Schaffner W, "Immunization of Adults," *N Engl J Med*, 1993, 328(17):1252-8.

♦ **Mebaral**® *see* Mephobarbital *on page 983*

Meclizine (MEK li zeen)

Medication Safety Issues
Sound-alike/look-alike issues:
Antivert® may be confused with Axert™

U.S. Brand Names Antivert®; Bonine® [OTC]; Dramamine® Less Drowsy Formula [OTC]

Canadian Brand Names Bonamine™; Bonine®

Index Terms Meclizine Hydrochloride; Meclozine Hydrochloride

Generic Available Yes

Pharmacologic Category Antiemetic; Antihistamine

Use Prevention and treatment of nausea, vomiting, and dizziness of motion sickness; management of vertigo with diseases affecting the vestibular system (only "possibly" effective)

Contraindications Hypersensitivity to meclizine or any component of the formulation

Warnings/Precautions Use with caution in patients with asthma, angle-closure glaucoma, prostatic hyperplasia, pyloric or duodenal obstruction, or bladder neck obstruction; elderly may be at risk for anticholinergic side effects such as glaucoma, prostatic hyperplasia, constipation, gastrointestinal obstructive disease; if vertigo does not respond in 1-2 weeks, it is advised to discontinue use. May be sedating, use with caution in disorders where CNS depression is a feature; patients must be cautioned about performing tasks which require mental alertness (eg, operating machinery or driving). Effects may be potentiated when used with other sedative drugs or ethanol.

Adverse Reactions (Reflective of adult population; not specific for elderly)
>10%:
Central nervous system: Slight to moderate drowsiness
Respiratory: Thickening of bronchial secretions
1% to 10%:
Central nervous system: Headache, fatigue, nervousness, dizziness
Gastrointestinal: Appetite increase, weight gain, nausea, diarrhea, abdominal pain, xerostomia
Respiratory: Pharyngitis

Overdosage/Toxicology Symptoms include CNS depression, confusion, nervousness, hallucinations, dizziness, blurred vision, nausea, vomiting, and hyperthermia. There is no specific treatment for antihistamine overdose, however, clinical toxicity is mostly due to anticholinergic effects. For anticholinergic overdose with severe life-threatening symptoms, physostigmine 1-2 mg slow I.V. may be given to reverse these effects.

Drug Interactions Increased toxicity: CNS depressants, neuroleptics, anticholinergics

Ethanol/Nutrition/Herb Interactions Ethanol: Avoid ethanol (may increase CNS depression).

Mechanism of Action Has central anticholinergic action by blocking chemoreceptor trigger zone; decreases excitability of the middle ear labyrinth and blocks conduction in the middle ear vestibular-cerebellar pathways

Pharmacodynamics
Onset of action: Oral: Within 30-60 minutes
Duration: 8-24 hours

Pharmacokinetics
Metabolism: Reportedly in the liver
Half-life: 6 hours
(Continued)

Meclizine *(Continued)*

Elimination: As metabolites in urine and as unchanged drug in feces

Dosage

Geriatrics & Adults:

Motion sickness: Oral: 12.5-25 mg 1 hour before travel, repeat dose every 12-24 hours if needed; doses up to 50 mg may be needed

Vertigo: Oral: 25-100 mg/day in divided doses

Monitoring Parameters Monitor for CNS anticholinergic side effects in older adults, relief of symptoms

Patient Information May impair ability to perform hazardous tasks and urinate; may also cause drowsiness, dry mouth, constipation, and dry eyes

Special Geriatric Considerations Due to anticholinergic action, use lowest dose in divided doses to avoid side effects and their inconvenience. Limit use if possible. May cause confusion or aggravate symptoms of confusion in those with dementia. If vertigo does not respond in 1-2 weeks, discontinue use.

Dosage Forms Excipient information presented when available (limited, particularly for generics); consult specific product labeling.

Tablet, as hydrochloride: 12.5 mg, 25 mg

Antivert®: 12.5 mg, 25 mg, 50 mg

Dramamine® Less Drowsy Formula: 25 mg

Tablet, chewable, as hydrochloride (Bonine®): 25 mg

♦ **Meclizine Hydrochloride** *see* Meclizine *on page 961*

Meclofenamate *(me kloe fen AM ate)*

Canadian Brand Names Meclomen®

Index Terms Meclofenamate Sodium

Generic Available Yes

Pharmacologic Category Nonsteroidal Anti-inflammatory Drug (NSAID), Oral

Use Treatment of inflammatory disorders such as rheumatoid arthritis, mild to moderate pain, osteoarthritis, pain of sunburn, migraine headaches (acute)

Restrictions An FDA-approved medication guide must be distributed when dispensing an oral outpatient prescription (new or refill) where this medication is to be used without direct supervision of a healthcare provider. Medication guides are available at http://www.fda.gov/cder/Offices/ODS/medication_guides.htm.

Contraindications Hypersensitivity to meclofenamate, aspirin, other NSAIDs, or any component of the formulation; perioperative pain in the setting of coronary artery bypass surgery (CABG); active GI bleeding, ulcer disease

Warnings/Precautions [U.S. Boxed Warning]: NSAIDs are associated with an increased risk of adverse cardiovascular events, including MI, stroke, and new onset or worsening of pre-existing hypertension. Risk may be increased with duration of use or pre-existing cardiovascular risk factors or disease. Carefully evaluate individual cardiovascular risk profiles prior to prescribing. Use caution with fluid retention, CHF or hypertension. Concurrent administration of ibuprofen, and potentially other nonselective NSAIDs, may interfere with aspirin's cardioprotective effect.

Use of NSAIDs can compromise existing renal function. Renal toxicity can occur in patient with impaired renal function, dehydration, heart failure, liver dysfunction, those taking diuretics and ACEI and the elderly. Rehydrate patient before starting therapy. Monitor renal function closely. Use caution in patients with advanced renal disease.

[U.S. Boxed Warning]: NSAIDs may increase risk of gastrointestinal irritation, ulceration, bleeding, and perforation. These events may occur at any time during therapy and without warning. Use caution with a history of GI disease (bleeding or ulcers), concurrent therapy with aspirin, anticoagulants and/or corticosteroids, smoking, use of alcohol, the elderly or debilitated patients.

Use the lowest effective dose for the shortest duration of time, consistent with individual patient goals, to reduce risk of cardiovascular or GI adverse events. Alternate therapies should be considered for patients at high risk.

NSAIDs may cause serious skin adverse events including exfoliative dermatitis, Stevens-Johnson syndrome (SJS) and toxic epidermal necrolysis (TEN). Anaphylactoid reactions may occur, even without prior exposure; patients with "aspirin triad" (bronchial asthma, aspirin intolerance, rhinitis) may be at increased risk. Do not use in patients who experience bronchospasm, asthma, rhinitis, or urticaria with NSAID or aspirin therapy. Use caution in other forms of asthma.

Use with caution in patients with decreased hepatic function. Closely monitor patients with any abnormal LFT. Severe hepatic reactions (eg, fulminant hepatitis, liver failure) have occurred with NSAID use, rarely; discontinue if signs or symptoms of liver disease develop, or if systemic manifestations occur.

The elderly are at increased risk for adverse effects (especially peptic ulceration, CNS effects, renal toxicity) from NSAIDs even at low doses

Withhold for at least 4-6 half-lives prior to surgical or dental procedures.

Adverse Reactions (Reflective of adult population; not specific for elderly)
>10%:
Central nervous system: Dizziness
Dermatologic: Rash
Gastrointestinal: Abdominal cramps, heartburn, indigestion, nausea
1% to 10%:
Central nervous system: Headache, nervousness
Dermatologic: Itching
Endocrine & metabolic: Fluid retention
Gastrointestinal: Vomiting
Otic: Tinnitus

Overdosage/Toxicology Symptoms include drowsiness, lethargy, nausea, vomiting, seizures, paresthesia, headache, dizziness, GI bleeding, cerebral edema, cardiac arrest, and tinnitus. Management of nonsteroidal anti-inflammatory drug (NSAID) intoxication is primarily supportive and symptomatic. Fluid therapy is commonly effective in managing hypotension that may occur following an acute NSAID overdose, except when due to acute blood loss. Seizures tend to be very short-lived and often do not require drug treatment, although recurrent seizures should be treated with I.V. diazepam. Since many of NSAIDs undergo enterohepatic cycling, multiple doses of charcoal may be needed to reduce the potential for delayed toxicities.

Drug Interactions
ACE inhibitors: Antihypertensive effects may be decreased by concurrent therapy with NSAIDs; monitor blood pressure.
Angiotensin II antagonists: Antihypertensive effects may be decreased by concurrent therapy with NSAIDs; monitor blood pressure.
Anticoagulants (warfarin, heparin, LMWHs) in combination with NSAIDs can cause increased risk of bleeding.
Antiplatelet drugs (ticlopidine, clopidogrel, aspirin, abciximab, dipyridamole, eptifibatide, tirofiban) can cause an increased risk of bleeding.
Beta-blockers: NSAIDs may decrease the antihypertensive effect of beta-blockers. Monitor.
Cholestyramine (and other bile acid sequestrants): May decrease the absorption of NSAIDs. Separate by at least 2 hours.
Corticosteroids may increase the risk of GI ulceration; avoid concurrent use.
Cyclosporine: NSAIDs may increase serum creatinine, potassium, blood pressure, and cyclosporine levels; monitor cyclosporine levels and renal function carefully.
Fluoroquinolone antibiotics: Risk of seizures may be increased with concomitant quinolone use. Risk is considered quite low and may only be a factor with high serum levels of either agent and/or in patients with additional predisposing factors (eg, renal dysfunction, history of seizure or other neurological disorder).
Gentamicin and amikacin serum concentrations are increased by indomethacin in premature infants. Results may apply to other aminoglycosides and NSAIDs.
Hydralazine's antihypertensive effect is decreased; avoid concurrent use.
Lithium levels can be increased; avoid concurrent use if possible or monitor lithium levels and adjust dose. Sulindac may have the least effect. When NSAID is stopped, lithium will need adjustment again.
Loop diuretics efficacy (diuretic and antihypertensive effect) is reduced. Indomethacin reduces this efficacy, however, it may be anticipated with any NSAID.
Methotrexate: Severe bone marrow suppression, aplastic anemia, and GI toxicity have been reported with concomitant NSAID therapy. Avoid use during moderate or high-dose methotrexate (increased and prolonged methotrexate levels). NSAID use during low-dose treatment of rheumatoid arthritis has not been fully evaluated; extreme caution is warranted.
Salicylates: NSAIDs (nonselective) may diminish the cardioprotective effect of acetylated salicylates. Avoid regular use of NSAIDs if possible; consider alternatives (eg, acetaminophen). Give salicylate before NSAID; for example ibuprofen should be given 30-120 minutes after aspirin (immediate release).
Thiazides antihypertensive effects are decreased; avoid concurrent use.
Verapamil plasma concentration is decreased by diclofenac; avoid concurrent use.
Warfarin's INRs may be increased by piroxicam. Other NSAIDs may have the same effect depending on dose and duration. Monitor INR closely. Use the lowest dose of NSAIDs possible and for the briefest duration.

Ethanol/Nutrition/Herb Interactions
Ethanol: Avoid ethanol (may enhance gastric mucosal irritation).
Herb/Nutraceutical: Avoid alfalfa, anise, bilberry, bladderwrack, bromelain, cat's claw, celery, coleus, cordyceps, dong quai, evening primrose, feverfew, fenugreek, garlic, ginger, ginkgo biloba, red clover, horse chestnut, grapeseed, green tea, ginseng, (Continued)

Meclofenamate *(Continued)*

guggul, horse chestnut seed, horseradish, licorice, prickly ash, red clover, reishi, SAMe, sweet clover, turmeric, white willow (all have additional antiplatelet activity).

Mechanism of Action Inhibits prostaglandin synthesis by decreasing the activity of the enzyme, cyclooxygenase, which results in decreased formation of prostaglandin precursors

Pharmacodynamics

Onset of analgesia: 30 minutes to 1 hour

Duration: 2-4 hours

Onset of anti-inflammatory action: 3-4 days

Peak effect: 2-3 weeks

Pharmacokinetics

Protein binding: 99%

Half-life: 2-3.3 hours

Time to peak serum concentration: Oral: Within 30-90 minutes

Elimination: Principally in urine and in feces as glucuronide conjugates

Dosage

Geriatrics & Adults:

Mild to moderate pain: Oral: 50 mg every 4-6 hours; increases to 100 mg may be required; maximum dose: 400 mg

Rheumatoid arthritis/osteoarthritis: Oral: 50 mg every 4-6 hours; increase, over weeks, to 200-400 mg/day in 3-4 divided doses; do not exceed 400 mg/day; maximal benefit for any dose may not be seen for 2-3 weeks

Monitoring Parameters Monitor response (pain, range of motion, grip strength, mobility, ADL function), inflammation; observe for weight gain, edema; monitor renal function; observe for bleeding, bruising; evaluate gastrointestinal effects (abdominal pain, bleeding, dyspepsia); mental confusion, disorientation, CBC, serum, creatinine, BUN, liver function tests

Test Interactions Increased chloride (S), increased sodium (S)

Patient Information Serious gastrointestinal bleeding can occur as well as ulceration and perforation. Pain may or may not be present. Avoid aspirin and aspirin-containing products while taking this medication. If gastric upset occurs, take with food, milk, or antacid. If gastric adverse effects persist, contact physician. May cause drowsiness, dizziness, blurred vision, and confusion. Use caution when performing tasks which require alertness (eg, driving). Do not take for more than 3 days for fever or 10 days for pain without physician advice.

Additional Information There are no clinical guidelines to predict which NSAID will give response in a particular patient. Trials with each must be initiated until response determined. If diarrhea develops, reduce dose or discontinue use of meclofenamate for a short time (until diarrhea stops). Some patients are not able to tolerate further use. Consider dose, patient convenience, and cost.

Special Geriatric Considerations Elderly are a high-risk population for adverse effects from NSAIDs. As much as 60% of elderly can develop peptic ulceration and/or hemorrhage asymptomatically. The concomitant use of H_2 blockers and sucralfate is not effective as prophylaxis with the exception of NSAID-induced duodenal ulcers which may be prevented by the use of ranitidine. Misoprostol and proton pump inhibitors are the only agents proven to help prevent the development of NSAID-induced ulcers. Also, concomitant disease and drug use contribute to the risk for GI adverse effects. Use lowest effective dose for shortest period possible. Consider renal function decline with age. Use of NSAIDs can compromise existing renal function especially when Cl_{cr} is ≤30 mL/minute. Tinnitus may be a difficult and unreliable indication of toxicity due to age-related hearing loss or eighth cranial nerve damage. CNS adverse effects such as confusion, agitation, and hallucination are generally seen in overdose or high dose situations, but elderly may demonstrate these adverse effects at lower doses than younger adults.

Dosage Forms Excipient information presented when available (limited, particularly for generics); consult specific product labeling.

Capsule, as sodium: 50 mg, 100 mg

Selected References

Brooks PM and Day RO, "Nonsteroidal Anti-inflammatory Drugs - Differences and Similarities," *N Engl J Med*, 1991, 324(24):1716-25.

Clinch D, Banerjee AK, and Ostick G, "Absence of Abdominal Pain in Elderly Patients With Peptic Ulcer," *Age Ageing*, 1984, 13(2):120-3.

Clive DM and Stoff JS, "Renal Syndromes Associated With Nonsteroidal Anti-inflammatory Drugs," *N Engl J Med*, 1984, 310(9):563-72.

Graham DY, "Prevention of Gastroduodenal Injury Induced by Chronic Nonsteroidal Anti-inflammatory Drug Therapy," *Gastroenterology*, 1989, 96(2 Pt 2 Suppl):675-81.

Gurwitz JH, Avorn J, Ross-Degnan D, et al, "Nonsteroidal Anti-Inflammatory Drug-Associated Azotemia in the Very Old," *JAMA*, 1990, 264(4):471-5.

Hawkey CJ, Karrasch JA, Szczepański L, et al, "Omeprazole Compared With Misoprostol for Ulcers Associated With Nonsteroidal Anti-inflammatory Drugs," *N Engl J Med*, 1998, 338(11):727-34.

Knodel LC, "Preventing NSAID-induced Ulcers: The Role of Misoprostol," *Consult Pharm*, 1989, 4:37-41.

Pounder R, "Silent Peptic Ulceration: Deadly Silence or Golden Silence?" *Gastroenterology*, 1989, 96(2 Pt 2 Suppl):626-31.

Yeomans ND, Tulassay Z, Juhasz L, et al, "A Comparison of Omeprazole With Ranitidine for Ulcers Associated With Nonsteroidal Anti-inflammatory Drugs," *N Engl J Med*, 1998, 338(11):719-26.

♦ **Meclofenamate Sodium** *see* Meclofenamate *on page 962*
♦ **Meclozine Hydrochloride** *see* Meclizine *on page 961*
♦ **Medicone® Suppositories [OTC]** *see* Phenylephrine *on page 1247*
♦ **Medi-Phenyl [OTC]** *see* Phenylephrine *on page 1247*
♦ **Mediplast® [OTC]** *see* Salicylic Acid *on page 1441*
♦ **Medrol®** *see* MethylPREDNISolone *on page 1017*

MedroxyPROGESTERone (me DROKS ee proe JES te rone)

Medication Safety Issues

Sound-alike/look-alike issues:

MedroxyPROGESTERone may be confused with hydroxyprogesterone, methylPREDNISolone, methylTESTOSTERone

Provera® may be confused with Covera®, Parlodel®, Premarin®

The injection dosage form is available in different formulations. Carefully review prescriptions to assure the correct formulation and route of administration.

U.S. Brand Names Depo-Provera®; Depo-Provera® Contraceptive; depo-subQ provera 104™; Provera®

Canadian Brand Names Alti-MPA; Apo-Medroxy®; Depo-Prevera®; Depo-Provera®; Gen-Medroxy; Novo-Medrone; Provera®; Provera-Pak

Index Terms Acetoxymethylprogesterone; Medroxyprogesterone Acetate; Methylacetoxyprogesterone; MPA

Generic Available Yes

Pharmacologic Category Contraceptive; Progestin

Use Endometrial carcinoma or renal carcinoma; secondary amenorrhea or abnormal uterine bleeding due to hormonal imbalance; reduction of endometrial hyperplasia in nonhysterectomized postmenopausal women receiving conjugated estrogens; management of endometriosis-associated pain

Unlabeled/Investigational Use Treatment of hypoventilation disorders, advanced breast cancer

Contraindications Hypersensitivity to medroxyprogesterone or any component of the formulation; cerebral apoplexy, undiagnosed vaginal bleeding, liver dysfunction; thrombophlebitis

Warnings/Precautions [U.S. Boxed Warning]: Prolonged use of medroxyprogesterone contraceptive injection may result in a loss of bone mineral density (BMD). Loss is related to the duration of use, and may not be completely reversible on discontinuation of the drug. **[U.S. Boxed Warning]: Long-term use (ie, >2 years) should be limited to situations where other birth control methods are inadequate.** Consider other methods of birth control in women with (or at risk for) osteoporosis.

Use caution with cardiovascular disease or dysfunction. MPA used in combination with estrogen may increase the risks of cardiovascular disease, myocardial infarction (MI), stroke, pulmonary emboli (PE), and deep vein thrombosis; incidence of these effects was shown to be significantly increased in postmenopausal women using conjugated equine estrogens (CEE) in combination with MPA. MPA in combination with estrogens should not be used to prevent coronary heart disease.

The risk of dementia may be increased in postmenopausal women; increased incidence was observed in women ≥65 years of age taking MPA in combination with CEE. An increased risk of invasive breast cancer was observed in postmenopausal women using MPA in combination with CEE. An increase in abnormal mammograms has also been reported with estrogen and progestin therapy.

Discontinue pending examination in cases of sudden partial or complete vision loss, sudden onset of proptosis, diplopia, or migraine; discontinue permanently if papilledema or retinal vascular lesions are observed on examination. Use with caution in patients with diseases that may be exacerbated by fluid retention (including asthma, epilepsy, migraine, diabetes, or renal dysfunction). Use caution with history of depression. Whenever possible, progestins in combination with estrogens should be discontinued at least 4-6 weeks prior to surgeries associated with an increased risk of thromboembolism or during periods of prolonged immobilization. Progestins used in combination with estrogen should be used for shortest duration possible consistent with treatment goals. Conduct periodic risk:benefit assessments.

Adverse Reactions (Reflective of adult population; not specific for elderly) Adverse effects as reported with any dosage form; percent ranges presented are noted with the MPA contraceptive injection:

(Continued)

MedroxyPROGESTERone *(Continued)*

>5%:
   Central nervous system: Dizziness, headache, nervousness
   Endocrine & metabolic: Libido decreased, menstrual irregularities (includes bleeding, amenorrhea, or both)
   Gastrointestinal: Abdominal pain/discomfort, weight changes (average 3-5 pounds after 1 year, 8 pounds after 2 years)
   Neuromuscular & skeletal: Weakness

1% to 5%:
   Cardiovascular: Edema
   Central nervous system: Depression, fatigue, insomnia, irritability, pain
   Dermatologic: Acne, alopecia, rash
   Endocrine & metabolic: Anorgasmia, breast pain, hot flashes
   Gastrointestinal: Bloating, nausea
   Genitourinary: Cervical smear abnormal, leukorrhea, menometrorrhagia, menorrhagia, pelvic pain, urinary tract infection, vaginitis, vaginal infection, vaginal hemorrhage
   Local: Injection site atrophy, injection site reaction, injection site pain
   Neuromuscular & skeletal: Arthralgia, backache, leg cramp
   Respiratory: Respiratory tract infections

Overdosage/Toxicology Toxicity is unlikely following single exposures of excessive doses. Supportive treatment is adequate in most cases.

Drug Interactions Substrate of CYP3A4 (major); **Induces** CYP3A4 (weak)
   Acitretin: May diminish the therapeutic effect of progestin contraceptives; contraceptive failure is possible.
   CYP3A4 inducers: CYP3A4 inducers may decrease the levels/effects of medroxyprogesterone. Example inducers include aminoglutethimide, carbamazepine, nafcillin, nevirapine, phenobarbital, phenytoin, and rifamycins.
   Griseofulvin: May diminish the therapeutic effect of progestin contraceptives; contraceptive failure is possible.
   Warfarin: Progestins may diminish the anticoagulant effect of coumarin derivatives. In contrast, enhanced anticoagulant effects have also been noted with some products.

Ethanol/Nutrition/Herb Interactions
   Ethanol: Avoid ethanol (may increase risk of osteoporosis).
   Food: Bioavailability of the oral tablet is increased when taken with food; half-life is unchanged.
   Herb/Nutraceutical: St John's wort may diminish the therapeutic effect of progestin contraceptives (contraceptive failure is possible).

Stability Store at controlled room temperature.

Mechanism of Action Inhibits secretion of pituitary gonadotropins, which prevents follicular maturation and ovulation; causes endometrial thinning

Pharmacokinetics
   Absorption: Oral: Well absorbed; I.M.: Slow
   Protein binding: 86% to 90% primarily to albumin; does not bind to sex hormone-binding globulin
   Metabolism: Extensively hepatic via hydroxylation and conjugation; forms metabolites
   Time to peak: Oral: 2-4 hours
   Half-life elimination: Oral: 12-17 hours; I.M. (Depo-Provera® Contraceptive): 50 days; SubQ: ~40 days
   Excretion: Urine

Dosage
  Geriatrics & Adults:
    Amenorrhea: Oral: 5-10 mg/day for 5-10 days
    Abnormal uterine bleeding: Oral: 5-10 mg for 5-10 days starting on day 16 or 21 of cycle
    Endometriosis: depo-subQ provera 104™: SubQ: 104 mg every 3 months (every 12-14 weeks)
    Endometrial or renal carcinoma (Depo-Provera®): I.M.: 400-1000 mg/week
    Accompanying cyclic estrogen therapy, postmenopausal: Oral: 5-10 mg for 12-14 consecutive days each month, starting on day 1 or day 16 of the cycle; lower doses may be used if given with estrogen continuously throughout the cycle
  Hepatic Impairment: Use is contraindicated with severe impairment. Consider lower dose or less frequent administration with mild-to-moderate impairment. Use of the contraceptive injection has not been studied in patients with hepatic impairment; consideration should be given to not readminister if jaundice develops

Monitoring Parameters Before starting therapy, a physical exam with reference to the breasts and pelvis are recommended, including a Papanicolaou smear. Monitor patient closely for loss of vision, sudden onset of proptosis, diplopia, migraine; signs and symptoms of thromboembolic disorders; signs or symptoms of depression; glucose in diabetics; blood pressure

Test Interactions

The following tests may be decreased: Steroid levels (plasma and urinary), gonado-tropin levels, SHBG concentration, T_3 uptake

The following tests may be increased: Protein-bound iodine, butanol extractable protein-bound iodine, Factors II, VII, VIII, IX, X

Pathologist should be advised of estrogen/progesterone therapy when specimens are submitted.

Patient Information Take this medicine only as directed; do not take more or for a longer period of time. Drug will induce menstrual bleeding in women with an intact uterus. When taken daily with estrogen, spotting will occur for the first 6-12 months of therapy. Take with food if GI upset occurs.

Dosage Forms Excipient information presented when available (limited, particularly for generics); consult specific product labeling.

Injection, suspension, as acetate: 150 mg/mL (1 mL)

Depo-Provera®: 400 mg/mL (2.5 mL)

Depo-Provera® Contraceptive: 150 mg/mL (1 mL) [prefilled syringe or vial]

depo-subQ provera 104™: 104 mg/0.65 mL (0.65 mL) [prefilled syringe]

Tablet, as acetate (Provera®): 2.5 mg, 5 mg, 10 mg

♦ **Medroxyprogesterone Acetate** *see* MedroxyPROGESTERone *on page 965*

♦ **Medroxyprogesterone and Estrogens (Conjugated)** *see* Estrogens (Conjugated/Equine) and Medroxyprogesterone *on page 568*

Mefenamic Acid (me fe NAM ik AS id)

Medication Safety Issues

Sound-alike/look-alike issues:

Ponstel® may be confused with Pronestyl®

U.S. Brand Names Ponstel®

Canadian Brand Names Apo-Mefenamic®; Dom-Mefenamic Acid; Mefenamic-250; Nu-Mefenamic; PMS-Mefenamic Acid; Ponstan®

Generic Available Yes

Pharmacologic Category Nonsteroidal Anti-inflammatory Drug (NSAID), Oral

Use Short-term relief of mild to moderate pain, sunburn, migraine headache (acute)

Restrictions An FDA-approved medication guide must be distributed when dispensing an oral outpatient prescription (new or refill) where this medication is to be used without direct supervision of a healthcare provider. Medication guides are available at http://www.fda.gov/cder/Offices/ODS/medication_guides.htm.

Contraindications Hypersensitivity to mefenamic acid, aspirin, other NSAIDs, or any component of the formulation; perioperative pain in the setting of coronary artery bypass surgery (CABG); active ulceration or chronic inflammation of the GI tract; renal disease

Warnings/Precautions [U.S. Boxed Warning]: NSAIDs are associated with an increased risk of adverse cardiovascular events, including MI, stroke, and new onset or worsening of pre-existing hypertension. Risk may be increased with duration of use or pre-existing cardiovascular risk factors or disease. Carefully evaluate individual cardiovascular risk profiles prior to prescribing. Use caution with fluid retention, CHF or hypertension. Concurrent administration of ibuprofen, and potentially other nonselective NSAIDs, may interfere with aspirin's cardioprotective effect.

Use of NSAIDs can compromise existing renal function. Renal toxicity can occur in patient with impaired renal function, dehydration, heart failure, liver dysfunction, those taking diuretics and ACEI and the elderly. Rehydrate patient before starting therapy. Monitor renal function closely. Mefenamic acid is not recommended for patients with advanced renal disease.

[U.S. Boxed Warning]: NSAIDs may increase risk of gastrointestinal irritation, ulceration, bleeding, and perforation. These events may occur at any time during therapy and without warning. Use caution with a history of GI disease (bleeding or ulcers), concurrent therapy with aspirin, anticoagulants and/or corticosteroids, smoking, use of alcohol, the elderly or debilitated patients.

Use the lowest effective dose for the shortest duration of time, consistent with individual patient goals, to reduce risk of cardiovascular or GI adverse events. Alternate therapies should be considered for patients at high risk.

NSAIDs may cause serious skin adverse events including exfoliative dermatitis, Stevens-Johnson syndrome (SJS) and toxic epidermal necrolysis (TEN). Anaphylac-toid reactions may occur, even without prior exposure; patients with "aspirin triad" (bronchial asthma, aspirin intolerance, rhinitis) may be at increased risk. Do not use in patients who experience bronchospasm, asthma, rhinitis, or urticaria with NSAID or aspirin therapy.

(Continued)

Mefenamic Acid *(Continued)*

Use with caution in patients with decreased hepatic function. Closely monitor patients with any abnormal LFT. Severe hepatic reactions (eg, fulminant hepatitis, liver failure) have occurred with NSAID use, rarely; discontinue if signs or symptoms of liver disease develop, or if systemic manifestations occur.

The elderly are at increased risk for adverse effects (especially peptic ulceration, CNS effects, renal toxicity) from NSAIDs even at low doses.

Withhold for at least 4-6 half-lives prior to surgical or dental procedures.

Adverse Reactions (Reflective of adult population; not specific for elderly)
1% to 10%:
Central nervous system: Headache, nervousness, dizziness (3% to 9%)
Dermatologic: Itching, rash
Endocrine & metabolic: Fluid retention
Gastrointestinal: Abdominal cramps, heartburn, indigestion, nausea (1% to 10%), vomiting (1% to 10%), diarrhea (1% to 10%), constipation (1% to 10%), abdominal distress/cramping/pain (1% to 10%), dyspepsia (1% to 10%), flatulence (1% to 10%), gastric or duodenal ulcer with bleeding or perforation (1% to 10%), gastritis (1% to 10%)
Hematologic: Bleeding (1% to 10%)
Hepatic: Elevated LFTs (1% to 10%)
Otic: Tinnitus (1% to 10%)

Overdosage/Toxicology Symptoms include CNS stimulation, agitation, and seizures. Management of nonsteroidal anti-inflammatory drug (NSAID) intoxication is primarily supportive and symptomatic. Fluid therapy is commonly effective in managing hypotension that may occur following an acute NSAID overdose, except when due to acute blood loss. Seizures tend to be very short-lived and often do not require drug treatment, although recurrent seizures should be treated with I.V. diazepam. Since many of the NSAIDs undergo enterohepatic cycling, multiple doses of charcoal may be needed to reduce the potential for delayed toxicities.

Drug Interactions Substrate of CYP2C9 (minor); **Inhibits** CYP2C9 (strong)
ACE inhibitors: Antihypertensive effects may be decreased by concurrent therapy with NSAIDs; monitor blood pressure.
Angiotensin II antagonists: Antihypertensive effects may be decreased by concurrent therapy with NSAIDs; monitor blood pressure.
Anticoagulants (warfarin, heparin, LMWHs) in combination with NSAIDs can cause increased risk of bleeding.
Antiplatelet drugs (ticlopidine, clopidogrel, aspirin, abciximab, dipyridamole, eptifibatide, tirofiban) can cause an increased risk of bleeding.
Beta-blockers: NSAIDs may decrease the antihypertensive effect of beta-blockers. Monitor.
Cholestyramine (and other bile acid sequestrants): May decrease the absorption of NSAIDs. Separate by at least 2 hours.
Corticosteroids may increase the risk of GI ulceration; avoid concurrent use.
Cyclosporine: NSAIDs may increase serum creatinine, potassium, blood pressure, and cyclosporine levels; monitor cyclosporine levels and renal function carefully.
CYP2C9 Substrates: Mefenamic acid may increase the levels/effects of CYP2C9 substrates. Example substrates include bosentan, dapsone, fluoxetine, glimepiride, glipizide, losartan, montelukast, nateglinide, paclitaxel, phenytoin, warfarin, and zafirlukast.
Fluoroquinolone antibiotics: Risk of seizures may be increased with concomitant quinolone use. Risk is considered quite low and may only be a factor with high serum levels of either agent and/or in patients with additional predisposing factors (eg, renal dysfunction, history of seizure or other neurological disorder).
Gentamicin and amikacin serum concentrations are increased by indomethacin in premature infants. Results may apply to other aminoglycosides and NSAIDs.
Hydralazine's antihypertensive effect is decreased; avoid concurrent use.
Lithium levels can be increased; avoid concurrent use if possible or monitor lithium levels and adjust dose. Sulindac may have the least effect. When NSAID is stopped, lithium will need adjustment again.
Loop diuretics efficacy (diuretic and antihypertensive effect) is reduced. Indomethacin reduces this efficacy, however, it may be anticipated with any NSAID.
Methotrexate: Severe bone marrow suppression, aplastic anemia, and GI toxicity have been reported with concomitant NSAID therapy. Avoid use during moderate or high-dose methotrexate (increased and prolonged methotrexate levels). NSAID use during low-dose treatment of rheumatoid arthritis has not been fully evaluated; extreme caution is warranted.
Salicylates: NSAIDs (nonselective) may diminish the cardioprotective effect of acetylated salicylates. Avoid regular use of NSAIDs if possible; consider alternatives (eg, acetaminophen). Give salicylate before NSAID; for example ibuprofen should be given 30-120 minutes after aspirin (immediate release).

Thiazides antihypertensive effects are decreased; avoid concurrent use.

Verapamil plasma concentration is decreased by diclofenac; avoid concurrent use.

Warfarin's INRs may be increased by piroxicam. Other NSAIDs may have the same effect depending on dose and duration. Monitor INR closely. Use the lowest dose of NSAIDs possible and for the briefest duration.

Ethanol/Nutrition/Herb Interactions

Ethanol: Avoid ethanol (may enhance gastric mucosal irritation).

Herb/Nutraceutical: Avoid alfalfa, anise, bilberry, bladderwrack, bromelain, cat's claw, celery, coleus, cordyceps, dong quai, evening primrose, feverfew, fenugreek, garlic, ginger, ginkgo biloba, red clover, horse chestnut, grapeseed, green tea, ginseng, guggul, horse chestnut seed, horseradish, licorice, prickly ash, red clover, reishi, SAMe, sweet clover, turmeric, white willow (all have additional antiplatelet activity).

Mechanism of Action Inhibits prostaglandin synthesis by decreasing the activity of the enzyme, cyclooxygenase, which results in decreased formation of prostaglandin precursors

Pharmacodynamics

Peak effect: Oral: Within 2-4 hours

Duration: Up to 6 hours

Pharmacokinetics

Protein binding: High (>90%)

Metabolism: Conjugated in the liver

Half-life: 3.5 hours

Elimination: In urine (50%) and feces as unchanged drug and metabolites

Dosage

Geriatrics & Adults: Mild-moderate pain: Oral: Initial: 500 mg; then 250 mg every 4 hours as needed; maximum therapy: 1 week

Renal Impairment: Not recommended for use

Monitoring Parameters Monitor for pain relief, gastric adverse effects, bleeding, confusion; renal function

Test Interactions Increased chloride (S), increased sodium (S), positive Coombs' [direct], false-positive urinary bilirubin

Patient Information Serious gastrointestinal bleeding can occur as well as ulceration and perforation. Pain may or may not be present. Avoid aspirin and aspirin-containing products while taking this medication. If gastric upset occurs, take with food, milk, or antacid. If gastric adverse effects persist, contact physician. May cause drowsiness, dizziness, blurred vision, and confusion. Use caution when performing tasks which require alertness (eg, driving). Do not take for more than 3 days for fever or 10 days for pain without physician advice.

Additional Information There are no clinical guidelines to predict which NSAID will give response in a particular patient. Trials with each must be initiated until response determined. If diarrhea develops, reduce dose or discontinue use of mefenamic acid for a short time (until diarrhea stops). Some patients may be unable to tolerate further use. Consider dose, patient convenience, and cost.

Special Geriatric Considerations Elderly are a high-risk population for adverse effects from NSAIDs. As much as 60% of elderly can develop peptic ulceration and/or hemorrhage asymptomatically. The concomitant use of H_2 blockers, omeprazole, and sucralfate is not effective as prophylaxis with the exception of NSAID-induced duodenal ulcers which may be prevented by the use of ranitidine. Misoprostol and proton pump inhibitors are the only agents proven to help prevent the development of NSAID-induced ulcers. Also, concomitant disease and drug use contribute to the risk for GI adverse effects. Use lowest effective dose for shortest period possible. Consider renal function decline with age. Use of NSAIDs can compromise existing renal function especially when Cl_{cr} is ≤30 mL/minute. Tinnitus may be a difficult and unreliable indication of toxicity due to age-related hearing loss or eighth cranial nerve damage. CNS adverse effects such as confusion, agitation, and hallucination are generally seen in overdose or high-dose situations, but elderly may demonstrate these adverse effects at lower doses than younger adults.

Dosage Forms Excipient information presented when available (limited, particularly for generics); consult specific product labeling.

Capsule: 250 mg

Ponstel®: 250 mg

Selected References

Brooks PM and Day RO, "Nonsteroidal Anti-inflammatory Drugs - Differences and Similarities," *N Engl J Med*, 1991, 324(24):1716-25.

Clinch D, Banerjee AK, and Ostick G, "Absence of Abdominal Pain in Elderly Patients With Peptic Ulcer," *Age Ageing*, 1984, 13(2):120-3.

Clive DM and Stoff JS, "Renal Syndromes Associated With Nonsteroidal Anti-inflammatory Drugs," *N Engl J Med*, 1984, 310(9):563-72.

Graham DY, "Prevention of Gastroduodenal Injury Induced by Chronic Nonsteroidal Anti-inflammatory Drug Therapy," *Gastroenterology*, 1989, 96(2 Pt 2 Suppl):675-81.

Gurwitz JH, Avorn J, Ross-Degnan D, et al, "Nonsteroidal Anti-Inflammatory Drug-Associated Azotemia in the Very Old," *JAMA*, 1990, 264(4):471-5.

(Continued)

Mefenamic Acid (Continued)

Hawkey CJ, Karrasch JA, Szczepański L, et al, "Omeprazole Compared With Misoprostol for Ulcers Associated With Nonsteroidal Anti-inflammatory Drugs," *N Engl J Med*, 1998, 338(11):727-34.

Knodel LC, "Preventing NSAID-induced Ulcers: The Role of Misoprostol," *Consult Pharm*, 1989, 4:37-41.

Pounder R, "Silent Peptic Ulceration: Deadly Silence or Golden Silence?" *Gastroenterology*, 1989, 96(2 Pt 2 Suppl):626-31.

Yeomans ND, Tulassay Z, Juhasz L, et al, "A Comparison of Omeprazole With Ranitidine for Ulcers Associated With Nonsteroidal Anti-inflammatory Drugs," *N Engl J Med*, 1998, 338(11):719-26.

♦ **Mefoxin**® see Cefoxitin on page 263
♦ **Megace**® see Megestrol on page 970
♦ **Megace**® **ES** see Megestrol on page 970
♦ **Megadophilus**® **[OTC]** see Lactobacillus on page 867

Megestrol (me JES trole)

Medication Safety Issues
Sound-alike/look-alike issues:
Megace® may be confused with Reglan®

U.S. Brand Names Megace®; Megace® ES
Canadian Brand Names Apo-Megestrol®; Megace®; Megace® OS; Nu-Megestrol
Index Terms 5071-1DL(6); Megestrol Acetate; NSC-71423
Generic Available Yes
Pharmacologic Category Antineoplastic Agent, Hormone; Appetite Stimulant; Progestin
Use Palliative treatment of breast and endometrial carcinoma; treatment of anorexia, cachexia, or unexplained significant weight loss in patients with AIDS
Unlabeled/Investigational Use Treatment of uterine bleeding
Contraindications Hypersensitivity to megestrol or any component of the formulation
Warnings/Precautions Hazardous agent - use appropriate precautions for handling and disposal. May suppress hypothalamic-pituitary-adrenal (HPA) axis during chronic administration; consider the possibility of adrenal suppression in any patient receiving or being withdrawn from chronic therapy when signs/symptoms suggestive of hypoadrenalism are noted (during stress or in unstressed state). Laboratory evaluation and replacement/stress doses of rapid-acting glucocorticoid should be considered. New-onset diabetes and exacerbation of pre-existing diabetes have been reported with long-term use. Use with caution in patients with a history of thromboembolic disease. Vaginal bleeding or discharge may occur in elderly females. Megace® ES suspension is not equivalent to other formulations on a mg per mg basis; Megace® ES suspension 625 mg/5 mL is equivalent to megestrol acetate suspension 800 mg/20 mL.

Adverse Reactions (Reflective of adult population; not specific for elderly)
Frequency not always defined.

Cardiovascular: Hypertension (≤8%), cardiomyopathy (1% to 3%), chest pain (1% to 3%), edema (1% to 3%), palpitation (1% to 3%), peripheral edema (1% to 3%), heart failure

Central nervous system: Headache (≤10%), insomnia (≤6%), fever (1% to 6%), pain (≤6%, similar to placebo), abnormal thinking (1% to 3%), confusion (1% to 3%), seizure (1% to 3%), depression (1% to 3%), hypoesthesia (1% to 3%), mood changes, malaise, lethargy

Dermatologic: Rash (2% to 12%), alopecia (1% to 3%), pruritus (1% to 3%), vesiculobullous rash (1% to 3%)

Endocrine & metabolic: Breakthrough bleeding and amenorrhea, spotting, changes in menstrual flow, changes in cervical erosion and secretions, increased breast tenderness, changes in vaginal bleeding pattern, hyperglycemia (≤6%), gynecomastia (1% to 3%), diabetes, HPA axis suppression, adrenal insufficiency, Cushing's syndrome, hypercalcemia, hot flashes

Gastrointestinal: Weight gain (not attributed to edema or fluid retention), diarrhea (6% to 15%, similar to placebo), flatulence (≤10%), vomiting (≤6%), nausea (≤5%), dyspepsia (≤4%), abdominal pain (1% to 3%), constipation (1% to 3%), salivation increased (1% to 3%), xerostomia (1% to 3%)

Genitourinary: Impotence (4% to 14%), decreased libido (≤5%), urinary incontinence (1% to 3%), urinary tract infection (1% to 3%), urinary frequency (≤2%)

Hematologic: Anemia (≤5%), leukopenia (1% to 3%)

Hepatic: Hepatomegaly (1% to 3%), LDH increased (1% to 3%), cholestatic jaundice, hepatotoxicity

Neuromuscular & skeletal: Carpal tunnel syndrome, weakness (2% to 8%), neuropathy (1% to 3%), paresthesia (1% to 3%)

Ocular: Amblyopia (1% to 3%)

Renal: Albuminuria (1% to 3%)

Respiratory: Dyspnea (1% to 3%), cough (1% to 3%), pharyngitis (1% to 3%), pneumonia (≤2%), hyperpnea

Miscellaneous: Diaphoresis (1% to 3%), herpes infection (1% to 3%), infection (1% to 3%), tumor flare

Overdosage/Toxicology Toxicity is unlikely following single exposures of excessive doses. Although not tested for dialyzability, dialysis would not likely be effective in treating an overdose.

Drug Interactions
Aminoglutethimide: May increase the metabolism, via CYP isoenzymes, of megestrol.
Cyclosporine: Megestrol may enhance the hepatotoxic effect of cyclosporine; megestrol may increase the serum concentration of cyclosporine.

Ethanol/Nutrition/Herb Interactions Herb/Nutraceutical: Avoid herbs with progestogenic properties (eg, bloodroot, chasteberry, damiana, oregano, and yucca); may enhance the adverse/toxic effect of megestrol.

Stability Store at 15°C to 30°C (59°F to 86°F).

Mechanism of Action A synthetic progestin with antiestrogenic properties which disrupt the estrogen receptor cycle. Megestrol interferes with the normal estrogen cycle and results in a lower LH titer. May also have a direct effect on the endometrium. Megestrol is an antineoplastic progestin thought to act through an antileutenizing effect mediated via the pituitary. May stimulate appetite by antagonizing the metabolic effects of catabolic cytokines.

Pharmacokinetics
Absorption: Well absorbed orally
Metabolism: Hepatic (to free steroids and glucuronide conjugates)
Time to peak, serum: 1-3 hours
Half-life elimination: 13-105 hours
Excretion: Urine (57% to 78%; 5% to 8% as metabolites); feces (8% to 30%)

Dosage
Geriatrics & Adults: Note: Megace® ES suspension is not equivalent to other formulations on a mg-per-mg basis.
Breast carcinoma (female): Refer to individual protocols: Oral: Tablet: 40 mg 4 times/day
Endometrial carcinoma: Refer to individual protocols: Oral: Tablet: 40-320 mg/day in divided doses; use for 2 months to determine efficacy; maximum doses used have been up to 800 mg/day.
HIV-related cachexia (male/female): Oral: Suspension:
Megace®: Initial dose: 800 mg/day; daily doses of 400 and 800 mg/day were found to be clinically effective
Megace® ES: 625 mg/day
Renal Impairment: No data available; however, the urinary excretion of megestrol acetate administered in doses of 4-90 mg ranged from 56% to 78% within 10 days.

Administration Megestrol acetate (Megace®) oral suspension is compatible with water, orange juice, apple juice, or Sustacal H.C. for immediate consumption.

Monitoring Parameters Observe for signs of thromboembolic phenomena; blood pressure, weight; serum glucose

Test Interactions Altered thyroid and liver function tests

Patient Information Report any calf pain, difficulty breathing, or vaginal bleeding to physician; may cause abdominal pain, headache, nausea, vomiting, breast tenderness; notify physician if these persist

Special Geriatric Considerations Elderly females may have vaginal bleeding or discharge and need to be forewarned of this side effect and inconvenience. No specific changes in dose are required for the elderly. Megestrol has been used in the treatment of the failure to thrive syndrome in cachectic elderly in addition to proper nutrition. Data does not support the use of megestrol for weight gain. The increase in weight tends to be mostly fat instead of lean body mass. Also, this agent is associated with DVTs.

Dosage Forms Excipient information presented when available (limited, particularly for generics); consult specific product labeling.
Suspension, oral, as acetate: 40 mg/mL (10 mL, 20 mL, 240 mL, 480 mL)
Megace®: 40 mg/mL (240 mL) [contains alcohol 0.06% and sodium benzoate; lemon-lime flavor]
Megace® ES: 125 mg/mL (150 mL) [contains alcohol 0.06% and sodium benzoate; lemon-lime flavor]
Tablet, as acetate: 20 mg, 40 mg

Selected References
Farrar DJ, "Megestrol Acetate: Promises and Pitfalls," *AIDS Patient Care STDS,* 1999, 13(3):149-52.

♦ **Megestrol Acetate** *see* Megestrol *on page 970*

Meloxicam (mel OKS i kam)

U.S. Brand Names Mobic®
Canadian Brand Names Apo-Meloxicam®; CO Meloxicam; Gen-Meloxicam; Mobic®; Mobicox®; Novo-Meloxicam; PMS-Meloxicam
(Continued)

Meloxicam *(Continued)*

Generic Available Yes

Pharmacologic Category Nonsteroidal Anti-inflammatory Drug (NSAID), Oral

Use Relief of signs and symptoms of osteoarthritis, rheumatoid arthritis, and juvenile rheumatoid arthritis (JRA)

Restrictions An FDA-approved medication guide must be distributed when dispensing an oral outpatient prescription (new or refill) where this medication is to be used without direct supervision of a healthcare provider. Medication guides are available at http://www.fda.gov/cder/Offices/ODS/medication_guides.htm.

Contraindications Hypersensitivity to meloxicam, aspirin, other NSAIDs, or any component of the formulation; perioperative pain in the setting of coronary artery bypass surgery (CABG)

Warnings/Precautions [U.S. Boxed Warning]: NSAIDs are associated with an increased risk of adverse cardiovascular events, including MI, stroke, and new onset or worsening of pre-existing hypertension. Risk may be increased with duration of use or pre-existing cardiovascular risk factors or disease. Carefully evaluate individual cardiovascular risk profiles prior to prescribing. Use caution with fluid retention, CHF or hypertension. Concurrent administration of ibuprofen, and potentially other nonselective NSAIDs, may interfere with aspirin's cardioprotective effect.

Use of NSAIDs can compromise existing renal function. Renal toxicity can occur in patient with impaired renal function, dehydration, heart failure, liver dysfunction, those taking diuretics, angiotensin antagonists, ACEIs, and the elderly. Rehydrate patient before starting therapy. Monitor renal function closely. Meloxicam is not recommended for patients with advanced renal disease

[U.S. Boxed Warning]: NSAIDs may increase risk of gastrointestinal irritation, ulceration, bleeding, and perforation. These events may occur at any time during therapy and without warning. Use caution with a history of GI disease (bleeding or ulcers), concurrent therapy with aspirin, anticoagulants and/or corticosteroids, smoking, use of alcohol, the elderly or debilitated patients.

Use the lowest effective dose for the shortest duration of time, consistent with individual patient goals, to reduce risk of cardiovascular or GI adverse events. Alternate therapies should be considered for patients at high risk.

NSAIDs may cause serious skin adverse events including exfoliative dermatitis, Stevens-Johnson syndrome (SJS) and toxic epidermal necrolysis (TEN). Anaphylactoid reactions may occur, even without prior exposure; patients with "aspirin triad" (bronchial asthma, aspirin intolerance, rhinitis) may be at increased risk. Do not use in patients who experience bronchospasm, asthma, rhinitis, or urticaria with NSAID or aspirin therapy. Use caution in other forms of asthma.

Use with caution in patients with decreased hepatic function. Closely monitor patients with any abnormal LFT. Severe hepatic reactions (eg, fulminant hepatitis, liver failure) have occurred with NSAID use, rarely; discontinue if signs or symptoms of liver disease develop, or if systemic manifestations occur.

The elderly are at increased risk for adverse effects (especially peptic ulceration, CNS effects, renal toxicity) from NSAIDs even at low doses.

Withhold for at least 4-6 half-lives prior to surgical or dental procedures.

Adverse Reactions (Reflective of adult population; not specific for elderly)
Percentages reported in adult patients; abdominal pain, diarrhea, headache, pyrexia, and vomiting were reported more commonly in pediatric patients

2% to 10%:

    Cardiovascular: Edema (<1% to 4%)

    Central nervous system: Headache (2% to 8%), dizziness (<1% to 4%), insomnia (<1% to 4%)

    Dermatologic: Pruritus (<1% to 2%), rash (<1% to 3%)

    Gastrointestinal: Diarrhea (3% to 8%), dyspepsia (4% to 9%), abdominal pain (2% to 5%), nausea (2% to 7%), constipation (<1% to 3%), flatulence (<1% to 3%), vomiting (<1% to 3%)

    Hematologic: Anemia (<1% to 4%)

    Neuromuscular & skeletal: Arthralgia (<1% to 5%), back pain (<1% to 3%)

    Respiratory: Cough (<1% to 2%), pharyngitis (<1% to 3%), upper respiratory infection (2% to 8%)

    Miscellaneous: Flu-like syndrome (2% to 6%), falls (3%)

Overdosage/Toxicology Symptoms include lethargy, drowsiness, nausea, vomiting, and epigastric pain. Rarely, severe symptoms have been associated with NSAID overdose including apnea, metabolic acidosis, coma, nystagmus, seizures, leukocytosis, and renal failure. Management of nonsteroidal anti-inflammatory (NSAID) intoxication is supportive and symptomatic. Since meloxicam undergoes enterohepatic cycling, multiple doses of charcoal may be needed to reduce the potential for delayed toxicities. Cholestyramine has been shown to increase meloxicam clearance. Meloxicam is not dialyzable,

Drug Interactions Substrate (minor) of CYP2C9, 3A4; **Inhibits** CYP2C9 (weak)

ACE inhibitors: Antihypertensive effects may be decreased by concurrent therapy with NSAIDs; renal adverse effects of NSAIDs may be increased; monitor blood pressure

Angiotensin II antagonists: Antihypertensive effects may be decreased by concurrent therapy with NSAIDs; renal adverse effects of NSAIDs may be increased; monitor blood pressure

Anticoagulants (warfarin, heparin, LMWHs) in combination with NSAIDs can cause increased risk of bleeding.

Antiplatelet drugs (ticlopidine, clopidogrel, aspirin, abciximab, dipyridamole, eptifibatide, tirofiban) can cause an increased risk of bleeding.

Aspirin increases serum concentrations (AUC) of meloxicam (in addition to potential for additive adverse effects); concurrent use is not recommended.

Beta-blockers: NSAIDs may decrease the antihypertensive effect of beta-blockers. Monitor.

Cholestyramine (and other bile acid sequestrants): May decrease the absorption of NSAIDs. Separate by at least 2 hours.

Corticosteroids may increase the risk of GI ulceration; avoid concurrent use.

Cyclosporine: NSAIDs may increase serum creatinine, potassium, blood pressure, and cyclosporine levels; monitor cyclosporine levels and renal function carefully.

Fluoroquinolone antibiotics: Risk of seizures may be increased with concomitant quinolone use. Risk is considered quite low and may only be a factor with high serum levels of either agent and/or in patients with additional predisposing factors (eg, renal dysfunction, history of seizure or other neurological disorder).

Hydralazine's antihypertensive effect is decreased; avoid concurrent use.

Lithium levels can be increased; avoid concurrent use if possible or monitor lithium levels and adjust dose. When NSAID is stopped, lithium will need adjustment again.

Loop diuretic's efficacy (diuretic and antihypertensive effect) may be reduced by NSAIDs.

Methotrexate: Severe bone marrow suppression, aplastic anemia, and GI toxicity have been reported with concomitant NSAID therapy. Avoid use during moderate or high-dose methotrexate (increased and prolonged methotrexate levels). NSAID use during low-dose treatment of rheumatoid arthritis has not been fully evaluated; extreme caution is warranted.

Salicylates: NSAIDs (nonselective) may diminish the cardioprotective effect of acetylated salicylates. Avoid regular use of NSAIDs if possible; consider alternatives (eg, acetaminophen). Give salicylate before NSAID; for example ibuprofen should be given 30-120 minutes after aspirin (immediate release).

Thiazide diuretics: Antihypertensive effects of thiazide diuretics are decreased; avoid concurrent use.

Warfarin INRs may be increased by meloxicam. Monitor INR closely, particularly during initiation or change in dose. May increase risk of bleeding. Use lowest possible dose for shortest duration possible.

Ethanol/Nutrition/Herb Interactions

Ethanol: Avoid ethanol (may enhance gastric mucosal irritation).

Herb/Nutraceutical: Avoid alfalfa, anise, bilberry, bladderwrack, bromelain, cat's claw, celery, coleus, cordyceps, dong quai, evening primrose, feverfew, fenugreek, garlic, ginger, ginkgo biloba, red clover, horse chestnut, grapeseed, green tea, ginseng, guggul, horse chestnut seed, horseradish, licorice, prickly ash, red clover, reishi, SAMe, sweet clover, turmeric, white willow (all have additional antiplatelet activity).

Stability Store at 25°C (77°F).

Mechanism of Action Inhibits prostaglandin synthesis by decreasing the activity of the enzyme, cyclooxygenase, which results in decreased formation of prostaglandin precursors

Pharmacokinetics

Distribution: 10 L

Protein binding: 99.4%

Metabolism: Hepatic via CYP2C9 and CYP3A4 (minor); forms 4 metabolites (inactive)

Bioavailability: 89%

Half-life: Adults: 15-20 hours

Time to peak: Initial: 5-10 hours; Secondary: 12-14 hours

Elimination: As inactive metabolites, in urine and feces (bile or enteral secretion)

Dosage

Geriatrics & Adults: Osteoarthritis, rheumatoid arthritis: Oral: Initial: 7.5 mg once daily; some patients may receive additional benefit from an increased dose of 15 mg once daily.

Renal Impairment:

Mild to moderate impairment: No specific dosage recommendations

Significant impairment (Cl_{cr} ≤15 mL/minute): Avoid use

Hemodialysis: Supplemental dose after dialysis not necessary.

(Continued)

Meloxicam *(Continued)*

Hepatic Impairment:

Mild (Child-Pugh class A) to moderate (Child-Pugh class B) hepatic dysfunction: No dosage adjustment is necessary

Severe hepatic impairment: Patients with severe hepatic impairment have not been adequately studied

Monitoring Parameters CBC, periodic liver function, renal function (serum BUN, and creatinine)

Patient Information If self-administered, use exactly as directed (do not increase dose or frequency); adverse reactions can occur with overuse. Take with food or milk to reduce GI upset. While using this medication, do not use alcohol, excessive amounts of vitamin C, or salicylate-containing foods (curry powder, prunes, raisins, tea, or licorice), other prescription or OTC medications containing aspirin or salicylate, or other NSAIDs without consulting prescriber. Maintain adequate hydration (2-3 L/day of fluids unless instructed to restrict fluid intake). You may experience nausea, vomiting, gastric discomfort (frequent mouth care, small frequent meals, chewing gum, sucking lozenges may help). GI bleeding, ulceration, or perforation can occur with or without pain. Stop taking medication and report ringing in ears; persistent cramping or pain in stomach; unresolved nausea or vomiting; difficulty breathing or shortness of breath; unusual bruising or bleeding (mouth, urine, stool); skin rash; unusual swelling of extremities; chest pain; or palpitations.

Special Geriatric Considerations Men ≥65 years of age exhibited steady-state plasma concentrations and pharmacokinetics similar to younger men. Elderly women (≥65 years of age) had nearly a 50% greater AUC and 32% higher C_{max} compared to younger women.

Dosage Forms Excipient information presented when available (limited, particularly for generics); consult specific product labeling.

Suspension: 7.5 mg/5 mL (100 mL)

Mobic®: 7.5 mg/5 mL (100 mL) [contains sodium benzoate; raspberry flavor]

Tablet: 7.5 mg, 15 mg

Mobic®: 7.5 mg, 15 mg

Selected References

MOBIC® [package insert], Final Draft Labeling, April 17, 2000.

Melphalan *(MEL fa lan)*

Medication Safety Issues

Sound-alike/look-alike issues:

Melphalan may be confused with Mephyton®, Myleran®

Alkeran® may be confused with Alferon®, Leukeran®

High alert medication: The Institute for Safe Medication Practices (ISMP) includes this medication among its list of drugs which have a heightened risk of causing significant patient harm when used in error.

U.S. Brand Names Alkeran®

Canadian Brand Names Alkeran®

Index Terms L-PAM; L-Sarcolysin; NSC-8806; Phenylalanine Mustard

Generic Available No

Pharmacologic Category Antineoplastic Agent, Alkylating Agent

Use Palliative treatment of multiple myeloma and nonresectable epithelial ovarian carcinoma

Unlabeled/Investigational Use Treatment of neuroblastoma, rhabdomyosarcoma, breast cancer; part of an induction regimen for marrow and stem cell transplantation

Contraindications Hypersensitivity to melphalan or any component of the formulation; severe bone marrow suppression; patients whose disease was resistant to prior therapy

Warnings/Precautions Hazardous agent - use appropriate precautions for handling and disposal. **[U.S. Boxed Warning]: Is potentially mutagenic, leukemogenic and carcinogenic.** Suppresses ovarian function and produces amenorrhea; may also cause testicular suppression. **[U.S. Boxed Warning]: Bone marrow suppression is common.** Use with caution in patients with prior bone marrow suppression, impaired renal function (consider dose reduction), or who have received prior chemotherapy or irradiation. Toxicity to immunosuppressives is increased in elderly; start with lowest recommended adult doses. Signs of infection, such as fever and WBC rise, may not occur. Lethargy and confusion may be more prominent signs of infection. **[U.S. Boxed Warning]: Hypersensitivity has been reported with I.V. administration** and oral melphalan; may occur after multiple treatment cycles. **[U.S. Boxed Warning]: Should be administered under the supervision of an experienced cancer chemotherapy physician.**

Adverse Reactions (Reflective of adult population; not specific for elderly)
>10%:

Gastrointestinal: Vomiting (oral low-dose: <10%; I.V.: 30% to 90%)

Hematologic: Myelosuppression, leukopenia (onset 7 days; nadir 14-35 days; recovery 28-56 days), thrombocytopenia (onset 7 days; nadir 14-35 days; recovery 28-56 days)

Miscellaneous: Secondary malignancy (<2% to 20%; cumulative dose and duration dependent)

1% to 10%: Miscellaneous: Hypersensitivity (I.V.: 2%)

Overdosage/Toxicology
Symptoms of overdose include hypocalcemia, hyponatremia, pulmonary fibrosis, severe nausea and vomiting, diarrhea, GI hemorrhage, mucositis, stomatitis, and bone marrow suppression (including pancytopenia). Deaths have been reported with I.V. overdoses. Monitor hematologic parameters closely for 3-6 weeks; consider growth factor support, transfusions, and antibiotics. Treatment is otherwise symptom-directed and supportive. Not removed by hemodialysis.

Drug Interactions
Cisplatin: May decrease I.V. melphalan clearance by altering renal function.

Cyclosporine: Risk of nephrotoxicity is increased by melphalan.

Digitalis glycosides: Melphalan may decrease plasma levels of digoxin.

Nalidixic acid: Concomitant use of I.V. melphalan with nalidixic acid may increase risk of necrotic enterocolitis (reported with pediatric patients).

Vaccine (live organism): Melphalan may increase the risk of vaccinal infection.

Ethanol/Nutrition/Herb Interactions
Ethanol: Avoid ethanol (due to GI irritation).

Food: Food interferes with oral absorption.

Stability
Tablet: Store in refrigerator at 2°C to 8°C (36°F to 46°F). Protect from light.

Injection: Store at room temperature (15°C to 30°C). Protect from light. Must be prepared fresh. **The time between reconstitution/dilution and administration of parenteral melphalan must be kept to a minimum (manufacturer recommends <60 minutes) because reconstituted and diluted solutions are unstable.** Dissolve powder initially with 10 mL of diluent to a concentration of 5 mg/mL. Shake vigorously to dissolve. This solution is chemically and physically stable for at least 90 minutes when stored at 25°C (77°F). **Immediately** dilute dose in 250-500 mL NS to a concentration of 0.1-0.45 mg/mL. This solution is physically and chemically stable for at least 60 minutes at 25°C (77°F). Do not refrigerate solution; precipitation occurs.

Mechanism of Action
Alkylating agent which is a derivative of mechlorethamine that inhibits DNA and RNA synthesis via formation of carbonium ions; cross-links strands of DNA; acts on both resting and rapidly dividing tumor cells.

Pharmacokinetics
Absorption: Oral: Variable and incomplete

Distribution: V_d: 0.5-0.6 L/kg throughout total body water

Protein binding: 60% to 90%; primarily to albumin, 20% to α_1-acid glycoprotein

Metabolism: Hepatic; chemical hydrolysis to monohydroxymelphalan and dihydroxymelphalan

Bioavailability: Unpredictable; 61% ± 26%, decreasing with repeated doses

Half-life elimination: Terminal: I.V.: 1.5 hours; oral: 1-1.25 hours

Time to peak, serum: ~1-2 hours

Excretion: Oral: Feces (20% to 50%); urine (10% to 30% as unchanged drug)

Dosage
Geriatrics & Adults: Refer to individual protocols; oral dose should always be adjusted to patient response and weekly blood counts.

Multiple myeloma:

Oral: Multiple regimens have been employed: **Note:** Response is gradual; may require repeated courses to realize benefit:

6 mg daily for 2-3 weeks initially, followed by up to 4 weeks rest, then a maintenance dose of 2 mg daily as hematologic recovery begins **or**

10 mg daily for 7-10 days; institute 2 mg daily maintenance dose after WBC >4000 cells/mcL and platelets >100,000 cells/mcL (~4-8 weeks); titrate maintenance dose to hematologic response **or**

0.15 mg/kg/day for 7 days, with a 2-6 week rest, followed by a maintenance dose of ≤0.05 mg/kg/day as hematologic recovery begins **or**

0.25 mg/kg/day for 4 days (or 0.2 mg/kg/day for 5 days); repeat at 4- to 6-week intervals as ANC and platelet counts return to normal

I.V.: 16 mg/m² administered at 2-week intervals for 4 doses, then administer at 4-week intervals after adequate hematologic recovery.

Ovarian carcinoma: Oral: 0.2 mg/kg/day for 5 days, repeat every 4-5 weeks

High dose BMT: I.V.: 140-240 mg/m² as a single dose or divided into 2-5 daily doses. Infuse over 20-60 minutes.

(Continued)

Melphalan (Continued)

Renal Impairment:

The manufacturer recommends the following adjustments for renal impairment based on route of administration:

Oral: Moderate-to-severe renal impairment: Consider a reduced dose initially

I.V.: BUN >30 mg/dL: Reduce dose by up to 50%

The following guidelines are also used by some clinicians:

Aronoff, 1999 (route of administration not specified):

Cl_{cr} 10-50 mL/minute: Administer at 75% of normal dose

Cl_{cr} <10 mL/minute: Administer at 50% of normal dose

Hemodialysis, CAPD effects: Unknown

CAVH effects: Dose for GFR 10-50 mL/minute

Kintzel, 1995:

Oral: Adjust dose in the presence of hematologic toxicity

I.V.:

Cl_{cr} 46-60 mL/minute: Administer 85% of normal dose

Cl_{cr} 31-45 mL/minute: Administer 75% of normal dose

Cl_{cr} <30 mL/minute: Administer 70% of normal dose

Administration

Oral: Administer on an empty stomach (1 hour prior to or 2 hours after meals).

Parenteral: Due to limited stability, complete administration of I.V. dose should occur within 60 minutes of reconstitution.

I.V. infusion: I.V. dose is FDA-approved for administration as a single infusion over 15-20 minutes

I.V. bolus: I.V. may be administered via central line and via peripheral vein as a rapid I.V. bolus; there have not been any unexpected or serious adverse events specifically related to rapid I.V. bolus administration; the most common adverse events were transient mild symptoms of hot flush and tingling sensation over the body

Central line: I.V. bolus doses of 17-200 mg/m² (reconstituted and not diluted) have been infused over 2-20 minutes

Peripheral line: I.V. bolus doses of 2-23 mg/m² (reconstituted and not diluted) have been infused over 1-4 minutes

Monitoring Parameters Observe for signs of infection or bleeding; monitor WBCs and platelets

Test Interactions False-positive Coombs' test [direct]

Patient Information Any signs of infection, easy bruising or bleeding, shortness of breath, or painful or burning urination should be brought to physician's attention. Nausea, vomiting, or hair loss sometimes occur.

Additional Information

Myelosuppressive effects:

WBC: Moderate

Platelets: Moderate

Onset (days): 7

Nadir (days): 10-18

Recovery (days): 42-50

Special Geriatric Considerations Toxicity to immunosuppressives is increased in the elderly. Start with lowest recommended adult doses. Signs of infection, such as fever and WBC rise, may not occur. Lethargy and confusion may be more prominent signs of infection.

Dosage Forms Excipient information presented when available (limited, particularly for generics); consult specific product labeling.

Injection, powder for reconstitution: 50 mg [diluent contains ethanol and propylene glycol]

Tablet: 2 mg

Selected References

Aronoff GR, Berns JS, Brier ME, et al, "Drug Prescribing in Renal Failure: Dosing Guidelines for Adults," 4th ed. Philadelphia, PA: American College of Physicians; 1999, p. 75.

Hutchins LF and Lipschitz DA, "Cancer, Clinical Pharmacology, and Aging," *Clin Geriatr Med*, 1987, 3(3):483-503.

Kaplan HG, "Use of Cancer Chemotherapy in the Elderly," *Drug Treatment in the Elderly*, Vestal RE, ed, Boston, MA: ADIS Health Science Press, 1984, 338-49.

Kintzel PE and Dorr RT, "Anticancer Drug Renal Toxicity and Elimination: Dosing Guidelines for Altered Renal Function," *Cancer Treat Rev*, 1995, 21(1):33-64.

Kyle RA and Rajkumar SV, "Multiple Myeloma," *N Engl J Med*, 2004, 351(18):1860-73.

NCCN (National Comprehensive Cancer Network) "Practice Guidelines in Oncology: Antiemesis Version 2.2006." Available at http://www.nccn.org/professionals/physician_gls/PDF/antiemesis.pdf

Seddon BM, Cassoni AM, Galloway MJ, et al, "Fatal Radiation Myelopathy After High-Dose Busulfan and Melphalan Chemotherapy and Radiotherapy for Ewing's Sarcoma: A Review of the Literature and Implications for Practice," *Clin Oncol*, 2005, 17(5):385-90.

Memantine (me MAN teen)

U.S. Brand Names Namenda™
Canadian Brand Names Ebixa®
Index Terms Memantine Hydrochloride
Generic Available No
Pharmacologic Category N-Methyl-D-Aspartate Receptor Antagonist
Use Treatment of moderate-to-severe dementia of the Alzheimer's type
Contraindications Hypersensitivity to memantine or any component of the formulation
Warnings/Precautions Use caution with seizure disorders or hepatic impairment. Caution with use in severe renal impairment; dose adjustment recommended. Clearance is significantly reduced by alkaline urine; use caution with medications, dietary changes, or patient conditions which may alter urine pH.
Adverse Reactions (Reflective of adult population; not specific for elderly)
1% to 10%:
  Cardiovascular: Hypertension (4%), cardiac failure, syncope, cerebrovascular accident, transient ischemic attack
  Central nervous system: Dizziness (7%), confusion (6%), headache (6%), hallucinations (3%), pain (3%), somnolence (3%), fatigue (2%), aggressive reaction, ataxia, vertigo
  Dermatologic: Rash
  Gastrointestinal: Constipation (5%), vomiting (3%), weight loss
  Genitourinary: Micturition
  Hematologic: Anemia
  Hepatic: Alkaline phosphatase increased
  Neuromuscular & skeletal: Back pain (3%), hypokinesia
  Ocular: Cataract, conjunctivitis
  Respiratory: Cough (4%), dyspnea (2%), pneumonia
Overdosage/Toxicology Loss of consciousness, psychosis, restlessness, somnolence, stupor, and visual hallucinations were reported following ingestion of memantine 400 mg. In case of overdose, treatment should be symptomatic and supportive. Elimination may be increased by acidifying the urine.
Drug Interactions
  Carbonic anhydrase inhibitors: Carbonic anhydrase inhibitors may alkalinize the urine; clearance of memantine is decreased 80% at urinary pH 8.
  Sodium bicarbonate: Sodium bicarbonate may alkalinize the urine; clearance of memantine is decreased 80% at urinary pH 8.
Stability Store at controlled room temperature of 15°C to 30°C (59°F to 86°F).
Mechanism of Action Glutamate, the primary excitatory amino acid in the CNS, may contribute to the pathogenesis of Alzheimer's disease (AD) by overstimulating various glutamate receptors leading to excitotoxicity and neuronal cell death. Memantine is an uncompetitive antagonist of the N-methyl-D-aspartate (NMDA) type of glutamate receptors, located ubiquitously throughout the brain. Under normal physiologic conditions, the (unstimulated) NMDA receptor ion channel is blocked by magnesium ions, which are displaced after agonist-induced depolarization. Pathologic or excessive receptor activation, as postulated to occur during AD, prevents magnesium from reentering and blocking the channel pore resulting in a chronically open state and excessive calcium influx. Memantine binds to the intra-pore magnesium site, but with longer dwell time, and thus functions as an effective receptor blocker only under conditions of excessive stimulation; memantine does not affect normal neurotransmission.
Pharmacokinetics
  Distribution: 9-11 L/kg
  Protein binding: 45%
  Metabolism: Forms three metabolites (minimal activity)
  Half-life elimination: Terminal: 60-80 hours; severe renal impairment (Cl$_{cr}$ 5-29 mL/minute): 117-156 hours
  Time to peak, serum: 3-7 hours
  Excretion: Urine (57% to 82% unchanged); excretion reduced by alkaline urine pH
Dosage
  Geriatrics & Adults:
    Alzheimer's disease: Oral: Initial: 5 mg/day; increase dose by 5 mg/day to a target dose of 20 mg/day; wait at least 1 week between dosage changes. Doses >5 mg/day should be given in 2 divided doses.
      Suggested titration: 5 mg/day for ≥1 week; 5 mg twice daily for ≥1 week; 15 mg/day given in 5 mg and 10 mg separated doses for ≥1 week; then 10 mg twice daily.
    Mild-to-moderate vascular dementia (unlabeled use): Oral: 10 mg twice daily
  Renal Impairment:
    Mild-to-moderate impairment: No adjustment required.
    Severe impairment: Cl$_{cr}$ 5-29 mL/minute): 5 mg twice daily
(Continued)

Memantine *(Continued)*

Patient Information Inform prescriber of any prescription, OTC medication, or herbal products you are using and any allergies you have. Do not take any new medications during therapy without consulting prescriber. Take as directed with or without food. May cause hypertension (monitor if recommended); headache (consult prescriber for analgesic); CNS changes (confusion, hallucinations, fatigue, aggressive reaction); consult prescriber if persistent. Report chest pain or palpitations, dizziness or fainting; difficulty breathing or tightness in chest; rash; alteration in elimination patterns, increase in any adverse CNS symptoms, or other persistent adverse reactions.

Special Geriatric Considerations In clinical trials, patients on memantine had less of a decline in cognitive function and activities of daily living (ADL) as compared to placebo. This was true for monotherapy with memantine, as well as combination therapy with donepezil, an acetylcholinesterase inhibitor.

Dosage Forms Excipient information presented when available (limited, particularly for generics); consult specific product labeling.

Solution, oral: 2 mg/mL (360 mL) [alcohol free, dye free, sugar free; peppermint flavor]

Tablet, as hydrochloride: 5 mg, 10 mg

Combination package [titration pack contains two separate tablet formulations]: Memantine hydrochloride 5 mg (28s) and memantine hydrochloride 10 mg (21s)

Selected References

Orgogozo JM, Rigaud AS, Stoffler A et al, "Efficacy and Safety of Memantine in Patients with Mild to Moderate Vascular Dementia: A Randomized, Placebo-Controlled Trial (MMM 300)," *Stroke,* 2002, 33:1834-39.

Reisberg B, Doody R, Stoffler A, et al, "Memantine in Moderate-to-Severe Alzheimer's Disease," *N Engl J Med,* 2003, 348(14):1333-41.

Tariot PN, Farlow MR, Grossberg GT, et al, "Memantine Treatment in Patients With Moderate to Severe Alzheimer Disease Already Receiving Donepezil: A Randomized Controlled Trial. The Memantine Study Group," *JAMA,* 2004, 291(3):317-24.

Wilcock G, Mobius HJ, Stoffler A et al, "A Double-Blind, Placebo-Controlled Multicentre Study of Memantine in Mild to Moderate Vascular Dementia (MMM 500)," *Int Clin Psychopharmacol,* 2002, 17(6):297-305.

♦ **Memantine Hydrochloride** *see* Memantine *on page 977*

♦ **Menactra®** *see* Meningococcal Polysaccharide (Groups A / C / Y and W-135) Diphtheria Toxoid Conjugate Vaccine *on page 978*

♦ **Menest®** *see* Estrogens (Esterified) *on page 572*

Meningococcal Polysaccharide (Groups A / C / Y and W-135) Diphtheria Toxoid Conjugate Vaccine

(me NIN joe kok al pol i SAK a ride groops aye, see, why & dubl yoo won thur tee fyve dif THEER ee a TOKS oyds KON joo gate vak SEEN)

Medication Safety Issues

Administration issue:

Menactra® (MCV4) should be administered by intramuscular (I.M.) injection only. Inadvertent subcutaneous (SubQ) administration has been reported; possibly due to confusion of this product with Menomune® (MPSV4), also a meningococcal polysaccharide vaccine, which is administered by the SubQ route.

U.S. Brand Names Menactra®

Index Terms MCV4; Quadrivalent Meningococcal Conjugate Vaccine

Generic Available No

Pharmacologic Category Vaccine

Use Provide active immunization of adolescents and adults (11-55 years of age) against invasive meningococcal disease caused by *N. meningitidis* serogroups A, C, Y and W-135

Dosage

Geriatrics: Safety and efficacy not established in patients >55 years.

Adults: Immunization: I.M.: Adults ≤55 years: 0.5 mL

Note: Revaccination: May be indicated in patients previously vaccinated with MPSV4 who remain at increased risk for infection. The ACIP recommends the use of MCV4 for revaccination in patients 11-55 years, however use of MPSV4 is also acceptable. Consider revaccination after 3-5 years. The need for revaccination in patients previously vaccinated with MCV4 is currently under study.

Special Geriatric Considerations

May be used though safety and efficacy have not been established in patients >55 years of age.

Dosage Forms Excipient information presented when available (limited, particularly for generics); consult specific product labeling.

Injection, solution:

Menactra®: 4 mcg each of polysaccharide antigen groups A, C, Y, and W-135 per 0.5 mL [conjugated to diphtheria toxoid protein 48 mcg; adjuvant and preservative free; vial stopper contains dry, natural latex rubber]

Meningococcal Polysaccharide Vaccine (Groups A / C / Y and W-135)

(me NIN joe kok al pol i SAK a ride vak SEEN groops aye, see, why & dubl yoo won thur tee fyve)

Related Information
Immunization Recommendations *on page 1787*

Medication Safety Issues
Administration issue:
Menomune® (MPSV4) should be administered by subcutaneous (SubQ) injection. Menactra® (MCV4), also a meningococcal polysaccharide vaccine, is to be administered by intramuscular (I.M.) injection only.

U.S. Brand Names Menomune®-A/C/Y/W-135

Index Terms MPSV4; Quadrivalent Meningococcal Conjugate Vaccine

Generic Available No

Pharmacologic Category Vaccine

Use Provide active immunity to meningococcal serogroups contained in the vaccine

The ACIP recommends routine vaccination for persons at increased risk for meningococcal disease. (Use of MPSV4 is recommended in children 2-10 years and adults > 55 years. MCV4 is preferred for persons aged 11-55 years; MPSV4 may be used if MCV4 is not available). Persons at increased risk include:
College freshmen living in dormitories
Microbiologists routinely exposed to isolates of *N. meningitides*
Military recruits
Persons traveling to or who reside in countries where *N. meningitides* is hyperendemic or epidemic, particularly if contact with local population will be prolonged
Persons with terminal complement component deficiencies
Persons with anatomic or functional asplenia
Use is also recommended during meningococcal outbreaks caused by vaccine preventable serogroups.

Contraindications Hypersensitivity to any component of the formulation; defer immunization during acute illness

Warnings/Precautions Patients who undergo splenectomy secondary to trauma or nonlymphoid tumors respond well; however, those asplenic patients with lymphoid tumors who receive either chemotherapy or irradiation respond poorly. Response may not be as great as desired in immunosuppressed patients. Use with caution in patients with latex sensitivity; the stopper to the vial contains dry, natural latex rubber. Some dosage forms contain thimerosal.

Adverse Reactions (Reflective of adult population; not specific for elderly)
All serious adverse reactions must be reported to the U.S. Department of Health and Human Services (DHHS) Vaccine Adverse Event Reporting System (VAERS) 1-800-822-7967. Percentages reported in adults; incidence of erythema, swelling, or tenderness may be higher in children
>10%: Local: Tenderness (9% to 36%)
1% to 10%:
Central nervous system: Headache (2% to 5%), malaise (2%), fever (100°F to 106°F: 3%), chills (2%)
Local: Pain at injection site (2% to 3%), erythema (1% to 4%), induration (1% to 4%)

Drug Interactions
Immunoglobulin: Decreased effect with administration of immunoglobulin within 1 month.
Vaccines: Should not be administered with whole-cell pertussis or whole-cell typhoid vaccines due to combined endotoxin content.

Stability Prior to and following reconstitution, store at 2°C to 8°C (35°F to 46°F). Reconstitute using provided diluent; shake well. Use single-dose vial within 30 minutes of reconstitution. Use multidose vial within 35 days of reconstitution.

Mechanism of Action Induces the formation of bactericidal antibodies to meningococcal antigens; the presence of these antibodies is strongly correlated with immunity to meningococcal disease caused by *Neisseria meningitidis* groups A, C, Y and W-135.

Pharmacodynamics
Onset of action: Antibody levels are achieved within 10-14 days after administration
Duration: Antibodies against group A and C polysaccharides decline markedly (to prevaccination levels) over the first 3 years following a single dose of vaccine

Dosage
Geriatrics & Adults: Immunization: SubQ: 0.5 mL; the need for booster is unknown, but may be considered in high-risk individuals. **Note:** Individuals who are sensitive to thimerosal should receive single-dose pack (reconstituted with 0.78 mL vial without preservative).
(Continued)

Meningococcal Polysaccharide Vaccine (Groups A / C / Y and W-135) *(Continued)*

Administration Administer by SubQ injection; do not administer intradermally, I.M., or I.V.

Monitoring Parameters Monitor for side effects, especially local effects at site of injection

Patient Information Report serious and unusual effects to physician

Additional Information Federal law requires that the date of administration, the vaccine manufacturer, lot number of vaccine, and the administering person's name, title, and address be entered into the patient's permanent medical record.

Special Geriatric Considerations No specific data; only recommended when traveling to highly endemic areas.

Dosage Forms Excipient information presented when available (limited, particularly for generics); consult specific product labeling.

Injection, powder for reconstitution: 50 mcg each of polysaccharide antigen groups A, C, Y, and W-135 [contains lactose; packaged with 0.78 mL preservative free diluent or 6 mL diluent containing thimerosal; vial stoppers contain dry, natural latex rubber]

♦ **Menomune®-A/C/Y/W-135** *see* Meningococcal Polysaccharide Vaccine (Groups A / C / Y and W-135) *on page 979*

♦ **Menostar™** *see* Estradiol *on page 549*

Meperidine *(me PER i deen)*

Related Information
Narcotic / Opioid Analgesics *on page 1763*
Potentially Inappropriate Medications for Geriatrics *on page 1824*

Medication Safety Issues
Sound-alike/look-alike issues:
Meperidine may be confused with meprobamate
Demerol® may be confused with Demulen®, Desyrel®, dicumarol, Dilaudid®, Dymelor®, Pamelor®

U.S. Brand Names Demerol®; Meperitab®

Canadian Brand Names Demerol®

Index Terms Isonipecaine Hydrochloride; Meperidine Hydrochloride; Pethidine Hydrochloride

Generic Available Yes

Pharmacologic Category Analgesic, Opioid

Use Management of moderate to severe pain; adjunct to anesthesia and preoperative sedation

Unlabeled/Investigational Use
Reduce postoperative shivering; reduce rigors from amphotericin

Restrictions C-II

Contraindications Hypersensitivity to meperidine or any component of the formulation; use with or within 14 days of MAO inhibitors

Warnings/Precautions Meperidine is not recommended for the management of chronic pain. When used for acute pain (in patients without renal or CNS disease), treatment should be limited to 48 hours and doses should not exceed 600 mg/24 hours. Oral meperidine is not recommended for acute pain management. Normeperidine (an active metabolite and CNS stimulant) may accumulate and precipitate anxiety, tremors, or seizures; risk increases with renal dysfunction and cumulative dose. Effects may be potentiated when used with other sedative drugs or ethanol.

May cause CNS depression, which may impair physical or mental abilities; patients must be cautioned about performing tasks which require mental alertness (eg, operating machinery or driving). Use only with extreme caution (if at all) in patients with head injury or increased intracranial pressure (ICP). Use caution with pulmonary, hepatic, or renal disorders, supraventricular tachycardias, acute abdominal conditions, hypothyroidism, toxic psychosis, kyphoscoliosis, morbid obesity, Addison's disease, BPH, or urethral stricture. Use with caution in patients with biliary tract dysfunction; acute pancreatitis may cause constriction of sphincter of Oddi. May cause hypotension; use with caution in patients with depleted blood volume or drugs which may exaggerate hypotensive effects (including phenothiazines or general anesthetics).

An opioid-containing analgesic regimen should be tailored to each patient's needs. The optimal analgesic dose varies widely among patients. Some preparations contain sulfites which may cause allergic reaction. Tolerance or drug dependence may result from extended use. Healthcare provider should be alert to problems of abuse, misuse, and diversion.Concurrent use of agonist/antagonist analgesics may precipitate withdrawal symptoms and/or reduced analgesic efficacy in patients following prolonged therapy with mu opioid agonists. Abrupt discontinuation following prolonged use may also lead to withdrawal symptoms. Use with caution in the elderly and debilitated patients; may be more sensitive to adverse effects.

Adverse Reactions (Reflective of adult population; not specific for elderly)
Frequency not defined.

Cardiovascular: Hypotension

Central nervous system: Fatigue, drowsiness, dizziness, nervousness, headache, restlessness, malaise, confusion, mental depression, hallucinations, paradoxical CNS stimulation, increased intracranial pressure, seizure (associated with metabolite accumulation), serotonin syndrome

Dermatologic: Rash, urticaria

Gastrointestinal: Nausea, vomiting, constipation, anorexia, stomach cramps, xerostomia, biliary spasm, paralytic ileus, sphincter of Oddi spasm

Genitourinary: Ureteral spasms, decreased urination

Local: Pain at injection site

Neuromuscular & skeletal: Weakness

Respiratory: Dyspnea

Miscellaneous: Histamine release, physical and psychological dependence

Overdosage/Toxicology Symptoms include CNS depression, respiratory depression, mydriasis, bradycardia, pulmonary edema, chronic tremors, CNS excitability, and seizures. Treatment of overdose includes airway support, establishment of an I.V. line, and administration of naloxone 2 mg I.V., with repeat administration as necessary, up to a total of 10 mg. Naloxone does not reverse the adverse effects of normeperidine.

Drug Interactions
Substrate (minor) of CYP2B6, 2C19, 3A4

Acyclovir: May increase meperidine metabolite concentrations. Use caution.

Barbiturates: May decrease analgesic efficacy and increase sedative and/or respiratory depressive effects of meperidine.

Cimetidine: May increase meperidine metabolite concentrations; use caution.

CNS depressants (including benzodiazepines): May potentiate the sedative and/or respiratory depressive effects of meperidine.

MAO inhibitors: May enhance the serotonergic effect of meperidine, which may cause serotonin syndrome. Concurrent use with or within 14 days of an MAO inhibitor is contraindicated.

Phenothiazines: May potentiate the sedative and/or respiratory depressive effects of meperidine; may increase the incidence of hypotension.

Phenytoin: May decrease the analgesic effects of meperidine

Ritonavir: May increase meperidine metabolite concentrations; use caution.

Serotonin agonists: Serotonin agonists and meperidine may enhance serotonin levels in the brain. Serotonin syndrome may occur.

Serotonin reuptake inhibitors: May potentiate the effects of meperidine, increasing serotonin levels in the brain. Serotonin syndrome may occur.

Sibutramine: May enhance the serotonergic effect of meperidine. Serotonin syndrome may occur.

Tricyclic antidepressants: May potentiate the sedative and/or respiratory depressive effects of meperidine. In addition, potentially may increase the risk of serotonin syndrome.

Ethanol/Nutrition/Herb Interactions
Ethanol: Avoid or limit ethanol (may increase CNS depression). Watch for sedation.

Herb/Nutraceutical: Avoid valerian, St John's wort, kava kava, gotu kola (may increase CNS depression).

Stability Meperidine injection should be stored at room temperature; do not freeze. Protect from light. Protect oral dosage forms from light.

Mechanism of Action Binds to opiate receptors in the CNS, causing inhibition of ascending pain pathways, altering the perception of and response to pain; produces generalized CNS depression

Pharmacodynamics
Onset of action: Analgesic: Oral, SubQ: 10-15 minutes; I.V.: ~5 minutes

Peak effect: SubQ.: ~1 hour; Oral: 2 hours

Duration: Oral, SubQ.: 2-4 hours; may be increased in older adults

Pharmacokinetics
Absorption: I.M.: Erratic and highly variable

Distribution: Crosses placenta; enters breast milk

Protein binding: 65% to 75%

Metabolism: Hepatic; hydrolyzed to meperidinic acid (inactive) or undergoes N-demethylation to normeperidine (active; has $1/2$ the analgesic effect and 2-3 times the CNS effects of meperidine)

Bioavailability: ~50% to 60%; increased with liver disease

Half-life elimination:
  Parent drug: Terminal phase: Adults: 2.5-4 hours, Liver disease: 7-11 hours
  Normeperidine (active metabolite): 15-30 hours; can accumulate with high doses or with decreased renal function

Excretion: Urine (as metabolites)

(Continued)

Meperidine *(Continued)*

Dosage

Geriatrics: Note: Doses should be titrated to necessary analgesic effect. When changing route of administration, note that oral doses are about half as effective as parenteral dose. Oral route not recommended for chronic pain. These are guidelines and do not represent the maximum doses that may be required in all patients.
Oral: 50 mg every 4 hours
I.M.: 25 mg every 4 hours

Adults: Note: Doses should be titrated to necessary analgesic effect. When changing route of administration, note that oral doses are about half as effective as parenteral dose. Not recommended for chronic pain. These are guidelines and do not represent the maximum doses that may be required in all patients. In patients with normal renal function, doses of ≤600 mg/24 hours and use for ≤48 hours are recommended (American Pain Society, 1999).

Pain (analgesic):
Oral: Initial: Opiate-naive: 50 mg every 3-4 hours as needed; usual dosage range: 50-150 mg every 2-4 hours as needed (manufacturers recommendation; oral route is not recommended for acute pain)
I.M., SubQ: Initial: Opiate-naive: 50-75 mg every 3-4 hours as needed; patients with prior opiate exposure may require higher initial doses.
Preoperatively: 50-100 mg given 30-90 minutes before the beginning of anesthesia
Slow I.V.: Initial: 5-10 mg every 5 minutes as needed
Patient-controlled analgesia (PCA): Usual concentration: 10 mg/mL
Initial dose: 10 mg
Demand dose: 1-5 mg (manufacturer recommendations); range 5-25 mg (American Pain Society, 1999).
Lockout interval: 5-10 minutes

Renal Impairment:
Cl_{cr} 10-50 mL/minute: Administer 75% of normal dose.
Cl_{cr} <10 mL/minute: Administer 50% of normal dose.
Note: Repeated use in renal impairment **should be avoided** due to potential accumulation of neuroexcitatory metabolite.

Hepatic Impairment: Increased narcotic effect in cirrhosis; reduction in dose is more important for oral than I.V. route.

Administration Meperidine may be administered I.M., SubQ, or I.V.; I.V. push should be administered slowly, use of a 10 mg/mL concentration has been recommended. For continuous I.V. infusions, a more dilute solution (eg, 1 mg/mL) should be used.
Oral: Administer syrup diluted in 1/2 glass of water; undiluted syrup may exert topical anesthetic effect on mucous membranes

Monitoring Parameters Pain relief, respiratory and mental status, blood pressure

Reference Range Therapeutic: 70-500 ng/mL (SI: 283-2020 nmol/L); Toxic: >1000 ng/mL (SI: >4043 nmol/L)

Test Interactions Increased amylase (S), increased BSP retention, increased CPK (I.M. injections)

Patient Information Will cause drowsiness; avoid alcoholic beverages.

Special Geriatric Considerations Meperidine is not recommended as a drug of first choice for the treatment of chronic pain in the elderly due to the accumulation of its metabolite, normeperidine, which leads to serious CNS side effects (eg, tremor, seizures). For acute pain, its use should be limited to 1-2 doses.

Dosage Forms Excipient information presented when available (limited, particularly for generics); consult specific product labeling.
Injection, solution, as hydrochloride [ampul]: 25 mg/0.5 mL (0.5 mL); 25 mg/mL (1 mL); 50 mg/mL (1 mL, 1.5 mL, 2 mL); 75 mg/mL (1 mL); 100 mg/mL (1 mL)
Injection, solution, as hydrochloride [prefilled syringe]: 25 mg/mL (1 mL); 50 mg/mL (1 mL); 75 mg/mL (1 mL); 100 mg/mL (1 mL)
Injection, solution, as hydrochloride [for PCA pump]: 10 mg/mL (30 mL, 50 mL, 60 mL)
Injection, solution, as hydrochloride [vial]: 25 mg/mL (1 mL); 50 mg/mL (1 mL, 30 mL); 75 mg/mL (1 mL); 100 mg/mL (1 mL, 20 mL) [may contain sodium metabisulfite]
Solution, oral, as hydrochloride: 50 mg/5 mL (500 mL)
Syrup, as hydrochloride:
Demerol®: 50 mg/5 mL (480 mL) [contains benzoic acid; banana flavor]
Tablet, as hydrochloride: 50 mg, 100 mg
Demerol®, Meperitab®: 50 mg, 100 mg

Selected References

AGS Panel on Persistent Pain in Older Persons, "The Management of Persistent Pain in Older Persons," *J Am Geriatr Soc*, 2002, 50(6 Suppl):S205-24.
Clark RF, Wei EM, and Anderson PO, "Meperidine: Therapeutic Use and Toxicity," *J Emerg Med*, 1995,13(6):797-802.
Ferrell BA, "Pain Management in Elderly People," *J Am Geriatr Soc*, 1991, 39(1):64-73.
Golembiewski J, "Safety Concerns With Meperidine," *J Perianesth Nurs*, 2002, 17(2):123-5.
Latta KS, Ginsberg B, and Barkin RL, "Meperidine: A Critical Review," *Am J Ther*, 2002, 9(1):53-68.

♦ **Meperidine Hydrochloride** *see* Meperidine *on page 980*

♦ **Meperitab**® *see* Meperidine *on page 980*

Mephobarbital (me foe BAR bi tal)

Medication Safety Issues
Sound-alike/look-alike issues:
Mephobarbital may be confused with methocarbamol
Mebaral® may be confused with Medrol®, Mellaril®, Tegretol®

U.S. Brand Names Mebaral®

Canadian Brand Names Mebaral®

Index Terms Methylphenobarbital

Generic Available No

Pharmacologic Category Barbiturate

Use Sedation; treatment of grand mal and petit mal epilepsy

Restrictions C-IV

Contraindications Hypersensitivity to mephobarbital, other barbiturates, or any component of the formulation; pre-existing CNS depression; respiratory depression; severe uncontrolled pain; history of porphyria

Warnings/Precautions Use with caution in patients with renal impairment, pulmonary insufficiency, or hepatic dysfunction; abrupt withdrawal may precipitate status epilepticus; use with caution in patients with depression, suicidal threats, or history of drug abuse; use cautiously in patients with pain as signs may be masked by barbiturate; vitamin D requirements may be increased (increased metabolism); use cautiously in older adults. See Special Geriatric Considerations.

Use with caution in patients with myxedema or myasthenia gravis. Barbiturates may be habit forming; abrupt withdrawal in patients with seizure disorders may precipitate status epilepticus.

Adverse Reactions (Reflective of adult population; not specific for elderly)
>10%: Central nervous system: Dizziness, lightheadedness, drowsiness, "hangover" effect

1% to 10%:
Central nervous system: Confusion, mental depression, unusual excitement, nervousness, faint feeling, headache, insomnia, nightmares
Gastrointestinal: Constipation, nausea, vomiting

Drug Interactions Substrate of CYP2B6 (minor), 2C9 (minor), 2C19 (major); **Inhibits** CYP2C19 (weak); **Induces** CYP2A6 (weak)

Acetaminophen: Barbiturates may enhance the hepatotoxic potential of acetaminophen overdoses

CNS depressants: Sedative effects and/or respiratory depression with barbiturates may be additive with other CNS depressants; monitor for increased effect; includes ethanol, sedatives, antidepressants, opioid analgesics, and benzodiazepines

Cyclosporine: Levels may be decreased by barbiturates; monitor

CYP2C19 inducers: May decrease the levels/effects of mephobarbital. Example inducers include aminoglutethimide, carbamazepine, phenytoin, and rifampin.

CYP2C19 inhibitors: May increase the levels/effects of mephobarbital. Example inhibitors include delavirdine, fluconazole, fluvoxamine, gemfibrozil, isoniazid, omeprazole, and ticlopidine.

Griseofulvin: Barbiturates may impair the absorption of griseofulvin, and griseofulvin metabolism may be increased by barbiturates, decreasing clinical effect

Guanfacine: Effect may be decreased by barbiturates

MAO inhibitors: Metabolism of barbiturates may be inhibited, increasing clinical effect or toxicity of the barbiturates

Methoxyflurane: Barbiturates may enhance the nephrotoxic effects of methoxyflurane

Valproic acid: Metabolism of barbiturates may be inhibited by valproic acid; monitor for excessive sedation; a dose reduction may be needed

Mechanism of Action Increases seizure threshold in the motor cortex; depresses monosynaptic and polysynaptic transmission in the CNS

Pharmacodynamics
Onset of action: 20-60 minutes
Duration: 10-16 hours

Pharmacokinetics
Absorption: Oral: ~50%
Metabolism: By the liver to phenobarbital
Half-life: 34 hours
Elimination: In urine
(Continued)

Mephobarbital *(Continued)*

Dosage
  Geriatrics: Refer to adult dosing. Start at lowest recommended doses.
  Adults:
    Epilepsy: Oral: 200-600 mg/day in 2-4 divided doses
    Sedation: Oral: 32-100 mg 3-4 times/day
  Renal Impairment: Use with caution and reduce dose.

Reference Range Phenobarbital level should be in the range of 15-40 mcg/mL.

Patient Information May cause drowsiness, may impair coordination and judgment; do not discontinue abruptly; notify physician of dark urine, pale stools, jaundice, abdominal pain, persistent nausea, and vomiting; do not skip doses

Additional Information May use in combination with phenobarbital or phenytoin. When using with phenobarbital, both agents should be started at ½ dose. When mephobarbital is used with phenytoin, the dose of phenytoin must be reduced. Full doses of mephobarbital may be given.

Special Geriatric Considerations Using barbiturates in the elderly may induce paradoxical stimulation, cause or aggravate depression and confusion. Due to mephobarbital's long half-life and risk of dependence, it is not a drug of choice in the elderly as a sedative/hypnotic. Interpretive guidelines from Centers for Medicare and Medicaid Services (CMS) OBRA regulations discourage the use of barbiturates as sedative/hypnotics in nursing home patients.

Dosage Forms Excipient information presented when available (limited, particularly for generics); consult specific product labeling.
  Tablet: 32 mg, 50 mg, 100 mg

Selected References
Pond SM, Olson KR, Osterloh JD, et al, "Randomized Study of the Treatment of Phenobarbital Overdose With Repeated Doses of Activated Charcoal," *JAMA*, 1984, 251(23):3104-8.

Zawada ET, Nappi J, Done G, et al, "Advances in the Hemodialysis Management of Phenobarbital Overdose," *South Med J*, 1983, 76(1):6-8.

♦ **Mephyton®** *see Phytonadione on page 1257*

Meprobamate *(me proe BA mate)*

Related Information
  Potentially Inappropriate Medications for Geriatrics *on page 1824*

Medication Safety Issues
  Sound-alike/look-alike issues:
    Meprobamate may be confused with Mepergan, meperidine
    Equanil may be confused with Elavil®

U.S. Brand Names Miltown® [DSC]

Canadian Brand Names Novo-Mepro

Index Terms Equanil

Generic Available Yes

Pharmacologic Category Antianxiety Agent, Miscellaneous

Use Management of anxiety disorders

Unlabeled/Investigational Use Demonstrated value for muscle contraction, headache, premenstrual tension, external sphincter spasticity, muscle rigidity, opisthotonos-associated with tetanus

Restrictions C-IV

Contraindications Hypersensitivity to meprobamate, related compounds (including carisoprodol), or any component of the formulation; acute intermittent porphyria; pre-existing CNS depression; narrow-angle glaucoma; severe uncontrolled pain

Warnings/Precautions Physical and psychological dependence and abuse may occur; abrupt cessation may precipitate withdrawal. Use with caution in patients with depression or suicidal tendencies, or in patients with a history of drug abuse. May cause CNS depression, which may impair physical or mental abilities. Patients must be cautioned about performing tasks which require mental alertness (eg, operating machinery or driving). Effects with other sedative drugs or ethanol may be potentiated. Allergic reaction may occur in patients with history of dermatological condition (usually by fourth dose). Use with caution in patients with renal or hepatic impairment, or with a history of seizures. Use caution in the elderly as it may cause confusion, cognitive impairment, or excessive sedation.

Adverse Reactions (Reflective of adult population; not specific for elderly)
  Frequency not defined.
  Cardiovascular: Syncope, peripheral edema, palpitation, tachycardia, arrhythmia
  Central nervous system: Drowsiness, ataxia, dizziness, paradoxical excitement, confusion, slurred speech, headache, euphoria, chills, vertigo, paresthesia, overstimulation
  Dermatologic: Rashes, purpura, dermatitis, Stevens-Johnson syndrome, petechiae, ecchymosis

Gastrointestinal: Diarrhea, vomiting, nausea

Hematologic: Leukopenia, eosinophilia, agranulocytosis, aplastic anemia

Neuromuscular & skeletal: Weakness

Ocular: Blurred vision, impairment of accommodation

Renal: Renal failure

Respiratory: Wheezing, dyspnea, bronchospasm, angioneurotic edema

Overdosage/Toxicology Symptoms include drowsiness, lethargy, ataxia, coma, hypotension, shock, and death. Treatment is supportive following attempts to enhance drug elimination. Hypotension should be treated with I.V. fluids and/or Trendelenburg positioning. Dialysis and hemoperfusion have not demonstrated significant reductions in blood drug concentrations.

Drug Interactions CNS depressants: Sedative effects may be additive with other CNS depressants; monitor for increased effect; includes barbiturates, benzodiazepines, opioid analgesics, ethanol, and other sedative agents

Ethanol/Nutrition/Herb Interactions

Ethanol: Avoid ethanol (may increase CNS depression).

Herb/Nutraceutical: Avoid valerian, St John's wort, kava kava, gotu kola (may increase CNS depression).

Mechanism of Action Affects the thalamus and limbic system; also appears to inhibit multineuronal spinal reflexes

Pharmacodynamics Onset of sedation: Oral: Within 60 minutes

Pharmacokinetics

Metabolism: Promptly in the liver

Half-life: 10 hours

Elimination: In urine (8% to 20% as unchanged drug) and in feces (10% as metabolites)

Dosage

Geriatrics: Oral (use lowest effective dose): Initial: 200 mg 2-3 times/day

Adults: Oral: 400 mg 3-4 times/day, up to 2400 mg/day

Renal Impairment:

Cl_{cr} 10-50 mL/minute: Administer every 9-12 hours.

Cl_{cr} <10 mL/minute: Administer every 12-18 hours.

Moderately dialyzable (20% to 50%)

Hepatic Impairment: Probably necessary in patients with liver disease; no specific recommendations.

Monitoring Parameters Mental status

Reference Range Therapeutic: 6-12 mcg/mL (SI: 28-55 μmol/L); Toxic: >60 mcg/mL (SI: >275 μmol/L)

Patient Information May cause drowsiness; avoid alcoholic beverages

Special Geriatric Considerations Meprobamate is not considered a drug of choice in the elderly because of its potential to cause physical and psychological dependence. Interpretive guidelines from the Centers for Medicare and Medicaid Services (CMS) strongly discourage the use of meprobamate in residents of long-term care facilities.

Dosage Forms Excipient information presented when available (limited, particularly for generics); consult specific product labeling. [DSC] = Discontinued product

Tablet: 200 mg, 400 mg

Miltown®: 200 mg, 400 mg [DSC]

Mercaptopurine (mer kap toe PYOOR een)

Medication Safety Issues

Sound-alike/look-alike issues:

Purinethol® may be confused with propylthiouracil

High alert medication: The Institute for Safe Medication Practices (ISMP) includes this medication among its list of drugs which have a heightened risk of causing significant patient harm when used in error.

To avoid potentially serious dosage errors, the terms "6-mercaptopurine" or "6-MP" should be avoided; use of these terms has been associated with sixfold overdosages.

Azathioprine is metabolized to mercaptopurine; concurrent use of these commercially-available products has resulted in profound myelosuppression.

U.S. Brand Names Purinethol®

Canadian Brand Names Purinethol®

Index Terms 6-Mercaptopurine (error-prone abbreviation); 6-MP (error-prone abbreviation); NSC-755

Generic Available Yes

Pharmacologic Category Antineoplastic Agent, Antimetabolite; Immunosuppressant Agent

Use Treatment (maintenance and induction) of acute lymphoblastic leukemia (ALL)

(Continued)

Mercaptopurine *(Continued)*

Unlabeled/Investigational Use Steroid-sparing agent for corticosteroid-dependent Crohn's disease (CD) and ulcerative colitis (UC); maintenance of remission in CD; fistulizing Crohn's disease

Contraindications Hypersensitivity to mercaptopurine or any component of the formulation; patients whose disease showed prior resistance to mercaptopurine or thioguanine; severe liver disease, severe bone marrow suppression

Warnings/Precautions Hazardous agent - use appropriate precautions for handling and disposal. Adjust dosage in patients with renal impairment or hepatic failure; use with caution in patients with prior bone marrow suppression; patients may be at risk for pancreatitis. Toxicity to immunosuppressives is increased in elderly. Start with lowest recommended adult doses. Signs of infection, such as fever and WBC rise, may not occur. Lethargy and confusion may be more prominent signs of infection. Use caution with other hepatotoxic drugs or in dosages >2.5 mg/kg/day; hepatotoxicity may occur. Patients with genetic deficiency of thiopurine methyltransferase (TPMT) or concurrent therapy with drugs which may inhibit TPMT (eg, olsalazine) or xanthine oxidase (eg, allopurinol) may be sensitive to myelosuppressive effects. Azathioprine is metabolized to mercaptopurine; concomitant use may result in profound myelosuppression and should be avoided. Immune response to vaccines may be diminished.

To avoid potentially serious dosage errors, the terms "6-mercaptopurine" or "6-MP" should be avoided; use of these terms has been associated with sixfold overdosages.

Adverse Reactions (Reflective of adult population; not specific for elderly)

>10%:

Hematologic: Myelosuppression; leukopenia, thrombocytopenia, anemia

Onset: 7-10 days

Nadir: 14-16 days

Recovery: 21-28 days

Hepatic: Intrahepatic cholestasis and focal centralobular necrosis (40%), characterized by hyperbilirubinemia, increased alkaline phosphatase and AST, jaundice, ascites, encephalopathy; more common at doses >2.5 mg/kg/day. Usually occurs within 2 months of therapy but may occur within 1 week, or be delayed up to 8 years.

1% to 10%:

Central nervous system: Drug fever

Dermatologic: Hyperpigmentation, rash

Endocrine & metabolic: Hyperuricemia

Gastrointestinal: Nausea, vomiting, diarrhea, stomatitis, anorexia, stomach pain, mucositis

Renal: Renal toxicity

Overdosage/Toxicology Immediate symptoms are nausea and vomiting. Delayed symptoms include bone marrow suppression, hepatic necrosis, and gastroenteritis. Efforts to minimize absorption (charcoal, gastric lavage) may be ineffective unless instituted within 60 minutes of ingestion.

Drug Interactions

Allopurinol: Can cause increased levels of mercaptopurine by inhibition of xanthine oxidase; decrease dose of mercaptopurine by 75% when both drugs are used concomitantly; may potentiate effect of bone marrow suppression (reduce mercaptopurine to 25% of dose).

Aminosalicylates (olsalazine, mesalamine, sulfasalazine): May inhibit TPMT, increasing toxicity/myelosuppression of mercaptopurine. Use caution.

Azathioprine: Metabolized to mercaptopurine, concomitant use may result in profound myelosuppression and should be avoided

Doxorubicin: Synergistic liver toxicity with mercaptopurine in >50% of patients, which resolved with discontinuation of the mercaptopurine.

Hepatotoxic drugs: Any agent which could potentially alter the metabolic function of the liver could produce higher drug levels and greater toxicities from either mercaptopurine or 6-TG.

Warfarin: mercaptopurine inhibits the anticoagulation effect of warfarin by an unknown mechanism.

Stability Store at room temperature of 15°C to 25°C (59°F to 77°F). Protect from moisture.

Mechanism of Action Purine antagonist which inhibits DNA and RNA synthesis; acts as false metabolite and is incorporated into DNA and RNA, eventually inhibiting their synthesis; specific for the S phase of the cell cycle

Pharmacokinetics

Absorption: Variable and incomplete (16% to 50%)

Protein binding: 19%

Metabolism: Hepatic and in GI mucosa; hepatically via xanthine oxidase and methylation via TPMT to sulfate conjugates, 6-thiouric acid, and other inactive compounds; first-pass effect

Half-life (adults): 47 minutes
Time to peak concentration: Within 2 hours
Elimination: Prompt excretion in urine

Dosage
  Geriatrics: Due to renal decline with age, start with lower recommended doses for adults.
  Adults: Refer to individual protocols.
    ALL:
      Induction: Oral: 2.5-5 mg/kg/day (100-200 mg)
      Maintenance: Oral: 1.5-2.5 mg/kg/day **or** 80-100 mg/m^2/day given once daily
    Note: In ALL, administration in the evening (vs morning administration) may lower the risk of relapse.
    Reduction of steroid use in CD or UC, maintenance of remission in CD or fistulizing disease (unlabeled uses): Oral: Initial: 50 mg daily; may increase by 25 mg/day every 1-2 weeks as tolerated to target dose of 1-1.5 mg/kg/day
    Dosage adjustment with concurrent allopurinol: Reduce mercaptopurine dosage to $^1/_4$ to $^1/_3$ the usual dose.
    Dosage adjustment in TPMT-deficiency: Not established; substantial reductions are generally required only in homozygous deficiency.
  Renal Impairment: Dose should be reduced to avoid accumulation, but specific guidelines are not available.
    Hemodialysis: Removed; supplemental dosing is usually required
  Hepatic Impairment: Dose should be reduced to avoid accumulation, but specific guidelines are not available.
Administration Administer by slow I.V. continuous infusion.
Monitoring Parameters CBC with differential and platelet count, liver function tests, uric acid, urinalysis; TPMT genotyping may identify individuals at risk for toxicity
  For use as immunomodulatory therapy in CD or UC, monitor CBC with differential weekly for 1 month, then biweekly for 1 month, followed by monitoring every 1-2 months throughout the course of therapy. LFT's should be assessed every 3 months.
Patient Information Do not take with meals; nausea and vomiting are rare with usual doses; report to physician if fever, sore throat, bleeding, bruising, shortness of breath, or painful urination occurs; hair loss occurs sometimes
Special Geriatric Considerations Toxicity to immunosuppressives is increased in the elderly. Start with lowest recommended adult doses. Signs of infection, such as fever and WBC rise, may not occur. Lethargy and confusion may be more prominent signs of infection.
Dosage Forms Excipient information presented when available (limited, particularly for generics); consult specific product labeling.
  Tablet [scored]: 50 mg

Selected References
Hutchins LF and Lipschitz DA, "Cancer, Clinical Pharmacology, and Aging," *Clin Geriatr Med*, 1987, 3(3):483-503.
Kaplan HG, "Use of Cancer Chemotherapy in the Elderly," *Drug Treatment in the Elderly*, Vestal RE, ed, Boston, MA: ADIS Health Science Press, 1984, 338-49.
Lichtenstein GR, Abreu MT, Cohen R, et al, "American Gastroenterological Association Institute Medical Position Statement on Corticosteroids, Immunomodulators, and Infliximab in Inflammatory Bowel Disease," *Gastroenterology*, 2006, 130(3):935-9.
Sandborn WJ, "A Review of Immune Modifier Therapy for Inflammatory Bowel Disease: Azathioprine, 6-mercaptopurine, Cyclosporine, and Methotrexate," *Am J Gastroenterol*, 1996, 91(3):423-33.

♦ **6-Mercaptopurine (error-prone abbreviation)** *see* Mercaptopurine *on page 985*

Meropenem (mer oh PEN em)

U.S. Brand Names Merrem® I.V.
Canadian Brand Names Merrem®
Generic Available No
Pharmacologic Category Antibiotic, Carbapenem
Use Treatment of intra-abdominal infections (complicated appendicitis and peritonitis); treatment of complicated skin and skin structure infections caused by susceptible organisms
Unlabeled/Investigational Use Febrile neutropenia, urinary tract infections
Contraindications Hypersensitivity to meropenem, any component of the formulation, or other carbapenems (eg, imipenem); patients who have experienced anaphylactic reactions to other beta-lactams
Warnings/Precautions Serious hypersensitivity reactions, including anaphylaxis, have been reported (some without a history of previous allergic reactions to beta-lactams). Has been associated with CNS adverse effects, including confusional states and seizures; use caution with CNS disorders (eg, brain lesions, history of seizures, or renal impairment). Prolonged *(Continued)*

Meropenem *(Continued)*

use may result in fungal or bacterial superinfection, including *C. difficile*-associated diarrhea and pseudomembranous colitis. Use with caution in patients with renal impairment; dosage adjustment required in patients with moderate-to-severe renal dysfunction. Thrombocytopenia has been reported in patients with significant renal dysfunction. Lower doses (based upon renal function) are often required in the elderly.

Adverse Reactions (Reflective of adult population; not specific for elderly)

1% to 10%:

Cardiovascular: Peripheral vascular disorder (<1%)

Central nervous system: Headache (2% to 8%), pain (5%)

Dermatologic: Rash (2% to 3%, includes diaper-area moniliasis in pediatrics), pruritus (1%)

Gastrointestinal: Diarrhea (4% to 5%), nausea/vomiting (1% to 8%), constipation (1% to 7%), oral moniliasis (up to 2% in pediatric patients), glossitis

Hematologic: Anemia (up to 6%)

Local: Inflammation at the injection site (2%), phlebitis/thrombophlebitis (1%), injection site reaction (1%)

Respiratory: Apnea (1%)

Miscellaneous: Sepsis (2%), septic shock (1%)

Overdosage/Toxicology No cases of acute overdosage are reported which have resulted in symptoms. Supportive therapy is recommended. Meropenem and its metabolite are removable by dialysis.

Drug Interactions

Probenecid: May increase meropenem serum concentrations; use caution.

Valproic acid: Meropenem may decrease valproic acid serum concentrations to subtherapeutic levels; monitor.

Stability Dry powder should be stored at controlled room temperature 20°C to 25°C (68°F to 77°F). Meropenem infusion vials may be reconstituted with SWFI or a compatible diluent (eg, NS). The 500 mg vials should be reconstituted with 10 mL, and 1 g vials with 20 mL. May be further diluted with compatible solutions for infusion. Consult detailed reference/product labeling for compatibility.

Injection reconstitution: Stability in vial when constituted (up to 50 mg/mL) with:

SWFI: Stable for up to 2 hours at room temperature and for up to 12 hours under refrigeration.

Sodium chloride: Stable for up to 2 hours at room temperature or for up to 18 hours under refrigeration.

Dextrose 5% injection: Stable for 1 hour at room temperature or for 8 hours under refrigeration.

Infusion admixture (1-20 mg/mL): Solution stability when diluted in NS is 4 hours at room temperature or 24 hours under refrigeration. Stability in D_5W is 1 hour at room temperature and 4 hours under refrigeration.

Mechanism of Action Inhibits bacterial cell wall synthesis by binding to several of the penicillin-binding proteins, which in turn inhibit the final transpeptidation step of peptidoglycan synthesis in bacterial cell walls, thus inhibiting cell wall biosynthesis; bacteria eventually lyse due to ongoing activity of cell wall autolytic enzymes (autolysins and murein hydrolases) while cell wall assembly is arrested

Pharmacokinetics

Distribution: V_d: ~0.3 L/kg in adults; penetrates well into most body fluids and tissues; CSF concentrations approximate those of the plasma

Protein binding: 2%

Metabolism: Hepatic; metabolizes to open beta-lactam form (inactive); not metabolized by same enzyme as imipenem which results in toxic metabolite

Half-life:

Normal renal function: 1-1.5 hours

Cl_{cr} 30-80 mL/minute: 1.9-3.3 hours

Cl_{cr} 2-30 mL/minute: 3.82-5.7 hours

Time to peak tissue concentration: 1 hour following infusion

Elimination: Renal, ~25% as the inactive metabolite

Dosage

Geriatrics & Adults:

Burkholderia pseudomallei (melioidosis) (unlabeled use), *Pseudomonas:* 1 g every 8 hours

Cholangitis, intra-abdominal infections, febrile neutropenia: 1 g every 8 hours

Pneumonia, otitis externa (unlabeled use): 1 g every 8 hours

Liver abscess (unlabeled use): I.V.: 1 g every 8 hours for 2-3 weeks, then oral therapy for duration of 4-6 weeks

Mild-to-moderate infection, other severe infections (unlabeled use): 1.5-3 g/day divided every 8 hours

Skin and skin structure infections (complicated): I.V.: 500 mg every 8 hours; diabetic foot: 1 g every 8 hours

Urinary tract infections, complicated (unlabeled use): I.V.: 500 mg to 1 g every 8 hours

Renal Impairment:
Cl_{cr} 26-50 mL/minute: Administer recommended dose based on indication every 12 hours
Cl_{cr} 10-25 mL/minute: Administer one-half recommended dose every 12 hours
Cl_{cr} <10 mL/minute: Administer one-half recommended dose every 24 hours
Dialysis: Meropenem and its metabolites are readily dialyzable
Continuous arteriovenous or venovenous hemodiafiltration effects: Dose as Cl_{cr} 10-50 mL/minute

Additional Information 1 g of meropenem contains 90.2 mg of sodium as sodium carbonate (3.92 mEq).

Special Geriatric Considerations Adjust dose based on renal function.

Dosage Forms Excipient information presented when available (limited, particularly for generics); consult specific product labeling.

Injection, powder for reconstitution: 500 mg [contains sodium 45.1 mg as sodium carbonate (1.96 mEq)]; 1 g [contains sodium 90.2 mg as sodium carbonate (3.92 mEq)]

Selected References
Ljungberg B and Nilsson-Ehle I, "Pharmacokinetics of Meropenem an Its Metabolites in Young and Elderly Healthy Men," *Antimicrob Agents Chemother*, 1992, 36(7):1437-40.
Wiseman LR, Wagstaff AJ, Brogden RN, et al, "Meropenem. A Review of Its Antibacterial Activity, Pharmacokinetic Properties and Clinical Efficacy," *Drugs*, 1995, 50(1):73-101.

♦ **Merrem® I.V.** *see* Meropenem *on page 987*
♦ **Meruvax® II** *see* Rubella Virus Vaccine (Live) *on page 1436*

Mesalamine (me SAL a meen)

Medication Safety Issues
Sound-alike/look-alike issues:
Mesalamine may be confused with mecamylamine
Asacol® may be confused with Ansaid®, Os-Cal®
Lialda™ may be confused with Aldara™

U.S. Brand Names Asacol®; Canasa™; Lialda™; Pentasa®; Rowasa®

Canadian Brand Names Asacol®; Asacol® 800; Mesasal®; Novo-5 ASA; Pendo-5 ASA; Pentasa®; Quintasa®; Rowasa®; Salofalk®

Index Terms 5-Aminosalicylic Acid; 5-ASA; Fisalamine; Mesalazine

Generic Available Yes: Rectal suspension

Pharmacologic Category 5-Aminosalicylic Acid Derivative

Use Treatment of ulcerative colitis, proctosigmoiditis, proctitis

Contraindications Hypersensitivity to mesalamine, sulfasalazine, salicylates, or any component of the formulation; Canasa™ suppositories contain saturated vegetable fatty acid esters (contraindicated in patients with allergy to these components)

Warnings/Precautions May cause an acute intolerance syndrome (cramping, acute abdominal pain, bloody diarrhea; sometimes fever, headache, rash); discontinue if this occurs. Patients with pyloric stenosis may have prolonged gastric retention of tablets, delaying the release of mesalamine in the colon. Pericarditis or myocarditis should be considered in patients with chest pain; use with caution in patients predisposed to these conditions. Pancreatitis should be considered in patients with new abdominal complaints. Symptomatic worsening of colitis/IBD may occur following initiation of therapy. Oligospermia (rare) has been reported in males. Use caution in patients with impaired renal or hepatic function. Renal impairment (including minimal change nephropathy and acute/chronic interstitial nephritis) has been reported; use caution with other medications converted to mesalamine. Postmarketing reports suggest an increased incidence of blood dyscrasias in patients >65 years of age. In addition, elderly may have difficulty administering and retaining rectal suppositories and decreased renal function; use with caution and monitor.

Canasa™ suppositories contain saturated vegetable fatty acid esters (contraindicated in patients with allergy to these components). Rowasa® enema contains potassium metabisulfite; may cause severe hypersensitivity reactions (ie, anaphylaxis) in patients with sulfite allergies.

Adverse Reactions (Reflective of adult population; not specific for elderly) Adverse effects vary depending upon dosage form. Effects as reported with tablets, unless otherwise noted:
>10%:
Central nervous system: Headache (4% to 35% [capsule 2%; enema 7%; suppository 14%]), pain (14%)
Gastrointestinal: Abdominal pain (3% to 18% [capsule 1%; enema 8%; suppository 5%]), eructation (16%), nausea (13% [capsule 3%; enema 6%; suppository 3%])
Respiratory: Pharyngitis (11%)
(Continued)

Mesalamine (Continued)

1% to 10%:

Cardiovascular: Chest pain (3%), peripheral edema (3%)

Central nervous system: Chills (3%), dizziness (8% [enema 2%; suppository 3%]), fever (6% [capsule 1%; enema 3%; suppository 1%]), insomnia (2%), malaise (2% [enema 3%])

Dermatologic: Rash (6% [capsule 1%; enema 3%; suppository 1%]), pruritus (1% to 3%), acne (2% [suppository 1%]), alopecia (1%)

Gastrointestinal: Colitis exacerbation (3% [suppository 1%]), constipation (5%), diarrhea (7% [capsule 4%; enema 2%; suppository 3%]), dyspepsia (6%), flatulence (3% [enema 6%; suppository 5%]), hemorrhoids (enema 1%), rectal pain (enema 1%; suppository 2%), vomiting (5% [capsule 1%])

Hepatic: ALT increased (1%)

Local: Pain on insertion of enema tip (enema 1%)

Neuromuscular & skeletal: Back pain (7% [enema 1%]), arthralgia (5%), hypertonia (5%), myalgia (3%), arthritis (2%), leg/joint pain (enema 2%)

Ocular: Conjunctivitis (2%)

Respiratory: Flu-like syndrome (3% [enema 5%]), cough increased (2%)

Miscellaneous: Diaphoresis (3%), intolerance syndrome (3%)

Overdosage/Toxicology Symptoms include decreased motor activity, diarrhea, vomiting, and renal function impairment. Treatment is supportive following emesis, gastric lavage, and activated charcoal slurry.

Drug Interactions

Azathioprine, mercaptopurine, thioguanine: Risk of myelosuppression may be increased by aminosalicylates (due to inhibition of TPMT).

Digoxin: Mesalamine may decrease digoxin bioavailability.

Stability

Capsule: Store at controlled room temperature of 15°C to 30°C (59°F to 86°F).

Enema: Store at controlled room temperature. Use promptly once foil wrap is removed. Contents may darken with time (do not use if dark brown).

Suppository: Store at controlled room temperature; do not refrigerate. Protect from direct heat, light, and humidity.

Tablet: Store at controlled room temperature:

Asacol®: 20°C to 25°C (68°F to 77°F).

Lialda™: 15°C to 30°C (59°F to 86°F).

Mechanism of Action Mesalamine (5-aminosalicylic acid) is the active component of sulfasalazine; the specific mechanism of action of mesalamine is unknown; however, it is thought that it modulates local chemical mediators of the inflammatory response, especially leukotrienes, and is also postulated to be a free radical scavenger or an inhibitor of tumor necrosis factor (TNF); action appears topical rather than systemic

Pharmacokinetics

Absorption: Rectal: Variable and dependent upon retention time, underlying GI disease, and colonic pH; Oral: Tablet: ~21% to 28%, Capsule: ~20% to 30%

Protein binding: 43%

Metabolism: Hepatic and via GI tract to acetyl-5-aminosalicylic acid

Half-life elimination: 5-ASA: 0.5-1.5 hours; acetyl-5-ASA: 5-12 hours

Time to peak, serum:

Capsule: Pentasa®: 3 hours

Rectal: 4-7 hours

Tablet: Asacol®: 4-12 hours; Lialda™: 9-12 hours

Excretion: Urine (primarily as metabolites, <8% as unchanged drug); feces (<2%)

Dosage

Geriatrics & Adults:

Treatment of ulcerative colitis: Oral:

Capsule: 1 g 4 times/day

Tablet:

Asacol®: 800 mg 3 times/day for 6 weeks

Lialda™ (once-daily formulation): 2.4"4.8 g/day for up to 8 weeks (treatment only)

Maintenance of remission of ulcerative colitis: Oral:

Capsule: 1 g 4 times/day

Tablet (Asacol®): 1.6 g/day in divided doses

Distal ulcerative colitis, proctosigmoiditis, or proctitis: Rectal: Retention enema: 60 mL (4 g) at bedtime, retained overnight, approximately 8 hours

Active ulcerative proctitis: Rectal: Rectal suppository (Canasa™):

500 mg: Insert 1 suppository in rectum twice daily; may increase to 3 times/day if inadequate response is seen after 2 weeks

1000 mg: Insert 1 suppository in rectum daily at bedtime

Note: Suppositories should be retained for at least 1-3 hours to achieve maximum benefit.

Note: Some patients may require rectal and oral therapy concurrently.

Administration
Oral: Swallow capsules or tablets whole, do not chew or crush. Do not break outer coating of Asacol® or Lialda™ tablets. Lialda™ should be taken with a meal.
Rectal enema: Shake bottle well. Retain enemas for 8 hours or as long as practical.
Suppository: Remove foil wrapper; avoid excessive handling. Should be retained for at least 1-3 hours to achieve maximum benefit.

Monitoring Parameters Renal status (serum creatinine); stool frequency; GI symptoms; sigmoidoscopy

Patient Information Take as directed. Oral: Do not chew or break tablets. Enemas: Shake well before using, retain for 8 hours or as long as possible. Suppository: After removing foil wrapper, insert high in rectum without excessive handling (warmth will melt suppository). Retain suppositories for at least 1-3 hours to achieve maximum benefit. Report severe abdominal pain, unresolved diarrhea, jaundice, severe headache, or chest pain.
Enema and suppository: May cause staining of clothing, undergarments; lubricating gel may be used if needed to assist insertion.
Tablet: Notify prescriber if whole or partial tablets repeatedly are found in stool.

Additional Information Patients hypersensitive to sulfasalazine may tolerate mesalamine rectally; however, use with caution.

Special Geriatric Considerations Use with caution. Elderly may have difficulty administering and retaining rectal suppositories. Given renal function decline with aging, monitor serum creatinine often during therapy.

Dosage Forms Excipient information presented when available (limited, particularly for generics); consult specific product labeling.
Capsule, controlled release:
Pentasa®: 250 mg, 500 mg
Suppository, rectal:
Canasa™: 1000 mg [contains saturated vegetable fatty acid esters]
Suspension, rectal: 4 g/60 mL (7s, 28s) [contains potassium metabisulfite and sodium benzoate]
Rowasa®: 4 g/60 mL (7s, 28s) [contains potassium metabisulfite and sodium benzoate]
Tablet, delayed release [enteric coated]:
Asacol®: 400 mg
Lialda™: 1.2 g

Metaproterenol (met a proe TER e nol)

Related Information
Inhalant Agents *on page 1760*

Medication Safety Issues
Sound-alike/look-alike issues:
Metaproterenol may be confused with metipranolol, metoprolol
Alupent® may be confused with Atrovent®

U.S. Brand Names Alupent®

Canadian Brand Names Apo-Orciprenaline®; Ratio-Orciprenaline®; Tanta-Orciprenaline®

Index Terms Metaproterenol Sulfate; Orciprenaline Sulfate

Generic Available Yes: Excludes inhaler

Pharmacologic Category Beta$_2$-Adrenergic Agonist

Use Bronchodilator in reversible airway obstruction due to asthma or COPD

Contraindications Hypersensitivity to metaproterenol or any component of the formulation; pre-existing cardiac arrhythmias associated with tachycardia

Warnings/Precautions Optimize anti-inflammatory treatment before initiating maintenance treatment with metaproterenol. Do not use as a component of chronic therapy without an anti-inflammatory agent. Only the mildest form of asthma (Step 1 and/or exercise-induced) would not require concurrent use based upon asthma guidelines. Patient must be instructed to seek medical attention in cases where acute symptoms are not relieved or a previous level of response is diminished. The need to increase
(Continued)

Metaproterenol *(Continued)*

frequency of use may indicate deterioration of asthma, and treatment must not be delayed.

Use caution in patients with cardiovascular disease (arrhythmia or hypertension or CHF), convulsive disorders, diabetes, glaucoma, hyperthyroidism, or hypokalemia. Beta-agonists may cause elevation in blood pressure, heart rate, and result in CNS stimulation/excitation. Beta$_2$-agonists may increase risk of arrhythmia, increase serum glucose, or decrease serum potassium.

Immediate hypersensitivity reactions (urticaria, angioedema, rash, bronchospasm) have been reported. Do not exceed recommended dose; serious adverse events including fatalities, have been associated with excessive use of inhaled sympathomimetics. Rarely, paradoxical bronchospasm may occur with use of inhaled bronchodilating agents; this should be distinguished from inadequate response. All patients should utilize a spacer device when using a metered-dose inhaler.

Metaproterenol has more beta$_1$ activity than beta$_2$-selective agents such as albuterol and, therefore, may no longer be the beta-agonist of first choice. Oral use should be avoided due to the increased incidence of adverse effects.

Adverse Reactions (Reflective of adult population; not specific for elderly)
>10%:
  Cardiovascular: Tachycardia (<17%)
  Central nervous system: Nervousness (3% to 14%)
  Endocrine & metabolic: Serum glucose increased, serum potassium decreased
  Neuromuscular & skeletal: Tremor (1% to 33%)
1% to 10%:
  Cardiovascular: Palpitation (<4%)
  Central nervous system: Headache (<4%), dizziness (1% to 4%), insomnia (2%)
  Gastrointestinal: Nausea, vomiting, bad taste, heartburn (≥4%), xerostomia
  Neuromuscular & skeletal: Trembling, muscle cramps, weakness (1%)
  Respiratory: Coughing, pharyngitis (≤4%)
  Miscellaneous: Diaphoresis (increased) (≤4%)

Overdosage/Toxicology Symptoms of overdose include tachycardia, tremor, hypertension, angina, and seizures. Hypokalemia also may occur. Cardiac arrest and death may be associated with abuse of beta-agonist bronchodilators. Treatment includes immediate discontinuation and symptomatic and supportive therapies. Cautious use of beta-adrenergic blocking agents may be considered in severe cases.

Drug Interactions
  Beta-adrenergic blockers (eg, propranolol) antagonize metaproterenol's effects; avoid concurrent use.
  Inhaled ipratropium may increase duration of bronchodilation.
  MAO inhibitors may increase side effects; monitor heart rate and blood pressure.
  TCAs may increase side effects; monitor heart rate and blood pressure.
  Sympathomimetics may increase side effects; monitor heart rate and blood pressure.
  Halothane may increase risk of malignant arrhythmias; avoid concurrent use.

Stability Store in tight, light-resistant container. Do not use if brown solution or contains a precipitate.

Mechanism of Action Relaxes bronchial smooth muscle by action on beta$_2$-receptors with very little effect on heart rate

Pharmacodynamics
  Onset of action: Oral: Bronchodilation occurs within 15 minutes; following inhalation these effects occur within 5 minutes
  Peak effect: Within 1 hour
  Duration: Similar (~3-4 hours) regardless of route administered

Pharmacokinetics
  Absorption: Oral: 40% from GI tract
  Metabolism: In the liver
  Elimination: Via kidneys as metabolites

Dosage
  Geriatrics: Oral: Initial: 10 mg 3-4 times/day; increase as necessary up to 20 mg 3-4 times/day.
  Adults:
    Bronchoconstriction (Asthma, COPD):
      Oral: 20 mg 3-4 times/day
      Inhalation: 2-3 inhalations every 3-4 hours, up to 12 inhalations in 24 hours
      Nebulizer: 5-20 breaths of full strength 5% metaproterenol **or** 0.2 to 0.3 mL 5% metaproterenol in 2.5-3 mL normal saline until nebulized every 4-6 hours (can be given more frequently according to need)

Administration Inhalation: Do not use solutions for nebulization if they are brown or contain a precipitate. Shake inhaler well before using.

Monitoring Parameters Pulmonary function, blood pressure, pulse

Test Interactions Increased potassium (S)

Patient Information Do not exceed recommended dosage - excessive use may lead to adverse effects or loss of effectiveness. Follow instructions accompanying inhaler. If more than one inhalation per dose is necessary, wait at least 1 full minute between inhalations - second inhalation is best delivered after 10 minutes for Alupent®. May cause nervousness, restlessness, insomnia - if these effects continue after dosage reduction, notify physician. Also notify physician if palpitations, tachycardia, chest pain, muscle tremors, dizziness, headache, flushing, or if breathing difficulty persists.

Additional Information Metaproterenol has more beta$_1$ activity than other sympathomimetics such as albuterol and, therefore, may no longer be the beta agonist of first choice

Special Geriatric Considerations Elderly may find it useful to utilize a spacer device when using a metered dose inhaler. Oral use should be avoided due to the increased incidence of adverse effects.

Dosage Forms Excipient information presented when available (limited, particularly for generics); consult specific product labeling.

Aerosol for oral inhalation, as sulfate (Alupent®): 0.65 mg/inhalation (14 g) [200 doses]

Solution for nebulization, as sulfate [preservative free]: 0.4% [4 mg/mL] (2.5 mL); 0.6% [6 mg/mL] (2.5 mL)

Syrup, as sulfate: 10 mg/5 mL (480 mL) [may contain sodium benzoate]

Tablet, as sulfate: 10 mg, 20 mg

♦ **Metaproterenol Sulfate** see Metaproterenol on page 991

Metformin (met FOR min)

Medication Safety Issues

Sound-alike/look-alike issues:

Metformin may be confused with metronidazole

Glucophage® may be confused with Glucotrol®, Glutofac®

U.S. Brand Names Fortamet®; Glucophage®; Glucophage® XR; Glumetza™; Riomet™

Canadian Brand Names Alti-Metformin; Apo-Metformin®; BCI-Metformin; Gen-Metformin; Glucophage®; Glumetza®; Glycon; Novo-Metformin; Nu-Metformin; PMS-Metformin; RAN™-Metformin; ratio-Metformin; Rho®-Metformin; Sandoz-Metformin FC

Index Terms Metformin Hydrochloride

Generic Available Yes: Excludes solution

Pharmacologic Category Antidiabetic Agent, Biguanide

Use Treatment of nonketosis-prone patients with noninsulin-dependent diabetes mellitus who have been unable to control their blood glucose with diet and exercise. Metformin has also been used in combination with a sulfonylurea when a sulfonylurea alone, or metformin and diet have not provided adequate glucose control. Limited information is available on the efficacy of the drug in insulin-dependent diabetes mellitus.

Unlabeled/Investigational Use Treatment of HIV lipodystrophy syndrome

Contraindications Hypersensitivity to metformin or any component of the formulation; renal disease or renal dysfunction (serum creatinine ≥1.5 mg/dL in males or ≥1.4 mg/dL in females or abnormal creatinine clearance from any cause, including shock, acute myocardial infarction, or septicemia); acute or chronic metabolic acidosis with or without coma (including diabetic ketoacidosis)

Note: Temporarily discontinue in patients undergoing radiologic studies in which intravascular iodinated contrast materials are utilized.

Warnings/Precautions [U.S. Boxed Warning]: Lactic acidosis is a rare, but potentially severe consequence of therapy with metformin. Lactic acidosis should be suspected in any diabetic patient receiving metformin who has evidence of acidosis when evidence of ketoacidosis is lacking. Discontinue metformin in clinical situations predisposing to hypoxemia, including conditions such as cardiovascular collapse, respiratory failure, acute myocardial infarction, acute congestive heart failure, and septicemia. Use caution in patients with congestive heart failure requiring pharmacologic management, particularly in patients with unstable or acute CHF; risk of lactic acidosis may be increased secondary to hypoperfusion.

Metformin is substantially excreted by the kidney. The risk of accumulation and lactic acidosis increases with the degree of impairment of renal function. Patients with renal function below the limit of normal for their age should not receive metformin. In elderly patients, renal function should be monitored regularly; should not be used in any patient ≥80 years of age unless measurement of creatinine clearance verifies normal renal function. Use of concomitant medications that may affect renal function (ie, affect tubular secretion) may also affect metformin disposition. Metformin should be suspended in patients with dehydration and/or prerenal azotemia. Therapy should be suspended for any surgical procedures (resume only after normal intake resumed and normal renal function is verified). Metformin should also be temporarily discontinued for (Continued)

Metformin (Continued)

48 hours in patients undergoing radiologic studies involving the intravascular administration of iodinated contrast materials (potential for acute alteration in renal function). It
may be necessary to discontinue metformin and administer insulin if the patient is
exposed to stress (fever, trauma, infection, surgery).

Avoid use in patients with impaired liver function. Patient must be instructed to avoid
excessive acute or chronic ethanol use. Administration of oral antidiabetic drugs has
been reported to be associated with increased cardiovascular mortality; metformin
does not appear to share this risk.

Adverse Reactions (Reflective of adult population; not specific for elderly)
>10%:
  Gastrointestinal: Nausea/vomiting (6% to 25%), diarrhea (10% to 53%), flatulence
    (12%)
  Neuromuscular & skeletal: Weakness (9%)
1% to 10%:
  Cardiovascular: Chest discomfort, flushing, palpitation
  Central nervous system: Headache (6%), chills, dizziness, lightheadedness
  Dermatologic: Rash
  Endocrine & metabolic: Hypoglycemia
  Gastrointestinal: Indigestion (7%), abdominal discomfort (6%), abdominal distention,
    abnormal stools, constipation, dyspepsia/ heartburn, taste disorder
  Neuromuscular & skeletal: Myalgia
  Respiratory: Dyspnea, upper respiratory tract infection
  Miscellaneous: Decreased vitamin B_{12} levels (7%), increased diaphoresis, flu-like
    syndrome, nail disorder

Overdosage/Toxicology Hypoglycemia (10% of cases) or lactic acidosis (~32% of
cases) may occur. Metformin is dialyzable with a clearance of up to 170 mL/minute.
Hemodialysis may be useful for removal of accumulated drug from patients in whom
metformin overdose is suspected. Treatment is supportive.

Drug Interactions
  Drugs which tend to produce hyperglycemia (eg, diuretics, corticosteroids, phenothi-
    azines, thyroid products, estrogens, oral contraceptives, phenytoin, nicotinic acid,
    sympathomimetics, calcium channel blocking drugs, isoniazid) may lead to a loss of
    glycemic control
  Cationic drugs (eg, amiloride, digoxin, morphine, procainamide, quinidine, quinine,
    ranitidine, triamterene, trimethoprim, and vancomycin) which are eliminated by renal
    tubular secretion could have the potential for interaction with metformin by
    competing for common renal tubular transport systems
  Cimetidine increases (by 60%) peak metformin plasma and whole blood concentra-
    tions
  Contrast agents: May increase the risk of metformin-induced lactic acidosis. Discon-
    tinue metformin prior to exposure and withhold for 48 hours.
  Furosemide increased the metformin plasma and blood C_{max} without altering metformin
    renal clearance in a single dose study

Ethanol/Nutrition/Herb Interactions
  Ethanol: Avoid or limit ethanol (incidence of lactic acidosis may be increased; may
    cause hypoglycemia).
  Food: Food decreases the extent and slightly delays the absorption. May decrease
    absorption of vitamin B_{12} and/or folic acid.
  Herb/Nutraceutical: Caution with chromium, garlic, gymnema (may cause hypogly-
    cemia).

Stability Store tablets and oral solution at 15°C to 30°C (59°F to 86°F).

Mechanism of Action Decreases hepatic glucose production, decreasing intestinal
absorption of glucose and improves insulin sensitivity (increases peripheral glucose
uptake and utilization).

Pharmacokinetics
  Distribution: V_d: 654 L (mean)
  Protein binding: Negligible
  Bioavailability: 50% to 60%
  Half-life:
    Normal renal function: 1.5 hours
    Renal dysfunction: 4.9 hours
  Time to reach steady state: 24-48 hours
  Elimination: Unchanged in urine by renal tubular secretion
  Dialyzable

Dosage
  Geriatrics: The initial and maintenance dosing should be conservative, due to the
    potential for decreased renal function. Generally, elderly patients should **not** be
    titrated to the maximum dose of metformin. See Special Geriatric Considerations.

Adults: Management of type 2 diabetes mellitus: Oral: **Note:** Allow 1-2 weeks between dose titrations: Generally, clinically significant responses are not seen at doses <1500 mg daily; however, a lower recommended starting dose and gradual increased dosage is recommended to minimize gastrointestinal symptoms.

Immediate release tablet or solution: Adults ≥17 years: Initial: 500 mg twice daily (give with the morning and evening meals) **or** 850 mg once daily; increase dosage incrementally.

Incremental dosing recommendations based on dosage form:

500 mg tablet: One tablet/day at weekly intervals

850 mg tablet: One tablet/day every other week

Oral solution: 500 mg twice daily every other week

Doses of up to 2000 mg/day may be given twice daily. If a dose >2000 mg/day is required, it may be better tolerated in three divided doses. Maximum recommended dose 2550 mg/day.

Extended release tablet: **Note:** If glycemic control is not achieved at maximum dose, may divide dose and administer twice daily.

Fortamet®: Initial: 1000 mg once daily; dosage may be increased by 500mg weekly; maximum dose: 2500 mg once daily

Glucophage® XR: Initial: 500 mg once daily (with the evening meal); dosage may be increased by 500 mg weekly; maximum dose: 2000 mg once daily

Glumetza™: Initial: 1000 mg once daily; dosage may be increased by 500 mg weekly; maximum dose: 2000 mg once daily

Transfer from other antidiabetic agents: No transition period is generally necessary except when transferring from chlorpropamide. When transferring from chlorpropamide, care should be exercised during the first 2 weeks because of the prolonged retention of chlorpropamide in the body, leading to overlapping drug effects and possible hypoglycemia.

Concomitant metformin and oral sulfonylurea therapy: If patients have not responded to 4 weeks of the maximum dose of metformin monotherapy, consider a gradual addition of an oral sulfonylurea, even if prior primary or secondary failure to a sulfonylurea has occurred. Continue metformin at the maximum dose.

Failed sulfonylurea therapy: Patients with prior failure on glyburide may be treated by gradual addition of metformin. Initiate with glyburide 20 mg and metformin 500 mg daily. Metformin dosage may be increased by 500 mg/day at weekly intervals, up to a maximum metformin dose (dosage of glyburide maintained at 20 mg/day).

Concomitant metformin and insulin therapy: Initial: 500 mg metformin once daily, continue current insulin dose; increase by 500 mg metformin weekly until adequate glycemic control is achieved

Maximum daily dose: Immediate release and solution: 2550 mg metformin; Extended release: 2000-2500 mg (varies by product)

Decrease insulin dose 10% to 25% when FPG <120 mg/dL; monitor and make further adjustments as needed

Renal Impairment: The plasma and blood half-life of metformin is prolonged and the renal clearance is decreased in proportion to the decrease in creatinine clearance. Per the manufacturer, metformin is contraindicated in the presence of renal dysfunction defined as a serum creatinine >1.5 mg/dL in males, or >1.4 mg/dL in females and in patients with abnormal clearance. Clinically, it has been recommended that metformin be avoided in patients with Cl_{cr} <60-70 mL/minute (DeFronzo, 1999).

Hepatic Impairment: Avoid metformin; liver disease is a risk factor for the development of lactic acidosis during metformin therapy.

Monitoring Parameters Urine for glucose and ketones, fasting blood glucose, hemoglobin A_{1c}, and fructosamine. Initial and periodic monitoring of hematologic parameters (eg, hemoglobin/hematocrit and red blood cell indices) and renal function should be performed, at least annually. While megaloblastic anemia has been rarely seen with metformin, if suspected, vitamin B_{12} deficiency should be excluded.

Reference Range Glucose:

Adults: 60-110 mg/dL

Older adults: 100-180 mg/dL

Patient Information May cause lactic acidosis; stop immediately and call physician if unexplained difficulty breathing/rapid breathing, muscle aches, malaise, dizziness or lightheadedness, unexpected stomach discomfort, or unusual sedation occur; avoid excessive alcohol ingestion, either acutely or chronically; take with meals to minimize gastrointestinal symptoms; notify physician if you develop an illness that causes severe vomiting, diarrhea, and/or fever, or if normal fluid intake is significantly reduced; extended release dosage form should be swallowed whole; do not crush, break, or chew

Additional Information May be used in combination with oral sulfonylureas if indicated for glycemic control; gradual dose titration should minimize gastrointestinal side effects. This agent does not cause weight gain and may actually decrease adipose tissue mass; may be preferred for obese patients.

(Continued)

Metformin *(Continued)*

Special Geriatric Considerations Limited data suggest that metformin's total body clearance may be decreased and AUC and half-life increased in elderly patients; presumably due to decreased renal clearance. Metformin has been well tolerated by the elderly but lower doses and frequent monitoring are recommended. In one study of elderly subjects, its effects could not be distinguished from tolbutamide, except for weight loss. The initial and maintenance dosing should be conservative, due to the potential for decreased renal function. Generally, elderly patients should not be titrated to the maximum dose of metformin. Do not use in patients ≥80 years of age unless normal renal function has been established.

Dosage Forms Excipient information presented when available (limited, particularly for generics); consult specific product labeling.

Solution, oral, as hydrochloride:
Riomet™: 100 mg/mL (118 mL, 473 mL) [contains saccharin; cherry flavor]
Tablet, as hydrochloride: 500 mg, 850 mg, 1000 mg
Glucophage®: 500 mg, 850 mg, 1000 mg
Tablet, extended release, as hydrochloride: 500 mg, 750 mg
Fortamet®: 500 mg, 1000 mg
Glucophage® XR: 500 mg, 750 mg
Glumetza™: 500 mg

Selected References

Bailey CJ and Turner RC, "Metformin," *N Engl J Med*, 1996, 334(9):574-9.
Dunn CJ and Peters DH, "Metformin: A Review of Its Pharmacologic Properties and Therapeutic Use in Diabetes Mellitus," *Drugs*, 1995, 49(5):721-49.
Josephkutty S and Potter JM, "Comparison of Tolbutamide and Metformin in Elderly Diabetic Patients," *Diabet Med*, 1990, 7(16):510-4.
Lalau JD, Vermersch A, Hary L, et al, "Type 2 Diabetes in the Elderly: An Assessment of Metformin," *Int J Clin Pharmacol Ther Toxicol*, 1990, 28(8):329-32.

- ◆ **Metformin and Glipizide** *see* Glipizide and Metformin *on page 712*
- ◆ **Metformin and Glyburide** *see* Glyburide and Metformin *on page 717*
- ◆ **Metformin and Rosiglitazone** *see* Rosiglitazone and Metformin *on page 1431*
- ◆ **Metformin and Sitagliptin** *see* Sitagliptin and Metformin *on page 1472*
- ◆ **Metformin Hydrochloride** *see* Metformin *on page 993*
- ◆ **Metformin Hydrochloride and Pioglitazone Hydrochloride** *see* Pioglitazone and Metformin *on page 1269*
- ◆ **Metformin Hydrochloride and Rosiglitazone Maleate** *see* Rosiglitazone and Metformin *on page 1431*

Methadone *(METH a done)*

Related Information
Narcotic / Opioid Analgesics *on page 1763*

Medication Safety Issues
Sound-alike/look-alike issues:
Methadone may be confused with Mephyton®, methylphenidate, Metadate®, and Metadate® ER

U.S. Brand Names Dolophine®; Methadone Diskets®; Methadone Intensol™; Methadose®

Canadian Brand Names Metadol™

Index Terms Methadone Hydrochloride

Generic Available Yes

Pharmacologic Category Analgesic, Opioid

Use Management of moderate-to-severe pain; detoxification and maintenance treatment of opioid addiction (if used for detoxification and maintenance treatment of narcotic addiction, it must be part of an FDA-approved program)

Restrictions C-II

When used for treatment of opioid addiction: May only be dispensed in accordance to guidelines established by the Substance Abuse and Mental Health Services Administration's (SAMHSA) Center for Substance Abuse Treatment (CSAT). Regulations regarding methadone use may vary by state and/or country. Obtain advice from appropriate regulatory agencies and/or consult with pain management/palliative care specialists.

Note: Regulatory Exceptions to the General Requirement to Provide Opioid Agonist Treatment (per manufacturer's labeling):
1. During inpatient care, when the patient was admitted for any condition other than concurrent opioid addiction, to facilitate the treatment of the primary admitting diagnosis.
2. During an emergency period of no longer than 3 days while definitive care for the addiction is being sought in an appropriately licensed facility.

Contraindications Hypersensitivity to methadone or any component of the formulation; respiratory depression (in the absence of resuscitative equipment or in an unmonitored setting); acute bronchial asthma or hypercarbia; paralytic ileus; concurrent use of selegiline

Warnings/Precautions An opioid-containing analgesic regimen should be tailored to each patient's needs and based upon the type of pain being treated (acute versus chronic), the route of administration, degree of tolerance for opioids (naive versus chronic user), age, weight, and medical condition. The optimal analgesic dose varies widely among patients. Doses should be titrated to pain relief/prevention. Patients maintained on stable doses of methadone may need higher and/or more frequent doses in case of acute pain (eg, postoperative pain, physical trauma). Methadone is ineffective for the relief of anxiety.

[U.S. Boxed Warning]: May prolong the QT interval; use caution in patients at risk for QT prolongation, with medications known to prolong the QT interval, or history of conduction abnormalities. QT interval prolongation and torsade de pointes may be associated with doses >200 mg/day, but have also been observed with lower doses. Correct potassium and magnesium abnormalities prior to initiation. May cause severe hypotension; use caution with severe volume depletion or other conditions which may compromise maintenance of normal blood pressure. Use caution with cardiovascular disease or patients predisposed to dysrhythmias.

[U.S. Boxed Warning]: May cause respiratory depression. Use caution in patients with respiratory disease or pre-existing respiratory conditions (eg, severe obesity, asthma, COPD, sleep apnea, CNS depression). Because the respiratory effects last longer than the analgesic effects, slow titration is required. Use extreme caution during treatment initiation, dose titration and conversion from other opioid agonists. Incomplete cross tolerance may occur; patients tolerant to other mu opioid agonists may not be tolerant to methadone. Abrupt cessation may precipitate withdrawal symptoms.

May cause CNS depression, which may impair physical or mental abilities. Patients must be cautioned about performing tasks which require mental alertness (eg, operating machinery or driving). Effects with other sedative drugs or ethanol may be potentiated. Use with caution in patients with depression or suicidal tendencies, or in patients with a history of drug abuse. Tolerance or psychological and physical dependence may occur with prolonged use.

Use with caution in patients with head injury or increased intracranial pressure. May obscure diagnosis or clinical course of patients with acute abdominal conditions. Elderly may be more susceptible to adverse effects (eg, CNS, respiratory, gastrointestinal). Decrease initial dose and use caution in the elderly or debilitated; with hyper/hypothyroidism, morbid obesity, adrenal insufficiency, prostatic hyperplasia, or urethral stricture; or with severe renal or hepatic failure. Use with caution in patients with biliary tract dysfunction; acute pancreatitis may cause constriction of sphincter of Oddi. **[U.S. Boxed Warning]: For oral administration only;** excipients to deter use by injection are contained in tablets.

[U.S. Boxed Warning]: When used for treatment of narcotic addiction: May only be dispensed by opioid treatment programs certified by the Substance Abuse and Mental Health Services Administration (SAMHSA) and certified by the designated state authority. Exceptions include inpatient treatment of other conditions and emergency period (not >3 days) while definitive substance abuse treatment is being sought.

Adverse Reactions (Reflective of adult population; not specific for elderly) Frequency not defined. During prolonged administration, adverse effects may decrease over several weeks; however, constipation and sweating may persist.

Cardiovascular: Bradycardia, peripheral vasodilation, cardiac arrest, syncope, faintness, shock, hypotension, edema, arrhythmia, bigeminal rhythms, extrasystoles, tachycardia, torsade de pointes, ventricular fibrillation, ventricular tachycardia, ECG changes, QT interval prolonged, T-wave inversion, cardiomyopathy, flushing, heart failure, palpitation, phlebitis, orthostatic hypotension

Central nervous system: Euphoria, dysphoria, hallucination, headache, insomnia, agitation, disorientation, drowsiness, dizziness, lightheadedness, sedation, confusion, seizure

Dermatologic: Pruritus, urticaria, rash, hemorrhagic urticaria

Endocrine & metabolic: Libido decreased, hypokalemia, hypomagnesemia, antidiuretic effect, amenorrhea

Gastrointestinal: Nausea, vomiting, constipation, anorexia, stomach cramps, xerostomia, biliary tract spasm, abdominal pain, glossitis, weight gain

Genitourinary: Urinary retention or hesitancy, impotence

Hematologic: Thrombocytopenia (reversible, reported in patients with chronic hepatitis)

Neuromuscular & skeletal: Weakness

Local: I.M./SubQ injection: Pain, erythema, swelling; I.V. injection: pruritus, urticaria, rash, hemorrhagic urticaria (rare)

Ocular: Miosis, visual disturbances

Respiratory: Respiratory depression, respiratory arrest, pulmonary edema

(Continued)

Methadone *(Continued)*

Miscellaneous: Physical and psychological dependence, death, diaphoresis

Overdosage/Toxicology Symptoms include respiratory depression, CNS depression, miosis, hypothermia, circulatory collapse, and convulsions. Treatment includes naloxone 2 mg I.V., with repeat administration as necessary, up to a total of 10 mg, or as a continuous infusion. Nalmefene may also be used to reverse signs of intoxication. Patient should be monitored for depressant effects of methadone for 36-48 hours and other supportive measures should be employed as needed. Forced diuresis, peritoneal dialysis, hemodialysis, or charcoal hemoperfusion have not been established as beneficial for increasing methadone or metabolite elimination.

Drug Interactions Substrate of CYP2C9 (minor), 2C19 (minor), 2D6 (minor), 3A4 (major); **Inhibits** CYP2D6 (moderate), 3A4 (weak)

Agonist/antagonist analgesics (buprenorphine, butorphanol, nalbuphine, pentazocine): May decrease analgesic effect of methadone and precipitate withdrawal symptoms; use is not recommended.

Antiretroviral agents, NNRTI: May decrease levels of methadone, opioid withdrawal syndrome has been reported. Effect reported with efavirenz and nevirapine.

Antiretroviral agents, NRTI: Methadone may increase bioavailability and toxic effects of zidovudine. Methadone may decrease bioavailability of didanosine and stavudine.

Antiretroviral agent, PI: Ritonavir (and combinations) may decrease levels of methadone; withdrawal symptoms have inconsistently been observed, monitor.

CNS depressants (including but not limited to opioid analgesics, general anesthetics, sedatives, hypnotics, ethanol): May cause respiratory depression, hypotension, profound sedation, or coma.

CYP2D6 substrates: Methadone may increase the levels/effects of CYP2D6 substrates. Example substrates include amphetamines, selected beta-blockers, dextromethorphan, fluoxetine, lidocaine, mirtazapine, nefazodone, paroxetine, risperidone, ritonavir, thioridazine, tricyclic antidepressants, and venlafaxine.

CYP2D6 prodrug substrates: Methadone may decrease the levels/effects of CYP2D6 prodrug substrates. Example prodrug substrates include codeine, hydrocodone, oxycodone, and tramadol.

CYP3A4 inducers: CYP3A4 inducers may decrease the levels/effects of methadone. Example inducers include aminoglutethimide, carbamazepine, nafcillin, nevirapine, phenobarbital, phenytoin, and rifamycins.

CYP3A4 inhibitors: May increase the levels/effects of methadone. Example inhibitors include azole antifungals, clarithromycin, diclofenac, doxycycline, erythromycin, imatinib, isoniazid, nefazodone, nicardipine, propofol, protease inhibitors, quinidine, telithromycin, and verapamil.

Desipramine: Levels of desipramine may be increased by methadone.

Pegvisomant: Methadone may diminish the therapeutic effect of pegvisomant.

QT_c interval-prolonging agents (including but may not be limited to amitriptyline, astemizole, bepridil, disopyramide, erythromycin, haloperidol, imipramine, quinidine, pimozide, procainamide, sotalol, and thioridazine): Effect/toxicity increased; use with caution.

Ritonavir: May increase levels/effects of methadone shortly after initiation. May decrease levels/effects of methadone with continued dosing.

Selegiline: Methadone may enhance the serotonergic effects of selegiline. Concurrent use is contraindicated.

Somatostatin: Therapeutic effect of methadone may be decreased; limited documentation; monitor

SSRIs: May increase the levels/effects of methadone; methadone may enhance the serotonergic effects of SSRIs; use caution.

Zidovudine: serum concentrations may be increased by methadone; monitor

Ethanol/Nutrition/Herb Interactions

Ethanol: Avoid ethanol (may increase CNS effects). Watch for sedation.

Herb/Nutraceutical: Avoid St John's wort (may decrease methadone levels; may increase CNS depression). Avoid valerian, kava kava, gotu kola (may increase CNS depression). Methadone is metabolized by CYP3A4 in the intestines; avoid concurrent use of grapefruit juice.

Stability

Injection: Store at controlled room temperature of 15°C to 30°C (59°F to 86°F). Protect from light.

Oral concentrate, oral solution, tablet: Store at controlled room temperature of 15°C to 30°C (59°F to 86°F).

Mechanism of Action Binds to opiate receptors in the CNS, causing inhibition of ascending pain pathways, altering the perception of and response to pain; produces generalized CNS depression

Pharmacodynamics

Onset of action: Parenteral: Within 10-20 minutes; Oral: Within 30-60 minutes

Peak effect: Parenteral: 1-2 hours; Oral: continuous dosing: 3-5 days

Duration of analgesia: Oral: 4-8 hours, increases to 22-48 hours with repeated doses

Pharmacokinetics

Distribution: V_{dss}: 1-8 L/kg

Protein binding: 85% to 90%

Metabolism: Hepatic; N-demethylation primarily via CYP3A4, CYP2B6, and CYP2C19 to inactive metabolites

Bioavailability: Oral: 36% to 100%

Half-life:

Older adults: >36 hours

Adults: 7-59 hours; half-life may be prolonged with alkaline pH; half-life increases with repeated dosing

Time to peak, plasma: 1-7.5 hours

Elimination: In urine (<10% as unchanged drug); increased renal excretion with urine pH <6

Dosage

Geriatrics: Oral, I.M.: 2.5 mg every 8-12 hours; refer to adult dosing.

Adults: Regulations regarding methadone use may vary by state and/or country. Obtain advice from appropriate regulatory agencies and/or consult with pain management/palliative care specialists. **Note:** These are guidelines and do not represent the maximum doses that may be required in all patients. Methadone accumulates with repeated doses and dosage may need reduction after 3-5 days to prevent CNS depressant effects. Some patients may benefit from every 8-12 hour dosing interval for chronic pain management. Doses should be titrated to appropriate effects.

Acute pain (moderate-to-severe):

Opioid-naive: *Oral:* Initial: 2.5-10 mg every 8-12 hours; more frequent administration may be required during initiation to maintain adequate analgesia. Dosage interval may range from 4-12 hours, since duration of analgesia is relatively short during the first days of therapy, but increases substantially with continued administration.

Chronic pain (opioid-tolerant): Conversion from oral morphine to oral methadone:

Daily oral morphine dose <100 mg: Estimated daily oral methadone dose: 20% to 30% of total daily morphine dose

Daily oral morphine dose 100-300 mg: Estimated daily oral methadone dose: 10% to 20% of total daily morphine dose

Daily oral morphine dose 300-600 mg: Estimated daily oral methadone dose: 8% to 12% of total daily morphine dose

Daily oral morphine dose 600-1000 mg: Estimated daily oral methadone dose: 5% to 10% of total daily morphine dose

Daily oral morphine dose >1000 mg: Estimated daily oral methadone dose: <5% of total daily morphine dose.

Note: The total daily methadone dose should then be divided to reflect the intended dosing schedule.

I.V.: Manufacturers labeling: Initial: 2.5-10 mg every 8-12 hours in opioid-naive patients; titrate slowly to effect; may also be administered by SubQ or I.M. injection

Conversion from oral to parenteral dose: Initial dose: Parenteral:Oral ratio: 1:2 (eg, 5 mg parenteral methadone equals 10 mg oral methadone)

Detoxification: *Oral:*

Initial: A single dose of 20-30 mg is usually sufficient to suppress symptoms. Should not exceed 30 mg; lower doses should be considered in patients with low tolerance at initiation (eg, absence of opioids ≥5 days); an additional 5-10 mg of methadone may be provided if withdrawal symptoms have not been suppressed or if symptoms reappear after 2-4 hours; total daily dose on the first day should not exceed 40 mg, unless the program physician documents in the patient's record that 40 mg did not control opiate abstinence symptoms.

Maintenance: Titrate to a dosage which prevents craving, attenuates euphoric effect of self-administered opiates, and tolerance to sedative effects of methadone. Usual range: 80-120 mg/day (titration should occur cautiously)

Withdrawal: Dose reductions should be <10% of the maintenance dose, every 10-14 days

Detoxification (short-term): *Oral:*

Initial: Titrate to ~40 mg/day in divided doses to achieve stabilization. May continue 40 mg dose for 2-3 days

Maintenance: Titrate to a dosage which prevents/attenuates euphoric effects of self-administered opioids, reduces drug craving, and withdrawal symptoms are prevented for 24 hours.

Withdrawal: Requires individualization. Decrease daily or every other day, keeping withdrawal symptoms tolerable; hospitalized patients may tolerate a 20% reduction/day; ambulatory patients may require a slower reduction

(Continued)

Methadone *(Continued)*

Renal Impairment: Cl_{cr} <10 mL/minute: Administer 50% to 75% of normal dose.

Hepatic Impairment: Avoid in severe liver disease.

Administration Oral dose for detoxification and maintenance may be administered in fruit juice or water. Dispersible tablet should not be chewed or swallowed; add to liquid and allow to dissolve before administering. May rinse if residual remains.

Monitoring Parameters Pain relief, respiratory and mental status, blood pressure

Reference Range Prevention of opiate withdrawal: Therapeutic: 100-400 ng/mL (SI: 0.32-1.29 µmol/L); Toxic: >2 mcg/mL (SI: >6.46 µmol/L)

Test Interactions Some quinolones may produce a false-positive urine screening result for opiates using commercially-available immunoassay kits. This has been demonstrated most consistently for levofloxacin and ofloxacin, but other quinolones have shown cross-reactivity in certain assay kits. Confirmation of positive opiate screens by more specific methods should be considered.

Patient Information May cause drowsiness, avoid alcohol and other CNS depressants

Special Geriatric Considerations Because of it's long half-life and risk of accumulation, methadone is difficult to titrate and is not considered a drug of first choice. It should be prescribed only by physicians who are experienced in using it. Elderly may be particularly susceptible to the CNS depressant and constipating effects of narcotics.

Dosage Forms Excipient information presented when available (limited, particularly for generics); consult specific product labeling.

Injection, solution, as hydrochloride: 10 mg/mL (20 mL)

Solution, oral, as hydrochloride: 5 mg/5 mL (500 mL); 10 mg/5 mL (500 mL) [contains alcohol 8%; citrus flavor]

Solution, oral, as hydrochloride [concentrate]: 10 mg/mL (946 mL)

  Methadone Intensol™: 10 mg/mL (30 mL)

  Methadose®: 10 mg/mL (1000 mL) [cherry flavor]

  Methadose®: 10 mg/mL (1000 mL) [dye free, sugar free, unflavored]

Tablet, as hydrochloride: 5 mg, 10 mg

  Dolophine®: 5 mg, 10 mg

  Methadose®: 5 mg, 10 mg [DSC]

Tablet, dispersible, as hydrochloride: 40 mg

  Methadose®: 40 mg

  Methadone Diskets®: 40 mg [orange-pineapple flavor]

Selected References

AGS Panel on Persistent Pain in Older Persons, "The Management of Persistent Pain in Older Persons," *J Am Geriatr Soc*, 2002, 50(6 Suppl):S205-24.

Department of Health and Human Services: Substance Abuse and Mental Health Services Administration, "Opioid Drugs in Maintenance and Detoxification of Opiate Addiction; Final Rule," *Fed Regist*, 2001, 66(11):4075-102.

Ferrell BA, "Pain Management in Elderly People," *J Am Geriatr Soc*, 1991, 39(1):64-73.

Gazelle G and Fine PG, "Methadone for the Treatment of Pain #75," *J Palliat Med*, 2003, 6(4):620-1.

♦ **Methadone Diskets®** *see* Methadone *on page 996*

♦ **Methadone Hydrochloride** *see* Methadone *on page 996*

♦ **Methadone Intensol™** *see* Methadone *on page 996*

♦ **Methadose®** *see* Methadone *on page 996*

♦ **Methaminodiazepoxide Hydrochloride** *see* Chlordiazepoxide *on page 290*

Methazolamide *(meth a ZOE la mide)*

Related Information

Glaucoma Drug Therapy *on page 1758*

Medication Safety Issues

Sound-alike/look-alike issues:

Methazolamide may be confused with methenamine, metolazone

Neptazane® may be confused with Nesacaine®

Canadian Brand Names Apo-Methazolamide®

Generic Available Yes

Pharmacologic Category Carbonic Anhydrase Inhibitor; Diuretic, Carbonic Anhydrase Inhibitor; Ophthalmic Agent, Antiglaucoma

Use Adjunctive treatment of open-angle or secondary glaucoma; short-term therapy of narrow-angle glaucoma when delay of surgery is desired

Contraindications Hypersensitivity to methazolamide or any component of the formulation; marked kidney or liver dysfunction; severe pulmonary obstruction

Warnings/Precautions May impair mental alertness and/or physical coordination. Use with caution in patients with prediabetes or diabetes mellitus; may see a change in glucose control. Use with caution in patients with respiratory acidosis. Use with caution in the elderly; may be more sensitive to side effects.

Chemical similarities are present among sulfonamides, sulfonylureas, carbonic anhydrase inhibitors, thiazides, and loop diuretics (except ethacrynic acid). Use in patients with sulfonylurea allergy is specifically contraindicated in product labeling, however, a risk of cross-reaction exists in patients with allergy to any of these compounds; avoid use when previous reaction has been severe. Discontinue if signs of hypersensitivity are noted.

Adverse Reactions (Reflective of adult population; not specific for elderly)
Frequency not defined.

Central nervous system: Malaise, fever, mental depression, drowsiness, dizziness, nervousness, headache, confusion, seizure, fatigue, trembling, unsteadiness

Dermatologic: Urticaria, pruritus, photosensitivity, rash, Stevens-Johnson syndrome

Endocrine & metabolic: Hyperchloremic metabolic acidosis, hypokalemia, hyperglycemia

Gastrointestinal: Metallic taste, anorexia, nausea, vomiting, diarrhea, constipation, weight loss, GI irritation, xerostomia, black tarry stools

Genitourinary: Polyuria, crystalluria, hematuria, polyuria, renal calculi, impotence

Hematologic: Bone marrow depression, thrombocytopenia, thrombocytopenic purpura, hemolytic anemia, leukopenia, pancytopenia, agranulocytosis

Hepatic: Hepatic insufficiency

Neuromuscular & skeletal: Weakness, ataxia, paresthesia

Miscellaneous: Hypersensitivity

Drug Interactions
Increased toxicity:
May induce hypokalemia which would sensitize a patient to digitalis toxicity
May increase the potential for salicylate toxicity
Hypokalemia may be compounded with concurrent diuretic use or steroids
Primidone absorption may be delayed

Decreased effect: Increased lithium excretion and altered excretion of other drugs by alkalinization of the urine, such as amphetamines, quinidine, procainamide, methenamine, phenobarbital, salicylates

Mechanism of Action Noncompetitive inhibition of the enzyme carbonic anhydrase; thought that carbonic anhydrase is located at the luminal border of cells of the proximal tubule. When the enzyme is inhibited, there is an increase in urine volume and a change to an alkaline pH with a subsequent decrease in the excretion of titratable acid and ammonia.

Pharmacodynamics
Onset of action: 2-4 hours
Peak effect: 6-8 hours
Duration: 10-18 hours

Pharmacokinetics
Absorption: Slow from GI tract
Distribution: Well into tissue
Protein binding: ~55%
Half-life: ~14 hours
Elimination: ~25% excreted unchanged in urine

Dosage
Geriatrics & Adults: Glaucoma: Oral: 50-100 mg 2-3 times/day

Monitoring Parameters Intraocular pressure, serum potassium, serum bicarbonate, serum sodium

Patient Information Take with food; ability to perform tasks requiring mental alertness and/or physical coordination may be impaired; report numbness or tingling of extremities to physician

Special Geriatric Considerations Malaise and complaints of tiredness and myalgia are signs of excessive dosing and acidosis in the elderly.

Dosage Forms Excipient information presented when available (limited, particularly for generics); consult specific product labeling.
Tablet: 25 mg, 50 mg

Methenamine (meth EN a meen)

Medication Safety Issues
Sound-alike/look-alike issues:
Methenamine may be confused with methazolamide, methionine
Urex® may be confused with Eurax®, Serax®

International issues:
Urex®: Brand name for furosemide in Australia

U.S. Brand Names Hiprex®; Mandelamine®; Urex®

Canadian Brand Names Dehydral®; Hiprex®; Mandelamine®; Urasal®; Urex®

Index Terms Hexamethylenetetramine; Methenamine Hippurate; Methenamine Mandelate

Generic Available Yes
(Continued)

Methenamine *(Continued)*

Pharmacologic Category Antibiotic, Miscellaneous

Use Prophylaxis or suppression of recurrent urinary tract infections; urinary tract discomfort secondary to hypermotility

Contraindications Hypersensitivity to methenamine or any component of the formulation; severe dehydration, renal insufficiency, hepatic insufficiency in patients receiving hippurate salt; concurrent treatment with sulfonamides

Warnings/Precautions Methenamine should not be used to treat infections outside of the lower urinary tract. Use with caution in patients with hepatic disease, gout, and the elderly; doses of 8 g/day for 3-4 weeks may cause bladder irritation. Use care to maintain an acid pH of the urine, especially when treating infections due to urea splitting organisms (eg, *Proteus* and strains of *Pseudomonas*); reversible increases in LFTs have occurred during therapy especially in patients with hepatic dysfunction. Prolonged use may result in fungal or bacterial superinfection, including *C. difficile*-associated diarrhea and pseudomembranous colitis. Hiprex® contains tartrazine dye.

Adverse Reactions (Reflective of adult population; not specific for elderly)
1% to 10%:
Dermatologic: Rash (<4%)
Gastrointestinal: Nausea, dyspepsia (<4%)
Genitourinary: Dysuria (<4%)

Overdosage/Toxicology Well tolerated. Treatment includes GI decontamination, if possible, and supportive care.

Drug Interactions
Sulfonamides: Concurrent therapy may result in precipitation of sulfonamides in the urine; concurrent use is contraindicated.
Urinary alkalinizers: Sodium bicarbonate and acetazolamide will decrease effect secondary to alkalinization of urine.

Ethanol/Nutrition/Herb Interactions Food: Foods/diets which alkalinize urine pH >5.5 decrease therapeutic effect of methenamine.

Stability Protect from excessive heat.

Mechanism of Action Methenamine is hydrolyzed to formaldehyde and ammonia in acidic urine; formaldehyde has nonspecific bactericidal action

Pharmacokinetics
Absorption: Readily from GI tract; 10% to 30% of drug will be hydrolyzed by gastric juices unless it is protected by an enteric coating
Metabolism: ~10% to 25% is metabolized in the liver
Half-life: 3-6 hours
Elimination: Occurs via glomerular filtration and tubular secretion with ~70% to 90% of dose excreted unchanged in urine within 24 hours; a urinary formaldehyde concentration >25 mcg/mL is necessary for antibacterial activity

Dosage
Geriatrics & Adults: Urinary tract infection: Oral:
Hippurate: 0.5-1 g twice daily
Mandelate: 1 g 4 times/day after meals and at bedtime
Renal Impairment: Cl$_{cr}$ <50 mL/minute: Avoid use.

Monitoring Parameters Urinalysis, periodic liver function tests in patients, temperature

Test Interactions Increased catecholamines and VMA (U); decreased HIAA (U)

Patient Information Take with ascorbic acid to acidify urine and avoid intake of alkalinizing agents (sodium bicarbonate, antacids); take with food to minimize GI upset; drink plenty of fluids to ensure adequate urine flow; complete full course of therapy; notify physician of rash or if side effects persist or are bothersome

Additional Information Hippurate salt should not be used to treat infections outside of the lower urinary tract.

Special Geriatric Considerations Methenamine has little, if any, role in the treatment or prevention of infections in patients with indwelling urinary (Foley) catheters. Furthermore, in noncatheterized patients, more effective antibiotics are available for the prevention or treatment of urinary tract infections. The influence of decreased renal function on the pharmacologic effects of methenamine results are unknown.

Dosage Forms Excipient information presented when available (limited, particularly for generics); consult specific product labeling.
Tablet, as hippurate (Hiprex®, Urex®): 1 g [Hiprex® contains tartrazine dye]
Tablet, enteric coated, as mandelate (Mandelamine®): 500 mg, 1 g

Selected References
Vainrub B and Musher DM, "Lack of Effect of Methenamine in Suppression of, or Prophylaxis Against, Chronic Urinary Tract Infection," *Antimicrob Agents Chemother*, 1977, 12:625-9.

♦ **Methenamine Hippurate** see Methenamine *on page 1001*
♦ **Methenamine Mandelate** see Methenamine *on page 1001*

Methimazole (meth IM a zole)

Medication Safety Issues
Sound-alike/look-alike issues:
Methimazole may be confused with metolazone
U.S. Brand Names Tapazole®
Canadian Brand Names Dom-Methimazole; PHL-Methimazole; Tapazole®
Index Terms Thiamazole
Generic Available Yes
Pharmacologic Category Antithyroid Agent
Use Palliative treatment of hyperthyroidism, to return the hyperthyroid patient to a normal metabolic state prior to thyroidectomy; control of thyrotoxic crisis that may accompany thyroidectomy
Contraindications Hypersensitivity to methimazole or any component of the formulation
Warnings/Precautions Use with extreme caution in patients receiving other drugs known to cause myelosuppression particularly agranulocytosis, patients >40 years of age; avoid doses >40 mg/day (increased myelosuppression); may cause acneiform eruptions or worsen the condition of the thyroid
Adverse Reactions (Reflective of adult population; not specific for elderly)
Frequency not defined.
Cardiovascular: Edema
Central nervous system: Headache, vertigo, drowsiness, CNS stimulation, depression
Dermatologic: Skin rash, urticaria, pruritus, erythema nodosum, skin pigmentation, exfoliative dermatitis, alopecia
Endocrine & metabolic: Goiter
Gastrointestinal: Nausea, vomiting, stomach pain, abnormal taste, constipation, weight gain, salivary gland swelling
Hematologic: Leukopenia, agranulocytosis, granulocytopenia, thrombocytopenia, aplastic anemia, hypoprothrombinemia
Hepatic: Cholestatic jaundice, jaundice, hepatitis
Neuromuscular & skeletal: Arthralgia, paresthesia
Renal: Nephrotic syndrome
Miscellaneous: SLE-like syndrome
Overdosage/Toxicology Symptoms include nausea, vomiting, epigastric distress, headache, fever, arthralgia, pruritus, edema, pancytopenia, and signs of hypothyroidism. Management of overdose is supportive.
Drug Interactions Inhibits CYP1A2 (weak), 2A6 (weak), 2B6 (weak), 2C9 (weak), 2C19 (weak), 2D6 (moderate), 2E1 (weak), 3A4 (weak)
Beta-blockers: Methimazole may decrease beta-blocker clearance due to changes in thyroid function.
Digoxin: Methimazole may increase digoxin levels due to changes in thyroid function.
CYP2D6 substrates: Methimazole may increase the levels/effects of CYP2D6 substrates. Example substrates include amphetamines, selected beta-blockers, dextromethorphan, fluoxetine, lidocaine, mirtazapine, nefazodone, paroxetine, risperidone, ritonavir, thioridazine, tricyclic antidepressants, and venlafaxine.
CYP2D6 prodrug substrates: Methimazole may decrease the levels/effects of CYP2D6 prodrug substrates. Example prodrug substrates include codeine, hydrocodone, oxycodone, and tramadol.
Theophylline: Methimazole may decrease theophylline clearance due to changes in thyroid function.
Warfarin: Anticoagulant effect of warfarin may be decreased.
Stability Protect from light.
Mechanism of Action Inhibits the synthesis of thyroid hormones by blocking the oxidation of iodine in the thyroid gland, blocking iodine's ability to combine with tyrosine to form thyroxine and triiodothyronine (T_3), does not inactivate circulating T_4 and T_3
Pharmacodynamics
Onset of action: Oral: Within 30-40 minutes
Duration: 2-4 hours
Pharmacokinetics
Half-life: 4-13 hours
Elimination: Renally with ~12% excreted in urine within 24 hours and remainder hepatically metabolized
Dosage
Geriatrics & Adults:
Hyperthyroidism: Oral: Administer in 3 equally divided doses at approximately 8-hour intervals
Initial: 15 mg/day for mild hyperthyroidism; 30-40 mg/day in moderately severe hyperthyroidism; 60 mg/day in severe hyperthyroidism; maintenance: 5-15 mg/day
(Continued)

Methimazole (Continued)

Adjustment: Adjust dosage as required to achieve and maintain serum T_3, T_4, and TSH levels in the normal range. An elevated T_3 may be the sole indicator of inadequate treatment. An elevated TSH indicates excessive antithyroid treatment.

Monitoring Parameters Monitor signs of hypo- and hyperthyroidism, T_4, T_3, TSH, CBC

Patient Information Always take with meals; do not exceed prescribed dosage; take at regular intervals around-the-clock; notify physician or pharmacist if fever, sore throat, unusual bleeding or bruising, headache, or general malaise occurs

Additional Information Periodic blood counts are recommended with chronic therapy. See Warnings/Precautions.

Special Geriatric Considerations The use of antithyroid thioamides is as effective in the elderly as they are in younger adults; however, the expense, potential adverse effects, and inconvenience (compliance, monitoring) make them undesirable. The use of radioiodine due to ease of administration and less concern for long-term side effects and reproduction problems (some elderly males) makes it a more appropriate therapy.

Dosage Forms Excipient information presented when available (limited, particularly for generics); consult specific product labeling.

Tablet: 5 mg, 10 mg, 20 mg

Tapazole® 5 mg, 10 mg

Selected References

Johnson DG and Campbell S, "Hormonal and Metabolic Agents," *Geriatric Pharmacology*, Bressler R and Katz MD, eds, New York, NY: McGraw-Hill, 1993, 427-50.

Raby C, Lagorce JF, Jambut-Absil AC, et al, "The Mechanism of Action of Synthetic Antithyroid Drugs: Iodine Complexation During Oxidation of Iodide," *Endocrinology*, 1990, 126(3):1683-91.

♦ **Methitest**™ *see* MethylTESTOSTERone *on page 1020*

Methocarbamol (meth oh KAR ba mole)

Related Information

Potentially Inappropriate Medications for Geriatrics *on page 1824*

Medication Safety Issues

Sound-alike/look-alike issues:

Methocarbamol may be confused with mephobarbital

Robaxin® may be confused with Rubex®

U.S. Brand Names Robaxin®

Canadian Brand Names Robaxin®

Generic Available Yes: Tablet

Pharmacologic Category Skeletal Muscle Relaxant

Use Treatment of muscle spasm associated with acute painful musculoskeletal conditions; supportive therapy in tetanus

Contraindications Hypersensitivity to methocarbamol or any component of the formulation; renal impairment (injection formulation)

Warnings/Precautions

May cause CNS depression, which may impair physical or mental abilities; patients must be cautioned about performing tasks which require mental alertness (eg, operating machinery or driving). Effects may be potentiated when used with other sedative drugs or ethanol.

Oral: Use caution with renal and hepatic impairment.

Injection: Rate of injection should not exceed 3 mL/minute; solution is hypertonic; avoid extravasation. Use with caution in patients with a history of seizures. Use caution with hepatic impairment. Vial stopper contains latex.

Adverse Reactions (Reflective of adult population; not specific for elderly)

Frequency not defined.

Cardiovascular: Flushing of face, bradycardia, hypotension, syncope

Central nervous system: Drowsiness, dizziness, lightheadedness, convulsion, vertigo, headache, fever, amnesia, confusion, insomnia, sedation, coordination impaired (mild)

Dermatologic: Allergic dermatitis, urticaria, pruritus, rash, angioneurotic edema

Gastrointestinal: Nausea, vomiting, metallic taste, dyspepsia

Hematologic: Leukopenia

Hepatic: Jaundice

Local: Pain at injection site, thrombophlebitis

Ocular: Nystagmus, blurred vision, diplopia, conjunctivitis

Renal: Renal impairment

Respiratory: Nasal congestion

Miscellaneous: Allergic manifestations, anaphylactic reaction

Overdosage/Toxicology Symptoms include cardiac arrhythmias, nausea, vomiting, drowsiness, and coma. Treatment is supportive following attempts to enhance drug elimination. Hypotension should be treated with I.V. fluids and/or Trendelenburg positioning. Dialysis, hemoperfusion, and osmotic diuresis have all been useful in reducing serum drug concentrations. The patient should be observed for possible relapses due to incomplete gastric emptying.

Drug Interactions Increased effect/toxicity with CNS depressants; pyridostigmine (a single case of worsening myasthenia has been reported following methocarbamol administration)

Ethanol/Nutrition/Herb Interactions

Ethanol: Avoid ethanol (may increase CNS depression).

Herb/Nutraceutical: Avoid valerian, St John's wort, kava kava, gotu kola (may increase CNS depression).

Stability

Injection: Prior to dilution, store at controlled room temperature of 20°C to 25°C (68°F to 77°F). Injection when diluted to 4 mg/mL in sterile water, 5% dextrose, or 0.9% saline is stable for 6 days at room temperature. Do **not** refrigerate after dilution.

Tablet: Store at controlled room temperature of 20°C to 25°C (68°F to 77°F).

Mechanism of Action Causes skeletal muscle relaxation by general CNS depression

Pharmacodynamics Onset of action: Oral: Muscle relaxation reportedly occurs within 30 minutes.

Pharmacokinetics

Metabolism: In the liver

Half-life: 1-2 hours

Time to peak serum concentration: ~2 hours

Elimination: Renal

Dosage

Geriatrics: Muscle spasm: Oral: Initial: 500 mg 4 times/day; titrate to response

Adults:

Muscle spasm:

Oral: 1.5 g 4 times/day for 2-3 days (up to 8 g/day may be given in severe conditions), then decrease to 4-4.5 g/day in 3-6 divided doses

I.M., I.V.: 1 g every 8 hours if oral not possible; injection should not be used for more than 3 consecutive days. If condition persists, may repeat course of therapy after a drug-free interval of 48 hours.

Tetanus: I.V.: Initial dose: 1-3 g; may repeat dose every 6 hours until oral dosing is possible; injection should not be used for more than 3 consecutive days

Renal Impairment: Do not administer parenteral formulation to patients with renal dysfunction.

Hepatic Impairment: Specific dosing guidelines are not available. Plasma protein binding and clearance are decreased; half-life is increased.

Administration

Injection:

I.M.: A maximum of 5 mL can be administered into each gluteal region.

I.V.: Maximum rate: 3 mL/minute; should not be used for more than 3 consecutive days; may be administered undiluted. Monitor closely for extravasation. Administer I.V. while in recumbent position. Maintain position 15-30 minutes following infusion.

Tablet: May be crushed and mixed with food or liquid if needed. Avoid alcohol.

Monitoring Parameters Relief of symptoms, mental status; blood pressure, pulse in I.V. administration

Test Interactions May cause color interference in certain screening tests for 5-HIAA using nitrosonaphthol reagent and in screening tests for urinary VMA using the Gitlow method.

Patient Information May cause drowsiness, impair judgment or coordination; avoid alcohol or other CNS depressants; notify physician of rash, itching, or nasal congestion

Special Geriatric Considerations There is no specific information on the use of skeletal muscle relaxants in the elderly. Methocarbamol has a short half-life, so it may be considered one of the safer agents in this class.

Dosage Forms Excipient information presented when available (limited, particularly for generics); consult specific product labeling.

Injection, solution: 100 mg/mL (10 mL) [in polyethylene glycol; vial stopper contains latex]

Tablet: 500 mg, 750 mg

Methotrexate (meth oh TREKS ate)

Medication Safety Issues

Sound-alike/look-alike issues:

Methotrexate may be confused with metolazone, mitoxantrone

MTX is an error-prone abbreviation (mistaken as mitoxantrone)

(Continued)

Methotrexate *(Continued)*

High alert medication: The Institute for Safe Medication Practices (ISMP) includes this medication among its list of drugs which have a heightened risk of causing significant patient harm when used in error.

Errors have occurred (resulting in death) when methotrexate was administered as "daily" dose instead of the recommended "weekly" dose.

International issues:

Trexall™ may be confused with Truxal® which is a brand name for chlorprothixene in Belgium

Trexall™ may be confused with Trexol® which is a brand name for tramadol in Mexico

U.S. Brand Names Rheumatrex®; Trexall™

Canadian Brand Names Apo-Methotrexate®; ratio-Methotrexate

Index Terms Amethopterin; Methotrexate Sodium; MTX (error-prone abbreviation); NSC-740

Generic Available Yes

Pharmacologic Category Antineoplastic Agent, Antimetabolite (Antifolate); Antirheumatic, Disease Modifying

Use Treatment of trophoblastic neoplasms, leukemias, psoriasis, rheumatoid arthritis (RA); treatment of the following types of carcinoma: breast, head and neck, lung, gastrointestinal tract, esophagus, and testes; treatment of lymphomas, osteosarcoma, soft-tissue sarcoma

Unlabeled/Investigational Use Treatment and maintenance of remission in Crohn's disease

Contraindications Hypersensitivity to methotrexate or any component of the formulation; severe renal or hepatic impairment; pre-existing profound bone marrow suppression in patients with psoriasis or rheumatoid arthritis, alcoholic liver disease, AIDS, pre-existing blood dyscrasias

Warnings/Precautions Hazardous agent - use appropriate precautions for handling and disposal.

[U.S. Boxed Warning]: Methotrexate has been associated with acute (elevated transaminases) and potentially fatal chronic (fibrosis, cirrhosis) hepatotoxicity. Risk is related to cumulative dose and prolonged exposure. Monitor closely (with liver function tests, including serum albumin) for liver toxicities. Liver enzyme elevations may be noted, but may not be predictive of hepatic disease in long term treatment for psoriasis (but generally is predictive in rheumatoid arthritis [RA] treatment). With long-term use, liver biopsy may show histologic changes, fibrosis or cirrhosis; periodic liver biopsy is recommended with long-term use for psoriasis and for persistent abnormal liver function tests with RA; discontinue methotrexate with moderate-to-severe change in liver biopsy. Ethanol abuse, obesity, advanced age, and diabetes may increase the risk of hepatotoxic reactions. Use caution with preexisting liver impairment; may require dosage reduction. Use caution when used with other hepatotoxic agents (azathioprine, retinoids, sulfasalazine). **[U.S. Boxed Warning]: Methotrexate elimination is reduced in patients with ascites;** may require dose reduction or discontinuation. Monitor closely for toxicity.

[U.S. Boxed Warning]: May cause renal damage leading to acute renal failure, especially with high-dose methotrexate; monitor renal function and methotrexate levels closely, maintain adequate hydration and urinary alkalinization. Use caution in osteosarcoma patients treated with high-dose methotrexate in combination with nephrotoxic chemotherapy (eg, cisplatin). **[U.S. Boxed Warning]: Methotrexate elimination is reduced in patients with renal impairment;** may require dose reduction or discontinuation; monitor closely for toxicity. **[U.S. Boxed Warning]: Tumor lysis syndrome may occur in patients with high tumor burden;** use appropriate prevention and treatment.

[U.S. Boxed Warning]: May cause potentially life-threatening pneumonitis (may occur at any time during therapy and at any dosage); monitor closely for pulmonary symptoms, particularly dry, nonproductive cough. Other potential symptoms include fever, dyspnea, hypoxemia, or pulmonary infiltrate. **[U.S. Boxed Warning]: Methotrexate elimination is reduced in patients with pleural effusions;** may require dose reduction or discontinuation. Monitor closely for toxicity.

[U.S. Boxed Warning]: Bone marrow suppression may occur, resulting in anemia, aplastic anemia, pancytopenia, leukopenia, neutropenia, and/or thrombocytopenia. Use caution in patients with pre-existing bone marrow suppression. Discontinue therapy in RA or psoriasis if a significant decrease in hematologic components is noted. **[U.S. Boxed Warning]: Use of low dose methotrexate has been associated with the development of malignant lymphomas;** may regress upon discontinuation of therapy; treat lymphoma appropriately if regression is not induced by cessation of methotrexate.

[U.S. Boxed Warning]: Diarrhea and ulcerative stomatitis may require interruption of therapy; death from hemorrhagic enteritis or intestinal perforation has been reported. Use with caution in patients with peptic ulcer disease, ulcerative colitis.

May cause neurotoxicity including seizures, leukoencephalopathy (usually with concurrent cranial irradiation) and stroke-like encephalopathy (usually with high-dose regimens). Chemical arachnoiditis (headache, back pain, nuchal rigidity, fever), myelopathy and chronic leukoencephalopathy may result from intrathecal administration.

[U.S. Boxed Warning]: Any dose level or route of administration may cause severe and potentially fatal dermatologic reactions, including toxic epidermal necrolysis, Stevens-Johnson syndrome, exfoliative dermatitis, skin necrosis, and erythema multiforme. Radiation dermatitis and sunburn may be precipitated by methotrexate administration. Psoriatic lesions may be worsened by concomitant exposure to ultraviolet radiation.

[U.S. Boxed Warning]: Concomitant administration with NSAIDs may cause severe bone marrow suppression, aplastic anemia, and GI toxicity. Do not administer NSAIDs prior to or during high dose methotrexate therapy; may increase and prolong serum methotrexate levels. Doses used for psoriasis may still lead to unexpected toxicities; use caution when administering NSAIDs or salicylates with lower doses of methotrexate for RA. Methotrexate may increase the levels and effects of mercaptopurine; may require dosage adjustments. Vitamins containing folate may decrease response to systemic methotrexate; folate deficiency may increase methotrexate toxicity. **[U.S. Boxed Warning]: Concomitant methotrexate administration with radiotherapy may increase the risk of soft tissue necrosis and osteonecrosis.**

[U.S. Boxed Warnings]: Should be administered under the supervision of a physician experienced in the use of antimetabolite therapy; serious and fatal toxicities have occurred at all dose levels. Immune suppression may lead to potentially fatal opportunistic infections. For rheumatoid arthritis and psoriasis, immunosuppressive therapy should only be used when disease is active and less toxic, traditional therapy is ineffective. Methotrexate formulations and/or diluents containing preservatives should not be used for intrathecal or high-dose therapy. May cause impairment of fertility, oligospermia, and menstrual dysfunction. Toxicity from methotrexate or any immunosuppressive is increased in the elderly.

Adverse Reactions (Reflective of adult population; not specific for elderly)
Note: Adverse reactions vary by route and dosage. Hematologic and/or gastrointestinal toxicities may be common at dosages used in chemotherapy; these reactions are much less frequent when used at typical dosages for rheumatic diseases.

>10%:
Central nervous system (with I.T. administration or very high-dose therapy):
Arachnoiditis: Acute reaction manifested as severe headache, nuchal rigidity, vomiting, and fever; may be alleviated by reducing the dose
Subacute toxicity: 10% of patients treated with 12-15 mg/m^2 of I.T. methotrexate may develop this in the second or third week of therapy; consists of motor paralysis of extremities, cranial nerve palsy, seizure, or coma. This has also been seen in pediatric cases receiving very high-dose I.V. methotrexate.
Demyelinating encephalopathy: Seen months or years after receiving methotrexate; usually in association with cranial irradiation or other systemic chemotherapy
Dermatologic: Reddening of skin
Endocrine & metabolic: Hyperuricemia, defective oogenesis or spermatogenesis
Gastrointestinal: Ulcerative stomatitis, glossitis, gingivitis, nausea, vomiting, diarrhea, anorexia, intestinal perforation, mucositis (dose dependent; appears in 3-7 days after therapy, resolving within 2 weeks)
Hematologic: Leukopenia, thrombocytopenia
Renal: Renal failure, azotemia, nephropathy
Respiratory: Pharyngitis

1% to 10%:
Cardiovascular: Vasculitis
Central nervous system: Dizziness, malaise, encephalopathy, seizure, fever, chills
Dermatologic: Alopecia, rash, photosensitivity, depigmentation or hyperpigmentation of skin
Endocrine & metabolic: Diabetes
Genitourinary: Cystitis
Hematologic: Hemorrhage
Myelosuppressive: This is the primary dose-limiting factor (along with mucositis) of methotrexate; occurs about 5-7 days after methotrexate therapy, and should resolve within 2 weeks
WBC: Mild
(Continued)

Methotrexate *(Continued)*

Platelets: Moderate

Onset: 7 days

Nadir: 10 days

Recovery: 21 days

Hepatic: Cirrhosis and portal fibrosis have been associated with chronic methotrexate therapy; acute elevation of liver enzymes are common after high-dose methotrexate, and usually resolve within 10 days.

Neuromuscular & skeletal: Arthralgia

Ocular: Blurred vision

Renal: Renal dysfunction: Manifested by an abrupt rise in serum creatinine and BUN and a fall in urine output; more common with high-dose methotrexate, and may be due to precipitation of the drug.

Respiratory: Pneumonitis: Associated with fever, cough, and interstitial pulmonary infiltrates; treatment is to withhold methotrexate during the acute reaction; interstitial pneumonitis has been reported to occur with an incidence of 1% in patients with RA (dose 7.5-15 mg/week)

Overdosage/Toxicology Symptoms include nausea, vomiting, alopecia, melena, and renal failure.

Antidote: Leucovorin; administer as soon as toxicity is seen. Administer 10 mg/m^2 orally or parenterally; follow with 10 mg/m^2 orally every 6 hours for 72 hours. After 24 hours following methotrexate administration, if the serum creatinine is ≥50% of premethotrexate serum creatinine, increase leucovorin dose to 100 mg/m^2 every 3 hours until serum methotrexate level is <5 x 10^{-8} M. Hydration and alkalinization may be used to prevent precipitation of methotrexate or methotrexate metabolites in the renal tubules. Toxicity in low dose range is negligible, but may present mucositis and mild bone marrow suppression. Severe bone marrow toxicity can result from overdose. Generally, neither peritoneal nor hemodialysis have been shown to increase elimination. However, effective clearance of methotrexate has been reported with acute, intermittent hemodialysis using a high-flux dialyzer. Leucovorin should be administered intravenously, never intrathecally, for overdoses of intrathecal methotrexate.

Drug Interactions

Acitretin: May enhance the hepatotoxic effect of methotrexate. Avoid concurrent use.

Cholestyramine: May decrease levels of methotrexate.

Corticosteroids: May decrease uptake of methotrexate into leukemia cells. Administration of these drugs should be separated by 12 hours. Dexamethasone has been reported to not affect methotrexate influx into cells.

Cyclosporine: Concomitant administration with methotrexate may increase levels and toxicity of each.

Cytarabine: Methotrexate, when administered prior to cytarabine, may enhance the efficacy and toxicity of cytarabine. Some combination treatment regimens (eg, hyper-CVAD) have been designed to take advantage of this interaction.

Hepatotoxic agents (azathioprine, retinoids, sulfasalazine) may increase the risk of hepatotoxic reactions

Mercaptopurine: Methotrexate may increase mercaptopurine levels. Dosage adjustment may be required.

NSAIDs: Severe bone marrow suppression, aplastic anemia, and GI toxicity have been reported with concomitant therapy. Should not be used during moderate or high-dose methotrexate due to increased and prolonged methotrexate levels (may increase toxicity); NSAID use during treatment of rheumatoid arthritis has not been fully explored, but continuation of prior regimen has been allowed in some circumstances, with cautious monitoring

Penicillins: May increase methotrexate concentrations (due to a reduction in renal tubular secretion). Primarily a concern with high doses of penicillins and higher dosages of methotrexate.

Probenecid: May increase methotrexate concentrations (due to a reduction in renal tubular secretion). Primarily a concern with higher dosages of methotrexate.

Salicylates: May increase the serum concentration of Methotrexate. Salicylate doses used for prophylaxis of cardiovascular events are not likely to be of concern.

Sulfonamides: May increase methotrexate concentrations (due to a reduction in renal tubular secretion). In addition, sulfonamides may reduce folate levels, increasing the risk/severity of bone marrow suppression. Particularly a concern with higher dosages of methotrexate.

Tetracyclines: May increase methotrexate toxicity; monitor

Theophylline: Methotrexate may increase theophylline levels.

Vaccines (live virus): Concurrent use with methotrexate may result in vaccinia infections.

Ethanol/Nutrition/Herb Interactions

Ethanol: Avoid ethanol (may be associated with increased liver injury).

Food: Methotrexate peak serum levels may be decreased if taken with food. Milk-rich foods may decrease methotrexate absorption. Folate may decrease drug response.

Herb/Nutraceutical: Avoid echinacea (has immunostimulant properties).

Stability Store tablets and intact vials at room temperature (15°C to 25°C). Protect from light. Dilute powder with D_5W or NS to a concentration of ≤25 mg/mL (20 mg and 50 mg vials) and 50 mg/mL (1 g vial). Intrathecal solutions may be reconstituted to 2.5-5 mg/mL with NS, D_5W, lactated Ringer's, or Elliott's B solution. **Use preservative free preparations for intrathecal or high-dose administration.** Further dilution in D_5W or NS is stable for 24 hours at room temperature (21°C to 25°C). Reconstituted solutions with a preservative may be stored under refrigeration for up to 3 months, and up to 4 weeks at room temperature. Intrathecal dilutions are stable at room temperature for 7 days, but it is generally recommended that they be used within 4-8 hours.

Mechanism of Action Methotrexate is a folate antimetabolite that inhibits DNA synthesis. Methotrexate irreversibly binds to dihydrofolate reductase, inhibiting the formation of reduced folates, and thymidylate synthetase, resulting in inhibition of purine and thymidylic acid synthesis. Methotrexate is cell cycle specific for the S phase of the cycle.

The MOA in the treatment of rheumatoid arthritis is unknown, but may affect immune function. In psoriasis, methotrexate is thought to target rapidly proliferating epithelial cells in the skin.

In Crohn's disease, it may have immune modulator and anti-inflammatory activity.

Pharmacokinetics

Absorption: Oral: Rapid; well absorbed orally at low doses (<30 mg/m^2); incomplete absorption after large doses; completely absorbed after I.M. injection

Protein binding: 50%; does not achieve therapeutic concentrations in the CSF; sustained concentrations are retained in the kidney and liver

Half-life: 8-15 hours with high doses (>30 mg/m^2) and 3-10 hours with low doses (<30 mg/m^2)

Time to peak serum concentration:

Oral: Within 1-2 hours

Parenteral: 30-60 minutes

Elimination: Small amounts excreted in feces; primarily excreted in urine (90%) via glomerular filtration and active transport

Dosage

Geriatrics: Refer to individual protocols; adjust for renal impairment.

Rheumatoid arthritis/psoriasis: Oral: Initial: 5-7.5 mg/week, not to exceed 20 mg/week

Adults: Refer to individual protocols.

Note: Doses between 100-500 mg/m^2 **may require** leucovorin rescue. Doses >500 mg/m^2 **require** leucovorin rescue: I.V., I.M., Oral: Leucovorin 10-15 mg/m^2 every 6 hours for 8 or 10 doses, starting 24 hours after the start of methotrexate infusion. Continue until the methotrexate level is ≤0.1 micromolar (10^{-7}M). Some clinicians continue leucovorin until the methotrexate level is <0.05 micromolar (5 x 10^{-8}M) or 0.01 micromolar (10^{-8}M).

If the 48-hour methotrexate level is >1 micromolar (10^{-7}M) or the 72-hour methotrexate level is >0.2 micromolar (2 x 10^{-7}M): I.V., I.M, Oral: Leucovorin 100 mg/m^2 every 6 hours until the methotrexate level is ≤0.1 micromolar (10^{-7}M). Some clinicians continue leucovorin until the methotrexate level is <0.05 micromolar (5 x 10^{-8}M) or 0.01 micromolar (10^{-8}M).

Antineoplastic dosage range: I.V.: Range is wide from 30-40 mg/m^2/week to 100-12,000 mg/m^2 with leucovorin rescue

Trophoblastic neoplasms:

Oral, I.M.: 15-30 mg/day for 5 days; repeat in 7 days for 3-5 courses

I.V.: 11 mg/m^2 days 1 through 5 every 3 weeks

Head and neck cancer: Oral, I.M., I.V.: 25-50 mg/m^2 once weekly

Mycosis fungoides (cutaneous T-cell lymphoma): Oral, I.M.: Initial (early stages):

5-50 mg once weekly **or**

15-37.5 mg twice weekly

Bladder cancer: I.V.:

30 mg/m^2 day 1 and 8 every 3 weeks **or**

30 mg/m^2 day 1, 15, and 22 every 4 weeks

Breast cancer: I.V.: 30-60 mg/m^2 Day 1 and 8 every 3-4 weeks

Gastric cancer: I.V.: 1500 mg/m^2 every 4 weeks

Lymphoma, non-Hodgkin's: I.V.:

30 mg/m^2 days 3 and 10 every 3 weeks **or**

120 mg/m^2 day 8 and 15 every 3-4 weeks **or**

200 mg/m^2 day 8 and 15 every 3 weeks **or**

400 mg/m^2 every 4 weeks for 3 cycles **or**

1 g/m^2 every 3 weeks **or**

1.5 g/m^2 every 4 weeks

(Continued)

Methotrexate *(Continued)*

Sarcoma: I.V.: 8-12 g/m^2 weekly for 2-4 weeks

Rheumatoid arthritis: Oral: 7.5 mg once weekly **or** 2.5 mg every 12 hours for 3 doses/week, not to exceed 20 mg/week

Psoriasis: Oral: 2.5-5 mg/dose every 12 hours for 3 doses given weekly **or** Oral, I.M.: 10-25 mg/dose given once weekly

Active Crohn's disease (unlabeled use): Induction of remission: I.M., SubQ: 15-25 mg once weekly; remission maintenance: 15 mg once weekly

Note: Oral dosing has been reported as effective but oral absorption is highly variable. If patient relapses after a switch to oral, may consider returning to injectable.

Renal Impairment:

Cl$_{cr}$ 61-80 mL/minute: Reduce dose to 75%.

Cl$_{cr}$ 51-60 mL/minute: Reduce dose to 70%.

Cl$_{cr}$ 10-50 mL/minute: Reduce dose to 30% to 50%.

Cl$_{cr}$ <10 mL/minute: Avoid use.

Hemodialysis effects: Not dialyzable (0% to 5%)

Supplemental dose is not necessary.

Peritoneal dialysis effects: Supplemental dose is not necessary.

CAVH effects: Unknown

Hepatic Impairment:

Bilirubin 3.1-5 mg/dL or AST >180 units: Administer 75% of dose.

Bilirubin >5 mg/dL: Do not use.

Administration Methotrexate may be administered I.M., I.V., or I.T.; I.V. administration may be as slow push, short bolus infusion, or 24- to 42-hour continuous infusion. Specific dosing schemes vary, but high dose should be followed by leucovorin calcium to prevent toxicity.

Monitoring Parameters For prolonged use (especially rheumatoid arthritis, psoriasis); liver biopsies are recommended in patients with a history of cirrhosis or alcohol abuse or if liver function test increase; WBC and platelet counts every 4 weeks; CBC and creatinine, LFTs every 3-4 months; chest x-ray, pulmonary function tests prior to starting therapy; liver biopsies are recommended in patients with a history of cirrhosis or alcohol abuse or if liver function tests increase

Reference Range Therapeutic levels: Variable; Toxic concentration: Variable; therapeutic range is dependent upon therapeutic approach.

High-dose regimens produce drug levels that are between 10^{-6} Molar and 10^{-7} Molar 24-72 hours after drug infusion

10^{-6} Molar unit = 1 microMolar unit

Toxic: Low-dose therapy: >9.1 ng/mL; high-dose therapy: >454 ng/mL

Patient Information Do not take any new medication during therapy unless approved by prescriber. **Infusion/injection:** Report immediately any redness, swelling, pain, or burning at infusion/injection site. It is very important to maintain adequate hydration (2-3 L/day of fluids) unless instructed to restrict fluid intake and nutrition (small frequent meals may help). Avoid alcohol to prevent serious side effects. You will be more susceptible to infection (avoid crowds and exposure to infection and do not have any vaccinations without consulting prescriber). May cause sensitivity to sunlight (use sunscreen, wear protective clothing, and eyewear); nausea or vomiting (small frequent meals, frequent mouth care, sucking lozenges, or chewing gum may help; if unresolved, contact prescriber); drowsiness, dizziness, numbness, or blurred vision (use caution when driving or engaging in tasks that require alertness until response to drug is known); loss of hair (may be reversible); color change of skin; permanent sterility; or mouth sores (frequent mouth care with soft toothbrush or cotton swabs and frequent rinses may help). Report immediately any rash, excessive or unusual fatigue, or respiratory difficulty. Report rapid heartbeat or palpitations, black or tarry stools, fever, chills, unusual bleeding or bruising, shortness of breath, persistent GI disturbances, diarrhea, constipation, pain on urination or change in urinary patterns, or any other persistent adverse effects.

Additional Information Sodium content: 100 mg injection: 20 mg (0.86 mEq) 100 mg (low sodium) injection: 15 mg (0.65 mEq)

Special Geriatric Considerations Toxicity to methotrexate or any immunosuppressive is increased in the elderly. Must monitor carefully. For rheumatoid arthritis and psoriasis, immunosuppressive therapy should only be used when disease is active and less toxic, traditional therapy is ineffective. Recommended doses should be reduced when initiating therapy in the elderly due to possible decreased metabolism, reduced renal function, and presence of interacting diseases and drugs. Adjust dose as needed for renal function (Cl$_{cr}$).

Dosage Forms Excipient information presented when available (limited, particularly for generics); consult specific product labeling.

Injection, powder for reconstitution [preservative free]: 20 mg, 1 g

Injection, solution: 25 mg/mL (2 mL, 10 mL) [contains benzyl alcohol]

Injection, solution [preservative free]: 25 mg/mL (2 mL, 4 mL, 8 mL, 10 mL)
Tablet: 2.5 mg
  Trexall™: 5 mg, 7.5 mg, 10 mg, 15 mg
Tablet, as sodium [dose pack] (Rheumatrex® Dose Pack): 2.5 mg (4 cards with 2, 3, 4, 5, or 6 tablets each)

Selected References
Egan LJ, Sandborn WJ, Tremaine WJ, et al, "A Randomized Dose-Response and Pharmacokinetic Study of Methotrexate for Refractory Inflammatory Crohn's Disease and Ulcerative Colitis," *Aliment Pharmacol Ther*, 1999, 13(12):1597-604.

Feagan BG, Fedorak RN, Irvine EJ, et al, "A Comparison of Methotrexate With Placebo for the Maintenance of Remission in Crohn's Disease. North American Crohn's Study Group Investigators." *N Engl J Med*, 2000, 342(22):1627-32.

Hutchins LF and Lipschitz DA, "Cancer, Clinical Pharmacology, and Aging," *Clin Geriatr Med*, 1987, 3(3):483-503.

Kaplan HG, "Use of Cancer Chemotherapy in the Elderly," *Drug Treatment in the Elderly*, Vestal RE, ed, Boston, MA: ADIS Health Science Press, 1984, 338-49.

Tugwell P, Pincus T, Yocum D, et al, "Combination Therapy With Cyclosporine and Methotrexate in Severe Rheumatoid Arthritis," *N Engl J Med*, 1995, 333(3):137-41.

♦ **Methotrexate Sodium** see Methotrexate on page 1005

♦ **Methscopolamine Nitrate and Chlordiazepoxide Hydrochloride** see Chlordiazepoxide and Methscopolamine on page 293

Methsuximide (meth SUKS i mide)

Medication Safety Issues
Sound-alike/look-alike issues:
  Methsuximide may be confused with ethosuximide

U.S. Brand Names Celontin®

Canadian Brand Names Celontin®

Generic Available No

Pharmacologic Category Anticonvulsant, Succinimide

Use Control of absence (petit mal) seizures that are refractory to other drugs

Unlabeled/Investigational Use Treatment of partial complex (psychomotor) seizures

Contraindications Hypersensitivity to succinimides or any component of the formulation

Warnings/Precautions Use with caution in patients with hepatic or renal disease. Abrupt withdrawal of the drug may precipitate absence status. Methsuximide may increase tonic-clonic seizures in patients with mixed seizure disorders. Methsuximide must be used in combination with other anticonvulsants in patients with both absence and tonic-clonic seizures. Effects with other sedative drugs or ethanol may be potentiated. Consider evaluation of blood counts in patients with signs/symptoms of infection. Succinimides have been associated with severe blood dyscrasias and cases of systemic lupus erythematosus.

Adverse Reactions (Reflective of adult population; not specific for elderly)
Frequency not defined.
Cardiovascular: Hyperemia
Central nervous system: Ataxia, dizziness, drowsiness, headache, aggressiveness, mental depression, irritability, nervousness, insomnia, confusion, psychosis, suicidal behavior, auditory hallucinations
Dermatologic: Stevens-Johnson syndrome, rash, urticaria, pruritus
Gastrointestinal: Anorexia, nausea, vomiting, weight loss, diarrhea, epigastric and abdominal pain, constipation
Genitourinary: Proteinuria, hematuria (microscopic); cases of blood dyscrasias have been reported with succinimides
Hematologic: Leukopenia, pancytopenia, eosinophilia, monocytosis
Neuromuscular & skeletal: Cases of systemic lupus erythematosus have been reported
Ocular: Blurred vision, photophobia, peripheral edema

Drug Interactions Substrate of CYP2C19 (major); **Inhibits** CYP2C19 (weak)
CNS depressants: Sedative effects and/or respiratory depression may be additive with CNS depressants; includes ethanol, benzodiazepines, barbiturates, opioid analgesics, and other sedative agents; monitor for increased effect
CYP2C19 inducers: May decrease the levels/effects of methsuximide. Example inducers include aminoglutethimide, carbamazepine, phenytoin, and rifampin.
CYP2C19 inhibitors: May increase the levels/effects of methsuximide. Example inhibitors include delavirdine, fluconazole, fluvoxamine, gemfibrozil, isoniazid, omeprazole, and ticlopidine.
Phenobarbital: Methsuximide may increase phenobarbital concentration.
Phenytoin: Methsuximide may increase phenytoin concentration.

Stability Protect from high temperature.
(Continued)

Methsuximide *(Continued)*

Mechanism of Action Increases the seizure threshold and suppresses paroxysmal spike-and-wave pattern in absence seizures; depresses nerve transmission in the motor cortex

Pharmacokinetics
Rapidly demethylated in the liver to the active metabolite N-desmethylmethsuximide
Half-life: 2-4 hours
Time to peak serum concentration: Oral: Within 1-3 hours
Elimination: <1% excreted in urine as unchanged drug

Dosage
Geriatrics & Adults: Anticonvulsant: Oral: 300 mg/day for the first week; may increase by 300 mg/day at weekly intervals up to 1.2 g/day in 2-4 divided doses/day

Monitoring Parameters Monitor serum concentrations, CBC, renal function, LFTs

Reference Range Therapeutic: 10-40 mcg/mL (SI: 53-212 μmol/L); Toxic: >40 mcg/mL (SI: >212 μmol/L)

Patient Information May cause drowsiness; periodic blood test monitoring required; if stomach upset occurs, take with food; do not stop medication without physician's advice; notify physician if skin rash, joint pain, fever, sore throat, dizziness, or blurred vision occur

Special Geriatric Considerations No specific data available for the elderly. This drug is rarely used in the elderly, however, if it is used for partial complex seizure control, monitor closely.

Dosage Forms Excipient information presented when available (limited, particularly for generics); consult specific product labeling.
Capsule: 150 mg, 300 mg

♦ **Methylacetoxyprogesterone** *see MedroxyPROGESTERone on page 965*

Methyldopa (meth il DOE pa)

Related Information
Potentially Inappropriate Medications for Geriatrics *on page 1824*

Medication Safety Issues
Sound-alike/look-alike issues:
Methyldopa may be confused with L-dopa, levodopa

Canadian Brand Names Apo-Methyldopa®; Nu-Medopa

Index Terms Aldomet; Methyldopate Hydrochloride

Generic Available Yes

Pharmacologic Category Alpha-Adrenergic Inhibitor; Alpha$_2$-Adrenergic Agonist

Use Management of moderate to severe hypertension

Contraindications Hypersensitivity to methyldopa or any component of the formulation; active hepatic disease; liver disorders previously associated with use of methyldopa; on MAO inhibitors; bisulfite allergy if using oral suspension or injectable

Warnings/Precautions May rarely produce hemolytic anemia and liver disorders; positive Coombs' test occurs in 10% to 20% of patients (perform periodic CBCs); sedation usually transient may occur during initial therapy or whenever the dose is increased. Use with caution in patients with previous liver disease or dysfunction, the active metabolites of methyldopa accumulate in uremia. Patients with impaired renal function may respond to smaller doses. Elderly patients may experience syncope (avoid by giving smaller doses). Tolerance may occur usually between the second and third month of therapy. Adding a diuretic or increasing the dosage of methyldopa frequently restores blood pressure control. Because of its CNS effects, methyldopa is not considered a drug of first choice in the elderly.

Adverse Reactions (Reflective of adult population; not specific for elderly)
>10%: Cardiovascular: Peripheral edema
1% to 10%:
Central nervous system: Drug fever, mental depression, anxiety, nightmares, drowsiness, headache
Gastrointestinal: Dry mouth

Overdosage/Toxicology Symptoms include hypotension, sedation, bradycardia, dizziness, constipation or diarrhea, flatus, nausea, and vomiting. Hypotension usually responds to I.V. fluids, Trendelenburg positioning, or vasoconstrictors. Treatment is primarily supportive and symptomatic; can be removed by hemodialysis.

Drug Interactions
Barbiturates and TCAs may reduce response to methyldopa.
Beta-blockers, MAO inhibitors, phenothiazines, and sympathomimetics: Hypertension, sometimes severe, may occur.
Iron supplements can interact and cause a significant **increase** in blood pressure.
Lithium: Methyldopa may increase lithium toxicity; monitor lithium levels.

Tolbutamide, haloperidol, anesthetics, and levodopa effects/toxicity are increased with methyldopa.

Ethanol/Nutrition/Herb Interactions Herb/Nutraceutical: Avoid dong quai if using for hypertension (has estrogenic activity). Avoid ephedra, yohimbe, ginseng (may worsen hypertension). Avoid valerian, St John's wort, kava kava, gotu kola (may increase CNS depression). Avoid natural licorice (causes sodium and water retention and increases potassium loss). Avoid garlic (may have increased antihypertensive effect).

Stability Injectable dosage form is most stable at acid to neutral pH. Stability of parenteral admixture at room temperature (25°C) is 24 hours. Stability of parenteral admixture at refrigeration temperature (4°C) is 4 days.

Standard diluent: 250-500 mg/100 mL D_5W.

Mechanism of Action Stimulation of central alpha-adrenergic receptors by a false transmitter that results in a decreased sympathetic outflow to the heart, kidneys, and peripheral vasculature

Pharmacodynamics

Peak hypotensive effect: Oral, parenteral: Within 3-6 hours

Duration: 12-24 hours

Pharmacokinetics

Protein binding: <15%

Metabolism: Intestinally and in the liver with most (85%) metabolites appearing in urine within 24 hours

Half-life: 75-80 minutes

Elimination: Most (85%) metabolites appearing in urine within 24 hours

Dosage

Geriatrics: Oral: Initial: 125 mg 1-2 times/day; increase by 125 mg every 2-3 days as needed. Adjust for renal impairment. See Special Geriatric Considerations.

Adults: Hypertension:

Oral: Initial: 250 mg 2-3 times/day; increase every 2 days as needed (maximum dose: 3 g/day); usual dose range (JNC 7): 250-1000 mg/day in 2 divided doses

I.V.: 250-1000 mg every 6-8 hours; maximum: 1 g every 6 hours

Renal Impairment:

Cl_{cr} >50 mL/minute: Administer every 8 hours.

Cl_{cr} 10-50 mL/minute: Administer every 8-12 hours.

Cl_{cr} <10 mL/minute: Administer every 12-24 hours.

Slightly dialyzable (5% to 20%)

Administration Infuse over 30-60 minutes

Monitoring Parameters Blood pressure (standing and sitting/lying down), weight, symptoms of fluid retention

Reference Range Therapeutic: 1-5 mcg/mL (SI: 4.7-23.7 µmol/L); Toxic: >7 mcg/mL (SI: >33 µmol/L)

Test Interactions Methyldopa interferes with the following laboratory tests: urinary uric acid, serum creatinine (alkaline picrate method), AST (colorimetric method), and urinary catecholamines (falsely high levels)

Patient Information May cause transient drowsiness; may cause urine discoloration; notify physician of unexplained prolonged general tiredness, fever or jaundice; rise slowly from sitting/lying position

Special Geriatric Considerations Because of its CNS effects, methyldopa is not considered a drug of first choice in the elderly. Adjust dose for renal function.

Dosage Forms Excipient information presented when available (limited, particularly for generics); consult specific product labeling.

Injection, solution, as methyldopate hydrochloride: 50 mg/mL (5 mL) [contains sodium bisulfite]

Tablet: 250 mg, 500 mg

- ♦ **Methyldopate Hydrochloride** *see* Methyldopa *on page 1012*
- ♦ **Methylin®** *see* Methylphenidate *on page 1013*
- ♦ **Methylin® ER** *see* Methylphenidate *on page 1013*
- ♦ **Methylmorphine** *see* Codeine *on page 356*

Methylphenidate (meth il FEN i date)

Medication Safety Issues

Sound-alike/look-alike issues:

Methylphenidate may be confused with methadone

Ritalin® may be confused with Ismelin®, Rifadin®

U.S. Brand Names Concerta®; Daytrana™; Metadate® CD; Metadate® ER; Methylin®; Methylin® ER; Ritalin®; Ritalin® LA; Ritalin-SR®

Canadian Brand Names Apo-Methylphenidate®; Apo-Methylphenidate® SR; Biphentin®; Concerta®; PMS-Methylphenidate; Riphenidate; Ritalin®; Ritalin® SR

Index Terms Methylphenidate Hydrochloride

Generic Available Yes: Immediate release tablet, extended release 20 mg tablet

(Continued)

Methylphenidate *(Continued)*

Pharmacologic Category Central Nervous System Stimulant

Use Symptomatic management of narcolepsy

Unlabeled/Investigational Use Treatment of depression (especially older adults or medically ill)

Restrictions C-II

An FDA-approved medication guide must be distributed when dispensing an outpatient prescription (new or refill) where this medication is to be used without direct supervision of a healthcare provider. Medication guides are available at http://www.fda.gov/cder/Offices/ODS/medication_guides.htm.

Contraindications Hypersensitivity to methylphenidate, any component of the formulation, or idiosyncratic reactions to sympathomimetic amines; marked anxiety, tension, and agitation; glaucoma; use during or within 14 days following MAO inhibitor therapy; Tourette's syndrome or tics

Metadate CD™ is contraindicated in patients with severe hypertension, heart failure, arrhythmia, hyperthyroidism, recent MI or angina.

Warnings/Precautions CNS stimulant use has been associated with serious cardiovascular events including sudden death in patients with pre-existing structural cardiac abnormalities or other serious heart problems (sudden death, stroke, and MI in adults). These products should be avoided in patients with known serious structural cardiac abnormalities, cardiomyopathy, serious heart rhythm abnormalities, or other serious cardiac problems that could increase the risk of sudden death that these conditions alone carry. Patients should be carefully evaluated for cardiac disease prior to initiation of therapy. Some products are contraindicated in patients with heart failure, arrhythmias or recent MI. Use of stimulants can cause an increase in blood pressure (average 2-4 mm Hg) and increases in heart rate (average 3-6 bpm), although some patients may have larger than average increases. Use caution with hypertension, hyperthyroidism, or other cardiovascular conditions that might be exacerbated by increases in blood pressure or heart rate. Some products are contraindicated in patients with severe hypertension, hyperthyroidism or angina.

Has demonstrated value as part of a comprehensive treatment program for ADHD. Use with caution in patients with bipolar disorder (may induce mixed/manic episode). May exacerbate symptoms of behavior and thought disorder in psychotic patients; new onset psychosis or mania may occur with stimulant use; observe for symptoms of aggression and/or hostility. Use caution with seizure disorders (may reduce seizure threshold). Use caution in patients with history of ethanol or drug abuse. May exacerbate symptoms of behavior and thought disorder in psychotic patients. **[U.S. Boxed Warning]: Potential for drug dependency exists - avoid abrupt discontinuation in patients who have received for prolonged periods.** Visual disturbances have been reported (rare). Concerta® should not be used in patients with esophageal motility disorders or pre-existing severe gastrointestinal narrowing (small bowel disease, short gut syndrome, history of peritonitis, cystic fibrosis, chronic intestinal pseudo-obstruction, Meckel's diverticulum). Transdermal system may cause allergic contact sensitization, characterized by intense local reactions (edema, papules); sensitization may subsequently manifest systemically with other routes of methylphenidate administration; monitor closely. Avoid exposure of application site to any direct external heat sources (eg, heating pads, electric blankets). Efficacy of transdermal methylphenidate therapy for >7 weeks has not been established.

Adverse Reactions (Reflective of adult population; not specific for elderly)

Transdermal system: Frequency of adverse events as reported in trials of 7-week duration. Incidence of some events reportedly higher with extended use.

>10%:
  Central nervous system: Insomnia (13%)
  Endocrine & metabolic: Appetite decreased (26%)
  Gastrointestinal: Nausea (12%)

1% to 10%:
  Central nervous system: Tic (7%), emotional instability (6%)
  Gastrointestinal: Vomiting (10%), anorexia (5%)
  Respiratory: Nasal congestion (6%), nasopharyngitis (5%)
  Endocrine & metabolic: Weight loss (9%)

All dosage forms: Frequency not defined:
Cardiovascular: Angina, cardiac arrhythmia, cerebral arteritis, cerebral occlusion, hyper-/hypotension, MI, necrotizing vasculitis, palpitation, pulse increase/decrease, tachycardia
Central nervous system: Depression, dizziness, drowsiness, fever, headache, insomnia, nervousness, neuroleptic malignant syndrome (NMS), Tourette's syndrome, toxic psychosis
Dermatologic: Erythema multiforme, exfoliative dermatitis, hair loss, rash, urticaria
Endocrine & metabolic: Growth retardation

Gastrointestinal: Abdominal pain, anorexia, diarrhea, nausea, vomiting, weight loss

Hematologic: Anemia, leukopenia, thrombocytopenic purpura, thrombocytopenia

Hepatic: Liver function tests abnormal, hepatic coma, transaminases increased

Neuromuscular & skeletal: Arthralgia, dyskinesia

Ocular: Blurred vision, visual accommodation disturbance

Renal: Necrotizing vasculitis

Respiratory: Cough increased, pharyngitis, sinusitis, upper respiratory tract infection

Miscellaneous: Accidental injury, hypersensitivity reactions

Overdosage/Toxicology Symptoms include vomiting, agitation, tremors, hyperpyrexia, muscle twitching, hallucinations, tachycardia, mydriasis, sweating, and palpitations. There is no specific antidote for methylphenidate intoxication and the bulk of the treatment is symptom-directed and supportive. Hyperactivity and agitation usually respond to reduced sensory input or benzodiazepines, however, with extreme agitation haloperidol (2-5 mg I.M. for adults) may be required. Hyperthermia is best treated with external cooling measures, or when severe or unresponsive, muscle paralysis with pancuronium may be needed. Hypertension is usually transient and generally does not require treatment unless severe. For diastolic blood pressures >110 mm Hg, a nitroprusside infusion should be initiated. Seizures usually respond to diazepam I.V. and/or phenytoin maintenance regimens. Transdermal system: Remove patch and thoroughly cleanse area; consider that absorption may continue in absence of patch.

Drug Interactions Substrate of CYP2D6 (major); **Inhibits** CYP2D6 (weak)

Antihypertensive agents: Effectiveness of antihypertensive agent may be decreased; use with caution

Carbamazepine: Carbamazepine may decrease the serum concentration of methylphenidate.

Clonidine: Severe toxic reactions have been reported in combined use with methylphenidate.

CYP2D6 inhibitors: May increase the levels/effects of methylphenidate. Example inhibitors include chlorpromazine, delavirdine, fluoxetine, miconazole, paroxetine, pergolide, quinidine, quinine, ritonavir, and ropinirole.

Linezolid: Due to MAO inhibition (see note on MAO inhibitors), concurrent use with methylphenidate should generally be avoided.

MAO inhibitors: Severe hypertensive episodes have occurred with amphetamine when used in patients receiving nonselective MAO inhibitors; methylphenidate may be less likely to interact, or reactions may be less severe; use with caution only when warranted; wait 14 days following discontinuation of MAO inhibitor.

Phenytoin: Serum levels may be increased by methylphenidate (in some patients); monitor

Selegiline: When selegiline is used at low dosages (<10 mg/day), an interaction with methylphenidate is less likely than with nonselective MAO inhibitors (see MAO inhibitor information), but theoretically possible; monitor

Sibutramine: Potential for reactions noted with amphetamines (severe hypertension and tachycardia) appears to be low; use with caution

Tricyclic antidepressants: Methylphenidate may increase serum concentrations of some tricyclic agents; clinical reports of toxicity are limited; dosage reduction of tricyclic antidepressants may be required; monitor

Ethanol/Nutrition/Herb Interactions

Ethanol: Avoid ethanol (may cause CNS depression).

Food: Food may increase oral absorption; Concerta® formulation is not affected. Food delays early peak and high-fat meals increase C_{max} and AUC of Metadate® CD formulation.

Herb/Nutraceutical: Avoid ephedra (may cause hypertension or arrhythmias) and yohimbe (also has CNS stimulatory activity).

Stability

Chewable tablet: Store at room temperature of 20°C to 25°C (68°F to 77°F). Protect from moisture.

Extended release capsule: Store in dose pack provided at 25°C (77°F).

Immediate release tablet: Do not store above 30°C (86°F). Protect from light.

Osmotic controlled release tablet (Concerta®): Store at 25°C (77°F). Protect from humidity.

Solution: Store at room temperature of 20°C to 25°C (68°F to 77°F).

Sustained release tablet: Do not store above 30°C (86°F). Protect from moisture.

Transdermal system: Store at 15°C to 30°C (59°F to 86°F). Keep patches stored in protective pouch. Once tray is opened, use patches within 2 months.

Mechanism of Action Mild CNS stimulant; blocks the reuptake of norepinephrine and dopamine into presynaptic neurons; appears to stimulate the cerebral cortex and subcortical structures similar to amphetamines

Pharmacodynamics

Onset of action: Peak effect:

Immediate release tablet: Cerebral stimulation: ~2 hours

Sustained release tablet: 4-7 hours

Transdermal: ~2 hours

(Continued)

Methylphenidate *(Continued)*

Duration: Immediate release tablet: 3-6 hours; Sustained release tablet: 8 hours

Pharmacokinetics

Absorption:

Oral: Readily absorbed

Transdermal: Absorption increased when applied to inflamed skin or exposed to heat.

Metabolism: Hepatic via de-esterification to minimally active metabolite

Half-life elimination: *d*-methylphenidate: 3-4 hours; *l*-methylphenidate: 1-3 hours

Time to peak: Concerta®: C_{max}: 6-8 hours; Daytrana™: 7.5-10.5 hours

Excretion: Urine (90% as metabolites and unchanged drug)

Dosage

Geriatrics & Adults:

Narcolepsy: Oral: 10 mg 2-3 times/day, up to 60 mg/day

Depression: Oral: Initial: 2.5 mg every morning before 9 AM; dosage may be increased by 2.5-5 mg every 2-3 days as tolerated to a maximum of 20 mg/day. May be divided (eg, 7 AM and 12 noon), but should not be given after noon. Do not use sustained release product.

Note: Discontinue periodically to re-evaluate or if no improvement occurs within 1 month.

Administration

Oral: Do not crush or allow patient to chew sustained release dosage form. To effectively avoid insomnia, dosing should be completed by noon.

Topical: Transdermal (Daytrana™): Apply to clean, dry, non-oily, intact skin to the hip area, avoiding the waistline. Apply at the same time each day to alternating hips. Press firmly for 30 seconds to ensure proper adherence. Avoid exposure of application site to external heat source, which may increase the amount of drug absorbed. If patch should dislodge, may replace with new patch (to different site) but total wear time should not exceed 9 hours. Patch may be removed early if a shorter duration of effect is desired or if late day side effects occur. Wash hands with soap and water after handling. Avoid touching the sticky side of the patch. Dispose of used patch by folding adhesive side onto itself, and discard in toilet or appropriate lidded container.

Monitoring Parameters Blood pressure, heart rate, signs and symptoms of depression, CBC, differential and platelet counts, signs of central nervous system stimulation

Transdermal: Signs of worsening erythema, blistering or edema which does not improve within 24 hours of patch removal, or spreads beyond patch site.

Patient Information Should be taken 30-45 minutes before meals. Concerta® is not affected by food and may be taken with or without meals. Metadate® CD should be taken before breakfast. Metadate® ER should be taken before breakfast and lunch. Last daily dose should be given several hours before retiring; notify physician if headache, palpitations, nervousness, dizziness, or skin rash occurs; do not crush or chew sustained release form

Transdermal: Apply to clean, dry skin, immediately after removing from package. Firmly press in place and hold for 30 seconds. Avoid exposing application site to external heat sources (eg, heating pad, electric blanket, hot tub, heat lamp).

Special Geriatric Considerations Methylphenidate is often useful in treating elderly patients who are discouraged, withdrawn, apathetic, or disinterested in their activities. In particular, it is useful in patients who are starting a rehabilitation program but have resigned themselves to fail; these patients may not have a major depressive disorder; will not improve memory or cognitive function; use with caution in patients with dementia who may have increased agitation and confusion.

Dosage Forms Excipient information presented when available (limited, particularly for generics); consult specific product labeling.

Capsule, extended release, as hydrochloride:

Metadate® CD: 10 mg, 20 mg, 30 mg, 40 mg, 50 mg, 60 mg

Ritalin® LA: 10 mg, 20 mg, 30 mg, 40 mg

Solution, oral, as hydrochloride:

Methylin®: 5 mg/5 mL (500 mL) [grape flavor]; 10 mg/5 mL (500 mL) [grape flavor]

Tablet, as hydrochloride: 5 mg, 10 mg, 20 mg

Methylin®, Ritalin®: 5 mg, 10 mg, 20 mg

Tablet, chewable, as hydrochloride:

Methylin®: 2.5 mg [contains phenylalanine 0.42 mg; grape flavor]; 5 mg [contains phenylalanine 0.84 mg; grape flavor]; 10 mg [contains phenylalanine 1.68 mg; grape flavor]

Tablet, extended release, as hydrochloride: 20 mg

Concerta®: 18 mg, 27 mg, 36 mg, 54 mg [osmotic controlled release]

Metadate® ER, Methylin® ER: 10 mg, 20 mg

Tablet, sustained release, as hydrochloride:

Ritalin-SR®: 20 mg [dye free]

Transdermal system [once-daily patch]:

Daytrana™: 10 mg/9 hours (10s, 30s) [12.5 cm^2, total methylphenidate 27.5 mg]; 15 mg/9 hours (10s, 30s) [18.75 cm^2, total methylphenidate 41.3 mg]; 20 mg/9 hours (10s, 30s) [25 cm^2, total methylphenidate 55 mg]; 30 mg/9 hours (10s, 30s) [37.5 cm^2, total methylphenidate 82.5 mg]

Selected References

Emptage RE and Semla TP, "Depression in the Medically Ill Elderly: A Focus on Methylphenidate," *Ann Pharmacother*, 1996, 30(2):151-7.

Lazarus LW, Moberg PJ, Langsley PR, et al, "Methylphenidate and Nortriptyline in the Treatment of Post-stroke Depression: A Retrospective Comparison," *Arch Phys Med Rehabil*, 1994, 75(4):403-6.

Nissen SE, "ADHD and Cardiovascular Risk," *New Eng J Med*, 2006, 354:1445-8.

Wallace AE, Kofoed LL and West AN, "Double-Blind, Placebo-Controlled Trial of Methylphenidate in Older, Depressed, Medically Ill Patients," *Am J Psychiatry*, 1995, 152(6):929-31.

♦ **Methylphenidate Hydrochloride** *see* Methylphenidate *on page 1013*

♦ **Methylphenobarbital** *see* Mephobarbital *on page 983*

♦ **Methylphenyl Isoxazolyl Penicillin** *see* Oxacillin *on page 1168*

♦ **Methylphytyl Napthoquinone** *see* Phytonadione *on page 1257*

MethylPREDNISolone (meth il pred NIS oh lone)

Related Information

Corticosteroids *on page 1755*

Medication Safety Issues

Sound-alike/look-alike issues:

MethylPREDNISolone may be confused with medroxyPROGESTERone, predniSONE

Depo-Medrol® may be confused with Solu-Medrol®

Medrol® may be confused with Mebaral®

Solu-Medrol® may be confused with Depo-Medrol®

International issues:

Medor® may be confused with Medral® which is a brand name for omeprazole in Mexico

U.S. Brand Names Depo-Medrol®; Medrol®; Solu-Medrol®

Canadian Brand Names Depo-Medrol®; Medrol®; Methylprednisolone Acetate; Solu-Medrol®

Index Terms 6-α-Methylprednisolone; A-Methapred; Methylprednisolone Acetate; Methylprednisolone Sodium Succinate

Generic Available Yes: Sodium succinate injection, tablet

Pharmacologic Category Corticosteroid, Systemic

Use Primarily an anti-inflammatory or immunosuppressant agent in the treatment of a variety of diseases including those of hematologic, allergic, inflammatory, neoplastic, and autoimmune origin

Unlabeled/Investigational Use Treatment of fibrosing-alveolitis phase of adult respiratory distress syndrome (ARDS)

Contraindications Hypersensitivity to methylprednisolone or any component of the formulation; viral, fungal, or tubercular skin lesions; administration of live virus vaccines; serious infections, except septic shock or tuberculous meningitis

Warnings/Precautions Use with caution in patients with thyroid disease, hepatic impairment, renal impairment, cardiovascular disease, diabetes, glaucoma, cataracts, myasthenia gravis, patients at risk for osteoporosis, patients at risk for seizures, or GI diseases (diverticulitis, peptic ulcer, ulcerative colitis) due to perforation risk. Use caution following acute MI (corticosteroids have been associated with myocardial rupture). Because of the risk of adverse effects, systemic corticosteroids should be used cautiously in the elderly in the smallest possible effective dose for the shortest duration. Withdraw therapy with gradual tapering of dose.

May cause hypercorticism or suppression of hypothalamic-pituitary-adrenal (HPA) axis, particularly in patients receiving high doses for prolonged periods. HPA axis suppression may lead to adrenal crisis. Withdrawal and discontinuation of a corticosteroid should be done slowly and carefully. Particular care is required when patients are transferred from systemic corticosteroids to inhaled products due to possible adrenal insufficiency or withdrawal from steroids, including an increase in allergic symptoms. Patients receiving >20 mg per day of prednisone (or equivalent) may be most susceptible. Fatalities have occurred due to adrenal insufficiency in asthmatic patients during and after transfer from systemic corticosteroids to aerosol steroids; aerosol steroids do not provide the systemic steroid needed to treat patients having trauma, surgery, or infections.

Acute myopathy has been reported with high dose corticosteroids, usually in patients with neuromuscular transmission disorders; may involve ocular and/or respiratory muscles; monitor creatine kinase; recovery may be delayed. Corticosteroid use may cause psychiatric disturbances, including depression, euphoria, insomnia, mood (Continued)

MethylPREDNISolone *(Continued)*

swings, and personality changes. Pre-existing psychiatric conditions may be exacerbated by corticosteroid use. Prolonged use of corticosteroids may also increase the incidence of secondary infection, mask acute infection (including fungal infections), prolong or exacerbate viral infections, or limit response to vaccines. Exposure to chickenpox should be avoided; corticosteroids should not be used to treat ocular herpes simplex. Corticosteroids should not be used for cerebral malaria. Close observation is required in patients with latent tuberculosis and/or TB reactivity; restrict use in active TB (only in conjunction with antituberculosis treatment). Prolonged treatment with corticosteroids has been associated with the development of Kaposi's sarcoma (case reports); if noted, discontinuation of therapy should be considered.

Adverse Reactions (Reflective of adult population; not specific for elderly)
Frequency not defined.
Cardiovascular: Edema, hypertension, arrhythmia
Central nervous system: Insomnia, nervousness, vertigo, seizure, psychoses, pseudotumor cerebri, headache, mood swings, delirium, hallucinations, euphoria
Dermatologic: Hirsutism, acne, skin atrophy, bruising, hyperpigmentation
Endocrine & metabolic: Diabetes mellitus, adrenal suppression, hyperlipidemia, Cushing's syndrome, pituitary-adrenal axis suppression, growth suppression, glucose intolerance, hypokalemia, alkalosis, amenorrhea, sodium and water retention, hyperglycemia
Gastrointestinal: Increased appetite, indigestion, peptic ulcer, nausea, vomiting, abdominal distention, ulcerative esophagitis, pancreatitis
Hematologic: Transient leukocytosis
Neuromuscular & skeletal: Arthralgia, muscle weakness, osteoporosis, fractures
Ocular: Cataracts, glaucoma
Miscellaneous: Infections, hypersensitivity reactions, avascular necrosis, secondary malignancy, intractable hiccups

Overdosage/Toxicology Arrhythmias and cardiovascular collapse are possible with rapid intravenous infusion of high dose methylprednisolone. Symptoms include cushingoid appearance (systemic), muscle weakness (systemic), and osteoporosis (systemic) - all with long-term use only. When consumed in excessive quantities for prolonged periods, systemic hypercorticism and adrenal suppression may occur; in those cases, discontinuation and withdrawal of the corticosteroid should be done judiciously.

Drug Interactions Substrate of CYP3A4 (major); **Inhibits** CYP2C8 (weak), 3A4 (weak)

Aminoglutethimide: May reduce the serum levels/effects of corticosteroids; likely via induction of microsomal isoenzymes.
Amphotericin: Corticosteroids may increase the hypokalemic effects of amphotericin B; monitor.
Antacids: May decrease the absorption of corticosteroids; separate administration by 2 hours.
Antidiabetic agents: Corticosteroids may decrease the hypoglycemic effects of antidiabetic agents; monitor.
Anticholinesterases: Concurrent use may lead to severe weakness in patients with myasthenia gravis.
Aprepitant: May increase the serum levels/effects of corticosteroids; monitor.
Antifungal agents (azole): May increase the serum levels/effects of corticosteroids; monitor.
Barbiturates: May decrease the levels/effects of corticosteroids.
Bile acid sequestrants: May reduce the absorption of corticosteroids; separate administration by 2 hours.
Calcium channel blockers (nondihydropyridine): May increase the serum levels/effects of corticosteroids; monitor.
Cyclosporine: Corticosteroids may increase the serum levels/effects of cyclosporine. In addition, cyclosporine may increase levels of corticosteroids.
CYP3A4 Inducers may decrease the levels/effects of corticosteroids. Example inducers include aminoglutethimide, carbamazepine, nafcillin, nevirapine, phenobarbital, phenytoin, and rifamycins.
CYP3A4 Inhibitors may increase the levels/effects of corticosteroids. Example inhibitors include azole antifungals, clarithromycin, diclofenac, doxycycline, erythromycin, imatinib, isoniazid, nefazodone, nicardipine, propofol, protease inhibitors, quinidine, telithromycin, and verapamil.
Diuretics, potassium-wasting (loop or thiazide): Hypokalemic effects may be increased by corticosteroids; monitor.
Estrogens: May increase the serum levels/effects of corticosteroids; monitor.
Fluoroquinolones: Concurrent use may increase the risk of tendinopathies (including tendonitis and rupture), particularly in elderly patients (overall incidence rare)
Isoniazid: Serum levels/effects may be decreased by corticosteroids.
Macrolide antibiotics: May increase the serum levels/effects of corticosteroids.

Neuromuscular-blocking agents: Concurrent use with corticosteroids may increase the risk of myopathy.

Nonsteroidal anti-inflammatory drugs (NSAIDs): Concurrent use with corticosteroids may lead to an increased incidence of gastrointestinal adverse effects; use caution.

Salicylates: Salicylates may increase the gastrointestinal adverse effects of corticosteroids.

Vaccine (dead organism): Corticosteroids may decrease the effect of vaccines (dead organisms). In patients receiving high doses of systemic corticosteroids for ≥14 days, wait at least 1 month between discontinuing steroid therapy and administering immunization.

Vaccine (live organism): Corticosteroids may increase the risk of vaccinal infection. The use of live vaccines is contraindicated in immunosuppressed patients.

Warfarin: Corticosteroids may increase the anticoagulant effects of warfarin; monitor INR.

Ethanol/Nutrition/Herb Interactions

Ethanol: Avoid ethanol (may increase gastric mucosal irritation).

Food: Methylprednisolone interferes with calcium absorption. Limit caffeine.

Herb/Nutraceutical: St John's wort may decrease methylprednisolone levels. Avoid cat's claw, echinacea (have immunostimulant properties).

Stability

Intact vials of methylprednisolone sodium succinate should be stored at controlled room temperature.

Reconstituted solutions of methylprednisolone sodium succinate should be stored at room temperature (15°C to 30°C) and used within 48 hours.

Stability of parenteral admixture at room temperature (25°C) and at refrigeration temperature (4°C) is 48 hours.

Standard diluent (Solu-Medrol®): 40 mg/50 mL D_5W; 125 mg/50 mL D_5W.

Minimum volume (Solu-Medrol®): 50 mL D_5W.

Mechanism of Action In a tissue-specific manner, corticosteroids regulate gene expression subsequent to binding specific intracellular receptors and translocation into the nucleus. Corticosteroids exert a wide array of physiologic effects including modulation of carbohydrate, protein, and lipid metabolism and maintenance of fluid and electrolyte homeostasis. Moreover cardiovascular, immunologic, musculoskeletal, endocrine, and neurologic physiology are influenced by corticosteroids. Decreases inflammation by suppression of migration of polymorphonuclear leukocytes and reversal of increased capillary permeability.

Pharmacodynamics Time to obtain peak effects and the duration of these effects is dependent upon the route of administration. See table.

Methylprednisolone

Route	Peak Effect	Duration
P.O.	1-2 h	30-36 h
I.M.	4-8 d	1-4 wk
Intra-articular	1 wk	1-5 wk

Pharmacokinetics A single dose study found a slower methylprednisolone clearance in older volunteers compared to younger ones.

Distribution: V_d: 0.7-1.5 L/kg

Half-life: 3-3.5 hours; clearance reduced in obese patients

Dosage

Geriatrics: Only sodium succinate salt may be given I.V. Use the lowest effective adult dose.

Adults: Only sodium succinate may be given I.V.; methylprednisolone sodium succinate is highly soluble and has a rapid effect by I.M. and I.V. routes. Methylprednisolone acetate has a low solubility and has a sustained I.M. effect.

Anti-inflammatory or immunosuppressive:

Oral: 2-60 mg/day in 1-4 divided doses to start, followed by gradual reduction in dosage to the lowest possible level consistent with maintaining an adequate clinical response.

I.M. (sodium succinate): 10-80 mg/day once daily

I.M. (acetate): 10-80 mg every 1-2 weeks

I.V. (sodium succinate): 10-40 mg over a period of several minutes and repeated I.V. or I.M. at intervals depending on clinical response; when high dosages are needed, give 30 mg/kg over a period ≥30 minutes and may be repeated every 4-6 hours for 48 hours.

Status asthmaticus: I.V. (sodium succinate): Loading dose: 2 mg/kg/dose, then 0.5-1 mg/kg/dose every 6 hours for up to 5 days

Acute spinal cord injury: I.V. (sodium succinate): 30 mg/kg over 15 minutes, followed in 45 minutes by a continuous infusion of 5.4 mg/kg/hour for 23 hours

(Continued)

MethylPREDNISolone *(Continued)*

Lupus nephritis: High-dose "pulse" therapy: I.V. (sodium succinate): 1 g/day for 3 days

Aplastic anemia: I.V. (sodium succinate): 1 mg/kg/day or 40 mg/day (whichever dose is higher), for 4 days. After 4 days, change to oral and continue until day 10 or until symptoms of serum sickness resolve, then rapidly reduce over approximately 2 weeks.

Pneumonia in AIDS patients due to *Pneumocystis:* I.V.: 40-60 mg every 6 hours for 7-10 days

Arthritis: Intra-articular (acetate): Administer every 1-5 weeks.
Large joints: 20-80 mg
Small joints: 4-10 mg

Intralesional (acetate): 20-60 mg every 1-5 weeks

Renal Impairment:
Hemodialysis effects: Slightly dialyzable (5% to 20%)
Administer dose posthemodialysis.

Administration Succinate: I.V. push over 1-15 minutes; intermittent infusion over 15-60 minutes; maximum concentration: IVP: 125 mg/mL

Monitoring Parameters Blood pressure, blood glucose, electrolytes, symptoms of fluid retention

Test Interactions Interferes with skin tests

Patient Information Do not discontinue or decrease the drug without contacting your physician; carry an identification card or bracelet advising that you are on steroids; may take with meals to decrease GI upset; apply topical product sparingly

Additional Information Sodium content of 1 g sodium succinate injection: 2.01 mEq; 53 mg of sodium succinate salt is equivalent to 40 mg of methylprednisolone base

Methylprednisolone acetate: Depo-Medrol®; methylprednisolone sodium succinate: Solu-Medrol®

Withdrawal/tapering of therapy: Corticosteroid tapering following short-term use is limited primarily by the need to control the underlying disease state; tapering may be accomplished over a period of days. Following longer-term use, tapering over weeks to months may be necessary to avoid signs and symptoms of adrenal insufficiency and to allow recovery of the HPA axis. Testing of HPA axis responsiveness may be of value in selected patients. Subtle deficits in HPA response may persist for months after discontinuation of therapy, and may require supplemental dosing during periods of acute illness or surgical stress.

Special Geriatric Considerations Because of the risk of adverse effects, systemic corticosteroids should be used cautiously in the elderly, in the smallest possible dose, and for the shortest possible time.

Dosage Forms Excipient information presented when available (limited, particularly for generics); consult specific product labeling.

Injection, powder for reconstitution, as sodium succinate: 125 mg [strength expressed as base]
Solu-Medrol®: 40 mg, 125 mg, 500 mg, 1 g, 2 g [packaged with diluent; diluent contains benzyl alcohol; strength expressed as base]
Solu-Medrol®: 500 mg, 1 g

Injection, suspension, as acetate (Depo-Medrol®): 20 mg/mL (5 mL); 40 mg/mL (5 mL); 80 mg/mL (5 mL) [contains benzyl alcohol; strength expressed as base]

Injection, suspension, as acetate [single-dose vial] (Depo-Medrol®): 40 mg/mL (1 mL, 10 mL); 80 mg/mL (1 mL)

Tablet: 4 mg
Medrol®: 2 mg, 4 mg, 8 mg, 16 mg, 32 mg

Tablet, dose-pack: 4 mg (21s)
Medrol® Dosepack™: 4 mg (21s)

Selected References

Tornatore KM, Logue G, Venuto RC, et al, "Pharmacokinetics of Methylprednisolone in Elderly and Young Healthy Males," *J Am Geriatr Soc*, 1994, 42(10):1118-22.

◆ **6-α-Methylprednisolone** *see* MethylPREDNISolone *on page 1017*

◆ **Methylprednisolone Acetate** *see* MethylPREDNISolone *on page 1017*

◆ **Methylprednisolone Sodium Succinate** *see* MethylPREDNISolone *on page 1017*

MethylTESTOSTERone *(meth il tes TOS te rone)*

Related Information
Potentially Inappropriate Medications for Geriatrics *on page 1824*

Medication Safety Issues
Sound-alike/look-alike issues:
MethylTESTOSTERone may be confused with medroxyPROGESTERone
Virilon® may be confused with Verelan®

U.S. Brand Names Android®; Methitest™; Testred®; Virilon®

Generic Available No

Pharmacologic Category Androgen

Use

Male: Treatment of hypogonadism, impotence, climacteric symptoms

Female: Palliative treatment of metastatic breast cancer

Restrictions C-III

Contraindications Hypersensitivity to methyltestosterone or any component of the formulation; in males, known or suspected carcinoma of the breast or the prostate

Warnings/Precautions Prolonged use and/or high doses may cause peliosis hepatis or liver cell tumors which may not be apparent until liver failure or intra-abdominal hemorrhage develops. Discontinue in case of cholestatic hepatitis with jaundice or abnormal liver function tests. Use with caution in patients with breast cancer; may cause hypercalcemia by stimulating osteolysis. Use with caution in patients with diabetes mellitus; monitor carefully. Use with caution in patients with conditions influenced by edema (eg, cardiovascular disease, migraine, seizure disorder, renal impairment); may cause fluid retention. Discontinue with evidence of mild virilization in women. Use with caution in hepatic impairment. Use with caution in elderly. Product may contain tartrazine.

Adverse Reactions (Reflective of adult population; not specific for elderly)

Frequency not defined.

Male: Virilism, priapism, prostatic hyperplasia, prostatic carcinoma, impotence, testicular atrophy, gynecomastia

Female: Virilism, menstrual problems (amenorrhea), breast soreness, hirsutism (increase in pubic hair growth), atrophy

Cardiovascular: Edema

Central nervous system: Headache, anxiety, depression

Dermatologic: Acne, "male pattern" baldness, seborrhea

Endocrine & metabolic: Hypercalcemia, hypercholesterolemia

Gastrointestinal: GI irritation, nausea, vomiting

Hematologic: Leukopenia, polycythemia

Hepatic: Hepatic dysfunction, hepatic necrosis, cholestatic hepatitis

Miscellaneous: Hypersensitivity reactions

Overdosage/Toxicology Abnormal liver function tests.

Drug Interactions

Anticoagulants, oral: May have increased effect; monitor INR

Cyclosporine: Toxicity may occur; avoid concurrent use

Hypoglycemics, oral: May have increased effect; monitor blood glucose

Mechanism of Action Stimulates receptors in organs and tissues to promote growth and development of male sex organs and maintains secondary sex characteristics in androgen-deficient males

Pharmacokinetics

Absorption: From GI tract and oral mucosa

Metabolism: Hepatic

Elimination: In urine

Dosage

Geriatrics & Adults: Note: Buccal absorption produces twice the androgenic activity of oral tablets.

Hypogonadism; impotence and climacteric symptoms (Males):

Oral: 10-40 mg/day

Buccal: 5-25 mg/day

Breast pain/engorgement (Female):

Oral: 80 mg/day for 3-5 days

Buccal: 40 mg/day for 3-5 days

Breast cancer (Female):

Oral: 50-200 mg/day

Buccal: 25-100 mg/day

Monitoring Parameters Cholesterol, PSA, electrolyte changes

Patient Information Men should report overly frequent or persistent penile erections; women should report menstrual irregularities; all patients should report persistent GI distress, diarrhea, or jaundice; buccal tablet should not be chewed or swallowed

Special Geriatric Considerations Since elderly males have prostate changes with age, it would be best to obtain a PSA initially and periodically. Retention of sodium and water could be a problem in patients with CHF and hypertension.

Dosage Forms Excipient information presented when available (limited, particularly for generics); consult specific product labeling.

Capsule (Android®, Testred®, Virilon®): 10 mg

Tablet (Methitest™): 10 mg

Metipranolol (met i PRAN oh lol)

Related Information
Glaucoma Drug Therapy *on page 1758*

Medication Safety Issues
Sound-alike/look-alike issues:
Metipranolol may be confused with metaproterenol

International issues:
Betanol® [Monaco] may be confused with Beta-Val® which is a brand name for betamethasone in the U.S.
Betanol® [Monaco] may be confused with Patanol® which is a brand name for olopatadine in the U.S.
Betanol® [Monaco] may be confused with Betimol® which is a brand name for timolol in the U.S.

U.S. Brand Names OptiPranolol®
Canadian Brand Names OptiPranolol®
Index Terms Metipranolol Hydrochloride
Generic Available Yes
Pharmacologic Category Beta-Adrenergic Blocker, Nonselective; Ophthalmic Agent, Antiglaucoma
Use Treatment of elevated intraocular pressure in patients with chronic open-angle glaucoma
Contraindications Hypersensitivity to metipranolol or any component of the formulation; bronchial asthma, sinus bradycardia, second- and third-degree AV block, cardiac failure, cardiogenic shock
Warnings/Precautions Consider pre-existing conditions such as sick sinus syndrome before initiating. Use with caution in patients with bronchospastic disease, cardiac failure, diabetes mellitus, myasthenia gravis, peripheral vascular disease, or psychiatric disease. Systemic absorption and adverse effects may occur with ophthalmic use, including bradycardia and/or hypotension. Beta-blocker therapy should not be withdrawn abruptly (particularly in patients with CAD), but gradually tapered to avoid acute tachycardia, hypertension, and/or ischemia. Some products may contain benzalkonium chloride which may be absorbed by soft contact lenses; do not administer while wearing soft contact lenses.
Adverse Reactions (Reflective of adult population; not specific for elderly)
>10%: Ocular: Mild ocular stinging and discomfort, eye irritation
1% to 10%: Ocular: Blurred vision, browache
Drug Interactions No data reported
Mechanism of Action Beta-adrenoceptor-blocking agent; lacks intrinsic sympathomimetic activity and membrane-stabilizing effects and possesses only slight local anesthetic activity; mechanism of action of metipranolol in reducing intraocular pressure appears to be via reduced production of aqueous humor. This effect may be related to a reduction in blood flow to the iris root-ciliary body. It remains unclear if the reduction in intraocular pressure observed with beta-blockers is actually secondary to beta-adrenoceptor blockade.
Pharmacodynamics
Onset of action: ≤30 minutes
Maximum effects: ~2 hours
Duration: Intraocular pressure reduction has persisted for 24 hours following ocular instillation
Pharmacokinetics
Metabolism: Rapid and complete to deacetyl metipranolol, an active metabolite
Half-life, elimination: ~3 hours
Dosage
Geriatrics & Adults: Glaucoma: Ophthalmic: Instill 1 drop in the affected eye(s) twice daily
Monitoring Parameters Intraocular pressure, funduscopic exam, visual field testing
Patient Information May sting on instillation; do not touch dropper to eye; visual acuity may be decreased after administration; distance vision may be altered; assess patient's or caregiver's ability to administer; apply gentle pressure to lacrimal sac during and immediately following instillation (1 minute) to avoid systemic absorption; stop drug if breathing difficulty occurs
Special Geriatric Considerations Because systemic absorption occurs with ophthalmic administration, elderly patients with other disease states or syndromes that may be affected by a beta-blocker (ie, CHF, COPD, etc) should be closely monitored.
Dosage Forms Excipient information presented when available (limited, particularly for generics); consult specific product labeling.
Solution, ophthalmic: 0.3% (5 mL, 10 mL) [contains benzalkonium chloride]

♦ **Metipranolol Hydrochloride** *see* Metipranolol *on page 1022*

Metoclopramide (met oh KLOE pra mide)

Medication Safety Issues
Sound-alike/look-alike issues:
Metoclopramide may be confused with metolazone
Reglan® may be confused with Megace®, Regonol®, Renagel®
U.S. Brand Names Reglan®
Canadian Brand Names Apo-Metoclop®; Metoclopramide Hydrochloride Injection; Nu-Metoclopramide
Generic Available Yes
Pharmacologic Category Antiemetic; Gastrointestinal Agent, Prokinetic
Use
Oral: Symptomatic treatment of diabetic gastric stasis; gastroesophageal reflux
I.V., I.M.: Symptomatic treatment of diabetic gastric stasis; postpyloric placement of enteral feeding tubes; prevention and/or treatment of nausea and vomiting associated with chemotherapy, or postsurgery; to stimulate gastric emptying and intestinal transit of barium during radiological examination
Contraindications Hypersensitivity to metoclopramide or any component of the formulation; GI obstruction, perforation or hemorrhage; pheochromocytoma; history of seizure disorder
Warnings/Precautions Use caution with a history of mental illness; has been associated with extrapyramidal symptoms (EPS) and depression; risk is increased at higher dosages. Extrapyramidal reactions typically occur within the initial 24-48 hours of treatment. Use caution with concurrent use of other drugs associated with EPS. Use caution in the elderly and with Parkinson's disease; may have increased risk of tardive dyskinesia. Neuroleptic malignant syndrome (NMS) has been reported (rarely) with metoclopramide. Use lowest recommended doses initially; may cause transient increase in serum aldosterone; use caution in patients who are at risk of fluid overload (CHF, cirrhosis). Use caution in patients with hypertension or following surgical anastomosis/closure. Patients with NADH-cytochrome b5 reductase deficiency are at increased risk of methemoglobinemia and/or sulfhemoglobinemia. Abrupt discontinuation may (rarely) result in withdrawal symptoms (dizziness, headache, nervousness). Use caution and adjust dose in renal impairment.
Adverse Reactions (Reflective of adult population; not specific for elderly)
Frequency not always defined.
Cardiovascular: AV block, bradycardia, CHF, fluid retention, flushing (following high I.V. doses), hyper-/hypotension, supraventricular tachycardia
Central nervous system: Drowsiness (~10% to 70%; dose related), fatigue (~10%), restlessness (~10%), acute dystonic reactions (<1%; dose and age related), akathisia, confusion, depression, dizziness, hallucinations (rare), headache, insomnia, neuroleptic malignant syndrome (rare), Parkinsonian-like symptoms, suicidal ideation, seizure, tardive dyskinesia
Dermatologic: Angioneurotic edema (rare), rash, urticaria
Endocrine & metabolic: Amenorrhea, galactorrhea, gynecomastia, impotence
Gastrointestinal: Diarrhea, nausea
Genitourinary: Incontinence, urinary frequency
Hematologic: Agranulocytosis, leukopenia, neutropenia, porphyria
Hepatic: Hepatotoxicity (rare)
Ocular: Visual disturbance
Respiratory: Bronchospasm, laryngeal edema (rare)
Miscellaneous: Allergic reactions, methemoglobinemia, sulfhemoglobinemia
Overdosage/Toxicology Symptoms of overdose include drowsiness, ataxia, extrapyramidal symptoms, seizures. Disorientation, muscle hypertonia, irritability, and agitation are common. Metoclopramide often causes extrapyramidal symptoms (eg, dystonic reactions) requiring management with diphenhydramine 1-2 mg/kg up to a maximum of 50-100 mg I.M. or I.V. slow push followed by a maintenance dose (25-50 mg orally every 4-6 hours) for 48-72 hours. When these reactions are unresponsive to diphenhydramine, benztropine mesylate I.V. 1-2 mg may be effective. These agents are generally effective within 2-5 minutes. Methylene blue is not recommended in patients with G6PD deficiency who experience methemoglobinemia.
Drug Interactions Substrate (minor) of CYP1A2, 2D6; **Inhibits** CYP2D6 (weak)
Anticholinergic agents antagonize metoclopramide's actions
Antipsychotic agents: Metoclopramide may increase extrapyramidal symptoms (EPS) or risk when used concurrently.
Cyclosporine: Metoclopramide may increase cyclosporine levels.
Opiate analgesics may increase CNS depression
Ethanol/Nutrition/Herb Interactions Ethanol: Avoid ethanol (may increase CNS depression).
Stability
Injection: Store intact vial at controlled room temperature. Injection is photosensitive and should be protected from light during storage. Parenteral admixtures in D_5W or (Continued)

Metoclopramide *(Continued)*

NS are stable for at least 24 hours and do not require light protection if used within 24 hours.

Tablet: Store at controlled room temperature.

Mechanism of Action Blocks dopamine receptors and (when given in higher doses) also blocks serotonin receptors in chemoreceptor trigger zone of the CNS; enhances the response to acetylcholine of tissue in upper GI tract causing enhanced motility and accelerated gastric emptying without stimulating gastric, biliary, or pancreatic secretions; increases lower esophageal sphincter tone

Pharmacodynamics

Onset of action: Oral: Within 30-60 minutes; I.V.: Within 1-3 minutes; I.M.: 10-15 minutes

Duration: 1-2 hours, regardless of route administered

Pharmacokinetics

Distribution: V_d: 2-4 L/kg

Protein binding: 30%

Half-life elimination: Normal renal function: 4-6 hours (may be dose dependent)

Bioavailability: Oral: 65% to 95%

Time to peak, serum: Oral: 1-2 hours

Excretion: Urine (~85%)

Dosage

Geriatrics:

Gastroesophageal reflux: Oral: 5 mg 4 times/day (30 minutes before meals or food and at bedtime); increase dose to 10 mg 4 times/day if no response at lower dose

Gastrointestinal hypomotility:

Oral: Initial: 5 mg 30 minutes before meals and at bedtime; increase if necessary to 10 mg doses

I.V.: Initiate at 5 mg over 1-2 minutes; increase to 10 mg if necessary

Postoperative nausea and vomiting: I.M., I.V.: 5 mg near end of surgery; may repeat dose if necessary

Adults:

Gastroesophageal reflux: Oral: 10-15 mg/dose up to 4 times/day 30 minutes before meals or food and at bedtime; single doses of 20 mg are occasionally needed for provoking situations. Treatment >12 weeks has not been evaluated.

Diabetic gastric stasis:

Oral: 10 mg 30 minutes before each meal and at bedtime

I.M., I.V. (for severe symptoms): 10 mg over 1-2 minutes; 10 days of I.V. therapy may be necessary for best response

Chemotherapy-induced emesis:

I.V.: 1-2 mg/kg 30 minutes before chemotherapy and repeated every 2 hours for 2 doses, then every 3 hours for 3 doses (manufacturer labeling)

Alternate dosing (with or without diphenhydramine):

Moderate emetic risk chemotherapy: 0.5 mg/kg every 6 hours on days 2-4

Low and minimal risk chemotherapy: 1-2 mg/kg every 3-4 hours

Breakthrough treatment: 1-2 mg/kg every 3-4 hours

Oral (unlabeled use; with or without diphenhydramine):

Moderate emetic risk chemotherapy: 0.5 mg/kg every 6 hours or 20 mg 4 times/ day on days 2-4

Low and minimal risk chemotherapy: 20-40 mg every 4-6 hours

Breakthrough treatment: 20-40 mg every 4-6 hours

Postoperative nausea and vomiting: I.M., I.V.: 10-20 mg near end of surgery

Postpyloric feeding tube placement, radiological exam: I.V.: 10 mg

Renal Impairment:

Cl_{cr} <40 mL/minute: Administer 50% of normal dose.

Not dialyzable (0% to 5%); supplemental dose is not necessary.

Administration Injection solution may be given I.M., direct I.V. push, short infusion (15-30 minutes), or continuous infusion; lower doses (≤10 mg) of metoclopramide can be given I.V. push undiluted over 1-2 minutes; higher doses to be given IVPB over at least 15 minutes; continuous SubQ infusion and rectal administration have been reported. **Note:** Rapid I.V. administration may be associated with a transient (but intense) feeling of anxiety and restlessness, followed by drowsiness.

Monitoring Parameters Monitor for dystonic reactions; monitor for signs of hypoglycemia in patients using insulin and those being treated for gastroparesis; monitor for agitation and irritable confusion

Test Interactions Increased aminotransferase [ALT/AST] (S), increased amylase (S)

Patient Information May impair mental alertness or physical coordination; produces drowsiness, dizziness; avoid alcohol, barbiturates or other CNS depressants; take medication 30 minutes before meals; notify physician if any abnormal muscle movements occur

Special Geriatric Considerations Elderly are more likely to develop tardive dyskinesia syndrome (especially elderly females) reactions than younger adults. Use lowest recommended doses initially. Must consider renal function (estimate creatinine clearance). It is recommended to do involuntary movement assessments on elderly using this medication at high doses and for long-term therapy.

Dosage Forms Excipient information presented when available (limited, particularly for generics); consult specific product labeling.

Injection, solution (Reglan®): 5 mg/mL (2 mL, 10 mL, 30 mL)

Syrup: 5 mg/5 mL (10 mL, 480 mL)

Tablet (Reglan®): 5 mg, 10 mg

Extemporaneously Prepared

Reglan® suppository: 5 pulverized tablets in polyethylene glycol; administer 1 suppository 30-60 minutes before meals and at bedtime; use ½ for older adults.

Metoclophen nausea suppository:
Metoclopramide powder (USP) 40 mg
Haloperidol powder (USP) 1 mg
Dexamethasone powder (USP) 10 mg
Diphenhydramine HCl (USP) 25 mg
Benztropine mesylate (USP) 1 mg
Silica gel powder 200 mg
Fatty base (emulsifying type) qs 2.2 g

Metoclophen-modified nausea suppository:
Metoclopramide powder (USP) 40 mg
Haloperidol powder (USP) 1 mg
Lorazepam (USP) 1 mg
Benztropine mesylate (USP) 1 mg
Fatty base (emulsifying type) qs 2.2 g

Grind all powders (and/or tablets) into a fine uniform powder. Melt the fatty base on low temperature, then add the powder. Stir the mixture until uniform. With continuous stirring, draw up part of the mixture and instill into calibrated suppository molds. Refrigerate.

Francom M, "Compounding Nausea Aid," *Am Pharm*, 1991, NS31(7):7.

Selected References

Bruera E, Seifert L, Watanabe S, et al, "Chronic Nausea in Advanced Cancer Patients: A Retrospective Assessment of a Metoclopramide-Based Antiemetic Regimen," *J Pain Symptom Manage*, 1996, 11(3):147-53.

DiPalma JR, "Metoclopramide: A Dopamine Receptor Antagonist," *Am Fam Physician*, 1990, 41(3):919-24.

Harrington RA, Hamilton CW, Brogden RN, et al, "Metoclopramide. An Updated Review of Its Pharmacological Properties and Clinical Use," *Drugs*, 1983, 25(5):451-94.

Karadsheh NS, Shaker Q, and Ratroat B, "Metoclopramide-induced Methemoglobinemia in a Patient With Co-Existing Deficiency of Glucose-6-Phosphate Dehydrogenase and NADH-Cytochrome b5 Reductase: Failure of Methylene Blue Treatment," *Haematologica*, 2001, 86(6):659-60.

Mary AM and Bhupalam L, "Metoclopramide-induced Methemoglobinemia in an Adult," *J KY Med Assoc*, 2000, 98(6):245-7.

"National Comprehensive Cancer Network Practice Guidelines in Oncology," (version 1.2005); available at: http://www.nccn.org/professionals/physician_gls/PDF/antiemesis.pdf

Parrish RH and Bonzo SM, "Use of Metoclopramide Suppositories," *Clin Pharm*, 1983, 2:395-6.

Patterson JF, "Neuroleptic Malignant Syndrome Associated With Metoclopramide," *South Med J*, 1988, 81(5):674-5.

Schulze-Delrieu K, "Drug Therapy. Metoclopramide," *N Engl J Med*, 1981, 305(1):28-33.

Van Veldhuizen PJ and Wyatt A, "Metoclopramide-induced Sulfhemoglobinemia," *Am J Gastroenterol*, 1995, 90(6):1010-1.

Metolazone (me TOLE a zone)

Medication Safety Issues

Sound-alike/look-alike issues:
Metolazone may be confused with metaxalone, methazolamide, methimazole, methotrexate, metoclopramide, metoprolol, minoxidil
Zaroxolyn® may be confused with Zarontin®

U.S. Brand Names Zaroxolyn®

Canadian Brand Names Zaroxolyn®

Generic Available Yes

Pharmacologic Category Diuretic, Thiazide-Related

Use Management of mild to moderate hypertension; treatment of edema in congestive heart failure and nephrotic syndrome, impaired renal function

Contraindications Hypersensitivity to metolazone, any component of the formulation, other thiazides, and sulfonamide derivatives; anuria; hepatic coma

Warnings/Precautions Electrolyte disturbances (hypokalemia, hypochloremic alkalosis, hyponatremia) can occur. Large or prolonged fluid and electrolyte losses may occur with concomitant furosemide administration. Use with caution in severe hepatic dysfunction; hepatic encephalopathy can be caused by electrolyte disturbances. Gout can be precipitate in certain patients with a history of gout, a familial predisposition to gout, or chronic renal failure. Cautious use in patients with prediabetes or diabetes; may see a change in glucose control. Can cause SLE exacerbation or activation. Use (Continued)

Metolazone *(Continued)*

caution in severe renal impairment. Use with caution in patients with moderate or high cholesterol concentrations. Photosensitization may occur.

Chemical similarities are present among sulfonamides, sulfonylureas, carbonic anhydrase inhibitors, thiazides, and loop diuretics (except ethacrynic acid). Use in patients with thiazide or sulfonamide allergy is specifically contraindicated in product labeling, however, a risk of cross-reaction exists in patients with allergy to any of these compounds; avoid use when previous reaction has been severe. Discontinue if signs of hypersensitivity are noted.

Adverse Reactions (Reflective of adult population; not specific for elderly)
Frequency not defined.

Cardiovascular: Chest pain/discomfort, necrotizing angiitis, orthostatic hypotension, palpitation, syncope, venous thrombosis, vertigo, volume depletion

Central nervous system: chills, depression, dizziness, drowsiness, fatigue, headache, lightheadedness, restlessness

Dermatologic: Petechiae, photosensitivity, pruritus, purpura, rash, skin necrosis, Stevens-Johnson syndrome, toxic epidermal necrolysis, urticaria

Endocrine & metabolic: Gout attacks, hypercalcemia, hyperglycemia, hyperuricemia, hypochloremia, hypochloremic alkalosis, hypokalemia, hypomagnesemia, hyponatremia, hypophosphatemia

Gastrointestinal: Abdominal bloating, abdominal pain, anorexia, constipation, diarrhea, epigastric distress, nausea, pancreatitis, vomiting, xerostomia

Genitourinary: Impotence

Hematologic: Agranulocytosis, aplastic/hypoplastic anemia, hemoconcentration, leukopenia, thrombocytopenia

Hepatic: Cholestatic jaundice, hepatitis

Neuromuscular & skeletal: Joint pain, muscle cramps/spasm, neuropathy, paresthesia, weakness

Ocular: Blurred vision (transient)

Renal: BUN increased, glucosuria

Overdosage/Toxicology Symptoms include hypermotility, diuresis, lethargy, confusion, and muscle weakness. Following GI decontamination, therapy is supportive with I.V. fluids, electrolytes, and I.V. pressors if needed.

Drug Interactions

ACE inhibitors: Thiazide diuretics may enhance the hypotensive effect of ACE inhibitors. Thiazide diuretics may enhance the nephrotoxic effect of ACE inhibitors.

Bile acid sequestrants: May decrease metolazone absorption.

Diazoxide: Diazoxide may enhance the hyperglycemic effect of thiazide diuretics.

Dofetilide: Thiazide diuretics may enhance the serum concentration and QT_c-prolonging effect of dofetilide.

Lithium:Thiazide diuretics may decrease the excretion of lithium; monitor lithium concentration and adjust as needed.

Ethanol/Nutrition/Herb Interactions

Ethanol: May potentiate hypotensive effect of metazolone.

Herb/Nutraceutical: Avoid dong quai if using for hypertension (has estrogenic activity). Avoid dong quai, St John's wort (may also cause photosensitization). Avoid ephedra, yohimbe, ginseng (may worsen hypertension). Avoid natural licorice. Avoid garlic (may have increased antihypertensive effect).

Mechanism of Action Inhibits sodium reabsorption in the distal tubules causing increased excretion of sodium and water, as well as, potassium and hydrogen ions

Pharmacodynamics

Onset of action: Diuresis: ~60 minutes

Duration: ≥24 hours

Pharmacokinetics

Absorption: Oral: Incomplete

Protein binding: 95%

Half-life: 20 hours

Excretion: Urine (80%); bile (10%)

Dosage

Geriatrics: Oral: Initial: 2.5 mg/day or every other day

Adults:

Edema: Oral: 2.5-20 mg/dose every 24 hours (ACC/AHA 2005 Heart Failure Guidelines)

Hypertension: Oral: 2.5-5 mg/dose every 24 hours

Renal Impairment: Not dialyzable (0% to 5%) via hemo- or peritoneal dialysis; supplemental dose is not necessary

Monitoring Parameters Blood pressure both standing and sitting/supine, serum electrolytes, renal function, weight, I & O

Patient Information Take in the morning, may be taken with food or milk; take the last dose of multiple doses no later than 6 PM unless instructed otherwise; may cause increased sensitivity to sunlight

Additional Information 5 mg is approximately equivalent to 50 mg of hydrochlorothiazide; may be effective in patients with glomerular filtration rate <20 mL/minute; metolazone is often used in combination with a loop diuretic in patients who are unresponsive to the loop diuretic alone

Special Geriatric Considerations When metolazone is used in combination with other diuretics, there is an increased risk of azotemia and electrolyte depletion, particularly in the elderly, monitor closely. May be effective in patients with glomerular filtration rate <20 mL/minute. Metolazone is often used in combination with a loop diuretic in patients who are unresponsive to the loop diuretic alone.

Dosage Forms Excipient information presented when available (limited, particularly for generics); consult specific product labeling.
Tablet: 2.5 mg, 5 mg, 10 mg
Zaroxolyn®: 2.5 mg, 5 mg, 10 mg

Metoprolol (me toe PROE lole)

Related Information
Beta-Blockers *on page 1751*
Medication Safety Issues
Sound-alike/look-alike issues:
Metoprolol may be confused with metaproterenol, metolazone, misoprostol
Toprol-XL® may be confused with Tegretol®, Tegretol®-XR, Topamax®

High alert medication: The Institute for Safe Medication Practices (ISMP) includes this medication among its list of drugs which have a heightened risk of causing significant patient harm when used in error.

Significant differences exist between oral and I.V. dosing. Use caution when converting from one route of administration to another.

U.S. Brand Names Lopressor®; Toprol-XL®
Canadian Brand Names Apo-Metoprolol®; Betaloc®; Betaloc® Durules®; Lopressor®; Metoprolol Tartrate Injection, USP; Novo-Metoprolol; Nu-Metop; PMS-Metoprolol; Sandoz-Metoprolol; Toprol-XL®
Index Terms Metoprolol Succinate; Metoprolol Tartrate
Generic Available Yes
Pharmacologic Category Beta Blocker, Beta$_1$ Selective
Use Treatment of hypertension and angina pectoris; prevention of myocardial infarction, atrial fibrillation, flutter, symptomatic treatment of hypertrophic subaortic stenosis
Extended release: To reduce mortality/hospitalization in patients with congestive heart failure (stable NYHA Class II or III) in patients already receiving ACE inhibitors, diuretics, and/or digoxin
Unlabeled/Investigational Use Treatment of ventricular arrhythmias, atrial ectopy, migraine prophylaxis, essential tremor, aggressive behavior
Contraindications Hypersensitivity to metoprolol or any component of the formulation; sinus bradycardia; heart block greater than first degree (except in patients with a functioning artificial pacemaker); cardiogenic shock; uncompensated cardiac failure
Warnings/Precautions [U.S. Boxed Warning]: Beta-blocker therapy should not be withdrawn abruptly (particularly in patients with CAD), but gradually tapered to avoid acute tachycardia, hypertension, and/or ischemia. Consider pre-existing conditions such as sick sinus syndrome before initiating. Use caution in patients with PVD (can aggravate arterial insufficiency). Use caution with concurrent use of beta-blockers and either verapamil or diltiazem; bradycardia or heart block can occur; avoid concurrent I.V. use of both agents. In general, beta-blockers should be avoided in patients with bronchospastic disease. Metoprolol, with B$_1$ selectivity, should be used cautiously in bronchospastic disease with close monitoring. Use cautiously in diabetics because it can mask prominent hypoglycemic symptoms. Use caution with hepatic dysfunction. Use with caution in patients with myasthenia gravis or psychiatric disease (may cause CNS depression). Use care with anesthetic agents which decrease myocardial function. Use of beta-blockers may unmask cardiac failure in patients without a history of dysfunction. Adequate alpha-blockade is required prior to use of any beta-blocker for patients with untreated pheochromocytoma.

Extended release: Use care in compensated heart failure and monitor closely for a worsening of the condition.

Adverse Reactions (Reflective of adult population; not specific for elderly)
Frequency may not be defined.
Cardiovascular: Bradycardia (2% to 16%), hypotension (1% to 2%), arterial insufficiency (usually Raynaud type; 1%), chest pain (1%), CHF (1%), edema (peripheral; 1%), palpitation (1%), syncope (1%), gangrene (rare)
(Continued)

Metoprolol *(Continued)*

Central nervous system: Dizziness (2% to 10%), fatigue (10%), depression (5%), confusion, headache, insomnia, memory loss (short-term), nightmares, somnolence

Dermatology: Pruritus (5%), rash (5%), psoriasis increased, alopecia (reversible; rare)

Endocrine & metabolic: Libido decreased, Peyronie's disease (<1%)

Gastrointestinal: Diarrhea (5%), constipation (1%), flatulence (1%), gastrointestinal pain (1%), heartburn (1%), nausea (1%), xerostomia (1%)

Hematologic: Agranulocytosis (rare)

Neuromuscular & skeletal: Musculoskeletal pain

Ocular: Blurred vision, dry eyes (rare), oculomucocutaneous syndrome

Otic: Tinnitus

Respiratory: Dyspnea (1% to 3%), bronchospasm (1%), wheezing (1%), rhinitis

Miscellaneous: Cold extremities (1%)

Other events reported with beta-blockers: AV block increased, catatonia, emotional lability, fever, hypersensitivity reactions, laryngospasm, nonthrombocytopenic purpura, respiratory distress, thrombocytopenic purpura

Overdosage/Toxicology Symptoms of intoxication include cardiac disturbances, CNS toxicity, bronchospasm, hypoglycemia and hyperkalemia. The most common cardiac symptoms include hypotension and bradycardia. Atrioventricular block, intraventricular conduction disturbances, cardiogenic shock, and asystole may occur with severe overdose, especially with membrane-depressant drugs (eg, propranolol). CNS effects include convulsions, coma, and respiratory arrest. Treatment is symptomatic for seizures, hypotension, hyperkalemia and hypoglycemia. Bradycardia and hypotension resistant to atropine, isoproterenol, or pacing may respond to glucagon. Wide QRS defects caused by membrane-depressant poisoning may respond to hypertonic sodium bicarbonate. Repeat-dose charcoal, hemoperfusion, or hemodialysis may be helpful in removal of only those beta-blockers with a small V_d, long half-life, or low intrinsic clearance (acebutolol, atenolol, nadolol, sotalol).

Drug Interactions Substrate of CYP2C19 (minor), 2D6 (major); **Inhibits** CYP2D6 (weak)

Acetylcholinesterase inhibitors (eg, donepezil, galantamine, neostigmine): May enhance the bradycardic effect of beta-blockers.

Alpha-/beta-agonists: Beta-blockers may enhance the vasopressor effect of alpha-/beta-agonists (direct-acting).

Alpha₁-blockers (prazosin, terazosin): Concurrent use of beta-blockers may increase risk of orthostasis.

Alpha₂-agonists: Beta-blockers may enhance the rebound hypertensive effect of alpha₂-agonists. This effect can occur when the alpha₂-agonist is abruptly withdrawn.

Aminoquinolines (antimalarial): May decrease the metabolism, via CYP isoenzymes, of beta-blockers.

Amiodarone: May enhance the bradycardic effect of beta-blockers.

Antipsychotic agents (phenothiazines): May enhance the hypotensive effect of beta-blockers. Beta-blockers may decrease the metabolism, via CYP isoenzymes, of antipsychotic agents (phenothiazines).

Barbiturates: May increase the metabolism, via CYP isoenzymes, of beta-blockers.

Beta₂-agonists: May diminish the bradycardic effect of beta-blockers (beta₁ selective).

Bupropion: Concomitant therapy may result in bradycardia; monitor.

Calcium channel blockers (nondihydropyridine): May enhance the hypotensive effect of beta-blockers. Bradycardia and signs of heart failure have also been reported.

Cardiac glycosides: Beta-blockers may enhance the bradycardic effect of cardiac glycosides.

CYP2D6 inhibitors: May increase the levels/effects of metoprolol. Example inhibitors include chlorpromazine, delavirdine, fluoxetine, miconazole, paroxetine, pergolide, quinidine, quinine, ritonavir, and ropinirole.

Dipyridamole: May enhance the bradycardic effect of beta-blockers.

Disopyramide: May enhance the bradycardic effect of beta-blockers.

Insulin: Beta-blockers may enhance the hypoglycemic effect of insulin. Tachycardia may be masked as a symptom of hypoglycemia.

Lidocaine: Beta-blockers may decrease the metabolism of lidocaine.

Nonsteroidal anti-inflammatory agents (NSAIDs): May diminish the antihypertensive effect of beta-blockers.

Propafenone: May decrease the metabolism, via CYP isoenzymes, of beta-blockers. Propafenone possesses some independent beta-blocking activity.

Propoxyphene: May decrease the metabolism, via CYP isoenzymes, of beta-blockers.

Quinidine: May decrease the metabolism, via CYP isoenzymes, of beta-blockers.

Rifamycin derivatives: May increase the metabolism, via CYP isoenzymes, of beta-blockers.

Selective serotonin reuptake inhibitors (SSRIs): May enhance the bradycardic effect of beta-blockers.

Sulfonylureas: Beta-blockers may enhance the hypoglycemic effect of sulfonylureas. Tachycardia may be masked as a symptom of hypoglycemia.

Theophylline: Beta-blockers (beta$_1$ selective) may diminish the bronchodilatory effect of theophylline derivatives.

Ethanol/Nutrition/Herb Interactions

Food: Food increases absorption. Metoprolol serum levels may be increased if taken with food.

Herb/Nutraceutical: Avoid dong quai if using for hypertension (has estrogenic activity). Avoid bayberry, blue cohosh, cayenne, ephedra, ginger, ginseng (american), gotu kola, licorice, yohimbe (may worsen hypertension). Avoid black cohosh, california poppy, coleus, garlic, golden seal, hawthorn, mistletoe, periwinkle, quinine, shepherd's purse (have antihypertensive activity, may cause hypotension).

Stability

Injection: Do not store above 30°C (86°F). Protect from light.

Tablet: Store between 15°C to 30°C (59°F to 86°F).

Mechanism of Action Selective inhibitor of beta$_1$-adrenergic receptors; competitively blocks beta$_1$-receptors, with little or no effect on beta$_2$-receptors at doses <100 mg; does not exhibit any membrane stabilizing or intrinsic sympathomimetic activity

Pharmacodynamics

Onset of Action: Peak effect: Antihypertensive: Oral: Within 1.5-4 hours

Duration: 10-20 hours

Pharmacokinetics

Absorption: 95%

Protein binding: 12%

Metabolism: Extensively hepatic via CYP2D6; significant first-pass effect

Bioavailability: Oral: 40% to 50%

Half-life elimination: 3-8 hours

Elimination: In urine (3% to 10% as unchanged drug)

Dosage

Geriatrics: Oral: Initial: 25 mg/day; usual dose range: 25-300 mg/day; increase at 1- to 2-week intervals.

Extended release: 25-50 mg/day initially as a single dose; increase at 1- to 2-week intervals.

Adults:

Hypertension: Oral: 100-450 mg/day in 2-3 divided doses, begin with 50 mg twice daily and increase doses at weekly intervals to desired effect; usual dosage range (JNC 7): 50-100 mg/day

Extended release: Initial: 25-100 mg/day (maximum: 400 mg/day)

Angina, SVT, MI prophylaxis: Oral: 100-450 mg/day in 2-3 divided doses, begin with 50 mg twice daily and increase doses at weekly intervals to desired effect

Extended release: Initial: 100 mg/day (maximum: 400 mg/day)

Hypertension/ventricular rate control: I.V. (in patients having nonfunctioning GI tract): Initial: 1.25-5 mg every 6-12 hours; titrate initial dose to response. Initially, low doses may be appropriate to establish response; however, up to 15 mg every 3-6 hours has been employed.

Congestive heart failure: Oral (extended release): Initial: 25 mg once daily (reduce to 12.5 mg once daily in NYHA class higher than class II); may double dosage every 2 weeks as tolerated, up to 200 mg/day

Myocardial infarction (acute): I.V.: 5 mg every 2 minutes for 3 doses in early treatment of myocardial infarction; thereafter give 50 mg orally every 6 hours 15 minutes after last I.V. dose and continue for 48 hours; then administer a maintenance dose of 100 mg twice daily.

Note: When switching from immediate release metoprolol to extended release, the same total daily dose of metoprolol should be used.

Hepatic Impairment: Reduced dose is probably necessary.

Administration

Oral: Extended release tablets: May be divided in half; do not crush or chew.

I.V.: When administered acutely for cardiac treatment, monitor ECG and blood pressure. May administer by rapid infusion (I.V. push) over 1 minute or by slow infusion (ie, 5-10 mg of metoprolol in 50 mL of fluid) over ~30 minutes. Necessary monitoring for surgical patients who are unable to take oral beta-blockers (prolonged ileus) has not been defined. Some institutions require monitoring of baseline and postinfusion heart rate and blood pressure when a patient's response to beta-blockade has not been characterized (ie, the patient's initial dose or following a change in dose). Consult individual institutional policies and procedures.

Monitoring Parameters Blood pressure, orthostatic hypotension, heart rate, CNS effects

Patient Information I.V. use in emergency situations: Patient information is appropriate to patient condition.

Oral: Inform prescriber of all prescriptions, OTC medications, or herbal products you are taking, and any allergies you have. Do not take any new medication during therapy unless approved by prescriber. Take exactly as directed. Do not change dosage or (Continued)

Metoprolol *(Continued)*

discontinue without consulting prescriber. Take pulse daily, prior to medication and follow prescriber's instruction about holding medication. Do not take with antacids. If you have diabetes, monitor serum sugar closely (drug may alter glucose tolerance or mask signs of hypoglycemia). May cause fatigue, dizziness, or postural hypotension (use caution when changing position from lying or sitting to standing, when driving, or when climbing stairs until response to medication is known); or alteration in sexual performance (reversible). Report unresolved swelling of extremities, respiratory difficulty or new cough, unresolved fatigue, unusual weight gain, unresolved constipation, or unusual muscle weakness.

Special Geriatric Considerations Due to alterations in the beta-adrenergic autonomic nervous system, beta-adrenergic blockade may result in less hemodynamic response than seen in younger adults. Studies indicate that despite decreased sensitivity to the chronotropic effects of beta-blockade with age, there appears to be an increased myocardial sensitivity to the negative inotropic effect during stress (ie, exercise). Controlled trials have shown the overall response rate for propranolol to be only 20% to 50% in the elderly populations. Therefore, all beta-adrenergic blocking drugs may result in a decreased response as compared to younger adults.

Dosage Forms Excipient information presented when available (limited, particularly for generics); consult specific product labeling.

Injection, solution, as tartrate: 1 mg/mL (5 mL)
  Lopressor®: 1 mg/mL (5 mL)
Tablet, as tartrate: 25 mg, 50 mg, 100 mg
  Lopressor®: 50 mg, 100 mg
Tablet, extended release, as succinate: 25 mg, 50 mg, 100 mg, 200 mg [expressed as mg equivalent to tartrate]
  Toprol-XL®: 25 mg, 50 mg, 100 mg, 200 mg [expressed as mg equivalent to tartrate]

Extemporaneously Prepared A mixture of metoprolol 10 mg/mL plus hydrochlorothiazide 5 mg/mL was found to be stable for 60 days in a refrigerator in a 1:1 preparation of Ora-Sweet® and Ora-Plus®, in Ora-Sweet® SF and Ora-Plus®, and in cherry syrup

Allen LV and Erickson III MA, "Stability of Labetalol Hydrochloride, Metoprolol Tartrate, Verapamil Hydrochloride, and Spironolactone With Hydrochlorothiazide in Extemporaneously Compounded Oral Liquids," *Am J Health Syst Pharm*, 1996, 53:2304-9.

Selected References

Aagaard GN, "Treatment of Hypertension in the Elderly," *Drug Treatment in the Elderly*, Vestal RE, ed, Boston, MA: ADIS Health Science Press, 1984, 77.

Fleisher LA, Beckman JA, Brown KA, et al, "ACC/AHA 2006 Guideline Update on Perioperative Cardiovascular Evaluation for Noncardiac Surgery: Focused Update on Perioperative Beta-Blocker Therapy. A Report of the American College of Cardiology/American Heart Association Task Force on Practice Guidelines (Writing Committee to Update the 2002 Guidelines on Perioperative Cardiovascular Evaluation for Noncardiac Surgery) Developed in Collaboration With the American Society of Echocardiography, American Society of Nuclear Cardiology, Heart Rhythm Society, Society of Cardiovascular Anesthesiologists, Society for Cardiovascular Angiography and Interventions, and Society for Vascular Medicine and Biology," *J Am Coll Cardiol*, 2006, 47(11):2343-55.

Juul AB, Wetterslev J, Gluud C, et al, "Effect of Perioperative Beta Blockade in Patients With Diabetes Undergoing Major Non-Cardiac Surgery: Randomized Placebo Controlled, Blinded Multicentre Trial. DIPOM Trial Group," *BMJ*, 2006, 332(7556):1482.

Metoprolol and Hydrochlorothiazide

(me toe PROE lole & hye droe klor oh THYE a zide)

U.S. Brand Names Lopressor HCT®

Index Terms Hydrochlorothiazide and Metoprolol; Hydrochlorothiazide and Metoprolol Tartrate; Metoprolol Tartrate and Hydrochlorothiazide

Generic Available Yes

Pharmacologic Category Beta Blocker, Beta$_1$ Selective; Diuretic, Thiazide

Dosage

Geriatrics & Adults: Hypertension: Oral: Dosage should be determined by titration of the individual agents and the combination product substituted based upon the daily requirements.

Usual dose: Metoprolol 50-100 mg and hydrochlorothiazide 25-50 mg administered daily as single or divided doses (twice daily)

Note: Hydrochlorothiazide >50 mg/day is not recommended.

Concomitant therapy: It is recommended that if an additional antihypertensive agent is required, gradual titration should occur using $^1/_2$ the usual starting dose of the other agent to avoid hypotension.

Special Geriatric Considerations See individual agents.

Dosage Forms Excipient information presented when available (limited, particularly for generics); consult specific product labeling.

Tablet:
  50/25: Metoprolol tartrate 50 mg and hydrochlorothiazide 25 mg
  100/25: Metoprolol tartrate 100 mg and hydrochlorothiazide 25 mg
  100/50: Metoprolol tartrate 100 mg and hydrochlorothiazide 50 mg

♦ **Metoprolol Succinate** *see* Metoprolol *on page 1027*

♦ **Metoprolol Tartrate** *see* Metoprolol *on page 1027*

♦ **Metoprolol Tartrate and Hydrochlorothiazide** *see* Metoprolol and Hydrochlorothiazide *on page 1030*

♦ **MetroCream®** *see* Metronidazole *on page 1031*

♦ **MetroGel®** *see* Metronidazole *on page 1031*

♦ **MetroGel-Vaginal®** *see* Metronidazole *on page 1031*

♦ **MetroLotion®** *see* Metronidazole *on page 1031*

Metronidazole (met roe NYE da zole)

Related Information
Antimicrobial Activity Against Selected Organisms *on page 1728*
Helicobacter pylori Treatment *on page 1759*

Medication Safety Issues
Sound-alike/look-alike issues:
Metronidazole may be confused with metformin.

U.S. Brand Names Flagyl®; Flagyl ER®; MetroCream®; MetroGel®; MetroGel-Vaginal®; MetroLotion®; Noritate®; Vandazole™

Canadian Brand Names Apo-Metronidazole®; Flagyl®; Florazole® ER; MetroCream®; Metrogel®; Nidagel™; Noritate®; Trikacide

Index Terms Metronidazole Hydrochloride

Generic Available Yes: Capsule, cream, gel, infusion, lotion, tablet

Pharmacologic Category Amebicide; Antibiotic, Miscellaneous; Antibiotic, Topical; Antiprotozoal, Nitroimidazole

Use Treatment of susceptible anaerobic bacterial and protozoal infections in the following conditions: Amebiasis, symptomatic and asymptomatic trichomoniasis; skin and skin structure infections; CNS infections; intra-abdominal infections (as part of combination regimen); systemic anaerobic infections; treatment of antibiotic-associated pseudomembranous colitis (AAPC), bacterial vaginosis; as part of a multidrug regimen for *H. pylori* eradication to reduce the risk of duodenal ulcer recurrence; also used in Crohn's disease and hepatic encephalopathy

Orphan drug: MetroGel® Topical: Treatment of acne rosacea

Contraindications Hypersensitivity to metronidazole, nitroimidazole derivatives, or any component of the formulation

Warnings/Precautions Use with caution in patients with liver impairment due to potential accumulation, blood dyscrasias; history of seizures, CHF, or other sodium retaining states; reduce dosage in patients with severe liver impairment, CNS disease, and consider dosage reduction in longer-term therapy with severe renal failure; seizures and neuropathies have been reported especially with increased doses and chronic treatment; if this occurs, discontinue therapy. **[U.S. Boxed Warning]: Possibly carcinogenic based on animal data.** Prolonged use may result in fungal or bacterial superinfection, including *C. difficile*-associated diarrhea and pseudomembranous colitis.

Adverse Reactions (Reflective of adult population; not specific for elderly)
Systemic: Frequency not defined:
Cardiovascular: Flattening of the T-wave, flushing
Central nervous system: Ataxia, confusion, coordination impaired, dizziness, fever, headache, insomnia, irritability, seizure, vertigo
Dermatologic: Erythematous rash, urticaria
Endocrine & metabolic: Disulfiram-like reaction, dysmenorrhea, libido decreased
Gastrointestinal: Nausea (~12%), anorexia, abdominal cramping, constipation, diarrhea, furry tongue, glossitis, proctitis, stomatitis, unusual/metallic taste, vomiting, xerostomia
Genitourinary: Cystitis, darkened urine (rare), dysuria, incontinence, polyuria, vaginitis
Hematologic: Neutropenia (reversible), thrombocytopenia (reversible, rare)
Neuromuscular & skeletal: Peripheral neuropathy, weakness
Respiratory: Nasal congestion, rhinitis, sinusitis, pharyngitis
Miscellaneous: Flu-like syndrome, moniliasis

Topical: Frequency not defined:
Central nervous system: Headache
Dermatologic: Burning, contact dermatitis, dryness, erythema, irritation, pruritus, rash
Gastrointestinal: Unusual/metallic taste, nausea, constipation
Local: Local allergic reaction
Neuromuscular & skeletal: Tingling/numbness of extremities
Ocular: Eye irritation
(Continued)

Metronidazole *(Continued)*

Vaginal:
>10%: Genitourinary: Vaginal discharge (12%)
1% to 10%:
Central nervous system: Headache (5%), dizziness (2%)
Gastrointestinal: Gastrointestinal discomfort (7%), nausea and/or vomiting (4%), unusual/metallic taste (2%), diarrhea (1%)
Genitourinary: Vaginitis (10%), vulva/vaginal irritation (9%), pelvic discomfort (3%)
Hematologic: WBC increased (2%)

Overdosage/Toxicology Symptoms include nausea, vomiting, ataxia, seizures, and peripheral neuropathy. Treatment is symptomatic and supportive.

Drug Interactions Inhibits CYP2C9 (weak), 3A4 (moderate)
Cimetidine may increase metronidazole levels.
Cisapride: May inhibit metabolism of cisapride, causing potential arrhythmias; avoid concurrent use
CYP3A4 substrates: Metronidazole may increase the levels/effects of CYP3A4 substrates. Example substrates include benzodiazepines, calcium channel blockers, cyclosporine, mirtazapine, nateglinide, nefazodone, sildenafil (and other PDE-5 inhibitors), tacrolimus, and venlafaxine. Selected benzodiazepines (midazolam and triazolam), cisapride, ergot alkaloids, selected HMG-CoA reductase inhibitors (lova-statin and simvastatin), and pimozide are generally contraindicated with strong CYP3A4 inhibitors.
Ethanol: Ethanol results in disulfiram-like reactions.
Lithium: Metronidazole may increase lithium levels/toxicity; monitor lithium levels.
Phenytoin, phenobarbital may increase metabolism of metronidazole, potentially decreasing its effect.
Warfarin: Metronidazole increases P-T prolongation with warfarin.

Ethanol/Nutrition/Herb Interactions
Ethanol: The manufacturer recommends to avoid all ethanol or any ethanol-containing drugs (may cause disulfiram-like reaction characterized by flushing, headache, nausea, vomiting, sweating or tachycardia).
Food: Peak antibiotic serum concentration lowered and delayed, but total drug absorbed not affected.

Stability Metronidazole injection should be stored at 15°C to 30°C and protected from light. Product may be refrigerated but crystals may form. Crystals redissolve on warming to room temperature. Prolonged exposure to light will cause a darkening of the product. However, short-term exposure to normal room light does not adversely affect metronidazole stability. Direct sunlight should be avoided. Stability of parenteral admixture at room temperature (25°C): Out of overwrap stability: 30 days.
Standard diluent: 500 mg/100 mL NS.

Mechanism of Action After diffusing into the organism, interacts with DNA to cause a loss of helical DNA structure and strand breakage resulting in inhibition of protein synthesis and cell death in susceptible organisms

Pharmacokinetics
Absorption: Oral: Well absorbed
Protein binding: <20%
Metabolism: 30% to 60% in the liver
Half-life, normal: 6-8 hours (half-life increases with hepatic impairment)
Time to peak serum concentration: Within 1-2 hours
Elimination: Final excretion via urine (20% as unchanged drug) and feces (6% to 15%).
Following a single 500 mg oral dose, serum concentration and AUCs were increased, total clearance and V_d reduced in subject >70 years compared to younger subjects (20-25 years); the decreased V_d was attributed to a significant decrease in red blood cell binding

Dosage
Geriatrics: Use the lower end of the dosing recommendations for adults; do not administer as single dose as efficacy has not been established.
Adults:
Anaerobic infections (diverticulitis, intra-abdominal, peritonitis, cholangitis, or abscess): Oral, I.V.: 500 mg every 6-8 hours, not to exceed 4 g/day
Acne rosacea: Topical:
0.75%: Apply and rub a thin film twice daily, morning and evening, to entire affected areas after washing. Significant therapeutic results should be noticed within 3 weeks. Clinical studies have demonstrated continuing improvement through 9 weeks of therapy.
1%: Apply thin film to affected area once daily
Amebiasis: Oral: 500-750 mg every 8 hours for 5-10 days
Antibiotic-associated pseudomembranous colitis: Oral: 250-500 mg 3-4 times/day for 10-14 days
Giardiasis: 500 mg twice daily for 5-7 days

Peptic ulcer disease: *Helicobacter pylori* **eradication:** Oral: 250-500 mg with meals and at bedtime for 14 days; requires combination therapy with at least one other antibiotic and an acid-suppressing agent (proton pump inhibitor or H$_2$ blocker)

Bacterial vaginosis or vaginitis due to *Gardnerella, Mobiluncus*:

Oral: 500 mg twice daily (regular release) or 750 mg once daily (extended release tablet) for 7 days

Vaginal: 1 applicatorful (~37.5 mg metronidazole) intravaginally once or twice daily for 5 days; apply once in morning and evening if using twice daily, if daily, use at bedtime

Trichomoniasis: Oral: 250 mg every 8 hours for 7 days **or** 375 mg twice daily for 7 days **or** 2 g as a single dose

Renal Impairment:

Cl$_{cr}$ <10 mL/minute, but not on dialysis: Recommendations vary: To reduce possible accumulation in patients receiving multiple doses, consider reduction to 50% of dose or every 12 hours; **Note:** Dosage reduction is unnecessary in short courses of therapy. Clinical recommendations and practice vary. Some references do not recommend reduction at any level of renal impairment (Lamp, 1999).

Hemodialysis effects: Extensively removed by hemodialysis and peritoneal dialysis (50% to 100%); dosage reduction not recommended; administer full dose posthemodialysis. During peritoneal dialysis, dose as for Cl$_{cr}$ <10 mL/minute.

Continuous arteriovenous or venovenous hemofiltration: Dose as for normal renal function

Hepatic Impairment: Unchanged in mild liver disease; reduce dosage in severe liver disease.

Monitoring Parameters Signs and symptoms of infection; diarrhea

Test Interactions May interfere with AST, ALT, triglycerides, glucose, and LDH testing

Patient Information Urine may be discolored to a dark or reddish-brown. Do not ingest alcohol for at least 24 hours after the last dose. Avoid beverage alcohol during therapy. May cause metallic taste; may be taken with food to minimize stomach upset.

Additional Information Sodium content of 500 mg (I.V.): 322 mg (14 mEq)

Special Geriatric Considerations Adjust dose based on renal function.

Dosage Forms Excipient information presented when available (limited, particularly for generics); consult specific product labeling.

Capsule: 375 mg

Flagyl®: 375 mg

Cream, topical: 0.75% (45 g)

MetroCream®: 0.75% (45 g) [contains benzyl alcohol]

Noritate®: 1% (60 g)

Gel, topical: 0.75% (45 g)

MetroGel®: 1% (46 g, 60 g) [60 g tube also packaged in a kit with Cetaphil® skin cleanser]

Gel, vaginal: 0.75% (70 g)

MetroGel-Vaginal®, Vandazole™: 0.75% (70 g)

Infusion [premixed iso-osmotic sodium chloride solution]: 500 mg (100 mL)

Lotion, topical: 0.75% (60 mL)

MetroLotion®: 0.75% (60 mL) [contains benzyl alcohol]

Tablet: 250 mg, 500 mg

Flagyl®: 250 mg, 500 mg

Tablet, extended release:

Flagyl® ER: 750 mg

Selected References

Lamp KC, Freeman CD, Klutman NE, et al, "Pharmacokinetics and Pharmacodynamics of the Nitroimidazole Antimicrobials," *Clin Pharmacokinet*, 1999, 36(5):353-73.

Ludwig E, Csiba A, Magyar T, et al, "Age-Associated Pharmacokinetic Changes of Metronidazole," *Int J Clin Pharmacol Ther Toxicol*, 1983, 21(2):87-91.

♦ **Metronidazole Hydrochloride** *see* Metronidazole *on page 1031*

♦ **Mevacor®** *see* Lovastatin *on page 936*

♦ **Mevinolin** *see* Lovastatin *on page 936*

♦ **Mexar™ Wash** *see* Sulfacetamide *on page 1496*

Mexiletine (meks IL e teen)

U.S. Brand Names Mexitil® [DSC]

Canadian Brand Names Novo-Mexiletine

Generic Available Yes

Pharmacologic Category Antiarrhythmic Agent, Class Ib

Use Management of life-threatening ventricular arrhythmias

Unlabeled/Investigational Use Treatment of diabetic neuropathy

(Continued)

Mexiletine *(Continued)*

Contraindications Hypersensitivity to mexiletine or any component of the formulation; cardiogenic shock; second- or third-degree AV block (except in patients with a functioning artificial pacemaker)

Warnings/Precautions [U.S. Boxed Warning]: In the Cardiac Arrhythmia Suppression Trial (CAST), recent (>6 days but <2 years ago) myocardial infarction patients with asymptomatic, nonlife-threatening ventricular arrhythmias did not benefit and may have been harmed by attempts to suppress the arrhythmia with flecainide or encainide. An increased mortality or non-fatal cardiac arrest rate (7.7%) was seen in the active treatment group compared with patients in the placebo group (3%). The applicability of the CAST results to other populations is unknown. Antiarrhythmic agents should be reserved for patients with life-threatening ventricular arrhythmias. Can be proarrhythmic. Electrolyte disturbances alter response; should be corrected before initiating therapy. Use cautiously in patients with first-degree block, pre-existing sinus node dysfunction, intraventricular conduction delays, significant hepatic dysfunction, hypotension, or severe CHF. Alterations in urinary pH may change urinary excretion. Rare hepatic toxicity may occur; may cause acute hepatic injury.

Adverse Reactions (Reflective of adult population; not specific for elderly)
>10%:
- Central nervous system: Lightheadedness (11% to 25%), dizziness (20% to 25%), nervousness (5% to 10%), incoordination (10%)
- Gastrointestinal: GI distress (41%), nausea/vomiting (40%)
- Neuromuscular & skeletal: Trembling, unsteady gait, tremor (13%), ataxia (10% to 20%)

1% to 10%:
- Cardiovascular: Chest pain (3% to 8%), premature ventricular contractions (1% to 2%), palpitation (4% to 8%), angina (2%), proarrhythmia (10% to 15% in patients with malignant arrhythmia)
- Central nervous system: Confusion, headache, insomnia (5% to 7%), depression (2%)
- Dermatologic: Rash (4%)
- Gastrointestinal: Constipation or diarrhea (4% to 5%), xerostomia (3%), abdominal pain (1%)
- Neuromuscular & skeletal: Weakness (5%), numbness of fingers or toes (2% to 4%), paresthesia (2%), arthralgia (1%)
- Ocular: Blurred vision (5% to 7%), nystagmus (6%)
- Otic: Tinnitus (2% to 3%)
- Respiratory: Dyspnea (3%)

Overdosage/Toxicology Has a narrow therapeutic index and severe toxicity may occur slightly above the therapeutic range, especially with other antiarrhythmic drugs. Acute ingestion of twice the daily therapeutic dose is potentially life-threatening. Symptoms include sedation, confusion, coma, seizures, respiratory arrest, and cardiac toxicity (sinus arrest, AV block, asystole, hypotension). The QRS and QT intervals are usually normal, although they may be prolonged after massive overdose. Other effects include dizziness, paresthesias, tremor, ataxia, and GI disturbance. Treatment is supportive, using conventional therapies (fluids, positioning, vasopressors, antiarrhythmics, anticonvulsants). Sodium bicarbonate may reverse QRS prolongation, bradyarrhythmias. and hypotension. Enhanced elimination with dialysis, hemoperfusion, or repeat charcoal is not effective.

Drug Interactions Substrate (major) of CYP1A2, 2D6; **Inhibits** CYP1A2 (strong)
CYP1A2 inducers: May decrease the levels/effects of mexiletine. Example inducers include aminoglutethimide, carbamazepine, phenobarbital, and rifampin.
CYP1A2 inhibitors: May increase the levels/effects of mexiletine. Example inhibitors include ciprofloxacin, ketoconazole, norfloxacin, ofloxacin, and rofecoxib.
CYP1A2 substrates: Mexiletine may increase the levels/effects of CYP1A2 substrates. Example substrates include aminophylline, fluvoxamine, mirtazapine, ropinirole, theophylline, and trifluoperazine.
CYP2D6 inhibitors: May increase the levels/effects of mexiletine. Example inhibitors include chlorpromazine, delavirdine, fluoxetine, miconazole, paroxetine, pergolide, quinidine, quinine, ritonavir, and ropinirole.
Fluvoxamine: Clearance of mexiletine was reduced by 38% following coadministration with fluvoxamine. If used concurrently, mexiletine levels should be monitored.
Quinidine may increase mexiletine blood levels.
Theophylline blood levels are increased by mexiletine.
Urinary alkalinizers (antacids, sodium bicarbonate, acetazolamide) may increase mexiletine blood levels.

Ethanol/Nutrition/Herb Interactions Food: Food may decrease the rate, but not the extent of oral absorption; diets which affect urine pH can increase or decrease excretion of mexiletine. Avoid dietary changes that alter urine pH.

Mechanism of Action Class IB antiarrhythmic, structurally related to lidocaine, which inhibits inward sodium current, decreases rate of rise of phase 0, increases effective refractory period/action potential duration ratio

Pharmacodynamics Onset of action: Oral: Within 30 minutes to 2 hours

Pharmacokinetics

Absorption: Older adults have a slightly slower rate of absorption but extent of absorption is the same as young adults.

Distribution: V_d: 5-7 L/kg

Protein binding: 50% to 70%

Metabolism: Low first-pass metabolism

Half-life: Adults: 10-14 hours (average: 14.4 hours older adults, 12 hours in younger adults); increase in half-life with hepatic or heart failure

Time to peak serum concentration: 2-3 hours

Elimination: 10% to 15% excreted unchanged in urine; urinary acidification increases excretion, alkalinization decreases excretion

Dosage

Geriatrics & Adults: Arrhythmias: Oral: Initial: 200 mg every 8 hours (may load with 400 mg if necessary); adjust dose every 2-3 days; usual dose: 200-300 mg every 8 hours; maximum: 1.2 g/day (some patients respond to every 12-hour dosing). When switching from another antiarrhythmic, initiate a 200 mg dose 6-12 hours after stopping former agents, 3-6 hours after stopping procainamide.

Hepatic Impairment: Patients with hepatic impairment or CHF may require dose reduction; reduce dose to 25% to 30% of usual dose

Administration Administer with food, around-the-clock rather than 3 times/day to promote less variation in peak and trough serum levels.

Monitoring Parameters EKG, blood pressure, pulse, serum concentrations

Reference Range Therapeutic: 0.5-2 mcg/mL; Potentially toxic: >2 mcg/mL

Test Interactions Abnormal liver function test, positive ANA, thrombocytopenia

Patient Information Take with food; notify physician of side effects such as jaundice, fever, palpitations, dizziness, tremor, heartburn, and sore throat

Additional Information I.V. form under investigation

Special Geriatric Considerations No specific changes in dose are necessary.

Dosage Forms Excipient information presented when available (limited, particularly for generics); consult specific product labeling. [DSC] = Discontinued product

Capsule, as hydrochloride: 150 mg, 200 mg, 250 mg

Mexitil®: 150 mg, 200 mg, 250 mg [DSC]

Selected References

Fenster PE and Nolan PE, "Antiarrhythmic Drugs," *Geriatric Pharmacology*, Bressler R and Katz MD, eds, New York, NY: McGraw-Hill, 1993, 6:105-49.

♦ **Mexitil® [DSC]** *see* Mexiletine *on page 1033*

♦ **MG217 Sal-Acid® [OTC]** *see* Salicylic Acid *on page 1441*

♦ **Mg-plus® [OTC]** *see* Magnesium Salts (Various Salts) *on page 952*

♦ **Miacalcin®** *see* Calcitonin *on page 209*

♦ **Mi-Acid [OTC]** *see* Aluminum Hydroxide, Magnesium Hydroxide, and Simethicone *on page 66*

♦ **Mi-Acid Maximum Strength [OTC]** *see* Aluminum Hydroxide, Magnesium Hydroxide, and Simethicone *on page 66*

♦ **Micaderm® [OTC]** *see* Miconazole *on page 1036*

Micafungin (mi ka FUN gin)

U.S. Brand Names Mycamine®

Index Terms Micafungin Sodium

Generic Available No

Pharmacologic Category Antifungal Agent, Parenteral; Echinocandin

Use Esophageal candidiasis; *Candida* prophylaxis in patients undergoing hematopoietic stem cell transplant

Unlabeled/Investigational Use Treatment of infections due to *Aspergillus* spp; prophylaxis of HIV-related esophageal candidiasis

Contraindications Hypersensitivity to micafungin or any component of the formulation

Warnings/Precautions Anaphylactic reactions, including shock have been reported; new onset or worsening hepatic failure has been reported; use caution in pre-existing mild-moderate hepatic impairment; safety in severe liver failure has not been evaluated; hemolytic anemia and hemoglobinuria have been reported; increased BUN, serum creatinine, renal dysfunction and/or acute renal failure has been reported; use with caution in patients with pre-existing renal impairment and monitor closely.

Adverse Reactions (Reflective of adult population; not specific for elderly)

1% to 10%:

Cardiovascular: Phlebitis (2%), hypertension (1%), flushing (1%)

(Continued)

Micafungin (Continued)

Central nervous system: Headache (2%), pyrexia (2%), delirium (1%), dizziness (1%), somnolence (1%)

Dermatologic: Rash (2%), pruritus (1%), febrile neutropenia (1%)

Endocrine & metabolic: Hypokalemia (1%), hypocalcemia (1%), hypomagnesemia (1%), hypophosphatemia (1%)

Gastrointestinal: Nausea (3%), diarrhea (2%), vomiting (2%), abdominal pain (1%), appetite decreased (1%), dysgeusia (1%), dyspepsia (1%)

Hematologic: Leukopenia (2%), neutropenia (1%), thrombocytopenia (1%), anemia (1%), lymphopenia (1%), eosinophilia (1%)

Hepatic: Transaminase increased (2% to 3%), serum alkaline phosphatase increased (2%), hyperbilirubinemia (1%)

Local: Infusion site inflammation (1%)

Neuromuscular & skeletal: Rigors (1%), lactate dehydrogenase increased (1%)

Renal: Serum creatinine increased (1%), serum urea increased (1%)

Overdosage/Toxicology Treatment should be symptom-directed and supportive. Not removed by dialysis.

Drug Interactions Substrate of CYP3A4 (minor); Inhibits CYP3A4 (weak)
No clinically-significant interactions have been identified.

Stability Store at 25°C (77°F). Reconstituted and diluted solutions are stable for 24 hours at room temperature. Protect from light. Aseptically add 5 mL of NS (preservative-free) to each 50 mg vial. Swirl to dissolve; do not shake. Further dilute 50-150 mg in 100 mL NS. Protect from light. Alternatively, D_5W may be used for reconstitution and dilution.

Mechanism of Action Concentration-dependent inhibition of 1,3-beta-D-glucan synthase resulting in reduced formation of 1,3-beta-D-glucan, an essential polysaccharide comprising 30% to 60% of *Candida* cell walls (absent in mammalian cells); decreased glucan content leads to osmotic instability and cellular lysis

Pharmacokinetics

Distribution: 0.28-0.5 L/kg

Protein binding: >99%

Metabolism: Hepatic; forms M-1 (catechol) and M-2 (methoxy) metabolites (activity unknown)

Half-life elimination: 11-21 hours

Excretion: Primarily feces (71%), urine (<15%, unchanged drug)

Dosage

Geriatrics & Adults:

Esophageal candidiasis: I.V.: 150 mg daily; median duration of therapy (from clinical trials) was 14 days

Prophylaxis of *Candida* infection in hematopoietic stem cell transplantation: 50 mg daily; median duration of therapy (from clinical trials) was 18 days

Administration For intravenous use only; infuse over 1 hour

Monitoring Parameters Liver function tests

Dosage Forms Excipient information presented when available (limited, particularly for generics); consult specific product labeling.

Injection, powder for reconstitution, as sodium [preservative-free]:
Mycamine®: 50 mg, 100 mg [contains lactose]

Selected References

Carver PL, "Micafungin," *Ann Pharmacother*, 2004, 38(10):1707-21.

de Wet N, Llanos-Cuentas A, Suleiman J, et al, "A Randomized, Double-Blind, Parallel-Group, Dose-Response Study of Micafungin Compared With Fluconazole for the Treatment of Esophageal Candidiasis in HIV-Positive Patients," *Clin Infect Dis*, 2004, 39(6):842-9.

Kohno S, Masaoka T, Yamaguchi H, et al, "A Multicenter, Open-Label Clinical Study of Micafungin (FK463) in the Treatment of Deep-Seated Mycosis in Japan," *Scand J Infect Dis*, 36(5):372-9.

Pettengell K, Mynhardt J, Kluyts T, et al, "Successful Treatment of Oesophageal Candidiasis by Micafungin: A Novel Systemic Antifungal Agent," *Aliment Pharmacol Ther*, 2004, 20(4):475-81.

Yokote T, Akioka T, Oka S, et al, "Successful Treatment With Micafungin of Invasive Pulmonary Aspergillosis in Acute Myeloid Leukemia, With Renal Failure Due to Amphotericin B Therapy," *Ann Hematol*, 2004, 83(1):64-6.

♦ **Micafungin Sodium** see Micafungin on page 1035
♦ **Micardis®** see Telmisartan on page 1526
♦ **Micardis® HCT** see Telmisartan and Hydrochlorothiazide on page 1527
♦ **Micatin® Athlete's Foot [OTC]** see Miconazole on page 1036
♦ **Micatin® Jock Itch [OTC]** see Miconazole on page 1036

Miconazole (mi KON a zole)

Medication Safety Issues

Sound-alike/look-alike issues:

Miconazole may be confused with Micronase®, Micronor®

Lotrimin® may be confused with Lotrisone®, Otrivin®

Micatin® may be confused with Miacalcin®

U.S. Brand Names Aloe Vesta® 2-n-1 Antifungal [OTC]; Baza® Antifungal [OTC]; Carrington Antifungal [OTC]; DermaFungal [OTC]; Dermagran® AF [OTC]; DiabetAid™ Antifungal Foot Bath [OTC]; Fungoid® Tincture [OTC]; Lotrimin® AF Jock Itch Powder Spray [OTC]; Lotrimin® AF Powder/Spray [OTC]; Micaderm® [OTC]; Micatin® Athlete's Foot [OTC]; Micatin® Jock Itch [OTC]; Micro-Guard® [OTC]; Mitrazol™ [OTC]; Monistat® 1 Combination Pack [OTC]; Monistat® 3 [OTC]; Monistat® 3 Combination Pack [OTC]; Monistat® 7 [OTC]; Monistat-Derm® [DSC]; Neosporin® AF [OTC]; Podactin Cream [OTC]; Secura® Antifungal [OTC]; Zeasorb®-AF [OTC]

Canadian Brand Names Dermazole; Micatin®; Micozole; Monistat®; Monistat® 3

Index Terms Miconazole Nitrate

Generic Available Yes

Pharmacologic Category Antifungal Agent, Topical; Antifungal Agent, Vaginal

Use

Topical: Treatment of vulvovaginal candidiasis and a variety of skin and mucous membrane fungal infections

I.V.: Treatment of severe systemic fungal infections and fungal meningitis that are refractory to standard treatment

Contraindications Hypersensitivity to miconazole or any component of the formulation

Warnings/Precautions For external use only; discontinue if sensitivity or irritation develop. Petrolatum-based vaginal products may damage rubber or latex condoms or diaphragms. Separate use by 3 days.

Adverse Reactions (Reflective of adult population; not specific for elderly)

Frequency not defined.

Topical: Allergic contact dermatitis, burning, maceration

Vaginal: Abdominal cramps, burning, irritation, itching

Drug Interactions Substrate of CYP3A4 (major); **Inhibits** CYP1A2 (moderate), 2A6 (strong), 2B6 (weak), 2C9 (strong), 2C19 (strong), 2D6 (strong), 2E1 (moderate), 3A4 (strong)

Note: The majority of reported drug interactions were observed following intravenous miconazole administration. Although systemic absorption following topical and/or vaginal administration is low, potential interactions due to CYP isoenzyme inhibition may occur (rarely). This may be particularly true in situations where topical absorption may be increased (eg, inflamed tissue).

Amphotericin B: Antifungal effects of both agents may be decreased

Cisapride: Risk of cardiotoxicity may be increased due to effect on metabolism; concurrent administration is contraindicated

CYP1A2 substrates: Miconazole may increase the levels/effects of CYP1A2 substrates. Example substrates include aminophylline, fluvoxamine, mexiletine, mirtazapine, ropinirole, theophylline, and trifluoperazine.

CYP2A6 substrates: Miconazole may increase the levels/effects of CYP2A6 substrates. Example substrates include dexmedetomidine and ifosfamide.

CYP2C9 Substrates: Miconazole may increase the levels/effects of CYP2C9 substrates. Example substrates include bosentan, dapsone, fluoxetine, glimepiride, glipizide, losartan, montelukast, nateglinide, paclitaxel, phenytoin, warfarin, and zafirlukast.

CYP2C19 substrates: Miconazole may increase the levels/effects of CYP2C19 substrates. Example substrates include citalopram, diazepam, methsuximide, phenytoin, propranolol, and sertraline.

CYP2D6 substrates: Miconazole may increase the levels/effects of CYP2D6 substrates. Example substrates include amphetamines, selected beta-blockers, dextromethorphan, fluoxetine, lidocaine, mirtazapine, nefazodone, paroxetine, risperidone, ritonavir, thioridazine, tricyclic antidepressants, and venlafaxine.

CYP2D6 prodrug substrates: Miconazole may decrease the levels/effects of CYP2D6 prodrug substrates. Example prodrug substrates include codeine, hydrocodone, oxycodone, and tramadol.

CYP2E1 substrates: Miconazole may increase the levels/effects of CYP2E1 substrates. Example substrates include inhalational anesthetics, theophylline, and trimethadione.

CYP3A4 inducers: CYP3A4 inducers may decrease the levels/effects of miconazole. Example inducers include aminoglutethimide, carbamazepine, nafcillin, nevirapine, phenobarbital, phenytoin, and rifamycins.

CYP3A4 substrates: Miconazole may increase the levels/effects of CYP3A4 substrates. Example substrates include benzodiazepines, calcium channel blockers, mirtazapine, nateglinide, nefazodone, tacrolimus, and venlafaxine. Selected benzodiazepines (midazolam and triazolam), cisapride, ergot alkaloids, selected HMG-CoA reductase inhibitors (lovastatin and simvastatin), and pimozide are generally contraindicated with strong CYP3A4 inhibitors.

Phenytoin: Serum concentration may be increased by miconazole

Sulfonylureas: Hypoglycemic effects may be increased

(Continued)

Miconazole *(Continued)*

Warfarin: An increased anticoagulant effect may occur with coadministration, including reports associated with short-term (3-day) intravaginal miconazole therapy

Ethanol/Nutrition/Herb Interactions Herb/Nutraceutical: St John's wort may decrease miconazole levels.

Mechanism of Action Inhibits biosynthesis of ergosterol, damaging the fungal cell wall membrane, which increases permeability causing leaking of nutrients

Pharmacokinetics Multiphasic degradation

Protein binding: 91% to 93%

Metabolism: Hepatic

Half-life:

Initial: 40 minutes

Secondary: 126 minutes

Terminal: 24 hours

Elimination: ~50% in feces and <1% in urine as unchanged drug

Dosage

Geriatrics & Adults:

Tinea corporis: Topical: Apply twice daily for 4 weeks

Tinea pedis: Topical: Apply twice daily for 4 weeks

Effervescent tablet: Dissolve 1 tablet in ~1 gallon of water; soak feet for 15-30 minutes; pat dry

Tinea cruris: Topical: Apply twice daily for 2 weeks

Vulvovaginal candidiasis: Vaginal:

Cream, 2%: Insert 1 applicatorful at bedtime for 7 days

Cream, 4%: Insert 1 applicatorful at bedtime for 3 days

Suppository, 100 mg: Insert 1 suppository at bedtime for 7 days

Suppository, 200 mg: Insert 1 suppository at bedtime for 3 days

Suppository, 1200 mg: Insert 1 suppository (a one-time dose); may be used at bedtime or during the day

Note: Many products are available as a combination pack, with a suppository for vaginal instillation and cream to relieve external symptoms. External cream may be used twice daily, as needed, for up to 7 days.

Administration Administer I.V. dose over 2 hours; administer around-the-clock rather than 4 times/day, 3 times/day, etc (ie, 12-6-12-6, not 9-1-5-9) to promote less variation in peak and trough serum concentration

Monitoring Parameters Signs and symptoms of infection

Patient Information Avoid contact with the eyes; if no response after several weeks of therapy, contact physician. Deodorant-free pads or panty shields may be used to protect clothing during use.

Special Geriatric Considerations No specific data for the elderly; use does not require alteration in dose or dose intervals. Assess patient's ability to self administer, may be difficult in patients with arthritis or limited range of motion.

Dosage Forms Excipient information presented when available (limited, particularly for generics); consult specific product labeling. [DSC] = Discontinued product

Combination products: Miconazole nitrate vaginal suppository 200 mg (3s) and miconazole nitrate external cream 2%

Monistat® 1 Combination Pack: Miconazole nitrate vaginal insert 1200 mg (1) and miconazole nitrate external cream 2% (5 g) [Note: Do not confuse with 1-Day™ (formerly Monistat® 1) which contains tioconazole]

Monistat® 3 Combination Pack:

Miconazole nitrate vaginal insert 200 mg (3s) and miconazole nitrate external cream 2%

Miconazole nitrate vaginal cream 4% and miconazole nitrate external cream 2%

Monistat® 7 Combination Pack:

Miconazole nitrate vaginal suppository 100 mg (7s) and miconazole nitrate external cream 2%

Miconazole nitrate vaginal cream 2% (7 prefilled applicators) and miconazole nitrate external cream 2%

Cream, topical, as nitrate: 2% (15 g, 30 g, 45 g)

Baza® Antifungal: 2% (4 g, 57 g, 142 g) [zinc oxide based formula]

Carrington Antifungal: 2% (150 g)

Micaderm®, Neosporin® AF, Podactin: 2% (30 g)

Micatin® Athlete's Foot, Micatin® Jock Itch: 2% (15 g)

Micro-Guard®, Mitrazol™: 2% (60 g)

Monistat-Derm®: 2% (15 g, 30 g, 85 g) [DSC]

Secura® Antifungal: 2% (60 g, 98 g)

Cream, vaginal, as nitrate [prefilled or refillable applicator]: 2% (45 g)

Monistat® 3: 4% (15 g, 25 g)

Monistat® 7: 2% (45 g)

Liquid, spray, topical, as nitrate:
Micatin® Athlete's Foot: 2% (90 mL) [contains alcohol]
Neosporin AF®: 2% (105 mL)
Lotion, powder, as nitrate (Zeasorb®-AF): 2% (56 g) [contains alcohol 36%]
Ointment, topical, as nitrate:
Aloe Vesta® 2-n-1 Antifungal: 2% (60 g, 150 g)
DermaFungal: 2% (113 g)
Dermagran® AF: (113 g) [contains vitamin A and zinc]
Powder, topical, as nitrate:
Lotrimin® AF: 2% (160 g)
Micro-Guard®: 2% (90 g)
Mitrazol™: 2% (30 g)
Zeasorb®-AF: 2% (70 g)
Powder spray, topical, as nitrate:
Lotrimin® AF, Lotrimin® AF Jock Itch: 2% (140 g)
Micatin® Athlete's Foot, Micatin® Jock Itch: 2% (90 g) [contains alcohol]
Neosporin® AF: 2% (85 g)
Suppository, vaginal, as nitrate: 100 mg (7s); 200 mg (3s)
Monistat® 3: 200 mg (3s)
Monistat® 7: 100 mg (7s)
Tablet, for solution, topical, as nitrate [effervescent]:
DiabetAid™ Antifungal Foot Bath: 2% (10s)
Tincture, topical, as nitrate (Fungoid®): 2% (30 mL, 473 mL) [contains isopropyl alcohol 30%]; 30 mL size also available in a treatment kit which contains nail scrub and nail brush]

♦ **Miconazole Nitrate** see Miconazole on page 1036
♦ **Micro-Guard® [OTC]** see Miconazole on page 1036
♦ **microK®** see Potassium Chloride on page 1288
♦ **microK® 10** see Potassium Chloride on page 1288
♦ **Micronase®** see GlyBURIDE on page 714
♦ **Microzide™** see Hydrochlorothiazide on page 756

Midazolam (MID aye zoe lam)

Related Information
Anxiolytic, Sedative / Hypnotic, and Miscellaneous Benzodiazepines on page 1750
Medication Safety Issues
Sound-alike/look-alike issues:
Versed may be confused with VePesid®, Vistaril®

High alert medication: The Institute for Safe Medication Practices (ISMP) includes this medication among its list of drugs which have a heightened risk of causing significant patient harm when used in error.
Canadian Brand Names Apo-Midazolam®; Midazolam Injection
Index Terms Midazolam Hydrochloride; Versed
Generic Available Yes
Pharmacologic Category Benzodiazepine
Use Preoperative sedation; conscious sedation prior to diagnostic or radiographic procedures; ICU sedation (continuous infusion); intravenous anesthesia (induction and maintenance)
Unlabeled/Investigational Use Treatment of anxiety, status epilepticus
Restrictions C-IV
Contraindications Hypersensitivity to midazolam or any component of the formulation, including benzyl alcohol (cross-sensitivity with other benzodiazepines may exist); parenteral form is not for intrathecal or epidural injection; narrow-angle glaucoma; concurrent use of potent inhibitors of CYP3A4 (amprenavir, atazanavir, or ritonavir)
Warnings/Precautions [U.S. Boxed Warning]: May cause severe respiratory depression, respiratory arrest, or apnea. Use with extreme caution, particularly in noncritical care settings. Appropriate resuscitative equipment and qualified personnel must be available for administration and monitoring. Initial dosing must be cautiously titrated and individualized, particularly in elderly or debilitated patients, patients with hepatic impairment (including alcoholics), or in renal impairment, particularly if other CNS depressants (including opiates) are used concurrently. **[U.S. Boxed Warning]: Initial doses in elderly or debilitated patients should be conservative; as little as 1 mg, but not to exceed 2.5 mg.** Use with caution in patients with respiratory disease or impaired gag reflex. Use during upper airway procedures may increase risk of hypoventilation. Prolonged responses have been noted following extended administration by continuous infusion (possibly due to metabolite accumulation) or in the presence of drugs which inhibit midazolam metabolism.
(Continued)

Midazolam *(Continued)*

Causes CNS depression (dose-related) resulting in sedation, dizziness, confusion, or ataxia which may impair physical and mental capabilities. Patients must be cautioned about performing tasks which require mental alertness (eg, operating machinery or driving). A minimum of 1 day should elapse after midazolam administration before attempting these tasks. Use with caution in patients receiving other CNS depressants or psychoactive agents. Effects with other sedative drugs or ethanol may be potentiated. Benzodiazepines have been associated with falls and traumatic injury and should be used with extreme caution in patients who are at risk of these events (especially the elderly).

May cause hypotension - hemodynamic events are more common in patients with hemodynamic instability. Hypotension and/or respiratory depression may occur more frequently in patients who have received opioid analgesics. Use with caution in obese patients, chronic renal failure, and HF. Does not protect against increases in heart rate or blood pressure during intubation. Should not be used in shock, coma, or acute alcohol intoxication. **[U.S. Boxed Warning]: Parenteral form contains benzyl alcohol; avoid rapid injection in prolonged infusions.** Avoid intra-arterial administration or extravasation of parenteral formulation.

Midazolam causes anterograde amnesia. Paradoxical reactions, including hyperactive or aggressive behavior have been reported with benzodiazepines, particularly in psychiatric patients. Does not have analgesic, antidepressant, or antipsychotic properties.

Benzodiazepines have been associated with dependence and acute withdrawal symptoms on discontinuation or reduction in dose. Acute withdrawal, including seizures, may be precipitated after administration of flumazenil to patients receiving long-term benzodiazepine therapy.

Adverse Reactions (Reflective of adult population; not specific for elderly)

>10%: Respiratory: Decreased tidal volume and/or respiratory rate decrease, apnea

1% to 10%:

Cardiovascular: Hypotension

Central nervous system: Drowsiness (1%), oversedation, headache (1%), seizure-like activity

Gastrointestinal: Nausea (3%), vomiting (3%)

Local: Pain and local reactions at injection site (4% I.M., 5% I.V.; severity less than diazepam)

Ocular: Nystagmus

Respiratory: Cough (1%)

Miscellaneous: Physical and psychological dependence with prolonged use, hiccups (4%), paradoxical reaction

Overdosage/Toxicology
Symptoms include respiratory depression, hypotension, coma, stupor, confusion, and apnea. Treatment for benzodiazepine overdose is supportive. Rarely is mechanical ventilation required. Flumazenil has been shown to selectively block the binding of benzodiazepines to CNS receptors, resulting in a reversal of benzodiazepine-induced CNS depression. Respiratory reaction to hypoxia may not be restored.

Drug Interactions Substrate of CYP2B6 (minor), 3A4 (major); Inhibits CYP2C8 (weak), 2C9 (weak), 3A4 (weak)

CNS depressants: Sedative effects and/or respiratory depression may be additive with CNS depressants; includes ethanol, barbiturates, opioid analgesics, and other sedative agents; monitor for increased effect. **If narcotics or other CNS depressants are administered concomitantly, the midazolam dose should be reduced by 30% if <65 years of age, or by at least 50% if >65 years of age.**

CYP3A4 inducers: CYP3A4 inducers may decrease the levels/effects of midazolam. Example inducers include aminoglutethimide, carbamazepine, nafcillin, nevirapine, phenobarbital, phenytoin, and rifamycins.

CYP3A4 inhibitors: May increase the levels/effects of midazolam. Example inhibitors include azole antifungals, clarithromycin, diclofenac, doxycycline, erythromycin, imatinib, isoniazid, nefazodone, nicardipine, propofol, protease inhibitors, quinidine, telithromycin, and verapamil.

Levodopa: Therapeutic effects may be diminished in some patients following the addition of a benzodiazepine; limited/inconsistent data

Oral contraceptives: May decrease the clearance of some benzodiazepines (those which undergo oxidative metabolism); monitor for increased benzodiazepine effect

Saquinavir: A 56% reduction in clearance and a doubling of midazolam's half-life were seen with concurrent administration with saquinavir.

Theophylline: May partially antagonize some of the effects of benzodiazepines; monitor for decreased response; may require higher doses for sedation

Ethanol/Nutrition/Herb Interactions

Ethanol: Avoid ethanol (may increase CNS depression).

Food: Grapefruit juice may increase serum concentrations of midazolam; avoid concurrent use with oral form.

Herb/Nutraceutical: Avoid concurrent use with St John's wort (may decrease midazolam levels, may increase CNS depression). Avoid concurrent use with valerian, kava kava, gotu kola (may increase CNS depression).

Stability The manufacturer states that midazolam, at a final concentration of 0.5 mg/mL, is stable for up to 24 hours when diluted with D_5W or NS. A final concentration of 1 mg/mL in NS has been documented to be stable for up to 10 days (McMullen, 1995). Admixtures do not require protection from light for short-term storage.

Mechanism of Action Binds to stereospecific benzodiazepine receptors on the postsynaptic GABA neuron at several sites within the central nervous system, including the limbic system, reticular formation. Enhancement of the inhibitory effect of GABA on neuronal excitability results by increased neuronal membrane permeability to chloride ions. This shift in chloride ions results in hyperpolarization (a less excitable state) and stabilization.

Pharmacodynamics

Sedation onset:

I.M.: Within 15 minutes

I.V. within 1-5 minutes

Peak effect: I.M.: 30-60 minutes

Duration: I.M.: Mean: 2 hours, up to 6 hours

Pharmacokinetics

Distribution: V_d: 0.8-2.5 L/kg; increased V_d with congestive heart failure and chronic renal failure; slightly increased V_d in older adults

Protein binding: 95%

Metabolism: Extensive in the liver (microsomally)

Half-life: Elimination: 1-4 hours; increased half-life with cirrhosis, congestive heart failure, obesity, older adults (5.6 ± 4.8 hours); some older adult males had a marked increase in elimination half-life

Elimination: Excreted as glucuronide conjugated metabolites in urine, ~2% to 10% is excreted in feces

Pharmacokinetics in older adult males were less predictable than in older adult females

Dosage

Geriatrics: The dose of midazolam needs to be individualized based on the patient's age, underlying diseases, and concurrent medications. Decrease dose (by ~30%) if narcotics or other CNS depressants are administered concomitantly. **Personnel and equipment needed for standard respiratory resuscitation should be immediately available during midazolam administration.**

I.V.: Conscious sedation: Initial: 0.5 mg slow I.V.; give no more than 1.5 mg in a 2-minute period. If additional titration is needed, give no more than 1 mg over 2 minutes, waiting another 2 or more minutes to evaluate sedative effect. A total dose >3.5 mg is rarely necessary.

Adults:

Note: The dose of midazolam needs to be individualized based on the patient's age, underlying diseases, and concurrent medications. Decrease dose (by ~30%) if narcotics or other CNS depressants are administered concomitantly. **Personnel and equipment needed for standard respiratory resuscitation should be immediately available during midazolam administration.**

Preoperative sedation:

I.M.: 0.07-0.08 mg/kg 30-60 minutes prior to surgery/procedure; usual dose: 5 mg; **Note:** Reduce dose in patients with COPD, high-risk patients, patients ≥60 years of age, and patients receiving other narcotics or CNS depressants

I.V.: 0.02-0.04 mg/kg; repeat every 5 minutes as needed to desired effect or up to 0.1-0.2 mg/kg

Intranasal (not an approved route): 0.2 mg/kg (up to 0.4 mg/kg in some studies); administer 30-45 minutes prior to surgery/procedure

Conscious sedation: I.V.: Initial: 0.5-2 mg slow I.V. over at least 2 minutes; slowly titrate to effect by repeating doses every 2-3 minutes if needed; usual total dose: 2.5-5 mg; use decreased doses in elderly.

Healthy Adults <60 years:

Initial: Some patients respond to doses as low as 1 mg; no more than 2.5 mg should be administered over a period of 2 minutes. Additional doses of midazolam may be administered after a 2-minute waiting period and evaluation of sedation after each dose increment. A total dose >5 mg is generally not needed. If narcotics or other CNS depressants are administered concomitantly, the midazolam dose should be reduced by 30%. *Refer to geriatric dosing for patients ≥60 years, debilitated, or chronically ill.*

Maintenance: 25% of dose used to reach sedative effect

(Continued)

Midazolam *(Continued)*

Anesthesia: I.V.:
Induction:
Unpremedicated patients: 0.3-0.35 mg/kg (up to 0.6 mg/kg in resistant cases)
Premedicated patients: 0.15-0.35 mg/kg
Maintenance: 0.05-0.3 mg/kg as needed, or continuous infusion 0.25-1.5 mcg/kg/minute

Sedation in mechanically-ventilated patients: I.V. continuous infusion: 100 mg in 250 mL D_5W or NS (if patient is fluid-restricted, may concentrate up to a maximum of 0.5 mg/mL); initial dose: 0.02-0.08 mg/kg (~1 mg to 5 mg in 70 kg adult) initially and either repeated at 5-15 minute intervals until adequate sedation is achieved or continuous infusion rates of 0.04-0.2 mg/kg/hour and titrate to reach desired level of sedation

Renal Impairment:
Hemodialysis: Supplemental dose is not necessary.
Peritoneal dialysis: Significant drug removal is unlikely based on physiochemical characteristics.

Administration See Dosage.

Monitoring Parameters Respiratory, cardiovascular and mental status

Patient Information May cause drowsiness; do not drive or operate hazardous machinery until the effects of the drug are gone or until the day after administration

Additional Information Healthy adults <60 years of age: Some patients respond to doses as low as 1 mg; no more than 2.5 mg should be administered over a period of 2 minutes. Additional doses of midazolam may be administered after a 2-minute waiting period and evaluation of sedation after each dose increment. A total dose >5 mg is generally not needed. If narcotics or other CNS depressants are administered concomitantly, the midazolam dose should be reduced by 30%.

Special Geriatric Considerations In the elderly if concomitant CNS depressant medications are used, the midazolam dose will be at least 50% less than doses used in healthy, young, unpremedicated patients.

Dosage Forms Excipient information presented when available (limited, particularly for generics); consult specific product labeling.
Injection, solution: 1 mg/mL (2 mL, 5 mL, 10 mL); 5 mg/mL (1 mL, 2 mL, 5 mL, 10 mL) [contains benzyl alcohol 1%]
Injection, solution [preservative free]: 1 mg/mL (2 mL, 5 mL); 5 mg/mL (1 mL, 2 mL)
Syrup: 2 mg/mL (118 mL) [contains sodium benzoate; cherry flavor]

Selected References
Kanto J, Aaltonen L, Himberg JJ, et al, "Midazolam as an Intravenous Induction Agent in the Elderly: A Clinical and Pharmacokinetic Study," *Anesth Analg*, 1986, 65(1):15-20.
Servin F, Enriquez I, Fournet M, et al, "Pharmacokinetics of Midazolam Used as an Intravenous Induction Agent for Patients Over 80 Years of Age," *Eur J Anaesthesiol*, 1987, 4(1):1-7.

♦ **Midazolam Hydrochloride** *see* Midazolam *on page 1039*

Midodrine *(MI doe dreen)*

Medication Safety Issues
Sound-alike/look-alike issues:
ProAmatine® may be confused with protamine

U.S. Brand Names Orvaten™; ProAmatine®
Canadian Brand Names Amatine®; Apo-Midodrine®
Index Terms Midodrine Hydrochloride
Generic Available Yes
Pharmacologic Category Alpha$_1$ Agonist
Use Treatment of symptomatic orthostatic hypotension
Unlabeled/Investigational Use Investigational: Management of urinary incontinence
Contraindications Hypersensitivity to midodrine or any component of the formulation; severe organic heart disease; urinary retention; pheochromocytoma; thyrotoxicosis; persistent and significant supine hypertension

Warnings/Precautions [U.S. Boxed Warning]: Indicated for patients for whom orthostatic hypotension significantly impairs their daily life despite standard clinical care. Use is not recommended with supine hypertension. Caution should be exercised in patients with diabetes, visual problems (especially if receiving fludrocortisone), urinary retention (reduce initial dose), or hepatic dysfunction; monitor renal and hepatic function prior to and periodically during therapy; discontinue and re-evaluate therapy if signs of bradycardia occur.

Adverse Reactions (Reflective of adult population; not specific for elderly)
>10%:
Cardiovascular: Supine hypertension (7% to 13%)
Dermatologic: Piloerection (13%), pruritus (12%)
Genitourinary: Urinary urgency, retention, or polyuria, dysuria (up to 13%)

Neuromuscular & skeletal: Paresthesia (18%)
1% to 10%:
  Central nervous system: Chills (5%), pain (5%)
  Dermatologic: Rash (2%)
  Gastrointestinal: Abdominal pain

Overdosage/Toxicology Symptoms include hypertension, piloerection, and urinary retention. Treatment is symptomatic following gastric decontamination. Alpha-sympatholytics and/or dialysis may be helpful.

Drug Interactions Increased effect: Concomitant fludrocortisone results in hypernatremia or an increase in intraocular pressure and glaucoma; bradycardia may be accentuated with concomitant administration of cardiac glycosides, psychotherapeutics, and beta-blockers; alpha-agonists may increase the pressure effects and alpha-antagonists may negate the effects of midodrine

Mechanism of Action Midodrine forms an active metabolite, desglymidodrine, that is an alpha$_1$-agonist. This agent increases arteriolar and venous tone resulting in a rise in standing, sitting, and supine systolic and diastolic blood pressure in patients with orthostatic hypotension. See table.

Causes of Orthostatic Hypotension

Primary Autonomic Causes
Pure autonomic failure (Bradbury-Eggleston syndrome, idiopathic orthostatic hypotension)
Autonomic failure with multiple system atrophy (Shy-Drager syndrome)
Familial dysautonomia (Riley-Day syndrome)
Dopamine beta-hydroxylase deficiency
Secondary Autonomic Causes
Chronic alcoholism
Parkinson's disease
Diabetes mellitus
Porphyria
Amyloidosis
Various carcinomas
Vitamin B$_1$ or B$_{12}$ deficiency
Nonautonomic Causes
Hypovolemia (such as associated with hemorrhage, burns, or hemodialysis) and dehydration
Diminished homeostatic regulation (such as associated with aging, pregnancy, fever, or prolonged bedrest)
Medications (eg, antihypertensives, insulin, tricyclic antidepressants)

Pharmacokinetics
Absorption: Rapid
Distribution: V$_d$ (desglymidodrine): <1.6 L/kg; poorly across membrane (eg, blood brain barrier)
Protein binding: Minimal
Metabolism: Hepatic; midodrine is a prodrug which undergoes rapid deglycination to desglymidodrine (active metabolite); metabolism occurs in many tissues and plasma
Bioavailability: Desglymidodrine: 93%
Half-life elimination: Desglymidodrine: ~3-4 hours; Midodrine: 25 minutes
Time to peak, serum: Desglymidodrine: 1-2 hours; Midodrine: 30 minutes
Elimination:
  Renal, midodrine: Insignificant
  Desglymidodrine: 80% by renal secretion

Dosage
Geriatrics & Adults: Orthostatic hypotension: Oral: 10 mg 3 times/day during daytime hours (every 3-4 hours) when patient is upright (maximum: 40 mg/day)
Renal Impairment: 2.5 mg 3 times/day; gradually increase as tolerated.
  Hemodialysis: Dialyzable

Monitoring Parameters Blood pressure (standing and sitting), renal and hepatic parameters, symptoms of orthostasis

Patient Information Use caution with over-the-counter medications which may affect blood pressure (cough and cold, diet, stay-awake medications). Avoid taking a particular dose if you are to be supine for any length of time. Take your last daily dose 3-4 hours before bedtime to minimize nighttime supine hypertension. May need to sleep with the head of the bed elevated.

Special Geriatric Considerations Adjust dosage for renal impairment.

Dosage Forms Excipient information presented when available (limited, particularly for generics); consult specific product labeling.
  Tablet, as hydrochloride: 2.5 mg, 5 mg, 10 mg

♦ **Midodrine Hydrochloride** *see Midodrine on page 1042*

♦ **Midol® Cramp and Body Aches [OTC]** *see Ibuprofen on page 784*

♦ **Midol® Extended Relief** *see Naproxen on page 1088*

♦ **Migergot** *see Ergotamine and Caffeine on page 530*

Miglitol (MIG li tol)

U.S. Brand Names Glyset®
Canadian Brand Names Glyset®
Generic Available No
Pharmacologic Category Antidiabetic Agent, Alpha-Glucosidase Inhibitor
Use Treatment of noninsulin-dependent diabetes mellitus (NIDDM); monotherapy adjunct to diet to improve glycemic control in patients with NIDDM whose hyperglycemia cannot be managed with diet alone; combination therapy with a sulfonylurea when diet plus either miglitol or a sulfonylurea alone do not result in adequate glycemic control (effect of miglitol to enhance glycemic control is additive to that of sulfonylureas when used in combination)
Contraindications Hypersensitivity to miglitol or any of component of the formulation; diabetic ketoacidosis; inflammatory bowel disease; colonic ulceration; partial intestinal obstruction or predisposition to intestinal obstruction; chronic intestinal diseases associated with marked disorders of digestion or absorption or with conditions that may deteriorate as a result of increased gas formation in the intestine
Warnings/Precautions GI symptoms are the most common reactions. The incidence of abdominal pain and diarrhea tend to diminish considerably with continued treatment. Long-term clinical trials in diabetic patients with significant renal dysfunction (serum creatinine >2 mg/dL) have not been conducted. Treatment of these patients is not recommended. In combination with a sulfonylurea will cause a further lowering of blood glucose and may increase the hypoglycemic potential of the sulfonylurea. It may be necessary to discontinue miglitol and administer insulin if the patient is exposed to stress (ie, fever, trauma, infection, surgery).
Adverse Reactions (Reflective of adult population; not specific for elderly)
>10%: Gastrointestinal: Flatulence (42%), diarrhea (29%), abdominal pain (12%)
1% to 10%: Dermatologic: Rash
Overdosage/Toxicology An overdose of miglitol will not result in hypoglycemia. An overdose may result in transient increases in flatulence, diarrhea, and abdominal discomfort. No serious systemic reactions are expected in the event of an overdose.
Drug Interactions Decreased effect:
Miglitol may decrease the absorption and bioavailability of digoxin, propranolol, ranitidine
Digestive enzymes (amylase, pancreatin, charcoal) may reduce the effect of miglitol and should **not** be taken concomitantly
Mechanism of Action In contrast to sulfonylureas, miglitol does not enhance insulin secretion; the antihyperglycemic action of miglitol results from a reversible inhibition of membrane-bound intestinal alpha-glucosidases which hydrolyze oligosaccharides and disaccharides to glucose and other monosaccharides in the brush border of the small intestine; in patients with diabetes, this enzyme inhibition results in delayed glucose absorption and lowering of postprandial hyperglycemia
Pharmacokinetics
Absorption: Saturable at high doses: 25% mg dose: Completely absorbed; 100 mg dose: 50% to 70% absorbed; Peak concentrations within 2-3 hours
Distribution: V_d: 0.18 L/kg
Protein binding: Negligible (<4%)
Metabolism: Not metabolized
Half-life, elimination: ~2 hours
Elimination: Renal as unchanged drug
Dosage
Geriatrics & Adults: Type 2 diabetes (noninsulin dependent, NIDDM): Oral: 25 mg 3 times/day with the first bite of food at each meal; the dose may be increased to 50 mg 3 times/day after 4-8 weeks; maximum recommended dose: 100 mg 3 times/day
Renal Impairment: Miglitol is primarily excreted by the kidneys; there is little information of miglitol in patients with a Cl_{cr} <25 mL/minute.
Hepatic Impairment: No adjustment necessary.
Monitoring Parameters Monitor therapeutic response by periodic blood glucose tests; measurement of glycosylated hemoglobin is recommended for the monitoring of long-term glycemic control
Patient Information Take this medication exactly as directed, with the first bite of each main meal. Do not change dosage or discontinue without first consulting prescriber. Do

not take other medications with or within 2 hours of this medication unless so advised by prescriber. It is important to follow dietary and lifestyle recommendations of prescriber. You will be instructed in signs of hypo-/hyperglycemia by prescriber or diabetic educator. If combining miglitol with other diabetic medication (eg, sulfonylureas, insulin), keep source of glucose (sugar) on hand in case hypoglycemia occurs. You may experience mild side effects during the first weeks of therapy (eg, bloating, flatulence, diarrhea, abdominal discomfort), these should diminish over time. Report severe or persistent side effects, fever, extended vomiting or flu, or change in color of urine or stool.

Special Geriatric Considerations In a double-blind randomized, placebo-controlled trial, glyburide caused significantly greater reductions in hemoglobin A_{1c} compared to miglitol 25 mg or 50 mg three times per day, but was associated with more weight gain. Diarrhea, soft stools, and flatulence were more common with miglitol.

Dosage Forms Excipient information presented when available (limited, particularly for generics); consult specific product labeling.
Tablet: 25 mg, 50 mg, 100 mg

Selected References
Johnston PS, Lebovitz HE, Coniff RF, et al, "Advantages of Alpha-Glucosidase Inhibition as Monotherapy in Elderly Type 2 Diabetic Patients," *J Clin Endocrinol Metab*, 1998, 83(5):1515-22.

◆ **Migranal**® see Dihydroergotamine *on page 437*
◆ **Mild-C**® [OTC] see Ascorbic Acid *on page 125*
◆ **Milkinol**® [OTC] see Mineral Oil *on page 1045*
◆ **Milk of Magnesia** see Magnesium Hydroxide *on page 946*
◆ **Miltown**® [DSC] see Meprobamate *on page 984*

Mineral Oil (MIN er al oyl)

Related Information
Potentially Inappropriate Medications for Geriatrics *on page 1824*

U.S. Brand Names Fleet® Mineral Oil Enema [OTC]; Kondremul® [OTC]; Milkinol® [OTC]; Neo-Cultol® [OTC]; Zymenol® [OTC]

Index Terms Heavy Mineral Oil; Liquid Paraffin; White Mineral Oil

Generic Available Yes

Pharmacologic Category Laxative, Lubricant

Use Temporary relief of constipation, relief of fecal impaction; preparation for bowel studies or surgery

Contraindications Patients with colostomy or an ileostomy, appendicitis, ulcerative colitis, diverticulitis

Warnings/Precautions Lipid pneumonitis results from aspiration of mineral oil. Aspiration risk increased in patients in prolonged supine position or conditions which interfere with swallowing or epiglottal function (eg, stroke, Parkinson's disease, Alzheimer's disease, esophageal dysmotility).

When used for self-medication (OTC): Healthcare provider should be contacted in case of sudden changes in bowel habits which last over 2 weeks; abdominal pain, nausea, vomiting; rectal bleeding following use; if needed for >1 week.

Adverse Reactions (Reflective of adult population; not specific for elderly)
Frequency not defined.
Gastrointestinal: Abdominal cramps, diarrhea, nausea, vomiting
Respiratory: Lipid pneumonitis with aspiration
Miscellaneous: Large doses may cause anal leakage causing anal itching, irritation, hemorrhoids, perianal discomfort, soiling of clothes

Drug Interactions May impair absorption of fat-soluble vitamins (A, D, K, E), coumarin, sulfonamides; administration of surfactants (docusate) with mineral oil may increase mineral oil absorption and therefore enhance toxic potential of mineral oil resulting in a foreign body reaction in lymphoid tissue

Mechanism of Action Eases passage of stool by decreasing water absorption and lubricating the intestine; retards colonic absorption of water

Pharmacodynamics Onset of action: ~6-8 hours; effect on bowel function is generally seen after 2-3 days of use

Pharmacokinetics
Distribution: Site of action is the colon
Elimination: In feces

Dosage
Geriatrics & Adults:
Constipation:
Oral: 15-45 mL/day
Kondremul®: 30-75 mL/day
Liqui-Doss®: 15-45 mL at bedtime
Rectal (Fleet® Mineral Oil): 118 mL as a single dose
(Continued)

Mineral Oil *(Continued)*

Fecal impaction or following barium studies: Rectal (Fleet® Mineral Oil): 118 mL as a single dose

Monitoring Parameters Monitor for response: Stool frequency, consistency. Avoid use in patients who may aspirate.

Patient Information Do not take with food or meals; do not use if experiencing abdominal pain, nausea, or vomiting; do not take while reclining in bed, sit up; do **not** administer just before bedtime; wear protective undergarments

Additional Information Do not administer with food or meals because of the risk of aspiration; prolonged administration of mineral oil may decrease absorption of lipid-soluble vitamins A, D, E, and K. Light sterile mineral oils are not for injection.

Special Geriatric Considerations Other therapies should be attempted before using mineral oil to relieve constipation to avoid complications with mineral oil; doses, if used, should begin low and should be used as infrequently as possible.

Dosage Forms

Emulsion: 1.4 g/5 mL (480 mL); 2.5 mL/5 mL (420 mL); 2.75 mL/5 mL (480 mL); 4.75 mL/5 mL (240 mL)

Jelly: 2.75 mL/5 mL (180 mL)

Liquid: 500 mL, 1000 mL, 4000 mL

Liquid, rectal: 133 mL

♦ **Minipress**® *see* Prazosin *on page 1301*

♦ **Minitran**™ *see* Nitroglycerin *on page 1129*

♦ **Minocin**® **PAC** *see* Minocycline *on page 1046*

Minocycline (mi noe SYE kleen)

Medication Safety Issues

Sound-alike/look-alike issues:

Dynacin® may be confused with Dyazide®, Dynabac®, DynaCirc®, Dynapen®

Minocin® may be confused with Indocin®, Lincocin®, Minizide®, Mithracin®, niacin

U.S. Brand Names Dynacin®; Minocin® PAC; myrac™; Solodyn™

Canadian Brand Names Alti-Minocycline; Apo-Minocycline®; Gen-Minocycline; Minocin®; Novo-Minocycline; PMS-Minocycline; Rhoxal-minocycline; Sandoz-Minocycline

Index Terms Minocycline Hydrochloride

Generic Available Yes: Excludes extended release tablet

Pharmacologic Category Antibiotic, Tetracycline Derivative

Use Treatment of susceptible bacterial infections of both gram-negative and gram-positive organisms; treatment of anthrax (inhalational, cutaneous, and gastrointestinal); acne, meningococcal carrier state

Dental: Treatment of periodontitis associated with presence of *Actinobacillus actinomycetemcomitans* (AA); as adjunctive therapy in recurrent aphthous ulcers

Contraindications Hypersensitivity to minocycline, other tetracyclines, or any component of the formulation

Warnings/Precautions May cause tissue hyperpigmentation or permanent tooth discoloration. May be associated with increases in BUN secondary to antianabolic effects; use caution in patients with renal impairment. Hepatotoxicity has been reported; use caution in patients with hepatic insufficiency. Autoimmune syndromes (eg, lupus-like, hepatitis, and vasculitis) have been reported; discontinue if symptoms. CNS effects (lightheadedness, vertigo) may occur; patients must be cautioned about performing tasks which require mental alertness (eg, operating machinery or driving). Has been associated (rarely) with pseudotumor cerebri. May cause photosensitivity; discontinue if skin erythema occurs. Prolonged use may result in fungal or bacterial superinfection, including *C. difficile*-associated diarrhea and pseudomembranous colitis.

Adverse Reactions (Reflective of adult population; not specific for elderly) Frequency not defined.

Cardiovascular: Myocarditis, pericarditis, vasculitis

Central nervous system: Bulging fontanels, dizziness, fatigue, fever, headache, hypoesthesia, malaise, mood changes, paresthesia, pseudotumor cerebri, sedation, seizure, somnolence, vertigo

Dermatologic: Alopecia, angioedema, erythema multiforme, erythema nodosum, erythematous rash, exfoliative dermatitis, hyperpigmentation of nails, maculopapular rash, photosensitivity, pigmentation of the skin and mucous membranes, pruritus, Stevens-Johnson syndrome, toxic epidermal necrolysis, urticaria

Endocrine & metabolic: Thyroid discoloration, thyroid dysfunction

Gastrointestinal: Anorexia, diarrhea, dyspepsia, dysphagia, enamel hypoplasia, enterocolitis, esophageal ulcerations, esophagitis, glossitis, inflammatory lesions (oral/

anogenital), moniliasis, nausea, oral cavity discoloration, pancreatitis, pseudomembranous colitis, stomatitis, tooth discoloration, vomiting, xerostomia

Genitourinary: Balanitis, vulvovaginitis

Hematologic: Agranulocytosis, eosinophilia, hemolytic anemia, leukopenia, neutropenia, pancytopenia, thrombocytopenia

Hepatic: Hepatic cholestasis, hepatic failure, hepatitis, hyperbilirubinemia, jaundice, liver enzyme increases

Neuromuscular & skeletal: Arthralgia, arthritis, bone discoloration, joint stiffness, joint swelling, myalgia

Otic: Hearing loss, tinnitus

Renal: Acute renal failure, BUN increased, interstitial nephritis

Respiratory: Asthma, bronchospasm, cough, dyspnea, pneumonitis, pulmonary infiltrate (with eosinophilia)

Miscellaneous: Anaphylaxis, hypersensitivity, lupus erythematosus, lupus-like syndrome, serum sickness

Overdosage/Toxicology Symptoms include diabetes insipidus, nausea, anorexia, dizziness, vomiting, and diarrhea. Following GI decontamination, care is symptom-directed and supportive. Fluid support may be required. Not dialyzable (0% to 5%).

Drug Interactions

Calcium-, magnesium-, or aluminum-containing antacids, bile acid sequestrants, bismuth, oral contraceptives, iron, zinc, sodium bicarbonate, penicillins, quinapril: May decrease absorption of tetracyclines.

Methoxyflurane anesthesia, when concurrent with tetracyclines, may cause fatal nephrotoxicity.

Penicillins: Tetracyclines may reduce bactericidal efficacy of penicillins and cephalosporins.

Retinoic acid derivatives: May increase risk of pseudotumor cerebri.

Typhoid vaccine: Antibacterial agents may decrease the therapeutic efficacy of the live, attenuated typhoid (Ty21a strain) vaccine

Warfarin: Hypoprothrombinemic response may be increased with tetracyclines; monitor INR closely during initiation or discontinuation.

Ethanol/Nutrition/Herb Interactions

Food: Minocycline serum concentrations are not significantly altered if taken with food or dairy products.

Herb/Nutraceutical: Avoid dong quai, St John's wort (may also cause photosensitization).

Stability

Capsule (including pellet-filled), tablet: Store at 20°C to 25°C (68°F to 77°F). Protect from light and moisture.

Extended release tablet: Store at 15°C to 30°C (59°F to 86°F). Protect from light, moisture, and heat.

Mechanism of Action Inhibits bacterial protein synthesis by binding with the 30S and possibly the 50S ribosomal subunit(s) of susceptible bacteria; cell wall synthesis is not affected

Pharmacokinetics

Absorption: Well absorbed

Protein binding: 70% to 75%

Half-life elimination: 16 hours (range: 11-23 hours)

Time to peak: Capsule, pellet filled: 1-4 hours; Extended release tablet: 3.5-4 hours

Elimination: Majority of dose deposits for extended periods in fat and eventually is cleared renally

Dosage

Geriatrics & Adults:

Usual dosage range: Oral: Initial: 200 mg, followed by 100 mg every 12 hours (maximum: 400 mg/day)

Acne: Oral: Capsule or immediate-release tablet: 50-100 mg daily

Inflammatory, non-nodular, moderate-to-severe acne (Solodyn™):

45-59 kg: 45 mg once daily

60-90 kg: 90 mg once daily

91-136 kg: 135 mg once daily

Note: Therapy should be continued for 12 weeks. Higher doses do not confer greater efficacy, and safety of use beyond 12 weeks has not been established.

Chlamydial or *Ureaplasma urealyticum* infection, uncomplicated: Urethral, endocervical, or rectal: Oral: 100 mg every 12 hours for at least 7 days

Gonococcal infection, uncomplicated (males): Oral:

Without urethritis or anorectal infection: Initial: 200 mg, followed by 100 mg every 12 hours for at least 4 days (cultures 2-3 days post-therapy)

Urethritis: 100 mg every 12 hours for 5 days

Meningococcal carrier state: Oral: 100 mg every 12 hours for 5 days

Mycobacterium marinum: Oral: 100 mg every 12 hours for 6-8 weeks

(Continued)

Minocycline (Continued)

Nocardiosis, cutaneous (non-CNS): Oral: 100 mg every 12 hours

Syphilis: Oral: Initial: 200 mg, followed by 100 mg every 12 hours for 10-15 days

Renal Impairment: Consider decreasing dose or increasing dosing interval; total daily dose should not exceed 200 mg.

Administration Infuse I.V. minocycline slowly, usually over a 6-hour period.

Monitoring Parameters Signs and symptoms of infection; monitor for CNS adverse effects

Test Interactions May cause interference with fluorescence test for urinary catecholamines (false elevations)

Patient Information Complete full course of therapy; use caution if vertigo, dizziness, and driving or operation of machinery; may be taken with food or milk; avoid prolonged exposure to sunlight or tanning equipment

Special Geriatric Considerations Minocycline has not been studied in the elderly but its CNS effects may limit its use. Dose reduction for renal function not necessary.

Dosage Forms Excipient information presented when available (limited, particularly for generics); consult specific product labeling.

Capsule: 50 mg, 75 mg, 100 mg
Dynacin®: 75 mg, 100 mg
Capsule, pellet filled: 50 mg, 100 mg
Minocin® PAC: 50 mg, 100 mg [packaged with wipes, serum, and masque]
Tablet: 50 mg, 75 mg, 100 mg
Dynacin®, myrac™: 50 mg, 75 mg, 100 mg
Tablet, extended release:
Solodyn™: 45 mg, 90 mg, 135 mg

♦ **Minocycline Hydrochloride** see Minocycline on page 1046

Minoxidil (mi NOKS i dil)

Medication Safety Issues

Sound-alike/look-alike issues:
Minoxidil may be confused with metolazone, Monopril®, Noxafil®

International issues:
Noxidil® [Thailand] may be confused with Noxafil® which is a brand name for posaconazole in the U.S.

U.S. Brand Names Rogaine® Extra Strength for Men [OTC]; Rogaine® for Men [OTC]; Rogaine® for Women [OTC]

Canadian Brand Names Apo-Gain®; Minox; Rogaine®

Generic Available Yes

Pharmacologic Category Topical Skin Product; Vasodilator

Use Management of severe hypertension; treatment of male pattern baldness (alopecia androgenetica)

Contraindications Hypersensitivity to minoxidil or any component of the formulation; pheochromocytoma; acute MI; dissecting aortic aneurysm

Warnings/Precautions [U.S. Boxed Warnings]: Minoxidil can cause pericardial effusion, occasionally progressing to tamponade and it can exacerbate angina pectoris; use with caution in patients with pulmonary hypertension, significant renal failure, or CHF; use with caution in patients with coronary artery disease or recent myocardial infarction; renal failure or dialysis patients may require smaller doses; usually used with a beta-blocker (to treat minoxidil-induced tachycardia) and a diuretic (for treatment of water retention/edema); may take 1-6 months for hypertrichosis to totally reverse after minoxidil therapy is discontinued. **[U.S. Boxed Warning]: Maximum therapeutic doses of a diuretic and two antihypertensives should be used before this drug is ever added. May need to add a diuretic to minimize fluid gain** and a beta-blocker (if no contraindications) to treat tachycardia. **[U.S. Boxed Warning]: Monitor patients who are receiving guanethidine concurrently (orthostasis can be problematic).**

Adverse Reactions (Reflective of adult population; not specific for elderly)

Oral: Incidence of reactions not always reported.

Cardiovascular: Peripheral edema (7%), sodium and water retention, CHF, tachycardia, angina pectoris, pericardial effusion with or without tamponade, pericarditis, ECG changes (T-wave changes, 60%), rebound hypertension (in children after a gradual withdrawal)

Central nervous system: Headache (rare), fatigue

Dermatologic: Hypertrichosis (common, 80%), transient pruritus, changes in pigmentation (rare), serosanguineous bullae (rare), rash (rare), Stevens-Johnson syndrome

Hepatic: Increased alkaline phosphatase

Renal: Transient increase in serum BUN and creatinine

Respiratory: Pulmonary edema
Topical: Incidence of adverse events is not always reported.

Cardiovascular: Increased left ventricular end-diastolic volume, increased cardiac output, increased left ventricular mass, dizziness, tachycardia, edema, transient chest pain, palpitation, increase or decrease in blood pressure, increase or decrease in pulse rate (1.5%, placebo 1.6%)

Central nervous system: Headache, dizziness, taste alterations, faintness, lightheadedness (3.4%, placebo 3.5%), vertigo (1.2%, placebo 1.2%), anxiety (rare), mental depression (rare), fatigue (rare 0.4%, placebo 1%)

Dermatologic: Local irritation, dryness, erythema, allergic contact dermatitis (7.4%, placebo 5.4%), pruritus, scaling/flaking, eczema, seborrhea, papular rash, folliculitis, local erythema, flushing, exacerbation of hair loss, alopecia, hypertrichosis, increased hair growth outside the area of application (face, beard, eyebrows, ear, arm)

Gastrointestinal: Diarrhea, nausea, vomiting (4.3%, placebo 6.6%), weight gain (1.2%, placebo 1.3%)

Neuromuscular & skeletal: Fractures, back pain, retrosternal chest pain of muscular origin, tendonitis (2.6%, placebo 2.2%), weakness

Ocular: Conjunctivitis, visual disturbances, decreased visual acuity

Respiratory: Bronchitis, upper respiratory infection, sinusitis (7.2%, placebo 8.6%)

Overdosage/Toxicology Symptoms include hypotension, tachycardia, headache, nausea, dizziness, weakness syncope, warm flushed skin and palpitations. Hypotension usually responds to I.V. fluids, Trendelenburg positioning or vasoconstrictor. Treatment is primarily supportive and symptomatic.

Drug Interactions
Antihypertensives: Effects may be additive.
Guanethidine can cause severe orthostasis; avoid concurrent use - discontinue 1-3 weeks prior to initiating minoxidil.

Ethanol/Nutrition/Herb Interactions Herb/Nutraceutical: Avoid natural licorice (causes sodium and water retention and increases potassium loss).

Stability Store at controlled room temperature of 20°C to 25°C (68°F to 77°F).

Mechanism of Action Produces vasodilation by directly relaxing arteriolar smooth muscle, with little effect on veins; effects may be mediated by cyclic AMP; stimulation of hair growth is secondary to vasodilation, increased cutaneous blood flow and stimulation of resting hair follicles

Pharmacodynamics
Onset of action: Oral: Hypotensive effects occur within 30 minutes
Peak effect: Within 2-8 hours
Duration: Up to 2-5 days

Pharmacokinetics
Protein binding: None
Metabolism: 88% primarily via glucuronidation
Bioavailability: Oral: 90%
Half-life: 3.5-4.2 hours
Elimination: 12% unchanged in urine

Dosage
Geriatrics: Hypertension: Initial: 2.5 mg once daily; increase gradually.
Adults:
  Hypertension: Oral: Initial: 5 mg once daily, increase gradually every 3 days (maximum: 100 mg/day); usual dose range (JNC 7): 2.5-80 mg/day in 1-2 divided doses
  Alopecia: Topical: Apply twice daily; 4 months of therapy may be necessary for hair growth.
  Note: Dosage adjustment is needed when added to concomitant therapy.
Renal Impairment: Dialysis: Supplemental dose is not necessary via hemo- or peritoneal dialysis.

Monitoring Parameters Blood pressure, standing and sitting/supine, fluid and electrolyte status, signs and symptoms of congestive heart failure, weight

Patient Information Topical product must be used every day. Minoxidil is usually taken with at least two other antihypertensive medications. Take all medications as prescribed; do not discontinue except on advice of physician. Notify the physician if any of the following occur: heart rate ≥20 beats/minute over normal; rapid weight gain >5 pounds (2 kg); unusual swelling of extremities, face, or abdomen; breathing difficulty, especially when lying down; new or aggravated angina symptoms (chest, arm or shoulder pain); severe indigestion; dizziness, lightheadedness, or fainting; nausea or vomiting may occur.

Additional Information Usually given in combination with a diuretic and beta-blocker

Dosage Forms Excipient information presented when available (limited, particularly for generics); consult specific product labeling.
Aerosol, topical [foam]:
  Men's Rogaine®: 5% (60 g)

(Continued)

Minoxidil (Continued)

Solution, topical: 2% (60 mL); 5% (60 mL)
Rogaine® for Men, Rogaine® for Women: 2% (60 mL) [supplied with dropper applicator]
Rogaine® Extra Strength for Men: 5% (60 mL) [supplied with dropper applicator]
Tablet: 2.5 mg, 10 mg

- ♦ **Mintab DM** see Guaifenesin and Dextromethorphan on page 730
- ♦ **Mintox Extra Strength [OTC]** see Aluminum Hydroxide, Magnesium Hydroxide, and Simethicone on page 66
- ♦ **Mintox Plus [OTC]** see Aluminum Hydroxide, Magnesium Hydroxide, and Simethicone on page 66
- ♦ **Miochol®-E** see Acetylcholine on page 36
- ♦ **Miostat®** see Carbachol on page 230
- ♦ **MiraLax® [OTC]** see Polyethylene Glycol 3350 on page 1283
- ♦ **Mirapex®** see Pramipexole on page 1295

Mirtazapine (mir TAZ a peen)

Related Information
Antidepressant Agents on page 1742

Medication Safety Issues
Sound-alike/look-alike issues:
Remeron® may be confused with Premarin®, Zemuron®

International issues:
Avanza® [Australia] may be confused with Albenza® which is a brand name for albendazole in the U.S.
Avanza® [Australia] may be confused with Avandia® which is a brand name for rosiglitazone in the U.S.
Remeron® my be confused with Reneuron® which is a brand name for fluoxetine in Spain

U.S. Brand Names Remeron®; Remeron SolTab®

Canadian Brand Names CO Mirtazapine; Gen-Mirtazapine; Novo-Mirtazapine; PMS-Mirtazapine; ratio-Mirtazapine; Remeron®; Remeron® RD; Rhoxal-mirtazapine; Rhoxal-mirtazapine FC; Riva-Mirtazapine; Sandoz-Mirtazapine; Sandoz-Mirtazapine FC

Generic Available Yes

Pharmacologic Category Antidepressant, Alpha-2 Antagonist

Use Treatment of depression

Restrictions An FDA-approved medication guide concerning the use of antidepressants in children, adolescents, and young adults must be distributed when dispensing an outpatient prescription (new or refill) where this medication is to be used without direct supervision of a healthcare provider. Medication guides are available at http://www.fda.gov/cder/Offices/ODS/medication_guides.htm. Dispense to parents or guardians of children and adolescents receiving this medication.

Contraindications Hypersensitivity to mirtazapine or any component of the formulation; use of MAO inhibitors within 14 days

Warnings/Precautions [U.S. Boxed Warning]: Antidepressants increase the risk of suicidal thinking and behavior in children, adolescents, and young adults (18-24 years of age) with major depressive disorder (MDD) and other psychiatric disorders; consider risk prior to prescribing. Short-term studies did not show an increased risk in patients >24 years of age and showed a decreased risk in patients ≥65 years. Closely monitor for clinical worsening, suicidality, or unusual changes in behavior; the patient's family or caregiver should be instructed to closely observe the patient and communicate condition with healthcare provider. A medication guide should be dispensed with each prescription.

The possibility of a suicide attempt is inherent in major depression and may persist until remission occurs. Monitor for worsening of depression or suicidality, especially during initiation of therapy (generally first 1-2 months) or with dose increases or decreases. Use caution in high-risk patients. Worsening depression and severe abrupt suicidality that are not part of the presenting symptoms may require discontinuation or modification of drug therapy. The patient's family or caregiver should be alerted to monitor patients for the emergence of suicidality and associated behaviors (such as agitation, irritability, hostility, impulsivity, and hypomania) and call healthcare provider.

May worsen psychosis in some patients or precipitate a shift to mania or hypomania in patients with bipolar disorder. Patients presenting with depressive symptoms should be screened for bipolar disorder. Monotherapy in patients with bipolar disorder should be avoided. **Mirtazapine is not FDA approved for the treatment of bipolar depression.**

Discontinue immediately if signs and symptoms of neutropenia/agranulocytosis occur. May cause sedation, resulting in impaired performance of tasks requiring alertness (eg, operating machinery or driving). Sedative effects may be additive with other CNS depressants and/or ethanol. The degree of sedation is moderate-high relative to other antidepressants. The risks of orthostatic hypotension or anticholinergic effects are low relative to other antidepressants. The incidence of sexual dysfunction with mirtazapine is generally lower than with SSRIs.

May increase appetite and stimulate weight gain. Weight gain of >7% of body weight reported in 7.5% of patients treated with mirtazapine compared to 0% for placebo; 8% of patients receiving mirtazapine discontinued treatment due to the weight gain. In an 8-week pediatric clinical trial, 49% of mirtazapine-treated patients had a weight gain of at least 7% (mean increase 4 kg) as compared to 5.7% of placebo-treated patients (mean increase 1 kg). May increase serum cholesterol and triglyceride levels.

Use caution in patients with a previous seizure disorder or condition predisposing to seizures such as brain damage, alcoholism, or concurrent therapy with other drugs which lower the seizure threshold. Use with caution in patients with hepatic or renal dysfunction and in elderly patients. SolTab® formulation contains phenylalanine.

Adverse Reactions (Reflective of adult population; not specific for elderly)
>10%:
  Central nervous system: Somnolence (54%)
  Endocrine & metabolic: Increased cholesterol
  Gastrointestinal: Constipation (13%), xerostomia (25%), increased appetite (17%), weight gain (12%; weight gain of >7% reported in 8% of adults, ≤49% of pediatric patients)
1% to 10%:
  Cardiovascular: Hypertension, vasodilatation, peripheral edema (2%), edema (1%)
  Central nervous system: Dizziness (7%), abnormal dreams (4%), abnormal thoughts (3%), confusion (2%), malaise
  Endocrine & metabolic: Increased triglycerides
  Gastrointestinal: Vomiting, anorexia, abdominal pain
  Genitourinary: Urinary frequency (2%)
  Neuromuscular & skeletal: Myalgia (2%), back pain (2%), arthralgia, tremor (2%), weakness (8%)
  Respiratory: Dyspnea (1%)
  Miscellaneous: Flu-like syndrome (5%), thirst

Drug Interactions Substrate of CYP1A2 (major), 2C9 (minor), 2D6 (major), 3A4 (major); **Inhibits** CYP1A2 (weak), 3A4 (weak)
  Clonidine: Antihypertensive effects of clonidine may be antagonized by mirtazapine (hypertensive urgency has been reported following addition of mirtazapine to clonidine); in addition, mirtazapine may potentially enhance the hypertensive response associated with abrupt clonidine withdrawal. Avoid this combination; consider an alternative agent.
  CNS depressants: Sedative effects may be additive with other CNS depressants; monitor for increased effect; includes barbiturates, benzodiazepines, opioid analgesics, ethanol and other sedative agents
  CYP1A2 inducers: May decrease the levels/effects of mirtazapine. Example inducers include aminoglutethimide, carbamazepine, phenobarbital, and rifampin.
  CYP1A2 inhibitors: May increase the levels/effects of mirtazapine. Example inhibitors include ciprofloxacin, fluvoxamine, ketoconazole, norfloxacin, ofloxacin, and rofecoxib.
  CYP2D6 inhibitors: May increase the levels/effects of mirtazapine. Example inhibitors include chlorpromazine, delavirdine, fluoxetine, miconazole, paroxetine, pergolide, quinidine, quinine, ritonavir, and ropinirole.
  CYP3A4 inducers: CYP3A4 inducers may decrease the levels/effects of mirtazapine. Example inducers include aminoglutethimide, carbamazepine, nafcillin, nevirapine, phenobarbital, phenytoin, and rifamycins.
  CYP3A4 inhibitors: May increase the levels/effects of mirtazapine. Example inhibitors include azole antifungals, clarithromycin, diclofenac, doxycycline, erythromycin, imatinib, isoniazid, nefazodone, nicardipine, propofol, protease inhibitors, quinidine, telithromycin, and verapamil.
  Linezolid: Due to MAO inhibition (see note on MAO inhibitors), this combination should be avoided
  MAO inhibitors: Possibly serious or fatal reactions can occur when given with or when given within 14 days of an MAO inhibitor; use is contraindicated.
  Selegiline: Interaction is less likely than with nonselective MAO inhibitors (see MAO inhibitor information), but theoretically possible; monitor
  Sibutramine: Potential for serotonin syndrome when used in combination

Ethanol/Nutrition/Herb Interactions
  Ethanol: Avoid ethanol (may increase CNS depression).
  Herb/Nutraceutical: Avoid St John's wort (may decrease mirtazapine levels). Avoid valerian, St John's wort, SAMe, kava kava (may increase CNS depression).
  (Continued)

Mirtazapine *(Continued)*

Stability Store at controlled room temperature.

SolTab®: Protect from light and moisture. Use immediately upon opening tablet blister.

Mechanism of Action Mirtazapine is a tetracyclic antidepressant that works by its central presynaptic alpha$_2$-adrenergic antagonist effects, which results in increased release of norepinephrine and serotonin. It is also a potent antagonist of 5-HT$_2$ and 5-HT$_3$ serotonin receptors and H1 histamine receptors and a moderate peripheral alpha$_1$-adrenergic and muscarinic antagonist; it does not inhibit the reuptake of norepinephrine or serotonin.

Pharmacokinetics

Absorption: Food has minimal effect

Distribution: V$_d$: 4.5 L/kg

Protein binding: 85%

Metabolism: Hepatic

Bioavailability: ~50%

Half-life:

Older adults: 31-39 hours

Adults: 21 hours (13-34 hours)

Dosage

Geriatrics: Initial: 7.5 mg/day as a single bedtime dose; increase by 7.5-15 mg/day every 1-2 weeks; usual dose: 15-30 mg/day; maximum dose: 45 mg/day

Adults: Depression: Oral: Initial: 15 mg nightly, titrate up to 15-45 mg/day with dose increases made no more frequently than every 1-2 weeks. There is an inverse relationship between dose and sedation.

Renal Impairment:

Cl$_{cr}$ 11-39 mL/minute: 30% decreased clearance

Cl$_{cr}$ <10 mL/minute: 50% decreased clearance

Hepatic Impairment: Clearance is decreased by 30%.

Monitoring Parameters Patients should be monitored for signs of agranulocytosis or severe neutropenia such as sore throat, stomatitis or other signs of infection or a low WBC; mental status for depression, suicidal ideation (especially at the beginning of therapy or when doses are increased or decreased), anxiety, social functioning, mania, panic attacks; lipid profile

Patient Information Take as a single bedtime dose; avoid alcohol and other sedating medications; impaired driving performance or delayed reaction times are possible; expect a delay in the onset of therapeutic effects; report side effects

Special Geriatric Considerations Limited published data specifically in the elderly or addressing *in vivo* drug interactions.

Dosage Forms Excipient information presented when available (limited, particularly for generics); consult specific product labeling.

Tablet (Remeron®): 15 mg, 30 mg, 45 mg

Tablet, orally disintegrating: 15 mg, 30 mg

Remeron SolTab®:

15 mg [contains phenylalanine 2.6 mg/tablet; orange flavor]

30 mg [contains phenylalanine 5.2 mg/tablet; orange flavor]

45 mg [contains phenylalanine 7.8 mg/tablet; orange flavor]

Selected References

"Mirtazapine - A New Antidepressant," *Med Lett Drugs Ther*, 1996, 38(990):113-4.

Stimmel GL, Dopheide JA, and Stahl SM, "Mirtazapine: An Antidepressant With Noradrenergic and Specific Serotonergic Effects," *Pharmacotherapy*, 1997, 17(1):10-21.

Misoprostol *(mye soe PROST ole)*

Medication Safety Issues

Sound-alike/look-alike issues:

Misoprostol may be confused with metoprolol

Cytotec® may be confused with Cytoxan®, Sytobex®

U.S. Brand Names Cytotec®

Canadian Brand Names Apo-Misoprostol®; Novo-Misoprostol

Generic Available Yes

Pharmacologic Category Prostaglandin

Use Prevention of NSAID-induced gastric ulcers

Unlabeled/Investigational Use Treatment of NSAID-induced nephropathy; fat malabsorption in cystic fibrosis

Contraindications Hypersensitivity to misoprostol, prostaglandins, or any component of the formulation

Warnings/Precautions Use with caution in patients with renal impairment, cardiovascular disease and the elderly.

Adverse Reactions (Reflective of adult population; not specific for elderly)

>10%: Gastrointestinal: Diarrhea, abdominal pain

1% to 10%:
Central nervous system: Headache
Gastrointestinal: Constipation, flatulence, nausea, dyspepsia, vomiting

Overdosage/Toxicology Symptoms include sedation, tremor, convulsions, dyspnea, abdominal pain, diarrhea, hypotension, and bradycardia.

Drug Interactions
Oxytocin: Misoprostol may increase the effect of oxytocin; wait 6-12 hours after misoprostol administration before initiating oxytocin.

Ethanol/Nutrition/Herb Interactions Food: Misoprostol peak serum concentrations may be decreased if taken with food (not clinically significant).

Stability Store at or below 25°C (77°F).

Mechanism of Action Misoprostol is a synthetic prostaglandin E_1 analog that replaces the protective prostaglandins consumed with prostaglandin-inhibiting therapies (eg, NSAIDs); has been shown to induce uterine contractions

Pharmacokinetics
Absorption: Oral: Rapid
Half-life (parent and metabolite combined): 1.5 hours; metabolite: 20-40 minutes
Time to peak serum concentration (active metabolite): Within 15-30 minutes
Rapidly de-esterified to misoprostol acid
Elimination: In urine (64% to 73% in 24 hours) and feces (15% in 24 hours)
Since older adults have decreased clearance (increased AUC), it may be necessary to reduce dose to 100 mcg 4 times/day

Dosage
Geriatrics: Oral: 100-200 mcg 4 times/day with food; if 200 mcg 4 times/day not tolerated, reduce to 100 mcg 4 times/day or 200 mcg twice daily with food. **Note:** To avoid the diarrhea potential, doses can be initiated at 100 mcg/day and increased 100 mcg/day at 3-day intervals until desired dose is achieved; also, recommend administering with food to decrease diarrhea incidence.

Adults: Prevention of NSAID-induced ulcers: Oral: 200 mcg 4 times/day with food; if not tolerated, may decrease dose to 100 mcg 4 times/day with food or 200 mcg twice daily with food. Last dose of the day should be taken at bedtime.

Administration Incidence of diarrhea may be lessened by having patient take dose right after meals. Therapy is usually begun on the second or third day of the next normal menstrual period.

Monitoring Parameters Monitor for diarrhea, stool occult blood; gastroscopy may be preferred

Patient Information May cause diarrhea when first being used (within 2 weeks); diarrhea incidence and severity may be decreased by taking with food and at bedtime Take as directed; continue taking your NSAIDs while taking this medication. Take with meals or after meals to prevent nausea, diarrhea, and flatulence. Avoid using antacids.

Additional Information Although food may decrease absorption, the clinical significance is unknown; administration with food may decrease diarrhea; diarrhea is normally a transient problem

Special Geriatric Considerations Elderly, due to extensive use of NSAIDs and the high percentage of asymptomatic hemorrhage and perforation from NSAIDs, are at risk for NSAID-induced ulcers and may be candidates for misoprostol use. However, routine use for prophylaxis is not justified. Patients must be selected upon demonstration that they are at risk for NSAID-induced lesions. Misoprostol should not be used as a first-line therapy for gastric or duodenal ulcers.

Dosage Forms Excipient information presented when available (limited, particularly for generics); consult specific product labeling.
Tablet: 100 mcg, 200 mcg

Selected References
Cleghorn GJ, Shepherd RW, and Holt TL, "The Use of a Synthetic Prostaglandin E1 Analogue (Misoprostol) as an Adjunct to Pancreatic Enzyme Replacement in Cystic Fibrosis," *Scand J Gastroenterol Suppl*, 1988, 143:142-7.

Robinson PJ, Smith AL, and Sly PD, "Duodenal pH in Cystic Fibrosis and Its Relationship to Fat Malabsorption," *Dig Dis Sci*, 1990, 35(10):1299-304.

Walt RP, "Misoprostol for the Treatment of Peptic Ulcer and Anti-inflammatory Drug-Induced Gastroduodenal Ulceration," *N Engl J Med*, 1992, 327(22):1575-80.

♦ **Mobic®** *see* Meloxicam *on page 971*
♦ **Mobidin®** *see* Salicylates (Various Salts) *on page 1439*
♦ **Modane® Bulk [OTC]** *see* Psyllium *on page 1347*
♦ **Modified Shohl's Solution** *see* Sodium Citrate and Citric Acid *on page 1477*

Moexipril (mo EKS i pril)

Related Information
Angiotensin Agents *on page 1737*

Medication Safety Issues
Sound-alike/look-alike issues:
Moexipril may be confused with Monopril®

U.S. Brand Names Univasc®

Index Terms Moexipril Hydrochloride

Generic Available Yes

Pharmacologic Category Angiotensin-Converting Enzyme (ACE) Inhibitor

Use Treatment of hypertension, alone or in combination with thiazide diuretics

Contraindications Hypersensitivity to moexipril, moexiprilat, or any component of the formulation; hypersensitivity or allergic reactions or angioedema related to previous treatment with an ACE inhibitor

Warnings/Precautions Use with caution and modify dosage in patients with renal impairment especially renal artery stenosis, severe CHF, or with coadministered diuretic therapy. Hyperkalemia may rarely occur. Severe hypotension may occur in patients who are sodium and/or volume depleted; initiate lower doses and monitor closely when starting therapy in these patients; ACE inhibitors may be preferred agents in elderly patients with CHF and diabetes mellitus (diabetic proteinuria is reduced, minimal CNS effects, and enhanced insulin sensitivity), however, due to decreased renal function, tolerance must be carefully monitored; if possible, discontinue the diuretic 2-3 days prior to initiating moexipril in patients receiving them to reduce the risk of symptomatic hypotension.

Anaphylactic reactions can occur. Angioedema can occur at any time during treatment (especially following first dose). It may involve head and neck (potentially affecting the airway) or the intestine (presenting with abdominal pain). Prolonged monitoring may be required especially if tongue, glottis, or larynx are involved as they are associated with airway obstruction. Those with a history of airway surgery in this situation have a higher risk. Use with caution in collagen vascular diseases; valvular stenosis (particularly aortic stenosis); hyperkalemia; or before, during, or immediately after anesthesia. Avoid rapid dosage escalation which may lead to renal insufficiency. Rare toxicities associated with ACE inhibitors include cholestatic jaundice (which may progress to hepatic necrosis) and neutropenia/agranulocytosis with myeloid hyperplasia. May be associated with deterioration of renal function and/or increases in serum creatinine, particularly in patients dependent on renin-angiotensin-aldosterone system. If patient has renal impairment then a baseline WBC with differential and serum creatinine should be evaluated and monitored closely during the first 3 months of therapy. Hypersensitivity reactions may be seen during hemodialysis with high-flux dialysis membranes (eg, AN69).

Adverse Reactions (Reflective of adult population; not specific for elderly)
1% to 10%:
Cardiovascular: Hypotension, peripheral edema
Central nervous system: Headache, dizziness, fatigue
Dermatologic: Rash, alopecia, flushing, rash
Endocrine & metabolic: Hyperkalemia, hyponatremia
Gastrointestinal: Diarrhea, nausea, heartburn
Genitourinary: Polyuria
Neuromuscular & skeletal: Myalgia
Renal: Reversible increases in creatinine or BUN
Respiratory: Cough, pharyngitis, upper respiratory infection, sinusitis

Overdosage/Toxicology Mild hypotension has been the only toxic effect seen with acute overdose; bradycardia may also occur. Hyperkalemia occurs even with therapeutic doses, especially in patients with renal insufficiency and those taking NSAIDs. Following initiation of essential overdose management, toxic symptom and supportive treatment should be initiated. Hypotension usually responds to I.V. fluids or Trendelenburg positioning.

Drug Interactions
ACE inhibitors: Potential for allergic reactions increased with moexipril.
Allopurinol: Potential for allergic reactions increased with moexipril.
Alpha₁ blockers: Hypotensive effect increased.
Antacids: May decrease the bioavailability of ACE inhibitors (may be more likely to occur with captopril); separate administration times by 1-2 hours.

Aspirin: The effects of ACE inhibitors may be blunted by aspirin administration, particularly at higher dosages; may increase potential for adverse renal effects.

Diuretics: Hypovolemia due to diuretics may precipitate acute hypotensive events or acute renal failure.

Gold sodium thiomalate: ACE inhibitors may enhance the adverse/toxic effects (nitritoid reaction) of gold sodium thiomalate. The reaction may include facial flushing, nausea, vomiting, hypotension, and syncope. If it is to occur, would be expected shortly after administration of gold compound in patients maintained on an ACEI.

Insulin: Risk of hypoglycemia may be increased.

Lithium: Risk of lithium toxicity may be increased; monitor lithium levels, especially the first 4 weeks of therapy.

Mercaptopurine: Risk of neutropenia may be increased.

NSAIDs: May attenuate hypertensive efficacy; effect has been seen with captopril and may occur with other ACE inhibitors; monitor blood pressure. May increase potential to alter renal function.

Potassium-sparing diuretics (amiloride, potassium, spironolactone, triamterene): Increased risk of hyperkalemia.

Potassium supplements may increase the risk of hyperkalemia.

Probenecid: Blood levels of moexipril are increased (may occur with other ACE inhibitors).

Trimethoprim (high dose) may increase the risk of hyperkalemia.

Ethanol/Nutrition/Herb Interactions

Food: Food may delay and reduce peak serum levels.

Herb/Nutraceutical: Avoid dong quai if using for hypertension (has estrogenic activity). Avoid ephedra, yohimbe, ginseng (may worsen hypertension). Avoid garlic (may have increased antihypertensive effect).

Mechanism of Action Competitive inhibitor of angiotensin-converting enzyme (ACE); prevents conversion of angiotensin I to angiotensin II, a potent vasoconstrictor; results in lower levels of angiotensin II which causes an increase in plasma renin activity and a reduction in aldosterone secretion

Pharmacodynamics

Onset of action: 2 hours after administration

Peak effect: 3-6 hours

Duration: 24 hours. See Additional Information.

Pharmacokinetics Moexipril is a prodrug and is converted to moexiprilat in the liver

Protein binding: 50% (moexiprilat)

Bioavailability: 13% (reduced with food)

Half-life:

Moexipril: 1 hour

Moexiprilat: 2-10 hours

Elimination: With oral administration, 52% of the dose is recovered in the feces as moexiprilat and 1% as moexipril; only 7% appears in the urine as moexiprilat and 1% as moexipril

In older adult male subjects, the AUC and peak serum concentrations were 30% greater than those of younger subjects; no difference in clinical effect was seen

Dosage

Geriatrics: Dose the same as adults; adjust for renal impairment. Tablet may be cut in half (3.75 mg) for starting therapy (see Renal Impairment).

Adults: Hypertension, LV dysfunction (post MI): Oral: Initial: 7.5 mg once daily (in patients **not** receiving diuretics), 1 hour prior to a meal **or** 3.75 mg once daily (when combined with thiazide diuretics); maintenance dose: 7.5-30 mg/day in 1 or 2 divided doses 1 hour before meals

Renal Impairment: $Cl_{cr} \leq 40$ mL/minute: Patients may be cautiously placed on 3.75 mg once daily, then upwardly titrated to a maximum of 15 mg/day.

Administration Administer on an empty stomach at least 1 hour before meals

Monitoring Parameters Blood pressure, serum potassium concentration, BUN, serum creatinine, renal function, WBCs

Test Interactions Increases BUN, creatinine, potassium, positive Coombs' [direct]; decreases cholesterol (S); may cause false-positive results in urine acetone determinations using sodium nitroprusside reagent

Patient Information Do not stop therapy except under prescriber advice; notify physician if you develop sore throat, fever, swelling of hands, feet, face, eyes, lips, and tongue; difficult breathing, irregular heartbeats, chest pains, or cough. May cause dizziness, fainting, and lightheadedness, especially in first week of therapy, sit and stand up slowly; may cause changes in taste or rash; do not add a salt substitute (potassium) without advice of physician.

Additional Information The antihypertensive effect of moexipril may decrease towards the end of the dosing interval; blood pressure should be monitored prior to dosing. If blood pressure control is not adequate, an increased dose or divided dose may be attempted. Moexipril offers no therapeutic advantage over other ACE inhibitors. To reduce the risk of hypotension, discontinue therapy 2-3 days prior to starting

(Continued)

Moexipril *(Continued)*

moexipril if possible. If diuretics cannot be stopped for a short period, initiate dose at 3.75 mg/day.

Special Geriatric Considerations Due to frequent decreases in glomerular filtration (also creatinine clearance) with aging, elderly patients may have exaggerated responses to ACE inhibitors; differences in clinical response due to hepatic changes are not observed. ACE inhibitors may be preferred agents in elderly patients with congestive heart failure and diabetes mellitus. Diabetic proteinuria is reduced and insulin sensitivity is enhanced. In general, the side effect profile is favorable in the elderly and causes little or no CNS confusion; use lowest dose recommendations initially; adjust dose for renal function in the elderly. Many elderly may be volume depleted due to diuretic use and/or blunted thirst reflex resulting in inadequate fluid intake.

Dosage Forms Excipient information presented when available (limited, particularly for generics); consult specific product labeling.

Tablet, as hydrochloride [scored]: 7.5 mg, 15 mg

Univasc®: 7.5 mg, 15 mg

Selected References

Konstam MA, Drakup K, Baker DW, et al, "Heart Failure: Evaluation and Care of Patients With Left Ventricular Systolic Dysfunction," *Clinical Practice Guideline No 11*, Rockville, MD: Agency for Health Care Policy and Research, Public Health Service, U.S. Department of Health and Human Services, 1994.

Lewis EJ, Hunsicker LG, Bain RP, et al, "The Effect of Angiotensin-Converting Enzyme Inhibition on Diabetic Nephropathy," *N Engl J Med*, 1993, 329(20):1456-62.

McAreavey D and Robertson JI, "Angiotensin Converting Enzyme Inhibitors and Moderate Hypertension," *Drugs*, 1990, 40(3):326-45.

Williams JF, Bristow MR, Fowler MB, et al, "Guidelines for the Evaluation and Management of Heart Failure: Report of the American College of Cardiology/American Heart Association Task Force on Practice Guidelines (Committee on Evaluation and Management of Heart Failure)," *J Am Coll Cardiol*, 1995, 26:1376-8.

♦ **Moexipril Hydrochloride** *see* Moexipril *on page 1054*

♦ **Moi-Stir® [OTC]** *see* Saliva Substitute *on page 1443*

♦ **Moisture® Eyes [OTC]** *see* Artificial Tears *on page 124*

♦ **Moisture® Eyes PM [OTC]** *see* Artificial Tears *on page 124*

Molindone *(moe LIN done)*

Related Information

Antipsychotic Agents *on page 1747*

Medication Safety Issues

Sound-alike/look-alike issues:

Molindone may be confused with Mobidin®

Moban® may be confused with Mobidin®, Modane®

U.S. Brand Names Moban®

Canadian Brand Names Moban®

Index Terms Molindone Hydrochloride

Generic Available No

Pharmacologic Category Antipsychotic Agent, Typical

Use Management of nonpsychotic symptoms associated with dementia (older adults), Tourette's syndrome, Huntington's chorea

See Special Geriatric Considerations.

Unlabeled/Investigational Use Management of psychotic disorders

Contraindications Hypersensitivity to molindone or any component of the formulation (cross-reactivity between phenothiazines may occur); severe CNS depression; coma

Warnings/Precautions May be sedating, use with caution in disorders where CNS depression is a feature. Use with caution in Parkinson's disease. Caution in patients with hemodynamic instability; bone marrow suppression; predisposition to seizures; subcortical brain damage; severe cardiac, hepatic, renal, or respiratory disease. Esophageal dysmotility and aspiration have been associated with antipsychotic use - use with caution in patients at risk of pneumonia (ie, Alzheimer's disease). Caution in breast cancer or other prolactin-dependent tumors (may elevate prolactin levels). May alter temperature regulation or mask toxicity of other drugs due to antiemetic effects. May alter cardiac conduction; life-threatening arrhythmias have occurred with therapeutic doses of neuroleptics. May cause orthostatic hypotension - use with caution in patients at risk of this effect or those who would tolerate transient hypotensive episodes (cerebrovascular disease, cardiovascular disease, or other medications which may predispose).

May cause anticholinergic effects (confusion, agitation, constipation, xerostomia, blurred vision, urinary retention); therefore, they should be used with caution in patients with decreased gastrointestinal motility, urinary retention, BPH, xerostomia, or visual problems. Conditions which also may be exacerbated by cholinergic blockade include narrow-angle glaucoma (screening is recommended) and worsening of myasthenia gravis. Relative to other neuroleptics, molindone has a low potency of cholinergic blockade.

May cause extrapyramidal reactions, including pseudoparkinsonism, acute dystonic reactions, akathisia, and tardive dyskinesia (risk of these reactions is moderate-high relative to other neuroleptics). May be associated with neuroleptic malignant syndrome (NMS) or pigmentary retinopathy.

Adverse Reactions (Reflective of adult population; not specific for elderly)
Frequency not defined.

Cardiovascular: Orthostatic hypotension, tachycardia, arrhythmia

Central nervous system: Extrapyramidal reactions (akathisia, pseudoparkinsonism, dystonia, tardive dyskinesia), mental depression, altered central temperature regulation, sedation, drowsiness, restlessness, anxiety, hyperactivity, euphoria, seizure, neuroleptic malignant syndrome (NMS)

Dermatologic: Pruritus, rash, photosensitivity

Endocrine & metabolic: Change in menstrual periods, edema of breasts, amenorrhea, galactorrhea, gynecomastia

Gastrointestinal: Constipation, xerostomia, nausea, salivation, weight gain (minimal compared to other antipsychotics), weight loss

Genitourinary: Urinary retention, priapism

Hematologic: Leukopenia, leukocytosis

Ocular: Blurred vision, retinal pigmentation

Miscellaneous: Diaphoresis (decreased)

Overdosage/Toxicology
Symptoms include deep sleep, extrapyramidal symptoms, cardiac arrhythmias, seizures, and hypotension. Following initiation of essential overdose management, toxic symptom and supportive treatment should be initiated. Hypotension usually responds to I.V. fluids or Trendelenburg positioning. If unresponsive to these measures, the use of a parenteral inotrope may be required (eg, norepinephrine 0.1-0.2 mcg/kg/minute titrated to response). Seizures commonly respond to diazepam (I.V. 5-10 mg bolus every 15 minutes, if needed up to a total of 30 mg) or to phenytoin or phenobarbital. Critical cardiac arrhythmias often respond to I.V. phenytoin (15 mg/kg up to 1 g), while other antiarrhythmics can be used. Neuroleptics often cause extrapyramidal symptoms (eg, dystonic reactions) requiring management with diphenhydramine 1-2 mg/kg (adults), up to a maximum of 50 mg I.M. or slow I.V. push, followed by a maintenance dose for 48-72 hours. When these reactions are unresponsive to diphenhydramine, anticholinergic agents such as benztropine mesylate I.V. 1-2 mg may be effective. These agents are generally effective within 2-5 minutes.

Drug Interactions
Acetylcholinesterase inhibitors (central): May increase the risk of antipsychotic-related extrapyramidal symptoms; monitor.

Aluminum salts: May decrease the absorption of antipsychotics; monitor

Amphetamines: Efficacy may be diminished by antipsychotics; in addition, amphetamines may increase psychotic symptoms; avoid concurrent use

Anticholinergics: May inhibit the therapeutic response to antipsychotics and excess anticholinergic effects may occur; includes benztropine, trihexyphenidyl, biperiden, and drugs with significant anticholinergic activity (TCAs, antihistamines, disopyramide)

Antihypertensives: Concurrent use of antipsychotics with an antihypertensive may produce additive hypotensive effects (particularly orthostasis)

Bromocriptine: Antipsychotics inhibit the ability of bromocriptine to lower serum prolactin concentrations

CNS depressants: Sedative effects may be additive with antipsychotics; monitor for increased effect; includes barbiturates, benzodiazepines, opioid analgesics, ethanol and other sedative agents

Epinephrine: Chlorpromazine (and possibly other low potency antipsychotics) may diminish the pressor effects of epinephrine

Guanethidine and guanadrel: Antihypertensive effects may be inhibited by antipsychotics

Levodopa: Antipsychotics may inhibit the antiparkinsonian effect of levodopa; avoid this combination

Lithium: Antipsychotics may produce neurotoxicity with lithium; this is a rare effect

Metoclopramide: May increase extrapyramidal symptoms (EPS) or risk.

Propranolol: Serum concentrations of antipsychotics may be increased; propranolol also increases antipsychotic concentrations

Sulfadoxine-pyrimethamine: May increase antipsychotics concentrations

Tricyclic antidepressants: Concurrent use may produce increased toxicity or altered therapeutic response

Trazodone: Antipsychotics and trazodone may produce additive hypotensive effects

Valproic acid: Serum levels may be increased by antipsychotics

Ethanol/Nutrition/Herb Interactions
Ethanol: Avoid ethanol (may increase CNS depression).
(Continued)

Molindone *(Continued)*

Herb/Nutraceutical: Avoid kava kava, gotu kola, valerian, St John's wort (may increase CNS depression).

Stability Protect from light. Dispense in amber or opaque vials.

Mechanism of Action Molindone is a dihydroindoline antipsychotic whose mechanism of action mimics that of chlorpromazine; however, it produces more extrapyramidal symptoms and less sedation than chlorpromazine

Pharmacodynamics Duration: 24-36 hours

Pharmacokinetics

Absorption: Oral: May be affected by the inherent anticholinergic action on the gastrointestinal tissue causing variable absorption. Absorption from tablets is erratic with less variation seen with solutions. These agents are widely distributed in tissues with CNS concentrations exceeding that of plasma due to their lipophilic characteristics.

Protein binding: Antipsychotic agents are bound 90% to 99% to plasma proteins; highly bound to brain and lung tissue and other tissues with a high blood perfusion.

Metabolism: Metabolized in the liver

Time to peak: Following oral administration peak serum concentrations occur within 90 minutes; peak concentrations between 2-4 hours

Elimination: Principally excreted in the urine and feces (90% within 24 hours); <2% to 3% excreted unmetabolized; eliminated through hepatic metabolism (oxidation) where numerous active metabolites are produced; active metabolites excreted in urine; elimination half-lives of antipsychotics ranges from 20-40 hours which may be extended in older adults due to decline in oxidative hepatic reactions (phase I) with age.

The biologic effect of a single dose persists for 24 hours. When the patient has accommodated to initial side effects (sedation), once daily dosing is possible due to the long half-life of antipsychotics.

Steady-state plasma concentrations are achieved in 4-7 days; therefore, if possible, do not make dose adjustments more than once in a 7-day period. Due to the long half-lives of antipsychotics, as needed (prn) use is ineffective since repeated doses are necessary to achieve therapeutic tissue concentrations in the CNS.

Dosage

Geriatrics: Behavioral symptoms associated with dementia in the elderly (unlabeled use): Oral: Initial: 5-10 mg 1-2 times/day; increase at 4- to 7-day intervals by 5-10 mg/day; increase dosing intervals (eg, twice daily, 3 times/day) as necessary to control response or side effects. Maximum dose: 112 mg/day. Gradual increases (titration) may prevent some side effects or decrease their severity.

Adults: Schizophrenia/psychoses: Oral: 50-75 mg/day increase at 3- to 4-day intervals up to 225 mg/day

Monitoring Parameters Monitor orthostatic blood pressures 3-5 days after initiation of therapy or a dose increase; tremors, gait changes, abnormal movement in trunk, neck, buccal area, or extremities; monitor target behaviors for which the agent is given

Patient Information May cause drowsiness; avoid alcoholic beverages; do not take within 1 hour of taking antacids; rise slowly from recumbent position; use of supportive stockings may prevent orthostatic hypotension

Special Geriatric Considerations Any changes in disease status in any organ system can result in behavior changes.

Many elderly patients receive antipsychotic medications for inappropriate nonpsychotic behavior. Before initiating antipsychotic medication, the clinician should investigate any possible reversible cause; any stress or stress from any disease can cause acute "confusion" or worsening of baseline nonpsychotic behavior. Most commonly acute changes in behavior are due to increases in drug dose or addition of new drug to regimen, fluid electrolyte loss, infections, and changes in environment.

In the treatment of agitated, demented, elderly patients, authors of meta-analysis of controlled trials of the response to the traditional antipsychotics (phenothiazines, butyrophenones) in controlling agitation have concluded that the use of neuroleptics results in a response rate of 18%. Clearly neuroleptic therapy for behavior control should be limited with frequent attempts to withdraw the agent given for behavior control.

Dosage Forms Excipient information presented when available (limited, particularly for generics); consult specific product labeling.

Tablet, as hydrochloride: 5 mg, 10 mg, 25 mg, 50 mg

Selected References

Peabody CA, Warner MD, Whiteford HA, et al, "Neuroleptics and the Elderly," *J Am Geriatr Soc*, 1987, 35(3):233-8.

Risse SC and Barnes R, "Pharmacologic Treatment of Agitation Associated With Dementia," *J Am Geriatr Soc*, 1986, 34(5):368-76.

Saltz BL, Woerner MG, Kane JM, et al, "Prospective Study of Tardive Dyskinesia Incidence in the Elderly," *JAMA*, 1991, 266(17):2402-6.

Seifert RD, "Therapeutic Drug Monitoring: Psychotropic Drugs," *J Pharm Pract*, 1984, 6:403-16.

♦ **Molindone Hydrochloride** *see* Molindone *on page 1056*

♦ **MOM** *see* Magnesium Hydroxide *on page 946*

Mometasone (moe MET a sone)

Related Information
Corticosteroids *on page 1755*

Medication Safety Issues
Sound-alike/look-alike issues:

Elocon® lotion may be confused with ophthalmic solutions. Manufacturer's labeling emphasizes the product is **NOT** for use in the eyes.

U.S. Brand Names Asmanex® Twisthaler®; Elocon®; Nasonex®

Canadian Brand Names Elocom®; Nasonex®; PMS-Mometasone; ratio-Mometasone; Taro-Mometasone

Index Terms Mometasone Furoate

Generic Available Yes: Cream, lotion, ointment

Pharmacologic Category Corticosteroid, Inhalant (Oral); Corticosteroid, Nasal; Corticosteroid, Topical

Use Relief of the inflammatory and pruritic manifestations of corticosteroid-responsive dermatoses (medium potency topical corticosteroid); treatment of nasal symptoms of seasonal and perennial allergic rhinitis; prevention of nasal symptoms associated with seasonal allergic rhinitis; treatment of nasal polyps in adults; maintenance treatment of asthma as prophylactic therapy or as a supplement in asthma patients requiring oral corticosteroids for the purpose of decreasing or eliminating the oral corticosteroid requirement

Contraindications Hypersensitivity to mometasone or any component of the formulation; treatment of acute bronchospasm (oral inhaler)

Warnings/Precautions

May cause hypercorticism or suppression of hypothalamic-pituitary-adrenal (HPA) axis, particularly in patients receiving high doses for prolonged periods. HPA axis suppression may lead to adrenal crisis. Withdrawal and discontinuation of a corticosteroid should be done slowly and carefully. Particular care is required when patients are transferred from systemic corticosteroids to inhaled products due to possible adrenal insufficiency or withdrawal from steroids, including an increase in allergic symptoms. Patients receiving >20 mg per day of prednisone (or equivalent) may be most susceptible. Fatalities have occurred due to adrenal insufficiency in asthmatic patients during and after transfer from systemic corticosteroids to aerosol steroids; aerosol steroids do not provide the systemic steroid needed to treat patients having trauma, surgery, or infections. When transferring to oral inhaler, previously-suppressed allergic conditions (rhinitis, conjunctivitis, eczema) may be unmasked.

Bronchospasm may occur with wheezing after inhalation; if this occurs stop steroid and treat with a fast-acting bronchodilator. Supplemental steroids (oral or parenteral) may be needed during stress or severe asthma attacks. Not to be used in status asthmaticus or for the relief of acute bronchospasm. Corticosteroid use may cause psychiatric disturbances, including depression, euphoria, insomnia, mood swings, and personality changes. Pre-existing psychiatric conditions may be exacerbated by corticosteroid use. Prolonged use of corticosteroids may also increase the incidence of secondary infection, mask acute infection (including fungal infections), prolong or exacerbate viral infections, or limit response to vaccines. Exposure to chickenpox should be avoided; corticosteroids should not be used to treat ocular herpes simplex. Corticosteroids should not be used for cerebral malaria. Close observation is required in patients with latent tuberculosis and/or TB reactivity; restrict use in active TB (only in conjunction with antituberculosis treatment). Prolonged treatment with corticosteroids has been associated with the development of Kaposi's sarcoma (case reports); if noted, discontinuation of therapy should be considered.

Use with caution in patients with thyroid disease, hepatic impairment, renal impairment, cardiovascular disease, diabetes, glaucoma, cataracts, myasthenia gravis, patients at risk for osteoporosis, patients at risk for seizures, or GI diseases (diverticulitis, peptic ulcer, ulcerative colitis) due to perforation risk. Use caution following acute MI (corticosteroids have been associated with myocardial rupture). Because of the risk of adverse effects, systemic corticosteroids should be used cautiously in the elderly in the smallest possible effective dose for the shortest duration. Avoid nasal corticosteroid use in patients with recent nasal septal ulcers, nasal surgery or nasal trauma until healing has occurred.

To minimize the systemic effects of orally-inhaled and intranasal corticosteroids, each patient should be titrated to the lowest effective dose. There have been reports of systemic corticosteroid withdrawal symptoms (eg, joint/muscle pain, lassitude, depression) when withdrawing oral inhalation therapy.
(Continued)

Mometasone *(Continued)*

Adverse Reactions (Reflective of adult population; not specific for elderly)
Nasal/oral inhalation:
>10%:
Central nervous system: Headache (17% to 22%), fatigue (oral inhalation 1% to 13%), depression (oral inhalation 11%)
Neuromuscular & skeletal: Musculoskeletal pain (1% to 22%), arthralgia (oral inhalation 13%)
Respiratory: Sinusitis (oral inhalation 22%), rhinitis (2% to 20%), upper respiratory infection (8% to 15%), pharyngitis (8% to 13%), cough (nasal inhalation 7% to 13%), epistaxis (1% to 11%)
Miscellaneous: Viral infection (nasal inhalation 8% to 14%), oral candidiasis (oral inhalation 4% to 22%)
1% to 10%:
Cardiovascular: Chest pain
Gastrointestinal: Abdominal pain, dry throat (oral inhalation), vomiting (1% to 5%), diarrhea, dyspepsia, flatulence, gastroenteritis, nausea, vomiting
Genitourinary: Dysmenorrhea
Neuromuscular & skeletal: Back pain, myalgia
Ocular: Conjunctivitis
Otic: Earache, otitis media
Respiratory: Asthma, bronchitis, dysphonia, epistaxis, nasal irritation, rhinitis, wheezing
Miscellaneous: Accidental injury, flu-like syndrome

Topical:
1% to 10%: Dermatologic: Bacterial skin infection, burning, furunculosis, pruritus, skin atrophy, tingling/stinging

Cataract formation, reduction in growth velocity, and HPA axis suppression have been reported with other corticosteroids

Drug Interactions Substrate of CYP3A4 (minor)
Amphotericin: Corticosteroids may increase the hypokalemic effects of amphotericin B; monitor.
Antidiabetic agents: Corticosteroids may decrease the hypoglycemic effects of antidiabetic agents; monitor.
Antifungal agents (imidazole): May increase the serum levels/effects of corticosteroids; monitor.
Diuretics, potassium-wasting (loop or thiazide): Hypokalemic effects may be increased by corticosteroids; monitor.
Fluoroquinolones: Concurrent use may increase the risk of tendinopathies (including tendonitis and rupture), particularly in elderly patients (overall incidence rare)

Stability
Cream: Store between 2°C to 25°C (36°F to 77°F).
Lotion: Store between 2°C to 30°C (36°F to 86°F).
Nasal spray: Store at room temperature of 15°C to 30°C (59°F to 86°F). Protect from light.
Ointment: Store at room temperature of 15°C to 30°C (59°F to 86°F).
Oral Inhaler: Store at room temperature of 15°C to 30°C (59°F to 86°F). Discard when oral dose counter reads "0" (or 45 days after opening the foil pouch).

Mechanism of Action May depress the formation, release, and activity of endogenous chemical mediators of inflammation (kinins, histamine, liposomal enzymes, prostaglandins). Leukocytes and macrophages may have to be present for the initiation of responses mediated by the above substances. Inhibits the margination and subsequent cell migration to the area of injury, and also reverses the dilatation and increased vessel permeability in the area resulting in decreased access of cells to the sites of injury.

Pharmacokinetics
Absorption:
Nasal inhalation: Mometasone furoate monohydrate: Undetectable in plasma
Ointment: 0.7%; increased by occlusive dressings
Oral inhalation: <1%
Protein binding: Mometasone furoate: 98% to 99%
Metabolism: Mometasone furoate: Hepatic via CYP3A4; forms metabolite
Half-life elimination: Oral inhalation: 5 hours
Excretion: Feces, bile, urine

Dosage
Geriatrics & Adults:
Treatment of seasonal and perennial allergic rhinitis: Nasal spray: 2 sprays (100 mcg) in each nostril daily
Prevention of seasonal and perennial allergic rhinitis: Nasal spray: 2 sprays (100 mcg) in each nostril daily beginning 2-4 weeks prior to pollen season

Treatment of corticosteroid-responsive dermatoses: Topical: Apply sparingly, do not use occlusive dressings. Therapy should be discontinued when control is achieved; if no improvement is seen in 2 weeks, reassessment of diagnosis may be necessary.

Cream, ointment: Apply a thin film to affected area once daily

Lotion: Apply a few drops to affected area once daily

Treatment of nasal polyps: Nasal spray: 2 sprays (100 mcg) in each nostril twice daily; 2 sprays (100 mcg) once daily may be effective in some patients

Asthma: Oral inhalation:

Bronchodilators or inhaled corticosteroids: Initial: 1 inhalation (220 mcg) daily (maximum 2 inhalations or 440 mcg/day); may be given in the evening or in divided doses twice daily

Oral corticosteroids: Initial: 440 mcg twice daily (maximum 880 mcg/day); prednisone should be reduced no faster than 2.5 mg/day on a weekly basis, beginning after at least 1 week of mometasone furoate use

Note: Maximum effects may not be evident for 1-2 weeks or longer; dose should be titrated to effect, using the lowest possible dose

Administration

Nasal spray: Prior to first use, prime pump by actuating 10 times or until fine spray appears; may store for a maximum of 1 week without repriming. Spray should be administered once or twice daily, at a regular interval. Shake well prior to use.

Oral inhalation: Exhale fully prior to bringing the Twisthaler® up to the mouth. Place between lips and inhale quickly and deeply. Do not breath out through the inhaler. Remove inhaler and hold breath for 10 seconds if possible.

Topical: Apply sparingly; avoid eyes, face, underarms, and groin. Do not wrap or bandage affected area.

Monitoring Parameters Relief of symptoms

Patient Information

Nasal: Shake well before using; protect from light. Before using a new bottle, the pump must be primed by actuating 10 times until a fine spray appears.

Oral inhalation: Read complete instructions in package. Not to be used for the relief of acute attacks. Use at regular intervals. **Do not** exceed prescribed dose. Record date of pouch opening on the cap label and discard the inhaler after 45 days or when the dose counter reads "00", whichever comes first.

Topical: Use only as prescribed and for no longer than the period prescribed; apply sparingly in a thin film and rub in lightly; avoid contact with eyes; notify physician if condition persists or worsens

Additional Information Considered a moderate-potency steroid; may be used for a limited time on the face; prolonged use may cause atrophic changes

Special Geriatric Considerations Due to age-related changes in skin, limit use of topical glucocorticosteroids.

Dosage Forms Excipient information presented when available (limited, particularly for generics); consult specific product labeling.

Cream, topical, as furoate: 0.1% (15 g, 45 g)

Elocon®: 0.1% (15 g, 45 g)

Lotion, topical, as furoate: 0.1% (30 mL, 60 mL)

Elocon®: 0.1% (30 mL, 60 mL) [contains isopropyl alcohol 40%]

Ointment, topical, as furoate: 0.1% (15 g, 45 g)

Elocon®: 0.1% (15 g, 45 g)

Powder for oral inhalation, as furoate:

Asmanex® Twisthaler®: 220 mcg (14 units, 30 units, 60 units, 120 units) [contains lactose]

Suspension, intranasal, as furoate [spray]:

Nasonex®: 50 mcg/spray (17 g) [delivers 120 sprays; contains benzalkonium chloride]

Montelukast (mon te LOO kast)

Medication Safety Issues
Sound-alike/look-alike issues:
Singulair® may be confused with Sinequan®

U.S. Brand Names Singulair®

Canadian Brand Names Singulair®

Index Terms Montelukast Sodium

Generic Available No

Pharmacologic Category Leukotriene-Receptor Antagonist

Use Prophylaxis and chronic treatment of asthma; relief of symptoms of seasonal allergic rhinitis and perennial allergic rhinitis; prevention of exercise-induced bronchospasm

Unlabeled/Investigational Use Acute asthma

Contraindications Hypersensitivity to montelukast or any component of the formulation

Warnings/Precautions Montelukast is not FDA approved for use in the reversal of bronchospasm in acute asthma attacks, including status asthmaticus; some clinicians, however, support its use (Cylly, 2003; Camargo, 2003; Ferreira, 2001). Advise patients to have appropriate rescue medication available. Appropriate clinical monitoring and caution are recommended when systemic corticosteroid reduction is considered in patients receiving montelukast. Inform phenylketonuric patients that the chewable tablet contains phenylalanine.

In rare cases, patients on therapy with montelukast may present with systemic eosinophilia, sometimes presenting with clinical features of vasculitis consistent with Churg-Strauss syndrome, a condition which is often treated with systemic corticosteroid therapy. Healthcare providers should be alert to eosinophilia, vasculitic rash, worsening pulmonary symptoms, cardiac complications, and/or neuropathy presenting in their patients. A causal association between montelukast and these underlying conditions has not been established. Montelukast will not interrupt bronchoconstrictor response to aspirin or other NSAIDs; aspirin sensitive asthmatics should continue to avoid these agents.

Adverse Reactions (Reflective of adult population; not specific for elderly)
1% to 10%:
Central nervous system: Dizziness (2%), fatigue (2%), fever (2%)
Dermatologic: Rash (2%)
Gastrointestinal: Abdominal pain (3%), dyspepsia (2%), dental pain (2%), gastroenteritis (2%)
Hepatic: AST increased (2%)
Neuromuscular & skeletal: Weakness (2%)
Respiratory: Cough (3%), nasal congestion (2%)

Overdosage/Toxicology Abdominal pain, headache, psychomotor hyperactivity, vomiting, somnolence, and thirst have been reported with doses as high as 1000 mg. Treatment is symptom-directed and supportive. It is not known if dialysis would be effective.

Drug Interactions Substrate (major) of CYP2C9, 3A4; **Inhibits** CYP2C8 (weak), 2C9 (weak)
CYP2C9 inducers: May decrease the levels/effects of montelukast. Example inducers include carbamazepine, phenobarbital, phenytoin, rifampin, rifapentine, and secobarbital.
CYP3A4 inducers: May decrease the levels/effects of montelukast. Example inducers include aminoglutethimide, carbamazepine, nafcillin, nevirapine, phenobarbital, phenytoin, and rifamycins.
CYP2C9 inhibitors: May increase the levels/effects of montelukast. Example inhibitors include delavirdine, fluconazole, flurbiprofen, gemfibrozil, ibuprofen, indomethacin, ketoconazole, mefenamic acid, miconazole, nicardipine, piroxicam, sulfadiazine, sulfisoxazole, and tolbutamide.

Ethanol/Nutrition/Herb Interactions Herb/Nutraceutical: St John's wort may decrease montelukast levels.

Stability Store at room temperature of 15°C to 30°C (59°F to 86°F). Protect from moisture and light.
Granules: Use within 15 minutes of opening packet.

Mechanism of Action Selective leukotriene receptor antagonist that inhibits the cysteinyl leukotriene receptor. Cysteinyl leukotrienes and leukotriene receptor occupation have been correlated with the pathophysiology of asthma, including airway edema, smooth muscle contraction, and altered cellular activity associated with the inflammatory process, which contribute to the signs and symptoms of asthma. Cysteinyl leukotrienes are also released from the nasal mucosa following allergen exposure leading to symptoms associated with allergic rhinitis.

Pharmacodynamics Duration: >24 hours

Pharmacokinetics

Absorption: Rapid

Distribution: V_d: 8-11 L

Protein binding, plasma: >99%

Metabolism: Extensively hepatic via CYP3A4 and 2C9

Bioavailability: Tablet: 10 mg: Mean: 64%; 5 mg: 63% to 73%

Half-life, plasma: Mean: 2.7-5.5 hours

Time to peak, serum: Tablet: 10 mg: 3-4 hours; 5 mg: 2-2.5 hours; 4 mg: 2 hours

Elimination: Feces (86%); urine (<0.2%)

Dosage

Geriatrics & Adults:

Asthma, allergic seasonal or perennial rhinitis: Oral: One 10 mg tablet daily in the evening

Asthma, acute (unlabeled use): 10 mg as a single dose administered with first-line therapy

Bronchoconstriction, exercise-induced (prevention): 10 mg at least 2 hours prior to exercise; additional doses should not be administered within 24 hours. Daily administration to prevent exercise-induced bronchoconstriction has not been evaluated.

Renal Impairment: No adjustment is necessary.

Hepatic Impairment: No adjustment necessary in mild-to-moderate hepatic disease. Patients with severe hepatic disease were **not** studied.

Administration When treating asthma, administer dose in the evening. Patients with allergic rhinitis may individualize administration time. Granules may be administered directly in the mouth or mixed with applesauce, carrots, rice, or ice cream; do not add to any other liquids. Administer within 15 minutes of opening packet.

Monitoring Parameters Pulmonary function tests and symptomatic effects

Patient Information This medication is not for an acute asthmatic attack; in acute attack, follow instructions of prescriber. Do not stop other asthma medication unless advised by prescriber. Chewable tablet contains phenylalanine. Take every evening on a continuous basis; do not discontinue even if feeling better (this medication may help reduce incidence of acute attacks). Granules may be administered directly in the mouth or mixed with applesauce, carrots, rice, or ice cream (do not mix in liquids); administer within 15 minutes of opening packet. You may experience mild headache (mild analgesic may help); fatigue or dizziness (use caution when driving). Report skin rash or itching, abdominal pain or persistent GI upset, unusual cough or congestion, or worsening of asthmatic condition.

Special Geriatric Considerations The pharmacokinetic profile in the elderly is similar to younger adults except the half-life is slightly longer in the elderly. Despite this difference, no adjustment in dose is necessary in the elderly. Elimination is mostly fecal and bile with insignificant amounts from renal elimination, which is an advantage for the elderly.

Dosage Forms Excipient information presented when available (limited, particularly for generics); consult specific product labeling.

Granules:

Singulair®: 4 mg/packet

Tablet:

Singulair®: 10 mg

Tablet, chewable:

Singulair®: 4 mg [contains phenylalanine 0.674 mg; cherry flavor]; 5 mg [contains phenylalanine 0.842 mg; cherry flavor]

Selected References

Camargo CA Jr, Smithline HA, Malice MP, et al, "A Randomized Controlled Trial of Intravenous Montelukast in Acute Asthma," *Am J Respir Crit Care Med*, 2003, 167(4):528-33.

Cylly A, Kara A, Ozdemir T, et al, "Effects of Oral Montelukast on Airway Function in Acute Asthma," *Respir Med*, 2003, 97(5):533-6.

♦ **Montelukast Sodium** *see* Montelukast *on page 1062*

♦ **More Attenuated Enders Strain** *see* Measles Virus Vaccine (Live) *on page 959*

♦ **MoreDophilus® [OTC]** *see* Lactobacillus *on page 867*

Moricizine (mor I siz een)

Medication Safety Issues

Sound-alike/look-alike issues:

Ethmozine® may be confused with Erythrocin®, erythromycin

U.S. Brand Names Ethmozine®

Canadian Brand Names Ethmozine®

Index Terms Moricizine Hydrochloride

Generic Available No

Pharmacologic Category Antiarrhythmic Agent, Class I

Use Treatment of ventricular tachycardia and life-threatening ventricular arrhythmias

(Continued)

Moricizine *(Continued)*

Unlabeled/Investigational Use Treatment of PVCs, complete and nonsustained ventricular tachycardia, atrial arrhythmias

Contraindications Hypersensitivity to moricizine or any component of the formulation; pre-existing second- or third-degree AV block (except in patients with a functioning artificial pacemaker); right bundle branch block when associated with left hemiblock or bifascicular block (unless functional pacemaker in place); cardiogenic shock

Warnings/Precautions Considering the known proarrhythmic properties and lack of evidence of improved survival for any antiarrhythmic drug in patients without life-threatening arrhythmias, it is prudent to reserve the use for patients with life-threatening ventricular arrhythmias. **[U.S. Boxed Warning]: The CAST II trial demonstrated a trend towards decreased survival for patients treated with moricizine.** Use with caution in patients with sick-sinus syndrome, hepatic, and renal impairment; correct electrolyte disturbances, especially hypokalemia or hypomagnesemia, prior to use and throughout therapy

Adverse Reactions (Reflective of adult population; not specific for elderly)
>10%: Central nervous system: Dizziness
1% to 10%:
Cardiovascular: Proarrhythmia, palpitation, cardiac death, ECG abnormalities, CHF
Central nervous system: Headache, fatigue, insomnia
Endocrine & metabolic: Decreased libido
Gastrointestinal: Nausea, diarrhea, ileus
Ocular: Blurred vision, periorbital edema
Respiratory: Dyspnea

Overdosage/Toxicology Has a narrow therapeutic index and severe toxicity may occur slightly above the therapeutic range, especially if combined with other antiarrhythmic drugs. Acute single ingestion of twice the daily therapeutic dose is life-threatening. Symptoms include increased PR, QRS, and QT intervals, amplitude of the T wave, AV block, bradycardia, hypotension, ventricular arrhythmias (monomorphic or polymorphic ventricular tachycardia), and asystole. Other symptoms include dizziness, blurred vision, headache, and GI upset. Treatment is supportive, using conventional treatment (fluids, positioning, anticonvulsants, antiarrhythmics). **Note:** Type Ia antiarrhythmic agents should not be used to treat cardiotoxicity caused by type Ic antiarrhythmic drugs. Sodium bicarbonate may reverse QRS prolongation, bradycardia and hypotension. Ventricular pacing may be needed.

Drug Interactions Substrate of CYP3A4 (major); **Induces** CYP1A2 (weak), 3A4 (weak)
Cimetidine increases moricizine levels by 50%.
CYP3A4 inducers: CYP3A4 inducers may decrease the levels/effects of moricizine. Example inducers include aminoglutethimide, carbamazepine, nafcillin, nevirapine, phenobarbital, phenytoin, and rifamycins.
CYP3A4 inhibitors: May increase the levels/effects of moricizine. Example inhibitors include azole antifungals, clarithromycin, diclofenac, doxycycline, erythromycin, imatinib, isoniazid, nefazodone, nicardipine, propofol, protease inhibitors, quinidine, telithromycin, and verapamil.
Digoxin may result in additive prolongation of the PR interval when combined with moricizine (but not rate of second- and third-degree AV block).
Diltiazem increases moricizine levels resulting in an increased incidence of side effects. Moricizine decreases diltiazem plasma levels and decreases its half-life.
Drugs which may prolong QT interval (including cisapride, erythromycin, phenothiazines, cyclic antidepressants, and some quinolones) are contraindicated with Type Ia antiarrhythmics. Moricizine has some type Ia activity, and caution should be used.
Theophylline levels are decreased by 50% with moricizine due to increased clearance.

Ethanol/Nutrition/Herb Interactions Food: Moricizine peak serum concentrations may be decreased if taken with food.

Mechanism of Action Class I antiarrhythmic agent; reduces the fast inward current carried by sodium ions, shortens Phase I and Phase II repolarization, resulting in decreased action potential duration and effective refractory period

Pharmacokinetics
Protein binding, plasma: 95%
Metabolism: Undergoes significant first-pass metabolism (38%)
Half-life:
Normal patients: 3-4 hours
Cardiac disease patients: 6-13 hours
Elimination: 56% excreted in feces and 39% in urine, some enterohepatic recycling occurs

Dosage
Geriatrics & Adults: Ventricular arrhythmias: Oral: 200-300 mg every 8 hours, adjust dosage at 150 mg/day at 3-day intervals. See table on next page for dosage recommendations of transferring from other antiarrhythmic agents to Ethmozine®. Hospitalization required to start therapy.

Moricizine

Transferred From	Start Ethmozine®
Encainide, propafenone, tocainide, or mexiletine	8-12 hours after last dose
Flecainide	12-24 hours after last dose
Procainamide	3-6 hours after last dose
Quinidine, disopyramide	6-12 hours after last dose

Renal Impairment: Start at 600 mg/day or less.

Hepatic Impairment: Start at 600 mg/day or less.

Monitoring Parameters Holter monitoring may be considered; monitor pulse, EKG, and blood pressure

Patient Information Take as directed; do not change dose except from advice of your physician; report any chest pain and irregular heartbeats

Additional Information For transferring a patient from another antiarrhythmic agent, discontinue previous antiarrhythmic for 1-2 half-lives before starting moricizine; if this cannot be done, hospitalize patient to make transfer

Special Geriatric Considerations Due to moricizine binding to plasma albumin and alpha-glycoprotein, other highly bound drugs may displace moricizine. Since elderly may require multiple drugs, caution with highly bound drugs is necessary. Consider changes in renal and hepatic function with age and monitor closely since half-life may be prolonged.

Dosage Forms Excipient information presented when available (limited, particularly for generics); consult specific product labeling.

Tablet, as hydrochloride: 200 mg, 250 mg, 300 mg

Selected References

Fenster PE and Nolan PE, "Antiarrhythmic Drugs," *Geriatric Pharmacology*, Bressler R and Katz MD, eds, New York, NY: McGraw-Hill, 1993, 6:105-49.

♦ **Moricizine Hydrochloride** *see* Moricizine *on page 1063*

Morphine Sulfate (MOR feen SUL fate)

Related Information

Narcotic / Opioid Analgesics *on page 1763*

Medication Safety Issues

Sound-alike/look-alike issues:

Morphine may be confused with hydromorphone

Morphine sulfate may be confused with magnesium sulfate

MSO_4 is an error-prone abbreviation (mistaken as magnesium sulfate)

Avinza® may be confused with Evista®, Invanz®

Roxanol™ may be confused with OxyFast®, Roxicet™

Use care when prescribing and/or administering morphine solutions. These products are available in different concentrations. Always prescribe dosage in mg; **not** by volume (mL).

Use caution when selecting a morphine formulation for use in neurologic infusion pumps (eg, Medtronic delivery systems). The product should be appropriately labeled as "preservative-free" and suitable for intraspinal use via continuous infusion. In addition, the product should be formulated in a pH range that is compatible with the device operation specifications.

Significant differences exist between oral and I.V. dosing. Use caution when converting from one route of administration to another.

U.S. Brand Names Astramorph/PF™; Avinza®; DepoDur™; Duramorph®; Infumorph®; Kadian®; MS Contin®; Oramorph SR®; RMS® [DSC]; Roxanol™

Canadian Brand Names Kadian®; M-Eslon®; Morphine HP®; Morphine LP® Epidural; M.O.S.® 10; M.O.S.® 20; M.O.S.® 30; M.O.S.-SR®; M.O.S.-Sulfate®; MS Contin®; MS-IR®; PMS-Morphine Sulfate SR; ratio-Morphine SR; Statex®; Zomorph®

Index Terms MSO_4 (error-prone abbreviation and should not be used)

Generic Available Yes: Excludes capsule, controlled release tablet, sustained release tablet, extended release liposomal suspension for injection

Pharmacologic Category Analgesic, Opioid

Use Relief of moderate to severe acute and chronic pain, pain of myocardial infarction, dyspnea of acute left ventricular failure and pulmonary edema; preanesthetic medication

DepoDur™: Epidural (lumbar) single-dose management of surgical pain

Infumorph®: Used in microinfusion devices for intraspinal administration in treatment of intractable chronic pain

Restrictions C-II

(Continued)

Morphine Sulfate *(Continued)*

Contraindications Hypersensitivity to morphine sulfate or any component of the formulation; increased intracranial pressure; severe respiratory depression (in absence of resuscitative equipment or ventilatory support); acute or severe asthma; known or suspected paralytic ileus (sustained release products only); sustained release products are not recommended in acute/postoperative pain

Warnings/Precautions An opioid-containing analgesic regimen should be tailored to each patient's needs and based upon the type of pain being treated (acute versus chronic), the route of administration, degree of tolerance for opioids (naive versus chronic user), age, weight, and medical condition. The optimal analgesic dose varies widely among patients. Doses should be titrated to pain relief/prevention. When used as an epidural injection, monitor for delayed sedation.

May cause respiratory depression; use with caution in patients (particularly elderly or debilitated) with impaired respiratory function, morbid obesity, adrenal insufficiency, prostatic hyperplasia, urinary stricture, renal impairment, or severe hepatic dysfunction and in patients with hypersensitivity reactions to other phenanthrene derivative opioid agonists (codeine, hydrocodone, hydromorphone, levorphanol, oxycodone, oxymorphone). Use with caution in patients with biliary tract dysfunction; acute pancreatitis may cause constriction of sphincter of Oddi. Some preparations contain sulfites which may cause allergic reactions. May cause CNS depression, which may impair physical or mental abilities; patients must be cautioned about performing tasks which require mental alertness (eg, operating machinery or driving). Effects may be potentiated when used with other sedative drugs or ethanol. May cause hypotension in patients with acute myocardial infarction, volume depletion, or concurrent drug therapy which may exaggerate vasodilation. Use with extreme caution in patients with head injury, intracranial lesions, or elevated intracranial pressure; exaggerated elevation of ICP may occur. May obscure diagnosis or clinical course of patients with acute abdominal conditions. Tolerance or drug dependence may result from extended use. Concurrent use of agonist/antagonist analgesics may precipitate withdrawal symptoms and/or reduced analgesic efficacy in patients following prolonged therapy with mu opioid agonists. Abrupt discontinuation following prolonged use may also lead to withdrawal symptoms. Elderly may be particularly susceptible to adverse effects of narcotics.

Extended or sustained-release formulations:

[U.S. Boxed Warning]: Extended or sustained release dosage forms should not be crushed or chewed. Controlled-, extended-, or sustained-release products are not intended for "as needed (PRN)" use. MS Contin® 100 or 200 mg tablets are for use only in opioid-tolerant patients requiring >400 mg/day.

[U.S. Boxed Warning]: Avinza®: Do not administer with alcoholic beverages or ethanol-containing products, which may disrupt extended-release characteristic of product.

Injections: Note: Products are designed for administration by specific routes (I.V., intrathecal, epidural). Use caution when prescribing, dispensing, or administering to use formulations only by intended route(s).

[U.S. Boxed Warning]: Duramorph®: Due to the risk of severe and/or sustained cardiopulmonary depressant effects of Duramorph® must be administered in a fully equipped and staffed environment. Naloxone injection should be immediately available. Patient should remain in this environment for at least 24 hours following the initial dose.

Infumorph® solutions are **for use in microinfusion devices only**; not for I.V., I.M., or SubQ administration.

Depo-Dur™: **For epidural administration only.** Intrathecal administration has resulted in prolonged respiratory depression. Freezing may adversely affect modified-release mechanism of drug; check freeze indicator within carton prior to administration.

Adverse Reactions (Reflective of adult population; not specific for elderly)

Note: Individual patient differences are unpredictable, and percentage may differ in acute pain (surgical) treatment.

Frequency not defined: Flushing, CNS depression, sedation, antidiuretic hormone release, physical and psychological dependence, diaphoresis

>10%:

Cardiovascular: Palpitation, hypotension, bradycardia

Central nervous system: Drowsiness (48%, tolerance usually develops to drowsiness with regular dosing for 1-2 weeks); dizziness (20%), confusion, headache (following epidural or intrathecal use)

Dermatologic: Pruritus (may be secondary to histamine release)

Note: Pruritus may be dose-related, but not confined to the site of administration.

Gastrointestinal: Nausea (28%, tolerance usually develops to nausea and vomiting with chronic use); constipation (40%, tolerance develops very slowly if at all); xerostomia (78%)

Genitourinary: Urinary retention (16%; may be prolonged, up to 20 hours, following epidural or intrathecal use)

Local: Pain at injection site

Neuromuscular & skeletal: Weakness

Miscellaneous: Histamine release

1% to 10%:

Cardiovascular: Atrial fibrillation (<3%), chest pain (<3%), edema (<3%), syncope (<3%), tachycardia (<3%)

Central nervous system: Amnesia, anxiety, apathy, ataxia, chills, depression, euphoria, false feeling of well being, fever, headache, hypoesthesia, insomnia, lethargy, malaise, restlessness, seizure, vertigo

Endocrine & metabolic: Gynecomastia (<3%), hyponatremia (<3%)

Gastrointestinal: Anorexia, biliary colic, dyspepsia, dysphagia, GERD, GI irritation, paralytic ileus, vomiting (9%)

Genitourinary: Decreased urination

Hematologic: Anemia (<3%), leukopenia (<3%), thrombocytopenia (<3%)

Neuromuscular & skeletal: Arthralgia, back pain, bone pain, paresthesia, trembling

Ocular: Vision problems

Respiratory: Asthma, atelectasis, dyspnea, hiccups, hypoxia, noncardiogenic pulmonary edema, respiratory depression, rhinitis

Miscellaneous: Diaphoresis, flu-like syndrome, withdrawal syndrome

Overdosage/Toxicology Symptoms include respiratory depression, miosis, hypotension, bradycardia, apnea, and pulmonary edema. Treatment includes airway support, establishment of an I.V. line, and administration of naloxone 2 mg I.V., with repeat administration as necessary, up to a total of 10 mg. Primary attention should be directed to ensuring adequate respiratory exchange.

Drug Interactions Substrate of CYP2D6 (minor)

Antipsychotic agents: May increase hypotensive effects of morphine; monitor.

CNS depressants: May increase the effects/toxicity of morphine; monitor.

MAO inhibitors: May increase the effects/toxicity of morphine; some manufacturers recommend avoiding use within 14 days of MAO inhibitors

Pegvisomant: Therapeutic efficacy may be decreased by concomitant opiates, possibly requiring dosage adjustment of pegvisomant.

Rifamycin derivatives: May decrease levels/effects of morphine; monitor.

Selective serotonin reuptake inhibitors (SSRIs) and meperidine: Serotonergic effects may be additive, leading to serotonin syndrome.

Ethanol/Nutrition/Herb Interactions

Ethanol: Avoid ethanol (may increase CNS depression).

Avinza®: Alcoholic beverages or ethanol-containing products may disrupt extended-release formulation resulting in rapid release of entire morphine dose.

Food: Administration of oral morphine solution with food may increase bioavailability (ie, a report of 34% increase in morphine AUC when morphine oral solution followed a high-fat meal). The bioavailability of Oramorph SR® or Kadian® does not appear to be affected by food.

Herb/Nutraceutical: Avoid valerian, St John's wort, kava kava, gotu kola (may increase CNS depression).

Stability

Capsule, sustained release (Kadian®): Store at controlled room temperature 15°C to 30°C (59°F to 86°F). Protect from light and moisture.

Suppositories: Store at controlled room temperature 25°C (77°F). Protect from light.

Injection: Store at controlled room temperature. Protect from light. Degradation depends on pH and presence of oxygen; relatively stable in pH ≤4; darkening of solutions indicate degradation. Usual concentration for continuous I.V. infusion: 0.1-1 mg/mL in D_5W.

DepoDur™: Store under refrigeration, 2°C to 8°C (36°F to 46°F); do not freeze. Check freeze indicator before administration; do not administer if bulb is pink or purple. May store at room temperature for up to 30 days in sealed, unopened vials. DepoDur™ may be diluted in preservative-free NS to a volume of 5 mL. Gently invert to suspend particles prior to removal from vial. Once vial is opened, use within 4 hours.

Mechanism of Action Binds to opiate receptors in the CNS, causing inhibition of ascending pain pathways, altering the perception of and response to pain; produces generalized CNS depression

Pharmacodynamics Enhanced analgesia has been seen in older adult patients on therapeutic doses of narcotics; duration of action may be prolonged in older adults. See table on next page.

Pharmacokinetics

Absorption: Oral: Variable

Distribution: V_d: Decreased in older adults

(Continued)

Morphine Sulfate *(Continued)*

Metabolism: In the liver via glucuronide conjugation
Half-life: 2-4 hours (immediate release forms)
Elimination: 6% to 10% excreted unchanged in urine; total body clearance decreased in older adults

Morphine Sulfate

Dosage Form/Route	Analgesia	
	Peak	Duration
Extended release epidural injection	1 h	>48 h
I.M. injection	30-60 min	4-5 h
I.V. injection	20 min	4-5 h
Long-acting tablets/capsules	1 h	8-12 h
Oral solution	1 h	4-5 h
Subcutaneous injection	50-90 min	4-5 h
Suppository	20-60 min	3-7 h
Tablets/capsules	1 h	4-5 h

Dosage

Geriatrics: Refer to adult dosing. Use with caution; may require reduced dosage in the elderly and debilitated patients.

Adults: Note: These are guidelines and do not represent the maximum doses that may be required in all patients. Doses should be titrated to pain relief/prevention.

Acute pain (moderate-to-severe):

Oral: Prompt release formulations: Opiate-naive: Initial: 10 mg every 3 to 4 hours as needed; patients with prior opiate exposure may require higher initial doses: usual dosage range: 10-30 mg every 3-4 hours as needed

Oral: Controlled-, extended-, or sustained-release formulations: **Note:** A patient's morphine requirement should be established using prompt-release formulations. Conversion to long-acting products may be considered when chronic, continuous treatment is required. Higher dosages should be reserved for use only in opioid-tolerant patients.

Capsules, extended release (Avinza™): Daily dose administered once daily (for best results, administer at same time each day)

Capsules, sustained release (Kadian®): Daily dose administered once daily or in 2 divided doses daily (every 12 hours)

Tablets, controlled release (MS Contin®), sustained release (Oramorph SR®), or extended release: Daily dose divided and administered every 8 or every 12 hours

I.V.: Initial: Opiate-naive: 2.5-5 mg every 3 to 4 hours; patients with prior opiate exposure may require higher initial doses. **Note:** Repeated doses (up to every 5 minutes if needed) in small increments (eg, 1-4 mg) may be preferred to larger and less frequent doses.

I.V., SubQ continuous infusion: 0.8-10 mg/hour; may increase depending on pain relief/adverse effects: usual range: up to 80 mg/hour although higher doses may be required

Mechanically-ventilated patients (based on 70 kg patient): 0.7-10 mg every 1-2 hours as needed; infusion: 5-35 mg/hour

Patient-controlled analgesia (PCA): (Opiate-naive: Consider lower end of dosing range):
Usual concentration: 1 mg/mL
Demand dose: Usual: 1 mg; range: 0.5-2.5 mg
Lockout interval: 5-10 minutes

Epidural: **Note:** Administer with extreme caution and in reduced dosage to geriatric or debilitated patients.

Infusion:
Bolus dose: 1-6 mg
Infusion rate: 0.1-1 mg/hour
Maximum dose: 10 mg/24 hours

Single-dose (extended release, DepoDur™): Lower abdominal/pelvic surgery: 10-15 mg
Note: Some patients may benefit from a 20 mg dose, however, the incidence of adverse effects may be increased.

Intrathecal (I.T.): One-tenth of epidural dose; **Note:** Administer with extreme caution and in reduced dosage to geriatric or debilitated patients.

Opiate-naive: 0.2-1 mg/dose (may provide adequate relief for 24 hours); repeat doses **not** recommended except to establish initial IT dose.

    I.M., SubQ: **Note:** Repeated SubQ administration causes local tissue irritation, pain, and induration.

      Initial: Opiate-naive: 5-10 mg every 3-4 hours as needed; patients with prior opiate exposure may require higher initial doses; usual dosage range: 5-20 mg every 3-4 hours as needed

    Rectal: 10-20 mg every 3-4 hours

    Chronic pain: Patients taking opioids chronically may become tolerant and require doses higher than the usual dosage range to maintain the desired effect. Tolerance can be managed by appropriate dose titration. There is no optimal or maximal dose for morphine in chronic pain. The appropriate dose is one that relieves pain throughout its dosing interval without causing unmanageable side effects.

Renal Impairment:
    Cl_{cr} 10-50 mL/minute: Administer 75% of normal dose.
    Cl_{cr} <10 mL/minute: Administer 50% of normal dose.

Hepatic Impairment: Unchanged in mild liver disease; substantial extrahepatic metabolism may occur. Excessive sedation may occur in cirrhosis.

Administration
    Oral: Do not crush controlled release drug product, swallow whole. Kadian® can be opened and sprinkled on applesauce. Avinza™ can also be opened and sprinkled on applesauce; do not crush or chew the beads. Administration of oral morphine solution with food may increase bioavailability (not observed with Oramorph SR®).

    I.V.: When giving morphine I.V. push, it is best to first dilute in 4-5 mL of sterile water, and then to administer slowly (eg, 15 mg over 3-5 minutes)

    Epidural: Use preservative-free solutions

    Epidural, extended release liposomal suspension (DepoDur™): May be administered undiluted or diluted up to 5 mL total volume in preservative-free NS. Do not use an in-line filter during administration. Not for I.V. or I.M. administration.

      Resedation may occur following epidural administration; this may be delayed ≥48 hours in patients receiving extended-release (DepoDur™) injections.

      Administration of an epidural test dose (lidocaine 1.5% and epinephrine 1:200,000) may affect the release of morphine from the liposomal preparation. Delaying the dose for an interval of at least 15 minutes following the test dose minimizes this pharmacokinetic interaction. Except for a test dose, other epidural local anesthetics should not be used before or after this product.

    Intrathecal: Use preservative-free solutions

Monitoring Parameters Pain relief, respiratory and mental status, blood pressure
    Infumorph®: Patients should be observed in a fully-equipped and staffed environment for at least 24 hours following initiation, and as appropriate for the first several days after catheter implantation.

    DepoDur™: Patient should be monitored for at least 48 hours following administration.

Reference Range Therapeutic: Surgical anesthesia: 65-80 ng/mL (SI: 227-280 nmol/L); Toxic: 200-5000 ng/mL (SI: 700-17,500 nmol/L)

Test Interactions Some quinolones may produce a false-positive urine screening result for opiates using commercially-available immunoassay kits. This has been demonstrated most consistently for levofloxacin and ofloxacin, but other quinolones have shown cross-reactivity in certain assay kits. Confirmation of positive opiate screens by more specific methods should be considered.

Patient Information May cause drowsiness; avoid alcoholic beverages; do not crush controlled release tablet

Additional Information Because of its variety of dosage forms, morphine is particularly useful in the treatment of terminal pain. Serum concentrations >20 ng/dL may cause seizures; when converting from immediate release to controlled release morphine, the conversion is on a mg for mg basis. Immediate release morphine (oral, I.M., or SubQ) may be used for breakthrough pain until the dosage is adjusted.

Special Geriatric Considerations The elderly may be particularly susceptible to the CNS depressant and constipating effects of narcotics. For chronic administration of narcotic analgesics, morphine is preferable in the elderly due to its pharmacokinetics and side effect profile as compared to meperidine and methadone.

Dosage Forms Excipient information presented when available (limited, particularly for generics); consult specific product labeling. [DSC] = Discontinued product
    Capsule, extended release:
      Avinza®: 30 mg, 60 mg, 90 mg, 120 mg
    Capsule, sustained release:
      Kadian®: 20 mg, 30 mg, 50 mg, 60 mg, 80 mg, 100 mg, 200 mg
    Infusion [premixed in D_5W]: 1 mg/mL (100 mL, 250 mL)
    Injection, extended release liposomal suspension [lumbar epidural injection, preservative free]:
      DepoDur™: 10 mg/mL (1 mL, 1.5 mL, 2 mL)
    Injection, solution: 2 mg/mL (1 mL); 4 mg/mL (1 mL); 5 mg/mL (1 mL); 8 mg/mL (1 mL); 10 mg/mL (1 mL, 10 mL); 15 mg/mL (1 mL, 20 mL); 25 mg/mL (4 mL, 10 mL, 20 mL, (Continued)

Morphine Sulfate *(Continued)*

40 mL, 50 mL, 100 mL, 250 mL); 50 mg/mL (20 mL, 40 mL) [some preparations contain sodium metabisulfite]

Injection, solution [epidural, intrathecal, or I.V. infusion; preservative free]:

Astramorph/PF™: 0.5 mg/mL (2 mL, 10 mL); 1 mg/mL (2 mL, 10 mL)

Duramorph®: 0.5 mg/mL (10 mL); 1 mg/mL (10 mL)

Injection, solution [epidural or intrathecal infusion via microinfusion device; preservative free]:

Infumorph®: 10 mg/mL (20 mL); 25 mg/mL (20 mL)

Injection, solution [I.V. infusion via PCA pump]: 0.5 mg/mL (30 mL); 1 mg/mL (30 mL, 50 mL); 2 mg/mL (30 mL); 5 mg/mL (30 mL, 50 mL)

Injection, solution [preservative free]: 0.5 mg/mL (10 mL); 1 mg/mL (10 mL); 25 mg/mL (4 mL, 10 mL, 20 mL)

Solution, oral: 10 mg/5 mL (5 mL, 10 mL, 100 mL, 500 mL); 20 mg/5 mL (100 mL, 500 mL); 20 mg/mL (30 mL, 120 mL, 240 mL)

Roxanol™: 20 mg/mL (30 mL, 120 mL); 100 mg/5 mL (240 mL) [with calibrated spoon]

Solution, oral [concentrate]: 5 mg/0.25 mL (0.25 mL); 10 mg/0.5 mL (0.5 mL); 20 mg/mL (1 mL)

Suppository, rectal: 5 mg (12s), 10 mg (12s), 20 mg (12s), 30 mg (12s)

RMS®: 5 mg (12s), 10 mg (12s), 20 mg (12s), 30 mg (12s) [DSC]

Tablet: 10 mg, 15 mg, 30 mg

Tablet, controlled release:

MS Contin®: 15 mg, 30 mg, 60 mg, 100 mg, 200 mg

Tablet, extended release: 15 mg, 30 mg, 60 mg, 100 mg, 200 mg

Tablet, sustained release:

Oramorph SR®: 15 mg, 30 mg, 60 mg, 100 mg

Selected References

AGS Panel on Persistent Pain in Older Persons, "The Management of Persistent Pain in Older Persons," *J Am Geriatr Soc*, 2002, 50(6 Suppl):S205-24.

Ferrell BA, "Pain Management in Elderly People," *J Am Geriatr Soc*, 1991, 39(1):64-73.

Kaiko RF, "Age and Morphine Analgesia in Cancer Patients With Postoperative Pain," *Clin Pharmacol Ther*, 1980, 28(6):823-6.

Kaiko RF, Wallenstein SL, Rogers AG, et al, "Narcotics in the Elderly," *Med Clin North Am*, 1982, 66(5):1079-89.

- ◆ Mosco® Corn and Callus Remover [OTC] *see* Salicylic Acid *on page 1441*
- ◆ Motrin® *see* Ibuprofen *on page 784*
- ◆ Motrin® Children's [OTC] *see* Ibuprofen *on page 784*
- ◆ Motrin® IB [OTC] *see* Ibuprofen *on page 784*
- ◆ Motrin® Infants' [OTC] *see* Ibuprofen *on page 784*
- ◆ Motrin® Junior Strength [OTC] *see* Ibuprofen *on page 784*
- ◆ Mouthkote® [OTC] *see* Saliva Substitute *on page 1443*

Moxifloxacin *(moxs i FLOKS a sin)*

Related Information

Antimicrobial Activity Against Selected Organisms *on page 1728*

Medication Safety Issues

Sound-alike/look-alike issues:

Avelox® may be confused with Avonex®

International issues:

Vigamox™ may be confused with Fisamox® which is a brand name for amoxicillin in Australia

U.S. Brand Names Avelox®; Avelox® I.V.; Vigamox™

Canadian Brand Names Avelox®; Avelox® I.V.; Vigamox™

Index Terms Moxifloxacin Hydrochloride

Generic Available No

Pharmacologic Category Antibiotic, Ophthalmic; Antibiotic, Quinolone

Use Treatment of mild to moderate community-acquired pneumonia, including multi-drug-resistant *Streptococcus pneumoniae* (MDRSP); acute bacterial exacerbation of chronic bronchitis; acute bacterial sinusitis; complicated and uncomplicated skin infections; complicated intra-abdominal infections; bacterial conjunctivitis (ophthalmic formulation)

Contraindications Hypersensitivity to moxifloxacin, other quinolone antibiotics, or any component of the formulation

Warnings/Precautions Use with caution in patients with significant bradycardia or acute myocardial ischemia. Moxifloxacin causes a concentration-dependent QT prolongation. Do not exceed recommended dose or infusion rate. Avoid use with uncorrected hypokalemia, with other drugs that prolong the QT interval or induce bradycardia, or with class IA or III antiarrhythmic agents. Use with caution in individuals at risk of seizures (CNS disorders or concurrent therapy with medications which may lower seizure threshold). Potential for seizures, although very rare, may be increased with concomitant NSAID therapy. Discontinue in patients who experience significant CNS adverse effects (dizziness, hallucinations, suicidal ideation or actions). Not recommended in patients with moderate to severe hepatic insufficiency. Use with caution in diabetes; glucose regulation may be altered. Tendon inflammation and/or rupture have been reported with quinolone antibiotics. Risk may be increased with concurrent corticosteroids, particularly in the elderly. Discontinue at first signs or symptoms of tendon pain.

Severe hypersensitivity reactions, including anaphylaxis, have occurred with quinolone therapy. If an allergic reaction occurs (itching, urticaria, dyspnea or facial edema, loss of consciousness, tingling, cardiovascular collapse) discontinue drug immediately. May cause photosensitivity. Prolonged use may result in fungal or bacterial superinfection, including *C. difficile*-associated diarrhea and pseudomembranous colitis. Quinolones may exacerbate myasthenia gravis. Peripheral neuropathy may rarely occur.

Ophthalmic: Eye drops should not be injected subconjunctivally or introduced directly into the anterior chamber of the eye. Contact lenses should not be worn during therapy.

Adverse Reactions (Reflective of adult population; not specific for elderly)
Systemic:
3% to 10%: Gastrointestinal: Nausea (6%), diarrhea (5%)
0.1% to 3%:
  Cardiovascular: Hypertension, palpitation, QT_c prolongation, tachycardia, vasodilation
  Central nervous system: Anxiety, chills, dizziness, headache, insomnia, nervousness, pain, somnolence, tremor, vertigo
  Dermatologic: Dry skin, pruritus, rash (maculopapular, purpuric, pustular)
  Endocrine & metabolic: Serum chloride increased ($\geq 2\%$), serum ionized calcium increased ($\geq 2\%$), serum glucose decreased ($\geq 2\%$)
  Gastrointestinal: Abdominal pain, amylase increased, amylase decreased ($\geq 2\%$), anorexia, constipation, dry mouth, dyspepsia, flatulence, glossitis, lactic dehydrogenase increased, stomatitis, taste perversion, vomiting
  Genitourinary: Vaginal moniliasis, vaginitis
  Hematologic: Eosinophilia, leukopenia, prothrombin time prolonged, increased INR, thrombocythemia
    Increased serum levels of the following ($\geq 2\%$): MCH, neutrophils, WBC
    Decreased serum levels of the following ($\geq 2\%$): Basophils, eosinophils, hemoglobin, RBC, neutrophils
  Hepatic: Bilirubin decreased or increased ($\geq 2\%$), GGTP increased, liver function test abnormal
  Local: Injection site reaction
  Neuromuscular & skeletal: Arthralgia, myalgia, weakness
  Renal: Kidney function abnormal, serum albumin increased ($\geq 2\%$)
  Respiratory: Pharyngitis, pneumonia, rhinitis, sinusitis, pO_2 increased ($\geq 2\%$)

Additional reactions with **ophthalmic** preparation: 1% to 6%: Conjunctivitis, dry eye, ocular discomfort, ocular hyperemia, ocular pain, ocular pruritus, subconjunctival hemorrhage, tearing, visual acuity decreased

Overdosage/Toxicology Potential symptoms of overdose may include CNS excitation, seizures, QT prolongation, and arrhythmias (including torsade de pointes). Patients should be monitored by continuous ECG in the event of an overdose. Management is supportive and symptomatic. Hemodialysis only removes ~9% of dose.

Drug Interactions
  Corticosteroids: Concurrent use may increase the risk of tendon rupture, particularly in elderly patients (overall incidence rare).
  Glyburide: Quinolones may increase the effect of glyburide; monitor
  Metal cations (aluminum, calcium, iron, magnesium, and zinc) bind quinolones in the gastrointestinal tract and inhibit absorption. Concurrent administration of most antacids, oral electrolyte supplements, quinapril, sucralfate, some didanosine formulations (pediatric powder for oral suspension), and other higly-buffered oral drugs, should be avoided. Moxifloxacin should be administered 4 hours before or 8 hours after these agents. Calcium products do not appear to significantly affect moxifloxacin absorption.
  NSAIDs: Risk of seizures may be increased with concomitant NSAID use. Risk is considered quite low and may only be a factor with high serum levels of either agent and/or in patients with additional predisposing factors (eg, renal dysfunction, history of seizure or other neurological disorder).
  QT_c-prolonging agents: Effects may be additive with moxifloxacin. Avoid concurrent use with Class Ia and Class III antiarrhythmics, erythromycin, cisapride, antipsychotics, and cyclic antidepressants.
  (Continued)

Moxifloxacin *(Continued)*

Typhoid vaccine: Antibiotics may decrease the therapeutic effect of live, attenuated Ty21a vaccine; delay vaccination for >24 hours after administration of antibacterial agents.

Warfarin: The hypoprothrombinemic effect of warfarin may be enhanced by some quinolone antibiotics; monitor INR.

Ethanol/Nutrition/Herb Interactions Food: Absorption is not affected by administration with a high-fat meal or yogurt.

Stability Store at 15°C to 30°C (59°F to 86°F). Do not refrigerate infusion solution.

Mechanism of Action Moxifloxacin is a DNA gyrase inhibitor, and also inhibits topoisomerase IV. DNA gyrase (topoisomerase II) is an essential bacterial enzyme that maintains the superhelical structure of DNA. DNA gyrase is required for DNA replication and transcription, DNA repair, recombination, and transposition; inhibition is bactericidal.

Pharmacokinetics

Absorption: Well absorbed; not affected by high fat meal or yogurt

Distribution: V_d: 1.7 to 2.7 L/kg; tissue concentrations often exceed plasma concentrations in respiratory tissues, alveolar macrophages, abdominal tissues/fluids, and sinus tissues

Protein binding: 30% to 50%

Metabolism: Hepatic (52% of dose) via glucuronide (14%) and sulfate (38%) conjugation

Bioavailability: 90%

Half-life: Oral: 12 hours; I.V.: 15 hours

Elimination: Approximately 45% of a dose is excreted in feces (25%) and urine (20%) as unchanged drug

Metabolites: Sulfate conjugates in feces, glucuronide conjugates in urine

Dosage

Geriatrics & Adults:

Acute bacterial sinusitis: Oral, I.V.: 400 mg every 24 hours for 10 days

Bacterial conjunctivitis: Ophthalmic: Instill 1 drop into affected eye(s) 3 times/day for 7 days

Chronic bronchitis, acute bacterial exacerbation: Oral, I.V.: 400 mg every 24 hours for 5 days

Note: Avelox® ABC Pack™ (Avelox® Bronchitis Course) contains five tablets of 400 mg each.

Intra-abdominal infections, complicated: Oral, I.V.: 400 mg every 24 hours for 5-14 days (initiate with I.V.)

Pneumonia, community-acquired (including MDRSP): Oral, I.V.: 400 mg every 24 hours for 7-14 days

Skin and skin structure infections: Oral, I.V.:
Complicated: 400 mg every 24 hours for 7-21 days
Uncomplicated: 400 mg every 24 hours for 7 days

Renal Impairment: No adjustment is necessary, including patients on hemodialysis or CAPD.

Hepatic Impairment: No dosage adjustment is required in mild to moderate hepatic insufficiency (Child-Pugh Classes A and B). Not recommended in patients with severe hepatic insufficiency.

Monitoring Parameters WBC, signs of infection

Test Interactions Some quinolones may produce a false-positive urine screening result for opiates using commercially-available immunoassay kits. This has been demonstrated most consistently for levofloxacin and ofloxacin, but other quinolones have shown cross-reactivity in certain assay kits. Confirmation of positive opiate screens by more specific methods should be considered.

Patient Information May be taken with or without food. Drink plenty of fluids. Avoid direct exposure to direct sunlight during therapy and for several days following. Do not take antacids within 4 hours before or 8 hours after dosing. Contact your physician immediately if signs of allergy, tendon inflammation, or pain occur. Do not discontinue therapy until your course has been completed. Take a missed dose as soon as possible, unless it is almost time for your next dose.

Ophthalmic: Wash hands before instilling solution. Sit or lie down to instill. Open eye, look at ceiling, and instill prescribed amount of solution as directed. Do not touch tip of applicator or let tip of applicator touch eye. Do not wear contact lenses during therapy. Temporary stinging or blurred vision, or dry eyes may occur. Report persistent pain, burning, excessive tearing, decreased visual acuity, swelling, itching, or worsening of condition.

Special Geriatric Considerations No dosage adjustments are required based on age. Assess patient's ability to self-administer eye drops.

Dosage Forms Excipient information presented when available (limited, particularly for generics); consult specific product labeling.

Infusion [premixed in sodium chloride 0.8%] (Avelox® I.V.): 400 mg (250 mL)

Solution, ophthalmic (Vigamox™): 0.5% (3 mL)
Tablet:
Avelox®: 400 mg
Avelox® ABC Pack [unit-dose pack]: 400 mg (5s)

Selected References

Balfour JA and Wiseman LR, "Moxifloxacin," *Drugs*, 1999, 57(3):363-73.

Blondeau JM, "Expanded Activity and Utility of the New Fluoroquinolones: A Review," *Clin Ther*, 1999, 21(1):3-40.

"Gatifloxacin and Moxifloxacin: Two New Fluoroquinolones," *Med Lett Drugs Ther*, 2000, 42(1072):15-7.

♦ **Moxifloxacin Hydrochloride** *see* Moxifloxacin *on page 1070*

♦ **MPA** *see* MedroxyPROGESTERone *on page 965*

♦ **MPA and Estrogens (Conjugated)** *see* Estrogens (Conjugated/Equine) and Medroxyprogesterone *on page 568*

♦ **6-MP (error-prone abbreviation)** *see* Mercaptopurine *on page 985*

♦ **MPSV4** *see* Meningococcal Polysaccharide Vaccine (Groups A / C / Y and W-135) *on page 979*

♦ **MS Contin®** *see* Morphine Sulfate *on page 1065*

♦ **MSO₄ (error-prone abbreviation and should not be used)** *see* Morphine Sulfate *on page 1065*

♦ **MTX (error-prone abbreviation)** *see* Methotrexate *on page 1005*

♦ **Mucinex® [OTC]** *see* Guaifenesin *on page 727*

♦ **Mucinex®, Children's [OTC]** *see* Guaifenesin *on page 727*

♦ **Mucinex® Children's Cough [OTC]** *see* Guaifenesin and Dextromethorphan *on page 730*

♦ **Mucinex®, Children's Mini-Melts™ [OTC]** *see* Guaifenesin *on page 727*

♦ **Mucinex® DM [OTC]** *see* Guaifenesin and Dextromethorphan *on page 730*

♦ **Mucinex® DM Maximum Strength [OTC]** *see* Guaifenesin and Dextromethorphan *on page 730*

♦ **Mucinex®, Junior Mini-Melts™ [OTC]** *see* Guaifenesin *on page 727*

♦ **Mucinex® Maximum Strength [OTC]** *see* Guaifenesin *on page 727*

♦ **Multidex® [OTC]** *see* Maltodextrin *on page 953*

♦ **Mumps, Measles and Rubella Vaccines, Combined** *see* Measles, Mumps, and Rubella Vaccines (Combined) *on page 957*

♦ **Mumpsvax®** *see* Mumps Virus Vaccine (Live/Attenuated) *on page 1073*

Mumps Virus Vaccine (Live/Attenuated)
(mumpz VYE rus vak SEEN, live, a ten YOO ate ed)

Related Information
Immunization Recommendations *on page 1787*
U.S. Brand Names Mumpsvax®
Generic Available No
Pharmacologic Category Vaccine
Use Mumps prophylaxis by promoting active immunity
  Note: Trivalent measles-mumps-rubella (MMR) vaccine is the preferred agent for most children and many adults; persons born prior to 1957 are generally considered immune and need not be vaccinated
Contraindications Hypersensitivity to mumps vaccine or any component of the formulation, including gelatin; febrile respiratory illness or active febrile infection; immunosuppressant therapy; primary or acquired immunodeficiency states; blood dyscrasias, leukemia, lymphoma or other malignant neoplasm affecting bone marrow or lymphatic systems; untreated tuberculosis
Warnings/Precautions Use caution with hypersensitivity to eggs or neomycin; patients with history of anaphylactic reaction may be at increased risk of immediate-type hypersensitivity reaction. Patients with minor illnesses (diarrhea, mild upper respiratory tract infection with or without low grade fever or other illnesses with low-grade fever) may receive vaccine. Leukemia patients who are in remission and who have not received chemotherapy for at least 3 months may be vaccinated. Patients with a history of congenital or hereditary immunodeficiency should not receive immunization until immune competence is demonstrated. Do not administer to severely immunocompromised persons. Corticosteroid replacement therapy is not a contraindication for vaccination. Use caution in patients with thrombocytopenia and those who develop thrombocytopenia after first dose; thrombocytopenia may worsen. Immediate treatment for anaphylactic/anaphylactoid reaction should be available during vaccine use.
Adverse Reactions (Reflective of adult population; not specific for elderly)
All serious adverse reactions must be reported to the U.S. Department of Health and Human Services (DHHS) Vaccine Adverse Event Reporting System (VAERS) 1-800-822-7967.
(Continued)

Mumps Virus Vaccine (Live/Attenuated) *(Continued)*

Frequency not defined.

Cardiovascular: Syncope, vasculitis

Central nervous system: Encephalitis, febrile seizure, fever, Guillain-Barré syndrome, irritability

Dermatologic: Angioneurotic edema, erythema multiforme, purpura, Stevens-Johnson syndrome, urticaria

Endocrine & metabolic: Diabetes mellitus, parotitis

Gastrointestinal: Diarrhea, pancreatitis

Genitourinary: Orchitis

Hematologic: Leukocytosis, thrombocytopenia

Local: Burning/stinging at injection site, wheal and flare at injection site

Ocular: Conjunctivitis, ocular palsies, optic neuritis, papillitis, retrobulbar neuritis

Otic: Nerve deafness, otitis media

Respiratory: Bronchial spasm, cough, rhinitis

Miscellaneous: Anaphylaxis, anaphylactoid reactions, lymphadenopathy

Drug Interactions

Corticosteroids: In patients receiving high doses of systemic corticosteroids for ≥14 days, wait at least 1 month between discontinuing steroid therapy and administering vaccine.

Immune globulin, whole blood, plasma: Do not administer together; immune response may be compromised. Defer vaccine administration for ≥3 months.

Immunosuppressant medications: The effect of the vaccine may be decreased.

Vaccines: May be administered with Varivax® and PedvaxHIB® using separate syringes and injection sites. Although data is limited concerning simultaneous administration of DTP, OPV, Hib, and hepatitis B vaccine, the ACIP supports the simultaneous use of all as recommended. Do not give within 1 month of other live virus vaccine.

Stability Product is shipped at ≤10°C (50°F). Prior to reconstitution, vaccine must be stored at ≤2°C to 8°C (36°F to 46°F). Reconstitute using entire contents of one vial of provided preservative free diluent. Following reconstitution, use as soon as possible, but may be stored at 2°C to 8°C (36°F to 46°F) for up to 8 hours. Protect from light prior to and after reconstitution.

Mechanism of Action Promotes active immunity to mumps virus by inducing specific antibodies.

Dosage

Geriatrics & Adults: Immunization: SubQ : 0.5 mL as a single dose

Administration For SubQ administration in outer asped of the upper arm using 25G 5/8" needle.

Monitoring Parameters Monitor for anaphylaxis after vaccination, having person remain in office for a period of 15-30 minutes would be more than adequate

Test Interactions Temporary suppression of tuberculosis skin test

Patient Information A little swelling of the glands in the cheeks and under the jaw may occur that lasts for a few days; this could appear from 1-2 weeks after receiving the mumps vaccine; this happens rarely

Additional Information Federal law requires that the date of administration, the vaccine manufacturer, lot number of vaccine, and the administering person's name, title, and address be entered into the patient's permanent medical record.

Acceptable presumptive evidence of immunity includes one of the following:
1. Documentation of adequate vaccination. Adequate vaccination for mumps is defined as 1 dose of a live mumps virus vaccine for adults not at high risk; 2 doses of a live mumps virus vaccine for high-risk adults. Healthcare workers, international travelers, and students in institutions of higher learning are considered high-risk adults.
2. Laboratory evidence of immunity to mumps
3. Birth prior to 1957
4. Documentation of physician-diagnosed mumps

During a mumps outbreak, additional doses of a mumps virus vaccine may need to be considered. MMR vaccine is recommended; refer to Measles Mumps Rubella Vaccine (Combined) monograph. Minimum interval between doses is 28 days.

Special Geriatric Considerations Most adults are immune to mumps and vaccination is not necessary for those born prior to 1957; elderly who have lived in isolated communities may have no immunity; for those who fail to demonstrate immunity by testing, vaccination would be desired if exposure is likely (travel to endemic area, etc); the trivalent MMR is preferred, however

Dosage Forms Excipient information presented when available (limited, particularly for generics); consult specific product labeling.

Injection, powder for reconstitution [preservative free]:

Mumpsvax®: TCID$_{50}$ 20,000 [contains human albumin, bovine serum, gelatin, neomycin; packaged with diluent]

Selected References

Centers for Disease Control and Prevention (CDC), "Notice to Readers: Updated Recommendations of the Advisory Committee on Immunization Practices (ACIP) for the Control and Elimination of Mumps," *MMWR Recomm Rep*, 2006, 55(early release):1-2. Available at http://www.cdc.gov/mmwr/pdf/wk/mm55e601.pdf

Centers for Disease Control, "Recommendations of the Advisory Committee on Immunization Practices (ACIP): General Recommendations on Immunization," *MMWR Recomm Rep*, 1994, 43(RR-1):23.

Watson JC, Hadler SC, Dykewicz CA, et al, "Measles, Mumps, and Rubella — Vaccine Use and Strategies for Elimination of Measles, Rubella, and Congenital Rubella Syndrome and Control of Mumps: Recommendations of the Advisory Committee on Immunization Practices (ACIP)," *MMWR Recomm Rep*, 1998, 47(RR-8):1-57.

Mupirocin (myoo PEER oh sin)

Medication Safety Issues
Sound-alike/look-alike issues:
Bactroban® may be confused with bacitracin, baclofen

U.S. Brand Names Bactroban®; Bactroban® Nasal; Centany™

Canadian Brand Names Bactroban®

Index Terms Mupirocin Calcium; Pseudomonic Acid A

Generic Available Yes: Topical ointment

Pharmacologic Category Antibiotic, Topical

Use Topical treatment of impetigo due to *Staphylococcus aureus*, beta-hemolytic *Streptococcus* and *S. pyogenes*; intranasally for the eradication of nasal colonization with methicillin-resistant *Staphylococcus aureus* in adult patients and healthcare workers during institutional outbreaks

Unlabeled/Investigational Use Intranasal: Surgical prophylaxis to prevent wound infections

Contraindications Hypersensitivity to mupirocin, polyethylene glycol, or any component of the formulation

Warnings/Precautions Potentially toxic amounts of polyethylene glycol contained in some topical products may be absorbed percutaneously in patients with extensive burns or open wounds; use caution with renal impairment. Prolonged use may result in over growth of nonsusceptible organisms. For external use only; avoid contact with eyes. Not for treatment of pressure sores.

Adverse Reactions (Reflective of adult population; not specific for elderly)
Frequency not defined.
Central nervous system: Dizziness, headache
Dermatologic: Cellulitis, dermatitis, dry skin, erythema, hives, pruritus, rash, ulcerative stomatitis
Gastrointestinal: Abdominal pain, diarrhea, nausea, taste perversion, xerostomia
Local: Burning, edema, pain, stinging, tenderness
Ocular: Blepharitis
Otic: Ear pain
Respiratory: Cough, pharyngitis, rhinitis, upper respiratory tract congestion
Miscellaneous: Secondary wound infection

Drug Interactions No data reported

Mechanism of Action Binds to bacterial isoleucyl transfer-RNA synthetase resulting in the inhibition of protein synthesis

Pharmacokinetics
Absorption: Topical: Penetrates outer layers of skin; systemic absorption is minimal through intact skin
Protein binding: 95%
Metabolism: Extensive, principally in the liver and skin to monic acid
Half-life: 17-36 minutes
Elimination: In urine

Dosage
Geriatrics & Adults:
Impetigo: Topical: Ointment: Apply to affected area 3 times/day; re-evaluate after 3-5 days if no clinical response
Secondary skin infections: Topical: Cream: Apply to affected area 3 times/day for 10 days; re-evaluate after 3-5 days if no clinical response
Elimination of MRSA colonization: Intranasal: Approximately one-half of the ointment from the single-use tube should be applied into one nostril and the other half into the other nostril twice daily for 5 days

Monitoring Parameters If no clinical response in 3-5 days, re-evaluate use

Patient Information For topical use only; do not apply into the eye

Additional Information Contains polyethylene glycol vehicle

Special Geriatric Considerations Not for treatment of pressure sores.

Dosage Forms Excipient information presented when available (limited, particularly for generics); consult specific product labeling.
Note: Strength expressed as base
(Continued)

Mupirocin (Continued)

Cream, topical, as calcium:
Bactroban®: 2% (15 g, 30 g) [contains benzyl alcohol]
Ointment, intranasal, as calcium:
Bactroban® Nasal: 2% (1 g) [single-use tube]
Ointment, topical: 2% (0.9 g, 22 g)
Bactroban®: 2% (22 g) [contains polyethylene glycol]
Centany™: 2% (15 g, 30 g)

Selected References

Goldfarb J, Crenshaw D, O'Horo J, et al, "Randomized Clinical Trial of Topical Mupirocin Versus Oral Erythromycin for Impetigo," *Antimicrob Agents Chemother*, 1988, 32(12):1780-3.

- ◆ **Mupirocin Calcium** *see* Mupirocin *on page 1075*
- ◆ **Murine® Ear Wax Removal System [OTC]** *see* Carbamide Peroxide *on page 235*
- ◆ **Murine® Tears [OTC]** *see* Artificial Tears *on page 124*
- ◆ **Murine® Tears Plus [OTC]** *see* Tetrahydrozoline *on page 1547*
- ◆ **Muro 128® [OTC]** *see* Sodium Chloride *on page 1475*
- ◆ **Murocel® [OTC]** *see* Artificial Tears *on page 124*
- ◆ **Muse®** *see* Alprostadil *on page 57*
- ◆ **Myambutol®** *see* Ethambutol *on page 581*
- ◆ **Mycamine®** *see* Micafungin *on page 1035*
- ◆ **Mycelex®** *see* Clotrimazole *on page 349*
- ◆ **Mycelex®-7 [OTC]** *see* Clotrimazole *on page 349*
- ◆ **Mycelex® Twin Pack [OTC]** *see* Clotrimazole *on page 349*
- ◆ **Mycinaire™ [OTC]** *see* Sodium Chloride *on page 1475*
- ◆ **Mycobutin®** *see* Rifabutin *on page 1400*
- ◆ **Mycocide® NS [OTC]** *see* Tolnaftate *on page 1596*
- ◆ **Mycolog®-II [DSC]** *see* Nystatin and Triamcinolone *on page 1143*
- ◆ **Mycostatin®** *see* Nystatin *on page 1142*
- ◆ **Mydfrin®** *see* Phenylephrine *on page 1247*
- ◆ **Mylanta® Gas [OTC]** *see* Simethicone *on page 1467*
- ◆ **Mylanta® Gas Maximum Strength [OTC]** *see* Simethicone *on page 1467*
- ◆ **Mylanta® Liquid [OTC]** *see* Aluminum Hydroxide, Magnesium Hydroxide, and Simethicone *on page 66*
- ◆ **Mylanta® Maximum Strength Liquid [OTC]** *see* Aluminum Hydroxide, Magnesium Hydroxide, and Simethicone *on page 66*
- ◆ **Mylanta® Soothing Antacids [OTC]** *see* Calcium Salts (Oral) *on page 220*
- ◆ **Myleran®** *see* Busulfan *on page 203*
- ◆ **Mylicon® Infants [OTC]** *see* Simethicone *on page 1467*
- ◆ **Mylocel™** *see* Hydroxyurea *on page 774*
- ◆ **Myobloc®** *see* Botulinum Toxin Type B *on page 181*
- ◆ **Myochrysine®** *see* Gold Sodium Thiomalate *on page 721*
- ◆ **myrac™** *see* Minocycline *on page 1046*
- ◆ **Mysoline®** *see* Primidone *on page 1312*
- ◆ **Mytussin® AC** *see* Guaifenesin and Codeine *on page 729*
- ◆ **N-0923** *see* Rotigotine *on page 1434*
- ◆ **Nabi-HB®** *see* Hepatitis B Immune Globulin *on page 748*

Nabumetone (na BYOO me tone)

U.S. Brand Names Relafen® [DSC]
Canadian Brand Names Apo-Nabumetone®; Gen-Nabumetone; Novo-Nabumetone; Relafen®; Rhoxal-nabumetone; Sandoz-Nabumetone
Generic Available Yes
Pharmacologic Category Nonsteroidal Anti-inflammatory Drug (NSAID), Oral
Use Management of osteoarthritis and rheumatoid arthritis
Unlabeled/Investigational Use Treatment of sunburn, mild to moderate pain
Restrictions An FDA-approved medication guide must be distributed when dispensing an oral outpatient prescription (new or refill) where this medication is to be used without direct supervision of a healthcare provider. Medication guides are available at http://www.fda.gov/cder/Offices/ODS/medication_guides.htm.
Contraindications Hypersensitivity to nabumetone, aspirin, other NSAIDs, or any component of the formulation; perioperative pain in the setting of coronary artery bypass surgery (CABG)
Warnings/Precautions [U.S. Boxed Warning]: NSAIDs are associated with an increased risk of adverse cardiovascular events, including MI, stroke, and new onset or worsening of pre-existing hypertension. Risk may be increased with

duration of use or pre-existing cardiovascular risk factors or disease. Carefully evaluate individual cardiovascular risk profiles prior to prescribing. Use caution with fluid retention, CHF or hypertension. Concurrent administration of ibuprofen, and potentially other nonselective NSAIDs, may interfere with aspirin's cardioprotective effect.

Use of NSAIDs can compromise existing renal function. Renal toxicity can occur in patient with impaired renal function, dehydration, heart failure, liver dysfunction, those taking diuretics and ACEI and the elderly. Rehydrate patient before starting therapy. Monitor renal function closely. Not recommended for use in patients with advanced renal disease.

[U.S. Boxed Warning]: NSAIDs may increase risk of gastrointestinal irritation, ulceration, bleeding, and perforation. These events may occur at any time during therapy and without warning. Use caution with a history of GI disease (bleeding or ulcers), concurrent therapy with aspirin, anticoagulants and/or corticosteroids, smoking, use of alcohol, the elderly or debilitated patients.

Use the lowest effective dose for the shortest duration of time, consistent with individual patient goals, to reduce risk of cardiovascular or GI adverse events. Alternate therapies should be considered for patients at high risk.

NSAIDs may cause serious skin adverse events including exfoliative dermatitis, Stevens-Johnson syndrome (SJS) and toxic epidermal necrolysis (TEN). Anaphylactoid reactions may occur, even without prior exposure; patients with "aspirin triad" (bronchial asthma, aspirin intolerance, rhinitis) may be at increased risk. Do not use in patients who experience bronchospasm, asthma, rhinitis, or urticaria with NSAID or aspirin therapy. Use caution in other forms of asthma.

Use with caution in patients with decreased hepatic function. Closely monitor patients with any abnormal LFT. Severe hepatic reactions (eg, fulminant hepatitis, liver failure) have occurred with NSAID use, rarely; discontinue if signs or symptoms of liver disease develop, or if systemic manifestations occur.

The elderly are at increased risk for adverse effects (especially peptic ulceration, CNS effects, renal toxicity) from NSAIDs even at low doses.

Withhold for at least 4-6 half-lives prior to surgical or dental procedures. May cause photosensitivity reactions.

Adverse Reactions (Reflective of adult population; not specific for elderly)
>10%: Gastrointestinal: Abdominal pain (12%), diarrhea (14%), dyspepsia (13%)
1% to 10%:
  Cardiovascular: Edema (3% to 9%)
  Central nervous system: Dizziness (3% to 9%), headache (3% to 9%), fatigue (1% to 3%), insomnia (1% to 3%), nervousness (1% to 3%), somnolence (1% to 3%)
  Dermatologic: Pruritus (3% to 9%), rash (3% to 9%)
  Gastrointestinal: Constipation (3% to 9%), flatulence (3% to 9%), guaic positive (3% to 9%), nausea (3% to 9%), gastritis (1% to 3%), stomatitis (1% to 3%), vomiting (1% to 3%), xerostomia (1% to 3%)
  Otic: Tinnitus
  Miscellaneous: Diaphoresis (1% to 3%)

Drug Interactions
  ACE inhibitors: Antihypertensive effects may be decreased by concurrent therapy with NSAIDs; monitor blood pressure.
  Angiotensin II antagonists: Antihypertensive effects may be decreased by concurrent therapy with NSAIDs; monitor blood pressure.
  Anticoagulants (warfarin, heparin, LMWHs) in combination with NSAIDs can cause increased risk of bleeding.
  Antiplatelet drugs (ticlopidine, clopidogrel, aspirin, abciximab, dipyridamole, eptifibatide, tirofiban) can cause an increased risk of bleeding.
  Beta-blockers: NSAIDs may decrease the antihypertensive effect of beta-blockers. Monitor.
  Cholestyramine (and other bile acid sequestrants): May decrease the absorption of NSAIDs. Separate by at least 2 hours.
  Corticosteroids may increase the risk of GI ulceration; avoid concurrent use.
  Cyclosporine: NSAIDs may increase serum creatinine, potassium, blood pressure, and cyclosporine levels; monitor cyclosporine levels and renal function carefully.
  Fluoroquinolone antibiotics: Risk of seizures may be increased with concomitant quinolone use. Risk is considered quite low and may only be a factor with high serum levels of either agent and/or in patients with additional predisposing factors (eg, renal dysfunction, history of seizure or other neurological disorder).
  Hydralazine's antihypertensive effect is decreased; avoid concurrent use.
  Lithium levels can be increased; avoid concurrent use if possible or monitor lithium levels and adjust dose. Sulindac may have the least effect. When NSAID is stopped, lithium will need adjustment again.
  Loop diuretics efficacy (diuretic and antihypertensive effect) is reduced.
(Continued)

Nabumetone *(Continued)*

Methotrexate: Severe bone marrow suppression, aplastic anemia, and GI toxicity have been reported with concomitant NSAID therapy. Avoid use during moderate or high-dose methotrexate (increased and prolonged methotrexate levels). NSAID use during low-dose treatment of rheumatoid arthritis has not been fully evaluated; extreme caution is warranted.

Salicylates: NSAIDs (nonselective) may diminish the cardioprotective effect of acetylated salicylates. Avoid regular use of NSAIDs if possible; consider alternatives (eg, acetaminophen). Give salicylate before NSAID; for example ibuprofen should be given 30-120 minutes after aspirin (immediate release).

Thiazides antihypertensive effects are decreased; avoid concurrent use.

Warfarin's INRs may be increased by nabumetone. Monitor INR closely. Use the lowest dose of NSAIDs possible and for the briefest duration.

Ethanol/Nutrition/Herb Interactions

Ethanol: Avoid ethanol (may enhance gastric mucosal irritation).

Food: Nabumetone peak serum concentrations may be increased if taken with food or dairy products.

Herb/Nutraceutical: Avoid alfalfa, anise, bilberry, bladderwrack, bromelain, cat's claw, celery, coleus, cordyceps, dong quai, evening primrose, feverfew, fenugreek, garlic, ginger, ginkgo biloba, red clover, horse chestnut, grapeseed, green tea, ginseng, guggul, horse chestnut seed, horseradish, licorice, prickly ash, red clover, reishi, SAMe, sweet clover, turmeric, white willow (all have additional antiplatelet activity).

Mechanism of Action Nabumetone is a nonacidic NSAID that is rapidly metabolized after absorption to a major active metabolite, 6-methoxy-2-naphthylacetic acid. As found with previous NSAIDs, nabumetone's active metabolite inhibits the cyclooxygenase enzyme which is indirectly responsible for the production of inflammation and pain during arthritis by way of enhancing the production of endoperoxides and prostaglandins E_2 and I_2 (prostacyclin). The active metabolite of nabumetone is felt to be the compound primarily responsible for therapeutic effect. Comparatively, the parent drug is a poor inhibitor of prostaglandin synthesis.

Pharmacokinetics

Absorption: Rapidly and completely

Distribution: Readily distributes into body fluids and tissues

Metabolism: Nabumetone is essentially a prodrug which is activated to its active metabolite (acetic acid metabolites) in the liver; these are subsequently eliminated by liver metabolism

Half-life: 22-30 hours for active metabolite

Time to peak: 2-4 hours

Dosage

Geriatrics: Refer to adult dosing; do not exceed 2000 mg/day.

Adults: Osteoarthritis, rheumatoid arthritis: Oral: 1000 mg/day; an additional 500-1000 mg may be needed in some patients to obtain more symptomatic relief; may be administered once or twice daily; maximum dose: 2000 mg/day

Note: Patients <50 kg are less likely to require doses >1000 mg/day

Renal Impairment: In general, NSAIDs are not recommended for use in patients with advanced renal disease, but the manufacturer of nabumetone does provide some guidelines for adjustment in renal dysfunction:

Moderate impairment (Cl_{cr} 30-49 mL/minute): Initial dose: 750 mg/day; maximum dose: 1500 mg/day

Severe impairment (Cl_{cr} <30 mL/minute): Initial dose: 500 mg/day; maximum dose: 1000 mg/day

Monitoring Parameters Monitor response (pain, range of motion, grip strength, mobility, ADL function), inflammation; observe for weight gain, edema; monitor renal function; observe for bleeding, bruising; evaluate gastrointestinal effects (abdominal pain, bleeding, dyspepsia); mental confusion, disorientation, CBC, serum, creatinine, BUN, liver function tests; perform baseline renal testing in patients with renal dysfunction and repeat in 1-2 weeks to determine if deterioration has occurred

Patient Information Serious gastrointestinal bleeding can occur as well as ulceration and perforation. Pain may or may not be present. Avoid aspirin and aspirin-containing products while taking this medication. If gastric upset occurs, take with food, milk, or antacid. If gastric adverse effects persist, contact physician. May cause drowsiness, dizziness, blurred vision, and confusion. Use caution when performing tasks which require alertness (eg, driving). Do not take for more than 3 days for fever or 10 days for pain without physician advice.

Additional Information There are no clinical guidelines to predict which NSAID will give response in a particular patient. Trials with each must be initiated until response determined. Consider dose, patient convenience, and cost.

Special Geriatric Considerations In trials with nabumetone, no significant differences were noted between young and the elderly in regards to efficacy and safety. However, the elderly are a high-risk population for adverse effects from NSAIDs. As much as 60% of elderly can develop peptic ulceration and/or hemorrhage asymptomatically. The concomitant use of H_2 blockers and sucralfate is not effective as prophylaxis with the exception of NSAID-induced duodenal ulcers which may be prevented by the use of ranitidine. Misoprostol and proton pump inhibitors are the only agents proven to help prevent the development of NSAID-induced ulcers. Also, concomitant disease and drug use contribute to the risk for GI adverse effects. Use lowest effective dose for shortest period possible. Consider renal function decline with age. Use of NSAIDs can compromise existing renal function especially when Cl_{cr} is ≤ 30 mL/minute. Tinnitus may be a difficult and unreliable indication of toxicity due to age-related hearing loss or eighth cranial nerve damage. CNS adverse effects such as confusion, agitation, and hallucination are generally seen in overdose or high dose situations, but the elderly may demonstrate these adverse effects at lower doses than younger adults.

Dosage Forms Excipient information presented when available (limited, particularly for generics); consult specific product labeling. [DSC] = Discontinued product

Tablet: 500 mg, 750 mg

Relafen®: 500 mg, 750 mg [DSC]

Selected References

Brooks PM and Day RO, "Nonsteroidal Anti-inflammatory Drugs - Differences and Similarities," *N Engl J Med*, 1991, 324(24):1716-25.

Clinch D, Banerjee AK, and Ostick G, "Absence of Abdominal Pain in Elderly Patients With Peptic Ulcer," *Age Ageing*, 1984, 13(2):120-3.

Clive DM and Stoff JS, "Renal Syndromes Associated With Nonsteroidal Anti-inflammatory Drugs," *N Engl J Med*, 1984, 310(9):563-72.

Graham DY, "Prevention of Gastroduodenal Injury Induced by Chronic Nonsteroidal Anti-inflammatory Drug Therapy," *Gastroenterology*, 1989, 96(2 Pt 2 Suppl):675-81.

Gurwitz JH, Avorn J, Ross-Degnan D, et al, "Nonsteroidal Anti-Inflammatory Drug-Associated Azotemia in the Very Old," *JAMA*, 1990, 264(4):471-5.

Hawkey CJ, Karrasch JA, Szczepański L, et al, "Omeprazole Compared With Misoprostol for Ulcers Associated With Nonsteroidal Anti-inflammatory Drugs," *N Engl J Med*, 1998, 338(11):727-34.

Knodel LC, "Preventing NSAID-induced Ulcers: The Role of Misoprostol," *Consult Pharm*, 1989, 4:37-41.

Pounder R, "Silent Peptic Ulceration: Deadly Silence or Golden Silence?" *Gastroenterology*, 1989, 96:(2 Pt 2 Suppl)626-31.

Yeomans ND, Tulassay Z, Juhasz L, et al, "A Comparison of Omeprazole With Ranitidine for Ulcers Associated With Nonsteroidal Anti-inflammatory Drugs," *N Engl J Med*, 1998, 338(11):719-26.

♦ **N-Acetyl-P-Aminophenol** see Acetaminophen on page 29

♦ **NaCl** see Sodium Chloride on page 1475

Nadolol (NAY doe lol)

Related Information

Beta-Blockers on page 1751

Medication Safety Issues

Sound-alike/look-alike issues:

Nadolol may be confused with Mandol®

Corgard® may be confused with Cognex®

U.S. Brand Names Corgard®

Canadian Brand Names Alti-Nadolol; Apo-Nadol®; Corgard®; Novo-Nadolol

Generic Available Yes

Pharmacologic Category Beta-Adrenergic Blocker, Nonselective

Use Treatment of hypertension and angina pectoris

Contraindications Hypersensitivity to nadolol or any component of the formulation; bronchial asthma; sinus bradycardia; sinus node dysfunction; heart block greater than first degree (except in patients with a functioning artificial pacemaker); cardiogenic shock; uncompensated cardiac failure

Warnings/Precautions Consider pre-existing conditions such as sick sinus syndrome before initiating. Administer only with extreme caution in patients with compensated heart failure, monitor for a worsening of the condition. Efficacy in heart failure has not been established for nadolol. **[U.S. Boxed Warning]: Beta-blocker therapy should not be withdrawn abruptly (particularly in patients with CAD), but gradually tapered to avoid acute tachycardia, hypertension, and/or ischemia.** Use caution with concurrent use of beta-blockers and either verapamil or diltiazem; bradycardia or heart block can occur. In general, patients with bronchospastic disease should not receive beta-blockers. Nadolol, if used at all, should be used cautiously in bronchospastic disease with close monitoring. Use cautiously in diabetics because it can mask prominent hypoglycemic symptoms. Use cautiously in the renally impaired (dosage adjustments are required). Use with caution in patients with myasthenia gravis, peripheral vascular disease, or psychiatric disease (may cause CNS depression). Use care with anesthetic agents which decrease myocardial function. Adequate alpha-blockade is required prior to use of any beta-blocker for patients with untreated pheochromocytoma.

Adverse Reactions (Reflective of adult population; not specific for elderly)

>10%:

Central nervous system: Drowsiness, insomnia

(Continued)

Nadolol *(Continued)*

Endocrine & metabolic: Decreased sexual ability

1% to 10%:

Cardiovascular: Bradycardia, palpitation, edema, CHF, reduced peripheral circulation

Central nervous system: Mental depression

Gastrointestinal: Diarrhea or constipation, nausea, vomiting, stomach discomfort

Respiratory: Bronchospasm

Miscellaneous: Cold extremities

Overdosage/Toxicology Symptoms of intoxication include cardiac disturbances, CNS toxicity, bronchospasm, hypoglycemia, and hyperkalemia. The most common cardiac symptoms include hypotension and bradycardia. Atrioventricular block, intraventricular conduction disturbances, cardiogenic shock, and asystole may occur with severe overdose, especially with membrane-depressant drugs (eg, propranolol). CNS effects include convulsions, coma, and respiratory arrest (commonly seen with propranolol and other membrane-depressant and lipid-soluble drugs). Treatment is symptomatic for seizures, hypotension, hyperkalemia, and hypoglycemia. Bradycardia and hypotension resistant to atropine, isoproterenol, or pacing may respond to glucagon. Wide QRS defects caused by membrane-depressant poisoning may respond to hypertonic sodium bicarbonate. Repeat-dose charcoal, hemoperfusion, or hemodialysis may be helpful in removal of only those beta-blockers with a small V_d, long half-life, or low intrinsic clearance (acebutolol, atenolol, nadolol, sotalol).

Drug Interactions

Albuterol (and other beta$_2$ agonists): Effects may be blunted by nonspecific beta-blockers.

Alpha-blockers (prazosin, terazosin): Concurrent use of beta-blockers may increase risk of orthostasis.

Clonidine: Hypertensive crisis after or during withdrawal of either agent.

Drugs which slow AV conduction (digoxin): Effects may be additive with beta-blockers.

Epinephrine (including local anesthetics with epinephrine): Propranolol may cause hypertension.

Glucagon: Nadolol may blunt the hyperglycemic action of glucagon.

Insulin and oral hypoglycemics: Nadolol may mask symptoms of hypoglycemia.

Nadolol increases antipyrine's half-life.

NSAIDs (ibuprofen, indomethacin, naproxen, piroxicam) may reduce the antihypertensive effects of beta-blockers.

Salicylates may reduce the antihypertensive effects of beta-blockers.

Sulfonylureas: Beta-blockers may alter response to hypoglycemic agents.

Verapamil or diltiazem may have synergistic or additive pharmacological effects when taken concurrently with beta-blockers.

Ethanol/Nutrition/Herb Interactions Herb/Nutraceutical: Avoid dong quai if using for hypertension (has estrogenic activity). Avoid ephedra, garlic, yohimbe, ginseng (may worsen hypertension). Avoid natural licorice (causes sodium and water retention and increases potassium loss).

Mechanism of Action Competitively blocks response to beta$_1$- and beta$_2$-adrenergic stimulation; does not exhibit any membrane stabilizing or intrinsic sympathomimetic activity

Pharmacodynamics Duration of effect: 24 hours

Pharmacokinetics

Absorption: Oral: 30% to 50%

Protein binding: 28%

Half-life: Adults: 20-24 hours; increased half-life with decreased renal function

Time to peak serum concentration: Oral: Within 2-4 hours and persist for 17-24 hours

Elimination: Renally eliminated unchanged. Since geriatric patients will have reduced renal function, correct for Cl_{cr}

Dosage

Geriatrics: Oral: Initial: 20 mg/day; increase doses by 20 mg increments at 3- to 7-day intervals; usual dosage range: 20-240 mg/day. Adjust for renal impairment.

Adults:

Hypertension, angina: Oral: Initial: 40-80 mg/day, increase dosage gradually by 40-80 mg increments at 3- to 7-day intervals until optimum clinical response is obtained with profound slowing of heart rate. Doses up to 160-240 mg/day in angina and 240-320 mg/day in hypertension may be necessary. Doses as high as 640 mg/day have been used.

Usual dosage range (JNC 7): 40-120 mg once daily

Renal Impairment:

Cl_{cr} 31-40 mL/minute: Administer every 24-36 hours or administer 50% of normal dose.

Cl_{cr} 10-30 mL/minute: Administer every 24-48 hours or administer 50% of normal dose.

Cl_{cr} <10 mL/minute: Administer every 40-60 hours or administer 25% of normal dose.

Hemodialysis effects: Moderately dialyzable (20% to 50%) via hemodialysis. Administer dose postdialysis or administer 40 mg supplemental dose. Supplemental dose is not necessary following peritoneal dialysis.

Hepatic Impairment: Reduced dose is probably necessary.

Monitoring Parameters Blood pressure, orthostatic hypotension, heart rate, CNS effects

Patient Information Do not discontinue medication abruptly, sudden stopping of medication may precipitate or cause angina; consult pharmacist or physician before taking with other adrenergic drugs (eg, cold medications); notify physician if any of the following symptoms occur: difficult breathing, night cough, swelling of extremities, slow pulse, dizziness, lightheadedness, confusion, depression, skin rash, fever, sore throat, unusual bleeding or bruising; may produce drowsiness, blurred vision; use with caution while driving or performing tasks requiring alertness; may mask signs of hypoglycemia in diabetics; may be taken without regard to meals

Special Geriatric Considerations Due to alterations in the beta-adrenergic autonomic nervous system, beta-adrenergic blockade may result in less hemodynamic response than seen in younger adults. Studies indicate that despite decreased sensitivity to the chronotropic effects of beta-blockade with age, there appears to be an increased myocardial sensitivity to the negative inotropic effect during stress (ie, exercise). Controlled trials have shown the overall response rate for propranolol to be only 20% to 50% in elderly populations. Therefore, all beta-adrenergic blocking drugs may result in a decreased response as compared to younger adults. Must adjust dose for renal function.

Dosage Forms Excipient information presented when available (limited, particularly for generics); consult specific product labeling. [DSC] = Discontinued product
Tablet: 20 mg, 40 mg, 80 mg, 120 mg, 160 mg
Corgard®: 20 mg, 40 mg, 80 mg, 120 mg [DSC], 160 mg [DSC]

Selected References

Aagaard GN, "Treatment of Hypertension in the Elderly," *Drug Treatment in the Elderly*, Vestal RE, ed, Boston, MA: ADIS Health Science Press, 1984, 77.

Chobanian AV, Bakris GL, Black HR, et al, "The Seventh Report of the Joint National Committee on Prevention, Detection, Evaluation, and Treatment of High Blood Pressure: The JNC 7 Report," *JAMA*, 2003, 289(19):2560-71.

Fleisher LA, Beckman JA, Brown KA, et al, "ACC/AHA 2006 Guideline Update on Perioperative Cardiovascular Evaluation for Noncardiac Surgery: Focused Update on Perioperative Beta-Blocker Therapy. A Report of the American College of Cardiology/American Heart Association Task Force on Practice Guidelines (Writing Committee to Update the 2002 Guidelines on Perioperative Cardiovascular Evaluation for Noncardiac Surgery) Developed in Collaboration With the American Society of Echocardiography, American Society of Nuclear Cardiology, Heart Rhythm Society, Society of Cardiovascular Anesthesiologists, Society for Cardiovascular Angiography and Interventions, and Society for Vascular Medicine and Biology," *J Am Coll Cardiol*, 2006, 47(11):2343-55.

Juul AB, Wetterslev J, Gluud C, et al, "Effect of Perioperative Beta Blockade in Patients With Diabetes Undergoing Major Non-Cardiac Surgery: Randomized Placebo Controlled, Blinded Multicentre Trial. DIPOM Trial Group," *BMJ*, 2006, 332(7556):1482.

Nafcillin (naf SIL in)

Related Information
Antibiotic Treatment of Adults With Infective Endocarditis *on page 1797*
Antimicrobial Activity Against Selected Organisms *on page 1728*

Canadian Brand Names Nallpen®; Unipen®

Index Terms Ethoxynaphthamido Penicillin Sodium; Nafcillin Sodium; Nallpen; Sodium Nafcillin

Generic Available Yes

Pharmacologic Category Antibiotic, Penicillin

Use Treatment of susceptible bacterial infections such as osteomyelitis, cellulitis, septicemia, endocarditis, and CNS infections due to penicillinase-producing strains of *Staphylococcus*

Contraindications Hypersensitivity to nafcillin, or any component of the formulation, or penicillins

Warnings/Precautions Serious and occasionally severe or fatal hypersensitivity (anaphylactoid) reactions have been reported in patients on penicillin therapy, especially with a history of beta-lactam hypersensitivity, history of sensitivity to multiple allergens, or previous IgE-mediated reactions (eg, anaphylaxis, angioedema, urticaria). Use with caution in asthmatic patients. Extravasation of I.V. infusions should be avoided; modification of dosage is necessary in patients with both severe renal and hepatic impairment. Prolonged use may result in fungal or bacterial superinfection, including *C. difficile*-associated diarrhea and pseudomembranous colitis.

Adverse Reactions (Reflective of adult population; not specific for elderly)
Frequency not defined.
Central nervous system: Pain, fever
Dermatologic: Rash
Gastrointestinal: Nausea, diarrhea, pseudomembranous colitis
Hematologic: Agranulocytosis, bone marrow depression, neutropenia
(Continued)

Nafcillin *(Continued)*

Local: Pain, swelling, inflammation, phlebitis, skin sloughing, and thrombophlebitis at the injection site; oxacillin (less likely to cause phlebitis) is often preferred in pediatric patients

Renal: Interstitial nephritis (acute)

Miscellaneous: Hypersensitivity reactions

Overdosage/Toxicology Symptoms of penicillin overdose include neuromuscular hypersensitivity (agitation, hallucinations, asterixis, encephalopathy, confusion, and seizures) and electrolyte imbalance (with potassium or sodium salts), especially in renal failure. Treatment is supportive or symptom-directed.

Drug Interactions Induces CYP3A4 (strong)

Calcium channel blockers: Nafcillin may increase the metabolism, via CYP isoenzymes, of calcium channel blockers.

Cyclosporine: Levels may be decreased by nafcillin

CYP3A4 substrates: Nafcillin may decrease the levels/effects of CYP3A4 substrates. Example substrates include benzodiazepines, calcium channel blockers, clarithromycin, cyclosporine, erythromycin, estrogens, mirtazapine, nateglinide, nefazodone, nevirapine, protease inhibitors, tacrolimus, and venlafaxine

Fusidic acid: May diminish the therapeutic effect of penicillins. Administer the penicillin at least 2 hours before fusidic acid.

Methotrexate: Penicillins may increase the exposure to methotrexate during concurrent therapy; monitor.

Oral contraceptives: Anecdotal reports suggesting decreased contraceptive efficacy with penicillins have been refuted by more rigorous scientific and clinical data.

Probenecid: May increase levels of penicillins (nafcillin)

Tetracycline derivatives: May diminish the therapeutic effect of penicillins.

Typhoid vaccine: Antibiotics may diminish the therapeutic effect of typhoid vaccine; only the live attenuated Ty21a strain is affected.

Warfarin: Nafcillin may diminish the anticoagulant effect of coumarin derivatives.

Stability Reconstituted parenteral solution is stable for 3 days at room temperature and 7 days when refrigerated or 12 weeks when frozen. For I.V. infusion in NS or D_5W, solution is stable for 24 hours at room temperature and 96 hours when refrigerated.

Mechanism of Action Interferes with bacterial cell wall synthesis during active multiplication, causing cell wall death and resultant bactericidal activity against susceptible bacteria

Pharmacokinetics

Absorption: Oral: Poor and erratic

Protein binding: 90%

Half-life: Adults with normal renal and hepatic function: 0.5-1.5 hours

Time to peak serum concentration:

Oral: Within 2 hours

I.M.: 30-60 minutes

Elimination: Primarily in bile, and 10% to 30% in urine as unchanged drug; undergoes enterohepatic recycling

Dosage

Geriatrics & Adults:

Susceptible infections:

I.M.: 500 mg every 4-6 hours

I.V.: 500-2000 mg every 4-6 hours

Endocarditis: MSSA:

Native valve: I.V.: 12 g/24 hours in 4-6 divided doses for 6 weeks

Prosthetic valve: I.V.: 12 g/24 hours in 4-6 divided doses for ≥6 weeks (use with rifampin and gentamicin)

Joint:

Bursitis, septic: I.V.: 2 g every 4 hours

Prosthetic: I.V.: 2 g every 4-6 hours with rifampin for 6 weeks

***Staphylococcus aureus*, methicillin-susceptible infections, including brain abscess, empyema, erysipelas, mastitis, myositis, osteomyelitis, pneumonia, toxic shock, urinary tract (perinephric abscess):** I.V.: 2 g every 4 hours

Renal Impairment: No adjustment is necessary.

Hemodialysis effects: Not dialyzable (0% to 5%) via hemodialysis. Supplemental dose is not necessary with hemo- or peritoneal dialysis or continuous arteriovenous or venovenous hemofiltration.

Hepatic Impairment: In patients with both hepatic and renal impairment, modification of dosage may be necessary; no data available.

Administration Administer around-the-clock rather than 4 times/day, 3 times/day, etc (ie, 12-6-12-6, not 9-1-5-9) to promote less variation in peak and trough serum concentrations; burning on I.V. administration may be decreased by further diluting the preparation to 250 mL NS or D_5W

Monitoring Parameters Watch for signs or symptoms of fluid overload or retention in patients with congestive heart failure; pain/burning with administration

Test Interactions Positive Coombs' test (direct), false-positive urinary and serum proteins; may inactivate aminoglycosides *in vitro*

Patient Information Report any diarrhea that develops within 2 weeks of completion of therapy to your physician or pharmacist; complete full course of therapy

Additional Information Sodium content of 1 g: 66.7 mg (2.9 mEq)

Special Geriatric Considerations Nafcillin has not been studied exclusively in the elderly, however, given its route of elimination, dosage adjustments based upon age and renal function is not necessary

Dosage Forms Excipient information presented when available (limited, particularly for generics); consult specific product labeling.
Infusion [premixed iso-osmotic dextrose solution]: 1 g (50 mL); 2 g (100 mL)
Injection, powder for reconstitution, as sodium: 1 g, 2 g, 10 g

♦ **Nafcillin Sodium** *see* Nafcillin *on page 1081*

Naftifine (NAF ti feen)

U.S. Brand Names Naftin®
Index Terms Naftifine Hydrochloride
Generic Available No
Pharmacologic Category Antifungal Agent, Topical
Use Topical treatment of tinea cruris (jock itch), tinea corporis (ring worm), and tinea pedis (athlete's foot)
Contraindications Hypersensitivity to any component
Warnings/Precautions For external use only
Adverse Reactions (Reflective of adult population; not specific for elderly)
>10%: Local: Burning, stinging
1% to 10%:
Dermatologic: Erythema, itching
Local: Dryness, irritation
Drug Interactions No data reported
Mechanism of Action Synthetic, broad-spectrum antifungal agent in the allylamine class; appears to have both fungistatic and fungicidal activity. Exhibits antifungal activity by selectively inhibiting the enzyme squalene epoxidase in a dose-dependent manner which results in the primary sterol, ergosterol, within the fungal membrane not being synthesized.
Pharmacokinetics
Absorption: Systemic, 6% for cream, ≤4% for gel
Half-life: 2-3 days
Elimination: Metabolites excreted in urine and feces
Dosage
Geriatrics & Adults: Tinea infection: Topical: Apply cream once daily and gel twice daily (morning and evening) for up to 4 weeks
Patient Information External use only; avoid eyes, mouth, and other mucous membranes; do not use occlusive dressings unless directed to do so; discontinue if irritation or sensitivity develops; wash hands after application
Special Geriatric Considerations No specific recommendations for use in the elderly.
Dosage Forms Excipient information presented when available (limited, particularly for generics); consult specific product labeling.
Cream, as hydrochloride:
Naftin®: 1% (15 g, 30 g, 60 g, 90 g) [contains benzyl alcohol]
Gel, as hydrochloride:
Naftin®: 1% (20 g, 40 g, 60 g) [contains alcohol 52%]

♦ **Naftifine Hydrochloride** *see* Naftifine *on page 1083*
♦ **Naftin®** *see* Naftifine *on page 1083*
♦ **NaHCO₃** *see* Sodium Bicarbonate *on page 1474*

Nalbuphine (NAL byoo feen)

Related Information
Narcotic / Opioid Analgesics *on page 1763*
Medication Safety Issues
Sound-alike/look-alike issues:
Nubain® may be confused with Navane®, Nebcin®
U.S. Brand Names Nubain®
Index Terms Nalbuphine Hydrochloride
Generic Available Yes
Pharmacologic Category Analgesic, Opioid
Use Relief of moderate to severe pain
(Continued)

Nalbuphine *(Continued)*

Unlabeled/Investigational Use Opioid-induced pruritus

Contraindications Hypersensitivity to nalbuphine or any component, including sulfites

Warnings/Precautions Use caution in CNS depression. Sedation and psychomotor impairment are likely, and are additive with other CNS depressants or ethanol. May cause respiratory depression. Ambulatory patients must be cautioned about performing tasks which require mental alertness (eg, operating machinery or driving). Effects may be potentiated when used with other sedative drugs or ethanol. Use with caution in patients with recent myocardial infarction, biliary tract impairment, morbid obesity, thyroid dysfunction, head trauma, or increased intracranial pressure. Use caution in patients with prostatic hyperplasia and/or urinary stricture, adrenal insufficiency, decreased hepatic or renal function. Use with caution in patients with pre-existing respiratory compromise (hypoxia and/or hypercapnia), COPD or other obstructive pulmonary disease; critical respiratory depression may occur, even at therapeutic dosages. May cause hypotension; use with caution in patients with hypovolemia, cardiovascular disease (including acute MI), or drugs which may exaggerate hypotensive effects (including phenothiazines or general anesthetics). May obscure diagnosis or clinical course of patients with acute abdominal conditions. May result in tolerance and/or drug dependence with chronic use; use with caution in patients with a history of drug dependence. Abrupt discontinuation following prolonged use may lead to withdrawal symptoms. May precipitate withdrawal symptoms in patients following prolonged therapy with mu opioid agonists. Use with caution in the elderly and debilitated patients; may be more sensitive to adverse effects.

Adverse Reactions (Reflective of adult population; not specific for elderly)

>10%: Central nervous system: Sedation (36%)

1% to 10%:

Central nervous system: Dizziness (5%), headache (3%)

Gastrointestinal: Nausea/vomiting (6%), xerostomia (4%)

Miscellaneous: Clamminess (9%)

Overdosage/Toxicology Symptoms include CNS depression, respiratory depression, miosis, hypotension, and bradycardia. Treatment of overdose includes airway support, establishment of an I.V. line, and administration of naloxone 2 mg I.V., with repeat administration as necessary, up to a total of 10 mg.

Drug Interactions Increased toxicity: Barbiturate anesthetics may increase CNS depression

Ethanol/Nutrition/Herb Interactions

Ethanol: Avoid ethanol (may increase CNS depression).

Herb/Nutraceutical: Avoid valerian, St John's wort, kava kava, gotu kola (may increase CNS depression).

Stability Store at room temperature of 15°C to 30°C (59°F to 86°F). Protect from light.

Mechanism of Action Agonist of kappa opiate receptors and partial antagonist of mu opiate receptors in the CNS, causing inhibition of ascending pain pathways, altering the perception of and response to pain; produces generalized CNS depression

Pharmacodynamics Onset of action: Peak effect: SubQ, I.M.: <15 minutes; I.V.: 2-3 minutes

Pharmacokinetics

Metabolism: In the liver

Half-life elimination: 5 hours

Elimination: Metabolites excreted primarily in feces (via bile) and in urine (~7%)

Dosage

Geriatrics: Refer to adult dosing; use with caution.

Adults:

Pain management: I.M., I.V., SubQ: 10 mg/70 kg every 3-6 hours; maximum single dose in nonopioid-tolerant patients: 20 mg; maximum daily dose: 160 mg

Surgical anesthesia supplement: I.V.: Induction: 0.3-3 mg/kg over 10-15 minutes; maintenance doses of 0.25-0.5 mg/kg may be given as required

Opioid-induced pruritus (unlabeled use): I.V. 2.5-5 mg; may repeat dose

Renal Impairment: Use with caution and reduce dose. Monitor.

Hepatic Impairment: Use with caution and reduce dose.

Monitoring Parameters Relief of pain, respiratory and mental status, blood pressure

Patient Information May cause drowsiness; avoid CNS depressants and alcohol

Special Geriatric Considerations The elderly may be particularly susceptible to CNS effects; monitor closely.

Dosage Forms Excipient information presented when available (limited, particularly for generics); consult specific product labeling. [DSC] = Discontinued product

Injection, solution, as hydrochloride: 10 mg/mL (10 mL); 20 mg/mL (10 mL)

Nubain®: 10 mg/mL (10 mL) [DSC]; 20 mg/mL (10 mL)

Injection, solution, as hydrochloride [preservative free]: 10 mg/mL (1 mL); 20 mg/mL (1 mL)

Nubain®: 10 mg/mL (1 mL); 20 mg/mL (1 mL)

Selected References
AGS Panel on Persistent Pain in Older Persons, "The Management of Persistent Pain in Older Persons," *J Am Geriatr Soc*, 2002, 50(6 Suppl):S205-24.
Cohen SE, Ratner EF, Kreitzman TR, et al, "Nalbuphine is Better Than Naloxone for Treatment of Side Effects After Epidural Morphine," *Anesth Analg*, 1992, 75(5):747-52.

♦ **Nalbuphine Hydrochloride** *see* Nalbuphine *on page 1083*
♦ **Nalfon®** *see* Fenoprofen *on page 606*
♦ **Nallpen** *see* Nafcillin *on page 1081*
♦ **N-allylnoroxymorphine Hydrochloride** *see* Naloxone *on page 1085*

Naloxone (nal OKS one)

Medication Safety Issues
Sound-alike/look-alike issues:
Naloxone may be confused with naltrexone
Narcan® may be confused with Marcaine®, Norcuron®

International issues:
Narcan® may be confused with Marcen® which is a brand name for ketazolam in Spain

Canadian Brand Names Naloxone Hydrochloride Injection®
Index Terms *N*-allylnoroxymorphine Hydrochloride; Naloxone Hydrochloride; Narcan
Generic Available Yes
Pharmacologic Category Antidote
Use Complete or partial reversal of opioid depression including respiratory depression induced by natural and synthetic opioids (eg, propoxyphene, methadone, and certain mixed agonist-antagonist analgesics: nalbuphine, pentazocine, and butorphanol); diagnosis of suspected opioid tolerance or acute opioid overdose; adjunctive agent to increase blood pressure in the management of septic shock
Unlabeled/Investigational Use PCP and ethanol ingestion; opioid-induced pruritus
Contraindications Hypersensitivity to naloxone or any component of the formulation
Warnings/Precautions Use with caution in patients with cardiovascular disease; excessive dosages should be avoided after use of opiates in surgery, because naloxone may cause an increase in blood pressure and reversal of anesthesia; may precipitate withdrawal symptoms in patients addicted to opiates, including pain, hypertension, sweating, agitation, irritability, shrill cry, failure to feed

Adverse Reactions (Reflective of adult population; not specific for elderly)
Frequency not defined.
Cardiovascular: Hyper-/hypotension, tachycardia, ventricular arrhythmia, cardiac arrest
Central nervous system: Irritability, anxiety, narcotic withdrawal, restlessness, seizure
Gastrointestinal: Nausea, vomiting, diarrhea
Neuromuscular & skeletal: Tremulousness
Respiratory: Dyspnea, pulmonary edema, runny nose, sneezing
Miscellaneous: Diaphoresis

Overdosage/Toxicology Naloxone is the drug of choice for respiratory depression that is known or suspected to be caused by an opiate or opioid overdose.

Caution: Naloxone's effects are due to its action on narcotic reversal, not due to direct effect upon opiate receptors. Therefore, adverse events occur secondarily to reversal (withdrawal) of narcotic analgesia and sedation, which can cause severe reactions.

Drug Interactions Opioid analgesics: Decreased effect of opioid analgesics; may precipitate acute withdrawal reaction in physically dependent patients
Stability Store at 25°C (77°F). Protect from light. Stable in 0.9% sodium chloride and D_5W at 4 mcg/mL for 24 hours.
Mechanism of Action Pure opioid antagonist that competes and displaces narcotics at opioid receptor sites

Pharmacodynamics
Onset of action:
I.V.: Within 2 minutes
SubQ, I.M., E.T.: Within 2-5 minutes
Duration of effect: 20-60 minutes; shorter than that of most opioids, therefore, repeated doses are usually needed

Pharmacokinetics
Metabolism: Primarily by glucuronidation in the liver
Half-life: 1-1.5 hours
Elimination: In urine as metabolites

Dosage
Geriatrics & Adults:
Narcotic overdose:
I.V. (preferred), I.M., intratracheal, SubQ: 0.4-2 mg every 2-3 minutes as needed; may need to repeat doses every 20-60 minutes. If no response is observed after 10 mg, question the diagnosis. **Note:** Use 0.1-0.2 mg increments in patients who
(Continued)

Naloxone *(Continued)*

are opioid dependent and in postoperative patients to avoid large cardiovascular changes.

Continuous infusion: I.V.: If continuous infusion is required, calculate dosage/hour based on effective intermittent dose used and duration of adequate response seen; adult dose typically 0.25-6.25 mg/hour (short-term infusions as high as 2.4 mg/kg/hour have been tolerated in adults during treatment for septic shock); alternatively, continuous infusion utilizes $2/3$ of the initial naloxone bolus on an hourly basis; add 10 times this dose to each liter of D_5W and infuse at a rate of 100 mL/hour; $1/2$ of the initial bolus dose should be readministered 15 minutes after initiation of the continuous infusion to prevent a drop in naloxone levels; increase infusion rate as needed to assure adequate ventilation

Opioid-induced pruritus (unlabeled use): I.V. infusion: 0.25 mcg/kg/hour; **Note:** Monitor pain control; verify that the naloxone is not reversing analgesia.

Monitoring Parameters Blood pressure, pulse, mental status

Additional Information Too rapid a reversal of narcotic depression may result in nausea, vomiting, sweating, tachycardia, increased blood pressure, and tremulousness

Special Geriatric Considerations In small trials, naloxone has shown temporary improvement in Alzheimer's disease; however, is not recommended for treatment.

Dosage Forms Excipient information presented when available (limited, particularly for generics); consult specific product labeling.

Injection, solution, as hydrochloride: 0.4 mg/mL (1 mL, 10 mL); 1 mg/mL (2 mL)

Selected References

Kendrick WD, Woods AM, Daly MY, et al, "Naloxone Versus Nalbuphine Infusion for Prophylaxis of Epidural Morphine-Induced Pruritus," *Anesth Analg*, 1996, 82(3):641-7.

Kjellberg F and Tramer MR, "Pharmacological Control of Opioid-Induced Pruritus: A Quantitative Systematic Review of Randomized Trials," *Eur J Anaesthesiol*, 2001, 18(6):346-57.

Waters C, "Cognitive Enhancing Agents: Current Status in the Treatment of Alzheimer's Disease," *Can J Neurol Sci*, 1988, 15(3):249-56.

♦ **Naloxone Hydrochloride** *see* Naloxone *on page 1085*

♦ **Naloxone Hydrochloride and Pentazocine Hydrochloride** *see* Pentazocine *on page 1229*

♦ **Namenda**™ *see* Memantine *on page 977*

Naphazoline *(naf AZ oh leen)*

U.S. Brand Names AK-Con™; Albalon®; Clear eyes® for Dry Eyes and ACR Relief [OTC]; Clear eyes® for Dry Eyes and Redness Relief [OTC]; Clear eyes® Redness Relief [OTC]; Clear eyes® Seasonal Relief [OTC]; Naphcon® [OTC]; Privine® [OTC]

Canadian Brand Names Naphcon Forte®; Vasocon®

Index Terms Naphazoline Hydrochloride

Generic Available No

Pharmacologic Category Alpha$_1$ Agonist; Imidazoline Derivative; Ophthalmic Agent, Vasoconstrictor

Use Topical ocular vasoconstrictor; temporarily relief of congestion, itching, and minor irritation; control pf hyperemia in patients with superficial corneal vascularity

Contraindications Hypersensitivity to naphazoline or any component of the formulation; narrow-angle glaucoma, prior to peripheral iridectomy (in patients susceptible to angle block)

Warnings/Precautions Rebound congestion may occur with extended use. Use with caution in the presence of hypertension, diabetes, hyperthyroidism, heart disease, coronary artery disease, cerebral arteriosclerosis, local infection or injury, benign prostatic hyperplasia, or long-standing bronchial asthma. Products may contain benzalkonium chloride which may be absorbed by soft contact lenses.

When used for self-medication (OTC): Patients should notify healthcare provider if symptoms last >72 hours or if condition worsens. In addition with ophthalmic products, contact prescriber in case of eye pain or if changes in vision occur.

Adverse Reactions (Reflective of adult population; not specific for elderly)

Frequency not defined.

Cardiovascular: Cardiac irregularities, hypertension

Central nervous system: Body temperature decreased, dizziness, drowsiness, headache, nervousness

Endocrine & metabolic: Hyperglycemia

Gastrointestinal: Nausea

Local: Transient stinging, nasal mucosa irritation, dryness, rebound congestion

Neuromuscular & skeletal: Weakness

Ocular: Blurred vision, discomfort, intraocular pressure increased, irritation, lacrimation, mydriasis, punctuate keratitis, redness

Respiratory: Sneezing

Miscellaneous: Diaphoresis

Overdosage/Toxicology Symptoms include CNS depression, hypothermia, brady-cardia, cardiovascular collapse, apnea, and coma. Following initiation of essential overdose management, toxic symptoms should be treated. The patient should be kept warm and monitored for alterations in vital functions. Seizures commonly respond to diazepam (5-10 mg I.V. bolus every 15 minutes, if needed, up to a total of 30 mg) or to phenytoin or phenobarbital. Hypotension should be treated with fluids.

Drug Interactions

Guanadrel: May enhance the therapeutic effect of alpha$_1$-agonists, in particular the mydriatic effects of ophthalmic products.

MAO inhibitors: MAO inhibitors may enhance the hypertensive effect of alpha$_1$-agonists; avoid use.

Methyldopa: May enhance the therapeutic effect of alpha$_1$-agonists, in particular the mydriatic effects of ophthalmic products.

Tricyclic antidepressants: Tricyclic antidepressants may enhance the vasopressor effect of alpha$_1$-agonists; avoid use.

Stability Store at controlled room temperature.

Mechanism of Action Stimulates alpha-adrenergic receptors in the arterioles of the conjunctiva and the nasal mucosa to produce vasoconstriction

Pharmacodynamics

Onset of action: Following topical administration, decongestion occurs within 10 minutes

Duration: 2-6 hours

Pharmacokinetics Elimination is not well defined

Dosage

Geriatrics & Adults:

Nasal congestion (decongestant): Nasal: 0.05%, instill 1-2 drops or sprays every 6 hours if needed; therapy should not exceed 3 days

Decrease in eye redness (vasoconstrictor): Ophthalmic:

0.1% (prescription): 1-2 drops into conjuctival sac every 3-4 hours as needed

0.012% or 0.025% (OTC): 1-2 drops into affected eye(s) up to 4 times a day; therapy should not exceed 3 days

Monitoring Parameters Blood pressure in hypertensives

Patient Information Do not use discolored solutions; discontinue eye drops if visual changes or ocular pain occur; do not use nasal products for >3 days without physician's consent

Special Geriatric Considerations Evaluate patient's ability to self-administer; use cautiously in patients with cardiovascular disease.

Dosage Forms Excipient information presented when available (limited, particularly for generics); consult specific product labeling.

Solution, intranasal, as hydrochloride [drops]:

Privine®: 0.05% (25 mL)

Solution, intranasal, as hydrochloride [spray]:

Privine®: 0.05% (20 mL)

Solution, ophthalmic, as hydrochloride:

AK-Con™, Albalon®: 0.1% (15 mL) [contains benzalkonium chloride]

Clear eyes® for Dry Eyes and ACR Relief: 0.025% (15 mL) [contains hypromellose, and zinc sulfate]

Clear eyes® for Dry Eyes and Redness Relief: 0.012% (15 mL) [contains hypromellose, glycerin and benzalkonium chloride]

Clear eyes® Redness Relief: 0.012% (6 mL, 15 mL, 30 mL) [contains glycerin and benzalkonium chloride]

Clear eyes® Seasonal Relief: 0.012% (15 mL, 30 mL) [contains glycerin, zinc sulfate and benzalkonium chloride]

Naphcon®: 0.012% (15 mL) [contains benzalkonium chloride]

Naphazoline and Pheniramine (naf AZ oh leen & fen NIR a meen)

Related Information

Naphazoline on page 1086

Medication Safety Issues

Sound-alike/look-alike issues:

Visine® may be confused with Visken®

U.S. Brand Names Naphcon-A® [OTC]; Opcon-A® [OTC]; Visine-A® [OTC]

Canadian Brand Names Naphcon-A®; Visine® Advanced Allergy

Index Terms Pheniramine and Naphazoline

Generic Available No

Pharmacologic Category Ophthalmic Agent, Vasoconstrictor

Use Treatment of ocular congestion, irritation, and itching

(Continued)

Naphazoline and Pheniramine *(Continued)*

Contraindications Hypersensitivity to naphazoline, pheniramine, or any component of the formulation

Warnings/Precautions Not for OTC use >72 hours. Notify healthcare provider of eye pain or vision changes. Not recommended for OTC use in patients with cardiovascular disease, hypertension, or narrow-angle glaucoma. Not for use with contact lenses.

Adverse Reactions (Reflective of adult population; not specific for elderly)
Frequency not defined.
Ocular: Pupillary dilation, increase in intraocular pressure
Systemic effects due to absorption:
Cardiovascular: Hypertension, cardiac irregularities
Endocrine & metabolic: Hyperglycemia

Drug Interactions
MAO inhibitors (exaggerated adrenergic effects may result)
Tricyclic antidepressants: Exaggerated response of naphazoline may occur.

Dosage
Geriatrics & Adults: Ophthalmic: 1-2 drops up to 4 times/day

Patient Information Discontinue drug and consult physician if ocular pain or visual changes occur, ocular redness or irritation, or condition worsens or persists more than 72 hours

Special Geriatric Considerations Evaluate patient's ability to self-administer; use cautiously in patients with cardiovascular disease.

Dosage Forms Excipient information presented when available (limited, particularly for generics); consult specific product labeling.
Solution, ophthalmic:
Naphcon-A®: Naphazoline hydrochloride 0.025% and pheniramine maleate 0.3% (5 mL) [contains benzalkonium chloride; 2 bottles/box], (15 mL) [contains benzalkonium chloride]
Opcon-A®: Naphazoline hydrochloride 0.027% and pheniramine maleate 0.3% (15 mL) [contains benzalkonium chloride]
Visine-A®: Naphazoline hydrochloride 0.025% and pheniramine maleate 0.3% (15 mL) [contains benzalkonium chloride]

+ **Naphazoline Hydrochloride** *see* Naphazoline *on page 1086*
+ **Naphcon®** [OTC] *see* Naphazoline *on page 1086*
+ **Naphcon-A®** [OTC] *see* Naphazoline and Pheniramine *on page 1087*
+ **Naprelan®** *see* Naproxen *on page 1088*
+ **Naprosyn®** *see* Naproxen *on page 1088*

Naproxen *(na PROKS en)*

Related Information
Potentially Inappropriate Medications for Geriatrics *on page 1824*
Medication Safety Issues
Sound-alike/look-alike issues:
Naproxen may be confused with Natacyn®, Nebcin®
Aleve® may be confused with Alesse®
Anaprox® may be confused with Anaspaz®, Avapro®
Naprelan® may be confused with Naprosyn®
Naprosyn® may be confused with Naprelan®, Natacyn®, Nebcin®

International issues:
Flogen® [Mexico] may be confused with Flovent® which is a brand name for fluticasone in the U.S.
Flogen® [Mexico] may be confused with Floxin® which is a brand name for ofloxacin in the U.S.

U.S. Brand Names Aleve® [OTC]; Anaprox®; Anaprox® DS; EC-Naprosyn®; Midol® Extended Relief; Naprelan®; Naprosyn®; Pamprin® Maximum Strength All Day Relief [OTC]

Canadian Brand Names Anaprox®; Anaprox® DS; Apo-Napro-Na®; Apo-Napro-Na DS®; Apo-Naproxen®; Apo-Naproxen EC®; Apo-Naproxen SR®; Gen-Naproxen EC; Naprosyn®; Naxen®; Naxen® EC; Novo-Naproc EC; Novo-Naprox; Novo-Naprox Sodium; Novo-Naprox Sodium DS; Novo-Naprox SR; Nu-Naprox; Riva-Naproxen

Index Terms Naproxen Sodium
Generic Available Yes
Pharmacologic Category Nonsteroidal Anti-inflammatory Drug (NSAID), Oral
Use Management of ankylosing spondylitis, osteoarthritis, and rheumatoid disorders; acute gout; mild to moderate pain; tendonitis, bursitis; dysmenorrhea; fever, migraine headache

Restrictions An FDA-approved medication guide must be distributed when dispensing an oral outpatient prescription (new or refill) where this medication is to be used without direct supervision of a healthcare provider. Medication guides are available at http://www.fda.gov/cder/Offices/ODS/medication_guides.htm.

Contraindications Hypersensitivity to naproxen, aspirin, other NSAIDs, or any component of the formulation; perioperative pain in the setting of coronary artery bypass surgery (CABG)

Warnings/Precautions [U.S. Boxed Warning]: NSAIDs are associated with an increased risk of adverse cardiovascular events, including MI, stroke, and new onset or worsening of pre-existing hypertension. Risk may be increased with duration of use or pre-existing cardiovascular risk factors or disease. Carefully evaluate individual cardiovascular risk profiles prior to prescribing. Use caution with fluid retention, CHF or hypertension. Use the lowest effective dose for the shortest duration of time, consistent with individual patient goals, to reduce risk of cardiovascular or GI adverse events. Alternate therapies should be considered for patients at high risk. Concurrent administration of ibuprofen, and potentially other nonselective NSAIDs, may interfere with aspirin's cardioprotective effect.

[U.S. Boxed Warning]: NSAIDs may increase risk of gastrointestinal irritation, ulceration, bleeding, and perforation. These events may occur at any time during therapy and without warning. Use caution with a history of GI disease (bleeding or ulcers), concurrent therapy with aspirin, anticoagulants and/or corticosteroids, smoking, use of alcohol, the elderly or debilitated patients.

Use of NSAIDs can compromise existing renal function. Renal toxicity can occur in patient with impaired renal function, dehydration, heart failure, liver dysfunction, those taking diuretics and ACEI and the elderly. Rehydrate patient before starting therapy. Monitor renal function closely. Naproxen is not recommended for patients with advanced renal disease.

NSAIDs may cause serious skin adverse events including exfoliative dermatitis, Stevens-Johnson Syndrome (SJS) and toxic epidermal necrolysis (TEN). Anaphylactoid reactions may occur, even without prior exposure; patients with "aspirin triad" (bronchial asthma, aspirin intolerance, rhinitis) may be at increased risk. Do not use in patients who experience bronchospasm, asthma, rhinitis, or urticaria with NSAID or aspirin therapy. Use caution in other forms of asthma.

Use with caution in patients with decreased hepatic function. Closely monitor patients with any abnormal LFT. Severe hepatic reactions (eg, fulminant hepatitis, liver failure) have occurred with NSAID use, rarely; discontinue if signs or symptoms of liver disease develop, or if systemic manifestations occur.

The elderly are at increased risk for adverse effects (especially peptic ulceration, CNS effects, renal toxicity) from NSAIDs even at low doses.

Withhold for at least 4-6 half-lives prior to surgical or dental procedures.

OTC labeling: Prior to self-medication, patients should contact healthcare provider if they have had recurring stomach pain or upset, ulcers, bleeding problems, high blood pressure, heart or kidney disease, other serious medical problems, are currently taking a diuretic, or are ≥60 years of age. Recommended dosages should not be exceeded, due to an increased risk of GI bleeding. Consuming ≥3 alcoholic beverages/day or taking longer than recommended may increase the risk of GI bleeding.

Adverse Reactions (Reflective of adult population; not specific for elderly)
1% to 10%:
Cardiovascular: Edema (3% to 9%), palpitations (<3%)
Central nervous system: Dizziness (3% to 9%), drowsiness (3% to 9%), headache (3% to 9%), lightheadedness (<3%), vertigo (<3%)
Dermatologic: Pruritus (3% to 9%), skin eruption (3% to 9%), ecchymosis (3% to 9%), purpura (<3%), rash
Endocrine & metabolic: Fluid retention (3% to 9%)
Gastrointestinal: Abdominal pain (3% to 9%), constipation (3% to 9%), nausea (3% to 9%), heartburn (3% to 9%), diarrhea (<3%), dyspepsia (<3%), stomatitis (<3%), flatulence, gross bleeding/perforation, indigestion, ulcers, vomiting
Genitourinary: Abnormal renal function
Hematologic: Hemolysis (3% to 9%), ecchymosis (3% to 9%), anemia, bleeding time increased
Hepatic: LFTs increased
Ocular: Visual disturbances (<3%)
Otic: Tinnitus (3% to 9%), hearing disturbances (<3%)
Respiratory: Dyspnea (3% to 9%)
Miscellaneous: Diaphoresis (<3%), thirst (<3%)

Overdosage/Toxicology Symptoms include drowsiness, heartburn, vomiting, CNS depression, leukocytosis, and renal failure. Management of nonsteroidal anti-inflammatory drug (NSAID) intoxication is primarily supportive and symptomatic. Fluid therapy is commonly effective in managing hypotension that may occur following an acute NSAID overdose, except when due to acute blood loss. Seizures tend to be very short-lived and often do not require drug treatment, although recurrent seizures
(Continued)

Naproxen *(Continued)*

should be treated with I.V. diazepam. Since many of NSAIDs undergo enterohepatic cycling, multiple doses of charcoal may be needed to reduce the potential for delayed toxicities.

Drug Interactions Substrate (minor) of CYP1A2, 2C9

ACE inhibitors: Antihypertensive effects may be decreased by concurrent therapy with NSAIDs; monitor blood pressure.

Angiotensin II antagonists: Antihypertensive effects may be decreased by concurrent therapy with NSAIDs; monitor blood pressure.

Anticoagulants (warfarin, heparin, LMWHs) in combination with NSAIDs can cause increased risk of bleeding.

Antiplatelet drugs (ticlopidine, clopidogrel, aspirin, abciximab, dipyridamole, eptifibatide, tirofiban) can cause an increased risk of bleeding.

Beta-blockers: NSAIDs may decrease the antihypertensive effect of beta-blockers. Monitor.

Cholestyramine (and other bile acid sequestrants): May decrease the absorption of NSAIDs. Separate by at least 2 hours.

Corticosteroids may increase the risk of GI ulceration; avoid concurrent use.

Cyclosporine: NSAIDs may increase serum creatinine, potassium, blood pressure, and cyclosporine levels; monitor cyclosporine levels and renal function carefully.

Fluoroquinolone antibiotics: Risk of seizures may be increased with concomitant quinolone use. Risk is considered quite low and may only be a factor with high serum levels of either agent and/or in patients with additional predisposing factors (eg, renal dysfunction, history of seizure or other neurological disorder).

Hydralazine's antihypertensive effect is decreased; avoid concurrent use.

Lithium levels can be increased; avoid concurrent use if possible or monitor lithium levels and adjust dose. Sulindac may have the least effect. When NSAID is stopped, lithium will need adjustment again.

Loop diuretics efficacy (diuretic and antihypertensive effect) is reduced. Indomethacin reduces this efficacy, however, it may be anticipated with any NSAID.

Methotrexate: Severe bone marrow suppression, aplastic anemia, and GI toxicity have been reported with concomitant NSAID therapy. Avoid use during moderate or high-dose methotrexate (increased and prolonged methotrexate levels). NSAID use during low-dose treatment of rheumatoid arthritis has not been fully evaluated; extreme caution is warranted.

Salicylates: NSAIDs (nonselective) may diminish the cardioprotective effect of acetylated salicylates. Avoid regular use of NSAIDs if possible; consider alternatives (eg, acetaminophen). Give salicylate before NSAID; for example ibuprofen should be given 30-120 minutes after aspirin (immediate release).

Thiazides antihypertensive effects are decreased; avoid concurrent use.

Warfarin's INRs may be increased by naproxen. Other NSAIDs may have the same effect depending on dose and duration. Monitor INR closely. Use the lowest dose of NSAIDs possible and for the briefest duration.

Ethanol/Nutrition/Herb Interactions

Ethanol: Avoid ethanol (may enhance gastric mucosal irritation).

Food: Naproxen absorption ratelevels may be decreased if taken with food.

Herb/Nutraceutical: Avoid alfalfa, anise, bilberry, bladderwrack, bromelain, cat's claw, celery, coleus, cordyceps, dong quai, evening primrose, feverfew, fenugreek, garlic, ginger, ginkgo biloba, red clover, horse chestnut, grapeseed, green tea, ginseng, guggul, horse chestnut seed, horseradish, licorice, prickly ash, red clover, reishi, SAMe, sweet clover, turmeric, white willow (all have additional antiplatelet activity).

Stability Store oral suspension and tablet at 15°C to 30°C (59°F to 86°F).

Mechanism of Action Inhibits prostaglandin synthesis by decreasing the activity of the enzyme, cyclooxygenase, which results in decreased formation of prostaglandin precursors

Pharmacodynamics

Analgesia:

Onset of action: 1 hour

Duration: Up to 7 hours

Anti-inflammatory:

Onset of action: Within 2 weeks

Peak effect: 2-4 weeks

Pharmacokinetics

Absorption: Oral: Almost 100%

Metabolism: Hepatic

Protein binding: >99%; increased free fraction in elderly

Half-life elimination: Normal renal function: 12-17 hours; End-stage renal disease: No change

Time to peak, serum: 1-4 hours

Dosage

Geriatrics: Refer to adult dosing and Special Geriatric Considerations.

OTC labeling: Pain/fever: Adults >65 years: 200 mg naproxen base every 12 hours

Adults: Note: Dosage expressed as naproxen base; 200 mg naproxen base is equivalent to 220 mg naproxen sodium.

Gout, acute: Oral: Initial: 750 mg, followed by 250 mg every 8 hours until attack subsides. **Note:** EC-Naprosyn® is not recommended.

Migraine, acute (unlabeled use): Initial: 500-750 mg; an additional 250-500 mg may be given if needed (maximum: 1250 mg in 24 hours). **Note:** EC-Naprosyn® is not recommended.

Pain (mild-to-moderate), dysmenorrhea, acute tendonitis, bursitis: Oral: Initial: 500 mg, then 250 mg every 6-8 hours; maximum: 1250 mg/day naproxen base

Rheumatoid arthritis, osteoarthritis, and ankylosing spondylitis: 500-1000 mg/day in 2 divided doses; may increase to 1.5 g/day of naproxen base for limited time period

OTC labeling: Pain/fever:

Adults ≤65 years: 200 mg naproxen base every 8-12 hours; if needed, may take 400 mg naproxen base for the initial dose; maximum: 600 mg naproxen base/24 hours

Adults >65 years: Refer to geriatric dosing.

Renal Impairment: Cl_{cr} <30 mL/minute: use is not recommended.

Administration Administer with food, milk, or antacids to decrease GI adverse effects

Monitoring Parameters Monitor response (pain, range of motion, grip strength, mobility, ADL function), inflammation; observe for weight gain, edema; monitor renal function (serum creatinine, BUN); observe for bleeding, bruising; evaluate gastrointestinal effects (abdominal pain, bleeding, dyspepsia); mental confusion, disorientation, CBC, liver function tests; urine output

Test Interactions Naproxen may interfere with 5-HIAA urinary assays; due to an interaction with m-di-nitrobenzene, naproxen should be discontinued 72 hours before adrenal function testing if the Porter-Silber test is used.

Patient Information Serious gastrointestinal bleeding can occur as well as ulceration and perforation. Pain may or may not be present. Avoid aspirin and aspirin-containing products while taking this medication. If gastric upset occurs, take with food, milk, or antacid. If gastric adverse effects persist, contact physician. May cause drowsiness, dizziness, blurred vision, and confusion. Use caution when performing tasks which require alertness (eg, driving). Do not take for more than 3 days for fever or 10 days for pain without physician's advice.

Special Geriatric Considerations Elderly are a high-risk population for adverse effects from NSAIDs. As much as 60% of the elderly can develop peptic ulceration and/or hemorrhage asymptomatically. The concomitant use of H_2 blockers and sucralfate is not effective as prophylaxis with the exception of NSAID-induced duodenal ulcers which may be prevented by the use of ranitidine. Misoprostol and proton pump inhibitors are the only agents proven to help prevent the development of NSAID-induced ulcers. Also, concomitant disease and drug use contribute to the risk for GI adverse effects. Use lowest effective dose for shortest period possible. Consider renal function decline with age. Use of NSAIDs can compromise existing renal function especially when Cl_{cr} is ≤30 mL/minute. Tinnitus may be a difficult and unreliable indication of toxicity due to age-related hearing loss or eighth cranial nerve damage. CNS adverse effects such as confusion, agitation, and hallucination are generally seen in overdose or high-dose situations, but elderly may demonstrate these adverse effects at lower doses than younger adults.

Dosage Forms Excipient information presented when available (limited, particularly for generics); consult specific product labeling.

Caplet, as sodium: 220 mg [equivalent to naproxen 200 mg and sodium 20 mg]

Aleve®, Midol® Extended Relief, Pamprin® Maximum Strength All Day Relief): 220 mg [equivalent to naproxen 200 mg and sodium 20 mg]

Capsule, liquid gel:

Aleve®: 220 mg [equivalent to naproxen 200 mg and sodium 20 mg]

Gelcap, as sodium:

Aleve®): 220 mg [equivalent to naproxen 200 mg and sodium 20 mg]

Suspension, oral: 125 mg/5 mL (500 mL)

Naprosyn®): 125 mg/5 mL (480 mL) [contains sodium 0.3 mEq/mL; orange-pineapple flavor]

Tablet: 250 mg, 375 mg, 500 mg

Naprosyn®): 250 mg, 375 mg, 500 mg

Tablet, as sodium: 220 mg [equivalent to naproxen 200 mg and sodium 20 mg]; 275 mg [equivalent to naproxen 250 mg and sodium 25 mg]; 550 mg [equivalent to naproxen 500 mg and sodium 50 mg]

Aleve®: 220 mg [equivalent to naproxen 200 mg and sodium 20 mg]

Anaprox®: 275 mg [equivalent to naproxen 250 mg and sodium 25 mg]

Anaprox® DS: 550 mg [equivalent to naproxen 500 mg and sodium 50 mg]

(Continued)

Naproxen *(Continued)*

Tablet, controlled release, as sodium: 550 mg [equivalent to naproxen 500 mg and sodium 50 mg]

Naprelan®: 421.5 mg [equivalent to naproxen 375 mg and sodium 37.5 mg]; 550 mg [equivalent to naproxen 500 mg and sodium 50 mg]

Tablet, delayed release: 375 mg, 500 mg

EC-Naprosyn®): 375 mg, 500 mg

Selected References

Brooks PM and Day RO, "Nonsteroidal Anti-inflammatory Drugs - Differences and Similarities," *N Engl J Med*, 1991, 324(24):1716-25.

Clinch D, Banerjee AK, Ostick G, "Absence of Abdominal Pain in Elderly Patients With Peptic Ulcer," *Age Ageing*, 1984, 13:120-3.

Clive DM and Stoff JS, "Renal Syndromes Associated With Nonsteroidal Anti-inflammatory Drugs," *N Engl J Med*, 1984, 310(9):563-72.

Graham DY, "Prevention of Gastroduodenal Injury Induced by Chronic Nonsteroidal Anti-inflammatory Drug Therapy," *Gastroenterology*, 1989, 96(2 Pt 2 Suppl):675-81.

Gurwitz JH, Avorn J, Ross-Degnan D, et al, "Nonsteroidal Anti-Inflammatory Drug-Associated Azotemia in the Very Old," *JAMA*, 1990, 264(4):471-5.

Hawkey CJ, Karrasch JA, Szczepański L, et al, "Omeprazole Compared With Misoprostol for Ulcers Associated With Nonsteroidal Anti-inflammatory Drugs," *N Engl J Med*, 1998, 338(11):727-34.

Knodel LC, "Preventing NSAID-induced Ulcers: The Role of Misoprostol," *Consult Pharm*, 1989, 4:37-41.

Pounder R, "Silent Peptic Ulceration: Deadly Silence or Golden Silence?" *Gastroenterology*, 1989, 96:(2 Pt 2 Suppl)626-31.

Snow V, Weiss K, Wall EM, et al, "Pharmacologic Management of Acute Attacks of Migraine and Prevention of Migraine Headache," *Ann Intern Med*, 2002, 137(10):840-9.

Yeomans ND, Tulassay Z, Juhasz L, et al, "A Comparison of Omeprazole With Ranitidine for Ulcers Associated With Nonsteroidal Anti-inflammatory Drugs," *N Engl J Med*, 1998, 338(11):719-26.

♦ **Naproxen Sodium** *see Naproxen on page 1088*

Naratriptan *(NAR a trip tan)*

Medication Safety Issues

Sound-alike/look-alike issues:

Amerge® may be confused with Altace®, Amaryl®

U.S. Brand Names Amerge®

Canadian Brand Names Amerge®

Index Terms Naratriptan Hydrochloride

Generic Available No

Pharmacologic Category Antimigraine Agent; Serotonin 5-HT$_{1B, 1D}$ Receptor Agonist

Use Treatment of acute migraine headache, with or without aura

Contraindications Hypersensitivity to naratriptan or any component of the formulation; cerebrovascular, peripheral vascular disease (ischemic bowel disease), ischemic heart disease (angina pectoris, history of myocardial infarction, or proven silent ischemia); or in patients with symptoms consistent with ischemic heart disease, coronary artery vasospasm, or Prinzmetal's angina; uncontrolled hypertension or patients who have received within 24 hours another 5-HT agonist (sumatriptan, zolmitriptan) or ergotamine-containing product; patients with known risk factors associated with coronary artery disease; patients with severe hepatic or renal disease (Cl$_{cr}$ <15 mL/minute); do not administer naratriptan to patients with hemiplegic or basilar migraine

Warnings/Precautions Use only if there is a clear diagnosis of migraine. Do not give to patients with risk factors for CAD until a cardiovascular evaluation has been performed; if evaluation is satisfactory, the healthcare provider should administer the first dose and cardiovascular status should be periodically re-evaluated. Cardiac events (coronary artery vasospasm, transient ischemia, myocardial infarction, ventricular tachycardia/fibrillation, cardiac arrest, and death), cerebral/subarachnoid hemorrhage, stroke, peripheral vascular ischemia, and colonic ischemia have been reported with 5-HT$_1$ agonist administration. Significant elevation in blood pressure, including hypertensive crisis, has also been reported on rare occasions in patients with and without a history of hypertension. If the patient does not respond to the first dose, re-evaluate the diagnosis of migraine before trying a second dose.

Adverse Reactions (Reflective of adult population; not specific for elderly)

1% to 10%:

Central nervous system: Dizziness, drowsiness, malaise/fatigue

Gastrointestinal: Nausea, vomiting

Neuromuscular & skeletal: Paresthesia

Miscellaneous: Pain or pressure in throat or neck

Drug Interactions

Ergot-containing drugs (dihydroergotamine or methysergide): May cause vasospastic reactions when taken with naratriptan. Avoid concomitant use with ergots; separate dose of naratriptan and ergots by at least 24 hours.

Oral contraceptives: May increase the levels/effects of naratriptan; monitor.

Serotonergic reuptake inhibitors (eg, SSRIs/SNRIs): Concurrent use of naratriptan with these agents may increase the risk of serotonin syndrome; monitor.

Serotonin agonists (eg, triptans): Concurrent use of naratriptan with these agents may increase the risk of serotonin syndrome; monitor.

Mechanism of Action The therapeutic effect for migraine is due to serotonin agonist activity

Pharmacokinetics

Protein binding, plasma: 28% to 31%

Metabolism: Hepatic

Bioavailability: 70%

Time to peak: 2-3 hours

Elimination: Urine

Dosage

Geriatrics: Not recommended for use in the elderly.

Adults: Migraine: Oral: 1 mg to 2.5 mg at the onset of headache. It is recommended to use the lowest possible dose to minimize adverse effects. If headache returns or dose not fully resolve, the dose may be repeated after 4 hours. Do not exceed 5 mg in 24 hours.

Renal Impairment:

Cl_{cr} 18-39 mL/minute: Initial: 1 mg; do not exceed 2.5 mg in 24 hours.

Cl_{cr} <15 mL/minute: Do not use.

Hepatic Impairment: Contraindicated in patients with severe liver failure. The maximum dose is 2.5 mg in 24 hours for patients with mild or moderate liver failure. The recommended starting dose is 1 mg.

Patient Information Do not crush or chew tablet; swallow whole with water. This drug is to be used to reduce migraine, not to prevent or reduce the number of attacks. If headache returns or is not fully resolved, the dose may be repeated after 4 hours. If no relief with first dose, do not take a second dose without consulting prescriber. Do not exceed 5 mg in 24 hours. Do not take within 24 hours of any other migraine medication without first consulting prescriber. You may experience some dizziness, fatigue, or drowsiness; use caution when driving or engaging in tasks that require alertness. Frequent mouth care and sucking on lozenges may relieve dry mouth. Report immediately any chest pain, heart throbbing, tightness in throat, skin rash or hives, hallucinations, anxiety, or panic.

Special Geriatric Considerations Naratriptan was not studied in patients >65 years of age. Use in elderly patients is not recommended because of the presence of risk factors associated with adverse effects. These include the presence of coronary artery disease, decreased liver or renal function, and the risk of pronounced blood pressure increases.

Dosage Forms Excipient information presented when available (limited, particularly for generics); consult specific product labeling.

Tablet: 1 mg, 2.5 mg

Natamycin (na ta MYE sin)

Medication Safety Issues

Sound-alike/look-alike issues:

Natacyn® may be confused with Naprosyn®

U.S. Brand Names Natacyn®

Canadian Brand Names Natacyn®

Index Terms Pimaricin

Generic Available No

Pharmacologic Category Antifungal Agent, Ophthalmic

Use Treatment of blepharitis, conjunctivitis, and keratitis caused by susceptible fungi (*Aspergillus, Candida*), *Cephalosporium, Curvularia, Fusarium, Penicillium, Microsporum, Epidermophyton, Blastomyces dermatitidis, Coccidioides immitis, Cryptococcus neoformans, Histoplasma capsulatum, Sporothrix schenckii*, and *Trichomonas vaginalis*

Contraindications Hypersensitivity to natamycin or any component of the formulation (Continued)

Natamycin *(Continued)*

Warnings/Precautions Failure to improve (keratitis) after 7-10 days of administration suggests infection caused by a microorganism not susceptible to natamycin; inadequate as a single agent in fungal endophthalmitis

Adverse Reactions (Reflective of adult population; not specific for elderly)
Frequency not defined: Ocular: Blurred vision, photophobia, eye pain, eye irritation not present before therapy

Drug Interactions Increased toxicity: Topical corticosteroids (concomitant use contraindicated)

Stability Store at room temperature (8°C to 24°C/46°F to 75°F); do not freeze. Protect from excessive heat and light.

Mechanism of Action Increases cell membrane permeability in susceptible fungi

Pharmacokinetics
Absorption: Ophthalmic: <2% systemically absorbed
Distribution: Adheres to cornea and is retained in the conjunctival fornices

Dosage
Geriatrics & Adults: Fungal infections: Ophthalmic: Instill 1 drop in conjunctival sac every 1-2 hours, after 3-4 days reduce to 1 drop 6-8 times/day; usual course of therapy is 2-3 weeks.

Monitoring Parameters Monitor tolerance to the drug at least twice weekly

Patient Information Shake well before using, do not touch dropper to eye; notify physician if condition worsens or does not improve after 3-4 days

Special Geriatric Considerations Assess patient's ability to self-administer ophthalmic drops.

Dosage Forms Excipient information presented when available (limited, particularly for generics); consult specific product labeling.
Suspension, ophthalmic: 5% (15 mL) [contains benzalkonium chloride]

Nateglinide *(na te GLYE nide)*

U.S. Brand Names Starlix®
Canadian Brand Names Starlix®
Generic Available No
Pharmacologic Category Antidiabetic Agent, Meglitinide Derivative
Use Management of type 2 diabetes mellitus (noninsulin dependent, NIDDM) as monotherapy when hyperglycemia cannot be managed by diet and exercise alone; in combination with metformin or a thiazolidinedione to lower blood glucose in patients whose hyperglycemia cannot be controlled by exercise, diet, or a single agent alone

Contraindications Hypersensitivity to nateglinide or any component of the formulation; diabetic ketoacidosis, with or without coma (treat with insulin); type 1 diabetes mellitus (insulin dependent, IDDM); patients not adequately controlled on oral agents which stimulate insulin release (eg, glyburide)

Warnings/Precautions Use with caution in patients with moderate-to-severe hepatic impairment. Use caution in severe renal dysfunction, elderly, malnourished, or patients with adrenal/pituitary dysfunction; may be more susceptible to glucose-lowering effects. All oral hypoglycemic agents are capable of producing hypoglycemia. Proper patient selection, dosage, and instructions to the patients are important to avoid hypoglycemic episodes. It may be necessary to discontinue nateglinide and administer insulin if the patient is exposed to stress (ie, fever, trauma, infection, surgery). Indicated for adjunctive therapy with metformin; not to be used as a substitute for metformin monotherapy. Combination treatment with sulfonylureas is not recommended (no additional benefit). Patients not adequately controlled on oral agents which stimulate insulin release (eg, glyburide) should not be switched to nateglinide or have nateglinide added to therapy.

Adverse Reactions (Reflective of adult population; not specific for elderly)
As reported with nateglinide monotherapy: 1% to 10%:
Central nervous system: Dizziness (4%)
Endocrine & metabolic: Hypoglycemia (2%), increased uric acid
Gastrointestinal: Weight gain
Neuromuscular & skeletal: Arthropathy (3%)
Respiratory: Upper respiratory infection (10%)
Miscellaneous: Flu-like syndrome (4%)

Overdosage/Toxicology In case of overdose, hypoglycemic symptoms would be expected. Severe hypoglycemic reactions should be treated with intravenous glucose. Dialysis is not effective.

Drug Interactions Substrate (major) of CYP2C9, 3A4; **Inhibits** CYP2C9 (weak)
Beta-blockers, nonselective: May potentiate hypoglycemic effect when given with nateglinide; monitor
Corticosteroids: May see poor glycemic control when given with nateglinide; monitor

CYP2C9 inducers: May decrease the levels/effects of nateglinide. Example inducers include carbamazepine, phenobarbital, phenytoin, rifampin, rifapentine, and secobarbital.

CYP2C9 inhibitors: May increase the levels/effects of nateglinide. Example inhibitors include delavirdine, fluconazole, gemfibrozil, ketoconazole, nicardipine, NSAIDs, sulfonamides and tolbutamide.

CYP3A4 inducers: CYP3A4 inducers may decrease the levels/effects of nateglinide. Example inducers include aminoglutethimide, carbamazepine, nafcillin, nevirapine, phenobarbital, phenytoin, and rifamycins.

CYP3A4 inhibitors: May increase the levels/effects of nateglinide. Example inhibitors include azole antifungals, clarithromycin, diclofenac, doxycycline, erythromycin, imatinib, isoniazid, nefazodone, nicardipine, propofol, protease inhibitors, quinidine, telithromycin, and verapamil.

Pegvisomant: May enhance the hypoglycemic effect of antidiabetic agents.

Thiazide diuretics: May see reduced effectiveness of nateglinide; monitor

Ethanol/Nutrition/Herb Interactions

Ethanol: Avoid ethanol (increased risk of hypoglycemia).

Food: Rate of absorption is decreased and time to T_{max} is delayed when taken with food. Food does not affect AUC. Multiple peak plasma concentrations may be observed if fasting. Not affected by composition of meal.

Herb/Nutraceutical: Avoid alfalfa, aloe, bilberry, bitter melon, burdock, celery, damiana, fenugreek, garcinia, garlic, ginger, ginseng (American), gymnema, marshmallow, and stinging nettle (may enhance the hypoglycemic effects of antidiabetic agents). St. John's wort may decrease the levels/effect of nateglinide.

Stability Store at 25°C (77°F).

Mechanism of Action A phenylalanine derivative, nonsulfonylurea hypoglycemic agent used in the management of type 2 diabetes mellitus (noninsulin dependent, NIDDM); stimulates insulin release from the pancreatic beta cells to reduce postprandial hyperglycemia; amount of insulin release is dependent upon existing glucose levels

Pharmacodynamics

Onset of action: Insulin secretion: ~20 minutes

Peak effect: 1 hour

Duration: 4 hours

Pharmacokinetics

Absorption: Rapid

Distribution: 10 L

Protein binding: 98%, primarily to albumin

Metabolism: Hepatic via hydroxylation followed by glucuronide conjugation

Bioavailability: 73%

Half-life: 1.5 hours

Time to peak: ≤1 hour

Elimination: Urine (83%, 16% as unchanged drug); feces (10%)

Dosage

Geriatrics & Adults: Management of type 2 diabetes mellitus: Oral: Initial and maintenance dose: 120 mg 3 times/day, 1-30 minutes before meals; may be given alone or in combination with metformin or a thiazolidinedione; patients close to Hb A_{1c} goal may be started at 60 mg 3 times/day

Renal Impairment: No specific dosage adjustment is recommended for patients with mild-to-severe renal disease. Patients on dialysis showed reduced medication exposure and plasma protein binding. Patients with severe renal dysfunction are more susceptible to glucose-lowering effect; use with caution.

Hepatic Impairment: Increased serum levels are seen with mild hepatic insufficiency; no dosage adjustment is needed. Has not been studied in patients with moderate to severe liver disease; use with caution.

Monitoring Parameters Glucose and Hb A_{1c} levels, weight, lipid profile

Reference Range Target range: Adults:

Fasting blood glucose: <110 mg/dL

Glycosylated hemoglobin: <6%

Patient Information Take this medication exactly as directed, 1-30 minutes before a meal. If you skip a meal (or add an extra meal) skip (or add) a dose for that meal. Do not change dosage or discontinue without first consulting prescriber. Follow dietary and lifestyle recommendations of provider. You will be instructed in signs of hypo- or hyperglycemia by healthcare provider or diabetic educator; be alert for adverse hypoglycemia (tachycardia, profuse perspiration, tingling of lips and tongue, seizures, or change in sensorium) and follow prescriber's instructions for intervention. Note that unusual strenuous exercise, excessive alcohol intake, or acute reduction in caloric intake may increase risk of hypoglycemia. Persistent nausea or vomiting, or severely decreased dietary intake, may increase risk of hyperglycemia. You may experience mild side effects during the first weeks of therapy (dizziness, weight gain, mild muscle
(Continued)

Nateglinide *(Continued)*

aches or pain, or flu-like symptoms); if these do not diminish, notify prescriber. Report signs of respiratory infection or other persistent adverse effect.

Additional Information An increase in weight was seen in nateglinide monotherapy, which was not seen when used in combination with metformin.

Special Geriatric Considerations No changes in safety and efficacy were seen in patients ≥65 years; however, some older adults may show increased sensitivity to dosing. How "tightly" a geriatric patient's blood glucose should be controlled is controversial; however, a fasting blood sugar of <150 mg/dL is now an acceptable endpoint. Such a decision should be based on the patient's functional and cognitive status, how well they recognize hypoglycemic or hyperglycemic symptoms, and how to respond to them and their other disease states.

Dosage Forms Excipient information presented when available (limited, particularly for generics); consult specific product labeling.
Tablet:
Starlix®: 60 mg, 120 mg

Selected References
"American Diabetes Association: Clinical Practice Recommendations 2000," *Diabetes Care*, 2000, 23(Suppl 1):S1-116.
Levien TL, Baker DE, Campbell RK, et al, "Nateglinide Therapy for Type 2 Diabetes Mellitus," *Ann Pharmacother*, 2001, 35(11):1426-34.

- ♦ **Natrecor®** *see* Nesiritide *on page 1106*
- ♦ **Natriuretic Peptide** *see* Nesiritide *on page 1106*
- ♦ **Natural Fiber Therapy [OTC]** *see* Psyllium *on page 1347*
- ♦ **Nature's Tears® [OTC]** *see* Artificial Tears *on page 124*
- ♦ **Nature-Throid® NT** *see* Thyroid *on page 1559*
- ♦ **Navane®** *see* Thiothixene *on page 1556*
- ♦ **Na-Zone® [OTC]** *see* Sodium Chloride *on page 1475*
- ♦ **NC-722665** *see* Bicalutamide *on page 169*

Nedocromil *(ne doe KROE mil)*

Related Information
Asthma *on page 1767*
Inhalant Agents *on page 1760*
U.S. Brand Names Alocril®; Tilade®
Canadian Brand Names Alocril®; Tilade®
Index Terms Nedocromil Sodium
Generic Available No
Pharmacologic Category Mast Cell Stabilizer
Use
Aerosol: Maintenance therapy in patients with mild to moderate bronchial asthma
Ophthalmic: Treatment of itching associated with allergic conjunctivitis
Contraindications Hypersensitivity to nedocromil or any component of the formulation
Warnings/Precautions
Aerosol: If systemic or inhaled steroid therapy is at all reduced, monitor patients carefully; nedocromil is **not** a bronchodilator and, therefore, should not be used for reversal of acute bronchospasm
Ophthalmic solution: Users of contact lenses should not wear them during periods of symptomatic allergic conjunctivitis
Adverse Reactions (Reflective of adult population; not specific for elderly)
Inhalation aerosol:
>10%: Gastrointestinal: Unpleasant taste
1% to 10%:
Cardiovascular: Chest pain
Central nervous system: Dizziness, dysphonia, headache, fatigue
Dermatologic: Rash
Gastrointestinal: Nausea, vomiting, dyspepsia, diarrhea, abdominal pain, xerostomia, unpleasant taste
Hepatic: Increased ALT
Neuromuscular & skeletal: Arthritis, tremor
Respiratory: Cough, pharyngitis, rhinitis, bronchitis, upper respiratory infection, bronchospasm, increased sputum production
Ophthalmic solution:
>10%:
Central nervous system: Headache (40%)
Gastrointestinal: Unpleasant taste
Ocular: Burning, irritation, stinging
Respiratory: Nasal congestion

1% to 10%:
Ocular: Conjunctivitis, eye redness, photophobia
Respiratory: Asthma, rhinitis

Stability Store at 2°C to 30°C/36°F to 86°F; do not freeze.

Mechanism of Action Inhibits the activation of and mediator release from a variety of inflammatory cell types associated with asthma including eosinophils, neutrophils, macrophages, mast cells, monocytes, and platelets; it inhibits the release of histamine, leukotrienes, and slow-reacting substance of anaphylaxis; it inhibits the development of early and late bronchoconstriction responses to inhaled antigen

Pharmacodynamics Duration of therapeutic effect: 2 hours

Pharmacokinetics
Protein binding, plasma: 89%
Bioavailability: 7% to 9%
Half-life elimination: 1.5-2 hours
Elimination: Urine (as unchanged drug)

Dosage
Geriatrics & Adults:
Asthma: Inhalation: 2 inhalations 4 times/day; may reduce dosage to 2-3 times/day once desired clinical response to initial dose is observed. Drug has no known therapeutic systemic activity when delivered by inhalation.
Allergic conjunctivitis: Ophthalmic: 1-2 drops in each eye twice daily

Administration If patient has aerosol (MDI) bronchodilators in their regimen, these should be used first, 5-10 minutes prior to use of nedocromil.

Monitoring Parameters Pulmonary function, spirometry

Patient Information An illustrated patient instruction packet is included with inhaler; must be used regularly to obtain benefit, even though symptoms may be absent; be aware of proper use.

Aerosol: Do not use during acute bronchospasm. Use exactly as directed; do not use more often than instructed or discontinue without consulting prescriber.

Inhaler: Review use with prescriber or follow package insert for directions. Prime with 3 activations prior to first use or if unused more than 7 days. Keep inhaler clean and unobstructed. Always rinse mouth and throat after use of inhaler to prevent advantageous infection. If you are also using a steroid bronchodilator, wait 10 minutes before using this aerosol.

Ophthalmic: Do not wear contact lenses with allergic conjunctivitis. For the eye only. Open eyes, look up, and pull lower lid down. Squeeze medicine into lower eyelid and close eye. Do not touch bottle tip to eye, eyelid, or other skin.

Additional Information Nedocromil has no known therapeutic systemic activity when delivered by inhalation.

Special Geriatric Considerations Elderly may have difficulty using inhaler delivery system, especially if they have physical or medical impairment (eg, Parkinson's disease, stroke). If this prophylactic modality is desired but patient cannot tolerate nedocromil inhalations, consider cromolyn sodium solution for nebulizer use.

Dosage Forms Excipient information presented when available (limited, particularly for generics); consult specific product labeling.
Aerosol for oral inhalation, as sodium (Tilade®): 1.75 mg/activation (16.2 g)
Solution, ophthalmic, as sodium (Alocril®): 2% (5 mL) [contains benzalkonium chloride]

♦ **Nedocromil Sodium** see Nedocromil on page 1096

Nefazodone (nef AY zoe done)

Related Information
Antidepressant Agents on page 1742
Medication Safety Issues
Sound-alike/look-alike issues:
Serzone® may be confused with selegiline, Serentil®, Seroquel®, sertraline
Index Terms Nefazodone Hydrochloride; Serzone
Generic Available Yes
Pharmacologic Category Antidepressant, Serotonin Reuptake Inhibitor/Antagonist
Use Treatment of depression
Unlabeled/Investigational Use Treatment of post-traumatic stress disorder
Restrictions An FDA-approved medication guide concerning the use of antidepressants in children, adolescents, and young adults must be distributed when dispensing an outpatient prescription (new or refill) where this medication is to be used without direct supervision of a healthcare provider. Medication guides are available at http://www.fda.gov/cder/Offices/ODS/medication_guides.htm. Dispense to parents or guardians of children and adolescents receiving this medication.
Contraindications Hypersensitivity to nefazodone, related compounds (phenylpiperazines), or any component of the formulation; liver injury due to previous nefazodone
(Continued)

Nefazodone *(Continued)*

treatment, active liver disease, or elevated serum transaminases; concurrent use or use of MAO inhibitors within previous 14 days; use in a patient during the acute recovery phase of MI; concurrent use with astemizole, carbamazepine, cisapride, or pimozide; concurrent therapy with triazolam or alprazolam is generally contraindicated (dosage must be reduced by 75% for triazolam and 50% for alprazolam; such reductions may not be possible with available dosage forms).

Warnings/Precautions [U.S. Boxed Warning]: Antidepressants increase the risk of suicidal thinking and behavior in children, adolescents, and young adults (18-24 years of age) with major depressive disorder (MDD) and other psychiatric disorders; consider risk prior to prescribing. Short-term studies did not show an increased risk in patients >24 years of age and showed a decreased risk in patients ≥65 years. Closely monitor for clinical worsening, suicidality, or unusual changes in behavior; the patient's family or caregiver should be instructed to closely observe the patient and communicate condition with healthcare provider. A medication guide should be dispensed with each prescription.

The possibility of a suicide attempt is inherent in major depression and may persist until remission occurs. Monitor for worsening of depression or suicidality, especially during initiation of therapy (generally first 1-2 months) or with dose increases or decreases. Use caution in high-risk patients. Worsening depression and severe abrupt suicidality that are not part of the presenting symptoms may require discontinuation or modification of drug therapy. The patient's family or caregiver should be alerted to monitor patients for the emergence of suicidality and associated behaviors (such as agitation, irritability, hostility, impulsivity, and hypomania) and call healthcare provider.

May worsen psychosis in some patients or precipitate a shift to mania or hypomania in patients with bipolar disorder. Patients presenting with depressive symptoms should be screened for bipolar disorder. Monotherapy in patients with bipolar disorder should be avoided. **Nefazodone is not FDA approved for the treatment of bipolar depression.**

Cases of life-threatening hepatic failure have been reported (risk should be considered when choosing an agent for the treatment of depression); discontinue if clinical signs or symptoms suggest liver failure. May cause sedation, resulting in impaired performance of tasks requiring alertness (eg, operating machinery or driving). May increase the risks associated with electroconvulsive therapy. Consider discontinuing, when possible, prior to elective surgery. Therapy should not be abruptly discontinued in patients receiving high doses for prolonged periods. Rare reports of priapism have occurred. The incidence of sexual dysfunction with nefazodone is generally lower than with SSRIs.

The risk of sedation, conduction disturbances, orthostatic hypotension, or anticholinergic effects are very low relative to other antidepressants. Use with caution in patients with a history of cardiovascular disease (including previous MI, stroke, tachycardia, or conduction abnormalities). Use with caution in patients with urinary retention, benign prostatic hyperplasia, narrow-angle glaucoma, xerostomia, visual problems, constipation, or history of bowel obstruction (due to anticholinergic effects).

Use caution in patients with a previous seizure disorder or condition predisposing to seizures such as brain damage, alcoholism, or concurrent therapy with other drugs which lower the seizure threshold. Use with caution in patients with renal dysfunction and in elderly patients.

Adverse Reactions (Reflective of adult population; not specific for elderly)
>10%:
  Central nervous system: Headache, drowsiness, insomnia, agitation, dizziness
  Gastrointestinal: Xerostomia, nausea, constipation
  Neuromuscular & skeletal: Weakness
1% to 10%:
  Cardiovascular: Bradycardia, hypotension, peripheral edema, postural hypotension, vasodilation
  Central nervous system: Chills, fever, incoordination, lightheadedness, confusion, memory impairment, abnormal dreams, decreased concentration, ataxia, psychomotor retardation, tremor
  Dermatologic: Pruritus, rash
  Endocrine & metabolic: Breast pain, impotence, libido decreased
  Gastrointestinal: Gastroenteritis, vomiting, dyspepsia, diarrhea, increased appetite, thirst, taste perversion
  Genitourinary: Urinary frequency, urinary retention
  Hematologic: Hematocrit decreased
  Neuromuscular & skeletal: Arthralgia, hypertonia, paresthesia, neck rigidity, tremor
  Ocular: Blurred vision (9%), abnormal vision (7%), eye pain, visual field defect
  Otic: Tinnitus
  Respiratory: Bronchitis, cough, dyspnea, pharyngitis

Miscellaneous: Flu syndrome, infection

Overdosage/Toxicology Symptoms include drowsiness, vomiting, hypotension, tachycardia, incontinence, and coma. Following initiation of essential overdose management, toxic symptoms should be treated. Ventricular arrhythmias often respond to lidocaine 1.5 mg/kg bolus followed by a 2 mg/minute infusion with concurrent systemic alkalinization (sodium bicarbonate 0.5-2 mEq/kg I.V.). Seizures usually respond to diazepam I.V. boluses (5-10 mg up to 30 mg). If seizures are unresponsive or recur, phenytoin or phenobarbital may be required. Hypotension is best treated by I.V. fluids and by Trendelenburg positioning.

Drug Interactions Substrate (major) of CYP2D6, 3A4; **Inhibits** CYP1A2 (weak), 2B6 (weak), 2C8 (weak), 2D6 (weak), 3A4 (strong)

Antiarrhythmics: Serum concentrations may be increased due to enzyme inhibition; monitor; includes amiodarone, lidocaine, propafenone, quinidine

Antipsychotics: Serum concentrations of some antipsychotics may be increased by nefazodone due to enzyme inhibition; includes clozapine, haloperidol, mesoridazine, pimozide, quetiapine, and risperidone

Benzodiazepines: Nefazodone inhibits the metabolism of triazolam (decrease dose by 75%) and alprazolam (decrease dose by 50%); triazolam is contraindicated per manufacturer

Buspirone: Concurrent use may result in serotonin syndrome; serum concentrations may be increased due to enzyme inhibition; these combinations are best avoided or limit buspirone to 2.5 mg/day

Calcium channel blockers: Serum concentrations may be increased due to enzyme inhibition; monitor for increased effect (hypotension)

Carbamazepine: Significantly reduces serum concentrations of nefazodone; coadministration is contraindicated

Cisapride: Nefazodone likely increases cisapride serum concentrations via CYP3A4 inhibition; this combination may lead to cardiac arrhythmias; concurrent use is contraindicated

Cyclosporine and tacrolimus: Serum levels and toxicity may be increased by nefazodone; monitor

CYP2D6 inhibitors: May increase the levels/effects of nefazodone. Example inhibitors include chlorpromazine, delavirdine, fluoxetine, miconazole, paroxetine, pergolide, quinidine, quinine, ritonavir, and ropinirole.

CYP3A4 inducers: CYP3A4 inducers may decrease the levels/effects of nefazodone. Example inducers include aminoglutethimide, carbamazepine (contraindicated), nafcillin, nevirapine, phenobarbital, phenytoin, and rifamycins.

CYP3A4 inhibitors: May increase the levels/effects of nefazodone. Example inhibitors include azole antifungals, clarithromycin, diclofenac, doxycycline, erythromycin, imatinib, isoniazid, nicardipine, propofol, protease inhibitors, quinidine, telithromycin, and verapamil.

CYP3A4 substrates: Nefazodone may increase the levels/effects of CYP3A4 substrates. Example substrates include benzodiazepines, calcium channel blockers, mirtazapine, nateglinide, nefazodone, tacrolimus, and venlafaxine. Selected benzodiazepines (midazolam and triazolam), cisapride, ergot alkaloids, selected HMG-CoA reductase inhibitors (lovastatin and simvastatin), and pimozide are generally contraindicated with strong CYP3A4 inhibitors.

Digoxin: Serum levels may be increased by nefazodone (modest increases); monitor for digoxin toxicity or increased serum levels

Donepezil: Serum concentrations may be increased due to enzyme inhibition; monitor

HMG-CoA reductase inhibitors (statins) have been associated with myositis and rhabdomyolysis when used in combination with nefazodone; this has been associated most strongly with lovastatin and simvastatin. Concomitant use of lovastatin with nefazodone should be avoided.

Linezolid: Due to MAO inhibition (see note on MAO inhibitors), this combination should be avoided

MAO inhibitors: Concurrent use may lead to serotonin syndrome; avoid concurrent use or use within 14 days

Meperidine: Combined use theoretically may increase the risk of serotonin syndrome

Methadone: Serum concentrations may be increased due to enzyme inhibition; monitor

Oral contraceptives: Serum concentrations may be increased due to enzyme inhibition; monitor

Pimozide: Serum concentrations may be increased due to enzyme inhibition; may result in life-threatening arrhythmias (also see note on antipsychotics); avoid use

Protease inhibitors: Indinavir, ritonavir saquinavir; serum concentrations may be increased due to enzyme inhibition; monitor

Quinidine: Metabolism is likely to be inhibited by nefazodone; avoid concurrent use

Selegiline: Concurrent use with nefazodone may be associated with a risk of serotonin syndrome, particularly at higher dosages (>10 mg/day)

Serotonin agonists: Theoretically may increase the risk of serotonin syndrome; includes sumatriptan, naratriptan, rizatriptan, and zolmitriptan

Sibutramine: Serum concentrations may be increased by nefazodone; monitor
(Continued)

Nefazodone *(Continued)*

Sildenafil, vardenafil: Serum concentrations may be increased by nefazodone via inhibition of CYP3A4; use caution. Specific dosage adjustment guidelines have not been established. Recommendations for other strong CYP3A4 inhibitors include single sildenafil dose not to exceed 25 mg in a 48-hour period, a single tadalafil dose not to exceed 10 mg in a 72-hour period, or a single vardenafil dose not to exceed 2.5 mg in a 24-hour period.

SSRIs: Combined use of nefazodone with an SSRI may produce serotonin syndrome; in addition, nefazodone may increase serum concentrations of some SSRIs due to enzyme inhibition (fluoxetine and citalopram)

Tricyclic antidepressants: Serum concentrations of some tricyclic antidepressants (amitriptyline, clomipramine) may be increased; monitor for increased effect or toxicity

Venlafaxine: Combined use with nefazodone may increase the risk of serotonin syndrome

Vinca alkaloids (vincristine and vinblastine): Serum concentrations may be increased due to enzyme inhibition; may result in increased toxicity

Zolpidem: Serum concentrations may be increased due to enzyme inhibition; monitor

Ethanol/Nutrition/Herb Interactions

Ethanol: Avoid ethanol (may increase CNS depression).

Food: Nefazodone absorption may be delayed and bioavailability may be decreased if taken with food.

Herb/Nutraceutical: Avoid valerian, St John's wort, SAMe, kava kava (may increase risk of serotonin syndrome and/or excessive sedation).

Stability Store at room temperature, below 40°C (104°F) in a tight container.

Mechanism of Action Inhibits neuronal reuptake of serotonin and norepinephrine; also blocks $5-HT_2$ and $alpha_1$ receptors; has no significant affinity for $alpha_2$, beta-adrenergic, $5-HT_{1A}$, cholinergic, dopaminergic, or benzodiazepine receptors

Pharmacokinetics

Absorption: Nearly complete with oral dosing, however, first-pass effect results in 20% systemic bioavailability

Protein binding: >99%

Metabolism: In the liver to 3 active metabolites; triazoledione, hydroxynefazodone and m-chlorophenylpiperazine (mCPP); hydroxynefazodone is equipotent $5-HT_2$ antagonist and 5-HT reuptake inhibitor as nefazodone

Half-life: 2-4 hours (parent compound), active metabolites persist longer

Time to peak serum concentration: 30 minutes, prolonged in presence of food

Elimination: Primarily as metabolites in urine and secondarily in feces

Dosage

Geriatrics: Oral: Initial: 50 mg twice daily; increase dose to 100 mg twice daily in 2 weeks; usual maintenance dose: 200-400 mg/day

Adults: Depression: Oral: 200 mg/day, administered in two divided doses initially, with a range of 300-600 mg/day in two divided doses thereafter.

Administration Dosing after meals may decrease lightheadedness and postural hypotension, but may also decrease absorption and therefore effectiveness.

Monitoring Parameters If AST/ALT increase >3 times ULN, the drug should be discontinued and not reintroduced; mental status for depression, suicidal ideation (especially at the beginning of therapy or when doses are increased or decreased), anxiety, social functioning, mania, panic attacks

Reference Range Therapeutic plasma concentrations have not yet been defined

Patient Information Take exactly as directed (do not increase dose or frequency); may take 2-3 weeks to achieve desired results; may cause physical and/or psychological dependence. Avoid alcohol, caffeine, and other prescription or OTC medications not approved by prescriber. Maintain adequate hydration (2-3 L/day of fluids unless instructed to restrict fluid intake). You may experience drowsiness, dizziness, or lightheadedness (use caution when driving or engaging in tasks requiring alertness until response to drug is known); nausea or vomiting (small frequent meals, frequent mouth care, chewing gum, or sucking lozenges may help); or orthostatic hypotension (use caution when climbing stairs or changing position from lying or sitting to standing). Report persistent insomnia or excessive daytime sedation; muscle cramping, tremors, weakness, tiredness, or change in gait; chest pain, palpitations, or rapid heartbeat; vision changes or eye pain; difficulty breathing or breathlessness; abdominal pain or blood in stool; yellowing of skin or eyes (jaundice); or worsening of condition.

Additional Information Experience with this drug has led some clinicians to realize that it may cause less insomnia, anxiety, and sexual dysfunction than the SSRIs; should consider this agent for patients who cannot tolerate the sexual dysfunction that may result from other antidepressants

Special Geriatric Considerations Data on nefazodone in the elderly are limited, specifically regarding efficacy; clinical trials in adult patients have found it superior to placebo and similar to imipramine; nefazodone's C_{max} and AUC have been reported to be increased twofold in the elderly and women after a single dose compared to younger patients, however, these differences were markedly reduced with multiple dosing with women having AUC values of nefazodone and its hydroxy metabolite remaining approximately 50% higher

Dosage Forms Excipient information presented when available (limited, particularly for generics); consult specific product labeling.

Tablet, as hydrochloride: 50 mg, 100 mg, 150 mg, 200 mg, 250 mg

Selected References

Barbhaiya RH, Buch AB, and Greene DS, "A Study of the Effect of Age and Gender on the Pharmacokinetics of Nefazodone After Single and Multiple Doses," *J Clin Psychopharmacol*, 1996, 16(1):19-25.

Fontaine R, Ontiveros A, Elie R, et al, "A Double-Blind Comparison of Nefazodone, Imipramine, and Placebo in Major Depression," *J Clin Psychiatry*, 1994, 55(6):234-41.

Rickels K, Schweizer E, Clary C, et al, "Nefazodone and Imipramine in Major Depression: A Placebo-Controlled Trial," *Br J Psychiatry*, 1994, 164(6):802-5.

Shea JP, Shulka UA, Rittman KA, "Single Dose Pharmacokinetics of Nefazodone in Elderly Subjects, Renally Impaired Patients, and Patients With Hepatic Cirrhosis in Comparison to Healthy Volunteers," *Clin Pharmacol Ther*, 1988, 43:146.

♦ **Nefazodone Hydrochloride** see Nefazodone on page 1097

♦ **Neo-Calglucon® [OTC]** see Calcium Salts (Oral) on page 220

♦ **NeoCeuticals™ Acne Spot Treatment [OTC]** see Salicylic Acid on page 1441

♦ **Neo-Cultol® [OTC]** see Mineral Oil on page 1045

♦ **Neofrin™** see Phenylephrine on page 1247

Neomycin and Polymyxin B (nee oh MYE sin & pol i MIKS in bee)

U.S. Brand Names Neosporin® G.U. Irrigant
Canadian Brand Names Neosporin® Irrigating Solution
Index Terms Polymyxin B and Neomycin
Generic Available Yes: Irrigation solution 1 mL package size
Pharmacologic Category Antibiotic, Topical; Genitourinary Irrigant
Use Short-term as a continuous irrigant or rinse in the urinary bladder to prevent bacteriuria and gram-negative rod septicemia associated with the use of indwelling catheters; to help prevent infection in minor cuts, scrapes, and burns
Contraindications Hypersensitivity to neomycin, polymyxin B, or any component of the formulation
Adverse Reactions (Reflective of adult population; not specific for elderly) Frequency not defined.
Dermatologic: Contact dermatitis, erythema, rash, urticaria
Genitourinary: Bladder irritation
Local: Burning
Neuromuscular & skeletal: Neuromuscular blockade
Otic: Ototoxicity
Renal: Nephrotoxicity
Drug Interactions No data reported
Stability Store irrigation solution in refrigerator. Aseptic prepared dilutions (1 mL/1 L) should be stored in the refrigerator and discarded after 48 hours.
Mechanism of Action See individual agents.
Pharmacokinetics Absorption: Topical: Not absorbed following application to intact skin; absorbed through denuded or abraded skin, peritoneum, wounds, or ulcers
Dosage
Geriatrics & Adults: Bladder irrigation: **Not for I.V. injection**; add 1 mL irrigant to 1 liter isotonic saline solution and connect container to the inflow of lumen of 3-way catheter. Continuous irrigant or rinse in the urinary bladder for up to a maximum of 10 days with administration rate adjusted to patient's urine output; usually no more than 1 L of irrigant is used per day.
Administration Bladder irrigant: Do not inject irrigant solution; concentrated irrigant solution must be diluted in 1 L normal saline before administration; connect irrigation container to the inflow lumen of a 3-way catheter to permit continuous irrigation of the urinary bladder
Patient Information Notify physician if condition worsens or if rash or irritation develops
Dosage Forms Excipient information presented when available (limited, particularly for generics); consult specific product labeling.
Solution, irrigant: Neomycin 40 mg and polymyxin B 200,000 units per mL (1 mL)
Neosporin® G.U. Irrigant: Neomycin 40 mg and polymyxin B 200,000 units per mL (1 mL, 20 mL)

Neomycin, Colistin, Hydrocortisone, and Thonzonium (nee oh MYE sin, koe LIS tin, hye droe KOR ti sone, & thon ZOE nee um)

Related Information
Hydrocortisone on page 762
U.S. Brand Names Coly-Mycin® S; Cortisporin®-TC
(Continued)

Neomycin, Colistin, Hydrocortisone, and Thonzonium
(Continued)

Index Terms Colistin, Neomycin, Hydrocortisone, and Thonzonium; Hydrocortisone, Neomycin, Colistin, and Thonzonium; Thonzonium, Neomycin, Colistin, and Hydrocortisone

Generic Available No

Pharmacologic Category Antibiotic/Corticosteroid, Otic

Use Treatment of superficial and susceptible bacterial infections of the external auditory canal and susceptible bacterial infections of mastoidectomy and fenestration cavities

Contraindications Hypersensitivity to any component of the formulation and/or aminoglycosides; herpes simplex, vaccinia, varicella

Warnings/Precautions Prolonged treatment may result in overgrowth of nonsusceptible organisms. Discontinue if irritation occurs. Use caution in longstanding otitis media or tympanic perforation; risk of ototoxicity is increased. Do not use for longer than 10 days.

Adverse Reactions (Reflective of adult population; not specific for elderly)
Frequency not defined.
Dermatologic: Hypersensitivity reaction, irritation
Otic: Ototoxicity (rare)

Drug Interactions Hydrocortisone: **Substrate** of CYP3A4 (minor); **Induces** CYP3A4 (weak)

Dosage
Geriatrics & Adults: Ear inflammation/infection: Otic:
Calibrated dropper: 5 drops in affected ear 3-4 times/day
Dropper bottle: 4 drops in affected ear 3-4 times/day
Note: Alternatively, a cotton wick may be inserted in the ear canal and saturated with suspension every 4 hours; wick should be replaced at least every 24 hours

Patient Information Shake well before using.

Special Geriatric Considerations Many elderly will overuse eye drops or use for nonindicated reasons; limit use.

Dosage Forms Excipient information presented when available (limited, particularly for generics); consult specific product labeling.
Suspension, otic [drops]:
Coly-Mycin® S: Neomycin 0.33%, colistin 0.3%, hydrocortisone acetate 1%, and thonzonium bromide 0.05% (5 mL) [contains thimerosal; packaged with dropper]
Cortisporin®-TC: Neomycin 0.33%, colistin 0.3%, hydrocortisone acetate 1%, and thonzonium bromide 0.05% (10 mL) [contains thimerosal; packaged with dropper]

Neomycin, Polymyxin B, and Dexamethasone
(nee oh MYE sin, pol i MIKS in bee, & deks a METH a sone)

Related Information
Dexamethasone *on page 413*

Medication Safety Issues
Sound-alike/look-alike issues:
AK-Trol® may be confused with AKTob®

U.S. Brand Names AK-Trol® [DSC]; Maxitrol®; Poly-Dex™

Canadian Brand Names Dioptrol®; Maxitrol®

Index Terms Dexamethasone, Neomycin, and Polymyxin B; Polymyxin B, Neomycin, and Dexamethasone

Generic Available Yes

Pharmacologic Category Antibiotic/Corticosteroid, Ophthalmic

Use Steroid-responsive inflammatory ocular conditions in which a corticosteroid is indicated and where bacterial infection or a risk of bacterial infection exists

Contraindications
Based on **neomycin** component: Hypersensitivity to neomycin or any component of the formulation, or other aminoglycosides
Based on **polymyxin B** component: Hypersensitivity to polymyxin B or any component of the formulation
Based on **dexamethasone** component: Hypersensitivity to dexamethasone or any component of the formulation; ophthalmic use in viral, fungal, or tuberculosis diseases of the eye

Warnings/Precautions Sensitivity to neomycin may develop; discontinue if sensitivity reaction occurs. Prolonged use of corticosteroids may result in glaucoma; damage to the optic nerve, defects in visual acuity and fields of vision, and posterior subcapsular cataract formation may occur. Prolonged use of corticosteroids may increase the incidence of secondary ocular infection or mask acute infection (including fungal infections); may prolong or exacerbate ocular viral infections; use following cataract surgery may delay healing or increase the incidence of bleb formation. A maximum of 8 g of ointment or 20 mL of suspension should be prescribed initially; patients should be evaluated prior to additional refills. Suspension contains benzalkonium chloride which may be adsorbed by contact lenses; contact lenses should not be worn during treatment of ophthalmic infections.

Adverse Reactions (Reflective of adult population; not specific for elderly)
Frequency not defined: Ocular: Allergic sensitivity, cutaneous sensitization, eye pain, development of glaucoma, cataract, increased intraocular pressure, optic nerve damage, wound healing delayed

Drug Interactions Dexamethasone: **Substrate** of CYP3A4 (minor); **Induces** CYP2A6 (weak), 2B6 (weak), 2C8 (weak), 2C9 (weak), 3A4 (weak)
Also see individual agents.

Mechanism of Action See individual agents.

Dosage
Geriatrics & Adults: Ocular inflammation/infection: Ophthalmic:
Ointment: Place a small amount (~½") in the affected eye 3-4 times/day or apply at bedtime as an adjunct with drops
Suspension: Instill 1-2 drops into affected eye(s) every 3-4 hours; in severe disease, drops may be used hourly and tapered to discontinuation

Administration Shake well before using; tilt head back, place medication in conjunctival sac, and close eyes; apply finger pressure on lacrimal sac for 1 minute following instillation

Monitoring Parameters Intraocular pressure with use >10 days

Patient Information For the eye; shake well before using; do not touch dropper to eye; notify physician if condition worsens or does not improve in 3-4 days

Special Geriatric Considerations Assess patients ability to self-administer.

Dosage Forms Excipient information presented when available (limited, particularly for generics); consult specific product labeling. [DSC] = Discontinued product
Ointment, ophthalmic (Maxitrol®, Poly-Dex™): Neomycin 3.5 mg, polymyxin B sulfate 10,000 units, and dexamethasone 0.1% per g (3.5 g)
Suspension, ophthalmic (AK-Trol® [DSC], Maxitrol®, Poly-Dex™): Neomycin 3.5 mg, polymyxin B sulfate 10,000 units, and dexamethasone 0.1% per mL (5 mL) [contains benzalkonium chloride]

Neomycin, Polymyxin B, and Gramicidin
(nee oh MYE sin, pol i MIKS in bee, & gram i SYE din)

U.S. Brand Names Neosporin® Ophthalmic Solution
Canadian Brand Names Neosporin®; Optimyxin Plus®
Index Terms Gramicidin, Neomycin, and Polymyxin B; Polymyxin B, Neomycin, and Gramicidin
Generic Available Yes
Pharmacologic Category Antibiotic, Ophthalmic
Use Treatment of superficial ocular infection
Contraindications Hypersensitivity to neomycin, polymyxin B, gramicidin or any component of the formulation
Warnings/Precautions Symptoms of neomycin sensitization include itching, reddening, edema, failure to heal; prolonged use may result in glaucoma, defects in visual acuity, posterior subcapsular cataract formation, and secondary ocular infections
Adverse Reactions (Reflective of adult population; not specific for elderly)
Frequency not defined: Ocular: Transient irritation, burning, stinging, itching, inflammation, angioneurotic edema, urticaria, vesicular and maculopapular dermatitis
Drug Interactions No data reported
Mechanism of Action Interferes with bacterial protein synthesis by binding to 30S ribosomal subunits; binds to phospholipids, alters permeability, and damages the bacterial cytoplasmic membrane permitting leakage of intracellular constituents
Dosage
Geriatrics & Adults: Ophthalmic: Instill 1-2 drops 4-6 times/day or more frequently as required for severe infections
Patient Information Tilt head back, place medication in conjunctival sac, and close eyes; apply finger pressure on lacrimal sac for 1 minute following instillation
Special Geriatric Considerations Assess patient's ability to self-administer ophthalmic drops.
Dosage Forms Excipient information presented when available (limited, particularly for generics); consult specific product labeling.
Solution, ophthalmic: Neomycin 1.75 mg, polymyxin B 10,000 units, and gramicidin 0.025 mg per mL (10 mL) [contains alcohol 0.5% and thimerosal]

♦ **Neoral**® see CycloSPORINE on page 380
♦ **Neosar** see Cyclophosphamide on page 376

- ◆ **Neosporin® AF [OTC]** *see* Miconazole *on page 1036*
- ◆ **Neosporin® G.U. Irrigant** *see* Neomycin and Polymyxin B *on page 1101*
- ◆ **Neosporin® Ophthalmic Solution** *see* Neomycin, Polymyxin B, and Gramicidin *on page 1103*

Neostigmine (nee oh STIG meen)

Medication Safety Issues
Sound-alike/look-alike issues:
Prostigmin® may be confused with physostigmine

U.S. Brand Names Prostigmin®

Canadian Brand Names Prostigmin®

Index Terms Neostigmine Bromide; Neostigmine Methylsulfate

Generic Available Yes: Injection

Pharmacologic Category Acetylcholinesterase Inhibitor

Use Diagnosis and treatment of myasthenia gravis and prevent and treat postoperative bladder distention and urinary retention; reversal of the effects of nondepolarizing neuromuscular blocking agents after surgery

Contraindications Hypersensitivity to neostigmine, bromides, or any component of the formulation; GI or GU obstruction

Warnings/Precautions Does **not** antagonize and may prolong the Phase I block of depolarizing muscle relaxants (eg, succinylcholine); use with caution in patients with epilepsy, asthma, bradycardia, hyperthyroidism, cardiac arrhythmias, or peptic ulcer; not generally recommended for use in patients with vagotonia; adequate facilities should be available for cardiopulmonary resuscitation when testing and adjusting dose for myasthenia gravis; have atropine and epinephrine ready to treat hypersensitivity reactions; overdosage may result in cholinergic crisis, this must be distinguished from myasthenic crisis; anticholinesterase insensitivity can develop for brief or prolonged periods

Adverse Reactions (Reflective of adult population; not specific for elderly)
Frequency not defined.

Cardiovascular: Arrhythmias (especially bradycardia), hypotension, tachycardia, AV block, nodal rhythm, nonspecific ECG changes, cardiac arrest, syncope, flushing

Central nervous system: Convulsions, dysarthria, dysphonia, dizziness, loss of consciousness, drowsiness, headache

Dermatologic: Skin rash, thrombophlebitis (I.V.), urticaria

Gastrointestinal: Hyperperistalsis, nausea, vomiting, salivation, diarrhea, stomach cramps, dysphagia, flatulence

Genitourinary: Urinary urgency

Neuromuscular & skeletal: Weakness, fasciculations, muscle cramps, spasms, arthralgia

Ocular: Small pupils, lacrimation

Respiratory: Increased bronchial secretions, laryngospasm, bronchiolar constriction, respiratory muscle paralysis, dyspnea, respiratory depression, respiratory arrest, bronchospasm

Miscellaneous: Diaphoresis (increased), anaphylaxis, allergic reactions

Overdosage/Toxicology Symptoms include muscle weakness, blurred vision, excessive sweating, tearing and salivation, nausea, vomiting, diarrhea, hypertension, bradycardia, muscle weakness, and paralysis. Atropine sulfate injection should be readily available as an antagonist for the effects of neostigmine.

Drug Interactions
Anticholinergics: Effects may be reduced with cholinesterase inhibitors; atropine antagonizes the muscarinic effects of cholinesterase inhibitors

Beta-blockers without ISA: Activity may increase risk of bradycardia

Calcium channel blockers (diltiazem or verapamil): May increase risk of bradycardia

Cholinergic agonists: Effects may be increased with cholinesterase inhibitors

Corticosteroids: May see increased muscle weakness and decreased response to anticholinesterases shortly after onset of corticosteroid therapy in the treatment of myasthenia gravis. Deterioration in muscle strength, including severe muscular depression, has been documented in patients with myasthenia gravis while receiving corticosteroids and anticholinesterases.

Digoxin: Increased risk of bradycardia with concurrent use

Neuromuscular blockers: Depolarizing neuromuscular blocking agents effects may be increased with cholinesterase inhibitors; nondepolarizing agents are antagonized by cholinesterase inhibitors

Mechanism of Action Inhibits destruction of acetylcholine by acetylcholinesterase which facilitates transmission of impulses across myoneural junction

Pharmacodynamics
Onset of effect:
I.M.: Within 20-30 minutes
I.V.: Within 1-20 minutes

Oral: 45-75 minutes
Duration:
    I.M.: 2.5-4 hours
    I.V.: 1-2 hours
    Oral: 2-4 hours

Pharmacokinetics
Absorption: Oral: Poor, <2%
Metabolism: In the liver
Half-life:
    Normal renal function: 0.5-2.1 hours
    End-stage renal disease: Prolonged
Elimination: 50% excreted renally as unchanged drug

Dosage
Geriatrics & Adults:
  Myasthenia gravis, diagnosis: I.M.: 0.02 mg/kg as a single dose
  Myasthenia gravis, treatment:
    Oral: 15 mg/dose every 3-4 hours up to 375 mg/day maximum
    I.M., I.V., SubQ: 0.5-2.5 mg every 1-3 hours up to 10 mg/24 hours maximum
  Reversal of nondepolarizing neuromuscular blockade after surgery in conjunction with atropine: I.V.: 0.5-2.5 mg; total dose not to exceed 5 mg; must administer atropine several minutes prior to neostigmine
  Bladder atony: I.M., SubQ:
    Prevention: 0.25 mg every 4-6 hours for 2-3 days
    Treatment: 0.5-1 mg every 3 hours for 5 doses after bladder has emptied
Renal Impairment:
  Cl_{cr} 10-50 mL/minute: Administer 50% of normal dose.
  Cl_{cr} <10 mL/minute: Administer 25% of normal dose.

Administration May be administered undiluted by slow I.V. injection over several minutes

Monitoring Parameters Respiratory rate, pulse, blood pressure, signs of cholinergic crisis. See Overdosage/Toxicology.

Patient Information Side effects are generally due to exaggerated pharmacologic effects; most common are salivation and muscle fasciculations; notify physician if nausea, vomiting, muscle weakness, severe abdominal pain, or difficulty breathing occurs

Additional Information
Neostigmine bromide: Prostigmin® tablet
Neostigmine methylsulfate: Prostigmin® injection
In the diagnosis of myasthenia gravis, all anticholinesterase medications should be discontinued for at least 8 hours before administering neostigmine.

Special Geriatric Considerations Many elderly will have diseases which may influence the use of neostigmine. Also, many elderly will need doses reduced 50% due to creatinine clearances in the 10-50 mL/minute range (common in the aged). Side effects or concomitant disease may warrant use of pyridostigmine.

Dosage Forms Excipient information presented when available (limited, particularly for generics); consult specific product labeling.
Injection, solution, as methylsulfate: 0.5 mg/mL (1 mL, 10 mL); 1 mg/mL (10 mL)
Tablet, as bromide: 15 mg

Selected References
Payne JP, Hughes R, and Al Azawi S, "Neuromuscular Blockade by Neostigmine in Anaesthetized Man," *Br J Anaesth*, 1980, 52(1):69-76.

♦ **Neostigmine Bromide** *see* Neostigmine *on page 1104*

♦ **Neostigmine Methylsulfate** *see* Neostigmine *on page 1104*

♦ **Neo-Synephrine® 12 Hour [OTC]** *see* Oxymetazoline *on page 1184*

♦ **Neo-Synephrine® 12 Hour Extra Moisturizing [OTC]** *see* Oxymetazoline *on page 1184*

♦ **Neo-Synephrine® Extra Strength [OTC]** *see* Phenylephrine *on page 1247*

♦ **Neo-Synephrine® Injection** *see* Phenylephrine *on page 1247*

♦ **Neo-Synephrine® Mild [OTC]** *see* Phenylephrine *on page 1247*

♦ **Neo-Synephrine® Regular Strength [OTC]** *see* Phenylephrine *on page 1247*

Nepafenac (ne pa FEN ak)

U.S. Brand Names Nevanac™
Generic Available No
Pharmacologic Category Nonsteroidal Anti-inflammatory Drug (NSAID), Ophthalmic
Use Treatment of pain and inflammation associated with cataract surgery
Contraindications Hypersensitivity to nepafenac, other NSAIDs, or any component of the formulation
(Continued)

Nepafenac *(Continued)*

Warnings/Precautions Use caution in patients with previous sensitivity to acetylsalicylic acid and phenylacetic acid derivatives, including patients who experience bronchospasm, asthma, rhinitis, or urticaria following NSAID or aspirin. May slow/delay healing or prolong bleeding time following surgery. Use caution in patients with a predisposition to bleeding (bleeding tendencies or medications which interfere with coagulation).

May cause keratitis; continued use of nepafenac in a patient with keratitis may cause severe corneal adverse reactions, potentially resulting in loss of vision. Immediately discontinue use in patients with evidence of corneal epithelial damage.

Use caution in patients with complicated ocular surgeries, corneal denervation, corneal epithelial defects, diabetes mellitus, ocular surface disease, rheumatoid arthritis, or repeat ocular surgeries (within a short timeframe); may be at risk of corneal adverse events, potentially resulting in loss of vision. Use more than 1 day prior to surgery or for 14 days beyond surgery may increase risk and severity of corneal adverse events. Patients using ophthalmic drops should not wear soft contact lenses.

Adverse Reactions (Reflective of adult population; not specific for elderly)
1% to 10%:
Cardiovascular: Hypertension (1% to 4%)
Central nervous system: Headache (1% to 4%)
Gastrointestinal: Nausea (1% to 4%), vomiting (1% to 4%)
Ocular: Capsular opacity (5% to 10%), foreign body sensation (5% to 10%), intraocular pressure increased (5% to 10%), sticky sensation (5% to 10%), visual acuity decreased (5% to 10%), conjunctival edema (1% to 5%), corneal edema (1% to 5%), dry eye (1% to 5%), lid margin crusting (1% to 5%), ocular discomfort (1% to 5%), ocular hyperemia (1% to 5%), ocular pain (1% to 5%), ocular pruritus (1% to 5%), photophobia (1% to 5%), tearing (1% to 5%), vitreous detachment (1% to 5%)
Respiratory: Sinusitis (1% to 4%)

Stability Store at 2°C to 25°C (36°F to 77°F).

Mechanism of Action Nepafenac is a prodrug which once converted to amfenac inhibits prostaglandin synthesis by decreasing the activity of the enzyme, cyclooxygenase, which results in decreased formation of prostaglandin precursors.

Pharmacokinetics
Absorption: Low levels (0.2-0.5 ng/mL) of nepafenac and amfenac are detected in the plasma following ophthalmic administration
Metabolism: Hydrolyzed in ocular tissue to amfenac (active)

Dosage
Geriatrics & Adults: Pain, inflammation associated with cataract surgery: Ophthalmic: Instill 1 drop into affected eye(s) 3 times/day, beginning 1 day prior to surgery, the day of surgery, and through the first 2 weeks of the postoperative period

Administration Shake well prior to use.

Patient Information Do not use nepafenac while wearing contact lenses. Report any abnormal sensations in eye, redness, severe headache, or pain.

Special Geriatric Considerations No differences in safety and efficacy noted between elderly and younger adults. No dosage adjustment necessary. Elderly may be taking other medications that will increase bleeding.

Dosage Forms Excipient information presented when available (limited, particularly for generics); consult specific product labeling.
Suspension, ophthalmic: 0.1% (3 mL) [contains benzalkonium chloride]

♦ **Nephro-Calci®** [OTC] *see* Calcium Salts (Oral) *on page 220*
♦ **Nephro-Fer®** [OTC] *see* Ferrous Fumarate *on page 618*

Nesiritide *(ni SIR i tide)*

Medication Safety Issues
High alert medication: The Institute for Safe Medication Practices (ISMP) includes this medication among its list of drugs which have a heightened risk of causing significant patient harm when used in error.

International issues:
Natrecor® may be confused with Nitrocor® which is a brand name for nitroglycerin in Chile and Italy

U.S. Brand Names Natrecor®
Index Terms B-type Natriuretic Peptide (Human); hBNP; Natriuretic Peptide
Generic Available No
Pharmacologic Category Natriuretic Peptide, B-Type, Human; Vasodilator
Use Treatment of acutely decompensated congestive heart failure (CHF) in patients with dyspnea at rest or with minimal activity

Contraindications Hypersensitivity to natriuretic peptide or any component of the formulation; cardiogenic shock (when used as primary therapy); hypotension (systolic blood pressure <90 mm Hg)

Warnings/Precautions May cause hypotension; administer in clinical situations when blood pressure may be closely monitored. Use caution in patients with systolic blood pressure <100 mm Hg (contraindicated if <90 mm Hg); more likely to experience hypotension. Effects may be additive with other agents capable of causing hypotension. Hypotensive effects may last for several hours.

Should not be used in patients with low cardiac filling pressures, or in patients with conditions which depend on venous return including significant valvular stenosis, restrictive or obstructive cardiomyopathy, constrictive pericarditis, and pericardial tamponade. May be associated with development of azotemia; use caution in patients with renal impairment or in patients where renal perfusion is dependent on renin-angiotensin-aldosterone system; avoid initiation at doses higher than recommended.

Monitor for allergic or anaphylactic reactions. Use caution with prolonged infusions; limited experience for infusions >48 hours.

Adverse Reactions (Reflective of adult population; not specific for elderly)
Note: Frequencies cited below were recorded in VMAC trial at dosages similar to approved labeling. Higher frequencies have been observed in trials using higher dosages of nesiritide. The percentages marked with an asterisk (*) indicate frequency less than or equal to placebo or other standard therapy.
>10%:
  Cardiovascular: Hypotension (total: 11%; symptomatic: 4% at recommended dose, up to 17% at higher doses)
  Renal: Increased serum creatinine (28% with >0.5 mg/dL increase over baseline)
1% to 10%:
  Cardiovascular: Ventricular tachycardia (3%)*, ventricular extrasystoles (3%)*, angina (2%)*, bradycardia (1%), tachycardia, atrial fibrillation, AV node conduction abnormalities
  Central nervous system: Headache (8%)*, dizziness (3%)*, insomnia (2%)*, anxiety (3%), fever, confusion, paresthesia, somnolence, tremor
  Dermatologic: Pruritus, rash
  Gastrointestinal: Nausea (4%)*, abdominal pain (1%)*, vomiting (1%)*
  Hematologic: Anemia
  Local: Injection site reaction
  Neuromuscular & skeletal: Back pain (4%), leg cramps
  Ocular: Amblyopia
  Respiratory: Cough (increased), hemoptysis, apnea
  Miscellaneous: Increased diaphoresis

Overdosage/Toxicology Symptoms of overdose would be expected to include excessive and/or prolonged hypotension. Treatment is symptom-directed and supportive.

Drug Interactions
  ACE inhibitors: An increased frequency of symptomatic hypotension was observed with concurrent administration.
  Diazoxide: Vasodilators may enhance the antihypertensive effect of diazoxide.
  Diuretics: Use caution in patients who may have decreased intravascular volume due to diuretic therapy (risk of hypotension and/or renal impairment may be increased).
  Hypotensive agents: Effects on blood pressure may be additive with nesiritide.

Ethanol/Nutrition/Herb Interactions Herb/Nutraceutical: Avoid bayberry, blue cohosh, cayenne, ephedra, ginger, ginseng (American), kola, and licorice (may increase blood pressure). Avoid black cohosh, California poppy, coleus, golden seal, hawthorn, mistletoe, periwinkle, quinine, and shepherd's purse (may enhance decreased blood pressure).

Stability Vials may be stored below 25°C (77°F); do not freeze. Protect from light. Following reconstitution, vials are stable at 2°C to 25°C (36°F to 77°F) for up to 24 hours. Use reconstituted solution within 24 hours.
Reconstitute 1.5 mg vial with 5 mL of diluent removed from a prefilled 250 mL plastic I.V. bag (compatible with D_5W, $D_5\frac{1}{2}NS$, $D_5\frac{1}{4}NS$, NS). Do not shake vial to dissolve (roll gently). Withdraw entire contents of vial and add to 250 mL I.V. bag. Invert several times to mix. Resultant concentration of solution is ~6 mcg/mL.

Mechanism of Action Binds to guanylate cyclase receptor on vascular smooth muscle and endothelial cells, increasing intracellular cyclic GMP, resulting in smooth muscle cell relaxation. Has been shown to produce dose-dependent reductions in pulmonary capillary wedge pressure (PCWP) and systemic arterial pressure.

Pharmacodynamics
  Onset of action: 15 minutes (60% of 3-hour effect achieved)
  Duration: >60 minutes (up to several hours) for systolic blood pressure. Hemodynamic effects persist longer than serum half-life would predict.

Pharmacokinetics
  Distribution: V_{ss}: 0.19 L/kg
(Continued)

Nesiritide *(Continued)*

Metabolism: Proteolytic cleavage by vascular endopeptidases and proteolysis following receptor binding and cellular internalization

Half-life: Initial (distribution) 2 minutes; Terminal: 18 minutes

Time to peak: 1 hour

Elimination: Renal (via filtration)

Dosage

Geriatrics & Adults:

Congestive heart failure: I.V.: Initial: 2 mcg/kg (bolus); followed by continuous infusion at 0.01 mcg/kg/minute. **Note:** Should not be initiated at a dosage higher than initial recommended dose. There is limited experience with larger doses; in one trial a limited number of patients received higher doses that were increased no faster than every 3 hours by 0.005 mcg/kg/minute (preceded by a bolus of 1 mcg/kg), up to a maximum of 0.03 mcg/kg/minute. Increases beyond the initial infusion rate should be limited to selected patients and accompanied by close hemodynamic and renal function monitoring.

Patients experiencing hypotension during the infusion: Infusion should be interrupted. May attempt to restart at a lower dose (reduce initial infusion dose by 30% and omit bolus).

Renal Impairment: No adjustment required but use cautiously in patients with renal impairment or those patients who rely on the renin-angiotensin-aldosterone system for renal perfusion. Monitor renal function closely.

Hepatic Impairment:

No dosage adjustment recommended.

Administration Do not administer through a heparin-coated catheter (concurrent administration of heparin via a separate catheter is acceptable, per manufacturer).

Prime I.V. tubing with 5 mL of infusion prior to connection with vascular access port and prior to administering bolus or starting the infusion. Withdraw bolus from the prepared infusion bag and administer over 60 seconds. Begin infusion immediately following administration of the bolus.

Monitoring Parameters Blood pressure, hemodynamic responses (PCWP, RAP, CI), BUN, creatinine; urine output

Additional Information The duration of symptomatic improvement with nesiritide following discontinuation of the infusion has been limited (generally lasting several days). Atrial natriuretic peptide, which is related to nesiritide, has been associated with increased vascular permeability. This has not been observed in clinical trials with nesiritide, but patients should be monitored for this effect.

Special Geriatric Considerations No specific data to date; elderly are liable to have hypotension, see Warnings/Precautions for blood pressure criteria. Elderly with reduced renal function should be monitored closely.

Dosage Forms Excipient information presented when available (limited, particularly for generics); consult specific product labeling.

Injection, powder for reconstitution:

Natrecor®: 1.5 mg

Selected References

Colucci WS, Elkayam U, Horton DP, et al, "Intravenous Nesiritide, A Natriuretic Peptide, in the Treatment of Decompensated Congestive Heart Failure. Nesiritide Study Group," *N Engl J Med*, 2000, 343(4):246-53.

Niacin (NYE a sin)

Related Information
Hyperlipidemia Management *on page 1773*

Medication Safety Issues
Sound-alike/look-alike issues:
Niacin may be confused with Minocin®, Niaspan®, Nispan®
Niaspan® may be confused with niacin
Nicobid® may be confused with Nitro-Bid®

International issues:
Niacor® may be confused with Nacor® which is a brand name for enalapril in Spain

U.S. Brand Names Niacin-Time®; Niacor®; Niaspan®; Slo-Niacin® [OTC]

Canadian Brand Names Niaspan®

Index Terms Nicotinic Acid; Vitamin B₃

Generic Available Yes

Pharmacologic Category Antilipemic Agent, Miscellaneous; Vitamin, Water Soluble

Use Adjunctive treatment of dyslipidemias (types IIa and IIb or primary hypercholesterolemia) to lower the risk of recurrent MI and/or slow progression of coronary artery disease, including combination therapy with other antidyslipidemic agents when additional triglyceride-lowering or HDL-increasing effects are desired; treatment of hypertriglyceridemia in patients at risk of pancreatitis; treatment of peripheral vascular disease and circulatory disorders; treatment of pellagra; dietary supplement

Contraindications Hypersensitivity to niacin, niacinamide, or any component of the formulation; active hepatic disease; active peptic ulcer; arterial hemorrhage

Warnings/Precautions Use caution in heavy ethanol users, unstable angina or MI, diabetes (interferes with glucose control), renal disease, active gallbladder disease (can exacerbate), gout, past history of hepatic disease, or with anticoagulants. Monitor glucose and liver function tests. Rare cases of rhabdomyolysis have occurred during concomitant use with HMG-CoA reductase inhibitors. With concurrent use or if symptoms suggestive of myopathy occur, monitor creatinine phosphokinase (CPK) and potassium. Immediate and extended or sustained release products should not be interchanged. Flushing is common and can be attenuated with a gradual increase in dose, and/or by taking aspirin 30-60 minutes before dosing. Compliance is enhanced with twice daily dosing.

Note: Formulations of niacin (regular release versus extended release) are not interchangeable.

Adverse Reactions (Reflective of adult population; not specific for elderly)
Frequency not defined.
Cardiovascular: Arrhythmias, atrial fibrillation, edema, flushing, hypotension, orthostasis, palpitation, syncope (rare), tachycardia
Central nervous system: Chills, dizziness, headache, insomnia, migraine
Dermatologic: Acanthosis nigricans, dry skin, hyperpigmentation, maculopapular rash, pruritus, rash, urticaria
Endocrine & metabolic: Glucose tolerance decreased, gout, phosphorous levels decreased, uric acid level increased
Gastrointestinal: Abdominal pain, dyspepsia, eructation, flatulence, nausea, peptic ulcers, vomiting
Hematologic: Platelet counts decreased, prothrombin time increased
Hepatic: Hepatic necrosis (rare), jaundice, liver enzymes increased
Neuromuscular & skeletal: Leg cramps, myalgia, myasthenia, myopathy (with concurrent HMG-CoA reductase inhibitor), pain, rhabdomyolysis (with concurrent HMG-CoA reductase inhibitor; rare), weakness
Ocular: Cystoid macular edema, toxic amblyopia
Respiratory: Dyspnea
Miscellaneous: Diaphoresis, hypersensitivity reactions (rare)

Overdosage/Toxicology Symptoms of acute overdose include flushing, GI distress, and pruritus. Chronic excessive use has been associated with hepatitis. Antihistamines may relieve niacin-induced histamine release, otherwise, treatment is symptomatic.

Drug Interactions Bile acid sequestrants: May decrease the absorption of niacin; separate administration by 4-6 hours.

Ethanol/Nutrition/Herb Interactions Ethanol: Avoid heavy use; avoid use around niacin dose.

Mechanism of Action Component of two coenzymes which is necessary for tissue respiration, lipid metabolism, and glycogenolysis; inhibits the synthesis of very low density lipoproteins

Pharmacodynamics
Onset of action: Vasodilation occurs within 20 minutes
Duration: 20-60 minutes (extended release preparations persist for 8-10 hours)
(Continued)

Niacin *(Continued)*

Pharmacokinetics

Absorption: Rapid and extensive (60% to 76%)

Distribution: Mainly to hepatic, renal, and adipose tissue

Metabolism: Extensive first-pass effects; converted to nicotinamide adenine dinucleotide, nicotinuric acid, and other metabolites

Half-life: 45 minutes

Time to peak serum concentration: Immediate release formulation: ~45 minutes; extended release formulation: 4-5 hours

Excretion: Urine 60% to 88% (unchanged drug and metabolites)

Dosage

Geriatrics & Adults: Note: Formulations of niacin (regular release versus extended release) are not interchangeable.

Recommended daily allowances:

Male: 25-50 years: 19 mg/day; >51 years: 15 mg/day

Female: 25-50 years: 15 mg/day; >51 years: 13 mg/day

Hyperlipidemia: Oral: Usual target dose: 1.5-6 g/day in 3 divided doses with or after meals using a dosage titration schedule; extended release: 375 mg to 2 g once daily at bedtime

Regular release formulation (Niacor®): Initial: 250 mg once daily (with evening meal); increase frequency and/or dose every 4-7 days to desired response or first-level therapeutic dose (1.5-2 g/day in 2-3 divided doses); after 2 months, may increase at 2- to 4-week intervals to 3 g/day in 3 divided doses

Extended release formulation (Niaspan®): 500 mg at bedtime for 4 weeks, then 1 g at bedtime for 4 weeks; adjust dose to response and tolerance; can increase to a maximum of 2 g/day, but only at 500 mg/day at 4-week intervals

Pellagra: Oral: 50-100 mg 3-4 times/day, maximum: 500 mg/day

Niacin deficiency: Oral: 10-20 mg/day, maximum: 100 mg/day

Renal Impairment: Use with caution.

Hepatic Impairment: Not recommended for use in patients with significant or unexplained hepatic dysfunction.

Administration Administer with food. Administer Niaspan® at bedtime. Niaspan® tablet strengths are not interchangeable. When switching from immediate release tablet, initiate Niaspan® at lower dose and titrate. Long-acting forms should not be crushed, broken, or chewed. Do not substitute long-acting forms for immediate release ones.

Monitoring Parameters Blood glucose; liver function tests (dyslipidemia, high dose, prolonged therapy) pretreatment and every 6-12 weeks for first year then periodically; lipid profile

Test Interactions False elevations in some fluorometric determinations of urinary catecholamines; false-positive urine glucose (Benedict's reagent)

Patient Information May experience transient cutaneous flushing and sensation of warmth, especially of face and upper body; itching or tingling, and headache may occur; may cause GI upset, take with food; if dizziness occurs, avoid sudden changes in posture

Additional Information If flushing is bothersome or persistent, 325 mg of aspirin 30 minutes before each dose or increasing the dose slowly with weekly increase may minimize this reaction; for explicit guidelines on the risk factors for CHD and when to treat high blood cholesterol. See Selected References. Due to liver function test abnormalities induced by sustained release niacin, these dosage forms are not currently recommended

Special Geriatric Considerations The definition of and, therefore, when to treat hyperlipidemia in the elderly is a controversial issue. The National Cholesterol Education Program recommends that all adults maintain a plasma cholesterol <160 mg/dL. Elderly with one additional risk factor, goal LDL would be <130 mg/dL. It is the authors' belief that pharmacologic treatment is reserved for those who are unable to obtain a desirable plasma cholesterol concentration by diet alone and for whom the benefits of treatment are believed to outweigh the potential adverse effects, drug interactions, and cost of treatment.

Dosage Forms Excipient information presented when available (limited, particularly for generics); consult specific product labeling.

Capsule, extended release: 125 mg, 250 mg, 400 mg, 500 mg

Capsule, timed release: 250 mg, 500 mg

Tablet: 50 mg, 100 mg, 250 mg, 500 mg

Niacor®: 500 mg

Tablet, controlled release (Slo-Niacin®): 250 mg, 500 mg, 750 mg

Tablet, extended release (Niaspan®): 500 mg, 750 mg, 1000 mg

Tablet, timed release: 250 mg, 500 mg, 750 mg, 1000 mg

Niacin-Time®: 500 mg

Selected References
"Executive Summary of The Third Report of The National Cholesterol Education Program (NCEP) Expert Panel on Detection, Evaluation, and Treatment of High Blood Cholesterol in Adults (Adult Treatment Panel III)," *JAMA*, 2001, 285(19):2486-97.

Niacinamide (nye a SIN a mide)

Medication Safety Issues
Sound-alike/look-alike issues:
Niacinamide may be confused with niCARdipine
U.S. Brand Names Nicomide-T™
Index Terms Nicotinamide; Nicotinic Acid Amide; Vitamin B_3
Generic Available Yes: Tablet
Pharmacologic Category Vitamin, Water Soluble
Use
Oral: Prophylaxis and treatment of pellagra
Topical: Improve the appearance of acne and decrease visible inflammation and irritation caused by acne medications
Contraindications Hypersensitivity to niacin, niacinamide, or any component of the formulation; liver disease; active peptic ulcer
Warnings/Precautions Large doses should be administered with caution to patients with gallbladder disease or diabetes; monitor blood glucose; may elevate uric acid levels; use with caution in patients predisposed to gout; some products may contain tartrazine
Adverse Reactions (Reflective of adult population; not specific for elderly)
Frequency not defined.
Cardiovascular: Tachycardia
Dermatologic: Increased sebaceous gland activity, rash
Endocrine & metabolic: Hyperglycemia, hyperuricemia
Gastrointestinal: Bloating, flatulence, nausea
Neuromuscular & skeletal: Paresthesia in extremities
Ocular: Blurred vision
Respiratory: Wheezing
Overdosage/Toxicology Symptoms include GI distress. Treatment is supportive.
Mechanism of Action Used by the body as a source of niacin; is a component of two coenzymes which is necessary for tissue respiration, lipid metabolism, and glycogenolysis; does not have hypolipidemia or vasodilating effects. Niacinamide has anti-inflammatory properties which are believed to help decrease inflammatory acne lesions.
Pharmacokinetics
Absorption: Oral: Rapid; Topical: Absorbed systemically
Metabolism: In the liver
Half-life: 45 minutes
Time to peak, serum concentration: 20-70 minutes
Excretion: Urine (as metabolites)
Dosage
Geriatrics & Adults:
Pellagra: Oral: 300-500 mg/day
Acne: Topical: Apply to affected area on face twice daily
Administration Topical: Prior to using cream or gel, wash face with mild cleanser. Apply thin layer to affected area. May apply under make-up or other acne medications. Re-evaluate after 8-12 weeks.
Test Interactions False elevations of urinary catecholamines in some fluorometric determinations
Special Geriatric Considerations Should not be confused with niacin.
Dosage Forms Excipient information presented when available (limited, particularly for generics); consult specific product labeling.
Cream (Nicomide-T™): 4% (30 g) [contains benzyl alcohol]
Gel (Nicomide-T™): 4% (30 g) [contains alcohol]
Tablet: 100 mg, 250 mg, 500 mg

Niacin and Lovastatin (NYE a sin & LOE va sta tin)

Related Information
Lovastatin *on page 936*
Niacin *on page 1109*
Medication Safety Issues
Sound-alike/look-alike issues:
Advicor® may be confused with Advair, Altocor™
(Continued)

Niacin and Lovastatin *(Continued)*

U.S. Brand Names Advicor®
Canadian Brand Names Advicor®
Index Terms Lovastatin and Niacin
Generic Available No
Pharmacologic Category Antilipemic Agent, HMG-CoA Reductase Inhibitor; Antilipemic Agent, Miscellaneous
Use Treatment of primary hypercholesterolemia (heterozygous familial and nonfamilial) and mixed dyslipidemia (Fredrickson types IIa and IIb) in patients previously treated with either agent alone (patients who require further lowering of triglycerides or increase in HDL cholesterol from addition of niacin or further lowering of LDL cholesterol from addition of lovastatin). Combination product; not intended for initial treatment.
Contraindications Hypersensitivity to lovastatin, niacin, or any component of the formulation; active liver disease; unexplained persistent elevations of serum transaminases; active peptic ulcer disease; arterial bleeding
Warnings/Precautions Liver function must be monitored by periodic laboratory assessment. Use with caution in patients who consume large amounts of ethanol or who have a history of liver disease.

Myopathy and/or rhabdomyolysis with acute renal failure has occurred with HMG-CoA reductase inhibitors. Combination with niacin may increase the risk of this event, and patients should be monitored closely, particularly at higher doses (niacin >1 g/day). Risk is increased with concurrent use of azole antifungals, clarithromycin, cyclosporine, danazol, diltiazem, erythromycin, fibric acid derivatives, fluvoxamine, indinavir, nefazodone, nelfinavir, ritonavir, troleandomycin, verapamil, or large quantities of grapefruit juice. Monitor closely if used with other drugs associated with myopathy (eg, colchicine). Weigh the risk versus benefit when combining any of these drugs with lovastatin. Temporarily discontinue for elective major surgery, acute medical or surgical conditions, or in any patient experiencing an acute or serious condition predisposing to renal failure secondary to rhabdomyolysis.

Use caution in unstable angina or CAD (risk of arrhythmias at high doses), diabetes (may interfere with glucose control), renal disease, active gallbladder disease (may exacerbate), or gout. Flushing is a common adverse effect of niacin and may be attenuated with a gradual increase in dose. Tablet strengths are not interchangeable.
Adverse Reactions (Reflective of adult population; not specific for elderly)
>10%: Cardiovascular: Flushing (71%)
1% to 10%:
  Central nervous system: Headache (9%), pain (8%)
  Dermatologic: Pruritus (7%), rash (5%)
  Endocrine & metabolic: Hyperglycemia (4%)
  Gastrointestinal: Nausea (7%), diarrhea (6%), abdominal pain (4%), dyspepsia (3%), vomiting (3%)
  Neuromuscular & skeletal: Back pain (5%), weakness (5%), myalgia (3%)
  Miscellaneous: Flu-like syndrome (6%)
Drug Interactions Lovastatin: **Substrate** of CYP3A4 (major); **Inhibits** CYP2C9 (weak), 2D6 (weak), 3A4 (weak)
Also see individual agents.
Ethanol/Nutrition/Herb Interactions
Ethanol: Consumption of large amounts of ethanol may increase the risk of liver damage with HMG-CoA reductase inhibitors.
Food: Lovastatin absorption may be decreased with food, however, the combination product is recommended to be taken with a low-fat snack at bedtime. Lovastatin serum concentrations may be increased if taken with grapefruit juice; avoid concurrent use. Red yeast rice contains an estimated 2.4 mg lovastatin per 600 mg rice.
Herb/Nutraceutical: St John's wort may decrease lovastatin levels.
Stability Store at 20°C to 25°C (68°F to 77°F).
Mechanism of Action Lovastatin acts by competitively inhibiting 3-hydroxyl-3-methylglutaryl-coenzyme A (HMG-CoA) reductase, the enzyme that catalyzes the rate-limiting step in cholesterol biosynthesis. Niacin is a component of two coenzymes which is necessary for tissue respiration, lipid metabolism, and glycogenolysis; inhibits the synthesis of very low density lipoproteins.
Pharmacokinetics See individual agents.
Dosage
  Geriatrics & Adults: Dosage forms are a fixed combination of niacin and lovastatin.
    Dyslipidemia: Oral: Lowest dose: Niacin 500 mg/lovastatin 20 mg; may increase by not more than 500 mg (niacin) at 4-week intervals (maximum dose: niacin 2000 mg/lovastatin 40 mg daily); should be taken at bedtime with a low-fat snack
    Note: Not for use as initial therapy of dyslipidemias. May be substituted for equivalent dose of Niaspan®, however, manufacturer does not recommend direct substitution with other niacin products.

Administration Tablet must be swallowed whole; do not crush or chew. Should be taken with a low-fat snack at bedtime.

Monitoring Parameters Obtain baseline LFTs and total cholesterol profile. LFTs should be performed before initiation of therapy, at 6- and 12 weeks after initiation or first dose, and periodically thereafter. Monitor blood glucose.

Test Interactions Niacin: False elevations in some fluorometric determinations of urinary catecholamines; false-positive urine glucose (Benedict's reagent)

Special Geriatric Considerations The definition of and, therefore, when to treat hyperlipidemia in the elderly is a controversial issue. The National Cholesterol Education Program recommends that all adults maintain a plasma cholesterol <160 mg/dL. Elderly with one additional risk factor, goal LDL would be <130 mg/dL. It is the authors' belief that pharmacologic treatment be reserved for those who are unable to obtain a desirable plasma cholesterol concentration by diet alone and for whom the benefits of treatment are believed to outweigh the potential adverse effects, drug interactions, and cost of treatment.

Dosage Forms Excipient information presented when available (limited, particularly for generics); consult specific product labeling.

Tablet, variable release (Advicor®):

500/20: Niacin 500 mg [extended release] and lovastatin 20 mg [immediate release] [contains polysorbate 80]

750/20: Niacin 750 mg [extended release] and lovastatin 20 mg [immediate release] [contains polysorbate 80]

1000/20: Niacin 1000 mg [extended release] and lovastatin 20 mg [immediate release] [contains polysorbate 80]

1000/40: Niacin 1000 mg [extended release] and lovastatin 40 mg [immediate release] [contains polysorbate 80]

♦ **Niacin-Time**® *see* Niacin *on page 1109*

♦ **Niacor**® *see* Niacin *on page 1109*

♦ **Niaspan**® *see* Niacin *on page 1109*

NiCARdipine (nye KAR de peen)

Related Information
Calcium Channel Blockers *on page 1753*

Medication Safety Issues

Sound-alike/look-alike issues:

NiCARdipine may be confused with niacinamide, NIFEdipine, nimodipine

Cardene® may be confused with Cardizem®, Cardura®, codeine

International issues:

Cardene® may be confused with Cardem® which is a brand name for celiprolol in Spain

Cardene® may be confused with Cardin® which is a brand name for methyldopa in Brazil and a brand name for simvastatin in Poland

Significant differences exist between oral and I.V. dosing. Use caution when converting from one route of administration to another.

U.S. Brand Names Cardene®; Cardene® I.V.; Cardene® SR

Index Terms Nicardipine Hydrochloride

Generic Available Yes: Capsule

Pharmacologic Category Calcium Channel Blocker

Use Treatment of chronic stable angina; management of essential hypertension

Unlabeled/Investigational Use Treatment of congestive heart failure

Contraindications Hypersensitivity to nicardipine or any component of the formulation; advanced aortic stenosis; severe hypotension; cardiogenic shock; ventricular tachycardia

Warnings/Precautions Symptomatic hypotension with or without syncope can rarely occur; blood pressure must be lowered at a rate appropriate for the patient's clinical condition. Reflex tachycardia may occur with use. The most common side effect is peripheral edema; occurs within 2-3 weeks of starting therapy. Use with caution in CAD (can cause increase in angina), CHF (can worsen heart failure symptoms), hypertrophic cardiomyopathy, and pheochromocytoma (limited clinical experience). Peripheral infusion sites (for I.V. therapy) should be changed ever 12 hours. Titrate I.V. dose cautiously in patients with CHF, renal, or hepatic dysfunction. Use the I.V. form cautiously in patients with portal hypertension (can cause increase in hepatic pressure gradient). Abrupt withdrawal may cause rebound angina in patients with CAD.

Adverse Reactions (Reflective of adult population; not specific for elderly)

1% to 10%:

Cardiovascular: Flushing (6% to 10%), palpitation (3% to 4%), tachycardia (1% to 4%), peripheral edema (dose related 7% to 8%), increased angina (dose related 6%), hypotension (I.V. 6%), orthostasis (I.V. 1%)

(Continued)

NiCARdipine *(Continued)*

Central nervous system: Headache (6% to 15%), dizziness (4% to 7%), somnolence (4% to 6%)

Dermatologic: Rash (1%)

Gastrointestinal: Nausea (2% to 5%), dry mouth (1%)

Genitourinary: Polyuria (1%)

Local: Injection site reaction (I.V. 1%)

Neuromuscular & skeletal: Weakness (4% to 6%), myalgia (1%), paresthesia (1%)

Miscellaneous: Diaphoresis

Overdosage/Toxicology Primary cardiac symptoms of calcium blocker overdose include hypotension and bradycardia. Hypotension is caused by peripheral vasodilation, myocardial depression, and bradycardia. Bradycardia results from sinus bradycardia, second- or third-degree atrioventricular block, or sinus arrest with junctional rhythm. Intraventricular conduction is usually not affected so the QRS duration is normal (verapamil prolongs the PR interval and bepridil prolongs the QT interval and may cause ventricular arrhythmias, including torsade de pointes).

Noncardiac symptoms include confusion, stupor, nausea, vomiting, metabolic acidosis, and hyperglycemia. Following initial gastric decontamination, if possible, repeated calcium administration may promptly reverse depressed cardiac contractility (but not sinus node depression or peripheral vasodilation). Glucagon, epinephrine, and inamrinone (amrinone) may treat refractory hypotension. Glucagon and epinephrine also increase the heart rate (outside the U.S., 4-aminopyridine may be available as an antidote). Dialysis and hemoperfusion are not effective in enhancing elimination, although repeat-dose activated charcoal may serve as an adjunct with sustained-release preparations.

In a few reported cases, overdose with calcium channel blockers has been associated with hypotension and bradycardia, initially refractory to atropine, but becoming more responsive to this agent when larger doses (approaching 1 g/hour for more than 24 hours) of calcium chloride were administered.

Drug Interactions Substrate of CYP1A2 (minor), 2C9 (minor), 2D6 (minor), 2E1 (minor), 3A4 (major); **Inhibits** CYP2C9 (strong), 2C19 (moderate), 2D6 (moderate), 3A4 (strong)

Azole antifungals may inhibit the calcium channel blocker's metabolism; avoid this combination. Try an antifungal like terbinafine (if appropriate) or monitor closely for altered effect of the calcium channel blocker.

Calcium may reduce the calcium channel blocker's effects, particularly hypotension.

Cyclosporine's serum concentrations are increased by nicardipine; avoid this combination. Use another calcium channel blocker or monitor cyclosporine trough levels and renal function closely. Tacrolimus may be affected similarly.

CYP2C9 Substrates: Nicardipine may increase the levels/effects of CYP2C9 substrates. Example substrates include bosentan, dapsone, fluoxetine, glimepiride, glipizide, losartan, montelukast, nateglinide, paclitaxel, phenytoin, warfarin, and zafirlukast.

CYP2C19 substrates: Nicardipine may increase the levels/effects of CYP2C19 substrates. Example substrates include citalopram, diazepam, methsuximide, phenytoin, propranolol, and sertraline.

CYP2D6 substrates: Nicardipine may increase the levels/effects of CYP2D6 substrates. Example substrates include amphetamines, selected beta-blockers, dextromethorphan, fluoxetine, lidocaine, mirtazapine, nefazodone, paroxetine, risperidone, ritonavir, thioridazine, tricyclic antidepressants, and venlafaxine.

CYP2D6 prodrug substrates: Nicardipine may decrease the levels/effects of CYP2D6 prodrug substrates. Example prodrug substrates include codeine, hydrocodone, oxycodone, and tramadol.

CYP3A4 inducers: CYP3A4 inducers may decrease the levels/effects of nicardipine. Example inducers include aminoglutethimide, carbamazepine, nafcillin, nevirapine, phenobarbital, phenytoin, and rifamycins.

CYP3A4 inhibitors: May increase the levels/effects of nicardipine. Example inhibitors include azole antifungals, clarithromycin, diclofenac, doxycycline, erythromycin, imatinib, isoniazid, nefazodone, propofol, protease inhibitors, quinidine, telithromycin, and verapamil.

CYP3A4 substrates: Nicardipine may increase the levels/effects of CYP3A4 substrates. Example substrates include benzodiazepines, calcium channel blockers, mirtazapine, nateglinide, nefazodone, tacrolimus, and venlafaxine. Selected benzodiazepines (midazolam and triazolam), cisapride, ergot alkaloids, selected HMG-CoA reductase inhibitors (lovastatin and simvastatin), and pimozide are generally contraindicated with strong CYP3A4 inhibitors.

Metoprolol: Concentration of metoprolol is increased by 25% with concurrent use.

Nafcillin decreases plasma concentration of nicardipine; avoid this combination.

Propranolol: May decrease the metabolism of nicardipine.

Protease inhibitor like amprenavir and ritonavir may increase nicardipine's serum concentration.

Rifampin increases the metabolism of the calcium channel blocker; adjust the dose of the calcium channel blocker to maintain efficacy.

Sildenafil, tadalafil, vardenafil: Blood pressure-lowering effects may be additive; use caution.

Vecuronium: Clearance of vecuronium is decreased by 25% with use of I.V. nicardipine; reduce dose of muscle relaxant.

Ethanol/Nutrition/Herb Interactions

Ethanol: Avoid ethanol (may increase CNS depression).

Food: Nicardipine average peak concentrations may be decreased if taken with food. Serum concentrations/toxicity of nicardipine may be increased by grapefruit juice; avoid concurrent use.

Herb/Nutraceutical: St John's wort may decrease levels. Avoid dong quai if using for hypertension (has estrogenic activity). Avoid ephedra, yohimbe, ginseng (may worsen hypertension). Avoid garlic (may have increased antihypertensive effect).

Stability Store at room temperature; stable for 24 hours at room temperature. Protect from light.

Mechanism of Action Inhibits calcium ion from entering the "slow channels" or select voltage-sensitive areas of vascular smooth muscle and myocardium during depolarization, producing a relaxation of coronary vascular smooth muscle and coronary vasodilation; increases myocardial oxygen delivery in patients with vasospastic angina

Pharmacokinetics

Absorption: Oral: Well absorbed, ~100%

Protein binding: 95%

Metabolism: Extensive first-pass metabolism; only metabolized in the liver

Bioavailability: Absolute, 35%

Half-life: 2-4 hours

Time to peak serum concentrations: Within 20-120 minutes and an onset of hypotension occurs within 20 minutes

Elimination: As metabolites in urine

Dosage

Geriatrics & Adults:

Angina: Immediate release: Oral: 20 mg 3 times/day; usual range: 60-120 mg/day; increase dose at 3-day intervals

Hypertension: Oral:

Immediate release: Initial: 20 mg 3 times/day; usual: 20-40 mg 3 times/day (allow 3 days between dose increases)

Sustained release: Initial: 30 mg twice daily, titrate up to 60 mg twice daily

Note: The total daily dose of immediate-release product may not automatically be equivalent to the daily sustained-release dose; use caution in converting.

Acute hypertension: I.V. (dilute to 0.1 mg/mL): Initial: 5 mg/hour increased by 2.5 mg/hour every 15 minutes to a maximum of 15 mg/hour; consider reduction to 3 mg/hour after response is achieved. Monitor and titrate to lowest dose necessary to maintain stable blood pressure.

Substitution for oral therapy (approximate equivalents):

20 mg every 8 hours oral, equivalent to 0.5 mg/hour I.V. infusion

30 mg every 8 hours oral, equivalent to 1.2 mg/hour I.V. infusion

40 mg every 8 hours oral, equivalent to 2.2 mg/hour I.V. infusion

Renal Impairment: Titrate dose beginning with 20 mg 3 times/day (immediate release) or 30 mg twice daily (sustained release). Specific guidelines for adjustment of I.V. nicardipine are not available, but careful monitoring/adjustment is warranted.

Hepatic Impairment: Starting dose: 20 mg twice daily (immediate release) with titration. Refer to "Note" in adult dosing. Specific guidelines for adjustment of I.V. nicardipine are not available, but careful monitoring/adjustment is warranted.

Administration

Oral: The total daily dose of immediate-release product may not automatically be equivalent to the daily sustained-release dose; use caution in converting. Do not chew or crush the sustained release formulation, swallow whole. Do not open or cut capsules.

I.V.: Ampuls must be diluted before use. Administer as a slow continuous infusion.

Monitoring Parameters Heart rate, signs and symptoms of CHF; monitor blood pressure 1, 2, and 8 hours after dosing; measure sustained release blood pressure at 2, 4, and 6 hours after dosing

Reference Range Therapeutic: 28-50 ng/mL

Patient Information Sustained release products should be taken with food and not crushed; limit caffeine intake; avoid alcohol; notify physician if angina pain is not reduced when taking this drug, irregular heartbeat, shortness of breath, swelling, dizziness, constipation, nausea, or hypotension occur; do not stop therapy without advice of physician

(Continued)

NiCARdipine *(Continued)*

Additional Information The FDA's Cardiovascular and Renal Drug Advisory Committee reviewed current data regarding the risk of heart attacks in patients treated with calcium channel blockers and determined that as a class, the calcium channel antagonists are safe; however, they warned that short-acting nifedipine could increase the risk of myocardial infarction in some patients. The committee was in agreement with a statement issued September, 1995 by the National Heart Lung, and Blood Institute of the National Institute of Health, that warned that short-acting nifedipine should be used with great caution especially at higher doses.

Special Geriatric Considerations Elderly may experience a greater hypotensive response. Constipation may be more of a problem in the elderly. Calcium channel blockers are no more effective in the elderly than other therapies; however, they do not cause significant CNS effects which is an advantage over some antihypertensive agents.

Dosage Forms Excipient information presented when available (limited, particularly for generics); consult specific product labeling.
Capsule (Cardene®): 20 mg, 30 mg
Capsule, sustained release (Cardene® SR): 30 mg, 45 mg, 60 mg
Injection, solution (Cardene® IV): 2.5 mg/mL (10 mL)

- ◆ **Nicardipine Hydrochloride** *see* NiCARdipine *on page 1113*
- ◆ **NicoDerm® CQ® [OTC]** *see* Nicotine *on page 1116*
- ◆ **Nicomide-T™** *see* Niacinamide *on page 1111*
- ◆ **Nicorette® [OTC]** *see* Nicotine *on page 1116*
- ◆ **Nicotinamide** *see* Niacinamide *on page 1111*

Nicotine *(nik oh TEEN)*

Medication Safety Issues
Sound-alike/look-alike issues:
NicoDerm® may be confused with Nitroderm
Nicorette® may be confused with Nordette®

Transdermal patch may contain conducting metal (eg, aluminum); remove patch prior to MRI.

U.S. Brand Names Commit® [OTC]; NicoDerm® CQ® [OTC]; Nicorette® [OTC]; Nicotrol® Inhaler; Nicotrol® NS

Canadian Brand Names Habitrol®; Nicoderm®; Nicorette®; Nicorette® Plus; Nicotrol®

Index Terms Habitrol

Generic Available Yes: Transdermal patch and gum

Pharmacologic Category Smoking Cessation Aid

Use Treatment aid to smoking cessation for the relief of nicotine withdrawal symptoms (including nicotine craving) while participating in a behavioral modification program under medical supervision

Unlabeled/Investigational Use Management of ulcerative colitis (transdermal)

Contraindications Hypersensitivity to nicotine or any component of the formulation; patients who are smoking during the postmyocardial infarction period; patients with life-threatening arrhythmias, or severe or worsening angina pectoris; active temporomandibular joint disease (gum)

Warnings/Precautions The risk versus the benefits must be weighed for each of these groups: patients with CAD, serious cardiac arrhythmias, vasospastic disease. Use caution in patients with hyperthyroidism, pheochromocytoma, or insulin-dependent diabetes. Use with caution in oropharyngeal inflammation and in patients with history of esophagitis, peptic ulcer, coronary artery disease, vasospastic disease, angina, hypertension, pheochromocytoma, severe renal dysfunction, and hepatic dysfunction. The inhaler should be used with caution in patients with bronchospastic disease (other forms of nicotine replacement may be preferred). Use of nasal product is not recommended with chronic nasal disorders (eg, allergy, rhinitis, nasal polyps, and sinusitis). Transdermal patch may contain conducting metal (eg, aluminum); remove patch prior to MRI. Cautious use of topical nicotine in patients with certain skin diseases. Hypersensitivity to the topical products can occur. Dental problems may be worsened by chewing the gum. Urge patients to stop smoking completely when initiating therapy.

Adverse Reactions (Reflective of adult population; not specific for elderly)
Nasal spray/inhaler:
>10%:
Central nervous system: Headache (18% to 26%)
Gastrointestinal: Inhaler: Mouth/throat irritation (66%), dyspepsia (18%)
Respiratory: Inhaler: Cough (32%), rhinitis (23%)
1% to 10%:
Dermatologic: Acne (3%)
Endocrine & metabolic: Dysmenorrhea (3%)

Gastrointestinal: Flatulence (4%), gum problems (4%), diarrhea, hiccup, nausea, taste disturbance, tooth disorder

Neuromuscular & skeletal: Back pain (6%), arthralgia (5%), jaw/neck pain

Respiratory: Sinusitis

Miscellaneous: Withdrawal symptoms

Adverse events previously reported in prescription labeling for chewing gum, lozenge and/or transdermal systems. Frequency not defined; may be product or dose specific:

Central nervous system: Concentration impaired, depression, dizziness, headache, insomnia, nervousness, pain

Gastrointestinal: Aphthous stomatitis, constipation, cough, diarrhea, dyspepsia, flatulence, gingival bleeding, glossitis, hiccups, jaw pain, nausea, salivation increased, stomatitis, taste perversion, tooth disorder, ulcerative stomatitis, xerostomia

Dermatologic: Rash

Local: Application site reaction, local edema, local erythema

Neuromuscular & skeletal: Arthralgia, myalgia, paresthesia

Respiratory: Cough, sinusitis

Miscellaneous: Allergic reaction, diaphoresis

Overdosage/Toxicology Symptoms include nausea, vomiting, abdominal pain, mental confusion, diarrhea, salivation, tachycardia, respiratory and cardiovascular collapse. Treatment after decontamination is symptomatic and supportive. Remove the patch, rinse the area with water and dry; do not use soap as this may increase absorption.

Nicotine nasal spray: Fatal dose: 40 mg

Drug Interactions Substrate (minor) of CYP1A2, 2A6, 2B6, 2C9, 2C19, 2D6, 2E1, 3A4; **Inhibits** CYP2A6 (weak), 2E1 (weak)

Adenosine: Nicotine increases the hemodynamic and AV blocking effects of adenosine; monitor

Bupropion: Monitor for treatment-emergent hypertension in patients treated with the combination of nicotine patch and bupropion

Cimetidine; May increases serum nicotine concentrations; therefore, may decrease amount of gum or patches needed

Ethanol/Nutrition/Herb Interactions Food: Lozenge: Acidic foods/beverages decrease absorption of nicotine.

Stability Nicotrol®: Store inhaler cartridge at room temperature not to exceed 30°C (86°F). Protect cartridges from light.

Mechanism of Action Nicotine is one of two naturally-occurring alkaloids which exhibit their primary effects via autonomic ganglia stimulation. The other alkaloid is lobeline which has many actions similar to those of nicotine but is less potent. Nicotine is a potent ganglionic and central nervous system stimulant, the actions of which are mediated via nicotine-specific receptors. Biphasic actions are observed depending upon the dose administered. The main effect of nicotine in small doses is stimulation of all autonomic ganglia; with larger doses, initial stimulation is followed by blockade of transmission. Biphasic effects are also evident in the adrenal medulla; discharge of catecholamines occurs with small doses, whereas prevention of catecholamines release is seen with higher doses as a response to splanchnic nerve stimulation. Stimulation of the central nervous system (CNS) is characterized by tremors and respiratory excitation. However, convulsions may occur with higher doses, along with respiratory failure secondary to both central paralysis and peripheral blockade to respiratory muscles.

Pharmacodynamics Duration: Transdermal: 24 hours

Pharmacokinetics Intranasal nicotine may more closely approximate the time course of plasma nicotine levels observed after cigarette smoking than other dosage forms

Absorption: Transdermal: Slow

Metabolism: In the liver, primarily to cotinine, which is ⅕ as active

Half-life, elimination: 4 hours

Time to peak serum concentration: Transdermal: 8-9 hours

Elimination: Via the kidneys; renal clearance is pH-dependent

Oral:

Absorption: Dependent upon the vigor and duration of chewing

Half-life: ~4 hours

Dosage

Geriatrics & Adults:

Tobacco cessation (patients should be advised to completely stop smoking upon initiation of therapy):

Gum: Chew 1 piece of gum when urge to smoke, up to 24 pieces/day. Patients who smoke <25 cigarettes/day should start with 2-mg strength; patients smoking

(Continued)

Nicotine (Continued)

≥25 cigarettes/day should start with the 4-mg strength. Use according to the following 12-week dosing schedule:

Weeks 1-6: Chew 1 piece of gum every 1-2 hours; to increase chances of quitting, chew at least 9 pieces/day during the first 6 weeks

Weeks 7-9: Chew 1 piece of gum every 2-4 hours

Weeks 10-12: Chew 1 piece of gum every 4-8 hours

Inhaler: Oral: Usually 6-16 cartridges per day; best effect was achieved by frequent continuous puffing (20 minutes); recommended duration of treatment is 3 months, after which patients may be weaned from the inhaler by gradual reduction of the daily dose over 6-12 weeks

Lozenge: Oral: Patients who smoke their first cigarette within 30 minutes of waking should use the 4-mg strength; otherwise the 2-mg strength is recommended. Use according to the following 12-week dosing schedule:

Weeks 1-6: One lozenge every 1-2 hours

Weeks 7-9: One lozenge every 2-4 hours

Weeks 10-12: One lozenge every 4-8 hours

Note: Use at least 9 lozenges/day during first 6 weeks to improve chances of quitting; do not use more than one lozenge at a time (maximum: 5 lozenges every 6 hours, 20 lozenges/day)

Spray: Nasal: 1-2 sprays/hour; do not exceed more than 5 doses (10 sprays) per hour [maximum: 40 doses/day (80 sprays); each dose (2 sprays) contains 1 mg of nicotine

Transdermal patch: Topical: Apply new patch every 24 hours to nonhairy, clean, dry skin on the upper body or upper outer arm; each patch should be applied to a different site. (**Note:** Adjustment may be required during initial treatment (move to higher dose if experiencing withdrawal symptoms; lower dose if side effects are experienced).

NicoDerm CQ®:

Patients smoking ≥10 cigarettes/day: Begin with step 1 (21 mg/day) for 4-6 weeks, **followed by** step 2 (14 mg/day) for 2 weeks; **finish with** step 3 (7 mg/day) for 2 weeks

Patients smoking <10 cigarettes/day: Begin with step 2 (14 mg/day) for 6 weeks, **followed by** step 3 (7 mg/day) for 2 weeks

Note: Initial starting dose for patients <100 pounds, history of cardiovascular disease: 14 mg/day for 4-6 weeks, **followed by** 7 mg/day for 2-4 weeks

Note: Patients who are receiving >600 mg/day of cimetidine: Decrease to the next lower patch size

Benefits of use of nicotine transdermal patches beyond 3 months have not been demonstrated

Ulcerative colitis (unlabeled use): Topical: Transdermal: Titrated to 22-25 mg/day

Administration

Gum: Should be chewed slowly to avoid jaw ache and to maximize benefit. Chew slowly until it tingles, then park gum between cheek and gum until tingle is gone; repeat process until most of tingle is gone (~30 minutes).

Lozenge: Should not be chewed or swallowed; allow to dissolve slowly (~20-30 minutes)

Transdermal patch: Do not cut patch; causes rapid evaporation, rendering the patch useless

Monitoring Parameters Smoking habit, blood pressure, pulse, sleeping, and mood; monitor skin for side effects if transdermal system used

Patient Information Instructions for the proper use of the patch should be given to the patient; notify physician if persistent rash, itching, or burning may occur with the patch; do not smoke while wearing patches

Special Geriatric Considerations Must evaluate benefit in the elderly who may have chronic diseases mentioned in Warning and Contraindications. The transdermal systems are as effective in the elderly as they are in younger adults; however, complaints of body aches, dizziness, and asthenia were reported more often in the elderly.

Dosage Forms Excipient information presented when available (limited, particularly for generics); consult specific product labeling.

Gum, chewing, as polacrilex: 2 mg (20s, 50s, 110s); 4 mg (20s, 50s, 110s)

Nicorette®:

2 mg (48s, 50s, 108s, 110s, 168s, 170s, 192s, 200s, 216s) [original and mint flavors]; (48s, 108s, 110s) [orange flavor]; (40s, 100s) [contains calcium 94 mg/gum and sodium 11 mg/gum; fresh mint and fruit chill flavors]

4 mg (48s, 50s, 108s, 110s, 168s, 170s, 192s, 200s, 216s) [original and mint flavors]; (48s, 108s, 110s) [orange flavor]; (40s, 100s) [contains calcium 94 mg/gum and sodium 13 mg/gum; fresh mint and fruit chill flavors]

Lozenge, as polacrilex:
Commit®:
2 mg (48s, 72s, 84s, 168s) [contains phenylalanine 3.4 mg/lozenge, sodium 18 mg/lozenge; mint flavor]; (108s) [contains phenylalanine 3.4 mg/lozenge, sodium 18 mg/lozenge; original flavor]
4 mg (48s, 72s, 84s, 168s, 192s) [contains phenylalanine 3.4 mg/lozenge, sodium 18 mg/lozenge; mint flavor]; (108s) [contains phenylalanine 3.4 mg/lozenge, sodium 18 mg/lozenge; original flavor]
Oral inhalation system:
Nicotrol® Inhaler: 10 mg cartridge (168s) [cartridge delivers nicotine 4 mg; each unit consists of 5 mouthpieces, 28 storage trays each containing 6 cartridges, and 1 storage case]
Patch, transdermal: 7 mg/24 (30s); 14 mg/24 hours (30s); 21 mg/24 hours (30s)
NicoDerm® CQ®: 7 mg/24 hours (14s) [step 3; available in tan or clear patch]; 14 mg/24 hours (14s) [step 2; available in tan or clear patch]; 21 mg/24 hours (7s, 14s) [step 1; available in tan or clear patch]
Solution, intranasal [spray]:
Nicotrol® NS: 10 mg/mL (10 mL) [delivers 0.5 mg/spray; 200 sprays]

Selected References

Benowitz NL, Jacob P 3rd, and Sachs DP, "Deficient C-oxidation of Nicotine," Clin Pharmacol Ther, 1995, 57(5):590-4.

Benowitz NL, "Pharmacologic Aspects of Cigarette Smoking and Nicotine Addiction," N Engl J Med, 1988, 319(20):1318-30.

Blanchard J, "Nicotine," Clin Toxicol Rev, 1993, 15:11-2.

Harchelroad F, Potts K, Burdick J, et al, "Oral Absorption of Nicotine From Transdermal Therapeutic Systems," Vet Hum Toxicol, 1992, 34:332.

Ottervanger JP, Festen JM, de Vries AG, et al, "Acute Myocardial Infarction While Using The Nicotine," Chest, 1995, 107(6):1765-6.

Ross MP, Revolinski D, and Taurman L, "Green Tobacco Sickness Among Adults in Kentucky," Vet Hum Toxicol, 1994, 36:360.

Svensson CK, "Clinical Pharmacokinetics of Nicotine," Clin Pharmacokinet, 1987, 12(1):30-40.

Thomas GA, Rhodes J, Mani V, et al, "Transdermal Nicotine as Maintenance Therapy for Ulcerative Colitis," N Engl J Med, 1995, 332(15):988-92.

♦ **Nicotinic Acid** see Niacin on page 1109
♦ **Nicotinic Acid Amide** see Niacinamide on page 1111
♦ **Nicotrol® Inhaler** see Nicotine on page 1116
♦ **Nicotrol® NS** see Nicotine on page 1116
♦ **Nifediac™ CC** see NIFEdipine on page 1119
♦ **Nifedical™ XL** see NIFEdipine on page 1119

NIFEdipine (nye FED i peen)

Related Information
Calcium Channel Blockers on page 1753
Potentially Inappropriate Medications for Geriatrics on page 1824

Medication Safety Issues
Sound-alike/look-alike issues:
NIFEdipine may be confused with niCARdipine, nimodipine, nisoldipine
Procardia XL® may be confused with Cartia® XT

International issues:
Nipin® [Italy and Singapore] may be confused with Nipent® which is a brand name for pentostatin in the U.S.

U.S. Brand Names Adalat® CC; Afeditab™ CR; Nifediac™ CC; Nifedical™ XL; Procardia®; Procardia XL®

Canadian Brand Names Adalat® XL®; Apo-Nifed®; Apo-Nifed PA®; Novo-Nifedin; Nu-Nifed; Procardia®

Generic Available Yes

Pharmacologic Category Calcium Channel Blocker

Use Treatment of angina (vasospastic, chronic stable), hypertrophic cardiomyopathy, hypertension (sustained release only), pulmonary hypertension

Contraindications Hypersensitivity to nifedipine or any component of the formulation; immediate release preparation for treatment of urgent or emergent hypertension; acute MI

Warnings/Precautions Symptomatic hypotension with or without syncope can rarely occur; blood pressure must be lowered at a rate appropriate for the patient's clinical condition. **The use of sublingual short-acting nifedipine in hypertensive emergencies and urgencies is neither safe nor effective and SHOULD BE ABANDONED!** Serious adverse events (eg, cerebrovascular ischemia, syncope, stroke, acute myocardial infarction, and fetal distress) have been reported in relation to such use.

Severe hypotension may occur in patients taking immediate release concurrently with beta-blockers when undergoing CABG with high dose fentanyl anesthesia. When (Continued)

NIFEdipine *(Continued)*

considering surgery with high dose fentanyl, may consider withdrawing nifedipine (>36 hours) before surgery if possible.

Increased angina may be seen upon starting or increasing doses; may increase frequency, duration, and severity of angina during initiation of therapy; use with caution in patients with CHF or aortic stenosis (especially with concomitant beta-adrenergic blocker); severe left ventricular dysfunction, hepatic or renal impairment, hypertrophic cardiomyopathy (especially obstructive), concomitant therapy with beta-blockers or digoxin, edema. The elderly may be more susceptible to adverse effects.

Mild and transient elevations in liver function enzymes may be apparent within 8 weeks of therapy initiation. The most common side effect is peripheral edema; occurs within 2-3 weeks of starting therapy. Reflex tachycardia may occur with use.

Avoid use of extended release tablets (Procardia XL®) in patients with known stricture/narrowing of the GI tract. Therapeutic potential of sustained-release formulation (elementary osmotic pump, gastrointestinal therapeutic system [GITS]) may be decreased in patients with certain GI disorders that accelerate intestinal transit time (eg, short bowel syndrome, inflammatory bowel disease, severe diarrhea).

Adverse Reactions (Reflective of adult population; not specific for elderly)
>10%:
  Cardiovascular: Flushing (10% to 25%), peripheral edema (dose related 7% to 10%; up to 50%)
  Central nervous system: Dizziness/lightheadedness/giddiness (10% to 27%), headache (10% to 23%)
  Gastrointestinal: Nausea/heartburn (10% to 11%)
  Neuromuscular & skeletal: Weakness (10% to 12%)
≥1% to 10%:
  Cardiovascular: Palpitation (≤2% to 7%), transient hypotension (dose related 5%), CHF (2%)
  Central nervous system: Nervousness/mood changes (≤2% to 7%), shakiness (≤2%), jitteriness (≤2%), sleep disturbances (≤2%), difficulties in balance (≤2%), fever (≤2%), chills (≤2%)
  Dermatologic: Dermatitis (≤2%), pruritus (≤2%), urticaria (≤2%)
  Endocrine & metabolic: Sexual difficulties (≤2%)
  Gastrointestinal: Diarrhea (≤2%), constipation (≤2%), cramps (≤2%), flatulence (≤2%), gingival hyperplasia (≤10%)
  Neuromuscular & skeletal: Muscle cramps/tremor (≤2% to 8%), inflammation (≤2%), joint stiffness (≤2%)
  Ocular: Blurred vision (≤2%)
  Respiratory: Dyspnea/cough/wheezing (6%), nasal congestion/sore throat (≤2% to 6%), chest congestion (≤2%), dyspnea (≤2%)
  Miscellaneous: Diaphoresis (≤2%)

Overdosage/Toxicology Primary cardiac symptoms of calcium blocker overdose include hypotension and bradycardia. Hypotension is caused by peripheral vasodilation, myocardial depression, and bradycardia. Bradycardia results from sinus bradycardia, second- or third-degree atrioventricular block, or sinus arrest with junctional rhythm. Intraventricular conduction is usually not affected so the QRS duration is normal.

Noncardiac symptoms include confusion, stupor, nausea, vomiting, metabolic acidosis and hyperglycemia. Following initial gastric decontamination, if possible, repeated calcium administration may promptly reverse depressed cardiac contractility (but not sinus node depression or peripheral vasodilation). Glucagon, epinephrine, and inamrinone (amrinone) may treat refractory hypotension. Glucagon and epinephrine also increase the heart rate (outside the U.S., 4-aminopyridine may be available as an antidote). Dialysis and hemoperfusion are not effective in enhancing elimination although repeat-dose activated charcoal may serve as an adjunct with sustained-release preparations.

In a few reported cases, overdose with calcium channel blockers has been associated with hypotension and bradycardia, initially refractory to atropine, but becoming more responsive to this agent when larger doses (approaching 1 g/hour for more than 24 hours) of calcium chloride were administered.

Drug Interactions Substrate of CYP2D6 (minor), 3A4 (major); **Inhibits** CYP1A2 (moderate), 2C9 (weak), 2D6 (weak), 3A4 (weak)
  Alpha 1-blockers: May enhance the effects of calcium channel blockers; monitor blood pressure.
  Azole antifungals: May inhibit the calcium channel blocker's metabolism; monitor for the toxic effects of calcium channel blocker and adjust accordingly.
  Barbiturates: May increase metabolism of calcium channel blocker. Consider therapy modification.
  Calcium may reduce the calcium channel blocker's effects.

Calcium channel blocker (nondihydropyridine): May enhance the hypotensive effects of calcium channel blocker (dihydropyridine).

Carbamazepine: May decrease nifedipine serum concentration.

Cimetidine: May increase nifedipine serum concentrations; monitor for toxic effects of calcium channel blocker or choose an alternative H_2 antagonist.

Cisapride: May increase nifedipine's effects; monitor blood pressure.

Cyclosporine: May decrease metabolism of calcium channel blocker (dihydropyridine); monitor for toxic effects of calcium channel blocker.

CYP1A2 substrates: Nifedipine may increase the levels/effects of CYP1A2 substrates. Example substrates include aminophylline, fluvoxamine, mexiletine, mirtazapine, ropinirole, theophylline, and trifluoperazine.

CYP3A4 inducers: CYP3A4 inducers may decrease the levels/effects of nifedipine. Example inducers include aminoglutethimide, carbamazepine, nafcillin, nevirapine, phenobarbital, phenytoin, and rifamycins.

CYP3A4 inhibitors: May increase the levels/effects of nifedipine. Example inhibitors include azole antifungals, clarithromycin, diclofenac, doxycycline, erythromycin, imatinib, isoniazid, nefazodone, nicardipine, propofol, protease inhibitors, quinidine, telithromycin, and verapamil.

Erythromycin: May increase nifedipine serum concentration; monitor blood pressure and adjust if necessary.

Grapefruit juice increases the bioavailability of nifedipine; avoid grapefruit juice.

Magnesium salts: Concurrent use may enhance the adverse/toxic effects of magnesium and enhance the hypotensive effects of the calcium channel blocker.

Nafcillin decreases plasma concentration of nifedipine; avoid this combination.

Neuromuscular-blocking agent (nondepolarizing): Calcium channel blockers may enhance the neuromuscular blocking effect; monitor.

Phenobarbital reduces the plasma concentration of nifedipine. May require much higher dose of nifedipine.

Phenytoin: May decrease nifedipine serum concentration; monitor and adjust if necessary.

Protease inhibitors like amprenavir and ritonavir may increase nifedipine's serum concentration.

Quinidine's serum concentration is reduced and nifedipine's is increased; adjust doses as needed.

Quinupristin/dalfopristin: May increase nifedipine serum concentration; monitor blood pressure and adjust if necessary.

Rifamycin derivatives: Increase the metabolism of the calcium channel blocker; adjust the dose of the calcium channel blocker to maintain efficacy.

Tacrolimus's serum concentrations are increased by nifedipine; monitor tacrolimus trough levels and renal function closely.

Vincristine's half-life is increased by nifedipine; monitor closely for vincristine dose adjustment.

Ethanol/Nutrition/Herb Interactions

Ethanol: Avoid ethanol (may increase CNS depression and may increase the effects of nifedipine). Monitor.

Food: Nifedipine serum levels may be decreased if taken with food. Food may decrease the rate but not the extent of absorption of Procardia XL®. Increased therapeutic and vasodilator side effects, including severe hypotension and myocardial ischemia, may occur if nifedipine is taken by patients ingesting grapefruit.

Herb/Nutraceutical: St John's wort may decrease nifedipine levels. Avoid dong quai if using for hypertension (has estrogenic activity). Avoid ephedra, yohimbe, ginseng (may worsen hypertension). Avoid garlic (may have increased antihypertensive effect).

Mechanism of Action Inhibits calcium ion from entering the "slow channels" or select voltage-sensitive areas of vascular smooth muscle and myocardium during depolarization, producing a relaxation of coronary vascular smooth muscle and coronary vasodilation; increases myocardial oxygen delivery in patients with vasospastic angina

Pharmacodynamics Onset of action: Immediate release: ~20 minutes

Pharmacokinetics

Protein binding (concentration dependent): 92% to 98%

Metabolism: Hepatic to inactive metabolites

Bioavailability: Capsule: 40% to 77%; Sustained release: 65% to 89% relative to immediate release capsules

Half-life: Adults: Healthy: 2-5 hours, Cirrhosis: 7 hours; Older adults: 6.7 hours

Excretion: Urine (as metabolites)

Dosage

Geriatrics & Adults: Hypertension: Oral: Initial: 10 mg 3 times/day as capsules or 30 mg once daily as sustained release

Usual dose: 10-30 mg 3 times/day as capsules or 30-60 mg once daily as sustained release

Maximum: 120-180 mg/day

(Continued)

NIFEdipine *(Continued)*

Note: Adjustment of sustained release formulations should be made at 7- to 14-day intervals

Hepatic Impairment: Reduce oral dose by 50% to 60% in patients with cirrhosis.

Administration Extended release tablets should be swallowed whole; do not crush or chew.

Monitoring Parameters Heart rate, blood pressure, signs and symptoms of CHF, peripheral edema

Reference Range Therapeutic: 25-100 ng/mL

Patient Information Take as directed; do not alter dosage regimen or increase, decrease, or discontinue without consulting prescriber. Do not crush or chew tablets or capsules. Consult prescriber before increasing exercise routine (decreased angina does not mean it is safe to increase exercise). Avoid grapefruit juice. Avoid alcohol. Change position slowly to prevent orthostatic events. May cause dizziness or fatigue; use caution when driving or engaging in tasks that require alertness until response to drug is known. Maintain good oral care and inspect gums for swelling or redness. May cause frequent urination at night. Report irregular heartbeat, swelling, difficulty breathing or new cough, unresolved fatigue, unusual weight gain, unresolved dizziness or constipation, and swollen or bleeding gums.

Special Geriatric Considerations Elderly may experience a greater hypotensive response. Theoretically, constipation may be more of a problem in elderly patients. The half-life of nifedipine is extended in elderly patients (6.7 hours) as compared to younger subjects (3.8 hours).

Dosage Forms Excipient information presented when available (limited, particularly for generics); consult specific product labeling.

Capsule, softgel: 10 mg, 20 mg
  Procardia®: 10 mg
Tablet, extended release: 30 mg, 60 mg, 90 mg
  Adalat® CC, Procardia XL®: 30 mg, 60 mg, 90 mg
  Afeditab™ CR, Nifedical™ XL: 30 mg, 60 mg
  Nifediac™ CC: 30 mg, 60 mg, 90 mg [90 mg tablet contains tartrazine]

Selected References

Messerli FH, Kowey P, and Grodzicki T, "Sublingual Nifedipine for Hypertensive Emergencies," *Lancet*, 1991, 338(8771):881.

Rosen WJ and Johnson CE, "Evaluation of Five Procedures for Measuring Nonstandard Doses of Nifedipine Liquid," *Am J Hosp Pharm*, 1989, 46(11):2313-7.

♦ **Niftolid** *see* Flutamide *on page 658*
♦ **Nilandron®** *see* Nilutamide *on page 1122*

Nilutamide *(ni LOO ta mide)*

U.S. Brand Names Nilandron®
Canadian Brand Names Anandron®
Index Terms NSC-684588; RU-23908
Generic Available No
Pharmacologic Category Antiandrogen; Antineoplastic Agent, Antiandrogen
Use Treatment of metastatic prostate cancer
Contraindications Hypersensitivity to nilutamide or any component of the formulation; severe hepatic impairment; severe respiratory insufficiency
Warnings/Precautions Hazardous agent - use appropriate precautions for handling and disposal. **[U.S. Boxed Warning]: Interstitial pneumonitis has been reported in 2% of patients exposed to nilutamide.** Patients typically experienced progressive exertional dyspnea, and possibly cough, chest pain and fever. X-rays showed interstitial or alveolo-interstitial changes. The suggestive signs of pneumonitis most often occurred within the first 3 months of nilutamide treatment.

Hepatitis or marked increases in liver enzymes leading to drug discontinuation occurred in 1% of nilutamide patients. Rare cases of elevated hepatic enzymes followed by death have been reported.

13% to 57% of patients receiving nilutamide reported a delay in adaptation to the dark, ranging from seconds to a few minutes. This effect sometimes does not abate as drug treatment is continued. Caution patients who experience this effect about driving at night or through tunnels. This effect can be alleviated by wearing tinted glasses.

Adverse Reactions (Reflective of adult population; not specific for elderly)
>10%:
  Central nervous system: Headache, insomnia
  Endocrine & metabolic: Hot flashes (30% to 67%), gynecomastia (10%)
  Gastrointestinal: Nausea (mild - 10% to 32%), abdominal pain (10%), constipation, anorexia
  Genitourinary: Testicular atrophy (16%), libido decreased

Hepatic: Transaminases increased (8% to 13%; transient)

Ocular: Impaired dark adaptation (13% to 57%), usually reversible with dose reduction, may require discontinuation of the drug in 1% to 2% of patients

Respiratory: Dyspnea (11%)

1% to 10%:

Cardiovascular: Chest pain, edema, heart failure, hypertension, syncope

Central nervous system: Dizziness, drowsiness, malaise, hypoesthesia, depression

Dermatologic: Pruritus, alopecia, dry skin, rash

Endocrine & metabolic: Disulfiram-like reaction (hot flashes, rash) (5%); Flu-like syndrome, fever

Gastrointestinal: Vomiting, diarrhea, dyspepsia, GI hemorrhage, melena, weight loss, xerostomia

Genitourinary: Hematuria, nocturia

Hematologic: Anemia

Hepatic: Hepatitis (1%)

Neuromuscular & skeletal: Arthritis, paresthesia

Ocular: Chromatopsia (9%), abnormal vision (6% to 7%), cataracts, photophobia

Respiratory: Interstitial pneumonitis (2% - typically exertional dyspnea, cough, chest pain, and fever; most often occurring within the first 3 months of treatment); rhinitis

Miscellaneous: Diaphoresis

Overdosage/Toxicology Management is supportive and there is no benefit from dialysis. Induce vomiting if the patient is alert. Administer general supportive care (including frequent monitoring of vital signs and close observation).

Drug Interactions Substrate of CYP2C19 (major); **Inhibits** CYP2C19 (weak)

CYP2C19 inducers: May decrease the levels/effects of nilutamide. Example inducers include aminoglutethimide, carbamazepine, phenytoin, and rifampin.

CYP2C19 inhibitors: May increase the levels/effects of nilutamide. Example inhibitors include delavirdine, fluconazole, fluvoxamine, gemfibrozil, isoniazid, omeprazole, and ticlopidine.

Ethanol/Nutrition/Herb Interactions

Ethanol: Avoid ethanol. Up to 5% of patients may experience a systemic reaction (flushing, hypotension, malaise) when combined with nilutamide.

Herb/Nutraceutical: St John's wort may decrease nilutamide levels.

Stability Store at room temperature of 15°C to 30°C (59°F to 86°F). Protect from light.

Mechanism of Action Nonsteroidal antiandrogen that inhibits androgen uptake or inhibits binding of androgen in target tissues. It specifically blocks the action of androgens by interacting with cytosolic androgen receptor F sites in target tissue

Pharmacokinetics

Absorption: Rapid and complete

Protein binding: 72% to 85%

Metabolism: Hepatic, forms active metabolites

Half-life: Terminal: 23-87 hours; Metabolites: 35-137 hours

Elimination: Urine (up to 78% at 120 hours; <1% as unchanged drug); feces (1% to 7%)

Dosage

Geriatrics & Adults: Refer to individual protocols. Prostate cancer: Oral: 300 mg daily for 30 days starting the same day or day after surgical castration, then 150 mg/day

Monitoring Parameters Obtain a chest x-ray if a patient reports dyspnea. If findings are suggestive of interstitial pneumonitis, discontinue nilutamide treatment. Measure serum hepatic enzyme levels at baseline and at regular intervals (3 months). If transaminases increase over 2-3 times the upper limit of normal, discontinue treatment. Perform appropriate laboratory testing at the first symptom/sign of liver injury (eg, jaundice, dark urine, fatigue, abdominal pain or unexplained GI symptoms).

Patient Information Take as prescribed; do not change dosing schedule or stop taking without consulting prescriber. May cause a severe reaction with alcohol. Use alcohol cautiously while taking this medication; if the reaction occurs, avoid alcohol. Periodic laboratory tests are necessary while taking this medication. You may experience dizziness, confusion, or blurred vision (avoid driving or engaging in tasks that require alertness until response to drug is known); loss of light accommodation (avoid night driving and use caution in poorly lighted or changing light situations); impotence; or loss of libido (discuss with prescriber). Report yellowing of skin or eyes; change in color of urine or stool; unusual bruising or bleeding; chest pain; difficult or painful voiding. Report immediately any shortness of breath, difficult breathing, or increased cough.

Special Geriatric Considerations Your eyes may be slow to adapt to darkness; be careful when driving at night; tinted glasses may help.

Dosage Forms Excipient information presented when available (limited, particularly for generics); consult specific product labeling.

Tablet: 150 mg

(Continued)

Nilutamide *(Continued)*

Selected References

Bertagna C, DeGery A, Hucher M, et al, "Efficacy of the Combination of Nilutamide Plus Orchidectomy in Patients With Metastatic Prostatic Cancer, A Meta-Analysis of Seven Randomized Double-Blind Trials (1056 Patients)," *Br J Urol*, 1994, 73(4):396-402.

Dijkman GA, Janknegt RA, De Reijke TM, et al, "Long-term Efficacy and Safety of Nilutamide Plus Castration in Advanced Prostate Cancer, and the Significance of Early Prostate Specific Antigen Normalization. International Anandron Study Group," *J Urol*, 1997, 158(1):160-3.

Dole EJ and Holdsworth MT, "Nilutamide: An Antiandrogen for the Treatment of Prostate Cancer," *Ann Pharmacother*, 1997, 31(1):65-75.

Du Plessis DJ, "Castration Plus Nilutamide vs Castration Plus Placebo in Advanced Prostate Cancer. A Review," *Urology*, 1991, 37(2 Suppl):20-4.

Harris MG, Coleman SG, Faulds D, et al, "Nilutamide. A Review of Its Pharmacodynamic and Pharmacokinetic Properties, and Therapeutic Efficacy in Prostate Cancer," *Drugs Aging*, 1993, 3(1):9-25.

Pendyala L, Creaven PJ, Huben R, et al, "Pharmacokinetics of Anandron in Patients With Advanced Carcinoma of the Prostate," *Cancer Chemother Pharmacol*, 1988, 22(1):69-76.

Nimodipine *(nye MOE di peen)*

Related Information
Calcium Channel Blockers *on page 1753*

Medication Safety Issues
Sound-alike/look-alike issues:
Nimodipine may be confused with niCARdipine, NIFEdipine

Administration issues: **For oral administration only.** For patients unable to swallow a capsule, the drug should be dispensed in an oral syringe labeled **"for oral use only."** Nimodipine has inadvertently been administered I.V. when withdrawn from capsules into a syringe for subsequent nasogastric administration. Severe cardiovascular adverse events, including fatalities, have resulted. Employ precautions against such an event.

U.S. Brand Names Nimotop®
Canadian Brand Names Nimotop®
Generic Available No
Pharmacologic Category Calcium Channel Blocker
Use Treatment of spasm following subarachnoid hemorrhage from ruptured intracranial aneurysms regardless of the patients neurological condition postictus (Hunt and Hess grades I-V)

Contraindications Hypersensitivity to nimodipine or any component of the formulation

Warnings/Precautions Increased angina and/or MI has occurred with initiation or dosage titration of calcium channel blockers. The most common side effect is peripheral edema; occurs within 2-3 weeks of starting therapy. Reflex tachycardia may occur with use. Symptomatic hypotension with or without syncope can rarely occur; blood pressure must be lowered at a rate appropriate for the patient's clinical condition. Use caution in hepatic impairment. Intestinal pseudo-obstruction and ileus have been reported during the use of nimodipine. Use caution in patients with decreased GI motility of a history of bowel obstruction. Use caution when treating patients with hypertrophic cardiomyopathy. Safety and efficacy have not been established in children.

[U.S. Boxed Warning]: Nimodipine has inadvertently been administered I.V. when withdrawn from capsules into a syringe for subsequent nasogastric administration. Severe cardiovascular adverse events, including fatalities, have resulted; precautions should be employed against such an event.

Adverse Reactions (Reflective of adult population; not specific for elderly)
1% to 10%:
Cardiovascular: Reductions in systemic blood pressure (1% to 8%)
Central nervous system: Headache (1% to 4%)
Dermatologic: Rash (1% to 2%)
Gastrointestinal: Diarrhea (2% to 4%), abdominal discomfort (2%)

Overdosage/Toxicology Primary cardiac symptoms of calcium blocker overdose include hypotension and bradycardia. Hypotension is caused by peripheral vasodilation, myocardial depression, and bradycardia. Bradycardia results from sinus bradycardia, second- or third-degree atrioventricular block, or sinus arrest with junctional rhythm. Intraventricular conduction is usually not affected so the QRS duration is normal.

Noncardiac symptoms include confusion, stupor, nausea, vomiting, metabolic acidosis and hyperglycemia. Following initial gastric decontamination, if possible, repeated calcium administration may promptly reverse the depressed cardiac contractility (but not sinus node depression or peripheral vasodilation). Glucagon, epinephrine, and inamrinone (amrinone) may treat refractory hypotension. Glucagon and epinephrine also increase the heart rate (outside the U.S., 4-aminopyridine may be available as an antidote). Dialysis and hemoperfusion are not effective in enhancing elimination although repeat-dose activated charcoal may serve as an adjunct with sustained-release preparations.

In a few reported cases, overdose with calcium channel blockers has been associated with hypotension and bradycardia, initially refractory to atropine, but becoming more responsive to this agent when larger doses (approaching 1 g/hour for more than 24 hours) of calcium chloride were administered.

Drug Interactions Substrate of CYP3A4 (major)

Antihypertensive agents: Effects may be potentiated by nimodipine.

Azole antifungals may inhibit the calcium channel blocker's metabolism; avoid this combination. Try an antifungal like terbinafine (if appropriate) or monitor closely for altered effect of the calcium channel blocker.

Calcium may reduce the calcium channel blocker's effects, particularly hypotension.

Calcium channel blockers: The effects of other calcium channel blockers may be potentiated by nimodipine.

CYP3A4 inducers: CYP3A4 inducers may decrease the levels/effects of nimodipine. Example inducers include aminoglutethimide, carbamazepine, nafcillin, nevirapine, phenobarbital, phenytoin, and rifamycins.

CYP3A4 inhibitors: May increase the levels/effects of nimodipine. Example inhibitors include azole antifungals, clarithromycin, diclofenac, doxycycline, erythromycin, imatinib, isoniazid, nefazodone, nicardipine, propofol, protease inhibitors, quinidine, telithromycin, and verapamil.

Grapefruit juice increases the bioavailability of nimodipine; monitor for altered nimodipine effects.

Protease inhibitor like amprenavir and ritonavir may increase nimodipine's serum concentration.

Rifampin increases the metabolism of the calcium channel blocker; adjust the dose of the calcium channel blocker to maintain efficacy.

Sildenafil, tadalafil, vardenafil: Blood pressure-lowering effects may be additive; use caution.

Valproic acid increased nimodipine's serum concentration; monitor altered effect of nimodipine.

Ethanol/Nutrition/Herb Interactions

Food: Nimodipine has shown a 1.5-fold increase in bioavailability when taken with grapefruit juice; avoid concurrent use.

Herb/Nutraceutical: St John's wort may decrease levels. Avoid dong quai if using for hypertension (has estrogenic activity). Avoid ephedra, yohimbe, ginseng (may worsen hypertension). Avoid garlic (may have increased antihypertensive effect).

Mechanism of Action Nimodipine shares the pharmacology of other calcium channel blockers; animal studies indicate that nimodipine has a greater effect on cerebral arterials than other arterials; this increased specificity may be due to the drug's increased lipophilicity and cerebral distribution as compared to nifedipine; inhibits calcium ion from entering the "slow channels" or select voltage sensitive areas of vascular smooth muscle and myocardium during depolarization

Pharmacokinetics

Protein binding: >95%

Metabolism: Extensive in the liver

Bioavailability: 13% absolute

Half-life: 3 hours, increases with reduced renal function

Time to peak serum concentration: Oral: Within 1 hour

Elimination: In feces (32%) and in urine (50% within 4 days)

Dosage

Geriatrics & Adults: Note: Capsules and contents are for oral administration **ONLY.** Subarachnoid hemorrhage: Oral: 60 mg every 4 hours for 21 days, start therapy within 96 hours after subarachnoid hemorrhage.

Renal Impairment: Not removed by hemo- or peritoneal dialysis; supplemental dose is not necessary.

Hepatic Impairment: Reduce dosage to 30 mg every 4 hours in patients with liver failure.

Administration If the capsules cannot be swallowed, the liquid may be removed by making a hole in each end of the capsule with an 18-gauge needle and extracting the contents into a syringe. If administered via NG tube, follow with a flush of 30 mL NS.

Monitoring Parameters CNS response, heart rate, blood pressure, signs and symptoms of congestive heart failure

Patient Information Do not crush or chew capsule; notify physician if you experience irregular heartbeat, shortness of breath, swelling, constipation, nausea, hypotension, or dizziness; do not stop or interrupt therapy without advice of physician

Additional Information The FDA's Cardiovascular and Renal Drug Advisory Committee reviewed current data regarding the risk of heart attacks in patients treated with calcium channel blockers and determined that as a class, the calcium channel antagonists are safe; however, they warned that short-acting nifedipine could increase the risk of myocardial infarction in some patients. The committee was in agreement (Continued)

Nimodipine *(Continued)*

with a statement issued September, 1995 by the National Heart Lung, and Blood Institute of the National Institute of Health, that warned that short-acting nifedipine should be used with great caution especially at higher doses.

Special Geriatric Considerations Elderly may experience a greater hypotensive response. Constipation may be more of a problem in the elderly. Studies in the treatment of Alzheimer's disease have not demonstrated clear clinical effect.

Dosage Forms Excipient information presented when available (limited, particularly for generics); consult specific product labeling.

Capsule, liquid filled: 30 mg

♦ **Nimotop**® *see Nimodipine on page 1124*

♦ **Niravam**™ *see Alprazolam on page 54*

Nisoldipine *(nye SOL di peen)*

Related Information
Calcium Channel Blockers *on page 1753*

Medication Safety Issues
Sound-alike/look-alike issues:
Nisoldipine may be confused with NIFEdipine

U.S. Brand Names Sular®

Generic Available No

Pharmacologic Category Calcium Channel Blocker

Use Management of hypertension, alone or in combination with other antihypertensive agents

Contraindications Hypersensitivity to nisoldipine, any component of the formulation, or other dihydropyridine calcium channel blockers

Warnings/Precautions Increased angina and/or myocardial infarction in patients with coronary artery disease. Use with caution in patients with CHF, hypertrophic cardiomyopathy, and hepatic impairment. The most common side effect is peripheral edema; occurs within 2-3 weeks of starting therapy. Reflex tachycardia may occur with use. Symptomatic hypotension with or without syncope can rarely occur; blood pressure must be lowered at a rate appropriate for the patient's clinical condition.

Adverse Reactions (Reflective of adult population; not specific for elderly)
>10%:
Cardiovascular: Peripheral edema (dose related 7% to 29%)
Central nervous system: Headache (22%)
1% to 10%:
Cardiovascular: Chest pain (2%), palpitation (3%), vasodilation (4%)
Central nervous system: Dizziness (3% to 10%)
Dermatologic: Rash (2%)
Gastrointestinal: Nausea (2%)
Respiratory: Pharyngitis (5%), sinusitis (3%), dyspnea (3%), cough (5%)

Overdosage/Toxicology Primary cardiac symptoms of calcium blocker overdose include hypotension and bradycardia. Hypotension is caused by peripheral vasodilation, myocardial depression, and bradycardia. Bradycardia results from sinus bradycardia, second- or third-degree atrioventricular block, or sinus arrest with junctional rhythm. Intraventricular conduction is usually not affected so the QRS duration is normal.

Noncardiac symptoms include confusion, stupor, nausea, vomiting, metabolic acidosis and hyperglycemia. Following initial gastric decontamination, if possible, repeated calcium administration may promptly reverse the depressed cardiac contractility (but not sinus node depression or peripheral vasodilation). Glucagon, epinephrine, and inamrinone (amrinone) may treat refractory hypotension. Glucagon and epinephrine also increase the heart rate (outside the U.S., 4-aminopyridine may be available as an antidote). Dialysis and hemoperfusion are not effective in enhancing elimination although repeat-dose activated charcoal may serve as an adjunct with sustained release preparations.

In a few reported cases, overdose with calcium channel blockers has been associated with hypotension and bradycardia, initially refractory to atropine, but becoming more responsive to this agent when larger doses (approaching 1 g/hour for more than 24 hours) of calcium chloride were administered.

Drug Interactions Substrate of CYP3A4 (major); **Inhibits** CYP1A2 (weak), 3A4 (weak)

Azole antifungals may inhibit the calcium channel blocker's metabolism; avoid this combination. Try an antifungal like terbinafine (if appropriate) or monitor closely for altered effect of the calcium channel blocker.

Beta-blockers may have increased pharmacokinetic or pharmacodynamic interactions with nisoldipine.

Calcium may reduce the calcium channel blocker's effects, particularly hypotension.

CYP3A4 inducers: CYP3A4 inducers may decrease the levels/effects of nisoldipine. Example inducers include aminoglutethimide, carbamazepine, nafcillin, nevirapine, phenobarbital, phenytoin, and rifamycins.

CYP3A4 inhibitors: May increase the levels/effects of nisoldipine. Example inhibitors include azole antifungals, clarithromycin, diclofenac, doxycycline, erythromycin, imatinib, isoniazid, nefazodone, nicardipine, propofol, protease inhibitors, quinidine, telithromycin, and verapamil.

Grapefruit juice increases the bioavailability of nisoldipine; monitor for altered nisoldipine effects.

Phenytoin decreases nisoldipine to undetectable levels. Avoid use of any CYP3A4 inducer with nisoldipine.

Rifampin increases the metabolism of the calcium channel blocker; adjust the dose of the calcium channel blocker to maintain efficacy.

Sildenafil, tadalafil, vardenafil: Blood pressure-lowering effects may be additive; use caution.

Ethanol/Nutrition/Herb Interactions

Food: Nisoldipine bioavailability may be increased if taken with high-lipid foods or with grapefruit juice. Avoid grapefruit products before and after dosing.

Herb/Nutraceutical: St John's wort may decrease nisoldipine levels. Avoid dong quai if using for hypertension (has estrogenic activity). Avoid ephedra, yohimbe, ginseng (may worsen hypertension). Avoid garlic (may have increased antihypertensive effect).

Mechanism of Action As a dihydropyridine calcium channel blocker, structurally similar to nifedipine, nisoldipine impedes the movement of calcium ions into vascular smooth muscle and cardiac muscle. Dihydropyridines are potent vasodilators and are not as likely to suppress cardiac contractility and slow cardiac conduction as other calcium antagonists such as verapamil and diltiazem; nisoldipine is 5-10 times as potent a vasodilator as nifedipine.

Pharmacokinetics

Absorption: Well absorbed

Metabolism: Extensive presystemic metabolism in the intestinal wall and the liver; hepatically metabolized to inactive metabolites

Bioavailability: 5%; T_{max}: 6-12 hours

Half-life: 7-12 hours

Elimination: Hepatic metabolism with metabolites excreted in the urine; only a trace of unchanged drug excreted in urine

Dosage

Geriatrics: Initial dose: 10 mg/day, increase by 10 mg/week (or longer intervals) to attain adequate blood pressure control. Those with hepatic disease should be started with 10 mg/day.

Adults:

Hypertension: Oral: Initial: 20 mg once daily, then increase by 10 mg/week (or longer intervals) to attain adequate control of blood pressure

Usual dose range (JNC 7): 10-40 mg once daily; doses >60 mg once daily are not recommended.

Hepatic Impairment: A starting dose not exceeding 10 mg/day is recommended for patients with hepatic impairment.

Administration Administer at the same time each day to ensure minimal fluctuation of serum levels. Avoid high-fat diet.

Monitoring Parameters Heart rate, blood pressure, signs and symptoms of CHF, peripheral edema

Patient Information Avoid grapefruit products before and after dosing; administration with a high fat meal can lead to excessive peak drug concentrations and should be avoided; do not crush tablets

Additional Information Initial data indicate that once daily doses of 10-40 mg are about as effective as hydrochlorothiazide, lisinopril, or amlodipine; doses of 20-60 mg are about as effective as twice daily verapamil in lowering blood pressure in patients with mild to moderate hypertension; although there are some initial data which may show increased risk of myocardial infarction following treatment of hypertension with calcium channel blockers, controlled trials (eg, ALL-HAT) are ongoing to examine the long-term effects of not only the calcium channel blockers, but also other antihypertensives in preventing heart disease. Until done, patients taking these agents should be encouraged to continue with prescribed antihypertension regimens although a switch from high-dose, short-acting agents to sustained release products may be warranted. Many practitioners agree to avoid calcium channel blockers as primary treatment for hypertension unless diuretics or beta-blockers are contraindicated.

The FDA's Cardiovascular and Renal Drug Advisory Committee reviewed current data regarding the risk of heart attacks in patients treated with calcium channel blockers and determined that as a class, the calcium channel antagonists are safe.

(Continued)

Nisoldipine *(Continued)*

Special Geriatric Considerations Elderly may experience a greater hypotensive response. Constipation may be more of a problem in the elderly. Calcium channel blockers are no more effective in the elderly than other therapies; however, they do not cause significant CNS effects which is an advantage over some antihypertensive agents.

Dosage Forms Excipient information presented when available (limited, particularly for generics); consult specific product labeling.

Tablet, extended release: 10 mg, 20 mg, 30 mg, 40 mg

Selected References

Chobanian AV, Bakris GL, Black HR, et al, "The Seventh Report of the Joint National Committee on Prevention, Detection, Evaluation, and Treatment of High Blood Pressure: The JNC 7 Report," *JAMA*, 2003, 289(19):2560-71.

♦ **Nitalapram** *see* Citalopram *on page 322*

♦ **Nitrek® [DSC]** *see* Nitroglycerin *on page 1129*

♦ **Nitro-Bid®** *see* Nitroglycerin *on page 1129*

♦ **Nitro-Dur®** *see* Nitroglycerin *on page 1129*

Nitrofurantoin *(nye troe fyoor AN toyn)*

Related Information

Antimicrobial Activity Against Selected Organisms *on page 1728*
Potentially Inappropriate Medications for Geriatrics *on page 1824*

Medication Safety Issues

International issues:

Macrobid® may be confused with Mikrozid® which is a brand name for ethanol/propanol combination in Great Britain

U.S. Brand Names Furadantin®; Macrobid®; Macrodantin®

Canadian Brand Names Apo-Nitrofurantoin®; Macrobid®; Macrodantin®; Novo-Furantoin

Generic Available Yes: Excludes suspension

Pharmacologic Category Antibiotic, Miscellaneous

Use Prevention and treatment of urinary tract infections caused by susceptible strains of *E. coli, S. aureus, Enterococcus, Klebsiella,* and *Enterobacter*

Contraindications Hypersensitivity to nitrofurantoin or any component of the formulation; renal impairment (anuria, oliguria, significantly elevated serum creatinine, or $Cl_{cr} <$ 60 mL/minute)

Warnings/Precautions Use with caution in patients with G6PD deficiency or in patients with anemia. Therapeutic concentrations of nitrofurantoin are not attained in urine of patients with $Cl_{cr} < 60$ mL/minute. Use with caution if prolonged therapy is anticipated due to possible pulmonary toxicity. Acute, subacute, or chronic (usually after 6 months of therapy) pulmonary reactions have been observed in patients treated with nitrofurantoin; if these occur, discontinue therapy immediately; monitor closely for malaise, dyspnea, cough, fever, radiologic evidence of diffuse interstitial pneumonitis or fibrosis. Rare, but severe hepatic reactions have been associated with nitrofurantoin (onset may be insidious); discontinue immediately if hepatitis occurs. Has been associated with peripheral neuropathy (rare); risk may be increased by renal impairment, diabetes, vitamin B deficiency, or electrolyte imbalance; use caution. Prolonged use may result in fungal or bacterial superinfection, including *C. difficile*-associated diarrhea and pseudomembranous colitis.

Adverse Reactions (Reflective of adult population; not specific for elderly)

Frequency not defined.

Cardiovascular: Chest pain, cyanosis, ECG changes

Central nervous system: Bulging fontanels (infants), chills, confusion, depression, dizziness, drowsiness, fever, headache, malaise, pseudotumor cerebri, psychotic reaction, vertigo

Dermatologic: Alopecia, angioedema, erythema multiforme, exfoliative dermatitis, pruritus, rash (eczematous, erythematous, maculopapular), Stevens-Johnson syndrome, urticaria

Gastrointestinal: Abdominal pain, *C. difficile* colitis, constipation, diarrhea, dyspepsia, flatulence, nausea, pancreatitis, sialadenitis, vomiting

Hematologic: Agranulocytosis, eosinophilia, granulocytopenia, hemolytic anemia, leukopenia, megaloblastic anemia, thrombocytopenia

Hepatic: Cholestasis, hepatitis, hepatic necrosis, transaminases increased, jaundice (cholestatic)

Neuromuscular & skeletal: Arthralgia, myalgia, numbness, paresthesia, peripheral neuropathy, weakness

Ocular: Amblyopia, nystagmus, optic neuritis

Respiratory: Cough, dyspnea, pneumonitis, pulmonary fibrosis (with long-term use), pulmonary infiltration

Miscellaneous: Anaphylaxis, hypersensitivity (including acute pulmonary hypersensitivity), lupus-like syndrome

Overdosage/Toxicology Symptoms include vomiting. Treatment is supportive. Nitrofurantoin is dialyzable.

Drug Interactions

Antacids: Magnesium trisilicate-containing antacids may decrease the absorption of nitrofurantoin.

Uricosuric agents (probenecid, sulfinpyrazone): May decrease renal excretion of nitrofurantoin.

Ethanol/Nutrition/Herb Interactions

Ethanol: Avoid ethanol (may increase CNS depression).

Food: Nitrofurantoin serum concentrations may be increased if taken with food.

Stability Store at room temperature 15°C to 30°C (59°F to 86°F).

Mechanism of Action Inhibits several bacterial enzyme systems including acetyl coenzyme A interfering with metabolism and possibly cell wall synthesis

Pharmacokinetics

Absorption: Well from the GI tract; the macrocrystalline form is absorbed more slowly due to slower dissolution, but causes less GI distress

Distribution: V_d: 0.8 L/kg

Protein binding: ~40%

Metabolism: 60% of the drug is metabolized by body tissues throughout the body, with the exception of plasma, to inactive metabolites

Bioavailability: Presence of food increases bioavailability

Half-life: 20-60 minutes and is prolonged with renal impairment

Elimination:

Suspension: Urine (40%) and feces (small amounts) as metabolites and unchanged drug

Macrocrystals: Urine (20% to 25% as unchanged drug)

Dosage

Geriatrics: Refer to adult dosing (see Special Geriatric Considerations).

Adults:

UTI treatment:

Furadantin®, Macrodantin®: Oral: 50-100 mg/dose every 6 hours; administer for 7 days or at least 3 days after obtaining sterile urine

Macrobid®: Oral: 100 mg twice daily for 7 days

UTI prophylaxis (Furadantin®, Macrodantin®): Oral: 50-100 mg/dose at bedtime

Renal Impairment:

Cl_{cr} <60 mL/minute: Contraindicated

Contraindicated in hemo- and peritoneal dialysis and continuous arteriovenous or venovenous hemofiltration.

Administration Administer with meals to improve absorption and decrease adverse effects; suspension may be mixed with water, milk, or fruit juice. Shake suspension well before use.

Monitoring Parameters Signs of pulmonary reaction, signs of numbness or tingling of the extremities; periodic liver function tests; signs and symptoms of infection

Test Interactions False-positive urine glucose (Benedict's and Fehling's methods); no false positives with enzymatic tests

Patient Information Take with food or milk; may discolor urine to a dark yellow or brown color; complete full course of therapy; notify physician or pharmacist if diarrhea, tingling in extremities, skin rash, or difficulty breathing occurs

Special Geriatric Considerations Because of nitrofurantoin's decreased efficacy in patients with a Cl_{cr} <60 mL/minute and its side effect profile, it is not an antibiotic of choice for acute or prophylactic treatment of urinary tract infections in the elderly. An increased rate of severe hepatic toxicity has been suggested by postmarketing reports.

Dosage Forms Excipient information presented when available (limited, particularly for generics); consult specific product labeling.

Capsule [macrocrystal]: 50 mg, 100 mg

Macrodantin®: 25 mg, 50 mg, 100 mg

Capsule [macrocrystal/monohydrate]: 100 mg [nitrofurantoin macrocrystal 25% and nitrofurantoin monohydrate 75%]

Macrobid®: 100 mg [nitrofurantoin macrocrystal 25% and nitrofurantoin monohydrate 75%]

Suspension, oral:

Furadantin®: 25 mg/5 mL (470 mL)

Nitroglycerin (nye troe GLI ser in)

Medication Safety Issues

Sound-alike/look-alike issues:

Nitroglycerin may be confused with nitroprusside

Nitro-Bid® may be confused with Nicobid®

(Continued)

Nitroglycerin *(Continued)*

Nitroderm may be confused with NicoDerm®
Nitrol® may be confused with Nizoral®
Nitrostat® may be confused with Hyperstat®, Nilstat®, nystatin

Nitroglycerin transdermal patches should be removed prior to defibrillation or MRI study.

International issues:

Nitrocor® [Chile and Italy] may be confused with Natrecor® which is a brand name for nesiritide in the U.S.

Nitrocor® [Chile and Italy] may be confused with Nutracort® which is a brand name for hydrocortisone in the U.S.

Nitro-Dur® may be confused with Nitrocor® [Chile and Italy]

U.S. Brand Names Minitran™; Nitrek® [DSC]; Nitro-Bid®; Nitro-Dur®; Nitrolingual®; NitroMist™; NitroQuick®; Nitrostat®; NitroTime®

Canadian Brand Names Gen-Nitro; Minitran™; Nitro-Dur®; Nitroglycerin Injection, USP; Nitrol®; Nitrostat™; Rho®-Nitro; Transderm-Nitro®; Trinipatch® 0.2; Trinipatch® 0.4; Trinipatch® 0.6

Index Terms Glyceryl Trinitrate; Nitroglycerol; NTG

Generic Available Yes: Capsule, injection, patch, tablet

Pharmacologic Category Vasodilator

Use Treatment of angina pectoris, congestive heart failure (especially when associated with acute myocardial infarction), pulmonary hypertension, hypertensive emergencies occurring perioperatively (especially during cardiovascular surgery)

Unlabeled/Investigational Use Esophageal spastic disorders (sublingual nitrate formulations)

Contraindications Hypersensitivity to organic nitrates; hypersensitivity to isosorbide, nitroglycerin, or any component of the formulation; concurrent use with sildenafil; angle-closure glaucoma (intraocular pressure may be increased); head trauma or cerebral hemorrhage (increase intracranial pressure); severe anemia; allergy to adhesive (transdermal product)

I.V. product: Hypotension; uncorrected hypovolemia; inadequate cerebral circulation; increased intracranial pressure; constrictive pericarditis; pericardial tamponade

Warnings/Precautions Severe hypotension can occur. Use with caution in volume depletion, hypotension, and right ventricular infarctions. Paradoxical bradycardia and increased angina pectoris can accompany hypotension. Orthostatic hypotension can also occur. Ethanol can accentuate this. Tolerance does develop to nitrates and appropriate dosing is needed to minimize this (drug-free interval). Avoid use of long-acting agents in acute MI or CHF; cannot easily reverse. Nitrate may aggravate angina caused by hypertrophic cardiomyopathy. Nitroglycerin transdermal patches should be removed prior to defibrillation or MRI study. Avoid concurrent use with PDE-5 inhibitors.

Overdosage/Toxicology Symptoms include hypotension, flushing, syncope, throbbing headache with reflex tachycardia, and methemoglobinemia with extremely large overdoses. I.V. overdose may additionally be associated with increased intracranial pressure, confusion, vertigo, palpitations, nausea, vomiting, dyspnea, diaphoresis, heart block, bradycardia, coma, seizures, and death. After gastric decontamination, treatment is supportive and symptomatic. Hypotension is treated with positioning, fluids, and careful use of low-dose pressors, if needed. Methylene blue may treat methemoglobinemia.

Drug Interactions

Diazoxide: Vasodilators may enhance the antihypertensive effect of diazoxide.

Ergot alkaloids: May diminish the vasodilatory effect of nitroglycerin. Of particular concern in patients being treated for angina. Avoid concurrent use.

Heparin: Effect may be reduced by I.V. nitroglycerin. May affect only a minority of patients.

Phosphodiesterase 5 inhibitors: May enhance the vasodilatory effect of organic nitrates; avoid concurrent use (contraindicated). Do not administer sildenafil, tadalafil, or vardenafil within 24 hours of a nitrate preparation.

Ethanol/Nutrition/Herb Interactions

Ethanol: Avoid ethanol (may increase the hypotensive effects of nitroglycerin). Monitor.

Herb/Nutraceutical: Avoid bayberry, blue cohosh, cayenne, ephedra, ginger, ginseng (american), kola, licorice (may worsen hypertension). Avoid black cohosh, California poppy, coleus, golden seal, hawthorn, mistletoe, periwinkle, quinine, shepherd's purse (may cause hypotension).

Stability Doses should be made in glass bottles, Excell® or PAB® containers. Adsorption occurs to soft plastic (ie, PVC).

Nitroglycerin diluted in D_5W or NS in glass containers is physically and chemically stable for 48 hours at room temperature and 7 days under refrigeration. In D_5W or

NS in Excell®/PAB® containers it is physically and chemically stable for 24 hours at room temperature and 14 days under refrigeration.

Premixed bottles are stable according to the manufacturer's expiration dating.

Standard diluent: 50 mg/250 mL D₅W; 50 mg/500 mL D₅W.

Minimum volume: 100 mg/250 mL D₅W; concentration should not exceed 400 mcg/mL.

Store sublingual tablets and ointment in tightly closed containers at 15°C to 30°C. Store spray and transdermal patch at 25°C; excursions permitted to 15°C to 30°C (59°F to 86°F).

Mechanism of Action Works by relaxation of smooth muscle, producing a vasodilator effect on the peripheral veins and arteries with more prominent effects on the veins. Primarily reduces cardiac oxygen demand by decreasing preload (left ventricular end-diastolic pressure); may modestly reduce afterload; dilates coronary arteries and improves collateral flow to ischemic regions

Pharmacodynamics Onset and duration of action is dependent upon dosage form administered. See table.

Nitroglycerin

Dosage Form	Onset of Effect	Peak Effect	Duration
Sublingual tablet	1-3 min	4-8 min	30-60 min
Translingual spray	2 min	4-10 min	30-60 min
Buccal tablet	2-5 min	4-10 min	2 h
Sustained release	20-45 min	45-120 min	4-8 h
Topical	15-60 min	30-120 min	2-12 h
Transdermal	40-60 min	60-180 min	18-24 h
I.V. drip	Immediate	Immediate	3-5 min

Pharmacokinetics
Protein binding: 60%
Metabolism: Extensive first-pass
Half-life: 1-4 minutes
Elimination: Excretion of inactive metabolites in urine

Dosage
Geriatrics & Adults: Note: Hemodynamic and antianginal tolerance often develop within 24-48 hours of continuous nitrate administration. Nitrate-free interval (10-12 hours/day) is recommended to avoid tolerance development; gradually decrease dose in patients receiving NTG for prolonged period to avoid withdrawal reaction.

Angina/coronary artery disease:
Oral: 2.5-9 mg 2-4 times/day (up to 26 mg 4 times/day)
I.V.: 5 mcg/minute, increase by 5 mcg/minute every 3-5 minutes to 20 mcg/minute. If no response at 20 mcg/minute increase by 10 mcg/minute every 3-5 minutes, up to 200 mcg/minute.
Topical ointment: Include a nitrate free interval, ~10 to 12 hours; Apply 0.5" to 2" every 6 hours with a nitrate free interval.
Topical patch, transdermal: 0.2-0.4 mg/hour initially and titrate to doses of 0.4-0.8 mg/hour. Tolerance is minimized by using a patch-on period of 12-14 hours and patch-off period of 10-12 hours.
Sublingual: 0.2-0.6 mg every 5 minutes for maximum of 3 doses in 15 minutes; may also use prophylactically 5-10 minutes prior to activities which may provoke an attack.
Esophageal spastic disorders (unlabeled use): 0.3-0.4 mg 5 minutes before meals
Translingual: 1-2 sprays into mouth under tongue every 5 minutes for maximum of 3 doses in 15 minutes, may also be used 5-10 minutes prior to activities which may provoke an attack prophylactically.

Administration
I.V.: I.V. must be prepared in glass bottles; use special sets intended for nitroglycerin. glass I.V. bottles and administration sets provided by manufacturer.
Sublingual: Do not crush sublingual product (tablet). Place under tongue and allow to dissolve.
Translingual spray: Prime prior to first use (5 sprays into the air). If unused for 6 weeks, a single priming spray should be completed. Priming sprays should be directed away from patient and others. The end of the pump should be covered by the fluid in the bottle.

Monitoring Parameters Orthostatic blood pressure, blood pressure, heart rate; therapeutic dose may be determined by observing for a decrease in systolic blood pressure by 15 mm Hg, diastolic reduction of 10 mm Hg or an increase in heart rate of 10 bpm

Patient Information Go to hospital or call 911 if no relief after 3 sublingual doses; do not swallow or chew sublingual form; keep in original container and tightly closed; remove and do not reinsert cotton plug; for the sublingual tablets, it is best to get a (Continued)

Nitroglycerin *(Continued)*

fresh bottle 3-6 months after opening. Get instructions on proper use of transdermal patches or ointment.

Additional Information I.V. preparations contain alcohol and/or propylene glycol; may need to use nitrate-free interval (10-12 hours/day) to avoid tolerance development. Tolerance may possibly be reversed with acetylcysteine; gradually decrease dose in patients receiving NTG for prolonged period to avoid withdrawal reaction.

Special Geriatric Considerations Caution should be used when using nitrate therapy in the elderly due to hypotension. Hypotension is enhanced in the elderly due to decreased baroreceptor response, decreased venous tone, and often hypovolemia (dehydration) or other hypotensive drugs.

Dosage Forms Excipient information presented when available (limited, particularly for generics); consult specific product labeling.

Capsule, extended release: 2.5 mg, 6.5 mg, 9 mg

Nitro-Time®: 2.5 mg, 6.5 mg, 9 mg

Infusion [premixed in D₅W]: 25 mg (250 mL) [0.1 mg/mL]; 50 mg (250 mL) [0.2 mg/mL]; 50 mg (500 mL) [0.1 mg/mL]; 100 mg (250 mL) [0.4 mg/mL]; 200 mg (500 mL) [0.4 mg/mL]

Injection, solution: 5 mg/mL (5 mL, 10 mL) [contains alcohol and propylene glycol]

Ointment, topical:

Nitro-Bid®: 2% [20 mg/g] (1 g, 30 g, 60 g)

Solution, translingual [spray]:

Nitrolingual®: 0.4 mg/metered spray (4.9 g) [contains alcohol 20%; 60 metered sprays]; (12 g) [contains alcohol 20%; 200 metered sprays]

NitroMist™:0.4 mg/metered spray (8.5 g) [230 metered sprays]

Tablet, sublingual:

NitroQuick®, Nitrostat®: 0.3 mg, 0.4 mg, 0.6 mg

Transdermal system [once-daily patch]: 0.1 mg/hour (30s); 0.2 mg/hour (30s); 0.4 mg/hour (30s); 0.6 mg/hour (30s)

Minitran™: 0.1 mg/hour (30s); 0.2 mg/hour (30s); 0.4 mg/hour (30s); 0.6 mg/hour (30s)

Nitrek®: 0.2 mg/hour (30s); 0.4 mg/hour (30s); 0.6 mg/hour (30s) [DSC]

Nitro-Dur®: 0.1 mg/hour (30s); 0.2 mg/hour (30s); 0.3 mg/hour (30s); 0.4 mg/hour (30s); 0.6 mg/hour (30s); 0.8 mg/hour (30s)

Selected References

Braunwald E, Antman EM, Beasley JW, et al, "ACC/AHA 2002 Guideline Update for the Management of Patients With Unstable Angina and Non-ST-Segment Elevation Myocardial Infarction - Summary Article: A Report of the American College of Cardiology/American Heart Association Task Force on Practice Guidelines (Committee on the Management of Patients With Unstable Angina)," *J Am Coll Cardiol*, 2002, 40(7):1366-74. Available at: http://www.acc.org/clinical/guidelines/unstable/incorporated/index.htm. Accessed May 20, 2003.

Elkayam U, "Tolerance to Organic Nitrates: Evidence, Mechanisms, Clinical Relevance, and Strategies for Prevention," *Ann Intern Med*, 1991, 114(8):667-77.

Gibbons RJ, Abrams J, Chatterjee K, et al, "ACC/AHA 2002 Guideline Update for the Management of Patients With Chronic Stable Angina - Summary Article: A Report of the American College of Cardiology/American Heart Association Task Force on Practice Guidelines (Committee on the Management of Patients With Chronic Stable Angina)," *J Am Coll Cardiol*, 2003, 41(1):159-68. Available at: http://http://www.acc.org/clinical/guidelines/stable/stable_clean.pdf. Accessed May 5, 2004.

Ryan TJ, Anderson JL, Antman EM, et al, "1999 Update: ACC/AHA Guidelines for the Management of Patients With Acute Myocardial Infarction: Executive Summary. A Report of the American College of Cardiology/American Heart Association Task Force on Practice Guidelines (Committee on Management of Acute Myocardial Infarction)," *Circulation*, 1999, 100(9):1016-30. Available at: http://216.185.112.5/presenter.jhtml?identifier=1829#primary. Accessed May 20, 2003.

♦ **Nitroglycerol** *see* Nitroglycerin *on page 1129*

♦ **Nitrolingual®** *see* Nitroglycerin *on page 1129*

♦ **NitroMist™** *see* Nitroglycerin *on page 1129*

♦ **Nitropress®** *see* Nitroprusside *on page 1132*

Nitroprusside *(nye troe PRUS ide)*

Medication Safety Issues

Sound-alike/look-alike issues:

Nitroprusside may be confused with nitroglycerin

High alert medication: The Institute for Safe Medication Practices (ISMP) includes this medication among its list of drugs which have a heightened risk of causing significant patient harm when used in error.

U.S. Brand Names Nitropress®

Index Terms Nitroprusside Sodium; Sodium Nitroferricyanide; Sodium Nitroprusside

Generic Available Yes

Pharmacologic Category Vasodilator

Use Management of hypertensive crises, congestive heart failure; controlled hypotension to reduce bleeding during surgery

Contraindications Hypersensitivity to nitroprusside or any component of the formulation; treatment of compensatory hypertension (aortic coarctation, arteriovenous shunting); high output failure; congenital optic atrophy or tobacco amblyopia

Warnings/Precautions [U.S. Boxed Warning]: Continuous blood pressure monitoring is needed. Except when used briefly or at low (<2 mcg/kg/minute) infusion rates, nitroprusside gives rise to large cyanide quantities. Do not use the maximum dose for more than 10 minutes; if blood pressure not controlled then discontinue infusion. Monitor for cyanide toxicity via acid-base balance and venous oxygen concentration. Use with caution in patients with increased intracranial pressure (head trauma, cerebral hemorrhage); severe renal impairment, hepatic failure, hypothyroidism. **[U.S. Boxed Warning]: Use only as an infusion with 5% dextrose in water.** Excessive amounts of nitroprusside can cause cyanide toxicity (usually in patients with decreased liver function) or thiocyanate toxicity (usually in patients with decreased renal function, or in patients with normal renal function but prolonged nitroprusside use).

Adverse Reactions (Reflective of adult population; not specific for elderly)
1% to 10%:
Cardiovascular: Excessive hypotensive response, palpitation, substernal distress
Central nervous system: Disorientation, psychosis, headache, restlessness
Endocrine & metabolic: Thyroid suppression
Gastrointestinal: Nausea, vomiting
Neuromuscular & skeletal: Weakness, muscle spasm
Otic: Tinnitus
Respiratory: Hypoxia
Miscellaneous: Diaphoresis, thiocyanate toxicity

Overdosage/Toxicology Symptoms include hypotension, vomiting, hyperventilation, tachycardia, muscular twitching, hypothyroidism, cyanide or thiocyanate toxicity. Thiocyanate toxicity includes psychosis, hyper-reflexia, confusion, weakness, tinnitus, seizures, and coma. Cyanide toxicity includes acidosis (decreased HCO_3, decreased pH, increased lactate), increase in mixed venous blood oxygen tension, tachycardia, altered consciousness, coma, convulsions, and almond smell on breath. Nitroprusside has been shown to release cyanide *in vivo* with hemoglobin. Cyanide toxicity does not usually occur because of the rapid uptake of cyanide by erythrocytes and its eventual incorporation into cyanocobalamin. However, prolonged administration of nitroprusside or its reduced elimination can lead to cyanide intoxication. In these situations, airway support with oxygen therapy is germane, followed closely with antidotal therapy of amyl nitrate perles, sodium nitrate 300 mg I.V., and sodium thiosulfate 12.5 g I.V.. Thiocyanate is dialyzable. May be mixed with sodium thiosulfate in I.V. to prevent cyanide toxicity.

Drug Interactions None noted

Stability
Nitroprusside sodium should be reconstituted freshly by diluting 50 mg in 250-1000 mL of D_5W.
Use only clear solutions; solutions of nitroprusside exhibit a color described as brownish, brown, brownish-pink, light orange, and straw. Solutions are highly sensitive to light. Exposure to light causes decomposition, resulting in a highly colored solution of orange, dark brown or blue. **A blue color indicates almost complete degradation and breakdown to cyanide.**
Solutions should be wrapped with aluminum foil or other opaque material to protect from light (do as soon as possible).
Stability of parenteral admixture at room temperature (25°C) and at refrigeration temperature (4°C) is 24 hours.

Mechanism of Action Causes peripheral vasodilation by direct action on venous and arteriolar smooth muscle, thus reducing peripheral resistance; will increase cardiac output by decreasing afterload; reduces aortal and left ventricular impedance

Pharmacodynamics
Onset of action: Hypotensive effects occur in <2 minutes
Duration: Following discontinuation of therapy, effects cease within 1-10 minutes

Pharmacokinetics
Metabolism: Converted to cyanide by erythrocyte and tissue sulfhydryl group interactions; cyanide is converted in the liver by rhodanese to thiocyanate
Half-life: <10 minutes; half-life (thiocyanate): 2.7-7 days
Elimination: In urine

Dosage
Geriatrics & Adults:
Acute hypertension: I.V.: Initial: 0.3-0.5 mcg/kg/minute; increase in increments of 0.5 mcg/kg/minute, titrating to the desired hemodynamic effect or the appearance of headache or nausea; usual dose: 3 mcg/kg/minute; rarely need >4 mcg/kg/minute; maximum: 10 mcg/kg/minute. When >500 mcg/kg is administered by prolonged infusion of faster than 2 mcg/kg/minute, cyanide is generated faster than an unaided patient can handle.
(Continued)

Nitroprusside *(Continued)*

Note: Administration requires the use of an infusion pump. Average dose: 5 mcg/kg/minute.

Renal Impairment: Limit use; accumulation of thiocyanate may occur.

Hepatic Impairment: Limit use; risk of cyanide toxicity.

Monitoring Parameters Blood pressure, cardiac status, thiocyanate levels

Reference Range Monitor thiocyanate levels if requiring prolonged infusion (>4 days) or ≥4 mcg/kg/minute; Therapeutic: 6-29 mcg/mL (SI: 103-499 μmol/L)

Additional Information Nitroprusside is converted to cyanide ions in the bloodstream; decomposes to prussic acid which in the presence of sulfur donor is converted to thiocyanate (liver and kidney rhodanase systems); thiocyanate is then renally eliminated

Special Geriatric Considerations Elderly patients may have an increased sensitivity to nitroprusside possibly due to a decreased baroreceptor reflex, altered sensitivity to vasodilating effects or a resistance of cardiac adrenergic receptors to stimulation by catecholamines.

Dosage Forms Excipient information presented when available (limited, particularly for generics); consult specific product labeling.

Injection, solution, as sodium: 25 mg/mL (2 mL)

♦ **Nitroprusside Sodium** *see Nitroprusside on page 1132*
♦ **NitroQuick®** *see Nitroglycerin on page 1129*
♦ **Nitrostat®** *see Nitroglycerin on page 1129*
♦ **NitroTime®** *see Nitroglycerin on page 1129*
♦ **4′-Nitro-3′-Trifluoromethylisobutyrantide** *see Flutamide on page 658*
♦ **Nix® [OTC]** *see Permethrin on page 1235*

Nizatidine *(ni ZA ti deen)*

Medication Safety Issues
Sound-alike/look-alike issues:
Axid® may be confused with Ansaid®

International issues:
Tazac® [Australia] may be confused with Tiazac® which is a brand name for diltiazem in the U.S.

U.S. Brand Names Axid®; Axid® AR [OTC]

Canadian Brand Names Apo-Nizatidine®; Axid®; Gen-Nizatidine; Novo-Nizatidine; Nu-Nizatidine; PMS-Nizatidine

Generic Available Yes: Capsule

Pharmacologic Category Histamine H_2 Antagonist

Use Treatment and maintenance of duodenal ulcer, benign gastric ulcer, GERD

Unlabeled/Investigational Use Part of a multidrug regimen for *H. pylori* eradication to reduce the risk of duodenal ulcer recurrence

Contraindications Hypersensitivity to nizatidine or any component of the formulation; hypersensitivity to other H_2 antagonists (cross-sensitivity has been observed)

Warnings/Precautions Relief of symptoms does not preclude the presence of a gastric malignancy. Use with caution in patients with liver and renal impairment; dosage modification required in patients with renal impairment

Adverse Reactions (Reflective of adult population; not specific for elderly)
>10%: Central nervous system: Headache (16%)
1% to 10%:
Central nervous system: Anxiety, dizziness, fever (reported in children), insomnia, irritability (reported in children), somnolence, nervousness
Dermatologic: Pruritus, rash
Gastrointestinal: Abdominal pain, anorexia, constipation, diarrhea, dry mouth, flatulence, heartburn, nausea, vomiting
Respiratory: Reported in children: Cough, nasal congestion, nasopharyngitis

Overdosage/Toxicology Symptoms include muscular tremors, vomiting, rapid respiration. LD_{50}: ~80 mg/kg. Treatment is primarily symptomatic and supportive.

Drug Interactions Inhibits 3A4 (weak)
Antifungal agents (imidazole): Nizatidine may decrease the absorption of itraconazole or ketoconazole.

Ethanol/Nutrition/Herb Interactions
Ethanol: Avoid ethanol (may cause gastric mucosal irritation).
Food: Administration with apple juice may decrease absorption.

Mechanism of Action Competitive inhibition of histamine at H_2-receptors of the gastric parietal cells resulting in reduced gastric acid secretion, gastric volume and hydrogen ion concentration reduced. In healthy volunteers, nizatidine suppresses gastric acid secretion induced by pentagastrin infusion or food.

Pharmacokinetics

Bioavailability: >90% (rapidly absorbed)
Protein binding: ~35%
Metabolism: Partially hepatic; forms metabolites
Time to peak serum concentration: 0.5-3 hours
Elimination:
Renal: Unchanged, 60%
Hepatic: <18%
Elimination: Urine (90%; ~60% as unchanged drug); feces (<6%)

Dosage

Geriatrics & Adults:

Duodenal ulcer: Oral:
Treatment of active ulcer: 300 mg at bedtime or 150 mg twice daily
Maintenance of healed ulcer: 150 mg/day at bedtime
Gastric ulcer: Oral: 150 mg twice daily or 300 mg at bedtime
GERD: Oral: 150 mg twice daily
Meal-induced heartburn, acid indigestion, and sour stomach (OTC labeling):
Oral: 75 mg tablet [OTC] twice daily, 30-60 minutes prior to consuming food or beverages
Eradication of *Helicobacter pylori* (unlabeled use): Oral: 150 mg twice daily; requires combination therapy

Renal Impairment:

Active treatment:
Cl_{cr} 20-50 mL/minute: 150 mg/day
Cl_{cr} <20 mL/minute: 150 mg every other day
Maintenance treatment:
Cl_{cr} 20-50 mL/minute: 150 mg every other day
Cl_{cr} <20 mL/minute: 150 mg every 3 days

Monitoring Parameters Signs and symptoms of peptic ulcer disease, occult blood with GI bleeding, gastric pH where necessary; monitor renal function to correct dose; monitor for side effects

Test Interactions False-positive urine protein using Multistix®, gastric acid secretion test, skin tests allergen extracts, serum creatinine and serum transaminase concentrations, urine protein test

Patient Information May take several days before relief of stomach pain occurs; take with or immediately after meals; inform pharmacist and physician (nurse practitioner) of any concomitant drug therapy; stagger doses with antacids with this medication by taking antacids 30-60 minutes before or after taking nizatidine

Additional Information Giving a dose at 6 PM may more effectively suppress nocturnal acid secretion than giving a dose at 10 PM.

Special Geriatric Considerations H_2 blockers are the preferred drugs for treating peptic ulcer disorder (PUD) in the elderly due to cost and ease of administration. These agents are no less or more effective than any other therapy. The preferred agents (due to side effects and drug interaction profile and pharmacokinetics) are ranitidine, famotidine, and nizatidine. Treatment for PUD in the elderly is recommended for 12 weeks since their lesions are larger, and therefore, take longer to heal. Always adjust dose based upon creatinine clearance.

Dosage Forms Excipient information presented when available (limited, particularly for generics); consult specific product labeling.
Capsule (Axid®): 150 mg, 300 mg
Solution, oral (Axid®): 15 mg/mL (120 mL, 480 mL) [bubble gum flavor]
Tablet (Axid® AR): 75 mg

Selected References

Fennerty MD and Higbee M, "Drug Therapy of Gastrointestinal Disease," *Geriatric Pharmacology*, Bressler R and Katz MD, eds, New York, NY: McGraw-Hill, 1993, 585-608.

- ♦ **Nizoral®** *see* Ketoconazole *on page 853*
- ♦ **Nizoral® A-D [OTC]** *see* Ketoconazole *on page 853*
- ♦ **Nolvadex® [DSC]** *see* Tamoxifen *on page 1515*
- ♦ **Norco®** *see* Hydrocodone and Acetaminophen *on page 759*
- ♦ **Nordeoxyguanosine** *see* Ganciclovir *on page 697*
- ♦ **Norflex™** *see* Orphenadrine *on page 1165*

Norfloxacin (nor FLOKS a sin)

Related Information

Antimicrobial Activity Against Selected Organisms *on page 1728*

Medication Safety Issues

Sound-alike/look-alike issues:
Norfloxacin may be confused with Norflex™, Noroxin®
Noroxin® may be confused with Neurontin®, Norflex™, norfloxacin

(Continued)

Norfloxacin *(Continued)*

U.S. Brand Names Noroxin®

Canadian Brand Names Apo-Norflox®; CO Norfloxacin; Norfloxacine®; Noroxin®; Novo-Norfloxacin; PMS-Norfloxacin; Riva-Norfloxacin

Generic Available No

Pharmacologic Category Antibiotic, Quinolone

Use Uncomplicated and complicated urinary tract infections caused by susceptible gram-negative and gram-positive bacteria; sexually-transmitted disease (eg, uncomplicated urethral and cervical gonorrhea) caused by *N. gonorrhoeae*; prostatitis due to *E. coli*

> **Note:** As of April 2007, the CDC no longer recommends the use of fluoroquinolones for the treatment of gonococcal disease.

Contraindications Hypersensitivity to norfloxacin, quinolones, or any component of the formulation; history of tendonitis or tendon rupture associated with quinolone use

Warnings/Precautions Use with caution in patients with known or suspected CNS disorders. Tendon inflammation and/or rupture have been reported with quinolone antibiotics. Risk may be increased with concurrent corticosteroids, particularly in the elderly. Discontinue at first sign of tendon inflammation or pain. CNS stimulation may occur which may lead to tremor, restlessness, confusion, and very rarely to hallucinations or convulsive seizures. Potential for seizures, although very rare, may be increased with concomitant NSAID therapy. Use with caution in individuals at risk of seizures. Use may be associated (rarely) with prolongation of QT_c interval; avoid concurrent use with class Ia and class III antiarrhythmics; use caution with other drugs may cause QT_c prolongation.

Severe hypersensitivity reactions, including anaphylaxis, have occurred with quinolone therapy. Reactions may present as typical allergic symptoms after a single dose, or may manifest as severe idiosyncratic dermatologic, vascular, pulmonary, renal, hepatic, and/or hematologic events, usually after multiple doses. Prompt discontinuation of drug should occur if skin rash or other symptoms arise. Prolonged use may result in fungal or bacterial superinfection, including *C. difficile*-associated diarrhea (CDAD) and pseudomembranous colitis; CDAD has been observed >2 months postantibiotic treatment. Avoid excessive exposure to sunlight; other quinolones have been associated with phototoxicity. May be associated with the development of peripheral neuropathy and/or paresthesias; discontinue in patients who develop symptoms consistent with neuropathy. Quinolones may exacerbate myasthenia gravis; use with caution (rare, potentially life-threatening weakness of respiratory muscles may occur). Use caution with renal impairment.

Adverse Reactions (Reflective of adult population; not specific for elderly) 1% to 10%:

Central nervous system: Headache (3%), dizziness (3%)

Gastrointestinal: Nausea (4%), abdominal cramping (2%)

Neuromuscular & skeletal: Weakness (1%)

Overdosage/Toxicology Symptoms include acute renal failure and seizures. Following GI decontamination, treatment should be symptom-directed and supportive.

Drug Interactions Inhibits CYP1A2 (strong), 3A4 (moderate)

Caffeine: Levels/effects may be increased by quinolones; monitor for CNS stimulation.

Corticosteroids: Concurrent use may increase the risk of tendon rupture, particularly in elderly patients (overall incidence rare).

Cyclosporine: Norfloxacin may increase serum cyclosporine concentrations; monitor

CYP1A2 substrates: Norfloxacin may increase the levels/effects of CYP1A2 substrates. Example substrates include aminophylline, fluvoxamine, mexiletine, mirtazapine, ropinirole, and trifluoperazine.

CYP3A4 substrates: Norfloxacin may increase the levels/effects of CYP3A4 substrates. Example substrates include benzodiazepines, calcium channel blockers, mirtazapine, nateglinide, nefazodone, sildenafil (and other PDE-5 inhibitors), tacrolimus, and venlafaxine. Selected benzodiazepines (midazolam and triazolam), cisapride, ergot alkaloids, selected HMG-CoA reductase inhibitors (lovastatin and simvastatin), and pimozide are generally contraindicated with strong CYP3A4 inhibitors.

Glyburide: Quinolones may increase the effect of glyburide; monitor.

Metal cations (aluminum, calcium, iron, magnesium, and zinc) bind quinolones in the gastrointestinal tract and inhibit absorption. Concurrent administration of most antacids, oral electrolyte supplements, quinapril, sucralfate, some didanosine formulations (pediatric powder for oral suspension), and other highly-buffered oral drugs, should be avoided. Norfloxacin should be administered 4 hours before or 8 hours after these agents.

Nitrofurantoin: May antagonize the activity of norfloxacin in treating UTIs.

NSAIDs: Risk of seizures may be increased with concomitant NSAID use. Risk is considered quite low and may only be a factor with high serum levels of either agent and/or in patients with additional predisposing factors (eg, renal dysfunction, history of seizure or other neurological disorder).

Probenecid: May decrease renal secretion of norfloxacin.

QT_c-prolonging agents: Effects may be additive with norfloxacin. Avoid concurrent use with Class Ia and Class III antiarrhythmics; use caution with other drugs known to prolong QT_c, including erythromycin, cisapride, antipsychotics, and cyclic antidepressants.

Theophylline: Norfloxacin may increase serum levels/effects of theophylline; monitor.

Typhoid vaccine: Antibiotics may decrease the therapeutic effect of live, attenuated Ty21a vaccine; delay vaccination for >24 hours after administration of antibacterial agents.

Warfarin: The hypoprothrombinemic effect of warfarin may be enhanced by some quinolone antibiotics; monitor INR.

Ethanol/Nutrition/Herb Interactions

Food: Norfloxacin average peak serum concentrations may be decreased if taken with dairy products. Use caution with caffeine-containing beverages/foods; quinolones may increase blood levels of caffeine.

Herb/Nutraceutical: Avoid dong quai, St John's wort (may also cause photosensitization); avoid administration within 2 hours of multivitamins or other supplements containing iron, zinc, magnesium, or aluminum.

Stability Store at 25°C (77°F). Keep container tightly closed.

Mechanism of Action Norfloxacin is a DNA gyrase inhibitor. DNA gyrase is an essential bacterial enzyme that maintains the superhelical structure of DNA. DNA gyrase is required for DNA replication and transcription, DNA repair, recombination, and transposition; bactericidal

Pharmacokinetics

Absorption: Oral: Rapid, up to 40%

Protein binding: 10% to 15%

Metabolism: Hepatic

Half-life: 4.8 hours (can be higher with reduced glomerular filtration rates)

Time to peak serum concentration: Within 1-2 hours

Excretion: Urine (26% to 32% as unchanged drug; 5% to 8% as metabolites); feces

Dosage

Geriatrics & Adults:

Dysenteric enterocolitis *(Shigella* unlabeled use): Oral: 400 mg twice daily for 5 days

Prostatitis: Oral: 400 mg every 12 hours for 4-6 weeks

Traveler's diarrhea (unlabeled use): Oral: 400 mg twice daily for 3 days, single dose may also be effective

Uncomplicated gonorrhea: Oral: 800 mg as a single dose. **Note:** As of April 2007, the CDC no longer recommends the use of fluoroquinolones for the treatment of uncomplicated gonococcal disease.

Urinary tract infections: Oral:

Uncomplicated: 400 mg twice daily for 3-14 days

Uncomplicated due to *E. coli, K. pneumoniae, P. mirabilis*: 400 mg twice daily for 7-10 days

Complicated: 400 mg twice daily for 10-21 days

Renal Impairment: Cl_{cr} ≤30 mL/minute/1.73 m^2: Administer 400 mg every 24 hours

Administration Hold antacids, sucralfate, or multivitamins/supplements containing iron, zinc, magnesium, or aluminum for 3-4 hours after giving norfloxacin; do not administer together. Best taken on an empty stomach with water (1 hour before or 2 hours after meals, milk, or other dairy products).

Monitoring Parameters Signs and symptoms of infection, WBC, mental status, culture, and sensitivity

Patient Information Take 1 hour before or 2 hours after meals; do not take with antacids, dairy products, iron, or zinc products; may cause dizziness, headache, or stimulation; avoid excess natural or artificial sunlight exposure; complete full course of therapy

Special Geriatric Considerations Adjust dose for renal function.

Dosage Forms Excipient information presented when available (limited, particularly for generics); consult specific product labeling.

Tablet:

Noroxin®: 400 mg

Selected References

Nilsson-Ehle I and Ljungberg B, "Quinolone Disposition in the Elderly: Practical Implications," *Drugs Aging*, 1991, 1(4):279-88.

♦ **Norgestimate and Estradiol** *see* Estradiol and Norgestimate *on page 554*

♦ **Noritate®** *see* Metronidazole *on page 1031*

♦ **Normal Saline** *see* Sodium Chloride *on page 1475*

♦ **Noroxin®** *see* Norfloxacin *on page 1135*

♦ **Norpace®** *see* Disopyramide *on page 455*

♦ **Norpace® CR** *see* Disopyramide *on page 455*

♦ **Norpramin®** *see* Desipramine *on page 406*

♦ **Nortemp Children's [OTC]** *see* Acetaminophen *on page 29*

Nortriptyline (nor TRIP ti leen)

Related Information
Antidepressant Agents *on page 1742*
Pharmacotherapy of Urinary Incontinence *on page 1822*
Serum Drug Concentrations Commonly Monitored Guidelines *on page 1862*

Medication Safety Issues
Sound-alike/look-alike issues:
Nortriptyline may be confused with amitriptyline, desipramine, Norpramin®
Aventyl® HCl may be confused with Bentyl®
Pamelor® may be confused with Demerol®, Dymelor®

U.S. Brand Names Pamelor®

Canadian Brand Names Alti-Nortriptyline; Apo-Nortriptyline®; Aventyl®; Gen-Nortriptyline; Norventyl; Novo-Nortriptyline; Nu-Nortriptyline; PMS-Nortriptyline

Index Terms Nortriptyline Hydrochloride

Generic Available Yes: Excludes solution

Pharmacologic Category Antidepressant, Tricyclic (Secondary Amine)

Use Treatment of various forms of depression, often in conjunction with psychotherapy

Unlabeled/Investigational Use Treatment of chronic pain, anxiety disorders, enuresis, attention-deficit/hyperactivity disorder (ADHD); adjunctive therapy for smoking cessation

Restrictions An FDA-approved medication guide concerning the use of antidepressants in children, adolescents, and young adults must be distributed when dispensing an outpatient prescription (new or refill) where this medication is to be used without direct supervision of a healthcare provider. Medication guides are available at http://www.fda.gov/cder/Offices/ODS/medication_guides.htm. Dispense to parents or guardians of children and adolescents receiving this medication.

Contraindications Hypersensitivity to nortriptyline and similar chemical class, or any component of the formulation; use of MAO inhibitors within 14 days; use in a patient during the acute recovery phase of MI

Warnings/Precautions [U.S. Boxed Warning]: Antidepressants increase the risk of suicidal thinking and behavior in children, adolescents, and young adults (18-24 years of age) with major depressive disorder (MDD) and other psychiatric disorders; consider risk prior to prescribing. Short-term studies did not show an increased risk in patients >24 years of age and showed a decreased risk in patients ≥65 years. Closely monitor for clinical worsening, suicidality, or unusual changes in behavior; the patient's family or caregiver should be instructed to closely observe the patient and communicate condition with healthcare provider. A medication guide should be dispensed with each prescription.

The possibility of a suicide attempt is inherent in major depression and may persist until remission occurs. Monitor for worsening of depression or suicidality, especially during initiation of therapy (generally first 1-2 months) or with dose increases or decreases. Use caution in high-risk patients. Worsening depression and severe abrupt suicidality that are not part of the presenting symptoms may require discontinuation or modification of drug therapy. The patient's family or caregiver should be alerted to monitor patients for the emergence of suicidality and associated behaviors (such as agitation, irritability, hostility, impulsivity, and hypomania) and call healthcare provider.

May worsen psychosis in some patients or precipitate a shift to mania or hypomania in patients with bipolar disorder. Patients presenting with depressive symptoms should be screened for bipolar disorder. Monotherapy in patients with bipolar disorder should be avoided. **Nortriptyline is not FDA approved for the treatment of bipolar depression.**

The risk of sedation and orthostatic effects are low relative to other antidepressants. However, nortriptyline may result in impaired performance of tasks requiring alertness (eg, operating machinery or driving). Sedative effects may be additive with other CNS depressants and/or ethanol. The degree of anticholinergic blockade produced by this agent is moderate relative to other cyclic antidepressants, however, caution should still be used in patients with urinary retention, benign prostatic hyperplasia, narrow-angle glaucoma, xerostomia, visual problems, constipation, or history of bowel obstruction. May cause orthostatic hypotension (risk is low relative to other antidepressants) or conduction disturbances. Use with caution in patients with a history of cardiovascular disease (including previous MI, stroke, tachycardia, or conduction abnormalities). The risk conduction abnormalities with this agent is moderate relative to other antidepressants.

Consider discontinuing, when possible, prior to elective surgery. Therapy should not be abruptly discontinued in patients receiving high doses for prolonged periods. May alter glucose regulation - use caution in patients with diabetes. Use caution in patients with a previous seizure disorder or condition predisposing to seizures such as brain damage, alcoholism, or concurrent therapy with other drugs which lower the seizure threshold. May increase the risks associated with electroconvulsive therapy. Use with caution in hyperthyroid patients or those receiving thyroid supplementation. Use with caution in patients with hepatic or renal dysfunction and in elderly patients.

Adverse Reactions (Reflective of adult population; not specific for elderly)
Frequency not defined.

Cardiovascular: Postural hypotension, arrhythmia, hypertension, heart block, tachycardia, palpitation, MI

Central nervous system: Confusion, delirium, hallucinations, restlessness, insomnia, disorientation, delusions, anxiety, agitation, panic, nightmares, hypomania, exacerbation of psychosis, incoordination, ataxia, extrapyramidal symptoms, seizure

Dermatologic: Alopecia, photosensitivity, rash, petechiae, urticaria, itching

Endocrine & metabolic: Sexual dysfunction, gynecomastia, breast enlargement, galactorrhea, increase or decrease in libido, increase in blood sugar, SIADH

Gastrointestinal: Xerostomia, constipation, vomiting, anorexia, diarrhea, abdominal cramps, black tongue, nausea, unpleasant taste, weight gain/loss

Genitourinary: Urinary retention, delayed micturition, impotence, testicular edema

Hematologic: Rarely agranulocytosis, eosinophilia, purpura, thrombocytopenia

Hepatic: Increased liver enzymes, cholestatic jaundice

Neuromuscular & skeletal: Tremor, numbness, tingling, paresthesia, peripheral neuropathy

Ocular: Blurred vision, eye pain, disturbances in accommodation, mydriasis

Otic: Tinnitus

Miscellaneous: Diaphoresis (excessive), allergic reactions

Overdosage/Toxicology Signs and symptoms include agitation, confusion, hallucinations, urinary retention, hypothermia, hypotension, seizures, ventricular and tachycardia. Following initiation of essential overdose management, toxic symptoms should be treated. Ventricular arrhythmias often respond to phenytoin 15-20 mg/kg with concurrent systemic alkalinization (sodium bicarbonate 0.5-2 mEq/kg I.V.). Arrhythmias unresponsive to this therapy may respond to lidocaine 1 mg/kg I.V. followed by a titrated infusion. Physostigmine (1-2 mg slow I.V.) may be indicated in reversing life-threatening cardiac arrhythmias. Seizures usually respond to diazepam I.V. boluses (5-10 mg up to 30 mg). If seizures are unresponsive or recur, phenytoin or phenobarbital may be required.

Drug Interactions Substrate of CYP1A2 (minor), 2C19 (minor), 2D6 (major), 3A4 (minor); **Inhibits** CYP2D6 (weak), 2E1 (weak)

Altretamine: Concurrent use may cause orthostatic hypertension

Amphetamines: TCAs may enhance the effect of amphetamines; monitor for adverse CV effects

Anticholinergics: Combined use with TCAs may produce additive anticholinergic effects

Antihypertensives: TCAs may inhibit the antihypertensive response to bethanidine, clonidine, debrisoquin, guanadrel, guanethidine, guanabenz, guanfacine; monitor BP; consider alternate antihypertensive agent

Beta-agonists: When combined with TCAs may predispose patients to cardiac arrhythmias

Bupropion: May increase the levels of tricyclic antidepressants; based on limited information; monitor response

Carbamazepine: Tricyclic antidepressants may increase carbamazepine levels; monitor

Cholestyramine and colestipol: May bind TCAs and reduce their absorption; monitor for altered response

Clonidine: Abrupt discontinuation of clonidine may cause hypertensive crisis, amitriptyline may enhance the response

CNS depressants: Sedative effects may be additive with TCAs; monitor for increased effect; includes benzodiazepines, barbiturates, antipsychotics, ethanol and other sedative medications

CYP2D6 inhibitors: May increase the levels/effects of nortriptyline. Example inhibitors include chlorpromazine, delavirdine, fluoxetine, miconazole, paroxetine, pergolide, quinidine, quinine, ritonavir, and ropinirole.

Epinephrine (and other direct alpha-agonists): Pressor response to I.V. epinephrine, norepinephrine, and phenylephrine may be enhanced in patients receiving TCAs (**Note:** Effect is unlikely with epinephrine or levonordefrin dosages typically administered as infiltration in combination with local anesthetics)

Fenfluramine: May increase tricyclic antidepressant levels/effects

Hypoglycemic agents (including insulin): TCAs may enhance the hypoglycemic effects of tolazamide, chlorpropamide, or insulin; monitor for changes in blood glucose levels; reported with chlorpropamide, tolazamide, and insulin

(Continued)

Nortriptyline *(Continued)*

Levodopa: Tricyclic antidepressants may decrease the absorption (bioavailability) of levodopa; rare hypertensive episodes have also been attributed to this combination

Linezolid: Hyperpyrexia, hypertension, tachycardia, confusion, seizures, and **deaths have been reported** with agents which inhibit MAO (serotonin syndrome); this combination should be avoided

Lithium: Concurrent use with a TCA may increase the risk for neurotoxicity

MAO inhibitors: Hyperpyrexia, hypertension, tachycardia, confusion, seizures, and **deaths have been reported** (serotonin syndrome); this combination should be avoided

Methylphenidate: Metabolism of TCAs may be decreased

Phenothiazines: Serum concentrations of some TCAs may be increased; in addition, TCAs may increase concentration of phenothiazines; monitor for altered clinical response

QT_c-prolonging agents: Concurrent use of tricyclic agents with other drugs which may prolong QT_c interval may increase the risk of potentially fatal arrhythmias; includes type Ia and type III antiarrhythmics agents, selected quinolones (moxifloxacin), cisapride, and other agents

Ritonavir: Combined use of high-dose tricyclic antidepressants with ritonavir may cause serotonin syndrome in HIV-positive patients; monitor

Sucralfate: Absorption of tricyclic antidepressants may be reduced with coadministration

Sympathomimetics, indirect-acting: Tricyclic antidepressants may result in a decreased sensitivity to indirect-acting sympathomimetics; includes dopamine and ephedrine; also see interaction with epinephrine (and direct-acting sympathomimetics)

Tramadol: Tramadol's risk of seizures may be increased with TCAs

Valproic acid: May increase serum concentrations/adverse effects of some tricyclic antidepressants

Warfarin (and other oral anticoagulants): TCAs may increase the anticoagulant effect in patients stabilized on warfarin; monitor INR

Ethanol/Nutrition/Herb Interactions

Ethanol: Avoid ethanol (may increase CNS depression).

Food: Grapefruit juice may inhibit the metabolism of some TCAs and clinical toxicity may result.

Herb/Nutraceutical: Avoid valerian, St John's wort, SAMe, kava kava (may increase risk of serotonin syndrome and/or excessive sedation).

Stability Protect from light.

Mechanism of Action Traditionally believed to increase the synaptic concentration of serotonin and/or norepinephrine in the central nervous system by inhibition of their reuptake by the presynaptic neuronal membrane. However, additional receptor effects have been found including desensitization of adenyl cyclase, down regulation of beta-adrenergic receptors, and down regulation of serotonin receptors.

Pharmacodynamics Onset of therapeutic effects: Takes 1-3 weeks before effects are seen; NE >5-HT

Pharmacokinetics

Distribution: V_d: 21 L/kg

Protein binding: 93% to 95%

Metabolism: Hepatic; undergoes significant first-pass metabolism

Half-life: 28-31 hours

Geriatrics: Single-dose pharmacokinetic studies have found the mean half-life to range from 37-45 hours in older subjects; the mean metabolic clearance was significantly lower compared to younger subjects, 20 vs 54 L/hour

Time to peak serum concentration: Oral: Within 7-8.5 hours

Elimination: Primarily detoxified in the liver and excreted as metabolites and small amounts of unchanged drug in the urine; small amounts of biliary elimination occurs.

Dosage

Geriatrics: Note: Nortriptyline is one of the best tolerated TCAs in the elderly.

Initial: 10-25 mg at bedtime

Dosage can be increased by 25 mg every 3 days for inpatients and weekly for outpatients if tolerated.

Usual maintenance dose: 75 mg as a single bedtime dose or 2 divided doses; however, lower or higher doses may be required to stay within the therapeutic window.

Adults:

Depression: Oral: 25 mg 3-4 times/day up to 150 mg/day

Chronic urticaria, angioedema, nocturnal pruritus (unlabeled use): Oral: 75 mg/day

Smoking cessation (unlabeled use): Oral: 25-75 mg/day beginning 10-14 days before "quit" day; continue therapy for ≥12 weeks after "quit" day

Hepatic Impairment: Lower doses and slower titration are recommended dependent on individualization of dosage.

Monitoring Parameters Blood pressure and pulse; serum concentration, target symptoms

Reference Range Therapeutic: 50-150 ng/mL (SI: 190-570 nmol/L); Toxic: >500 ng/mL (SI: >1900 nmol/L)

Patient Information Do not stop abruptly, rise slowly to avoid dizziness; may cause dry mouth, constipation, blurred vision; use sugarless hard candy for dry mouth

Additional Information Maximum antidepressant effect may not be seen for 2 or more weeks after initiation of therapy

Special Geriatric Considerations Since nortriptyline is the least likely of the tricyclic antidepressants (TCAs) to cause orthostatic hypotension and one of the least anticholinergic and sedating TCAs, it is a preferred agent when a TCA is indicated. Data from a clinical trial comparing fluoxetine to tricyclics suggests that fluoxetine is significantly less effective than nortriptyline in hospitalized elderly patients with unipolar affective disorder, especially those with melancholia and concurrent cardiovascular disease. Paroxetine has been shown to be an equally effective antidepressant compared to nortriptyline in patients with ischemic heart disease. However, nortriptyline was associated a significantly higher rate of adverse cardiac events (sustained increase in heart rate, sinus tachycardia, and asymptomatic increase in ventricular ectopy) compared to placebo.

Dosage Forms Excipient information presented when available (limited, particularly for generics); consult specific product labeling.

Capsule, as hydrochloride: 10 mg, 25 mg, 50 mg, 75 mg

Pamelor®: 10 mg, 25 mg, 50 mg, 75 mg [may contain benzyl alcohol; 50 mg may also contain sodium bisulfite]

Solution, as hydrochloride (Pamelor®): 10 mg/5 mL (473 mL) [contains alcohol 4% and benzoic acid]

Selected References

Dowling S, Crome P, and Braithwaite R, "Pharmacokinetics of Single Oral Doses of Nortriptyline in Depressed Elderly Hospital Patients and Young Healthy Volunteers," *Clin Pharmacokinet*, 1980, 5(4):394-401.

Prochazka AV, Kick S, Steinbrunn C, et al, "A Randomized Trial of Nortriptyline Combined With Transdermal Nicotine for Smoking Cessation," *Arch Intern Med*, 2004, 164(20):2229-33.

Roose SP, Glassman AH, Attia E, et al, "Comparative Efficacy of Selective Serotonin Reuptake Inhibitors and Tricyclics in the Treatment of Melancholia," *Am J Psychiatry*, 1994, 151(12):1735-9.

Roose SP, Laghrissi-Thode F, Kennedy JS, et al, "Comparison of Paroxetine and Nortriptyline in Depressed Patients With Ischemic Heart Disease," *JAMA*, 1998, 279(4):287-91.

Schneider LS, Cooper TB, Staples FR, et al, "Prediction of Individual Dosage of Nortriptyline in Depressed Elderly Outpatients," *J Clin Psychopharmacol*, 1987, 7(5):311-4.

Turbott J, Norman TR, Burrows GD, et al, "Pharmacokinetics of Nortriptyline in Elderly Volunteers," *Commun Psychopharmacol*, 1980, 4(3):225-31.

◆ **Nortriptyline Hydrochloride** *see* Nortriptyline *on page 1138*
◆ **Norvasc®** *see* Amlodipine *on page 88*
◆ **Novolin® 70/30** *see* Insulin NPH and Insulin Regular *on page 814*
◆ **Novolin® N** *see* Insulin NPH *on page 813*
◆ **Novolin® R** *see* Insulin Regular *on page 815*
◆ **NovoLog®** *see* Insulin Aspart *on page 808*
◆ **NovoLog® Mix 70/30** *see* Insulin Aspart Protamine and Insulin Aspart *on page 809*
◆ **Noxafil®** *see* Posaconazole *on page 1285*
◆ **NPH Insulin** *see* Insulin NPH *on page 813*
◆ **NPH Insulin and Regular Insulin** *see* Insulin NPH and Insulin Regular *on page 814*
◆ **NRS® [OTC]** *see* Oxymetazoline *on page 1184*
◆ **NSC-740** *see* Methotrexate *on page 1005*
◆ **NSC-750** *see* Busulfan *on page 203*
◆ **NSC-755** *see* Mercaptopurine *on page 985*
◆ **NSC-3088** *see* Chlorambucil *on page 287*
◆ **NSC-8806** *see* Melphalan *on page 974*
◆ **NSC-26271** *see* Cyclophosphamide *on page 376*
◆ **NSC-71423** *see* Megestrol *on page 970*
◆ **NSC-147834** *see* Flutamide *on page 658*
◆ **NSC-180973** *see* Tamoxifen *on page 1515*
◆ **NSC-367982** *see* Interferon Alfa-2a *on page 820*
◆ **NSC-377526** *see* Leuprolide *on page 883*
◆ **NSC-606864** *see* Goserelin *on page 722*
◆ **NSC-614629** *see* Filgrastim *on page 624*
◆ **NSC-684588** *see* Nilutamide *on page 1122*
◆ **NSC-706725** *see* Raloxifene *on page 1374*
◆ **NSC-714371** *see* Dalteparin *on page 388*
◆ **NSC-719344** *see* Anastrozole *on page 112*

- ◆ **NSC-719345** *see* Letrozole *on page 882*
- ◆ **NSC-721517** *see* Zoledronic Acid *on page 1704*
- ◆ **NSC-722623** *see* Ibandronate *on page 782*
- ◆ **NSC-724223** *see* Epoetin Alfa *on page 519*
- ◆ **NSC-725961** *see* Pegfilgrastim *on page 1212*
- ◆ **NSC-729969** *see* Darbepoetin Alfa *on page 397*
- ◆ **NTG** *see* Nitroglycerin *on page 1129*
- ◆ **Nubain®** *see* Nalbuphine *on page 1083*
- ◆ **NuLev™** *see* Hyoscyamine *on page 778*
- ◆ **Numoisyn™** *see* Saliva Substitute *on page 1443*
- ◆ **Numorphan® [DSC]** *see* Oxymorphone *on page 1186*
- ◆ **Nupercainal® Hydrocortisone Cream [OTC]** *see* Hydrocortisone *on page 762*
- ◆ **Nu-Tears® [OTC]** *see* Artificial Tears *on page 124*
- ◆ **Nu-Tears® II [OTC]** *see* Artificial Tears *on page 124*
- ◆ **Nutracort®** *see* Hydrocortisone *on page 762*
- ◆ **Nyamyc™** *see* Nystatin *on page 1142*
- ◆ **Nydrazid® [DSC]** *see* Isoniazid *on page 836*

Nystatin (nye STAT in)

Medication Safety Issues
Sound-alike/look-alike issues:
Nystatin may be confused with Nilstat®, Nitrostat®
Nilstat may be confused with Nitrostat®, nystatin

U.S. Brand Names Bio-Statin®; Mycostatin®; Nyamyc™; Nystat-Rx®; Nystop®; Pedi-Dri®

Canadian Brand Names Candistatin®; Nilstat; Nyaderm; PMS-Nystatin

Generic Available Yes: Cream, ointment, powder, suspension, tablet

Pharmacologic Category Antifungal Agent, Oral Nonabsorbed; Antifungal Agent, Topical; Antifungal Agent, Vaginal

Use Treatment of susceptible cutaneous, mucocutaneous, and oral cavity fungal infections normally caused by the *Candida* species

Contraindications Hypersensitivity to nystatin or any component of the formulation

Adverse Reactions (Reflective of adult population; not specific for elderly)
Frequency not defined: Dermatologic: Contact dermatitis, Stevens-Johnson syndrome
1% to 10%: Gastrointestinal: Nausea, vomiting, diarrhea, stomach pain

Overdosage/Toxicology Symptoms include nausea, vomiting, and diarrhea. Treatment is supportive.

Drug Interactions No data reported

Stability
Vaginal insert: Store in refrigerator. Protect from temperature extremes, moisture, and light.
Oral tablet, ointment, topical powder, and oral suspension: Store at controlled room temperature of 15°C to 25°C (59°F to 77°F).

Mechanism of Action Binds to sterols in fungal cell membrane, changing the cell wall permeability allowing for leakage of cellular contents

Pharmacokinetics
Absorption: Not absorbed through mucous membranes or intact skin; poorly absorbed from the GI tract
Elimination: In feces as unchanged drug

Dosage
Geriatrics & Adults:
Oral candidiasis: Suspension (swish and swallow orally): 400,000-600,000 units 4 times/day
Mucocutaneous infections: Topical: Apply 2-3 times/day to affected areas; very moist topical lesions are treated best with powder.
Intestinal infections: Oral tablets: 500,000-1,000,000 units every 8 hours
Vaginal infections: Vaginal tablets: Insert 1 tablet/day at bedtime for 2 weeks. (May also be given orally.)
Note: Powder for compounding: 1/8 teaspoon (500,000 units) to equal approximately 1/2 cup of water; give 4 times/day

Patient Information The oral suspension should be swished about the mouth and retained in the mouth for as long as possible (several minutes) before swallowing. Troches must be allowed to dissolve slowly and should not be chewed or swallowed whole. *Candida* infections should be treated for 48 hours after symptoms have disappeared. Avoid contact with the eyes.

Special Geriatric Considerations For oral infections, patients who wear dentures must have them removed and cleaned in order to eliminate source of reinfection.

Dosage Forms Excipient information presented when available (limited, particularly for generics); consult specific product labeling.

Capsule:

Bio-Statin®: 500,000 units, 1 million units

Cream: 100,000 units/g (15 g, 30 g)

Mycostatin®: 100,000 units/g (30 g)

Ointment, topical: 100,000 units/g (15 g, 30 g)

Powder, for prescription compounding: 50 million units (10 g); 150 million units (30 g); 500 million units (100 g); 2 billion units (400 g)

Nystat-Rx®: 50 million units (10 g); 150 million units (30 g); 500 million units (100 g); 1 billion units (190 g); 2 billion units (350 g)

Powder, topical:

Mycostatin®: 100,000 units/g (15 g) [contains talc]

Nyamyc™: 100,000 units/g (15 g, 30 g) [contains talc]

Nystop®: 100,000 units/g (15 g, 30 g, 60 g) [contains talc]

Pedi-Dri®: 100,000 units/g (56.7 g) [contains talc]

Suspension, oral: 100,000 units/mL (5 mL, 60 mL, 480 mL)

Tablet: 500,000 units

Tablet, vaginal: 100,000 units (15s) [packaged with applicator]

Selected References

Dismukes WE, Wade JS, Lee JY, et al, "A Randomized, Double-Blind Trial of Nystatin Therapy for the Candidiasis Hypersensitivity Syndrome," *N Engl J Med*, 1990, 323(25):1717-23.

Nystatin and Triamcinolone (nye STAT in & trye am SIN oh lone)

Related Information

Nystatin on page 1142
Triamcinolone on page 1619

Medication Safety Issues

Sound-alike/look-alike issues:

Mycolog®-II may be confused with Halog®

U.S. Brand Names Mycolog®-II [DSC]

Index Terms Triamcinolone and Nystatin

Generic Available Yes

Pharmacologic Category Antifungal Agent, Topical; Corticosteroid, Topical

Use Treatment of cutaneous candidiasis

Contraindications Hypersensitivity to nystatin, triamcinolone, or any component of the formulation

Warnings/Precautions

Concerns related to adverse effects:

- Adrenal suppression: Systemic absorption of topical corticosteroids may cause hypothalamic-pituitary-adrenal (HPA) axis suppression (reversible). HPA axis suppression may lead to adrenal crisis. Risk is increased when used over large surface areas, for prolonged periods, or with occlusive dressings.
- Contact dermatitis: Allergic contact dermatitis can occur, it is usually diagnosed by failure to heal rather than clinical exacerbation.
- Kaposi's sarcoma: Prolonged treatment with corticosteroids has been associated with the development of Kaposi's sarcoma (case reports); if noted, discontinuation of therapy should be considered.
- Systemic effects: Adverse systemic effects including hyperglycemia, glycosuria, fluid and electrolyte changes, and HPA suppression may occur when used on large surface areas, for prolonged periods, or with an occlusive dressing.

Adverse Reactions (Reflective of adult population; not specific for elderly)

1% to 10%:

Dermatologic: Dryness, folliculitis, hypertrichosis, acne, hypopigmentation, allergic dermatitis, maceration of the skin, skin atrophy

Local: Burning, itching, irritation

Miscellaneous: Increased incidence of secondary infection

Drug Interactions No data reported

Mechanism of Action Nystatin is an antifungal agent that binds to sterols in fungal cell membrane, changing the cell wall permeability allowing for leakage of cellular contents. Triamcinolone is a synthetic corticosteroid; it decreases inflammation by suppression of migration of polymorphonuclear leukocytes and reversal of increased capillary permeability. It suppresses the immune system reducing activity and volume of the lymphatic system. It suppresses adrenal function at high doses.

Dosage

Geriatrics & Adults: Cutaneous *Candida*: Topical: Apply sparingly 2-4 times/day

Administration External use only; do not use on open wounds; apply sparingly to occlusive dressings; should not be used in the presence of open or weeping lesions

(Continued)

Nystatin and Triamcinolone *(Continued)*

Patient Information Before applying, gently wash area to reduce risk of infection; apply a thin film to cleansed area and rub in gently and thoroughly until medication vanishes; avoid exposure to sunlight, severe sunburn may occur

Special Geriatric Considerations No specific dose adjustment or use consideration necessary in the elderly; for oral infections, patients who wear dentures must have them removed and cleaned in order to eliminate source of reinfection.

Dosage Forms Excipient information presented when available (limited, particularly for generics); consult specific product labeling. [DSC] = Discontinued product

Cream (Mycolog®-II [DSC]): Nystatin 100,000 units and triamcinolone acetonide 0.1% (15 g, 30 g, 60 g)

Ointment: Nystatin 100,000 units and triamcinolone acetonide 0.1% (15 g, 30 g, 60 g)

Mycolog®-II: Nystatin 100,000 units and triamcinolone acetonide 0.1% (15 g, 30 g, 60 g) [DSC]

- ♦ **Nystat-Rx®** *see Nystatin on page 1142*
- ♦ **Nystop®** *see Nystatin on page 1142*
- ♦ **Nytol® Quick Caps [OTC]** *see DiphenhydrAMINE on page 447*
- ♦ **Nytol® Quick Gels [OTC]** *see DiphenhydrAMINE on page 447*
- ♦ **NāSop™** *see Phenylephrine on page 1247*
- ♦ **Nöstrilla® [OTC]** *see Oxymetazoline on page 1184*
- ♦ **OCBZ** *see Oxcarbazepine on page 1174*
- ♦ **Occlusal®-HP [OTC]** *see Salicylic Acid on page 1441*
- ♦ **Ocean® [OTC]** *see Sodium Chloride on page 1475*
- ♦ **Oceant® for Kids [OTC]** *see Sodium Chloride on page 1475*
- ♦ **OcuCoat® [OTC]** *see Artificial Tears on page 124*
- ♦ **OcuCoat® PF [OTC]** *see Artificial Tears on page 124*
- ♦ **Ocufen®** *see Flurbiprofen on page 655*
- ♦ **Ocuflox®** *see Ofloxacin on page 1144*

Ocular Lubricant *(OK yoo lar LOO bri kant)*

U.S. Brand Names Akwa Tears® Ophthalmic Ointment [OTC]; Dry Eyes® Ophthalmic Ointment [OTC]; Duratears® Naturale® Ophthalmic Ointment [OTC]; HypoTears® Ophthalmic Ointment [OTC]; Lacri-Lube® NP Ophthalmic Ointment [OTC]; Lacri-Lube® S.O.P. Ophthalmic Ointment [OTC]; LubriTears® Ophthalmic Ointment [OTC]; Puralube® Ophthalmic Ointment [OTC]; Refresh PM® Ophthalmic Ointment [OTC]; Stye® Ophthalmic Ointment [OTC]; Tears Renewed® Ophthalmic Ointment [OTC]

Index Terms Petrolatum White and Mineral Oil Ophthalmic Ointment

Generic Available Yes

Pharmacologic Category Ophthalmic Agent, Miscellaneous

Use Ocular lubricant

Contraindications Known hypersensitivity to any of the components

Warnings/Precautions Discontinue if eye pain, vision change, redness or eye irritation occurs or if condition worsens or persists >72 hours; do not use with contact lenses

Stability Store away from heat

Mechanism of Action Forms an occlusive film on the surface of the eye to lubricate and protect the eye from drying

Patient Information If condition worsens or persists more than 72 hours, discontinue use and consult a physician; do not touch tip of tube or dropper to any surface to avoid contamination; do not use with contact lenses

Additional Information Ointment contains petrolatum and mineral oil

Special Geriatric Considerations Ointment is useful at bedtime; make sure patient is able to apply correctly

Dosage Forms Ointment, ophthalmic: 3.5 g

- ♦ **OcuNefrin™ [OTC]** *see Phenylephrine on page 1247*

Ofloxacin *(oh FLOKS a sin)*

Related Information

Antimicrobial Activity Against Selected Organisms *on page 1728*

Medication Safety Issues

Sound-alike/look-alike issues:

Floxin® may be confused with Flexeril®

Ocuflox® may be confused with Ocufen®

International issues:

Floxin® may be confused with Flogen® which is a brand name for naproxen in Mexico

Floxin® may be confused with Fluoxin® which is a brand name for fluoxetine in the Czech Republic and Romania

Floxin® may be confused with Flexin® which is a brand name for orphenadrine in Israel and indomethacin in Great Britain

U.S. Brand Names Floxin®; Ocuflox®

Canadian Brand Names Apo-Oflox®; Apo-Ofloxacin®; Floxin®; Novo-Ofloxacin; Ocuflox®; PMS-Ofloxacin

Index Terms Floxin Otic Singles

Generic Available Yes: Tablet, ophthalmic solution

Pharmacologic Category Antibiotic, Quinolone

Use

Quinolone antibiotic for skin and skin structure, lower respiratory, and urinary tract infections and sexually-transmitted diseases. Active against many gram-positive and gram-negative aerobic bacteria.

Note: As of April 2007, the CDC no longer recommends the use of fluoroquinolones for the treatment of gonococcal disease.

Ophthalmic: Treatment of superficial ocular infections involving the conjunctiva or cornea due to strains of susceptible organisms

Otic: Otitis externa, chronic suppurative otitis media, acute otitis media

Contraindications Hypersensitivity to ofloxacin or other members of the quinolone group such as nalidixic acid, oxolinic acid, cinoxacin, norfloxacin, and ciprofloxacin; hypersensitivity to any component of the formulation

Warnings/Precautions Use with caution in patients with epilepsy or other CNS diseases which could predispose seizures; potential for seizures, although very rare, may be increased with concomitant NSAID therapy. Tremor, restlessness, confusion, and very rarely hallucinations or seizures may occur; use with caution in patients with known or suspected CNS disorder. Discontinue in patients who experience significant CNS adverse effects (eg, dizziness, hallucinations, suicidal ideations or actions). Use with caution in patients with renal or hepatic impairment. Tendon inflammation and/or rupture have been reported with quinolone antibiotics, including ofloxacin. Risk may be increased with concurrent corticosteroids, particularly in the elderly. Discontinue at first sign of tendon inflammation or pain. Peripheral neuropathies have been linked to ofloxacin use; discontinue if numbness, tingling, or weakness develops.

Rare cases of torsade de pointes have been reported in patients receiving ofloxacin and other quinolones. Risk may be minimized by avoiding use in patients with known prolongation of the QT interval, bradycardia, hypokalemia, hypomagnesemia, cardiomyopathy, or in those receiving concurrent therapy with Class Ia or Class III antiarrhythmics.

Severe hypersensitivity reactions, including anaphylaxis, have occurred with quinolone therapy. If an allergic reaction occurs (itching, urticaria, dyspnea, facial edema, loss of consciousness, tingling, cardiovascular collapse), discontinue drug immediately. Prolonged use may result in fungal or bacterial superinfection, including *C. difficile*-associated diarrhea and pseudomembranous colitis. Quinolones may exacerbate myasthenia gravis. Avoid excessive sunlight; may cause moderate-to-severe phototoxicity reactions.

Adverse Reactions (Reflective of adult population; not specific for elderly)

Systemic:

1% to 10%:

Cardiovascular: Chest pain (1% to 3%)

Central nervous system: Headache (1% to 9%), insomnia (3% to 7%), dizziness (1% to 5%), fatigue (1% to 3%), somnolence (1% to 3%), sleep disorders (1% to 3%), nervousness (1% to 3%), pyrexia (1% to 3%)

Dermatologic: Rash/pruritus (1% to 3%)

Gastrointestinal: Diarrhea (1% to 4%), vomiting (1% to 4%), GI distress (1% to 3%), abdominal cramps (1% to 3%), flatulence (1% to 3%), abnormal taste (1% to 3%), xerostomia (1% to 3%), appetite decreased (1% to 3%), nausea (3% to 10%), constipation (1% to 3%)

Genitourinary: Vaginitis (1% to 5%), external genital pruritus in women (1% to 3%)

Ocular: Visual disturbances (1% to 3%)

Respiratory: Pharyngitis (1% to 3%)

Miscellaneous: Trunk pain

Ophthalmic: Frequency not defined:

Central nervous system: Dizziness

Gastrointestinal: Nausea

Ocular: Blurred vision, burning, chemical conjunctivitis/keratitis, discomfort, dryness, edema, eye pain, foreign body sensation, itching, photophobia, redness, stinging, tearing

Otic:

>10%: Local: Application site reaction (<1% to 17%)

(Continued)

Ofloxacin *(Continued)*

1% to 10%:
Central nervous system: Dizziness (≤1%), vertigo (≤1%)
Dermatologic: Pruritus (1% to 4%), rash (1%)
Gastrointestinal: Taste perversion (7%)
Neuromuscular & skeletal: Paresthesia (1%)

Overdosage/Toxicology Symptoms include acute renal failure, seizures, nausea, and vomiting. Treatment includes GI decontamination, if possible, and supportive care.

Drug Interactions Inhibits CYP1A2 (strong)

Corticosteroids: Concurrent use may increase the risk of tendon rupture, particularly in elderly patients (overall incidence rare).

CYP1A2 substrates: Ofloxacin may increase the levels/effects of CYP1A2 substrates. Example substrates include aminophylline, fluvoxamine, mexiletine, mirtazapine, ropinirole, and trifluoperazine.

Glyburide: Quinolones may increase the effect of glyburide; monitor.

Metal cations (aluminum, calcium, iron, magnesium, and zinc) bind quinolones in the gastrointestinal tract and inhibit absorption. Concurrent administration of most antacids, oral electrolyte supplements, quinapril, sucralfate, some didanosine formulations (pediatric powder for oral suspension), and other highly-buffered oral drugs, should be avoided. Ofloxacin should be administered 2 hours before or 2 hours after these agents.

NSAIDs: Risk of seizures may be increased with concomitant NSAID use. Risk is considered quite low and may only be a factor with high serum levels of either agent and/or in patients with additional predisposing factors (eg, renal dysfunction, history of seizure or other neurological disorder).

Probenecid: May decrease renal secretion of ofloxacin.

QT_c-prolonging agents: Effects may be additive with ofloxacin. Avoid concurrent use with Class Ia and Class III antiarrhythmics; use caution with other drugs known to prolong QT_c, including erythromycin, cisapride, antipsychotics, and cyclic antidepressants.

Theophylline: Ofloxacin may increase plasma levels of theophylline; monitor.

Typhoid vaccine: Antibiotics may decrease the therapeutic effect of live, attenuated Ty21a vaccine; delay vaccination for >24 hours after administration of antibacterial agents.

Warfarin: The hypoprothrombinemic effect of warfarin may be enhanced by some quinolone antibiotics; monitor INR.

Ethanol/Nutrition/Herb Interactions

Food: Ofloxacin average peak serum concentrations may be decreased by 20% if taken with food.

Herb/Nutraceutical: Avoid dong quai, St John's wort (may also cause photosensitization).

Stability

Ophthalmic and otic solution: Store at 15°C to 25°C (59°F to 77°F).

Otic Singles™: Store at 15°C to 30°C (59°F to 86°F). Store in pouch to protect from light.

Tablet: Store below 30°C (86°F).

Mechanism of Action Ofloxacin is a DNA gyrase inhibitor. DNA gyrase is an essential bacterial enzyme that maintains the superhelical structure of DNA. DNA gyrase is required for DNA replication and transcription, DNA repair, recombination, and transposition; bactericidal

Pharmacokinetics

Absorption: Fraction absorbed increases proportionately with the dose; age does not affect absorption

Half-life:
Young adults: 5 hours
Older adults with normal renal function: 6-8 hours
Sick, older, hospitalized adults: Between 9-13 hours
Time to peak serum concentration: Within 1-2 hours
Elimination: Primarily renal with ~5% excreted in feces

Dosage

Geriatrics: Oral: 200-400 mg every 12-24 hours (based on estimated renal function) for 7 days to 6 weeks depending on indication.

Adults:

Cervicitis/urethritis (nongonococcal):

Nongonococcal: 300 mg every 12 hours for 7 days

Gonococcal (acute, uncomplicated): 400 mg as a single dose; **Note:** As of April 2007, the CDC no longer recommends the use of fluoroquinolones for the treatment of uncomplicated gonococcal disease.

Chronic bronchitis (acute exacerbation), community-acquired pneumonia, skin and skin structure infections (uncomplicated): 400 mg every 12 hours for 10 days

Conjunctivitis: Ophthalmic: Instill 1-2 drops in affected eye(s) every 2-4 hours for the first 2 days, then use 4 times/day for an additional 5 days.

Corneal ulcer: Ophthalmic: Instill 1-2 drops every 30 minutes while awake and every 4-6 hours after retiring for the first 2 days; beginning on day 3, instill 1-2 drops every hour while awake for 4-6 additional days; thereafter, 1-2 drops 4 times/day until clinical cure.

Epididymitis, nongonococcal (unlabeled use): 300 mg twice daily for 10 days

Leprosy (unlabeled use): 400 mg once daily

Otitis media, chronic suppurative with perforated tympanic membranes: Otic: Instill 10 drops (or the contents of 2 single-dose containers) into affected ear twice daily for 14 days

Otitis externa: Otic: Instill 10 drops (or the contents of 2 single-dose containers) into affected ear(s) once daily for 7 days

Pelvic inflammatory disease (acute): 400 mg every 12 hours for 10-14 days; **Note:** The CDC recommends use only if standard cephalosporin therapy is not feasible and community prevalence of quinolone-resistant gonococcal organisms is low. Culture sensitivity must be confirmed.

Prostatitis:
Acute: 400 mg for 1 dose, then 300 mg twice daily for 10 days
Chronic: 200 mg every 12 hours for 6 weeks

Traveler's diarrhea (unlabeled use): 300 mg twice daily for 3 days

UTI:
Uncomplicated: 200 mg every 12 hours for 3-7 days
Complicated: 200 mg every 12 hours for 10 days

Renal Impairment: Adults: Oral: After a normal initial dose, adjust as follows:
Cl_{cr} 20-50 mL/minute: Administer usual dose every 24 hours
Cl_{cr} <20 mL/minute: Administer half the usual dose every 24 hours
Continuous arteriovenous or venovenous hemodiafiltration effects: Administer 300 mg every 24 hours

Hepatic Impairment: Severe impairment: Maximum dose: 400 mg/day

Administration

Ophthalmic: For ophthalmic use only; avoid touching tip of applicator to eye or other surfaces.

Oral: Do not take within 2 hours of food or any antacids which contain zinc, magnesium, or aluminum.

Otic: Prior to use, warm solution by holding container in hands for 1-2 minutes. Patient should lie down with affected ear upward and medication instilled. Pump tragus 4 times to ensure penetration of medication. Patient should remain in this position for 5 minutes.

Monitoring Parameters Signs and symptoms of infection; WBC, mental status

Test Interactions Some quinolones may produce a false-positive urine screening result for opiates using commercially-available immunoassay kits. This has been demonstrated most consistently for levofloxacin and ofloxacin, but other quinolones have shown cross-reactivity in certain assay kits. Confirmation of positive opiate screens by more specific methods should be considered.

Patient Information Do not take antacids or multivitamins with minerals within 6 hours before or 2 hours after taking drug; take 1 hour before or 2 hours after meals; do not take with dairy products, iron, or zinc products; may cause dizziness, headache, or stimulation; avoid excess natural or artificial sunlight exposure; complete full course of therapy

Otic: Wash hands before and after applying drops. Lie with affected ear up and instill prescribed number of drops into ear. Remain on side with ear up for 5 minutes.

Special Geriatric Considerations Dosage must be carefully adjusted to renal function. The half-life of ofloxacin may be prolonged and serum concentrations are elevated in elderly patients even in the absence of overt renal impairment. The risk of torsade de pointes and tendon inflammation and/or rupture associated with the concomitant use of corticosteroids and quinolones is increased in the elderly population.

Dosage Forms Excipient information presented when available (limited, particularly for generics); consult specific product labeling. [DSC] = Discontinued product
Solution, ophthalmic (Ocuflox®): 0.3% (5 mL; 10 mL [DSC]) [contains benzalkonium chloride]
Solution, otic:
Floxin®: 0.3% (5 mL, 10 mL) [contains benzalkonium chloride]
Floxin® Otic Singles™: 0.3% (0.25 mL) [contains benzalkonium chloride; packaged as 2 single-dose containers per pouch, 10 pouches per carton, total net volume 5 mL]
Tablet (Floxin®): 200 mg, 300 mg, 400 mg

Selected References
Nilsson-Ehle I and Ljungberg B, "Quinolone Disposition in the Elderly: Practical Implications," *Drugs Aging,* 1991, 1(4):279-88.

♦ **9-OH-risperidone** *see* Paliperidone *on page 1190*

Olanzapine (oh LAN za peen)

Related Information
Antipsychotic Agents *on page 1747*
Atypical Antipsychotics *on page 1749*

Medication Safety Issues
Sound-alike/look-alike issues:
Olanzapine may be confused with olsalazine
Zyprexa® may be confused with Celexa™, Zyrtec®

U.S. Brand Names Zyprexa®; Zyprexa® Zydis®

Canadian Brand Names Zyprexa®; Zyprexa® Zydis®

Index Terms LY170053; Zyprexa Zydis

Generic Available No

Pharmacologic Category Antipsychotic Agent, Atypical

Use Treatment of the manifestations of schizophrenia; treatment of acute mania episodes associated with bipolar I disorder (as monotherapy or in combination with lithium or valproate); maintenance treatment of bipolar disorder; acute agitation (patients with schizophrenia or bipolar mania)

Unlabeled/Investigational Use Treatment of psychosis/schizophrenia in children or adolescents; chronic pain

Contraindications Hypersensitivity to olanzapine or any component of the formulation

Warnings/Precautions [U.S. Boxed Warning]: Patients with dementia-related psychosis treated with atypical antipsychotics are at an increased risk of death compared to placebo. An increased incidence of cerebrovascular adverse events (including fatalities) has been reported in elderly patients with dementia-related psychosis. Risk may be increased by dehydration; use caution with concurrent diuretics. Olanzapine is not approved for this indication.

Moderate to highly sedating, use with caution in disorders where CNS depression is a feature; patients must be cautioned about performing tasks which require mental alertness (eg, operating machinery or driving). Use caution in patients with cardiac disease. Use with caution in Parkinson's disease, predisposition to seizures, or severe hepatic or renal disease. Life-threatening arrhythmias have occurred with therapeutic doses of some neuroleptics. May induce orthostatic hypotension; use caution with history of cardiovascular disease. Esophageal dysmotility and aspiration have been associated with antipsychotic use; use with caution in patients at risk of aspiration pneumonia. Caution in breast cancer or other prolactin-dependent tumors (elevates prolactin levels). Significant weight gain may occur; monitor waist circumference and BMI. Impaired core body temperature regulation may occur; caution with strenuous exercise, heat exposure, dehydration, and concomitant medication possessing anticholinergic effects.

May cause anticholinergic effects; use with caution in patients with decreased gastrointestinal motility, urinary retention, BPH, xerostomia, glaucoma, or myasthenia gravis. Relative to other neuroleptics, olanzapine has a moderate potency of cholinergic blockade. May cause extrapyramidal symptoms, although risk of these reactions is lower relative to other neuroleptics. May be associated with neuroleptic malignant syndrome (NMS). May cause extreme and life-threatening hyperglycemia; use with caution in patients with diabetes or other disorders of glucose regulation; monitor. Olanzapine levels may be lower in patients who smoke, requiring dosage adjustment.

The possibility of a suicide attempt is inherent in psychotic illness or bipolar disorder; use caution in high-risk patients during initiation of therapy. Prescriptions should be written for the smallest quantity consistent with good patient care.

Intramuscular administration: Patients should remain recumbent if drowsy/dizzy until hypotension, bradycardia and/or hypoventilation has been ruled out. Concurrent use of I.M./I.V. benzodiazepines is not recommended (fatalities have been reported, though causality not determined).

Adverse Reactions (Reflective of adult population; not specific for elderly)
>10%:
Central nervous system: Somnolence (6% to 39% dose dependent), extrapyramidal symptoms (15% to 32% dose dependent), insomnia (up to 12%), dizziness (4% to 18%)
Gastrointestinal: Dyspepsia (7% to 11%), constipation (9% to 11%), weight gain (5% to 6%, has been reported as high as 40%), xerostomia (9% to 22% dose dependent)
Neuromuscular & skeletal: Weakness (2% to 20% dose dependent)
Miscellaneous: Accidental injury (12%)

1% to 10%:

Cardiovascular: Postural hypotension (1% to 5%), tachycardia (up to 3%), peripheral edema (up to 3%), chest pain (up to 3%), hyper-/hypotension (up to 2%)

Central nervous system: Personality changes (8%), speech disorder (7%), fever (up to 6%), abnormal dreams, euphoria, amnesia, delusions, emotional lability, mania, schizophrenia

Dermatologic: Bruising (up to 5%)

Endocrine & metabolic: Cholesterol increased, prolactin increased

Gastrointestinal: Nausea (up to 9% dose dependent), appetite increased (3% to 6%), vomiting (up to 4%), flatulence, salivation increased, thirst

Genitourinary: Incontinence (up to 2%), UTI (up to 2%), vaginitis

Hepatic: ALT increased (2%)

Local: Injection site pain (I.M. administration)

Neuromuscular & skeletal: Tremor (1% to 7% dose dependent), abnormal gait (6%), back pain (up to 5%), joint/extremity pain (up to 5%), akathisia (3% to 5% dose dependent), hypertonia (up to 3%), articulation impairment (up to 2%), falling (particularly in older patients), joint stiffness, paresthesia, twitching

Ocular: Amblyopia (up to 3%), conjunctivitis

Respiratory: Rhinitis (up to 7%), cough (up to 6%), pharyngitis (up to 4%), dyspnea

Miscellaneous: Dental pain, diaphoresis, flu-like syndrome

Overdosage/Toxicology Signs and symptoms of overdose include CNS depression (ranging from drowsiness to coma), extrapyramidal movements, fasciculations, hypotension (possible, though not described), miosis, respiratory depression, rhinitis (10%), slurred speech, tachycardia, trismus, and possible NMS. Treatment is symptom-directed and supportive. Cardiac monitoring should be initiated, including continuous EEG monitoring. Activated charcoal (1 g) may reduce the C_{max} and AUC of olanzapine by ~60%.

Drug Interactions Substrate of CYP1A2 (major), 2D6 (minor); **Inhibits** CYP1A2 (weak), 2C9 (weak), 2C19 (weak), 2D6 (weak), 3A4 (weak)

Acetylcholinesterase inhibitors (central): May increase the risk of antipsychotic-related extrapyramidal symptoms; monitor.

Anticholinergics: Adverse effects/toxicity may be additive with olanzapine.

Benzodiazepines (parenteral): Concomitant parenteral administration may increase the risk of cardiopulmonary toxicity (fatalities have been reported, though causality not determined); manufacturer recommends avoiding concurrent use.

Carbamazepine: May decrease olanzapine levels/effects; monitor.

Ciprofloxacin; May increase the levels/effects of olanzapine.

CNS depressants: Sedative effects and may be additive with CNS depressants; includes ethanol, barbiturates, opioid analgesics, and other sedative agents; monitor for increased effect.

CYP1A2 inducers may decrease the levels/effects of olanzapine. Example inducers include aminoglutethimide, carbamazepine, phenobarbital, and rifampin.

CYP1A2 inhibitors: May increase the levels/effects of olanzapine. Example inhibitors include ciprofloxacin, fluvoxamine, ketoconazole, norfloxacin, ofloxacin, and rofecoxib.

Fluvoxamine: Increases olanzapine levels; consider using a lower dose of olanzapine in patients receiving concomitant treatment with fluvoxamine.

Lithium: Risk of extrapyramidal effects may be increased with concurrent therapy.

Pramlintide: Anticholinergic effects may be increased with concomitant therapy.

Ethanol/Nutrition/Herb Interactions

Ethanol: Avoid ethanol (may increase CNS depression).

Herb/Nutraceutical: Avoid dong quai, St John's wort (may also cause photosensitization). Avoid kava kava, gotu kola, valerian, St John's wort (may increase CNS depression).

Stability

Injection, powder for reconstitution: Store at room temperature 15°C to 30°C (59°F to 86°F); do not freeze. Protect from light. Reconstitute 10 mg vial with 2.1 mL SWFI. Resulting solution is ~5 mg/mL. Use immediately (within 1 hour) following reconstitution. Discard any unused portion.

Tablet and orally-disintegrating tablet: Store at room temperature of 15°C to 30°C (59°F to 86°F). Protect from light and moisture.

Mechanism of Action Olanzapine is a second generation thienobenzodiazepine antipsychotic which displays potent antagonist of serotonin 5-HT$_{2A}$ and 5-HT$_{2C}$, dopamine D_{1-4}, muscarinic M_{1-5}, histamine H_1- and alpha$_1$-adrenergic receptors. Olanzapine shows moderate antagonism of 5-HT$_3$ and muscarinic M_{1-5} receptors, and weak binding to GABA-A, BZD, and beta-adrenergic receptors. Although the precise mechanism of action in schizophrenia and bipolar disorder is not known, the efficacy of olanzapine is thought to be mediated through combined antagonism of dopamine and serotonin type 2 receptor sites.

Pharmacokinetics

Absorption:

I.M.: Rapidly absorbed

(Continued)

Olanzapine *(Continued)*

Oral: Well absorbed; not affected by food; tablets and orally-disintegrating tablets are bioequivalent

Distribution: V_d: 1000 L

Metabolism: Highly metabolized via direct glucuronidation and cytochrome P450 mediated oxidation (CYP1A2, CYP2D6); 40% removed via first pass metabolism

Peak serum concentrations: 6 hours

Half-life: 21-54 hours (mean half-life: 30 hours)

Time to peak, plasma: Maximum plasma concentrations after I.M. administration are 5 times higher than maximum plasma concentrations produced by an oral dose.

I.M.: 15-45 minutes

Oral: ~6 hours

Excretion: Urine (57%, 7% as unchanged drug); feces (30%)

Clearance: 40% increase in olanzapine clearance in smokers; 30% decrease in females

Dosage

Geriatrics: Refer to adult dosing. Consider lower starting dose of 2.5-5 mg/day for elderly or debilitated patients; may increase as clinically indicated and tolerated with close monitoring of orthostatic blood pressure.

Adults:

Schizophrenia: Initial: 5-10 mg once daily (increase to 10 mg once daily within 5-7 days); thereafter, adjust by 5 mg/day at 1-week intervals, up to a recommended maximum of 20 mg/day. Maintenance: 10-20 mg once daily. **Note:** Doses of 30-50 mg/day have been used; however, doses >10 mg/day have not demonstrated better efficacy, and safety and efficacy of doses >20 mg/day have not been evaluated.

Acute mania associated with bipolar disorder: Oral:

Monotherapy: Initial: 10-15 mg once daily; increase by 5 mg/day at intervals of not less than 24 hours. Maintenance: 5-20 mg/day; recommended maximum dose: 20 mg/day.

Combination therapy (with lithium or valproate): Initial: 10 mg once daily; dosing range: 5-20 mg/day

Agitation (acute, associated with bipolar disorder or schizophrenia): I.M.: Initial dose: 5-10 mg (a lower dose of 2.5 mg may be considered when clinical factors warrant); additional doses (2.5-10 mg) may be considered; however, 2-4 hours should be allowed between doses to evaluate response (maximum total daily dose: 30 mg, per manufacturer's recommendation)

Renal Impairment: No dosage adjustment required. Not removed by dialysis.

Hepatic Impairment: Dosage adjustment may be necessary, however, there are no specific recommendations. Monitor closely.

Administration

Injection: For I.M. administration only; do not administer injection intravenously; inject slowly, deep into muscle. If dizziness and/or drowsiness are noted, patient should remain recumbent until examination indicates postural hypotension and/or bradycardia are not a problem.

Tablet: May be administered with or without food/meals.

Orally-disintegrating: Remove from foil blister by peeling back (do not push tablet through the foil); place tablet in mouth immediately upon removal; tablet dissolves rapidly in saliva and may be swallowed with or without liquid. May be administered with or without food/meals.

Monitoring Parameters Vital signs; fasting lipid profile and fasting blood glucose/Hgb A_{1c} (prior to treatment, at 3 months, then annually); periodic assessment of hepatic transaminases (in patients with hepatic disease); BMI, personal/family history of obesity, waist circumference; orthostatic blood pressure; mental status, abnormal involuntary movement scale (AIMS), extrapyramidal symptoms (EPS). Weight should be assessed prior to treatment, at 4 weeks, 8 weeks, 12 weeks, and then at quarterly intervals. Consider titrating to a different antipsychotic agent for a weight gain ≥5% of the initial weight.

Monitor orthostatic blood pressures 3-5 days after initiation of therapy or a dose increase.

Patient Information There is a risk of hypotension, especially at the start of therapy. Other medications may induce hypotension and augment the orthostatic effects of olanzapine. Olanzapine may impair judgment, thinking, or motor skills making driving or operating hazardous equipment a risk. Therefore, use caution until the effects of the dose is experienced and known. Avoid overheating and dehydration.

Special Geriatric Considerations Elderly patients have an increased risk of adverse response to side effects or adverse reactions to antipsychotics. A higher incidence of falls has been reported in elderly patients, particularly in debilitated patients. Olanzapine half-life that was 1.5 times that of younger (<65 years of age) adults;

therefore, lower initial doses are recommended. Olanzapine is not indicated in dementia-related psychosis.

Studies with patients ≥65 years of age with schizophrenia showed no difference in tolerability compared to younger adults. Studies in the elderly with dementia-related psychosis suggested a different tolerability compared to younger patients with schizophrenia. In light of significant risks and adverse effects in the elderly population (compared with limited data demonstrating efficacy in the treatment of dementia-related psychosis, aggression, and agitation), an extensive risk:benefit analysis should be performed prior to use. Therefore, use with caution and at lower recommended doses.

Dosage Forms Excipient information presented when available (limited, particularly for generics); consult specific product labeling.

Injection, powder for reconstitution (Zyprexa® IntraMuscular): 10 mg [contains lactose 50 mg]

Tablet (Zyprexa®): 2.5 mg, 5 mg, 7.5 mg, 10 mg, 15 mg, 20 mg

Tablet, orally disintegrating (Zyprexa® Zydis®): 5 mg [contains phenylalanine 0.34 mg/tablet], 10 mg [contains phenylalanine 0.45 mg/tablet], 15 mg [contains phenylalanine 0.67 mg/tablet], 20 mg [contains phenylalanine 0.9 mg/tablet]

Selected References

American Diabetes Association; American Psychiatric Association; American Association of Clinical Endocrinologists; North American Association for the Study of Obesity, "Consensus Development Conference on Antipsychotic Drugs and Obesity and Diabetes," *Diabetes Care*, 2004, 27(2):596-601.

Baldwin DS and Montgomery SA, "First Clinical Experience With Olanzapine (LY 170053): Results of an Open-label Safety and Dose-Ranging Study in Patients With Schizophrenia," *Int Clin Psychopharmacol*, 1995, 10(4):239-44.

Carrillo JA, Herraiz AG, Ramos SI, et al, "Role of the Smoking-Induced Cytochrome P450 (CYP)1A2 and Polymorphic CYP2D6 in Steady-State Concentration of Olanzapine," *J Clin Psychopharmacol*, 23(2):119-27.

Goldberg RJ, "Managing Psychosis-Related Behavioral Problems in the Elderly," *Consult Pharm*, 1997, 12(Suppl C):4-10.

Farwell WR, Stump TE, Wang J, et al, "Weight Gain and New Onset Diabetes Associated With Olanzapine and Risperidone," *J Gen Intern Med*, 2004, 19(12):1200-5.

Littrell K, Peabody CD, and Littrell SH, "Olanzapine: A New Atypical Antipsychotic," *J Psychosoc Nurs Ment Health Serv*, 1996, 34(8):41-6.

"Olanzapine for Schizophrenia," *Med Lett Drugs Ther*, 1997, 39(992):5-6.

Schneider LS, Tariot PN, Dagerman KS, et al, "Effectiveness of Atypical Antipsychotic Drugs in Patients With Alzheimer's Disease," *N Engl J Med*, 2006, 355(15):1525-38.

Sorsaburu S, Hornbuckle K, Blake D, et al, "The First 21 Months of Safety Experience with Post-Marketing Use of Olanzapine's Intramuscular Formulation," College of Psychiatric and Neurologic Pharmacists, April, 2006, Baltimore, MD.

Tollefson GD, Beasley CM Jr, Tran PV, et al, "Olanzapine Versus Haloperidol in the Treatment of Schizophrenia and Schizoaffective and Schizophreniform Disorders: Results of an International Collaborative Trial," *Am J Psychiatry*, 1997, 154(4):457-65.

♦ **Oleum Ricini** *see* Castor Oil *on page 249*

Olmesartan (ole me SAR tan)

Related Information
Angiotensin Agents *on page 1737*
U.S. Brand Names Benicar®
Index Terms Olmesartan Medoxomil
Generic Available No
Pharmacologic Category Angiotensin II Receptor Blocker
Use Treatment of hypertension, alone or with other antihypertensive agents
Contraindications Hypersensitivity to olmesartan or any component of the formulation; hypersensitivity to other A-II receptor antagonists; primary hyperaldosteronism; bilateral renal artery stenosis
Warnings/Precautions May cause hyperkalemia; avoid potassium supplementation unless specifically required by healthcare provider. Avoid use or use a smaller dose in patients who are volume depleted; correct depletion first. May be associated with deterioration of renal function and/or increases in serum creatinine, particularly in patients dependent on renin-angiotensin-aldosterone system. Use with caution in unilateral renal artery stenosis and pre-existing renal insufficiency; significant aortic/mitral stenosis.

Adverse Reactions (Reflective of adult population; not specific for elderly)
1% to 10%:
Central nervous system: Dizziness (3%), headache
Endocrine & metabolic: Hyperglycemia, hypertriglyceridemia
Gastrointestinal: Diarrhea
Neuromuscular & skeletal: Back pain, CPK increased
Renal: Hematuria
Respiratory: Bronchitis, pharyngitis, rhinitis, sinusitis
Miscellaneous: Flu-like syndrome
(Continued)

Olmesartan *(Continued)*

Drug Interactions
Lithium: Risk of toxicity may be increased by olmesartan; monitor lithium levels.

NSAIDs: May decrease angiotensin II antagonist efficacy; effect has been seen with losartan, but may occur with other medications in this class; monitor blood pressure.

Potassium-sparing diuretics (amiloride, potassium, spironolactone, triamterene): Increased risk of hyperkalemia.

Potassium supplements may increase the risk of hyperkalemia.

Trimethoprim (high dose) may increase the risk of hyperkalemia.

Ethanol/Nutrition/Herb Interactions
Food: Does not affect olmesartan bioavailability.

Herb/Nutraceutical: Avoid ephedra, yohimbe, ginseng (may worsen hypertension). Avoid garlic (may have increased antihypertensive effect).

Stability Store at 20°C to 25°C (68°F to 77°F).

Mechanism of Action As a selective and competitive, nonpeptide angiotensin II receptor antagonist, olmesartan blocks the vasoconstrictor and aldosterone-secreting effects of angiotensin II; olmesartan interacts reversibly at the AT1 and AT2 receptors of many tissues and has slow dissociation kinetics; its affinity for the AT1 receptor is 12,500 times greater than the AT2 receptor. Angiotensin II receptor antagonists may induce a more complete inhibition of the renin-angiotensin system than ACE inhibitors, they do not affect the response to bradykinin, and are less likely to be associated with nonrenin-angiotensin effects (eg, cough and angioedema). Olmesartan increases urinary flow rate and, in addition to being natriuretic and kaliuretic, increases excretion of chloride, magnesium, uric acid, calcium, and phosphate.

Pharmacokinetics
Distribution: 17 L; does not cross the blood-brain barrier (animal studies)

Protein binding: 99%

Metabolism: Olmesartan medoxomil is hydrolyzed in the GI tract to active olmesartan. No further metabolism occurs.

Bioavailability: 26%

Half-life: Terminal: 13 hours

Time to peak: 1-2 hours

Elimination: All as unchanged drug: Feces (50% to 65%); urine (35% to 50%)

Dosage
Geriatrics: Initial: May start at 5-10 mg/day (due to concomitant disease or age changes).

Adults: Antihypertensive: Oral: Initial: Usual starting dose is 20 mg once daily; if initial response is inadequate, may be increased to 40 mg once daily after 2 weeks. May administer with other antihypertensive agents if blood pressure inadequately controlled with olmesartan. Consider lower starting dose in patients with possible depletion of intravascular volume (eg, patients receiving diuretics).

Renal Impairment: No specific guidelines for dosage adjustment; patients undergoing hemodialysis have not been studied.

Hepatic Impairment: No adjustment necessary.

Administration May be administered with or without food.

Monitoring Parameters Blood pressure, serum potassium

Patient Information Take exactly as directed; do not discontinue without consulting prescriber. Take first dose at bedtime. May be taken with or without food. Consult your prescriber before using NSAIDs, like ibuprofen or naproxen. This drug does not eliminate need for diet or exercise regimen as recommended by prescriber. May cause dizziness, fainting, lightheadedness (use caution when driving or engaging in tasks that require alertness until response to drug is known); diarrhea (buttermilk, boiled milk, yogurt may help). Report chest pain or palpitations; unrelenting headache; swelling of extremities, face, or tongue; difficulty in breathing or unusual cough; flu-like symptoms; or other persistent adverse reactions.

Special Geriatric Considerations No dosage adjustment is necessary when initiating angiotensin II receptor antagonists in the elderly. In clinical studies, no differences between younger adults and the elderly were demonstrated.

For age alone, consider hydration status to avoid hypotension; many elderly are volume depleted due to age-related blunting of the thirst reflex and diuretic use. May consider starting this medication at 5-10 mg once daily.

Dosage Forms Excipient information presented when available (limited, particularly for generics); consult specific product labeling.
Tablet, as medoxomil: 5 mg, 20 mg, 40 mg

Olmesartan and Hydrochlorothiazide
(ole me SAR tan & hye droe klor oh THYE a zide)

Related Information
Hydrochlorothiazide *on page 756*

Olmesartan *on page 1151*

U.S. Brand Names Benicar HCT®
Index Terms Hydrochlorothiazide and Olmesartan Medoxomil; Olmesartan Medoxomil and Hydrochlorothiazide
Generic Available No
Pharmacologic Category Angiotensin II Receptor Blocker Combination; Antihypertensive Agent, Combination; Diuretic, Thiazide
Use Treatment of hypertension (not recommended for initial treatment)
Dosage
Geriatrics & Adults:
    Hypertension: Oral: Dosage must be individualized; may be titrated at 2- to 4-week intervals.
      Replacement therapy: May be substituted for titrated components.
      Patients not controlled with single-agent therapy: Initiate by adding the lowest available dose of the alternative component (hydrochlorothiazide 12.5 mg or olmesartan 20 mg). Titrate to effect (maximum hydrochlorothiazide dose: 25 mg, maximum olmesartan dose: 40 mg).
  Renal Impairment: Not recommended in patients with Cl_{cr} <30 mL/minute.
Dosage Forms Excipient information presented when available (limited, particularly for generics); consult specific product labeling.
Tablet:
20/12.5: Olmesartan medoxomil 20 mg and hydrochlorothiazide 12.5 mg
40/12.5: Olmesartan medoxomil 40 mg and hydrochlorothiazide 12.5 mg
40/25: Olmesartan medoxomil 40 mg and hydrochlorothiazide 25 mg

♦ **Olmesartan Medoxomil** *see* Olmesartan *on page 1151*
♦ **Olmesartan Medoxomil and Hydrochlorothiazide** *see* Olmesartan and Hydrochlorothiazide *on page 1152*

Olopatadine (oh la PAT a deen)

Medication Safety Issues
  Sound-alike/look-alike issues:
    Patanol® may be confused with Platinol®

  International issues:
    Patanol® may be confused with Betanol® which is a brand name for metipranolol in Monaco and a brand name for atenolol in Bangladesh
U.S. Brand Names Pataday™; Patanol®
Canadian Brand Names Patanol®
Index Terms Olopatadine Hydrochloride
Generic Available No
Pharmacologic Category Antihistamine; Ophthalmic Agent, Miscellaneous
Use Treatment of the signs and symptoms of allergic conjunctivitis
Contraindications Hypersensitivity to olopatadine hydrochloride or any component of the formulation
Warnings/Precautions Contains benzalkonium chloride which may be absorbed by contact lenses; remove contact lens prior to administration and wait 10 minutes before reinserting; do not wear contact lenses if eyes are red. Not for use to treat contact lens-related irritation.
Adverse Reactions (Reflective of adult population; not specific for elderly)
>5%:
  Central nervous system: Cold syndrome (up to 10%), headache (up to 7%)
  Respiratory: Pharyngitis (up to 10%)
≤5%:
  Gastrointestinal: Nausea, taste perversion
  Neuromuscular & skeletal: Back pain, weakness
  Ocular: Blurred vision, burning, conjunctivitis, dry eyes, eye pain, eyelid edema, foreign body sensation, hyperemia, itching, keratitis, ocular pruritus, stinging
  Respiratory: Cough, rhinitis, sinusitis
  Miscellaneous: Flu-like syndrome, hypersensitivity, infection
Drug Interactions Studies evaluating drug interactions with olopatadine hydrochloride have not been conducted.
Stability Store at 2°C to 25°C (36°F to 77°F).
Mechanism of Action
Selective histamine H_1-antagonist; inhibits release of histamine from mast cells. Inhibits histamine induced effects on conjunctival epithelial cells. Has no effect on alpha-adrenergic, dopaminergic, and muscarinic type 1 and 2 receptors.
Pharmacokinetics
Absorption: Low systemic absorption following topical administration
Half-life elimination: ~3 hours
(Continued)

Olopatadine *(Continued)*

Excretion: Urine (60% to 70%)

Dosage

Geriatrics & Adults: Allergic conjunctivitis: Ophthalmic:

Patanol®: Instill 1drop into affected eye(s) twice daily (allowing 6-8 hours between doses); results from an environmental study demonstrated that olopatadine was effective when dosed twice daily for up to 6 weeks

Pataday™: Instill 1 drop into affected eye(s) once daily

Administration For topical ophthalmic use only. After instilling drops, wait at least 10 minutes before inserting contact lenses. Do not insert contacts if eyes are red.

Monitoring Parameters Relief of symptoms

Patient Information Instruct on proper use of ophthalmic product.

Special Geriatric Considerations No specific information in the elderly.

Dosage Forms Excipient information presented when available (limited, particularly for generics); consult specific product labeling.

Solution, ophthalmic:

Patanol®: 0.1% (5 mL) [contains benzalkonium chloride]

Pataday™: 0.2% (2.5 mL) [contains benzalkonium chloride]

♦ **Olopatadine Hydrochloride** *see* Olopatadine *on page 1153*

Olsalazine (ole SAL a zeen)

Medication Safety Issues

Sound-alike/look-alike issues:

Olsalazine may be confused with olanzapine

Dipentum® may be confused with Dilantin®

U.S. Brand Names Dipentum®

Canadian Brand Names Dipentum®

Index Terms Olsalazine Sodium

Generic Available No

Pharmacologic Category 5-Aminosalicylic Acid Derivative

Use Maintenance of remission of ulcerative colitis in patients intolerant to sulfasalazine

Contraindications Hypersensitivity to olsalazine, salicylates, or any component of the formulation

Warnings/Precautions Diarrhea is a common adverse effect of olsalazine; use with caution in patients with hypersensitivity to salicylates, sulfasalazine, or mesalamine. May exacerbate symptoms of colitis. Use with caution in patients with renal impairment.

Adverse Reactions (Reflective of adult population; not specific for elderly)

>10%: Gastrointestinal: Diarrhea, cramps, abdominal pain

1% to 10%:

Central nervous system: Headache, fatigue, depression

Dermatologic: Rash, itching

Gastrointestinal: Nausea, heartburn, bloating, anorexia

Neuromuscular & skeletal: Arthralgia

Overdosage/Toxicology Symptoms include decreased motor activity and diarrhea.

Drug Interactions

Azathioprine, mercaptopurine, thioguanine: Aminosalicylates may increase the risk of myelosuppression (due to TPMT inhibition).

Warfarin: Olsalazine has been reported to increase the prothrombin time in patients taking warfarin.

Mechanism of Action The mechanism of action appears to be topical rather than systemic

Pharmacokinetics

Absorption: 2% to 4%

Protein binding: 98%

Metabolism: 98% to 99% is converted to 5-aminosalicylic acid

Half-life: 0.9 hours; olsalazine-0-sulfate (olsalazine-S) accounts for 0.1% of the dose and has a half-life of 7 days

Time to peak serum concentration: Within 1 hour

Elimination: Primarily in feces

Dosage

Geriatrics & Adults: Ulcerative colitis: Oral: 1 g/day in 2 divided doses

Administration Take with food in evenly divided doses.

Monitoring Parameters Stool frequency

Reference Range Olsalazine: 0-4.3 mmol/L; olsalazine sodium: 3.3-12.4 mmol/L. These are not therapeutic guideline levels. These are reported levels after administration that have been observed on study. No correlation to response is known at this time.

Test Interactions Increased ALT, AST (S)

Patient Information Take with food in evenly divided doses; contact physician if rash or diarrhea occur

Special Geriatric Considerations No specific data is available on elderly to suggest the drug needs alterations in dose. Since so little is absorbed, dosing should not be changed for reasons of age. Diarrhea may pose a serious problem for elderly in that it may cause dehydration, electrolyte imbalance, hypotension, and confusion.

Dosage Forms Excipient information presented when available (limited, particularly for generics); consult specific product labeling.

Capsule, as sodium: 250 mg

♦ **Olsalazine Sodium** see Olsalazine on page 1154

♦ **Olux®** see Clobetasol on page 335

♦ **Olux-E™** see Clobetasol on page 335

♦ **Omacor®** see Omega-3-Acid Ethyl Esters on page 1155

Omega-3-Acid Ethyl Esters (oh MEG a three AS id ETH il ES ters)

Medication Safety Issues
Sound-alike/look-alike issues:
Omacor® may be confused with Amicar®

U.S. Brand Names Omacor®

Index Terms Ethyl Esters of Omega-3 Fatty Acids; Fish Oil

Pharmacologic Category Antilipemic Agent, Miscellaneous

Use Omacor®: Treatment of hypertriglyceridemia (≥500 mg/dL)

Note: A number of OTC formulations containing omega-3 fatty acids are marketed as nutritional supplements; these do not have FDA-approved indications.

Unlabeled/Investigational Use Omacor®: Treatment of IgA nephropathy

Contraindications Hypersensitivity to omega-3-acid ethyl esters or any component of the formulation

Warnings/Precautions Use with caution in patients with known allergy to fish. Should be used as an adjunct to diet and exercise only in those with very high triglyceride levels. Treatment of primary metabolic disorders (eg, diabetes, thyroid disease) and/or evaluation of the patient's medication regimen for possible etiologic agents should be completed prior to a decision to initiate therapy. If triglyceride levels do not adequately respond after 2 months of treatment with omega-3-acid ethyl esters, discontinue treatment. Prolongation of bleeding time has been observed in some clinical studies. Use caution in patients with coagulopathy or in those receiving therapeutic anticoagulation.

Adverse Reactions (Reflective of adult population; not specific for elderly)
Cardiovascular: Angina (1%)
Central nervous system: Pain (2%)
Dermatologic: Rash (2%)
Gastrointestinal: Eructation (5%), dyspepsia (3%), taste perversion (3%)
Neuromuscular and skeletal: Back pain (2%)
Miscellaneous: Flu-like syndrome (4%), infection (4%)

Drug Interactions
Anticoagulants: Omega-3-acid ethyl esters may prolong bleeding time. The effect of concurrent anticoagulant therapy has not been evaluated.
Antiplatelet agents, salicylates, and nonsteroidal anti-inflammatory agents: Omega-3-acid ethyl esters may prolong bleeding time. The effect of concurrent medications which may alter platelet function has not been evaluated.
Beta-blockers: May decrease the therapeutic effect of omega-3-acid ethyl esters. Omega-3-acid ethyl esters may augment the antihypertensive effect of beta-blockers.
Estrogens: May decrease the therapeutic effect of omega-3-acid ethyl esters.
Thiazide diuretics: May decrease the therapeutic effect of omega-3-acid ethyl esters. Thiazide diuretics may increase serum triglycerides. Omega-3-acid ethyl esters may augment the antihypertensive effect of thiazide diuretics.

Ethanol/Nutrition/Herb Interactions
Ethanol: Monitor ethanol use (alcohol use may increase triglycerides).

Stability Store at 25°C (77°F); excursions permitted to 15°C to 30°C (59°F to 86°F). Do not freeze.

Mechanism of Action Mechanism has not been completely defined. Possible mechanisms include inhibition of acyl CoA:1,2 diacylglycerol acyltransferase, increased hepatic beta-oxidation, or a reduction in the hepatic synthesis of triglycerides.

Dosage
Geriatrics & Adults:
Hypertriglyceridemia: Oral: 4 g/day as a single daily dose or in 2 divided doses.
Treatment of IgA nephropathy (unlabeled use): Oral: 4 g/day
Renal Impairment: No dosage adjustment required.

Administration May be administered with meals.
(Continued)

Omega-3-Acid Ethyl Esters *(Continued)*

Monitoring Parameters Triglycerides and other lipids (LDL-C) should be monitored at baseline and periodically. Hepatic transaminase levels, particularly ALT, should be monitored periodically.

Special Geriatric Considerations Specific information about the safety and efficacy of omega-3-acid ethyl esters is limited. The manufacturer states there were no apparent differences between persons <60 and >60 years of age.

Dosage Forms Excipient information presented when available (limited, particularly for generics); consult specific product labeling.

Capsule: 1 g [contains EPA ~465 mg and DHA ~375 mg]

Selected References

Donadio JV and Grande JP, "The Role of Fish Oil/Omega-3 Fatty Acids in the Treatment of IgA Nephropathy," *Semin Nephrol*, 2004, 24(3):225-43.

Donadio JV Jr, Larson TS, Bergstralh EJ, et al, "A Randomized Trial of High-Dose Compared With Low-Dose Omega-3 Fatty Acids in Severe IgA Nephropathy," *J Am Soc Nephrol*, 2001, 12(4):791-9.

Durrington PN, Bhatnagar D, Mackness MI, et al, "An Omega-3 Polyunsaturated Fatty Acid Concentrate Administered for One Year Decreased Triglycerides in Simvastatin Treated Patients With Coronary Heart Disease and Persisting Hypertriglyceridaemia," *Heart*, 2001, 85(5):544-8.

Harris WS, Ginsberg HN, Arunakul N, et al, "Safety and Efficacy of Omacor in Severe Hypertriglyceridemia," *J Cardiovasc Risk*, 1997, 4(5-6):385-91.

Stalenhoef AF, de Graaf J, Wittekoek ME, et al, "The Effect of Concentrated n-3 Fatty Acids Versus Gemfibrozil on Plasma Lipoproteins, Low Density Lipoprotein Heterogeneity and Oxidizability in Patients With Hypertriglyceridemia," *Atherosclerosis*, 2000, 153(1):129-38.

Omeprazole *(oh MEP ra zole)*

Related Information

Helicobacter pylori Treatment *on page 1759*

Medication Safety Issues

Sound-alike/look-alike issues:

Prilosec® may be confused with Plendil®, Prevacid®, predniSONE, prilocaine, Prinivil®, Proventil®, Prozac®

International issues:

Norpramin®: Brand name for desipramine in the U.S.

U.S. Brand Names Prilosec®; Prilosec OTC™ [OTC]

Canadian Brand Names Apo-Omeprazole®; Losec®; Losec MUPS®

Generic Available Yes: Delayed release capsule

Pharmacologic Category Proton Pump Inhibitor; Substituted Benzimidazole

Use Short-term (4-8 weeks) treatment of erosive esophagitis (grade ≥2), diagnosed by endoscopy; maintain healing of erosive esophagitis; short-term treatment of symptomatic gastroesophageal reflux disease (GERD) poorly responsive to customary medical treatment; short-term treatment of active duodenal ulcer; short-term treatment of active benign gastric ulcers; long-term treatment of pathological hypersecretory conditions; may be effective in treating gastric ulcers caused by NSAIDs, more studies may be necessary to clearly establish this use; treatment of *H. pylori* in combination with clarithromycin for the treatment of ulcers; heartburn (initial symptoms associated with GERD)

Unlabeled/Investigational Use Prevention and treatment of NSAID-induced ulcers

Contraindications Hypersensitivity to omeprazole, substituted benzimidazoles (ie, esomeprazole, lansoprazole, pantoprazole, rabeprazole), or any component of the formulation

Warnings/Precautions Relief of symptoms does not preclude the presence of a gastric malignancy. Atrophic gastritis (by biopsy) has been noted with long-term omeprazole therapy. In long-term (2-year) studies in rats, omeprazole produced a dose-related increase in gastric carcinoid tumors. While available endoscopic evaluations and histologic examinations of biopsy specimens from human stomachs have not detected a risk from short-term exposure to omeprazole, further human data on the effect of sustained hypochlorhydria and hypergastrinemia are needed to rule out the possibility of an increased risk for the development of tumors in humans receiving long-term therapy. Bioavailability may be increased in the elderly, Asian population, and with hepatic dysfunction. When used for self-medication (OTC), do not use for >14 days. Treatment should not be repeated more often than every 4 months.

Adverse Reactions (Reflective of adult population; not specific for elderly)

1% to 10%:

Central nervous system: Headache (3% to 7%), dizziness (2%)

Dermatologic: Rash (2%)

Gastrointestinal: Diarrhea (3% to 4%), abdominal pain (2% to 5%), nausea (2% to 4%), vomiting (2% to 3%), flatulence (≤3%), acid regurgitation (2%), constipation (1% to 2%), taste perversion

Neuromuscular & skeletal: Weakness (1%), back pain (1%)

Respiratory: Upper respiratory infection (2%), cough (1%)

Overdosage/Toxicology Limited experience with human overdose. Symptoms include confusion, drowsiness, blurred vision, tachycardia, nausea, flushing, diaphoresis, headache, and dry mouth. Treatment is symptom-directed and supportive.

Zegerid™: Also consider signs and symptoms of sodium bicarbonate overdose. Electrolytes (including sodium, potassium, calcium) may be altered; monitoring may be required.

Drug Interactions Substrate of CYP2A6 (minor), 2C9 (minor), 2C19 (major), 2D6 (minor), 3A4 (major); **Inhibits** CYP1A2 (weak), 2C9 (moderate), 2C19 (strong), 2D6 (weak), 3A4 (weak); **Induces** CYP1A2 (weak)

Antifungal agents (imidazole): Proton pump inhibitors may decrease the absorption of itraconazole and ketoconazole.

Benzodiazepines metabolized by oxidation (eg, diazepam, midazolam, triazolam): Esomeprazole and omeprazole may increase levels of benzodiazepines metabolized by oxidation.

Cilostazol: Omeprazole may enhance the adverse/toxic effect of cilostazol; dose reductions of cilostazol (50 mg twice daily) are recommended if coadministered.

Clozapine: Omeprazole may alter the concentrations/effects of clozapine; monitor.

CYP2C9 substrates: Omeprazole may increase the levels/effects of CYP2C9 substrates. Example substrates include bosentan, dapsone, fluoxetine, glimepiride, glipizide, losartan, montelukast, nateglinide, paclitaxel, phenytoin, warfarin, and zafirlukast.

CYP2C19 inducers: May decrease the levels/effects of omeprazole. Example inducers include aminoglutethimide, carbamazepine, phenytoin, and rifampin.

CYP2C19 substrates: Omeprazole may increase the levels/effects of CYP2C19 substrates. Example substrates include citalopram, diazepam, methsuximide, phenytoin, propranolol, and sertraline.

Dasatinib: Omeprazole may decrease the absorption of dasatinib.

HMG-CoA reductase inhibitors: Omeprazole may increase the levels/effects of HMG-CoA reductase inhibitors; monitor.

Iron salts (oral): Omeprazole may decrease the absorption of oral iron salts

Methotrexate: Concurrent use with omeprazole may decrease the excretion of methotrexate. **Note:** Antirheumatic doses of methotrexate probably hold minimal risk.

Nelfinavir: Omeprazole may decrease the serum concentration of nelfinavir.

Phenytoin: Elimination of phenytoin may be prolonged; monitor. Phenytoin may decrease omeprazole levels/effects.

Protease inhibitors: Proton pump inhibitors may decrease absorption of some protease inhibitors (atazanavir and indinavir); avoid concurrent use.

Warfarin: Proton pump inhibitors may increase the levels/effects or warfarin; monitor.

Ethanol/Nutrition/Herb Interactions

Ethanol: Avoid ethanol (may cause gastric mucosal irritation).

Food: Food delays absorption.

Stability Store at 15°C to 30°C (59°F to 86°F). Protect from light.

Mechanism of Action Proton pump inhibitor; suppresses gastric basal and stimulated acid secretion by inhibiting the parietal cell H+/K+ ATP pump

Pharmacodynamics

Onset of action: Antisecretory: ~1 hour

Peak effect: 0.5-3.5 hours

Duration: Up to 72 hours

Pharmacokinetics

Protein binding: ~95%

Metabolism: Extensively hepatic to inactive metabolites

Bioavailability: Oral: ~30% to 40%; increased in Asian patients and patients with hepatic dysfunction

Half-life elimination: Delayed release capsule: 0.5-1 hour

Excretion: Urine (77% as metabolites, very small amount as unchanged drug); feces

Dosage

Geriatrics & Adults:

Active duodenal ulcer: Oral: 20 mg/day for 4-8 weeks

Gastric ulcers: Oral: 40 mg/day for 4-8 weeks

Symptomatic GERD: Oral: 20 mg/day for up to 4 weeks

Erosive esophagitis: Oral: 20 mg/day for 4-8 weeks; maintenance of healing: 20 mg/day for up to 12 months total therapy (including treatment period of 4-8 weeks)

Peptic ulcer disease: Eradication of *Helicobacter pylori*: Oral: Dose varies with regimen: 20 mg once daily **or** 40 mg/day as single dose or in 2 divided doses; requires combination therapy with antibiotics

Pathological hypersecretory conditions: Oral: Initial: 60 mg once daily; doses up to 120 mg 3 times/day have been administered; administer daily doses >80 mg in divided doses

Frequent heartburn (OTC labeling): Oral: 20 mg/day for 14 days; treatment may be repeated after 4 months if needed

(Continued)

Omeprazole *(Continued)*

Renal Impairment: No adjustment is necessary.

Hepatic Impairment: Specific guidelines are not available; bioavailability is increased with chronic liver disease.

Administration

Capsule: Should be swallowed whole. Do not chew, crush, or open. Best if taken before breakfast. May be opened and contents added to applesauce. Administration via NG tube should be in an acidic juice.

Powder for oral suspension (Zegerid™):

Oral: Administer 1 hour before a meal. Mix with 2 tablespoons of water; stir well and drink immediately. Rinse cup with water and drink.

Nasogastric/orogastric tube: Mix well with 20 mL of water and administer immediately; flush tube with an additional 20 mL of water. Suspend enteral feeding for 3 hours before and 1 hour after administering Zegerid™.

Monitoring Parameters Monitor symptoms, occult blood; use of gastroscopy is preferred; INR for patients on warfarin

Patient Information Take before eating; do not chew, crush, or open capsule; if need to open capsule for ease of administration, place contents in acid juice (orange juice, tomato juice, etc); may take with antacids concomitantly

Special Geriatric Considerations In clinical trials, the incidence of side effects in the elderly is no different than that of younger adults (≤65 years) despite slight decrease in elimination and increase in bioavailability. Bioavailability may be increased in the elderly (≥65 years of age), however, dosage adjustments are not necessary.

Dosage Forms Excipient information presented when available (limited, particularly for generics); consult specific product labeling.

Capsule, delayed release: 10 mg, 20 mg

Prilosec®: 10 mg, 20 mg, 40 mg

Tablet, delayed release:

Prilosec OTC™: 20 mg

Selected References

Andersson T, Hasan-Alin M, Hasselgren G, et al, "Drug Interactions Studies With Esomeprazole, the (S)-Isomer of Omeprazole," *Clin Pharmacokinet*, 2001, 40(7):523-37.

Blume H, Donath F, Warnke A, et al, "Pharmacokinetic Drug Interaction Profiles of Proton Pump Inhibitors," *Drug Saf*, 2006, 29(9): 769-84.

Cockayne SE, Glet RJ, Gawkrodger DJ, et al, "Severe Erythrodermic Reactions to the Proton Pump Inhibitors Omeprazole and Lansoprazole," *Br J Dermatol*, 1999, 141(1):173-5.

Natsch S, Vinks MH, Voogt AK, et al, "Anaphylactic Reactions to Proton-Pump Inhibitors," *Ann Pharmacother*, 2000, 34(4):474-6.

Omeprazole and Sodium Bicarbonate

(oh MEP ra zole & SOW dee um bye KAR bun ate)

U.S. Brand Names Zegerid®

Generic Available No

Pharmacologic Category Proton Pump Inhibitor; Substituted Benzimidazole

Use Short-term (4-8 weeks) treatment of active duodenal ulcer disease or active benign gastric ulcer; treatment of heartburn and other symptoms associated with gastroesophageal reflux disease (GERD); short-term (4-8 weeks) treatment of endoscopically-diagnosed erosive esophagitis; maintenance healing of erosive esophagitis; reduction of risk of upper gastrointestinal bleeding in critically-ill patients

Contraindications Hypersensitivity to omeprazole, substituted benzimidazoles (eg, esomeprazole, lansoprazole, pantoprazole, rabeprazole), or any component of the formulation

Warnings/Precautions Relief of symptoms does not preclude the presence of a gastric malignancy. Atrophic gastritis (by biopsy) has been noted with long-term omeprazole therapy. In long-term (2-year) studies in rats, omeprazole produced a dose-related increase in gastric carcinoid tumors. While available endoscopic evaluations and histologic examinations of biopsy specimens from human stomachs have not detected a risk from short-term exposure to omeprazole, further human data on the effect of sustained hypochlorhydria and hypergastrinemia are needed to rule out the possibility of an increased risk for the development of tumors in humans receiving long-term therapy. Bioavailability may be increased in the elderly, Asian population, and with hepatic dysfunction. Use with caution in patients with Bartter's syndrome, hypocalcemia, hypokalemia, sodium-restricted diets, and respiratory alkalosis (contains sodium bicarbonate).

Adverse Reactions (Reflective of adult population; not specific for elderly)

Frequency of adverse events reported for 40 mg dose of oral powder for suspension. **Note:** Asterisked (*) percentages indicate frequency reported from a controlled clinical trial of 359 critically-ill patients.

>10%:

Central nervous system: Pyrexia (20%*)

Endocrine & metabolic: Hypokalemia (12%*), hyperglycemia (11%*)

Respiratory: Nosocomial pneumonia (11%*)
1% to 10%:
  Cardiovascular: Hypotension (10%*), hypertension (8%*), atrial fibrillation (6%*), ventricular tachycardia (5%*), bradycardia (4%*), tachycardia (3%*), supraventricular tachycardia (3%*), edema (3%*)
  Central nervous system: Hyperpyrexia (5%), agitation (3%), headache (2%)
  Dermatological: Rash (6%*), decubitus ulcer (3%)
  Endocrine & metabolic: Hypomagnesemia (10%*), hypocalcemia (6%*), hypophosphatemia (6%*), fluid overload (5%*), hypoglycemia (3%*), hyponatremia (4%*), hypernatremia (2%*), hyperkalemia (2%*)
  Gastrointestinal: Constipation (5%*), diarrhea (4%*), hypomotility (2%*)
  Genitourinary: Urinary tract infection (2%*)
  Hematological: Thrombocytopenia (10%*), anemia (8%*), anemia increased (2%*)
  Hepatic: LFTs increased (2%*)
  Respiratory: ARDS (3%*), respiratory failure (2%*), URI (2%), cough (1%)
  Miscellaneous: Sepsis (5%*), oral candidiasis (2%*), candidal infection (2%*)

Overdosage/Toxicology Limited experience with overdose in humans. Doses up to 2400 mg of omeprazole have been reported. Symptoms include confusion, drowsiness, blurred vision, tachycardia, nausea, flushing, diaphoresis, headache, and dry mouth. Also consider signs and symptoms of sodium bicarbonate overdose; electrolytes, including sodium, potassium, and calcium, may be altered (monitoring may be required). Treatment is symptom-directed and supportive. Not dialyzable.

Drug Interactions **Substrate** of CYP2A6 (minor), 2C9 (minor), 2C19 (major), 2D6 (minor), 3A4 (minor); **Inhibits** CYP1A2 (weak), 2C9 (moderate), 2C19 (strong), 2D6 (weak), 3A4 (weak); **Induces** CYP1A2 (weak)

Benzodiazepines metabolized by oxidation (eg, diazepam, midazolam, triazolam): Esomeprazole and omeprazole may increase levels of benzodiazepines metabolized by oxidation.

Carbamazepine: Esomeprazole and omeprazole may increase carbamazepine levels.

Clozapine: Omeprazole may alter the concentrations/effects of clozapine; monitor.

CYP2C9 substrates: Omeprazole may increase the levels/effects of CYP2C9 substrates. Example substrates include amiodarone, fluoxetine, glimepiride, glipizide, nateglinide, phenytoin, pioglitazone, rosiglitazone, sertraline, and warfarin.

CYP2C19 inducers: May decrease the levels/effects of omeprazole. Example inducers include aminoglutethimide, carbamazepine, phenytoin, and rifampin.

CYP2C19 substrates: Omeprazole may increase the levels/effects of CYP2C19 substrates. Example substrates include citalopram, diazepam, methsuximide, phenytoin, propranolol, and sertraline.

Itraconazole and ketoconazole: Proton pump inhibitors may decrease the absorption of itraconazole and ketoconazole.

Methotrexate: Concurrent use with omeprazole may decrease the excretion of methotrexate. **Note:** Antirheumatic doses of methotrexate probably hold minimal risk.

Phenytoin: Elimination of phenytoin may be prolonged; monitor. Phenytoin may decrease omeprazole levels/effects.

Protease inhibitors: Proton pump inhibitors may decrease absorption of some protease inhibitors (atazanavir and indinavir).

Warfarin: Elimination of warfarin may be prolonged; monitor.

Ethanol/Nutrition/Herb Interactions

Ethanol: Avoid ethanol (may cause gastric mucosal irritation).

Food: Food delays absorption. When given 1 hour after a meal, absorption is reduced.

Herb/Nutraceutical: St John's wort may decrease omeprazole levels.

Stability Store at 15°C to 30°C (59°F to 86°F).

Mechanism of Action Suppresses gastric basal and stimulated acid secretion by inhibiting the parietal cell H+/K+ ATP pump

Pharmacokinetics

Onset of action: Antisecretory: ~1 hour
  Peak effect: 2 hours
Duration: 72 hours
Protein binding: 95%
Metabolism: Extensively hepatic to inactive metabolites
Bioavailability: Oral: 30% to 40%; increased in Asian patients and patients with hepatic dysfunction
Half-life elimination: 0.4-3.2 hours
Excretion: Urine (77% as metabolites, very small amount as unchanged drug); feces

Dosage

Geriatrics & Adults:
  Active duodenal ulcer: Oral: 20 mg/day for 4-8 weeks
  Gastric ulcers: Oral: 40 mg/day for 4-8 weeks
  Symptomatic GERD: Oral: 20 mg/day for up to 4 weeks
  Erosive esophagitis: Oral: 20 mg/day for 4-8 weeks; maintenance of healing: 20 mg/day for up to 12 months total therapy (including treatment period of 4-8 weeks)

(Continued)

Omeprazole and Sodium Bicarbonate *(Continued)*

Risk reduction of upper GI bleeding in critically-ill patients (Zegerid® powder for oral suspension): Oral:

Loading dose: Day 1: 40 mg every 6-8 hours for two doses

Maintenance dose: 40 mg/day for up to 14 days; therapy >14 days has not been evaluated

Renal Impairment: No adjustment is necessary.

Hepatic Impairment: Specific guidelines are not available; bioavailability is increased with chronic liver disease.

Administration

Capsule: Should be swallowed whole; do not chew or crush. Capsules should **not** be opened, sprinkled on food, or administered via NG. Best if taken before breakfast.

Powder for oral suspension:

Oral: Administer 1 hour before a meal. Mix with 2 tablespoons of water; stir well and drink immediately. Rinse cup with water and drink.

Nasogastric/orogastric tube: Mix well with 20 mL of water and administer immediately; flush tube with an additional 20 mL of water. Suspend enteral feeding for 3 hours before and 1 hour after administering.

Patient Information Take as directed, before eating. Do not crush or chew capsules. Avoid alcohol. You may experience anorexia; small frequent meals may help to maintain adequate nutrition. Report changes in urination or pain on urination, unresolved severe diarrhea, testicular pain, or changes in respiratory status.

Special Geriatric Considerations The incidence of side effects in the elderly is no different than that of younger adults (≤65 years of age) despite slight decrease in elimination and increase in bioavailability. Dosage adjustments are not necessary. Use cautiously in patients requiring sodium restriction, hypertension, or congestive heart failure.

Dosage Forms Excipient information presented when available (limited, particularly for generics); consult specific product labeling.

Capsule, immediate release:

Zegerid®: 20 mg, 40 mg [both strengths contain sodium bicarbonate 1100 mg, equivalent to sodium 300 mg (13 mEq) per capsule]

Powder for oral suspension [packet]:

Zegerid®: 20 mg (30s), 40 mg (30s) [both strengths contain sodium bicarbonate 1680 mg, equivalent to sodium 460 mg per packet]

Selected References

Andersson T, "Omeprazole Drug Interaction Studies," *Clin Pharmacokinet*, 1991, 21(3):195-212.

Balian JD, Sukhova N, Harris JW, et al, "The Hydroxylation of Omeprazole Correlates With S-Mephenytoin Metabolism: A Population Study," *Clin Pharmacol Ther*, 1995, 57(6):662-9.

Berardi RR and Dunn-Kucharski VA, "Omeprazole: Defining Its Role in Gastroesophageal Reflux Disease," *Hosp Formul*, 1995, 30:216-25.

Beutler M, Hartmann K, Kuhn M, et al, "Arthralgias on Omeprazole," *BMJ*, 1994, 309(6969):1620.

Carvajal A and Martin Arias LH, "Gynecomastia and Sexual Disorders After the Administration of Omeprazole," *Am J Gastroenterol*, 1995, 90(6):1028-9.

Cockayne SE, Glet RJ, Gawkrodger DJ, et al, "Severe Erythrodermic Reactions to the Proton Pump Inhibitors Omeprazole and Lansoprazole," *Br J Dermatol*, 1999, 141(1):173-5.

Epelde Gonzalo FD, Boada Montagut L, and Tomas Vecina S, "Exfoliative Dermatitis Related to Omeprazole," *Ann Pharmacother*, 1995, 29(1):82-3.

Kane DL, "Administration of Omeprazole (Prilosec®) in the Atypical Patient," *Int J Pharm Compounding*, 1997, 1(1):13.

Kraus A and Flores-Suarez LF, "Acute Gout Associated With Omeprazole," *Lancet*, 1995, 345(8947):461-2.

Larner AJ and Lendrum R, "Oesophageal Candidiasis After Omeprazole Therapy," *Gut*, 1992, 33(6):860-1.

Lau JY, Sung JJ, Lee KK, et al, "Effect of Intravenous Omeprazole on Recurrent Bleeding After Endoscopic Treatment of Bleeding Peptic Ulcers," *N Engl J Med*, 2000, 343(5):310-6.

Lindquist M and Edwards IR, "Endocrine Adverse Effects of Omeprazole," *Br Med J*, 1992, 305(6851):451-2.

Natsch S, Vinks MH, Voogt AK, et al, "Anaphylactic Reactions to Proton-Pump Inhibitors," *Ann Pharmacother*, 2000, 34(4):474-6.

Ottervanger JP, Stricker BH, Kappelle JW, et al, "Omeprazole-Associated Agranulocytosis," *Eur J Haematol*, 1995, 54(4):279-80.

Soll AH, Weinstein WM, Kurata J, et al, "Nonsteroidal Anti-inflammatory Drugs and Peptic Ulcer Disease," *Ann Intern Med*, 1991, 114(4):307-19.

Wolfe MM and Sachs G, "Acid Suppression: Optimizing Therapy for Gastroduodenal Ulcer Healing, Gastroesophageal Reflux Disease, and Stress-Related Erosive Syndrome," *Gastroenterology*, 2000, 118(2 Suppl 1):9-31.

Woods DJ and McClintock AD, "Omeprazole Administration," *Ann Pharmacother*, 1993, 27(5):651.

♦ **Omnaris™** *see* Ciclesonide *on page 308*

♦ **Omnicef®** *see* Cefdinir *on page 254*

♦ **Omnii Gel™ [OTC]** *see* Fluoride *on page 642*

Ondansetron *(on DAN se tron)*

Medication Safety Issues

Sound-alike/look-alike issues:

Ondansetron may be confused with dolasetron, granisetron, palonosetron

Zofran® may be confused with Zantac®, Zosyn®

U.S. Brand Names Zofran®; Zofran® ODT
Canadian Brand Names Apo-Ondansetron®; Zofran®; Zofran® ODT
Index Terms GR38032R; Ondansetron Hydrochloride
Generic Available Yes
Pharmacologic Category Antiemetic; Selective 5-HT$_3$ Receptor Antagonist
Use Prevention of nausea and vomiting associated with moderately- to highly-emetogenic cancer chemotherapy; radiotherapy in patients receiving total body irradiation or fractions to the abdomen; prevention and treatment of postoperative nausea and vomiting

Generally **not** recommended for treatment of existing chemotherapy-induced emesis (CIE) or for prophylaxis of nausea from agents with a low emetogenic potential.
Unlabeled/Investigational Use Treatment of early-onset alcoholism; hyperemesis gravidarum
Contraindications Hypersensitivity to ondansetron, other selective 5-HT$_3$ antagonists, or any component of the formulation
Warnings/Precautions Ondansetron should be used on a scheduled basis, not on an "as needed" (PRN) basis, since data support the use of this drug only in the prevention of nausea and vomiting (due to antineoplastic therapy) and not in the rescue of nausea and vomiting. Ondansetron should only be used in the first 24-48 hours of chemotherapy. Data do not support any increased efficacy of ondansetron in delayed nausea and vomiting. Does not stimulate gastric or intestinal peristalsis; may mask progressive ileus and/or gastric distension. Use with caution in patients allergic to other 5-HT$_3$ receptor antagonists; cross-reactivity has been reported. Transient ECG changes (including QT interval prolongation) have been reported (rarely) with I.V. use. Orally-disintegrating tablets contain phenylalanine.
Adverse Reactions (Reflective of adult population; not specific for elderly)
Note: Percentages reported in adult patients.
>10%:
  Central nervous system: Headache (9% to 27%), malaise/fatigue (9% to 13%)
  Gastrointestinal: Constipation (6% to 11%)
1% to 10%:
  Central nervous system: Drowsiness (8%), fever (2% to 8%), dizziness (4% to 7%), anxiety (6%), cold sensation (2%)
  Dermatologic: Pruritus (2% to 5%), rash (1%)
  Gastrointestinal: Diarrhea (2% to 7%)
  Genitourinary: Gynecological disorder (7%), urinary retention (5%)
  Hepatic: ALT/AST increased (1% to 5%)
  Local: Injection site reaction (4%; pain, redness, burning)
  Neuromuscular & skeletal: Paresthesia (2%)
  Respiratory: Hypoxia (9%)
Overdosage/Toxicology Sudden transient blindness, severe constipation, hypotension, and vasovagal episode with transient secondary heart block have been reported in some cases of overdose. I.V. doses up to 252 mg/day have been inadvertently given without adverse effects. There is no specific antidote. Treatment is symptom-directed and supportive.
Drug Interactions Substrate of CYP1A2 (minor), 2C9 (minor), 2D6 (minor), 2E1 (minor), 3A4 (major); **Inhibits** CYP1A2 (weak), 2C9 (weak), 2D6 (weak)
  Apomorphine: Due to reports of profound hypotension during concomitant therapy, the manufacturer of apomorphine contraindicates its use with ondansetron.
  CYP3A4 inducers: CYP3A4 inducers may decrease the levels/effects of ondansetron. Example inducers include aminoglutethimide, carbamazepine, nafcillin, nevirapine, phenobarbital, phenytoin, and rifamycins. The manufacturer does not recommend dosage adjustment in patients receiving CYP3A4 inducers.
Ethanol/Nutrition/Herb Interactions
  Food: Food increases the extent of absorption. The C_{max} and T_{max} do not change much.
  Herb/Nutraceutical: St John's wort may decrease ondansetron levels.
Stability
  Oral solution: Store between 15°C and 30°C (59°F and 86°F). Protect from light.
  Premixed bag: Store between 2°C and 30°C (36°F and 86°F). Protect from light.
  Tablet: Store between 2°C and 30°C (36°F and 86°F).
  Vial: Store between 2°C and 30°C (36°F and 86°F). Protect from light. Prior to I.V. infusion, dilute in 50 mL D$_5$W or NS. Solution is stable for 48 hours at room temperature.
Mechanism of Action Selective 5-HT$_3$-receptor antagonist, blocking serotonin, both peripherally on vagal nerve terminals and centrally in the chemoreceptor trigger zone
Pharmacodynamics Onset of effect: Within 30 minutes
Pharmacokinetics
  Distribution: V_d: 2.2-2.5 L/kg
  Plasma protein binding: 70% to 76%
  Metabolism: Extensively in the liver by hydroxylation, followed by glucuronide or sulfate conjugation
  (Continued)

Ondansetron *(Continued)*

Bioavailability: Oral: 56% to 71%; Rectal: 58% to 74%
Half-life: Adults and Geriatrics <75 years of age: 3-6 hours
   Mild-to-moderate hepatic impairment: Adults: 12 hours
   Severe hepatic impairment: Adults: 20 hours
Time to peak: Oral: ~2 hours
Elimination: Urine (44% to 60% as metabolites, 5% to 10% as unchanged drug); feces (~25%)

Dosage

Geriatrics & Adults: Note: Studies in adults have shown a single daily dose of 8-12 mg I.V. or 8-24 mg orally to be as effective as mg/kg dosing, and should be considered for **all** patients whose mg/kg dose exceeds 8-12 mg I.V.; oral solution and ODT formulations are bioequivalent to corresponding doses of tablet formulation.

Prevention of chemotherapy-induced emesis:
  I.V.:
    0.15 mg/kg 3 times/day beginning 30 minutes prior to chemotherapy **or**
    0.45 mg/kg once daily **or**
    8-10 mg 1-2 times/day **or**
    24 mg or 32 mg once daily
  Highly-emetogenic agents/single-day therapy: Oral: 24 mg given 30 minutes prior to the start of therapy
  Moderately-emetogenic agents: Oral: 8 mg every 12 hours beginning 30 minutes before chemotherapy, continuously for 1-2 days after chemotherapy completed

Total body irradiation: Oral: 8 mg 1-2 hours before each daily fraction of radiotherapy

Single high-dose fraction radiotherapy to abdomen: Oral: 8 mg 1-2 hours before irradiation, then 8 mg every 8 hours after first dose for 1-2 days after completion of radiotherapy

Daily fractionated radiotherapy to abdomen: 8 mg 1-2 hours before irradiation, then 8 mg 8 hours after first dose for each day of radiotherapy

Postoperative nausea and vomiting (PONV):
  Oral: 16 mg given one hour prior to induction of anesthesia
  I.M., I.V.: 4 mg as a single dose immediately before induction of anesthesia, or shortly following procedure if vomiting occurs
    Note: Repeat doses given in response to inadequate control of nausea/vomiting from preoperative doses are generally ineffective.

Treatment of hyperemesis gravidum (unlabeled use):
  Oral: 8 mg every 12 hours
  I.V.: 8 mg administered over 15 minutes every 12 hours or 1 mg/hour infused continuously for up to 24 hours

Renal Impairment: No adjustment is necessary.

Hepatic Impairment: Severe liver disease (Child-Pugh C): Maximum daily dose: 8 mg

Administration

Oral: Oral dosage forms should be administered 30 minutes prior to chemotherapy; 1-2 hours before radiotherapy; 1 hour prior to the induction of anesthesia
  Orally-disintegrating tablets: Do not remove from blister until needed. Peel backing off the blister, do not push tablet through. Using dry hands, place tablet on tongue and allow to dissolve. Swallow with saliva.
I.M.: Should be administered undiluted
I.V.: Give first dose 30 minutes prior to beginning chemotherapy; the I.V. preparation has been successful when administered orally
IVPB: Dilute in 50 mL D₅W or NS. Infuse over 15-30 minutes; 24-hour continuous infusions have been reported, but are rarely used

Monitoring Parameters Emetic episodes, diarrhea, headache

Patient Information This drug may cause drowsiness; use caution when driving or engaging in tasks that require alertness until response to drug is known. You may experience fatigue, drowsiness, dizziness, diarrhea, constipation and headache (request appropriate treatment from healthcare provider). Do not change position rapidly (rise slowly). Good mouth care and sucking on lozenges may help relieve nausea. Report persistent headache, excessive drowsiness, fever, numbness or tingling, or severe changes in elimination patterns (constipation or diarrhea), chest pain, or palpitations.

Orally-disintegrating tablets: Do not remove from blister until needed. Peel backing off the blister, do not push tablet through. Using dry hands, place tablet on tongue and allow to dissolve. Swallow with saliva. Contains <0.03 mg phenylalanine/tablet.

Additional Information The I.V. product has been used orally successfully

Special Geriatric Considerations Elderly have a slightly decreased hepatic clearance rate. This does not, however, require a dose adjustment.

Dosage Forms Excipient information presented when available (limited, particularly for generics); consult specific product labeling.

Infusion [premixed in D_5W, preservative free]: 32 mg (50 mL)
Zofran®: 32 mg (50 mL)

Injection, solution: 2 mg/mL (2 mL, 20 mL)
Zofran®: 2 mg/mL (2 mL, 20 mL)

Solution, oral: 4 mg/5 mL (50 mL)
Zofran®: 4 mg/5 mL (50 mL) [contains sodium benzoate; strawberry flavor]

Tablet: 4 mg; 8 mg
Zofran®: 4 mg; 8 mg

Tablet, orally disintegrating: 4 mg; 8 mg
Zofran® ODT: 4 mg, 8 mg [each strength contains phenylalanine <0.03 mg/tablet; strawberry flavor]

Extemporaneously Prepared A 0.8 mg/mL syrup may be made by crushing ten 8 mg tablets; flaking of the tablet coating occurs. Mix thoroughly with 50 mL of the suspending vehicle, Ora-Plus® (Paddock), in 5 mL increments. Add sufficient volume of any of the following syrups: Cherry syrup USP, Syrpalta® (Humco), Ora-Sweet® (Paddock), or Ora-Sweet® Sugar-Free (Paddock) to make a final volume of 100 mL. Stability is 42 days refrigerated.

Trissel LA, "Trissel's Stability of Compounded Formulations," American Pharmaceutical Association, 1996.

Rectal suppositories: Calibrate a suppository mold for the base being used. Determine the displacement factor (DF) for ondansetron for the base being used (Fattibase® = 1.1; Polybase® = 0.6). Weigh the ondansetron tablet. Divide the tablet weight by the DF. Subtract the weight of base displaced from the calculated weight of base required for each suppository. Grind the ondansetron tablets to a fine powder in a mortar. Weigh out the appropriate weight of suppository base. Melt the base over a water bath (<55°C). Add the ondansetron powder to the suppository base and mix well. Pour the mixture into the suppository mold and cool. Stable for at least 30 days under refrigeration.

Allen LV, "Ondansetron Suppositories," *US Pharm*, 20(7):84-6.

♦ **Ondansetron Hydrochloride** *see* Ondansetron *on page 1160*
♦ **One Gram C [OTC]** *see* Ascorbic Acid *on page 125*
♦ **Opana®** *see* Oxymorphone *on page 1186*
♦ **Opana® ER** *see* Oxymorphone *on page 1186*
♦ **OPC-13013** *see* Cilostazol *on page 312*
♦ **OPC-14597** *see* Aripiprazole *on page 121*
♦ **Opcon-A® [OTC]** *see* Naphazoline and Pheniramine *on page 1087*
♦ **Optase™** *see* Trypsin, Balsam Peru, and Castor Oil *on page 1642*
♦ **Opticrom®** *see* Cromolyn *on page 369*
♦ **Optigene® 3 [OTC]** *see* Tetrahydrozoline *on page 1547*
♦ **OptiPranolol®** *see* Metipranolol *on page 1022*
♦ **Optivar®** *see* Azelastine *on page 143*
♦ **Oracea™** *see* Doxycycline *on page 479*
♦ **Oracit®** *see* Sodium Citrate and Citric Acid *on page 1477*
♦ **Orajel® Perioseptic® Spot Treatment [OTC]** *see* Carbamide Peroxide *on page 235*
♦ **Oramorph SR®** *see* Morphine Sulfate *on page 1065*
♦ **Oranyl [OTC]** *see* Pseudoephedrine *on page 1346*
♦ **Orap®** *see* Pimozide *on page 1261*
♦ **Orapred®** *see* PrednisoLONE *on page 1303*
♦ **Orapred ODT™** *see* PrednisoLONE *on page 1303*
♦ **OraRinse™ [OTC]** *see* Maltodextrin *on page 953*
♦ **Orazinc® [OTC]** *see* Zinc Sulfate *on page 1700*
♦ **Orciprenaline Sulfate** *see* Metaproterenol *on page 991*
♦ **Orencia®** *see* Abatacept *on page 22*
♦ **Organidin® NR** *see* Guaifenesin *on page 727*
♦ **Original Doan's® [OTC]** *see* Salicylates (Various Salts) *on page 1439*

Orlistat (OR li stat)

Medication Safety Issues
Sound-alike/look-alike issues:
Xenical® may be confused with Xeloda®
U.S. Brand Names Alli™ [OTC]; Xenical®
Canadian Brand Names Xenical®
Generic Available No
(Continued)

Orlistat *(Continued)*

Pharmacologic Category Lipase Inhibitor

Use Management of obesity, including weight loss and weight management when used in conjunction with a reduced-calorie and low-fat diet; reduction of risk of weight regain after prior weight loss; indicated for obese patients with an initial body mass index (BMI) ≥30 kg/m^2 or ≥27 kg/m^2 in the presence of other risk factors. See table.

Body Mass Index (BMI), kg/m^2 Height (feet, inches)

Weight (lb)	5'0"	5'3"	5'6"	5'9"	6'0"	6'3"
140	27	25	23	21	19	18
150	29	27	24	22	20	19
160	31	28	26	24	22	20
170	33	30	28	25	23	21
180	35	32	29	27	25	23
190	37	34	31	28	26	24
200	39	36	32	30	27	25
210	41	37	34	31	29	26
220	43	39	36	33	30	28
230	45	41	37	34	31	29
240	47	43	39	36	33	30
250	49	44	40	37	34	31

Contraindications Hypersensitivity to orlistat or any component of the formulation; chronic malabsorption syndrome or cholestasis

Warnings/Precautions Patients should be advised to adhere to dietary guidelines; gastrointestinal adverse events may increase if taken with a diet high in fat (>30% total daily calories from fat). The daily intake of fat should be distributed over three main meals. If taken with any one meal very high in fat, the possibility of gastrointestinal effects increases. Patients should be counseled to take a multivitamin supplement that contains fat-soluble vitamins to ensure adequate nutrition because orlistat has been shown to reduce the absorption of some fat-soluble vitamins and beta-carotene. Some patients may develop increased levels of urinary oxalate following treatment; caution should be exercised when prescribing it to patients with a history of hyperoxaluria or calcium oxalate nephrolithiasis. As with any weight-loss agent, the potential exists for misuse in appropriate patient populations (eg, patients with anorexia nervosa or bulimia). Safety and efficacy with >4 years of use have not been established.

OTC labeling: Prior to use, patients should contact their healthcare provider if they have ever had kidney stones, gall bladder disease, or pancreatitis. Patients taking medications for diabetes or thyroid disease, anticoagulants, or other weight-loss products should consult their healthcare provider or pharmacist. Patients who have had an organ transplant should not use orlistat. If severe and/or continuous abdominal pain occurs, use should be discontinued and healthcare provider consulted.

Adverse Reactions (Reflective of adult population; not specific for elderly)
>10%:
   Central nervous system: Headache (31%)
   Gastrointestinal: Oily spotting (27%), abdominal pain/discomfort (26%), flatus with discharge (24%), fecal urgency (22%), fatty/oily stool (20%), oily evacuation (12%), defecation increased (11%)
   Neuromuscular & skeletal: Back pain (14%)
   Respiratory: Upper respiratory infection (38%)
1% to 10%:
   Central nervous system: Fatigue (7%), anxiety (5%), sleep disorder (4%)
   Dermatologic: Dry skin (2%)
   Endocrine & metabolic: Menstrual irregularities (10%)
   Gastrointestinal: Fecal incontinence (8%), nausea (8%), infectious diarrhea (5%), rectal pain/discomfort (5%), vomiting (4%)
   Neuromuscular & skeletal: Arthritis (5%), myalgia (4%)
   Otic: Otitis (4%)

Overdosage/Toxicology Single doses of 800 mg and multiple doses up to 400 mg 3 times daily for 15 days have been studied in normal weight and obese patients, without significant adverse findings. In significant overdose, observation of the patient is recommended for 24 hours.

Drug Interactions
   Amiodarone: Orlistat may decrease amiodarone absorption; monitor.
   Cyclosporine: Cyclosporine serum levels may de decreased; administer cyclosporine 2 hours before or after orlistat; monitor.

Warfarin: Orlistat does not alter the pharmacokinetics of warfarin, however, vitamin K absorption may be decreased during orlistat therapy. Therefore, patients stabilized on warfarin should be monitored for changes in warfarin effects.

Ethanol/Nutrition/Herb Interactions
Fat-soluble vitamins: Absorption of vitamins A, D, E, and K may be decreased by orlistat. A multivitamin containing the fat-soluble vitamins (A, D, E, and K) should be administered once daily at least 2 hours before or after orlistat.

Stability Store at 15°C to 30°C (59°F to 86°F).

Mechanism of Action A reversible inhibitor of gastric and pancreatic lipases, thus inhibiting absorption of dietary fats by 30% (at doses of 120 mg 3 times/day).

Pharmacodynamics
Onset: 24-48 hours
Duration of action: 48-72 hours

Pharmacokinetics
Absorption: Minimal
Metabolism: Metabolized within the gastrointestinal wall; forms inactive metabolites
Excretion: Feces (97%, 83% as unchanged drug); urine (<2%)

Dosage
Geriatrics & Adults: Obesity: Oral:
Xenical®: 120 mg 3 times/day with each main meal containing fat (during or up to 1 hour after the meal); omit dose if meal is occasionally missed or contains no fat.
Alli™: OTC labeling: 60 mg 3 times/day with each main meal containing fat

Patient Information Patient should be on a nutritionally balanced, reduced-calorie diet that contains approximately 30% of calories from fat; daily intake of fat, carbohydrate, and protein should be distributed over the three main meals

Dosage Forms Excipient information presented when available (limited, particularly for generics); consult specific product labeling.
Capsule:
Alli™ [OTC]: 60 mg
Xenical®: 120 mg

Selected References
Cyr EE Jr, "Orlistat (Xenical®)," *Clin Toxicol Rev*, 2000, 22(4):1-2.
Davidson MH, Hauptman J, DiGirolamo M, et al, "Weight Control and Risk Factor Reduction in Obese Subjects Treated for 2 Years With Orlistat: A Randomized Controlled Trial," *JAMA*, 1999, 281(3):235-42.

Orphenadrine (or FEN a dreen)

Related Information
Potentially Inappropriate Medications for Geriatrics *on page 1824*

Medication Safety Issues
Sound-alike/look-alike issues:
Norflex™ may be confused with norfloxacin, Noroxin®

International issues:
Flexin® [Israel] may be confused with Floxin® which is a brand name for ofloxacin in the U.S.
Flexin® [Israel]: Brand name for indomethacin in Great Britain

U.S. Brand Names Norflex™

Canadian Brand Names Norflex™; Orphenace®; Rhoxal-orphendrine

Index Terms Orphenadrine Citrate

Generic Available Yes

Pharmacologic Category Anti-Parkinson's Agent, Anticholinergic; Skeletal Muscle Relaxant

Use Treatment of muscle spasm associated with acute painful musculoskeletal conditions

Contraindications Hypersensitivity to orphenadrine or any component of the formulation; glaucoma; GI obstruction, stenosing peptic ulcer; prostatic hypertrophy, bladder neck obstruction; cardiospasm; myasthenia gravis

Warnings/Precautions Use with caution in patients with CHF, cardiac decompensation, coronary insufficiency , tachycardia, or cardiac arrhythmias. May cause CNS depression, which may impair physical or mental abilities. Potential for abuse; use with caution in patients with history of drug abuse. Solution for injection contains sodium, bisulfite which may cause allergic reaction in some individuals. Has not been evaluated for continuous long-term use; monitor closely.

Adverse Reactions (Reflective of adult population; not specific for elderly)
Frequency not defined.
Cardiovascular: Palpitation, tachycardia
Central nervous system: Agitation, drowsiness, dizziness, euphoria, hallucination, headache, mental confusion
Dermatologic: Pruritus, urticaria
Gastrointestinal: Constipation, gastric irritation, nausea, vomiting, xerostomia
(Continued)

Orphenadrine *(Continued)*

Genitourinary: Urination hesitancy, urinary retention
Hematologic: Aplastic anemia (rare)
Neuromuscular & skeletal: Tremor, weakness
Ocular: Blurred vision, intraocular pressure increased, nystagmus, pupil dilation
Respiratory: Nasal congestion
Miscellaneous: Anaphylactic reaction (injection, rare), hypersensitivity

Overdosage/Toxicology Symptoms include blurred vision, tachycardia, confusion, seizures, respiratory arrest, and dysrhythmias. Doses of 2-3 g may be lethal in adults, however, the toxicity range is unpredictable. Although there is no specific treatment, clinical toxicity is due to blockade of cholinergic receptors. Anticholinesterase inhibitors may be useful by reducing acetylcholinesterase. Anticholinesterase inhibitors include physostigmine, neostigmine, pyridostigmine, and edrophonium. For anticholinergic overdose with severe life-threatening symptoms, physostigmine 1-2 mg slow I.V. may be given to reverse these effects. Treatment is otherwise symptom-directed and supportive; monitor closely.

Drug Interactions Substrate (minor) of CYP1A2, 2B6, 2D6, 3A4; **Inhibits** CYP1A2 (weak), 2A6 (weak), 2B6 (weak), 2C9 (weak), 2C19 (weak), 2D6 (weak), 2E1 (weak), 3A4 (weak)

Acetylcholinesterase inhibitors (donepezil, galantamine, rivastigmine, tacrine): May diminish the therapeutic effect of orphenadrine. If the anticholinergic action is a side effect of the agent, the result may be beneficial. Orphenadrine may diminish the therapeutic effect of centrally-acting acetylcholinesterase inhibitors.

Anticholinergic agents: May increase potential for anticholinergic adverse effects; includes drugs with high anticholinergic activity (diphenhydramine, TCAs, phenothiazines).

CNS depressants: Sedative effects may be additive; monitor.

Pramlintide: May enhance the anticholinergic effect of orphenadrine (these effects are specific to the GI tract).

Ethanol/Nutrition/Herb Interactions

Ethanol: Avoid ethanol (may increase CNS depression).

Herb/Nutraceutical: Avoid valerian, St John's wort, kava kava, gotu kola (may increase CNS depression).

Stability Store at 15°C to 30°C (59°F to 86°F). Protect injection solution from light.

Mechanism of Action Indirect skeletal muscle relaxant thought to work by central atropine-like effects; has some euphorigenic and analgesic properties

Pharmacodynamics

Peak effect: Oral: Within 2-4 hours
Duration: 4-6 hours

Pharmacokinetics

Protein binding: 20%
Metabolism: Extensive
Half-life: 14-16 hours
Elimination: Urine (8% as unchanged drug)

Dosage

Geriatrics: Use caution; generally not recommended for use in the elderly (see Special Geriatric Considerations).

Adults: Muscle spasms:
Oral: 100 mg twice daily
I.M., I.V.: 60 mg every 12 hours

Monitoring Parameters Relief of symptoms, mental status, anticholinergic effects

Patient Information May cause drowsiness, dizziness, blurred vision, or fainting; do not crush or chew sustained release product; avoid alcohol, may impair coordination and judgment

Special Geriatric Considerations Because of its anticholinergic side effects (eg, constipation, urinary retention, confusion), orphenadrine is not a drug of choice in the elderly.

Dosage Forms Excipient information presented when available (limited, particularly for generics); consult specific product labeling.

Injection, solution, as citrate: 30 mg/mL (2 mL)
Norflex™: 30 mg/mL (2 mL) [contains sodium bisulfite]
Tablet, extended release, as citrate: 100 mg
Norflex™: 100 mg

Selected References

Olanow CW, Watts RL, and Koller WC, "An Algorithm (Decision Tree) for the Management of Parkinson's Disease (2001): Treatment Guidelines," *Neurology*, 2001, 56(11 Suppl 5):S1-S88.

- ◆ **Orphenadrine Citrate** *see* Orphenadrine *on page 1165*
- ◆ **Ortho Prefest** *see* Estradiol and Norgestimate *on page 554*
- ◆ **Orudis® KT [OTC] [DSC]** *see* Ketoprofen *on page 856*
- ◆ **Orvaten™** *see* Midodrine *on page 1042*

♦ **Os-Cal® 500 [OTC]** *see* Calcium Salts (Oral) *on page 220*
♦ **Os-Cal® 500+D [OTC]** *see* Calcium and Vitamin D *on page 214*

Oseltamivir (oh sel TAM i vir)

Medication Safety Issues
Sound-alike/look-alike issues:
Tamiflu® may be confused with Thera-Flu®

U.S. Brand Names Tamiflu®

Canadian Brand Names Tamiflu®

Generic Available No

Pharmacologic Category Antiviral Agent; Neuraminidase Inhibitor

Use Treatment of uncomplicated acute illness due to influenza (A or B) infection in children ≥1 year of age and adults who have been symptomatic for no more than 2 days; prophylaxis against influenza (A or B) infection in children ≥1 year of age and adults

Contraindications Hypersensitivity to oseltamivir or any component of the formulation

Warnings/Precautions Oseltamivir is not a substitute for the influenza virus vaccine. Use caution with renal impairment; dosage adjustment is required for creatinine clearance between 10-30 mL/minute. Also consider primary or concomitant bacterial infections. Safety and efficacy for use in hepatic impairment or for treatment or prophylaxis in immunocompromised patients have not been established. Efficacy has not been established if treatment begins >40 hours after the onset of symptoms or in the treatment of patients with chronic cardiac and/or respiratory disease. Rare but severe hypersensitivity reactions (anaphylaxis, severe dermatologic reactions) have been associated with use.

Adverse Reactions (Reflective of adult population; not specific for elderly)
>10%: Gastrointestinal: Vomiting (2% to 15%)
1% to 10%: Gastrointestinal: Nausea (3% to 10%), abdominal pain (2% to 5%)

Overdosage/Toxicology Single doses of 1000 mg resulted in nausea and vomiting.

Drug Interactions Influenza virus vaccine nasal spray (fluMist™): Safety and efficacy for use with influenza virus vaccine nasal spray have not been established. Do not administer nasal spray until 48 hours after stopping antiviral; do not administer antiviral for 2 weeks after receiving influenza virus vaccine nasal spray.

Stability
Capsules: Store at 25°C (77°F).
Oral suspension: Store powder for suspension at 25°C (77°F). Reconstitute with 23 mL of water (to make 25 mL total suspension). Once reconstituted, store suspension under refrigeration at 2°C to 8°C (36°F to 46°F); do not freeze. Use within 10 days of preparation.

Mechanism of Action Oseltamivir, a prodrug, is hydrolyzed to the active form, oseltamivir carboxylate. It is thought to inhibit influenza virus neuraminidase, with the possibility of alteration of virus particle aggregation and release.

Pharmacokinetics
Absorption: Well absorbed
Distribution: V_d: 23-26 L (oseltamivir carboxylate)
Protein binding, plasma: Oseltamivir carboxylate: 3%; Oseltamivir: 42%
Metabolism: Hepatic (90%) to oseltamivir carboxylate; neither the parent drug nor active metabolite has any effect on CYP
Bioavailability: 75% as oseltamivir carboxylate
Half-life elimination: Oseltamivir: 1-3 hours; Oseltamivir carboxylate: 6-10 hours
Excretion: Urine (>90% as oseltamivir carboxylate); feces

Dosage
Geriatrics & Adults:
Influenza prophylaxis: Oral: 75 mg once daily; initiate treatment within 2 days of contact with an infected individual; duration of treatment: 10 days. During community outbreaks, dosing is 75 mg once daily. May be used for up to 6 weeks; duration of protection lasts for length of dosing period.
Influenza treatment: Oral: 75 mg twice daily initiated within 2 days of onset of symptoms; duration of treatment: 5 days

Renal Impairment: Adults:
Cl_{cr} 10-30 mL/minute:
Treatment: Reduce dose to 75 mg once daily for 5 days.
Prophylaxis: Administer 75 mg every other day or 30 mg once daily.
Cl_{cr} <10 mL/minute: Dosing recommendations are not available.

Hepatic Impairment: Dosing recommendations are not available.

Patient Information Take within 2 days of flu symptoms (fever, cough, headache, fatigue, muscular weakness, and sore throat). This is not a substitute for the flu shot. For best results, do not miss doses. Take with or without food; take with food to improve tolerance.
(Continued)

Oseltamivir *(Continued)*

Additional Information In clinical studies of the influenza virus, 1.3% of post-treatment isolates in adults had decreased neuraminidase susceptibility *in vitro* to oseltamivir carboxylate.

Dosage Forms Excipient information presented when available (limited, particularly for generics); consult specific product labeling.
Capsule, as phosphate:
Tamiflu®: 75 mg
Powder for oral suspension:
Tamiflu®: 12 mg/mL (25 mL) [contains sodium benzoate; tutti-frutti flavor]

Selected References
Bardsley-Elliot A and Noble S, "Oseltamivir," *Drugs*, 1999, 58(5):851-60.

Hayden FG, Atmar RL, Schilling M, et al, "Use of the Selective Oral Neuraminidase Inhibitor Oseltamivir to Prevent Influenza," *N Engl J Med*, 1999, 341(18):1336-43.

Hayden FG, Treanor JJ, Fritz RS, et al, "Use of the Oral Neuraminidase Inhibitor Oseltamivir in Experimental Human Influenza: Randomized Controlled Trials for Prevention and Treatment," *JAMA*, 1999, 282(13):1240-6.

He G, Massarella J, and Ward P, "Clinical Pharmacokinetics of the Prodrug Oseltamivir and Its Active Metabolite Ro 64-0802," *Clin Pharmacokinet*, 1999, 37(6):471-84.

"Neuraminidase Inhibitors for Treatment of Influenza A and B Infections," *MMWR*, 1999, 48(RR-14):1-9.

♦ **Osmoglyn® [DSC]** *see* Glycerin *on page 718*
♦ **OsmoPrep™** *see* Sodium Phosphates *on page 1478*
♦ **OTFC (Oral Transmucosal Fentanyl Citrate)** *see* Fentanyl *on page 609*
♦ **Otrivin® [OTC] [DSC]** *see* Xylometazoline *on page 1689*
♦ **Otrivin® Pediatric [OTC] [DSC]** *see* Xylometazoline *on page 1689*
♦ **Ovace®** *see* Sulfacetamide *on page 1496*
♦ **Ovace® Wash** *see* Sulfacetamide *on page 1496*

Oxacillin (oks a SIL in)

Related Information
Antibiotic Treatment of Adults With Infective Endocarditis *on page 1797*
Antimicrobial Activity Against Selected Organisms *on page 1728*

Index Terms Methylphenyl Isoxazolyl Penicillin; Oxacillin Sodium

Generic Available Yes

Pharmacologic Category Antibiotic, Penicillin

Use Treatment of susceptible bacterial infections such as osteomyelitis, septicemia, endocarditis, and CNS infections due to penicillinase-producing strains of *Staphylococcus* (except methicillin resistant)

Contraindications Hypersensitivity to oxacillin or other penicillins or any component of the formulation

Warnings/Precautions Modify dosage in patients with renal impairment and in the elderly. Serious and occasionally severe or fatal hypersensitivity (anaphylactoid) reactions have been reported in patients on penicillin therapy, especially with a history of beta-lactam hypersensitivity, history of sensitivity to multiple allergens, or previous IgE-mediated reactions (eg, anaphylaxis, angioedema, urticaria). Use with caution in asthmatic patients. Prolonged use may result in fungal or bacterial superinfection, including *C. difficile*-associated diarrhea and pseudomembranous colitis.

Adverse Reactions (Reflective of adult population; not specific for elderly)
Frequency not defined.
Central nervous system: Fever
Dermatologic: Rash
Gastrointestinal: Nausea, diarrhea, vomiting
Hematologic: Eosinophilia, leukopenia, neutropenia, thrombocytopenia, agranulocytosis
Hepatic: Hepatotoxicity, AST increased
Renal: Acute interstitial nephritis, hematuria
Miscellaneous: Serum sickness-like reactions

Overdosage/Toxicology Symptoms of penicillin overdose include neuromuscular hypersensitivity (agitation, hallucinations, asterixis, encephalopathy, confusion, and seizures) and electrolyte imbalance (with potassium or sodium salts), especially in renal failure. Hemodialysis may be helpful to aid in the removal of the drug from the blood, otherwise most treatment is supportive or symptom-directed.

Drug Interactions
Fusidic acid: May decrease the therapeutic effect of penicillins; administer the penicillin at least 2 hours before fusidic acid.
Methotrexate: Penicillins may increase the exposure to methotrexate during concurrent therapy; monitor.
Oral contraceptives: Anecdotal reports suggesting decreased contraceptive efficacy with penicillins have been refuted by more rigorous scientific and clinical data.
Probenecid, disulfiram: May increase levels of penicillins (oxacillin).

Warfarin: Effects of warfarin may be increased.

Stability Reconstituted parenteral solution is stable for 3 days at room temperature and 7 days when refrigerated. For I.V. infusion in NS or D_5W, solution is stable for 24 hours at room temperature.

Mechanism of Action Inhibits bacterial cell wall synthesis by binding to one or more of the penicillin-binding proteins (PBPs); which in turn inhibits the final transpeptidation step of peptidoglycan synthesis in bacterial cell walls, thus inhibiting cell wall biosynthesis. Bacteria eventually lyse due to ongoing activity of cell wall autolytic enzymes (autolysins and murein hydrolases) while cell wall assembly is arrested.

Pharmacokinetics
Distribution: Into bile, synovial and pleural fluids, bronchial secretions, peritoneal, and pericardial fluids; penetrates the blood-brain barrier only when meninges are inflamed
Protein binding: ~94%
Metabolism: Hepatic to active metabolites
Half-life: Adults: 23-60 minutes
Time to peak, serum: I.M.: 30-60 minutes
Elimination: Urine and feces (small amounts as unchanged drug and metabolites)

Dosage
Geriatrics & Adults:
Endocarditis: I.V.: 2 g every 4 hours with gentamicin
Mild-to-moderate infections: I.M., I.V.: 250-500 mg every 4-6 hours
Prosthetic joint infection: I.V.: 2 g every 4 hours with rifampin
Severe infections: I.M., I.V.: 1-2 g every 4-6 hours
***Staphylococcus aureus*, methicillin-susceptible infections, including brain abscess, bursitis, erysipelas, mastitis, mastoiditis, osteomyelitis, perinephric abscess, pneumonia, pyomyositis, scalded skin syndrome, toxic shock syndrome:** I.V.: 2 g every 4 hours

Renal Impairment:
Cl_{cr} <10 mL/minute: Clinical practice varies; some clinicians recommend adjustment to the lower range of the usual dosage as based on severity of infection.
Not dialyzable (0% to 5%)

Administration Administer around-the-clock to promote less variation in peak and trough serum concentrations. Administer IVP over 10 minutes. Administer IVPB over 30 minutes.

Monitoring Parameters Monitor signs and symptoms of infection, WBC, mental status; monitor periodic CBC, urinalysis, BUN, serum creatinine, AST and ALT

Test Interactions May interfere with urinary glucose tests using cupric sulfate (Benedict's solution, Clinitest®); may inactivate aminoglycosides *in vitro*; false-positive urinary and serum proteins

Patient Information Complete course of treatment as prescribed. You may experience nausea or vomiting; small frequent meals and good mouth care may help. If diabetic, drug may cause false tests with Clinitest® urine glucose monitoring; use of glucose oxidase methods (Clinistix®) or serum glucose monitoring is preferable. Report persistent fever, sore throat, sores in mouth, diarrhea, unusual bleeding or bruising, difficulty breathing, or skin rash. Notify prescriber if condition does not respond to treatment.

Additional Information Sodium content of 1 g: 2.5 mEq

Special Geriatric Considerations Oxacillin has not been studied in the elderly. Dosing adjustments are not necessary except in renal failure (eg, Cl_{cr} <10 mL/minute). Consider sodium content in patients who may be sensitive to volume expansion (ie, CHF).

Dosage Forms Excipient information presented when available (limited, particularly for generics); consult specific product labeling.
Infusion [premixed iso-osmotic dextrose solution]: 1 g (50 mL); 2 g (50 mL)
Injection, powder for reconstitution, as sodium: 1 g, 2 g, 10 g

Selected References
Yoshikawa TT, "Antimicrobial Therapy for the Elderly Patient," *J Am Geriatr Soc*, 1990, 38(12):1353-72.

♦ **Oxacillin Sodium** *see* Oxacillin *on page 1168*

Oxaprozin (oks a PROE zin)

Related Information
Potentially Inappropriate Medications for Geriatrics *on page 1824*
Medication Safety Issues
Sound-alike/look-alike issues:
Daypro® may be confused with Diupres®
Oxaprozin may be confused with oxazepam
U.S. Brand Names Daypro®
Canadian Brand Names Apo-Oxaprozin®; Daypro®
Generic Available Yes
(Continued)

Oxaprozin *(Continued)*

Pharmacologic Category Nonsteroidal Anti-inflammatory Drug (NSAID), Oral

Use Acute and long-term use in the management of signs and symptoms of osteoarthritis and rheumatoid arthritis

Restrictions An FDA-approved medication guide must be distributed when dispensing an oral outpatient prescription (new or refill) where this medication is to be used without direct supervision of a healthcare provider. Medication guides are available at http://www.fda.gov/cder/Offices/ODS/medication_guides.htm.

Contraindications Hypersensitivity to oxaprozin, aspirin, other NSAIDs, or any component of the formulation; perioperative pain in the setting of coronary artery bypass surgery (CABG)

Warnings/Precautions [U.S. Boxed Warning]: NSAIDs are associated with an increased risk of adverse cardiovascular events, including MI, stroke, and new onset or worsening of pre-existing hypertension. Risk may be increased with duration of use or pre-existing cardiovascular risk factors or disease. Carefully evaluate individual cardiovascular risk profiles prior to prescribing. Use caution with fluid retention, CHF, or hypertension. Concurrent administration of ibuprofen, and potentially other nonselective NSAIDs, may interfere with aspirin's cardioprotective effect.

Use of NSAIDs can compromise existing renal function. Renal toxicity can occur in patients with impaired renal function, dehydration, heart failure, liver dysfunction, those taking diuretics and ACEIs, and the elderly. Rehydrate patient before starting therapy. Monitor renal function closely. Oxaprozin is not recommended for patients with advanced renal disease.

[U.S. Boxed Warning]: NSAIDs may increase risk of gastrointestinal irritation, ulceration, bleeding, and perforation. These events may occur at any time during therapy and without warning. Use caution with a history of GI disease (bleeding or ulcers); concurrent therapy with aspirin, anticoagulants, and/or corticosteroids; smoking; use of alcohol; and the elderly or debilitated patients.

Use the lowest effective dose for the shortest duration of time, consistent with individual patient goals, to reduce risk of cardiovascular or GI adverse events. Alternate therapies should be considered for patients at high risk.

NSAIDs may cause serious skin adverse events including exfoliative dermatitis, Stevens-Johnson syndrome (SJS), and toxic epidermal necrolysis (TEN). Anaphylactoid reactions may occur, even without prior exposure; patients with "aspirin triad" (bronchial asthma, aspirin intolerance, rhinitis) may be at increased risk. Do not use in patients who experience bronchospasm, asthma, rhinitis, or urticaria with NSAID or aspirin therapy. Use caution in other forms of asthma.

Use with caution in patients with decreased hepatic function. Closely monitor patients with any abnormal LFT. Severe hepatic reactions (eg, fulminant hepatitis, liver failure) have occurred with NSAID use, rarely; discontinue if signs or symptoms of liver disease develop, or if systemic manifestations occur.

The elderly are at increased risk for adverse effects (especially peptic ulceration, CNS effects, renal toxicity) from NSAIDs even at low doses.

Withhold for at least 4-6 half-lives prior to surgical or dental procedures. May cause mild photosensitivity reactions.

Adverse Reactions (Reflective of adult population; not specific for elderly)
1% to 10%:
Cardiovascular: Edema
Central nervous system: Confusion, depression, dizziness, headache, sedation, sleep disturbance, somnolence
Dermatologic: Pruritus, rash
Gastrointestinal: Abdominal distress, abdominal pain, anorexia, constipation, diarrhea, flatulence, gastrointestinal ulcer, gross bleeding with perforation, heartburn, nausea, vomiting
Hematologic: Anemia, bleeding time increased
Hepatic: Liver enzyme elevation
Otic: Tinnitus
Renal: Dysuria, renal function abnormal, urinary frequency

Overdosage/Toxicology Symptoms include acute renal failure, vomiting, drowsiness, and leukocytosis. Management of nonsteroidal anti-inflammatory drug (NSAID) intoxication is primarily supportive and symptomatic. Fluid therapy is commonly effective in managing hypotension that may occur following an acute NSAID overdose, except when due to acute blood loss. Seizures tend to be very short-lived and often do not require drug treatment, although recurrent seizures should be treated with I.V. diazepam. Since many of NSAIDs undergo enterohepatic cycling, multiple doses of charcoal may be needed to reduce the potential for delayed toxicities.

Drug Interactions

ACE inhibitors: Antihypertensive effects may be decreased by concurrent therapy with NSAIDs; monitor blood pressure. Oxaprozin may decrease serum concentration of enalapril.

Angiotensin II antagonists: Antihypertensive effects may be decreased by concurrent therapy with NSAIDs; monitor blood pressure.

Anticoagulants (warfarin, heparin, LMWHs) in combination with NSAIDs can cause increased risk of bleeding.

Antiplatelet drugs (ticlopidine, clopidogrel, aspirin, abciximab, dipyridamole, eptifibatide, tirofiban) can cause an increased risk of bleeding.

Beta-blockers: NSAIDs may decrease the antihypertensive effect of beta-blockers; monitor.

Cholestyramine (and other bile acid sequestrants): May decrease the absorption of NSAIDs; separate by at least 2 hours.

Corticosteroids may increase the risk of GI ulceration; avoid concurrent use.

Cyclosporine: NSAIDs may increase serum creatinine, potassium, blood pressure, and cyclosporine levels; monitor cyclosporine levels and renal function carefully.

Fluoroquinolone antibiotics: Risk of seizures may be increased with concomitant quinolone use. Risk is considered quite low and may only be a factor with high serum levels of either agent and/or in patients with additional predisposing factors (eg, renal dysfunction, history of seizure or other neurological disorder).

Hydralazine's antihypertensive effect is decreased; avoid concurrent use.

Lithium levels can be increased; avoid concurrent use if possible or monitor lithium levels and adjust dose. Sulindac may have the least effect. When NSAID is stopped, lithium will need adjustment again.

Loop diuretics efficacy (diuretic and antihypertensive effect) may be reduced.

Methotrexate: Severe bone marrow suppression, aplastic anemia, and GI toxicity have been reported with concomitant NSAID therapy. Avoid use during moderate or high-dose methotrexate (increased and prolonged methotrexate levels). NSAID use during low-dose treatment of rheumatoid arthritis has not been fully evaluated; extreme caution is warranted.

Salicylates: NSAIDs (nonselective) may diminish the cardioprotective effect of acetylated salicylates. Avoid regular use of NSAIDs if possible; consider alternatives (eg, acetaminophen). Give salicylate before NSAID; for example ibuprofen should be given 30-120 minutes after aspirin (immediate release).

Thiazides antihypertensive effects are decreased; avoid concurrent use.

Warfarin's INRs may be increased by piroxicam. Other NSAIDs may have the same effect depending on dose and duration. Monitor INR closely. Use the lowest dose of NSAIDs possible and for the briefest duration.

Ethanol/Nutrition/Herb Interactions

Ethanol: Avoid ethanol (may enhance gastric mucosal irritation).

Herb/Nutraceutical: Avoid alfalfa, anise, bilberry, bladderwrack, bromelain, cat's claw, celery, coleus, cordyceps, dong quai, evening primrose, feverfew, fenugreek, garlic, ginger, ginkgo biloba, red clover, horse chestnut, grapeseed, green tea, ginseng, guggul, horse chestnut seed, horseradish, licorice, prickly ash, red clover, reishi, SAMe, sweet clover, turmeric, white willow (all have additional antiplatelet activity).

Stability Store at 25°C (77°F). Protect from light; keep bottle tightly closed.

Mechanism of Action Inhibits prostaglandin synthesis by decreasing the activity of the enzyme, cyclooxygenase, which results in decreased formation of prostaglandin precursors

Pharmacodynamics Onset of anti-inflammatory action: Up to 7 days

Pharmacokinetics

Absorption: Almost complete

Protein binding: >99%

Metabolism: Hepatic, forms metabolites

Half-life: 40-50 hours

Time to peak: 2-4 hours

Elimination: Urine (5% unchanged, 65% as metabolites); feces (35% as metabolites)

Dosage

Geriatrics & Adults:

Osteoarthritis: Oral: 600-1200 mg once daily; patients should be titrated to lowest dose possible; patients with low body weight should start with 600 mg daily

Rheumatoid arthritis: Oral: 1200 mg once daily; a one-time loading dose of up to 1800 mg/day or 26 mg/kg (whichever is lower) may be given

Maximum doses:

Patient <50 kg: Maximum: 1200 mg/day

Patient >50 kg with normal renal/hepatic function and low risk of peptic ulcer: Maximum: 1800 mg or 26 mg/kg (whichever is lower) in divided doses

Renal Impairment: In general, NSAIDs are not recommended for use in patients with advanced renal disease but the manufacturer of oxaprozin does provide some guidelines for adjustment in renal dysfunction.

(Continued)

Oxaprozin *(Continued)*

Severe renal impairment or on dialysis: 600 mg once daily; may increase cautiously to 1200 mg/day with close monitoring.

Hepatic Impairment: Use caution in patients with severe dysfunction.

Monitoring Parameters Monitor response (pain, range of motion, grip strength, mobility, ADL function), inflammation; observe for weight gain, edema; monitor renal function; observe for bleeding, bruising; evaluate gastrointestinal effects (abdominal pain, bleeding, dyspepsia); mental confusion, disorientation, CBC, serum, creatinine, BUN, liver function tests

Test Interactions False-positive urine immunoassay screening tests for benzodiazepines have been reported and may occur several days after discontinuing oxaprozin.

Patient Information Take this medication exactly as directed; do not increase dose without consulting prescriber. Do not crush tablets. Take with food or milk to reduce GI distress. Maintain adequate fluid intake (2-3 L/day of fluids unless instructed to restrict fluid intake). Do not use alcohol, aspirin, or aspirin-containing medication, and all other anti-inflammatory medications without consulting prescriber. You may experience drowsiness, dizziness, or nervousness (use caution when driving or engaging in tasks requiring alertness until response to drug is known); anorexia, nausea, vomiting, or heartburn (frequent small meals, frequent mouth care, sucking lozenges, or chewing gum may help). GI bleeding, ulceration, or perforation can occur with or without pain; discontinue medication and contact prescriber if persistent abdominal pain or cramping, or blood in stool occurs. Report vaginal bleeding; breathlessness, difficulty breathing, or unusual cough; chest pain, rapid heartbeat, palpitations; unusual bruising/bleeding; blood in urine, stool, mouth, or vomitus; swollen extremities; skin rash or itching; acute fatigue; or swelling of face, lips, tongue, or throat.

Additional Information There are no clinical guidelines to predict which NSAID will give response in a particular patient; trials with each must be initiated until response determined; consider dose, patient convenience, and cost

Special Geriatric Considerations Elderly are a high-risk population for adverse effects from NSAIDs. As much as 60% of the elderly can develop peptic ulceration and/or hemorrhage asymptomatically. The concomitant use of H_2 blockers and sucralfate is not generally effective as prophylaxis with the exception of NSAID-induced duodenal ulcers which may be prevented by the use of ranitidine. Misoprostol and proton pump inhibitors are the only agents proven to help prevent the development of NSAID-induced ulcers. Also, concomitant disease and drug use contribute to the risk for GI adverse effects. Use lowest effective dose for shortest period possible. Consider renal function decline with age. Use of NSAIDs can compromise existing renal function especially when Cl_{cr} is ≤30 mL/minute. Tinnitus may be a difficult and unreliable indication of toxicity due to age-related hearing loss or eighth cranial nerve damage. CNS adverse effects, such as confusion, agitation, and hallucination, are generally seen in overdose or high dose situations, but the elderly may demonstrate these adverse effects at lower doses than younger adults.

Dosage Forms Excipient information presented when available (limited, particularly for generics); consult specific product labeling.

Tablet: 600 mg

Selected References

Brooks PM and Day RO, "Nonsteroidal Anti-inflammatory Drugs - Differences and Similarities," *N Engl J Med*, 1991, 324(24):1716-25.

Clinch D, Banerjee AK, Ostick G, "Absence of Abdominal Pain in Elderly Patients With Peptic Ulcer," *Age Ageing*, 1984, 13(2):120-3.

Clive DM, Stoff JS, "Renal Syndromes Associated With Nonsteroidal Anti-inflammatory Drugs," *N Engl J Med*, 1984, 310(9):563-72.

Graham DY, "Prevention of Gastroduodenal Injury Induced by Chronic Nonsteroidal Anti-inflammatory Drug Therapy," *Gastroenterology*, 1989, 96(2 Pt 2 Suppl):675-81.

Gurwitz JH, Avorn J, Ross-Degnan D, et al, "Nonsteroidal Anti-Inflammatory Drug-Associated Azotemia in the Very Old," *JAMA*, 1990, 264(4):471-5.

Hawkey CJ, Karrasch JA, Szczepañski L, et al, "Omeprazole Compared With Misoprostol for Ulcers Associated With Nonsteroidal Anti-inflammatory Drugs," *N Engl J Med*, 1998, 338(11):727-34.

Heerdink ER, Leufkens HG, Herings RM, et al, "NSAIDs Associated With Increased Risk of Congestive Heart Failure in Elderly Patients Taking Diuretics," *Arch Intern Med*, 1998, 158(10):1108-12.

Knodel LC, "Preventing NSAID-induced Ulcers: The Role of Misoprostol," *Consult Pharm*, 1989, 4:37-41.

Morgan TO, Anderson A, and Bertram D, "Effect of Indomethacin on Blood Pressure in Elderly People With Essential Hypertension Well Controlled on Amlodipine or Enalapril," *Am J Hypertens*, 2000, 13:1161-7.

Page J and Henry D, "Consumption of NSAIDs and the Development of Congestive Heart Failure in Elderly Patients: An Underrecognized Public Health Problem," *Arch Intern Med*, 2000, 160(6):777-84.

Pope JE, Anderson JJ, and Felson DT, "A Meta-analysis of the Effects of Nonsteroidal Anti-inflammatory Drugs on Blood Pressure," *Arch Intern Med*, 1993, 153(4):477-84.

Pounder R, "Silent Peptic Ulceration: Deadly Silence or Golden Silence?" *Gastroenterology*, 1989, 96:(2 Pt 2 Suppl)626-31.

Yeomans ND, Tulassay Z, Juhasz L, et al, "A Comparison of Omeprazole With Ranitidine for Ulcers Associated With Nonsteroidal Anti-inflammatory Drugs," *N Engl J Med*, 1998, 338(11):719-26.

Oxazepam (oks A ze pam)

Related Information
Anxiolytic, Sedative / Hypnotic, and Miscellaneous Benzodiazepines *on page 1750*
Potentially Inappropriate Medications for Geriatrics *on page 1824*

Medication Safety Issues
Sound-alike/look-alike issues:
Oxazepam may be confused with oxaprozin, quazepam
Serax® may be confused with Eurax®, Urex®, Zyrtec®

International issues:
Murelax® [Australia] may be confused with Miralax™ which is a brand name for polyethylene glycol 3350 in the U.S.

U.S. Brand Names Serax®

Canadian Brand Names Apo-Oxazepam®; Novoxapram®; Oxpam®; Oxpram®; PMS-Oxazepam; Riva-Oxazepam

Generic Available Yes: Capsule

Pharmacologic Category Benzodiazepine

Use Treatment of anxiety; management of ethanol withdrawal

Unlabeled/Investigational Use Anticonvulsant in management of simple partial seizures; hypnotic

Restrictions C-IV

Contraindications Hypersensitivity to oxazepam or any component of the formulation (cross-sensitivity with other benzodiazepines may exist); narrow-angle glaucoma (not in product labeling, however, benzodiazepines are contraindicated); not indicated for use in the treatment of psychosis

Warnings/Precautions May cause hypotension (rare) - use with caution in patients with cardiovascular or cerebrovascular disease, or in patients who would not tolerate transient decreases in blood pressure. Serax® 15 contains tartrazine.

Use with caution in elderly or debilitated patients, patients with hepatic disease (including alcoholics), or renal impairment. Use with caution in patients with respiratory disease or impaired gag reflex. Avoid use in patients with sleep apnea.

Causes CNS depression (dose-related) resulting in sedation, dizziness, confusion, or ataxia which may impair physical and mental capabilities. Patients must be cautioned about performing tasks which require mental alertness (eg, operating machinery or driving). Use with caution in patients receiving other CNS depressants or psychoactive agents. Effects with other sedative drugs or ethanol may be potentiated. Benzodiazepines have been associated with falls and traumatic injury and should be used with extreme caution in patients who are at risk of these events (especially the elderly).

Use caution in patients with suicidal risk. Use with caution in patients with a history of drug dependence. Benzodiazepines have been associated with dependence and acute withdrawal symptoms on discontinuation or reduction in dose. Acute withdrawal, including seizures, may be precipitated after administration of flumazenil to patients receiving long-term benzodiazepine therapy.

Benzodiazepines have been associated with anterograde amnesia. Paradoxical reactions, including hyperactive or aggressive behavior have been reported with benzodiazepines, particularly in psychiatric patients. Does not have analgesic, antidepressant, or antipsychotic properties.

Adverse Reactions (Reflective of adult population; not specific for elderly)
Frequency not defined.
Cardiovascular: Syncope (rare), edema
Central nervous system: Drowsiness, ataxia, dizziness, vertigo, memory impairment, headache, paradoxical reactions (excitement, stimulation of effect), lethargy, amnesia, euphoria
Dermatologic: Rash
Endocrine & metabolic: Decreased libido, menstrual irregularities
Genitourinary: Incontinence
Hematologic: Leukopenia, blood dyscrasias
Hepatic: Jaundice
Neuromuscular & skeletal: Dysarthria, tremor, reflex slowing
Ocular: Blurred vision, diplopia
Miscellaneous: Drug dependence

Overdose/Toxicology Symptoms include somnolence, confusion, coma, hypoactive reflexes, dyspnea, hypotension, slurred speech, and impaired coordination. Treatment for benzodiazepine overdose is supportive. Rarely is mechanical ventilation required. Flumazenil has been shown to selectively block the binding of benzodiazepines to CNS receptors, resulting in reversal of benzodiazepine-induced CNS depression, but not respiratory depression due to toxicity.
(Continued)

Oxazepam *(Continued)*

Drug Interactions
Ethanol and other CNS depressants may increase the CNS effects of oxazepam

Levodopa: Therapeutic effects may be diminished in some patients following the addition of a benzodiazepine; limited/inconsistent data

Theophylline and other CNS stimulants may antagonize the sedative effects of oxazepam

Zidovudine: Increased incidence of headache with concurrent use.

Ethanol/Nutrition/Herb Interactions
Ethanol: Avoid ethanol (may increase CNS depression).

Herb/Nutraceutical: Avoid valerian, St John's wort, kava kava, gotu kola (may increase CNS depression).

Mechanism of Action Binds to stereospecific benzodiazepine receptors on the postsynaptic GABA neuron at several sites within the central nervous system, including the limbic system, reticular formation. Enhancement of the inhibitory effect of GABA on neuronal excitability results by increased neuronal membrane permeability to chloride ions. This shift in chloride ions results in hyperpolarization (a less excitable state) and stabilization.

Pharmacodynamics Studies have shown that older adults are more sensitive to the effects of benzodiazepines as compared to younger adults.

Pharmacokinetics No significant changes in pharmacokinetics are seen in older adults.

Absorption: Oral: Almost completely

Protein binding: 86% to 99%

Metabolism: In the liver to inactive compounds (primarily as glucuronides)

Half-life: 5-20 hours

Time to peak serum concentration: Within 2-4 hours

Elimination: Urinary excretion of unchanged drug (50%) and metabolites; excreted without need for liver metabolism

Dosage
Geriatrics: Oral: Anxiety: 10 mg 2-3 times/day; increase gradually as needed to a total of 30-45 mg/day. Dose titration should be slow to evaluate sensitivity.

Adults:
Anxiety: Oral: 10-30 mg 3-4 times/day
Ethanol withdrawal: Oral: 15-30 mg 3-4 times/day
Hypnotic: Oral: 15-30 mg

Renal Impairment: Not dialyzable (0% to 5%)

Monitoring Parameters Respiratory, cardiovascular and mental status, symptoms of anxiety

Reference Range Therapeutic: 0.2-1.4 mcg/mL (SI: 0.7-4.9 µmol/L)

Patient Information Avoid alcohol and other CNS depressants; may cause drowsiness; avoid activities needing good psychomotor coordination until CNS effects are known; may cause physical or psychological dependence; avoid abrupt discontinuation after prolonged use

Special Geriatric Considerations Because of its relatively short half-life and its lack of active metabolites, oxazepam is recommended for use in the elderly when a benzodiazepine is indicated.

Dosage Forms Excipient information presented when available (limited, particularly for generics); consult specific product labeling.

Capsule: 10 mg, 15 mg, 30 mg

Tablet: 15 mg [contains tartrazine]

Selected References
Hicks R, Dysken MW, Davis JM, et al, "The Pharmacokinetics of Psychotropic Medication in the Elderly: A Review," *J Clin Psychiatry*, 1981, 42(10)374-85.

Oxcarbazepine *(ox car BAZ e peen)*

U.S. Brand Names Trileptal®
Canadian Brand Names Trileptal®
Index Terms GP 47680; OCBZ
Generic Available No
Pharmacologic Category Anticonvulsant, Miscellaneous
Use Monotherapy or adjunctive therapy in the treatment of partial seizures in adults with epilepsy
Unlabeled/Investigational Use Bipolar disorder; treatment of neuropathic pain
Contraindications Hypersensitivity to oxcarbazepine or any component of the formulation
Warnings/Precautions Clinically-significant hyponatremia (sodium <125 mmol/L) can develop during oxcarbazepine use. Potentially serious, sometimes fatal, dermatologic

reactions (eg, Stevens-Johnson, toxic epidermal necrolysis) and multiorgan hypersensitivity reactions have been reported in adults and children; monitor for signs and symptoms of skin reactions and possible disparate manifestations associated with lymphatic, hepatic, renal, and/or hematologic organ systems; gradual discontinuation and conversion to alternate therapy may be required. As with all antiepileptic drugs, oxcarbazepine should be withdrawn gradually to minimize the potential of increased seizure frequency. Use of oxcarbazepine has been associated with CNS-related adverse events, most significant of these were cognitive symptoms including psychomotor slowing, difficulty with concentration, speech or language problems, somnolence or fatigue, and coordination abnormalities, including ataxia and gait disturbances. Effects with other sedative drugs or ethanol may be potentiated. Use caution in patients with previous hypersensitivity to carbamazepine (cross-sensitivity occurs in 25% to 30%). May reduce the efficacy of oral contraceptives (nonhormonal contraceptive measures are recommended).

Adverse Reactions (Reflective of adult population; not specific for elderly) As reported in adults with doses of up to 2400 mg/day (includes patients on monotherapy, adjunctive therapy, and those not previously on AEDs); incidence in children was similar.

>10%:
  Central nervous system: Dizziness (22% to 49%), somnolence (20% to 36%), headache (13% to 32%, placebo 23%), ataxia (5% to 31%), fatigue (12% to 15%), vertigo (6% to 15%)
  Gastrointestinal: Vomiting (7% to 36%), nausea (15% to 29%), abdominal pain (10% to 13%)
  Neuromuscular & skeletal: Abnormal gait (5% to 17%), tremor (3% to 16%)
  Ocular: Diplopia (14% to 40%), nystagmus (7% to 26%), abnormal vision (4% to 14%)

1% to 10%:
  Cardiovascular: Hypotension (1% to 2%), leg edema (1% to 2%, placebo 1%)
  Central nervous system: Nervousness (2% to 5%, placebo 1% to 2%), amnesia (4%), abnormal thinking (2% to 4%), insomnia (2% to 4%), speech disorder (1% to 3%), EEG abnormalities (2%), abnormal feelings (1% to 2%), agitation (1% to 2%, placebo 1%), confusion (1% to 2%, placebo 1%)
  Dermatologic: Rash (4%), acne (1% to 2%)
  Endocrine & metabolic: Hyponatremia (1% to 3%, placebo 1%)
  Gastrointestinal: Diarrhea (5% to 7%), dyspepsia (5% to 6%), constipation (2% to 6%, placebo 0% to 4%), gastritis (1% to 2%, placebo 1%), weight gain (1% to 2%, placebo 1%)
  Neuromuscular & skeletal: Weakness (3% to 6%, placebo 5%), back pain (4%), falling down (4%), abnormal coordination (1% to 4%, placebo 1% to 2%), dysmetria (1% to 3%), sprains/strains (2%), muscle weakness (1% to 2%)
  Ocular: Abnormal accommodation (2%)
  Respiratory: Upper respiratory tract infection (7%), rhinitis (2% to 5%, placebo 4%), chest infection (4%), epistaxis (4%), sinusitis (4%)

Overdosage/Toxicology Symptoms may include CNS depression (somnolence, ataxia). Treatment is symptomatic and supportive.

Drug Interactions Inhibits CYP2C19 (weak); **Induces** CYP3A4 (strong)
  Carbamazepine: Oxcarbazepine serum concentrations may be reduced by a mean 40%.
  CYP3A4 substrates: Oxcarbazepine may decrease the levels/effects of CYP3A4 substrates. Example substrates include benzodiazepines, calcium channel blockers, clarithromycin, cyclosporine, erythromycin, estrogens, mirtazapine, nateglinide, nefazodone, nevirapine, protease inhibitors, tacrolimus, and venlafaxine.
  Felodipine: Metabolism is increased due to enzyme induction; similar effects may be anticipated with other dihydropyridine calcium channel blockers.
  Hormonal contraceptives: Metabolism may be increased due to enzyme induction; use alternative contraceptive measures; oxcarbazepine with oral contraceptives has been shown to decrease plasma concentrations of the two hormonal components, ethinyl estradiol (48% and 52%) and levonorgestrel (32% and 52%).
  Phenobarbital: Phenobarbital levels are increased (average of 14%); oxcarbazepine levels are decreased (average of 25%).
  Phenytoin: Phenytoin levels may be increased (high dosages) by an average of 40%; oxcarbazepine levels may be decreased (by an average of 30%) during concurrent therapy; monitor phenytoin levels.
  Valproic acid decreases oxcarbazepine levels by an average of 18%.
  Verapamil's metabolism may be increased due to enzyme induction; verapamil may reduce blood levels of oxcarbazepine's active metabolite (MHD).

Ethanol/Nutrition/Herb Interactions
  Ethanol: Avoid ethanol (may increase CNS depression).
  (Continued)

Oxcarbazepine *(Continued)*

Herb/Nutraceutical: St John's wort may decrease oxcarbazepine levels. Avoid evening primrose (seizure threshold decreased). Avoid valerian, St John's wort, kava kava, gotu kola.

Stability Store tablets and suspension at 25°C (77°F). Use suspension within 7 weeks of first opening container.

Mechanism of Action Pharmacological activity results from both oxcarbazepine and its monohydroxy metabolite (MHD). Precise mechanism of anticonvulsant effect has not been defined. Oxcarbazepine and MHD block voltage-sensitive sodium channels, stabilizing hyperexcited neuronal membranes, inhibiting repetitive firing, and decreasing the propagation of synaptic impulses. These actions are believed to prevent the spread of seizures. Oxcarbazepine and MHD also increase potassium conductance and modulate the activity of high-voltage activated calcium channels.

Pharmacokinetics

Absorption: Completely absorbed and extensively metabolized to its pharmacologically active 10-monohydroxy metabolite (MHD); food has no effect on rate or extent

Distribution: MHD: V_d: 49 L

Protein binding: 40% of MHD is bound to serum proteins

Metabolism: Hepatic to 10-monohydroxy metabolite (MHD; active); MHD is further conjugated to DHD (inactive)

Bioavailability: Increased in older adults >60 years of age

Half-life elimination: Parent drug: 2 hours; MHD: 9 hours; renal impairment (Cl_{cr} 30 mL/minute): MHD: 19 hours

Elimination: Urine (95%: <1% as unchanged oxcarbazepine, 27% as unchanged MHD, 49% as MHD glucuronides); feces (<4%)

Dosage

Geriatrics & Adults:

Adjunctive therapy, partial seizures (epilepsy): Oral: Initial: 300 mg twice daily; dosage may be increased by 600 mg/day at approximate weekly intervals. Recommended daily dose is 1200 mg/day in 2 divided doses. Although daily doses >1200 mg/day demonstrated greater efficacy, most patients were unable to tolerate 2400 mg/day (due to CNS effects).

Conversion to monotherapy, partial seizures (epilepsy): Oral: Patients receiving concomitant antiepileptic drugs (AEDs): Initial: 300 mg twice daily while simultaneously reducing the dose of concomitant AEDs. Withdraw concomitant AEDs completely over 3-6 weeks, while increasing the oxcarbazine dose in increments of 600 mg/day at weekly intervals, reaching the maximum oxcarbazine dose (2400 mg/day) in about 2-4 weeks (lower doses have been effective in patients in whom monotherapy has been initiated).

Initiation of monotherapy, partial seizures (epilepsy): Oral: Patients not receiving prior AEDs: 300 mg twice daily (total dose 600 mg/day). Increase dose by 300 mg/day every third day to a dose of 1200 mg/day. Higher dosages (2400 mg/day) have been shown to be effective in patients converted to monotherapy from other AEDs.

Renal Impairment: Cl_{cr} <30 mL/minute: Therapy should be initiated at one-half the usual starting dose (300 mg/day in adults) and increased slowly to achieve the desired clinical response

Hepatic Impairment: No dosage adjustment recommended in mild-to-moderate hepatic impairment. Patients with severe hepatic impairment have not been evaluated.

Administration Suspension: Prior to using for the first time, firmly insert the plastic adapter provided with the bottle. Cover adapter with child-resistant cap when not in use. Shake bottle for at least 10 seconds, remove child-resistant cap and insert the oral dosing syringe provided to withdraw appropriate dose. Dose may be taken directly from oral syringe or may be mixed in a small glass of water immediately prior to swallowing. Rinse syringe with warm water after use and allow to dry thoroughly. Discard any unused portion after 7 weeks of first opening bottle.

Monitoring Parameters Seizure frequency, serum sodium (particularly during first 3 months of therapy), symptoms of CNS depression (dizziness, headache, somnolence). Additional serum sodium monitoring is recommended during maintenance treatment in patients receiving other medications known to decrease sodium levels, in patients with signs/symptoms of hyponatremia, and in patients with an increase in seizure frequency or severity.

Test Interactions Thyroid function tests may depress serum T_4 without affecting T_3 levels or TSH.

Patient Information Inform prescriber if you are allergic to carbamazepine. May be taken without regard to food. Take with food if medicine causes stomach upset. Avoid alcohol or other drugs which may cause sedation. Do not drive or operate heavy machinery until you see how this medication affects you. Report symptoms of excessive somnolence or allergic reaction to your healthcare provider. Report symptoms of nausea, malaise, headache, lethargy or confusion to your healthcare provider; blood levels of sodium may need to be checked. Do not stop medicine without healthcare provider's instruction; may cause an increase in seizures.

Special Geriatric Considerations Studies in elderly volunteers (60-82 years of age) with both single dose (300 mg) and multiple doses (600 mg/day) reported maximum plasma concentrations and AUC as being 30% to 60% higher than younger volunteers (18-32 years of age). These results were due to differences in creatinine clearance between the two groups. Since elderly may have Cl_{cr} <30 mL/minute, dose reductions may be needed.

Dosage Forms Excipient information presented when available (limited, particularly for generics); consult specific product labeling.

Suspension, oral: 300 mg/5 mL (250 mL) [contains ethanol; packaged with oral syringe]

Tablet: 150 mg, 300 mg, 600 mg

Selected References

Carrazana E and Mikoshiba I, "Rationale and Evidence for the Use of Oxcarbazepine in Neuropathic Pain," *J Pain Symptom Manage*, 2003, 25(5 Suppl):31-5. Suppl):S31-5.

Irving GA, "Contemporary Assessment and Management of Neuropathic Pain," *Neurology*, 2005, 28;64(12 Suppl 3):21-7.

♦ **Oxilapine Succinate** *see* Loxapine *on page 939*

♦ **Oxpentifylline** *see* Pentoxifylline *on page 1230*

♦ **Oxy Balance® [OTC]** *see* Salicylic Acid *on page 1441*

♦ **Oxy Balance® Deep Pore [OTC]** *see* Salicylic Acid *on page 1441*

Oxybutynin (oks i BYOO ti nin)

Related Information

Pharmacotherapy of Urinary Incontinence *on page 1822*
Potentially Inappropriate Medications for Geriatrics *on page 1824*

Medication Safety Issues

Sound-alike/look-alike issues:

Oxybutynin may be confused with OxyContin®
Ditropan® may be confused with Detrol®, diazepam, Diprivan®, dithranol

Transdermal patch may contain conducting metal (eg, aluminum); remove patch prior to MRI.

U.S. Brand Names Ditropan®; Ditropan® XL; Oxytrol®

Canadian Brand Names Apo-Oxybutynin®; Ditropan®; Ditropan® XL; Gen-Oxybutynin; Novo-Oxybutynin; Nu-Oxybutyn; Oxytrol®; PMS-Oxybutynin; Uromax®

Index Terms Oxybutynin Chloride

Generic Available Yes: Excludes transdermal patch

Pharmacologic Category Antispasmodic Agent, Urinary

Use Antispasmodic for bladder (urgency, frequency, urge incontinence) and uninhibited bladder

Contraindications Hypersensitivity to oxybutynin or any component of the formulation; untreated glaucoma; partial or complete GI obstruction; GU obstruction; urinary retention; megacolon; toxic megacolon

Warnings/Precautions Use with caution in patients with urinary tract obstruction, angle-closure glaucoma (treated), hyperthyroidism, reflux esophagitis (including concurrent therapy with oral bisphosphonates or drugs which may increase the risk of esophagitis), heart disease, hepatic or renal disease, prostatic hyperplasia, autonomic neuropathy, ulcerative colitis (may cause ileus and toxic megacolon), hypertension, hiatal hernia, myasthenia gravis, ulcerative colitis, or intestinal atony. Caution should be used in elderly due to anticholinergic activity (eg, confusion, constipation, blurred vision, and tachycardia). May increase the risk of heat prostration.

The extended release formulation consists of drug within a nondeformable matrix; following drug release/absorption, the matrix/shell is expelled in the stool. The use of nondeformable products in patients with known stricture/narrowing of the GI tract has been associated with symptoms of obstruction. Transdermal patch may contain conducting metal (eg, aluminum); remove patch prior to MRI.

Adverse Reactions (Reflective of adult population; not specific for elderly)

Oral:

>10%:

Central nervous system: Dizziness (6% to 16%), somnolence (12% to 13%)
Gastrointestinal: Xerostomia (61% to 71%), constipation (13%)
Genitourinary: Urination impaired (11%)

1% to 10%:

Cardiovascular: Palpitation (2% to <5%), peripheral edema (2% to <5%), hypertension (2% to <5%), vasodilation (2% to <5%)
Central nervous system: Headache (6% to 10%), pain (7%), confusion (2% to <5%), insomnia (2% to <5%), nervousness (2% to <5%)
Dermatologic: Dry skin (2% to <5%), skin rash (2% to <5%)

(Continued)

Oxybutynin *(Continued)*

Gastrointestinal: Nausea (9% to 10%), dyspepsia (7%), abdominal pain (2% to 6%), diarrhea (5% to 9%), flatulence (2% to <5%), gastrointestinal reflux (2% to <5%), taste perversion (2% to <5%)

Genitourinary: Postvoid residuals increased (2% to 9%), urinary tract infection (5%)

Neuromuscular & skeletal: Weakness (2% to 7%)

Ocular: Blurred vision (8% to 9%), dry eyes (2% to 6%)

Respiratory: Rhinitis (6%), dry nasal and sinus membranes (2% to <5%)

Transdermal:

>10%: Local: Application site reaction (17%), pruritus (14%)

1% to 10%:

Gastrointestinal: Xerostomia (4% to 10%), diarrhea (3%), constipation (3%)

Genitourinary: Dysuria (2%)

Local: Erythema (6% to 8%), vesicles (3%), rash (3%)

Ocular: Vision changes (3%)

Overdosage/Toxicology Symptoms include hypotension, circulatory failure, psychotic behavior, flushing, respiratory failure, paralysis, tremor, irritability, seizures, delirium, hallucinations, and coma. Treatment is symptomatic and supportive. Induce emesis or perform gastric lavage followed by charcoal and a cathartic. Physostigmine may be required. Treat hyperpyrexia with cooling techniques (ice bags, cold applications, alcohol sponges).

Drug Interactions Substrate of CYP3A4 (minor); **Inhibits** CYP2C8 (weak), 2D6 (weak), 3A4 (weak)

Anticholinergic agents: Additive anticholinergic effects may occur with concurrent antihistamines and anticholinergic agents.

CNS depressants: Additive sedation with CNS depressants and ethanol.

Ethanol/Nutrition/Herb Interactions Ethanol: Use ethanol with caution (may increase CNS depression and toxicity). Watch for sedation.

Stability Store at controlled room temperature. Protect syrup from light. Keep transdermal patch in sealed pouch.

Mechanism of Action Direct antispasmodic effect on smooth muscle, also inhibits the action of acetylcholine on smooth muscle (exhibits $1/5$ the anticholinergic activity of atropine, but is 4-10 times the antispasmodic activity); does not block effects at skeletal muscle or at autonomic ganglia; increases bladder capacity, decreases uninhibited contractions, and delays desire to void, therefore, decreases urgency and frequency

Pharmacodynamics

Onset of action: Oral: 30-60 minutes

Peak effect: 3-6 hours

Duration: 6-10 hours (up to 24 hours for extended release oral formulation)

Pharmacokinetics

Absorption: Oral: Rapid and well absorbed; Transdermal: High

Distribution: V_d: 193 L

Metabolism: Hepatic via CYP3A4; Oral: High first-pass metabolism (not with I.V. or transdermal use). Forms active and inactive metabolites

Half-life: I.V.: ~2 hours (parent drug), 7-8 hours (metabolites)

Time to peak, serum: Oral: ~60 minutes; Transdermal: 24-48 hours

Excretion: Urine, as metabolites (<0.1% as unchanged drug)

Dosage

Geriatrics:

Oral: 2.5-5 mg 2-3 times/day

Transdermal: Refer to adult dosing. **Note:** Should be discontinued periodically to determine whether the patient can manage without the drug and to minimize resistance to the drug.

Adults:

Bladder spasms:

Oral:

Regular release: 5 mg 2-3 times/day up to maximum of 5 mg 4 times/day

Extended release: Initial: 5-10 mg once daily, may increase in 5-10 mg increments; maximum: 30 mg daily

Transdermal: Apply one 3.9 mg/day patch twice weekly (every 3-4 days)

Note: Should be discontinued periodically to determine whether the patient can manage without the drug and to minimize resistance to the drug.

Administration

Oral: Immediate release tablets and solution should be administered on an empty stomach with water. Extended release tablets may be taken with or without food and must be swallowed whole; do not crush, divide, or chew.

Transdermal: Apply to clean, dry skin on abdomen, hip, or buttock. Select a new site for each new system (avoid reapplication to same site within 7 days).

Monitoring Parameters Monitor incontinence episodes, postvoid residual (PVR)

Test Interactions May suppress the wheal and flare reactions to skin test antigens.

Patient Information Take prescribed oral dose preferably on an empty stomach, 1 hour before or 2 hours after meals. Swallow extended-release tablets whole, do not chew or crush. You may experience dizziness, lightheadedness, or drowsiness (use caution when driving or engaging in tasks requiring alertness until response to drug is known); dry mouth or changes in appetite (small, frequent meals, frequent mouth care, sucking lozenges, or chewing gum may help); constipation (increased exercise, fluids, fruit, fiber, or stool softener may help); decreased sexual ability (reversible with discontinuance of drug); or decreased sweating (use caution in hot weather, avoid extreme exercise or activity). Report rapid heartbeat, palpitations, or chest pain; difficulty voiding; or vision changes.

Special Geriatric Considerations Caution should be used in the elderly due to anticholinergic activity (eg, confusion, constipation, blurred vision, and tachycardia). Start with lower doses. Transdermal dosage form may have less potential for these effects. Oxybutynin may cause memory problems in the elderly. A study of 12 healthy volunteers with an average age of 69 showed cognitive decline while taking the drug (*J Am Geriatr Soc*, 1998, L46:8-13). Studies using transdermal dosage form did not reveal any differences in safety or efficacy between elderly and younger adults.

Dosage Forms Excipient information presented when available (limited, particularly for generics); consult specific product labeling.

Syrup, as chloride: 5 mg/5 mL (473 mL)
  Ditropan®: 5 mg/5 mL (473 mL)
Tablet, as chloride: 5 mg
  Ditropan®: 5 mg
Tablet, extended release, as chloride: 5 mg, 10 mg, 15 mg
  Ditropan® XL: 5 mg, 10 mg, 15 mg
Transdermal system:
  Oxytrol®: 3.9 mg/day (8s) [39 cm^2; total oxybutynin 36 mg]

♦ **Oxybutynin Chloride** *see* Oxybutynin *on page 1177*

Oxycodone (oks i KOE done)

Related Information
  Narcotic / Opioid Analgesics *on page 1763*
Medication Safety Issues
  Sound-alike/look-alike issues:
    Oxycodone may be confused with OxyContin®, oxymorphone
    OxyContin® may be confused with oxybutynin
    OxyFast® may be confused with Roxanol™
U.S. Brand Names ETH-Oxydose™; OxyContin®; OxyFast®; OxyIR®; Roxicodone®
Canadian Brand Names OxyContin®; Oxy.IR®; Supeudol®
Index Terms Dihydrohydroxycodeinone; Oxycodone Hydrochloride
Generic Available Yes
Pharmacologic Category Analgesic, Opioid
Use Management of moderate-to-severe pain, normally used in combination with nonopioid analgesics

  OxyContin® is indicated for around-the-clock management of moderate-to-severe pain when an analgesic is needed for an extended period of time.
Restrictions C-II
Contraindications Hypersensitivity to oxycodone or any component of the formulation; significant respiratory depression; hypercarbia; acute or severe bronchial asthma; OxyContin® is also contraindicated in paralytic ileus (known or suspected)
Warnings/Precautions May cause CNS depression, which may impair physical or mental abilities; patients must be cautioned about performing tasks which require mental alertness (eg, operating machinery or driving). Effects may be potentiated when used with other sedative drugs or ethanol. Use with caution in patients with hypersensitivity reactions to other phenanthrene-derivative opioid agonists (morphine, hydrocodone, hydromorphone, levorphanol, oxymorphone), respiratory diseases including asthma, emphysema, or COPD. Use with caution in pancreatitis or biliary tract disease, acute alcoholism (including delirium tremens), morbid obesity, adrenocortical insufficiency, history of seizure disorders, CNS depression/coma, kyphoscoliosis (or other skeletal disorder which may alter respiratory function), hypothyroidism (including myxedema), prostatic hyperplasia, urethral stricture, and toxic psychosis. May obscure diagnosis or clinical course of patients with acute abdominal conditions.

Use with caution in the elderly, debilitated, severe hepatic or renal function. Hemodynamic effects (hypotension, orthostasis) may be exaggerated in patients with hypovolemia, concurrent vasodilating drugs, or in patients with head injury. Respiratory depressant effects and capacity to elevate CSF pressure may be exaggerated in presence of head injury, other intracranial lesion, or pre-existing intracranial pressure. (Continued)

Oxycodone *(Continued)*

Concurrent use of agonist/antagonist analgesics may precipitate withdrawal symptoms and/or reduced analgesic efficacy in patients following prolonged therapy with mu opioid agonists. Abrupt discontinuation following prolonged use may also lead to withdrawal symptoms.

[U.S. Boxed Warning]: Healthcare provider should be alert to problems of abuse, misuse, and diversion. Tolerance or drug dependence may result from extended use.

Controlled-release formulations:

[U.S. Boxed Warning]: OxyContin® is not intended for use as an "as needed" analgesic or for immediately-postoperative pain management (should be used postoperatively only if the patient has received it prior to surgery or if severe, persistent pain is anticipated). **[U.S. Boxed Warning]: Do NOT crush, break, or chew controlled-release tablets;** 60 mg, 80 mg, and 160 mg strengths are for use only in opioid-tolerant patients.

Adverse Reactions (Reflective of adult population; not specific for elderly)
>10%:
Central nervous system: Somnolence (23% to 24%), dizziness (13% to 16%)
Dermatologic: Pruritus (12% to 13%)
Gastrointestinal: Nausea (23% to 27%), constipation (23% to 26%), vomiting (12% to 14%)
1% to 10%:
Cardiovascular: Postural hypotension (1% to 5%)
Central nervous system: Headache (7% to 8%), abnormal dreams (1% to 5%), anxiety (1% to 5%), chills (1% to 5%), confusion (1% to 5%), euphoria (1% to 5%), fever (1% to 5%), insomnia (1% to 5%), nervousness (1% to 5%), thought abnormalities (1% to 5%)
Dermatologic: Rash (1% to 5%)
Gastrointestinal: Xerostomia (6% to 7%), abdominal pain (1% to 5%), anorexia (1% to 5%), diarrhea (1% to 5%), dyspepsia (1% to 5%), gastritis (1% to 5%)
Neuromuscular & skeletal: Weakness (6% to 7%), twitching (1% to 5%)
Respiratory: Dyspnea (1% to 5%), hiccups (1% to 5%)
Miscellaneous: Diaphoresis (5% to 6%)

Overdosage/Toxicology Symptoms of toxicity include CNS depression, respiratory depression, and miosis. Treatment is symptom-directed and supportive. Naloxone can reverse opioid-induced hypotension and respiratory depression. An initial I.V. dose of 0.2-0.4 mg can be administered. Lower initial doses should be considered in opioid-dependent patients or if suspected concurrent stimulant overdose. If no response in 2-3 minutes after initial dose, consider an additional 1-2 mg evey 2-3 minutes up to a total dose of 10 mg. There is no role for dialysis or hemoperfusion.

Drug Interactions Substrate (minor) of CYP2D6, 3A
Ammonium chloride: May increase the excretion of analgesics (opioid).
Antipsychotic agents (phenothiazines): May enhance the hypotensive effect of analgesics (opioid).
CNS depressants: May enhance the adverse/toxic effect of analgesics (opioids).
Pegvisomant: Analgesics (opioid) may diminish the therapeutic effect of pegvisomant.
Selective serotonin reuptake inhibitors (SSRIs): Analgesics (opioid) may enhance the serotonergic effect of selective serotonin reuptake inhibitors. This may cause serotonin syndrome.

Ethanol/Nutrition/Herb Interactions
Ethanol: Avoid ethanol (may increase CNS depression).
Food: When taken with a high-fat meal, peak concentration is 25% greater following a single OxyContin® 160 mg tablet as compared to two 80 mg tablets.
Herb/Nutraceutical: Avoid valerian, St John's wort, kava kava, gotu kola (may increase CNS depression).

Stability Store at 15°C to 30°C (59°F to 86°F). Protect from light.

Mechanism of Action Binds to opiate receptors in the CNS, causing inhibition of ascending pain pathways, altering the perception of and response to pain; produces generalized CNS depression

Pharmacodynamics
Onset of action: Oral: Pain relief occurs within 10-15 minutes
Peak effect: 30-60 minutes
Duration: 4-5 hours (immediate release), 12 hours (sustained release); enhanced analgesia has been seen in older adult patients on therapeutic doses of narcotics; duration of action may be increased in older adults

Pharmacokinetics
Distribution: V$_d$: 2.6 L/kg; distributed to skeletal muscle, liver, intestinal tract, lungs, spleen, and brain
Protein binding: ~45%

Metabolism: Hepatically via CYP2D6 to various metabolites including noroxycodone (weak analgesic activity), oxymorphone (has analgesic activity; low concentrations in plasma) and their glucuronides

Bioavailability: Controlled release, immediate release: 60% to 87%

Half-life elimination: Immediate release: 2-3 hours; controlled release: ~5 hours

Excretion: Urine (~19% as parent; > 64% as metabolites)

Dosage

Geriatrics & Adults: Management of pain: Oral:

Regular or immediate release formulations: 2.5-5 mg every 6 hours as needed

Controlled release:

Opioid naive: 10 mg every 12 hours

Concurrent CNS depressants: Reduce usual dose by $\frac{1}{3}$ to $\frac{1}{2}$

Conversion from transdermal fentanyl: For each 25 mcg/hour transdermal dose, substitute 10 mg controlled release oxycodone every 12 hours; should be initiated 18 hours after the removal of the transdermal fentanyl patch

Currently on opioids: Use standard conversion chart to convert daily dose to oxycodone equivalent. Divide daily dose in 2 (for twice-daily dosing, usually every 12 hours) and round down to nearest dosage form.

Note: 60 mg, 80 mg, or 160 mg tablets are for use **only** in opioid-tolerant patients. Special safety considerations must be addressed when converting to OxyContin® doses ≥160 mg every 12 hours. Dietary caution must be taken when patients are initially titrated to 160 mg tablets. Using different strengths to obtain the same daily dose is equivalent (eg, four 40 mg tablets, two 80 mg tablets, one 160 mg tablet); all produce similar blood levels.

Multiplication factors for converting the daily dose of current oral opioid to the daily dose of oral oxycodone:

Current opioid mg/day dose x factor = Oxycodone mg/day dose

Codeine mg/day oral dose **x** 0.15 = Oxycodone mg/day dose

Hydrocodone mg/day oral dose **x** 0.9 = Oxycodone mg/day dose

Hydromorphone mg/day oral dose **x** 4 = Oxycodone mg/day dose

Levorphanol mg/day oral dose **x** 7.5 = Oxycodone mg/day dose

Meperidine mg/day oral dose **x** 0.1 = Oxycodone mg/day dose

Methadone mg/day oral dose **x** 1.5 = Oxycodone mg/day dose

Morphine mg/day oral dose **x** 0.5 = Oxycodone mg/day dose

Note: Divide the oxycodone mg/day dose into the appropriate dosing interval for the specific form being used.

Hepatic Impairment: Reduce dosage in patients with severe liver disease.

Administration Do not crush, break, or chew controlled-release tablets; 60 mg, 80 mg, and 160 mg tablets are for use **only** in opioid-tolerant patients. Do not administer OxyContin® 160 mg tablet with a high-fat meal. Controlled release tablets are not indicated for rectal administration; increased risk of adverse events due to better rectal absorption.

Monitoring Parameters Pain relief, respiratory and mental status, blood pressure

Test Interactions Some quinolones may produce a false-positive urine screening result for opiates using commercially-available immunoassay kits. This has been demonstrated most consistently for levofloxacin and ofloxacin, but other quinolones have shown cross-reactivity in certain assay kits. Confirmation of positive opiate screens by more specific methods should be considered.

Patient Information If self-administered, use exactly as directed; do not increase dose or frequency. Drug may cause physical and/or psychological dependence. Do not crush or chew controlled-release tablets. While using this medication, do not use alcohol and other prescription or OTC medications (especially sedatives, tranquilizers, antihistamines, or pain medications) without consulting prescriber. Maintain adequate hydration (2-3 L/day of fluids) unless instructed to restrict fluid intake. May cause hypotension, dizziness, drowsiness, impaired coordination, or blurred vision (use caution when driving, climbing stairs, or changing position - rising from sitting or lying to standing, or when engaging in tasks requiring alertness until response to drug is known); nausea, vomiting, or dry mouth (frequent mouth care, small frequent meals, chewing gum, or sucking lozenges may help); or constipation (increased exercise, fluids, fruit, or fiber may help; if unresolved, consult prescriber about use of stool softeners). The wax matrix from OxyContin® tablets may appear in stool. Report persistent dizziness or headache; excessive fatigue or sedation; changes in mental status; changes in urinary elimination or pain on urination; weakness or trembling; blurred vision; or shortness of breath.

Special Geriatric Considerations The elderly may be particularly susceptible to the CNS depressant and constipating effects of narcotics. Prophylactic use of a laxative should be considered. Serum levels at a given dose may also be increased relative to concentrations in younger patients.

Dosage Forms Excipient information presented when available (limited, particularly for generics); consult specific product labeling.

Capsule, as hydrochloride: 5 mg

(Continued)

Oxycodone *(Continued)*

OxyIR®: 5 mg

Solution, oral, as hydrochloride: 5 mg/5 mL (500 mL)

    Roxicodone®: 5 mg/5 mL (5 mL, 500 mL) [contains alcohol]

Solution, oral, as hydrochloride [concentrate]: 20 mg/mL (30 mL)

    ETH-Oxydose™: 20 mg/mL (1 mL, 30 mL) [contains sodium benzoate; berry flavor]

    OxyFast®: 20 mg/mL (30 mL) [contains sodium benzoate and dry natural rubber]

    Roxicodone®: 20 mg/mL (30 mL) [contains sodium benzoate]

Tablet, as hydrochloride: 5 mg, 15 mg, 30 mg

    Roxicodone®: 5 mg, 15 mg, 30 mg

Tablet, controlled release, as hydrochloride:

    OxyContin®: 10 mg, 20 mg, 40 mg, 60 mg, 80 mg, 160 mg

Tablet, extended release, as hydrochloride: 10 mg, 20 mg, 40 mg, 80 mg

Selected References

AGS Panel on Persistent Pain in Older Persons, "The Management of Persistent Pain in Older Persons," *J Am Geriatr Soc*, 2002, 50(6 Suppl):S205-24.

Oxycodone and Acetaminophen

(oks i KOE done & a seet a MIN oh fen)

Related Information

Acetaminophen *on page 29*

Narcotic / Opioid Analgesics *on page 1763*

Oxycodone *on page 1179*

Medication Safety Issues

Sound-alike/look-alike issues:

Percocet® may be confused with Percodan®

Roxicet™ may be confused with Roxanol™

Tylox® may be confused with Trimox®, Tylenol®, Wymox®, Xanax®

Duplicate therapy issues: This product contains acetaminophen, which may be a component of other combination products. Do not exceed the maximum recommended daily dose of acetaminophen.

U.S. Brand Names Endocet®; Magnacet™; Percocet®; Roxicet™; Roxicet™ 5/500; Tylox®

Canadian Brand Names Endocet®; Oxycocet®; Percocet®; Percocet®-Demi; PMS-Oxycodone-Acetaminophen

Index Terms Acetaminophen and Oxycodone

Generic Available Yes: Excludes caplet and solution

Pharmacologic Category Analgesic, Opioid

Use Management of moderate to severe pain

Restrictions C-II

Contraindications Hypersensitivity to oxycodone, acetaminophen, or any component of the formulation; severe respiratory depression (in absence of resuscitative equipment or ventilatory support)

Warnings/Precautions Use with caution in patients with hypersensitivity reactions to other phenanthrene-derivative opioid agonists (morphine, codeine, hydrocodone, hydromorphone, levorphanol, oxymorphone); respiratory diseases including asthma, emphysema, COPD; severe liver or renal insufficiency; hypothyroidism; Addison's disease; seizure disorder; toxic psychosis; morbid obesity; CNS depression/coma; biliary tract impairment; prostatic hyperplasia; or urethral stricture. May obscure diagnosis or clinical course of patients with acute abdominal conditions. Some preparations contain sulfites which may cause allergic reactions. May be habit-forming. Causes sedation; caution must be used in performing tasks which require alertness (eg, operating machinery or driving). Effects may be potentiated when used with other sedative drugs or ethanol. May cause hypotension. Concurrent use of agonist/antagonist analgesics may precipitate withdrawal symptoms and/or reduced analgesic efficacy in patients following prolonged therapy with mu opioid agonists. Abrupt discontinuation following prolonged use may also lead to withdrawal symptoms.

Use with caution in patients with head injury and increased intracranial pressure (respiratory depressant effects increased and may also elevate CSF pressure).

Enhanced analgesia has been seen in elderly and debilitated patients on therapeutic doses of narcotics. Duration of action may be increased in the elderly. The elderly may be particularly susceptible to the CNS depressant and constipating effects of narcotics.

May cause severe hepatic toxicity on acute overdose; in addition, chronic daily dosing in adults has resulted in liver damage in some patients. Use with caution in patients with alcoholic liver disease; consuming ≥3 alcoholic drinks/day may increase the risk of liver damage. Use with caution in patients with known G6PD deficiency. Limit acetaminophen dose to <4 g/day.

Adverse Reactions (Reflective of adult population; not specific for elderly)
Frequency not defined (also see individual agents): Allergic reaction, constipation, dizziness, dysphoria, euphoria, lightheadedness, nausea, pruritus, respiratory depression, sedation, skin rash, vomiting

Drug Interactions Also see individual agents.
Oxycodone: **Substrate** (minor) of CYP2D6, 3A
Acetaminophen: **Substrate** (minor) of CYP1A2, 2A6, 2C9, 2D6, 2E1, 3A4
Anesthetics, general: May have additive CNS depression; consider lowering dose of one or both agents.
Anticholinergics: Concomitant use may lead to paralytic ileus.
CNS depressants: May have additive CNS depression; consider lowering dose of one or both agents.
Phenothiazines: May have additive CNS depression with phenothiazine and other tranquilizers; consider lowering dose of one or both agents.
Sedative hypnotics: May have additive CNS depression; consider lowering dose of one or both agents.

Ethanol/Nutrition/Herb Interactions Ethanol: May have additive CNS depression. In addition, excessive intake of ethanol may increase the risk of acetaminophen-induced hepatotoxicity. Avoid ethanol or limit to <3 drinks/day.

Stability Store at controlled room temperature of 20°C to 25°C (68°F to 77°F). Protect from moisture.

Mechanism of Action
Oxycodone, as with other narcotic (opiate) analgesics, blocks pain perception in the cerebral cortex by binding to specific receptor molecules (opiate receptors) within the neuronal membranes of synapses. This binding results in a decreased synaptic chemical transmission throughout the CNS thus inhibiting the flow of pain sensations into the higher centers. Mu and kappa are the two subtypes of the opiate receptor to which oxycodone binds to cause analgesia.
Acetaminophen inhibits the synthesis of prostaglandins in the CNS and peripherally blocks pain impulse generation; produces antipyresis from inhibition of hypothalamic heat-regulating center.

Dosage
Geriatrics: Doses should be titrated to appropriate analgesic effects: Oral: Initial dose, **based on oxycodone content:** 2.5-5 mg every 6 hours. Do not exceed 4 g/day of acetaminophen.
Adults:
  Note: Initial dose is based on the **oxycodone** content; however, the maximum daily dose is based on the **acetaminophen** content.
  Management of pain: Doses should be given every 4-6 hours as needed and titrated to appropriate analgesic effects.

  Maximum daily dose, based on acetaminophen content: Oral: 4 g/day.
  Mild-to-moderate pain: Oral: Initial dose, **based on oxycodone content:** 2.5-5 mg
  Severe pain: Oral: Initial dose, **based on oxycodone content:** 10-30 mg
Hepatic Impairment: Dose should be reduced in patients with severe liver disease.

Monitoring Parameters Pain relief, respiratory and mental status, blood pressure

Patient Information May cause drowsiness, avoid alcoholic beverages; do not exceed recommended dose

Special Geriatric Considerations Enhanced analgesia has been seen in elderly patients on therapeutic doses of narcotics; duration of action may be increased in the elderly. Elderly may be particularly susceptible to the CNS depressant and constipating effects of narcotics. If 1 tablet/dose is used, it may be useful to add an additional 325 mg of acetaminophen to maximize analgesic effect.

Dosage Forms Excipient information presented when available (limited, particularly for generics); consult specific product labeling.
Caplet:
  Roxicet™ 5/500: Oxycodone hydrochloride 5 mg and acetaminophen 500 mg
Capsule: 5/500: Oxycodone hydrochloride 5 mg and acetaminophen 500 mg
  Tylox® 5/500: Oxycodone hydrochloride 5 mg and acetaminophen 500 mg [contains sodium benzoate and sodium metabisulfite]
Solution, oral:
  Roxicet™: Oxycodone hydrochloride 5 mg and acetaminophen 325 mg per 5 mL (5 mL, 500 mL) [contains alcohol <0.5%]
Tablet: 5/325: Oxycodone hydrochloride 5 mg and acetaminophen 325 mg; 7.5/325: Oxycodone hydrochloride 7.5 mg and acetaminophen 325 mg; 7.5/500: Oxycodone hydrochloride 7.5 mg and acetaminophen 500 mg; 10/325: Oxycodone hydrochloride 10 mg and acetaminophen 325 mg; 10/650: Oxycodone hydrochloride 10 mg and acetaminophen 650 mg
  Endocet® 5/325 [scored]: Oxycodone hydrochloride 5 mg and acetaminophen 325 mg
  Endocet® 7.5/325: Oxycodone hydrochloride 7.5 mg and acetaminophen 325 mg
  Endocet® 7.5/500: Oxycodone hydrochloride 7.5 mg and acetaminophen 500 mg
(Continued)

Oxycodone and Acetaminophen *(Continued)*

Endocet® 10/325: Oxycodone hydrochloride 10 mg and acetaminophen 325 mg
Endocet® 10/650: Oxycodone hydrochloride 10 mg and acetaminophen 650 mg
Magnacet™ 2.5/400: Oxycodone hydrochloride 2.5 mg and acetaminophen 400 mg
Magnacet™ 5/400: Oxycodone hydrochloride 5 mg and acetaminophen 400 mg
Magnacet™ 7.5/400: Oxycodone hydrochloride 7.5 mg and acetaminophen 400 mg
Magnacet™ 10/400: Oxycodone hydrochloride 10 mg and acetaminophen 400 mg
Percocet® 2.5/325: Oxycodone hydrochloride 2.5 mg and acetaminophen 325 mg
Percocet® 5/325 [scored]: Oxycodone hydrochloride 5 mg and acetaminophen 325 mg
Percocet® 7.5/325: Oxycodone hydrochloride 7.5 mg and acetaminophen 325 mg
Percocet® 7.5/500: Oxycodone hydrochloride 7.5 mg and acetaminophen 500 mg
Percocet® 10/325: Oxycodone hydrochloride 10 mg and acetaminophen 325 mg
Percocet® 10/650: Oxycodone hydrochloride 10 mg and acetaminophen 650 mg
Roxicet™ [scored]: Oxycodone hydrochloride 5 mg and acetaminophen 325 mg

Selected References
AGS Panel on Persistent Pain in Older Persons, "The Management of Persistent Pain in Older Persons," *J Am Geriatr Soc*, 2002, 50(6 Suppl):S205-24.

Oxycodone and Aspirin (oks i KOE done & AS pir in)

Related Information
Aspirin *on page 127*
Narcotic / Opioid Analgesics *on page 1763*
Oxycodone *on page 1179*

Medication Safety Issues
Sound-alike/look-alike issues:
Percodan® may be confused with Decadron®, Percocet®, Percogesic®, Periactin®

U.S. Brand Names Endodan®; Percodan®
Canadian Brand Names Endodan®; Oxycodan®; Percodan®
Index Terms Aspirin and Oxycodone
Generic Available Yes
Pharmacologic Category Analgesic, Opioid
Use Relief of moderate to moderately severe pain
Restrictions C-II

Dosage
Geriatrics & Adults: Analgesic: Oral (based on oxycodone combined salts):
Percodan®: 1 tablet every 6 hours as needed for pain; maximum aspirin dose should not exceed 4 g/day.

Hepatic Impairment: Dose should be reduced in patients with severe liver disease.

Special Geriatric Considerations Enhanced analgesia has been seen in the elderly patients on therapeutic doses of narcotics; duration of action may be increased. Elderly may be particularly susceptible to the CNS depressant and constipating effects of narcotics. If 1 tablet/dose is used, it may be useful to add an additional 325 mg of aspirin to maximize analgesic effect.

Dosage Forms Excipient information presented when available (limited, particularly for generics); consult specific product labeling.
Tablet: Oxycodone hydrochloride 4.5 mg, oxycodone terephthalate 0.38 mg, and aspirin 325 mg
Endodan®, Percodan®: Oxycodone hydrochloride 4.8355 mg and aspirin 325 mg

♦ **Oxycodone Hydrochloride** *see* Oxycodone *on page 1179*
♦ **OxyContin®** *see* Oxycodone *on page 1179*
♦ **OxyFast®** *see* Oxycodone *on page 1179*
♦ **OxyIR®** *see* Oxycodone *on page 1179*

Oxymetazoline (oks i met AZ oh leen)

Medication Safety Issues
Sound-alike/look-alike issues:
Oxymetazoline may be confused with oxymetholone
Afrin® may be confused with aspirin
Visine® may be confused with Visken®

U.S. Brand Names Afrin® Extra Moisturizing [OTC]; Afrin® Original [OTC]; Afrin® Severe Congestion [OTC]; Afrin® Sinus [OTC]; Dristan™ 12-Hour [OTC]; Duramist® Plus [OTC]; Duration® [OTC]; Genasal [OTC]; Neo-Synephrine® 12 Hour [OTC]; Neo-Synephrine® 12 Hour Extra Moisturizing [OTC]; Nōstrilla® [OTC]; NRS® [OTC]; Vicks Sinex® 12 Hour [OTC]; Vicks Sinex® 12 Hour Ultrafine Mist [OTC]; Visine® L.R. [OTC]; 4-Way® 12 Hour [OTC]

Canadian Brand Names Claritin® Allergic Decongestant; Dristan® Long Lasting Nasal; Drixoral® Nasal

Index Terms Oxymetazoline Hydrochloride

Generic Available Yes: Nasal spray

Pharmacologic Category Adrenergic Agonist Agent; Imidazoline Derivative; Vasoconstrictor

Use Symptomatic relief of nasal mucosal congestion and adjunctive therapy of middle ear infections, associated with acute or chronic rhinitis, the common cold, sinusitis, hay fever, or other allergies (nasal); relief of redness of eye due to minor eye irritations (ophthalmic)

Contraindications Hypersensitivity to oxymetazoline or any component of the formulation

Warnings/Precautions
Nasal: Rebound congestion may occur with extended use (>3 days). Prior to self-medication (OTC use), contact healthcare provider in the presence of hypertension, diabetes, hyperthyroidism, heart disease, coronary artery disease, cerebral arteriosclerosis, or long-standing bronchial asthma.
Ophthalmic: Prior to OTC use, contact healthcare provider in the presence of glaucoma or if needed for >72 hours.

Adverse Reactions (Reflective of adult population; not specific for elderly)
Frequency not defined.
Cardiovascular: Hypertension, palpitation
Local: Transient burning, stinging
Respiratory: Dryness of the nasal mucosa, rebound congestion with prolonged use, sneezing

Drug Interactions Increased toxicity with MAO inhibitors.

Stability Store at room temperature.

Mechanism of Action Stimulates alpha-adrenergic receptors in the arterioles of the nasal mucosa to produce vasoconstriction

Pharmacodynamics
Onset of effect: Intranasal: Within 5-10 minutes
Duration: 5-6 hours

Pharmacokinetics Metabolism: Metabolic fate is unknown

Dosage
Geriatrics & Adults:
Nasal congestion: Intranasal (therapy should not exceed 3-5 days): 0.05% solution: Instill 2-3 drops or 2-3 sprays into each nostril twice daily
Relief of eye redness: Ophthalmic: 0.025% solution: Instill 1-2 drops in affected eye(s) every 6 hours as needed or as directed by healthcare provider

Monitoring Parameters Blood pressure in hypertensives

Patient Information Should not be used for self-medication for longer than 3 days, if symptoms persist, drug should be discontinued and a physician consulted; notify physician of insomnia, tremor, or irregular heartbeat; burning, stinging, or drying of the nasal mucosa may occur

Special Geriatric Considerations Evaluate the patient's ability to self-administer. Use with caution in patients with cardiovascular disease.

Dosage Forms Excipient information presented when available (limited, particularly for generics); consult specific product labeling.
Solution, intranasal, as hydrochloride [spray]: 0.05% (15 mL, 30 mL)
Afrin® Extra Moisturizing: 0.05% (15 mL) [contains benzyl alcohol and glycerin; regular or no drip formula]
Afrin® Original: 0.05% (15 mL, 30 mL) [contains benzalkonium chloride]
Afrin® Original: 0.05% (15 mL) [contains benzyl alcohol and benzalkonium chloride; no drip formula]
Afrin® Severe Congestion: 0.05% (15 mL) [contains benzyl alcohol and menthol; regular or no drip formula]
Afrin® Sinus: 0.05% (15 mL) [contains benzyl alcohol, benzalkonium chloride, camphor, phenol; regular or no drip formula]
Dristan™ 12-Hour: 0.05% (15 mL) [contains benzyl alcohol and benzalkonium chloride]
Duramist® Plus, Neo-Synephrine® 12 Hour, Nostrilla®, Vicks Sinex® 12 Hour Ultrafine Mist, Vicks Sinex® 12 Hour, 4-Way® 12 Hour: 0.05% (15 mL) [contains benzalkonium chloride]
Duration®: 0.05% (30 mL) [contains benzalkonium chloride]
Genasal, NRS®: 0.05% (15 mL, 30 mL) [contains benzalkonium chloride]
Neo-Synephrine® 12 Hour Extra Moisturizing: 0.05% (15 mL) [contains glycerin]
Solution, ophthalmic, as hydrochloride (Visine® L.R.): 0.025% (15 mL, 30 mL) [contains benzalkonium chloride]

♦ **Oxymetazoline Hydrochloride** *see* Oxymetazoline *on page 1184*

Oxymorphone (oks i MOR fone)

Related Information
Narcotic / Opioid Analgesics *on page 1763*

Medication Safety Issues
Sound-alike/look-alike issues:
Oxymorphone may be confused with oxycodone, oxymetholone

U.S. Brand Names Numorphan® [DSC]; Opana®; Opana® ER

Index Terms Oxymorphone Hydrochloride

Generic Available No

Pharmacologic Category Analgesic, Opioid

Use
Parenteral: Management of moderate-to-severe pain and preoperatively as a sedative and/or supplement to anesthesia
Oral, regular release: Management of moderate-to-severe pain
Oral, extended release: Management of moderate-to-severe pain in patients requiring around-the-clock opioid treatment for an extended period of time

Restrictions C-II

Contraindications Hypersensitivity to oxymorphone, other morphine analogs (phenanthrene derivatives) or any component of the formulation; paralytic ileus (known or suspected); increased intracranial pressure; severe respiratory depression (unless in monitored setting with resuscitative equipment); acute/severe bronchial asthma; hypercarbia
Note: Oral formulations are also contraindicated in moderate-to-severe hepatic impairment

Warnings/Precautions An opioid-containing analgesic regimen should be tailored to each patient's needs and based upon the type of pain being treated (acute versus chronic), the route of administration, degree of tolerance for opioids (naive versus chronic user), age, weight, and medical condition. The optimal analgesic dose varies widely among patients. Doses should be titrated to pain relief/prevention.

May cause CNS depression, which may impair physical or mental abilities; patients must be cautioned about performing tasks which require mental alertness (eg, operating machinery or driving). Effects may be potentiated when used with other sedative drugs or ethanol. Use with caution in patients with hypersensitivity reactions to other phenanthrene-derivative opioid agonists (codeine, hydrocodone, hydromorphone, levorphanol, oxycodone). May cause respiratory depression. Use extreme caution in patients with COPD or other chronic respiratory conditions characterized by hypoxia, hypercapnia, or diminished respiratory reserve (myxedema, cor pulmonale, kyphoscoliosis, obstructive sleep apnea, severe obesity). Use with caution in patients (particularly elderly or debilitated) with impaired respiratory function, adrenal disease, morbid obesity, thyroid dysfunction, prostatic hyperplasia, renal impairment, or severe hepatic dysfunction. Use only with extreme caution (if at all) in patients with head injury or increased intracranial pressure (ICP); potential to elevate ICP and/or blunt papillary response may be greatly exaggerated in these patients. Use with caution in biliary tract disease or acute pancreatitis (may cause constriction of sphincter of Oddi). May obscure diagnosis or clinical course of patients with acute abdominal conditions.

Oxymorphone shares the toxic potential of opiate agonists and usual precautions of opiate agonist therapy should be observed; may cause hypotension in patients with acute myocardial infarction, volume depletion, or concurrent drug therapy which may exaggerate vasodilation. The elderly may be particularly susceptible to adverse effects of narcotics.

[U.S. Boxed Warning]: Healthcare provider should be alert to problems of abuse, misuse, and diversion. Tolerance or drug dependence may result from extended use. Use caution in patients with a history of drug dependence or abuse. Abrupt discontinuation may precipitate withdrawal syndrome.

Extended release formulation:

[U.S. Boxed Warnings]: Opana® ER is an extended release oral formulation of oxymorphone and is not suitable for use as an "as needed" analgesic. Tablets should not be broken, chewed, dissolved, or crushed; tablets should be swallowed whole. Opana® ER is intended for use in long-term, continuous management of moderate to severe chronic pain. It is not indicated for use in the immediate postoperative period (12-24 hours). **[U.S. Boxed Warning]: The co-ingestion of ethanol or ethanol-containing medications with Opana® ER may result in accelerated release of drug from the dosage form, abruptly increasing plasma levels, which may have fatal consequences.**

Adverse Reactions (Reflective of adult population; not specific for elderly)
Frequency not defined.
Cardiovascular: Bradycardia, cardiac shock, flushing, hypotension, orthostatic hypotension, palpitation, peripheral vasodilation, shock, tachycardia

Central nervous system: Agitation, amnesia, anorexia, anxiety, CNS depression, coma, confusion, convulsion, dizziness, drowsiness, dysphoria, euphoria, fatigue, fever, hallucinations, headache, insomnia, intracranial pressure increased, malaise, mental depression, mental impairment, nervousness, restlessness, paradoxical CNS stimulation

Dermatologic: Pruritus, urticaria, rash

Endocrine & metabolic: Antidiuretic hormone release, weight loss

Gastrointestinal: Abdominal pain, appetite depression, biliary tract spasm, constipation, dehydration, dry mouth, dyspepsia, flatulence, nausea, paralytic ileus, stomach cramps, vomiting, xerostomia

Genitourinary: Urination decreased, urinary retention, urinary tract spasm

Local: Pain/reaction at injection site

Neuromuscular & skeletal: Weakness

Ocular: Blurred vision, diplopia, miosis

Renal: Oliguria

Respiratory: Apnea, bronchospasm, cyanosis, dyspnea, hypoventilation, laryngeal edema, laryngeal spasm, respiratory depression

Miscellaneous: Diaphoresis, histamine release, physical and psychological dependence

Overdosage/Toxicology Symptoms include respiratory depression, miosis, hypotension, bradycardia, apnea, and pulmonary edema. Treatment of overdose includes airway support, establishment of an I.V. line, and administration of naloxone 2 mg I.V., with repeat administration as necessary, up to a total of 10 mg.

Drug Interactions

CNS depressants (includes antipsychotics, benzodiazepines, barbiturates): May potentiate the CNS depressant effects of opiate agonists; reduce oxymorphone dosage in patients receiving other CNS depressants.

Dextroamphetamine: May enhance the analgesic effect of opiate agonists.

General anesthetics: May potentiate the CNS depressant effects of opiate agonists.

MAO inhibitors: May potentiate the CNS depressant effects of opiate agonists; monitor.

SSRIs: Analgesics (narcotic) may enhance the serotonergic effect of selective serotonin reuptake inhibitors. This may cause serotonin syndrome.

Tricyclic antidepressants: May potentiate the CNS depressant effects of opiate agonists; monitor.

Ethanol/Nutrition/Herb Interactions

Ethanol: Avoid ethanol (may increase CNS depression). Ethanol ingestion with extended-release tablets is specifically contraindicated due to possible accelerated release and potentially fatal overdose.

Food: When taken orally with a high-fat meal, peak concentration is 38% to 50% greater. Both immediate-release and extended-release tablets should be taken 1 hour before or 2 hours after eating.

Herb/Nutraceutical: Avoid valerian, St John's wort, kava kava, gotu kola (may increase CNS depression).

Stability Injection solution, tablet: Store at 15°C to 30°C (59°F to 86°F).

Mechanism of Action Oxymorphone hydrochloride (Numorphan®) is a potent narcotic analgesic with uses similar to those of morphine. The drug is a semisynthetic derivative of morphine (phenanthrene derivative) and is closely related to hydromorphone chemically (Dilaudid®).

Pharmacodynamics

Onset of action: Analgesic: I.V., I.M., SubQ: 5-10 minutes

Duration: Analgesic: Parenteral: 3-4 hours

Pharmacokinetics

Protein binding: 10% to 12%

Metabolism: Hepatic via glucuronidation to active and inactive metabolites

Bioavailability: Oral: 10%

Half-life elimination: Oral: Immediate release: 7-9 hours; Extended release: 9-11 hours

Excretion: Urine

Dosage

Geriatrics: Refer to adult dosing. **Note:** Initiate dosing at the lower end of the dosage range.

Adults: Analgesia: **Note:** Dosage must be individualized.

I.M., SubQ: Initial: 1-1.5 mg; may repeat every 4-6 hours as needed

Labor analgesia: I.M.: 0.5-1 mg

I.V.: Initial: 0.5 mg

Oral:

Immediate release:

Opioid-naive: 10-20 mg every 4-6 hours as needed. Initial dosages as low as 5 mg may be considered in selected patients and/or patients with renal impairment. Dosage adjustment should be based on level of analgesia, side effects, and pain intensity. Initiation of therapy with initial dose >20 mg is **not** recommended.

(Continued)

Oxymorphone *(Continued)*

Currently on stable dose of parenteral oxymorphone: ~10 times the daily parenteral requirement. The calculated amount should be divided and given in 4-6 equal doses.

Currently on other opioids: Use standard conversion chart to convert daily dose to oxymorphone equivalent. Generally start with $^1/_2$ the calculated daily oxymorphone dosage and administered in divided doses every 4-6 hours.

Extended release (Opana® ER):

Opioid-naive: Initial: 5 mg every 12 hours. Supplemental doses of immediate-release oxymorphone may be used as "rescue" medication as dosage is titrated.

Note: Continued requirement for supplemental dosing may be used to titrate the dose of extended-release continuous therapy. Adjust therapy incrementally, by 5-10 mg every 12 hours at intervals of every 3-7 days. Ideally, basal dosage may be titrated to generally mild pain or no pain with the regular use of fewer than 2 supplemental doses per 24 hours.

Currently on stable dose of parenteral oxymorphone: Approximately 10 times the daily parenteral requirement. The calculated amount should be given in 2 divided doses (every 12 hours).

Currently on opioids: Use conversion chart (see Note below) to convert daily dose to oxymorphone equivalent. Generally start with $^1/_2$ the calculated daily oxymorphone dosage. Divide daily dose in 2 (for every 12-hour dosing) and round down to nearest dosage form. **Note:** Per manufacturer, the following approximate oral dosages are equivalent to oxymorphone 10 mg:

Hydrocodone 20 mg
Oxycodone 20 mg
Methadone 20 mg
Morphine 30 mg

Conversion of stable dose of immediate-release oxymorphone to extended-release oxymorphone: Administer $^1/_2$ of the daily dose of immediate-release oxymorphone (Opana®) as the extended-release formulation (Opana® ER) every 12 hours

Renal Impairment: Cl_{cr} <50 mL/minute: Reduce initial dosage of oral formulations (bioavailability increased 57% to 65%). Begin therapy at lowest dose and titrate carefully.

Hepatic Impairment: Generally, contraindicated for use in patients with moderate-to-severe liver disease. Initiate with lowest possible dose and titrate slowly in mild impairment.

Administration Administer immediate release and extended release tablets 1 hour before or 2 hours after eating. Opana® ER tablet should be swallowed; do not break, crush. or chew.

Monitoring Parameters Pain relief, respiratory and mental status, blood pressure, pulse

Test Interactions

Some quinolones may produce a false-positive urine screening result for opiates using commercially-available immunoassay kits. This has been demonstrated most consistently for levofloxacin and ofloxacin, but other quinolones have shown cross-reactivity in certain assay kits. Confirmation of positive opiate screens by more specific methods should be considered. May cause elevation in amylase (due to constriction of the sphincter of Oddi).

Patient Information Take 1 hour before or 2 hours after meals. Do not crush, break, or chew the extended release tablet. If self-administered, use exactly as directed; do not increase dose or frequency or discontinue without consulting prescriber. Drug may cause physical and/or psychological dependence. While using this medication, do not use alcohol and other prescription or OTC medications (especially sedatives, tranquilizers, antihistamines, or pain medications) without consulting prescriber. Maintain adequate hydration (2-3 L/day of fluids) unless instructed to restrict fluid intake. May cause hypotension, dizziness, drowsiness, impaired coordination, or blurred vision (use caution when driving, climbing stairs, or changing position - rising from sitting or lying to standing, or when engaging in tasks requiring alertness until response to drug is known); nausea, vomiting or dry mouth (frequent mouth care, small frequent meals, chewing gum, or sucking lozenges may help); or constipation (increased exercise, fluids, fruit, or fiber may help; if unresolved, consult prescriber about use of stool softeners). Report persistent dizziness or headache; excessive fatigue or sedation; changes in mental status; changes in urinary elimination or pain on urination; weakness or trembling; blurred vision; or shortness of breath.

Special Geriatric Considerations Elderly may be particularly susceptible to the CNS depressant and constipating effects of narcotics. Plasma levels of oxymorphone were about 40% higher in elderly patients as compared to younger patients.

Dosage Forms Excipient information presented when available (limited, particularly for generics); consult specific product labeling.

Injection, solution, as hydrochloride:
Numorphan® [DSC], Opana®: 1 mg (1 mL)
Tablet, as hydrochloride:
Opana®: 5 mg, 10 mg
Tablet, extended release, as hydrochloride:
Opana®: ER: 5 mg, 10 mg, 20 mg, 40 mg

Selected References

Adams MP and Ahdieh H, "Pharmacokinetics and Dose-Proportionality of Oxymorphone Extended Release and its Metabolites: Results of a Randomized Crossover Study," *Pharmacotherapy*, 2004, 24(4):468-76.

Adams MP and Ahdieh H, "Single- and Multiple-Dose Pharmacokinetic and Dose-Proportionality Study of Oxymorphone Immediate-Release Tablets," *Drugs R D*, 2005, 6(2):91-9.

Carr DB, Jacox AK, Chapman RC, et al, "Acute Pain Management," Guideline Technical Report, No. 1. Rockville, MD: U.S. Department of Health and Human Services, Public Health Service, Agency for Health Care Policy and Research. AHCPR Publication No. 95-0034. February 1995.

"Drugs for Pain," *Med Lett Drugs Ther*, 2000, 42(1085):73-8.

Gabrail NY, Dvergsten C, and Ahdieh H, "Establishing the Dosage Equivalency of Oxymorphone Extended Release and Oxycodone Controlled Release in Patients With Cancer Pain: A Randomized Controlled Study," *Curr Med Res Opin*, 2004, 20(6):911-8.

Gimbel J and Ahdieh H, "The Efficacy and Safety of Oral Immediate-Release Oxymorphone for Postsurgical Pain," *Anesth Analg*, 2004, 99(5):1472-7.

Gimbel J, Walker D, Ma T, et al, "Efficacy and Safety of Oxymorphone Immediate Release for the Treatment of Mild to Moderate Pain After Ambulatory Orthopedic Surgery: Results of a Randomized, Double-Blind, Placebo-Controlled Trial," *Arch Phys Med Rehabil*, 2005, 86(12):2284-9

Matsumoto AK, Babul N, and Ahdieh H, "Oxymorphone Extended-Release Tablets Relieve Moderate to Severe Pain and Improve Physical Function in Osteoarthritis: Results of a Randomized, Double-Blind, Placebo- and Active-Controlled Phase III Trial," *Pain Med*, 2005, 6(5):357-66.

McIlwain H and Ahdieh H, "Safety, Tolerability, and Effectiveness of Oxymorphone Extended Release for Moderate to Severe Osteoarthritis Pain: A One-Year Study," *Am J Ther*, 2005, 12(2):106-12.

Mokhlesi B, Leikin JB, Murray P, et al, "Adult Toxicology in Critical Care: Part II: Specific Poisonings," *Chest*, 2003, 123(2):897-922.

"Principles of Analgesic Use in the Treatment of Acute Pain and Chronic Cancer Pain," 4th ed, Glenview, IL: American Pain Society, 1999.

Prommer E, "Oxymorphone: A Review," *Support Care Cancer*, 2006, 14(2):109-15.

Sinatra RS and Harrison DM, "Oxymorphone in Patient-Controlled Analgesia," *Clin Pharm*, 1989, 8(8):541, 544.

Zacher JL and Givone DM, "False-Positive Urine Opiate Screening Associated With Fluoroquinolone Use," *Ann Pharmacother*, 2004, 38:1525-28.

♦ **Oxymorphone Hydrochloride** *see* Oxymorphone *on page 1186*

Oxytetracycline (oks i tet ra SYE kleen)

Medication Safety Issues
Sound-alike/look-alike issues:
Terramycin® may be confused with Garamycin®

U.S. Brand Names Terramycin® I.M. [DSC]
Canadian Brand Names Terramycin®
Index Terms Oxytetracycline Hydrochloride
Generic Available No
Pharmacologic Category Antibiotic, Tetracycline Derivative
Use Treatment of susceptible bacterial infections; both gram-positive and gram-negative, as well as *Rickettsia* and *Mycoplasma* organisms
Contraindications Hypersensitivity to tetracycline or any component of the formulation
Warnings/Precautions Photosensitivity can occur with oxytetracycline.
Adverse Reactions (Reflective of adult population; not specific for elderly)
Frequency not defined; also refer to Tetracycline monograph
Cardiovascular: Pericarditis
Central nervous system: Bulging fontanels (infants), intracranial hypertension (adults)
Dermatologic: Angioneurotic edema, erythematous rash, exfoliative dermatitis (uncommon), maculopapular rash, photosensitivity, urticaria
Gastrointestinal: Anogenital inflammatory lesions, diarrhea, dysphagia, enamel hypoplasia, enterocolitis, glossitis, nausea, tooth discoloration, vomiting
Hematologic: Anemia, eosinophilia, neutropenia, thrombocytopenia
Local: Irritation
Renal: BUN increased
Miscellaneous: Anaphylactoid purpura, anaphylaxis, hypersensitivity reaction, SLE exacerbation
Overdosage/Toxicology Symptoms include nausea, anorexia, and diarrhea. Treatment following GI decontamination is supportive care only.
Drug Interactions
Barbiturates, phenytoin, and carbamazepine decrease serum levels of tetracyclines.
Oral contraceptives: Anecdotal reports suggesting decreased contraceptive efficacy with tetracyclines have been refuted by more rigorous scientific and clinical data.
Increased effect of warfarin.
Mechanism of Action Inhibits bacterial protein synthesis by binding with the 30S and possibly the 50S ribosomal subunit(s) of susceptible bacteria, cell wall synthesis is not affected
(Continued)

Oxytetracycline *(Continued)*

Pharmacokinetics
Absorption: Poor
Metabolism: Hepatic (small amounts)
Half-life: 8.5-9.6 hours; prolonged with renal impairment
Elimination: Urine; feces

Dosage
Geriatrics & Adults: I.M.: Usual dosage: 250 mg every 24 hours or 300 mg/day divided every 8-12 hours
Renal Impairment: Cl_{cr} <10 mL/minute: Administer every 24 hours or avoid use if possible
Hepatic Impairment: Avoid use in patients with severe liver disease.

Administration Injection for intramuscular use only.

Monitoring Parameters Signs and symptoms of infection, WBC, mental status

Patient Information You may be sensitive to sunlight; use sunblock, wear protective clothing, or avoid direct sun. If diabetic, drug may cause false tests with Clinitest® urine glucose monitoring; use of glucose oxidase methods (Clinistix®) or serum glucose monitoring is preferable. Report rash, difficulty breathing, yellowing of skin or eyes, change in color of urine or stool, easy bruising or bleeding, fever, chills, perianal itching, purulent vaginal discharge, white plaques in mouth, or persistent diarrhea.

Dosage Forms Excipient information presented when available (limited, particularly for generics); consult specific product labeling. [DSC] = Discontinued product
Injection, solution:
Terramycin® I.M: 5% [50 mg/mL] (10 mL) [contains lidocaine hydrochloride 2%] [DSC]

- ♦ **Oxytetracycline Hydrochloride** *see* Oxytetracycline *on page 1189*
- ♦ **Oxytrol®** *see* Oxybutynin *on page 1177*
- ♦ **Oysco D [OTC]** *see* Calcium and Vitamin D *on page 214*
- ♦ **Oysco 500+D [OTC]** *see* Calcium and Vitamin D *on page 214*
- ♦ **Oyst-Cal-D [OTC]** *see* Calcium and Vitamin D *on page 214*
- ♦ **Oyst-Cal 500 [OTC]** *see* Calcium Salts (Oral) *on page 220*
- ♦ **Oyst-Cal-D 500 [OTC]** *see* Calcium and Vitamin D *on page 214*
- ♦ **Oystercal® 500** *see* Calcium Salts (Oral) *on page 220*
- ♦ **P-071** *see* Cetirizine *on page 283*
- ♦ **Pacerone®** *see* Amiodarone *on page 80*
- ♦ **Pain Eze [OTC]** *see* Acetaminophen *on page 29*
- ♦ **Palcaps** *see* Pancrelipase *on page 1196*
- ♦ **Palgic®-D [DSC]** *see* Carbinoxamine and Pseudoephedrine *on page 239*
- ♦ **Palgic®-DS [DSC]** *see* Carbinoxamine and Pseudoephedrine *on page 239*

Paliperidone *(pal ee PER i done)*

Related Information
Antipsychotic Agents *on page 1747*
Atypical Antipsychotics *on page 1749*

U.S. Brand Names Invega™

Index Terms 9-hydroxy-risperidone; 9-OH-risperidone

Generic Available No

Pharmacologic Category Antipsychotic Agent, Atypical

Use Treatment of schizophrenia

Contraindications Hypersensitivity to paliperidone, risperidone, or any component of the formulation

Warnings/Precautions [U.S. Boxed Warning]: Patients with dementia-related psychosis treated with atypical antipsychotics are at an increased risk of death compared to placebo. An increased incidence of cerebrovascular adverse events (including fatalities) has been reported in elderly patients with dementia-related psychosis. Paliperidone has not been studied in this clinical population and is not approved for the treatment of dementia-related psychosis.

Compared with risperidone, paliperidone is low to moderately sedating; use with caution in disorders where CNS depression is a feature. Use caution in patients with predisposition to seizures. Use with caution in renal dysfunction; dose reduction recommended. Esophageal dysmotility and aspiration have been associated with antipsychotic use; use with caution in patients at risk of aspiration pneumonia (eg, Alzheimer's disease). Elevates prolactin levels; use with caution in breast cancer or other prolactin-dependent tumors. May alter temperature regulation. May mask toxicity of other drugs or conditions (eg intestinal obstruction, Reyes syndrome, brain tumor) due to antiemetic effects.

May cause orthostasis. Use with caution in patients with cardiovascular diseases (eg, heart failure, history of myocardial infarction or ischemia, cerebrovascular disease, conduction abnormalities). Use caution in patients receiving medications for hypertension (orthostatic effects may be exacerbated) or in patients with hypovolemia or dehydration. May alter cardiac conduction (low risk relative to other neuroleptics); life-threatening arrhythmias have occurred with therapeutic doses of neuroleptics. Avoid use in combination with QT_c-prolonging drugs. Avoid use in patients with congenital long-QT syndrome and in patients with history of cardiac arrhythmia.

May cause extrapyramidal symptoms, including pseudoparkinsonism, acute dystonic reactions, akathisia, and tardive dyskinesia (risk of these reactions is low relative to other neuroleptics, and is dose dependent). Risk of neuroleptic malignant syndrome (NMS) may be increased in patients with Parkinson's disease or Lewy body dementia; monitor for symptoms of confusion, obtundation, postural instability and extrapyramidal symptoms. May cause hyperglycemia; in some cases may be extreme and associated with ketoacidosis, hyperosmolar coma, or death. Use with caution in patients with diabetes (or risk factors) or other disorders of glucose regulation; monitor for worsening of glucose control. Significant weight gain has been observed with antipsychotic therapy; incidence varies with product. Monitor waist circumference and BMI.

The possibility of a suicide attempt is inherent in psychotic illness or bipolar disorder; use caution in high-risk patients during initiation of therapy. Prescriptions should be written for the smallest quantity consistent with good patient care.

Formulation consists of drug within a nonabsorbable shell that is expelled and may be visible in the stool. The use of nondeformable products is not recommended in patients with known stricture/narrowing of the GI tract or other GI motility/transit disorders. Do not use in patients unable to swallow the tablet whole.

Adverse Reactions (Reflective of adult population; not specific for elderly)
>10%:
  Cardiovascular: Tachycardia (12% to 14%)
  Central nervous system: Headache (11% to 14%), somnolence (6% to 11% dose dependent)
1% to 10%:
  Cardiovascular: QT_c interval prolongation (3% to 5%), orthostatic hypotension (1% to 4% dose dependent), bundle branch block (<1% to 3%), AV block (first degree, up to 2%), arrhythmia (<1% to 2%), blood pressure increased (<1% to 2%), T-wave abnormality (1% to 2%), palpitation
  Central nervous system: Akathisia (3% to 10% dose dependent), anxiety (5% to 9%), EPS (2% to 7% dose dependent), parkinsonism (up to 7% dose dependent), dizziness (4% to 6%), dystonia (1% to 5% dose dependent), hypertonia (1% to 4% dose dependent), fatigue (1% to 2%), fever (<1% to 2%)
  Endocrine & metabolic: Weight gain (6% to 9% dose dependent), insulin increased (<1% to 2%)
  Gastrointestinal: Nausea (4% to 6%), dyspepsia (2% to 5%), salivation increased (up to 4% dose dependent), xerostomia (2% to 3%), abdominal pain (1% to 3%)
  Neuromuscular & skeletal: Hyperkinesia (3% to 10% dose dependent), dyskinesia (3% to 9% dose dependent), tremor (3% to 5%), back pain (1% to 2%), weakness (<1% to 2%), extremity pain (up to 2%)
  Ocular: Vision blurred (up to 2%)
  Respiratory: Cough (2% to 3%), dyspnea

Overdosage/Toxicology Ingestion of doses as high as 405 mg have been reported. Symptoms of overdose may include drowsiness, sedation, tachycardia, hypotension, extrapyramidal symptoms (EPS), and prolonged QT interval. Treatment is symptom-directed and supportive. Gastric decontamination and cardiac monitoring should be initiated immediately. Consider risk of aspiration. Avoid antiarrhythmic therapy known to prolong the QT interval. Avoid vasopressors (eg, epinephrine or dopamine) which may worsen hypotensive effects in the setting of paliperidone's alpha-blocking effects.

Drug Interactions
  Acetylcholinesterase inhibitors (central): May increase the risk of antipsychotic-related extrapyramidal symptoms; monitor.
  Carbamazepine: May decrease levels/effects of paliperidone; monitor for reduced antipsychotic efficacy.
  CNS depressants: May increase adverse effects/toxicity of other CNS depressants.
  Itraconazole: May increase the levels/effects of paliperidone; monitor.
  Levodopa: Paliperidone may decrease effects of levodopa and other dopamine agonists.
  Lithium: May increase the neurotoxic effects (eg, EPS) of paliperidone; monitor.

Ethanol/Nutrition/Herb Interactions
  Ethanol: Avoid ethanol (may increase CNS depression).
  Herb/Nutraceutical: Avoid kava kava, gotu kola, valerian, St John's wort (may increase CNS depression).

Stability Store at 15°C to 30°C (59°F to 86°F). Protect from moisture.
  (Continued)

Paliperidone *(Continued)*

Mechanism of Action Paliperidone is considered a benzisoxazole atypical antipsychotic as it is the primary active metabolite of risperidone. As with other atypical antipsychotics, it's therapeutic efficacy is believed to result from mixed central serotonergic and dopaminergic antagonism. The addition of serotonin antagonism to dopamine antagonism (classic neuroleptic mechanism) is thought to improve negative symptoms of psychoses and reduce the incidence of extrapyramidal side effects. Similar to risperidone, paliperidone demonstrates high affinity to α_1, D_2, H_1, and $5\text{-}HT_{2C}$ receptors, and low affinity for muscarinic and $5\text{-}HT_{1A}$ receptors. In contrast to risperidone, paliperidone displays nearly 10-fold lower affinity for α_2 and $5\text{-}HT_{2A}$ receptors, and nearly three- to fivefold less affinity for $5\text{-}HT_{1A}$ and $5\text{-}HT_{1D}$, respectively.

Pharmacokinetics

Distribution: V_d: 487 L

Protein binding: 74%

Metabolism: Hepatic via CYP2D6 and 3A4

Bioavailability: 28%

Half-life elimination: 23 hours; 24-51 hours with renal impairment (Cl_{cr} <80 mL/minute)

Time to peak, plasma: ~24 hours

Excretion: Urine (80%); feces (11%)

Dosage

Geriatrics: Refer to adult dosing. Additional monitoring of renal function and orthostatic blood pressure may be warranted.

Adults: Schizophrenia: Oral: Initial: 6 mg once daily in the morning; titration not required, though some may benefit from higher or lower doses. If exceeding 6 mg/day, increases of 3 mg/day are recommended no more frequently than every 5 days, up to a maximum of 12 mg/day.

Renal Impairment:

Mild impairment (Cl_{cr} ≥50 mL/minute to <80 mL/minute): Maximal dose: 6 mg/day

Moderate-to-severe impairment (Cl_{cr} 10-49 mL/minute): Maximal dose: 3 mg/day

Hepatic Impairment: No adjustment necessary for mild-to-moderate (Child-Pugh class A and B) impairment. Not studied in severe impairment.

Administration May be administered with or without food. Extended release tablets should be swallowed whole with liquids; do not crush, chew, or divide.

Monitoring Parameters Vital signs; fasting lipid profile and fasting blood glucose/Hgb A_{1c} (prior to treatment, at 3 months, then annually); BMI, personal/family history of obesity, diabetes, waist circumference; blood pressure; mental status, abnormal involuntary movement scale (AIMS), extrapyramidal symptoms; orthostatic blood pressure changes for 3-5 days after starting or increasing dose. Weight should be assessed prior to treatment, at 4 weeks, 8 weeks, 12 weeks, and then at quarterly intervals. Consider titrating to a different antipsychotic agent for a weight gain ≥5% of the initial weight.

Patient Information Do not take any new prescription or over-the-counter medications or herbal products without consulting prescriber. Take exactly as directed with liquids. Do not chew, crush, or break tablet; swallow whole with liquids. Do not increase dose or frequency or discontinue without consulting prescriber; may take several weeks to achieve desired results. Avoid alcohol or stimulants unless approved by prescriber. Maintain adequate hydration (2-3 L/day of fluids) unless instructed to restrict fluid intake. If you are diabetic you should monitor glucose levels closely; this medication may affect glucose control (notify prescriber of any change in glucose levels). This medication comes in a nonabsorbable shell; after release of the drug the shell is expelled and may be visible in the stool (normal). You may experience fatigue, dizziness, restlessness, or blurred vision (use caution when driving or engaging in tasks requiring alertness until response to drug in known); orthostatic hypotension (use caution climbing stairs or when changing position from lying or sitting to standing); nausea, abdominal pain, dry or sore mouth (small, frequent meals, frequent mouth care, chewing gum, or sucking lozenges may help); difficulty on urination (void before taking medication). Report immediately any chest pain, rapid or irregular heart beat; difficulty breathing; weight gain >5 pounds; muscle or bone pain, tremors, or unusual movements; altered gait or balance; CNS changes (unusual anxiety or nervousness, abnormal thoughts, excessive sleepiness, dizziness, confusion, or suicidal ideation); or other adverse effects.

Additional Information Invega™ is an extended release tablet based on the OROS® osmotic delivery system. Water from the GI tract enters through a semipermeable membrane coating the tablet, solubilizing the drug into a gelatinous form which, through hydrophilic expansion, is then expelled through laser-drilled holes in the coating.

Special Geriatric Considerations Any changes in disease status in any organ system can result in behavior changes. Extrapyramidal syndrome symptoms occur less with this agent when total daily dose remains ≤6 mg as compared with phenothiazines and butyrophenone classes of antipsychotics.

In the treatment of agitated, demented, elderly patients, authors of meta-analysis of controlled trials of the response to the traditional antipsychotics (phenothiazines, butyrophenones) in controlling agitation have concluded that the use of neuroleptics results in a response rate of 18%. Clearly neuroleptic therapy for behavior control should be limited with frequent attempts to withdraw the agent given for behavior control. In light of significant risks and adverse effects in elderly population compared with limited data demonstrating efficacy in the treatment of dementia related psychosis, aggression, and agitation, an extensive risk:benefit analysis should be performed prior to use.

Dosage Forms Excipient information presented when available (limited, particularly for generics); consult specific product labeling.

Tablet, extended-release:
Invega™: 3 mg, 6 mg, 9 mg [osmotic controlled release]

Selected References

Jung SM, Kim K-A, Cho H-K, et al, "Cytochrome P450 3A Inhibitor Itraconazole Affects Plasma Concentrations of Risperidone and 9-Hydroxyrisperidone in Schizophrenic Patients," *Clin Pharmacol Ther*, 2005, 78(5):520-8.

Richelson E and Souder T, "Binding of Antipsychotic Drugs to Human Brain Receptors. Focus on Newer Generation Compounds," *Life Sci*, 2000, 68(1):29-39.

Spina E, Avenoso A, Facciola G, et al, "Plasma Concentrations of Risperidone and 9-Hydroxyrisperidone: Effect of Comedication with Carbamazepine or Valproate," *Ther Drug Monit*, 2000, 22:481-5.

♦ **Palmer's® Skin Success Acne Cleanser [OTC]** *see* Salicylic Acid *on page 1441*

♦ **Pamelor®** *see* Nortriptyline *on page 1138*

Pamidronate (pa mi DROE nate)

Medication Safety Issues
Sound-alike/look-alike issues:
Aredia® may be confused with Adriamycin, Meridia®

International issues:
Linoten® [Spain] may be confused with Lidopen® which is a brand name for lidocaine in the U.S.

U.S. Brand Names Aredia®
Canadian Brand Names Aredia®; Pamidronate Disodium®; Rhoxal-pamidronate
Index Terms Pamidronate Disodium
Generic Available Yes
Pharmacologic Category Antidote; Bisphosphonate Derivative
Use Treatment of hypercalcemia associated with malignancy with or without bone metastases
Contraindications Hypersensitivity to pamidronate, other bisphosphonates, or any component of the formulation
Warnings/Precautions Bisphosphonate therapy has been associated with osteonecrosis, primarily of the jaw; this has been observed mostly in cancer patients, but also in patients with postmenopausal osteoporosis and other diagnoses. Dental exams and preventative dentistry should be performed prior to placing patients with risk factors on chronic bisphosphonate therapy. Invasive dental procedures should be avoided during treatment.

Infrequently, severe (and occasionally debilitating) bone, joint, and/or muscle pain have been reported during bisphosphonate treatment. The onset of pain ranged from a single day to several months. Symptoms usually resolve upon discontinuation. Some patients experienced recurrence when rechallenged with same drug or another bisphosphonate; avoid use in patients with a history of these symptoms in association with bisphosphonate therapy.

May cause deterioration in renal function. Use caution in patients with renal impairment and avoid in severe renal impairment. Assess serum creatinine prior to each dose; withhold dose in patients with bone metastases who experience deterioration in renal function. Use has been associated with asymptomatic electrolyte abnormalities (including hypophosphatemia, hypokalemia, hypomagnesemia, and hypocalcemia). Rare cases of symptomatic hypocalcemia, including tetany have been reported. Leukopenia has been observed with oral pamidronate and monitoring of white blood cell counts is suggested. Patients with pre-existing anemia, leukopenia, or thrombocytopenia should be closely monitored during the first 2 weeks of treatment.

Vein irritation and thrombophlebitis may occur with infusions.

Adverse Reactions (Reflective of adult population; not specific for elderly)
Percentage of adverse effect varies upon dose and duration of infusion.
>10%:
Central nervous system: Fatigue (12% to 40%), fever (18% to 39%), headache (24% to 27%), anxiety (8% to 18%), insomnia (1% to 25%), pain (13% to 15%)
Endocrine & metabolic: Hypophosphatemia (9% to 18%), hypokalemia (4% to 18%), hypomagnesemia (4% to 12%), hypocalcemia (1% to 12%)
(Continued)

Pamidronate *(Continued)*

Gastrointestinal: Nausea (4% to 64%), vomiting (4% to 46%), anorexia (1% to 31%), abdominal pain (1% to 24%), dyspepsia (4% to 23%)

Genitourinary: Urinary tract infection (15% to 20%)

Hematologic: Anemia (6% to 48%), leukopenia (4% to 21%)

Local: Infusion site reaction (4% to 18%)

Neuromuscular & skeletal: Weakness (16% to 26%), myalgia (1% to 26%), arthralgia (11% to 15%)

Renal: Serum creatinine increased (19%)

Respiratory: Dyspnea (22% to 35%), cough (25% to 26%), upper respiratory tract infection (3% to 20%), sinusitis (15% to 16%), pleural effusion (3% to 15%)

1% to 10%:

Cardiovascular: Atrial fibrillation (6%), hypertension (6%), syncope (6%), tachycardia (6%), atrial flutter (1%), cardiac failure (1%), edema (1%)

Central nervous system: Somnolence (1% to 6%), psychosis (4%)

Endocrine & metabolic: Hypothyroidism (6%)

Gastrointestinal: Constipation (4% to 6%), gastrointestinal hemorrhage (6%), diarrhea (1%), stomatitis (1%)

Hematologic: Neutropenia (1%), thrombocytopenia (1%)

Neuromuscular & skeletal: Back pain (5%), bone pain (5%)

Renal: Uremia (4%)

Respiratory: Rales (6%), rhinitis (6%)

Miscellaneous: Moniliasis (6%)

Overdosage/Toxicology Symptoms include hypocalcemia, hypotention, ECG changes, seizures, bleeding, paresthesias, carpopedal spasm, and fever. Treat with I.V. calcium gluconate and general supportive care. Fever and hypotension can be treated with corticosteroids.

Drug Interactions

Aminoglycosides: May lower serum calcium levels with prolonged administration. Concomitant use may have an additive hypocalcemic effect.

Antacids: May decrease the absorption of bisphosphonate derivatives; should be administered at a different time of the day. Antacids containing aluminum, calcium, or magnesium are of specific concern.

Calcium salts: May decrease the absorption of bisphosphonate derivatives. Separate oral dosing in order to minimize risk of interaction.

Iron salts: May decrease the absorption of bisphosphonate derivatives. Only oral iron salts and oral bisphosphonates are of concern.

Magnesium salts: May decrease the absorption of bisphosphonate derivatives. Only oral magnesium salts and oral bisphosphonates are of concern.

Nonsteroidal anti-inflammatory drugs (NSAIDs): May enhance the gastrointestinal adverse/toxic effects (increased incidence of GI ulcers) of bisphosphonate derivatives.

Phosphate supplements: Bisphosphonate derivatives may enhance the hypocalcemic effect of phosphate supplements.

Stability

Powder for injection: Store below 30°C (86°F). Reconstitute by adding 10 mL of SWFI to each vial of lyophilized pamidronate disodium powder; the resulting solution will be 30 mg/10 mL or 90 mg/10 mL. The reconstituted solution is stable for 24 hours stored under refrigeration at 2°C to 8°C (36°F to 46°F).

Solution for injection: Store below 25°C (77°F).

Pamidronate may be further diluted in 250-1000 mL of 0.45% or 0.9% sodium chloride or 5% dextrose. Pamidronate solution for infusion is stable at room temperature for up to 24 hours.

Mechanism of Action A bisphosphonate which inhibits bone resorption via actions on osteoclasts or on osteoclast precursors. Does not appear to produce any significant effects on renal tubular calcium handling and is poorly absorbed following oral administration (high oral doses have been reported effective); therefore, I.V. therapy is preferred.

Pharmacokinetics Limited data in humans

Half-life elimination: 21-35 hours

Elimination, biphasic: ~50% excreted unchanged in urine within 72 hours

Dosage

Geriatrics: Refer to adult dosing. Begin at lower end of adult dosing range.

Adults: Note: Drug must be diluted properly before administration and infused intravenously slowly. Due to risk of nephrotoxicity, doses should not exceed 90 mg.

Hypercalcemia of malignancy: I.V.:

Moderate cancer-related hypercalcemia (corrected serum calcium: 12-13.5 mg/dL): 60-90 mg, as a single dose

Severe cancer-related hypercalcemia (corrected serum calcium: >13.5 mg/dL): 90 mg, as a single dose

Repeat dosing: A period of 7 days should elapse before the use of second course; repeat infusions every 2-3 weeks have been suggested, however, could be administered every 2-3 months according to the degree and of severity of hypercalcemia and/or the type of malignancy.

Osteolytic bone lesions with multiple myeloma: I.V.: 90 mg monthly

Osteolytic bone lesions with metastatic breast cancer: I.V.: 90 mg repeated every 3-4 weeks

Paget's disease: I.V.: 30 mg daily for 3 consecutive days

Renal Impairment: Not recommended in severe renal impairment (patients with bone metastases). Safety and efficacy have not been established in patients with serum creatinine >5 mg/dL. Studies are limited in multiple myeloma patients with serum creatinine ≥3 mg/dL.

Dosing adjustment in renal toxicity: In patients with bone metastases, treatment should be withheld in patients who experience deterioration in renal function (increase of serum creatinine ≥0.5 mg/dL in patients with normal baseline or ≥1.0 mg/dL in patients with abnormal baseline). Resumption of therapy may be considered when serum creatinine returns to within 10% of baseline.

Administration Drug must be properly diluted before administration and slowly infused intravenously (over at least 2 hours).

Monitoring Parameters Serum calcium, electrolytes, phosphate, magnesium, CBC with differential; monitor for hypocalcemia for at least 2 weeks after therapy; monitor serum creatinine prior to each dose; dental exam and preventative dentistry for patients at risk for osteonecrosis; patients with pre-existing anemia, leukopenia or thrombocytopenia should be closely monitored during the first 2 weeks of treatment

Reference Range Calcium (total): Adults: 9.0-11.0 mg/dL (2.05-2.54 mmol/L), may slightly decrease with aging; phosphorus: 2.5-4.5 mg/dL (0.81-1.45 mmol/L)

Test Interactions Bisphosphonates may interfere with diagnostic imaging agents such as technetium-99m-diphosphonate in bone scans.

Patient Information Maintain adequate intake of calcium and vitamin D; report any fever, sore throat, or unusual bleeding to your physician. Maintain adequate hydration while receiving this medication.

Additional Information Do not mix with calcium containing solutions (ie, lactated Ringer's solution); reconstitute in 10 mL sterile water for injection USP for each vial (results in 30 mg/10 mL); dilute in 0.45% NS, 0.9% NS, or D_5W to administer

Special Geriatric Considerations Has not been studied exclusively in the elderly. Monitor serum electrolytes periodically since the elderly are often receiving diuretics which can result in decreases in serum calcium, potassium, and magnesium.

Dosage Forms Excipient information presented when available (limited, particularly for generics); consult specific product labeling.

Injection, powder for reconstitution, as disodium: 30 mg, 90 mg

Aredia®: 30 mg, 90 mg

Injection, solution: 3 mg/mL (10 mL); 6 mg/mL (10 mL); 9 mg/mL (10 mL)

Selected References

Drug Facts and Comparisons, St Louis, MO: JB Lippincott Co, 1992, 134f-134m.

Kellihan MJ and Mangino PD, "Pamidronate," *Ann Pharmacother*, 1992, 26(10):1262-9.

♦ **Pamidronate Disodium** *see Pamidronate on page 1193*

♦ **p-Aminoclonidine** *see Apraclonidine on page 116*

♦ **Pamprin® Maximum Strength All Day Relief [OTC]** *see Naproxen on page 1088*

♦ **Pan-2400™ [OTC]** *see Pancreatin on page 1195*

♦ **Panafil®** *see Chlorophyllin, Papain, and Urea on page 293*

♦ **Panafil® SE** *see Chlorophyllin, Papain, and Urea on page 293*

♦ **Pancrease® MT** *see Pancrelipase on page 1196*

Pancreatin (PAN kree a tin)

Medication Safety Issues

Sound-alike/look-alike issues:

Pancreatin may be confused with Panretin®

U.S. Brand Names Dygase; Hi-Vegi-Lip [OTC]; kutrase®; ku-zyme®; Lapase; Pan-2400™ [OTC]; Pancreatin 4X [OTC]; Pancreatin 8X [OTC]; Veg-Pancreatin 4X [OTC]

Generic Available Yes

Pharmacologic Category Enzyme

Use Relief of functional indigestion due to enzyme deficiency or imbalance

Contraindications Hypersensitivity to pork protein or any component of the formulation; acute pancreatitis or acute exacerbations of chronic pancreatic disease

Warnings/Precautions Some products are made from pork protein and should not be used if allergic to pork.

Adverse Reactions (Reflective of adult population; not specific for elderly)

Frequency not defined.

(Continued)

Pancreatin *(Continued)*

Gastrointestinal: Loose stools (decrease dose)

Respiratory: Mucous membrane irritation or precipitation of asthma attack (due to inhalation of airborne powder)

Overdosage/Toxicology Overdose may lead to laxative effect. Treatment should be supportive.

Stability Store at controlled room temperature of 15°C to 30°C (59°F to 86°F). Protect from humidity.

Mechanism of Action An enzyme supplement, not a replacement, which contains a combination of lipase, amylase and protease. Enhances the digestion of proteins, starch and fat in the stomach and intestines.

Pharmacokinetics

Absorption: Not absorbed, acts locally in GI tract

Elimination: In feces

Dosage

Geriatrics & Adults: Actual dose varies with condition of patient and is usually given with each meal or snack.

Malabsorption: Oral:

ku-zyme®: 1-2 capsules with each meal or snack

kutrase®: 1 capsule with each meal or snack

Administration Oral: Swallow capsules/tablets whole; retention in the mouth before swallowing may cause mucosal irritation and stomatitis. Capsules may also be opened and sprinkled on soft food (do not chew).

Monitoring Parameters Stool frequency and fat content

Patient Information To be taken with a meal or a snack. Swallow tablets and capsules whole, do not chew, crush, or dissolve. Do not let dissolve in mouth. Capsules may also be opened and sprinkled on soft food (do not chew). Notify prescriber if diarrhea or loose stools develop

Additional Information These products are not bioequivalent and, therefore, cannot be interchanged (substituted) without consulting the physician.

Special Geriatric Considerations No special considerations necessary since drug is dosed to response; however, drug-induced diarrhea can result in unwanted side effects (confusion, hypotension, lethargy, fluid electrolyte loss).

Dosage Forms Excipient information presented when available (limited, particularly for generics); consult specific product labeling.

Capsule: Lipase 8500 units, protease 50,000 units, amylase 50,000 units [pancreatin 500 mg]

Dygase, kutrase®: Lipase 2400 units, protease 30,000 units, amylase 30,000 units

ku-zyme®: Lipase 1200 units, protease 15,000 units, amylase 15,000 units

Lapase: Lipase 1200 units, protease 15,000 units, and amylase 15,000 units [contains tartrazine]

Pan-2400™: Lipase 9816 units, protease 60,214 units, amylase 75,900 units [pancreatin 2400 mg]

Tablet: Lipase 565 units, protease 8200 units, amylase 8200 units [pancreatin 325 mg]; lipase 2400 units, protease 30,000 units, amylase 30,000 units [pancreatin 1200 mg]

Hi-Vegi-Lip: Lipase 4800 units, protease 60,000 units, amylase 60,000 units [pancreatin 2400 mg; vegetable source]

Pancreatin 4X: Lipase 4800 units, protease 60,000 units, amylase 60,000 units [pancreatin 600 mg]

Pancreatin 8X: Lipase 14,400 units, protease 180,000 units, amylase 180,000 units [pancreatin 900 mg]

Veg-Pancreatin 4X: Lipase 5500 units, protease 690,000 units, amylase 690,000 units [pancreatin 690 mg; vegetable source]

♦ **Pancreatin 4X [OTC]** *see* Pancreatin *on page 1195*

♦ **Pancreatin 8X [OTC]** *see* Pancreatin *on page 1195*

♦ **Pancrecarb MS®** *see* Pancrelipase *on page 1196*

Pancrelipase *(pan kre LYE pase)*

U.S. Brand Names Creon®; ku-zyme® HP; Lipram 4500; Lipram-CR; Lipram-PN; Lipram-UL; Palcaps; Pancrease® MT; Pancrecarb MS®; Pangestyme™ CN; Pangestyme™ EC; Pangestyme™ MT; Pangestyme™ UL; Panocaps; Panocaps MT; Panokase®; Panokase® 16; Plaretase® 8000; Ultracaps MT; Ultrase®; Ultrase® MT; Viokase®

Canadian Brand Names Cotazym®; Creon®; Pancrease®; Pancrease® MT; Ultrase®; Ultrase® MT; Viokase®

Index Terms Lipancreatin

Generic Available Yes: Excludes powder

Pharmacologic Category Enzyme

Use Replacement therapy in symptomatic treatment of malabsorption syndrome caused by pancreatic insufficiency secondary to disease or surgery; presumptive test for pancreatic function in patients with suspected pancreatic insufficiency

Contraindications Hypersensitivity to pork protein or any component of the formulation; acute pancreatitis or acute exacerbations of chronic pancreatic disease

Warnings/Precautions Pancrelipase is inactivated by acids; do not crush or chew, some capsules may be opened and sprinkled on food. Fibrotic strictures in the colon, some requiring surgery, have been reported with high doses; use caution. Use caution when adjusting doses or changing brands. Avoid inhalation of powder; may cause nasal and respiratory tract irritation.

Adverse Reactions (Reflective of adult population; not specific for elderly)
Frequency not defined; occurrence of events may be dose related.

Central nervous system: Pain

Dermatologic: Rash

Endocrine & metabolic: Hyperuricemia

Gastrointestinal: Nausea, cramps, constipation, diarrhea, perianal irritation/inflammation (large doses), irritation of the mouth, abdominal pain, intestinal obstruction, vomiting, flatulence, melena, weight loss, fibrotic strictures, greasy stools

Ocular: Lacrimation

Renal: Hyperuricosuria

Respiratory: Sneezing, dyspnea, bronchospasm

Miscellaneous: Allergic reactions

Overdosage/Toxicology Symptoms include diarrhea, other transient intestinal upset, hyperuricosuria, and hyperuricemia.

Ethanol/Nutrition/Herb Interactions Food: Avoid placing contents of opened capsules on alkaline food (pH >5.5); pancrelipase may impair absorption of oral iron and folic acid.

Stability Store between 15°C to 25°C (59°F to 77°F); do not refrigerate. Keep in a dry place.

Mechanism of Action Pancrelipase is a natural product harvested from the hog pancreas. It contains a combination of lipase, amylase, and protease. Products are formulated to dissolve in the more basic pH of the duodenum so that they may act locally to break down fats, protein, and starch.

Pharmacokinetics
Absorption: Not absorbed, acts locally in GI tract
Elimination: In feces

Dosage
Geriatrics & Adults:
Malabsorption: Oral:
Powder: Actual dose depends on the condition being treated and the digestive requirements of the patient: 0.7 g (1/4 teaspoonful) with meals
Capsules/tablets: The following dosage recommendations are only an approximation for initial dosages. The actual dosage will depend on the condition being treated and the digestive requirements of the individual patient.
Note: Dosage adjustment: Adjust dose based on body weight and stool fat content. Total daily dose reflects ~3 meals/day and 2-3 snacks/day, with half the mealtime dose given with a snack. Older patients may need less units/kg due to increased weight, but decreased ingestion of fat/kg. Maximum dose: 2500 units of lipase/kg/meal (10,000 units of lipase/kg/day): 4000-48,000 units of lipase with meals and with snacks
Occluded feeding tubes (unlabeled use): One tablet of Viokase® crushed with one 325 mg tablet of sodium bicarbonate (to activate the Viokase®) in 5 mL of water can be instilled into the nasogastric tube and clamped for 5 minutes; then, flushed with 50 mL of tap water

Administration Oral: Administer with meals or snacks and swallow whole with a generous amount of liquid. Do not crush or chew; retention in the mouth before swallowing may cause mucosal irritation and stomatitis. Delayed-release capsules containing enteric-coated microspheres or microtablets may also be opened and the contents sprinkled on soft food with a low pH that does not require chewing, such as applesauce, gelatin; apricot, banana, or sweet potato baby food; baby formula. Dairy products such as milk, custard, or ice cream may have a high pH and should be avoided. Avoid inhalation of powder, may cause nasal and respiratory tract irritation.

Monitoring Parameters Abdominal symptoms, nutritional intake, stool character, fecal fat; monitor stool fat and frequency (3-4 stools daily in acceptable)

Patient Information Take before or with meals. Dairy products such as milk, custard or ice cream may have a high pH and should be avoided. Do not chew, crush, or dissolve delayed release capsules; swallow whole. Do not inhale powder when preparing. You may experience some gastric discomfort. Report unusual joint pain or swelling, respiratory difficulty, or persistent GI upset.
(Continued)

Pancrelipase *(Continued)*

Additional Information These products are not bioequivalent and, therefore, cannot be interchanged (substituted) without consulting the physician. Should be used as part of a high-calorie diet, appropriate for age and clinical status.

Special Geriatric Considerations No special considerations are necessary since drug is dosed to response; however, drug-induced diarrhea can result in unwanted side effects (eg, confusion, hypotension, lethargy, fluid and electrolyte loss).

Dosage Forms Excipient information presented when available (limited, particularly for generics); consult specific product labeling. [DSC] = Discontinued product

Capsule:

ku-zyme® HP: Lipase 8000 units, protease 30,000 units, and amylase 30,000 units

Capsule, delayed release, enteric coated granules:

Pangestyme™ CN-10: Lipase 10,000 units, protease 37,500 units, amylase 33,200 units

Pangestyme™ CN-20: Lipase 20,000 units, protease 75,000 units, amylase 66,400 units

Pangestyme™ EC: Lipase 4500 units, protease 25,000 units, and amylase 20,000 units

Pangestyme™ MT16: Lipase 16,000 units, protease 48,000 units, and amylase 48,000 units

Pangestyme™ UL 12: Lipase 12,000 units, protease 39,000 units, and amylase 39,000 units

Pangestyme™ UL 18: Lipase 18,000 units, protease 58,500 units, and amylase 58,500 units

Pangestyme™ UL 20: Lipase 20,000 units, protease 65,000 units, and amylase 65,000 units

Capsule, delayed release, enteric coated microspheres: Lipase 4500 units, protease 25,000 units, and amylase 20,000 units

Creon® 5: Lipase 5000 units, protease 18,750 units, and amylase 16,600 units

Creon® 10, Palcaps 10: Lipase 10,000 units, protease 37,500 units, and amylase 33,200 units

Creon® 20, Palcaps 20: Lipase 20,000 units, protease 75,000 units, and amylase 66,400 units

Lipram 4500, Panocaps: Lipase 4500 units, protease 25,000 units, and amylase 20,000 units

Lipram-CR10: Lipase 10,000 units, protease 37,500 units, and amylase 33,200 units

Lipram-CR20: Lipase 20,000 units, protease 75,000 units, and amylase 66,400 units

Lipram-PN10: Lipase 10,000 units, protease 30,000 units, and amylase 30,000 units

Lipram-PN16, Panocap MT 16: Lipase 16,000 units, protease 48,000 units, and amylase 48,000 units

Lipram-PN20, Panocap MT 20: Lipase 20,000 units, protease 44,000 units, and amylase 56,000 units

Lipram-UL20, Ultracaps MT 20: Lipase 20,000 units, protease 65,000 units, and amylase 65,000 units

Pancrecarb MS-4®: Lipase 4000 units, protease 25,000 units, and amylase 25,000 units [buffered]

Pancrecarb MS-8®: Lipase 8000 units, protease 45,000 units, and amylase 40,000 units [buffered]

Pancrecarb MS-16® Lipase 16,000 units, protease 52,000 units, and amylase 52,000 units [buffered]

Capsule, enteric coated microspheres:

Ultrase®: Lipase 4500 units, protease 25,000 units, and amylase 20,000 units

Capsule, enteric coated microtablets:

Pancrease® MT 4: Lipase 4000 units, protease 12,000 units, and amylase 12,000 units

Pancrease® MT 10: Lipase 10,000 units, protease 30,000 units, and amylase 30,000 units

Pancrease® MT 16: Lipase 16,000 units, protease 48,000 units, and amylase 48,000 units

Pancrease® MT 20: Lipase 20,000 units, protease 44,000 units, and amylase 56,000 units

Capsule, enteric coated minitablets:

Ultrase® MT12: Lipase 12,000 units, protease 39,000 units, and amylase 39,000 units

Ultrase® MT18: Lipase 18,000 units, protease 58,500 units, and amylase 58,500 units

Ultrase® MT20: Lipase 20,000 units, protease 65,000 units, and amylase 65,000 units

Powder (Viokase®): Lipase 16,800 units, protease 70,000 units, and amylase 70,000 units per 0.7 g (227 g)

Tablet: Lipase 8000 units, protease 30,000 units, and amylase 30,000 units

Panokase®: Lipase 8000 units, protease 30,000 units, and amylase 30,000 units
Panokase® 16: Lipase 16,000 units, protease 60,000 units, and amylase 60,000 units
Plaretase™ 8000: Lipase 8000 units, protease 30,000 units, and amylase 30,000 units
Viokase® 8: Lipase 8000 units, protease 30,000 units, and amylase 30,000 units
Viokase® 16: Lipase 16,000 units, protease 60,000 units, and amylase 60,000 units

♦ **Pandel**® see Hydrocortisone on page 762
♦ **Pangestyme™ CN** see Pancrelipase on page 1196
♦ **Pangestyme™ EC** see Pancrelipase on page 1196
♦ **Pangestyme™ MT** see Pancrelipase on page 1196
♦ **Pangestyme™ UL** see Pancrelipase on page 1196
♦ **Panocaps** see Pancrelipase on page 1196
♦ **Panocaps MT** see Pancrelipase on page 1196
♦ **Panokase**® see Pancrelipase on page 1196
♦ **Panokase**® **16** see Pancrelipase on page 1196

Pantoprazole (pan TOE pra zole)

Medication Safety Issues
Sound-alike/look-alike issues:
Protonix® may be confused with Lotronex®, Lovenox®, protamine

Vials containing Protonix® I.V. for injection are not recommended for use with spiked I.V. system adaptors. Nurses and pharmacists have reported breakage of the glass vials during attempts to connect spiked I.V. system adaptors, which may potentially result in injury to healthcare professionals.

International issues:
Protonix® may be confused with Pretanix® which is a brand name for indapamide in Hungary

U.S. Brand Names Protonix®

Canadian Brand Names Panto™ IV; Pantoloc®; Pantoloc® M; PMS-Pantoprazole; Protonix®

Generic Available No

Pharmacologic Category Proton Pump Inhibitor; Substituted Benzimidazole

Use
Oral: Treatment and maintenance of healing of erosive esophagitis associated with GERD; reduction in relapse rates of daytime and nighttime heartburn symptoms in GERD; hypersecretory disorders associated with Zollinger-Ellison syndrome or other neoplastic disorders

I.V.: Short-term treatment (7-10 days) of patients with gastroesophageal reflux disease (GERD) and a history of erosive esophagitis; hypersecretory disorders associated with Zollinger-Ellison syndrome or other neoplastic disorders

Unlabeled/Investigational Use Treatment of peptic ulcer disease, active ulcer bleeding (parenteral formulation); adjunct treatment with antibiotics for *Helicobacter pylori* eradication

Contraindications Hypersensitivity to pantoprazole or any component of the formulation

Warnings/Precautions Relief of symptoms does not preclude the presence of a gastric malignancy. Long-term omeprazole therapy has caused atrophic gastritis (by biopsy); this may also occur with pantoprazole. No reports of enterochromaffin-like (ECL) cell carcinoids, dysplasia, or neoplasia has occurred. Not indicated for maintenance therapy; safety and efficacy for use beyond 16 weeks have not been established. Prolonged treatment (typically >3 years) may lead to vitamin B_{12} malabsorption. Intravenous preparation contains edetate sodium (EDTA); use caution in patients who are risk for zinc deficiency if other EDTA-containing solutions are coadministered.

Adverse Reactions (Reflective of adult population; not specific for elderly)
≥1%:
Cardiovascular: Chest pain
Central nervous system: Headache (5% to 9%), insomnia (<1% to 1%), dizziness, migraine, anxiety
Dermatologic: Rash (<1% to 2%)
Endocrine and metabolic: Hyperglycemia (<1% to 1%), hyperlipidemia
Gastrointestinal: Diarrhea (4% to 6%), flatulence (2% to 4%), abdominal pain (1% to 4%), nausea (≤2%), vomiting (≤2%), eructation (≤1%), constipation, dyspepsia, gastroenteritis, rectal disorder
Genitourinary: Urinary frequency, UTI
Hepatic: Liver function abnormal (up to 2%)
Local: Injection site reaction (includes thrombophlebitis and abscess)
Neuromuscular & skeletal: Arthralgia, back pain, hypertonia, neck pain, weakness
(Continued)

Pantoprazole *(Continued)*

Respiratory: Bronchitis, cough, dyspnea, pharyngitis, rhinitis, sinusitis, upper respiratory tract infection

Miscellaneous: Flu syndrome, infection, pain

Overdosage/Toxicology Treatment of an overdose would include appropriate supportive treatment. No adverse events were seen with ingestions of 400 mg and 600 mg. Pantoprazole is not removed by hemodialysis.

Drug Interactions Substrate of CYP2C19 (major), 3A4 (minor); **Inhibits** 2C9 (moderate); **Induces** CYP1A2 (weak), 3A4 (weak)

CYP2C9 Substrates: Pantoprazole may increase the levels/effects of CYP2C9 substrates. Example substrates include bosentan, dapsone, fluoxetine, glimepiride, glipizide, losartan, montelukast, nateglinide, paclitaxel, phenytoin, warfarin, and zafirlukast.

CYP2C19 inducers: May decrease the levels/effects of pantoprazole. Example inducers include aminoglutethimide, carbamazepine, phenytoin, and rifampin.

Iron salts: Oral absorption may be reduced by pantoprazole.

Itraconazole and ketoconazole: Proton pump inhibitors may decrease the absorption of itraconazole and ketoconazole.

Protease inhibitors: Proton pump inhibitors may decrease absorption of some protease inhibitors (atazanavir and indinavir).

Warfarin: Increased anticoagulant effects/INR have been reported with concurrent use (postmarketing case reports); monitor INR closely.

Ethanol/Nutrition/Herb Interactions

Ethanol: Avoid ethanol (may cause gastric mucosal irritation).

Herb/Nutraceutical: Prolonged treatment (typically >3 years) may lead to vitamin B_{12} malabsorption.

Stability

Oral: Store tablet at 15°C to 30°C (59°F to 77°F).

I.V.:

EDTA-stabilized formulation: Prior to use: Store at 15°C to 30°C (59°F to 86°F). Protect from light. When reconstituted with 10 mL NS (final concentration 4 mg/mL), solution is stable up to 24 hours at room temperature. If further diluting in 100 mL of D_5W, LR, or NS, dilute within 6 hours of reconstitution. Diluted solution is stable at room temperature for up to 24 hours from the time of initial reconstitution; protection from light is not required.

Original formulation (discontinued): Store at 2°C to 8°C (36°F to 46°F). Protect from light. When reconstituted with 10 mL NS (final concentration 4 mg/mL), solution is stable up to 2 hours at room temperature; protection from light is not required. When diluted in 100 mL D_5W, LR, or NS, may be stored at room temperature for up to 12 hours.

Mechanism of Action Suppresses gastric acid secretin by inhibiting the parietal cell H^+/K^+ ATP pump

Pharmacokinetics

Absorption: Well absorbed

Distribution: V_d: 11-24 L

Protein binding: 98% primarily to albumin

Metabolism: Extensively metabolized; no evidence that metabolites have pharmacologic activity

Bioavailability: 77%

Half-life: 1 hour

Time to peak: 2.5 hours after oral ingestion

Elimination: Urine (71%) and feces (18%)

Dosage

Geriatrics & Adults:

Erosive esophagitis associated with GERD:

Oral:

Treatment: 40 mg once daily for up to 8 weeks; an additional 8 weeks may be used in patients who have not healed after an 8-week course

Maintenance of healing: 40 mg once daily

Note: Lower doses (20 mg once daily) have been used successfully in mild GERD treatment and maintenance of healing

I.V.: 40 mg once daily for 7-10 days

Peptic ulcer disease: Eradication of *Helicobacter pylori* (unlabeled use): Oral: Doses up to 40 mg twice daily have been used as part of combination therapy

Hypersecretory disorders (including Zollinger-Ellison):

Oral: Initial: 40 mg twice daily; adjust dose based on patient needs; doses up to 240 mg/day have been administered

I.V.: 80 mg twice daily; adjust dose based on acid output measurements; 160-240 mg/day in divided doses has been used for a limited period (up to 7 days)

Prevention of rebleeding in peptic ulcer bleed (unlabeled use): I.V.: 80 mg, followed by 8 mg/hour infusion for 72 hours. **Note:** A daily infusion of 40 mg does not raise gastric pH sufficiently to enhance coagulation in active GI bleeds.

Renal Impairment: No adjustment is required. Pantoprazole is not removed by hemodialysis.

Hepatic Impairment: No adjustment is required.

Administration

I.V.: Flush I.V. line before and after administration. Solutions prepared from original formulation must be infused through an inline filter. Solutions prepared from the EDTA-stabilized formulation do not require an in-line filter (per manufacturer).

2-minute infusion: The volume of reconstituted solution (4 mg/mL) to be injected may be administered intravenously over at least 2 minutes.

15-minute infusion: Infuse over 15 minutes at a rate not to exceed 7 mL/minute (3 mg/minute).

Oral: Tablets should be swallowed whole, do not crush or chew. Best if taken before breakfast.

Monitoring Parameters Hypersecretory disorders: Acid output measurements, target level <10 mEq/hour (<5 mEq/hour if prior gastric acid-reducing surgery)

Test Interactions False-positive urine screening tests for tetrahydrocannabinol (THC) have been noted in patients receiving proton pump inhibitors, including pantoprazole.

Patient Information Take as directed; do not alter dosage without consulting prescriber. Take at similar time each day. Swallow tablet whole (do not crush or chew). Avoid alcohol. You may experience dizziness, headache, or anxiety (use caution when driving or engaging in dangerous activities until response to medication is known); vomiting or loss of appetite (small, frequent meals, frequent mouth care, sucking lozenges, or chewing gum may help); or diarrhea (boiled milk, yogurt, or buttermilk may help). Report persistent abdominal discomfort; chest pain or palpitations; acute headache; unresolved diarrhea; excessive fatigue; increased muscle, joint, or body pain; shortness of breath or wheezing; cold or flu symptoms; changes in urinary pattern; or other persistent adverse reactions.

Special Geriatric Considerations Dosage adjustment not required.

Dosage Forms Excipient information presented when available (limited, particularly for generics); consult specific product labeling. [CAN] = Canadian brand name

Note: Strength expressed as base

Injection, powder for reconstitution, as sodium:

Protonix®: 40 mg [contains edetate sodium 1 mg]

Tablet, delayed release, as sodium:

Protonix®: 20 mg, 40 mg

Tablet, enteric coated, as magnesium (Pantoloc® M) [CAN]: 40 mg [not available in the U.S.]

Papain and Urea (pa PAY in & yoor EE a)

U.S. Brand Names Accuzyme®; Allanzyme; Allanzyme 650; Ethezyme™; Ethezyme™ 830; Gladase®; Kovia®

Generic Available Yes: Ointment

Pharmacologic Category Enzyme, Topical Debridement

Use Debridement of necrotic tissue and liquefaction of slough in acute and chronic lesions such as pressure ulcers, varicose and diabetic ulcers, burns, postoperative wounds, pilonidal cyst wounds, carbuncles, and miscellaneous traumatic or infected wounds

Dosage

Geriatrics & Adults: Topical: Apply with each dressing change. Daily or twice daily dressing changes are preferred, but may be every 2-3 days. Cover with dressing following application.

Ointment: Apply $1/8$-inch thickness over the wound with clean applicator.

Spray: Completely cover the wound site so that the wound is not visible.

Special Geriatric Considerations Preventive skin care should be instituted in all older patients at high risk for pressure ulcers.

Dosage Forms Excipient information presented when available (limited, particularly for generics); consult specific product labeling.

Ointment, topical:

Accuzyme®: Papain 6.5×10^5 units/g and urea 10% (6 g, 30 g)

Allanzyme 650: Papain 6.5×10^5 units/g and urea 10% (30 g)

Ethezyme™: Papain 1.1×10^6 units and urea 10% (30 g)

Ethezyme™ 830: Papain 8.3×10^5 units/g and urea 10% (30 g)

Gladase®: Papain 8.3×10^5 units/g and urea 10% (6 g, 30 g)

Kovia®: Papain 8.3×10^5 units/g and urea 10% (3.5 g) [single-dose packet]; 30 g

Spray, topical:

Accuzyme®, Allanzyme: Papain 6.5×10^5 units/g and urea 10% (33 mL)

♦ **Papain, Urea, and Chlorophyllin** *see* Chlorophyllin, Papain, and Urea *on page 293*

Papaverine (pa PAV er een)

U.S. Brand Names Para-Time SR®
Index Terms Papaverine Hydrochloride; Pavabid [DSC]
Generic Available Yes
Pharmacologic Category Vasodilator
Use Papaverine has been used for many conditions where vasodilatation is felt to be of some benefit; however, to date, insufficient scientific evidence exists for any therapeutic value to its use except in testing for impotence.
Unlabeled/Investigational Use Investigational: Parenteral: Various vascular spasms associated with muscle spasms as in myocardial infarction, angina, peripheral and pulmonary embolism, peripheral vascular disease, angiospastic states, and visceral spasm (ureteral, biliary, and GI colic); testing for impotence

Papaverine has been used for many conditions where vasodilatation is felt to be of some benefit; however, to date, insufficient scientific evidence exists for any therapeutic value to its use except in testing for impotence.
Contraindications Hypersensitivity to papaverine or any component of the formulation
Warnings/Precautions Use with caution in patients with glaucoma. Administer I.V. cautiously since apnea and arrhythmias may result. May, in large doses, depress cardiac conduction (eg, AV node) leading to arrhythmias. May interfere with levodopa therapy of Parkinson's disease. Hepatic hypersensitivity has been noted with jaundice, eosinophilia, and abnormal LFTs.
Adverse Reactions (Reflective of adult population; not specific for elderly)
Frequency not defined.
Cardiovascular: Arrhythmias (with rapid I.V. use), flushing of the face, mild hypertension, tachycardia
Central nervous system: Drowsiness, headache, lethargy, sedation, vertigo
Gastrointestinal: Abdominal distress, anorexia, constipation, diarrhea, nausea
Hepatic: Chronic hepatitis, hepatic hypersensitivity
Respiratory: Apnea (with rapid I.V. use)
Drug Interactions
Decreased effect: Papaverine decreases the effects of levodopa
Increased toxicity: Additive effects with CNS depressants
Ethanol/Nutrition/Herb Interactions Ethanol: Avoid ethanol (may increase CNS depression).
Stability Refrigerate injection at 2°C to 8°C (35°F to 46°F); do not freeze. Protect from heat. Solutions should be clear to pale yellow; precipitates with lactated Ringer's.
Mechanism of Action Smooth muscle spasmolytic producing a generalized smooth muscle relaxation including: vasodilatation, gastrointestinal sphincter relaxation, bronchiolar muscle relaxation, and potentially a depressed myocardium (with large doses); muscle relaxation may occur due to inhibition or cyclic nucleotide phosphodiesterase, increasing cyclic AMP; muscle relaxation is unrelated to nerve innervation; papaverine increases cerebral blood flow in normal subjects; oxygen uptake is unaltered
Pharmacodynamics Peak concentrations: 1-2 hours
Pharmacokinetics
Absorption: Sustained preparations erratically absorbed
Protein binding: 90%
Metabolism: Rapidly in the liver
Bioavailability: Oral: ~54%
Half-life: 30-120 minutes
Elimination: Primarily as metabolites in urine
Dosage
Geriatrics & Adults: Arterial spasm:
Oral, sustained release: 150-300 mg every 12 hours; in difficult cases: 150 mg every 8 hours
I.M., I.V.: 30-65 mg (rarely up to 120 mg); may repeat every 3 hours
Administration Rapid I.V. administration may result in arrhythmias and fatal apnea
Monitoring Parameters Monitor blood pressure
Patient Information Inform your physician of dizziness, hypotension, drowsiness; alcohol may enhance these effects; may cause flushing, sweating, headache, tiredness, jaundice, skin rash, nausea, anorexia, abdominal discomfort, constipation, or diarrhea
Additional Information Therapeutic value is lacking
Special Geriatric Considerations Vasodilators have been used to treat dementia upon the premise that dementia is secondary to a cerebral blood flow insufficiency. The hypothesis is that if blood flow could be increased, cognitive function would be increased. This hypothesis is no longer valid. The use of vasodilators for cognitive dysfunction is not recommended or proven by appropriate scientific study.

Dosage Forms Excipient information presented when available (limited, particularly for generics); consult specific product labeling.

Capsule, sustained release, as hydrochloride: 150 mg

Para-Time SR®: 150 mg

Injection, solution, as hydrochloride: 30 mg/mL (2 mL, 10 mL)

Selected References

Erwin WG, "Senile Dementia of the Alzheimer Type," *Clin Pharm,* 1984, 3(5):497-504.

Higbee MD, "Noncholinergic Approaches to Treating Senile Dementia of the Alzheimer's Type," *Consult Pharm,* 1992, 7(6):635-41.

Waters C, "Cognitive Enhancing Agents: Current Status in the Treatment of Alzheimer's Disease," *Can J Neurol Sci,* 1988, 15(3):249-56.

Yesavage JA, Tinklenberg JR, Hollister LE, et al, "Vasodilators in Senile Dementias: A Review of the Literature," *Arch Gen Psychiatry,* 1979, 36:220-3.

♦ **Papaverine Hydrochloride** *see* Papaverine *on page 1202*

♦ **Para-Aminosalicylate Sodium** *see* Aminosalicylic Acid *on page 79*

♦ **Paracetamol** *see* Acetaminophen *on page 29*

♦ **Parafon Forte® DSC** *see* Chlorzoxazone *on page 303*

♦ **Parathyroid Hormone (1-34)** *see* Teriparatide *on page 1535*

♦ **Para-Time SR®** *see* Papaverine *on page 1202*

♦ **Parcopa™** *see* Levodopa and Carbidopa *on page 892*

Paricalcitol (pah ri KAL si tole)

U.S. Brand Names Zemplar®

Canadian Brand Names Zemplar®

Generic Available No

Pharmacologic Category Vitamin D Analog

Use

I.V.: Prevention and treatment of secondary hyperparathyroidism associated with stage 5 chronic kidney disease (CKD)

Oral: Prevention and treatment of secondary hyperparathyroidism associated with stage 3 and 4 CKD

Contraindications Hypersensitivity to paricalcitol or any component of the formulation; patients with evidence of vitamin D toxicity; hypercalcemia

Warnings/Precautions Excessive administration may lead to over suppression of PTH, hypercalcemia, hypercalciuria, hyperphosphatemia and adynamic bone disease. Acute hypercalcemia may increase risk of cardiac arrhythmias and seizures; use caution with cardiac glycosides as toxicity may be increased. Chronic hypercalcemia may lead to generalized vascular and other soft-tissue calcification. Phosphate and vitamin D (and its derivatives) should be withheld during therapy to avoid hypercalcemia.

Adverse Reactions (Reflective of adult population; not specific for elderly)

>10%: Gastrointestinal: Nausea (6% to 13%)

1% to 10%:

Cardiovascular: Edema (7%), hypertension (7%), hypotension (5%), palpitation (3%), chest pain (3%), syncope (3%), cardiomyopathy (2%), MI (2%), postural hypotension (2%)

Central nervous system: Pain (8%), chills (5%), dizziness (5%), headache (5%), lightheadedness (5%), vertigo (5%), fever (3% to 5%), depression (3%), insomnia (2%)

Dermatologic: Rash (2% to 6%), skin ulcer (3%), pruritus (3%), skin hypertrophy (2%)

Endocrine & metabolic: Dehydration (3%), acidosis (2%), hypokalemia (2%)

Gastrointestinal: Vomiting (6% to 8%), diarrhea (7%), GI bleeding (5%), abdominal pain (5%), xerostomia (3%), constipation (4%), gastroenteritis (3%), dyspepsia (2%), gastritis (2%), rectal disorder (2%)

Genitourinary: Urinary tract infection (3%), kidney function abnormal (2%)

Neuromuscular & skeletal: Arthritis (5%), back pain (4%), leg cramps (3%), weakness (3%), neuropathy (2%)

Ocular: Amblyopia (2%), retinal disorder (2%)

Respiratory: Pneumonia (2% to 5%), rhinitis (5%), sinusitis (3%), bronchitis (3%), cough (3%), epistaxis (2%)

Miscellaneous: Infection (bacterial, fungal, viral: 2% to 8%); allergic reaction (6%), flu-like syndrome (2% to 5%), sepsis (5%), cyst (2%)

Overdosage/Toxicology Acute overdose may cause hypercalcemia. Monitor serum calcium and phosphorus closely during titration of paricalcitol. Dosage reduction/interruption may be required if hypercalcemia develops. Chronic use may predispose to metastatic calcification. Bone lesions may develop if parathyroid hormone is suppressed below normal.

Drug Interactions

Substrate of CYP3A4 (major)

(Continued)

Paricalcitol *(Continued)*

CYP3A4 inhibitors (strong): May increase the levels/effects of paricalcitol. Example CYP3A4 inhibitors include azole antifungals, ciprofloxacin, clarithromycin, diclofenac, doxycycline, erythromycin, imatinib, isoniazid, nefazodone, nicardipine, propofol, protease inhibitors, quinidine, and verapamil.

Ketoconazole: May increase paricalcitol levels/effects; monitor.

Mechanism of Action Decreased renal conversion of vitamin D to its primary active metabolite (1,25-hydroxyvitamin D) in chronic renal failure leads to reduced activation of vitamin D receptor (VDR), which subsequently removes inhibitory suppression of parathyroid hormone (PTH) release; increased serum PTH (secondary hyperparathyroidism) reduces calcium excretion and enhances bone resorption. Paricalcitol is a synthetic vitamin D analog which binds to and activates the VDR in kidney, parathyroid gland, intestine and bone, thus reducing PTH levels and improving calcium and phosphate homeostasis.

Pharmacokinetics

Distribution: V_d:
Healthy subjects: Oral: 34 L; I.V.: 24 L
Stage 3 and 4 CKD: Oral: 44-46 L;
Stage 5 CKD: I.V.: 31-35 L

Protein binding: >99%

Metabolism: Hydroxylation and glucuronidation via hepatic and nonhepatic enzymes, including CYP24, CYP3A4, UGT1A4; forms metabolites (at least one active)

Bioavailability: Oral: ~72% in healthy subjects

Half-life elimination:
Healthy subjects: Oral: 4-6 hours
Stage 3 and 4 CKD: Oral: 17-20 hours
Stage 5 CKD: I.V.: 14-15 hours

Excretion: Healthy subjects: Feces (oral: 70% to 74%; I.V.: 63%); urine (oral: 16% to 18%, I.V.: 19%); 51% to 59% as metabolites

Dosage

Geriatrics & Adults: Note: If hypercalcemia or Ca x P >75 is observed, reduce or interrupt dosing until parameters are normalized.

Secondary hyperparathyroidism associated with chronic renal failure (stage 5 CKD): I.V.: 0.04-0.1 mcg/kg (2.8-7 mcg) given as a bolus dose no more frequently than every other day at any time during dialysis; dose may be increased by 2-4 mcg every 2-4 weeks; doses as high as 0.24 mcg/kg (16.8 mcg) have been administered safely; the dose of paricalcitol should be adjusted based on serum intact PTH (iPTH) levels, as follows:
Same or increasing iPTH level: Increase paricalcitol dose
iPTH level decreased by <30%: Increase paricalcitol dose
iPTH level decreased by >30% and <60%: Maintain paricalcitol dose
iPTH level decrease by >60%: Decrease paricalcitol dose
iPTH level 1.5-3 times upper limit of normal: Maintain paricalcitol dose

Secondary hyperparathyroidism associated with stage 3 and 4 CKD: Oral: Initial dose based on baseline serum iPTH:
iPTH ≤500 pg/mL: 1 mcg/day or 2 mcg 3 times/week
iPTH >500 pg/mL: 2 mcg/day or 4 mcg 3 times/week

Dosage adjustment based on iPTH level relative to baseline, adjust dose at 2-4 week intervals:
iPTH same or increased: Increase paricalcitol dose by 1 mcg/day or 2 mcg 3 times/week
iPTH decreased by <30%: Increase paricalcitol dose by 1 mcg/day or 2 mcg 3 times//week
iPTH decreased by ≥30% or ≤60%: Maintain paricalcitol dose
iPTH decreased by >60%: Decrease paricalcitol dose by 1 mcg/day* or 2 mcg 3 times/week
iPTH <60 pg/mL: Decrease paricalcitol dose by 1 mcg/day* or 2 mcg 3 times/week

*If patient is taking the lowest dose on a once-daily regimen, but further dose reduction is needed, decrease dose to 1 mcg 3 times/week. If further dose reduction is required, withhold drug as needed and restart at a lower dose. If applicable, calcium-phosphate binder dosing may also be adjusted or withheld, or switch to noncalcium-based binder

Renal Impairment: Refer to adult dosing.

Hepatic Impairment: Adjustment not needed for mild-to-moderate impairment. Paricalcitol has not been evaluated in severe hepatic impairment.

Administration

Oral: May be administered with or without food. With the 3 times/week dosing schedule, doses should not be given more frequently than every other day.

I.V.: Administered as a bolus dose at anytime during dialysis. Doses should not be administered more often than every other day.

Monitoring Parameters
Signs and symptoms of vitamin D intoxication
Serum calcium and phosphorus:
I.V.: Twice weekly during initial phase, then at least monthly once dose established
Oral: At least every 2 weeks for 3 months or following dose adjustment, then monthly for 3 months, then every 3 months
Serum or plasma intact PTH (iPTH):
I.V.: Every 3 months
Oral: At least every 2 weeks for 3 months or following dose adjustment, then monthly for 3 months, then every 3 months
In trials, a mean PTH level reduction of 30% was achieved within 6 weeks with I.V. administration

Reference Range
CKD (definition of stages; chronic disease is kidney damage or GFR <60 mL/minute/1.73 m^2 for ≥3 months)
Stage 3: GFR 30-59 mL/minute/1.73 m^2 (moderate decrease GFR)
Stage 4: GFR 15-29 mL/minute/1.73 m^2 (severe decreased GFR)
Stage 5: GFR <15 mL/minute/1.73 m^2 or dialysis (kidney failure)
Target range for iPTH:
Stage 3 CKD: 35-70 pg/mL
Stage 4 CKD: 70-110 pg/mL
Stage 5 CKD: 150-300 pg/mL
Serum phosphorous:
Stage 3 and 4 CKD: ≥2.7 to <4.6 mg/dL
Stage 5 CKD: 3.5-5.5 mg/dL

Patient Information To ensure effectiveness of therapy, it is important to adhere to a dietary regimen of calcium supplementation and phosphorous restriction; avoid excessive use of aluminum-containing compounds

Special Geriatric Considerations No specific dose changes necessary. Monitor closely. It may be advised to obtain baseline electrolytes, calcium, phosphorous, and digoxin serum concentrations, if applicable.

Dosage Forms Excipient information presented when available (limited, particularly for generics); consult specific product labeling.
Capsule, gelatin: 1 mcg, 2 mcg, 4 mcg [contains alcohol and coconut or palm kernel oil]
Injection, solution: 2 mcg/mL (1 mL); 5 mcg/mL (1 mL, 2 mL) [contains alcohol 20% v/v and propylene glycol 30% v/v]

Selected References
"K/DOQI Clinical Practice Guidelines for Bone Metabolism and Disease in Chronic Kidney Disease. Guideline 1. Evaluation of Calcium and Phosphorus Metabolism," *Am J Kidney Dis*, 2003, 42(4 Suppl 3):52-7.
"K/DOQI Clinical Practice Guidelines for Bone Metabolism and Disease in Chronic Kidney Disease. Guideline 3. Evaluation of Serum Phosphorus Levels," *Am J Kidney Dis*, 2003, 42(4 Suppl 3):62-3.
"K/DOQI Clinical Practice Guidelines for Chronic Kidney Disease: Evaluation, Classification, and Stratification, Part 4. Definition and Classification of Stages of Chronic Kidney Disease," *Am J Kidney Dis*, 2002, 39(2 Suppl 1):46-75.

♦ **Pariprazole** *see* Rabeprazole *on page 1370*
♦ **Parlodel**® *see* Bromocriptine *on page 186*
♦ **Parlodel**® **SnapTabs**® *see* Bromocriptine *on page 186*
♦ **Parnate**® *see* Tranylcypromine *on page 1612*

Paroxetine (pa ROKS e teen)

Related Information
Antidepressant Agents *on page 1742*

Medication Safety Issues
Sound-alike/look-alike issues:
Paroxetine may be confused with paclitaxel, pyridoxine
Paxil® may be confused with Doxil®, paclitaxel, Plavix®, Taxol®

U.S. Brand Names Paxil®; Paxil CR®; Pexeva®

Canadian Brand Names Apo-Paroxetine®; CO Paroxetine; Gen-Paroxetine; Novo-Paroxetine; Paxil®; Paxil CR®; PMS-Paroxetine; ratio-Paroxetine; Rhoxal-paroxetine; Sandoz-Paroxetine

Index Terms Paroxetine Hydrochloride; Paroxetine Mesylate

Generic Available Yes: Tablet, as hydrochloride

Pharmacologic Category Antidepressant, Selective Serotonin Reuptake Inhibitor

Use Treatment of major depressive disorder (MDD); treatment of panic disorder with or without agoraphobia; obsessive-compulsive disorder (OCD); social anxiety disorder (social phobia); generalized anxiety disorder (GAD); post-traumatic stress disorder (PTSD)
(Continued)

Paroxetine *(Continued)*

Unlabeled/Investigational Use May be useful in eating disorders, impulse control disorders, self-injurious behavior; vasomotor symptoms of menopause

Restrictions An FDA-approved medication guide concerning the use of antidepressants in children, adolescents, and young adults must be distributed when dispensing an outpatient prescription (new or refill) where this medication is to be used without direct supervision of a healthcare provider. Medication guides are available at http://www.fda.gov/cder/Offices/ODS/medication_guides.htm. Dispense to parents or guardians of children and adolescents receiving this medication.

Contraindications Hypersensitivity to paroxetine or any component of the formulation; use with or within 14 days of MAO inhibitors; concurrent use with thioridazine or pimozide

Warnings/Precautions [U.S. Boxed Warning]: Antidepressants increase the risk of suicidal thinking and behavior in children, adolescents, and young adults (18-24 years of age) with major depressive disorder (MDD) and other psychiatric disorders; consider risk prior to prescribing. Short-term studies did not show an increased risk in patients >24 years of age and showed a decreased risk in patients ≥65 years. Closely monitor patients for clinical worsening, suicidality, or unusual changes in behavior, particularly during the initial 1-2 months of therapy or during periods of dosage adjustments (increases or decreases); the patient's family or caregiver should be instructed to closely observe the patient and communicate condition with healthcare provider. A medication guide concerning the use of antidepressants should be dispensed with each prescription.

The possibility of a suicide attempt is inherent in major depression and may persist until remission occurs. Patients treated with antidepressants (for any indication) should be observed for clinical worsening and suicidality, especially during the initial few months of a course of drug therapy, or at times of dose changes, either increases or decreases. Use caution in high-risk patients. Worsening depression and severe abrupt suicidality that are not part of the presenting symptoms may require discontinuation or modification of drug therapy. The patient's family or caregiver should be alerted to monitor patients for the emergence of suicidality and associated behaviors (such as agitation, irritability, hostility, impulsivity, and hypomania) and call healthcare provider.

May worsen psychosis in some patients or precipitate a shift to mania or hypomania in patients with bipolar disorder. Patients presenting with depressive symptoms should be screened for bipolar disorder. Monotherapy in patients with bipolar disorder should be avoided. **Paroxetine is not FDA approved for the treatment of bipolar depression.**

Potential for severe reaction when used with MAO inhibitors, SSRIs/SNRIs or triptans; serotonin syndrome (hyperthermia, muscular rigidity, mental status changes/agitation, autonomic instability) may occur; concurrent use with MAO inhibitors contraindicated. May increase the risks associated with electroconvulsive therapy. Has a low potential to impair cognitive or motor performance - caution operating hazardous machinery or driving. Symptoms of agitation and/or restlessness may occur during initial few weeks of therapy. Low potential for sedation or anticholinergic effects relative to cyclic antidepressants.

Use caution in patients with a previous seizure disorder or condition predisposing to seizures such as brain damage, alcoholism, or concurrent therapy with other drugs which lower the seizure threshold. Use with caution in patients with hepatic dysfunction and in elderly patients. May cause hyponatremia/SIADH. Use with caution in patients at risk of bleeding or receiving anticoagulant therapy - may cause impairment in platelet aggregation. Use with caution in patients with renal insufficiency or other concurrent illness (due to limited experience); dose reduction recommended with severe renal impairment. May cause or exacerbate sexual dysfunction. Use caution in patients with narrow-angle glaucoma.

Upon discontinuation of paroxetine therapy, gradually taper dose and monitor for discontinuation symptoms (eg, dizziness, dysphoric mood, irritability, agitation, confusion, paresthesias). If intolerable symptoms occur following a decrease in dosage or upon discontinuation of therapy, then resuming the previous dose with a more gradual taper should be considered.

Adverse Reactions (Reflective of adult population; not specific for elderly)
Frequency varies by dose and indication. Adverse reactions reported as a composite of all indications.

>10%:

Central nervous system: Somnolence (15% to 24%), insomnia (11% to 24%), headache (17% to 18%), dizziness (6% to 14%)

Endocrine & metabolic: Libido decreased (3% to 15%)

Gastrointestinal: Nausea (19% to 26%), xerostomia (9% to 18%), constipation (5% to 16%), diarrhea (9% to 12%)

Genitourinary: Ejaculatory disturbances (10% to 28%)

Neuromuscular & skeletal: Weakness (12% to 22%), tremor (4% to 11%)

Miscellaneous: Diaphoresis (5% to 14%)

1% to 10%:

Cardiovascular: Vasodilation (2% to 4%), chest pain (3%), palpitation (2% to 3%), hypertension (≥1%), tachycardia (≥1%)

Central nervous system: Nervousness (4% to 9%), anxiety (5%), agitation (3% to 5%), abnormal dreams (3% to 4%), concentration impaired (3% to 4%), yawning (2% to 4%), depersonalization (up to 3%), amnesia (2%), emotional lability (≥1%), vertigo (≥1%), confusion (1%), chills (2%)

Dermatologic: Rash (2% to 3%), pruritus (≥1%)

Endocrine & metabolic: Orgasmic disturbance (2% to 9%), dysmenorrhea (5%)

Gastrointestinal: Anorexia, appetite decreased (5% to 9%), dyspepsia (2% to 5%), flatulence (4%), abdominal pain (4%), appetite increased (2% to 4%), vomiting (2% to 3%), taste perversion (2%), weight gain (≥1%)

Genitourinary: Impotence (2% to 9%), genital disorder (female 2% to 9%), urinary frequency (2% to 3%), urinary tract infection (2%)

Neuromuscular & skeletal: Paresthesia (4%), myalgia (2% to 4%), back pain (3%), myoclonus (2% to 3%), myopathy (2%), myasthenia (1%), arthralgia (≥1%)

Ocular: Blurred vision (4%), abnormal vision (2% to 4%)

Otic: Tinnitus (≥1%)

Respiratory: Respiratory disorder (up to 7%), pharyngitis (4%), sinusitis (up to 4%), rhinitis (3%)

Miscellaneous: Infection (5% to 6%)

Overdosage/Toxicology Symptoms include somnolence, nausea, vomiting, hepatic dysfunction, drowsiness, sinus tachycardia, urinary retention, renal failure (acute), and dilated pupils. Convulsions, status epilepticus, and ventricular arrhythmias (including torsade de pointes) have been reported, as well as serotonin syndrome and manic reaction. There are no specific antidotes. Following attempts at decontamination, treatment is supportive and symptom-directed. Cardiac monitoring is recommended. Forced diuresis, dialysis, and hemoperfusion are unlikely to be beneficial.

Drug Interactions Substrate of CYP2D6 (major); **Inhibits** CYP1A2 (weak), 2B6 (moderate), 2C9 (weak), 2C19 (weak), 2D6 (strong), 3A4 (weak)

Amphetamines: SSRIs may increase the sensitivity to amphetamines, and amphetamines may increase the risk of serotonin syndrome.

Aspirin (and other antiplatelet drugs): Concomitant use of paroxetine and NSAIDs, aspirin, or other drugs affecting coagulation has been associated with an increased risk of bleeding; monitor.

Atomoxetine: Paroxetine may increase the levels/effects of atomoxetine; dose reduction of atomoxetine may be required.

Beta-adrenergic blockers: Concomitant use with paroxetine may enhance the bradycardic effect of beta-blockers.

Buspirone: Combined use with SSRIs may cause serotonin syndrome.

Carbamazepine: May increase levels/effects of paroxetine; monitor.

Carvedilol: Serum concentrations may be increased; monitor carefully for increased carvedilol effect (hypotension and bradycardia).

Cimetidine: Cimetidine may reduce the first-pass metabolism of paroxetine resulting in elevated paroxetine serum concentrations; consider an alternative H₂antagonist.

Clozapine: Paroxetine may increase serum levels of clozapine; monitor for increased effect/toxicity.

CNS depressants: Paroxetine may enhance the adverse/toxic effect of other CNS depressants; monitor.

CYP2B6 substrates: Paroxetine may increase the levels/effects of CYP2B6 substrates. Example substrates include bupropion, promethazine, propofol, selegiline, and sertraline.

CYP2D6 inhibitors: May increase the levels/effects of paroxetine. Example inhibitors include chlorpromazine, delavirdine, fluoxetine, miconazole, pergolide, quinidine, quinine, ritonavir, and ropinirole.

CYP2D6 substrates: Paroxetine may increase the levels/effects of CYP2D6 substrates. Example substrates include amphetamines, selected beta-blockers, dextromethorphan, fluoxetine, lidocaine, mirtazapine, nefazodone, risperidone, ritonavir, thioridazine, tricyclic antidepressants, and venlafaxine.

CYP2D6 prodrug substrates: Paroxetine may decrease the levels/effects of CYP2D6 prodrug substrates. Example prodrug substrates include codeine, hydrocodone, oxycodone, and tramadol.

Cyproheptadine: May inhibit the effects of serotonin reuptake inhibitors; monitor for altered antidepressant response; cyproheptadine acts as a serotonin agonist.

Dextromethorphan: Metabolism of dextromethorphan may be inhibited; visual hallucinations occurred; monitor.

Duloxetine: Concomitant use may increase the levels/effects of duloxetine; monitor.

Galantamine: Paroxetine may increase levels/effects of galantamine; monitor.

Haloperidol: Metabolism may be inhibited and cause extrapyramidal symptoms (EPS); monitor patients for EPS if combination is utilized.

(Continued)

Paroxetine *(Continued)*

Lithium: Patients receiving SSRIs and lithium have developed neurotoxicity; if combination is used; monitor for neurotoxicity.

Loop diuretics: SSRIs may cause hyponatremia; additive hyponatremic effects may be seen with combined use of a loop diuretic (bumetanide, furosemide, torsemide); monitor for hyponatremia.

MAO inhibitors: SSRIs should not be used with nonselective MAO inhibitors (isocarboxazid, phenelzine); fatal reactions have been reported; this combination should be avoided.

Mexiletine: Paroxetine may increase the levels/effects of mexiletine; monitor.

Meperidine: Combined use may cause serotonin syndrome; monitor.

Nefazodone and trazodone: May increase the risk of serotonin syndrome with SSRIs; monitor.

NSAIDs: Concomitant use of paroxetine and NSAIDs, aspirin, or other drugs affecting coagulation has been associated with an increased risk of bleeding; monitor.

Phenytoin: May decrease the levels/effects of paroxetine; monitor.

Pimozide: Paroxetine may increase the levels/effects of pimozide; concomitant use contraindicated.

Procyclidine: Paroxetine may increase the levels/effects of procyclidine; monitor for increased anticholinergic effects; procyclidine dose reduction may be necessary.

Propafenone: Paroxetine may increase the levels/effects of propafenone; monitor.

Risperidone: Paroxetine may increase the levels/effects of risperidone; monitor.

Ritonavir: May increase the levels/effects of paroxetine increasing the risk of serotonin syndrome; conversely, concomitant use of paroxetine with fosamprenavir/ritonavir has been reported to cause decreased levels/effects of paroxetine; monitor.

Selegiline: SSRIs have been reported to cause mania or hypertension when combined with selegiline; this combination is best avoided; concurrent use with SSRIs has also been reported to cause serotonin syndrome; as an MAO type B inhibitor, the risk of serotonin syndrome may be less than with nonselective MAO inhibitors.

Serotonin agonists (eg, triptans): Concurrent use of paroxetine with these agents may increase the risk of serotonin syndrome; monitor.

Serotonergic reuptake inhibitors (eg, SSRIs/SNRIs): Concurrent use of paroxetine with these agents may increase the risk of serotonin syndrome; monitor.

Sibutramine: May increase the risk of serotonin syndrome with SSRIs; avoid coadministration.

Sympathomimetics: May increase the risk of serotonin syndrome with SSRIs.

Thioridazine: Paroxetine may inhibit the metabolism of thioridazine, resulting in increased plasma levels and increasing the risk of QT_c interval prolongation. Concurrent use is contraindicated.

Tramadol: Combined use may cause serotonin syndrome; monitor.

Tricyclic antidepressants: The metabolism of tricyclic antidepressants (amitriptyline, desipramine, imipramine, nortriptyline) may be inhibited by SSRIs resulting is elevated serum levels; if combination is warranted, a low dose of TCA (10-25 mg/day) should be utilized.

Tryptophan: May increase serotonergic effects; concomitant use not recommended.

Venlafaxine: Combined use with paroxetine may increase the risk of serotonin syndrome.

Warfarin: May alter the hypoprothrombinemic response to warfarin; monitor INR.

Ethanol/Nutrition/Herb Interactions

Ethanol: Avoid ethanol (may increase CNS depression).

Food: Peak concentration is increased, but bioavailability is not significantly altered by food.

Herb/Nutraceutical: Avoid valerian, St John's wort, SAMe, kava kava.

Stability

Suspension: Store at ≤25°C (≤77°F).

Tablet: Store at 15°C to 30°C (59°F to 86°F).

Mechanism of Action
Paroxetine is a selective serotonin reuptake inhibitor, chemically unrelated to tricyclic, tetracyclic, or other antidepressants; presumably, the inhibition of serotonin reuptake from brain synapse stimulated serotonin activity in the brain

Pharmacodynamics
Maximum antidepressant effect usually seen after 4 weeks

Pharmacokinetics

Absorption: Completely absorbed following oral administration

Metabolism: Extensively hepatic via CYP enzymes via oxidation and methylation; nonlinear pharmacokinetics may be seen with higher doses and longer duration of therapy. Saturation of CYP2D6 appears to account for the nonlinearity. C_{min} concentrations 70% to 80% greater in the elderly compared to nonelderly patients; clearance is also decreased.

Metabolism: Hepatic

Half-life: 21 hours

Geriatrics: Half-life and steady-state concentration increase disproportionately to dose with single and multiple dosing.

Excretion: Urine (64%, 2% as unchanged drug); feces (36% primarily via bile, <1% as unchanged drug)

Dosage

Geriatrics:

MDD, obsessive compulsive disorder, panic attack, social anxiety disorder:

Paxil®, Pexeva®: Oral: Initial: 10 mg/day; increase if needed by 10 mg/day increments at intervals of at least 1 week; maximum dose: 40 mg/day

Paxil CR®: Initial: 12.5 mg/day; increase if needed by 12.5 mg/day increments at intervals of at least 1 week; maximum dose: 50 mg/day

Note: Upon discontinuation of paroxetine therapy, gradually taper dose:

Paxil®, Pexeva®: 10 mg/day at weekly intervals; when 20 mg/day dose is reached, continue for 1 week before treatment is discontinued. Some patients may need to be titrated to 10 mg/day for 1 week before discontinuation.

Paxil CR®: Patients receiving 37.5 mg/day in clinical trials had their dose decreased by 12.5 mg/day to a dose of 25 mg/day and remained at a dose of 25 mg/day for 1 week before treatment was discontinued.

Adults:

MDD: Oral:

Paxil®, Pexeva®: Initial: 20 mg once daily, preferably in the morning; increase if needed by 10 mg/day increments at intervals of at least 1 week; maximum dose: 50 mg/day

Paxil CR®: Initial: 25 mg once daily; increase if needed by 12.5 mg/day increments at intervals of at least 1 week; maximum dose: 62.5 mg/day

GAD (Paxil®, Pexeva®): Oral: Initial: 20 mg once daily, preferably in the morning (if dose is increased, adjust in increments of 10 mg/day at 1-week intervals); doses of 20-50 mg/day were used in clinical trials, however, no greater benefit was seen with doses >20 mg.

OCD (Paxil®, Pexeva®): Oral: Initial: 20 mg once daily, preferably in the morning; increase if needed by 10 mg/day increments at intervals of at least 1 week; recommended dose: 40 mg/day; range: 20-60 mg/day; maximum dose: 60 mg/day

Panic disorder: Oral:

Paxil®, Pexeva®: Initial: 10 mg once daily, preferably in the morning; increase if needed by 10 mg/day increments at intervals of at least 1 week; recommended dose: 40 mg/day; range: 10-60 mg/day; maximum dose: 60 mg/day

Paxil CR®: Initial: 12.5 mg once daily; increase if needed by 12.5 mg/day at intervals of at least 1 week; maximum dose: 75 mg/day

PTSD (Paxil®): Oral: Initial: 20 mg once daily, preferably in the morning; increase if needed by 10 mg/day increments at intervals of at least 1 week; range: 20-50 mg. Limited data suggest doses of 40 mg/day were not more efficacious than 20 mg/day.

Social anxiety disorder: Oral:

Paxil®: Initial: 20 mg once daily, preferably in the morning; recommended dose: 20 mg/day; range: 20-60 mg/day; doses >20 mg may not have additional benefit

Paxil CR®: Initial: 12.5 mg once daily, preferably in the morning; may be increased by 12.5 mg/day at intervals of at least 1 week; maximum dose: 37.5 mg/day

Menopause-associated vasomotor symptoms (unlabeled use, Paxil CR®): Oral: 12.5-25 mg/day

Note: Upon discontinuation of paroxetine therapy, gradually taper dose:

Paxil®, Pexeva®: 10 mg/day at weekly intervals; when 20 mg/day dose is reached, continue for 1 week before treatment is discontinued. Some patients may need to be titrated to 10 mg/day for 1 week before discontinuation.

Paxil CR®: Patients receiving 37.5 mg/day in clinical trials had their dose decreased by 12.5 mg/day to a dose of 25 mg/day and remained at a dose of 25 mg/day for 1 week before treatment was discontinued.

Renal Impairment:

Cl_{cr} <30 mL/minute: Mean plasma concentrations ~4 times that seen in normal function.

Cl_{cr} 30-60 mL/minute: Plasma concentrations 2 times that seen in normal function.

Paxil®, Pexeva®: Adults: Initial: 10 mg/day; increase if needed by 10 mg/day increments at intervals of at least 1 week; maximum dose: 40 mg/day

Paxil CR®: Initial: 12.5 mg/day; increase if needed by 12.5 mg/day increments at intervals of at least 1 week; maximum dose: 50 mg/day

Hepatic Impairment: In hepatic dysfunction, plasma concentration is 2 times that seen in normal function.

Paxil®, Pexeva®: Initial: 10 mg/day; increase if needed by 10 mg/day increments at intervals of at least 1 week; maximum dose: 40 mg/day

Paxil CR®: Initial: 12.5 mg/day; increase if needed by 12.5 mg/day increments at intervals of at least 1 week; maximum dose: 50 mg/day

Administration Best given in the morning unless too sedating; then administer as divided dose or at bedtime

(Continued)

Paroxetine *(Continued)*

Monitoring Parameters Mental status for depression, suicidal ideation (especially at the beginning of therapy or when doses are increased or decreased), anxiety, social functioning, mania, panic attacks; akathisia

Reference Range Not established

Patient Information If currently on another antidepressant, notify physician; refrain from alcohol; if taking warfarin, anticonvulsants, or other drugs with CNS effects, notify physician; avoid abrupt discontinuation

Additional Information Paxil CR™ incorporates a degradable polymeric matrix (Geomatrix™) to control dissolution rate over a period of 4-5 hours. An enteric coating delays the start of drug release until tablets have left the stomach.

Special Geriatric Considerations Paroxetine is the most sedating and anticholinergic of the selective serotonin reuptake inhibitors. Paroxetine has been shown to be an equally effective antidepressant compared to nortriptyline in patients with ischemic heart disease. However, nortriptyline was associated with a significantly higher rate of adverse cardiac events (sustained increase in heart rate, sinus tachycardia, and asymptomatic increase in ventricular ectopy) compared to placebo.

Dosage Forms Excipient information presented when available (limited, particularly for generics); consult specific product labeling.

Note: Strength expressed as base:

Suspension, oral, as hydrochloride:

Paxil®: 10 mg/5 mL (250 mL) [orange flavor]

Tablet, as hydrochloride: 10 mg, 20 mg, 30 mg, 40 mg

Paxil®: 10 mg, 20 mg, 30 mg, 40 mg

Tablet, as mesylate:

Pexeva®: 10 mg, 20 mg, 30 mg, 40 mg

Tablet, controlled release, as hydrochloride:

Paxil CR®: 12.5 mg, 25 mg, 37.5 mg

Selected References

Grimsley SR and Jann MW, "Paroxetine, Sertraline, and Fluvoxamine: New Selective Serotonin Reuptake Inhibitors," *Clin Pharm*, 1992, 11(11):930-57.

Hebenstreit GF, Fellerer K, Zochling R, et al, "A Pharmacokinetic Dose Titration Study in Adult and Elderly Depressed Patients," *Acta Psychiatr Scand Suppl*, 1989, 350:81-4.

Lundmark J, Scheel Thomsen I, Fjord-Larsen T, et al, "Paroxetine: Pharmacokinetic and Antidepressant Effect in the Elderly," *Acta Psychiatr Scand Suppl*, 1989, 350:76-80.

Roose SP, Glassman AH, Attia E, et al, "Comparative Efficacy of Selective Serotonin Reuptake Inhibitors and Tricyclics in the Treatment of Melancholia," *Am J Psychiatry*, 1994, 151(12):1735-9.

Roose SP, Laghrissi-Thode F, Kennedy JS, et al, "Comparison of Paroxetine and Nortriptyline in Depressed Patients With Ischemic Heart Disease," *JAMA*, 1998, 279(4):287-91.

Schone W and Ludwig M, "A Double-Blind Study of Paroxetine Compared With Fluoxetine in Geriatric Patients With Major Depression," *J Clin Psychopharmacol*, 1993, 13(6 Suppl 2):34S-9S.

Pegaptanib (peg AP ta nib)

U.S. Brand Names Macugen®
Canadian Brand Names Macugen®
Index Terms EYE001; Pegaptanib Sodium
Generic Available No
Pharmacologic Category Ophthalmic Agent; Vascular Endothelial Growth Factor (VEGF) Inhibitor
Use Treatment of neovascular (wet) age-related macular degeneration (AMD)
Contraindications Hypersensitivity to pegaptanib or any component of the formulation; ocular or periocular infection
Warnings/Precautions Intravitreous injections may be associated with endophthalmitis; patients should be instructed to report any signs of infection immediately. Intraocular pressure may increase following injection. Safety and efficacy for administration into both eyes concurrently have not been studied. Safety and efficacy have not been established with hepatic impairment, or in patients requiring hemodialysis. Rare hypersensitivity reactions (including anaphylaxis) have been associated with pegaptanib, occurring within several hours of use; monitor closely. Equipment and appropriate personnel should be available for monitoring and treatment of anaphylaxis.
Adverse Reactions (Reflective of adult population; not specific for elderly)
10% to 40%:
  Cardiovascular: Hypertension
  Ocular: Anterior chamber inflammation, blurred vision, cataract, conjunctival hemorrhage, corneal edema, eye discharge, eye irritation, eye pain, intraocular pressure increased, ocular discomfort, punctate keratitis, visual acuity decreased, visual disturbance, vitreous floaters, vitreous opacities
1% to 10%:
  Cardiovascular: Carotid artery occlusion (1% to 5%), cerebrovascular accident (1% to 5%), chest pain (1% to 5%), transient ischemic attack (1% to 5%)
  Central nervous system: Dizziness (6% to 10%), headache (6% to 10%), vertigo (1% to 5%)
  Dermatologic: Contact dermatitis (1% to 5%)
  Endocrine & metabolic: Diabetes mellitus (1% to 5%)
  Gastrointestinal: Diarrhea (6% to 10%), nausea (6% to 10%), dyspepsia (1% to 5%), vomiting (1% to 5%)
  Genitourinary: Urinary retention (1% to 5%)
  Neuromuscular & skeletal: Arthritis (1% to 5%), bone spur (1% to 5%)
  Ocular: Blepharitis (6% to 10%), conjunctivitis (6% to 10%), photopsia (6% to 10%), vitreous disorder (6% to 10%), allergic conjunctivitis (1% to 5%), conjunctival edema (1% to 5%), corneal abrasion (1% to 5%), corneal deposits (1% to 5%), corneal epithelium disorder (1% to 5%), endophthalmitis (1% to 5%), eye inflammation (1% to 5%), eye swelling (1% to 5%), eyelid irritation (1% to 5%), meibomianitis (1% to 5%), mydriasis (1% to 5%), periorbital hematoma (1% to 5%), retinal edema (1% to 5%), vitreous hemorrhage (1% to 5%)
  Otic: Hearing loss (1% to 5%)
  Renal: Urinary tract infection (6% to 10%)
  Respiratory: Bronchitis (6% to 10%), pleural effusion (1% to 5%)
  Miscellaneous: Contusion (1% to 5%)
Overdosage/Toxicology No additional adverse events were observed with doses up to 3 mg.
Stability Store under refrigeration at 2°C to 8°C (36°F to 46°F); do not freeze. Do not shake vigorously.
Mechanism of Action Pegaptanib is an apatamer, an oligonucleotide covalently bound to polyethylene glycol, which can adopt a three-dimensional shape and bind to vascular endothelial growth factor (VEGF). Pegaptanib binds to extracellular VEGF, inhibiting VEGF from binding to its receptors and thereby suppressing neovascularization and slowing vision loss.
Pharmacokinetics
  Absorption: Slow systemic absorption following intravitreous injection
  Metabolism: Metabolized by endo- and exonucleases
  Half-life elimination: Plasma: 6-14 days
Dosage
  Geriatrics & Adults: AMD: Intravitreous injection: 0.3 mg into affected eye every 6 weeks
  Renal Impairment: Adjustment not required with renal impairment; information not available for patients requiring hemodialysis.
Administration For intravitreous injection only; adequate anesthesia and a broad spectrum antibiotic should be administered prior to injection
pH: 6-7
(Continued)

Pegaptanib *(Continued)*

Monitoring Parameters Intraocular pressure (within 30 minutes and 2-7 days after injection); endophthalmitis

Patient Information Report eye pain, redness, light sensitivity, or change in vision to ophthalmologist immediately.

Special Geriatric Considerations In studies, 94% of patients treated with pegaptanib were ≥65 years of age. No difference in efficacy was seen as compared to younger adults.

Dosage Forms Excipient information presented when available (limited, particularly for generics); consult specific product labeling.

Injection, solution [preservative free]: 0.3 mg/90 µL (90 µL) [prefilled syringe]

Selected References

Gragoudas ES, Adamis AP, Cunningham ET, et al, "Pegaptanib for Neovascular Age-Related Macular Degeneration," *N Engl J Med*, 2004, 351(27):2805-16.

♦ **Pegaptanib Sodium** *see* Pegaptanib *on page 1211*

Pegfilgrastim (peg fil GRA stim)

Medication Safety Issues

Sound-alike/look-alike issues:

Neulasta® may be confused with Neumega® and Lunesta™

U.S. Brand Names Neulasta®

Canadian Brand Names Neulasta®

Index Terms G-CSF (PEG Conjugate); Granulocyte Colony Stimulating Factor (PEG Conjugate); NSC-725961; SD/01

Generic Available No

Pharmacologic Category Colony Stimulating Factor

Use Decrease the incidence of infection, by stimulation of granulocyte production, in patients with nonmyeloid malignancies receiving myelosuppressive therapy associated with a significant risk of febrile neutropenia

Contraindications Hypersensitivity to pegfilgrastim, filgrastim, *E. coli*-derived proteins, or any component of the formulation; concurrent myelosuppressive, chemotherapy, or radiation therapy

Warnings/Precautions Do not use pegfilgrastim in the period 14 days before to 24 hours after administration of cytotoxic chemotherapy because of the potential sensitivity of rapidly dividing myeloid cells to cytotoxic chemotherapy. Pegfilgrastim can potentially act as a growth factor for any tumor type, particularly myeloid malignancies. Precaution should be exercised in the usage of pegfilgrastim in any malignancy with myeloid characteristics. Tumors of nonhematopoietic origin may have surface receptors for pegfilgrastim. Pegfilgrastim has not been evaluated with patients receiving radiation therapy, or with chemotherapy associated with delayed myelosuppression (nitrosoureas, mitomycin C). Safety and efficacy have not been evaluated for peripheral blood progenitor cell (PBPC) mobilization.

Allergic-type reactions (anaphylaxis, skin rash, urticaria) have occurred primarily with the initial dose and may recur after discontinuation; close follow up for several days and permanent discontinuation are recommended for severe reactions. Rare cases of splenic rupture have been reported; patients must be instructed to report left upper quadrant pain or shoulder tip pain. Adult respiratory distress syndrome (ARDS) has been associated with the parent compound, filgrastim; withhold pegfilgrastim and evaluate patients with symptoms of ARDS (fever, lung infiltrates, respiratory distress). May precipitate sickle cell crises in patients with sickle cell disease; carefully evaluate potential risks and benefits. The packaging (needle cover) contains latex.

Adverse Reactions (Reflective of adult population; not specific for elderly)

>10%:

Cardiovascular: Peripheral edema (12%)

Central nervous system: Headache (16%)

Gastrointestinal: Vomiting (13%), constipation (12%)

Neuromuscular & skeletal: Bone pain (31% to 57%), myalgia (21%), arthralgia (16%), weakness (13%)

Overdosage/Toxicology No clinical adverse effects have been seen with high doses producing ANC >10,000/mm^3. The duration of leukocytosis has ranged from 6-13 days. Leukapheresis may be considered in symptomatic individuals.

Drug Interactions No formal drug interactions studies have been conducted.

Stability Store under refrigeration 2°C to 8°C (36°F to 46°F); do not freeze. If inadvertently frozen, allow to thaw in refrigerator; discard if frozen more than one time. Protect from light. Do not shake. Allow to reach room temperature prior to injection. May be kept at room temperature for 48 hours.

Mechanism of Action Stimulates the production, maturation, and activation of neutrophils, pegfilgrastim activates neutrophils to increase both their migration and cytotoxicity. Pegfilgrastim has a prolonged duration of effect relative to filgrastim and a reduced renal clearance.

Pharmacokinetics Half-life: SubQ: 15-80 hours

Dosage

Geriatrics & Adults: Myelosuppressive therapy: SubQ: 6 mg once per chemotherapy cycle; do not administer in the period between 14 days before and 24 hours after administration of cytotoxic chemotherapy

Renal Impairment: No adjustment necessary.

Administration Engage/activate needle guard following use to prevent accidental needlesticks.

Monitoring Parameters Complete blood count and platelet count should be obtained prior to chemotherapy. Leukocytosis (white blood cell counts 100,000/mm^3) has been observed in <1% of patients receiving pegfilgrastim. Monitor platelets and hematocrit regularly.

Reference Range No clinical benefit seen with ANC >10,000/mm^3.

Test Interactions May interfere with bone imaging studies; increased hematopoietic activity of the bone marrow may appear as transient positive bone imaging changes

Patient Information Follow directions for proper storage and administration of SubQ medication. Never reuse syringes or needles. You may experience bone pain (request analgesic). Report unusual fever or chills; unhealed sores; severe bone pain; pain, redness, or swelling at injection site; pain in the upper abdomen or shoulder tip; unusual swelling of extremities or difficulty breathing; or chest pain and palpitations.

Special Geriatric Considerations Not for patients <45 kg.

Dosage Forms Excipient information presented when available (limited, particularly for generics); consult specific product labeling.

Injection, solution [preservative free]:

Neulasta®: 10 mg/mL (0.6 mL) [prefilled syringe; needle cover contains latex]

Selected References

Holmes FA, O'Shaughnessy JA, Vukelja S, et al, "Blinded, Randomized, Multicenter Study to Evaluate Single Administration Pegfilgrastim Once Per Cycle Versus Daily Filgrastim as an Adjunct to Chemotherapy in Patients With High-Risk Stage II or Stage III/IV Breast Cancer," *J Clin Oncol*, 2002, 20(3): 727-31.

Peginterferon Alfa-2b (peg in ter FEER on AL fa too bee)

U.S. Brand Names PEG-Intron®

Canadian Brand Names PEG-Intron®

Index Terms Interferon Alfa-2b (PEG Conjugate); Pegylated Interferon Alfa-2b

Generic Available No

Pharmacologic Category Interferon

Use Treatment of chronic hepatitis C (as monotherapy or in combination with ribavirin) in adult patients who have never received interferon alpha and have compensated liver disease

Restrictions An FDA-approved medication guide must be distributed when dispensing an outpatient prescription (new or refill) where this medication is to be used without direct supervision of a healthcare provider. Medication guides are available at http://www.fda.gov/cder/Offices/ODS/medication_guides.htm.

Contraindications Hypersensitivity to polyethylene glycol (PEG), interferon alfa, or any component of the formulation; autoimmune hepatitis; decompensated liver disease; previous treatment with interferon; severe psychiatric disorder

Warnings/Precautions [U.S. Boxed Warning]: Severe psychiatric adverse effects, including depression, suicidal ideation, and suicide attempt, may occur; use caution with a history of depression. Avoid use in severe psychiatric disorders and discontinue if worsening or persistently severe signs/symptoms of neuropsychiatric disorders (including depression and/or suicidal thoughts/behavior) occur. Use with caution in patients who are chronically immunosuppressed, with low peripheral blood counts or myelosuppression, including concurrent use of myelosuppressive therapy. Discontinue therapy when significant decreases in neutrophil (<0.5 x 10^9/L) or platelet counts (<50,000/mm^3 occur).

[U.S. Boxed Warning]: Use with caution in patients with prior cardiovascular disease, endocrine disorders, autoimmune disorders, and pulmonary dysfunction; may cause or aggravate fatal or life-threatening conditions. Discontinue therapy if colitis develops or known or suspected pancreatitis develops. Patients with renal dysfunction should be monitored for signs/symptoms of toxicity (dosage adjustment required if toxicity occurs); avoid use of combination therapy with ribavirin in renal dysfunction (Cl$_{cr}$ <50 mL/minute). Ophthalmologic disorders (including retinal hemorrhages, cotton wool spots, and retinal artery or vein obstruction) have occurred in patients using other alpha interferons. Prior to start of therapy, visual exams are (Continued)

Peginterferon Alfa-2b *(Continued)*

recommended for patients with diabetes mellitus or hypertension. Transient rashes do not necessitate interruption of therapy.

Due to differences in dosages, patients should not change brands. Safety and efficacy have not been established in patients who have failed other alpha interferon (including peginterferon alfa-2b) therapy, received organ transplants, been infected with HIV or hepatitis B, or received treatment for >48 weeks. Use caution in geriatric patients.

Adverse Reactions (Reflective of adult population; not specific for elderly)

>10%:

Central nervous system: Headache (56%), fatigue (52%), depression (16% to 29%), anxiety/emotional liability/irritability (28%), insomnia (23%), fever (22%), dizziness (12%), impaired concentration (5% to 12%), pain (12%)

Dermatologic: Alopecia (22%), pruritus (12%), dry skin (11%)

Gastrointestinal: Nausea (26%), anorexia (20%), diarrhea (18%), abdominal pain (15%), weight loss (11%)

Local: Injection site inflammation/reaction (47%)

Neuromuscular & skeletal: Musculoskeletal pain (56%), myalgia (38% to 42%), rigors (23% to 45%)

Respiratory: Epistaxis (14%), nasopharyngitis (11%)

Miscellaneous: Flu-like syndrome (46%), viral infection (11%)

>1% to 10%:

Cardiovascular: Flushing (6%)

Central nervous system: Malaise (8%)

Dermatologic: Rash (6%), dermatitis (7%)

Endocrine & metabolic: Hypothyroidism (5%)

Gastrointestinal: Vomiting (7%), dyspepsia (6%), taste perversion

Hematologic: Neutropenia, thrombocytopenia

Hepatic: Hepatomegaly (6%), transaminases increased (10%; transient)

Local: Injection site pain (2%)

Neuromuscular & skeletal: Hypertonia (5%)

Respiratory: Pharyngitis (10%), sinusitis (7%), cough (6%)

Miscellaneous: Diaphoresis (6%)

Overdosage/Toxicology Limited experience with accidental doses ≥2.5 times the intended dose. No serious side effects have been noted. Treatment is symptom-directed and supportive.

Drug Interactions Inhibits CYP1A2 (weak)

ACE inhibitors: Interferons may increase the risk of neutropenia. Risk: Monitor

Clozapine: A case report of agranulocytosis with concurrent use.

Erythropoietin: Case reports of decreased hematopoietic effect

Fluorouracil: Concentrations of fluorouracil doubled in patients with gastrointestinal carcinoma who received interferon alfa-2b.

Melphalan: Interferon alfa may decrease the serum concentrations of melphalan; monitor.

Prednisone: Prednisone may decrease the therapeutic effects of interferon alfa. Risk: Moderate.

Ribavirin: Concurrent therapy may increase the risk of hemolytic anemia.

Theophylline: Interferon alfa may decrease the P450 isoenzyme metabolism of theophylline. Risk: Moderate.

Warfarin: Interferons may increase the anticoagulant effects of warfarin; monitor.

Zidovudine: Interferons may decrease the metabolism of zidovudine; monitor.

Ethanol/Nutrition/Herb Interactions Ethanol: Avoid use in patients with hepatitis C virus.

Stability Prior to reconstitution, store Redipen™ at 2°C to 8°C (36°F to 46°F) and store vials at 15°C to 30°C (59°F to 86°F).

Redipen™: Hold cartridge upright and press the two halves together until there is a "click". Gently invert to mix; do not shake.

Vial: Add 0.7 mL of sterile water for injection, USP (supplied diluent) to the vial. Gently swirl. Do not re-enter vial after dose removed. Discard unused portion.

Once reconstituted each product should be used immediately or may be stored for ≤24 hours at 2°C to 8°C (36°F to 46°F); do not freeze. Products do not contain preservative.

Mechanism of Action Alpha interferons are a family of proteins, produced by nucleated cells, that have antiviral, antiproliferative, and immune-regulating activity. There are 16 known subtypes of alpha interferons. Interferons interact with cells through high affinity cell surface receptors. Following activation, multiple effects can be detected including induction of gene transcription. Inhibits cellular growth, alters the state of cellular differentiation, interferes with oncogene expression, alters cell surface antigen expression, increases phagocytic activity of macrophages, and augments cytotoxicity of lymphocytes for target cells.

Pharmacokinetics

Bioavailability: Increases with chronic dosing

Half-life: 40 hours
Time to peak: 15 to 44 hours
Elimination: Renal (30%)

Dosage

Geriatrics: May require dosage reduction based upon renal dysfunction, but no established guidelines are available.

Adults:

Chronic hepatitis C: SubQ: Administer dose once weekly; **Note:** Treatment duration may vary. Consult current guidelines and literature.

Monotherapy: Initial:

≤45 kg: 40 mcg
46-56 kg: 50 mcg
57-72 kg: 64 mcg
73-88 kg: 80 mcg
89-106 kg: 96 mcg
107-136 kg: 120 mcg
137-160 kg: 150 mcg

Combination therapy with ribavirin (400 mg twice daily): Initial: 1.5 mcg/kg/week

<40 kg: 50 mcg
40-50 kg: 64 mcg
51-60 kg: 80 mcg
61-75 kg: 96 mcg
76-85 kg: 120 mcg
>85 kg: 150 mcg

Dose adjustment if serious adverse event occurs: Depression (severity based upon DSM-IV criteria):

Mild depression: No dosage adjustment required; evaluate once weekly by visit/phone call. If depression remains stable, continue weekly visits. If depression improves, resume normal visit schedule.

Moderate depression: Decrease interferon dose by 50%; evaluate once weekly with an office visit at least every other week. If depression remains stable, consider psychiatric evaluation and continue with reduced dosing. If symptoms improve and remain stable for 4 weeks, resume normal visit schedule; continue reduced dosing or return to normal dose.

Severe depression: Discontinue interferon and ribavirin permanently. Obtain immediate psychiatric consultation.

Renal Impairment: Monitor for signs and symptoms of toxicity and if toxicity occurs then adjust dose. Do not use in patients with Cl_{cr} <50 mL/minute. Patients were excluded from the clinical trials if serum creatinine >1.5 times the upper limits of normal.

Hepatic Impairment: Contraindicated in decompensated liver disease

Administration For SubQ administration; rotate injection site

Monitoring Parameters Baseline and periodic TSH, hematology (including CBC with differential, platelets), and chemistry (including LFTs) testing. Evaluate for depression and other psychiatric symptoms before and after initiation of therapy; baseline eye examination in diabetic and hypertensive patients; baseline echocardiogram in patients with cardiac disease; serum HCV RNA levels after 24 weeks of treatment

Patient Information You may be taught to give yourself the injection if you are willing and able to learn. Blood work will be done before the start of this medicine and during its use. Other tests may be needed depending on your medical history. If you are diabetic or have high blood pressure, get an eye examination before starting treatment. Maintain adequate hydration (2-3 L/day of fluids unless instructed to restrict fluid intake). Avoid alcohol. You may experience flu-like syndrome (giving the medicine at bedtime or using acetaminophen may help), nausea and vomiting (frequent small meals, frequent mouth care, sucking lozenges, or chewing gum may help), feeling tired (use caution when driving or engaging in tasks requiring alertness until response to drug is known), or headache. Report persistent abdominal pain, bloody diarrhea, and fever; symptoms of depression, suicidal ideas; unusual bruising or bleeding, any signs or symptoms of infection, unusual fatigue, chest pain or palpitations, difficulty breathing, wheezing, severe nausea or vomiting.

Special Geriatric Considerations May require dosage reduction based upon renal dysfunction, but no established guidelines are available. Geriatric patients often have Cl_{cr} <50 mL/minute, as well as, many diseases that put them at risk for adverse effects with this agent. Calculation and measuring creatinine clearance must be done prior to initiating this drug.

Dosage Forms Excipient information presented when available (limited, particularly for generics); consult specific product labeling.

Injection, powder for reconstitution [prefilled syringe]:

PEG-Intron® Redipen®: 50 mcg, 80 mcg, 120 mcg, 150 mcg [contains polysorbate 80 and sucrose; packaged with alcohol swabs and needle for injection]

(Continued)

Peginterferon Alfa-2b (Continued)

Injection, powder for reconstitution [vial]:
PEG-Intron®: 50 mcg, 80 mcg, 120 mcg, 150 mcg [contains polysorbate 80 and sucrose; packaged with SWFI, alcohol swabs, and syringes]

Selected References

Heathcote EJ, Shiffman ML, Cooksley GE, et al, "Peginterferon Alfa-2a in Patients With Chronic Hepatitis C and Cirrhosis," *N Engl J Med*, 2000, 343(23):1673-80.

Zeuzem S, Feinman SV, Rasenack J, et al, "Peginterferon Alfa-2a in Patients With Chronic Hepatitis C," *N Engl J Med*, 2000, 343(23):1666-72.

♦ **PEG-Intron®** see Peginterferon Alfa-2b on page 1213

Pegvisomant (peg VI soe mant)

U.S. Brand Names Somavert®
Index Terms B2036-PEG
Generic Available No
Pharmacologic Category Growth Hormone Receptor Antagonist
Use Treatment of acromegaly in patients resistant to or unable to tolerate other therapies
Contraindications Hypersensitivity to polyethylene glycol or any component of the formulation
Warnings/Precautions Use caution with hepatic or renal disease, or in the elderly. Growth hormone (GH)-secreting tumor size and liver function should be carefully monitored. Interferes with commercially available GH assays; IGF-I levels not GH levels, should be used to adjust therapy. The manufacturer recommends the initial dose be administered under the supervision of prescribing healthcare provider.
Adverse Reactions (Reflective of adult population; not specific for elderly)
>10%:
  Central nervous system: Pain (4% to 14%; placebo: 6%)
  Gastrointestinal: Diarrhea (4% to 14%), nausea (8% to 14%)
  Hepatic: Liver function tests abnormal (4% to 12%)
  Local: Injection site reaction (4% to 11%)
  Miscellaneous: Infection (23%), non-neutralizing anti-GH antibodies (17%; relevance unknown), flu-like syndrome (4% to 12%)
1% to 10%:
  Cardiovascular: Hypertension (8%), chest pain (4% to 8%), peripheral edema (4% to 8%)
  Central nervous system: Dizziness (4% to 8%; placebo: 6%)
  Neuromuscular & skeletal: Back pain (4% to 8%), paresthesia (7%)
  Respiratory: Sinusitis (4% to 8%)
Overdosage/Toxicology No specific experience with overdose. Fatigue reported at a dose of 80 mg/day for 7 days. In case of overdose, discontinue until IGF-I levels return to normal.
Drug Interactions
  Hypoglycemic agents (insulin, oral agents): Pegvisomant may increase glucose tolerance; dose reduction of hypoglycemic agent may be needed.
  Opioids: Increased doses of pegvisomant may be needed.
Stability Store intact vials under refrigeration at 2°C to 8°C (36°F to 46°F); protect from freezing. Reconstitute with SWFI. Gently roll in order to dissolve powder; do not shake. Following reconstitution, use within 6 hours. Do not use solution if cloudy.
Mechanism of Action An analogue of human growth hormone, pegvisomant selectively binds to growth hormone (GH) receptors, blocking the binding of endogenous GH, leading to decreased serum concentrations of insulin-like growth factor-I (IGF-I) and other GH-responsive proteins. Pegvisomant is made up of a recombinant DNA protein covalently bound to polyethylene glycol (PEG) polymers.
Pharmacokinetics
  Absorption: 57%
  Distribution: 7 L
  Half-life: 6 days
  Time to peak, serum: 33-77 hours
  Elimination: Urine (<1%)
Dosage
  Geriatrics & Adults: Acromegaly: SubQ: Initial loading dose: 40 mg; maintenance dose: 10 mg once daily; doses may be adjusted by 5 mg in 4- to 6-week intervals based on IGF-I concentrations (maximum dose: 30 mg/day)
  Hepatic Impairment:
    Baseline liver function tests (LFT) >3 times ULN: Do not initiate treatment without comprehensive work-up to determine cause; monitor closely if treatment is started.
    LFT ≥3 times but <5 times ULN: Continue treatment, but monitor weekly if no signs or symptoms of hepatitis or liver injury; perform comprehensive hepatic work-up

LFT ≥5 times ULN or transaminase >3 times ULN associated with any increase in total bilirubin: Discontinue immediately and perform comprehensive hepatic work-up. If LFTs return to normal, may cautiously consider restarting therapy with frequent monitoring.

Signs or symptoms of hepatitis or hepatic injury: Evaluate liver function tests; discontinue if liver injury is confirmed

Administration For SubQ administration only; rotate injection site daily; may administer in upper arm, upper thigh, abdomen, or buttocks; do not rub injection site. The manufacturer recommends the initial dose be administered under the supervision of prescribing healthcare provider.

Monitoring Parameters GH-secreting tumor size, serum glucose, signs and symptoms of growth hormone deficiency, serum IGF-I (every 4-6 weeks after initial dose and dosage change, every 6 months when normalized)

Liver function tests:

Normal at baseline: Monthly for first 6 months, quarterly for next 6 months, biannually for the next year

Elevated, but ≤3 times ULN: Monitor monthly for at least 1 year, then biannually the next year

Test Interactions Interferes with measurement of serum GH concentrations by available GH assays.

Dosage Forms Excipient information presented when available (limited, particularly for generics); consult specific product labeling.

Injection, powder for reconstitution [preservative free]: 10 mg, 15 mg, 20 mg [vial stopper contains latex; packaged with SWFI]

♦ **Pegylated Interferon Alfa-2b** *see* Peginterferon Alfa-2b *on page 1213*

Penbutolol (pen BYOO toe lole)

Related Information
Beta-Blockers *on page 1751*
Medication Safety Issues
Sound-alike/look-alike issues:
Levatol® may be confused with Lipitor®

International issues:
Levatol® may be confused with Lovacol® which is a brand name for lovastatin in Chile, Finland, and France
U.S. Brand Names Levatol®
Canadian Brand Names Levatol®
Index Terms Penbutolol Sulfate
Generic Available No
Pharmacologic Category Beta Blocker With Intrinsic Sympathomimetic Activity
Use Treatment of mild to moderate arterial hypertension
Contraindications Hypersensitivity to penbutolol or any component of the formulation; uncompensated congestive heart failure; cardiogenic shock; bradycardia or heart block (except in patients with a functioning artificial pacemaker); sinus node dysfunction; asthma; bronchospastic disease; COPD; pulmonary edema
Warnings/Precautions Consider pre-existing conditions such as sick sinus syndrome before initiating. Beta-blocker therapy should not be withdrawn abruptly (particularly in patients with CAD), but gradually tapered to avoid acute tachycardia, hypertension, and/or ischemia. In general, patients with bronchospastic disease should not receive beta-blockers; if used at all, should be used cautiously with close monitoring. Use with caution in patients receiving anesthetic agents which decrease myocardial function. Use caution with concurrent use of beta-blockers and either verapamil or diltiazem; bradycardia or heart block can occur. Use caution in patients with PVD (can aggravate arterial insufficiency), psychiatric disease (may cause CNS depression), or myasthenia gravis. Use cautiously in patients with diabetes because it can mask prominent hypoglycemic symptoms. Beta-blockers with intrinsic sympathomimetic activity (including penbutolol) do not appear to be of benefit in CHF. Adequate alpha-blockade is required prior to use of any beta-blocker for patients with untreated pheochromocytoma.
Adverse Reactions (Reflective of adult population; not specific for elderly)
1% to 10%:
Cardiovascular: CHF, arrhythmia
Central nervous system: Mental depression, headache, dizziness, fatigue
Gastrointestinal: Nausea, diarrhea, dyspepsia
Neuromuscular & skeletal: Arthralgia
Drug Interactions
Alpha-blockers (prazosin, terazosin): Concurrent use of beta-blockers may increase risk of orthostasis.
Albuterol (and other beta$_2$ agonists): Effects may be blunted by nonspecific beta-blockers.
(Continued)

Penbutolol *(Continued)*

Clonidine: Hypertensive crisis after or during withdrawal of either agent.

Drugs which slow AV conduction (digoxin): Effects may be additive with beta-blockers.

Epinephrine (including local anesthetics with epinephrine): Penbutolol may cause hypertension.

Glucagon: Penbutolol may blunt the hyperglycemic action.

Insulin and oral hypoglycemics: May mask symptoms of hypoglycemia.

NSAIDs (ibuprofen, indomethacin, naproxen, piroxicam) may reduce the antihypertensive effects of beta-blockers.

Penbutolol masks the tachycardia that usually accompanies insulin-induced hypoglycemia.

Salicylates may reduce the antihypertensive effects of beta-blockers.

Sulfonylureas: Beta-blockers may alter response to hypoglycemic agents.

Verapamil or diltiazem may have synergistic or additive pharmacological effects when taken concurrently with beta-blockers.

Mechanism of Action Blocks both beta$_1$- and beta$_2$-receptors and has mild intrinsic sympathomimetic activity; has negative inotropic and chronotropic effects and can significantly slow AV nodal conduction

Pharmacokinetics

Absorption: Well absorbed, ~100%

Protein binding: 80% to 98%

Metabolism: Extensive in the liver (oxidation and conjugation)

Bioavailability: Oral: ~100%

Half-life: 5 hours

Elimination: Hepatic oxidation and conjugation with metabolites; excreted renally

Dosage

Geriatrics & Adults: Hypertension: Oral: Initial: 20 mg once daily, full effect of a 20 or 40 mg dose is seen by the end of a 2-week period, doses of 40-80 mg have been tolerated but have shown little additional antihypertensive effects; usual dose range (JNC 7): 10-40 mg once daily

Monitoring Parameters Blood pressure, orthostatic hypotension, heart rate, CNS effects

Patient Information Do not discontinue medication abruptly, sudden stopping of medication may precipitate or cause angina; consult pharmacist or physician before taking with other adrenergic drugs (eg, cold medications); notify physician if any of the following symptoms occur: difficult breathing, night cough, swelling of extremities, slow pulse, dizziness, lightheadedness, confusion, depression, skin rash, fever, sore throat, unusual bleeding or bruising; may produce drowsiness, dizziness, lightheadedness, blurred vision, confusion; use with caution while driving or performing tasks requiring alertness; may mask signs of hypoglycemia in diabetics; may be taken without regard to meals

Special Geriatric Considerations Due to alterations in the beta-adrenergic autonomic nervous system, beta-adrenergic blockade may result in less hemodynamic response than seen in younger adults. Studies indicate that despite decreased sensitivity to the chronotropic effects of beta-blockade with age, there appears to be an increased myocardial sensitivity to the negative inotropic effect during stress (ie, exercise). Controlled trials have shown the overall response rate for propranolol to be only 20% to 50% in elderly populations. Therefore, all beta-adrenergic blocking drugs may result in a decreased response as compared to younger adults.

Dosage Forms Excipient information presented when available (limited, particularly for generics); consult specific product labeling.

Tablet, as sulfate: 20 mg

Selected References

Chobanian AV, Bakris GL, Black HR, et al, "The Seventh Report of the Joint National Committee on Prevention, Detection, Evaluation, and Treatment of High Blood Pressure: The JNC 7 Report," *JAMA*, 2003, 289(19):2560-71.

♦ **Penbutolol Sulfate** *see* Penbutolol *on page 1217*

Penicillamine *(pen i SIL a meen)*

Medication Safety Issues

Sound-alike/look-alike issues:

Penicillamine may be confused with penicillin

Depen® may be confused with Endal®

International issues:

Depen® may be confused with Depon® which is a brand name for acetaminophen in Greece

Depen® may be confused with Dipen® which is a brand name for diltiazem in Greece

Pemine® [Italy] may be confused with Pamine® which is a brand name for methscopolamine in the U.S.

U.S. Brand Names Cuprimine®; Depen®

Canadian Brand Names Cuprimine®; Depen®

Index Terms β,β-Dimethylcysteine; D-3-Mercaptovaline; D-Penicillamine

Generic Available No

Pharmacologic Category Chelating Agent

Use Treatment of Wilson's disease, cystinuria; adjunctive treatment of rheumatoid arthritis

Unlabeled/Investigational Use Lead, mercury, copper, arsenic, and possibly gold poisoning (**Note:** Oral succimer [DMSA] is preferable for lead or mercury poisoning)

Contraindications Hypersensitivity to penicillamine or any component of the formulation; renal insufficiency (in patients with rheumatoid arthritis); patients with previous penicillamine-related aplastic anemia or agranulocytosis

Warnings/Precautions Cross-sensitivity with penicillin is possible; therefore, should be used cautiously in patients with a history of penicillin allergy. Once instituted for Wilson's disease or cystinuria, continue treatment on a daily basis; interruptions of even a few days have been followed by hypersensitivity with reinstitution of therapy. Penicillamine has been associated with fatalities due to agranulocytosis, aplastic anemia, thrombocytopenia, Goodpasture's syndrome, and myasthenia gravis. **[U.S. Boxed Warning]: Patients should be warned to report promptly any symptoms suggesting toxicity (fever, sore throat, chills, bruising, or bleeding);** approximately 33% of patients will experience an allergic reaction; toxicity may be dose related, use caution in the elderly. Use caution with other hematopoietic-depressant drugs (eg, gold, immunosuppressants, antimalarials, phenylbutazone); hematologic and renal adverse reactions are similar. Proteinuria or hematuria may develop; monitor for membranous glomerulopathy which can lead to nephrotic syndrome. In rheumatoid arthritis patients, discontinue if gross hematuria or persistent microscopic hematuria develop. Monitor liver function tests periodically due to rare reports of intrahepatic cholestasis or toxic hepatitis. **[U.S. Boxed Warning]: Should be administered under the close supervision of a physician familiar with the toxicity and dosage considerations.**

Adverse Reactions (Reflective of adult population; not specific for elderly) Frequency not defined, may vary by indication. Adverse effects requiring discontinuation of treatment have been reported in 20% to 30% of patients with Wilson's disease.

Cardiovascular: Vasculitis

Central nervous system: Anxiety, agitation, fever, hyperpyrexia, psychiatric disturbances; worsening neurologic symptoms (10% to 50% patients with Wilson's disease)

Dermatologic: Alopecia, cheilosis, dermatomyositis, exfoliative dermatitis, lichen planus, rash (early and late 5%), pemphigus, pruritus, skin friability increased, toxic epidermal necrolysis, urticaria, wrinkling (excessive), yellow nail syndrome

Endocrine & metabolic: Hypoglycemia, thyroiditis

Gastrointestinal: Anorexia, diarrhea (17%), epigastric pain, gingivostomatitis, glossitis, nausea, oral ulcerations, pancreatitis, peptic ulcer reactivation, taste alteration (12%), vomiting

Hematologic: Eosinophilia, hemolytic anemia, leukocytosis, leukopenia (2% to 5%), monocytosis, red cell aplasia, thrombocytopenia (4% to 5%), thrombotic thrombocytopenia purpura, thrombocytosis

Hepatic: Alkaline phosphatase increased, hepatic failure, intrahepatic cholestasis, toxic hepatitis

Local: Thrombophlebitis, white papules at venipuncture and surgical sites

Neuromuscular & skeletal: Arthralgia, dystonia, myasthenia gravis, muscle weakness, neuropathies, polyarthralgia (migratory, often with objective synovitis), polymyositis

Ocular: Diplopia, extraocular muscle weakness, optic neuritis, ptosis, visual disturbances

Otic: Tinnitus

Renal: Goodpasture's syndrome, hematuria, nephrotic syndrome, proteinuria (6%), renal failure, renal vasculitis

Respiratory: Asthma, interstitial pneumonitis, pulmonary fibrosis, obliterative bronchiolitis

Miscellaneous: Allergic alveolitis, anetoderma, elastosis perforans serpiginosa, lupus-like syndrome, lactic dehydrogenase increased, lymphadenopathy, mammary hyperplasia, positive ANA test

Overdosage/Toxicology Symptoms include nausea and vomiting. Following GI decontamination, treatment is supportive.

Drug Interactions

Antacids: May decrease the effects of penicillamine.

Digoxin: Penicillamine may decrease the levels of digoxin; monitor.

Iron salts: May decrease the effects of penicillamine.

Ethanol/Nutrition/Herb Interactions

Ethanol: Avoid or limit ethanol.

(Continued)

Penicillamine *(Continued)*

Food: Penicillamine serum levels may be decreased if taken with food. Do not administer with milk.

Stability Store in tight, well-closed containers.

Mechanism of Action Chelates with lead, copper, mercury and other heavy metals to form stable, soluble complexes that are excreted in urine; depresses circulating IgM rheumatoid factor, depresses T-cell but not B-cell activity; combines with cystine to form a compound which is more soluble, thus cystine calculi are prevented

Pharmacodynamics

Onset of action: Rheumatoid arthritis: 2-3 months; Wilson's disease: 1-3 months

Pharmacokinetics

Absorption: Oral: 40% to 70%

Protein binding: 80% bound to albumin

Half-life: 1.7-3.2 hours

Time to peak serum concentration: Within 1 hour

Elimination: Primarily (30% to 60%) in urine as unchanged drug with small amounts of hepatic metabolism

Dosage

Geriatrics & Adults:

Rheumatoid arthritis: Oral: 125-250 mg/day, may increase dose at 1- to 3-month intervals up to 1-1.5 g/day (maximum in older adults: 750 mg/day)

Wilson's disease: Oral: 250 mg 4 times/day (maximum in older adults: 750 mg/day). **Note:** Dose titrated to maintain urinary copper excretion >2 mg/day; decrease dose for surgery

Cystinuria: Note: Adjust dose to limit cystine excretion to 100-200 mg/day (<100 mg/day with history of stone formation): Oral: 1-4 g/day in divided doses every 6 hours; usual dose: 2 g/day

Lead poisoning (unlabeled use): Oral: 250-500 mg/dose every 8-12 hours. **Note:** In acute poisoning, continue until blood lead level is <15 mcg/dL; may also be used in other heavy metal poisoning.

Renal Impairment: Cl_{cr} <50 mL/minute: Avoid use.

Hemodialysis: Dialyzable; a dosing decrease from 250 mg/day to 250 mg 3 times/week after dialysis has been suggested in the treatment of rheumatoid arthritis.

Administration For patients who cannot swallow, contents of capsules may be administered in 15-30 mL of chilled puréed fruit or fruit juice. Give on an empty stomach (1 hour before meals and at bedtime).

Cystinuria: If administering 4 equal doses is not feasible, administer the larger dose at bedtime.

Rheumatoid arthritis: Doses ≤500 mg/day may be given as a single dose; >500 mg administer in divided doses

Monitoring Parameters Urinalysis, CBC with differential, platelet count, skin, lymph nodes, and body temperature twice weekly during the first month of therapy, then every 2 weeks for 5 months, then monthly; LFTs every 6 months

Cystinuria: Urinary cystine, annual X-ray for renal stones

Lead poisoning: Serum lead concentration

Wilson's disease: Serum copper, 24-hour urinary copper excretion, LFTs every 3 months during the first year of treatment

CBC: WBC <3500/mm³, neutrophils <2000/mm³, or monocytes >500/mm³ indicate need to stop therapy immediately; platelet counts <100,000/mm³ indicate need to stop therapy until numbers of platelets increase

Urinalysis: Monitor for proteinuria and hematuria. A quantitative 24-hour urine protein at 1- to 2-week intervals initially (first 2-3 months) is recommended if proteinuria develops; in patients with rheumatoid arthritis, discontinue or decrease dose with proteinuria >1 g/24 hours, progressively increasing proteinuria or hematuria.

Patient Information Take at least 1 hour before a meal; loss of taste may occur; probable severe allergic reaction if patient allergic to penicillin; report any signs of toxicity to physician; patients with cystinuria should drink copious amounts of water; report any unusual bleeding, bruising, persistent fever, fatigue, sore throat, shortness of breath

Additional Information Approximately 33% of patients will experience an allergic reaction

Special Geriatric Considerations Close monitoring of elderly is necessary; since steady-state serum/tissue concentrations rise slowly, "go slow" with dose increase intervals; steady-state concentrations decline slowly after discontinuation suggesting extensive tissue distribution. Skin rashes and taste abnormalities occur more frequently in the elderly than in young adults; leukopenia, thrombocytopenia, and proteinuria occur with equal frequency in both younger adults and elderly. Since toxicity may be dose related, it is recommended not to exceed 750 mg/day in the elderly.

Dosage Forms Excipient information presented when available (limited, particularly for generics); consult specific product labeling. [DSC] = Discontinued product

Capsule (Cuprimine®): 125 mg [DSC], 250 mg
Tablet (Depen®): 250 mg

Selected References

Roberts EA and Schilsky ML, "A Practice Guideline on Wilson Disease," *Hepatology*, 2003, 37(6):1475-92.

Stein HB, Patterson AC, Offer RC, et al, "Adverse Effects of D-Penicillamine in Rheumatoid Arthritis," *Ann Intern Med*, 1980, 92(1):24-9.

Swarup A, Sachdeva N, and Schumacher Jr HP, "Dosing of Antirheumatic Drugs in Renal Disease and Dialysis," *J Clin Rheumatol*, 2004, 10(4):190-204.

Penicillin G Benzathine (pen i SIL in jee BENZ a theen)

Related Information
Antimicrobial Activity Against Selected Organisms *on page 1728*

Medication Safety Issues
Sound-alike/look-alike issues:

Penicillin may be confused with penicillamine

Bicillin® may be confused with Wycillin®

Bicillin® C-R (penicillin G benzathine and penicillin G procaine) may be confused with Bicillin® L-A (penicillin G benzathine). Penicillin G benzathine is the only product currently approved for the treatment of syphilis. Administration of penicillin G benzathine and penicillin G procaine combination instead of Bicillin® L-A may result in inadequate treatment response.

Penicillin G benzathine may only be administered by deep intramuscular injection; intravenous administration of penicillin G benzathine has been associated with cardiopulmonary arrest and death.

U.S. Brand Names Bicillin® L-A

Canadian Brand Names Bicillin® L-A

Index Terms Benzathine Benzylpenicillin; Benzathine Penicillin G; Benzylpenicillin Benzathine

Generic Available No

Pharmacologic Category Antibiotic, Penicillin

Use Active against most gram-positive organisms; some gram-negative organisms such as *Neisseria gonorrhoeae* and some anaerobes and spirochetes; used only for the treatment of mild to moderately severe infections caused by organisms susceptible to low concentrations of penicillin G, or for prophylaxis of infections caused by these organisms

Contraindications Hypersensitivity to penicillin or any component of the formulation

Warnings/Precautions Use with caution in patients with impaired renal function, seizure disorder, or history of hypersensitivity to other beta-lactams; CDC and AAP do not currently recommend the use of penicillin G benzathine to treat congenital syphilis or neurosyphilis due to reported treatment failures and lack of published clinical data on its efficacy. Prolonged use may result in fungal or bacterial superinfection, including *C. difficile*-associated diarrhea and pseudomembranous colitis. Extended duration of therapy or use associated with high serum concentrations may be associated with an increased risk for some adverse reactions.

Adverse Reactions (Reflective of adult population; not specific for elderly)
Frequency not defined.

Central nervous system: Convulsions, confusion, drowsiness, myoclonus, fever

Dermatologic: Rash

Endocrine & metabolic: Electrolyte imbalance

Hematologic: Positive Coombs' reaction, hemolytic anemia

Local: Pain, thrombophlebitis

Renal: Acute interstitial nephritis

Miscellaneous: Anaphylaxis, hypersensitivity reactions, Jarisch-Herxheimer reaction

Overdosage/Toxicology Symptoms of penicillin overdose include neuromuscular hypersensitivity (agitation, hallucinations, asterixis, encephalopathy, confusion, seizures) and electrolyte imbalance with potassium or sodium salts, especially in renal failure. Hemodialysis may be helpful to aid in removal of the drug from the blood, otherwise, most treatment is supportive or symptom-directed.

Drug Interactions
Aminoglycosides: May be synergistic against selected organisms

Fusidic acid: May decrease the therapeutic effect of penicillins; administer the penicillin at least 2 hours before fusidic acid.

Heparin: Heparin and parenteral penicillins may result in increased bleeding

Methotrexate: Penicillins may increase the exposure to methotrexate during concurrent therapy; monitor.

Oral contraceptives: Anecdotal reports suggesting decreased contraceptive efficacy with penicillins have been refuted by more rigorous scientific and clinical data.

Probenecid, disulfiram: May increase penicillin levels

Tetracyclines: May decrease penicillin effectiveness

Warfarin: Effects of warfarin may be increased

(Continued)

Penicillin G Benzathine *(Continued)*

Stability Refrigerate

Mechanism of Action Interferes with bacterial cell wall synthesis during active multiplication, causing cell wall death and resultant bactericidal activity against susceptible bacteria

Pharmacokinetics

Absorption: I.M.: Slow

Time to peak serum concentration: Within 12-24 hours; serum concentrations are usually detectable for 1-4 weeks depending on the dose; larger doses result in more sustained concentrations rather than higher concentrations; following equal, simple I.M. injections, older adults have serum penicillin concentrations approximately twice that of younger adults 48, 96, and 144 hours postadministration

Dosage

Geriatrics & Adults: Note: Not indicated as single drug therapy for neurosyphilis, but may be given 1 time/week for 3 weeks following I.V. treatment (refer to Penicillin G monograph for dosing)

Group A streptococcal upper respiratory infection: I.M.: 1.2 million units as a single dose

Prophylaxis of recurrent rheumatic fever: I.M.: 1.2 million units every 3-4 weeks or 600,000 units twice monthly

Syphilis:

Early: I.M.: 2.4 million units as a single dose in 2 injection sites

More than 1-year duration: I.M.: 2.4 million units in 2 injection sites once weekly for 3 doses

Neurosyphilis: Not indicated as single-drug therapy, but may be given once weekly for 3 weeks following I.V. treatment; refer to Penicillin G Parenteral/Aqueous monograph for dosing

Administration I.M. Administer undiluted injection by deep injection in the upper outer quadrant of the buttock do **not** administer I.V., intra-arterially, or SubQ

Monitoring Parameters Signs and symptoms of infection

Test Interactions Positive Coombs' [direct], false-positive urinary and/or serum proteins; false-positive or negative urinary glucose using Clinitest®

Additional Information A single dose of 600,000 to 1,200,000 units is effective in the prevention of rheumatic fever secondary to streptococcal pharyngitis; used when patient cannot be kept in a hospital environment and neurosyphilis has been ruled out

Special Geriatric Considerations Not indicated as single drug therapy for neurosyphilis, but may be given 1 time/week for 3 weeks following I.V. treatment with Penicillin G (Parenteral/Aqueous). No adjustment for renal function or age is necessary.

Dosage Forms Excipient information presented when available (limited, particularly for generics); consult specific product labeling.

Injection, suspension [prefilled syringe]: 600,000 units/mL (1 mL, 2 mL, 4 mL)

Selected References

Collart P, Poitevin M, Milovanovic A, et al, "Kinetic Study of Serum Penicillin Concentrations After Single Doses of Benzathine and Benethamine Penicillins in Young and Old People," *Br J Vener Dis*, 1980, 56(6):355-62.

WHO Study Group, "Rheumatic Fever and Rheumatic Heart Disease," *World Health Organ Tech Rep Ser*, 1988, 764:1-58.

Penicillin G Benzathine and Penicillin G Procaine
(pen i SIL in jee BENZ a theen & pen i SIL in jee PROE kane)

Related Information

Antimicrobial Activity Against Selected Organisms *on page 1728*
Penicillin G Benzathine *on page 1221*
Penicillin G Procaine *on page 1226*

Medication Safety Issues

Bicillin® C-R (penicillin G benzathine and penicillin G procaine) may be confused with Bicillin® L-A (penicillin G benzathine). Penicillin G benzathine is the only product currently approved for the treatment of syphilis. Administration of penicillin G benzathine and penicillin G procaine combination instead of Bicillin® L-A may result in inadequate treatment response.

Penicillin G benzathine may only be administered by deep intramuscular injection; intravenous administration of penicillin G benzathine has been associated with cardiopulmonary arrest and death.

Sound-alike/look-alike issues:

Penicillin may be confused with penicillamine

Bicillin® may be confused with Wycillin®

U.S. Brand Names Bicillin® C-R; Bicillin® C-R 900/300

Index Terms Penicillin G Procaine and Benzathine Combined

Generic Available No

Pharmacologic Category Antibiotic, Penicillin

Use Active against most gram-positive organisms; some gram-negative such as *Neisseria gonorrhoeae* and some anaerobes and spirochetes

Contraindications Hypersensitivity to penicillin or any component of the formulation

Warnings/Precautions Use with caution in patients with impaired renal function. Serious and occasionally severe or fatal hypersensitivity (anaphylactoid) reactions have been reported in patients on penicillin therapy, especially with a history of beta-lactam hypersensitivity, history of sensitivity to multiple allergens, or previous IgE-mediated reactions (eg, anaphylaxis, angioedema, urticaria). Use with caution in asthmatic patients. Prolonged use may result in fungal or bacterial superinfection, including *C. difficile*-associated diarrhea and pseudomembranous colitis. **[U.S. Boxed Warning]: Not for intravenous use; cardiopulmonary arrest and death have occurred from inadvertent I.V. administration.** Extended duration of therapy or use associated with high serum concentrations may be associated with an increased risk for some adverse reactions.

Adverse Reactions (Reflective of adult population; not specific for elderly) Frequency not defined.

Central nervous system: CNS toxicity (convulsions, confusion, drowsiness, myoclonus)

Hematologic: Positive Coombs' reaction, hemolytic anemia

Renal: Interstitial nephritis

Miscellaneous: Hypersensitivity reactions, Jarisch-Herxheimer reaction

Overdosage/Toxicology Many beta-lactam-containing antibiotics have the potential to cause neuromuscular hyperirritability or convulsive seizures. Hemodialysis may be helpful to aid in removal of the drug from the blood, otherwise, most treatment is supportive or symptom-directed.

Drug Interactions

Aminoglycosides: May be synergistic against selected organisms

Fusidic acid: May decrease the therapeutic effect of penicillins; administer the penicillin at least 2 hours before fusidic acid.

Methotrexate: Penicillins may increase the exposure to methotrexate during concurrent therapy; monitor.

Oral contraceptives: Anecdotal reports suggesting decreased contraceptive efficacy with penicillins have been refuted by more rigorous scientific and clinical data.

Probenecid, disulfiram: May increase penicillin levels

Tetracyclines: May decrease penicillin effectiveness

Warfarin: Effects of warfarin may be increased

Stability Refrigerate

Mechanism of Action Inhibits bacterial cell wall synthesis by binding to one or more of the penicillin binding proteins (PBPs); which in turn inhibits the final transpeptidation step of peptidoglycan synthesis in bacterial cell walls, thus inhibiting cell wall biosynthesis. Bacteria eventually lyse due to ongoing activity of cell wall autolytic enzymes (autolysins and murein hydrolases) while cell wall assembly is arrested.

Dosage

Geriatrics & Adults: Streptococcal infections: I.M.: 2.4 million units in a single dose

Administration Administer by deep I.M. injection in the upper outer quadrant of the buttock do **not** administer I.V., intravascularly, or intra-arterially

Test Interactions May interfere with urinary glucose tests using cupric sulfate (Benedict's solution, Clinitest®); may inactivate aminoglycosides *in vitro*; positive Coombs' [direct], increased protein

Special Geriatric Considerations No adjustment for renal function or age is necessary.

Dosage Forms Excipient information presented when available (limited, particularly for generics); consult specific product labeling.

Injection, suspension [prefilled syringe]:

Bicillin® C-R:

600,000 units: Penicillin G benzathine 300,000 units and penicillin G procaine 300,000 units per 1 mL (1 mL)

1,200,000 units: Penicillin G benzathine 600,000 units and penicillin G procaine 600,000 units per 2 mL (2 mL)

2,400,000 units: Penicillin G benzathine 1,200,000 units and penicillin G procaine 1,200,000 units per 4 mL (4 mL)

Bicillin® C-R 900/300: 1,200,000 units: Penicillin G benzathine 900,000 units and penicillin G procaine 300,000 units per 2 mL (2 mL)

Penicillin G (Parenteral/Aqueous)
(pen i SIL in jee, pa REN ter al, AYE kwee us)

Related Information
Antibiotic Treatment of Adults With Infective Endocarditis *on page 1797*
Antimicrobial Activity Against Selected Organisms *on page 1728*

Medication Safety Issues
Sound-alike/look-alike issues:
Penicillin may be confused with penicillamine

U.S. Brand Names Pfizerpen®

Canadian Brand Names Pfizerpen®

Index Terms Benzylpenicillin Potassium; Benzylpenicillin Sodium; Crystalline Penicillin; Penicillin G Potassium; Penicillin G Sodium

Generic Available Yes

Pharmacologic Category Antibiotic, Penicillin

Use Active against most gram-positive organisms except *Staphylococcus aureus*; some gram-negative such as *Neisseria gonorrhoeae* and some anaerobes and spirochetes; although ceftriaxone is now the drug of choice for lyme disease and gonorrhea

Contraindications Hypersensitivity to penicillin or any component of the formulation

Warnings/Precautions Avoid intra-arterial administration or injection into or near major peripheral nerves or blood vessels since such injections may cause severe and/ or permanent neurovascular damage; use with caution in patients with renal impairment (dosage reduction required), pre-existing seizure disorders, or with a history of hypersensitivity to cephalosporins. Prolonged use may result in fungal or bacterial superinfection, including *C. difficile*-associated diarrhea and pseudomembranous colitis. Serious and occasionally severe or fatal hypersensitivity (anaphylactoid) reactions have been reported in patients on penicillin therapy, especially with a history of beta-lactam hypersensitivity, history of sensitivity to multiple allergens, or previous IgE-mediated reactions (eg, anaphylaxis, angioedema, urticaria). Use with caution in asthmatic patients. Extended duration of therapy or use associated with high serum concentrations may be associated with an increased risk for some adverse reactions.

Adverse Reactions (Reflective of adult population; not specific for elderly)
Frequency not defined.
Central nervous system: Convulsions, confusion, drowsiness, myoclonus, fever
Dermatologic: Rash
Endocrine & metabolic: Electrolyte imbalance
Hematologic: Positive Coombs' reaction, hemolytic anemia
Local: Injection site reaction, thrombophlebitis
Renal: Acute interstitial nephritis
Miscellaneous: Anaphylaxis, hypersensitivity reactions, Jarisch-Herxheimer reaction

Overdosage/Toxicology Symptoms of penicillin overdose include neuromuscular hypersensitivity (agitation, hallucinations, asterixis, encephalopathy, confusion, seizures) and electrolyte imbalance with potassium or sodium salts, especially in renal failure. Hemodialysis may be helpful to aid in removal of the drug from the blood, otherwise, most treatment is supportive or symptom-directed.

Drug Interactions
Aminoglycosides: May be synergistic against selected organisms
Fusidic acid: May decrease the therapeutic effect of penicillins; administer the penicillin at least 2 hours before fusidic acid.
Methotrexate: Penicillins may increase the exposure to methotrexate during concurrent therapy; monitor.
Oral contraceptives: Anecdotal reports suggesting decreased contraceptive efficacy with penicillins have been refuted by more rigorous scientific and clinical data.
Probenecid, disulfiram: May increase penicillin levels
Tetracyclines: May decrease penicillin effectiveness
Warfarin: Effects of warfarin may be increased

Stability
Penicillin G potassium powder for injection should be stored below 86°F (30°C). Following reconstitution, solution may be stored for up to 7 days under refrigeration. Premixed bags for infusion should be stored in the freezer (-20°C to -4°F); frozen bags may be thawed at room temperature or in refrigerator. Once thawed, solution is stable for 14 days if stored in refrigerator or for 24 hours when stored at room temperature. Do not refreeze once thawed.
Penicillin G sodium powder for injection should be stored at controlled room temperature. Reconstituted solution may be stored under refrigeration for up to 3 days.

Mechanism of Action Interferes with bacterial cell wall synthesis during active multiplication, causing cell wall death and resultant bactericidal activity against susceptible bacteria

Pharmacokinetics

Distribution: Penetration across the blood-brain barrier is poor, despite inflamed meninges

Protein binding: 65%

Metabolism: In the liver (30%) to penicilloic acid

Half-life: 20-50 minutes; prolonged half-life reported in some older adults (~1 hour) compared to younger subjects presumably due to decreased renal function

Time to peak serum concentration: I.V.: Within 1 hour

Elimination: In urine

Dosage

Geriatrics & Adults:

***Actinomyces* species:** I.V.: 10-20 million units/day divided every 4-6 hours for 4-6 weeks

Anthrax (cutaneous): I.V.: 2 million units every 3 hours for 5-7 days

Clostridium perfringens: I.V.: 24 million units/day divided every 4-6 hours with clindamycin

Corynebacterium diptheriae: I.V.: 25,000-50,000 units/kg to maximum 1.2 million units every 12 hours, until oral therapy tolerated

Erysipelas: I.V.: 1-2 million units every 4-6 hours

Erysipelothrix: I.V.: 2-4 million units every 4 hours

Fascial space infections: I.V.: 2-4 million units every 4-6 hours with metronidazole

Leptospirosis: I.V.: 1.5 million units every 6 hours for 7 days

Listeria: I.V.: 300,000 units/kg/day every 4 hours

Lyme disease (meningitis): I.V.: 20 million units/day in divided doses

Neurosyphilis: I.M., I.V.: 18-24 million units/day in divided doses every 4 hours (or by continuous infusion) for 10-14 days

Streptococcus:

Brain abscess: I.V.: 20-24 million units/day in divided doses with metronidazole

Endocarditis or osteomyelitis: I.V.: 3-4 million units every 4 hours for at least 4 weeks

Meningitis: I.V.: 3-4 million units every 4 hours for 2-3 weeks

Skin and soft tissue: I.V.: 3-4 million units every 4 hours for 10 days

Toxic shock: I.V.: 24 million units/day in divided doses with clindamycin

Streptococcal pneumonia:

Meningitis: I.V.: 2-4 million units every 2-4 hours

Nonmeningitis: I.V.: 2-3 million units every 4 hours

Whipple's disease: I.V.: 2 million units every 4 hours (with streptomycin) for 10-14 days, followed by oral trimethoprim/sulfamethoxazole or doxycycline for 1 year

Renal Impairment: Dosage modification is required in patients with renal insufficiency.

Cl_{cr} >10 mL/minute: Administer full loading dose followed by $^{1}/_{2}$ loading dose given every 4-5 hours

Cl_{cr} <10 mL/minute: Administer full loading dose followed by $^{1}/_{2}$ loading dose given every 8-10 hours

Monitoring Parameters Fever, mental status, WBC count, appetite

Test Interactions False-positive or negative urinary glucose determination using Clinitest®; positive Coombs' [direct]; false-positive urinary and/or serum proteins

Patient Information Complete full course of treatment; notify physician if rash, itching, hives, diarrhea, or any other unusual finding

Additional Information 1 million units is approximately equal to 625 mg.

Special Geriatric Considerations Despite a reported prolonged half-life, it is usually not necessary to adjust the dose of penicillin G or VK in elderly to account for renal function changes with age, however, it is advised to calculate an estimated creatinine clearance and adjust dose accordingly.

Dosage Forms Excipient information presented when available (limited, particularly for generics); consult specific product labeling.

Infusion, as potassium [premixed iso-osmotic dextrose solution, frozen]: 1 million units (50 mL), 2 million units (50 mL), 3 million units (50 mL) [contains sodium 1.02 mEq and potassium 1.7 mEq per 1 million units]

Injection, powder for reconstitution, as potassium (Pfizerpen®): 5 million units, 20 million units [contains sodium 6.8 mg (0.3 mEq) and potassium 65.6 mg (1.68 mEq) per 1 million units]

Injection, powder for reconstitution, as sodium: 5 million units [contains sodium 1.68 mEq per 1 million units]

Selected References

Centers for Disease Control and Prevention, "Sexually Transmitted Diseases Treatment Guidelines - 2002," *MMWR Recomm Rep*, 2002, 51(RR-6):1-78. Available at: http://www.cdc.gov/mmwr/preview/mmwrhtml/rr5106a1.htm.

Hansen JM, Kampmann J, and Laursen H, "Renal Excretion of Drugs in the Elderly," *Lancet*, 1970, 1(657):1170.

Leikola E and Vartia KO, "On Penicillin Levels in Young and Geriatric Subjects," *J Gerontol*, 1957, 12:48-52.

Yoshikawa TT, "Antimicrobial Therapy for the Elderly Patient," *J Am Geriatr Soc*, 1990, 38(12):1353-72.

◆ **Penicillin G Potassium** *see* Penicillin G (Parenteral/Aqueous) *on page 1224*

Penicillin G Procaine (pen i SIL in jee PROE kane)

Related Information
Antimicrobial Activity Against Selected Organisms *on page 1728*

Medication Safety Issues
Sound-alike/look-alike issues:
Penicillin G procaine may be confused with penicillin V potassium
Wycillin® may be confused with Bicillin®

Canadian Brand Names Pfizerpen-AS®; Wycillin®

Index Terms APPG; Aqueous Procaine Penicillin G; Procaine Benzylpenicillin; Procaine Penicillin G; Wycillin [DSC]

Generic Available Yes

Pharmacologic Category Antibiotic, Penicillin

Use Moderately severe infections due to *Treponema pallidum* and other penicillin G-sensitive microorganisms that are susceptible to low, but prolonged serum penicillin concentrations; anthrax due to *Bacillus anthracis* (postexposure) to reduce the incidence or progression of disease following exposure to aerolized *Bacillus anthracis*

Contraindications Hypersensitivity to penicillin, procaine, or any component of the formulation

Warnings/Precautions May need to modify dosage in patients with severe renal impairment or seizure disorders; avoid I.V., intravascular, or intra-arterial administration of penicillin G procaine since severe and/or permanent neurovascular damage may occur. Serious and occasionally severe or fatal hypersensitivity (anaphylactoid) reactions have been reported in patients on penicillin therapy, especially with a history of beta-lactam hypersensitivity, history of sensitivity to multiple allergens, or previous IgE-mediated reactions (eg, anaphylaxis, angioedema, urticaria). Use with caution in asthmatic patients. Extended duration of therapy or use associated with high serum concentrations may be associated with an increased risk for some adverse reactions. Prolonged use may result in fungal or bacterial superinfection, including *C. difficile*-associated diarrhea and pseudomembranous colitis.

Adverse Reactions (Reflective of adult population; not specific for elderly)
Frequency not defined.
Cardiovascular: Myocardial depression, vasodilation, conduction disturbances
Central nervous system: Confusion, drowsiness, myoclonus, CNS stimulation, seizure
Hematologic: Positive Coombs' reaction, hemolytic anemia, neutropenia
Local: Pain at injection site, thrombophlebitis, sterile abscess at injection site
Renal: Interstitial nephritis
Miscellaneous: Pseudoanaphylactic reactions, hypersensitivity reactions, Jarisch-Herxheimer reaction, serum sickness

Overdosage/Toxicology Symptoms of penicillin overdose include neuromuscular hypersensitivity (agitation, hallucinations, asterixis, encephalopathy, confusion, seizures) and electrolyte imbalance with potassium or sodium salts, especially in renal failure. Hemodialysis may be helpful to aid in removal of the drug from the blood, otherwise, most treatment is supportive or symptom-directed.

Drug Interactions
Aminoglycosides: May be synergistic against selected organisms
Fusidic acid: May decrease the therapeutic effect of penicillins; administer the penicillin at least 2 hours before fusidic acid.
Methotrexate: Penicillins may increase the exposure to methotrexate during concurrent therapy; monitor.
Oral contraceptives: Anecdotal reports suggesting decreased contraceptive efficacy with penicillins have been refuted by more rigorous scientific and clinical data.
Probenecid, disulfiram: May increase penicillin levels
Tetracyclines: May decrease penicillin effectiveness
Warfarin: Effects of warfarin may be increased

Stability Refrigerate

Mechanism of Action Inhibits bacterial cell wall synthesis by binding to one or more of the penicillin binding proteins (PBPs); which in turn inhibits the final transpeptidation step of peptidoglycan synthesis in bacterial cell walls, thus inhibiting cell wall biosynthesis. Bacteria eventually lyse due to ongoing activity of cell wall autolytic enzymes (autolysins and murein hydrolases) while cell wall assembly is arrested.

Pharmacokinetics
Absorption: I.M.: Slow
Distribution: Penetration across the blood-brain barrier is poor, despite inflamed meninges
Protein binding: 65%
Half-life: 20-50 minutes
Time to peak serum concentration: Within 1-4 hours and can persist within the therapeutic range for 15-24 hours

Elimination: 60% to 90% of drug is excreted unchanged via renal tubular excretion; ~30% of dose inactivated in the liver

Renal clearance is delayed in patients with impaired renal function

Dosage

Geriatrics & Adults:

Anthrax:

Inhalational (postexposure prophylaxis): I.M.: 1,200,000 units every 12 hours

Note: Overall treatment duration should be 60 days. Available safety data suggest continued administration of penicillin G procaine for longer than 2 weeks may incur additional risk of adverse reactions. Clinicians may consider switching to effective alternative treatment for completion of therapy beyond 2 weeks.

Cutaneous (treatment): I.M.: 600,000-1,200,000 units/day; alternative therapy is recommended in severe cutaneous or other forms of anthrax infection

Endocarditis caused by susceptible viridans *Streptococcus* (when used in conjunction with an aminoglycoside): I.M.: 1.2 million units every 6 hours for 2-4 weeks

Gonorrhea (uncomplicated): 4.8 million units as a single dose divided in 2 sites given 30 minutes after probenecid 1 g orally

Neurosyphilis: I.M.: 2.4 million units/day with 500 mg probenecid by mouth 4 times/day for 10-14 days; **penicillin G aqueous I.V. is the preferred agent**

Whipple's disease: I.M.: 1.2 million units/day (with streptomycin) for 10-14 days, followed by oral trimethoprim/sulfamethoxazole or doxycycline for 1 year

Renal Impairment:

Cl_{cr} 10-30 mL/minute: Administer every 8-12 hours.

Cl_{cr} <10 mL/minute: Administer every 12-18 hours.

Moderately dialyzable (20% to 50%)

Administration Procaine suspension for deep I.M. injection only; administer around-the-clock rather than 4 times/day, 3 times/day, etc (ie, 12-6-12-6, not 9-1-5-9) to promote less variation in peak and trough serum concentrations; when doses are repeated, rotate the injection site; avoid I.V., intravascular, or intra-arterial administration of penicillin G procaine since severe and/or permanent neurovascular damage may occur; renal and hematologic systems should be evaluated periodically during prolonged therapy

Monitoring Parameters Fever, mental status, WBC count, appetite

Test Interactions Positive Coombs' [direct], false-positive urinary and/or serum proteins

Patient Information Notify physician if skin rash, itching, hives or severe diarrhea occurs; complete full course of therapy

Special Geriatric Considerations Dosage does not usually need to be adjusted in the elderly, however, if multiple doses are to be given, adjust dose for renal function.

Dosage Forms Excipient information presented when available (limited, particularly for generics); consult specific product labeling.

Injection, suspension: 600,000 units/mL (1 mL, 2 mL)

Selected References

Yoshikawa TT, "Antimicrobial Therapy for the Elderly Patient," *J Am Geriatr Soc*, 1990, 38(12):1353-72.

♦ **Penicillin G Procaine and Benzathine Combined** *see* Penicillin G Benzathine and Penicillin G Procaine *on page 1222*

♦ **Penicillin G Sodium** *see* Penicillin G (Parenteral/Aqueous) *on page 1224*

Penicillin V Potassium (pen i SIL in vee poe TASS ee um)

Related Information

Antimicrobial Activity Against Selected Organisms *on page 1728*

Medication Safety Issues

Sound-alike/look-alike issues:

Penicillin V procaine may be confused with penicillin G potassium

Canadian Brand Names Apo-Pen VK®; Novo-Pen-VK; Nu-Pen-VK

Index Terms Pen VK; Phenoxymethyl Penicillin

Generic Available Yes

Pharmacologic Category Antibiotic, Penicillin

Use Treatment of moderate to severe susceptible bacterial infections; no longer recommended for dental procedure prophylaxis; prophylaxis in rheumatic fever; infections caused by susceptible organisms involving the respiratory tract, otitis media, sinusitis, skin, and urinary tract

Contraindications Hypersensitivity to penicillin or any component of the formulation

Warnings/Precautions Use with caution in patients with severe renal impairment (modify dosage) or history of seizures. Serious and occasionally severe or fatal hypersensitivity (anaphylactoid) reactions have been reported in patients on penicillin therapy, especially with a history of beta-lactam hypersensitivity, history of sensitivity to

(Continued)

Penicillin V Potassium *(Continued)*

multiple allergens, or previous IgE-mediated reactions (eg, anaphylaxis, angioedema, urticaria). Use with caution in asthmatic patients. Extended duration of therapy or use associated with high serum concentrations may be associated with an increased risk for some adverse reactions. Prolonged use may result in fungal or bacterial superinfection, including *C. difficile*-associated diarrhea and pseudomembranous colitis.

Adverse Reactions (Reflective of adult population; not specific for elderly)
>10%: Gastrointestinal: Mild diarrhea, vomiting, nausea, oral candidiasis

Overdosage/Toxicology Symptoms of penicillin overdose include neuromuscular hypersensitivity (agitation, hallucinations, asterixis, encephalopathy, confusion, seizures) and electrolyte imbalance with potassium or sodium salts, especially in renal failure. Hemodialysis may be helpful to aid in removal of the drug from the blood, otherwise, most treatment is supportive or symptom-directed.

Drug Interactions
Aminoglycosides: May be synergistic against selected organisms
Fusidic acid: May decrease the therapeutic effect of penicillins; administer the penicillin at least 2 hours before fusidic acid.
Methotrexate: Penicillins may increase the exposure to methotrexate during concurrent therapy; monitor.
Oral contraceptives: Anecdotal reports suggesting decreased contraceptive efficacy with penicillins have been refuted by more rigorous scientific and clinical data.
Probenecid, disulfiram: May increase penicillin levels
Tetracyclines: May decrease penicillin effectiveness
Warfarin: Effects of warfarin may be increased

Ethanol/Nutrition/Herb Interactions Food: Decreases drug absorption rate; decreases drug serum concentration.

Stability Refrigerate suspension after reconstitution; discard after 14 days

Mechanism of Action Inhibits bacterial cell wall synthesis by binding to one or more of the penicillin binding proteins (PBPs); which in turn inhibits the final transpeptidation step of peptidoglycan synthesis in bacterial cell walls, thus inhibiting cell wall biosynthesis. Bacteria eventually lyse due to ongoing activity of cell wall autolytic enzymes (autolysins and murein hydrolases) while cell wall assembly is arrested.

Pharmacokinetics
Absorption: Oral: 60% to 73% from GI tract
Protein binding: 80%
Half-life: 30 minutes, prolonged in patients with renal impairment
Time to peak serum concentration: Oral: Within 30-60 minutes
Elimination: Penicillin V and its metabolites are excreted in urine mainly by tubular secretion

Dosage
Geriatrics & Adults:
Acintomycosis:
Mild: 2-4 g/day in 4 divided doses for 8 weeks
Surgical: 2-4 g/day in 4 divided doses for 6-12 months (after I.V. penicillin G therapy of 4-6 weeks)
Erysipelas: 500 mg 4 times/day
Pharyngitis (streptococcal): 500 mg 3-4 times/day for 10 days
Prophylaxis of pneumococcal or recurrent rheumatic fever infections: 250 mg twice daily
Renal Impairment:
Cl_{cr} 10-50 mL/minute: Administer every 8-12 hours.
Cl_{cr} <10 mL/minute: Administer every 12-16 hours.

Administration Administer on an empty stomach (ie, 1 hour prior to, or 2 hours after meals) to increase total absorption; administer around-the-clock rather than 4 times/day, 3 times/day, etc (ie, 12-6-12-6, not 9-1-5-9) to promote less variation in peak and trough serum concentrations

Monitoring Parameters Fever, WBC count, mental status, appetite

Test Interactions False-positive or negative urinary glucose determination using Clinitest®; positive Coombs' [direct]; false-positive urinary and/or serum proteins

Patient Information Take on an empty stomach 1 hour before or 2 hours after meals; complete full course of therapy, do not skip doses

Additional Information 0.7 mEq of potassium per 250 mg penicillin V; 250 mg equals 400,000 units of penicillin); each gram contains 2.6 mEq of potassium

Special Geriatric Considerations Dosage adjustment in the elderly is usually not necessary.

Dosage Forms Excipient information presented when available (limited, particularly for generics); consult specific product labeling.
Note: 250 mg = 400,000 units
Powder for oral solution: 125 mg/5 mL (100 mL, 200 mL); 250 mg/5 mL (100 mL, 200 mL)
Tablet: 250 mg, 500 mg

♦ **Penlac**® *see* Ciclopirox *on page 311*
♦ **Pentasa**® *see* Mesalamine *on page 989*

Pentazocine (pen TAZ oh seen)

Related Information
Narcotic / Opioid Analgesics *on page 1763*
Potentially Inappropriate Medications for Geriatrics *on page 1824*
U.S. Brand Names Talwin®; Talwin® NX

Canadian Brand Names Talwin®

Index Terms Naloxone Hydrochloride and Pentazocine Hydrochloride; Pentazocine Hydrochloride; Pentazocine Hydrochloride and Naloxone Hydrochloride; Pentazocine Lactate

Generic Available Yes: Tablet

Pharmacologic Category Analgesic, Opioid

Use Relief of moderate to severe pain; preoperative sedative; supplement to surgical anesthesia

Restrictions C-IV

Contraindications Hypersensitivity to pentazocine, naloxone, or any component of the formulation; increased intracranial pressure (unless the patient is mechanically ventilated)

Warnings/Precautions May cause CNS depression, which may impair physical or mental abilities; patients must be cautioned about performing tasks which require mental alertness (eg, operating machinery or driving). Effects may be potentiated when used with other sedative drugs or ethanol. Use with caution in seizure-prone patients, acute myocardial infarction, patients undergoing biliary tract impairment, thyroid dysfunction, prostatic hyperplasia/urinary stricture, patients with respiratory, adrenal insufficiency, morbid obesity, renal and hepatic dysfunction, head trauma, increased intracranial pressure, and patients with a history of prior opioid dependence or abuse; pentazocine may precipitate opiate withdrawal symptoms in patients who have been receiving opiates regularly; injection contains sulfites which may cause allergic reaction; tolerance or drug dependence may result from extended use. May cause hypotension; use with caution in patients with hypovolemia, cardiovascular disease (including acute MI), or drugs which may exaggerate hypotensive effects (including phenothiazines or general anesthetics). May obscure diagnosis or clinical course of patients with acute abdominal conditions. **[U.S. Boxed Warning]: Talwin® NX is intended for oral administration only - severe vascular reactions have resulted from misuse by injection.** Severe sclerosis has occurred at the injection-site following multiple injections; rotate sites of injection. Use with caution in the elderly and debilitated patients; may be more sensitive adverse effects.

Adverse Reactions (Reflective of adult population; not specific for elderly)
Frequency not defined.
Cardiovascular: Circulatory depression, facial edema, flushing, hypotension, shock, syncope, tachycardia
Central nervous system: Chills, CNS depression, confusion, disorientation, dizziness, drowsiness, euphoria, excitement, hallucinations, headache, insomnia, irritability, lightheadedness, malaise, nightmares, sedation
Dermatologic: Dermatitis, erythema multiforme, pruritus, rash, Stevens-Johnson syndrome, toxic epidermal necrolysis, urticaria
Gastrointestinal: Abdominal distress, anorexia, constipation, diarrhea, nausea, vomiting, xerostomia
Genitourinary: Urinary retention
Hematologic: Decreased WBCs, eosinophilia
Local: Tissue damage and irritation with I.M./SubQ use
Neuromuscular & skeletal: Paresthesia, tremor, weakness
Ocular: Blurred vision, miosis
Otic: Tinnitus
Respiratory: Dyspnea, respiratory depression (rare)
Miscellaneous: Anaphylaxis, diaphoresis, physical and psychological dependence

Overdosage/Toxicology Symptoms include drowsiness, sedation, respiratory depression, and coma. Treatment consists of naloxone 2 mg I.V., with repeat administration as necessary, up to a total of 10 mg.

Drug Interactions
May potentiate or reduce analgesic effect of opiate agonist (eg, morphine) depending on patients tolerance to opiates can precipitate withdrawal in narcotic addicts
Increased effect/toxicity with tripelennamine (can be lethal), CNS depressants (phenothiazines, tranquilizers, anxiolytics, sedatives, hypnotics, or alcohol)

Ethanol/Nutrition/Herb Interactions Ethanol: Avoid ethanol (may increase CNS depression).
(Continued)

Pentazocine *(Continued)*

Stability Injection: Store at room temperature; do not freeze. Protect from heat.

Mechanism of Action Binds to opiate receptors in the CNS, causing inhibition of ascending pain pathways, altering the perception of and response to pain; produces generalized CNS depression; partial agonist-antagonist

Pharmacodynamics
Onset of action:
Oral, I.M., SubQ: Within 15-30 minutes
I.V.: Within 2-3 minutes
Duration:
Parenteral: 2-3 hours
Oral: 4-5 hours

Pharmacokinetics
Protein binding: 60%
Bioavailability: Oral: ~20% due to large first-pass effect; increased oral bioavailability to 60% to 70% in patients with cirrhosis
Metabolism: In liver via oxidative and glucuronide conjugation pathways
Half-life: 2-3 hours, increased half-life with decreased hepatic function
Elimination: Excreted unchanged in urine

Dosage
Geriatrics: See Special Geriatric Considerations. Initial dose:
Oral: 50 mg every 4 hours
I.M.: 30 mg every 4 hours
Adults: Analgesic:
Oral: 50 mg every 3-4 hours; may increase to 100 mg/dose if needed, but should not exceed 600 mg/day
I.M., SubQ: 30-60 mg every 3-4 hours; do **not** exceed 60 mg/dose (maximum: 360 mg/day)
I.V.: 30 mg every 3-4 hours; do **not** exceed 30 mg/dose (maximum: 360 mg/day)
Renal Impairment:
Cl_{cr} 10-50 mL/minute: Administer 75% of normal dose.
Cl_{cr} <10 mL/minute: Administer 50% of normal dose.
Hepatic Impairment: Reduce dose or avoid use in patients with liver disease.

Administration
Rotate injection site for I.M., SubQ use; avoid intra-arterial injection.

Monitoring Parameters Relief of pain, respiratory and mental status, blood pressure

Patient Information May cause drowsiness; avoid alcohol and CNS depressants; may be addicting if used for prolonged periods; will cause withdrawal in patients currently dependent on narcotics

Additional Information
Pentazocine hydrochloride: Talwin® NX tablet (with naloxone); naloxone is used to prevent abuse by dissolving tablets in water and using as injection
Pentazocine lactate: Talwin® injection

Special Geriatric Considerations Pentazocine is not recommended for use in the elderly because of its propensity to cause delirium and agitation. If pentazocine must be used, be sure to adjust dose for renal function.

Dosage Forms Excipient information presented when available (limited, particularly for generics); consult specific product labeling.
Injection, solution:
Talwin®: 30 mg/mL (1 mL, 10 mL) [10 mL size contains sodium bisulfite]
Tablet: Pentazocine 50 mg and naloxone 0.5 mg
Talwin® NX: Pentazocine 50 mg and naloxone 0.5 mg

Selected References
AGS Panel on Persistent Pain in Older Persons, "The Management of Persistent Pain in Older Persons," *J Am Geriatr Soc*, 2002, 50(6 Suppl):S205-24.

- ♦ **Pentazocine Hydrochloride** *see* Pentazocine *on page 1229*
- ♦ **Pentazocine Hydrochloride and Naloxone Hydrochloride** *see* Pentazocine *on page 1229*
- ♦ **Pentazocine Lactate** *see* Pentazocine *on page 1229*

Pentoxifylline *(pen toks IF i lin)*

Medication Safety Issues
Sound-alike/look-alike issues:
Pentoxifylline may be confused with tamoxifen
Trental® may be confused with Bentyl®, Tegretol®, Trandate®

U.S. Brand Names Pentoxil®; Trental®

Canadian Brand Names Albert® Pentoxifylline; Apo-Pentoxifylline SR®; Nu-Pentoxifylline SR; ratio-Pentoxifylline; Trental®

Index Terms Oxpentifylline

Generic Available Yes

Pharmacologic Category Blood Viscosity Reducer Agent

Use Symptomatic management of peripheral vascular disease, mainly intermittent claudication

Unlabeled/Investigational Use Treatment of AIDS patients with increased TNF, CVA, cerebrovascular diseases, diabetic atherosclerosis, diabetic neuropathy, gangrene, hemodialysis shunt thrombosis, vascular impotence, cerebral malaria, septic shock, sickle cell syndromes, and vasculitis

Contraindications Hypersensitivity to pentoxifylline, xanthines (eg, caffeine, theophylline), or any component of the formulation; recent cerebral and/or retinal hemorrhage

Warnings/Precautions Use with caution in patients with renal and hepatic impairment; start with lower doses in elderly patients and monitor renal function. Use caution in patients receiving anticoagulant therapy or at risk for bleeding complications; monitor PT/INR, hematocrit and/or hemoglobin as necessary. May lower blood pressure; monitor with concomitant antihypertensive agent use.

Adverse Reactions (Reflective of adult population; not specific for elderly)
1% to 10%: Gastrointestinal: Nausea (2%), vomiting (1%)

Overdosage/Toxicology Symptoms of overdose have been reported to occur 4-5 hours postingestion and last approximately 12 hours. Symptoms may include hypotension, flushing, convulsions, deep sleep, agitation, bradycardia, and AV block. Treatment should be symptom-directed and supportive.

Drug Interactions
Theophylline: Increased toxicity

Ethanol/Nutrition/Herb Interactions Food: Food may decrease rate but not extent of absorption. Pentoxifylline peak serum levels may be decreased if taken with food.

Stability Store between 15°C to 30°C (59°F to 86°F).

Mechanism of Action Reduces blood viscosity via increased leukocyte and erythrocyte deformability and decreased neutrophil adhesion/activation; improves peripheral tissue oxygenation presumably through enhanced blood flow.

Pharmacokinetics
Absorption: Oral: Well absorbed
Half-life: 24-48 minutes (metabolites half-life: 60-96 minutes)
Time to peak serum concentration: Within 1 hour
Metabolism: Undergoes first-pass metabolism; metabolized in the liver and
Excretion: Primarily urine (active metabolites); feces (4%)

Dosage
Geriatrics & Adults: Peripheral vascular disease: Oral: 400 mg 3 times/day with meals; maximal therapeutic benefit may take 2-4 weeks to develop; recommended to maintain therapy for at least 8 weeks. May reduce to 400 mg twice daily if GI or CNS side effects occur.

Monitoring Parameters PT, PTT if used in conjunction with other agents that may affect coagulation or platelet aggregation, clotting time

Test Interactions Decreased calcium (S), magnesium (S); false-positive theophylline levels

Patient Information Take with food or meals; if GI or CNS side effects continue, contact physician; while effects may be seen in 2-4 weeks, continue treatment for at least 8 weeks

Special Geriatric Considerations Pentoxifylline's value in the treatment of intermittent claudication is controversial. Walking distance improved statistically in some clinical trials, but the actual distance was minimal when applied to improving physical activity.

Dosage Forms Excipient information presented when available (limited, particularly for generics); consult specific product labeling.
Tablet, controlled release:
Trental®: 400 mg
Tablet, extended release: 400 mg
Pentoxil®: 400 mg

Selected References
Luke DR, Rocci ML Jr, and Hoholick C, "Inhibition of Pentoxifylline Clearance by Cimetidine," *J Pharm Sci*, 1986, 75(2):155-7.
Mauro VF, Mauro LS, and Hageman JH, "Alteration of Pentoxifylline Pharmacokinetics by Cimetidine," *Clin Pharmacol*, 1988, 28(7):649-54.

♦ **Pepto-Bismol® [OTC]** see Bismuth on page 174
♦ **Pepto-Bismol® Maximum Strength [OTC]** see Bismuth on page 174
♦ **Pepto Relief [OTC]** see Bismuth on page 174
♦ **Percocet®** see Oxycodone and Acetaminophen on page 1182
♦ **Percodan®** see Oxycodone and Aspirin on page 1184
♦ **Perdiem® Overnight Relief [OTC]** see Senna on page 1456
♦ **Periactin** see Cyproheptadine on page 386
♦ **Peri-Colace® [OTC]** see Docusate and Senna on page 461

Perindopril Erbumine (per IN doe pril er BYOO meen)

Related Information
Angiotensin Agents on page 1737
U.S. Brand Names Aceon®
Canadian Brand Names Apo-Perindopril®; Coversyl®
Generic Available No
Pharmacologic Category Angiotensin-Converting Enzyme (ACE) Inhibitor
Use Treatment of essential hypertension; reduction of cardiovascular mortality or nonfatal myocardial infarction in patients with stable coronary artery disease
Unlabeled/Investigational Use As a class, ACE inhibitors are recommended in the treatment of congestive heart failure with left ventricular dysfunction.
Contraindications Hypersensitivity to perindopril or any component of the formulation; angioedema related to previous treatment with an ACE inhibitor; bilateral renal artery stenosis; primary hyperaldosteronism
Warnings/Precautions Anaphylactic reactions can occur. Angioedema can occur at any time during treatment (especially following first dose). It may involve head and neck (potentially affecting the airway) or the intestine (presenting with abdominal pain). Prolonged monitoring may be required especially if tongue, glottis, or larynx are involved as they are associated with airway obstruction. Those with a history of airway surgery in this situation have a higher risk. Careful blood pressure monitoring with first dose (hypotension can occur especially in volume- and/or salt-depleted patients); caution in patients receiving hypotensive-inducing anesthesia. Dosage adjustment needed in renal impairment. Avoid rapid dosage escalation, which may lead to renal insufficiency.

Use with caution in hypovolemia; collagen vascular diseases; valvular stenosis (particularly aortic stenosis); concomitant use with potassium-sparing agents, potassium supplements or salt substitutes not recommended; risk of hyperkalemia may be increased with renal insufficiency. Rare toxicities associated with ACE inhibitors include cholestatic jaundice (which may progress to hepatic necrosis) and neutropenia/agranulocytosis with myeloid hyperplasia. May be associated with deterioration of renal function and/or increases in serum creatinine, particularly in patients dependent on renin-angiotensin-aldosterone system. Use with caution in unilateral renal artery stenosis and pre-existing renal insufficiency; if patient has renal impairment then a baseline WBC with differential and serum creatinine should be evaluated and monitored closely during the first 3 months of therapy. Hypersensitivity reactions may be seen during hemodialysis with high-flux dialysis membranes (eg, AN69).

Adverse Reactions (Reflective of adult population; not specific for elderly)
>10%:
 Central nervous system: Headache (24%)
 Respiratory: Cough (incidence is higher in women, 3:1) (12%)
1% to 10%:
 Cardiovascular: Edema (4%), chest pain (2%)), ECG abnormal (2%), palpitation (1%)
 Central nervous system: Dizziness (8%, less than placebo), sleep disorders (3%), depression (2%), fever (2%), nervousness (1%), somnolence (1%)
 Dermatologic: Rash (2%)
 Endocrine & metabolic: Hyperkalemia (1%, less than placebo), triglycerides increased (1%), menstrual disorder (1%)
 Gastrointestinal: Nausea (2%), diarrhea (4%), vomiting (2%), dyspepsia (2%), abdominal pain (3%), flatulence (1%)
 Genitourinary: Urinary tract infection (3%), sexual dysfunction (male 1%)
 Hepatic: Increased ALT (2%)
 Neuromuscular & skeletal: Weakness (8%), back pain (6%), lower extremity pain (5%), upper extremity pain (3%), hypertonia (3%), paresthesia (2%), joint pain (1%), myalgia (1%), arthritis (1%), neck pain (1%)
 Renal: Proteinuria (2%)
 Respiratory: Upper respiratory tract infection (9%), sinusitis (5%), rhinitis (5%), pharyngitis (3%)
 Otic: Tinnitus (2%), ear infection (1%)
 Miscellaneous: Viral infection (3%), allergy (2%)

Note: Some reactions occurred at an incidence >1% but ≤ placebo.

Additional adverse effects that have been reported with **ACE inhibitors** include agranulocytosis (especially in patients with renal impairment or collagen vascular disease), neutropenia, anemia, bullous pemphigus, cardiac arrest, eosinophilic pneumonitis, exfoliative dermatitis, hepatic failure, hyponatremia, jaundice, pancreatitis (acute), pancytopenia, thrombocytopenia; decreases in creatinine clearance in some elderly hypertensive patients or those with chronic renal failure, and worsening of renal function in patients with bilateral renal artery stenosis or hypovolemic patients (diuretic therapy). In addition, a syndrome which may include fever, myalgia, arthralgia, interstitial nephritis, vasculitis, rash, eosinophilia and positive ANA, and elevated ESR has been reported with ACE inhibitors.

Overdosage/Toxicology Mild hypotension has been the primary toxic effect seen with acute overdose. Bradycardia may also occur. Hyperkalemia occurs even with therapeutic doses, especially in patients with renal insufficiency and those taking NSAIDs. Treatment is symptom-directed and supportive. Hemodialysis may be beneficial.

Drug Interactions

Allopurinol: ACE inhibitors may increase hypersensitivity reactions to allopurinol; monitor for at least 5 weeks following initiation of allopurinol.

Alpha$_1$ blockers: Hypotensive effect increased.

Aspirin: The effects of ACE inhibitors may be blunted by aspirin administration, particularly at higher dosages and/or increase adverse renal effects.

Cyclosporine: ACE inhibitors may increase nephrotoxicity of cyclosporine; monitor.

Diuretics: Hypovolemia due to diuretics may precipitate acute hypotensive events or acute renal failure.

Gold sodium thiomalate: ACE inhibitors may enhance the adverse/toxic effects (nitritoid reaction) of gold sodium thiomalate. The reaction may include facial flushing, nausea, vomiting, hypotension, and syncope. If it is to occur, would be expected shortly after administration of gold compound in patients maintained on an ACEI.

Insulin: Risk of hypoglycemia may be increased.

Lithium: Risk of lithium toxicity may be increased; monitor lithium levels, especially the first 4 weeks of therapy.

Mercaptopurine: Risk of neutropenia may be increased.

NSAIDs: May attenuate hypertensive efficacy; effect has been seen with captopril and may occur with other ACE inhibitors; monitor blood pressure. May increase risk of renal effects.

Potassium-sparing diuretics (amiloride, eplerenone, spironolactone, triamterene): Increased risk of hyperkalemia.

Potassium supplements may increase the risk of hyperkalemia.

Trimethoprim (high dose) may increase the risk of hyperkalemia.

Ethanol/Nutrition/Herb Interactions

Food: Perindopril active metabolite concentrations may be lowered if taken with food.

Herb/Nutraceutical: Avoid dong quai if using for hypertension (has estrogenic activity). Avoid ephedra, yohimbe, ginseng (may worsen hypertension). Avoid garlic (may have increased antihypertensive effect).

Stability Store at room temperature of 20°C to 25°C (68°F to 77°F). Protect from moisture.

Mechanism of Action Perindopril is a prodrug for perindoprilat, which acts as a competitive inhibitor of angiotensin-converting enzyme (ACE); prevents conversion of angiotensin I to angiotensin II, a potent vasoconstrictor; results in lower levels of angiotensin II which, in turn, causes an increase in plasma renin activity and a reduction in aldosterone secretion

Pharmacodynamics Onset of action: Peak effect: 1-2 hours

Pharmacokinetics

Protein binding: Perindopril: 60%; Perindoprilat: 10% to 20%

Metabolism: Hepatically hydrolyzed to active metabolite, perindoprilat (~17% to 20% of a dose) and other inactive metabolites

Bioavailability: Perindopril: 75%; Perindoprilat ~25% (~16% with food)

Half-life: Parent drug: 1.5-3 hours; Metabolite: Effective: 3-10 hours, Terminal: 30-120 hours

Time to peak: Chronic therapy: Perindopril: 1 hour; Perindoprilat: 3-7 hours (maximum perindoprilat serum concentrations are 2-3 times higher and T_{max} is shorter following chronic therapy); CHF: Perindoprilat: 6 hours

Excretion: Urine (75%, 4% to 12% as unchanged drug)

Dosage

Geriatrics:

Essential hypertension: >65 years of age: Initial: 4 mg/day; maintenance: 8 mg/day

Stable coronary artery disease: >70 years of age: Initial: 2 mg/day for 1 week; increase as tolerated to 4 mg/day for 1 week; then increase as tolerated to 8 mg/day

(Continued)

Perindopril Erbumine *(Continued)*

Adults:

Essential hypertension: Oral: Initial: 4 mg/day but may be titrated to response; usual range: 4-8 mg/day (may be given in 2 divided doses); increase at 1- to 2-week intervals (maximum: 16 mg/day)

Concomitant therapy with diuretics: To reduce the risk of hypotension, discontinue diuretic, if possible, 2-3 days prior to initiating perindopril. If unable to stop diuretic, initiate perindopril at 2-4 mg/day and monitor blood pressure closely for the first 2 weeks of therapy, and after any dose adjustment of perindopril or diuretic.

Stable coronary artery disease: Oral: Initial: 4 mg once daily for 2 weeks; increase as tolerated to 8 mg once daily.

Congestive heart failure (unlabeled use): Oral: Initial: 2 mg once daily; increase at 1- to 2-week intervals; target dose: 8-16 mg once daily (ACC/AHA 2005 Heart Failure Guidelines)

Renal Impairment:

Cl_{cr} >30 mL/minute: Initial: 2 mg/day; maintenance dosing not to exceed 8 mg/day

Cl_{cr} <30 mL/minute: Safety and efficacy not established.

Hemodialysis: Perindopril and its metabolites are dialyzable

Hepatic Impairment: No adjustment required.

Monitoring Parameters Serum creatinine, electrolytes; urinalysis for protein

Patient Information This medication does not replace the need to follow exercise and diet recommendations for hypertension. Take as directed; do not miss doses, alter dosage, or discontinue without consulting prescriber. Consult prescriber for appropriate diet. Do not use NSAIDs (like indomethacin or naproxen), potassium supplements, or salt substitutes containing potassium without consulting prescriber. Change position slowly when rising from sitting or lying. May cause transient drowsiness; avoid driving or engaging in tasks that require alertness until response to drug is known. Small frequent meals may help reduce any nausea, vomiting, or epigastric pain. You may experience persistent cough; contact prescriber. Report unusual weight gain or swelling of ankles and hands; persistent fatigue; dry cough; difficulty breathing; palpitations; or swelling of face, eyes, or lips.

Special Geriatric Considerations Due to frequent decreases in glomerular filtration (also creatinine clearance) with aging, elderly patients may have exaggerated responses to ACE inhibitors; differences in clinical response due to hepatic changes are not observed. ACE inhibitors may be preferred agents in elderly patients with congestive heart failure and diabetes mellitus. Diabetic proteinuria is reduced and insulin sensitivity is enhanced. In general, the side effect profile is favorable in elderly and causes little or no CNS confusion; use lowest dose recommendations initially. Many elderly may be volume depleted due to diuretic use and/or blunted thirst reflex resulting in inadequate fluid intake.

Dosage Forms Excipient information presented when available (limited, particularly for generics); consult specific product labeling.

Tablet: 2 mg, 4 mg, 8 mg

Selected References

Braunwald E, Antman EM, Beasley JW, et al, "ACC/AHA Guidelines for the Management of Patients With Unstable Angina and Non-ST-Segment Elevation Myocardial Infarction. A Report of the American College of Cardiology/American Heart Association Task Force on Practice Guidelines (Committee on the Management of Patients With Unstable Angina)," *J Am Coll Cardiol*, 2000, 36(3):970-1062.

Conlin P, Moore T, Swartz S, et al, "Effect of Indomethacin on Blood Pressure Lowering by Captopril and Losartan in Hypertensive Patients," *Hypertension*, 2000, 36:461-5.

"Consensus Recommendations for the Management of Chronic Heart Failure. On Behalf of the Membership of the Advisory Council to Improve Outcomes Nationwide in Heart Failure," *Am J Cardiol*, 1999, 83(2A):1A-38A.

Fox KM and EURopean Trial on Reduction of Cardiac Events With Perindopril in Stable Coronary Artery Disease Investigators, "Efficacy of Perindopril in Reduction of Cardiovascular Events Among Patients With Stable Coronary Artery Disease: Randomised, Double-Blind, Placebo-Controlled, Multicentre Trial (The EUROPA Study)," *Lancet*, 2003, 362(9386):782-8.

Hunt SA, Abraham WT, Chin MH, et al, "ACC/AHA 2005 Guideline Update for the Diagnosis and Management of Chronic Heart Failure in the Adult-Summary Article A Report of the American College of Cardiology/American Heart Association Task Force on Practice Guidelines (Writing Committee to Update the 2001 Guidelines for the Evaluation and Management of Heart Failure)," *J Am Coll Cardiol*, 2005, 46(6):1116-43.

"K/DOQI Clinical Practice Guidelines for Chronic Kidney Disease: Evaluation, Classification, and Stratification. Kidney Disease Outcome Quality Initiative," Am J Kidney Dis, 2002, 39(2 Suppl 2):1-246. Available at: http://www.kidney.org/professionals/doqi/kdoqi/toc.htm. Accessed August 1, 2003.

Packer M, Poole-Wilson PA, Armstrong PW, et al, "Comparative Effects of Low and High Doses of the Angiotensin-Converting Enzyme Inhibitor, Lisinopril, on Morbidity and Mortality in Chronic Heart Failure," *Circulation*, 1999, 100(23):2312-8.

Pfeffer MA, Greaves SC, Arnold JM, et al, "Early Versus Delayed Angiotensin-Converting Enzyme Inhibition Therapy in Acute Myocardial Infarction. The Healing and Early Afterload Reducing Therapy Trial," *Circulation*, 1997, 95(12):2643-51.

Ryan TJ, Anderson JL, Antman EM, et al, "ACC/AHA Guidelines for the Management of Patients With Acute Myocardial Infarction. A Report of the American College of Cardiology/American Heart Association Task Force on Practice Guidelines (Committee on Management of Acute Myocardial Infarction)," *J Am Coll Cardiol*, 1996, 28(5):1328-428.

♦ **PerioMed**™ *see* Fluoride *on page 642*

♦ **Periostat®** *see* Doxycycline *on page 479*

Permethrin (per METH rin)

U.S. Brand Names A200® Lice [OTC]; Acticin®; Elimite®; Nix® [OTC]; Rid® Spray [OTC]
Canadian Brand Names Kwellada-P™; Nix®
Generic Available Yes: Excludes spray
Pharmacologic Category Antiparasitic Agent, Topical; Scabicidal Agent
Use Single application treatment of infestation with *Pediculus humanus capitis* (head louse) and its nits, or *Sarcoptes scabiei* (scabies)
Contraindications Hypersensitivity to pyrethroid, pyrethrin, chrysanthemums, or any component of the formulation
Warnings/Precautions Treatment may temporarily exacerbate the symptoms of itching, redness, swelling; for external use only.
Adverse Reactions (Reflective of adult population; not specific for elderly)
1% to 10%:
Dermatologic: Pruritus, erythema, rash of the scalp
Local: Burning, stinging, tingling, numbness or scalp discomfort, edema
Drug Interactions No data reported
Mechanism of Action Inhibits sodium ion influx through nerve cell membrane channels in parasites resulting in delayed repolarization and thus paralysis and death of the pest
Pharmacokinetics
Absorption: Topical: Minimal, <2%
Metabolism: In the liver
Elimination: In urine
Dosage
Geriatrics & Adults:
Head lice: Topical: After hair has been washed with shampoo, rinsed with water and towel dried, apply a sufficient volume of creme rinse to saturate the hair and scalp; also apply behind the ears and at the base of the neck; leave on hair for 10 minutes before rinsing off with water; remove remaining nits. May repeat in 1 week if lice or nits still present; in areas of head lice resistance to 1% permethrin, 5% permethrin has been applied to clean, dry hair and left on overnight (8-14 hours) under a shower cap.
Scabies: Topical: Apply cream from head to toe; leave on for 8-14 hours before washing off with water; may reapply in 1 week if live mites appear. Time of application was limited to 6 hours before rinsing with soap and water.
Administration Because scabies and lice are so contagious, use caution to avoid spreading or infecting oneself; wear gloves when applying. See Dosage.
Patient Information Avoid contact with eyes during application; shake well before using; notify physician if irritation persists; clothing and bedding should be washed in hot water or dry cleaned to kill the scabies mite
Special Geriatric Considerations Because of its minimal absorption, permethrin is a drug of choice and is preferred over lindane.
Dosage Forms Excipient information presented when available (limited, particularly for generics); consult specific product labeling.
Cream, topical (Acticin®, Elimite®): 5% (60 g) [contains coconut oil]
Lotion, topical: 1% (59 mL)
Liquid, topical [creme rinse formulation] (Nix®): 1% (60 mL) [contains isopropyl alcohol 20%]
Solution, spray [for bedding and furniture]:
A200® Lice: 0.5% (180 mL)
Nix®: 0.25% (148 mL)
Rid®: 0.5% (150 mL)

Perphenazine (per FEN a zeen)

Related Information
Antipsychotic Agents *on page 1747*
Medication Safety Issues
Sound-alike/look-alike issues:
Trilafon® may be confused with Tri-Levlen®
Canadian Brand Names Apo-Perphenazine®
Generic Available Yes
Pharmacologic Category Antipsychotic Agent, Typical, Phenothiazine
Use Treatment of severe schizophrenia, nausea, vomiting
Unlabeled/Investigational Use Treatment of ethanol withdrawal, dementia in older adults, Tourette's syndrome, Huntington's chorea, spasmodic torticollis, Reye's syndrome, psychosis
(Continued)

Perphenazine *(Continued)*

Contraindications Hypersensitivity to perphenazine or any component of the formulation (cross-reactivity between phenothiazines may occur); severe CNS depression; subcortical brain damage; bone marrow suppression; blood dyscrasias; coma

Warnings/Precautions May cause hypotension. May be sedating, use with caution in disorders where CNS depression is a feature. Use with caution in Parkinson's disease. Caution in patients with hemodynamic instability; predisposition to seizures; severe cardiac, hepatic, renal, or respiratory disease. Esophageal dysmotility and aspiration have been associated with antipsychotic use - use with caution in patients at risk of pneumonia (ie, Alzheimer's disease). Caution in breast cancer or other prolactin-dependent tumors (may elevate prolactin levels). May alter temperature regulation or mask toxicity of other drugs due to antiemetic effects. May alter cardiac conduction - life-threatening arrhythmias have occurred with therapeutic doses of phenothiazines. May cause orthostatic hypotension - use with caution in patients at risk of this effect or those who would tolerate transient hypotensive episodes (cerebrovascular disease, cardiovascular disease, or other medications which may predispose). Check blood counts periodically and discontinue at first signs of blood dyscrasias; use is contraindicated in patients with bone marrow suppression.

Phenothiazines may cause anticholinergic effects (confusion, agitation, constipation, xerostomia, blurred vision, urinary retention); therefore, they should be used with caution in patients with decreased gastrointestinal motility, urinary retention, BPH, xerostomia, or visual problems. Conditions which also may be exacerbated by cholinergic blockade include narrow-angle glaucoma (screening is recommended) and worsening of myasthenia gravis. Relative to other neuroleptics, perphenazine has a low potency of cholinergic blockade.

May cause extrapyramidal reactions, including pseudoparkinsonism, acute dystonic reactions, akathisia, and tardive dyskinesia (risk of these reactions is moderate-high relative to other neuroleptics). May be associated with neuroleptic malignant syndrome (NMS) or pigmentary retinopathy. May cause photosensitization.

Adverse Reactions (Reflective of adult population; not specific for elderly)
Frequency not defined.

Cardiovascular: Hyper-/hypotension, orthostatic hypotension, tachycardia, bradycardia, dizziness, cardiac arrest

Central nervous system: Extrapyramidal symptoms (pseudoparkinsonism, akathisia, dystonias, tardive dyskinesia), dizziness, cerebral edema, seizure, headache, drowsiness, paradoxical excitement, restlessness, hyperactivity, insomnia, neuroleptic malignant syndrome (NMS), impairment of temperature regulation

Dermatologic: Rash, discoloration of skin (blue-gray), photosensitivity

Endocrine & metabolic: Hypoglycemia, hyperglycemia, galactorrhea, lactation, breast enlargement, gynecomastia, menstrual irregularity, amenorrhea, SIADH, libido (changes in)

Gastrointestinal: Constipation, weight gain, vomiting, stomach pain, nausea, xerostomia, salivation, diarrhea, anorexia, ileus

Genitourinary: Difficulty in urination, ejaculatory disturbances, incontinence, polyuria, ejaculating dysfunction, priapism

Hematologic: Agranulocytosis, leukopenia, eosinophilia, hemolytic anemia, thrombocytopenic purpura, pancytopenia

Hepatic: Cholestatic jaundice, hepatotoxicity

Neuromuscular & skeletal: Tremor

Ocular: Pigmentary retinopathy, blurred vision, cornea and lens changes

Respiratory: Nasal congestion

Miscellaneous: Diaphoresis

Overdosage/Toxicology Symptoms include deep sleep, dystonia, agitation, coma, abnormal involuntary muscle movements, hypotension, and arrhythmias. Following initiation of essential overdose management, toxic symptom and supportive treatment should be initiated. Hypotension usually responds to I.V. fluids or Trendelenburg positioning. If unresponsive to these measures, the use of a parenteral inotrope may be required (eg, norepinephrine 0.1-0.2 mcg/kg/minute titrated to response). Seizures commonly respond to diazepam (I.V. 5-10 mg bolus every 15 minutes, if needed, up to a total of 30 mg) or to phenytoin or phenobarbital. Extrapyramidal symptoms (eg, dystonic reactions) may be managed with diphenhydramine. When these reactions are unresponsive to diphenhydramine, benztropine mesylate may be effective.

Drug Interactions Substrate of CYP1A2 (minor), 2C9 (minor), 2C19 (minor), 2D6 (major), 3A4 (minor); **Inhibits** CYP1A2 (weak), 2D6 (weak)

Acetylcholinesterase inhibitors (central): May increase the risk of antipsychotic-related extrapyramidal symptoms; monitor

Aluminum salts: May decrease the absorption of phenothiazines; monitor

Amphetamines: Efficacy may be diminished by antipsychotics; in addition, amphetamines may increase psychotic symptoms; avoid concurrent use

Anticholinergics: May inhibit the therapeutic response to phenothiazines and excess anticholinergic effects may occur; includes benztropine, trihexyphenidyl, biperiden, and drugs with significant anticholinergic activity (TCAs, antihistamines, disopyramide)

Antihypertensives: Concurrent use of phenothiazines with an antihypertensive may produce additive hypotensive effects (particularly orthostasis)

Bromocriptine: Phenothiazines inhibit the ability of bromocriptine to lower serum prolactin concentrations

CNS depressants: Sedative effects may be additive with phenothiazines; monitor for increased effect; includes barbiturates, benzodiazepines, opioid analgesics, ethanol, and other sedative agents

CYP2D6 inhibitors: May increase the levels/effects of perphenazine. Example inhibitors include chlorpromazine, delavirdine, fluoxetine, miconazole, paroxetine, pergolide, quinidine, quinine, ritonavir, and ropinirole.

Epinephrine: Chlorpromazine (and possibly other low potency antipsychotics) may diminish the pressor effects of epinephrine

Guanethidine and guanadrel: Antihypertensive effects may be inhibited by phenothiazines

Levodopa: Phenothiazines may inhibit the antiparkinsonian effect of levodopa; avoid this combination

Lithium: Phenothiazines may produce neurotoxicity with lithium; this is a rare effect

Metoclopramide: May increase extrapyramidal symptoms (EPS) or risk.

Phenytoin: May reduce serum levels of phenothiazines; phenothiazines may increase phenytoin serum levels

Propranolol: Serum concentrations of phenothiazines may be increased; propranolol also increases phenothiazine concentrations

Polypeptide antibiotics: Rare cases of respiratory paralysis have been reported with concurrent use of phenothiazines

QT_c-prolonging agents: Effects on QT_c interval may be additive with phenothiazines, increasing the risk of malignant arrhythmias; includes type Ia antiarrhythmics, TCAs, and some quinolone antibiotics (moxifloxacin).

Sulfadoxine-pyrimethamine: May increase phenothiazine concentrations

Tricyclic antidepressants: Concurrent use may produce increased toxicity or altered therapeutic response

Trazodone: Phenothiazines and trazodone may produce additive hypotensive effects

Valproic acid: Serum levels may be increased by phenothiazines

Ethanol/Nutrition/Herb Interactions

Ethanol: Avoid ethanol (may increase CNS depression).

Herb/Nutraceutical: Avoid kava kava, gotu kola, valerian, St John's wort (may increase CNS depression).

Stability Store at 2°C to 25°C (36°F to 77°F). Protect from light.

Mechanism of Action Perphenazine is a piperazine phenothiazine antipsychotic which blocks postsynaptic mesolimbic dopaminergic receptors in the brain; exhibits alpha-adrenergic blocking effect and depresses the release of hypothalamic and hypophyseal hormones

Pharmacokinetics

Absorption: Oral: Well absorbed; absorption may be affected by the inherent anticholinergic action on the gastrointestinal tissue causing variable absorption. Absorption from tablets is erratic with less variation seen with solutions. These agents are widely distributed in tissues with CNS concentrations exceeding that of plasma due to their lipophilic characteristics.

Protein binding: Antipsychotic agents are bound 90% to 99% to plasma or proteins; highly bound to brain and lung tissue and other tissues with a high blood perfusion

Metabolism: Extensively hepatic to metabolites via sulfoxidation, hydroxylation, dealkylation, and glucuronidation

Time to peak: Peak serum concentrations occur within 4-8 hours; peak concentrations between 2-4 hours

Elimination: Excreted in urine and bile; excretion occurs through hepatic metabolism (oxidation) where numerous active metabolites are produced; active metabolites excreted in urine; elimination half-lives of antipsychotics ranges from 20-40 hours which may be extended in older adults due to decline in oxidative hepatic reactions (phase I) with age.

The biologic effect of a single dose persists for 24 hours. When the patient has accommodated to initial side effects (sedation), once daily dosing is possible due to the long half-life of antipsychotics.

Steady-state plasma concentrations are achieved in 4-7 days; therefore, if possible, do not make dose adjustments more than once in a 7-day period. Due to the long half-lives of antipsychotics, as needed (prn) use is ineffective since repeated doses are necessary to achieve therapeutic tissue concentrations in the CNS.

Dosage

Geriatrics: Behavioral symptoms associated with dementia (unlabeled use): Oral: Initial: 2-4 mg 1-2 times/day; increase at 4- to 7-day intervals by 2-4 mg/day. (Continued)

Perphenazine *(Continued)*

Increase dose intervals (bid, tid, etc) as necessary to control behavior response or side effects. Maximum daily dose: 32 mg; gradual increase (titration) and bedtime administration may prevent some side effects or decrease their severity.

Adults:

Schizophrenia/psychoses: Oral: 4-16 mg 2-4 times/day not to exceed 64 mg/day

Nausea/vomiting: Oral: 8-16 mg/day in divided doses up to 24 mg/day

Renal Impairment: Not dialyzable (0% to 5%)

Hepatic Impairment: Dosage reductions should be considered in patients with liver disease although no specific guidelines are available.

Monitoring Parameters Orthostatic blood pressures; tremors, gait changes, abnormal movement in trunk, neck, buccal area, or extremities; monitor target behaviors for which the agent is given

Reference Range 0.8-1.2 ng/mL; serum concentrations are controversial and dosing to response is recommended

Patient Information Oral concentrate must be diluted in 2-4 oz of liquid (water, fruit juice, carbonated drinks, milk, or pudding); do not take antacid within 1 hour of taking drug; avoid alcohol; avoid excess sun exposure (use sun block); may cause drowsiness, rise slowly from recumbent position; use of supportive stockings may help prevent orthostatic hypotension

Special Geriatric Considerations Any changes in disease status in any organ system can result in behavior changes.

Many elderly patients receive antipsychotic medications for inappropriate nonpsychotic behavior. Before initiating antipsychotic medication, the clinician should investigate any possible reversible cause; any stress or stress from any disease can cause acute "confusion" or worsening of baseline nonpsychotic behavior. Most commonly acute changes in behavior are due to increases in drug dose or addition of new drug to regimen; fluid electrolyte loss; infections; and changes in environment.

In the treatment of agitated, demented, elderly patients, authors of meta-analysis of controlled trials of the response to the traditional antipsychotics (phenothiazines, butyrophenones) in controlling agitation have concluded that the use of neuroleptics results in a response rate of 18%. Clearly neuroleptic therapy for behavior control should be limited with frequent attempts to withdraw the agent given for behavior control.

Dosage Forms Excipient information presented when available (limited, particularly for generics); consult specific product labeling.

Tablet: 2 mg, 4 mg, 8 mg, 16 mg

Selected References

Peabody CA, Warner MD, Whiteford HA, et al, "Neuroleptics and the Elderly," *J Am Geriatr Soc*, 1987, 35(3):233-8.

Risse SC and Barnes R, "Pharmacologic Treatment of Agitation Associated With Dementia," *J Am Geriatr Soc*, 1986, 34(5):368-76.

Saltz BL, Woerner MG, Kane JM, et al, "Prospective Study of Tardive Dyskinesia Incidence in the Elderly," *JAMA*, 1991, 266(17):2402-6.

Seifert RD, "Therapeutic Drug Monitoring: Psychotropic Drugs," *J Pharm Pract*, 1984, 6:403-16.

- ♦ **Persantine®** *see* Dipyridamole *on page 454*
- ♦ **Pethidine Hydrochloride** *see* Meperidine *on page 980*
- ♦ **Petrolatum White and Mineral Oil Ophthalmic Ointment** *see* Ocular Lubricant *on page 1144*
- ♦ **Pexeva®** *see* Paroxetine *on page 1205*
- ♦ **Pfizerpen®** *see* Penicillin G (Parenteral/Aqueous) *on page 1224*
- ♦ **PGE₁** *see* Alprostadil *on page 57*
- ♦ **Phanasin® [OTC]** *see* Guaifenesin *on page 727*
- ♦ **Phanasin® Diabetic Choice [OTC]** *see* Guaifenesin *on page 727*
- ♦ **Phanatuss® DM [OTC]** *see* Guaifenesin and Dextromethorphan *on page 730*
- ♦ **Pharmaflur®** *see* Fluoride *on page 642*
- ♦ **Pharmaflur® 1.1** *see* Fluoride *on page 642*
- ♦ **Phazyme® Quick Dissolve [OTC]** *see* Simethicone *on page 1467*
- ♦ **Phazyme® Ultra Strength [OTC]** *see* Simethicone *on page 1467*
- ♦ **Phenadoz™** *see* Promethazine *on page 1327*

Phenazopyridine *(fen az oh PEER i deen)*

Medication Safety Issues

Sound-alike/look-alike issues:

Pyridium® may be confused with Dyrenium®, Perdiem®, pyridoxine, pyrithione

U.S. Brand Names AZO-Gesic® [OTC]; AZO-Standard® [OTC]; AZO-Standard® Maximum Strength [OTC]; Baridium® [OTC]; Prodium® [OTC]; Pyridium®; ReAzo [OTC]; Uristat® [OTC]; UTI Relief® [OTC]

Canadian Brand Names Phenazo™

Index Terms Phenazopyridine Hydrochloride; Phenylazo Diamino Pyridine Hydrochloride

Generic Available Yes

Pharmacologic Category Analgesic, Urinary

Use Symptomatic relief of urinary burning, itching, frequency and urgency in association with urinary tract infection or following urologic procedures

Contraindications Hypersensitivity to phenazopyridine or any component of the formulation; kidney or liver disease; patients with a Cl_{cr} <50 mL/minute

Warnings/Precautions Does not treat urinary infection, acts only as an analgesic; drug should be discontinued if skin or sclera develop a yellow color; use with caution in patients with renal impairment. Use of this agent in the elderly is limited since accumulation of phenazopyridine can occur in patients with renal insufficiency. Use is contraindicated in patients with a Cl_{cr} <50 mL/minute.

Adverse Reactions (Reflective of adult population; not specific for elderly)
1% to 10%:
Central nervous system: Headache, dizziness
Gastrointestinal: Stomach cramps

Overdosage/Toxicology Symptoms include methemoglobinemia, hemolytic anemia, skin pigmentation, and renal and hepatic impairment. The antidote for methemoglobinemia is methylene blue 1-2 mg/kg I.V.

Drug Interactions No data reported

Mechanism of Action An azo dye which exerts local anesthetic or analgesic action on urinary tract mucosa through an unknown mechanism

Pharmacokinetics
Metabolism: In the liver and other tissues
Elimination: In urine (where it exerts its action); renal excretion (as unchanged drug) is rapid and accounts for 65% of the drug's elimination

Dosage
Geriatrics & Adults: Urinary analgesic: Oral: 100-200 mg 3 times/day after meals for 2 days when used concomitantly with an antibacterial agent
Renal Impairment:
Cl_{cr} 50-80 mL/minute: Administer every 8-16 hours.
Cl_{cr} <50 mL/minute: Avoid use.

Monitoring Parameters Relief of urinary discomfort

Test Interactions Phenazopyridine may cause delayed reactions with glucose oxidase reagents (Clinistix®, Tes-Tape®); occasional false-positive tests occur with Tes-Tape®; cupric sulfate tests (Clinitest®) are not affected; interference may also occur with urine ketone tests (Acetest®, Ketostix®) and urinary protein tests; tests for urinary steroids and porphyrins may also occur

Patient Information Take by mouth after meals; tablets may color the urine orange or red and may stain clothing. This medication treats the painful symptoms of a urinary tract infection but does not cure the infection.

Special Geriatric Considerations Use of this agent in older adults is limited since accumulation of phenazopyridine can occur in patients with renal insufficiency.

Dosage Forms Excipient information presented when available (limited, particularly for generics); consult specific product labeling.
Tablet, as hydrochloride: 100 mg, 200 mg
AZO-Gesic®, AZO-Standard®, Prodium®, ReAzo, Uristat®: 95 mg
AZO Standard® Maximum Strength: 97.5 mg
Baridium®, UTI Relief®: 97.2 mg
Pyridium®: 100 mg, 200 mg

♦ **Phenazopyridine Hydrochloride** see Phenazopyridine on page 1238

Phenelzine (FEN el zeen)

Related Information
Antidepressant Agents on page 1742
Medication Safety Issues
Sound-alike/look-alike issues:
Phenelzine may be confused with phenytoin
Nardil® may be confused with Norinyl®
U.S. Brand Names Nardil®
Canadian Brand Names Nardil®
Index Terms Phenelzine Sulfate
Generic Available No
Pharmacologic Category Antidepressant, Monoamine Oxidase Inhibitor
Use Symptomatic treatment of depressed patients refractory to or intolerant to other antidepressants or electroconvulsive therapy
(Continued)

PHENELZINE

Phenelzine *(Continued)*

Unlabeled/Investigational Use Treatment of selective mutism

Restrictions An FDA-approved medication guide concerning the use of antidepressants in children, adolescents, and young adults must be distributed when dispensing an outpatient prescription (new or refill) where this medication is to be used without direct supervision of a healthcare provider. Medication guides are available at http://www.fda.gov/cder/Offices/ODS/medication_guides.htm. Dispense to parents or guardians of children and adolescents receiving this medication.

Contraindications Hypersensitivity to phenelzine or any component of the formulation; congestive heart failure; pheochromocytoma; hepatic disease or abnormal liver function tests; renal disease or severe renal impairment

Concurrent use of sympathomimetics (including amphetamines, cocaine, dopamine, epinephrine, methylphenidate, norepinephrine, or phenylephrine) and related compounds (methyldopa, levodopa, phenylalanine, tryptophan, or tyrosine), as well as ophthalmic alpha$_2$-agonists (apraclonidine, brimonidine); may result in hypertensive reactions

CNS depressants, cyclobenzaprine, dextromethorphan, ethanol, meperidine, bupropion, buspirone, or guanethidine [DSC]; may result in delirium, excitation, hyperpyrexia, seizures, and coma.

Serotonergic drugs (including dexfenfluramine, tricyclics, and SSRIs) — do not use within 5 weeks of fluoxetine discontinuation or 2 weeks of other antidepressant discontinuation, including MAO inhibitors

General anesthesia, spinal anesthesia (hypotension may be exaggerated). Use caution with local anesthetics containing sympathomimetic agents.

Foods high in tyramine or dopamine content; foods and/or supplements containing tyrosine, phenylalanine, tryptophan, or caffeine; may result in hypertensive reactions

Warnings/Precautions [U.S. Boxed Warning]: Antidepressants increase the risk of suicidal thinking and behavior in children, adolescents, and young adults (18-24 years of age) with major depressive disorder (MDD) and other psychiatric disorders; consider risk prior to prescribing. Short-term studies did not show an increased risk in patients >24 years of age and showed a decreased risk in patients ≥65 years. Closely monitor for clinical worsening, suicidality, or unusual changes in behavior; the patient's family or caregiver should be instructed to closely observe the patient and communicate condition with healthcare provider. Such observation would generally include at least weekly face-to-face contact with patients or their family members or caregivers during the first 4 weeks of treatment, then every other week visits for the next 4 weeks, then at 12 weeks, and as clinically indicated beyond 12 weeks. Additional contact by telephone may be appropriate between face-to-face visits. Adults treated with antidepressants should be observed similarly for clinical worsening and suicidality, especially during the initial few months of a course of drug therapy, or at times of dose changes, either increases or decreases. A medication guide should be dispensed with each prescription.

The possibility of a suicide attempt is inherent in major depression and may persist until remission occurs. Monitor for worsening of depression or suicidality, especially during initiation of therapy (generally first 1-2 months) or with dose increases or decreases. Worsening depression and severe abrupt suicidality that are not part of the presenting symptoms may require discontinuation or modification of drug therapy. Use caution in high-risk patients during initiation of therapy. Prescriptions should be written for the smallest quantity consistent with good patient care. The patient's family or caregiver should be alerted to monitor patients for the emergence of suicidality and associated behaviors such as anxiety, agitation, panic attacks, insomnia, irritability, hostility, impulsivity, akathisia, hypomania, and mania; patients should be instructed to notify their healthcare provider if any of these symptoms or worsening depression occur.

May worsen psychosis in some patients or precipitate a shift to mania or hypomania in patients with bipolar disorder. Monotherapy in patients with bipolar disorder should be avoided. Patients presenting with depressive symptoms should be screened for bipolar disorder. Phenelzine is not FDA approved for the treatment of bipolar depression.

Sensitization to the effects of insulin may occur; monitor blood glucose closely in patients with diabetes. Use with caution in patients who are hyperactive, hyperexcitable, or who have glaucoma, or hyperthyroidism. Hypertensive crisis may occur with tyramine-, tryptophan-, or dopamine-containing foods. Should not be used in combination with other antidepressants. Hypotensive effects of antihypertensives (beta-blockers, thiazides) may be exaggerated. May cause orthostatic hypotension - use with caution in patients with hypotension or patients who would not tolerate transient hypotensive episodes (cardiovascular or cerebrovascular disease) - effects may be additive with other agents which cause orthostasis. Use with caution in patients at risk of seizures, or in patients receiving other drugs which may lower seizure threshold. Discontinue at least 48 hours prior to myelography. May increase the risks associated with electroconvulsive therapy. Consider discontinuing, when possible, prior to elective surgery.

Adverse Reactions (Reflective of adult population; not specific for elderly)

Frequency not defined.

Cardiovascular: Edema, orthostatic hypotension

Central nervous system: Anxiety (acute), ataxia, coma, delirium, dizziness, drowsiness, fatigue, fever, headache, hyper-reflexia, mania, seizure, sleep disturbances, twitching

Dermatologic: Pruritus, rash

Endocrine & metabolic: Decreased sexual ability (anorgasmia, ejaculatory disturbances, impotence), hypermetabolic syndrome, hypernatremia

Gastrointestinal: Constipation, weight gain, xerostomia

Genitourinary: Urinary retention

Hematologic: Leukopenia

Hepatic: Hepatitis, jaundice, necrotizing hepatocellular necrosis (rare)

Neuromuscular & skeletal: Lupus-like syndrome, myoclonia, tremor, weakness

Ocular: Blurred vision, glaucoma

Miscellaneous: Diaphoresis, transient cardiac or respiratory depression (following ECT), withdrawal syndrome (nausea, vomiting, malaise)

Respiratory: Edema (glottis)

Overdosage/Toxicology

Symptoms include tachycardia, palpitations, muscle twitching, seizures, insomnia, restlessness, transient hypertension, hypotension, drowsiness, hyperpyrexia, and coma. Competent supportive care is the most important treatment for overdose with a monoamine oxidase (MAO) inhibitor. Both hypertension or hypotension can occur with intoxication. Hypotension may respond to I.V. fluids or vasopressors and hypertension usually responds to an alpha-adrenergic blocker. While treating the hypertension, care is warranted to avoid sudden drops in blood pressure, since this may worsen MAO inhibitor toxicity. Muscle irritability and seizures often respond to diazepam, while hyperthermia is best treated with antipyretics and cooling blankets.

Drug Interactions

Amphetamines: MAO inhibitors in combination with amphetamines may result in severe hypertensive reaction; concurrent use is contraindicated.

Anorexiants: Concurrent use of anorexiants may result in serotonin syndrome; these combinations are best avoided; includes dexfenfluramine, fenfluramine, or sibutramine

Barbiturates: MAO inhibitors may inhibit the metabolism of barbiturates and prolong their effect

Bupropion: Concurrent use is contraindicated; allow at least 14 days between discontinuing MAO inhibitor and starting bupropion.

Buspirone: May cause hypertension; wait at least 10 days between discontinuing one agent and starting the other.

CNS stimulants: MAO inhibitors in combination with stimulants (methylphenidate) may result in severe hypertensive reaction; concurrent use is contraindicated.

Dextromethorphan: Concurrent use of MAO inhibitors may result in serotonin syndrome; concurrent use is contraindicated.

Disulfiram: MAO inhibitors may produce delirium in patients receiving disulfiram; monitor.

Duloxetine: Concurrent use is contraindicated, allow 5 days after discontinuing duloxetine before initiating therapy with a MAO inhibitor.

Guanadrel and guanethidine: MAO inhibitors inhibit the antihypertensive response to guanadrel or guanethidine; concurrent use is contraindicated; use an alternative antihypertensive agent.

Hypoglycemic agents: MAO inhibitors may produce hypoglycemia in patients with diabetes; monitor.

Levodopa: MAO inhibitors in combination with levodopa may result in hypertensive reactions; monitor.

Lithium: MAO inhibitors in combination with lithium have resulted in malignant hyperpyrexia; this combination is best avoided.

Meperidine: May cause serotonin syndrome when combined with an MAO inhibitor; concurrent use is contraindicated; avoid use of meperidine within 2 weeks of phenelzine use.

Nefazodone: Concurrent use of MAO inhibitors may result in serotonin syndrome; these combinations are best avoided

Norepinephrine: MAO inhibitors may increase the pressor response of norepinephrine (effect is generally small); monitor

Reserpine: MAO inhibitors in combination with reserpine may result in hypertensive reactions; monitor

Serotonin agonists: Theoretically may increase the risk of serotonin syndrome; includes sumatriptan, naratriptan, rizatriptan, and zolmitriptan

SSRIs: May cause serotonin syndrome when combined with an MAO inhibitor; avoid this combination. Allow 5 weeks between discontinuing fluoxetine and starting an

(Continued)

Phenelzine *(Continued)*

MAO inhibitor; allow at least 10 days after discontinuing MAO inhibitor and starting fluoxetine.

Succinylcholine: MAO inhibitors may prolong the muscle relaxation produced by succinylcholine via decreased plasma pseudocholinesterase

Sympathomimetics (indirect-acting): MAO inhibitors in combination with sympathomimetics such as dopamine, metaraminol, phenylephrine, and decongestants (pseudoephedrine) may result in severe hypertensive reaction; concurrent use is contraindicated.

Tramadol: May increase the risk of seizures and serotonin syndrome in patients receiving an MAO inhibitor

Trazodone: Concurrent use of MAO inhibitors may result in serotonin syndrome; these combinations are best avoided

Tricyclic antidepressants: May cause serotonin syndrome when combined with an MAO inhibitor; avoid this combination

Venlafaxine: Concurrent use of MAO inhibitors may result in serotonin syndrome; these combinations are best avoided

Ethanol/Nutrition/Herb Interactions

Ethanol: Avoid ethanol (based on CNS depressant effects and potential tyramine content)

Food: Concurrent ingestion of foods rich in tyramine may cause sudden and severe high blood pressure (hypertensive crisis). Avoid tyramine-containing foods with MAOIs. Food's freshness is also an important concern; improperly stored or spoiled food can create an environment where tyramine concentrations may increase.

Herb/Nutraceuticals: Avoid supplements containing caffeine, tyrosine, tryptophan or phenylalanine. Ingestion of large quantities may increase the risk of severe side effects (eg, hypertensive reactions, serotonin syndrome).

Stability Protect from light.

Mechanism of Action Thought to act by increasing endogenous concentrations of norepinephrine, dopamine, and serotonin through inhibition of the enzyme (monoamine oxidase) responsible for the breakdown of these neurotransmitters

Pharmacodynamics

Onset of action: Expect to see some clinical response in 2-4 weeks, provided that the dosing is adequate

Duration: May continue to have a therapeutic effect and interactions 2 weeks after discontinuing therapy

Geriatric patients receiving an average of 55 mg/day developed a mean platelet MAO activity inhibition of about 85%

Pharmacokinetics

Absorption: Oral: Well absorbed; undergoes acetylation in the liver

Older patients have been reported to have higher blood concentrations than younger adults after 2 weeks of continuous treatment

Metabolism: Oxidized via monoamine oxidase (primary pathway) and acetylation (minor pathway)

Half-life elimination: 11 hours

Elimination: In urine primarily as metabolites and unchanged drug

Dosage

Geriatrics: Oral: Initial: 7.5 mg/day; increase by 7.5-15 mg/day every 3-4 days as tolerated; usual therapeutic dose: 15-60 mg/day in 3-4 divided doses.

Adults: Depression: Oral: 15 mg 3 times/day; may increase to 60-90 mg/day during early phase of treatment, then reduce dose for maintenance therapy slowly after maximum benefit is obtained. Takes 2-4 weeks for a significant response to occur.

Monitoring Parameters Blood pressure, heart rate; diet; weight; mood if depressive symptoms

Reference Range Inhibition of platelet monoamine oxidase (≥80%) correlates with clinical response

Patient Information Avoid tyramine-containing foods: red wine, aged cheese (except cottage, ricotta, and cream), smoked or pickled fish, beef or chicken liver, dried sausage, fava or broad bean pods, yeast, vitamin supplements. Report severe headaches, irregular heartbeats, skin rash, insomnia, sedation, changes in strength, sensations of pain, burning, touch, or vibration, or any other unusual symptoms to your physician; avoid alcohol; get up slowly from chair or bed.

Special Geriatric Considerations The MAO inhibitors are effective and generally well tolerated by elderly patients. It is their potential interactions with tyramine or tryptophan-containing food and other drugs and their effects on blood pressure that have limited their use. The MAO inhibitors are usually reserved for patients who do not tolerate or respond to the traditional "cyclic" or "second generation" antidepressants. The brain activity of monoamine oxidase increases with age and even more so in patients with Alzheimer's disease. Therefore, the MAO inhibitors may have an increased role in patients with Alzheimer's disease who are depressed. Phenelzine is less stimulating than tranylcypromine.

Dosage Forms Excipient information presented when available (limited, particularly for generics); consult specific product labeling.

Tablet: 15 mg

Selected References

Alexopoulos GS, "Treatment of Depression," *Clinical Geriatric Psychopharmacology*, 2nd ed, Salzman C, ed, Baltimore, MD: Williams & Wilkins, 1992, 137-74.

Georgotas A, Friedman E, McCarthy M, et al, "Resistant Geriatric Depression and Therapeutic Response to Monoamine-Oxidase Inhibitors," *Biol Psychiatry*, 1983, 18:195-205.

Goff DC and Jenike MA, "Treatment-Resistant Depression in the Elderly," *J Am Geriatr Soc*, 1986, 34(1):63-70.

Jenike MA, "MAO Inhibitors as Treatment for Depressed Patients With Primary Degenerative Dementia (Alzheimer's Disease)," *Am J Psychiatry*, 1985, 142:763.

♦ **Phenelzine Sulfate** *see* Phenelzine *on page 1239*

♦ **Phenergan**® *see* Promethazine *on page 1327*

♦ **Pheniramine and Naphazoline** *see* Naphazoline and Pheniramine *on page 1087*

Phenobarbital (fee noe BAR bi tal)

Related Information

Serum Drug Concentrations Commonly Monitored Guidelines *on page 1862*

Medication Safety Issues

Sound-alike/look-alike issues:

Phenobarbital may be confused with pentobarbital

Luminal® may be confused with Tuinal®

U.S. Brand Names Luminal® Sodium

Canadian Brand Names PMS-Phenobarbital

Index Terms Phenobarbital Sodium; Phenobarbitone; Phenylethylmalonylurea

Generic Available Yes

Pharmacologic Category Anticonvulsant, Barbiturate; Barbiturate

Use Management of generalized tonic-clonic (grand mal) and partial seizures; sedation; hypnosis; reduction of bilirubin in chronic cholestasis

Unlabeled/Investigational Use Management of sedative/hypnotic withdrawal

Restrictions C-IV

Contraindications Hypersensitivity to barbiturates or any component of the formulation; marked hepatic impairment; dyspnea or airway obstruction; porphyria

Warnings/Precautions Use with caution in patients with hypovolemic shock, CHF, hepatic impairment, respiratory dysfunction or depression, previous addiction to the sedative/hypnotic group, chronic or acute pain, renal dysfunction, and the elderly, due to its long half-life and risk of dependence, phenobarbital is not recommended as a sedative in the elderly; tolerance or psychological and physical dependence may occur with prolonged use. Use with caution in patients with depression or suicidal tendencies, or in patients with a history of drug abuse. **Abrupt withdrawal in patients with epilepsy may precipitate status epilepticus.**

Adverse Reactions (Reflective of adult population; not specific for elderly)

Frequency not defined.

Cardiovascular: Bradycardia, hypotension, syncope

Central nervous system: Drowsiness, lethargy, CNS excitation or depression, impaired judgment, "hangover" effect, confusion, somnolence, agitation, hyperkinesia, ataxia, nervousness, headache, insomnia, nightmares, hallucinations, anxiety, dizziness

Dermatologic: Rash, exfoliative dermatitis, Stevens-Johnson syndrome

Gastrointestinal: Nausea, vomiting, constipation

Hematologic: Agranulocytosis, thrombocytopenia, megaloblastic anemia

Local: Pain at injection site, thrombophlebitis with I.V. use

Renal: Oliguria

Respiratory: Laryngospasm, respiratory depression, apnea (especially with rapid I.V. use), hypoventilation

Miscellaneous: Gangrene with inadvertent intra-arterial injection

Overdosage/Toxicology Symptoms include unsteady gait, slurred speech, confusion, jaundice, hypothermia, hypotension, respiratory depression, and coma. If hypotension occurs, administer I.V. fluids and place in Trendelenburg position. If unresponsive, an I.V. vasopressor (eg, dopamine, epinephrine) may be required. Repeat oral doses of activated charcoal significantly reduce the half-life of phenobarbital resulting from enhancement of nonrenal elimination. The usual dose is 0.1-1 g/kg every 4-6 hours for 3-4 days, unless the patient has no bowel movement, causing charcoal to remain in the GI tract. Assure adequate hydration and renal function. Urinary alkalinization with I.V. sodium bicarbonate also helps enhance elimination. Hemodialysis or hemoperfusion is of uncertain value. Patients in stage IV coma, due to high serum barbiturate levels, may require charcoal hemoperfusion.

Drug Interactions Substrate of CYP2C9 (minor), 2C19 (major), 2E1 (minor); **Induces** CYP1A2 (strong), 2A6 (strong), 2B6 (strong), 2C8 (strong), 2C9 (strong), 3A4 (strong)

(Continued)

Phenobarbital *(Continued)*

Acetaminophen: Barbiturates may enhance the hepatotoxic potential of acetaminophen overdoses

Antiarrhythmics: Barbiturates may increase the metabolism of antiarrhythmics, decreasing their clinical effect; includes disopyramide, propafenone, and quinidine

Anticonvulsants: Barbiturates may increase the metabolism of anticonvulsants; includes ethosuximide, felbamate (possibly), lamotrigine, phenytoin, tiagabine, topiramate, and zonisamide; does not appear to affect gabapentin or levetiracetam

Antineoplastics: Limited evidence suggests that enzyme-inducing anticonvulsant therapy may reduce the effectiveness of some chemotherapy regimens (specifically in ALL); teniposide and methotrexate may be cleared more rapidly in these patients

Antipsychotics: Barbiturates may enhance the metabolism (decrease the efficacy) of antipsychotics; monitor for altered response; dose adjustment may be needed

Beta-blockers: Metabolism of beta-blockers may be increased and clinical effect decreased; atenolol and nadolol are unlikely to interact given their renal elimination

Calcium channel blockers: Barbiturates may enhance the metabolism of calcium channel blockers, decreasing their clinical effect

Chloramphenicol: Barbiturates may increase the metabolism of chloramphenicol and chloramphenicol may inhibit barbiturate metabolism; monitor for altered response

Cimetidine: Barbiturates may enhance the metabolism of cimetidine, decreasing its clinical effect

CNS depressants: Sedative effects and/or respiratory depression with barbiturates may be additive with other CNS depressants; monitor for increased effect; includes ethanol, sedatives, antidepressants, opioid analgesics, and benzodiazepines

Corticosteroids: Barbiturates may enhance the metabolism of corticosteroids, decreasing their clinical effect

Cyclosporine: Levels may be decreased by barbiturates; monitor

CYP1A2 substrates: Phenobarbital may decrease the levels/effects of CYP1A2 substrates. Example substrates include aminophylline, estrogens, fluvoxamine, mirtazapine, ropinirole, and theophylline.

CYP2A6 substrates: Phenobarbital may decrease the levels/effects of CYP2A6 substrates. Example substrates include ifosfamide and rifampin.

CYP2B6 substrates: Phenobarbital may decrease the levels/effects of CYP2B6 substrates. Example substrates include bupropion, efavirenz, promethazine, selegiline, and sertraline.

CYP2C8 Substrates: Phenobarbital may decrease the levels/effects of CYP2C8 substrates. Example substrates include amiodarone, paclitaxel, pioglitazone, repaglinide, and rosiglitazone.

CYP2C9 Substrates: Phenobarbital may decrease the levels/effects of CYP2C9 substrates. Example substrates include bosentan, celecoxib, dapsone, fluoxetine, glimepiride, glipizide, losartan, montelukast, nateglinide, paclitaxel, phenytoin, sulfonamides, trimethoprim, warfarin, and zafirlukast.

CYP2C19 inducers: May decrease the levels/effects of phenobarbital. Example inducers include aminoglutethimide, carbamazepine, phenytoin, and rifampin.

CYP2C19 inhibitors: May increase the levels/effects of phenobarbital. Example inhibitors include delavirdine, fluconazole, fluvoxamine, gemfibrozil, isoniazid, omeprazole, and ticlopidine.

CYP3A4 substrates: Phenobarbital may decrease the levels/effects of CYP3A4 substrates. Example substrates include benzodiazepines, calcium channel blockers, clarithromycin, cyclosporine, erythromycin, estrogens, mirtazapine, nateglinide, nefazodone, nevirapine, protease inhibitors, tacrolimus, and venlafaxine.

Doxycycline: Barbiturates may enhance the metabolism of doxycycline, decreasing its clinical effect; higher dosages may be required

Estrogens: Barbiturates may increase the metabolism of estrogens and reduce their efficacy

Felbamate may inhibit the metabolism of barbiturates and barbiturates may increase the metabolism of felbamate

Griseofulvin: Barbiturates may impair the absorption of griseofulvin, and griseofulvin metabolism may be increased by barbiturates, decreasing clinical effect

Guanfacine: Effect may be decreased by barbiturates

Immunosuppressants: Barbiturates may enhance the metabolism of immunosuppressants, decreasing its clinical effect; includes both cyclosporine and tacrolimus

Loop diuretics: Metabolism may be increased and clinical effects decreased; established for furosemide, effect with other loop diuretics not established

MAO inhibitors: Metabolism of barbiturates may be inhibited, increasing clinical effect or toxicity of the barbiturates

Methadone: Barbiturates may enhance the metabolism of methadone resulting in methadone withdrawal

Methoxyflurane: Barbiturates may enhance the nephrotoxic effects of methoxyflurane

Oral contraceptives: Barbiturates may enhance the metabolism of oral contraceptives, decreasing their clinical effect; an alternative method of contraception should be considered

Theophylline: Barbiturates may increase metabolism of theophylline derivatives and decrease their clinical effect

Tricyclic antidepressants: Barbiturates may increase metabolism of tricyclic antidepressants and decrease their clinical effect; sedative effects may be additive

Valproic acid: Metabolism of barbiturates may be inhibited by valproic acid; monitor for excessive sedation; a dose reduction may be needed

Warfarin: Barbiturates inhibit the hypoprothrombinemic effects of oral anticoagulants via increased metabolism; this combination should generally be avoided

Ethanol/Nutrition/Herb Interactions

Ethanol: Avoid ethanol (may increase CNS depression).

Food: May cause decrease in vitamin D and calcium.

Herb/Nutraceutical: Avoid evening primrose (seizure threshold decreased). Avoid valerian, St John's wort, kava kava, gotu kola (may increase CNS depression).

Stability Protect elixir from light. Not stable in aqueous solutions; use only clear solutions. Do not add to acidic solutions; precipitation may occur.

Mechanism of Action Short-acting barbiturate with sedative, hypnotic, and anticonvulsant properties. Barbiturates depress the sensory cortex, decrease motor activity, alter cerebellar function, and produce drowsiness, sedation, and hypnosis. In high doses, barbiturates exhibit anticonvulsant activity; barbiturates produce dose-dependent respiratory depression.

Pharmacodynamics

Hypnosis after oral dose:

Onset of action: Within 20-60 minutes

Duration: 6-10 hours

I.V.:

Onset of action: Within 5 minutes

Peak effect: Within 30 minutes

Duration: 4-10 hours; older adults may be more sensitive to the sedative effects of phenobarbital

Pharmacokinetics

Absorption: Oral: 70% to 90%

Protein binding: 20% to 45%

Metabolism: In liver via hydroxylation and glucuronide conjugation

Half-life: 53-140 hours; half-life may be increased in older adults; clearance can be increased with alkalinization of urine or with oral multiple dose activated charcoal

Time to peak serum concentration: Oral: Within 1-6 hours

Elimination: 20% to 50% excreted unchanged in urine

Dosage

Geriatrics: Geriatric patients should be started at the lowest recommended dose. Refer to adult dosing.

Adults:

Sedation: Oral, I.M.: 30-120 mg/day in 2-3 divided doses

Hypnotic: Oral, I.M., I.V., SubQ: 100-320 mg at bedtime

Preoperative sedation: I.M.: 100-200 mg 1-1.5 hours before procedure

Anticonvulsant/status epilepticus:

Loading dose: I.V.: 300-800 mg initially followed by 120-240 mg/dose at 20-minute intervals until seizures are controlled or a total dose of 1-2 g

Maintenance dose: Oral, I.V.: 1-3 mg/kg/day in divided doses or 50-100 mg 2-3 times/day

Sedative/hypnotic withdrawal (unlabeled use): Initial daily requirement is determined by substituting phenobarbital 30 mg for every 100 mg pentobarbital used during tolerance testing; then daily requirement is decreased by 10% of initial dose.

Renal Impairment:

Cl_{cr} <10 mL/minute: Administer every 12-16 hours.

Moderately dialyzable (20% to 50%)

Hepatic Impairment: Increased side effects may occur in severe liver disease. Monitor plasma levels and adjust dose accordingly.

Monitoring Parameters Phenobarbital serum concentrations, mental status, CBC, LFTs, seizure activity

Reference Range Adults: Therapeutic: 15-40 mcg/mL (SI: 65-172 μmol/L); Toxic: >40 mcg/mL (SI: >172 μmol/L)

Test Interactions Assay interference of LDH

Patient Information May cause drowsiness, avoid alcohol and other CNS depressants

Additional Information Sodium content of injection (65 mg, 1 mL): 6 mg (0.3 mEq)

Phenobarbital: Barbita®, Solfoton®

Phenobarbital sodium: Luminal®

(Continued)

Phenobarbital *(Continued)*

Special Geriatric Considerations Using barbiturates in elderly may induce paradoxical stimulation, cause or aggravate depression and confusion. Due to its long half-life and risk of dependence, phenobarbital is not recommended as a sedative or hypnotic in the elderly. Interpretive guidelines from the Centers for Medicare and Medicaid Services (CMS) discourage the use of this agent as a sedative/hypnotic in long-term care residents.

Dosage Forms Excipient information presented when available (limited, particularly for generics); consult specific product labeling.

Elixir: 20 mg/5 mL (5 mL, 7.5 mL, 15 mL, 480 mL) [contains alcohol]

Injection, solution, as sodium: 65 mg/mL (1 mL); 130 mg/mL (1 mL) [contains alcohol and propylene glycol]

Luminal® Sodium: 60 mg/mL (1 mL); 130 mg/mL (1 mL) [contains alcohol 10% and propylene glycol]

Tablet: 15 mg, 30 mg, 60 mg, 100 mg

Extemporaneously Prepared An alcohol-free phenobarbital 10 mg/mL suspension can be prepared as follows: Levigate ten phenobarbital 60 mg tablets in a glass mortar into a fine powder. Mix 30 mL of Ora-Plus® and 30 mL of either Ora-Sweet® or Ora-Sweet® SF; stir vigorously. Add 15 mL of the Ora-Plus®/Ora-Sweet® (or Ora-Sweet® SF) mixture to the powder; triturate well. Transfer to a 2 ounce amber plastic bottle; qs to a final volume of 60 mL. Stable for up to 115 days at room temperature. Shake well prior to use.

May mix dose with chocolate syrup (1:1 volume) immediately before administration to mask the bitter aftertaste.

Cober M and Johnson CE, "Stability of an Extemporaneously Prepared Alcohol-Free Phenobarbital Suspension," *Am J Health Syst Pharm*, 2007, 64(6):644-6.

♦ **Phenobarbital, Hyoscyamine, Atropine, and Scopolamine** *see* Hyoscyamine, Atropine, Scopolamine, and Phenobarbital *on page 780*

♦ **Phenobarbital Sodium** *see* Phenobarbital *on page 1243*

♦ **Phenobarbitone** *see* Phenobarbital *on page 1243*

Phenoxybenzamine (fen oks ee BEN za meen)

U.S. Brand Names Dibenzyline®

Canadian Brand Names Dibenzyline®

Index Terms Phenoxybenzamine Hydrochloride

Generic Available No

Pharmacologic Category Alpha$_1$ Blocker

Use Symptomatic management of pheochromocytoma; treatment of hypertensive crisis caused by sympathomimetic amines

Unlabeled/Investigational Use Treatment of micturition problems associated with neurogenic bladder, functional outlet obstruction, and partial prostate obstruction

Contraindications Hypersensitivity to phenoxybenzamine or any component of the formulation; conditions in which a fall in blood pressure would be undesirable (eg, shock)

Warnings/Precautions Use with caution in patients with renal impairment, cerebral, or coronary arteriosclerosis, can exacerbate symptoms of respiratory tract infections. Discontinue if symptoms of angina occur or worsen. Because of the risk of adverse effects, avoid the use of this medication in the elderly if possible.

Adverse Reactions (Reflective of adult population; not specific for elderly)
Frequency not defined.

Cardiovascular: Postural hypotension, shock, syncope, tachycardia

Central nervous system: Confusion, fatigue headache, lethargy

Gastrointestinal: Diarrhea, nausea, vomiting, xerostomia

Genitourinary: Inhibition of ejaculation

Neuromuscular & skeletal: Weakness

Ocular: Miosis

Respiratory: Nasal congestion

Overdosage/Toxicology Symptoms include hypotension, tachycardia, lethargy, dizziness, and shock. Hypotension and shock should be treated with fluids and Trendelenburg positioning. Only alpha-adrenergic pressors, such as norepinephrine should be used. Mixed agents such as epinephrine, may cause more hypotension.

Drug Interactions

Alpha-adrenergic agonists decrease the effect of phenoxybenzamine.

Beta-blockers may result in increased toxicity (hypotension, tachycardia).

Sildenafil, tadalafil, vardenafil: Blood pressure-lowering effects are additive. Use of vardenafil or tadalafil is contraindicated by the manufacturer. Use sildenafil with extreme caution (dose ≤25 mg).

Ethanol/Nutrition/Herb Interactions Ethanol: Avoid ethanol.

Mechanism of Action Produces long-lasting noncompetitive alpha-adrenergic blockade of postganglionic synapses in exocrine glands and smooth muscle; relaxes urethra and increases opening of the bladder

Pharmacodynamics
Onset of action: Oral: Within 2 hours
Peak effect: Within 4-6 hours
Duration: 4 or more days

Pharmacokinetics
Half-life: 24 hours
Elimination: Primarily in urine and feces

Dosage
Geriatrics & Adults:
Pheochromocytoma, hypertension: Oral: Initial: 10 mg twice daily, increase by 10 mg every other day until optimum dose is achieved; usual range: 20-40 mg 2-3 times/day
Urinary incontinence: 10 mg 1-3 times/day

Monitoring Parameters Blood pressure, pulse, urine output

Patient Information Avoid alcoholic beverages; if dizziness occurs, avoid sudden changes in posture; may cause nasal congestion and constricted pupils; may inhibit ejaculation; avoid cough, cold or allergy medications containing sympathomimetics

Special Geriatric Considerations Because of the risk of adverse effects, avoid the use of this medication in the elderly if possible.

Dosage Forms Excipient information presented when available (limited, particularly for generics); consult specific product labeling.
Capsule, as hydrochloride: 10 mg [contains benzyl alcohol]

♦ **Phenoxybenzamine Hydrochloride** see Phenoxybenzamine on page 1246
♦ **Phenoxymethyl Penicillin** see Penicillin V Potassium on page 1227
♦ **Phenylalanine Mustard** see Melphalan on page 974
♦ **Phenylazo Diamino Pyridine Hydrochloride** see Phenazopyridine on page 1238

Phenylephrine (fen il EF rin)

Medication Safety Issues
Sound-alike/look-alike issues:
Mydfrin® may be confused with Midrin®

High alert medication: The Institute for Safe Medication Practices (ISMP) includes this medication among its list of drugs which have a heightened risk of causing significant patient harm when used in error.

U.S. Brand Names Ah-Chew D®; AK-Dilate®; Altafrin; Anu-Med [OTC]; Dimetapp® Toddler's [OTC]; Formulation R™ [OTC]; LuSonal™; Medicone® Suppositories [OTC]; Medi-Phenyl [OTC]; Mydfrin®; NāSop™; Neofrin™; Neo-Synephrine® Extra Strength [OTC]; Neo-Synephrine® Injection; Neo-Synephrine® Mild [OTC]; Neo-Synephrine® Regular Strength [OTC]; OcuNefrin™ [OTC]; Preparation H® [OTC]; Rectacaine [OTC]; Relief® [OTC]; Rhinall [OTC]; Sudafed PE™ [OTC]; Triaminic® Infant Thin Strips® Decongestant [OTC]; Triaminic® Thin Strips® Cold [OTC]; Tronolane® Suppository [OTC]; Tur-bi-kal® [OTC]; Vicks® Sinex® Nasal Spray [OTC]; Vicks® Sinex® UltraFine Mist [OTC]; 4 Way® Fast Acting [OTC]; 4 Way® Menthol [OTC]; 4 Way® No Drip [OTC]

Canadian Brand Names Dionephrine®; Mydfrin®; Neo-Synephrine®

Index Terms Phenylephrine Hydrochloride; Phenylephrine Tannate

Generic Available Yes: Excludes cream, filmstrip, liquid, suspension

Pharmacologic Category Alpha/Beta Agonist; Ophthalmic Agent, Antiglaucoma; Ophthalmic Agent, Mydriatic

Use Treatment of hypotension, vascular failure in shock; vasoconstrictor in regional analgesia; mydriatic in ophthalmic procedures and treatment of wide-angle glaucoma; supraventricular tachycardia

OTC: Symptomatic relief of nasal and nasopharyngeal mucosal congestion; treatment of hemorrhoids; relief of redness of the eye due to irritation

Contraindications Hypersensitivity to phenylephrine or any component of the formulation; hypertension; ventricular tachycardia
Oral: Use with or within 14 days of MAO inhibitor therapy
Ophthalmic: Narrow-angle glaucoma

Warnings/Precautions Some products contain sulfites which may cause allergic reactions in susceptible individuals. Use with extreme caution in patients taking MAO inhibitors.

Intravenous: Use with caution in the elderly, patients with hyperthyroidism, bradycardia, partial heart block, myocardial disease, or severe CAD. Assure adequate circulatory volume to minimize need for vasoconstrictors. Avoid hypertension; monitor blood pressure closely and adjust infusion rate. Avoid extravasation; infuse into a large vein if possible. Avoid infusion into leg veins. Watch I.V. site closely. If extravasation (Continued)

Phenylephrine *(Continued)*

occurs, infiltrate the area with diluted phentolamine (5-10 mg in 10-15 mL of saline) with a fine hypodermic needle. Phentolamine should be administered as soon as possible after extravasation is noted. **[U.S. Boxed Warning]: Should be administered by adequately trained individuals familiar with its use.**

Nasal, oral, rectal: Use caution with hyperthyroidism, diabetes mellitus, cardiovascular disease, ischemic heart disease, increased intraocular pressure, prostatic hyperplasia or in the elderly. Rebound congestion may occur when nasal products are discontinued after chronic use. When used for self-medication (OTC), notify healthcare provider if symptoms do not improve within 7 days (oral, rectal) or 3 days (nasal), are accompanied by fever (oral), or if bleeding occurs (rectal).

Ophthalmic: When used for self-medication (OTC), notify healthcare provider in case of vision changes, continued redness, or if symptoms worsen or do not improve within 3 days.

Adverse Reactions (Reflective of adult population; not specific for elderly) Frequency not defined.

Cardiovascular: Reflex bradycardia, excitability, restlessness, arrhythmia (rare), precordial pain or discomfort, pallor, hypertension, severe peripheral and visceral vasoconstriction, decreased cardiac output

Central nervous system: Headache, anxiety, dizziness, tremor, paresthesia, restlessness

Endocrine & metabolic: Metabolic acidosis

Local: I.V.: Extravasation which may lead to necrosis and sloughing of surrounding tissue, blanching of skin

Neuromuscular & skeletal: Pilomotor response, weakness

Renal: Decreased renal perfusion, reduced urine output, reduced urine output

Respiratory: Respiratory distress

Overdosage/Toxicology Symptoms include vomiting, hypertension, palpitations, paresthesia, and ventricular extrasystoles. Treatment is supportive. In extreme cases, I.V. phentolamine may be used.

Drug Interactions

Beta-blockers (nonselective) may increase hypertensive effect; avoid concurrent use.

MAO inhibitors: May potentiate hypertension and hypertensive crisis; avoid concurrent use.

Methyldopa can increase the pressor response; be aware of patient's drug regimen.

Tricyclic antidepressants: May enhance the vasopressor effect phenylephrine; avoid concurrent use.

Ethanol/Nutrition/Herb Interactions Herb/Nutraceutical: Avoid ephedra, yohimbe (may cause CNS stimulation).

Stability

Solution for injection: Store vials at controlled room temperature of 15°C to 30°C (59°F to 86°F). Protect from light. Do not use solution if brown or contains a precipitate.

I.V. infusion: May dilute 10 mg in 500 mL NS or D_5W.

I.V. injection: Dilute with SWFI to a concentration of 1 mg/mL.

Ophthalmic solution:

0.12%: Store at controlled room temperature. Protect from light and excessive heat.

2.5% and 10%: Refer to product labeling. Some products are labeled to store at room temperature, others should be stored under refrigeration at 2°C to 8°C (36°F to 46°F). Do not use solution if brown or contains a precipitate.

Mechanism of Action Potent, direct-acting alpha-adrenergic stimulator with weak beta-adrenergic activity; causes vasoconstriction of the arterioles of the nasal mucosa and conjunctiva; activates the dilator muscle of the pupil to cause contraction; produces vasoconstriction of arterioles in the body; produces systemic arterial vasoconstriction

Pharmacodynamics

Onset of action: Parenteral injection: Effects occur immediately

Duration:

I.M., SubQ: 45-60 minutes

I.V.: 20-30 minutes

Pharmacokinetics

Half-life: 2.5 hours

Metabolism: To phenolic conjugates

Elimination: Urine (90%)

Dosage

Geriatrics:

Nasal decongestant: Administer 2-3 drops or 1-2 sprays every 4 hours of 0.125% to 0.25% solution as needed; do not use more than 3 days.

Ophthalmic preparations for pupil dilation: Instill 1 drop of 2.5% solution, may repeat in 1 hour if necessary.

Refer to adult dosing for other uses and Geriatric Considerations for cautions on I.V. use.

Adults:

Hemorrhoids: Rectal:
Cream/ointment: Apply to clean dry area, up to 4 times/day; may be used externally or inserted rectally using applicator.
Suppository: Insert 1 suppository rectally, up to 4 times/day

Hypotension/shock:
I.V. bolus: 0.1-0.5 mg/dose every 10-15 minutes as needed (initial dose should not exceed 0.5 mg)
I.V. infusion: Initial dose: 100-180 mcg/minute; when blood pressure is stabilized, maintenance rate: 40-60 mcg/minute; rates up to 360 mcg/minute have been reported; dosing range: 0.4-9.1 mcg/kg/minute

Nasal congestion:
Intranasal: Instill 1-2 sprays or instill 1-2 drops every 4 hours of 0.25% to 0.5% solution as needed; 1% solution may be used in adult in cases of extreme nasal congestion; do not use nasal solutions more than 3 days
Oral:
Hydrochloride salt: 10-20 mg every 4 hours
Tannate salt (NāSop™ suspension): 7.5-15 mg every 12 hours

Ocular procedures: Ophthalmic: Instill 1 drop of 2.5% or 10% solution, may repeat in 10-60 minutes as needed.

Paroxysmal supraventricular tachycardia: I.V.: 0.25-0.5 mg/dose over 20-30 seconds

Reduction in ocular redness (OTC formulation): Ophthalmic: Instill 1-2 drops 0.12% solution into affected eye, up to 4 times/day; do not use for >72 hours

Administration

I.V.: May cause necrosis or sloughing tissue if extravasation occurs during I.V. administration or SubQ administration.
Extravasation management: Use phentolamine as antidote; mix 5 mg with 9 mL of NS. Inject a small amount of this dilution into extravasated area. Blanching should reverse immediately. Monitor site. If blanching should recur, additional injections of phentolamine may be needed.

Oral: NāSop™: Place tablet on tongue and allow to dissolve

Monitoring Parameters Blood pressure, pulse, EKG (systemic), relief of symptoms (topical)

Patient Information Nasal decongestant should not be used for >3 days in a row, hereby reducing problems of rebound congestion. Consult physician or pharmacist before using. Notify physician of insomnia, weakness, dizziness, tremor, or irregular heartbeat.

Special Geriatric Considerations Elderly are more predisposed to the adverse effects of sympathomimetics since they frequently have cardiovascular disease and diabetes mellitus, and are on multiple medications. Since oral and topical phenylephrine can be obtained OTC, elderly patients should be counseled about their proper use and in what disease states they should be avoided. Phenylephrine I.V. should be used with extreme caution in the elderly. The 10% ophthalmic solution has caused increased blood pressure in elderly patients and its use should, therefore, be avoided.

Dosage Forms Excipient information presented when available (limited, particularly for generics); consult specific product labeling. [DSC] = Discontinued product
Cream, rectal, as hydrochloride:
Formulation R™: 0.25% (54 g) [contains sodium benzoate]
Filmstrip, orally disintegrating, as hydrochloride:
Sudafed PE™: 10 mg (5s, 10s) [contains phenylalanine 1 mg/strip; cherry menthol flavor]
Triaminic® Infant Thin Strips® Decongestant: 1.25 mg [mixed berry flavor]
Triaminic® Thin Strips® Cold: 2.5 mg [raspberry flavor]
Injection, solution, as hydrochloride: 1% [10 mg/mL] (1 mL, 5 mL, 10 mL) [may contain sodium metabisulfite]
Neo-Synephrine®: 1% (1 mL) [contains sodium metabisulfite]
Liquid, oral, as hydrochloride:
LuSonal™: 7.5 mg/5 mL (480 mL) [contains phenylalanine; strawberry flavor]
Liquid, oral, as hydrochloride [drops]:
Dimetapp® Toddler's: 1.25 mg/0.8 mL (15 mL) [alcohol free; contains sodium benzoate; grape flavor]
Ointment, rectal, as hydrochloride:
Formulation R™, Preparation H®: 0.25% (30 g, 60 g) [contains benzoic acid]
Rectacaine: 0.25% (30 g)
Solution, intranasal, as hydrochloride [drops]:
Neo-Synephrine® Extra Strength: 1% (15 mL) [contains benzalkonium chloride]
Neo-Synephrine® Regular Strength: 0.5% (15 mL) [contains benzalkonium chloride]
Rhinall: 0.25% (30 mL) [contains benzalkonium chloride and sodium bisulfite]
(Continued)

Phenylephrine (Continued)

Tur-bi-kal®: 0.17% (30 mL) [contains benzalkonium choride]
Solution, intranasal, as hydrochloride [spray]:
4 Way® Fast Acting: 1% (15 mL, 30 mL) [contains benzalkonium chloride]
4 Way® Menthol: 1% (15 mL) [contains benzalkonium chloride and menthol]
4 Way® No Drip: 1% (15 mL) [contains benzalkonium chloride]
Neo-Synephrine® Extra Strength: 1% (15 mL) [contains benzalkonium chloride]
Neo-Synephrine® Mild: 0.25% (15 mL) [contains benzalkonium chloride]
Neo-Synephrine® Regular Strength: 0.5% (15 mL) [contains benzalkonium chloride]
Rhinall: 0.25% (40 mL) [contains benzalkonium chloride and sodium bisulfite]
Vicks® Sinex®, Vicks® Sinex® UltraFine Mist: 0.5% (15 mL) [contains benzalkonium chloride]
Solution, ophthalmic, as hydrochloride: 2.5% (2 mL, 3 mL, 5 mL, 15 mL) [may contain sodium bisulfite]
AK-Dilate®: 2.5% (2 mL, 15 mL); 10% (5 mL) [contains benzyl alcohol]
Altrafrin: 0.12% (15 mL) [OTC]; 2.5% (15 mL) [RX; contains benzalkonium chloride]; 10% (5 mL) [RX; contains benzalkonium chloride]
Mydfrin®: 2.5% (3 mL, 5 mL) [contains sodium bisulfite]
Neofrin™: 2.5% (15 mL); 10% (15 mL)
OcuNefrin™: 0.12% (15 mL)
Relief®: 0.12% (15 mL) [contains benzalkonium chloride]
Suppository, rectal, as hydrochloride: 0.25% (12s)
Anu-Med: 0.25% (12s)
Formulation R™, Preparation H®: 0.25% (12s, 24s, 48s)
Medicone®, Tronolane®: 0.25% (12s, 24s)
Rectacaine: 0.25% (12s)
Suspension, oral, as tannate:
Ah-Chew D®: Phenylephrine tannate (120 mL) [equivalent to phenylephrine hydro-chloride 10 mg/5 mL]
NāSop™: 7.5 mg/5 mL (120 mL) [orange flavor]
Tablet, as hydrochloride: 10 mg
Medi-Phenyl: 5 mg
Sudafed PE™: 10 mg
Tablet, orally dissolving, as hydrochloride:
NāSop™: 10 mg [contains phenylalanine 4 mg/tablet; bubble gum flavor]

♦ **Phenylephrine Hydrochloride** see Phenylephrine on page 1247
♦ **Phenylephrine Tannate** see Phenylephrine on page 1247
♦ **Phenylethylmalonylurea** see Phenobarbital on page 1243
♦ **Phenytek®** see Phenytoin on page 1250

Phenytoin (FEN i toyn)

Related Information
Serum Drug Concentrations Commonly Monitored Guidelines on page 1862
Medication Safety Issues
Sound-alike/look-alike issues:
Phenytoin may be confused with phenelzine, phentermine
Dilantin® may be confused with Dilaudid®, diltiazem, Dipentum®

International issues:
Dilantin® may be confused with Dolantine® which is a brand name for pethidine in Belgium and Switzerland
U.S. Brand Names Dilantin®; Phenytek®
Canadian Brand Names Dilantin®
Index Terms Diphenylhydantoin; DPH; Phenytoin Sodium; Phenytoin Sodium, Extended; Phenytoin Sodium, Prompt
Generic Available Yes: Excludes chewable tablet
Pharmacologic Category Antiarrhythmic Agent, Class Ib; Anticonvulsant, Hydantoin
Use Management of generalized tonic-clonic (grand mal), simple partial and complex partial seizures; prevention of seizures following head trauma/neurosurgery; ventric-ular arrhythmias, including those associated with digitalis intoxication, also used for epidermolysis bullosa; trigeminal neuralgia
Unlabeled/Investigational Use Treatment of ventricular arrhythmias (including those associated with digitalis intoxication, and prolonged QT interval), epidermolysis bullosa
Contraindications Hypersensitivity to phenytoin, other hydantoins, or any component of the formulation
Warnings/Precautions May increase frequency of petit mal seizures; I.V. form may cause hypotension, skin necrosis at I.V. site; avoid I.V. administration in small veins; use with caution in patients with porphyria; discontinue if rash or lymphadenopathy

occurs; a spectrum of hematologic effects have been reported with use (eg, neutropenia, leukopenia, thrombocytopenia, pancytopenia, and anemias); use with caution in patients with hepatic dysfunction, sinus bradycardia, S-A block, or AV block; use with caution in elderly or debilitated patients, or in any condition associated with low serum albumin levels, which will increase the free fraction of phenytoin in the serum and, therefore, the pharmacologic response. Sedation, confusional states, or cerebellar dysfunction (loss of motor coordination) may occur at higher total serum concentrations, or at lower total serum concentrations when the free fraction of phenytoin is increased. Effects with other sedative drugs or ethanol may be potentiated. Abrupt withdrawal may precipitate status epilepticus.

Adverse Reactions (Reflective of adult population; not specific for elderly)
I.V. effects: Hypotension, bradycardia, cardiac arrhythmia, cardiovascular collapse (especially with rapid I.V. use), venous irritation and pain, thrombophlebitis

Effects not related to plasma phenytoin concentrations: Hypertrichosis, gingival hypertrophy, thickening of facial features, carbohydrate intolerance, folic acid deficiency, peripheral neuropathy, vitamin D deficiency, osteomalacia, systemic lupus erythematosus

Concentration-related effects: Nystagmus, blurred vision, diplopia, ataxia, slurred speech, dizziness, drowsiness, lethargy, coma, rash, fever, nausea, vomiting, gum tenderness, confusion, mood changes, folic acid depletion, osteomalacia, hyperglycemia

Related to elevated concentrations:
>20 mcg/mL: Far lateral nystagmus
>30 mcg/mL: 45° lateral gaze nystagmus and ataxia
>40 mcg/mL: Decreased mentation
>100 mcg/mL: Death

Cardiovascular: Hypotension, bradycardia, cardiac arrhythmia, cardiovascular collapse
Central nervous system: Psychiatric changes, slurred speech, dizziness, drowsiness, headache, insomnia
Dermatologic: Rash
Gastrointestinal: Constipation, nausea, vomiting, gingival hyperplasia, enlargement of lips
Hematologic: Leukopenia, thrombocytopenia, agranulocytosis
Hepatic: Hepatitis
Local: Thrombophlebitis
Neuromuscular & skeletal: Tremor, peripheral neuropathy, paresthesia
Ocular: Diplopia, nystagmus, blurred vision
Rarely seen effects: SLE-like syndrome, lymphadenopathy, hepatitis, Stevens-Johnson syndrome, blood dyscrasias, dyskinesias, pseudolymphoma, lymphoma, venous irritation and pain, coarsening of the facial features, hypertrichosis

Overdosage/Toxicology Symptoms include unsteady gait, slurred speech, confusion, nausea, hypothermia, fever, hypotension, respiratory depression, and coma. Treatment is supportive for hypotension. Treat with I.V. fluids and place in Trendelenburg position. Seizures may be controlled with diazepam 5-10 mg.

Drug Interactions Substrate of CYP2C9 (major), 2C19 (major), 3A4 (minor); **Induces** CYP2B6 (strong), 2C8 (strong), 2C9 (strong), 2C19 (strong), 3A4 (strong)
Acetaminophen: Phenytoin may enhance the hepatotoxic potential of acetaminophen overdoses
Acetazolamide: Concurrent use with phenytoin may result in an increased risk of osteomalacia
Acyclovir: May decrease phenytoin serum levels; limited documentation; monitor
Allopurinol: May increase phenytoin serum concentrations; monitor
Antacids: May decrease absorption of phenytoin; separate oral doses by several hours
Antiarrhythmics: Phenytoin may increase the metabolism of antiarrhythmics, decreasing their clinical effect; includes disopyramide, propafenone, and quinidine; amiodarone also may increase phenytoin concentrations (see CYP inhibitors)
Anticonvulsants: Phenytoin may increase the metabolism of anticonvulsants; includes barbiturates, carbamazepine, ethosuximide, felbamate, lamotrigine, tiagabine, topiramate, and zonisamide; does not appear to affect gabapentin or levetiracetam; felbamate and gabapentin may increase phenytoin levels; monitor
Antineoplastics: Several chemotherapeutic agents have been associated with a decrease in serum phenytoin levels; includes cisplatin, bleomycin, carmustine, methotrexate, and vinblastine; monitor phenytoin serum levels. Limited evidence also suggest that enzyme-inducing anticonvulsant therapy may reduce the effectiveness of some chemotherapy regimens (specifically in ALL). Teniposide and methotrexate may be cleared more rapidly in these patients.
Antipsychotics: Phenytoin may enhance the metabolism (decrease the efficacy) of antipsychotics; monitor for altered response; dose adjustment may be needed; also see note on clozapine
Benzodiazepines: Phenytoin may decrease the serum concentrations of some benzodiazepines; monitor for decreased benzodiazepine effect
(Continued)

Phenytoin *(Continued)*

Beta-blockers: Metabolism of beta-blockers may be increased and clinical effect decreased; atenolol and nadolol are unlikely to interact given their renal elimination

Calcium channel blockers: Phenytoin may enhance the metabolism of calcium channel blockers, decreasing their clinical effect; calcium channel blockers (diltiazem, nifedipine) have been reported to increase phenytoin levels (case report); monitor.

Capecitabine: May increase the serum concentrations of phenytoin; monitor

Chloramphenicol: Phenytoin may increase the metabolism of chloramphenicol and chloramphenicol may inhibit phenytoin metabolism; monitor for altered response

Cimetidine: May increase the serum concentrations of phenytoin; monitor.

Ciprofloxacin: May decrease serum phenytoin concentrations; monitor.

Clozapine: Phenytoin may decrease levels/effects of clozapine; monitor.

CNS depressants: Sedative effects may be additive with other CNS depressants; monitor for increased effect; includes ethanol, barbiturates, sedatives, antidepressants, opioid analgesics, and benzodiazepines

Corticosteroids: Phenytoin may increase the metabolism of corticosteroids, decreasing their clinical effect; also see dexamethasone

Cyclosporine and tacrolimus: Levels may be decreased by phenytoin; monitor

CYP2B6 substrates: Phenytoin may decrease the levels/effects of CYP2B6 substrates. Example substrates include bupropion, efavirenz, promethazine, selegiline, and sertraline.

CYP2C9 inducers: May decrease the levels/effects of phenytoin. Example inducers include carbamazepine, phenobarbital, rifampin, rifapentine, and secobarbital.

CYP2C9 Inhibitors may increase the levels/effects of phenytoin. Example inhibitors include delavirdine, fluconazole, gemfibrozil, ketoconazole, nicardipine, NSAIDs, sulfonamides and tolbutamide.

CYP2C8 Substrates: Phenytoin may decrease the levels/effects of CYP2C8 substrates. Example substrates include amiodarone, paclitaxel, pioglitazone, repaglinide, and rosiglitazone.

CYP2C9 Substrates: Phenytoin may decrease the levels/effects of CYP2C9 substrates. Example substrates include bosentan, celecoxib, dapsone, fluoxetine, glimepiride, glipizide, losartan, montelukast, nateglinide, paclitaxel, sulfonamides, trimethoprim, warfarin, and zafirlukast.

CYP2C19 inducers: May decrease the levels/effects of phenytoin. Example inducers include aminoglutethimide, carbamazepine, phenytoin, and rifampin.

CYP2C19 inhibitors: May increase the levels/effects of phenytoin. Example inhibitors include delavirdine, fluconazole, fluvoxamine, gemfibrozil, isoniazid, omeprazole, and ticlopidine.

CYP2C19 substrates: Phenytoin may decrease the levels/effects of CYP2C19 substrates. Example substrates include citalopram, diazepam, methsuximide, propranolol, proton pump inhibitors, sertraline, and voriconazole.

CYP3A4 substrates: Phenytoin may decrease the levels/effects of CYP3A4 substrates. Example substrates include benzodiazepines, calcium channel blockers, clarithromycin, cyclosporine, erythromycin, estrogens, mirtazapine, nateglinide, nefazodone, nevirapine, protease inhibitors, tacrolimus, and venlafaxine.

Digoxin: Effects and/or levels of digitalis glycosides may be decreased by phenytoin

Disulfiram: May increase serum phenytoin concentrations; monitor

Dopamine: Phenytoin (I.V.) may increase the effect of dopamine (enhanced hypotension)

Doxycycline: Phenytoin may enhance the metabolism of doxycycline, decreasing its clinical effect; higher dosages may be required

Estrogens: Phenytoin may increase the metabolism of estrogens, decreasing their clinical effect; monitor

Folic acid: Replacement of folic acid has been reported to increase the metabolism of phenytoin, decreasing its serum concentrations and/or increasing seizures

HMG-CoA reductase inhibitors: Phenytoin may increase the metabolism of these agents, reducing their clinical effect; monitor

Itraconazole: Phenytoin may decrease the effect of itraconazole

Levodopa: Phenytoin may inhibit the anti-Parkinson effect of levodopa

Lithium: Concurrent use of phenytoin and lithium has resulted in lithium intoxication

Methadone: Phenytoin may enhance the metabolism of methadone resulting in methadone withdrawal

Methylphenidate: May increase serum phenytoin concentrations; monitor

Metronidazole: May increase the serum concentrations of phenytoin; monitor.

Neuromuscular-blocking agents: Duration of effect may be decreased by phenytoin

Omeprazole: May increase serum phenytoin concentrations; monitor

Oral contraceptives: Phenytoin may enhance the metabolism of oral contraceptives, decreasing their clinical effect; an alternative method of contraception should be considered

Primidone: Phenytoin enhances the conversion of primidone to phenobarbital resulting in elevated phenobarbital serum concentrations

Quetiapine: Serum concentrations may be substantially reduced by phenytoin, potentially resulting in a loss of efficacy; limited documentation; monitor

SSRIs: May increase phenytoin serum concentrations; fluoxetine and fluvoxamine are known to inhibit metabolism via CYP enzymes; sertraline and paroxetine have also been shown to increase concentrations in some patients; monitor

Sucralfate: May reduce the GI absorption of phenytoin; monitor

Theophylline: Phenytoin may increase metabolism of theophylline derivatives and decrease their clinical effect; theophylline may also increase phenytoin concentrations

Thyroid hormones (including levothyroxine): Phenytoin may alter the metabolism of thyroid hormones, reducing its effect; there is limited documentation of this interaction, but monitoring should be considered

Ticlopidine: May increase serum phenytoin concentrations and/or toxicity; monitor

Tricyclic antidepressants: Phenytoin may increase metabolism of tricyclic antidepressants and decrease their clinical effect; sedative effects may be additive; tricyclics may also increase phenytoin concentrations

Topiramate: Phenytoin may decrease serum levels of topiramate; topiramate may increase the effect of phenytoin

Trazodone: Serum levels of phenytoin may be increased; limited documentation; monitor

Trimethoprim: May increase serum phenytoin concentrations; monitor

Valproic acid (and sulfisoxazole): May displace phenytoin from binding sites; valproic acid may increase, decrease, or have no effect on phenytoin serum concentrations

Vigabatrin: May reduce phenytoin serum concentrations; monitor

Warfarin: Phenytoin transiently increased the hypothrombinemia response to warfarin initially; this is followed by an inhibition of the hypoprothrombinemic response

Ethanol/Nutrition/Herb Interactions

Ethanol:

Acute use: Avoid or limit ethanol (inhibits metabolism of phenytoin). Watch for sedation.

Chronic use: Avoid or limit ethanol (stimulates metabolism of phenytoin).

Food: Phenytoin serum concentrations may be altered if taken with food. If taken with enteral nutrition, phenytoin serum concentrations may be decreased. Tube feedings decrease bioavailability; hold tube feedings 1-2 hours before and 1-2 hours after phenytoin administration. May decrease calcium, folic acid, and vitamin D levels.

Herb/Nutraceutical: Avoid evening primrose (seizure threshold decreased). Avoid valerian, St John's wort, kava kava, gotu kola (may increase CNS depression).

Stability

Capsule, tablet: Store below 30°C (86°F). Protect from light and moisture.

Oral suspension: Store at room temperature of 20°C to 25°C (68°F to 77°F); do not freeze. Protect from light.

Solution for injection: Store at room temperature of 15°C to 30°C (59°F to 86°F). Use only clear solutions free of precipitate and haziness; slightly yellow solutions may be used. Precipitation may occur if solution is refrigerated and may dissolve at room temperature.

Further dilution of the solution for I.V. infusion is controversial and no consensus exists as to the optimal concentration and length of stability. Stability is concentration and pH dependent. Based on limited clinical consensus, NS or LR are recommended diluents. Dilutions of 1-10 mg/mL have been used and should be administered as soon as possible after preparation (some recommend to discard if not used within 4 hours). Do not refrigerate.

Mechanism of Action Stabilizes neuronal membranes and decreases seizure activity by increasing efflux or decreasing influx of sodium ions across cell membranes in the motor cortex during generation of nerve impulses; prolongs effective refractory period and suppresses ventricular pacemaker automaticity, shortens action potential in the heart

Pharmacodynamics Onset of action: I.V.: ~0.5-1 hour

Pharmacokinetics

Absorption: Oral: Slow

Distribution: V_d: Adults: 0.6-0.7 L/kg

Protein binding:

Adults: 90% to 95%

Others: Decreased protein binding

Disease states resulting in a decrease in serum albumin concentration: Burns, hepatic cirrhosis, nephrotic syndrome, cystic fibrosis

Disease states resulting in an apparent decrease in affinity of phenytoin for serum albumin: Renal failure, jaundice (severe), other drugs (displacers), hyperbilirubinemia (total bilirubin >15 mg/dL), Cl_{cr} <25 mL/minute (unbound fraction is increased two- to threefold in uremia)

Metabolism: Follows dose-dependent capacity-limited (Michaelis-Menten) pharmacokinetics with increased V_{max} in infants >6 months of age and children versus adults; major metabolite (via oxidation), HPPA, undergoes enterohepatic recirculation

(Continued)

Phenytoin *(Continued)*

Bioavailability: Form dependent

Half-life elimination: Oral: 22 hours (range: 7-42 hours)

Time to peak, serum (form dependent): Oral: Extended-release capsule: 4-12 hours; Immediate release preparation: 2-3 hours

Excretion: Urine (<5% as unchanged drug); as glucuronides

Clearance: Highly variable, dependent upon intrinsic hepatic function and dose administered; increased clearance and decreased serum concentrations with febrile illness

Dosage

Geriatrics & Adults:

Status epilepticus: I.V.: Loading dose: Manufacturer recommends 10-15 mg/kg, however, 15-25 mg/kg has been used clinically; maintenance dose: 300 mg/day or 5-6 mg/kg/day in 3 divided doses or 1-2 divided doses using extended release

Anticonvulsant: Oral: Loading dose: 15-20 mg/kg; based on phenytoin serum concentrations and recent dosing history; administer oral loading dose in 3 divided doses given every 2-4 hours to decrease GI adverse effects and to ensure complete oral absorption; maintenance dose: 300 mg/day or 5-6 mg/kg/day in 3 divided doses or 1-2 divided doses using extended release (range 200-1200 mg/day)

Renal Impairment: Phenytoin level in serum may be difficult to interpret in renal failure. Monitoring of free (unbound) concentrations or adjustment to allow interpretation is recommended.

Hepatic Impairment: Safe in usual doses in mild liver disease; clearance may be substantially reduced in cirrhosis and plasma level monitoring with dose adjustment advisable. Free phenytoin levels should be monitored closely.

Administration

Oral: Suspension: Shake well prior to use. Absorption is impaired when phenytoin suspension is given concurrently to patients who are receiving continuous nasogastric feedings. A method to resolve this interaction is to divide the daily dose of phenytoin and withhold the administration of nutritional supplements for 1-2 hours before and after each phenytoin dose.

I.M.: Although approved for I.M. use, I.M. administration is not recommended due to erratic absorption and pain on injection. Fosphenytoin may be considered.

I.V.: Vesicant. Fosphenytoin may be considered for loading in patients who are in status epilepticus, hemodynamically unstable, or develop hypotension/bradycardia with I.V. administration of phenytoin. Phenytoin may be administered by IVP or IVPB administration. The maximum rate of I.V. administration is 50 mg/minute. Highly sensitive patients (eg, elderly, patients with pre-existing cardiovascular conditions) should receive phenytoin more slowly (eg, 20 mg/minute). An in-line 0.22-5 micron filter is recommended for IVPB solutions due to the high potential for precipitation of the solution. Avoid extravasation. Following I.V. administration, NS should be injected through the same needle or I.V. catheter to prevent irritation.

pH: 10.0-12.3

SubQ: SubQ administration is not recommended because of the possibility of local tissue damage, due to the high pH.

Monitoring Parameters Monitor serum concentration and note time for serum assays; gait, CNS effects, speech; free concentrations for patients with low serum albumin. See Reference Range.

Reference Range Timing of serum samples: Because it is slowly absorbed, peak blood levels may occur 4-8 hours after ingestion of an oral dose. The serum half-life varies with the dosage and the drug follows Michaelis-Menten kinetics. The average adult half-life is about 24 hours. Steady-state concentrations are reached in 5-10 days.

Adults: Toxicity is measured clinically, and some patients require levels outside the suggested therapeutic range

Therapeutic range:

Total phenytoin: 10-20 mcg/mL

Concentrations of 5-10 mcg/mL may be therapeutic for some patients but concentrations <5 mcg/mL are not likely to be effective

50% of patients show decreased frequency of seizures at concentrations >10 mcg/mL

86% of patients show decreased frequency of seizures at concentrations >15 mcg/mL

Add another anticonvulsant if satisfactory therapeutic response is not achieved with a phenytoin concentration of 20 mcg/mL

Free phenytoin: 1-2.5 mcg/mL

Toxic: >30 mcg/mL (SI: <120-200 μmol/L)

Lethal: >100 mcg/mL (SI: >400 μmol/L)

When to draw levels: This is dependent on the disease state being treated and the clinical condition of the patient

Key points:
Slow absorption of extended capsules and prolonged half-life minimize fluctuations between peak and trough concentrations, timing of sampling not crucial

Trough concentrations are generally recommended for routine monitoring. Daily levels are not necessary and may result in incorrect dosage adjustments. If it is determined essential to monitor free phenytoin concentrations, concomitant monitoring of total phenytoin concentrations is not necessary and expensive.

After a loading dose: Draw level within 48-96 hours

Rapid achievement: Draw within 2-3 days of therapy initiation to ensure that the patient's metabolism is not remarkably different from that which would be predicted by average literature-derived pharmacokinetic parameters; early levels should be used cautiously in design of new dosing regimens

Second concentration: Draw within 6-7 days with subsequent doses of phenytoin adjusted accordingly

If plasma concentrations have not changed over a 3- to 5-day period, monitoring interval may be increased to once weekly in the acute clinical setting

In stable patients requiring long-term therapy, generally monitor levels at 3- to 12-month intervals

Adjustment of serum concentration: See tables.

Adjustment of Serum Concentration in Patients With Low Serum Albumin

Measured Total Phenytoin Concentration (mcg/mL)	Patient's Serum Albumin (g/dL)			
	3.5	3	2.5	2
	Adjusted Total Phenytoin Concentration (mcg/mL)[1]			
5	6	7	8	10
10	13	14	17	20
15	19	21	25	30

[1]Adjusted concentration = measured total concentration divided by [(0.2 x albumin) + 0.1].

Adjustment of Serum Concentration in Patients With Renal Failure (Cl$_{cr}$ ≤10 mL/min)

Measured Total Phenytoin Concentration (mcg/mL)	Patient's Serum Albumin (g/dL)				
	4	3.5	3	2.5	2
	Adjusted Total Phenytoin Concentration (mcg/mL)[1]				
5	10	11	13	14	17
10	20	22	25	29	33
15	30	33	38	43	50

[1]Adjusted concentration = measured total concentration divided by [(0.1 x albumin) + 0.1].

Patient Information Do not take any new medication during therapy without consulting prescriber. Take exactly as directed, preferably on an empty stomach. Do not alter dose or discontinue without consulting prescriber. Do not crush, break, or chew extended release capsules. Shake liquid suspension well before using. Follow recommended diet, avoid alcohol, and maintain adequate hydration (2-3 L/day of fluids) unless instructed to restrict fluid intake. May cause gum or mouth soreness (use good oral hygiene and have frequent dental exams); drowsiness, dizziness, nervousness, or headache (use caution when driving or engaging in tasks that require alertness until response to drug is known); or nausea or vomiting (small frequent meals, frequent mouth care, chewing gum, or sucking lozenges may help). Report chest pain, irregular heartbeat, or palpitations; slurred speech, unsteady gait, coordination difficulties, or change in mentation; skin rash; unresolved nausea, vomiting, or constipation; swollen glands; swollen, sore, or bleeding gums; unusual bruising or bleeding; acute persistent fatigue; vision changes; or other persistent adverse effects.

Additional Information Not recommended to be given I.M. unless no other route exists due to erratic absorption; best to not switch brands once stabilized

Special Geriatric Considerations Elderly may have reduced hepatic clearance due to age decline in phase I metabolism. Elderly may have low albumin which will increase free fraction and, therefore, pharmacologic response. Monitor closely in those who are hypoalbuminemic. Free fraction measurements advised, also elderly may display a higher incidence of adverse effects (cardiovascular) when using the I.V. loading regimen; therefore, recommended to decrease loading I.V. dose to 25 mg/minute.

Dosage Forms Excipient information presented when available (limited, particularly for generics); consult specific product labeling.
Capsule, extended release, as sodium: 100 mg
Dilantin®: 30 mg [contains sodium benzoate], 100 mg
(Continued)

Phenytoin (Continued)

Phenytek®: 200 mg, 300 mg
Capsule, prompt release, as sodium: 100 mg
Injection, solution, as sodium: 50 mg/mL (2 mL, 5 mL) [contains alcohol and propylene glycol]
Suspension, oral: 100 mg/4 mL (4 mL); 125 mg/5 mL (240 mL)
  Dilantin®: 125 mg/5 mL (240 mL) [contains alcohol <0.6%, sodium benzoate; orange vanilla flavor]
Tablet, chewable:
  Dilantin®: 50 mg

♦ **Phenytoin Sodium** see Phenytoin on page 1250
♦ **Phenytoin Sodium, Extended** see Phenytoin on page 1250
♦ **Phenytoin Sodium, Prompt** see Phenytoin on page 1250
♦ **Phillips'® M-O [OTC]** see Magnesium Hydroxide and Mineral Oil on page 948
♦ **Phillips'® Chews [OTC]** see Magnesium Hydroxide on page 946
♦ **Phillips'® Milk of Magnesia [OTC]** see Magnesium Hydroxide on page 946
♦ **Phillips'® Stool Softener Laxative [OTC]** see Docusate on page 459
♦ **Phlemex** see Guaifenesin and Dextromethorphan on page 730
♦ **Phos-Flur®** see Fluoride on page 642
♦ **Phos-Flur® Rinse [OTC]** see Fluoride on page 642
♦ **PhosLo®** see Calcium Acetate on page 213
♦ **Phos-NaK** see Potassium Phosphate and Sodium Phosphate on page 1293
♦ **Phospha 250™ Neutral** see Potassium Phosphate and Sodium Phosphate on page 1293
♦ **Phosphate, Potassium** see Potassium Phosphate on page 1291
♦ **Phospholine Iodide®** see Echothiophate Iodide on page 498
♦ **p-Hydroxyampicillin** see Amoxicillin on page 95
♦ **Phylloquinone** see Phytonadione on page 1257

Physostigmine (fye zoe STIG meen)

Related Information
  Glaucoma Drug Therapy on page 1758
Medication Safety Issues
  Sound-alike/look-alike issues:
    Physostigmine may be confused with Prostigmin®, pyridostigmine
Canadian Brand Names Eserine®; Isopto® Eserine
Index Terms Eserine Salicylate; Physostigmine Salicylate; Physostigmine Sulfate
Generic Available Yes
Pharmacologic Category Acetylcholinesterase Inhibitor
Use Reversal of toxic CNS effects caused by anticholinergic drugs; miotic in treatment of glaucoma
Contraindications Hypersensitivity to physostigmine or any component of the formulation; GI or GU obstruction; physostigmine therapy of drug intoxications should be used with extreme caution in patients with asthma, gangrene, severe cardiovascular disease, or mechanical obstruction of the GI tract or urogenital tract. In these patients, physostigmine should be used only to treat life-threatening conditions.
Warnings/Precautions Use with caution in patients with epilepsy, asthma, diabetes, gangrene, cardiovascular disease, bradycardia. Discontinue if excessive salivation or emesis, frequent urination or diarrhea occur. Reduce dosage if excessive sweating or nausea occurs. Administer I.V. slowly or at a controlled rate not faster than 1 mg/minute. Due to the possibility of hypersensitivity or overdose/cholinergic crisis, atropine should be readily available; not intended as a first-line agent for anticholinergic toxicity or Parkinson's disease. Products may contain benzyl alcohol. Products may contain sodium bisulfate.
Adverse Reactions (Reflective of adult population; not specific for elderly)
  Frequency not defined.
  Cardiovascular: Palpitation, bradycardia
  Central nervous system: Restlessness, nervousness, hallucinations, seizure
  Gastrointestinal: Nausea, salivation, diarrhea, stomach pain
  Genitourinary: Frequent urge to urinate
  Neuromuscular & skeletal: Muscle twitching
  Ocular: Lacrimation, miosis
  Respiratory: Dyspnea, bronchospasm, respiratory paralysis, pulmonary edema
  Miscellaneous: Diaphoresis
Overdosage/Toxicology Symptoms include muscle weakness, blurred vision, excessive sweating, tearing and salivation, nausea, vomiting, bronchospasm, and seizures. If physostigmine is used in excess or in the absence of an anticholinergic overdose,

patients may manifest signs of cholinergic toxicity. At this point, an anticholinergic agent (eg, atropine 0.015-0.05 mg/kg) may be necessary.

Drug Interactions Increased toxicity: Bethanechol, methacholine, succinylcholine may increase neuromuscular blockade with systemic administration

Stability Do not use solution if cloudy or dark brown.

Mechanism of Action Inhibits destruction of acetylcholine by acetylcholinesterase which facilitates transmission of impulses across myoneural junction and prolongs the central and peripheral effects of acetylcholine

Pharmacodynamics
Onset of action: ~5 minutes
Duration: 0.5-5 hours

Pharmacokinetics
Absorption: I.M., SubQ: Readily absorbed
Distribution: Crosses blood-brain barrier readily and reverses both central and peripheral anticholinergic effects
Metabolism: Hepatic and via hydrolysis by cholinesterases
Half-life: 15-40 minutes

Dosage
Geriatrics & Adults:
Anticholinergic drug overdose:
I.M., I.V., SubQ: 0.5-2 mg to start; repeat every 20 minutes until response occurs or adverse effect occurs.
Repeat 1-4 mg every 30-60 minutes as life-threatening signs (arrhythmias, seizures, deep coma) recur; maximum I.V. rate: 1 mg/minute.

Administration Too rapid administration (I.V. rate not to exceed 1 mg/minute) can cause bradycardia, hypersalivation leading to respiratory difficulties and seizures

Monitoring Parameters Blood pressure, pulse, intraocular pressure

Test Interactions Increased aminotransferase [ALT/AST] (S), increased amylase (S)

Special Geriatric Considerations Studies on the use of physostigmine in Alzheimer's disease have reported variable results. Doses generally were in the range of 2-4 mg 4 times/day. Limitations to the use of physostigmine include a short half-life requiring frequent dosing, variable absorption from the GI tract, and no commercially available oral product; therefore, not recommended for treatment of Alzheimer's disease.

Dosage Forms Excipient information presented when available (limited, particularly for generics); consult specific product labeling.
Injection, solution, as salicylate: 1 mg/mL (2 mL) [contains benzyl alcohol and sodium metabisulfite]

Selected References
Jenike MA, Albert MS, Heller H, et al, "Oral Physostigmine Treatment for Patients With Presenile and Senile Dementia of the Alzheimer's Type: A Double-Blind Placebo-Controlled Trial," *J Clin Psychiatry*, 1990, 51(1):3-7.
Theesen KA, Boyd JA, "Dementia of the Alzheimer's Type: An Update," *Consult Pharm*, 1990, 5:535-40.

♦ **Physostigmine Salicylate** *see* Physostigmine *on page 1256*
♦ **Physostigmine Sulfate** *see* Physostigmine *on page 1256*
♦ **Phytomenadione** *see* Phytonadione *on page 1257*

Phytonadione (fye toe na DYE one)

Medication Safety Issues
Sound-alike/look-alike issues:
Mephyton® may be confused with melphalan, methadone

U.S. Brand Names Mephyton®

Canadian Brand Names AquaMEPHYTON®; Konakion; Mephyton®

Index Terms Methylphytyl Napthoquinone; Phylloquinone; Phytomenadione; Vitamin K₁

Generic Available Yes

Pharmacologic Category Vitamin, Fat Soluble

Use Prevention and treatment of hypoprothrombinemia caused by coumarin derivative-induced or other drug-induced vitamin K deficiency, hypoprothrombinemia caused by malabsorption or inability to synthesize vitamin K; hemorrhagic disease of the newborn

Contraindications Hypersensitivity to phytonadione or any component of the formulation

Warnings/Precautions [U.S. Boxed Warning]: Severe reactions resembling hypersensitivity (eg, anaphylaxis) reactions have occurred rarely during or immediately after I.V. administration. Allergic reactions have also occurred with I.M. and SubQ injections; oral administration is the safest. In obstructive jaundice or with biliary fistulas concurrent administration of bile salts is necessary. Manufacturers recommend the SubQ route over other parenteral routes. SubQ is less predictable (Continued)

Phytonadione *(Continued)*

when compared to the oral route. The American College of Chest Physicians recommends the I.V. route in patients with serious or life-threatening bleeding secondary to warfarin. The I.V. route should be restricted to emergency situations where oral phytonadione cannot be used. Efficacy is delayed regardless of route of administration; patient management may require other treatments in the interim. Administer a dose that will quickly lower the INR into a safe range without causing resistance to warfarin. Some dosage forms contain benzyl alcohol. In liver disease, if initial doses do not reverse coagulopathy then higher doses are unlikely to have any effect. Ineffective in hereditary hypoprothrombinemia. Use caution with renal dysfunction. Injectable products may contain aluminum.

Adverse Reactions (Reflective of adult population; not specific for elderly)
Parenteral administration: Frequency not defined.
Cardiovascular: Cyanosis, flushing, hypotension
Central nervous system: Dizziness
Dermatologic: Scleroderma-like lesions
Endocrine & metabolic: Hyperbilirubinemia (newborn; greater than recommended doses)
Gastrointestinal: Abnormal taste
Local: Injection site reactions
Respiratory: Dyspnea
Miscellaneous: Anaphylactoid reactions, diaphoresis, hypersensitivity reactions

Drug Interactions
Coumarin derivatives: Phytonadione may diminish the anticoagulant effect; monitor INR.
Orlistat: Phytonadione (oral) may not be properly absorbed when administered concurrently; separate doses by at least 2 hours.

Management of Elevated INR

INR	Symptom	Action
Above therapeutic range to <5	No significant bleeding	Lower or hold the next dose and monitor frequently; when INR approaches desired range, may resume dosing with a lower dose if INR was significantly above therapeutic range.
≥ 5 and <9	No significant bleeding	Omit the next 1 or 2 doses; monitor INR and resume with a lower dose when the INR approaches the desired range.
		Alternatively, if there are other risk factors for bleeding, omit the next dose and give vitamin K_1 orally ≤ 5 mg; resume with a lower dose when the INR approaches the desired range.
		If rapid reversal is required for surgery, then given vitamin K_1 orally 2-4 mg and hold warfarin. Expect a response within 24 hours; another 1-2 mg may be given orally if needed.
≥ 9	No significant bleeding	Hold warfarin, give vitamin K_1 orally 5-10 mg, expect the INR to be reduced within 24-48 hours; monitor INR and administer additional vitamin K if necessary. Resume warfarin at lower doses when INR is in the desired range.
Any INR elevation	Serious bleeding	Hold warfarin, give vitamin K_1 (10 mg by slow I.V. infusion), and supplement with fresh plasma transfusion or prothrombin complex concentrate (Factor X complex); recombinant factor VIIa is an alternative to prothrombin complex concentrate. Vitamin K_1 injection can be repeated every 12 hours.
Any INR elevation	Life-threatening bleeding	Hold warfarin, give prothrombin complex concentrate, supplemented with vitamin K_1 (10 mg by slow I.V. infusion); repeat if necessary. Recombinant factor VIIa is an alternative to prothrombin complex concentrate.

Note: Use of high doses of vitamin K_1 (10-15 mg) may cause resistance to warfarin for up to a week. Heparin or low molecular weight heparin can be given until the patient becomes responsive to warfarin.

Reference: Ansell J, Hirsh J, Poller L et al. "The Pharmacology and Management of the Vitamin K Antagonists," *Chest*, 2004, 126 (3 Suppl):204-33.

Stability

Injection: Store at 15°C to 30°C (59°F to 86°F). Dilute in preservative-free NS, D$_5$W, or D$_5$NS.

Note: Store Hospira product at 20°C to 25°C (68°F to 77°F).

Oral: Store tablets at 15°C to 30°C (59°F to 86°F). Protect from light.

Mechanism of Action
Promotes liver synthesis of clotting factors (II, VII, IX, X); however, the exact mechanism as to this stimulation is unknown. Menadiol is a water soluble form of vitamin K; phytonadione has a more rapid and prolonged effect than menadione; menadiol sodium diphosphate (K$_4$) is half as potent as menadione (K$_3$).

Pharmacodynamics
Onset of action: Increased coagulation factors: Oral: 6-10 hours; I.V.: 1-2 hours

Peak effect: INR values return to normal: Oral: 24-48 hours; I.V.: 12-14 hours

Pharmacokinetics
Absorption: Oral: From intestines in presence of bile; SubQ: Variable

Metabolism: Rapidly hepatic

Excretion: Urine and feces

Dosage

Geriatrics & Adults:

Adequate intake: Males: 120 mcg/day; Females: 90 mcg/day

Hypoprothrombinemia due to drugs (other than coumarin derivatives) or factors limiting absorption or synthesis: Oral, SubQ, I.M., I.V.: Initial: 2.5-25 mg (rarely up to 50 mg)

Vitamin K deficiency secondary to coumarin derivative: See table on previous page:

Administration
I.V. administration: Infuse slowly; rate of infusion should not exceed 1 mg/minute. The injectable route should be used only if the oral route is not feasible or there is a greater urgency to reverse anticoagulation.

Monitoring Parameters
PT, INR

Additional Information
Injection contains benzyl alcohol 0.9% as preservative

Dosage Forms
Excipient information presented when available (limited, particularly for generics); consult specific product labeling.

Injection, aqueous colloidal: 2 mg/mL (0.5 mL); 10 mg/mL (1 mL)

Tablet: 100 mcg [OTC]

Mephyton®: 5 mg

Selected References

Ansell J, Hirsh J, Poller L, et al, "The Pharmacology and Management of the Vitamin K Antagonists: The Seventh ACCP Conference on Antithrombotic and Thrombolytic Therapy," *Chest*, 2004, 126(3 Suppl):204-33.

Barash P, Kitahata LM, and Mandel S, "Acute Cardiovascular Collapse After Intravenous Phytonadione," *Anesth Analg*, 1976, 55(2):304-6.

Crowther MA, Douketis JD, Schnurr T, et al, "Oral Vitamin K Lowers the International Normalized Ratio More Rapidly Than Subcutaneous Vitamin K in the Treatment of Warfarin-Associated Coagulopathy. A Randomized, Controlled Trial," *Ann Intern Med*, 2002, 137(4):251-4.

"Dietary Reference Intakes for Vitamin A, Vitamin K, Arsenic, Boron, Chromium, Copper, Iodine, Iron, Manganese, Molybdenum, Nickel, Silicon, Vanadium, and Zinc," Food and Nutrition Board, Institute of Medicine. National Academy of Sciences, Washington, DC: National Academy Press, 2001, 162-84.

Fiore LD, Scola MA, Cantillon CE, et al, "Anaphylactoid Reactions to Vitamin K," *J Thromb Thrombolysis*, 2001, 11(2):175-83.

Harrell CC and Kline SS, "Oral Vitamin K1: An Option to Reduce Warfarin's Activity," *Ann Pharmacother*, 1995, 29(12):1228-32.

Hopkins CS, "Adverse Reaction to a Cremophor-Containing Preparation of Intravenous Vitamin K," *Intensive Therapy Clin Monit*, 1988, 9:254-5.

Martinez-Abad M, Delgado F, Palop V, et al, "Vitamin K$_1$ and Anaphylactic Shock," *DICP*, 1991, 25(7-8):871-2.

Weibert RT, Le DT, Kayser SR, et al, "Correction of Excessive Anticoagulation With Low-Dose Oral Vitamin K1," *Ann Intern Med*, 1997, 126(12):959-62.

Pilocarpine (pye loe KAR peen)

Related Information

Glaucoma Drug Therapy *on page 1758*

Medication Safety Issues

Sound-alike/look-alike issues:

Isopto® Carpine may be confused with Isopto® Carbachol

Salagen® may be confused with Salacid®, selegiline

International issues:

Salagen® may be confused with Poagen® which is a brand name for grass pollen extract in Portugal

U.S. Brand Names Isopto® Carpine; Pilopine HS®; Salagen®

Canadian Brand Names Diocarpine; Isopto® Carpine; Pilopine HS®; Salagen®

Index Terms Pilocarpine Hydrochloride

Generic Available Yes: Hydrochloride solution, tablet

Pharmacologic Category Cholinergic Agonist; Ophthalmic Agent, Antiglaucoma; Ophthalmic Agent, Miotic

(Continued)

Pilocarpine *(Continued)*

Use

Ophthalmic: Management of chronic simple glaucoma, chronic and acute angle-closure glaucoma

Oral: Symptomatic treatment of xerostomia caused by salivary gland hypofunction resulting from radiotherapy for cancer of the head and neck or Sjögren's syndrome

Unlabeled/Investigational Use Counter effects of cycloplegics

Contraindications Hypersensitivity to pilocarpine or any component of the formulation; acute inflammatory disease of the anterior chamber of the eye; in addition, tablets are also contraindicated in patients with uncontrolled asthma, angle-closure glaucoma, severe hepatic impairment

Warnings/Precautions Use with caution in patients with corneal abrasion, CHF, asthma, peptic ulcer, urinary tract obstruction, Parkinson's disease, or narrow-angle glaucoma

Adverse Reactions (Reflective of adult population; not specific for elderly)

Ophthalmic: Frequency not defined:

Cardiovascular: Hypertension, tachycardia

Gastrointestinal: Diarrhea, nausea, salivation, vomiting

Ocular: Burning, ciliary spasm, conjunctival vascular congestion, corneal granularity (gel 10%), lacrimation, lens opacity, myopia, retinal detachment, supraorbital or temporal headache, visual acuity decreased

Respiratory: Bronchial spasm, pulmonary edema

Miscellaneous: Diaphoresis

Oral (frequency varies by indication and dose):

>10%:

Cardiovascular: Flushing (8% to 13%)

Central nervous system: Chills (3% to 15%), dizziness (5% to 12%), headache (11%)

Gastrointestinal: Nausea (6% to 15%)

Genitourinary: Urinary frequency (9% to 12%)

Neuromuscular & skeletal: Weakness (2% to 12%)

Respiratory: Rhinitis (5% to 14%)

Miscellaneous: Diaphoresis (29% to 68%)

1% to 10%:

Cardiovascular: Edema (<1% to 5%), facial edema, hypertension (3%), palpitation, tachycardia

Central nervous system: Pain (4%), fever, somnolence

Dermatologic: Pruritus, rash

Gastrointestinal: Diarrhea (4% to 7%), dyspepsia (7%), vomiting (3% to 4%), constipation, flatulence, glossitis, salivation increased, stomatitis, taste perversion

Genitourinary: Vaginitis, urinary incontinence

Neuromuscular & skeletal: Myalgias, tremor

Ocular: Lacrimation (6%), amblyopia (4%), abnormal vision, blurred vision, conjunctivitis

Otic: Tinnitus

Respiratory: Cough increased, dysphagia, epistaxis, sinusitis

Miscellaneous: Allergic reaction, voice alteration

Overdosage/Toxicology Symptoms include bronchospasm, bradycardia, involuntary urination, vomiting, hypotension, and tremors. Atropine is the treatment of choice for intoxications manifesting with significant muscarinic symptoms. Atropine I.V. 2-4 mg every 3-60 minutes should be repeated to control symptoms and then continued as needed for 1-2 days following acute ingestion. Epinephrine 0.1-1 mg SubQ may be useful in reversing severe cardiovascular or pulmonary sequelae.

Drug Interactions Inhibits CYP2A6 (weak), 2E1 (weak), 3A4 (weak)

Concurrent use with beta-blockers may cause conduction disturbances; pilocarpine may antagonize the effects of anticholinergic drugs

Ethanol/Nutrition/Herb Interactions Food: Avoid administering oral formulation with high-fat meal; fat decreases the rate of absorption, maximum concentration and increases the time it takes to reach maximum concentration.

Stability

Gel: Store at room temperature of 2°C to 27°C (36°F to 80°F); do not freeze. Avoid excessive heat.

Tablets: Store at controlled room temperature of 15°C to 30°C (59°F to 86°F).

Mechanism of Action Directly stimulates cholinergic receptors in the eye causing miosis (by contraction of the iris sphincter), loss of accommodation (by constriction of ciliary muscle), and lowering of intraocular pressure (with decreased resistance to aqueous humor outflow)

Pharmacodynamics

Onset of action:
Ophthalmic: Miosis: 10-30 minutes; Intraocular pressure reduction: 1 hour
Oral: 20 minutes
Duration:
Ophthalmic: Miosis: 4-8 hours; Intraocular pressure reduction: 4-12 hours
Oral: 3-5 hours

Pharmacokinetics

Half-life: Oral: 0.76-1.35 hours; increased with hepatic impairment
Elimination: Urine

Dosage

Geriatrics & Adults:

Glaucoma: Ophthalmic:
Solution: Instill 1-2 drops up to 6 times/day; adjust the concentration and frequency as required to control elevated intraocular pressure.
Gel: Instill 0.5" ribbon into lower conjunctival sac once daily at bedtime.

To counteract the mydriatic effects of sympathomimetic agents (unlabeled use): Ophthalmic solution: Instill 1 drop of a 1% solution in the affected eye.

Xerostomia: Oral:
Following head and neck cancer: 5 mg 3 times/day, titration up to 10 mg 3 times/day may be considered for patients who have not responded adequately; do not exceed 2 tablets/dose

Sjögren's syndrome: 5 mg 4 times/day

Hepatic Impairment: Oral: Patients with moderate impairment: 5 mg 2 times/day regardless of indication; adjust dose based on response and tolerability. Do not use with severe impairment (Child-Pugh score 10-15)

Administration

Oral: Avoid administering with a high-fat meal. Fat decreases the rate of absorption, maximum concentration, and increases the time it takes to reach maximum concentration.

Ophthalmic: If both solution and gel are used, the solution should be applied first, then the gel at least 5 minutes later. Following administration of the solution, finger pressure should be applied on the lacrimal sac for 1-2 minutes.

Monitoring Parameters Intraocular pressure, fundoscopic exam, visual field testing

Patient Information May sting on instillation, do not touch dropper to eye; visual acuity may be decreased after administration; night vision may be decreased; distance vision may be altered. Do not leave damaged Ocusert® system in the eye; read package instructions for insertion; after topical instillation, finger pressure should be applied to lacrimal sac to decrease drainage into the nose and throat and minimize possible systemic absorption.

Special Geriatric Considerations Assure the patient or a caregiver can adequately administer ophthalmic medication dosage form.

Dosage Forms Excipient information presented when available (limited, particularly for generics); consult specific product labeling.
Gel, ophthalmic, as hydrochloride (Pilopine HS®): 4% (4 g) [contains benzalkonium chloride]
Solution, ophthalmic, as hydrochloride: 0.5% (15 mL); 1% (2 mL, 15 mL); 2% (2 mL, 15 mL); 3% (15 mL); 4% (2 mL, 15 mL); 6% (15 mL) [may contain benzalkonium chloride]
Isopto® Carpine: 1% (15 mL); 2% (15 mL); 4% (15 mL) [contains benzalkonium chloride]
Tablet, as hydrochloride: 5 mg, 7.5 mg
Salagen®: 5 mg, 7.5 mg

♦ **Pilocarpine Hydrochloride** *see* Pilocarpine *on page 1259*
♦ **Pilopine HS®** *see* Pilocarpine *on page 1259*
♦ **Pimaricin** *see* Natamycin *on page 1093*

Pimozide (PI moe zide)

Related Information

Antipsychotic Agents *on page 1747*

U.S. Brand Names Orap®

Canadian Brand Names Apo-Pimozide®; Orap®

Generic Available No

Pharmacologic Category Antipsychotic Agent, Typical

Use Suppression of severe motor and phonic tics in patients with Tourette's disorder who have failed to respond to other standard treatment

Unlabeled/Investigational Use Treatment of Huntington's chorea, psychosis; reported use in individuals with delusions focused on physical symptoms (ie, preoccupation with parasitic infestation)

(Continued)

Pimozide *(Continued)*

Contraindications Hypersensitivity to pimozide or any component of the formulation; severe CNS depression; coma; history of dysrhythmia; prolonged QT syndrome; concurrent use with QT_c-prolonging agents; hypokalemia or hypomagnesemia; concurrent use of drugs that are inhibitors of CYP3A4, including concurrent use of azole antifungals, fluvoxamine, macrolide antibiotics (such as clarithromycin or erythromycin), mesoridazine, nefazodone, protease inhibitors (ie, atazanavir, indinavir, nelfinavir, ritonavir, saquinavir), sertraline, thioridazine, zileuton, and ziprasidone; simple tics other than Tourette's

Warnings/Precautions Sudden, unexpected deaths have been known to occur in patients taking high doses (>10 mg) of pimozide. One possible explanation is prolongation of QT intervals predisposing the patients to arrhythmias. Monitor ECG at baseline and periodically during dosage titration. May alter cardiac conduction - life-threatening arrhythmias have occurred with therapeutic doses of phenothiazines. May cause hypotension, use with caution in patients with autonomic instability. Moderately sedating, use with caution in disorders where CNS depression is a feature. Use with caution in Parkinson's disease. Caution in patients with hemodynamic instability; bone marrow suppression; predisposition to seizures; subcortical brain damage; severe cardiac, hepatic, renal, or respiratory disease. Esophageal dysmotility and aspiration have been associated with antipsychotic use; use with caution in patients at risk of pneumonia (ie, Alzheimer's disease). Caution in breast cancer or other prolactin-dependent tumors (may elevate prolactin levels). May alter temperature regulation or mask toxicity of other drugs due to antiemetic effects. May cause orthostatic hypotension; use with caution in patients at risk of this effect or those who would tolerate transient hypotensive episodes (cerebrovascular disease, cardiovascular disease, or other medications which may predispose).

May cause anticholinergic effects (confusion, agitation, constipation, xerostomia, blurred vision, urinary retention); therefore, use with caution in patients with decreased gastrointestinal motility, urinary retention, BPH, xerostomia, or visual problems. Conditions which also may be exacerbated by cholinergic blockade include narrow-angle glaucoma (screening is recommended) and worsening of myasthenia gravis. Relative to neuroleptics, pimozide has a moderate potency of cholinergic blockade.

May cause extrapyramidal symptoms, including pseudoparkinsonism, acute dystonic reactions, akathisia, and tardive dyskinesia (risk of these reactions is high relative to other neuroleptics). May be associated with neuroleptic malignant syndrome (NMS) or pigmentary retinopathy.

Avoid concurrent grapefruit juice, macrolide antibiotics, azole antifungal agents, protease inhibitors, nefazodone, and zileuton due to their potential inhibition of pimozide metabolism, leading to the accumulation of active compound and the increased chance of serious arrhythmias

Adverse Reactions (Reflective of adult population; not specific for elderly)
Frequencies >1% reported in adults (limited data) with Tourette's disorder:
Cardiovascular: Abnormal ECG (3%)
Central nervous system: Somnolence, sedation (14%), akathisia (8%), drowsiness (7%), hyperkinesias (6%), insomnia (2%), depression(2%), headache (1%), nervousness (1% to 8%)
Dermatologic: Rash (8%)
Gastrointestinal: Xerostomia (25%), constipation (20%), increased salivation (14%), diarrhea (5%), thirst (5%), appetite increased (5%), taste disturbance (5%), dysphagia (3%)
Genitourinary: Impotence (15%)
Neuromuscular & skeletal: Weakness (22%), muscle tightness (15%), rigidity (10%), myalgia (3%), torticollis (3%), tremor (3%)
Ocular: Visual disturbance (6% to 20%), accommodation decreased (20%)
Miscellaneous: Speech disorder (10%)
Frequency not established (reported in disorders other than Tourette's disorder): Blood dyscrasias, breast edema, chest pain, dizziness, extrapyramidal symptoms (akathisia, akinesia, dystonia, pseudoparkinsonism, tardive dyskinesia); facial edema, gingival hyperplasia (case report), hyper-/hypotension, hyponatremia, jaundice, libido decreased, neuroleptic malignant syndrome, orthostatic hypotension, palpitation, periorbital edema, postural hypotension, QT_c prolongation, seizure, tachycardia, ventricular arrhythmia, vomiting, weight gain/loss

Overdosage/Toxicology Symptoms include hypotension, respiratory depression, ECG abnormalities, and extrapyramidal symptoms. Following attempts at decontamination, treatment is supportive and symptomatic. Seizures can be treated with diazepam, phenytoin, or phenobarbital. Epinephrine should not be used (consider norepinephrine or phenylephrine for hypotension).

Drug Interactions Substrate (major) of CYP1A2, 3A4; **Inhibits** CYP2C19 (weak), 2D6 (weak), 2E1 (weak), 3A4 (weak)

Acetylcholinesterase inhibitors (central): May increase the risk of antipsychotic-related extrapyramidal symptoms; monitor.

Aluminum salts: May decrease the absorption of antipsychotics; monitor

Amphetamines: Efficacy may be diminished by antipsychotics; in addition, amphetamines may increase psychotic symptoms; avoid concurrent use

Anticholinergics: May inhibit the therapeutic response to antipsychotics and excess anticholinergic effects may occur; includes benztropine, trihexyphenidyl, biperiden, and drugs with significant anticholinergic activity (TCAs, antihistamines, disopyramide)

Antihypertensives: Concurrent use of antipsychotics with an antihypertensive may produce additive hypotensive effects (particularly orthostasis)

Bromocriptine: Antipsychotics inhibit the ability of bromocriptine to lower serum prolactin concentrations

CNS depressants: Sedative effects may be additive with antipsychotics; monitor for increased effect; includes barbiturates, benzodiazepines, opioid analgesics, ethanol, and other sedative agents

CYP1A2 inducers: May decrease the levels/effects of pimozide. Example inducers include aminoglutethimide, carbamazepine, phenobarbital, and rifampin.

CYP1A2 inhibitors: May increase the levels/effects of pimozide. Example inhibitors include ciprofloxacin, fluvoxamine, ketoconazole, norfloxacin, ofloxacin, and rofecoxib.

CYP3A4 inducers: CYP3A4 inducers may decrease the levels/effects of pimozide. Example inducers include aminoglutethimide, carbamazepine, nafcillin, nevirapine, phenobarbital, phenytoin, and rifamycins.

CYP3A4 inhibitors: May increase the levels/effects of pimozide. Example inhibitors include azole antifungals, clarithromycin, diclofenac, doxycycline, erythromycin, imatinib, isoniazid, nefazodone, nicardipine, propofol, protease inhibitors, quinidine, telithromycin, and verapamil. Concurrent use of strong CYP3A4 inhibitors with pimozide is contraindicated.

Epinephrine: Chlorpromazine (and possibly other low potency antipsychotics) may diminish the pressor effects of epinephrine

Guanethidine and guanadrel: Antihypertensive effects may be inhibited by antipsychotics

Levodopa: Antipsychotics may inhibit the antiparkinsonian effect of levodopa; avoid this combination

Lithium: Antipsychotics may produce neurotoxicity with lithium; this is a rare effect

Macrolide antibiotics: Concurrent use is contraindicated due to CYP inhibition and QT_c-prolonging effects. **Note:** The manufacturer lists azithromycin and dirithromycin in its list of contraindicated macrolides; however, these drugs do not inhibit CYP3A4 and are not expected to interact with pimozide.

Mesoridazine: Concurrent use with pimozide is contraindicated due to potential arrhythmias.

Metoclopramide: May increase extrapyramidal symptoms (EPS) or risk.

Phenytoin: May reduce serum levels of antipsychotics; antipsychotics may increase phenytoin serum levels

Propranolol: Serum concentrations of antipsychotics may be increased; propranolol also increases antipsychotics concentrations

QT_c-prolonging agents: Effects on QT_c interval may be additive with antipsychotics, increasing the risk of malignant arrhythmias; includes Class Ia and Class III antiarrhythmics, arsenic trioxide, chlorpromazine, dolasetron, droperidol, levomethadyl, mefloquine, pentamidine, probucol, tacrolimus, ziprasidone, tricyclic antidepressants, and some quinolone antibiotics (moxifloxacin).

Sertraline: Concurrent use is contraindicated; may produce increased toxicity or attenuate therapeutic response.

Sulfadoxine-pyrimethamine: May increase antipsychotics concentrations

Thioridazine: Concurrent use with pimozide is contraindicated due to potential arrhythmias.

Tricyclic antidepressants: Concurrent use may produce increased toxicity or altered therapeutic response (also see note under QT_c prolonging agents)

Trazodone: Antipsychotics and trazodone may produce additive hypotensive effects

Valproic acid: Serum levels may be increased by antipsychotics

Ziprasidone: Concurrent use with pimozide is contraindicated due to potential arrhythmias.

Ethanol/Nutrition/Herb Interactions

Ethanol: Avoid ethanol (may increase CNS depression).

Food: Pimozide serum concentration may be increased when taken with grapefruit juice; avoid concurrent use.

Herb/Nutraceutical: St John's wort may decrease pimozide levels. Avoid kava kava, gotu kola, valerian, St John's wort (may increase CNS depression).

Mechanism of Action Pimozide, a diphenylbutylperidine antipsychotic, is a potent centrally-acting dopamine-receptor antagonist resulting in its characteristic neuroleptic effects

(Continued)

Pimozide *(Continued)*

Pharmacokinetics
Absorption: Oral: 50%
Protein binding: 99%
Metabolism: In the liver with significant first-pass metabolism
Half-life: 50 hours
Time to peak serum concentration: Within 6-8 hours
Elimination: Metabolites excreted in urine

Dosage
Geriatrics: Recommend initial dose of 1 mg/day; periodically attempt gradual reduction of dose to determine if tic persists; follow up for 1-2 weeks before concluding the tic is a persistent disease phenomenon and not a manifestation of drug withdrawal.
Note: An ECG should be performed baseline and periodically thereafter, especially during dosage adjustment.

Adults:
Tourette's disorder: Oral: Initial: 1-2 mg/day, then increase dosage as needed every other day; range is usually 7-16 mg/day; maximum: 10 mg/day or 0.2 mg/kg/day are not generally recommended.
Note: Sudden unexpected deaths have occurred in patients taking doses >10 mg.
Note: An ECG should be performed baseline and periodically thereafter, especially during dosage adjustment.

Hepatic Impairment: Reduced dose is necessary.

Monitoring Parameters Monitor EKG, blood pressure, and CNS side effects. ECG should be performed baseline and periodically thereafter, especially during dosage adjustment.

Patient Information May cause drowsiness; use caution when driving or performing tasks which require alertness; do not stop medication without physician advice

Additional Information Treatment with pimozide exposes the patient to serious risks; a decision to use pimozide chronically in Tourette's disorder is one that deserves full consideration by the patient (or patient's family) as well as by the treating physician. Because the goal of treatment is symptomatic improvement, the patient's view of the need for treatment and assessment of response are critical in evaluating the impact of therapy and weighing its benefits against the risks.

Special Geriatric Considerations No specific clinical studies in the use of this drug in elderly; use with extreme caution in elderly due to cardiovascular effects. Consider cardiovascular effects of drugs an elderly patient may be receiving.

In the treatment of agitated, demented, older adult patients, authors of meta-analysis of controlled trials of the response to the traditional antipsychotics (phenothiazines, butyrophenones) in controlling agitation have concluded that the use of neuroleptics results in a response rate of 18%. Clearly neuroleptic therapy for behavior control should be limited with frequent attempts to withdraw the agent given for behavior control.

Dosage Forms Excipient information presented when available (limited, particularly for generics); consult specific product labeling.
Tablet: 1 mg, 2 mg

Selected References
Peabody CA, Warner MD, Whiteford HA, et al, "Neuroleptics and the Elderly," *J Am Geriatr Soc*, 1987, 35(3):233-8.
Risse SC and Barnes R, "Pharmacologic Treatment of Agitation Associated With Dementia," *J Am Geriatr Soc*, 1986, 34(5):368-76.
Saltz BL, Woerner MG, Kane JM, et al, "Prospective Study of Tardive Dyskinesia Incidence in the Elderly," *JAMA*, 1991, 266(17):2402-6.
Seifert RD, "Therapeutic Drug Monitoring: Psychotropic Drugs," *J Pharm Pract*, 1984, 6:403-16.

Pindolol *(PIN doe lole)*

Related Information
Beta-Blockers *on page 1751*

Medication Safety Issues
Sound-alike/look-alike issues:
Pindolol may be confused with Parlodel®, Plendil®
Visken® may be confused with Visine®

Canadian Brand Names Apo-Pindol®; Gen-Pindolol; Novo-Pindol; Nu-Pindol; PMS-Pindolol; Visken®

Generic Available Yes

Pharmacologic Category Beta Blocker With Intrinsic Sympathomimetic Activity

Use Management of hypertension

Unlabeled/Investigational Use Potential augmenting agent for antidepressants; treatment of ventricular arrhythmias/tachycardia, antipsychotic-induced akathisia, situational anxiety, aggressive behavior associated with dementia

Contraindications Hypersensitivity to pindolol, beta-blockers, or any component of the formulation; uncompensated congestive heart failure; cardiogenic shock; bradycardia, sinus node dysfunction, or heart block (2nd or 3rd degree) except in patients with a functioning artificial pacemaker; pulmonary edema; severe hyperactive airway disease (asthma or COPD); Raynaud's disease

Warnings/Precautions Consider pre-existing conditions such as sick sinus syndrome before initiating. Use with caution in patients with inadequate myocardial function, undergoing anesthesia, bronchospastic disease, myasthenia gravis, peripheral vascular disease, renal impairment, psychiatric disease (may cause CNS depression) or impaired hepatic function. Use with caution in patients with diabetes mellitus; may potentiate hypoglycemia and/or mask signs and symptoms. Beta-blockers with intrinsic sympathomimetic activity (including pindolol) do not appear to be of benefit in CHF. Beta-blocker therapy should not be withdrawn abruptly (particularly in patients with CAD), but gradually tapered to avoid acute tachycardia, hypertension, and/or ischemia. Adequate alpha-blockade is required prior to use of any beta-blocker for patients with untreated pheochromocytoma.

Adverse Reactions (Reflective of adult population; not specific for elderly) 1% to 10%:

Cardiovascular: Chest pain (3%), edema (6%)

Central nervous system: Nightmares/vivid dreams (5%), dizziness (9%), insomnia (10%), fatigue (8%), nervousness (7%), anxiety (<2%)

Dermatologic: Rash, itching (4%)

Gastrointestinal: Nausea (5%), abdominal discomfort (4%)

Neuromuscular & skeletal: Weakness (4%), paresthesia (3%), arthralgia (7%), muscle pain (10%)

Respiratory: Dyspnea (5%)

Overdosage/Toxicology Symptoms of intoxication include cardiac disturbances, CNS toxicity, bronchospasm, hypoglycemia, and hyperkalemia. The most common cardiac symptoms include hypotension and bradycardia. Atrioventricular block, intraventricular conduction disturbances, cardiogenic shock, and asystole may occur with severe overdose, especially with membrane-depressant drugs (eg, propranolol). CNS effects include convulsions, coma, and respiratory arrest and are commonly seen with propranolol and other membrane-depressant and lipid-soluble drugs. Treatment is symptomatic for seizures, hypotension, hyperkalemia and hypoglycemia; bradycardia and hypotension resistant to atropine, isoproterenol or pacing may respond to glucagon. Wide QRS defects caused by membrane-depressant poisoning may respond to hypertonic sodium bicarbonate. Repeat-dose charcoal, hemoperfusion, or hemodialysis may be helpful in removal of only those beta-blockers with a small V_d, long half-life, or low intrinsic clearance (acebutolol, atenolol, nadolol, sotalol).

Drug Interactions **Substrate** of CYP2D6 (major); **Inhibits** CYP2D6 (weak)

Albuterol (and other beta$_2$ agonists): Effects may be blunted by nonspecific beta-blockers

Alpha-blockers (prazosin, terazosin): Concurrent use of beta-blockers may increase risk of orthostasis

AV conduction-slowing agents (digoxin): Effects may be additive with beta-blockers.

Calcium channel blockers (diltiazem, verapamil): May have synergistic or additive pharmacological effects when taken concurrently with beta-blockers

Clonidine: Hypertensive crisis after or during withdrawal of either agent

CYP2D6 inhibitors: May increase the levels/effects of pindolol. Example inhibitors include chlorpromazine, delavirdine, fluoxetine, miconazole, paroxetine, pergolide, quinidine, quinine, ritonavir, and ropinirole.

Epinephrine (including local anesthetics with epinephrine): Pindolol may cause hypertension

Glucagon: Pindolol may blunt the hyperglycemic action

Insulin and oral hypoglycemics: May mask symptoms of hypoglycemia

NSAIDs (ibuprofen, indomethacin, naproxen, piroxicam): May reduce the antihypertensive effects of beta-blockers

Salicylates: May reduce the antihypertensive effects of beta-blockers

Sulfonylureas: Beta-blockers may alter response to hypoglycemic agents

Ethanol/Nutrition/Herb Interactions Herb/Nutraceutical: Avoid dong quai if using for hypertension (has estrogenic activity). Avoid ephedra, yohimbe, ginseng (may worsen hypertension).

Stability Protect from light.

Mechanism of Action Blocks both beta$_1$- and beta$_2$-receptors and has mild intrinsic sympathomimetic activity; pindolol has negative inotropic and chronotropic effects and can significantly slow AV nodal conduction. Augmentive action of antidepressants thought to be mediated via a serotonin 1A autoreceptor antagonism.

Pharmacodynamics One study found that beta blockade lasted longer in older adult patients as compared to younger patients

Pharmacokinetics

Absorption: Oral: Rapid, 50% to 95%

Protein binding: 50%

Metabolism: In the liver (60% to 65%) to conjugates

(Continued)

Pindolol (Continued)

Half-life: 2.5-4 hours (increased with renal insufficiency, and cirrhosis); half-life is not significantly prolonged in older adults, though some accumulation of drug may occur (related to renal function)

Time to peak: Within 1-2 hours

Elimination: In urine (35% to 50% unchanged drug)

Dosage

Geriatrics: Oral: Initial: 5 mg once daily; increase as necessary by 5 mg/day every 3-4 weeks.

Adults:

Hypertension: Oral: Initial: 5 mg twice daily, increase as necessary by 10 mg/day every 3-4 weeks (maximum daily dose: 60 mg); usual dose range (JNC 7): 10-40 mg twice daily.

Antidepressant augmentation (unlabeled use): Oral: 2.5 mg 3 times/day

Renal Impairment: Reduction is necessary in severe impairment.

Hepatic Impairment: Reduce dose in severely impaired.

Monitoring Parameters Blood pressure, standing and sitting/supine, pulse, respiratory function, signs of congestive heart failure

Patient Information Do not discontinue medication abruptly; consult pharmacist or physician before taking over-the-counter cold preparations

Special Geriatric Considerations Due to alterations in the beta-adrenergic autonomic nervous system, beta-adrenergic blockade may result in less hemodynamic response than seen in younger adults. Studies indicate that despite decreased sensitivity to the chronotropic effects of beta-blockade with age, there appears to be an increased myocardial sensitivity to the negative inotropic effect during stress (eg, exercise). Controlled trials have shown the overall response rate for propranolol to be only 20% to 50% in elderly populations. Therefore, all beta-adrenergic blocking drugs may result in a decreased response as compared to younger adults.

Dosage Forms Excipient information presented when available (limited, particularly for generics); consult specific product labeling.

Tablet: 5 mg, 10 mg

Selected References

Gretzer I, Alvan G, Duner H, et al, "Beta-Blocking Effect and Pharmacokinetics of Pindolol in Young and Elderly Hypertensive Patients," *Eur J Clin Pharmacol*, 1986, 31(4):415-8.

♦ **Pink Bismuth** see Bismuth on page 174

Pioglitazone (pye oh GLI ta zone)

Medication Safety Issues

Sound-alike/look-alike issues:

Actos® may be confused with Actidose®, Actonel®

U.S. Brand Names Actos®

Canadian Brand Names Actos®

Generic Available No

Pharmacologic Category Antidiabetic Agent, Thiazolidinedione

Use

Type 2 diabetes, monotherapy: Adjunct to diet and exercise, to improve glycemic control

Type 2 diabetes, combination therapy with sulfonylurea, metformin, or insulin: When diet, exercise, and a single agent alone does not result in adequate glycemic control

Contraindications Hypersensitivity to pioglitazone or any component of the formulation; active liver disease (transaminases >2.5 times the upper limit of normal at baseline); patients who have experienced jaundice during troglitazone therapy

Warnings/Precautions Should not be used in diabetic ketoacidosis. Mechanism requires the presence of insulin, therefore use in type 1 diabetes is not recommended. May potentiate hypoglycemia when used in combination with sulfonylureas or insulin. Use with caution in patients with anemia (may reduce hemoglobin and hematocrit). Use with caution in patients with edema; may increase plasma volume and/or increase cardiac hypertrophy. Monitor closely for signs and symptoms of heart failure (including weight gain, edema, or dyspnea). Not recommended for use in patients with NYHA Class III or IV heart failure. In patients with NYHA class II (systolic) heart failure, initiate at lowest dosage and monitor closely. Discontinue if heart failure develops.

Use with caution in patients with minor elevations in transaminases (AST or ALT). Idiosyncratic hepatotoxicity has been reported with another thiazolidinedione agent (troglitazone) and postmarketing case reports of hepatitis (with rare hepatic failure) have been received for pioglitazone. Monitoring should include periodic determinations of liver function. Use caution with pre-existing macular edema or diabetic retinopathy. Postmarketing reports of new-onset or worsening diabetic macular edema with decreased visual acuity has been reported.

Adverse Reactions (Reflective of adult population; not specific for elderly)

>10%:

Cardiovascular: Edema (5%; in combination trials with sulfonylureas or insulin, the incidence of edema was as high as 15%)

Respiratory: Upper respiratory tract infection (13%)

1% to 10%:

Cardiovascular: Heart failure (requiring hospitalization; up to 6% in patients with prior macrovascular disease)

Central nervous system: Headache (9%), fatigue (4%)

Gastrointestinal: Tooth disorder (5%)

Hematologic: Anemia ($\leq$2%)

Neuromuscular & skeletal: Myalgia (5%)

Respiratory: Sinusitis (6%), pharyngitis (5%)

Frequency not defined: HDL-cholesterol increased, hypoglycemia (in combination trials with sulfonylureas or insulin), serum triglycerides decreased, weight gain/loss

Overdosage/Toxicology Experience in overdose is limited. Symptoms may include hypoglycemia. Treatment is symptom-directed and supportive.

Drug Interactions Substrate of CYP2C8 (major); 3A4 (minor); **Inhibits** CYP2C8 (moderate), 2C9 (weak), 2C19 (weak), 2D6 (moderate); **Induces** CYP3A4 (weak)

Bile acid sequestrants: May decrease pioglitazone levels.

CYP2C8 inducers: May decrease the levels/effects of pioglitazone. Example inducers include carbamazepine, phenobarbital, phenytoin, rifampin, rifapentine, and secobarbital.

CYP2C8 inhibitors: May increase the levels/effects of pioglitazone. Example inhibitors include atazanavir, gemfibrozil, and ritonavir.

CYP2C8 substrates: Pioglitazone may increase the levels/effects of CYP2C8 substrates. Example substrates include amiodarone, paclitaxel, and repaglinide.

CYP2D6 substrates: Pioglitazone may increase the levels/effects of CYP2D6 substrates. Example substrates include amphetamines, selected beta-blockers, dextromethorphan, fluoxetine, lidocaine, mirtazapine, nefazodone, paroxetine, risperidone, ritonavir, thioridazine, tricyclic antidepressants, and venlafaxine.

CYP2D6 prodrug substrates: Pioglitazone may decrease the levels/effects of CYP2D6 prodrug substrates. Example prodrug substrates include codeine, hydrocodone, oxycodone, and tramadol.

Gemfibrozil: Gemfibrozil may increase pioglitazone levels.

Pregabalin: Pioglitazone effect on fluid retention may be enhanced with pregabalin.

Rifampin: Pioglitazone level/effect may be decreased.

Thioridazine: Pioglitazone may increase thioridazine levels; concomitant use is contraindicated.

Trimethoprim: Pioglitazone level/effect may be increased if trimethoprim is initiated, and level/effect may be decreased if trimethoprim is discontinued.

Ethanol/Nutrition/Herb Interactions

Ethanol: Caution with ethanol (may cause hypoglycemia).

Food: Peak concentrations are delayed when administered with food, but the extent of absorption is not affected. Pioglitazone may be taken without regard to meals.

Herb/Nutraceutical: Caution with alfalfa, aloe, bilberry, bitter melon, burdock, celery, damiana, fenugreek, garcinia, garlic, ginger, ginseng (American), gymnema, marshmallow, and stinging nettle (may cause hypoglycemia).

Mechanism of Action Thiazolidinedione antidiabetic agent that lowers blood glucose by improving target cell response to insulin, without increasing pancreatic insulin secretion. It has a mechanism of action that is dependent on the presence of insulin for activity. Pioglitazone is a potent and selective agonist for peroxisome proliferator-activated receptor-gamma (PPARgamma). Activation of nuclear PPARgamma receptors influences the production of a number of gene products involved in glucose and lipid metabolism. PPARgamma is abundant in the cells within the renal collecting tubules; fluid retention results from stimulation by thiazolidinediones which increases sodium reabsorption.

Pharmacodynamics Onset of action: Delayed, may require several weeks to maximal effect

Pharmacokinetics

Absorption: Time to peak: Within 2 hours

Distribution: Protein binding: 99.8% V_{ss} (apparent): 0.63 L/kg

Metabolism: Hepatic (99%) to both active and inactive metabolites

Half-life: 3-7 hours (parent); 16-24 hours (total)

Elimination: As metabolites, in urine (15% to 30%) and feces

Dosage

Geriatrics & Adults: Type 2 diabetes: Oral:

Monotherapy: Initial: 15-30 mg once daily; if response is inadequate, the dosage may be increased in increments up to 45 mg once daily; maximum recommended dose: 45 mg once daily

Combination therapy:

Note: Maximum recommended dose: 45 mg/day

(Continued)

Pioglitazone *(Continued)*

With sulfonylureas: Initial: 15-30 mg once daily; dose of sulfonylurea should be reduced if the patient reports hypoglycemia

With metformin: Initial: 15-30 mg once daily; it is unlikely that the dose of metformin will need to be reduced due to hypoglycemia

With insulin: Initial: 15-30 mg once daily; dose of insulin should be reduced by 10% to 25% if the patient reports hypoglycemia or if the plasma glucose falls to below 100 mg/dL.

Dosage adjustment in patients with CHF (NYHA Class II) in mono- or combination therapy: Oral: Initial: 15 mg once daily; may be increased after several months of treatment, with close attention to heart failure symptoms

Renal Impairment: No adjustment is necessary.

Hepatic Impairment: Clearance is significantly lower in hepatic impairment (Child-Pugh Grade B/C). Therapy should not be initiated if the patient exhibits active liver disease or increased transaminases (>2.5 times ULN) at baseline. During treatment if ALT levels elevate >3 times ULN, the test should be repeated as soon as possible. If ALT levels remain >3 times ULN or if the patient is jaundiced, therapy should be discontinued.

Administration Oral: May be taken without regard to meals

Monitoring Parameters Hemoglobin A_{1c}, serum glucose; signs and symptoms of heart failure; liver enzymes prior to initiation and periodically during treatment (per clinician judgment). If the ALT is increased to >2.5 times the upper limit of normal, liver function testing should be performed more frequently until the levels return to normal or pretreatment values. Patients with an elevation in ALT >3 times the upper limit of normal should be rechecked as soon as possible. If the ALT levels remain >3 times the upper limit of normal, therapy with pioglitazone should be discontinued. Routine ophthalmic exams are recommended; patients reporting visual deterioration should have a prompt referral to an ophthalmologist and consideration should be given to discontinuing pioglitazone.

Patient Information May be taken without regard to meals. Follow directions of prescriber. Monitor urine or serum glucose as recommended by prescriber. More frequent monitoring is required during periods of stress, trauma, surgery, increased activity or exercise. Avoid alcohol. Report chest pain, rapid heartbeat or palpitations, abdominal pain, fever, rash, hypoglycemia reactions, yellowing of skin or eyes, dark urine or light stool, unusual fatigue, or nausea/vomiting.

Special Geriatric Considerations No dosage adjustment is recommended in elderly patients.

Dosage Forms Excipient information presented when available (limited, particularly for generics); consult specific product labeling.
Tablet:
Actos®: 15 mg, 30 mg, 45 mg

Pioglitazone and Glimepiride *(pye oh GLI ta zone & GLYE me pye ride)*

Medication Safety Issues
High alert medication: The Institute for Safe Medication Practices (ISMP) includes this medication among its list of drugs which have a heightened risk of causing significant patient harm when used in error.

U.S. Brand Names Duetact™
Index Terms Glimepiride and Pioglitazone; Glimepiride and Pioglitazone Hydrochloride
Generic Available No
Pharmacologic Category Antidiabetic Agent, Sulfonylurea; Antidiabetic Agent, Thiazolidinedione; Hypoglycemic Agent, Oral
Use Management of type 2 diabetes mellitus (noninsulin dependent, NIDDM) as an adjunct to diet and exercise
Dosage
Geriatrics: Initial: Glimepiride 1 mg/day prior to initiating Duetact™; dose titration and maintenance dosing should be conservative to avoid hypoglycemia. Refer to adult dosing.

Adults: Type 2 diabetes mellitus: Oral: Initial dose should be based on current dose of pioglitazone and/or sulfonylurea.
Patients inadequately controlled on **glimepiride** alone: Initial dose: 30 mg/2 mg or 30 mg/4 mg once daily
Patients inadequately controlled on **pioglitazone** alone: Initial dose: 30 mg/2 mg once daily
Patients with systolic dysfunction (eg, NYHA Class I and II): Initiate only after patient has been safely titrated to 30 mg of pioglitazone. Initial dose: 30 mg/2 mg or 30 mg/4 mg once daily
Note: No exact dosing relationship exists between glimepiride and other sulfonlyureas. Dosing should be limited to less than or equal to the maximum initial dose

of glimepiride (2 mg). When converting patients from other sulfonylureas with longer half lives (eg, chlorpropamide) to glimepiride, observe patient carefully for 1-2 weeks due to overlapping hypoglycemic effects.

Dosing adjustment: Dosage may be increased up to max dose and formulation strengths available; tablet should not be given more than once daily; see individual agents for frequency of adjustments. Dosage adjustments in patients with systolic dysfunction should be done carefully and patient monitored for symptoms of worsening heart failure.

Maximum dose: Pioglitazone 45 mg/glimepiride 8 mg daily

Renal Impairment: Cl_{cr} <22 mL/minute: Initial dose should be 1 mg of glimepiride and dosage increments should be based on fasting blood glucose levels.

Hepatic Impairment: Do not initiate treatment with active liver disease or ALT >2.5 times ULN. During treatment, if ALT levels elevate >3 times ULN, the test should be repeated as soon as possible. If ALT levels remain >3 times ULN or if the patient is jaundiced, Duetact™ should be discontinued.

Special Geriatric Considerations Rapid and prolonged hypoglycemia (>12 hours) despite hypertonic glucose injections have been reported with glimepiride. Age, hepatic impairment, and renal impairment are independent risk factors for hypoglycemia; dosage titration should be made at weekly intervals. How "tightly" a geriatric patient's blood glucose should be controlled is controversial; however, a fasting blood sugar of <150 mg/dL is now an acceptable endpoint. Such a decision should be based on the patient's functional and cognitive status, how well they recognize hypoglycemic or hyperglycemic symptoms, and how to respond to them and their other disease states.

Dosage Forms Excipient information presented when available (limited, particularly for generics); consult specific product labeling.

Tablet:
Duetact™:
30 mg/2 mg: Pioglitazone 30 mg and glimepiride 2 mg
30 mg/4 mg: Pioglitazone 30 mg and glimepiride 4 mg

Pioglitazone and Metformin (pye oh GLI ta zone & met FOR min)

U.S. Brand Names Actoplus Met™
Index Terms Metformin Hydrochloride and Pioglitazone Hydrochloride
Generic Available No
Pharmacologic Category Antidiabetic Agent, Biguanide; Antidiabetic Agent, Thiazolidinedione
Use Management of type 2 diabetes mellitus (noninsulin dependent, NIDDM)
Dosage

Geriatrics: Refer to adult dosing. The initial and maintenance dosing should be conservative, due to the potential for decreased renal function (monitor). Generally, elderly patients should not be titrated to the maximum; do not use in patients ≥80 years of age unless normal renal function has been established.

Adults: Type 2 diabetes mellitus: Oral: Initial dose should be based on current dose of pioglitazone and/or metformin; daily dose should be divided and given with meals.
Patients inadequately controlled on **metformin alone:** Initial dose: Pioglitazone 15-30 mg/day plus current dose of metformin
Patients inadequately controlled on **pioglitazone alone**: Initial dose: Metformin 1000-1700 mg/day plus current dose of pioglitazone
Note: When switching from combination pioglitazone and metformin as separate tablets: Use current dose.

Dosing adjustment: Doses may be increased as increments of pioglitazone 15 mg and/or metformin 500-850 mg, up to the maximum dose; doses should be titrated gradually. Guidelines for frequency of adjustment (adapted from rosiglitazone/metformin combination labeling):
After a change in the **metformin** dosage, titration can be done after 1-2 weeks
After a change in the **pioglitazone** dosage, titration can be done after 8-12 weeks
Maximum dose: Pioglitazone 45 mg/metformin 2550 mg daily

Renal Impairment: Do not use with renal disease or renal dysfunction (serum creatinine ≥1.5 mg/dL in males or ≥1.4 mg/dL in females or abnormal clearance).

Hepatic Impairment: Do not initiate treatment with active liver disease or ALT >2.5 times ULN. During treatment if ALT levels elevate >3 times ULN, the test should be repeated as soon as possible. If ALT levels remain >3 times ULN or if the patient is jaundiced, therapy should be discontinued.

Dosage Forms Excipient information presented when available (limited, particularly for generics); consult specific product labeling.

Tablet:
Actoplus Met™:
15/500: Pioglitazone 15 mg and metformin hydrochloride 500 mg
15/850: Pioglitazone 15 mg and metformin hydrochloride 850 mg

Piperacillin (pi PER a sil in)

Related Information
Antimicrobial Activity Against Selected Organisms *on page 1728*

Canadian Brand Names Piperacillin for Injection, USP

Index Terms Piperacillin Sodium

Generic Available Yes

Pharmacologic Category Antibiotic, Penicillin

Use Treatment of *Pseudomonas aeruginosa* infections in combination with an aminoglycoside which are susceptible to piperacillin; also effective against other gram-negative microorganisms and nonpenicillinase-producing anaerobes (including *B. fragilis*) and gram-positive organisms; normally used with other antibiotics (ie, aminoglycosides)

Contraindications Hypersensitivity to piperacillin, other penicillins, or any component of the formulation

Warnings/Precautions Serious and occasionally severe or fatal hypersensitivity (anaphylactoid) reactions have been reported in patients on penicillin therapy, especially with a history of beta-lactam hypersensitivity, history of sensitivity to multiple allergens, or previous IgE-mediated reactions (eg, anaphylaxis, angioedema, urticaria). Use with caution in asthmatic patients. Bleeding disorders have been observed, particularly in patients with renal impairment; discontinue if thrombocytopenia or bleeding occurs. Due to sodium load and adverse effects (anemia, neuropsychological changes), use with caution and modify dosage in patients with renal impairment. Use caution in patients with history of seizure activity. Leukopenia and neutropenia have been reported (during prolonged therapy). An increased frequency of fever and rash has been reported in patients with cystic fibrosis. Prolonged use may result in fungal or bacterial superinfection, including *C. difficile*-associated diarrhea and pseudomembranous colitis.

Adverse Reactions (Reflective of adult population; not specific for elderly)
Frequency not defined.

Central nervous system: Confusion, convulsions, drowsiness, fever, Jarisch-Herxheimer reaction

Dermatologic: Rash, toxic epidermal necrolysis, urticaria

Endocrine & metabolic: Electrolyte imbalance, hypokalemia

Hematologic: Abnormal platelet aggregation and prolonged PT (high doses), agranulocytosis, Coombs' reaction (positive), hemolytic anemia, pancytopenia

Local: Thrombophlebitis

Neuromuscular & skeletal: Myoclonus

Renal: Acute interstitial nephritis, acute renal failure

Miscellaneous: Anaphylaxis, hypersensitivity reactions

Overdosage/Toxicology Symptoms of penicillin overdose include neuromuscular hypersensitivity (agitation, hallucinations, asterixis, encephalopathy, confusion, and seizures) and electrolyte imbalance (with potassium or sodium salts), especially in renal failure. Hemodialysis may be helpful to aid in the removal of the drug from the blood, otherwise, most treatment is supportive or symptom-directed.

Drug Interactions
Aminoglycosides: May be synergistic against selected organisms; physical inactivation of aminoglycosides in the presence of high concentrations of piperacillin and potential toxicity in patients with mild to moderate renal dysfunction

Fusidic acid: May decrease the therapeutic effect of penicillins; administer the penicillin at least 2 hours before fusidic acid.

Heparin: Concomitant use with high-dose parenteral penicillins may result in increased risk of bleeding

Methotrexate: Penicillins may increase the exposure to methotrexate during concurrent therapy; monitor.

Neuromuscular blockers: May increase duration of blockade

Oral contraceptives: Anecdotal reports suggesting decreased contraceptive efficacy with penicillins have been refuted by more rigorous scientific and clinical data.

Probenecid: May increase levels of penicillins (piperacillin)

Tetracyclines: May decrease effectiveness of penicillins (piperacillin)

Warfarin: Effects of warfarin may be increased

Stability Reconstituted solution is stable (I.V. infusion) in NS or D_5W for 24 hours at room temperature, 7 days when refrigerated, or 4 weeks when frozen. After freezing, thawed solution is stable for 24 hours at room temperature or 48 hours when refrigerated. 40 g bulk vial should **not** be frozen after reconstitution.

Mechanism of Action Inhibits bacterial cell wall synthesis by binding to one or more of the penicillin binding proteins (PBPs); which in turn inhibits the final transpeptidation

step of peptidoglycan synthesis in bacterial cell walls, thus inhibiting cell wall biosynthesis. Bacteria eventually lyse due to ongoing activity of cell wall autolytic enzymes (autolysins and murein hydrolases) while cell wall assembly is arrested.

Pharmacokinetics
Absorption: I.M.: 70% to 80%
Protein binding: 22%
Half-life: Adults: 36-80 minutes (dose-dependent), prolonged with moderately severe renal or hepatic impairment
Time to peak serum concentration: Within 30-50 minutes
Elimination: Principally in urine and partially in feces (via bile)

Dosage
Geriatrics: Adjust dose for renal impairment:
I.M.: 1-2 g every 8-12 hours
I.V.: 2-4 g every 6-8 hours
Adults:
Usual dosage range:
I.M.: 2-3 g/dose every 6-12 hours; maximum: 24 g/24 hours
I.V.: 3-4 g/dose every 4-6 hours; maximum: 24 g/24 hours
Burn wound sepsis: I.V.: 4 g every 4 hours with vancomycin and amikacin
Cholangitis, acute: I.V.: 4 g every 6 hours
Keratitis (Pseudomonas): Ophthalmic: 6-12 mg/mL every 15-60 minutes around the clock for 24-72 hours, then slow reduction
Malignant otitis externa: I.V.: 4-6 g every 4-6 hours with tobramycin
Moderate infections: I.M., I.V.: 2-3 g/dose every 6-12 hours (maximum: 2 g I.M./ site)
Prosthetic joint (Pseudomonas): I.V.: 3 g every 6 hours with aminoglycoside
Pseudomonas infections: I.V.: 4 g every 4 hours
Severe infections: I.M., I.V.: 3-4 g/dose every 4-6 hours (maximum: 24 g/24 hours)
Urinary tract infections: I.M., I.V.: 2-3 g/dose every 6-12 hours
Uncomplicated gonorrhea: I.M.: 2 g in a single dose accompanied by 1 g probenecid 30 minutes prior to injection
Renal Impairment:
Cl$_{cr}$ 10-50 mL/minute: Administer every 6-8 hours.
Cl$_{cr}$ <10 mL/minute: Administer every 8 hours.
Moderately dialyzable (20% to 50%)
Continuous arteriovenous or venovenous hemofiltration: Dose as for Cl$_{cr}$ 10-50 mL/ minute.

Monitoring Parameters Temperature, WBC count, mental status, appetite; bleeding time, especially in patients with renal impairment

Test Interactions May interfere with urinary glucose tests using cupric sulfate (Benedict's solution, Clinitest®); false-positive urinary and serum proteins, positive Coombs' test [direct]. False-positive Platelia® Aspergillus EIA test (Bio-Rad Laboratories) has been reported.
Some penicillin derivatives may accelerate the degradation of aminoglycosides *in vitro*, leading to a potential underestimation of aminoglycoside serum concentration.

Additional Information Sodium content of 1 g: 1.85 mEq. Administer 1 hour apart from aminoglycosides.

Special Geriatric Considerations Antipseudomonal penicillins should not be used alone and are often combined with an aminoglycoside as empiric therapy for lower respiratory infection and sepsis in which gram-negative (including *Pseudomonas*) and/ or anaerobes are of a high probability. Because of piperacillin's lower sodium content, it is preferred over ticarcillin in patients with a history of heart failure and/or renal or hepatic disease. Adjust dose for renal function.

Dosage Forms Excipient information presented when available (limited, particularly for generics); consult specific product labeling.
Injection, powder for reconstitution: 2 g, 3 g, 4 g, 40 g

Selected References
Donowitz GR and Mandell GL, "Drug Therapy. Beta-Lactam Antibiotics (1)," *N Engl J Med*, 1988, 318(7):419-26.
Donowitz GR and Mandell GL, "Drug Therapy. Beta-Lactam Antibiotics (2)," *N Engl J Med*, 1988, 318(8):490-500.
Yoshikawa TT, "Antimicrobial Therapy for the Elderly Patient," *J Am Geriatr Soc*, 1990, 38(12):1353-72.

Piperacillin and Tazobactam Sodium
(pi PER a sil in & ta zoe BAK tam SOW dee um)

Related Information
Antimicrobial Activity Against Selected Organisms *on page 1728*
Piperacillin *on page 1270*
Medication Safety Issues
Sound-alike/look-alike issues:
Zosyn® may be confused with Zofran®, Zyvox®
(Continued)

Piperacillin and Tazobactam Sodium *(Continued)*

U.S. Brand Names Zosyn®

Canadian Brand Names Tazocin®

Index Terms Piperacillin Sodium and Tazobactam Sodium; Tazobactam and Piperacillin

Generic Available No

Pharmacologic Category Antibiotic, Penicillin

Use Treatment of moderate-to-severe infections caused by susceptible organisms, including infections of the lower respiratory tract (community-acquired pneumonia, nosocomial pneumonia); urinary tract; uncomplicated and complicated skin and skin structures; gynecologic (endometritis, pelvic inflammatory disease); bone and joint infections; intra-abdominal infections (appendicitis with rupture/abscess, peritonitis); and septicemia. Tazobactam expands activity of piperacillin to include beta-lactamase producing strains of *S. aureus*, *H. influenzae*, *Bacteroides*, and other gram-negative bacteria.

Contraindications Hypersensitivity to penicillins, beta-lactamase inhibitors, or any component of the formulation

Warnings/Precautions Bleeding disorders have been observed, particularly in patients with renal impairment; discontinue if thrombocytopenia or bleeding occurs. Due to sodium load and to the adverse effects of high serum concentrations of penicillins, dosage modification is required in patients with impaired or underdeveloped renal function; use with caution in patients with seizures or in patients with history of beta-lactam allergy; associated with an increased incidence of rash and fever in cystic fibrosis patients. Prolonged use may result in fungal or bacterial superinfection, including *C. difficile*-associated diarrhea and pseudomembranous colitis.

Adverse Reactions (Reflective of adult population; not specific for elderly)

>10%: Gastrointestinal: Diarrhea (7% to 11%)

>1% to 10%:

    Cardiovascular: Hypertension (2%)

    Central nervous system: Insomnia (7%), headache (8%), fever (2% to 5%), agitation (2%), pain (2%)

    Dermatologic: Rash (4%), pruritus (3%)

    Gastrointestinal: Constipation (1% to 8%), nausea (7%), vomiting (3% to 4%), dyspepsia (3%), stool changes (2%), abdominal pain (1% to 2%)

    Hepatic: Transaminases increased

    Local: Local reaction (3%), abscess (2%)

    Respiratory: Pharyngitis (2%)

    Miscellaneous: Moniliasis (2%), sepsis (2%), infection (2%)

Overdosage/Toxicology Symptoms of penicillin overdose include neuromuscular hypersensitivity (agitation, hallucinations, asterixis, encephalopathy, confusion, and seizures) and electrolyte imbalance (with potassium or sodium salts), especially in renal dysfunction. Hemodialysis may be helpful to aid in the removal of the drug from the blood, otherwise, most treatment is supportive or symptom-directed.

Drug Interactions

    Aminoglycosides: May be synergistic against selected organisms; physical inactivation of aminoglycosides in the presence of high concentrations of piperacillin and potential toxicity in patients with mild to moderate renal dysfunction

    Fusidic acid: May decrease the therapeutic effect of penicillins; administer the penicillin at least 2 hours before fusidic acid.

    Heparin: Concomitant use with high-dose parenteral penicillins may result in increased risk of bleeding

    Methotrexate: Penicillins may increase the exposure to methotrexate during concurrent therapy; monitor.

    Neuromuscular blockers: May increase duration of blockade

    Oral contraceptives: Anecdotal reports suggesting decreased contraceptive efficacy with penicillins have been refuted by more rigorous scientific and clinical data.

    Probenecid: May increase levels of penicillins (piperacillin)

    Tetracyclines: May decrease effectiveness of penicillins (piperacillin)

    Warfarin: Effects of warfarin may be increased

Stability

    Vials: Store at controlled room temperature of 20°C to 25°C (68°F to 77°F). Use single-dose vials immediately after reconstitution (discard unused portions after 24 hours at room temperature and 48 hours if refrigerated). Reconstitute with 5 mL of diluent per 1 g of piperacillin and then further dilute. After reconstitution, vials or solution are stable in NS or D$_5$W for 24 hours at room temperature and 48 hours (vials) or 7 days (solution) when refrigerated.

    Premixed solution: Store frozen at -20°C (-4°F). Thawed solution is stable for 24 hours at room temperature or 14 days under refrigeration; do not refreeze.

Mechanism of Action Inhibits bacterial cell wall synthesis by binding to one or more of the penicillin binding proteins (PBPs); which in turn inhibits the final transpeptidation step of peptidoglycan synthesis in bacterial cell walls, thus inhibiting cell wall biosynthesis. Bacteria eventually lyse due to ongoing activity of cell wall autolytic enzymes (autolysins and murein hydrolases) while cell wall assembly is arrested. Tazobactam inhibits many beta-lactamases, including staphylococcal penicillinase and Richmond and Sykes types II, III, IV, and V, including extended spectrum enzymes; it has only limited activity against class I beta-lactamases other than class Ic types.

Pharmacokinetics Both AUC and peak concentrations are dose proportional; hepatic impairment does not affect kinetics

  Distribution: Well into lungs, intestinal mucosa, skin, muscle, uterus, ovary, prostate, gallbladder, and bile; penetration into CSF is low in subject with noninflamed meninges

  Protein binding: Piperacillin and tazobactam: ~30%

  Metabolism:

    Piperacillin: 6% to 9% to desethyl metabolite (weak activity)

    Tazobactam: ~26% to inactive metabolite

  Half-life elimination: Piperacillin and tazobactam: 0.7-1.2 hours

  Time to peak, plasma: Immediately following infusion of 30 minutes

  Excretion: Clearance of both piperacillin and tazobactam are directly proportional to renal function

    Piperacillin: Urine (68% as unchanged drug); feces (10% to 20%)

    Tazobactam: Urine (80% as inactive metabolite)

Dosage

  Geriatrics & Adults:

    Diverticulitis, intra-abdominal abscess, peritonitis: I.V.: 3.375 g every 6 hours; **Note:** Some clinicians use 4.5 g every 8 hours for empiric coverage since the %time>MIC is similar between the regimens for most pathogens; however, this regimen is NOT recommended for nosocomial pneumonia or *Pseudomonas* coverage.

    Pneumonia (nosocomial): I.V.: 4.5 g every 6 hours for 7-14 days (when used empirically, combination with an aminoglycoside is recommended; consider discontinuation of aminoglycoside if *P. aeruginosa* is not isolated)

    Severe infections: I.V.: 3.375 g every 6 hours for 7-10 days; **Note:** Some clinicians use 4.5 g every 8 hours for empiric coverage since the %time>MIC is similar between the regimens for most pathogens; however, this regimen is NOT recommended for nosocomial pneumonia or *Pseudomonas* coverage.

  Renal Impairment:

    Cl_{cr} 20-40 mL/minute: Administer 2.25 g every 6 hours (3.375 g every 6 hours for nosocomial pneumonia)

    Cl_{cr} <20 mL/minute: Administer 2.25 g every 8 hours (2.25 g every 6 hours for nosocomial pneumonia)

    Hemodialysis/CAPD: Administer 2.25 g every 12 hours (2.25 g every 8 hours for nosocomial pneumonia) with an additional dose of 0.75 g after each dialysis

  Hepatic Impairment: Hepatic impairment does not affect the kinetics of piperacillin or tazobactam significantly.

Administration Administer by I.V. infusion over 30 minutes

  Some penicillins (eg, carbenicillin, ticarcillin and piperacillin) have been shown to inactivate aminoglycosides *in vitro*. This has been observed to a greater extent with tobramycin and gentamicin, while amikacin has shown greater stability against inactivation. Concurrent use of these agents may pose a risk of reduced antibacterial efficacy *in vivo*, particularly in the setting of profound renal impairment. However, definitive clinical evidence is lacking. If combination penicillin/aminoglycoside therapy is desired in a patient with renal dysfunction, separation of doses (if feasible), and routine monitoring of aminoglycoside levels, CBC, and clinical response should be considered. **Note:** Reformulated Zosyn® containing EDTA has been shown to be compatible *in vitro* for Y-site infusion with amikacin and gentamicin, but not compatible with tobramycin.

Monitoring Parameters Signs and symptoms of infection, mental status, WBC; bleeding time, especially in patients with renal impairment

Test Interactions Positive Coombs' [direct] test; false positive reaction for urine glucose using copper-reduction method (Clinitest®); may result in false positive results with the Platelia® *Aspergillus* enzyme immunoassay (EIA)

  Some penicillin derivatives may accelerate the degradation of aminoglycosides *in vitro*, leading to a potential underestimation of aminoglycoside serum concentration. **Note:** Reformulated Zosyn® containing EDTA has been shown to be compatible *in vitro* for Y-site infusion with amikacin and gentamicin, but not compatible with tobramycin.

Additional Information

  Administer 1 hour apart from aminoglycosides.

Special Geriatric Considerations Has not been studied exclusively in the elderly.

Dosage Forms Excipient information presented when available (limited, particularly for generics); consult specific product labeling.

  Note: 8:1 ratio of piperacillin sodium/tazobactam sodium

  (Continued)

Piperacillin and Tazobactam Sodium *(Continued)*

Infusion [premixed iso-osmotic solution, frozen]:

2.25 g: Piperacillin 2 g and tazobactam 0.25 g (50 mL) [contains sodium 5.58 mEq (128 mg) and EDTA]

3.375 g: Piperacillin 3 g and tazobactam 0.375 g (50 mL) [contains sodium 8.38 mEq (192 mg) and EDTA]

4.5 g: Piperacillin 4 g and tazobactam 0.5 g (50 mL) [contains sodium 11.17 mEq (256 mg) and EDTA]

Injection, powder for reconstitution:

2.25 g: Piperacillin 2 g and tazobactam 0.25 g [contains sodium 5.58 mEq (128 mg) and EDTA]

3.375 g: Piperacillin 3 g and tazobactam 0.375 g [contains sodium 8.38 mEq (192 mg) and EDTA]

4.5 g: Piperacillin 4 g and tazobactam 0.5 g [contains sodium 11.17 mEq (256 mg) and EDTA]

40.5 g: Piperacillin 36 g and tazobactam 4.5 g [contains sodium 100.4 mEq (2304 mg) and EDTA; bulk pharmacy vial]

♦ **Piperacillin Sodium** *see* Piperacillin *on page 1270*
♦ **Piperacillin Sodium and Tazobactam Sodium** *see* Piperacillin and Tazobactam Sodium *on page 1271*

Piperazine *(PI per a zeen)*

Canadian Brand Names Entacyl®
Index Terms Piperazine Citrate
Generic Available Yes
Pharmacologic Category Anthelmintic
Use Treatment of pinworm and roundworm infections (used as an alternative to first-line agents, mebendazole, or pyrantel pamoate)
Contraindications Hypersensitivity to piperazine or any component of the formulation; seizure disorders; liver or kidney impairment
Warnings/Precautions Use with caution in patients with anemia or malnutrition
Drug Interactions Pyrantel pamoate (antagonistic mode of action)
Mechanism of Action Causes muscle paralysis of the roundworm by blocking the effects of acetylcholine at the neuromuscular junction
Pharmacokinetics
Absorption: Well absorbed from GI tract
Time to peak plasma concentration: 1 hour
Elimination: In urine as metabolites and unchanged drug
Dosage
Geriatrics & Adults:
Pinworm eradication: Oral: 65 mg/kg/day (not to exceed 2.5 g/day) as a single daily dose for 7 days; in severe infections, repeat course after a 1-week interval
Roundworm eradication: Oral: 3.5 g/day for 2 days (in severe infections, repeat course, after a 1-week interval)
Monitoring Parameters Stool exam for worms and ova
Patient Information Take on an empty stomach; contact physician if headache, dizziness, poor coordination, muscle weakness, seizures, nausea, vomiting, diarrhea, or rash occur; wash bed clothes, towels, night clothes, and maintain good hygiene to prevent spread or reinfection
Special Geriatric Considerations Not a drug of choice. Monitor closely in the elderly.
Dosage Forms Excipient information presented when available (limited, particularly for generics); consult specific product labeling.
Piperazine citrate is available from Panorama Pharmacy (1-800-247-9767).

♦ **Piperazine Citrate** *see* Piperazine *on page 1274*

Pirbuterol *(peer BYOO ter ole)*

Related Information
Inhalant Agents *on page 1760*
U.S. Brand Names Maxair™ Autohaler™
Index Terms Pirbuterol Acetate
Generic Available No
Pharmacologic Category Beta$_2$-Adrenergic Agonist
Use Prevention and treatment of reversible bronchospasm including asthma
Contraindications Hypersensitivity to pirbuterol, albuterol, or any component of the formulation

Warnings/Precautions Optimize anti-inflammatory treatment before initiating maintenance treatment with pirbuterol. Do not use as a component of chronic therapy without an anti-inflammatory agent. Only the mildest form of asthma (Step 1 and/or exercise-induced) would not require concurrent use based upon asthma guidelines. Patient must be instructed to seek medical attention in cases where acute symptoms are not relieved or a previous level of response is diminished. The need to increase frequency of use may indicate deterioration of asthma, and treatment must not be delayed.

Use caution in patients with cardiovascular disease (arrhythmia or hypertension or CHF), convulsive disorders, diabetes, glaucoma, hyperthyroidism, or hypokalemia. Beta-agonists may cause elevation in blood pressure, heart rate, and result in CNS stimulation/excitation. Beta₂-agonists may increase risk of arrhythmia, increase serum glucose, or decrease serum potassium.

Do not exceed recommended dose; serious adverse events including fatalities, have been associated with excessive use of inhaled sympathomimetics. Rarely, paradoxical bronchospasm may occur with use of inhaled bronchodilating agents; this should be distinguished from inadequate response. All patients should utilize a spacer device when using a metered-dose inhaler.

Adverse Reactions (Reflective of adult population; not specific for elderly)
>10%:
 Central nervous system: Nervousness (7%)
 Endocrine & metabolic: Serum glucose increased, serum potassium decreased
 Neuromuscular & skeletal: Trembling (6%)
1% to 10%:
 Cardiovascular: Palpitation (2%), tachycardia (1%)
 Central nervous system: Headache (2%), dizziness (1%)
 Gastrointestinal: Nausea (2%)
 Respiratory: Cough (1%)

Overdosage/Toxicology Symptoms of overdose include tachycardia, tremor, hypertension, angina, and seizures. Hypokalemia also may occur. Cardiac arrest and death may be associated with abuse of beta-agonist bronchodilators. Treatment includes immediate discontinuation and symptomatic and supportive therapies. Cautious use of beta-adrenergic blocking agents may be considered in severe cases.

Drug Interactions
 Decreased effect with beta-blockers
 Increased toxicity with other beta-agonists, MAO inhibitors, TCAs

Stability Store between 15°C and 30°C (59°F and 86°F).

Mechanism of Action Pirbuterol is a beta₂-adrenergic agonist with a similar structure to albuterol, specifically a pyridine ring has been substituted for the benzene ring in albuterol. The increased beta₂ selectivity of pirbuterol results from the substitution of a tertiary butyl group on the nitrogen of the side chain, which additionally imparts resistance of pirbuterol to degradation by monoamine oxidase and provides a lengthened duration of action in comparison to the less selective previous beta-agonist agents.

Pharmacodynamics
 Onset of action: Within 5 minutes
 Peak effect: 30-60 minutes
 Duration: 3-5 hours

Pharmacokinetics
 Metabolism: In the liver
 Elimination: Urine as unchanged drug and metabolites

Dosage
 Geriatrics & Adults: Bronchospasm: Inhalation: 2 inhalations every 4-6 hours for prevention; 2 inhalations at an interval of at least 1-3 minutes, followed by a third inhalation in treatment of bronchospasm, not to exceed 12 inhalations/day

Monitoring Parameters Pulmonary function, blood pressure, pulse

Patient Information Patient instructions are available with product. Do not exceed recommended dosage; rinse mouth with water following each inhalation to help with dry throat and mouth. May cause nervousness, restlessness, insomnia - if these effects continue after dosage reduction, notify physician. Also notify physician if palpitations, tachycardia, chest pain, muscle tremors, dizziness, headache, flushing, or if breathing difficulty persists. Autohaler™ is breath-activated; follow instructions with product.

Special Geriatric Considerations Elderly patients may find it beneficial to utilize a spacer device when using a metered dose inhaler. Difficulty in using the inhaler often limits its effectiveness. The Maxair™ Autohaler™ may be easier for the elderly to use.

Dosage Forms Excipient information presented when available (limited, particularly for generics); consult specific product labeling.
 Aerosol for oral inhalation, as acetate:
  Maxair™ Autohaler™: 200 mcg/actuation (14 g) [400 actuations; contains chlorofluorocarbons]

♦ **Pirbuterol Acetate** see Pirbuterol on page 1274

Piroxicam (peer OKS i kam)

Related Information
Potentially Inappropriate Medications for Geriatrics *on page 1824*
Medication Safety Issues
International issues:
Flogene® [Brazil] may be confused with Florone® which is a brand name for diflora-sone in the U.S.
U.S. Brand Names Feldene®
Canadian Brand Names Apo-Piroxicam®; Gen-Piroxicam; Novo-Pirocam; Nu-Pirox; Pexicam®
Generic Available Yes
Pharmacologic Category Nonsteroidal Anti-inflammatory Drug (NSAID), Oral
Use Management of inflammatory disorders; symptomatic treatment of acute and chronic rheumatoid arthritis, osteoarthritis, and sunburn
Restrictions An FDA-approved medication guide must be distributed when dispensing an oral outpatient prescription (new or refill) where this medication is to be used without direct supervision of a healthcare provider. Medication guides are available at http://www.fda.gov/cder/Offices/ODS/medication_guides.htm.
Contraindications Hypersensitivity to piroxicam, aspirin, other NSAIDs or any component of the formulation; perioperative pain in the setting of coronary artery bypass surgery (CABG)
Warnings/Precautions [U.S. Boxed Warning]: NSAIDs are associated with an increased risk of adverse cardiovascular events, including MI, stroke, and new onset or worsening of pre-existing hypertension. Risk may be increased with duration of use or pre-existing cardiovascular risk factors or disease. Carefully evaluate individual cardiovascular risk profiles prior to prescribing. Use caution with fluid retention, CHF or hypertension. Concurrent administration of ibuprofen, and potentially other nonselective NSAIDs, may interfere with aspirin's cardioprotective effect.

Use of NSAIDs can compromise existing renal function. Renal toxicity can occur in patient with impaired renal function, dehydration, heart failure, liver dysfunction, those taking diuretics and ACEI and the elderly. Rehydrate patient before starting therapy. Monitor renal function closely. Not recommended for use in patients with advanced renal disease.

[U.S. Boxed Warning]: NSAIDs may increase risk of gastrointestinal irritation, ulceration, bleeding, and perforation. These events may occur at any time during therapy and without warning. Use caution with a history of GI disease (bleeding or ulcers), concurrent therapy with aspirin, anticoagulants and/or corticosteroids, smoking, use of alcohol, the elderly or debilitated patients.

Use the lowest effective dose for the shortest duration of time, consistent with individual patient goals, to reduce risk of cardiovascular or GI adverse events. Alternate therapies should be considered for patients at high risk.

NSAIDs may cause serious skin adverse events including exfoliative dermatitis, Stevens-Johnson syndrome (SJS) and toxic epidermal necrolysis (TEN). Anaphylactoid reactions may occur, even without prior exposure; patients with "aspirin triad" (bronchial asthma, aspirin intolerance, rhinitis) may be at increased risk. Do not use in patients who experience bronchospasm, asthma, rhinitis, or urticaria with NSAID or aspirin therapy. Use caution with other forms of asthma. A serum sickness-like reaction can rarely occur; watch for arthralgias, pruritus, fever, fatigue, and rash.

Use with caution in patients with decreased hepatic function. Closely monitor patients with any abnormal LFT. Severe hepatic reactions (eg, fulminant hepatitis, liver failure) have occurred with NSAID use, rarely; discontinue if signs or symptoms of liver disease develop, or if systemic manifestations occur.

The elderly are at increased risk for adverse effects (especially peptic ulceration, CNS effects, renal toxicity) from NSAIDs even at low doses

Withhold for at least 4-6 half-lives prior to surgical or dental procedures.
Adverse Reactions (Reflective of adult population; not specific for elderly)
>10%:
Central nervous system: Dizziness
Dermatologic: Rash
Gastrointestinal: Abdominal cramps, heartburn, indigestion, nausea
1% to 10%:
Central nervous system: Headache, nervousness
Dermatologic: Itching
Endocrine & metabolic: Fluid retention
Gastrointestinal: Vomiting
Otic: Tinnitus

Overdosage/Toxicology Symptoms include nausea, epigastric distress, CNS depression, leukocytosis, and renal failure. Management of nonsteroidal anti-inflammatory drug (NSAID) intoxication is primarily supportive and symptomatic. Fluid therapy is commonly effective in managing hypotension that may occur following an acute NSAID overdose, except when due to acute blood loss. Seizures tend to be very short-lived and often do not require drug treatment; although, recurrent seizures should be treated with I.V. diazepam. Since many of the NSAIDs undergo enterohepatic cycling, multiple doses of charcoal may be needed to reduce the potential for delayed toxicities.

Drug Interactions Substrate of CYP2C9 (minor); **Inhibits** CYP2C9 (strong)

ACE inhibitors: Antihypertensive effects may be decreased by concurrent therapy with NSAIDs; monitor blood pressure.

Angiotensin II antagonists: Antihypertensive effects may be decreased by concurrent therapy with NSAIDs; monitor blood pressure.

Anticoagulants (warfarin, heparin, LMWHs) in combination with NSAIDs can cause increased risk of bleeding.

Antiplatelet drugs (ticlopidine, clopidogrel, aspirin, abciximab, dipyridamole, eptifibatide, tirofiban) can cause an increased risk of bleeding.

Beta-blockers: NSAIDs may decrease the antihypertensive effect of beta-blockers. Monitor.

Cholestyramine (and other bile acid sequestrants): May decrease the absorption of NSAIDs. Separate by at least 2 hours.

Corticosteroids may increase the risk of GI ulceration; avoid concurrent use.

Cyclosporine: NSAIDs may increase serum creatinine, potassium, blood pressure, and cyclosporine levels; monitor cyclosporine levels and renal function carefully.

CYP2C9 Substrates: Piroxicam may increase the levels/effects of CYP2C9 substrates. Example substrates include bosentan, dapsone, fluoxetine, glimepiride, glipizide, losartan, montelukast, nateglinide, paclitaxel, phenytoin, warfarin, and zafirlukast.

Fluoroquinolone antibiotics: Risk of seizures may be increased with concomitant quinolone use. Risk is considered quite low and may only be a factor with high serum levels of either agent and/or in patients with additional predisposing factors (eg, renal dysfunction, history of seizure or other neurological disorder).

Hydralazine's antihypertensive effect is decreased; avoid concurrent use.

Lithium levels can be increased; avoid concurrent use if possible or monitor lithium levels and adjust dose.

Loop diuretics efficacy (diuretic and antihypertensive effect) is reduced. Indomethacin reduces this efficacy, however, it may be anticipated with any NSAID.

Methotrexate: Severe bone marrow suppression, aplastic anemia, and GI toxicity have been reported with concomitant NSAID therapy. Avoid use during moderate or high-dose methotrexate (increased and prolonged methotrexate levels). NSAID use during low-dose treatment of rheumatoid arthritis has not been fully evaluated; extreme caution is warranted.

Salicylates: NSAIDs (nonselective) may diminish the cardioprotective effect of acetylated salicylates. Avoid regular use of NSAIDs if possible; consider alternatives (eg, acetaminophen). Give salicylate before NSAID; for example ibuprofen should be given 30-120 minutes after aspirin (immediate release).

Thiazides antihypertensive effects are decreased; avoid concurrent use.

Warfarin's INRs may be increased by piroxicam. Other NSAIDs may have the same effect depending on dose and duration. Monitor INR closely. Use the lowest dose of NSAIDs possible and for the briefest duration.

Ethanol/Nutrition/Herb Interactions

Ethanol: Avoid ethanol (may enhance gastric mucosal irritation).

Food: Onset of effect may be delayed if piroxicam is taken with food.

Herb/Nutraceutical: Avoid alfalfa, anise, bilberry, bladderwrack, bromelain, cat's claw, celery, coleus, cordyceps, dong quai, evening primrose, feverfew, fenugreek, garlic, ginger, ginkgo biloba, red clover, horse chestnut, grapeseed, green tea, ginseng, guggul, horse chestnut seed, horseradish, licorice, prickly ash, red clover, reishi, SAMe, sweet clover, turmeric, white willow (all have additional antiplatelet activity).

Mechanism of Action Inhibits prostaglandin synthesis, acts on the hypothalamus heat-regulating center to reduce fever, blocks prostaglandin synthetase action which prevents formation of the platelet-aggregating substance thromboxane A_2; decreases pain receptor sensitivity. Other proposed mechanisms of action for salicylate anti-inflammatory action are lysosomal stabilization, kinin and leukotriene production, alteration of chemotactic factors, and inhibition of neutrophil activation. This latter mechanism may be the most significant pharmacologic action to reduce inflammation.

Pharmacodynamics

Onset of action:

Analgesia: Oral: Within 1 hour

Anti-inflammatory effect: 7-12 days

Duration of analgesia: 2-3 days

Peak anti-inflammatory effect: 2-3 weeks

Pharmacokinetics

Protein binding: 99%

(Continued)

Piroxicam (Continued)

Metabolism: Hepatic

Half-life: 45-50 hours

Time to peak serum concentration: 3-5 hours after ingestion

Elimination: Excreted as unchanged drug (5%) and metabolites primarily in urine and to a small degree in feces

Dosage

Geriatrics: Refer to adult dosing. **Note:** Some clinicians have used 10 mg every other day to initiate therapy in the elderly to help avoid side effects and produce therapeutic effect at minimal dose. Maximum dose: 20 mg/day.

Adults: Inflammation, rheumatoid arthritis: Oral: 10-20 mg/day once daily; although associated with increase in GI adverse effects, doses >20 mg/day have been used (ie, 30-40 mg/day); maximum dose: 20 mg/day

Renal Impairment: Not recommended in patients with advanced renal disease.

Hepatic Impairment: Reduced dose is necessary.

Monitoring Parameters Monitor response (pain, range of motion, grip strength, mobility, ADL function), inflammation; observe for weight gain, edema; monitor renal function; observe for bleeding, bruising; evaluate gastrointestinal effects (abdominal pain, bleeding, dyspepsia); mental confusion, disorientation, CBC, serum, creatinine, BUN, liver function tests

Test Interactions Increased chloride (S), increased sodium (S), increased bleeding time

Patient Information Serious gastrointestinal bleeding can occur as well as ulceration and perforation. Pain may or may not be present. Avoid aspirin and aspirin-containing products while taking this medication. If gastric upset occurs, take with food, milk, or antacid. If gastric adverse effects persist, contact physician. May cause drowsiness, dizziness, blurred vision, and confusion. Use caution when performing tasks which require alertness (eg, driving). Do not take for more than 3 days for fever or 10 days for pain without physician's advice.

Additional Information Because of its long half-life, may be dosed once daily. There are no clinical guidelines to predict which NSAID will give response in a particular patient. Trials with each must be initiated until response determined. Consider dose, patient convenience, and cost.

Special Geriatric Considerations Elderly are a high-risk population for adverse effects from NSAIDs. As much as 60% of elderly can develop peptic ulceration and/or hemorrhage asymptomatically. The concomitant use of H_2 blockers and sucralfate is not generally effective as prophylaxis with the exception of NSAID-induced duodenal ulcers which may be prevented by the use of ranitidine. Misoprostol and proton pump inhibitors are the only agents proven to help prevent the development of NSAID-induced ulcers. Also, concomitant disease and drug use contribute to the risk for GI adverse effects. Use lowest effective dose for shortest period possible. Consider renal function decline with age. Use of NSAIDs can compromise existing renal function especially when Cl_{cr} is ≤30 mL/minute. Tinnitus may be a difficult and unreliable indication of toxicity due to age-related hearing loss or eighth cranial nerve damage. CNS adverse effects such as confusion, agitation, and hallucination are generally seen in overdose or high dose situations, but elderly may demonstrate these adverse effects at lower doses than younger adults.

Dosage Forms Excipient information presented when available (limited, particularly for generics); consult specific product labeling.

Capsule: 10 mg, 20 mg

Selected References

Brooks PM and Day RO, "Nonsteroidal Anti-inflammatory Drugs - Differences and Similarities," *N Engl J Med*, 1991, 324(24):1716-25.

Clinch D, Banerjee AK, and Ostick G, "Absence of Abdominal Pain in Elderly Patients With Peptic Ulcer," *Age Ageing*, 1984, 13(2):120-3.

Clive DM and Stoff JS, "Renal Syndromes Associated With Nonsteroidal Anti-inflammatory Drugs," *N Engl J Med*, 1984, 310(9):563-72.

Graham DY, "Prevention of Gastroduodenal Injury Induced by Chronic Nonsteroidal Anti-inflammatory Drug Therapy," *Gastroenterology*, 1989, 96(2 Pt 2 Suppl):675-81.

Gurwitz JH, Avorn J, Ross-Degnan D, et al, "Nonsteroidal Anti-Inflammatory Drug-Associated Azotemia in the Very Old," *JAMA*, 1990, 264(4):471-5.

Hawkey CJ, Karrasch JA, Szczepański L, et al, "Omeprazole Compared With Misoprostol for Ulcers Associated With Nonsteroidal Anti-inflammatory Drugs," *N Engl J Med*, 1998, 338(11):727-34.

Knodel LC, "Preventing NSAID-induced Ulcers: The Role of Misoprostol," *Consult Pharm*, 1989, 4:37-41.

Pounder R, "Silent Peptic Ulceration: Deadly Silence or Golden Silence?" *Gastroenterology*, 1989, 96(2 Pt 2 Suppl):626-31.

Yeomans ND, Tulassay Z, Juhasz L, et al, "A Comparison of Omeprazole With Ranitidine for Ulcers Associated With Nonsteroidal Anti-inflammatory Drugs," *N Engl J Med*, 1998, 338(11):719-26.

♦ *p*-**Isobutylhydratropic Acid** *see* Ibuprofen *on page 784*

♦ **Pitressin**® *see* Vasopressin *on page 1665*

♦ **Plantago Seed** *see* Psyllium *on page 1347*

♦ **Plantain Seed** *see* Psyllium *on page 1347*

♦ **Plaquenil**® *see* Hydroxychloroquine *on page 772*

♦ **Plaretase**® **8000** *see* Pancrelipase *on page 1196*
♦ **Plavix**® *see* Clopidogrel *on page 345*
♦ **Plendil**® *see* Felodipine *on page 602*
♦ **Pletal**® *see* Cilostazol *on page 312*

Pneumococcal Polysaccharide Vaccine (Polyvalent)
(noo moe KOK al pol i SAK a ride vak SEEN, pol i VAY lent)

Related Information
Immunization Recommendations *on page 1787*

U.S. Brand Names Pneumovax® 23

Canadian Brand Names Pneumo 23™; Pneumovax® 23

Index Terms PPV23; 23PS; 23-Valent Pneumococcal Polysaccharide Vaccine

Generic Available No

Pharmacologic Category Vaccine

Use Immunity to pneumococcal lobar pneumonia and bacteremia in individuals ≥2 years of age who are at high risk of morbidity and mortality from pneumococcal infection; patients with a chronic disease which predisposes them to pneumococcal pneumonia (pulmonary, cardiovascular disease, diabetes, alcoholism, liver disease); patients with immunodeficiency due to drugs and/or disease; persons whose living environments place them at risk (nursing homes, hospitals, community epidemics)

Contraindications Hypersensitivity to pneumococcal vaccine or any component of the formulation. **Note:** Epinephrine injection (1:1000) must be immediately available in the case of anaphylaxis.

Warnings/Precautions Use caution in patients with severe cardiovascular or pulmonary disease where a systemic reaction may pose a significant risk. Use caution and consider delay of vaccination in any active infection. Use caution in individuals who have had episodes of pneumococcal infection within the preceding 3 years (pre-existing pneumococcal antibodies may result in increased reactions to vaccine); may cause relapse in patients with stable idiopathic thrombocytopenia purpura. Epinephrine injection (1:1000) must be immediately available in the case of anaphylaxis.

Patients who will be receiving immunosuppressive therapy (including Hodgkin's disease, cancer chemotherapy, or transplantation) should be vaccinated at least 2 weeks prior to the initiation of therapy. Immune responses may be impaired for several months following intensive immunosuppressive therapy (up to 2 years in Hodgkin's disease patients). Patients who undergo splenectomy should also be vaccinated 2 weeks prior to surgery, if possible. Patients with HIV should be vaccinated as soon as possible (following confirmation of the diagnosis).

Adverse Reactions (Reflective of adult population; not specific for elderly)
All serious adverse reactions must be reported to the U.S. Department of Health and Human Services (DHHS) Vaccine Adverse Event Reporting System (VAERS) 1-800-822-7967.

Frequency not defined.
Cardiovascular: Malaise
Central nervous system: Guillain-Barré syndrome, fever ≤102°F*, fever >102°F, headache, radiculoneuropathy
Dermatologic: Angioneurotic edema, cellulitis, rash, urticaria
Gastrointestinal: Nausea, vomiting
Hematologic: Hemolytic anemia (in patients with other hematologic disorders), thrombocytopenia (in patients with stabilized ITP)
Local: Injection site reaction* (erythema, induration, swelling, soreness, warmth)
Neuromuscular & skeletal: Arthralgia, arthritis, myalgia, paresthesia, weakness
Miscellaneous: Anaphylactoid reaction, lymphadenitis, serum sickness
*Reactions most commonly reported in clinical trials.

Drug Interactions Immunosuppressant medications: The effect of the vaccine may be decreased.
Vaccines: May be administered at the same time as influenza vaccine, by separate injection and injection site.

Stability Store under refrigeration at 2°C to 8°C (36°F to 46°F).

Mechanism of Action Although there are more than 80 known pneumococcal capsular types, pneumococcal disease is mainly caused by only a few types of pneumococci. Pneumococcal vaccine contains capsular polysaccharides of 23 pneumococcal types of *Streptococcal pneumoniae* which represent at least 85% to 90% of pneumococcal disease isolates in the United States. The pneumococcal vaccine with 23 pneumococcal capsular polysaccharide types became available in 1983. The 23 capsular pneumococcal vaccine contains purified capsular polysaccharides of pneumococcal types 1, 2, 3, 4, 5, 6B, 7F, 8, 9N, 9V, 10A, 11A, 12F, 14, 15B, 17F, 18C, 19F, 19A, 20, 22F, 23F, and 33F. These are the main pneumococcal types associated with serious infections in the United States.
(Continued)

Pneumococcal Polysaccharide Vaccine (Polyvalent)
(Continued)

Dosage

Geriatrics & Adults: Immunization: I.M., SubQ:

Adults: 0.5 mL

Previously vaccinated with PCV7 vaccine: Adults:

With sickle cell disease, asplenia, immunocompromised or HIV infection: 0.5 mL ≥2 months after last dose of PCV7; revaccination with PPV23 should be given ≥5 years

With chronic illness: 0.5 mL ≥2 months after last dose of PCV7; revaccination with PPV23 is not recommended

Following bone marrow transplant (use of PCV7 under study): Administer one dose PPV23 at 12- and 24-months following BMT

Revaccination should be considered:

1. If ≥6 years since initial vaccination has elapsed, or
2. In patients who received 14-valent pneumococcal vaccine and are at highest risk (asplenic) for fatal infection or
3. At ≥6 years in patients with nephrotic syndrome, renal failure, or transplant recipients

Administration Do not inject I.V., avoid intradermal, administer SubQ or I.M. (deltoid muscle or lateral midthigh)

For patients at risk of hemorrhage following intramuscular injection, the ACIP recommends "it should be administered intramuscularly if, in the opinion of the physician familiar with the patients bleeding risk, the vaccine can be administered with reasonable safety by this route. If the patient receives antihemophilia or other similar therapy, intramuscular vaccination can be scheduled shortly after such therapy is administered. A fine needle (23 gauge or smaller) can be used for the vaccination and firm pressure applied to the site (without rubbing) for at least 2 minutes. The patient should be instructed concerning the risk of hematoma from the injection."

Patient Information Be aware of adverse effects

Additional Information Inactivated bacteria vaccine. Federal law requires that the date of administration, the vaccine manufacturer, lot number of vaccine, and the administering person's name, title, and address be entered into the patient's permanent medical record.

Special Geriatric Considerations Elderly have ~3 times the incidence of pneumococcal pneumonia than younger adults and 30% of all pneumococcal meningitis occurs in persons >50 years of age with a 20% mortality. Limited data on the elderly; however, elderly, compared to young adults, develop slightly lower antibody titers; provides 60% to 70% protection for bacterial pneumonia. 90% protection for pneumococcal pneumonia strains; 20% of the elderly with pneumococcal pneumonia have an associated bacteremia with a 17% to 40% fatality. All persons ≥65 years of age should receive the pneumococcal vaccine including previously unvaccinated persons and persons who have not been vaccinated within 5 years. All persons of unknown vaccination status should receive once dose of vaccine.

Dosage Forms Excipient information presented when available (limited, particularly for generics); consult specific product labeling.

Injection, solution: 25 mcg each of 23 polysaccharide isolates/0.5 mL (0.5 mL, 2.5 mL)

Selected References

Advisory Committee on Immunization Practices, "Prevention of Pneumococcal Disease," *MMWR*, 1997, 46(RR-8):1-31.

Centers for Disease Control, "Recommendations of the Advisory Committee on Immunization Practices (ACIP): General Recommendations on Immunization," *MMWR*, 1994, 43(RR-1):23.

Davidson M, Bulkow LR, Grabman J, et al, "Immunogenicity of Pneumococcal Revaccination in Patients With Chronic Disease," *Arch Intern Med*, 1994, 154(19):2209-14.

Gardner P and Schaffner W, "Immunization of Adults," *N Engl J Med*, 1993, 328(17):1252-8.

U.S. Department of Health and Human Services, "Prevention of Pneumococcal Disease. Recommendations of the Advisory Committee on Immunization Practices (ACIP)," *MMWR*, 1997, 46(RR-8):1-24.

- ◆ **Pneumovax® 23** *see* Pneumococcal Polysaccharide Vaccine (Polyvalent) *on page 1279*
- ◆ **Podactin Cream [OTC]** *see* Miconazole *on page 1036*
- ◆ **Podactin Powder [OTC]** *see* Tolnaftate *on page 1596*

Poliovirus Vaccine (Inactivated)
(POE lee oh VYE rus vak SEEN, in ak ti VAY ted)

Related Information

Immunization Recommendations *on page 1787*

U.S. Brand Names IPOL®

Canadian Brand Names IPOL®

Index Terms Enhanced-potency Inactivated Poliovirus Vaccine; IPV; Salk Vaccine

Generic Available No

Pharmacologic Category Vaccine

Use Active immunization against poliomyelitis caused by poliovirus types 1, 2 and 3. Routine immunization of adults in the United States is generally not recommended. Adults with previous wild poliovirus disease, who have never been immunized, or those who are incompletely immunized may receive inactivated poliovirus vaccine if they fall into one of the following categories:

- Travelers to regions or countries where poliomyelitis is endemic or epidemic
- Healthcare workers in close contact with patients who may be excreting poliovirus
- Laboratory workers handling specimens that may contain poliovirus
- Members of communities or specific population groups with diseases caused by wild poliovirus
- Incompletely vaccinated or unvaccinated adults in a household or with other close contact with children receiving oral poliovirus (may be at increased risk of vaccine associated paralytic poliomyelitis)

Contraindications Hypersensitivity to any component including neomycin, strepto- mycin, or polymyxin B; defer vaccination for persons with acute febrile illness until recovery

Warnings/Precautions Patients with prior clinical poliomyelitis, incomplete immuniza- tion with oral poliovirus vaccine (OPV), HIV infection, severe combined immunodefi- ciency, hypogammaglobulinemia, agammaglobulinemia, or altered immunity (due to corticosteroids, alkylating agents, antimetabolites or radiation) may receive inactivated poliovirus vaccine (IPV). Immune response may be decreased in patients receiving immune globulin. Vaccination may be deferred with an acute febrile illness; minor illnesses with or without a low-grade fever are not reasons to postpone vaccination. Immediate treatment for anaphylactic/anaphylactoid reaction should be available during vaccine use.

The injection contains 2-phenoxyethanol, calf serum protein, formaldehyde, neomycin, streptomycin, and polymyxin B; the packaging contains natural latex rubber.

Adverse Reactions (Reflective of adult population; not specific for elderly)
All serious adverse reactions must be reported to the U.S. Department of Health and Human Services (DHHS) Vaccine Adverse Event Reporting System (VAERS) 1-800-822-7967.

1% to 10%:

Percentages noted with concomitant administration of DTP or DTaP vaccine and observed within 48 hours of injection.

>10%:

Central nervous system: Irritability (7% to 65%), tiredness (4% to 61%), fever ≥39°C (≤38%)

Gastrointestinal: Anorexia (1% to 17%)

Local: Injection Site: Tenderness (≤29%), pain (13%), swelling (≤11%)

1% to 10%:

Gastrointestinal: Vomiting (1% to 3%)

Local: Injection site: Erythema (≤3%), induration (1%)

Miscellaneous: Persistent crying (up to 1% reported within 72 hours)

Drug Interactions

Immunosuppressant medications: The effect of the vaccine may be decreased; consider deferring vaccination for 3 months after immunosuppressant therapy is discontinued.

Vaccines: May be administered with DTaP, Hib, HepB, varicella (chickenpox) vaccine, and measles-mumps-rubella vaccine.

Stability Store under refrigeration 2°C to 8°C (35°F to 46°F); do not freeze.

Dosage

Geriatrics & Adults: Immunization: I.M., SubQ:

Previously unvaccinated: Two 0.5 mL doses administered at 1- to 2-month intervals, followed by a third dose 6-12 months later. If <3 months, but at least 2 months are available before protection is needed, 3 doses may be administered at least 1 month apart. If administration must be completed within 1-2 months, give 2 doses at least 1 month apart. If <1 month is available, give 1 dose.

Incompletely vaccinated: Adults with at least 1 previous dose of OPV, <3 doses of IPV, or a combination of OPV and IPV equaling <3 doses, administer at least one 0.5 mL dose of IPV. Additional doses to complete the series may be given if time permits.

Completely vaccinated: One 0.5 mL dose

Administration Do not administer I.V.; for I.M. or SubQ administration. Administer in the deltoid area.

Reference Range >1:8 titer

Patient Information Be aware of adverse reactions

(Continued)

Poliovirus Vaccine (Inactivated) *(Continued)*

Additional Information Federal law requires that the date of administration, the vaccine manufacturer, lot number of vaccine, and the administering person's name, title, and address be entered into the patient's permanent medical record.

As the global eradication of poliomyelitis continues, the risk for importation of wild-type poliovirus into the United States decreases dramatically. To eliminate the risk for vaccine-associated paralytic poliomyelitis (VAPP), an all-IPV schedule is recommended for routine childhood vaccination in the United States. Oral poliovirus vaccine (OPV), is not commercially available in the United States, but has been stockpiled for use in the following special circumstances:

Mass vaccination campaigns to control outbreaks of paralytic polio

Unvaccinated children who will be traveling within 4 weeks to areas where polio is endemic or epidemic

Children of parents who do not accept the recommended number of vaccine injections; these children may receive OPV only for the third or fourth dose or both. In this situation, healthcare providers should administer OPV only after discussing the risk for VAPP with parents or caregivers.

Currently, the primary risk for paralytic polio in U.S. residents is through travel to countries where polio remains endemic or where polio outbreaks are occurring. Unvaccinated persons traveling to countries that use OPV should be aware of the risk caused by OPV and should consider polio vaccination prior to travel.

Special Geriatric Considerations For the elderly who cannot document a primary immunization series or at risk due to contact or travel, administer the initial series. Boosters may be necessary for travel since antibody titers may diminish with age.

Dosage Forms Excipient information presented when available (limited, particularly for generics); consult specific product labeling.

Injection, suspension:

IPOL®: Type 1 poliovirus 40 D antigen units, type 2 poliovirus 8 D antigen units, and type 3 poliovirus 32 D antigen units per 0.5 mL (0.5 mL, 5 mL) [contains 2-phenoxyethanol, formaldehyde, calf serum protein, neomycin, streptomycin, and polymyxin B; packaging contains natural latex rubber]

Selected References

Centers for Disease Control and Prevention, "Imported Vaccine-Associated Paralytic Poliomyelitis -- United States," *MMWR Recomm Rep*, 2005, 55(RR 4);97-9.

Centers for Disease Control and Prevention, "Poliomyelitis Prevention in the United States: Updated Recommendations of the Advisory Committee on Immunization Practices (ACIP)," *MMWR Recomm Rep*, 2000, 49(RR-5):14.

Centers for Disease Control, "Recommendations of the Advisory Committee on Immunization Practices (ACIP): General Recommendations on Immunization," *MMWR Recomm Rep*, 1994, 43(RR-1):23.

Gardner P and Schaffner W, "Immunization of Adults," *N Engl J Med*, 1993, 328(17):1252-8.

Polycarbophil (pol i KAR boe fil)

U.S. Brand Names Equalactin® [OTC]; FiberCon® [OTC]; Fiber-Lax® [OTC]; Fiber-Tabs™ [OTC]; Konsyl® Fiber Caplets [OTC]

Generic Available Yes

Pharmacologic Category Antidiarrheal; Laxative, Bulk-Producing

Use Treatment of constipation or acute nonspecific diarrhea (production of more normal moisture level, source of bulk in the patient's intestinal tract), constipation or diarrhea associated with irritable bowel syndrome and diverticulosis (approved substitute whenever a bulk-forming laxative is ordered in a tablet, capsule, wafer, or other oral solid dosage form)

Contraindications Hypersensitivity to any component; do not use if patient is experiencing nausea, vomiting, appendicitis, fecal impaction, acute surgical abdomen, intestinal obstruction, undiagnosed abdominal pain

Warnings/Precautions Use caution in patients who have difficulty swallowing; taking products without adequate fluid may cause it to swell and block throat or esophagus

Adverse Reactions (Reflective of adult population; not specific for elderly)
Frequency not defined: Gastrointestinal: Abdominal fullness

Drug Interactions Decreased absorption of oral anticoagulants, digoxin, potassium-sparing diuretics, salicylates, tetracycline, and ciprofloxacin

Mechanism of Action Restoring a more normal moisture level and providing bulk in the patient's intestinal tract

Pharmacodynamics

Onset of action: 12-24 hours; can be up to 72 hours

Site of action: Small and large intestines

Dosage

Geriatrics & Adults: Constipation or diarrhea: General dosing guidelines (OTC labeling): Oral: 1250 mg calcium polycarbophil 1-4 times/day

Administration Patient should drink adequate fluids (8 oz of water or other fluids) with each dose.

Monitoring Parameters Monitor for diarrhea, abdominal pain, bowel obstruction, or impaction

Patient Information Drink a full glass of liquid with each dose; must drink fluids throughout the day to be effective and avoid impaction; report bleeding or failure to respond to physician, pharmacist, or nurse; do not use for acute constipation

Additional Information Each calcium polycarbophil tablet contains ~100 mg of absorbable elemental calcium; chewable tablets are available

Special Geriatric Considerations Elderly may have insufficient fluid intake which may predispose them to fecal impaction and bowel obstruction. Bloating and flatulence may be a problem when used short-term. Use cautiously in patients with a history of bowel impaction/obstruction.

Dosage Forms Excipient information presented when available (limited, particularly for generics); consult specific product labeling.
Caplet: Calcium polycarbophil 625 mg [equivalent to polycarbophil 500 mg]
  FiberCon®: Calcium polycarbophil 625 mg [equivalent to polycarbophil 500 mg; contains calcium 122 mg/caplet]
  Konsyl® Fiber: Calcium polycarbophil 625 mg [equivalent to polycarbophil 500 mg; contains calcium 125 mg/caplet]
Captab:
  Fiber-Lax®: Calcium polycarbophil 625 mg [equivalent to polycarbophil 500 mg; contains calcium 170 mg/captab]
Tablet: Calcium polycarbophil 625 mg [equivalent to polycarbophil 500 mg]
  Fiber-Tabs™: Calcium polycarbophil 625 mg [equivalent to polycarbophil 500 mg]
Tablet, chewable:
  Equalactin®: Calcium polycarbophil 625 mg [equivalent to polycarbophil 500 mg; citrus flavor]

♦ **Polycitra®** see Citric Acid, Sodium Citrate, and Potassium Citrate on page 325
♦ **Polycitra®-LC** see Citric Acid, Sodium Citrate, and Potassium Citrate on page 325
♦ **Poly-Dex™** see Neomycin, Polymyxin B, and Dexamethasone on page 1102

Polyethylene Glycol 3350 (pol i ETH i leen GLY kol 3350)

Medication Safety Issues
Sound-alike/look-alike issues:
  MiraLax™ may be confused with Mirapex®

International issues:
  MiraLax™ may be confused with Murelax® which is a brand name for oxazepam in Australia

U.S. Brand Names GlycoLax®; MiraLax® [OTC]

Index Terms PEG

Generic Available Yes

Pharmacologic Category Laxative, Osmotic

Use Treatment of occasional constipation in adults

Contraindications Hypersensitivity to polyethylene glycol or any component of the formulation; gastrointestinal obstruction

Warnings/Precautions Evaluate patients with symptoms of bowel obstruction (nausea, vomiting, abdominal pain or distension) prior to use. Do not use for longer than 2 weeks; 2-4 days may be required to produce bowel movement. Not intended for use as a bowel evacuant prior to GI examination.

Adverse Reactions (Reflective of adult population; not specific for elderly)
Frequency not defined.
Dermatologic: Urticaria
Gastrointestinal: Abdominal bloating, cramping, diarrhea, flatulence, nausea

Stability Store at room temperature of 15°C to 30°C (59°F to 86°F) before reconstitution. Dissolve powder in 8 ounces of water, juice, cola, or tea.

Mechanism of Action An osmotic agent, polyethylene glycol 3350 causes water retention in the stool; increases stool frequency and consistency

Pharmacodynamics Onset of action: Oral: 48-96 hours

Dosage
Geriatrics & Adults: Occasional constipation: Oral: 17 g of powder (~1 heaping tablespoon) dissolved in 8 oz of water, once daily; do not use for >2 weeks.

Special Geriatric Considerations Elderly are more likely to show CNS signs of dehydration and electrolyte loss than younger adults. Therefore, monitor closely for fluid and electrolyte loss with chronic use.

Dosage Forms Excipient information presented when available (limited, particularly for generics); consult specific product labeling. [DSC] = Discontinued product
Powder, for oral solution: PEG 3350 17 g/packet (12s); PEG 3350 255 g (14 oz); PEG 3350 527 g (26 oz)
(Continued)

Polyethylene Glycol 3350 *(Continued)*

GlycoLax®: PEG 3350 17 g/packet (14s); PEG 3350 255 g (16 oz); PEG 3350 527 g (24 oz)

MiraLax®: PEG 3350 17 g/packet (12s) [DSC]; PEG 3350 255 g (14 oz); PEG 3350 527 g (26 oz) [DSC]

Polyethylene Glycol-Electrolyte Solution and Bisacodyl

(pol i ETH i leen GLY kol ee LEK troe lite soe LOO shun & bis a KOE dil)

U.S. Brand Names HalfLytely® and Bisacodyl

Index Terms Electrolyte Lavage Solution

Generic Available No

Pharmacologic Category Laxative, Bowel Evacuant; Laxative, Stimulant

Use Bowel cleansing prior to GI examination

Contraindications Hypersensitivity to bisacodyl, polyethylene glycol or any component of the formulation; ileus, gastrointestinal obstruction, gastric retention, bowel perforation, toxic colitis, or toxic megacolon

Warnings/Precautions Do not add flavorings or additional ingredients to the polyethylene glycol-electrolyte solution. Use with caution in patients with severe ulcerative colitis. Observe unconscious or semiconscious patients with impaired gag reflex or those who are prone to regurgitation or aspiration during administration. Closely monitor patients with impaired water handling who develop nausea and vomiting.

Adverse Reactions (Reflective of adult population; not specific for elderly)
>10%: Gastrointestinal: Fullness (22%), nausea (17%),
1% to 10%: Gastrointestinal: Cramping (9%), vomiting (6%)

Overdosage/Toxicology Treatment is symptom-directed and supportive.

Drug Interactions

Antacids: Prevent absorption of bisacodyl; avoid bisacodyl within 1 hour of taking an antacid.

Oral medications: Polyethylene glycol-electrolyte solution may decrease absorption of other medications because of decreased transit time through the GI tract; other medications should not be administered within 1 hour of start of therapy and for the duration of therapy.

Ethanol/Nutrition/Herb Interactions Food: Take clear liquid diet during bowel preparation.

Stability Polyethylene glycol-electrolyte solution: Store at 15°C to 30°C (59°F to 86°F). Fill the container with water to the fill mark. Shake well. When reconstituted, may refrigerate. Use within 48 hours.

Mechanism of Action Bisacodyl acts on the colonic mucosa to increase peristalsis throughout the large intestine. Polyethylene glycol-electrolyte solution induces catharsis through strong electrolyte and osmotic effects.

Pharmacokinetics See individual agents.

Dosage

Geriatrics & Adults: Bowel cleansing: Oral:

Bisacodyl: 4 tablets as a single dose. After bowel movement or 6 hours (whichever occurs first), initiate polyethylene glycol-electrolyte solution

Polyethylene glycol-electrolyte solution: 8 ounces every 10 minutes until 2 L are consumed

Administration Do not chew or crush bisacodyl tablets. Rapidly drinking the polyethylene glycol-electrolyte solution is preferred to drinking small amount continuously.

Monitoring Parameters Bowel movements

Special Geriatric Considerations Studies of this combination preparation drug included 28% of patients >65 years of age with 9.1% being >75 years. No differences in safety or efficacy were observed. No adjustments in dose are necessary.

Dosage Forms Excipient information presented when available (limited, particularly for generics); consult specific product labeling.

Kit (HalfLytely® and Bisacodyl) [each kit contains]:

Powder for oral solution (HalfLytely®): PEG 3350 210 g, sodium bicarbonate 2.86 g, sodium chloride 5.6 g, potassium chloride 0.74 g (2000 mL) [sulfate-free, regular, cherry, lemon-lime, orange flavor]

Tablet, delayed release (Bisacodyl): 5 mg (4s)

Selected References

DiPalma JA, Wolff BG, Meagher A, et al, "Comparison of Reduced Volume Versus Four Liters Sulfate-Free Electrolyte Lavage Solutions for Colonoscopy Colon Cleansing," *Am J Gastroenterol*, 2003, 98(10):2187-91.

♦ **Polymyxin B and Neomycin** *see* Neomycin and Polymyxin B *on page 1101*

♦ **Polymyxin B, Neomycin, and Dexamethasone** *see* Neomycin, Polymyxin B, and Dexamethasone *on page 1102*

♦ **Polymyxin B, Neomycin, and Gramicidin** *see* Neomycin, Polymyxin B, and Gramicidin *on page 1103*

♦ **Polyvinyl Alcohol** *see* Artificial Tears *on page 124*
♦ **Ponstel®** *see* Mefenamic Acid *on page 967*

Posaconazole (poe sa KON a zole)

Medication Safety Issues
Sound-alike/look-alike issues:
Noxafil® may be confused with minoxidil

International issues:
Noxafil® may be confused with Noxidil® which is a brand name for minoxidil in Thailand

U.S. Brand Names Noxafil®
Index Terms SCH 56592
Generic Available No
Pharmacologic Category Antifungal Agent, Oral
Use Prophylaxis of invasive *Aspergillus* and *Candida* infections in severely-immunocompromised patients [eg, hematopoietic stem cell transplant (HSCT) recipients with graft-versus-host disease (GVHD) or those with prolonged neutropenia secondary to chemotherapy for hematologic malignancies]; treatment of oropharyngeal candidiasis (including patients refractory to itraconazole and/or fluconazole)
Unlabeled/Investigational Use Salvage therapy of refractory invasive fungal infections
Contraindications Hypersensitivity to posaconazole or any component of the formulation; coadministration of cisapride, pimozide, quinidine, or ergot alkaloids
Warnings/Precautions Use caution in hepatic impairment; hepatic dysfunction has occurred, ranging from mild/moderate increases of ALT/AST, alkaline phosphatase, and/or clinical hepatitis to severe reactions (cholestasis, hepatic failure including death). Use caution in patients with an increased risk of arrhythmia (concurrent QT_c-prolonging drugs, hypokalemia). Correct electrolyte abnormalities (eg, potassium, magnesium, and calcium) before initiating therapy.

Use caution in hypersensitivity with other azole antifungal agents; cross-reaction may occur, but has not been established. Alternative antifungal therapy should be considered in any patient unable to eat or tolerate an oral liquid nutritional supplement. Use caution in severe renal impairment; monitor for breakthrough fungal infections.

Adverse Reactions (Reflective of adult population; not specific for elderly)
Note: A higher frequency of adverse reactions was observed in studies with refractory oropharyngeal candidiasis patients and percentages are included below.
>10%: Gastrointestinal: Diarrhea (3% to 11%)
1% to 10%:
Cardiovascular: QT_c prolongation (up to 4%), hypertension (1%)
Central nervous system: Headache (1% to 8%), dizziness (1% to 3%), fatigue (1% to 3%), insomnia (1% to 3%), fever (up to 3%), somnolence (1%)
Dermatologic: Rash (1% to 4%), pruritus (1% to 2%)
Endocrine & metabolic: Hypokalemia (3%)
Gastrointestinal: Nausea (5% to 8%), vomiting (4% to 7%), abdominal pain (1% to 5%), flatulence (1% to 5%), anorexia (1% to 3%), mucositis (2%), dyspepsia (1% to 2%), xerostoma (1% to 2%), taste perversion (1%), constipation (up to 1%)
Hematologic: Neutropenia (2% to 8%), anemia (up to 3%), thrombocytopenia (up to 2%)
Hepatic: Bilirubin increased (2% to 3%), ALT increased (2% to 3%), AST increased (2% to 3%), GGT increased (2% to 3%), alkaline phosphatase increased (2%), hepatocellular damage (1%)
Neuromuscular & skeletal: Weakness (1% to 3%), myalgia (up to 2%), tremor (1%)
Ocular: Blurred vision (1%)
Renal: Serum creatinine increased (2%)
Overdosage/Toxicology Experience with overdosage is limited; treatment is symptom-directed and supportive. Posaconazole is not removed by hemodialysis.
Drug Interactions Inhibits CYP3A4 (moderate)
Calcium channel blockers: Posaconazole may increase the levels/effects of calcium channel blockers (applies to those agents metabolized by CYP3A4, including felodipine, nifedipine, and verapamil).
Cimetidine: May decrease the levels/effects of posaconazole. If needed, monitor for breakthrough fungal infections.
Cyclosporine: Posaconazole may increase the levels/effects of cyclosporine. Reduce cyclosporine dose to approximately 75% of original dose and monitor. Readjust dose when posaconazole is discontinued.
CYP3A4 substrates: Posaconazole may increase the levels/effects of CYP3A4 substrates. Examples substrates include benzodiazepines, calcium channel blockers, cyclosporine, mirtazapine, nateglinide, nefazodone, sildenafil (and other (Continued)

Posaconazole (Continued)

PDE-5 inhibitors), tacrolimus, and venlafaxine. Selected benzodiazepines (midazolam and triazolam), cisapride, ergot alkaloids, selected HMG-CoA reductase inhibitors (lovastatin and simvastatin), and pimozide are generally contraindicated with strong CYP3A4 inhibitors.

Ergot alkaloids: Posaconazole may increase the levels/effects of ergot alkaloids, leading to ergotism; concurrent use is contraindicated.

Glipizide: Posaconazole may increase level/effect of glipizide; monitor glucose concentrations.

HMG-CoA reductase inhibitors: Posaconazole may increase the levels/effects of HMG-CoA reductase inhibitors; consider reducing HMG-CoA dose.

Midazolam: Posaconazole may increase the levels/effects of midazolam. Monitor for midazolam adverse effects and/or consider reducing midazolam dose.

Phenytoin: Posaconazole may increase the levels/effects of phenytoin. Monitor phenytoin concentrations and/or consider reducing phenytoin dose. Phenytoin may decrease the levels/effects of posaconazole. Avoid concurrent use; if given, monitor for breakthrough fungal infections.

QT_c"prolonging agents: Risk of arrhythmia (torsade de pointes) may be increased. Posaconazole use with cisapride, pimozide or quinidine is contraindicated.

Rifabutin: Posaconazole may increase the levels/effects of rifabutin. If coadministered, monitor for rifabutin adverse effects (eg, uveitis, leukopenia). Rifabutin may decrease the levels/effects of posaconazole. Avoid concurrent use; if given, monitor for breakthrough fungal infections.

Sirolimus: Posaconazole may increase the levels/effects of sirolimus. Monitor sirolimus concentrations and reduce dose accordingly.

Tacrolimus: Posaconazole may increase the levels/effects of tacrolimus. Reduce tacrolimus dose to approximately $1/3$ of original dose and monitor. Readjust dose when posaconazole is discontinued.

Vinca alkaloids: Posaconazole may increase the levels/effects of vinca alkaloids (eg, vincristine, vinblastine), leading to neurotoxicity; consider reducing vinca alkaloid dose.

Ethanol/Nutrition/Herb Interactions Food: Bioavailability increased ~3-4 times when posaconazole administered with a meal or an oral liquid nutritional supplement.

Stability Store at 15°C to 30°C (59°F to 86°F); do not freeze.

Mechanism of Action Interferes with fungal cytochrome P450 activity, decreasing ergosterol synthesis (principal sterol in fungal cell membrane) and inhibiting fungal cell membrane formation.

Pharmacokinetics

Absorption: Food and/or liquid nutritional supplements increase absorption; fasting states do not provide sufficient absorption to ensure adequate plasma concentrations

Distribution: V_d: 465-1774 L

Protein binding: ≥97%; predominantly bound to albumin

Metabolism: Not significantly metabolized; ~15% to 17% undergoes non-CYP-mediated metabolism, primarily via hepatic glucuronidation into metabolites

Half-life elimination: 35 hours (range: 20-66 hours)

Time to peak, plasma: 3-5 hours

Excretion: Feces 71% to 77% (~66% as unchanged drug); urine 13% to 14% (<0.2% as unchanged drug)

Dosage

Geriatrics & Adults:

Aspergillus and *Candida* prophylaxis in high-risk immunocompromised patients: Oral: 200 mg 3 times/day

Treatment of oropharyngeal candidiasis: Oral: Initial: 100 mg twice daily for 1 day; maintenance: 100 mg once daily for 13 days

Treatment of refractory oropharyngeal candidiasis: Oral: 400 mg twice daily

Treatment of refractory invasive fungal infections (unlabeled use): Oral: 800 mg/day in divided doses

Renal Impairment: No adjustment necessary; use caution in severe renal impairment and monitor for breakthrough fungal infections. Variability in posaconazole exposure observed with Cl_{cr}<20 mL/minute.

Hepatic Impairment: No adjustment necessary; use with caution.

Administration Must be administered with a full meal or an oral liquid nutritional supplement.

Monitoring Parameters Hepatic function (eg, SGOT, SGPT, alkaline phosphatase and bilirubin) prior to initiation and during treatment; renal function; electrolyte disturbances (eg, calcium, magnesium, potassium)

Patient Information It is important to inform prescriber of any other prescription or herbal products you are taking. Do not take any new medication during therapy without consulting prescriber. Must be taken with a full meal or an oral liquid nutritional supplement. Take full course of medication as directed; some infections may require long periods of therapy. May cause nausea and vomiting (small, frequent meals, frequent mouth care, sucking lozenges, or chewing gum may help); headache (mild analgesic may be necessary); or dizziness (use caution when driving). Report chest pain or palpitations; unresolved headache; rash or itching; yellowing of eyes or skin or changes in color of urine or stool; unusual muscle or skeletal weakness or tremor, or changes in vision.

Special Geriatric Considerations Dosage adjustment not necessary.

Dosage Forms Excipient information presented when available (limited, particularly for generics); consult specific product labeling.

Suspension, oral:

Noxafil®: 40 mg/mL (123 mL) [contains sodium benzoate; delivers 105 mL of suspension; cherry flavor; packaged with calibrated dosing spoon]

Selected References

Herbrecht R, "Posaconazole: A Potent, Extended-Spectrum Triazole Anti-Fungal for the Treatment of Serious Fungal Infections," *Int J Clin Pract*, 2004, 58(6): 612-24.

Keating G, "Posaconazole," *Drugs*, 2005, 65(11):1553-67.

Krieter P, Flannery B, Musick T, et al, "Disposition of Posaconazole Following Single-Dose Oral Administration in Healthy Subjects," *Antimicrob Agents Chemother*, 2004, 48(9):3543-51.

Raad II, Graybill JR, Bustamante AB, "Safety of Long-Term Oral Posaconazole Use in the Treatment of Refractory Invasive Fungal Infections," *Clin Infect Dis*, 2006, 42(12):1726-34.

♦ **Post Peel Healing Balm [OTC]** *see* Hydrocortisone *on page 762*

♦ **Posture® [OTC]** *see* Calcium Salts (Oral) *on page 220*

Potassium Acid Phosphate (poe TASS ee um AS id FOS fate)

U.S. Brand Names K-Phos® Original

Generic Available No

Pharmacologic Category Urinary Acidifying Agent

Use Acidification of urine and reduction of urinary calcium concentration; reduction of odor and rash caused by ammoniacal urine; increased antibacterial activity of methenamine

Contraindications Severe renal impairment; hyperkalemia, hyperphosphatemia; infected magnesium ammonium phosphate stones

Warnings/Precautions Use with caution in patients receiving other potassium supplementation and in patients with renal insufficiency, or severe tissue breakdown (eg, chemotherapy or hemodialysis)

Adverse Reactions (Reflective of adult population; not specific for elderly)

>10%: Gastrointestinal: Diarrhea, nausea, stomach pain, flatulence, vomiting

1% to 10%:

Cardiovascular: Bradycardia

Endocrine & metabolic: Hyperkalemia

Local: Local tissue necrosis with extravasation

Neuromuscular & skeletal: Weakness

Respiratory: Dyspnea

Overdosage/Toxicology Symptoms include muscle weakness, paralysis, peaked T waves, flattened P waves, prolongation of QRS complex, and ventricular arrhythmias. Removal of potassium can be accomplished by various means such as through the GI tract with Kayexalate® administration, by way of the kidney through diuresis, mineralocorticoid administration or increased sodium intake, by hemodialysis or peritoneal dialysis, or by shifting potassium back into the cells by insulin and glucose infusion or sodium bicarbonate. Calcium chloride will reverse cardiac effects.

Drug Interactions

Increased effect/levels with potassium-sparing diuretics, salt substitutes, salicylates, ACE inhibitors

Decreased effect with antacids containing magnesium, calcium or aluminum (bind phosphate and decreased its absorption)

Mechanism of Action The principal intracellular cation; involved in transmission of nerve impulses, muscle contractions, enzyme activity, and glucose utilization

Pharmacokinetics

Absorption: Absorbed well from upper GI tract

Distribution: Enters cells via active transport from extracellular fluid

Elimination: Largely by the kidneys, but also small amount via the skin and feces, with most intestinal potassium being reabsorbed

Dosage

Geriatrics & Adults: Urine acidification: Oral: 1000 mg dissolved in 6-8 oz of water 4 times/day with meals and at bedtime; for best results, soak tablets in water for 2-5 minutes, then stir and swallow

Monitoring Parameters Serum potassium, sodium, phosphate, calcium; serum salicylates (if taking salicylates); signs of muscle weakness, cramps

(Continued)

Potassium Acid Phosphate *(Continued)*

Test Interactions Decreased ammonia (B)

Patient Information Dissolve tablets completely before drinking; avoid taking magnesium, calcium, or aluminum antacids at the same time; patients may pass old kidney stones when starting therapy; notify physician if experiencing nausea, vomiting, or abdominal pain, muscle weakness, or cramps

Special Geriatric Considerations A complete drug history should be taken to rule out potential drug interactions since the elderly frequently may be taking potassium and potassium-sparing diuretics, salicylates, or antacids. Use with caution in renal impairment (low Cl$_{cr}$).

Dosage Forms Excipient information presented when available (limited, particularly for generics); consult specific product labeling.

Tablet [scored]: 500 mg [phosphorus 114 mg and potassium 144 mg (3.7 mEq) per tablet; sodium free]

Potassium Chloride (poe TASS ee um KLOR ide)

Medication Safety Issues

Sound-alike/look-alike issues:

Kaon-Cl-10® may be confused with kaolin

KCl may be confused with HCl

K-Dur® may be confused with Cardura®, Imdur®

K-Lor® may be confused with Kaochlor®, Klor-Con®

Klor-Con® may be confused with Klaron®, K-Lor®

Klotrix® may be confused with liotrix

microK® may be confused with Micronase®

High alert medication: The Institute for Safe Medication Practices (ISMP) includes this medication (I.V. formulation) among its list of drugs which have a heightened risk of causing significant patient harm when used in error.

Per JCAHO recommendations, concentrated electrolyte solutions should not be available in patient care areas.

Consider special storage requirements for intravenous potassium salts; I.V. potassium salts have been administered IVP in error, leading to fatal outcomes.

U.S. Brand Names Kaon-Cl-10®; Kaon-Cl® 20; Kay Ciel®; K-Dur® 10; K-Dur® 20; K-Lor®; Klor-Con®; Klor-Con® 8; Klor-Con® 10; Klor-Con®/25; Klor-Con® M; K+ Potassium; K-Tab®; microK®; microK® 10; Rum-K®

Canadian Brand Names Apo-K®; K-10®; K-Dur®; K-Lor®; K-Lyte®/Cl; Micro-K Extencaps®; Roychlor®; Slo-Pot®; Slow-K®

Index Terms KCl

Generic Available Yes

Pharmacologic Category Electrolyte Supplement, Oral; Electrolyte Supplement, Parenteral

Use Treatment or prevention of hypokalemia

Contraindications Severe renal impairment, untreated Addison's disease, heat cramps, hyperkalemia, severe tissue trauma; solid oral dosage forms are contraindicated in patients in whom there is a structural, pathological, and/or pharmacologic cause for delay or arrest in passage through the GI tract; an oral liquid potassium preparation should be used in patients with esophageal compression or delayed gastric emptying time

Warnings/Precautions Use with caution in patients with cardiac disease, severe renal impairment, hyperkalemia

Adverse Reactions (Reflective of adult population; not specific for elderly)

>10%: Gastrointestinal: Diarrhea, nausea, stomach pain, flatulence, vomiting (oral)

1% to 10%:

Cardiovascular: Bradycardia

Endocrine & metabolic: Hyperkalemia

Local: Local tissue necrosis with extravasation, pain at the site of injection

Neuromuscular & skeletal: Weakness

Respiratory: Dyspnea

Overdosage/Toxicology Symptoms include muscle weakness, paralysis, peaked T waves, flattened P waves, prolongation of QRS complex, and ventricular arrhythmias. Removal of potassium can be accomplished by various means such as through the GI tract with Kayexalate® administration, by way of the kidney through diuresis, mineralocorticoid administration or increased sodium intake, by hemodialysis or peritoneal dialysis, or by shifting potassium back into the cells by insulin and glucose infusion or sodium bicarbonate. Calcium chloride reverses cardiac effects.

Drug Interactions Increased effect/levels with potassium-sparing diuretics, salt substitutes, ACE inhibitors

Stability Store at room temperature; do not freeze. Use only clear solutions. Use admixtures within 24 hours.

Mechanism of Action Potassium is the major cation of intracellular fluid and is essential for the conduction of nerve impulses in heart, brain, and skeletal muscle; contraction of cardiac, skeletal and smooth muscles; maintenance of normal renal function, acid-base balance, carbohydrate metabolism, and gastric secretion

Pharmacokinetics

Absorption: Well from upper GI tract; enters cells via active transport from extracellular fluid

Elimination: Largely by the kidneys, but also small amount via skin and feces, with most intestinal potassium being reabsorbed

Dosage

Geriatrics & Adults: I.V. doses should be incorporated into the patient's maintenance I.V. fluids; intermittent I.V. potassium administration should be reserved for severe depletion situations in patients undergoing ECG monitoring.

Normal daily requirements: Oral, I.V.: 40-80 mEq/day

Prevention of hypokalemia during diuretic therapy: Oral: 20-40 mEq/day in 1-2 divided doses

Treatment of hypokalemia (guidelines):

Potassium >2.5 mEq/L:

Oral: 60-80 mEq/day plus additional amounts if needed

I.V.: 10 mEq over 1 hour with additional doses if needed

Potassium <2.5 mEq/L:

Oral: Up to 40-60 mEq initial dose, followed by further doses based on lab values

I.V.: Up to 40 mEq over 1 hour, with doses based on frequent lab monitoring; deficits at a plasma level of 2 mEq/L may be as high as 400-800 mEq of potassium

Acute hypokalemia:

I.V. intermittent infusion: 5-10 mEq/hour (continuous cardiac monitor recommended for rates >5 mEq/hour), not to exceed 40 mEq/hour; usual adult maximum per 24 hours: 400 mEq/day.

Potassium dosage/rate of infusion guidelines:

Serum potassium >2.5 mEq/L: Maximum infusion rate: 10 mEq/hour; maximum concentration: 40 mEq/L; maximum 24-hour dose: 200 mEq

Serum potassium <2.5 mEq/L: Maximum infusion rate: 40 mEq/hour; maximum concentration: 80 mEq/L; maximum 24-hour dose: 400 mEq

Administration Potassium must be diluted prior to parenteral administration; maximum recommended concentration (peripheral line): 80 mEq/L; maximum recommended concentration (central line): 150 mEq/L or 15 mEq/100 mL; in severely fluid-restricted patients (with central lines): 200 mEq/L or 20 mEq/100 mL has been used; maximum rate of infusion, see Dosage, I.V. intermittent infusion

Monitoring Parameters Serum potassium, blood pressure, pulse, EKG (as needed), signs of muscle weakness, cramps

Reference Range 3.5-5.0 mEq/L (3.5-5.0 mmol/L)

Patient Information Long acting and wax matrix tablets should be swallowed whole, do not crush or chew; powder must be dissolved in water before use; take with food; liquid can be diluted or dissolved in water or juice.

Special Geriatric Considerations Elderly may require less potassium than younger adults due to decreased renal function. For the elderly who do not respond to replacement therapy, check serum magnesium. Long-term use of diuretics may result in hypomagnesemic.

Dosage Forms Excipient information presented when available (limited, particularly for generics); consult specific product labeling. [DSC] = Discontinued product

Capsule, extended release: 10 mEq [750 mg]

microK® [microencapsulated]: 8 mEq [600 mg]

microK® 10 [microencapsulated]: 10 mEq [750 mg]

Infusion [premixed in D₅W]: 20 mEq (1000 mL); 30 mEq (1000 mL); 40 mEq (1000 mL)

Infusion [premixed in D₅W and LR]: 20 mEq (1000 mL); 30 mEq (1000 mL); 40 mEq (1000 mL)

Infusion [premixed in D₅W and ¼NS]: 10 mEq (500 mL, 1000 mL); 20 mEq (250 mL, 500 mL, 1000 mL); 30 mEq (1000 mL); 40 mEq (1000 mL)

Infusion [premixed in D₅W and ½NS]: 10 mEq (500 mL, 1000 mL); 20 mEq (500 mL, 1000 mL); 30 mEq (1000 mL); 40 mEq (1000 mL)

Infusion [premixed in D₅ and NS]: 20 mEq (1000 mL); 40 mEq (1000 mL)

Infusion [premixed in D₅W and sodium chloride 0.3%]: 10 mEq (500 mL); 20 mEq (1000 mL); 30 mEq (1000 mL); 40 mEq (1000 mL)

Infusion [premixed in D₁₀W and sodium chloride 0.2%]: 20 mEq (250 mL)

Infusion [premixed in NS]: 20 mEq (1000 mL); 40 mEq (1000 mL)

Infusion [premixed in SWFI; concentrate]: 10 mEq (50 mL, 100 mL); 20 mEq (50 mL, 100 mL); 30 mEq (100 mL); 40 mEq (100 mL)

Injection, solution [concentrate]: 2 mEq/mL (5 mL, 10 mL, 15 mL, 20 mL, 30 mL, 250 mL, 500 mL)

(Continued)

Potassium Chloride *(Continued)*

Powder, for oral solution: 20 mEq/packet (30s, 100s, 1000s)
   K-Lor™: 20 mEq/packet (30s, 100s) [fruit flavor]
   K+ Potassium: 20 mEq/packet (30s) [orange flavor]
   Kay Ciel® 10%: 20 mEq/packet (30s, 100s) [sugar free]
   Klor-Con®: 20 mEq/packet (30s, 100s) [sugar free; fruit flavor]
   Klor-Con®/25: 25 mEq/packet (30s, 100s) [sugar free; fruit flavor]
Solution, oral: 20 mEq/15 mL (480 mL, 3840 mL); 40 mEq/15 mL (480 mL)
   Kaon-Cl® 20: 40 mEq/15 mL (480 mL) [sugar free; contains alcohol; cherry flavor]
   Kay Ciel® 10%: 20 mEq/15 mL (480 mL) [sugar free; contains alcohol] [DSC]
   Rum-K®: 20 mEq/10 mL (480 mL) [alcohol free, sugar free; butter/rum flavor]
Tablet, extended release: 8 mEq [600 mg]; 10 mEq [750 mg]; 20 mEq [1500 mg]
   K-Dur® 10 [microencapsulated]: 10 mEq [750 mg]
   K-Dur® 20 [microencapsulated]: 20 mEq [1500 mg; scored]
   K-Tab®: 10 mEq [750 mg]
   Kaon-Cl® 10: 10 mEq [750 mg]
   Klor-Con® 8: 8 mEq [600 mg; wax matrix]
   Klor-Con® 10: 10 mEq [750 mg; wax matrix]
   Klor-Con® M10 [microencapsulated]: 10 mEq [750 mg]
   Klor-Con® M15 [microencapsulated]: 15 mEq [1125 mg; scored]
   Klor-Con® M20 [microencapsulated]: 20 mEq [1500 mg; scored]

♦ **Potassium Citrate, Citric Acid, and Sodium Citrate** *see* Citric Acid, Sodium Citrate, and Potassium Citrate *on page 325*

Potassium Gluconate *(poe TASS ee um GLOO coe nate)*

Generic Available Yes

Pharmacologic Category Electrolyte Supplement, Oral

Use Treatment of potassium deficiency (hypokalemia) or prevention of hypokalemia

Contraindications Severe renal impairment, untreated Addison's disease, heat cramps, hyperkalemia, severe tissue trauma; solid oral dosage forms are contraindicated in patients in whom there is a structural, pathological, and/or pharmacologic cause for delay or arrest in passage through the GI tract

Warnings/Precautions Use with caution in patients with cardiac disease, severe renal impairment, hyperkalemia; patients must be on a cardiac monitor during intermittent infusions

Adverse Reactions (Reflective of adult population; not specific for elderly)
>10%: Gastrointestinal: Diarrhea, nausea, stomach pain, flatulence, vomiting (oral)
1% to 10%:
   Cardiovascular: Bradycardia
   Endocrine & metabolic: Hyperkalemia
   Neuromuscular & skeletal: Weakness
   Respiratory: Dyspnea

Overdosage/Toxicology Symptoms of hyperkalemia include muscle weakness, paralysis, peaked T waves, flattened P waves, prolongation of QRS complex, and ventricular arrhythmias. Removal of potassium can be accomplished by various means such as through the GI tract with Kayexalate® administration, by way of the kidney through diuresis, mineralocorticoid administration or increased sodium intake, by hemodialysis or peritoneal dialysis, or by shifting potassium back into the cells by insulin, glucose infusion, or sodium bicarbonate. Calcium chloride reverses cardiac effects.

Drug Interactions Increased effect/levels with potassium-sparing diuretics, salt substitutes, ACE inhibitors; increased effect of digitalis

Stability Store at room temperature.

Mechanism of Action Potassium is the major cation of intracellular fluid and is essential for the conduction of nerve impulses in heart, brain, and skeletal muscle; contraction of cardiac, skeletal and smooth muscles; maintenance of normal renal function, acid-base balance, carbohydrate metabolism, and gastric secretion

Pharmacokinetics
   Absorption: Well from upper GI tract
   Distribution: Enters cells via active transport from extracellular fluid
   Elimination: Largely by the kidneys, but also small amount via skin and feces, with most intestinal potassium being reabsorbed

Dosage
   Geriatrics & Adults: Note: Doses listed as mEq of potassium:
      Normal daily requirement: Oral: 40-80 mEq/day
      Prevention of hypokalemia during diuretic therapy: Oral: 16-24 mEq/day in 1-2 divided doses
      Treatment of hypokalemia: Oral: 40-100 mEq/day in 2-4 divided doses

Monitoring Parameters Serum potassium, blood pressure, pulse, EKG (as needed), signs of muscle weakness, cramps; serum magnesium for failure to respond to replacement

Reference Range 3.5-5 mEq/L (3.5-5 mmol/L)

Test Interactions Decreased ammonia (B)

Patient Information Take with food, water, or fruit juice; swallow tablets whole; do not crush or chew

Additional Information 9.4 g potassium gluconate is approximately equal to 40 mEq potassium (4.3 mEq potassium/g salt)

Special Geriatric Considerations Elderly may require less potassium than younger adults due to decreased renal function. For the elderly who do not respond to replacement therapy, check serum magnesium. Long-term use of diuretics may result in hypomagnesemia.

Dosage Forms Excipient information presented when available (limited, particularly for generics); consult specific product labeling.

Caplet: 595 mg [equivalent to potassium 99 mg]

Capsule: 99 mg [strength expressed as base]

Tablet: 99 mg [strength expressed as base]; 550 mg [equivalent to potassium 90 mg]; 595 mg [equivalent to potassium 99 mg]

Tablet, timed release: 95 mg [strength expressed as base]

Potassium Iodide and Iodine (poe TASS ee um EYE oh dide & EYE oh dine)

Medication Safety Issues

Sound-alike/look-alike issues:

Potassium iodide and iodine (Strong Iodide Solution or Lugol's solution) may be confused with potassium iodide products, including saturated solution of potassium iodide (SSKI®)

Index Terms Lugol's Solution; Strong Iodine Solution

Generic Available Yes

Pharmacologic Category Antithyroid Agent

Use Reduce thyroid vascularity prior to thyroidectomy and management of thyrotoxic crisis; block thyroidal uptake of radioactive isotopes of iodine in a radiation emergency or other exposure to radioactive iodine

Dosage

Geriatrics & Adults: RDA, Adults: 150 mcg (iodine)

Preoperative thyroidectomy: Oral: 0.1-0.3 mL (3-5 drops) of strong iodine (Lugol's solution) 3 times/day; administer for 10 days before surgery

Thyrotoxic crisis: Oral: 1 mL strong iodine (Lugol's solution) 3 times/day

Special Geriatric Considerations

Elderly may have reduced renal function and require close monitoring of serum potassium. May be also recommended to check serum magnesium.

Dosage Forms Excipient information presented when available (limited, particularly for generics); consult specific product labeling.

Solution, oral (Lugol's solution, strong iodine): Potassium iodide 100 mg/mL and iodine 50 mg/mL (15 mL, 480 mL)

Potassium Phosphate (poe TASS ee um FOS fate)

Medication Safety Issues

Sound-alike/look-alike issues:

Neutra-Phos®-K may be confused with K-Phos Neutral®

High alert medication: The Institute for Safe Medication Practices (ISMP) includes this medication (I.V. formulation) among its list of drugs which have a heightened risk of causing significant patient harm when used in error.

Per JCAHO recommendations, concentrated electrolyte solutions should not be available in patient care areas.

Consider special storage requirements for intravenous potassium salts; I.V. potassium salts have been administered IVP in error, leading to fatal outcomes.

U.S. Brand Names Neutra-Phos®-K [OTC]

Index Terms Phosphate, Potassium

Generic Available Yes: Injection

Pharmacologic Category Electrolyte Supplement, Oral; Electrolyte Supplement, Parenteral

Use Source of potassium and phosphorus in parenteral nutrition and large volume I.V. fluids; treatment of conditions associated with excessive renal phosphate and potassium loss, inadequate GI absorption of these electrolytes, or inadequate phosphate and potassium in the diet

(Continued)

Potassium Phosphate *(Continued)*

Contraindications Hyperphosphatemia, hyperkalemia, hypocalcemia, hypomagnesemia, renal failure

Warnings/Precautions Use with caution in patients with renal insufficiency, cardiac disease, metabolic alkalosis; admixture of phosphate and calcium in I.V. fluids can result in calcium phosphate precipitation

Adverse Reactions (Reflective of adult population; not specific for elderly)
>10%: Gastrointestinal: Diarrhea, nausea, stomach pain, flatulence, vomiting
1% to 10%:
  Cardiovascular: Bradycardia
  Endocrine & metabolic: Hyperkalemia
  Neuromuscular & skeletal: Weakness
  Respiratory: Dyspnea

Overdosage/Toxicology Symptoms include muscle weakness, paralysis, peaked T waves, flattened P waves, prolongation of QRS complex, ventricular arrhythmias, tetany, and calcium-phosphate precipitation. Removal of potassium can be accomplished by various means such as through the GI tract with Kayexalate® administration, by way of the kidney through diuresis, mineralocorticoid administration or increased sodium intake, by hemodialysis or peritoneal dialysis, or by shifting potassium back into the cells by insulin, glucose infusion, or sodium bicarbonate. Calcium chloride reverses cardiac effects.

Drug Interactions
Decreased effect/levels with aluminum and magnesium-containing antacids or sucralfate which can act as phosphate binders
Increased effect/levels with potassium-sparing diuretics, salt substitutes, or ACE inhibitors; increased effect of digitalis

Ethanol/Nutrition/Herb Interactions Food: Avoid administering with oxalate (berries, nuts, chocolate, beans, celery, tomato) or phytate-containing foods (bran, whole wheat).

Stability Store at room temperature; do not freeze. Use only clear solutions. Up to 10-15 mEq of calcium may be added per liter before precipitate may occur.

Stability of parenteral admixture at room temperature (25°C) is 24 hours.

Phosphate salts may precipitate when mixed with calcium salts. Solubility is improved in amino acid parenteral nutrition solutions. Check with a pharmacist to determine compatibility.

Dosage
Geriatrics & Adults:
Normal requirements elemental phosphorus: Oral: 800 mg

I.V.: Doses listed as mmol of phosphate.**Caution: With orders for I.V. phosphate, there is considerable confusion associated with the use of millimoles (mmol) versus milliequivalents (mEq) to express the phosphate requirement.** The most reliable method of ordering I.V. phosphate is by millimoles, then specifying the potassium or sodium salt (see Additional Information).

Acute treatment of hypophosphatemia: It is recommended that repletion of severe hypophosphatemia be done I.V. because large doses of oral phosphate may cause diarrhea and intestinal absorption may be unreliable. Intermittent I.V. infusion should be reserved for severe depletion situations; requires continuous cardiac monitoring. Guidelines differ based on degree of illness, need/use of TPN, and severity of hypophosphatemia. If potassium >4.0 mEq/L consider phosphate replacement strategy without potassium (eg, sodium phosphates). Obese patients and/or severe renal impairment were excluded from phosphate supplement trials.

General replacement guidelines (Lentz, 1978):
Low dose: 0.08 mmol/kg over 6 hours; use if losses are recent and uncomplicated
Intermediate dose: 0.16-0.24 mmol/kg over 4-6 hours; use if serum phosphorus level 0.5-1 mg/dL (0.16-0.32 mmoles/L)
  Note: The initial dose may be increased by 25% to 50% if the patient is symptomatic secondary to hypophosphatemia and lowered by 25% to 50% if the patient is hypercalcemic.
Patients receiving TPN; supplemental dose (Clark, 1995):
Low dose: 0.16 mmol/kg over 4-6 hours; use if serum phosphorus level 2.3-3 mg/dL (0.73-0.96 mmoles/L)
Intermediate dose: 0.32 mmol/kg over 4-6 hours; use if serum phosphorus level 1.6-2.2 mg/dL (0.51-0.72 mmoles/L)
High dose: 0.64 mmol/kg over 8-12 hours; use if serum phosphorus <1.5 mg/dL (<0.5 mmoles/L)

Critically-ill adult trauma patients receiving TPN (Brown, 2006):

Low dose: 0.32 mmol/kg over 4-6 hours; use if serum phosphorus level 2.3-3 mg/dL (0.73-0.96 mmoles/L)

Intermediate dose: 0.64 mmol/kg over 4-6 hours; use if serum phosphorus level 1.6-2.2 mg/dL (0.51-0.72 mmoles/L)

High dose: 1 mmol/kg over 8-12 hours; use if serum phosphorus <1.5 mg/dL (<0.5 mmoles/L)

Maintenance:

I.V. solutions: 15-30 mmol/24 hours I.V. or 50-150 mmol/24 hours orally in divided doses

Oral: 1-2 capsules (250-500 mg phosphorus/8-16 mmol) 4 times/day; dilute as instructed

Administration Injection must be diluted in appropriate I.V. solution and volume prior to administration and administered over a minimum of 4 hours

Monitoring Parameters Serum potassium, phosphate, magnesium (failure to respond), calcium, EKG, salicylate serum concentrations if patient is taking salicylates; signs of muscle weakness, cramps

Reference Range Geriatrics and Adults: 2.5-5 mg/dL

Test Interactions Decreased ammonia (B)

Additional Information Because inorganic phosphate exists as monobasic and dibasic anions, with the mixture of valences dependent on pH, ordering by mEq amounts is unreliable and may lead to large dosing errors. In addition, I.V. phosphate is available in the sodium and potassium salt; therefore, the content of these cations must be considered when ordering phosphate. The most reliable method of ordering I.V. phosphate is by millimoles, then specifying the potassium or sodium salt. For example, an order for 15 mmol of phosphate as potassium phosphate in one liter of normal saline. The dosing of phosphate should be 0.2-0.3 mmol/kg with a usual daily requirement of 30-60 mmol/day or 15 mmol of phosphate per liter of TPN or 15 mmol phosphate per 1000 calories of dextrose. Would also provide 22 mEq of potassium.

Special Geriatric Considerations A complete drug history should be taken to rule out potential drug interactions since elderly frequently may be taking potassium and potassium-sparing diuretics or salicylates as antacids. Elderly may require less potassium than younger adults due to decreased renal function. Elderly who do not respond to replacement therapy, check serum magnesium. Long-term use of diuretics may result in hypomagnesemia. Monitor closely in elderly with Cl_{cr} <30 mL/minute.

Dosage Forms Excipient information presented when available (limited, particularly for generics); consult specific product labeling.

Injection, solution: Potassium 4.4 mEq and phosphorus 3 mmol per mL (5 mL, 15 mL, 50 mL) [equivalent to potassium 170 mg and phosphate 285 mg per mL]

Powder for oral solution [packet] (Neutra-Phos®-K): Monobasic potassium phosphate and dibasic potassium phosphate/packet (100s) [equivalent to elemental potassium 556 mg (14.2 mEq) and phosphorus 250 mg per packet; sodium and sugar free; fruit flavor]

Selected References

Brown KA, Dickerson RN, Morgan LM, et al, "A New Graduated Dosing Regimen for Phosphorus Replacement in Patients Receiving Nutrition Support," *JPEN J Parenter Enteral Nutr*, 2006, 30(3):209-14.

Clark CL, Sacks GS, Dickerson RN, et al, "Treatment of Hypophosphatemia in Patients Receiving Specialized Nutrition Support Using a Graduated Dosing Scheme: Results From a Prospective Clinical Trial," *Crit Care Med*, 1995, 23(9):1504-1.

Potassium Phosphate and Sodium Phosphate

(poe TASS ee um FOS fate & SOW dee um FOS fate)

Related Information

Potassium Phosphate *on page 1291*
Sodium Phosphates *on page 1478*

Medication Safety Issues

Sound-alike/look-alike issues:

K-Phos® Neutral may be confused with Neutra-Phos-K®

U.S. Brand Names K-Phos® MF; K-Phos® Neutral; K-Phos® No. 2; Neutra-Phos® [OTC]; Phos-NaK; Phospha 250™ Neutral; Uro-KP-Neutral®

Index Terms Sodium Phosphate and Potassium Phosphate

Generic Available Yes

Pharmacologic Category Electrolyte Supplement, Oral

Use Treatment of conditions associated with excessive renal phosphate loss or inadequate GI absorption of phosphate; acidification of urine; reduction of urinary calcium concentrations; increased antibacterial activity of methenamine; reduction of odor and rash caused by ammonia in urine

Contraindications Addison's disease, hyperkalemia, hyperphosphatemia, infected urolithiasis or struvite stone formation, patients with severely impaired renal function

(Continued)

Potassium Phosphate and Sodium Phosphate *(Continued)*

Warnings/Precautions Use with caution in patients with renal disease, cardiac disease, metabolic alkalosis, acute dehydration, hepatic impairment, hypernatremia, and hypotension. Products also contain potassium and sodium.

Adverse Reactions (Reflective of adult population; not specific for elderly)
Frequency not defined.
Cardiovascular: Bradycardia, arrhythmia, chest pain, edema, tachycardia
Central nervous system: Mental confusion, tetany (with large doses of phosphate), headache, dizziness, seizure
Endocrine & metabolic: Hyperkalemia, alkalosis
Gastrointestinal: Diarrhea, nausea, stomach pain, flatulence, vomiting, throat pain, weight gain
Genitourinary: Urine output decreased
Local: Phlebitis
Neuromuscular & skeletal: Weakness, arthralgia, bone pain, paralysis, paresthesia, pain/weakness of extremities, muscle cramps
Renal: Acute renal failure
Respiratory: Dyspnea
Miscellaneous: Thirst

Overdosage/Toxicology Symptoms include muscle weakness, paralysis, peaked T waves, flattened P waves, prolongation of QRS complex, ventricular arrhythmias, tetany, and calcium phosphate precipitation. Removal of potassium can be accomplished by various means such as through the GI tract with Kayexalate® administration, by way of the kidney through diuresis, mineralocorticoid administration or increased sodium intake, by hemodialysis or peritoneal dialysis, or by shifting potassium back into the cells by insulin and glucose infusion. Calcium chloride reverses cardiac effects.

Drug Interactions
Decreased effect/levels with aluminum and magnesium-containing antacids or sucralfate which can act as phosphate binders
Increased effect/levels with potassium-sparing diuretics or ACE inhibitors; salicylates

Dosage
Geriatrics & Adults: Note: All dosage forms to be mixed in 6-8 oz of water prior to administration
Phosphate supplement: Oral: Elemental phosphorus 250-500 mg 4 times/day after meals and at bedtime

Administration
Powder: Following dilution of powder, solution may be chilled to increase palatability.
Tablet: Should be taken with a full glass of water.

Monitoring Parameters Serum potassium, sodium, magnesium (failure to respond to replacement), calcium, phosphate, EKG; signs of muscle weakness, cramps

Patient Information Powder packets are to be mixed in 6-8 oz of water; following dilution, solution may be chilled to increase palatability. Tablets should be taken with a full glass of water.

Special Geriatric Considerations A complete drug history should be taken to rule out potential drug interactions since elderly frequently may be taking potassium and potassium-sparing diuretics or salicylates as antacids. Elderly may require less potassium than younger adults due to decreased renal function. Elderly who do not respond to replacement therapy, check serum magnesium. Long-term use of diuretics may result in hypomagnesemia.

Dosage Forms Excipient information presented when available (limited, particularly for generics); consult specific product labeling.
Caplet:
Uro-KP-Neutral®: Sodium phosphate monobasic, dipotassium phosphate, and disodium phosphate [equivalent to elemental phosphorus 258 mg, sodium 262.4 mg (10.8 mEq), and potassium 49.4 mg (1.3 mEq)]
Powder, for oral solution:
Neutra-Phos®, Phos-NaK): Monobasic sodium, dibasic sodium, and potassium phosphate/packet (100s) [equivalent to elemental phosphorus 250 mg, sodium 164 mg (7.1 mEq), and potassium 278 mg (7.1 mEq) per packet]
Tablet:
K-Phos® MF: Potassium acid phosphate 155 mg and sodium acid phosphate 350 mg [equivalent to elemental phosphorus 125.6 mg, sodium 67 mg (2.9 mEq), and potassium 44.5 mg (1.1 mEq)]
K-Phos® Neutral: Dibasic sodium phosphate 852 mg, monobasic potassium phosphate 155 mg, and monobasic sodium phosphate 130 mg [equivalent to elemental phosphorus 250 mg, sodium 298 mg (13 mEq), and potassium 45 mg (1.1 mEq)]
K-Phos® No. 2: Potassium acid phosphate 305 mg and sodium acid phosphate 700 mg [equivalent to elemental phosphorus 250 mg, sodium 134 mg (5.8 mEq), and potassium 88 mg (2.3 mEq)]
Phospha 250™ Neutral: Dibasic sodium phosphate 852 mg, monobasic potassium phosphate 155 mg, and monobasic sodium phosphate 130 mg [equivalent to

elemental phosphorus 250 mg, sodium 298 mg (13 mEq), and potassium 45 mg (1.1 mEq)]

- ♦ **PPD** *see* Tuberculin Tests *on page 1643*
- ♦ **PPV23** *see* Pneumococcal Polysaccharide Vaccine (Polyvalent) *on page 1279*

Pramipexole (pra mi PEKS ole)

Related Information
Antiparkinsonian Agents *on page 1745*
Medication Safety Issues
Sound-alike/look-alike issues:
Mirapex® may be confused with Mifeprex®, MiraLax™
U.S. Brand Names Mirapex®
Canadian Brand Names Apo-Pramipexole; Mirapex®; Novo-Pramipexole; PMS-Pramipexole
Generic Available No
Pharmacologic Category Anti-Parkinson's Agent, Dopamine Agonist
Use Treatment of the signs and symptoms of idiopathic Parkinson's disease; treatment of moderate-to-severe primary Restless Legs Syndrome (RLS)
Unlabeled/Investigational Use Treatment of depression
Contraindications Hypersensitivity to pramipexole or any component of the formulation
Warnings/Precautions Caution should be taken in patients with renal insufficiency; dose adjustment necessary. Caution in patients with pre-existing dyskinesias; may be exacerbated. May cause orthostatic hypotension; Parkinson's disease patients appear to have an impaired capacity to respond to a postural challenge. Use with caution in patients at risk of hypotension or where transient hypotensive episodes would be poorly tolerated. Parkinson's patients being treated with dopaminergic agonists ordinarily require careful monitoring for signs and symptoms of postural hypotension, especially during dose escalation. May cause hallucinations.

Dopaminergic agents have been associated with a syndrome resembling neuroleptic malignant syndrome on abrupt withdrawal or significant dosage reduction after long-term use. Ergot-derived dopamine agonists have also been associated with fibrotic complications (eg, retroperitoneal fibrosis, pleural thickening, and pulmonary infiltrates). Although pramipexole is not an ergot, there have been postmarketing reports of possible fibrotic complications with pramipexole; monitor closely for signs and symptoms of fibrosis.

Pramipexole has been associated with somnolence, particularly at higher dosages (>1.5 mg/day). In addition, patients have been reported to fall asleep during activities of daily living, including driving, while taking this medication. Whether these patients exhibited somnolence prior to these events is not clear. Patients should be advised of this issue and factors which may increase risk (sleep disorders, other sedating medications, or concomitant medications which increase pramipexole concentrations) and instructed to report daytime somnolence or sleepiness to the prescriber. Patients should use caution in performing activities which require alertness (driving or operating machinery), and to avoid other medications which may cause CNS depression, including ethanol.

Pathologic degenerative changes were observed in the retinas of albino rats during studies with this agent, but were not observed in the retinas of albino mice or in other species. The significance of these data for humans remains uncertain. Augmentation (earlier onset of symptoms in the evening/afternoon, increase and/or spread of symptoms to other extremities) or rebound (shifting of symptoms to early morning hours) may occur in some RLS patients.

Adverse Reactions (Reflective of adult population; not specific for elderly)
Parkinson's disease (PD) unless identified as RLS:
>10%:
  Cardiovascular: Postural hypotension (dose related; PD 53%)
  Central nervous system: Dizziness (PD 25%), headache (RLS 16%), somnolence (dose related; RLS 6%; PD 9% to 22%), insomnia (RLS 13%; PD 17% to 27%), hallucinations (PD 9% to 17%), abnormal dreams (RLS up to 8%)
  Gastrointestinal: Nausea (dose related; RLS: 5% to 27%; PD 28%), constipation (dose related; RLS: 4%; PD 10% to 14%)
  Neuromuscular & skeletal: Weakness (PD 10% to 14%), dyskinesia (PD 47%), EPS
1% to 10%:
  Cardiovascular: Edema, syncope, tachycardia, chest pain
  Central nervous system: Malaise, confusion (PD 4% to 10%), amnesia (dose related), dystonias, akathisia, thinking abnormalities, myoclonus, hyperesthesia, paranoia, fever
  Endocrine & metabolic: Decreased libido
(Continued)

Pramipexole *(Continued)*

Gastrointestinal: Anorexia, diarrhea (RLS 3% to 7%), dysphagia, weight loss, xerostomia (up to 7%)

Genitourinary: Urinary frequency (PD 6%), impotence, urinary incontinence

Neuromuscular & skeletal: Muscle twitching, leg cramps, arthritis, bursitis, myasthenia, gait abnormalities, hypertonia

Ocular: Vision abnormalities

Respiratory: Dyspnea, nasal congestion (RLS up to 6%), rhinitis

Miscellaneous: Influenza (RLS 3%)

Overdosage/Toxicology Treatment is symptom-directed and supportive. Negligible amounts removed by dialysis.

Drug Interactions

Antipsychotics (typical): May diminish the therapeutic effect of anti-Parkinson's agents (dopamine agonist).

CNS depressants: May enhance the adverse/toxic effect of pramipexole.

Cimetidine: May increase level/effects of pramipexole.

Metoclopramide: May decrease the efficacy of pramipexole due to dopamine antagonism

Ethanol/Nutrition/Herb Interactions

Ethanol: Avoid ethanol (may increase CNS depression).

Food: Food intake does not affect the extent of drug absorption, although the time to maximal plasma concentration is delayed by 60 minutes when taken with a meal.

Herb/Nutraceutical: Avoid valerian, St John's wort, SAMe, kava kava (may increase risk of serotonin syndrome and/or excessive sedation).

Stability Store at 15°C to 30°C (59°F to 86°F). Protect from light.

Mechanism of Action Pramipexole is a nonergot dopamine agonist with specificity for the D_2 subfamily dopamine receptor, and has also been shown to bind to D_3 and D_4 receptors. By binding to these receptors, it is thought that pramipexole can stimulate dopamine activity on the nerves of the striatum and substantia nigra.

Pharmacokinetics

Absorption: Rapid

Distribution: V_d: 500 L

Metabolism: Minimal

Bioavailability: >90%

Half-life: Adults: 8 hours; older adults: 12 hours

Elimination: 90% eliminated unchanged in the urine

Clearance is decreased in older adults, likely due to decreased renal function. Clearance in Parkinson's patients was 30% less than healthy older adult volunteers. Clearance is decreased 60% when creatinine clearance is 40 mL/minute; 75% when clearance is 20 mL/minute.

Dosage

Geriatrics & Adults: **Parkinson's disease:** Oral: Initial: 0.375 mg/day given in 3 divided doses; increase gradually by 0.125 mg/dose every 5-7 days; range: 1.5-4.5 mg/day.

Restless legs syndrome: Oral: Initial: 0.125 mg once daily 2-3 hours before bedtime. Dose may be doubled every 4-7 days up to 0.5 mg/day. Maximum dose: 0.5 mg/day (manufacturer's recommendation).

Note: Most patients require <0.5 mg/day, but higher doses have been used (2 mg/day). If augmentation occurs, dose earlier in the day.

Renal Impairment: Use caution; renally-eliminated

Parkinson's disease:

Cl_{cr} 35-59 mL/minute: Initial: 0.125 mg twice daily (maximum dose: 1.5 mg twice daily)

Cl_{cr} 15-34 mL/minute: Initial: 0.125 mg once daily (maximum dose: 1.5 mg once daily)

Cl_{cr} <15 mL/minute (or hemodialysis patients): Not adequately studied.

Restless legs syndrome:

Cl_{cr} 20-60 mL/minute: Duration between titration should be increased to 14 days

Cl_{cr} <20 mL/minute: Not adequately studied

Monitoring Parameters Blood pressure, standing and sitting/lying down; mental status

Patient Information If pramipexole causes nausea, may take with food; rise slowly from sitting/lying down position; drowsiness may occur, use caution when driving until used to the effects of pramipexole; avoid alcohol and other CNS depressants

Dosage Forms Excipient information presented when available (limited, particularly for generics); consult specific product labeling.

Tablet, as dihydrochloride monohydrate:

Mirapex®: 0.125 mg, 0.25 mg, 0.5 mg, 1 mg, 1.5 mg

Additional formulations available in Canada: With the exception of the 0.125 mg tablet, generic formulations are also available in Canada

Selected References

Lieberman A, Ranhosky A, and Korts D, "Clinical Evaluation of Pramipexole in Advanced Parkinson's Disease: Results of a Double-Blind, Placebo-Controlled, Parallel-Group Study," *Neurology*, 1997, 49(1):162-8.

Olanow CW, Watts RL, and Koller WC, "An Algorithm (Decision Tree) for the Management of Parkinson's Disease (2001): Treatment Guidelines," *Neurology*, 2001, 56(11 Suppl 5):S1-S88.

"RLS Medical Bulletin," Restless Legs Syndrome Foundation, 2005, 1-34. Available at www.rls.org. Last accessed December 13, 2006.

"Safety and Efficacy of Pramipexole in Early Parkinson Disease. Parkinson Study Group," *JAMA*, 1997, 278(2):125-30.

Silber MH, Girish M, and Izurieta R, "Pramipexole in the Management of Restless Legs Syndrome: An Extended Study," *Sleep*, 2003, 26(7):819-21.

Stern MB, "Contemporary Approaches to the Pharmacotherapeutic Management of Parkinson's Disease: An Overview," *Neurology*, 1997, 49(1 Suppl 1):S2-9.

Watts RL, "The Role of Dopamine Agonists in Early Parkinson's Disease," *Neurology*, 1997, 49(1 Suppl 1):S34-48.

Winkelman JW and Johnston L, "Augmentation and Tolerance With Long-Term Pramipexole Treatment of Restless Legs Syndrome (RLS)," *Sleep Med*, 2004, 5(1):9-14.

Pramlintide (PRAM lin tide)

Medication Safety Issues

Dosing: The concentration of this product is 600 micrograms (mcg)/mL. Manufacturer recommended dosing ranges from 15 mcg to 120 mcg, which corresponds to injectable volumes of 0.025 mL to 0.2 mL. Patients and healthcare providers should exercise caution when administering this product to avoid inadvertent calculation of the dose based on "units," which could result in a sixfold overdose.

U.S. Brand Names Symlin®

Index Terms Pramlintide Acetate

Generic Available No

Pharmacologic Category Amylinomimetic; Antidiabetic Agent

Use

Adjunctive treatment with mealtime insulin in type 1 diabetes mellitus (insulin dependent, IDDM) patients who have failed to achieve desired glucose control despite optimal insulin therapy

Adjunctive treatment with mealtime insulin in type 2 diabetes mellitus (noninsulin dependent, NIDDM) patients who have failed to achieve desired glucose control despite optimal insulin therapy, with or without concurrent sulfonylurea and/or metformin

Restrictions An FDA-approved medication guide must be distributed when dispensing an outpatient prescription (new or refill) where this medication is to be used without direct supervision of a healthcare provider. Medication guides are available at http://www.fda.gov/cder/Offices/ODS/medication_guides.htm.

Contraindications Hypersensitivity to pramlintide or any component of the formulation; confirmed diagnosis of gastroparesis; hypoglycemia unawareness

Warnings/Precautions [U.S. Boxed Warning]: Coadministration with insulin may induce severe hypoglycemia (usually within 3 hours following administration); coadministration with insulin therapy is an approved indication but does require an initial dosage reduction of insulin and frequent pre and post blood glucose monitoring to reduce risk of severe hypoglycemia. Concurrent use of other glucose-lowering agents may increase risk of hypoglycemia. Avoid use in patients with poor compliance with their insulin regimen and/or blood glucose monitoring. Do not use in patients with Hb A_{1c} levels >9% or recent, recurrent episodes of hypoglycemia; obtain detailed history of glucose control (eg, Hb A_{1c}, incidence of hypoglycemia, glucose monitoring, and medication compliance) and body weight before initiating therapy. Use caution when driving or operating heavy machinery until effects on blood sugar are known. Use caution with certain antihypertensive agents (eg, beta-adrenergic blockers) or neuropathic conditions which may mask signs/symptoms of hypoglycemia. Use caution in patients with history of nausea; avoid use in patients with conditions or concurrent medications likely to impair gastric motility (eg, anticholinergics); do not use in patients requiring medication(s) to stimulate gastric emptying.

Adverse Reactions (Reflective of adult population; not specific for elderly)

>10%:

Central nervous system: Headache (5% to 13%)

Gastrointestinal: Nausea (28% to 48%), vomiting (7% to 11%), anorexia (<1% to 17%)

Endocrine & metabolic: Severe hypoglycemia (type 1 diabetes): <1% to 17%)

Miscellaneous: Inflicted injury (8% to 14%)

1% to 10%:

Central nervous system: Fatigue (3% to 7%), dizziness (2% to 6%)

Endocrine & metabolic: Severe hypoglycemia (type 2 diabetes): <1% to 8%)

Gastrointestinal: Abdominal pain (2% to 8%)

Respiratory: Pharyngitis (3% to 5%), cough (2% to 6%)

Neuromuscular & skeletal: Arthralgia (2% to 7%)

(Continued)

Pramlintide (Continued)

Miscellaneous: Allergic reaction (<1% to 6%)

Overdosage/Toxicology Severe nausea and vomiting likely to occur, possibly accompanied by diarrhea, vasodilatation and dizziness. Treatment should be symptom-directed and supportive.

Drug Interactions Pramlintide may delay absorption of concomitantly administered medication due to increased gastric emptying time; coadministration with agents in which a rapid onset of action is desired (eg, analgesics) may delay drug response.

Anticholinergic agents: May cause synergistic impairment of gastric motility.

Beta-blockers, nonselective: May delay recovery from hypoglycemic episodes and mask signs/symptoms of hypoglycemia.

Medications which may induce or exacerbate hypoglycemia include ACE inhibitors, alcohol, alpha-blockers, anabolic steroids, beta-blockers, clofibrate, clonidine, disopyramide, fenfluramine, fibrates, fluoxetine, guanethidine, MAO inhibitors, pentamidine, pentoxifylline, phenylbutazone, propoxyphene, reserpine, salicylates, sulfinpyrazone, sulfonamides, and tetracyclines.

Ethanol/Nutrition/Herb Interactions

Ethanol: Use caution with ethanol (may increase hypoglycemia).

Herb/Nutraceutical: Use caution with garlic, chromium, gymnema (may increase hypoglycemia).

Stability Store unopened vials at 2°C to 8°C (36°F to 46°F); do not freeze. Opened vials may be kept refrigerated or at room temperature ≤25°C (≤77°F). Discard opened vial after 28 days. Protect from light.

Mechanism of Action Synthetic analog of human amylin cosecreted with insulin by pancreatic beta cells; reduces postprandial glucose increases via the following mechanisms: 1) prolongation of gastric emptying time, 2) reduction of postprandial glucagon secretion, and 3) reduction of caloric intake through centrally-mediated appetite suppression

Pharmacodynamics Duration: 3 hours

Pharmacokinetics Note: Pharmacokinetic studies have not been conducted in the elderly.

Protein binding: 60%

Metabolism: Primarily renal to des-lys^1 pramlintide (active metabolite)

Bioavailability: 30% to 40%

Half-life elimination: 48 minutes

Time to peak, plasma: 20 minutes

Excretion: Primarily urine

Dosage

Geriatrics & Adults: Note: When initiating pramlintide, reduce current insulin dose (including rapidly- and mixed-acting preparations) by 50% to avoid hypoglycemia. If pramlintide is discontinued for any reason, restart therapy with same initial titration protocol.

Type 1 diabetes mellitus (insulin dependent, IDDM): SubQ: Initial: 15 mcg immediately prior to meals; titrate in 15 mcg increments every 3 days (if no significant nausea occurs) to target dose of 30-60 mcg (consider discontinuation if intolerant of 30 mcg dose)

Type 2 diabetes mellitus (noninsulin dependent, NIDDM): SubQ: Initial: 60 mcg immediately prior to meals; after 3-7 days, increase to 120 mcg prior to meals if no significant nausea occurs (if nausea occurs at 120 mcg dose, reduce to 60 mcg)

Renal Impairment: No dosage adjustment required; not evaluated in dialysis patients

Administration Do not mix with insulins; administer subcutaneously into abdominal or thigh areas at sites distinct from concomitant insulin injections (do not administer into arm due to variable absorption); rotate injection sites frequently. For oral medications in which a rapid onset of action is desired, administer 1 hour before, or 2 hours after pramlintide, if possible.

Monitoring Parameters Prior to initiating therapy: Hb A_{1c}, hypoglycemic history, body weight. During therapy: urine sugar and acetone, pre- and postprandial and bedtime serum glucose, electrolytes, Hb A_{1c}, lipid profile

Special Geriatric Considerations Patients must be able to adhere to their insulin regimen and self-monitor their blood glucose. In premarketing studies, the change in the Hb A_{1c} values and hypoglycemia frequencies did not differ by age. Monitor regimen closely.

Dosage Forms Excipient information presented when available (limited, particularly for generics); consult specific product labeling.

Injection, solution: Pramlintide acetate 0.6 mg/mL (5 mL) [contains phenol-derivative metacresol]

♦ **Pramlintide Acetate** see Pramlintide on page 1297

♦ **Prandin**® see Repaglinide on page 1390

♦ **Pravachol**® see Pravastatin on page 1299

Pravastatin (prav a STAT in)

Related Information
Hyperlipidemia Management *on page 1773*
Medication Safety Issues
Sound-alike/look-alike issues:
Pravachol® may be confused with Prevacid®, Prinivil®, propranolol
U.S. Brand Names Pravachol®
Canadian Brand Names Apo-Pravastatin®; CO Pravastatin; Novo-Pravastatin; PMS-Pravastatin; Pravachol®; ratio-Pravastatin; Riva-Pravastatin; Sandoz-Pravastatin
Index Terms Pravastatin Sodium
Generic Available Yes
Pharmacologic Category Antilipemic Agent, HMG-CoA Reductase Inhibitor
Use
"Primary prevention" in hypercholesterolemic patients without clinically-evident coronary heart disease to reduce the risk of myocardial infarction, reduce the risk of undergoing myocardial revascularization procedures, reduce the risk of cardiovascular mortality with no increase in death from noncardiovascular causes

"Secondary prevention" in hypercholesterolemic patients with clinically-evident coronary artery disease, including prior myocardial infarction, to slow the progression of coronary atherosclerosis, and reduce the risk of acute coronary events

"Secondary prevention" in patients with previous myocardial infarction, and normal cholesterol levels; to reduce the risk of recurrent myocardial infarction; reduce the risk of undergoing myocardial revascularization procedures; and reduce the risk of stroke or transient ischemic attack (TIA)

Adjunct to diet to reduce elevated total cholesterol, LDL cholesterol, apolipoprotein B (apo-B) and triglyceride levels, and increasing HDL-C in patients with primary hypercholesterolemia and mixed dyslipidemia (Frederickson types IIa and IIb); Frederickson type IV, type III (who do not respond adequately to diet)

Contraindications Hypersensitivity to pravastatin or any component of the formulation; active liver disease; unexplained persistent elevations of serum transaminases

Warnings/Precautions Secondary causes of hyperlipidemia should be ruled out prior to therapy. Liver function must be monitored by periodic laboratory assessment. Rhabdomyolysis with acute renal failure has occurred. Risk may be increased with concurrent use of other drugs which may cause rhabdomyolysis (including colchicine, gemfibrozil, fibric acid derivatives, or niacin at doses ≥1 g/day). Temporarily discontinue in any patient experiencing an acute or serious condition predisposing to renal failure secondary to rhabdomyolysis. Use with caution in patients with advanced age, these patients are predisposed to myopathy. Use caution in patients with previous liver disease or heavy ethanol use.

Adverse Reactions (Reflective of adult population; not specific for elderly)
As reported in short-term trials; safety and tolerability with long-term use were similar to placebo
1% to 10%:
Cardiovascular: Chest pain (4%)
Central nervous system: Headache (2% to 6%), fatigue (4%), dizziness (1% to 3%)
Dermatologic: Rash (4%)
Gastrointestinal: Nausea/vomiting (7%), diarrhea (6%), heartburn (3%)
Hepatic: Transaminases increased (>3x normal on two occasions - 1%)
Neuromuscular & skeletal: Myalgia (2%)
Respiratory: Cough (3%)
Miscellaneous: Influenza (2%)
Additional class-related events or case reports (not necessarily reported with pravastatin therapy): Angioedema, cataracts, depression, dyspnea, eosinophilia, erectile dysfunction, facial paresis, hypersensitivity reaction, impaired extraocular muscle movement, impotence, leukopenia, malaise, memory loss, ophthalmoplegia, paresthesia, peripheral neuropathy, photosensitivity, psychic disturbance, skin discoloration, thrombocytopenia, thyroid dysfunction, toxic epidermal necrolysis, transaminases increased, vomiting

Overdosage/Toxicology Treatment is symptomatic.

Drug Interactions Substrate of CYP3A4 (minor); **Inhibits** CYP2C9 (weak), 2D6 (weak), 3A4 (weak)
Cholestyramine: Reduces pravastatin absorption; separate administration times by at least 4 hours.
Clofibrate and fenofibrate: May increase the risk of myopathy and rhabdomyolysis.
Colchicine: Concomitant therapy with an HMG-CoA reductase inhibitor may increase risk of myopathy/rhabdomyolysis; use caution
Colestipol: Reduces pravastatin absorption; separate administration by 1 hour.
Cyclosporine: Concurrent use may increase the risk of myopathy and rhabdomyolysis.
Gemfibrozil: Increased risk of myopathy and rhabdomyolysis.
(Continued)

Pravastatin *(Continued)*

Imidazole antifungals (itraconazole, ketoconazole): May modestly increase pravastatin concentrations (AUC).

Niacin: May increase the risk of myopathy and rhabdomyolysis.

P-glycoprotein inhibitors (eg, amiodarone, cyclosporine, ketoconazole): May increase pravastatin concentrations.

Ethanol/Nutrition/Herb Interactions

Ethanol: Consumption of large amounts of ethanol may increase the risk of liver damage with HMG-CoA reductase inhibitors.

Food: Red yeast rice contains an estimated 2.4 mg lovastatin per 600 mg rice.

Herb/Nutraceutical: St John's wort may decrease pravastatin levels.

Stability Store at 25°C (77°F); excursions permitted to 15°C to 30°C (59°F to 86°F). Protect from moisture and light.

Mechanism of Action Pravastatin is a competitive inhibitor of 3-hydroxy-3-methylglutaryl coenzyme A (HMG-CoA) reductase, which is the rate-limiting enzyme involved in *de novo* cholesterol synthesis.

Pharmacodynamics

Onset of action: Several days

Peak effect: 4 weeks

Pharmacokinetics

Absorption: Rapidly absorbed; average absorption 34%

Protein binding: 50%

Metabolism: Hepatic to at least two metabolites

Bioavailability: 17%

Half-life: ~2-3 hours

Time to peak, serum: 1-1.5 hours

Elimination: Feces (70%); urine (≤20%, 8% as unchanged drug)

Dosage

Geriatrics & Adults:

Hyperlipidemias, primary prevention of coronary events, secondary prevention of cardiovascular events: Oral: Initial: 40 mg once daily; titrate dosage to response (usual range: 10-80 mg) (maximum dose: 80 mg once daily)

Dosage adjustment based on concomitant cyclosporine: Oral: Initial: 10 mg/day, titrate with caution (maximum dose: 20 mg/day)

Note: Doses should be individualized according to the baseline LDL-cholesterol levels, the recommended goal of therapy, and patient response; adjustments should be made at intervals of 4 weeks or more; doses may need adjusted based on concomitant medications

Renal Impairment: Initial: 10 mg/day

Hepatic Impairment: Initial: 10 mg/day

Monitoring Parameters Obtain baseline LFTs and total cholesterol profile; creatine phosphokinase due to possibility of myopathy. Repeat LFTs prior to elevation of dose. May be measured when clinically indicated and/or periodically thereafter.

Patient Information Promptly report any unexplained muscle pain, tenderness or weakness, especially if accompanied by malaise or fever; follow prescribed diet

Additional Information May be taken without regard to meals. Before initiation of therapy, patients should be placed on a standard cholesterol-lowering diet for 6 weeks and the diet should be continued during drug therapy.

Special Geriatric Considerations Effective and well tolerated in the elderly. No specific dosage recommendations. Clearance is reduced in elderly, resulting in an increase in AUC between 25% to 50%. However, substantial accumulation is not expected.

The definition of and, therefore, when to treat hyperlipidemia in elderly is a controversial issue. The National Cholesterol Education Program recommends that all adults maintain a plasma cholesterol <160 mg/dL. Elderly with one additional risk factor, goal LDL would be <130 mg/dL. It is the authors' belief that pharmacologic treatment be reserved for those who are unable to obtain a desirable plasma cholesterol concentration by diet alone and for whom the benefits of treatment are believed to outweigh the potential adverse effects, drug interactions, and cost of treatment.

Dosage Forms Excipient information presented when available (limited, particularly for generics); consult specific product labeling.

Tablet, as sodium: 10 mg, 20 mg, 40 mg

Pravachol®: 10 mg, 20 mg, 40 mg, 80 mg

Selected References

"Executive Summary of The Third Report of The National Cholesterol Education Program (NCEP) Expert Panel on Detection, Evaluation, And Treatment of High Blood Cholesterol In Adults (Adult Treatment Panel III)," *JAMA*, 2001, 285(19):2486-97.

Lintott CJ and Scott RS, "HMG-CoA Reductase Inhibitor Use in the Aged: A Review of Clinical Experience," *Drugs Aging*, 1992, 2(6):518-29.

♦ **Pravastatin Sodium** *see* Pravastatin *on page 1299*

Prazosin (PRAZ oh sin)

Medication Safety Issues
Sound-alike/look-alike issues:
Prazosin may be confused with predniSONE

International issues:
Prazac® [Denmark] may be confused with Prozac® which is a brand name for fluoxetine in the U.S.
Prazepam [multiple international markets] may be confused with prazosin.

U.S. Brand Names Minipress®
Canadian Brand Names Apo-Prazo®; Minipress®; Novo-Prazin; Nu-Prazo
Index Terms Furazosin; Prazosin Hydrochloride
Generic Available Yes
Pharmacologic Category Alpha₁ Blocker
Use Treatment of hypertension
Unlabeled/Investigational Use Post-traumatic stress disorder (PTSD); benign prostatic hyperplasia; Raynaud's syndrome
Contraindications Hypersensitivity to quinazolines (doxazosin, prazosin, terazosin) or any component of the formulation
Warnings/Precautions May cause significant orthostatic hypotension and syncope, especially with first dose; anticipate a similar effect if therapy is interrupted for a few days, if dosage is rapidly increased, or if another antihypertensive drug (particularly vasodilators) or a PDE-5 inhibitor is introduced. Patients should be cautioned about performing hazardous tasks when starting new therapy or adjusting dosage upward. Discontinue if symptoms of angina occur or worsen. Should rule out prostatic carcinoma before beginning therapy.

Adverse Reactions (Reflective of adult population; not specific for elderly)
>10%: Central nervous system: Dizziness (10%)
1% to 10%:
Cardiovascular: Palpitation (5%), edema, orthostatic hypotension, syncope (1%)
Central nervous system: Headache (8%), drowsiness (8%), weakness (7%), vertigo, depression, nervousness
Dermatologic: Rash (1% to 4%)
Endocrine & metabolic: Decreased energy (7%)
Gastrointestinal: Nausea (5%), vomiting, diarrhea, constipation
Genitourinary: Urinary frequency (1% to 5%)
Ocular: Blurred vision, reddened sclera, xerostomia
Respiratory: Dyspnea, epistaxis, nasal congestion

Overdosage/Toxicology Symptoms include hypotension and drowsiness. Hypotension usually responds to I.V. fluids, Trendelenburg positioning, or vasoconstrictors. Treatment is otherwise supportive and symptomatic.

Drug Interactions
ACE inhibitors: Hypotensive effect may be increased.
Beta-blockers: Hypotensive effect may be increased.
Calcium channel blockers: Hypotensive effect may be increased.
NSAIDs may reduce antihypertensive efficacy.
Sildenafil, tadalafil, vardenafil: Blood pressure-lowering effects are additive. Use of tadalafil or vardenafil is contraindicated by the manufacturer. Use sildenafil with extreme caution (dose ≤25 mg).
Tricyclic antidepressants (TCAs) and low-potency antipsychotics: May increase risk of orthostasis.

Ethanol/Nutrition/Herb Interactions
Ethanol: Avoid ethanol (may increase vasodilation).
Food: Food has variable effects on absorption.
Herb/Nutraceutical: Avoid dong quai if using for hypertension (has estrogenic activity). Avoid ephedra, yohimbe, ginseng (may worsen hypertension). Avoid saw palmetto (due to limited experience with this combination). Avoid garlic (may have increased antihypertensive effect).

Stability Store in airtight container. Protect from light.
Mechanism of Action Competitively inhibits postsynaptic alpha-adrenergic receptors which results in vasodilation of veins and arterioles and a decrease in total peripheral resistance and blood pressure

Pharmacodynamics
Onset of hypotensive effect: Within 2 hours; maximum decrease: 2-4 hours
Duration: 10-24 hours

Pharmacokinetics
Distribution: V_d: 0.5 L/kg (hypertensive adults)
Protein binding: 92% to 97%
Metabolism: Extensive in the liver; metabolites may be active
Bioavailability: Oral: 43% to 82%
(Continued)

Prazosin *(Continued)*

Half-life: 2-4 hours; increased half-life with congestive heart failure

Elimination: 6% to 10% excreted renally as unchanged drug

In older adults, half-life and volume of distribution may be increased and the oral absorption decreased, though the clinical significance is unknown

Dosage

Geriatrics: Oral (first dose given at bedtime): Initial: 1 mg 1-2 times/day

Adults:

Hypertension: Oral: Initial: 1 mg/dose 2-3 times/day; usual maintenance dose: 3-15 mg/day in divided doses 2-4 times/day; maximum daily dose: 20 mg

Hypertensive urgency: Oral: 10-20 mg once, may repeat in 30 minutes

PTSD (unlabeled use): Oral: Initial: 2 mg at bedtime; titrate as tolerated to 10-15 mg at bedtime

Raynaud's (unlabeled use): Oral: 0.5-3 mg twice daily

Benign prostatic hyperplasia (unlabeled use): Oral: 2 mg twice daily

Monitoring Parameters Blood pressure, standing and sitting/supine

Test Interactions Increased urinary VMA 17%, norepinephrine metabolite 42%

Patient Information Rise from sitting/lying carefully, may cause dizziness; take first dose at bedtime

Special Geriatric Considerations Adverse effects such as dry mouth and urinary problems can be particularly bothersome in elderly.

Dosage Forms Excipient information presented when available (limited, particularly for generics); consult specific product labeling.

Capsule, as hydrochloride: 1 mg, 2 mg, 5 mg

Selected References

Chobanian AV, Bakris GL, Black HR, et al, "The Seventh Report of the Joint National Committee on Prevention, Detection, Evaluation, and Treatment of High Blood Pressure: The JNC 7 Report," *JAMA*, 2003, 289(19):2560-71.

Peskind ER, Bonner LT, Hoff DJ, et al, "Prazosin Reduces Trauma-Related Nightmares in Older Men With Chronic Posttraumatic Stress Disorder," *J Geriatr Psychiatry Neurol*, 2003, 16(3):165-71.

Rubin PC, Scott PJ, and Reid JL, "Prazosin Disposition in Young and Elderly Subjects," *Br J Clin Pharmacol*, 1981, 12(3):401-4.

♦ **Prazosin Hydrochloride** *see* Prazosin *on page 1301*

♦ **Precose®** *see* Acarbose *on page 25*

♦ **Pred Forte®** *see* PrednisoLONE *on page 1303*

♦ **Pred-G®** *see* Prednisolone and Gentamicin *on page 1306*

♦ **Pred Mild®** *see* PrednisoLONE *on page 1303*

Prednicarbate *(pred ni KAR bate)*

Related Information

Corticosteroids *on page 1755*

Medication Safety Issues

Sound-alike/look-alike issues:

Dermatop® may be confused with Dimetapp®

U.S. Brand Names Dermatop®

Canadian Brand Names Dermatop®

Generic Available Yes: Cream

Pharmacologic Category Corticosteroid, Topical

Use Relief of the inflammatory and pruritic manifestations of corticosteroid-responsive dermatoses

Contraindications Hypersensitivity to prednicarbate or any component of the formulation; fungal, viral, or tubercular skin lesions, herpes simplex or zoster

Warnings/Precautions Systemic absorption of topical corticosteroids may cause hypothalamic-pituitary-adrenal (HPA) axis suppression (reversible). HPA axis suppression may lead to adrenal crisis. Risk is increased when used over large surface areas, for prolonged periods, or with occlusive dressings. Allergic contact dermatitis can occur, it is usually diagnosed by failure to heal rather than clinical exacerbation. Prolonged treatment with corticosteroids has been associated with the development of Kaposi's sarcoma (case reports); if noted, discontinuation of therapy should be considered. Adverse systemic effects including hyperglycemia, glycosuria, fluid and electrolyte changes, and HPA suppression may occur when used on large surface areas, for prolonged periods, or with an occlusive dressing.

Adverse Reactions (Reflective of adult population; not specific for elderly)

1% to 10%: Dermatologic: Skin atrophy, shininess, thinness, mild telangiectasia

Drug Interactions No data reported

Mechanism of Action Topical corticosteroids have anti-inflammatory, antipruritic, vasoconstrictive, and antiproliferative actions

Dosage

Geriatrics & Adults: Steroid-responsive dermatoses: Topical: Apply a thin film to affected area twice daily. Therapy should be discontinued when control is achieved; if no improvement is seen, reassessment of diagnosis may be necessary.

Monitoring Parameters Relief of symptoms

Patient Information Use only as prescribed and for no longer than the period prescribed; apply sparingly in a thin film and rub in lightly; avoid contact with eyes; notify physician if condition persists or worsens

Additional Information Considered a moderate-potency steroid; has been shown that the atrophic activity of prednicarbate is many times less than agents with similar clinical potency, nevertheless, avoid prolonged use on the face

Special Geriatric Considerations Due to age-related changes in skin, limit use of topical corticosteroids.

Dosage Forms Excipient information presented when available (limited, particularly for generics); consult specific product labeling.

Cream: 0.1% (15 g, 60 g)
Dermatop®: 0.1% (15 g, 60 g)
Ointment:
Dermatop®: 0.1% (15 g, 60 g)

Selected References
Rumbaugh MM, "High Potency Topical Corticosteroids," *U.S. Pharmacist*, 1993, 18(6):30-41.

PrednisoLONE (pred NISS oh lone)

Related Information
Corticosteroids *on page 1755*

Medication Safety Issues
Sound-alike/look-alike issues:
PrednisoLONE may be confused with predniSONE
Pediapred® may be confused with Pediazole®

U.S. Brand Names Econopred® Plus; Orapred®; Orapred ODT™; Pediapred®; Pred Forte®; Pred Mild®; Prelone®

Canadian Brand Names Diopred®; Hydeltra T.B.A.®; Inflamase® Mild; Novo-Prednisolone; Ophtho-Tate®; Pediapred®; Pred Forte®; Pred Mild®; Sab-Prenase

Index Terms Deltahydrocortisone; Metacortandralone; Prednisolone Acetate; Prednisolone Acetate, Ophthalmic; Prednisolone Sodium Phosphate; Prednisolone Sodium Phosphate, Ophthalmic

Generic Available Yes

Pharmacologic Category Corticosteroid, Ophthalmic; Corticosteroid, Systemic

Use Treatment of palpebral and bulbar conjunctivitis; corneal injury from chemical, radiation, thermal burns, or foreign body penetration; endocrine disorders, rheumatic disorders, collagen diseases, dermatologic diseases, allergic states, ophthalmic diseases, respiratory diseases, hematologic disorders, neoplastic diseases, edematous states, and gastrointestinal diseases; resolution of acute exacerbations of multiple sclerosis; management of fulminating or disseminated tuberculosis and trichinosis; acute or chronic solid organ rejection

Contraindications Hypersensitivity to prednisolone or any component of the formulation; acute superficial herpes simplex keratitis; live or attenuated virus vaccines; systemic fungal infections; varicella

Warnings/Precautions May cause hypercorticism or suppression of hypothalamic-pituitary-adrenal (HPA) axis, particularly in patients receiving high doses for prolonged periods. HPA axis suppression may lead to adrenal crisis. Withdrawal and discontinuation of a corticosteroid should be done slowly and carefully. Particular care is required when patients are transferred from systemic corticosteroids to inhaled products due to possible adrenal insufficiency or withdrawal from steroids, including an increase in allergic symptoms. Patients receiving >20 mg per day of prednisone (or equivalent) may be most susceptible. Fatalities have occurred due to adrenal insufficiency in asthmatic patients during and after transfer from systemic corticosteroids to aerosol steroids; aerosol steroids do **not** provide the systemic steroid needed to treat patients having trauma, surgery, or infections.

Acute myopathy has been reported with high dose corticosteroids, usually in patients with neuromuscular transmission disorders; may involve ocular and/or respiratory muscles; monitor creatine kinase; recovery may be delayed. Corticosteroid use may cause psychiatric disturbances, including depression, euphoria, insomnia, mood swings, and personality changes. Pre-existing psychiatric conditions may be exacerbated by corticosteroid use. Prolonged use of corticosteroids may also increase the incidence of secondary infection, mask acute infection (including fungal infections), prolong or exacerbate viral infections, or limit response to vaccines. Exposure to chickenpox should be avoided; corticosteroids should not be used to treat ocular herpes simplex. Corticosteroids should not be used for cerebral malaria. Close observation is required in patients with latent tuberculosis and/or TB reactivity; restrict use in (Continued)

PrednisoLONE *(Continued)*

active TB (only in conjunction with antituberculosis treatment). Prolonged use of corticosteroids may result in glaucoma; damage to the optic nerve (not indicated for treatment of optic neuritis), defects in visual acuity and fields of vision, and posterior subcapsular cataract formation may occur. Use following cataract surgery may delay healing or increase the incidence of bleb formation. Prolonged treatment with corticosteroids has been associated with the development of Kaposi's sarcoma (case reports); if noted, discontinuation of therapy should be considered.

Use with caution in patients with thyroid disease, hepatic impairment, renal impairment, cardiovascular disease, diabetes, glaucoma, cataracts, myasthenia gravis, patients at risk for osteoporosis, patients at risk for seizures, or GI diseases (diverticulitis, peptic ulcer, ulcerative colitis) due to perforation risk. Use caution following acute MI (corticosteroids have been associated with myocardial rupture). Because of the risk of adverse effects, systemic corticosteroids should be used cautiously in the elderly in the smallest possible effective dose for the shortest duration. Do not use occlusive dressings on weeping or exudative lesions and general caution with occlusive dressings should be observed; adverse effects may be increased. Discontinue if skin irritation or contact dermatitis should occur; do not use in patients with decreased skin circulation. Withdraw therapy with gradual tapering of dose.

Adverse Reactions (Reflective of adult population; not specific for elderly)
Frequency not defined.
Ophthalmic formulation:
  Endocrine & metabolic: Hypercorticoidism (rare)
  Ocular: Conjunctival hyperemia, conjunctivitis, corneal ulcers, delayed wound healing, glaucoma, intraocular pressure increased, keratitis, loss of accommodation, optic nerve damage, mydriasis, posterior subcapsular cataract formation, ptosis, secondary ocular infection
Oral formulation:
  Cardiovascular: Cardiomyopathy, CHF, edema, facial edema, hypertension
  Central nervous system: Convulsions, headache, insomnia, malaise, nervousness, pseudotumor cerebri, psychic disorders, vertigo
  Dermatologic: Bruising, facial erythema, hirsutism, petechiae, skin test reaction suppression, thin fragile skin, urticaria
  Endocrine & metabolic: Carbohydrate tolerance decreased, Cushing's syndrome, diabetes mellitus, growth suppression, hyperglycemia, hypernatremia, hypokalemia, hypokalemic alkalosis, menstrual irregularities, negative nitrogen balance, pituitary adrenal axis suppression
  Gastrointestinal: Abdominal distention, increased appetite, indigestion, nausea, pancreatitis, peptic ulcer, ulcerative esophagitis, weight gain
  Hepatic: LFTs increased (usually reversible)
  Neuromuscular & skeletal: Arthralgia, aseptic necrosis (humeral/femoral heads), fractures, muscle mass decreased, muscle weakness, osteoporosis, steroid myopathy, tendon rupture, weakness
  Ocular: Cataracts, exophthalmus, eyelid edema, glaucoma, intraocular pressure increased, irritation
  Respiratory: Epistaxis
  Miscellaneous: Diaphoresis increased, impaired wound healing

Overdosage/Toxicology When consumed in excessive quantities for prolonged periods, systemic hypercorticism and adrenal suppression may occur; in those cases, discontinuation and withdrawal of the corticosteroid should be done judiciously.

Drug Interactions Substrate of CYP3A4 (minor); **Inhibits** CYP3A4 (weak)

Aminoglutethimide: May reduce the serum levels/effects of corticosteroids; likely via induction of microsomal isoenzymes.
Amphotericin: Corticosteroids may increase the hypokalemic effects of amphotericin B; monitor.
Antacids: May decrease the absorption of corticosteroids; separate administration by 2 hours.
Anticholinesterases: Concurrent use may lead to severe weakness in patients with myasthenia gravis.
Antidiabetic agents: Corticosteroids may decrease the hypoglycemic effects of antidiabetic agents; monitor.
Aprepitant: May increase the serum levels/effects of corticosteroids; monitor.
Antifungal agents (azole): May increase the serum levels/effects of corticosteroids; monitor.
Barbiturates: May decrease the levels/effects of corticosteroids.
Bile acid sequestrants: May reduce the absorption of corticosteroids; separate administration by 2 hours.
Calcium channel blockers (nondihydropyridine): May increase the serum levels/effects of corticosteroids; monitor.

Cyclosporine: Corticosteroids may increase the serum levels/effects of cyclosporine. In addition, cyclosporine may increase levels of corticosteroids.

Diuretics, potassium-wasting (loop or thiazide): Hypokalemic effects may be increased by corticosteroids; monitor.

Estrogens: May increase the serum levels/effects of corticosteroids; monitor.

Fluoroquinolones: Concurrent use may increase the risk of tendinopathies (including tendonitis and rupture), particularly in elderly patients (overall incidence rare)

Isoniazid: Serum levels/effects may be decreased by corticosteroids.

Ketoconazole: May decrease metabolism of certain corticosteroids leading to increased levels (up to 60%) and increased risk of adverse effects; monitor.

Macrolide antibiotics: May increase the serum levels/effects of corticosteroids.

Neuromuscular-blocking agents: Concurrent use with corticosteroids may increase the risk of myopathy.

Nonsteroidal anti-inflammatory drugs (NSAIDs): Concurrent use with corticosteroids may lead to an increased incidence of gastrointestinal adverse effects; use caution. NSAID (ophthalmic) may enhance the adverse/toxic effect of prednisolone (ophthalmic).

Rifamycin derivatives: May decrease the levels/effects of corticosteroids (systemic); monitor.

Salicylates: Salicylates may increase the gastrointestinal adverse effects of corticosteroids.

Vaccine (dead organism): Corticosteroids may decrease the effect of vaccines (dead organisms). In patients receiving high doses of systemic corticosteroids for ≥14 days, wait at least 1 month between discontinuing steroid therapy and administering immunization.

Vaccine (live organism): Corticosteroids may increase the risk of vaccinal infection. The use of live vaccines is contraindicated in immunosuppressed patients.

Warfarin: Corticosteroids may increase the anticoagulant effects of warfarin; monitor INR.

Ethanol/Nutrition/Herb Interactions
Ethanol: Avoid ethanol (may increase gastric mucosal irritation).
Food: Prednisolone interferes with calcium absorption. Limit caffeine.
Herb/Nutraceutical: St John's wort may decrease prednisolone levels. Avoid cat's claw, echinacea (have immunostimulant properties).

Stability Store Orapred ODT™ at 20°C to 25°C (68°F to 77°F) in blister pack. Protect from moisture.

Mechanism of Action Decreases inflammation by suppression of migration of polymorphonuclear leukocytes and reversal of increased capillary permeability; suppresses the immune system by reducing activity and volume of the lymphatic system

Pharmacokinetics
Half-life: 3.6 hours; biologic: 18-36 hours
Protein binding: 65% to 91% (concentration dependent); decreased in elderly. However, the elderly subjects still had higher AUCs of cortisol, suggesting a decreased sensitivity to suppression of endogenous cortisol compared to younger adults. Plasma prednisolone concentrations were higher in elderly subjects. Elderly subjects had higher AUCs for total and unbound prednisolone.
Metabolism: Primarily in the liver, but also metabolized in most tissues, to inactive compounds
Elimination: In urine principally as glucuronides, sulfates, and unconjugated metabolites

Dosage
Geriatrics: Use lowest effective adult dose. Dose depends upon condition being treated and response of patient; alternate day dosing may be attempted in some disease states.

Adults: Dose depends upon condition being treated and response of patient. Consider alternate day therapy for long-term therapy. Discontinuation of long-term therapy requires gradual withdrawal by tapering the dose. Patients undergoing unusual stress while receiving corticosteroids, should receive increased doses prior to, during, and after the stressful situation.

Usual dose (range): Oral: 5-60 mg/day
Rheumatoid arthritis: Oral: Initial: 5-7.5 mg/day, adjust dose as necessary
Multiple sclerosis: Oral: 200 mg/day for 1 week followed by 80 mg every other day for 1 month
Conjunctivitis: Ophthalmic (suspension/solution): Instill 1-2 drops into conjunctival sac every hour during day, every 2 hours at night until favorable response is obtained, then use 1 drop every 4 hours.
Dosing adjustment in hyperthyroidism: Prednisolone dose may need to be increased to achieve adequate therapeutic effects.
Renal Impairment: Slightly dialyzable (5% to 20%)

Administration Administer oral formulation with food or milk to decrease GI effects.
(Continued)

PrednisoLONE *(Continued)*

Orapred ODT™: Do not break or use partial tablet. Remove tablet from blister pack just prior to use. May swallow whole or allow to dissolve on tongue.

Monitoring Parameters Blood pressure; blood glucose, electrolytes; intraocular pressure (use >6 weeks); bone mineral density

Test Interactions Response to skin tests

Patient Information Take oral form after meals or with food or milk; do not abruptly discontinue if on long-term therapy; carry an identification card or bracelet advising that you are on steroids; notify physician of any signs of infection

Additional Information Withdrawal/tapering of therapy: Corticosteroid tapering following short-term use is limited primarily by the need to control the underlying disease state; tapering may be accomplished over a period of days. Following longer-term use, tapering over weeks to months may be necessary to avoid signs and symptoms of adrenal insufficiency and to allow recovery of the HPA axis. Testing of HPA axis responsiveness may be of value in selected patients. Subtle deficits in HPA response may persist for months after discontinuation of therapy, and may require supplemental dosing during periods of acute illness or surgical stress.

Special Geriatric Considerations Useful in patients with inability to activate prednisone (liver disease). Because of the risk of adverse effects, systemic corticosteroids should be used cautiously in the elderly, in the smallest possible dose, and for the shortest possible time. For long-term use, monitor bone mineral density and institute fracture prevention strategies.

Dosage Forms Excipient information presented when available (limited, particularly for generics); consult specific product labeling.

Solution, ophthalmic, as sodium phosphate: 1% (5 mL, 10 mL, 15 mL) [contains benzalkonium chloride]

Solution, oral, as sodium phosphate: Prednisolone base 5 mg/5 mL (120 mL)
Orapred®: 20 mg/5 mL (20 mL, 240 mL) [equivalent to prednisolone base 15 mg/5 mL; dye free; contains alcohol 2%, sodium benzoate; grape flavor]
Pediapred®: 6.7 mg/5 mL (120 mL) [equivalent to prednisolone base 5 mg/5 mL; dye free; raspberry flavor]

Suspension, ophthalmic, as acetate: 1% (5 mL, 10 mL, 15 mL)
Econopred® Plus: 1% (5 mL, 10 mL) [contains benzalkonium chloride]
Pred Forte®: 1% (1 mL, 5 mL, 10 mL, 15 mL) [contains benzalkonium chloride and sodium bisulfite]
Pred Mild®: 0.12% (5 mL, 10 mL) [contains benzalkonium chloride and sodium bisulfite]

Syrup, as base: 5 mg/5 mL (120 mL); 15 mg/5 mL (240 mL, 480 mL)
Prelone®: 15 mg/5 mL (240 mL, 480 mL) [contains alcohol 5%, benzoic acid; cherry flavor]

Tablet, as base: 5 mg

Tablet, orally disintegrating, as base:
Orapred ODT™: 10 mg, 15 mg, 30 mg [grape flavor]

♦ **Prednisolone Acetate** *see* PrednisoLONE *on page 1303*
♦ **Prednisolone Acetate, Ophthalmic** *see* PrednisoLONE *on page 1303*

Prednisolone and Gentamicin (pred NIS oh lone & jen ta MYE sin)

Related Information
Gentamicin *on page 705*
PrednisoLONE *on page 1303*

U.S. Brand Names Pred-G®

Index Terms Gentamicin and Prednisolone

Generic Available No

Pharmacologic Category Antibiotic/Corticosteroid, Ophthalmic

Use Treatment of steroid responsive inflammatory conditions and superficial ocular infections due to microorganisms susceptible to gentamicin

Dosage
Geriatrics & Adults: Inflammatory conditions and superficial ocular infections:
Ophthalmic:
Ointment: Apply ½ inch ribbon in the conjunctival sac 1-3 times/day
Suspension: 1 drop 2-4 times/day; during the initial 24-48 hours, the dosing frequency may be increased if necessary up to 1 drop every hour

Special Geriatric Considerations No specific recommendations for use in the elderly necessary.

Dosage Forms Excipient information presented when available (limited, particularly for generics); consult specific product labeling.
Ointment, ophthalmic:
Pred-G®: Prednisolone acetate 0.6% and gentamicin sulfate 0.3% (3.5 g)

Suspension, ophthalmic:
Pred-G®: Prednisolone acetate 1% and gentamicin sulfate 0.3% (5 mL, 10 mL) [contains benzalkonium chloride]

♦ **Prednisolone and Sulfacetamide** *see* Sulfacetamide and Prednisolone *on page 1497*
♦ **Prednisolone Sodium Phosphate** *see* PrednisoLONE *on page 1303*
♦ **Prednisolone Sodium Phosphate, Ophthalmic** *see* PrednisoLONE *on page 1303*

PredniSONE (PRED ni sone)

Related Information
Corticosteroids *on page 1755*

Medication Safety Issues
Sound-alike/look-alike issues:
PredniSONE may be confused with methylPREDNISolone, Pramosone®, prazosin, prednisoLONE, Prilosec®, primidone, promethazine

U.S. Brand Names Prednisone Intensol™; Sterapred®; Sterapred® DS

Canadian Brand Names Apo-Prednisone®; Novo-Prednisone; Winpred™

Index Terms Deltacortisone; Deltadehydrocortisone

Generic Available Yes

Pharmacologic Category Corticosteroid, Systemic

Use Treatment of adrenocortical insufficiency, hypercalcemia, rheumatic and collagen disorders, and a variety of diseases including those of hematologic, allergic, inflammatory, dermatologic, ocular, respiratory, gastrointestinal, neoplastic, and autoimmune origin; organ transplantation

Unlabeled/Investigational Use Investigational: Prevention of postherpetic neuralgia and relief of acute pain in the early stages

Contraindications Hypersensitivity to prednisone or any component of the formulation; serious infections, except tuberculous meningitis; systemic fungal infections; varicella

Warnings/Precautions May cause hypercorticism or suppression of hypothalamic-pituitary-adrenal (HPA) axis, particularly in patients receiving high doses for prolonged periods. HPA axis suppression may lead to adrenal crisis. Withdrawal and discontinuation of a corticosteroid should be done slowly and carefully. Particular care is required when patients are transferred from systemic corticosteroids to inhaled products due to possible adrenal insufficiency or withdrawal from steroids, including an increase in allergic symptoms. Patients receiving >20 mg per day of prednisone (or equivalent) may be most susceptible. Fatalities have occurred due to adrenal insufficiency in asthmatic patients during and after transfer from systemic corticosteroids to aerosol steroids; aerosol steroids do **not** provide the systemic steroid needed to treat patients having trauma, surgery, or infections.

Acute myopathy has been reported with high dose corticosteroids, usually in patients with neuromuscular transmission disorders; may involve ocular and/or respiratory muscles; monitor creatine kinase; recovery may be delayed. Corticosteroid use may cause psychiatric disturbances, including depression, euphoria, insomnia, mood swings, and personality changes. Pre-existing psychiatric conditions may be exacerbated by corticosteroid use. Prolonged use of corticosteroids may also increase the incidence of secondary infection, mask acute infection (including fungal infections), prolong or exacerbate viral infections, or limit response to vaccines. Exposure to chickenpox should be avoided; corticosteroids should not be used to treat ocular herpes simplex. Corticosteroids should not be used for cerebral malaria. Close observation is required in patients with latent tuberculosis and/or TB reactivity; restrict use in active TB (only in conjunction with antituberculosis treatment). Prolonged treatment with corticosteroids has been associated with the development of Kaposi's sarcoma (case reports); if noted, discontinuation of therapy should be considered.

Use with caution in patients with thyroid disease, hepatic impairment, renal impairment, cardiovascular disease, diabetes, glaucoma, cataracts, myasthenia gravis, patients at risk for osteoporosis, patients at risk for seizures, or GI diseases (diverticulitis, peptic ulcer, ulcerative colitis) due to perforation risk. Use caution following acute MI (corticosteroids have been associated with myocardial rupture). Because of the risk of adverse effects, systemic corticosteroids should be used cautiously in the elderly in the smallest possible effective dose for the shortest duration. Withdraw therapy with gradual tapering of dose.

Adverse Reactions (Reflective of adult population; not specific for elderly)
>10%:
Central nervous system: Insomnia, nervousness
Gastrointestinal: Increased appetite, indigestion
1% to 10%:
Dermatologic: Hirsutism
Endocrine & metabolic: Diabetes mellitus, glucose intolerance, hyperglycemia
Neuromuscular & skeletal: Arthralgia
(Continued)

PredniSONE *(Continued)*

Ocular: Cataracts, glaucoma

Respiratory: Epistaxis

Overdosage/Toxicology When consumed in excessive quantities for prolonged periods, systemic hypercorticism and adrenal suppression may occur; in those cases, discontinuation and withdrawal of the corticosteroid should be done judiciously.

Drug Interactions Substrate of CYP3A4 (minor); **Induces** CYP2C19 (weak), 3A4 (weak)

Aminoglutethimide: May reduce the serum levels/effects of corticosteroids; likely via induction of microsomal isoenzymes.

Amphotericin: Corticosteroids may increase the hypokalemic effects of amphotericin B; monitor.

Antacids: May decrease the absorption of corticosteroids; separate administration by 2 hours.

Anticholinesterases: Concurrent use may lead to severe weakness in patients with myasthenia gravis.

Antidiabetic agents: Corticosteroids may decrease the hypoglycemic effects of antidiabetic agents; monitor.

Aprepitant: May increase the serum levels/effects of corticosteroids; monitor.

Antifungal agents (azole): May increase the serum levels/effects of corticosteroids; monitor.

Barbiturates: May decrease the levels/effects of corticosteroids.

Bile acid sequestrants: May reduce the absorption of corticosteroids; separate administration by 2 hours.

Calcium channel blockers (nondihydropyridine): May increase the serum levels/effects of corticosteroids; monitor.

Cyclosporine: Corticosteroids may increase the serum levels/effects of cyclosporine. In addition, cyclosporine may increase levels of corticosteroids.

Diuretics, potassium-wasting (loop or thiazide): Hypokalemic effects may be increased by corticosteroids; monitor.

Estrogens: May increase the serum levels/effects of corticosteroids; monitor.

Fluoroquinolones: Concurrent use may increase the risk of tendinopathies (including tendonitis and rupture), particularly in elderly patients (overall incidence rare)

Isoniazid: Serum levels/effects may be decreased by corticosteroids.

Macrolide antibiotics: May increase the serum levels/effects of corticosteroids.

Neuromuscular-blocking agents: Concurrent use with corticosteroids may increase the risk of myopathy.

Nonsteroidal anti-inflammatory drugs (NSAIDs): Concurrent use with corticosteroids may lead to an increased incidence of gastrointestinal adverse effects; use caution.

Rifamycin derivatives: May decrease the levels/effects of corticosteroids (systemic); monitor.

Salicylates: Salicylates may increase the gastrointestinal adverse effects of corticosteroids.

Vaccine (dead organism): Corticosteroids may decrease the effect of vaccines (dead organisms). In patients receiving high doses of systemic corticosteroids for ≥14 days, wait at least 1 month between discontinuing steroid therapy and administering immunization.

Vaccine (live organism): Corticosteroids may increase the risk of vaccinal infection. The use of live vaccines is contraindicated in immunosuppressed patients.

Warfarin: Corticosteroids may increase the anticoagulant effects of warfarin; monitor INR.

Ethanol/Nutrition/Herb Interactions

Ethanol: Avoid ethanol (may increase gastric mucosal irritation)

Food: Prednisone interferes with calcium absorption. Limit caffeine.

Herb/Nutraceutical: St John's wort may decrease prednisone levels. Avoid cat's claw, echinacea (have immunostimulant properties).

Mechanism of Action Decreases inflammation by suppression of migration of polymorphonuclear leukocytes and reversal of increased capillary permeability; suppresses the immune system by reducing activity and volume of the lymphatic system; suppresses adrenal function at high doses. Antitumor effects may be related to inhibition of glucose transport, phosphorylation, or induction of cell death in immature lymphocytes. Antiemetic effects are thought to occur due to blockade of cerebral innervation of the emetic center via inhibition of prostaglandin synthesis.

Pharmacokinetics Converted rapidly to prednisolone in the liver (active). See PrednisoLONE *on page 1303* for full kinetic information.

Dosage

Geriatrics: Refer to adult dosing; use the lowest effective dose. Oral dose depends upon condition being treated and response of patient. Alternate day dosing may be attempted.

Adults: Dose depends upon condition being treated and response of patient; consider alternate day therapy for long-term therapy. Discontinuation of long-term therapy requires gradual withdrawal by tapering the dose.

Physiologic replacement: Oral: 4-5 mg/m^2/day

Immunosuppression/chemotherapy adjunct: Oral: Range: 5-60 mg/day in divided doses 1-4 times/day

Allergic reaction (contact dermatitis): Oral:

Day 1: 30 mg divided as 10 mg before breakfast, 5 mg at lunch, 5 mg at dinner, 10 mg at bedtime

Day 2: 5 mg at breakfast, 5 mg at lunch, 5 mg at dinner, 10 mg at bedtime

Day 3: 5 mg 4 times/day (with meals and at bedtime)

Day 4: 5 mg 3 times/day (breakfast, lunch, bedtime)

Day 5: 5 mg 2 times/day (breakfast, bedtime)

Day 6: 5 mg before breakfast

Acute asthma: 1-2 mg/kg/day in divided doses 1-2 times/day for 3-5 days

Asthma maintenance:

Moderate persistent: Inhaled corticosteroid (medium dose) or inhaled corticosteroid (low-medium dose) with a long-acting bronchodilator

Severe persistent: Inhaled corticosteroid (high dose) and corticosteroid tablets or syrup long term: 2 mg/kg/day, generally not to exceed 60 mg/day

Pneumonia due to *Pneumocystis carinii*: Oral:

40 mg twice daily for 5 days **followed by**

40 mg once daily for 5 days **followed by**

20 mg once daily for 11 days or until antimicrobial regimen is completed

Thyrotoxicosis: Oral: 60 mg/day

Note: Dosing adjustment in hyperthyroidism: Prednisone dose may need to be increased to achieve adequate therapeutic effects

Chemotherapy (refer to individual protocols): Oral: Range: 20 mg/day to 100 mg/m^2/day

Rheumatoid arthritis: Oral: Use lowest possible daily dose (often ≤7.5 mg/day)

Idiopathic thrombocytopenia purpura (ITP): Oral: 60 mg daily for 4-6 weeks, gradually tapered over several weeks

Systemic lupus erythematosus (SLE): Oral:

Acute: 1-2 mg/kg/day in 2-3 divided doses

Maintenance: Reduce to lowest possible dose, usually <1 mg/kg/day as single dose (morning)

Renal Impairment: Hemodialysis effects: Supplemental dose is not necessary.

Monitoring Parameters Blood pressure, blood glucose, electrolytes, symptoms of fluid retention

Test Interactions Response to skin tests

Patient Information Take with food or milk or after meals; do not discontinue or decrease the drug without contacting your physician; carry an identification card or bracelet advising that you are on steroids; notify physician if signs of infection occur

Additional Information Not available in injectable form, prednisolone must be used.

Withdrawal/tapering of therapy: Corticosteroid tapering following short-term use is limited primarily by the need to control the underlying disease state; tapering may be accomplished over a period of days. Following longer-term use, tapering over weeks to months may be necessary to avoid signs and symptoms of adrenal insufficiency and to allow recovery of the HPA axis. Testing of HPA axis responsiveness may be of value in selected patients. Subtle deficits in HPA response may persist for months after discontinuation of therapy, and may require supplemental dosing during periods of acute illness or surgical stress.

Special Geriatric Considerations Because of the risk of adverse effects, systemic corticosteroids should be used cautiously in the elderly, in the smallest possible dose, and for the shortest possible time.

Dosage Forms Excipient information presented when available (limited, particularly for generics); consult specific product labeling.

Solution, oral: 1 mg/mL (5 mL, 120 mL, 500 mL) [contains alcohol 5%, sodium benzoate; vanilla flavor]

Solution, oral concentrate (Prednisone Intensol™): 5 mg/mL (30 mL) [contains alcohol 30%]

Tablet: 1 mg, 2.5 mg, 5 mg, 10 mg, 20 mg, 50 mg

Sterapred®: 5 mg [supplied as 21 tablet 6-day unit-dose package or 48 tablet 12-day unit-dose package]

Sterapred® DS: 10 mg [supplied as 21 tablet 6-day unit-dose package or 48 tablet 12-day unit-dose package]

♦ **Prednisone Intensol**™ *see* PredniSONE *on page 1307*

♦ **Prefest**™ *see* Estradiol and Norgestimate *on page 554*

Pregabalin (pre GAB a lin)

U.S. Brand Names Lyrica®
Canadian Brand Names Lyrica®
Index Terms CI-1008; S-(+)-3-isobutylgaba
Generic Available No
Pharmacologic Category Analgesic, Miscellaneous; Anticonvulsant, Miscellaneous
Use Management of pain associated with diabetic peripheral neuropathy; management of postherpetic neuralgia; adjunctive therapy for partial-onset seizure disorder in adults; management of fibromyalgia
Restrictions C-V
Contraindications Hypersensitivity to pregabalin or any component of the formulation
Warnings/Precautions Angioedema has been reported; may be life threatening; use with caution in patients with a history of angioedema episodes. Concurrent use with other drugs known to cause angioedema (eg, ACE inhibitors) may increase risk. Hypersensitivity reactions, including skin redness, blistering, hives, rash, dyspnea and wheezing have been reported; discontinue treatment of hypersensitivity occurs. May cause CNS depression and/or dizziness, which may impair physical or mental abilities. Patients must be cautioned about performing tasks which require mental alertness (eg, operating machinery or driving). Effects with other sedative drugs or ethanol may be potentiated. Visual disturbances (blurred vision, decreased acuity and visual field changes) have been associated with pregabalin therapy; patients should be instructed to notify their physician if these effects are noted.

Pregabalin has been associated with increases in CPK and rare cases of rhabdomyolysis. Patients should be instructed to notify their prescriber if unexplained muscle pain, tenderness, or weakness, particularly if fever and/or malaise are associated with these symptoms. Use may be associated with weight gain and peripheral edema; use caution in patients with congestive heart failure, hypertension, or diabetes. Effect on weight gain/edema may be additive to thiazolidinedione antidiabetic agent; particularly in patients with prior cardiovascular disease. May decrease platelet count or prolong PR interval.

Has been noted to be tumorigenic (increased incidence of hemangiosarcoma) in animal studies; significance of these findings in humans is unknown. Pregabalin has been associated with discontinuation symptoms following abrupt cessation, and increases in seizure frequency (when used as an antiepileptic) may occur. Should not be discontinued abruptly; dosage tapering over at least 1 week is recommended. Use caution in renal impairment; dosage adjustment required.

Adverse Reactions (Reflective of adult population; not specific for elderly)
Note: Frequency of adverse effects may be influenced by dose or concurrent therapy. In add-on trials in epilepsy, frequency of CNS and visual adverse effects were higher than those reported in pain management trials. Range noted below is inclusive of all trials.
>10%:
  Cardiovascular: Peripheral edema (up to 16%)
  Central nervous system: Dizziness (8% to 45%), somnolence (4% to 28%), ataxia (up to 20%), headache (up to 14%)
  Gastrointestinal: Weight gain (up to 16%), xerostomia (1% to 15%)
  Neuromuscular & skeletal: Tremor (up to 11%)
  Ocular: Blurred vision (1% to 12%), diplopia (up to 12%)
  Miscellaneous: Infection (up to 14%), accidental injury (2% to 11%)
1% to 10%:
  Cardiovascular: Chest pain (up to 4%), edema (up to 6%)
  Central nervous system: Neuropathy (up to 9%), thinking abnormal (up to 9%), fatigue (up to 8%), confusion (up to 7%), euphoria (up to 7%), speech disorder (up to 7%), attention disturbance (up to 6%), incoordination (up to 6%), amnesia (up to 6%), pain (up to 5%), memory impaired (up to 4%), vertigo (up to 4%), feeling abnormal (up to 3%), hypoesthesia (up to 3%), anxiety (up to 2%), depression (up to 2%), disorientation (up to 2%), lethargy (up to 2%), fever (≥1%), depersonalization (≥1%), hypertonia (≥1%), stupor (≥1%), nervousness (up to 1%)
  Dermatologic: Facial edema (up to 3%), bruising (≥1%), pruritus (≥1%)
  Endocrine & metabolic: Fluid retention (up to 3%), hypoglycemia (up to 3%), libido decreased (≥1%)
  Gastrointestinal: Constipation (up to 10%), appetite increased (up to 7%), flatulence (up to 3%), vomiting (up to 3%), abdominal distension (up to 2%), abdominal pain (≥1%), gastroenteritis (≥1%)
  Genitourinary: Incontinence (up to 2%), anorgasmia (≥1%), impotence (≥1%), urinary frequency (≥1%)
  Hematologic: Thrombocytopenia (3%)

Neuromuscular & skeletal: Balance disorder (up to 9%), abnormal gait (up to 8%), weakness (up to 7%), arthralgia (up to 6%), twitching (up to 5%), back pain (up to 4%), muscle spasm (up to 4%), myoclonus (up to 4%), paresthesia (>2%), CPK increased (2%), leg cramps (≥1%), myalgia (≥1%), myasthenia (up to 1%)

Ocular: Visual abnormalities (up to 5%), visual field defect (≥2%), eye disorder (up to 2%), nystagmus (>2%), conjunctivitis (≥1%)

Otic: Otitis media (≥1%), tinnitus (≥1%)

Respiratory: Sinusitis (up to 7%), dyspnea (up to 3%), bronchitis (up to 3%), pharyngolaryngeal pain (up to 3%)

Miscellaneous: Flu-like syndrome (up to 2%), allergic reaction (≥1%)

Overdosage/Toxicology Symptoms are similar to those experienced at therapeutic doses (somnolence). Treatment is symptom-directed and supportive. A 4-hour hemodialysis procedure reduces plasma concentrations by ~50%.

Drug Interactions

CNS depressants: Sedative effects may be additive with CNS depressants; includes ethanol, barbiturates, opioid analgesics, and other sedative agents; monitor for increased effect.

Thiazolidinediones: Pregabalin's effect on weight gain/edema may be additive with thiazolidinedione antidiabetic agents (includes pioglitazone, rosiglitazone).

Ethanol/Nutrition/Herb Interactions

Ethanol: Avoid ethanol (may increase CNS depression).

Herb/Nutraceutical: Avoid valerian, St John's wort, kava kava, gotu kola (may increase CNS depression).

Stability Store at 15°C to 30°C (59°F to 86°F).

Mechanism of Action Binds to alpha₂-delta subunit of voltage-gated calcium channels within the CNS, inhibiting excitatory neurotransmitter release. Although structurally related to GABA, it does not bind to GABA or benzodiazepine receptors. Exerts antinociceptive and anticonvulsant activity. Decreases symptoms of painful peripheral neuropathies and, as adjunctive therapy in partial seizures, decreases the frequency of seizures.

Pharmacokinetics

Onset: Pain management: Effects may be noted as early as the first week of therapy.

Distribution: V_d: 0.5 L/kg

Protein binding: 0%

Metabolism: Negligible

Bioavailability: >90%

Half-life elimination: 6.3 hours

Time to peak, plasma: 1.5 hours (3 hours with food)

Excretion: Urine (90% as unchanged drug; minor metabolites)

Pregabalin Renal Impairment Dosing

Cl_{cr} (mL/ minute)	Total Pregabalin Daily Dose (mg/day)				Dosing Frequency
≥60	150	300	450	600	2-3 divided doses
30-60	75	150	225	300	2-3 divided doses
15-30	25-50	75	100-150	150	1-2 divided doses
<15	25	25-50	50-75	75	single daily dose

Posthemodialysis supplementary dosage (as a single additional dose):
25 mg/day schedule: Single supplementary dose of 25 mg **or** 50 mg
25-50 mg/day schedule: Single supplementary dose of 50 mg **or** 75 mg
50-75 mg/day schedule: Single supplementary dose of 75 mg **or** 100 mg
75 mg/day schedule: Single supplementary dose of 100 mg **or** 150 mg

Dosage

Geriatrics & Adults:

Fibromyalgia: Oral: Initial: 150 mg/day in divided doses (75 mg 2 times/day); may be increased to 300 mg/day (150 mg 2 times/day) within 1 week based on tolerability and effect; may be further increased to 450 mg/day (225 mg 2 times/day). Maximum dose: 450 mg/day (dosages up to 600 mg/day were evaluated with no significant additional benefit and an increase in adverse effects)

Neuropathic pain (diabetes-associated): Oral: Initial: 150 mg/day in divided doses (50 mg 3 times/day); may be increased within 1 week based on tolerability and effect; maximum dose: 300 mg/day (dosages up to 600 mg/day were evaluated with no significant additional benefit and an increase in adverse effects)

Postherpetic neuralgia: Oral: Initial: 150 mg/day in divided doses (75 mg 2 times/day or 50 mg 3 times/day); may be increased to 300 mg/day within 1 week based

(Continued)

Pregabalin *(Continued)*

on tolerability and effect; further titration (to 600 mg/day) after 2-4 weeks may be considered in patients who do not experience sufficient relief of pain provided they are able to tolerate pregabalin. Maximum dose: 600 mg/day

Partial onset seizures (adjunctive therapy): Oral: Initial: 150 mg per day in divided doses (75 mg 2 times/day or 50 mg 3 times/day); may be increased based on tolerability and effect (optimal titration schedule has not been defined). Maximum dose: 600 mg/day

Note: Discontinuing therapy: Pregabalin should not be abruptly discontinued; taper dosage over at least 1 week

Renal Impairment: See table on previous page.

Administration May be administered with or without food.

Monitoring Parameters Measures of efficacy (pain intensity/seizure frequency); degree of sedation; symptoms of myopathy or ocular disturbance; weight gain/edema; CPK; skin integrity (in diabetic patients).

Patient Information Do not discontinue use abruptly. Pregabalin should be tapered gradually over a minimum of 1 week.

Special Geriatric Considerations In clinical studies, no differences in safety and efficacy were noted between elderly. Since pregabalin is primarily excreted renally, dosage adjustment, based on Cl_{cr}, is necessary.

Dosage Forms Excipient information presented when available (limited, particularly for generics); consult specific product labeling.

Capsule:
Lyrica®: 25 mg, 50 mg, 75 mg, 100 mg, 150 mg, 200 mg, 225 mg, 300 mg

Selected References

Hill CM, Balkenohl M, Thomas DW, et al, "Pregabalin in Patients With Postoperative Dental Pain," *Eur J Pain*, 2001, 5(2):119-24.

Primidone *(PRI mi done)*

Related Information

Serum Drug Concentrations Commonly Monitored Guidelines *on page 1862*

Medication Safety Issues

Sound-alike/look-alike issues:
Primidone may be confused with predniSONE

U.S. Brand Names Mysoline®

Canadian Brand Names Apo-Primidone®

Index Terms Desoxyphenobarbital; Primaclone

Generic Available Yes

Pharmacologic Category Anticonvulsant, Miscellaneous; Barbiturate

Use Management of grand mal, complex partial, and psychomotor or focal seizures

Unlabeled/Investigational Use Treatment of benign familial tremor (essential tremor)

Contraindications Hypersensitivity to primidone, phenobarbital, or any component of the formulation; porphyria

Warnings/Precautions Use with caution in patients with renal or hepatic impairment, pulmonary insufficiency; abrupt withdrawal may precipitate status epilepticus. Potential for drug dependency exists. Do not administer to patients in acute pain. Use caution in elderly or debilitated patients; may cause paradoxical responses. May cause CNS depression, which may impair physical or mental abilities. Patients must be cautioned about performing tasks which require mental alertness (eg, operating machinery or driving). Effects with other sedative drugs or ethanol may be potentiated. Use with caution in patients with depression or suicidal tendencies, or in patients with a history of drug abuse. Tolerance or psychological and physical dependence may occur with prolonged use. Use with caution in patients with hypoadrenalism.

Adverse Reactions (Reflective of adult population; not specific for elderly)
Frequency not defined.

Central nervous system: Drowsiness, vertigo, ataxia, lethargy, behavior change, fatigue, hyperirritability

Dermatologic: Rash

Gastrointestinal: Nausea, vomiting, anorexia

Genitourinary: Impotence

Hematologic: Agranulocytopenia, agranulocytosis, anemia

Ocular: Diplopia, nystagmus

Overdosage/Toxicology Symptoms include unsteady gait, slurred speech, confusion, jaundice, hypothermia, fever, hypotension, coma, and respiratory arrest. Assure adequate hydration and renal function. Urinary alkalinization with I.V. sodium bicarbonate also helps enhance elimination. Repeat oral doses of activated charcoal significantly reduce the half-life of primidone resulting from enhancement of nonrenal elimination. The usual dose is 0.1-1 g/kg every 4-6 hours for 3-4 days, unless the patient has no bowel movement, causing charcoal to remain in the GI tract. Hemodialysis or hemoperfusion is of uncertain value. Patients in stage IV coma, due to high serum drug levels, may require charcoal hemoperfusion.

Drug Interactions Metabolized to phenobarbital; **Induces** CYP1A2 (strong), 2B6 (strong), 2C8 (strong), 2C9 (strong), 3A4 (strong)

Acetaminophen: Barbiturates may enhance the hepatotoxic potential of acetaminophen overdoses

Antiarrhythmics: Barbiturates may increase the metabolism of antiarrhythmics, decreasing their clinical effect; includes disopyramide, propafenone, and quinidine

Anticonvulsants: Barbiturates may increase the metabolism of anticonvulsants; includes ethosuximide, felbamate (possibly), lamotrigine, phenytoin, tiagabine, topiramate, and zonisamide; does not appear to affect gabapentin or levetiracetam

Antineoplastics: Limited evidence suggests that enzyme-inducing anticonvulsant therapy may reduce the effectiveness of some chemotherapy regimens (specifically in ALL); teniposide and methotrexate may be cleared more rapidly in these patients

Antipsychotics: Barbiturates may enhance the metabolism (decrease the efficacy) of antipsychotics; monitor for altered response; dose adjustment may be needed

Beta-blockers: Metabolism of beta-blockers may be increased and clinical effect decreased; atenolol and nadolol are unlikely to interact given their renal elimination

Calcium channel blockers: Barbiturates may enhance the metabolism of calcium channel blockers, decreasing their clinical effect

Chloramphenicol: Barbiturates may increase the metabolism of chloramphenicol and chloramphenicol may inhibit barbiturate metabolism; monitor for altered response

Cimetidine: Barbiturates may enhance the metabolism of cimetidine, decreasing its clinical effect

CNS depressants: Sedative effects and/or respiratory depression with barbiturates may be additive with other CNS depressants; monitor for increased effect. Includes ethanol, sedatives, antidepressants, opioid analgesics, and benzodiazepines

Corticosteroids: Barbiturates may enhance the metabolism of corticosteroids, decreasing their clinical effect

Cyclosporine: Levels may be decreased by barbiturates; monitor

CYP1A2 substrates: Primidone may decrease the levels/effects of CYP1A2 substrates. Example substrates include aminophylline, estrogens, fluvoxamine, mirtazapine, ropinirole, and theophylline.

CYP2B6 substrates: Primidone may decrease the levels/effects of CYP2B6 substrates. Example substrates include bupropion, efavirenz, promethazine, selegiline, and sertraline.

CYP2C8 Substrates: Primidone may decrease the levels/effects of CYP2C8 substrates. Example substrates include amiodarone, paclitaxel, pioglitazone, repaglinide, and rosiglitazone.

CYP2C9 Substrates: Primidone may decrease the levels/effects of CYP2C9 substrates. Example substrates include bosentan, celecoxib, dapsone, fluoxetine, glimepiride, glipizide, losartan, montelukast, nateglinide, paclitaxel, phenytoin, sulfonamides, trimethoprim, warfarin, and zafirlukast.

(Continued)

Primidone *(Continued)*

CYP3A4 substrates: Primidone may decrease the levels/effects of CYP3A4 substrates. Example substrates include benzodiazepines, calcium channel blockers, clarithromycin, cyclosporine, erythromycin, estrogens, mirtazapine, nateglinide, nefazodone, nevirapine, protease inhibitors, tacrolimus, and venlafaxine.

Doxycycline: Barbiturates may enhance the metabolism of doxycycline, decreasing its clinical effect; higher dosages may be required

Estrogens: Barbiturates may increase the metabolism of estrogens and reduce their efficacy

Felbamate may inhibit the metabolism of barbiturates and barbiturates may increase the metabolism of felbamate

Griseofulvin: Barbiturates may impair the absorption of griseofulvin, and griseofulvin metabolism may be increased by barbiturates, decreasing clinical effect

Guanfacine: Effect may be decreased by barbiturates

Immunosuppressants: Barbiturates may enhance the metabolism of immunosuppressants, decreasing its clinical effect; includes both cyclosporine and tacrolimus

Loop diuretics: Metabolism may be increased and clinical effects decreased; established for furosemide, effect with other loop diuretics not established

MAO inhibitors: Metabolism of barbiturates may be inhibited, increasing clinical effect or toxicity of the barbiturates

Methadone: Barbiturates may enhance the metabolism of methadone resulting in methadone withdrawal

Methoxyflurane: Barbiturates may enhance the nephrotoxic effects of methoxyflurane

Oral contraceptives: Barbiturates may enhance the metabolism of oral contraceptives, decreasing their clinical effect; an alternative method of contraception should be considered

Theophylline: Barbiturates may increase metabolism of theophylline derivatives and decrease their clinical effect

Tricyclic antidepressants: Barbiturates may increase metabolism of tricyclic antidepressants and decrease their clinical effect; sedative effects may be additive

Valproic acid: Metabolism of barbiturates may be inhibited by valproic acid; monitor for excessive sedation; a dose reduction may be needed

Warfarin: Barbiturates inhibit the hypoprothrombinemic effects of oral anticoagulants via increased metabolism; this combination should generally be avoided

Ethanol/Nutrition/Herb Interactions

Ethanol: Avoid ethanol (may increase CNS depression).

Food: Protein-deficient diets increase duration of action of primidone.

Herb/Nutraceutical: Avoid valerian, St John's wort, kava kava, gotu kola (may increase CNS depression).

Stability Protect from light.

Mechanism of Action Decreases neuron excitability, raises seizure threshold similar to phenobarbital; primidone has two active metabolites, phenobarbital and phenylethylmalonamide (PEMA); PEMA may enhance the activity of phenobarbital

Pharmacokinetics

Distribution: V_d: 2-3L/kg (adults)

Protein binding: 99%

Metabolism: In the liver to phenobarbital (active) and phenylethylmalonamide (PEMA)

Bioavailability: 60% to 80%

Half-life:

Primidone: 10-12 hours

PEMA: 16 hours

Phenobarbital: 52-118 hours (age-dependent with older adults generally having the longer half-life)

Time to peak serum concentration: Oral: Within 4 hours

Elimination: Urinary excretion of both active metabolites and unchanged primidone (15% to 25%)

Dosage

Geriatrics & Adults:

Essential tremor (unlabeled use): 750 mg early in divided doses

Seizure disorders (grand mal, psychomotor, and focal): Oral: Initial: 125-250 mg/day at bedtime; increase by 125-250 mg/day every 3-7 days; usual dose: 750-1500 mg/day in divided doses 3-4 times/day with maximum dosage of 2 g/day.

Renal Impairment:

Cl_{cr} 50-80 mL/minute: Administer every 8 hours.

Cl_{cr} 10-50 mL/minute: Administer every 8-12 hours.

Cl_{cr} <10 mL/minute: Administer every 12-24 hours.

Moderately dialyzable (20% to 50%)

Administer dose postdialysis or administer supplemental 30% dose.

Hepatic Impairment: Increased side effects may occur in severe liver disease. Monitor plasma levels and adjust dose accordingly.

Monitoring Parameters Monitor CBC, serum concentrations of primidone, and if applicable, other anticonvulsants when given concomitantly

Reference Range

Therapeutic: Adults: 5-12 mcg/mL (SI: 23-55 µmol/L); Toxic effects rarely present with serum concentrations <10 mcg/mL (SI: 46 µmol/L) if phenobarbital concentrations are low

Dosage of primidone is adjusted with reference mostly to the phenobarbital serum concentration

Toxic: >15 mcg/mL (SI: >69 µmol/L)

Patient Information May cause drowsiness; if stomach upset occurs, take with food; do not stop therapy without consulting physician

Additional Information Bioequivalence problems have been noted with primidone from one manufacturer to another, therefore, brand interchange is not recommended

Special Geriatric Considerations Due to CNS effects, monitor closely when initiating drug in elderly. Monitor CBC at 6-month intervals to compare with baseline obtained at start of therapy. Since elderly metabolize phenobarbital at a slower rate than younger adults, it is suggested to measure both primidone and phenobarbital serum concentrations together. Adjust dose for renal function in elderly when initiating or changing dose.

Dosage Forms Excipient information presented when available (limited, particularly for generics); consult specific product labeling.

Tablet: 50 mg, 250 mg [generic tablet may contain sodium benzoate]

Dosage forms available in Canada: Tablet: 125 mg, 250 mg. **Note:** 50 mg tablet is **not** available in Canada.

- ♦ **Primsol**® *see* Trimethoprim *on page 1634*
- ♦ **Prinivil**® *see* Lisinopril *on page 917*
- ♦ **Prinzide**® *see* Lisinopril and Hydrochlorothiazide *on page 920*
- ♦ **Pristinamycin** *see* Quinupristin and Dalfopristin *on page 1368*
- ♦ **Privine**® **[OTC]** *see* Naphazoline *on page 1086*
- ♦ **ProAir**™ **HFA** *see* Albuterol *on page 40*
- ♦ **ProAmatine**® *see* Midodrine *on page 1042*

Probenecid (proe BEN e sid)

Medication Safety Issues

Sound-alike/look-alike issues:

Probenecid may be confused with Procanbid®

Canadian Brand Names Benuryl™

Index Terms Benemid [DSC]

Generic Available Yes

Pharmacologic Category Uricosuric Agent

Use Prevention of hyperuricemia associated with gout or gouty arthritis; prolongation and elevation of beta-lactam plasma levels

Contraindications Hypersensitivity to probenecid or any component of the formulation; high-dose aspirin therapy; blood dyscrasias; uric acid kidney stones

Warnings/Precautions Use with caution in patients with peptic ulcer. Salicylates may diminish the therapeutic effect of probenecid. This effect may be more pronounced with high, chronic doses, however, the manufacturer recommends the use of an alternative analgesic even in place of small doses of aspirin. Use of probenecid with penicillin in patients with renal insufficiency is not recommended. Probenecid monotherapy may not be effective in patients with a creatinine clearance <30 mL/minute. May cause exacerbation of acute gouty attack.

Adverse Reactions (Reflective of adult population; not specific for elderly)

Frequency not defined.

Cardiovascular: Flushing

Central nervous system: Dizziness, fever, headache

Dermatologic: Alopecia, dermatitis, pruritus, rash

Gastrointestinal: Anorexia, nausea, sore gums, vomiting

Genitourinary: Hematuria, polyuria

Hematologic: Anemia, aplastic anemia, hemolytic anemia, leukopenia

Hepatic: Hepatic necrosis

Neuromuscular & skeletal: Costovertebral pain, gouty arthritis (acute)

Renal: Nephrotic syndrome, renal colic

Miscellaneous: Anaphylaxis, hypersensitivity

Drug Interactions Inhibits CYP2C19 (weak)

Carbapenems (ertapenem, imipenem, meropenem): Probenecid may decrease the excretion of carbapenem antibiotics.

Cephalosporins: Probenecid may decrease the excretion of cephalosporin antibiotics. This effect is used advantageously in selected cases to increase serum antibiotic concentrations.

(Continued)

Probenecid *(Continued)*

Dapsone: Probenecid may decrease the excretion of dapsone.

Methotrexate: Probenecid may decrease the excretion of methotrexate; concomitant use should be avoided. If used concomitantly, the methotrexate dosage will likely need reduced. Monitor for evidence of methotrexate toxicity.

Nonsteroidal anti-inflammatory agents: Probenecid may increase the serum concentration of NSAIDs. The manufacturer of ketorolac contraindicates concomitant use.

Penicillins: Probenecid may decrease the excretion of penicillin antibiotics. This effect is used advantageously in selected cases to increase serum antibiotic concentrations.

Salicylates: Salicylates may diminish the therapeutic effect of probenecid.

Thiopental: Probenecid may enhance the therapeutic effect of thiopental.

Zidovudine: Probenecid may decrease the metabolism of zidovudine.

Mechanism of Action Competitively inhibits the reabsorption of uric acid at the proximal convoluted tubule, thereby promoting its excretion and reducing serum uric acid levels; increases plasma levels of weak organic acids (penicillins, cephalosporins, or other beta-lactam antibiotics) by competitively inhibiting their renal tubular secretion

Pharmacodynamics Onset of action: Effect on penicillin levels: 2 hours

Pharmacokinetics

Absorption: Rapid and complete

Metabolism: Hepatic

Half-life elimination (dose dependent): Normal renal function: 6-12 hours

Time to peak, serum: 2-4 hours

Excretion: Urine

Dosage

Geriatrics & Adults:

Hyperuricemia with gout: Oral: 250 mg twice daily for 1 week; increase to 250-500 mg/day; may increase by 500 mg/month, if needed, to maximum of 2-3 g/day (dosages may be increased by 500 mg every 6 months if serum urate concentrations are controlled)

Prolong penicillin serum levels: Oral: 500 mg 4 times/day

Gonorrhea: CDC guidelines (alternative regimen): Probenecid 1 g orally with cefoxitin 2 g I.M.

Pelvic inflammatory disease: CDC guidelines: Cefoxitin 2 g I.M. plus probenecid 1 g orally as a single dose

Neurosyphilis: CDC guidelines (alternative regimen): Procaine penicillin 2.4 million units/day I.M. plus probenecid 500 mg orally 4 times/day; both administered for 10-14 days

Renal Impairment: Cl_{cr} <30 mL/minute: Avoid use.

Administration Administer with food or antacids to minimize GI effects

Monitoring Parameters Uric acid, renal function, CBC

Test Interactions False-positive glucosuria with Clinitest®, a falsely high determination of theophylline has occurred and the renal excretion of phenolsulfonphthalein 17-ketosteroids and bromsulfophthalein (BSP) may be inhibited

Patient Information Take as directed; do not discontinue without consulting prescriber. May take 6-12 months to reduce gouty attacks (attacks may increase in frequency and severity for first few months of therapy). Take with food or antacids or alkaline ash foods (milk, nuts, beets, spinach, turnip greens). Maintain adequate hydration (2-3 L/day of fluids) unless instructed to restrict fluid intake. Avoid aspirin or aspirin-containing substances. If you have diabetes, use serum glucose monitoring. If you experience severe headache, contact prescriber for medication. You may experience dizziness or lightheadedness (use caution when driving, changing position, or engaging in tasks requiring alertness until response to drug is known); or nausea, vomiting, indigestion, or loss of appetite (small frequent meals, frequent mouth care, chewing gum, or sucking lozenges may help). Report skin rash or itching, persistent headache, blood in urine or painful urination, excessive tiredness or easy bruising or bleeding, or sore gums.

Additional Information Avoid fluctuation in uric acid (increase or decrease); may precipitate gout attack. Use of sodium bicarbonate or potassium citrate is suggested until serum uric acid normalizes and tophaceous deposits disappear.

Special Geriatric Considerations Since probenecid loses its effectiveness when the Cl_{cr} is <30 mL/minute, its usefulness in the elderly is limited.

Dosage Forms Excipient information presented when available (limited, particularly for generics); consult specific product labeling.

Tablet: 500 mg

Selected References

Centers for Disease Control and Prevention, "Sexually Transmitted Diseases Treatment Guidelines 2002," *MMWR Recomm Rep*, 2002, 51(RR-6):1-84.

♦ **Probenecid and Colchicine** see Colchicine and Probenecid *on page 360*

Procainamide (pro KANE a mide)

Related Information
Serum Drug Concentrations Commonly Monitored Guidelines *on page 1862*

Medication Safety Issues
Sound-alike/look-alike issues:
Procanbid® may be confused with probenecid
Pronestyl® may be confused with Ponstel®

High alert medication: The Institute for Safe Medication Practices (ISMP) includes this medication among its list of drugs which have a heightened risk of causing significant patient harm when used in error.

PCA is an error-prone abbreviation (mistaken as patient controlled analgesia)

U.S. Brand Names Procanbid®

Canadian Brand Names Apo-Procainamide®; Procainamide Hydrochloride Injection, USP; Procan® SR; Pronestyl®-SR

Index Terms PCA (error-prone abbreviation); Procainamide Hydrochloride; Procaine Amide Hydrochloride

Generic Available Yes

Pharmacologic Category Antiarrhythmic Agent, Class Ia

Use Ventricular tachycardia, premature ventricular contractions considered life-threatening, paroxysmal atrial tachycardia, and atrial fibrillation; to prevent recurrence of ventricular tachycardia, paroxysmal supraventricular tachycardia, atrial fibrillation or flutter

Unlabeled/Investigational Use ACLS guidelines:
Stable monomorphic VT (EF >40%, no CHF)
Stable wide complex tachycardia, likely VT (EF >40%, no CHF, patient stable)
Atrial fibrillation or flutter, including pre-excitation syndrome (EF >40%, no CHF)
AV reentrant, narrow complex tachycardia (eg, reentrant SVT) [preserved ventricular function]
PALS guidelines: Tachycardia with pulses and poor perfusion (possible VT)

Contraindications Hypersensitivity to procaine, other ester-type local anesthetics, or any component of the formulation; complete heart block (except in patients with a functioning artificial pacemaker); second-degree AV block (without a functional pacemaker); various types of hemiblock (without a functional pacemaker); SLE; torsade de pointes; concurrent cisapride use; QT prolongation

Warnings/Precautions Use with caution in patients with marked AV conduction disturbances, myasthenia gravis, bundle-branch block, or severe cardiac glycoside intoxication, ventricular arrhythmias with organic heart disease or coronary occlusion, CHF supraventricular tachyarrhythmias unless adequate measures are taken to prevent marked increases in ventricular rates; concurrent therapy with other class Ia drugs may accumulate in patients with renal or hepatic dysfunction; correct electrolyte disturbances, especially hypokalemia or hypomagnesemia, prior to use and throughout therapy; some tablets contain tartrazine; injection may contain bisulfite (allergens). **[U.S. Boxed Warning]: Long-term administration leads to the development of a positive antinuclear antibody (ANA) test in 50% of patients which may result in a lupus erythematosus-like syndrome (in 20% to 30% of patients);** discontinue procainamide with SLE symptoms and choose an alternative agent; elderly have reduced clearance and frequent drug interactions. **[U.S. Boxed Warning]: Potentially fatal blood dyscrasias have occurred with therapeutic doses;** close monitoring is recommended during the first 3 months of therapy.

[U.S. Boxed Warning] In the Cardiac Arrhythmia Suppression Trial (CAST), recent (>6 days but <2 years ago) myocardial infarction patients with asymptomatic, nonlife-threatening ventricular arrhythmias did not benefit and may have been harmed by attempts to suppress the arrhythmia with flecainide or encainide. An increased mortality or nonfatal cardiac arrest rate (7.7%) was seen in the active treatment group compared with patients in the placebo group (3%). The applicability of the CAST results to other populations is unknown. Antiarrhythmic agents should be reserved for patients with life-threatening ventricular arrhythmias.

Adverse Reactions (Reflective of adult population; not specific for elderly)
>1%:
Cardiovascular: Hypotension (I.V., up to 5%)
Dermatologic: Rash
Gastrointestinal: Diarrhea (3% to 4%), nausea, vomiting, taste disorder, GI complaints (3% to 4%)

Overdosage/Toxicology Has a low toxic:therapeutic ratio and may easily produce fatal intoxication (acute toxic dose: 5 g). Symptoms of include sinus bradycardia, sinus node arrest or asystole; PR, QRS or QT interval prolongation; torsade de pointes (polymorphous ventricular tachycardia); and depressed myocardial contractility, which (Continued)

Procainamide *(Continued)*

along with alpha-adrenergic or ganglionic blockade, may result in hypotension and pulmonary edema. Other effects are seizures, coma, and respiratory arrest.

Treatment is primarily symptomatic and effects usually respond to conventional therapies (fluids, positioning, vasopressors, anticonvulsants, antiarrhythmics). **Note**: Do not use other type 1a or 1c antiarrhythmic agents to treat ventricular tachycardia. Sodium bicarbonate may treat wide QRS intervals or hypotension. Markedly impaired conduction or high degree AV block, unresponsive to bicarbonate, indicates consideration of a pacemaker is needed.

Drug Interactions Substrate of CYP2D6 (major)

Amiodarone increases procainamide and NAPA blood levels; consider reducing procainamide dosage by 25% with concurrent use.

Cimetidine increases procainamide and NAPA blood concentrations; monitor blood levels closely or use an alternative H_2 antagonist.

Cisapride and procainamide may increase the risk of malignant arrhythmia; concurrent use is contraindicated.

CYP2D6 inhibitors: May increase the levels/effects of procainamide. Example inhibitors include chlorpromazine, delavirdine, fluoxetine, miconazole, paroxetine, pergolide, quinidine, quinine, ritonavir, and ropinirole.

Neuromuscular blocking agents: Procainamide may potentiate neuromuscular blockade.

Ofloxacin may increase procainamide levels due to an inhibition of renal secretion; monitor levels for procainamide closely.

QT_c-prolonging agents (eg, amiodarone, amitriptyline, bepridil, disopyramide, erythromycin, haloperidol, imipramine, pimozide, quinidine, sotalol, and thioridazine): Effects/toxicity may be increased; use with caution.

Moxifloxacin may result in additional prolongation of the QT interval; concurrent use is contraindicated.

Trimethoprim increases procainamide and NAPA blood levels; closely monitor levels.

Ethanol/Nutrition/Herb Interactions

Ethanol: Avoid ethanol (acute ethanol administration reduces procainamide serum concentrations).

Herb/Nutraceutical: Avoid ephedra (may worsen arrhythmia).

Stability Procainamide may be stored at room temperature up to 27°C; however, refrigeration retards oxidation, which causes color formation. The solution is initially colorless but may turn slightly yellow on standing. Injection of air into the vial causes the solution to darken. Solutions darker than a light amber should be discarded.

Minimum volume: 1 g/250 mL NS/D_5W.

Stability of admixture at room temperature in D_5W or NS: 24 hours.

Some information indicates that procainamide may be subject to greater decomposition in D_5W unless the admixture is refrigerated or the pH is adjusted. Procainamide is believed to form an association complex with dextrose - the bioavailability of procainamide in this complex is not known and the complex formation is reversible.

Mechanism of Action Decreases myocardial excitability and conduction velocity and may depress myocardial contractility, by increasing the electrical stimulation threshold of ventricle, His-Purkinje system and through direct cardiac effects

Pharmacodynamics Onset of action: I.M.: 10-30 minutes

Pharmacokinetics

Protein binding: 15% to 20%

Distribution: V_d: 2 L/kg, decreased V_d in congestive heart failure or shock

Metabolism: By acetylation in the liver to produce N-acetyl procainamide (NAPA) (active metabolite)

Bioavailability: 75% to 95% orally

Half-life (PCA):

Adults with normal renal function: 2.5-4.7 hours; half-life dependent upon hepatic acetylator phenotype, cardiac function, and renal function

NAPA (adults with normal renal function): 6-8 hours

Anephric half-life (procainamide): 11 hours

NAPA: 42 hours; half-life for procainamide and NAPA increases with age; clearance is 4.3 L/minute/kg for patients >60 years, whereas those younger have a clearance of procainamide of 7.7 L/minute/kg

Time to peak:

Capsule: Within 45 minutes to 2.5 hours

I.M.: 15-60 minutes

Elimination: Urinary excretion (25% as NAPA)

Dosage

Geriatrics & Adults: Dose must be titrated to patient's response.

Antiarrhythmic:

Oral: Usual dose: 50 mg/kg/24 hours: maximum: 5 g/24 hours (**Note:** Twice-daily dosing approved for Procanbid®.)

Immediate release formulation: 250-500 mg/dose every 3-6 hours

Extended release formulation: 500 mg to 1 g every 6 hours; Procanbid®: 1000-2500 mg every 12 hours

I.M.: 0.5-1 g every 4-8 hours until oral therapy is possible

I.V. (infusion requires use of an infusion pump):

Loading dose: 15-18 mg/kg administered as slow infusion over 25-30 minutes **or** 100-200 mg/dose repeated every 5 minutes as needed to a total dose of 1 g. Reduce loading dose to 12 mg/kg in severe renal or cardiac impairment.

Maintenance dose: 1-4 mg/minute by continuous infusion. Maintenance infusions should be reduced by one-third in patients with moderate renal or cardiac impairment and by two-thirds in patients with severe renal or cardiac impairment.

ACLS guidelines: Infuse 20 mg/minute until arrhythmia is controlled, hypotension occurs, QRS complex widens by 50% of its original width, or total of 17 mg/kg is given.

Renal Impairment:

Oral:

Cl_{cr} 10-50 mL/minute: Administer every 6-12 hours.

Cl_{cr} <10 mL/minute: Administer every 8-24 hours.

I.V.:

Loading dose: Reduce dose to 12 mg/kg in severe renal impairment.

Maintenance infusion: Reduce dose by one-third in patients with mild renal impairment. Reduce dose by two-thirds in patients with severe renal impairment.

Dialysis:

Procainamide: Moderately hemodialyzable (20% to 50%): 200 mg supplemental dose posthemodialysis is recommended.

N-acetylprocainamide: Not dialyzable (0% to 5%)

Procainamide/N-acetylprocainamide: Not peritoneal dialyzable (0% to 5%)

Procainamide/N-acetylprocainamide: Replace by blood level during continuous arteriovenous or venovenous hemofiltration

Hepatic Impairment: Reduce dose by 50%.

Administration

Oral: Do **not** crush or chew extended release drug products.

Must dilute prior to I.V. administration; maximum rate: 50 mg/minute; administer around-the-clock rather than 4 times/day to promote less variation in peak and trough serum levels.

Infusion rate: **2 g/250 mL** (I.V. infusion requires use of an infusion pump):

1 mg/minute: 7.5 mL/hour

2 mg/minute: 15 mL/hour

3 mg/minute: 22.5 mL/hour

4 mg/minute: 30 mL/hour

5 mg/minute: 37.5 mL/hour

6 mg/minute: 45 mL/hour

Monitoring Parameters Blood pressure, apical pulse, pulse, EKG; monitor for SLE, obtain CBC to monitor WBC every 2 weeks for first 3 months of treatment

Reference Range Optimal ranges must be ascertained for individual patients, with EKG monitoring.

Therapeutic: 4.9-12 mcg/mL (SI: 15-37 μmol/L) for procainamide, <30 mcg/mL (SI: <127 μmol/L) for sum of procainamide and NAPA

Toxic: >10-12 mcg/mL (SI: >42-51 μmol/L)

Patient Information Do not discontinue therapy unless instructed by physician; notify physician or pharmacist if soreness of mouth, throat or gums, unexplained fever, symptoms of upper respiratory tract infection. Do not break or chew sustained release tablets. Sustained release tablets contain a wax core that slowly releases the drug. When this process is complete, the empty, nonabsorbable wax core is eliminated.

Special Geriatric Considerations Monitor closely since clearance is reduced in those >60 years of age. If clinically possible, start doses at lowest recommended dose. Also, elderly frequently have drug therapy which may interfere with the use of procainamide. Adjust dose for renal function in the elderly.

Dosage Forms Excipient information presented when available (limited, particularly for generics); consult specific product labeling.

Capsule, as hydrochloride: 250 mg, 500 mg

Injection, solution, as hydrochloride: 100 mg/mL (10 mL); 500 mg/mL (2 mL) [contains sodium metabisulfite]

Tablet, extended release, as hydrochloride: 500 mg, 750 mg, 1000 mg

Procanbid®: 500 mg, 1000 mg

Selected References

"2005 American Heart Association Guidelines for Cardiopulmonary Resuscitation and Emergency Cardiovascular Care," *Circulation*, 2005, 112(24 Suppl):1-211.

Coyle JD and Lima JJ, "Procainamide" in Applied Pharmacokinetics: *Principles of Therapeutic Drug Monitoring*, 3rd Ed. Evans WE, Schentag JJ, and Jusko W (eds). Applied Therapeutics, Inc: Spokane, WA, 1992, 22-1-33.

(Continued)

Procainamide *(Continued)*

Fenster PE and Nolan PE, "Antiarrhythmic Drugs," *Geriatric Pharmacology*, Bressler R and Katz MD, eds, New York, NY: McGraw-Hill, 1993, 6:105-49.

Prochlorperazine (proe klor PER a zeen)

Medication Safety Issues

Sound-alike/look-alike issues:

Prochlorperazine may be confused with chlorproMAZINE

Compazine® may be confused with Copaxone®, Coumadin®

CPZ (occasional abbreviation for Compazine®) is an error-prone abbreviation (mistaken as chlorpromazine)

U.S. Brand Names Compro™

Canadian Brand Names Apo-Prochlorperazine®; Compazine®; Nu-Prochlor; Stemetil®

Index Terms Chlormeprazine; Compazine; Prochlorperazine Edisylate; Prochlorperazine Maleate

Generic Available Yes: Injection, tablet, suppository

Pharmacologic Category Antiemetic; Antipsychotic Agent, Typical, Phenothiazine

Use Management of nausea and vomiting; psychotic disorders including schizophrenia; anxiety

Unlabeled/Investigational Use Treatment of behavioral syndromes in dementia

Contraindications Hypersensitivity to prochlorperazine or any component of the formulation (cross-reactivity between phenothiazines may occur); severe CNS depression; coma

Warnings/Precautions May be sedating; use with caution in disorders where CNS depression is a feature. May obscure intestinal obstruction or brain tumor. May impair physical or mental abilities. Effects with other sedative drugs or ethanol may be potentiated. Use with caution in Parkinson's disease; hemodynamic instability; bone marrow suppression; predisposition to seizures; subcortical brain damage; and in severe cardiac, hepatic, renal or respiratory disease. Caution in breast cancer or other prolactin-dependent tumors. May alter temperature regulation or mask toxicity of other drugs. Use caution with exposure to heat. May alter cardiac conduction. May cause orthostatic hypotension. Hypotension may occur following administration, particularly when parenteral form is used or in high dosages. Antipsychotic use has been associated with esophageal dysmotility and aspiration; use with caution in patients at risk of pneumonia (ie, Alzheimer's disease). May be associated with pigmentary retinopathy.

Phenothiazines may cause anticholinergic effects; therefore, they should be used with caution in patients with decreased gastrointestinal motility, urinary retention, BPH, xerostomia, or visual problems. Conditions which also may be exacerbated by cholinergic blockade include narrow-angle glaucoma (screening is recommended) and worsening of myasthenia gravis. May cause extrapyramidal symptoms. Use caution in the elderly. May be associated with neuroleptic malignant syndrome (NMS).

Adverse Reactions (Reflective of adult population; not specific for elderly)

Reported with prochlorperazine or other phenothiazines. Frequency not defined

Cardiovascular: Cardiac arrest, hypotension, peripheral edema, Q-wave distortions, T-wave distortions

Central nervous system: Agitation, catatonia, cerebral edema, cough reflex suppressed, dizziness, drowsiness, fever (mild - I.M.), headache, hyperactivity, hyperpyrexia, impairment of temperature regulation, insomnia, neuroleptic malignant syndrome (NMS), paradoxical excitement, restlessness, seizure

Dermatologic: Angioedema, contact dermatitis, discoloration of skin (blue-gray), epithelial keratopathy, erythema, eczema, exfoliative dermatitis (injectable), itching, photosensitivity, rash, skin pigmentation, urticaria

Endocrine & metabolic: Amenorrhea, breast enlargement, galactorrhea, gynecomastia, glucosuria, hyperglycemia, hypoglycemia, lactation, libido (changes in), menstrual irregularity, SIADH

Gastrointestinal: Appetite increased, atonic colon, constipation, ileus, nausea, weight gain, xerostomia

Genitourinary: Ejaculating dysfunction, ejaculatory disturbances, impotence, incontinence, polyuria, priapism, urinary retention, urination difficulty

Hematologic: Agranulocytosis, aplastic anemia, eosinophilia, hemolytic anemia, leukopenia, pancytopenia, thrombocytopenic purpura

Hepatic: Biliary stasis, cholestatic jaundice, hepatotoxicity

Neuromuscular & skeletal: Dystonias (torticollis, opisthotonos, carpopedal spasm, trismus, oculogyric crisis, protusion of tongue); extrapyramidal symptoms (pseudoparkinsonism, akathisia, dystonias, tardive dyskinesia); SLE-like syndrome, tremor

Ocular: blurred vision, cornea and lens changes, lenticular/corneal deposits, miosis, mydriasis, pigmentary retinopathy

Respiratory: Asthma, laryngeal edema, nasal congestion

Miscellaneous: Allergic reactions, diaphoresis

Overdosage/Toxicology Symptoms include deep sleep, coma, extrapyramidal symptoms, abnormal involuntary muscle movements, and hypotension. Following initiation of essential overdose management, toxic symptom and supportive treatment should be initiated. Hypotension usually responds to I.V. fluids or Trendelenburg positioning. If unresponsive to these measures, the use of a parenteral medication may be required (eg, norepinephrine 0.1-0.2 mcg/kg/minute titrated to response). Seizures commonly respond to diazepam (I.V. 5-10 mg bolus in adults every 15 minutes, if needed, up to a total of 30 mg) or to phenytoin or phenobarbital. Critical cardiac arrhythmias often respond to I.V. phenytoin (15 mg/kg up to 1 g), while other antiarrhythmics can be used. Extrapyramidal symptoms (eg, dystonic reactions) may require management with diphenhydramine 1-2 mg/kg (adults) up to a maximum of 50 mg I.M. or slow I.V. push followed by a maintenance dose for 48-72 hours. When these reactions are unresponsive to diphenhydramine, anticholinergic agents such as benztropine mesylate I.V. 1-2 mg (adults) may be effective. These agents are generally effective within 2-5 minutes.

Drug Interactions

Acetylcholinesterase inhibitors (central): May increase the risk of antipsychotic-related extrapyramidal symptoms; monitor.

Alpha-/Beta- agonists: May enhance the arrhythmogenic effect of phenothiazines.

Analgesics (opioid): Phenothiazines may enhance the hypotensive effect of opioid analgesics.

Antacids: May decrease the absorption of phenothiazines; monitor.

Antidepressants (serotonin reuptake inhibitors/antagonist): Concurrent use may produce increased hypotension.

Anticholinergics: May inhibit the therapeutic response to phenothiazines and excess anticholinergic effects may occur; includes benztropine, trihexyphenidyl, biperiden, and drugs with significant anticholinergic activity (TCAs, antihistamines, disopyramide)

Antihistamines: May enhance the arrhythmogenic effect of phenothiazines.

Antimalarial agents: May increase phenothiazine concentrations.

Antiparkinson's Agents (dopamine agonists such as levodopa): Phenothiazines may inhibit the antiparkinsonian effect of levodopa; avoid this combination.

Attapulgite: May decrease absorption of phenothiazines.

Beta-blockers: Serum concentrations of phenothiazines may be increased; phenothiazines may increase hypotensive effects of beta-blockers.

CNS depressants: Sedative effects may be additive with phenothiazines; monitor for increased effect; includes barbiturates, benzodiazepines, opioid analgesics, ethanol and other sedative agents.

Epinephrine: Chlorpromazine (and possibly other low potency antipsychotics) may diminish the pressor effects of epinephrine.

False neurotransmitters (guanadrel, methyldopa): Antihypertensive effects may be inhibited by phenothiazines.

Lithium: Phenothiazines may produce neurotoxicity with lithium; this is a rare effect.

Phenytoin: Concurrent use may increase CNS depression.

Polypeptide antibiotics: Rare cases of respiratory paralysis have been reported with concurrent use of phenothiazines.

Pramlintide: May enhance the anticholinergic effects of phenothiazines.

QT_c-prolonging agents: Effects on QT_c interval may be additive with phenothiazines, increasing the risk of malignant arrhythmias; includes type Ia antiarrhythmics, TCAs, and some quinolone antibiotics (moxifloxacin).

Ethanol/Nutrition/Herb Interactions

Ethanol: Avoid ethanol (may increase CNS depression).

Food: Limit caffeine.

Herb/Nutraceutical: Avoid dong quai, St John's wort (may also cause photosensitization). Avoid kava kava, gotu kola, valerian, St John's wort (may increase CNS depression).

Stability

Injection: Store at <30°C (<86°F); do not freeze. Protect from light. Clear or slightly yellow solutions may be used.

(Continued)

Prochlorperazine *(Continued)*

I.V. infusion: Injection may be diluted in 50-100 mL NS or D₅W.

Suppository, tablet: Store at 15°C to 30°C (59°F to 86°F). Protect from light.

Mechanism of Action Prochlorperazine is a piperazine phenothiazine antipsychotic which blocks postsynaptic mesolimbic dopaminergic D_1 and D_2 receptors in the brain, including the chemoreceptor trigger zone; exhibits a strong alpha-adrenergic and anticholinergic blocking effect and depresses the release of hypothalamic and hypophyseal hormones; believed to depress the reticular activating system, thus affecting basal metabolism, body temperature, wakefulness, vasomotor tone and emesis

Pharmacodynamics

Onset of action:

Oral: Within 30-40 minutes

I.M.: Within 10-20 minutes

Rectal: Within 60 minutes

Duration: Rectal: 12 hours; Oral: 3-4 hours; I.M., I.V.: 4-6 hours

Pharmacokinetics

Distribution: V_d: 1400-1548 L

Metabolism: Primarily hepatic; N-desmethyl prochlorperazine (major active metabolite)

Bioavailability: Oral: 12.5%

Half-life: Oral: 3-5 hours; I.V.: ~7 hours

Dosage

Geriatrics: Dementia behavior (nonpsychotic, unlabeled use): Initial: 2.5-5 mg 1-2 times/day; increase dose at 4- to 7-day intervals by 2.5-5 mg/day. Increase dosing intervals (twice daily, 3 times/day, etc) as necessary to control response or side effects. Maximum daily dose should probably not exceed 75 mg in the elderly. Gradual increases (titration) may prevent some side effects or decrease their severity. See Special Geriatric Considerations.

Adults:

Antiemetic:

Oral (tablet): 5-10 mg 3-4 times/day; usual maximum: 40 mg/day; larger doses may rarely be required

I.M. (deep): 5-10 mg every 3-4 hours; usual maximum: 40 mg/day

I.V.: 2.5-10 mg; maximum 10 mg/dose or 40 mg/day; may repeat dose every 3-4 hours as needed

Rectal: 25 mg twice daily

Surgical nausea/vomiting: Note: Should not exceed 40 mg/day

I.M.: 5-10 mg 1-2 hours before induction or to control symptoms during or after surgery; may repeat once if necessary

I.V. (administer slow IVP <5 mg/minute): 5-10 mg 15-30 minutes before induction or to control symptoms during or after surgery; may repeat once if necessary

Rectal (unlabeled use): 25 mg

Antipsychotic:

Oral: 5-10 mg 3-4 times/day; titrate dose slowly every 2-3 days; doses up to 150 mg/day may be required in some patients for treatment of severe disturbances

I.M.: Initial: 10-20 mg; if necessary repeat initial dose every 1-4 hours to gain control; more than 3-4 doses are rarely needed. If parenteral administration is still required; give 10-20 mg every 4-6 hours; change to oral as soon as possible.

Nonpsychotic anxiety: *Oral (tablet):* Usual dose: 15-20 mg/day in divided doses; do not give doses >20 mg/day or for longer than 12 weeks

Administration May be administered orally, I.M., or I.V.

I.M.: Inject by deep IM into outer quadrant of buttocks.

I.V.: Doses should be given as a short (~30 minute) infusion to avoid orthostatic hypotension; administer at ≤5 mg/minute

Monitoring Parameters Orthostatic blood pressures; tremors, gait changes, abnormal movement in trunk, neck, buccal area, or extremities; monitor target behaviors for which the agent is given; CBC with differential and periodic ophthalmic exams (if chronically used); baseline and periodic hepatic and renal function tests; monitor orthostatic blood pressures 3-5 days after initiation of therapy or a dose increase

Test Interactions False-positives for phenylketonuria, urinary amylase, uroporphyrins, urobilinogen

Patient Information Do not take antacid within 1 hour of taking drug; avoid alcohol; avoid excess sun exposure (use sun block); may cause drowsiness, rise slowly from recumbent position; use of supportive stockings may help prevent orthostatic hypotension

Special Geriatric Considerations Due to side effect profile (dystonias, EPS) this is not a preferred drug in the elderly for antiemetic therapy.

Many elderly patients receive antipsychotic medications for inappropriate nonpsychotic behavior. Before initiating antipsychotic medication, the clinician should investigate any possible reversible cause; any stress or stress from any disease can cause acute "confusion" or worsening of baseline nonpsychotic behavior. Most commonly acute changes in behavior are due to increases in drug dose or addition of new drug to regimen, fluid electrolyte loss, infections, and changes in environment.

Any changes in disease status in any organ system can result in behavior changes.

In the treatment of agitated, demented, older adult patients, authors of meta-analysis of controlled trials of the response to the traditional antipsychotics (phenothiazines, butyrophenones) in controlling agitation have concluded that the use of neuroleptics results in a response rate of 18%. Clearly neuroleptic therapy for behavior control should be limited with frequent attempts to withdraw the agent given for behavior control.

Dosage Forms Excipient information presented when available (limited, particularly for generics); consult specific product labeling.

Injection, solution, as edisylate: 5 mg/mL (2 mL, 10 mL) [contains benzyl alcohol]

Suppository, rectal: 2.5 mg (12s), 5 mg (12s), 25 mg (12s) [may contain coconut and palm oil]

Compro™: 25 mg (12s) [contains coconut and palm oils]

Tablet, as maleate: 5 mg, 10 mg

Selected References

Ernst AA, Weiss SJ, Park S, et al, "Prochlorperazine Versus Promethazine for Uncomplicated Nausea and Vomiting in the Emergency Department: A Randomized, Double-Blind Clinical Trial," *Ann Emerg Med*, 2000, 36 (2):89-94.

Golembiewski J, Chernin E, and Chopra T, "Prevention and Treatment of Postoperative Nausea and Vomiting," *Am J Health-Syst Pharm* , 2005, 62:1247-60.

Peabody CA, Warner MD, Whiteford HA, et al, "Neuroleptics and the Elderly," *J Am Geriatr Soc*, 1987, 35(3):233-8.

Risse SC and Barnes R, "Pharmacologic Treatment of Agitation Associated With Dementia," *J Am Geriatr Soc*, 1986, 34(5):368-76.

Saltz BL, Woerner MG, Kane JM, et al, "Prospective Study of Tardive Dyskinesia Incidence in the Elderly," *JAMA*, 1991, 266(17):2402-6.

Seifert RD, "Therapeutic Drug Monitoring: Psychotropic Drugs," *J Pharm Pract*, 1984, 6:403-16.

♦ **Prochlorperazine Edisylate** see Prochlorperazine on page 1320

♦ **Prochlorperazine Maleate** see Prochlorperazine on page 1320

♦ **Procrit®** see Epoetin Alfa on page 519

♦ **Proctocort®** see Hydrocortisone on page 762

♦ **ProctoCream® HC** see Hydrocortisone on page 762

♦ **Proctofene** see Fenofibrate on page 604

♦ **Procto-Kit™** see Hydrocortisone on page 762

♦ **Procto-Pak™** see Hydrocortisone on page 762

♦ **Proctosert** see Hydrocortisone on page 762

♦ **Proctosol-HC®** see Hydrocortisone on page 762

♦ **Proctozone-HC™** see Hydrocortisone on page 762

Procyclidine (proe SYE kli deen)

Medication Safety Issues
Sound-alike/look-alike issues:
Kemadrin® may be confused with Coumadin®

U.S. Brand Names Kemadrin®

Canadian Brand Names PMS-Procyclidine

Index Terms Procyclidine Hydrochloride

Generic Available No

Pharmacologic Category Anti-Parkinson's Agent, Anticholinergic; Anticholinergic Agent

Use Relief of parkinsonian syndrome symptoms and drug-induced extrapyramidal symptoms

Contraindications Hypersensitivity to procyclidine or any component of the formulation; angle-closure glaucoma; myasthenia gravis

Warnings/Precautions Use with caution in hot weather or during exercise. Elderly patients frequently develop increased sensitivity and require strict dosage regulation; side effects may be more severe in elderly patients with atherosclerotic changes. Use with caution in patients with tachycardia, cardiac arrhythmias, hypertension, hypotension, prostatic hyperplasia (especially in the elderly) or any tendency toward urinary retention, liver or kidney disorders and obstructive disease of the GI or GU tract. When given in large doses or to susceptible patients, may cause weakness and inability to move particular muscle groups. May be associated with confusion or hallucinations (generally at higher dosages); intensification of symptoms or toxic psychosis may occur in patients with mental disorders. May cause CNS depression, which may impair physical or mental abilities; patients must be cautioned about performing tasks which require mental alertness (eg, operating machinery or driving).

Adverse Reactions (Reflective of adult population; not specific for elderly)
Frequency not defined.
(Continued)

Procyclidine *(Continued)*

Cardiovascular: Palpitation, tachycardia

Central nervous system: Ataxia, confusion, drowsiness, fatigue, giddiness, headache, lightheadedness, loss of memory

Dermatologic: Dry skin, photosensitivity, rash

Gastrointestinal: Constipation, dry throat, epigastric distress, nausea, vomiting, xerostomia

Genitourinary: Difficult urination

Neuromuscular & skeletal: Weakness

Ocular: Blurred vision, increased intraocular pain, mydriasis

Respiratory: Dry nose

Miscellaneous: Diaphoresis decreased

Overdosage/Toxicology Symptoms include disorientation, hallucinations, delusions, blurred vision, dysphagia, absent bowel sounds, hyperthermia, hypertension, and urinary retention. Anticholinergic toxicity is caused by strong binding of the drug to cholinergic receptors. Anticholinesterase inhibitors reduce acetylcholinesterase, the enzyme that breaks down acetylcholine and thereby allows acetylcholine to accumulate and compete for receptor binding with the offending anticholinergic. For anticholinergic overdose with severe life-threatening symptoms, physostigmine 1-2 mg SubQ or slow I.V. may be given to reverse these effects.

Drug Interactions

Amantadine, rimantadine: Central and/or peripheral anticholinergic syndrome can occur when administered with amantadine or rimantadine

Anticholinergic agents: Central and/or peripheral anticholinergic syndrome can occur when administered with opioid analgesics, phenothiazines and other antipsychotics (especially with high anticholinergic activity), tricyclic antidepressants, quinidine and some other antiarrhythmics, and antihistamines

Atenolol: Anticholinergics may increase the bioavailability of atenolol (and possibly other beta-blockers); monitor for increased effect

Cholinergic agents: Anticholinergics may antagonize the therapeutic effect of cholinergic agents; includes tacrine and donepezil

Digoxin: Anticholinergics may decrease gastric degradation and increase the amount of digoxin absorbed by delaying gastric emptying

Levodopa: Anticholinergics may increase gastric degradation and decrease the amount of levodopa absorbed by delaying gastric emptying

Neuroleptics: Anticholinergics may antagonize the therapeutic effects of neuroleptics

Ethanol/Nutrition/Herb Interactions Ethanol: Avoid ethanol.

Mechanism of Action Thought to act by blocking excess acetylcholine at cerebral synapses; many of its effects are due to its pharmacologic similarities with atropine; it exerts an antispasmodic effect on smooth muscle, is a potent mydriatic; inhibits salivation

Pharmacodynamics

Onset of action: Oral: Within 30-40 minutes

Duration: 4-6 hours; effects may still be seen at 12 hours after the dose

Pharmacokinetics

Half-life: 12 hours

Metabolism: In the liver

Elimination: In urine

Dosage

Geriatrics: Oral: Initial: 2.5 mg once or twice daily, gradually increasing as necessary. Avoid use if possible (see Special Geriatric Considerations).

Adults: Parkinson's disease or treatment of EPS: Oral: 2.5 mg 3 times/day after meals; if tolerated, gradually increase dose, to a maximum of 20 mg/day if necessary.

Hepatic Impairment: Decrease dose to a twice daily dosing regimen.

Monitoring Parameters Symptoms of EPS or Parkinson's, pulse, anticholinergic effects (ie, CNS < bowel and bladder function)

Patient Information Take after meals or with food if GI upset occurs; do not discontinue drug abruptly; notify physician if adverse GI effects, rapid or pounding heartbeat, confusion, eye pain, rash, fever, or heat intolerance occurs. Observe caution when performing hazardous tasks or those that require alertness such as driving, as may cause drowsiness. Avoid alcohol and other CNS depressants. May cause dry mouth which adequate fluid intake or hard sugar-free candy may relieve. Difficult urination or constipation may occur, notify physician if effects persist; may increase susceptibility to heat stroke.

Special Geriatric Considerations Anticholinergic agents are generally not well tolerated in the elderly and their use should be avoided when possible. In the elderly, anticholinergic agents should not be used as prophylaxis against extrapyramidal symptoms. Elderly patients frequently develop increased sensitivity and require strict dosage regulation - side effects may be more severe in elderly patients with atherosclerotic changes.

Dosage Forms Excipient information presented when available (limited, particularly for generics); consult specific product labeling.
Tablet, as hydrochloride [scored]: 5 mg

Selected References
Feinberg M, "The Problems of Anticholinergic Adverse Effects in Older Patients," *Drugs Aging*, 1993, 3(4):335-48.
Olanow CW, Watts RL, and Koller WC, "An Algorithm (Decision Tree) for the Management of Parkinson's Disease (2001): Treatment Guidelines," *Neurology*, 2001, 56(11 Suppl 5):S1-S88.

♦ **Procyclidine Hydrochloride** *see* Procyclidine *on page 1323*
♦ **Prodium® [OTC]** *see* Phenazopyridine *on page 1238*

Progesterone (proe JES ter one)

U.S. Brand Names Crinone®; Endometrin®; Prochieve®; Prometrium®
Canadian Brand Names Crinone®; Prometrium®
Index Terms Pregnenedione; Progestin
Generic Available Yes: Injection
Pharmacologic Category Progestin
Use Treatment of endometrial carcinoma, renal carcinoma, secondary amenorrhea, abnormal uterine bleeding due to hormonal imbalance
Contraindications Hypersensitivity to progesterone or any component of the formulation; undiagnosed abnormal vaginal bleeding; history of or current thrombophlebitis or venous thromboembolic disorders (including DVT, PE); active or recent (within 1 year) arterial thromboembolic disease (eg, stroke, MI); carcinoma of the breast or genital organs; hepatic dysfunction or disease
The following are also contraindicated in patients with allergies to their inactive ingredient:
Crinone® and Prochieve™ vaginal gels contain palm oil
Prometrium® capsules contain peanut oil
Oil for injection contains sesame oil
Warnings/Precautions Use caution with cardiovascular disease or dysfunction. Progestins used in combination with estrogen may increase the risks of hypertension, myocardial infarction (MI), stroke, pulmonary emboli (PE), and deep vein thrombosis; incidence of these effects was shown to be significantly increased in postmenopausal women using conjugated equine estrogens (CEE) in combination with medroxyprogesterone acetate (MPA). Similar risk should be assumed with other progestins. Progestins in combination with estrogens should not be used to prevent coronary heart disease.

The risk of dementia may be increased in postmenopausal women; increased incidence was observed in women ≥65 years of age taking CEE in combination with MPA. An increased risk of invasive breast cancer was observed in postmenopausal women using CEE in combination with MPA. An increase in abnormal mammograms has also been reported with estrogen and progestin therapy.

Discontinue pending examination in cases of sudden partial or complete vision loss, sudden onset of proptosis, diplopia, or migraine; discontinue permanently if papilledema or retinal vascular lesions are observed on examination. Use with caution in patients with diseases that may be exacerbated by fluid retention, including asthma, epilepsy, migraine, diabetes or renal dysfunction. Use caution with history of depression. Patients should be warned that progesterone might cause transient dizziness or drowsiness during initial therapy. Whenever possible, progestins in combination with estrogens should be discontinued at least 4-6 weeks prior to surgeries associated with an increased risk of thromboembolism or during periods of prolonged immobilization. Progestins used in combination with estrogen should be used for shortest duration possible consistent with treatment goals. Conduct periodic risk:benefit assessments.

Products may contain palm oil, peanut oil, sesame oil, or benzyl alcohol.

Adverse Reactions (Reflective of adult population; not specific for elderly)
Injection (I.M.):
Cardiovascular: Cerebral edema, cerebral thrombosis, edema
Central nervous system: Depression, fever, insomnia, somnolence
Dermatologic: Acne, allergic rash (rare), alopecia, hirsutism, pruritus, rash, urticaria
Endocrine & metabolic: Amenorrhea, breakthrough bleeding, breast tenderness, galactorrhea, menstrual flow changes, spotting
Gastrointestinal: Nausea, weight gain/loss
Genitourinary: Cervical erosion changes, cervical secretion changes
Hepatic: Cholestatic jaundice
Local: Injection site: Irritation, pain, redness
Ocular: Optic neuritis, retinal thrombosis
Respiratory: Pulmonary embolism
Miscellaneous: Anaphylactoid reactions
(Continued)

Progesterone *(Continued)*

Oral capsule (percentages reported when used in combination with or cycled with conjugated estrogens):

>10%:

Central nervous system: Headache (10% to 31%), dizziness (15% to 24%), depression (19%)

Endocrine & metabolic: Breast tenderness (27%), breast pain (6% to 16%)

Gastrointestinal: Abdominal pain (6% to 12%), abdominal bloating (10% to 20%)

Genitourinary: Urinary problems (11%)

Neuromuscular & skeletal: Joint pain (20%), musculoskeletal pain (6% to 12%)

Miscellaneous: Viral infection (7% to 12%)

5% to 10%:

Cardiovascular: Chest pain (7%)

Central nervous system: Fatigue (8% to 9%), emotional lability (6%), irritability (5% to 8%), worry (8%)

Gastrointestinal: Nausea/vomiting (8%), diarrhea (8%)

Respiratory: Upper respiratory tract infection (5%), cough (8%)

Miscellaneous: Night sweats (7%)

Vaginal gel (percentages reported with ART); also refer to oral capsule reactions listing for additional effects noted with progesterone:

>10%:

Central nervous system: Somnolence (27%), headache (13% to 17%), nervousness (16%), depression (11%)

Endocrine & metabolic: Breast enlargement (40%), breast pain (13%), libido decreased (11%)

Gastrointestinal: Constipation (27%), nausea (7% to 22%), cramps (15%), abdominal pain (12%)

Genitourinary: Perineal pain (17%), nocturia (13%)

5% to 10%:

Central nervous system: Pain (8%), dizziness (5%)

Gastrointestinal: Diarrhea (8%), bloating (7%), vomiting (5%)

Genitourinary: Vaginal discharge (7%), dyspareunia (6%), genital moniliasis (5%), genital pruritus (5%)

Neuromuscular & skeletal: Arthralgia (8%)

Vaginal tablet (percentages reported with ART); also refer to oral capsule reactions listing for additional effects noted with progesterone:

>10%:

Gastrointestinal: Abdominal pain (12%)

Miscellaneous: Post-oocyte retrieval pain (25% to 28%)

1% to 10%:

Central nervous system: Headache (3% to 4%), fatigue (2% to 3%)

Endocrine & metabolic: Ovarian hyperstimulation syndrome (7%)

Gastrointestinal: Nausea (7% to 8%), abdominal distension (4%), constipation (2% to 3%), vomiting (2% to 3%)

Genitourinary: Uterine spasm (3% to 4%), vaginal bleeding (3%), urinary tract infection (1% to 2%)

Overdosage/Toxicology Toxicity is unlikely following single exposures of excessive doses. Supportive treatment is adequate in most cases.

Drug Interactions Substrate of CYP1A2 (minor), 2A6 (minor), 2C9 (minor), 2C19 (major), 2D6 (minor), 3A4 (major); **Inhibits** CYP2C9 (weak), 2C19 (weak), 3A4 (weak)

Cyclosporine: Progestins may enhance the hepatotoxic effects of cyclosporine and may increase the serum concentration of cyclosporine; monitor.

CYP2C19 inducers: May decrease the levels/effects of progesterone. Example inducers include aminoglutethimide, carbamazepine, phenytoin, and rifampin.

CYP3A4 inducers: CYP3A4 inducers may decrease the levels/effects of progesterone. Example inducers include aminoglutethimide, carbamazepine, nafcillin, nevirapine, phenobarbital, phenytoin, and rifamycins.

Estrogen: Plasma concentrations of estrogen may be increased by progesterone.

Intravaginal medications: Do not use progesterone gel within 6 hours of any other intravaginal medications. Do not use the intravaginal tablet with other intravaginal medications (eg antifungals); may alter progesterone release and absorption

Ethanol/Nutrition/Herb Interactions

Food: Food increases oral bioavailability.

Herb/Nutraceutical: St John's wort may decrease progesterone levels. Herbs with progestogenic properties may enhance the adverse/toxic effects of progestin; example herbs include bloodroot, chasteberry, damiana, oregano, yucca.

Stability Store at controlled room temperature.

Mechanism of Action Natural steroid hormone that induces secretory changes in the endometrium, promotes mammary gland development, relaxes uterine smooth muscle

Pharmacodynamics Duration: 24 hours

Pharmacokinetics
 Absorption: Vaginal gel: Prolonged
  Absorption half-life: 25-50 hours
 Protein binding: 96% to 99%
 Metabolism: Hepatic to metabolites
 Half-life elimination: Vaginal gel: 5-20 minutes
 Time to peak: Oral: Within 3 hours
 Excretion: Urine, bile, feces

Dosage
 Geriatrics & Adults: Female:
  Endometrial hyperplasia prevention (in postmenopausal women with a uterus who are receiving daily conjugated estrogen tablets): Oral: 200 mg as a single daily dose every evening for 12 days sequentially per 28-day cycle
  Functional uterine bleeding: I.M.: 5-10 mg/day for 6 doses

Administration Administer deep I.M. only

Monitoring Parameters Before starting therapy, a physical exam including the breasts and pelvis are recommended, also a Pap smear; signs or symptoms of depression, glucose in diabetics

Test Interactions Thyroid function, metyrapone, liver function, coagulation tests, endocrine function tests

Patient Information It is important that you you have an annual physical assessment, Pap smear, and vision assessment while taking this medication. You may experience increased facial hair or loss of head hair (reversible); loss of appetite (small frequent meals will help); constipation (increased fluids, exercise, dietary fiber, or stool softeners may help). Diabetics should use accurate serum glucose testing to identify any changes in glucose tolerance. Report immediately pain or muscle soreness; swelling, heat, or redness in calves; shortness of breath; sudden loss of vision; unresolved leg or foot swelling; breast tenderness that does not go away; acute abdominal cramping; signs of vaginal infection (drainage, pain, itching); or changes in CNS (eg, blurred vision, confusion, acute anxiety, or unresolved depression).

Additional Information May be used to prepare suppositories

Special Geriatric Considerations Not a progestin of choice in the elderly for hormonal cycling.

Dosage Forms Excipient information presented when available (limited, particularly for generics); consult specific product labeling.
 Capsule:
  Prometrium®: 100 mg, 200 mg [contains peanut oil]
 Gel, vaginal:
  Crinone®, Prochieve®: 4% (45 mg); 8% (90 mg) [contains palm oil; prefilled applicators]
 Injection, oil: 50 mg/mL (10 mL) [contains benzyl alcohol 10%, sesame oil]
 Tablet, vaginal:
  Endometrin®: 100 mg (21s) [packaged with applicators]

- ♦ **Progestin** see Progesterone on page 1325
- ♦ **Prolixin® [DSC]** see Fluphenazine on page 649
- ♦ **Prolixin Decanoate®** see Fluphenazine on page 649
- ♦ **Proloprim®** see Trimethoprim on page 1634

Promethazine (proe METH a zeen)

Related Information
 Potentially Inappropriate Medications for Geriatrics on page 1824

Medication Safety Issues
 Sound-alike/look-alike issues:
  Promethazine may be confused with chlorproMAZINE, predniSONE, promazine
  Phenergan® may be confused with Phenaphen®, Phrenilin®, Theragran®

 High alert medication: The Institute for Safe Medication Practices (ISMP) includes this medication among its list of drugs which have a heightened risk of causing significant patient harm when used in error.

 Administration issues:
  To prevent or minimize tissue damage during I.V. administration, the Institute for Safe Medication Practices (ISMP) has the following recommendations:
   Limit concentration available to the 25 mg/mL product
   Consider limiting initial doses to 6.25-12.5 mg
   Further dilute the 25 mg/mL strength into 10-20 mL NS
   Administer through a large bore vein (not hand or wrist)
   Administer via running I.V. line at port furthest from patient's vein
   Consider administering over 10-15 minutes
   Instruct patients to report immediately signs of pain or burning
(Continued)

Promethazine *(Continued)*

U.S. Brand Names Phenadoz™; Phenergan®; Promethegan™

Canadian Brand Names Phenergan®

Index Terms Promethazine Hydrochloride

Generic Available Yes

Pharmacologic Category Antiemetic; Antihistamine; Phenothiazine Derivative; Sedative

Use Symptomatic treatment of various allergic conditions, motion sickness; sedation; antiemetic

Contraindications Hypersensitivity to promethazine or any component of the formulation (cross-reactivity between phenothiazines may occur); severe CNS depression; coma; intra-arterial or subcutaneous injection; treatment of lower respiratory tract symptoms, including asthma

Warnings/Precautions Not for SubQ or intra-arterial administration. Injection may contain sodium metabisulfite. I.M. is the preferred route of parenteral administration. I.V. use has been associated with severe tissue damage; discontinue immediately if burning or pain occurs with administration. May be sedating; use with caution in disorders where CNS depression is a feature. May impair physical or mental abilities; patients must be cautioned about performing tasks which require mental alertness. Use with caution in Parkinson's disease; hemodynamic instability; bone marrow suppression; subcortical brain damage; and in severe cardiac, hepatic, renal, or respiratory disease. Avoid use in Reye's syndrome. May lower seizure threshold; use caution in persons with seizure disorders or in persons using narcotics or local anesthetics which may also affect seizure threshold. May alter temperature regulation or mask toxicity of other drugs due to antiemetic effects. May alter cardiac conduction (life-threatening arrhythmias have occurred with therapeutic doses of phenothiazines). May cause orthostatic hypotension; use with caution in patients at risk of hypotension or where transient hypotensive episodes would be poorly tolerated (cardiovascular disease or cerebrovascular disease).

Phenothiazines may cause anticholinergic effects; therefore, they should be used with caution in patients with decreased gastrointestinal motility, urinary retention, BPH, xerostomia, or visual problems. Conditions which also may be exacerbated by cholinergic blockade include narrow-angle glaucoma (screening is recommended) and worsening of myasthenia gravis. May cause extrapyramidal symptoms, including pseudoparkinsonism, acute dystonic reactions, akathisia, and tardive dyskinesia. May be associated with neuroleptic malignant syndrome (NMS).

Adverse Reactions (Reflective of adult population; not specific for elderly)

Cardiovascular: Bradycardia, hypertension, nonspecific QT changes, postural hypotension, tachycardia

Central nervous system: Akathisia, catatonic states, confusion, delirium, disorientation, dizziness, drowsiness, dystonias, euphoria, excitation, extrapyramidal symptoms, fatigue, hallucinations, hysteria, insomnia, lassitude, nervousness, neuroleptic malignant syndrome, nightmares, pseudoparkinsonism, sedation, seizure, somnolence, tardive dyskinesia

Dermatologic: Angioneurotic edema, dermatitis, photosensitivity, skin pigmentation (slate gray), urticaria

Endocrine & metabolic: Amenorrhea, breast engorgement, gynecomastia, hyper-/hypoglycemia, lactation

Gastrointestinal: Constipation, nausea, vomiting, xerostomia

Genitourinary: Ejaculatory disorder, impotence, urinary retention

Hematologic: Agranulocytosis, aplastic anemia, eosinophilia, hemolytic anemia, leukopenia, thrombocytopenia, thrombocytopenic purpura

Hepatic: Jaundice

Local: Venous thrombosis; injection site reactions (burning, erythema, pain, edema)

Neuromuscular & skeletal: Incoordination, tremor

Ocular: Blurred vision, corneal and lenticular changes, diplopia, epithelial keratopathy, pigmentary retinopathy

Otic: Tinnitus

Respiratory: Apnea, asthma, nasal congestion, respiratory depression

Overdosage/Toxicology Symptoms include CNS depression, respiratory depression, possible CNS stimulation, dry mouth, fixed and dilated pupils, and hypotension. Following initiation of essential overdose management, toxic symptom and supportive treatment should be initiated. Hypotension usually responds to I.V. fluids or Trendelenburg positioning. If unresponsive to these measures, norepinephrine 0.1-0.2 mcg/kg/minute titrated to response may be tried. Seizures commonly respond to diazepam (I.V. 5-10 mg bolus every 15 minutes if needed up to a total of 30 mg) or to phenytoin or phenobarbital. Critical cardiac arrhythmias often respond to I.V. phenytoin (15 mg/kg up to 1 g), while other antiarrhythmics can be used. Neuroleptics often cause extrapyramidal symptoms (eg, dystonic reactions) requiring management with diphenhydramine 1-2 mg/kg up to a maximum of 50 mg I.M. or slow I.V. push followed by a maintenance dose for 48-72 hours. When these reactions are unresponsive to diphenhydramine, anticholinergic agents such as benztropine mesylate I.V. 1-2 mg may be effective. These agents are generally effective within 2-5 minutes. Epinephrine should not be used. Hemodialysis: Not dialyzable (0% to 5%)

Drug Interactions Substrate (major) of CYP2B6, 2D6; **Inhibits** CYP2D6 (weak)

Acetylcholinesterase inhibitors, central (donepezil, galantamine, rivastigmine, tacrine): May diminish the therapeutic effect of promethazine. Promethazine may diminish the therapeutic effect of centrally acting acetylcholinesterase inhibitors.

Anticholinergics: May inhibit the therapeutic response to phenothiazines and excess anticholinergic effects may occur; includes benztropine, trihexyphenidyl, biperiden, and drugs with significant anticholinergic activity (TCAs, antihistamines, disopyramide).

CYP2B6 inducers: May decrease the levels/effects of promethazine. Example inducers include carbamazepine, nevirapine, phenobarbital, phenytoin, and rifampin.

CYP2B6 inhibitors: May increase the levels/effects of promethazine. Example inhibitors include desipramine, paroxetine, and sertraline.

CYP2D6 inhibitors: May increase the levels/effects of promethazine. Example inhibitors include chlorpromazine, delavirdine, fluoxetine, miconazole, paroxetine, pergolide, quinidine, quinine, ritonavir, and ropinirole.

Pramlintide: May enhance the gastrointestinal anticholinergic effects of promethazine.

Ethanol/Nutrition/Herb Interactions

Ethanol: Avoid ethanol (may increase CNS depression).

Herb/Nutraceutical: Avoid valerian, St John's wort, kava kava, gotu kola (may increase CNS depression).

Stability

Injection: Prior to dilution, store at room temperature. Protect from light. Solutions in NS or D_5W are stable for 24 hours at room temperature.

Suppositories: Store refrigerated at 2°C to 8°C (36°F to 46°F).

Tablets: Store at room temperature. Protect from light.

Mechanism of Action Blocks postsynaptic mesolimbic dopaminergic receptors in the brain; exhibits a strong alpha-adrenergic blocking effect and depresses the release of hypothalamic and hypophyseal hormones; competes with histamine for the H_1-receptor; reduces stimuli to the brainstem reticular system

Pharmacodynamics

Onset of action: Within 20 minutes (3-5 minutes with I.V. injection)

Duration: 4-6 hours

Pharmacokinetics

Metabolism: In the liver

Elimination: Principally as inactive metabolites in urine and feces

Dosage

Geriatrics & Adults:

Allergic conditions (including allergic reactions to blood or plasma):

Oral, rectal: 25 mg at bedtime **or** 12.5 mg before meals and at bedtime (range: 6.25-12.5 mg 3 times/day)

I.M., I.V.: 25 mg, may repeat in 2 hours when necessary; switch to oral route as soon as feasible

Antiemetic: Oral, I.M., I.V., rectal: 12.5-25 mg every 4-6 hours as needed

Motion sickness: Oral, rectal: 25 mg 30-60 minutes before departure, then every 12 hours as needed

Sedation: Oral, I.M., I.V., rectal: 12.5-50 mg/dose

Administration Formulations available for oral, rectal, I.M./I.V.; not for SubQ or intra-arterial administration. Administer I.M. into deep muscle (preferred route of administration). I.V. administration is **not** the preferred route; severe tissue damage may occur. Solution for injection should be administered in a maximum concentration of 25 mg/mL (more dilute solutions are recommended). Administer via running I.V. line at port furthest from patient's vein, or through a large bore vein (not hand or wrist). Consider administering over 10-15 minutes (maximum:25 mg/minute). Discontinue immediately if burning or pain occurs with administration. Rapid I.V. administration may produce a transient fall in blood pressure; slow I.V. administration may produce a slightly elevated blood pressure.

Monitoring Parameters Relief of symptoms, mental status; monitor for EPS

Test Interactions Alters the flare response in intradermal allergen tests; increased serum glucose may be seen with glucose tolerance tests

Patient Information May cause drowsiness; avoid the use of alcohol and other CNS depressants; may cause photosensitivity

Additional Information Promethazine is available in various combinations; these include codeine, phenylephrine, phenylephrine and codeine

(Continued)

Promethazine *(Continued)*

Special Geriatric Considerations Because promethazine is a phenothiazine (and can, therefore, cause side effects such as extrapyramidal symptoms), it is not considered an antihistamine of choice in the elderly.

Dosage Forms Excipient information presented when available (limited, particularly for generics); consult specific product labeling. [DSC] = Discontinued product

Injection, solution, as hydrochloride: 25 mg/mL (1 mL); 50 mg/mL (1 mL)
  Phenergan®: 25 mg/mL (1 mL); 50 mg/mL (1 mL) [contains sodium metabisulfite]
Suppository, rectal, as hydrochloride: 12.5 mg, 25 mg, 50 mg
  Phenadoz™: 12.5 mg, 25 mg
  Phenergan®: 25 mg, 50 mg [DSC]
  Promethegan™: 12.5 mg, 25 mg, 50 mg
Syrup, as hydrochloride: 6.25 mg/5 mL (120 mL, 480 mL) [contains alcohol]
Tablet, as hydrochloride: 12.5 mg, 25 mg, 50 mg
  Phenergan®: 25 mg [DSC]

Selected References
http://www.ismp.org/Newsletters/acutecare/articles/20060810.asp

♦ **Promethazine Hydrochloride** see Promethazine on page 1327
♦ **Promethegan™** see Promethazine on page 1327
♦ **Prometrium®** see Progesterone on page 1325
♦ **Pronap-100®** see Propoxyphene and Acetaminophen on page 1335

Propafenone *(pro PAF en one)*

U.S. Brand Names Rythmol®; Rythmol® SR
Canadian Brand Names Apo-Propafenone®; Rythmol® Gen-Propafenone
Index Terms Propafenone Hydrochloride
Generic Available Yes: Tablet
Pharmacologic Category Antiarrhythmic Agent, Class Ic
Use Treatment of life-threatening ventricular arrhythmias
  Rythmol® SR: Maintenance of normal sinus rhythm in patients with symptomatic atrial fibrillation
Unlabeled/Investigational Use Treatment of supraventricular tachycardias, including those patients with Wolff-Parkinson-White syndrome
Contraindications Hypersensitivity to propafenone or any component of the formulation; sinoatrial, AV, and intraventricular disorders of impulse generation and/or conduction (except in patients with a functioning artificial pacemaker); sinus bradycardia; cardiogenic shock; uncompensated cardiac failure; hypotension; bronchospastic disorders; uncorrected electrolyte abnormalities; concurrent use of amprenavir, cimetidine, metoprolol, propranolol quinidine, and ritonavir (see Drug Interactions)
Warnings/Precautions Monitor for proarrhythmic events. May prolong QT$_c$ interval; use caution with other QT$_c$-prolonging drugs. **[U.S. Boxed Warning]: In the Cardiac Arrhythmia Suppression Trial (CAST), recent (>6 days but <2 years ago) myocardial infarction patients with asymptomatic, nonlife-threatening ventricular arrhythmias did not benefit and may have been harmed by attempts to suppress the arrhythmia with flecainide or encainide. An increased mortality or nonfatal cardiac arrest rate (7.7%) was seen in the active treatment group compared with patients in the placebo group (3%). The applicability of the CAST results to other populations is unknown. Antiarrhythmic agents should be reserved for patients with life-threatening ventricular arrhythmias.** Can cause or unmask a variety of conduction disturbances. May alter pacing and sensing thresholds of artificial pacemakers. Patients with bronchospastic disease should generally not receive this drug. Monitor for worsening CHF if patient has underlying condition. Correct electrolyte disturbances, especially hypokalemia or hypomagnesemia, prior to use and throughout therapy. Administer cautiously in significant hepatic dysfunction. Use with caution in patients with myasthenia gravis; may exacerbate condition.
Adverse Reactions (Reflective of adult population; not specific for elderly)
1% to 10%:
  Cardiovascular: New or worsened arrhythmia (proarrhythmic effect) (2% to 10%), angina (2% to 5%), CHF (1% to 4%), ventricular tachycardia (1% to 3%), palpitation (1% to 3%), AV block (first-degree) (1% to 3%), syncope (1% to 2%), increased QRS interval (1% to 2%), chest pain (1% to 2%), PVCs (1% to 2%), bradycardia (1% to 2%), edema (0% to 1%), bundle branch block (0% to 1%), atrial fibrillation (1%), hypotension (0% to 1%), intraventricular conduction delay (0% to 1%)
  Central nervous system: Dizziness (4% to 15%), fatigue (2% to 6%), headache (2% to 5%), ataxia (0% to 2%), insomnia (0% to 2%), anxiety (1% to 2%), drowsiness (1%)
  Dermatologic: Rash (1% to 3%)
  Gastrointestinal: Nausea/vomiting (2% to 11%), unusual taste (3% to 23%), constipation (2% to 7%), dyspepsia (1% to 3%), diarrhea (1% to 3%), xerostomia (1% to 2%), anorexia (1% to 2%), abdominal pain (1% to 2%), flatulence (0% to 1%)

Neuromuscular & skeletal: Tremor (0% to 1%), arthralgia (0% to 1%), weakness (1% to 2%)

Ocular: Blurred vision (1% to 6%)

Respiratory: Dyspnea (2% to 5%)

Miscellaneous: Diaphoresis (1%)

Overdosage/Toxicology Has a narrow therapeutic index and severe toxicity may occur slightly above the therapeutic range, especially if combined with other antiarrhythmic drugs. Acute single ingestion of twice the daily therapeutic dose is life-threatening. Symptoms include increases in PR, QRS, QT intervals and amplitude of the T wave, as well as AV block, bradycardia, hypotension, ventricular arrhythmias (monomorphic or polymorphic ventricular tachycardia), and asystole. Other symptoms include dizziness, blurred vision, headache, and GI upset. Treatment is supportive, using conventional treatment (fluids, positioning, anticonvulsants, antiarrhythmics). **Note:** Type Ia antiarrhythmic agents should not be used to treat cardiotoxicity caused by type 1c antiarrhythmic drugs. Sodium bicarbonate may reverse QRS prolongation, bradycardia and hypotension; ventricular pacing may be needed. Hemodialysis is only of possible benefit for tocainide or flecainide overdose in patients with renal failure.

Drug Interactions Substrate of CYP1A2 (minor), 2D6 (major), 3A4 (minor); **Inhibits** CYP1A2 (weak), 2D6 (weak)

Cimetidine: May increase propafenone levels.

CYP2D6 inhibitors: May increase the levels/effects of propafenone. Example inhibitors include chlorpromazine, delavirdine, fluoxetine, miconazole, paroxetine, pergolide, quinidine, quinine, ritonavir, and ropinirole.

Digoxin: Propafenone may increase digoxin levels; monitor for toxicity.

Metoprolol: Propafenone may increase metoprolol levels.

Phenobarbital: May decrease propafenone levels.

Propranolol: Propafenone may increase propranolol levels.

QT_c-prolonging agents: Effects may be additive with propafenone. Use caution with Class Ia and Class III antiarrhythmics, erythromycin, cisapride, antipsychotics, and cyclic antidepressants.

Quinidine: May increase propafenone levels.

Rifampin: May decrease propafenone levels.

Ritonavir: May increase propafenone levels; concurrent use is contraindicated.

Theophylline: Propafenone may increase theophylline levels.

Warfarin: Propafenone may increase warfarin levels/effects. Monitor INR closely.

Ethanol/Nutrition/Herb Interactions

Food: Propafenone serum concentrations may be increased if taken with food.

Herb/Nutraceutical: St John's wort may decrease propafenone levels. Avoid ephedra (may worsen arrhythmia).

Stability Store at 25°C (77°F); excursions permitted to 15°C to 30°C (59°F to 86°F).

Mechanism of Action Propafenone is a class 1c antiarrhythmic agent which possesses local anesthetic properties, blocks the fast inward sodium current, and slows the rate of increase of the action potential. Prolongs conduction and refractoriness in all areas of the myocardium, with a slightly more pronounced effect on intraventricular conduction; it prolongs effective refractory period, reduces spontaneous automaticity and exhibits some beta-blockade activity.

Pharmacokinetics

Absorption: Well absorbed

Metabolism: Two genetically determined metabolism groups exist: fast or slow metabolizers; 10% of Caucasians are slow metabolizers

Half-life after a single dose (100-300 mg): 2-8 hours; half-life after chronic dosing ranges from 10-32 hours

Time to peak serum concentration: 2 hours with a 150 mg dose and 3 hours after a 300 mg dose; this agent exhibits nonlinear pharmacokinetics; when dose is increased from 300-900 mg/day, serum concentrations increase tenfold; this nonlinearity is thought to be due to saturable first-pass hepatic enzyme metabolism

Dosage

Geriatrics & Adults: Note: Patients who exhibit significant widening of QRS complex or second- or third-degree AV block may need dose reduction.

Ventricular arrhythmias: Oral:

Immediate release tablet: Initial: 150 mg every 8 hours, increase at 3- to 4-day intervals up to 300 mg every 8 hours.

Extended release capsule: Initial: 225 mg every 12 hours; dosage increase may be made at a minimum of 5-day intervals; may increase to 325 mg every 12 hours; if further increase is necessary, may increase to 425 mg every 12 hours

Paroxysmal atrial fibrillation (unlabeled dose): Oral: *Immediate release:* Outpatient: "Pill-in-the-pocket" dose: 450 mg (weight <70 kg); 600 mg (weight ≥70 kg). May not repeat in ≤24 hours. **Note:** An initial inpatient conversion trial should have been successful before sending patient home on this approach. Patient must be taking an AV nodal-blocking agent (eg, beta-blocker, nondihydropyridine calcium channel blocker) prior to initiation of antiarrhythmic.

(Continued)

Propafenone *(Continued)*

Hepatic Impairment: Reduction is necessary; however, specific guidelines are not available.

Monitoring Parameters EKG, blood pressure, pulse (particularly at initiation of therapy), signs and symptoms of CHF; titrate dose according to response and tolerance

Patient Information Take dose the same way each day, either with or without food; very important to take drug correctly, do not double the next dose if present dose is missed; report any palpitations, chest pain, difficult breathing, blurred vision, fever, sore throat, bleeding, bruising, or drowsiness; may impair coordination and judgment

Additional Information An oral sodium channel blocker similar to flecainide; in clinical trials was used effectively to treat atrial flutter, atrial fibrillation, and other arrhythmias, but are not labeled indications; can worsen or even cause new ventricular arrhythmias (proarrhythmic effect)

Special Geriatric Considerations Elderly may have age-related decreases in hepatic Phase I metabolism. Propafenone is dependent upon liver metabolism, therefore, monitor closely in the elderly and adjust dose more gradually during initial treatment. No differences in clearance noted with impaired renal function and, therefore, no adjustment for renal function in the elderly is necessary.

Dosage Forms Excipient information presented when available (limited, particularly for generics); consult specific product labeling.

Capsule, extended release, as hydrochloride (Rythmol® SR): 225 mg, 325 mg, 425 mg [contains soy lecithin]

Tablet, as hydrochloride (Rythmol®): 150 mg, 225 mg, 300 mg

Selected References

Fenster PE and Nolan PE, "Antiarrhythmic Drugs," *Geriatric Pharmacology*, Bressler R and Katz MD, eds, New York, NY: McGraw-Hill, 1993, 6:105-49.

♦ **Propafenone Hydrochloride** *see* Propafenone *on page 1330*

Propantheline *(proe PAN the leen)*

Related Information

Pharmacotherapy of Urinary Incontinence *on page 1822*
Potentially Inappropriate Medications for Geriatrics *on page 1824*

Index Terms Propantheline Bromide

Generic Available Yes

Pharmacologic Category Anticholinergic Agent

Use Adjunctive treatment of peptic ulcer, irritable bowel syndrome, pancreatitis, ureteral and urinary bladder spasm; reduction of duodenal motility during diagnostic radiologic procedures

Contraindications Hypersensitivity to propantheline or any component of the formulation; ulcerative colitis, toxic megacolon, obstructive disease of the GI or urinary tract; narrow-angle glaucoma; myasthenia gravis

Warnings/Precautions Use with caution in febrile patients, patients with hyperthyroidism, hepatic, cardiac, or renal disease, hypertension, GI infections

Adverse Reactions (Reflective of adult population; not specific for elderly)
Frequency not defined.
Dermatologic: Dry skin
Gastrointestinal: Constipation, dry mouth and throat, dysphagia
Respiratory: Dry nose
Miscellaneous: Diaphoresis (decreased)

Drug Interactions

Decreased effect with antacids (decreased absorption); decreased effect of sustained release dosage forms (decreased absorption)

Increased effect/toxicity with anticholinergics, disopyramide, opioid analgesics, bretylium, type I antiarrhythmics, antihistamines, phenothiazines, TCAs, corticosteroids (increased IOP), CNS depressants (sedation), adenosine, amiodarone, beta-blockers, amoxapine

Mechanism of Action Competitively blocks the action of acetylcholine at postganglionic parasympathetic receptor sites

Pharmacodynamics
Onset of action: Oral: Within 30-45 minutes
Duration: 4-6 hours

Pharmacokinetics
Metabolism: In the liver and GI tract
Elimination: In urine, bile, and other body fluids

Dosage
Geriatrics: Antisecretory: 7.5 mg 3 times/day before meals and at bedtime; increase as necessary to a maximum of 30 mg 3 times/day

Adults:
Antisecretory: Oral: 15 mg 3 times/day before meals or food and 30 mg at bedtime
Antispasmodic: Oral: 15 mg 3 times/day before meals or food and 30 mg at bedtime

Monitoring Parameters Anticholinergic effects, blood pressure, pulse, urinary output, postvoid residual, GI symptoms

Patient Information Take 30 minutes before meals and at bedtime. Maintain good oral hygiene habits, because lack of saliva may increase chance of cavities. Observe caution while driving or performing other tasks requiring alertness, as may cause drowsiness, dizziness, or blurred vision. Notify physician if skin rash, flushing or eye pain occurs; or if difficulty in urinating, constipation or sensitivity to light becomes severe or persists.

Additional Information Because propantheline is a quaternary ammonium compound, it does not cross the blood-brain barrier and is less likely to cause CNS effects as compared to atropine

Special Geriatric Considerations The primary use of propantheline in the geriatric population is for treatment of urinary incontinence due to detrusor instability. Even though it does not cross the blood-brain barrier, CNS effects have been reported. Orthostatic hypotension may also occur, therefore, avoid long-term use in the elderly.

Dosage Forms Excipient information presented when available (limited, particularly for generics); consult specific product labeling.
Tablet, as bromide: 15 mg [contains lactose 23.2 mg]

- ♦ **Propantheline Bromide** *see* Propantheline *on page 1332*
- ♦ **Propa pH [OTC]** *see* Salicylic Acid *on page 1441*
- ♦ **Propecia®** *see* Finasteride *on page 626*
- ♦ **Propine®** *see* Dipivefrin *on page 453*

Propoxyphene (proe POKS i feen)

Related Information
Narcotic / Opioid Analgesics *on page 1763*
Potentially Inappropriate Medications for Geriatrics *on page 1824*

Medication Safety Issues
Sound-alike/look-alike issues:
Propoxyphene may be confused with proparacaine
Darvon® may be confused with Devrom®, Diovan®
Darvon-N® may be confused with Darvocet-N®

U.S. Brand Names Darvon®; Darvon-N®

Canadian Brand Names Darvon-N®; 642® Tablet

Index Terms Dextropropoxyphene; Propoxyphene Hydrochloride; Propoxyphene Napsylate

Generic Available Yes: Capsule

Pharmacologic Category Analgesic, Opioid

Use Management of mild to moderate pain

Restrictions C-IV

Contraindications Hypersensitivity to propoxyphene or any component of the formulation

Warnings/Precautions [U.S. Boxed Warning]: When given in excessive doses, either alone or in combination with other CNS depressants (including alcohol), propoxyphene is a major cause of drug-related deaths; recommended dosage must not be exceeded and alcohol intake should be limited. Avoid use in severely depressed or suicidal patients. Should not be prescribed in patients who are addiction prone or suicidal. Use caution in patients taking CNS depressant medications or antidepressants, and in patients who use alcohol in excess. Use with caution in patients with CNS depression coma, head trauma, thyroid dysfunction, adrenal insufficiency, morbid obesity, and prostatic hyperplasia/urinary stricture. Use with caution in patients with biliary tract dysfunction; acute pancreatitis may cause constriction of sphincter of Oddi. May cause hypotension; use with caution in patients with hypovolemia, cardiovascular disease (including acute MI), or drugs which may exaggerate hypotensive effects (including phenothiazines or general anesthetics). May obscure diagnosis or clinical course of patients with acute abdominal conditions.

May cause CNS depression, which may impair physical or mental abilities; patients must be cautioned about performing tasks which require mental alertness (eg, operating machinery or driving). Effects may be potentiated when used with other sedative drugs or ethanol. Use caution in patients dependent on opiates, substitution may result in acute opiate withdrawal symptoms. Tolerance or drug dependence may result from extended use. Propoxyphene should be used with caution in patients with renal or hepatic dysfunction, debilitated patients or in the elderly; consider dosing adjustment.
(Continued)

Propoxyphene *(Continued)*

An opioid-containing analgesic regimen should be tailored to each patient's needs and based upon the type of pain being treated (acute versus chronic), the route of administration, degree of tolerance for opioids (naive versus chronic user), age, weight, and medical condition. The optimal analgesic dose varies widely among patients; doses should be titrated to pain relief/prevention.

Adverse Reactions (Reflective of adult population; not specific for elderly)
Frequency not defined.

Cardiovascular: Bundle branch block, hypotension

Central nervous system: Confusion, dizziness, dysphoria, drowsiness, fatigue, hallucinations, headache, increased intracranial pressure, lightheadedness, malaise, mental depression, nervousness, paradoxical CNS stimulation, paradoxical excitement and insomnia, restlessness, sedation, vertigo

Dermatologic: Rash, urticaria

Endocrine & metabolic: Decreased urinary 17-OHCS, hypoglycemia

Gastrointestinal: Abdominal pain, anorexia, biliary spasm, constipation, nausea, paralytic ileus, stomach cramps, vomiting, xerostomia

Genitourinary: Decreased urination, ureteral spasms

Hepatic: LFTs increased, jaundice

Neuromuscular & skeletal: Weakness

Ocular: Visual disturbances

Respiratory: Dyspnea

Miscellaneous: Histamine release, hypersensitivity reaction psychologic and physical dependence with prolonged use

Overdosage/Toxicology Symptoms include CNS and respiratory depression, hypotension, pulmonary edema, and seizures. Treatment includes airway support, establishment of an I.V. line, and administration of naloxone 2 mg I.V., with repeat administration as necessary, up to a total of 10 mg. Emesis is not indicated as overdose may cause seizures. Charcoal is very effective (>95%) at binding propoxyphene.

Drug Interactions Inhibits CYP2C9 (weak), 2D6 (weak), 3A4 (weak)

Decreased effect with charcoal, cigarette smoking

Increased toxicity: CNS depressants may potentiate pharmacologic effects; propoxyphene may inhibit the metabolism and increase the serum concentrations of carbamazepine, phenobarbital, MAO inhibitors, tricyclic antidepressants, and warfarin

Ethanol/Nutrition/Herb Interactions

Ethanol: Avoid or limit ethanol (may increase CNS depression). Watch for sedation.

Food: May decrease rate of absorption, but may slightly increase bioavailability.

Stability Store at controlled room temperature of 15°C to 30°C (59°F to 86°F).

Mechanism of Action Propoxyphene is a weak narcotic analgesic which acts through binding to opiate receptors to inhibit ascending pain pathways. Propoxyphene, as with other narcotic (opiate) analgesics, blocks pain perception in the cerebral cortex by binding to specific receptor molecules (opiate receptors) within the neuronal membranes of synapses. This binding results in a decreased synaptic chemical transmission throughout the CNS thus inhibiting the flow of pain sensations into the higher centers. Mu and kappa are the two subtypes of the opiate receptor which propoxyphene binds to cause analgesia.

Pharmacodynamics

Onset of effect: Oral: Within 30-60 minutes

Duration: 4-6 hours

Pharmacokinetics

Bioavailability: Oral: 30% to 70% due to first-pass effect

Metabolism: In the liver to an active metabolite (norpropoxyphene) and inactive metabolites; metabolism is decreased in older adults and hepatic dysfunction; propoxyphene and norpropoxyphene accumulate in renal failure

Half-life: 8-24 hours (mean: ~15 hours); norpropoxyphene: 34 hours

Dosage

Geriatrics: Pain management: Oral:

Hydrochloride: 65 mg every 4-6 hours as needed for pain

Napsylate: 100 mg every 4-6 hours as needed for pain

Adults: Pain management: Oral:

Hydrochloride: 65 mg every 3-4 hours as needed for pain; maximum: 390 mg/day

Napsylate: 100 mg every 4 hours as needed for pain; maximum: 600 mg/day

Renal Impairment: Serum concentrations of propoxyphene may be increased or elimination may be delayed. Avoid use in Cl$_{cr}$ <10 mL/minute. Specific dosing recommendations not available for less severe impairment.

Not dialyzable (0% to 5%)

Hepatic Impairment: Serum concentrations of propoxyphene may be increased or elimination may be delayed. Specific dosing recommendations not available.

Monitoring Parameters Pain relief, respiratory and mental status, blood pressure

Reference Range Therapeutic: 0.1-0.4 mcg/mL (SI: 0.3-1.2 µmol/L) (therapeutic ranges published vary between laboratories and may not correlate with clinical effect); Toxic: >0.5 mcg/mL (SI: >1.5 µmol/L)

Test Interactions False-positive methadone test

Patient Information May cause drowsiness, dizziness, or blurring of vision; avoid alcohol and other sedatives; may take with food

Additional Information Some studies have found no significant difference in pain relief between propoxyphene and aspirin or acetaminophen

Propoxyphene hydrochloride: Darvon®

Propoxyphene napsylate: Darvon-N®

Special Geriatric Considerations Elderly may be particularly susceptible to the CNS depressant and constipating effects of narcotics. Propoxyphene is not considered the analgesic of choice in the elderly when mild to moderate pain requires a narcotic analgesic. This is due to the higher incidence of adverse CNS effects seen in the elderly population. Also a concern is the addiction potential in elderly; avoid use, if possible.

Dosage Forms Excipient information presented when available (limited, particularly for generics); consult specific product labeling.

Capsule, as hydrochloride (Darvon®): 65 mg

Tablet, as napsylate (Darvon-N®): 100 mg

Selected References

AGS Panel on Persistent Pain in Older Persons, "The Management of Persistent Pain in Older Persons," *J Am Geriatr Soc*, 2002, 50(6 Suppl):S205-24.

Ferrell BA, "Pain Management in Elderly People," *J Am Geriatr Soc*, 1991, 39(1):64-73.

Miller RR, "Propoxyphene: A Review," *Am J Hosp Pharm*, 1977, 34(4):413-23.

Propoxyphene and Acetaminophen

(proe POKS i feen & a seet a MIN oh fen)

Related Information

Acetaminophen *on page 29*

Narcotic / Opioid Analgesics *on page 1763*

Propoxyphene *on page 1333*

Medication Safety Issues

Sound-alike/look-alike issues:

Darvocet-N® may be confused with Darvon-N®

Duplicate therapy issues: This product contains acetaminophen, which may be a component of other combination products. Do not exceed the maximum recommended daily dose of acetaminophen.

U.S. Brand Names Balacet 325™; Darvocet A500™; Darvocet-N® 50; Darvocet-N® 100; Pronap-100®

Canadian Brand Names Darvocet-N® 50; Darvocet-N® 100

Index Terms Acetaminophen and Propoxyphene; Propoxyphene Hydrochloride and Acetaminophen; Propoxyphene Napsylate and Acetaminophen

Generic Available Yes

Pharmacologic Category Analgesic Combination (Opioid)

Use Management of mild to moderate pain

Restrictions C-IV

Contraindications Hypersensitivity to propoxyphene, acetaminophen, or any component of the formulation

Warnings/Precautions [U.S. Boxed Warning]: When given in excessive doses, either alone or in combination with other CNS depressants (including alcohol), propoxyphene is a major cause of drug-related deaths; recommended dosage must not be exceeded and alcohol intake should be limited. Avoid use in severely depressed or suicidal patients. Should not be prescribed in patients who are addiction prone or suicidal. Use caution in patients taking CNS depressant medications or antidepressants, and in patients who use alcohol in excess.

Use caution in patients dependent on opiates, substitution may result in acute opiate withdrawal symptoms. Tolerance or drug dependence may result from extended use. Propoxyphene should be used with caution in patients with renal or hepatic dysfunction or in the elderly; consider dosing adjustment.

Propoxyphene should be used with caution in patients with renal or hepatic dysfunction or in the elderly; consider dosing adjustment. Acetaminophen should be used with caution in patients with liver disease; consuming ≥3 alcoholic drinks/day may increase risk of liver damage. Use caution in patients with known G6PD deficiency.

Adverse Reactions (Reflective of adult population; not specific for elderly) See individual agents.

Drug Interactions

Propoxyphene: **Inhibits** CYP2C9 (weak), 2D6 (weak), 3A4 (weak)

(Continued)

Propoxyphene and Acetaminophen *(Continued)*

Acetaminophen: **Substrate** (minor) of CYP1A2, 2A6, 2C9, 2D6, 2E1, 3A4; **Inhibits** CYP3A4 (weak)

Also see individual agents.

Ethanol/Nutrition/Herb Interactions

Based on **propoxyphene** component:

Ethanol: Avoid or limit ethanol (may increase CNS depression). Watch for sedation.

Food: May decrease rate of absorption, but may slightly increase bioavailability.

Based on **acetaminophen** component:

Ethanol: Excessive intake of ethanol may increase the risk of acetaminophen-induced hepatotoxicity. Avoid ethanol or limit to <3 drinks/day.

Food: Rate of absorption may be decreased when given with food.

Herb/Nutraceutical: St John's wort may decrease acetaminophen levels.

Stability Store at controlled room temperature.

Mechanism of Action See individual agents.

Dosage

Geriatrics & Adults:

Pain management: Oral:

Darvocet A500™, Darvocet-N® 100: 1 tablet every 4 hours as needed; maximum: 600 mg propoxyphene napsylate/day

Darvocet-N® 50: 1-2 tablets every 4 hours as needed; maximum: 600 mg propoxyphene napsylate/day

Propoxyphene hydrochloride 65 mg and acetaminophen 650 mg: 1 tablet every 4 hours as needed; maximum: 390 mg/day propoxyphene hydrochloride, 4 g/day acetaminophen)

Note: Formulations contain significant amounts of acetaminophen; intake should be limited to <4 g acetaminophen/day (less in patients with hepatic impairment/ethanol abuse)

Renal Impairment: Serum concentrations of propoxyphene may be increased or elimination may be delayed; specific dosing recommendations not available.

Hepatic Impairment: Serum concentrations of propoxyphene may be increased or elimination may be delayed; specific dosing recommendations not available.

Administration Should be administered with water on an empty stomach.

Monitoring Parameters Pain relief, respiratory and mental status, blood pressure

Patient Information See individual agents.

Additional Information Some studies have found no significant difference in pain relief between propoxyphene and aspirin or acetaminophen.

Special Geriatric Considerations The elderly may be particularly susceptible to the CNS depressant and constipating effects of narcotics; do not exceed 4 g/day of acetaminophen. See Warnings/Precautions and Dosage. Propoxyphene is not considered the analgesic of choice in the elderly patient when mild-to-moderate pain requires a narcotic analgesic. This is due to the higher incidence of adverse CNS effects seen in this population group. The addiction potential is also a concern; avoid use, if possible.

Dosage Forms Excipient information presented when available (limited, particularly for generics); consult specific product labeling.

Tablet: Propoxyphene hydrochloride 65 mg and acetaminophen 650 mg, propoxyphene napsylate 100 mg, and acetaminophen 650 mg

Balacet 325™: Propoxyphene napsylate 100 mg and acetaminophen 325 mg

Darvocet A500™: Propoxyphene napsylate 100 mg and acetaminophen 500 mg [contains lactose]

Darvocet-N® 50: Propoxyphene napsylate 50 mg and acetaminophen 325 mg

Darvocet-N® 100, Pronap-100®: Propoxyphene napsylate 100 mg and acetaminophen 650 mg

♦ **Propoxyphene Hydrochloride** *see* Propoxyphene *on page 1333*

♦ **Propoxyphene Hydrochloride and Acetaminophen** *see* Propoxyphene and Acetaminophen *on page 1335*

♦ **Propoxyphene Napsylate** *see* Propoxyphene *on page 1333*

♦ **Propoxyphene Napsylate and Acetaminophen** *see* Propoxyphene and Acetaminophen *on page 1335*

Propranolol *(proe PRAN oh lole)*

Related Information

Beta-Blockers *on page 1751*

Medication Safety Issues

Sound-alike/look-alike issues:

Propranolol may be confused with Pravachol®, Propulsid®

Inderal® may be confused with Adderall®, Enduron®, Enduronyl®, Imdur®, Imuran®, Inderide®, Isordil®, Toradol®

Inderal® 40 may be confused with Endouronyl® Forte

High alert medication: The Institute for Safe Medication Practices (ISMP) includes this medication among its list of drugs which have a heightened risk of causing significant patient harm when used in error.

Significant differences exist between oral and I.V. dosing. Use caution when converting from one route of administration to another.

International issues:
Inderal® may be confused with Indiaral® which is a brand name for loperamide in France

U.S. Brand Names Inderal®; Inderal® LA; InnoPran XL™

Canadian Brand Names Apo-Propranolol®; Inderal®; Inderal®-LA; Novo-Pranol; Nu-Propranolol; Propranolol Hydrochloride Injection, USP

Index Terms Propranolol Hydrochloride

Generic Available Yes

Pharmacologic Category Antiarrhythmic Agent, Class II; Beta-Adrenergic Blocker, Nonselective

Use Management of hypertension; angina pectoris; pheochromocytoma; essential tremor; supraventricular arrhythmias (such as atrial fibrillation and flutter, AV nodal re-entrant tachycardias); ventricular tachycardias (catecholamine-induced arrhythmias, digoxin toxicity); prevention of myocardial infarction; migraine headache prophylaxis; symptomatic treatment of hypertrophic subaortic stenosis

Unlabeled/Investigational Use Tremor due to Parkinson's disease; ethanol withdrawal; aggressive behavior; antipsychotic-induced akathisia; prevention of bleeding esophageal varices; anxiety; schizophrenia; acute panic; gastric bleeding in portal hypertension; thyrotoxicosis; tetralogy of Fallot (TOF) hypercyanotic spells

Contraindications Hypersensitivity to propranolol, beta-blockers, or any component of the formulation; uncompensated congestive heart failure (unless the failure is due to tachyarrhythmias being treated with propranolol), cardiogenic shock, bradycardia or heart block (2nd or 3rd degree), pulmonary edema, severe hyperactive airway disease (asthma or COPD), Raynaud's disease

Warnings/Precautions Consider pre-existing conditions such as sick sinus syndrome before initiating. Administer cautiously in compensated heart failure and monitor for a worsening of the condition (efficacy of propranolol in CHF has not been demonstrated). Beta-blocker therapy should not be withdrawn abruptly (particularly in patients with CAD), but gradually tapered to avoid acute tachycardia, hypertension, and/or ischemia. Use caution in patient with peripheral vascular disease (PVD). Use caution with concurrent use of beta-blockers and either verapamil or diltiazem; bradycardia or heart block can occur. Avoid concurrent I.V. use of both agents. Use cautiously in diabetics because it can mask prominent hypoglycemic symptoms. Use with caution in myasthenia gravis or psychiatric disease (may cause CNS depression). Use cautiously in renal and hepatic dysfunction; dosage adjustment required in hepatic impairment. Use care with anesthetic agents which decrease myocardial function. In general, patients with bronchospastic disease should not receive beta-blockers; if used at all, should be used cautiously with close monitoring. Not indicated for hypertensive emergencies. Adequate alpha-blockade is required prior to use of any beta-blocker for patients with untreated pheochromocytoma.

Adverse Reactions (Reflective of adult population; not specific for elderly) Frequency not defined.

Cardiovascular: Arterial insufficiency, AV conduction disturbance increased, bradycardia, cardiogenic shock, CHF, chest pain, hypotension, impaired myocardial contractility, mesenteric thrombosis (rare), Raynaud's syndrome, syncope

Central nervous system: Amnesia, cognitive dysfunction, cold extremities, confusion, depression, dizziness, emotional lability, fatigue, hallucinations, hypersomnolence, insomnia, lethargy, lightheadedness, memory loss (short-term), psychosis, vertigo, vivid dreams

Dermatologic: Alopecia, contact dermatitis, eczematous eruptions, erythema multiforme, exfoliative dermatitis, hyperkeratosis, nail changes, oculomucocutaneous reactions, pruritus, psoriasiform eruptions, rash, Stevens-Johnson syndrome, toxic epidermal necrolysis, ulcers, ulcerative lichenoid, urticaria

Endocrine & metabolic: Hyper-/hypoglycemia, hyperkalemia, hyperlipidemia

Gastrointestinal: Anorexia, cramping, constipation, diarrhea, ischemic colitis, mesenteric arterial thrombosis, nausea, stomach discomfort, vomiting

Genitourinary: Impotence, interstitial nephritis (rare), oliguria (rare), Peyronie's disease, proteinuria (rare)

Hematologic: Agranulocytosis, nonthrombocytopenic purpura, thrombocytopenia, thrombocytopenic purpura

Neuromuscular & skeletal: Arthropathy, carpal tunnel syndrome (rare), myotonus, paresthesia, polyarthritis, weakness

Ocular: Hyperemia of the conjunctiva, mydriasis, tear production decreased, visual acuity decreased

(Continued)

Propranolol *(Continued)*

Respiratory: Bronchospasm, laryngospasm, pharyngitis, pulmonary edema, respiratory distress, wheezing

Miscellaneous: Anaphylactic/anaphylactoid allergic reaction, lupus-like syndrome (rare)

Overdosage/Toxicology Symptoms of intoxication include cardiac disturbances, CNS toxicity, bronchospasm, hypoglycemia, and hyperkalemia. The most common cardiac symptoms include hypotension and bradycardia. Atrioventricular block, intraventricular conduction disturbances, cardiogenic shock, and asystole may occur with severe overdose, especially with membrane-depressant drugs (eg, propranolol). CNS effects include convulsions, coma, and respiratory arrest and are commonly seen with propranolol and other membrane-depressant and lipid-soluble drugs. Treatment is symptomatic for seizures, hypotension, hyperkalemia, and hypoglycemia. Bradycardia and hypotension resistant to atropine, isoproterenol, or pacing may respond to glucagon. Wide QRS defects caused by membrane-depressant poisoning may respond to hypertonic sodium bicarbonate. Repeat-dose charcoal, hemoperfusion, or hemodialysis may be helpful in removal of only those beta-blockers with a small V_d, long half-life, or low intrinsic clearance (acebutolol, atenolol, nadolol, sotalol). Atropine can be administered for symptomatic bradycardia; glucagon can reverse the negative inotropy/chronotropy. Norepinephrine is the preferred vasopressor. Propranolol is not dialyzable. Avoid epinephrine because it may cause uncontrolled hypertension.

Drug Interactions Substrate of CYP1A2 (major), 2C19 (minor), 2D6 (major), 3A4 (minor); **Inhibits** CYP1A2 (weak), 2D6 (weak)

Acetylcholinesterase inhibitors (eg, donepezil, galantamine): May enhance the bradycardic effect of beta-blockers.

Alpha-/Beta-agonists: Beta-blockers may enhance the vasopressor effect of alpha-/beta-agonists (direct-acting).

Alpha$_1$-blockers (eg, prazosin, terazosin): Concurrent use of beta-blockers may increase risk of orthostasis.

Alpha$_2$-agonists: Beta-blockers may enhance the rebound hypertensive effect of alpha$_2$-agonists. This effect can occur when the alpha$_2$-agonist is abruptly withdrawn.

Aminoquinolines (antimalarial): May decrease the metabolism, via CYP isoenzymes, of beta-blockers.

Amiodarone: May enhance the bradycardic effect of beta-blockers.

Antipsychotic agents (phenothiazines): May enhance the hypotensive effect of beta-blockers. Beta-blockers may decrease the metabolism, via CYP isoenzymes, of antipsychotic agents (phenothiazines).

Barbiturates: May increase the metabolism, via CYP isoenzymes, of beta-blockers.

Beta$_2$-agonists: May diminish the bradycardic effect of beta-blockers (nonselective).

Calcium channel blockers (nondihydropyridine; diltiazem, verapamil): May enhance the hypotensive effect of beta-blockers. Bradycardia and signs of heart failure have also been reported.

Cardiac glycosides: Beta-blockers may enhance the bradycardic effect of cardiac glycosides.

CYP1A2 inducers: May decrease the levels/effects of propranolol. Example inducers include aminoglutethimide, carbamazepine, phenobarbital, and rifampin.

CYP1A2 inhibitors: May increase the levels/effects of propranolol. Example inhibitors include amiodarone, ciprofloxacin, fluvoxamine, ketoconazole, norfloxacin, ofloxacin, and rofecoxib.

CYP2D6 inhibitors: May increase the levels/effects of propranolol. Example inhibitors include chlorpromazine, delavirdine, fluoxetine, miconazole, paroxetine, pergolide, quinidine, quinine, ritonavir, and ropinirole.

Dipyridamole: May enhance the bradycardic effect of beta-blockers.

Disopyramide: May enhance the bradycardic effect of beta-blockers.

Insulin: Beta-blockers may enhance the hypoglycemic effect of insulin. Tachycardia may be masked as a symptom of hypoglycemia.

Lidocaine: Beta-blockers may decrease the metabolism of lidocaine.

NSAIDs: May diminish the antihypertensive effects of beta-blockers.

Propafenone: May decrease the metabolism, via CYP isoenzymes, of beta-blockers. Propafenone possesses some independent beta-blocking activity.

Propoxyphene: May increase the levels/effects, via CYP isoenzymes, of beta-blockers.

Quinidine: May increase the levels/effects, via CYP isoenzymes, of beta-blockers.

Rifamycin derivatives: May decrease the levels/effects, via CYP isoenzymes, of beta-blockers.

Rizatriptan: Propranolol may increase the serum concentration of rizatriptan.

Selective serotonin reuptake inhibitors (SSRIs): May enhance the bradycardic effect of beta-blockers.

Sulfonylureas: Beta-blockers enhance the hypoglycemic effect of sulfonylureas Tachycardia may be masked as a symptom of hypoglycemia.

Theophylline: Beta-blockers (nonselective) may diminish the bronchodilatory effect of theophylline derivatives.

Warfarin: Propranolol may increase bioavailability of warfarin and PT may be increased.

Zileuton: May increase the serum concentration of propranolol.

Ethanol/Nutrition/Herb Interactions

Ethanol: Ethanol may increase or decrease plasma levels of propranolol. Reports are variable and have shown both enhanced as well as inhibited hepatic metabolism (of propranolol). Caution advised with consumption of alcohol and monitor for heart rate and/or blood pressure changes.

Food: Propranolol serum levels may be increased if taken with food. Protein-rich foods may increase bioavailability; a change in diet from high carbohydrate/low protein to low carbohydrate/high protein may result in increased oral clearance.

Cigarette: Smoking may decrease plasma levels of propranolol by increasing metabolism.

Herb/Nutraceutical: Avoid dong quai if using for hypertension (has estrogenic activity). Avoid bayberry, blue cohosh, cayenne, ephedra, ginger, ginseng (american), gotu kola, licorice, yohimbe (may worsen hypertension). Avoid black cohosh, california poppy, coleus, garlic, golden seal, hawthorn, mistletoe, periwinkle, quinine, shepherd's purse (have antihypertensive activity, may cause hypotension).

Stability

Injection: Propranolol is stable for 24 hours at room temperature in D$_5$W or NS. Protect injection from light. Solution has a maximum stability at pH of 3 and decomposes rapidly in alkaline pH.

Capsule, tablet: Store at controlled room temperature; protect from light, moisture, freezing, or excessive heat

Mechanism of Action Nonselective beta-adrenergic blocker (class II antiarrhythmic); competitively blocks response to beta$_1$- and beta$_2$-adrenergic stimulation which results in decreases in heart rate, myocardial contractility, blood pressure, and myocardial oxygen demand

Pharmacodynamics

Onset of action: Oral: Beta blockade occurs within 1-2 hours

Duration: ~6 hours

Pharmacokinetics Extensive first-pass effect

Distribution: V$_d$: 3.9 L/kg

Protein binding: 93%

Metabolism: In the liver to active and inactive compounds

Bioavailability: 30% to 40%

Half-life: 4-6 hours

Elimination: Primarily in urine (96% to 99%)

Dosage

Geriatrics: I.V.: Use caution; initiate at lower end of the dosing range.

Oral: Tachyarrhythmias: Initial: 10 mg twice daily; increase dosage every 3-7 days; usual dose range: 10-320 mg given 1-2 times/day. Refer to adult dosing for additional uses.

Adults:

Akathisia (unlabeled use): Oral: 30-120 mg/day in 2-3 divided doses

Essential tremor: Oral: 20-40 mg twice daily initially; maintenance doses: usually 120-320 mg/day

Hypertension: Oral: 40 mg twice daily; increase dosage every 3-7 days; usual dose: ≤320 mg divided in 2-3 doses/day; maximum daily dose: 640 mg; usual dosage range (JNC 7): 40-160 mg/day in 2 divided doses

Long-acting formulation: Initial: 80 mg once daily; usual maintenance: 120-160 mg once daily; maximum daily dose: 640 mg; usual dosage range (JNC 7): 60-180 mg/day once daily

Hypertrophic subaortic stenosis: Oral: 20-40 mg 3-4 times/day

Long-acting formulation: 80-160 mg once daily

Migraine headache prophylaxis: Oral: Initial: 80 mg/day divided every 6-8 hours; increase by 20-40 mg/dose every 3-4 weeks to a maximum of 160-240 mg/day given in divided doses every 6-8 hours; if satisfactory response not achieved within 6 weeks of starting therapy, drug should be withdrawn gradually over several weeks

Long-acting formulation: Initial: 80 mg once daily; effective dose range: 160-240 mg once daily

Pheochromocytoma: Oral: 30-60 mg/day in divided doses

Post-MI mortality reduction: Oral: 180-240 mg/day in 3-4 divided doses

Stable angina: Oral: 80-320 mg/day in doses divided 2-4 times/day

Long-acting formulation: Initial: 80 mg once daily; maximum dose: 320 mg once daily

Tachyarrhythmias:

Oral: 10-30 mg/dose every 6-8 hours

I.V. (in patients having nonfunctional GI tract): 1 mg/dose slow IVP; repeat every 5 minutes up to a total of 5 mg; titrate initial dose to desired response

(Continued)

Propranolol *(Continued)*

Thyrotoxicosis (unlabeled use):
Oral: 10-40 mg/dose every 6 hours
I.V.: 1-3 mg/dose slow IVP as a single dose

Renal Impairment:
Not dialyzable (0% to 5%); supplemental dose is not necessary.
Peritoneal dialysis effects: Supplemental dose is not necessary.

Hepatic Impairment: Marked slowing of heart rate may occur in chronic liver disease with conventional doses; low initial dose and regular heart rate monitoring.

Administration I.V. administration should not exceed 1 mg/minute; I.V. dose much smaller than oral dose; monitor EKG and CV

Monitoring Parameters Blood pressure, orthostatic hypotension, heart rate, CNS effects

Reference Range Therapeutic: 50-100 ng/mL (SI: 190-390 nmol/L) at end of dose interval

Patient Information Do not discontinue abruptly, sudden stopping of medication may precipitate or cause angina; consult pharmacist or physician before taking with other adrenergic drugs (eg, cold medications); notify physician if any of the following symptoms occur: difficult breathing, night cough, swelling of extremities, slow pulse, dizziness, lightheadedness, confusion, depression, skin rash, fever, sore throat, unusual bleeding, or bruising; may produce drowsiness, dizziness, lightheadedness, blurred vision, confusion; use with caution while driving or performing tasks requiring alertness; take at the same time each day, may be taken without regard to meals; may mask signs of hypoglycemia in diabetes

Special Geriatric Considerations Since bioavailability increased in about twofold in elderly patients, geriatrics may require lower maintenance doses. Also, as serum and tissue concentrations increase beta₁ selectivity diminishes. Beta-adrenergic blockade may result in less hemodynamic response than seen in younger adults due to alerations in the beta-adrenergic autonomic system. Studies indicate that despite decreased sensitivity to the chronotropic effects of beta-blockade with age, there appears to be an increased myocardial sensitivity to the negative inotropic effect during stress (ie, exercise). Controlled trials have shown the overall response rate for propranolol to be only 20% to 50% in elderly populations. Therefore, all beta-adrenergic blocking drugs may result in a decreased response as compared to younger adults. Due to propranolol's CNS penetration and nonselective action, it may not be the beta-blocker of choice for use in elderly.

Dosage Forms Excipient information presented when available (limited, particularly for generics); consult specific product labeling. [DSC] = Discontinued product
Capsule, extended release, as hydrochloride: 60 mg, 80 mg, 120 mg, 160 mg
InnoPran XL™: 80 mg, 120 mg
Capsule, sustained release, as hydrochloride:
Inderal® LA: 60 mg, 80 mg, 120 mg, 160 mg
Injection, solution, as hydrochloride: 1 mg/mL (1 mL)
Inderal®: 1 mg/mL (1 mL)
Solution, oral, as hydrochloride: 4 mg/mL (500 mL); 8 mg/mL (500 mL) [strawberry-mint flavor; contains alcohol 0.6%]
Tablet, as hydrochloride: 10 mg, 20 mg, 40 mg, 80 mg
Inderal®: 40 mg, 60 mg; 80 mg [DSC]

Selected References

Aagaard GN, "Treatment of Hypertension in the Elderly," *Drug Treatment in the Elderly*, Vestal RE, ed, Boston, MA: ADIS Health Science Press, 1984, 77.

Adler LA, Peselow E, Rosenthal M, et al, "A Controlled Comparison of the Effects of Propranolol, Benztropine, and Placebo on Akathisia: An Interim Analysis," *Psychopharmacol Bull*, 1993, 29(2):283-6.

Chobanian AV, Bakris GL, Black HR, et al, "The Seventh Report of the Joint National Committee on Prevention, Detection, Evaluation, and Treatment of High Blood Pressure: The JNC 7 Report," *JAMA*, 2003, 289(19):2560-71.

Fleisher LA, Beckman JA, Brown KA, et al, "ACC/AHA 2006 Guideline Update on Perioperative Cardiovascular Evaluation for Noncardiac Surgery: Focused Update on Perioperative Beta-Blocker Therapy. A Report of the American College of Cardiology/American Heart Association Task Force on Practice Guidelines (Writing Committee to Update the 2002 Guidelines on Perioperative Cardiovascular Evaluation for Noncardiac Surgery) Developed in Collaboration With the American Society of Echocardiography, American Society of Nuclear Cardiology, Heart Rhythm Society, Society of Cardiovascular Anesthesiologists, Society for Cardiovascular Angiography and Interventions, and Society for Vascular Medicine and Biology," *J Am Coll Cardiol*, 2006, 47(11):2343-55.

Juul AB, Wetterslev J, Gluud C, et al, "Effect of Perioperative Beta Blockade in Patients With Diabetes Undergoing Major Non-Cardiac Surgery: Randomized Placebo Controlled, Blinded Multicentre Trial. DIPOM Trial Group," *BMJ*, 2006, 332(7556):1482.

Propranolol and Hydrochlorothiazide
(proe PRAN oh lole & hye droe klor oh THYE a zide)

Related Information
Hydrochlorothiazide *on page 756*
Propranolol *on page 1336*

Medication Safety Issues
Sound-alike/look-alike issues:
Inderide® may be confused with Inderal®
U.S. Brand Names Inderide®
Index Terms Hydrochlorothiazide and Propranolol
Generic Available Yes
Pharmacologic Category Antihypertensive Agent, Combination
Use Management of hypertension
Dosage
  Geriatrics & Adults:
    Hypertension: Oral: Dose is individualized; typical dosages of **hydrochlorothia-zide**: 12.5-50 mg/day; initial dose of **propranolol** 80 mg/day
    Note: Daily dose of tablet form should be divided into 2 daily doses; may be used to maximum dosage of up to 160 mg of propranolol; higher dosages would result in higher than optimal thiazide dosages.
Special Geriatric Considerations Combination products are not recommended for first-line therapy and divided doses of diuretics may increase the incidence of nocturia in the elderly.
Dosage Forms Excipient information presented when available (limited, particularly for generics); consult specific product labeling.
    Tablet: Propranolol hydrochloride 40 mg and hydrochlorothiazide 25 mg; propranolol hydrochloride 80 mg and hydrochlorothiazide 25 mg
    Inderide®: 40/25: Propranolol hydrochloride 40 mg and hydrochlorothiazide 25 mg

◆ **Propranolol Hydrochloride** *see* Propranolol *on page 1336*
◆ **Proprinal [OTC]** *see* Ibuprofen *on page 784*
◆ **2-Propylpentanoic Acid** *see* Valproic Acid and Derivatives *on page 1652*

Propylthiouracil (proe pil thye oh YOOR a sil)

Medication Safety Issues
Sound-alike/look-alike issues:
Propylthiouracil may be confused with Purinethol®
PTU is an error-prone abbreviation (mistaken as mercaptopurine [Purinethol®; 6-MP])
Canadian Brand Names Propyl-Thyracil®
Index Terms PTU (error-prone abbreviation)
Generic Available Yes
Pharmacologic Category Antithyroid Agent
Use Palliative treatment of hyperthyroidism as an adjunct to ameliorate hyperthyroidism in preparation for surgical treatment or radioactive iodine therapy and in the management of thyrotoxic crisis
Contraindications Hypersensitivity to propylthiouracil or any component of the formulation
Warnings/Precautions Use with caution in patients >40 years of age because PTU may cause hypoprothrombinemia and bleeding; use with extreme caution in patients receiving other drugs known to cause agranulocytosis; may cause agranulocytosis, thyroid hyperplasia, thyroid carcinoma (usage >1 year). Discontinue in the presence of agranulocytosis, aplastic anemia, ANCA-positive vasculitis, hepatitis, unexplained fever, or exfoliative dermatitis.
Adverse Reactions (Reflective of adult population; not specific for elderly)
Frequency not defined.
    Cardiovascular: ANCA-positive vasculitis, cutaneous vasculitis, edema, leukocytoclastic vasculitis
    Central nervous system: Dizziness, drowsiness, drug fever, fever, headache, neuritis, vertigo
    Dermatologic: Alopecia, erythema nodosum, exfoliative dermatitis, pruritus, skin rash, urticaria
    Endocrine & metabolic: Goiter, swollen salivary glands, weight gain
    Gastrointestinal: Constipation, loss of taste perception, nausea, stomach pain, vomiting
    Hematologic: Agranulocytosis, aplastic anemia, bleeding, leukopenia, thrombocytopenia
    Hepatic: Cholestatic jaundice, hepatitis
    Neuromuscular & skeletal: Arthralgia, paresthesia
    Renal: Acute renal failure, glomerulonephritis, nephritis
    Respiratory: Alveolar hemorrhage, interstitial pneumonitis
    Miscellaneous: SLE-like syndrome
Overdosage/Toxicology Symptoms include nausea, vomiting, epigastric pain, headache, fever, arthralgia, pruritus, edema, pancytopenia, epigastric distress, headache, fever, CNS stimulation or depression. Treatment is supportive and includes monitoring (Continued)

Propylthiouracil *(Continued)*

bone marrow response, forced diuresis, peritoneal and hemodialysis, as well as charcoal hemoperfusion.

Drug Interactions

Anticoagulants: Activity of oral anticoagulants is decreased until a new stable level of thyroid function is reached. Conversely, anticoagulants may be potentiated by an antivitamin K effect of propylthiouracil, though this is relatively uncommon.

Correction of hyperthyroidism may alter disposition of beta-blockers, digoxin, and theophylline, necessitating a dose reduction of these agents.

Ethanol/Nutrition/Herb Interactions Food: Propylthiouracil serum levels may be altered if taken with food.

Mechanism of Action Inhibits the synthesis of thyroid hormones by blocking the oxidation of iodine in the thyroid gland; blocks synthesis of thyroxine and triiodothyronine

Pharmacodynamics For significant therapeutic effects, 24-36 hours are required and remissions of hyperthyroidism do not usually occur before 4 months of continued therapy

Pharmacokinetics

Protein binding: 75% to 80%

Metabolism: Hepatic

Half-life: 1-2 hours

Time to peak serum concentration: Oral: Within 1 hour and persist for 2-3 hours

Elimination: 35% in urine

Dosage

Geriatrics: Use lower dose recommendations; adjust for renal impairment.

Initial: 150-300 mg/day in divided doses every 8 hours

Maintenance: 100-150 mg/day in divided doses every 8-12 hours

Adults:

Hyperthyroidism: Oral: Initial: 300-450 mg/day in divided doses every 8 hours (severe hyperthyroidism may require 600-1200 mg/day); maintenance: 100-150 mg/day in divided doses every 8-12 hours

Note: Administer in 3 equally divided doses at approximately 8-hour intervals. Adjust dosage to maintain T_3, T_4, and TSH levels in normal range; elevated T_3 may be sole indicator of inadequate treatment. Elevated TSH indicates excessive antithyroid treatment.

Renal Impairment:

Cl_{cr} 10-50 mL/minute: Administer 75% of normal dose.

Cl_{cr} <10 mL/minute: Administer 50% of normal dose.

Monitoring Parameters Monitor signs of hypo- and hyperthyroidism, T_4, T_3, TSH, CBC, prothrombin time. See Warnings/Precautions.

Patient Information Do not exceed prescribed dosage; take at regular intervals around-the-clock; notify physician or pharmacist if fever, sore throat, unusual bleeding or bruising, headache, or general malaise occurs

Additional Information Periodic blood counts are recommended with chronic therapy. See Warnings/Precautions.

Special Geriatric Considerations The use of antithyroid thioamides is as effective in the elderly as they are in younger adults; however, the expense, potential adverse effects, and inconvenience (compliance, monitoring) make them undesirable. The use of radioiodine, due to ease of administration and less concern for long-term side effects and reproduction problems, makes it a more appropriate therapy.

Dosage Forms Excipient information presented when available (limited, particularly for generics); consult specific product labeling.

Tablet: 50 mg

Selected References

Johnson DG and Campbell S, "Hormonal and Metabolic Agents," *Geriatric Pharmacology*, Bressler R and Katz MD, eds, New York, NY: McGraw-Hill, 1993, 427-50.

Raby C, Lagorce JF, Jambut-Absil AC, et al, "The Mechanism of Action of Synthetic Antithyroid Drugs: Iodine Complexation During Oxidation of Iodide," *Endocrinology*, 1990, 126(3):1683-91.

Protriptyline (proe TRIP ti leen)

Related Information
Antidepressant Agents *on page 1742*

Medication Safety Issues
Sound-alike/look-alike issues:
Vivactil® may be confused with Vyvanse™

U.S. Brand Names Vivactil®

Index Terms Protriptyline Hydrochloride

Generic Available No

Pharmacologic Category Antidepressant, Tricyclic (Secondary Amine)

Use Treatment of various forms of depression, often in conjunction with psychotherapy

Restrictions An FDA-approved medication guide concerning the use of antidepressants in children, adolescents, and young adults must be distributed when dispensing an outpatient prescription (new or refill) where this medication is to be used without direct supervision of a healthcare provider. Medication guides are available at http://www.fda.gov/cder/Offices/ODS/medication_guides.htm. Dispense to parents or guardians of children and adolescents receiving this medication.

Contraindications Hypersensitivity to protriptyline (cross-reactivity to other cyclic antidepressants may occur) or any component of the formulation; use of MAO inhibitors within 14 days; use of cisapride; use in a patient during the acute recovery phase of MI

Warnings/Precautions [U.S. Boxed Warning]: Antidepressants increase the risk of suicidal thinking and behavior in children, adolescents, and young adults (18-24 years of age) with major depressive disorder (MDD) and other psychiatric disorders; consider risk prior to prescribing. Short-term studies did not show an increased risk in patients >24 years of age and showed a decreased risk in patients ≥65 years. Closely monitor for clinical worsening, suicidality, or unusual changes in behavior; the patient's family or caregiver should be instructed to closely observe the patient and communicate condition with healthcare provider. A medication guide should be dispensed with each prescription.

The possibility of a suicide attempt is inherent in major depression and may persist until remission occurs. Monitor for worsening of depression or suicidality, especially during initiation of therapy (generally first 1-2 months) or with dose increases or decreases. Use caution in high-risk patients. Worsening depression and severe abrupt suicidality that are not part of the presenting symptoms may require discontinuation or modification of drug therapy. The patient's family or caregiver should be alerted to monitor patients for the emergence of suicidality and associated behaviors (such as agitation, irritability, hostility, impulsivity, and hypomania) and call healthcare provider.

May worsen psychosis in some patients or precipitate a shift to mania or hypomania in patients with bipolar disorder. Patients presenting with depressive symptoms should be screened for bipolar disorder. Monotherapy in patients with bipolar disorder should be avoided. **Protriptyline is not FDA approved for the treatment of bipolar depression.**

Although the degree of sedation is low relative to other antidepressant agents, protriptyline may cause sedation, resulting in impaired performance of tasks requiring alertness (eg, operating machinery or driving). Sedative effects may be additive with other CNS depressants and/or ethanol. Protriptyline may aggravate aggressive behavior. Consider discontinuing, when possible, prior to elective surgery. Therapy should not be abruptly discontinued in patients receiving high doses for prolonged periods. May alter glucose regulation - use with caution in patients with diabetes.

May cause orthostatic hypotension or conduction abnormalities (risks are moderate relative to other antidepressants). Use with caution in patients with a history of cardiovascular disease (including previous MI, stroke, tachycardia, or conduction abnormalities). The degree of anticholinergic blockade produced by this agent is moderate relative to other cyclic antidepressants, however, caution should still be used in patients with urinary retention, benign prostatic hyperplasia, narrow-angle glaucoma, xerostomia, visual problems, constipation, or history of bowel obstruction.

Use caution in patients with a previous seizure disorder or condition predisposing to seizures such as brain damage, alcoholism, or concurrent therapy with other drugs which lower the seizure threshold. May increase the risks associated with electroconvulsive therapy. Use with caution in hyperthyroid patients or those receiving thyroid supplementation. Use with caution in patients with hepatic or renal dysfunction and in elderly patients.

Adverse Reactions (Reflective of adult population; not specific for elderly)
Frequency not defined.
Cardiovascular: Arrhythmias, heart block, hyper-/hypotension, MI, palpitation, stroke, tachycardia
(Continued)

Protriptyline *(Continued)*

Central nervous system: agitation, anxiety, ataxia, confusion, delirium, delusions, dizziness, drowsiness, EPS, exacerbation of psychosis, fatigue, hallucinations, headache, hypomania, incoordination, insomnia, nightmares, panic, restlessness, seizure

Dermatologic: Alopecia, itching, petechiae, photosensitivity, rash, urticaria

Endocrine & metabolic: Breast enlargement, galactorrhea, gynecomastia, increased or decreased libido, syndrome of inappropriate ADH secretion (SIADH)

Gastrointestinal: Anorexia, constipation, decreased lower esophageal sphincter tone may cause GE reflux, diarrhea, heartburn, increased appetite, nausea, trouble with gums, unpleasant taste, vomiting, weight gain/loss, xerostomia

Genitourinary: Difficult urination, impotence, testicular edema

Hematologic: Agranulocytosis, eosinophilia, leukopenia, purpura, thrombocytopenia

Hepatic: Cholestatic jaundice, increased liver enzymes

Neuromuscular & skeletal: Fine muscle tremor, numbness, tingling, tremor, weakness

Ocular: Blurred vision, eye pain, increased intraocular pressure

Otic: Tinnitus

Miscellaneous: Allergic reactions, excessive diaphoresis

Overdosage/Toxicology Symptoms include confusion, hallucinations, urinary retention, hypotension, tachycardia, seizures, and hyperthermia. Following initiation of essential overdose management, toxic symptoms should be treated. Sodium bicarbonate is indicated when the QRS interval is >0.10 seconds or the QT_c >0.42 seconds. Ventricular arrhythmias often respond to systemic alkalinization (sodium bicarbonate 0.5-2 mEq/kg I.V.). Arrhythmias unresponsive to this therapy may respond to lidocaine 1 mg/kg I.V. followed by a titrated infusion. Physostigmine (1-2 mg I.V. slowly) may be indicated in reversing life-threatening cardiac arrhythmias. Seizures usually respond to diazepam I.V. boluses (5-10 mg up to 30 mg). If seizures are unresponsive or recur, phenytoin or phenobarbital may be required.

Drug Interactions Substrate of CYP2D6 (major)

Altretamine: Concurrent use may cause orthostatic hypertension

Amphetamines: TCAs may enhance the effect of amphetamines; monitor for adverse CV effects

Anticholinergics: Combined use with TCAs may produce additive anticholinergic effects

Antihypertensives: Cyclic antidepressants may inhibit the antihypertensive response to bethanidine, clonidine, debrisoquin, guanadrel, guanethidine, guanabenz, guanfacine; monitor BP; consider alternate antihypertensive agent

Beta-agonists: When combined with TCAs may predispose patients to cardiac arrhythmias

Bupropion: May increase the levels of tricyclic antidepressants; based on limited information; monitor response

Carbamazepine: Tricyclic antidepressants may increase carbamazepine levels; monitor

Cholestyramine and colestipol: May bind TCAs and reduce their absorption; monitor for altered response

Clonidine: Abrupt discontinuation of clonidine may cause hypertensive crisis, cyclic antidepressants may enhance the response

CNS depressants: Sedative effects may be additive with TCAs; monitor for increased effect; includes benzodiazepines, barbiturates, antipsychotics, ethanol, and other sedative medications

CYP2D6 inhibitors: May increase the levels/effects of protriptyline. Example inhibitors include chlorpromazine, delavirdine, fluoxetine, miconazole, paroxetine, pergolide, quinidine, quinine, ritonavir, and ropinirole.

Epinephrine (and other direct alpha-agonists): Pressor response to I.V. epinephrine, norepinephrine, and phenylephrine may be enhanced in patients receiving TCAs (**Note:** Effect is unlikely with epinephrine or levonordefrin dosages typically administered as infiltration in combination with local anesthetics)

Fenfluramine: May increase tricyclic antidepressant levels/effects

Hypoglycemic agents (including insulin): TCAs may enhance the hypoglycemic effects of tolazamide, chlorpropamide, or insulin; monitor for changes in blood glucose levels; reported with chlorpropamide, tolazamide, and insulin

Levodopa: tricyclic antidepressants may decrease the absorption (bioavailability) of levodopa; rare hypertensive episodes have also been attributed to this combination

Linezolid: Hyperpyrexia, hypertension, tachycardia, confusion, seizures, and **deaths have been reported** with agents which inhibit MAO (serotonin syndrome); this combination should be avoided

Lithium: Concurrent use with a TCA may increase the risk for neurotoxicity

MAO inhibitors: Hyperpyrexia, hypertension, tachycardia, confusion, seizures, and **deaths have been reported** (serotonin syndrome); this combination should be avoided

Methylphenidate: Metabolism of tricyclic antidepressants may be decreased

Phenothiazines: Serum concentrations of some TCAs may be increased; in addition, TCAs may increase concentration of phenothiazines; monitor for altered clinical response

QT_c-prolonging agents: Concurrent use of tricyclic agents with other drugs which may prolong QT_c interval may increase the risk of potentially fatal arrhythmias; includes type Ia and type III antiarrhythmics agents, selected quinolones (moxifloxacin), cisapride, and other agents

Ritonavir: Combined use of high-dose tricyclic antidepressants with ritonavir may cause serotonin syndrome in HIV-positive patients; monitor

Sucralfate: Absorption of tricyclic antidepressants may be reduced with coadministration

Sympathomimetics, indirect-acting: Tricyclic antidepressants may result in a decreased sensitivity to indirect-acting sympathomimetics; includes dopamine and ephedrine; also see interaction with epinephrine (and direct-acting sympathomimetics)

Tramadol: Tramadol's risk of seizures may be increased with TCAs

Valproic acid: May increase serum concentrations/adverse effects of some tricyclic antidepressants

Warfarin (and other oral anticoagulants): Tricyclic antidepressants may increase the anticoagulant effect in patients stabilized on warfarin; monitor INR

Ethanol/Nutrition/Herb Interactions

Ethanol: Avoid ethanol (may increase CNS depression).

Food: Grapefruit juice may inhibit the metabolism of some TCAs and clinical toxicity may result.

Herb/Nutraceutical: Avoid valerian, St John's wort, SAMe, kava kava (may increase risk of serotonin syndrome and/or excessive sedation).

Mechanism of Action Increases the synaptic concentration of serotonin and/or norepinephrine in the central nervous system by inhibition of their reuptake by the presynaptic neuronal membrane

Pharmacodynamics Onset of therapeutic effects: Takes 1-3 weeks before effects are seen; effects on norepinephrine are much greater than on serotonin.

Pharmacokinetics

Protein binding: 92%

Metabolism: Undergoes first-pass metabolism (10% to 25%); extensively metabolized in the liver by N-oxidation, hydroxylation and glucuronidation

Half-life: 54-92 hours, averaging 74 hours

Time to peak serum concentration: Oral: Within 24-30 hours

Elimination: In urine

Dosage

Geriatrics: Oral: Initial: 5-10 mg/day; increase every 3-7 days by 5-10 mg; usual dose: 15-20 mg/day

Adults: Depression: Oral: 15-60 mg/day in 3-4 divided doses

Monitoring Parameters Blood pressure, pulse, target symptoms, mental status; occasional use of serum concentrations may be necessary in cases where response or toxicity are in question

Reference Range Therapeutic: 70-250 ng/mL (SI: 266-950 nmol/L); Toxic: >500 ng/mL (SI: >1900 nmol/L)

Patient Information Do not drink alcoholic beverages, may cause dry mouth, constipation, blurred vision, dizziness, avoid sudden changes in position

Special Geriatric Considerations Little data on its use in the elderly. Strong anticholinergic properties which may limit its use; more often stimulating rather than sedating. Data from a clinical trial comparing fluoxetine to tricyclics suggest that fluoxetine is significantly less effective than nortriptyline in hospitalized elderly patients with unipolar major affective disorder, especially those with melancholia and concurrent cardiovascular diseases.

Dosage Forms Excipient information presented when available (limited, particularly for generics); consult specific product labeling.

Tablet, as hydrochloride: 5 mg, 10 mg

Selected References

Roose SP, Glassman AH, Attia E, et al, "Comparative Efficacy of Selective Serotonin Reuptake Inhibitors and Tricyclics in the Treatment of Melancholia," Am J Psychiatry, 1994, 151(12):1735-9.

♦ **Protriptyline Hydrochloride** see Protriptyline on page 1343

♦ **Proventil®** see Albuterol on page 40

♦ **Proventil® HFA** see Albuterol on page 40

♦ **Provera®** see MedroxyPROGESTERone on page 965

♦ **Prozac®** see Fluoxetine on page 644

♦ **Prozac® Weekly™** see Fluoxetine on page 644

♦ **Prudoxin™** see Doxepin on page 473

♦ **23PS** see Pneumococcal Polysaccharide Vaccine (Polyvalent) on page 1279

Pseudoephedrine (soo doe e FED rin)

Related Information
Pharmacotherapy of Urinary Incontinence *on page 1822*

Medication Safety Issues
Sound-alike/look-alike issues:
Dimetapp® may be confused with Dermatop®, Dimetabs®, Dimetane®
Sudafed® may be confused with Sufenta®

U.S. Brand Names Contac® Cold [OTC] [DSC]; Dimetapp® 12-Hour Non-Drowsy Extentabs® [OTC] [DSC]; Dimetapp® Decongestant Infant [OTC] [DSC]; Genaphed® [OTC]; Kidkare Decongestant [OTC]; Kodet SE [OTC]; Oranyl [OTC]; PediaCare® Decongestant Infants [OTC]; Silfedrine Children's [OTC]; Simply Stuffy™ [OTC] [DSC]; Sudafed® 12 Hour [OTC]; Sudafed® 24 Hour [OTC]; Sudafed® Children's [OTC]; Sudafed® Maximum Strength Nasal Decongestant [OTC]; Sudodrin [OTC]; SudoGest [OTC]; Sudo-Tab® [OTC]

Canadian Brand Names Balminil Decongestant; Benylin® D for Infants; Contac® Cold 12 Hour Relief Non Drowsy; Drixoral® ND; Eltor®; PMS-Pseudoephedrine; Pseudofrin; Robidrine®; Sudafed® Decongestant

Index Terms *d*-Isoephedrine Hydrochloride; Pseudoephedrine Hydrochloride; Pseudo-ephedrine Sulfate

Generic Available Yes: Liquid, tablet

Pharmacologic Category Alpha/Beta Agonist

Use Temporary symptomatic relief of nasal congestion due to common cold, upper respiratory allergies, and sinusitis; promotion of nasal or sinus drainage

Contraindications Hypersensitivity to pseudoephedrine or any component of the formulation; MAO inhibitor therapy

Warnings/Precautions Use with caution in patients >60 years of age; administer with caution to patients with hypertension, hyperthyroidism, diabetes mellitus, cardiovascular disease, ischemic heart disease, increased intraocular pressure, or prostatic hyperplasia. Elderly patients are more likely to experience adverse reactions to sympathomimetics. Overdosage may cause hallucinations, seizures, CNS depression, and death. When used for self-medication (OTC), notify healthcare provider if symptoms do not improve within 7 days or are accompanied by fever.

Adverse Reactions (Reflective of adult population; not specific for elderly)
Frequency not defined.
Cardiovascular: Arrhythmia, palpitaion, tachycardia
Central nervous system: Convulsion, dizziness, drowsiness, excitability, hallucination, headache, insomnia, nervousness, transient stimulation
Gastrointestinal: Nausea, vomiting
Genitourinary: Dysuria
Neuromuscular & skeletal: Tremor, weakness
Respiratory: Dyspnea
Miscellaneous: Diaphoresis

Overdosage/Toxicology Symptoms include seizures, nausea, vomiting, cardiac arrhythmias, hypertension, and agitation. There is no specific antidote. The bulk of treatment is supportive. Hyperactivity and agitation usually respond to reduced sensory input; however, with extreme agitation, haloperidol (2-5 mg I.M.) may be required. Hyperthermia is best treated with external cooling measures; or when severe or unresponsive, muscle paralysis with pancuronium may be needed. Hypertension is usually transient and generally does not require treatment unless severe. For diastolic blood pressures >110 mm Hg, a nitroprusside infusion should be initiated. Seizures usually respond to diazepam I.V. and/or phenytoin maintenance regimens.

Drug Interactions
Decreased effect of methyldopa, reserpine
Increased toxicity: MAO inhibitors may increase blood pressure effects of pseudoephedrine; propranolol, sympathomimetic agents may increase toxicity

Ethanol/Nutrition/Herb Interactions
Food: Onset of effect may be delayed if pseudoephedrine is taken with food.
Herb/Nutraceutical: Avoid ephedra, yohimbe (may cause hypertension).

Mechanism of Action Directly stimulates alpha-adrenergic receptors of respiratory mucosa causing vasoconstriction; directly stimulates beta-adrenergic receptors causing bronchial relaxation, increased heart rate and contractility

Pharmacodynamics
Onset of action: Oral: Decongestant effects occur within 15-30 minutes
Duration: 4-6 hours (up to 12 hours with extended release formulation administration)

Pharmacokinetics
Metabolism: Partially in liver
Half-life: 9-16 hours

Elimination: 70% to 90% of dose excreted in urine as unchanged drug and 1% to 6% as norpseudoephedrine (active); renal elimination is dependent on urine pH and flow rate; alkaline urine decreases renal elimination of pseudoephedrine

Dosage
Geriatrics: Nasal congestion: 30-60 mg every 6 hours as needed
Adults: Nasal congestion: Oral: 30-60 mg every 4-6 hours, sustained release: 120 mg every 12 hours; maximum: 240 mg/24 hours
Renal Impairment: Reduce dose.

Monitoring Parameters Blood pressure, pulse, relief of symptoms, urinary output, episodes of incontinence

Test Interactions Interferes with urine detection of amphetamine (false-positive)

Patient Information Do not crush sustained release products; consult pharmacist or physician before using; do not exceed recommended dose; notify physician of insomnia, weakness, dizziness, tremor, or irregular heartbeat

Additional Information Pseudoephedrine is found in many combination cough and cold products

Special Geriatric Considerations Elderly patients should be counseled about the proper use of over-the-counter cough and cold preparations. Elderly are more predisposed to adverse effects of sympathomimetics since they frequently have cardiovascular diseases and diabetes mellitus as well as multiple drug therapies. It may be advisable to treat with a short-acting/immediate-release formulation before initiating sustained-release/long-acting formulations.

Dosage Forms Excipient information presented when available (limited, particularly for generics); consult specific product labeling. [DSC] = Discontinued product
Caplet, extended release, as hydrochloride:
Contac® Cold [DSC], Sudafed® 12 Hour: 120 mg
Liquid, as hydrochloride: 30 mg/5 mL (120 mL, 480 mL)
Silfedrine Children's: 15 mg/5 mL (120 mL, 480 mL) [alcohol and sugar free; grape flavor]
Simply Stuffy™: 15 mg/5 mL (120 mL) [alcohol free; contains sodium benzoate; cherry berry flavor] [DSC]
Sudafed® Children's: 15 mg/5 mL (120 mL) [alcohol and sugar free; contains sodium benzoate; grape flavor]
Liquid, oral, as hydrochloride [drops]:
Dimetapp® Decongestant Infant Drops: 7.5 mg/0.8 mL (15 mL) [alcohol free; contains sodium benzoate; grape flavor] [DSC]
Kidkare Decongestant: 7.5 mg/0.8 mL (30 mL) [alcohol free; contains benzoic acid and sodium benzoate; cherry flavor]
PediaCare® Decongestant: 7.5 mg/0.8 mL (15 mL) [alcohol free, dye free; contains benzoic acid, sodium benzoate; fruit flavor]
Tablet, as hydrochloride: 30 mg, 60 mg
Genaphed®, Kodet SE, Oranyl, Sudafed®, Sudodrin, Sudo-Tab®: 30 mg
SudoGest: 30 mg, 60 mg
Tablet, chewable, as hydrochloride:
Sudafed® Children's: 15 mg [sugar free; contains phenylalanine 0.78 mg/tablet; orange flavor]
Tablet, extended release, as hydrochloride:
Dimetapp® 12-Hour Non-Drowsy Extentabs®: 120 mg [DSC]
Sudafed® 24 Hour: 240 mg

♦ **Pseudoephedrine and Carbinoxamine** see Carbinoxamine and Pseudoephedrine on page 239
♦ **Pseudoephedrine and Triprolidine** see Triprolidine and Pseudoephedrine on page 1638
♦ **Pseudoephedrine Hydrochloride** see Pseudoephedrine on page 1346
♦ **Pseudoephedrine Sulfate** see Pseudoephedrine on page 1346
♦ **Pseudomonic Acid A** see Mupirocin on page 1075

Psyllium (SIL i yum)

Medication Safety Issues
Sound-alike/look-alike issues:
Fiberall® may be confused with Feverall®
Hydrocil® may be confused with Hydrocet®
Modane® may be confused with Matulane®, Moban®
Perdiem® may be confused with Pyridium®

U.S. Brand Names Fiberall®; Fibro-Lax [OTC]; Fibro-XL [OTC]; Genfiber® [OTC]; Hydrocil® Instant [OTC]; Konsyl® [OTC]; Konsyl-D® [OTC]; Konsyl® Easy Mix [OTC]; Konsyl® Orange [OTC]; Metamucil® [OTC]; Metamucil® Plus Calcium [OTC]; Metamucil® Smooth Texture [OTC]; Modane® Bulk [OTC]; Natural Fiber Therapy [OTC]; Reguloid® [OTC]; Serutan® [OTC]
(Continued)

Psyllium *(Continued)*

Canadian Brand Names Metamucil®

Index Terms Plantago Seed; Plantain Seed; Psyllium Hydrophilic Mucilloid

Generic Available Yes: Capsule, powder

Pharmacologic Category Antidiarrheal; Laxative, Bulk-Producing

Use Treatment of chronic atonic or spastic constipation and in constipation associated with rectal disorders; management of irritable bowel syndrome; labeled for OTC use as fiber supplement, treatment of constipation

Contraindications Hypersensitivity to psyllium or any component of the formulation; fecal impaction; GI obstruction

Warnings/Precautions Products must be taken with adequate fluid. Use with caution in patients with esophageal strictures, ulcers, stenosis, or intestinal adhesions; elderly may have insufficient fluid intake which may predispose them to fecal impaction and bowel obstruction.

Adverse Reactions (Reflective of adult population; not specific for elderly)
Frequency not defined.

Gastrointestinal: Abdominal cramps, constipation, diarrhea, esophageal or bowel obstruction

Respiratory: Bronchospasm

Miscellaneous: Anaphylaxis upon inhalation in susceptible individuals, rhinoconjunctivitis

Overdosage/Toxicology Symptoms include abdominal pain, diarrhea, and constipation.

Drug Interactions Decreased effect of warfarin, digitalis, potassium-sparing diuretics, salicylates, tetracyclines, nitrofurantoin

Mechanism of Action Adsorbs water in the intestine to form a viscous liquid which promotes peristalsis and reduces transit time

Pharmacodynamics Onset of action: 12-24 hours, but full effect may take 2-3 days; considered the safest and most physiologic laxative agent

Pharmacokinetics Absorption: Oral: Generally not absorbed, small amounts of grain extracts present in the preparation have been reportedly absorbed following colonic hydrolysis

Dosage

Geriatrics & Adults:

Constipation, IBS: Oral (administer at least 2 hours before or after other drugs): Take 1 dose up to 3 times/day; all doses should be followed with 8 oz of water or liquid

Capsule: 4 capsules/dose (range: 2-6); swallow capsules one at a time

Powder: 1 rounded tablespoonful/dose (1 teaspoonful/dose for many sugar free or select concentrated products) mixed in 8 oz liquid

Tablet: 1 tablet/dose

Wafer: 2 wafers/dose

Administration Inhalation of psyllium dust may cause sensitivity to psyllium (eg, runny nose, watery eyes, wheezing). Drink a full glass of liquid with each dose. Powder must be mixed in a glass of water or juice. Separate dose from other drug therapies.

Monitoring Parameters Monitor for diarrhea, abdominal pain, bowel obstruction, or impaction

Patient Information Must be mixed in a glass of water or juice; drink a full glass of liquid with each dose; must drink fluids throughout the day to be effective and avoid impaction; report bleeding or failure to respond to physician, pharmacist, or nurse; do not use for acute constipation

Additional Information 3.4 g psyllium hydrophilic mucilloid per 7 g powder is equivalent to a rounded teaspoonful or one packet; fiber therapy results in increased frequency of defecation. Diabetic patients may need or prefer sugar-free products; psyllium using aspartame is available for diabetic patients. Bloating and flatulence are mostly a problem in first 4 weeks of therapy.

Special Geriatric Considerations Elderly may have insufficient fluid intake which may predispose them to fecal impaction and bowel obstruction. Patients should have a 1 month trial, with at least 14 g/day, before effects in bowel function are determined. Bloating and flatulence are mostly a problem in first 4 weeks of therapy.

Dosage Forms Excipient information presented when available (limited, particularly for generics); consult specific product labeling.

Capsule:

Fibro XL: 675 mg

Metamucil®: 0.52 g [contains potassium 5 mg/capsule; provides 3 g dietary fiber 2.4 g per 6 capsules]

Metamucil® Plus Calcium: 0.42 g [contains potassium 6 mg/capsule; provides dietary fiber 2.1 g and calcium 300 mg per 5 capsules]

Granules (Serutan®): 2.5 g/teaspoon (510 g) [contains sodium benzoate]

Powder: 3.4 g/dose (390 g, 570 g)

Bulk-K: 4.725 g/dose (392 g)

Fiberall®: 3.5 g/dose (454 g) [sugar free; contains phenylalanine; orange flavor]

Fibro-Lax: 4.725 g /dose (140 g, 392g)

Genfiber®: 3.4 g/dose (397 g, 595 g) [regular flavor]

Genfiber®: 3.5 g/dose (283 g) [sugar free; orange flavor]

Hydrocil® Instant: 3.5 g/dose (3.7 g unit-dose packets, 300 g) [sugar free]

Konsyl®: 6 g/dose (6 g unit-dose packets, 300 g, 450 g) [sugar free; contains sodium 4.1 mg/dose; regular flavor]

Konsyl-D®: 3.4 g/dose (6.5 g unit-dose packets, 325 g, 397 g, 500 g) [contains sodium 2.3 mg/dose and dextrose]

Konsyl® Easy Mix: 6 g/dose (6 g unit-dose packets, 250 g) [sugar free; contains sodium 4.4 mg/dose]

Konsyl® Orange: 3.4 g/dose (12 g unit-dose packets, 538 g) [contains sodium 2.3 mg/dose and sucrose; orange flavor]

Konsyl® Orange: 3.4 g/dose (425 g) [sugar free; contains sodium 2.3 mg/dose; orange flavor]

Metamucil®: 3.4 g/dose:
(390 g, 570 g, 870 g) [contains sodium 3 mg and potassium 30 mg per dose; regular flavor]
(570 g, 870 g, 1254 g) [contains sodium 5 mg and potassium 30 mg per dose; orange flavor]

Metamucil® Smooth Texture: 3.4 g/dose:
(unit-dose packets, 609 g, 912 g, 1446 g) [contains sodium 5 mg and potassium 30 mg per dose; orange flavor]
(300 g, 450 g, 690 g) [contains sodium 4 mg and potassium 30 mg per dose; regular flavor]
(unit-dose packets, 183 g, 300 g, 450 g, 699 g, 1104 g) [sugar free; contains phenylalanine 25 mg, sodium 5 mg, and potassium 30 mg per dose; orange flavor]

Modane® Bulk: 3.4 g/dose (390 g) [contains dextrose; flavor free]

Natural Fiber Therapy: 3.4 g/dose (369 g, 539 g) [natural and orange flavors]

Reguloid®: 3.4 g/dose (300 g, 450 g) [sugar free; regular or orange flavors]; (390 g, 570g) [regular or orange flavors]

Wafers (Metamucil®): 3.4 g/dose (24s) [one dose = 2 wafers; contains sodium 20 mg and potassium 60 mg per dose; apple crisp and cinnamon spice flavors]

- ♦ **Psyllium Hydrophilic Mucilloid** *see* Psyllium *on page 1347*
- ♦ **Pteroylglutamic Acid** *see* Folic Acid *on page 673*
- ♦ **PTU (error-prone abbreviation)** *see* Propylthiouracil *on page 1341*
- ♦ **Pulmicort Flexhaler®** *see* Budesonide *on page 190*
- ♦ **Pulmicort Respules®** *see* Budesonide *on page 190*
- ♦ **Pulmicort Turbuhaler®** *see* Budesonide *on page 190*
- ♦ **Puralube® Ophthalmic Ointment [OTC]** *see* Ocular Lubricant *on page 1144*
- ♦ **Puralube® Tears [OTC]** *see* Artificial Tears *on page 124*
- ♦ **Purified Chick Embryo Cell** *see* Rabies Virus Vaccine *on page 1372*
- ♦ **Purinethol®** *see* Mercaptopurine *on page 985*

Pyrazinamide (peer a ZIN a mide)

Canadian Brand Names Tebrazid™

Index Terms Pyrazinoic Acid Amide

Generic Available Yes

Pharmacologic Category Antitubercular Agent

Use Adjunctive treatment of tuberculosis when primary and secondary agents cannot be used or have failed

Contraindications Hypersensitivity to pyrazinamide or any component of the formulation; acute gout; severe hepatic damage

Warnings/Precautions Use with caution in patients with renal failure, chronic gout, diabetes mellitus, or porphyria

Adverse Reactions (Reflective of adult population; not specific for elderly)
1% to 10%:
Central nervous system: Malaise
Gastrointestinal: Anorexia, nausea, vomiting
Neuromuscular & skeletal: Arthralgia, myalgia

Overdosage/Toxicology Symptoms include gout, gastric upset, and hepatic damage (mild). Treatment following GI decontamination is supportive.

Drug Interactions Combination therapy with rifampin and pyrazinamide has been associated with severe and fatal hepatotoxic reactions.
(Continued)

Pyrazinamide *(Continued)*

Mechanism of Action Converted to pyrazinoic acid in susceptible strains of *Mycobacterium* which lowers the pH of the environment; exact mechanism of action has not been elucidated

Pharmacodynamics Bacteriostatic or bactericidal depending on the drug's concentration at the site of infection

Pharmacokinetics

Absorption: Oral: Well absorbed

Distribution: Widely distributed into body tissues and fluids including the liver, lung, and CSF

Protein binding: 50%

Metabolism: In the liver

Half-life: 9-10 hours, increased with reduced renal or hepatic function

Time to peak serum concentration: Within 2 hours

Elimination: In urine (4% as unchanged drug)

Dosage

Geriatrics: Start with a lower daily dose (15 mg/kg) and increase as tolerated.

Adults:

Tuberculosis treatment: Oral (dosing is based on lean body weight):

Daily therapy: 15-30 mg/kg/day

40-55 kg: 1000 mg

56-75 kg: 1500 mg

76-90 kg: 2000 mg (maximum dose regardless of weight)

Twice weekly directly observed therapy (DOT): 50 mg/kg

40-55 kg: 2000 mg

56-75 kg: 3000 mg

76-90 kg: 4000 mg (maximum dose regardless of weight)

Three times/week DOT: 25-30 mg/kg (maximum: 2.5 g)

40-55 kg: 1500 mg

56-75 kg: 2500 mg

76-90 kg: 3000 mg (maximum dose regardless of weight)

Note: Used as part of a multidrug regimen. Treatment regimens consist of an initial 2-month phase, followed by a continuation phase of 4 or 7 additional months; frequency of dosing may differ depending on phase of therapy.

Renal Impairment:

Cl_{cr} <50 mL/minute: Avoid use or reduce dose to 12-20 mg/kg/day.

Avoid use in hemo- and peritoneal dialysis as well as continuous arteriovenous or venovenous hemofiltration.

Hepatic Impairment: Reduce dose.

Monitoring Parameters Periodic liver function tests, serum uric acid, sputum culture, chest x-ray 2-3 months into treatment and at completion

Test Interactions Reacts with Acetest® and Ketostix® to produce pinkish-brown color

Patient Information Compliance must be stressed; inform physician if fever, malaise, weakness, nausea or vomiting, darkened urine, skin or eye discoloration (yellow), or swollen or painful joints develop

Special Geriatric Considerations Pyrazinamide is used in the 2-month intensive treatment phase of a 6-month treatment plan. Most elderly acquired their *Mycobacterium tuberculosis* infection before effective chemotherapy was available; however, older persons with new infections (not reactivation), or who are from areas where drug-resistant *M. tuberculosis* is endemic, or who are HIV-infected should receive 3-4 drug therapies including pyrazinamide.

Dosage Forms Excipient information presented when available (limited, particularly for generics); consult specific product labeling.

Tablet: 500 mg

Selected References

American Thoracic Society, "Targeted Tuberculin Testing and Treatment of Latent Tuberculosis Infection," *MMWR*, 2000, 49(RR-6):1-51.

Bass JB Jr, Farer LS, Hopewell PC, et al, "Treatment of Tuberculosis and Tuberculosis Infection in Adults and Children," *Am J Respir Crit Care Med*, 1994, 149(5):1359-74.

Blumberg HM, Burman WJ, Chaisson RE, et al, "American Thoracic Society/Centers for Disease Control and Prevention/Infectious Diseases Society of America: Treatment of Tuberculosis," *Am J Respir Crit Care Med*, 2003, 167(4):603-62.

Centers for Disease Control and Prevention (CDC) and American Thoracic Society, "Update: Adverse Event Data and Revised American Thoracic Society/CDC Recommendations Against the Use of Rifampin and Pyrazinamide for Treatment of Latent Tuberculosis Infection - United States, 2003," *MMWR*, 2003, 52(31):735-9. Available at http://www.cdc.gov/mmwr/preview/mmwrhtml/mm5231a4.htm. Last accessed February 16, 2005.

"Treatment of Latent Tuberculosis Infection (LTBI), Last Updated: April 8, 2004," available at http://www.cdc.gov/nchstp/tb/pubs/tbfactsheets/250110.htm. Last accessed February 16, 2005.

Van Scoy RE and Wilkowske CJ, "Antituberculous Agents: Isoniazid, Rifampin, Streptomycin, Ethambutol, and Pyrazinamide," *Mayo Clin Proc*, 1983, 58(4):233-40.

Yoshikawa TT, "Tuberculosis in Aging Adults," *J Am Geriatr Soc*, 1992, 40(2):178-87.

♦ **Pyrazinoic Acid Amide** *see* Pyrazinamide *on page 1349*

Pyridostigmine (peer id oh STIG meen)

Medication Safety Issues
Sound-alike/look-alike issues:
Pyridostigmine may be confused with physostigmine
Mestinon® may be confused with Metatensin®
Regonol® may be confused with Reglan®, Renagel®

U.S. Brand Names Mestinon®; Mestinon® Timespan®; Regonol®

Canadian Brand Names Mestinon®; Mestinon®-SR

Index Terms Pyridostigmine Bromide

Generic Available Yes: Tablet

Pharmacologic Category Acetylcholinesterase Inhibitor

Use Symptomatic treatment of myasthenia gravis; antidote for nondepolarizing neuromuscular blockers

Contraindications Hypersensitivity to pyridostigmine, bromides, or any component of the formulation; GI or GU obstruction

Warnings/Precautions Use with caution in patients with epilepsy, asthma, bradycardia, hyperthyroidism, cardiac arrhythmias, or peptic ulcer; adequate facilities should be available for cardiopulmonary resuscitation when testing and adjusting dose for myasthenia gravis; have atropine and epinephrine ready to treat hypersensitivity reactions; overdosage may result in cholinergic crisis, this must be distinguished from myasthenic crisis; anticholinesterase insensitivity can develop for brief or prolonged periods. Regonol® injection contains 1% benzyl alcohol as the preservative (not intended for use in newborns). **[U.S. Boxed Warning]: Regonol® injection must be administered by trained personnel.**

Adverse Reactions (Reflective of adult population; not specific for elderly) Frequency not defined.

Cardiovascular: Arrhythmias (especially bradycardia), AV block, cardiac arrest, decreased carbon monoxide, flushing, hypotension, nodal rhythm, nonspecific ECG changes, syncope, tachycardia

Central nervous system: Convulsions, dizziness, drowsiness, dysphonia, headache, loss of consciousness

Dermatologic: Skin rash, thrombophlebitis (I.V.), urticaria

Gastrointestinal: Abdominal pain, diarrhea, dysphagia, flatulence, hyperperistalsis, nausea, salivation, stomach cramps, vomiting

Genitourinary: Urinary urgency

Neuromuscular & skeletal: Arthralgia, dysarthria, fasciculations, muscle cramps, myalgia, spasms, weakness

Ocular: Amblyopia, lacrimation, small pupils

Respiratory: Bronchial secretions increased, bronchiolar constriction, bronchospasm, dyspnea, laryngospasm, respiratory arrest, respiratory depression, respiratory muscle paralysis

Miscellaneous: Allergic reactions, anaphylaxis, diaphoresis increased

Overdosage/Toxicology Symptoms include muscle weakness, blurred vision, excessive sweating, tearing and salivation, nausea, vomiting, diarrhea, hypertension, bradycardia, and paralysis. Atropine is the treatment of choice for intoxications manifesting with significant muscarinic symptoms. Atropine I.V. 2-4 mg every 3-60 minutes should be repeated to control symptoms and then continued as needed for 1-2 days following the acute ingestion.

Drug Interactions
Aminoglycosides (gentamicin, kanamycin, neomycin, streptomycin): Use of high parenteral doses may intensify/prolong neuromuscular blockade, or lead to resistance of neuromuscular blockade reversal, especially if used with other nondepolarizing neuromuscular-blocking drugs.

Antibiotics (bacitracin, colistin, polymyxin B, sodium colistimethate, tetracycline): Use of high parenteral doses may intensify/prolong neuromuscular blockade, or lead to resistance of neuromuscular blockade reversal, especially if used with other nondepolarizing neuromuscular-blocking drugs.

Beta-blockers: Pyridostigmine and beta-blockers may both cause bradycardia and hypotension, effect may be additive; monitor.

Depolarizing neuromuscular-blocking agents (succinylcholine): Increased neuromuscular blocking effect with concomitant use.

Edrophonium: Increased toxicity with concomitant use.

Magnesium: Patients with elevated serum magnesium concentrations may experience enhanced neuromuscular blockage with blocking agents. The reversing effect of pyridostigmine may be compensated.

(Continued)

Pyridostigmine *(Continued)*

Quinidine: Recurrent paralysis may occur when quinidine is administered with nonde-polarizing neuromuscular-blocking drugs. This may complicate attempts to reverse blockade with pyridostigmine.

Quinolone antibiotics (ciprofloxacin, norfloxacin): Case reports suggest these drugs may exhibit neuromuscular-blocking effects (especially in some patients with myas-thenia gravis); monitor.

Stability

Injection: Protect from light.

Tablet:

30 mg: Store under refrigeration at 2°C to 8°C (36°F to 46°F). Protect from light. Stable at room temperature for up to 3 months.

Mestinon®: Store at 25°C (77°F). Protect from moisture.

Mechanism of Action
Inhibits destruction of acetylcholine by acetylcholinesterase which facilitates transmission of impulses across myoneural junction

Pharmacodynamics

Onset of action:

Oral, I.M.: Within 15-30

I.V.: Within 2-5 minutes

Duration:

Oral: 3-6 hours

I.M., I.V.: 2-4 hours

Pharmacokinetics

Absorption: Oral: Very poor (10% to 20%) from GI tract

Metabolism: In the liver (to a small extent)

Dosage

Geriatrics & Adults:

Myasthenia gravis:

Oral: Highly individualized dosing ranges: 60-1500 mg/day, usually 600 mg/day divided into 5-6 doses, spaced to provide maximum relief

Sustained release formulation: Highly individualized dosing ranges: 180-540 mg once or twice daily (doses separated by at least 6 hours); **Note:** Most clinicians reserve sustained release dosage form for bedtime dose only.

I.M. or slow I.V. Push: To supplement oral dosage pre- and postoperatively, during myasthenic crisis, or when oral therapy is impractical): ~1/30th of oral dose; observe patient closely for cholinergic reactions

I.V. infusion: To supplement oral dosage pre- and postoperatively, during myas-thenic crisis, or when oral therapy is impractical): Initial: 2 mg/hour with gradual titration in increments of 0.5-1 mg/hour, up to a maximum rate of 4 mg/hour

Pretreatment for Soman nerve gas exposure (military use): Oral: 30 mg every 8 hours beginning several hours prior to exposure; discontinue at first sign of nerve agent exposure, then begin atropine and pralidoxime

Reversal of nondepolarizing muscle relaxants: I.V.: 0.1-0.25 mg/kg/dose; 10-20 mg is usually sufficient (full recovery usually occurs ≤15 minutes, but ≥30 minutes may be required).

Note: Atropine sulfate (0.6-1.2 mg) I.V. immediately prior to pyridostigmine to minimize side effects:

Renal Impairment: Lower dosages may be required due to prolonged elimination; no specific recommendations have been published.

Administration
When giving for reversal of neuromuscular blockade, keep patient well ventilated until recovered

Monitoring Parameters
Symptoms of myasthenia gravis, blood pressure, pulse, respi-ratory rate, signs of cholinergic crisis. See Overdosage/Toxicology.

Test Interactions
Increased aminotransferase [ALT/AST] (S), increased amylase (S)

Patient Information
Side effects are generally due to exaggerated pharmacologic effects; most common are salivation and muscle fasciculations; notify physician if nausea, vomiting, muscle weakness, severe abdominal pain, or difficulty breathing occurs; take drug as ordered; take with food; report adverse reactions to physician promptly; do not chew or crush sustained release tablets

Additional Information
Not a cure; patient may develop resistance to the drug; normally, sustained release dosage form is used at bedtime for patients who complain of morning weakness

Special Geriatric Considerations
Many elderly may have pulmonary or cardiovas-cular diseases which will require cautious use of pyridostigmine.

Dosage Forms
Excipient information presented when available (limited, particularly for generics); consult specific product labeling.

Injection, solution, as bromide:

Regonol®: 5 mg/mL (2 mL) [contains benzyl alcohol]

Syrup, as bromide:
Mestinon®: 60 mg/5 mL (480 mL) [raspberry flavor; contains alcohol 5%, sodium benzoate]
Tablet, as bromide: 60 mg
Mestinon®: 60 mg
Tablet, sustained release, as bromide:
Mestinon® Timespan®: 180 mg

♦ **Pyridostigmine Bromide** *see* Pyridostigmine *on page 1351*

Pyridoxine (peer i DOKS een)

Medication Safety Issues
Sound-alike/look-alike issues:
Pyridoxine may be confused with paroxetine, pralidoxime, Pyridium®
U.S. Brand Names Aminoxin [OTC]; Pyri-500 [OTC]
Index Terms Pyridoxine Hydrochloride; Vitamin B$_6$
Generic Available Yes
Pharmacologic Category Vitamin, Water Soluble
Use Prevention and treatment of vitamin B$_6$ deficiency; adjunct to treatment of acute toxicity from isoniazid, cycloserine, or hydrazine overdose
Contraindications Hypersensitivity to pyridoxine or any component of the formulation
Warnings/Precautions Dependence and withdrawal may occur with doses >200 mg/day. Single vitamin deficiency is rare; evaluate for other deficiencies. Some parenteral products contain aluminum; use caution in patients with impaired renal function.
Adverse Reactions (Reflective of adult population; not specific for elderly)
Frequency not defined.
Central nervous system: Headache, seizure (following very large I.V. doses), sensory neuropathy
Endocrine & metabolic: Decreased serum folic acid secretions
Gastrointestinal: Nausea
Hepatic: Increased AST
Neuromuscular & skeletal: Paresthesia
Miscellaneous: Allergic reactions
Overdosage/Toxicology Symptoms include ataxia and sensory neuropathy with doses of 50 mg to 2 g daily over prolonged periods. Acute doses of 70-357 mg/kg have been well tolerated.
Drug Interactions Decreased serum levels of levodopa, phenobarbital, and phenytoin
Stability Protect from light.
Mechanism of Action Precursor to pyridoxal, which functions in the metabolism of proteins, carbohydrates, and fats; pyridoxal also aids in the release of liver and muscle-stored glycogen and in the synthesis of GABA (within the central nervous system) and heme
Pharmacokinetics
Absorption: Enteral, parenteral: Well absorbed
Metabolism: In 4-pyridoxic acid, and other metabolites
Half-life: 2-3 weeks
Elimination: Urinary excretion
Dosage
Geriatrics & Adults:
Recommended daily allowance (RDA):
Male: 1.7-2.0 mg
Female: 1.4-1.6 mg
Dietary deficiency: Oral: 10-20 mg/day for 3 weeks
Drug-induced neuritis (eg, isoniazid, hydralazine, penicillamine, cycloserine):
Oral:
Treatment: 100-200 mg/24 hours
Prophylaxis: 25-100 mg/24 hours
Treatment of seizures and/or coma from acute isoniazid toxicity: A dose of pyridoxine hydrochloride equal to the amount of INH ingested can be given I.M./I.V. in divided doses together with other anticonvulsants; if the amount INH ingested is not known, administer 5 g I.V. pyridoxine.
Treatment of acute hydrazine toxicity: A pyridoxine dose of 25 mg/kg in divided doses I.M./I.V. has been used.
Administration Administer slow I.V. Burning may occur at the injection site after I.M. or SubQ administration; seizures have occurred following I.V. administration of very large doses
Monitoring Parameters When administering large I.V. doses, monitor respiratory rate, heart rate, and blood pressure
(Continued)

Pyridoxine *(Continued)*

Reference Range >50 ng/mL (SI: 243 nmol/L) (varies considerably with method). A broad range is ~25-80 ng/mL (SI: 122-389 nmol/L). HPLC method for pyridoxal phosphate has normal range of 3.5-18 ng/mL (SI: 17-88 nmol/L).

Test Interactions Urobilinogen

Patient Information Take exactly as directed. Do not take more than recommended. Do not exceed recommended intake of dietary B$_6$ (eg, red meat, bananas, potatoes, yeast, lima beans, and whole grain cereals). You may experience burning or pain at injection site; notify prescriber if this persists.

Additional Information

For the treatment of seizures and/or coma from acute isoniazid toxicity, a dose of pyridoxine hydrochloride equal to the amount of INH ingested can be given I.M./I.V. in divided doses together with other anticonvulsants

For the treatment of acute hydrazine toxicity, pyridoxine 25 mg/kg/dose I.M./I.V. has been used

Special Geriatric Considerations Use with caution in patients with Parkinson's disease treated with levodopa.

Dosage Forms Excipient information presented when available (limited, particularly for generics); consult specific product labeling.

Capsule, as hydrochloride: 50 mg, 250 mg

Aminoxin: 20 mg

Injection, solution, as hydrochloride: 100 mg/mL (1 mL)

Liquid, oral, as hydrochloride: 200 mg/5 mL (120 mL)

Tablet, as hydrochloride: 25 mg, 50 mg, 100 mg, 250 mg, 500 mg

Tablet, sustained release, as hydrochloride:

Pyri-500: 500 mg

Selected References

Schnyder G, Roffi M, Flammer Y, et al, "Effect of Homocysteine-Lowering Therapy With Folic Acid, Vitamin B12, and Vitamin B6 on Clinical Outcome After Percutaneous Coronary Intervention: The Swiss Heart Study: A Randomized Controlled Trial," *JAMA*, 2002, 288(8):973-9.

- ◆ **Pyridoxine Hydrochloride** *see* Pyridoxine *on page 1353*
- ◆ **QDALL® AR** *see* Chlorpheniramine *on page 296*
- ◆ **Q-Naftate [OTC]** *see* Tolnaftate *on page 1596*
- ◆ **Quadrivalent Meningococcal Conjugate Vaccine** *see* Meningococcal Polysaccharide (Groups A / C / Y and W-135) Diphtheria Toxoid Conjugate Vaccine *on page 978*
- ◆ **Quadrivalent Meningococcal Conjugate Vaccine** *see* Meningococcal Polysaccharide Vaccine (Groups A / C / Y and W-135) *on page 979*
- ◆ **Qualaquin™** *see* Quinine *on page 1366*

Quazepam *(KWAZ e pam)*

Related Information

Anxiolytic, Sedative / Hypnotic, and Miscellaneous Benzodiazepines *on page 1750*

Potentially Inappropriate Medications for Geriatrics *on page 1824*

Medication Safety Issues

Sound-alike/look-alike issues:

Quazepam may be confused with oxazepam

U.S. Brand Names Doral®

Canadian Brand Names Doral®

Generic Available No

Pharmacologic Category Benzodiazepine

Use Short-term treatment of insomnia

Restrictions C-IV

Contraindications Hypersensitivity to quazepam or any component of the formulation (cross-sensitivity with other benzodiazepines may exist); narrow-angle glaucoma (not in product labeling, however, benzodiazepines are contraindicated)

Warnings/Precautions Should be used only after evaluation of potential causes of sleep disturbance. Failure of sleep disturbance to resolve after 7-10 days may indicate psychiatric or medical illness. A worsening of insomnia or the emergence of new abnormalities of thought or behavior may represent unrecognized psychiatric or medical illness and requires immediate and careful evaluation. Use with caution in elderly or debilitated patients, patients with hepatic disease (including alcoholics), or renal impairment. Use with caution in patients with respiratory disease or impaired gag reflex. Avoid use in patients with sleep apnea.

Causes CNS depression (dose related) resulting in sedation, dizziness, confusion, or ataxia which may impair physical and mental capabilities. Patients must be cautioned about performing tasks which require mental alertness (operating machinery or driving). Use with caution in patients receiving other CNS depressants or psychoactive agents. Postmarketing studies have indicated that the use of hypnotic/sedative agents for sleep has been associated with hypersensitivity reactions including anaphylaxis as well as angioedema. An increased risk for hazardous sleep-related activities such as sleep-driving; cooking and eating food, and making phone calls while asleep have also been noted. Effects with other sedative drugs or ethanol may be potentiated. Benzodiazepines have been associated with falls and traumatic injury and should be used with extreme caution in patients who are at risk of these events (especially the elderly).

Use caution in patients with depression, particularly if suicidal risk may be present. Use with caution in patients with a history of drug dependence. Benzodiazepines have been associated with dependence and acute withdrawal symptoms on discontinuation or reduction in dose. Acute withdrawal, including seizures, may be precipitated after administration of flumazenil to patients receiving long-term benzodiazepine therapy.

Benzodiazepines have been associated with anterograde amnesia. Paradoxical reactions, including hyperactive or aggressive behavior have been reported with benzodiazepines, particularly in psychiatric patients. Does not have analgesic, antidepressant, or antipsychotic properties.

Adverse Reactions (Reflective of adult population; not specific for elderly)
Frequency not defined.
Cardiovascular: Palpitation
Central nervous system: Abnormal thinking, agitation, anxiety, ataxia, confusion, depression, dizziness, drowsiness, euphoria, fatigue, headache, hyper-/hypokinesia, incoordination, memory impairment, nervousness, nightmare, paranoid reaction
Dermatologic: Dermatitis, pruritus, rash
Endocrine & metabolic: Libido decreased, menstrual irregularities
Gastrointestinal: Abdominal pain, abnormal taste perception, anorexia, appetite increased/decreased, constipation, diarrhea, dyspepsia, nausea, xerostomia
Genitourinary: Impotence, incontinence
Hematologic: Blood dyscrasias
Neuromuscular & skeletal: Dysarthria, muscle cramps, reflex slowing, rigidity, tremor
Ocular: Blurred vision
Miscellaneous: Drug dependence

Drug Interactions Substrate of CYP3A4 (minor)
CNS depressants: Sedative effects and/or respiratory depression may be additive with CNS depressants; includes ethanol, barbiturates, opioid analgesics, and other sedative agents; monitor for increased effect.
Levodopa: Therapeutic effects may be diminished in some patients following the addition of a benzodiazepine; limited/inconsistent data.
Oral contraceptives: May decrease the clearance of some benzodiazepines (those which undergo oxidative metabolism); monitor for increased benzodiazepine effect.
Theophylline: May partially antagonize some of the effects of benzodiazepines; monitor for decreased response; may require higher doses for sedation.

Ethanol/Nutrition/Herb Interactions Ethanol: Avoid ethanol (may increase CNS depression).

Mechanism of Action Binds to stereospecific benzodiazepine receptors on the postsynaptic GABA neuron at several sites within the central nervous system, including the limbic system, reticular formation. Enhancement of the inhibitory effect of GABA on neuronal excitability results by increased neuronal membrane permeability to chloride ions. This shift in chloride ions results in hyperpolarization (a less excitable state) and stabilization.

Pharmacodynamics Studies have shown that older adults are more sensitive to the effects of benzodiazepines as compared to younger adults.

Pharmacokinetics
Absorption: Oral: Rapidly absorbed
Protein binding: 95%.
Metabolism: In the liver to at least one active compound
Half-life:
  Geriatrics:
    Parent: 53 hours
    Active metabolite: 190 hours
  Adults:
    Parent: 25-41 hours
    Active metabolite: 40-114 hours

Dosage
Geriatrics: Dosing should be cautious; begin at lower end of dosing range (ie, 7.5 mg)
Adults: Hypnotic: Oral: Initial: 15 mg at bedtime; in some patients, the dose may be reduced to 7.5 mg after a few nights
Hepatic Impairment: Dose reduction may be necessary.

Monitoring Parameters Respiratory, cardiovascular and mental status

Patient Information Avoid alcohol and other CNS depressants; may cause drowsiness; avoid activities needing good psychomotor coordination until CNS effects are
(Continued)

Quazepam (Continued)

known; may cause physical or psychological dependence; avoid abrupt discontinuation after prolonged use; may cause "hangover" effect

Additional Information More likely than short-acting benzodiazepine to cause daytime sedation and fatigue; is classified as a long-acting benzodiazepine hypnotic (like flurazepam - Dalmane®), this long duration of action may prevent withdrawal symptoms when therapy is discontinued.

Special Geriatric Considerations Two short-term placebo controlled studies found minimal daytime drowsiness or other side effects with quazepam in elderly patients. There is little clinical experience with this drug in the elderly, but because of its long duration of action, it is probably not a drug of choice. Long-acting benzodiazepines have been associated with falls in the elderly. Interpretive guidelines from the Centers for Medicare and Medicaid Services (CMS) discourage the use of this agent in residents of long-term care facilities.

Dosage Forms Excipient information presented when available (limited, particularly for generics); consult specific product labeling.
Tablet: 7.5 mg, 15 mg

Selected References
Martinez HT and Serna CT, "Short-Term Treatment With Quazepam of Insomnia in Geriatric Patients," *Clin Ther*, 1982, 5(2):174-8.
Winsauer HJ and O'Hair DE, "Quazepam: Short-Term Treatment of Insomnia in Geriatric Outpatients," *Curr Ther Res*, 1984, 35(2):228-34.

♦ **Questran®** *see* Cholestyramine Resin *on page 305*
♦ **Questran® Light** *see* Cholestyramine Resin *on page 305*

Quetiapine (kwe TYE a peen)

Related Information
Antipsychotic Agents *on page 1747*
Atypical Antipsychotics *on page 1749*
Medication Safety Issues
Sound-alike/look-alike issues:
Seroquel® may be confused with Serentil®, Serzone®, Sinequan®
U.S. Brand Names Seroquel®; Seroquel® XR
Canadian Brand Names Seroquel®
Index Terms Quetiapine Fumarate
Generic Available No
Pharmacologic Category Antipsychotic Agent, Atypical
Use Treatment of schizophrenia; treatment of acute manic episodes associated with bipolar disorder (as monotherapy or in combination with lithium or valproate); treatment of depressive episodes associated with bipolar disorder
Unlabeled/Investigational Use Treatment of mania, bipolar disorder, autism
Restrictions An FDA-approved medication guide concerning the use of antidepressants in children, adolescents, and young adults must be distributed when dispensing an outpatient prescription (new or refill) where this medication is to be used without direct supervision of a healthcare provider. Medication guides are available at http://www.fda.gov/cder/drug/antidepressants/MG_template.pdf. Dispense to parents or guardians of children and adolescents receiving this medication.
Contraindications Hypersensitivity to quetiapine or any component of the formulation; severe CNS depression; bone marrow suppression; blood dyscrasias; severe hepatic disease; coma
Warnings/Precautions [U.S. Boxed Warning]: Antidepressants increase the risk of suicidal thinking and behavior in children, adolescents, and young adults (18-24 years of age) with major depressive disorder (MDD) and other psychiatric disorders; consider risk prior to prescribing. Short-term studies did not show an increased risk in patients >24 years of age and showed a decreased risk in patients ≥65 years. Closely monitor all patients for clinical worsening, suicidality, or unusual changes in behavior; particularly during the initial 1-2 months of therapy or during periods of dosage adjustments (increased or decreases); the patient's family or caregiver should be instructed to closely observe the patient and communicate condition with healthcare provider. A medication guide concerning the use of antidepressants should be dispensed with each prescription.

May be sedating, use with caution in disorders where CNS depression is a feature. Use with caution in Parkinson's disease. May induce orthostatic hypotension associated with dizziness, tachycardia, and, in some cases, syncope, especially during the initial dose titration period. Should be used with particular caution in patients with known cardiovascular disease (history of MI or ischemic heart disease, heart failure, or conduction abnormalities), cerebrovascular disease, or conditions that predispose to hypotension. Esophageal dysmotility and aspiration have been associated with antipsychotic use; use with caution in patients at risk of aspiration pneumonia (eg,

Alzheimer's disease). Development of cataracts has been observed in animal studies, therefore, lens examinations should be made upon initiation of therapy and every 6 months thereafter.

Due to anticholinergic effects, use with caution in patients with decreased gastrointestinal motility, urinary retention, BPH, xerostomia, visual problems, narrow-angle glaucoma (screening is recommended), and myasthenia gravis. Relative to other antipsychotics, quetiapine has a moderate potency of cholinergic blockade. May cause extrapyramidal symptoms, pseudoparkinsonism, and/or tardive dyskinesia. Impaired core body temperature regulation may occur; caution with strenuous exercise, heat exposure, dehydration, and concomitant medication possessing anticholinergic effects. Neuroleptic malignant syndrome (NMS) is a potentially fatal symptom complex that has been reported in association with administration of antipsychotic drugs. Clinical manifestations of NMS are hyperpyrexia, muscle rigidity, altered mental status, and evidence of autonomic instability (irregular pulse or blood pressure, tachycardia, diaphoresis, and cardiac dysrhythmia). Management of NMS should include immediate discontinuation of antipsychotic drugs and other drugs not essential to concurrent therapy, intensive symptomatic treatment and medication monitoring, and treatment of any concomitant medical problems for which specific treatment are available.

Use caution in patients with a history of seizures. May cause decreases in total free thyroxine, elevations of liver enzymes, cholesterol levels, and/or triglyceride increases.

May cause hyperglycemia; in some cases may be extreme and associated with ketoacidosis, hyperosmolar coma, or death. Use with caution in patients with diabetes or other disorders of glucose regulation; monitor for worsening of glucose control. Significant weight gain has been observed with antipsychotic therapy; incidence varies with product. Monitor waist circumference and BMI.

Adverse Reactions (Reflective of adult population; not specific for elderly)
>10%:
  Cardiovascular: Hypotension (<5% to 19%)
  Central nervous system: Somnolence (12% to 34%), sedation (13% to 30%), headache (17% to 21%), agitation (6% to 20%), dizziness (9% to 18%), extrapyramidal symptoms (8% to 12%)
  Endocrine & metabolic: Triglycerides increased (14% to 23%), cholesterol increased (9% to 16%)
  Gastrointestinal: Xerostomia (9% to 44%), weight gain (dose-related; <5% to 23%)
1% to 10%:
  Cardiovascular: Orthostatic hypotension (4% to 7%), tachycardia (≤6%), syncope (<5%)
  Central nervous system: Fatigue (10%), pain (7%), lethargy (5%), akathisia (<5%), fever (2% to <5%), dystonia (<5%), tardive dyskinesia (<5%), anxiety (4%)
  Dermatologic: Rash (4% to <5%)
  Gastrointestinal: Constipation (6% to 10%), dyspepsia (dose-related; 5% to 7%), abdominal pain (dose-related; 4% to 7%), vomiting (5% to 6%), appetite increased (≤5%), drooling (<5%), dysphagia (<5%), gastroenteritis (2%)
  Hematologic: Leukopenia (<5%), neutropenia (2%)
  Hepatic: Transaminases increased (1% to 6%), GGT increased (1%)
  Neuromuscular & skeletal: Weakness (5% to 10%), tremor (≤8%), back pain (3% to 5%), dysarthria (<5%), hypertonia (≥1%)
  Ocular: Blurred vision (<5%), amblyopia (2%)
  Respiratory: Pharyngitis (4% to 6%), nasal congestion (5%), rhinitis (3%)

Overdosage/Toxicology Symptoms of overdose include drowsiness, sedation, tachycardia and hypotension. Initiate cardiac monitoring; patients with pre-existing cardiovascular disease may have an increased risk for adverse events with overdose. Intravenous hydration may be useful in the management of hypotension. Anticholinergics may be used to manage severe extrapyramidal symptoms. Treatment is otherwise symptom-directed and supportive.

Drug Interactions Substrate of CYP2D6 (minor), 3A4 (major)
  Acetylcholinesterase inhibitors (central): May increase the risk of antipsychotic-related extrapyramidal symptoms; monitor.
  Anticholinergics: May enhance the anticholinergic adverse/toxic effects of quetiapine.
  Antihypertensives: Concurrent use with an antihypertensive may produce additive hypotensive effects (particularly orthostasis).
  Azole antifungals (fluconazole, itraconazole, ketoconazole): Administration with ketoconazole increases serum concentration of quetiapine by 335%; use with caution.
  Cimetidine: May increase levels/effects of quetiapine; monitor.
  Ciprofloxacin: May enhance the QT_c-prolonging effect of quetiapine.
  CNS depressants: Quetiapine may enhance the sedative effects of other CNS depressants; includes antidepressants, benzodiazepines, barbiturates, ethanol, opioid analgesics, and other sedative agents; monitor for increased effect.
(Continued)

Quetiapine (Continued)

CYP3A4 inducers: CYP3A4 inducers may decrease the levels/effects of quetiapine. Example inducers include aminoglutethimide, carbamazepine, nafcillin, nevirapine, phenobarbital, phenytoin, and rifamycins. Higher maintenance doses of quetiapine may be required.

CYP3A4 inhibitors: May increase the levels/effects of quetiapine. Example inhibitors include azole antifungals, clarithromycin, diclofenac, doxycycline, erythromycin, imatinib, isoniazid, nefazodone, nicardipine, propofol, protease inhibitors, quinidine, telithromycin, and verapamil.

Phenytoin: Metabolism/clearance of quetiapine may be increased; fivefold changes have been noted. Higher maintenance doses of quetiapine may be required.

Pramlintide: May enhance the gastrointestinal anticholinergic effects of quetiapine.

QT_c-prolonging agents: Concurrent use of quetiapine with other agents known to cause QT_c prolongation may increase the risk of serious arrhythmias.

Thioridazine: May decrease the levels/effects of quetiapine. Also, concomitant treatment may increase risk of QT_c prolongation. Avoid concurrent use.

Ethanol/Nutrition/Herb Interactions

Ethanol: Avoid ethanol (may cause excessive impairment in cognition/motor function).

Food: In healthy volunteers, administration of quetiapine with food resulted in an increase in the peak serum concentration and AUC (each by ~15%) compared to the fasting state.

Herb/Nutraceutical: St John's wort may decrease quetiapine levels. Avoid valerian, St John's wort, kava kava, gotu kola (may increase CNS depression).

Stability Store at 15°C to 30°C (59°F to 86°F).

Mechanism of Action Quetiapine is a dibenzothiazepine atypical antipsychotic. It has been proposed that this drug's antipsychotic activity is mediated through a combination of dopamine type 2 (D_2) and serotonin type 2 (5-HT_2) antagonism. It is an antagonist at multiple neurotransmitter receptors in the brain: serotonin 5-HT_{1A} and 5-HT_2, dopamine D_1 and D_2, histamine H_1, and adrenergic alpha$_1$- and alpha$_2$- receptors; but appears to have no appreciable affinity at cholinergic muscarinic and benzodiazepine receptors.

Antagonism at receptors other than dopamine and 5-HT_2 with similar receptor affinities may explain some of the other effects of quetiapine. The drug's antagonism of histamine H_1-receptors may explain the somnolence observed with it. The drug's antagonism of adrenergic alpha$_1$-receptors may explain the orthostatic hypotension observed with it.

Pharmacokinetics

Absorption: Rapidly absorbed following oral administration

Distribution: V_d: 10 ± 4 L/kg; V_{dss}: ~2 days

Protein binding, plasma: 83%

Metabolism: Primarily hepatic; via CYP3A4; forms the metabolite N-desalkyl quetiapine (active) and two inactive metabolites

Bioavailability: Tablet is 100% bioavailable relative to solution; marginally affected by administration with food, with C_{max} and AUC values increased by 25% and 15% respectively

Half-life elimination: Mean: Terminal: Quetiapine: ~7 hours; N-desalkyl quetiapine: 9-12 hours

Time to peak plasma concentrations: 1.5 hours

Elimination: Mainly via hepatic metabolism; reduced clearance seen in older adults when compared to younger adults (40% reduction)

Dosage

Geriatrics: Lower clearance in elderly patients (40%), resulting in higher concentrations. Usual dosage requirement is 50-200 mg/day with a slower titration schedule. Begin titration with immediate release formulation, increase dose by 25-50 mg/day to effective dose, based on clinical response and tolerability. May transition to extended release formulation (at equivalent total daily dose) when effective dose has been reached.

Adults:

Bipolar depression: Oral: Immediate release tablet: Initial: 50 mg/day the first day; increase to 100 mg/day on day 2, further increasing by 100 mg/day each day to a target of 300 mg/day by day 4. Further increases up to 600 mg/day by day 8 have been evaluated in clinical trials, but no additional antidepressant efficacy was noted.

Bipolar mania: Oral: Immediate release tablet: Initial: 50 mg twice daily on day 1, increase dose in increments of 100 mg/day to 200 mg twice daily on day 4; may increase to a target dose of 800 mg/day by day 6 at increments ≤200 mg/day. Usual dosage range: 400-800 mg/day.

Schizophrenia/psychoses: Oral:

Immediate release tablet: Initial: 25 mg twice daily; increase in increments of 25-50 mg 2-3 times/day on the second and third day, if tolerated, to a target dose of 300-400 mg in 2-3 divided doses by day 4. Make further adjustments as needed at intervals of at least 2 days in adjustments of 25-50 mg twice daily. Usual maintenance range: 300-800 mg/day.

Extended-release tablet: Initial: 300 mg once daily; increase in increments of up to 300 mg/day (in intervals of ≥1 day). For dosage requirements <200 mg during initial titration, the immediate release formulation should be used. Usual maintenance range: 400-800 mg/day.

Note: Dose reductions should be attempted periodically to establish lowest effective dose in patients with psychosis. Patients being restarted after 1 week of no drug need to be titrated as above.

Renal Impairment: No dosage adjustment required: 25% lower mean oral clearance of quetiapine than normal subjects; however, plasma concentrations similar to normal subjects receiving the same dose.

Hepatic Impairment: Lower clearance in hepatic impairment (30%), may result in higher concentrations. Dosage adjustment may be required.

Oral: Initial: 25 mg/day, increase dose by 25-50 mg/day to effective dose, based on clinical response and tolerability to patient. Begin titration with immediate release formulation; may transition to extended release formulation (at equivalent total daily dose) when effective dose has been reached.

Monitoring Parameters Vital signs; fasting lipid profile and fasting blood glucose/Hgb A_{1c} (prior to treatment, at 3 months, then annually); BMI, personal/family history of obesity, waist circumference; blood pressure; mental status, abnormal involuntary movement scale (AIMS); Weight should be assessed prior to treatment, at 4 weeks, 8 weeks, 12 weeks, and then at quarterly intervals. Consider titrating to a different antipsychotic agent for a weight gain ≥5% of the initial weight. Patients should have eyes checked for cataracts every 6 months while on this medication. Observe for new or worsening depression, anxiety, irritability, aggression, or other symptoms of unusual behavior or mood.

Patient Information May cause drowsiness, dizziness, and/or headache; might increase risk of cataracts; care should be exercised when operating machinery/cars

Special Geriatric Considerations Any changes in disease status in any organ system can result in behavior changes.

Extrapyramidal syndrome symptoms occur less often than with traditional antipsychotics from the phenothiazine and butyrophenone classes. Many elderly patients receive antipsychotic medications for inappropriate nonpsychotic behavior. Before initiating antipsychotic medication, the clinician should investigate any possible reversible cause; any stress or stress from any disease can cause acute "confusion" or worsening of baseline nonpsychotic behavior. Most commonly acute changes in behavior are due to increases in drug dose or addition of new drug to regimen; fluid electrolyte loss; infections; and changes in environment.

In the treatment of agitated, demented elderly patients, authors of meta-analyses of controlled trials of the response to the traditional antipsychotics (eg, phenothiazines, butyrophenones) in controlling agitation, have concluded that the use of neuroleptics results in a response rate of 18%. Clearly neuroleptic therapy for behavior control should be limited with frequent attempts to withdraw the agent given for behavior control. In light of significant risks and adverse effects in elderly population compared with limited data demonstrating efficacy in the treatment of dementia related psychosis, aggression, and agitation, an extensive risk:benefit analysis should be performed prior to use.

Dosage Forms Excipient information presented when available (limited, particularly for generics); consult specific product labeling.

Tablet, as fumarate:

Seroquel®: 25 mg, 50 mg, 100 mg, 200 mg, 300 mg, 400 mg

Tablet, extended release, as fumarate:

Seroquel® XR: 200 mg, 300 mg, 400 mg

Selected References

American Diabetes Association; American Psychiatric Association; American Association of Clinical Endocrinologists; North American Association for the Study of Obesity, "Consensus Development Conference on Antipsychotic Drugs and Obesity and Diabetes," *Diabetes Care*, 2004, 27(2):596-601.

Goldberg RJ, "Managing Psychosis-Related Behavioral Problems in the Elderly," *Consult Pharm*, 1997, 12(Suppl C):4-10.

Schneider LS, Tariot PN, Dagerman KS, et al, "Effectiveness of Atypical Antipsychotic Drugs in Patients With Alzheimer's Disease," *N Engl J Med*, 2006, 355(15):1525-38.

♦ **Quetiapine Fumarate** see Quetiapine on page 1356

♦ **Quibron®-T [DSC]** see Theophylline on page 1548

♦ **Quibron®-T/SR [DSC]** see Theophylline on page 1548

Quinapril (KWIN a pril)

Related Information

Angiotensin Agents on page 1737

(Continued)

Quinapril *(Continued)*

Medication Safety Issues

Sound-alike/look-alike issues:

Accupril® may be confused with Accolate®, Accutane®, AcipHex®, Monopril®

International issues:

Accupril® may be confused with Acepril® which is a brand name for lisinopril in Denmark, a brand name for enalapril in Hungary and Switzerland, and a brand name for captopril in Great Britain

U.S. Brand Names Accupril®

Canadian Brand Names Accupril®; GD-Quinapril

Index Terms Quinapril Hydrochloride

Generic Available Yes

Pharmacologic Category Angiotensin-Converting Enzyme (ACE) Inhibitor

Use Management of hypertension; treatment of systolic congestive heart failure

Unlabeled/Investigational Use Treatment of left ventricular dysfunction after myocardial infarction

Contraindications Hypersensitivity to quinapril or any component of the formulation; angioedema related to previous treatment with an ACE inhibitor; bilateral renal artery stenosis; primary hyperaldosteronism; patients with idiopathic or hereditary angioedema

Warnings/Precautions Anaphylactic reactions can occur. Use with caution in patients with renal insufficiency, autoimmune disease, renal artery stenosis; excessive hypotension may be more likely in volume-depleted patients, the elderly, and following the first dose (first dose phenomenon); quinapril should be discontinued if laryngeal stridor or angioedema is observed. Angioedema can occur at any time during treatment (especially following first dose). It may involve head and neck (potentially affecting the airway) or the intestine (presenting with abdominal pain). Prolonged monitoring may be required, especially if tongue, glottis, or larynx are involved as they are associated with airway obstruction. Those with a history of airway surgery in this situation have a higher risk. Rare toxicities associated with ACE inhibitors include cholestatic jaundice (which may progress to hepatic necrosis) and neutropenia/agranulocytosis with myeloid hyperplasia. Hyperkalemia may rarely occur. May be associated with deterioration of renal function and/or increases in serum creatinine, particularly in patients dependent on renin-angiotensin-aldosterone system. Use with caution in unilateral renal artery stenosis and pre-existing renal insufficiency; if patient has renal impairment, then a baseline WBC with differential and serum creatinine should be evaluated and monitored closely during the first 3 months of therapy. Hypersensitivity reactions may be seen during hemodialysis with high-flux dialysis membranes (eg, AN69).

Adverse Reactions (Reflective of adult population; not specific for elderly)

Note: Frequency ranges include data from hypertension and heart failure trials. Higher rates of adverse reactions have generally been noted in patients with CHF. However, the frequency of adverse effects associated with placebo is also increased in this population.

1% to 10%:

Cardiovascular: Hypotension (3%), chest pain (2%), first-dose hypotension (up to 3%)

Central nervous system: Dizziness (4% to 8%), headache (2% to 6%), fatigue (3%)

Dermatologic: Rash (1%)

Endocrine & metabolic: Hyperkalemia (2%)

Gastrointestinal: Vomiting/nausea (1% to 2%), diarrhea (2%)

Neuromuscular & skeletal: Myalgias (2% to 5%), back pain (1%)

Renal: BUN/serum creatinine increased (2%, transient elevations may occur with a higher frequency), worsening of renal function (in patients with bilateral renal artery stenosis or hypovolemia)

Respiratory: Upper respiratory symptoms, cough (2% to 4%; up to 13% in some studies), dyspnea (2%)

Overdosage/Toxicology Mild hypotension has been the only toxic effect seen with acute overdose; bradycardia may also occur. Hyperkalemia occurs even with therapeutic doses, especially in patients with renal insufficiency and those taking NSAIDs. Following initiation of essential overdose management, toxic symptom and supportive treatment should be initiated. Hypotension usually responds to I.V. fluids or Trendelenburg positioning.

Drug Interactions

Alpha$_1$ blockers: Hypotensive effect increased.

Aspirin: The effects of ACE inhibitors may be blunted by aspirin administration, particularly at higher dosages and/or increased adverse renal effects.

Diuretics: Hypovolemia due to diuretics may precipitate acute hypotensive events or acute renal failure.

Gold sodium thiomalate: ACE inhibitors may enhance the adverse/toxic effects (nitritoid reaction) of gold sodium thiomalate. The reaction may include facial flushing, nausea, vomiting, hypotension, and syncope. If it is to occur, would be expected shortly after administration of gold compound in patients maintained on an ACEI.

Insulin: Risk of hypoglycemia may be increased.

Lithium: Risk of lithium toxicity may be increased; monitor lithium levels, especially the first 4 weeks of therapy.

Mercaptopurine: Risk of neutropenia may be increased.

NSAIDs: May attenuate hypertensive efficacy; effect has been seen with captopril and may occur with other ACE inhibitors; monitor blood pressure. May increase risk of adverse renal effects.

Potassium-sparing diuretics (amiloride, spironolactone, triamterene): Increased risk of hyperkalemia.

Potassium supplements may increase the risk of hyperkalemia.

Quinolones: Absorption may be decreased by quinapril; separate administration by at least 2-4 hours.

Tetracyclines: Absorption may be reduced by quinapril; separate administration by at least 2-4 hours.

Trimethoprim (high dose) may increase the risk of hyperkalemia.

Ethanol/Nutrition/Herb Interactions Herb/Nutraceutical: Avoid dong quai if using for hypertension (has estrogenic activity). Avoid ephedra, yohimbe, ginseng (may worsen hypertension). Avoid garlic (may have increased antihypertensive effect).

Stability Store at room temperature. To prepare solution for oral administration, mix prior to administration and use within 10 minutes.

Mechanism of Action Competitive inhibitor of angiotensin-converting enzyme (ACE); prevents conversion of angiotensin I to angiotensin II, a potent vasoconstrictor; results in lower levels of angiotensin II which causes an increase in plasma renin activity and a reduction in aldosterone secretion; a CNS mechanism may also be involved in hypotensive effect as angiotensin II increases adrenergic outflow from CNS; vasoactive kallikreins may be decreased in conversion to active hormones by ACE inhibitors, thus reducing blood pressure

Pharmacodynamics

Onset of action: Within 1 hour

Duration: 24 hours; data demonstrate excellent tissue penetration with a long tissue half-life

Pharmacokinetics

Absorption: Quinapril: ≥60%

Protein binding: Quinapril: 97%; Quinaprilat: 97%

Metabolism: Rapidly hydrolyzed to quinaprilat, the active metabolite

Half-life elimination: Quinapril: 0.8 hours; Quinaprilat: 3 hours; increases as Cl_{cr} decreases

Time to peak, serum: Quinapril: 1 hour; Quinaprilat: ~2 hours

Elimination: Urine (50% to 60% primarily as quinaprilat)

Dosage

Geriatrics: Oral: Initial: 2.5-5 mg/day; increase dosage at increments of 2.5-5 mg at 1- to 2-week intervals; adjust for renal impairment.

Adults:

Hypertension: Oral: Initial: 10-20 mg once daily, adjust according to blood pressure response at peak and trough blood levels; initial dose may be reduced to 5 mg in patients receiving diuretic therapy if the diuretic is continued.

Usual dose range (JNC 7): 10-40 mg once daily

Congestive heart failure or post-MI: Oral: Initial: 5 mg once or twice daily, titrated at weekly intervals to 20-40 mg daily in 2 divided doses; target dose (heart failure): 20 mg twice daily (ACC/AHA 2005 Heart Failure Guidelines)

Renal Impairment: Lower initial doses should be used; after initial dose (if tolerated), administer initial dose twice daily; may be increased at weekly intervals to optimal response:

Hypertension: Oral: Initial:

Cl_{cr} >60 mL/minute: Administer 10 mg/day

Cl_{cr} 30-60 mL/minute: Administer 5 mg/day

Cl_{cr} 10-30 mL/minute: Administer 2.5 mg/day

Congestive heart failure: Oral: Initial:

Cl_{cr} >30 mL/minute: Administer 5 mg/day

Cl_{cr} 10-30 mL/minute: Administer 2.5 mg/day

Hepatic Impairment: In patients with alcoholic cirrhosis, hydrolysis of quinapril to quinaprilat is impaired; however, the subsequent elimination of quinaprilat is unaltered.

Monitoring Parameters BUN, serum creatinine, renal function, WBC, and potassium

Patient Information Inform prescriber of all prescriptions, OTC medications, or herbal products you are taking, and any allergies you have. Do not take any new medication during therapy unless approved by prescriber. Take as directed; do not alter dose or discontinue without consulting prescriber. Take first dose at bedtime or when sitting down (hypotension may occur). This drug does not eliminate need for diet or exercise (Continued)

Quinapril *(Continued)*

regimen as recommended by prescriber. May cause increased cough (if persistent or bothersome, contact prescriber); postural hypotension (use caution when rising from lying or sitting position or climbing stairs); headache (consult prescriber for approved analgesic); dizziness (use caution when driving or engaging in tasks that require alertness until response to drug is known); nausea or vomiting (small, frequent meals, frequent mouth care, sucking lozenges, or chewing gum may help); or muscle or back pain (consult prescriber for approved analgesic). Immediately report swelling of face, mouth, lips, tongue or throat; chest pain or respiratory difficulty. Report persistent cough; persistent pain in muscles, joints, or back; skin rash; or other persistent adverse reactions.

Additional Information Patients taking diuretics are at risk for developing hypotension on initial dosing; to prevent this, discontinue diuretics 2-3 days prior to initiating quinapril; may restart diuretics if blood pressure is not controlled by quinapril alone

Special Geriatric Considerations Due to frequent decreases in glomerular filtration (also creatinine clearance) with aging, elderly patients may have exaggerated responses to ACE inhibitors; differences in clinical response due to hepatic changes are not observed. ACE inhibitors may be preferred agents in elderly patients with CHF and diabetes mellitus. Diabetic proteinuria is reduced and insulin sensitivity is enhanced. In general, the side effect profile is favorable in elderly and causes little or no CNS confusion; use lowest dose recommendations initially. Adjust for renal function. Many elderly may be volume depleted due to diuretic use and/or blunted thirst reflex resulting in inadequate fluid intake.

Dosage Forms Excipient information presented when available (limited, particularly for generics); consult specific product labeling.

Tablet: 5 mg, 10 mg, 20 mg, 40 mg

Accupril®: 5 mg, 10 mg, 20 mg, 40 mg

Selected References

Chobanian AV, Bakris GL, Black HR, et al, "The Seventh Report of the Joint National Committee on Prevention, Detection, Evaluation, and Treatment of High Blood Pressure: The JNC 7 Report," *JAMA*, 2003, 289(19):2560-71.

Konstam MA, Drakup K, Baker DW, et al, "Heart Failure: Evaluation and Care of Patients With Left Ventricular Systolic Dysfunction," *Clinical Practice Guideline No 11*, Rockville, MD: Agency for Health Care Policy and Research, Public Health Service, U.S. Department of Health and Human Services, 1994.

Lewis EJ, Hunsicker LG, Bain RP, et al, "The Effect of Angiotensin-Converting Enzyme Inhibition on Diabetic Nephropathy," *N Engl J Med*, 1993, 329(20):1456-62.

McAreavey D and Robertson JI, "Angiotensin Converting Enzyme Inhibitors and Moderate Hypertension," *Drugs*, 1990, 40(3):326-45.

Williams JF, Bristow MR, Fowler MB, et al, "Guidelines for the Evaluation and Management of Heart Failure: Report of the American College of Cardiology/American Heart Association Task Force on Practice Guidelines (Committee on Evaluation and Management of Heart Failure)," *J Am Coll Cardiol*, 1995, 26:1376-8.

Quinapril and Hydrochlorothiazide

(KWIN a pril & hye droe klor oh THYE a zide)

Related Information

Hydrochlorothiazide *on page 756*

Quinapril *on page 1359*

U.S. Brand Names Accuretic®; Quinaretic

Canadian Brand Names Accuretic®

Index Terms Hydrochlorothiazide and Quinapril

Generic Available Yes

Pharmacologic Category Angiotensin-Converting Enzyme (ACE) Inhibitor; Antihypertensive; Diuretic, Thiazide

Use Treatment of hypertension (not for initial therapy)

Dosage

Geriatrics: If previous response to individual components is unknown, initial dose selection should be cautious, at the low end of adult dosage range; titration should occur at 1- to 2-week intervals.

Adults:

Hypertension: Oral:

Patients with inadequate response to quinapril monotherapy: Quinapril 10 mg/hydrochlorothiazide 12.5 mg **or** quinapril 20 mg/hydrochlorothiazide 12.5 mg once daily

Patients with adequate blood pressure control on hydrochlorothiazide 25 mg/day, but significant potassium loss: Quinapril 10 mg/hydrochlorothiazide 12.5 mg **or** quinapril 20 mg/hydrochlorothiazide 12.5 mg once daily

Note: Clinical trials of quinapril/hydrochlorothiazide combinations used quinapril doses of 2.5-40 mg/day and hydrochlorothiazide doses of 6.25-25 mg/day.

Renal Impairment: Cl_{cr} <30 mL/minute/1.73 m^2 or serum creatinine ≤3 mg/dL: Use is not recommended.

Special Geriatric Considerations Combination products are not recommended for first-line treatment. Hydrochlorothiazide is not effective in patients with a Cl_{cr} <30 mL/minute, therefore, it may not be a useful agent in many elderly patients. Due to frequent decreases in glomerular filtration (also creatinine clearance) with aging, elderly patients may have exaggerated responses to ACE inhibitors; differences in clinical response due to hepatic changes are not observed. ACE inhibitors may be preferred agents in elderly patients with CHF and diabetes mellitus. Diabetic proteinuria is reduced and insulin sensitivity is enhanced. In general, the side effect profile is favorable in the elderly and causes little or no CNS confusion; use lowest dose recommendations initially. Adjust for renal function. Many elderly may be volume depleted due to diuretic use and/or blunted thirst reflex resulting in inadequate fluid intake.

Dosage Forms Excipient information presented when available (limited, particularly for generics); consult specific product labeling.

Tablet:
10/12.5: Quinapril 10 mg and hydrochlorothiazide 12.5 mg
20/12.5: Quinapril 20 mg and hydrochlorothiazide 12.5 mg
20/25: Quinapril 20 mg and hydrochlorothiazide 25 mg
Accuretic® 10/12.5, Quinaretic 10/12.5: Quinapril 10 mg and hydrochlorothiazide 12.5 mg
Accuretic® 20/12.5, Quinaretic 20/12.5: Quinapril 20 mg and hydrochlorothiazide 12.5 mg
Accuretic® 20/25, Quinaretic 20/25: Quinapril 20 mg and hydrochlorothiazide 25 mg

♦ **Quinapril Hydrochloride** see Quinapril on page 1359
♦ **Quinaretic** see Quinapril and Hydrochlorothiazide on page 1362

Quinidine (KWIN i deen)

Related Information
Serum Drug Concentrations Commonly Monitored Guidelines on page 1862
Medication Safety Issues
Sound-alike/look-alike issues:
Quinidine may be confused with clonidine, quinine, Quinora®
Canadian Brand Names Apo-Quinidine®; BioQuin® Durules™; Novo-Quinidin; Quinate®
Index Terms Quinidine Gluconate; Quinidine Polygalacturonate; Quinidine Sulfate
Generic Available Yes
Pharmacologic Category Antiarrhythmic Agent, Class Ia
Use Prophylaxis after cardioversion of atrial fibrillation and/or flutter to maintain normal sinus rhythm; also used to prevent recurrence of paroxysmal supraventricular tachycardia, paroxysmal AV junctional rhythm, paroxysmal ventricular tachycardia, paroxysmal atrial fibrillation, and atrial or ventricular premature contractions; also has activity against *Plasmodium falciparum* malaria
Contraindications Hypersensitivity to quinidine or any component of the formulation; thrombocytopenia; thrombocytopenic purpura; myasthenia gravis; heart block greater than first degree; idioventricular conduction delays (except in patients with a functioning artificial pacemaker); those adversely affected by anticholinergic activity; concurrent use of quinolone antibiotics which prolong QT interval, cisapride, amprenavir, or ritonavir
Warnings/Precautions Monitor and adjust dose to prevent QT_c prolongation. Watch for proarrhythmic effects. Correct hypokalemia before initiating therapy. Hypokalemia may worsen toxicity. **[U.S. Boxed Warning]: Antiarrhythmic drugs have not been shown to enhance survival in nonlife-threatening ventricular arrhythmias and may increase mortality; the risk is greatest with structural heart disease. Quinidine may increase mortality in treatment of atrial fibrillation/flutter.** May precipitate or exacerbate CHF. Reduce dosage in hepatic impairment. Use may cause digoxin-induced toxicity (adjust digoxin's dose). Use caution with concurrent use of other antiarrhythmics. Hypersensitivity reactions can occur. Can unmask sick sinus syndrome (causes bradycardia); use with caution in patients with heart block. Has been associated with severe hepatotoxic reactions, including granulomatous hepatitis. Hemolysis may occur in patients with G6PD (glucose-6-phosphate dehydrogenase) deficiency. Different salt products are not interchangeable.
Adverse Reactions (Reflective of adult population; not specific for elderly)
Frequency not defined: Hypotension, syncope
>10%:
Cardiovascular: QT_c prolongation (modest prolongation is common, however, excessive prolongation is rare and indicates toxicity)
Central nervous system: Lightheadedness (15%)
Gastrointestinal: Diarrhea (35%), upper GI distress, bitter taste, diarrhea, anorexia, nausea, vomiting, stomach cramping (22%)
(Continued)

Quinidine (Continued)

1% to 10%:

Cardiovascular: Angina (6%), palpitation (7%), new or worsened arrhythmia (proarrhythmic effect)

Central nervous system: Syncope (1% to 8%), headache (7%), fatigue (7%), sleep disturbance (3%), tremor (2%), nervousness (2%), incoordination (1%)

Dermatologic: Rash (5%)

Neuromuscular & skeletal: Weakness (5%)

Ocular: Blurred vision

Otic: Tinnitus

Respiratory: Wheezing

Note: Cinchonism, a syndrome which may include tinnitus, high-frequency hearing loss, deafness, vertigo, blurred vision, diplopia, photophobia, headache, confusion, and delirium has been associated with quinidine use. Usually associated with chronic toxicity, this syndrome has also been described after brief exposure to a moderate dose in sensitive patients. Vomiting and diarrhea may also occur as isolated reactions to therapeutic quinidine levels.

Overdosage/Toxicology Has a low toxic:therapeutic ratio and may easily produce fatal intoxication (acute toxic dose: 1 g); symptoms include sinus bradycardia, sinus node arrest or asystole, PR, QRS, or QT interval prolongation, torsade de pointes (polymorphic ventricular tachycardia) and depressed myocardial contractility, which along with alpha-adrenergic or ganglionic blockade, may result in hypotension and pulmonary edema. Other effects are anticholinergic (dry mouth, dilated pupils, and delirium) as well as seizures, coma and respiratory arrest.

Treatment is primarily symptomatic and effects usually respond to conventional therapies (fluids, positioning, vasopressors, anticonvulsants, antiarrhythmics). **Note:** Do not use other type 1a or 1c antiarrhythmic agents to treat ventricular tachycardia. Sodium bicarbonate may treat wide QRS intervals or hypotension. Markedly impaired conduction or high degree AV block, unresponsive to bicarbonate, indicates consideration of a pacemaker is needed.

Drug Interactions Substrate of CYP2C9 (minor), 2E1 (minor), 3A4 (major); **Inhibits** CYP2C9 (weak), 2D6 (strong), 3A4 (strong)

Amiloride may cause prolonged ventricular conduction leading to arrhythmias.

Amiodarone may increase quinidine blood levels; monitor quinidine levels.

Cimetidine: Increases quinidine blood levels; closely monitor levels or use an alternative H_2 antagonist.

Cisapride and quinidine may increase risk of malignant arrhythmias; concurrent use is contraindicated.

Codeine: Analgesic efficacy may be reduced.

CYP2D6 substrates: Quinidine may increase the levels/effects of CYP2D6 substrates. Example substrates include amphetamines, selected beta-blockers, dextromethorphan, fluoxetine, lidocaine, mirtazapine, nefazodone, paroxetine, risperidone, ritonavir, thioridazine, tricyclic antidepressants, and venlafaxine.

CYP2D6 prodrug substrates: Quinidine may decrease the levels/effects of CYP2D6 prodrug substrates. Example prodrug substrates include codeine, hydrocodone, oxycodone, and tramadol.

CYP3A4 inducers: CYP3A4 inducers may decrease the levels/effects of quinidine. Example inducers include aminoglutethimide, carbamazepine, nafcillin, nevirapine, phenobarbital, phenytoin, and rifamycins.

CYP3A4 inhibitors: May increase the levels/effects of quinidine. Example inhibitors include azole antifungals, clarithromycin, diclofenac, doxycycline, erythromycin, imatinib, isoniazid, nefazodone, nicardipine, propofol, protease inhibitors, telithromycin, and verapamil.

CYP3A4 substrates: Quinidine may increase the levels/effects of CYP3A4 substrates. Example substrates include benzodiazepines, calcium channel blockers, mirtazapine, nateglinide, nefazodone, tacrolimus, and venlafaxine. Selected benzodiazepines (midazolam and triazolam), cisapride, ergot alkaloids, selected HMG-CoA reductase inhibitors (lovastatin and simvastatin), and pimozide are generally contraindicated with strong CYP3A4 inhibitors.

Digoxin blood levels may be increased; monitor digoxin blood levels.

Metoprolol: Increased metoprolol blood levels.

Mexiletine blood levels may be increased.

Nifedipine blood levels may be increased by quinidine; nifedipine may decrease quinidine blood levels.

Propafenone blood levels may be increased.

Propranolol blood levels may be increased.

QT_c-prolonging agents (eg, amiodarone, amitriptyline, bepridil, disopyramide, erythromycin, haloperidol, imipramine, pimozide, procainamide, sotalol, thioridazine): Effects may be additive; use with caution.

Ritonavir, nelfinavir, and amprenavir may increase quinidine levels and toxicity; concurrent use is contraindicated.

Moxifloxacin may result in additional prolongation of the QT interval; concurrent use is contraindicated.

Timolol blood levels may be increased.

Urinary alkalinizers (antacids, sodium bicarbonate, acetazolamide) increase quinidine blood levels.

Verapamil and diltiazem increase quinidine blood levels.

Warfarin effects may be increased by quinidine; monitor INR closely during addition or withdrawal of quinidine.

Ethanol/Nutrition/Herb Interactions

Food: Dietary salt intake may alter the rate and extent of quinidine absorption. A decrease in dietary salt may lead to an increase in quinidine serum concentrations. Avoid changes in dietary salt intake. Quinidine serum levels may be increased if taken with food. Food has a variable effect on absorption of sustained release formulation. The rate of absorption of quinidine may be decreased following the ingestion of grapefruit juice. In addition, CYP3A4 metabolism of quinidine may be reduced by grapefruit juice. Grapefruit juice should be avoided. Excessive intake of fruit juices or vitamin C may decrease urine pH and result in increased clearance of quinidine with decreased serum concentration. Alkaline foods may result in increased quinidine serum concentrations.

Herb/Nutraceutical: St John's wort may decrease quinidine levels. Avoid ephedra (may worsen arrhythmia).

Stability Do not use discolored parenteral solution.

Mechanism of Action Class Ia antiarrhythmic agent; depresses phase O of the action potential; decreases myocardial excitability and conduction velocity, and myocardial contractility by decreasing sodium influx during depolarization and potassium efflux in repolarization; also reduces calcium transport across cell membrane

Pharmacokinetics

Distribution: V_d: 2-3.5 L/kg, decreased V_d with congestive heart failure, malaria; increased V_d with cirrhosis; V_d is not significantly changed with age

Protein binding: 80% to 90% (younger adults); decreased protein binding with cyanotic congenital heart disease, cirrhosis, or acute myocardial infarction

Metabolism: Extensive in the liver (50% to 90%) to inactive compounds

Bioavailability: 80% (sulfate), 70% (gluconate); 87% (older adults)

Half-life, plasma: 6-8 hours (average 5.7 hours) in young adults, increased half-life with older adults (average 9.7 hours), cirrhosis and congestive heart failure

Elimination: In urine (15% to 25% as unchanged drug)

Dosage

Geriatrics & Adults:

Note: Dosage expressed in terms of the salt: 267 mg of quinidine gluconate = 275 mg of quinidine polygalacturonate = 200 mg of quinidine sulfate.

Test dose for idiosyncratic reaction: Oral, I.M.: 200 mg administered several hours before full dosage (to determine possibility of idiosyncratic reaction)

Antiarrhythmic:

Oral:

Sulfate: 100-600 mg/dose every 4-6 hours; begin at 200 mg/dose and titrate to desired effect (maximum daily dose: 3-4 g)

Gluconate: 324-972 mg every 8-12 hours

I.M.: 400 mg/dose every 4-6 hours

I.V.: 200-400 mg/dose diluted and given at a rate ≤10 mg/minute

Renal Impairment:

Cl_{cr} <10 mL/minute: Administer 75% of normal dose.

Hemodialysis effects: Slightly hemodialyzable (5% to 20%); 200 mg supplemental dose posthemodialysis is recommended; not dialyzable (0% to 5%) by peritoneal dialysis.

Hepatic Impairment: Larger loading dose may be indicated; reduce maintenance doses by 50% and monitor serum levels closely.

Administration Administer around-the-clock to promote less variation in peak and trough serum levels

Oral: Do not crush, chew, or break sustained release dosage forms.

Parenteral: When injecting I.M., aspirate carefully to avoid injection into a vessel; maximum I.V. infusion rate: 10 mg/minute

Monitoring Parameters EKG, apical pulse, heart rate, serum concentrations; monitor for syncope initially, diarrhea, periodic CBC, renal and liver function tests

Reference Range Therapeutic: 2-5 mcg/mL (SI: 6.2-15.4 µmol/L). Patient-dependent therapeutic response occurs at levels of 3-6 mcg/mL (SI: 9.2-18.5 µmol/L). Optimal therapeutic serum concentration is method dependent: >6 mcg/mL (SI: >18 µmol/L).

Patient Information Take exactly as directed, around-the-clock; do not take additional doses or discontinue without consulting prescriber. Do not crush, chew, or break sustained release dosage forms. Do not take with grapefruit juice. You will need (Continued)

Quinidine *(Continued)*

regular cardiac checkups and blood tests while taking this medication. You may experience dizziness, drowsiness, or visual changes (use caution when driving or engaging in tasks requiring alertness until response to drug is known); abnormal taste, nausea or vomiting, or loss of appetite (small frequent meals, frequent mouth care, chewing gum, or sucking lozenges may help); headaches (prescriber may recommend mild analgesic); or diarrhea (yogurt or boiled milk may help - if persistent consult prescriber). Report chest pain, palpitation, or erratic heartbeat; difficulty breathing or wheezing; CNS changes (confusion, delirium, fever, consistent dizziness); skin rash; sense of fullness or ringing in ears; or changes in vision.

Additional Information Sulfate form is the standard dosage preparation

Special Geriatric Considerations Clearance may be decreased with a resultant increased half-life. Must individualize dose. Bioavailability and half-life are increased in the elderly due to decreases in both renal and hepatic function with age.

Dosage Forms Excipient information presented when available (limited, particularly for generics); consult specific product labeling.

Injection, solution, as gluconate: 80 mg/mL (10 mL) [equivalent to quinidine base 50 mg/mL]

Tablet, as sulfate: 200 mg, 300 mg

Tablet, extended release, as gluconate: 324 mg [equivalent to quinidine base 202 mg]

Tablet, extended release, as sulfate: 300 mg [equivalent to quinidine base 249 mg]

Selected References

Fenster PE and Nolan PE, "Antiarrhythmic Drugs," *Geriatric Pharmacology*, Bressler R and Katz MD, eds, New York, NY: McGraw-Hill, 1993, 6:105-49.

♦ **Quinidine Gluconate** *see* Quinidine *on page 1363*

♦ **Quinidine Polygalacturonate** *see* Quinidine *on page 1363*

♦ **Quinidine Sulfate** *see* Quinidine *on page 1363*

Quinine *(KWYE nine)*

Medication Safety Issues

Sound-alike/look-alike issues:

Quinine may be confused with quinidine

U.S. Brand Names Qualaquin™

Canadian Brand Names Apo-Quinine®; Novo-Quinine; Quinine-Odan™

Index Terms Quinine Sulfate

Generic Available No

Pharmacologic Category Antimalarial Agent

Use In conjunction with other antimalarial agents, treatment of uncomplicated chloroquine-resistant *P. falciparum* malaria

Unlabeled/Investigational Use Treatment of *Babesia microti* infection in conjunction with clindamycin

Note: Prevention/treatment of nocturnal leg cramps (unapproved) removed following FDA-issued warning regarding severe adverse events (eg, cardiac arrhythmias, thrombocytopenia, and severe hypersensitivity reactions) and potentially serious drug interactions associated with quinine; use not justified in this condition.

Contraindications Hypersensitivity to quinine or any component of the formulation; tinnitus, optic neuritis, G6PD deficiency; history of black water fever; thrombocytopenia with quinine or quinidine

Warnings/Precautions Use caution with medications or clinical conditions which may prolong the QT interval or cause cardiac arrhythmias. Use may cause significant hypoglycemia. Use caution with atrial fibrillation or flutter, renal or hepatic impairment. Quinine interacts with many medications due to its hepatic metabolism; use caution with other medications metabolized via the CYP3A4 isoenzyme system. Severe hypersensitivity reactions (eg, Stevens-Johnson syndrome, anaphylactic shock) have occurred; discontinue following any signs of sensitivity. Other events, including thrombocytopenia and hemolytic uremic syndrome, may also be attributed to hypersensitivity reactions. Because of the potential for severe and/or life-threatening side effects, as well as the absence of clinical effectiveness, quinine is no longer recommended for the treatment of nocturnal leg cramps.

Adverse Reactions (Reflective of adult population; not specific for elderly)

Frequency not defined.

Cardiovascular: Atrial fibrillation, atrioventricular block, bradycardia, cardiac arrest, chest pain, hypotension, irregular rhythm, nodal escape beats, palpitation, postural hypotension, QT prolongation, syncope, tachycardia, torsade de pointes, unifocal premature ventricular contractions, U waves, vasodilation, ventricular fibrillation, ventricular tachycardia

Central nervous system: Aphasia, ataxia, chills, coma, confusion, disorientation, dizziness, dystonic reaction, fever, flushing, headache, mental status altered, restlessness, seizure, suicide, vertigo

Dermatologic: Acral necrosis, allergic contact dermatitis, bullous dermatitis, bruising, cutaneous rash (urticaria, papular, scarlatinal), cutaneous vasculitis, diaphoresis, exfoliative dermatitis, erythema multiforme, petechiae, photosensitivity, pruritus, Stevens-Johnson syndrome, toxic epidermal necrolysis

Endocrine & metabolic: Hypoglycemia

Gastrointestinal: Abdominal pain, anorexia, diarrhea, esophagitis, gastric irritation, nausea, vomiting

Hematologic: Agranulocytosis, aplastic anemia, coagulopathy, disseminated intravascular coagulation, hemolytic anemia, hemolytic uremic syndrome, hemorrhage, hypoprothrombinemia, leukopenia, neutropenia, pancytopenia, thrombocytopenia, thrombotic thrombocytopenic purpura

Hepatic: Granulomatous hepatitis, hepatitis, jaundice, liver function test abnormalities

Neuromuscular & skeletal: Myalgia, tremor, weakness

Ocular: Blindness, blurred vision (with or without scotomata), color vision disturbance, diminished visual fields, diplopia, night blindness, optic neuritis, photophobia, pupillary dilation, vision loss (sudden)

Otic: Deafness, hearing impaired, tinnitus

Respiratory: Asthma, dyspnea, pulmonary edema

Renal: Acute interstitial nephritis, hemoglobinuria, renal failure, renal impairment

Miscellaneous: Black water fever, hypersensitivity syndrome, lupus anticoagulant, lupus-like syndrome

Overdosage/Toxicology Symptoms of mild toxicity include nausea, vomiting, and cinchonism. Severe intoxication may cause ataxia, obtundation, convulsions, coma, and respiratory arrest. With massive intoxication quinidine-like cardiotoxicity (hypotension, QRS and QT interval prolongation, AV block, and ventricular arrhythmias) may be fatal. Retinal toxicity occurs 9-10 hours after ingestion (blurred vision, impaired color perception, constriction of visual fields, blindness). Other toxic effects include hypokalemia, hypoglycemia, and hemolysis. Treatment includes symptomatic therapy with conventional agents (anticonvulsants, fluids, positioning, vasoconstrictors, antiarrhythmias). **Note:** Avoid type 1a and 1c antiarrhythmic drugs. Treat cardiotoxicity with sodium bicarbonate. Dialysis and hemoperfusion procedures are ineffective in enhancing elimination. Activated charcoal may enhance elimination if administered repeatedly (every 4 hours) and within a reasonable period of time after quinine ingestion (≤4 hours).

Drug Interactions Substrate of CYP1A2 (minor), 2C19 (minor), 3A4 (major); **Inhibits** CYP2C8 (moderate), 2C9 (moderate), 2D6 (strong), 3A4 (weak)

Antacids: Products containing aluminum or magnesium may decrease absorption of quinine; avoid concurrent administration.

Cardiac glycosides (digoxin): Quinine may increase the serum concentration of cardiac glycosides.

CYP2C8 substrates: Quinine may increase the levels/effects of CYP2C8 substrates. Example substrates include amiodarone, paclitaxel, pioglitazone, repaglinide, and rosiglitazone.

CYP2C9 substrates: Quinine may increase the levels/effects of CYP2C9 substrates. Example substrates include bosentan, dapsone, fluoxetine, glimepiride, glipizide, losartan, montelukast, nateglinide, paclitaxel, phenytoin, warfarin, and zafirlukast.

CYP2D6 substrates: Quinine may increase the levels/effects of CYP2D6 substrates. Example substrates include amphetamines, selected beta-blockers, dextromethorphan, fluoxetine, lidocaine, mirtazapine, nefazodone, paroxetine, risperidone, ritonavir, thioridazine, tricyclic antidepressants, and venlafaxine.

CYP2D6 prodrug substrates: Quinine may decrease the levels/effects of CYP2D6 prodrug substrates. Example prodrug substrates include codeine, hydrocodone, oxycodone, and tramadol.

CYP3A4 inducers: CYP3A4 inducers may decrease the levels/effects of quinine. Example inducers include aminoglutethimide, carbamazepine, nafcillin, nevirapine, phenobarbital, phenytoin, and rifamycins.

Phenothiazines: Quinine may increase the serum concentration of phenothiazine antipsychotic agents.

QT$_c$-prolonging agents (eg, amiodarone, amitriptyline, bepridil, disopyramide, erythromycin, haloperidol, imipramine, pimozide, procainamide, sotalol, thioridazine): Effects may be additive; use with caution.

Urinary alkalinizers (sodium bicarbonate, acetazolamide): May increase quinine blood levels.

Ethanol/Nutrition/Herb Interactions Herb/Nutraceutical: St John's wort may decrease quinine levels. Black cohosh, California poppy, coleus, golden seal, hawthorn, mistletoe, periwinkle, and shepherd's purse may cause excessive decreases in blood pressure.

Stability Store at 25°C to 30°C (77°F to 86°F); do not refrigerate or freeze.

(Continued)

Quinine *(Continued)*

Mechanism of Action Depresses oxygen uptake and carbohydrate metabolism; intercalates into DNA, disrupting the parasite's replication and transcription; cardiovascular effects similar to quinidine

Pharmacokinetics

Absorption: Readily, mainly from upper small intestine

Distribution: 2.5-7.1 L/kg; varies with severity of infection

Intraerythrocytic levels are ~30% to 50% of the plasma concentration; distributes poorly to the CSF (~2% to 7% of plasma concentration)

Protein binding: 69% to 92% in healthy subjects; 78% to 95% with malaria

Metabolism: Primarily hepatic via CYP450 enzymes, including CYP3A4 and 2C19; forms metabolites

Bioavailability: 76% to 88% in healthy subjects; increased with malaria

Half-life elimination: Healthy adults: 10-13 hours

Time to peak, serum: Adults: 1-3 hours in healthy subjects; 1.2-11 hours with malaria

Excretion: Urine (<20% as unchanged drug)

Dosage

Geriatrics & Adults:

Treatment of chloroquine-resistant malaria: 648 mg every 8 hours for 7 days with tetracycline, doxycycline, or clindamycin

Note: Actual duration of treatment for malaria may be dependent upon the geographic region or pathogen.

Babesiosis (unlabeled use): 650 mg every 8 hours for 7 days with clindamycin

Renal Impairment:

Cl_{cr} 10-50 mL/minute: Administer every 8-12 hours

Cl_{cr} <10 mL/minute: Administer every 24 hours

Severe chronic renal failure not on dialysis: Initial dose: 648 mg followed by 324 mg every 12 hours

Dialysis: Administer dose after dialysis

Not removed by hemo- or peritoneal dialysis; dose as for Cl_{cr} <10 mL/minute. Continuous arteriovenous or hemodialysis: Dose as for Cl_{cr} 10-50 mL/minute.

Hepatic Impairment:

Child-Pugh Class B: No dosing adjustment required; monitor closely

Child-Pugh Class C: Data not available

Administration Avoid use of aluminum- or magnesium-containing antacids because of drug absorption problems. Swallow dose whole to avoid bitter taste. May be administered with food.

Reference Range Toxic: >10 mcg/mL

Test Interactions Positive Coombs' [direct]; false elevation of urinary steroids (when assayed by Zimmerman method) and catecholamines

Patient Information Avoid use of aluminum-containing antacids because of drug absorption problems; swallow dose whole to avoid bitter taste; take with food; notify physician if diarrhea, nausea, and other GI complaints or blurred vision, vertigo, confusion or dizziness occurs

Additional Information Parenteral dosage form may be obtained from Centers for Disease Control if needed

Special Geriatric Considerations Quinine's efficacy as a treatment for nocturnal leg cramps is not well supported in the medical and pharmacy literature. The FDA's decision to remove all quinine products (except one that is indicated for the treatment of malaria) indicates that quinine's benefits for nocturnal leg cramps do not out weigh its risks.

Dosage Forms Excipient information presented when available (limited, particularly for generics); consult specific product labeling. [DSC] = Discontinued product

Capsule, as sulfate: 325 mg [DSC]

Qualaquin™: 324 mg

Tablet, as sulfate: 260 mg [DSC]

♦ **Quinine Sulfate** *see* Quinine *on page 1366*

Quinupristin and Dalfopristin *(kwi NYOO pris tin & dal FOE pris tin)*

Related Information

Antimicrobial Activity Against Selected Organisms *on page 1728*

U.S. Brand Names Synercid®

Canadian Brand Names Synercid®

Index Terms Pristinamycin; RP-59500

Generic Available No

Pharmacologic Category Antibiotic, Streptogramin

Use Treatment of serious or life-threatening infections associated with vancomycin-resistant *Enterococcus faecium* bacteremia; treatment of complicated skin and skin structure infections caused by methicillin-susceptible *Staphylococcus aureus* or *Streptococcus pyogenes*

Contraindications Hypersensitivity to quinupristin, dalfopristin, pristinamycin, or virginiamycin, or any component of the formulation

Warnings/Precautions Use with caution in patients with hepatic or renal dysfunction. May cause pain and phlebitis when infused through a peripheral line (not relieved by hydrocortisone or diphenhydramine). Prolonged use may result in fungal or bacterial superinfection, including *C. difficile*-associated diarrhea and pseudomembranous colitis. May cause arthralgias, myalgias, and hyperbilirubinemia. May inhibit the metabolism of many drugs metabolized by CYP3A4. Concurrent therapy with cisapride (which may prolong QT_c interval and lead to arrhythmias) should be avoided.

Adverse Reactions (Reflective of adult population; not specific for elderly)
>10%:
  Hepatic: Hyperbilirubinemia (3% to 35%)
  Local: Inflammation at infusion site (38% to 42%), local pain (40% to 44%), local edema (17% to 18%), infusion site reaction (12% to 13%)
  Neuromuscular & skeletal: Arthralgia (up to 47%), myalgia (up to 47%)
1% to 10%:
  Central nervous system: Pain (2% to 3%), headache (2%)
  Dermatologic: Pruritus (2%), rash (3%)
  Endocrine & metabolic: Hyperglycemia (1%)
  Gastrointestinal: Nausea (3% to 5%), diarrhea (3%), vomiting (3% to 4%)
  Hematologic: Anemia (3%)
  Hepatic: GGT increased (2%), LDH increased (3%)
  Local: Thrombophlebitis (2%)
  Neuromuscular & skeletal: CPK increased (2%)

Overdosage/Toxicology Symptoms may include dyspnea, emesis, tremors, and ataxia. Treatment is supportive. Not removed by hemodialysis or peritoneal dialysis.

Drug Interactions Quinupristin: **Inhibits** CYP3A4 (weak)
  Cisapride: The manufacturer states that quinupristin/dalfopristin may increase cisapride concentrations and cause QT_c prolongation, and recommends to avoid concurrent use with cisapride.
  Cyclosporine: Quinupristin/dalfopristin may increase cyclosporine concentrations; monitor.

Stability Store unopened vials under refrigeration (2°C to 8°C/36°F to 46°F). Reconstitute single dose vial with 5 mL of 5% dextrose in water or sterile water for injection. Swirl gently to dissolve; do not shake (to limit foam formation). The reconstituted solution should be diluted within 30 minutes. Stability of the diluted solution prior to the infusion is established as 5 hours at room temperature or 54 hours if refrigerated at 2°C to 8°C. Reconstituted solution should be added to at least 250 mL of 5% dextrose in water for peripheral administration (increase to 500 mL or 750 mL if necessary to limit venous irritation). An infusion volume of 100 mL may be used for central line infusions. Do not freeze solution.

Mechanism of Action Quinupristin/dalfopristin inhibits bacterial protein synthesis by binding to different sites on the 50S bacterial ribosomal subunit thereby inhibiting protein synthesis

Pharmacokinetics
  Distribution: Quinupristin: 0.45 L/kg; dalfopristin: 0.24 L/kg
  Protein binding: Moderate
  Metabolism: To active metabolites via nonenzymatic reactions
  Half-life: Quinupristin: 0.85 hour, dalfopristin: 0.7 hour (mean elimination half-lives, including metabolites: 3 and 1 hours, respectively), no change in older adults
  Elimination: Primarily by biliary excretion and fecal elimination (parent drug and metabolites 75% to 77%). Renal elimination accounts for 15% to 19% of a dose.

Dosage
  Geriatrics & Adults:
    Vancomycin-resistant *Enterococcus faecium*: I.V.: 7.5 mg/kg every 8 hours
    Complicated skin and skin structure infection: I.V.: 7.5 mg/kg every 12 hours
  Renal Impairment: No adjustment is necessary in renal failure, hemodialysis, or peritoneal dialysis.
  Hepatic Impairment: Pharmacokinetic data suggest dosage adjustment may be necessary; however, specific recommendations have not been proposed.

Administration Line should be flushed with 5% dextrose in water prior to and following administration. Incompatible with saline. Infusion should be completed over 60 minutes (toxicity may be increased with shorter infusion). Compatible (Y-site injection) with aztreonam, ciprofloxacin, haloperidol, metoclopramide or potassium chloride when admixed in 5% dextrose in water. Also compatible (Y-site injection) with fluconazole (used as undiluted solution). If severe venous irritation occurs following peripheral administration of quinupristin/dalfopristin diluted in 250 mL 5% dextrose in water, consideration should be given to increasing the infusion volume to 500 mL or 750 mL,
(Continued)

Quinupristin and Dalfopristin *(Continued)*

changing the infusion site, or infusing by a peripherally inserted central catheter (PICC) or a central venous catheter.

Monitoring Parameters Signs of infection, mental status

Special Geriatric Considerations No pharmacokinetic changes in the elderly in one study. No dose adjustment necessary.

Dosage Forms Excipient information presented when available (limited, particularly for generics); consult specific product labeling.

Injection, powder for reconstitution:

500 mg: Quinupristin 150 mg and dalfopristin 350 mg

600 mg: Quinupristin 180 mg and dalfopristin 420 mg

Selected References

Bryson HM and Spencer CM, "Quinupristin/Dalfopristin," *Drugs,* 1996, 52(3):406-15.

Chant C and Rybak MH, "Quinupristin/Dalfopristin (RP 59500): A New Streptogramin Antibiotic," *Ann Pharmacother,* 1995, 29(10):1022-7.

Cupo-Abbott J, Holton P, Rho JP, "Focus on Quinupristin/Dalfopristin: An Investigational Streptogramin Antibiotic for the Treatment of Multiresistant Gram-Positive Infections," *Formulary,* 33:841-57.

Griswold MW, Lomaestro BM, and Briceland LL, "Quinupristin-Dalfopristin (RP 59500): An Injectable Streptogramin Combination," *Am J Health Syst Pharm,* 1996, 53(17):2045-53.

♦ **Quixin**™ *see* Levofloxacin *on page 896*

♦ **QVAR**® *see* Beclomethasone *on page 153*

♦ **RabAvert**® *see* Rabies Virus Vaccine *on page 1372*

Rabeprazole *(ra BEP ra zole)*

Related Information

Helicobacter pylori Treatment *on page 1759*

Medication Safety Issues

Sound-alike/look-alike issues:

AcipHex® may be confused with Acephen®, Accupril®, Aricept®

Rabeprazole may be confused with aripiprazole

U.S. Brand Names AcipHex®

Canadian Brand Names AcipHex®; Pariet®

Index Terms Pariprazole

Generic Available No

Pharmacologic Category Proton Pump Inhibitor; Substituted Benzimidazole

Use Short-term (4-8 weeks) treatment and maintenance of erosive or ulcerative gastroesophageal reflux disease (GERD), symptomatic GERD; short-term (up to 4 weeks) treatment of duodenal ulcers; long-term treatment of pathological hypersecretory conditions, including Zollinger-Ellison syndrome; *H. pylori* eradication (in combination with amoxicillin and clarithromycin)

Unlabeled/Investigational Use Maintenance of duodenal ulcer

Contraindications Hypersensitivity to rabeprazole, substituted benzimidazoles, or any component of the formulation

Warnings/Precautions Use caution in severe hepatic impairment; relief of symptoms with rabeprazole does not preclude the presence of a gastric malignancy

Adverse Reactions (Reflective of adult population; not specific for elderly)

1% to 10%: Central nervous system: Headache

Overdosage/Toxicology There has been no experience with large overdoses. Seven reports of accidental overdosage have been reported. The maximum reported overdose was 80 mg. There were no clinical signs or symptoms associated with any reported overdose. Patients with Zollinger-Ellison syndrome have been treated with up to 120 mg/day. No specific antidote is known. A single oral dose of 2000 mg/kg was not lethal to dogs.

Drug Interactions Substrate (major) of CYP2C19, 3A4; **Inhibits** CYP2C8 (moderate), 2C19 (moderate), 2DC (weak), 3A4 (weak)

CYP2C8 Substrates: Rabeprazole may increase the levels/effects of CYP2C8 substrates. Example substrates include amiodarone, paclitaxel, pioglitazone, repaglinide, and rosiglitazone.

CYP2C19 inducers: May decrease the levels/effects of rabeprazole. Example inducers include aminoglutethimide, carbamazepine, phenytoin, and rifampin.

CYP2C19 substrates: Rabeprazole may increase the levels/effects of CYP2C19 substrates. Example substrates include citalopram, diazepam, methsuximide, phenytoin, propranolol, and sertraline.

CYP3A4 inducers: CYP3A4 inducers may decrease the levels/effects of rabeprazole. Example inducers include aminoglutethimide, carbamazepine, nafcillin, nevirapine, phenobarbital, phenytoin, and rifamycins.

Iron Salts (oral): Rabeprazole may decrease the absorption of oral iron salts.

Itraconazole and ketoconazole: Proton pump inhibitors may decrease the absorption of itraconazole and ketoconazole; concurrent use is contraindicated.

Protease inhibitors: Proton pump inhibitors may decrease absorption of some protease inhibitors (atazanavir and indinavir).

Ethanol/Nutrition/Herb Interactions
Ethanol: Avoid ethanol (may cause gastric mucosal irritation).
Food: High-fat meals may delay absorption, but C_{max} and AUC are not altered.

Stability Rapidly degraded in acid conditions.

Mechanism of Action Potent proton pump inhibitor; suppresses gastric acid secretion by inhibiting the parietal cell H+/K+ ATP pump

Pharmacodynamics
Onset of action: 1 hour
Duration: 24 hours

Pharmacokinetics
Absorption: Oral: Well absorbed within 1 hour
Distribution: 96.3%
Protein binding, serum: 94.8% to 97.5%
Metabolism: Hepatic; inactive metabolites
Bioavailability: Oral: 52%
Half-life (dose dependent): 0.85-2 hours
Time to peak, plasma: 2-5 hours
Elimination: Urine (90% primarily as thioether carboxylic acid); remainder in feces

Dosage
Geriatrics & Adults:
GERD: Oral: 20 mg once daily for 4-8 weeks; maintenance: 20 mg once daily
Duodenal ulcer: Oral: 20 mg/day before breakfast for 4 weeks
Eradication of *H. pylori*: Oral: 20 mg twice daily for 7 days; to be administered with amoxicillin 1000 mg and clarithromycin 500 mg, also given twice daily for 7 days.
Hypersecretory conditions: Oral: 60 mg once daily; dose may need to be adjusted as necessary. Doses as high as 100 mg once daily and 60 mg twice daily have been used.
Renal Impairment: No dosage adjustment required.
Hepatic Impairment:
Mild to moderate: Elimination decreased; no dosage adjustment required.
Severe: Use caution.

Administration May be administered with or without food. Do not crush, split, or chew tablet. May be administered with an antacid.

Monitoring Parameters Symptom relief, mucosal healing

Patient Information Take as directed. Swallow whole, do not crush, split, or chew. Follow recommended diet and activity instructions. Avoid alcohol. You may experience headache (use of mild analgesic may help) or other side effects. Report these to prescriber if they persist.

Special Geriatric Considerations No difference in efficacy or safety was noted in elderly subjects as compared to younger subjects. No dosage adjustment is necessary in the elderly.

Dosage Forms Excipient information presented when available (limited, particularly for generics); consult specific product labeling.
Tablet, delayed release, enteric coated, as sodium: 20 mg

Rabies Immune Globulin (Human)
(RAY beez i MYUN GLOB yoo lin, HYU man)

Related Information
Immunization Recommendations *on page 1787*
U.S. Brand Names HyperRAB™ S/D; Imogam® Rabies-HT
Canadian Brand Names HyperRAB™ S/D; Imogam® Rabies Pasteurized
Index Terms RIG
Generic Available No
Pharmacologic Category Immune Globulin
Use Part of postexposure prophylaxis of persons with rabies exposure who lack a history or pre-exposure or postexposure prophylaxis with rabies vaccine or a recently documented neutralizing antibody response to previous rabies vaccination; although it is preferable to administer RIG with the first dose of vaccine, it can be given up to 8 days after vaccination
Contraindications Hypersensitivity to thimerosal or any component of the formulation
Warnings/Precautions Hypersensitivity and anaphylactic reactions can occur; immediate treatment (including epinephrine 1:1000) should be available. Use with caution in patients with isolated immunoglobulin A deficiency or a history of systemic hypersensitivity to human immunoglobulins. Use with caution in patients with thrombocytopenia or coagulation disorders; I.M. injections may be contraindicated. Product of human plasma; may potentially contain infectious agents which could transmit disease. Screening of donors, as well as testing and/or inactivation or removal of certain
(Continued)

Rabies Immune Globulin (Human) *(Continued)*

viruses, reduces the risk. Infections thought to be transmitted by this product should be reported to the manufacturer. Not for intravenous administration.

Adverse Reactions (Reflective of adult population; not specific for elderly)
1% to 10%:
Central nervous system: Fever (mild)
Local: Soreness at injection site

Drug Interactions Decreased effect: Live virus vaccines (eg, MMR, rabies) may have delayed or diminished antibody response with immune globulin administration; should not be administered within 3 months unless antibody titers dictate as appropriate

Stability Refrigerate

Mechanism of Action Rabies immune globulin is a solution of globulins dried from the plasma or serum of selected adult human donors who have been immunized with rabies vaccine and have developed high titers of rabies antibody. It generally contains 10% to 18% of protein of which not less than 80% is monomeric immunoglobulin G.

Dosage
Geriatrics & Adults: Postexposure prophylaxis: Local wound infiltration: 20 units/kg in a single dose. RIG should always be administered as part of rabies vaccine (HDCV) regimen (as soon as possible after the first dose of vaccine, up to 8 days). If anatomically feasible, the full rabies immune globulin dose should be infiltrated around and into the wound(s); remaining volume should be administered I.M. at a site distant from the vaccine administration site. If rabies vaccine was initiated without rabies immune globulin, rabies immune globulin may be administered through the seventh day after the first vaccine dose.

Note: Persons known to have an adequate titer or who have been completely immunized with rabies vaccine should not receive RIG, only booster doses of HDCV

Administration Intramuscular injection only; injection should be made into the gluteal muscle

Monitoring Parameters Monitor for adverse effects

Special Geriatric Considerations No special considerations are needed for initiating therapy. No specific data relevant to the elderly to date.

Dosage Forms Excipient information presented when available (limited, particularly for generics); consult specific product labeling.
Injection, solution [preservative free]:
HyperRAB™ S/D: 150 int. units/mL (2 mL, 10 mL) [solvent/detergent treated]
Imogam® Rabies-HT: 150 int. units/mL (2 mL, 10 mL) [heat treated]

Rabies Virus Vaccine (RAY beez VYE rus vak SEEN)

Related Information
Immunization Recommendations *on page 1787*

U.S. Brand Names Imovax® Rabies; RabAvert®

Canadian Brand Names Imovax® Rabies; RabAvert®

Index Terms HDCV; Human Diploid Cell Cultures Rabies Vaccine; PCEC; Purified Chick Embryo Cell

Generic Available No

Pharmacologic Category Vaccine

Use Pre-exposure immunization: Vaccinate persons with greater than usual risk due occupation or avocation including veterinarians, rangers, animal handlers, certain laboratory workers, and persons living in or visiting countries for longer than 1 month where rabies is a constant threat.

Postexposure prophylaxis: If a bite from a carrier animal is unprovoked, if it is not captured and rabies is present in that species and area, administer rabies immune globulin (RIG) and the vaccine as indicated

The Food and Drug Administration has not approved the I.D. use of rabies vaccine for postexposure prophylaxis (only I.M.). The type of and schedule for postexposure prophylaxis depends upon the previous rabies vaccination status or the result of a previous or current serologic test for rabies antibody.

Contraindications Hypersensitivity to neomycin, gentamicin, or amphotericin B or any component of the formulation; developing febrile illness (during pre-exposure therapy only); life-threatening allergic reactions to rabies vaccine or any components of the formulation (however, carefully consider a patient's risk of rabies before continuing therapy)

Warnings/Precautions Report serious reactions to the State Health Department or the manufacturer/distributor, an immune complex reaction is possible 2-21 days following booster doses of HDCV; hypersensitivity reactions may be treated with antihistamines or epinephrine, if severe. Immune response may be decreased in immunosuppressed patients. Imovax® Rabies contains albumin and neomycin. RabAvert® contains amphotericin B, bovine gelatin, chicken protein, chlortetracycline, and neomycin. For I. M. administration only.

Adverse Reactions (Reflective of adult population; not specific for elderly)
All serious adverse reactions must be reported to the U.S. Department of Health and Human Services (DHHS) Vaccine Adverse Event Reporting System (VAERS) 1-800-822-7967.
Frequency not defined.
Cardiovascular: Edema
Central nervous system: Dizziness, malaise, encephalomyelitis, transverse myelitis, fever, pain, headache, neuroparalytic reactions
Gastrointestinal: Nausea, abdominal pain
Local: Local discomfort, pain at injection site, itching, erythema, swelling or pain
Neuromuscular & skeletal: Myalgia

Drug Interactions Decreased effect with immunosuppressive agents, corticosteroids, antimalarial drugs (ie, chloroquine); persons on these drugs should receive RIG (3 doses/1 mL each) by the I.M. route

Stability Store under refrigeration at 2°C to 8°C (36°F to 46°F); do not freeze. Protect from light.

Mechanism of Action Rabies vaccine is an inactivated virus vaccine which promotes immunity by inducing an active immune response. The production of specific antibodies requires about 7-10 days to develop. Rabies immune globulin or antirabies serum, equine (ARS) is given in conjunction with rabies vaccine to provide immune protection until an antibody response can occur.

Pharmacodynamics
Onset of effect: I.M.: Rabies antibody appears in the serum within 7-10 days
Peak effect: Within 30-60 days and persists for at least 1 year

Dosage
Geriatrics & Adults:
Pre-exposure prophylaxis: I.M.: 1 mL on days 0, 7, and 21 to 28.
Note: Prolonging the interval between doses does not interfere with immunity achieved after the concluding dose of the basic series.
Postexposure prophylaxis: All postexposure treatment should begin with immediate cleansing of the wound with soap and water
Persons not previously immunized as above: I.M.: 5 doses (1 mL each) on days 0, 3, 7, 14, 28. In addition, patients should receive rabies immune globulin 20 units/kg body weight, half infiltrated at bite site if possible, remainder I.M.)
Persons who have previously received postexposure prophylaxis with rabies vaccine, received a recommended I.M. pre-exposure series of rabies vaccine or have a previously documented rabies antibody titer considered adequate: I.M.: 1 mL of either vaccine only on days 0 and 3; do not administer RIG
Booster (for occupational or other continuing risk): I.M.: 1 mL every 2-5 years or based on antibody titers

Administration HDCV and RVA administered I.M.; administer I.M. injections in the the outer aspect of the thigh in adults.

For patients at risk of hemorrhage following intramuscular injection, the ACIP recommends "it should be administered intramuscularly if, in the opinion of the physician familiar with the patients bleeding risk, the vaccine can be administered with reasonable safety by this route. If the patient receives antihemophilia or other similar therapy, intramuscular vaccination can be scheduled shortly after such therapy is administered. A fine needle (23 gauge or smaller) can be used for the vaccination and firm pressure applied to the site (without rubbing) for at least 2 minutes. The patient should be instructed concerning the risk of hematoma from the injection."

Monitoring Parameters Monitor for local adverse effects

Reference Range Antibody titers ≥115 as determined by rapid fluorescent-focus inhibition test are indicative of adequate response; collect titers on day 28 postexposure

Additional Information Federal law requires that the date of administration, the vaccine manufacturer, lot number of vaccine, and the administering person's name, title, and address be entered into the patient's permanent medical record.

Special Geriatric Considerations No specific data for use in the elderly. Use as recommended in elderly patients for whom this vaccine would be indicated.

Dosage Forms Injection, powder for reconstitution:
Imovax® Rabies: 2.5 int. units [HDCV; grown in human diploid cell culture; contains albumin <100 mg, neomycin <150 mcg]
RabAvert®: 2.5 int. units [PCEC; grown in chicken fibroblasts; contains amphotericin <2 ng, chlortetracycline <20 ng, and neomycin <1 mcg]

Selected References
"A New Rabies Vaccine," Med Lett Drugs Ther, 1998, 40(1029):64-5.
Centers for Disease Control, "Recommendations of the Advisory Committee on Immunization Practices (ACIP): General Recommendations on Immunization," MMWR, 1994, 43(RR-1):23.
Dreesen DW and Hanlon CA, "Current Recommendations for the Prophylaxis and Treatment of Rabies," Drugs, 1998, 56(5):801-9.
(Continued)

Rabies Virus Vaccine *(Continued)*

Strady A, Lang J, Lienard M, et al, "Antibody Persistence Following Pre-exposure Regimens of Cell-Culture Rabies Vaccines: 10-Year Follow-up and Proposal for a New Booster Policy," *J Infect Dis*, 1998, 177(5):1290-5.

♦ **Racepinephrine** *see* Epinephrine *on page 514*
♦ **R-albuterol** *see* Levalbuterol *on page 887*

Raloxifene (ral OKS i feen)

Related Information
Osteoporosis Management *on page 1779*
Medication Safety Issues
Sound-alike/look-alike issues:
Evista® may be confused with Avinza™
U.S. Brand Names Evista®
Canadian Brand Names Evista®
Index Terms Keoxifene Hydrochloride; NSC-706725; Raloxifene Hydrochloride
Generic Available No
Pharmacologic Category Selective Estrogen Receptor Modulator (SERM)
Use Prevention and treatment of osteoporosis in postmenopausal women
Unlabeled/Investigational Use Risk reduction for invasive breast cancer in postmenopausal women at increased risk for breast cancer
Contraindications Hypersensitivity to raloxifene or any component of the formulation; active or history of venous thromboembolic events
Warnings/Precautions Use caution in patients at high risk for venous thromboembolism (deep vein thrombosis, pulmonary embolism); patients with cardiovascular disease; history of cervical/uterine carcinoma; renal/hepatic insufficiency (however, pharmacokinetic data are lacking); concurrent use of estrogens; women with a history of elevated triglycerides in response to treatment with oral estrogens (or estrogen/ progestin). Safety and efficacy in premenopausal women or men have not been established.
Adverse Reactions (Reflective of adult population; not specific for elderly)
Note: Raloxifene has been associated with increased risk of thromboembolism (DVT, PE) and superficial thrombophlebitis; risk is similar to reported risk of HRT
>10%:
Endocrine & metabolic: Hot flashes (10% to 29%)
Neuromuscular & skeletal: Arthralgia (11% to 16%)
Miscellaneous: Flu syndrome (14% to 15%), infection (11% to 15%)
1% to 10%:
Cardiovascular: Peripheral edema (3% to 5%), chest pain (3% to 4%), syncope (2%), varicose vein (2%), venous thromboembolism (1%)
Central nervous system: Headache (9%), depression (6%), insomnia (6%), vertigo (4%), fever (3% to 4%), migraine (2%), hypoesthesia (≤2%)
Dermatologic: Rash (6%)
Endocrine & metabolic: Breast pain (4%)
Gastrointestinal: Nausea (8% to 9%), weight gain (9%), abdominal pain (7%), diarrhea (7%), dyspepsia (6%), vomiting (3% to 5%), flatulence (2% to 3%), gastroenteritis (≤3%)
Genitourinary: Vaginal bleeding (6%), cystitis (3% to 5%), urinary tract infection (4%), vaginitis (4%), leukorrhea (3%), urinary tract disorder (3%), uterine disorder (3%), vaginal hemorrhage (3%), endometrial disorder (≤3%)
Neuromuscular & skeletal: Myalgia (8%), leg cramps (6% to 7%), arthritis (4%), tendon disorder (4%), neuralgia (≤2%)
Ocular: Conjunctivitis (2%)
Respiratory: Bronchitis (10%), rhinitis (10%), sinusitis (8% to 10%), cough (6% to 9%), pharyngitis (5% to 8%), pneumonia (3%), laryngitis (≤2%)
Miscellaneous: Diaphoresis (3%)
Overdosage/Toxicology Incidence of overdose in humans has not been reported. In an 8-week study of postmenopausal women, a dose of raloxifene 600 mg/day was safely tolerated. No mortality was seen after a single oral dose in rats or mice (at 810 times the human dose for rats and 405 times the human dose for mice). There is no specific antidote for raloxifene. Treatment is symptom-directed and supportive.
Drug Interactions
Cholestyramine: May decrease the absorption of raloxifene; separate doses by at least 2 hours.
Levothyroxine: Raloxifene may decrease levothyroxine absorption; separate doses by several hours.
Ethanol/Nutrition/Herb Interactions Ethanol: Avoid ethanol (may increase risk of osteoporosis).
Stability Store between 15°C to 30°C (59°F to 86°F).

Mechanism of Action A selective estrogen receptor modulator, meaning that it affects some of the same receptors that estrogen does, but not all, and in some instances, it antagonizes or blocks estrogen; it acts like estrogen to prevent bone loss and improve lipid profiles (decreases total and LDL-cholesterol but does not raise triglycerides), but it has the potential to block some estrogen effects such as those that lead to breast cancer and uterine cancer. Raloxifene decreases bone resorption, increasing bone mineral density and decreasing fracture incidence.

Pharmacokinetics
Absorption: ~60%
Distribution: V_d: 2348 L/kg
Protein binding: >95% to albumin and alpha$_1$-acid glycoprotein
Metabolism: Hepatic, extensive first-pass effect; metabolized to glucuronide conjugates
Half-life: 28-32.5 hours
Elimination: Feces; <0.2% as unchanged drug in the urine
Note: No age-related differences in raloxifene pharmacokinetics have been identified

Dosage
Geriatrics & Adults:
Osteoporosis: Female: Oral: 60 mg/day
Invasive breast cancer risk reduction (investigational use): Female: Oral: 60 mg/day for 5 years
Hepatic Impairment: Child-Pugh class A: Plasma concentrations were higher and correlated with total bilirubin. Safety and efficacy in hepatic insufficiency have not been established

Administration May be administered any time of the day without regard to meals.

Monitoring Parameters INR if on warfarin, lipid profile, bone mineral density

Patient Information Take without regard to meals; will not reduce hot flashes or flushes associated with estrogen deficiency; supplement calcium and vitamin D if indicated

Additional Information The decrease in estrogen-related adverse effects with the selective estrogen-receptor modulators in general and raloxifene in particular should improve compliance and decrease the incidence of cardiovascular events and fractures while not increasing breast cancer

Special Geriatric Considerations No need to cycle with progesterone.

Dosage Forms Excipient information presented when available (limited, particularly for generics); consult specific product labeling.
Tablet, as hydrochloride:
Evista®: 60 mg

Selected References
Chlebowski RT, Col N, Winer EP, et al, "American Society of Clinical Oncology Technology Assessment of Pharmacologic Interventions for Breast Cancer Risk Reduction Including Tamoxifen, Raloxifene, and Aromatase Inhibition," *J Clin Oncol*, 2002, 20(15):3328-43.

Cummings SR, Eckert S, Krueger KA, et al, "The Effect of Raloxifene on Risk of Breast Cancer in Postmenopausal Women: Results from the MORE Randomized Trial," *JAMA*, 1999, 281(23) 2189-97.

Delmas PD, Bjarnason NH, Mitlak BH, et al, "Effects of Raloxifene on Bone Mineral Density, Serum Cholesterol Concentrations, and Uterine Endometrium in Postmenopausal Women," *N Engl J Med*, 1997, 337(23):1641-7.

Martino S, Cauley JA, Barrett-Connor E, et al, "Continuing Outcomes Relevant to Evista: Breast Cancer Incident in Postmenopausal Women in a Randomized Trial of Raloxifene," *J Natl Cancer Inst*, 2004, 96(23):1751-61.

♦ **Raloxifene Hydrochloride** *see* Raloxifene *on page 1374*

Ramelteon (ra MEL tee on)

Medication Safety Issues
Sound-alike/look-alike issues:
Rozerem™ may be confused with Razadyne™

U.S. Brand Names Rozerem™

Index Terms TAK-375

Generic Available No

Pharmacologic Category Hypnotic, Nonbenzodiazepine

Use Treatment of insomnia characterized by difficulty with sleep onset

Contraindications Hypersensitivity to ramelteon or any component of the formulation; severe hepatic impairment; concurrent use with fluvoxamine

Warnings/Precautions
Symptomatic treatment of insomnia should be initiated only after careful evaluation of potential causes of sleep disturbance. Failure of sleep disturbance to resolve after a reasonable period of treatment may indicate psychiatric and/or medical illness. Because of the rapid onset of action, administer immediately prior to bedtime or after the patient has gone to bed and is having difficulty falling asleep. Hypnotics/sedatives have been associated with abnormal thinking and behavior changes including
(Continued)

Ramelteon (Continued)

decreased inhibition, aggression, bizarre behavior, agitation, hallucinations, and depersonalization. These changes may occur unpredictably and may indicate previously unrecognized psychiatric disorders; evaluate appropriately. Postmarketing studies have indicated that the use of hypnotic/sedative agents for sleep has been associated with hypersensitivity reactions including anaphylaxis as well as angioedema. An increased risk for hazardous sleep-related activities such as sleep-driving; cooking and eating food, and making phone calls while asleep have also been noted. Use caution with pre-existing depression or other psychiatric conditions. Caution when using with other CNS depressants; avoid engaging in hazardous activities or activities requiring mental alertness. Not recommended for use in patients with severe sleep apnea or COPD. Use caution with moderate hepatic impairment. May cause disturbances of hormonal regulation. Use caution when administered concomitantly with strong CYP1A2 inhibitors.

Adverse Reactions (Reflective of adult population; not specific for elderly)
1% to 10%:

Central nervous system: Headache (7%, same as placebo), somnolence (5%), dizziness (5%), fatigue (4%), insomnia worsened (3%), depression (2%)

Endocrine & metabolic: Serum cortisol decreased (1%)

Gastrointestinal: Nausea (3%), diarrhea (2%, same as placebo), taste perversion (2%)

Neuromuscular & skeletal: Myalgia (2%), arthralgia (2%)

Respiratory: Upper respiratory infection (3%; 2 % with placebo)

Miscellaneous: Influenza (1%)

Overdosage/Toxicology Single doses of up to 160 mg have been administered, with no safety or tolerability concerns noted. Treatment should be symptom-directed and supportive. Hemodialysis is not effective in removing ramelteon.

Drug Interactions

Substrate of CYP1A2 (major), CYP3A4 (minor), CYP2C family (minor)

CNS depressants: Sedative effects and/or respiratory depression may be additive with CNS depressants; includes ethanol, barbiturates, opioid analgesics, and other sedative agents; monitor for increased effect.

CYP1A2 Inhibitors may increase the levels/effects of ramelteon. Example inhibitors include ciprofloxacin, fluvoxamine, ketoconazole, norfloxacin, ofloxacin, and rofecoxib.

Fluconazole: May increase the levels of ramelteon leading to increased toxicity. Monitor for excessive somnolence.

Fluvoxamine: May markedly increase the levels of ramelteon leading to increased toxicity. Concomitant use not recommended.

Ketoconazole: May increase the levels of ramelteon leading to increased toxicity. Monitor for excessive somnolence.

Rifampin: May decrease levels/effects of ramelteon; monitor.

Ethanol/Nutrition/Herb Interactions

Ethanol: Avoid ethanol (may increase CNS depression).

Food: Taking with high-fat meal delays T_{max} and increases AUC (~31%); do not take with high-fat meal.

Stability Store at 15°C to 30°C (59°F to 86°F).

Mechanism of Action Potent, selective agonist of melatonin receptors MT_1 and MT_2 (with little affinity for MT_3) within the suprachiasmic nucleus of the hypothalamus, an area responsible for determination of circadian rhythms and synchronization of the sleep-wake cycle. Agonism of MT_1 is thought to preferentially induce sleepiness, while MT_2 receptor activation preferentially influences regulation of circadian rhythms. Ramelteon is eightfold more selective for MT_1 than MT_2 and exhibits nearly sixfold higher affinity for MT_1 than melatonin, presumably allowing for enhanced effects on sleep induction.

Pharmacokinetics

Onset of action: 30 minutes

Absorption: Rapid

Distribution: 74 L

Protein binding: 82%

Metabolism: Extensive first-pass effect; oxidative metabolism primarily through CYP1A2 and to a lesser extent through CYP2C and CYP3A4; forms active metabolite (M-II)

Bioavailability: Absolute: 1.8%

Half-life elimination: Ramelteon: 1-2.6 hours; M-II: 2-5 hours

Time to peak, plasma: Median: 0.5-1.5 hours

Excretion: Primarily as metabolites: Urine (84%); feces (4%)

Dosage
Geriatrics & Adults: Insomnia: Oral: One 8 mg tablet within 30 minutes of bedtime
Renal Impairment: No dosage adjustment required
Hepatic Impairment: No adjustment required for mild-to-moderate impairment. Avoid use with severe impairment.

Monitoring Parameters Mental status

Patient Information
Take within 30 minutes of going to bed. Avoid engaging in hazardous activities after taking. Do not take after a high fat meal.

Special Geriatric Considerations Although the C_{max} and AUC of ramelteon were increased in elderly patients, in clinical trials there were no significant differences in safety or efficacy between elderly and younger adult subjects.

Dosage Forms Excipient information presented when available (limited, particularly for generics); consult specific product labeling.
Tablet: 8 mg

Selected References
Kato K, Hirai K, Nishiyama K, et al, "Neurochemical Properties of Ramelteon (TAK-375), A Selective MT1/MT2 Receptor Agonist," *Neuropharmacology.* 2005, 48(2):301-10.
Nguyen NN, Uy SS, and Song JC, "Ramelteon: A Novel Melatonin Receptor Agonist for the Treatment of Insomnia," *Formulary,* 2005, 40:146-55.

Ramipril (RA mi pril)

Related Information
Angiotensin Agents *on page 1737*

Medication Safety Issues
Sound-alike/look-alike issues:
Ramipril may be confused with enalapril, Monopril®
Altace® may be confused with alteplase, Amaryl®, Amerge®, Artane®

International issues:
Altace® may be confused with Altace® HCT which is a brand name for ramipril/hydrochlorothiazide combination product in Canada

U.S. Brand Names Altace®

Canadian Brand Names Altace®; Apo-Ramipril®

Generic Available No

Pharmacologic Category Angiotensin-Converting Enzyme (ACE) Inhibitor

Use Treatment of hypertension (alone or in combination with thiazide diuretics), congestive heart failure, left ventricular dysfunction after myocardial infarction; reduction of risk of heart attack, stroke, and death in patients at increased risk for these disease entities

Contraindications Hypersensitivity to ramipril or any component of the formulation; prior hypersensitivity (including angioedema) to ACE inhibitors; bilateral renal artery stenosis; primary hyperaldosteronism

Warnings/Precautions Anaphylactic or anaphylactoid reactions can occur. Use with caution and modify dosage in patients with renal impairment (especially renal artery stenosis), severe CHF. Severe hypotension may occur in the elderly and patients who are sodium and/or volume depleted, initiate lower doses and monitor closely when starting therapy in these patients. Angioedema can occur at any time during treatment (especially following first dose). It may involve head and neck (potentially affecting the airway) or the intestine (presenting with abdominal pain). Prolonged monitoring may be required especially if tongue, glottis, or larynx are involved as they are associated with airway obstruction. Those with a history of airway surgery in this situation have a higher risk. Careful blood pressure monitoring with first dose (hypotension can occur especially in volume-depleted patients). Use with caution in hypovolemia; collagen vascular diseases; valvular stenosis (particularly aortic stenosis); hyperkalemia; or before, during, or immediately after anesthesia. Avoid rapid dosage escalation, which may lead to renal insufficiency. Hyperkalemia may rarely occur. Rare toxicities associated with ACE inhibitors include cholestatic jaundice (which may progress to hepatic necrosis) and neutropenia/agranulocytosis with myeloid hyperplasia. May be associated with deterioration of renal function and/or increases in serum creatinine, particularly in patients dependent on renin-angiotensin-aldosterone system. Use with caution in unilateral renal artery stenosis and pre-existing renal insufficiency; if patient has renal impairment then a baseline WBC with differential and serum creatinine should be evaluated and monitored closely during the first 3 months of therapy. Hypersensitivity reactions may be seen during hemodialysis with high-flux dialysis membranes (eg, AN69).

Adverse Reactions (Reflective of adult population; not specific for elderly)
Note: Frequency ranges include data from hypertension and heart failure trials. Higher rates of adverse reactions have generally been noted in patients with CHF. However, the frequency of adverse effects associated with placebo is also increased in this population.
(Continued)

Ramipril *(Continued)*

>10%: Respiratory: Cough (increased) (7% to 12%)

1% to 10%:

Cardiovascular: Hypotension (11%), angina (3%), postural hypotension (2%), syncope (2%)

Central nervous system: Headache (1% to 5%), dizziness (2% to 4%), fatigue (2%), vertigo (2%)

Endocrine & metabolic: Hyperkalemia (1% to 10%)

Gastrointestinal: Nausea/vomiting (1% to 2%)

Neuromuscular & skeletal: Chest pain (noncardiac) (1%)

Renal: Renal dysfunction (1%), elevation in serum creatinine (1% to 2%), increased BUN (<1% to 3%); transient elevations of creatinine and/or BUN may occur more frequently

Respiratory: Cough (estimated 1% to 10%)

Worsening of renal function may occur in patients with bilateral renal artery stenosis or in hypovolemia. In addition, a syndrome which may include fever, myalgia, arthralgia, interstitial nephritis, vasculitis, rash, eosinophilia and positive ANA, and elevated ESR has been reported with ACE inhibitors. Risk of pancreatitis and agranulocytosis may be increased in patients with collagen vascular disease or renal impairment.

Overdosage/Toxicology Mild hypotension has been the only toxic effect seen with acute overdose; bradycardia may also occur. Mild hyperkalemia may occur even with therapeutic doses, especially in patients with renal insufficiency and those taking NSAIDs. Following initiation of essential overdose management, toxic symptom and supportive treatment should be initiated. Hypotension usually responds to I.V. fluids or Trendelenburg positioning.

Drug Interactions

Alpha$_1$ blockers: Hypotensive effect increased.

Aspirin: The effects of ACE inhibitors may be blunted by aspirin administration, particularly at higher dosages and/or increase adverse renal effects.

Diuretics: Hypovolemia due to diuretics may precipitate acute hypotensive events or acute renal failure.

Gold sodium thiomalate: ACE inhibitors may enhance the adverse/toxic effects (nitritoid reaction) of gold sodium thiomalate. The reaction may include facial flushing, nausea, vomiting, hypotension, and syncope. If it is to occur, would be expected shortly after administration of gold compound in patients maintained on an ACEI.

Insulin: Risk of hypoglycemia may be increased.

Lithium: Risk of lithium toxicity may be increased; monitor lithium levels, especially the first 4 weeks of therapy.

Mercaptopurine: Risk of neutropenia may be increased.

NSAIDs: May attenuate hypertensive efficacy; effect has been seen with captopril and may occur with other ACE inhibitors; monitor blood pressure. May increase risk of adverse renal effects or hyperkalemia.

Potassium-sparing diuretics (amiloride, spironolactone, triamterene): Increased risk of hyperkalemia.

Potassium supplements may increase the risk of hyperkalemia.

Trimethoprim (high dose) may increase the risk of hyperkalemia.

Ethanol/Nutrition/Herb Interactions Herb/Nutraceutical: Avoid dong quai if using for hypertension (has estrogenic activity). Avoid ephedra, yohimbe, ginseng (may worsen hypertension). Avoid garlic (may have increased antihypertensive effect).

Stability Store at controlled room temperature.

Mechanism of Action Ramipril is an ACE inhibitor which prevents the formation of angiotensin II from angiotensin I and exhibits pharmacologic effects that are similar to captopril. Ramipril must undergo enzymatic saponification by esterases in the liver to its biologically active metabolite, ramiprilat. The pharmacodynamic effects of ramipril result from the high-affinity, competitive, reversible binding of ramiprilat to angiotensin-converting enzyme thus preventing the formation of the potent vasoconstrictor angiotensin II. This isomerized enzyme-inhibitor complex has a slow rate of dissociation, which results in high potency and a long duration of action; a CNS mechanism may also be involved in the hypotensive effect as angiotensin II increases adrenergic outflow from CNS; vasoactive kallikreins may be decreased in conversion to active hormones by ACE inhibitors, thus reducing blood pressure

Pharmacodynamics

Onset of action: Reduction of blood pressure occurs in 2 hours

Duration: 24 hours

Pharmacokinetics

Absorption: Well absorbed from GI tract (50% to 60%)

Distribution: Plasma concentrations decline in a triphasic fashion; rapid decline is a distribution phase to peripheral compartment, plasma protein and tissue ACE (half-life 2-4 hours); 2nd phase is an apparent elimination phase representing the clearance of free ramiprilat (half-life: 9-18 hours); and final phase is the terminal elimination phase representing the equilibrium phase between tissue binding and dissociation (half-life: >50 hours)

Metabolism: Hepatic to the active form, ramiprilat

Half-life: Ramiprilat: Effective: 13-17 hours, terminal: >50 hours

Time to peak serum concentration: ~1 hour

Elimination: Ramipril and its metabolites are eliminated primarily through the kidneys (60%) and feces (40%)

Dosage

Geriatrics: Refer to adult dosing (see Special Geriatric Considerations). Adjust for renal function for elderly since glomerular filtration rates are decreased; may see exaggerated hypotensive effects if renal clearance is not considered.

Adults:

Hypertension: Oral: 2.5-5 mg once daily, maximum: 20 mg/day

To reduce the risk of MI, stroke, and death from cardiovascular causes: Oral: Initial: 2.5 mg once daily for 1 week, then 5 mg once daily for the next 3 weeks, then increase as tolerated to 10 mg once daily (may be given as divided dose)

Left ventricular dysfunction postmyocardial infarction: Oral: Initial: 2.5 mg twice daily titrated upward, if possible, to 5 mg twice daily.

Heart failure (unlabeled use): Initial: 1.25-2.5 mg once daily; target dose: 10 mg once daily (ACC/AHA 2005 Heart Failure Guidelines)

Note: The dose of any concomitant diuretic should be reduced. If the diuretic cannot be discontinued, initiate therapy with 1.25 mg. After the initial dose, the patient should be monitored carefully until blood pressure has stabilized.

Renal Impairment:

Cl_{cr} <40 mL/minute: Administer 25% of normal dose.

Renal failure and hypertension: Administer 1.25 mg once daily, titrated upward as possible.

Renal failure and heart failure: Administer 1.25 mg once daily, increasing to 1.25 mg twice daily up to 2.5 mg twice daily as tolerated.

Administration Capsule is usually swallowed whole, but may be may be mixed in water, apple juice, or applesauce.

Monitoring Parameters BUN, serum creatinine, renal function, WBC, and potassium

Test Interactions Increases BUN, creatinine, potassium, positive Coombs' [direct]; decreases cholesterol (S); may cause false-positive results in urine acetone determinations using sodium nitroprusside reagent

Patient Information Notify physician if vomiting, diarrhea, excessive perspiration, or dehydration should occur; also if swelling of face, lips, tongue, or difficulty in breathing occurs or if persistent cough develops; do not stop therapy or use potassium salt substitutes without physician's advice; may be taken with food

Additional Information Some patients may have a decreased hypotensive effect between 12 and 16 hours; consider dividing total daily dose into 2 doses 12 hours apart. If patient is receiving a diuretic, a potential for first-dose hypotension is increased. To decrease this potential, stop diuretic for 2-3 days prior to initiating ramipril. If diuretic cannot be stopped temporarily, then initiate therapy with 1.25 mg daily. Continue diuretic if needed to control blood pressure. Capsules should be swallowed whole; if this cannot be done, capsule contents may be mixed with applesauce; also, contents may be mixed with apple juice or water. Mixtures in juice and water are stable for 24 hours at room temperature or 48 hours with refrigeration.

Special Geriatric Considerations Due to frequent decreases in glomerular filtration (also creatinine clearance) with aging, elderly patients may have exaggerated responses to ACE inhibitors; differences in clinical response due to hepatic changes are not observed. ACE inhibitors may be preferred agents in elderly patients with CHF and diabetes mellitus. Diabetic proteinuria is reduced and insulin sensitivity is enhanced. In general, the side effect profile is favorable in the elderly and causes little or no CNS confusion; use lowest dose recommendations initially. Many elderly may be volume depleted due to diuretic use and/or blunted thirst reflex resulting in inadequate fluid intake.

Dosage Forms Excipient information presented when available (limited, particularly for generics); consult specific product labeling.

Capsule:

Altace®: 1.25 mg, 2.5 mg, 5 mg, 10 mg

Selected References

Konstam MA, Drakup K, Baker DW, et al, "Heart Failure: Evaluation and Care of Patients With Left Ventricular Systolic Dysfunction," *Clinical Practice Guideline No 11*, Rockville, MD: Agency for Health Care Policy and Research, Public Health Service, U.S. Department of Health and Human Services, 1994.

McAreavey D and Robertson JI, "Angiotensin Converting Enzyme Inhibitors and Moderate Hypertension," *Drugs*, 1990, 40(3):326-45.

Williams JF, Bristow MR, Fowler MB, et al, "Guidelines for the Evaluation and Management of Heart Failure: Report of the American College of Cardiology/American Heart Association Task Force on Practice Guidelines (Committee on Evaluation and Management of Heart Failure)," *J Am Coll Cardiol*, 1995, 26:1376-8.

Yusuf S, Sleight P, Pogue J, et al, "Effects of an Angiotensin-Converting-Enzyme Inhibitor, Ramipril, on Cardiovascular Events in High-Risk Patients. The Heart Outcomes Prevention Evaluation Study Investigators," *N Engl J Med*, 2000, 342(3):145-53.

Ramipril and Hydrochlorothiazide
(RA mi pril & hye droe klor oh THYE a zide)

Related Information
  Hydrochlorothiazide *on page 756*
  Ramipril *on page 1377*
Medication Safety Issues
  Sound-alike/look-alike issues:
    Altace® HCT may be confused with alteplase, Artane®, Altace®
Canadian Brand Names Altace® HCT
Index Terms Hydrochlorothiazide and Ramipril
Generic Available No
Pharmacologic Category Angiotensin-Converting Enzyme (ACE) Inhibitor; Antihypertensive Agent, Combination; Diuretic, Thiazide
Use Treatment of essential hypertension (not for initial therapy)
Restrictions Not available in U.S.
Dosage
  Geriatrics & Adults: Hypertension: Oral: **Note:** Not for initial therapy; titration of individual agents to an appropriate clinical response is required before patient is converted over to an equivalent dose of the combination product.
    Usual dosage: Ramipril 2.5 mg/hydrochlorothiazide 12.5 mg once daily; titrate to maximum ramipril 10 mg/hydrochlorothiazide 50 mg once daily
  Renal Impairment:
    Cl_{cr} 30-60 mL/minute: Use caution; maximum dose: Ramipril 5 mg/hydrochlorothiazide 25 mg once daily
    Cl_{cr} <30 mL/minute: Hydrochlorothiazide is usually ineffective
  Hepatic Impairment: No specific dosing available.
Special Geriatric Considerations See individual agents.
Dosage Forms Excipient information presented when available (limited, particularly for generics); consult specific product labeling. [CAN] = Canadian brand name
  Tablet:
    Altace® HCT 2.5/12.5 [CAN]: Ramipril 2.5 mg and hydrochlorothiazide 12.5 mg [not available in the U.S.]
    Altace® HCT 5/12.5 [CAN]: Ramipril 5 mg and hydrochlorothiazide 12.5 mg [not available in the U.S.]
    Altace® HCT 5/25 [CAN]: Ramipril 5 mg and hydrochlorothiazide 25 mg [not available in the U.S.]
    Altace® HCT 10/12.5 [CAN]: Ramipril 10 mg and hydrochlorothiazide 12.5 mg [not available in the U.S.]
    Altace® HCT 10/25 [CAN]: Ramipril 10 mg and hydrochlorothiazide 25 mg [not available in the U.S.]

♦ **Ranexa**™ *see Ranolazine on page 1384*

Ranibizumab (ra ni BIZ oo mab)

U.S. Brand Names Lucentis®
Index Terms rhuFabV2
Generic Available No
Pharmacologic Category Monoclonal Antibody; Ophthalmic Agent; Vascular Endothelial Growth Factor (VEGF) Inhibitor
Use Treatment of neovascular (wet) age-related macular degeneration (AMD)
Contraindications Hypersensitivity to ranibizumab or any component of the formulation; ocular or periocular infection
Warnings/Precautions Intravitreous injections may be associated with endophthalmitis and retinal detachments. Proper aseptic injection techniques should be used and patients should be instructed to report any signs of infection immediately. Intraocular pressure may increase following injection. Use for >24 months has not been evaluated.

Risk of thromboembolic events, particularly stroke, may be increased following intravitreal administration of VEGF inhibitors. Rare hypersensitivity reactions (including anaphylaxis) have been associated with another VEGF inhibitor, pegaptanib, occurring within several hours of use; monitor closely. Equipment and appropriate personnel should be available for monitoring and treatment of anaphylaxis.
Adverse Reactions (Reflective of adult population; not specific for elderly)
  Note: Rates of ocular adverse reactions reported for control group when percentages overlapped with treatment group.
  >10%:
    Central nervous system: Headache (2% to 15%)
    Neuromuscular & skeletal: Arthralgia (3% to 11%)

Ocular: Conjunctival hemorrhage (43% to 77%; control: 29% to 66%), eye pain (17% to 37%; control 11% to 33%), vitreous floaters (3% to 32%), retinal hemorrhage (15% to 26%; control 37% to 56%), intraocular pressure increased (8% to 24%), vitreous detachment (7% to 22%; control 13% to 18%), intraocular inflammation (5% to 18%; control 3% to 11%), eye irritation (4% to 19%; control 6% to 20%), visual disturbance (up to 14%), blepharitis (3% to 13%)

Note: Cataract, foreign body sensation, lacrimation increased, pruritus, and subretinal fibrosis occurred in >10% of patients, but also occurred in similar percentages to the control; visual acuity blurred/decreased occurred more often in the control.

Respiratory: Nasopharyngitis (5% to 16%), upper respiratory tract infection (2% to 15%):

1% to 10%:

Cardiovascular: Arterial thromboembolic events (up to 5%; stroke up to 3%)

Gastrointestinal: Nausea (2% to 9%)

Ocular: Conjunctival hyperemia (up to 9%), posterior capsule opacification (up to 8%)

Note: Ocular hyperemia, maculopathy, dry eye, and ocular discomfort occurred in 1% to 10% of patients, but also occurred in similar percentages to the control; retinal exudates occurred more often in the control.

Respiratory: Bronchitis (3% to 10%), cough (3% to 10%), sinusitis (2% to 8%)

Miscellaneous: Influenza (2% to 10%), ranibizumab antibodies (1% to 6%)

Overdosage/Toxicology Significant intraocular inflammation was noted with initial doses of 1 mg; when using escalating regimens, doses up to 2 mg have been tolerated

Stability Store in original carton under refrigeration at 2°C to 8°C (36°F to 46°F); protect from light. Do not freeze.

Mechanism of Action Ranibizumab is a recombinant humanized monoclonal antibody fragment which binds to and inhibits human vascular endothelial growth factor A (VEGF-A). Ranibizumab inhibits VEGF from binding to its receptors and thereby suppressing neovascularization and slowing vision loss.

Pharmacokinetics

Absorption: Low levels are detected in the serum following intravitreal injection

Half-life elimination: Vitreous: 9 days

Dosage

Geriatrics & Adults: AMD: Intravitreal injection: 0.5 mg once a month. Although not as effective, frequency may be reduced after the first 4 injections to once every 3 months if monthly injections are not feasible. Dosing every 3 months will lead to an ~5 letter (1 line) loss of visual acuity over 9 months, as compared to monthly dosing.

Renal Impairment: Dose adjustment not expected.

Hepatic Impairment: Dose adjustment not expected.

Administration For ophthalmic intravitreal injection only. Remove contents from vial using a 5 micron 19-gauge filter needle attached to a tuberculin syringe. Discard filter needle and replace with a sterile 30 gauge ½ inch needle for injection. Adequate anesthesia and a broad-spectrum antimicrobial agent should be administered prior to the procedure.

Monitoring Parameters Intraocular pressure (within 30 minutes and between 2-7 days following administration); retinal perfusion, endophthalmitis

Patient Information This medication can only be administered by injection. You will be monitored closely during and following injection procedure. Report immediately any acute pain, difficulty breathing or swallowing, chest pain; heart palpitations, or other acute reactions. In the days following injection you may experience headache (consult prescriber for approved analgesic); mild cough, or flu symptoms (consult prescriber if persistent); foreign body sensation and increased tearing or visual blurring (use caution when driving or engaged in potentially hazardous tasks). Report immediately is your eye becomes red, painful, swollen, sensitive to light, or if there is a change in your vision, or any other adverse effects.

Special Geriatric Considerations

In clinical trials, ~94% of the the patients were >65 years and 68% were >75 years of age. No differences were seen in efficacy with increasing age. After correcting for creatinine clearance, age did not effect systemic exposure of ranibizumab.

Dosage Forms Excipient information presented when available (limited, particularly for generics); consult specific product labeling.

Injection, solution [preservative free]:

Lucentis®: 10 mg/mL (0.05 mL)

Selected References

Gaudreault J, Fei D, Rusit J, et al, "Preclinical Pharmacokinetics of Ranibizumab (rhuFabV2) After a Single Intravitreal Administration," *Invest Ophthalmol Vis Sci*, 2005, 46(2):726-33.

Heier JS, Antoszyk AN, Pavan PR, et al, "Ranibizumab for Treatment of Neovascular Age-Related Macular Degeneration: A Phase I/II Multicenter, Controlled, Multidose Study," *Ophthalmology*, 2006, 113(4):633-42.

Rosenfeld PJ, Brown DM, Heier JS, et al, "Ranibizumab for Neovascular Age-Related Macular Degeneration," *N Engl J Med*, 2006, 355(14):1419-31.

Rosenfeld PJ, Rich RM and Lalwani, "Ranibizumab: Phase III Clinical Trial Results," *Ophthalmol Clin North Am*, 2006, 19(3):361-72.

◆ **Raniclor**™ *see Cefaclor on page 250*

Ranitidine (ra NI ti deen)

Medication Safety Issues
Sound-alike/look-alike issues:
Ranitidine may be confused with amantadine, rimantadine
Zantac® may be confused with Xanax®, Zarontin®, Zofran®, Zyrtec®
International issues:
Antagon®: Brand name for astemizole in Mexico; brand name for ganirelix in the U.S.

U.S. Brand Names Zantac®; Zantac 75® [OTC]; Zantac 150™ [OTC]; Zantac® EFFER-dose®

Canadian Brand Names Alti-Ranitidine; Apo-Ranitidine®; BCI-Ranitidine; CO Raniti-dine; Gen-Ranidine; Novo-Ranidine; Nu-Ranit; PMS-Ranitidine; Ranitidine Injection, USP; Rhoxal-ranitidine; Sandoz-Ranitidine; Zantac®; Zantac 75®

Index Terms Ranitidine Hydrochloride

Generic Available Yes: Excludes effervescent tablet

Pharmacologic Category Histamine H_2 Antagonist

Use
Short-term and maintenance therapy of duodenal ulcer, gastric ulcer, gastroesopha-geal reflux, active benign ulcer, erosive esophagitis, and pathological hypersecretory conditions

OTC: Relief of heartburn, acid indigestion, and sour stomach

Unlabeled/Investigational Use Treatment of recurrent postoperative ulcer, upper GI bleeding; prevention of acid-aspiration pneumonitis during surgery, stress-induced ulcers

Contraindications Hypersensitivity to ranitidine or any component of the formulation

Warnings/Precautions Ranitidine has been associated with confusional states (rare). Use with caution in patients with hepatic impairment; use with caution in renal impair-ment, dosage modification required. Avoid use in patients with history of acute porphyria (may precipitate attacks); long-term therapy may be associated with vitamin B_{12} deficiency. Symptoms of GI distress may be associated with a variety of conditions; symptomatic response to H_2 antagonists does not rule out the potential for significant pathology (eg, malignancy). EFFERdose® formulations contain phenylalanine.

Adverse Reactions (Reflective of adult population; not specific for elderly)
Frequency not defined.
Cardiovascular: Atrioventricular block, bradycardia, premature ventricular beats, tachy-cardia, vasculitis
Central nervous system: Agitation, dizziness, depression, hallucinations, headache, insomnia, malaise, mental confusion, somnolence, vertigo
Dermatologic: Alopecia, erythema multiforme, rash
Endocrine & metabolic: Increased prolactin levels
Gastrointestinal: Abdominal discomfort/pain, constipation, diarrhea, nausea, pancrea-titis, vomiting
Hematologic: Acquired hemolytic anemia, agranulocytosis, aplastic anemia, granulocy-topenia, leukopenia, pancytopenia, thrombocytopenia
Hepatic: Hepatic failure, hepatitis
Local: Transient pain, burning or itching at the injection site
Neuromuscular & skeletal: Arthralgia, involuntary motor disturbance, myalgia
Ocular: Blurred vision
Renal: Increased serum creatinine
Respiratory: Pneumonia (causal relationship not established)
Miscellaneous: Anaphylaxis, angioneurotic edema, hypersensitivity reactions

Overdosage/Toxicology Symptoms include abnormal gait, hypotension, and adverse effects seen with normal use. Treatment is primarily symptomatic and supportive.

Drug Interactions Substrate (minor) of CYP1A2, 2C19, 2D6; **Inhibits** CYP1A2 (weak), 2D6 (weak)
Atazanavir: Ranitidine may reduce the absorption of atazanavir.
Cefuroxime, cefpodoxime: The absorption of some cephalosporins may be reduced by ranitidine (separate administrations times by at least 2 hours).
Itraconazole, ketoconazole: Ranitidine may reduce the absorption of itraconazole or ketoconazole.
Warfarin: May increase or decrease prothrombin time when used concomitantly; monitor.

Ethanol/Nutrition/Herb Interactions
Ethanol: Avoid ethanol (may cause gastric mucosal irritation).
Food: Does not interfere with absorption of ranitidine.

Stability
Injection: Vials: Store between 4°C to 30°C (39°F to 86°F). Protect from light. Solution is a clear, colorless to yellow solution; slight darkening does not affect potency.

Premixed bag: Store between 2°C to 25°C (36°F to 77°F). Protect from light.
EFFERdose® formulations: Store between 2°C to 30°C (36°F to 86°F).
Syrup: Store between 4°C to 25°C (39°F to 77°F). Protect from light.
Tablet: Store in dry place, between 15°C to 30°C (59°F to 86°F). Protect from light.

Vials can be mixed with NS or D_5W; solutions are stable for 48 hours at room temperature.
Intermittent bolus injection: Dilute to maximum of 2.5 mg/mL.
Intermittent infusion: Dilute to maximum of 0.5 mg/mL.

Mechanism of Action Competitive inhibition of histamine at H_2-receptors of the gastric parietal cells, which inhibits gastric acid secretion, gastric volume, and hydrogen ion concentration are reduced. Does not affect pepsin secretion, pentagastrin-stimulated intrinsic factor secretion, or serum gastrin.

Pharmacodynamics
Efficacy of healing rate: 63% to 77% at 4 weeks; 82% to 95% at 8 weeks
Duration of effect: Oral: 12 hours; I.V.: 6-8 hours

Pharmacokinetics
Absorption: Oral: 50%
Distribution: V_d: 1.4 L/kg in patients with normal renal function; 1.76 L/kg in patients with Cl_{cr} 25-35 mL/minute; minimally penetrates the blood-brain barrier
Protein binding: 15%
Metabolism: Hepatic, to 3 primary metabolites
Bioavailability: Oral: 48%
Half-life:
  Oral: 2.5-3 hours in patients with normal renal function (3-4 hours in older adults); 4.8 hours in patients with Cl_{cr} 25-35 mL/minute
  I.V.: 2-2.5 hours in patients with normal renal function
Time to peak serum concentration:
  Oral: 2-3 hours
  I.M.: ≤15 minutes
Elimination: Renal (amount dependent on route of administration): 30% (oral), 70% (I.V.) eliminated as unchanged drug in the urine; also in feces (as metabolites)

Dosage
Geriatrics & Adults:
  Duodenal ulcer: Oral: Treatment: 150 mg twice daily, or 300 mg once daily after the evening meal or at bedtime; maintenance: 150 mg once daily at bedtime
  Eradication of *Helicobacter pylori*: Oral: 150 mg twice daily; requires combination therapy
  Pathological hypersecretory conditions:
    Oral: 150 mg twice daily; adjust dose or frequency as clinically indicated; doses of up to 6 g/day have been used
    I.V.: Continuous infusion for Zollinger-Ellison: 1 mg/kg/hour; measure gastric acid output at 4 hours, if >10 mEq or if patient is symptomatic, increase dose in increments of 0.5 mg/kg/hour; doses of up to 2.5 mg/kg/hour have been used
  Gastric ulcer, benign: *Oral:* 150 mg twice daily; maintenance: 150 mg once daily at bedtime
  Erosive esophagitis: *Oral:* Treatment: 150 mg 4 times/day; maintenance: 150 mg twice daily
  Prevention of heartburn: *Oral:* Zantac®75 [OTC]: 75 mg 30-60 minutes before eating food or drinking beverages which cause heartburn; maximum: 150 mg in 24 hours; do not use for more than 14 days
  Patients not able to take oral medication:
    I.M.: 50 mg every 6-8 hours
    I.V.: Intermittent bolus or infusion: 50 mg every 6-8 hours
    Continuous I.V. infusion: 6.25 mg/hour
  Renal Impairment: Adults: Cl_{cr} <50 mL/minute:
    Oral: 150 mg every 24 hours; adjust dose cautiously if needed
    I.V.: 50 mg every 18-24 hours; adjust dose cautiously if needed
    Hemodialysis: Adjust dosing schedule so that dose coincides with the end of hemodialysis.
  Hepatic Impairment: Patients with hepatic impairment may have minor changes in ranitidine half-life, distribution, clearance, and bioavailability; dosing adjustments are not necessary; monitor patient.

Administration
Ranitidine injection may be administered I.M. or I.V.:
  I.M.: Injection is administered undiluted
  I.V.: Must be diluted; may be administered IVP or IVPB or continuous I.V. infusion
    IVP: Ranitidine (usually 50 mg) should be diluted to a total of 20 mL with NS or D_5W and administered over at least 5 minutes
    IVPB: Administer over 15-20 minutes
    Continuous I.V. infusion: Administer at 6.25 mg/hour and titrate dosage based on gastric pH by continuous infusion over 24 hours
(Continued)

Ranitidine (Continued)

EFFERdose®:
25 mg tablet: Dissolve in at least 5 mL (1 teaspoonful) of water; wait until completely dissolved before administering
150 mg tablet: Dissolve each dose in 6-8 ounces of water before drinking

Monitoring Parameters Signs and symptoms of peptic ulcer disease, occult blood with GI bleeding, gastric pH where necessary; monitor renal function to correct dose; monitor for side effects

Test Interactions False-positive urine protein using Multistix®, gastric acid secretion test, skin test allergen extracts, serum creatinine, urine protein test

Patient Information It may take several days before this medicine begins to relieve stomach pain; antacids may be taken with ranitidine unless your physician has told you not to use them; wait 30-60 minutes between taking the antacid and ranitidine; inform prescribers of any concomitant medications
Zantac® 75 [OTC]: Do not take maximum dose for more than 14 days continuously unless directed by physician

Additional Information Giving dose at 6 PM may be better than 10 PM bedtime, the highest acid production usually starts at approximately 7 PM, thus giving at 6 PM controls acid secretion better; administer I.V. administration over a 30 minute period to avoid bradycardia; causes fewer adverse reactions and interactions than cimetidine; most patient's ulcers have healed within 4 weeks, however, older adults require 12 weeks of therapy; long-term therapy may cause vitamin B_{12} deficiency

Special Geriatric Considerations Ulcer healing rates and incidence of adverse effects are similar in the elderly, when compared to younger patients; dosing adjustments not necessary based on age alone. Always adjust dose based upon creatinine clearance. Serum half-life is increased to 3-4 hours in elderly patients. H_2 blockers are the preferred drugs for treating PUD in the elderly due to cost and ease of administration. These agents are no less or more effective than any other therapy. The preferred agents, due to side effects and drug interaction profile and pharmacokinetics are ranitidine, famotidine, and nizatidine. Treatment for PUD in the elderly is recommended for 12 weeks since their lesions are larger; therefore, take longer to heal. This drug is substantially cleared renally, and elderly, having decreased renal function in general, should be monitored closely for adverse effects, especially CNS.

Dosage Forms Excipient information presented when available (limited, particularly for generics); consult specific product labeling. [DSC] = Discontinued product
Capsule 150 mg, 300 mg
Infusion [premixed in NaCl 0.45%; preservative free]:
Zantac®: 50 mg (50 mL)
Injection, solution: 25 mg/mL (2 mL, 6 mL)
Zantac®: 25 mg/mL (2 mL, 6 mL, 40 mL) [contains phenol 0.5% as preservative]
Syrup: 15 mg/mL (5 mL, 10 mL)
Zantac®: 15 mg/mL (473 mL) [contains alcohol 7.5%; peppermint flavor]
Tablet: 75 mg [OTC], 150 mg, 300 mg
Zantac®: 150 mg, 300 mg
Zantac 75®: 75 mg
Zantac 150™: 150 mg
Tablet, effervescent:
Zantac® EFFERdose®: 25 mg [contains sodium 1.33 mEq/tablet, phenylalanine 2.81 mg/tablet, and sodium benzoate]; 150 mg [contains sodium 7.96 mEq/tablet, phenylalanine 16.84 mg/tablet, and sodium benzoate] [DSC]

Selected References
Fennerty MD and Higbee M, "Drug Therapy of Gastrointestinal Disease," *Geriatric Pharmacology*, Bressler R and Katz MD, eds, New York, NY: McGraw-Hill, 1993, 585-608.
Morris DL, Markham SJ, Beechey A, et al, "Ranitidine-Bolus or Infusion Prophylaxis for Stress Ulcer," *Crit Care Med*, 1988, 16(3):229-32.
Roberts CJ, "Clinical Pharmacokinetics of Ranitidine," *Clin Pharmacokinet*, 1984, 9(3):211-21.

♦ **Ranitidine Hydrochloride** *see* Ranitidine *on page 1382*

Ranolazine (ra NOE la zeen)

Medication Safety Issues
Sound-alike/look-alike issues:
Ranexa™ may be confused with Celexa®
U.S. Brand Names Ranexa™
Generic Available No
Pharmacologic Category Cardiovascular Agent, Miscellaneous
Use Treatment of chronic angina in combination with amlodipine, beta-blockers, or nitrates
Contraindications Hypersensitivity to ranolazine or any component of the formulation; pre-existing QT prolongation (including congenital long-QT syndrome, uncorrected hypokalemia); known history of ventricular tachycardia; hepatic dysfunction (of any

degree); concurrent QT$_c$-prolonging drugs; concurrent strong or moderate CYP3A4 inhibitors (including diltiazem and grapefruit juice)

Warnings/Precautions Ranolazine will not relieve acute angina attacks. Has been shown to prolong QT$_c$ interval in a dose/plasma concentration-related manner. Hepatically-impaired patients may have a more significant increase in QT$_c$. Use caution in patients ≥75 years of age; they may experience more adverse events. Use caution in patients with renal dysfunction. In general, avoid use in severe renal dysfunction. Monitor blood pressure in patients with renal dysfunction.

Adverse Reactions (Reflective of adult population; not specific for elderly)

>10%: Gastrointestinal: Constipation (5% to 8%; 19% in the elderly)

>0.5% to 10%:

Cardiovascular: Syncope (0.7%), palpitation, peripheral edema

Central nervous system: Dizziness (5% to 6%), headache (3% to 6%), vertigo

Gastrointestinal: Nausea (4% to 6%), abdominal pain, vomiting, xerostomia

Hematologic: Hematocrit decreased

Neuromuscular & skeletal: Weakness

Respiratory: Dyspnea

Overdosage/Toxicology Symptoms may include dizziness, nausea, vomiting, diplopia, paresthesias, confusion, syncope, and prolonged loss of consciousness. QT prolongation may occur and continuous ECG monitoring may be warranted. Treatment is symptom-directed and supportive. Complete clearance of ranolazine by hemodialysis is unlikely.

Drug Interactions Substrate of CYP3A4 (major), 2D6 (minor); **Inhibits** CYP3A4 (weak), 2D6 (weak)

CYP3A4 inducers: CYP3A4 inducers may decrease the levels/effects of ranolazine. Example inducers include aminoglutethimide, carbamazepine, nafcillin, nevirapine, phenobarbital, phenytoin, and rifamycins.

CYP3A4 inhibitors: May increase the levels/effects of ranolazine. Example inhibitors include azole antifungals, clarithromycin, diclofenac, diltiazem, doxycycline, erythromycin, imatinib, isoniazid, nefazodone, nicardipine, propofol, protease inhibitors, quinidine, telithromycin, and verapamil. Ranolazine is contraindicated for use with strong or moderately-strong CYP3A4 inhibitors (including diltiazem).

Digoxin: May cause an increase in digoxin concentrations. Concurrent use may require a decrease in digoxin dose.

Diltiazem: May increase ranolazine serum concentration. Ranolazine is contraindicated for use with diltiazem.

Ketoconazole: May increase ranolazine serum concentration. Ranolazine is contraindicated for use with ketoconazole.

QT$_c$-prolonging agents: May increase the effects of ranolazine on QT prolongation. Some examples of QT$_c$-prolonging agents include abarelix, amiodarone, amitriptyline, apomorphine, arsenic trioxide, bretylium, chlorpromazine, cisapride, clarithromycin, disopyramide, dofetilide, dolasetron, domperidone, droperidol, erythromycin, flecainide, fluoxetine, flupenthixol, foscarnet, haloperidol, ibutilide, imipramine, indapamide, isradipine, levofloxacin, loxapine, mesoridazine, moxifloxacin, norfloxacin, octreotide, pentamidine, pimozide, probucol, procainamide, propafenone, quetiapine, quinidine, sotalol, telithromycin, thioridazine, thiothixene, voriconazole, ziprasidone, and zuclopenthixol. Ranolazine is contraindicated with QT$_c$-prolonging drugs.

Simvastatin: Ranolazine may increase simvastatin serum levels. The manufacturer suggests that the dose of simvastatin may need to be reduced.

Verapamil: May result in increased toxicity of ranolazine by inhibition of the P-glycoprotein pump and/or CYP3A4 inhibition. Ranolazine is contraindicated for use with verapamil.

Stability Store at 15°C to 30°C (59°F to 86°F).

Mechanism of Action A proposed mechanism suggests ranolazine is a partial fatty acid oxidation inhibitor; may change myocardial energy metabolism from fatty acids to glucose, increasing the efficiency of ATP production under hypoxic conditions. Exerts antianginal and anti-ischemic effects without changing hemodynamic parameters. In addition, it is a late sodium channel inhibitor.

Pharmacokinetics

Absorption: Highly variable; ranolazine is a substrate of P-glycoprotein; concurrent use of P-glycoprotein inhibitors may increase absorption

Protein binding: 62%

Metabolism: Hepatic via CYP3A (major) and 2D6 (minor)

Half-life elimination: Terminal: 7 hours

Time to peak, plasma: 2-5 hours

Excretion: Primarily urine (75% mostly as metabolites, <5% to 7% excreted unchanged); feces (25% mostly as metabolites)

Dosage

Geriatrics: Refer to adult dosing. Select dose cautiously, starting at the lower end of the dosing range.

(Continued)

Ranolazine *(Continued)*

Adults: Chronic angina: Oral: Initial: 500 mg twice daily; maximum recommended dose: 1000 mg twice daily

Renal Impairment: Dosage adjustment recommendations have not been established. However, plasma ranolazine levels increased ~50% in patients with varying degrees of renal dysfunction. Patients with severe renal dysfunction had an increase in mean diastolic blood pressure of 10-15 mm Hg. Monitor blood pressure closely in these patients. Patients on dialysis have not been studied. Avoid use in severe renal dysfunction.

Hepatic Impairment: Use is contraindicated.

Administration May be taken with or without meals. Swallow tablet whole; do not crush, break, or chew.

Monitoring Parameters Baseline and follow up ECG to evaluate QT interval; blood pressure in patients with renal dysfunction; correct and maintain serum potassium in normal limits

Special Geriatric Considerations

Elderly comprised 48% of study group participants. For those elderly, no overall difference in efficacy was observed between younger and older adults. There was, however, a higher incidence of adverse effects for those ≥75 years of age, resulting in drug discontinuations. The most common adverse effects were constipation (19%), nausea (6%), and dizziness (6%). Therefore, start dosing at lower end of range.

Dosage Forms Excipient information presented when available (limited, particularly for generics); consult specific product labeling.

Tablet, extended release: 500 mg

Selected References

Abdallah H and Jerling M, "Effect of Hepatic Impairment on the Multiple-Dose Pharmacokinetics of Ranolazine Sustained Release Tablets," *J Clin Pharmacol*, 2005, 45(7):802-9.

Chaitman BR, Pepine CJ, Parker JO, et al, "Effects of Ranolazine With Atenolol, Amlodipine, or Diltiazem on Exercise Tolerance and Angina Frequency in Patients With Severe Chronic Angina. A Randomized Controlled Trial," *JAMA*, 2004, 291(3):309-16.

Jerling M and Abdallah H, "Effect of Renal Impairment on Multiple-Dose Pharmacokinetics of Extended Release Ranolazine," *Clin Pharmacol Ther*, 2005, 78(3):288-97.

♦ **Raphon [OTC]** *see* Epinephrine *on page 514*

Rasagiline (ra SA ji leen)

Related Information

Antiparkinsonian Agents *on page 1745*

Medication Safety Issues

Sound-alike/look-alike issues:

Azilect® may be confused with Aricept®

U.S. Brand Names Azilect®

Index Terms AGN 1135; Rasagiline Mesylate; TVP-1012

Generic Available No

Pharmacologic Category Anti-Parkinson's Agent, MAO Type B Inhibitor

Use Initial monotherapy or as adjunct to levodopa in the treatment of idiopathic Parkinson's disease

Contraindications Hypersensitivity to rasagiline or any component of the formulation; concomitant use of amphetamine, tramadol, propoxyphene, methadone, dextromethorphan, St John's wort, mirtazapine, cyclobenzaprine, or sympathomimetic amines (eg, pseudoephedrine, ephedrine); use of meperidine or other MAO inhibitor within 14 days of rasagiline; elective surgery requiring general anesthesia, local anesthesia containing sympathomimetic vasoconstrictors; patients with pheochromocytoma

Warnings/Precautions

Cardiovascular system: Hypertensive crisis may occur with tyramine, tryptophan, or dopamine-containing foods; avoid for at least 2 weeks following discontinuation of rasagiline. May cause orthostatic hypotension, particularly in combination with levodopa; use with caution in patients with hypotension or patients who would not tolerate transient hypotensive episodes (cardiovascular or cerebrovascular disease); orthostasis is usually most problematic during first 2 months of therapy and tends to abate thereafter. Due to the potential for hemodynamic instability, patients should not undergo elective surgery requiring general anesthesia and should avoid local anesthesia containing sympathomimetic vasoconstrictors within 14 days of discontinuing rasagiline. If surgery is required, benzodiazepines, mivacurium, fentanyl, morphine or codeine may be used cautiously.

Central nervous system: May cause hallucinations; signs of severe CNS toxicity (some fatal), including hyperpyrexia, hyperthermia, rigidity, altered mental status, seizure and coma have been reported with selective and nonselective MAO inhibitor use in combination with antidepressants; Do not use within 5 weeks of fluoxetine discontinuation; do not initiate tricyclic, SSRI or SNRI therapy within 2 weeks of discontinuing rasagiline. Addition to levodopa therapy may result in exacerbation of dyskinesias, requiring a reduction in levodopa dosage.

Dermatologic: Risk of melanoma may be increased with rasagiline, although increased risk has been associated with Parkinson's disease itself; patients should have regular and frequent skin examinations.

Organ dysfunction: Use caution in mild hepatic impairment; dose reduction recommended. Do not use with moderate to severe hepatic impairment.

Adverse Reactions (Reflective of adult population; not specific for elderly)

Unless otherwise noted, the following adverse reactions are as reported for monotherapy. Spectrum of adverse events was generally similar with adjunctive (levodopa) therapy, though the incidence tended to be higher.

>10%:

Central nervous system: Dyskinesia (18% adjunct therapy), headache (14%)

Gastrointestinal: Nausea (10% to 12% adjunct therapy)

1% to 10%:

Cardiovascular: Postural hypotension (6% to 9% adjunct therapy; dose dependent), bundle branch block angina, chest pain, syncope

Central nervous system: Depression (5%), hallucinations (4% to 5% adjunct therapy), fever (3%), malaise (2%), vertigo (2%), anxiety, dizziness

Dermatologic: Bruising (2%), alopecia, skin carcinoma, vesiculobullous rash

Endocrine & metabolic: Impotence, libido decreased

Gastrointestinal: Constipation (4% to 9% adjunct therapy; dose dependent), weight loss (2% to 9% adjunct therapy; dose dependent), dyspepsia (7%), xerostomia (2% to 6% adjunct therapy; dose dependent), gastroenteritis (3%), anorexia, diarrhea, gastrointestinal hemorrhage, vomiting

Genitourinary: Hematuria, urinary incontinence

Hematologic: Leukopenia

Hepatic: Liver function tests increased

Neuromuscular & skeletal: Arthralgia (7%), neck pain (2%), arthritis (2%), paresthesia (2%), abnormal gait, hyperkinesias, hypertonia, neuropathy, tremor, weakness

Ocular: Conjunctivitis (3%)

Renal: Albuminuria

Respiratory: Rhinitis (3%), asthma, cough increased

Miscellaneous: Fall (5%), flu-like syndrome (5%), allergic reaction

Overdosage/Toxicology No reports of overdose have been documented. Symptoms of overdose would be expected to present similar to other MAO inhibitors, including cardiovascular events (eg, arrhythmia, rapid blood pressure changes), altered mental status, muscle twitching or seizure and respiratory failure. Treatment should be symptom-directed and supportive.

Drug Interactions Substrate of CYP1A2 (major)

Amphetamines: MAO inhibitors in combination with amphetamines may result in severe hypertensive reaction or serotonin syndrome; these combinations are best avoided.

Anorexiants: Concurrent use of rasagiline in combination with CNS stimulants or anorexiants may result in serotonin syndrome; these combinations are best avoided (eg, dexfenfluramine, fenfluramine, or sibutramine).

Atomoxetine: MAO inhibitors may increase the toxicity of atomoxetine; avoid concomitant use.

Bupropion: MAO inhibitors may increase the toxicity of bupropion; avoid concomitant use.

Buspirone: Concomitant use with rasagiline may cause increased blood pressure; avoid combination.

CNS stimulants: MAO inhibitors in combination with stimulants (methylphenidate) may result in serotonin syndrome; these combinations are best avoided

COMT inhibitors (eg, entacapone, tolcapone): May increase toxicity of MAO inhibitors; avoid concomitant use.

Ciprofloxacin: May increase the levels/effects of rasagiline; monitor.

Cyclobenzaprine: Concurrent use of rasagiline may result in serotonin syndrome; this combination is contraindicated.

CYP1A2 inducers may decrease the levels/effects of rasagiline. Example inducers include aminoglutethimide, carbamazepine, phenobarbital, and rifampin.

CYP1A2 inhibitors may increase the levels/effects of rasagiline. Example inhibitors include amiodarone, ciprofloxacin, fluvoxamine, ketoconazole, norfloxacin, and ofloxacin.

Dextromethorphan: Concurrent use of rasagiline may result in psychosis and bizarre behavior; concomitant use contraindicated.

Guanadrel and guanethidine: MAO inhibitors inhibit the antihypertensive response to guanadrel or guanethidine; use an alternative antihypertensive agent.

(Continued)

Rasagiline *(Continued)*

Levodopa: MAO inhibitors in combination with levodopa may result in hypertensive or (orthostatic) hypotensive reactions; monitor.

Lithium: MAO inhibitors in combination with lithium have resulted in malignant hyperpyrexia; this combination is best avoided.

MAO inhibitors (eg, phenelzine, tranylcypromine): Concurrent use with other MAO inhibitors may result in hypertensive crisis; combination use contraindicated.

Meperidine: Use with rasagiline may result in coma, severe hypertension or hypotension, respiratory depression, convulsions, hyperpyrexia, excitation, and death; concurrent use contraindicated.

Methadone: Concomitant use with an MAO inhibitor may increase the risk of coma, severe hypertension or hypotension, respiratory depression, convulsions, hyperpyrexia, excitation, and death; this combination is contraindicated.

Mirtazapine: Concurrent use of rasagiline may result in serotonin syndrome; this combination is contraindicated.

Propoxyphene: Concomitant use with an MAO inhibitor may increase the risk of coma, severe hypertension or hypotension, respiratory depression, convulsions, hyperpyrexia, vascular collapse, and death; this combination is contraindicated.

Reserpine: MAO inhibitors in combination with reserpine may result in hypertensive reactions; monitor.

Sibutramine: May cause serotonin syndrome when combined with an MAO inhibitor; avoid this combination.

SSRIs/SNRIs: Concurrent use of rasagiline with a selective serotonin or serotonin/norepinephrine reuptake inhibitor may result in mania or hypertension. It is generally best to avoid these combinations.

St John's wort: May cause hypertensive crisis or serotonin syndrome when combined with an MAO inhibitor; this combination is contraindicated.

Sympathomimetics (indirect-acting): MAO inhibitors in combination with sympathomimetics such as dopamine, metaraminol, phenylephrine, and decongestants (pseudoephedrine) may result in severe hypertensive reaction; these combinations are contraindicated.

Tramadol: May increase the risk of seizures and coma, severe hypertension or hypotension, respiratory depression, convulsions, hyperpyrexia, vascular collapse, and death in patients receiving an MAO inhibitor; concurrent use contraindicated.

Trazodone: Concurrent use of rasagiline may result in serotonin syndrome; these combinations are best avoided.

Tricyclic antidepressants: May cause serotonin syndrome when combined with an MAO inhibitor; this combination is contraindicated.

Venlafaxine: Concurrent use of rasagiline may result in serotonin syndrome; these combinations are best avoided.

Ethanol/Nutrition/Herb Interactions

Ethanol: Avoid ethanol. Avoid beverages containing tyramine (hearty red wine and beer).

Food: Concurrent ingestion of foods rich in tyramine may cause sudden and severe high blood pressure (hypertensive crisis). Avoid tyramine-containing foods with MAOIs. Food's freshness is also an important concern; improperly stored or spoiled food can create an environment where tyramine concentrations may increase.

Herb/Nutraceutical: Avoid valerian, St John's wort, SAMe, kava kava (may increase risk of serotonin syndrome and/or excessive sedation); Avoid supplements containing caffeine, tyrosine, tryptophan or phenylalanine. Ingestion of large quantities may increase the risk of severe side effects (eg, hypertensive reactions, serotonin syndrome).

Stability Store at 15°C to 30°C (59°F to 86°F).

Mechanism of Action Potent, irreversible and selective inhibitor of brain monoamine oxidase (MAO) type B, which plays a major role in the catabolism of dopamine. Inhibition of dopamine depletion in the striatal region of the brain reduces the symptomatic motor deficits of Parkinson's disease. There is also experimental evidence of rasagiline conferring neuroprotective effects (antioxidant, antiapoptotic), which may delay onset of symptoms and progression of neuronal deterioration.

Pharmacodynamics

Onset of action: Therapeutic: Within 1 hour

Duration: ~1 week (irreversible inhibition); may require ~14-40 days for complete restoration of (brain) MAO-B activity

Pharmacokinetics

Absorption: Rapid

Protein binding: 88% to 94%

Metabolism: Hepatic N-dealkylation and/or hydroxylation via CYP1A2 to multiple inactive metabolites (nonamphetamine derivatives)

Distribution: V_{dss}: 87 L

Bioavailability: 36%

Half-life elimination: ~1.3-3 hours (no correlation with biologic effect due to irreversible inhibition)

Time to peak, plasma: 30 minutes to 1 hour

Excretion: Urine (62%, >99% as metabolites); feces (7%)

Dosage

Geriatrics & Adults: Parkinson's disease: Oral:

Monotherapy: 1 mg once daily

Adjunctive therapy with levodopa: Initial: 0.5 mg once daily; may increase to 1 mg once daily based on response and tolerability

Note: When added to existing levodopa therapy, a dose reduction of levodopa may be required to avoid exacerbation of dyskinesias; typical dose reductions of ~9% to 13% were employed in clinical trials.

Dose reduction with concomitant ciprofloxacin or other CYP1A2 inhibitors: 0.5 mg once daily

Renal Impairment:

Mild impairment: No adjustment necessary.

Moderate-to-severe impairment: No data available.

Hepatic Impairment:

Mild impairment (Child-Pugh ≤6): 0.5 mg once daily

Moderate-to-severe impairment: Not recommended.

Monitoring Parameters Blood pressure; symptoms of parkinsonism; general mood and behavior (increased anxiety, or presence of mania or agitation); skin examination for presence of melanoma (higher incidence in Parkinson's patients- drug causation not established)

Patient Information Take exactly as directed (may be prescribed in conjunction with levodopa/carbidopa); do not change dosage or discontinue without consulting prescriber. Therapeutic effects may take several weeks or months to achieve and you may need frequent monitoring during first weeks of therapy. Take with meals if GI upset occurs, before meals if dry mouth occurs, or after eating if drooling or if nausea occurs. Take at the same time each day. Avoid tyramine-containing foods and for two weeks once the medication had been stopped. Maintain adequate hydration (2-3 L/day of fluids) unless instructed to restrict fluid intake. Do not use alcohol and prescription or OTC sedatives or CNS depressants without consulting prescriber. You may experience drowsiness, dizziness, confusion, or vision changes (use caution when driving, climbing stairs, or engaging in tasks requiring alertness until response to drug is known); orthostatic hypotension (use caution when changing position - rising to standing from sitting or lying); constipation (increased exercise, fluids, fruit, or fiber may help); runny nose or flu-like symptoms (consult prescriber for appropriate relief); or nausea, vomiting, loss of appetite, or stomach discomfort (small frequent meals, frequent mouth care, chewing gum, or sucking lozenges may help). You are at an increased risk of melanoma. Have skin monitored by a qualified professional. Report any skin changes or suspicious areas. Report unresolved constipation or vomiting; chest pain, palpitations, irregular heartbeat; CNS changes (hallucination, loss of memory, seizures, acute headache, nervousness, thoughts of suicide, etc); painful or difficult urination; increased muscle spasticity, rigidity, or involuntary movements; skin rash; or significant worsening of condition.

Additional Information When adding rasagiline to levodopa/carbidopa, the dose of the latter can usually be decreased. Studies are investigating the use of rasagiline in early Parkinson's disease to slow the progression of the disease.

Special Geriatric Considerations In clinical trials, no significant differences in the safety profile were seen between elderly and younger adults.

Dosage Forms Excipient information presented when available (limited, particularly for generics); consult specific product labeling.

Tablet, as mesylate:

Azilect®: 0.5 mg, 1 mg

Selected References

Chen JJ and Ly A-V, "Rasagiline: A Second-Generation Monoamine Oxidase Type-B Inhibitor for the Treatment of Parkinson's Disease," Am J Health-Syst Pharm, 2006, 63(10):915-28.

Parkinson Study Group, "A Randomized Placebo-Controlled Trial of Rasagiline in Levodopa-Treated Patients with Parkinson Disease and Motor Fluctuations. The PRESTO Study," Arch Neurol, 2005 62(2):241-8.

Parkinson Study Group, "A Controlled, Randomized, Delayed-Start Study of Rasagiline in Early Parkinson Disease," Arch Neurol, 2004, 6(4):561-66.

Parkinson Study Group, "A Controlled Trial of Rasagiline in Early Parkinson Disease: the TEMPO Study," Arch Neurol, 2002, 59(12):1937-43.

Rascol O, Brooks DJ, Melamed E et al, "Rasagiline as an Adjunct to Levodopa in Patients with Parkinson's Disease and Motor Fluctuations (LARGO, Lasting effect in Adjunct therapy With Rasagiline Given Once Daily, Study): A Randomized, Double-Blind, Parallel-Group Trial," Lancet, 2005, 365(9463):947-54.

Shulman KI and Walker SE, "A Reevaluation of Dietary Restrictions for Irreversible Monoamine Oxidase Inhibitors," Psychiatr Ann, 2001, 31(6):378-84.

Shulman KI and Walker SE, "Refining the MAOI Diet: Tyramine Content of Pizzas and Soy Products," J Clin Psychiatry, 1999, 60(3):191-3.

Walker SE, Shulman KI, Tailor SA, et al, "Tyramine Content of Previously Restricted Foods in Monoamine Oxidase Inhibitor Diets," J Clin Psychopharmacol, 1996, 16(5):383-8.

◆ **Rasagiline Mesylate** see Rasagiline on page 1386

+ **Razadyne**™ *see* Galantamine *on page 695*
+ **Razadyne**™ **ER** *see* Galantamine *on page 695*
+ **ReAzo [OTC]** *see* Phenazopyridine *on page 1238*
+ **Rebetol**® *see* Ribavirin *on page 1397*
+ **Reclast**® *see* Zoledronic Acid *on page 1704*
+ **Recombinant Human Parathyroid Hormone (1-34)** *see* Teriparatide *on page 1535*
+ **Recombinant Human Platelet-Derived Growth Factor B** *see* Becaplermin *on page 152*
+ **Recombinant Plasminogen Activator** *see* Reteplase *on page 1395*
+ **Recombivax HB**® *see* Hepatitis B Vaccine *on page 750*
+ **Rectacaine [OTC]** *see* Phenylephrine *on page 1247*
+ **Refresh**® **[OTC]** *see* Artificial Tears *on page 124*
+ **Refresh Plus**® **[OTC]** *see* Artificial Tears *on page 124*
+ **Refresh PM**® **Ophthalmic Ointment [OTC]** *see* Ocular Lubricant *on page 1144*
+ **Refresh Tears**® **[OTC]** *see* Artificial Tears *on page 124*
+ **Reglan**® *see* Metoclopramide *on page 1023*
+ **Regonol**® *see* Pyridostigmine *on page 1351*
+ **Regranex**® *see* Becaplermin *on page 152*
+ **Regular Insulin** *see* Insulin Regular *on page 815*
+ **Reguloid**® **[OTC]** *see* Psyllium *on page 1347*
+ **Relafen**® **[DSC]** *see* Nabumetone *on page 1076*
+ **Relenza**® *see* Zanamivir *on page 1694*
+ **Relief**® **[OTC]** *see* Phenylephrine *on page 1247*
+ **Relpax**® *see* Eletriptan *on page 501*
+ **Remeron**® *see* Mirtazapine *on page 1050*
+ **Remeron SolTab**® *see* Mirtazapine *on page 1050*
+ **Reminyl**® **[DSC]** *see* Galantamine *on page 695*
+ **Renagel**® *see* Sevelamer *on page 1461*

Repaglinide (re PAG li nide)

Medication Safety Issues
Sound-alike/look-alike issues:
Prandin® may be confused with Avandia®
U.S. Brand Names Prandin®
Canadian Brand Names GlucoNorm®; Prandin®
Generic Available No
Pharmacologic Category Antidiabetic Agent, Meglitinide Derivative
Use Management of noninsulin-dependent diabetes mellitus (type II)
As an adjunct to diet and exercise to lower the blood glucose in patients with type II diabetes mellitus whose hyperglycemia cannot be controlled satisfactorily by diet and exercise alone

In combination with metformin to lower blood glucose in patients whose hyperglycemia cannot be controlled by exercise, diet, and either agent alone
Contraindications Hypersensitivity to repaglinide or any component of the formulation; diabetic ketoacidosis, with or without coma (treat with insulin); type 1 diabetes (insulin dependent, IDDM)
Warnings/Precautions Use with caution in patients with moderate-to-severe hepatic impairment. Use caution in severe renal dysfunction, elderly, malnourished, or patients with adrenal/pituitary dysfunction; may be more susceptible to glucose-lowering effects. May cause hypoglycemia; appropriate patient selection, dosage, and patient education are important to avoid hypoglycemic episodes. It may be necessary to discontinue repaglinide and administer insulin if the patient is exposed to stress (fever, trauma, infection, surgery). Not indicated for use in combination with NPH insulin due to potential cardiovascular events.
Adverse Reactions (Reflective of adult population; not specific for elderly)
>10%:
    Central nervous system: Headache (9% to 11%)
    Endocrine & metabolic: Hypoglycemia (16% to 31%)
    Respiratory: Upper respiratory tract infection (10% to 16%)
1% to 10%:
    Cardiovascular: Ischemia (4%), chest pain (2% to 3%)
    Gastrointestinal: Diarrhea (4% to 5%), constipation (2% to 3%), tooth disorder (<1% to 2%)
    Genitourinary: Urinary tract infection (2% to 3%)
    Neuromuscular & skeletal: Arthralgia (3% to 6%), back pain (5% to 6%)
    Respiratory: Sinusitis (3% to 6%), bronchitis (2% to 6%)
    Miscellaneous: Allergy (1% to 2%)

Overdosage/Toxicology Symptoms include severe hypoglycemia, seizures, cerebral damage, tingling of lips and tongue, nausea, yawning, confusion, agitation, tachycardia, sweating, convulsions, stupor, and coma. Intoxications are best managed with glucose administration (oral for milder hypoglycemia or by injection in more severe forms) and symptomatic management.

Drug Interactions Substrate of CYP2C8 (major), 3A4 (major)

CYP2C8 inducers: May decrease the levels/effects of repaglinide. Example inducers include carbamazepine, phenobarbital, phenytoin, rifampin, rifapentine, and secobarbital.

CYP2C8 Inhibitors may increase the levels/effects of repaglinide. Example inhibitors include atazanavir, gemfibrozil, and ritonavir.

CYP3A4 inducers: CYP3A4 inducers may decrease the levels/effects of repaglinide. Example inducers include aminoglutethimide, carbamazepine, nafcillin, nevirapine, phenobarbital, phenytoin, and rifamycins.

CYP3A4 inhibitors: May increase the levels/effects of repaglinide. Example inhibitors include azole antifungals, clarithromycin, diclofenac, doxycycline, erythromycin, imatinib, isoniazid, nefazodone, nicardipine, propofol, protease inhibitors, quinidine, telithromycin, and verapamil.

Gemfibrozil: Gemfibrozil may increase the serum concentration of repaglinide (prolonged, severe hypoglycemia has been reported). The addition of itraconazole may augment the effects of gemfibrozil on repaglinide. Consider alternative therapy.

HMG-CoA reductase inhibitors (eg, atorvastatin, fluvastatin, lovastatin, pravastatin, simvastatin): May increase repaglinide concentrations by decreasing metabolism.

Macrolide antibiotics (eg, clarithromycin, erythromycin, troleandomycin): May increase repaglinide concentrations by decreasing metabolism.

Oral contraceptives (estrogens, such as estradiol, ethinyl estradiol, mestranol): May increase repaglinide concentrations. Repaglinide may increase oral contraceptive (estrogens) serum concentration.

Oral contraceptives (progestins): May increase repaglinide concentrations. Repaglinide may increase oral contraceptive (progestins) serum concentration.

Rifampin: May decrease levels/effects of repaglinide; monitor serum glucose.

Trimethoprim: May increase repaglinide concentrations; monitor serum glucose carefully.

Ethanol/Nutrition/Herb Interactions

Ethanol: Avoid ethanol (may cause hypoglycemia).

Food: When given with food, the AUC of repaglinide is decreased.

Herb/Nutraceutical: St John's wort may decrease repaglinide levels. Avoid gymnema, garlic (may cause hypoglycemia).

Stability Do not store above 25°C (77°F). Protect from moisture.

Mechanism of Action Nonsulfonylurea hypoglycemic agent of the meglitinide class (the nonsulfonylurea moiety of glyburide) used in the management of type 2 diabetes mellitus; stimulates insulin release from the pancreatic beta cells

Pharmacodynamics

Onset of action: Oral: Insulin levels in the serum begin to increase within 15-60 minutes after a single dose

Duration: Up to 24 hours

Pharmacokinetics

Absorption: Rapidly and completely from the GI tract with peak plasma drug levels within 1 hour

Distribution: V_d: 31 L

Protein binding, plasma: >98%

Metabolism: Hepatic; completely metabolized by oxidative biotransformation and direct conjugation with glucuronic acid

Bioavailability, mean absolute: ~56%

Half-life: 1 hour

Elimination: ~90% in the feces and ~8% within 96 hours

Dosage

Geriatrics & Adults:

Type 2 diabetes: Oral:

Note: Doses should be taken within 15 minutes of the meal, but time may vary from immediately preceding the meal to as long as 30 minutes before the meal

Patients not previously treated or whose Hb A_{1c} is <8%: Initial: 0.5 mg before each meal

Patients previously treated with blood glucose-lowering agents whose Hb A_{1c} is ≥8%: Initial: 1 or 2 mg before each meal.

Dose adjustment: Determine dosing adjustments by blood glucose response, usually fasting blood glucose. Double the preprandial dose up to 4 mg until satisfactory blood glucose response is achieved. At least 1 week should elapse to assess response after each dose adjustment.

Dose range: 0.5-4 mg taken with meals. Repaglinide may be dosed preprandial 2, 3, or 4 times/day in response to changes in the patient's meal pattern. Maximum recommended daily dose: 16 mg.

(Continued)

Repaglinide (Continued)

Patients receiving other oral hypoglycemic agents: When repaglinide is used to replace therapy with other oral hypoglycemic agents, it may be started the day after the final dose is given. Observe patients carefully for hypoglycemia because of potential overlapping of drug effects. When transferred from longer half-life sulfonylureas (eg, chlorpropamide), close monitoring may be indicated for up to ≥1 week.

Note: Combination therapy: If repaglinide monotherapy does not result in adequate glycemic control, metformin or a thiazolidinedione may be added. Or, if metformin or thiazolidinedione therapy does not provide adequate control, repaglinide may be added. The starting dose and dose adjustments for combination therapy are the same as repaglinide monotherapy. Carefully adjust the dose of each drug to determine the minimal dose required to achieve the desired pharmacologic effect. Failure to do so could result in an increase in the incidence of hypoglycemic episodes. Use appropriate monitoring of FPG and Hb A_{1c} measurements to ensure that the patient is not subjected to excessive drug exposure or increased probability of secondary drug failure. If glucose is not achieved after a suitable trial of combination therapy, consider discontinuing these drugs and using insulin.

Renal Impairment:

Cl_{cr} 40-80 mL/minute (mild to moderate renal dysfunction): Initial dosage adjustment does not appear to be necessary.

Cl_{cr} 20-40 mL/minute: Initiate 0.5 mg with meals; titrate carefully.

Hepatic Impairment: Use conservative initial and maintenance doses. Use longer intervals between dosage adjustments.

Monitoring Parameters Periodically monitor fasting blood glucose and glycosylated hemoglobin (Hb A_{1c}) levels or fructosamine with a goal of decreasing these levels towards the normal range. During dose adjustment, fasting glucose can be used to determine response.

Reference Range Target range:

Geriatrics: 100-150 mg/dL

Adults: Fasting blood glucose: <120 mg/dL

Patient Information Do not take any new medication during therapy without consulting prescriber. Take this medication exactly as directed (3-4 times a day) 15-30 minutes prior to a meal. If you skip a meal (or add an extra meal), skip (or add) a dose for that meal. Do not change dosage or discontinue without consulting prescriber. Follow dietary and lifestyle directions of prescriber or diabetic educator. Avoid alcohol. You will be instructed in signs of hypo- or hyperglycemia by prescriber or diabetic educator; be alert for adverse hypoglycemia (lightheadedness, tachycardia or palpitations, sweaty palms or profuse perspiration, yawning, tingling of lips and tongue, seizures, or change in sensorium) and follow prescriber's instructions for intervention. May cause headache or mild GI effects during first weeks of therapy (nausea, vomiting, diarrhea, constipation, heartburn); if these do not diminish, consult prescriber for approved medication. Report chest pain; respiratory difficulty or symptoms of upper respiratory infection; urinary tract infection (burning or itching on urination); muscle pain or back pain; or other adverse effects.

Special Geriatric Considerations Repaglinide has not been studied exclusively in the elderly; information from the manufacturer states that no differences in its effectiveness or adverse effects had been identified between persons younger than and older than 65 years of age. How "tightly" a geriatric patient's blood glucose should be controlled is controversial; however, a fasting blood glucose <150 mg/dL is now an acceptable endpoint. Such a decision should be based on the patient's functional status, how well he/she recognizes hypoglycemic or hyperglycemic symptoms, and how to respond to them and their other disease states.

Dosage Forms Excipient information presented when available (limited, particularly for generics); consult specific product labeling.

Tablet:

Prandin®: 0.5 mg, 1 mg, 2 mg

♦ **Requip®** *see* Ropinirole *on page 1425*

Reserpine (re SER peen)

Related Information

Potentially Inappropriate Medications for Geriatrics *on page 1824*

Medication Safety Issues

Sound-alike/look-alike issues:

Reserpine may be confused with Risperdal®, risperidone

Generic Available Yes

Pharmacologic Category Central Monoamine-Depleting Agent; Rauwolfia Alkaloid

Use Management of mild-to-moderate hypertension; treatment of agitated psychotic states (schizophrenia)

Unlabeled/Investigational Use Management of tardive dyskinesia

Contraindications Hypersensitivity to reserpine or any component of the formulation; active peptic ulcer disease, ulcerative colitis; history of mental depression (especially with suicidal tendencies); patients receiving electroconvulsive therapy (ECT)

Warnings/Precautions

Use with caution in patients with impaired renal function, inflammatory bowel disease, asthma, Parkinson's disease, gallstones, or history of peptic ulcer disease, and the elderly. At high doses, significant mental depression, anxiety, or psychosis may occur (uncommon at dosages <0.25 mg/day). May cause orthostatic hypotension; use with caution in patients at risk of hypotension or in patients where transient hypotensive episodes would be poorly tolerated (cardiovascular disease or cerebrovascular disease). Avoid concurrent use of MAO inhibitors and/or drugs with MAO-inhibiting properties. Some products may contain tartrazine.

Adverse Reactions (Reflective of adult population; not specific for elderly)

Frequency not defined.

Cardiovascular: Peripheral edema, arrhythmia, bradycardia, chest pain, PVC, hypotension, syncope

Central nervous system: Dizziness, headache, nightmares, nervousness, drowsiness, fatigue, mental depression, parkinsonism, dull sensorium, paradoxical anxiety

Dermatologic: Rash, pruritus, flushing of skin, purpura

Endocrine & metabolic: Gynecomastia, weight gain

Gastrointestinal: Anorexia, diarrhea, dry mouth, nausea, vomiting, increased salivation, increased gastric acid secretion

Genitourinary: Impotence, decreased libido

Hematologic: Thrombocytopenia purpura

Neuromuscular & skeletal: Muscle ache

Ocular: Blurred vision, optic atrophy

Respiratory: Nasal congestion, dyspnea, epistaxis

Drug Interactions

Antihypertensives: Hypotensive effects may be increased.

CNS depressants, ethanol: Additive CNS effects may occur.

Digitalis glycosides: Concomitant administration may predispose some patients to cardiac arrhythmias.

MAO inhibitors: Reserpine may cause hypertensive reactions; concurrent use is not recommended. Theoretically, risk is decreased if reserpine is initiated several days prior to MAO inhibitors.

Quinidine, procainamide: Reserpine may increase the risk of cardiac arrhythmias effects.

Sympathomimetics: The effects of direct-acting sympathomimetics (eg, epinephrine, norepinephrine) may be modestly increased/prolonged. However, the effects of indirect-acting sympathomimetics (amphetamines, dopamine) may be blocked by reserpine.

Ethanol/Nutrition/Herb Interactions

Ethanol: Avoid ethanol (may increase CNS depression).

Herb/Nutraceutical: Avoid dong quai if using for hypertension (has estrogenic activity). Avoid ephedra, yohimbe (may worsen hypertension). Avoid valerian, St John's wort, kava kava, gotu kola (may increase CNS depression). Avoid garlic (may have increased antihypertensive effect).

Stability Protect oral dosage forms from light.

Mechanism of Action Reduces blood pressure via depletion of sympathetic biogenic amines (norepinephrine and dopamine); this also commonly results in sedative effects

Pharmacodynamics

Onset of action: Within 3-6 days

Duration: 2-6 weeks

Pharmacokinetics

Absorption: Oral: ~40%

Protein binding: 96%

Metabolism: Extensive in the liver (>90%)

Half-life: 50-100 hours

Elimination: Principal excretion in feces (30% to 60%) and small amounts in urine (10%)

Dosage

Geriatrics: Oral: Initial: 0.05 mg once daily increasing by 0.05 mg every week as necessary (full antihypertensive effects may take as long as 3 weeks).

Adults:

Hypertension:

Manufacturer's labeling: Initial: 0.5 mg/day for 1-2 weeks; maintenance: 0.1-0.25 mg/day

(Continued)

Reserpine *(Continued)*

Note: Clinically, the need for a "loading" period (as recommended by the manufacturer) is not well supported, and alternative dosing is preferred.

Alternative dosing (unlabeled): Initial: 0.1 mg once daily; adjust as necessary based on response.

Usual dose range (JNC 7): 0.05-0.25 mg once daily; 0.1 mg every other day may be given to achieve 0.05 mg once daily

Schizophrenia (labeled use) or tardive dyskinesia (unlabeled use): Dosing recommendations vary; initial dose recommendations generally range from 0.05-0.25 mg (although manufacturer recommends 0.5 mg once daily initially in schizophrenia). May be increased in increments of 0.1-0.25 mg; maximum dose in tardive dyskinesia: 5 mg/day.

Renal Impairment:

Cl_{cr} <10 mL/minute: Avoid use.

Not removed by hemo- or peritoneal dialysis; supplemental dose is not necessary.

Monitoring Parameters Blood pressure, standing and sitting/supine, symptoms of depression

Patient Information Take with food or milk; impotency is reversible; notify physician if a weight gain of more than 5 pounds has taken place during therapy; may cause drowsiness

Additional Information Full antihypertensive effects may take as long as 3 weeks; at high doses, mental depression is possible and might lead to suicide

Special Geriatric Considerations Some studies advocate the use of reserpine because of its low cost, long half-life, and efficacy, but it is generally not considered a first-line drug.

Dosage Forms Excipient information presented when available (limited, particularly for generics); consult specific product labeling.

Tablet: 0.1 mg, 0.25 mg

Selected References

Adelman AM, Daly MP, and Michocki RJ, "Alternate Drugs," *Clin Geriatr Med*, 1990, 6(2):423-44.

Chobanian AV, Bakris GL, Black HR, et al, "The Seventh Report of the Joint National Committee on Prevention, Detection, Evaluation, and Treatment of High Blood Pressure: The JNC 7 Report," *JAMA*, 2003, 289(19):2560-71.

♦ **Respa-DM**® *see* Guaifenesin and Dextromethorphan *on page 730*

♦ **Restasis**® *see* CycloSPORINE *on page 380*

♦ **Restoril**® *see* Temazepam *on page 1528*

Retapamulin (re te PAM ue lin)

U.S. Brand Names Altabax™

Generic Available No

Pharmacologic Category Antibiotic, Pleuromutilin; Antibiotic, Topical

Use Treatment of impetigo caused by susceptible strains of *S. pyogenes* or methicillin-susceptible *S. aureus*

Contraindications Hypersensitivity to retapamulin or any component of the formulation

Warnings/Precautions For treatment of impetigo covering up to 100 cm^2 total area in adults. For external use only; not for intranasal, intravaginal, ophthalmic, oral, or mucosal application. May cause superinfection. Concomitant use with other topical products to the same treatment area has not been evaluated.

Adverse Reactions (Reflective of adult population; not specific for elderly)

1% to 10%:

Central nervous system: Headache (1% to 2%), pyrexia (1%)

Dermatologic: Pruritus (2%), eczema (1%)

Gastrointestinal: Diarrhea (1% to 2%), nausea (1%)

Local: Application site irritation (2%), application site pruritus (2%)

Respiratory: Nasopharyngitis (1% to 2%)

Overdosage/Toxicology Overdose has not been reported. Treatment should be symptom-directed and supportive.

Stability Store at room temperature of 15°C to 30°C (59°F to 86°F).

Mechanism of Action Primarily bacteriostatic. Inhibits normal bacterial protein biosynthesis by binding at a unique site (protein L3) on the ribosomal 50S subunit; prevents formation of active 50S ribosomal subunits by inhibiting peptidyl transfer and blocking P-site interactions at this site

Pharmacokinetics

Absorption: Topical: Low; increased when applied to abraded skin

Protein binding: 94%

Metabolism: Hepatic via CYP 3A4; extensively metabolized by mono-oxygenation and di-oxygenation to multiple metabolites

Dosage

Adults: Impetigo: Topical: Apply to affected area twice daily for 5 days. Total treatment area should not exceed 100 cm² total body surface area.

Administration Topical: May cover treatment area with sterile bandage or gauze dressing if needed. Concomitant use with other topical products to the same treatment area has not been evaluated.

Patient Information This medication is for external use only; do not swallow, and do not use in the eyes, on the mouth or lips, inside the nose, or inside the female genital area. Do not take any other prescription or over-the-counter medications or herbal products during therapy unless approved by prescriber. Use for the full time recommended by prescriber, even if symptoms have improved. Apply to affected area as directed; may cover treatment area with sterile bandage or gauze dressing. Wash hands thoroughly after applying (if hands are not the area for treatment). Report immediately if the application area worsens with increased irritation, redness, itching, burning, swelling, blistering, or oozing. Notify prescriber if there is no improvement in symptoms within 3-4 days after starting use.

Special Geriatric Considerations No specific recommendations for elderly patients.

Dosage Forms

Ointment, topical:

Altabax™: 1% (5 g, 10 g, 15 g)

Selected References

Parish LC, Jorizzo JL, Breton JJ, et al, "Topical Retapamulin Ointment (1%, wt/wt) Twice Daily for 5 Days Versus Oral Cephalexin Twice Daily for 10 Days in the Treatment of Secondarily Infected Dermatitis: Results of a Randomized Controlled Trial," *J Am Acad Dermatol*, 2006, 55(6):1003-13.

♦ **Retavase®** *see* Reteplase *on page 1395*

Reteplase (RE ta plase)

Medication Safety Issues

High alert medication: The Institute for Safe Medication Practices (ISMP) includes this medication (I.V.) among its list of drugs which have a heightened risk of causing significant patient harm when used in error.

U.S. Brand Names Retavase®

Canadian Brand Names Retavase®

Index Terms Recombinant Plasminogen Activator; r-PA

Generic Available No

Pharmacologic Category Thrombolytic Agent

Use Improvement of ventricular function following acute myocardial infarction, for the reduction of the incidence of CHF and the reduction of mortality associated with acute myocardial infarction

Contraindications Hypersensitivity to reteplase or any component of the formulation; active internal bleeding; history of cerebrovascular accident; recent intracranial or intraspinal surgery or trauma; intracranial neoplasm, arteriovenous malformations, or aneurysm; known bleeding diathesis; severe uncontrolled hypertension

Warnings/Precautions Concurrent heparin anticoagulation can contribute to bleeding; careful attention to all potential bleeding sites. I.M. injections and nonessential handling of the patient should be avoided. Venipunctures should be performed carefully and only when necessary. If arterial puncture is necessary, use an upper extremity vessel that can be manually compressed. If serious bleeding occurs then the infusion of anistreplase and heparin should be stopped.

For the following conditions the risk of bleeding is higher with use of reteplase and should be weighed against the benefits of therapy: recent major surgery (eg, CABG, obstetrical delivery, organ biopsy, previous puncture of noncompressible vessels), cerebrovascular disease, recent gastrointestinal or genitourinary bleeding, recent trauma including CPR, hypertension (systolic BP >180 mm Hg and/or diastolic BP >110 mm Hg), high likelihood of left heart thrombus (eg, mitral stenosis with atrial fibrillation), acute pericarditis, subacute bacterial endocarditis, hemostatic defects including ones caused by severe renal or hepatic dysfunction, significant hepatic dysfunction, diabetic hemorrhagic retinopathy or other hemorrhagic ophthalmic conditions, septic thrombophlebitis or occluded AV cannula at seriously infected site, advanced age (eg, >75 years), patients receiving oral anticoagulants, any other condition in which bleeding constitutes a significant hazard or would be particularly difficult to manage because of location.

Coronary thrombolysis may result in reperfusion arrhythmias. Follow standard MI management. Rare anaphylactic reactions can occur.

Adverse Reactions (Reflective of adult population; not specific for elderly)
Bleeding is the most frequent adverse effect associated with reteplase. Heparin and aspirin have been administered concurrently with reteplase in clinical trials. The incidence of adverse events is a reflection of these combined therapies, and are comparable with comparison thrombolytics.

(Continued)

Reteplase *(Continued)*

>10%: Local: Injection site bleeding (4.6% to 48.6%)

1% to 10%:

Gastrointestinal: Bleeding (1.8% to 9.0%)

Genitourinary: Bleeding (0.9% to 9.5%)

Hematologic: Anemia (0.9% to 2.6%)

Other adverse effects noted are frequently associated with MI (and therefore may or may not be attributable to Retavase®) and include arrhythmia, hypotension, cardiogenic shock, pulmonary edema, cardiac arrest, reinfarction, pericarditis, tamponade, thrombosis, and embolism.

Overdosage/Toxicology Symptoms include increased incidence of intracranial bleeding.

Drug Interactions

Aminocaproic acid (antifibrinolytic agent) may decrease effectiveness.

Drugs which affect platelet function (eg, NSAIDs, dipyridamole, ticlopidine, clopidogrel, IIb/IIIa antagonists) may potentiate the risk of hemorrhage; use with caution.

Heparin and aspirin: Use with aspirin and heparin may increase bleeding. However, aspirin and heparin were used concomitantly with reteplase in the majority of patients in clinical studies.

Warfarin or oral anticoagulants: Risk of bleeding may be increased during concurrent therapy.

Stability Dosage kits should be stored at 2°C to 25°C (36°F to 77°F) and remain sealed until use in order to protect from light. Reteplase should be reconstituted using the diluent, syringe, needle, and dispensing pin provided with each kit.

Mechanism of Action Reteplase is a nonglycosylated form of tPA produced by recombinant DNA technology using *E. coli*; it initiates local fibrinolysis by binding to fibrin in a thrombus (clot) and converts entrapped plasminogen to plasmin

Pharmacodynamics Onset of action: 30-90 minutes

Pharmacokinetics

Half-life: 13-16 minutes

Elimination: Hepatic and renal, cleared from the plasma at a rate of 250-450 mL/minute

Dosage

Geriatrics & Adults:

Acute MI (thrombolysis): I.V.: 10 units I.V. over 2 minutes, followed by a second dose 30 minutes later of 10 units I.V. over 2 minutes; withhold second dose if serious bleeding or anaphylaxis occurs.

Administration Reteplase should be reconstituted using the diluent, syringe, needle, and dispensing pin provided with each kit and the each reconstituted dose should be given I.V. over 2 minutes; no other medication should be added to the injection solution

Monitoring Parameters Monitor for signs of bleeding (hematuria, GI bleeding, gingival bleeding)

Additional Information The dosage of reteplase in clinical trials was expressed in terms of million unit (MU); however, reteplase is being marketed in units (U) with 1 unit equivalent to 1 million units, reteplase units are expressed using a reference standard specific for reteplase and are not comparable with units used for other thrombolytic agents, 10 units is equivalent to 17.4 mg

Special Geriatric Considerations No specific changes in use in the elderly are necessary.

Dosage Forms Excipient information presented when available (limited, particularly for generics); consult specific product labeling.

Injection, powder for reconstitution [preservative free]: 10.4 units [equivalent to reteplase 18.1 mg; contains sucrose and polysorbate 80; packaged with sterile water for injection]

Ribavirin (rye ba VYE rin)

Medication Safety Issues
Sound-alike/look-alike issues:
Ribavirin may be confused with riboflavin

U.S. Brand Names Copegus®; Rebetol®; RibaPak™; Ribasphere™; Virazole®

Canadian Brand Names Virazole®

Index Terms RTCA; Tribavirin

Generic Available Yes: Capsule, tablet

Pharmacologic Category Antiviral Agent

Use

Inhalation: Treatment of patients with respiratory syncytial virus (RSV) infections; may also be used in other viral infections including influenza A and B and adenovirus; specially indicated for treatment of severe lower respiratory tract RSV infections in patients with an underlying compromising condition (prematurity, bronchopulmonary dysplasia and other chronic lung conditions, congenital heart disease, immunodeficiency, immunosuppression), and recent transplant recipients

Oral capsule:

In combination with interferon alfa-2b (Intron® A) injection for the treatment of chronic hepatitis C in patients with compensated liver disease who have relapsed after alpha interferon therapy or were previously untreated with alpha interferons

In combination with peginterferon alfa-2b (PEG-Intron™) injection for the treatment of chronic hepatitis C in patients with compensated liver disease who were previously untreated with alpha interferons

Oral solution: In combination with interferon alfa 2b (Intron® A) injection for the treatment of chronic hepatitis C in patients ≥18 years of age who have relapsed after alpha interferon therapy

Oral tablet: In combination with peginterferon alfa-2a (Pegasys®) injection for the treatment of chronic hepatitis C in patients with compensated liver disease who were previously untreated with alpha interferons (includes patients with histological evidence of cirrhosis [Child-Pugh class A] and patients with clinically-stable HIV disease)

Unlabeled/Investigational Use Treatment of West Nile virus; hemorrhagic fever virus infections with renal syndrome (Lassa, Venezuelan, Korean hemorrhagic fever, Sabia, Argentian hemorrhagic fever, Bolivian hemorrhagic fever, Junin, Machupa)

Restrictions An FDA-approved medication guide must be distributed when dispensing an outpatient prescription (new or refill) for treatment of hepatitis C where this medication is to be used without direct supervision of a healthcare provider. Medication guides are available at http://www.fda.gov/cder/Offices/ODS/medication_guides.htm.

Contraindications Hypersensitivity to ribavirin or any component of the formulation

Additional contraindications for oral formulation: Male partners of pregnant women; $Cl_{cr} < 50$ mL/minute; hemoglobinopathies (eg, thalassemia major, sickle cell anemia); as monotherapy for treatment of chronic hepatitis C; patients with autoimmune hepatitis

Refer to individual monographs for Interferon Alfa-2b (Intron® A) and Peginterferon Alfa-2a (Pegasys®) for additional contraindication information.

Warnings/Precautions

Oral: Elderly patients are more susceptible to adverse effects; use caution. Safety and efficacy have not been established in patients who have failed other alpha interferon therapy, received organ transplants, or been coinfected with hepatitis B or HIV (Copegus® may be used in HIV coinfected patients unless CD4+ cell count is <100 cells/microL). **[U.S. Boxed Warning]: Monotherapy not effective for chronic hepatitis C infection.** Severe psychiatric events have occurred including depression and suicidal behavior during combination therapy. Avoid use in patients with a psychiatric history; discontinue if severe psychiatric symptoms occur.

[U.S. Boxed Warning]: Hemolytic anemia is a significant toxicity; usually occurring within 1-2 weeks; observed in ~10% of treated patients in clinical trials when alfa interferons were combined with ribavirin. Assess cardiac disease before initiation. Anemia may worsen underlying cardiac disease; avoid use in patients with significant/unstable cardiac disease. If deterioration in cardiovascular status occurs, discontinue therapy. Patients with renal dysfunction and/or those >50 years of age should be carefully assessed for development of anemia. Use caution in pulmonary disease; pulmonary symptoms have been associated with administration. Discontinue therapy in suspected/confirmed pancreatitis or if hepatic decompensation occurs. Use caution in patients with sarcoidosis (exacerbation reported). Dental and periodontal disorders have been reported with ribavirin and interferon therapy; patients should be instructed to brush teeth twice daily and have regular dental exams.

Inhalation: **[U.S. Boxed Warning]: Use with caution in patients requiring assisted ventilation because precipitation of the drug in the respiratory equipment may**
(Continued)

Ribavirin *(Continued)*

interfere with safe and effective patient ventilation; sudden deterioration of respiratory function has been observed; monitor carefully in patients with COPD and asthma for deterioration of respiratory function. Ribavirin is potentially mutagenic, tumor-promoting, and gonadotoxic. Although anemia has not been reported with inhalation therapy, consider monitoring for anemia 1-2 weeks post-treatment. Pregnant healthcare workers may consider unnecessary occupational exposure; ribavirin has been detected in healthcare workers' urine. Healthcare professionals or family members who are pregnant (or may become pregnant) should be counseled about potential risks of exposure and counseled about risk reduction strategies.

Adverse Reactions (Reflective of adult population; not specific for elderly)

Inhalation:

1% to 10%:

Central nervous system: Fatigue, headache, insomnia

Gastrointestinal: Nausea, anorexia

Hematologic: Anemia

Note: Incidence of adverse effects (approximate) in healthcare workers: Headache (51%); conjunctivitis (32%); rhinitis, nausea, rash, dizziness, pharyngitis, and lacrimation (10% to 20%)

Oral (all adverse reactions are documented while receiving combination therapy with interferon alpha-2b or interferon alpha-2a; percentages as reported in adults):

>10%:

Central nervous system: Fatigue (60% to 70%)*, headache (43% to 66%)*, fever (32% to 46%)*, insomnia (26% to 41%), depression (20% to 36%)*, irritability (23% to 32%), dizziness (14% to 26%), impaired concentration (10% to 14%)*, emotional lability (7% to 12%)*

Dermatologic: Alopecia (27% to 36%), pruritus (13% to 29%), dry skin (13% to 24%), rash (5% to 28%), dermatitis (up to 16%)

Gastrointestinal: Nausea (33% to 47%), anorexia (21% to 32%), weight decrease (10% to 29%), diarrhea (10% to 22%), dyspepsia (8% to 16%), vomiting (9% to 14%)*, abdominal pain (8% to 13%), xerostomia (up to 12%), RUQ pain (up to 12%)

Hematologic: Neutropenia (8% to 27%; 40% with HIV coinfection), hemoglobin decreased (25% to 36%), hyperbilirubinemia (24% to 34%), anemia (11% to 17%), lymphopenia (12% to 14%), absolute neutrophil count <0.5 x 10^9/L (5% to 11%), thrombocytopenia (<1% to 14%), hemolytic anemia (10% to 13%), WBC decreased

Neuromuscular & skeletal: Myalgia (40% to 64%)*, rigors (40% to 48%), arthralgia (22% to 34%)*, musculoskeletal pain (19% to 28%)

Respiratory: Dyspnea (13% to 26%), cough (7% to 23%), pharyngitis (up to 13%), sinusitis (up to 12%)*, nasal congestion

Miscellaneous: Flu-like syndrome (13% to 18%)*, viral infection (up to 12%), diaphoresis increased (up to 11%)

*Similar to interferon alone

1% to 10%:

Cardiovascular: Chest pain (5% to 9%)*, flushing (up to 4%)

Central nervous system: Mood alteration (up to 6%; 9% with HIV coinfection), memory impairment (up to 6%), malaise (up to 6%), nervousness (~5%)*

Dermatologic: Eczema (4% to 5%)

Endocrine & metabolic: Hypothyroidism (up to 5%)

Gastrointestinal: Taste perversion (4% to 9%), constipation (up to 5%)

Genitourinary: Menstrual disorder (up to 7%)

Hepatic: Hepatomegaly (up to 4%)

Neuromuscular & skeletal: Weakness (9% to 10%), back pain (5%)

Ocular: Conjunctivitis (up to 6%), blurred vision (up to 5%)

Respiratory: Rhinitis (up to 8%), exertional dyspnea (up to 7%)

Miscellaneous: Fungal infection (up to 6%)

*Similar to interferon alone

Note: Incidence of anorexia, headache, fever, suicidal ideation, and vomiting are higher in children.

Drug Interactions

Antiretroviral (nucleoside): Concomitant use of ribavirin and nucleoside analogues may increase the risk of developing lactic acidosis (includes adefovir, didanosine, lamivudine, stavudine, zalcitabine, zidovudine). Concurrent use with didanosine has been noted to increase the risk of pancreatitis, peripheral neuropathy in addition to lactic acidosis. Suspend therapy if signs/symptoms of toxicity are present.

Interferons (alfa): Concurrent therapy may increase the risk of hemolytic anemia.

Lamivudine, stavudine: Antagonistic *in vitro*; use with caution (per manufacturer)

Zidovudine: Antagonistic *in vitro*; use with caution (per manufacturer). Concurrent therapy with ribavirin/interferon alfa-2a may cause increased risk of severe anemia and/or severe neutropenia.

Ethanol/Nutrition/Herb Interactions Food: Oral: High-fat meal increases the AUC and C_{max}.

Stability

Inhalation: Store vials in a dry place at 15°C to 25°C (59°F to 78°F). Do not use any water containing an antimicrobial agent to reconstitute drug. Reconstituted solution is stable for 24 hours at room temperature. Should not be mixed with other aerosolized medication.

Oral: Store at 15°C to 30°C (59°F to 86°F). Solution may also be refrigerated at 2°C to 8°C (36°F to 46°F).

Mechanism of Action Inhibits replication of RNA and DNA viruses; inhibits influenza virus RNA polymerase activity and inhibits the initiation and elongation of RNA fragments resulting in inhibition of viral protein synthesis

Pharmacokinetics

Absorption: Rapidly and extensively absorbed

Distribution: V_d 2825 L (single dose)

Protein binding: None

Metabolism: Occurs intracellularly (reversible phosphorylation in nucleated cells); metabolized by the liver to deribosylated ribavirin (active metabolite)

Bioavailability: 64%

Half-life elimination, plasma:

Adults: Oral:

Capsule, single dose (Rebetol®, Ribasphere™): 24 hours in healthy adults, 44 hours with chronic hepatitis C infection (increases to ~298 hours at steady state)

Tablet, single dose (Copegus®): 120-170 hours

Time to peak: 3 hours (multiple dose)

Elimination: Urine (61%), feces (12%)

Dosage

Geriatrics & Adults:

Chronic hepatitis C (in combination with peginterferon alfa-2a): Oral tablet (Copegus®):

Monoinfection, genotype 1,4:

<75 kg: 1000 mg/day, in 2 divided doses

≥75 kg: 1200 mg/day, in 2 divided doses

Monoinfection, genotype 2,3: 800 mg/day, in 2 divided doses

Coinfection with HIV: 800 mg/day in 2 divided doses

Note: Treatment duration may vary. Consult current guidelines and literature.

Chronic hepatitis C (in combination with interferon alfa-2b): Oral capsule (Rebetol®, Ribasphere™):

≤75 kg: 400 mg in the morning, then 600 mg in the evening

>75 kg: 600 mg in the morning, then 600 mg in the evening

Note: Treatment duration may vary. Consult current guidelines and literature.

Chronic hepatitis C (in combination with peginterferon alfa-2b): Oral capsule (Rebetol®, Ribasphere™): 400 mg twice daily

Note: Treatment duration may vary. Consult current guidelines and literature.

Renal Impairment: Cl_{cr} <50 mL/minute: Oral is route contraindicated.

Administration Oral: Administer concurrently with interferon alfa injection.

Capsule, in combination with interferon alfa-2b: May be administered with or without food, but always in a consistent manner in regard to food intake.

Capsule, in combination with peginterferon alfa 2b: Administer with food.

Solution, in combination with interferon alfa-2b: May be administered with or without food, but always in a consistent manner in regard to food intake.

Tablet: Should be administered with food.

Healthcare professionals who are pregnant (or may become pregnant) should **not** handle the product.

Monitoring Parameters

Inhalation: Respiratory function, hemoglobin, reticulocyte count, CBC, I & O

Oral: Hemoglobin and hematocrit (pretreatment, 2 and 4 weeks after initiation); LFTs, TSH, serum HCV RNA ; pretreatment ECG in patients with pre-existing cardiac disease; dental exams

Reference Range

Early viral response (EVR): >2 log decrease in HCV RNA after 12 weeks of treatment

End of treatment response (ETR): Absence of detectable HCV RNA at end of the recommended treatment period

Sustained treatment response (STR): Absence of HCV RNA in the serum 6 months following completion of full treatment course

Patient Information Take as directed, for full course of therapy; do not discontinue even if you are feeling better. Use aerosol device as instructed. Maintain adequate fluid intake and report any swelling of ankles or feet, difficulty breathing, persistent lethargy, acute headache, insomnia, severe nausea or anorexia, confusion, fever, chills, sore throat, easy bruising or bleeding, mouth sores, or worsening of respiratory condition. (Continued)

Ribavirin *(Continued)*

Additional Information RSV season is usually December to April; viral shedding period for RSV is usually 3-8 days

Special Geriatric Considerations No specific recommendations are necessary in the elderly.

Dosage Forms Excipient information presented when available (limited, particularly for generics); consult specific product labeling.

Capsule: 200 mg
  Rebetol®, Ribasphere™: 200 mg
Powder for solution, inhalation [for aerosol administration]:
  Virazole®: 6 g [reconstituted product provides 20 mg/mL]
Solution, oral:
  Rebetol®: 40 mg/mL (100 mL) [contains sodium benzoate; bubble-gum flavor]
Tablet: 200 mg
  Copegus®: 200 mg
Tablet [dose pack]:
  RibaPak™: 400 mg (14s), 600 mg (14s)

♦ **Ridaura**® *see* Auranofin *on page 139*
♦ **Rid**® **Spray [OTC]** *see* Permethrin *on page 1235*

Rifabutin (rif a BYOO tin)

Medication Safety Issues
Sound-alike/look-alike issues:
  Rifabutin may be confused with rifampin

U.S. Brand Names Mycobutin®

Canadian Brand Names Mycobutin®

Index Terms Ansamycin

Generic Available No

Pharmacologic Category Antibiotic, Miscellaneous; Antitubercular Agent

Use Prevention of disseminated *Mycobacterium avium* complex (MAC) in patients with advanced HIV infection; included in multiple drug regimens for treatment of MAC

Contraindications Hypersensitivity to rifabutin, any other rifamycins, or any component of the formulation; rifabutin is contraindicated in patients with a WBC <1000/mm^3 or a platelet count <50,000/mm^3

Warnings/Precautions Rifabutin as a single agent must not be administered to patients with active tuberculosis since its use may lead to the development of tuberculosis that is resistant to both rifabutin and rifampin; rifabutin should be discontinued in patients with AST >500 units/L or if total bilirubin is >3 mg/dL. Use with caution in patients with liver impairment; modification of dosage should be considered in patients with renal impairment. Prolonged use may result in fungal or bacterial superinfection, including *C. difficile*-associated diarrhea and pseudomembranous colitis.

Adverse Reactions (Reflective of adult population; not specific for elderly)
>10%:
  Dermatologic: Rash (11%)
  Genitourinary: Discoloration of urine (30%)
  Hematologic: Neutropenia (25%), leukopenia (17%)
1% to 10%:
  Central nervous system: Headache (3%)
  Gastrointestinal: Vomiting/nausea (3%), abdominal pain (4%), diarrhea (3%), anorexia (2%), flatulence (2%), eructation (3%)
  Hematologic: Anemia, thrombocytopenia (5%)
  Hepatic: Increased AST/ALT (7% to 9%)
  Neuromuscular & skeletal: Myalgia

Overdosage/Toxicology Symptoms include nausea, vomiting, hepatotoxicity, lethargy, and CNS depression. Treatment is supportive. Hemodialysis will remove rifabutin, its effect on outcome is unknown.

Drug Interactions Substrate of CYP3A4 (major); **Induces** CYP3A4 (strong)

Alfentanil: Rifamycin derivatives may increase the metabolism, via CYP isoenzymes, of alfentanil.

Amiodarone: Rifamycin derivatives may increase the metabolism, via CYP isoenzymes, of amiodarone.

Angiotensin II receptor blockers (irbesartan, losartan): Rifamycin derivatives may increase the metabolism, via CYP isoenzymes, of angiotensin II receptor blockers.

Antiemetics (5-HT$_3$ antagonists): Rifamycin derivatives may increase the metabolism, via CYP isoenzymes, of antiemetics (5-HT$_3$ antagonists).

Antifungal agents (imidazole): Rifamycin derivatives may increase the metabolism, via CYP isoenzymes, of antifungal agents (imidazole). Antifungal agents (imidazole) may decrease the metabolism, via CYP isoenzymes, of rifabutin.

Aprepitant: Rifamycin derivatives may increase the metabolism, via CYP isoenzymes, of aprepitant.

Barbiturates: Rifamycin derivatives may increase the metabolism, via CYP isoenzymes, of barbiturates.

Benzodiazepines (metabolized by oxidation): Rifamycin derivatives may increase the metabolism, via CYP isoenzymes, of benzodiazepines (metabolized by oxidation).

Beta-blockers: Rifamycin derivatives may increase the metabolism, via CYP isoenzymes, of beta-blockers.

Buspirone: Rifamycin derivatives may increase the metabolism, via CYP isoenzymes, of buspirone.

Calcium channel blockers: Rifamycin derivatives may increase the metabolism, via CYP isoenzymes, of calcium channel blockers.

Clopidogrel: Rifamycin derivatives may enhance the therapeutic effect of clopidogrel.

Corticosteroids (systemic): Rifamycin derivatives may increase the metabolism, via CYP isoenzymes, of corticosteroids (systemic).

Cyclosporine: Rifamycin derivatives may increase the metabolism, via CYP isoenzymes, of cyclosporine.

CYP3A4 inducers: CYP3A4 inducers may decrease the levels/effects of rifabutin. Example inducers include aminoglutethimide, carbamazepine, nafcillin, nevirapine, phenobarbital, and phenytoin.

CYP3A4 substrates: Rifabutin may decrease the levels/effects of CYP3A4 substrates. Example substrates include benzodiazepines, calcium channel blockers, clarithromycin, cyclosporine, erythromycin, estrogens, mirtazapine, nateglinide, nefazodone, nevirapine, protease inhibitors, tacrolimus, and venlafaxine.

Dapsone: Rifamycin derivatives may increase the metabolism, via CYP isoenzymes, of dapsone.

Disopyramide: Rifamycin derivatives may increase the metabolism, via CYP isoenzymes, of disopyramide.

Estrogens (oral contraceptives): Rifamycin derivatives may decrease the serum concentration of oral contraceptive (estrogens); contraceptive failure is possible.

Fluconazole: Rifamycin derivatives may increase the metabolism, via CYP isoenzymes, of fluconazole. Fluconazole may decrease the metabolism, via CYP isoenzymes, of rifabutin.

Gefitinib: Rifamycin derivatives may increase the metabolism, via CYP isoenzymes, of gefitinib.

HMG-CoA reductase inhibitors: Rifamycin derivatives may increase the metabolism, via CYP isoenzymes, of HMG-CoA reductase inhibitors.

Isoniazid: Rifamycin derivatives may enhance the hepatotoxic effect of isoniazid; however, this is a frequently employed combination regimen.

Macrolide antibiotics: Macrolide antibiotics may decrease the metabolism, via CYP isoenzymes, of rifamycin derivatives.

Morphine: Rifamycin derivatives may decrease the serum concentration of morphine sulfate.

Phenytoin: Rifamycin derivatives may increase the metabolism, via CYP isoenzymes, of phenytoin.

Progestins (contraceptives): Rifamycin derivatives may decrease the serum concentration of contraceptives (progestins); contraceptive failure is possible.

Propafenone: Rifamycin derivatives may increase the metabolism, via CYP isoenzymes, of propafenone.

Protease inhibitors: Rifamycin derivatives may increase the metabolism, via CYP isoenzymes, of protease inhibitors. Protease inhibitors may decrease the metabolism, via CYP isoenzymes, of rifabutin. Dosage adjustments of both rifabutin and the protease inhibitors are necessary if used together.

Quinidine: Rifamycin derivatives may increase the metabolism, via CYP isoenzymes, of quinidine.

Repaglinide: Rifamycin derivatives may increase the metabolism, via CYP isoenzymes, of repaglinide.

Reverse transcriptase inhibitors (non-nucleoside): Rifamycin derivatives may increase the metabolism, via CYP isoenzymes, of reverse transcriptase inhibitors (non-nucleoside).

Tacrolimus: Rifamycin derivatives may increase the metabolism, via CYP isoenzymes, of tacrolimus.

Tamoxifen: Rifamycin derivatives may increase the metabolism, via CYP isoenzymes, of tamoxifen.

Terbinafine: Rifamycin derivatives may increase the metabolism of terbinafine.

Tocainide: Rifamycin derivatives may increase the metabolism, via CYP isoenzymes, of tocainide.

Tricyclic antidepressants: Rifamycin derivatives may increase the metabolism, via CYP isoenzymes, of tricyclic antidepressants.

Warfarin: Rifamycin derivatives may increase the metabolism, via CYP isoenzymes, of warfarin.

(Continued)

Rifabutin *(Continued)*

Zaleplon: Rifamycin derivatives may increase the metabolism, via CYP isoenzymes, of zaleplon.

Zolpidem: Rifamycin derivatives may increase the metabolism, via CYP isoenzymes, of zolpidem.

Ethanol/Nutrition/Herb Interactions Food: High-fat meal may decrease the rate but not the extent of absorption.

Mechanism of Action Inhibits DNA-dependent RNA polymerase at the beta subunit which prevents chain initiation

Pharmacokinetics

Absorption: Oral: Readily absorbed 53%

Distribution: V_d: 9.32 L/kg; distributes to body tissues including the lungs, liver, spleen, eyes, and kidneys

Protein binding: 85%

Metabolism: Hepatic to active and inactive metabolites

Bioavailability: Absolute, 20% in HIV patients

Half-life, terminal: 45 hours (range: 16-69 hours)

Peak serum concentration: Within 2-4 hours

Elimination: Renal and biliary clearance of unchanged drug is 10%; 30% excreted in feces; 53% in urine unchanged

Dosage

Geriatrics & Adults:

Disseminated MAC in advanced HIV infection:

Prophylaxis: Oral: 300 mg once daily (alone or in combination with azithromycin)

Treatment (unlabeled use): Oral:

Patients not receiving NNRTIs or protease inhibitors:

Initial phase: 5 mg/kg daily (maximum: 300 mg)

Second phase: 5 mg/kg daily or twice weekly

Dosage adjustment for concurrent nelfinavir, amprenavir, indinavir: Reduce rifabutin dose to 150 mg/day; no change in dose if administered twice weekly

Dosage adjustment for concurrent efavirenz (no concomitant protease inhibitor): Increase rifabutin dose to 450-600 mg daily, or 600 mg 3 times/week

Renal Impairment: Cl_{cr} <30 mL/minute: Reduce dose by 50%

Administration May be mixed with food (ie, applesauce)

Monitoring Parameters Periodic liver function tests, CBC with differential, platelet count, hemoglobin, hematocrit

Patient Information May discolor urine, tears, sweat, or other body fluids to a red-orange color; soft contact lenses may be permanently stained; report to physician any severe or persistent flu-like symptoms, nausea, vomiting, dark urine or pale stools, or unusual bleeding or bruising; can be taken with meals or sprinkled on applesauce

Special Geriatric Considerations No specific recommendations for the elderly.

Dosage Forms Excipient information presented when available (limited, particularly for generics); consult specific product labeling.

Capsule: 150 mg

Extemporaneously Prepared Rifabutin is insoluble in water and ethanol; prepare powder packets or compound with a suspending agent and shake well before using

- ◆ **Rifadin**® *see* Rifampin *on page 1402*
- ◆ **Rifampicin** *see* Rifampin *on page 1402*

Rifampin *(rif AM pin)*

Related Information

Antibiotic Treatment of Adults With Infective Endocarditis *on page 1797*

Antimicrobial Activity Against Selected Organisms *on page 1728*

Medication Safety Issues

Sound-alike/look-alike issues:

Rifampin may be confused with rifabutin, Rifamate®, rifapentine, rifaximin

Rifadin® may be confused with Ritalin®

U.S. Brand Names Rifadin®

Canadian Brand Names Rifadin®; Rofact™

Index Terms Rifampicin

Generic Available Yes

Pharmacologic Category Antibiotic, Miscellaneous; Antitubercular Agent

Use Management of active tuberculosis; eliminate meningococci from the nasopharnx in asymptomatic carriers; prophylaxis of *Haemophilus influenzae* type b infection; used in combination therapy against *Staphylococcus aureus*; used with oral vancomycin for resistant *C. difficile* diarrhea

Contraindications Hypersensitivity to rifampin, any rifamycins, or any component of the formulation; concurrent use of amprenavir, saquinavir/ritonavir (possibly other protease inhibitors)

Warnings/Precautions Use with caution and modify dosage in patients with liver impairment; observe for hyperbilirubinemia; discontinue therapy if this in conjunction with clinical symptoms or any signs of significant hepatocellular damage develop; since rifampin has enzyme-inducing properties, porphyria exacerbation is possible; use with caution in patients with porphyria; do not use for meningococcal disease, only for short-term treatment of asymptomatic carrier states

Monitor for compliance and effects including hypersensitivity, thrombocytopenia in patients on intermittent therapy; urine, feces, saliva, sweat, tears, and CSF may be discolored to red/orange; do not administer I.V. form via I.M. or SubQ routes; restart infusion at another site if extravasation occurs; remove soft contact lenses during therapy since permanent staining may occur; regimens of 600 mg once or twice weekly have been associated with a high incidence of adverse reactions including a flu-like syndrome. Prolonged use may result in fungal or bacterial superinfection, including *C. difficile*-associated diarrhea and pseudomembranous colitis.

Adverse Reactions (Reflective of adult population; not specific for elderly)
Frequency not defined:
Cardiovascular: Edema, flushing
Central nervous system: Ataxia, behavioral changes, concentration impaired, confusion, dizziness, drowsiness, fatigue, fever, headache, numbness, psychosis
Dermatologic: Pemphigoid reaction, pruritus, urticaria
Endocrine & metabolic: Adrenal insufficiency, menstrual disorders
Hematologic: Agranulocytosis (rare), DIC, eosinophilia, hemoglobin decreased, hemolysis, hemolytic anemia, leukopenia, thrombocytopenia (especially with high-dose therapy)
Hepatic: Hepatitis (rare), jaundice
Neuromuscular & skeletal: Myalgia, osteomalacia, weakness
Ocular: Exudative conjunctivitis, visual changes
Renal: Acute renal failure, BUN increased, hemoglobinuria, hematuria, interstitial nephritis, uric acid increased
Miscellaneous: Flu-like syndrome
1% to 10%:
Dermatologic: Rash (1% to 5%)
Gastrointestinal (1% to 2%): Anorexia, cramps, diarrhea, epigastric distress, flatulence, heartburn, nausea, pseudomembranous colitis, pancreatitis vomiting
Hepatic: LFTs increased (up to 14%)

Overdosage/Toxicology Symptoms include nausea, vomiting, and hepatotoxicity. Treatment is supportive. Lavage with activated charcoal is preferred to ipecac, as emesis is frequently present with overdose. Hemodialysis will remove rifampin, but its effect on outcome is unknown.

Drug Interactions Induces CYP1A2 (strong), 2A6 (strong), 2B6 (strong), 2C8 (strong), 2C9 (strong), 2C19 (strong), 3A4 (strong)
Acetaminophen: Rifampin may increase the metabolism of acetaminophen.
Alfentanil: Rifamycin derivatives may increase the metabolism, via CYP isoenzymes, of alfentanil.
Amiodarone: Rifamycin derivatives may increase the metabolism, via CYP isoenzymes, of amiodarone
Angiotensin II receptor blockers (irbesartan, losartan): Rifamycin derivatives may increase the metabolism, via CYP isoenzymes, of angiotensin II receptor blockers.
Antiemetics (5-HT$_3$ antagonists): Rifamycin derivatives may increase the metabolism, via CYP isoenzymes, of antiemetics (5-HT$_3$ antagonists).
Antifungal Agents (imidazole): Rifamycin derivatives may increase the metabolism, via CYP isoenzymes, of antifungal agents (imidazole).
Aprepitant: Rifamycin derivatives may increase the metabolism, via CYP isoenzymes, of aprepitant.
Barbiturates: Rifamycin derivatives may increase the metabolism, via CYP isoenzymes, of barbiturates.
Benzodiazepines (metabolized by oxidation): Rifamycin derivatives may increase the metabolism, via CYP isoenzymes, of benzodiazepines (metabolized by oxidation).
Beta-blockers: Rifamycin derivatives may increase the metabolism, via CYP isoenzymes, of beta-blockers.
Buspirone: Rifamycin derivatives may increase the metabolism, via CYP isoenzymes, of buspirone.
Calcium channel blockers: Rifamycin derivatives may increase the metabolism, via CYP isoenzymes, of calcium channel blockers.
Chloramphenicol: Rifampin may increase the metabolism, via CYP isoenzymes, of chloramphenicol.
Clopidogrel: Rifamycin derivatives may enhance the therapeutic effect of Clopidogrel.
(Continued)

Rifampin *(Continued)*

Corticosteroids (systemic): Rifamycin derivatives may increase the metabolism, via CYP isoenzymes, of corticosteroids (systemic).

Cyclosporine: Rifamycin derivatives may increase the metabolism, via CYP isoenzymes, of cyclosporine.

CYP1A2 substrates: Rifampin may decrease the levels/effects of CYP1A2 substrates. Example substrates include aminophylline, estrogens, fluvoxamine, mirtazapine, ropinirole, and theophylline.

CYP2A6 substrates: Rifampin may decrease the levels/effects of CYP2A6 substrates (eg, ifosfamide).

CYP2B6 substrates: Rifampin may decrease the levels/effects of CYP2B6 substrates. Example substrates include bupropion, efavirenz, promethazine, selegiline, and sertraline.

CYP2C8 substrates: Rifampin may decrease the levels/effects of CYP2C8 substrates. Example substrates include amiodarone, paclitaxel, pioglitazone, repaglinide, and rosiglitazone.

CYP2C9 substrates: Rifampin may decrease the levels/effects of CYP2C9 substrates. Example substrates include bosentan, celecoxib, dapsone, fluoxetine, glimepiride, glipizide, losartan, montelukast, nateglinide, paclitaxel, phenytoin, sulfonamides, trimethoprim, warfarin, and zafirlukast.

CYP2C19 substrates: Rifampin may decrease the levels/effects of CYP2C19 substrates. Example substrates include citalopram, diazepam, methsuximide, phenytoin, propranolol, proton pump inhibitors, sertraline, and voriconazole.

CYP3A4 substrates: Rifampin may decrease the levels/effects of CYP3A4 substrates. Example substrates include benzodiazepines, calcium channel blockers, clarithromycin, cyclosporine, erythromycin, estrogens, mirtazapine, nateglinide, nefazodone, nevirapine, protease inhibitors, tacrolimus, and venlafaxine.

Dapsone: Rifamycin derivatives may increase the metabolism, via CYP isoenzymes, of dapsone.

Disopyramide: Rifamycin derivatives may increase the metabolism, via CYP isoenzymes, of disopyramide.

Estrogens (oral contraceptives): Rifamycin derivatives may decrease the serum concentration of oral contraceptive (estrogens); contraceptive failure is possible.

Fexofenadine: Rifampin may decrease the serum concentration of fexofenadine.

Fluconazole: Rifamycin derivatives may increase the metabolism, via CYP isoenzymes, of fluconazole.

Fusidic Acid: Rifampin may decrease the excretion of fusidic acid.

Gefitinib: Rifamycin derivatives may increase the metabolism, via CYP isoenzymes, of gefitinib.

HMG-CoA reductase inhibitors: Rifamycin derivatives may increase the metabolism, via CYP isoenzymes, of HMG-CoA reductase inhibitors.

Isoniazid: Rifamycin derivatives may enhance the hepatotoxic effect of isoniazid; however, this is a frequently employed combination regimen.

Macrolide antibiotics: Macrolide antibiotics may decrease the metabolism, via CYP isoenzymes, of rifamycin derivatives.

Methadone: Rifamycin derivatives may increase the metabolism, via CYP isoenzymes, of methadone.

Morphine: Rifamycin derivatives may decrease the serum concentration of morphine sulfate.

Phenytoin: Rifamycin derivatives may increase the metabolism, via CYP isoenzymes, of phenytoin.

Progestins (contraceptives): Rifamycin derivatives may decrease the serum concentration of contraceptive (progestins); contraceptive failure is possible.

Propafenone: Rifamycin derivatives may increase the metabolism, via CYP isoenzymes, of propafenone.

Protease inhibitors: Rifamycin derivatives may increase the metabolism, via CYP isoenzymes, of protease inhibitors. Concurrent use with saquinavir/ritonavir increases risk of hepatotoxicity. Rifampin administration should be avoided.

Pyrazinamide: Pyrazinamide may enhance the hepatotoxic effect of rifampin.

Quinidine: Rifamycin derivatives may increase the metabolism, via CYP isoenzymes, of quinidine.

Repaglinide: Rifamycin derivatives may increase the metabolism, via CYP isoenzymes, of repaglinide.

Reverse transcriptase inhibitors (non-nucleoside): Rifamycin derivatives may increase the metabolism, via CYP isoenzymes, of reverse transcriptase inhibitors (non-nucleoside).

Sulfonylureas: Rifampin may increase the metabolism, via CYP isoenzymes, of sulfonylureas.

Tacrolimus: Rifamycin derivatives may increase the metabolism, via CYP isoenzymes, of tacrolimus.

Tamoxifen: Rifamycin derivatives may increase the metabolism, via CYP isoenzymes, of tamoxifen.

Terbinafine: Rifamycin derivatives may increase the metabolism of terbinafine.

Tocainide: Rifamycin derivatives may increase the metabolism, via CYP isoenzymes, of tocainide.

Tricyclic antidepressants: Rifamycin derivatives may increase the metabolism, via CYP isoenzymes, of tricyclic antidepressants.

Warfarin: Rifamycin derivatives may increase the metabolism, via CYP isoenzymes, of warfarin.

Zaleplon: Rifamycin derivatives may increase the metabolism, via CYP isoenzymes, of zaleplon.

Zidovudine: Rifamycin derivatives may increase the metabolism, via CYP isoenzymes, of zidovudine.

Zolpidem: Rifamycin derivatives may increase the metabolism, via CYP isoenzymes, of zolpidem.

Ethanol/Nutrition/Herb Interactions

Ethanol: Avoid ethanol (may increase risk of hepatotoxicity).

Food: Food decreases the extent of absorption; rifampin concentrations may be decreased if taken with food.

Herb/Nutraceutical: St John's wort may decrease rifampin levels.

Stability Rifampin powder is reddish brown. Intact vials should be stored at room temperature and protected from excessive heat and light. Reconstitute powder for injection with SWFI. Prior to injection, dilute in appropriate volume of compatible diluent (eg, 100 mL D$_5$W). Reconstituted vials are stable for 24 hours at room temperature.

Stability of parenteral admixture at room temperature (25°C) is 4 hours for D$_5$W and 24 hours for NS.

Mechanism of Action Inhibits bacterial RNA synthesis by binding to the beta subunit of DNA-dependent RNA polymerase, blocking RNA transcription

Pharmacodynamics

Peak serum concentrations: Within 2-4 hours

Duration: Up to 24 hours

Pharmacokinetics

Absorption: Oral: Well absorbed

Half-life: 3-4 hours, prolonged with hepatic impairment

Protein binding: 80%

Metabolism: Hepatic

Highly lipophilic; crosses the blood-brain barrier well, undergoes enterohepatic recycling

Time to peak serum concentration: Within 2-4 hours; food may delay or slightly reduce peak serum concentration

Elimination: Principally in feces (60% to 65%) and urine (~30%)

Plasma rifampin concentrations are not significantly affected by hemodialysis or peritoneal dialysis

In a small (n=6) single-dose study, rifampin's pharmacokinetic parameters in older adult subjects were not significantly different compared to values of younger subjects reported in the literature

Dosage

Geriatrics & Adults:

Tuberculosis therapy (drug susceptible): Oral, I.V.: **Note:** A four-drug regimen (isoniazid, rifampin, pyrazinamide, and ethambutol) is preferred for the initial, empiric treatment of TB. When the drug susceptibility results are available, the regimen should be altered as appropriate.

Daily therapy: 10 mg/kg/day (maximum: 600 mg/day)

Twice weekly directly observed therapy (DOT): 10 mg/kg (maximum: 600 mg); 3 times/week: 10 mg/kg (maximum: 600 mg)

Latent tuberculosis infection (LTBI): As an alternative to isoniazid: Oral, I.V.: 10 mg/kg/day (maximum: 600 mg/day) for 4 months. **Note:** Combination with pyrazinamide should not generally be offered (*MMWR*, Aug 8, 2003).

H. influenzae **prophylaxis (unlabeled use):** Oral, I.V.: 600 mg every 24 hours for 4 days

Leprosy (unlabeled use): Oral, I.V.:

Multibacillary: 600 mg once monthly for 24 months in combination with ofloxacin and minocycline

Paucibacillary: 600 mg once monthly for 6 months in combination with dapsone

Single lesion: 600 mg as a single dose in combination with ofloxacin 400 mg and minocycline 100 mg

Meningococcal meningitis prophylaxis: Oral, I.V.: 600 mg every 12 hours for 2 days

Meningitis (*Pneumococcus* or *Staphylococcus*): I.V.: 600 mg once daily

Nasal carriers of *Staphylococcus aureus* (unlabeled use): Oral, I.V.: 600 mg/day for 5-10 days in combination with other antibiotics

(Continued)

Rifampin *(Continued)*

Synergy for *Staphylococcus aureus* infections (unlabeled use): Oral, I.V.: 300-600 mg twice daily with other antibiotics

Renal Impairment: Plasma rifampin concentrations are not significantly affected by hemodialysis or peritoneal dialysis.

Hepatic Impairment: Dose reductions are necessary to reduce hepatotoxicity.

Administration Administer on an empty stomach (ie, 1 hour prior to, or 2 hours after meals) to increase total absorption

Monitoring Parameters Periodic (baseline and every 2-4 weeks during therapy) monitoring of liver function (AST, ALT, bilirubin), CBC; hepatic status and mental status, sputum culture, chest x-ray 2-3 months into treatment

Test Interactions Positive Coombs' reaction [direct], rifampin inhibits standard assay's ability to measure serum folate and B_{12}; transient increase in LFTs and decreased biliary excretion of contrast media

Patient Information May discolor urine, tears, sweat, or other body fluids to a red-orange color; take 1 hour before or 2 hours after a meal on an empty stomach; soft contact lenses may be permanently stained

Additional Information Since resistant strains occur rapidly, is normally used with other anti-TB drugs

Special Geriatric Considerations Rifampin, in combination with isoniazid, is the foundation of tuberculosis treatment. Since most older patients acquired their *Mycobacterium tuberculosis* infection before effective chemotherapy was available, either a 9-month regimen of isoniazid and rifampin or a 6-month regimen of isoniazid and rifampin with pyrazinamide (the first 2 months) should be effective.

Dosage Forms Excipient information presented when available (limited, particularly for generics); consult specific product labeling.

Capsule: 150 mg, 300 mg

Injection, powder for reconstitution: 600 mg

Selected References

Advenier C, Gobert C, Houin G, et al, "Pharmacokinetic Studies of Rifampicin in the Elderly," *Ther Drug Monit*, 1983, 5(1):61-5.

American Thoracic Society, "Targeted Tuberculin Testing and Treatment of Latent Tuberculosis Infection," *MMWR*, 2000, 49(RR-6):1-51.

Bass JB Jr, Farer LS, Hopewell PC, et al, "Treatment of Tuberculosis and Tuberculosis Infection in Adults and Children," *Am J Respir Crit Care Med*, 1994, 149(5):1359-74.

Blumberg HM, Burman WJ, Chaisson RE, et al, "American Thoracic Society/Centers for Disease Control and Prevention/Infectious Diseases Society of America: Treatment of Tuberculosis," *Am J Respir Crit Care Med*, 2003, 167(4):603-62.

Centers for Disease Control, "Update: Adverse Event Data and Revised American Thoracic Society/CDC Recommendations Against the Use of Rifampin and Pyrazinamide for Treatment of Latent Tuberculosis Infection - United States, 2003," *MMWR*, 52(31);735-9. Available at http://www.cdc.gov/mmwr/preview/mmwrhtml/mm5231a4.htm. Last accessed February 16, 2005.

"Treatment of Latent Tuberculosis Infection (LTBI), Last Updated: April 8, 2004," available at http://www.cdc.gov/nchstp/tb/pubs/tbfactsheets/250110.htm. Last accessed February 16, 2005.

Van Scoy RE and Wilkowske CJ, "Antituberculosis Agents," *Mayo Clin Proc*, 1992, 67(2):179-87.

Yoshikawa TT, "Tuberculosis in Aging Adults," *J Am Geriatr Soc*, 1992, 40(2):178-87.

Rifapentine *(rif a PEN teen)*

Medication Safety Issues

Sound-alike/look-alike issues:

Rifapentine may be confused with rifampin

U.S. Brand Names Priftin®

Canadian Brand Names Priftin®

Generic Available No

Pharmacologic Category Antitubercular Agent

Use Treatment of pulmonary tuberculosis (indication is based on the 6-month follow-up treatment outcome observed in controlled clinical trial). Rifapentine must always be used in conjunction with at least one other antituberculosis drug to which the isolate is susceptible; it may also be necessary to add a third agent (either streptomycin or ethambutol) until susceptibility is known.

Contraindications Hypersensitivity to rifapentine, rifampin, rifabutin, any rifamycin analog, or any component of the formulation

Warnings/Precautions Patients with abnormal liver tests and/or liver disease should only be given rifapentine when absolutely necessary and under strict medical supervision. If signs of liver disease occur or worsen, rifapentine should be discontinued. Experience in treating TB in HIV-infected patients is limited.

Rifapentine may produce a red-orange discoloration of body tissues/fluids including skin, teeth, tongue, urine, feces, saliva, sputum, tears, sweat, and cerebral spinal fluid. Contact lenses may become permanently stained. All patients treated with rifapentine should have baseline measurements of liver function tests and enzymes, bilirubin, and a complete blood count. Patients should be seen and monitored monthly and specifically questioned regarding symptoms associated with adverse reactions. Routine laboratory monitoring in people with normal baseline measurements is generally not necessary.

Adverse Reactions (Reflective of adult population; not specific for elderly)

>10%: Endocrine & metabolic: Hyperuricemia (most likely due to pyrazinamide from initiation phase combination therapy)

1% to 10%:

Cardiovascular: Hypertension

Central nervous system: Headache, dizziness

Dermatologic: Rash, pruritus, acne

Gastrointestinal: Anorexia, nausea, vomiting, dyspepsia, diarrhea

Hematologic: Neutropenia, lymphopenia, anemia, leukopenia, thrombocytosis

Hepatic: Increased ALT/AST

Neuromuscular & skeletal: Arthralgia, pain

Renal: Pyuria, proteinuria, hematuria, urinary casts

Respiratory: Hemoptysis

Overdosage/Toxicology There is no experience with treatment of acute overdose. Experience with other rifamycins suggests that gastric lavage, followed by activated charcoal, may help adsorb any remaining drug from the GI tract. Hemodialysis or forced diuresis is not expected to enhance elimination of unchanged rifapentine in an overdose.

Drug Interactions Induces CYP2C8 (strong), 2C9 (strong), 3A4 (strong)

Alfentanil: Rifamycin derivatives may increase the metabolism, via CYP isoenzymes, of alfentanil.

Amiodarone: Rifamycin derivatives may increase the metabolism, via CYP isoenzymes, of amiodarone.

Angiotensin II receptor blockers (irbesartan and losartan): Rifamycin derivatives may increase the metabolism, via CYP isoenzymes, of angiotensin II receptor blockers.

Antiemetics (5-HT$_3$ antagonists): Rifamycin derivatives may increase the metabolism, via CYP isoenzymes, of Antiemetics (5-HT$_3$ antagonists).

Antifungal agents (imidazole): Rifamycin derivatives may increase the metabolism, via CYP isoenzymes, of antifungal agents (imidazole).

Aprepitant: Rifamycin derivatives may increase the metabolism, via CYP isoenzymes, of aprepitant.

Barbiturates: Rifamycin derivatives may increase the metabolism, via CYP isoenzymes, of barbiturates.

Benzodiazepines (metabolized by oxidation): Rifamycin derivatives may increase the metabolism, via CYP isoenzymes, of benzodiazepines (metabolized by oxidation).

Beta-blockers: Rifamycin derivatives may increase the metabolism, via CYP isoenzymes, of beta-blockers.

Buspirone: Rifamycin derivatives may increase the metabolism, via CYP isoenzymes, of buspirone.

Calcium channel blockers: Rifamycin derivatives may increase the metabolism, via CYP isoenzymes, of calcium channel blockers.

Clopidogrel: Rifamycin derivatives may enhance the therapeutic effect of clopidogrel.

Corticosteroids (systemic): Rifamycin derivatives may increase the metabolism, via CYP isoenzymes, of corticosteroids (systemic).

Cyclosporine: Rifamycin derivatives may increase the metabolism, via CYP isoenzymes, of cyclosporine.

CYP2C8 Substrates: Rifapentine may decrease the levels/effects of CYP2C8 substrates. Example substrates include amiodarone, paclitaxel, pioglitazone, repaglinide, and rosiglitazone.

CYP2C9 Substrates: Rifapentine may decrease the levels/effects of CYP2C9 substrates. Example substrates include bosentan, celecoxib, dapsone, fluoxetine, glimepiride, glipizide, losartan, montelukast, nateglinide, paclitaxel, phenytoin, sulfonamides, trimethoprim, warfarin, and zafirlukast.

CYP3A4 substrates: Rifapentine may decrease the levels/effects of CYP3A4 substrates. Example substrates include benzodiazepines, calcium channel blockers, clarithromycin, cyclosporine, erythromycin, estrogens, mirtazapine, nateglinide, nefazodone, nevirapine, protease inhibitors, tacrolimus, and venlafaxine.

Dapsone: Rifamycin derivatives may increase the metabolism, via CYP isoenzymes, of dapsone.

Disopyramide: Rifamycin derivatives may increase the metabolism, via CYP isoenzymes, of disopyramide.

Estrogens (oral contraceptives): Rifamycin derivatives may decrease the serum concentration of oral contraceptive (estrogens); contraceptive failure is possible.

Fluconazole: Rifamycin derivatives may increase the metabolism, via CYP isoenzymes, of fluconazole.

Gefitinib: Rifamycin derivatives may increase the metabolism, via CYP isoenzymes, of gefitinib.

(Continued)

Rifapentine *(Continued)*

HMG-CoA reductase inhibitors: Rifamycin derivatives may increase the metabolism, via CYP isoenzymes, of HMG-CoA reductase inhibitors.

Isoniazid: Rifamycin derivatives may enhance the hepatotoxic effect of isoniazid; however, this is a frequently employed combination regimen.

Methadone: Rifamycin derivatives may increase the metabolism, via CYP isoenzymes, of methadone.

Morphine: Rifamycin derivatives may decrease the serum concentration of morphine sulfate.

Phenytoin: Rifamycin derivatives may increase the metabolism, via CYP isoenzymes, of phenytoin.

Progestins (contraceptives): Rifamycin derivatives may decrease the serum concentration of contraceptive (progestins); contraceptive failure is possible.

Propafenone: Rifamycin derivatives may increase the metabolism, via CYP isoenzymes, of propafenone.

Protease inhibitors: Rifamycin derivatives may increase the metabolism, via CYP isoenzymes, of protease inhibitors.

Quinidine: Rifamycin derivatives may increase the metabolism, via CYP isoenzymes, of quinidine.

Repaglinide: Rifamycin derivatives may increase the metabolism, via CYP isoenzymes, of repaglinide.

Reverse Transcriptase inhibitors (non-nucleoside): Rifamycin derivatives may increase the metabolism, via CYP isoenzymes, of reverse transcriptase inhibitors (non-nucleoside).

Tacrolimus: Rifamycin derivatives may increase the metabolism, via CYP isoenzymes, of tacrolimus.

Tamoxifen: Rifamycin derivatives may increase the metabolism, via CYP isoenzymes, of tamoxifen.

Terbinafine: Rifamycin derivatives may increase the metabolism of terbinafine.

Tocainide: Rifamycin derivatives may increase the metabolism, via CYP isoenzymes, of tocainide.

Tricyclic antidepressants: Rifamycin derivatives may increase the metabolism, via CYP isoenzymes, of tricyclic antidepressants.

Ethanol/Nutrition/Herb Interactions Food: Food increases AUC and maximum serum concentration by 43% and 44% respectively as compared to fasting conditions.

Stability Store at room temperature (15°C to 30°C; 59°F to 86°F). Protect from excessive heat and humidity.

Mechanism of Action Inhibits DNA-dependent RNA polymerase in susceptible strains of *Mycobacterium tuberculosis* (but not in mammalian cells). Rifapentine is bactericidal against both intracellular and extracellular MTB organisms. MTB resistant to other rifamycins including rifampin are likely to be resistant to rifapentine. Cross-resistance does not appear between rifapentine and other nonrifamycin antimycobacterial agents.

Pharmacokinetics

Absorption: Food increases AUC and C_{max} by 43% and 44% respectively.

Distribution: V_d: ~70.2 L

Metabolism: Hydrolyzed by an esterase and esterase enzyme to form the active metabolite 25-desacetyl rifapentine

Protein binding: Rifapentine and 25-desacetyl metabolite were 97.7% and 93.2% protein bound (mainly to albumin). Rifapentine and metabolite accumulate in human monocyte-derived macrophages with intracellular/extracellular ratios of 24:1 and 7:1 respectively.

Half-life: Rifapentine: 14-17 hours; 25-desacetyl rifapentine: 13 hours

Bioavailability: ~70%

Time to peak serum concentration: 5-6 hours

Elimination: Extent of renal excretion is unknown; excreted as parent drug and metabolite; 17% of administered dose is excreted via the kidneys

Dosage

Geriatrics & Adults: Note: Rifapentine should not be used alone; initial phase should include a 3- to 4-drug regimen.

Tuberculosis, intensive phase (initial 2 months) of short-term therapy: 600 mg (four 150 mg tablets) given twice weekly (with an interval of not less than 72 hours between doses); following the intensive phase, treatment should continue with rifapentine 600 mg once weekly for 4 months in combination with INH or appropriate agent for susceptible organisms.

Monitoring Parameters Patients with pre-existing hepatic problems should have liver function tests monitored every 2-4 weeks during therapy

Test Interactions Rifampin has been shown to inhibit standard microbiological assays for serum folate and vitamin B_{12}; this should be considered for rifapentine; therefore, alternative assay methods should be considered.

Patient Information May produce a reddish coloration of urine, sweat, sputum, tears; contact lenses may be permanently stained. Administration of rifapentine with food may decrease GI intolerance. Notify physician if experiencing fever, decreased appetite, malaise, nausea/vomiting, darkened urine, yellowish discoloration of skin or eyes, and pain or swelling of joints. Adherence to the full course of therapy is essential; no doses of therapy should be missed.

Additional Information Rifapentine has only been studied in patients with tuberculosis receiving a 6-month short-course intensive regimen approval; outcomes have been based on 6-month follow-up treatment observed in clinical trial 008 as a surrogate for the 2-year follow-up generally accepted as evidence for efficacy in the treatment of pulmonary tuberculosis

Dosage Forms Excipient information presented when available (limited, particularly for generics); consult specific product labeling.
Tablet: 150 mg

Selected References

Grosser J, Lounis N, Truffot-Pernot C, et al, "Once Weekly Rifapentine-Containing Regimens for Treatment of Tuberculosis in Mice," *Am J Respir Crit Care Med*, 1998, 157:1436-40.

Keung AC, Eller MG, and Weir SJ, "Pharmacokinetics of Rifapentine in Patients With Varying Degrees of Hepatic Dysfunction," *J Clin Pharmacol*, 1998, 38(6):517-24.

Moghazeh SL, Pan X, Arain T, et al, "Comparative Antimycobacterial Activities of Rifampin, Rifapentine, and KRM-1648 Against a Collection of Rifampin-Resistant *Mycobacterium* tuberculosis Isolates With Known rpoβ Mutations," *Antimicrob Agents Chemother*, 1996, 40(11):2655-7.

Tam CM, Chan SL, Lam CW, et al, "Rifapentine and Isoniazid in the Continuation Phase of Treating Pulmonary Tuberculosis, Initial Report," *Am J Respir Crit Care Med*, 1998, 157:1726-33.

Rifaximin (rif AX i min)

Medication Safety Issues
Sound-alike/look-alike issues:
Rifaximin may be confused with rifampin
U.S. Brand Names Xifaxan™
Generic Available No
Pharmacologic Category Antibiotic, Miscellaneous
Use Treatment of travelers' diarrhea caused by noninvasive strains of *E. coli*
Dosage
Geriatrics & Adults: Travelers' diarrhea: Oral: 200 mg 3 times/day for 3 days
Special Geriatric Considerations Rifaximin has not been studied in the elderly.
Dosage Forms Excipient information presented when available (limited, particularly for generics); consult specific product labeling.
Tablet: 200 mg

♦ **rIFN-A** *see* Interferon Alfa-2a *on page 820*
♦ **rIFN beta-1b** *see* Interferon Beta-1b *on page 824*
♦ **RIG** *see* Rabies Immune Globulin (Human) *on page 1371*
♦ **Rilutek®** *see* Riluzole *on page 1409*

Riluzole (RIL yoo zole)

U.S. Brand Names Rilutek®
Canadian Brand Names Rilutek®
Index Terms 2-Amino-6-Trifluoromethoxy-benzothiazole; RP-54274
Generic Available No
Pharmacologic Category Glutamate Inhibitor
Use Treatment of amyotrophic lateral sclerosis (ALS); riluzole can extend survival or time to tracheostomy
Contraindications Severe hypersensitivity reactions to riluzole or any component of the formulation
Warnings/Precautions Among 4000 patients given riluzole for ALS, there were 3 cases of marked neutropenia (ANC <500/mm³), all seen within the first 2 months of treatment. Use with caution in patients with concomitant renal insufficiency. Use with caution in patients with current evidence or history of abnormal liver function; do not administer if baseline liver function tests are elevated. The elderly, female, or Japanese patients may have decreased clearance of riluzole; use with caution. May cause dizziness or somnolence; caution should be used performing tasks which require alertness (operating machinery or driving).
Adverse Reactions (Reflective of adult population; not specific for elderly)
>10%:
Gastrointestinal: Nausea (12% to 21%)
Neuromuscular & skeletal: Weakness (15% to 20%)
Respiratory: Lung function decreased (10% to 16%)
1% to 10%:
Cardiovascular: Edema, hypertension, tachycardia
(Continued)

Riluzole *(Continued)*

Central nervous system: Agitation, circumoral paresthesia, depression, dizziness, headache, insomnia, malaise, somnolence, tremor, vertigo

Dermatologic: Alopecia, eczema, pruritus

Gastrointestinal: Abdominal pain, anorexia, diarrhea, dyspepsia, flatulence, oral moniliasis, stomatitis, vomiting

Hepatic: Liver function tests increased

Neuromuscular & skeletal: Arthralgia, back pain

Respiratory: Cough increased, rhinitis, sinusitis

Miscellaneous: Aggravation reaction

Overdosage/Toxicology No specific antidote or treatment information is available. Treatment should be supportive and directed toward alleviating symptoms.

Drug Interactions Substrate of CYP1A2 (major)

CYP1A2 inducers: May decrease the levels/effects of riluzole. Example inducers include aminoglutethimide, carbamazepine, phenobarbital, and rifampin.

CYP1A2 inhibitors: May increase the levels/effects of riluzole. Example inhibitors include amiodarone, ciprofloxacin, fluvoxamine, ketoconazole, norfloxacin, ofloxacin, and rofecoxib.

Ethanol/Nutrition/Herb Interactions

Ethanol: Avoid ethanol (due to CNS depression and possible risk of liver toxicity).

Food: A high-fat meal decreases absorption of riluzole (decreasing AUC by 20% and peak blood levels by 45%). Charbroiled food may increase riluzole elimination.

Stability Store at 20°C to 25°C (68°F to 77°F). Protect from bright light.

Mechanism of Action Mechanism of action is not known. Pharmacologic properties include inhibitory effect on glutamate release, inactivation of voltage-dependent sodium channels; and ability to interfere with intracellular events that follow transmitter binding at excitatory amino acid receptors

Pharmacokinetics

Absorption: Well absorbed (90%); a high fat meal decreases absorption of riluzole (decreasing AUC by 20% and peak blood concentrations by 45%)

Protein binding: 96% bound to plasma proteins, mainly albumin and lipoproteins

Metabolism: Extensively hepatic to six major and a number of minor metabolites via CYP1A2 dependent hydroxylation and glucuronidation

Bioavailability: Oral: Absolute (50%)

Dosage

Geriatrics & Adults:

ALS treatment: Oral: 50 mg every 12 hours; no increased benefit can be expected from higher daily doses, but adverse events are increased.

Dosage adjustment in smoking: Cigarette smoking is known to induce CYP1A2; patients who smoke cigarettes would be expected to eliminate riluzole faster. There is no information, however, on the effect of, or need for, dosage adjustment in these patients.

Dosage adjustment in special populations: Females and Japanese patients may possess a lower metabolic capacity to eliminate riluzole compared with male and Caucasian subjects, respectively.

Renal Impairment: Use with caution in patients with concomitant renal insufficiency.

Hepatic Impairment: Use with caution in patients with current evidence or history of abnormal liver function indicated by significant abnormalities in serum transaminase, bilirubin or GGT levels. Baseline elevations of several LFTs (especially elevated bilirubin) should preclude use of riluzole.

Administration Administer at the same time each day, 1 hour before or 2 hours after a meal.

Monitoring Parameters Monitor serum aminotransferases including ALT levels before and during therapy. Evaluate serum ALT levels every month during the first 3 months of therapy, every 3 months during the remainder of the first year and periodically thereafter. Evaluate ALT levels more frequently in patients who develop elevations. Maximum increases in serum ALT usually occurred within 3 months after the start of therapy and were usually transient when <5 x ULN.

In trials, if ALT levels were <5 x ULN, treatment continued and ALT levels usually returned to below 2 x ULN within 2-6 months. There is no experience with continued treatment of ALS patients once ALT values exceed 5 x ULN.

If a decision is made to continue treatment in patients when the ALT exceeds 5 x ULN, frequent monitoring (at least weekly) of complete liver function is recommended. Discontinue treatment if ALT exceeds 10 x ULN or if clinical jaundice develops. Monitor temperature, especially during first 2 months of therapy.

Patient Information Take at least 1 hour before or 2 hours after a meal to avoid decreased bioavailability. Report any febrile illness to your physician. Take riluzole at the same time of the day each day. If a dose is missed, take the next tablet as originally planned.

Avoid alcohol. You may experience increased spasticity, dizziness, or sleepiness; use caution when driving or engaging in tasks requiring alertness until response to drug is known.

Additional Information May be obtained through Rhone-Poulenc Rorer Inc (Collegeville, PA) for compassionate use (through treatment IND process) by calling 800-727-6737 for treatment of amyotrophic lateral sclerosis; may be more effective for amyotrophic lateral sclerosis of bulbar onset; in animal models, riluzole was a potent inhibitor of seizures induced by ouabain

Special Geriatric Considerations In clinical trials, no difference was demonstrated between elderly and younger adults. However, renal and hepatic changes with age can be expected to result in higher serum concentrations of the parent drug and its metabolites.

Dosage Forms Excipient information presented when available (limited, particularly for generics); consult specific product labeling.
Tablet: 50 mg

Selected References
Bensimon G, Lacomblez L, Meininger V, et al, "A Controlled Trial of Riluzole in Amyotrophic Lateral Sclerosis. ALS/Riluzole Study Group," *N Engl J Med*, 1994, 330(9):585-91.

Rimantadine (ri MAN ta deen)

Medication Safety Issues
Sound-alike/look-alike issues:
Rimantadine may be confused with amantadine, ranitidine, Rimactane®
Flumadine® may be confused with fludarabine, flunisolide, flutamide

U.S. Brand Names Flumadine®
Canadian Brand Names Flumadine®
Index Terms Rimantadine Hydrochloride
Generic Available Yes: Tablet
Pharmacologic Category Antiviral Agent, Adamantane
Use Prophylaxis and treatment of influenza A viral infection
Contraindications Hypersensitivity to drugs of the adamantine class, including rimantadine and amantadine, or any component of the formulation
Warnings/Precautions Use with caution in patients with renal and hepatic dysfunction; avoid use, if possible, in patients with recurrent and eczematoid dermatitis, uncontrolled psychosis, or severe psychoneurosis. An increase in seizure incidence may occur in patients with seizure disorders; discontinue drug if seizures occur; resistance may develop during treatment; viruses exhibit cross-resistance between amantadine and rimantadine. Due to increased resistance, in June 2006, the CDC recommended that rimantadine no longer be used for the treatment or prophylaxis of influenza A in the United States until susceptibility has been re-established.
Adverse Reactions (Reflective of adult population; not specific for elderly)
1% to 10%:
Central nervous system: Dizziness (1% to 2%), insomnia (2% to 3%), concentration impaired (2%), anxiety (1%), fatigue (1%), headache (1%), nervousness (1% to 2%)
Gastrointestinal: Nausea (3%), anorexia (2%), vomiting (2%), xerostomia (2%), abdominal pain (1%)
Neuromuscular & skeletal: Weakness (1%)
Overdosage/Toxicology Agitation, hallucinations, ventricular cardiac arrhythmias (torsade de pointes and PVCs), slurred speech, anticholinergic effects (dry mouth, urinary retention and mydriasis), ataxia, tremor, myoclonus, seizures, and death have been reported with amantadine (a related drug). Treatment is symptomatic (do not use physostigmine). Tachyarrhythmias may be treated with beta-blockers such as propranolol. Dialysis is not recommended except possibly in renal failure.
Drug Interactions Influenza virus vaccine (live organism): Rimantadine may decrease the efficacy of vaccine. Administer vaccine at least 48 hours after rimantadine. Do not give rimantadine within 2 weeks of live virus vaccine.
Ethanol/Nutrition/Herb Interactions Food: Food does not affect rate or extent of absorption
Stability Store at 15°C to 30°C (59°F to 86°F).
Mechanism of Action Exerts its inhibitory effect on three antigenic subtypes of influenza A virus (H1N1, H2N2, H3N2) early in the viral replicative cycle, possibly inhibiting the uncoating process; it has no activity against influenza B virus and is two- to eightfold more active than amantadine
Pharmacokinetics
Absorption: Tablet and syrup essentially completely absorbed
Distribution: 40% bound to plasma protein
Metabolism: 90%
Half-life:
Adults: Mean: 25.4 hours
Older adults (healthy): Mean: 32 hours
(Continued)

Rimantadine *(Continued)*

At steady-state, AUC, plasma concentration, and half-life are 20% to 30% greater in persons >60 years of age; older adult nursing home residents were found to have steady-state plasma concentrations 2-4 times greater than older adults community residents

Dosage

Geriatrics:

Prophylaxis of influenza A: Oral: 100 mg/day in nursing home patients or all elderly patients who may experience adverse effects using the adult dose

Treatment of influenza A: Oral: 100 mg once daily in patients ≥65 years

Adults:

Prophylaxis of influenza A: Oral: 100 mg twice daily

Treatment of influenza A: Oral: 100 mg twice daily

Renal Impairment:

Cl_{cr} >10 mL/minute: Dose adjustment not required

Cl_{cr} ≤10 mL/minute: 100 mg/day

Hepatic Impairment: Severe dysfunction: 100 mg/day

Monitoring Parameters Signs and symptoms of toxicity, especially CNS

Reference Range No relationship between plasma concentration and antiviral effects has been established

Special Geriatric Considerations Adverse CNS and GI effects occur frequently if dosage is not adjusted. Monitor GI effects in the elderly or patients with renal or hepatic impairment. Dosing must be individualized (100 mg 1-2 times/day). It is recommended that nursing home patients receive 100 mg/day.

Dosage Forms Excipient information presented when available (limited, particularly for generics); consult specific product labeling.

Syrup, as hydrochloride:

Flumadine®: 50 mg/5 mL (240 mL) [raspberry flavor]

Tablet, as hydrochloride: 100 mg

Flumadine®: 100 mg

Selected References

Centers for Disease Control, "Recommendations of the Advisory Committee on Immunization Practices (ACIP): Prevention and Control of Influenza," *MMWR Recomm Rep*, 2005, 54:1-43. Available at: http://www.cdc.gov/mmwr/pdf/rr/rr54e713.pdf

Douglas RG Jr, "Prophylaxis and Treatment of Influenza," *N Engl J Med*, 1990, 322(7):443-50.

Guay DR, "Amantadine and Rimantadine Prophylaxis of Influenza A in Nursing Homes," *Drugs Aging*, 1994, 5(1):8-19.

Patriarca PA, Kater NA, Kendal AP, et al, "Safety of Prolonged Administration of Rimantadine Hydrochloride in the Prophylaxis of Influenza A Virus Infections in Nursing Homes," *Antimicrob Agents Chemother*, 1984, 26(1):101-3.

♦ **Rimantadine Hydrochloride** *see* Rimantadine *on page 1411*

Rimexolone *(ri MEKS oh lone)*

Medication Safety Issues

Sound-alike/look-alike issues:

Vexol® may be confused with VoSol®

U.S. Brand Names Vexol®

Canadian Brand Names Vexol®

Generic Available No

Pharmacologic Category Corticosteroid, Ophthalmic

Use Treatment of inflammation after ocular surgery, anterior uveitis

Contraindications Hypersensitivity to rimexolone or any component of the formulation; fungal, viral, or untreated pus-forming bacterial ocular infections

Warnings/Precautions Prolonged use has been associated with the development of corneal or scleral perforation and posterior subcapsular cataracts; may mask or enhance the establishment of acute purulent untreated infections of the eye; may delay healing after cataract surgery; intraocular pressure should be monitored if this product is used >10 days.

Adverse Reactions (Reflective of adult population; not specific for elderly)

1% to 10%: Ocular: Temporary mild blurred vision

Mechanism of Action Decreases inflammation by suppression of migration of polymorphonuclear leukocytes and reversal of increased capillary permeability

Pharmacokinetics

Absorption: Through aqueous humor

Metabolism: Any drug absorbed is metabolized in the liver

Elimination: By the kidneys and feces

Dosage

Geriatrics & Adults: Anti-inflammatory: Ophthalmic: Instill 1 drop in conjunctival sac 2-4 times/day up to every 4 hours; may use every 1-2 hours during first 1-2 days

Monitoring Parameters Intraocular pressure and periodic examination of lens (with prolonged use)

Patient Information Shake well before using, do not touch dropper to the eye

Special Geriatric Considerations No special considerations; must limit the time steroids are used to prevent adverse effects.

Dosage Forms Excipient information presented when available (limited, particularly for generics); consult specific product labeling.

Suspension, ophthalmic: 1% (5 mL, 10 mL) [contains benzalkonium chloride]

♦ **Riomet**™ see Metformin on page 993

♦ **Riopan Plus®** [OTC] [DSC] see Magaldrate and Simethicone on page 943

♦ **Riopan Plus® Double Strength** [OTC] [DSC] see Magaldrate and Simethicone on page 943

Risedronate (ris ED roe nate)

Related Information
Osteoporosis Management on page 1779

U.S. Brand Names Actonel®

Canadian Brand Names Actonel®

Index Terms Risedronate Sodium

Generic Available No

Pharmacologic Category Bisphosphonate Derivative

Use Paget's disease of the bone; treatment and prevention of glucocorticoid-induced osteoporosis; treatment and prevention of osteoporosis in postmenopausal women; treatment of osteoporosis in men

Contraindications Hypersensitivity to risedronate, bisphosphonates, or any component of the formulation; hypocalcemia; abnormalities of the esophagus which delay esophageal emptying such as stricture or achalasia; inability to stand or sit upright for at least 30 minutes; severe renal impairment (Cl$_{cr}$ <30 mL/minute)

Warnings/Precautions Bisphosphonates may cause upper gastrointestinal disorders such as dysphagia, esophagitis, esophageal ulcer, and gastric ulcer. Use caution in patients with renal impairment (not recommended in patients with a Cl$_{cr}$ <30 mL/minute). Hypocalcemia must be corrected before therapy initiation with risedronate. Ensure adequate calcium and vitamin D intake, especially for patients with Paget's disease in whom the pretreatment rate of bone turnover may be greatly elevated.

Bisphosphonate therapy has been associated with osteonecrosis, primarily of the jaw; this has been observed mostly in cancer patients, but also in patients with postmenopausal osteoporosis and other diagnoses. Dental exams and preventative dentistry should be performed prior to placing patients with risk factors on chronic bisphosphonate therapy. Invasive dental procedures should be avoided during treatment.

Infrequently, severe (and occasionally debilitating) bone, joint, and/or muscle pain have been reported during bisphosphonate treatment. The onset of pain ranged from a single day to several months. Symptoms usually resolve upon discontinuation. Some patients experienced recurrence when rechallenged with same drug or another bisphosphonate; avoid use in patients with a history of these symptoms in association with bisphosphonate therapy.

Adverse Reactions (Reflective of adult population; not specific for elderly)
Frequency may vary with dose and indication.
>10%:
 Central nervous system: Headache (18%), pain (14%)
 Dermatologic: Rash (8% to 12%)
 Gastrointestinal: Diarrhea (11% to 20%), abdominal pain (12%)
 Genitourinary: Urinary tract infection (11%)
 Neuromuscular & skeletal: Arthralgia (14% to 33%), back pain (26%)
1% to 10%:
 Cardiovascular: Hypertension (10%), peripheral edema (8%), chest pain (5% to 7%), cardiovascular disorder (3%), angina (3%), arrhythmia (2%)
 Central nervous system: Depression (7%), dizziness (6% to 7%), insomnia (5%), anxiety (4%)
 Dermatologic: Pruritus (3%)
 Endocrine & metabolic: Hypophosphatemia (<3%)
 Gastrointestinal: Constipation (7%), nausea (7%), flatulence (5%), belching (3%), colitis (3%), gastritis (3%)
 Genitourinary: Prostatic hyperplasia (5%), cystitis (4%), nephrolithiasis (3%)
 Hematologic: Anemia (2%)
 Neuromuscular & skeletal: Joint disorder (7%), myalgia (5% to 7%), neck pain (5%), bone pain (5%), weakness (5%), neuralgia (4%), leg cramps (4%), myasthenia (3%), tendon disorder (3%)

(Continued)

Risedronate *(Continued)*

   Ocular: Cataract (6%), dry eyes (3%)

   Respiratory: Pharyngitis (6%), rhinitis (6%), sinusitis (5%), dyspnea (4%), bronchitis (3%)

   Miscellaneous: Flu symptoms (10%), neoplasm (3%), hernia (3%)

Overdosage/Toxicology Symptoms include hypophosphatemia and upper GI adverse events (upset stomach, heartburn, esophagitis, gastritis, or ulcer). Signs and symptoms of hypocalcemia may also occur in some patients. Milk or antacids containing calcium should be given to bind Actonel® and reduce absorption of the drug. Decreases in serum calcium and phosphorus following substantial overdose may be expected in some patients. In cases of substantial overdose, use of gastric lavage to remove unabsorbed drug and I.V. calcium may be required. Dialysis would not be beneficial. Standard procedures that are effective for treating hypocalcemia, including the administration of calcium intravenously, would be expected to restore physiologic amounts of ionized calcium and to relieve signs and symptoms of hypocalcemia.

Drug Interactions

   Aminoglycosides: May lower serum calcium levels with prolonged administration. Concomitant use may have an additive hypocalcemic effect.

   Antacids: May decrease the absorption of bisphosphonate derivatives; should be administered at a different time of the day. Antacids containing aluminum, calcium, or magnesium are of specific concern.

   Calcium salts: May decrease the absorption of bisphosphonate derivatives. Separate oral dosing in order to minimize risk of interaction.

   Iron salts: May decrease the absorption of bisphosphonate derivatives. Only oral iron salts and oral bisphosphonates are of concern.

   Magnesium salts: May decrease the absorption of bisphosphonate derivatives. Only oral magnesium salts and oral bisphosphonates are of concern.

   Nonsteroidal anti-inflammatory drugs (NSAIDs): May enhance the gastrointestinal adverse/toxic effects (increased incidence of GI ulcers) of bisphosphonate derivatives.

   Phosphate supplements: Bisphosphonate derivatives may enhance the hypocalcemic effect of phosphate supplements.

Ethanol/Nutrition/Herb Interactions

   Ethanol: Avoid ethanol (may increase risk of osteoporosis).

   Food: Food reduces absorption (similar to other bisphosphonates); mean oral bioavailability is decreased when given with food.

Stability Store at room temperature of 20°C to 25°C (68°F to 77°F).

Mechanism of Action A bisphosphonate which inhibits bone resorption via actions on osteoclasts or on osteoclast precursors; decreases the rate of bone resorption, leading to an indirect increase in bone mineral density. In Paget's disease, characterized by disordered resorption and formation of bone, inhibition of resorption leads to an indirect decrease in bone formation; but the newly-formed bone has a more normal architecture.

Pharmacodynamics Onset of action may require weeks.

Pharmacokinetics

   Absorption: Rapid

   Distribution: V_d: 6.3 L/kg

   Protein binding: ~24%

   Metabolism: None

   Bioavailability: Poor, ~0.54% to 0.75%

   Half-life: Initial: 1.5 hours; Terminal: 480 hours

   Time to peak, serum: 1 hour

   Elimination: Urine (up to 80%); feces (as unabsorbed drug)

Dosage

   Geriatrics & Adults:

   Paget's disease of bone: Oral: 30 mg once daily for 2 months

   Note: Retreatment may be considered (following post-treatment observation of at least 2 months) if relapse occurs, or if treatment fails to normalize serum alkaline phosphatase. For retreatment, the dose and duration of therapy are the same as for initial treatment. No data are available on more than one course of retreatment.

   Osteoporosis (postmenopausal) prevention and treatment: Oral: 5 mg once daily **or** 35 mg once weekly **or** one 75 mg tablet taken on 2 consecutive days once a month (total of 2 tablets/month)

   Osteoporosis (male) treatment: 35 mg once weekly

   Osteoporosis (glucocorticoid-induced) prevention and treatment: Oral: 5 mg once daily

   Renal Impairment: Cl_{cr} <30 mL/minute: Not recommended

Administration It is imperative to administer risedronate 30-60 minutes before the patient takes any food, drink, or other medications orally to avoid interference with absorption. The patient should take risedronate on an empty stomach with a full glass

(8 oz) of **plain water** (not mineral water) and avoid lying down for 30 minutes after swallowing tablet to help delivery to stomach. Tablet should be swallowed whole; do not crush or chew.

Monitoring Parameters Alkaline phosphatase should be periodically measured; serum calcium, phosphorus, and possibly potassium due to its drug class; use of absorptiometry may assist in evaluating benefit in osteoporosis; monitor pain and fracture rate

Reference Range Calcium (total): Adults: 9.0-11.0 mg/dL (2.05-2.54 mmol/L), may slightly decrease with aging; phosphorus: 2.5-4.5 mg/dL (0.81-1.45 mmol/L)

Test Interactions Bisphosphonates may interfere with diagnostic imaging agents such as technetium-99m-diphosphonate in bone scans.

Patient Information The expected benefits of risedronate may only be obtained when each tablet is taken with plain water the first thing in the morning and at least 30 minutes before the first food, beverage, or medication of the day. Wait >30 minutes to improve risedronate absorption. Even dosing with orange juice or coffee markedly reduces the absorption of risedronate.

Take supplemental calcium and vitamin D if dietary intake is inadequate. Consider weight-bearing exercise along with the modification of certain behavioral factors, such as excessive cigarette smoking or alcohol consumption if these factors exist.

Additional Information Esophageal irritation and gastric pain have been reported frequently. Proper administration may prevent or decrease this common adverse effect. Patients need to take supplemental calcium while treated with risedronate appropriate for age and hormonal status; vitamin D supplements suggested if patient is deficient in this vitamin.

Special Geriatric Considerations No dosage adjustment required if Cl_{cr} ≥30 mL/minute. Since elderly often receive diuretics, evaluate electrolyte status periodically due to the drug class (bisphosphonates). Should assure that immobile patients are sitting up for at least 30 minutes after swallowing tablets.

Dosage Forms Excipient information presented when available (limited, particularly for generics); consult specific product labeling.
Tablet, as sodium:
Actonel®: 5 mg, 30 mg, 35 mg, 75 mg

Risedronate and Calcium (ris ED roe nate & KAL see um)

U.S. Brand Names Actonel® and Calcium

Index Terms Calcium and Risedronate; Risedronate Sodium and Calcium Carbonate

Generic Available No

Pharmacologic Category Bisphosphonate Derivative; Calcium Salt

Use Treatment and prevention of osteoporosis in postmenopausal women

Contraindications Hypersensitivity to risedronate, bisphosphonates, or any component of the formulation; hypocalcemia, hypercalcemia; abnormalities of the esophagus which delay esophageal emptying (eg, stricture or achalasia); inability to stand or sit upright for at least 30 minutes; severe renal impairment (Cl_{cr} <30 mL/minute)

Warnings/Precautions Bisphosphonates may cause upper gastrointestinal disorders such as dysphagia, esophageal ulcer, and gastric ulcer. Use caution in patients with renal impairment (not recommended in patients with a Cl_{cr} <30 mL/minute). Hypocalcemia must be corrected before therapy initiation. Ensure adequate vitamin D intake. Severe bone pain has been reported (rare) with the use of bisphosphonates; onset varied from 1 day to several months following the onset of therapy.

Bisphosphonate therapy has been associated with osteonecrosis, primarily of the jaw; this has been observed mostly in cancer patients, but also in patients with postmenopausal osteoporosis and other diagnoses. Dental exams and preventative dentistry should be performed prior to placing patients with risk factors on chronic bisphosphonate therapy. Invasive dental procedures should be avoided during treatment.

Infrequently, severe (and occasionally debilitating) bone, joint, and/or muscle pain have been reported during bisphosphonate treatment. The onset of pain ranged from a single day to several months. Symptoms usually resolve upon discontinuation. Some patients experienced recurrence when rechallenged with same drug or another bisphosphonate; avoid use in patients with a history of these symptoms in association with bisphosphonate therapy.

Calcium carbonate absorption is impaired in achlorhydria (common in elderly); administer calcium component with food. Calcium should be used with caution in patients with a history of kidney stones or hypercalciuria.

Safety and efficacy using the combination as packaged have not been established for the treatment of primary osteoporosis in men.

Adverse Reactions (Reflective of adult population; not specific for elderly) See individual agents.
(Continued)

Risedronate and Calcium *(Continued)*

Overdosage/Toxicology See individual agents.

Drug Interactions See individual agents.

Ethanol/Nutrition/Herb Interactions

Ethanol: Avoid ethanol (may increase risk of osteoporosis).

Food:

Risedronate: Food may reduce absorption (similar to other bisphosphonates); mean oral bioavailability is decreased when given with food.

Calcium: Food increases absorption. Calcium may decrease iron absorption. Bran, foods high in oxalates, or whole grain cereals may decrease calcium absorption

Stability Store at room temperature of 15°C to 30°C (59°F to 86°F).

Mechanism of Action

Risedronate inhibits bone resorption via actions on osteoclasts or on osteoclast precursors; decreases the rate of bone resorption, leading to an indirect increase in bone mineral density.

Calcium helps to prevent or decrease the rate of bone loss.

Pharmacokinetics See individual agents.

Dosage

Geriatrics:

Refer to adult dosing.

Adults: Osteoporosis in postmenopausal females: Oral:

Risedronate: 35 mg once weekly on day 1 of 7-day treatment cycle

Calcium carbonate: 1250 mg (elemental calcium 500 mg) once daily on days 2 through 7 of 7-day treatment cycle

Renal Impairment: Cl_{cr} <30 mL/minute: Not recommended for use.

Administration Risedronate should be administered ≥30 minutes before the first food or drink of the day other than water. Risedronate should be taken in an upright position with a full glass (6-8 oz) of plain water and the patient should avoid lying down for 30 minutes to minimize the possibility of GI side effects. Calcium should be taken with food. If additional calcium is needed (other than what is provided in blister package), it should be taken at a separate time of the day.

Monitoring Parameters Pain and fracture rate, bone mineral density, height

Reference Range Calcium (total): Adults: 9.0-11.0 mg/dL (2.05-2.54 mmol/L), may slightly decrease with aging; phosphorus: 2.5-4.5 mg/dL (0.81-1.45 mmol/L)

Test Interactions Bisphosphonates may interfere with diagnostic imaging agents such as technetium-99m-diphosphonate in bone scans.

Special Geriatric Considerations See individual agents.

Dosage Forms Excipient information presented when available (limited, particularly for generics); consult specific product labeling.

Combination package [each package contains]:

Tablet (Actonel®): Risedronate 35 mg (4s)

Tablet: Calcium carbonate 1250 mg (24s) [equivalent to elemental calcium 500 mg]

Selected References

Ruggiero SL, Mehrotra B, Rosenberg TJ, et al, "Osteonecrosis of the Jaws Associated With the Use of Bisphosphonates: A Review of 63 Cases," *J Oral Maxillofac Surg*, 2004, 62(5):527-34.

♦ **Risedronate Sodium** *see* Risedronate *on page 1413*

♦ **Risedronate Sodium and Calcium Carbonate** *see* Risedronate and Calcium *on page 1415*

♦ **Risperdal®** *see* Risperidone *on page 1416*

♦ **Risperdal M-Tab** *see* Risperidone *on page 1416*

♦ **Risperdal® M-Tab®** *see* Risperidone *on page 1416*

♦ **Risperdal® Consta®** *see* Risperidone *on page 1416*

Risperidone *(ris PER i done)*

Related Information

Antipsychotic Agents *on page 1747*
Atypical Antipsychotics *on page 1749*
Liquid Compatibility of Antipsychotics and Mood Stabilizers *on page 1851*

Medication Safety Issues

Sound-alike/look-alike issues:

Risperidone may be confused with reserpine

Risperdal® may be confused with lisinopril, reserpine

U.S. Brand Names Risperdal®; Risperdal® Consta®; Risperdal® M-Tab®

Canadian Brand Names Apo-Risperidone®; PMS-Risperidone ODT; Risperdal®; Risperdal® Consta®; Risperdal® M-Tab®; Sandoz Risperidone

Index Terms Risperdal M-Tab

Generic Available No

Pharmacologic Category Antipsychotic Agent, Atypical

Use Treatment of schizophrenia; treatment of acute mania or mixed episodes associated with bipolar I disorder (as monotherapy or in combination with lithium or valproate); treatment of irritability/aggression associated with autistic disorder

Unlabeled/Investigational Use Behavioral symptoms associated with dementia in elderly; treatment of Tourette's disorder; treatment of pervasive developmental disorder

Contraindications Hypersensitivity to risperidone or any component of the formulation

Warnings/Precautions [U.S. Boxed Warning]: Patients with dementia-related psychosis treated with atypical antipsychotics are at an increased risk of death compared to placebo. An increased incidence of cerebrovascular adverse events (including fatalities) has been reported in elderly patients with dementia-related psychosis. Risk may be increased by dehydration; use caution with concurrent diuretics. Risperidone is not approved for the treatment of dementia-related psychosis.

Low- to moderately-sedating, use with caution in disorders where CNS depression is a feature. Use with caution in Parkinson's disease. Caution in patients with predisposition to seizures; or severe cardiac disease. Use with caution in renal or hepatic dysfunction; dose reduction recommended. Esophageal dysmotility and aspiration have been associated with antipsychotic use; use with caution in patients at risk of aspiration pneumonia (eg, Alzheimer's disease). Elevates prolactin levels; effects seen in adults. Use with caution in breast cancer or other prolactin-dependent tumors. May alter temperature regulation. May mask toxicity of other drugs or conditions (eg intestinal obstruction, Reyes syndrome, brain tumor) due to antiemetic effects.

Use with caution in patients with cardiovascular diseases (eg, heart failure, history of myocardial infarction or ischemia, cerebrovascular disease, conduction abnormalities). May cause orthostatic hypotension; use with caution in patients at risk of this effect (eg, concurrent medication use which may predispose to hypotension/bradycardia or presence of hypovolemia) or in those who would not tolerate transient hypotensive episodes. May alter cardiac conduction (low risk relative to other neuroleptics); life-threatening arrhythmias have occurred with therapeutic doses of neuroleptics.

May cause anticholinergic effects (confusion, agitation, constipation, xerostomia, blurred vision, urinary retention); therefore, they should be used with caution in patients with decreased gastrointestinal motility, urinary retention, BPH, xerostomia, or visual problems. Conditions which also may be exacerbated by cholinergic blockade include narrow-angle glaucoma (screening is recommended) and worsening of myasthenia gravis. Relative to other neuroleptics, risperidone has a low potency of cholinergic blockade.

May cause extrapyramidal symptoms, including pseudoparkinsonism, acute dystonic reactions, akathisia, and tardive dyskinesia (risk of these reactions is low relative to other neuroleptics, and is dose dependent). Risk of neuroleptic malignant syndrome (NMS) may be increased in patients with Parkinson's disease or Lewy body dementia; monitor for symptoms of confusion, obtundation, postural instability and extrapyramidal symptoms. May cause hyperglycemia; in some cases may be extreme and associated with ketoacidosis, hyperosmolar coma, or death. Use with caution in patients with diabetes or other disorders of glucose regulation; monitor for worsening of glucose control. Significant weight gain has been observed with antipsychotic therapy; incidence varies with product. Monitor waist circumference and BMI.

The possibility of a suicide attempt is inherent in psychotic illness or bipolar disorder; use caution in high-risk patients during initiation of therapy. Prescriptions should be written for the smallest quantity consistent with good patient care.

Adverse Reactions (Reflective of adult population; not specific for elderly)

The frequency of adverse effects is reported as absolute percentages and is not based upon net frequencies as compared to placebo. Unless otherwise noted, frequency of adverse effects is reported for the oral formulation in adults.

>10%:

Central nervous system: Fatigue (adults 4%; children 42%), extrapyramidal symptoms (adults 17% to 34%; children 28%), somnolence (adults 3% to 28%; children 67%), insomnia (23% to 26%), agitation (8% to 26%), anxiety (4% to 20%), dystonia (adults 18%; children 12%), akathisia (16%), headache (12% to 14%), dizziness (4% to 11%)

Gastrointestinal: Appetite increased (children 49%), salivation increased (adults up to 5%; children 22%), weight gain (adults 2% to 18%; children 5%), constipation (adults 7% to 13%; children 21%), xerostomia (adults 3% to ≥5%; children 13%), dyspepsia (5% to 11%), nausea (4% to 11%)

Neuromuscular & skeletal: Tremor (children 12%)

Respiratory: Upper respiratory infection (adults 3%; children 34%)

1% to 10%:

Cardiovascular: Tachycardia (adults 3% to 5%; children 7%), hypertension (3%), chest pain (2% to 3%), hypotension (2%; especially orthostatic)

(Continued)

1417

Risperidone *(Continued)*

Central nervous system: Mania (8%), automatism (children 7%), pseudoparkin-sonism (adults 6%; children 7%), dreaming increased (≥5%), sleep prolonged (≥5%), confusion (children 5%), pain (5%), fever (2% to 3%), aggressiveness (1% to 3%), concentration impaired (2%), hypoesthesia (2%), tardive dyskinesia, neuroleptic malignant syndrome, altered central temperature regulation, nervous-ness, sleep duration increased

Dermatologic: Rash (2% to 5%), dry skin (2% to 4%), acne (2%), pruritus (2%), seborrhea (up to 1%), pigmentation increased, photosensitivity

Endocrine & metabolic: Sexual dysfunction (3%), menorrhagia (≥5%), galactorrhea (children 1%), gynecomastia (children 2%)

Gastrointestinal: Vomiting (5% to 9%), diarrhea (≥5%), abdominal pain (1% to 4%), toothache (up to 2%), anorexia

Genitourinary: Micturition disturbances (≥5%)

Hematologic: Anemia (≥1% I.M. injection)

Hepatic: Transaminases increased (≥1% I.M. injection)

Neuromuscular & skeletal: Dyskinesia (children 7%), myalgia (5%), arthralgia (2% to 3%), skeletal pain (2%), back pain (up to 2%)

Ocular: Abnormal vision (1% to 6%), accommodation disturbances (≥5%)

Renal: Polydipsia, polyuria

Respiratory: Rhinitis (3% to 10%), sinusitis (1% to 4%), cough (2% to 3%), pharyn-gitis (2% to 3%), dyspnea (up to 1%)

Miscellaneous: Injury (2%)

Overdosage/Toxicology Ingestion of doses as high as 360 mg have been reported. Symptoms of overdose are commonly drowsiness, sedation, tachycardia, hypotension, and extrapyramidal symptoms (EPS). Other reactions reported include torsade de pointes, prolonged QT interval, seizures, and cardiopulmonary arrest. Treatment should be symptom-directed and supportive. Gastric lavage and activated charcoal should be initiated. Risk of aspiration should be considered; cardiac monitoring should be initiated. Avoid antiarrhythmic therapy with agents known to prolong the QT interval (eg, disopyramide or procainamide) Avoid use of epinephrine and dopamine as vaso-pressors which may worsen hypotensive effects of risperidone. Anticholinergics may be used for severe EPS.

Drug Interactions Substrate of CYP2D6 (major), 3A4 (minor); **Inhibits** CYP2D6 (weak), 3A4 (weak)

Acetylcholinesterase inhibitors (central): May increase the risk of antipsychotic-related extrapyramidal symptoms; monitor.

Anticholinergics: May enhance the effects of other anticholinergics.

Carbamazepine: Plasma concentrations of risperidone and 9-hydroxyrisperidone were decreased by ~50% with concomitant use. The dose of risperidone may need to be titrated accordingly when carbamazepine is added or discontinued.

Clozapine: Decreases clearance of risperidone, increasing its serum concentrations

CNS depressants: May increase adverse effects/toxicity of other CNS depressants.

CYP2D6 inhibitors: May increase the levels/effects of risperidone. Example inhibitors include chlorpromazine, delavirdine, fluoxetine, miconazole, paroxetine, pergolide, quinidine, quinine, ritonavir, and ropinirole.

Lithium: May increase the neurotoxic effects (eg, EPS) of risperidone; monitor.

Pramlintide: May enhance the anticholinergic effect of risperidone. These effects are specific to the GI tract.

SSRIs: May increase the levels/effects of risperidone; monitor.

Valproic acid: Valproic acid may enhance the adverse/toxic effect of risperidone.

Verapamil: May increase the levels and effects of risperidone.

Ethanol/Nutrition/Herb Interactions

Ethanol: Avoid ethanol (may increase CNS depression).

Herb/Nutraceutical: Avoid kava kava, gotu kola, valerian, St John's wort (may increase CNS depression).

Stability

Injection: Risperdal® Consta®: Store in refrigerator at 2°C to 8°C (36°F to 46°F) and protect from light. May be stored at room temperature of 25°C (77°F) for up to 7 days prior to administration. Bring to room temperature prior to reconstitution. Reconsti-tute with provided diluent only. Shake vigorously to mix; will form thick, milky suspen-sion. Following reconstitution, store at room temperature and use within 6 hours. If suspension settles prior to use, shake vigorously to resuspend.

Oral solution, tablet: Store at 15°C to 25°C (59°F to 77°F). Protect from light and moisture. Keep orally-disintegrating tablets sealed in foil pouch until ready to use. Do not freeze solution.

Mechanism of Action Risperidone is a benzisoxazole atypical antipsychotic with mixed serotonin-dopamine antagonist activity that binds to 5-HT$_2$-receptors in the CNS and in the periphery with a very high affinity; binds to dopamine-D$_2$ receptors with less affinity. The binding affinity to the dopamine-D$_2$ receptor is 20 times lower than the 5-HT$_2$ affinity. The addition of serotonin antagonism to dopamine antagonism (classic neuroleptic mechanism) is thought to improve negative symptoms of psychoses and reduce the incidence of extrapyramidal side effects. Alpha$_1$, alpha$_2$ adrenergic, and histaminergic receptors are also antagonized with high affinity. Risperidone has low to moderate affinity for 5-HT$_{1C}$, 5-HT$_{1D}$, and 5-HT$_{1A}$ receptors, weak affinity for D$_1$ and no affinity for muscarinics or beta$_1$ and beta$_2$ receptors

Pharmacokinetics

Absorption:

Oral: Rapid and well absorbed; food does not affect rate or extent

Injection: <1% absorbed initially; main release occurs at ~3 weeks and is maintained from 4-6 weeks

Protein binding, plasma: Risperidone 90%; 9-hydroxyrisperidone: 77%

Metabolism: Extensively hepatic to 9-hydroxyrisperidone (equieffective with risperidone); N-dealkylation is a second minor pathway

Bioavailability: Solution: 70%; Tablet: 66%; orally-disintegrating tablets and oral solution are bioequivalent to tablets

Half-life elimination: Active moiety (risperidone and its active metabolite 9-hydroxyrisperidone)

Oral: 20 hours (mean)

Extensive metabolizers: Risperidone: 3 hours; 9-hydroxyrisperidone: 21 hours

Poor metabolizers: Risperidone: 20 hours; 9-hydroxyrisperidone: 30 hours

Injection: 3-6 days; related to microsphere erosion and subsequent absorption of risperidone

Time to peak, plasma: Oral: Risperidone: Within 1 hour; 9-hydroxyrisperidone: 3 hours in extensive metabolizers and 17 hours in poor metabolizers

Dosage

Geriatrics:

Oral: A starting dose of 0.5 mg twice daily, and titration should progress slowly in increments of no more than 0.5 mg twice daily; increases to dosages >1.5 mg twice daily should occur at intervals of ≥1 week.

I.M. (Risperdal® Consta®): A lower initial dose of 12.5 mg may be appropriate.

Additional monitoring of renal function and orthostatic blood pressure may be warranted. If once-a-day dosing in the elderly or debilitated patient is considered, a twice daily regimen should be used to titrate to the target dose, and this dose should be maintained for 2-3 days prior to attempts to switch to a once-daily regimen.

Adults:

Bipolar mania: Oral: Recommended starting dose: 2-3 mg once daily; if needed, adjust dose by 1 mg/day in intervals ≥24 hours; dosing range: 1-6 mg/day.

Schizophrenia:

Oral: Initial: 1 mg twice daily; may be increased by 2 mg/day to a target dose of 6 mg/day; usual range: 4-8 mg/day; may be given as a single daily dose once maintenance dose is achieved; daily dosages >6 mg do not appear to confer any additional benefit, and the incidence of extrapyramidal symptoms is higher than with lower doses. Further dose adjustments should be made in increments/ decrements of 1-2 mg/day on a weekly basis. Dose range studied in clinical trials: 4-16 mg/day. Maintenance: Target dose: 4 mg once daily (range 2-8 mg/ day)

I.M. (Risperdal® Consta®): 25 mg every 2 weeks; some patients may benefit from larger doses; maximum dose not to exceed 50 mg every 2 weeks. Dosage adjustments should not be made more frequently than every 4 weeks. A lower initial dose of 12.5 mg may be appropriate in some patients.

Note: Oral risperidone (or other antipsychotic) should be administered with the initial injection of Risperdal® Consta® and continued for 3 weeks (then discontinued) to maintain adequate therapeutic plasma concentrations prior to main release phase of risperidone from injection site.

Tourette's disorder (unlabeled use): Oral: Initial: 0.5 mg; titrate to 2-4 mg/day

Renal Impairment:

Oral: Starting dose of 0.5 mg twice daily; clearance of the active moiety is decreased by 60% in patients with moderate to severe renal disease compared to healthy subjects.

I.M.: An initial dose of 12.5 mg may be considered

Hepatic Impairment:

Oral: Starting dose of 0.5 mg twice daily; the mean free fraction of risperidone in plasma was increased by 35% compared to healthy subjects.

I.M.: An initial dose of 12.5 mg may be considered

Administration

Oral: Oral solution can be mixed with water, coffee, orange juice, or low-fat milk, but is not compatible with cola or tea. May be administered with or without food.

Risperdal® M-Tabs® should not be removed from blister pack until administered. Using dry hands, place immediately on tongue. Tablet will dissolve within seconds, and may be swallowed with or without liquid. Do not split or chew.

(Continued)

Risperidone *(Continued)*

I.M.: Risperdal® Consta® should be administered into the upper outer quadrant of the gluteal area. Avoid inadvertent injection into vasculature. Injection should alternate between the two buttocks. Do not combine two different dosage strengths into one single administration. Do not substitute any components of the dose-pack; administer with needle provided.

Monitoring Parameters Vital signs; fasting lipid profile and fasting blood glucose/Hgb A$_{1c}$ (prior to treatment, at 3 months, then annually); BMI, personal/family history of obesity, waist circumference; blood pressure; mental status, abnormal involuntary movement scale (AIMS), extrapyramidal symptoms; orthostatic blood pressure changes for 3-5 days after starting or increasing dose. Weight should be assessed prior to treatment, at 4 weeks, 8 weeks, 12 weeks, and then at quarterly intervals. Consider titrating to a different antipsychotic agent for a weight gain ≥5% of the initial weight.

Patient Information Explain to patients that orthostatic hypotension may occur at initiation of therapy; may cause impairment of alertness and judgment; enhanced sedation will occur with the ingestion of alcohol; photosensitivity may occur; use sunscreen or avoid exposure to sunlight and ultraviolet light

Use exactly as directed (do not increase dose or frequency). It may take 2-3 weeks to achieve desired results; do not discontinue without consulting prescriber. Dilute solution with water, milk, or orange juice; do not dilute with beverages containing tannin or pectinate (eg, colas, tea). Avoid concurrent grapefruit juice. Avoid alcohol or caffeine and other prescription or OTC medications not approved by prescriber. Maintain adequate hydration (2-3 L/day of fluids unless instructed to restrict fluid intake). You may experience excess sedation, drowsiness, restlessness, dizziness, or blurred vision (use caution driving or when engaging in tasks requiring alertness until response to drug is known); dry mouth, nausea, or GI upset (small frequent meals, frequent mouth care, chewing gum, or sucking lozenges may help); postural hypotension (use caution climbing stairs or when changing position from lying or sitting to standing); or urinary retention (void before taking medication). Report persistent CNS effects (eg, trembling fingers, altered gait or balance, excessive sedation, seizures, unusual muscle or skeletal movements, anxiety, abnormal thoughts, confusion, personality changes); chest pain, palpitations, rapid heartbeat, severe dizziness; swelling or pain in breasts (male and female), altered menstrual pattern, sexual dysfunction; pain or difficulty on urination; vision changes; skin rash or yellowing of skin; difficulty breathing; or worsening of condition.

Additional Information Risperdal Consta™ is an injectable formulation of risperidone using the extended release Medisorb® drug-delivery system; small polymeric microspheres degrade slowly, releasing the medication at a controlled rate.

Special Geriatric Considerations Any changes in disease status in any organ system can result in behavior changes.

Extrapyramidal syndrome symptoms occur less with this agent when total daily dose remains <6 mg as compared with phenothiazines and butyrophenone classes of antipsychotics. Many elderly patients receive antipsychotic medications for inappropriate nonpsychotic behavior. Before initiating antipsychotic medication, the clinician should investigate any possible reversible cause; any stress or stress from any disease can cause acute "confusion" or worsening of baseline nonpsychotic behavior. Most commonly acute changes in behavior are due to increases in drug dose or addition of new drug to regimen; fluid electrolyte loss; infections; and changes in environment.

In the treatment of agitated, demented, elderly patients, authors of meta-analysis of controlled trials of the response to the traditional antipsychotics (phenothiazines, butyrophenones) in controlling agitation have concluded that the use of neuroleptics results in a response rate of 18%. Clearly neuroleptic therapy for behavior control should be limited with frequent attempts to withdraw the agent given for behavior control. In light of significant risks and adverse effects in elderly population compared with limited data demonstrating efficacy in the treatment of dementia related psychosis, aggression, and agitation, an extensive risk:benefit analysis should be performed prior to use.

Dosage Forms Excipient information presented when available (limited, particularly for generics); consult specific product labeling.

Injection, microspheres for reconstitution, extended release:

Risperdal® Consta®: 12.5 mg, 25 mg, 37.5 mg, 50 mg [supplied in a dose-pack containing vial with active ingredient in microsphere formulation, prefilled syringe with diluent, needle-free vial access device, and safety needle]

Solution, oral:

Risperdal®: 1 mg/mL (30 mL) [contains benzoic acid]

Tablet:

Risperdal®: 0.25 mg, 0.5 mg, 1 mg, 2 mg, 3 mg, 4 mg

Tablet, orally disintegrating:
Risperdal® M-Tabs®: 0.5 mg [contains phenylalanine 0.14 mg]; 1 mg [contains phenylalanine 0.28 mg]; 2 mg [contains phenylalanine 0.42 mg]; 3 mg [contains phenylalanine 0.63 mg]; 4 mg [contains phenylalanine 0.84 mg]

Selected References

American Diabetes Association; American Psychiatric Association; American Association of Clinical Endocrinologists; North American Association for the Study of Obesity, "Consensus Development Conference on Antipsychotic Drugs and Obesity and Diabetes," *Diabetes Care*, 2004, 27(2):596-601.

Cohen LJ, "Risperidone," *Pharmacotherapy*, 1994, 14(3):253-65.

Schneider LS, Tariot PN, Dagerman KS, et al, "Effectiveness of Atypical Antipsychotic Drugs in Patients With Alzheimer's Disease," *N Engl J Med*, 2006, 355(15):1525-38.

♦ **Ritalin®** *see* Methylphenidate *on page 1013*

♦ **Ritalin® LA** *see* Methylphenidate *on page 1013*

♦ **Ritalin-SR®** *see* Methylphenidate *on page 1013*

Rivastigmine (ri va STIG meen)

U.S. Brand Names Exelon®
Canadian Brand Names Exelon®
Index Terms ENA 713; Rivastigmine Tartrate; SDZ ENA 713
Generic Available No
Pharmacologic Category Acetylcholinesterase Inhibitor (Central)
Use Treatment of mild-to-moderate dementia associated with Alzheimer's disease and Parkinson's disease
Contraindications Hypersensitivity to rivastigmine, other carbamate derivatives (eg, neostigmine, pyridostigmine, physostigmine), or any component of the formulation
Warnings/Precautions Significant nausea, vomiting, anorexia, and weight loss are associated with use; occurs more frequently in women and during the titration phase. Nausea and/or vomiting may be severe, particularly at doses higher than recommended. Monitor weight during therapy. Therapy should be initiated at lowest dose and titrated; if treatment is interrupted for more than several days, reinstate at the lowest daily dose. Cholinesterase inhibitors may have vagotonic effects which may cause bradycardia and/or heart block with or without a history of cardiac disease. Use caution in patients with a history of peptic ulcer disease or concurrent NSAID use. Use caution in patients undergoing anesthesia who will receive succinylcholine-type muscle relaxation, patients with sick-sinus syndrome, bradycardia or supraventricular conduction conditions, urinary obstruction, seizure disorders, or pulmonary conditions such as asthma or COPD. Use caution in patients with low body weight (<50 kg) due to increased risk of adverse reactions.
Adverse Reactions (Reflective of adult population; not specific for elderly)
Note: Many concentration-related effects are reported at a lower frequency by transdermal route.
>10%:
Central nervous system: Dizziness (2% to 21%), headache (3% to 17%)
Gastrointestinal: Nausea (7% to 47%), vomiting (6% to 31%), diarrhea (5% to 19%), anorexia (3% to 17%), abdominal pain (1% to 13%)
1% to 10%:
Cardiovascular: Syncope (3%), hypertension (3%)
Central nervous system: Fatigue (2% to 9%), insomnia (1% to 9%), confusion (8%), depression (4% to 6%), anxiety (2% to 5%), malaise (5%), somnolence (4% to 5%), hallucinations (4%), aggressiveness (3%), parkinsonism symptoms worsening (2% to 3%), vertigo (≤2%)
Gastrointestinal: Dyspepsia (9%), constipation (5%), flatulence (4%), weight loss (3% to 8%), eructation (2%), dehydration (2%)
Genitourinary: Urinary tract infection (1% to 7%)
Neuromuscular & skeletal: Weakness (2% to 6%), tremor (1%; up to 10% in Parkinson's patients)
Respiratory: Rhinitis (4%)
Miscellaneous: Diaphoresis (4%), flu-like syndrome (3%)
Overdosage/Toxicology In cases of asymptomatic overdoses, rivastigmine should be held for 24 hours. Cholinergic crisis, caused by significant acetylcholinesterase inhibition, is characterized by severe nausea, vomiting, salivation, sweating, bradycardia, hypotension, respiratory depression, cardiovascular collapse, and convulsions. Treatment is supportive and symptomatic. Dialysis would not be helpful.
Drug Interactions
Anticholinergics: Effects may be reduced with rivastigmine.
Antipsychotic agents: Acetylcholinesterase inhibitors (central) may increase the risk of antipsychotic-related extrapyramidal symptoms; monitor.
Beta-blockers without ISA activity: May increase risk of bradycardia.
Calcium channel blockers (diltiazem or verapamil): May increase risk of bradycardia.
Cholinergic agonists: Effects may be increased with rivastigmine.
(Continued)

Rivastigmine *(Continued)*

Corticosteroids (systemic): May enhance the adverse effects (muscle weakness) of rivastigmine.

Digoxin: Increased risk of bradycardia with concurrent use

Neuromuscular blockers, nondepolarizing: Rivastigmine may decrease the effects of nondepolarizing neuromuscular-blocking agents. Rivastigmine may decrease the metabolism of mivacurium.

Neuromuscular blockers (succinylcholine): Depolarizing neuromuscular blocking agents effects may be increased with rivastigmine.

NSAIDs: Although not seen in clinical studies, patients may be at increased risk for peptic ulcers or gastrointestinal bleeding with concomitant use; monitor

Ethanol/Nutrition/Herb Interactions

Smoking: Nicotine increases the clearance of rivastigmine by 23%.

Ethanol: Avoid ethanol (due to risk of sedation; may increase GI irritation).

Food: Food delays absorption by 90 minutes, lowers C_{max} by 30% and increases AUC by 30%.

Herb/Nutraceutical: Avoid ginkgo biloba (may increase cholinergic effects).

Stability

Oral: Store at 15°C to 30°C (59°F to 86°F); do not freeze. Store solution in an upright position.

Transdermal patch: Store at 15°C to 30°C (59°F to 86°F). Patches should be kept in sealed pouch until use.

Mechanism of Action A deficiency of cortical acetylcholine is thought to account for some of the symptoms of Alzheimer's disease and the dementia of Parkinson's disease; rivastigmine increases acetylcholine in the central nervous system through reversible inhibition of its hydrolysis by cholinesterase

Pharmacodynamics Duration: Anticholinesterase activity (CSF): ~10 hours (6 mg dose)

Pharmacokinetics

Absorption: Rapid and complete within 1 hour when administered in the fasting state. Food delays absorption.

Distribution: V_d: 1.8-2.7 L/kg

Protein binding: 40%

Metabolism: Extensively metabolized by cholinesterase-mediated hydrolysis in the brain. The metabolite undergoes N-demethylation and/or sulfate conjugation in the liver. Linear kinetics at 3 mg twice daily, but nonlinear at higher doses.

Bioavailability: 36% to 40%

Half-life: 1.5 hours

Time to peak: 1 hour

Elimination: 97% recovered in urine as metabolites; 0.4% in feces. Mean oral clearance was 30% lower in older adult patients as compared to younger patients.

Dosage

Geriatrics: Following oral administration, clearance is significantly lower in patients >60 years of age, but dosage adjustments are not recommended. Age was not associated with exposure in patients treated transdermally. Titrate dose to individual's tolerance. Refer to adult dosing.

Adults: Note: Exelon® oral solution and capsules are bioequivalent.

Mild-to-moderate Alzheimer's dementia:

Oral: Initial: 1.5 mg twice daily; may increase by 3 mg/day (1.5 mg/dose) every 2 weeks based on tolerability (maximum recommended dose: 6 mg twice daily)

Note: If GI adverse events occur, discontinue treatment for several doses then restart at the same or next lower dosage level; antiemetics have been used to control GI symptoms. If treatment is interrupted for longer than several days, restart the treatment at the lowest dose and titrate as previously described.

Transdermal patch: Initial: 4.6 mg/24 hours; if well tolerated, may be increased (after at least 4 weeks) to 9.5 mg/24 hours (recommended effective dose). Maintenance: 9.5 mg/24 hours (maximum dose: 9.5 mg/24 hours).

Note: If intolerance is noted (nausea, vomiting), patch should be removed and treatment interrupted for several days and restarted at the same or lower dosage. If interrupted for more than several days, reinitiate at lowest dosage and increase to maintenance dose after 4 weeks.

Conversion from oral therapy: If oral daily dose <6 mg, switch to 4.6 mg/24 hours patch; if oral daily dose 6-12 mg, switch to 9.5 mg/24 hours patch. Apply patch on the next day following last oral dose.

Mild-to-moderate Parkinson's-related dementia:

Oral: Initial: 1.5 mg twice daily; may increase by 3 mg/day (1.5 mg/dose) every 4 weeks based on tolerability (maximum recommended dose: 6 mg twice daily)

Transdermal patch: See transdermal dosing for Alzheimer's dementia.

Renal Impairment: Dosage adjustments are not recommended, however, titrate the dose to the individual's tolerance.

Hepatic Impairment: Clearance is significantly reduced in mild to moderately impaired patients. Although dosage adjustments are not recommended, use lowest possible dose and titrate according to individual's tolerance. Consider intervals of >2 weeks between dosage adjustments.

Administration Should be administered with meals (breakfast or dinner). Capsule should be swallowed whole. Liquid form is available for patients who cannot swallow capsules (can be swallowed directly from syringe or mixed with water, soda, or cold fruit juice). Stir well and drink within 4 hours of mixing.

Monitoring Parameters Cognitive function at periodic intervals

Patient Information Take with meals at breakfast and dinner. Swallow capsule whole. Do not chew, break, or crush capsule. A liquid (solution) is available for patients who cannot swallow capsules. Notify healthcare provider if nausea, vomiting, loss of appetite, or weight loss occur. See instructions for use of oral solution. Can swallow solution directly from syringe or mix with water, juice, or soda. Stir well and drink all of mixture within 4 hours of mixing. Do not mix with other liquids. Avoid concurrent ethanol use.

Special Geriatric Considerations Titrate dose to tolerance.

Dosage Forms Excipient information presented when available (limited, particularly for generics); consult specific product labeling.
Capsule:
Exelon®: 1.5 mg, 3 mg, 4.5 mg, 6 mg
Solution, oral:
Exelon®: 2 mg/mL (120 mL) [contains sodium benzoate]
Transdermal system [once-daily patch]:
Exelon®: 4.6 mg/24 hours (30s) [5 cm²; contains rivastigmine 9 mg]; 9.5 mg/24 hours (30s) [5 cm²; contains rivastigmine 18 mg]

♦ **Rivastigmine Tartrate** see Rivastigmine on page 1421

Rizatriptan (rye za TRIP tan)

U.S. Brand Names Maxalt®; Maxalt-MLT®
Canadian Brand Names Maxalt™; Maxalt RPD™
Index Terms MK462
Generic Available No
Pharmacologic Category Antimigraine Agent; Serotonin 5-HT$_{1B, 1D}$ Receptor Agonist
Use Acute treatment of migraine, with or without aura
Contraindications Hypersensitivity to rizatriptan or any component of the formulation; documented ischemic heart disease or Prinzmetal's angina; uncontrolled hypertension; basilar or hemiplegic migraine; during or within 2 weeks of MAO inhibitors; during or within 24 hours of treatment with another 5-HT$_1$ agonist, or an ergot-containing or ergot-type medication (eg, methysergide, dihydroergotamine)
Warnings/Precautions Use only in patients with a clear diagnosis of migraine. May cause vasospastic reactions resulting in colonic, peripheral, or coronary ischemia. Use with caution in elderly or patients with hepatic or renal impairment (including dialysis patients), history of hypersensitivity to sumatriptan or adverse effects from sumatriptan, and in patients at risk of coronary artery disease (as predicted by presence of risk factors) unless cardiovascular evaluation provides evidence that the patient is free of cardiovascular disease. In patients with risk factors for coronary artery disease, following adequate evaluation to establish the absence of coronary artery disease, the initial dose should be administered in a setting where response may be evaluated (physician's office or similarly staffed setting). ECG monitoring may be considered. May increase blood pressure transiently; may cause coronary vasospasm (less than sumatriptan); avoid in patients with signs/symptoms suggestive of reduced arterial flow (ischemic bowel, Raynaud's) which could be exacerbated by vasospasm. Cerebral/subarachnoid hemorrhage and stroke have been reported with 5-HT$_1$ agonist administration.

Patients who experience sensations of chest pain/pressure/tightness or symptoms suggestive of angina following dosing should be evaluated for coronary artery disease or Prinzmetal's angina before receiving additional doses. Symptoms of agitation, confusion, hallucinations, hyper-reflexia, myoclonus, shivering, and tachycardia (serotonin syndrome) may occur with concomitant proserotonergic drugs (ie, SSRIs/SNRIs or triptans) or agents which reduce rizatriptan's metabolism. Concurrent use of serotonin precursors (eg, tryptophan) is not recommended.

Reconsider diagnosis of migraine if no response to initial dose. Long-term effects on vision have not been evaluated. Maxalt-MLT® tablets contain phenylalanine.

Adverse Reactions (Reflective of adult population; not specific for elderly)
1% to 10%:
Cardiovascular: Systolic/diastolic blood pressure increases (5-10 mm Hg), chest pain (5%), palpitation
Central nervous system: Dizziness, drowsiness, fatigue (13% to 30%, dose related)
Dermatologic: Skin flushing
(Continued)

Rizatriptan *(Continued)*

Endocrine & metabolic: Mild increase in growth hormone, hot flashes
Gastrointestinal: Abdominal pain, dry mouth (<5%), nausea
Respiratory: Dyspnea

Drug Interactions Use within 24 hours of another selective 5-HT$_1$ agonist or ergot-containing drug should be avoided due to possible additive vasoconstriction

MAO inhibitors and nonselective MAO inhibitors increase concentration of rizatriptan
Propranolol: Plasma concentration of rizatriptan increased 70%

Serotonergic reuptake inhibitors (eg, SSRIs/SNRIs): Concurrent use of rizatriptan with these agents may increase the risk of serotonin syndrome; monitor.

Serotonin agonists (eg, triptans): Concurrent use of rizatriptan with these agents may increase the risk of serotonin syndrome; monitor.

Ethanol/Nutrition/Herb Interactions Food: Food delays absorption.

Stability Store in blister pack until administration.

Mechanism of Action Selective agonist for serotonin (5-HT$_{1D}$ receptor) in cranial arteries to cause vasoconstriction and reduce sterile inflammation associated with antidromic neuronal transmission correlating with relief of migraine

Pharmacodynamics
Onset of action: Within 30 minutes
Duration: 14-16 hours

Pharmacokinetics
Protein binding: Minimal (14%)
Metabolism: Substantial nonrenal clearance by monoamine oxidase-A; undergoes first-pass metabolism
Bioavailability: 40% to 50%
Half-life: 2-3 hours
Time to peak concentration: 1-1.5 hours
Elimination: 8% to 16% excreted unchanged in urine; parent and metabolites eliminated (82%)

Dosage
Geriatrics & Adults: Note: In patients with risk factors for coronary artery disease, following adequate evaluation to establish the absence of coronary artery disease, the initial dose should be administered in a setting where response may be evaluated (physician's office or similarly staffed setting). ECG monitoring may be considered.

Migraine: Oral: 5-10 mg, repeat after 2 hours if significant relief is not attained; maximum: 30 mg in a 24-hour period (use 5 mg dose in patients receiving propranolol with a maximum of 15 mg in 24 hours)

Note: For orally-disintegrating tablets (Maxalt-MLT®): Patient should be instructed to place tablet on tongue and allow to dissolve. Dissolved tablet will be swallowed with saliva.

Monitoring Parameters Headache severity, signs/symptoms suggestive of angina; consider monitoring blood pressure, heart rate, and/or EKG with first dose in patients with likelihood of unrecognized coronary disease, such as patients with significant hypertension, hypercholesterolemia, obese patients, diabetics, smokers with other risk factors or strong family history of coronary artery disease

Patient Information For orally disintegrating tablets: Do not remove blister from outer pouch until just before dosing; open blister with dry hands, place tablet on tongue and allow to dissolve. Dissolved tablet will be swallowed with saliva.

For all dosage forms: May repeat dose anytime after 2 hours of the first dose. Do not take a second dose without first consulting your physician. Do not take more than 30 mg in a 24-hour period (15 mg maximum in 24 hours if taking propranolol).

Special Geriatric Considerations Since the elderly often have cardiovascular disease, careful evaluation of the use of 5-HT agonists is needed to avoid complications with the use of these agents. The pharmacokinetic disposition of these agents is similar to that seen in younger adults.

Dosage Forms Excipient information presented when available (limited, particularly for generics); consult specific product labeling.
Tablet, as benzoate:
Maxalt®: 5 mg, 10 mg
Tablet, orally disintegrating, as benzoate:
Maxalt-MLT®: 5 mg [contains phenylalanine 1.05 mg/tablet; peppermint flavor]; 10 mg [contains phenylalanine 2.1 mg/tablet; peppermint flavor]

- **Robinul® Forte** *see* Glycopyrrolate *on page 719*
- **Robitussin® [OTC]** *see* Guaifenesin *on page 727*
- **Robitussin® Cough and Congestion [OTC]** *see* Guaifenesin and Dextromethorphan *on page 730*
- **Robitussin® CoughGels™ [OTC]** *see* Dextromethorphan *on page 419*
- **Robitussin® DM [OTC]** *see* Guaifenesin and Dextromethorphan *on page 730*
- **Robitussin® DM Infant [OTC]** *see* Guaifenesin and Dextromethorphan *on page 730*
- **Robitussin® Maximum Strength Cough [OTC]** *see* Dextromethorphan *on page 419*
- **Robitussin® Pediatric Cough [OTC]** *see* Dextromethorphan *on page 419*
- **Robitussin® Sugar Free Cough [OTC]** *see* Guaifenesin and Dextromethorphan *on page 730*
- **Rocaltrol®** *see* Calcitriol *on page 210*
- **Rocephin®** *see* Ceftriaxone *on page 272*
- **Roferon®-A** *see* Interferon Alfa-2a *on page 820*
- **Rogaine® Extra Strength for Men [OTC]** *see* Minoxidil *on page 1048*
- **Rogaine® for Men [OTC]** *see* Minoxidil *on page 1048*
- **Rogaine® for Women [OTC]** *see* Minoxidil *on page 1048*
- **Rolaids® Calcium Rich [OTC]** *see* Calcium Salts (Oral) *on page 220*
- **Romilar® AC** *see* Guaifenesin and Codeine *on page 729*
- **Romycin®** *see* Erythromycin *on page 533*

Ropinirole (roe PIN i role)

Related Information
Antiparkinsonian Agents *on page 1745*
Medication Safety Issues
Sound-alike/look-alike issues:
Ropinirole may be confused with ropivacaine
U.S. Brand Names Requip®
Canadian Brand Names Requip®
Index Terms Ropinirole Hydrochloride
Generic Available No
Pharmacologic Category Anti-Parkinson's Agent, Dopamine Agonist
Use Treatment of idiopathic Parkinson's disease; in patients with early Parkinson's disease who were not receiving concomitant levodopa therapy as well as in patients with advanced disease on concomitant levodopa; treatment of moderate-to-severe primary Restless Legs Syndrome (RLS)
Contraindications Hypersensitivity to ropinirole or any component of the formulation
Warnings/Precautions Syncope, sometimes associated with bradycardia, was observed in association with ropinirole in both early Parkinson's disease (without levodopa) patients and advanced Parkinson's disease (with levodopa) patients. Dopamine agonists appear to impair the systemic regulation of blood pressure resulting in postural hypotension, especially during dose escalation. Parkinson's disease patients appear to have an impaired capacity to respond to a postural challenge; use with caution in patients at risk of hypotension (ie, those receiving antihypertensive drugs) or where transient hypotensive episodes would be poorly tolerated (cardiovascular disease or cerebrovascular disease). Parkinson's patients being treated with dopaminergic agonists ordinarily require careful monitoring for signs and symptoms of postural hypotension, especially during dose escalation, and should be informed of this risk. May cause hallucinations. Use with caution in patients with pre-existing dyskinesia, severe hepatic or renal dysfunction.

Patients treated with ropinirole have reported falling asleep while engaging in activities of daily living; this has been reported to occur without significant warning signs. Monitor for daytime somnolence or pre-existing sleep disorder; caution with concomitant sedating medication; discontinue if significant daytime sleepiness or episodes of falling asleep occur. Patients must be cautioned about performing tasks which require mental alertness (eg, operating machinery or driving). Use with caution in patients receiving other CNS depressants or psychoactive agents. Effects with other sedative drugs or ethanol may be potentiated.

Some patients treated for RLS may experience worsening of symptoms in the early morning hours (rebound) or an increase and/or spread of daytime symptoms (augmentation); clinical management of these phenomena has not been evaluated in controlled clinical trials. Pathologic degenerative changes were observed in the retinas of albino rats during studies with this agent, but were not observed in the retinas of albino mice or in other species. The significance of these data for humans remains uncertain.

Other dopaminergic agents have been associated with a syndrome resembling neuroleptic malignant syndrome on withdrawal or significant dosage reduction after (Continued)

Ropinirole *(Continued)*

long-term use. Risk of fibrotic complications (eg, pleural effusion/fibrosis, interstitial lung disease) and melanoma has been reported in patients receiving ropinirole; drug causation has not been established.

Adverse Reactions (Reflective of adult population; not specific for elderly)

Data inclusive of trials in early Parkinson's disease (without levodopa) and Restless Legs Syndrome:

>10%:

Cardiovascular: Syncope (1% to 12%)

Central nervous system: Somnolence (12% to 40%), dizziness (11% to 40%), fatigue (8% to 11%)

Gastrointestinal: Nausea (40% to 60%), vomiting (12%)

Miscellaneous: Viral infection (11%)

1% to 10%:

Cardiovascular: Dependent/leg edema (2% to 7%), orthostasis (1% to 6%), hypertension (5%), chest pain (4%), flushing (3%), palpitation (3%), peripheral ischemia (3%), hypotension (2%), tachycardia (2%)

Central nervous system: Pain (3% to 8%), confusion (5%), hallucinations (up to 5%, dose related), hypoesthesia (4%), amnesia (3%), malaise (3%), paresthesia (3%), vertigo (2%), yawning (3%)

Gastrointestinal: Constipation (>5%), dyspepsia (4% to 10%), abdominal pain (3% to 6%), xerostomia (3% to 5%), diarrhea (5%), anorexia (4%), flatulence (3%)

Genitourinary: Urinary tract infection (5%), impotence (3%)

Hepatic: Alkaline phosphatase increased (3%)

Neuromuscular & skeletal: Weakness (6%), arthralgia (4%), muscle cramps (3%)

Ocular: Abnormal vision (6%), xerophthalmia (2%)

Respiratory: Pharyngitis (6% to 9%), rhinitis (4%), sinusitis (4%), dyspnea (3%), influenza (3%), cough (3%), nasal congestion (2%)

Miscellaneous: Diaphoresis increased (3% to 6%)

Advanced Parkinson's disease (with levodopa):

>10%:

Central nervous system: Dizziness (26%), somnolence (20%), headache (17%)

Gastrointestinal: Nausea (30%)

Neuromuscular & skeletal: Dyskinesias (34%)

1% to 10%:

Cardiovascular: Syncope (3%), hypotension (2%)

Central nervous system: Hallucinations (10%, dose related), aggravated parkinsonism, confusion (9%), pain (5%), paresis (3%), amnesia (5%), anxiety (6%), abnormal dreaming (3%), insomnia

Gastrointestinal: Abdominal pain (9%), vomiting (7%), constipation (6%), diarrhea (5%), dysphagia (2%), flatulence (2%), increased salivation (2%), xerostomia, weight loss (2%)

Genitourinary: Urinary tract infection

Hematologic: Anemia (2%)

Neuromuscular & skeletal: Falls (10%), arthralgia (7%), tremor (6%), hypokinesia (5%), paresthesia (5%), arthritis (3%)

Respiratory: Upper respiratory tract infection (9%), dyspnea (3%)

Miscellaneous: Injury, diaphoresis increased (7%), viral infection, increased drug level (7%)

Other adverse effects (all phase 2/3 trials):

1% to 10%:

Central nervous system: Neuralgia (>1%)

Renal: BUN increased (>1%)

Overdosage/Toxicology There have been no reports of intentional overdose. Symptoms reported with accidental overdosage included agitation, increased dyskinesia, sedation, orthostatic hypotension, chest pain, confusion, nausea, and vomiting. It is anticipated that the symptoms of overdose will be related to its dopaminergic activity. General supportive measures are recommended. Vital signs should be maintained, if necessary. Removal of any unabsorbed material (eg, by gastric lavage) should be considered.

Drug Interactions Substrate of CYP1A2 (major), 3A4 (minor); **Inhibits** CYP1A2 (weak), 2D6 (strong)

Antipsychotics: May reduce the effect of ropinirole due to dopamine antagonism

CYP1A2 inducers: May decrease the levels/effects of ropinirole. Example inducers include aminoglutethimide, carbamazepine, phenobarbital, and rifampin.

CYP1A2 inhibitors: May increase the levels/effects of ropinirole. Example inhibitors include fluvoxamine, ketoconazole, and rofecoxib.

CYP2D6 substrates: Ropinirole may increase the levels/effects of CYP2D6 substrates. Example substrates include amphetamines, selected beta-blockers, dextromethorphan, fluoxetine, lidocaine, mirtazapine, nefazodone, paroxetine, risperidone, ritonavir, thioridazine, tricyclic antidepressants, and venlafaxine.

CYP2D6 prodrug substrates: Ropinirole may decrease the levels/effects of CYP2D6 prodrug substrates. Example prodrug substrates include codeine, hydrocodone, oxycodone, and tramadol.

Estrogens: May reduce the metabolism of ropinirole; dosage adjustments may be needed; clearance may be reduced by 36%

Metoclopramide: May reduce the effect of ropinirole due to dopamine antagonism

Quinolone antibiotics (specifically ciprofloxacin, norfloxacin, ofloxacin): May increase the levels/effects of ropinirole.

Ethanol/Nutrition/Herb Interactions

Ethanol: Avoid ethanol (may increase CNS depression).

Herb/Nutraceutical: Avoid kava kava, gotu kola, valerian, St John's wort (may increase CNS depression).

Mechanism of Action Ropinirole has a high relative *in vitro* specificity and full intrinsic activity at the D_2 and D_3 dopamine receptor subtypes, binding with higher affinity to D_3 than to D_2 or D_4 receptor subtypes; relevance of D_3 receptor binding in Parkinson's disease is unknown. Ropinirole has moderate *in vitro* affinity for opioid receptors. Ropinirole and its metabolites have negligible *in vitro* affinity for dopamine D_1, 5-HT_1, 5-HT_2, benzodiazepine, GABA, muscarinic, alpha$_1$-, alpha$_2$-, and beta-adrenoreceptors. Although precise mechanism of action of ropinirole is unknown, it is believed to be due to stimulation of postsynaptic dopamine D_2-type receptors within the caudate putamen in the brain. Ropinirole caused decreases in systolic and diastolic blood pressure at doses >0.25 mg. The mechanism of ropinirole-induced postural hypotension is believed to be due to D_2-mediated blunting of the noradrenergic response to standing and subsequent decrease in peripheral vascular resistance.

Pharmacokinetics

Absorption: Not affected by food; T_{max} increased by 2.5 hours when drug taken with a meal; absolute bioavailability was 55%, indicating first-pass effect

Distribution: V_d: 525 L; removal of drug by hemodialysis is unlikely

Metabolism: Extensively by liver to inactive metabolites

Half-life, elimination: ~6 hours

Time to peak concentration: ~1-2 hours

Clearance of ropinirole is reduced by 30% in patients >65 years of age

Dosage

Geriatrics & Adults:

Parkinson's disease: Oral: The dosage should be increased to achieve a maximum therapeutic effect, balanced against the principal side effects of nausea, dizziness, somnolence and dyskinesia. Recommended starting dose is 0.25 mg 3 times/day; based on individual patient response, the dosage should be titrated with weekly increments as described below:

- Week 1: 0.25 mg 3 times/day; total daily dose: 0.75 mg
- Week 2: 0.5 mg 3 times/day; total daily dose: 1.5 mg
- Week 3: 0.75 mg 3 times/day; total daily dose: 2.25 mg
- Week 4: 1 mg 3 times/day; total daily dose: 3 mg

Note: After week 4, if necessary, daily dosage may be increased by 1.5 mg per day on a weekly basis up to a dose of 9 mg/day, and then by up to 3 mg/day weekly to a total of 24 mg/day

Parkinson's disease discontinuation taper: Ropinirole should be gradually tapered over 7 days as follows: reduce frequency of administration from 3 times daily to twice daily for 4 days, then reduce to once daily for remaining 3 days.

Restless Legs Syndrome: Initial: 0.25 mg once daily 1-3 hours before bedtime. Dose may be increased after 2 days to 0.5 mg daily, and after 7 days to 1 mg daily. Dose may be further titrated upward in 0.5 mg increments every week until reaching a daily dose of 3 mg during week 6. If symptoms persist or reappear, the daily dose may be increased to a maximum of 4 mg beginning week 7.

Note: Doses up to 4 mg per day may be discontinued without tapering.

Renal Impairment: Removal by hemodialysis is unlikely.

Monitoring Parameters Blood pressure (orthostatic); daytime alertness

Patient Information Ropinirole can be taken with or without food. Hallucinations can occur and older adults are at a higher risk than younger patients with Parkinson's disease. Postural hypotension may develop with or without symptoms such as dizziness, nausea, syncope, and sometimes sweating. Hypotension and/or orthostatic symptoms may occur more frequently during initial therapy or with an increase in dose at any time. Use caution when rising rapidly after sitting or lying down, especially after having done so for prolonged periods and especially at the initiation of treatment with ropinirole. Ropinirole can cause sedation and patients have reported falling asleep while involved in activities of daily living. Patients should be advised about the potential for drowsiness or sleepiness and should not drive if they note new-onset sleepiness. (Continued)

Ropinirole (Continued)

Because of additive sedative effects, caution should be used when taking CNS depressants (eg, benzodiazepines, antipsychotics, antidepressants) in combination with ropinirole.

Additional Information If ropinirole needs to be discontinued, it should be done so gradually over a 7-day period. Decrease dosing to twice daily for 4 days and then once daily for 3 days.

Special Geriatric Considerations Since the dose is titrated to clinical response, no specific dosage adjustment is necessary in the elderly.

Dosage Forms Excipient information presented when available (limited, particularly for generics); consult specific product labeling. [DSC] = Discontinued product
Combination package:
  Requip® [starter kit; contents per each administration card]: Tablet: 0.25 mg (2s), 0.5 mg (5s), 1 mg (7s) [DSC]
Tablet:
  Requip®: 0.25 mg, 0.5 mg, 1 mg, 2 mg, 3 mg, 4 mg, 5 mg

Selected References
Olanow CW, Watts RL, and Koller WC, "An Algorithm (Decision Tree) for the Management of Parkinson's Disease (2001): Treatment Guidelines," *Neurology*, 2001, 56(11 Suppl 5):S1-S88.
Stern MB, "Contemporary Approaches to the Pharmacotherapeutic Management of Parkinson's Disease: An Overview," *Neurology*, 1997, 49(1 Suppl 1):S2-9.
Watts RL, "The Role of Dopamine Agonists in Early Parkinson's Disease," *Neurology*, 1997, 49(1 Suppl 1):S34-48.

♦ **Ropinirole Hydrochloride** see Ropinirole on page 1425

Rosiglitazone (roh si GLI ta zone)

Medication Safety Issues
Sound-alike/look-alike issues:
  Avandia® may be confused with Avalide®, Coumadin®, Prandin®

International issues:
  Avandia® may be confused with Avanza® which is a brand name for mirtazapine in Australia

U.S. Brand Names Avandia®
Canadian Brand Names Avandia®
Generic Available No
Pharmacologic Category Antidiabetic Agent, Thiazolidinedione
Use Treatment of Type 2 diabetes mellitus (noninsulin dependent, NIDDM):
  Monotherapy: Improve glycemic control as an adjunct to diet and exercise
  Combination therapy: In combination with a sulfonylurea, metformin, or insulin or sulfonylurea plus metformin when diet, exercise, and a single agent do not result in adequate glycemic control

Contraindications Hypersensitivity to rosiglitazone or any component of the formulation; active liver disease (transaminases >2.5 times the upper limit of normal at baseline); contraindicated in patients who previously experienced jaundice during troglitazone therapy

Warnings/Precautions Should not be used in diabetic ketoacidosis. Mechanism requires the presence of insulin; therefore, use in type 1 diabetes (insulin dependent, IDDM) is not recommended.

May increase plasma volume and/or increase cardiac hypertrophy. Use with caution in patients with edema. Assess for fluid accumulation in patients with unusually rapid weight gain. Monitor closely for signs and symptoms of heart failure. Drug discontinuation is recommended if cardiovascular status worsens. A higher frequency of cardiovascular events has been noted in patients with NYHA Class I or II heart failure; up to 33% require adjustment of medications. Not recommended for use in patients with NYHA class III or IV heart failure. In patients with NYHA class II (systolic) heart failure, initiate at lowest dosage and monitor closely. Discontinue if heart failure develops. Use caution in patients with CAD or at risk for CAD; may be associated with an increased risk. Use with caution in patients with anemia or depressed leukocyte counts (may reduce hemoglobin, hematocrit, and/or WBC).

Use with caution in patients with elevated transaminases (AST or ALT). Idiosyncratic hepatotoxicity has been reported with another thiazolidinedione agent (troglitazone) and (rarely) with rosiglitazone; discontinue if jaundice occurs. Monitoring should include periodic determinations of liver function. Rosiglitazone has been associated with new onset and/or worsening of macular edema in diabetic patients. Rosiglitazone should be used with caution in patients with a pre-existing macular edema or diabetic retinopathy. Discontinuation of rosiglitazone should be considered in any patient who reports visual deterioration. In addition, ophthalmological consultation should be initiated in these patients. May result in hormonal imbalance; development of menstrual irregularities should prompt reconsideration of therapy.

Adverse Reactions (Reflective of adult population; not specific for elderly)
Rare cases of hepatocellular injury have been reported in men in their 60s within 2-3 weeks after initiation of rosiglitazone therapy. LFTs in these patients revealed severe hepatocellular injury which responded with rapid improvement of liver function and resolution of symptoms upon discontinuation of rosiglitazone. Patients were also receiving other potentially hepatotoxic medications (*Ann Intern Med*, 2000, 132:121-4; 132:164-6). The rate of certain adverse reactions (eg, anemia, edema, hypoglycemia) may be higher with some combination therapies. Patients with Class I or II heart failure (EF ≤45%) have a higher frequency of cardiovascular adverse events (edema, dyspnea in ≥25%).

>10%: Endocrine & metabolic: Weight gain, increase in total cholesterol, increased LDL-cholesterol, increased HDL-cholesterol

1% to 10%:
    Cardiovascular: Edema (5%), heart failure/CHF (up to 2% to 3% in patients receiving insulin; incidence likely higher in patients with pre-existing CHF or macrovascular disease)
    Central nervous system: Headache (6%), fatigue (4%)
    Endocrine & metabolic: Hyperglycemia (4%), hypoglycemia (1%; increased with insulin to 12% to 14%)
    Gastrointestinal: Diarrhea (2%)
    Hematologic: Anemia (2%)
    Neuromuscular & skeletal: Back pain (4%)
    Respiratory: Upper respiratory tract infection (10%), sinusitis (3%)
    Miscellaneous: Injury (8%)

Overdosage/Toxicology Experience in overdose is limited. Symptoms may include hypoglycemia. Treatment is symptom-directed and supportive.

Drug Interactions Substrate of CYP2C8 (major), 2C9 (minor); **Inhibits** CYP2C8 (moderate), 2C9 (weak), 2C19 (weak), 2D6 (weak)

Bile acid sequestrants: May decrease rosiglitazone levels; separate dosing by 2 hours.
Corticosteroids (systemic): May diminish the hypoglycemic effect of rosiglitazone.
CYP2C8 inducers: May decrease the levels/effects of rosiglitazone. Example inducers include carbamazepine, phenobarbital, phenytoin, rifampin, rifapentine, and secobarbital.
CYP2C8 inhibitors: May increase the levels/effects of rosiglitazone. Example inhibitors include atazanavir, gemfibrozil, and ritonavir.
CYP2C8 substrates: Rosiglitazone may increase the levels/effects of CYP2C8 substrates. Example substrates include amiodarone, paclitaxel, pioglitazone, repaglinide, and rosiglitazone.
Gemfibrozil: Gemfibrozil may increase rosiglitazone levels; a decreased rosiglitazone dose may be warranted
Insulin: May enhance the fluid-retaining effect of antidiabetic agents (thiazolidinedione).
Pegvisomant: May enhance the hypoglycemic effect of antidiabetic agents.
Pregabalin: May enhance the fluid-retaining effect of antidiabetic agents (thiazolidinedione).
Rifampin: May decrease rosiglitazone levels/effects.
Trimethoprim: May decrease the metabolism, via CYP isoenzymes, of rosiglitazone.

Ethanol/Nutrition/Herb Interactions
Ethanol: Avoid ethanol (may cause hypoglycemia).
Food: Peak concentrations are lower by 28% and delayed when administered with food, but these effects are not believed to be clinically significant.
Herb/Nutraceutical: Avoid alfalfa, aloe, bilberry, bitter melon, burdock, celery, damiana, fenugreek, garcinia, garlic, ginger, ginseng (American), gymnema, marshmallow, stinging nettle (may cause hypoglycemia).

Stability Store at 15°C to 30°C (59°F to 86°F). Protect from light.

Mechanism of Action Thiazolidinedione antidiabetic agent that lowers blood glucose by improving target cell response to insulin, without increasing pancreatic insulin secretion. It has a mechanism of action that is dependent on the presence of insulin for activity. Rosiglitazone is an agonist for peroxisome proliferator-activated receptor-gamma (PPARgamma). Activation of nuclear PPARgamma receptors influences the production of a number of gene products involved in glucose and lipid metabolism. Thiazolidinedione antidiabetic agent that lowers blood glucose by improving target cell response to insulin, without increasing pancreatic insulin secretion. It has a mechanism of action that is dependent on the presence of insulin for activity. PPARgamma is abundant in the cells within the renal collecting tubules; fluid retention results from stimulation by thiazolidinediones which increases sodium reabsorption.

Pharmacodynamics Onset of action: Delayed, may require up to 12 weeks to achieve maximal effect

Pharmacokinetics
Distribution: V_{dss} (apparent): 17.6 L
(Continued)

Rosiglitazone *(Continued)*

Protein binding: 99.8%

Metabolism: Hepatic (99%)

Bioavailability: 99%

Half-life: 3-4 hours

Time to peak, plasma: 1 hour; delayed with food

Excretion: Urine (64%) and feces (23%) as metabolites

Dosage

Geriatrics & Adults: Type 2 diabetes: Oral: **Note:** All patients should be initiated at the lowest recommended dose.

Monotherapy: Initial: 4 mg daily as a single daily dose or in divided doses twice daily. If response is inadequate after 8-12 weeks of treatment, the dosage may be increased to 8 mg daily as a single daily dose or in divided doses twice daily. In clinical trials, the 4 mg twice-daily regimen resulted in the greatest reduction in fasting plasma glucose and Hb A_{1c}.

Combination therapy: When adding rosiglitazone to existing therapy, continue current dose(s) of previous agents:

With sulfonylureas or metformin (or sulfonylurea plus metformin): Initial: 4 mg daily as a single daily dose or in divided doses twice daily. If response is inadequate after 8-12 weeks of treatment, the dosage may be increased to 8 mg daily as a single daily dose or in divided doses twice daily. Reduce dose of sulfonylurea if hypoglycemia occurs. It is unlikely that the dose of metformin will need to be reduced to hypoglycemia.

With insulin: Initial: 4 mg daily as a single daily dose or in divided doses twice daily. Dose of insulin should be reduced by 10% to 25% if the patient reports hypoglycemia or if the plasma glucose falls to <100 mg/dL. Doses of rosiglitazone >4 mg/day are not indicated in combination with insulin.

Renal Impairment: No adjustment is necessary.

Hepatic Impairment: Clearance is significantly lower in hepatic impairment. Therapy should not be initiated if the patient exhibits active liver disease of increased transaminases (>2.5 times the upper limit of normal) at baseline.

Monitoring Parameters Hemoglobin A_{1c}, serum glucose; signs and symptoms of fluid retention or heart failure; liver enzymes (prior to initiation of therapy, then periodically thereafter). Patients with an elevation in ALT >3 times the upper limit of normal should be rechecked as soon as possible. If the ALT levels remain >3 times the upper limit of normal, therapy with rosiglitazone should be discontinued.

Patient Information May be taken without regard to meals. Follow directions of prescriber. Monitor urine or serum glucose as recommended by prescriber. More frequent monitoring is required during periods of stress, trauma, surgery, increased activity, or exercise. Avoid alcohol. Report chest pain, rapid heartbeat or palpitations, abdominal pain, fever, rash, hypoglycemia reactions, yellowing of skin or eyes, dark urine or light stool, unusual fatigue, or nausea/vomiting.

Special Geriatric Considerations No dosage adjustment required.

Dosage Forms Excipient information presented when available (limited, particularly for generics); consult specific product labeling.

Tablet:

Avandia®: 2 mg, 4 mg, 8 mg

Rosiglitazone and Glimepiride (roh si GLI ta zone & GLYE me pye ride)

Related Information

Glimepiride *on page 708*

Rosiglitazone *on page 1428*

Medication Safety Issues

High alert medication: The Institute for Safe Medication Practices (ISMP) includes this medication among its list of drugs which have a heightened risk of causing significant patient harm when used in error.

U.S. Brand Names Avandaryl™

Index Terms Glimepiride and Rosiglitazone Maleate

Generic Available No

Pharmacologic Category Antidiabetic Agent, Sulfonylurea; Antidiabetic Agent, Thiazolidinedione

Use Management of type 2 diabetes mellitus (noninsulin dependent, NIDDM) in patients who are already treated with the combination of rosiglitazone and a sulfonylurea, or who are not adequately controlled on a sulfonylurea alone, or who initially responded to rosiglitazone alone and require additional glycemic control; used as an adjunct to diet and exercise to lower the blood glucose when hyperglycemia cannot be controlled satisfactorily by diet and exercise alone

Dosage

Geriatrics: Rosiglitazone 4 mg and glimepiride 1 mg once daily. Carefully titrate dose.

Adults: Type 2 diabetes mellitus: Oral: Initial: Rosiglitazone 4 mg and glimepiride 1 mg once daily **or** rosiglitazone 4 mg and glimepiride 2 mg once daily (for patients previously treated with sulfonylurea or thiazolidinedione monotherapy)

Patients switching from combination rosiglitazone and glimepiride as separate tablets: Use current dose. Maximum: Rosiglitazone 8 mg and glimepiride 4 mg once daily

Titration:

Dose adjustment in patients previously on sulfonylurea monotherapy: May take 2 weeks to observe decreased blood glucose and 2-3 months to see full effects of rosiglitazone component. If not adequately controlled after 8-12 weeks, increase daily dose of rosiglitazone component. Maximum: Rosiglitazone 8 mg and glimepiride 4 mg once daily

Dose adjustment in patients previously on thiazolidinedione monotherapy: If not adequately controlled after 1-2 weeks, increase daily dose of glimepiride component in ≤2 mg increments in 1-2 week intervals. Maximum: Rosiglitazone 8 mg and glimepiride 4 mg once daily

Renal Impairment: Rosiglitazone 4 mg and glimepiride 1 mg once daily. Carefully titrate dose.

Hepatic Impairment: Rosiglitazone 4 mg and glimepiride 1 mg once daily. Carefully titrate dose.

ALT ≤2.5 times ULN: Use with caution.

ALT >2.5 times ULN: Do not initiate therapy.

ALT >3 times ULN or jaundice: Discontinue.

Special Geriatric Considerations Rapid and prolonged hypoglycemia (>12 hours) despite hypertonic glucose injections have been reported; age, hepatic, and renal impairment are independent risk factors for hypoglycemia; dosage titration should be made at weekly intervals. How "tightly" a geriatric patient's blood glucose should be controlled is controversial; however, a fasting blood sugar of <150 mg/dL is now an acceptable endpoint. Such a decision should be based on the patient's functional and cognitive status, how well they recognize hypoglycemic or hyperglycemic symptoms, and how to respond to them and their other disease states.

Dosage Forms Excipient information presented when available (limited, particularly for generics); consult specific product labeling.

Tablet:

Avandaryl™ 4 mg/1 mg: Rosiglitazone 4 mg and glimepiride 1 mg

Avandaryl™ 4 mg/2 mg: Rosiglitazone 4 mg and glimepiride 2 mg

Avandaryl™ 4 mg/4 mg: Rosiglitazone 4 mg and glimepiride 4 mg

Rosiglitazone and Metformin (roh si GLI ta zone & met FOR min)

Related Information
Metformin *on page 993*
Rosiglitazone *on page 1428*

U.S. Brand Names Avandamet®

Canadian Brand Names Avandamet®

Index Terms Metformin and Rosiglitazone; Metformin Hydrochloride and Rosiglitazone Maleate; Rosiglitazone Maleate and Metformin Hydrochloride

Generic Available No

Pharmacologic Category Antidiabetic Agent, Biguanide; Antidiabetic Agent, Thiazolidinedione

Use Management of type 2 diabetes mellitus (noninsulin dependent, NIDDM) as an adjunct to diet and exercise in patients where dual rosiglitazone and metformin therapy is appropriate

Dosage

Geriatrics: The initial and maintenance dosing should be conservative, due to the potential for decreased renal function (monitor). Generally, elderly patients should not be titrated to the maximum. Do not use in patients ≥80 years unless normal renal function has been established.

Adults: Type 2 diabetes mellitus: Oral:

First-line therapy (drug-naive patients): Initial: Rosiglitazone 2 mg and metformin 500 mg once or twice daily; may increase by 2 mg/500 mg per day after 4 weeks to a maximum of 8 mg/2000 mg per day.

Second-line therapy:

Patients inadequately controlled on metformin alone: Initial dose: Rosiglitazone 4 mg/day plus current dose of metformin

Patients inadequately controlled on rosiglitazone alone: Initial dose: Metformin 1000 mg/day plus current dose of rosiglitazone

Note: When switching from combination rosiglitazone and metformin as separate tablets: Use current dose

(Continued)

Rosiglitazone and Metformin *(Continued)*

Dose adjustment: Doses may be increased as increments of rosiglitazone 4 mg and/or metformin 500 mg, up to the maximum dose; doses should be titrated gradually.

After a change in the metformin dosage, titration can be done after 1-2 weeks

After a change in the rosiglitazone dosage, titration can be done after 8-12 weeks

Maximum dose: Rosiglitazone 8 mg/metformin 2000 mg daily

Renal Impairment: Do not use with renal disease or renal dysfunction (serum creatinine ≥1.5 mg/dL in males or ≥1.4 mg/dL in females or abnormal clearance).

Hepatic Impairment: Do not use with active liver disease or ALT >2.5 times the upper limit of normal.

Dosage Forms Excipient information presented when available (limited, particularly for generics); consult specific product labeling. [DSC] = Discontinued product

Tablet:

Avandamet®: 1/500: Rosiglitazone 1 mg and metformin hydrochloride 500 mg [DSC]

Avandamet®: 2/500: Rosiglitazone 2 mg and metformin hydrochloride 500 mg

Avandamet®: 4/500: Rosiglitazone 4 mg and metformin hydrochloride 500 mg

Avandamet®: 2/1000: Rosiglitazone 2 mg and metformin hydrochloride 1000 mg

Avandamet®: 4/1000: Rosiglitazone 4 mg and metformin hydrochloride 1000 mg

♦ **Rosiglitazone Maleate and Metformin Hydrochloride** *see* Rosiglitazone and Metformin *on page 1431*

♦ **Rosula® NS** *see* Sulfacetamide *on page 1496*

Rosuvastatin *(roe soo va STAT in)*

Related Information

Hyperlipidemia Management *on page 1773*

U.S. Brand Names Crestor®

Canadian Brand Names Crestor®

Index Terms Rosuvastatin Calcium

Generic Available No

Pharmacologic Category Antilipemic Agent, HMG-CoA Reductase Inhibitor

Use In conjunction with dietary therapy for hyperlipidemias to reduce elevations in total cholesterol (TC), LDL-C, apolipoprotein B, and triglycerides (TG) in patients with primary hypercholesterolemia (elevations of 1 or more components are present in Fredrickson type IIa, IIb, and IV hyperlipidemias); treatment of homozygous familial hypercholesterolemia (FH)

Contraindications Hypersensitivity to rosuvastatin or any component of the formulation; active liver disease; unexplained persistent elevations of serum transaminases (>3 times ULN)

Warnings/Precautions Secondary causes of hyperlipidemia should be ruled out prior to therapy. Liver function must be monitored by periodic laboratory assessment. Use with caution in patients who consume large amounts of ethanol or have a history of liver disease. Rhabdomyolysis with acute renal failure has occurred. Discontinue in any patient in which CPK levels are markedly elevated (>10 times ULN) or if myopathy is suspected/diagnosed. An increased incidence of rosuvastatin-associated myopathy has been reported during concomitant therapy with fibric acid derivatives, niacin, cyclosporine, and in certain subgroups of the Asian population. Monitor closely if used with other drugs associated with myopathy (eg, colchicine). Risk is also elevated at higher dosages of rosuvastatin. Patients should be instructed to report unexplained muscle pain, tenderness, or weakness, particularly if associated with fever and/or malaise. Use caution in patients predisposed to myopathy (eg, renal failure, advanced age, inadequately treated hypothyroidism). Temporarily withhold in patients experiencing an acute or serious condition predisposing to renal failure secondary to rhabdomyolysis (sepsis, hypotension, major surgery, trauma, severe metabolic or endocrine or electrolyte disorders, uncontrolled seizures). Use with caution in patients with advanced age, these patients are predisposed to myopathy.

Adverse Reactions (Reflective of adult population; not specific for elderly)

1% to 10%:

Cardiovascular: Chest pain, hypertension, palpitation, peripheral edema

Central nervous system: Headache (6%), anxiety, depression, dizziness, insomnia, neuralgia, pain, vertigo

Dermatologic: Rash

Gastrointestinal: Pharyngitis (9%), abdominal pain, constipation, diarrhea, dyspepsia, gastroenteritis, nausea, vomiting

Hematologic: Anemia, bruising

Neuromuscular & skeletal: Myalgia (3%), arthralgia, arthritis, back pain, hypertonia, paresthesia, weakness

Respiratory: Bronchitis, cough, rhinitis, sinusitis

Miscellaneous: Flu-like syndrome

Adverse reactions reported with other HMG-CoA reductase inhibitors include a hypersensitivity syndrome (symptoms may include anaphylaxis, angioedema, arthralgia, erythema multiforme, eosinophilia, hemolytic anemia, lupus syndrome, photosensitivity, polymyalgia rheumatica, positive ANA, purpura, Stevens-Johnson syndrome, toxic epidermal necrolysis, urticaria, vasculitis)

Overdosage/Toxicology CNS vascular lesions and corneal opacities have been reported following high-dose, long-term exposure to HMG-CoA reductase inhibitors in animal studies. The relationship to human exposures has not been established. No specific experience in overdose. Treatment is supportive. Rosuvastatin is not removed by hemodialysis.

Drug Interactions Substrate (minor) of CYP2C9, 3A4

Antacids: Plasma concentrations may be decreased when given with magnesium/aluminum hydroxide-containing antacids. Antacids should be administered at least 2 hours after rosuvastatin.

Cholestyramine and colestipol (bile acid sequestrants): Reduce absorption of several HMG-CoA reductase inhibitors; separate administration times by at least 4 hours. Cholesterol-lowering effects are additive.

Clofibrate and fenofibrate may increase the risk of myopathy and rhabdomyolysis with HMG-CoA reductase inhibitors. Effects on lipid levels may be additive.

Colchicine: Concomitant therapy with an HMG-CoA reductase inhibitor may increase risk of myopathy/rhabdomyolysis; use caution.

Cyclosporine: May increase serum concentrations of rosuvastatin (up to 10 times usual concentrations). Limit dose to 5 mg/day.

Gemfibrozil: Serum concentrations of rosuvastatin may be increased (doubled) during concurrent administration; combination should be avoided. Limit dose to 10 mg/day.

Hormonal contraceptives: Rosuvastatin increases serum concentrations of ethinyl estradiol and norgestrel.

Lopinavir/ritonavir: May increase levels/toxicity of rosuvastatin. Limit dose to 10 mg/day.

Niacin: May increase the risk of myopathy and rhabdomyolysis with HMG-CoA reductase inhibitors.

Protease inhibitors: May decrease the metabolism, via CYP isoenzymes, of HMG-CoA reductase inhibitors.

Warfarin: Effects may be increased by rosuvastatin. Monitor.

Ethanol/Nutrition/Herb Interactions Ethanol: Avoid excessive ethanol consumption (due to potential hepatic effects).

Food: Red yeast rice contains an estimated 2.4 mg lovastatin per 600 mg rice.

Stability Store between 20°C and 25°C (68°F to 77°F). Protect from moisture.

Mechanism of Action Inhibitor of 3-hydroxy-3-methylglutaryl coenzyme A (HMG-CoA) reductase, the rate-limiting enzyme in cholesterol synthesis (reduces the production of mevalonic acid from HMG-CoA); this then results in a compensatory increase in the expression of LDL receptors on hepatocyte membranes and a stimulation of LDL catabolism

Pharmacodynamics

Onset of action: Within 1 week; maximal at 4 weeks

Pharmacokinetics

Distribution: V_d: 134 L

Protein binding: 90%

Metabolism: Hepatic (10%); 1 active metabolite identified

Bioavailability: 20% (high first-pass extraction by liver)

Half-life: 19 hours

Time to peak, plasma: 3-5 hours

Elimination: Feces (90%), primarily as unchanged drug

Dosage

Geriatrics & Adults:

Heterozygous familial and nonfamilial hypercholesterolemia; mixed dyslipidemia: Oral:

Initial dose:

General dosing: 10 mg once daily (20 mg in patients with severe hypercholesterolemia)

Conservative dosing: Patients requiring less aggressive treatment or predisposed to myopathy (including patients of Asian descent): 5 mg once daily

Titration: After 2 weeks, may be increased by 5-10 mg once daily; dosing range: 5-40 mg/day (maximum dose: 40 mg once daily)

Note: The 40 mg dose should be reserved for patients who have not achieved goal cholesterol levels on a dose of 20 mg/day, including patients switched from another HMG-CoA reductase inhibitor.

Homozygous familial hypercholesterolemia (HFH): Oral: Initial: 20 mg once daily (maximum dose: 40 mg/day)

Dosage adjustment with concomitant medications: Oral:

Cyclosporine: Rosuvastatin dose should not exceed 5 mg/day

(Continued)

Rosuvastatin *(Continued)*

Gemfibrozil or lopinavir and ritonavir combination: Rosuvastatin dose should not exceed 10 mg/day

Dosage adjustment for persistent, unexplained proteinuria while on 40 mg/ day: Reduce dose and evaluate causes.

Renal Impairment:

Mild to moderate impairment: No dosage adjustment required.

Cl_{cr} <30 mL/minute/1.73 m^2: Initial: 5 mg/day; do not exceed 10 mg once daily

Monitoring Parameters Total cholesterol, LDL, and HDL cholesterol; liver function tests should be determined at baseline (prior to initiation), 3 months following initiation, and 3 months after any increase in dose; baseline CPK (recheck CPK in any patient with symptoms suggestive of myopathy)

Special Geriatric Considerations Effective and well tolerated in the elderly. The definition of and, therefore, when to treat hyperlipidemia in geriatrics is a controversial issue. The National Cholesterol Education Program recommends that all adults maintain a plasma cholesterol <160 mg/dL. Elderly with one additional risk factor, goal LDL would be <130 mg/dL. It is the authors' belief that pharmacologic treatment be reserved for those who are unable to obtain a desirable plasma cholesterol concentration by diet alone and for whom the benefits of treatment are believed to outweigh the potential adverse effects, drug interactions, and cost of treatment.

Dosage Forms Excipient information presented when available (limited, particularly for generics); consult specific product labeling.

Tablet, as calcium: 5 mg, 10 mg, 20 mg, 40 mg

Selected References

Pasternak RC, Smith SC Jr, Bairey-Merz CN, et al, "ACC/AHA/NHLBI Clinical Advisory on the Use and Safety of Statins," *J Am Coll Cardiol*, 2002, 40(3):567-72, viewable at http://www.nhlbi.nih.gov/guidelines/cholesterol/statins.pdf, last accessed March 14, 2003.

♦ **Rosuvastatin Calcium** *see* Rosuvastatin *on page 1432*

Rotigotine *(roe TIG oh teen)*

Medication Safety Issues

Sound-alike/look-alike issues:

Neupro® may be confused with Neupogen®

Transdermal patch contains metal (eg, aluminum); remove patch prior to MRI.

U.S. Brand Names Neupro®

Index Terms N-0923

Generic Available No

Pharmacologic Category Anti-Parkinson's Agent, Dopamine Agonist

Use Treatment of the signs and symptoms of early-stage idiopathic Parkinson's disease

Contraindications Hypersensitivity to rotigotine or any component of the formulation

Warnings/Precautions Use commonly associated with somnolence. In addition, patients falling asleep during activities of daily living, including driving, have also been reported and may occur without significant warning signs. Monitor for daytime somnolence or pre-existing sleep disorder. Patients must be cautioned about performing tasks which require mental alertness (eg, operating machinery or driving). Use with caution in patients receiving other CNS depressants or psychoactive agents; discontinue if significant daytime sleepiness or episodes of falling asleep occur. Effects with other sedative drugs or ethanol may be potentiated.

Dopamine agonists may cause orthostatic hypotension and syncope; Parkinson's disease patients appear to have an impaired capacity to respond to a postural challenge. Use with caution in patients at risk of hypotension (such as those receiving antihypertensive drugs) or where transient hypotensive episodes would be poorly tolerated (cardiovascular disease or cerebrovascular disease). Parkinson's patients being treated with dopaminergic agonists ordinarily require careful monitoring for signs and symptoms of postural hypotension, especially during dose escalation, and should be informed of this risk. Therapy has also been associated with inconsistent increases in blood pressure, increased heart rate (average increase of 2-4 bpm), and fluid retention.

Use with caution in patients with pre-existing dyskinesia; therapy may exacerbate. Therapy may also cause hallucinations. Risk for melanoma development is increased in Parkinson's disease patients; drug causation or factors contributing to risk have not been established. Other dopaminergic agents have been associated with a syndrome resembling neuroleptic malignant syndrome on withdrawal and/or significant dosage reduction. Taper treatment when discontinuing therapy; do not stop abruptly. Rare cases of pleural, retroperitoneal fibrosis and/or cardiac valvulopathy have been reported in patients treated with ergot-derived dopamine agonists, generally with prolonged use. The potential of rotigotine, a nonergot-derived dopamine agonist, to cause similar fibrotic complications is unknown.

Patch contains aluminum; remove patch prior to magnetic resonance imaging or cardioversion to avoid skin burns. Patch also contains sodium metabisulfite which may cause allergic reaction in susceptible individuals. Patients should be instructed to rotate application sites to reduce incidence of application site reactions. Reactions increasing in severity, spreading outside of application site or persistent reactions (lasting longer than several days) prompt assessment and any generalized skin reaction require discontinuation of therapy. Patients should be instructed to avoid patch exposure to heat sources; heat application may result in several fold increases in drug absorption.

Adverse Reactions (Reflective of adult population; not specific for elderly)
>10%:
    Central nervous system: Somnolence (13% to 25%), dizziness (18%), headache (14%), insomnia (6% to 14%)
    Gastrointestinal: Nausea (34% to 48%), vomiting (10% to 20%)
    Local: Application site reactions (21% to 37%)
1% to 10%:
    Cardiovascular: Sinus tachycardia (9%), peripheral edema (7%), orthostatic hypotension (5% to 7%), hypertension (3%), syncope
    Central nervous system: Fatigue (8%), abnormal dreams (2% to 5%), hallucination (≤3%), vertigo (3%), ataxia, confusion, fever, hypoesthesia, malaise
    Dermatologic: Erythematous rash (2% to 6%), contact dermatitis, pruritus, purpura
    Endocrine and metabolic: Hypoglycemia (7%)
    Gastrointestinal: Constipation (dose related; 5%), dyspepsia (4%), anorexia (dose related; 3%), xerostomia (3%), weight gain (3%), weight loss (≤2%)
    Genitourinary: Urinary tract infection (3%), urinary incontinence
    Hematologic: Hemoglobin decreased
    Hepatic: Albumin decreased, GGT increased
    Neuromuscular & skeletal: Back pain (6%), arthralgia (4%), myalgia (≤2%), abnormal gait, hypertonia, leg pain, neuralgia, paresthesia
    Ocular: Vision changes (dose related; 3%)
    Respiratory: Sinusitis (3%)
    Miscellaneous: Accident (5%), diaphoresis increased (4%)

Overdosage/Toxicology Signs and symptoms expected with overdosage include nausea, vomiting, hypotension, hallucinations, and confusion. Dialysis is not likely to provide benefit. Treatment is symptom-directed and supportive.

Drug Interactions
    Antipsychotics (typical): May decrease the therapeutic effect of anti-Parkinson's agent (dopamine agonist).
    CNS depressants: May enhance the adverse/toxic effect of rotigotine.
    Metoclopramide: May decrease the efficacy of rotigotine due to dopamine antagonism.

Ethanol/Nutrition/Herb Interactions Ethanol: Avoid ethanol (may increase CNS depression).

Stability Store at 15°C to 30°C (59°F to 86°F). Store in original pouch until application.

Mechanism of Action Rotigotine is a nonergot dopamine agonist with specificity for D_3-, D_2-, and D_1-dopamine receptors. Although the precise mechanism of action of rotigotine is unknown, it is believed to be due to stimulation of postsynaptic dopamine D_2-type auto receptors within the substantia nigra in the brain, leading to improved dopaminergic transmission in the motor areas of the basal ganglia, notably the caudate nucleus/putamen regions.

Pharmacokinetics
    Distribution: V_d: 84 L/kg
    Protein binding: ~90%
    Metabolism: Extensive conjugation and N-dealkylation
    Half-life elimination: After removal of patch: ~5-7 hours
    Time to peak, plasma: 15-18 hours; can occur 4-27 hours post application
    Excretion: Urine (~71% as metabolites, <1% as unchanged drug); feces (~11%)

Dosage
    Geriatrics & Adults: Parkinson's disease: Topical: Transdermal: Initial: Apply 2 mg/24 hours patch once daily; may increase by 2 mg/24 hours weekly, based on clinical response and tolerability (maximum: 6 mg/24 hours)
    Dosage reductions or discontinuation: Decrease by 2 mg/24 hours every other day
    Note: In clinical trials, the lowest effective dose was 4 mg/24 hours and doses >6 mg/24 hours did not provide any additional therapeutic benefit and increased incidence of adverse effects
    Renal Impairment: Severe impairment (Cl_{cr} 15-29 mL/minute): No dosage adjustment required
    Hepatic Impairment:
    Moderate hepatic impairment (Child-Pugh class B): No dosage adjustment required
    Severe hepatic impairment: Not studied

Administration Apply to clean, dry, hairless area of skin on the front of the abdomen, thigh, hip, flank, shoulder, or upper arm at approximately the same time daily. Remove
(Continued)

Rotigotine *(Continued)*

from pouch immediately before use and press patch firmly in place on skin for 20-30 seconds. Application sites should be rotated on a daily basis. Do not apply to same application site for more than once every 14 days or apply patch to oily, irritated or damaged skin. Avoid exposing patch to external heat sources (eg, heating pad, electric blanket, heat lamp, hot tub). If applied to hairy area, shave ≥3 days prior to applying patch. If patch detaches, immediately apply a new one to a new site.

Monitoring Parameters Blood pressure (orthostatic); daytime alertness; periodic skin evaluations (melanoma development)

Dosage Forms Excipient information presented when available (limited, particularly for generics); consult specific product labeling.

Transdermal system [once-daily patch]:

Neupro®:

2 mg/24 hours (7s, 30s) [10 cm^2, total rotigotine 4.5 mg; contains sodium metabisulfite]

4 mg/24 hours (7s, 30s) [20 cm^2, total rotigotine 9 mg; contains sodium metabisulfite]

6 mg/24 hours (7s, 30s) [30 cm^2, total rotigotine 13.5 mg; contains sodium metabisulfite]

Selected References

Reichmann H, Bilsing A, Ehret R, et al, "Ergoline and Non-Ergoline Derivatives in the Treatment of Parkinson's Disease," *J Neurol*, 2006, 253(Suppl 4):36-8.

Reynolds NA, Wellington K, and Easthope SE, "Rotigotine in Parkinson's Disease," *CNS Drugs*, 2005, 19(11):973-81.

Rubella Virus Vaccine (Live) (rue BEL a VYE rus vak SEEN, live)

Related Information

Immunization Recommendations *on page 1787*

Medication Safety Issues

Sound-alike/look-alike issues:

Meruvax® II may be confused with Attenuvax®

U.S. Brand Names Meruvax® II

Index Terms German Measles Vaccine

Generic Available No

Pharmacologic Category Vaccine

Use Selective active immunization against rubella

Note: Trivalent measles - mumps - rubella (MMR) vaccine is the preferred immunizing agent for most children and many adults.

Contraindications Hypersensitivity to rubella vaccine or any component of the vaccine; history of anaphylactic reactions to neomycin; individuals with blood dyscrasias, leukemia, lymphomas, or other malignant neoplasms affecting the bone marrow or lymphatic systems; concurrent immunosuppressive therapy (not including steroid replacement); primary and acquired immunodeficiency states; family history of congenital or hereditary immunodeficiency; active/untreated tuberculosis; current febrile illness

Warnings/Precautions Immediate treatment for anaphylactic/anaphylactoid reaction should be available during vaccine use. Use with caution in patients with thrombocytopenia and those who develop thrombocytopenia after first dose; thrombocytopenia may worsen. Defer vaccine following blood, plasma, or immune globulin (human) administration. The manufacturer contraindicates use with febrile infections; however, the ACIP notes that patients with minor illnesses with or without fever (diarrhea, mild upper respiratory tract infection, otitis media) may receive vaccines. Leukemia patients who are in remission and who have not received chemotherapy for at least 3 months may be vaccinated; patients with HIV infection, who are asymptomatic and not severely immunosuppressed may be vaccinated. Therapy to treat tuberculosis should be started prior to administering vaccine to patients with untreated, active tuberculosis. Contains gelatin, human albumin, neomycin, sorbitol and sucrose. A history of contact dermatitis to neomycin is not a contraindication to use, however, do not use with previous anaphylactic reaction to neomycin. Vaccination is recommended for individuals in certain high-risk groups (students entering institutions of higher learning, healthcare workers, travelers to endemic areas, etc).

Adverse Reactions (Reflective of adult population; not specific for elderly)
All serious adverse reactions must be reported to the U.S. Department of Health and Human Services (DHHS) Vaccine Adverse Event Reporting System (VAERS) 1-800-822-7967.
Frequency not defined.
Cardiovascular: Syncope, vasculitis
Central nervous system: Dizziness, encephalitis, fever, Guillain-Barré syndrome, headache, irritability, malaise, polyneuritis, polyneuropathy
Dermatologic: Angioneurotic edema, erythema multiforme, pruritus, purpura, rash, Stevens-Johnson syndrome, urticaria
Gastrointestinal: Diarrhea, nausea, sore throat, vomiting
Hematologic: Leukocytosis, thrombocytopenia
Local: Injection site reactions which include burning, induration, pain, redness, stinging, wheal and flare
Neuromuscular & skeletal: Arthralgia/arthritis (variable; highest rates in women, 12% to 26% versus children, up to 3%), myalgia, paresthesia
Ocular: Conjunctivitis, optic neuritis, papillitis, retrobulbar neuritis
Otic: Nerve deafness, otitis media
Respiratory: Bronchial spasm, cough, rhinitis
Miscellaneous: Anaphylactoid reactions, anaphylaxis, regional lymphadenopathy

Drug Interactions
Corticosteroids: In patients receiving high doses of systemic corticosteroids for ≥14 days, wait at least 1 month between discontinuing steroid therapy and administering immunization.
Immune globulin, whole blood, plasma: Do not administer together; immune response may be compromised. Defer vaccine administration for ≥3 months.
Immunosuppressant medications: The effect of the vaccine may be decreased, increasing the risk of rubella disease in individuals who are receiving immunosuppressant drugs.
Vaccines: Using separate sites and syringes, may be administered concurrently with *Haemophilus* b conjugate vaccine or varicella virus vaccine. Unless otherwise specified, should be given 1 month before or 1 month after live virus vaccines.

Stability Vaccine is to be shipped at 10°C (50°F). May use dry ice. Protect from light at all times. Prior to reconstitution, store at 2°C to 8°C (36°F to 46°F) or colder. Discard reconstituted vaccine after 8 hours.

Mechanism of Action Rubella vaccine is a live attenuated vaccine that contains the Wistar Institute RA 27/3 strain, which is adapted to and propagated in human diploid cell culture. Promotes active immunity by inducing rubella hemagglutination-inhibiting antibodies.

Dosage
Geriatrics & Adults: Immunization: SubQ: 0.5 mL
Adults without documentation of immunity: Vaccination is recommended for healthcare workers and for international travelers who visit endemic areas.

Administration SubQ injection only in outer aspect of upper arm; avoid injection into blood vessel. **Not for I.V. administration.** Federal law requires that the date of administration, the vaccine manufacturer, lot number of vaccine, and the administering person's name, title and address be entered into the patient's permanent medical record.

Monitoring Parameters See Adverse Reactions.

Test Interactions May depress tuberculin skin test sensitivity

Patient Information This medication is only given by injection. You may experience burning or stinging at the injection site; joint pain usually occurs 1-10 weeks after vaccination and persists 1-3 days. Notify your healthcare provider immediately if these effects continue or are severe, or for a high fever, seizures or allergic reaction (difficulty breathing, hives, weakness, dizziness, fast heart beat).

Additional Information Live virus vaccine. Federal law requires that the date of administration, the vaccine manufacturer, lot number of vaccine, and the administering person's name, title, and address be entered into the patient's permanent record.
Acceptable presumptive evidence of immunity includes one of the following:
1. Documentation of adequate vaccination
2. Laboratory evidence of immunity
3. Documentation of physician-diagnosed disease
(Continued)

Rubella Virus Vaccine (Live) (Continued)

Special Geriatric Considerations Not a vaccine necessary for most adults and elderly; however, necessary to protect persons without immunity traveling into endemic or epidemic countries. May need to test for rubella immunity if no record of disease of vaccination is available.

Dosage Forms Excipient information presented when available (limited, particularly for generics); consult specific product labeling.

Injection, powder for reconstitution [preservative free]:

Meruvax® II: ≥1000 TCID$_{50}$ (Wistar RA 27/3 Strain) [contains gelatin, human albumin, sorbitol, sucrose, and neomycin]

Selected References

Centers for Disease Control, "Recommendations of the Advisory Committee on Immunization Practices (ACIP): General Recommendations on Immunization," *MMWR Recomm Rep*, 2006, 55(RR-15):1-48.
Gardner P and Schaffner W, "Immunization of Adults," *N Engl J Med*, 1993, 328(17):1252-8.

♦ **Rubeola Vaccine** *see* Measles Virus Vaccine (Live) *on page 959*

♦ **Rulox [OTC]** *see* Aluminum Hydroxide and Magnesium Hydroxide *on page 65*

♦ **Rulox No. 1 [DSC]** *see* Aluminum Hydroxide and Magnesium Hydroxide *on page 65*

♦ **Rum-K®** *see* Potassium Chloride *on page 1288*

♦ **Rythmol®** *see* Propafenone *on page 1330*

♦ **Rythmol® SR** *see* Propafenone *on page 1330*

♦ **Rēv-Eyes™** *see* Dapiprazole *on page 394*

♦ **S2® [OTC]** *see* Epinephrine *on page 514*

♦ **S-(+)-3-isobutylgaba** *see* Pregabalin *on page 1310*

Saccharomyces boulardii (sak roe MYE sees boo LAR dee)

U.S. Brand Names Florastor® [OTC]; Florastor® Kids [OTC]

Index Terms *Saccharomyces boulardii lyo; S. boulardii*

Generic Available No

Pharmacologic Category Dietary Supplement; Probiotic

Use Promote maintenance of normal microflora in the gastrointestinal tract; used in management of bloating, gas, and diarrhea, particularly to decrease the incidence of diarrhea associated with antibiotic use

Contraindications Hypersensitivity to *Saccharomyces boulardii* or any component of the formulation

Warnings/Precautions *S. boulardii*, a nonpathogenic yeast, has been associated with case reports of invasive fungemias in immunocompromised, debilitated, or critically ill patients; use caution or avoid use in these patients, particularly those with a central venous catheter and/or previous or current antibiotic therapy. Use caution in patients allergic to yeast; *S. boulardii* is a live yeast preparation and a subtype of the species, *S. cervasiae*, which is also referred to as "baker's yeast" or "brewer's yeast." Avoid use in patients on systemic antifungal therapy; *S. boulardii* may be susceptible. Probiotic products are classified as dietary supplements; therefore, there are no safety reviews or approved therapeutic indications by the FDA. There is no conclusive evidence to support widespread use in the treatment of diarrhea. Significant differences may exist from one preparation of *S. boulardii* compared to another with respect to biologic activity and composition. Some products may contain lactose.

Adverse Reactions (Reflective of adult population; not specific for elderly)
Frequency not defined.

Gastrointestinal: Constipation, flatulence

Miscellaneous: Thirst

Drug Interactions Antifungals: *S. boulardii* effect may be diminished when given concurrently with systemic antifungals.

Stability Some preparations may need to be refrigerated or stored in freezer; consult individual product labeling.

Florastor®, Florastor® Kids: Store at ≤25°C (≤77°F); refrigeration not necessary.

Mechanism of Action *S. boulardii*, a nonpathogenic live yeast probiotic, acts as temporary flora to help re-establish the normal gastrointestinal microflora. May also modulate the immune system by inducing cytokines and suppress pathogenic bacteria growth.

Pharmacodynamics

Onset of action: Yeast cell release from capsules/powder: 30 minutes

Duration: Yeast cells cleared in 5-7 days

Dosage

Geriatrics:

Refer to adult dosing. Use caution in debilitated patients.

Adults: Dietary supplement: Oral: Dosing varies by manufacturer; consult product labeling.

Florastor®: 250 mg twice daily

Administration
Florastor®: Swallow capsule whole or capsules may be opened and emptied on tongue (wash down with water or juice) or sprinkled on semi-solid food (eg, applesauce, sour cream, yogurt) or added to a drink (eg, water, apple or orange juice, milk or formula); may be administered with or without food.
Florastor® Kids: Add powder to a drink or sprinkle on semi-solid food; may be administered with or without food.

Special Geriatric Considerations Use caution in debilitated patients.

Dosage Forms Excipient information presented when available (limited, particularly for generics); consult specific product labeling.
Capsule:
Florastor®: *S. boulardii lyo* 250 mg [provides 5 billion live cells; contains lactose 32.5 mg and magnesium 2.85 mg]
Powder:
Florastor® Kids: *S. boulardii lyo* 250 mg [provides 5 billion live cells; contains lactose 32.5 mg and magnesium 2.85 mg; tutti frutti flavor]

Selected References
Enache-Angoulvant A and Hennequin C, "Invasive Saccharomyces Infection: A Comprehensive Review," *Clin Infect Dis*, 2005, 41(11):1559-68.

♦ **Saccharomyces boulardii lyo** *see Saccharomyces boulardii on page 1438*
♦ **Safe Tussin**® [OTC] *see Guaifenesin and Dextromethorphan on page 730*
♦ **SalAc**® [OTC] *see Salicylic Acid on page 1441*
♦ **Sal-Acid**® [OTC] *see Salicylic Acid on page 1441*
♦ **Salactic**® [OTC] *see Salicylic Acid on page 1441*
♦ **Salagen**® *see Pilocarpine on page 1259*
♦ **Salbutamol** *see Albuterol on page 40*
♦ **Salbutamol and Ipratropium** *see Ipratropium and Albuterol on page 828*
♦ **Salbutamol Sulphate** *see Albuterol on page 40*

Salicylates (Various Salts) (sa LIS i lates)

U.S. Brand Names Arthropan®; Asproject®; Extra Strength Doan's® [OTC]; Magan®; Mobidin®; Original Doan's® [OTC]; Rexolate®; Tusal®

Index Terms Choline Salicylate; Magnesium Salicylate; Sodium Salicylate; Sodium Thiosalicylate

Generic Available Yes

Pharmacologic Category Analgesic, Nonopioid; Anti-inflammatory Agent; Anti-platelet Agent; Antipyretic; Nonsteroidal Anti-inflammatory Drug (NSAID), Oral; Salicylate

Use Treatment of mild to moderate pain, inflammation, and fever; management of rheumatic fever, rheumatoid arthritis, osteoarthritis, gout
See Mechanism of Action.

Contraindications Bleeding disorders (factor VII or IX deficiencies), hypersensitivity to salicylates or other nonsteroidal anti-inflammatory drugs (NSAIDs); tartrazine dye and asthma

Warnings/Precautions Tinnitus or impaired hearing may indicate toxicity; discontinue use 1 week prior to surgical procedures. Use with caution in patients with platelet and bleeding disorders, renal dysfunction, hepatic disease, history of salicylate-induced gastric irritation, peptic ulcer disease, erosive gastritis, bleeding disorders, hypopro-thrombinemia, and vitamin K deficiency; use cautiously in asthmatics, especially those with aspirin intolerance and nasal polyps

Drug Interactions
May increase nephrotoxicity of cyclosporin; diclofenac + K^+ sparing diuretics may increase serum K^+
Concomitant insulin or oral hypoglycemic agents may increase or decrease serum glucose
May increase digoxin, methotrexate, and lithium serum concentrations
Aspirin or other salicylates may decrease NSAID serum concentrations
Other NSAIDs may increase adverse GI effects
Increased prothrombin time with anticoagulants
Decreased antihypertensive effects of ACE inhibitors, beta-blockers, and thiazide diuretics
Increased response to sympathomimetics
Probenecid may increase toxicity of NSAIDs by increase in serum concentrations
Effects of loop diuretics may decrease; concomitant use with loop diuretics may enhance azotemia in older adults

Stability Keep suppositories in refrigerator, do not freeze; hydrolysis of aspirin occurs upon exposure to water or moist air, resulting in salicylate and acetate, which possess a vinegar-like odor; do not use if a strong odor is present

(Continued)

Salicylates (Various Salts) *(Continued)*

Mechanism of Action Inhibits prostaglandin synthesis; acts on the hypothalamus heat-regulating center to reduce fever through vasodilation of peripheral vessels; decreases pain receptor sensitivity. Other proposed mechanisms of action for salicylate anti-inflammatory action are lysosomal stabilization, inhibition of kinin and leukotriene production, alteration of chemotactic factors, and inhibition of neutrophil activation. This latter mechanism may be the most significant pharmacologic action to reduce inflammation. Nonacetylated salicylates are **not** as potent in prostaglandin synthesis inhibition and, therefore, tend to have less adverse effects on gastrointestinal and renal tissues. They do not inhibit platelet function as aspirin does since they are not acetylated and, therefore, cannot acetylate platelet cyclooxygenase.

Pharmacokinetics

Absorption: From the stomach and small intestine

Distribution: Readily into most body fluids and tissues

Aspirin is hydrolyzed to salicylate (active) by esterases in the GI mucosa, red blood cells, synovial fluid and blood

Metabolism: Metabolism of salicylate occurs primarily by hepatic microsomal enzymes

Half-life, aspirin: 15-20 minutes; metabolic pathways are saturable such that salicylate half-life is dose-dependent ranging from 3 hours at lower doses (300-600 mg), 5-6 hours (after 1 g) and 15-30 hours with higher doses; in therapeutic anti-inflammatory doses, half-lives generally range from 6-12 hours

Time to peak plasma concentration: ~1-2 hours

Monitoring Parameters Serum concentrations, renal function; hearing changes or tinnitus; monitor for response (ie, pain, inflammation, range of motion, grip strength); observe for abnormal bleeding, bruising, weight gain

Reference Range Timing of serum samples: Peak serum concentrations usually occur 2 hours after ingestion; the half-life increases with the dosage (eg, the half-life after 300 mg is 3 hours, and after 1 g is 5-6 hours, and after 8-10 g is 10-15 hours).

Salicylate serum concentrations correlate with the pharmacological actions and adverse effects observed. Anti-inflammatory therapeutic serum concentrations 150-300 mcg/mL. See table.

Serum Salicylate: Clinical Correlations

Serum Salicylate Concentration (mcg/mL)	Desired Effects	Adverse Effects / Intoxication
~100	Antiplatelet Antipyresis Analgesia	GI intolerance and bleeding, hypersensitivity, hemostatic defects
150-300	Anti-inflammatory	Mild salicylism
250-400	Treatment of rheumatic fever	Nausea/vomiting, hyperventilation, salicylism, flushing, sweating, thirst, headache, diarrhea, and tachycardia
>400-500		Respiratory alkalosis, hemorrhage, excitement, confusion, asterixis, pulmonary edema, convulsions, tetany, metabolic acidosis, fever, coma, cardiovascular collapse, renal and respiratory failure

Test Interactions False-negative results for glucose oxidase urinary glucose tests (Clinistix®); false-positives using the cupric sulfate method (Clinitest®); also, interferes with Gerhardt test (urinary ketone analysis), VMA determination; 5-HIAA, xylose tolerance test, and T_3 and T_4; increased PBI; increased uric acid

Patient Information Watch for any signs of bleeding (stool); take with food to minimize GI distress; report ringing in ears, persistent GI pain to physician or pharmacist

Additional Information Liquid dosage form may be useful for those who have difficulty swallowing tablets or caplets. These agents do not appear to inhibit platelet aggregation. Nonacetylated salicylates have less GI toxicity and renal effects than aspirin and other NSAIDs. They also do not cause reactions in aspirin sensitive patients.

Choline salicylate: Arthropan®

Sodium thiosalicylate: Asproject®; Rexolate®; Tusal®

Magnesium salicylate: Extra Strength Doan's® [OTC]; Magan®; Mobidin®; Original Doan's® [OTC]

Special Geriatric Considerations Elderly are a high-risk population for adverse effects from NSAIDs. As much as 60% of elderly can develop peptic ulceration and/or hemorrhage asymptomatically. The concomitant use of H_2 blockers, omeprazole, and sucralfate is not effective as prophylaxis with the exception of NSAID-induced duodenal ulcers which may be prevented by the use of ranitidine. Misoprostol and proton pump inhibitors are the only agents proven to help prevent the development of NSAID-induced ulcers. Also, concomitant disease and drug use contribute to the risk for GI adverse effects. Use lowest effective dose for shortest period possible. Consider renal function decline with age. Use of NSAIDs can compromise existing renal function especially when Cl_{cr} is ≤30 mL/minute. Tinnitus may be a difficult and unreliable indication of toxicity due to age-related hearing loss or eighth cranial nerve damage. CNS adverse effects such as confusion, agitation, and hallucination are generally seen in overdose or high dose situations, but elderly may demonstrate these adverse effects at lower doses than younger adults.

Dosage Forms

Injection: 50 mg/mL

Liquid: 870 mg/mL (choline salicylate)

Tablet, enteric coated: 325 mg, 545 mg, 600 mg, 650 mg

Selected References

AGS Panel on Persistent Pain in Older Persons, "The Management of Persistent Pain in Older Persons," *J Am Geriatr Soc*, 2002, 50(6 Suppl):S205-24.

Emmerson BT, "The Management of Gout," *N Engl J Med*, 1996, 334(7):445-51.

Gurwitz JH, Avorn J, Ross-Degnan D, et al, "Nonsteroidal Anti-Inflammatory Drug-Associated Azotemia in the Very Old," *JAMA*, 1990, 264(4):471-5.

Hawkey CJ, Karrasch JA, Szczepański L, et al, "Omeprazole Compared With Misoprostol for Ulcers Associated With Nonsteroidal Anti-inflammatory Drugs," *N Engl J Med*, 1998, 338(11):727-34.

Weissmann G, "Aspirin," *Sci Am*, 1991, 264(1):84-90.

Yeomans ND, Tulassay Z, Juhasz L, et al, "A Comparison of Omeprazole With Ranitidine for Ulcers Associated With Nonsteroidal Anti-inflammatory Drugs," *N Engl J Med*, 1998, 338(11):719-26.

♦ **Salicylazosulfapyridine** *see* Sulfasalazine *on page 1501*

Salicylic Acid (sal i SIL ik AS id)

Medication Safety Issues

Transdermal patch may contain conducting metal (eg, aluminum); remove patch prior to MRI.

U.S. Brand Names Compound W® [OTC]; Compound W® One Step Wart Remover [OTC]; DHS™ Sal [OTC]; Dr. Scholl's® Callus Remover [OTC]; Dr. Scholl's® Clear Away [OTC]; DuoFilm® [OTC]; DuoPlant® [DSC] [OTC]; Freezone® [OTC]; Fung-O® [OTC]; Gordofilm® [OTC]; Hydrisalic™ [OTC]; Ionil® [OTC]; Ionil® Plus [OTC]; Keralyt® [OTC]; LupiCare™ Dandruff [OTC]; LupiCare™ II Psoriasis [OTC]; LupiCare™ Psoriasis [OTC]; Mediplast® [OTC]; MG217 Sal-Acid® [OTC]; Mosco® Corn and Callus Remover [OTC]; NeoCeuticals™ Acne Spot Treatment [OTC]; Neutrogena® Acne Wash [OTC]; Neutrogena® Body Clear™ [OTC]; Neutrogena® Clear Pore [OTC]; Neutrogena® Clear Pore Shine Control [OTC]; Neutrogena® Healthy Scalp [OTC]; Neutrogena® Maximum Strength T/Sal® [OTC]; Neutrogena® On The Spot® Acne Patch [OTC]; Occlusal®-HP [OTC]; Oxy Balance® [OTC]; Oxy Balance® Deep Pore [OTC]; Palmer's® Skin Success Acne Cleanser [OTC]; Pedisilk® [OTC]; Propa pH [OTC]; SalAc® [OTC]; Sal-Acid® [OTC]; Salactic® [OTC]; Sal-Plant® [OTC]; Stri-dex® [OTC]; Stri-dex® Body Focus [OTC]; Stri-dex® Facewipes To Go™ [OTC]; Stri-dex® Maximum Strength [OTC]; Tinamed® [OTC]; Tiseb® [OTC]; Trans-Ver-Sal® [OTC]; Wart-Off® Maximum Strength [OTC]; Zapzyt® Acne Wash [OTC]; Zapzyt® Pore Treatment [OTC]

Canadian Brand Names Duofilm®; Duoforte® 27; Occlusal™-HP; Sebcur®; Soluver®; Soluver® Plus; Trans-Plantar®; Trans-Ver-Sal®

Generic Available Yes: Gel, soap

Pharmacologic Category Acne Products; Keratolytic Agent; Topical Skin Product, Acne

Use Topically for its keratolytic effect in controlling seborrheic dermatitis or psoriasis of body and scalp, dandruff, and other scaling dermatoses; removal of warts, corns, and calluses

Contraindications Hypersensitivity to salicylic acid or any component of the formulation

Warnings/Precautions Prior to OTC use, consult with healthcare provider if diabetic or have poor circulation. Not for application to areas that are irritated, infected, reddened, birthmarks, genital or facial warts, or mucous membranes. Avoid contact with eyes.

Adverse Reactions (Reflective of adult population; not specific for elderly) Frequency not defined.

Central nervous system: Dizziness, mental confusion, headache

Local: Burning and irritation at site of exposure on normal tissue, peeling, scaling

Otic: Tinnitus

Respiratory: Hyperventilation

Drug Interactions No data reported

Mechanism of Action Produces desquamation of hyperkeratotic epithelium via dissolution of the intercellular cement which causes the cornified tissue to swell, soften, macerate, and desquamate. Salicylic acid is keratolytic at concentrations of 3% to 6%; it becomes destructive to tissue at concentrations >6%. Concentrations of 6% to 60% are used to remove corns and warts and in the treatment of psoriasis and other hyperkeratotic disorders.

(Continued)

Salicylic Acid *(Continued)*

Pharmacokinetics

Absorption: Absorbed percutaneously, but systemic toxicity is unlikely with normal use

Time to peak serum concentration: Topical: Within 5 hours of application with occlusion

Elimination: Salicyluric acid (52%), salicylate glucuronides (42%), and salicylic acid (6%) are major metabolites identified in urine after percutaneous absorption

Dosage

Geriatrics & Adults:

Acne:

Cream, cloth, foam, or liquid cleansers (2%): Use to cleanse skin once or twice daily. Massage gently into skin, work into lather and rinse thoroughly. Cloths should be wet with water prior to using and disposed of (not flushed) after use.

Gel (0.5% or 2%): Apply small amount to face in the morning or evening; if peeling occurs, may be used every other day. Some products may be labeled for OTC use up to 3 or 4 times per day. Apply to clean, dry skin

Pads (0.5% or 2%): Use pad to cover affected area with thin layer of salicylic acid one to three times a day. Apply to clean, dry skin. Do not leave pad on skin.

Patch (2%): At bedtime, after washing face, allow skin to dry at least 5 minutes. Apply patch directly over pimple being treated. Remove in the morning.

Shower/bath gels or soap (2%): Use once daily in shower or bath to massage over skin prone to acne. Rinse well.

Callus, corns, or warts:

Gel or liquid (17%): Apply to each wart and allow to dry. May repeat once or twice daily, up to 12 weeks. Apply to clean dry area.

Gel (6%): Apply to affected area once daily, generally used at night and rinsed off in the morning.

Plaster or transdermal patch (40%): Apply directly over affected area, leave in place for 48 hours. Some products may be cut to fit area or secured with adhesive strips. May repeat procedure for up to 12 weeks. Apply to clean, dry skin

Transdermal patch (15%): Apply directly over affected area at bedtime, leave in place overnight and remove in the morning. Patch should be trimmed to cover affected area. May repeat daily for up to 12 weeks.

Dandruff, psoriasis, or seborrheic dermatitis:

Cream (2.5%): Apply to affected area 3-4 times daily. Apply to clean, dry skin. Some products may be left in place overnight.

Ointment (3%): Apply to scales or plaques on skin up to 4 times per day (not for scalp or face)

Shampoo (1.8% to 3%): Massage into wet hair or affected area; leave in place for several minutes; rinse thoroughly. Labeled for OTC use 2-3 times a week, or as directed by healthcare provider. Some products may be left in place overnight.

Administration For warts: Before applying product, soak area in warm water for 5 minutes; dry area thoroughly, then apply medication

Patient Information When applying in concentrations >10%, protect surrounding tissue with petrolatum; do not use on open skin, avoid contact with eyes, mouth, and other mucous membranes

Special Geriatric Considerations No specific considerations are needed if used according to recommended doses and duration of use. Many elderly may have diabetes or impaired circulation and avoidance of topical salicylic acid would be advised.

Dosage Forms Excipient information presented when available (limited, particularly for generics); consult specific product labeling. [DSC] = Discontinued product

Cream:

LupiCare™ Dandruff, LupiCare™ Psoriasis: 2.5% (120 g, 240 g) [contains alcohol]

LupiCare™ II Psoriasis: 2.5% (60 g, 240 g) [contains alcohol]

Neutrogena® Acne Wash: 2% (200 mL) [contains alcohol]

Cloths (Neutrogena® Acne Wash): 2% (30s) [disposable cloths]

Foam:

Neutrogena® Acne Wash: 2% (150 mL) [foaming cleanser]

SalAc®: 2% (100 g)

Gel: 17% (15 g)

Compound W®: 17% (7 g) [contains alcohol]

DuoPlant® [DSC]: 17% (15 g)

Hydrisalic™: 6% (28 g) [contains alcohol and propylene glycol]

Keralyt®: 6% (30 g) [contains alcohol and propylene glycol]

NeoCeuticals™ Acne Spot Treatment: 2% (15 g) [contains alcohol]

Neutrogena® Clear Pore: 2% (60 g) [contains alcohol]

Neutrogena® Clear Pore Shine Control: 0.5% (10 g)

Oxy Balance®: 2% (240 mL) [shower gel]

Sal-Plant®: 17% (14 g) [contains alcohol]

Stri-dex® Body Focus™: 2% (300 mL)

Zapzyt® Acne Wash: 2% (190 g) [alcohol free]
Zapzyt® Pore Treatment: 2% (23 g) [alcohol free]
Liquid, topical:
  Compound W®: 17% (9 mL) [contains alcohol]
  DuoFilm®: 17% (15 mL) [contains alcohol]
  Freezone®: 17.6% (9.3 mL) [contains alcohol]
  Fung-O®: 17% (15 mL)
  Gordofilm®: 16.7% (15 mL)
  Mosco® Corn and Callus Remover: 17.6% (10 mL)
  NeoCeuticals™ Acne Spot Treatment: 2% (60 mL) [contains alcohol]
  Neutrogena® Acne Wash: 2% (180 mL) [contains tartrazine]
  Neutrogena® Body Clear™ [body scrub with microbeads]: 2% (250 mL) [contains tartrazine]
  Neutrogena® Body Clear™ [body wash]: 2% (250 mL) [contains tartrazine]
  Occlusal®-HP: 17% (10 mL)
  Palmer's® Skin Success Acne Cleanser: 0.5% (240 mL)
  Pedisilk®: 17% (15 mL)
  Propa pH: 2% (80 mL) [alcohol free; contains aloe vera]
  SalAc®: 2% (180 mL)
  Salactic®: 17% (15 mL) [contains alcohol]
  Tinamed®: 17% (15 mL)
  Wart-Off®: 17% (13 mL) [contains alcohol]
Ointment (MG217 Sal-Acid®): 3% (56 g) [contains vitamin E]
Pads:
  Oxy Balance®, Oxy Balance® Deep Pore: 0.5% (55s, 90s) [contains alcohol]
  Stri-dex®: 0.5% (55s)
  Stri-dex® Facewipes To Go™: 0.5% (32s) [contains alcohol]
  Stri-dex® Maximum Strength: 2% (32s, 55s, 90s)
Patch, transdermal:
  Compound W® One Step Wart Remover: 40% (12s, 14s)
  Dr. Scholl's® Callus Remover: 40% (4s)
  Dr. Scholl's® Clear Away: 40% (14s, 16s, 18s, 24s)
  DuoFilm®: 40% (18s)
  Neutrogena® On The Spot® Acne Patch: 2% (27s)
  Trans-Ver-Sal®: 15% [6 mm PediaPatch, 12 mm AdultPatch, 20 mm PlantarPatch] (10s, 12s, 15s, 25s, 40s)
Plaster:
  Mediplast®: 40% (25s)
  Sal-Acid®: 40% (14s)
  Tinamed®: 40% (24s)
Shampoo:
  DHS™ Sal: 3% (120 mL)
  Ionil®: 2% (240 mL, 480 mL, 960 mL)
  Ionil® Plus: 2% (240 mL) [conditioning shampoo]
  LupiCare™ Dandruff, LupiCare™ Psoriasis: 2% (120 mL, 240 mL)
  Neutrogena® Healthy Scalp: 1.8% (90 mL, 180 mL)
  Neutrogena® Maximum Strength T/Sal®: 3% (135 mL)
  Tiseb®: 2% (240 mL)
Soap: 2% (114 g)

♦ **Salicylsalicylic Acid** *see* Salsalate *on page 1446*
♦ **SalineX® [OTC]** *see* Sodium Chloride *on page 1475*
♦ **Salivart® [OTC]** *see* Saliva Substitute *on page 1443*

Saliva Substitute (sa LYE va SUB stee tute)

U.S. Brand Names Aquoral™; Caphosol; Entertainer's Secret® [OTC]; Moi-Stir® [OTC]; Mouthkote® [OTC]; Numoisyn™; Salivart® [OTC]; Saliva Substitute™ [OTC]; SalivaSure™ [OTC]
Generic Available No
Pharmacologic Category Gastrointestinal Agent, Miscellaneous
Use Relief of dry mouth and throat in xerostomia
Dosage
  Geriatrics & Adults: Xerostomia: Oral: Use as needed
Special Geriatric Considerations Saliva production has not been shown to change with aging, however, many drugs used by elderly can cause dry mouth. These patients may benefit from a saliva substitute.
Dosage Forms Excipient information presented when available (limited, particularly for generics); consult specific product labeling. [DSC] = Discontinued product
(Continued)

Saliva Substitute *(Continued)*

Liquid:

Numoisyn™: Water, sorbitol, linseed extract, *Chondrus crispus*, methylparaben, sodium benzoate, potassium sorbate, dipotassium phosphate, propylparaben (300 mL)

Lozenge:

Numoisyn™: Sorbitol 0.3 g/lozenge, polyethylene glycol, malic acid, sodium citrate, calcium phosphate dibasic, hydrogenated cottonseed oil, citric acid, magnesium stearate, silicon dioxide (100s)

SalivaSure™: Xylitol, citric acid, apple acid, sodium citrate dihydrate, sodium carboxymethylcellulose, dibasic calcium phosphate, silica colloidal, magnesium stearate, stearic acid (90s)

Solution, oral:

Caphosol: Dibasic sodium phosphate 0.032%, monobasic sodium phosphate 0.009%, calcium chloride 0.052%, sodium chloride 0.569%, purified water (30 mL) [packaged in two 15 mL ampuls when mixed together provide one 30 mL dose]

Entertainer's Secret®: Sodium carboxymethylcellulose, aloe vera gel, glycerin (60 mL) [honey-apple flavor]

Saliva Substitute®: Sorbitol, sodium carboxymethylcellulose, methylparaben (120 mL)

Solution, oral [spray]:

Aquora™: Oxidized glycerol triesters and silicon dioxide (40 mL) [contains aspartame; delivers 400 sprays]

Moi-Stir®: Water, sorbitol, sodium carboxymethylcellulose, methylparaben, propylparaben, potassium chloride, dibasic sodium phosphate, calcium chloride, magnesium chloride, sodium chloride (120 mL)

Mouthkote®: Water, xylitol, sorbitol, yerba santa, citric acid, ascorbic acid, sodium saccharin, sodium benzoate (5 mL, 60 mL, 240 mL) [alcohol free, sugar free; lemon-lime flavor]

Salivart®: Water, sodium carboxymethylcellulose, sorbitol, sodium chloride, potassium chloride, calcium chloride, magnesium chloride, potassium phosphate (70 mL) [alcohol free]

♦ **Saliva Substitute™ [OTC]** *see* Saliva Substitute *on page 1443*
♦ **SalivaSure™ [OTC]** *see* Saliva Substitute *on page 1443*
♦ **Salk Vaccine** *see* Poliovirus Vaccine (Inactivated) *on page 1280*

Salmeterol *(sal ME te role)*

Related Information
Inhalant Agents *on page 1760*
Medication Safety Issues
Sound-alike/look-alike issues:
Salmeterol may be confused with Salbutamol
Serevent® may be confused with Serentil®
U.S. Brand Names Serevent® Diskus®
Canadian Brand Names Serevent®
Index Terms Salmeterol Xinafoate
Generic Available No
Pharmacologic Category Beta$_2$-Adrenergic Agonist
Use Maintenance treatment of asthma and in prevention of bronchospasm with reversible obstructive airway disease, including patients with symptoms of nocturnal asthma; prevention of exercise-induced bronchospasm; maintenance treatment of bronchospasm associated with COPD
Restrictions An FDA-approved medication guide must be distributed when dispensing an outpatient prescription (new or refill) where this medication is to be used without direct supervision of a healthcare provider. Medication guides are available at http://www.fda.gov/cder/Offices/ODS/medication_guides.htm.
Contraindications Hypersensitivity to salmeterol, adrenergic amines, or any component of the formulation; need for acute bronchodilation
Warnings/Precautions
Asthma treatment: [U.S. Boxed Warning]: Long-acting beta$_2$-agonists may increase the risk of asthma-related deaths. In a large, randomized clinical trial (SMART, 2006), salmeterol was associated with an increase in asthma-related deaths (when added to usual asthma therapy); risk may be greater in African-American patients versus Caucasians. Should only be used as adjuvant therapy in patients not adequately controlled on inhaled corticosteroids or whose disease requires two maintenance therapies. Salmeterol is not meant to relieve acute asthmatic symptoms, should not be initiated in patients with significantly worsening or acutely deteriorating asthma, and is not a substitute for inhaled or oral corticosteroids. Short-acting beta$_2$-agonist should be used for acute symptoms and symptoms occurring between

treatments. Corticosteroids should not be stopped or reduced when salmeterol is initiated. During the initiation of salmeterol watch for signs of worsening asthma.

Concurrent diseases: Use caution in patients with cardiovascular disease (eg, arrhythmia, hypertension, or CHF), seizure disorders, diabetes, glaucoma, hyperthyroidism, hepatic impairment, or hypokalemia. Beta-agonists may cause elevation in blood pressure, heart rate, CNS stimulation/excitation, increased risk of arrhythmia, increase serum glucose, or decrease serum potassium.

Adverse events: Immediate hypersensitivity reactions (urticaria, angioedema, rash, bronchospasm) have been reported. There have been reports of laryngeal spasm, irritation, swelling (stridor, choking) with use. Salmeterol should not be used more than twice daily; do not exceed recommended dose; do not use with other long-acting beta$_2$-agonists; serious adverse events including fatalities, have been associated with excessive use of inhaled sympathomimetics. Rarely, paradoxical bronchospasm may occur; distinguished from inadequate response. Powder for oral inhalation contains lactose; very rare anaphylactic reactions have been reported in patients with severe milk protein allergy.

Adverse Reactions (Reflective of adult population; not specific for elderly)
>10%:
  Central nervous system: Headache (13% to 17%)
  Neuromuscular & skeletal: Pain (1% to 12%)
1% to 10%:
  Cardiovascular: Hypertension (4%), edema (1% to <3%)
  Central nervous system: Dizziness (4%), sleep disturbance (1% to 3%), fever (1% to 3%), anxiety (1% to <3%), migraine (1% to <3%)
  Dermatologic: Rash (1% to 4%), contact dermatitis (1% to 3%), eczema (1% to 3%), urticaria (3%), photodermatitis (1% to 2%)
  Endocrine & metabolic: Hyperglycemia (1% to <3%)
  Gastrointestinal: Nausea (1% to 3%), dyspepsia (1% to <3%), dental pain (1% to <3%), infections (1% to <3%), oropharyngeal candidiasis (1% to <3%), xerostomia (1% to <3%)
  Neuromuscular & skeletal: Muscular cramps/spasm (3%), paresthesia (1% to 3%), arthralgia (1% to <3%), muscular stiffness, rigidity (1% to <3%)
  Ocular: Keratitis/conjunctivitis (1% to <3%)
  Respiratory: Tracheitis/bronchitis (7%), pharyngitis (up to 6%), cough (5%), influenza (5%), infection (5%), sinusitis (4% to 5%), rhinitis (4% to 5%), nasal congestion (4%), asthma (3% to 4%)

Overdosage/Toxicology Symptoms of overdose include tachycardia, tremor, hypertension, angina, and seizures. Hypokalemia also may occur. Cardiac arrest and death may be associated with abuse of beta-agonist bronchodilators. Treatment includes immediate discontinuation and symptomatic and supportive therapies. Cautious use of beta-adrenergic blocking agents may be considered in severe cases.

Drug Interactions Substrate of CYP3A4 (major)
  Atomoxetine: May enhance the tachycardia effect of beta$_2$-agonists.
  Beta$_2$-agonists: May diminish the bradycardia effect of beta-blockers (beta$_1$ selective).
  Beta-blockers (nonselective): May diminish the bronchodilator effect of beta$_2$-agonists.
  Sympathomimetics: May enhance the adverse/toxic effect of salmeterol.

Stability Inhalation powder: Store at controlled room temperature 20°C to 25°C (68°F to 77°F) in a dry place away from direct heat or sunlight. Stable for 6 weeks after removal from foil pouch.

Mechanism of Action Relaxes bronchial smooth muscle by selective action on beta$_2$-receptors with little effect on heart rate; because salmeterol acts locally in the lung, therapeutic effect is not predicted by plasma levels

Pharmacodynamics
  Onset of action: Asthma: 30-48 minutes, COPD: 2 hours
    Peak effect: 2-4 hours, COPD: 3.27-4.75 hours
  Duration: 12 hours

Pharmacokinetics
  Protein binding: 96%
  Metabolism: Hepatically hydroxylated
  Half-life elimination: 5.5 hours
  Excretion: Feces (60%), urine (25%)

Dosage
Geriatrics & Adults:
  Asthma, maintenance and prevention: Inhalation, powder (Serevent® Diskus®): One inhalation (50 mcg) twice daily (~12 hours apart); maximum: 1 inhalation twice daily
  Exercise-induced asthma, prevention: One inhalation (50 mcg) at least 30 minutes prior to exercise; additional doses should not be used for 12 hours; should not be used in individuals already receiving salmeterol twice daily
  COPD (maintenance treatment of associated bronchospasm): One inhalation (50 mcg) twice daily (~12 hours apart); maximum: 1 inhalation twice daily

(Continued)

Salmeterol *(Continued)*

Hepatic Impairment: Systemic absorption is poor from inhalation therapy; therefore, no dosage adjustment recommended. Manufacturer suggests close monitoring of patients with hepatic impairment.

Administration Inhalation: **Not** to be used for the relief of acute attacks. Not for use with a spacer device. Administer with Diskus® in a level, horizontal position. Do not wash mouthpiece; Diskus® should be kept dry.

Monitoring Parameters FEV_1, peak flow, and/or other pulmonary function tests; blood pressure, heart rate; CNS stimulation; serum glucose, serum potassium. Monitor for increased use of short-acting beta$_2$-agonist inhalers; may be marker of a deteriorating asthma condition.

Patient Information Not to be used for the relief of acute attacks; do not exceed recommended dosage; rinse mouth with water following each inhalation to help with dry throat and mouth; follow specific instructions accompanying inhaler. Do not use a spacer with inhalation powder. Keep device dry - do not wash mouthpiece. May cause nervousness, restlessness, insomnia - if these effects continue after dosage reduction, notify physician; also notify physician if palpitations, tachycardia, chest pain, muscle tremors, dizziness, headache, flushing or if breathing difficulty persists.

Special Geriatric Considerations Geriatric patients were included in four clinical studies of salmeterol; no apparent differences in efficacy and safety were noted in geriatric patients compared to younger adults. Because salmeterol is only to be used for prevention of bronchospasm, patients also need a short-acting beta-agonist to treat acute attacks. Elderly patients should be carefully counseled about which inhaler to use and the proper scheduling of doses.

Dosage Forms Excipient information presented when available (limited, particularly for generics); consult specific product labeling.

Powder for oral inhalation: 50 mcg (28s, 60s) [delivers 50 mcg/inhalation; contains lactose]

Selected References

Nelson HS, Weiss ST, Bleecker ER, et al, "The Salmeterol Multicenter Asthma Research Trial: A Comparison of Usual Pharmacotherapy for Asthma or Usual Pharmacotherapy Plus Salmeterol," *Chest*, 2006, 129(1):15-26.

◆ **Salmeterol and Fluticasone** *see* Fluticasone and Salmeterol *on page 663*

◆ **Salmeterol Xinafoate** *see* Salmeterol *on page 1444*

◆ **Sal-Plant® [OTC]** *see* Salicylic Acid *on page 1441*

Salsalate *(SAL sa late)*

Medication Safety Issues

Sound-alike/look-alike issues:

Salsalate may be confused with sucralfate, sulfasalazine

U.S. Brand Names Amigesic®

Canadian Brand Names Amigesic®; Salflex®

Index Terms Disalicylic Acid; Salicylsalicylic Acid

Generic Available Yes

Pharmacologic Category Salicylate

Use Treatment of mild to moderate pain, inflammation and fever; management of rheumatic fever, rheumatoid arthritis, osteoarthritis, gout

See Mechanism of Action.

Contraindications Hypersensitivity to salsalate or any component of the formulation; GI ulcer or bleeding

Warnings/Precautions Use with caution in patients with platelet and bleeding disorders, dehydration, renal dysfunction, erosive gastritis, or peptic ulcer disease; patients with sensitivity to tartrazine dyes, nasal polyps, and asthma may have an increased risk of salicylate sensitivity, previous nonreaction does not guarantee future safe taking of medication. Changes in behavior (along with nausea and vomiting) may be an early sign of Reye's syndrome; patients should be instructed to contact their healthcare provider if these occur.

Adverse Reactions (Reflective of adult population; not specific for elderly)

>10%: Gastrointestinal: Nausea, heartburn, stomach pain, dyspepsia

1% to 10%:

Central nervous system: Fatigue

Dermatologic: Rash

Gastrointestinal: Gastrointestinal ulceration

Hematologic: Hemolytic anemia

Neuromuscular & skeletal: Weakness

Respiratory: Dyspnea

Miscellaneous: Anaphylactic shock

Overdosage/Toxicology Symptoms include respiratory alkalosis, hyperpnea, tachypnea, tinnitus, headache, hyperpyrexia, metabolic acidosis, hypoglycemia, and coma.

The "Done" nomogram is very helpful for estimating the severity of aspirin poisoning and directing treatment using serum salicylate levels. Treatment can also be based upon symptomatology.

Drug Interactions

Decreased effect with urinary alkalinizers, antacids, corticosteroids; decreased effect of uricosurics, spironolactone; ACE inhibitor effects may be decreased by concurrent therapy with NSAIDs

Increased effect/toxicity of oral anticoagulants, hypoglycemics, methotrexate

Ethanol/Nutrition/Herb Interactions

Ethanol: Avoid ethanol (may enhance gastric mucosal irritation).

Food: Salsalate peak serum levels may be delayed if taken with food.

Herb/Nutraceutical: Avoid cat's claw, dong quai, evening primrose, feverfew, garlic, ginger, ginkgo, red clover, horse chestnut, green tea, ginseng (all have additional antiplatelet activity).

Mechanism of Action Inhibits prostaglandin synthesis, acts on the hypothalamus heat-regulating center to reduce fever, blocks prostaglandin synthetase action which prevents formation of the platelet-aggregating substance thromboxane A_2

Pharmacodynamics Onset of action: Within 3-4 days of continuous dosing

Pharmacokinetics

Absorption: Oral: Completely from the small intestine; insoluble in gastric acid secretions and, therefore, is not absorbed until it reaches the small intestine

Protein binding: 90%

Half-life: 7-8 hours; half-life increases with dose, 15-30 hours with higher doses hydrolyzed in the liver to 2 moles of salicylic acid (active)

Elimination: Almost totally excreted renally

Dosage

Geriatrics & Adults: Pain, inflammation (arthritis): Oral: 3 g/day in 2-3 divided doses

Renal Impairment: Patients with end-stage renal disease undergoing hemodialysis: Administer 750 mg twice daily with an additional 500 mg after dialysis.

Monitoring Parameters Serum concentrations, renal function; hearing changes or tinnitus; monitor for response (ie, pain, inflammation, range of motion, grip strength); observe for abnormal bleeding, bruising, weight gain

Reference Range

Sample size: 1.5-2 mL blood (purple top tube)

Timing of serum samples: Peak serum concentrations usually occur 2 hours after ingestion; the half-life increases with the dosage (eg, the half-life after 300 mg is 3 hours; and after 1 g is 5-6 hours, and after 8-10 g is 10-15 hours).

Salicylate serum concentrations correlate with the pharmacological actions and adverse effects observed. Anti-inflammatory therapeutic serum concentrations 150-300 mcg/mL. See table.

Serum Salicylate: Clinical Correlations

Serum Salicylate Concentration (mcg/mL)	Desired Effects	Adverse Effects / Intoxication
~100	Antiplatelet Antipyresis Analgesia	GI intolerance and bleeding, hypersensitivity, hemostatic defects
150-300	Anti-inflammatory	Mild salicylism
250-400	Treatment of rheumatic fever	Nausea/vomiting, hyperventilation, salicylism, flushing, sweating, thirst, headache, diarrhea, and tachycardia
>400-500		Respiratory alkalosis, hemorrhage, excitement, confusion, asterixis, pulmonary edema, convulsions, tetany, metabolic acidosis, fever, coma, cardiovascular collapse, renal and respiratory failure

Test Interactions False-negative results for glucose oxidase urinary glucose tests (Clinistix®); false-positives using the cupric sulfate method (Clinitest®); also, interferes with Gerhardt test, VMA determination; 5-HIAA, xylose tolerance test and T_3 and T_4

Patient Information Avoid alcohol; do not self-medicate with other drug products containing aspirin; use antacids to relieve upset stomach; watch for any signs of bleeding (stool); take with food to minimize GI distress; report ringing in ears, persistent GI pain to physician or pharmacist

Additional Information Does not appear to inhibit platelet aggregation; salsalate causes less GI and renal toxicity than aspirin and other NSAIDs. See Mechanism of Action.

Special Geriatric Considerations Elderly are a high-risk population for adverse effects from NSAIDs. As much as 60% of the elderly can develop peptic ulceration and/ (Continued)

Salsalate *(Continued)*

or hemorrhage asymptomatically. The concomitant use of H_2 blockers and sucralfate is not effective as prophylaxis with the exception of NSAID-induced duodenal ulcers which may be prevented by the use of ranitidine. Misoprostol and proton pump inhibitors are the only agents proven to help prevent the development of NSAID-induced ulcers. Also, concomitant disease and drug use contribute to the risk for GI adverse effects. Use lowest effective dose for shortest period possible. Consider renal function decline with age. Use of NSAIDs can compromise existing renal function especially when Cl_{cr} is ≤30 mL/minute. Tinnitus may be a difficult and unreliable indication of toxicity due to age-related hearing loss or eighth cranial nerve damage. CNS adverse effects such as confusion, agitation, and hallucinations are generally seen in overdose or high dose situations, but elderly may demonstrate these adverse effects at lower doses than younger adults.

Dosage Forms Excipient information presented when available (limited, particularly for generics); consult specific product labeling.

Tablet: 500 mg, 750 mg

Amigesic®: 500 mg, 750 mg

Selected References

Gurwitz JH, Avorn J, Ross-Degnan D, et al, "Nonsteroidal Anti-Inflammatory Drug-Associated Azotemia in the Very Old," *JAMA*, 1990, 264(4):471-5.

Hawkey CJ, Karrasch JA, Szczepański L, et al, "Omeprazole Compared With Misoprostol for Ulcers Associated With Nonsteroidal Anti-inflammatory Drugs," *N Engl J Med*, 1998, 338(11):727-34.

Weissmann G, "Aspirin," *Sci Am*, 1991, 264(1):84-90.

Yeomans ND, Tulassay Z, Juhasz L, et al, "A Comparison of Omeprazole With Ranitidine for Ulcers Associated With Nonsteroidal Anti-inflammatory Drugs," *N Engl J Med*, 1998, 338(11):719-26.

♦ **Salt** *see* Sodium Chloride *on page 1475*

♦ **Sal-Tropine**™ *see* Atropine *on page 137*

♦ **Sanctura®** *see* Trospium *on page 1641*

♦ **Sandimmune®** *see* CycloSPORINE *on page 380*

♦ **Sani-Supp® [OTC]** *see* Glycerin *on page 718*

♦ **Santyl®** *see* Collagenase *on page 363*

♦ **Sarafem®** *see* Fluoxetine *on page 644*

♦ **Sarnol®-HC [OTC]** *see* Hydrocortisone *on page 762*

♦ **SB-265805** *see* Gemifloxacin *on page 702*

♦ **S. boulardii** *see* Saccharomyces boulardii *on page 1438*

♦ **SCH 13521** *see* Flutamide *on page 658*

♦ **SCH 56592** *see* Posaconazole *on page 1285*

♦ **SCIG** *see* Immune Globulin (Subcutaneous) *on page 796*

♦ **S-Citalopram** *see* Escitalopram *on page 539*

♦ **Scopace**™ *see* Scopolamine Derivatives *on page 1448*

♦ **Scopolamine Base** *see* Scopolamine Derivatives *on page 1448*

♦ **Scopolamine Butylbromide** *see* Scopolamine Derivatives *on page 1448*

Scopolamine Derivatives (skoe POL a meen dah RIV ah tives)

Medication Safety Issues

Transdermal patch may contain conducting metal (eg, aluminum); remove patch prior to MRI.

U.S. Brand Names Isopto® Hyoscine; Maldemar™; Scopace™; Transderm Scōp®

Canadian Brand Names Buscopan®; Transderm-V®

Index Terms Hyoscine Butylbromide; Hyoscine Hydrobromide; Scopolamine Base; Scopolamine Butylbromide; Scopolamine Hydrobromide

Generic Available Yes: Injection

Pharmacologic Category Anticholinergic Agent

Use

Scopolamine base:

Transdermal: Prevention of nausea/vomiting associated with motion sickness and recovery from anesthesia and surgery

Scopolamine hydrobromide:

Injection: Preoperative medication to produce amnesia, sedation, tranquilization, antiemetic effects, and decrease salivary and respiratory secretions

Ophthalmic: Produce cycloplegia and mydriasis; treatment of iridocyclitis

Oral: Symptomatic treatment of postencephalitic parkinsonism and paralysis agitans; in spastic states; inhibits excessive motility and hypertonus of the gastro-intestinal tract in such conditions as the irritable colon syndrome, mild dysentery, diverticulitis, pylorospasm, and cardiospasm

Scopolamine butylbromide [not available in the U.S.]:

Oral/injection: Treatment of smooth muscle spasm of the genitourinary or gastrointestinal tract; injection may also be used to prior to radiological/diagnostic procedures to prevent spasm

Contraindications Hypersensitivity to scopolamine, other belladonna alkaloids, or any component of the formulation; narrow-angle glaucoma; acute hemorrhage; paralytic ileus; tachycardia secondary to cardiac insufficiency; myasthenia gravis

Tablet formulations are contraindicated in patients with prostatic hyperplasia, pyloric obstruction, or patients with an idiosyncrasy to anticholinergic drugs.

Injectable formulations are contraindicated in patients with chronic lung disease (repeated administration).

Warnings/Precautions Use with caution with hepatic or renal impairment; adverse CNS effects occur more often in these patients. Use with caution in patients with GI obstruction, prostatic hyperplasia (nonobstructive), or urinary retention. Discontinue if patient reports unusual visual disturbances or pain within the eye. Use caution in hiatal hernia, reflux esophagitis, and ulcerative colitis. Use with caution in patients with a history of seizure or psychosis; may exacerbate these conditions. Patients with idiosyncratic reaction to anticholinergics, including scopolamine, may experience disorientation, delirium and/or marked somnolence; may be accompanied by dilated pupils, rapid pulse and xerostomia. May cause CNS depression, which may impair physical or mental abilities; patients must be cautioned about performing tasks which require mental alertness (eg, operating machinery or driving).

Transdermal patch may contain conducting metal (eg, aluminum); remove patch prior to MRI. Ophthalmic products may contain benzalkonium chloride which may be absorbed by contact lenses; remove contacts prior to administration and wait 15 minutes before reinserting. Scopolamine (hyoscine) hydrobromide should not be interchanged with scopolamine butylbromide formulations; dosages are not equivalent.

Adverse Reactions (Reflective of adult population; not specific for elderly)

Frequency not defined.

Ophthalmic: Note: Systemic adverse effects have been reported following ophthalmic administration.

Cardiovascular: Vascular congestion, edema

Central nervous system: Drowsiness

Dermatologic: Eczematoid dermatitis

Ocular: Blurred vision, photophobia, local irritation, increased intraocular pressure, follicular conjunctivitis, exudate

Respiratory: Congestion

Systemic:

Cardiovascular: Orthostatic hypotension, ventricular fibrillation, tachycardia, palpitation

Central nervous system: Confusion, drowsiness, headache, loss of memory, ataxia, fatigue

Dermatologic: Dry skin, increased sensitivity to light, rash

Endocrine & metabolic: Decreased flow of breast milk

Gastrointestinal: Constipation, xerostomia, dry throat, dysphagia, bloated feeling, nausea, vomiting

Genitourinary: Dysuria

Local: Irritation at injection site

Neuromuscular & skeletal: Weakness

Ocular: Increased intraocular pain, blurred vision

Respiratory: Dry nose

Miscellaneous: Diaphoresis (decreased)

Overdosage/Toxicology Symptoms include dilated pupils, flushed skin, tachycardia, hypertension, ECG abnormalities, and CNS manifestations resembling acute psychosis. CNS depression, circulatory collapse, hyperpyrexia, respiratory failure, and death can occur. Artificial respiration with oxygen may be necessary; fever may be managed with ice or alcohol sponges. Pure scopolamine intoxication is extremely rare. However, for a scopolamine overdose with severe life-threatening symptoms, physostigmine 1-2 mg SubQ or slow I.V. should be given to reverse the toxic effects; repeat administration after 2 hours may be necessary. Treatment is otherwise symptom-directed and supportive.

Drug Interactions

Acetylcholinesterase inhibitors (donepezil, galantamine, rivastigmine, tacrine): May diminish the therapeutic effect of scopolamine. If the anticholinergic action is a side effect of the agent, the result may be beneficial. Scopolamine may diminish the therapeutic effect of acetylcholinesterase inhibitors.

Anticholinergic agents: Adverse anticholinergic effects may be additive with other anticholinergic agents (includes tricyclic antidepressants, antihistamines, and phenothiazines).

CNS depressants: Sedative effects may be additive with scopolamine; use caution. (Continued)

Scopolamine Derivatives *(Continued)*

Pramlintide: May enhance the anticholinergic effect of scopolamine (these effects are specific to the GI tract).

Ethanol/Nutrition/Herb Interactions Ethanol: Avoid ethanol (may increase CNS depression).

Stability

Injection: Store at room temperature of 15°C to 30°C (58°F to 86°F). Protect from light.
  Hydrobromide injection: Avoid acid solutions, hydrolysis occurs at pH <3.
  Butylbromide injection: Stable in D_5W, NS, $D_{10}W$, and LR for up to 8 hours.
Ophthalmic solution: Store at 8°C to 27°C (46°F to 80°F). Protect from light.
Tablet: Store at room temperature of 15°C to 30°C (58°F to 86°F).
Transdermal system: Store at 20°C to 25°C (68°F to 77°F).

Mechanism of Action Blocks the action of acetylcholine at parasympathetic sites in smooth muscle, secretory glands and the CNS; increases cardiac output, dries secretions, antagonizes histamine and serotonin; dilates pupils

Pharmacodynamics Peak effect: 20-60 minutes; may take 3-7 days for full recovery; transdermal: 24 hours

Pharmacokinetics

Absorption: Tertiary salts (hydrobromide) are well absorbed; quaternary salts (butylbromide) are poorly absorbed (local concentrations in the GI tract following oral dosing may be high)
Half-life elimination: 4.8 hours
Excretion: Urine (<10%, as parent drug and metabolites)

Dosage

Geriatrics & Adults: Note: Scopolamine (hyoscine) hydrobromide should not be interchanged with scopolamine butylbromide formulations. Dosages are not equivalent.

Scopolamine base:
Preoperative: Transdermal patch: Apply 1 patch to hairless area behind ear the night before surgery; remove 24 hours after surgery
Motion sickness: Transdermal patch: Apply 1 patch behind the ear at least 4 hours prior to exposure and every 3 days as needed; effective if applied as soon as 2-3 hours before anticipated need, best if 12 hours before

Scopolamine hydrobromide:
Antiemetic: SubQ: 0.6-1 mg
Preoperative: I.M., I.V., SubQ: 0.3-0.65 mg
Sedation, tranquilization: I.M., I.V., SubQ: 0.6 mg 3-4 times/day
Refraction: Ophthalmic: Instill 1-2 drops of 0.25% to eye(s) 1 hour before procedure
Iridocyclitis: Ophthalmic: Instill 1-2 drops of 0.25% to eye(s) up to 4 times/day
Parkinsonism, spasticity, motion sickness: Oral: 0.4-0.8 mg. May repeat every 8-12 hours as needed; the dosage may be cautiously increased in parkinsonism and spastic states. For motion sickness, administration at least 1 hour before exposure is recommended.

Scopolamine butylbromide:
Gastrointestinal/genitourinary spasm (Buscopan® [CAN]; not available in the U.S.):
  Oral: 10-20 mg daily (1-2 tablets); maximum: 6 tablets/day
  I.M., I.V., SubQ: 10-20 mg; maximum: 100 mg/day. Intramuscular injections should be administered 10-15 minutes prior to radiological/diagnostic procedures

Administration

I.V.:
  Hydrobromide: Dilute with an equal volume of sterile water and administer by direct I.V.; inject over 2-3 minutes
  Butylbromide: No dilution is necessary prior to injection; inject at a rate of 1 mL/minute
Ophthalmic: Remove contact lenses prior to administration; wait 15 minutes before reinserting if using products containing benzalkonium chloride. Wash hands following administration.
Transdermal: Topical patch is programmed to deliver 1 mg over 3 days. Once applied, do not remove the patch for 3 full days. Apply to hairless area of skin behind the ear. Wash hands before and after applying the disc to avoid drug contact with eyes.

Monitoring Parameters Body temperature, heart rate, urinary output, intraocular pressure

Test Interactions Interferes with gastric secretion test

Patient Information Report any changes of vision; wait 5 minutes after instilling ophthalmic preparation before using any other drops, do not blink excessively; after instilling ophthalmic preparation, apply pressure to the side of the nose near the eye to minimize systemic absorption; put patch on at least 4 hours before traveling; once applied, do not remove the patch for 3 full days. May cause dry mouth, drowsiness, blurred vision. If eye pain, blurred vision, dizziness, or rapid pulse occurs, remove patch and consult physician. Wash hands thoroughly after handling the patch.

Special Geriatric Considerations Because of its long duration of action as a mydriatic agent, it should be avoided in elderly patients. Anticholinergic agents are not well tolerated in the elderly and their use should be avoided when possible.

Dosage Forms Excipient information presented when available (limited, particularly for generics); consult specific product labeling. [CAN] = Canadian brand name

Injection, solution, as hydrobromide: 0.4 mg/mL (1 mL)

Injection, solution, as hyoscine-N-butylbromide:
Buscopan® [CAN]: 20 mg/mL [not available in U.S.]

Solution, ophthalmic, as hydrobromide:
Isopto® Hyoscine: 0.25% (5 mL, 15 mL) [contains benzalkonium chloride]

Tablet, as hyoscine-N-butylbromide:
Buscopan® [CAN]: 10 mg [not available in U.S.]

Tablet, soluble, as hydrobromide:
Maldemar™, Scopace™: 0.4 mg

Transdermal system:
Transderm Scōp®: 1.5 mg (4s, 10s, 24s) [releases ~1 mg over 72 hours]

Selected References

Feinberg M, "The Problems of Anticholinergic Adverse Effects in Older Patients," *Drugs Aging*, 1993, 3(4):335-48.

♦ **Scopolamine Hydrobromide** *see* Scopolamine Derivatives *on page 1448*

♦ **Scopolamine, Hyoscyamine, Atropine, and Phenobarbital** *see* Hyoscyamine, Atropine, Scopolamine, and Phenobarbital *on page 780*

♦ **Scot-Tussin DM® Cough Chasers [OTC]** *see* Dextromethorphan *on page 419*

♦ **Scot-Tussin® Expectorant [OTC]** *see* Guaifenesin *on page 727*

♦ **Scot-Tussin® Senior [OTC]** *see* Guaifenesin and Dextromethorphan *on page 730*

♦ **SD/01** *see* Pegfilgrastim *on page 1212*

♦ **SDZ ENA 713** *see* Rivastigmine *on page 1421*

♦ **Sectral®** *see* Acebutolol *on page 27*

♦ **Secura® Antifungal [OTC]** *see* Miconazole *on page 1036*

Selegiline (se LE ji leen)

Related Information
Antiparkinsonian Agents *on page 1745*

Medication Safety Issues
Sound-alike/look-alike issues:
Selegiline may be confused with Salagen®, Serentil®, sertraline, Serzone®, Stelazine®
Eldepryl® may be confused with Elavil®, enalapril
Zelapar™ may be confused with zaleplon, Zemplar®

U.S. Brand Names Eldepryl®; Emsam®; Zelapar™

Canadian Brand Names Apo-Selegiline®; Gen-Selegiline; Novo-Selegiline; Nu-Selegiline

Index Terms Deprenyl; L-Deprenyl; Selegiline Hydrochloride

Generic Available Yes: Capsule, tablet

Pharmacologic Category Anti-Parkinson's Agent, MAO Type B Inhibitor; Antidepressant, Monoamine Oxidase Inhibitor

Use Adjunct in the management of parkinsonian patients in which levodopa/carbidopa therapy is deteriorating (oral products); treatment of major depressive disorder (transdermal product)

Unlabeled/Investigational Use Early Parkinson's disease; attention-deficit/hyperactivity disorder (ADHD); negative symptoms of schizophrenia; extrapyramidal symptoms; Alzheimer's disease (studies have shown some improvement in behavioral and cognitive performance)

Restrictions An FDA-approved medication guide concerning the use of antidepressants in children, adolescents, and young adults must be distributed when dispensing a transdermal selegiline outpatient prescription (new or refill) where this medication is to be used without direct supervision of a healthcare provider. Medication guides are available at http://www.fda.gov/cder/Offices/ODS/medication_guides.htm. Dispense to parents or guardians of children and adolescents receiving this medication.

Contraindications Hypersensitivity to selegiline or any component of the formulation; concomitant use of meperidine

Orally disintegrating tablet: Additional contraindications: Concomitant use of dextromethorphan, methadone, propoxyphene, tramadol, oral selegiline, other MAO inhibitors

Transdermal: Additional contraindications: Pheochromocytoma; concomitant use of bupropion, selective or dual serotonin reuptake inhibitors (including SSRIs and SNRIs), tricyclic antidepressants, buspirone, tramadol, propoxyphene, methadone, (Continued)

Selegiline *(Continued)*

dextromethorphan, St. John's wort, mirtazapine, cyclobenzaprine, oral selegiline and other MAO inhibitors; carbamazepine, and oxcarbazepine; elective surgery requiring general anesthesia, local anesthesia containing sympathomimetic vasoconstrictors; sympathomimetics (and related compounds); foods high in tyramine content; supplements containing tyrosine, phenylalanine, tryptophan, or caffeine

Warnings/Precautions

Oral: MAO-B selective inhibition should not pose a problem with tyramine-containing products as long as the typical oral doses are employed, however, rare reactions have been reported. Increased risk of nonselective MAO inhibition occurs with oral capsule/tablet doses >10 mg/day or orally disintegrating tablet doses >2.5 mg/day. Use of oral selegiline with tricyclic antidepressants and SSRIs has also been associated with rare reactions and should generally be avoided. Addition to levodopa therapy may result in exacerbation of levodopa adverse effects, requiring a reduction in levodopa dosage.

Transdermal: Nonselective MAO inhibition occurs with transdermal delivery and is necessary for antidepressant efficacy. Hypertensive crisis as a result of ingesting tyramine-rich foods is always a concern with nonselective MAO inhibition. Although transdermal delivery minimizes inhibition of MAO-A in the gut, there is limited data with higher transdermal doses; dietary restrictions are recommended with doses >6 mg/24hours.

Transdermal: **[U.S. Boxed Warning]: Antidepressants increase the risk of suicidal thinking and behavior in children, adolescents, and young adults (18-24 years of age) with major depressive disorder (MDD) and other psychiatric disorders;** consider risk prior to prescribing. Short-term studies did not show an increased risk in patients >24 years of age and showed a decreased risk in patients ≥65 years. Closely monitor patients for worsening of depression, suicidality and/or associated behaviors, particularly during the initial 1-2 months of therapy or during periods of dosage adjustments (increases or decreases); the patient's family or caregiver should be instructed to closely observe the patient and communicate condition with healthcare provider. A medication guide concerning the use of antidepressants should be dispensed with each prescription.

Transdermal: The possibility of a suicide attempt is inherit in major depression and may persist until remission occurs. Patients treated with antidepressants (for any indication) should be observed for clinical worsening and suicidality, especially during the initial few months of a course of drug therapy, or at times of dose changes, either increases or decreases. Use caution in high-risk patients. Worsening depression and severe abrupt suicidality that are not part of the presenting symptoms may require discontinuation or modification of drug therapy. Use caution in high-risk patients during initiation of therapy. The patient's family or caregiver should be alerted to monitor patients for the emergence of suicidality and associated behaviors (such as agitation, irritability, hostility, and hypomania) and call healthcare provider.

Transdermal selegiline may worsen psychosis in some patients or precipitate a shift to mania or hypomania in patients with bipolar disorder. Monotherapy in patients with bipolar disorder should be avoided. Patients presenting with depressive symptoms should be screened for bipolar disorder. **Selegiline is not FDA approved for the treatment of bipolar depression.**

Adverse Reactions (Reflective of adult population; not specific for elderly)

Unless otherwise noted, the percentage of adverse events is reported for the transdermal patch (**Note:** ODT = orally disintegrating tablet, Oral = capsule/tablet)

>10%:
Central nervous system: Headache (18%; ODT 7%; oral 2%), insomnia (12%; ODT 7%), dizziness (ODT 11%; oral 7%)
Gastrointestinal: Nausea (ODT 11%; oral 10%)
Local: Application site reaction (24%)

1% to 10%:
Cardiovascular: Hypotension (including postural 3% to 10%), chest pain (≥1%; ODT 2%), hypertension (≥1%), peripheral edema (≥1%)
Central nervous system: Pain (ODT 8%), hallucinations (ODT 4%; oral 3%), confusion (ODT 4%; oral 3%), headache (ODT 7%; oral 2%), ataxia (ODT 3%), somnolence (ODT 3%), agitation (≥1%), amnesia (≥1%), paresthesia (≥1%), thinking abnormal (≥1%), depression (<1%; ODT 2%)
Dermatologic: Rash (4%), ecchymosis (ODT 2%), bruising (≥1%), pruritus (≥1%), acne (≥1%)
Endocrine and metabolic: Weight loss (5%), hypokalemia (ODT 2%), sexual side effects (≤1%)
Gastrointestinal: Diarrhea (9%; ODT 2%), xerostomia (8%; ODT 4%), stomatitis (ODT 5%), abdominal pain (oral 4%), dyspepsia (4%; ODT 5%), constipation (≥1%; ODT 4%), flatulence (≥1%; ODT 2%), anorexia (≥1%), gastroenteritis (≥1%), taste perversion (≥1%; ODT 2%), vomiting (≥1%; ODT 3%), tooth disorder (ODT 2%), dysphagia (ODT 2%)

Genitourinary: Dysmenorrhea (≥1%), metrorrhagia (≥1%), UTI (≥1%), urinary frequency (≥1%)

Neuromuscular & skeletal: Dyskinesia (ODT 6%), back pain (ODT 5%), ataxia (<1%; ODT 3%), leg cramps (ODT 3%), myalgia (≥1%; ODT 3%), neck pain (≥1%), tremor (<1%; ODT 3%)

Otic: Tinnitus (≥1%)

Respiratory: Rhinitis (ODT 7%), pharyngitis (3%; ODT 4%), sinusitis (3%), cough (≥1%), bronchitis (≥1%), dyspnea (<1%; ODT 3%)

Miscellaneous: Diaphoresis (≥1%)

Overdosage/Toxicology Symptoms include tachycardia, palpitations, muscle twitching, and seizures. Competent supportive care is the most important treatment. Both hypertension or hypotension can occur with intoxication. Hypotension may respond to I.V. fluids or vasopressors, and hypertension usually responds to an alpha-adrenergic blocker. While treating the hypertension, care is warranted to avoid sudden drops in blood pressure, since this may worsen MAO inhibitor toxicity. Muscle irritability and seizures often respond to diazepam, while hyperthermia is best treated with antipyretics and cooling blankets. Cardiac arrhythmias are best treated with phenytoin or procainamide. Restrict dietary tyramine for several weeks after overdose.

Drug Interactions Substrate of CYP1A2 (minor), 2A6 (minor), 2B6 (major), 2C8 (minor), 2C19 (minor), 2D6 (minor), 3A4 (minor); **Inhibits** CYP1A2 (weak), 2A6 (weak), 2C9 (weak), 2C19 (weak), 2D6 (weak), 2E1 (weak), 3A4 (weak)

Note: Many drug interactions involving selegiline are theoretical, primarily based on interactions with nonspecific MAO inhibitors; at oral (capsule/tablet) doses <10 mg/day and orally disintegrating tablet doses <2.5 mg, the risk of these interactions with selegiline may be very low. Transdermal selegiline results in higher plasma levels and nonselective MAO inhibition.

Amphetamines: MAO inhibitors in combination with amphetamines may result in severe hypertensive reaction or serotonin syndrome; these combinations are best avoided (contraindicated with transdermal selegiline).

Anorexiants: Concurrent use of selegiline (high dose) in combination with CNS stimulants or anorexiants may result in serotonin syndrome; these combinations are best avoided; includes dexfenfluramine, fenfluramine, or sibutramine

Atomoxetine: MAO inhibitors may increase the toxicity of atomoxetine; avoid concomitant use.

Barbiturates: MAO inhibitors may inhibit the metabolism of barbiturates and prolong their effect

Bupropion: MAO inhibitors may increase the toxicity of bupropion; avoid concomitant use.

Buspirone: Concomitant use with selegiline may cause increased blood pressure; avoid combination.

Carbamazepine: May increase levels/effects of selegiline; concomitant use of transdermal selegiline is contraindicated.

CNS stimulants: MAO inhibitors in combination with stimulants (methylphenidate, dexmethylphenidate) may result in serotonin syndrome; these combinations are best avoided (contraindicated with transdermal selegiline).

COMT inhibitors (eg, entacapone, tolcapone): May increase to toxicity of MAO inhibitors; avoid concomitant use.

CYP2B6 inducers: May decrease the levels/effects of selegiline. Example inducers include carbamazepine, nevirapine, phenobarbital, phenytoin, and rifampin.

CYP2B6 inhibitors: May increase the levels/effects of selegiline. Example inhibitors include desipramine, paroxetine, and sertraline.

Dextromethorphan: Concurrent use of selegiline (high dose) may result in serotonin syndrome; these combinations are best avoided (contraindicated with transdermal and orally disintegrating tablet selegiline).

Disulfiram: MAO inhibitors may produce delirium in patients receiving disulfiram; monitor.

False neurotransmitters (eg, guanadrel and guanethidine): MAO inhibitors inhibit the antihypertensive response to guanadrel or guanethidine; use an alternative antihypertensive agent.

Hypoglycemic agents: MAO inhibitors may produce hypoglycemia in patients with diabetes; monitor.

Levodopa: MAO inhibitors in combination with levodopa may result in hypertensive reactions; monitor.

Lithium: MAO inhibitors in combination with lithium have resulted in malignant hyperpyrexia; this combination is best avoided.

Meperidine: Use with selegiline (high dose) may result in serotonin syndrome; concurrent use contraindicated.

Methadone: Concomitant use with an MAO inhibitor may increase the risk of serotonin syndrome (contraindicated with transdermal and orally disintegrating tablet selegiline).

(Continued)

Selegiline *(Continued)*

Mirtazapine, nefazodone: Concurrent use of selegiline (high dose) may result in serotonin syndrome; these combinations are best avoided (contraindicated with transdermal selegiline).

Norepinephrine: MAO inhibitors may increase the pressor response of norepinephrine (effect is generally small); monitor (contraindicated with transdermal selegiline).

Oral contraceptives: Increased selegiline levels have been noted with concurrent administration; monitor

Propoxyphene: Concomitant use with an MAO inhibitor may increase the risk of serotonin syndrome (contraindicated with transdermal and orally disintegrating tablet selegiline).

Reserpine: MAO inhibitors in combination with reserpine may result in hypertensive reactions; monitor.

Sibutramine: May cause serotonin syndrome when combined with an MAO inhibitor; avoid this combination.

SSRIs/SNRIs: Concurrent use of selegiline with a selective serotonin or serotonin/ norepinephrine reuptake inhibitor may result in mania or hypertension. It is generally best to avoid these combinations (contraindicated with transdermal selegiline).

St John's wort: May cause serotonin syndrome when combined with an MAO inhibitor; avoid this combination.

Sympathomimetics (indirect-acting): MAO inhibitors in combination with sympathomimetics such as dopamine, metaraminol, phenylephrine, and decongestants (pseudoephedrine) may result in severe hypertensive reaction; these combinations are best avoided (contraindicated with transdermal selegiline).

Tramadol: May increase the risk of seizures and serotonin syndrome in patients receiving an MAO inhibitor (contraindicated with transdermal and orally disintegrating tablet selegiline).

Trazodone: Concurrent use of selegiline (high dose) may result in serotonin syndrome; these combinations are best avoided.

Tricyclic antidepressants: May cause serotonin syndrome when combined with an MAO inhibitor; avoid this combination (contraindicated with transdermal selegiline).

Venlafaxine: Concurrent use of selegiline (high dose) may result in serotonin syndrome; these combinations are best avoided (contraindicated with transdermal selegiline).

Ethanol/Nutrition/Herb Interactions

Ethanol: Avoid ethanol (based on CNS depressant effects and potential tyramine content)

Food: Concurrent ingestion of foods rich in tyramine may cause sudden and severe high blood pressure (hypertensive crisis). Avoid tyramine-containing foods with MAOIs. Food's freshness is also an important concern; improperly stored or spoiled food can create an environment where tyramine concentrations may increase.

Herb/Nutraceuticals: Avoid valerian, St John's wort, SAMe, kava kava. Avoid supplements containing caffeine, tryptophan, or phenylalanine. Ingestion of large quantities may increase the risk of severe side effects (eg, hypertensive reactions, serotonin syndrome).

Stability

Capsule, tablet: Store at controlled room temperature 15°C to 30°C (59°F to 86°F).

Orally-disintegrating tablet: Store at controlled room temperature 15°C to 30°C (59°F to 86°F). Use within 3 months of opening pouch and immediately after opening individual blister.

Transdermal: Store at 20°C to 25°C (68°F to 77°F).

Mechanism of Action Potent, irreversible inhibitor of monoamine oxidase (MAO). Plasma concentrations achieved via administration of oral dosage forms in recommended doses confer selective inhibition of MAO type B, which plays a major role in the metabolism of dopamine; selegiline may also increase dopaminergic activity by interfering with dopamine reuptake at the synapse. When administered transdermally in recommended doses, selegiline achieves higher blood levels and effectively inhibits both MAO-A and MAO-B, which blocks catabolism of other centrally-active biogenic amine neurotransmitters.

Pharmacodynamics

Onset of action: Therapeutic: Oral: Within 1 hour

Duration: Oral: 24-72 hours

Pharmacokinetics

Absorption:

Orally disintegrating tablet: Rapid; greater bioavailability than capsule/tablet

Transdermal: 25% to 30% (of total selegiline content) over 24 hours

Protein binding: ~90%

Metabolism: Hepatic, primarily via CYP2B6 to active (N-desmethylselegiline, amphetamine, methamphetamine) and inactive metabolites

Half-life elimination: Oral: 10 hours; Transdermal: 18-25 hours

Excretion: Urine (primarily metabolites); feces

Dosage

Geriatrics:

Parkinson's disease:

Capsule/tablet: Initial: 5 mg in the morning; may increase to a total of 10 mg/day.

Orally disintegrating tablet (Zelapar™): Initial 1.25 mg daily for at least 6 weeks; may increase to 2.5 mg daily based on clinical response (maximum: 2.5 mg daily)

Depression: Transdermal (Emsam®): 6 mg/24 hours

Adults:

Parkinson's disease:

Capsule/tablet: 5 mg twice daily with breakfast and lunch or 10 mg in the morning

Orally disintegrating tablet (Zelapar™): Initial 1.25 mg daily for at least 6 weeks; may increase to 2.5 mg daily based on clinical response (maximum: 2.5 mg daily)

Depression: Transdermal (Emsam®): Initial: 6 mg/24 hours once daily; may titrate based on clinical response in increments of 3 mg/day every 2 weeks up to a maximum of 12 mg/24 hours

Renal Impairment: No adjustment necessary.

Hepatic Impairment: No adjustment necessary in mild-moderate hepatic impairment.

Administration

Oral: Orally disintegrating tablet (Zelapar™): Take in morning before breakfast; place on top of tongue and allow to dissolve. Avoid food or liquid 5 minutes before and after administration.

Topical: Transdermal (Emsam®): Apply to clean, dry, intact skin to the upper torso (below the neck and above the waist), upper thigh, or outer surface of the upper arm. Avoid exposure of application site to external heat source, which may increase the amount of drug absorbed. Apply at the same time each day and rotate application sites. Wash hands with soap and water after handling. Avoid touching the sticky side of the patch.

Monitoring Parameters Blood pressure; symptoms of parkinsonism; general mood and behavior (increased anxiety, presence of mania or agitation, or suicidal ideation/tendencies)

Patient Information Take exactly as directed (may be prescribed in conjunction with levodopa/carbidopa); do not change dosage or discontinue without consulting prescriber. Therapeutic effects may take several weeks or months to achieve and you may need frequent monitoring during first weeks of therapy. Take oral capsule/tablet with meals if GI upset occurs, before meals if dry mouth occurs, or after eating if drooling or if nausea occurs. Do not take food or liquid for 5 five minutes before or after administering orally disintegrating tablets. Do not swallow orally disintegrating tablet; allow to dissolve on tongue. Take at the same time each day. Avoid tyramine-containing foods (low potential for reaction) with oral products. Maintain adequate hydration (2-3 L/day of fluids) unless instructed to restrict fluid intake. Do not use alcohol and prescription or OTC sedatives or CNS depressants without consulting prescriber. You may experience drowsiness, dizziness, confusion, or vision changes (use caution when driving, climbing stairs, or engaging in tasks requiring alertness until response to drug is known); orthostatic hypotension (use caution when changing position - rising to standing from sitting or lying); constipation (increased exercise, fluids, fruit, or fiber may help); runny nose or flu-like symptoms (consult prescriber for appropriate relief); or nausea, vomiting, loss of appetite, or stomach discomfort (small frequent meals, frequent mouth care, chewing gum, or sucking lozenges may help). Report unresolved constipation or vomiting; chest pain, palpitations, irregular heartbeat; CNS changes (hallucination, loss of memory, seizures, acute headache, nervousness, thoughts of suicide, etc); painful or difficult urination; increased muscle spasticity, rigidity, or involuntary movements; skin rash; or significant worsening of condition.

Additional Information Selegiline is a monoamine oxidase inhibitor type "B"; there should not be a problem with tyramine-containing products as long as the typical doses are employed. When adding selegiline to levodopa/carbidopa, the dose of the latter can usually be decreased.

Special Geriatric Considerations Do not use capsule/tablet at doses >10 mg/day or orally disintegrating tablet at doses >2.5 mg/day because of the risks associated with nonselective inhibition of MAO.

Orally-disintegrating tablets: In clinical trials, adverse effects were seen more frequently in the elderly compared to younger adults. This is particularly of concern for hypertension, orthostatic hypotension, dizziness, and somnolence. If using the orally disintegrating tablets, administer at the lowest dose and monitor for side effects.

Dosage Forms Excipient information presented when available (limited, particularly for generics); consult specific product labeling.

Capsule, as hydrochloride: 5 mg

Eldepryl®: 5 mg

(Continued)

Selegiline *(Continued)*

Tablet, as hydrochloride: 5 mg

Tablet, orally-disintegrating:

Zelapar™: 1.25 mg [contains phenylalanine 1.25 mg/tablet]

Transdermal system [once-daily patch]:

Emsam®: 6 mg/24 hours (30s); 9 mg/24 hours (30s); 12 mg/24 hours (30s)

Selected References

Lawlor BA, Aisen PS, and Green C, "Selegiline in the Treatment of Behavioural Disturbances in Alzheimer's Disease," *Int J Geriatr Psychiatry*, 1997, 12(3):319-22.

Olanow CW, Watts RL, and Koller WC, "An Algorithm (Decision Tree) for the Management of Parkinson's Disease (2001): Treatment Guidelines," *Neurology*, 2001, 56(11 Suppl 5):S1-S88.

Sano M, Ernesto C, Thomas RG, et al, "A Controlled Trial of Selegiline, Alpha-Tocopherol, or Both as Treatment for Alzheimer's Disease," *N Engl J Med*, 1997, 336(17):1216-22.

Stern MB, "Contemporary Approaches to the Pharmacotherapeutic Management of Parkinson's Disease: An Overview," *Neurology*, 1997, 49(1 Suppl 1):S2-9.

The Parkinson Study Group, "Effects of Tocopherol and Deprenyl on the Progression of Disability in Early Parkinson's Disease," *N Engl J Med*, 1993, 328(3):176-83.

♦ **Selegiline Hydrochloride** *see* Selegiline *on page 1451*

♦ **Senexon [OTC]** *see* Senna *on page 1456*

Senna *(SEN na)*

Related Information

Treatment Options for Constipation *on page 1785*

Medication Safety Issues

Sound-alike/look-alike issues:

Senexon® may be confused with Cenestin®

Senokot® may be confused with Depakote®

U.S. Brand Names Black-Draught Tablets [OTC]; Evac-U-Gen [OTC]; ex-lax® [OTC]; ex-lax® Maximum Strength [OTC]; Fletcher's® [OTC]; Perdiem® Overnight Relief [OTC]; Senexon [OTC]; Senna-Gen® [OTC]; Sennatural™ [OTC]; Senokot® [OTC]; SenokotXTRA® [OTC]; Uni-Senna [OTC]

Generic Available Yes

Pharmacologic Category Laxative, Stimulant

Use Short-term treatment of constipation; evacuation of the colon for bowel or rectal examinations

Contraindications Per Commission E: Intestinal obstruction, acute intestinal inflammation (eg, Crohn's disease), colitis ulcerosa, appendicitis, abdominal pain of unknown origin

Warnings/Precautions Not recommended for over-the-counter (OTC) use in patients experiencing stomach pain, nausea, vomiting, or a sudden change in bowel movements which lasts >2 weeks.

Adverse Reactions (Reflective of adult population; not specific for elderly)

Frequency not defined: Gastrointestinal: Nausea, vomiting, diarrhea, abdominal cramps

Pharmacodynamics Onset of action: Oral: Within 6-10 hours

Pharmacokinetics

Metabolism: In the liver

Elimination: In feces (via bile) and urine

Dosage

Geriatrics & Adults:

Bowel evacuation: Oral: OTC labeling: Usual dose: Sennosides 130 mg (X-Prep® 75 mL) between 2-4 PM the afternoon of the day prior to procedure

Constipation: Oral: OTC ranges: Sennosides 15 mg once daily (maximum: 70-100 mg/day, divided twice daily)

Administration Oral: Once daily doses should be taken at bedtime. Granules may be eaten plain, sprinkled on food, or mixed in liquids

Monitoring Parameters Monitor stools daily for consistency, occult or gross blood; also with chronic use, monitor serum electrolytes; monitor for dehydration and hypotension

Patient Information May discolor urine or feces (yellow-brown); do not use in presence of nausea, vomiting, or abdominal pain; stimulant laxative use should be limited; notify physician if unrelieved by laxative, rectal bleeding occurs, or signs of electrolyte imbalance develop (dizziness, weakness, muscle cramps); take with a full glass of water

Additional Information Long-term, chronic use should be avoided; patients should be encouraged to increase fluid intake, fiber intake, and exercise

Special Geriatric Considerations Elderly are often predisposed to constipation due to disease, immobility, drugs, and a decreased "thirst reflex" with age enhancing the possibility of dehydration. Avoid stimulant cathartic use on a chronic basis if possible. Use osmotic, lubricant, stool softeners, and bulk agents as prophylaxis. Patients should be instructed for proper dietary fiber and fluid intake as well as regular exercise. Monitor closely for fluid/electrolyte imbalance, CNS signs of fluid/electrolyte loss, and hypotension.

Dosage Forms Excipient information presented when available (limited, particularly for generics); consult specific product labeling.

Liquid:

Senexon: Sennosides 8.8 mg/5 mL (240 mL)

Liquid [concentrate]:

Fletcher's®: Senna concentrate 33.3 mg/mL (75 mL) [alcohol free; contains sodium benzoate; root beer flavor]

Syrup: Sennosides 8.8 mg/5 mL (240 mL)

Tablet: Sennosides 8.6 mg

ex-lax®: Sennosides USP 15 mg

ex-lax® Maximum Strength: Sennosides USP 25 mg

Perdiem® Overnight Relief: Sennosides USP 15 mg

Sennatural™, Senokot®, Senexon®, Senna-Gen®, Uni-Senna: Sennosides 8.6 mg

SenokotXTRA®: Sennosides 17 mg

Tablet, chewable:

Black-Draught™: Sennosides 10 mg

ex-lax®: Sennosides USP 15 mg [chocolate flavor]

Evac-U-Gen: Sennosides 10 mg

♦ **Senna and Docusate** *see Docusate and Senna on page 461*

♦ **Senna-Gen®** [OTC] *see Senna on page 1456*

♦ **Senna-S** *see Docusate and Senna on page 461*

♦ **Sennatural™** [OTC] *see Senna on page 1456*

♦ **Senokot®** [OTC] *see Senna on page 1456*

♦ **Senokot-S®** [OTC] *see Docusate and Senna on page 461*

♦ **SenokotXTRA®** [OTC] *see Senna on page 1456*

♦ **SenoSol™-SS** [OTC] *see Docusate and Senna on page 461*

♦ **Septra®** *see Sulfamethoxazole and Trimethoprim on page 1498*

♦ **Septra® DS** *see Sulfamethoxazole and Trimethoprim on page 1498*

♦ **Serax®** *see Oxazepam on page 1173*

♦ **Serevent® Diskus®** *see Salmeterol on page 1444*

♦ **Seromycin®** *see CycloSERINE on page 379*

♦ **Seroquel®** *see Quetiapine on page 1356*

♦ **Seroquel® XR** *see Quetiapine on page 1356*

Sertraline (SER tra leen)

Related Information
Antidepressant Agents *on page 1742*

Medication Safety Issues
Sound-alike/look-alike issues:
Sertraline may be confused with selegiline, Serentil®
Zoloft® may be confused with Zocor®

U.S. Brand Names Zoloft®

Canadian Brand Names Apo-Sertraline®; Gen-Sertraline; GMD-Sertraline; Novo-Sertraline; Nu-Sertraline; PMS-Sertraline; ratio-Sertraline; Rhoxal-sertraline; Sandoz-Sertraline; Zoloft®

Index Terms Sertraline Hydrochloride

Generic Available Yes

Pharmacologic Category Antidepressant, Selective Serotonin Reuptake Inhibitor

Use Treatment of major depression, obsessive-compulsive disorder (OCD), panic disorder, post-traumatic stress disorder (PTSD), social anxiety disorder

Unlabeled/Investigational Use Treatment of eating disorders, generalized anxiety disorder (GAD), impulse control disorders

Restrictions An FDA-approved medication guide concerning the use of antidepressants in children, adolescents, and young adults must be distributed when dispensing an outpatient prescription (new or refill) where this medication is to be used without direct supervision of a healthcare provider. Medication guides are available at http://www.fda.gov/cder/Offices/ODS/medication_guides.htm. Dispense to parents or guardians of children and adolescents receiving this medication.

Contraindications Hypersensitivity to sertraline or any component of the formulation; use of MAO inhibitors within 14 days; concurrent use of pimozide; concurrent use of sertraline oral concentrate with disulfiram

Warnings/Precautions [U.S. Boxed Warning]: Antidepressants increase the risk of suicidal thinking and behavior in children, adolescents, and young adults (18-24 years of age) with major depressive disorder (MDD) and other psychiatric disorders; consider risk prior to prescribing. Short-term studies did not show an
(Continued)

Sertraline *(Continued)*

increased risk in patients >24 years of age and showed a decreased risk in patients ≥65 years. Closely monitor patients for clinical worsening, suicidality, or unusual changes in behavior, particularly during the initial 1-2 months of therapy or during periods of dosage adjustments (increases or decreases); the patient's family or caregiver should be instructed to closely observe the patient and communicate condition with healthcare provider. A medication guide concerning the use of antidepressants should be dispensed with each prescription.

The possibility of a suicide attempt is inherent in major depression and may persist until remission occurs. Use caution in high-risk patients. Worsening depression and severe abrupt suicidality that are not part of the presenting symptoms may require discontinuation or modification of drug therapy. The patient's family or caregiver should be alerted to monitor patients for the emergence of suicidality and associated behaviors (such as agitation, irritability, hostility, impulsivity, and hypomania) and call healthcare provider.

May worsen psychosis in some patients or precipitate a shift to mania or hypomania in patients with bipolar disorder. Patients presenting with depressive symptoms should be screened for bipolar disorder. Monotherapy in patients with bipolar disorder should be avoided. **Sertraline is not FDA approved for the treatment of bipolar depression.**

The potential for severe reaction exists when used with MAO inhibitors, SSRIs/SNRIs or triptans; serotonin syndrome (hyperthermia, muscular rigidity, mental status changes/agitation, autonomic instability) may occur; concomitant use with MAO inhibitors is contraindicated. Has a very low potential to impair cognitive or motor performance. However, caution patients regarding activities requiring alertness until response to sertraline is known. Does not appear to potentiate the effects of alcohol, however, ethanol use is not advised.

Use caution in patients with a previous seizure disorder or condition predisposing to seizures such as brain damage, alcoholism, or concurrent therapy with other drugs which lower the seizure threshold. May increase the risks associated with electroconvulsive therapy. Use with caution in patients with hepatic or renal dysfunction and in elderly patients. May cause hyponatremia/SIADH. Use with caution in patients with renal insufficiency or other concurrent illness (due to limited experience). Sertraline acts as a mild uricosuric; use with caution in patients at risk of uric acid nephropathy. Use with caution in patients at risk of bleeding or receiving anticoagulant therapy; may cause impairment in platelet aggregation. Use with caution in patients where weight loss is undesirable. May cause or exacerbate sexual dysfunction.

Use oral concentrate formulation with caution in patients with latex sensitivity; dropper dispenser contains dry natural rubber. Discontinuation symptoms (eg, dysphoric mood, irritability, agitation, confusion, anxiety, insomnia, hypomania) may occur upon abrupt discontinuation. Taper dose when discontinuing therapy.

Adverse Reactions (Reflective of adult population; not specific for elderly)
>10%:
  Central nervous system: Dizziness, fatigue, headache, insomnia, somnolence
  Endocrine & metabolic: Libido decreased
  Gastrointestinal: Anorexia, diarrhea, nausea, xerostomia
  Genitourinary: Ejaculatory disturbances
  Neuromuscular & skeletal: Tremors
  Miscellaneous: Diaphoresis
1% to 10%:
  Cardiovascular: Chest pain, palpitation
  Central nervous system: Agitation, anxiety, hypoesthesia, malaise, nervousness, pain
  Dermatologic: Rash
  Endocrine & metabolic: Impotence
  Gastrointestinal: Appetite increased, constipation, dyspepsia, flatulence, vomiting, weight gain
  Neuromuscular & skeletal: Back pain, hypertonia, myalgia, paresthesia, weakness
  Ocular: Visual difficulty, abnormal vision
  Otic: Tinnitus
  Respiratory: Rhinitis
  Miscellaneous: Yawning

Additional adverse reactions reported in pediatric patients (frequency >2%): Aggressiveness, epistaxis, hyperkinesia, purpura, sinusitis, urinary incontinence

Overdosage/Toxicology Among 634 patients who overdosed on sertraline alone, 8 resulted in a fatal outcome. Symptoms include somnolence, vomiting, tachycardia, nausea, dizziness, agitation, and tremor. Treatment is symptomatic and supportive.

Drug Interactions Substrate of CYP2B6 (minor), 2C9 (minor), 2C19 (major), 2D6 (major), 3A4 (minor); **Inhibits** CYP1A2 (weak), 2B6 (moderate), 2C8 (weak), 2C9 (weak), 2C19 (moderate), 2D6 (moderate), 3A4 (moderate)

Amphetamines: SSRIs may increase the sensitivity to amphetamines, and amphetamines may increase the risk of serotonin syndrome

Benzodiazepines: Sertraline may inhibit the metabolism of alprazolam and diazepam resulting in elevated serum levels; monitor for increased sedation and psychomotor impairment

Buspirone: Sertraline inhibits the reuptake of serotonin; combined use with a serotonin agonist (buspirone) may cause serotonin syndrome

Carbamazepine: Sertraline may inhibit the metabolism of carbamazepine resulting in increased carbamazepine levels and toxicity; monitor for altered carbamazepine response

Cimetidine: Concurrent use resulted in an increase in sertraline's AUC, C_{max}, and half-life; monitor.

Clozapine: Sertraline may increase serum levels of clozapine; monitor for increased effect/toxicity

Cyclosporine: Sertraline may increase serum levels of cyclosporine (and possibly tacrolimus); monitor

CYP2B6 substrates: Sertraline may increase the levels/effects of CYP2B6 substrates. Example substrates include bupropion, promethazine, propofol, and selegiline.

CYP2C19 inducers: May decrease the levels/effects of sertraline. Example inducers include aminoglutethimide, carbamazepine, phenytoin, and rifampin.

CYP2C19 inhibitors: May increase the levels/effects of sertraline. Example inhibitors include delavirdine, fluconazole, fluvoxamine, gemfibrozil, isoniazid, omeprazole, and ticlopidine.

CYP2C19 substrates: Sertraline may increase the levels/effects of CYP2C19 substrates. Example substrates include citalopram, diazepam, methsuximide, phenytoin, and propranolol.

CYP2D6 inhibitors: May increase the levels/effects of sertraline. Example inhibitors include chlorpromazine, delavirdine, fluoxetine, miconazole, paroxetine, pergolide, quinidine, quinine, ritonavir, and ropinirole.

CYP2D6 substrates: Sertraline may increase the levels/effects of CYP2D6 substrates. Example substrates include amphetamines, selected beta-blockers, dextromethorphan, fluoxetine, lidocaine, mirtazapine, nefazodone, paroxetine, risperidone, ritonavir, thioridazine, tricyclic antidepressants, and venlafaxine.

CYP2D6 prodrug substrates: Sertraline may decrease the levels/effects of CYP2D6 prodrug substrates. Example prodrug substrates include codeine, hydrocodone, oxycodone, and tramadol.

CYP3A4 substrates: Sertraline may increase the levels/effects of CYP3A4 substrates. Example substrates include benzodiazepines, calcium channel blockers, cyclosporine, mirtazapine, nateglinide, nefazodone, sildenafil (and other PDE-5 inhibitors), tacrolimus, and venlafaxine. Selected benzodiazepines (midazolam and triazolam), cisapride, ergot alkaloids, selected HMG-CoA reductase inhibitors (lovastatin and simvastatin), and pimozide are generally contraindicated with strong CYP3A4 inhibitors.

Cyproheptadine: May inhibit the effects of serotonin reuptake inhibitors (fluoxetine); monitor for altered antidepressant response; cyproheptadine acts as a serotonin agonist

Dextromethorphan: Some SSRIs inhibit the metabolism of dextromethorphan; visual hallucinations occurred; monitor for serotonin syndrome

Erythromycin: Serotonin syndrome has been reported when added to sertraline; limited documentation

Haloperidol: Serum concentrations may be increased by sertraline (small increase); monitor

HMG-CoA reductase inhibitors: Sertraline may inhibit the metabolism of lovastatin and simvastatin (metabolized by CYP3A4) resulting in myositis and rhabdomyolysis; although its inhibition is weak, these combinations are best avoided

Lamotrigine: Toxicity has been reported following the addition of sertraline; monitor

Lithium: Patients receiving SSRIs and lithium have developed neurotoxicity; if combination is used, monitor for neurotoxicity

Loop diuretics: Sertraline may cause hyponatremia; additive hyponatremic effects may be seen with combined use of a loop diuretic (bumetanide, furosemide, torsemide); monitor for hyponatremia

MAO inhibitors: Sertraline should not be used with nonselective MAO inhibitors (isocarboxazid, phenelzine); fatal reactions have been reported; this combination is contraindicated.

Meperidine: Concurrent use may result in serotonin syndrome; these combinations are best avoided

Nefazodone: May increase the risk of serotonin syndrome

NSAIDs: Concomitant use of sertraline and NSAIDs, aspirin, or other drugs affecting coagulation has been associated with an increased risk of bleeding; monitor.

Phenothiazines: Sertraline may inhibit metabolism of thioridazine or mesoridazine, potentially leading to malignant ventricular arrhythmias. Avoid concurrent use. Wait at least 5 weeks after discontinuing sertraline prior to starting thioridazine.

(Continued)

Sertraline *(Continued)*

Phenytoin: Sertraline may inhibit the metabolism of phenytoin and may result in phenytoin toxicity. Studies have demonstrated minimal impact with concurrent dosing, however, monitoring of levels/effects is recommended.

Pimozide: Sertraline may increase serum levels of pimozide. Concurrent use is contraindicated.

Ritonavir: Combined use of sertraline with ritonavir may cause serotonin syndrome in HIV-positive patients; monitor

Selegiline: SSRIs have been reported to cause mania or hypertension when combined with selegiline; this combination is best avoided. Concurrent use with SSRIs has been reported to cause serotonin syndrome. As an MAO type B inhibitor, the risk of serotonin syndrome may be less than with nonselective MAO inhibitors.

Sibutramine: May increase the risk of serotonin syndrome with SSRIs; monitor.

Serotonin agonists (eg, triptans): Concurrent use of sertraline with these agents may increase the risk of serotonin syndrome; monitor.

Serotonergic reuptake inhibitors (eg, SSRIs/SNRIs): Concurrent use of sertraline with these agents may increase the risk of serotonin syndrome; monitor.

Sympathomimetics: May increase the risk of serotonin syndrome with SSRIs

Tolbutamide: Sertraline may decrease the metabolism of tolbutamide; monitor for changes in glucose control.

Tramadol: Sertraline combined with tramadol (serotonergic effects) may cause serotonin syndrome; monitor

Trazodone: Sertraline may inhibit the metabolism of trazodone resulting in increased toxicity; monitor

Tricyclic antidepressants: Sertraline may inhibit the metabolism of tricyclic antidepressants (amitriptyline, desipramine, imipramine, nortriptyline) resulting is elevated serum levels; if combination is warranted, a low dose of TCA (10-25 mg/day) should be utilized

Tryptophan: Sertraline may inhibit the reuptake of serotonin; combination with tryptophan, a serotonin precursor, may cause agitation and restlessness; this combination is best avoided

Venlafaxine: Sertraline may increase the risk of serotonin syndrome

Warfarin: Sertraline may alter the hypoprothrombinemic response to warfarin; monitor

Zolpidem: Onset of hypnosis may be shortened in patients receiving sertraline; monitor

Ethanol/Nutrition/Herb Interactions

Ethanol: Avoid ethanol (may increase CNS depression).

Food: Sertraline average peak serum levels may be increased if taken with food.

Herb/Nutraceutical: Avoid valerian, St John's wort, kava kava, gotu kola (may increase CNS depression).

Stability Tablets and oral solution should be stored at controlled room temperature of 15°C to 30°C (59°F to 86°F).

Mechanism of Action Antidepressant with selective inhibitory effects on presynaptic serotonin (5-HT) reuptake and only very weak effects on norepinephrine and dopamine neuronal uptake. *In vitro* studies demonstrate no significant affinity for adrenergic, cholinergic, GABA, dopaminergic, histaminergic, serotonergic, or benzodiazepine receptors.

Pharmacodynamics Maximum antidepressant effects usually seen after 4 weeks

Pharmacokinetics

Protein binding: 98%

Metabolism: Hepatic; extensive first-pass metabolism; principle metabolite, N-desmyethylsertraline, is 8 times less active as a serotonin reuptake inhibitor and 4 times less active in its inhibition of norepinephrine and dopamine, and is considered to have little or no clinical activity.

Half-life, elimination: 26 hours

Time to peak plasma concentration: 4.5-8.4 hours after single daily doses of 50-200 mg for 14 days; food appears to increase both the area under the curve and peak plasma concentrations, while decreasing time to peak plasma concentration

Elimination: Both sertraline and N-desmyethylsertraline are further metabolized to ketones and hydroxylates which are eliminated in the urine and feces

Sertraline's clearance has been found to be reduced by 40% in older adults

Dosage

Geriatrics: Oral: Initial: 25 mg/day in the morning; increase by 25 mg/day increments every 2-3 days if tolerated to 50-100 mg/day; additional increases may be necessary; maximum: 200 mg/day.

Adults:

Depression/OCD: Oral: Initial: 50 mg/day

Note: May increase daily dose, at intervals of not less than 1 week, to a maximum of 200 mg/day. If somnolence is noted, give at bedtime.

Panic disorder, PTSD, social anxiety disorder: Oral: Initial: 25 mg once daily; increased after 1 week to 50 mg once daily (see "Note" above)

Renal Impairment: Multiple-dose pharmacokinetics are unaffected by renal impairment.

Hemodialysis effect: Not removed by hemodialysis

Hepatic Impairment: Sertraline is extensively metabolized by the liver. Caution should be used in patients with hepatic impairment. A lower dose or less frequent dosing should be used.

Monitoring Parameters Monitor nutritional intake and weight; mental status for depression, suicidal ideation, anxiety, social functioning, mania, panic attacks; akathisia

Patient Information If currently on another antidepressant drug, patients should notify their physician. Although sertraline has not been shown to increase the effects of alcohol, it is recommended to refrain from drinking while on this medication. May experience some weight loss, but it is usually minimal. If on warfarin, digoxin, an oral hypoglycemic drug, or a drug having an effect on the central nervous system, such as a medication for insomnia or anxiety, patients should notify physician. There are no known interactions between sertraline and over-the-counter medications; however, these should be used with caution and the directions for their use should be followed carefully.

Special Geriatric Considerations Sertraline's favorable side effect profile makes it a useful alternative to the traditional tricyclic antidepressants; its potential stimulation effect and anorexia may be bothersome. Has the shortest half-life of the currently marketed serotonin-reuptake inhibitors. Data from a clinical trial comparing fluoxetine to tricyclics suggest that fluoxetine is significantly less effective than nortriptyline in hospitalized elderly patients with unipolar major affective disorder, especially those with melancholia and concurrent cardiovascular diseases.

Dosage Forms Excipient information presented when available (limited, particularly for generics); consult specific product labeling.

Solution, oral [concentrate]: 20 mg/mL (60 mL)

Zoloft®: 20 mg/mL (60 mL) [contains alcohol 12%; dropper contains dry natural rubber]

Tablet: 25 mg, 50 mg, 100 mg

Zoloft®: 25 mg, 50 mg, 100 mg

Selected References

Cohn CK, Shrivastava R, Mendels J, et al, "Double-Blind, Multicenter Comparison of Sertraline and Amitriptyline in Elderly Depressed Patients," *J Clin Psychiatry*, 1990, 51(Suppl B):28-33.

Grimsley SR and Jann MW, "Paroxetine, Sertraline, and Fluvoxamine: New Selective Serotonin Reuptake Inhibitors," *Clin Pharm*, 1992, 11(11):930-57.

Reimherr FW, Chouinard G, Cohn CK, et al, "Antidepressant Efficacy of Sertraline: A Double-Blind Placebo- and Amitriptyline-Controlled, Multicenter Comparison Study in Outpatients With Major Depression," *J Clin Psychiatry*, 1990, 51(Suppl B):18-27.

Roose SP, Glassman AH, Attia E, et al, "Comparative Efficacy of Selective Serotonin Reuptake Inhibitors and Tricyclics in the Treatment of Melancholia," *Am J Psychiatry*, 1994, 151(12):1735-9.

♦ **Sertraline Hydrochloride** *see* Sertraline *on page 1457*

♦ **Serutan® [OTC]** *see* Psyllium *on page 1347*

♦ **Serzone** *see* Nefazodone *on page 1097*

Sevelamer (se VEL a mer)

Medication Safety Issues

Sound-alike/look-alike issues:

Renagel® may be confused with Reglan®, Regonol®

International issues:

Renagel® may be confused with Remegel® which is a brand name for calcium carbonate in Ireland, Italy, and Great Britain

U.S. Brand Names Renagel®

Canadian Brand Names Renagel®

Index Terms Sevelamer Hydrochloride

Generic Available No

Pharmacologic Category Phosphate Binder

Use Reduction of serum phosphorous in patients with chronic kidney disease on hemodialysis

Contraindications Hypersensitivity to sevelamer or any component of the formulation; hypophosphatemia; bowel obstruction

Warnings/Precautions Use with caution in patients with gastrointestinal disorders including dysphagia, swallowing disorders, severe gastrointestinal motility disorders, or major gastrointestinal surgery. May cause reductions in vitamin D, E, K, and folic acid absorption. Long-term studies of carcinogenic potential have not been completed. Tablets should not be taken apart or chewed; broken or crushed tablets will rapidly expand in water/saliva and may be a choking hazard.

(Continued)

Sevelamer *(Continued)*

Adverse Reactions (Reflective of adult population; not specific for elderly)
>10%:
- Dermatologic: Rash (13%)
- Gastrointestinal: Vomiting (22%), nausea (7% to 20%), diarrhea (4% to 19%), dyspepsia (5% to 16%)
- Neuromuscular & skeletal: Limb pain (13%), arthralgia (12%)
- Respiratory: Nasopharyngitis (14%), bronchitis (11%)

1% to 10%:
- Cardiovascular: Hypertension (10%)
- Central nervous system: Headache (9%), pyrexia (5%)
- Gastrointestinal: Constipation (2% to 8%), flatulence (4%)
- Neuromuscular & skeletal: Back pain (4%)
- Respiratory: Dyspnea (10%), cough (7%), upper respiratory tract infection (5%)

Postmarketing and/or case reports: Abdominal pain

Overdosage/Toxicology
Sevelamer is not absorbed systemically. Doses up to 14 g/day for 8 days have been administered without adverse effects. There are no reports of overdosage in patients.

Drug Interactions
Ciprofloxacin: Sevelamer may decrease the bioavailability of ciprofloxacin by 50%.

Sevelamer: May bind to some drugs in the gastrointestinal tract and decrease their absorption. When changes in absorption of oral medications may have significant clinical consequences (such as antiarrhythmic and antiseizure medications), these medications should be taken at least 1 hour before or 3 hours after a dose of sevelamer.

Stability
Store at controlled room temperature of 15°C to 30°C (59°F to 86°F).

Mechanism of Action
Sevelamer (a polymeric compound) binds phosphate within the intestinal lumen, limiting absorption and decreasing serum phosphate concentrations without altering calcium, aluminum, or bicarbonate concentrations

Pharmacokinetics
Absorption: Not absorbed systemically
Elimination: Feces

Dosage
Geriatrics & Adults: Reduction of serum phosphorous: Oral:
Patients not taking a phosphate binder: 800-1600 mg 3 times/day with meals; the initial dose may be based on serum phosphorous levels:
>5.5 mg/dL to <7.5 mg/dL: 800 mg 3 times/day
≥7.5 mg/dL to <9.0 mg/dL: 1200-1600 mg 3 times/day
≥9.0 mg/dL: 1600 mg 3 times/day

Maintenance dose adjustment based on serum phosphorous concentration (goal of lowering to <5.5 mg/dL; maximum daily dose studied was equivalent to 13 g/day):
>5.5 mg/dL: Increase by 1 tablet per meal every 2 weeks
3.5-5.5 mg/dL: Maintain current dose
<3.5 mg/dL: Decrease by 1 tablet per meal

Dosage adjustment when switching between phosphate binder products: 667 mg of calcium acetate is equivalent to 800 mg sevelamer

Administration
Must be administered with meals

Monitoring Parameters
Serum phosphorus, calcium, bicarbonate, chloride

Patient Information
Take as directed, with meals. Do not break or chew capsules or tablets (contents will expand in water). You may experience headache or dizziness; upset stomach, nausea, or vomiting (frequent small meals, frequent mouth care, or sucking hard candy may help); diarrhea; hypotension (use caution when rising from sitting or lying position or when climbing stairs or bending over). Report persistent adverse reactions.

Additional Information
Switching patients from calcium acetate to sevelamer: 667 mg of calcium acetate is equivalent to 800 mg sevelamer

Special Geriatric Considerations
No specific dose changes needed for the elderly. Since electrolyte changes (ie, phosphorus, calcium) can have dramatic effects in the elderly, monitor closely.

Dosage Forms
Excipient information presented when available (limited, particularly for generics); consult specific product labeling.
Tablet, as hydrochloride: 400 mg, 800 mg

♦ **Sildec [DSC]** *see* Carbinoxamine and Pseudoephedrine *on page 239*

Sildenafil (sil DEN a fil)

Medication Safety Issues
Sound-alike/look-alike issues:
Viagra® may be confused with Allegra®, Vaniqa™
U.S. Brand Names GD-Sildenafil; Revatio™; Viagra®
Canadian Brand Names Viagra®
Index Terms UK92480
Generic Available No
Pharmacologic Category Phosphodiesterase-5 Enzyme Inhibitor
Use Treatment of erectile dysfunction; treatment of pulmonary arterial hypertension
Unlabeled/Investigational Use Psychotropic-induced sexual dysfunction; pulmonary arterial hypertension in children
Contraindications Hypersensitivity to sildenafil or any component of the formulation; concurrent use of organic nitrates (nitroglycerin) in any form (potentiates the hypotensive effects)
Warnings/Precautions Decreases in blood pressure may occur due to vasodilator effects; use caution in patients with resting hypotension (BP <90/50), hypertension (BP >170/110), fluid depletion, severe left ventricular outflow obstruction, or autonomic dysfunction, and patients receiving alpha-blockers or other antihypertensive medication. Not recommended for use with pulmonary veno-occlusive disease.

Use caution in patients with cardiovascular disease, including cardiac failure, unstable angina, or a recent history (within the last 6 months) of myocardial infarction, stroke, or life-threatening arrhythmia. Use caution in patients receiving concurrent bosentan. Use caution in patients with bleeding disorders or with active peptic ulcer disease; safety and efficacy have not been established.

There is a degree of cardiac risk associated with sexual activity; therefore, physicians may wish to consider the cardiovascular status of their patients prior to initiating any treatment for erectile dysfunction. Sildenafil should be used with caution in patients with anatomical deformation of the penis (angulation, cavernosal fibrosis, or Peyronie's disease), or in patients who have conditions which may predispose them to priapism (sickle cell anemia, multiple myeloma, leukemia).

Rare cases of nonarteritic ischemic optic neuropathy (NAION) have been reported; risk may be increased with history of vision loss. Other risk factors for NAION include low cup-to-disc ratio ("crowded disc"), coronary artery disease, diabetes, hypertension, hyperlipidemia, smoking, and age >50 years.

The safety and efficacy of sildenafil with other treatments for erectile dysfunction have not been established; use is not recommended. May cause dose-related impairment of color discrimination. Use caution in patients with retinitis pigmentosa; a minority have genetic disorders of retinal phosphodiesterases (no safety information available). Use with caution in patients taking strong CYP3A4 inhibitors. All patients should be instructed to seek medical attention if erection persists >4 hours.
Adverse Reactions (Reflective of adult population; not specific for elderly) Based upon normal doses. (Adverse effects such as flushing, diarrhea, myalgia, and visual disturbances may be increased with doses >100 mg/24 hours.)
>10%:
Central nervous system: Headache (16% to 46%)
Gastrointestinal: Dyspepsia (7% to 17%)
1% to 10%:
Cardiovascular: Flushing (10%)
Central nervous system: Dizziness, insomnia, pyrexia
Dermatologic: Erythema, rash
Gastrointestinal: Diarrhea (3% to 9%), gastritis
Genitourinary: Urinary tract infection
Hematologic: Anemia, leukopenia
Hepatic: LFTs increased
Neuromuscular & skeletal: Myalgia, paresthesia
Ocular: Abnormal vision (color changes, blurred or increased sensitivity to light 3%; up to 11% with doses >100 mg)
Respiratory: Dyspnea exacerbated, epistaxis, nasal congestion, rhinitis, sinusitis
Overdosage/Toxicology In studies of healthy volunteers with single doses up to 800 mg, adverse events were similar to those seen at lower doses, but incidence rates were increased. Dialysis not likely to be beneficial due to protein binding.
Drug Interactions Substrate of CYP2C9 (minor), 3A4 (major); **Inhibits** CYP1A2 (weak), 2C9 (weak), 2C19 (weak), 2D6 (weak), 2E1 (weak), 3A4 (weak)
Azole antifungals: May increase the serum concentrations of sildenafil; reduce starting dose to 25 mg.
(Continued)

Sildenafil *(Continued)*

Alpha-blockers (doxazosin): Concomitant use may lead to symptomatic hypotension in some patients. Patient should be stable on an alpha-blocker prior to initiation of PDE-5 inhibitor. Sildenafil should be started at 25 mg. If patient is taking an optimal dose of PDE-5 inhibitor, alpha-blocker should be initiated at lowest dose.

Bosentan: May decrease serum concentration and effect of sildenafil.

CYP3A4 inhibitors: May increase the levels/effects of sildenafil. Example inhibitors include azole antifungals, clarithromycin, diclofenac, doxycycline, erythromycin, imatinib, isoniazid, nefazodone, nicardipine, propofol, protease inhibitors, quinidine, telithromycin, and verapamil.

Macrolide antibiotics: May increase serum concentrations of sildenafil; reduce starting dose of Viagra® to 25 mg if used with clarithromycin, erythromycin, telithromycin, or troleandomycin. No adjustments with Revatio™ are required.

Nitroglycerin (other nitrates): Concurrent use with sildenafil is contraindicated due to the potential for severe, potentially fatal, hypotensive responses.

Protease inhibitors: May increase the serum concentrations of sildenafil; reduce dose of Viagra® to 25 mg/24 hours; use of Revatio™ is not recommended.

Ethanol/Nutrition/Herb Interactions

Food: Amount and rate of absorption of sildenafil is reduced when taken with a high-fat meal. Serum concentrations/toxicity may be increased with grapefruit juice; avoid concurrent use.

Herb/Nutraceutical: St John's wort may decrease sildenafil levels.

Stability Store tablets at controlled room temperature of 15°C to 30°C (59°F to 86°F).

Mechanism of Action

Erectile dysfunction: Does not directly cause penile erections, but affects the response to sexual stimulation. The physiologic mechanism of erection of the penis involves release of nitric oxide (NO) in the corpus cavernosum during sexual stimulation. NO then activates the enzyme guanylate cyclase, which results in increased levels of cyclic guanosine monophosphate (cGMP), producing smooth muscle relaxation and inflow of blood to the corpus cavernosum. Sildenafil enhances the effect of NO by inhibiting phosphodiesterase type 5 (PDE-5), which is responsible for degradation of cGMP in the corpus cavernosum; when sexual stimulation causes local release of NO, inhibition of PDE-5 by sildenafil causes increased levels of cGMP in the corpus cavernosum, resulting in smooth muscle relaxation and inflow of blood to the corpus cavernosum; at recommended doses, it has no effect in the absence of sexual stimulation.

Pulmonary arterial hypertension (PAH): Inhibits phosphodiesterase type 5 (PDE-5) in smooth muscle of pulmonary vasculature where PDE-5 is responsible for the degradation of cyclic guanosine monophosphate (cGMP). Increased cGMP concentration results in pulmonary vasculature relaxation; vasodilation in the pulmonary bed and the systemic circulation (to a lesser degree) may occur.

Pharmacokinetics

Absorption: Rapid; slower with a high-fat meal

Distribution: V_{dss}: 105 L

Bioavailability: 40%

Protein binding: 96%

Half-life: 4 hours

Time to peak: 30-120 minutes; delayed by 60 minutes with a high-fat meal

Metabolism: Hepatic

Elimination: Feces (80%), urine (13%)

Dosage

Geriatrics: Initial: 25 mg, 1 hour before sexual activity. Age >65 years was associated with increased serum sildenafil concentrations which may increase side effects and efficacy.

Adults:

Erectile dysfunction (Viagra®): Oral: For most patients, the recommended dose is 25-50 mg taken as needed, approximately 1 hour before sexual activity. However, sildenafil may be taken anywhere from 30 minutes to 4 hours before sexual activity. Based on effectiveness and tolerance, the dose may be increased to a maximum recommended dose of 100 mg or decreased to 25 mg. The maximum recommended dosing frequency is once daily.

Pulmonary arterial hypertension (Revatio™): Oral: 20 mg 3 times/day, taken 4-6 hours apart

Dosage adjustment for patients >65 years of age: Hepatic impairment (cirrhosis), severe renal impairment (creatinine clearance <30 mL/minute): Higher plasma levels have been associated which may result in increase in efficacy and adverse effects; Viagra®: Starting dose of 25 mg should be considered

Dosage considerations for patients stable on alpha-blockers: Viagra®: Initial: 25 mg

Dosage adjustment for concomitant use of potent CYP34A inhibitors:
Revatio™:
Erythromycin, saquinavir: No dosage adjustment
Itraconazole, ketoconazole, ritonavir: Not recommended
Viagra®:
Erythromycin, itraconazole, ketoconazole, saquinavir: Starting dose of 25 mg should be considered
Ritonavir: Maximum: 25 mg every 48 hours

Renal Impairment: Cl_{cr} <30 mL/minute: Initial: 25 mg, 1 hour before sexual activity.

Hepatic Impairment: Hepatic impairment; cirrhosis: Initial: 25 mg, 1 hour before sexual activity.

Administration
Revatio™: Administer tablets at least 4-6 hours apart
Viagra®: Administer orally ~1 hour before sexual activity (may be used anytime from 4 hours to 30 minutes before).

Monitoring Parameters Monitor for response and adverse reactions.

Patient Information Discuss with your physician the contraindication of sildenafil citrate with concurrent organic nitrates. The use of sildenafil offers no protection against sexually transmitted diseases. Counseling of patients about the protective measures necessary to guard against transmitted diseases, including the human immunodeficiency virus (HIV), may be considered. Patients who experience adverse effects (eg, cardiac) should report these to their physician and refrain from sexual activity. Patients should not take more than one dose per day. Sildenafil has no effect without sexual stimulation.

Special Geriatric Considerations
Since the elderly often have concomitant diseases, many of which may contraindicate the use of sildenafil, a thorough knowledge of diseases and medications used must be assessed. Adjust dose for renal/hepatic function.

Dosage Forms Excipient information presented when available (limited, particularly for generics); consult specific product labeling.
Tablet:
Revatio™: 20 mg
Viagra®: 25 mg, 50 mg, 100 mg

Extemporaneously Prepared A stable suspension of sildenafil citrate (2.5 mg/mL) may be prepared as follows: Triturate thirty (30) sildenafil 25 mg tablets (Viagara®) to a fine powder in a mortar and pestle. Create a uniform paste by stirring in a small volume of suspending agent (1:1 mixture of methylcellulose 1% and simple syrup NF or a 1:1 mixture of Ora-Sweet® and Ora-Plus®). Continue adding vehicle to the paste in a geometric manner, with mixing, until near the desired volume. Transfer suspension to a graduated cylinder and QS to 300 mL with vehicle. Final suspension should be transferred to amber plastic bottles, labeled with "shake well" and dated for 90-day expiration at room temperature (25°C) or under refrigeration (4°C).

Nahata MC, Morosco RS, and Brady MT, "Extemporaneous Sildenafil Citrate Oral Suspensions for the Treatment of Pulmonary Hypertension in Children," *Am J Health-Syst Pharm*, 2006, 63:254-7.

Selected References
Cheitlin MD, Hutter AM Jr, Brindis RG, et al, "Use of Sildenafil (Viagra®) in Patients With Cardiovascular Disease," *J Am Coll Cardiol*, 1999, 33:273-82.

"Erythromycin (E-Mycin®) and Sildenafil (Viagra®)," in *Hansten and Horn's Drug Interactions Analysis and Management*, Seattle, WA: Applied Therapeutics, Inc, 1998, 2:3N109.

Galie N, Ghofrani HA, Torbicki A, et al, "Sildenafil Citrate Therapy for Pulmonary Arterial Hypertension," *N Engl J Med*, 2005, 353(20):2148-57.

Geelen P, Drolet B, Rail J, et al, "Sildenafil (Viagra) Prolongs Cardiac Repolarization by Blocking the Rapid Component of the Delayed Rectifier Potassium Current," *Circulation*, 2000, 102(3):275-7.

Goldstein I, Lue TF, Padma-Nathan H, et al, "Oral Sildenafil in the Treatment of Erectile Dysfunction. Sildenafil Study Group," *N Engl J Med*, 1998, 338(20):1397-404.

Humpl T, Reyes JT, Holtby H, et al, "Beneficial Effect of Oral Sildenafil Therapy in Childhood Pulmonary Arterial Hypertension: Twelve-Month Clinical Trial of a Single-Drug, Open-Label, Pilot Study," *Circulation*, 2005, 111(24):3274-80.

Ishikura F, Beppu S, Hamada T, et al, "Effects of Sildenafil Citrate (Viagra) Combined With Nitrate on the Heart," *Circulation*, 2000, 102(20):2516-21.

Phillips BG, Kato M, Pesek CA, et al, "Sympathetic Activation by Sildenafil," *Circulation*, 2000, 102(25):3068-73.

Rendell MS, Rajfer J, Wicker PA, et al, "Sildenafil for Treatment of Erectile Dysfunction in Men With Diabetes: A Randomized Controlled Trial. Sildenafil Diabetes Study Group," *JAMA*, 1999, 281(5):421-6.

Traverse JH, Chen YJ, Du R, et al, "Cyclic Nucleotide Phosphodiesterase Type 5 Activity Limits Blood Flow to Hypoperfused Myocardium During Exercise," *Circulation*, 2000, 102(24):2997-3002.

- **Silexin [OTC]** *see* Guaifenesin and Dextromethorphan *on page 730*
- **Silfedrine Children's [OTC]** *see* Pseudoephedrine *on page 1346*
- **Silphen® [OTC]** *see* DiphenhydrAMINE *on page 447*
- **Silphen DM® [OTC]** *see* Dextromethorphan *on page 419*
- **Siltussin DAS [OTC]** *see* Guaifenesin *on page 727*
- **Siltussin DM [OTC]** *see* Guaifenesin and Dextromethorphan *on page 730*

♦ **Siltussin DM DAS [OTC]** *see* Guaifenesin and Dextromethorphan *on page 730*

♦ **Siltussin SA [OTC]** *see* Guaifenesin *on page 727*

♦ **Silvadene®** *see* Silver Sulfadiazine *on page 1466*

Silver Sulfadiazine (SIL ver sul fa DYE a zeen)

U.S. Brand Names Silvadene®; SSD®; SSD® AF; Thermazene®

Canadian Brand Names Flamazine®

Generic Available Yes

Pharmacologic Category Antibiotic, Topical

Use Adjunct in the prevention and treatment of infection in second and third degree burns

Contraindications Hypersensitivity to silver sulfadiazine or any component of the formulation

Warnings/Precautions Use with caution in patients with G6PD deficiency, renal impairment, or history of allergy to other sulfonamides; sulfadiazine may accumulate in patients with impaired hepatic or renal function. Prolonged use may result in fungal or bacterial superinfection, including *C. difficile*-associated diarrhea and pseudomembranous colitis. Use of analgesic might be needed before application; systemic absorption is significant and adverse reactions may occur.

Adverse Reactions (Reflective of adult population; not specific for elderly) Frequency not defined.

Dermatologic: Itching, rash, erythema multiforme, discoloration of skin, photosensitivity

Hematologic: Hemolytic anemia, leukopenia, agranulocytosis, aplastic anemia

Hepatic: Hepatitis

Renal: Interstitial nephritis

Miscellaneous: Allergic reactions may be related to sulfa component

Drug Interactions Decreased effect: Topical proteolytic enzymes are inactivated

Stability Silvadene® cream will occasionally darken either in the jar or after application to the skin. This color change results from a light catalyzed reaction which is a common characteristic of all silver salts. A similar analogy is the oxidation of silverware. The product of this color change reaction is silver oxide which ranges in color from gray to black. Silver oxide has rarely been associated with permanent skin discoloration. Additionally, the antimicrobial activity of the product is not substantially diminished because the color change reaction involves such a small amount of the active drug and is largely a surface phenomenon.

Mechanism of Action Acts upon the bacterial cell wall and cell membrane. Bactericidal for many gram-negative and gram-positive bacteria and is effective against yeast. Active against *Pseudomonas aeruginosa, Pseudomonas maltophilia, Enterobacter* species, *Klebsiella* species, *Serratia* species, *Escherichia coli, Proteus mirabilis, Morganella morganii, Providencia rettgeri, Proteus vulgaris, Providencia* species, *Citrobacter* species, *Acinetobacter calcoaceticus, Staphylococcus aureus, Staphylococcus epidermidis, Enterococcus* species, *Candida albicans, Corynebacterium diphtheriae,* and *Clostridium perfringens*

Pharmacokinetics

Absorption: Significant percutaneous absorption of sulfadiazine can occur especially when applied to extensive burns

Half-life: 10 hours, prolonged in patients with renal insufficiency

Time to peak serum concentration: Within 3-11 days of continuous therapy

Elimination: ~50% excreted unchanged in urine

Dosage

Geriatrics & Adults: Antiseptic, burns: Topical: Apply once or twice daily

Administration See Patient Information.

Patient Information Bathe daily to aid in debridement (if not contraindicated); apply liberally to burned areas; for external use only; notify physician if condition persists or worsens

Additional Information Contains methylparaben and propylene glycol; use of analgesic might be needed before application

Special Geriatric Considerations No specific recommendations for use in the elderly.

Dosage Forms Excipient information presented when available (limited, particularly for generics); consult specific product labeling.

Cream, topical: 1% (25 g, 50 g, 85 g, 400 g)

Silvadene®, Thermazene®: 1% (20 g, 50 g, 85 g, 400 g, 1000 g)

SSD®: 1% (25 g, 50 g, 85 g, 400 g)

SSD® AF: 1% (50 g, 400 g)

Simethicone (sye METH i kone)

Medication Safety Issues
Sound-alike/look-alike issues:
Simethicone may be confused with cimetidine
Mylanta® may be confused with Mynatal®
Mylicon® may be confused with Modicon®, Myleran®
Phazyme® may be confused with Pherazine®

U.S. Brand Names Equalizer Gas Relief [OTC]; GasAid [OTC]; Gas-X® [OTC]; Gas-X® Extra Strength [OTC]; Gas-X® Maximum Strength [OTC]; Genasyme® [OTC]; Infantaire Gas Drops [OTC]; Mylanta® Gas [OTC]; Mylanta® Gas Maximum Strength [OTC]; Mylicon® Infants [OTC]; Phazyme® Quick Dissolve [OTC]; Phazyme® Ultra Strength [OTC]

Canadian Brand Names Ovol®; Phazyme™

Index Terms Activated Dimethicone; Activated Methylpolysiloxane

Generic Available Yes

Pharmacologic Category Antiflatulent

Use Relief of flatulence, functional gastric bloating, postoperative gas pains, painful distention due to air swallowing; treatment of peptic ulcer, diverticulitis, irritable (spastic) colon, functional dyspepsia

Contraindications Hypersensitivity to simethicone or any component of the formulation

Adverse Reactions (Reflective of adult population; not specific for elderly)
No data reported

Drug Interactions No data reported

Ethanol/Nutrition/Herb Interactions Food: Avoid carbonated beverages and gas-forming foods.

Stability Protect from light.

Mechanism of Action Decreases the surface tension of gas bubbles thereby disperses and prevents gas pockets in the GI system

Pharmacokinetics Elimination: In feces

Dosage
Geriatrics & Adults: Flatulence/bloating: Oral: 40-120 mg after meals and at bedtime as needed, not to exceed 500 mg/day

Administration Shake oral suspension (drops) before using; mix with water or other liquids.

Monitoring Parameters Monitor for feelings of relief, decreased pain, bloating

Patient Information Chew tablets thoroughly before swallowing; shake drops well before using

Additional Information Drops have small amount of saccharin calcium and sodium benzoate

Special Geriatric Considerations Before treating excess gas or pain due to gas accumulation, a thorough evaluation must be made to determine cause since many bowel diseases may present with flatulence and bloating.

Dosage Forms Excipient information presented when available (limited, particularly for generics); consult specific product labeling.
Softgels: 125 mg
GasAid, Gas-X® Extra Strength, Mylanta® Gas Maximum Strength: 125 mg
Gas-X® Maximum Strength: 166 mg
Phazyme® Ultra Strength: 180 mg
Suspension, oral drops: 40 mg/0.6 mL (30 mL)
Equalizer Gas Relief, Genasyme®, Infantaire Gas: 40 mg/0.6 mL (30 mL)
Mylicon® Infants: 40 mg/0.6 mL (15 mL, 30 mL) [alcohol free; contains sodium benzoate; available in a nonstaining formula]
Tablet, chewable: 80 mg, 125 mg
Gas-X®: 80 mg [sodium free; peppermint crème or cherry crème flavor]
Gas-X® Extra Strength: 125 mg [peppermint crème or cherry crème flavor]
Genasyme®: 80 mg
Mylanta® Gas: 80 mg [mint flavor]
Mylanta® Gas Maximum Strength: 125 mg [cherry and mint flavors]
Phazyme® Quick Dissolve: 125 mg [contains phenylalanine 0.4 mg per tablet; mint flavor]

♦ **Simethicone, Aluminum Hydroxide, and Magnesium Hydroxide** see Aluminum Hydroxide, Magnesium Hydroxide, and Simethicone on page 66
♦ **Simethicone and Loperamide Hydrochloride** see Loperamide and Simethicone on page 926
♦ **Simethicone and Magaldrate** see Magaldrate and Simethicone on page 943
♦ **Simply Cough® [OTC] [DSC]** see Dextromethorphan on page 419
♦ **Simply Saline® [OTC]** see Sodium Chloride on page 1475

♦ **Simply Saline® Baby [OTC]** see Sodium Chloride on page 1475
♦ **Simply Saline® Nasal Moist® [OTC]** see Sodium Chloride on page 1475
♦ **Simply Sleep® [OTC]** see DiphenhydrAMINE on page 447
♦ **Simply Stuffy™ [OTC] [DSC]** see Pseudoephedrine on page 1346
♦ **Simuc-DM** see Guaifenesin and Dextromethorphan on page 730

Simvastatin (sim va STAT in)

Related Information
Hyperlipidemia Management on page 1773

Medication Safety Issues
Sound-alike/look-alike issues:
Zocor® may be confused with Cozaar®, Yocon®, Zoloft®

International issues:
Cardin® [Poland] may be confused with Cardene® which is a brand name for nicardipine in the U.S.
Cardin® [Poland] may be confused with Cardem® which is a brand name for celiprolol in Spain

U.S. Brand Names Zocor®

Canadian Brand Names Apo-Simvastatin®; BCI-Simvastatin; CO Simvastatin; Gen-Simvastatin; Novo-Simvastatin; PMS-Simvastatin; ratio-Simvastatin; Riva-Simvastatin; Sandoz-Simvastatin; Taro-Simvastatin; Zocor®

Generic Available Yes

Pharmacologic Category Antilipemic Agent, HMG-CoA Reductase Inhibitor

Use Used with dietary therapy for the following:
Secondary prevention of cardiovascular events in hypercholesterolemic patients with established coronary heart disease (CHD) or at high risk for CHD: To reduce cardiovascular morbidity (myocardial infarction, coronary revascularization procedures) and mortality; to reduce the risk of stroke and transient ischemic attacks
Hyperlipidemias: To reduce elevations in total cholesterol, LDL-C, apolipoprotein B, and triglycerides in patients with primary hypercholesterolemia (elevations of 1 or more components are present in Fredrickson type IIa, IIb, III, and IV hyperlipidemias); treatment of homozygous familial hypercholesterolemia

Contraindications Hypersensitivity to simvastatin or any component of the formulation; acute liver disease; unexplained persistent elevations of serum transaminases

Warnings/Precautions Secondary causes of hyperlipidemia should be ruled out prior to therapy. Liver function must be monitored by laboratory assessment. Rhabdomyolysis with acute renal failure has occurred. Risk is dose-related and is increased with concurrent use of lipid-lowering agents which may cause rhabdomyolysis (gemfibrozil, fibric acid derivatives, or niacin at doses ≥1 g/day), during concurrent use with danazol or strong CYP3A4 inhibitors (including amiodarone, clarithromycin, cyclosporine, erythromycin, telithromycin, itraconazole, ketoconazole, nefazodone, grapefruit juice in large quantities, verapamil, or protease inhibitors such as indinavir, nelfinavir, or ritonavir). Monitor closely if used with other drugs associated with myopathy (eg, colchicine). Weigh the risk versus benefit when combining any of these drugs with simvastatin. Do not initiate simvastatin-containing treatment in a patient with pre-existing therapy of cyclosporine or danazol, unless the patient has previously demonstrated tolerance to ≥5 mg/day simvastatin. Temporarily discontinue in any patient experiencing an acute or serious major medical or surgical condition which may increase the risk of rhabdomyolysis. Discontinue temporarily for elective surgical procedures. Use caution in patients with renal insufficiency. Use with caution in patients with advanced age, these patients are predisposed to myopathy. Use with caution in patients who consume large amounts of ethanol or have a history of liver disease.

Adverse Reactions (Reflective of adult population; not specific for elderly)
1% to 10%:
Gastrointestinal: Constipation (2%), dyspepsia (1%), flatulence (2%)
Neuromuscular & skeletal: CPK elevation (>3x normal on one or more occasions - 5%)
Respiratory: Upper respiratory infection (2%)

Additional class-related events or case reports (not necessarily reported with simvastatin therapy): Alopecia, alteration in taste, anaphylaxis, angioedema, anorexia, anxiety, arthritis, cataracts, chills, cholestatic jaundice, cirrhosis, decreased libido, depression, dermatomyositis, dryness of skin/mucous membranes, dyspnea, elevated transaminases, eosinophilia, erectile dysfunction/impotence, erythema multiforme, facial paresis, fatty liver, fever, flushing, fulminant hepatic necrosis, gynecomastia, hemolytic anemia, hepatitis, hepatoma, hyperbilirubinemia, hypersensitivity reaction, impaired extraocular muscle movement, increased alkaline phosphatase, increased CPK (>10x normal), increased ESR, increased GGT, leukopenia, malaise, memory loss, myopathy, nail changes, nodules, ophthalmoplegia, pancreatitis, paresthesia, peripheral nerve palsy, peripheral neuropathy, photosensitivity, polymyalgia rheumatica, positive ANA, pruritus, psychic disturbance, purpura, rash, renal failure (secondary to rhabdomyolysis), rhabdomyolysis, skin discoloration, Stevens-Johnson syndrome, systemic lupus erythematosus-like syndrome, thrombocytopenia, thyroid dysfunction, toxic epidermal necrolysis, tremor, urticaria, vasculitis, vertigo, vomiting

Overdosage/Toxicology Very few adverse events. Treatment is symptomatic.

Drug Interactions Substrate of CYP3A4 (major); **Inhibits** CYP2C8 (weak), 2C9 (weak), 2D6 (weak)

Amiodarone may increase the risk of myopathy and rhabdomyolysis; dose of simvastatin should not exceed 20 mg/day.

Antacids: Plasma concentrations may be decreased when given with magnesium-aluminum hydroxide containing antacids (reported with atorvastatin and pravastatin). Clinical efficacy is not altered, no dosage adjustment is necessary

Cholestyramine reduces absorption of several HMG-CoA reductase inhibitors. Separate administration times by at least 4 hours.

Cholestyramine and colestipol (bile acid sequestrants): Cholesterol-lowering effects are additive.

Clofibrate and fenofibrate may increase the risk of myopathy and rhabdomyolysis; dose of simvastatin should not exceed 10 mg/day

Colchicine: Concomitant therapy with an HMG-CoA reductase inhibitor may increase risk of myopathy/rhabdomyolysis; use caution.

Cyclosporine: Concurrent use may increase the risk of myopathy and rhabdomyolysis; dose of simvastatin should not exceed 10 mg/day

CYP3A4 inhibitors: May increase the levels/effects of simvastatin. Example inhibitors include azole antifungals, clarithromycin, diclofenac, doxycycline, erythromycin, imatinib, isoniazid, nefazodone, nicardipine, propofol, protease inhibitors, quinidine, telithromycin, and verapamil.

Danazol: May increase risk of myopathy and rhabdomyolysis; dose of simvastatin should not exceed 10 mg/day.

Diltiazem: May increase levels/effects of simvastatin.

Gemfibrozil: Increased risk of myopathy and rhabdomyolysis; dose of simvastatin should not exceed 10 mg/day.

Grapefruit juice may inhibit metabolism of simvastatin via CYP3A4; avoid high dietary intakes of grapefruit juice.

Niacin (≥1 g/day): Concurrent use may increase the risk of myopathy and rhabdomyolysis; dose of simvastatin should not exceed 10 mg/day.

Verapamil may increase the risk of myopathy and rhabdomyolysis; dose of simvastatin should not exceed 20 mg/day.

Warfarin effects (hypoprothrombinemic response) may be increased; monitor INR closely when simvastatin is initiated or discontinued.

Ethanol/Nutrition/Herb Interactions

Ethanol: Avoid excessive ethanol consumption (due to potential hepatic effects).

Food: Simvastatin serum concentration may be increased when taken with grapefruit juice; avoid concurrent intake of large quantities (>1 quart/day). Red yeast rice contains an estimated 2.4 mg lovastatin per 600 mg rice.

Herb/Nutraceutical: St John's wort may decrease simvastatin levels.

Stability Tablets should be stored in tightly-closed containers at temperatures between 5°C to 30°C (41°F to 86°F).

Mechanism of Action Simvastatin is a methylated derivative of lovastatin that acts by competitively inhibiting 3-hydroxy-3-methylglutaryl-coenzyme A (HMG-CoA) reductase, the enzyme that catalyzes the rate-limiting step in cholesterol biosynthesis

Pharmacodynamics

Onset of action: >3 days

Peak effect: 2 weeks

Pharmacokinetics

Absorption: 85%

Protein binding: ~95%

Metabolism: Hepatic; extensive first-pass effect

Bioavailability: <5%

Half-life: Unknown

Time to peak: 1.3-2.4 hours

Elimination: Feces (60%); urine (13%)

Dosage

Geriatrics: Oral: Initial: Maximum reductions in LDL-cholesterol may be achieved with daily dose ≤20 mg.

Adults: Note: Doses should be individualized according to the baseline LDL-cholesterol levels, the recommended goal of therapy, and the patient's response; adjustments should be made at intervals of 4 weeks or more; doses may need adjusted based on concomitant medications

Homozygous familial hypercholesterolemia: Oral: 40 mg once daily in the evening **or** 80 mg/day (given as 20 mg, 20 mg, and 40 mg evening dose)

(Continued)

Simvastatin *(Continued)*

Prevention of cardiovascular events, hyperlipidemias: Oral: 20-40 mg once daily in the evening; range: 5-80 mg/day

Patients requiring only moderate reduction of LDL-cholesterol: May be started at 10 mg once daily

Patients requiring reduction of >45% in low-density lipoprotein (LDL) cholesterol: May be started at 40 mg once daily in the evening

Patients with CHD or at high risk for CHD: Dosing should be started at 40 mg once daily in the evening; simvastatin may be started simultaneously with diet

Dosage adjustment for simvastatin with concomitant medications:

Cyclosporine or danazol: Patient must first demonstrate tolerance to simvastatin ≥5 mg once daily; Initial: 5 mg, should **not** exceed 10 mg/day

Fibrates or niacin: Dose should **not** exceed 10 mg/day

Amiodarone or verapamil: Dose should **not** exceed 20 mg/day

Renal Impairment: Because simvastatin does not undergo significant renal excretion, modification of dose should not be necessary in patients with mild to moderate renal insufficiency.

Severe renal impairment: Cl_{cr} <10 mL/minute: Initial: 5 mg/day with close monitoring.

Monitoring Parameters Serum cholesterol (total and fractionated), CPK serum concentrations

Patient Information Take as directed without regard to meals. You may experience nausea, flatulence, dyspepsia (small frequent meals may help), and headache. Report severe and unresolved acute muscle pain or weakness, gastric upset, vision changes, changes in color of urine or stool, yellowing of skin or eyes, and unusual bruising. This drug may cause severe fetal defects; do not donate blood during therapy or for 1 month following discontinuation.

Special Geriatric Considerations Effective and well tolerated in the elderly. The definition and, therefore, when to treat hyperlipidemia in the elderly is a controversial issue. The National Cholesterol Education Program recommends that all adults maintain a plasma cholesterol <160 mg/dL. In elderly with one additional risk factor, goal LDL would be <130 mg/dL. It is the authors' belief that pharmacologic treatment be reserved for those who are unable to obtain a desirable plasma cholesterol concentration by diet alone and for whom the benefits of treatment are believed to outweigh the potential adverse effects, drug interactions, and cost of treatment.

Dosage Forms Excipient information presented when available (limited, particularly for generics); consult specific product labeling.
Tablet: 5 mg, 10 mg, 20 mg, 40 mg, 80 mg
Zocor®: 5 mg, 10 mg, 20 mg, 40 mg, 80 mg

Selected References
Bach LA, Cooper ME, O'Brien RC, et al, "The Use of Simvastatin, an HMG-CoA Reductase Inhibitor, in Older Patients With Hypercholesterolemia and Atherosclerosis," *J Am Geriatr Soc*, 1990, 38(1):10-4.
"Executive Summary of The Third Report of The National Cholesterol Education Program (NCEP) Expert Panel on Detection, Evaluation, And Treatment of High Blood Cholesterol In Adults (Adult Treatment Panel III)," *JAMA*, 2001, 285(19):2486-97.
Lintott CJ and Scott RS, "HMG-CoA Reductase Inhibitor Use in the Aged: A Review of Clinical Experience," *Drugs Aging*, 1992, 2(6):518-29.

♦ **Sinemet®** *see* Levodopa and Carbidopa *on page 892*

♦ **Sinemet® CR** *see* Levodopa and Carbidopa *on page 892*

♦ **Sinequan® [DSC]** *see* Doxepin *on page 473*

♦ **Singulair®** *see* Montelukast *on page 1062*

♦ **Sirdalud®** *see* Tizanidine *on page 1581*

Sitagliptin *(sit a GLIP tin)*

Medication Safety Issues
Sound-alike/look-alike issues:
Januvia™ may be confused with Jantoven™

U.S. Brand Names Januvia™

Index Terms MK-0431; Sitagliptin Phosphate

Generic Available No

Pharmacologic Category Antidiabetic Agent, Dipeptidyl Peptidase IV (DPP-IV) Inhibitor

Use Management of type 2 diabetes mellitus (noninsulin dependent, NIDDM) as an adjunct to diet and exercise as monotherapy or in combination therapy with metformin or a peroxisome proliferator-activated receptor (PPAR) gamma agonist (eg, a thiazolidinedione)

Contraindications Hypersensitivity to sitagliptin or any component of the formulation

Warnings/Precautions Use with caution in patients with moderate-to-severe renal dysfunction and end-stage renal disease (ESRD) requiring hemodialysis or peritoneal dialysis; dosing adjustment required.

Adverse Reactions (Reflective of adult population; not specific for elderly)
1% to 10%:
Central nervous system: Headache (5%)
Gastrointestinal: Diarrhea (3%)
Respiratory: Upper respiratory tract infection (6%), nasopharyngitis (5%)
Incidence less than or equal to placebo: Abdominal pain (2%), hypoglycemia (1%), nausea (1%), neutrophils increased, serum creatinine increased

Overdosage/Toxicology
Experience in overdose is limited. Treatment should be symptom-directed and supportive. QT_c prolongation, reported as not clinically significant, occurred in one study using doses of 800 mg. Sitagliptin is modestly dialyzable by hemodialysis ($\sim$14% of dose removed after a 3-4 hour hemodialysis session); unknown if dialyzable by peritoneal dialysis.

Drug Interactions
Substrate (minor) of CYP2C8, 3A4

Stability
Store at 20°C to 25°C (68°F to 77°F).

Mechanism of Action
Sitagliptin inhibits dipeptidyl peptidase IV (DPP-IV) enzyme resulting in increased active incretin levels. Incretin hormones [eg, glucagon-like peptide-1 (GLP-1) and glucose-dependent insulinotropic polypeptide (GIP)] regulate glucose homeostasis by increasing insulin synthesis and release from pancreatic beta cells and decreasing glucagon secretion from pancreatic alpha cells. Decreased glucagon secretion results in decreased hepatic glucose production. Under normal physiologic circumstances, incretin hormones are released by the intestine throughout the day and levels are increased in response to a meal; incretin hormones are rapidly inactivated by the DPP-IV enzyme.

Pharmacokinetics
Absorption: Rapid
Distribution: 198 L
Protein binding: 38%
Metabolism: Not extensively metabolized; minor metabolism via CYP3A4 and 2C8 to metabolites (inactive) suggested by *in vitro* studies
Bioavailability: 87%
Half-life elimination: 12 hours
Time to peak, plasma: 1-4 hours
Excretion: Urine 87% (79% as unchanged drug, 16% as metabolites); feces 13%

Dosage
Adults: Type 2 diabetes: Oral: 100 mg once daily
Renal Impairment:
$Cl_{cr} \geq 30$ to <50 mL/minute: 50 mg once daily
S_{cr}: Males: >1.7 to ≤3.0 mg/dL; Females: >1.5 to ≤2.5 mg/dL: 50 mg once daily
Cl_{cr}<30 mL/minute: 25 mg once daily
S_{cr}: Males: >3.0 mg/dL; Females: >2.5 mg/dL: 25 mg once daily
ESRD requiring hemodialysis or peritoneal dialysis: 25 mg once daily; administered without regard to timing of hemodialysis
Hepatic Impairment:
Mild-to-moderate impairment (Child-Pugh score 7-9): No dosage adjustment required
Severe impairment (Child-Pugh score >9): Not studied

Administration
May be administered with or without food.

Monitoring Parameters
Hgb A_{1c} and serum glucose; renal function prior to initiation and periodically during treatment.

Reference Range
Target range: Adults:
Fasting blood glucose: 90-130 mg/dL
Glycosylated hemoglobin: <7%

Patient Information
This medication will not cure diabetes and may be prescribed in conjunction with another antidiabetic medication. Do not take any new medications during therapy unless approved by prescriber. Take as directed; do not chew or crush tablets. May be taken with or without food. It is important to follow dietary and lifestyle recommendations and glucose monitoring instructions of prescriber or diabetic educator. You will be instructed in signs of hyper- or hypoglycemia; always carry a source of glucose with you in event of hypoglycemia. You may experience mild headache, upper respiratory infection, stuffy or runny nose, sore throat, or diarrhea when beginning treatment. Notify prescriber of any persistent or acute reactions.

Special Geriatric Considerations
Sitagliptin has not been studied exclusively in the elderly. The manufacturer reports that 725 out of 3884 patients in clinical trials were >65 years (only 61 were age 75 years and older), with no difference in safety or efficacy compared to younger patients. How "tightly" a geriatric patient's blood glucose should be controlled is controversial; however, a fasting blood sugar of <150 mg/dL is now an acceptable endpoint. Such a decision should be based on the patient's functional and cognitive status, how well they recognize hypoglycemic or hyperglycemic symptoms, and how to respond to them and their other disease states.

Dosage Forms
Excipient information presented when available (limited, particularly for generics); consult specific product labeling.
Tablet: Januvia™: 25 mg, 50 mg, 100 mg

Sitagliptin and Metformin (sit a GLIP tin & met FOR min)

U.S. Brand Names Janumet™

Index Terms Metformin and Sitagliptin; Sitagliptin Phosphate and Metformin Hydrochloride

Generic Available No

Pharmacologic Category Antidiabetic Agent, Biguanide; Antidiabetic Agent, Dipeptidyl Peptidase IV (DPP-IV) Inhibitor; Hypoglycemic Agent, Oral

Use Management of type 2 diabetes mellitus (noninsulin dependent, NIDDM) as an adjunct to diet and exercise

Contraindications Hypersensitivity to sitagliptin, metformin, or any component of the formulation; type 1 diabetes (insulin dependant, IDDM); renal disease or renal dysfunction (serum creatinine ≥1.5 mg/dL in males or ≥1.4 mg/dL in females, or abnormal creatinine clearance which may also result from conditions such as cardiovascular collapse, acute myocardial infarction, and septicemia); acute or chronic metabolic acidosis including diabetic ketoacidosis (with or without coma).

Warnings/Precautions [U.S. Boxed Warning]: Lactic acidosis is a rare, but potentially severe consequence of therapy with metformin. Lactic acidosis should be suspected in any diabetic patient receiving metformin who has evidence of acidosis when evidence of ketoacidosis is lacking. Discontinue metformin in clinical situations predisposing to hypoxemia, including conditions such as cardiovascular collapse, respiratory failure, acute myocardial infarction, acute congestive heart failure, and septicemia. Use caution in patients with congestive heart failure requiring pharmacologic management, particularly in patients with unstable or acute CHF; risk of lactic acidosis may be increased secondary to hypoperfusion. Avoid use in patients with impaired liver function due to potential for lactic acidosis. Patients should be instructed to avoid excessive acute or chronic ethanol use.

Sitagliptin and metformin are substantially excreted by the kidney; patients with renal function below the limit of normal for their age should not receive therapy. In elderly patients, renal function should be monitored regularly; should not be used in any patient ≥80 years of age unless measurement of creatinine clearance verifies normal renal function. The risk of accumulation and lactic acidosis increases with the degree of impairment of renal function. Use of concomitant medications that may affect renal function (eg, affect tubular secretion) may also affect metformin disposition. Metformin should be suspended in patients with dehydration and/or prerenal azotemia. Therapy should be temporarily discontinued for 48 hours in patients undergoing radiologic studies involving the intravascular administration of iodinated contrast materials (potential for acute alteration in renal function). Therapy should be suspended for any surgical procedures (resume only after normal intake resumed and normal renal function is verified). It may be necessary to discontinue metformin and administer insulin if the patient is exposed to stress (fever, trauma, infection, surgery).

Adverse Reactions (Reflective of adult population; not specific for elderly)
See individual agents.

Drug Interactions Sitagliptin: Substrate (minor) of CYP3A4 and CYP2C8
See individual agents.

Ethanol/Nutrition/Herb Interactions See individual agents.

Stability Store at 15°C to 30°C (59°F to 86°F).

Mechanism of Action Sitagliptin inhibits dipeptidyl peptidase IV (DPP-IV) enzymes resulting in prolonged active incretin levels. Incretin hormones [eg, glucagon-like peptide-1 (GLP-1) and glucose-dependent insulinotropic polypeptide (GIP)] regulate glucose homeostasis by increasing insulin synthesis and release from pancreatic beta cells and decreasing glucagon secretion from pancreatic alpha cells. Decreased glucagon secretion results in decreased hepatic glucose production. Under normal physiologic circumstances, incretin hormones are released by the intestine throughout the day and levels are increased in response to a meal; incretin hormones are rapidly inactivated by DPP-IV enzymes.

Metformin decreases hepatic glucose production, decreasing intestinal absorption of glucose, and improves insulin sensitivity (increases peripheral glucose uptake and utilization).

Pharmacokinetics See individual agents.

Dosage
Geriatrics: Refer to adult dosing. The initial and maintenance dosing should be conservative, due to the potential for decreased renal function (monitor). Do not use in patients ≥80 years of age unless normal renal function has been established.

Adults: Type 2 diabetes mellitus: Oral: Initial doses should be based on current dose of sitagliptin and metformin; daily doses should be divided and given twice daily with meals. Maximum: Sitagliptin 100 mg/metformin 2000 mg daily

Patients inadequately controlled on metformin alone: Initial dose: Sitagliptin 100 mg/day plus current dose of metformin. **Note:** Per manufacturer labeling, patients currently receiving metformin 850 mg twice daily should receive an initial dose of sitagliptin 50 mg and metformin 1000 mg twice daily

Patients inadequately controlled on sitagliptin alone: Initial dose: Metformin 1000 mg/day plus sitagliptin 100 mg/day. **Note:** Patients currently receiving a renally adjusted dose of sitagliptin should not be switched to combination product.

Dosing adjustment: Metformin component may be gradually increased up to the maximum dose. Maximum dose: Sitagliptin 100 mg/metformin 2000 mg daily

Renal Impairment: Do not use with renal disease or renal dysfunction (serum creatinine ≥1.5 mg/dL in males or ≥1.4 mg/dL in females or abnormal clearance).

Hepatic Impairment: Avoid metformin; liver disease is a risk factor for the development of lactic acidosis during metformin therapy.

Administration Administer with meals.

Monitoring Parameters Hgb A_{1c} and serum glucose, hematologic parameters (eg, hemoglobin/hematocrit, red blood cell indices), renal function; vitamin B_{12} and folate (if megaloblastic anemia is suspected)

Reference Range Recommendations for glycemic control in adults with diabetes:

Hb A_{1c}: <7%

Preprandial capillary plasma glucose: 90-130 mg/dL

Peak postprandial capillary blood glucose: <180 mg/dL

Blood pressure: <130/80 mm Hg

Patient Information Refer to individual agents.

Special Geriatric Considerations Sitagliptin has not been studied exclusively in the elderly. The manufacturer reports that 725 out of 3884 patients in clinical trials were >65 years of age (only 61 were ≥75 years), with no difference in safety or efficacy compared to younger patients. Limited data suggest that metformin's total body clearance may be decreased and AUC and half-life increased in elderly patients; presumably due to decreased renal clearance. Metformin has been well tolerated by the elderly but lower doses and frequent monitoring are recommended. In one study of elderly subjects, its effects could not be distinguished from tolbutamide, except for weight loss. The initial and maintenance dosing should be conservative, due to the potential for decreased renal function. Generally, elderly patients should not be titrated to the maximum dose of metformin. Do not use in patients ≥80 years of age unless normal renal function has been established. How "tightly" an elderly patient's blood glucose should be controlled is controversial; however, a fasting blood sugar of <150 mg/dL is now an acceptable endpoint. Such a decision should be based on the patient's functional and cognitive status, how well they recognize hypoglycemic or hyperglycemic symptoms, and how to respond to them and their other disease states.

Dosage Forms Excipient information presented when available (limited, particularly for generics); consult specific product labeling.

Tablet:

Janumet™:

50/500: Sitagliptin 50 mg and metformin hydrochloride 500 mg

50/1000: Sitagliptin 50 mg and metformin hydrochloride 1000 mg

Selected References

American Diabetes Association, "Standards of Medical Care in Diabetes — 2007," *Diabetes Care*, 2007, 30(Suppl 1):4-41.

Sodium Bicarbonate (SOW dee um bye KAR bun ate)

U.S. Brand Names Brioschi® [OTC]; Neut®

Index Terms Baking Soda; NaHCO$_3$; Sodium Acid Carbonate; Sodium Hydrogen Carbonate

Generic Available Yes

Pharmacologic Category Alkalinizing Agent; Antacid; Electrolyte Supplement, Oral; Electrolyte Supplement, Parenteral

Use Management of metabolic acidosis; gastric hyperacidity; as an alkalinization agent for the urine; treatment of hyperkalemia; management of overdose of certain drugs, including tricyclic antidepressants and aspirin

Contraindications Alkalosis, hypernatremia, severe pulmonary edema, hypocalcemia, unknown abdominal pain

Warnings/Precautions Use of I.V. NaHCO$_3$ should be reserved for documented metabolic acidosis and for hyperkalemia-induced cardiac arrest. Routine use in cardiac arrest is not recommended. Avoid extravasation, tissue necrosis can occur due to the hypertonicity of NaHCO$_3$. May cause sodium retention especially if renal function is impaired; not to be used in treatment of peptic ulcer; use with caution in patients with CHF, edema, cirrhosis, or renal failure. Not the antacid of choice for the elderly because of sodium content and potential for systemic alkalosis.

Adverse Reactions (Reflective of adult population; not specific for elderly)
Frequency not defined.
Cardiovascular: Cerebral hemorrhage, CHF (aggravated), edema
Central nervous system: Tetany
Gastrointestinal: Belching, flatulence (with oral), gastric distension
Endocrine & metabolic: Hypernatremia, hyperosmolality, hypocalcemia, hypokalemia, increased affinity of hemoglobin for oxygen-reduced pH in myocardial tissue necrosis when extravasated, intracranial acidosis, metabolic alkalosis, milk-alkali syndrome (especially with renal dysfunction)
Respiratory: Pulmonary edema

Overdosage/Toxicology Symptoms include hypocalcemia, hypokalemia, hypernatremia, and seizures. Seizures can be treated with diazepam 0.1-0.25 mg/kg. Hypernatremia is resolved through the use of diuretics and free water replacement.

Drug Interactions
Decreased effect/levels of lithium, chlorpropamide, methotrexate, tetracyclines, and salicylates due to urinary alkalinization
Increased toxicity/levels of amphetamines, anorexiants, mecamylamine, ephedrine, pseudoephedrine, flecainide, quinidine, quinine due to urinary alkalinization

Ethanol/Nutrition/Herb Interactions Herb/Nutraceutical: Concurrent doses with iron may decrease iron absorption.

Stability Store injection at room temperature; do not freeze. Protect from heat. Use only clear solutions.

Mechanism of Action Dissociates to provide bicarbonate ion which neutralizes hydrogen ion concentration and raises blood and urinary pH

Pharmacodynamics
Oral:
Onset of action: Rapid
Duration: of 8-10 minutes
I.V.:
Onset of action: 15 minutes
Duration: 1-2 hours

Pharmacokinetics
Absorption: Oral: Well absorbed
Elimination: Reabsorbed by kidney and <1% excreted by urine

Dosage
Geriatrics & Adults:
Cardiac arrest: I.V.: Initial: 1 mEq/kg/dose one time; maintenance: 0.5 mEq/kg/dose every 10 minutes or as indicated by arterial blood gases
Note: Routine use of NaHCO$_3$ is not recommended and should be given only after adequate alveolar ventilation has been established and effective cardiac compressions are provided
Metabolic acidosis: I.V.: Dosage should be based on the following formula if blood gases and pH measurements are available:
HCO$_3^-$(mEq) = 0.2 x weight (kg) x base deficit (mEq/L)
Administer ¹/₂ dose initially, then remaining ¹/₂ dose over the next 24 hours; monitor pH, serum HCO$_3^-$, and clinical status
Note: If acid-base status is not available: 2-5 mEq/kg I.V. infusion over 4-8 hours; subsequent doses should be based on patient's acid-base status
Hyperkalemia: I.V.: 1 mEq/kg over 5 minutes

Chronic renal failure: Oral: Initiate when plasma HCO_3^- <15 mEq/L Start with 20-36 mEq/day in divided doses, titrate to bicarbonate level of 18-20 mEq/L

Renal tubular acidosis: Oral:

Distal: 0.5-2 mEq/kg/day in 4-5 divided doses

Proximal: Initial: 5-10 mEq/kg/day; maintenance: Increase as required to maintain serum bicarbonate in the normal range

Urine alkalinization: Oral: Initial: 48 mEq (4 g), then 12-24 mEq (1-2 g) every 4 hours; dose should be titrated to desired urinary pH; doses up to 16 g/day (200 mEq) in patients <60 years and 8 g (100 mEq) in patients >60 years

Antacid: Oral: 325 mg to 2 g 1-4 times/day

Administration

Observe for extravasation when giving I.V.

Reference Range Therapeutic (sodium): 135-145 mmol/L (SI: 135-145 mmol/L)

Patient Information Avoid chronic use as an antacid (<2 weeks)

Additional Information May cause sodium retention especially if renal function is impaired; not to be used in treatment of peptic ulcer

Sodium content of injection 50 mL, 8.4%: 1150 mg (50 mEq); each 6 mg of $NaHCO_3$ contains 12 mEq sodium; 1 mEq $NaHCO_3$ = 84 mg; 1 mEq $NaHCO_3$ = 0.3 x body weight (kg) x base deficit (mEq/L)

Each 84 mg of sodium bicarbonate provides 1 mEq of sodium and bicarbonate ions; each gram of sodium bicarbonate provides 12 mEq of sodium and bicarbonate ions

Special Geriatric Considerations Not the antacid of choice for the elderly because of sodium content and potential for systemic alkalosis (see maximum daily dose under Dosage).

Dosage Forms Excipient information presented when available (limited, particularly for generics); consult specific product labeling.

Granules, effervescent (Brioschi®): 2.69 g/packet (6 g) [unit-dose packets; contains sodium 770 mg/packet; lemon flavor]; 2.69 g/capful (120 g, 240 g) [contains sodium 770 mg/capful; lemon flavor]

Infusion [premixed in sterile water]: 5% (500 mL)

Injection, solution:

4.2% [42 mg/mL = 5 mEq/10 mL] (10 mL)

7.5% [75 mg/mL = 8.92 mEq/10 mL] (50 mL)

8.4% [84 mg/mL = 10 mEq/10 mL] (10 mL, 50 mL)

Neut®: 4% [40 mg/mL = 2.4 mEq/5 mL] (5 mL)

Powder: Sodium bicarbonate USP (120 g, 480 g) [contains sodium 30 mEq per ½ teaspoon]

Tablet: 325 mg [3.8 mEq]; 650 mg [7.6 mEq]

Sodium Chloride (SOW dee um KLOR ide)

Medication Safety Issues

Per JCAHO recommendations, concentrated electrolyte solutions (eg, NaCl >0.9%) should not be available in patient care areas.

High alert medication: The Institute for Safe Medication Practices (ISMP) includes this medication (I.V. formulation) among its list of drugs which have a heightened risk of causing significant patient harm when used in error.

U.S. Brand Names Altachlore [OTC]; Altamist [OTC]; Ayr® Baby Saline [OTC]; Ayr® Saline [OTC]; Ayr® Saline No-Drip [OTC]; Breathe Right® Saline [OTC]; Broncho Saline® [OTC] [DSC]; Deep Sea [OTC]; Entsol® [OTC]; Muro 128® [OTC]; Mycinaire™ [OTC]; NaSal™ [OTC]; Nasal Moist® [OTC]; Na-Zone® [OTC]; Ocean® [OTC]; Oceant® for Kids [OTC]; Pretz® [OTC]; SalineX® [OTC]; Simply Saline® [OTC]; Simply Saline® Baby [OTC]; Simply Saline® Nasal Moist® [OTC]; Syrex; 4-Way® Saline Moisturizing Mist [OTC]; Wound Wash Saline™ [OTC]

Index Terms NaCl; Normal Saline; Salt

Generic Available Yes

Pharmacologic Category Electrolyte Supplement, Parenteral; Genitourinary Irrigant; Irrigant; Lubricant, Ocular; Sodium Salt

Use Prevention of muscle cramps and heat prostration; restoration of sodium ion in hyponatremia and moisture to nasal membranes; GU irrigant; reduction of corneal edema; source of electrolytes and water for expansion of the extracellular fluid compartment

Contraindications Hypersensitivity to sodium chloride or any component of the formulation; hypertonic uterus, hypernatremia, fluid retention

Warnings/Precautions Use with caution in patients with CHF, renal insufficiency, liver cirrhosis, hypertension, edema; sodium toxicity is almost exclusively related to how fast a sodium deficit is corrected; both rate and magnitude are extremely important; do not use bacteriostatic sodium chloride in newborns since benzyl alcohol preservatives have been associated with toxicity.

(Continued)

Sodium Chloride *(Continued)*

Irrigants: For external use only; not for parenteral use. Do not use during electrosurgical procedures. Irrigating fluids may be absorbed into systemic circulation; monitor for fluid or solute overload.

Adverse Reactions (Reflective of adult population; not specific for elderly)
Frequency not defined.
Cardiovascular: Congestive conditions
Endocrine & metabolic: Extravasation, hypervolemia, hypernatremia, dilution of serum electrolytes, overhydration, hypokalemia
Local: Thrombosis, phlebitis, extravasation
Respiratory: Pulmonary edema

Overdosage/Toxicology Symptoms include nausea, vomiting, diarrhea, abdominal cramps, hypocalcemia, hypokalemia, and hypernatremia. Hypernatremia is resolved through the use of diuretics and free water replacement.

Drug Interactions Lithium: Sodium chloride may decrease levelseffects of lithium.

Stability Store injection at room temperature; do not freeze. Protect from heat. Use only clear solutions.

Mechanism of Action Principal extracellular cation; functions in fluid and electrolyte balance, osmotic pressure control, and water distribution

Pharmacokinetics
Absorption: Oral, I.V.: Rapid
Distribution: Widely distributed
Elimination: Mainly in urine but also in sweat, tears, and saliva

Dosage
Geriatrics & Adults:
GU irrigant: Irrigation: 1-3 L/day by intermittent irrigation
Heat cramps: Oral: 0.5-1 g with full glass of water, up to 4.8 g/day
Replacement: I.V.: Determined by laboratory determinations mEq
Hyponatremia: Sodium deficiency (mEq/kg) = [% dehydration (L/kg)/100 x 70 (mEq/L)] + [0.6 (L/kg) x (140 - serum sodium) (mEq/L)]
To correct acute, serious hyponatremia: mEq sodium = [desired sodium (mEq/L) - actual sodium (mEq/L)] x [0.6 x wt (kg)]; for acute correction use 125 mEq/L as the desired serum sodium; acutely correct serum sodium in 5 mEq/L/dose increments; more gradual correction in increments of 10 mEq/L/day is indicated in the asymptomatic patient
Chloride maintenance electrolyte requirement in parenteral nutrition: 2-4 mEq/kg/24 hours or 25-40 mEq/1000 kcals/24 hours; maximum: 100-150 mEq/24 hours
Sodium maintenance electrolyte requirement in parenteral nutrition: 3-4 mEq/kg/24 hours or 25-40 mEq/1000 kcals/24 hours; maximum: 100-150 mEq/24 hours.
Ophthalmic:
Ointment: Apply once daily or more often
Solution: Instill 1-2 drops into affected eye(s) every 3-4 hours
Bronchodilator diluent: Inhalation: 1-3 sprays (1-3 mL) to dilute bronchodilator solution in nebulizer before administration
Nasal congestion: Intranasal: 2-3 sprays in each nostril as needed
Irrigation: Spray affected area

Monitoring Parameters I & O, weight, presence or worsening of rales and degree of peripheral edema with infusions, electrolyte levels

Reference Range Serum/plasma concentration: 135-145 mEq/L

Patient Information Blurred vision is common with ophthalmic ointment; may sting eyes when first applied

Dosage Forms Excipient information presented when available (limited, particularly for generics); consult specific product labeling. [DSC] = Discontinued product
Gel, intranasal:
Ayr® Saline No-Drip: 0.5% (22 mL) [spray gel; contains benzalkonium chloride, benzyl alcohol and soybean oil]
Ayr® Saline: 0.5% (14 g) [contains soybean oil]
Entsol®: 3% (20 g) [contains aloe, benzalkonium chloride, and vitamin E]
Simply Saline® Nasal Moist®: 0.65% (30 g)
Injection, solution [preservative free]: 0.9% (2 mL, 5 mL, 10 mL, 20 mL, 100 mL)
Injection, solution [preservative free, prefilled I.V. flush syringe]: 0.9% (2 mL, 2.5 mL, 3 mL, 5 mL, 10 mL)
Injection, solution: 0.45% (25 mL, 50 mL, 100 mL, 250 mL, 500 mL, 1000 mL); 0.9% (3 mL, 5 mL, 10 mL, 20 mL, 25 mL, 30 mL, 50 mL, 100 mL, 150 mL, 250 mL, 500 mL, 1000 mL); 3% (500 mL); 5% (500 mL)
Syrex: 0.9% (2.5 mL, 5 mL, 10 mL) [prefilled syringe]
Injection, solution [bacteriostatic]: 0.9% (10 mL, 20 mL, 30 mL) [contains benzyl alcohol]
Injection, solution [concentrate]: 14.6% (2.5 mEq/mL) (20 mL, 40 mL); 23.4% (4 mEq/mL) (30 mL, 100 mL, 200 mL, 250 mL)
Ointment, ophthalmic: 5% (3.5 g)

Altachlore, Muro 128®: 5% (3.5 g)

Powder for nasal solution (Entsol®): 3% (10.5 g)

Solution for inhalation: 0.45% (3 mL, 5 mL); 0.9% (3 mL, 5 mL, 15 mL); 3% (15 mL); 10% (15 mL)

Broncho® Saline: 0.9% (90 mL, 240 mL) [for dilution of bronchodilator solutions] [DSC]

Solution, intranasal: 0.65% (45 mL)

Altamist: 0.65% (60 mL) [spray; contains benzalkonium chloride]

Ayr® Baby Saline: 0.65% (30 mL) [spray/drops; contains benzalkonium chloride]

Ayr® Saline: 0.65% (50 mL) [drops; contains benzalkonium chloride]

Ayr® Saline: 0.65% (50 mL) [mist, contains benzalkonium chloride]

Breathe Right® Saline: 0.65% (44 mL) [spray; contains benzalkonium chloride]

Deep Sea: 0.65% (45 mL) [spray; contains benzalkonium chloride]

Entsol® Mist: 3% (30 mL) [spray; contains benzalkonium chloride]

Entsol® [preservative free]: 3% (100 mL) [spray]

Entsol® [preservative free]: 3% (240 mL) [nasal wash]

Mycinaire™: 0.65% (30 mL) [mist; contains benzalkonium chloride]

Na-Zone®: 0.65% (60 mL) [spray; contains benzalkonium chloride]

NaSal™: 0.65% (15 mL) [drops; contains benzalkonium chloride], (30 mL) [spray; contains benzalkonium chloride]

Nasal Moist®: 0.65% (45 mL) [spray]

Ocean®: 0.65% (45 mL) [mist/spray/drops; contains benzalkonium chloride]; (473 mL) [refill bottle; contains benzalkonium chloride]

Ocean® for Kids: 0.65% (37.5 mL) [drops/spray/stream; contains benzalkonium chloride]

Pretz®: 0.75% (50 mL) [spray; contains benzalkonium chloride and yerba santa]; (240 mL) [irrigation; contains benzalkonium chloride and yerba santa]; (960 mL) [refill bottle; contains benzalkonium chloride and yerba santa]

SalineX®: 0.4% (15 mL) [drops]; (50 mL) [spray]

Simply Saline®: 0.9% (44 mL, 90 mL) [mist]

Simply Saline® Baby: 0.9% (45 mL) [mist]

4-Way® Saline Moisturizing Mist: 0.74% (30 mL) [alcohol free; contains benzalkonium chloride, eucalyptol, and menthol]

Solution for irrigation: 0.45% (1500 mL, 2000 mL); 0.9% (250 mL, 500 mL, 1000 mL, 1500 mL, 2000 mL, 3000 mL, 4000 mL, 5000 mL)

Wound Wash Saline™: 0.9% (90 mL, 210 mL)

Solution, ophthalmic: 5% (15 mL)

Altachlore: 5% (15 mL, 30 mL)

Muro 128®: 2% (15 mL); 5% (15 mL, 30 mL)

Sodium Citrate and Citric Acid (SOW dee um SIT rate & SI trik AS id)

U.S. Brand Names Bicitra®; Cytra-2; Oracit®

Canadian Brand Names PMS-Dicitrate

Index Terms Modified Shohl's Solution

Generic Available Yes

Pharmacologic Category Alkalinizing Agent, Oral

Use Treatment of metabolic acidosis; alkalinizing agent in conditions where long-term maintenance of an alkaline urine is desirable

Contraindications Hypersensitivity to sodium citrate, citric acid, or any component of the formulation; severe renal insufficiency; sodium-restricted diet

Warnings/Precautions Conversion to bicarbonate may be impaired in patients with hepatic failure, in shock, or who are severely ill. Use caution with cardiac failure, hypertension, impaired renal function, and peripheral or pulmonary edema.

Adverse Reactions (Reflective of adult population; not specific for elderly)
Frequency not defined. Generally well tolerated with normal renal function.

Central nervous system: Tetany

Endocrine & metabolic: Metabolic alkalosis, hyperkalemia

Gastrointestinal: Diarrhea, nausea, vomiting

Overdosage/Toxicology Symptoms include hypokalemia, hypernatremia, tetany, and seizures. Hypernatremia is resolved through the use of diuretics and free water replacement.

Drug Interactions

Decreased effect/levels of lithium, chlorpropamide, salicylates due to urinary alkalinization

Increased toxicity/levels of amphetamines, ephedrine, pseudoephedrine, flecainide, quinidine, quinine due to urinary alkalinization

Stability Store at controlled room temperature of 15°C to 30°C (59°F to 86°F); do not freeze. Protect from excessive heat.

(Continued)

Sodium Citrate and Citric Acid (Continued)

Dosage

Geriatrics & Adults: Systemic alkalization: Oral: 10-30 mL with water after meals and at bedtime

Monitoring Parameters Blood gas for pH and bicarbonate; serum bicarbonate

Patient Information Palatability is improved by chilling solution, dilute each dose with 1-3 oz of water and follow with additional water (will also minimize laxative effect); take after meals to prevent saline laxative effect

Additional Information 1 mL of solution contains 1 mEq of sodium and is metabolized to form the equivalent of 1 mEq of bicarbonate/mL

Dosage Forms Excipient information presented when available (limited, particularly for generics); consult specific product labeling. **Note:** Contains sodium 1 mEq/mL and the equivalent to bicarbonate 1 mEq/mL

Solution, oral: Sodium citrate 500 mg and citric acid 334 mg per 5 mL (480 mL)

Bicitra®: Sodium citrate 500 mg and citric acid 334 mg per 5 mL (480 mL) [sugar free; grape flavor]

Cytra-2: Sodium citrate 500 mg and citric acid 334 mg per 5 mL (480 mL) [alcohol free, dye free, sugar free; grape flavor]

Oracit®: Sodium citrate 490 mg and citric acid 640 mg per 5 mL (15 mL, 30 mL, 500 mL, 3840 mL)

♦ **Sodium Citrate, Citric Acid, and Potassium Citrate** see Citric Acid, Sodium Citrate, and Potassium Citrate on page 325

♦ **Sodium Etidronate** see Etidronate Disodium on page 585

♦ **Sodium Ferric Gluconate** see Ferric Gluconate on page 616

♦ **Sodium Fluoride** see Fluoride on page 642

♦ **Sodium Hydrogen Carbonate** see Sodium Bicarbonate on page 1474

♦ **Sodium Nafcillin** see Nafcillin on page 1081

♦ **Sodium Nitroferricyanide** see Nitroprusside on page 1132

♦ **Sodium Nitroprusside** see Nitroprusside on page 1132

♦ **Sodium PAS** see Aminosalicylic Acid on page 79

♦ **Sodium Phosphate and Potassium Phosphate** see Potassium Phosphate and Sodium Phosphate on page 1293

Sodium Phosphates (SOW dee um FOS fates)

Related Information

Treatment Options for Constipation on page 1785

Medication Safety Issues

Sound-alike/look-alike issues:

Visicol® may be confused with VESIcare®

Enemas and oral solution are available in pediatric and adult sizes; prescribe by "volume" not by "bottle."

U.S. Brand Names Fleet® Accu-Prep® [OTC]; Fleet® Enema [OTC]; Fleet® Phospho-Soda® [OTC]; OsmoPrep™; Visicol®

Canadian Brand Names Fleet Enema®; Fleet® Phospho-Soda® Oral Laxative

Generic Available Yes: Enema, injection

Pharmacologic Category Cathartic; Electrolyte Supplement, Oral; Electrolyte Supplement, Parenteral; Laxative, Bowel Evacuant

Use Short-term treatment of constipation, evacuation of the colon for rectal and bowel exams; source of sodium and phosphorus; treatment and prevention of hypophosphatemia

Contraindications Hypersensitivity to sodium phosphate salts or any component of the formulation; congenital megacolon, toxic megacolon, bowel obstruction, bowel perforation, imperforate anus (enema), congestive heart failure, ascites

Additional product-specific contraindications:

Intravenous phosphate preparation: Should not be used in diseases with high phosphate levels, low calcium levels or hypernatremia.

Oral: Should not be used in patients with kidney disease, unstable angina pectoris, gastric retention, ileus, acute obstruction or pseudo-obstruction, severe chronic constipation, acute colitis, or hypomotility syndrome (ie, hypothyroidism, scleroderma). Should not be used in patients on a sodium-restricted diet.

Warnings/Precautions Use with caution in patients with impaired renal dysfunction, pre-existing electrolyte imbalances, risk of electrolyte disturbance (hypocalcemia, hyperphosphatemia, hypernatremia), dehydration, chronic inflammatory bowel disease, gastric bypass or stapling surgery.

Acute phosphate nephropathy may rarely occur during use as a bowel cleanser. Risk factors for acute phosphate nephropathy may include increased age (>62 years of age), renal dysfunction or dehydration, use of medicines that affect renal perfusion or function (eg, ACE inhibitors, angiotensin receptor blockers, diuretics, NSAIDs). Other preventive measures may include avoid excessive doses and concurrent use of other laxatives containing sodium phosphate; encourage patients to drink sufficient quantities of clear fluids during bowel cleansing; obtain baseline and post-procedure labs in patients at risk; consider hospitalization and intravenous hydration during bowel cleansing for patients unable to hydrate themselves.

Use caution in inflammatory bowel disease; may induce colonic aphthous ulceration. Use with caution in patients with a history of seizures and those at higher risk of seizures. Use with caution in patients with or at risk for arrhythmias. Prolongation of the QT interval has been reported; use caution with concurrent use of other QT prolonging medications. If using as a bowel evacuant, correct electrolyte abnormalities before administration. Inadequate fluid intake may lead to hypovolemia. Use with caution in debilitated patients. Use with caution in geriatric patients. Laxatives and purgatives have the potential for abuse by bulimia nervosa patients. Other oral medications may not be well absorbed when given during bowel evacuation. Enemas and oral solution are available in adult sizes; prescribe by "volume" not by "bottle."

Visicol®: Use caution with history of swallowing difficulties or esophageal narrowing. Tablet particles may be seen in the stool.

Adverse Reactions (Reflective of adult population; not specific for elderly)
Frequency not defined.
Cardiovascular: Edema, hypotension
Central nervous system: Dizziness, headache
Endocrine & metabolic: Hypocalcemia, hypernatremia, hyperphosphatemia, calcium phosphate precipitation
Gastrointestinal: Nausea, vomiting, diarrhea, abdominal bloating, abdominal pain, mucosal bleeding, superficial mucosal ulcerations
Renal: Acute renal failure
Postmarketing and/or case reports: Atrial fibrillation following severe vomiting (tablet formulation); nephrocalcinosis (oral solution)

Drug Interactions
ACE inhibitors or angiotensin-receptor antagonists: May increase the risk of electrolyte disorders or nephrocalcinosis when oral phosphates solution is used as a bowel evacuant. Use caution.
Antacids: Do not give with magnesium- and aluminum-containing antacids which can bind with phosphate.
Bisphosphonates: Increased risk of hypoglycemia with concurrent use.
Diuretics: May increase the risk of electrolyte disorders or nephrocalcinosis when oral phosphates solution is used as a bowel evacuant. Use caution.
Sucralfate: Do not give with sucralfate which can bind phosphate.
Oral preparations: May affect absorption of other medications due to rapid intestinal peristalsis and watery diarrhea caused by agent
Intravenous preparation: Use caution with thiazide diuretics, may lead to renal damage

Stability Store at 15°C to 30°C (59°F to 86°F).

Mechanism of Action As a laxative, exerts osmotic effect in the small intestine by drawing water into the lumen of the gut, producing distention and promoting peristalsis and evacuation of the bowel; phosphorous participates in bone deposition, calcium metabolism, utilization of B complex vitamins, and as a buffer in acid-base equilibrium

Pharmacodynamics Onset of action:
Cathartic: 3-6 hours
Rectal: 2-5 minutes

Pharmacokinetics
Absorption: Oral: ~1% to 20%
Elimination:
Oral phosphate: In feces
I.V. phosphate: In urine with over 80% of dose reabsorbed by the kidney

Dosage
Geriatrics & Adults:
Normal requirements elemental phosphorus: Oral:
≥19 years: RDA: 700 mg

Hypophosphatemia: It is difficult to provide concrete guidelines for the treatment of severe hypophosphatemia because the extent of total body deficits and response to therapy are difficult to predict. Aggressive doses of phosphate may result in a transient serum elevation followed by redistribution into intracellular compartments or bone tissue. Intermittent I.V. infusion should be reserved for severe depletion situations (<1 mg/dL in adults); large doses of oral phosphate may cause diarrhea and intestinal absorption may be unreliable. I.V. solutions should be infused slowly. Use caution when mixing with calcium and magnesium, precipitate may form. The following dosages are empiric guidelines. **Note:** 1 mmol phosphate = 31 mg phosphorus; 1 mg phosphorus = 0.032 mmol phosphate
(Continued)

Sodium Phosphates *(Continued)*

Hypophosphatemia treatment: Doses listed as mmol of phosphate:

Intermittent I.V. infusion: Acute repletion or replacement:

Varying dosages: 0.15-0.3 mmol/kg/dose over 12 hours; may repeat as needed to achieve desired serum level **or**

15 mmol/dose over 2 hours; use if serum phosphorus <2 mg/dL **or**

Low dose: 0.16 mmol/kg over 4-6 hours; use if serum phosphorus level 2.3-3 mg/dL

Intermediate dose: 0.32 mmol/kg over 4-6 hours; use if serum phosphorus level 1.6-2.2 mg/dL

High dose: 0.64 mmol/kg over 8-12 hours; use if serum phosphorus <1.5 mg/dL

Oral: 0.5-1 g elemental phosphorus 2-3 times/day may be used when serum phosphorus level is 1-2.5 mg/dL

Maintenance: Doses listed as mmol of phosphate:

Oral: 50-150 mmol/day in divided doses

I.V.: 50-70 mmol/day

Laxative (Fleet®): Rectal: Contents of one 4.5-ounce enema as a single dose, may repeat

Laxative (Fleet® Phospho-Soda®): Oral: Take on an empty stomach; dilute dose with 8 ounces cool water, then follow dose with 8 ounces water; **do not repeat dose within 24 hours**

15-45 mL as a single dose; maximum daily dose: 45 mL

Bowel cleansing prior to colonoscopy: Note: Each dose should be taken with a minimum of 8 ounces of clear liquids. Do not repeat treatment within 7 days. Do not use additional agents, especially sodium phosphate products.

Fleet® Phospho-Soda®: Oral: Prior to procedure (timing of doses determined by prescriber): One dose is equal to 45 mL (2 doses are recommended): Each dose is diluted as follows:

Mix 45 mL with 120 mL clear liquid; drink, then follow with at least 240 mL of clear liquid; **or**

Mix 15 mL with 240 mL clear liquid; drink, then follow with 240 mL clear liquid; repeat every 10 minutes for a total of 45 mL

Visicol™: Oral: Adults: A total of 40 tablets divided as follows:

Evening before colonoscopy: 3 tablets every 15 minutes for 6 doses, then 2 additional tablets in 15 minutes (total of 20 tablets)

3-5 hours prior to colonoscopy: 3 tablets every 15 minutes for 6 doses, then 2 additional tablets in 15 minutes (total of 20 tablets)

OsmoPrep™: A total of 32 tablets divided as follows:

Evening before colonoscopy: 4 tablets every 15 minutes for 5 doses (total of 20 tablets)

3-5 hours prior to colonoscopy: 4 tablets every 15 minutes for 3 doses (total of 12 tablets)

Renal Impairment: Use with caution; ionized inorganic phosphate is excreted by the kidneys. Oral solution is contraindicated in patients with kidney disease.

Administration For intermittent I.V. infusion, dilute at a maximum concentration of 0.12 mmol/mL and infuse over 4-6 hours; maximum, rate of infusion: 0.06 mmol/kg/hour

Monitoring Parameters

I.V.: Serum calcium and phosphate levels; renal function

Oral solution: Patients receiving >45 mL of oral solution may develop severe electrolyte shifts, even in the absence of medical contraindications.

Reference Range Phosphorous serum concentrations; it should be noted that serum concentrations do not accurately reflect intracellular phosphorous concentrations or extent of total body depletion

Adults: 3-4.5 mg/dL

Patient Information May cause diarrhea with the oral preparation; excessive or prolonged use as a laxative may cause dependence

Special Geriatric Considerations The use of laxatives should be limited in the elderly since abuse could lead to fluid/electrolyte deficiencies. Since elderly often have reduced renal function, or disease that could predispose them to adverse effects, caution must be used with parenteral sodium phosphate.

Dosage Forms Excipient information presented when available (limited, particularly for generics); consult specific product labeling.

Kit:

Fleet® Accu-Prep®:

Solution, oral (Fleet® Phosph-Soda®): Monobasic sodium phosphate monohydrate 2.4 g and dibasic sodium phosphate heptahydrate 0.9 g per 5 mL (15 mL) [contains contains sodium 556 mg/5 mL, phosphate 62.25 mEq/5 mL and sodium benzoate; kit contains six 15 mL unit-dose containers (equal to two 45 mL doses)]

Pads, anorectal (Fleet® Relief™): Pramoxine hydrochloride 1% and glycerin 12% (4s)

Injection, solution [preservative free]: Phosphorus 3 mmol and sodium 4 mEq per mL (5 mL, 15 mL, 50 mL)

Solution, oral:

Fleet® Phospho-Soda®: Monobasic sodium phosphate monohydrate 2.4 g and dibasic sodium phosphate heptahydrate 0.9 g per 5 mL (45 mL) [sugar free; contains sodium 556 mg/5 mL, sodium benzoate, and phosphate 62.25 mEq/5 mL; unflavored or ginger-lemon flavor]

Solution, rectal [enema]: Monobasic sodium phosphate 19 g and dibasic sodium phosphate 7 g per 118 mL delivered dose (135 mL)

Fleet® Enema: Monobasic sodium phosphate 19 g and dibasic sodium phosphate 7 g per 118 mL delivered dose (135 mL)

Fleet® Enema for Children: Monobasic sodium phosphate 9.5 g and dibasic sodium phosphate 3.5 g per 59 mL delivered dose (68 mL)

Tablet, oral:

OsmoPrep™: Sodium phosphate monobasic monohydrate 1.102 g and sodium phosphate dibasic anhydrous 0.398 g [sodium phosphate 1.5 g per tablet; gluten free]

Visicol®: Sodium phosphate monobasic monohydrate 1.102 g and sodium phosphate dibasic anhydrous 0.398 g [sodium phosphate 1.5 g per tablet]

Selected References

Lentz RD, Brown BM, and Kjellstrand CM, "Treatment of Severe Hypophosphatemia," *Ann Intern Med*, 1978, 89(6):941-4.

Lloyd CW and Johnson CE, "Management of Hypophosphatemia," *Clin Pharm*, 1988, 7(2):123-8.

Sodium Polystyrene Sulfonate
(SOW dee um pol ee STYE reen SUL fon ate)

Medication Safety Issues

Sound-alike/look-alike issues:

Kayexalate® may be confused with Kaopectate®

Always prescribe either one-time doses or as a specific number of doses (eg, 15 g q6h x 2 doses). Scheduled doses with no dosage limit could be given for days leading to dangerous hypokalemia.

International issues:

Kionex™ may be confused with Kinex® which is a brand name for biperiden in Mexico

U.S. Brand Names Kayexalate®; Kionex™; SPS®

Canadian Brand Names Kayexalate®; PMS-Sodium Polystyrene Sulfonate

Generic Available Yes

Pharmacologic Category Antidote

Use Treatment of hyperkalemia

Contraindications Hypersensitivity to sodium polystyrene sulfonate or any component of the formulation; hypernatremia, hypokalemia, obstructive bowel disease

Warnings/Precautions Use with caution in patients with severe CHF, hypertension, edema, or renal failure; large oral doses may cause fecal impaction (especially in elderly); enema will reduce the serum potassium faster than oral administration, but the oral route will result in a greater reduction over several hours.

Adverse Reactions (Reflective of adult population; not specific for elderly)
Frequency not defined.

Endocrine & metabolic: Hypernatremia, hypokalemia, hypocalcemia, hypomagnesemia

Gastrointestinal: Anorexia, colonic necrosis (rare), constipation, fecal impaction, intestinal obstruction (due to concretions in association with aluminum hydroxide), nausea, vomiting

Overdosage/Toxicology Symptoms include hypokalemia including cardiac dysrhythmias, confusion, irritability, ECG changes, muscle weakness, and gastrointestinal effects. Treatment is supportive and is limited to management of fluid and electrolytes.

Drug Interactions Systemic alkalosis and seizure has occurred after cation-exchange resins were administered with nonabsorbable cation-donating antacids and laxatives (eg, magnesium hydroxide, aluminum carbonate). Digitalis toxicity may occur with hypokalemia.

Stability Store prepared suspensions at 15°C to 30°C (59°F to 86°F). Store repackaged product in refrigerator and use within 14 days. Freshly prepared suspensions should be used within 24 hours. Do not heat resin suspension.

Mechanism of Action Removes potassium by exchanging sodium ions for potassium ions in the intestine before the resin is passed from the body
(Continued)

Sodium Polystyrene Sulfonate *(Continued)*

Pharmacodynamics Onset of action: Within 2-12 hours
Exchange capacity is ~1 mEq/g *in vivo*; *in vitro* capacity is 3.1 mEq/g; therefore, a wide range of exchange capacity exists such that close monitoring of serum electrolytes is necessary.

Pharmacokinetics Remains in the GI tract to be completely excreted in the feces (primarily as potassium polystyrene sulfonate)

Dosage
Geriatrics & Adults: Hyperkalemia:
Oral: 15 g (60 mL) 1-4 times/day
Rectal: 30-50 g every 6 hours

Administration Administer oral (or NG) as ~25% sorbitol solution, never mix in orange juice; enema route is less effective than oral administration; retain enema in colon for at least 30-60 minutes and for several hours, if possible

Monitoring Parameters Monitor serum electrolytes (potassium, sodium) frequently/24 hours; occasional serum calcium and magnesium is recommended; monitor for constipation and bowel obstruction; EKG monitoring for hypokalemia

Additional Information 1 gram of resin binds ~1 mEq of potassium; chilling the oral mixture will increase palatability
Sodium content of 1 g: 31 mg (1.3 mEq)

Special Geriatric Considerations Large doses in the elderly may cause fecal impaction and intestinal obstruction. Best to administer using sorbitol 70% as vehicle.

Dosage Forms Excipient information presented when available (limited, particularly for generics); consult specific product labeling.
Powder for suspension, oral/rectal:
Kayexalate®: 15 g/4 level teaspoons (480 g) [contains sodium 100 mg (4.1 mEq)/g]
Kionex™: 15 g/4 level teaspoons (454 g) [contains sodium 100 mg (4.1 mEq)/g]
Suspension, oral/rectal: 15 g/60 mL (60 mL, 120 mL, 200 mL, 500 mL) [contains sodium 1500 mg (65 mEq)/60 mL, sorbitol, and alcohol 0.1%; cherry/caramel flavor]
SPS®: 15 g/60 mL (60 mL, 120 mL, 480 mL) [contains alcohol 0.3%, sodium 1500 mg (65 mEq)/60 mL, and sorbitol; cherry flavor]

♦ **Sodium Salicylate** *see* Salicylates (Various Salts) *on page 1439*
♦ **Sodium Sulfacetamide** *see* Sulfacetamide *on page 1496*

Sodium Tetradecyl *(SOW dee um tetra DEK il)*

U.S. Brand Names Sotradecol®
Canadian Brand Names Trombovar®
Index Terms Sodium Tetradecyl Sulfate
Generic Available No
Pharmacologic Category Sclerosing Agent
Use Treatment of small, uncomplicated varicose veins of the lower extremities
Dosage
Geriatrics & Adults: Sclerosing agent: I.V.: Test dose: 0.5 mL given several hours prior to administration of larger dose; 0.5-2 mL (preferred maximum: 1 mL) in each vein, maximum: 10 mL per treatment session; 3% solution reserved for large varices

Special Geriatric Considerations Due to possible contraindications with disease states that may be "out of control," the elderly patient's medical condition must be thoroughly evaluated before use. No specific geriatric data available.

Dosage Forms Excipient information presented when available (limited, particularly for generics); consult specific product labeling.
Injection, as sulfate: 1% [10 mg/mL] (2 mL) [contains benzyl alcohol]; 3% [30 mg/mL] (2 mL) [contains benzyl alcohol]

♦ **Sodium Tetradecyl Sulfate** *see* Sodium Tetradecyl *on page 1482*
♦ **Sodium Thiosalicylate** *see* Salicylates (Various Salts) *on page 1439*
♦ **Solaraze®** *see* Diclofenac *on page 424*
♦ **Solarcaine® Aloe Extra Burn Relief [OTC]** *see* Lidocaine *on page 904*

Solifenacin *(sol i FEN a sin)*

Related Information
Pharmacotherapy of Urinary Incontinence *on page 1822*
Medication Safety Issues
Sound-alike/look-alike issues:
VESIcare® may be confused with Visicol®
U.S. Brand Names VESIcare®
Index Terms Solifenacin Succinate
Generic Available No

Pharmacologic Category Anticholinergic Agent

Use Treatment of overactive bladder with symptoms of urinary frequency, urgency, or urge incontinence

Contraindications Hypersensitivity to solifenacin or any component of the formulation; urinary retention; gastric retention; uncontrolled narrow-angle glaucoma.

Warnings/Precautions Use with caution in patients with bladder outflow obstruction, gastrointestinal obstructive disorders, and decreased gastrointestinal motility. Use with caution in patients with controlled (treated) narrow-angle glaucoma. Dosage adjustment is required for patients with renal or hepatic impairment. Patients on potent CYP3A4 inhibitors require lower dose.

Adverse Reactions (Reflective of adult population; not specific for elderly)
Adverse reactions are dose related.
>10%: Gastrointestinal: Xerostomia (11% to 28%), constipation (5% to 13%)
1% to 10%:
    Cardiovascular: Edema (up to 1%), hypertension (up to 1%)
    Central nervous system: Dizziness (2%), fatigue (1% to 2%), depression (up to 1%)
    Gastrointestinal: Nausea (2% to 3%), dyspepsia (1% to 4%), upper abdominal pain (1% to 2%), vomiting (up to 1%)
    Genitourinary: Urinary tract infection (3% to 5%), urinary retention (up to 1%)
    Ocular: Blurred vision (4% to 5%), dry eyes (up to 2%)
    Respiratory: Cough (up to 1%), pharyngitis (up to 1%)
    Miscellaneous: Influenza (1% to 2%)

Overdosage/Toxicology Overdosage can potentially result in severe central anticholinergic effects. Treatment should include gastric lavage and supportive measures.

Drug Interactions Substrate of CYP3A4 (major)
    CYP3A4 inducers: May decrease the levels/effects of solifenacin. Example inducers include aminoglutethimide, carbamazepine, nafcillin, nevirapine, phenobarbital, and phenytoin.
    CYP3A4 inhibitors: May increase the levels/effects of solifenacin. Example inhibitors include azole antifungals, clarithromycin, diclofenac, doxycycline, erythromycin, imatinib, isoniazid, nefazodone, nicardipine, propofol, protease inhibitors, quinidine, telithromycin, and verapamil. Solifenacin dose should not exceed 5 mg/day; monitor.
    Ketoconazole: May increase serum concentrations of solifenacin. Solifenacin dose should not exceed 5 mg/day; monitor.

Ethanol/Nutrition/Herb Interactions
    Food: Grapefruit juice may increase the serum level effects of solifenacin.
    Herb/Nutraceutical: St John's wort (*Hypericum*) may decrease the levels/effects of solifenacin.

Stability Store at room temperature between 15°C to 30°C (59°F to 86°F).

Mechanism of Action Inhibits muscarinic receptors resulting in decreased urinary bladder contraction, increased residual urine volume, and decreased detrusor muscle pressure.

Pharmacokinetics
    Distribution: V_d: 600 L
    Protein binding: 98% bound to alpha$_1$-acid glycoprotein
    Metabolism: Extensively hepatic; via N-oxidation and 4 R-hydroxylation, forms one active and three inactive metabolites; primary pathway for elimination is via CYP3A4 route
    Bioavailability: 90%
    Half-life elimination: 45-68 hours following chronic dosing
    Time to peak, plasma: 3-8 hours
    Excretion: Urine 69% (<15% as unchanged drug); feces 23%

Dosage
    Geriatrics: Base dosing on renal/hepatic function.
    Adults: Overactive bladder: Oral: 5 mg/day; if tolerated, may increase to 10 mg/day.
    Renal Impairment: Use with caution in reduced renal function; Cl$_{cr}$ <30 mL/minute: 5 mg/day
    Hepatic Impairment: Use with caution in reduced hepatic function: Moderate: 5 mg/day; Severe: Not recommended

Administration Swallow tablet whole; may take with liquids, without regard to food.

Monitoring Parameters Anticholinergic effects (eg, fixed and dilated pupils, blurred vision, tremors or dry skin)

Patient Information Do not take more than 1 dose/day. May cause blurred vision, dry mouth and constipation.

Special Geriatric Considerations In patients with Cl$_{cr}$ <30 mL/minute, doses >5 mg/day are not recommended.

Dosage Forms Excipient information presented when available (limited, particularly for generics); consult specific product labeling.
    Tablet: 5 mg, 10 mg

◆ **Solifenacin Succinate** *see* Solifenacin *on page 1482*

♦ **Solodyn**™ *see* Minocycline *on page 1046*
♦ **Soltamox**™ *see* Tamoxifen *on page 1515*
♦ **Solu-Cortef**® *see* Hydrocortisone *on page 762*
♦ **Solu-Medrol**® *see* MethylPREDNISolone *on page 1017*
♦ **Soma**® *see* Carisoprodol *on page 240*
♦ **Somavert**® *see* Pegvisomant *on page 1216*
♦ **Sominex**® **[OTC]** *see* DiphenhydrAMINE *on page 447*
♦ **Sominex**® **Maximum Strength [OTC]** *see* DiphenhydrAMINE *on page 447*
♦ **Somnote**® *see* Chloral Hydrate *on page 285*
♦ **Sonata**® *see* Zaleplon *on page 1693*
♦ **Soothe**® **[OTC]** *see* Artificial Tears *on page 124*

Sorbitol (SOR bi tole)

Related Information
  Treatment Options for Constipation *on page 1785*
Generic Available Yes
Pharmacologic Category Genitourinary Irrigant; Laxative, Osmotic
Use Genitourinary irrigant in transurethral prostatic resection or other transurethral resection or other transurethral surgical procedures; diuretic; humectant; sweetening agent; hyperosmotic laxative; facilitate the passage of sodium polystyrene sulfonate through the intestinal tract
Contraindications Anuria
Warnings/Precautions Use with caution in patients with severe cardiopulmonary or renal impairment and in patients unable to metabolize sorbitol; large volumes may result in fluid overload and/or electrolyte changes.
Adverse Reactions (Reflective of adult population; not specific for elderly)
  Frequency not defined.
  Cardiovascular: Edema
  Endocrine & metabolic: Fluid and electrolyte losses, hyperglycemia, lactic acidosis
  Gastrointestinal: Diarrhea, nausea, vomiting, abdominal discomfort, xerostomia
Overdosage/Toxicology Symptoms include nausea, diarrhea, fluid and electrolyte loss. Treatment is supportive to ensure fluid and electrolyte balance.
Stability Avoid storage in temperatures >150°F; do not freeze.
Mechanism of Action A polyalcoholic sugar with osmotic cathartic actions
Pharmacodynamics Onset of action: ~15-60 minutes
Pharmacokinetics
  Absorption: Oral, rectal: Poor
  Metabolism: Mainly in the liver to carbon dioxide (70%) and dextrose (30%)
  Elimination: In kidneys
Dosage
  Geriatrics & Adults:
    Hyperosmotic laxative (as single dose, at infrequent intervals):
      Oral: 30-150 mL (as 70% solution)
      Rectal enema: 120 mL as 25% to 30% solution
    Adjunct to sodium polystyrene sulfonate: 15 mL as 70% solution orally until diarrhea occurs (10-20 mL/2 hours) or 20-100 mL as an oral vehicle for the sodium polystyrene sulfonate resin
    When administered with charcoal:
      Oral: 4.3 mL/kg of 70% sorbitol with 1 g/kg of activated charcoal every 4 hours until first stool containing charcoal is passed
    Transurethral surgical procedures: Irrigation: Topical: 3% to 3.3% as transurethral surgical procedure irrigation
Monitoring Parameters Blood pressure, serum electrolytes, number of stools per day; when used as an irrigant in TURP. See Warnings/Precautions.
Patient Information Take with a full glass of water. When used as a cathartic, report failure of laxative effect, dizziness, weakness, and dehydration to physician, pharmacist, or nurse. Contact physician if more than 3-5 stools per day are produced.
Special Geriatric Considerations Causes for constipation must be evaluated prior to initiating treatment. Nonpharmacological dietary treatment should be initiated before laxative use. Sorbitol is as effective as lactulose but is much less expensive.
Dosage Forms Excipient information presented when available (limited, particularly for generics); consult specific product labeling.
  Solution, genitourinary irrigation: 3% (3000 mL, 5000 mL); 3.3% (2000 mL, 4000 mL)
  Solution, oral: 70% (30 mL, 480 mL, 3840 mL)
Selected References
  Lederle FA, Busch DL, Mattox KM, et al, "Cost-Effective Treatment of Constipation in the Elderly: A Randomized Double-Blend Comparison of Sorbitol and Lactulose," *Am J Med*, 1990, 89(5):597-601.

♦ **Sorine**® *see* Sotalol *on page 1485*

Sotalol (SOE ta lole)

Related Information
Beta-Blockers *on page 1751*

Medication Safety Issues
Sound-alike/look-alike issues:
Sotalol may be confused with Stadol®
Betapace® may be confused with Betapace AF®
Betapace AF® may be confused with Betapace®

U.S. Brand Names Betapace®; Betapace AF®; Sorine®

Canadian Brand Names Alti-Sotalol; Apo-Sotalol®; Betapace AF®; CO Sotalol; Gen-Sotalol; Lin-Sotalol; Novo-Sotalol; Nu-Sotalol; PMS-Sotalol; Rho®-Sotalol; Riva-Sotalol; Rylosol; Sotacor®

Index Terms Sotalol Hydrochloride

Generic Available Yes

Pharmacologic Category Antiarrhythmic Agent, Class II; Antiarrhythmic Agent, Class III; Beta-Adrenergic Blocker, Nonselective

Use Treatment of documented ventricular arrhythmias (ie, sustained ventricular tachycardia), that in the judgment of the physician are life-threatening; maintenance of normal sinus rhythm in patients with symptomatic atrial fibrillation and atrial flutter who are currently in sinus rhythm. Manufacturer states substitutions should not be made for Betapace AF™ since Betapace AF™ is distributed with a patient package insert specific for atrial fibrillation/flutter.

Contraindications Hypersensitivity to sotalol or any component of the formulation; bronchial asthma; sinus bradycardia; second- and third-degree AV block (unless a functioning pacemaker is present); congenital or acquired long QT syndromes; cardiogenic shock; uncontrolled congestive heart failure. Betapace AF® is contraindicated in patients with significantly reduced renal filtration (Cl_{cr} <40 mL/minute).

Warnings/Precautions [U.S. Boxed Warning] Manufacturer recommends initiation (or reinitiation) and doses increased in a hospital setting with continuous monitoring and staff familiar with the recognition and treatment of life-threatening arrhythmias. Dosage of sotalol should be adjusted gradually with 3 days between dosing increments to achieve steady-state concentrations, and to allow time to monitor QT intervals. Some experts will initiate therapy on an outpatient basis in a patient without heart disease or bradycardia, who has a baseline uncorrected QT interval <450 msec, and normal serum potassium and magnesium levels; close EKG monitoring during this time is necessary. ACC/AHA guidelines for management of atrial fibrillation also recommend that for outpatient initiation the patient not have risk factors predisposing to drug-induced ventricular proarrhythmia (Fuster, 2001). Creatinine clearance must be calculated prior to dosing. Use cautiously in the renally-impaired (dosage adjustment required).

Monitor and adjust dose to prevent QT_c prolongation. Concurrent use with other QT_c-prolonging drugs (including Class I and Class III antiarrhythmics) is generally not recommended; withhold for 3 half-lives. Watch for proarrhythmic effects. Correct electrolyte imbalances before initiating (especially hypokalemia and hypomagnesemia). Consider pre-existing conditions such as sick sinus syndrome before initiating. Conduction abnormalities can occur particularly sinus bradycardia. Use cautiously within the first 2 weeks post-MI (experience limited). Administer cautiously in compensated heart failure and monitor for a worsening of the condition. Use caution in patients with PVD (can aggravate arterial insufficiency). Beta-blocker therapy should not be withdrawn abruptly (particularly in patients with CAD), but gradually tapered to avoid acute tachycardia, hypertension, and/or ischemia. Use caution with concurrent use of beta-blockers and either verapamil or diltiazem; bradycardia or heart block can occur. Use cautiously in diabetics because it can mask prominent hypoglycemic symptoms. Use with caution in patients with bronchospastic disease, myasthenia gravis, peripheral vascular disease, or psychiatric disease. Use care with anesthetic agents which decrease myocardial function. Adequate alpha-blockade is required prior to use of any beta-blocker for patients with untreated pheochromocytoma.

[U.S. Boxed Warning]: Betapace® should not be substituted for Betapace® AF; Betapace® AF is distributed with an educational insert specifically for patients with atrial fibrillation/flutter.

Adverse Reactions (Reflective of adult population; not specific for elderly)
>10%:
Cardiovascular: Bradycardia (16%), chest pain (16%), palpitation (14%)
Central nervous system: Fatigue (20%), dizziness (20%), lightheadedness (12%)
Neuromuscular & skeletal: Weakness (13%)
Respiratory: Dyspnea (21%)
1% to 10%:
Cardiovascular: CHF (5%), peripheral vascular disorders (3%), edema (8%), abnormal ECG (7%), hypotension (6%), proarrhythmia (5%), syncope (5%)
(Continued)

Sotalol *(Continued)*

Central nervous system: Mental confusion (6%), anxiety (4%), headache (8%), sleep problems (8%), depression (4%)

Dermatologic: Itching/rash (5%)

Endocrine & metabolic: Sexual ability decreased (3%)

Gastrointestinal: Diarrhea (7%), nausea/vomiting (10%), stomach discomfort (3% to 6%), flatulence (2%)

Genitourinary: Impotence (2%)

Hematologic: Bleeding (2%)

Neuromuscular & skeletal: Paresthesia (4%), extremity pain (7%), back pain (3%)

Ocular: Visual problems (5%)

Respiratory: Upper respiratory problems (5% to 8%), asthma (2%)

Overdosage/Toxicology Symptoms of intoxication include cardiac disturbances, CNS toxicity, bronchospasm, hypoglycemia and hyperkalemia. The most common cardiac symptoms include hypotension and bradycardia. Atrioventricular block, intraventricular conduction disturbances, cardiogenic shock, and asystole may occur with severe overdose, especially with membrane-depressant drugs (eg, propranolol). CNS effects include convulsions, coma, and respiratory arrest and are commonly seen with propranolol and other membrane-depressant and lipid-soluble drugs. Treatment is symptomatic for seizures, hypotension, hyperkalemia and hypoglycemia. Bradycardia and hypotension resistant to atropine, isoproterenol or pacing may respond to glucagon. Wide QRS defects caused by membrane-depressant poisoning may respond to hypertonic sodium bicarbonate. Repeat-dose charcoal, hemoperfusion, or hemodialysis may be helpful in removal of only those beta-blockers with a small V_d, long half-life, or low intrinsic clearance (acebutolol, atenolol, nadolol, sotalol).

Drug Interactions

Amiodarone: May cause additive effects on QT_c prolongation as well as decreased heart rate, and has been associated with cardiac arrest in patients receiving beta-blockers.

Antacids (aluminum/magnesium) decrease sotalol blood levels; separate administration by 2 hours.

Antiarrhythmics: Concurrent use of Class Ia or Class III antiarrhythmics may result in additive QT_c prolongation; concurrent use is not recommended.

Beta$_2$ agonists: Effects may be diminished by concurrent sotalol; use caution.

Beta-blockers: Due to shared pharmacological effects, heart rate reductions may be additive; concurrent use is not recommended.

Calcium channel blockers: Concurrent use may lead to additive effects on AV conduction, ventricular contractility, and/or hypotension; use caution.

Cisapride: Concurrent use with sotalol increases malignant arrhythmias; contraindicated.

Clonidine: Sotalol may cause rebound hypertension after discontinuation of clonidine.

QT_c-prolonging drugs: Concurrent use may result in additive QT_c prolongation, potentially increasing the risk of malignant arrhythmias. Use of cisapride, mesoridazine, thioridazine, and pimozide with other QT_c-prolonging agents is contraindicated. Concurrent use of sotalol with Class I and Class III antiarrhythmics is not recommended; withhold for 3 half-lives. Use caution with other QT_c-prolonging agents (including bepridil, erythromycin, clarithromycin), fluoroquinolones (including moxifloxacin), haloperidol, and TCAs.

Phenothiazines (mesoridazine and thioridazine): Concurrent use may result in additive QT_c prolongation, potentially increasing the risk of malignant arrhythmias; contraindicated.

Pimozide: Concurrent use may result in additive QT_c prolongation, potentially increasing the risk of malignant arrhythmias; contraindicated.

Ethanol/Nutrition/Herb Interactions

Food: Sotalol peak serum concentrations may be decreased if taken with food.

Herb/Nutraceutical: Avoid ephedra (may worsen arrhythmia).

Stability Store at 25°C (77°F); excursions permitted to 15°C to 30°C (59°F to 86°F).

Mechanism of Action

Beta-blocker which contains both beta-adrenoreceptor-blocking (Vaughan Williams Class II) and cardiac action potential duration prolongation (Vaughan Williams Class III) properties

Class II effects: Increased sinus cycle length, slowed heart rate, decreased AV nodal conduction, and increased AV nodal refractoriness

Class III effects: Prolongation of the atrial and ventricular monophasic action potentials, and effective refractory prolongation of atrial muscle, ventricular muscle, and atrioventricular accessory pathways in both the antegrade and retrograde directions

Sotalol is a racemic mixture of *d*- and *l*-sotalol; both isomers have similar Class III antiarrhythmic effects while the *l*-isomer is responsible for virtually all of the beta-blocking activity

Sotalol has both beta$_1$- and beta$_2$-receptor blocking activity

The beta-blocking effect of sotalol is a noncardioselective [half maximal at about 80 mg/day and maximal at doses of 320-640 mg/day]. Significant beta-blockade occurs at oral doses as low as 25 mg/day.

The Class III effects are seen only at oral doses ≥160 mg/day

Pharmacodynamics
  Onset of action: Rapid, 1-2 hours
  Peak effect: 2.5-4 hours
  Duration: 8-16 ours

Pharmacokinetics
  Absorption: Decreased 20% to 30% by meals
  Distribution: Low lipid solubility
  Protein binding: Not protein bound
  Metabolism: Sotalol is not metabolized
  Bioavailability: 90% to 100%
  Half-life: 12 hours
  Elimination: Unchanged through kidney

Dosage
  Geriatrics & Adults: Sotalol should be initiated and doses increased in a hospital with facilities for cardiac rhythm monitoring and assessment. Proarrhythmic events can occur after initiation of therapy and with each upward dosage adjustment.

  Ventricular arrhythmias (Betapace®, Sorine®): Oral:
    Initial: 80 mg twice daily; dose may be increased gradually to 240-320 mg/day; allow 3 days between dosing increments (to attain steady-state plasma concentrations and to allow monitoring of QT intervals).
    Usual range: Most patients respond to 160-320 mg/day in 2-3 divided doses.
    Maximum: Some patients, with life-threatening refractory ventricular arrhythmias, may require doses as high as 480-640 mg/day; prescribed ONLY when the potential benefit outweighs the increased of adverse events.

  Atrial fibrillation or atrial flutter (Betapace AF®): Oral: Initial: 80 mg twice daily
    Note: If the initial dose does not reduce the frequency of relapses of atrial fibrillation/flutter and is tolerated without excessive QT prolongation (not >520 msec) after 3 days, the dose may be increased to 120 mg twice daily. This may be further increased to 160 mg twice daily if response is inadequate and QT prolongation is not excessive.

  Renal Impairment: Adults: Impaired renal function can increase the terminal half-life, resulting in increased drug accumulation. Sotalol (Betapace AF®) is contraindicated per the manufacturer for treatment of atrial fibrillation/flutter in patients with a Cl_{cr} <40 mL/minute.
    Ventricular arrhythmias (Betapace®, Sorine®):
      Cl_{cr} >60 mL/minute: Administer every 12 hours.
      Cl_{cr} 30-60 mL/minute: Administer every 24 hours.
      Cl_{cr} 10-30 mL/minute: Administer every 36-48 hours.
      Cl_{cr} <10 mL/minute: Individualize dose.
    Atrial fibrillation/flutter (Betapace AF®):
      Cl_{cr} >60 mL/minute: Administer every 12 hours.
      Cl_{cr} 40-60 mL/minute: Administer every 24 hours.
      Cl_{cr} <40 mL/minute: Use is contraindicated.

    Dialysis: Hemodialysis would be expected to reduce sotalol plasma concentrations because sotalol is not bound to plasma proteins and does not undergo extensive metabolism. Administer dose postdialysis or administer supplemental 80 mg dose. Peritoneal dialysis does not remove sotalol; supplemental dose is not necessary.

Administration Food may decrease adsorption

Monitoring Parameters Serum magnesium, potassium, EKG, pulse

Patient Information Seek emergency help if palpitations occur; do not discontinue abruptly or change dose without notifying physician; take on an empty stomach

Additional Information If patients are receiving another antiarrhythmic, it is best to withdraw the agent, with careful monitoring, for at least 2-3 half-lives of the agent if clinical condition allows before initiating sotalol; treatment with sotalol has been initiated in some with patients receiving I.V. lidocaine without problems; if patients are receiving amiodarone, **do not** start sotalol until QT interval is normal

Special Geriatric Considerations Since elderly frequently have Cl_{cr} <60 mL/minute, attention to dose, creatinine clearance, and monitoring is important. Make dosage adjustments at 3-day intervals or after 5-6 doses at any dosage.

Dosage Forms Excipient information presented when available (limited, particularly for generics); consult specific product labeling.
  Tablet, as hydrochloride: 80 mg, 80 mg [AF], 120 mg, 120 mg [AF], 160 mg, 160 mg [AF], 240 mg
    Betapace® [light blue]: 80 mg, 120 mg, 160 mg, 240 mg
    Betapace AF® [white]: 80 mg, 120 mg, 160 mg
    Sorine® [white]: 80 mg, 120 mg, 160 mg, 240 mg
(Continued)

Sotalol *(Continued)*

Extemporaneously Prepared To make a 5 mg/mL oral solution, using a 6-ounce amber plastic prescription bottle, add five sotalol 120 mg tablets to 120 mL of simple syrup containing 0.1% sodium benzoate (tablets do not need to be crushed). Shake well. Allow tablets to hydrate for ~2 hours; shake intermittently until tablets completely disintegrate. Store at room temperature; shake well before use. Stable for 3 months. (Refer to manufacturer's current labeling.)

Selected References

Fuster V, Ryden LE, Asinger RW, et al, "ACC/AHA/ESC Guidelines for the Mangement of Patients with ATrial Fibrillation. A Report of the American College of Cardiology/ American Heart Associateion Task Force on Practice Guidelines and the European Society of Cardiology Committee for Practice Guidelines and Policy Conferences (Committee to Develop Guidelines for the Management of Patients With Atrial Fibrillation)," *J Am Coll Cardiol*, 2001, 38(4):1231-66.

♦ **Sotalol Hydrochloride** *see Sotalol on page 1485*
♦ **Sotradecol®** *see Sodium Tetradecyl on page 1482*
♦ **Spacol [DSC]** *see Hyoscyamine on page 778*
♦ **Spacol T/S [DSC]** *see Hyoscyamine on page 778*
♦ **SPD417** *see Carbamazepine on page 231*
♦ **Spectracef®** *see Cefditoren on page 255*
♦ **SPI 0211** *see Lubiprostone on page 942*
♦ **Spiriva®** *see Tiotropium on page 1578*

Spironolactone *(speer on oh LAK tone)*

Medication Safety Issues
Sound-alike/look-alike issues:
Aldactone® may be confused with Aldactazide®

International issues:
Aldactone®: Brand name for potassium canrenoate in Austria, Czech Republic, Germany, and Hungary

U.S. Brand Names Aldactone®
Canadian Brand Names Aldactone®; Novo-Spiroton
Generic Available Yes
Pharmacologic Category Diuretic, Potassium-Sparing; Selective Aldosterone Blocker
Use Management of edema associated with excessive aldosterone excretion; hypertension; congestive heart failure; primary hyperaldosteronism; hypokalemia; treatment of hirsutism; cirrhosis of liver accompanied by edema or ascites
Contraindications Hypersensitivity to spironolactone or any component of the formulation; anuria; acute renal insufficiency; significant impairment of renal excretory function; hyperkalemia
Warnings/Precautions Avoid potassium supplements, potassium-containing salt substitutes, a diet rich in potassium, or other drugs that can cause hyperkalemia. Excess amounts can lead to profound diuresis with fluid and electrolyte loss; close medical supervision and dose evaluation are required. Watch for and correct electrolyte disturbances; adjust dose to avoid dehydration. In cirrhosis, avoid electrolyte and acid/base imbalances that might lead to hepatic encephalopathy. Gynecomastia is related to dose and duration of therapy. Discontinue use prior to adrenal vein catheterization. When evaluating a heart failure patient for spironolactone treatment, creatinine should be ≤2.5 mg/dL in men or ≤2 mg/dL in women and potassium <5 mEq/L. **[U.S. Boxed Warning]: Shown to be a tumorigen in chronic toxicity animal studies. Avoid unnecessary use.**
Adverse Reactions (Reflective of adult population; not specific for elderly)
Incidence of adverse events is not always reported. (Mean daily dose: 26 mg)

Cardiovascular: Edema (2%, placebo 2%)
Central nervous system: Disorders (23%, placebo 21%) which may include drowsiness, lethargy, headache, mental confusion, drug fever, ataxia, fatigue
Dermatologic: Maculopapular, erythematous cutaneous eruptions, urticaria, hirsutism, eosinophilia
Endocrine & metabolic: Gynecomastia (men 9%; placebo 1%), breast pain (men 2%; placebo 0.1%), serious hyperkalemia (2%, placebo 1%), hyponatremia, dehydration, hyperchloremic metabolic acidosis in decompensated hepatic cirrhosis, inability to achieve or maintain an erection, irregular menses, amenorrhea, postmenopausal bleeding
Gastrointestinal: Disorders (29%, placebo 29%) which may include anorexia, nausea, cramping, diarrhea, gastric bleeding, ulceration, gastritis, vomiting
Genitourinary: Disorders (12%, placebo 11%)
Hematologic: Agranulocytosis
Hepatic: Cholestatic/hepatocellular toxicity

Renal: Increased BUN concentration

Respiratory: Disorders (32%, placebo 34%)

Miscellaneous: Deepening of the voice, anaphylactic reaction, breast cancer

Overdosage/Toxicology Symptoms include drowsiness, confusion, clinical signs of dehydration and electrolyte imbalance, and hyperkalemia. Ingestion of large amounts of potassium-sparing diuretics, may result in life-threatening hyperkalemia. This can be treated with I.V. glucose, with concurrent regular insulin. Sodium bicarbonate may also be used as a temporary measure. If needed, Kayexalate® oral or rectal solutions in sorbitol may also be used.

Drug Interactions

ACE inhibitors can cause hyperkalemia, especially in patients with renal impairment, potassium-rich diets, or on other drugs causing hyperkalemia; avoid concurrent use or monitor closely.

Cholestyramine can cause hyperchloremic acidosis in cirrhotic patients; avoid concurrent use.

Digoxin's positive inotropic effect may be reduced; serum levels of digoxin may increase.

Mitotane loses its effect; avoid concurrent use.

Potassium supplements may increase potassium retention and cause hyperkalemia; avoid concurrent use.

Salicylates and NSAIDs may interfere with the natriuretic action of spironolactone.

Ethanol/Nutrition/Herb Interactions

Food: Food increases absorption.

Herb/Nutraceutical: Avoid natural licorice (due to mineralocorticoid activity)

Stability Protect from light.

Mechanism of Action Competes with aldosterone for receptor sites in the distal renal tubules, increasing sodium chloride and water excretion while conserving potassium and hydrogen ions; may block the effect of aldosterone on arteriolar smooth muscle as well

Pharmacodynamics Duration of action: 2-3 days

Pharmacokinetics

Protein binding: 91% to 98%

Metabolism: In the liver to multiple metabolites, including canrenone (active)

Half-life: 78-84 minutes

Time to peak serum concentrations: Oral: Within 1-3 hours (primarily as the active metabolite)

Elimination: Urinary and biliary

In older adults, levels of the metabolites were found to be twice as high as in younger patients

Dosage

Geriatrics: Oral: Initial: 25-50 mg/day in 1-2 divided doses; increase by 25-50 mg every 5 days as needed. Adjust for renal impairment.

Adults: To reduce delay in onset of effect, a loading dose of 2 or 3 times the daily dose may be administered on the first day of therapy. Oral:

Edema, hypokalemia: 25-200 mg/day in 1-2 divided doses

Hypertension (JNC 7): 25-50 mg/day in 1-2 divided doses

Diagnosis of primary aldosteronism: 100-400 mg/day in 1-2 divided doses

Acne in women (unlabeled use): 25-200 mg once daily

Hirsutism in women (unlabeled use): 50-200 mg/day in 1-2 divided doses

CHF, severe (with ACE inhibitor and a loop diuretic ± digoxin): 12.5-25 mg/day; maximum daily dose: 50 mg (higher doses may occasionallly be used). In the RALES trial, 25 mg every other day was the lowest maintenance dose possible. **Note:** If potassium >5.4 mEq/L, consider dosage reduction.

Renal Impairment:

Cl_{cr} 10-50 mL/minute: Administer every 12-24 hours.

Cl_{cr} <10 mL/minute: Avoid use.

Monitoring Parameters Blood pressure, serum electrolytes (potassium, sodium), renal function, I & O ratios and daily weight throughout therapy

CHF: Potassium levels and renal function should be checked in 3 days and 1 week after initiation, then every 2-4 weeks for 3-12 months, then every 3-6 months.

Test Interactions May cause false elevation in serum digoxin concentrations measured by RIA

Patient Information Avoid hazardous activity such as driving, until response to drug is known (may cause lethargy or confusion); take with meals or milk; avoid excessive ingestion of foods high in potassium or use of salt substitutes. Take in the morning; take the last dose of multiple doses no later than 6 PM unless instructed otherwise.

Additional Information A recent study found that 25 mg of spironolactone added to a regimen of a loop diuretic, ACE inhibitor with or without digoxin, decreased morbidity and mortality in NYHA Class III or IV heart failure.

(Continued)

Spironolactone *(Continued)*

To reduce delay in onset of effect, a loading dose of 2 or 3 times the daily dose may be administered on the first day of therapy; it is recommended the drug be discontinued several days prior to adrenal vein catheterization; adverse reactions are dose related and usually disappear upon drug withdrawal, except possibly gynecomastia.

Diuretic effect may be delayed 2-3 days and maximum hypertensive may be delayed 2-3 weeks.

Special Geriatric Considerations When used in combination with ACE inhibitors, monitor patient for hyperkalemia.

Dosage Forms Excipient information presented when available (limited, particularly for generics); consult specific product labeling.
Tablet: 25 mg, 50 mg, 100 mg

Selected References

Bozkurt B, Agoston I, and Knowlton AA, "Complications of Inappropriate Use of Spironolactone in Heart Failure: When an Old Medicine Spirals Out of New Guidelines," *J Am Coll Cardiol*, 2003, 41(2):211-4.

Hunt SA, Abraham WT, Chin MH, et al, "ACC/AHA 2005 Guideline Update for the Diagnosis and Management of Chronic Heart Failure in the Adult-Summary Article A Report of the American College of Cardiology/ American Heart Association Task Force on Practice Guidelines (Writing Committee to Update the 2001 Guidelines for the Evaluation and Management of Heart Failure)," *J Am Coll Cardiol*, 2005, 46(6):1116-43.

Hunter MH and Carek PJ, "Evaluation and Treatment of Women With Hirsutism," *Am Fam Physician*, 2003, 67(12):2565-72.

Juurlink DN, Mamdani MM, Lee DS, et al, "Rates of Hyperkalemia After Publication of the Randomized Aldactone Evaluation Study," *N Engl J Med*, 2004, 351(6):543-51.

Pitt B, Zannad F, Remme WJ, et al, "The Effect of Spironolactone on Morbidity and Mortality in Patients With Severe Heart Failure," *N Engl J Med*, 1999, 341(10):709-17.

Streptokinase *(strep toe KYE nase)*

Medication Safety Issues
High alert medication: The Institute for Safe Medication Practices (ISMP) includes this medication (I.V.) among its list of drugs which have a heightened risk of causing significant patient harm when used in error.

U.S. Brand Names Streptase®
Canadian Brand Names Streptase®
Index Terms SK
Generic Available No
Pharmacologic Category Thrombolytic Agent
Use Thrombolytic agent used in treatment of recent severe or massive deep vein thrombosis, pulmonary emboli, myocardial infarction, and occluded arteriovenous cannulas

Contraindications Hypersensitivity to anistreplase, streptokinase, or any component of the formulation; active internal bleeding; history of CVA; recent (within 2 months) intracranial or intraspinal surgery or trauma; intracranial neoplasm, arteriovenous malformation, or aneurysm; known bleeding diathesis; severe uncontrolled hypertension

Warnings/Precautions Concurrent heparin anticoagulation can contribute to bleeding; careful attention to all potential bleeding sites. I.M. injections and nonessential handling of the patient should be avoided. Venipunctures should be performed carefully and only when necessary. If arterial puncture is necessary, use an upper extremity vessel that can be manually compressed. If serious bleeding occurs then the infusion of streptokinase and heparin should be stopped. Use with caution in patients >75 years of age, patients with a history of cardiac arrhythmias, septic thrombophlebitis or occluded AV cannula at seriously infected site, patients with a high likelihood of left heart thrombus (eg, mitral stenosis with atrial fibrillation), major surgery within last 10 days, GI bleeding, diabetic hemorrhagic retinopathy, subacute bacterial endocarditis, cerebrovascular disease, recent trauma including cardiopulmonary resuscitation, or severe hypertension (systolic BP >180 mm Hg and/or diastolic BP >110 mm Hg); antibodies to streptokinase remain for 3-6 months after initial dose, use another thrombolytic enzyme (ie, alteplase) if thrombolytic therapy is indicated in patients with prior streptokinase therapy.

Coronary thrombolysis may result in reperfusion arrhythmias. Hypotension, occasionally severe, can occur (not from bleeding or anaphylaxis). Follow standard MI management. Rare anaphylactic reactions can occur. Cautious repeat administration in patients who have received anistreplase or streptokinase within 1 year (streptokinase antibody may decrease effectiveness or risk of allergic reactions).

Streptokinase is not indicated for restoration of patency of intravenous catheters. Serious adverse events relating to the use of streptokinase in the restoration of patency of occluded intravenous catheters have involved the use of high doses of streptokinase in small volumes (250,000 international units in 2 mL). Uses of lower doses of streptokinase in infusions over several hours, generally into partially occluded catheters, or local instillation into the catheter lumen and subsequent aspiration, have been described in the medical literature. Healthcare providers should consider the risk for potentially life-threatening reactions (eg, hypotension, hypersensitivity reactions, apnea, bleeding) associated with the use of streptokinase in the management of occluded intravenous catheters.

Adverse Reactions (Reflective of adult population; not specific for elderly) As with all drugs which may affect hemostasis, bleeding is the major adverse effect associated with streptokinase. Hemorrhage may occur at virtually any site. Risk is dependent on multiple variables, including the dosage administered, concurrent use of multiple agents which alter hemostasis, and patient predisposition (including hypertension). Rapid lysis of coronary artery thrombi by thrombolytic agents may be associated with reperfusion-related atrial and/or ventricular arrhythmia.

>10%:
  Cardiovascular: Hypotension
  Local: Injection site bleeding
1% to 10%:
  Central nervous system: Fever (1% to 4%)
  Dermatologic: Bruising, rash, pruritus
  Gastrointestinal: Gastrointestinal hemorrhage, nausea, vomiting
  Genitourinary: Genitourinary hemorrhage
  Hematologic: Anemia
  Neuromuscular & skeletal: Muscle pain
  Ocular: Eye hemorrhage, periorbital edema
  Respiratory: Bronchospasm, epistaxis
  Miscellaneous: Diaphoresis hemorrhage, gingival hemorrhage

Additional cardiovascular events associated with use in MI: Asystole, AV block, cardiac arrest, cardiac tamponade, cardiogenic shock, electromechanical dissociation, heart failure, mitral regurgitation, myocardial rupture, pericardial effusion, pericarditis, pulmonary edema, recurrent ischemia/infarction, thromboembolism, ventricular tachycardia

Overdosage/Toxicology Symptoms include epistaxis, bleeding gums, hematoma, spontaneous ecchymoses, and oozing at catheter site. If uncontrollable bleeding occurs, discontinue infusion; whole blood or blood products may be used to reverse bleeding.

Drug Interactions
  Aminocaproic acid (antifibrinolytic agent) may decrease effectiveness of thrombolytic agents.
  Drugs which affect platelet function (eg, NSAIDs, dipyridamole, ticlopidine, clopidogrel, IIb/IIIa antagonists) may potentiate the risk of hemorrhage; use with caution.
  Heparin and aspirin: Use with aspirin and heparin may increase bleeding over aspirin and heparin alone. However, aspirin and heparin were used concurrently in the majority of patients in some major clinical studies of streptokinase.
  Warfarin or oral anticoagulants: Risk of bleeding may be increased during concurrent therapy.

Ethanol/Nutrition/Herb Interactions Herb/Nutraceutical: Avoid cat's claw, dong quai, evening primrose, feverfew, red clover, horse chestnut, garlic, green tea, ginseng, ginkgo (all have additional antiplatelet activity).
(Continued)

Streptokinase *(Continued)*

Stability Streptokinase, a white lyophilized powder, may have a slight yellow color in solution due to the presence of albumin. Intact vials should be stored at room temperature. Reconstituted solutions should be refrigerated and are stable for 24 hours.

Stability of parenteral admixture at room temperature (25°C) is 8 hours; 24 hours when refrigerated (4°C).

Mechanism of Action Activates the conversion of plasminogen to plasmin by forming a complex, exposing plasminogen-activating site, and cleaving a peptide bond that converts plasminogen to plasmin; plasmin degrades fibrin, fibrinogen and other procoagulant proteins into soluble fragments; effective both outside and within the formed thrombus/embolus

Pharmacodynamics

Onset of effect: Following injection, activation of plasminogen occurs almost immediately

Duration: Fibrinolytic effects last only a few hours, while anticoagulant effects can persist for 12-24 hours

Pharmacokinetics

Half-life: 83 minutes

Elimination: By circulating antibodies and via the reticuloendothelial system

Dosage

Geriatrics & Adults: I.V.:

Note: Antibodies to streptokinase remain for at least 3-6 months after initial dose: See Warnings/Precautions. An intradermal skin test of 100 units has been suggested to predict allergic response to streptokinase. If a positive reaction is not seen after 15-20 minutes, a therapeutic dose may be administered.

Guidelines for acute myocardial infarction (AMI): I.V.: 1.5 million units over 60 minutes

Administration:

Dilute two 750,000 unit vials of streptokinase with 5 mL dextrose 5% in water (D_5W) each, gently swirl to dissolve.

Add this dose of the 1.5 million units to 150 mL D_5W.

This should be infused over 60 minutes; an in-line filter ≥0.45 micron should be used.

Monitor for the first few hours for signs of anaphylaxis or allergic reaction. **Infusion should be slowed if lowering of 25 mm Hg in blood pressure or terminated if asthmatic symptoms appear**.

Note: If heparin is administered, start when aPTT is less than 2 times the upper limit of control; do not use a bolus, but initiate infusion adjusted to a target a PTT of 1.5-2 times the upper limit of control. If heparin is not administered by infusion, initiate 7500-12,500 units SubQ every 12 hours.

Guidelines for acute pulmonary embolism (APE): I.V.: 3 million unit dose over 24 hours

Administration:

Dilute four 750,000 unit vials of streptokinase with 5 mL dextrose 5% in water (D_5W) each, gently swirl to dissolve.

Add this dose of 3 million units to 250 mL D_5W, an in-line filter ≥0.45 micron should be used.

Administer 250,000 units (23 mL) over 30 minutes followed by 100,000 units/ hour (9 mL/hour) for 24 hours.

Monitor for the first few hours for signs of anaphylaxis or allergic reaction. **Infusion should be slowed if blood pressure is lowered by 25 mm Hg or if asthmatic symptoms appear**.

Begin heparin 1000 units/hour about 3-4 hours after completion of streptokinase infusion or when PTT is <100 seconds.

Guidelines for thromboses: I.V.: Administer 250,000 units to start, then 100,000 units/hour for 24-72 hours depending on location.

Cannula occlusion: 250,000 units into cannula, clamp for 2 hours, then aspirate contents and flush with normal saline; **Not recommended; see Warnings/ Precautions**

Administration

For I.V. or intracoronary use only; do not administer by I.M. injections

Monitoring Parameters Before therapy, hematocrit, platelet count, PT, APTT, thrombin time (TT), fibrinogen concentration; check PT, APTT, TT, or fibrinogen level every 4 hours after starting therapy; monitor for bleeding every 15 minutes for the first hour of therapy

Special Geriatric Considerations Investigators applied analysis to data for patients ≥75 years of age from two large trials studying the impact of streptokinase on patient outcome after acute myocardial infarction. Their conclusion was that age alone is not a contraindication to the use of streptokinase and that thrombolytic therapy is cost-effective and is beneficial toward the survival of elderly patients. Additional studies are needed to determine if a weight-adjusted dose will maintain efficacy but decrease adverse events such as stroke.

Dosage Forms Excipient information presented when available (limited, particularly for generics); consult specific product labeling. [DSC] = Discontinued product

Injection, powder for reconstitution: 250,000 int. units; 750,000 int. units; 1,500,000 int. units [DSC]

Selected References

Krumholz HM, Pasternak RC, Weinstein MC, et al, "Cost Effectiveness of Thrombolytic Therapy With Streptokinase in Elderly Patients With Suspected Acute Myocardial Infarction," *N Engl J Med*, 1992, 327(1):7-13.

Streptomycin (strep toe MYE sin)

Related Information
Antimicrobial Activity Against Selected Organisms *on page 1728*

Medication Safety Issues
Sound-alike/look-alike issues:
Streptomycin may be confused with streptozocin

Index Terms Streptomycin Sulfate

Generic Available Yes

Pharmacologic Category Antibiotic, Aminoglycoside; Antitubercular Agent

Use Combination therapy of active tuberculosis; used in combination with other agents for treatment of streptococcal or enterococcal endocarditis, mycobacterial infections, plague, tularemia, and brucellosis

Contraindications Hypersensitivity to streptomycin or any component of the formulation

Warnings/Precautions [U.S. Boxed Warning]: May cause neurotoxicity, nephrotoxicity, and/or neuromuscular blockade and respiratory paralysis; usual risk factors include pre-existing renal impairment, concomitant neuro-/nephrotoxic medications, advanced age and dehydration. The drug's neurotoxicity can result in respiratory paralysis from neuromuscular blockade, especially when the drug is given soon after anesthesia or muscle relaxants. Use with caution in patients with pre-existing vertigo, tinnitus, hearing loss, neuromuscular disorders, or renal impairment; modify dosage in patients with renal impairment; ototoxicity is directly proportional to the amount of drug given and the duration of treatment; tinnitus or vertigo are indications of vestibular injury and impending bilateral irreversible damage; renal damage is usually reversible. **[U.S. Boxed Warning]: Parenteral form should be used only where appropriate audiometric and laboratory testing facilities are available.** Prolonged use may result in fungal or bacterial superinfection, including *C. difficile*-associated diarrhea and pseudomembranous colitis.

Adverse Reactions (Reflective of adult population; not specific for elderly)
Frequency not defined.
Cardiovascular: Hypotension
Central nervous system: Neurotoxicity, drowsiness, headache, drug fever, paresthesia
Dermatologic: Skin rash
Gastrointestinal: Nausea, vomiting
Hematologic: Eosinophilia, anemia
Neuromuscular & skeletal: Arthralgia, weakness, tremor
Otic: Ototoxicity (auditory), ototoxicity (vestibular)
Renal: Nephrotoxicity
Respiratory: Difficulty in breathing

Overdosage/Toxicology Symptoms include ototoxicity, nephrotoxicity, and neuromuscular toxicity. The treatment of choice following a single acute overdose appears to be the maintenance of urine output of at least 3 mL/kg/hour. Dialysis is of questionable value in the enhancement of aminoglycoside elimination. If required, hemodialysis is preferred over peritoneal dialysis in patients with normal renal function. Careful hydration may be all that is required to promote diuresis and therefore enhance elimination.

Drug Interactions
Increased/prolonged effect: Depolarizing and nondepolarizing neuromuscular blocking agents
Increased toxicity: Concurrent use of amphotericin may increase nephrotoxicity

Stability Depending upon manufacturer, reconstituted solution remains stable for 2-4 weeks when refrigerated. Exposure to light causes darkening of solution without apparent loss of potency.

Mechanism of Action Inhibits bacterial protein synthesis by binding directly to the 30S ribosomal subunits causing faulty peptide sequence to form in the protein chain

Pharmacodynamics Bactericidal at an alkaline pH

Pharmacokinetics
Protein binding: 34%; CNS penetration is fair
Half-life: 2-4.7 hours and is prolonged with renal impairment (up to 100 hours)
Time to peak serum concentration: I.M.: Within 1 hour
(Continued)

Streptomycin *(Continued)*

Elimination: Almost completely (90%) as unchanged drug in urine, with small amounts (1%) excreted in bile, saliva, sweat, and tears

Dosage

Geriatrics: I.M.: 10 mg/kg/day, not to exceed 750 mg/day; dosing interval should be adjusted for renal function. Some authors suggest not to give more than 5 days/week or give as 20-25 mg/kg/dose twice weekly.

Adults:

Brucellosis: I.M.: 1 g/day for 14-21 days (with doxycycline, 100 mg twice daily for 6 weeks)

Endocarditis: I.M.:

Enterococcal: 1 g every 12 hours for 2 weeks, 500 mg every 12 hours for 4 weeks in combination with penicillin

Streptococcal: 1 g every 12 hours for 1 week

***Mycobacterium avium* complex:** I.M.: Adjunct therapy (with macrolide, rifamycin, and ethambutol): 15 mg/kg 3 times/week for first 2-3 months for severe disease

Plague: I.M.: 15 mg/kg (or 1 g) every 12 hours until the patient is afebrile for at least 3 days

Tuberculosis: I.M.:

Daily therapy: 15 mg/kg/day (maximum: 1 g)

Directly observed therapy (DOT), twice weekly: 25-30 mg/kg (maximum: 1.5 g)

Directly observed therapy (DOT), 3 times/week: 25-30 mg/kg (maximum: 1.5 g)

Tularemia: I.M.: 10-15 mg/kg every 12 hours (maximum: 2 g/day) for 7-10 days or until patient is afebrile for 5-7 days

Renal Impairment:

Cl_{cr} 10-50 mL/minute: Administer every 24-72 hours.

Cl_{cr} <10 mL/minute: Administer every 72-96 hours.

Removed by hemo- and peritoneal dialysis: Administer dose postdialysis.

Administration

Inject deep I.M. into large muscle mass; I.V. administration is not recommended

Monitoring Parameters BUN and serum creatinine, hearing (if appropriate); in tuberculosis patients, monitor sputum culture and chest x-ray 2-3 months into treatment and at its completion

Reference Range

Therapeutic: Peak: 20-30 mcg/mL; trough: <5 mcg/mL

Toxic: Peak: >50 mcg/mL; trough: >10 mcg/mL

Test Interactions False-positive urine glucose with Benedict's solution or Clinitest®; penicillin may decrease aminoglycoside serum concentrations *in vitro*

Patient Information Report any unusual symptom

Additional Information Eighth cranial nerve damage is usually preceded by high-pitched tinnitus, roaring noises, sense of fullness in ears, or impaired hearing and may persist for weeks after drug is discontinued.

Special Geriatric Considerations Streptomycin is indicated for persons from endemic areas of drug-resistant *Mycobacterium tuberculosis* or who are HIV infected. Since most older patients acquired the *M. tuberculosis* infection prior to the availability of effective chemotherapy, isoniazid and rifampin are usually effective unless resistant organisms are suspected or the patient is HIV infected. Adjust dose interval for renal function.

Dosage Forms Excipient information presented when available (limited, particularly for generics); consult specific product labeling.

Injection, powder for reconstitution: 1 g

Selected References

Bass JB Jr, Farer LS, Hopewell PC, et al, "Treatment of Tuberculosis and Tuberculosis Infection in Adults and Children," *Am J Respir Crit Care Med*, 1994, 149(5):1359-74.

Stead WW and Dutt AK, "Tuberculosis: A Special Problem in the Elderly," *Principles of Geriatric Medicine and Gerontology*, 2nd ed, 1990, 522.

Yoshikawa TT, "Tuberculosis in Aging Adults," *J Am Geriatr Soc*, 1992, 40(2):178-87.

◆ **Streptomycin Sulfate** *see* Streptomycin *on page 1493*

◆ **Striant®** *see* Testosterone *on page 1537*

◆ **Stri-dex® [OTC]** *see* Salicylic Acid *on page 1441*

◆ **Stri-dex® Body Focus [OTC]** *see* Salicylic Acid *on page 1441*

◆ **Stri-dex® Facewipes To Go™ [OTC]** *see* Salicylic Acid *on page 1441*

◆ **Stri-dex® Maximum Strength [OTC]** *see* Salicylic Acid *on page 1441*

◆ **Strong Iodine Solution** *see* Potassium Iodide and Iodine *on page 1291*

◆ **Stye® Ophthalmic Ointment [OTC]** *see* Ocular Lubricant *on page 1144*

◆ **Sublimaze®** *see* Fentanyl *on page 609*

◆ **Subutex®** *see* Buprenorphine *on page 195*

Sucralfate (soo KRAL fate)

Medication Safety Issues
Sound-alike/look-alike issues:
Sucralfate may be confused with salsalate
Carafate® may be confused with Cafergot®

U.S. Brand Names Carafate®

Canadian Brand Names Novo-Sucralate; Nu-Sucralate; PMS-Sucralate; Sulcrate®; Sulcrate® Suspension Plus

Index Terms Aluminum Sucrose Sulfate, Basic

Generic Available Yes

Pharmacologic Category Gastrointestinal Agent, Miscellaneous

Use Short-term management of duodenal ulcers

Unlabeled/Investigational Use Treatment of gastric ulcers, stomatitis due to cancer chemotherapy and other causes of esophageal and gastric erosions (suspension), GERD, esophagitis, NSAID mucosal damage; prevention of stress ulcers; postsclerotherapy for esophageal variceal bleeding

Contraindications Hypersensitivity to sucralfate or any component of the formulation

Warnings/Precautions Successful therapy with sucralfate should not be expected to alter the posthealing frequency of recurrence or the severity of duodenal ulceration; use with caution in patients with chronic renal failure who have an impaired excretion of absorbed aluminum. Because of the potential for sucralfate to alter the absorption of some drugs, separate administration (take other medication 2 hours before sucralfate) should be considered when alterations in bioavailability are believed to be critical.

Adverse Reactions (Reflective of adult population; not specific for elderly)
1% to 10%: Gastrointestinal: Constipation

Overdosage/Toxicology Toxicity is minimal. May cause constipation.

Drug Interactions Decreased effect: Digoxin, phenytoin (hydantoins), warfarin, ketoconazole, quinidine, ciprofloxacin, norfloxacin (quinolones), tetracycline, theophylline; because of the potential for sucralfate to alter the absorption of some drugs, separate administration (take other medications 2 hours before sucralfate) should be considered when alterations in bioavailability are believed to be critical
Note: When given with aluminum-containing antacids, may increase serum/body aluminum concentrations (see Warnings/Precautions)

Ethanol/Nutrition/Herb Interactions Food: Sucralfate may interfere with absorption of vitamin A, vitamin D, vitamin E, and vitamin K.

Stability Suspension: Shake well. Refrigeration is **not** necessary; do **not** freeze.

Mechanism of Action Forms a complex by binding with positively charged proteins in exudates, forming a viscous paste-like, adhesive substance. This selectively forms a protective coating that protects the lining against peptic acid, pepsin, and bile salts.

Pharmacodynamics
Onset of paste formation and ulcer adhesion: within 1-2 hours
Duration: Up to 6 hours

Pharmacokinetics
Absorption: Oral: <5% of dose
Metabolism: Not metabolized
Protein binding: Unbound in GI tract to aluminum and sucrose octasulfate
Elimination: Small amounts that are absorbed are excreted in urine as unchanged compounds

Dosage
Geriatrics & Adults:
Stress ulcer prophylaxis: Oral: 1 g 4 times/day
Stress ulcer treatment: Oral: 1 g every 4 hours
Treatment of duodenal ulcer: Oral:
Initial treatment: 1 g 4 times/day, 1 hour before meals or food and at bedtime for 4-8 weeks, or alternatively 2 g twice daily; treatment is recommended for 4-8 weeks in adults, the elderly will require 12 weeks.
Maintenance/prophylaxis of duodenal ulcer: 1 g twice daily
Stomatitis (unlabeled use): Oral: 1 g/10 mL suspension; swish and spit or swish and swallow 4 times/day.

Renal Impairment: Aluminum salt is minimally absorbed (<5%), however, may accumulate in renal failure.

Administration Tablet may be broken or dissolved in water before ingestion. Administer with water on an empty stomach.

Monitoring Parameters Monitor signs and symptoms of disease process and adverse effects; evaluate by endoscopic examination or x-ray

Patient Information Take 1 hour before meals or on an empty stomach; may allow tablet to disintegrate in ~1 oz of room temperature water and drink the resulting suspension, if unable to swallow tablets whole; do not take within 30 minutes of (Continued)

Sucralfate *(Continued)*

antacids (before or after). Administer 2 hours before or after administration of other oral drugs.

Additional Information May decrease gastric emptying; many trials have demonstrated sucralfate is equivalent in efficacy to antacids and H_2 blockers; equivalence of sucralfate suspension to sucralfate tablets has not been established in studies

Special Geriatric Considerations Caution should be used in the elderly due to reduced renal function. Patients with Cl_{cr} <30 mL/minute may be at risk for aluminum intoxication. Due to low side effect profile, this may be an agent of choice in the elderly with PUD.

Dosage Forms Excipient information presented when available (limited, particularly for generics); consult specific product labeling.
Suspension, oral: 1 g/10 mL (10 mL)
    Carafate®: 1 g/10 mL (420 mL)
Tablet: 1 g
    Carafate®: 1 g

♦ **Sudafed® 12 Hour [OTC]** *see* Pseudoephedrine *on page 1346*
♦ **Sudafed® 24 Hour [OTC]** *see* Pseudoephedrine *on page 1346*
♦ **Sudafed® Children's [OTC]** *see* Pseudoephedrine *on page 1346*
♦ **Sudafed® Maximum Strength Nasal Decongestant [OTC]** *see* Pseudoephedrine *on page 1346*
♦ **Sudafed® Maximum Strength Sinus Nighttime [OTC] [DSC]** *see* Triprolidine and Pseudoephedrine *on page 1638*
♦ **Sudafed PE™ [OTC]** *see* Phenylephrine *on page 1247*
♦ **Sudodrin [OTC]** *see* Pseudoephedrine *on page 1346*
♦ **SudoGest [OTC]** *see* Pseudoephedrine *on page 1346*
♦ **Sudo-Tab® [OTC]** *see* Pseudoephedrine *on page 1346*
♦ **Sular®** *see* Nisoldipine *on page 1126*
♦ **Sulbactam and Ampicillin** *see* Ampicillin and Sulbactam *on page 108*

Sulfacetamide *(sul fa SEE ta mide)*

Medication Safety Issues
Sound-alike/look-alike issues:
    Bleph®-10 may be confused with Blephamide®
    Klaron® may be confused with Klor-Con®
U.S. Brand Names Bleph®-10; Carmol® Scalp; Klaron®; Mexar™ Wash; Ovace®; Ovace® Wash; Rosula® NS
Canadian Brand Names Cetamide™; Diosulf™
Index Terms Sodium Sulfacetamide; Sulfacetamide Sodium
Generic Available Yes: Ointment, solution, suspension
Pharmacologic Category Acne Products; Antibiotic, Ophthalmic; Antibiotic, Sulfonamide Derivative; Topical Skin Product, Acne
Use Treatment and prophylaxis of conjunctivitis due to susceptible organisms; corneal ulcers; adjunctive treatment with systemic sulfonamides for therapy of trachoma
Contraindications Hypersensitivity to sulfacetamide, sulfonamides, or any component of the formulation
Warnings/Precautions Severe reactions to sulfonamides have been reported, regardless of route of administration; reactions may include Stevens-Johnson syndrome, toxic epidermal necrolysis, fulminant hepatic necrosis, or blood dyscrasias. Chemical similarities are present among sulfonamides, sulfonylureas, carbonic anhydrase inhibitors, thiazides, and loop diuretics (except ethacrynic acid). Use in patients with sulfonamide allergy is specifically contraindicated in product labeling; however, a risk of cross-reaction exists in patients with allergy to any of these compounds; avoid use when previous reaction has been severe.

Ophthalmic: Inactivated by purulent exudates containing PABA; use with caution in severe dry eye; ointment may retard corneal epithelial healing. For topical application to the eye only; not for injection.

Dermatologic: Use caution if applied to denuded or abraded skin. Some products contain sodium metabisulfite which may cause allergic reactions in certain individuals. For external use only; avoid contact with eyes.

Adverse Reactions (Reflective of adult population; not specific for elderly)
Frequency not defined.
Cardiovascular: Edema
Dermatologic: Burning, erythema, irritation, itching, stinging, Stevens-Johnson syndrome
Ocular (following ophthalmic application): Burning, conjunctivitis, conjunctival hyperemia, corneal ulcers, irritation, stinging

Miscellaneous: Allergic reactions, systemic lupus erythematosus

Drug Interactions Decreased effect: Silver, gentamicin (antagonism)

Stability Store at controlled room temperature.

Ophthalmic solution: Solution may be used if yellow; do not use if darkened.

Carmol® Scalp treatment: Do not freeze. May be used if slightly discolored.

Mechanism of Action Interferes with bacterial growth by inhibiting bacterial folic acid synthesis through competitive antagonism of PABA

Pharmacokinetics Unknown

Dosage

Geriatrics & Adults:

Conjunctivitis: Ophthalmic:

Ointment: Apply to lower conjunctival sac 1-4 times/day and at bedtime

Solution: Instill 1-2 drops several times daily up to every 2-3 hours in lower conjunctival sac during waking hours and less frequently at night; increase dosing interval as condition responds. Usual duration of treatment: 7-10 days

Trachoma: Instill 2 drops into the conjunctival sac every 2 hours; must be used in conjunction with systemic therapy

Seborrheic dermatitis: Topical: Apply at bedtime and allow to remain overnight; in severe cases, may apply twice daily. Duration of therapy is usually 8-10 applications; dosing interval may be increased as eruption subsides. Applications once or twice weekly, or every other week may be used to prevent eruptions.

Secondary cutaneous bacterial infections: Topical: Apply 2-4 times/day until infection clears

Monitoring Parameters Response to therapy

Patient Information Eye drops will burn upon instillation; wait at least 10 minutes before using another eye preparation; ointment may sting eyes when first applied and blur vision; do not touch dropper to eye to maintain sterility

Additional Information Course of therapy is usually short-term; if infection does not clear in 7-10 days, need to reassess

Special Geriatric Considerations Assess whether patient can adequately instill drops or ointment.

Dosage Forms Excipient information presented when available (limited, particularly for generics); consult specific product labeling.

Cream, topical, as sodium:

Ovace®: 10% (30 g, 60 g)

Foam, topical, as sodium:

Ovace®: 10% (50 g, 100 g)

Gel, topical, as sodium:

Ovace®: 10% (30 g, 60 g)

Lotion, as sodium:

Carmol® Scalp: 10% (85 g) [contains urea 10%]

Klaron®: 10% (120 mL) [contains sodium metabisulfite]

Ovace® Wash: 10% (180 mL, 360 mL)

Ointment, ophthalmic, as sodium: 10% (3.5 g)

Pad, topical:

Rosula® NS: 10% (30s) [contains urea 10%]

Soap, topical:

Mexar™ Wash: 10% (170 mL)

Solution, ophthalmic, as sodium: 10% (15 mL)

Bleph®-10: 10% (5 mL) [contains benzalkonium chloride]

Suspension, topical: 10% (118 mL)

Sulfacetamide and Prednisolone
(sul fa SEE ta mide & pred NIS oh lone)

Related Information

PrednisoLONE *on page 1303*

Sulfacetamide *on page 1496*

Medication Safety Issues

Sound-alike/look-alike issues:

Blephamide® may be confused with Bleph®-10

Vasocidin® may be confused with Vasodilan®

U.S. Brand Names Blephamide®

Canadian Brand Names Blephamide®; Dioptimyd®

Index Terms Prednisolone and Sulfacetamide

Generic Available Yes: Solution

Pharmacologic Category Antibiotic/Corticosteroid, Ophthalmic

Use Steroid-responsive inflammatory ocular conditions where infection is present or there is a risk of infection

(Continued)

Sulfacetamide and Prednisolone *(Continued)*

Dosage
Geriatrics & Adults: Conjunctivitis: Ophthalmic:
Ointment: Apply to lower conjunctival sac 1-4 times/day
Solution, suspension: Instill 1-3 drops every 2-3 hours while awake
Special Geriatric Considerations Assess whether patient can adequately instill drops or ointment.

Dosage Forms Excipient information presented when available (limited, particularly for generics); consult specific product labeling.
Ointment, ophthalmic (Blephamide®): Sulfacetamide sodium 10% and prednisolone acetate 0.2% (3.5 g)
Solution, ophthalmic: Sulfacetamide sodium 10% and prednisolone sodium phosphate 0.25% (5 mL, 10 mL)
Suspension, ophthalmic (Blephamide®): Sulfacetamide sodium 10% and prednisolone acetate 0.2% (5 mL, 10 mL) [contains benzalkonium chloride]

♦ **Sulfacetamide Sodium** *see Sulfacetamide on page 1496*

Sulfamethoxazole and Trimethoprim
(sul fa meth OKS a zole & trye METH oh prim)

Related Information
Antimicrobial Activity Against Selected Organisms *on page 1728*
Trimethoprim *on page 1634*
Medication Safety Issues
Sound-alike/look-alike issues:
Bactrim™ may be confused with bacitracin, Bactine®
Co-trimoxazole may be confused with clotrimazole
Septra® may be confused with Ceptaz®, Sectral®, Septa®
U.S. Brand Names Bactrim™; Bactrim™ DS; Septra®; Septra® DS
Canadian Brand Names Apo-Sulfatrim®; Apo-Sulfatrim® DS; Apo-Sulfatrim® Pediatric; Novo-Trimel; Novo-Trimel D.S.; Nu-Cotrimox; Septra® Injection
Index Terms Co-Trimoxazole; SMZ-TMP; Sulfatrim; TMP-SMZ; Trimethoprim and Sulfamethoxazole
Generic Available Yes
Pharmacologic Category Antibiotic, Miscellaneous; Antibiotic, Sulfonamide Derivative
Use
Oral treatment of urinary tract infections; acute exacerbations of chronic bronchitis in adults; treatment and prophylaxis of *Pneumocystis carinii* pneumonitis (PCP); treatment of enteritis caused by *Shigella flexneri* or *Shigella sonnei*
I.V. treatment of documented PCP, empiric treatment of highly suspected PCP in immune compromised patients; treatment of documented or suspected shigellosis, typhoid fever, or *Nocardia asteroides* infection in patients who are NPO
Unlabeled/Investigational Use Treatment of cholera and *Salmonella*-type infections and nocardiosis; chronic prostatitis; as prophylaxis in neutropenic patients with *P. carinii* infections, in leukemics, and in patients following renal transplantation, to decrease incidence of gram-negative rod infections; treatment of *Cyclospora* infection, typhoid fever, *Nocardia asteroides* infection
Contraindications Hypersensitivity to any sulfa drug, trimethoprim, or any component of the formulation; porphyria; megaloblastic anemia due to folate deficiency; marked hepatic damage; severe renal disease
Warnings/Precautions Use with caution in patients with G6PD deficiency, impaired renal or hepatic function or potential folate deficiency (malnourished, chronic anticonvulsant therapy, or elderly); maintain adequate hydration to prevent crystalluria; adjust dosage in patients with renal impairment. Injection vehicle contains benzyl alcohol and sodium metabisulfite.

Chemical similarities are present among sulfonamides, sulfonylureas, carbonic anhydrase inhibitors, thiazides, and loop diuretics (except ethacrynic acid). Use in patients with sulfonamide allergy is specifically contraindicated in product labeling, however, a risk of cross-reaction exists in patients with allergy to any of these compounds; avoid use when previous reaction has been severe.

Fatalities associated with severe reactions including Stevens-Johnson syndrome, toxic epidermal necrolysis, hepatic necrosis, agranulocytosis, aplastic anemia and other blood dyscrasias; discontinue use at first sign of rash. Elderly patients appear at greater risk for more severe adverse reactions. May cause hypoglycemia, particularly in malnourished, or patients with renal or hepatic impairment. Use with caution in patients with porphyria or thyroid dysfunction. Slow acetylators may be more prone to adverse reactions. Caution in patients with allergies or asthma. May cause hyperkalemia (associated with high doses of trimethoprim). Incidence of adverse effects appears to be increased in patients with AIDS. Prolonged use may result in fungal or bacterial superinfection, including *C. difficile*-associated diarrhea and pseudomembranous colitis.

Adverse Reactions (Reflective of adult population; not specific for elderly)
The most common adverse reactions include gastrointestinal upset (nausea, vomiting, anorexia) and dermatologic reactions (rash or urticaria). Rare, life-threatening reactions have been associated with co-trimoxazole, including severe dermatologic reactions and hepatotoxic reactions. Most other reactions listed are rare, however, frequency cannot be accurately estimated.

Cardiovascular: Allergic myocarditis

Central nervous system: Confusion, depression, hallucinations, seizure, aseptic meningitis, peripheral neuritis, fever, ataxia, kernicterus in neonates

Dermatologic: Rashes, pruritus, urticaria, photosensitivity; rare reactions include erythema multiforme, Stevens-Johnson syndrome, toxic epidermal necrolysis, exfoliative dermatitis, and Henoch-Schönlein purpura

Endocrine & metabolic: Hyperkalemia (generally at high dosages), hypoglycemia

Gastrointestinal: Nausea, vomiting, anorexia, stomatitis, diarrhea, pseudomembranous colitis, pancreatitis

Hematologic: Thrombocytopenia, megaloblastic anemia, granulocytopenia, eosinophilia, pancytopenia, aplastic anemia, methemoglobinemia, hemolysis (with G6PD deficiency), agranulocytosis

Hepatic: Hepatotoxicity (including hepatitis, cholestasis, and hepatic necrosis), hyperbilirubinemia, transaminases increased

Neuromuscular & skeletal: Arthralgia, myalgia, rhabdomyolysis

Renal: Interstitial nephritis, crystalluria, renal failure, nephrotoxicity (in association with cyclosporine), diuresis

Respiratory: Cough, dyspnea, pulmonary infiltrates

Miscellaneous: Serum sickness, angioedema, periarteritis nodosa (rare), systemic lupus erythematosus (rare)

Overdosage/Toxicology Symptoms of acute overdose include nausea, vomiting, GI distress, hematuria, and crystalluria. Following GI decontamination, treatment is supportive. Adequate fluid intake is essential. Peritoneal dialysis is not effective and hemodialysis is only moderately effective in removing sulfamethoxazole and trimethoprim.

Drug Interactions
Sulfamethoxazole: **Substrate** of CYP2C9 (major), 3A4 (minor); **Inhibits** CYP2C9 (moderate)

Trimethoprim: **Substrate** (major) of CYP2C9, 3A4; **Inhibits** CYP2C8 (moderate) 2C9 (moderate)

ACE Inhibitors and angiotensin receptor antagonists: May increase the risk of hyperkalemia with sulfamethoxazole/trimethoprim.

Amantadine: Concurrent use with sulfamethoxazole/trimethoprim has been associated with toxic delirium (rare).

Cyclosporine: May result in an increased risk of nephrotoxicity when used with sulfamethoxazole/trimethoprim. Sulfonamides may decrease the serum concentrations of cyclosporine.

CYP2C9 inducers: May decrease the levels/effects of sulfamethoxazole and trimethoprim. Example inducers include carbamazepine, phenobarbital, phenytoin, rifampin, rifapentine, and secobarbital.

CYP2C8 Substrates: Trimethoprim may increase the levels/effects of CYP2C8 substrates. Example substrates include amiodarone, paclitaxel, pioglitazone, repaglinide, and rosiglitazone.

CYP2C9 Substrates: Sulfmethoxazole and trimethoprim may increase the levels/effects of CYP2C9 substrates. Example substrates include bosentan, dapsone, fluoxetine, glimepiride, glipizide, losartan, montelukast, nateglinide, paclitaxel, phenytoin, warfarin, and zafirlukast.

Dapsone: Trimethoprim may increase the serum concentration of dapsone.

Diuretics, potassium-sparing: May increase the risk of hyperkalemia with sulfamethoxazole/trimethoprim.

Leucovorin: Although occasionally recommended to limit or reverse hematologic toxicity of high-dose sulfamethoxazole/trimethoprim, concurrent use has been associated with a decreased effectiveness in treating *Pneumocystis carinii*.

Methotrexate: Sulfamethoxazole/trimethoprim may increase toxicity of methotrexate (due to displacement from binding sites and/or decreased renal secretion).

Phenytoin: Sulfamethoxazole/trimethoprim may increase phenytoin levels/toxicity. Phenytoin may decrease sulfamethoxazole/trimethoprim levels.

Procainamide: Trimethoprim may decrease the excretion of procainamide.

Pyrimethamine: Concurrent therapy with pyrimethamine (in doses >25 mg/week) may be at increased risk of megaloblastic anemia.

Sulfonylureas: Sulfamethoxazole/trimethoprim may increase the hypoglycemic effect of sulfonylureas; monitor.

(Continued)

Sulfamethoxazole and Trimethoprim *(Continued)*

Warfarin: Sulfamethoxazole/trimethoprim may increase the hypoprothrombinemic effect of warfarin; monitor INR closely.

Ethanol/Nutrition/Herb Interactions Herb/Nutraceutical: Avoid dong quai, St John's wort (may also cause photosensitization).

Stability

Injection: Store at room temperature; do not refrigerate. Less soluble in more alkaline pH. Protect from light. Solution must be diluted prior to administration. Following dilution, store at room temperature; do not refrigerate. Manufacturer recommended dilutions and stability of parenteral admixture at room temperature (25°C):

5 mL/125 mL D_5W; stable for 6 hours.

5 mL/100 mL D_5W; stable for 4 hours.

5 mL/75 mL D_5W; stable for 2 hours.

Studies have also confirmed limited stability in NS; detailed references should be consulted.

Suspension, tablet: Store at room temperature. Protect from light.

Mechanism of Action Sulfamethoxazole interferes with bacterial folic acid synthesis and growth via inhibition of dihydrofolic acid formation from para-aminobenzoic acid; trimethoprim inhibits dihydrofolic acid reduction to tetrahydrofolate resulting in sequential inhibition of enzymes of the folic acid pathway

Pharmacokinetics

Absorption: Oral: Almost completely, 90% to 100%

Protein binding:

SMX: 68%

TMP: 45%

Metabolism:

SMX is N-acetylated and glucuronidated

TMP is metabolized to oxide and hydroxylated metabolites

Half-life:

SMX: 9 hours

TMP: 6-17 hours, both are prolonged in renal failure

Time to peak serum concentration: Within 1-4 hours

Elimination: Both are excreted in urine as metabolites and unchanged drug

Effects of aging on the pharmacokinetics of both agents has been variable; increase in half-life and decreases in clearance have been associated with reduced creatinine clearance

Dosage

Geriatrics & Adults: Dosage recommendations are based on the trimethoprim component. Double-strength tablets are equivalent to sulfamethoxazole 800 mg and trimethoprim 160 mg.

Urinary tract infection:

Oral: One double-strength tablet every 12 hours for 10-14 days

Duration of therapy: Uncomplicated: 3-5 days; Complicated: 7-10 days

Pyelonephritis: 14 days

Prostatitis: Acute: 2 weeks; Chronic: 2-3 months

I.V.: 8-10 mg TMP/kg/day in divided doses every 6, 8, or 12 hours for up to 14 days with severe infections

Chronic bronchitis: Oral: One double-strength tablet every 12 hours for 10-14 days

Meningitis (bacterial): I.V.: 10-20 mg TMP/kg/day in divided doses every 6-12 hours

Shigellosis:

Oral: One double strength tablet every 12 hours for 5 days

I.V.: 8-10 mg TMP/kg/day in divided doses every 6, 8, or 12 hours for up to 5 days

Travelers' diarrhea: Oral: One double strength tablet every 12 hours for 5 days

Sepsis: I.V.: 20 TMP/kg/day divided every 6 hours

Pneumocystis jiroveci:

Prophylaxis: Oral: 1 double strength tablet daily or 3 times/week

Treatment: Oral, I.V.: 15-20 mg TMP/kg/day in 3-4 divided doses

Cyclospora (unlabeled use): Oral, I.V.: 160 mg TMP twice daily for 7-10 days

Nocardia (unlabeled use): Oral, I.V.:

Cutaneous infections: 5 mg TMP/kg/day in 2 divided doses

Severe infections (pulmonary/cerebral): 10-15 mg TMP/kg/day in 2-3 divided doses. Treatment duration is controversial; an average of 7 months has been reported.

Note: Therapy for severe infection may be initiated I.V. and converted to oral therapy (frequently converted to approximate dosages of oral solid dosage forms: 2 DS tablets every 8-12 hours). Although not widely available, sulfonamide levels should be considered in patients with questionable absorption, at risk for dose-related toxicity, or those with poor therapeutic response.

Renal Impairment:

Cl_{cr} 15-30 mL/minute: Administer 50% of recommended dose.

Cl_{cr} <15 mL/minute: Not recommended

Administration Infuse over 60-90 minutes, must dilute well before giving; not for I.M. injection

Monitoring Parameters Signs and symptoms of infection including mental status

Test Interactions Increased creatinine (Jaffé alkaline picrate reaction); increased serum methotrexate by dihydrofolate reductase method

Patient Information Take oral medication with 8 oz of water on an empty stomach (1 hour before or 2 hours after meals) for best absorption; report any skin rashes immediately; complete full course of therapy

Additional Information Do not use NS as a diluent; injection vehicle contains benzyl alcohol and sodium metabisulfite; the 5:1 ratio (SMX to TMP) remains constant in all dosage forms.

Special Geriatric Considerations Elderly patients appear at greater risk for more severe adverse reactions.

Dosage Forms Excipient information presented when available (limited, particularly for generics); consult specific product labeling. **Note:** The 5:1 ratio (SMX:TMP) remains constant in all dosage forms.

Injection, solution: Sulfamethoxazole 80 mg and trimethoprim 16 mg per mL (5 mL, 10 mL, 30 mL)

Suspension, oral: Sulfamethoxazole 200 mg and trimethoprim 40 mg per 5 mL (480 mL)

Tablet: Sulfamethoxazole 400 mg and trimethoprim 80 mg
    Bactrim™: Sulfamethoxazole 400 mg and trimethoprim 80 mg
    Septra®: Sulfamethoxazole 400 mg and trimethoprim 80 mg

Tablet, double strength: Sulfamethoxazole 800 mg and trimethoprim 160 mg
    Bactrim™ DS: Sulfamethoxazole 800 mg and trimethoprim 160 mg
    Septra® DS: Sulfamethoxazole 800 mg and trimethoprim 160 mg

Selected References

Naber K, Vergin H, and Weigand W, "Pharmacokinetics of Co-trimoxazole and Co-tetroxazine in Geriatric Patients," *Infection*, 1981, 9(5):239-43.

Varoquaux O, Lajoie D, Gobert C, et al, "Pharmacokinetics of the Trimethoprim-Sulfamethoxazole Combination in the Elderly," *Br J Clin Pharmacol*, 1985, 20(6):575-81.

Sulfasalazine (sul fa SAL a zeen)

Medication Safety Issues
Sound-alike/look-alike issues:

Sulfasalazine may be confused with salsalate, sulfaDIAZINE, sulfiSOXAZOLE

Azulfidine® may be confused with Augmentin®, azathioprine

U.S. Brand Names Azulfidine®; Azulfidine® EN-tabs®; Sulfazine; Sulfazine EC

Canadian Brand Names Alti-Sulfasalazine; Salazopyrin®; Salazopyrin En-Tabs®

Index Terms Salicylazosulfapyridine

Generic Available Yes

Pharmacologic Category 5-Aminosalicylic Acid Derivative

Use Management of ulcerative colitis, rheumatoid arthritis

Unlabeled/Investigational Use Treatment of ankylosing spondylitis, collagenous colitis, Crohn's disease, psoriasis, psoriatic arthritis

Contraindications Hypersensitivity to sulfasalazine, sulfa drugs, salicylates, or any component of the formulation; porphyria; GI or GU obstruction

Warnings/Precautions Use with caution in patients with renal impairment; impaired hepatic function or urinary obstruction, blood dyscrasias severe allergies or asthma, or G6PD deficiency; may cause folate deficiency (consider providing 1 mg/day folate supplement). Deaths from irreversible neuromuscular, central nervous system, fibrosing alveolitis, agranulocytosis, aplastic anemia, and other blood dyscrasias have been reported. In males, oligospermia (rare) has been reported. Chemical similarities are present among sulfonamides, sulfonylureas, carbonic anhydrase inhibitors, thiazides, and loop diuretics (except ethacrynic acid). Use in patients with sulfonamide allergy is specifically contraindicated in product labeling, however, a risk of cross-reaction exists in patients with allergy to any of these compounds; avoid use when previous reaction has been severe.

Adverse Reactions (Reflective of adult population; not specific for elderly)

>10%:

Central nervous system: Headache (33%)

Dermatologic: Photosensitivity

Gastrointestinal: Anorexia, nausea, vomiting, diarrhea (33%), gastric distress

Genitourinary: Reversible oligospermia (33%)

<3%:

Dermatologic: Urticaria/pruritus (<3%)

Hematologic: Hemolytic anemia (<3%), Heinz body anemia (<3%)

Additional events reported with sulfonamides and/or 5-ASA derivatives: Cholestatic jaundice, eosinophilia pneumonitis, erythema multiforme, fibrosing alveolitis, hepatic

(Continued)

Sulfasalazine *(Continued)*

necrosis, Kawasaki-like syndrome, SLE-like syndrome, pericarditis, seizure, transverse myelitis

Overdosage/Toxicology Symptoms include drowsiness, dizziness, anorexia, abdominal pain, nausea, vomiting, hemolytic anemia, acidosis, jaundice, fever, and agranulocytosis. The aniline radical is responsible for hematologic toxicity. High volume diuresis may aid in elimination and prevention of renal failure, gastric lavage or emesis plus catharsis, alkalinize urine. Dialysis may be helpful.

Drug Interactions

Azathioprine, mercaptopurine, sulfasalazine: May increase the risk of myelosuppression (due to TPMT inhibition).

Cyclosporine concentrations may be decreased; monitor levels and renal function

Digoxin's absorption may be decreased

Folic acid's absorption may be decreased

Hydantoin levels may be increased; monitor levels and adjust as necessary

Hypoglycemics: Increased effect of oral hypoglycemics (rare, but severe); monitor blood sugar

Methenamine: Combination may result in crystalluria; avoid use

Methotrexate-induced bone marrow suppression may be increased

NSAIDs and salicylates: May increase sulfonamide concentrations

PABA (para-aminobenzoic acid - may be found in some vitamin supplements): Interferes with the antibacterial activity of sulfonamides; avoid concurrent use

Sulfinpyrazone: May increase sulfonamide concentrations

Thiazide diuretics: May increase the incidence of thrombocytopenia purpura

Thiopental's effect may be enhanced; monitor for possible dosage reduction

Uricosuric agents: Actions of these agents are potentiated

Warfarin and other oral anticoagulants: Anticoagulant effect may be increased; decrease dose and monitor INR closely

Ethanol/Nutrition/Herb Interactions

Food: May impair folate absorption.

Herb/Nutraceutical: Avoid dong quai, St John's wort (may also cause photosensitization)

Stability Protect from light.

Mechanism of Action Acts locally in the colon to decrease the inflammatory response and systemically interferes with secretion by inhibiting prostaglandin synthesis

Pharmacokinetics

Absorption: Oral: Up to 33% as unchanged drug from the small intestine

Metabolism: Following absorption, both components are metabolized in the liver

Half-life: 5.7-10 hours; upon administration, the drug is split into sulfapyridine and 5-aminosalicylic acid (5-ASA) in the colon

Time to peak serum concentration:

5-aminosalicylic acid (active metabolite): Within 1.5-6 hours

Serum sulfapyridine (active metabolite): 6-24 hours

Elimination: Primary excretion in urine (as unchanged drug, components, and acetylated metabolites)

Dosage

Geriatrics & Adults:

Ulcerative colitis: Oral: Initial: 1 g 3-4 times/day, 2 g/day maintenance in divided doses; may initiate therapy with 0.5-1 g/day

Rheumatoid arthritis: Oral (enteric coated tablet): Initial: 0.5-1 g/day; increase weekly to maintenance dose of 2 g/day in 2 divided doses; maximum: 3 g/day (if response to 2 g/day is inadequate after 12 weeks of treatment)

Renal Impairment:

Cl_{cr} 10-30 mL/minute: Administer twice daily.

Cl_{cr} <10 mL/minute: Administer once daily.

Hepatic Impairment: Avoid use.

Monitoring Parameters Response to therapy, GI complaints

Patient Information Maintain adequate fluid intake; may cause orange-yellow discoloration of urine and skin; take after meals or with food; do not take with antacids; may permanently stain soft contact lenses yellow; avoid prolonged exposure to sunlight (wear sunscreen); do not chew or crush enteric coated tablets; report sore throat, fever, or other signs of infection to your physician. Missed doses should be taken as soon as remembered. If the forgotten dose is remembered at the next dosing interval, do not double the dose.

Additional Information This drug should be administered after food to reduce GI irritation. Sulfasalazine can be used as a disease-modifying agent (DMARD) in the treatment of progressive rheumatoid arthritis that has not responded adequately to anti-inflammatory agents.

Special Geriatric Considerations Adjust dose for renal function.

Dosage Forms Excipient information presented when available (limited, particularly for generics); consult specific product labeling.
Tablet: 500 mg
Azulfidine®, Sulfazine: 500 mg
Tablet, delayed release, enteric coated: 500 mg
Azulfidine® EN-tabs®, Sulfazine EC: 500 mg

♦ **Sulfatrim** *see* Sulfamethoxazole and Trimethoprim *on page 1498*
♦ **Sulfazine** *see* Sulfasalazine *on page 1501*
♦ **Sulfazine EC** *see* Sulfasalazine *on page 1501*

Sulfinpyrazone (sul fin PEER a zone)

Canadian Brand Names Apo-Sulfinpyrazone®; Nu-Sulfinpyrazone
Index Terms Anturane
Generic Available Yes
Pharmacologic Category Uricosuric Agent
Use Treatment of chronic gouty arthritis and intermittent gouty arthritis
Unlabeled/Investigational Use Reduction in incidence of sudden death postmyocardial infarction
Restrictions Not available in U.S.
Contraindications Hypersensitivity to sulfinpyrazone, phenylbutazone, other pyrazoles, or any component of the formulation; active peptic ulcer; GI inflammation; blood dyscrasias
Warnings/Precautions Use with caution in patients with impaired renal function and urolithiasis.
Adverse Reactions (Reflective of adult population; not specific for elderly)
Frequency not defined.
Cardiovascular: Flushing
Central nervous system: Dizziness, headache
Dermatologic: Dermatitis, rash
Gastrointestinal (most frequent adverse effects): Nausea, vomiting, stomach pain
Genitourinary: Polyuria
Hematologic: Anemia, leukopenia, increased bleeding time (decreased platelet aggregation)
Hepatic: Hepatic necrosis
Renal: Nephrotic syndrome, uric acid stones
Overdosage/Toxicology Symptoms include drowsiness, dizziness, anorexia, abdominal pain, nausea, vomiting, hemolytic anemia, acidosis, jaundice, fever, and agranulocytosis. The aniline radical is responsible for hematologic toxicity. High volume diuresis may aid in elimination and prevention of renal failure. Leucovorin 5-15 mg/day has been used to speed recovery of bone marrow.
Drug Interactions Substrate of CYP2C9 (major), 3A4 (minor); **Inhibits** CYP2C9 (moderate); **Induces** CYP3A4 (weak)
CYP2C9 inducers: May decrease the levels/effects of sulfinpyrazone. Example inducers include carbamazepine, phenobarbital, phenytoin, rifampin, rifapentine, and secobarbital.
CYP2C9 Substrates: Sulfinpyrazone may increase the levels/effects of CYP2C9 substrates. Example substrates include bosentan, dapsone, fluoxetine, glimepiride, glipizide, losartan, montelukast, nateglinide, paclitaxel, phenytoin, warfarin, and zafirlukast.
Salicylates: May decrease the effects of sulfinpyrazone.
Warfarin: Sulfinpyrazone may increase the levels/effects of warfarin; monitor.
Ethanol/Nutrition/Herb Interactions Herb/Nutraceutical: Avoid dong quai, St John's wort (may also cause photosensitization).
Mechanism of Action Acts by increasing the urinary excretion of uric acid, thereby decreasing serum urate levels; this effect is therapeutically useful in treating patients with acute intermittent gout, chronic tophaceous gout, and acts to promote resorption of tophi; also has antithrombic and platelet inhibitory effects
Pharmacokinetics
Absorption: Oral: Well absorbed
Protein binding: 98% to 99%
Metabolism: Hepatic to two active metabolites
Half-life: 2.2-3 hours
Elimination: ~50% of dose appears in urine unchanged
Dosage
Geriatrics & Adults: Gouty arthritis: Oral: 100-200 mg twice daily increasing to 400 mg twice daily, monitoring uric acid concentrations; decrease to 200 mg/day as a maintenance dose; maximum daily dose: 800 mg
Renal Impairment: Cl$_{cr}$ <50 mL/minute: Avoid use.
Monitoring Parameters Serum and urinary uric acid; CBC, renal function
(Continued)

Sulfinpyrazone *(Continued)*

Test Interactions Decreased uric acid (S)

Patient Information Take with food or milk; drink adequate fluids; avoid aspirin containing products

Additional Information This drug should only be used when other treatments for hyperuricemia or gout have failed or were not tolerated

Special Geriatric Considerations Since sulfinpyrazone loses its effectiveness when the Cl_{cr} is <50 mL/minute and since many elderly have reduced creatinine clearances, its usefulness in elderly is limited.

Dosage Forms Excipient information presented when available (limited, particularly for generics); consult specific product labeling.
Tablet: 100 mg

Selected References
Emmerson BT, "The Management of Gout," *N Engl J Med*, 1996, 334(7):445-51.

SulfiSOXAZOLE (sul fi SOKS a zole)

Medication Safety Issues
Sound-alike/look-alike issues:
SulfiSOXAZOLE may be confused with sulfaDIAZINE, sulfamethoxazole, sulfasalazine
Gantrisin® may be confused with Gastrosed™

U.S. Brand Names Gantrisin®

Canadian Brand Names Novo-Soxazole; Sulfizole®

Index Terms Sulfisoxazole Acetyl; Sulphafurazole

Generic Available Yes: Tablet

Pharmacologic Category Antibiotic, Sulfonamide Derivative

Use Treatment of urinary tract infections, otitis media, *Chlamydia*, nocardiosis; often used in combination with trimethoprim

Contraindications Hypersensitivity to sulfisoxazole, any sulfa drug, or any component of the formulation; porphyria; patients with urinary obstruction; sunscreens containing PABA

Warnings/Precautions Use with caution in patients with G6PD deficiency (hemolysis may occur), hepatic or renal impairment; dosage modification required in patients with renal impairment; risk of crystalluria should be considered in patients with impaired renal function. Chemical similarities are present among sulfonamides, sulfonylureas, carbonic anhydrase inhibitors, thiazides, and loop diuretics (except ethacrynic acid). Use in patients with sulfonamide allergy is specifically contraindicated in product labeling, however, a risk of cross-reaction exists in patients with allergy to any of these compounds; avoid use when previous reaction has been severe.

Adverse Reactions (Reflective of adult population; not specific for elderly)
Frequency not defined.
Cardiovascular: Vasculitis
Central nervous system: Dizziness, fever, headache
Dermatologic: Itching, Lyell's syndrome, rash, photosensitivity, Stevens-Johnson syndrome
Endocrine & metabolic: Thyroid function disturbance
Gastrointestinal: Anorexia, diarrhea, nausea, vomiting
Genitourinary: Crystalluria, hematuria
Hematologic: Aplastic anemia, granulocytopenia, hemolytic anemia, leukopenia, thrombocytopenia
Hepatic: Hepatitis, jaundice
Renal: Interstitial nephritis
Miscellaneous: Serum sickness-like reactions

Overdosage/Toxicology Symptoms include drowsiness, dizziness, anorexia, abdominal pain, nausea, vomiting, hemolytic anemia, acidosis, jaundice, fever, and agranulocytosis. Doses of as little as 2-5 g/day may produce toxicity. The aniline radical is responsible for hematologic toxicity. High volume diuresis may aid in elimination and prevention of renal failure.

Drug Interactions Substrate of CYP2C9 (major); **Inhibits** CYP2C9 (strong)
Cyclosporine concentrations may be decreased; monitor levels and renal function
CYP2C9 Inducers may decrease the levels/effects of Sulfisoxazole. Example inducers include carbamazepine, phenobarbital, phenytoin, rifampin, rifapentine, and secobarbital.
CYP2C9 Substrates: Sulfisoxazole may increase the levels/effects of CYP2C9 substrates. Example substrates include bosentan, dapsone, fluoxetine, glimepiride, glipizide, losartan, montelukast, nateglinide, paclitaxel, phenytoin, warfarin, and zafirlukast.
Hydantoin levels may be increased; monitor levels and adjust as necessary

Hypoglycemics: Increased effect of oral hypoglycemics (rare, but severe); monitor blood sugar

Methenamine: Combination may result in crystalluria; avoid use

Methotrexate-induced bone marrow suppression may be increased

NSAIDs and salicylates: May increase sulfonamide concentrations

PABA (para-aminobenzoic acid - may be found in some vitamin supplements): Interferes with the antibacterial activity of sulfonamides; avoid concurrent use

Sulfinpyrazone: May increase sulfonamide concentrations

Thiazide diuretics: May increase the incidence of thrombocytopenia purpura

Thiopental's effect may be enhanced; monitor for possible dosage reduction

Uricosuric agents: Actions of these agents are potentiated

Warfarin and other oral anticoagulants: Anticoagulant effect may be increased; decrease dose and monitor INR closely

Ethanol/Nutrition/Herb Interactions

Food: Interferes with folate absorption.

Herb/Nutraceutical: Avoid dong quai, St John's wort (may also cause photosensitization).

Stability Protect from light.

Mechanism of Action Interferes with bacterial growth by inhibiting bacterial folic acid synthesis through competitive antagonism of PABA

Pharmacokinetics

Absorption: Sulfisoxazole acetyl is hydrolyzed in the GI tract to sulfisoxazole which is readily absorbed

Protein binding: 85% to 88%

Metabolism: Metabolized in the liver by acetylation and glucuronide conjugation to inactive compounds

Half-life: 4-7 hours, prolonged with renal impairment

Time to peak serum concentration: Within 2-3 hours

Elimination: Primarily in urine (95% within 24 hours), 40% to 60% as unchanged drug

In a single dose study, absorption and peak serum concentrations were similar in older adults and younger subjects; in older adults, half-life was prolonged and renal and nonrenal clearance decreased

Dosage

Geriatrics & Adults: Susceptible infections: Oral: 2-4 g stat, 4-8 g/day in divided doses every 4-6 hours

Renal Impairment:

Cl_{cr} 10-50 mL/minutes: Administer every 8-12 hours.

Cl_{cr} <10 mL/minute: Administer every 12-24 hours.

Hemodialysis effects: >50% is removed by hemodialysis.

Administration

Administer around-the-clock rather than 4 times/day, 3 times/day, etc (ie, 12-6-12-6, not 9-1-5-9) to promote less variation in peak and trough serum concentrations; maintain adequate fluid intake

Monitoring Parameters Temperature, WBC, urine analysis and culture, appetite, mental status

Reference Range Therapeutic: 5-15 mg/dL; Toxic: >20 mg/dL (not routinely monitored)

Test Interactions False-positive protein in urine; false-positive urine glucose with Clinitest®

Patient Information Take with a glass of water on an empty stomach; avoid prolonged exposure to sunlight (wear sunscreen); report to physician any sore throat, mouth sores, rash, unusual bleeding, or fever; complete full course of therapy

Additional Information Routine alkalinization of urine is normally not required.

Special Geriatric Considerations Sulfisoxazole is an effective anti-infective agent. Most prescribers prefer the combination of sulfamethoxazole and trimethoprim for its dual mechanism of action. Trimethoprim penetrates the prostate. Adjust dose for renal function.

Dosage Forms Excipient information presented when available (limited, particularly for generics); consult specific product labeling.

Suspension, oral, pediatric, as acetyl (Gantrisin®): 500 mg/5 mL (480 mL) [contains alcohol 0.3%; raspberry flavor]

Tablet: 500 mg

Selected References

Boisvert A, Barbeau G, and Belanger PM, "Pharmacokinetics of Sulfisoxazole in Young and Elderly Subjects," *Gerontology*, 1984, 30(2):125-31.

♦ **Sulfisoxazole Acetyl** *see* SulfiSOXAZOLE *on page 1504*

♦ **Sulfisoxazole and Erythromycin** *see* Erythromycin and Sulfisoxazole *on page 538*

Sulindac (SUL in dak)

Medication Safety Issues
Sound-alike/look-alike issues:
Clinoril® may be confused with Cleocin®, Clozaril®, Oruvail®
U.S. Brand Names Clinoril®
Canadian Brand Names Apo-Sulin®; Novo-Sundac; Nu-Sundac
Generic Available Yes
Pharmacologic Category Nonsteroidal Anti-inflammatory Drug (NSAID), Oral
Use Management of inflammatory disease, osteoarthritis, rheumatoid disorders, acute gouty arthritis, ankylosing spondylitis, bursitis/tendonitis of shoulder
Restrictions An FDA-approved medication guide must be distributed when dispensing an oral outpatient prescription (new or refill) where this medication is to be used without direct supervision of a healthcare provider. Medication guides are available at http://www.fda.gov/cder/Offices/ODS/medication_guides.htm.
Contraindications Hypersensitivity to sulindac, aspirin, other NSAIDs, or any component of the formulation; perioperative pain in the setting of coronary artery bypass surgery (CABG)
Warnings/Precautions [U.S. Boxed Warning]: NSAIDs are associated with an increased risk of adverse cardiovascular events, including MI, stroke, and new onset or worsening of pre-existing hypertension. Use caution with fluid retention, CHF or hypertension. Concurrent administration of ibuprofen, and potentially other nonselective NSAIDs, may interfere with aspirin's cardioprotective effect. Use of NSAIDs can compromise existing renal function. Sulindac is not recommended for patients with advanced renal disease. Use caution in patients with renal lithiasis; sulindac metabolites have been reported as components of renal stones. Use hydration in patients with a history of renal stones. Use with caution in patients with decreased hepatic function. May require dosage adjustment in hepatic dysfunction; sulfide and sulfone metabolites may accumulate.

[U.S. Boxed Warning]: NSAIDs may increase risk of gastrointestinal irritation, ulceration, bleeding, and perforation. Use the lowest effective dose for the shortest duration of time, consistent with individual patient goals, to reduce risk of cardiovascular or GI adverse events.

NSAIDs may cause serious skin adverse events including exfoliative dermatitis, Stevens-Johnson syndrome (SJS) and toxic epidermal necrolysis (TEN). Anaphylactoid reactions may occur. Do not use in patients who experience bronchospasm, asthma, rhinitis, or urticaria with NSAID or aspirin therapy. Use caution in other forms of asthma.

Withhold for at least 4-6 half-lives prior to surgical or dental procedures.
Adverse Reactions (Reflective of adult population; not specific for elderly)
1% to 10%:
Cardiovascular: Edema (1% to 3%)
Central nervous system: Dizziness (3% to 9%), headache (3% to 9%), nervousness (1% to 3%)
Dermatologic: Rash (3% to 9%), pruritus (1% to 3%)
Gastrointestinal: GI pain (10%), constipation (3% to 9%), diarrhea (3% to 9%), dyspepsia (3% to 9%), nausea (3% to 9%), abdominal cramps (1% to 3%), anorexia (1% to 3%), flatulence (1% to 3%), vomiting (1% to 3%)
Otic: Tinnitus (1% to 3%)
Overdosage/Toxicology Symptoms include dizziness, vomiting, nausea, abdominal pain, hypotension, coma, stupor, metabolic acidosis, leukocytosis, and renal failure. Management of nonsteroidal anti-inflammatory drug (NSAID) intoxication is primarily supportive and symptomatic. Fluid therapy is commonly effective managing hypotension that may occur following an acute NSAID overdose, except when due to acute blood loss. Seizures tend to be very short-lived and often do not require drug treatment; although, recurrent seizures should be treated with I.V. diazepam.
Drug Interactions
ACE inhibitors: Antihypertensive effects may be decreased by concurrent therapy with NSAIDs; monitor blood pressure.
Aminoglycosides: NSAIDs may decrease the excretion of aminoglycosides.
Angiotensin II antagonists: Antihypertensive effects may be decreased by concurrent therapy with NSAIDs; monitor blood pressure.
Anticoagulants (warfarin, heparin, LMWHs): When used with NSAIDs can cause increased risk of bleeding.
Antiplatelet drugs (ticlopidine, clopidogrel, aspirin, abciximab, dipyridamole, eptifibatide, tirofiban): Concurrent use may cause an increased risk of bleeding.
Beta-blockers: NSAIDs may decrease the antihypertensive effect of beta-blockers. Monitor.
Bisphosphonates: NSAIDs may increase the risk of gastrointestinal ulceration.

Cholestyramine (and other bile acid sequestrants): May decrease the absorption of NSAIDs. Separate by at least 2 hours.

Corticosteroids: May increase the risk of GI ulceration; avoid concurrent use.

Cyclosporine: NSAIDs may increase serum creatinine, potassium, blood pressure, and cyclosporine levels; monitor cyclosporine levels and renal function carefully.

Dimethyl sulfoxide: May reduce plasma levels of sulindac's active metabolite. Combination may cause peripheral neuropathy; avoid concurrent use.

Fluoroquinolone antibiotics: Risk of seizures may be increased with concomitant quinolone use. Risk is considered quite low and may only be a factor with high serum levels of either agent and/or in patients with additional predisposing factors (eg, renal dysfunction, history of seizure or other neurological disorder).

Hydralazine's antihypertensive effect is decreased; avoid concurrent use.

Lithium: NSAIDs may increase lithium levels; avoid concurrent use if possible or monitor lithium levels and adjust dose. Sulindac may have the least effect. When NSAID is stopped, lithium will need adjustment again.

Loop diuretic: NSAIDs may decrease the efficacy (diuretic and antihypertensive effect) of loop diuretics.

Methotrexate: Severe bone marrow suppression, aplastic anemia, and GI toxicity have been reported with concomitant NSAID therapy. Avoid use during moderate or high-dose methotrexate (increased and prolonged methotrexate levels). NSAID use during low-dose treatment of rheumatoid arthritis has not been fully evaluated; extreme caution is warranted.

Pemetrexed: NSAIDs may decrease the excretion of pemetrexed. Patients with Cl_{cr} 45-79 mL/minute should avoid long-acting NSAIDs for 5 days before and 2 days after pemetrexed treatment.

Salicylates: NSAIDs (nonselective) may diminish the cardioprotective effect of acetylated salicylates. Avoid regular use of NSAIDs if possible; consider alternatives (eg, acetaminophen). Give salicylate before NSAID; for example give ibuprofen 30-120 minutes after aspirin (immediate release).

Thiazides antihypertensive effects are decreased; avoid concurrent use.

Treprostinil: May enhance the risk of bleeding with concurrent use.

Vancomycin: NSAIDs may decrease the excretion of vancomycin.

Ethanol/Nutrition/Herb Interactions

Ethanol: Avoid ethanol (may enhance gastric mucosal irritation).

Food: Food may decrease the rate but not the extent of oral absorption. The therapeutic effect of sulindac may be decreased if taken with food.

Herb/Nutraceutical: Avoid alfalfa, anise, bilberry, bladderwrack, bromelain, cat's claw, celery, coleus, cordyceps, dong quai, evening primrose, feverfew, fenugreek, garlic, ginger, ginkgo biloba, red clover, horse chestnut, grapeseed, green tea, ginseng, guggul, horse chestnut seed, horseradish, licorice, prickly ash, red clover, reishi, SAMe, sweet clover, turmeric, white willow (all have additional antiplatelet activity).

Mechanism of Action Inhibits prostaglandin synthesis by decreasing the activity of the enzyme, cyclooxygenase, which results in decreased formation of prostaglandin precursors

Pharmacodynamics

Onset of anti-inflammatory action: Within 7 days

Maximum response: 2-3 weeks

Pharmacokinetics

Absorption: Oral: 90%; sulindac is a prodrug and therefore requires metabolic activation

Protein binding: >90%

Half-life elimination: Parent drug: ~8 hours; Active metabolite: ~16 hours

Requires hepatic metabolism to sulfide metabolite (active) for therapeutic effects

Metabolism: Hepatic; prodrug metabolized to sulfide metabolite (active) for therapeutic effects and to sulfone metabolites (inactive)

Time to peak serum concentration: 2-4 hours

Excretion: Urine (50%, primarily as inactive metabolites); feces (25%, primarily as metabolites)

Dosage

Geriatrics & Adults: Note: Maximum daily dose: 400 mg

Osteoarthritis, rheumatoid arthritis, ankylosing spondylitis: 150 mg twice/daily

Bursitis/tendonitis: 200 mg twice daily; usual treatment: 7-14 days

Acute gouty arthritis: 200 mg twice daily; usual treatment: 7 days

Renal Impairment: Not recommended with advanced renal impairment; if required, decrease dose and monitor closely.

Hepatic Impairment: Dose reduction is necessary; discontinue if abnormal liver function tests occur.

Administration Should be administered with food or milk.

Monitoring Parameters Monitor response (pain, range of motion, grip strength, mobility, ADL function), inflammation; observe for weight gain, edema; monitor renal function; observe for bleeding, bruising; evaluate gastrointestinal effects (abdominal (Continued)

Sulindac *(Continued)*

pain, bleeding, dyspepsia); mental confusion, disorientation, CBC, serum, creatinine, BUN, liver function tests

Test Interactions Increased chloride (S), increased sodium (S), increased bleeding time

Patient Information Serious gastrointestinal bleeding can occur as well as ulceration and perforation. Pain may or may not be present. Avoid aspirin and aspirin-containing products while taking this medication. If gastric upset occurs, take with food, milk, or antacid. If gastric adverse effects persist, contact physician. May cause drowsiness, dizziness, blurred vision, and confusion. Use caution when performing tasks which require alertness (eg, driving). Do not take for more than 3 days for fever or 10 days for pain without physician's advice.

Additional Information Structurally similar to indomethacin but acts like aspirin; associated with the highest (one study) incidence of upper GI bleeds among NSAIDs; safest NSAID for use in mild renal impairment; maximum therapeutic response may not be realized for up to 3 weeks. There are no clinical guidelines to predict which NSAID will give which response in a particular patient. Trials with each must be initiated until response determined. Consider dose, patient convenience, and cost.

Special Geriatric Considerations Elderly are a high-risk population for adverse effects from NSAIDs. As much as 60% of the elderly who develop GI complications can develop peptic ulceration and/or hemorrhage asymptomatically. The concomitant use of H_2 blockers and sucralfate is not effective as prophylaxis with the exception of NSAID-induced duodenal ulcers which may be prevented by the use of ranitidine. Misoprostol and proton pump inhibitors are the only agents proven to help prevent the development of NSAID-induced ulcers. Also, concomitant disease and drug use contribute to the risk for GI adverse effects. Use lowest effective dose for shortest period possible. Consider renal function decline with age. Use of NSAIDs can compromise existing renal function especially when Cl_{cr} is ≤30 mL/minute. Tinnitus may be a difficult and unreliable indication of toxicity due to age-related hearing loss or eighth cranial nerve damage. CNS adverse effects such as confusion, agitation, and hallucination are generally seen in overdose or high-dose situations, but the elderly may demonstrate these adverse effects at lower doses than younger adults.

Dosage Forms Excipient information presented when available (limited, particularly for generics); consult specific product labeling.

Tablet: 150 mg, 200 mg

Clinoril®: 200 mg

Selected References

Brooks PM and Day RO, "Nonsteroidal Anti-inflammatory Drugs - Differences and Similarities," *N Engl J Med*, 1991, 324(24):1716-25.

Clinch D, Banerjee AK, and Ostick G, "Absence of Abdominal Pain in Elderly Patients With Peptic Ulcer," *Age Ageing*, 1984, 13(2):120-3.

Clive DM and Stoff JS, "Renal Syndromes Associated With Nonsteroidal Anti-inflammatory Drugs," *N Engl J Med*, 1984, 310(9):563-72.

Graham DY, "Prevention of Gastroduodenal Injury Induced by Chronic Nonsteroidal Anti-inflammatory Drug Therapy," *Gastroenterology*, 1989, 96(2 Pt 2 Suppl):675-81.

Gurwitz JH, Avorn J, Ross-Degnan D, et al, "Nonsteroidal Anti-Inflammatory Drug-Associated Azotemia in the Very Old," *JAMA*, 1990, 264(4):471-5.

Hawkey CJ, Karrasch JA, Szczepañski L, et al, "Omeprazole Compared With Misoprostol for Ulcers Associated With Nonsteroidal Anti-inflammatory Drugs," *N Engl J Med*, 1998, 338(11):727-34.

Hunt SA, Abraham WT, Chin MH , et al, "ACC/AHA 2005 Guideline Update for the Diagnosis and Management of Chronic Heart Failure in the Adult: A Report of the American College of Cardiology/American Heart Association Task Force on Practice Guidelines (Writing Committee to Update the 2001 Guidelines for the Evaluation and Management of Heart Failure)," available at: http://www.acc.org/clinical/guidelines/failure//index.pdf

Knodel LC, "Preventing NSAID-induced Ulcers: The Role of Misoprostol," *Consult Pharm*, 1989, 4:37-41.

Pounder R, "Silent Peptic Ulceration: Deadly Silence or Golden Silence?" *Gastroenterology*, 1989, 96:(2 Pt 2 Suppl)626-31.

Yeomans ND, Tulassay Z, Juhasz L, et al, "A Comparison of Omeprazole With Ranitidine for Ulcers Associated With Nonsteroidal Anti-inflammatory Drugs," *N Engl J Med*, 1998, 338(11):719-26.

♦ **Sulphafurazole** *see* SulfiSOXAZOLE *on page 1504*

Sumatriptan *(soo ma TRIP tan)*

Medication Safety Issues

Sound-alike/look-alike issues:

Sumatriptan may be confused with somatropin, zolmitriptan

International issues:

Imitrex® may be confused with Nitrex® which is a brand name for isosorbide mononitrate in Italy

U.S. Brand Names Imitrex®

Canadian Brand Names Apo-Sumatriptan®; CO Sumatriptan; Dom-Sumatriptan; Gen-Sumatriptan; Imitrex®; Imitrex® DF; Imitrex® Nasal Spray; Novo-Sumatriptan;

PHL-Sumatriptan; PMS-Sumatriptan; ratio-Sumatriptan; Rhoxal-sumatriptan; Riva-Sumatriptan; Sandoz-Sumatriptan; Sumatryx

Index Terms Sumatriptan Succinate

Generic Available No

Pharmacologic Category Antimigraine Agent; Serotonin 5-HT$_{1B, 1D}$ Receptor Agonist

Use

Oral, SubQ: Acute treatment of migraine with or without aura

SubQ: Acute treatment of cluster headache episodes

Contraindications Hypersensitivity to sumatriptan or any component of the formulation; patients with ischemic heart disease or signs or symptoms of ischemic heart disease (including Prinzmetal's angina, angina pectoris, myocardial infarction, silent myocardial ischemia); cerebrovascular syndromes (including strokes, transient ischemic attacks); peripheral vascular syndromes (including ischemic bowel disease); uncontrolled hypertension; use within 24 hours of ergotamine derivatives; use with in 24 hours of another 5-HT$_1$ agonist; concurrent administration or within 2 weeks of discontinuing an MAO inhibitor, specifically MAO type A inhibitors; management of hemiplegic or basilar migraine; prophylactic treatment of migraine; severe hepatic impairment; not for I.V. administration

Warnings/Precautions Sumatriptan is indicated only in patients ≥18 years of age with a clear diagnosis of migraine or cluster headache. Cardiac events (coronary artery vasospasm, transient ischemia, myocardial infarction, ventricular tachycardia/fibrillation, cardiac arrest and death), cerebral/subarachnoid hemorrhage, and stroke have been reported with 5-HT$_1$ agonist administration. Do not give to patients with risk factors for CAD until a cardiovascular evaluation has been performed; if evaluation is satisfactory, the healthcare provider should administer the first dose and cardiovascular status should be periodically evaluated.

Significant elevation in blood pressure, including hypertensive crisis, has also been reported on rare occasions in patients with and without a history of hypertension. Vasospasm-related reactions have been reported other than coronary artery vasospasm. Peripheral vascular ischemia and colonic ischemia with abdominal pain and bloody diarrhea have occurred. Use with caution in patients with a history of seizure disorder or in patients with a lowered seizure threshold. Use with caution in patients with hepatic impairment. Symptoms of agitation, confusion, hallucinations, hyper-reflexia, myoclonus, shivering, and tachycardia (serotonin syndrome) may occur with concomitant proserotonergic drugs (ie, SSRIs/SNRIs or triptans) or agents which reduce sumatriptan's metabolism. Concurrent use of serotonin precursors (eg, tryptophan) is not recommended.

Adverse Reactions (Reflective of adult population; not specific for elderly)

Injection:

>10%:

Central nervous system: Dizziness (12%), warm/hot sensation (11%)

Local: Pain at injection site (59%)

Neuromuscular & skeletal: Paresthesia (14%)

1% to 10%:

Cardiovascular: Chest pain/tightness/heaviness/pressure (2% to 3%), hyper-/hypotension (1%)

Central nervous system: Burning (7%), feeling of heaviness (7%), flushing (7%), pressure sensation (7%), feeling of tightness (5%), drowsiness (3%), malaise/fatigue (1%), feeling strange (2%), headache (2%), tight feeling in head (2%), cold sensation (1%), anxiety (1%)

Gastrointestinal: Abdominal discomfort (1%), dysphagia (1%)

Neuromuscular & skeletal: Neck, throat, and jaw pain/tightness/pressure (2% to 5%), mouth/tongue discomfort (5%), weakness (5%), myalgia (2%); muscle cramps (1%), numbness (5%)

Ocular: Vision alterations (1%)

Respiratory: Throat discomfort (3%), nasal disorder/discomfort (2%)

Miscellaneous: Diaphoresis (2%)

Nasal spray:

>10%: Gastrointestinal: Bad taste (13% to 24%), nausea (11% to 13%), vomiting (11% to 13%)

1% to 10%:

Central nervous system: Dizziness (1% to 2%)

Respiratory: Nasal disorder/discomfort (2% to 4%), throat discomfort (1% to 2%)

Tablet:

1% to 10%:

Cardiovascular: Chest pain/tightness/heaviness/pressure (1% to 2%), hyper-/hypotension (1%), palpitation (1%), syncope (1%)

Central nervous system: Burning (1%), dizziness (>1%), drowsiness (>1%), malaise/fatigue (2% to 3%), headache (>1%), nonspecified pain (1% to 2%, placebo 1%), vertigo (<1% to 2%), migraine (>1%), sleepiness (>1%)

(Continued)

Sumatriptan *(Continued)*

Gastrointestinal: Diarrhea (1%), nausea (>1%), vomiting (>1%), hyposalivation (>1%)

Genitourinary: Hematuria (1%)

Hematologic: Hemolytic anemia (1%)

Neuromuscular & skeletal: Neck, throat, and jaw pain/tightness/pressure (2% to 3%), paresthesia (3% to 5%), myalgia (1%), numbness (1%)

Otic: Ear hemorrhage (1%), hearing loss (1%), sensitivity to noise (1%), tinnitus (1%)

Respiratory: Allergic rhinitis (1%), dyspnea (1%), nasal inflammation (1%), nose/throat hemorrhage (1%), sinusitis (1%), upper respiratory inflammation (1%)

Miscellaneous: Hypersensitivity reactions (1%), nonspecified pressure/tightness/heaviness (1% to 3%, placebo 2%); warm/cold sensation (2% to 3%, placebo 2%)

Overdosage/Toxicology Single oral doses up to 400 mg, injectable doses up to 16 mg, and nasal doses of 40 mg have been reported without adverse effects. Treatment should be supportive and symptomatic. Monitor for at least 12 hours or until signs and symptoms subside. It is not known if hemodialysis or peritoneal dialysis is effective.

Drug Interactions Note: Use cautiously in patients receiving concomitant medications that can lower the seizure threshold.

Ergot-containing drugs: Prolong vasospastic reactions; do not use sumatriptan or ergot-containing drugs within 24 hours of each other.

MAO inhibitors (MAO type A inhibitors, nonspecific MAO inhibitors): Reduce sumatriptan clearance; concurrent use is contraindicated; wait at least 2 weeks after discontinuing MAO type A inhibitor to start sumatriptan.

Selegiline: Selegiline is a selective MAO type B inhibitor; while not specifically contraindicated, combination may best be avoided until further study.

Serotonergic reuptake inhibitors (eg, SSRIs/SNRIs): Concurrent use of sumatriptan with these agents may increase the risk of serotonin syndrome; monitor.

Serotonin agonists (eg, triptans): Concurrent use of sumatriptan with these agents may increase the risk of serotonin syndrome; monitor.

Stability Store at 2°C to 20°C (36°F to 86°F). Protect from light.

Mechanism of Action Selective agonist for serotonin (5-HT$_{1D}$ receptor) in cranial arteries to cause vasoconstriction and reduces sterile inflammation associated with antidromic neuronal transmission correlating with relief of migraine

Pharmacodynamics

Onset of action: ~30 minutes

Pharmacokinetics

Distribution: V$_d$: 2.4 L/kg

Protein binding: 14% to 21%

Metabolism: Hepatic, primarily via MAO-A isoenzyme

Bioavailability: SubQ: 97% ± 16% of that following I.V. injection; Oral: 15%

Half-life elimination: Injection, tablet: 2.5 hours; Nasal spray: 2 hours

Time to peak, serum: 5-20 minutes

Excretion:

Injection: Urine (38% as indole acetic acid metabolite, 22% as unchanged drug)

Nasal spray: Urine (42% as indole acetic acid metabolite, 3% as unchanged drug)

Tablet: Urine (60% as indole acetic acid metabolite, 3% as unchanged drug); feces (40%)

Dosage

Geriatrics & Adults:

Migraine:

Oral: A single dose of 25 mg, 50 mg, or 100 mg (taken with fluids). If a satisfactory response has not been obtained at 2 hours, a second dose may be administered. Results from clinical trials show that initial doses of 50 mg and 100 mg are more effective than doses of 25 mg, and that 100 mg doses do not provide a greater effect than 50 mg and may have increased incidence of side effects. Although doses of up to 300 mg/day have been studied, the total daily dose should not exceed 200 mg. The safety of treating an average of >4 headaches in a 30-day period have not been established.

Intranasal: Single dose of 5, 10, or 20 mg administered in one nostril; a 10 mg dose may be achieved by administration of a single 5 mg dose in each nostril; if headache returns, the dose may be repeated once after 2 hours, not to exceed a total daily dose of 40 mg. The safety of treating an average of >4 headaches in a 30-day period has not been established.

SubQ: Up to 6 mg; if side effects are dose-limiting, lower doses may be used. A second injection may be administered at least 1 hour after the initial dose, but not more than 2 injections in a 24-hour period.

Cluster headache: Refer to dosing under "Migraine, SubQ"

Renal Impairment: Dosage adjustment is not necessary.

Hepatic Impairment: Bioavailability of oral sumatriptan is increased with liver disease. If treatment is needed, do not exceed single doses of 50 mg. The nasal spray has not been studied in patients with hepatic impairment, however, because the spray does not undergo first-pass metabolism, levels would not be expected to alter. Use of all dosage forms is contraindicated with severe hepatic impairment.

Administration
Oral: Should be taken with fluids as soon as symptoms to appear
Injection solution: For SubQ administration; do not administer I.V.; may cause coronary vasospasm

Monitoring Parameters Monitor blood pressure, signs and symptoms of coronary vasospasm, response (resolution of migraine)

Patient Information If pain or tightness in chest or throat occurs, notify physician; pain at injection site lasts <1 hour

Special Geriatric Considerations Use cautiously in the elderly, particularly since many elderly have cardiovascular disease which would put them at risk for cardiovascular adverse effects. Safety and efficacy in the elderly (>65 years) have not been established. Pharmacokinetic disposition is, however, similar to that in young adults.

Dosage Forms Excipient information presented when available (limited, particularly for generics); consult specific product labeling. **Note:** Strength expressed as sumatriptan base
Injection, solution, as succinate: 8 mg/mL (0.5 mL) [disposable cartridge for use with STATdose System®]; 12 mg/mL (0.5 mL) [disposable cartridge for use with STAT-dose System® or vial]
Solution, intranasal spray: 5 mg (100 μL unit dose spray device); 20 mg (100 μL unit dose spray device)
Tablet, as succinate: 25 mg, 50 mg, 100 mg

- ◆ **Sumatriptan Succinate** see Sumatriptan on page 1508
- ◆ **Summer's Eve® SpecialCare™ Medicated Anti-Itch Cream [OTC] [DSC]** see Hydrocortisone on page 762
- ◆ **Sumycin® [DSC]** see Tetracycline on page 1545
- ◆ **Superdophilus® [OTC]** see Lactobacillus on page 867
- ◆ **Suprax®** see Cefixime on page 258
- ◆ **Surfak® [OTC]** see Docusate on page 459
- ◆ **Surmontil®** see Trimipramine on page 1635
- ◆ **Su-Tuss DM** see Guaifenesin and Dextromethorphan on page 730
- ◆ **Symax SL** see Hyoscyamine on page 778
- ◆ **Symax SR** see Hyoscyamine on page 778
- ◆ **Symlin®** see Pramlintide on page 1297
- ◆ **Symmetrel®** see Amantadine on page 68
- ◆ **Synalar®** see Fluocinolone on page 639
- ◆ **Synera™** see Lidocaine and Tetracaine on page 908
- ◆ **Synercid®** see Quinupristin and Dalfopristin on page 1368
- ◆ **Synthroid®** see Levothyroxine on page 901
- ◆ **Syrex** see Sodium Chloride on page 1475
- ◆ **Syrup of Ipecac** see Ipecac Syrup on page 826
- ◆ **Systane® [OTC]** see Artificial Tears on page 124
- ◆ **Systane® Free [OTC]** see Artificial Tears on page 124
- ◆ **T₃ Sodium (error-prone abbreviation)** see Liothyronine on page 912
- ◆ **T₃/T₄ Liotrix** see Liotrix on page 915
- ◆ **T₄** see Levothyroxine on page 901

Tacrine (TAK reen)

Medication Safety Issues
Sound-alike/look-alike issues:
Cognex® may be confused with Corgard®

International issues:
Cognex® may be confused with Codex® which is a brand name for *Saccharomyces boulardii* in Italy

U.S. Brand Names Cognex®
Index Terms Tacrine Hydrochloride; Tetrahydroaminoacrine; THA
Generic Available No
Pharmacologic Category Acetylcholinesterase Inhibitor (Central)
Use Treatment of mild to moderate dementia of the Alzheimer's type
Contraindications Hypersensitivity to tacrine, acridine derivatives, or any component of the formulation; patients previously treated with tacrine who developed jaundice
Warnings/Precautions The use of tacrine has been associated with elevations in serum transaminases; serum transaminases (specifically ALT) must be monitored throughout therapy; use extreme caution in patients with current evidence of a history of abnormal liver function tests; cholinesterase inhibitors may have vagotonic effects
(Continued)

Tacrine *(Continued)*

which may cause bradycardia and/or heart block with or without a history of cardiac disease; use caution in patients with urinary tract obstruction (bladder outlet obstruction or prostatic hyperplasia), asthma, and sick-sinus syndrome, bradycardia, or conduction abnormalities (tacrine may cause bradycardia and/or heart block). Also, patients with cardiovascular disease, asthma, or peptic ulcer should use cautiously. Use with caution in patients with a history of seizures. May cause nausea, vomiting, or loose stools. Abrupt discontinuation or dosage decrease may worsen cognitive function. May be associated with neutropenia. May exaggerate neuromuscular blockade effects of depolarizing neuromuscular-blocking agents like succinylcholine.

Adverse Reactions (Reflective of adult population; not specific for elderly)
>10%:
    Central nervous system: Dizziness, headache
    Gastrointestinal: Diarrhea, nausea, vomiting
    Miscellaneous: Transaminases increased
1% to 10%:
    Cardiovascular: Flushing
    Central nervous system: Ataxia, confusion, depression, fatigue, insomnia, somnolence
    Dermatologic: Rash
    Gastrointestinal: Abdominal pain, anorexia, constipation, dyspepsia, flatulence, weight loss
    Neuromuscular & skeletal: Myalgia, tremor
    Respiratory: Rhinitis

Overdosage/Toxicology Symptoms included cholinergic crisis characterized by severe nausea, vomiting, salivation, sweating, bradycardia, hypotension, cardiovascular collapse, and convulsions. Increased muscle weakness is a possibility and may result in death if respiratory muscles are involved. Treatments includes general supportive measures. Tertiary anticholinergics, such as atropine, may be used as an antidote. I.V. atropine sulfate titrated to effect is recommended. Atypical increases in blood pressure and heart rate have been reported with other cholinomimetics when coadministered with quaternary anticholinergics such as glycopyrrolate.

Drug Interactions Substrate of CYP1A2 (major); **Inhibits** CYP1A2 (weak)
Anticholinergic agents: Tacrine may antagonize the therapeutic effect of anticholinergic agents (benztropine, trihexyphenidyl); a peripherally-acting agent (glycopyrrolate) has been reported to reduce tacrine-associated gastrointestinal complaints
Antipsychotic agents: Acetylcholinesterase inhibitors (central) may increase the risk of antipsychotic-related extrapyramidal symptoms; monitor.
Beta-blockers: Tacrine in combination with beta-blockers may produce additive bradycardia
Calcium channel blockers: Tacrine in combination with heart rate lowering calcium channel blockers (diltiazem and verapamil) may produce additive bradycardia
Cholinergic agents: Tacrine in combination with other cholinergic agents (eg, ambenonium, edrophonium, neostigmine, pyridostigmine, bethanechol), will likely produce additive cholinergic effects
CYP1A2 inducers: May decrease the levels/effects of tacrine. Example inducers include aminoglutethimide, carbamazepine, phenobarbital, and rifampin.
CYP1A2 inhibitors: May increase the levels/effects of tacrine. Example inhibitors include ciprofloxacin, fluvoxamine, ketoconazole, norfloxacin, ofloxacin, and rofecoxib.
Digoxin: Tacrine, in combination with digoxin, may produce additive bradycardia
Haloperidol: Tacrine may worsen Parkinson's disease and inhibit the effects of haloperidol.
Levodopa: Tacrine may worsen Parkinson's disease and inhibit the effects of levodopa
Neuromuscular blocking agents (nondepolarizing): Theoretically, tacrine may antagonize the effect of nondepolarizing neuromuscular blocking agents
Succinylcholine: Tacrine may prolong the effect of succinylcholine
Theophylline: Tacrine may inhibit the metabolism of theophylline resulting in elevated plasma levels; dose adjustment will likely be needed

Ethanol/Nutrition/Herb Interactions Food: Food decreases bioavailability.

Mechanism of Action Centrally-acting cholinesterase inhibitor. It elevates acetylcholine in cerebral cortex by slowing the degradation of acetylcholine.

Pharmacokinetics
    Absorption: Reduced with food
    Protein binding: 55%
    Metabolism: Extensive; saturable at relatively low doses
    Bioavailability, absolute: 17%
    Half-life: 2-4 hours
    No clinically relevant age-related changes in pharmacokinetics have been found

Dosage
Geriatrics & Adults:
Alzheimer's disease: Oral: Initial: 10 mg 4 times/day; may increase by 40 mg/day adjusted every 6 weeks; maximum: 160 mg/day; best administered separate from meal times.

Dose adjustment based upon transaminase elevations:

ALT ≤3 times ULN: Continue titration

ALT >3 to ≤5 times ULN: Decrease dose by 40 mg/day, resume when ALT returns to normal

ALT >5 times ULN: Stop treatment, may rechallenge upon return of ALT to normal

*ULN = upper limit of normal

Note: Patients with clinical jaundice confirmed by elevated total bilirubin (>3 mg/dL) should not be rechallenged with tacrine.

Hepatic Impairment: Patients with clinical jaundice confirmed by elevated total bilirubin (>3 mg/dL) should not be rechallenged with tacrine.

Monitoring Parameters Serum ALT every other week for 16 weeks, then every month for 2 months, and then every 3 months thereafter

Reference Range In clinical trials, serum concentrations >20 ng/mL were associated with a much higher risk of development of symptomatic adverse effects

Patient Information Effect of tacrine therapy is thought to depend upon its administration at regular intervals, as directed; take between meals if possible; if GI upset occurs, may take with meals; inform physician of the emergence of new events or any increase in the severity of existing adverse effects (those that occur upon initiation of therapy or an increase in dose, ie, nausea, vomiting, loose stools, diarrhea; and those that can occur later in therapy, ie, rash, jaundice, very light stools, or black stools); abrupt discontinuation of the drug or a large reduction in total daily dose (≥80 mg/day) may cause a decline in cognitive function and behavioral disturbances; unsupervised increases in the dose may also have serious consequences; do not change dose without consulting physician; be compliant with required liver tests

Special Geriatric Considerations Tacrine is not a cure for Alzheimer's disease. At least 25% of patients may not tolerate the drug and only 50% of patients demonstrate some improvement in symptoms or a slowing of deterioration. While worth a trial in mild-to-moderate dementia of the Alzheimer's type, patients and their families must be counseled about the limitations of the drug and the importance of regular monitoring of liver function tests. No specific dosage adjustments are necessary due to age.

Dosage Forms Excipient information presented when available (limited, particularly for generics); consult specific product labeling.

Capsule, as hydrochloride: 10 mg, 20 mg, 30 mg, 40 mg

Selected References

Crismon ML, "Tacrine: First Drug Approved for Alzheimer's Disease," *Ann Pharmacother*, 1994, 28(6):744-51.

Davis KL, Thal LJ, Gamzu ER, et al, "A Double-Blind, Placebo-Controlled Multicenter Study of Tacrine for Alzheimer's Disease," *N Engl J Med*, 1992, 327(18):1253-9.

Farlow M, Gracon SI, Hershey LA, et al, "A Controlled Trial of Tacrine in Alzheimer's Disease," *JAMA*, 1992, 268(18):2523-9.

Knapp MJ, Knopman DS, Solomon PR, et al, "A 30-Week Randomized Controlled Trial of High-Dose Tacrine in Patients With Alzheimer's Disease," *JAMA*, 1994, 271(13):985-91.

♦ **Tacrine Hydrochloride** *see* Tacrine *on page 1511*

Tadalafil (tah DA la fil)

U.S. Brand Names Cialis®
Canadian Brand Names Cialis®
Index Terms GF196960
Generic Available No
Pharmacologic Category Phosphodiesterase-5 Enzyme Inhibitor
Use Treatment of erectile dysfunction
Contraindications Hypersensitivity to tadalafil or any component of the formulation; concurrent use of organic nitrates (nitroglycerin) in any form
Warnings/Precautions There is a degree of cardiac risk associated with sexual activity; therefore, physicians may wish to consider the cardiovascular status of their patients prior to initiating any treatment for erectile dysfunction. Use caution in patients with left ventricular outflow obstruction (aortic stenosis or IHSS); may be more sensitive to hypotensive actions. Concurrent use with alpha-adrenergic antagonist therapy may cause symptomatic hypotension; patients should be hemodynamically stable prior to initiating tadalafil therapy at the lowest possible dose. Use caution in patients receiving strong CYP3A4 inhibitors, the elderly, or those with hepatic impairment or renal impairment; dosage adjustment/limitation is needed. Use caution in patients with peptic ulcer disease.

Agents for the treatment of erectile dysfunction should be used with caution in patients with anatomical deformation of the penis (angulation, cavernosal fibrosis, or Peyronie's disease), or in patients who have conditions which may predispose them to priapism (Continued)

Tadalafil *(Continued)*

(sickle cell anemia, multiple myeloma, leukemia). All patients should be instructed to seek medical attention if erection persists >4 hours. The safety and efficacy of tadalafil with other treatments for erectile dysfunction have not been studied and are, therefore, not recommended as combination therapy.

Rare cases of nonarteritic ischemic optic neuropathy (NAION) have been reported; risk may be increased with history of vision loss. Other risk factors for NAION include heart disease, diabetes, hypertension, smoking, age >50 years, or history of certain eye problems.

Safety and efficacy have not been studied in patients with the following conditions, therefore, use in these patients is not recommended: Arrhythmias, hypotension, uncontrolled hypertension, unstable angina or angina during intercourse, cardiac failure (NYHA Class II or greater), myocardial infarction within the last 3 months, or stroke within the last 6 months. A minority of patients with retinitis pigmentosa have genetic disorders of retinal phosphodiesterases; use is not recommended.

Adverse Reactions (Reflective of adult population; not specific for elderly)
>10%: Central nervous system: Headache (11% to 15%)
2% to 10%:
Cardiovascular: Flushing (2% to 3%)
Gastrointestinal: Dyspepsia (4% to 10%)
Neuromuscular & skeletal: CPK increased (2%), back pain (3% to 6%), myalgia (1% to 4%), limb pain (1% to 3%)
Respiratory: Nasal congestion (2% to 3%)

Overdosage/Toxicology Symptoms similar to those seen at lower doses (headache, back pain, myalgias). Treatment is symptomatic and supportive.

Drug Interactions Substrate of CYP3A4 (major)
Alpha$_1$-blockers: Phosphodiesterase-5 inhibitors may enhance the hypotensive effect of alpha$_1$-blockers.
Antifungal agents (imidazole): May decrease the metabolism, via CYP isoenzymes, of phosphodiesterase-5 inhibitors. Ketoconazole significantly increased tadalafil levels.
CYP3A4 inhibitors: May increase the levels/effects of tadalafil. Dose reduction of tadalafil is recommended with strong CYP3A4 inhibitors. The dose of tadalafil should not exceed 10 mg, and tadalafil should not be taken more frequently than once every 72 hours. Example inhibitors include azole antifungals, clarithromycin, diclofenac, doxycycline, erythromycin, grapefruit juice, imatinib, isoniazid, nefazodone, nicardipine, propofol, protease inhibitors, quinidine, telithromycin, and verapamil.
Macrolide antibiotics (clarithromycin, erythromycin, telithromycin, troleandomycin): May decrease the metabolism, via cyp isoenzymes, of phosphodiesterase-5 inhibitors.
Protease inhibitors (amprenavir, atazanavir, fosamprenavir, indinavir, lopinavir, nelfinavir, ritonavir, saquinavir): May decrease the metabolism, via cyp isoenzymes, of phosphodiesterase-5 inhibitors. Ritonavir increased tadalafil levels.
Vasodilators (organic nitrates): Concomitant use is contraindicated due to the potential for severe, life-threatening hypotension; separate doses by 48 hours.

Ethanol/Nutrition/Herb Interactions
Ethanol: Substantial consumption of ethanol may increase the risk of hypotension and orthostasis. Lower ethanol consumption has not been associated with significant changes in blood pressure or increase in orthostatic symptoms.
Food: Rate and extent of absorption are not affected by food. Grapefruit juice may increase serum levels/toxicity of tadalafil. Do not give more than a single 10 mg dose of tadalafil more frequently than every 72 hours in patients who regularly consume grapefruit juice.

Stability Store at controlled room temperature of 15°C to 30°C (59°F to 86°F).

Mechanism of Action Does not directly cause penile erections, but affects the response to sexual stimulation. The physiologic mechanism of erection of the penis involves release of nitric oxide (NO) in the corpus cavernosum during sexual stimulation. NO then activates the enzyme guanylate cyclase, which results in increased levels of cyclic guanosine monophosphate (cGMP), producing smooth muscle relaxation and inflow of blood to the corpus cavernosum. Tadalafil enhances the effect of NO by inhibiting phosphodiesterase type 5 (PDE-5), which is responsible for degradation of cGMP in the corpus cavernosum; when sexual stimulation causes local release of NO, inhibition of PDE-5 by tadalafil causes increased levels of cGMP in the corpus cavernosum, resulting in smooth muscle relaxation and inflow of blood to the corpus cavernosum. At recommended doses, it has no effect in the absence of sexual stimulation.

Pharmacokinetics
Onset: Within 1 hour
Duration: Up to 36 hours
Distribution: V$_d$: 63 L
Protein binding: 94%
Metabolism: Hepatic, via CYP3A4 to metabolites (inactive)
Half-life elimination: 17.5 hours

Time to peak, plasma: 2 hours

Elimination: Feces (61%, as metabolites); urine (36%, as metabolites)

Dosage

Geriatrics: Dosage is based on renal function; refer to dosing in renal impairment.

Adults:

Erectile dysfunction: Oral: 10 mg prior to anticipated sexual activity (dosing range: 5-20 mg); to be given as one single dose and not given more than once daily. **Note:** Erectile function may be improved for up to 36 hours following a single dose; adjust dose.

Dosing adjustment with concomitant medications:

Alpha$_1$-blockers: If stabilized on either alpha-blockers or tadalafil therapy, initiate new therapy with the other agent at the lowest possible dose.

CYP3A4 inhibitors: Dose reduction of tadalafil is recommended with strong CYP3A4 inhibitors. The dose of tadalafil should not exceed 10 mg, and tadalafil should not be taken more frequently than once every 72 hours. Examples of such inhibitors include amprenavir, atazanavir, clarithromycin, conivaptan, delavirdine, diclofenac, fosamprenavir, imatinib, indinavir, isoniazid, itraconazole, ketoconazole, miconazole, nefazodone, nelfinavir, nicardipine, propofol, quinidine, ritonavir, and telithromycin.

Renal Impairment:

Cl$_{cr}$ 31-50 mL/minute: Initial dose 5 mg once daily; maximum dose 10 mg not to be given more frequently than every 48 hours.

Cl$_{cr}$ <30 mL/minute or hemodialysis: Maximum dose 5 mg.

Hepatic Impairment:

Mild-to-moderate hepatic impairment (Child-Pugh class A or B): Dose should not exceed 10 mg once daily.

Severe hepatic impairment: Use is not recommended.

Administration May be administered with or without food, prior to anticipated sexual activity.

Monitoring Parameters Monitor for response and adverse effects.

Patient Information Discuss with your physician the contraindications of tadalafil, particularly the use of nitrates. Report all adverse effects to your physician including erections lasting >4 hours. Do not take more than the prescribed dose. Take the dose 30-60 minutes before sexual activity; effects may last up to 3 days. Tadalafil has no effect without sexual stimulation. Do not drink excessive alcohol while taking tadalafil.

Special Geriatric Considerations No significant differences in pharmacokinetics were seen in elderly men versus younger men. Dosing should be adjusted for renal function. Since older adults often have concomitant diseases, many of which may be contraindicated with the use of tadalafil, prescriber should complete a thorough review of diseases and medications prior to prescribing tadalafil.

Dosage Forms Excipient information presented when available (limited, particularly for generics); consult specific product labeling.

Tablet: 5 mg, 10 mg, 20 mg

Selected References

Curran M and Keating G, "Tadalafil," *Drugs*, 2003, 63(20):2203-12; discussion 2213-4.

♦ **Tagamet**® **[DSC]** *see* Cimetidine *on page 313*

♦ **Tagamet**® **HB 200 [OTC]** *see* Cimetidine *on page 313*

♦ **TAK-375** *see* Ramelteon *on page 1375*

♦ **Talwin**® *see* Pentazocine *on page 1229*

♦ **Talwin**® **NX** *see* Pentazocine *on page 1229*

♦ **TAM** *see* Tamoxifen *on page 1515*

♦ **Tambocor**™ *see* Flecainide *on page 629*

♦ **Tamiflu**® *see* Oseltamivir *on page 1167*

Tamoxifen (ta MOKS i fen)

Medication Safety Issues

Sound-alike/look-alike issues:

Tamoxifen may be confused with pentoxifylline, Tambocor™

U.S. Brand Names Nolvadex® [DSC]; Soltamox™

Canadian Brand Names Apo-Tamox®; Gen-Tamoxifen; Nolvadex®; Nolvadex®-D; Novo-Tamoxifen; Tamofen®

Index Terms ICI-46474; NSC-180973; TAM; Tamoxifen Citrate

Generic Available Yes: Tablet

Pharmacologic Category Antineoplastic Agent, Estrogen Receptor Antagonist

Use Palliative or adjunctive treatment of advanced breast cancer; reduction of the incidence of breast cancer in women at high risk; reduction of risk of invasive breast cancer in women with ductal carcinoma *in situ* (DCIS); metastatic female and male breast cancer

(Continued)

Tamoxifen *(Continued)*

Unlabeled/Investigational Use Treatment of mastalgia, gynecomastia, pancreatic carcinoma, melanoma and desmoid tumors

Restrictions An FDA-approved medication guide must be distributed when dispensing the outpatient prescription (new or refill) to females for breast cancer prevention or treatment of ductal carcinoma *in situ* where this medication is to be used without direct supervision of a healthcare provider. Medication guides are available at http://www.fda.gov/cder/Offices/ODS/medication_guides.htm.

Contraindications Hypersensitivity to tamoxifen or any component of the formulation; concurrent warfarin therapy or history of deep vein thrombosis or pulmonary embolism (when tamoxifen is used for cancer risk reduction)

Warnings/Precautions Hazardous agent; use appropriate precautions for handling and disposal. **[U.S. Boxed Warning]: Serious and life-threatening events (including stroke, pulmonary emboli, and uterine malignancy) have occurred at an incidence greater than placebo during use for cancer risk reduction;** these events are rare, but require consideration in risk:benefit evaluation. An increased incidence of thromboembolic events has been associated with use for breast cancer; risk may increase with chemotherapy addition; use caution in individuals with a history of thromboembolic events. Use with caution in patients with leukopenia, thrombocytopenia, or hyperlipidemias. Decreased visual acuity, retinopathy, corneal changes, and increased incidence of cataracts have been reported. Hypercalcemia has occurred in patients with bone metastasis. Significant bone loss of the lumbar spine and hip was associated with use in premenopausal women. Liver abnormalities such as cholestasis, fatty liver, hepatitis, and hepatic necrosis have occurred. Hepatocellular carcinomas have been reported in some studies; relationship to treatment is unclear. Endometrial hyperplasia, polyps, endometriosis, uterine fibroids, and ovarian cysts have occurred. Increased risk of uterine or endometrial cancer; monitor.

Adverse Reactions (Reflective of adult population; not specific for elderly)

>10%:

Cardiovascular: Flushing (33% to 41%), hypertension (11%), peripheral edema (11%)

Central nervous system: Pain (3% to 16%), mood changes (12% to 18%), depression (2% to 12%)

Dermatologic: Skin changes (6% to 19%), rash (13%)

Endocrine & metabolic: Hot flashes (3% to 80%), fluid retention (32%), altered menses (13% to 25%), amenorrhea (16%)

Gastrointestinal: Nausea (5% to 26%), weight loss (23%)

Genitourinary: Vaginal bleeding (2% to 23%), vaginal discharge (13% to 55%)

Neuromuscular & skeletal: Weakness (19%), arthritis (14%), arthralgia (11%)

Respiratory: Pharyngitis (14%)

1% to 10%:

Cardiovascular: Chest pain (5%), venous thrombotic events (5%), edema (4%), cardiovascular ischemia (3%), cerebrovascular ischemia (3%), angina (2%), deep venous thrombus (2%), MI (1%)

Central nervous system: Insomnia (9%), dizziness (8%), headache (8%), anxiety (6%), fatigue (4%)

Dermatologic: Alopecia (<1% to 5%)

Endocrine & metabolic: Oligomenorrhea (9%), breast pain (6%), menstrual disorder (6%), breast neoplasm (5%), hypercholesterolemia (4%)

Gastrointestinal: Abdominal pain (9%), weight gain (9%), throat irritation (oral solution 5%), constipation (4% to 8%), diarrhea (7%), dyspepsia (6%), abdominal cramps (1%), anorexia (1%)

Genitourinary: Urinary tract infection (10%), leukorrhea (9%), vaginal hemorrhage (6%), vaginitis (5%), ovarian cyst (3%)

Hematologic: Thrombocytopenia (<1% to 10%), anemia (5%)

Hepatic: AST increased (5%), serum bilirubin increased (2%)

Neuromuscular & skeletal: Bone pain (6% to 10%), osteoporosis (7%), fracture (7%), arthrosis (5%), myalgia (5%), paresthesia (5%), musculoskeletal pain (3%)

Ocular: Cataract (7%)

Renal: Serum creatinine increased (up to 2%)

Respiratory: Cough (4% to 9%), dyspnea (8%), bronchitis (5%), sinusitis (5%)

Miscellaneous: Infection/sepsis (up to 9%), diaphoresis (6%), flu-like syndrome (6%), allergic reaction (3%)

Overdosage/Toxicology Overdose produced respiratory difficulties and seizure in animal studies. In humans, loading doses of 400 mg/m^2 followed by 150 mg/m^2 twice daily produced reversible neurotoxicity (tremor, hyperreflexia, unsteady gait, and dizziness). Loading doses of >250 mg/m^2 followed by 80 mg/m^2 twice daily produced QT prolongation in some patients. In the case of an overdose, treatment is symptom-directed and supportive.

Drug Interactions Substrate of CYP2A6 (minor), 2B6 (minor), 2C9 (major), 2D6 (major), 2E1 (minor), 3A4 (major); **Inhibits** CYP2B6 (weak), 2C8 (moderate), 2C9 (weak), 3A4 (weak)

Anastrozole: Tamoxifen may reduce the levels/effects of anastrozole. Concurrent therapy is not recommended (per manufacturer).

CYP2C8 substrates: Tamoxifen may increase the levels/effects of CYP2C8 substrates. Example substrates include amiodarone, paclitaxel, pioglitazone, repaglinide, and rosiglitazone.

CYP2C9 inducers: May decrease the levels/effects of tamoxifen. Example inducers include carbamazepine, phenobarbital, phenytoin, rifampin, rifapentine, and secobarbital.

CYP2C9 inhibitors: May increase the levels/effects of tamoxifen. Example inhibitors include delavirdine, fluconazole, gemfibrozil, ketoconazole, nicardipine, NSAIDs, sulfonamides, and tolbutamide.

CYP2D6 inhibitors: May increase the levels/effects of tamoxifen. Example inhibitors include chlorpromazine, delavirdine, fluoxetine, miconazole, paroxetine, pergolide, quinidine, quinine, ritonavir, and ropinirole.

CYP3A4 inducers: CYP3A4 inducers may decrease the levels/effects of tamoxifen. Example inducers include aminoglutethimide, carbamazepine, nafcillin, nevirapine, phenobarbital, phenytoin, and rifamycins.

CYP3A4 inhibitors: May increase the levels/effects of tamoxifen. Example inhibitors include azole antifungals, clarithromycin, diclofenac, doxycycline, erythromycin, imatinib, isoniazid, nefazodone, nicardipine, propofol, protease inhibitors, quinidine, telithromycin, and verapamil.

Rifamycins: Rifamycin derivatives may increase the metabolism (via CYP isoenzymes) of tamoxifen.

Warfarin: Concomitant use is contraindicated when used for risk reduction; results in significant enhancement of the anticoagulant effects of warfarin

Ethanol/Nutrition/Herb Interactions Herb/Nutraceutical: Avoid black cohosh, dong quai in estrogen-dependent tumors. Avoid St John's wort (may decrease levels/effects of tamoxifen).

Stability

Solution: Store at room temperature at or below 25°C (77°F); do not refrigerate or freeze. Protect from light. Use within 3 months of opening.

Tablet: Store at room temperature of 20°C to 25°C (68°F to 77°F).

Mechanism of Action Competitively binds to estrogen receptors on tumors and other tissue targets, producing a nuclear complex that decreases DNA synthesis and inhibits estrogen effects; nonsteroidal agent with potent antiestrogenic properties which compete with estrogen for binding sites in breast and other tissues; cells accumulate in the G_0 and G_1 phases; therefore, tamoxifen is cytostatic rather than cytocidal.

Pharmacokinetics

Absorption: Well absorbed; tablet and oral solution are bioequivalent

Distribution: High concentrations found in uterus, endometrial and breast tissue

Protein binding: 99%

Metabolism: Hepatic (via CYP3A4) to major metabolites, N-desmethyl tamoxifen (major) and 4-hydroxytamoxifen (minor), and a tamoxifen derivative (minor); undergoes enterohepatic recirculation

Half-life: Distribution: 7-14 hours; Elimination: 5-7 days; Metabolites: 14 days

Time to peak, serum: 5 hours

Elimination: Feces (26% to 51%); urine (9% to 13%)

Dosage

Geriatrics & Adults: Refer to individual protocols.

Breast cancer treatment:

Metastatic (males and females) or adjuvant therapy (females): Oral: 20-40 mg/day; daily doses >20 mg should be given in 2 divided doses (morning and evening)

DCIS (females): Oral: 20 mg once daily for 5 years

Breast cancer prevention (high-risk females): Oral: 20 mg/day for 5 years

Note: Higher dosages (up to 700 mg/day) have been investigated for use in modulation of multidrug resistance (MDR), but are not routinely used in clinical practice.

Monitoring Parameters CBC with platelets, serum calcium, LFTs; abnormal vaginal bleeding; annual gynecologic exams, mammogram

Test Interactions T_4 elevations (which may be explained by increases in thyroid-binding globulin) have been reported; not accompanied by clinical hyperthyroidism

Patient Information Take as directed, morning and night and maintain adequate hydration (2-3 L/day of fluids unless instructed to restrict fluid intake). You may experience hot flashes, hair loss, loss of libido (these will subside when treatment is completed). Bone pain may indicate a good therapeutic response (consult prescriber for mild analgesics). For nausea and vomiting - small frequent meals, chewing gum, or sucking lozenges may help. You may experience photosensitivity (use sunscreen, wear protective clothing and eyewear, and avoid direct sunlight). Notify prescriber if (Continued)

Tamoxifen *(Continued)*

vaginal bleeding occurs. Report unusual bleeding or bruising, new lumps, severe weakness, sedation, mental changes, swelling or pain in calves, difficulty breathing, or any vision change.

Additional Information Oral clonidine is being studied for the treatment of tamoxifen-induced "hot flashes." Tumor flare reaction may indicate a good therapeutic response and is often considered a good prognostic factor.

Special Geriatric Considerations Studies have shown tamoxifen to be effective in the treatment of primary breast cancer in elderly women. Comparative studies with other antineoplastic agents in elderly women with breast cancer had more favorable survival rates with tamoxifen. Initiation of hormone therapy rather than chemotherapy is justified for elderly patients with metastatic breast cancer who are responsive. Reduction of mortality and recurrence was greater in those studies that used tamoxifen for ≥2 years than those that use it for <2 years.

Dosage Forms Excipient information presented when available (limited, particularly for generics); consult specific product labeling.

Solution, oral:

Soltamox™: 10 mg/5 mL (150 mL) [licorice flavor]

Tablet: 10 mg, 20 mg

Nolvadex®: 10 mg, 20 mg [DSC]

Selected References

Allan SG, Rodger A, Smyth JF, et al, "Tamoxifen as Primary Treatment of Breast Cancer in Elderly or Frail Patients: a Practical Management," *Br Med J (Clin Res Ed)*, 1985, 290(6465):358.

Taylor SG 4th, Gelman RS, Falkson G, et al "Combination Chemotherapy Compared to Tamoxifen as Initial Therapy for Stage IV Breast Cancer in Elderly Women," *Ann Intern Med*, 1986, 104(4):455-61.

Winer EP, Hudis C, Burstein HJ, et al, "American Society of Clinical Oncology Technology Assessment on the Use of Aromatase Inhibitors as Adjuvant Therapy for Postmenopausal Women With Hormone Receptor-Positive Breast Cancer: Status Report 2004," *J Clin Oncol*, 2005, 23(3):619-29.

♦ **Tamoxifen Citrate** *see* Tamoxifen *on page 1515*

Tamsulosin *(tam SOO loe sin)*

Related Information

Pharmacotherapy of Urinary Incontinence *on page 1822*

Medication Safety Issues

Sound-alike/look-alike issues:

Flomax® may be confused with Fosamax®, Volmax®

International issues:

Flomax®: Brand name for morniflumate in Italy

Flomax® may be confused with Flomox® which is a brand name for cefcapene in Japan

U.S. Brand Names Flomax®

Canadian Brand Names Flomax®; Flomax® CR

Index Terms Tamsulosin Hydrochloride

Generic Available No

Pharmacologic Category Alpha₁ Blocker

Use Treatment of signs and symptoms of benign prostatic hyperplasia (BPH); **not** indicated for the treatment of hypertension

Unlabeled/Investigational Use Symptomatic treatment of bladder outlet obstruction or dysfunction

Contraindications Hypersensitivity to tamsulosin or any component of the formulation

Warnings/Precautions Not intended for use as an antihypertensive drug. May cause significant orthostatic hypotension and syncope, especially with first dose; anticipate a similar effect if therapy is interrupted for a few days, if dosage is rapidly increased, or if another antihypertensive drug (particularly vasodilators) or a PDE-5 inhibitor is introduced. "First-dose" orthostatic hypotension may occur 4-8 hours after dosing; may be dose related. Patients should be cautioned about performing hazardous tasks when starting new therapy or adjusting dosage upward. Discontinue if symptoms of angina occur or worsen. Rule out prostatic carcinoma before beginning therapy with tamsulosin. Intraoperative floppy iris syndrome has been observed in cataract surgery patients who were on or were previously treated with alpha₁-blockers; causality has not been established and there appears to be no benefit in discontinuing alpha-blocker therapy prior to surgery. Priapism has been associated with use (rarely). Rarely, patients with a sulfa allergy have also developed an allergic reaction to tamsulosin; avoid use when previous reaction has been severe.

Adverse Reactions (Reflective of adult population; not specific for elderly)

>10%:

Cardiovascular: Orthostatic hypotension (6 % to 19%)

Central nervous system: Headache (19% to 21%), dizziness (15% to 17%)

Genitourinary: Abnormal ejaculation (8% to 18%)

Respiratory: Rhinitis (13% to 18%)
Miscellaneous: Infection (9% to 11%)
1% to 10%:
Cardiovascular: Chest pain (4%)
Central nervous system: Somnolence (3% to 4%), insomnia (1% to 2%), vertigo (≤1%)
Endocrine & metabolic: Libido decreased (1% to 2%)
Gastrointestinal: Diarrhea (4% to 6%), nausea (3% to 4%), tooth disorder (1% to 2%)
Neuromuscular & skeletal: Weakness (8% to 9%), back pain (7% to 8%)
Ocular: Blurred vision (up to 2%)
Respiratory: Pharyngitis (5% to 6%), cough (3% to 5%), sinusitis (2% to 4%)

Overdosage/Toxicology Symptoms of overdose include headache and hypotension. To maintain blood pressure, patient should be in supine position; consider I.V. hydration; vasopressors may be necessary. Treatment is otherwise symptom-directed and supportive. Dialysis is not likely to benefit.

Drug Interactions Substrate (major) of CYP2D6, 3A4
Alpha-adrenergic blockers: Risk of hypotension may increase in combination with other alpha-adrenergic blocking agents.
Beta-blockers: Beta-blockers may increase risk of first-dose orthostatic hypotension of tamsulosin
Calcium channel blockers: Risk of hypotension may increase
Cimetidine: Cimetidine may decrease tamsulosin clearance.
CYP2D6 inhibitors: May increase the levels/effects of tamsulosin. Example inhibitors include chlorpromazine, delavirdine, fluoxetine, miconazole, paroxetine, pergolide, quinidine, quinine, ritonavir, and ropinirole.
CYP3A4 inducers: CYP3A4 inducers may decrease the levels/effects of tamsulosin. Example inducers include aminoglutethimide, carbamazepine, nafcillin, nevirapine, phenobarbital, phenytoin, and rifamycins.
CYP3A4 inhibitors: May increase the levels/effects of tamsulosin. Example inhibitors include azole antifungals, clarithromycin, diclofenac, doxycycline, erythromycin, imatinib, isoniazid, nefazodone, nicardipine, propofol, protease inhibitors, quinidine, telithromycin, and verapamil.
Phosphodiesterase-5 inhibitors (eg, sildenafil, tadalafil, vardenafil): Blood pressure-lowering effects are additive. Use of vardenafil is contraindicated by the manufacturer. Use sildenafil with extreme caution (dose ≤25 mg). Tadalafil may be used when tamsulosin dose is ≤0.4 mg/day.

Ethanol/Nutrition/Herb Interactions
Food: Fasting increases bioavailability by 30% and peak concentration 40% to 70%.
Herb/Nutraceutical: St John's wort: May decrease the levels/effects of tamsulosin. Avoid herbs with hypotensive properties (black cohosh, California poppy, coleus, golden seal, hawthorn, mistletoe, periwinkle, quinine, Shepherd's purse); may enhance the hypotensive effect of tamsulosin. Avoid saw palmetto (due to limited experience with this combination).

Stability Store at room temperature at 15°C to 30°C (59°F to 86°F).

Mechanism of Action Tamsulosin is an antagonist of alpha$_{1A}$-adrenoreceptors in the prostate. Smooth muscle tone in the prostate is mediated by alpha$_{1A}$-adrenoreceptors; blocking them leads to relaxation of smooth muscle in the bladder neck and prostate causing an improvement of urine flow and decreased symptoms of BPH. Approximately 75% of the alpha$_1$-receptors in the prostate are of the alpha$_{1A}$ subtype.

Pharmacokinetics
Absorption: >90% under fasting conditions
Protein binding: 94% to 99% to alpha$_1$-glycoprotein
Metabolism: Hepatic via CYP3A4 and 2D6; metabolites undergo extensive conjugation to glucuronide or sulfate
Bioavailability: Fasting: 30% increase
Half-life:
Healthy volunteers: 9-13 hours
Target population: 14-15 hours
Geriatrics: Slightly prolonged and AUC is increased by 40%
Elimination: 76% in urine as metabolites

Dosage
Geriatrics & Adults:
BPH: Oral: 0.4 mg once daily ~30 minutes after the same meal each day; dose may be increased after 2-4 weeks to 0.8 mg once daily in patients who fail to respond. If therapy is interrupted for several days, restart with 0.4 mg once daily.
Bladder outlet obstruction (unlabeled use): Oral: 0.4 mg once daily ~30 minutes after the same meal each day
Renal Impairment:
Cl$_{cr}$ ≥10 mL/minute: No adjustment needed.
Cl$_{cr}$ <10 mL/minute: Not studied.

Monitoring Parameters Relief of symptoms, blood pressure
(Continued)

Tamsulosin *(Continued)*

Patient Information Take approximately 30 minutes after the same meal each day. Do not chew, crush, or open the capsules. Though the incidence of orthostatic hypotension is minimal, patients should be instructed to rise slowly from a sitting or lying position. May cause dizziness, use caution when driving until you see how the medication affects you.

Additional Information If therapy with tamsulosin is discontinued or interrupted for several days, restart therapy at the 0.4 mg once daily dose

Special Geriatric Considerations Metabolism of tamsulosin may be slower, and older patients may be more sensitive to the orthostatic hypotension caused by this medication. A 40% higher exposure (AUC) is anticipated in patients between 55 and 75 years of age as compared to younger subjects (20-32 years).

Dosage Forms Excipient information presented when available (limited, particularly for generics); consult specific product labeling.
Capsule, as hydrochloride:
Flomax®: 0.4 mg

Selected References
Goldman HB and Zimmern PE, "The Treatment of Female Bladder Outlet Obstruction," *BJU Int*, 2006, 98(Suppl 1):17-23.
Pischedda A, Pirozzi Farina F, Madonia M, et al, "Use of Alpha₁-Blockers in Female Functional Bladder Neck Obstruction," *Urol Int*, 2005, 74(3):256-61.
Rossi C, Kortmann BB, Sonke GS, et al, "Alpha-Blockade Improves Symptoms Suggestive of Bladder Outlet Obstruction But Fails to Relieve It," *J Urol*, 2001, 165(1):38-41.

Tegaserod *(teg a SER od)*

U.S. Brand Names Zelnorm®
Canadian Brand Names Zelnorm® [DSC]
Index Terms HTF919; Tegaserod Maleate
Generic Available No
Pharmacologic Category Serotonin 5-HT₄ Receptor Agonist
Use Short-term treatment of constipation-predominate irritable bowel syndrome (IBS) in women

Restrictions Available in U.S. under a treatment investigational new drug (IND) protocol. Physicians must evaluate specific inclusion and exclusion protocol prior to enrolling qualifying patients. Physicians may contact Novartis (888-669-6682) or find additional information at http://www.zelnorm.com. The FDA may also offer assistance with potential alternatives in those patients not meeting specific criteria (888-463-6332 or 301-827-4570).

Contraindications Hypersensitivity to tegaserod or any component of the formulation; severe renal impairment; moderate or severe hepatic impairment; history of bowel obstruction, symptomatic gallbladder disease, suspected sphincter of Oddi dysfunction, or abdominal adhesions. Treatment should **not** be started in patients with diarrhea or in those who experience diarrhea frequently.

Warnings/Precautions Serious cardiovascular events (eg, MI, stroke, unstable angina) may occur; patients should seek emergency care following any sign and symptom suggestive of a serious cardiac event. Use extreme caution or avoid in patients with ischemic cardiovascular disease or a history of a MI, stroke, or unstable angina. Has been associated with rare intestinal ischemic events. Discontinue immediately with new or sudden worsening abdominal pain or rectal bleeding. Diarrhea may occur after the start of treatment, most cases reported as a single episode within the first week of therapy, and may resolve with continued dosing. However, serious consequences of diarrhea (hypovolemia, syncope) have been reported. Patients should be warned to contact healthcare provider immediately if they develop severe diarrhea, or diarrhea with severe cramping, abdominal pain, or dizziness. Use caution with mild hepatic impairment; not recommended with moderate or severe impairment.

Adverse Reactions (Reflective of adult population; not specific for elderly)
>10%:
    Central nervous system: Headache (15%)
    Gastrointestinal: Abdominal pain (12%)
1% to 10%:
    Central nervous system: Dizziness (4%), migraine (2%)
    Gastrointestinal: Diarrhea (9%; severe <1%), nausea (8%), flatulence (6%)
    Neuromuscular & skeletal: Back pain (5%), arthropathy (2%), leg pain (1%)

Overdosage/Toxicology Treatment should be symptom-directed and supportive. Diarrhea, headache, abdominal pain, orthostatic hypotension, nausea, and vomiting were reported in healthy volunteers with doses of 90-180 mg. Unlikely to be removed by dialysis.

Ethanol/Nutrition/Herb Interactions Food: Bioavailability is decreased by 40% to 65% and C_{max} is decreased by 20% to 40% when taken with food. T_{max} is prolonged from 1 hour up to 2 hours when taken following a meal, but decreased to 0.7 hours when taken 30 minutes before a meal.

Stability Store at controlled room temperature of 15°C to 30°C (59°F to 86°F). Protect from moisture.

Mechanism of Action Tegaserod is a partial neuronal 5-HT$_4$ receptor agonist. Its action at the receptor site leads to stimulation of the peristaltic reflex and intestinal secretion, and moderation of visceral sensitivity.

Pharmacokinetics
    Distribution: V_d: 368 ± 223 L
    Protein binding: 98% primarily to α_1-acid glycoprotein
    Metabolism: GI: Hydrolysis in the stomach; Hepatic: Oxidation, conjugation, and glucuronidation; metabolite (negligible activity); significant first-pass effect
    Bioavailability: Fasting: 10%
    Half-life: I.V.: 11 ± 5 hours
    Time to peak: 1 hour
    Elimination: Feces (~66% as unchanged drug); urine (~33% as metabolites)

Dosage
    Geriatrics: Use in elderly women (≥55 years of age) is contraindicated.
    Adults:
        IBS with constipation: Females <55 years of age: Oral: 6 mg twice daily, before meals, for 4-6 weeks; may consider continuing treatment for an additional 4-6 weeks in patients who respond initially
        Chronic idiopathic constipation: Females <55 years of age: Oral: 6 mg twice daily, before meals; the need for continued therapy should be reassessed periodically
    Renal Impairment: C_{max} and AUC of the inactive metabolite are increased with renal impairment.
        Mild to moderate impairment: No dosage adjustment recommended
        Severe impairment: Use is contraindicated
    Hepatic Impairment: C_{max} and AUC of tegaserod are increased with hepatic impairment.
        Mild impairment: No dosage adjustment recommended; however, user caution
        Moderate to severe impairment: Use is contraindicated

Administration Administer 30 minutes before meals.

Patient Information Diarrhea may occur during therapy, usually within the first week of treatment, and should resolve. Notify physician for severe diarrhea; diarrhea with severe cramping, or dizziness; new or worsening abdominal pain. Do not take if having diarrhea or if you experience diarrhea frequently.

Additional Information In clinical trials, constipation was defined as <3 bowel movements per week, hard or lumpy stools, or straining with a bowel movement.

Special Geriatric Considerations No dosing adjustment is required.

Dosage Forms Excipient information presented when available (limited, particularly for generics); consult specific product labeling.
    Tablet:
        Zelnorm®: 2 mg, 6 mg

♦ **Tegaserod Maleate** see Tegaserod on page 1520

♦ **Tegretol®** *see* Carbamazepine *on page 231*

♦ **Tegretol®-XR** *see* Carbamazepine *on page 231*

♦ **Tekturna®** *see* Aliskiren *on page 48*

Telbivudine (tel Bl vyoo deen)

U.S. Brand Names Tyzeka™

Canadian Brand Names Sebivo™

Index Terms L-Deoxythymidine

Generic Available No

Pharmacologic Category Antiretroviral Agent, Reverse Transcriptase Inhibitor (Nucleoside)

Use Treatment of chronic hepatitis B with evidence of viral replication and either persistent transaminase elevations or histologically-active disease

Contraindications Hypersensitivity to telbivudine or any component of the formulation

Warnings/Precautions [U.S. Boxed Warnings]: Cases of lactic acidosis and severe hepatomegaly with steatosis, some fatal, have been reported with the use of nucleoside analogues. Severe, acute exacerbation of hepatitis B may occur upon discontinuation. Monitor liver function several months after stopping treatment; reinitiation of antihepatitis B therapy may be required. Myopathy (eg, unexplained muscle aches and/or muscle weakness in conjunction with increases serum creatine kinase) has been reported with telbivudine initiation after several weeks to months; therapy should be interrupted if myopathy suspected and discontinued if diagnosed. Use caution in patients with renal impairment or patients receiving concomitant therapy which may reduce renal function; dosage adjustment required (Cl_{cr} <50 mL/minute). Monitor renal function before and during treatment in liver transplant patients receiving concurrent therapy of cyclosporine or tacrolimus; telbivudine may need to be adjusted. Safety and efficacy in liver transplant patients have not been established. Cross-resistance among other antivirals for hepatitis B may occur; use caution in patients failing previous therapy with lamivudine. Telbivudine does not exhibit any clinically-relevant activity against human immunodeficiency virus (HIV type 1). Safety and efficacy have not been studied in patients coinfected with HIV, hepatitis C virus (HCV), or hepatitis D virus (HDV).

Adverse Reactions (Reflective of adult population; not specific for elderly)

>10%:

Central nervous system: Fatigue (12%), malaise (12%), headache (11%)

Gastrointestinal: Abdominal pain (12%)

Neuromuscular & skeletal: CPK increased (72%; grades 3/4: 9%)

Respiratory: Upper respiratory tract infection (14%), nasopharyngitis (11%)

1% to 10%:

Central nervous system: Dizziness (4%), fever (4%), insomnia (3%)

Dermatologic: Rash (4%)

Endocrine & metabolic: Lipase increased (2%)

Gastrointestinal: Nausea (7%), vomiting (7%), diarrhea (7%), dyspepsia (3%)

Hematologic: Neutropenia (2%)

Hepatic: ALT increased (grades 3/4: 3% to 4%), AST increased (grades 3/4: 3%)

Neuromuscular & skeletal: Arthralgia (4%), back pain (4%), myalgia (3%)

Respiratory: Cough (7%), pharyngolaryngeal pain (5%)

Miscellaneous: Flu-like syndrome (7%), postprocedural pain (7%)

Overdosage/Toxicology Limited experience in acute overdose. Treatment should be symptom-directed and supportive. Hemodialysis (4 hours) will remove ~23% of dose.

Drug Interactions No interactions identified.

Ethanol/Nutrition/Herb Interactions

Ethanol: Should be avoided in hepatitis B infection due to potential hepatic toxicity.

Food: Does not have a significant effect on telbivudine absorption.

Stability Store at 15°C to 30°C (59°F to 86°F).

Mechanism of Action Telbivudine, a synthetic thymidine nucleoside analogue, is intracellularly phosphorylated to the active triphosphate form, which competes with the natural substrate, thymidine 5'-triphosphate, to inhibit hepatitis B viral DNA polymerase; enzyme inhibition blocks reverse transcriptase activity thereby reducing viral DNA replication.

Pharmacokinetics

Distribution: V_d > total body water

Protein binding: 3%

Metabolism: No metabolites detected

Half-life elimination: Terminal: 40-49 hours

Time to peak, plasma: 1-4 hours

Excretion: Urine (as unchanged drug)

Dosage

Adults: Chronic hepatitis B: Oral: 600 mg once daily

Renal Impairment:

Cl$_{cr}$ 30-49 mL/minute: 600 mg every 48 hours

Cl$_{cr}$ <30 mL/minute (not requiring dialysis): 600 mg every 72 hours

End stage renal disease: 600 mg every 96 hours

Hemodialysis: Administer after dialysis session

Hepatic Impairment: No adjustment necessary.

Administration May be administered without regard to food.

Monitoring Parameters LFTs (eg, AST and ALT) periodically during therapy and for several months following discontinuation of therapy; renal function prior to initiation and periodically during treatment; signs and symptoms of myopathy (eg, unexplained muscle pain, tenderness or weakness and serum creatine kinase)

Patient Information Do not take any new prescription or OTC medications, or herbal products during therapy without consulting prescriber. This medication does not stop you from spreading HBV to others; consult prescriber about safe sex practices and do not share needles or personal items that may have blood or body fluids on them. Take as directed with or without food. Do not discontinue without consulting prescriber (symptoms may worsen and/or become very serious). Avoid alcohol (may increase potential for liver damage). Maintain adequate hydration (2-3 L/day of fluids, unless instructed to restrict fluid intake). This medication may be prescribed with a combination of other medications; time these medications as directed by prescriber. Frequent blood tests may be required with prolonged therapy. May cause nausea or vomiting (small frequent meals, frequent mouth care, chewing gum, or sucking lozenges may help); dizziness or fatigue (use caution when driving or engaging in tasks that require alertness until response to drug is known); headache, fever, or muscle pain (an analgesic may be recommended). Report immediately any signs of lactic acidosis (eg, persistent lethargy or fatigue, unusual muscle pain or weakness, feel cold [especially in arms and legs], rapid or irregular heart beat, or difficulty breathing) or liver toxicity (eg, yellowing of eyes or skin, pale stool and dark urine); upper respiratory infection or other persistent adverse effects.

Additional Information Telbivudine is the L-enantiomer of thymidine

Special Geriatric Considerations Insufficient clinical data in elderly to determine differences between aged patients and younger patients. Since elderly often have Cl$_{cr}$ <50 mL/minute, dosage should be determined accordingly.

Dosage Forms Excipient information presented when available (limited, particularly for generics); consult specific product labeling.

Tablet:

Tyzeka™: 600 mg

Selected References

Kim JW, Park SH, and Louie SG, "Telbivudine: A Novel Nucleoside Analog for Chronic Hepatitis B," *Ann Pharmacother*, 2006, 40(3):472-8.

Yang H, Qi X, Sabogal A, et al, "Cross-Resistance Testing of Next-Generation Nucleoside and Nucleotide Analogues Against Lamivudine-Resistant HBV," *Antivir Ther*, 2005, 10(5):625-33.

♦ **Teldrin® HBP [OTC]** *see* Chlorpheniramine *on page 296*

Telithromycin (tel ith roe MYE sin)

U.S. Brand Names Ketek®

Canadian Brand Names Ketek®

Index Terms HMR 3647

Generic Available No

Pharmacologic Category Antibiotic, Ketolide

Use Treatment of community-acquired pneumonia (mild-to-moderate) caused by susceptible strains of *Streptococcus pneumoniae* (including multidrug-resistant isolates), *Haemophilus influenzae*, *Chlamydophila pneumoniae*, *Moraxella catarrhalis*, and *Mycoplasma pneumoniae*

Unlabeled/Investigational Use Approved in Canada for use in the treatment of tonsillitis/pharyngitis due to *S. pyogenes* (as an alternative to beta-lactam antibiotics when necessary/appropriate)

Restrictions

An FDA-approved Medication Guide is available and must be dispensed with every prescription. Copies may be found at: http://www.fda.gov/cder/foi/label/2007/021144s012medg.pdf

Contraindications Hypersensitivity to telithromycin, macrolide antibiotics, or any component of the formulation; myasthenia gravis; history of hepatitis and/or jaundice associated with telithromycin or other macrolide antibiotic use; concurrent use of cisapride or pimozide

Warnings/Precautions Acute hepatic failure and severe liver injury, including hepatitis and hepatic necrosis (leading to some fatalities) have been reported, in some cases (Continued)

Telithromycin *(Continued)*

after only a few doses; if signs/symptoms of hepatitis or liver damage occur, discontinue therapy and initiate liver function tests. **[U.S. Boxed Warning]: Life-threatening (including fatal) respiratory failure has occurred in patients with myasthenia gravis;** use in these patients is contraindicated. May prolong QT_c interval, leading to a risk of ventricular arrhythmias; closely-related antibiotics have been associated with malignant ventricular arrhythmias and torsade de pointes. Avoid in patients with prolongation of QTc interval due to congenital causes, history of long QT syndrome, uncorrected electrolyte disturbances (hypokalemia or hypomagnesemia), significant bradycardia (<50 bpm), or concurrent therapy with QT_c-prolonging drugs (eg, class Ia and class III antiarrhythmics). Avoid use in patients with a prior history of confirmed cardiogenic syncope or ventricular arrhythmias while receiving macrolide antibiotics or other QT_c-prolonging drugs. May cause severe visual disturbances (eg, changes in accommodation ability, diplopia, blurred vision). May cause loss of consciousness (possibly vagal-related); caution patients that these events may interfere with ability to operate machinery or drive, and to use caution until effects are known. Use caution in renal impairment; severe impairment (Cl_{cr} <30 mL/minute) requires dosage adjustment. Pseudomembranous colitis has been reported.

Adverse Reactions (Reflective of adult population; not specific for elderly)
>10%: Gastrointestinal: Diarrhea (10% to 11%)
2% to 10%:
  Central nervous system: Headache (2% to 6%), dizziness (3% to 4%)
  Gastrointestinal: Nausea (7% to 8%), vomiting (2% to 3%), loose stools (2%), dysgeusia (2%)
≥0.2% to <2%:
  Central nervous system: Vertigo, fatigue, somnolence, insomnia
  Dermatologic: Rash
  Gastrointestinal: Abdominal distension, abdominal pain, anorexia, constipation, dyspepsia, flatulence, gastritis, gastroenteritis, GI upset, glossitis, stomatitis, watery stools, xerostomia
  Genitourinary: Vaginal candidiasis
  Hematologic: Platelets increased
  Hepatic: Transaminases increased
  Ocular: Blurred vision, accommodation delayed, diplopia
  Miscellaneous: Candidiasis, diaphoresis increased

Overdosage/Toxicology Treatment should be symptomatic and supportive. Gastric lavage recommended. ECG and electrolytes should be monitored. Effectiveness of dialysis unknown. Maintain adequate hydration.

Drug Interactions Substrate of CYP1A2 (minor), 3A4 (major); **Inhibits** CYP2D6 (weak), 3A4 (strong)
Alfentanil: Telithromycin may increase the levels/effects of alfentanil.
Antiarrhythmics (class Ia and class III): Effect on QT_c prolongation may be additive; serious arrhythmias may occur; use caution.
Antipsychotic agents (mesoridazine and thioridazine): Risk of QT_c prolongation and malignant arrhythmias may be increased.
Benzodiazepines (those metabolized by CYP3A4, including alprazolam, midazolam, triazolam): Serum levels may be increased by telithromycin
Buspirone: Telithromycin may increase the levels/effects of buspirone; consider noninteracting macrolide.
Calcium channel blockers (felodipine, verapamil, and potentially others metabolized by CYP3A4): Serum levels may be increased by telithromycin; monitor.
Carbamazepine: Serum levels may be increased by telithromycin; consider noninteracting macrolide; monitor closely.
Cilostazol: Telithromycin may increase the levels/effects of cilostazol; consider reducing dose of cilostazol to 50 mg twice daily during concomitant use.
Cisapride: Serum levels may be increased by telithromycin; serious arrhythmias may occur; concurrent use is contraindicated.
Clopidogrel: Telithromycin may decrease the levels/effects of clopidogrel; monitor.
Clozapine: Telithromycin may increase the levels/effects of clozapine; consider noninteracting macrolide.
Colchicine: Serum levels/effects may be increased by telithromycin. Avoid use, if possible.
Corticosteroids: Telithromycin may increase the levels/effects of corticosteroids; monitor.
CYP3A4 inhibitors: May increase the levels/effects of telithromycin. Example inhibitors include azole antifungals, clarithromycin, diclofenac, doxycycline, erythromycin, imatinib, isoniazid, nefazodone, nicardipine, propofol, protease inhibitors, quinidine, and verapamil.
CYP3A4 inducers: CYP3A4 inducers may decrease the levels/effects of telithromycin. Example inducers include aminoglutethimide, carbamazepine, nafcillin, nevirapine, phenobarbital, phenytoin, and rifamycins.

CYP3A4 substrates: Telithromycin may increase the levels/effects of CYP3A4 substrates. Example substrates include benzodiazepines, calcium channel blockers, mirtazapine, nateglinide, nefazodone, tacrolimus, and venlafaxine. Selected benzodiazepines (midazolam and triazolam), cisapride, ergot alkaloids, selected HMG-CoA reductase inhibitors (atorvastatin and lovastatin and simvastatin), and pimozide are generally contraindicated with strong CYP3A4 inhibitors.

Digoxin: Serum levels may be increased by telithromycin; monitor digoxin levels.

Disopyramide: Telithromycin may increase the QT-prolonging effects of disopyramide; avoid concurrent use.

Eletriptan: Telithromycin may increase the levels/effects of eletriptan; consider noninteracting macrolide.

Eplerenone: Telithromycin may increase the levels/effects of eplerenone; consider noninteracting macrolide.

Ergot alkaloids: Concurrent use may lead to acute ergot toxicity (severe peripheral vasospasm and dysesthesia); concurrent use not recommended

HMG-CoA reductase inhibitors (atorvastatin, lovastatin, and simvastatin): Telithromycin may increase serum levels of "statins" metabolized by CYP3A4, increasing the risk of myopathy/rhabdomyolysis (does not include fluvastatin, pravastatin, and rosuvastatin). Switch to noninteracting drug or suspend treatment during course of telithromycin therapy.

Immunosuppressants (cyclosporine, pimecrolimus, sirolimus, tacrolimus): Serum levels may be increased by telithromycin; monitor serum levels.

Itraconazole, ketoconazole: May increase telithromycin levels; risk of telithromycin toxicity (eg, QT_c prolongation) may increase. No dosage adjustment recommended by manufacturer.

Neuromuscular-blocking agents: May be potentiated by telithromycin.

Pimozide: Serum levels may be increased by telithromycin; serious arrhythmias may occur; concurrent use contraindicated.

QT_c-prolonging agents: Concurrent use of telithromycin with other drugs which may prolong QT_c interval may increase the risk of potentially-fatal arrhythmias; includes type Ia and type III antiarrhythmic agents, selected quinolones, cisapride (concurrent use contraindicated), dolasetron, palonosetron, thioridazine, and other agents.

Quinolone antibiotics: Concurrent use may increase the risk of malignant arrhythmias.

Repaglinide: Telithromycin may increase the levels/effects of repaglinide; monitor.

Rifampin: Rifampin may decrease the serum concentrations/effect of telithromycin; avoid concurrent use if possible.

Sildenafil, tadalafil, vardenafil: Serum levels may be increased by telithromycin. Do not exceed single sildenafil doses of 25 mg in 48 hours or single vardenafil dose of 2.5 mg in 24 hours. The dose of tadalafil should not exceed 10 mg, and tadalafil should not be taken more frequently than once every 72 hours.

SSRIs: Telithromycin may increase the QT_c-prolonging effects of SSRIs; consider noninteracting macrolide; monitor for serotonin syndrome.

Thioridazine: Telithromycin may increase the QT_c-prolonging effects of thioridazine; avoid combination.

Typhoid vaccine: Telithromycin may diminish the therapeutic effect of the live, attenuated Ty21a strain of typhoid vaccine.

Warfarin: Telithromycin may increase the effect of warfarin (limited data); monitor.

Ethanol/Nutrition/Herb Interactions Herb/nutraceutical: St John's wort: May decrease the levels/effects of telithromycin.

Stability Store at 15°C to 30°C (59°F to 86°F).

Mechanism of Action Inhibits bacterial protein synthesis by binding to two sites on the 50S ribosomal subunit. Telithromycin has also been demonstrated to alter secretion of IL-1alpha and TNF-alpha; the clinical significance of this immunomodulatory effect has not been evaluated.

Pharmacokinetics
Absorption: Rapid
Distribution: 2.9 L/kg
Protein binding: 60% to 70%
Metabolism: Hepatic, via CYP3A4 (50%) and non-CYP-mediated pathways
Bioavailability: 57% (significant first-pass metabolism)
Half-life elimination: 10 hours
Time to peak, plasma: 1 hour
Elimination: Urine (13% unchanged drug, remainder as metabolites); feces (7%)

Dosage
Geriatrics & Adults:
Community-acquired pneumonia: Oral: 800 mg once daily for 7-10 days
Renal Impairment:
Cl_{cr} <30 mL/minute, including dialysis:
U.S. product labeling: 600 mg once daily; when renal impairment is accompanied by hepatic impairment, reduce dosage to 400 mg once daily
Canadian product labeling: Reduce dose to 400 mg once daily
Hemodialysis: Administer following dialysis
(Continued)

Telithromycin *(Continued)*

Hepatic Impairment: No adjustment recommended, unless concurrent severe renal impairment is present.

Administration May be administered with or without food.

Monitoring Parameters Liver function tests; signs/symptoms of liver failure (eg, jaundice, fatigue, malaise, anorexia, nausea, bilirubinemia, acholic stools, liver tenderness, hepatomegaly); visual acuity

Patient Information Inform prescriber of any prescription, OTC medication, or herbal products you are using, and any allergies you have. Do not take any new medications during therapy without consulting prescriber. Take as directed, with or without food. Do not chew or crush tablets. Take complete prescription even if you are feeling better. May cause dizziness or blurred vision (use caution when driving or engaging in tasks that require alertness until response to drug is known); nausea, vomiting, abdominal pain (frequent small meals and frequent mouth care may help), constipation (increased dietary fluid and fibers may help), diarrhea (consult prescribed if persistent). Report palpitations, irregular heart beat, flushing or facial swelling; CNS disturbance (dizziness, headache, anxiety, abnormal dreams, tremor); usual muscle weakness or cramping; rash; or other persistent adverse effects.

Special Geriatric Considerations Bioavailability (57%) equivalent in persons ≥65 years compared to younger adults; although a 1.4- to 2-fold increase in AUC found in older adults. No dosage adjustment required.

Dosage Forms Excipient information presented when available (limited, particularly for generics); consult specific product labeling.

Tablet:

Ketek®: 300 mg [not available in Canada], 400 mg

Ketek Pak™ [blister pack]: 400 mg (10s) [packaged as 10 tablets/card; 2 tablets/blister]

Selected References

Araujo FG, Slifer TL, and Remington JS, "Inhibition of Secretion of Interleukin-1alpha and Tumor Necrosis Factor Alpha by the Ketolide Antibiotic Telithromycin," *Antimicrob Agents Chemother*, 2002, 46(10):3327-30.

Bhargava V, Lenfant B, Perret C, et al, "Lack of Effect of Food on the Bioavailability of a New Ketolide Antibacterial, Telithromycin," *Scand J Infect Dis*, 2002, 34(11):823-6.

Cantalloube C, Bhargava V, Sultan E, et al, "Pharmacokinetics of the Ketolide Telithromycin After Single and Repeated Doses in Patients With Hepatic Impairment," *Int J Antimicrob Agents*, 2003, 22(2):112-21.

Carbon C, "A Pooled Analysis of Telithromycin in the Treatment of Community-Acquired Respiratory Tract Infections in Adults," *Infection*, 2003, 31(5):308-17.

Clay KD, Hanson JS, Pope SD, et al, "Brief Communication: Severe Hepatotoxicity of Telithromycin: Three Case Reports and Literature Review," *Ann Int Med*, 2006, 144(6):451-20.

Perret C, Lenfant B, Weinling E, et al, "Pharmacokinetics and Absolute Oral Bioavailability of an 800-mg Oral Dose of Telithromycin in Healthy Young and Elderly Volunteers," *Chemotherapy*, 2002, 48(5):217-23.

Telmisartan *(tel mi SAR tan)*

Related Information

Angiotensin Agents *on page 1737*

U.S. Brand Names Micardis®

Canadian Brand Names Micardis®

Generic Available No

Pharmacologic Category Angiotensin II Receptor Blocker

Use Treatment of essential hypertension, alone or in combination with other antihypertensive agents

Contraindications Hypersensitivity to telmisartan or any component of the formulation; hypersensitivity to other A-II receptor antagonists; primary hyperaldosteronism; bilateral renal artery stenosis

Warnings/Precautions May cause hyperkalemia; avoid potassium supplementation unless specifically required by healthcare provider. Avoid use or use a smaller dose in patients who are volume depleted; correct depletion first. May be associated with deterioration of renal function and/or increases in serum creatinine, particularly in patients dependent on renin-angiotensin-aldosterone system. Use with caution in unilateral renal artery stenosis and pre-existing renal insufficiency; significant aortic/mitral stenosis. Use with caution in patients who have biliary obstructive disorders or hepatic dysfunction.

Adverse Reactions (Reflective of adult population; not specific for elderly) May be associated with worsening of renal function in patients dependent on renin-angiotensin-aldosterone system.

1% to 10%:

Cardiovascular: Hypertension (1%), chest pain (1%), peripheral edema (1%)

Central nervous system: Headache (1%), dizziness (1%), pain (1%), fatigue (1%)

Gastrointestinal: Diarrhea (3%), dyspepsia (1%), nausea (1%), abdominal pain (1%)

Genitourinary: Urinary tract infection (1%)

Neuromuscular & skeletal: Back pain (3%), myalgia (1%)

Respiratory: Upper respiratory infection (7%), sinusitis (3%), pharyngitis (1%), cough (2%)

Miscellaneous: Flu-like syndrome (1%)

Overdosage/Toxicology Signs and symptoms of overdose include hypotension, dizziness, and tachycardia. Treatment is supportive. Vagal stimulation may result in bradycardia.

Drug Interactions Inhibits CYP2C19 (weak)

Digoxin levels may be increased.

Eplerenone: May enhance the hyperkalemic effect of angiotensin II receptor blockers.

Lithium: Risk of toxicity may be increased by telmisartan; monitor lithium levels.

NSAIDs: May decrease angiotensin II antagonist efficacy; effect has been seen with losartan, but may occur with other medications in this class; monitor blood pressure

Potassium-sparing diuretics (amiloride, potassium, spironolactone, triamterene): Increased risk of hyperkalemia.

Potassium supplements may increase the risk of hyperkalemia.

Trimethoprim (high dose) may increase the risk of hyperkalemia.

Ethanol/Nutrition/Herb Interactions Herb/Nutraceutical: Avoid dong quai if using for hypertension (has estrogenic activity). Avoid ephedra, yohimbe, ginseng (may worsen hypertension). Avoid garlic (may have increased antihypertensive effect).

Mechanism of Action Angiotensin II acts as a vasoconstrictor. In addition to causing direct vasoconstriction, angiotensin II also stimulates the release of aldosterone. Once aldosterone is released, sodium as well as water are reabsorbed. The end result is an elevation in blood pressure. Telmisartan is a nonpeptide AT1 angiotensin II receptor antagonist. This binding prevents angiotensin II from binding to the receptor thereby blocking the vasoconstriction and the aldosterone secreting effects of angiotensin II.

Pharmacodynamics Telmisartan does not require prodrug conversion prior to drug action

Onset of action: 1-2 hours

Duration: Up to 24 hours

Pharmacokinetics

Protein binding: >99.5%

Metabolism: Hepatic, via conjugation to inactive metabolites

Bioavailability: 42% to 58% (dose-dependent)

Half-life, terminal: 24 hours

Time to peak: 0.5-1 hours

Elimination: Total body clearance: 800 mL/minute; 97% of a dose is excreted in the feces via extensive biliary secretion

Dosage

Geriatrics: Initial: 20 mg/day; usual maintenance dose range: 20-80 mg/day

Adults: Hypertension: Oral: Initial: 40 mg once daily; usual maintenance dose range: 20-80 mg/day. Patients with volume depletion should be initiated on the lower dosage with close supervision.

Renal Impairment: No adjustment required; hemodialysis patients are more susceptible to orthostatic hypotension

Hepatic Impairment: Supervise patients closely.

Administration May administer with food. See Dosage.

Monitoring Parameters Supine blood pressure, electrolytes, serum creatinine, BUN, urinalysis, symptomatic hypotension, and tachycardia

Patient Information Patients should report episodes of hypotension (lightheadedness, dizziness, etc) and any evidence of edema or other perceived changes in health or disease status.

Special Geriatric Considerations No initial dose adjustment is required. There appear to be no significant differences in response between the elderly and younger adults (limited data available). Monitor closely during initiation phase. Many elderly may be volume depleted due to diuretics and/or blunted thirst reflex resulting in inadequate fluid intake.

Dosage Forms Excipient information presented when available (limited, particularly for generics); consult specific product labeling.

Tablet: 20 mg, 40 mg, 80 mg

Telmisartan and Hydrochlorothiazide

(tel mi SAR tan & hye droe klor oh THYE a zide)

Related Information

Hydrochlorothiazide *on page 756*

Telmisartan *on page 1526*

U.S. Brand Names Micardis® HCT

Canadian Brand Names Micardis® Plus

Index Terms Hydrochlorothiazide and Telmisartan

Generic Available No

(Continued)

Telmisartan and Hydrochlorothiazide *(Continued)*

Pharmacologic Category Angiotensin II Receptor Blocker Combination; Antihypertensive Agent, Combination; Diuretic, Thiazide

Use Treatment of hypertension; combination product should not be used for initial therapy

Dosage

Geriatrics: Refer to adult dosing. Monitor renal function.

Adults: Hypertension: Oral: Replacement therapy: Combination product can be substituted for individual titrated agents. Initiation of combination therapy when monotherapy has failed to achieve desired effects:

Patients currently on telmisartan: Initial dose if blood pressure is not currently controlled on monotherapy of 80 mg telmisartan: Telmisartan 80 mg/hydrochlorothiazide 12.5 mg once daily; may titrate up to telmisartan 160 mg/hydrochlorothiazide 25 mg if needed.

Patients currently on HCTZ: Initial dose if blood pressure is not currently controlled on monotherapy of 25 mg once daily: Telmisartan 80 mg/hydrochlorothiazide 12.5 mg once daily or telmisartan 80 mg/hydrochlorothiazide 25 mg once daily; may titrate up to telmisartan 160 mg/hydrochlorothiazide 25 mg if blood pressure remains uncontrolled after 2-4 weeks of therapy. Patients who develop hypokalemia may be switched to telmisartan 80 mg/hydrochlorothiazide 12.5 mg.

Renal Impairment:

Cl_{cr} >30 mL/minute: Usual recommended dose

Cl_{cr} ≤30 mL/minute: Not recommended

Hepatic Impairment: Dosing should be started at telmisartan 40 mg/hydrochlorothiazide 12.5 mg. Do **not** use in patients with severe hepatic impairment.

Special Geriatric Considerations No dosing adjustment needed based on age. Monitor renal function.

Dosage Forms Excipient information presented when available (limited, particularly for generics); consult specific product labeling. [CAN] = Canadian brand name

Tablet:

Micardis® HCT [available in U.S.]:

40/12.5: Telmisartan 40 mg and hydrochlorothiazide 12.5 mg

80/12.5: Telmisartan 80 mg and hydrochlorothiazide 12.5 mg

80/25: Telmisartan 80 mg and hydrochlorothiazide 25 mg

Micardis® Plus [CAN]: 80/25: Telmisartan 80 mg and hydrochlorothiazide 25 mg [Not available in U.S.]

Temazepam *(te MAZ e pam)*

Related Information

Anxiolytic, Sedative / Hypnotic, and Miscellaneous Benzodiazepines *on page 1750*

Potentially Inappropriate Medications for Geriatrics *on page 1824*

Medication Safety Issues

Sound-alike/look-alike issues:

Temazepam may be confused with flurazepam, lorazepam

Restoril® may be confused with Vistaril®, Zestril®

U.S. Brand Names Restoril®

Canadian Brand Names Apo-Temazepam®; CO Temazepam; Gen-Temazepam; Novo-Temazepam; Nu-Temazepam; PMS-Temazepam; ratio-Temazepam; Restoril®

Generic Available Yes

Pharmacologic Category Hypnotic, Benzodiazepine

Use Short-term treatment of insomnia

Unlabeled/Investigational Use Treatment of anxiety; adjunct in the treatment of depression; management of panic attacks

Restrictions C-IV

Contraindications Hypersensitivity to temazepam or any component of the formulation (cross-sensitivity with other benzodiazepines may exist); narrow-angle glaucoma (not in product labeling, however, benzodiazepines are contraindicated)

Warnings/Precautions Should be used only after evaluation of potential causes of sleep disturbance. Failure of sleep disturbance to resolve after 7-10 days may indicate psychiatric or medical illness. A worsening of insomnia or the emergence of new abnormalities of thought or behavior may represent unrecognized psychiatric or medical illness and requires immediate and careful evaluation.

Use with caution in elderly or debilitated patients, patients with hepatic disease (including alcoholics), or renal impairment. Use with caution in patients with respiratory disease, or impaired gag reflex. Avoid use inpatients with sleep apnea.

Causes CNS depression (dose-related) resulting in sedation, dizziness, confusion, or ataxia which may impair physical and mental capabilities. Patients must be cautioned about performing tasks which require mental alertness (eg, operating machinery or driving). Use with caution in patients receiving other CNS depressants or psychoactive agents. Postmarketing studies have indicated that the use of hypnotic/sedative agents for sleep has been associated with hypersensitivity reactions including anaphylaxis as well as angioedema. An increased risk for hazardous sleep-related activities such as sleep-driving; cooking and eating food, and making phone calls while asleep have also been noted. Effects with other sedative drugs or ethanol may be potentiated. Benzodiazepines have been associated with falls and traumatic injury and should be used with extreme caution in patients who are at risk of these events (especially the elderly).

Use caution in patients with suicidal risk. Use with caution in patients with a history of drug dependence. Benzodiazepines have been associated with dependence and acute withdrawal symptoms on discontinuation or reduction in dose (may occur after as little as 10 days). Acute withdrawal, including seizures, may be precipitated after administration of flumazenil to patients receiving long-term benzodiazepine therapy.

Benzodiazepines have been associated with anterograde amnesia. Paradoxical reactions, including hyperactive or aggressive behavior, have been reported with benzodiazepines, particularly in psychiatric patients. Does not have analgesic, antidepressant, or antipsychotic properties.

Adverse Reactions (Reflective of adult population; not specific for elderly)
1% to 10%:
  Central nervous system: Confusion, dizziness, drowsiness, fatigue, anxiety, headache, lethargy, hangover, euphoria, vertigo
  Dermatologic: Rash
  Endocrine & metabolic: Decreased libido
  Gastrointestinal: Diarrhea
  Neuromuscular & skeletal: Dysarthria, weakness
  Ocular: Blurred vision
  Miscellaneous: Diaphoresis

Overdosage/Toxicology Symptoms include somnolence, confusion, coma, hypoactive reflexes, dyspnea, hypotension, slurred speech, and impaired coordination. Treatment for benzodiazepine overdose is supportive. Rarely is mechanical ventilation required. Flumazenil has been shown to selectively block the binding of benzodiazepines to CNS receptors, resulting in reversal of benzodiazepine-induced CNS depression.

Drug Interactions Substrate (minor) of CYP2B6, 2C9, 2C19, 3A4
  CNS depressants: Sedative effects and/or respiratory depression may be additive with CNS depressants; includes ethanol, barbiturates, opioid analgesics, and other sedative agents; monitor for increased effect
  Theophylline: May partially antagonize some of the effects of benzodiazepines; monitor for decreased response; may require higher doses for sedation

Ethanol/Nutrition/Herb Interactions
  Ethanol: Avoid ethanol (may increase CNS depression).
  Food: Serum levels may be increased by grapefruit juice.
  Herb/Nutraceutical: St John's wort may decrease temazepam levels. Avoid valerian, St John's wort, kava kava, gotu kola (may increase CNS depression).

Mechanism of Action Binds to stereospecific benzodiazepine receptors on the postsynaptic GABA neuron at several sites within the central nervous system, including the limbic system, reticular formation. Enhancement of the inhibitory effect of GABA on neuronal excitability results by increased neuronal membrane permeability to chloride ions. This shift in chloride ions results in hyperpolarization (a less excitable state) and stabilization.

Pharmacodynamics Onset of hypnotic effect: 30 minutes to 1 hour; considered an intermediate-acting benzodiazepine; studies have shown that older adults are more sensitive to the effects of benzodiazepines as compared to younger adults

Pharmacokinetics
  Protein binding: 96%
  Metabolism: In the liver
  Half-life: 3.5-18.4 hours (mean: 8.8 hours)
  Time to peak serum concentrations: Oral: Approximately 1.5 hours
  Elimination: 80% to 90% in urine as inactive metabolites
  Pharmacokinetics are not significantly affected by aging

Dosage
  Geriatrics: 15 mg in elderly or debilitated patients
  Adults: Insomnia: Oral: 15-30 mg at bedtime

Monitoring Parameters Respiratory, cardiovascular and mental status

Reference Range Therapeutic: 26 ng/mL after 24 hours

Patient Information Avoid alcohol and other CNS depressants; may cause daytime drowsiness; avoid activities needing good psychomotor coordination until CNS effects are known; may cause physical or psychological dependence; avoid abrupt discontinuation after prolonged use; may be taken 30 minutes before bedtime
(Continued)

Temazepam *(Continued)*

Additional Information Causes minimal change in REM sleep patterns; reformulation of the commercial product now allows for a faster onset

Special Geriatric Considerations Because of its lack of active metabolites, temazepam is recommended in the elderly when a benzodiazepine hypnotic is indicated. Hypnotic use should be limited to 10-14 days. If insomnia persists, the patient should be evaluated for etiology.

Dosage Forms Excipient information presented when available (limited, particularly for generics); consult specific product labeling.
　　Capsule: 15 mg, 30 mg
　　　　Restoril®: 7.5 mg, 15 mg, 30 mg

Selected References
Divoll M, Greenblatt DJ, Harmatz JS, et al, "Effect of Age and Gender on Disposition of Temazepam," *J Pharm Sci*, 1981, 70(10):1104-7.
Scharf MB, Berkowitz DV, and Brannen DE, "Effectiveness of Low-Dose Temazepam on Sleep Patterns in Geriatric Insomniac Subjects," *Consult Pharm*, 1993, 8(12):1367-73.

◆ **Temovate**® *see* Clobetasol *on page 335*
◆ **Temovate E**® *see* Clobetasol *on page 335*
◆ **Tenex**® *see* Guanfacine *on page 734*
◆ **Tenormin**® *see* Atenolol *on page 132*
◆ **Terazol**® **3** *see* Terconazole *on page 1535*
◆ **Terazol**® **7** *see* Terconazole *on page 1535*

Terazosin *(ter AY zoe sin)*

Related Information
　　Pharmacotherapy of Urinary Incontinence *on page 1822*
U.S. Brand Names Hytrin® [DSC]
Canadian Brand Names Alti-Terazosin; Apo-Terazosin®; Hytrin®; Novo-Terazosin; Nu-Terazosin; PMS-Terazosin
Generic Available Yes
Pharmacologic Category Alpha$_1$ Blocker
Use Management of mild to moderate hypertension; treatment of symptomatic benign prostatic hyperplasia (BPH)
Contraindications Hypersensitivity to quinazolines (doxazosin, prazosin, terazosin) or any component of the formulation
Warnings/Precautions Can cause significant orthostatic hypotension and syncope, especially with first dose; anticipate a similar effect if therapy is interrupted for a few days, if dosage is rapidly increased, or if another antihypertensive drug (particularly vasodilators) or a PDE5 inhibitor is introduced. Discontinue if symptoms of angina occur or worsen. Patients should be cautioned about performing hazardous tasks when starting new therapy or adjusting dosage upward. Prostate cancer should be ruled out before starting for BPH. Use with caution in hepatic impairment. Intraoperative floppy iris syndrome has been observed in cataract surgery patients who were on or were previously treated with alpha$_1$-blockers. Causality has not been established and there appears to be no benefit in discontinuing alpha-blocker therapy prior to surgery.

Adverse Reactions (Reflective of adult population; not specific for elderly)
Asthenia, postural hypotension, dizziness, somnolence, nasal congestion/rhinitis, and impotence were the only events noted in clinical trials to occur at a frequency significantly greater than placebo (p <0.05).

>10%:
　　Central nervous system: Dizziness, headache
　　Neuromuscular & skeletal: Muscle weakness
1% to 10%:
　　Cardiovascular: Edema, palpitation, chest pain, peripheral edema (3%), orthostatic hypotension (3% to 4%), tachycardia
　　Central nervous system: Fatigue, nervousness, drowsiness
　　Gastrointestinal: Dry mouth
　　Genitourinary: Urinary incontinence
　　Ocular: Blurred vision
　　Respiratory: Dyspnea, nasal congestion

Overdosage/Toxicology Symptoms include hypotension, drowsiness, and shock (but very unusual). Hypotension usually responds to I.V. fluids or Trendelenburg positioning. If unresponsive to these measures, the use of a parenteral vasoconstrictor may be required. Treatment is primarily supportive and symptomatic.

Drug Interactions
　　ACE inhibitors: Hypotensive effect may be increased.
　　Beta-blockers: Hypotensive effect may be increased.

Calcium channel blockers: Hypotensive effect may be increased.

NSAIDs may reduce antihypertensive efficacy.

Sildenafil, tadalafil, vardenafil: Blood pressure-lowering effects are additive. Use of tadalafil or vardenafil is contraindicated by the manufacturer. Use sildenafil with extreme caution (dose ≤25 mg).

Ethanol/Nutrition/Herb Interactions Herb/Nutraceutical: Avoid dong quai if using for hypertension (has estrogenic activity). Avoid ephedra, yohimbe, ginseng (may worsen hypertension). Avoid saw palmetto. Avoid garlic (may have increased antihypertensive effect).

Mechanism of Action Alpha$_1$-specific blocking agent with minimal alpha$_2$ effects; this allows peripheral postsynaptic blockade, with the resultant decrease in arterial tone, while preserving the negative feedback loop which is mediated by the peripheral presynaptic alpha$_2$-receptors; terazosin relaxes the smooth muscle of the bladder neck, thus reducing bladder outlet obstruction

Pharmacokinetics

Absorption: Oral: Rapid

Protein binding: 90% to 95%

Metabolism: Extensive in the liver

Half-life: 9.2-12 hours; half-life is not significantly prolonged in older adults

Time to peak: Within 60 minutes

Elimination: In feces (60%) and urine (40%)

Dosage

Geriatrics & Adults:

Hypertension: Oral: Initial: 1 mg at bedtime; slowly increase dose to achieve desired blood pressure, up to 20 mg/day; usual dose range (JNC 7): 1-20 mg once daily

Benign prostatic hyperplasia: Oral: Initial: 1 mg at bedtime, increasing as needed; most patients require 10 mg day. If no response after 4-6 weeks of 10 mg/day, may increase to 20 mg/day.

Monitoring Parameters Blood pressure, standing and sitting/supine, urinary symptoms

Patient Information Report any gain of body weight; fainting sometimes occurs after the first dose, take first dose at bedtime; rise from sitting/lying carefully, may cause dizziness

Additional Information

Syncope may occur usually within 90 minutes of the initial dose; administer initial dose at bedtime.

Special Geriatric Considerations Adverse reactions such as dry mouth and urinary problems can be particularly bothersome in the elderly.

Dosage Forms Excipient information presented when available (limited, particularly for generics); consult specific product labeling. [DSC] = Discontinued product

Capsule: 1 mg, 2 mg, 5 mg, 10 mg

Hytrin®: 1 mg, 2 mg, 5 mg, 10 mg [DSC]

Terbinafine (TER bin a feen)

Medication Safety Issues

Sound-alike/look-alike issues:

Terbinafine may be confused with terbutaline

Lamisil® may be confused with Lamictal®, Lomotil®

International issues:

Lamisil® may be confused with Lemesil® which is a brand name for nimesulide in Greece and Romania

U.S. Brand Names Lamisil®; Lamisil® AT™ [OTC]

Canadian Brand Names Apo-Terbinafine®; CO Terbinafine; Gen-Terbinafine; Lamisil®; Novo-Terbinafine; PMS-Terbinafine

Index Terms Terbinafine Hydrochloride

Generic Available Yes: Excludes solution

Pharmacologic Category Antifungal Agent, Oral; Antifungal Agent, Topical

Use Treatment of onychomycosis of the toenail or fingernail due to susceptible dermatophytes (oral); topical antifungal for treatment of tinea pedis (athlete's foot), tinea cruris (jock itch), tinea corporis (ringworm), tinea versicolor [prescription formulations]; active against most strains of *Trichophyton mentagrophytes*, *Trichophyton rubrum*; may be effective for infections of *Microsporum gypseum* and *M. nanum*, *Trichophyton verrucosum*, *Epidermophyton floccosum*, *Candida albicans*, and *Scopulariopsis brevicaulis*

Unlabeled/Investigational Use Topical: Treatment of cutaneous candidiasis, pityriasis versicolor

Contraindications Hypersensitivity to terbinafine, naftifine, or any component of the formulation

(Continued)

Terbinafine *(Continued)*

Warnings/Precautions While rare, the following complications have been reported and may require discontinuation of therapy: Changes in the ocular lens and retina, pancytopenia, neutropenia, Stevens-Johnson syndrome, toxic epidermal necrolysis. Precipitation or exacerbation of cutaneous or systemic lupus erythematosus has been observed; discontinue if signs and/or symptoms develop. Rare cases of hepatic failure (including fatal cases) have been reported following oral treatment of onychomycosis. Not recommended for use in patients with active or chronic liver disease. Discontinue if symptoms or signs of hepatobiliary dysfunction or cholestatic hepatitis develop. If irritation/sensitivity develop with topical use, discontinue therapy. Oral products are not recommended for use with pre-existing liver or renal disease (Cl_{cr} ≤50 mL/minute).

Adverse Reactions (Reflective of adult population; not specific for elderly)

Oral: 1% to 10%:

Central nervous system: Headache, dizziness, vertigo

Dermatologic: Rash, pruritus, urticaria

Gastrointestinal: Diarrhea, dyspepsia, abdominal pain, appetite decrease, taste disturbance

Hematologic: Lymphocytopenia

Hepatic: Liver enzymes increased

Ocular: Visual disturbance

Topical: 1% to 10%:

Dermatologic: Pruritus, contact dermatitis, irritation, burning, dryness

Local: Irritation, stinging

Drug Interactions Substrate (minor) of 1A2, 2C9, 2C19, 3A4; **Inhibits** CYP2D6 (strong); **Induces** CYP3A4 (weak)

Effects of drugs metabolized by CYP2D6 (including beta-blockers, SSRIs, MAO inhibitors, tricyclic antidepressants) may be increased; warfarin effects may be increased

CYP2D6 substrates: Terbinafine may increase the levels/effects of CYP2D6 substrates. Example substrates include amphetamines, selected beta-blockers, dextromethorphan, fluoxetine, lidocaine, mirtazapine, nefazodone, paroxetine, risperidone, ritonavir, thioridazine, tricyclic antidepressants, and venlafaxine.

CYP2D6 prodrug substrates: Terbinafine may decrease the levels/effects of CYP2D6 prodrug substrates. Example prodrug substrates include codeine, hydrocodone, oxycodone, and tramadol.

Rifampin: Rifampin increases terbinafine clearance (100%).

Stability

Cream: Store at 5°C to 30°C (41°F to 86°F).

Solution: Store at 5°C to 25°C (41°F to 77°F); do not refrigerate.

Tablet: Store below 25°C (77°F). Protect from light.

Mechanism of Action Synthetic allylamine derivative which inhibits squalene epoxidase, a key enzyme in sterol biosynthesis in fungi. This results in a deficiency in ergosterol within the fungal cell wall and results in fungal cell death.

Pharmacokinetics

Absorption: Topical: Limited (<5%); Oral: >70%

Distribution: V_d: 2000 L; distributed to sebum and skin predominantly

Protein binding, plasma: >99%

Metabolism: Hepatic; no active metabolites; first-pass effect

Bioavailability: Oral: 40%

Half-life:

Topical: 22-26 hours

Oral: Terminal half-life: 200-400 hours; very slow release of drug from skin and adipose tissues occurs; effective half-life: ~36 hours

Time to peak plasma concentration: 1-2 hours

Elimination: Urine (70% to 75%)

Dosage

Geriatrics & Adults:

Superficial mycoses (onychomycosis): Oral:

Fingernail: 250 mg/day for up to 6 weeks; may be given in two divided doses

Toenail: 250 mg/day for 12 weeks; may be given in two divided doses

Systemic mycosis: Oral: 250-500 mg/day for up to 16 months

Athlete's foot (tinea pedis): Topical:

Cream: Apply to affected area twice daily for at least 1 week, not to exceed 4 weeks [OTC/prescription formulations]

Solution: Apply to affected area twice daily for 7 days [OTC/prescription formulations]:

Ringworm and jock itch (tinea corporis, tinea cruris): Topical:

Cream: Apply to affected area once or twice daily for at least 1 week, not to exceed 4 weeks [OTC formulations]

Solution: Apply to affected area once daily for 7 days in tinea corporis and tinea cruris [OTC formulations]; apply to affected area twice daily for 7 days in tinea versicolor [prescription formulation]

Renal Impairment: Cl$_{cr}$ <50 mL/minute: Oral administration is not recommended.

Hepatic Impairment: Clearance is decreased by ~50% with hepatic cirrhosis; use is not recommended.

Monitoring Parameters Oral: CBC and LFTs at baseline and repeated if use is for >6 weeks

Patient Information

Topical: Avoid contact with eyes, nose, or mouth. Advise physician if eyes or skin becomes yellow or if irritation, itching, or burning develops. Do not use occlusive dressings concurrent with therapy.

Oral: Full clinical effect may require several months due to the time required for a new nail to grow.

Additional Information Due to potential toxicity, the manufacturer recommends confirmation of diagnosis testing of nail specimens prior to treatment of onychomycosis.

A meta-analysis of efficacy studies for toenail infections revealed that weighted average mycological cure rates for continuous therapy were 36.7% (griseofulvin), 54.7% (itraconazole), and 77% (terbinafine). Cure rate for 4-month pulse therapy for itraconazole and terbinafine were 73.3% and 80%. Additionally, the final outcome measure of final costs per cured infections for continuous therapy was significantly lower for terbinafine.

Special Geriatric Considerations No specific information on the systemic use of terbinafine in the elderly is available; however, since many elderly will have creatinine clearances <50 mL/minute, this drug is not a drug of choice for elderly with onychomycosis.

Dosage Forms Excipient information presented when available (limited, particularly for generics); consult specific product labeling.

Cream, as hydrochloride: 1% (12 g, 24 g)
Lamisil® AT™: 1% (12 g) [contains benzyl alcohol]
Solution, as hydrochloride [topical spray]:
Lamisil® AT™: 1% (30 mL)
Tablet: 250 mg
Lamisil®: 250 mg

Selected References

Abdel-Rahman SM and Nahata MC, "Oral Terbinafine: A New Antifungal Agent," *Ann Pharmacother*, 1997, 31(4):445-56.

Gupta AK, Sibbald RG, Knowles SR, et al, "Terbinafine Therapy May Be Associated With the Development of Psoriasis De Novo or Its Exacerbation: Four Case Reports and a Review of Drug Induced Psoriasis," *J Am Acad Dermatol*, 1997, 36(5 Part 2):858-62.

Trepanier EF and Amsden GW, "Current Issues in Onychomycosis," *Ann Pharmacother*, 1998, 32(2):204-14.

♦ **Terbinafine Hydrochloride** *see* Terbinafine *on page 1531*

Terbutaline (ter BYOO ta leen)

Related Information

Inhalant Agents *on page 1760*

Medication Safety Issues

Sound-alike/look-alike issues:
Terbutaline may be confused with terbinafine, TOLBUTamide

Canadian Brand Names Bricanyl®

Index Terms Brethaire [DSC]; Bricanyl [DSC]

Generic Available Yes

Pharmacologic Category Beta$_2$-Adrenergic Agonist

Use Bronchodilator in reversible airway obstruction and bronchial asthma

Contraindications Hypersensitivity to terbutaline or any component of the formulation; cardiac arrhythmias associated with tachycardia; tachycardia caused by digitalis intoxication

Warnings/Precautions When used for tocolysis, there is some risk of maternal pulmonary edema, which has been associated with the following risk factors, excessive hydration, multiple gestation, occult sepsis and underlying cardiac disease. To reduce risk, limit fluid intake to 2.5-3 L/day, limit sodium intake, maintain maternal pulse to <130 beats/minute.

Use caution in patients with cardiovascular disease (arrhythmia or hypertension or CHF), convulsive disorders, diabetes, glaucoma, hyperthyroidism, or hypokalemia. Beta-agonists may cause elevation in blood pressure, heart rate, and result in CNS stimulation/excitation. Beta$_2$-agonists may increase risk of arrhythmia, increase serum glucose, or decrease serum potassium.

When used as a bronchodilator, optimize anti-inflammatory treatment before initiating maintenance treatment with terbutaline. Do not use as a component of chronic therapy without an anti-inflammatory agent. Only the mildest form of asthma (Step 1 and/or exercise-induced) would not require concurrent use based upon asthma guidelines. Patient must be instructed to seek medical attention in cases where acute symptoms (Continued)

Terbutaline *(Continued)*

are not relieved or a previous level of response is diminished. The need to increase frequency of use may indicate deterioration of asthma, and treatment must not be delayed.

Immediate hypersensitivity reactions (urticaria, angioedema, rash, bronchospasm) have been reported. Do not exceed recommended dose; serious adverse events including fatalities, have been associated with excessive use of inhaled sympathomimetics. Rarely, paradoxical bronchospasm may occur with use of inhaled bronchodilating agents; this should be distinguished from inadequate response.

Adverse Reactions (Reflective of adult population; not specific for elderly)

>10%:

Central nervous system: Nervousness, restlessness

Endocrine & metabolic: Serum glucose increased, serum potassium decreased

Neuromuscular & skeletal: Trembling

1% to 10%:

Cardiovascular: Tachycardia, hypertension

Central nervous system: Dizziness, drowsiness, headache, insomnia

Gastrointestinal: Xerostomia, nausea, vomiting, bad taste in mouth

Neuromuscular & skeletal: Muscle cramps, weakness

Miscellaneous: Diaphoresis

Overdosage/Toxicology Symptoms of overdose include tachycardia, tremor, hypertension, angina, and seizures. Hypokalemia also may occur. Cardiac arrest and death may be associated with abuse of beta-agonist bronchodilators. Treatment includes immediate discontinuation and symptomatic and supportive therapies. Cautious use of beta-adrenergic blocking agents may be considered in severe cases.

Drug Interactions

Decreased effect with beta-blockers

Increased toxicity with MAO inhibitors, TCAs

Ethanol/Nutrition/Herb Interactions Herb/Nutraceutical: Avoid ephedra, yohimbe (may cause CNS stimulation).

Stability Store injection at room temperature; do not freeze. Protect from heat and light. Use only clear solutions. Store powder for inhalation (Bricanyl® Turbuhaler [CAN]) at room temperature between 15°C and 30°C (58°F and 86°F).

Mechanism of Action Relaxes bronchial smooth muscle by action on beta$_2$-receptors with less effect on heart rate

Pharmacodynamics SubQ doses are more bioavailable and of quicker onset than oral doses.

Onset of action:

Oral: Within 30-45 minutes

Inhalation: 5-30 minutes

SubQ: Within 6-15 minutes

Duration:

Oral: 4-8 hours

Inhalation: 3-6 hours

SubQ: 1.5-4 hours

Pharmacokinetics

Protein binding: 25%

Metabolism: In the liver to inactive sulfate conjugates

Half-life: 11-16 hours

Elimination: In urine

Dosage

Geriatrics & Adults: Asthma or bronchoconstriction:

Oral: 5 mg/dose every 6 hours 3 times/day; if side effects occur, reduce dose to 2.5 mg every 6 hours; not to exceed 15 mg in 24 hours.

SubQ: 0.25 mg/dose repeated in 15-30 minutes for one time only; a total dose of 0.5 mg should not be exceeded within a 4-hour period.

Renal Impairment:

Cl_{cr} 10-50 mL/minute: Administer 50% of normal dose.

Cl_{cr} <10 mL/minute: Avoid use.

Monitoring Parameters Pulmonary function, blood pressure, pulse

Patient Information May cause nervousness, restlessness, insomnia - if these effects continue after dosage reduction, notify physician. Also notify physician if palpitations, tachycardia, chest pain, muscle tremors, dizziness, headache, flushing, or if breathing difficulty persists.

Special Geriatric Considerations Oral terbutaline should be avoided in the elderly due to the increased incidence of adverse effects as compared to the inhaled form.

Dosage Forms Excipient information presented when available (limited, particularly for generics); consult specific product labeling. [CAN] = Canadian brand name

Injection, solution, as sulfate: 1 mg/mL (1 mL)

Powder for oral inhalation:
Bricanyl® Turbuhaler [CAN]: 500 mcg/actuation [50 or 200 metered actuations] [not available in U.S.]
Tablet, as sulfate: 2.5 mg, 5 mg

Terconazole (ter KONE a zole)

Medication Safety Issues
Sound-alike/look-alike issues:
Terconazole may be confused with tioconazole
International issues:
Terazol® may be confused with Theradol® which is a brand name for tramadol in the Netherlands

U.S. Brand Names Terazol® 3; Terazol® 7; Zazole™
Canadian Brand Names Terazol®
Index Terms Triaconazole
Generic Available Yes: Cream
Pharmacologic Category Antifungal Agent, Vaginal
Use Local treatment of vulvovaginal candidiasis
Contraindications Hypersensitivity to terconazole or any component of the formulation
Warnings/Precautions Should be discontinued if sensitization or irritation occurs. Microbiological studies (KOH smear and/or cultures) should be repeated in patients not responding to terconazole in order to confirm the diagnosis and rule out other pathogens.
Adverse Reactions (Reflective of adult population; not specific for elderly)
1% to 10%:
Central nervous system; Fever, chills
Gastrointestinal: Abdominal pain
Genitourinary: Vulvar/vaginal burning, dysmenorrhea
Drug Interactions No data reported
Stability Store at room temperature of 13°C to 30°C (59°F to 86°F).
Mechanism of Action Triazole ketal antifungal agent; involves inhibition of fungal cytochrome P450. Specifically, terconazole inhibits cytochrome P450-dependent 14-alpha-demethylase which results in accumulation of membrane disturbing 14-alpha-demethylsterols and ergosterol depletion.
Pharmacokinetics Absorption: Extent of systemic absorption after vaginal administration may be dependent on the presence of a uterus; 5% to 8% in women who had a hysterectomy versus 12% to 16% in nonhysterectomized women
Dosage
Geriatrics & Adults: Vulvovaginal candidiasis: Intravaginal:
Terazol® 3, Zazole™ (0.8%) vaginal cream: Insert 1 applicatorful intravaginally at bedtime for 3 consecutive days.
Terazol® 7, Zazole™ (0.4%) vaginal cream: Insert 1 applicatorful intravaginally at bedtime for 7 consecutive days.
Terazol® 3 vaginal suppository: Insert 1 suppository intravaginally at bedtime for 3 consecutive days.
Monitoring Parameters Response to treatment
Patient Information Follow directions included with products; complete full course of therapy; notify physician if irritating; use sanitary napkin to protect clothing
Special Geriatric Considerations Assess patient's ability to self-administer; may be difficult in patients with arthritis or limited range of motion.
Dosage Forms Excipient information presented when available (limited, particularly for generics); consult specific product labeling.
Cream, vaginal: 0.4% (45 g); 0.8% (20 g)
Terazol® 7: 0.4% (45 g) [packaged with measured-dose applicator]
Terazol® 3: 0.8% (20 g) [packaged with measured-dose applicator]
Zazole™: 0.4% (45 g) [packaged with measured-dose applicator]; 0.8% (20 g) [packaged with measured-dose applicator]
Suppository, vaginal:
Terazol® 3: 80 mg (3s) [may contain coconut and/or palm kernel oil]
Selected References
Drug Facts and Comparisons, St Louis, MO: 1989, 528-9.

Teriparatide (ter i PAR a tide)

Related Information
Osteoporosis Management *on page 1779*
U.S. Brand Names Forteo™
(Continued)

Teriparatide *(Continued)*

Canadian Brand Names Forteo™

Index Terms Parathyroid Hormone (1-34); Recombinant Human Parathyroid Hormone (1-34); rhPTH(1-34)

Generic Available No

Pharmacologic Category Parathyroid Hormone Analog

Use Treatment of osteoporosis in postmenopausal women at high risk of fracture; treatment of primary or hypogonadal osteoporosis in men at high risk of fracture

Restrictions An FDA-approved medication guide must be distributed when dispensing an outpatient prescription (new or refill) where this medication is to be used without direct supervision of a healthcare provider. Medication guides are available at http://www.fda.gov/cder/Offices/ODS/medication_guides.htm.

Contraindications Hypersensitivity to teriparatide or any component of the formulation

Warnings/Precautions [U.S. Boxed Warning]: In animal studies, teriparatide has been associated with an increase in osteosarcoma; risk was dependent on both dose and duration. Use of teriparatide for longer than 2 years is not recommended. Avoid use in patients with an increased risk of osteosarcoma (including Paget's disease, prior radiation, unexplained elevation of alkaline phosphatase, or in patients with open epiphyses). Do not use in patients with a history of skeletal metastases, hyperparathyroidism, or pre-existing hypercalcemia. Exclude metabolic bone disease other than osteoporosis prior to initiating therapy. Use caution in patients with active or recent urolithiasis. Use caution in patients at risk of orthostasis (including concurrent antihypertensive therapy), or in patients who may not tolerate transient hypotension (cardiovascular or cerebrovascular disease). Use caution in patients with renal or hepatic impairment (limited data available concerning safety and efficacy).

Adverse Reactions (Reflective of adult population; not specific for elderly)
1% to 10%:
Cardiovascular: Chest pain (3%), syncope (3%)
Central nervous system: Dizziness (8%), depression (4%), vertigo (4%)
Dermatologic: Rash (5%)
Endocrine & metabolic: Hypercalcemia (transient increases noted 4-6 hours postdose in 11% of women and 6% of men)
Gastrointestinal: Nausea (9%), dyspepsia (5%), vomiting (3%), tooth disorder (2%)
Genitourinary: Hyperuricemia (3%)
Neuromuscular & skeletal: Arthralgia (10%), weakness (9%), leg cramps (3%)
Respiratory: Rhinitis (10%), pharyngitis (6%), dyspnea (4%), pneumonia (4%)
Miscellaneous: Antibodies to teriparatide (3% of women in long-term treatment; hypersensitivity reactions or decreased efficacy were not associated in preclinical trials)

Overdosage/Toxicology No specific experience in overdose. Symptoms may include hypercalcemia, hypotension, headache, nausea, vomiting, and hypotension. Treatment is supportive (monitor serum calcium and phosphorus).

Drug Interactions Digitalis: No effect on digitalis serum concentrations noted, however, transient hypercalcemia may increase risk of digitalis toxicity (case reports).

Ethanol/Nutrition/Herb Interactions
Ethanol: Excessive intake may increase risk of osteoporosis.
Herb/Nutraceutical: Ensure adequate calcium and vitamin D intake.

Stability Store at 2°C to 8°C (36°F to 46°F); do not freeze. Protect from light. Discard pen 28 days after first injection.

Mechanism of Action Teriparatide is a recombinant formulation of endogenous parathyroid hormone (PTH), containing a 34-amino-acid sequence which is identical to the N-terminal portion of this hormone. The pharmacologic activity of teriparatide is similar to the physiologic activity of PTH, stimulating osteoblast function, increasing gastrointestinal calcium absorption, increasing renal tubular reabsorption of calcium. Treatment with teriparatide increases bone mineral density, bone mass, and strength. In postmenopausal women, it has been shown to decrease osteoporosis-related fractures.

Pharmacokinetics
Distribution: V_d: 0.12 L/kg
Metabolism: Hepatic (nonspecific proteolysis)
Bioavailability: 95%
Half-life elimination: Serum: I.V.: 5 minutes; SubQ: 1 hour
Elimination: Urine (as metabolites)

Dosage
Geriatrics & Adults: Osteoporosis: SubQ: 20 mcg once daily; **Note:** Initial administration should occur under circumstances in which the patient may sit or lie down, in the event of orthostasis.
Renal Impairment: No dosage adjustment required. Bioavailability and half-life increase with Cl_{cr} <30 mL/minute.

Monitoring Parameters Serum calcium, serum phosphorus; blood pressure; bone mineral density; uric acid

Patient Information Inform prescriber of all prescriptions, OTC medications, or herbal products you are taking, and any allergies you have. Do not take any new medication during therapy without consulting prescriber. Use injector pen and dispose of pen exactly as instructed (refer to Forteo™ user manual dispensed with the medication); rotate injection sites in thigh or abdominal wall. Sit when administering to reduce possibility of falling or injury. Avoid excess alcohol and follow dietary instructions of prescriber. May cause dizziness (use caution when driving or engaged in potentially hazardous tasks until response to drug is known); nausea, vomiting, or upset stomach (small, frequent meals or frequent mouth care may help); muscle or skeletal pain, weakness, or cramping (consult prescriber for approved analgesic). Report chest pain or palpitations; respiratory difficulty; or other persistent adverse effects.

Additional Information Teriparatide was formerly marketed as a diagnostic agent (Perithar™); that agent was withdrawn from the market in 1997. Teriparatide (Forteo™) is manufactured through recombinant DNA technology using a strain of *E. coli*.

Special Geriatric Considerations No age-related differences in pharmacokinetics have been seen. In studies, no significant difference was seen in either efficacy or adverse effects between older patients and younger patients. Teriparatide should be considered as a last resort in patents who cannot tolerate or have not responded to other treatments for osteoporosis.

Dosage Forms Excipient information presented when available (limited, particularly for generics); consult specific product labeling.

Injection, solution: 250 mcg/mL (3 mL) [prefilled syringe, delivers teriparatide 20 mcg/dose]

Selected References

Body JJ, Gaich GA, Scheele WH, et al, "A Randomized Double-blind Trial to Compare the Efficacy of Teriparatide [Recombinant Human Parathyroid Hormone (1-34)] With Alendronate in Postmenopausal Women With Osteoporosis," *J Clin Endocrinol Metab*, 2002, 87(10):4528-35.

Neer RM, Arnaud CD, Zanchetta JR, et al, "Effect of Parathyroid Hormone (1-34) on Fractures and Bone Mineral Density in Postmenopausal Women With Osteoporosis," *N Engl J Med*, 2001, 344(19):1434-41.

Reeve, J, "Recombinant Human Parathyroid Hormone," *BMJ*, 2002, 324(7335):435-6.

♦ **Terramycin® I.M. [DSC]** *see* Oxytetracycline *on page 1189*

♦ **Tessalon®** *see* Benzonatate *on page 158*

♦ **Testim®** *see* Testosterone *on page 1537*

♦ **Testopel®** *see* Testosterone *on page 1537*

Testosterone (tes TOS ter one)

Medication Safety Issues

Sound-alike/look-alike issues:

Testosterone may be confused with testolactone

Testoderm® may be confused with Estraderm®

Transdermal patch may contain conducting metal (eg, aluminum); remove patch prior to MRI.

U.S. Brand Names Androderm®; AndroGel®; Delatestryl®; Depo®-Testosterone; First® Testosterone; First® Testosterone MC; Striant®; Testim®; Testopel®

Canadian Brand Names Andriol®; Androderm®; AndroGel®; Andropository; Delatestryl®; Depotest® 100; Everone® 200; Virilon® IM

Index Terms Testosterone Cypionate; Testosterone Enanthate

Generic Available Yes: Injection

Pharmacologic Category Androgen

Use

Injection: Androgen replacement therapy in the treatment of delayed male puberty; male hypogonadism (primary or hypogonadotropic); inoperable metastatic female breast cancer (enanthate only)

Pellet: Androgen replacement therapy in the treatment of delayed male puberty; male hypogonadism (primary or hypogonadotropic)

Topical (buccal system, gel, transdermal system): Male hypogonadism (primary or hypogonadotropic)

Capsule (not available in U.S.): Androgen replacement therapy in the treatment of delayed male puberty; male hypogonadism (primary or hypogonadotropic); replacement therapy in impotence or for male climacteric symptoms due to androgen deficiency

Unlabeled/Investigational Use Androgen deficiency in men with AIDS wasting; postmenopausal women with decreased sexual desire (in combination with estrogen therapy)

Restrictions C-III

Contraindications Hypersensitivity to testosterone or any component of the formulation; males with carcinoma of the breast or prostate

Depo®-Testosterone: Also contraindicated in serious hepatic, renal, or cardiac disease

(Continued)

Testosterone *(Continued)*

Andriol®: Also contraindicated in hepatic, renal, or cardiac disease; hypercalcemia; nephrosis or nephritic phase of nephritis; prepubertal males; patients who are easily sexually stimulated

Warnings/Precautions When used to treat delayed male puberty, perform radiographic examination of the hand and wrist every 6 months to determine the rate of bone maturation. May cause hypercalcemia in patients with prolonged immobilization. May accelerate bone maturation without producing compensating gain in linear growth. Has both androgenic and anabolic activity, the anabolic action may enhance hypoglycemia. May alter serum cholesterol; use caution with history of MI or coronary artery disease. Use caution in elderly patients or patients with other demographic factors which may increase the risk of prostatic carcinoma; careful monitoring is required. Urethral obstruction may develop in patients with BPH; treatment should be discontinued if this should occur (use lower dose if restarted). Withhold treatment pending urological evaluation if PSA >3 ng/mL. May cause fluid retention; use caution in patients with cardiovascular disease or other edematous conditions.

Prolonged use of high doses of androgens has been associated with serious hepatic effects (peliosis hepatis, hepatic neoplasms, cholestatic hepatitis, jaundice). May potentiate sleep apnea in some male patients (obesity or chronic lung disease). Testosterone may be transferred to another person following skin-to-skin contact with the application site; virilization of female sexual partners has been reported with male use of the topical gel. Transdermal patch may contain conducting metal (eg, aluminum); remove patch prior to MRI. Some testosterone products may be chemically synthesized from soy. Some products may contain benzyl alcohol.

Adverse Reactions (Reflective of adult population; not specific for elderly)
Frequency rarely defined.

Cardiovascular: Edema, hypertension, vasodilation

Central nervous system: Aggressive behavior, amnesia, anxiety, dizziness, emotional lability, excitation, headache, mental depression, nervousness, sleeplessness

Dermatologic: Acne, alopecia, dry skin, hirsutism (increase in pubic hair growth), pruritus, rash, seborrhea

Endocrine & metabolic: Breast soreness, gonadotropin secretion decreased, growth acceleration, gynecomastia, hot flashes, hypercalcemia, hyperchloremia, hypercholesterolemia, hyper-/hypokalemia, hyperlipidemia, hypernatremia, hypoglycemia, inorganic phosphate retention, libido changes, menstrual problems (including amenorrhea), virilism, water retention

Gastrointestinal: GI bleeding, GI irritation, nausea, taste disorder, vomiting

Following buccal administration (most common): Bitter taste, gum edema, gum or mouth irritation, gum pain, gum tenderness, taste perversion

Genitourinary: Bladder irritability, epididymitis, impotence, oligospermia, priapism, prostatic carcinoma, prostatic hyperplasia, PSA increased, testicular atrophy, urination impaired

Hepatic: Bilirubin increased, cholestatic hepatitis, cholestatic jaundice, hepatic dysfunction, hepatic necrosis, hepatocellular neoplasms, liver function test changes, peliosis hepatis

Hematologic: Bleeding, hematocrit/hemoglobin increased, leukopenia, polycythemia, suppression of clotting factors

Local: Application site reaction (gel), injection site pain

Transdermal system: Pruritus at application site (37%), burn-like blisters under system (12%), erythema at application site (7%), vesicles at application site (6%), allergic contact dermatitis to system (4%), burning at application site (3%), induration at application site (3%)

Neuromuscular & skeletal: Paresthesia, weakness

Ocular: Lacrimation increased

Renal: Creatinine increased

Miscellaneous: Anaphylactoid reactions, diaphoresis, hypersensitivity reactions, smell disorder

Postmarketing and/or case reports: Injection: Cough, coughing fits, respiratory distress

Drug Interactions Substrate (minor) of CYP2B6, 2C9, 2C19, 3A4; **Inhibits** CYP3A4 (weak)

Coumarin derivatives: Androgens may enhance the anticoagulant effect of coumarin derivatives.

Cyclosporine: Androgens may enhance the serum concentration and hepatotoxic effect of cyclosporine; avoid concurrent use, monitor closely.

Ethanol/Nutrition/Herb Interactions Herb/Nutraceutical: St John's wort may decrease testosterone levels.

Stability

Androderm®: Store at room temperature. Do not store outside of pouch. Excessive heat may cause system to burst.

AndroGel®, Delatestryl®, Striant®, Testim®: Store at room temperature.

Depo® Testosterone: Store at room temperature. Protect from light.

Testopel®: Store in a cool location.

Mechanism of Action Principal endogenous androgen responsible for promoting the growth and development of the male sex organs and maintaining secondary sex characteristics in androgen-deficient males

Pharmacodynamics Duration (route and ester dependent): I.M.: Cypionate and enanthate esters have longest duration, ≤2-4 weeks; gel: 24-48 hours

Pharmacokinetics

Absorption: Transdermal gel: ~10% of dose

Protein binding: 98% to transcortin and albumin

Metabolism: Hepatic; forms metabolites

Half-life: 10-100 minutes

Elimination: Urine (90%); feces (6%)

Dosage

Geriatrics & Adults:

Inoperable metastatic breast cancer (females): *I.M. (testosterone enanthate):* 200-400 mg every 2-4 weeks

Hypogonadism:

I.M. (testosterone enanthate or testosterone cypionate): 50-400 mg every 2-4 weeks (FDA-approved dosing range); 75-100 mg/week or 150-200 mg every 2 weeks (per practice guidelines)

Pellet (for subcutaneous implantation): 150-450 mg every 3-6 months

Hypogonadism or hypogonadotropic hypogonadism (males):

Oral capsule (Andriol®; not available in U.S.): Initial: 120-160 mg/day in 2 divided doses for 2-3 weeks; adjust according to individual response; usual maintenance dose: 40-120 mg/day (in divided doses)

Topical:

Buccal: 30 mg twice daily (every 12 hours) applied to the gum region above the incisor tooth

Transdermal system: Androderm®: Initial: Apply 5 mg/day once nightly to clean, dry area on the back, abdomen, upper arms, or thighs (do **not** apply to scrotum); dosing range: 2.5-7.5 mg/day; in nonvirilized patients, dose may be initiated at 2.5 mg/day

Gel: AndroGel®, Testim®: 5 g (to deliver 50 mg of testosterone with 5 mg systemically absorbed) applied once daily (preferably in the morning) to clean, dry, intact skin of the shoulder and upper arms. AndroGel® may also be applied to the abdomen. Dosage may be increased to a maximum of 10 g (100 mg). **Do not apply testosterone gel to the genitals.**

Hepatic Impairment: Reduce dose.

Administration

I.M.: Warm to room temperature; shaking vial will help redissolve crystals that have formed after storage. Administer by deep I.M. injection into the upper outer quadrant of the gluteus maximus.

Oral, buccal application (Striant®): One mucoadhesive for buccal application (buccal system) should be applied to a comfortable area above the incisor tooth. Apply flat side of system to gum. Rotate to alternate sides of mouth with each application. Hold buccal system firmly in place for 30 seconds to ensure adhesion. The buccal system should adhere to gum for 12 hours. If the buccal system falls out, replace with a new system. If the system falls out within 4 hours of next dose, the new buccal system should remain in place until the time of the following scheduled dose. System will soften and mold to shape of gum as it absorbs moisture from mouth. Do not chew or swallow the buccal system. The buccal system will not dissolve; gently remove by sliding downwards from gum; avoid scratching gum.

Oral, capsule (Andriol®; not available in the U.S.): Should be administered with meals. Should be swallowed whole; do not crush or chew.

Transdermal patch (Androderm®): Apply patch to clean, dry area of skin on the arm, back, or upper buttocks. Following patch removal, mild skin irritation may be treated with OTC hydrocortisone cream. A small amount of triamcinolone acetonide 0.1% cream may be applied under the system to decrease irritation; do not use ointment. Patch should be applied nightly. Rotate administration sites, allowing 7 days between applying to the same site.

Topical gel: AndroGel®, Testim®: Apply (preferably in the morning) to clean, dry, intact skin of the shoulder and upper arms (AndroGel® may also be applied to the abdomen). Apply at the same time each day. Upon opening the packet(s), the entire contents should be squeezed into the palm of the hand and immediately applied to the application site(s). Alternatively, a portion may be squeezed onto palm of hand and applied, repeating the process until entire packet has been applied. Application sites should be allowed to dry for a few minutes prior to dressing. Hands should be washed with soap and water after application. **Do not apply testosterone gel to the genitals.** For optimal absorption, after application wait at least 5-6 hours prior to showering or swimming; however waiting at least 1 hour should have minimal affect on absorption if done infrequently. Alcohol-based gels are flammable; avoid fire or smoking until gel has dried. Testosterone may be transferred to another person

(Continued)

Testosterone *(Continued)*

following skin-to-skin contact with the application site. Thoroughly wash hands after application and cover application site with clothing (ie shirt) once gel has dried, or clean application site thoroughly with soap and water prior to contact in order to minimize transfer.

AndroGel® multidose pump: Prime pump 3 times (and discard this portion of product) prior to initial use.

Monitoring Parameters Periodic liver function tests, PSA and prostate exam (prior to therapy, at 3 months, then as based on current guidelines), cholesterol, hemoglobin and hematocrit (prior to therapy, at 3 months, then annually). Withhold initial treatment with hematocrit >50%, hyperviscosity, untreated obstructive sleep apnea, or uncontrolled severe heart failure. Monitor urine and serum calcium and signs of virilization in women treated for breast cancer.

PSA: Withhold initial treatment if PSA >3 ng/mL, or with palpable prostate nodule or induration without further urological evaluation. Do not treat with severe untreated BPH with IPSS symptom score >19.

Serum testosterone: Monitor 3 months after initiating treatment, then annually.

Injection: Measure midway between injections

AndroGel®: Morning serum testosterone levels 14 days after start of therapy

Androderm®: Morning serum testosterone levels following application the previous evening

Striant®: Application area of gums; total serum testosterone 4-12 weeks after initiating treatment, prior to morning dose

Reference Range Testosterone, urine: Male: 100-1500 ng/24 hours; Female: 100-500 ng/24 hours

Test Interactions May cause a decrease in thyroid function tests

Patient Information Diabetics should monitor serum glucose closely and notify prescriber of changes; this medication may alter hypoglycemic requirements. You may experience acne, growth of body hair, loss of libido, impotence, or menstrual irregularity (usually reversible); nausea or vomiting (small frequent meals, frequent mouth care, sucking lozenges, or chewing gum may help). Report changes in menstrual pattern; enlarged or painful breasts; deepening of voice or unusual growth of body hair; persistent penile erection; fluid retention (swelling of ankles, feet, or hands, difficulty breathing or sudden weight gain); unresolved changes in CNS (nervousness, chills, insomnia, depression, aggressiveness); altered urinary patterns; change in color of urine or stool; yellowing of eyes or skin; unusual bruising or bleeding; or other persistent adverse reactions.

Transdermal:

Androderm®: Apply patch to clean, dry area of skin on the arm, back, or upper buttocks.

AndroGel®, Testim™: Apply gel (preferably in the morning) to clean, dry, intact skin of the shoulder and upper arms (AndroGel® may also be applied to the abdomen). Upon opening the packet(s), the entire contents should be squeezed into the palm of the hand and immediately applied to the application site(s). Alternatively, a portion may be squeezed onto palm of hand and applied, repeating the process until entire packet has been applied. Application sites should be allowed to dry for a few minutes prior to dressing. Hands should be washed with soap and water after application. **Do not apply testosterone gel to the genitals.**

Additional Information

Testosterone (aqueous): Andro®, Histerone®, Tesamone®

Testosterone cypionate: Andro-Cyp®, Andronate®, Depotest®, Depo®-Testosterone, Duratest®

Testosterone enanthate: Andro-L.A.®, Andropository®, Delatestryl®, Durathate®, Everone®, Testrin® P.A.

Testosterone propionate: Testex®

Special Geriatric Considerations Elderly males treated with androgens may be at increased risk of developing prostatic hyperplasia and prostatic carcinoma. Increase in libido may occur.

Dosage Forms Excipient information presented when available (limited, particularly for generics); consult specific product labeling. [CAN] = Canadian brand name

Capsule, gelatin, as undecanoate:

Andriol™ [CAN]: 40 mg (10s) [not available in U.S.]

Gel, topical:

AndroGel®:

1.25 g/actuation (75 g) [1% metered-dose pump; delivers 5 g/4 actuations; provides 60 1.25 g actuations; contains ethanol; may be chemically synthesized from soy]

2.5 g (30s) [1% unit dose packets; contains ethanol; may be chemically synthesized from soy]

5 g (30s) [1% unit dose packets; contains ethanol; may be chemically synthesized from soy]

Testim®: 5 g (30s) [1% unit-dose tube; contains ethanol; may be chemically synthesized from soy]

Injection, in oil, as cypionate: 100 mg/mL (10 mgL); 200 mg/mL (1 mL, 10 mL)

Depo®-Testosterone: 100 mg/mL (10 mL); 200 mg/mL (1 mL, 10 mL) [contains benzyl alcohol, benzyl benzoate, and cottonseed oil]

Injection, in oil, as enanthate: 200 mg/mL (5 mL)

Delatestryl®: 200 mg/mL (1 mL) [prefilled syringe; contains sesame oil]; (5 mL) [multidose vial; contains sesame oil]

Kit [for prescription compounding testosterone 2%; kits also contain mixing jar and stirrer]:

First® Testosterone:

Injection, in oil: Testosterone propionate 100 mg/mL (12 mL) [contains sesame oil and benzyl alcohol]

Ointment: White petroleum (48 g)

First® Testosterone MC:

Injection, in oil: Testosterone propionate 100 mg/mL (12 mL) [contains sesame oil and benzyl alcohol]

Cream: Moisturizing cream (48 g)

Mucoadhesive, for buccal application [buccal system]:

Striant®: 30 mg (10s) [may be chemically synthesized from soy]

Pellet, for subcutaneous implantation:

Testopel®: 75 mg

Transdermal system, topical:

Androderm®: 2.5 mg/day (60s) [contains ethanol]; 5 mg/day (30s) [contains ethanol]

Selected References

Bhasin S, Cunningham GR, Hayes FJ, et al, "Testosterone Therapy in Adult Men With Androgen Deficiency Syndromes: An Endocrine Society Clinical Practice Guideline," *J Clin Endocrinol Metab*, 2006, 91(6):1995-2010.

NAMS Board of Trustees, "The Role of Testosterone Therapy in Postmenopausal Women: Position Statement of The North American Menopause Society," *Menopause*, 2005, 12(5):497-511.

♦ **Testosterone Cypionate** *see* Testosterone *on page 1537*

♦ **Testosterone Enanthate** *see* Testosterone *on page 1537*

♦ **Testred®** *see* MethylTESTOSTERone *on page 1020*

♦ **Tetanus and Diphtheria Toxoid** *see* Diphtheria and Tetanus Toxoid *on page 451*

Tetanus Immune Globulin (Human)
(TET a nus i MYUN GLOB yoo lin HYU man)

Related Information

Immunization Recommendations *on page 1787*

U.S. Brand Names HyperTET™ S/D

Canadian Brand Names HyperTET™ S/D

Index Terms TIG

Generic Available No

Pharmacologic Category Immune Globulin

Use Passive immunization against tetanus

Contraindications Hypersensitivity to tetanus immune globulin, thimerosal, or any component of the formulation

Warnings/Precautions Hypersensitivity and anaphylactic reactions can occur; immediate treatment (including epinephrine 1:1000) should be available. Use caution in patients with isolated immunoglobulin A deficiency or a history of systemic hypersensitivity to human immunoglobulins. Use with caution in patients with thrombocytopenia or coagulation disorders; I.M. injections may be contraindicated. Product of human plasma; may potentially contain infectious agents which could transmit disease. Screening of donors, as well as testing and/or inactivation or removal of certain viruses, reduces the risk. Infections thought to be transmitted by this product should be reported to the manufacturer. Skin testing should not be performed as local irritation can occur and be misinterpreted as a positive reaction. Not for intravenous administration.

Adverse Reactions (Reflective of adult population; not specific for elderly)

>10%: Local: Pain, tenderness, erythema at injection site

1% to 10%:

Central nervous system: Fever (mild)

Dermatologic: Urticaria, angioedema

Neuromuscular & skeletal: Muscle stiffness

Miscellaneous: Anaphylaxis reaction

Drug Interactions Never administer tetanus toxoid and TIG in same syringe (toxoid will be neutralized); toxoid may be given at a separate site; concomitant administration with Td may decrease its immune response, especially in individuals with low prevaccination antibody titers

Stability Refrigerate

(Continued)

Tetanus Immune Globulin (Human) *(Continued)*

Mechanism of Action Passive immunity toward tetanus

Pharmacokinetics Half-life (tetanus toxoids): 3.5-4.5 weeks

Dosage
Geriatrics & Adults:
Prophylaxis of tetanus: I.M.: 250 units
Treatment of tetanus: I.M.: 3000-6000 units

Administration Do not administer I.V.; I.M. use only

Monitoring Parameters Monitor for hypersensitivity reactions

Patient Information Be aware of adverse reactions

Additional Information Tetanus immune globulin is preferred over tetanus antitoxin for treatment of active tetanus.

Special Geriatric Considerations Tetanus is a rare disease in U.S. with <100 cases annually; 66% of cases occur in persons >50 years of age; protective tetanus and diphtheria antibodies decline with age; it is estimated that <50% of the elderly are protected.

Elderly are at risk because:
Many lack proper immunization maintenance
Higher case fatality ratio
Immunizations are not available from childhood
Indications for vaccination:
Primary series with combined tetanus-diphtheria (Td) should be given to all elderly lacking a clear history of vaccination
Boosters should be given at 10-year intervals; earlier for wounds
Elderly are more likely to require tetanus immune globulin with infection of tetanus due to lower antibody titer.

Dosage Forms Excipient information presented when available (limited, particularly for generics); consult specific product labeling.
Injection, solution [preservative free]:
HyperTET™ S/D: 250 units/mL (1 mL) [prefilled syringe]

Tetanus Toxoid (Adsorbed) (TET a nus TOKS oyd, ad SORBED)

Related Information
Immunization Recommendations *on page 1787*

Medication Safety Issues
Sound-alike/look-alike issues:
Tetanus toxoid products may be confused with influenza virus vaccine and tuberculin products. Medication errors have occurred when tetanus toxoid products have been inadvertently administered instead of tuberculin skin tests (PPD) and influenza virus vaccine. These products are refrigerated and often stored in close proximity to each other.

Generic Available No

Pharmacologic Category Toxoid

Use Active immunization against tetanus when combination antigen preparations are not indicated. **Note:** Tetanus and diphtheria toxoids for adult use (Td) is the preferred immunizing agent for most adults.

Contraindications Hypersensitivity to tetanus toxoid or any component of the formulation

Warnings/Precautions Not equivalent to tetanus toxoid fluid; the tetanus toxoid adsorbed is the preferred toxoid for immunization and Td, TD or DTaP are the preferred adsorbed forms; avoid injection into a blood vessel; allergic reactions may occur; epinephrine 1:1000 must be available; elderly may not mount adequate antibody titers following immunization. Patients who are immunocompromised may have reduced response; may be used in patients with HIV infection. May defer elective immunization during febrile illness or acute infection; defer elective immunization during outbreaks of poliomyelitis. In patients with a history of severe local reaction (Arthus-type) or temperature of >39.4°C (>103°F) following previous dose, do not give further routine or emergency doses of tetanus and diphtheria toxoids for 10 years. Use caution in patients on anticoagulants, with thrombocytopenia, or bleeding disorders (bleeding may occur following intramuscular injection). Contains thimerosal; vial stopper may contain natural latex rubber.

Adverse Reactions (Reflective of adult population; not specific for elderly)
All serious adverse reactions must be reported to the U.S. Department of Health and Human Services (DHHS) Vaccine Adverse Event Reporting System (VAERS) 1-800-822-7967.
Frequency not defined.
Cardiovascular: Hypotension
Central nervous system: Brachial neuritis, fever, malaise, pain
Gastrointestinal: Nausea

Local: Edema, induration (with or without tenderness), rash, redness, urticaria, warmth

Neuromuscular: Arthralgia, Guillain-Barré syndrome

Miscellaneous: Anaphylactic reaction, Arthus-type hypersensitivity reaction

Drug Interactions

Corticosteroids: When used in greater than physiologic doses, corticosteroids lead to decreased effect of vaccine; consider deferring immunization for 1 month after steroid is discontinued.

Immunosuppressive agents: Decreased response to vaccine; consider deferring immunization for 1 month after immunosuppressive agent is discontinued.

Stability Refrigerate; do not freeze.

Mechanism of Action Tetanus toxoid preparations contain the toxin produced by virulent tetanus bacilli (detoxified growth products of *Clostridium tetani*). The toxin has been modified by treatment with formaldehyde so that it has lost toxicity but still retains ability to act as antigen and produce active immunity; the aluminum salt, a mineral adjuvant, delays the rate of absorption and prolongs and enhances its properties; duration ~10 years.

Dosage

Geriatrics & Adults:

Primary immunization: I.M.: 0.5 mL; repeat 0.5 mL at 4-8 weeks after first dose and at 6-12 months after second dose

Routine booster dose: Recommended every 10 years

Note: In most patients, Td is the recommended product for primary immunization, booster doses, and tetanus immunization in wound management.

Administration Inject intramuscularly in the area of the vastus lateralis (midthigh laterally) or deltoid. Do not inject into gluteal area. Shake well prior to withdrawing dose; do not use if product does not form a suspension.

For patients at risk of hemorrhage following intramuscular injection, the ACIP recommends "it should be administered intramuscularly if, in the opinion of the physician familiar with the patients bleeding risk, the vaccine can be administered with reasonable safety by this route. If the patient receives antihemophilia or other similar therapy, intramuscular vaccination can be scheduled shortly after such therapy is administered. A fine needle (23 gauge or smaller) can be used for the vaccination and firm pressure applied to the site (without rubbing) for at least 2 minutes. The patient should be instructed concerning the risk of hematoma from the injection."

Patient Information Be aware of adverse reactions

Additional Information Routine booster doses are recommended only every 10 years.

Federal law requires that the date of administration, the vaccine manufacturer, lot number of vaccine, and the administering person's name, title, and address be entered into the patient's permanent medical record.

Special Geriatric Considerations Tetanus is a rare disease in U.S. with <100 cases annually; 66% of cases occur in persons >50 years of age; protective tetanus and diphtheria antibodies decline with age; it is estimated that <50% of elderly are protected.

Elderly are at risk because:

Many lack proper immunization maintenance

Higher case fatality ratio

Immunizations are not available from childhood

Indications for vaccination:

Primary series with combined tetanus-diphtheria (Td) should be given to all elderly lacking a clean history of vaccination

Boosters should be given at 10-year intervals; earlier for wounds

Elderly are more likely to require tetanus immune globulin with infection of tetanus due to lower antibody titer.

Dosage Forms Excipient information presented when available (limited, particularly for generics); consult specific product labeling.

Injection, suspension: Tetanus 5 Lf units per 0.5 mL (0.5 mL) [contains trace amounts of thimerosal]; (5 mL) [contains thimerosal; vial stopper contains latex]

Selected References

Bentley DW, "Vaccinations," *Clin Geriatr Med*, 1992, 8(4):745-60.

Centers for Disease Control, "Recommendations of the Advisory Committee on Immunization Practices (ACIP): General Recommendations on Immunization," *MMWR*, 1994, 43(RR-1):23.

Gardner P and Schaffner W, "Immunization of Adults," *N Engl J Med*, 1993, 328(17):1252-8.

Tetanus Toxoid (Fluid) (TET a nus TOKS oyd FLOO id)

Related Information

Immunization Recommendations *on page 1787*
(Continued)

Tetanus Toxoid (Fluid) *(Continued)*

Medication Safety Issues
Sound-alike/look-alike issues:
Tetanus toxoid products may be confused with influenza virus vaccine and tuberculin products. Medication errors have occurred when tetanus toxoid products have been inadvertently administered instead of tuberculin skin tests (PPD) and influenza virus vaccine. These products are refrigerated and often stored in close proximity to each other.

Index Terms Tetanus Toxoid Plain

Generic Available No

Pharmacologic Category Toxoid

Use Active immunization against tetanus in adults

Unlabeled/Investigational Use Anergy testing (no longer recommended)

Contraindications Hypersensitivity to tetanus toxoid or any component of the formulation

Warnings/Precautions Epinephrine 1:1000 should be readily available; skin test responsiveness may be delayed or reduced in elderly patients. Patients who are immunocompromised may have reduced response; may be used in patients with HIV infection. May defer elective immunization during febrile illness or acute infection; defer elective immunization during outbreaks of poliomyelitis. In patients with a history of severe local reaction (Arthus-type) following previous dose, do not give further routine or emergency doses of tetanus and diphtheria toxoids for 10 years. Use caution in patients on anticoagulants, with thrombocytopenia, or bleeding disorders (bleeding may occur following intramuscular injection). Contains thimerosal; vial stopper contains natural latex rubber.

Adverse Reactions (Reflective of adult population; not specific for elderly)
All serious adverse reactions must be reported to the U.S. Department of Health and Human Services (DHHS) Vaccine Adverse Event Reporting System (VAERS) 1-800-822-7967.

Frequency not defined.
Cardiovascular: Hypotension
Central nervous system: Brachial neuritis, fever, Guillain-Barré syndrome, malaise
Dermatologic: Rash, urticaria
Gastrointestinal: Nausea
Local: Edema, induration (with or without tenderness), redness, warmth
Neuromuscular & skeletal: Arthralgia
Miscellaneous: Anaphylaxis, Arthus-type hypersensitivity reactions (severe local reaction developing 2-8 hours following injection)

Drug Interactions
Anticoagulants: Increased bleeding and bruising from intramuscular injection; subcutaneous administration is preferred.
Corticosteroids: When used in greater than physiologic doses, corticosteroids lead to decreased effect of vaccine; consider deferring immunization for 1 month after steroid is discontinued.
Immunosuppressive agents: Decreased response to vaccine; consider deferring immunization for 1 month after immunosuppressive agent is discontinued.

Stability Refrigerate 2°C to 8°C (35°F to 46°F); do not freeze.

Mechanism of Action Tetanus toxoid preparations contain the toxin produced by virulent tetanus bacilli (detoxified growth products of *Clostridium tetani*). The toxin has been modified by treatment with formaldehyde so that is has lost toxicity but still retains ability to act as antigen and produce active immunity.

Dosage
Geriatrics & Adults:
Primary immunization: Not indicated for this use.
Booster doses: I.M., SubQ: 0.5 mL every 10 years
Anergy testing (unlabeled use; no longer recommended for this indication): Intradermal: 0.1 mL; doses that have been used range from 0.1 mL of a 1:10 dilution to 0.1 mL of the undiluted product

Administration
I.M. Shake well prior to use. Administer I.M. in lateral aspect of midthigh or deltoid muscle of upper arm
For patients at risk of hemorrhage following intramuscular injection, the ACIP recommends "it should be administered intramuscularly if, in the opinion of the physician familiar with the patients bleeding risk, the vaccine can be administered with reasonable safety by this route. If the patient receives antihemophilia or other similar therapy, intramuscular vaccination can be scheduled shortly after such therapy is administered. A fine needle (23 gauge or smaller) can be used for the vaccination and firm pressure applied to the site (without rubbing) for at least 2 minutes. The patient should be instructed concerning the risk of hematoma from the injection."

SubQ: Shake well prior to use. Administer in area of the lateral aspect of midthigh or deltoid. SubQ route may be preferred in patients with thrombocytopenia or coagulation disorders.

Patient Information A nodule may be palpable at the injection site for a few weeks; be aware of adverse reactions

Additional Information Tetanus toxoid, adsorbed is preferred for all basic immunizing and recall reactions because of more persistent antitoxin titer induction.

Federal law requires that the date of administration, the vaccine manufacturer, lot number of vaccine, and the administering person's name, title, and address be entered into the patient's permanent medical record.

Special Geriatric Considerations Tetanus is a rare disease in U.S. with <100 cases annually; 66% of cases occur in persons >50 years of age; protective tetanus and diphtheria antibodies decline with age; it is estimated that <50% of elderly are protected.

Elderly are at risk because:
Many lack proper immunization maintenance
Higher case fatality ratio
Immunizations are not available from childhood
Indications for vaccination:
Primary series with combined tetanus-diphtheria (Td) should be given to all elderly lacking a clean history of vaccination
Boosters should be given at 10-year intervals; earlier for wounds
Elderly are more likely to require tetanus immune globulin with infection of tetanus due to lower antibody titer.

Dosage Forms Excipient information presented when available (limited, particularly for generics); consult specific product labeling.
Injection, solution: Tetanus 4 Lf units per 0.5 mL (7.5 mL) [contains thimerosal; vial stopper contains dry natural latex rubber]

Selected References
Centers for Disease Control, "Recommendations of the Advisory Committee on Immunization Practices (ACIP): General Recommendations on Immunization," *MMWR*, 1994, 43(RR-1):23.
Gardner P and Schaffner W, "Immunization of Adults," *N Engl J Med*, 1993, 328(17):1252-8.

◆ **Tetanus Toxoid Plain** see Tetanus Toxoid (Fluid) on page 1543
◆ **Tetracaine and Lidocaine** see Lidocaine and Tetracaine on page 908

Tetracycline (tet ra SYE kleen)

Related Information
Antimicrobial Activity Against Selected Organisms on page 1728
Helicobacter pylori Treatment on page 1759

Medication Safety Issues
Sound-alike/look-alike issues:
Tetracycline may be confused with tetradecyl sulfate
Achromycin may be confused with actinomycin, Adriamycin PFS®

U.S. Brand Names Sumycin® [DSC]

Canadian Brand Names Apo-Tetra®; Nu-Tetra

Index Terms Achromycin; TCN; Tetracycline Hydrochloride

Generic Available Yes: Capsule

Pharmacologic Category Antibiotic, Tetracycline Derivative

Use Treatment of susceptible bacterial infections of gram-positive and gram-negative organisms; infections due to *Mycoplasma*, *Chlamydia*, and *Rickettsia*; acne; exacerbations of chronic bronchitis; gonorrhea and syphilis (in patients allergic to penicillin); *H. pylori* (to reduce the risk of duodenal ulcer recurrence; part of a multidrug regimen)

Contraindications Hypersensitivity to tetracycline or any component of the formulation

Warnings/Precautions Use of tetracyclines during tooth development may cause permanent discoloration of the teeth and enamel, hypoplasia and retardation of skeletal development and bone growth with risk being the greatest for those receiving high doses; use with caution in patients with renal or hepatic impairment (eg, elderly); dosage modification required in patients with renal impairment since it may increase BUN as an antianabolic agent; pseudotumor cerebri has been reported with tetracycline use (usually resolves with discontinuation); outdated drug can cause nephropathy; use protective measure to avoid photosensitivity. Prolonged use may result in fungal or bacterial superinfection, including *C. difficile*-associated diarrhea and pseudomembranous colitis.

Adverse Reactions (Reflective of adult population; not specific for elderly)
Frequency not defined.
Cardiovascular: Pericarditis
Central nervous system: Intracranial pressure increased, bulging fontanels in infants, pseudotumor cerebri, paresthesia
Dermatologic: Photosensitivity, pruritus, pigmentation of nails, exfoliative dermatitis
(Continued)

Tetracycline *(Continued)*

Endocrine & metabolic: Diabetes insipidus syndrome

Gastrointestinal: Discoloration of teeth and enamel hypoplasia (young children), nausea, diarrhea, vomiting, esophagitis, anorexia, abdominal cramps, antibiotic-associated pseudomembranous colitis, staphylococcal enterocolitis, pancreatitis

Hematologic: Thrombophlebitis

Hepatic: Hepatotoxicity

Renal: Acute renal failure, azotemia, renal damage

Miscellaneous: Superinfection, anaphylaxis, hypersensitivity reactions, candidal superinfection

Overdosage/Toxicology Symptoms include nausea, anorexia, and diarrhea. Following GI decontamination, supportive care only.

Drug Interactions Substrate of CYP3A4 (major); **Inhibits** CYP3A4 (moderate)

Antacids: May decrease tetracycline absorption; separate doses.

Calcium supplements (oral): May decrease tetracycline absorption; separate doses.

CYP3A4 inducers: CYP3A4 inducers may decrease the levels/effects of tetracycline. Example inducers include aminoglutethimide, carbamazepine, nafcillin, nevirapine, phenobarbital, phenytoin, and rifamycins.

CYP3A4 substrates: Tetracycline may increase the levels/effects of CYP3A4 substrates. Example substrates include benzodiazepines, calcium channel blockers, cyclosporine, mirtazapine, nateglinide, nefazodone, sildenafil (and other PDE-5 inhibitors), tacrolimus, and venlafaxine. Selected benzodiazepines (midazolam and triazolam), cisapride, ergot alkaloids, selected HMG-CoA reductase inhibitors (lovastatin and simvastatin), and pimozide are generally contraindicated with strong CYP3A4 inhibitors.

Didanosine: May decrease tetracycline absorption; separate doses.

Digoxin: Tetracyclines may rarely increase digoxin serum levels.

Iron: May decrease tetracycline absorption; separate doses.

Methoxyflurane anesthesia when concurrent with tetracycline may cause fatal nephrotoxicity.

Oral contraceptives: Anecdotal reports suggesting decreased contraceptive efficacy with tetracyclines have been refuted by more rigorous scientific and clinical data.

Quinapril: May decrease tetracycline absorption; separate doses.

Warfarin with tetracyclines may result in increased anticoagulation.

Ethanol/Nutrition/Herb Interactions

Food: Tetracycline serum concentrations may be decreased if taken with dairy products.

Herb/Nutraceutical: Avoid dong quai, St John's wort (may also cause photosensitization)

Stability Outdated tetracyclines have caused a Fanconi-like syndrome. Protect oral dosage forms from light.

Mechanism of Action Inhibits bacterial protein synthesis by binding with the 30S and possibly the 50S ribosomal subunit(s) of susceptible bacteria; may also cause alterations in the cytoplasmic membrane

Pharmacodynamics Bacteriostatic

Pharmacokinetics

Absorption: Oral: 75%

Protein binding: ~65%

Half-life: Normal renal function: 8-11 hours

Time to peak serum concentration: Oral: 2-4 hours

Elimination: Primary route of elimination is the kidney, with 60% of a dose excreted as unchanged drug in urine; small amount appears in bile; feces (as active form)

Dosage

Geriatrics & Adults:

Usual dosage range: Oral: 250-500 mg every 6 hours

Acne: Oral: 250-500 twice daily

Chronic bronchitis, acute exacerbation: Oral: 500 mg 4 times/day

Erlichiosis: Oral: 500 mg 4 times/day for 7-14 days

Peptic ulcer disease: Eradication of *Helicobacter pylori*: Oral: 500 mg 2-4 times/day depending on regimen; requires combination therapy with at least one other antibiotic and an acid-suppressing agent (proton pump inhibitor or H_2 blocker)

Periodontitis: Oral: 250 mg every 6 hours until improvement (usually 10 days)

Vibrio cholerae: Oral: 500 mg 4 times/day for 3 days

Renal Impairment:

Cl_{cr} 50-80 mL/minute: Administer every 8-12 hours.

Cl_{cr} 10-50 mL/minute: Administer every 12-24 hours.

Cl_{cr} <10 mL/minute: Administer every 24 hours.

Slightly dialyzable (5% to 20%) via hemo- and peritoneal dialysis or via continuous arteriovenous or venovenous hemofiltration; supplemental dose is not necessary.

Hepatic Impairment: Avoid use or maximum dose is 1 g/day.

Monitoring Parameters Temperature, WBC, cultures and sensitivity (if applicable), appetite, mental status

Reference Range Therapeutic: Not established; Toxic: >16 mcg/mL

Test Interactions False-negative urine glucose with Clinistix®

Patient Information Take 1 hour before or 2 hours after meals with adequate amounts of fluid; avoid prolonged exposure to sunlight or sunlamps; avoid taking antacids, iron, or dairy products with tetracyclines

Additional Information Use of tetracycline in animal feed has caused emergence of resistant organisms

Tetracycline: Achromycin® V oral suspension, Sumycin® syrup, Tetralan® syrup

Tetracycline hydrochloride: Achromycin® injection, Achromycin® V capsule, Nor-tet® capsule, Panmycin® capsule, Robitet® capsule, Sumycin® capsule and tablet, Teline® capsule, Tetracyn® capsule, Tetralan® capsule

Special Geriatric Considerations The role of tetracycline has decreased because of the emergence of resistant organisms. Doxycycline is the tetracycline of choice when one is indicated because of its better GI absorption, less interactions with divalent cations, longer half-life, and the fact that the majority is cleared by nonrenal mechanisms.

Dosage Forms Excipient information presented when available (limited, particularly for generics); consult specific product labeling.

Capsule, as hydrochloride: 250 mg, 500 mg

Suspension, oral, as hydrochloride:
Sumycin®: 125 mg/5 mL (480 mL) [contains sodium benzoate and sodium metabisulfite; fruit flavor] [DSC]

Tablet, as hydrochloride:
Sumycin®: 250 mg, 500 mg [DSC]

Selected References
Yoshikawa TT, "Antimicrobial Therapy for the Elderly Patient," *J Am Geriatr Soc*, 1990, 38(12):1353-72.

Tetrahydrozoline (tet ra hye DROZ a leen)

Medication Safety Issues
Sound-alike/look-alike issues:
Visine® may be confused with Visken®

U.S. Brand Names Eye-Sine™ [OTC]; Geneye® [OTC]; Murine® Tears Plus [OTC]; Optigene® 3 [OTC]; Tyzine®; Tyzine® Pediatric; Visine® Advanced Relief [OTC]; Visine® Original [OTC]

Index Terms Tetrahydrozoline Hydrochloride; Tetryzoline

Generic Available Yes: Ophthalmic solution

Pharmacologic Category Adrenergic Agonist Agent; Imidazoline Derivative; Ophthalmic Agent, Vasoconstrictor

Use Symptomatic relief of nasal congestion and conjunctival congestion

Contraindications Narrow-angle glaucoma, patients receiving MAO inhibitors, known hypersensitivity to tetrahydrozoline

Warnings/Precautions Discontinue use prior to the use of anesthetics which sensitize the myocardium to the systemic effects of sympathomimetics. Use caution in patients with hypertension, diabetes, thyroid disorders, heart disease, and asthma.

Adverse Reactions (Reflective of adult population; not specific for elderly)
>10%:
Local: Transient stinging
Respiratory: Sneezing
1% to 10%:
Cardiovascular: Tachycardia, palpitation, hypertension, heart rate
Central nervous system: Headache
Neuromuscular & skeletal: Tremor
Ocular: Blurred vision

Drug Interactions Increased toxicity: MAO inhibitors can cause an exaggerated adrenergic response if taken concurrently or within 21 days of discontinuing MAO inhibitor; beta-blockers can cause hypertensive episodes and increased risk of intracranial hemorrhage; anesthetics

Stability Do not use if solution changes color or becomes cloudy.

Mechanism of Action Stimulates alpha-adrenergic receptors in the arterioles of the conjunctiva and the nasal mucosa to produce vasoconstriction

Pharmacodynamics
Onset of action: Intranasal: Decongestant effects occur within 4-8 hours
Duration: Ophthalmic vasoconstriction lasts 2-3 hours
(Continued)

Tetrahydrozoline *(Continued)*

Pharmacokinetics Absorption: Topical: Systemic absorption sometimes occurs

Dosage

Geriatrics & Adults:

Nasal congestion: Intranasal: Instill 2-4 drops or 3-4 sprays of 0.1% solution every 3-4 hours as needed, no more frequent than every 3 hours

Conjunctival congestion: Ophthalmic: Instill 1-2 drops in each eye 2-4 times/day

Administration See Patient Information and package instructions.

Monitoring Parameters Blood pressure, heart rate, symptom response

Patient Information Remove contact lenses before using in eye; do not use >72 hours; consult physician of changes in vision or visual acuity occur; do not exceed recommended dose or duration to avoid rebound congestion

Special Geriatric Considerations Use with caution in patients with cardiovascular disease.

Dosage Forms Excipient information presented when available (limited, particularly for generics); consult specific product labeling.

Solution, intranasal, as hydrochloride:

Tyzine®: 0.1% (15 mL) [spray bottle; contains benzalkonium chloride]; (30 mL) [dropper bottle; contains benzalkonium chloride]

Tyzine® Pediatric: 0.05% (15 mL) [spray bottle; contains benzalkonium chloride]

Solution, ophthalmic, as hydrochloride: 0.05% (15 mL)

Eye-Sine™, Geneye®, Optigene® 3: 0.05% (15 mL) [may contain benzalkonium chloride]

Murine® Tears Plus: 0.05% (15 mL, 30 mL) [contains benzalkonium chloride]

Visine® Advanced Relief: 0.05% (30 mL) [contains benzalkonium chloride and polyethylene glycol]

Visine® Original: 0.05% (15 mL, 30 mL) [contains benzalkonium chloride; 15 mL size also available with dropper]

Theophylline *(thee OFF i lin)*

Related Information

Asthma *on page 1767*

Serum Drug Concentrations Commonly Monitored Guidelines *on page 1862*

Medication Safety Issues

Sound-alike/look-alike issues:

Theolair™ may be confused with Thiola®, Thyrolar®

U.S. Brand Names Elixophyllin®; Quibron®-T [DSC]; Quibron®-T/SR [DSC]; Theo-24®; TheoCap™; Theochron®; Uniphyl®

Canadian Brand Names Apo-Theo LA®; Novo-Theophyl SR; PMS-Theophylline; Pulmophylline; ratio-Theo-Bronc; Theochron® SR; Theolair™; Uniphyl® SRT

Index Terms Theophylline Anhydrous

Generic Available Yes: Extended release capsule and tablet, infusion

Pharmacologic Category Theophylline Derivative

Use Bronchodilator in reversible bronchospasm due to asthma, chronic bronchitis, and emphysema

Contraindications Hypersensitivity to theophylline or any component of the formulation; premixed injection may contain corn-derived dextrose and its use is contraindicated in patients with allergy to corn-related products

Warnings/Precautions May precipitate or worsen pre-existing arrhythmias; use with caution in patients with peptic ulcer, hyperthyroidism, hypertension, and patients with compromised cardiac function; hepatic function, esophageal reflux disease, alcoholism, and older adults

Adverse Reactions (Reflective of adult population; not specific for elderly)

Adverse reactions/theophylline serum level: (Adverse effects do not necessarily occur according to serum levels. Arrhythmia and seizure can occur without seeing the other adverse effects).

15-25 mcg/mL: GI upset, diarrhea, nausea/vomiting, abdominal pain, nervousness, headache, insomnia, agitation, dizziness, muscle cramp, tremor

25-35 mcg/mL: Tachycardia, occasional PVC

>35 mcg/mL: Ventricular tachycardia, frequent PVC, seizure

Uncommon at serum theophylline concentrations ≤20 mcg/mL:

1% to 10%:

Cardiovascular: Tachycardia

Central nervous system: Nervousness, restlessness

Gastrointestinal: Nausea, vomiting

Drug Interactions Substrate of CYP1A2 (major), 2C9 (minor), 2D6 (minor), 2E1 (major), 3A4 (major); **Inhibits** CYP1A2 (weak)

CYP1A2 inducers: May decrease the levels/effects of theophylline. Example inducers include aminoglutethimide, carbamazepine, phenobarbital, and rifampin.

CYP1A2 inhibitors: May increase the levels/effects of theophylline. Example inhibitors include ciprofloxacin, fluvoxamine, ketoconazole, norfloxacin, ofloxacin, and rofecoxib.

CYP2E1 inhibitors: May increase the levels/effects of theophylline. Example inhibitors include disulfiram, isoniazid, and miconazole.

CYP3A4 inducers: CYP3A4 inducers may decrease the levels/effects of theophylline. Example inducers include aminoglutethimide, carbamazepine, nafcillin, nevirapine, phenobarbital, phenytoin, and rifamycins.

CYP3A4 inhibitors: May increase the levels/effects of theophylline. Example inhibitors include azole antifungals, clarithromycin, diclofenac, doxycycline, erythromycin, imatinib, isoniazid, nefazodone, nicardipine, propofol, protease inhibitors, quinidine, telithromycin, and verapamil.

Ethanol/Nutrition/Herb Interactions Food: Food does not appreciably affect the absorption of liquid, fast-release products, and most sustained release products; however, food may induce a sudden release (dose-dumping) of once-daily sustained release products resulting in an increase in serum drug levels and potential toxicity. Avoid excessive amounts of caffeine. Avoid extremes of dietary protein and carbohydrate intake. Changes in diet may affect the elimination of theophylline; charbroiled foods may increase elimination, reducing half-life by 50%.

Mechanism of Action Causes bronchodilatation, diuresis, CNS and cardiac stimulation, and gastric acid secretion by blocking phosphodiesterase which increases tissue concentrations of cyclic adenine monophosphate (cAMP) which in turn promotes catecholamine stimulation of lipolysis, glycogenolysis, and gluconeogenesis and induces release of epinephrine from adrenal medulla cells

Pharmacokinetics

Absorption: Oral: Up to 100%, depending upon the formulation used

Distribution: V_d: 0.45 L/kg

Metabolism: In the liver by demethylation

Half-life:

Normal, nonsmoking, healthy Geriatrics and Adults: 3-15 hours

Smokers (1-2 packs/day): 4-5 hours

Severe congestive heart failure: 18-24 hours

Cirrhosis: 29 hours

Time to peak plasma concentration: 1-2 hours, 4 hours for sustained release

Elimination: In urine; adults excrete 10% in urine as unchanged drug

Dosage

Geriatrics: Elderly patients should be started with a 25% reduction in the adult dose.

Adults: Bronchodilation/respiratory stimulant:

Initial dosage recommendation: Loading dose (to achieve a serum concentration of about 10 mcg/mL; loading doses should be given using a rapidly absorbed oral product **not** a sustained release product):

If no theophylline has been administered in the previous 24 hours: 4-6 mg/kg theophylline

If theophylline has been administered in the previous 24 hours: Administer ½ loading dose; 2-3 mg/kg theophylline can be given in emergencies when serum concentrations are not available

Maintenance Dose for Acute Symptoms

Population Group	Oral Theophylline (mg/kg/day)	I.V. Aminophylline
Otherwise healthy nonsmoking adults (including elderly patients)	10 (not to exceed 900 mg/day)	0.5 mg/kg/h
Cardiac decompensation, cor pulmonale, and/or liver dysfunction	5 (not to exceed 400 mg/day)	0.25 mg/kg/h

Note: For continuous I.V. infusion, divide total daily dose by 24 = mg/kg/h.

(Continued)

Theophylline *(Continued)*

> *On the average, for every 1 mg/kg theophylline given, blood concentrations will rise 2 mcg/mL*

Maintenance dose: See table on previous page.

Bronchodilation: Oral:

Nonsustained release: 16-20 mg/kg/day divided into 4 doses/day

Sustained release: 9-13 mg/kg/day divided into 2-3 doses/day

Note: These recommendations, based on mean clearance rates for age or risk factors, were calculated to achieve a serum concentration of 10 mcg/mL. In healthy adults, a slow-release product can be used (9-13 mg/kg in divided dose). The total daily dose can be divided every 8-12 hours.

Dosage in obese patients: Use ideal body weight for obese patients. Dose should be adjusted further based on serum concentrations.

Administration Oral: Long-acting preparations should be taken with a full glass of water, swallowed whole, or cut in half if scored. Do **not** crush. Extended release capsule forms may be opened and the contents sprinkled on soft foods; do **not** chew beads.

Monitoring Parameters Heart rate, CNS effects (insomnia, irritability); respiratory rate (COPD patients often have resting controlled respiratory rates in low 20's)

Reference Range

Sample size: 0.5-1 mL serum (red top tube)

Therapeutic: 10-20 mcg/mL; Toxic: >20 mcg/mL; some patients may have adequate clinical response with serum concentrations from 5-10 mcg/mL

Timing of serum samples: If toxicity is suspected, obtain a concentration any time during a continuous I.V. infusion, or 2 hours after an oral dose; if lack of therapeutic is affected, draw a trough immediately before the next oral dose or intermittent I.V. dose

Patient Information Oral preparations should be taken with a full glass of water; avoid drinking or eating large quantities of caffeine-containing beverages or food; take at regular intervals; take sustained release tablets whole; sustained release capsule forms may be opened and sprinkled on soft foods; do not chew beads; take with food if GI upset occurs; notify physician if nausea, vomiting, insomnia, nervousness, irritability, palpitations, seizures occur; do not change from one brand to another without consulting physician and pharmacist; do not change doses without consulting your physician

Additional Information Saliva levels are approximately equal to 60% of plasma concentrations. Charcoal-broiled foods may increase elimination, reducing half-life by 50%; cigarette smoking may require an increase of dosage by 50% to 100%. Because different salts of theophylline have different theophylline content, various salts are equivalent. The following are percent content of theophylline for various salts:

Theophylline anhydrous: 100%

Theophylline monohydrate: 91%

Aminophylline anhydrous: 86%

Oxtriphylline: 64%

Most preparations are now labeled with actual milligram content delivered by the particular product.

Theophylline immediate release tablet/capsule: Bronkodyl®, Elixophyllin®, Quibron®-T, Slo-Phyllin®, Somophyllin®-T, Theolair™

Theophylline liquid: Accurbron®, Aerolate®, Aquaphyllin®, Asmalix®, Elixicon®, Elixophyllin®, Lixolin®, Theon®

Theophylline timed release capsule: Aerolate III®, Aerolate JR®, Aerolate SR®, Elixophyllin® SR, Lodrane®, Slo-bid™ Gyrocaps®, Slo-Phyllin® Gyrocaps®, Somophyllin®-CRT, Theobid®, Theoclear® L.A., Theophyl-SR®, Theospan®-SR, Theospan®-SR

Theophylline timed release tablet: Constant-T®, Duraphyl™, LaBID®, Quibron®-T/S, Respbid®, Sustaire®, Theochron®, Theo-Dur®, Theolair™-SR, Theo-Time®, Uniphyl®

Special Geriatric Considerations Although there is a great intersubject variability for half-lives of methylxanthines (2-10 hours), elderly as a group have slower hepatic clearance. Therefore, use lower initial doses and monitor closely for response and adverse reactions. Additionally, elderly are at greater risk for toxicity due to concomitant disease (eg, CHF, arrhythmias), and drug use (eg, cimetidine, ciprofloxacin).

Dosage Forms Excipient information presented when available (limited, particularly for generics); consult specific product labeling.

Capsule, extended release: 100 mg, 125 mg, 200 mg, 300 mg

TheoCap™: 125 mg, 200 mg, 300 mg [12 hour]

Theo-24®: 100 mg, 200 mg, 300 mg, 400 mg [24 hours]

Elixir:

Elixophyllin®: 80 mg/15 mL (480 mL) [contains alcohol 20%; fruit flavor]

Infusion [premixed in D_5W]: 200 mg (50 mL, 100 mL); 400 mg (100 mL, 250 mL, 500 mL); 800 mg (250 mL, 500 mL, 1000 mL)

Tablet, controlled release:
Uniphyl®: 400 mg, 600 mg [24 hours; contains cetostearyl alcohol]
Tablet, extended release: 100 mg, 200 mg, 300 mg, 450 mg
Theochron®: 100 mg, 200 mg, 300 mg, 450 mg [12-24 hours]
Tablet, immediate release:
Quibron®-T: 300 mg [DSC]
Tablet, sustained release:
Quibron®-T/SR: 300 mg [8-12 hours] [DSC]

Selected References

Kearney TE, Manoguerra AS, Curtis GP, et al, "Theophylline Toxicity and the Beta-Adrenergic System," *Ann Intern Med*, 1985, 102(6):766-9.

Mahler DA, Barlow PB, and Matthay RA, "Chronic Obstructive Pulmonary Disease," *Clin Geriatr Med*, 1986, 2(2):285-312.

Upton RA, "Pharmacokinetic Interactions Between Theophylline and Other Medication (Part I)," *Clin Pharmacokinet*, 1991, 20(1):66-80.

Weinberger M and Hendeles L, "Theophylline in Asthma," *N Engl J Med*, 1996, 334(21):1380-8.

♦ **Theophylline Anhydrous** see Theophylline on page 1548
♦ **Theophylline Ethylenediamine** see Aminophylline on page 77
♦ **Thera-Flur-N®** see Fluoride on page 642
♦ **Thermazene®** see Silver Sulfadiazine on page 1466
♦ **Thiamazole** see Methimazole on page 1003
♦ **Thiamin** see Thiamine on page 1551

Thiamine (THYE a min)

Medication Safety Issues

Sound-alike/look-alike issues:
Thiamine may be confused with Tenormin®, Thorazine®

International issues:
Doxal® [Brazil] may be confused with Doxil® which is a brand name for doxorubicin in the U.S.
Doxal® [Brazil]: Brand name for doxycycline in Austria; brand name for pyridoxine in Brazil; brand name for doxepin in Finland

Canadian Brand Names Betaxin®

Index Terms Aneurine Hydrochloride; Thiamin; Thiamine Hydrochloride; Thiaminium Chloride Hydrochloride; Vitamin B₁

Generic Available Yes

Pharmacologic Category Vitamin, Water Soluble

Use Treatment of thiamine deficiency including beriberi, Wernicke's encephalopathy, Korsakoff's syndrome, neuritis associated with pregnancy, or in alcoholic patients; dietary supplement

Contraindications Hypersensitivity to thiamine or any component of the formulation

Warnings/Precautions Use with caution with parenteral route (especially I.V.) of administration. Hypersensitivity reactions have been reported following repeated parenteral doses; consider skin test in individuals with history of allergic reactions. Single vitamin deficiency is rare; evaluate for other deficiencies. Dextrose administration may precipitate acute symptoms of thiamine deficiency; use caution when thiamine status is marginal or suspect. Some parenteral products contain aluminum; use caution in patients with impaired renal function.

Adverse Reactions (Reflective of adult population; not specific for elderly)
Adverse reactions reported with injection. Frequency not defined.
Cardiovascular: Cyanosis
Central nervous system: Restlessness
Dermatologic: Angioneurotic edema, pruritus, urticaria
Gastrointestinal: Hemorrhage into GI tract, nausea, tightness of the throat
Local: Induration and/or tenderness at the injection site (following I.M. administration)
Neuromuscular & skeletal: Weakness
Respiratory: Pulmonary edema
Miscellaneous: Anaphylactic/hypersensitivity reactions (following I.V. administration), diaphoresis, warmth

Overdosage/Toxicology Anorexia, headache, insomnia, irritability, nausea, nervousness, palpitations, tremor, and vomiting have been rarely reported as an overdose response.

Ethanol/Nutrition/Herb Interactions
Ethanol: May decrease thiamine absorption.
Food: High carbohydrate diets may increase thiamine requirement.

Stability Injection: Store at 15°C to 30°C (59°F to 86°F). Protect from light

Mechanism of Action An essential coenzyme in carbohydrate metabolism by combining with adenosine triphosphate to form thiamine pyrophosphate
(Continued)

Thiamine *(Continued)*

Pharmacokinetics

Absorption:

Oral: Adequate

I.M.: Rapid and complete

Distribution: Highest concentrations found in brain, heart, kidney, liver

Elimination: Renally as unchanged drug, and as pyrimidine after body storage sites become saturated

Dosage

Geriatrics & Adults:

Recommended daily intake: Female: 1.1 mg; Male: 1.2 mg

Parenteral nutrition supplementation: 6 mg/day; may be increased to 25-50 mg/day with history of alcohol abuse

Thiamine deficiency (beriberi): 5-30 mg/dose I.M. or I.V. 3 times/day (if critically ill); then orally 5-30 mg/day in single or divided doses 3 times/day for 1 month

Alcohol withdrawal syndrome: 100 mg/day I.M. or I.V. for several days, followed by 50-100 mg/day orally

Wernicke's encephalopathy: Treatment: Initial: 100 mg I.V., then 50-100 mg/day I.M. or I.V. until consuming a regular, balanced diet. Larger doses may be needed in patients with alcohol abuse.

Administration Parenteral form may be administered by I.M. or I.V. injection. Various rates of administration have been reported. Local injection reactions may be minimized by slow administration (~30 minutes) into larger, more proximal veins. Thiamine should be administered prior to parenteral glucose solutions to prevent the precipitation of heart failure.

Reference Range Normal, serum: 1.1-1.6 mg/dL

Test Interactions False-positive for uric acid using the phosphotungstate method and for urobilinogen using the Ehrlich's reagent; large doses may interfere with the spectrophotometric determination of serum theophylline concentration

Patient Information Dietary sources include legumes, pork, beef, whole grains, yeast, fresh vegetables; a deficiency state can occur in as little 3 weeks following total dietary absence

Additional Information Thiamine (vitamin B_1) is unstable in alkaline or neutral solutions, therefore, do not mix with carbonates, citrates, barbiturates. Also, any solution containing sulfites is incompatible with thiamine. Recommended thiamine intake is 0.5 mg/1000 Kcal.

Special Geriatric Considerations No special recommendations are necessary. Elderly are treated the same as younger adults.

Dosage Forms Excipient information presented when available (limited, particularly for generics); consult specific product labeling.

Injection, solution, as hydrochloride: 100 mg/mL (2 mL)

Tablet, as hydrochloride: 50 mg, 100 mg, 250 mg, 500 mg

Selected References

Bayard M, McIntyre J, Hill K, et al, "Alcohol Withdrawal Syndrome," *Am Fam Physician*, 2004, 69(6):1443-50.

Diamond I and Messing R, "Neurologic Effects of Alcoholism," *West J Med*, 1994, 161(3):279-87.

Doyon S and Roberts JR, "Reappraisal of the "Coma Cocktail": Dextrose, Flumazenil, Naloxone, and Thiamine," *Emerg Med Clin North Am*, 1994, 12(2):301-16.

"Dietary Reference Intakes for Thiamin, Riboflavin, Niacin, Vitamin B_6, Folate, Vitamin B_{12}, Pantothenic Acid, Biotin and Choline. Standing Committee on the Scientific Evaluation of Dietary Reference Intakes, Food and Nutrition Board, Institute of Medicine," National Academy of Sciences, Washington, DC: National Academy Press, 1999. Available at: http://www.nap.edu.

Hoffman RS and Goldfrank LR, "The Poisoned Patient With Altered Consciousness. Controversies in the Use of a 'Coma Cocktail'," *JAMA*, 1995, 274(7):562-9.

Mirtallo J, Canada T, Johnson D, et al, "Safe Practices for Parenteral Nutrition. Task Force for the Revision of Safe Practices for Parenteral Nutrition," *JPEN J Parenter Enteral Nutr*, 2004, 28(6):39-70.

Petrie WM and Ban TA, "Vitamins in Psychiatry. Do They Have a Role?" *Drugs*, 1985, 30(1):58-65.

Proebstle TM, Gall H, and Jugert FK, "Specific IgE and IgG Serum Antibodies to Thiamine Associated With Anaphylactic Reaction," *J Allergy Clin Immunol*, 1995, 95(5 Pt 1):1059-60.

Reuler JB, Girard DE, and Cooney TG, "Current Concepts: Wernicke's Encephalopathy," *N Engl J Med*, 1985, 312(16):1035-39.

Stephen JM, Grant R, and Veh CS, "Anaphylaxis From Administration of Intravenous Thiamine," *Am J Emerg Med*, 1992, 10(1):61-3.

Thomson AD, Cook CC, Touquet R, et al, "The Royal College of Physicians Report on Alcohol: Guidelines for Managing Wernicke's Encephalopathy in the Accident and Emergency Department," *Alcohol, Alcohol*, 2002, 37(6):513-21.

Van Haecke P, Ramaekers D, Vanderwegen L, et al, "Thiamine-Induced Anaphylactic Shock," *Am J Emerg Med*, 1995, 13(3):371-2.

Wrenn KD, Murphy F, and Slovis CM, "A Toxicity Study of Parenteral Thiamine Hydrochloride," *Ann Emerg Med*, 1989, 18(8):867-70.

◆ **Thiamine Hydrochloride** *see* Thiamine *on page 1551*

◆ **Thiaminium Chloride Hydrochloride** *see* Thiamine *on page 1551*

Thioridazine (thye oh RID a zeen)

Related Information
Antipsychotic Agents *on page 1747*
Liquid Compatibility of Antipsychotics and Mood Stabilizers *on page 1851*
Potentially Inappropriate Medications for Geriatrics *on page 1824*

Medication Safety Issues
Sound-alike/look-alike issues:
  Thioridazine may be confused with thiothixene, Thorazine®
  Mellaril® may be confused with Elavil®, Mebaral®

Canadian Brand Names Mellaril®

Index Terms Thioridazine Hydrochloride

Generic Available Yes

Pharmacologic Category Antipsychotic Agent, Typical, Phenothiazine

Use
Management of schizophrenia (in patients who fail to respond adequately to treatment with other antipsychotic drugs, either because of insufficient effectiveness or the inability to achieve an effective dose due to intolerable adverse effects from those medications), manifestations of psychotic disorders, depressive neurosis, alcohol withdrawal, nausea and vomiting, nonpsychotic symptoms associated with dementia (older adults), Tourette's syndrome, Huntington's chorea, spasmodic torticollis, Reye's syndrome
See Special Geriatric Considerations.

Unlabeled/Investigational Use Treatment of psychosis

Contraindications
Hypersensitivity to thioridazine or any component of the formulation (cross-reactivity between phenothiazines may occur); severe CNS depression; circulatory collapse; severe hypotension; bone marrow suppression; blood dyscrasias; coma; in combination with other drugs that are known to prolong the QT_c interval; in patients with congenital long QT syndrome or a history of cardiac arrhythmias; concurrent use with medications that inhibit the metabolism of thioridazine (fluoxetine, paroxetine, fluvoxamine, propranolol, pindolol); patients known to have genetic defect leading to reduced levels of activity of CYP2D6

Warnings/Precautions
Oral formulations may cause stomach upset; may cause thermoregulatory changes; use caution in patients with narrow-angle glaucoma; doses of 1 g/day frequently cause pigmentary retinopathy. **[U.S. Boxed Warning]: Thioridazine has dose-related effects on ventricular repolarization leading to QT_c prolongation, a potentially life-threatening effect.** As a result, it should be reserved for patients whose schizophrenia has failed to respond to adequate trials of other antipsychotic drugs. Use with caution in Parkinson's disease; hemodynamic instability; predisposition to seizures; subcortical brain damage; severe cardiac, hepatic, renal, or respiratory disease. Esophageal dysmotility and aspiration have been associated with antipsychotic use; use with caution in patients at risk of pneumonia (ie, Alzheimer's disease). Caution in breast cancer or other prolactin-dependent tumors (may elevate prolactin levels). May alter temperature regulation or mask toxicity of other drugs due to antiemetic effects. Check blood counts periodically and discontinue at first signs of blood dyscrasias; use is contraindicated in patients with bone marrow suppression.

Phenothiazines may cause anticholinergic effects (confusion, agitation, constipation, xerostomia, blurred vision, urinary retention); therefore, they should be used with caution in patients with decreased gastrointestinal motility, urinary retention, BPH, xerostomia, or visual problems. Conditions which also may be exacerbated by cholinergic blockade include narrow-angle glaucoma (screening is recommended) and worsening of myasthenia gravis. Relative to other neuroleptics, thioridazine has a high potency of cholinergic blockade.

May cause extrapyramidal reactions, including pseudoparkinsonism, acute dystonic reactions, akathisia, and tardive dyskinesia (risk of these reactions is low relative to other neuroleptics). Use caution in the elderly. May be associated with neuroleptic malignant syndrome (NMS).

Adverse Reactions (Reflective of adult population; not specific for elderly)
Frequency not defined.
Cardiovascular: Hypotension, orthostatic hypotension, peripheral edema, ECG changes
Central nervous system: EPS (pseudoparkinsonism, akathisia, dystonias, tardive dyskinesia), dizziness, drowsiness, neuroleptic malignant syndrome (NMS), impairment of temperature regulation, lowering of seizure threshold, seizure
Dermatologic: Increased sensitivity to sun, rash, discoloration of skin (blue-gray)
Endocrine & metabolic: Changes in menstrual cycle, libido (changes in), breast pain, galactorrhea, amenorrhea
Gastrointestinal: Constipation, weight gain, nausea, vomiting, stomach pain, xerostomia, nausea, vomiting, diarrhea
Genitourinary: Difficulty in urination, ejaculatory disturbances, urinary retention, priapism
(Continued)

Thioridazine *(Continued)*

Hematologic: Agranulocytosis, leukopenia

Hepatic: Cholestatic jaundice, hepatotoxicity

Neuromuscular & skeletal: Tremor

Ocular: Pigmentary retinopathy, blurred vision, cornea and lens changes

Respiratory: Nasal congestion

Overdosage/Toxicology Symptoms include deep sleep, coma, extrapyramidal symptoms, abnormal involuntary muscle movements, hypotension, and arrhythmias. Immediate cardiovascular monitoring, including continuous ECG monitoring, to detect arrhythmias.

Following initiation of essential overdose management, toxic symptom treatment and supportive treatment should be initiated. **Avoid use of other medications that may also prolong the QT$_c$ interval, such as disopyramide, procainamide and quinidine.** Hypotension usually responds to I.V. fluids or Trendelenburg positioning. If unresponsive to these measures, the use of a parenteral inotrope may be required (eg, norepinephrine 0.1-0.2 mcg/kg/minute titrated to response); do not use epinephrine. Seizures commonly respond to diazepam (I.V. 5-10 mg bolus every 15 minutes if needed up to a total of 30 mg) or to phenytoin. Neuroleptics often cause extrapyramidal symptoms (eg, dystonic reactions) requiring management with diphenhydramine 1-2 mg/kg up to a maximum of 50 mg I.M. or slow I.V. push followed by a maintenance dose for 48-72 hours. When these reactions are unresponsive to diphenhydramine, anticholinergic agents such as benztropine mesylate I.V. 1-2 mg may be effective. These agents are generally effective within 2-5 minutes. Avoid barbiturates; may potentiate respiratory depression.

Drug Interactions Substrate of CYP2C19 (minor), 2D6 (major); **Inhibits** CYP1A2 (weak), 2C9 (weak), 2D6 (moderate), 2E1 (weak)

Acetylcholinesterase inhibitors (central): May increase the risk of antipsychotic-related extrapyramidal symptoms; monitor.

Aluminum salts: May decrease the absorption of phenothiazines; monitor

Amphetamines: Efficacy may be diminished by antipsychotics; in addition, amphetamines may increase psychotic symptoms; avoid concurrent use

Anticholinergics: May inhibit the therapeutic response to phenothiazines and excess anticholinergic effects may occur; includes benztropine, trihexyphenidyl, biperiden, and drugs with significant anticholinergic activity (TCAs, antihistamines, disopyramide)

Antihypertensives: Concurrent use of phenothiazines with an antihypertensive may produce additive hypotensive effects (particularly orthostasis)

Beta-blockers: May increase the risk of arrhythmia; propranolol and pindolol are **contraindicated**

Bromocriptine: Phenothiazines inhibit the ability of bromocriptine to lower serum prolactin concentrations

Carvedilol: Serum concentrations may be increased, leading to hypotension and bradycardia; avoid concurrent use

CNS depressants: Sedative effects may be additive with phenothiazines; monitor for increased effect; includes barbiturates, benzodiazepines, opioid analgesics, ethanol, and other sedative agents

CYP2D6 inhibitors: May increase the levels/effects of thioridazine. Example inhibitors include chlorpromazine, delavirdine, fluoxetine, miconazole, paroxetine, pergolide, quinidine, quinine, ritonavir, and ropinirole. **Thioridazine is contraindicated with inhibitors of this enzyme.**

CYP2D6 substrates: Thioridazine may increase the levels/effects of CYP2D6 substrates. Example substrates include amphetamines, selected beta-blockers, dextromethorphan, fluoxetine, lidocaine, mirtazapine, nefazodone, paroxetine, risperidone, ritonavir, tricyclic antidepressants, and venlafaxine.

CYP2D6 prodrug substrates: Thioridazine may decrease the levels/effects of CYP2D6 prodrug substrates. Example prodrug substrates include codeine, hydrocodone, oxycodone, and tramadol.

Epinephrine: Chlorpromazine (and possibly other low potency antipsychotics) may diminish the pressor effects of epinephrine

Guanethidine and guanadrel: Antihypertensive effects may be inhibited by phenothiazines

Levodopa: Phenothiazines may inhibit the antiparkinsonian effect of levodopa; avoid this combination

Lithium: Phenothiazines may produce neurotoxicity with lithium; this is a rare effect

Metoclopramide: May increase extrapyramidal symptoms (EPS) or risk.

Phenytoin: May reduce serum levels of phenothiazines; phenothiazines may increase phenytoin serum levels

Polypeptide antibiotics: Rare cases of respiratory paralysis have been reported with concurrent use of phenothiazines

Potassium-depleting agents: May increase the risk of serious arrhythmias with thioridazine; includes many diuretics, aminoglycosides, and amphotericin; monitor serum potassium closely

Propranolol: Serum concentrations of phenothiazines may be increased; propranolol also increases phenothiazine concentrations; may also occur with pindolol. **These agents are contraindicated with thioridazine.**

QT_c-prolonging agents: Effects on QT_c interval may be additive with phenothiazines, increasing the risk of malignant arrhythmias; includes type Ia antiarrhythmics, TCAs, and some quinolone antibiotics (moxifloxacin). **These agents are contraindicated with thioridazine.**

Sulfadoxine-pyrimethamine: May increase phenothiazine concentrations

Trazodone: Phenothiazines and trazodone may produce additive hypotensive effects

Tricyclic antidepressants: Concurrent use may produce increased toxicity or altered therapeutic response

Valproic acid: Serum levels may be increased by phenothiazines

Ethanol/Nutrition/Herb Interactions

Ethanol: Avoid ethanol (may increase CNS depression).

Herb/Nutraceutical: Avoid kava kava, valerian, St John's wort, gotu kola (may increase CNS depression). Avoid dong quai, St John's wort (may also cause photosensitization).

Stability Protect from light.

Mechanism of Action Thioridazine is a piperidine phenothiazine which blocks postsynaptic mesolimbic dopaminergic receptors in the brain; exhibits a strong alpha-adrenergic blocking effect and depresses the release of hypothalamic and hypophyseal hormones

Pharmacokinetics

Absorption: May be affected by the inherent anticholinergic action on the gastrointestinal tissue causing variable absorption. Absorption from tablets is erratic with less variation seen with solutions. These agents are widely distributed in tissues with CNS concentrations exceeding that of plasma due to their lipophilic characteristics.

Protein binding: Antipsychotic agents are bound 90% to 99% to plasma proteins; highly bound to brain and lung tissue and other tissues with a high blood perfusion.

Metabolism: Hepatic

Time to peak concentration: Oral: 2-4 hours

Elimination: Occurs through hepatic metabolism (oxidation) where numerous active metabolites are produced; active metabolites excreted in urine; elimination half-lives of antipsychotics ranges from 20-40 hours which may be extended in older adults due to decline in oxidative hepatic reactions (phase I) with age.

The biologic effect of a single dose persists for 24 hours. When the patient has accommodated to initial side effects (sedation), once daily dosing is possible due to the long half-life of antipsychotics.

Steady-state plasma concentrations are achieved in 4-7 days; therefore, if possible, do not make dose adjustments more than once in a 7-day period. Due to the long half-lives of antipsychotics, as needed (prn) use is ineffective since repeated doses are necessary to achieve therapeutic tissue concentrations in the CNS.

Dosage

Geriatrics: Behavioral symptoms associated with dementia (unlabeled use): Oral: Initial: 10-25 mg 1-2 times/day; increase at 4- to 7-day intervals by 10-25 mg/day; increase dose intervals (once daily, twice daily, etc) as necessary to control response or side effects. Maximum daily dose: 400 mg; gradual increases (titration) may prevent some side effects or decrease their severity.

Adults:

Schizophrenia/psychosis: Oral: Initial: 50-100 mg 3 times/day with gradual increments as needed and tolerated; maximum: 800 mg/day in 2-4 divided doses

Depressive disorders, dementia (unlabeled use): Oral: Initial: 25 mg 3 times/day; maintenance dose: 20-200 mg/day

Renal Impairment: Not dialyzable (0% to 5%)

Administration Oral concentrate must be diluted in 2-4 oz of liquid (eg, water, fruit juice, carbonated drinks, milk, or pudding) before administration. Do not take antacid within 2 hours of taking drug. Thioridazine concentrate is not compatible with carbamazepine suspension; schedule dosing at least 1-2 hours apart from each other. **Note:** Avoid skin contact with oral suspension or solution; may cause contact dermatitis.

Monitoring Parameters Orthostatic blood pressures; tremors, gait changes, abnormal movement in trunk, neck, buccal area, or extremities; monitor target behaviors for which the agent is given. Baseline and periodic EKG and serum potassium; periodic eye exam, CBC with differential, blood pressure, liver enzyme tests; do not initiate if QT_c >450 msec

Reference Range Therapeutic: 1.0-1.5 mcg/mL (SI: 2.7-4.1 µmol/L); Toxic: >1 mg/mL; lethal: 2-8 mg/dL

Test Interactions False-positives for phenylketonuria, urinary amylase, uroporphyrins, urobilinogen

(Continued)

Thioridazine *(Continued)*

Patient Information See Administration. Do not take antacid within 1 hour of taking drug. Avoid alcohol and excess sun exposure (use sun block). May cause drowsiness, rise slowly from recumbent position. Use of supportive stockings may help prevent orthostatic hypotension.

Additional Information Oral formulations may cause stomach upset; may cause thermoregulatory changes.

Special Geriatric Considerations Any changes in disease status in any organ system can result in behavior changes.

Many elderly patients receive antipsychotic medications for inappropriate nonpsychotic behavior. Before initiating antipsychotic medication, the clinician should investigate any possible reversible cause; any stress or stress from any disease can cause acute "confusion" or worsening of baseline nonpsychotic behavior. Most commonly acute changes in behavior are due to increases in drug dose or addition of new drug to regimen; fluid electrolyte loss; infections; and changes in environment.

In the treatment of agitated, demented, older adult patients, authors of meta-analysis of controlled trials of the response to the traditional antipsychotics (phenothiazines, butyrophenones) in controlling agitation have concluded that the use of neuroleptics results in a response rate of 18%. Clearly neuroleptic therapy for behavior control should be limited with frequent attempts to withdraw the agent given for behavior control.

Dosage Forms Excipient information presented when available (limited, particularly for generics); consult specific product labeling.

Tablet, as hydrochloride: 10 mg, 15 mg, 25 mg, 50 mg, 100 mg, 150 mg, 200 mg

Selected References

Appell RA, Shield DE, and McGuire EJ, "Thioridazine-Induced Priapism," *Br J Urol*, 1977, 49(2):160.

Baker PB, Merigian KS, Roberts JR, et al, "Hyperthermia, Hypertension, Hypertonia, and Coma in Massive Thioridazine Overdose," *Am J Emerg Med*, 1988, 6(4):346-9.

Buckley NA, Whyte IM, and Dawson AH, "Cardiotoxicity More Common in Thioridazine Overdose Than With Other Neuroleptics," *J Toxicol Clin Toxicol*, 1995, 33(3):199-204.

Burgess KR, Jefferis RW, and Stevenson IF, "Fatal Thioridazine Cardiotoxicity," *Med J Aust*, 1979, 2(4):177-8.

Cowen TD and Meythaler JM, "Hypotensive Effects of Thioridazine in an Elderly Patient With Traumatic Brain Injury," *Brain Inj*, 1994, 8(8):735-7.

Goss JB, "Concomitant Use of Thioridazine With Risperidone," *Am J Health Syst Pharm*, 1995, 52(9):1012.

Oshika T, "Ocular Adverse Effects of Neuropsychiatric Agents. Incidence and Management," *Drug Saf*, 1995, 12(4):256-63.

Peabody CA, Warner MD, Whiteford HA, et al, "Neuroleptics and the Elderly," *J Am Geriatr Soc*, 1987, 35(3):233-8.

Risse SC and Barnes R, "Pharmacologic Treatment of Agitation Associated With Dementia," *J Am Geriatr Soc*, 1986, 34(5):368-76.

Saltz BL, Woerner MG, Kane JM, et al, "Prospective Study of Tardive Dyskinesia Incidence in the Elderly," *JAMA*, 1991, 266(17):2402-6.

Seifert RD, "Therapeutic Drug Monitoring: Psychotropic Drugs," *J Pharm Pract*, 1984, 6:403-16.

Weisdorf D, Kramer J, Goldbarg A, et al, "Physostigmine for Cardiac and Neurologic Manifestations of Phenothiazine Poisoning," *Clin Pharmacol Ther*, 1978, 24(6):663-7.

♦ **Thioridazine Hydrochloride** *see* Thioridazine *on page 1553*

Thiothixene *(thye oh THIKS een)*

Related Information
Antipsychotic Agents *on page 1747*
Liquid Compatibility of Antipsychotics and Mood Stabilizers *on page 1851*

Medication Safety Issues
Sound-alike/look-alike issues:
Thiothixene may be confused with thioridazine
Navane® may be confused with Norvasc®, Nubain®

U.S. Brand Names Navane®

Canadian Brand Names Navane®

Index Terms Tiotixene

Generic Available Yes

Pharmacologic Category Antipsychotic Agent, Typical

Use Management of nonpsychotic symptoms associated with dementia (older adults), Tourette's syndrome, Huntington's chorea, schizophrenia

Unlabeled/Investigational Use Treatment of psychotic disorders

Contraindications Hypersensitivity to thiothixene or any component of the formulation; severe CNS depression; circulatory collapse; blood dyscrasias; coma

Warnings/Precautions Watch for hypotension when administering I.M. or I.V.; use with caution in patients with cardiovascular disease, seizures, and Parkinson's disease.

Tardive dyskinesia: Prevalence rate may be 40% in older adults; older adult women especially at risk; embarrassment from dyskinesias may lead to greater social isolation; development of the syndrome and the irreversible nature are proportional to duration and total cumulative dose over time. May be reversible if diagnosed early in therapy;

intermittent use of antipsychotics (not proven use) helps decrease total cumulative dose.

EPS: Extrapyramidal reactions are more common in older adults with up to 50% developing these reactions after age 60. These reactions may be more common in dementia patients. Drug-induced **Parkinson's syndrome** occurs often. Discontinuation usually resolves symptoms but may take weeks to months (12+) to clear. **Akathisia** is the most common EPS reaction in older adults. The symptoms of motor restlessness are difficult to diagnose in demented older adults; increased nervousness, assertiveness, restlessness with constant movement may indicate this adverse event. Consider decreasing dose if antipsychotic to treat as well as diagnose problem; usually see this reaction within 2-3 months of initiating antipsychotic drug.

Anticholinergic effects: These side effects most common with low potency antipsychotics (eg, thioridazine, chlorpromazine). CNS toxicity occurs more frequently and severely in older adults; increased confusion, memory loss, psychotic behavior, and agitation frequently occur as a consequence of anticholinergic effects to antipsychotic agents. Peripheral anticholinergic action troublesome to older adults; most peripheral anticholinergic effects last only 2-3 weeks. See Adverse Reactions.

Orthostatic hypotension: More common with low potency agents (eg, thioridazine, chlorpromazine, and clozapine) but of concern with all antipsychotic agents; orthostasis due to alpha-receptor blockade by antipsychotic agents. Older adults present many risk factors for orthostatic hypotension: Blunted baroreceptor reflexes, decreased vascular tone, decreased vascular volume, and possible presence of cardiac diseases which result in decreased cardiac output.

Sedation: Common side effect with antipsychotic therapy; should not be used as a hypnotic unless insomnia is associated with target behavior symptoms treated with antipsychotic medications. See Special Geriatric Considerations. Anecdotal reports suggesting antipsychotic sedation in nonpsychotic patients is extremely unpleasant due to feelings of depersonalization, derealization, and dysphoria. Due to the long duration of action with antipsychotic drugs, these reactions may last up to 24 hours and result in decreased daytime function.

Cardiac toxicity: Life-threatening arrhythmias have occurred at therapeutic doses of antipsychotics. Thioridazine more commonly demonstrates EKG changes than other antipsychotics; suggested to use high potency antipsychotic agents (ie, haloperidol) in patients with cardiac conduction defects.

Adverse Reactions (Reflective of adult population; not specific for elderly)
Frequency not defined.
Cardiovascular: Hypotension, nonspecific ECG changes, syncope, tachycardia
Central nervous system: Agitation, dizziness, drowsiness, extrapyramidal symptoms (akathisia, dystonias, lightheadedness, pseudoparkinsonism, tardive dyskinesia), insomnia restlessness
Dermatologic: Discoloration of skin (blue-gray), photosensitivity, pruritus, rash, urticaria
Endocrine & metabolic: Amenorrhea, breast pain, libido (changes in), changes in menstrual cycle, galactorrhea, gynecomastia, hyper-/hypoglycemia, lactation
Gastrointestinal: Constipation, nausea, salivation increased, stomach pain, vomiting, weight gain, xerostomia
Genitourinary: Difficulty in urination, ejaculatory disturbances, impotence
Hematologic: Leukocytes, leukopenia
Neuromuscular & skeletal: Tremors
Ocular: Blurred vision, pigmentary retinopathy
Respiratory: Nasal congestion
Miscellaneous: Diaphoresis

Overdosage/Toxicology Symptoms include muscle twitching, drowsiness, dizziness, rigidity, tremor, hypotension, and cardiac arrhythmias. Following initiation of essential overdose management, toxic symptom treatment and supportive treatment should be initiated. Hypotension usually responds to I.V. fluids or Trendelenburg positioning. If unresponsive to these measures, the use of a parenteral inotrope may be required (eg, norepinephrine 0.1-0.2 mcg/kg/minute titrated to response). Seizures commonly respond to diazepam (I.V. 5-10 mg bolus every 15 minutes if needed up to a total of 30 mg) or to phenytoin or phenobarbital. Neuroleptics often cause extrapyramidal symptoms (eg, dystonic reactions) requiring management with diphenhydramine 1-2 mg/kg up to a maximum of 50 mg I.M. or slow I.V. push, followed by a maintenance dose for 48-72 hours. When these reactions are unresponsive to diphenhydramine, anticholinergic agents such as benztropine mesylate I.V. 1-2 mg may be effective. These agents are generally effective within 2-5 minutes.

Drug Interactions Substrate of CYP1A2 (major); **Inhibits** CYP2D6 (weak)
Acetylcholinesterase inhibitors (central): May increase the risk of antipsychotic-related extrapyramidal symptoms; monitor.
Aluminum salts: May decrease the absorption of antipsychotics; monitor.
Amphetamines: Efficacy may be diminished by antipsychotics; in addition, amphetamines may increase psychotic symptoms; avoid concurrent use.
(Continued)

Thiothixene *(Continued)*

Anticholinergics: May inhibit the therapeutic response to antipsychotics and excess anticholinergic effects may occur; includes benztropine, trihexyphenidyl, biperiden, and drugs with significant anticholinergic activity (TCAs, antihistamines, disopyramide).

Antihypertensives: Concurrent use of antipsychotics with an antihypertensive may produce additive hypotensive effects (particularly orthostasis).

Bromocriptine: Antipsychotics inhibit the ability of bromocriptine to lower serum prolactin concentrations.

CNS depressants: Sedative effects may be additive with antipsychotics; monitor for increased effect; includes barbiturates, benzodiazepines, opioid analgesics, ethanol, and other sedative agents.

CYP1A2 inducers: May decrease the levels/effects of thiothixene. Example inducers include aminoglutethimide, carbamazepine, phenobarbital, and rifampin.

CYP1A2 inhibitors: May increase the levels/effects of thiothixene. Example inhibitors include ciprofloxacin, fluvoxamine, ketoconazole, norfloxacin, ofloxacin, and rofecoxib.

Epinephrine: Chlorpromazine (and possibly other low potency antipsychotics) may diminish the pressor effects of epinephrine.

Guanethidine and guanadrel: Antihypertensive effects may be inhibited by antipsychotics.

Levodopa: Antipsychotics may inhibit the antiparkinsonian effect of levodopa; avoid this combination.

Lithium: Antipsychotics may produce neurotoxicity with lithium; this is a rare effect.

Metoclopramide: May increase extrapyramidal symptoms (EPS) or risk.

Propranolol: Serum concentrations of antipsychotics may be increased; propranolol also increases antipsychotics concentrations.

QT_c-prolonging agents: Effects on QT_c interval may be additive with antipsychotics, increasing the risk of malignant arrhythmias; includes type Ia antiarrhythmics, TCAs, and some quinolone antibiotics (moxifloxacin).

Sulfadoxine-pyrimethamine: May increase antipsychotics concentrations.

Trazodone: Antipsychotics and trazodone may produce additive hypotensive effects.

Tricyclic antidepressants: Concurrent use may produce increased toxicity or altered therapeutic response.

Valproic acid: Serum levels may be increased by antipsychotics.

Ethanol/Nutrition/Herb Interactions

Ethanol: Avoid ethanol (may increase CNS depression).

Herb/Nutraceutical: Avoid kava kava, valerian, St John's wort, gotu kola (may increase CNS depression).

Mechanism of Action Thiothixene is a thioxanthene antipsychotic which elicits antipsychotic activity by postsynaptic blockade of CNS dopamine receptors resulting in inhibition of dopamine-mediated effects; also has alpha-adrenergic blocking activity

Pharmacokinetics

Absorption: May be affected by the inherent anticholinergic action on the gastrointestinal tissue causing variable absorption. Absorption from tablets is erratic with less variation seen with solutions. These agents are widely distributed in tissues with CNS concentrations exceeding that of plasma due to their lipophilic characteristics.

Protein binding: Antipsychotic agents are bound 90% to 99% to plasma proteins; highly bound to brain and lung tissue and other tissues with a high blood perfusion.

Metabolism: Extensive in the liver

Half-life: >24 hours with chronic use

Time to peak serum concentration: Oral: 2-4 hours

Elimination: Occurs through hepatic metabolism (oxidation) where numerous active metabolites are produced; active metabolites excreted in urine; elimination half-lives of antipsychotics ranges from 20-40 hours which may be extended in older adults due to decline in oxidative hepatic reactions (phase I) with age.

The biologic effect of a single dose persists for 24 hours. When the patient has accommodated to initial side effects (sedation), once daily dosing is possible due to the long half-life of antipsychotics.

Steady-state plasma concentrations are achieved in 4-7 days; therefore, if possible, do not make dose adjustments more than once in a 7-day period. Due to the long half-lives of antipsychotics, as needed (prn) use is ineffective since repeated doses are necessary to achieve therapeutic tissue concentrations in the CNS.

Dosage

Geriatrics: Nonpsychotic patient, dementia behavior (unlabeled use): Initial: 1-2 mg 1-2 times/day; increase dose at 4- to 7-day intervals by 1-2 mg/day. Increase dosing intervals (bid, tid, etc) as necessary to control response or side effects; maximum daily dose: 30 mg. Gradual increases in dose may prevent some side effects or decrease their severity.

Adults:

Mild to moderate psychosis: Oral: 2 mg 3 times/day, up to 20-30 mg/day; more severe psychosis: Initial: 5 mg 2 times/day, may increase gradually, if necessary; maximum: 60 mg/day

Rapid tranquilization of the agitated patient (administered every 30-60 minutes): Oral: 5-10 mg; average total dose for tranquilization: 15-30 mg

Renal Impairment: Not dialyzable (0% to 5%)

Administration Oral (concentrate) solution: Dilute immediately before administration with water, fruit juice, milk, etc. **Note:** Avoid skin contact with oral medication; may cause contact dermatitis.

Monitoring Parameters Orthostatic blood pressures; tremors, gait changes, abnormal movement in trunk, neck, buccal area, or extremities; monitor target behaviors for which the agent is given. Monitor orthostatic blood pressures 3-5 days after initiation of therapy or a dose increase.

Reference Range Serum concentration: 2-57 ng/mL; concentrations do not always correspond to response and are controversial; dose to response for efficacy and safety

Patient Information Oral concentrate must be diluted in 2-4 oz of liquid (water, fruit juice, carbonated drinks, milk, or pudding); do not take antacid within 1 hour of taking drug; avoid alcohol; avoid excess sun exposure (use sun block); may cause drowsiness, rise slowly from recumbent position; use of supportive stockings may help prevent orthostatic hypotension

Special Geriatric Considerations Any changes in disease status in any organ system can result in behavior changes.

Many elderly patients receive antipsychotic medications for inappropriate nonpsychotic behavior. Before initiating antipsychotic medication, the clinician should investigate any possible reversible cause; any stress or stress from any disease can cause acute "confusion" or worsening of baseline nonpsychotic behavior. Most commonly acute changes in behavior are due to increases in drug dose or addition of new drug to regimen; fluid electrolyte loss; infections; and changes in environment.

In the treatment of agitated, demented, elderly patients, authors of meta-analysis of controlled trials of the response to the traditional antipsychotics (phenothiazines, butyrophenones) in controlling agitation have concluded that the use of neuroleptics results in a response rate of 18%. Clearly neuroleptic therapy for behavior control should be limited with frequent attempts to withdraw the agent given for behavior control.

Dosage Forms Excipient information presented when available (limited, particularly for generics); consult specific product labeling. [DSC] = Discontinued product

Capsule: 1 mg, 2 mg, 5 mg, 10 mg
 Navane®: 1 mg [DSC], 2 mg, 5 mg, 10 mg, 20 mg

Selected References

Peabody CA, Warner MD, Whiteford HA, et al, "Neuroleptics and the Elderly," *J Am Geriatr Soc*, 1987, 35(3):233-8.

Risse SC and Barnes R, "Pharmacologic Treatment of Agitation Associated With Dementia," *J Am Geriatr Soc*, 1986, 34(5):368-76.

Saltz BL, Woerner MG, Kane JM, et al, "Prospective Study of Tardive Dyskinesia Incidence in the Elderly," *JAMA*, 1991, 266(17):2402-6.

Seifert RD, "Therapeutic Drug Monitoring: Psychotropic Drugs," *J Pharm Pract*, 1984, 6:403-16.

♦ **Thonzonium, Neomycin, Colistin, and Hydrocortisone** *see* Neomycin, Colistin, Hydrocortisone, and Thonzonium *on page 1101*

Thyroid (THYE roid)

U.S. Brand Names Armour® Thyroid; Nature-Throid™ NT; Westhroid®

Index Terms Desiccated Thyroid; Thyroid Extract; Thyroid USP

Generic Available Yes

Pharmacologic Category Thyroid Product

Use Replacement or supplemental therapy in hypothyroidism; pituitary TSH suppressants (thyroid nodules, thyroiditis, multinodular goiter, thyroid cancer), thyrotoxicosis, diagnostic suppression tests

Contraindications Hypersensitivity to beef or pork or any component of the formulation; recent myocardial infarction; thyrotoxicosis uncomplicated by hypothyroidism; uncorrected adrenal insufficiency

Warnings/Precautions [U.S. Boxed Warning]: Ineffective and potentially toxic for weight reduction. High doses may produce serious or even life-threatening toxic effects particularly when used with some anorectic drugs. Use with caution and reduce dosage in patients with angina pectoris or other cardiovascular disease and elderly since they may be more likely to have compromised cardiovascular function; chronic hypothyroidism predisposes patients to coronary artery disease. Use with caution in patients with adrenal insufficiency, diabetes mellitus or insipidus, and myxedema; symptoms may be exaggerated or aggravated. Desiccated thyroid contains variable amounts of T_3, T_4, and other triiodothyronine compounds which are more likely to cause cardiac signs or symptoms due to fluctuating levels. Should avoid use in the (Continued)

Thyroid *(Continued)*

elderly for this reason. Many clinicians consider levothyroxine to be the drug of choice for thyroid replacement.

Drug Interactions
Decreased effect:
Beta-blocker effect is decreased when patients become euthyroid
Thyroid hormones increase the therapeutic need for oral hypoglycemics or insulin
Estrogens increase TBG, thereby decreasing effect of thyroid replacement
Cholestyramine and colestipol decrease the effect of orally administered thyroid replacement
Serum digitalis concentrations are reduced in hyperthyroidism or when hypothyroid patients are converted to a euthyroid state
Theophylline levels decrease when hypothyroid patients converted to a euthyroid state
Increased toxicity: Thyroid may potentiate the hypoprothrombinemic effect of oral anticoagulants

Mechanism of Action The primary active compound is T_3 (triiodothyronine), which may be converted from T_4 (thyroxine) and then circulates throughout the body to influence growth and maturation of various tissues; exact mechanism of action is unknown; however, it is believed the thyroid hormone exerts its many metabolic effects through control of DNA transcription and protein synthesis; involved in normal metabolism, growth, and development; promotes gluconeogenesis, increases utilization and mobilization of glycogen stores and stimulates protein synthesis, increases basal metabolic rate

Pharmacodynamics
Onset of therapeutic effects: May be seen in 3-5 days
Maximum effects: 4-6 weeks may be required for any given dose

Pharmacokinetics
Absorption: T_4 is 48% to 79% absorbed; T_3 is 95% absorbed; desiccated thyroid contains thyroxine, liothyronine, and iodine (primarily bound); following absorption thyroxine is largely converted to liothyronine
Protein binding: 99% (bound to albumin, thyroxine-binding globulin, and thyroxine-binding prealbumin)
Metabolism: Liothyronine is metabolized in the liver, kidneys, and other tissues to inactive compounds
Half-life:
Liothyronine: 1-2 days
Thyroxine: 6-7 days
Elimination: In urine as conjugated forms

Dosage
Geriatrics: Not recommended for use in the elderly (see Special Geriatric Considerations).
Adults: Hypothyroidism: Oral: Initial: 15-30 mg; increase with 15 mg increments every 2-4 weeks; use 15 mg in patients with cardiovascular disease or myxedema. Maintenance dose: Usually 60-120 mg/day; monitor TSH and clinical symptoms.
Note: Thyroid cancer requires larger amounts than replacement therapy.

Monitoring Parameters T_4, TSH, heart rate, blood pressure, clinical signs of hypo- and hyperthyroidism; TSH is the most reliable guide for evaluating adequacy of thyroid replacement dosage. TSH may be elevated during the first few months of thyroid replacement despite patients being clinically euthyroid. In cases where T_4 remains low and TSH is within normal limits, an evaluation of "free" (unbound) T_4 is needed to evaluate further increase in dosage.

Reference Range
TSH 0.4-10 (for those ≥80 years) mIU/L
T_4: 4-12 mcg/dL (51-154 mmol:/L)
T_3 (RIA) (total T_3): 80-230 ng/dL (1.2-3.5 mmol/L)
T_4 free (Free T_4): 0.7-1.8 ng/dL (9-23 pmol/L)

Patient Information Do not change brands without physician's knowledge; report immediately to physician any chest pain, increased pulse, palpitations, heat intolerance, excessive sweating; do not stop use without physician's advice; replacement therapy will be for life; take as a single dose before breakfast

Additional Information Equivalent levothyroxine dose: Thyroid USP 60 mg = levothyroxine 0.05-0.06 mg; liothyronine: 15-37.5 mcg; liotrix: 60 mg

Special Geriatric Considerations Desiccated thyroid contains variable amounts of T_3, T_4, and other triiodothyronine compounds which are more likely to cause cardiac signs or symptoms due to fluctuating levels. Should avoid use in the elderly for this reason. Many clinicians consider levothyroxine to be the drug of choice.

Dosage Forms Excipient information presented when available (limited, particularly for generics); consult specific product labeling.
Tablet: 30 mg, 32.5 mg, 60 mg, 65 mg, 90 mg, 120 mg, 130 mg, 180 mg, 240 mg, 300 mg

Armour® Thyroid: 15 mg, 30 mg, 60 mg, 90 mg, 120 mg, 180 mg, 240 mg, 300 mg

Nature-Throid® NT, Westhroid®: 32.5 mg, 65 mg, 130 mg, 195 mg

Selected References

Helfand M and Crapo LM, "Monitoring Therapy in Patients Taking Levothyroxine," *Ann Intern Med*, 1990, 113(6):450-4.

Johnson DG and Campbell S, "Hormonal and Metabolic Agents," *Geriatric Pharmacology*, Bressler R and Katz MD, eds, New York, NY: McGraw-Hill, 1993, 427-50.

Sanders LR, "Pituitary, Thyroid, Adrenal and Parathyroid Diseases in the Elderly," *Geriatric Medicine*, 1990, 475-87.

Sawin CT, Geller A, Hershman JM, et al, "The Aging Thyroid. The Use of Thyroid Hormone in Older Persons," *JAMA*, 1989, 261(18):2653-5.

Watts NB, "Use of a Sensitive Thyrotropin Assay for Monitoring Treatment With Levothyroxine," *Arch Intern Med*, 1989, 149(2):309-12.

♦ **Thyroid Extract** *see* Thyroid *on page 1559*

♦ **Thyroid USP** *see* Thyroid *on page 1559*

♦ **Thyrolar®** *see* Liotrix *on page 915*

♦ ***L*-Thyroxine Sodium** *see* Levothyroxine *on page 901*

Tiagabine (tye AG a been)

Medication Safety Issues

Sound-alike/look-alike issues:

Tiagabine may be confused with tizanidine

U.S. Brand Names Gabitril®

Canadian Brand Names Gabitril®

Index Terms Tiagabine Hydrochloride

Generic Available No

Pharmacologic Category Anticonvulsant, Miscellaneous

Use Adjunctive therapy in the treatment of partial seizures

Contraindications Hypersensitivity to tiagabine or any component of the formulation

Warnings/Precautions New-onset seizures and status epilepticus have been associated with tiagabine use when taken for unlabeled indications. Often these seizures have occurred shortly after the initiation of treatment or shortly after a dosage increase. Seizures have also occurred with very low doses or after several months of therapy. In most cases, patients were using concomitant medications (eg, antidepressants, antipsychotics, stimulants, narcotics). In these instances, the discontinuation of tiagabine, followed by an evaluation for an underlying seizure disorder, is suggested. Use for unapproved indications, however, has not been proven to be safe or effective and is not recommended. When tiagabine is used as an adjunct in partial seizures (an FDA-approved indication), it should not be abruptly discontinued because of the possibility of increasing seizure frequency, unless safety concerns require a more rapid withdrawal. Rarely, nonconvulsive status epilepticus has been reported following abrupt discontinuation or dosage reduction.

Use with caution in patients with hepatic impairment. Experience in patients not receiving enzyme-inducing drugs has been limited; caution should be used in treating any patient who is not receiving one of these medications (decreased dose and slower titration may be required). Weakness, sedation, and confusion may occur with tiagabine use. Patients must be cautioned about performing tasks which require mental alertness (eg, operating machinery or driving). Effects with other sedative drugs or ethanol may be potentiated. May cause serious rash, including Stevens-Johnson syndrome.

Adverse Reactions (Reflective of adult population; not specific for elderly)

>10%:

Central nervous system: Concentration decreased, dizziness, nervousness, somnolence

Gastrointestinal: Nausea

Neuromuscular & skeletal: Weakness, tremor

1% to 10%:

Cardiovascular: Chest pain, edema, hypertension, palpitation, peripheral edema, syncope, tachycardia, vasodilation

Central nervous system: Agitation, ataxia, chills, confusion, difficulty with memory, confusion, depersonalization, depression, euphoria, hallucination, hostility, insomnia, malaise, migraine, paranoid reaction, personality disorder, speech disorder

Dermatologic: Alopecia, bruising, dry skin, pruritus, rash

Gastrointestinal: Abdominal pain, diarrhea, gingivitis, increased appetite, mouth ulceration, stomatitis, vomiting, weight gain/loss

Neuromuscular & skeletal: Abnormal gait, arthralgia, dysarthria, hyper-/hypokinesia, hyper-/hypotonia, myasthenia, myalgia, myoclonus, neck pain, paresthesia, reflexes decreased, stupor, twitching, vertigo

Ocular: Abnormal vision, amblyopia, nystagmus

Otic: Ear pain, hearing impairment, otitis media, tinnitus

(Continued)

Tiagabine *(Continued)*

Respiratory: Bronchitis, cough, dyspnea, epistaxis, pneumonia

Miscellaneous: Allergic reaction, cyst, diaphoresis, flu-like syndrome, lymphadenopathy

Drug Interactions Substrate of 3A4 (major)

CNS depressants: Sedative effects may be additive with other CNS depressants; monitor for increased effect; includes ethanol, sedatives, antidepressants, opioid analgesics, other anticonvulsants, and benzodiazepines

CYP3A4 inducers: CYP3A4 inducers may decrease the levels/effects of tiagabine. Example inducers include aminoglutethimide, carbamazepine, nafcillin, nevirapine, phenobarbital, phenytoin, and rifamycins.

CYP3A4 inhibitors: May increase the levels/effects of tiagabine. Example inhibitors include azole antifungals, clarithromycin, diclofenac, doxycycline, erythromycin, imatinib, isoniazid, nefazodone, nicardipine, propofol, protease inhibitors, quinidine, telithromycin, and verapamil.

Valproate: Increased free tiagabine concentrations (*in vitro*) by 40%

Ethanol/Nutrition/Herb Interactions

Ethanol: Avoid ethanol (may increase CNS depression).

Food: Food reduces the rate but not the extent of absorption.

Herb/Nutraceutical: St John's wort may decrease tiagabine levels. Avoid valerian, St John's wort, kava kava, gotu kola (may increase CNS depression).

Mechanism of Action The exact mechanism by which tiagabine exerts antiseizure activity is not definitively known; however, *in vitro* experiments demonstrate that it enhances the activity of gamma aminobutyric acid (GABA), the major neuroinhibitory transmitter in the nervous system; it is thought that binding to the GABA uptake carrier inhibits the uptake of GABA into presynaptic neurons, allowing an increased amount of GABA to be available to postsynaptic neurons; based on *in vitro* studies, tiagabine does not inhibit the uptake of dopamine, norepinephrine, serotonin, glutamate, or choline

Pharmacokinetics

Absorption: Rapid (45 minutes); food prolongs absorption

Protein binding: 96%

Half-life elimination: 2-5 hours when administered with enzyme inducers; 7-9 hours when administered without enzyme inducers

Time to peak, plasma: 45 minutes

Excretion: Feces (63%); urine (25%); 2% as unchanged drug; primarily as metabolites

Dosage

Geriatrics & Adults: Partial seizures (adjunct): Oral:

Patients receiving enzyme-inducing AED regimens: 4 mg once daily for 1 week; may increase by 4-8 mg weekly to response or up to 56 mg daily in 2-4 divided doses; usual maintenance: 32-56 mg/day

Patients **not** receiving enzyme-inducing AED regimens: The estimated plasma concentrations of tiagabine in patients not taking enzyme-inducing medications is twice that of patients receiving enzyme-inducing AEDs. Lower doses are required; slower titration may be necessary.

Monitoring Parameters Seizure frequency

Reference Range Maximal plasma concentration after a 24 mg/dose: 552 ng/mL

Patient Information Contact physician if dizziness, headache, mood changes, stomach pain, memory difficulties, or excessive sedation occur

Special Geriatric Considerations No special recommendations are made for the elderly; dose according to response.

Dosage Forms Excipient information presented when available (limited, particularly for generics); consult specific product labeling.

Tablet, as hydrochloride:

Gabitril®: 2 mg, 4 mg, 12 mg, 16 mg

Selected References

Patsalos PN and Sander JW, "Newer Antiepileptic Drugs: Towards an Improved Risk-Benefit Ratio," *Drug Saf,* 1994, 11(1):37-67.

◆ **Tiagabine Hydrochloride** *see* Tiagabine *on page 1561*

◆ **Tiazac®** *see* Diltiazem *on page 441*

◆ **Ticar®** *see* Ticarcillin *on page 1562*

Ticarcillin *(tye kar SIL in)*

Medication Safety Issues

Sound-alike/look-alike issues:

Ticar® may be confused with Tigan®

U.S. Brand Names Ticar®

Index Terms Ticarcillin Disodium

Generic Available No

Pharmacologic Category Antibiotic, Penicillin

Use Treatment of susceptible infections such as septicemia, acute and chronic respiratory tract infections, skin and soft tissue infections, and urinary tract infections due to susceptible strains of *Pseudomonas*, *Proteus*, and *Escherichia coli* and *Enterobacter*

Contraindications Hypersensitivity to ticarcillin, any component of the formulation, or penicillins

Warnings/Precautions Due to sodium load and adverse effects (anemia, neuropsychological changes), use with caution and modify dosage in patients with renal impairment; serious and occasionally severe or fatal hypersensitivity (anaphylactoid) reactions have been reported in patients on penicillin therapy (especially with a history of beta-lactam hypersensitivity and/or a history of sensitivity to multiple allergens); use with caution in patients with seizures. Prolonged use may result in fungal or bacterial superinfection, including *C. difficile*-associated diarrhea and pseudomembranous colitis.

Adverse Reactions (Reflective of adult population; not specific for elderly) Frequency not defined.

Central nervous system: Confusion, convulsions, drowsiness, fever, Jarisch-Herxheimer reaction

Dermatologic: Rash

Endocrine & metabolic: Electrolyte imbalance

Gastrointestinal: *Clostridium difficile* colitis

Hematologic: Bleeding, eosinophilia, hemolytic anemia, leukopenia, neutropenia, positive Coombs' reaction, thrombocytopenia

Hepatic: Hepatotoxicity, jaundice

Local: Thrombophlebitis

Neuromuscular & skeletal: Myoclonus

Renal: Interstitial nephritis (acute)

Miscellaneous: Anaphylaxis, hypersensitivity reactions

Overdosage/Toxicology Symptoms of penicillin overdose include neuromuscular hypersensitivity (agitation, hallucinations, asterixis, encephalopathy, confusion, and seizures) and electrolyte imbalance (with potassium or sodium salts), especially in renal failure. Hemodialysis may be helpful to aid in the removal of the drug from the blood, otherwise most treatment is supportive or symptom-directed.

Drug Interactions

Aminoglycosides: May be synergistic against selected organisms; physical inactivation of aminoglycosides in the presence of high concentrations of piperacillin and potential toxicity in patients with mild to moderate renal dysfunction

Fusidic acid: May decrease the therapeutic effect of penicillins; administer the penicillin at least 2 hours before fusidic acid.

Heparin: Concomitant use with high-dose parenteral penicillins may result in increased risk of bleeding

Methotrexate: Penicillins may increase the exposure to methotrexate during concurrent therapy; monitor.

Neuromuscular blockers: May increase duration of blockade

Oral contraceptives: Anecdotal reports suggesting decreased contraceptive efficacy with penicillins have been refuted by more rigorous scientific and clinical data.

Probenecid: May increase levels of penicillins (ticarcillin)

Tetracyclines: May decrease effectiveness of penicillins (ticarcillin)

Warfarin: Effects of warfarin may be increased

Stability Reconstituted solution is stable for 72 hours at room temperature and 14 days when refrigerated. For I.V. infusion in NS or D_5W, solution is stable for 72 hours at room temperature, 14 days when refrigerated, or 30 days when frozen. After freezing, thawed solution is stable for 72 hours at room temperature or 14 days when refrigerated.

Mechanism of Action Inhibits bacterial cell wall synthesis by binding to one or more of the penicillin binding proteins (PBPs); which in turn inhibits the final transpeptidation step of peptidoglycan synthesis in bacterial cell walls, thus inhibiting cell wall biosynthesis. Bacteria eventually lyse due to ongoing activity of cell wall autolytic enzymes (autolysins and murein hydrolases) while cell wall assembly is arrested.

Pharmacokinetics

Absorption: I.M.: 86%

Protein binding: 45% to 65%

Half-life: 66-72 minutes, prolonged with renal impairment and/or hepatic impairment

Time to peak serum concentration: I.M.: Within 30-75 minutes

Elimination: Almost entirely in urine as unchanged drug and its metabolites with small amounts excreted in feces (3.5%); CNS distribution is low and increased when the meninges are inflamed

(Continued)

Ticarcillin *(Continued)*

Dosage

Geriatrics: I.V.: 3 g every 4-6 hours; adjust dosing interval for renal impairment

Adults: Note: Ticarcillin is generally given I.V., I.M. injection is only for the treatment of uncomplicated urinary tract infections and dose should not exceed 2 g/injection when administered I.M.

Usual dosage range: I.M., I.V.: 1-4 g every 4-6 hours, usual dose: 3 g I.V. every 4-6 hours

Otitis externa (malignant): I.V.: 3 g every 4 hours with tobramycin

Pseudomonas **infections:** I.V.: 3 g every 4 hours

Renal Impairment:

Cl_{cr} 30-60 mL/minute: 2 g every 4 hours or 3 g every 8 hours

Cl_{cr} 10-30 mL/minute: 2 g every 8 hours or 3 g every 12 hours

Cl_{cr} <10 mL/minute: 2 g every 12 hours

Moderately dialyzable (20% to 50%)

Continuous arteriovenous or venovenous hemodiafiltration effects: Dose as for Cl_{cr} 10-50 mL/minute

Administration Administer 1 hour apart from aminoglycosides; do not administer I.M.

Monitoring Parameters Temperature, WBC, respiratory rate; cultures and sensitivity (if applicable), mental status, appetite

Test Interactions May interfere with urinary glucose tests using cupric sulfate (Benedict's solution, Clinitest®); false-positive urinary or serum protein, positive Coombs' test

Some penicillin derivatives may accelerate the degradation of aminoglycosides *in vitro*, leading to a potential underestimation of aminoglycoside serum concentration.

Additional Information Sodium content of 1 g: 5.2 to 6.5 mEq; normally used with other antibiotics (ie, aminoglycosides)

Special Geriatric Considerations When used as empiric therapy or for documented pseudomonal pneumonia, it is best to combine with an aminoglycoside such as gentamicin or tobramycin. High sodium may limit use in patients with congestive heart failure. Adjust dose for renal function.

Dosage Forms Excipient information presented when available (limited, particularly for generics); consult specific product labeling.

Injection, powder for reconstitution, as disodium: 3 g

Selected References

Brogden RN, Heel RC, Speight TM, et al, "Ticarcillin: A Review of Its Pharmacological Properties and Therapeutic Efficacy," *Drugs*, 1980, 20(5):325-52.

Yoshikawa TT, "Antimicrobial Therapy for the Elderly Patient," *J Am Geriatr Soc*, 1990, 38(12):1353-72.

Ticarcillin and Clavulanate Potassium

(tye kar SIL in & klav yoo LAN ate poe TASS ee um)

Related Information

Antimicrobial Activity Against Selected Organisms *on page 1728*

Ticarcillin *on page 1562*

U.S. Brand Names Timentin®

Canadian Brand Names Timentin®

Index Terms Ticarcillin and Clavulanic Acid

Generic Available No

Pharmacologic Category Antibiotic, Penicillin

Use Treatment of lower respiratory tract, urinary tract, skin and skin structures, bone and joint, gynecologic (endometritis) and intra-abdominal (peritonitis) infections, and septicemia caused by susceptible organisms. Clavulanate expands activity of ticarcillin to include beta-lactamase producing strains of *S. aureus, H. influenzae, Bacteroides* species, and some other gram-negative bacilli

Contraindications Hypersensitivity to ticarcillin, clavulanate, any penicillin, or any component of the formulation

Warnings/Precautions Use with caution and modify dosage in patients with renal impairment; serious and occasionally severe or fatal hypersensitivity (anaphylactoid) reactions have been reported in patients on penicillin therapy (especially with a history of beta-lactam hypersensitivity and/or a history of sensitivity to multiple allergens); use with caution in patients with seizures and in patients with CHF due to high sodium load. Particularly in patients with renal impairment, bleeding disorders have been observed; discontinue if thrombocytopenia or bleeding occurs. Prolonged use may result in fungal or bacterial superinfection, including *C. difficile*-associated diarrhea and pseudomembranous colitis.

Adverse Reactions (Reflective of adult population; not specific for elderly)

Frequency not defined.

Central nervous system: Confusion, drowsiness, fever, headache, Jarisch-Herxheimer reaction, seizure

Dermatologic: Erythema multiforme, pruritus, rash, Stevens-Johnson syndrome, toxic epidermal necrolysis, urticaria

Endocrine & metabolic: Electrolyte imbalance

Gastrointestinal: *Clostridium difficile* colitis, diarrhea, nausea, vomiting

Hematologic: Bleeding, eosinophilia, hemolytic anemia, leukopenia, neutropenia, positive Coombs' reaction, prothrombin time prolonged, thrombocytopenia

Hepatic: Hepatotoxicity, jaundice

Local: Injection site reaction (pain, burning, induration); thrombophlebitis

Neuromuscular & skeletal: Myoclonus

Renal: BUN increased, interstitial nephritis (acute), serum creatinine increased

Miscellaneous: Anaphylaxis, hypersensitivity reactions

Overdosage/Toxicology Symptoms include neuromuscular hypersensitivity and seizures. Many beta-lactam containing antibiotics have the potential to cause neuromuscular hyperirritability or convulsive seizures. Hemodialysis may be helpful to aid in removal of the drug from the blood, otherwise most treatment is supportive or symptom-directed.

Drug Interactions

Aminoglycosides: May be synergistic against selected organisms; physical inactivation of aminoglycosides in the presence of high concentrations of piperacillin and potential toxicity in patients with mild to moderate renal dysfunction.

Fusidic acid: May decrease the therapeutic effect of penicillins; administer the penicillin at least 2 hours before fusidic acid.

Methotrexate: Penicillins may increase the exposure to methotrexate during concurrent therapy; monitor.

Tetracyclines: May decrease the therapeutic effect of penicillins (ticarcillin).

Typhoid vaccines: Antibiotics may decrease the therapeutic effect of typhoid vaccine. Only the live, attenuated Ty21a strain is affected.

Uricosuric agents (eg, probenecid, sulfinpyrazone): Uricosuric agents may decrease the excretion of penicillins (ticarcillin).

Stability

Vials: Store intact vials at <24°C (<75°F). Reconstituted solution is stable for 6 hours at room temperature and 72 hours when refrigerated. I.V. infusion in NS or LR is stable for 24 hours at room temperature, 7 days when refrigerated, or 30 days when frozen. I.V. infusion in D_5W solution is stable for 24 hours at room temperature, 3 days when refrigerated, or 7 days when frozen. After freezing, thawed solution is stable for 8 hours at room temperature. Darkening of drug indicates loss of potency of clavulanate potassium.

Premixed solution: Store frozen at ≤-20°C (-4°F). Thawed solution is stable for 24 hours at room temperature or 7 days under refrigeration; do not refreeze.

Mechanism of Action Inhibits bacterial cell wall synthesis by binding to one or more of the penicillin binding proteins (PBPs); which in turn inhibits the final transpeptidation step of peptidoglycan synthesis in bacterial cell walls, thus inhibiting cell wall biosynthesis. Bacteria eventually lyse due to ongoing activity of cell wall autolytic enzymes (autolysins and murein hydrolases) while cell wall assembly is arrested.

Pharmacokinetics

Distribution: Low concentrations of ticarcillin distribute into the CSF and increase when meninges are inflamed

Protein binding:

Ticarcillin: 45% to 65%

Clavulanic acid: 9% to 30%

Metabolism: Clavulanic acid is metabolized in the liver

Half-life:

Clavulanate: 66-90 minutes

Ticarcillin: 66-72 minutes in patients with normal renal function

Clavulanic acid does not affect the clearance of ticarcillin

Elimination: 45% of clavulanic acid is excreted unchanged in urine, whereas 60% to 90% of ticarcillin is excreted unchanged in urine

Removed by hemodialysis

Dosage

Geriatrics: I.V.: 3.1 g every 4-6 hours; adjust for renal function.

Adults: Note: Timentin® (ticarcillin/clavulanate) is a combination product; each 3.1 g dosage form contains 3 g ticarcillin disodium and 0.1 g clavulanic acid.

Systemic infections: I.V.: 3.1 g (ticarcillin 3 g plus clavulanic acid 0.1 g) every 4-6 hours (maximum: 24 g of ticarcillin component/day)

Amnionitis, cholangitis, diverticulitis, endometritis, epididymo-orchitis, mastoiditis, orbital cellulitis, peritonitis, pneumonia (aspiration): I.V.: 3.1 g every 4 hours

Liver abscess, parafascial space infections, septic thrombophlebitis: I.V.: 3.1 g every 4 hours

***Pseudomonas* infections:** I.V.: 3.1 g every 4 hours

Urinary tract infections: I.V.: 3.1 g every 6-8 hours

(Continued)

Ticarcillin and Clavulanate Potassium *(Continued)*

Renal Impairment:

Loading dose: I.V.: 3.1 g one dose, followed by maintenance dose based on creatinine clearance:

Cl_{cr} 30-60 mL/minute: Administer 2 g of ticarcillin component every 4 hours or 3.1 g every 8 hours

Cl_{cr} 10-30 mL/minute: Administer 2 g of ticarcillin component every 8 hours or 3.1 g every 12 hours

Cl_{cr} <10 mL/minute: Administer 2 g of ticarcillin component every 12 hours

Cl_{cr} <10 mL/minute with concomitant hepatic dysfunction: 2 g of ticarcillin component every 24 hours

Moderately dialyzable (20% to 50%)

Continuous arteriovenous or venovenous hemodiafiltration effects: Dose as for Cl_{cr} 10-50 mL/minute

Peritoneal dialysis: 3.1 g every 12 hours

Hemodialysis: 2 g of ticarcillin component every 12 hours; supplemented with 3.1 g after each dialysis

Hepatic Impairment: With concomitant renal dysfunction (Cl_{cr} <10 mL/minute): 2 g of ticarcillin component every 24 hours.

Administration Infuse over 30 minutes. Administer 1 hour apart from aminoglycosides. Give around-the-clock. Rapid administration may lead to seizures.

Monitoring Parameters Temperature, WBC, respiratory rate; culture and sensitivity (if applicable), mental status, appetite

Test Interactions Positive Coombs' test, false-positive urinary proteins

Some penicillin derivatives may accelerate the degradation of aminoglycosides *in vitro*, leading to a potential underestimation of aminoglycoside serum concentration.

Additional Information Usually given for at least for 2 days after symptoms have disappeared

Special Geriatric Considerations When used as empiric therapy or for a documented pseudomonal pneumonia, it is best to combine with an aminoglycoside such as gentamicin or tobramycin. High sodium content may limit use in patients with congestive heart failure. Adjust dose for renal function.

Dosage Forms Excipient information presented when available (limited, particularly for generics); consult specific product labeling.

Infusion [premixed, frozen]: Ticarcillin 3 g and clavulanic acid 0.1 g (100 mL) [contains sodium 4.51 mEq and potassium 0.15 mEq per g]

Injection, powder for reconstitution: Ticarcillin 3 g and clavulanic acid 0.1 g (3.1 g, 31 g) [contains sodium 4.51 mEq and potassium 0.15 mEq per g]

- ◆ **Ticarcillin and Clavulanic Acid** *see* Ticarcillin and Clavulanate Potassium *on page 1564*
- ◆ **Ticarcillin Disodium** *see* Ticarcillin *on page 1562*
- ◆ **Ticlid®** *see* Ticlopidine *on page 1566*

Ticlopidine *(tye KLOE pi deen)*

Related Information

Potentially Inappropriate Medications for Geriatrics *on page 1824*

U.S. Brand Names Ticlid®

Canadian Brand Names Alti-Ticlopidine; Apo-Ticlopidine®; Gen-Ticlopidine; Novo-Ticlopidine; Nu-Ticlopidine; Rhoxal-ticlopidine; Sandoz-Ticlopidine; Ticlid®

Index Terms Ticlopidine Hydrochloride

Generic Available Yes

Pharmacologic Category Antiplatelet Agent

Use Platelet aggregation inhibitor; reduction of the risk of thrombotic stroke in patients who have had a stroke or stroke precursors; due to its association with life-threatening hematologic disorders (neutropenia), ticlopidine should be reserved for patients who are intolerant to aspirin, or who have failed aspirin therapy; adjunctive therapy (with aspirin) following successful coronary stent implantation to reduce the incidence of subacute stent thrombosis

Unlabeled/Investigational Use Protection of aortocoronary bypass grafts, diabetic microangiopathy, ischemic heart disease, prevention of postoperative DVT, reduction of graft loss following renal transplant

Contraindications Hypersensitivity to ticlopidine or any component of the formulation; active pathological bleeding such as PUD or intracranial hemorrhage; severe liver dysfunction; hematopoietic disorders (neutropenia, thrombocytopenia, a past history of TTP)

Warnings/Precautions Use with caution in patients who may be at risk of increased bleeding. Consider discontinuing 10-14 days before elective surgery (except in patients with cardiac stents that have not completed their full course of dual antiplatelet therapy;

patient-specific situations need to be discussed with cardiologist; AHA/ACC/SCAI/ ACS/ADA Science Advisory provides recommendations). Use caution in mixing with other antiplatelet drugs. Use with caution in patients with severe liver disease (experience is limited). **[U.S. Boxed Warning]: May cause life-threatening hematologic reactions, including neutropenia, agranulocytosis, thrombotic thrombocytopenia purpura (TTP), and aplastic anemia.** Routine monitoring is required (see Monitoring Parameters). Monitor for signs and symptoms of neutropenia including WBC count. Discontinue if the absolute neutrophil count falls to <1200/mm^3 or if the platelet count falls to <80,000/mm^3.

Adverse Reactions (Reflective of adult population; not specific for elderly)

As with all drugs which may affect hemostasis, bleeding is associated with ticlopidine. Hemorrhage may occur at virtually any site. Risk is dependent on multiple variables, including the use of multiple agents which alter hemostasis and patient susceptibility.

>10%:
 Endocrine & metabolic: Increased total cholesterol (increases of ~8% to 10% within 1 month of therapy)
 Gastrointestinal: Diarrhea (13%)
1% to 10%:
 Central nervous system: Dizziness (1%)
 Dermatologic: Rash (5%), purpura (2%), pruritus (1%)
 Gastrointestinal: Nausea (7%), dyspepsia (7%), gastrointestinal pain (4%), vomiting (2%), flatulence (2%), anorexia (1%)
 Hematologic: Neutropenia (2%)
 Hepatic: Abnormal liver function test (1%)

Overdosage/Toxicology
Symptoms include ataxia, seizures, vomiting, abdominal pain, and hematologic abnormalities. Specific treatments are lacking; after decontamination. Treatment is symptomatic and supportive.

Drug Interactions
Substrate of CYP3A4 (major); Inhibits CYP1A2 (weak), 2C9 (weak), 2C19 (strong), 2D6 (moderate), 2E1 (weak), 3A4 (weak)

Antacids reduce absorption of ticlopidine (~18%).
Anticoagulants or other antiplatelet agents may increase the risk of bleeding; use with caution.
Carbamazepine blood levels may be increased by ticlopidine.
Cimetidine increases ticlopidine levels.
Cyclosporine blood levels may be reduced by ticlopidine.
CYP2C19 substrates: Ticlopidine may increase the levels/effects of CYP2C19 substrates. Example substrates include citalopram, diazepam, methsuximide, phenytoin, propranolol, and sertraline.
CYP2D6 substrates: Ticlopidine may increase the levels/effects of CYP2D6 substrates. Example substrates include amphetamines, selected beta-blockers, dextromethorphan, fluoxetine, lidocaine, mirtazapine, nefazodone, paroxetine, risperidone, ritonavir, thioridazine, tricyclic antidepressants, and venlafaxine.
CYP2D6 prodrug substrates: Ticlopidine may decrease the levels/effects of CYP2D6 prodrug substrates. Example prodrug substrates include codeine, hydrocodone, oxycodone, and tramadol.
CYP3A4 inducers: CYP3A4 inducers may decrease the levels/effects of ticlopidine. Example inducers include aminoglutethimide, carbamazepine, nafcillin, nevirapine, phenobarbital, phenytoin, and rifamycins.
Digoxin blood levels may be decreased by ticlopidine.
Phenytoin blood levels may be increased by ticlopidine (case reports).
Theophylline blood levels may be increased by ticlopidine.

Ethanol/Nutrition/Herb Interactions
Food: Ticlopidine bioavailability may be increased (20%) if taken with food. High-fat meals increase absorption, antacids decrease absorption.
Herb/Nutraceutical: Avoid cat's claw, dong quai, evening primrose, feverfew, garlic, ginkgo, ginger, red clover, horse chestnut, green tea, ginseng (all have additional antiplatelet activity).

Mechanism of Action
Ticlopidine is an inhibitor of platelet function with a mechanism which is different from other antiplatelet drugs. The drug significantly increases bleeding time. This effect may not be solely related to ticlopidine's effect on platelets. The prolongation of the bleeding time caused by ticlopidine is further increased by the addition of aspirin in *ex vivo* experiments. Although many metabolites of ticlopidine have been found, none have been shown to account for *in vivo* activity.

Pharmacodynamics
Onset of action: Within 6 hours
Peak effect: Oral: Achieved after 3-5 days of therapy
Because the duration of inhibition of platelet function corresponds to the normal life span of the platelet, these effects usually reverse 1-2 weeks after stopping the drug
(Continued)

Ticlopidine *(Continued)*

Pharmacokinetics

Absorption: Following administration, 80% to 90% absorbed from GI tract with an average peak plasma steady-state concentration of 0.9 mg/mL ~2 hours after a 250 mg dose

Protein binding: 98% bound to plasma proteins, primarily albumin and lipoproteins, with ≤15% bound to alpha$_1$-acid glycoprotein

Metabolism: Metabolized in the liver extensively, principally by N-dealkylation and oxidation of the thiophene ring; four metabolites have been identified in humans

Half-life: 12-36 hours increasing to 4-5 days after continuous dosing; clearance decreases in older subjects; mean area under the serum concentration time curve was 2-3 times that in younger adults and trough concentrations were twice as high as compared to younger adults; at steady-state there were no significant differences in time to peak or elimination half-life between young and older adults subjects, but the average plasma concentration in older adults was twice that of the younger group. It is unknown whether these differences are due to increased absorption, decreased clearance, or a change in plasma protein binding.

Elimination: <1% excreted unchanged in urine

Dosage

Geriatrics: 250 mg twice daily with food; dosage in older patients has not been determined; however, in two large clinical trials, the average age of subjects was 63 and 66 years. A dosage decrease may be necessary if bleeding develops.

Adults:

Stroke prevention: Oral: 250 mg twice daily with food

Coronary artery stenting (initiate after successful implantation): Oral: 250 mg twice daily with food (in combination with antiplatelet doses of aspirin) for up to 30 days

Administration Oral: Administer with food.

Monitoring Parameters Signs of bleeding; CBC with differential every 2 weeks starting the second week through the third month of treatment; more frequent monitoring is recommended for patients whose absolute neutrophil counts have been consistently declining or are 30% less than baseline values. Liver function tests (alkaline phosphatase and transaminases) should be performed in the first 4 months of therapy if liver dysfunction is suspected.

Reference Range Serum concentrations do not correlate with clinical antiplatelet activity

Test Interactions Increased cholesterol (S), increased alkaline phosphatase, increased transaminases (S)

Patient Information Possibility of signs and symptoms of neutropenia, thrombocytopenia, and abnormal bleeding; comply with biweekly blood tests; report any symptoms of infection such as fever, chills, sore throat; report unusual bleeding; tell all physicians and dentists that you are on ticlopidine; take with food to minimize GI complaints

Special Geriatric Considerations Because of the risk of neutropenia and its relative expense as compared with aspirin, ticlopidine should only be used in patients with a documented intolerance to aspirin.

Dosage Forms Excipient information presented when available (limited, particularly for generics); consult specific product labeling.

Tablet, as hydrochloride: 250 mg

Selected References

Ito MK, Smith AR, and Lee ML, "Ticlopidine: A New Platelet Aggregation Inhibitor," *Clin Pharm*, 1992, 11(7):603-17.

Schömig A, Neumann, FJ, Kastrati A, et al, "A Randomized Comparison of Antiplatelet and Anticoagulant Therapy After the Placement of Coronary-Artery Stents," *N Engl J Med*, 1996, 334(17):1084-9.

Shah J, Teitelbaum P, Molony B, et al, "Single and Multiple Dose Pharmacokinetics of Ticlopidine in Young and Elderly Subjects," *Br J Clin Pharmacol*, 1991, 32:761-4.

Teitelbaum P, Gabzuda TG, Koretz SH, et al, "Pharmacokinetics of Ticlopidine Hydrochloride in Young and Old Normal Adult Subjects Following Single and Multiple Dosing," *J Pharm Sci*, 1987, 76:S99.

♦ **Ticlopidine Hydrochloride** *see* Ticlopidine *on page 1566*

♦ **TIG** *see* Tetanus Immune Globulin (Human) *on page 1541*

♦ **Tigan**® *see* Trimethobenzamide *on page 1633*

Tigecycline *(tye ge SYE kleen)*

U.S. Brand Names Tygacil™

Index Terms GAR-936

Generic Available No

Pharmacologic Category Antibiotic, Glycylcycline

Use Treatment of complicated skin and skin structure infections caused by susceptible organisms, including methicillin-resistant *Staphylococcus aureus* and vancomycin-sensitive *Enterococcus faecalis*; treatment of complicated intra-abdominal infections

Contraindications Hypersensitivity to tigecycline or any component of the formulation

Warnings/Precautions Due to structural similarity with tetracyclines, use caution in patients with prior hypersensitivity and/or severe adverse reactions associated with tetracycline use. Due to structural similarities with tetracyclines, may be associated with photosensitivity, pseudotumor cerebri, pancreatitis, and antianabolic effects (including increased BUN, azotemia, acidosis, and hyperphosphatemia) observed with this class. Use caution in hepatic impairment; dosage adjustment may be required with severe impairment.

Prolonged use may result in fungal or bacterial superinfection, including *C. difficile*-associated diarrhea and pseudomembranous colitis. Use with caution if using as monotherapy for patients with intestinal perforation (in the small sample of available cases, septic shock occurred more frequently than patients treated with imipenem/cilastatin comparator).

Adverse Reactions (Reflective of adult population; not specific for elderly)
Note: Frequencies relative to placebo are not available; some frequencies are lower than those experienced with comparator drugs.
>10%: Gastrointestinal: Nausea (25% to 30%; severe in 1%), vomiting (20%; severe in 1%), diarrhea (13%)
2% to 10%:
Cardiovascular: Hypertension (5%), peripheral edema (3%), hypotension (2%), phlebitis (2%)
Central nervous system: Fever (7%), headache (6%), dizziness (4%), pain (4%), insomnia (2%)
Dermatologic: Pruritus (3%), rash (2%)
Endocrine & metabolic: Hypoproteinemia (5%), hyperglycemia (2%), hypokalemia (2%)
Gastrointestinal: Abdominal pain (7%), constipation (3%), dyspepsia (3%)
Hematologic: Thrombocythemia (6%), anemia (4%), leukocytosis (4%)
Hepatic: ALT increased (6%), AST increased (4%), alkaline phosphatase increased (4%), amylase increased (3%), bilirubin increased (2%), LDH increased (4%)
Local: Reaction to procedure (9%)
Neuromuscular & skeletal: Weakness (3%)
Renal: BUN increased (2%)
Respiratory: Cough increased (4%), dyspnea (3%), pulmonary physical finding (2%)
Miscellaneous: Abnormal healing (4%), infection (8%), abscess (3%), diaphoresis increased (2%)

Overdosage/Toxicology No specific experience in overdose. May experience increased nausea/vomiting. Not significantly removed by hemodialysis.

Drug Interactions
Oral contraceptives: Anecdotal reports suggesting decreased contraceptive efficacy with tetracyclines have been refuted by more rigorous scientific and clinical data.
Retinoic acid derivatives: May increase risk of pseudotumor cerebri (reported with tetracyclines).
Warfarin: Hypoprothrombinemic response may be increased with tigecycline; monitor INR closely during initiation or discontinuation.

Stability Store at 15°C to 30°C (59°F to 86°F) prior to reconstitution. Add 5.3 mL NS or D₅W to each 50 mg vial. Swirl gently to dissolve. Resulting solution is 10 mg/mL. Reconstituted solution must be further diluted to allow I.V. administration. Transfer to 100 mL I.V. bag for infusion (final concentration should not exceed 1 mg/mL). Once reconstituted, may be stored at room temperature for up to 24 hours (up to 6 hours in the vial and after further dilution, in the I.V. bag). Alternatively, may be refrigerated for up to 45 hours following immediate transfer of the reconstituted solution into the I.V. bag. Reconstituted solution is red-orange.

Mechanism of Action Binds to the 30S ribosomal subunit of susceptible bacteria, inhibiting protein synthesis.

Pharmacokinetics Note: Systemic clearance is reduced by 55% and half-life increased by 43% in moderate hepatic impairment.
Distribution: V_d: 7-9 L/kg; extensive tissue distribution
Protein binding: 71% to 89%
Metabolism: Hepatic, via glucuronidation, N-acetylation, and epimerization to several metabolites, each <10% of the dose
Half-life elimination: Single dose: 27 hours; following multiple doses: 42 hours
Excretion: Urine (33%; with 22% as unchanged drug); feces (59%; primarily as unchanged drug)

Dosage
Geriatrics & Adults: Complicated skin/skin structure or intra-abdominal infections: I.V.:
Initial: 100 mg as a single dose
Maintenance dose: 50 mg every 12 hours
Recommended duration of therapy: Intra-abdominal infections or complicated skin/skin structure infections: 5-14 days.
(Continued)

Tigecycline *(Continued)*

Renal Impairment: No dosage adjustment required in renal impairment or after hemodialysis.

Hepatic Impairment:
Mild-to-moderate hepatic disease: No dosage adjustment required
Severe hepatic impairment (Child-Pugh class C): Initial dose of 100 mg should be followed with 25 mg every 12 hours

Administration
Infuse over 30-60 minutes through dedicated line or via Y-site

Special Geriatric Considerations The manufacturer reports no significant differences in tigecycline's pharmacokinetics in small numbers of healthy older adults 65-75 years of age and >75 years compared to younger adults following a single 100 mg dose. No dosage adjustment is recommended.

Dosage Forms Excipient information presented when available (limited, particularly for generics); consult specific product labeling.
Injection, powder for reconstitution:
Tygacil®: 50 mg [contains 100 mg lactose]

Selected References
Conte JE Jr, Golden JA, Kelly MG, et al, "Steady-State Serum and Intrapulmonary Pharmacokinetics and Pharmacodynamics of Tigecycline," *Int J Antimicrob Agents*, 2005, 25(6):523-9.
Fritsche TR and Jones RN, "Antimicrobial Activity of Tigecycline (GAR-936) Tested Against 3498 Recent Isolates of *Staphylococcus aureus* Recovered From Nosocomial and Community-Acquired Infections," *Int J Antimicrob Agents*, 2004, 24(6):567-71.
Jacobus NV, McDermott LA, Ruthazer R, et al, "In Vitro Activities of Tigecycline Against the *Bacteroides fragilis* Group," *Antimicrob Agents Chemother*, 2004, 48(3):1034-6.
Muralidharan G, Micalizzi M, Speth J, et al, "Pharmacokinetics of Tigecycline After Single and Multiple Doses in Healthy Subjects," *Antimicrob Agents Chemother*, 2005, 49(1):220-9.
Zhanel GG, Homenuik K, Nichol K, et al, "The Glycylcyclines: A Comparative Review With the Tetracyclines," *Drugs*, 2004, 64(1):63-88.

♦ **Tikosyn®** see Dofetilide *on page 461*
♦ **Tilade®** see Nedocromil *on page 1096*

Tiludronate *(tye LOO droe nate)*

Medication Safety Issues
International issues:
Skelid® may be confused with Skaelud® which is a brand name for pyrithione zinc in Denmark

U.S. Brand Names Skelid®

Index Terms Tiludronate Disodium

Generic Available No

Pharmacologic Category Bisphosphonate Derivative

Use Treatment of Paget's disease of the bone

Contraindications Hypersensitivity to bisphosphonates or any component of the formulation

Warnings/Precautions Not recommended in patients with severe renal impairment (Cl_{cr} <30 mL/minute). Use with caution in patients with active upper GI problems (eg, dysphagia, symptomatic esophageal diseases, gastritis, duodenitis, ulcers).

Bisphosphonate therapy has been associated with osteonecrosis, primarily of the jaw; this has been observed mostly in cancer patients, but also in patients with postmenopausal osteoporosis and other diagnoses. Dental exams and preventative dentistry should be performed prior to placing patients with risk factors on chronic bisphosphonate therapy. Invasive dental procedures should be avoided during treatment.

Infrequently, severe (and occasionally debilitating) bone, joint, and/or muscle pain have been reported during bisphosphonate treatment. The onset of pain ranged from a single day to several months. Symptoms usually resolve upon discontinuation. Some patients experienced recurrence when rechallenged with same drug or another bisphosphonate; avoid use in patients with a history of these symptoms in association with bisphosphonate therapy.

Adverse Reactions (Reflective of adult population; not specific for elderly)
The following events occurred >2% and at a frequency greater than placebo:
1% to 10%:
Cardiovascular: Chest pain (3%), edema (3%)
Central nervous system: Dizziness (4%), paresthesia (4%)
Dermatologic: Rash (3%), skin disorder (3%)
Gastrointestinal: Nausea (9%), diarrhea (9%), heartburn (5%), vomiting (4%), flatulence (3%)
Neuromuscular & skeletal: Arthrosis (3%)
Ocular: cataract (3%), conjunctivitis (3%), glaucoma (3%)
Respiratory: Rhinitis (5%), sinusitis (5%), cough (3%), pharyngitis (3%)

Overdosage/Toxicology Hypocalcemia is a potential consequence of tiludronate overdose. No specific information on overdose treatment is available. Dialysis would not be beneficial. Standard medical practices may be used to manage renal insufficiency or hypocalcemia, if signs of these occur.

Drug Interactions

Aminoglycosides: May lower serum calcium levels with prolonged administration. Concomitant use may have an additive hypocalcemic effect.

Antacids: May decrease the absorption of bisphosphonate derivatives; should be administered at a different time of the day. Antacids containing aluminum, calcium, or magnesium are of specific concern.

Calcium salts: May decrease the absorption of bisphosphonate derivatives. Separate oral dosing in order to minimize risk of interaction.

Iron salts: May decrease the absorption of bisphosphonate derivatives. Only oral iron salts and oral bisphosphonates are of concern.

Magnesium salts: May decrease the absorption of bisphosphonate derivatives. Only oral magnesium salts and oral bisphosphonates are of concern.

Nonsteroidal anti-inflammatory drugs (NSAIDs): May enhance the gastrointestinal adverse/toxic effects (increased incidence of GI ulcers) of bisphosphonate derivatives.

Phosphate supplements: Bisphosphonate derivatives may enhance the hypocalcemic effect of phosphate supplements.

Ethanol/Nutrition/Herb Interactions Food: In single-dose studies, the bioavailability of tiludronate was reduced by 90% when an oral dose was administered with, or 2 hours after, a standard breakfast compared to the same dose administered after an overnight fast and 4 hours before a standard breakfast.

Stability Do not remove tablets from foil strips until they are to be used.

Mechanism of Action Inhibition of normal and abnormal bone resorption. Inhibits osteoclasts through at least two mechanisms: disruption of the cytoskeletal ring structure, possibly by inhibition of protein-tyrosine-phosphatase, thus leading to the detachment of osteoclasts from the bone surface area and the inhibition of the osteoclast proton pump.

Pharmacodynamics Initial response in Paget's disease: 2 days to 1 month

Pharmacokinetics

Bioavailability: 4% to 8%

Distribution: 90% bound to plasma proteins, bone

Half-life: 43-150 hours

Elimination: Kidney (60%)

Dosage

Geriatrics & Adults: Paget's disease: Oral: 400 mg (2 tablets of tiludronic acid) daily for a period of 3 months

Renal Impairment: Tiludronate is excreted renally. It is not recommended for use in patients with severe renal impairment (Cl_{cr} <30 mL/minute) and is not removed by dialysis.

Monitoring Parameters Alkaline phosphatase, urinary hydroxyproline, adjusted calcium, serum osteocalcin

Test Interactions Bisphosphonates may interfere with diagnostic imaging agents such as technetium-99m-diphosphonate in bone scans.

Patient Information Take with 6-8 ounces of plain water; do not take other medications or food for 2 hours before or after dose; do not double dose if a dose is missed

Additional Information Three months of treatment is recommended; because of bioavailability problems, tiludronate should not be taken with beverages other than water or within 2 hours of food, calcium or mineral supplements, aspirin, or indomethacin; aluminum- or magnesium-containing antacids should be taken at least 2 hours after tiludronate

Special Geriatric Considerations No dose adjustment necessary.

Dosage Forms Excipient information presented when available (limited, particularly for generics); consult specific product labeling.

Tablet, tiludronic acid: 200 mg [equivalent to 240 mg tiludronate disodium]

♦ **Tiludronate Disodium** *see* Tiludronate *on page 1570*

♦ **Time-C [OTC]** *see* Ascorbic Acid *on page 125*

♦ **Time-C-Bio [OTC]** *see* Ascorbic Acid *on page 125*

♦ **Timentin®** *see* Ticarcillin and Clavulanate Potassium *on page 1564*

Timolol (TIM oh lol)

Related Information

Beta-Blockers *on page 1751*

Glaucoma Drug Therapy *on page 1758*

(Continued)

Timolol *(Continued)*

Medication Safety Issues

Sound-alike/look-alike issues:

Timolol may be confused with atenolol, Tylenol®

Timoptic® may be confused with Talacen®, Viroptic®

Bottle cap color change:

Timoptic®: Both the 0.25% and 0.5% strengths are now packaged in bottles with yellow caps; previously, the color of the cap on the product corresponded to different strengths.

International issues:

Betimol® may be confused with Betanol® which is a brand name for metipranolol in Monaco

U.S. Brand Names Betimol®; Blocadren®; Istalol™; Timolol GFS; Timoptic®; Timoptic® in OcuDose®; Timoptic-XE®

Canadian Brand Names Alti-Timolol; Apo-Timol®; Apo-Timop®; Gen-Timolol; Nu-Timolol; Phoxal-timolol; PMS-Timolol; Sandoz-Timolol; Tim-AK; Timoptic®; Timoptic-XE®

Index Terms Timolol Hemihydrate; Timolol Maleate

Generic Available Yes: Excludes hemihydrate ophthalmic solutions

Pharmacologic Category Beta-Adrenergic Blocker, Nonselective; Ophthalmic Agent, Antiglaucoma

Use

Ophthalmic: Treatment of elevated intraocular pressure such as glaucoma or ocular hypertension

Oral: Treatment of hypertension and angina and reduce mortality following myocardial infarction, hypertrophic subaortic stenosis, and prophylaxis of migraine; treatment of the postmyocardial infarction patient

Contraindications Hypersensitivity to timolol or any component of the formulation; sinus bradycardia; sinus node dysfunction; heart block greater than first degree (except in patients with a functioning artificial pacemaker); cardiogenic shock; uncompensated cardiac failure; bronchospastic disease

Warnings/Precautions Consider pre-existing conditions such as sick sinus syndrome before initiating. Administer cautiously in compensated heart failure and monitor for a worsening of the condition. **[U.S. Boxed Warning]: Beta-blocker therapy should not be withdrawn abruptly (particularly in patients with CAD), but gradually tapered to avoid acute tachycardia, hypertension, and/or ischemia.** Use caution with concurrent use of beta-blockers and either verapamil or diltiazem; bradycardia or heart block can occur. Beta-blockers can aggravate symptoms in patients with PVD. Patients with bronchospastic disease should generally not receive beta-blockers - monitor closely if used in patients with potential risk of bronchospasm. Use cautiously in diabetics because it can mask prominent hypoglycemic symptoms. Use cautiously in severe renal impairment: marked hypotension can occur in patients maintained on hemodialysis. Use care with anesthetic agents which decrease myocardial function. Can worsen myasthenia gravis. Use with caution in patients with a history of psychiatric illness; may cause or exacerbate CNS depression. Similar reactions found with systemic administration may occur with topical administration. Adequate alpha-blockade is required prior to use of any beta-blocker for patients with untreated pheochromocytoma.

Ophthalmic: Systemic absorption and adverse effects may occur, including bradycardia and/or hypotension. Should not be used alone in angle-closure glaucoma (has no effect on pupillary constriction). Multidose vials have been associated with development of bacterial keratitis; avoid contamination. Some product do contain benzalkonium chloride which may be absorbed by soft contact lenses; do not administer while wearing soft contact lenses.

Adverse Reactions (Reflective of adult population; not specific for elderly)

Ophthalmic:

>10%: Ocular: Burning, stinging

1% to 10%:

Cardiovascular: Hypertension

Central nervous system: Headache

Ocular: Blepharitis, blurred vision, cataract, conjunctival injection, conjunctivitis, foreign body sensation, hyperemia, itching, tearing, visual acuity decreased

Miscellaneous: Infection

Systemic:

1% to 10%:

Cardiovascular: Bradycardia

Central nervous system: Fatigue, dizziness

Respiratory: Dyspnea

Frequency not defined (reported with any dosage form):

Cardiovascular: Angina pectoris, arrhythmia, bradycardia, cardiac failure, cardiac arrest, cerebral vascular accident, cerebral ischemia, edema, hypotension, heart block, palpitation, Raynaud's phenomenon

Central nervous system: Anxiety, confusion, depression, disorientation, dizziness, hallucinations, insomnia, memory loss, nervousness, nightmares, somnolence

Dermatologic: Alopecia, angioedema, pseudopemphigoid, psoriasiform rash, psoriasis exacerbation, rash, urticaria

Endocrine & metabolic: Hypoglycemia masked, libido decreased

Gastrointestinal: Anorexia, diarrhea, dyspepsia, nausea, xerostomia

Genitourinary: Impotence, retoperitoneal fibrosis

Hematologic: Claudication

Neuromuscular & skeletal: Myasthenia gravis exacerbation, paresthesia

Ocular: Blepharitis, conjunctivitis, corneal sensitivity decreased, cystoid macular edema, diplopia, dry eyes, foreign body sensation, keratitis, ocular discharge, ocular pain, ptosis, refractive changes, tearing, visual disturbances

Otic: Tinnitus

Respiratory: Bronchospasm, cough, dyspnea, nasal congestion, pulmonary edema, respiratory failure

Miscellaneous: Allergic reactions, cold hands/feet, Peyronie's disease, systemic lupus erythematosus

Overdosage/Toxicology Symptoms of intoxication include cardiac disturbances, CNS toxicity, bronchospasm, hypoglycemia, and hyperkalemia. The most common cardiac symptoms include hypotension and bradycardia. Atrioventricular block, intraventricular conduction disturbances, cardiogenic shock, and asystole may occur with severe overdose, especially with membrane-depressant drugs (eg, propranolol). CNS effects include convulsions, coma, and respiratory arrest (commonly seen with propranolol and other membrane-depressant and lipid-soluble drugs). Treatment is symptomatic for seizures, hypotension, hyperkalemia, and hypoglycemia. Bradycardia and hypotension resistant to atropine, isoproterenol or pacing may respond to glucagon. Wide QRS defects caused by membrane-depressant poisoning may respond to hypertonic sodium bicarbonate. Repeat-dose charcoal, hemoperfusion, or hemodialysis may be helpful in removal of only those beta-blockers with a small V_d, long half-life, or low intrinsic clearance (acebutolol, atenolol, nadolol, sotalol).

Drug Interactions Substrate of CYP2D6 (major); **Inhibits** CYP2D6 (weak)

Albuterol (and other beta$_2$ agonists): Effects may be blunted by nonspecific beta-blockers.

Alpha-blockers (prazosin, terazosin): Concurrent use of beta-blockers may increase risk of orthostasis.

AV conduction-slowing agents (digoxin): Effects may be additive with beta-blockers.

Clonidine: Hypertensive crisis after or during withdrawal of either agent (not reported with timolol ophthalmic solution)

CYP2D6 inhibitors: May increase the levels/effects of timolol. Example inhibitors include chlorpromazine, delavirdine, fluoxetine, miconazole, paroxetine, pergolide, quinidine, quinine, ritonavir, and ropinirole.

Epinephrine (including local anesthetics with epinephrine): Timolol may cause hypertension.

Glucagon: Timolol may blunt hyperglycemic action.

Insulin and oral hypoglycemics: May mask symptoms of hypoglycemia.

NSAIDs (ibuprofen, indomethacin, naproxen, piroxicam) may reduce the antihypertensive effects of beta-blockers.

Salicylates may reduce the antihypertensive effects of beta-blockers.

Sulfonylureas: Beta-blockers may alter response to hypoglycemic agents.

Verapamil or diltiazem may have synergistic or additive pharmacological effects when taken concurrently with beta-blockers.

Stability Ophthalmic drops: Store at room temperature; do not freeze. Protect from light.

Timolol GFS: Store at 2°C to 25°C (36°F to 77°F). Protect from light.

Timoptic® in OcuDose®: Store in the protective foil wrap and use within 1 month after opening foil package.

Mechanism of Action Blocks both beta$_1$- and beta$_2$-adrenergic receptors, reduces intraocular pressure by reducing aqueous humor production or possibly outflow; reduces blood pressure by blocking adrenergic receptors and decreasing sympathetic outflow, produces a negative chronotropic and inotropic activity through an unknown mechanism

Pharmacodynamics

Onset of action:

Hypotensive: Oral: 15-45 minutes

Peak effect: 0.5-2.5 hours

Intraocular pressure reduction: Ophthalmic: 30 minutes

Peak effect: 1-2 hours

Duration: ~4 hours; intraocular effects persist for 24 hours after ophthalmic instillation

(Continued)

Timolol *(Continued)*

Pharmacokinetics

Protein binding: 60%

Metabolism: Extensive in the liver; extensive first-pass effect

Half-life: 2-2.7 hours; half-life prolonged with reduced renal function

Elimination: Urinary (15% to 20% as unchanged drug)

Dosage

Geriatrics & Adults:

Glaucoma: Ophthalmic:

Solution: Initial: 0.25% solution, instill 1 drop twice daily into affected eye(s); increase to 0.5% solution if response not adequate; decrease to 1 drop/day if controlled; do not exceed 1 drop twice daily of 0.5% solution.

Istalol™: Instill 1 drop (0.5% solution) once daily in the morning.

Gel-forming solution (Timolol GFS, Timoptic-XE®): Instill 1 drop (either 0.25% or 0.5%) once daily

Hypertension: Oral: Initial: 10 mg twice daily, increase gradually every 7 days, usual dosage: 20-40 mg/day in 2 divided doses; maximum: 60 mg/day.

Prevention of myocardial infarction: Oral: 10 mg twice daily initiated within 1-4 weeks after infarction.

Migraine prophylaxis: Oral: Initial: 10 mg twice daily, increase to maximum of 30 mg/day.

Administration Administer other topically-applied ophthalmic medications at least 10 minutes before Timoptic-XE®; wash hands before use; invert closed bottle and shake once before use; remove cap carefully so that tip does not touch anything; hold bottle between thumb and index finger; use index finger of other hand to pull down the lower eyelid to form a pocket for the eye drop and tilt head back; place the dispenser tip close to the eye and gently squeeze the bottle to administer 1 drop; remove pressure after a single drop has been released; **do not allow the dispenser tip to touch the eye**; replace cap and **store** bottle in an upright position in a clean area; do **not** enlarge hole of dispenser; do **not** wash tip with water, soap, or any other cleaner. Some ophthalmic solutions contain benzalkonium chloride; wait at least 10 minutes after instilling solution before inserting soft contact lenses.

Monitoring Parameters Intraocular pressure, heart rate, blood pressure, respiratory rate, funduscopic exam, visual field tests

Patient Information May sting on instillation; do not touch dropper to eye; visual acuity may be decreased after administration; distance vision may be altered; assess patient's or caregiver's ability to administer; apply gentle pressure to lacrimal sac during and immediately following instillation (1 minute) to avoid systemic absorption; stop drug if breathing difficulty occurs; administer other ophthalmics at least 10 minutes before the gel

Additional Information Does not cause night blindness

Special Geriatric Considerations Since bioavailability increased in about twofold in elderly patients, geriatrics may require lower maintenance doses. Also, as serum and tissue concentrations increase beta$_1$ selectivity diminishes. Beta-adrenergic blockade may result in less hemodynamic response than seen in younger adults due to alterations in the beta-adrenergic autonomic system. Studies indicate that despite decreased sensitivity to the chronotropic effects of beta-blockade with age, there appears to be an increased myocardial sensitivity to the negative inotropic effect during stress (ie, exercise). Controlled trials have shown the overall response rate for propranolol to be only 20% to 50% in elderly populations. Therefore, all beta-adrenergic blocking drugs may result in a decreased response as compared to younger adults. Due to propranolol's CNS penetration and nonselective action, it may not be the beta-blocker of choice for use in elderly.

Dosage Forms Excipient information presented when available (limited, particularly for generics); consult specific product labeling.

Note: Unless otherwise specified, strength expressed as base.

Gel-forming solution, ophthalmic, as maleate: 0.25% (5 mL); 0.5% (2.5 mL, 5 mL)

Timolol GFS: 0.25% (2.5 mL, 5 mL); 0.5% (2.5 mL, 5 mL) [contains benzododecinium bromide]

Timoptic-XE®: 0.25% (5 mL); 0.5% (5 mL)

Solution, ophthalmic, as hemihydrate:

Betimol®: 0.25% (5 mL, 10 mL, 15 mL); 0.5% (5 mL, 10 mL, 15 mL) [contains benzalkonium chloride]

Solution, ophthalmic, as maleate: 0.25% (5 mL, 10 mL, 15 mL); 0.5% (5 mL, 10 mL, 15 mL) [contains benzalkonium chloride]

Istalol™: 0.5% (10 mL) [contains benzalkonium chloride and potassium sorbate]

Timoptic®: 0.25% (5 mL); 0.5% (5 mL, 10 mL) [contains benzalkonium chloride]

Solution, ophthalmic, as maleate [preservative free]:

Timoptic® in OcuDose®: 0.25% (0.2 mL); 0.5% (0.2 mL) [single use]

Tablet, as maleate: 5 mg, 10 mg, 20 mg [strength expressed as salt]

Blocadren®: 20 mg [strength expressed as salt]

Selected References

Fleisher LA, Beckman JA, Brown KA, et al, "ACC/AHA 2006 Guideline Update on Perioperative Cardiovascular Evaluation for Noncardiac Surgery: Focused Update on Perioperative Beta-Blocker Therapy. A Report of the American College of Cardiology/American Heart Association Task Force on Practice Guidelines (Writing Committee to Update the 2002 Guidelines on Perioperative Cardiovascular Evaluation for Noncardiac Surgery) Developed in Collaboration With the American Society of Echocardiography, American Society of Nuclear Cardiology, Heart Rhythm Society, Society of Cardiovascular Anesthesiologists, Society for Cardiovascular Angiography and Interventions, and Society for Vascular Medicine and Biology," *J Am Coll Cardiol*, 2006, 47(11):2343-55.

Juul AB, Wetterslev J, Gluud C, et al, "Effect of Perioperative Beta Blockade in Patients With Diabetes Undergoing Major Non-Cardiac Surgery: Randomized Placebo Controlled, Blinded Multicentre Trial. DIPOM Trial Group," *BMJ*, 2006, 332(7556):1482.

Kligman EW and Higbee MD, "Drug Therapy for Hypertension in the Elderly," *J Fam Pract*, 1989, 28(1):81-7.

Levison SP, "Treating Hypertension in the Elderly," *Clin Geriatr Med*, 1988, 4(1):1-12.

Passo MS, Palmer EA, and Van Buskirk EM, "Plasma Timolol in Glaucoma Patients," *Ophthalmology*, 1984, 91(11):1361-3.

Vestal RE, Wood AJ, and Shand DG, "Reduced Beta-Adrenoceptor Sensitivity in the Elderly," *Clin Pharmacol Ther*, 1979, 26(2):181-6.

Yin FC, Raizes GS, Guarnieri T, et al, "Age-Associated Decrease in Ventricular Response to Haemodynamic Stress During Beta-Adrenergic Blockade," *Br Heart J*, 1978, 40(12):1349-55.

Tinzaparin (tin ZA pa rin)

Related Information
Anticoagulants, Injectable *on page 1741*
U.S. Brand Names Innohep®
Canadian Brand Names Innohep®
Index Terms Tinzaparin Sodium
Generic Available No
Pharmacologic Category Low Molecular Weight Heparin
Use Treatment of acute symptomatic deep vein thrombosis, with or without pulmonary embolism, in conjunction with warfarin sodium
Contraindications Hypersensitivity to tinzaparin sodium, heparin, sulfites, benzyl alcohol, pork products, or any component of the formulation; active major bleeding; heparin-induced thrombocytopenia (current or history of)
Warnings/Precautions [U.S. Boxed Warning]: Patients with recent or anticipated neuraxial anesthesia (epidural or spinal anesthesia) are at risk of spinal or epidural hematoma and subsequent paralysis. Consider risk versus benefit prior to neuraxial anesthesia; risk is increased by concomitant agents that may alter hemostasis, as well as traumatic or repeated epidural or spinal puncture, and indwelling epidural catheters. Patient should be observed closely for signs and symptoms of neurological impairment. Not to be used interchangeably (unit for unit) with heparin or any other low molecular weight heparins.

Monitor patient closely for signs or symptoms of bleeding. Certain patients are at increased risk of bleeding. Risk factors include bacterial endocarditis; congenital or acquired bleeding disorders; active ulcerative or angiodysplastic GI diseases; severe uncontrolled hypertension; hemorrhagic stroke; use shortly after brain, spinal, or ophthalmologic surgery; patients treated concomitantly with platelet inhibitors; recent GI bleeding; thrombocytopenia or platelet defects; severe liver disease; hypertensive or diabetic retinopathy; or in patients undergoing invasive procedures. Monitor platelet count closely. Rare cases of thrombocytopenia have occurred. Manufacturer recommends discontinuation of therapy if platelets are <100,000/mm³. Rare cases of thrombocytopenia with thrombosis have occurred.

Use with caution in the elderly (delayed elimination may occur). Patients with severe renal impairment may show reduced elimination of tinzaparin

Heparin can cause hyperkalemia by affecting aldosterone; similar reactions could occur with LMWHs. Monitor for hyperkalemia. Do not administer intramuscularly or (Continued)

Tinzaparin *(Continued)*

intravenously. Clinical experience is limited in patients with BMI >40 kg/m^2. Derived from porcine intestinal mucosa. Contains benzyl alcohol and sodium metabisulfite

Adverse Reactions (Reflective of adult population; not specific for elderly)
As with all anticoagulants, bleeding is the major adverse effect of tinzaparin. Hemorrhage may occur at virtually any site. Risk is dependent on multiple variables.

>10%:

Hepatic: Increased ALT (13%)

Local: Injection site hematoma (16%)

1% to 10%:

Cardiovascular: Angina pectoris, chest pain (2%), hyper-/hypotension, tachycardia

Central nervous system: Confusion, dizziness, fever (2%), headache (2%), insomnia, pain (2%)

Dermatologic: Bullous eruption, pruritus, rash (1%), skin disorder

Gastrointestinal: Constipation (1%), dyspepsia, flatulence, nausea (2%), nonspecified gastrointestinal disorder, vomiting (1%)

Genitourinary: Dysuria, urinary retention, urinary tract infection (4%)

Hematologic: Anemia, hematoma, hemorrhage (2%), thrombocytopenia (1%)

Hepatic: Increased AST (9%)

Local: Thrombophlebitis (deep)

Neuromuscular & skeletal: Back pain (2%)

Renal: Hematuria (1%)

Respiratory: Dyspnea (1%), epistaxis (2%), pneumonia, pulmonary embolism (2%), respiratory disorder

Miscellaneous: Impaired healing, infection, unclassified reactions

Overdosage/Toxicology Overdose may lead to bleeding; bleeding may occur at any site. In case of overdose, discontinue medication, apply pressure to the bleeding site if possible, and replace volume and hemostatic blood elements as required. If these measures are ineffective, or if bleeding is severe, protamine sulfate may be administered by slow infusion at 1 mg per every 100 anti-Xa int. units of tinzaparin administered. However, protamine does not completely neutralize tinzaparin anti-Xa activity.

Drug Interactions

Drugs which affect platelet function (eg, aspirin, NSAIDs, dipyridamole, ticlopidine, clopidogrel, sulfinpyrazone, dextran) may potentiate the risk of hemorrhage.

Thrombolytic agents increase the risk of hemorrhage.

Warfarin: Risk of bleeding may be increased during concurrent therapy. Tinzaparin is commonly continued during the initiation of warfarin therapy to assure anticoagulation and to protect against possible transient hypercoagulability

Stability Store at 15°C to 30°C (59°F to 86°F).

Mechanism of Action Standard heparin consists of components with molecular weights ranging from 4000-30,000 daltons with a mean of 16,000 daltons. Heparin acts as an anticoagulant by enhancing the inhibition rate of clotting proteases by antithrombin III, impairing normal hemostasis and inhibition of factor Xa. Low molecular weight heparins have a small effect on the activated partial thromboplastin time and strongly inhibit factor Xa. The primary inhibitory activity of tinzaparin is through antithrombin. Tinzaparin is derived from porcine heparin that undergoes controlled enzymatic depolymerization. The average molecular weight of tinzaparin ranges between 5500 and 7500 daltons which is distributed as (<10%) 2000 daltons (60% to 72%) 2000-8000 daltons, and (22% to 36%) >8000 daltons. The antifactor Xa activity is approximately 100 int. units/mg.

Pharmacodynamics Onset of action: 2-3 hours

Pharmacokinetics

Distribution: 3-5 L

Metabolism: Partially metabolized by desulphation and depolymerization

Bioavailability: 87%

Half-life: 3-4 hours

Time to peak: 4-5 hours

Elimination: Renal

Dosage

Geriatrics & Adults: Treatment of DVT: SubQ: 175 anti-Xa int. units/kg of body weight once daily. Warfarin sodium should be started when appropriate. Administer tinzaparin for at least 6 days and until patient is adequately anticoagulated with warfarin.

Note: To calculate the volume of solution to administer per dose: Volume to be administered (mL) = patient weight (kg) x 0.00875 mL/kg (may be rounded off to the nearest 0.05 mL)

Renal Impairment: Patients with severe renal impairment (Cl$_{cr}$ <30 mL/minute) had a 24% decrease in clearance, use with caution.

Hepatic Impairment: No adjustment necessary.

Administration Patient should be lying down or sitting. Administer by deep SubQ injection, alternating between the left and right anterolateral and left and right postero-lateral abdominal wall. Vary site daily. The entire needle should be introduced into the skin fold formed by the thumb and forefinger. Hold the skin fold until injection is complete. To minimize bruising, do not rub the injection site.

Monitoring Parameters CBC including platelet count and hematocrit or hemoglobin, and stool for occult blood; the monitoring of PT and/or aPTT is not of clinical value. Patients receiving both warfarin and tinzaparin should have their INR drawn just prior to the next scheduled dose of tinzaparin.

Patient Information This drug can only be administered by SubQ injection. You may have a tendency to bleed easily while taking this drug; brush teeth with a soft brush; floss with waxed floss; use electric razor; avoid scissors or sharp knives and potentially harmful activities. Report chest pain, persistent constipation, persistent erection, unusual bleeding or bruising (bleeding gums, nosebleed, blood in urine, dark stool), pain in joints or back; or numbness, tingling, swelling, or pain at injection site.

Additional Information Contains sodium metabisulfite and benzyl alcohol, 10 mg/mL

Special Geriatric Considerations No significant differences in safety or response were seen when used in patients ≥65 years of age. However, increased sensitivity to tinzaparin in elderly patients may be possible due to a decline in renal function.

Dosage Forms Excipient information presented when available (limited, particularly for generics); consult specific product labeling.
Injection, solution, as sodium:
Innohep®: 20,000 anti-Xa int. units/mL (2 mL) [contains benzyl alcohol and sodium metabisulfite]

♦ **Tinzaparin Sodium** *see* Tinzaparin *on page 1575*

Tioconazole (tye oh KONE a zole)

Medication Safety Issues
Sound-alike/look-alike issues: Tioconazole may be confused with terconazole

U.S. Brand Names 1-Day™ [OTC]; Vagistat®-1 [OTC]

Generic Available No

Pharmacologic Category Antifungal Agent, Vaginal

Use Local treatment of vulvovaginal candidiasis

Contraindications Hypersensitivity to tioconazole or any component of the formulation

Warnings/Precautions For vaginal use only. Petrolatum-based vaginal products may damage rubber or latex condoms or diaphragms. Separate use by 3 days.

Adverse Reactions (Reflective of adult population; not specific for elderly)
Frequency not defined.
Central nervous system: Headache
Gastrointestinal: Abdominal pain
Dermatologic: Burning, desquamation
Genitourinary: Discharge, dyspareunia, dysuria, irritation, itching, nocturia, vaginal pain, vaginitis, vulvar swelling

Drug Interactions Inhibits CYP1A2 (weak), 2A6 (weak), 2C9 (weak), 2C19 (weak), 2D6 (weak), 2E1 (weak)
No drug interaction data reported.

Stability Store at room temperature.

Mechanism of Action A 1-substituted imidazole derivative with a broad antifungal spectrum against a wide variety of dermatophytes and yeasts, including *Trichophyton mentagrophytes*, *T. rubrum*, *T. erinacei*, *T. tonsurans*, *Microsporum canis*, *Microsporum gypseum*, and *Candida albicans*. Both agents appear to be similarly effective against *Epidermophyton floccosum*.

Pharmacodynamics Onset of action: Some improvement may be seen in a single day; complete relief within 7 days.

Pharmacokinetics
Absorption: Intravaginal: Following application small amounts of drug are absorbed systemically (25%) within 2-8 hours; therapeutic levels persist for 3-5 days after single dose
Half-life: 21-24 hours
Elimination: Urine and feces in approximate equal amounts

Dosage
Geriatrics & Adults: Vulvovaginal candidiasis: Vaginal: Insert 1 applicatorful in vagina, just prior to bedtime, as a single dose

Patient Information Insert high into vagina; contact physician if itching or burning continues; Vagistat®-1 may interact with condoms (ie, weaken latex)

Dosage Forms Excipient information presented when available (limited, particularly for generics); consult specific product labeling.
Ointment, vaginal: 6.5% (4.6 g) [with applicator]

♦ **Tiotixene** see Thiothixene on page 1556

Tiotropium (ty oh TRO pee um)

Medication Safety Issues
Sound-alike/look-alike issues:
Spiriva® may be confused with Inspra™
Spiriva® capsules for inhalation are for administration via HandiHaler® device and are not for oral use

U.S. Brand Names Spiriva®

Canadian Brand Names Spiriva®

Index Terms Tiotropium Bromide Monohydrate

Generic Available No

Pharmacologic Category Anticholinergic Agent

Use Maintenance treatment of bronchospasm associated with COPD (bronchitis and emphysema)

Contraindications Hypersensitivity to tiotropium, its derivatives, or any component of the formulation (contains lactose); not for use as an acute ("rescue") bronchodilator

Warnings/Precautions Not indicated for the initial treatment of acute episodes of bronchospasm; use with caution in patients with myasthenia gravis, narrow-angle glaucoma, prostatic hyperplasia, or bladder neck obstruction; avoid inadvertent instillation of powder into the eyes. Immediate hypersensitivity reactions may occur. Use caution in renal impairment.

Adverse Reactions (Reflective of adult population; not specific for elderly)
>10%:
  Gastrointestinal: Xerostomia (16%)
  Respiratory: Upper respiratory tract infection (41% vs 37% with placebo), sinusitis (11% vs 9% with placebo), pharyngeal irritation (frequency not specified)
1% to 10%:
  Cardiovascular: Angina, edema (dependent, 5%)
  Central nervous system: Paresthesia, depression
  Dermatologic: Rash (4%)
  Endocrine & metabolic: Hypercholesterolemia, hyperglycemia
  Gastrointestinal: Dyspepsia (6%), abdominal pain (5%), constipation (4%), vomiting (4%), reflux, ulcerative stomatitis
  Genitourinary: Urinary tract infection (7%)
  Neuromuscular & skeletal: Myalgia (4%), leg pain, skeletal pain
  Ocular: Cataract
  Respiratory: Pharyngitis (9%), rhinitis (6%), epistaxis (4%), dysphonia, laryngitis
  Miscellaneous: Infection (4%), moniliasis (4%), allergic reaction, herpes zoster

Overdosage/Toxicology Conjunctivitis and xerostomia have been observed with doses up to 141 micrograms. Other symptoms of overdose include drying of respiratory secretions, cough, nausea, GI distress, blurred vision or impaired visual accommodation, headache, and nervousness. Acute overdose with tiotropium by inhalation is unlikely since it is so poorly absorbed. However, if poisoning occurs, it can be treated like any other anticholinergic toxicity. An anticholinergic overdose with severe life-threatening symptoms may be treated with physostigmine 1-2 mg SubQ or I.V. slowly.

Drug Interactions Substrate (minor) of CYP2D6, 3A4
Acetylcholinesterase inhibitors (central): May diminish the therapeutic effect of anticholinergics. Anticholinergics may diminish the therapeutic effect of acetylcholinesterase inhibitors (central).
Anticholinergic agents: Increased toxicity with anticholinergics or drugs with anticholinergic properties.

Stability Store between 15°C and 25°C. Do not store capsules in HandiHaler® device. Capsules should be stored in the blister pack and only removed immediately before use. After first capsule in the strip is used, the two remaining capsules should be used over the next 2 days.

Mechanism of Action Blocks the action of acetylcholine at parasympathetic sites in bronchial smooth muscle causing bronchodilation

Pharmacokinetics
Absorption: Poorly absorbed from GI tract, systemic absorption may occur from lung
Distribution: V_d: 32 L/kg
Protein binding: 72%
Metabolism: Hepatic (minimal), via CYP2D6 and CYP3A4
Bioavailability: Following inhalation, 19.5%; oral solution: 2% to 3%
Half-life elimination: 5-6 days
Time to peak, plasma: 5 minutes (following inhalation)

Elimination: Urine (74% as unchanged drug)

Dosage

    Geriatrics & Adults: COPD: Oral inhalation: Contents of 1 capsule (18 mcg) inhaled once daily using HandiHaler® device

    Renal Impairment: Plasma concentrations increase in renal impairment. Use caution; no specific dosage adjustment recommended.

Administration Administer once daily at the same time each day. Remove capsule from foil blister immediately before use. Place capsule in the capsule-chamber in the base of the HandiHaler® Inhaler. Must only use the HandiHaler® Inhaler. Close mouthpiece until a click is heard, leaving dustcap open. Exhale fully. Do not exhale into inhaler. Tilt head slightly back and inhale (rapidly, steadily and deeply); the capsule vibration may be heard within the device. Hold breath as long as possible. If any powder remains in capsule, exhale and inhale again. Repeat until capsule is empty. Throw away empty capsule; do not leave in inhaler. Do not use a spacer with the HandiHaler® Inhaler. Always keep capsules and inhaler dry.

Delivery of dose: Instruct patient to place mouthpiece gently between teeth, closing lips around inhaler. Instruct patient to inhale deeply and hold breath held for 5-10 seconds. The amount of drug delivered is small, and the individual will not sense the medication as it is inhaled. Remove mouthpiece prior to exhalation. Patient should not breathe out through the mouthpiece. After use of the inhaler, patient should rinse mouth/oropharynx with water and spit out rinse solution.

Monitoring Parameters FEV_1, peak flow (or other pulmonary function studies)

Special Geriatric Considerations Assess patient's ability to use the HandiHaler®. In elderly patients, renal clearance of tiotropium was decreased and plasma concentrations were increased, due to decreased renal function. No significant difference in adverse effects were seen in young vs elderly patients. No dosage adjustments are recommended due to age or renal function. However, the manufacturer recommends monitoring patients with moderate-to-severe renal impairment.

Dosage Forms Excipient information presented when available (limited, particularly for generics); consult specific product labeling.

    Powder for oral inhalation [capsule]:

        Spiriva®: 18 mcg/capsule (5s, 30s) [contains lactose; packaged with HandiHaler® device]

♦ **Tiotropium Bromide Monohydrate** *see* Tiotropium *on page 1578*

Tirofiban (tye roe FYE ban)

Medication Safety Issues

    Sound-alike/look-alike issues:

        Aggrastat® may be confused with Aggrenox®, argatroban

    High alert medication: The Institute for Safe Medication Practices (ISMP) includes this medication among its list of drugs which have a heightened risk of causing significant patient harm when used in error.

U.S. Brand Names Aggrastat®

Canadian Brand Names Aggrastat®

Index Terms MK383; Tirofiban Hydrochloride

Generic Available No

Pharmacologic Category Antiplatelet Agent, Glycoprotein IIb/IIIa Inhibitor

Use In combination with heparin, is indicated for the treatment of acute coronary syndrome, including patients who are to be managed medically and those undergoing PTCA or atherectomy. In this setting, it has been shown to decrease the rate of a combined endpoint of death, new myocardial infarction, or refractory ischemia/repeat cardiac procedure.

Contraindications Hypersensitivity to tirofiban or any component of the formulation; active internal bleeding or a history of bleeding diathesis within the previous 30 days; history of intracranial hemorrhage, intracranial neoplasm, arteriovenous malformation, or aneurysm; history of thrombocytopenia following prior exposure; history of CVA within 30 days or any history of hemorrhagic stroke; major surgical procedure or severe physical trauma within the previous month; history, symptoms, or findings suggestive of aortic dissection; severe hypertension (systolic BP >180 mm Hg and/or diastolic BP >110 mm Hg); concomitant use of another parenteral GP IIb/IIIa inhibitor; acute pericarditis

Warnings/Precautions Bleeding is the most common complication encountered during this therapy; most major bleeding occurs at the arterial access site for cardiac catheterization. Caution in patients with platelets <150,000/mm³; patients with hemorrhagic retinopathy; chronic dialysis patients; when used in combination with other drugs impacting on coagulation. To minimize bleeding complications, care must be taken in sheath insertion/removal. Sheath hemostasis should be achieved at least 4 hours before hospital discharge. Other trauma and vascular punctures should be

(Continued)

Tirofiban *(Continued)*

minimized. Avoid obtaining vascular access through a noncompressible site (eg, subclavian or jugular vein). Patients with severe renal insufficiency require dosage reduction.

Adverse Reactions (Reflective of adult population; not specific for elderly)
Bleeding is the major drug-related adverse effect. Patients received background treatment with aspirin and heparin. Major bleeding was reported in 1.4% to 2.2%; minor bleeding in 10.5% to 12%; transfusion was required in 4% to 4.3%.

>1% (nonbleeding adverse events):
Cardiovascular: Bradycardia (4%), coronary artery dissection (5%), edema (2%)
Central nervous system: Dizziness (3%), fever (>1%), headache (>1%), vasovagal reaction (2%)
Gastrointestinal: Nausea (>1%)
Genitourinary: Pelvic pain (6%)
Hematologic: Thrombocytopenia: <90,000/mm^3 (1.5%), <50,000/mm^3 (0.3%)
Neuromuscular & skeletal: Leg pain (3%)
Miscellaneous: Diaphoresis (2%)

Overdosage/Toxicology The most frequent manifestation of overdose is bleeding. Treatment is cessation of therapy and assessment of transfusion. Tirofiban has a relatively short half-life and its platelet effects dissipate rather quickly. However, when immediate reversal is required, platelet transfusions can be useful. Tirofiban is dialyzable.

Drug Interactions

Cephalosporins which contain the MTT side chain may theoretically increase the risk of hemorrhage.

Drugs which affect platelet function (eg, aspirin, NSAIDs, dipyridamole, ticlopidine, clopidogrel) may potentiate the risk of hemorrhage.

Heparin and aspirin: Use with aspirin and heparin is associated with an increase in bleeding over aspirin and heparin alone. However, the concurrent use of aspirin and heparin has also improved the efficacy of tirofiban.

Levothyroxine and omeprazole increase tirofiban clearance; however, the clinical significance of this interaction remains to be demonstrated.

Thrombolytic agents theoretically may increase the risk of hemorrhage.

Warfarin and oral anticoagulants: Risk of bleeding may be increased during concurrent therapy.

Other IIb/IIIa antagonists: Concomitant use of other injectable glycoprotein IIb/IIIa antagonists is contraindicated (see Contraindications).

Stability Store at 25°C (77°F); do not freeze. Protect from light during storage.

Mechanism of Action A reversible antagonist of fibrinogen binding to the GP IIb/IIIa receptor, the major platelet surface receptor involved in platelet aggregation. When administered intravenously, it inhibits *ex vivo* platelet aggregation in a dose- and concentration-dependent manner. When given according to the recommended regimen, >90% inhibition is attained by the end of the 30-minute infusion. Platelet aggregation inhibition is reversible following cessation of the infusion.

Pharmacokinetics

Distribution: 35% unbound
Metabolism: Minimal
Elimination: Primarily unchanged drug; 65% in urine, 25% in feces; clearance is reduced in older adult patients by 19% to 26%

Dosage

Geriatrics & Adults: Acute coronary syndromes: I.V.: Initial rate of 0.4 mcg/kg/minute for 30 minutes and then continued at 0.1 mcg/kg/minute. Dosing should be continued through angiography and for 12-24 hours after angioplasty or atherectomy.

Renal Impairment: Cl$_{cr}$ <30 mL/minute: Reduce dose to 50% of normal rate.

Administration Intended for intravenous delivery using sterile equipment and technique. Do not add other drugs or remove solution directly from the bag with a syringe. Do not use plastic containers in series connections; such use can result in air embolism by drawing air from the first container if it is empty of solution. Discard unused solution 24 hours following the start of infusion. May be administered through the same catheter as heparin. Tirofiban injection must be diluted to a concentration of 50 mcg/mL (premixed solution does not require dilution). Infuse over 30 minutes.

Monitoring Parameters Platelet count. Hemoglobin and hematocrit should be monitored prior to treatment, within 6 hours following loading infusion, and at least daily thereafter during therapy. Platelet count may need to be monitored earlier in patients who received prior glycoprotein IIb/IIIa antagonists. Persistent reductions of platelet counts <90,000/mm^3 may require interruption or discontinuation of infusion. Because tirofiban requires concurrent heparin therapy, aPTT levels should also be followed. Monitor vital signs and laboratory results prior to, during, and after therapy. Assess infusion insertion site during and after therapy (every 15 minutes or as institutional policy). Observe and teach patient bleeding precautions (avoid invasive procedures and activities that could result in injury). Monitor closely for signs of unusual or excessive bleeding (eg, CNS changes, blood in urine, stool, or vomitus, unusual bruising or bleeding).

Special Geriatric Considerations Elderly patients receiving tirofiban with heparin or heparin alone had a higher incidence of bleeding in clinical trials. Caution must be used when using other drugs affecting hemostasis, which are commonly used in elderly.

Dosage Forms Excipient information presented when available (limited, particularly for generics); consult specific product labeling.

Infusion [premixed in sodium chloride]: 50 mcg/mL (100 mL, 250 mL)

Injection, solution: 250 mcg/mL (50 mL)

Selected References

"A Comparison of Aspirin Plus Tirofiban With Aspirin Plus Heparin for Unstable Angina. Platelet Receptor Inhibition in Ischemic Syndrome Management (PRISM) Study Investigators," *N Engl J Med*, 1998, 338(21):1498-505.

Antman EM, Giugliano RP, Gibson CM, et al, "Abciximab Facilitates the Rate and Extent of Thrombolysis: Results of the Thrombolysis in Myocardial Infarction (TIMI) 14 Trial. The TIMI 14 Investigators," *Circulation*, 1999, 99(21):2720-32.

Brener SJ, Barr LA, Burchenal JE, et al, "Randomized, Placebo-Controlled Trial of Platelet Glycoprotein IIb/IIIa Blockade With Primary Angioplasty for Acute Myocardial Infarction. ReoPro and Primary PTCA Organization and Randomized Trial (RAPPORT) Investigators, *Circulation*, 1998, 98(8):734-41.

Braunwald E, Antman EM, Beasley JW, et al, "ACC/AHA Guidelines for the Management of Patients With Unstable Angina and Non-ST-Segment Elevation Myocardial Infarction. A Report of the American College of Cardiology/American Heart Association Task Force on Practice Guidelines (Committee on the Management of Patients With Unstable Angina)," *J Am Coll Cardiol*, 2000, 36(3):970-1062.

"Effects of Platelet Glycoprotein IIb/IIIa Blockade With Tirofiban on Adverse Cardiac Events in Patients With Unstable Angina or Acute Myocardial Infarction Undergoing Coronary Angioplasty. The RESTORE Investigators. Randomized Efficacy Study of Tirofiban for Outcomes and Restenosis," *Circulation*, 1997, 96(5):1445-53.

Hamm CW, Heeschen C, Goldmann B, et al, "Benefit of Abciximab in Patients With Refractory Unstable Angina in Relation to Serum Troponin T Levels. c7E3 Fab Antiplatelet Therapy in Unstable Refractory Angina (CAPTURE) Study Investigators," *N Engl J Med*, 1999, 340(21):1623-9.

"Inhibition of the Platelet Glycoprotein IIb/IIIa Receptor With Tirofiban in Unstable Angina and Non-Q-Wave Myocardial Infarction. Platelet Receptor Inhibition in Ischemic Syndrome Management in Patients Limited by Unstable Signs and Symptoms (PRISM-PLUS) Study Investigators," *N Engl J Med*, 1998, 338(21):1488-97.

"Inhibition of Platelet Glycoprotein IIb/IIIa With Eptifibatide in Patients With Acute Coronary Syndromes. The PURSUIT Trial Investigators. Platelet Glycoprotein IIb/IIIa in Unstable Angina: Receptor Suppression Using Integrilin Therapy," *N Engl J Med*, 1998, 339(7):436-43.

Lincoff AM, Califf RM, Anderson KM, et al, "Evidence for Prevention of Death and Myocardial Infarction With Platelet Membrane Glycoprotein IIb/IIIa Receptor Blockade by Abciximab (c7E3 Fab) Among Patients With Unstable Angina Undergoing Percutaneous Coronary Revascularization. EPIC Investigators. Evaluation of 7E3 in Preventing Ischemic Complications," *J Am Coll Cardiol*, 1997, 30(1):149-56.

Lincoff AM, Califf RM, Moliterno DJ, et al, "Complementary Clinical Benefits of Coronary-Artery Stenting and Blockade of Platelet Glycoprotein IIb/IIIa Receptors. Evaluation of Platelet IIb/IIIa Inhibition in Stenting Investigators," *N Engl J Med*, 1999, 341(5):319-27.

Lincoff AM, Tcheng JE, Califf RM, et al, "Sustained Suppression of Ischemic Complications of Coronary Intervention by Platelet GP IIb/IIIa Blockade With Abciximab: One-Year Outcome in the EPILOG Trial. Evaluation in PTCA to Improve Long-Term Outcome With Abciximab GP IIb/IIIa Blockade," *Circulation*, 1999, 99(15):1951-8.

Topol EJ, Ferguson JJ, Weisman HF, et al, "Long-Term Protection From Myocardial Ischemic Events in a Randomized Trial of Brief Integrin Beta₃ Blockade With Percutaneous Coronary Intervention. EPIC Investigator Group. Evaluation of Platelet IIb/IIIa Inhibition for Prevention of Ischemic Complication," *JAMA*, 1997, 278(6):479-84.

van den Merkhof LF, Zijlstra F, Olsson H, et al, "Abciximab in the Treatment of Acute Myocardial Infarction Eligible for Primary Percutaneous Transluminal Coronary Angioplasty. Results of the Glycoprotein Receptor Antagonist Patency Evaluation (GRAPE) Pilot Study," *J Am Coll Cardiol*, 1999, 33(6):1528-32.

♦ **Tirofiban Hydrochloride** *see* Tirofiban *on page 1579*

♦ **Tiseb® [OTC]** *see* Salicylic Acid *on page 1441*

♦ **Titralac® Plus Liquid [OTC]** *see* Calcium Salts (Oral) *on page 220*

Tizanidine (tye ZAN i deen)

Medication Safety Issues

Sound-alike/look-alike issues:

Tizanidine may be confused with tiagabine

U.S. Brand Names Zanaflex®

Canadian Brand Names Apo-Tizanidine®; Gen-Tizanidine; Zanaflex®

Index Terms Sirdalud®

Generic Available Yes: Tablet

Pharmacologic Category Alpha₂-Adrenergic Agonist

Use Skeletal muscle relaxant used for treatment of muscle spasticity

Unlabeled/Investigational Use Treatment of tension headaches, low back pain, trigeminal neuralgia

Contraindications Hypersensitivity to tizanidine or any component of the formulation; concomitant therapy with ciprofloxacin or fluvoxamine or other potent inhibitors of CYP1A2

Warnings/Precautions Significant hypotension (possibly with bradycardia or orthostatic hypotension) and sedation may occur; use caution in patients with cardiac *(Continued)*

Tizanidine *(Continued)*

disease or those at risk for severe hypotensive or sedative effects. Avoid concomitant administration with CYP1A2 inhibitors; increased tizanidine levels/effects (severe hypotension and sedation) may occur. These effects may also be increased with concomitant administration with other CNS depressants and/or antihypertensives; use caution. Elderly patients are particularly at risk; clearance is reduced by >50% in elderly patients with renal insufficiency (Cl_{cr} <25 mL/minute) compared to healthy elderly subjects; this may lead to a longer duration of effects. Use caution in any patient with renal impairment; consider dose reductions or increased dosing intervals. Use with extreme caution in hepatic impairment due to extensive hepatic metabolism and potential hepatotoxicity; AST/ALT elevations (≥2 baseline) and rarely hepatic failure have occurred. Use has been associated with visual hallucinations or delusions in first 6 weeks of therapy; use caution in patients with psychiatric disorders. Withdrawal resulting in rebound hypertension, tachycardia, and hypertonia may occur upon discontinuation; doses should be decreased slowly, particularly in patients receiving high doses for prolonged periods.

Adverse Reactions (Reflective of adult population; not specific for elderly)
>10%:
    Cardiovascular: Hypotension (16% to 33%)
    Central nervous system: Somnolence (48%), dizziness (16%)
    Gastrointestinal: Xerostomia (49%)
    Neuromuscular & skeletal: Weakness (41%)
1% to 10%:
    Cardiovascular: Bradycardia (2% to 10%)
    Central nervous system: Nervousness (3%), speech disorder (3%), visual hallucinations/delusions (3%; occurring in first 6 weeks of therapy)
    Gastrointestinal: Constipation (4%), vomiting (3%), pharyngitis (3%)
    Genitourinary: UTI (10%), urinary frequency (3%)
    Hepatic: Liver enzymes increased (3% to 5%)
    Neuromuscular & skeletal: Dyskinesia (3%)
    Ocular: Blurred vision (3%)
    Respiratory: Rhinitis (3%)
    Miscellaneous: Infection (6%), flu-like syndrome (3%)

Overdosage/Toxicology Symptoms include dry mouth, bradycardia, and hypotension. Lavage (within 2 hours of ingestion) with activated charcoal; benzodiazepines for seizure control. Atropine can be given for treatment of bradycardia. Flumazenil has been used to reverse coma successfully. Forced diuresis is not helpful. Multiple dosing of activated charcoal may be helpful. Following attempts to enhance drug elimination, hypotension should be treated with I.V. fluids and/or Trendelenburg positioning.

Drug Interactions Substrate of CYP1A2 (major)
    Baclofen: Additive CNS depression may occur.
    Beta-blockers: May potentiate bradycardia in patients receiving tizanidine and may increase the rebound hypertension of withdrawal; if possible, discontinue beta-blocker several days before tizanidine is tapered.
    CYP1A2 inhibitors: May increase the levels/effects of tizanidine. Example inhibitors include amiodarone, ciprofloxacin, fluvoxamine, ketoconazole, norfloxacin, ofloxacin, and rofecoxib. Avoid concomitant use; concurrent use of ciprofloxacin or fluvoxamine is contraindicated.
    Ciprofloxacin: May increase the levels/effects (eg, hypotension) of tizanidine. Concurrent use is contraindicated.
    Clonidine: Hypotensive effects may be enhanced with concurrent use.
    CNS depressants: Sedative effects may be additive; monitor for increased effect; includes barbiturates, benzodiazepines, opioid analgesics, ethanol, and other sedative agents.
    Diuretics, other alpha adrenergic agonists, antihypertensives: Additive hypotensive effects may occur.
    Fluvoxamine: May increase the levels/effects (eg, hypotension, sedation) of tizanidine. Concurrent use is contraindicated.
    Hormonal contraceptives: May increase the levels/effects of tizanidine.
    Mirtazapine: May antagonize the alpha-agonist effects of tizanidine.

Ethanol/Nutrition/Herb Interactions
    Ethanol: Avoid ethanol (may increase CNS depression).
    Food: The tablet and capsule dosage forms are not bioequivalent when administered with food. Food increases both the time to peak concentration and the extent of absorption for both the tablet and capsule. However, maximal concentrations of tizanidine achieved when administered with food were increased by 30% for the tablet, but decreased by 20% for the capsule. Under fed conditions, the capsule is approximately 80% bioavailable relative to the tablet.
    Herb/Nutraceutical: Avoid valerian, St John's wort, kava kava, gotu kola (may increase CNS depression). Avoid black cohosh, California poppy, coleus, golden seal,

hawthorn, mistletoe, periwinkle, quinine, shepherd's purse (may increase hypotensive effects).

Mechanism of Action An alpha$_2$-adrenergic agonist agent which decreases excitatory input to alpha motor neurons; an imidazole derivative chemically-related to clonidine, which acts as a centrally acting muscle relaxant with alpha$_2$-adrenergic agonist properties; acts on the level of the spinal cord

Pharmacodynamics
Peak effect: 1-2 hours
Duration: 3-6 hours

Pharmacokinetics
Absorption: Tablets and capsules are bioequivalent under fasting conditions, but not under nonfasting conditions.
Tablets administered with food: Peak plasma concentration is increased by ~30%; time to peak increased by 25 minutes; extent of absorption increased by ~30%.
Capsules administered with food: Peak plasma concentration decreased by 20%; time to peak increased by 2-3 hours; extent of absorption increased by ~10%.
Capsules opened and sprinkled on applesauce are not bioequivalent to administration of intact capsules under fasting conditions. Peak plasma concentration and AUC are increased by 15% to 20%.
Distribution: V$_d$: 204 L/kg
Metabolism: Extensively hepatic
Half-life elimination: 2 hours
Time to peak serum:
Fasting state: Capsule, tablet: 1 hour
Fed state: Capsule: 3-4 hours, Tablet: 1.5 hours
Excretion: Urine (60%); feces (20%)

Dosage
Geriatrics & Adults: Spasticity: Usual initial dose: 4 mg, may increase by 2-4 mg as needed for satisfactory reduction of muscle tone every 6-8 hours to a maximum of three doses in any 24 hour period
Range: 2-4 mg 3 times/day
Maximum dose: 36 mg/day
Renal Impairment: May require dose reductions or less frequent dosing
Hepatic Impairment: Avoid use in hepatic impairment; if used, lowest possible dose should be used initially with close monitoring for adverse effects (eg, hypotension).

Administration Capsules may be opened and contents sprinkled on food; however, extent of absorption is increased up to 20% relative to administration of the capsule under fasted conditions.

Monitoring Parameters Monitor liver function (aminotransferases) at baseline, 1, 3, 6 months and then periodically thereafter; monitor for orthostatic hypotension

Patient Information May cause hypotension, sedation, impaired coordination which affects operating hazardous machinery (ie, automobiles); other CNS depressants will be additive to sedation of tizanidine

Additional Information Single doses of 8 mg reduce muscle tone for a period of several hours; the effect peaks in 1-2 hours and lasts 3-6 hours; effects are dose-related, however, it is prudent to start at lower doses as above.

Special Geriatric Considerations Since elderly commonly have renal function of Cl$_{cr}$<30 mL/minute, creatinine clearance should be estimated before dosing this medication. Low doses should be started initially because of the possibility of CNS effects.

Dosage Forms Excipient information presented when available (limited, particularly for generics); consult specific product labeling.
Capsule:
Zanaflex®: 2 mg, 4 mg, 6 mg
Tablet: 2 mg, 4 mg
Zanaflex®: 2 mg [DSC], 4 mg

♦ **TMP** *see* Trimethoprim *on page 1634*
♦ **TMP-SMZ** *see* Sulfamethoxazole and Trimethoprim *on page 1498*
♦ **TOBI®** *see* Tobramycin *on page 1583*
♦ **TobraDex®** *see* Tobramycin and Dexamethasone *on page 1587*

Tobramycin (toe bra MYE sin)

Related Information
Aminoglycoside Dosing and Monitoring *on page 1794*
Antimicrobial Activity Against Selected Organisms *on page 1728*
Serum Drug Concentrations Commonly Monitored Guidelines *on page 1862*
Medication Safety Issues
Sound-alike/look-alike issues:
Tobramycin may be confused with Trobicin®
AKTob® may be confused with AK-Trol®
(Continued)

Tobramycin *(Continued)*

Nebcin® may be confused with Inapsine®, Naprosyn®, Nubain®

Tobrex® may be confused with TobraDex®

U.S. Brand Names AKTob®; TOBI®; Tobrex®

Canadian Brand Names PMS-Tobramycin; Sandoz-Tobramycin; TOBI®; Tobramycin Injection, USP; Tobrex®

Index Terms Tobramycin Sulfate

Generic Available Yes: Excludes ophthalmic ointment, solution for nebulization

Pharmacologic Category Antibiotic, Aminoglycoside; Antibiotic, Ophthalmic

Use Treatment of documented or suspected *Pseudomonas aeruginosa* infection; infection with a nonpseudomonal enteric bacillus which is more sensitive to tobramycin than gentamicin based on susceptibility tests; empiric therapy in cystic fibrosis and immunocompromised patients; topically used to treat superficial ophthalmic infections caused by susceptible bacteria

Contraindications Hypersensitivity to tobramycin, other aminoglycosides, or any component of the formulation

Warnings/Precautions [U.S. Boxed Warning]: Aminoglycosides may cause neurotoxicity and/or nephrotoxicity; usual risk factors include pre-existing renal impairment, concomitant neuro-/nephrotoxic medications, advanced age and dehydration. Ototoxicity may be directly proportional to the amount of drug given and the duration of treatment; tinnitus or vertigo are indications of vestibular injury and impending hearing loss; renal damage is usually reversible. May cause neuromuscular blockade and respiratory paralysis; especially when given soon after anesthesia or muscle relaxants.

Not intended for long-term therapy due to toxic hazards associated with extended administration; use caution in pre-existing renal insufficiency, vestibular or cochlear impairment, myasthenia gravis, hypocalcemia, conditions which depress neuromuscular transmission. Dosage modification required in patients with impaired renal function. Prolonged use may result in fungal or bacterial superinfection, including *C. difficile*-associated diarrhea and pseudomembranous colitis. Solution may contain sodium metabisulfate; use caution in patients with sulfite allergy.

Adverse Reactions (Reflective of adult population; not specific for elderly)

Injection: Frequency not defined:

Central nervous system: Confusion, disorientation, dizziness, fever, headache, lethargy, vertigo

Dermatologic: Exfoliative dermatitis, itching, rash, urticaria

Endocrine & metabolic: Serum calcium, magnesium, potassium, and/or sodium decreased

Gastrointestinal: Diarrhea, nausea, vomiting

Hematologic: Anemia, eosinophilia, granulocytopenia, leukocytosis, leukopenia, thrombocytopenia

Hepatic: ALT, AST, bilirubin, and/or LDH increased

Local: Pain at the injection site

Otic: Hearing loss, tinnitus, ototoxicity (auditory), ototoxicity (vestibular), roaring in the ears

Renal: BUN increased, cylindruria, serum creatinine increased, oliguria, proteinuria

Inhalation:

>10%:

Gastrointestinal: Sputum discoloration (21%)

Respiratory: Voice alteration (13%)

1% to 10%:

Central nervous system: Malaise (6%)

Otic: Tinnitus (3%)

Overdosage/Toxicology Symptoms include ototoxicity, nephrotoxicity, and neuromuscular toxicity. The treatment of choice following a single acute overdose appears to be the maintenance of urine output of at least 3 mL/kg/hour. Dialysis is of questionable value in the enhancement of aminoglycoside elimination. If required, hemodialysis is preferred over peritoneal dialysis in patients with normal renal function. Careful hydration may be all that is required to promote diuresis and therefore enhance elimination.

Drug Interactions

Increased effect: Extended spectrum penicillins (synergistic)

Increased toxicity:

Aminoglycosides may potentiate the effects of neuromuscular-blocking agents

Amphotericin B, cephalosporins, loop diuretics, and vancomycin may increase risk of nephrotoxicity

Decreased effect: Tobramycin's efficacy reduced when given concurrently with carbenicillin, ticarcillin, or piperacillin to patients with severe renal impairment (inactivation). Separate administration.

Stability

Injection: Stable at room temperature both as the clear, colorless solution and as the dry powder. Reconstituted solutions remain stable for 24 hours at room temperature and 96 hours when refrigerated. Dilute in 50-100 mL NS, D_5W for I.V. infusion.

Separate administration of extended-spectrum penicillins (eg, carbenicillin, ticarcillin, piperacillin) from tobramycin in patients with severe renal impairment; tobramycin's efficacy may be reduced if given concurrently.

Ophthalmic solution: Store at 8°C to 27°C (46°F to 80°F).

Solution, for inhalation (TOBI®): Store under refrigeration at 2°C to 8°C (36°F to 46°F). May be stored in foil pouch at room temperature of 25°C (77°F) for up to 28 days. Avoid intense light. Solution may darken over time; however, do not use if cloudy or contains particles.

Mechanism of Action
Interferes with bacterial protein synthesis by binding to 30S and 50S ribosomal subunits resulting in a defective bacterial cell membrane

Pharmacokinetics

Absorption: I.M.: Rapid and complete

Distribution: V_d: 0.2-0.3 L/kg

Half-life: 2-3 hours, directly dependent upon glomerular filtration rate; half-life (impaired renal function): 5-70 hours

Time to peak serum concentration:
I.M.: Within 30-60 minutes
I.V.: Within 30 minutes

Elimination: With normal renal function, about 90% to 95% of dose is excreted in urine within 24 hours

The pharmacokinetics of the aminoglycosides are heterogeneous in older adults. It is best to assume that clearance is reduced and half-life prolonged in older adults, while volume of distribution is usually unchanged. The establishment of each patient's pharmacokinetic parameters is important for proper dosing in order to achieve an optimal therapeutic benefit and minimize the risks of toxicity. Following I.M. administration, the time to peak serum concentration was delayed in older adults.

Dosage

Geriatrics: Dosage should be based on an estimate of ideal body weight.

I.M., I.V.: 1.5-5 mg/kg/day in 1-2 divided doses

I.V.: Once daily or extended interval: 5-7 mg/kg/dose given every 24, 36, or 48 hours based on Cl_{cr} (see Dosage: Renal Impairment and Special Geriatric Considerations).

Adults: Note: Individualization is **critical** because of the low therapeutic index.

Use of ideal body weight (IBW) for determining the mg/kg/dose appears to be more accurate than dosing on the basis of total body weight (TBW). In morbid obesity, dosage requirement may best be estimated using a dosing weight of IBW + 0.4 (TBW - IBW).

Initial and periodic plasma drug levels (eg, peak and trough with conventional dosing) should be determined, particularly in critically-ill patients with serious infections or in disease states known to significantly alter aminoglycoside pharmacokinetics (eg, cystic fibrosis, burns, or major surgery).

Severe life-threatening infections: I.M., I.V.:
Conventional: 1-2.5 mg/kg/dose every 8-12 hours; to ensure adequate peak concentrations early in therapy, higher initial dosage may be considered in selected patients when extracellular water is increased (edema, septic shock, postsurgical, and/or trauma)

Once-daily: 4-7 mg/kg/dose once daily; some clinicians recommend this approach for all patients with normal renal function; this dose is at least as efficacious with similar, if not less, toxicity than conventional dosing.

Brucellosis: I.M., I.V.: 240 mg (I.M.) daily or 5 mg/kg (I.V.) daily for 7 days; either regimen recommended in combination with doxycycline

Cholangitis: I.M., I.V.: 4-6 mg/kg once daily with ampicillin

Diverticulitis, complicated: I.M., I.V.: 1.5-2 mg/kg every 8 hours (with ampicillin and metronidazole)

Endocarditis prophylaxis (dental, oral, upper respiratory procedures, GI/GU procedures): I.M., I.V.: 1.5 mg/kg with ampicillin (50 mg/kg) 30 minutes prior to procedure

Endocarditis or synergy (for gram-positive infections): I.M., I.V.: 1 mg/kg/dose every 8 hours (with ampicillin)

Meningitis *(Enterococcus or Pseudomonas aeruginosa)*: I.V.: 5 mg/kg/day in divided doses every 8 hours (administered with another bacteriocidal drug)

Ocular infections: Ophthalmic:
Ointment: Apply 2-3 times/day; for severe infections, apply every 3-4 hours
Solution: Instill 1-2 drops every 4 hours; for severe infections, instill 2 drops every 30-60 minutes initially, then reduce to less frequent intervals

(Continued)

Tobramycin *(Continued)*

Pelvic inflammatory disease: I.M., I.V.: Loading dose: 2 mg/kg, then 1.5 mg/kg every 8 hours **or** 4.5 mg/kg once daily

Plague *(Yersinia pestis):* I.M., I.V.: Treatment: 5 mg/kg/day, followed by postexposure prophylaxis with doxycycline

Pneumonia, hospital- or ventilator-associated: I.M., I.V.: 7 mg/kg/day (with antipseudomonal beta-lactam or carbapenem)

Pulmonary infections: Inhalation:
Standard aerosolized tobramycin: 60-80 mg 3 times/day
High-dose regimen: 300 mg every 12 hours (do not administer doses <6 hours apart); administer in repeated cycles of 28 days on drug followed by 28 days off drug

Tularemia: I.M., I.V.: 5 mg/kg/day divided every 8 hours for 1-2 weeks

Urinary tract infection: I.M., I.V.: 1.5 mg/kg/dose every 8 hours

Renal Impairment: I.M., I.V.:
Conventional dosing:
Cl_{cr} ≥60 mL/minute: Administer every 8 hours.
Cl_{cr} 40-60 mL/minute: Administer every 12 hours.
Cl_{cr} 20-40 mL/minute: Administer every 24 hours.
Cl_{cr} 10-20 mL/minute: Administer every 48 hours.
Cl_{cr} <10 mL/minute: Administer every 72 hours.

High-dose therapy: Interval may be extended (eg, every 48 hours) in patients with moderate renal impairment (Cl_{cr} 30-59 mL/minute) and/or adjusted based on serum level determinations.

Dialyzable; 30% removal of aminoglycosides occurs during 4 hours of HD - administer dose after dialysis and follow levels.

Continuous arteriovenous or venovenous hemofiltration: Dose as for Cl_{cr} of 10-40 mL/minute and follow levels.

Administration via CAPD fluid:
Gram-negative infection: 4-8 mg/L (4-8 mcg/mL) of CAPD fluid
Gram-positive infection (ie, synergy): 3-4 mg/L (3-4 mcg/mL) of CAPD fluid
Administration IVPB/I.M.: Dose as for Cl_{cr} <10 mL/minute and follow levels.

Hepatic Impairment: Monitor plasma concentrations.

Administration

I.V.: Infuse over 30-60 minutes; give penicillins or cephalosporins at least 1 hour apart from tobramycin. Flush with saline before and after administration.

Inhalation (TOBI®): To be inhaled over ~15 minutes using a handheld nebulizer.

Ophthalmic: Contact lenses should not be worn during treatment of ophthalmic infections.
Ointment: Do not touch tip of tube to eye. Instill ointment into pocket between eyeball and lower lid; patient should look downward before closing eye.
Solution: Allow 5 minutes between application of "multiple-drop" therapy.
Suspension: Shake well before using; Tilt head back, instill suspension in conjunctival sac and close eye(s). Do not touch dropper to eye. Apply light finger pressure on lacrimal sac for 1 minute following instillation.

Monitoring Parameters Draw peak concentrations 30 minutes after the end of a 30-minute infusion; the trough is drawn just before the next dose; urine output; serum BUN and creatinine, signs and symptoms of infection; culture and sensitivities

Reference Range
Therapeutic:
Peak: 5-10 mcg/mL (SI: 11-21 μmol/L)
Trough: 1-1.5 mcg/mL (SI: 2-3 μmol/L)
Once daily or extended interval: Trough: <0.5 mcg/mL
Toxic:
Peak: >12 mcg/mL (SI: >21 μmol/L)
Trough: >2 mcg/mL (SI: >9 μmol/L)

Test Interactions Some penicillin derivatives may accelerate the degradation of aminoglycosides *in vitro*, leading to a potential underestimation of aminoglycoside serum concentration.

Patient Information Report symptoms of superinfection; for eye drops - no other eye drops 5-10 minutes before or after tobramycin

Additional Information Once-daily dosing: Higher peak serum drug concentration to MIC ratios, demonstrated aminoglycoside postantibiotic effect, decreased renal cortex drug uptake, and improved cost-time efficiency are supportive reasons for the use of once daily dosing regimens for aminoglycosides. Current research indicates these regimens to be as effective for nonlife-threatening infections, with no higher incidence of nephrotoxicity, than those requiring multiple daily doses. Doses are determined by calculating the entire day's dose via usual multiple dose calculation techniques and administering this quantity as a single dose. Doses are then adjusted to maintain mean serum concentrations above the MIC(s) of the causative organism(s). (Example: 2.5-5 mg/kg as a single dose; expected Cp_{max}: 10-20 mcg/mL and Cp_{min}: <1 mcg/mL).

Further research is needed for universal recommendation in all patient populations and gram-negative disease; exceptions may include those with known high clearance (eg, patients with cystic fibrosis or burns who may require shorter dosage intervals) and patients with renal function impairment for whom longer than conventional dosage intervals are usually required.

Special Geriatric Considerations The aminoglycosides are an important therapeutic intervention for susceptible organisms and as empiric therapy in seriously ill patients. Their use is not without risk of toxicity; however, these risks can be minimized if initial dosing is adjusted for estimated renal function and appropriate monitoring is performed. High dose, once daily aminoglycosides have been advocated as an alternative to traditional dosing regimens. Once daily or extended interval dosing is as effective and may be safer than traditional dosing. Interval must be adjusted for renal function.

Dosage Forms Excipient information presented when available (limited, particularly for generics); consult specific product labeling.

Infusion [premixed in NS]: 60 mg (50 mL); 80 mg (100 mL)

Injection, powder for reconstitution: 1.2 g

Injection, solution: 10 mg/mL (2 mL, 8 mL); 40 mg/mL (2 mL, 30 mL, 50 mL) [may contain sodium metabisulfite]

Ointment, ophthalmic (Tobrex®): 0.3% (3.5 g)

Solution for nebulization [preservative free] (TOBI®): 60 mg/mL (5 mL)

Solution, ophthalmic (AKTob®, Tobrex®): 0.3% (5 mL) [contains benzalkonium chloride]

Selected References

Bauer LA and Blouin RA, "Influence of Age on Tobramycin. Pharmacokinetics in Patients With Normal Renal Function," *Antimicrob Agents Chemother*, 1981, 20(5):587-9.

Matzke GR, Jameson JJ, and Halstenson CE, "Gentamicin Disposition in Young and Elderly Patients With Various Degrees of Renal Function," *J Clin Pharmacol*, 1987, 27(3):216-20.

Mayer PR, Brown CH, Carter RA, et al, "Intramuscular Tobramycin Pharmacokinetics in Geriatric Patients," *Drug Intell Clin Pharm*, 1986, 20(7-8):611-5.

Nicolau DP, Freeman CD, Belliveau PP, et al, "Experience With a Once-Daily Aminoglycoside Program Administered to 2184 Adult Patients," *Antimicrob Agents Chemother*, 1995, 39(3):650-5.

Preston SL and Briceland LL, "Single Daily Dosing of Aminoglycosides," *Pharmacotherapy*, 1995, 15(3):297-316.

Zaske DE, Irvine P, Strand LM, et al, "Wide Interpatient Variations in Gentamicin Dose Requirements for Geriatric Patients," *JAMA*, 1982, 248(23):3122-6.

Tobramycin and Dexamethasone
(toe bra MYE sin & deks a METH a sone)

Related Information
Dexamethasone *on page 413*
Tobramycin *on page 1583*

Medication Safety Issues
Sound-alike/look-alike issues:
TobraDex® may be confused with Tobrex®

U.S. Brand Names TobraDex®

Canadian Brand Names Tobradex®

Index Terms Dexamethasone and Tobramycin

Generic Available No

Pharmacologic Category Antibiotic/Corticosteroid, Ophthalmic

Use Treatment of external ocular infection caused by susceptible gram-negative bacteria and steroid responsive inflammatory conditions of the palpebral and bulbar conjunctiva, lid, cornea, and anterior segment of the globe

Dosage
Geriatrics & Adults: Ocular infection/inflammation: Ophthalmic: Instill 1-2 drops of solution every 4 hours; apply ointment 2-3 times/day; for severe infections apply ointment every 3-4 hours, or solution 2 drops every 30-60 minutes initially, then reduce to less frequent intervals

Special Geriatric Considerations Assess patient's ability to correctly self-administer eye drops.

Dosage Forms Excipient information presented when available (limited, particularly for generics); consult specific product labeling.

Ointment, ophthalmic: Tobramycin 0.3% and dexamethasone 0.1% (3.5 g)

Suspension, ophthalmic: Tobramycin 0.3% and dexamethasone 0.1% (2.5 mL, 5 mL, 10 mL) [contains benzalkonium chloride]

♦ **Tobramycin and Loteprednol Etabonate** *see* Loteprednol and Tobramycin *on page 936*

♦ **Tobramycin Sulfate** *see* Tobramycin *on page 1583*

♦ **Tobrex®** *see* Tobramycin *on page 1583*

♦ **Tofranil®** *see* Imipramine *on page 792*

♦ **Tofranil-PM®** *see* Imipramine *on page 792*

TOLAZamide (tole AZ a mide)

Medication Safety Issues
Sound-alike/look-alike issues:
TOLAZamide may be confused with tolazoline, TOLBUTamide
Tolinase® may be confused with Orinase®

High alert medication: The Institute for Safe Medication Practices (ISMP) includes this medication among its list of drugs which have a heightened risk of causing significant patient harm when used in error.

Canadian Brand Names Tolinase®

Generic Available Yes

Pharmacologic Category Antidiabetic Agent, Sulfonylurea

Use Adjunct to diet for the management of mild to moderately severe, stable, noninsulin-dependent (type II) diabetes mellitus

Contraindications Hypersensitivity to tolazamide, sulfonylureas, or any component of the formulation; type 1 diabetes mellitus (insulin dependent, IDDM) therapy; diabetic ketoacidosis

Warnings/Precautions All sulfonylurea drugs are capable of producing severe hypoglycemia. Hypoglycemia is more likely to occur when caloric intake is deficient, after severe or prolonged exercise, when ethanol is ingested, or when more than one glucose-lowering drug is used. It is also more likely in elderly patients, malnourished patients and in patients with impaired renal or hepatic function; use with caution.

Chemical similarities are present among sulfonamides, sulfonylureas, carbonic anhydrase inhibitors, thiazides, and loop diuretics (except ethacrynic acid). Use in patients with sulfonylurea allergy is specifically contraindicated in product labeling, however, a risk of cross-reaction exists in patients with allergy to any of these compounds; avoid use when previous reaction has been severe.

Product labeling states oral hypoglycemic drugs may be associated with an increased cardiovascular mortality as compared to treatment with diet alone or diet plus insulin. Data to support this association are limited, and several studies, including a large prospective trial (UKPDS) have not supported an association.

It may be necessary to discontinue therapy and administer insulin if the patient is exposed to stress (fever, trauma, infection, surgery).

Adverse Reactions (Reflective of adult population; not specific for elderly)
Frequency not defined.
Central nervous system: Dizziness, fatigue, headache, malaise, vertigo
Dermatologic: Maculopapular eruptions, morbilliform eruptions, photosensitivity, pruritus, rash, urticaria
Endocrine & metabolic: Disulfiram-like reaction, hypoglycemia, hyponatremia, SIADH
Gastrointestinal: Anorexia, constipation, diarrhea, epigastric fullness, heartburn, nausea, vomiting
Hematologic: Agranulocytosis, aplastic anemia, hemolytic anemia, leukopenia, pancytopenia, porphyria cutanea tarda, thrombocytopenia
Hepatic: Cholestatic jaundice, hepatic porphyria
Neuromuscular & skeletal: Weakness
Renal: Diuretic effect

Drug Interactions
Beta-blockers: Beta-blockers may enhance the hypoglycemic effect of tolazamide and mask tachycardia as an initial symptom of hypoglycemia.
Chloramphenicol: Chloramphenicol may decrease the metabolism of tolazamide.
Cimetidine: Cimetidine may decrease the metabolism, via CYP isoenzymes, of tolazamide.
Cyclic antidepressants: Cyclic antidepressants may enhance the hypoglycemic effect of tolazamide.
Cyclosporine: Tolazamide may increase the serum concentration of cyclosporine.
Fibric acid derivatives: Fibric acid derivatives may enhance the hypoglycemic effect of tolazamide.
Fluconazole: Fluconazole may increase the serum concentration of tolazamide.
Pegvisomant: Pegvisomant may enhance the hypoglycemic effect of tolazamide.
Rifampin: Rifampin may increase the metabolism, via CYP isoenzymes, of tolazamide.
Salicylates: Salicylates may enhance the hypoglycemic effect of tolazamide. Of concern with regular, higher doses of salicylates, not sporadic, low doses.
Sulfonamide derivatives (sulfadiazine, sulfadoxine, sulfamethoxazole, sulfisoxazole): Sulfonamide derivatives (except sulfacetamide) may enhance the hypoglycemic effect of tolazamide.

Ethanol/Nutrition/Herb Interactions
Ethanol: Avoid ethanol (possible disulfiram-like reaction).
Herb/Nutraceutical: Herbs with hypoglycemic properties may enhance the hypoglycemic effect of tolazamide. This includes alfalfa, aloe, bilberry, bitter melon, burdock,

celery, damiana, fenugreek, garcinia, garlic, ginger, ginseng (American), gymnema, marshmallow, stinging nettle.

Mechanism of Action Stimulates insulin release from the pancreatic beta cells; reduces glucose output from the liver; insulin sensitivity is increased at peripheral target sites

Pharmacodynamics

Onset of hypoglycemic effect: 20 minutes
Peak hypoglycemic effect: 4-6 hours
Duration: 10-24 hours

Pharmacokinetics

Absorption: Rapid
Protein binding: 94%
Metabolism: Extensively hepatic to 5 metabolites (activity 0% to 70%)
Half-life elimination: 7 hours
Time to peak, serum: 3-4 hours
Excretion: Urine (85%); feces (7%)

Dosage

Geriatrics & Adults:

Type 2 diabetes: Oral (doses >500 mg/day should be given in 2 divided doses):
Initial: 100-250 mg/day with breakfast or the first main meal of the day
Fasting blood sugar <200 mg/dL: 100 mg/day
Fasting blood sugar >200 mg/dL: 250 mg/day
Patient is malnourished, underweight, elderly, or not eating properly: 100 mg/day
Adjustment/titration: Increase in increments of 100-250 mg/day at weekly intervals to response; maximum daily dose: 1 g (doses >1 g/day are not likely to improve control)

Conversion from insulin to tolazamide
<20 units day = 100 mg/day
21- <40 units/day = 250 mg/day
≥40 units/day = 250 mg/day and 50% of insulin dose

Renal Impairment: Conservative initial and maintenance doses are recommended because tolazamide is metabolized to active metabolites, which are eliminated in the urine.

Hepatic Impairment: Conservative initial and maintenance doses and careful monitoring of blood glucose are recommended.

Monitoring Parameters Fasting blood glucose; hemoglobin A_{1c}, or fructosamine

Reference Range Recommendations for glycemic control in adults with diabetes:
Hb A_{1c}: <7%
Preprandial capillary plasma glucose: 90-130 mg/dL
Peak postprandial capillary blood glucose: <180 mg/dL
Blood pressure: <130/80 mm Hg

Patient Information Tablets may be crushed; take drug at the same time each day; avoid alcohol; recognize signs and symptoms of hypoglycemia; avoid hypoglycemia, eat regularly, do not skip meals; carry a quick sugar source; medical alert bracelet

Additional Information Transferring a patient from one sulfonylurea to another does not require a priming dose; doses >1000 mg/day normally do not improve diabetic control.

Special Geriatric Considerations Has not been studied in elderly patients, however, except for drug interactions it appears to have a safe profile and decline in renal function does not affect its pharmacokinetics. How "tightly" an elderly patient's blood glucose should be controlled is controversial; however, a fasting blood sugar of <150 mg/dL is now an acceptable endpoint. Such a decision should be based on the patient's functional and cognitive status, how well they recognize hypoglycemic or hyperglycemic symptoms, and how to respond to them and their other disease states.

Dosage Forms Excipient information presented when available (limited, particularly for generics); consult specific product labeling.
Tablet: 100 mg, 250 mg, 500 mg

Selected References
"Standards of Medical Care for Patients With Diabetes Mellitus. American Diabetes Association," *Diabetes Care,* 2007, 30(Suppl 1):4-41.

TOLBUTamide (tole BYOO ta mide)

Medication Safety Issues

Sound-alike/look-alike issues:
TOLBUTamide may be confused with terbutaline, TOLAZamide
Orinase® may be confused with Orabase®, Ornex®, Tolinase®

High alert medication: The Institute for Safe Medication Practices (ISMP) includes this medication among its list of drugs which have a heightened risk of causing significant patient harm when used in error.
(Continued)

TOLBUTamide (Continued)

Canadian Brand Names Apo-Tolbutamide®

Index Terms Tolbutamide Sodium

Generic Available Yes

Pharmacologic Category Antidiabetic Agent, Sulfonylurea

Use Adjunct to diet for the management of mild to moderately severe, stable, noninsulin-dependent (type II) diabetes mellitus

Contraindications Hypersensitivity to tolbutamide, sulfonylureas, or any component of the formulation; treatment of type 1 diabetes; diabetic ketoacidosis

Warnings/Precautions All sulfonylurea drugs are capable of producing severe hypoglycemia. Hypoglycemia is more likely to occur when caloric intake is deficient, after severe or prolonged exercise, when ethanol is ingested, or when more than one glucose-lowering drug is used. It is also more likely in elderly patients, malnourished patients and in patients with impaired renal or hepatic function; use with caution.

Chemical similarities are present among sulfonamides, sulfonylureas, carbonic anhydrase inhibitors, thiazides, and loop diuretics (except ethacrynic acid). Use in patients with sulfonylurea allergy is specifically contraindicated in product labeling, however, a risk of cross-reaction exists in patients with allergy to any of these compounds; avoid use when previous reaction has been severe.

Product labeling states oral hypoglycemic drugs may be associated with an increased cardiovascular mortality as compared to treatment with diet alone or diet plus insulin. Data to support this association are limited, and several studies, including a large prospective trial (UKPDS) have not supported an association.

It may be necessary to discontinue therapy and administer insulin if the patient is exposed to stress (fever, trauma, infection, surgery).

Adverse Reactions (Reflective of adult population; not specific for elderly) Frequency not defined.

Central nervous system: Headache

Dermatologic: Erythema, maculopapular rash, morbilliform rash, pruritus, urticaria, photosensitivity

Endocrine & metabolic: Disulfiram-like reactions, hypoglycemia, hyponatremia, SIADH

Gastrointestinal: Epigastric fullness, heartburn, nausea, taste alteration

Hematologic: Agranulocytosis, aplastic anemia, hemolytic anemia, leukopenia, pancytopenia, thrombocytopenia

Hepatic: Cholestatic jaundice, hepatic porphyria, porphyria cutanea tarda

Miscellaneous: Hypersensitivity reaction

Overdosage/Toxicology Symptoms include low blood sugar, tingling of lips and tongue, nausea, yawning, confusion, agitation, tachycardia, sweating, convulsions, stupor, and coma. Treatment includes I.V. glucose (12.5-25 g) for decrease in glucose and epinephrine for anaphylaxis.

Drug Interactions Substrate of CYP2C9 (major), 2C19 (minor); **Inhibits** CYP2C8 (weak), 2C9 (strong)

Beta-blockers: Beta-blockers may enhance the hypoglycemic effect of tolbutamide and mask tachycardia as an initial symptom of hypoglycemia.

Chloramphenicol: Chloramphenicol may decrease the metabolism of tolbutamide.

Cimetidine: Cimetidine may decrease the metabolism, via CYP isoenzymes, of tolbutamide.

Cyclic antidepressants: Cyclic antidepressants may enhance the hypoglycemic effect of tolbutamide.

Cyclosporine: tolbutamide may increase the serum concentration of cyclosporine.

CYP2C9 inducers: May decrease the levels/effects of tolbutamide. Example inducers include carbamazepine, phenobarbital, phenytoin, rifampin, rifapentine, and secobarbital.

CYP2C9 inhibitors may increase the levels/effects of tolbutamide. Example inhibitors include delavirdine, fluconazole, gemfibrozil, ketoconazole, nicardipine, NSAIDs, and sulfonamides.

CYP2C9 substrates: Tolbutamide may increase the levels/effects of CYP2C9 substrates. Example substrates include bosentan, dapsone, fluoxetine, glimepiride, glipizide, losartan, montelukast, nateglinide, paclitaxel, phenytoin, warfarin, and zafirlukast.

Fibric acid derivatives: Fibric acid derivatives may enhance the hypoglycemic effect of tolbutamide.

Fluconazole: Fluconazole may increase the serum concentration of tolbutamide.

Pegvisomant: Pegvisomant may enhance the hypoglycemic effect of tolbutamide.

Rifampin: Rifampin may increase the metabolism, via CYP isoenzymes, of tolbutamide.

Salicylates: Salicylates may enhance the hypoglycemic effect of tolbutamide. Of concern with regular, higher doses of salicylates, not sporadic, low doses.

Sulfonamide derivatives (sulfadiazine, sulfadoxine, sulfamethoxazole, sulfisoxazole): Sulfonamide derivatives (except sulfacetamide) may enhance the hypoglycemic effect of tolbutamide.

Ethanol/Nutrition/Herb Interactions

Ethanol: Avoid ethanol (possible disulfiram-like reaction).

Herb/Nutraceutical: Herbs with hypoglycemic properties may enhance the hypoglycemic effect of tolbutamide. This includes alfalfa, aloe, bilberry, bitter melon, burdock, celery, damiana, fenugreek, garcinia, garlic, ginger, ginseng (American), gymnema, marshmallow, stinging nettle.

Mechanism of Action Stimulates insulin release from the pancreatic beta cells; reduces glucose output from the liver; insulin sensitivity is increased at peripheral target sites, suppression of glucagon may also contribute

Pharmacodynamics

Onset of action: 1 hour

Duration: Oral: 6-24 hours

Pharmacokinetics

Absorption: Oral: Rapid

Distribution: V_d: 0.15 L/kg

Protein binding: ~95% (concentration dependent)

Metabolism: Hepatic via CYP2C9 to hydroxymethyltolbutamide (mildly active) and carboxytolbutamide (inactive); metabolism does not appear to be affected by age

Half-life elimination: 4.5-6.5 hours (range: 4-25 hours)

Time to peak, serum: 3-4 hours

Excretion: Urine (75% to 85% primarily as metabolites); feces

Dosage

Geriatrics: Initial: 250 mg 1-3 times/day; usual: 500-2000 mg; maximum: 3 g/day

Adults:

Type 2 diabetes: Oral: Initial: 1-2 g/day as a single dose in the morning or in divided doses throughout the day. Maintenance dose: 0.25-3 g/day; however, a maintenance dose >2 g/day is seldom required. **Note:** Divided doses may improve gastrointestinal tolerance

Renal Impairment: Adjustment is not necessary.

Hemodialysis: Not dialyzable (0% to 5%)

Hepatic Impairment: Reduced dose may be necessary.

Administration Oral: Entire dose can be administered in AM, divided doses may improve GI tolerance

Monitoring Parameters Blood glucose, hemoglobin A_{1c}; signs and symptoms of hypoglycemia

Reference Range Recommendations for glycemic control in adults with diabetes:

Hb A_{1c}: <7%

Preprandial capillary plasma glucose: 90-130 mg/dL

Peak postprandial capillary blood glucose: <180 mg/dL

Blood pressure: <130/80 mm Hg

Patient Information Fast the night before the test

Special Geriatric Considerations Because of its low potency and short duration, it is a useful agent in elderly if drug interactions can be avoided. How "tightly" an elderly patient's blood glucose should be controlled is controversial; however, a fasting blood sugar <150 mg/dL is now an acceptable endpoint. Such a decision should be based on the patient's functional and cognitive status, how well they recognize hypoglycemic or hyperglycemic symptoms, and how to respond to them and their other disease states.

Dosage Forms Excipient information presented when available (limited, particularly for generics); consult specific product labeling.

Tablet: 500 mg

Selected References

Miller AK, Adir J, and Vestal RE, "Effect of Age on the Pharmacokinetics of Tolbutamide in Man," *Pharmacologist,* 1977, 19:128.

Miller AK, Adir J, and Vestal RE, "Tolbutamide Binding to Plasma Proteins of Young and Old Human Subjects," *J Pharm Sci,* 1978, 67(8):1192-3.

"Standards of Medical Care for Patients With Diabetes Mellitus. American Diabetes Association," *Diabetes Care,* 2007, 30(Suppl 1):4-41.

♦ **Tolbutamide Sodium** see TOLBUTamide on page 1589

Tolcapone (TOLE ka pone)

Related Information

Antiparkinsonian Agents on page 1745

U.S. Brand Names Tasmar®

Generic Available No

(Continued)

Tolcapone *(Continued)*

Pharmacologic Category Anti-Parkinson's Agent, COMT Inhibitor

Use Adjunct to levodopa and carbidopa for the treatment of signs and symptoms of idiopathic Parkinson's disease in patients with motor fluctuations not responsive to other therapies

Restrictions A patient signed consent form acknowledging the risks of hepatic injury should be obtained by the treating physician.

Contraindications Hypersensitivity to tolcapone or any component of the formulation; history of liver disease or tolcapone-induced hepatocellular injury; nontraumatic rhabdomyolysis or hyperpyrexia and confusion

Warnings/Precautions [U.S. Boxed Warning]: Due to reports of fatal liver injury associated with use of this drug, the manufacturer is advising that tolcapone be reserved for patients who are experiencing inadequate symptom control or who are not appropriate candidates for other available treatments. Patients must provide written consent acknowledging the risks of hepatic injury. Liver disease should be excluded prior to initiation; laboratory monitoring is recommended. Discontinue if signs and/or symptoms of hepatic injury are noted (eg, transaminases >2 times upper limit of normal) or if clinical improvement is not evident after 3 weeks of therapy. Use with caution in patients with pre-existing dyskinesias; exacerbation of pre-existing dyskinesia and severe rhabdomyolysis has been reported. Levodopa dosage reduction may be required, particularly in patients with levodopa dosages >600 mg daily or with moderate-to-severe dyskinesia prior to initiation.

May cause orthostatic hypotension and syncope; Parkinson's disease patients appear to have an impaired capacity to respond to a postural challenge; use with caution in patients at risk of hypotension (such as those receiving antihypertensive drugs) or where transient hypotensive episodes would be poorly tolerated (cardiovascular disease or cerebrovascular disease). Parkinson's patients being treated with dopaminergic agonists ordinarily require careful monitoring for signs and symptoms of postural hypotension, especially during dose escalation, and should be informed of this risk. May cause hallucinations, which may improve with reduction in levodopa therapy. Use with caution in patients with lower gastrointestinal disease or an increased risk of dehydration; tolcapone has been associated with delayed development of diarrhea (onset after 2-12 weeks).

Tolcapone, in conjunction with other drug therapy that alters brain biogenic amine concentrations (eg, MAO inhibitors, SSRIs), has been associated with a syndrome resembling neuroleptic malignant syndrome (hyperpyrexia and confusion - some fatal) on abrupt withdrawal or dosage reduction. Concomitant use of tolcapone and nonselective MAO inhibitors should be avoided. Selegiline is a selective MAO type B inhibitor (when given orally at ≤10 mg/day) and can be taken with tolcapone. Dopaminergic agents from the ergot class have also been associated with fibrotic complications, such as retroperitoneal fibrosis, pulmonary infiltrates or effusion and pleural thickening. Use caution in patients with hepatic impairment or severe renal impairment.

Adverse Reactions (Reflective of adult population; not specific for elderly)
>10%:
  Cardiovascular: Orthostatic hypotension (17%)
  Central nervous system: Sleep disorder (24% to 25%), excessive dreaming (16% to 21%), somnolence (14% to 32%), hallucinations (8% to 24%) dizziness (6% to 13%), headache (10% to 11%), confusion (10% to 11%)
  Gastrointestinal: Nausea (28% to 50%), anorexia (19% to 23%), diarrhea (16% to 34%; approximately 3% to 4% severe)
  Neuromuscular & skeletal: Dyskinesia (42% to 51%), dystonia (19% to 22%), muscle cramps (17% to 18%)
1% to 10%:
  Cardiovascular: Syncope (4% to 5%), chest pain (1% to 3%), hypotension (2%), palpitation
  Central nervous system: Fatigue (3% to 7%), loss of balance (2% to 3%), agitation (1%), euphoria (1%), hyperactivity (1%), malaise (1%), panic reaction (1%), irritability (1%), mental deficiency (1%), fever (1%), depression, hypoesthesia, tremor, speech disorder, vertigo, emotional lability, hyperkinesia
  Dermatologic: Alopecia (1%), bleeding (1%), tumor (1%), rash
  Gastrointestinal: Vomiting (8% to 10%), constipation (6% to 8%), xerostomia (5% to 6%), abdominal pain (5% to 6%), dyspepsia (3% to 4%), flatulence (2% to 4%), tooth disorder
  Genitourinary: UTI (5%), hematuria (4% to 5%), urine discoloration (2% to 3%), urination disorder (1% to 2%), uterine tumor (1%), incontinence, impotence
  Hepatic: Transaminases increased (1% to 3%; 3 times ULN, usually with first 6 months of therapy)
  Neuromuscular & skeletal: Paresthesia (1% to 3%), hyper-/hypokinesia (1% to 3%), arthritis (1% to 2%), neck pain (2%), stiffness (2%), myalgia, rhabdomyolysis
  Ocular: Cataract (1%), eye inflammation (1%)

Otic: Tinnitus

Respiratory: Upper respiratory infection (5% to 7%), dyspnea (3%), sinus congestion (1% to 2%), bronchitis, pharyngitis

Miscellaneous: Diaphoresis (4% to 7%), influenza (3% to 4%), burning (1% to 2%), flank pain, injury, infection

Overdosage/Toxicology No information is available regarding intentional overdose with tolcapone. The highest dose evaluated clinically was 800 mg 3 times/day, with side effects consisting primarily of nausea/vomiting, and dizziness. Treatment should be supportive and symptom-directed. Dialysis not likely to benefit.

Drug Interactions Inhibits CYP2C9 (weak)

COMT substrates (eg, apomorphine, bitolterol, dobutamine, dopamine, epinephrine, norepinephrine, isoproterenol, isoetharine, and methyldopa): Tolcapone may decrease the metabolism and increase the side effects of these agents.

CNS depressants: Effects on mental status may be additive with other CNS depressants; includes barbiturates, benzodiazepines, TCAs, antipsychotics, ethanol, opioid analgesics, and other sedative-hypnotics.

MAO inhibitors: Concurrent use of nonselective MAO inhibitors with tolcapone may increase the risk of cardiovascular side effects; selective MAO inhibitors (eg, oral selegiline ≤10 mg/day) appear to pose limited risk.

Ethanol/Nutrition/Herb Interactions

Ethanol: Avoid ethanol (may increase CNS depression).

Food: Tolcapone, taken with food within 1 hour before or 2 hours after the dose, decreases bioavailability by 10% to 20%.

Avoid valerian, St John's wort, kava kava, gotu kola (may increase CNS depression).

Stability Store at 20°C to 25°C (68°F to 77°F).

Mechanism of Action Tolcapone is a selective and reversible inhibitor of catechol-o-methyltransferase (COMT). In the presence of a decarboxylase inhibitor (eg, carbidopa), COMT is the major degradation pathway for levodopa. Inhibition of COMT leads to more sustained plasma levels of levodopa and enhanced central dopaminergic activity.

Pharmacokinetics

Absorption: Rapid

Distribution: 9 L

Protein binding: >99.0%

Metabolism: Hepatic, via glucuronidation, to inactive metabolite (>99%)

Bioavailability: Oral: 65%

Half-life: 2-3 hours

Time to peak serum: Within 2 hours

Excretion: Urine (60% as metabolites, 0.5% as unchanged drug); feces (40%)

Dosage

Geriatrics & Adults: Note: If clinical improvement is not observed after 3 weeks of therapy (regardless of dose), tolcapone treatment should be discontinued.

Parkinson's Disease: Oral: Initial: 100 mg 3 times/day; may increase as tolerated to 200 mg 3 times/day. **Note:** Levodopa dose may need to be decreased upon initiation of tolcapone (average reduction in clinical trials was 30%). As many as 70% of patients receiving levodopa doses >600 mg daily required levodopa dosage reduction in clinical trials. Patients with moderate-to-severe dyskinesia prior to initiation are also more likely to require dosage reduction.

Renal Impairment: No adjustment necessary for mild-moderate impairment. Use caution with severe impairment; no safety information available in patients with Cl_{cr}<25 mL/minute.

Hepatic Impairment: Do not use. Discontinue immediately if signs/symptoms of hepatic impairment develop.

Administration May be administered with or without food. In clinical studies, the first dose of the day was given with levodopa/carbidopa and the subsequent doses were given 6 hours and 12 hours later.

Monitoring Parameters Blood pressure, symptoms of Parkinson's disease, liver enzymes at baseline and then every 2-4 weeks for the first 6 months of therapy; thereafter, periodic monitoring should be conducted as deemed clinically relevant. If the dose is increased to 200 mg 3 times/day, reinitiate LFT monitoring every 2-4 weeks for 6 months, and then resume periodic monitoring. Discontinue therapy if the ALT or AST exceeds 2 times ULN or if the clinical signs and symptoms suggest the onset of liver failure.

Patient Information Report persistent nausea, fatigue, lethargy, anorexia, jaundice, itching, right upper quadrant pain, or dark urine to physician. Report hypotension, falls, difficulty with movement and abnormal muscle, head, neck, or trunk contractions. Use extreme caution when driving a car or operating machinery.

Additional Information If no significant response in 3 weeks, discontinue tolcapone. Patient informed consent forms can be obtained from the manufacturer.

Special Geriatric Considerations No specific data in elderly patients, but based on the pharmacokinetic profile, no dosage adjustment appears necessary.

(Continued)

Tolcapone *(Continued)*

Dosage Forms Excipient information presented when available (limited, particularly for generics); consult specific product labeling.
Tablet:
Tasmar®: 100 mg, 200 mg

Selected References

Olanow CW, Watts RL, and Koller WC, "An Algorithm (Decision Tree) for the Management of Parkinson's Disease (2001): Treatment Guidelines," *Neurology,* 2001, 56(11 Suppl 5):S1-S88.

Pahwa R, Factor SA, Lyons KE, et al, "Practice Parameter: Treatment of Parkinson Disease With Motor Fluctuations and Dyskinesia (An Evidence-Based Review): Report of the Quality Standards Subcommittee of the American Academy of Neurology," *Neurology,* 2006, 66(7):983-95.

♦ Tolectin® *see* Tolmetin *on page 1594*

Tolmetin *(TOLE met in)*

U.S. Brand Names Tolectin®
Index Terms Tolmetin Sodium
Generic Available Yes
Pharmacologic Category Nonsteroidal Anti-inflammatory Drug (NSAID), Oral
Use Treatment of rheumatoid arthritis and osteoarthritis, juvenile rheumatoid arthritis, sunburn, mild to moderate pain
Restrictions An FDA-approved medication guide must be distributed when dispensing an oral outpatient prescription (new or refill) where this medication is to be used without direct supervision of a healthcare provider. Medication guides are available at http://www.fda.gov/cder/Offices/ODS/medication_guides.htm.
Contraindications Hypersensitivity to tolmetin, aspirin, other NSAIDs, or any component of the formulation; perioperative pain in the setting of coronary artery bypass surgery (CABG)
Warnings/Precautions [U.S. Boxed Warning]: NSAIDs are associated with an increased risk of adverse cardiovascular events, including MI, stroke, and new onset or worsening of pre-existing hypertension. Risk may be increased with duration of use or pre-existing cardiovascular risk factors or disease. Carefully evaluate individual cardiovascular risk profiles prior to prescribing. Use caution with fluid retention, CHF or hypertension. Concurrent administration of ibuprofen, and potentially other nonselective NSAIDs, may interfere with aspirin's cardioprotective effect.

Use of NSAIDs can compromise existing renal function. Renal toxicity can occur in patient with impaired renal function, dehydration, heart failure, liver dysfunction, those taking diuretics and ACEI and the elderly. Rehydrate patient before starting therapy. Monitor renal function closely. Use caution in patients with advanced renal disease.

[U.S. Boxed Warning]: NSAIDs may increase risk of gastrointestinal irritation, ulceration, bleeding, and perforation. These events may occur at any time during therapy and without warning. Use caution with a history of GI disease (bleeding or ulcers), concurrent therapy with aspirin, anticoagulants and/or corticosteroids, smoking, use of alcohol, the elderly or debilitated patients.

Use the lowest effective dose for the shortest duration of time, consistent with individual patient goals, to reduce risk of cardiovascular or GI adverse events. Alternate therapies should be considered for patients at high risk.

NSAIDs may cause serious skin adverse events including exfoliative dermatitis, Stevens-Johnson syndrome (SJS) and toxic epidermal necrolysis (TEN). Anaphylactoid reactions may occur, even without prior exposure; patients with "aspirin triad" (bronchial asthma, aspirin intolerance, rhinitis) may be at increased risk. Do not use in patients who experience bronchospasm, asthma, rhinitis, or urticaria with NSAID or aspirin therapy.

Use with caution in patients with decreased hepatic function. Closely monitor patients with any abnormal LFT. Severe hepatic reactions (eg, fulminant hepatitis, liver failure) have occurred with NSAID use, rarely; discontinue if signs or symptoms of liver disease develop, or if systemic manifestations occur.

The elderly are at increased risk for adverse effects (especially peptic ulceration, CNS effects, renal toxicity) from NSAIDs even at low doses.

Withhold for at least 4-6 half-lives prior to surgical or dental procedures.
Adverse Reactions (Reflective of adult population; not specific for elderly)
1% to 10%:
Cardiovascular: Chest pain, hypertension, edema
Central nervous system: Headache, dizziness, drowsiness, depression
Dermatologic: Skin irritation
Endocrine & metabolic: Weight gain/loss
Gastrointestinal: Heartburn, abdominal pain, diarrhea, flatulence, vomiting, constipation, gastritis, peptic ulcer, nausea

Genitourinary: Urinary Tract Infection
Hematologic: Elevated BUN, transient decreases in hemoglobin/hematocrit
Ocular: Visual disturbances
Otic: Tinnitus

Overdosage/Toxicology Symptoms include lethargy, mental confusion, dizziness, leukocytosis, and renal failure. Management of nonsteroidal anti-inflammatory drug (NSAID) intoxication is primarily supportive and symptomatic. Fluid therapy is commonly effective in managing hypotension that may occur following an acute NSAID overdose, except when due to acute blood loss. Seizures tend to be very short-lived and often do not require drug treatment; although, recurrent seizures should be treated with I.V. diazepam. Since many of the NSAIDs undergo enterohepatic cycling, multiple doses of charcoal may be needed to reduce the potential for delayed toxicities.

Drug Interactions

ACE inhibitors: Antihypertensive effects may be decreased by concurrent therapy with NSAIDs; monitor blood pressure.

Angiotensin II antagonists: Antihypertensive effects may be decreased by concurrent therapy with NSAIDs; monitor blood pressure.

Anticoagulants (warfarin, heparin, LMWHs) in combination with NSAIDs can cause increased risk of bleeding.

Antiplatelet drugs (ticlopidine, clopidogrel, aspirin, abciximab, dipyridamole, eptifibatide, tirofiban) can cause an increased risk of bleeding.

Beta-blockers: NSAIDs may decrease the antihypertensive effect of beta-blockers. Monitor.

Cholestyramine (and other bile acid sequestrants): May decrease the absorption of NSAIDs. Separate by at least 2 hours.

Corticosteroids may increase the risk of GI ulceration; avoid concurrent use.

Cyclosporine: NSAIDs may increase serum creatinine, potassium, blood pressure, and cyclosporine levels; monitor cyclosporine levels and renal function carefully.

Fluoroquinolone antibiotics: Risk of seizures may be increased with concomitant quinolone use. Risk is considered quite low and may only be a factor with high serum levels of either agent and/or in patients with additional predisposing factors (eg, renal dysfunction, history of seizure or other neurological disorder).

Hydralazine's antihypertensive effect is decreased; avoid concurrent use.

Lithium levels can be increased; avoid concurrent use if possible or monitor lithium levels and adjust dose. Sulindac may have the least effect. When NSAID is stopped, lithium will need adjustment again.

Loop diuretics efficacy (diuretic and antihypertensive effect) may be reduced.

Methotrexate: Severe bone marrow suppression, aplastic anemia, and GI toxicity have been reported with concomitant NSAID therapy. Avoid use during moderate or high-dose methotrexate (increased and prolonged methotrexate levels). NSAID use during low-dose treatment of rheumatoid arthritis has not been fully evaluated; extreme caution is warranted.

Salicylates: NSAIDs (nonselective) may diminish the cardioprotective effect of acetylated salicylates. Avoid regular use of NSAIDs if possible; consider alternatives (eg, acetaminophen). Give salicylate before NSAID; aspirin (immediate release) should be given 30-120 minutes before ibuprofen for example.

Thiazides antihypertensive effects are decreased; avoid concurrent use.

Warfarin's INRs may be increased by piroxicam. Other NSAIDs may have the same effect depending on dose and duration. Monitor INR closely. Use the lowest dose of NSAIDs possible and for the briefest duration.

Ethanol/Nutrition/Herb Interactions

Ethanol: Avoid ethanol (may enhance gastric mucosal irritation).

Food: Tolmetin peak serum concentrations may be decreased if taken with food or milk.

Herb/Nutraceutical: Avoid alfalfa, anise, bilberry, bladderwrack, bromelain, cat's claw, celery, coleus, cordyceps, dong quai, evening primrose, feverfew, fenugreek, garlic, ginger, ginkgo biloba, red clover, horse chestnut, grapeseed, green tea, ginseng, guggul, horse chestnut seed, horseradish, licorice, prickly ash, red clover, reishi, SAMe, sweet clover, turmeric, white willow (all have additional antiplatelet activity).

Mechanism of Action Inhibits prostaglandin synthesis by decreasing the activity of the enzyme, cyclooxygenase, which results in decreased formation of prostaglandin precursors

Pharmacodynamics

Onset of analgesic action: 0.5-1 hour
Duration: 4-6 hours
Onset of anti-inflammatory action: Within 7 days; Maximum benefit: 1-2 weeks

Pharmacokinetics

Absorption: Oral: Well absorbed
Protein binding: >90%
Half-life: 1-2 hours
Time to peak serum concentration: Within 30-60 minutes
(Continued)

Tolmetin *(Continued)*

Dosage
Geriatrics & Adults:
Inflammation, arthritis: Oral: 400 mg 3 times/day; usual dose: 600 mg to 1.8 g/day; maximum: 2 g/day

Monitoring Parameters Monitor response (pain, range of motion, grip strength, mobility, ADL function), inflammation; observe for weight gain, edema; monitor renal function; observe for bleeding, bruising; evaluate gastrointestinal effects (abdominal pain, bleeding, dyspepsia); mental confusion, disorientation, CBC, serum, creatinine, BUN, liver function tests

Patient Information Serious gastrointestinal bleeding can occur as well as ulceration and perforation. Pain may or may not be present. Avoid aspirin and aspirin-containing products while taking this medication. If gastric upset occurs, take with food, milk, or antacid. If gastric adverse effects persist, contact physician. May cause drowsiness, dizziness, blurred vision, and confusion. Use caution when performing tasks which require alertness (eg, driving). Do not take for more than 3 days for fever or 10 days for pain without physician's advice.

Additional Information Only NSAID affected by food/milk, which decreases total bioavailability by 16%. If GI upset occurs with tolmetin, take with antacids other than sodium bicarbonate. Each 200 mg of tolmetin contains 0.8 mEq of sodium. There are no clinical guidelines to predict which NSAID will give response in a particular patient. Trials with each must be initiated until response determined. Consider dose, patient convenience, and cost.

Special Geriatric Considerations Elderly are a high-risk population for adverse effects from NSAIDs. As much as 60% of the elderly can develop peptic ulceration and/or hemorrhage asymptomatically. The concomitant use of H_2 blockers and sucralfate is not effective as prophylaxis with the exception of NSAID-induced duodenal ulcers which may be prevented by the use of ranitidine. Misoprostol and proton pump inhibitors are the only agents proven to help prevent the development of NSAID-induced ulcers. Also, concomitant disease and drug use contribute to the risk for GI adverse effects. Use lowest effective dose for shortest period possible. Consider renal function decline with age. Use of NSAIDs can compromise existing renal function especially when Cl_{cr} is ≤30 mL/minute. Tinnitus may be a difficult and unreliable indication of toxicity due to age-related hearing loss or eighth cranial nerve damage. CNS adverse effects such as confusion, agitation, and hallucination are generally seen in overdose or high dose situations, but elderly may demonstrate these adverse effects at lower doses than younger adults.

Dosage Forms Excipient information presented when available (limited, particularly for generics); consult specific product labeling.
Capsule: 400 mg
Tablet: 200 mg, 600 mg
Tolectin®: 600 mg [contains sodium 54 mg (2.35 mEq)]

Selected References
Brooks PM and Day RO, "Nonsteroidal Anti-inflammatory Drugs - Differences and Similarities," *N Engl J Med*, 1991, 324(24):1716-25.

Clinch D, Banerjee AK, and Ostick G, "Absence of Abdominal Pain in Elderly Patients With Peptic Ulcer," *Age Ageing*, 1984, 13(2):120-3.

Clive DM and Stoff JS, "Renal Syndromes Associated With Nonsteroidal Anti-inflammatory Drugs," *N Engl J Med*, 1984, 310(9):563-72.

Graham DY, "Prevention of Gastroduodenal Injury Induced by Chronic Nonsteroidal Anti-inflammatory Drug Therapy," *Gastroenterology*, 1989, 96(2 Pt 2 Suppl):675-81.

Gurwitz JH, Avorn J, Ross-Degnan D, et al, "Nonsteroidal Anti-inflammatory Drug-Associated Azotemia in the Very Old," *JAMA*, 1990, 264(4):471-5.

Hawkey CJ, Karrasch JA, Szczepański L, et al, "Omeprazole Compared With Misoprostol for Ulcers Associated With Nonsteroidal Anti-inflammatory Drugs," *N Engl J Med*, 1998, 338(11):727-34.

Knodel LC, "Preventing NSAID-induced Ulcers: The Role of Misoprostol," *Consult Pharm*, 1989, 4:37-41.

Pounder R, "Silent Peptic Ulceration: Deadly Silence or Golden Silence?" *Gastroenterology*, 1989, 96(2 Pt 2 Suppl):626-31.

Yeomans ND, Tulassay Z, Juhasz L, et al, "A Comparison of Omeprazole With Ranitidine for Ulcers Associated With Nonsteroidal Anti-inflammatory Drugs," *N Engl J Med*, 1998, 338(11):719-26.

♦ **Tolmetin Sodium** *see* Tolmetin on page 1594

Tolnaftate *(tole NAF tate)*

Medication Safety Issues
Sound-alike/look-alike issues:
Tolnaftate may be confused with Tornalate®
Tinactin® may be confused with Talacen®

U.S. Brand Names Blis-To-Sol® [OTC]; Fungi-Guard [OTC]; Gold Bond® Antifungal [OTC] [DSC]; Mycocide® NS [OTC]; Podactin Powder [OTC]; Q-Naftate [OTC]; Tinactin® Antifungal [OTC]; Tinactin® Antifungal Jock Itch [OTC]; Tinaderm [OTC]; Ting® Cream [OTC]; Ting® Spray Liquid [OTC]

Canadian Brand Names Pitrex

Generic Available Yes: Cream, powder, solution

Pharmacologic Category Antifungal Agent, Topical

Use Treatment of tinea pedis, tinea cruris, tinea corporis

Contraindications Hypersensitivity to tolnaftate or any component of the formulation; nail and scalp infections

Warnings/Precautions For external use only; apply to clean, dry skin; keep away from eyes

Adverse Reactions (Reflective of adult population; not specific for elderly) Frequency not defined.

Dermatologic: Pruritus, contact dermatitis

Local: Irritation, stinging

Drug Interactions No data reported

Mechanism of Action Distorts the hyphae and stunts mycelial growth in susceptible fungi

Pharmacodynamics Onset of action: Response may be seen 24-72 hours after initiation of therapy

Dosage

Geriatrics & Adults: Tinea infection: Topical: Wash and dry affected area; spray aerosol or apply 1-3 drops of solution or a small amount of cream, or powder and rub into the affected areas 2 times/day

Note: May use for up to 4 weeks for tinea pedis or tinea corporis, and up to 2 weeks for tinea cruris.

Monitoring Parameters Resolution of skin infection

Patient Information Avoid contact with the eyes; apply to clean dry area; consult the physician if a skin irritation develops or if the skin infection worsens or does not improve after 10 days of therapy; does not stain skin or clothing

Additional Information Usually not effective alone for the treatment of infections involving hair follicles or nails

Special Geriatric Considerations No specific recommendations for use in the elderly.

Dosage Forms Excipient information presented when available (limited, particularly for generics); consult specific product labeling. [DSC] = Discontinued product

Aerosol, liquid, topical:

Tinactin® Antifungal: 1% (60 mL, 150 mL) [contains alcohol]

Ting®: 1% (90 mL)

Aerosol, powder, topical:

Tinactin® Antifungal: 1% (133 g) [contains alcohol]

Tinactin® Antifungal Jock Itch: 1% (100 g, 133 g) [contains alcohol]

Cream, topical: 1% (15 g, 30 g)

Fungi-Guard, Tinactin® Antifungal Jock Itch, Ting®: 1% (15 g)

Q-Naftate, Tinactin® Antifungal: 1% (15 g, 30 g)

Liquid, topical:

Blis-To-Sol®: 1% (30 mL, 55 mL)

Fungi-Guard: 1% (30 mL) [contains vitamin E and aloe; brush applicator provided]

Powder, topical: 1% (45 g)

Podactin: 1% (45 g)

Tinactin® Antifungal: 1% (108 g)

Solution, topical: 1% (10 mL)

Mycocide® NS: 1% (30 mL)

Tinaderm: 1% (10 mL)

Swab, topical [liquid-filled swabstick]:

Gold Bond® Antifungal: 1% (24s) [DSC]

Tolterodine (tole TER oh deen)

Related Information

Pharmacotherapy of Urinary Incontinence *on page 1822*

Medication Safety Issues

Sound-alike/look-alike issues:

Detrol® may be confused with Ditropan®

International issues:

Detrol® may be confused with Desurol® which is a brand name for oxolinic acid in the Czech Republic

U.S. Brand Names Detrol®; Detrol® LA

Canadian Brand Names Detrol®; Detrol® LA; Unidet®

Index Terms Tolterodine Tartrate

Generic Available No

(Continued)

Tolterodine *(Continued)*

Pharmacologic Category Anticholinergic Agent

Use Treatment of patients with an overactive bladder with symptoms of urinary frequency, urgency, or urge incontinence

Contraindications Hypersensitivity to tolterodine or any component of the formulation; urinary retention; gastric retention; uncontrolled narrow-angle glaucoma; myasthenia gravis

Warnings/Precautions Use with caution in patients with bladder flow obstruction, may increase the risk of urinary retention. Use with caution in patients with gastrointestinal obstructive disorders (ie, pyloric stenosis), may increase the risk of gastric retention. Use with caution in patients with controlled (treated) narrow-angle glaucoma; metabolized in the liver and excreted in the urine and feces, dosage adjustment is required for patients with renal or hepatic impairment. Tolterodine has been associated with QT_c prolongation at high (supratherapeutic) doses. The manufacturer recommends caution in patients with congenital prolonged QT or in patients receiving concurrent therapy with QT_c-prolonging drugs (class Ia or III antiarrhythmics). However, the mean change in QT_c even at supratherapeutic dosages was less than 15 msec. Individuals who are poor metabolizers via CYP2D6 or in the presence of inhibitors of CYP2D6 and CYP3A4 may be more likely to exhibit prolongation. Dosage adjustment is recommended in patients receiving CYP3A4 inhibitors (a lower dose of tolterodine is recommended).

Adverse Reactions (Reflective of adult population; not specific for elderly)
As reported with immediate release tablet, unless otherwise specified

>10%: Gastrointestinal: Dry mouth (35%; extended release capsules 23%)

1% to 10%:

Cardiovascular: Chest pain (2%)

Central nervous system: Headache (7%; extended release capsules 6%), somnolence (3%; extended release capsules 3%), fatigue (4%; extended release capsules 2%), dizziness (5%; extended release capsules 2%), anxiety (extended release capsules 1%)

Dermatologic: Dry skin (1%)

Gastrointestinal: Abdominal pain (5%; extended release capsules 4%), constipation (7%; extended release capsules 6%), dyspepsia (4%; extended release capsules 3%), diarrhea (4%), weight gain (1%)

Genitourinary: Dysuria (2%; extended release capsules 1%)

Neuromuscular & skeletal: Arthralgia (2%)

Ocular: Abnormal vision (2%; extended release capsules 1%), dry eyes (3%; extended release capsules 3%)

Respiratory: Bronchitis (2%), sinusitis (extended release capsules 2%)

Miscellaneous: Flu-like syndrome (3%), infection (1%)

Overdosage/Toxicology Overdosage can potentially result in severe central anticholinergic effects and should be treated accordingly. ECG monitoring is recommended in the event of overdosage. QT_c prolongation has been observed at supratherapeutic doses, particularly in CYP2D6 poor metabolizers.

Drug Interactions Substrate of CYP2C9 (minor), 2C19 (minor), 2D6 (major), 3A4 (major)

Acetylcholinesterase inhibitors (central): May reduce the therapeutic efficacy of tolterodine.

Anticholinergic agents: Concomitant use with tolterodine may increase the risk of anticholinergic side effects.

Antifungal agents (eg, ketoconazole, fluconazole): May increase the levels/effects of tolterodine; monitor.

CYP2D6 inhibitors: May increase the levels/effects of tolterodine, which may include QT_c prolongation. Example inhibitors include chlorpromazine, delavirdine, fluoxetine, miconazole, paroxetine, pergolide, quinidine, quinine, ritonavir, and ropinirole.

CYP3A4 inducers: CYP3A4 inducers may decrease the levels/effects of tolterodine. Example inducers include aminoglutethimide, carbamazepine, nafcillin, nevirapine, phenobarbital, phenytoin, and rifamycins.

CYP3A4 inhibitors: May increase the levels/effects of tolterodine, which may include QT_c prolongation. Example inhibitors include azole antifungals, clarithromycin, diclofenac, doxycycline, erythromycin, imatinib, isoniazid, nefazodone, nicardipine, propofol, protease inhibitors, quinidine, telithromycin, and verapamil.

Pramlintide: Concomitant use with tolterodine may increase the risk of anticholinergic gastrointestinal adverse effects (eg, reduced gut motility).

Warfarin: Tolterodine may increase the effects of warfarin.

Ethanol/Nutrition/Herb Interactions

Food: Increases bioavailability (~53% increase) of tolterodine tablets, but does not affect the pharmacokinetics of tolterodine extended release capsules; adjustment of dose is not needed. As a CYP3A4 inhibitor, grapefruit juice may increase the serum level and/or toxicity of tolterodine, but unlikely secondary to high oral bioavailability.

Herb/Nutraceutical: St John's wort (*Hypericum*) appears to induce CYP3A enzymes.

Stability Store at 15°C to 30°C (59°F to 86°F). Protect from light.

Mechanism of Action Tolterodine is a competitive antagonist of muscarinic receptors. In animal models, tolterodine demonstrates selectivity for urinary bladder receptors over salivary receptors. Urinary bladder contraction is mediated by muscarinic receptors. Tolterodine increases residual urine volume and decreases detrusor muscle pressure.

Pharmacokinetics
Distribution: Highly bound to alpha$_1$-acid glycoprotein
Metabolism: Extensive in the liver
Bioavailability: 77%; C_{max}: 1-2 hours after dose; food increases bioavailability
Elimination: <1% excreted unchanged in urine; 5% to 14% excreted as active metabolite
Note: Mean serum concentrations of tolterodine and its 5-hydroxy metabolite were 20% and 50% higher respectively in older adult patients as compared to young healthy volunteers

Dosage
Geriatrics & Adults: Treatment of overactive bladder: Oral:
Immediate release tablet: 2 mg twice daily; the dose may be lowered to 1 mg twice daily based on individual response and tolerability
Dosing adjustment in patients concurrently taking CYP3A4 inhibitors: 1 mg twice daily
Extended release capsule: 4 mg once a day; dose may be lowered to 2 mg daily based on individual response and tolerability
Dosing adjustment in patients concurrently taking CYP3A4 inhibitors: 2 mg daily
Renal Impairment: Use with caution (studies conducted in patients with Cl_{cr} 10-30 mL/minute):
Immediate release tablet: 1 mg twice daily
Extended release capsule: 2 mg daily
Hepatic Impairment:
Immediate release tablet: 1 mg twice daily
Extended release capsule: 2 mg daily

Monitoring Parameters Monitor incontinence episodes, postvoid residual (PVR)

Patient Information May cause blurred vision, dry eyes, dry mouth, constipation; report confusion or change in mental status

Additional Information
Tolterodine can be included in a bladder retraining program.

Special Geriatric Considerations No difference in safety has been noted between elderly and younger patients, therefore, no dosage adjustment is recommended.

Dosage Forms Excipient information presented when available (limited, particularly for generics); consult specific product labeling.
Capsule, extended release, as tartrate (Detrol® LA): 2 mg, 4 mg
Tablet, as tartrate (Detrol®): 1 mg, 2 mg

♦ **Tolterodine Tartrate** *see* Tolterodine *on page 1597*
♦ **Topamax**® *see* Topiramate *on page 1599*
♦ **Topicaine**® **[OTC]** *see* Lidocaine *on page 904*

Topiramate (toe PYRE a mate)

Medication Safety Issues
Sound-alike/look-alike issues:
Topamax® may be confused with Tegretol®, Tegretol®-XR, Toprol-XL®

U.S. Brand Names Topamax®

Canadian Brand Names Dom-Topiramate; Gen-Topiramate; Novo-Topiramate; PHL-Topiramate; PMS-Topiramate; ratio-Topiramate; Rhoxal-topiramate; Sandoz-Topiramate; Topamax®

Generic Available No

Pharmacologic Category Anticonvulsant, Miscellaneous

Use Monotherapy or adjunctive therapy for partial onset seizures and primary generalized tonic-clonic seizures; adjunctive treatment of seizures associated with Lennox-Gastaut syndrome; prophylaxis of migraine headache

Unlabeled/Investigational Use Infantile spasms, neuropathic pain, cluster headache

Contraindications Hypersensitivity to topiramate or any component of the formulation

Warnings/Precautions Use with caution in patients with hepatic, respiratory, or renal impairment. Topiramate may decrease serum bicarbonate concentrations (up to 67% of patients); treatment-emergent metabolic acidosis is less common. Risk may be increased in patients with a predisposing condition (organ dysfunction, ketogenic diet, or concurrent treatment with other drugs which may cause acidosis). Metabolic acidosis may occur at dosages as low as 50 mg/day. Monitor serum bicarbonate as well as potential complications of chronic acidosis (nephrolithiasis and osteomalacia). (Continued)

Topiramate *(Continued)*

The risk of kidney stones is about 2-4 times that of the untreated population, the risk of this event may be reduced by increasing fluid intake.

Cognitive dysfunction, psychiatric disturbances (mood disorders), and sedation (somnolence or fatigue) may occur with topiramate use; incidence may be related to rapid titration and higher doses. Topiramate may also cause paresthesia and ataxia. Topiramate has been associated with secondary angle-closure glaucoma in adults, typically within 1 month of initiation; discontinue in patients with acute onset of decreased visual acuity or ocular pain. Hyperammonemia with or without encephalopathy may occur with concomitant valproate administration; use with caution in patients with inborn errors of metabolism or decreased hepatic mitochondrial activity. Topiramate may be associated (rarely) with severe oligohydrosis and hyperthermia; use caution and monitor closely during strenuous exercise, during exposure to high environmental temperature, or in patients receiving drugs with anticholinergic activity.

Avoid abrupt withdrawal of topiramate therapy, it should be withdrawn/tapered slowly to minimize the potential of increased seizure frequency. Effects with other sedative drugs or ethanol may be potentiated.

Adverse Reactions (Reflective of adult population; not specific for elderly)
Adverse events are reported for placebo-controlled trials of adjunctive therapy in adult and pediatric patients. Unless otherwise noted, the percentages refer to incidence in epilepsy trials. Note: A wide range of dosages were studied; incidence of adverse events was frequently lower in the pediatric population studied.

>10%:
Central nervous system: Dizziness (4% to 32%), ataxia (6% to 16%), somnolence (15% to 29%), psychomotor slowing (3% to 21%), nervousness (9% to 19%), memory difficulties (2% to 14%), speech problems (2% to 13%), fatigue (9% to 30%), difficulty concentrating (5% to 14%), depression (9% to 13%), confusion (4% to 14%)
Endocrine & metabolic: Serum bicarbonate decreased (dose-related: 7% to 67%; marked reductions [to <17 mEq/L] 1% to 11%)
Gastrointestinal: Nausea (6% to 12%; migraine trial: 14%), weight loss (8% to 13%), anorexia (4% to 24%)
Neuromuscular & skeletal: Paresthesia (1% to 19%; migraine trial: 35% to 51%)
Ocular: Nystagmus (10% to 11%), abnormal vision (<1% to 13%)
Respiratory: Upper respiratory infection (migraine trial: 12% to 13%)
Miscellaneous: Injury (6% to 14%)

1% to 10%:
Cardiovascular: Chest pain (2% to 4%), edema (1% to 2%), bradycardia (1%), pallor (up to 1%), hypertension (1% to 2%)
Central nervous system: Abnormal coordination (4%), hypoesthesia (1% to 2%; migraine trial: 8%), convulsions (1%), depersonalization (1% to 2%), apathy (1% to 3%), cognitive problems (3%), emotional lability (3%), agitation (3%), aggressive reactions (2% to 9%), tremor (3% to 9%), stupor (1% to 2%), mood problems (4% to 9%), anxiety (2% to 10%), insomnia (4% to 8%), neurosis (1%), vertigo (1% to 2%)
Dermatologic: Pruritus (migraine trial: 2% to 4%), skin disorder (1% to 3%), alopecia (2%), dermatitis (up to 2%), hypertrichosis (up to 2%), rash erythematous (up to 2%), eczema (up to 1%), seborrhea (up to 1%), skin discoloration (up to 1%)
Endocrine & metabolic: Hot flashes (1% to 2%); metabolic acidosis (hyperchloremia, nonanion gap), dehydration, breast pain (up to 4%), menstrual irregularities (1% to 2%), hypoglycemia (1%), libido decreased (<1% to 2%)
Gastrointestinal: Dyspepsia (2% to 7%), abdominal pain (5% to 7%), constipation (3% to 5%), xerostomia (2% to 4%), fecal incontinence (1%), gingivitis (1%), diarrhea (2%; migraine trial: 11%), vomiting (1% to 3%), gastroenteritis (1% to 3%), appetite increased (1%), GI disorder (1%), dysgeusia (2% to 4%; migraine trial: 12% to 15%), dysphagia (1%), flatulence (1%), GERD (1%), glossitis (1%), gum hyperplasia (1%), weight increase (1%)
Genitourinary: Impotence, dysuria/incontinence (<1% to 4%), prostatic disorder (2%), UTI (2% to 3%), premature ejaculation (migraine trial: 3%), cystitis (2%)
Hematologic: Leukopenia (1% to 2%), purpura (8%), hematoma (1%), prothrombin time increased (1%), thrombocytopenia (1%)
Neuromuscular & skeletal: Myalgia (2%), weakness (3% to 6%), back pain (1% to 5%), leg pain (2% to 4%), rigors (1%), hypertonia, arthralgia (1% to 7%), gait abnormal (2% to 8%), involuntary muscle contractions (2%; migraine trial: 4%), hyperkinesia (up to 5%), skeletal pain (1% to 2%), hyporeflexia (up to 2%)
Ocular: Conjunctivitis (1%), diplopia (2% to 10%), myopia (up to 1%)
Otic: Hearing decreased (1% to 2%), tinnitus (1% to 2%), otitis media (migraine trial: 1% to 2%)
Renal: Nephrolithiasis, renal calculus (1% to 2%), hematuria (<1% to 2%)

Respiratory: Pharyngitis (3% to 6%), sinusitis (4% to 6%; migraine trial: 8% to 10%), epistaxis (1% to 4%), rhinitis (4% to 7%), dyspnea (1% to 2%), pneumonia (5%), coughing (migraine trial: 2% to 3%), bronchitis (migraine trial: 3%)

Miscellaneous: Flu-like syndrome (3% to 7%), allergy (2% to 3%), body odor (up to 1%), fever (migraine trial: 1% to 2%), viral infection (migraine trial: 3% to 4%), infection (<1% to 2%), diaphoresis (≤1%), thirst (2%)

Overdosage/Toxicology Signs and symptoms of overdose include convulsions, drowsiness, speech disturbance, blurred vision, diplopia, impaired mentation, lethargy, and metabolic acidosis. Activated charcoal has not been shown to adsorb topiramate and is, therefore, not recommended; gastric contents should be emptied via lavage or emesis. Hemodialysis can remove approximately ~30% of the drug; however, most cases do not require removal and instead are best treated with supportive measures.

Drug Interactions Inhibits CYP2C19 (weak); **Induces** CYP3A4 (weak)

Acetazolamide: Coadministration may increase the risk of nephrolithiasis.

Anticholinergic drugs: Concurrent administration may increase the risk of oligohydrosis and/or hyperthermia; includes drugs with high anticholinergic activity such as antihistamines, cyclic antidepressants, and antipsychotics; use caution

Carbamazepine: May decrease the levels/effects of topiramate.

CNS depressants: Sedative effects may be additive with topiramate; monitor for increased effect; includes barbiturates, benzodiazepines, opioid analgesics, ethanol, and other sedative agents.

Estrogens: Blood levels of estrogens are decreased when coadministered with topiramate, this may lead to a loss of efficacy.

Hormonal contraceptives: See interaction with Estrogens; use of alternative nonhormonal contraception is recommended.

Phenytoin: May decrease topiramate levels by as much as 48%; topiramate may increase phenytoin concentration by up to 25%

Valproic acid: Topiramate may enhance the hepatotoxic effects of valproic acid; hyperammonemia with or without encephalopathy has been reported in patients who tolerated either drug alone. These drugs may modestly decrease the serum concentrations of the other drug.

Ethanol/Nutrition/Herb Interactions

Ethanol: Avoid ethanol (may increase CNS depression).

Food: Ketogenic diet may increase the possibility of acidosis and/or kidney stones.

Herb/Nutraceutical: Avoid evening primrose (seizure threshold decreased).

Stability Store at room temperature of 15°C to 30°C (59°F to 86°F). Protect from moisture.

Mechanism of Action Anticonvulsant activity may be due to a combination of potential mechanisms: Blocks neuronal voltage-dependent sodium channels, enhances GABA(A) activity, antagonizes AMPA/kainate glutamate receptors, and weakly inhibits carbonic anhydrase.

Pharmacokinetics

Absorption: Good; rapid; unaffected by food

Protein binding: 15% to 41% (inversely related to plasma concentrations)

Metabolism: Hepatic (minimal, primarily excreted unchanged), via hydroxylation, hydrolysis, glucuronidation

Bioavailability: 80%

Time to peak serum concentration: ~2-4 hours

Elimination: Urine (70%)

Dialyzable: ~30%

Dosage

Geriatrics: Most older adults have creatinine clearances <70 mL/min; obtain a serum creatinine and calculate creatinine clearance prior to initiation of therapy. An initial dose of 25 mg/day may be recommended, followed by incremental increases of 25 mg at weekly intervals until an effective dose is reached; refer to adult dosing for titration schedule.

Adults: Note: Do not abruptly discontinue therapy; taper dosage gradually to prevent rebound effects. (In clinical trials, adult doses were withdrawn by decreasing in weekly intervals of 50-100 mg/day gradually over 2-8 weeks for seizure treatment, and by decreasing in weekly intervals by 25-50 mg/day for migraine prophylaxis.)

Partial onset seizure (monotherapy) and primary generalized tonic-clonic seizure (monotherapy): Oral: Initial: 25 mg twice daily; may increase weekly by 50 mg/day up to 100 mg twice daily (week 4 dose); thereafter, may further increase weekly by 100 mg/day up to the recommended maximum of 200 mg twice daily.

Migraine prophylaxis: Oral: Initial: 25 mg/day (in the evening), titrated at weekly intervals in 25 mg increments, up to the recommended total daily dose of 100 mg/day given in 2 divided doses

Partial onset seizures (adjunctive therapy): Oral: Initial: 25-50 mg/day (given in 2 divided doses) for 1 week; increase at weekly intervals by 25-50 mg/day until response; usual maintenance dose: 100-200 mg twice daily. Doses >1600 mg/day have not been studied.

(Continued)

Topiramate *(Continued)*

Primary generalized tonic-clonic seizures (adjunctive therapy): Oral: Use initial dose as listed above for partial onset seizures, but use slower initial titration rate; titrate upwards to recommended dose by the end of 8 weeks; usual maintenance dose: 200 mg twice daily. Doses >1600 mg/day have not been studied.

Cluster headache (unlabeled use): Oral: Initial: 25 mg/day, titrated at weekly intervals in 25 mg increments, up to 200 mg/day

Neuropathic pain (unlabeled use): Oral: Initial: 25 mg/day, titrated at weekly intervals in 25-50 mg increments to target dose of 400 mg daily in 2 divided doses. Reported dosage range studied: 25-800 mg/day

Renal Impairment: Cl_{cr} <70 mL/minute: Administer 50% dose and titrate more slowly.

Hemodialysis: Supplemental dose may be needed during hemodialysis

Dialyzable: ~30%

Hepatic Impairment: Clearance may be reduced.

Administration Oral: May be administered without regard to meals

Capsule sprinkles: May be swallowed whole or opened to sprinkle the contents on soft food (drug/food mixture should not be chewed).

Tablet: Because of bitter taste, tablets should not be broken.

Monitoring Parameters Seizure frequency, hydration status; electrolytes (recommended monitoring includes serum bicarbonate at baseline and periodically during treatment); monitor for symptoms of acute acidosis and complications of long-term acidosis (nephrolithiasis, osteomalacia); ammonia level in patients with unexplained lethargy, vomiting, or mental status changes; symptoms of secondary angle closure glaucoma

Patient Information Take exactly as directed; do not increase dose or frequency or discontinue without consulting prescriber. While using this medication, do not use alcohol and other prescription or OTC medications (especially pain medications, sedatives, antihistamines, or hypnotics) without consulting prescriber. Maintain adequate hydration (2-3 L/day of fluids unless instructed to restrict fluid intake). You may experience drowsiness, dizziness, disturbed concentration, memory changes, or blurred vision (use caution when driving or engaging in tasks requiring alertness until response to drug is known); mouth sores, nausea, vomiting, or loss of appetite (small frequent meals, frequent mouth care, chewing gum, or sucking lozenges may help). Wear identification of epileptic status and medications. Adults should be aware of and follow state laws about driving with a seizure disorder. Report behavioral or CNS changes; skin rash; muscle cramping, weakness, tremors, changes in gait; chest pain, irregular heartbeat, or palpitations; hearing loss; cough or difficulty breathing; worsening of seizure activity, or loss of seizure control. Seek immediate medical evaluation if you experience sudden changes in vision and/or periorbital pain.

Special Geriatric Considerations This drug may not be a drug of choice in the elderly until all other therapies for seizures have been exhausted. Follow the recommended titration schedule and adjust time intervals to meet patient's needs. Since most elderly will have a Cl_{cr} <70 mL/minute, it is important to either measure or estimate by calculation the Cl_{cr} prior to initiating therapy.

Dosage Forms Excipient information presented when available (limited, particularly for generics); consult specific product labeling.

Capsule, sprinkle:

Topamax®: 15 mg, 25 mg

Tablet:

Topamax®: 25 mg, 50 mg, 100 mg, 200 mg

Selected References

Carroll DG, Kline KM, and Malnar KF, "Role of Topiramate for the Treatment of Painful Diabetic Peripheral Neuropathy," *Pharmacotherapy*, 2004, 24(9):1186-93.

Chong MS and Libretto SE, " The Rationale and Use of Topiramate for Treating Neuropathic Pain," *Clin J Pain*, 2003, 19(1):59-68.

Dib JG, "Focus on Topiramate in Neuropathic Pain," *Curr Med Res Opin*, 2004, 20(12):1857-61.

Doose DR, Walker SA, Gisclon LG, et al, "Single-Dose Pharmacokinetics and Effect of Food on the Bioavailability of Topiramate, a Novel Antiepileptic Drug," *J Clin Pharmacol*, 1996, 36(10):884-91.

Sachdeo RC, "Topiramate. Clinical Profile in Epilepsy," *Clin Pharmacokinet*, 1998, 34(5):335-46.

♦ **Toprol-XL**® *see* Metoprolol *on page 1027*
♦ **Toradol**® *see* Ketorolac *on page 859*

Toremifene *(tore EM i feen)*

U.S. Brand Names Fareston®
Canadian Brand Names Fareston®
Index Terms FC1157a; Toremifene Citrate
Generic Available No

Pharmacologic Category Antineoplastic Agent, Estrogen Receptor Antagonist

Use Treatment of advanced breast cancer; management of desmoid tumors and endometrial carcinoma

Contraindications Hypersensitivity to toremifene or any component of the formulation

Warnings/Precautions Hypercalcemia and tumor flare have been reported in some breast cancer patients with bone metastases during the first weeks of treatment. Tumor flare is a syndrome of diffuse musculoskeletal pain and erythema with increased size of tumor lesions that later regress. It is often accompanied by hypercalcemia. Tumor flare does not imply treatment failure or represent tumor progression. Institute appropriate measures if hypercalcemia occurs, and if severe, discontinue treatment. Drugs that decrease renal calcium excretion (eg, thiazide diuretics) may increase the risk of hypercalcemia in patients receiving toremifene. Patients with pre-existing endometrial hyperplasia should not be given long-term toremifene treatment as endometrial hyperplasia has occurred with the drug. Patients with a history of thromboembolic disease should generally not be treated with toremifene.

Adverse Reactions (Reflective of adult population; not specific for elderly)
>10%:
    Endocrine & metabolic: Vaginal discharge, hot flashes
    Gastrointestinal: Nausea, vomiting
    Miscellaneous: Diaphoresis
1% to 10%:
    Cardiovascular: Thromboembolism: Toremifene has been associated with the occurrence of venous thrombosis and pulmonary embolism; arterial thrombosis has also been described in a few case reports; cardiac failure, MI, edema
    Central nervous system: Dizziness
    Endocrine & metabolic: Hypercalcemia may occur in patients with bone metastases; galactorrhea and vitamin deficiency, menstrual irregularities
    Genitourinary: Vaginal bleeding or discharge, endometriosis, priapism, possible endometrial cancer
    Ocular: Ophthalmologic effects (visual acuity changes, cataracts, or retinopathy), corneal opacities, dry eyes

Overdosage/Toxicology Theoretically, overdose may be manifested as an increase of antiestrogenic effects such as hot flashes; estrogenic effects such as vaginal bleeding; or nervous system disorders such as vertigo, dizziness, ataxia and nausea. No specific antidote exists and treatment is symptomatic.

Drug Interactions Substrate of CYP1A2 (minor), 3A4 (major)
    CYP3A4 inducers: CYP3A4 inducers may decrease the levels/effects of toremifene. Example inducers include aminoglutethimide, carbamazepine, nafcillin, nevirapine, phenobarbital, phenytoin, and rifamycins.
    Warfarin results in significant enhancement of the anticoagulant effects of warfarin; has been speculated that a decrease in antitumor effect of tamoxifen may also occur due to alterations in the percentage of active tamoxifen metabolites

Stability Store at 25°C (77°F); excursions permitted to 15°C to 30°C (59°F to 86°F). Protect from heat and light.

Mechanism of Action Nonsteroidal, triphenylethylene derivative. Competitively binds to estrogen receptors on tumors and other tissue targets, producing a nuclear complex that decreases DNA synthesis and inhibits estrogen effects. Nonsteroidal agent with potent antiestrogenic properties which compete with estrogen for binding sites in breast and other tissues; cells accumulate in the G_0 and G_1 phases; therefore, toremifene is cytostatic rather than cytocidal.

Pharmacokinetics
    Absorption: Well absorbed from GI tract
    Distribution: V_d: 580 L
        Protein binding: Plasma: Extensive, >99.5%, mainly to albumin
    Metabolism: Extensively, principally by N-demethyltoremifene, which is also antiestrogenic but with weak *in vivo* antitumor potency
    Half-life: ~5 days
    Time to peak serum concentration: Oral: Within 3 hours
    Elimination: Primarily as metabolite in the feces with about 10% excreted in the urine during a 1-week period
    Note: In older adult women, increases in half-life and V_d were seen with no change in AUC or clearance.

Dosage
    Geriatrics & Adults: Refer to individual protocols.
        Metastatic breast carcinoma: Oral: 60 mg once daily, generally continued until disease progression is observed
    Renal Impairment: No adjustment is necessary.
    Hepatic Impairment: Toremifene is extensively metabolized in the liver and dosage adjustments may be indicated in patients with liver disease; however, no specific guidelines have been developed.
    (Continued)

Toremifene *(Continued)*

Monitoring Parameters Obtain periodic complete blood counts, calcium levels, and liver function tests. Closely monitor patients with bone metastases for hypercalcemia during the first few weeks of treatment. Leukopenia and thrombocytopenia have been reported rarely; monitor leukocyte and platelet counts during treatment.

Patient Information This drug will cause an initial "flare" of this disease (increased bone pain and hot flashes) which will subside. Report any vomiting that occurs after taking dose; women should notify their physician of vaginal bleeding, weakness, or mental confusion. Patients with bone metastases should review symptoms of hypercalcemia (ie, confusion) and contact physician if they occur.

Additional Information Increase of bone pain usually indicates a good therapeutic response

Special Geriatric Considerations No specific information concerning elderly patients.

Dosage Forms Excipient information presented when available (limited, particularly for generics); consult specific product labeling.
Tablet: 60 mg

Selected References

Gams R, "Phase III Trials of Toremifene vs Tamoxifen," *Oncology*, 1997, 11(5 Suppl 4): 23-8.

Hamm JT, "Phase I and II Studies of Toremifene," *Oncology*, 1997, 11(5 Suppl 4):19-22.

Holli K, "Evolving Role of Toremifene in the Adjuvant Setting," *Oncology*, 1997, 11(5 Suppl 4):48-51.

Kangas L, "Review of the Pharmacological Properties of Toremifene," *J Steroid Biochem*, 1990, 36(3):191-5.

Pyrhönen S, Valavaara R, Modig H, et al, "Comparison of Toremifene and Tamoxifen in Postmenopausal Patients With Advanced Breast Cancer: A Randomized Double-Blind, the "Nordic" Phase III Study," *Br J Cancer*, 1997, 76(2):270-7.

Williams GM and Jeffrey AM, "Safety Assessment of Tamoxifen and Toremifene," *Oncology*, 1997, 11(5 Suppl 4):41-7.

♦ **Toremifene Citrate** *see* Toremifene *on page 1602*

Torsemide *(TORE se mide)*

Medication Safety Issues

Sound-alike/look-alike issues:

Torsemide may be confused with furosemide

Demadex® may be confused with Denorex®

U.S. Brand Names Demadex®

Generic Available Yes: Tablet

Pharmacologic Category Diuretic, Loop

Use Management of edema associated with congestive heart failure and hepatic or renal disease; alone or in combination with antihypertensives in treatment of hypertension

Contraindications Hypersensitivity to torsemide, any component of the formulation, or any sulfonylureas; anuria

Warnings/Precautions Loop diuretics are potent diuretics; excess amounts can lead to profound diuresis with fluid and electrolyte loss; close medical supervision and dose evaluation are required. Watch for and correct electrolyte disturbances; adjust dose to avoid dehydration. In cirrhosis, avoid electrolyte and acid/base imbalances that might lead to hepatic encephalopathy. Coadministration of antihypertensives may increase the risk of hypotension.

Monitor fluid status and renal function in an attempt to prevent oliguria, azotemia, and reversible increases in BUN and creatinine; close medical supervision of aggressive diuresis required. Rapid I.V. administration (associated with other loop diuretics), renal impairment, excessive doses, and concurrent use of other ototoxins is associated with ototoxicity; has been seen with oral torsemide.

Chemical similarities are present among sulfonamides, sulfonylureas, carbonic anhydrase inhibitors, thiazides, and loop diuretics (except ethacrynic acid). Use in patients with sulfonylurea allergy is specifically contraindicated in product labeling, however, a risk of cross-reaction exists in patients with allergy to any of these compounds; avoid use when previous reaction has been severe. Discontinue if signs of hypersensitivity are noted.

Adverse Reactions (Reflective of adult population; not specific for elderly)

1% to 10%:

Cardiovascular: Edema (1.1%), ECG abnormality (2%), chest pain (1.2%)

Central nervous system: Headache (7.3%), dizziness (3.2%), insomnia (1.2%), nervousness (1%)

Endocrine & metabolic: Hyperglycemia, hyperuricemia, hypokalemia

Gastrointestinal: Diarrhea (2%), constipation (1.8%), nausea (1.8%), dyspepsia (1.6%), sore throat (1.6%)

Genitourinary: Excessive urination (6.7%)

Neuromuscular & skeletal: Weakness (2%), arthralgia (1.8%), myalgia (1.6%)

Respiratory: Rhinitis (2.8%), cough increase (2%)

Overdosage/Toxicology Symptoms include electrolyte depletion, volume depletion, hypotension, dehydration, and circulatory collapse. Electrolyte depletion may be manifested by weakness, dizziness, mental confusion, anorexia, lethargy, vomiting, and cramps. Following GI decontamination, treatment is supportive. Hypotension responds to fluids and Trendelenburg positioning.

Drug Interactions **Substrate** of CYP2C8 (minor), 2C9 (major); **Inhibits** CYP2C19 (weak)

ACE inhibitors: Hypotensive effects and/or renal effects are potentiated by hypovolemia.

Aminoglycosides: Ototoxicity may be increased.

Anticoagulant activity is enhanced.

Antidiabetic agents: Glucose tolerance may be decreased.

Antihypertensive agents: Effects may be enhanced.

Beta-blockers: Plasma concentrations of beta-blockers may be increased with torsemide.

Chloral hydrate: Transient diaphoresis, hot flashes, hypertension may occur.

Cisplatin: Ototoxicity may be increased.

CYP2C9 inducers: May decrease the levels/effects of torsemide. Example inducers include carbamazepine, phenobarbital, phenytoin, rifampin, rifapentine, and secobarbital.

Digitalis: Arrhythmias may occur with diuretic-induced electrolyte disturbances.

Lithium: Plasma concentrations of lithium may be increased; monitor lithium levels.

NSAIDs: Torsemide efficacy may be decreased.

Probenecid: Torsemide action may be reduced.

Salicylates: Diuretic action may be impaired in patients with cirrhosis and ascites.

Thiazides: Synergistic effects may result.

Ethanol/Nutrition/Herb Interactions Herb/Nutraceutical: Avoid dong quai if using for hypertension (has estrogenic activity). Avoid ephedra, yohimbe, ginseng (may worsen hypertension). Avoid garlic (may have increased antihypertensive effect).

Stability If torsemide is to be administered via continuous infusion, stability has been demonstrated through 24 hours at room temperature in plastic containers for the following fluids and concentrations:

200 mg torsemide (10 mg/mL) added to 250 mL D_5W, 250 mL NS or 500 mL 0.45% sodium chloride.

50 mg torsemide (10 mg/mL) added to 500 mL D_5W, 250 mL NS or 500 mL 0.45% sodium chloride.

Mechanism of Action Inhibits reabsorption of sodium and chloride in the ascending loop of Henle and distal renal tubule, interfering with the chloride-binding cotransport system, thus causing increased excretion of water, sodium, chloride, magnesium, and calcium; does not alter GFR, renal plasma flow, or acid-base balance

Pharmacodynamics

Onset of diuresis: 30-60 minutes

Peak effect: 1-4 hours

Duration: ~6 hours

Pharmacokinetics

Absorption: Oral: Rapid

Protein binding: Plasma: ~97% to 99%

Metabolism: Hepatic (80%)

Bioavailability: 80% to 90%

Half-life: 2-4; 7-8 hours in cirrhosis (dose modification appears unnecessary)

Elimination: 20% excreted unchanged in urine

Dosage

Geriatrics: Usual starting dose should be 5 mg; refer to adult dosing.

Adults:

Note: The oral form may be given regardless of meal times. Patients may be switched from the I.V. form to the oral and vice-versa with no change in dose.

Congestive heart failure: Oral, I.V.: 10-20 mg once daily; may increase gradually for chronic treatment by doubling dose until the diuretic response is apparent (for acute treatment. I.V. dose may be repeated every 2 hours with double the dose as needed). **Note:** ACC/AHA 2005 guidelines for chronic heart failure recommend a maximum daily oral dose of 200 mg; maximum single I.V. dose 100-200 mg

Continuous I.V. infusion: 20 mg I.V. load then 5-20 mg/hour

Chronic renal failure: Oral, I.V.: 20 mg once daily; increase as above.

Hepatic cirrhosis: Oral, I.V.: 5-10 mg once daily with an aldosterone antagonist or a potassium-sparing diuretic; increase as above.

Hypertension: Oral, I.V.: 2.5-5 mg once daily; increase to 10 mg after 4-6 weeks if an adequate hypotensive response is not apparent. If still not effective, an additional antihypertensive agent may be added.

Administration Administer the I.V. dose slowly over 2 minutes

Monitoring Parameters Blood pressure, both standing and sitting/supine, serum electrolytes, weight, I & O; in high doses, monitor auditory function

(Continued)

Torsemide *(Continued)*

Patient Information May be taken with food or milk; rise slowly from a lying or sitting position to minimize dizziness, lightheadedness or fainting; also use extra care when exercising, standing for long periods of time, and during hot weather; take in the morning

Additional Information 10-20 mg torsemide is approximately equivalent to:
Furosemide 40 mg
Bumetanide 1 mg

Special Geriatric Considerations Loop diuretics are potent diuretics, excess amounts can lead to profound diuresis with fluid and electrolyte loss. Close medical supervision and dose evaluation is required, particularly in elderly.

Dosage Forms Excipient information presented when available (limited, particularly for generics); consult specific product labeling.
Injection, solution: 10 mg/mL (2 mL, 5 mL)
Tablet: 5 mg, 10 mg, 20 mg, 100 mg

♦ **Touro® DM** *see* Guaifenesin and Dextromethorphan *on page 730*

♦ **tPA** *see* Alteplase *on page 60*

Tramadol (TRA ma dole)

Medication Safety Issues
Sound-alike/look-alike issues:
Tramadol may be confused with Toradol®, Trandate®, Voltaren®
Ultram® may be confused with Ultane®, Voltaren®

International issues:
Theradol® [Netherlands] may be confused with Foradil® which is a brand name for formoterol in the U.S.
Theradol® [Netherlands] may be confused with Terazol® which is a brand name for terconazole in the U.S.
Theradol® [Netherlands] may be confused with Toradol® which is a brand name for ketorolac in the U.S.

U.S. Brand Names Ultram®; Ultram® ER

Canadian Brand Names Ultram®; Zytram® XL

Index Terms Tramadol Hydrochloride

Generic Available Yes: Excludes extended release tablet

Pharmacologic Category Analgesic, Nonopioid

Use Relief of moderate to moderately-severe pain

Contraindications Hypersensitivity to tramadol, opioids, or any component of the formulation; opioid-dependent patients; acute intoxication with alcohol, hypnotics, centrally-acting analgesics, opioids, or psychotropic drugs

Extended release formulations (Ultram® ER and Zytram® XL [CAN]): Additional contraindications: Severe (Cl_{cr} <30 mL/minute) renal dysfunction, severe (Child-Pugh Class C) hepatic dysfunction

Note: Based on Canadian product labeling, tramadol is contraindicated during or within 14 days following MAO inhibitor therapy

Warnings/Precautions May cause CNS depression, which may impair physical or mental abilities; patients must be cautioned about performing tasks which require mental alertness (eg, operating machinery or driving). Should be used only with extreme caution in patients receiving MAO inhibitors. May cause CNS depression and/or respiratory depression, particularly when combined with other CNS depressants. Use with caution and reduce dosage when administered to patients receiving other CNS depressants. An increased risk of seizures may occur in patients receiving serotonin reuptake inhibitors (SSRIs or anorectics), tricyclic antidepressants, other cyclic compounds (including cyclobenzaprine, promethazine), neuroleptics, MAO inhibitors (contraindicated in Canadian product labeling), or drugs which may lower seizure threshold. Patients with a history of seizures, or with a risk of seizures (head trauma, metabolic disorders, CNS infection, or malignancy, or during ethanol/drug withdrawal) are also at increased risk.

Elderly, debilitated patients and patients with chronic respiratory disorders may be at greater risk of adverse events. Use with caution in patients with increased intracranial pressure or head injury. Avoid use in patients who are suicidal or addiction prone. Use caution in heavy alcohol users. Use caution in treatment of acute abdominal conditions; may mask pain. Use tramadol with caution and reduce dosage in patients with liver disease or renal dysfunction. Tolerance or drug dependence may result from extended use (withdrawal symptoms have been reported); abrupt discontinuation should be avoided. Tapering of dose at the time of discontinuation limits the risk of withdrawal symptoms.

Adverse Reactions (Reflective of adult population; not specific for elderly)

>10%:

Cardiovascular: Flushing (8% to 16%)

Central nervous system: Dizziness (16% to 33%), headache (8% to 32%), insomnia (7% to 11%), somnolence (7% to 25%)

Dermatologic: Pruritus (6% to 12%)

Gastrointestinal: Constipation (12% to 46%), nausea (15% to 40%)

Neuromuscular & skeletal: Weakness (4% to 12%)

1% to 10%:

Cardiovascular: Chest pain (1% to <5%), postural hypotension (2% to 5%), vasodilation (1% to <5%)

Central nervous system: Agitation, anxiety (1% to <5%), confusion (1% to <5%), coordination impaired (1% to <5%), depression (1% to <5%), emotional lability, euphoria, hallucinations, hypoesthesia, lethargy, malaise, nervousness (1% to <5%), pain, pyrexia, restlessness

Dermatologic: Dermatitis, rash

Endocrine & metabolic: Hot flashes (2% to 9%), menopausal symptoms (1% to <5%)

Gastrointestinal: Abdominal pain, anorexia (<6%), diarrhea (5% to 10%), dry mouth (5% to 10%), dyspepsia, flatulence, vomiting (5% to 9%), weight loss

Genitourinary: Urinary frequency (1% to <5%), urinary retention (1% to <5%), urinary tract infection (1% to <5%)

Neuromuscular & skeletal: Arthralgia (1% to <5%), hypertonia (1% to <5%), rigors (<4%), paresthesia (1% to <5%), spasticity (1% to <5%), tremor (1% to <5%), creatinine phosphokinase increased

Ocular: Blurred vision (1% to <5%), miosis (1% to <5%)

Respiratory: Bronchitis (1% to <5%), cough (1% to <5%), dyspnea (1% to <5%), pharyngitis (1% to <5%), rhinorrhea (1% to <5%), sinusitis (1% to <5%)

Miscellaneous: Diaphoresis (2% to 6%), flu-like syndrome (<2%)

A withdrawal syndrome may occur with abrupt discontinuation; includes anxiety, diarrhea, hallucinations (rare), nausea, pain, piloerection, rigors, sweating, and tremor. Uncommon discontinuation symptoms may include severe anxiety, panic attacks, or paresthesia.

Overdosage/Toxicology
Symptoms of overdose include CNS and respiratory depression, lethargy, coma, miosis, seizure, cardiac arrest, and death. Treatment may be symptom-directed and supportive. Naloxone may reverse some overdose symptoms, but may increase the risk of seizures. Hemodialysis is not helpful in removal of tramadol.

Drug Interactions
Substrate of CYP2B6 (minor), 2D6 (major), 3A4 (minor)

Carbamazepine: Tramadol metabolism is increased by carbamazepine. Avoid concurrent use; increases risk of seizures.

Cyclobenzaprine: May enhance the neuroexcitatory and/or seizure-potentiating effect of tramadol.

CYP2D6 inhibitors: May decrease the effects of tramadol. Example inhibitors include chlorpromazine, delavirdine, fluoxetine, miconazole, paroxetine, pergolide, quinidine, quinine, ritonavir, and ropinirole.

Ethanol: Tramadol may enhance the CNS depressant effect of ethanol.

MAO inhibitors: May increase the neuroexcitatory effects or risk of seizures. Examples of inhibitors include isocarboxazid, linezolid, phenelzine, selegiline, and tranylcypromine.

Naloxone: May increase the risk of seizures (if administered in tramadol overdose).

Quinidine: May increase the tramadol serum concentrations and decrease serum concentrations of M1

SSRIs: May increase the neuroexcitatory effects or risk of seizures with tramadol. Examples of SSRIs include citalopram, escitalopram, fluoxetine, fluvoxamine, paroxetine, sertraline.

Serotonin modulators: May enhance the adverse/toxic effects of tramadol. The development of serotonin syndrome may occur.

Sibutramine: May enhance the serotonergic effects of tramadol. Avoid concurrent use.

Tricyclic antidepressants: May increase the risk of seizures.

Ethanol/Nutrition/Herb Interactions

Ethanol: Avoid ethanol (may increase CNS depression).

Food:

Immediate release: Does not affect the rate or extent of absorption.

Extended release: Reduced C_{max} and AUC and T_{max} occurred 3 hours earlier when taken with a high-fat meal.

Herb/Nutraceutical: Avoid valerian, St John's wort, kava kava, gotu kola (may increase CNS depression).

Stability
Store at 15°C to 30°C (59°F to 86°F).

Mechanism of Action
Binds to μ-opiate receptors in the CNS causing inhibition of ascending pain pathways, altering the perception of and response to pain; also inhibits the reuptake of norepinephrine and serotonin, which also modifies the ascending pain pathway

(Continued)

Tramadol *(Continued)*

Pharmacodynamics
Onset of action: ~1 hour
Peak serum concentrations: 2 hours
Duration: 9 hours

Pharmacokinetics
Absorption: Rapid and complete

Distribution: V_d: 2.5-3 L/kg

Protein binding:, plasma: 20%

Metabolism: Extensively hepatic via demethylation, glucuronidation, and sulfation; has pharmacologically active metabolite formed by CYP2D6 (M1; O-desmethyl tramadol)

Bioavailability: Immediate release: 75%; Extended release: 85% to 90% as compared to immediate release (Zytram® XL: 70%)

Half-life elimination: Tramadol: ~6-8 hours; Active metabolite: 7-9 hours; prolonged in elderly, hepatic or renal impairment; Zytram® XL: ~16 hours

Time to peak: Immediate release: 2 hours; Extended release: 12 hours

Excretion: Urine (30% as unchanged drug; 60% as metabolites)

Note: In subjects >75 years of age, peak serum concentrations were slightly elevated and the half-life was slightly prolonged (7 hours); no significant changes in the 65-75 year age group were noted as compared to younger adults

Dosage
Geriatrics: Oral: >75 years:

Immediate release: 50 mg every 6 hours (not to exceed 300 mg/day); see dosing adjustments for renal and hepatic impairment.

Extended release: Use with great caution. Refer to adult dosing.

Adults: Moderate-to-severe chronic pain: Oral:

Immediate release formulation: 50-100 mg every 4-6 hours (not to exceed 400 mg/day)

For patients not requiring rapid onset of effect, tolerability may be improved by starting dose at 25 mg/day and titrating dose by 25 mg every 3 days, until reaching 25 mg 4 times/day. Dose may then be increased by 50 mg every 3 days as tolerated, to reach dose of 50 mg 4 times/day.

Extended release formulation:

Ultram® ER: 100 mg once daily; titrate every 5 days (maximum: 300 mg/day)

Zytram® XL [per Canadian labeling: Not available in U.S.]: 150 mg once daily; if pain relief is not achieved may titrate by increasing dosage incrementally, with sufficient time to evaluate effect of increased dosage; generally not more often than every 7 days (maximum: 400 mg/day)

Renal Impairment:

Immediate release: Cl_{cr} <30 mL/minute: Administer 50-100 mg dose every 12 hours (maximum: 200 mg/day).

Extended release: Should not be used in patients with Cl_{cr} <30 mL/minute.

Hepatic Impairment:

Immediate release: Cirrhosis: Recommended dose: 50 mg every 12 hours.

Extended release: Should not be used in patients with severe (Child-Pugh Class C) hepatic dysfunction.

Administration Do not crush or chew extended release tablet.

Monitoring Parameters Monitor patient for pain, respiratory rate, and signs of tolerance and, therefore, abuse potential; monitor blood pressure and pulse rate, especially in patients on higher doses

Reference Range 100-300 ng/mL; however, serum concentration monitoring is not required

Patient Information If self-administered, use exactly as directed (do not increase dose or frequency); may cause physical and/or psychological dependence. While using this medication, do not use alcohol and other prescription or OTC medications (especially pain medications, sedatives, antihistamines, or cough preparations) without consulting prescriber. Maintain adequate hydration (2-3 L/day of fluids unless instructed to restrict fluid intake). You may experience drowsiness, dizziness, or blurred vision (use caution when driving or engaging in tasks requiring alertness until response to drug is known); nausea, vomiting, or loss of appetite (small frequent meals, frequent mouth care, chewing gum, or sucking lozenges may help); constipation (increased exercise, fluids, or dietary fruit and fiber may help). Report severe unresolved constipation; difficulty breathing or shortness of breath; excessive sedation or increased insomnia and restlessness; changes in urinary pattern; seizures; muscle weakness or tremors; or chest pain or palpitations.

Special Geriatric Considerations One study in the elderly found that tramadol 50 mg was similar in efficacy as acetaminophen 300 mg with codeine 30 mg. In Ultram® ER trials, elderly patients experienced more adverse effects than younger adults, particularly constipation, fatigue, weakness, postural hypotension, and dyspepsia. For this reason, the extended release formultaiton should probably be avoided in the elderly, or only used with great caution.

Dosage Forms Excipient information presented when available (limited, particularly for generics); consult specific product labeling. [CAN] = Canadian brand name
Tablet, as hydrochloride: 50 mg
  Ultram®: 50 mg
Tablet, extended release, as hydrochloride:
  Ultram® ER: 100 mg, 200 mg, 300 mg
  Zytram® XL [CAN]: 150 mg, 200 mg, 300 mg, 400 mg [not available in the U.S.]

Selected References
AGS Panel on Persistent Pain in Older Persons, "The Management of Persistent Pain in Older Persons," *J Am Geriatr Soc*, 2002, 50(6 Suppl):S205-24.

Gibson TP, "Pharmacokinetics, Efficacy, and Safety of Analgesia With a Focus on Tramadol HCl," *Am J Med*, 1996, 101(1A):47S-53S.

Rauck RL, Ruoff GE, and McGillen, "Comparison of Tramadol and Acetaminophen With Codeine for Long-Term Pain Management in Elderly Patients," *Curr Ther Res*, 1994, 556:1417-31.

♦ **Tramadol Hydrochloride** *see* Tramadol *on page 1606*

♦ **Trandate®** *see* Labetalol *on page 864*

Trandolapril (tran DOE la pril)

Related Information
Angiotensin Agents *on page 1737*
U.S. Brand Names Mavik®
Canadian Brand Names Mavik™
Generic Available Yes
Pharmacologic Category Angiotensin-Converting Enzyme (ACE) Inhibitor

Use Management of hypertension (alone or in combination with other antihypertensive agents), postmyocardial infarction heart failure, postmyocardial infarction left ventricular dysfunction

Unlabeled/Investigational Use As a class, ACE inhibitors are recommended in the treatment of systolic congestive heart failure.

Contraindications Hypersensitivity to trandolapril or any component of the formulation; history of angioedema-related to previous treatment with an ACE inhibitor; bilateral renal artery stenosis; primary hyperaldosteronism

Warnings/Precautions Anaphylactic reactions can occur. Angioedema can occur at any time during treatment (especially following first dose). It may involve head and neck (potentially affecting the airway) or the intestine (presenting with abdominal pain). Prolonged monitoring may be required especially if tongue, glottis, or larynx are involved as they are associated with airway obstruction. Those with a history of airway surgery in this situation have a higher risk. Careful blood pressure monitoring with first dose (hypotension can occur especially in volume-depleted patients). Dosage adjustment needed in severe renal dysfunction (Cl_{cr} <30 mL/minute) or in hepatic cirrhosis. Use with caution in hypovolemia; collagen vascular diseases; valvular stenosis (particularly aortic stenosis); hyperkalemia; or before, during, or immediately after anesthesia. Avoid rapid dosage escalation, which may lead to renal insufficiency. Hyperkalemia may rarely occur. Rare toxicities associated with ACE inhibitors include cholestatic jaundice (which may progress to hepatic necrosis) and neutropenia/agranulocytosis with myeloid hyperplasia. May be associated with deterioration of renal function and/or increases in serum creatinine, particularly in patients dependent on renin-angiotensin-aldosterone system. Use with caution in unilateral renal artery stenosis and pre-existing renal insufficiency; if patient has renal impairment then a baseline WBC with differential and serum creatinine should be evaluated and monitored closely during the first 3 months of therapy.

Adverse Reactions (Reflective of adult population; not specific for elderly)
Note: Frequency ranges include data from hypertension and heart failure trials. Higher rates of adverse reactions have generally been noted in patients with CHF. However, the frequency of adverse effects associated with placebo is also increased in this population.

>1%:
  Cardiovascular: Hypotension (<1% to 11%), bradycardia (<1% to 4.7%), intermittent claudication (3.8%), stroke (3.3%)
  Central nervous system: Dizziness (1.3% to 23%), syncope (5.9%), asthenia (3.3%)
  Endocrine & metabolic: Elevated uric acid (15%), hyperkalemia (5.3%), hypocalcemia (4.7%)
  Gastrointestinal: Dyspepsia (6.4%), gastritis (4.2%)
  Neuromuscular & skeletal: Myalgia (4.7%)
  Renal: Elevated BUN (9%), elevated serum creatinine (1.1% to 4.7%) Respiratory: Cough (1.9% to 35%)

Overdosage/Toxicology Symptoms may include hypotension, bradycardia, vertigo, and dizziness. Hyperkalemia occurs even with therapeutic doses, especially in patients with renal insufficiency and those taking NSAIDs. Following initiation of essential
(Continued)

Trandolapril *(Continued)*

overdose management, toxic symptom treatment and supportive treatment should be initiated.

Hypotension usually responds to I.V. fluids or Trendelenburg positioning. If unresponsive to these measures, the use of a parenteral vasopressor may be required (eg, norepinephrine 0.1-0.2 mcg/kg/minute titrated to response). Seizures commonly respond to diazepam (I.V. 5-10 mg bolus in adults every 15 minutes, if needed, up to a total of 30 mg) or to phenytoin or phenobarbital.

Drug Interactions

Alpha$_1$ blockers: Hypotensive effect increased.

Aspirin: The effects of ACE inhibitors may be blunted by aspirin administration, particularly at higher dosages and/or increase adverse renal effects.

Diuretics: Hypovolemia due to diuretics may precipitate acute hypotensive events or acute renal failure.

Gold sodium thiomalate: ACE inhibitors may enhance the adverse/toxic effects (nitritoid reaction) of gold sodium thiomalate. The reaction may include facial flushing, nausea, vomiting, hypotension, and syncope. If it is to occur, would be expected shortly after administration of gold compound in patients maintained on an ACEI.

Insulin: Risk of hypoglycemia may be increased.

Lithium: Risk of lithium toxicity may be increased; monitor lithium levels, especially the first 4 weeks of therapy.

Mercaptopurine: Risk of neutropenia may be increased.

NSAIDs: May attenuate hypertensive efficacy; effect has been seen with captopril and may occur with other ACE inhibitors; monitor blood pressure. May increase adverse renal effects.

Potassium-sparing diuretics (amiloride, potassium, spironolactone, triamterene): Increased risk of hyperkalemia.

Potassium supplements may increase the risk of hyperkalemia.

Trimethoprim (high dose) may increase the risk of hyperkalemia.

Ethanol/Nutrition/Herb Interactions Herb/Nutraceutical: Avoid dong quai if using for hypertension (has estrogenic activity). Avoid ephedra, yohimbe, ginseng (may worsen hypertension). Avoid garlic (may have increased antihypertensive effect).

Mechanism of Action Trandolapril is an ACE inhibitor which prevents the formation of angiotensin II from angiotensin I. Trandolapril must undergo enzymatic hydrolysis, mainly in liver, to its biologically active metabolite, trandolaprilat. A CNS mechanism may also be involved in the hypotensive effect as angiotensin II increases adrenergic outflow from the CNS. Vasoactive kallikrein's may be decreased in conversion to active hormones by ACE inhibitors, thus reducing blood pressure.

Pharmacodynamics

Peak reduction in blood pressure: 6 hours postdose

Peak concentrations: 6 hours

Trandolaprilat (active metabolite) is very lipophilic in comparison to other ACE inhibitors which may contribute to its prolonged duration of action (72 hours after a single dose).

Pharmacokinetics

Absorption: Rapid

Metabolism: Hydrolyzed, mainly in liver, to the active metabolite, trandolaprilat

Half-life:

Trandolapril: 6 hours

Trandolaprilat: Effective: 10 hours; terminal: 24 hours

Elimination: As metabolites in urine; reduce dose in renal failure; creatinine clearances ≤30 mL/minute result in accumulation of active metabolite

Dosage

Geriatrics & Adults:

Hypertension: Oral; Initial dose in patients not receiving a diuretic: 1 mg/day (2 mg/day in black patients). Adjust dosage according to the blood pressure response. Make dosage adjustments at intervals of ≥1 week. Most patients have required dosages of 2-4 mg/day. There is a little experience with doses >8 mg/day. Patients inadequately treated with once daily dosing at 4 mg may be treated with twice daily dosing. If blood pressure is not adequately controlled with trandolapril monotherapy, a diuretic may be added.

Usual dose range (JNC 7): 1-4 mg once daily

Heart failure postmyocardial infarction or left ventricular dysfunction postmyocardial infarction: Oral: Initial: 1 mg/day; titrate patients (as tolerated) towards the target dose of 4 mg/day. If a 4 mg dose is not tolerated, patients can continue therapy with the greatest tolerated dose.

Renal Impairment: Cl$_{cr}$ ≤30 mL/minute: Administer lowest doses, starting at 0.5 mg/day.

Hepatic Impairment: Patients with hepatic cirrhosis: Start dose at 0.5 mg.

Monitoring Parameters Serum potassium, renal function, serum creatinine, BUN, CBC

Patient Information Do not discontinue medication without advice of physician; notify physician if sore throat, swelling, palpitations, cough, chest pains, difficulty swallowing, swelling of face, eyes, tongue, lips, hoarseness, sweating, vomiting, or diarrhea occurs; may cause dizziness, lightheadedness during first few days; may also cause changes in taste perception; do not use salt substitutes containing potassium without consulting a physician

Additional Information Patients taking diuretics are at risk for developing hypotension on initial dosing; to prevent this, discontinue diuretics 2-3 days prior to initiating trandolapril; may restart diuretics if blood pressure is not controlled by trandolapril alone. Watch for hypotensive effect within 1-3 hours of first dose or new higher dose.

Special Geriatric Considerations Due to frequent decreases in glomerular filtration (also creatinine clearance) with aging, elderly patients may have exaggerated responses to ACE inhibitors; differences in clinical response due to hepatic changes are not observed. ACE inhibitors may be preferred agents in elderly patients with CHF and diabetes mellitus. Diabetic proteinuria is reduced and insulin sensitivity is enhanced. In general, the side effect profile is favorable in the elderly and causes little or no CNS confusion; use lowest dose recommendations initially. Adjust for renal function. Many elderly may be volume depleted due to diuretic use and/or blunted thirst reflex resulting in inadequate fluid intake.

Dosage Forms Excipient information presented when available (limited, particularly for generics); consult specific product labeling.
    Tablet: 1 mg, 2 mg, 4 mg
    Mavik®: 1 mg, 2 mg, 4 mg

Selected References

Bevan EG, McInnes GT, Aldigier JC, et al, "Effect of Renal Function on the Pharmacokinetics and Pharmaco-dynamics of Trandolapril," *Br J Clin Pharmacol*, 1993, 35(2):128-35.

Chobanian AV, Bakris GL, Black HR, et al, "The Seventh Report of the Joint National Committee on Prevention, Detection, Evaluation, and Treatment of High Blood Pressure: The JNC 7 Report," *JAMA*, 2003, 289(19):2560-71.

Conen H and Brunner HR, "Pharmacologic Profile of Trandolapril, A New Angiotensin-Converting Enzyme Inhibitor," *Am Heart J*, 1993, 125(5 Pt 2):1525-31.

Zannad F, "Trandolapril: How Does It Differ From Other Angiotensin-Converting Enzyme Inhibitors?" *Drugs*, 1993, 46(Suppl 2):172-81.

Trandolapril and Verapamil (tran DOE la pril & ver AP a mil)

Related Information
    Trandolapril *on page 1609*
    Verapamil *on page 1671*

U.S. Brand Names Tarka®

Canadian Brand Names Tarka®

Index Terms Verapamil and Trandolapril

Generic Available No

Pharmacologic Category Antihypertensive Agent, Combination

Use Combination drug for the treatment of hypertension; see individual agents

Dosage

    Geriatrics: Refer to dosing in individual monographs.

    Adults: Hypertension: Oral: Individualize dose. Patients receiving trandolapril (up to 8 mg) and verapamil (up to 240 mg) in separate tablets may wish to receive Tarka® at equivalent dosages once daily.

    Renal Impairment: Usual regimen need not be adjusted unless patient's creatinine clearance is <30 mL/minute. Titration of individual components must be done prior to switching to combination product

    Hepatic Impairment: Has not been evaluated in hepatic impairment. Verapamil is hepatically metabolized, adjustment of dosage in hepatic impairment is recommended.

Dosage Forms Excipient information presented when available (limited, particularly for generics); consult specific product labeling.
    Tablet, variable release:
        1/240: Trandolapril 1 mg [immediate release] and verapamil hydrochloride 240 mg [sustained release]
        2/180: Trandolapril 2 mg [immediate release] and verapamil hydrochloride 180 mg [sustained release]
        2/240: Trandolapril 2 mg [immediate release] and verapamil hydrochloride 240 mg [sustained release]
        4/240: Trandolapril 4 mg [immediate release] and verapamil hydrochloride 240 mg [sustained release]

♦ **Transamine Sulphate** *see* Tranylcypromine *on page 1612*

♦ **Transderm Scōp®** *see* Scopolamine Derivatives *on page 1448*

♦ **Trans-Ver-Sal®** [OTC] *see* Salicylic Acid *on page 1441*

♦ **Tranxene® SD™** *see* Clorazepate *on page 347*

♦ **Tranxene® SD™-Half Strength** *see* Clorazepate *on page 347*

♦ **Tranxene T-Tab®** *see* Clorazepate *on page 347*

♦ **Tranxene® T-Tab®** *see* Clorazepate *on page 347*

Tranylcypromine (tran il SIP roe meen)

Related Information
Antidepressant Agents *on page 1742*

U.S. Brand Names Parnate®

Canadian Brand Names Parnate®

Index Terms Transamine Sulphate; Tranylcypromine Sulfate

Generic Available No

Pharmacologic Category Antidepressant, Monoamine Oxidase Inhibitor

Use Symptomatic treatment of depressed patients refractory to or intolerant to tricyclic antidepressants or electroconvulsive therapy

Unlabeled/Investigational Use Treatment of post-traumatic stress disorder

Restrictions An FDA-approved medication guide concerning the use of antidepressants in children, adolescents, and young adults must be distributed when dispensing an outpatient prescription (new or refill) where this medication is to be used without direct supervision of a healthcare provider. Medication guides are available at http://www.fda.gov/cder/Offices/ODS/medication_guides.htm. Dispense to parents or guardians of children and adolescents receiving this medication.

Contraindications Hypersensitivity to tranylcypromine, other MAO inhibitors, dibenzazepine derivatives, or any component of the formulation; antiparkinson drugs; cardiovascular disease; cerebrovascular defect; headache history; hepatic disease; hypertension; pheochromocytoma; renal disease; concurrent use of antihistamines, antihypertensives, bupropion, buspirone, CNS depressants, dexfenfluramine, dextromethorphan, diuretics, ethanol, meperidine, SSRIs, and sympathomimetics; general anesthesia (discontinue 10 days prior to elective surgery); local vasoconstrictors; spinal anesthesia (hypotension may be exaggerated); foods which are high in tyramine, tryptophan, or dopamine, chocolate, or caffeine

Warnings/Precautions Risk of suicide: [U.S. Boxed Warning]: Antidepressants increase the risk of suicidal thinking and behavior in children, adolescents, and young adults (18-24 years of age) with major depressive disorder (MDD) and other psychiatric disorders; consider risk prior to prescribing. Short-term studies did not show an increased risk in patients >24 years of age and showed a decreased risk inpatients >65 years. Closely monitor for clinical worsening, suicidality, or unusual changes in behavior such as anxiety, agitation, panic attacks, insomnia, irritability, hostility, impulsivity, akathisia, hypomania, and mania. The patient's family or caregiver should be instructed to closely observe the patient and communicate condition with healthcare provider. Such observation would generally include at least weekly face-to-face contact with patients or their family members or caregivers during the first 4 weeks of treatment, then every other week visits for the next 4 weeks, then at 12 weeks, and as clinically indicated beyond 12 weeks. Additional contact by telephone may be appropriate between face-to-face visits. A medication guide should be dispensed with each prescription.

All patients treated with antidepressants should be observed similarly for clinical worsening and suicidality, especially during the initial few months of a course of drug therapy, or at times of dose changes, either increases or decreases. The possibility of a suicide attempt is inherent in major depression and may persist until remission occurs. Worsening depression and severe abrupt suicidality that are not part of the presenting symptoms may require discontinuation or modification of drug therapy. Use caution in high-risk patients during initiation of therapy. Prescriptions should be written for the smallest quantity consistent with good patient care.

Disease state precautions: Use with caution in patients who are hyperactive, hyperexcitable, or who have glaucoma, hyperthyroidism, diabetes or hypotension. May cause orthostatic hypotension (especially at dosages >30 mg/day). Use with caution in patients at risk of seizures, or in patients receiving other drugs which may lower seizure threshold. Discontinue at least 48 hours prior to myelography. May increase the risks associated with electroconvulsive therapy. Consider discontinuing, when possible, prior to elective surgery. Use with caution in patients with renal impairment. May worsen psychosis in some patients or precipitate a shift to mania or hypomania in patients with bipolar disorder. **Tranylcypromine is not FDA approved for the treatment of bipolar depression.**

Elderly patients: Interactions with tyramine or tryptophan-containing foods and orthostasis have limited tranylcypromine's use.

Adverse Reactions (Reflective of adult population; not specific for elderly)
Frequency not defined.

Cardiovascular: Edema, orthostatic hypotension, palpitation, tachycardia

Central nervous system: Agitation, akinesia, anxiety, ataxia, chills, confusion, disorientation, dizziness, drowsiness, fatigue, headache, hyper-reflexia, insomnia, mania, memory loss, restlessness, sleep disturbances, twitching

Dermatologic: Alopecia, cystic acne (flare), pruritus, rash, urticaria, scleroderma (localized)

Endocrine & metabolic: Hypernatremia, hypermetabolic syndrome; sexual dysfunction (anorgasmia, ejaculatory disturbances, impotence); SIADH

Gastrointestinal: Abdominal pain, anorexia, constipation, diarrhea, nausea, vomiting, weight gain, xerostomia

Genitourinary: Incontinence, urinary retention

Hematologic: Agranulocytosis, anemia, leukopenia, thrombocytopenia

Hepatic: Hepatitis

Neuromuscular & skeletal: Akinesis, muscle spasm, myoclonus, numbness, paresthesia, tremor, weakness

Ocular: Blurred vision, glaucoma

Otic: Tinnitus

Miscellaneous: Diaphoresis

Overdosage/Toxicology Symptoms of overdose include headache, tachycardia or bradycardia, neck stiffness, nausea, vomiting, chest pain, sweating, photophobia, palpitations, muscle twitching, seizures, insomnia, orthostatic hypotension, hypertension, hypertensive crisis, hyperpyrexia, and coma. Treatment is symptom-directed and supportive. The manufacturer suggests phentolamine (5 mg given slowly I.V.) for treatment of hypertensive crisis. Other useful agents may be labetalol or nitroprusside.

Drug Interactions Inhibits CYP1A2 (moderate), 2A6 (strong), 2C8 (weak), 2C9 (weak), 2C19 (moderate), 2D6 (moderate), 2E1 (weak), 3A4 (weak)

Acetylcholinesterase inhibitors: May diminish the anticholinergic side effects of tranylcypromine.

Alpha-/beta-agonists: MAO inhibitors may enhance the vasopressor effect. Alpha-/beta-agonists (indirect-acting): MAO inhibitors may enhance the vasopressor effect.

Alpha₁-agonist: MAO inhibitors may enhance the hypertensive effects.

Altretamine: May enhance the orthostatic effect of MAO inhibitors.

Amphetamines: MAO inhibitors in combination with amphetamines may result in severe hypertensive reaction; these combinations are best avoided.

Anesthetics, general: Discontinue tranylcypromine 10 days prior to elective surgery.

Anorexiants: Concurrent use of anorexiants may result in serotonin syndrome; contraindicated with dexfenfluramine; avoid use with fenfluramine or sibutramine.

Anticholinergics: May enhance the adverse/toxic anticholinergic effects of tranylcypromine.

Atomoxetine: MAO Inhibitors may enhance the neurotoxic (central) effect of atomoxetine. Avoid combination. Atomoxetine should not be used within 14 days of an MAO inhibitor.

Bupropion: May cause hypertensive crisis; at least 14 days should elapse before initiating bupropion; concurrent use with an MAO inhibitor is contraindicated.

Buspirone: May cause increased blood pressure; concurrent use with an MAO inhibitor should be avoided.

COMT Inhibitors: May enhance the adverse/toxic effect of MAO inhibitors. Avoid concurrent use.

Cyclobenzaprine: May enhance the serotonergic effect of MAO Inhibitors. This could result in serotonin syndrome. Avoid combination.

CYP1A2 substrates: Tranylcypromine may increase the levels/effects of CYP1A2 substrates. Example substrates include aminophylline, fluvoxamine, mexiletine, mirtazapine, ropinirole, theophylline, and trifluoperazine.

CYP2A6 substrates: Tranylcypromine may increase the levels/effects of CYP2A6 substrates. Example substrates include dexmedetomidine and ifosfamide.

CYP2C19 substrates: Tranylcypromine may increase the levels/effects of CYP2C19 substrates. Example substrates include citalopram, diazepam, methsuximide, phenytoin, and trimipramine.

CYP2D6 substrates: Tranylcypromine may increase the levels/effects of CYP2D6 substrates. Example substrates include amphetamines, selected beta-blockers, dextromethorphan, fluoxetine, lidocaine, mirtazapine, nefazodone, paroxetine, risperidone, thioridazine, tricyclic antidepressants, and venlafaxine.

CYP2D6 prodrug substrates: Tranylcypromine may decrease the levels/effects of CYP2D6 prodrug substrates. Example prodrug substrates include codeine, hydrocodone, oxycodone, and tramadol.

Dexmethylphenidate: MAO inhibitors may enhance the hypertensive effect of dexmethylphenidate; avoid concurrent use.

Dextromethorphan: Concurrent use of MAO inhibitors may result in serotonin syndrome; concurrent use is contraindicated.

(Continued)

Tranylcypromine *(Continued)*

Disulfiram: MAO inhibitors may produce delirium in patients receiving disulfiram; monitor.

Ethanol: Tranylcypromine may enhance CNS depressant effect of ethanol.

False neurotransmitters: MAO inhibitors inhibit the antihypertensive response to guanadrel or methyldopa; monitor therapy.

Levodopa: MAO inhibitors in combination with levodopa may result in hypertensive reactions; monitor.

Lithium: MAO inhibitors in combination with lithium have resulted in CNS toxicity (malignant hyperpyrexia, tardive dyskinesias); monitor therapy.

Meperidine: May cause serotonin syndrome when combined with an MAO inhibitor; concurrent use is contraindicated; should not be used within 14 days of an MAO inhibitor.

Methylphenidate: MAO inhibitors may enhance the hypertensive effect of methylphenidate. Avoid combination.

Mirtazapine: MAO inhibitors may enhance the neurotoxic (central) effect of mirtazapine. Avoid combination.

Pramlintide: Pramlintide may enhance the anticholinergic effect of tranylcypromine. Additive effects on reduced GI motility may occur.

Rauwolfia alkaloids: MAO inhibitors may enhance the adverse/toxic effect of rauwolfia alkaloids. If a rauwolfia alkaloid is added to existing MAOI therapy, a burst of catecholamine stimulation (eg, excitation, hypertension) may occur.

Serotonin/norepinephrine reuptake inhibitors (SNRIs): MAO inhibitors may enhance the serotonergic effect of SNRI antidepressants. This may cause serotonin syndrome.

Selective serotonin reuptake inhibitors (SSRIs): MAO Inhibitors may enhance the serotonergic effect of SSRIs. This may cause serotonin syndrome. Avoid concurrent use. Do not use within 5 weeks of fluoxetine discontinuation or 2 weeks of other antidepressant discontinuation.

Serotonin 5-HT$_{1D}$ receptor agonists: May increase the risk of serotonin syndrome. The manufacturers of rizatriptan, sumatriptan, and zolmitriptan state that concurrent use (or use within 2 weeks of MAO therapy) is contraindicated.

Serotonin modulators: May enhance the adverse/toxic effect of other serotonin modulators, such as tranylcypromine. The development of serotonin syndrome may occur.

Sibutramine: May enhance the serotonergic effect of tranylcypromine. This may cause serotonin syndrome. Avoid concurrent use.

Thioridazine: Tranylcypromine may decrease the metabolism of thioridazine. Avoid concurrent use.

Tramadol: May enhance the neuroexcitatory and/or seizure-potentiating effect of MAO Inhibitors.

Tricyclic antidepressants: MAO inhibitors may enhance the serotonergic effect of tricyclic antidepressants. This may cause serotonin syndrome. Avoid concurrent use.

Ethanol/Nutrition/Herb Interactions

Ethanol: Avoid ethanol (based on CNS depressant effects and potential tyramine content)

Food: Concurrent ingestion of foods rich in tyramine may cause sudden and severe high blood pressure (hypertensive crisis). Avoid tyramine-containing foods with MAOIs. Food's freshness is also an important concern; improperly stored or spoiled food can create an environment where tyramine concentrations may increase.

Herb/Nutraceuticals: Avoid valerian, St John's wort, SAMe. Avoid supplements containing caffeine, gingko, yohimbime, ephedra, tyrosine, tryptophan or phenylalanine. Ingestion of large quantities may increase the risk of severe side effects (eg, hypertensive reactions, serotonin syndrome).

Mechanism of Action Tranylcypromine is a nonhydrazine monoamine oxidase inhibitor. It increases endogenous concentrations of epinephrine, norepinephrine, dopamine, and serotonin through inhibition of the enzyme (monoamine oxidase) responsible for the breakdown of these neurotransmitters.

Pharmacodynamics Onset of action: Therapeutic: 2 days to 3 weeks continued dosing

Pharmacokinetics

Half-life: 90-190 minutes

Time to peak serum concentration: Oral: Within 2 hours

Elimination: In urine

Dosage

Geriatrics & Adults: Depression: Oral: 10 mg twice daily, increase by 10 mg increments at 1- to 3-week intervals; maximum: 60 mg/day; usual effective dose: 30 mg/day

Administration Administer second dose before 4 PM to avoid insomnia

Monitoring Parameters Blood pressure, heart rate, diet, mood and depressive symptoms, weight

Reference Range Inhibition of platelet monoamine oxidase (≥80%) correlated with clinical response

Patient Information Tablets may be crushed; avoid alcohol; do not discontinue abruptly; avoid foods high in tyramine (eg, cheese [except cottage, ricotta, and cream], smoked or pickled fish, beef or chicken liver, dried sausage, fava or broad bean pods, yeast, vitamin supplements); change positions slowly; discuss list of drugs and foods to avoid with pharmacist or physician; take second dose no later than 4 PM to avoid insomnia

Additional Information Has a more rapid onset of therapeutic effect than other MAO inhibitors, but causes more severe hypertensive reactions

Special Geriatric Considerations MAO inhibitors are effective and generally well tolerated by older patients. Potential interactions with tyramine- or trypto-phan-containing foods, other drugs, and adverse effects on blood pressure have limited use of MAO inhibitors. They are usually reserved for patients who do not tolerate or respond to traditional "cyclic" or "second generation" antidepressants. Tranylcypromine is the preferred MAO inhibitor because its enzymatic-blocking effects are more rapidly reversed. The brain activity of monoamine oxidase increases with age and even more so in patients with Alzheimer's disease. Therefore, MAO inhibitors may have an increased role in treating depressed patients with Alzheimer's disease.

Dosage Forms Excipient information presented when available (limited, particularly for generics); consult specific product labeling.
Tablet: 10 mg

Selected References
Georgotas A, Friedman E, McCarthy M, et al, "Resistant Geriatric Depression and Therapeutic Response to Monoamine-Oxidase Inhibitors," *Biol Psychiatry*, 1983, 18:195-205.

Goff DC and Jenike MA, "Treatment-Resistant Depression in the Elderly," *J Am Geriatr Soc*, 1986, 34(1):63-70.

Jenike MA, "MAO Inhibitors as Treatment for Depressed Patients With Primary Degenerative Dementia (Alzheimer's Disease)," *Am J Psychiatry* 1985, 142:763.

♦ **Tranylcypromine Sulfate** *see* Tranylcypromine *on page 1612*
♦ **Travatan®** *see* Travoprost *on page 1615*
♦ **Travatan® Z** *see* Travoprost *on page 1615*

Travoprost (TRA voe prost)

Related Information
Glaucoma Drug Therapy *on page 1758*
Medication Safety Issues
Sound-alike/look-alike issues:
Travatan® may be confused with Xalatan®
U.S. Brand Names Travatan®; Travatan® Z
Canadian Brand Names Travatan®
Generic Available No
Pharmacologic Category Ophthalmic Agent, Antiglaucoma; Prostaglandin, Ophthalmic

Use Reduction of elevated intraocular pressure in patients with open-angle glaucoma or ocular hypertension who are intolerant of the other IOP-lowering medications or insufficiently responsive (failed to achieve target IOP determined after multiple measurements over time) to another IOP-lowering medication

Contraindications Hypersensitivity to travoprost or any component of the formulation

Warnings/Precautions May permanently change/increase brown pigmentation of the iris, the eyelid skin, and eyelashes. In addition, may increase the length and/or number of eyelashes (may vary between eyes); changes occur slowly and may not be noticeable for months or years. Bacterial keratitis, caused by inadvertent contamination of multiple-dose ophthalmic solutions, has been reported. Use caution in patients with intraocular inflammation, aphakic patients, pseudophakic patients with a torn posterior lens capsule, or patients with risk factors for macular edema. Contact with contents of vial should be avoided in women who are pregnant or attempting to become pregnant; in case of accidental exposure to the skin, wash the exposed area with soap and water immediately. Safety and efficacy have not been determined for use in patients with renal or hepatic impairment, angle-closure-, inflammatory-, or neovascular glaucoma.

Travatan®: Contains benzalkonium chloride which may be adsorbed by contact lenses; remove contacts prior to administration and wait 15 minutes before reinserting.

Adverse Reactions (Reflective of adult population; not specific for elderly)
>10%: Ocular: Hyperemia (35% to 50%)
5% to 10%: Ocular: Decreased visual acuity, eye discomfort, foreign body sensation, pain, pruritus
1% to 5%:
Cardiovascular: Angina pectoris, bradycardia, hyper-/hypotension
Central nervous system: Depression, pain, anxiety, headache
Endocrine & metabolic: Hypercholesterolemia
Gastrointestinal: Dyspepsia
Genitourinary: Prostate disorder, urinary incontinence
(Continued)

Travoprost *(Continued)*

Neuromuscular & skeletal: Arthritis, back pain, chest pain

Ocular (1% to 4%): Abnormal vision, blepharitis, blurred vision, conjunctivitis, dry eye, iris discoloration, keratitis, lid margin crusting, photophobia, subconjunctival hemorrhage, cataract, tearing, periorbital skin discoloration (darkening), eyelash darkening, eyelash growth increased

Respiratory: Bronchitis, sinusitis

Stability Store between 2°C to 25°C (36°F to 77°F).

Mechanism of Action A selective FP prostanoid receptor agonist which lowers intraocular pressure by increasing trabecular meshwork and outflow

Pharmacodynamics

Onset of action: ~2 hours

Peak effect: After 12 hours

Pharmacokinetics

Absorption: Absorbed via cornea, plasma concentrations ≤25 pg/mL within 30 minutes

Metabolism: Hydrolyzed by esterases in the cornea to active free acid; systemically, the free acid is metabolized to inactive metabolites

Elimination: Rapid, plasma levels decrease to <10 pg/mL within 1 hour

Dosage

Geriatrics & Adults: Glaucoma (open angle) or ocular hypertension: Ophthalmic: Instill 1 drop into affected eye(s) once daily in the evening; do not exceed once-daily dosing (may decrease IOP-lowering effect). If used with other topical ophthalmic agents, separate administration by at least 5 minutes.

Administration May be used with other eye drops to lower intraocular pressure. If using more than one ophthalmic product, wait at least 5 minutes in between application of each medication. Travatan®: Remove contact lenses prior to administration and wait 15 minutes before reinserting.

Patient Information For use in eyes only. Wash hands before instilling. Sit or lie down to instill. Open eye, look at ceiling, and instill prescribed amount of solution. Apply gentle pressure to inner corner of eye. Do not let tip of applicator touch eye; do not contaminate tip of applicator (may cause eye infection, eye damage, or vision loss). Contact prescriber concerning continued use of drops if eye infection develops, trauma occurs to the eye, and prior to eye surgery. Travatan® contains benzalkonium chloride which may be adsorbed by contact lenses; remove contacts prior to administration and wait 15 minutes before reinserting. May cause permanent changes in eye color (increases the amount of brown pigment in the iris), eyelid, and eyelashes. May also increase the length and/or number of eyelashes. Changes may occur slowly (months to years). May be used with other eye drops to lower intraocular pressure. If using more than one eye medicine, wait at least 5 minutes in between application of each medication. Notify prescriber if conjunctivitis or eyelid reactions occur with use of this product. In case of accidental contact with the solution, wash skin with soap and water immediately.

Additional Information The IOP-lowering effect was shown to be 7-8 mm Hg in clinical studies. The mean IOP reduction in African-American patients was up to 1.8 mm Hg greater than in non-African-American patients. The reason for this effect is unknown.

Healthcare professionals who are pregnant (or attempting to become pregnant) and accidentally come into contact with the solution, should wash skin with soap and water immediately.

Special Geriatric Considerations Evaluate patient's ability to self-administer eye drops.

Dosage Forms Excipient information presented when available (limited, particularly for generics); consult specific product labeling.

Solution, ophthalmic:

Travatan®: 0.004% (2.5 mL, 5 mL) [contains benzalkonium chloride]

Travatan® Z: 0.004% (2.5 mL, 5 mL)

Trazodone *(TRAZ oh done)*

Related Information

Antidepressant Agents *on page 1742*

Medication Safety Issues

Sound-alike/look-alike issues:

Desyrel® may be confused with Demerol®, Delsym®, Zestril®

International issues:

Desyrel® may be confused with Deseril® which is a brand name for methysergide in multiple international markets

U.S. Brand Names Desyrel® [DSC]
Canadian Brand Names Alti-Trazodone; Apo-Trazodone®; Apo-Trazodone D®; Desyrel®; Gen-Trazodone; Novo-Trazodone; Nu-Trazodone; PMS-Trazodone; ratio-Trazodone; Trazorel®
Index Terms Trazodone Hydrochloride
Generic Available Yes
Pharmacologic Category Antidepressant, Serotonin Reuptake Inhibitor/Antagonist
Use Treatment of depression
Unlabeled/Investigational Use Potential augmenting agent for antidepressants; hypnotic
Restrictions An FDA-approved medication guide concerning the use of antidepressants in children, adolescents, and young adults must be distributed when dispensing an outpatient prescription (new or refill) where this medication is to be used without direct supervision of a healthcare provider. Medication guides are available at http://www.fda.gov/cder/Offices/ODS/medication_guides.htm. Dispense to parents or guardians of children and adolescents receiving this medication.
Contraindications Hypersensitivity to trazodone or any component of the formulation
Warnings/Precautions [U.S. Boxed Warning]: Antidepressants increase the risk of suicidal thinking and behavior in children, adolescents, and young adults (18-24 years of age) with major depressive disorder (MDD) and other psychiatric disorders; consider risk prior to prescribing. Short-term studies did not show an increased risk in patients >24 years of age and showed a decreased risk in patients ≥65 years. Closely monitor for clinical worsening, suicidality, or unusual changes in behavior; the patient's family or caregiver should be instructed to closely observe the patient and communicate condition with healthcare provider. A medication guide should be dispensed with each prescription.

The possibility of a suicide attempt is inherent in major depression and may persist until remission occurs. Monitor for worsening of depression or suicidality, especially during initiation of therapy (generally first 1-2 months) or with dose increases or decreases. Use caution in high-risk patients. Worsening depression and severe abrupt suicidality that are not part of the presenting symptoms may require discontinuation or modification of drug therapy. The patient's family or caregiver should be alerted to monitor patients for the emergence of suicidality and associated behaviors (such as agitation, irritability, hostility, impulsivity, and hypomania) and call healthcare provider.

May worsen psychosis in some patients or precipitate a shift to mania or hypomania in patients with bipolar disorder. Patients presenting with depressive symptoms should be screened for bipolar disorder. Monotherapy in patients with bipolar disorder should be avoided. **Trazodone is not FDA approved for the treatment of bipolar depression.**

Priapism, including cases resulting in permanent dysfunction, has occurred with the use of trazodone. Not recommended for use in a patient during the acute recovery phase of MI. Trazodone should be initiated with caution in patients who are receiving concurrent or recent therapy with a MAO inhibitor.

The risks of sedation and/or postural hypotension are high relative to other antidepressants. Trazodone frequently causes sedation, which may result in impaired performance of tasks requiring alertness (eg, operating machinery or driving). Sedative effects may be additive with other CNS depressants and ethanol. Use with caution in patients with a history of cardiovascular disease (including previous MI, stroke, tachycardia, or conduction abnormalities). The risk of conduction abnormalities with this agent is low relative to other antidepressants.

Consider discontinuing, when possible, prior to elective surgery. Therapy should not be abruptly discontinued in patients receiving high doses for prolonged periods. Use caution in patients with a previous seizure disorder or condition predisposing to seizures such as brain damage, alcoholism, or concurrent therapy with other drugs which lower the seizure threshold. Use with caution in patients with hepatic or renal dysfunction and in elderly patients.

Adverse Reactions (Reflective of adult population; not specific for elderly)
>10%:
  Central nervous system: Dizziness, headache, sedation
  Gastrointestinal: Nausea, xerostomia
  Ocular: Blurred vision
1% to 10%:
  Cardiovascular: Syncope, hyper-/hypotension, edema
  Central nervous system: Confusion, decreased concentration, fatigue, incoordination
  Gastrointestinal: Diarrhea, constipation, weight gain/loss
  Neuromuscular & skeletal: Tremor, myalgia
  Respiratory: Nasal congestion
Overdosage/Toxicology Symptoms include drowsiness, vomiting, hypotension, tachycardia, incontinence, coma, and priapism. Following initiation of essential overdose management, toxic symptoms should be treated. Ventricular arrhythmias often
(Continued)

Trazodone *(Continued)*

respond to lidocaine 1.5 mg/kg bolus, followed by 2 mg/minute infusion with concurrent systemic alkalinization (sodium bicarbonate 0.5-2 mEq/kg I.V.). Seizures usually respond to diazepam I.V. boluses (5-10 mg up to 30 mg). If seizures are unresponsive or recur, phenytoin or phenobarbital may be required. Hypotension is best treated by I.V. fluids and by Trendelenburg positioning.

Drug Interactions Substrate of CYP2D6 (minor), 3A4 (major); **Inhibits** CYP2D6 (moderate), 3A4 (weak)

Antipsychotics: Trazodone, in combination with other psychotropics (low potency antipsychotics), may result in additional hypotension (isolated case reports); monitor.

Azole antifungals: Serum concentrations of trazodone may be increased by azole antifungals, via inhibition of CYP3A4. Ketoconazole has been specifically studied. Consider a lower dose of trazodone.

Buspirone: Serotonergic effects may be additive (limited documentation); monitor.

Carbamazepine: Serum concentrations of trazodone may be decreased by carbamazepine, due to induction of CYP3A4. Other CYP inducers are likely to share this effect.

CNS depressants: Sedative effects may be additive with CNS depressants. Includes ethanol, barbiturates, benzodiazepines, opioid analgesics, and other sedative agents; monitor for increased effect

CYP2D6 substrates: Trazodone may increase the levels/effects of CYP2D6 substrates. Example substrates include amphetamines, selected beta-blockers, dextromethorphan, fluoxetine, lidocaine, mirtazapine, nefazodone, paroxetine, risperidone, ritonavir, thioridazine, tricyclic antidepressants, and venlafaxine.

CYP2D6 prodrug substrates: Trazodone may decrease the levels/effects of CYP2D6 prodrug substrates. Example prodrug substrates include codeine, hydrocodone, oxycodone, and tramadol.

CYP3A4 inducers: CYP3A4 inducers may decrease the levels/effects of trazodone. Example inducers include aminoglutethimide, carbamazepine, nafcillin, nevirapine, phenobarbital, phenytoin, and rifamycins.

CYP3A4 inhibitors: May increase the levels/effects of trazodone. Example inhibitors include azole antifungals, clarithromycin, diclofenac, doxycycline, erythromycin, imatinib, isoniazid, nefazodone, nicardipine, propofol, protease inhibitors, quinidine, telithromycin, and verapamil.

Linezolid: Due to MAO inhibition (see note on MAO inhibitors), this combination should be avoided

MAO inhibitors: Concurrent use may lead to serotonin syndrome; avoid concurrent use or use within 14 days

Meperidine: Combined use, theoretically, may increase the risk of serotonin syndrome

Protease inhibitors: Serum concentrations of trazodone may be increased by protease inhibitors, via inhibition of CYP3A4. Consider a lower dose of trazodone.

Serotonin agonists: Theoretically, may increase the risk of serotonin syndrome; includes sumatriptan, naratriptan, rizatriptan, and zolmitriptan

SSRIs: Combined use of trazodone with an SSRI may, theoretically, increase the risk of serotonin syndrome; in addition, some SSRIs may inhibit the metabolism of trazodone resulting in elevated plasma levels and increased sedation; includes fluoxetine and fluvoxamine (see CYP inhibition); low doses of trazodone appear to represent little risk

Venlafaxine: Combined use with trazodone may increase the risk of serotonin syndrome

Ethanol/Nutrition/Herb Interactions

Ethanol: Avoid ethanol (may increase CNS depression).

Food: Time to peak serum levels may be increased if trazodone is taken with food.

Herb/Nutraceutical: Avoid valerian, St John's wort, SAMe, kava kava (may increase risk of serotonin syndrome and/or excessive sedation).

Mechanism of Action Inhibits reuptake of serotonin, causes adrenoreceptor subsensitivity, and induces significant changes in 5-HT presynaptic receptor adrenoreceptors. Trazodone also significantly blocks histamine (H_1) and alpha$_1$-adrenergic receptors.

Pharmacodynamics Onset of action: Therapeutic (antidepressant): 1-3 weeks; sleep aid: 1-3 hours

Pharmacokinetics

Protein binding: 85% to 95%

Metabolism: Hepatic via CYP3A4 to an active metabolite (mCPP)

Half-life: 4-7.5 hours, 2 compartment kinetics

Elimination: Geriatrics: 11.6 hours, nearly twice that of younger patients

Time to peak serum concentration: Oral: Within 30-100 minutes, prolonged in the presence of food (up to 2.5 hours)

Elimination: Primarily in urine and secondarily in feces

Dosage

Geriatrics: Oral: 25-50 mg at bedtime with 25-50 mg/day dose increase every 3 days for inpatients and weekly for outpatients, if tolerated; usual dose: 75-150 mg/day

Adults:

Depression: Oral: Initial: 150 mg/day in 3 divided doses (may increase by 50 mg/day every 3-7 days); maximum: 600 mg/day

Note: Therapeutic effects may take up to 6 weeks. Therapy is normally maintained for 6-12 months after optimum response is reached to prevent recurrence of depression.

Sedation/hypnotic (unlabeled use): Oral: 25-50 mg at bedtime (often in combination with daytime SSRIs). May increase up to 200 mg at bedtime.

Monitoring Parameters Blood pressure, pulse, target symptoms

Reference Range Therapeutic: 0.5-2.5 mcg/mL (SI: 1-6 μmol/L); not well established

Patient Information Take shortly after a meal or light snack, can be given as bedtime dose if drowsiness occurs; avoid alcohol; be aware of possible photosensitivity reaction; may cause painful erections; avoid sudden changes of position

Special Geriatric Considerations Very sedating, but little anticholinergic effects.

Dosage Forms Excipient information presented when available (limited, particularly for generics); consult specific product labeling. [DSC] = Discontinued product

Tablet: 50 mg, 100 mg, 150 mg, 300 mg

Desyrel®: 50 mg, 100 mg, 150 mg, 300 mg [DSC]

Selected References

Bayer AJ, Pathy MS, and Ankier SI, "Pharmacokinetic and Pharmacodynamic Characteristics of Trazodone in the Elderly," *Br J Clin Pharmacol*, 1983, 16(4):371-6.

Gerson SC, Plotkin DA, and Jarvik LF, "Antidepressant Drug Studies, 1964-1986: Empirical Evidence for Aging Patients," *J Clin Psychopharmacol*, 1988, 8(5):311-21.

- ♦ **Trazodone Hydrochloride** see Trazodone on page 1616
- ♦ **Trecator®** see Ethionamide on page 583
- ♦ **Trelstar™ Depot** see Triptorelin on page 1640
- ♦ **Trelstar™ LA** see Triptorelin on page 1640
- ♦ **Trental®** see Pentoxifylline on page 1230
- ♦ **Tretinoin and Clindamycin** see Clindamycin and Tretinoin on page 334
- ♦ **Trexall™** see Methotrexate on page 1005
- ♦ **Triaconazole** see Terconazole on page 1535

Triamcinolone (trye am SIN oh lone)

Related Information

Asthma on page 1767

Corticosteroids on page 1755

Inhalant Agents on page 1760

Medication Safety Issues

Sound-alike/look-alike issues:

Kenalog® may be confused with Ketalar®

Nasacort® may be confused with NasalCrom®

TAC (occasional abbreviation for triamcinolone) is an error-prone abbreviation (mistaken as tetracaine-adrenaline-cocaine)

U.S. Brand Names Aristospan®; Azmacort®; Kenalog®; Kenalog-10®; Kenalog-40®; Nasacort® AQ; Triderm®; Tri-Nasal®

Canadian Brand Names Aristospan®; Kenalog®; Kenalog® in Orabase; Nasacort® AQ; Oracort; Triaderm; Trinasal®

Index Terms Triamcinolone Acetonide, Aerosol; Triamcinolone Acetonide, Parenteral; Triamcinolone Diacetate, Oral; Triamcinolone Diacetate, Parenteral; Triamcinolone Hexacetonide; Triamcinolone, Oral

Generic Available Yes: Cream, lotion, ointment, paste

Pharmacologic Category Corticosteroid, Adrenal; Corticosteroid, Inhalant (Oral); Corticosteroid, Nasal; Corticosteroid, Systemic; Corticosteroid, Topical

Use

Nasal inhalation: Management of seasonal and perennial allergic rhinitis

Oral inhalation: Control of bronchial asthma and related bronchospastic conditions

Oral topical: Adjunctive treatment and temporary relief of symptoms associated with oral inflammatory lesions and ulcerative lesions resulting from trauma

Systemic: Treatment of adrenocortical insufficiency, rheumatic disorders, allergic states, respiratory diseases, systemic lupus erythematosus, and other diseases requiring anti-inflammatory or immunosuppressive effects

Topical: Treatment of inflammatory dermatosis responsive to steroids

Contraindications Hypersensitivity to triamcinolone or any component of the formulation; systemic fungal infections; serious infections (except septic shock or tuberculous meningitis); primary treatment of status asthmaticus; fungal, viral, or bacterial infections of the mouth or throat (oral topical formulation)

Warnings/Precautions May cause hypercorticism or suppression of hypothalamic-pituitary-adrenal (HPA) axis, particularly in patients receiving high doses for prolonged periods. HPA axis suppression may lead to adrenal crisis. Withdrawal and (Continued)

Triamcinolone *(Continued)*

discontinuation of a corticosteroid should be done slowly and carefully. Particular care is required when patients are transferred from systemic corticosteroids to inhaled products due to possible adrenal insufficiency or withdrawal from steroids, including an increase in allergic symptoms. Patients receiving >20 mg per day of prednisone (or equivalent) may be most susceptible. Fatalities have occurred due to adrenal insufficiency in asthmatic patients during and after transfer from systemic corticosteroids to aerosol steroids; aerosol steroids do not provide the systemic steroid needed to treat patients having trauma, surgery, or infections.

Bronchospasm may occur with wheezing after inhalation; if this occurs stop steroid and treat with a fast-acting bronchodilator. Supplemental steroids (oral or parenteral) may be needed during stress or severe asthma attacks. Not to be used in status asthmaticus or for the relief of acute bronchospasm. Acute myopathy has been reported with high dose corticosteroids, usually in patients with neuromuscular transmission disorders; may involve ocular and/or respiratory muscles; monitor creatine kinase; recovery may be delayed. Corticosteroid use may cause psychiatric disturbances, including depression, euphoria, insomnia, mood swings, and personality changes. Pre-existing psychiatric conditions may be exacerbated by corticosteroid use. Prolonged use of corticosteroids may also increase the incidence of secondary infection, mask acute infection (including fungal infections), prolong or exacerbate viral infections, or limit response to vaccines. Exposure to chickenpox should be avoided; corticosteroids should not be used to treat ocular herpes simplex. Corticosteroids should not be used for cerebral malaria. Close observation is required in patients with latent tuberculosis and/or TB reactivity; restrict use in active TB (only in conjunction with antituberculosis treatment). Prolonged treatment with corticosteroids has been associated with the development of Kaposi's sarcoma (case reports); if noted, discontinuation of therapy should be considered.

Use with caution in patients with thyroid disease, hepatic impairment, renal impairment, cardiovascular disease, diabetes, glaucoma, cataracts, myasthenia gravis, patients at risk for osteoporosis, patients at risk for seizures, or GI diseases (diverticulitis, peptic ulcer, ulcerative colitis) due to perforation risk. Use caution following acute MI (corticosteroids have been associated with myocardial rupture). Because of the risk of adverse effects, systemic corticosteroids should be used cautiously in the elderly in the smallest possible effective dose for the shortest duration. Azmacort® (metered dose inhaler) comes with its own spacer device attached and may be easier to use in older patients. Avoid nasal corticosteroid use in patients with recent nasal septal ulcers, nasal surgery or nasal trauma until healing has occurred. Do not use occlusive dressings on weeping or exudative lesions and general caution with occlusive dressings should be observed; discontinue if skin irritation or contact dermatitis should occur; do not use in patients with decreased skin circulation; avoid the use of high potency steroids on the face.

Intravitreal injection has been associated with endophthalmitis and visual disturbances. Blindness has been reported following injection into nasal turbinates and intralesional injections into the head. Safety of intraturbinal, subconjunctival, subtenons, retrobulbar, or intravitreal injection has not been demonstrated.

To minimize the systemic effects of orally-inhaled and intranasal corticosteroids, each patient should be titrated to the lowest effective dose. Withdraw systemic therapy with gradual tapering of dose. There have been reports of systemic corticosteroid withdrawal symptoms (eg, joint/muscle pain, lassitude, depression) when withdrawing oral inhalation therapy. Injection suspension contains benzyl alcohol.

Oral topical: Discontinue if local irritation or sensitization should develop. If significant regeneration or repair of oral tissues has not occurred in seven days, re-evaluation of the etiology of the oral lesion is advised.

Adverse Reactions (Reflective of adult population; not specific for elderly)

Systemic: Frequency not defined:

Cardiovascular: Angioedema, bradycardia, CHF, hypertension, myocardial rupture (following recent MI), thrombophlebitis, vasculitis

Central nervous system: Convulsions, depression, emotional instability, fever, headache, intracranial pressure increased, neuropathy, paresthesia, personality changes, vertigo

Dermatologic: Acne, allergic dermatitis, bruising, cutaneous atrophy, dry/scaly skin, ecchymoses, facial erythema, petechiae, photosensitivity, rash, striae, thin/fragile skin, wound healing impaired

Endocrine & metabolic: Adrenocortical/pituitary unresponsiveness (particularly during stress), carbohydrate tolerance decreased, cushingoid state, diabetes mellitus (manifestations of latent disease), fluid retention, growth suppression (children), hirsutism, hypokalemic alkalosis, menstrual irregularities, negative nitrogen balance, potassium loss, sodium retention

Gastrointestinal: Abdominal distention, bowel perforation, diarrhea, dyspepsia, nausea, oral *Monilia* (oral inhaler), pancreatitis, peptic ulcer, ulcerative esophagitis, weight gain

Hepatic: Hepatomegaly

Local: Skin atrophy (at the injection site)

Neuromuscular & skeletal: Calcinosis (following intra-articular or intralesional injection), Charcot-like arthropathy, femoral/humeral head aseptic necrosis, muscle mass decreased, muscle weakness, osteoporosis, pathologic fracture of long bones, steroid myopathy, tendon rupture, vertebral compression fractures

Ocular: Blindness (periocular injections), cataracts, intraocular pressure increased, exophthalmos, glaucoma, subcapsular cataract

Respiratory: Cough increased (nasal spray), epistaxis (nasal inhaler/spray), pharyngitis (nasal spray/oral inhaler), sinusitis (oral inhaler), voice alteration (oral inhaler)

Miscellaneous: Abnormal fat deposition (moon face), anaphylactoid reaction, anaphylaxis, diaphoresis increased, suppression to skin tests

Topical: Frequency not defined:

Dermatologic: Itching, allergic contact dermatitis, dryness, folliculitis, skin infection (secondary), itching, hypertrichosis, acneiform eruptions, hypopigmentation, skin maceration, skin atrophy, striae, miliaria, perioral dermatitis, atrophy of oral mucosa

Local: Burning, irritation

Overdosage/Toxicology When consumed in excessive quantities, systemic hypercorticism and adrenal suppression may occur; in those cases, discontinuation and withdrawal of the corticosteroid should be done judiciously.

Drug Interactions

Aminoglutethimide: May reduce the serum levels/effects of corticosteroids; likely via induction of microsomal isoenzymes.

Amphotericin: Corticosteroids may increase the hypokalemic effects of amphotericin B; monitor.

Antacids: May decrease the absorption of corticosteroids; separate administration by 2 hours.

Anticholinesterases: Concurrent use may lead to severe weakness in patients with myasthenia gravis.

Antidiabetic agents: Corticosteroids may decrease the hypoglycemic effects of antidiabetic agents; monitor.

Aprepitant: May increase the serum levels/effects of corticosteroids; monitor.

Antifungal agents (azole): May increase the serum levels/effects of corticosteroids; monitor.

Barbiturates: May decrease the levels/effects of corticosteroids.

Bile acid sequestrants: May reduce the absorption of corticosteroids; separate administration by 2 hours.

Calcium channel blockers (nondihydropyridine): May increase the serum levels/effects of corticosteroids; monitor.

Cyclosporine: Corticosteroids may increase the serum levels/effects of cyclosporine. In addition, cyclosporine may increase levels of corticosteroids.

Diuretics, potassium-wasting (loop or thiazide): Hypokalemic effects may be increased by corticosteroids; monitor.

Estrogens: May increase the serum levels/effects of corticosteroids; monitor.

Fluoroquinolones: Concurrent use may increase the risk of tendinopathies (including tendonitis and rupture), particularly in elderly patients (overall incidence rare)

Isoniazid: Serum levels/effects may be decreased by corticosteroids.

Macrolide antibiotics: May increase the serum levels/effects of corticosteroids.

Neuromuscular-blocking agents: Concurrent use with corticosteroids may increase the risk of myopathy.

Nonsteroidal anti-inflammatory drugs (NSAIDs): Concurrent use with corticosteroids may lead to an increased incidence of gastrointestinal adverse effects; use caution.

Rifamycin derivatives: May decrease the levels/effects of corticosteroids (systemic); monitor.

Salicylates: Salicylates may increase the gastrointestinal adverse effects of corticosteroids.

Vaccine (dead organism): Corticosteroids may decrease the effect of vaccines (dead organisms). In patients receiving high doses of systemic corticosteroids for ≥14 days, wait at least 1 month between discontinuing steroid therapy and administering immunization.

Vaccine (live organism): Corticosteroids may increase the risk of vaccinal infection. The use of live vaccines is contraindicated in immunosuppressed patients.

Warfarin: Corticosteroids may increase the anticoagulant effects of warfarin; monitor INR.

Ethanol/Nutrition/Herb Interactions

Ethanol: Avoid ethanol (may enhance gastric mucosal irritation).

Food: Triamcinolone interferes with calcium absorption.

(Continued)

Triamcinolone *(Continued)*

Herb/Nutraceutical: Avoid cat's claw, echinacea (have immunostimulant properties).

Stability Store at room temperature; do not freeze.

Injection, suspension: Shake well prior to use.

Hexacetonide suspension: Avoid diluents containing parabens or preservatives (may cause flocculation). Diluted suspension stable ~1 week. Suspension for intralesional use may be diluted with D_5NS, $D_{10}NS$ or SWFI to a 1:1, 1:2, or 1:4 concentration. Solutions for intra-articular use, may be diluted with lidocaine 1% or 2%.

Topical spray: Avoid excessive heat.

Mechanism of Action Decreases inflammation by suppression of migration of polymorphonuclear leukocytes and reversal of increased capillary permeability; suppresses the immune system by reducing activity and volume of the lymphatic system; suppresses adrenal function at high doses

Pharmacodynamics Duration: Oral: 8-12 hours

Pharmacokinetics

Time to peak serum concentration: I.M.: Within 8-10 hours

Half-life, biologic: 18-36 hours

Dosage

Geriatrics & Adults: The lowest possible dose should be used to control the condition; when dose reduction is possible, the dose should be reduced gradually. Parenteral dose is usually $1/3$ to $1/2$ the oral dose given every 12 hours. In life-threatening situations, parenteral doses larger than the oral dose may be needed.

Allergic rhinitis (perennial or seasonal):

Nasal spray: 220 mcg/day as 2 sprays in each nostril once daily

Nasal inhaler: Initial: 220 mcg/day as 2 sprays in each nostril once daily; may increase dose to 440 mcg/day (given once daily or divided and given 2 or 4 times/day)

Asthma:

Oral inhalation: 200 mcg 3-4 times/day **or** 400 mcg twice daily; maximum dose: 1600 mcg/day

Carditis (acute rheumatic): Oral: Initial: 20-60 mg/day; reduce dose during maintenance therapy

Dermatoses (steroid-responsive, including contact/atopic dermatitis):

Injection:

Acetonide: Intradermal: Initial: 1 mg

Hexacetonide: Intralesional, sublesional: up to 0.5 mg/square inch of affected skin

Topical:

Cream, ointment: Apply thin film to affected areas 2-4 times/day

Spray: Apply to affected area 3-4 times/day

Ophthalmic disorders: Oral: 12-40 mg/day

Oral inflammatory lesions/ulcers: Oral topical: Press a small dab (about $1/4$ inch) to the lesion until a thin film develops; a larger quantity may be required for coverage of some lesions. For optimal results, use only enough to coat the lesion with a thin film; do not rub in.

Triamcinolone Dosing

	Acetonide	Hexacetonide
Intrasynovial	5-40 mg	
Intralesional	1-30 mg (usually 1 mg per injection site); 10 mg/mL suspension usually used	Up to 0.5 mg/sq inch affected area
Sublesional	1-30 mg	
Systemic I.M.	2.5-60 mg/dose (usual adult dose: 60 mg; may repeat with 20-100 mg dose when symptoms recur)	
Intra-articular	2.5-40 mg	2-20 mg average
large joints	5-15 mg	10-20 mg
small joints	2.5-5 mg	2-6 mg
Tendon sheaths	2.5-10 mg	
Intradermal	1 mg/site	

Rheumatic or arthritic disorders:
Intra-articular (or similar injection as designated):
Acetonide: Intra-articular, intrabursal, tendon sheaths: Initial: Smaller joints: 2.5-5 mg, larger joints: 5-15 mg
Hexacetonide: Intra-articular: Initial range: 2-20 mg/day
I.M.:
Acetonide: Range: 2.5-60 mg/day; Initial: 60 mg
See table on previous page.

Administration
Injection: Avoid injecting into a previously infected joint; do not inject into unstable joints
I.M.: Inject deep in large muscle mass, avoid deltoid.
SubQ: Avoid subcutaneous administration.
Nasal spray, inhalation: Shake well prior to use. Gently blow nose to clear nostrils.
Oral inhalation: Shake well prior to use. Rinse mouth and throat after using inhaler to prevent candidiasis. Use spacer device provided with Azmacort®.
Oral topical: Apply small dab to lesion until a thin film develops; do not rub in. Apply at bedtime or after meals if applications are needed throughout the day.
Topical: Apply a thin film sparingly and avoid topical application on the face. Do not use on open skin or wounds. Do not occlude area unless directed.

Monitoring Parameters Blood pressure, blood glucose, electrolytes

Patient Information Report any change in body weight. Do not discontinue or decrease the drug without contacting your prescriber. Carry an identification card or bracelet advising that you are on steroids. May take with meals to decrease GI upset.

Nasal inhaler: Do not use intranasal product if you have a nasal infection, nasal injury, or recent nasal surgery. If using two products, consult prescriber in which order to use the two products. Clear nasal passages before administration (use decongestant as needed). Follow package insert instructions for use. Do not exceed maximum dosage. Report unusual cough or spasm; persistent nasal bleeding, burning, or irritation; or worsening of condition.

Oral inhaler: Shake gently before use. Use at regular intervals, no more frequently than directed. Not for use during acute asthmatic attack. Follow directions that accompany product. Rinse mouth and throat after use to prevent candidiasis. Sit when using. Take deep breaths for 3-5 minutes. Hold breath for 5-10 seconds after use, and wait 1-3 minutes between inhalations. Follow package insert instructions for use. Do not exceed maximum dosage. If also using inhaled bronchodilator, use before triamcinolone.

Oral topical: Dab small amount to lesion, do not rub in. Notify health care provider if improvement is not seen within 7 days.

Topical: For external use only. Not for eyes or mucous membranes or open wounds. Apply in very thin layer to occlusive dressing. Apply dressing to area being treated. Avoid prolonged or excessive use around sensitive tissues, genital, or rectal areas. Inform prescriber if condition worsens (swelling, redness, irritation, pain, open sores) or fails to improve.

Additional Information Systemic absorption may occur after topical application; 16 mg triamcinolone is equivalent to 100 mg cortisone (no mineralocorticoid activity).

Special Geriatric Considerations Because of the risk of adverse effects, systemic corticosteroids should be used cautiously in the elderly, in the smallest possible dose, and for the shortest possible time. Azmacort® (metered dose inhaler) comes with its own spacer device attached and may be easier to use in older patients.

Dosage Forms Excipient information presented when available (limited, particularly for generics); consult specific product labeling.
Aerosol for oral inhalation, as acetonide:
Azmacort®: 100 mcg per actuation (20 g) [240 actuations]
Aerosol, topical, as acetonide:
Kenalog®: 0.2 mg/2-second spray (63 g)
Cream, as acetonide: 0.025% (15 g, 80 g, 454 g); 0.1% (15 g, 80 g, 454 g, 2270 g); 0.5% (15 g)
Triderm®: 0.1% (30 g, 85 g)
Injection, suspension, as acetonide:
Kenalog-10®: 10 mg/mL (5 mL) [contains benzyl alcohol; not for I.V. or I.M. use]
Kenalog-40®: 40 mg/mL (1 mL, 5 mL, 10 mL) [contains benzyl alcohol; not for I.V. or intradermal use]
Injection, suspension, as hexacetonide:
Aristospan®: 5 mg/mL (5 mL); 20 mg/mL (1 mL, 5 mL) [contains benzyl alcohol; not for I.V. use]
Lotion, as acetonide: 0.025% (60 mL); 0.1% (60 mL)
Ointment, topical, as acetonide: 0.025% (15 g, 80 g, 454 g); 0.1% (15 g, 80 g, 454 g); 0.5% (15 g)
Paste, oral, topical, as acetonide: 0.1% (5 g)
(Continued)

Triamcinolone *(Continued)*

Solution, intranasal, as acetonide [spray]:
Tri-Nasal®: 50 mcg/inhalation (15 mL) [120 actuations]
Suspension, intranasal, as acetonide [spray]:
Nasacort® AQ: 55 mcg/inhalation (16.5 g) [120 actuations]

◆ **Triamcinolone Acetonide, Aerosol** *see* Triamcinolone *on page 1619*
◆ **Triamcinolone Acetonide, Parenteral** *see* Triamcinolone *on page 1619*
◆ **Triamcinolone and Nystatin** *see* Nystatin and Triamcinolone *on page 1143*
◆ **Triamcinolone Diacetate, Oral** *see* Triamcinolone *on page 1619*
◆ **Triamcinolone Diacetate, Parenteral** *see* Triamcinolone *on page 1619*
◆ **Triamcinolone Hexacetonide** *see* Triamcinolone *on page 1619*
◆ **Triamcinolone, Oral** *see* Triamcinolone *on page 1619*
◆ **Triaminic® Allerchews™ [OTC]** *see* Loratadine *on page 928*
◆ **Triaminic® Infant Thin Strips® Decongestant [OTC]** *see* Phenylephrine *on page 1247*
◆ **Triaminic® Thin Strips® Cold [OTC]** *see* Phenylephrine *on page 1247*
◆ **Triaminic® Thin Strips™ Cough and Runny Nose [OTC]** *see* DiphenhydrAMINE *on page 447*
◆ **Triaminic® Thin Strips™ Long Acting Cough [OTC]** *see* Dextromethorphan *on page 419*

Triamterene *(trye AM ter een)*

Medication Safety Issues
Sound-alike/look-alike issues:
Triamterene may be confused with trimipramine
Dyrenium® may be confused with Pyridium®
U.S. Brand Names Dyrenium®
Generic Available No
Pharmacologic Category Diuretic, Potassium-Sparing
Use Alone or in combination with other diuretics to treat edema and hypertension; reduction of potassium excretion caused by kaliuretic diuretics
Contraindications Hypersensitivity to triamterene or any component of the formulation; patients receiving other potassium-sparing diuretics; anuria; severe hepatic disease; hyperkalemia or history of hyperkalemia; severe or progressive renal disease
Warnings/Precautions [U.S. Boxed Warning]: Hyperkalemia can occur; patients at risk include those with renal impairment, diabetes, the elderly, and the severely ill. Serum potassium levels must be monitored at frequent intervals especially when dosages are changed or with any illness that may cause renal dysfunction. Avoid potassium supplements, potassium-containing salt substitutes, a diet rich in potassium, or other drugs that can cause hyperkalemia. Monitor for fluid and electrolyte imbalances. Diuretic therapy should be carefully used in severe hepatic dysfunction; electrolyte and fluid shifts can cause or exacerbate encephalopathy. Use cautiously in patients with history of kidney stones and diabetes. Can cause photosensitivity.
Adverse Reactions (Reflective of adult population; not specific for elderly)
1% to 10%:
Cardiovascular: Hypotension, edema, CHF, bradycardia
Central nervous system: Dizziness, headache, fatigue
Gastrointestinal: Constipation, nausea
Respiratory: Dyspnea
Overdosage/Toxicology Symptoms include drowsiness, confusion, clinical signs of dehydration, electrolyte imbalance, and hypotension. Chronic or acute ingestion of large amounts of potassium-sparing diuretics, may result in life-threatening hyperkalemia, especially with decreased renal function. If the EKG shows no widening of the QRS or an arrhythmia, discontinue triamterene and any potassium supplement and substitute a thiazide. Consider Kayexalate® to increase potassium excretion. If an abnormal cardiac status is obvious, treat with calcium or sodium bicarbonates as needed, pacing dialysis and/or Kayexalate®. Infusions of glucose and insulin are also useful.
Drug Interactions
ACE inhibitors can cause hyperkalemia, especially in patients with renal impairment, potassium-rich diets, or on other drugs causing hyperkalemia; avoid concurrent use or monitor closely.
Potassium supplements may further increase potassium retention and cause hyperkalemia; avoid concurrent use.
Mechanism of Action Interferes with potassium/sodium exchange (active transport) in the distal tubule, cortical collecting tubule and collecting duct by inhibiting sodium, potassium-ATPase; decreases calcium excretion; increases magnesium loss

Pharmacodynamics
Onset of action: Within 2-4 hours
Duration: 7-9 hours

Pharmacokinetics
Absorption: Oral: Unreliably absorbed
Time to peak serum concentration: One study found that peak serum concentrations in older adults were approximately twice those in younger patients

Dosage
Geriatrics & Adults: Edema, hypertension: Oral: 100-300 mg/day in 1-2 divided doses; maximum dose: 300 mg/day; usual dosage range (JNC 7): 50-100 mg/day
Renal Impairment: Cl_{cr} <10 mL/minute: Avoid use.
Hepatic Impairment: Dose reduction is recommended in patients with cirrhosis.

Monitoring Parameters Blood pressure, serum electrolytes, renal function, weight, I & O

Test Interactions Interferes with fluorometric assay of quinidine

Patient Information Take in the morning; take the last dose of multiple doses no later than 6 PM unless instructed otherwise; take after meals; notify physician if weakness, headache or nausea occurs; avoid excessive ingestion of food high in potassium or use of salt substitute; may increase blood glucose; may impart a blue fluorescent color to urine

Special Geriatric Considerations Monitor serum potassium.

Dosage Forms Excipient information presented when available (limited, particularly for generics); consult specific product labeling.
Capsule: 50 mg, 100 mg [contains benzyl alcohol]

♦ **Triamterene and Hydrochlorothiazide** see Hydrochlorothiazide and Triamterene on page 759

Triazolam (trye AY zoe lam)

Related Information
Anxiolytic, Sedative / Hypnotic, and Miscellaneous Benzodiazepines on page 1750
Potentially Inappropriate Medications for Geriatrics on page 1824

Medication Safety Issues
Sound-alike/look-alike issues:
Triazolam may be confused with alprazolam
Halcion® may be confused with halcinonide, Haldol®

U.S. Brand Names Halcion® [DSC]

Canadian Brand Names Apo-Triazo®; Gen-Triazolam; Halcion®

Generic Available Yes

Pharmacologic Category Hypnotic, Benzodiazepine

Use Short-term treatment of insomnia

Restrictions C-IV

Contraindications Hypersensitivity to triazolam or any component of the formulation (cross-sensitivity with other benzodiazepines may exist); concurrent therapy with atazanavir, ketoconazole, itraconazole, nefazodone, and ritonavir

Warnings/Precautions Should be used only after evaluation of potential causes of sleep disturbance. Failure of sleep disturbance to resolve after 7-10 days may indicate psychiatric or medical illness. A worsening of insomnia or the emergence of new abnormalities of thought or behavior may represent unrecognized psychiatric or medical illness and requires immediate and careful evaluation. Prescription should be written for a maximum of 7-10 days and should not be prescribed in quantities exceeding a 1-month supply. Abrupt discontinuation after sustained use (generally >10 days) may cause withdrawal symptoms.

An increase in daytime anxiety may occur after as few as 10 days of continuous use, which may be related to withdrawal reaction in some patients. Anterograde amnesia may occur at a higher rate with triazolam than with other benzodiazepines. Use with caution in elderly or debilitated patients, patients with hepatic disease (including alcoholics), or renal impairment. Use with caution in patients with respiratory disease or impaired gag reflex. Avoid use in patients with sleep apnea.

Causes CNS depression (dose-related) resulting in sedation, dizziness, confusion, or ataxia which may impair physical and mental capabilities. Patients must be cautioned about performing tasks which require mental alertness (eg, operating machinery or driving). Use with caution in patients receiving other CNS depressants or psychoactive agents. Postmarketing studies have indicated that the use of hypnotic/sedative agents for sleep has been associated with hypersensitivity reactions including anaphylaxis as well as angioedema. An increased risk for hazardous sleep-related activities such as sleep-driving; cooking and eating food, and making phone calls while asleep have also (Continued)

Triazolam *(Continued)*

been noted. Effects with other sedative drugs or ethanol may be potentiated. Benzodiazepines have been associated with falls and traumatic injury and should be used with extreme caution in patients who are at risk of these events (especially the elderly).

Use caution with potent CYP3A4 inhibitors, as they may significantly decreased the clearance of triazolam. Use caution in patients with suicidal risk. Use with caution in patients with a history of drug dependence. Benzodiazepines have been associated with dependence and acute withdrawal symptoms on discontinuation or reduction in dose. Acute withdrawal, including seizures, may be precipitated after administration of flumazenil to patients receiving long-term benzodiazepine therapy.

Paradoxical reactions, including hyperactive or aggressive behavior have been reported with benzodiazepines, particularly in psychiatric patients. Does not have analgesic, antidepressant, or antipsychotic properties.

Adverse Reactions (Reflective of adult population; not specific for elderly)

>10%: Central nervous system: Drowsiness, anteriograde amnesia

1% to 10%:

Central nervous system: Headache, dizziness, nervousness, lightheadedness, ataxia

Gastrointestinal: Nausea, vomiting

Overdosage/Toxicology
Symptoms include somnolence, confusion, coma, diminished reflexes, dyspnea, and hypotension. Treatment for benzodiazepine overdose is supportive. Rarely is mechanical ventilation required. Flumazenil has been shown to selectively block the binding of benzodiazepines to CNS receptors, resulting in reversal of benzodiazepine-induced CNS depression, but not always respiratory depression.

Drug Interactions
Substrate of CYP3A4 (major); **Inhibits** CYP2C8 (weak), 2C9 (weak)

Clozapine: Benzodiazepines may enhance the adverse/toxic effect of clozapine.

CNS depressants: Sedative effects and/or respiratory depression may be additive with CNS depressants; includes ethanol, barbiturates, opioid analgesics, and other sedative agents; monitor for increased effect

CYP3A4 inducers: CYP3A4 inducers may decrease the levels/effects of triazolam. Example inducers include aminoglutethimide, carbamazepine, nafcillin, nevirapine, phenobarbital, phenytoin, and rifamycins.

CYP3A4 inhibitors: May increase the levels/effects of triazolam. Example inhibitors include azole antifungals, clarithromycin, diclofenac, doxycycline, erythromycin, imatinib, isoniazid, nefazodone, nicardipine, propofol, protease inhibitors, quinidine, telithromycin, and verapamil.

Disulfiram: May decrease the metabolism, via CYP isoenzymes, of triazolam.

Isoniazid: Isoniazid may increase triazolam levels.

Oral contraceptives: May decrease the clearance and increase the half-life of triazolam; monitor for increased triazolam effect

Proton Pump Inhibitors: May increase the serum concentration of triazolam.

Theophylline: May partially antagonize some of the effects of benzodiazepines; monitor for decreased response; may require higher doses for sedation

Ethanol/Nutrition/Herb Interactions

Ethanol: Avoid ethanol (may increase CNS depression).

Food: Food may decrease the rate of absorption. Triazolam serum concentration may be increased by grapefruit juice; avoid concurrent use.

Herb/Nutraceutical: St John's wort may decrease levels. Avoid valerian, St John's wort, kava kava, gotu kola (may increase CNS depression).

Mechanism of Action
Binds to stereospecific benzodiazepine receptors on the postsynaptic GABA neuron at several sites within the central nervous system, including the limbic system, reticular formation. Enhancement of the inhibitory effect of GABA on neuronal excitability results by increased neuronal membrane permeability to chloride ions. This shift in chloride ions results in hyperpolarization (a less excitable state) and stabilization.

Pharmacodynamics
Hypnotic effects:

Onset of action: Within 15-30 minutes

Duration: 6-7 hours; studies have shown that older adults are more sensitive to the effects of benzodiazepines as compared to younger adults

Pharmacokinetics

Distribution: V_d: 0.8-1.8 L/kg

Protein binding: 89%

Metabolism: Extensive in the liver

Half-life: 1.7-5 hours

Elimination: In urine as unchanged drug and metabolites; triazolam clearance is lower in older adults

Note: In older adults, peak plasma concentrations and AUC are increased

Dosage

Geriatrics: Oral: Insomnia (short-term use): 0.0625-0.125 mg at bedtime; maximum dose: 0.25 mg/day (see Special Geriatric Considerations)

Adults: Note: Onset of action is rapid, patient should be in bed when taking medication.

Insomnia (short-term): Oral: 0.125-0.25 mg at bedtime (maximum dose: 0.5 mg/day)

Dental (preprocedure): Oral: 0.25 mg taken the evening before oral surgery; or 0.25 mg 1 hour before procedure

Hepatic Impairment: Reduce dose or avoid use in cirrhosis.

Monitoring Parameters Respiratory, cardiovascular and mental status

Patient Information Avoid alcohol and other CNS depressants; may cause drowsiness; avoid activities needing good psychomotor coordination until CNS effects are known; may cause physical or psychological dependence; avoid abrupt discontinuation after prolonged use; **for short-term use only; do not exceed prescribed dose**

Additional Information Onset of action is rapid, patient should take triazolam right before going to bed

Special Geriatric Considerations Due to the higher incidence of CNS adverse reactions and its short half-life, this benzodiazepine is not a drug of first choice. For short-term only.

Dosage Forms Excipient information presented when available (limited, particularly for generics); consult specific product labeling.
Tablet: 0.125 mg, 0.25 mg
Halcion®: 0.125 mg, 0.25 mg [DSC]

Selected References
Greenblatt DJ, Harmatz JS, Shapiro L, et al, "Sensitivity to Triazolam in the Elderly," *N Engl J Med*, 1991, 324(24):1691-8.

- ♦ **Tribavirin** see Ribavirin *on page 1397*
- ♦ **Trichloroacetaldehyde Monohydrate** see Chloral Hydrate *on page 285*
- ♦ **TriCor®** see Fenofibrate *on page 604*
- ♦ **Tricosal** see Choline Magnesium Trisalicylate *on page 307*
- ♦ **Triderm®** see Triamcinolone *on page 1619*

Triethanolamine Polypeptide Oleate-Condensate
(trye eth a NOLE a meen pol i PEP tide OH lee ate-KON den sate)

U.S. Brand Names Cerumenex® [DSC]
Canadian Brand Names Cerumenex®
Generic Available No
Pharmacologic Category Otic Agent, Cerumenolytic
Use Removal of ear wax (cerumen)
Contraindications Hypersensitivity to triethanolamine polypeptide oleate-condensate or any component of the formulation; perforated tympanic membrane or otitis media
Warnings/Precautions Avoid undue exposure to peridural skin during administration and the flushing out of ear canal; discontinue if sensitization or irritation occurs
Drug Interactions No data reported
Mechanism of Action Emulsifies and disperses accumulated cerumen
Pharmacodynamics Onset of effect: Produces slight disintegration of very hard ear wax by 24 hours
Dosage
Geriatrics & Adults: Ear wax removal: Otic: Fill ear canal, insert cotton plug; allow to remain 15-30 minutes; flush ear with lukewarm water as a single treatment; if a second application is needed for unusually hard impactions, repeat the procedure
Monitoring Parameters Evaluate hearing before and after instillation of medication
Patient Information For external use in the ear only; warm to body temperature before using to improve effect; avoid touching dropper to any surface; hold ear lobe up and back; lie on your side or tilt the affected ear up for ease of administration; fill ear canal, let stand for 15-30 minutes, then flush
Special Geriatric Considerations Avoid contact with hearing aids.
Dosage Forms Excipient information presented when available (limited, particularly for generics); consult specific product labeling. [DSC] = Discontinued product
Solution, otic: 10% (6 mL, 12 mL) [DSC]

Trifluoperazine (trye floo oh PER a zeen)

Related Information
Antipsychotic Agents *on page 1747*
Liquid Compatibility of Antipsychotics and Mood Stabilizers *on page 1851*
(Continued)

Trifluoperazine *(Continued)*

Medication Safety Issues
Sound-alike/look-alike issues:
Trifluoperazine may be confused with triflupromazine, trihexyphenidyl
Stelazine® may be confused with selegiline

Canadian Brand Names Apo-Trifluoperazine®; Novo-Trifluzine; PMS-Trifluoperazine;
Terfluzine

Index Terms Trifluoperazine Hydrochloride

Generic Available Yes

Pharmacologic Category Antipsychotic Agent, Typical, Phenothiazine

Use Management of depressive neurosis, schizophrenia alcohol withdrawal, nausea and
vomiting, nonpsychotic symptoms associated with dementia (older adults), Tourette's
syndrome, Huntington's chorea, spasmodic torticollis, Reye's syndrome
See Special Geriatric Considerations.

Unlabeled/Investigational Use Management of psychotic disorders

Contraindications Hypersensitivity to trifluoperazine or any component of the formulation (cross-reactivity between phenothiazines may occur); severe CNS depression;
bone marrow suppression; blood dyscrasias; severe hepatic disease; coma

Warnings/Precautions Use with caution in patients with cardiovascular disease,
seizures, hepatic dysfunction, narrow-angle glaucoma, or bone marrow suppression;
use with caution in patients with myasthenia gravis or Parkinson's disease

Adverse Reactions (Reflective of adult population; not specific for elderly)
Frequency not defined.
Cardiovascular: Hypotension, orthostatic hypotension, cardiac arrest
Central nervous system: Extrapyramidal signs (pseudoparkinsonism, akathisia,
dystonias, tardive dyskinesia), dizziness, headache, neuroleptic malignant syndrome
(NMS), impairment of temperature regulation, lowering of seizure threshold
Dermatologic: Increased sensitivity to sun, rash, discoloration of skin (blue-gray),
photosensitivity
Endocrine & metabolic: Changes in menstrual cycle, libido (changes in), breast pain,
hyperglycemia, hypoglycemia, gynecomastia, lactation, galactorrhea
Gastrointestinal: Constipation, weight gain, nausea, vomiting, stomach pain, xero-
stomia
Genitourinary: Difficulty in urination, ejaculatory disturbances, urinary retention, pria-
pism
Hematologic: Agranulocytosis, leukopenia, pancytopenia, thrombocytopenic purpura,
eosinophilia, hemolytic anemia, aplastic anemia
Hepatic: Cholestatic jaundice, hepatotoxicity
Neuromuscular & skeletal: Tremor
Ocular: Pigmentary retinopathy, cornea and lens changes
Respiratory: Nasal congestion

Overdosage/Toxicology Symptoms include deep sleep, coma, extrapyramidal symptoms, abnormal involuntary muscle movements, hypo- or hypertension, and cardiac
arrhythmias. Following initiation of essential overdose management, toxic symptom
treatment and supportive treatment should be initiated. Hypotension usually responds
to I.V. fluids or Trendelenburg positioning. If unresponsive to these measures, the use
of a parenteral inotrope may be required (eg, norepinephrine 0.1-0.2 mcg/kg/minute
titrated to response). Seizures commonly respond to diazepam (I.V. 5-10 mg bolus
every 15 minutes if needed up to a total of 30 mg) or to phenytoin or phenobarbital.
Neuroleptics often cause extrapyramidal symptoms (eg, dystonic reactions) requiring
management with diphenhydramine 1-2 mg/kg up to a maximum of 50 mg I.M. or slow
I.V. push followed by a maintenance dose for 48-72 hours. When these reactions are
unresponsive to diphenhydramine, anticholinergic agents such as benztropine mesylate I.V. 1-2 mg may be effective. These agents are generally effective within 2-5
minutes. Cardiac arrhythmias are treated with lidocaine 1-2 mg/kg bolus followed by a
maintenance infusion.

Drug Interactions Substrate of CYP1A2 (major)
Acetylcholinesterase inhibitors (central): May increase the risk of antipsychotic-related
extrapyramidal symptoms; monitor.
Aluminum salts: May decrease the absorption of phenothiazines; monitor
Amphetamines: Efficacy may be diminished by antipsychotics; in addition, amphetamines may increase psychotic symptoms; avoid concurrent use
Anticholinergics: May inhibit the therapeutic response to phenothiazines and excess
anticholinergic effects may occur; includes benztropine, trihexyphenidyl, biperiden,
and drugs with significant anticholinergic activity (TCAs, antihistamines, disopyramide)
Antihypertensives: Concurrent use of phenothiazines with an antihypertensive may
produce additive hypotensive effects (particularly orthostasis)
Bromocriptine: Phenothiazines inhibit the ability of bromocriptine to lower serum
prolactin concentrations

CNS depressants: Sedative effects may be additive with phenothiazines; monitor for increased effect; includes barbiturates, benzodiazepines, opioid analgesics, ethanol, and other sedative agents

CYP1A2 inducers: May decrease the levels/effects of trifluoperazine. Example inducers include aminoglutethimide, carbamazepine, phenobarbital, and rifampin.

CYP1A2 inhibitors: May increase the levels/effects of trifluoperazine. Example inhibitors include ciprofloxacin, fluvoxamine, ketoconazole, norfloxacin, ofloxacin, and rofecoxib.

Epinephrine: Chlorpromazine (and possibly other low potency antipsychotics) may diminish the pressor effects of epinephrine

Guanethidine and guanadrel: Antihypertensive effects may be inhibited by phenothiazines

Levodopa: Phenothiazines may inhibit the antiparkinsonian effect of levodopa; avoid this combination

Lithium: Phenothiazines may produce neurotoxicity with lithium; this is a rare effect.

Metoclopramide: May increase extrapyramidal symptoms (EPS) or risk.

Polypeptide antibiotics: Rare cases of respiratory paralysis have been reported with concurrent use of phenothiazines

Propranolol: Serum concentrations of phenothiazines may be increased; propranolol also increases phenothiazine concentrations

QT_c-prolonging agents: Effects on QT_c interval may be additive with phenothiazines, increasing the risk of malignant arrhythmias; includes type Ia antiarrhythmics, TCAs, and some quinolone antibiotics (moxifloxacin).

Sulfadoxine-pyrimethamine: May increase phenothiazine concentrations

Trazodone: Phenothiazines and trazodone may produce additive hypotensive effects

Tricyclic antidepressants: Concurrent use may produce increased toxicity or altered therapeutic response

Valproic acid: Serum levels may be increased by phenothiazines

Ethanol/Nutrition/Herb Interactions

Ethanol: Avoid ethanol (may increase CNS depression).

Herb/Nutraceutical: Avoid kava kava, gotu kola, valerian, St John's wort (may increase CNS depression). Avoid dong quai, St John's wort (may also cause photosensitization).

Mechanism of Action Trifluoperazine is a piperazine phenothiazine antipsychotic which blocks postsynaptic mesolimbic dopaminergic receptors in the brain; exhibits alpha-adrenergic blocking effect and depresses the release of hypothalamic and hypophyseal hormones

Pharmacokinetics

Absorption: May be affected by the inherent anticholinergic action on the gastrointestinal tissue causing variable absorption. Absorption from tablets is erratic with less variation seen with solutions. These agents are widely distributed in tissues with CNS concentrations exceeding that of plasma due to their lipophilic characteristics.

Protein binding: Antipsychotic agents are bound 90% to 99% to plasma proteins; highly bound to brain and lung tissue and other tissues with a high blood perfusion.

Half-life: >24 hours with chronic use

Time to peak concentration: Oral: 2-4 hours

Elimination: Occurs through hepatic metabolism (oxidation) where numerous active metabolites are produced; active metabolites excreted in urine; elimination half-lives of antipsychotics ranges from 20-40 hours which may be extended in older adults due to decline in oxidative hepatic reactions (phase I) with age.

Biologic effect of a single dose persists for 24 hours. When the patient has accommodated to initial side effects (sedation), once daily dosing is possible due to the long half-life of antipsychotics.

Steady-state plasma concentrations are achieved in 4-7 days; therefore, if possible, do not make dose adjustments more than once in a 7-day period. Due to the long half-lives of antipsychotics, as needed (prn) use is ineffective since repeated doses are necessary to achieve therapeutic tissue concentrations in the CNS.

Dosage

Geriatrics:

Schizophrenia/psychoses: Oral: Refer to adult dosing. Dose selection should start at the low end of the dosage range and titration must be gradual.

Behavioral symptoms associated with dementia behavior (unlabeled use): Oral: Initial: 0.5-1 mg 1-2 times/day; increase dose at 4- to 7-day intervals by 0.5-1 mg/day; increase dosing intervals (bid, tid, etc) as necessary to control response or side effects. Maximum daily dose: 40 mg. Gradual increases (titration) may prevent some side effects or decrease their severity.

Adults:

Schizophrenia/psychoses: Oral:

Outpatients: 1-2 mg twice daily

Hospitalized or well supervised patient: Initial: 2-5 mg twice daily with optimum response in the 15-20 mg/day range; do not exceed 40 mg/day.

(Continued)

Trifluoperazine *(Continued)*

Nonpsychotic anxiety: Oral: 1-2 mg twice daily; maximum: 6 mg/day; therapy for anxiety should not exceed 12 weeks; do not exceed 6 mg/day for longer than 12 weeks when treating anxiety; agitation, jitteriness, or insomnia may be confused with original neurotic or psychotic symptoms.

Renal Impairment: Not dialyzable (0% to 5%)

Administration Administer I.M. injection deep in upper outer quadrant of buttock

Monitoring Parameters Orthostatic blood pressures; tremors, gait changes, abnormal movement in trunk, neck, buccal area, or extremities; monitor target behaviors for which the agent is given. Monitor orthostatic blood pressures 3-5 days after initiation of therapy or a dose increase.

Test Interactions False-positive for phenylketonuria

Patient Information Oral concentrate must be diluted in 2-4 oz of liquid (water, fruit juice, carbonated drinks, milk, or pudding); do not take antacid within 1 hour of taking drug; avoid alcohol; avoid excess sun exposure (use sun block); may cause drowsiness, rise slowly from recumbent position; use of supportive stockings may help prevent orthostatic hypotension

Additional Information Do not exceed 6 mg/day for longer than 12 weeks when treating anxiety; drug-induced agitation, jitteriness, or insomnia may be confused with original anxious or psychotic symptoms

Special Geriatric Considerations Elderly are more susceptible to hypotension and neuromuscular reactions.

Many elderly patients receive antipsychotic medications for inappropriate nonpsychotic behavior. Before initiating antipsychotic medication, the clinician should investigate any possible reversible cause; any stress or stress from any disease can cause acute "confusion" or worsening of baseline nonpsychotic behavior. Most commonly acute changes in behavior are due to increases in drug dose or addition of new drug to regimen; fluid electrolyte loss; infections; and changes in environment.

Any changes in disease status in any organ system can result in behavior changes.

In the treatment of agitated, demented, elderly patients, authors of meta-analysis of controlled trials of the response to the traditional antipsychotics (phenothiazines, butyrophenones) in controlling agitation have concluded that the use of neuroleptics results in a response rate of 18%. Clearly neuroleptic therapy for behavior control should be limited with frequent attempts to withdraw the agent given for behavior control.

Dosage Forms Excipient information presented when available (limited, particularly for generics); consult specific product labeling.

Tablet: 1 mg, 2 mg, 5 mg, 10 mg

Selected References

Peabody CA, Warner MD, Whiteford HA, et al, "Neuroleptics and the Elderly," *J Am Geriatr Soc*, 1987, 35(3):233-8.

Risse SC and Barnes R, "Pharmacologic Treatment of Agitation Associated With Dementia," *J Am Geriatr Soc*, 1986, 34(5):368-76.

Saltz BL, Woerner MG, Kane JM, et al, "Prospective Study of Tardive Dyskinesia Incidence in the Elderly," *JAMA*, 1991, 266(17):2402-6.

Seifert RD, "Therapeutic Drug Monitoring: Psychotropic Drugs," *J Pharm Pract*, 1984, 6:403-16.

♦ **Trifluoperazine Hydrochloride** *see* Trifluoperazine *on page 1627*
♦ **Trifluorothymidine** *see* Trifluridine *on page 1630*

Trifluridine *(trye FLURE i deen)*

Medication Safety Issues
Sound-alike/look-alike issues:
Viroptic® may be confused with Timoptic®

U.S. Brand Names Viroptic®

Canadian Brand Names SAB-Trifluridine; Sandoz-Trifluridine; Viroptic®

Index Terms F_3T; Trifluorothymidine

Generic Available Yes

Pharmacologic Category Antiviral Agent, Ophthalmic

Use Treatment of primary keratoconjunctivitis and recurrent epithelial keratitis caused by herpes simplex virus types I and II

Contraindications Hypersensitivity to trifluridine or any component of the formulation

Warnings/Precautions Mild local irritation of conjunctival and cornea may occur when instilled but usually transient effects

Adverse Reactions (Reflective of adult population; not specific for elderly)
1% to 10%: Local: Burning, stinging

Drug Interactions No data reported

Stability Refrigerate at 2°C to 8°C (36°F to 46°F). Storage at room temperature may result in a solution altered pH which could result in ocular discomfort upon administration and/or decreased potency.

Mechanism of Action Interferes with viral replication by incorporating into viral DNA in place of thymidine, inhibiting thymidylate synthetase resulting in the formation of defective proteins

Pharmacokinetics Absorption: Ophthalmic instillation: Systemic absorption is negligible, while corneal penetration is adequate

Dosage
Geriatrics & Adults: Herpes keratoconjunctivitis, keratitis: Ophthalmic: Instill 1 drop into affected eye every 2 hours while awake, to a maximum of 9 drops/day, until re-epithelialization of corneal ulcer occurs. Then use 1 drop every 4 hours for another 7 days. Do **not** exceed 21 days of treatment. If improvement has not taken place in 7-14 days, consider another form of therapy.

Monitoring Parameters Ophthalmologic exam (test for corneal staining with fluorescein or Rose Bengal)

Patient Information Notify physician if improvement is not seen after 7 days, condition worsens, or if irritation occurs; do not discontinue without notifying the physician, do not exceed recommended dosage

Special Geriatric Considerations Assess ability to self-administer.

Dosage Forms Excipient information presented when available (limited, particularly for generics); consult specific product labeling.
Solution, ophthalmic: 1% (7.5 mL)

♦ Triglide™ *see* Fenofibrate *on page 604*

Trihexyphenidyl (trye heks ee FEN i dil)

Related Information
Antiparkinsonian Agents *on page 1745*
Medication Safety Issues
Sound-alike/look-alike issues:
Trihexyphenidyl may be confused with trifluoperazine
Artane may be confused with Altace®, Anturane®, Aramine®
Canadian Brand Names Apo-Trihex®
Index Terms Artane; Benzhexol Hydrochloride; Trihexyphenidyl Hydrochloride
Generic Available Yes
Pharmacologic Category Anti-Parkinson's Agent, Anticholinergic; Anticholinergic Agent
Use Adjunctive treatment of Parkinson's disease; treatment of drug-induced extrapyramidal effects and acute dystonic reactions
Contraindications Hypersensitivity to trihexyphenidyl or any component of the formulation; narrow-angle glaucoma; pyloric or duodenal obstruction; stenosing peptic ulcers; bladder neck obstructions; achalasia; myasthenia gravis
Warnings/Precautions Use with caution in hot weather or during exercise, especially when administered concomitantly with other atropine-like drugs to chronically-ill patients, alcoholics, patients with CNS disease, or persons doing manual labor in a hot environment. Elderly patients require strict dosage regulation. Use with caution in patients with tachycardia, cardiac arrhythmias, hypertension, hypotension, glaucoma, prostatic hyperplasia or any tendency toward urinary retention, liver or kidney disorders, and obstructive disease of the GI or GU tract. May exacerbate mental symptoms when used to treat extrapyramidal symptoms. When given in large doses or to susceptible patients, may cause weakness.
Adverse Reactions (Reflective of adult population; not specific for elderly)
Frequency not defined.
Cardiovascular: Tachycardia
Central nervous system: Confusion, agitation, euphoria, drowsiness, headache, dizziness, nervousness, delusions, hallucinations, paranoia
Dermatologic: Dry skin, increased sensitivity to light, rash
Gastrointestinal: Constipation, xerostomia, dry throat, ileus, nausea, vomiting, parotitis
Genitourinary: Urinary retention
Neuromuscular & skeletal: Weakness
Ocular: Blurred vision, mydriasis, increase in intraocular pressure, glaucoma, blindness (long-term use in narrow-angle glaucoma)
Respiratory: Dry nose
Miscellaneous: Diaphoresis (decreased)
Overdosage/Toxicology Symptoms include blurred vision, urinary retention, and tachycardia. Anticholinergic toxicity is caused by strong binding of the drug to cholinergic receptors. Anticholinesterase inhibitors reduce acetylcholinesterase. For anticholinergic overdose with severe life-threatening symptoms, physostigmine 1-2 mg SubQ or slow I.V. may be given to reverse these effects.
Drug Interactions
Amantadine, rimantadine: Central and/or peripheral anticholinergic syndrome can occur when administered with amantadine or rimantadine
(Continued)

Trihexyphenidyl *(Continued)*

Anticholinergic agents: Central and/or peripheral anticholinergic syndrome can occur when administered with opioid analgesics, phenothiazines and other antipsychotics (especially with high anticholinergic activity), tricyclic antidepressants, MAO inhibitors, quinidine and some other antiarrhythmics, and antihistamines

Atenolol: Anticholinergics may increase the bioavailability of atenolol (and possibly other beta-blockers); monitor for increased effect

Cholinergic agents: Anticholinergics may antagonize the therapeutic effect of cholinergic agents (includes tacrine, donepezil, rivastigmine, and galantamine).

CNS depressants (cannabinoids, ethanol, barbiturates, and opioid analgesics): May have additive effects with trihexyphenidyl; an abuse potential exits.

Digoxin: Anticholinergics may decrease gastric degradation and increase the amount of digoxin absorbed by delaying gastric emptying

Levodopa: Anticholinergics may increase gastric degradation and decrease the amount of levodopa absorbed by delaying gastric emptying

Neuroleptics: Anticholinergics may antagonize the therapeutic effects of neuroleptics

Ethanol/Nutrition/Herb Interactions Ethanol: Avoid ethanol (may increase CNS depression).

Mechanism of Action Exerts a direct inhibitory effect on the parasympathetic nervous system. It also has a relaxing effect on smooth musculature; exerted both directly on the muscle itself and indirectly through parasympathetic nervous system (inhibitory effect)

Pharmacodynamics Peak effect: Within 60 minutes

Pharmacokinetics

Half-life: 5.6-10.2 hours

Time to peak serum concentrations: Oral: Within 60-90 minutes

Elimination: Primarily in urine

Dosage

Geriatrics: Parkinsonism: Oral: 1 mg on first day, increase by 2 mg every 3-5 days as needed until a total of 6-10 mg/day (in 3-4 divided doses) is reached. If the patient is on concomitant levodopa therapy, the daily dose is reduced to 1-2 mg 3 times/day. Avoid use if possible (see Special Geriatric Considerations).

Adults: Parkinson's disease or drug-induced EPS: Oral: Initial: 1-2 mg/day, increase by 2 mg increments at intervals of 3-5 days; usual dose: 5-15 mg/day in 3-4 divided doses

Administration Tolerated best if given in 3 daily doses and with food; high doses may be divided into 4 doses, at meal times and at bedtime

Monitoring Parameters Symptoms of EPS, Parkinson's, pulse, anticholinergic effects (ie, CNS, bowel and bladder function)

Patient Information Take after meals or with food if GI upset occurs; do not discontinue drug abruptly; notify physician if adverse GI effects, rapid or pounding heartbeat, confusion, eye pain, rash, fever or heat intolerance occurs. Observe caution when performing hazardous tasks or those that require alertness such as driving, as may cause drowsiness. Avoid alcohol and other CNS depressants. May cause dry mouth - adequate fluid intake or hard sugar-free candy may relieve. Difficult urination or constipation may occur - notify physician if effects persist; may increase susceptibility to heat stroke

Additional Information Incidence and severity of side effects are dose related; patients may be switched to sustained-action capsules when stabilized on conventional dosage forms

Special Geriatric Considerations Anticholinergic agents are generally not well tolerated in the elderly (eg, confusion, constipation, urinary retention) and their use should be avoided when possible. In elderly, anticholinergic agents should not be used as prophylaxis against extrapyramidal symptoms.

Dosage Forms Excipient information presented when available (limited, particularly for generics); consult specific product labeling.

Elixir, as hydrochloride: 2 mg/5 mL (480 mL)

Tablet, as hydrochloride: 2 mg, 5 mg

Selected References

Feinberg M, "The Problems of Anticholinergic Adverse Effects in Older Patients," *Drugs Aging*, 1993, 3(4):335-48.

Olanow CW, Watts RL, and Koller WC, "An Algorithm (Decision Tree) for the Management of Parkinson's Disease (2001): Treatment Guidelines," *Neurology*, 2001, 56(11 Suppl 5):S1-S88.

♦ **Trihexyphenidyl Hydrochloride** *see* Trihexyphenidyl *on page 1631*

♦ **Trileptal®** *see* Oxcarbazepine *on page 1174*

♦ **Trilisate® [DSC]** *see* Choline Magnesium Trisalicylate *on page 307*

Trimethobenzamide (trye meth oh BEN za mide)

Related Information
Potentially Inappropriate Medications for Geriatrics *on page 1824*
Medication Safety Issues
Sound-alike/look-alike issues:
Tigan® may be confused with Tiazac®, Ticar®
U.S. Brand Names Tigan®
Canadian Brand Names Tigan®
Index Terms Trimethobenzamide Hydrochloride
Generic Available Yes: Injection
Pharmacologic Category Anticholinergic Agent; Antiemetic
Use Treatment of nausea and vomiting
Contraindications Hypersensitivity to trimethobenzamide, benzocaine (or similar local anesthetics), or any component of the formulation
Warnings/Precautions May mask emesis due to Reye's syndrome or mimic CNS effects of Reye's syndrome in patients with emesis of other etiologies; use in patients with acute vomiting should be avoided. Risk of adverse effects (eg, EPS, seizure) may be increased in patients with acute febrile illness, dehydration, or electrolyte imbalance; use caution.
Adverse Reactions (Reflective of adult population; not specific for elderly)
Frequency not defined.
Cardiovascular: Hypotension
Central nervous system: Coma, depression, disorientation, dizziness, drowsiness, EPS, headache, opisthotonos, Parkinson-like syndrome, seizure
Gastrointestinal: Diarrhea
Hematologic: Blood dyscrasias
Hepatic: Jaundice
Neuromuscular & skeletal: Muscle cramps
Ocular: Blurred vision
Miscellaneous: Hypersensitivity reactions
Overdosage/Toxicology Symptoms include hypotension, seizures, CNS depression, cardiac arrhythmias, disorientation, and confusion. Following initiation of essential overdose management, toxic symptom and supportive treatment should be initiated. Hypotension usually responds to I.V. fluids or Trendelenburg positioning. If unresponsive to these measures, the use of a parenteral inotrope may be required (eg, norepinephrine 0.1-0.2 mcg/kg/minute titrated to response). Seizures commonly respond to diazepam (I.V. 5-10 mg bolus every 15 minutes, if needed, up to a total of 30 mg) or to phenytoin or phenobarbital. Critical cardiac arrhythmias often respond to lidocaine 1-2 mg/kg bolus followed by a maintenance infusion. Extrapyramidal symptoms (eg, dystonic reactions) may be managed with diphenhydramine 1-2 mg/kg up to a maximum of 50 mg I.M. or slow I.V. push followed by a maintenance dose for 48-72 hours. When these reactions are unresponsive to diphenhydramine, anticholinergic agents such as benztropine mesylate I.V. 1-2 mg may be effective. These agents are generally effective within 2-5 minutes.
Ethanol/Nutrition/Herb Interactions Ethanol: Concomitant use should be avoided (sedative effects may be additive).
Stability Store capsules and injection solution at room temperature.
Mechanism of Action Acts centrally to inhibit the medullary chemoreceptor trigger zone
Pharmacodynamics
Onset of action: Antiemetic: Oral: 10-40 minutes; I.M.: 15-35 minutes
Duration: 3-4 hours
Pharmacokinetics
Absorption: Rectal: ~60%
Bioavailability: Oral: 60% to 100%
Half-life: 7-9 hours
Time to peak: Oral: 45 minutes; I.M.: 30 minutes
Elimination: Urine (30% to 50%)
Dosage
Geriatrics & Adults:
Nausea, vomiting:
Oral: 300 mg 3-4 times/day
I.M.: 200 mg 3-4 times/day
Postoperative nausea and vomiting (PONV): I.M.: 200 mg, followed 1 hour later by a second 200 mg dose
Administration Administer I.M. only; not for I.V. administration. Inject deep into upper outer quadrant of gluteal muscle.
Monitoring Parameters See Adverse Reactions.
(Continued)

Trimethobenzamide *(Continued)*

Patient Information Take as directed before meals; do not increase dose and do not discontinue without consulting prescriber. You may experience drowsiness or blurred vision (use caution when driving or engaging in tasks that require alertness until response to drug is known). Report persistent dizziness or blurred vision, or CNS changes (disorientation, depression, confusion).

Additional Information Note: Less effective than phenothiazines but may be associated with fewer side effects; rectal is ~60% absorbed

Special Geriatric Considerations No specific data for use in the elderly have been established; as with any drug which has EPS adverse effects and possibility of confusion, caution should be used when administering to elderly.

Dosage Forms Excipient information presented when available (limited, particularly for generics); consult specific product labeling.
Capsule, as hydrochloride:
  Tigan®: 300 mg
Injection, solution, as hydrochloride: 100 mg/mL (2 mL)
  Tigan®: 100 mg/mL (2 mL [preservative free], 20 mL)

♦ **Trimethobenzamide Hydrochloride** *see* Trimethobenzamide *on page 1633*

Trimethoprim (trye METH oh prim)

Medication Safety Issues
Sound-alike/look-alike issues:
  Trimethoprim may be confused with trimethaphan
  Proloprim® may be confused with Prolixin®, Protropin®
U.S. Brand Names Primsol®; Proloprim®
Canadian Brand Names Apo-Trimethoprim®
Index Terms TMP
Generic Available Yes: Tablet
Pharmacologic Category Antibiotic, Miscellaneous
Use Treatment of uncomplicated urinary tract infections due to susceptible organisms (*Escherichia coli*, *Proteus mirabilis*, *Klebsiella pneumoniae*, *Enterobacter* sp, and coagulase-negative *Staphylococcus* sp); acute exacerbations of chronic bronchitis
Contraindications Hypersensitivity to trimethoprim or any component of the formulation; megaloblastic anemia due to folate deficiency
Warnings/Precautions Use with caution in patients with impaired renal or hepatic function or with possible folate deficiency. Prolonged use may result in fungal or bacterial superinfection, including *C. difficile*-associated diarrhea and pseudomembranous colitis.
Adverse Reactions (Reflective of adult population; not specific for elderly)
Frequency not defined.
Central nervous system: Aseptic meningitis (rare), fever
Dermatologic: Maculopapular rash (3% to 7% at 200 mg/day; incidence higher with larger daily doses), erythema multiforme (rare), exfoliative dermatitis (rare), pruritus (common), phototoxic skin eruptions, Stevens-Johnson syndrome (rare), toxic epidermal necrolysis (rare)
Endocrine & metabolic: Hyperkalemia, hyponatremia
Gastrointestinal: Epigastric distress, glossitis, nausea, vomiting
Hematologic: Leukopenia, megaloblastic anemia, methemoglobinemia, neutropenia, thrombocytopenia
Hepatic: Liver enzyme elevation, cholestatic jaundice (rare)
Renal: BUN and creatinine increased
Miscellaneous: Anaphylaxis, hypersensitivity reactions
Overdosage/Toxicology Symptom of acute toxicity includes nausea, vomiting, confusion, and dizziness. Chronic overdose results in bone marrow suppression. Treatment of acute overdose is supportive following GI decontamination. Treatment of chronic overdose includes the use of oral leucovorin 5-15 mg/day. Hemodialysis is only moderately effective in eliminating drug.
Drug Interactions Substrate (major) of CYP2C9, 3A4; **Inhibits** CYP2C8 (moderate), 2C9 (moderate)
ACE inhibitors: Concurrent therapy increases the risk of hyperkalemia.
CYP2C9 inducers: May decrease the levels/effects of trimethoprim. Example inducers include carbamazepine, phenobarbital, phenytoin, rifampin, rifapentine, and secobarbital.
CYP2C8 substrates: Trimethoprim may increase the levels/effects of CYP2C8 substrates. Example substrates include amiodarone, paclitaxel, pioglitazone, repaglinide, and rosiglitazone.
CYP2C9 substrates: Trimethoprim may increase the levels/effects of CYP2C9 substrates. Example substrates include bosentan, dapsone, fluoxetine, glimepiride,

glipizide, losartan, montelukast, nateglinide, paclitaxel, phenytoin, warfarin, and zafirlukast.

CYP3A4 inducers: CYP3A4 inducers may decrease the levels/effects of trimethoprim. Example inducers include aminoglutethimide, carbamazepine, nafcillin, nevirapine, phenobarbital, phenytoin, and rifamycins.

Dapsone: Trimethoprim may increase dapsone concentration/toxicity.

Digoxin: Trimethoprim may increase digoxin concentrations.

Methotrexate: Trimethoprim may increase methotrexate toxicity.

Phenytoin: Trimethoprim may increase phenytoin concentration/toxicity.

Procainamide: Trimethoprim may increase procainamide concentrations.

Stability Protect the 200 mg tablet from light.

Mechanism of Action Inhibits folic acid reduction to tetrahydrofolate, and thereby inhibits microbial growth

Pharmacokinetics

Absorption: Oral: Readily and extensively

Protein binding: 42% to 46%

Metabolism: Partially in the liver

Half-life: 8-14 hours, prolonged with renal impairment

Time to peak serum concentration: Within 1-4 hours

Elimination: Significantly in urine (60% to 80% as unchanged drug); in older adults, the area under the curve and peak concentration have been reported to be greater compared to younger subjects

Dosage

Geriatrics & Adults: Susceptible infections: Oral: 100 mg every 12 hours or 200 mg every 24 hours for 10 days; longer treatment periods may be necessary for prostatitis (ie, 4-16 weeks)

Renal Impairment:

Cl_{cr} 15-30 mL/minute: Administer 100 mg every 18 hours or 50 mg every 12 hours.

Cl_{cr} <15 mL/minute: Administer 100 mg every 24 hours or avoid use.

Moderately dialyzable (20% to 50%)

Monitoring Parameters Obtain culture and sensitivity results; repeat after treatment has concluded

Reference Range Therapeutic: Peak: 5-15 mg/L; Trough: 2-8 mg/L

Patient Information Complete full course of treatment; notify physician if sore throat, bleeding, or fever develops

Special Geriatric Considerations Trimethoprim is often used in combination with sulfamethoxazole; it can be used alone in patients who are allergic to sulfonamides; adjust dose for renal function (see Pharmacokinetics and Dosage).

Dosage Forms Excipient information presented when available (limited, particularly for generics); consult specific product labeling. [DSC] = Discontinued product

Solution, oral (Primsol®): 50 mg (base)/5 mL (480 mL) [contains sodium benzoate; bubble gum flavor]

Tablet: 100 mg

Proloprim®: 100 mg, 200 mg [DSC]

Selected References

Varoquaux O, Lajoie D, Gobert C, et al, "Pharmacokinetics of the Trimethoprim-Sulfamethoxazole Combination in the Elderly," Br J Clin Pharmacol, 1985, 20(6):575-81.

♦ **Trimethoprim and Sulfamethoxazole** see Sulfamethoxazole and Trimethoprim on page 1498

Trimipramine (trye MI pra meen)

Related Information

Antidepressant Agents on page 1742

Medication Safety Issues

Sound-alike/look-alike issues:

Trimipramine may be confused with triamterene, trimeprazine

U.S. Brand Names Surmontil®

Canadian Brand Names Apo-Trimip®; Nu-Trimipramine; Rhotrimine®; Surmontil®

Index Terms Trimipramine Maleate

Generic Available No

Pharmacologic Category Antidepressant, Tricyclic (Tertiary Amine)

Use Treatment of various forms of depression, often in conjunction with psychotherapy

Restrictions An FDA-approved medication guide concerning the use of antidepressants in children, adolescents, and young adults must be distributed when dispensing an outpatient prescription (new or refill) where this medication is to be used without direct supervision of a healthcare provider. Medication guides are available at http://www.fda.gov/cder/Offices/ODS/medication_guides.htm. Dispense to parents or guardians of children and adolescents receiving this medication.

(Continued)

Trimipramine *(Continued)*

Contraindications Hypersensitivity to trimipramine, any component of the formulation, or other dibenzodiazepines; use of MAO inhibitors within 14 days; use in a patient during the acute recovery phase of MI

Warnings/Precautions [U.S. Boxed Warning]: Antidepressants increase the risk of suicidal thinking and behavior in children, adolescents, and young adults (18-24 years of age) with major depressive disorder (MDD) and other psychiatric disorders; consider risk prior to prescribing. Short-term studies did not show an increased risk in patients >24 years of age and showed a decreased risk in patients ≥65 years. Closely monitor for clinical worsening, suicidality, or unusual changes in behavior; the patient's family or caregiver should be instructed to closely observe the patient and communicate condition with healthcare provider. A medication guide should be dispensed with each prescription.

The possibility of a suicide attempt is inherent in major depression and may persist until remission occurs. Monitor for worsening of depression or suicidality, especially during initiation of therapy (generally first 1-2 months) or with dose increases or decreases. Use caution in high-risk patients. Worsening depression and severe abrupt suicidality that are not part of the presenting symptoms may require discontinuation or modification of drug therapy. The patient's family or caregiver should be alerted to monitor patients for the emergence of suicidality and associated behaviors (such as agitation, irritability, hostility, impulsivity, and hypomania) and call healthcare provider.

May worsen psychosis in some patients or precipitate a shift to mania or hypomania in patients with bipolar disorder. Patients presenting with depressive symptoms should be screened for bipolar disorder. Monotherapy in patients with bipolar disorder should be avoided. **Trimipramine is not FDA approved for the treatment of bipolar depression.**

The degree of sedation, anticholinergic effects, orthostasis, and conduction abnormalities are high relative to other antidepressants. Trimipramine often causes drowsiness/sedation, resulting in impaired performance of tasks requiring alertness (eg, operating machinery or driving). Sedative effects may be additive with other CNS depressants and/or ethanol. Use with caution in patients with a history of cardiovascular disease (including previous MI, stroke, tachycardia, or conduction abnormalities). Use with caution in patients with urinary retention, benign prostatic hyperplasia, narrow-angle glaucoma, xerostomia, visual problems, constipation, or a history of bowel obstruction.

May alter glucose control - use with caution in patients with diabetes. Consider discontinuing, when possible, prior to elective surgery. Therapy should not be abruptly discontinued in patients receiving high doses for prolonged periods. May lower seizure threshold - use caution in patients with a previous seizure disorder or condition predisposing to seizures such as brain damage, alcoholism, or concurrent therapy with other drugs which lower the seizure threshold. May increase the risks associated with electroconvulsive therapy. Use with caution in hyperthyroid patients or those receiving thyroid supplementation. Use with caution in patients with hepatic or renal dysfunction and in elderly patients.

Adverse Reactions (Reflective of adult population; not specific for elderly)
Frequency not defined.
Cardiovascular: Arrhythmias, hyper-/hypotension, tachycardia, palpitation, heart block, stroke, MI
Central nervous system: Headache, exacerbation of psychosis, confusion, delirium, hallucinations, nervousness, restlessness, delusions, agitation, insomnia, nightmares, anxiety, seizure, drowsiness
Dermatologic: Photosensitivity, rash, petechiae, itching
Endocrine & metabolic: Sexual dysfunction, breast enlargement, galactorrhea, SIADH
Gastrointestinal: Xerostomia, constipation, increased appetite, nausea, unpleasant taste, weight gain, diarrhea, heartburn, vomiting, anorexia, trouble with gums, decreased lower esophageal sphincter tone may cause GE reflux
Genitourinary: Difficult urination, urinary retention, testicular edema
Hematologic: Agranulocytosis, eosinophilia, purpura, thrombocytopenia
Hepatic: Cholestatic jaundice, increased liver enzymes
Neuromuscular & skeletal: Tremors, numbness, tingling, paresthesia, incoordination, ataxia, peripheral neuropathy, extrapyramidal symptoms
Ocular: Blurred vision, eye pain, disturbances in accommodation, mydriasis, increased intraocular pressure
Otic: Tinnitus
Miscellaneous: Allergic reactions

Overdosage/Toxicology Symptoms include agitation, confusion, hallucinations, urinary retention, hypothermia, hypotension, tachycardia, and cardiac arrhythmias. Following initiation of essential overdose management, toxic symptoms should be treated. Sodium bicarbonate is indicated when the QRS interval is >0.10 seconds or the QT_c >0.42 seconds. Ventricular arrhythmias and ECG changes (QRS widening) often respond to systemic alkalinization (sodium bicarbonate 0.5-2 mEq/kg I.V.).

Arrhythmias unresponsive to this therapy may respond to lidocaine 1 mg/kg I.V. followed by a titrated infusion. Physostigmine (1-2 mg slow I.V.) may be indicated in reversing life-threatening cardiac arrhythmias. Seizures usually respond to diazepam I.V. boluses (5-10 mg up to 30 mg). If seizures are unresponsive or recur, phenytoin or phenobarbital may be required.

Drug Interactions Substrate (major) of CYP2C19, 2D6, 3A4

Altretamine: Concurrent use may cause orthostatic hypertension

Amphetamines: TCAs may enhance the effect of amphetamines; monitor for adverse CV effects

Anticholinergics: Combined use with TCAs may produce additive anticholinergic effects

Antihypertensives: TCAs may inhibit the antihypertensive response to bethanidine, clonidine, debrisoquin, guanadrel, guanethidine, guanabenz, guanfacine; monitor BP; consider alternate antihypertensive agent

Beta-agonists: When combined with TCAs may predispose patients to cardiac arrhythmias

Bupropion: May increase the levels of tricyclic antidepressants; based on limited information; monitor response

Carbamazepine: Tricyclic antidepressants may increase carbamazepine levels; monitor

Cholestyramine and colestipol: May bind TCAs and reduce their absorption; monitor for altered response

Clonidine: Abrupt discontinuation of clonidine may cause hypertensive crisis, amitriptyline may enhance the response (also see note on antihypertensives)

CNS depressants: Sedative effects may be additive with TCAs; monitor for increased effect; includes benzodiazepines, barbiturates, antipsychotics, ethanol, and other sedative medications

CYP2D6 inhibitors: May increase the levels/effects of trimipramine. Example inhibitors include chlorpromazine, delavirdine, fluoxetine, miconazole, paroxetine, pergolide, quinidine, quinine, ritonavir, and ropinirole.

CYP2C19 inducers: May decrease the levels/effects of trimipramine. Example inducers include aminoglutethimide, carbamazepine, phenytoin, and rifampin.

CYP2C19 inhibitors: May increase the levels/effects of trimipramine. Example inhibitors include delavirdine, fluconazole, fluvoxamine, gemfibrozil, isoniazid, omeprazole, and ticlopidine.

CYP3A4 inducers: CYP3A4 inducers may decrease the levels/effects of trimipramine. Example inducers include aminoglutethimide, carbamazepine, nafcillin, nevirapine, phenobarbital, phenytoin, and rifamycins.

CYP3A4 inhibitors: May increase the levels/effects of trimipramine. Example inhibitors include azole antifungals, clarithromycin, diclofenac, doxycycline, erythromycin, imatinib, isoniazid, nefazodone, nicardipine, propofol, protease inhibitors, quinidine, telithromycin, and verapamil.

Epinephrine (and other direct alpha-agonists): Pressor response to I.V. epinephrine, norepinephrine, and phenylephrine may be enhanced in patients receiving TCAs (**Note:** Effect is unlikely with epinephrine or levonordefrin dosages typically administered as infiltration in combination with local anesthetics).

Fenfluramine: May increase tricyclic antidepressant levels/effects

Hypoglycemic agents (including insulin): TCAs may enhance the hypoglycemic effects of tolazamide, chlorpropamide, or insulin; monitor for changes in blood glucose levels; reported with chlorpropamide, tolazamide, and insulin

Levodopa: Tricyclic antidepressants may decrease the absorption (bioavailability) of levodopa; rare hypertensive episodes have also been attributed to this combination

Linezolid: Hyperpyrexia, hypertension, tachycardia, confusion, seizures, and **deaths have been reported** with agents which inhibit MAO (serotonin syndrome); this combination should be avoided

Lithium: Concurrent use with a TCA may increase the risk for neurotoxicity

MAO inhibitors: Hyperpyrexia, hypertension, tachycardia, confusion, seizures, and **deaths have been reported** (serotonin syndrome); this combination should be avoided

Methylphenidate: Metabolism of TCAs may be decreased

Phenothiazines: Serum concentrations of some TCAs may be increased; in addition, TCAs may increase concentration of phenothiazines; monitor for altered clinical response

QT_c-prolonging agents: Concurrent use of tricyclic agents with other drugs which may prolong QT_c interval may increase the risk of potentially fatal arrhythmias; includes type Ia and type III antiarrhythmics agents, selected quinolones (sparfloxacin, gatifloxacin, moxifloxacin, grepafloxacin), cisapride, and other agents

Ritonavir: Combined use of high-dose tricyclic antidepressants with ritonavir may cause serotonin syndrome in HIV-positive patients; monitor

Sucralfate: Absorption of tricyclic antidepressants may be reduced with coadministration

(Continued)

Trimipramine *(Continued)*

Sympathomimetics, indirect-acting: Tricyclic antidepressants may result in a decreased sensitivity to indirect-acting sympathomimetics; includes dopamine and ephedrine; also see interaction with epinephrine (and direct-acting sympathomimetics)

Valproic acid: May increase serum concentrations/adverse effects of some tricyclic antidepressants

Warfarin (and other oral anticoagulants): TCAs may increase the anticoagulant effect in patients stabilized on warfarin; monitor INR

Ethanol/Nutrition/Herb Interactions

Ethanol: Avoid ethanol (may increase CNS depression).

Food: Grapefruit juice may inhibit the metabolism of some TCAs and clinical toxicity may result.

Herb/Nutraceutical: Avoid valerian, St John's wort, SAMe, kava kava (may increase risk of serotonin syndrome and/or excessive sedation).

Stability Solutions stable at a pH of 4-5. Turns yellowish or reddish on exposure to light. Slight discoloration does not affect potency; marked discoloration is associated with loss of potency. Capsules stable for 3 years following date of manufacture.

Mechanism of Action Increases the synaptic concentration of serotonin and/or norepinephrine in the central nervous system by inhibition of their reuptake by the presynaptic neuronal membrane

Pharmacodynamics Onset of therapeutic effects: May take 1-3 weeks to appear; serotonin greater than norepinephrine

Pharmacokinetics

Protein binding: 95%

Metabolism: Hepatic; undergoes significant first-pass metabolism

Half-life: 20-26 hours

Time to peak: Oral: Therapeutic plasma concentrations occur within 6 hours

Elimination: In urine

Dosage

Geriatrics: Oral: Initial: 25 mg at bedtime; increase by 25 mg/day every 3 days for inpatients and weekly for outpatients, as tolerated, to a maximum of 100 mg/day (see Special Geriatric Considerations).

Adults: Depression: Oral: 50-150 mg/day as a single bedtime dose up to a maximum of 200 mg/day for outpatients and 300 mg/day for inpatients

Monitoring Parameters Blood pressure, pulse, target symptoms

Patient Information May be taken with food to decrease GI distress. To prevent dizziness, avoid abrupt changes of position, may cause dry mouth, dizziness, blurred vision, constipation, sedation

Additional Information May cause alterations in bleeding time

Special Geriatric Considerations Similar to doxepin in its side effect profile; has not been well studied in the elderly; very anticholinergic and, therefore, not considered a drug of first choice in the elderly when selecting an antidepressant. Data from a clinical trial comparing fluoxetine to tricyclics suggest that fluoxetine is significantly less effective than nortriptyline in hospitalized elderly patients with unipolar major affective disorder, especially those with melancholia and concurrent cardiovascular diseases.

Dosage Forms Excipient information presented when available (limited, particularly for generics); consult specific product labeling.

Capsule: 25 mg, 50 mg, 100 mg

Selected References

Roose SP, Glassman AH, Attia E, et al, "Comparative Efficacy of Selective Serotonin Reuptake Inhibitors and Tricyclics in the Treatment of Melancholia," *Am J Psychiatry*, 1994, 151(12):1735-9.

♦ **Trimipramine Maleate** *see* Trimipramine *on page 1635*

♦ **Tri-Nasal®** *see* Triamcinolone *on page 1619*

♦ **Triostat®** *see* Liothyronine *on page 912*

Triprolidine and Pseudoephedrine

(trye PROE li deen & soo doe e FED rin)

Related Information

Pseudoephedrine *on page 1346*

Medication Safety Issues

Sound-alike/look-alike issues:

Aprodine® may be confused with Aphrodyne®

U.S. Brand Names Allerfrim® [OTC]; Aprodine® [OTC]; Genac® [OTC]; Silafed® [OTC]; Sudafed® Maximum Strength Sinus Nighttime [OTC] [DSC]; Tri-Sudo® [OTC] [DSC]; Zymine®-D

Canadian Brand Names Actifed®
Index Terms Pseudoephedrine and Triprolidine
Generic Available Yes
Pharmacologic Category Alpha/Beta Agonist; Antihistamine
Use Temporary relief of nasal congestion, runny nose, sneezing, itchy nose or throat, and itchy, watery eyes due to common cold, hay fever, or other upper respiratory allergies
Contraindications Hypersensitivity to pseudoephedrine or any component of the formulation; MAO therapy, hypertension, coronary artery disease
Warnings/Precautions Not recommended for OTC use for longer than 7 days or if symptoms are accompanied by fever. Consult healthcare provider prior to OTC use with heart disease, hypotension, thyroid disease, diabetes, emphysema, chronic bronchitis, glaucoma, or enlarged prostate.
Adverse Reactions (Reflective of adult population; not specific for elderly)
Frequency not defined.
Cardiovascular: Tachycardia
Central nervous system: Drowsiness, nervousness, insomnia, transient stimulation, headache, fatigue, dizziness
Respiratory: Thickening of bronchial secretions, pharyngitis
Gastrointestinal: Appetite increase, weight gain, nausea, diarrhea, abdominal pain, xerostomia
Genitourinary: Dysuria
Neuromuscular & skeletal: Arthralgia, weakness
Miscellaneous: Diaphoresis
Drug Interactions Triprolidine: **Inhibits** CYP2D6 (weak)
Decreased effect of guanethidine, reserpine, methyldopa
Increased toxicity with MAO inhibitors (hypertensive crisis), sympathomimetics, CNS depressants, ethanol (sedation)
Mechanism of Action Refer to Pseudoephedrine monograph
Triprolidine is a member of the propylamine (alkylamine) chemical class of H_1-antagonist antihistamines. As such, it is considered to be relatively less sedating than traditional antihistamines of the ethanolamine, phenothiazine, and ethylenediamine classes of antihistamines. Triprolidine has a shorter half-life and duration of action than most of the other alkylamine antihistamines. Like all H_1-antagonist antihistamines, the mechanism of action of triprolidine is believed to involve competitive blockade of H_1-receptor sites resulting in the inability of histamine to combine with its receptor sites and exert its usual effects on target cells. Antihistamines do not interrupt any effects of histamine which have already occurred. Therefore, these agents are used more successfully in the prevention rather than the treatment of histamine-induced reactions.
Dosage
Geriatrics & Adults: Cold, allergy symptoms: Oral:
Liquid (Zymine®-D): 5-10 mL every 4-6 hours (maximum pseudoephedrine: 240 mg/24 hours)
Syrup (Allerfrim®, Aprodine®): 10 mL every 4-6 hours; do not exceed 4 doses in 24 hours
Tablet (Aprodine®): One tablet every 4-6 hours; do not exceed 4 doses in 24 hours
Monitoring Parameters Relief of symptoms, blood pressure, pulse
Patient Information Do not exceed recommended dosage; do not crush or chew extended release capsule
Special Geriatric Considerations Use with caution in patients with cardiovascular disease; the anticholinergic action of triprolidine may cause confusion, constipation, or urinary retention in the elderly. Also refer to Pseudoephedrine *on page 1346.*
Dosage Forms Excipient information presented when available (limited, particularly for generics); consult specific product labeling. [DSC] = Discontinued product
Liquid:
Zymine®-D: Triprolidine hydrochloride 1.25 mg and pseudoephedrine hydrochloride 45 mg per 5 mL (480 mL)
Syrup: Triprolidine hydrochloride 1.25 mg and pseudoephedrine hydrochloride 30 mg per 5 mL (120 mL)
Allerfrim®: Triprolidine hydrochloride 1.25 mg and pseudoephedrine hydrochloride 30 mg per 5 mL (120 mL, 480 mL) [contains sodium benzoate]
Aprodine®: Triprolidine hydrochloride 1.25 mg and pseudoephedrine hydrochloride 30 mg per 5 mL (120 mL)
Silafed®: Triprolidine hydrochloride 1.25 mg and pseudoephedrine hydrochloride 30 mg per 5 mL (120 mL, 240 mL)
Tablet:
Allerfrim® [DSC], Aprodine®, Genac®, Sudafed® Maximum Strength Sinus Nighttime, Tri-Sudo® [DSC]: Triprolidine hydrochloride 2.5 mg and pseudoephedrine hydrochloride 60 mg

♦ **TripTone® [OTC] [DSC]** *see* DimenhyDRINATE *on page 445*

♦ **Triptoraline** *see* Triptorelin *on page 1640*

Triptorelin (trip toe REL in)

U.S. Brand Names Trelstar™ Depot; Trelstar™ LA

Canadian Brand Names Trelstar™; Trelstar™ Depot; Trelstar™ LA

Index Terms AY-25650; CL-118,532; D-Trp(6)-LHRH; Triptoraline; Triptorelin Pamoate; Tryptoreline

Generic Available No

Pharmacologic Category Gonadotropin Releasing Hormone Agonist

Use Palliative treatment of advanced prostate cancer as an alternative to orchiectomy or estrogen administration

Unlabeled/Investigational Use Treatment of endometriosis, hyperandrogenism, *in vitro* fertilization, ovarian carcinoma, pancreatic carcinoma, uterine leiomyomata

Contraindications Hypersensitivity to triptorelin or any component of the formulation, other LHRH agonists or LHRH

Warnings/Precautions Hazardous agent - use appropriate precautions for handling and disposal. Transient increases in testosterone can lead to worsening symptoms (bone pain, hematuria, bladder outlet obstruction) of prostate cancer during the first few weeks of therapy. Cases of spinal cord compression have been reported with LHRH agonists. Hypersensitivity reactions including angioedema and anaphylaxis have rarely occurred. Rare cases of pituitary apoplexy (frequently secondary to pituitary adenoma) have been observed with leuprolide administration (onset from 1 hour to usually <2 weeks); may present as sudden headache, vomiting, visual or mental status changes, and infrequently cardiovascular collapse; immediate medical attention required.

Adverse Reactions (Reflective of adult population; not specific for elderly)
As reported with Trelstar™ Depot and Trelstar™ LA; frequency of effect may vary by product:

>10%:
  Central nervous system: Headache (30% to 60%)
  Endocrine & metabolic: Hot flashes (95% to 100%), glucose increased
  Hematologic: Hemoglobin decreased, RBC count decreased
  Hepatic: Alkaline phosphatase increased, ALT increased, AST increased
  Neuromuscular & skeletal: Skeletal pain (12% to 13%)
  Renal: BUN increased

1% to 10%:
  Cardiovascular: Leg edema (6%), hypertension (4%), chest pain (2%), peripheral edema (1%)
  Central nervous system: Dizziness (1% to 3%), pain (2% to 3%), emotional lability (1%), fatigue (2%), insomnia (2%)
  Dermatologic: Rash (2%), pruritus (1%)
  Endocrine & metabolic: Alkaline phosphatase increased (2%), breast pain (2%), gynecomastia (2%), libido decreased (2%), tumor flare (8%)
  Gastrointestinal: Nausea (3%), anorexia (2%), constipation (2%), dyspepsia (2%), vomiting (2%), abdominal pain (1%), diarrhea (1%)
  Genitourinary: Dysuria (5%), impotence (2% to 7%), urinary retention (1%), urinary tract infection (1%)
  Hematologic: Anemia (1%)
  Local: Injection site pain (4%)
  Neuromuscular & skeletal: Leg pain (2% to 5%), back pain (3%), arthralgia (2%), leg cramps (2%), myalgia (1%), weakness (1%)
  Ocular: Conjunctivitis (1%), eye pain (1%)
  Respiratory: Cough (2%), dyspnea (1%), pharyngitis (1%)
Postmarketing and/or case reports: Anaphylaxis, angioedema, hypersensitivity reactions, spinal cord compression, renal dysfunction

Overdosage/Toxicology Accidental or intentional overdose unlikely. If it were to occur, supportive and symptomatic treatment would be indicated.

Drug Interactions Not studied. Hyperprolactinemic drugs (dopamine antagonists such as antipsychotics, and metoclopramide) are contraindicated.

Stability
Trelstar™ Depot: Store at 15°C to 30°C (59°F to 86°F).
Trelstar™ LA: Store at 20°C to 25°C (68°F to 77°F).

Reconstitution: Reconstitute with 2 mL sterile water for injection. Shake well to obtain a uniform suspension.
Debioclip™: Follow manufacturer's instructions for mixing prior to use.

Mechanism of Action Causes suppression of ovarian and testicular steroidogenesis due to decreased levels of LH and FSH with subsequent decrease in testosterone (male) and estrogen (female) levels. After chronic and continuous administration, usually 2-4 weeks after initiation, a sustained decrease in LH and FSH secretion occurs.

Pharmacokinetics
Absorption: Not active when administered orally
Distribution: V_d: 30-33 L
Protein binding: Not bound to plasma proteins
Metabolism: Unknown; no known metabolites
Half-life: 2.8 ± 1.2 hours
    Moderate to severe renal impairment: 6.5 ± 1.2 to 7.7 ± 1.3 hours
    Hepatic impairment: 7.6 ± 1.2 hours
Time to peak: T_{max}: 1-3 hours
Elimination: Renal (42% as intact peptide) and hepatic

Dosage
Geriatrics & Adults: Advanced prostate carcinoma:
    Trelstar™ Depot: 3.75 mg once every 28 days
    Trelstar™ LA: 11.25 mg once every 84 days
Renal Impairment: Specific guidelines are not available.
Hepatic Impairment: Specific guidelines are not available.

Administration Must be administered under the supervision of a physician. Administer by I.M. injection into the buttock; alternate injection sites.
Debioclip™: Follow manufacturer's instructions for mixing prior to use.

Monitoring Parameters Serum testosterone levels, prostate-specific antigen; blood pressure; monitor for bone pain and spinal symptoms of compression; urinary retention

Test Interactions Pituitary-gonadal function may be suppressed with chronic administration and for up to 8 weeks after triptorelin therapy has been discontinued.

Patient Information Use as directed. Do not miss monthly appointment for injection. You may experience disease flare (increased bone pain), blood in urine, and urinary retention during early treatment (usually resolves within 1 week). Hot flashes are common; you may feel flushed and hot (wearing layers of clothes or summer clothes and cool environment may help). If it becomes annoying and bothersome, let healthcare provider know. Report irregular or rapid heartbeat, unresolved nausea or vomiting, numbness of extremities, breast swelling or pain, difficulty breathing, or infection at injection sites.

Special Geriatric Considerations Since many elderly men may have hypertension, blood pressure needs be monitored closely for the first 4-8 weeks.

Dosage Forms Excipient information presented when available (limited, particularly for generics); consult specific product labeling.
Injection, powder for reconstitution, as pamoate [also available packaged with Debioclip™ (prefilled syringe containing sterile water)]:
    Trelstar™ Depot: 3.75 mg
    Trelstar™ LA: 11.25 mg

Selected References
Anonymous, "Triptorelin Pamoate. Phase III Drug Profiles," 1993, 3:1-8.
Filicor M, "Gonadotrop24-in-Releasing Hormone Agonists. A Guide to Use and Selection," *Drugs*, 1994, 48(1):41-58.
Swanson LJ, Seely JH, and Garnick MB, "Gonadotropin-Releasing Hormone Analogs and Prostatic Cancer," *Crit Rev Oncol Hematol*, 1988, 8(1):1-26.

♦ **Triptorelin Pamoate** *see* Triptorelin *on page 1640*

♦ **Tri-Sudo® [OTC] [DSC]** *see* Triprolidine and Pseudoephedrine *on page 1638*

♦ **Trivalent Inactivated Influenza Vaccine (TIV)** *see* Influenza Virus Vaccine *on page 803*

♦ **Tronolane® Suppository [OTC]** *see* Phenylephrine *on page 1247*

Trospium (TROSE pee um)

Related Information
Pharmacotherapy of Urinary Incontinence *on page 1822*
U.S. Brand Names Sanctura®
Canadian Brand Names Trosec
Index Terms Trospium Chloride
Generic Available No
Pharmacologic Category Anticholinergic Agent
Use Treatment of overactive bladder with symptoms of urgency, incontinence, and urinary frequency
Contraindications Hypersensitivity to trospium or any component of the formulation; urinary retention; gastric retention; uncontrolled narrow-angle glaucoma; myasthenia gravis
Warnings/Precautions Use with caution in patients with bladder flow obstruction, may increase the risk of urinary retention. Use with caution in patients with gastrointestinal obstructive disorders (eg, pyloric stenosis); may increase the risk of gastric retention. Use caution in patients with decreased GI motility (eg, myasthenia gravis, ulcerative (Continued)

Trospium *(Continued)*

colitis). Use with caution in renal dysfunction; dosage adjustment is required. Active tubular secretion (ATS) is a route of elimination; use caution with other medications that are eliminated by ATS (eg, procainamide, pancuronium, vancomycin, morphine). Use with extreme caution in patients with controlled (treated) narrow-angle glaucoma. Use caution in patients with moderate-to-severe hepatic dysfunction. Use caution in Alzheimer's patients. Use caution in the elderly (≥75 years); increased anticholinergic side effects are seen.

Adverse Reactions (Reflective of adult population; not specific for elderly)
>10%: Gastrointestinal: Xerostomia (20%)
1% to 10%:
Cardiovascular: Tachycardia, heart rate increase
Central nervous system: Headache (4%), fatigue (2%)
Dermatologic: Dry skin
Gastrointestinal: Constipation (10%), abdominal pain (2%), dyspepsia (1%), flatulence (1%), abdominal distention, vomiting, dysgeusia
Genitourinary: Urinary retention (1%)
Ocular: Dry eyes (1%), blurred vision

Overdosage/Toxicology ECG monitoring is recommended. Treatment is symptom-directed and supportive.

Drug Interactions
Acetylcholinesterase inhibitors (central): Trospium anticholinergic effect may be diminished with acetylcholinesterase inhibitors (central) via opposing effects. Trospium may diminish the therapeutic effect of acetylcholinesterase inhibitors.
Anticholinergics: Trospium anticholinergic effect may be increased with other anticholinergics.
Pramlintide: Trospium anticholinergic effect may be enhanced by pramlintide effect on delayed gastric emptying.

Ethanol/Nutrition/Herb Interactions
Ethanol: Avoid use.
Food: Administration with a fatty meal reduced absorption 70% to 80%.

Stability Store at 20°C to 25°C (68°F to 77°F).

Mechanism of Action Trospium antagonizes the effects of acetylcholine on muscarinic receptors in cholinergically innervated organs. It reduces the smooth muscle tone of the bladder.

Pharmacokinetics
Absorption: <10%
Distribution: V_d: 395 L, primarily in plasma
Protein binding: 50% to 85% *in vitro*
Metabolism: Hypothesized to be via esterase hydrolysis and conjugation; forms metabolites
Bioavailability: ~10%
Half-life elimination: 20 hours; severe renal insufficiency (Cl_{cr} <30 mL/minute): ~33 hours
Time to peak, plasma: 5-6 hours
Elimination: Feces primarily (85%); urine (~6%; mostly as unchanged drug)

Dosage
Geriatrics: ≥75 years: Consider initial dose of 20 mg once daily (based on tolerability) at bedtime
Adults: Overactive bladder: Oral: 20 mg twice daily
Renal Impairment: Cl_{cr} ≤30 mL/minute: 20 mg once daily at bedtime

Administration Administer 1 hour before meals or on an empty stomach.

Monitoring Parameters Monitor incontinence episodes, postvoid residual (PVR)

Patient Information Take on an empty stomach or 1 hour before meals. May cause dry mouth and constipation.

Special Geriatric Considerations In studies, the incidence of anticholinergic side effects was higher in patients ≥75 years of age as compared to younger adults.

Dosage Forms Excipient information presented when available (limited, particularly for generics); consult specific product labeling.
Tablet, as chloride:
Sanctura™: 20 mg

♦ **Trospium Chloride** see Trospium *on page 1641*
♦ **Trusopt®** see Dorzolamide *on page 470*

Trypsin, Balsam Peru, and Castor Oil
(TRIP sin, BAL sam pe RUE, & KAS tor oyl)

Related Information
Castor Oil *on page 249*

Medication Safety Issues
Sound-alike/look-alike issues:
Granulex® may be confused with Regranex®

U.S. Brand Names Granulex®; Optase™; Xenaderm™

Index Terms Balsam Peru, Trypsin, and Castor Oil; Castor Oil, Trypsin, and Balsam Peru

Generic Available Yes: Aerosol

Pharmacologic Category Protectant, Topical

Use Treatment of decubitus ulcers, varicose ulcers, debridement of eschar, dehiscent wounds and sunburn

Warnings/Precautions Do not apply to fresh arterial clots. Wound healing may be retarded in the presence of hemoglobin or zinc deficiency.

Adverse Reactions (Reflective of adult population; not specific for elderly)
Frequency not defined: Local: Temporary stinging at application site

Stability Store at controlled room temperature; do not freeze. Do not expose spray to fire, open flame, or temperatures >120°F.

Mechanism of Action Trypsin is used to debride necrotic tissue; balsam peru stimulates circulation at the wound site and may be mildly bactericidal; castor oil improves epithelialization, acts as a protectant covering and helps reduce pain

Dosage
Geriatrics & Adults: Dermatologic conditions: Topical: Apply a minimum of twice daily or as often as necessary

Administration Clean wound prior to application and at each redressing; shake well before spraying; hold can upright ~12" from area to be treated.

Monitoring Parameters Size of the ulcer, skin integrity

Patient Information Avoid contact with eyes; for external use only; shake well before spraying

Special Geriatric Considerations Preventive skin care should be instituted in all elderly patients at high risk for decubitus ulcers. Practical experience with Granulex® has found that it is not as effective in debriding wounds as compared to other enzymatic products. Therefore, Granulex® may be more appropriately used on stage 1 and 2 decubiti.

Dosage Forms Excipient information presented when available (limited, particularly for generics); consult specific product labeling.
Aerosol, topical: Trypsin 0.12 mg, balsam Peru 87 mg, and castor oil 788 mg per gram (120 g)
Granulex®: Trypsin 0.12 mg, balsam Peru 87 mg, and castor oil 788 mg per gram (60 g, 120 g)
Gel, topical:
Optase™: Trypsin 0.12 mg, balsam Peru 87 mg, and castor oil 788 mg per gram (95 g)
Ointment, topical:
Xenaderm™: Trypsin 90 USP units, balsam Peru 87 mg, and castor oil 788 mg per gram (30 g, 60 g)

Selected References
Chamberlain TM, Cali TJ, Cuzzell J, et al, "Assessment and Management of Pressure Sores in Long-Term Care Facilities," *Consult Pharm*, 1992, 7(12):1328-40.

♦ **Tryptoreline** see Triptorelin on page 1640
♦ **TST** see Tuberculin Tests on page 1643
♦ **Tuberculin Purified Protein Derivative** see Tuberculin Tests on page 1643
♦ **Tuberculin Skin Test** see Tuberculin Tests on page 1643

Tuberculin Tests (too BER kyoo lin tests)

Medication Safety Issues
Sound-alike/look-alike issues:
Aplisol® may be confused with Anusol®, A.P.L.®, Aplitest®, Atropisol®

Administration issues:
Tuberculin products may be confused with tetanus toxoid products and influenza virus vaccine. Medication errors have occurred when tuberculin skin tests (PPD) have been inadvertently administered instead of tetanus toxoid products and influenza virus vaccine. These products are refrigerated and often stored in close proximity to each other.

U.S. Brand Names Aplisol®; Tubersol®

Index Terms Mantoux; PPD; TB Skin Test; TST; Tuberculin Purified Protein Derivative; Tuberculin Skin Test

Generic Available No

Pharmacologic Category Diagnostic Agent

Use Skin test in diagnosis of tuberculosis
(Continued)

Tuberculin Tests *(Continued)*

Contraindications Hypersensitivity to tuberculin purified protein derivative (PPD) or any component of the formulation; previous severe reaction to tuberculin PPD skin test (TST)

Warnings/Precautions Patients with a previous severe reaction to TST (vesiculation, ulceration, necrosis) at the injection site should not receive tuberculin PPD again. Do not administer to persons with documented tuberculosis or a clear history of treatment for tuberculosis; persons with extensive burns or eczema. Skin testing may be deferred with major viral infections or live-virus vaccination within 1 month. Tuberculous or other bacterial infections, viral infection, live virus vaccination, malignancy, immunosuppressive agents, and conditions which impair immune response may cause a decreased response to test. For intradermal administration only; do not administer I.V., I.M., or SubQ. Epinephrine (1:1000) should be available to treat possible allergic reactions.

Adverse Reactions (Reflective of adult population; not specific for elderly)
Suspected adverse reactions should be reported to the Food and Drug Administration (FDA) MedWatch Program at 1-800-332-1088

Frequency not defined:

Dermatologic: Rash

Local: Injection site reactions: Bleeding, bruising, discomfort, erythematous reaction, hematoma, necrosis, pain, pruritus, redness, scarring, ulceration, vesiculation

Miscellaneous: Anaphylaxis

Drug Interactions

Corticosteroids: May depress or suppress reactivity to test for up to 5-6 weeks.

Immunosuppressants: May depress or suppress reactivity to test for up to 5-6 weeks.

Live viral vaccines: May depress or suppress reactivity to test for up to 5-6 weeks.

Stability Aplisol®, Tubersol®: Store under refrigeration at 2°C to 8°C (36°F to 46°F); do not freeze. Protect from light. Opened vials should be discarded after 30 days.

Mechanism of Action Tuberculosis results in individuals becoming sensitized to certain antigenic components of the *M. tuberculosis* organism. Culture extracts called tuberculins are contained in tuberculin skin test preparations. Upon intracutaneous injection of these culture extracts, a classic delayed (cellular) hypersensitivity reaction occurs. This reaction is characteristic of a delayed course (peak occurs >24 hours after injection, induration of the skin secondary to cell infiltration, and occasional vesiculation and necrosis). Delayed hypersensitivity reactions to tuberculin may indicate infection with a variety of nontuberculosis mycobacteria, or vaccination with the live attenuated mycobacterial strain of *M. bovis* vaccine, BCG, in addition to previous natural infection with *M. tuberculosis*.

Pharmacodynamics

Onset of action: Delayed hypersensitivity reactions to tuberculin usually occur within 5-6 hours following injection

Peak effect: Becomes maximal at 48-72 hours

Duration: Reactions subside over a few days

Dosage

Geriatrics & Adults:

Diagnosis of tuberculosis, cell-mediated immunodeficiencies: Intradermal: 0.1 mL

TST interpretation: Criteria for positive TST read at 48-72 hours (see Note below for healthcare workers):

Induration ≥5 mm: Persons with HIV infection (or risk factors for HIV infection, but unknown status), recent close contact to person with known active TB, persons with chest x-ray consistent with healed TB, persons who are immunosuppressed

Induration ≥10 mm: Persons with clinical conditions which increase risk of TB infection, recent immigrants, I.V. drug users, residents and employees of high-risk settings

Induration ≥15 mm: Persons who do not meet any of the above criteria (no risk factors for TB)

Note: A two-step test is recommended when testing will be performed at regular intervals (eg, for healthcare workers). If the first test is negative, a second TST should be administered 1-3 weeks after the first test was read.

TST interpretation (CDC guidelines) in a healthcare setting:

Baseline test: ≥10 mm is positive (either first or second step)

Serial testing without known exposure: Increase of ≥10 mm is positive

Known exposure:

≥5 mm is positive in patients with baseline of 0 mm

≥10 mm is positive in patients with negative baseline or previous screening result of ≥0mm

Read test at 48-72 hours following placement. Test results with 0 mm induration or measured induration less than the defined cutoff point are considered to signify absence of infection with *M. tuberculosis*. Test results should be documented in millimeters even if classified as negative. Erythema and redness of skin are not indicative of a positive test result.

Administration For intradermal administration only. Administer to upper third of forearm (palm up) ≥2 inches from elbow, wrist, or other injection site. If neither arm can be used, may administer to back of shoulder. Administer using inch ¼ to½ inch 27-gauge needle or finer tuberculin syringe. Should form wheal (6-10 mm in diameter) as liquid is injected which will remain ~10 minutes. Avoid pressure or bandage at injection site. Document date and time of injection, person placing TST, location of injection site and lot number of solution.

Monitoring Parameters Monitor for immediate hypersensitivity reactions for ~15 minutes following injection.

Test Interactions False-positive reactions may occur with BCG vaccination or previous mycobacteria (nonTB) infection (previous BCG vaccination is not a contraindication to testing). False-negative reactions may occur with impaired cell mediated immunity.

Patient Information Return to physician or nurse for reaction interpretation at 48-72 hours

Additional Information Situations where risk of tuberculosis infection may be increased are with contacts of recently-diagnosed persons with active disease, contact with immigrants from countries where tuberculosis is still common, or reactivation with impaired immunity (HIV infection, diabetes, renal failure, immunosuppressant use, pulmonary silicosis). Healthcare workers, staff of correctional facilities, and travelers at high risk of exposure should have routine testing. Patients with HIV infection should be tested as soon as possible following diagnosis.

The date of administration, the product manufacturer, and lot number of product must be entered into the patient's permanent medical record. Results should be recorded in millimeters (even if 0), not "negative" or "positive".

Special Geriatric Considerations Due to changes in the immune system with age, skin test response may be delayed or reduced in magnitude; therefore when testing, use a two-step test procedure; repeat test 2-4 weeks after reading first test dose; this elicits a "booster effect".

Dosage Forms Excipient information presented when available (limited, particularly for generics); consult specific product labeling.
Injection, solution:
Aplisol®, Tubersol®: 5 TU/0.1 mL (1 mL, 5 mL) [contains polysorbate 80]

Selected References
Dutt AK and Stead WW, "Tuberculosis," *Clin Geriatr Med*, 1992, 8(4):761-75.

♦ **Tylox**® *see* Oxycodone and Acetaminophen *on page 1182*
♦ **Typhim Vi**® *see* Typhoid Vaccine *on page 1646*

Typhoid Vaccine (TYE foid vak SEEN)

Related Information
   Immunization Recommendations *on page 1787*
U.S. Brand Names Typhim Vi®; Vivotif®
Index Terms Ty21a Vaccine; Typhoid Vaccine Live Oral Ty21a; Vi Vaccine
Generic Available No
Pharmacologic Category Vaccine
Use Active immunization against typhoid fever caused by *Salmonella typhi*
   Not for routine vaccination. In the United States, use should be limited to:
      — Travelers to areas with risk of exposure to *S. typhi*
      — Persons with intimate exposure to a *S. typhi* carrier
      — Laboratory technicians with exposure to *S. typhi*
Contraindications Hypersensitivity to any component of the vaccine. In addition, the
   oral vaccine is contraindicated with congenital or acquired immunodeficient state,
   acute febrile illness, acute GI illness
Warnings/Precautions Not all recipients of typhoid vaccine will be fully protected
   against typhoid fever. Travelers should take all necessary precautions to avoid contact
   or ingestion of potentially contaminated food or water sources. Should not be used to
   treat typhoid fever.

   Injection: Administer at least 2 weeks prior to expected exposure. Vaccination may be
   deferred during acute infection or febrile illness. Immune response may be decreased
   in those receiving immunosuppressive therapy or are otherwise immunocompromised.
   Use caution with coagulation disorders (including thrombocytopenia) where intramuscular injections should not be used. Epinephrine 1:1000 should be readily available.

   Oral: Full immunization schedule should be completed at least 1 week prior to
   expected exposure. The complete immunization schedule must be followed to achieve
   optimum immune response. Vaccination may be deferred with persistent diarrhea or
   vomiting.
Adverse Reactions (Reflective of adult population; not specific for elderly)
   **All serious adverse reactions must be reported to the U.S. Department of Health
   and Human Services (DHHS) Vaccine Adverse Event Reporting System (VAERS)
   1-800-822-7967.**

   Oral:
      1% to 10%:
         Central nervous system: Headache (5%), fever (3%)
         Dermatologic: Rash (1%)
         Gastrointestinal: Abdominal pain (6%), diarrhea (3%), nausea (6%), vomiting (2%)
   Injection:
      >10%:
         Central nervous system: Headache (16% to 20%), fever <100°F (3% to 11%),
            malaise (4% to 24%)
         Local: Tenderness (97% to 98%), induration (5% to 15%), pain at injection site
            (27% to 41%)
      1% to 10%:
         Central nervous system: Fever ≥100°F (2%)
         Gastrointestinal: Nausea (2% to 8%), vomiting (2%)
         Local: Erythema at injection site (4% to 5%)
         Neuromuscular & skeletal: Myalgia (3% to 7%)
Drug Interactions
   Antibiotics (systemic): May decrease the effect of oral live attenuated Ty21a vaccine
      (Vivotif®); delay vaccine administration for at least 24 hours after administration of
      any systemic antibiotic.
   Immune globulins: Immune globulins may diminish the therapeutic effect of live
      vaccines.
   Immunosuppressants: Immunosuppressants may enhance the adverse/toxic effect of
      live vaccines. Vaccinial infections may develop.
   Mefloquine: May decrease the effect of oral live attenuated Ty21a vaccine (Vivotif®).
      The CDC recommends delaying vaccine administration for at least 24 hours after
      administration of mefloquine. The manufacturer notes that no delay is needed.
   Proguanil: May decrease the effect of oral live attenuated Ty21a vaccine (Vivotif®);
      separate dosing by at least 10 days.
Ethanol/Nutrition/Herb Interactions Ethanol: Avoid alcohol within 2 hours of taking
   the capsule; may disrupt the enteric coating
Stability
   Typhim Vi®: Store between 2°C to 8°C (35°F to 46°F); do not freeze.
   Vivotif®: Store between 2°C to 8°C (35°F to 46°F).

Mechanism of Action Virulent strains of *Salmonella typhi* cause disease by penetrating the intestinal mucosa and entering the systemic circulation via the lymphatic vasculature. One possible mechanism of conferring immunity may be the provocation of a local immune response in the intestinal tract induced by oral ingesting of a live strain with subsequent aborted infection. The ability of *Salmonella typhi* to produce clinical disease (and to elicit an immune response) is dependent on the bacteria having a complete lipopolysaccharide. The live attenuate Ty21a strain lacks the enzyme UDP-4-galactose epimerase so that lipopolysaccharide is only synthesized under conditions that induce bacterial autolysis. Thus, the strain remains avirulent despite the production of sufficient lipopolysaccharide to evoke a protective immune response. Despite low levels of lipopolysaccharide synthesis, cells lyse before gaining a virulent phenotype due to the intracellular accumulation of metabolic intermediates.

Pharmacodynamics

Onset of action: Immunity to *Salmonella typhi*: Oral: ~1 week

Duration: Immunity: Oral: ~4-7 years; Parenteral: >17-21 months

Dosage

Geriatrics & Adults: Immunization:

Oral:

Primary immunization: One capsule on alternate days (day 1, 3, 5, and 7) for a total of 4 doses; all doses should be complete at least 1 week prior to potential exposure

Booster immunization: Repeat full course of primary immunization every 5 years

I.M.:

Initial: 0.5 mL given at least 2 weeks prior to expected exposure

Reimmunization: 0.5 mL; optimal schedule has not been established; a single dose every 2 years is currently recommended for repeated or continued exposure

Administration Injection: Typhim Vi® may be given I.M.; administer as a single 0.5 mL (25 mcg) injection in deltoid muscle. **Note:** For patients at risk of hemorrhage following intramuscular injection, the ACIP recommends "it should be administered intramuscularly if, in the opinion of the physician familiar with the patients bleeding risk, the vaccine can be administered with reasonable safety by this route. If the patient receives antihemophilia or other similar therapy, intramuscular vaccination can be scheduled shortly after such therapy is administered. A fine needle (23 gauge or smaller) can be used for the vaccination and firm pressure applied to the site (without rubbing) for at least 2 minutes. The patient should be instructed concerning the risk of hematoma from the injection."

Oral: Swallow capsule whole soon after placing into mouth; do not chew or open capsule. Capsule should be taken with a cold or lukewarm beverage (≤37°C/98.6°F). Take one hour prior to a meal. Avoid alcohol within 2 hours of administration.

Patient Information Oral capsule should be taken 1 hour before a meal with cold or lukewarm drink; systemic adverse effects may persist for 1-2 days

Additional Information Federal law requires that the date of administration, the vaccine manufacturer, lot number of vaccine, and the administering person's name, title, and address be entered into the patient's permanent medical record.

Special Geriatric Considerations Vaccinating elderly is often overlooked; if no record of immunization can be recalled, repeat primary series.

Dosage Forms Excipient information presented when available (limited, particularly for generics); consult specific product labeling.

Capsule, enteric coated:

Vivotif®: Viable *S. typhi* Ty21a 2-6 x 10⁹ colony-forming units and nonviable *S. typhi* Ty21a 5-50 x 10⁹ bacterial cells [contains lactose and sucrose]

Injection, solution:

Typhim Vi®: Purified Vi capsular polysaccharide 25 mcg/0.5 mL (0.5 mL, 10 mL) [derived from *S. typhi* Ty2 strain]

Selected References

Begier EM, Burewn DR, Haber P, et al, "Postmarketing Safety Surveillance for Typhoid Fever Vaccines From the Vaccine Adverse Event Reporting System, July 1990 Through June 2002," *Clin Infect Dis*, 2004, 38(6):771-9.

Centers for Disease Control, "Recommendations of the Advisory Committee on Immunization Practices (ACIP): General Recommendations on Immunization," *MMWR Recomm Rep*, 2006, 55(RR-15):1-48.

Gardner P and Schaffner W, "Immunization of Adults," *N Engl J Med*, 1993, 328(17):1252-8.

Guzman CA, Borsutzky S, Griot-Wenk M, et al, "Vaccines Against Typhoid Fever," *Vaccine*, 2006, 24(18):3804-11.

Parry CM, Hien TT, Dougan G, et al, "Typhoid Fever," *N Engl J Med*, 2002, 347(22):1770-82.

Unoprostone (yoo noe PROS tone)

Related Information
Glaucoma Drug Therapy *on page 1758*
Canadian Brand Names Rescula®
Index Terms Unoprostone Isopropyl
Generic Available No
Pharmacologic Category Ophthalmic Agent, Antiglaucoma; Prostaglandin, Ophthalmic
Use Reduction of intraocular pressure (IOP) in patients with open-angle glaucoma or ocular hypertension; should be used in patients who are not tolerant of, or failed treatment with other IOP-lowering medications
Restrictions Not available in U.S.
Contraindications Hypersensitivity to unoprostone, benzalkonium chloride, or any component of the formulation
Warnings/Precautions May cause permanent change in eye color (increases the amount of brown pigment in the iris); long-term consequences and potential injury to eye are not known. Bacterial keratitis, caused by inadvertent contamination of multiple-dose ophthalmic solutions, has been reported. Use caution in patients with intraocular inflammation. Contains benzalkonium chloride which may be adsorbed by contact lenses; remove contacts prior to administration and wait 15 minutes before reinserting. Safety and efficacy have not been determined for use in patients with renal or hepatic impairment, angle closure, inflammatory or neovascular glaucoma.
Adverse Reactions (Reflective of adult population; not specific for elderly)
>10%: Ocular: Burning/stinging (10% to 25%), dry eyes (10% to 25%), injection (10% to 25%), ophthalmic itching (10% to 25%), increased length of eyelashes (10% to 14%)
1% to 10%:
Cardiovascular: Hypertension
Central nervous system: Dizziness, headache, insomnia, pain
Endocrine & metabolic: Diabetes mellitus
Neuromuscular & skeletal: Back pain
Ocular: Abnormal vision (5% to 10%), eyelid disorder (5% to 10%), foreign body sensation (5% to 10%), lacrimation disorder (5% to 10%), decreased length of eyelashes (7%), blepharitis, cataract, conjunctivitis, corneal lesion, eye discharge, eye hemorrhage, eye pain, irritation, keratitis, photophobia, vitreous disorder
Respiratory: Bronchitis, increased cough, pharyngitis, rhinitis, sinusitis
Miscellaneous: Flu-like syndrome (6%), accidental injury, allergic reaction
Overdosage/Toxicology No data available. If overdose occurs, treatment should be symptomatic.
Drug Interactions Specific drug interactions have not been reported. When using more than one ophthalmic product, wait at least 5 minutes between application of each medication.
Stability Store between 2°C to 25°C (36°F to 77°F).
Mechanism of Action The exact mechanism of action is unknown; however, unoprostone decreases IOP by increasing the outflow of aqueous humor. Cardiovascular and pulmonary function were not affected in clinical studies. IOP was decreased by 3-4 mm Hg in patients with a mean baseline IOP of 23 mm Hg.
Pharmacokinetics
Absorption: Absorbed through the cornea and conjunctival epithelium
Metabolism: Hydrolyzed by esterases to a metabolite, unoprostone-free acid

Half-life: 14 minutes
Elimination: Metabolite excreted in the urine

Dosage
 Geriatrics & Adults: Glaucoma or ocular hypertension: Ophthalmic: Instill 1 drop into affected eye(s) twice daily
 Renal Impairment: Use with caution, no dosing adjustment reported.
 Hepatic Impairment: Use with caution, no dosing adjustment reported.

Administration May be used with other eye drops to lower intraocular pressure; if using more than one product, wait at least 5 minutes between application of each medication. Remove contact lenses prior to administration and wait 15 minutes before reinserting.

Patient Information Wash hands before instilling solution. Sit or lie down to instill. Open eye, look at ceiling, and instill prescribed amount of solution. Apply gentle pressure to inner corner of eye. Do not let tip of applicator touch eye; do not contaminate tip of applicator (contamination may cause eye infection leading to possible eye damage or vision loss). Contact prescriber concerning continued use of drops if eye infection develops, trauma occurs to the eye, and prior to eye surgery. This product contains benzalkonium chloride which may be adsorbed by contact lenses; remove contacts prior to administration and wait 15 minutes before reinserting. May cause permanent changes in eye color (increases the amount of brown pigment in the iris); long-term consequences and potential injury to eye are not known. Changes to eye color may occur slowly (months to years). May be used with other eye drops to lower intraocular pressure; if using more than one product, wait at least 5 minutes between application of each medication. Notify prescriber if conjunctivitis or eyelid reactions occur with use of this product.

Additional Information Contains benzalkonium chloride 0.015% as a preservative

Special Geriatric Considerations No differences in safety and efficacy have been reported in the elderly. Assess patient's ability to self-administer eye drops.

Dosage Forms Excipient information presented when available (limited, particularly for generics); consult specific product labeling. [DSC] = Discontinued product
 Solution, ophthalmic: 0.15% (5 mL) [contains benzalkonium chloride] [DSC]

Ursodiol (ur soe DYE ol)

U.S. Brand Names Actigall®; Urso 250™; Urso Forte™
Canadian Brand Names Urso®; Urso® DS
Index Terms Ursodeoxycholic Acid
Generic Available Yes: Capsule
Pharmacologic Category Gallstone Dissolution Agent
Use
 Actigall®: Gallbladder stone dissolution in patients with radiolucent, noncalcified stones <20 mm in greatest diameter with an increased risk for surgical removal; prevention of gallstones in obese patients experiencing rapid weight loss
 Urso®: Treatment of primary biliary cirrhosis

Unlabeled/Investigational Use Liver transplantation

Contraindications Hypersensitivity to ursodiol, bile acids, or any component of the formulation; not to be used with cholesterol, radiopaque, bile pigment stones, or stones >20 mm in diameter; allergy to bile acids

Warnings/Precautions Gallbladder stone dissolution may take several months of therapy. Complete dissolution may not occur and recurrence of stones within 5 years has been observed in 50% of patients. Use with caution in patients with a nonvisualizing gallbladder and those with chronic liver disease.

Adverse Reactions (Reflective of adult population; not specific for elderly)
 >10%:
  Central nervous system: Headache (up to 25%), dizziness (up to 17%)
  Gastrointestinal: In treatment of primary biliary cirrhosis: Constipation (up to 26%)
 1% to 10%:
  Dermatologic: Rash (<1% to 3%), alopecia (<1% to 5%)
(Continued)

Ursodiol *(Continued)*

Gastrointestinal:
In gallstone dissolution: Most GI events (diarrhea, nausea, vomiting) are similar to placebo and attributable to gallstone disease.
In treatment of primary biliary cirrhosis: Diarrhea (1%)
Hematologic: Leukopenia (3%)
Miscellaneous: Allergy (5%)

Overdosage/Toxicology Symptom include diarrhea. No specific therapy for diarrhea or overdose.

Stability Do not store above 30°C (86°F).

Mechanism of Action Decreases the cholesterol content of bile and bile stones by reducing the secretion of cholesterol from the liver and the fractional reabsorption of cholesterol by the intestines. Mechanism of action in primary biliary cirrhosis is not clearly defined.

Pharmacokinetics

Metabolism: Undergoes extensive enterohepatic recycling; following hepatic conjugation and biliary secretion, the drug is hydrolyzed to active ursodiol, where it is recycled or transformed to lithocholic acid by colonic microbial flora
Half-life: 100 hours
Elimination: In feces via bile

Dosage

Geriatrics & Adults:

Gallstone dissolution: Oral: 8-10 mg/kg/day in 2-3 divided doses; use beyond 24 months is not established; obtain ultrasound images at 6-month intervals for the first year of therapy; 30% of patients have stone recurrence after dissolution

Gallstone prevention: Oral: 300 mg twice daily

Primary biliary cirrhosis: Oral: 13-15 mg/kg/day in 2-4 divided doses (with food)

Administration Oral: Do not administer with aluminum-based antacids. If aluminum-based antacids are needed, administer 2 hours after ursodiol.

Monitoring Parameters

Gallstone disease: ALT, ALP, AST at initiation, 1 and 3 months and every 6 months thereafter, sonogram
Hepatic disease: Monitor hepatic function tests frequently

Patient Information Urso® should be taken with food. Frequent blood work necessary to follow drug effects; report any persistent nausea, vomiting, abdominal pain

Special Geriatric Considerations No specific clinical studies in the elderly. Would recommend starting at lowest recommended dose with scheduled monitoring.

Dosage Forms Excipient information presented when available (limited, particularly for generics); consult specific product labeling.
Capsule (Actigall®): 300 mg
Tablet:
Urso 250™: 250 mg
Urso Forte™: 500 mg

♦ **Urso Forte™** *see* Ursodiol *on page 1649*
♦ **UTI Relief® [OTC]** *see* Phenazopyridine *on page 1238*
♦ **Vagifem®** *see* Estradiol *on page 549*
♦ **Vagistat®-1 [OTC]** *see* Tioconazole *on page 1577*

Valacyclovir *(val ay SYE kloe veer)*

Medication Safety Issues

Sound-alike/look-alike issues:
Valtrex® may be confused with Valcyte™
Valacyclovir may be confused with valganciclovir

U.S. Brand Names Valtrex®

Canadian Brand Names Valtrex®

Index Terms Valacyclovir Hydrochloride

Generic Available No

Pharmacologic Category Antiviral Agent, Oral

Use Treatment of herpes zoster (shingles) in immunocompetent patients; treatment of first-episode genital herpes; episodic treatment of recurrent genital herpes; suppression of recurrent genital herpes and reduction of heterosexual transmission of genital herpes in immunocompetent patients; suppression of genital herpes in HIV-infected individuals; treatment of herpes labialis (cold sores)

Contraindications Hypersensitivity to valacyclovir, acyclovir, or any component of the formulation

Warnings/Precautions Hazardous agent - use appropriate precautions for handling and disposal. Thrombotic thrombocytopenic purpura/hemolytic uremic syndrome has occurred in immunocompromised patients; use caution and adjust the dose in elderly patients or those with renal insufficiency.

Adverse Reactions (Reflective of adult population; not specific for elderly)
>10%: Central nervous system: Headache (14% to 35%)
1% to 10%:
Central nervous system: Dizziness (2% to 4%), depression (0% to 7%)
Endocrine: Dysmenorrhea (≤1% to 8%)
Gastrointestinal: Abdominal pain (2% to 11%), vomiting (<1% to 6%), nausea (6% to 15%)
Hematologic: Leukopenia (≤1%), thrombocytopenia (≤1%)
Hepatic: AST increased (1% to 4%)
Neuromuscular & skeletal: Arthralgia (≤1 to 6%)

Overdosage/Toxicology Symptoms include elevated serum creatinine, renal failure, encephalitis, and precipitation in renal tubules. Hemodialysis has resulted in up to 60% reduction in serum acyclovir levels after administration of acyclovir.

Drug Interactions
Cimetidine: Decreased renal clearance of acyclovir; no dosage adjustment needed in patients with normal renal function.
Probenecid: Decreased renal clearance of acyclovir; no dosage adjustment needed in patients with normal renal function.

Stability Store at 15°C to 25°C (59°F to 77°F).

Mechanism of Action Valacyclovir is rapidly and nearly completely converted to acyclovir by intestinal and hepatic metabolism. Acyclovir is converted to acyclovir monophosphate by virus-specific thymidine kinase then further converted to acyclovir triphosphate by other cellular enzymes. Acyclovir triphosphate inhibits DNA synthesis and viral replication by competing with deoxyguanosine triphosphate for viral DNA polymerase and being incorporated into viral DNA.

Pharmacokinetics
Absorption: Rapid
Distribution: Acyclovir is widely distributed throughout the body including brain, kidney, lungs, liver, spleen, muscle, uterus, vagina, and CSF
Protein binding: Valacyclovir is 13.5% to 17.9% bound to human plasma proteins
Metabolism: Hepatic; valacyclovir is rapidly and nearly completely converted to acyclovir and L-valine by first pass intestinal and/or hepatic metabolism; acyclovir is hepatically metabolized to a very small extent by aldehyde oxidase and by alcohol and aldehyde dehydrogenase (inactive metabolites)
Bioavailability: After administration of valacyclovir, bioavailability of acyclovir is ~55%
Half-life: Normal renal function: Adults: 2.5-3.3 hours (acyclovir), ~30 minutes (valacyclovir); end-stage renal disease: 14-20 hours (acyclovir)
Elimination: Urine: Acyclovir (88%); valacyclovir (46%); Feces: Valacyclovir (47%)

Dosage
Geriatrics & Adults:
Herpes labialis (cold sores): Oral: 2 g twice daily for 1 day (separate doses by ~12 hours)
Herpes zoster (shingles): Oral: 1 g 3 times/day for 7 days
Genital herpes: Oral:
Initial episode: 1 g twice daily for 10 days
Recurrent episode: 500 mg twice daily for 3 days
Reduction of transmission: 500 mg once daily (source partner)
Suppressive therapy:
Immunocompetent patients: 1000 mg once daily (500 mg once daily in patients with <9 recurrences per year)
HIV-infected patients (CD4 ≥100 cells/mm³): 500 mg twice daily
Renal Impairment:
Herpes zoster: Adults:
Cl_{cr} 30-49 mL/minute: 1 g every 12 hours
Cl_{cr} 10-29 mL/minute: 1 g every 24 hours
Cl_{cr} <10 mL/minute: 500 mg every 24 hours
Genital herpes: Adults:
Initial episode:
Cl_{cr} 10-29 mL/minute: 1 g every 24 hours
Cl_{cr} <10 mL/minute: 500 mg every 24 hours
Recurrent episode: Cl_{cr} <10-29 mL/minute: 500 mg every 24 hours
Suppressive therapy: Cl_{cr} <10-29 mL/minute:
For usual dose of 1 g every 24 hours, decrease dose to 500 mg every 24 hours
For usual dose of 500 mg every 24 hours, decrease dose to 500 mg every 48 hours
HIV-infected patients: 500 mg every 24 hours
Herpes labialis: Adults:
Cl_{cr} 30-49 mL/minute: 1 g every 12 hours for 2 doses
Cl_{cr} 10-29 mL/minute: 500 mg every 12 hours for 2 doses
Cl_{cr} <10 mL/minute: 500 mg as a single dose
(Continued)

Valacyclovir *(Continued)*

Hemodialysis: Dialyzable (~33% removed during 4-hour session); administer dose postdialysis

Chronic ambulatory peritoneal dialysis/continuous arteriovenous hemofiltration dialysis: Pharmacokinetic parameters are similar to those in patients with ESRD; supplemental dose not needed following dialysis

Monitoring Parameters Urinalysis, BUN, serum creatinine, liver enzymes, CBC

Patient Information Begin use as soon as possible following development of signs of herpes zoster. Take with plenty of fluids. May take without regard to meals. This medication is not a cure for genital herpes; it is not known if it will prevent transmission to others.

Special Geriatric Considerations More convenient dosing and increased bioavailability, without increasing side effects, make valacyclovir a favorable choice compared to acyclovir; has been shown to accelerate resolution of postherpetic pain. See Warnings/Precautions and Dosage. Also see Acyclovir *on page 37.*

Dosage Forms Excipient information presented when available (limited, particularly for generics); consult specific product labeling.
Caplet: 500 mg, 1000 mg

Selected References
Beutner KR, Friedman DJ, Forszpaniak C, et al, "Valacyclovir Compared With Acyclovir for Improved Therapy for Herpes Zoster in Immunocompetent Adults," *Antimicrob Agents Chemother,* 1995, 39(7):1546-53.

- ◆ **Valacyclovir Hydrochloride** *see* Valacyclovir *on page 1650*
- ◆ **23-Valent Pneumococcal Polysaccharide Vaccine** *see* Pneumococcal Polysaccharide Vaccine (Polyvalent) *on page 1279*
- ◆ **Valium®** *see* Diazepam *on page 420*
- ◆ **Valorin [OTC]** *see* Acetaminophen *on page 29*
- ◆ **Valorin Extra [OTC]** *see* Acetaminophen *on page 29*
- ◆ **Valproate Semisodium** *see* Valproic Acid and Derivatives *on page 1652*
- ◆ **Valproate Sodium** *see* Valproic Acid and Derivatives *on page 1652*
- ◆ **Valproic Acid** *see* Valproic Acid and Derivatives *on page 1652*

Valproic Acid and Derivatives *(val PROE ik AS id & dah RIV ah tives)*

Related Information
Liquid Compatibility of Antipsychotics and Mood Stabilizers *on page 1851*
Serum Drug Concentrations Commonly Monitored Guidelines *on page 1862*

Medication Safety Issues
Sound-alike/look-alike issues:
Depakene® may be confused with Depakote®
Depakote® may be confused with Depakene®, Depakote® ER, Senokot®

U.S. Brand Names Depacon®; Depakene®; Depakote®; Depakote® ER; Depakote® Sprinkle

Canadian Brand Names Alti-Divalproex; Apo-Divalproex®; Apo-Valproic®; Depakene®; Epival® I.V.; Gen-Divalproex; Novo-Divalproex; Nu-Divalproex; PMS-Valproic Acid; PMS-Valproic Acid E.C.; Rhoxal-valproic; Sandoz-Valproic

Index Terms Dipropylacetic Acid; Divalproex Sodium; DPA; 2-Propylpentanoic Acid; 2-Propylvaleric Acid; Valproate Semisodium; Valproate Sodium; Valproic Acid

Generic Available Yes: Capsule (excluding sprinkle), injection, syrup

Pharmacologic Category Anticonvulsant, Miscellaneous

Use
Depacon®, Depakene®, Depakote®, Depakote® ER, Depakote® Sprinkle: Monotherapy and adjunctive therapy in the treatment of patients with complex partial seizures; monotherapy and adjunctive therapy of simple and complex absence seizures; adjunctive therapy in patients with multiple seizure types that include absence seizures

Depakote®, Depakote® ER: Mania associated with bipolar disorder; migraine prophylaxis

Unlabeled/Investigational Use Status epilepticus

Contraindications Hypersensitivity to valproic acid, derivatives, or any component of the formulation; hepatic dysfunction; urea cycle disorders

Warnings/Precautions
[U.S. Boxed Warning]: Hepatic failure resulting in fatalities has occurred in patients. Other risk factors include organic brain disease, mental retardation with severe seizure disorders, congenital metabolic disorders, and patients on multiple anticonvulsants. Hepatotoxicity has been reported within 6 months of therapy. Monitor patients closely for appearance of malaise, weakness, facial edema, anorexia, jaundice, and vomiting.

[U.S. Boxed Warning]: Cases of life-threatening pancreatitis, occurring at the start of therapy or following years of use, have been reported. Some cases have been hemorrhagic with rapid progression of initial symptoms to death. Evaluate symptoms of abdominal pain, nausea, vomiting, and/or anorexia.

May cause severe thrombocytopenia, inhibition of platelet aggregation, and bleeding. Tremors may indicate overdosage; use with caution in patients receiving other anticonvulsants. Hypersensitivity reactions affecting multiple organs have been reported in association with valproic acid use; may include dermatologic and/or hematologic changes (eosinophilia, neutropenia, thrombocytopenia) or symptoms of organ dysfunction.

Hyperammonemia and/or encephalopathy, sometimes fatal, have been reported following the initiation of valproic acid therapy and may be present with normal transaminase levels. Ammonia levels should be measured in patients who develop unexplained lethargy and vomiting, or changes in mental status. Discontinue therapy if ammonia levels are increased and evaluate for possible urea cycle disorder (UCD). Although rare genetic disorders, UCD evaluation should be considered for the following patients prior to the start of therapy: History of unexplained encephalopathy or coma; encephalopathy associated with protein load; unexplained mental retardation; history of elevated plasma ammonia or glutamine; history of cyclical vomiting and lethargy; episodic extreme irritability, ataxia; low BUN or protein avoidance; family history of UCD or unexplained infant deaths (particularly male); or signs or symptoms of UCD (hyperammonemia, encephalopathy, respiratory alkalosis).

In vitro studies have suggested valproic acid stimulates the replication of HIV and CMV viruses under experimental conditions. The clinical consequence of this is unknown, but should be considered when monitoring affected patients.

Use of Depacon® injection is not recommended for post-traumatic seizure prophylaxis following acute head trauma. Anticonvulsants should not be discontinued abruptly because of the possibility of increasing seizure frequency; valproic acid should be withdrawn gradually to minimize the potential of increased seizure frequency, unless safety concerns require a more rapid withdrawal. Concomitant use with clonazepam may induce absence status. Patients treated for bipolar disorder should be monitored closely for clinical worsening or suicidality; prescriptions should be written for the smallest quantity consistent with good patient care.

CNS depression may occur with valproic acid use. Patients must be cautioned about performing tasks which require mental alertness (operating machinery or driving). Effects with other sedative drugs or ethanol may be potentiated. Use with caution in the elderly.

Adverse Reactions (Reflective of adult population; not specific for elderly)

Adverse reactions reported when used as monotherapy for complex partial seizure:

>10%:
  Central nervous system: Somnolence (18% to 30%), dizziness (13% to 18%), insomnia (9% to 15%), nervousness (7% to 11%)
  Dermatologic: Alopecia (13% to 24%)
  Gastrointestinal: Nausea (26% to 34%), vomiting (15% to 23%), diarrhea (19% to 23%), abdominal pain (9% to 12%), dyspepsia (10% to 11%), anorexia (4% to 11%)
  Hematologic: Thrombocytopenia (1% to 24%)
  Neuromuscular & skeletal: Tremor (19% to 57%), weakness (10% to 21%)
  Miscellaneous: Infection (13% to 20%)

1% to 10%:
  Cardiovascular: Chest pain, hypertension, palpitation, peripheral edema, tachycardia
  Central nervous system: Abnormal dreams, amnesia, anxiety, confusion, coordination abnormal, depression, headache, malaise, personality disorder
  Dermatologic: Bruising, dry skin, petechia, pruritus, rash
  Endocrine & metabolic: Amenorrhea, dysmenorrhea
  Gastrointestinal: Appetite increased, eructation, flatulence, hematemesis, pancreatitis, periodontal abscess, taste perversion, weight gain
  Genitourinary: Urinary frequency, urinary incontinence, vaginitis
  Hepatic: AST/ALT increased
  Neuromuscular & skeletal: Abnormal gait, arthralgia, back pain, hypertonia, leg cramps, myalgia, myasthenia, paresthesia, twitching
  Ocular: Abnormal vision, amblyopia/blurred vision, nystagmus
  Otic: Deafness, otitis media, tinnitus
  Respiratory: Cough increased, dyspnea, epistaxis, pharyngitis, pneumonia, sinusitis

Additional adverse effects: Frequency not defined:
  Cardiovascular: Bradycardia, edema
  Central nervous system: Aggression, ataxia, behavioral deterioration, cerebral atrophy (reversible), coma (rare), dementia, encephalopathy (rare), fever, hallucinations, hostility, hyperactivity, hypoesthesia, hypothermia, parkinsonism, psychosis, sedation, vertigo

(Continued)

Valproic Acid and Derivatives *(Continued)*

Dermatologic: Cutaneous vasculitis, erythema multiforme, photosensitivity, Stevens-Johnson syndrome, toxic epidermal necrolysis (rare)

Endocrine & metabolic: Breast enlargement, galactorrhea, hyperammonemia, hyponatremia, inappropriate ADH secretion, parotid gland swelling, polycystic ovary disease (rare), abnormal thyroid function tests

Gastrointestinal: Abdominal cramps, constipation, indigestion, weight loss

Genitourinary: Enuresis, urinary tract infection

Hematologic: Agranulocytosis, anemia, aplastic anemia, bone marrow suppression, eosinophilia, hematoma formation, hemorrhage, hypofibrinogenemia, intermittent porphyria, leukopenia, lymphocytosis, macrocytosis, pancytopenia

Hepatic: Bilirubin increased, hyperammonemic encephalopathy (in patients with UCD)

Neuromuscular & skeletal: Asterixis, bone pain, dysarthria

Ocular: Diplopia, seeing "spots before the eyes"

Otic: Ear pain

Renal: Fanconi-like syndrome (rare, in children)

Miscellaneous: Allergic reaction, anaphylaxis, carnitine decreased, hyperglycinemia, lupus

Overdosage/Toxicology Symptoms include coma, deep sleep, motor restlessness, heart block, and visual hallucinations. Naloxone has been used to reverse CNS depressant effects, but may block the action of other anticonvulsants. In overdose, the fraction of unbound valproate is high. Hemodialysis or tandem hemodialysis plus hemoperfusion may lead to significant removal of the drug.

Drug Interactions For valproic acid: **Substrate** (minor) of CYP2A6, 2B6, 2C9, 2C19, 2E1; **Inhibits** CYP2C9 (weak), 2C19 (weak), 2D6 (weak), 3A4 (weak); **Induces** CYP2A6 (weak)

Carbamazepine: Valproic acid may increase, decrease, or have no effect on carbamazepine levels; valproic acid may increase serum concentrations of carbamazepine - epoxide (active metabolite); valproic acid may induce the metabolism of carbamazepine; monitor.

Carbapenem antibiotics (ertapenem, imipenem, meropenem): May decrease valproic acid concentrations to subtherapeutic levels; monitor.

Felbamate: May increase the levels/effects of valproic acid; monitor.

Isoniazid: May decrease valproic acid metabolism (limited documentation).

Lamotrigine: Valproic acid inhibits the metabolism of lamotrigine; combination therapy has been proposed to increase the risk of toxic epidermal necrolysis; monitor.

Macrolide antibiotics: May decrease valproic acid metabolism (limited documentation); includes clarithromycin, erythromycin, troleandomycin; monitor.

Oxcarbazepine: Valproic acid may decrease the serum concentration of oxcarbazepine; monitor.

Primidone, phenobarbital: Valproic acid appears to inhibit the metabolism of phenobarbital; monitor for increased effect.

Risperidone: Valproic acid may enhance the adverse/toxic effect of risperidone. Monitor for the development of peripheral edema during concomitant use; a reduction in the dose of risperidone may be needed.

Salicylates: May displace valproic acid from plasma proteins, leading to acute toxicity.

Topiramate: Hyperammonemia with or without encephalopathy has been reported in patients who tolerated either drug alone. These drugs may modestly decrease the serum concentrations of the other drug.

Tricyclic antidepressants (eg, amitriptyline, nortriptyline): Valproic acid may increase the levels/effects of some tricyclic antidepressants. This has been specifically observed with amitriptyline, nortriptyline, and clomipramine. Monitor levels and consider dose reduction of tricyclic agent.

Zidovudine: Valproic acid may increase the levels/effects of zidovudine; monitor.

Ethanol/Nutrition/Herb Interactions

Ethanol: Avoid ethanol (may increase CNS depression).

Food: Food may delay but does not affect the extent of absorption. Valproic acid serum concentrations may be decreased if taken with food. Milk has no effect on absorption.

Herb/Nutraceutical: Avoid evening primrose (seizure threshold decreased).

Stability

Depakote® tablet, Depakene® solution: Store below 30°C (86°F).

Depakote® Sprinkles: Store below 25°C (77°F).

Depakote® ER: Store at 15°C to 30°C (59°F to 86°F).

Depakene® capsule: Store at 15°C to 25°C (59°F to 77°F).

Depacon®: Store vial at room temperature of 15°C to 30°C (59°F to 86°F). Injection should be diluted in 50 mL of a compatible diluent. Stable in D_5W, NS, and LR for at least 24 hours when stored in glass or PVC.

Mechanism of Action Causes increased availability of gamma-aminobutyric acid (GABA), an inhibitory neurotransmitter, to brain neurons or may enhance the action of GABA or mimic its action at postsynaptic receptor sites

Pharmacokinetics

Distribution: Total valproate: 11 L/1.73 m^2; free valproate 92 L/1.73 m^2

Protein binding (dose dependent): 80% to 90%; decreased in the elderly and with hepatic or renal dysfunction

Metabolism: Extensively hepatic via glucuronide conjugation and mitochondrial beta-oxidation. The relationship between dose and total valproate concentration is nonlinear; concentration does not increase proportionally with the dose, but increases to a lesser extent due to saturable plasma protein binding. The kinetics of unbound drug are linear.

Bioavailability: Depakote® ER: 90% of I.V. dose and ~89% of delayed release formulation

Half-life elimination: 9-16 hours

Time to peak, serum: Depakote® tablet: ~4 hours; Depakote® ER: 4-17 hours

Excretion: Urine (30% to 50% as glucuronide conjugate, 3% as unchanged drug)

Dosage

Geriatrics & Adults:

Seizures: Administer doses >250 mg/day in divided doses.

Oral:

Simple and complex absence seizure: Initial: 15 mg/kg/day; increase by 5-10 mg/kg/day at weekly intervals until therapeutic levels are achieved; maximum: 60 mg/kg/day.

Complex partial seizure: Initial: 10-15 mg/kg/day; increase by 5-10 mg/kg/day at weekly intervals until therapeutic levels are achieved; maximum: 60 mg/kg/day.

Note: Regular release and delayed release formulations are usually given in 2-4 divided doses/day; extended release formulation (Depakote® ER) is usually given once daily. Conversion to Depakote® ER from a stable dose of Depakote® may require an increase in the total daily dose between 8% and 20% to maintain similar serum concentrations.

I.V.: Administer as a 60-minute infusion (≤20 mg/minute) with the same frequency as oral products; switch patient to oral products as soon as possible. Rapid infusions ≤15 mg/kg over 5-10 minutes (1.5-3 mg/kg/minute) were generally well tolerated in a clinical trial.

Rectal (unlabeled): Dilute syrup 1:1 with water for use as a retention enema; loading dose: 17-20 mg/kg one time; maintenance: 10-15 mg/kg/dose every 8 hours

Status epilepticus (unlabeled use):

Loading dose: I.V.: 15-25 mg/kg administered at 3 mg/kg/minute

Maintenance dose: I.V. infusion: 1-4 mg/kg/hour; titrate dose as needed based upon patient response and evaluation of drug-drug interactions

Mania:

Oral: Initial: 750 mg/day in divided doses; dose should be adjusted as rapidly as possible to desired clinical effect; maximum recommended dosage: 60 mg/kg/day

Depakote® ER: Initial: 25 mg/kg/day given once daily; dose should be adjusted as rapidly as possible to desired clinical effect; maximum recommended dose: 60 mg/kg/day.

Migraine prophylaxis:

Depakote® ER: 500 mg once daily for 7 days, then increase to 1000 mg once daily; adjust dose based on patient response; usual dosage range 500-1000 mg/day

Depakote® tablet: 250 mg twice daily; adjust dose based on patient response, up to 1000 mg/day

Renal Impairment: A 27% reduction in clearance of unbound valproate is seen in patients with Cl$_{cr}$ <10 mL/minute. Hemodialysis reduces valproate concentrations by 20%, therefore, no dose adjustment is needed in patients with renal failure. Protein binding is reduced, monitoring only total valproate concentrations may be misleading.

Hepatic Impairment: Dosage reduction is required. Clearance is decreased with liver impairment. Hepatic disease is also associated with decreased albumin concentrations and 2- to 2.6-fold increase in the unbound fraction. Free concentrations of valproate may be elevated while total concentrations appear normal.

Administration

Depakote® ER: Swallow whole, do not crush or chew. Patients who need dose adjustments smaller than 500 mg/day for migraine prophylaxis should be changed to Depakote® delayed release tablets.

(Continued)

Valproic Acid and Derivatives *(Continued)*

Depakote® Sprinkle capsules may be swallowed whole or open capsule and sprinkle on small amount (1 teaspoonful) of soft food and use immediately (do not store or chew).

Depacon®: Following dilution to final concentration, administer over 60 minutes at a rate of ≤20 mg/minute. Alternatively, single doses up to 15 mg/kg have been administered as a rapid infusion over 5-10 minutes (1.5-3 mg/kg/minute).

Depakene® capsule: Swallow whole; do not chew

Monitoring Parameters Liver enzymes (at baseline and during therapy), CBC with platelets, PT/PTT (especially prior to surgery), serum ammonia (with symptoms of lethargy, mental status change), serum valproate levels

Reference Range

Therapeutic:

Epilepsy: 50-100 mcg/mL (SI: 350-690 µmol/L)

Mania: 50-125 mcg/mL (SI: 350-860 µmol/L)

Toxic: Some laboratories may report >200 mcg/mL (SI: >1390 µmol/L) as a toxic threshold, although clinical toxicity can occur at lower concentrations. Probability of thrombocytopenia increases with total valproate levels of ≥110 mcg/mL in females or ≥135 mcg/mL in males.

Seizure control: May improve at levels >100 mcg/mL (SI: 690 µmol/L), but toxicity may occur at levels of 100-150 mcg/mL (SI: 690-1040 µmol/L)

Mania: Clinical response seen with trough levels between 50-125 mcg/mL; risk of toxicity increases at levels >125 mcg/mL

Test Interactions False-positive result for urine ketones; accuracy of thyroid function tests

Patient Information Take with food or milk; do not chew, break or crush the tablet or capsule; do not administer with carbonated drinks; report any sore throat, fever, or fatigue

Additional Information Tremors may indicate overdosage. The most frequent side effects to valproic acid use are anorexia, vomiting, and nausea; taking doses with meals or changing to the enteric coated product may reduce these side effects

Sodium content of valproate sodium syrup (5 mL): 23 mg (1 mEq)

Divalproex sodium: Depakote®

Valproate sodium: Depakene® syrup

Valproic acid: Depakene® capsule

Special Geriatric Considerations Although there is little data in elderly for the use of valproic acid in the treatment of seizures, there are a number of studies which demonstrate its benefit in the treatment of agitation and dementia and other psychiatric disorders. It is important that the clinician understand that serum concentrations do not correlate with behavior response; likewise, it is imperative to monitor LFTs and CBC during the first 6 months of therapy. See Warnings/Precautions, Monitoring Parameters, and Additional Information.

Elimination is decreased in elderly. Studies of older adults with dementia show a high incidence of somnolence. In some patients, this was associated with weight loss. Starting doses should be lower and increased slowly, with careful monitoring of nutritional intake and dehydration. Safety and efficacy for use in patients >65 years of age have not been studied for migraine prophylaxis.

Dosage Forms Excipient information presented when available (limited, particularly for generics); consult specific product labeling. **Note:** Strength expressed as valproic acid

Capsule, as valproic acid: 250 mg

Depakene®: 250 mg

Capsule, sprinkles, as divalproex sodium:

Depakote® Sprinkle: 125 mg

Injection, solution, as valproate sodium: 100 mg/mL (5 mL)

Depacon®: 100 mg/mL (5 mL) [contains edetate disodium]

Syrup, as valproic acid: 250 mg/5 mL (5 mL, 480 mL)

Depakene®: 250 mg/5 mL (480 mL)

Tablet, delayed release, as divalproex sodium:

Depakote®: 125 mg, 250 mg, 500 mg

Tablet, extended release, as divalproex sodium:

Depakote® ER: 250 mg, 500 mg

Selected References

Dreifuss FE, Santilli N, Langer DH, et al, "Valproic Acid Hepatic Fatalities: A Retrospective Review," *Neurology*, 1987, 37(3):379-85.

Kunik ME, Puryear L, Orengo CA, et al, "The Efficacy and Tolerability of Divalproex Sodium in Elderly Demented Patients With Behavioral Disturbances," *Int J Geriatr Psychiatry*, 1998, 13(1):29-34.

Loy R and Tariot PN, "Neuroprotective Properties of Valproate: Potential Benefit for AD and Tauopathies,'" *J Mol Neurosci*, 2002, 19(3):303-7.

Mazure CM, Druss BG, and Cellar JS, "Valproate Treatment of Older Psychotic Patients With Organic Mental Syndromes and Behavioral Dyscontrol," *J Am Geriatr Soc*, 1992, 40(9):914-6.

Mellow AM, Solano-Lopez C, and Davis S, "Sodium Valproate in the Treatment of Behavioral Disturbance in Dementia," *J Geriatr Psychiatry Neurol*, 1993, 6(4):205-9.

Pratt CE and Davis SM, "Divalproex Sodium Therapy in Elderly with Dementia-Related Agitation," *Ann Pharmacother*, 2002, 36:1625-28.

Raskind MA, "Evaluation and Management of Aggressive Behavior in the Elderly Demented Patient," *J Clin Psychiatry*, 1999, 60(Suppl 15):45-9.

Sink KM, Holden KF, and Yaffe K, "Pharmacological Treatment of Neuropsychiatric Symptoms of Dementia. A Review of Evidence," *JAMA*, 2005, 293(5):596-608.

Swan AC, "Treatment of Aggression in Patients With Bipolar Disorder," *J Clin Psychiatry*, 1999, 60(Suppl 15):25-8.

Tariot PN, Raman R, Jakimovich L, et al, "Divalproex Sodium in Nursing Home Residents With Possible or Probable Alzheimer Disease Complicated by Agitation: A Randomized, Controlled Trial," *Am J Geriatr Psychiatry*, 2005, 13(11):942-49.

Valsartan (val SAR tan)

Related Information
Angiotensin Agents *on page 1737*

Medication Safety Issues
Sound-alike/look-alike issues:
Valsartan may be confused with losartan, Valstar™
Diovan® may be confused with Darvon®, Dioval®, Zyban®

U.S. Brand Names Diovan®

Canadian Brand Names Diovan®

Generic Available No

Pharmacologic Category Angiotensin II Receptor Blocker

Use Alone or in combination with other antihypertensive agents in the treatment of essential hypertension; treatment of heart failure (NYHA Class II-IV); reduction of cardiovascular mortality in patients with left ventricular dysfunction postmyocardial infarction

Contraindications Hypersensitivity to valsartan or any component of the formulation; hypersensitivity to other A-II receptor antagonists; primary hyperaldosteronism; bilateral renal artery stenosis

Warnings/Precautions May cause hyperkalemia; avoid potassium supplementation unless specifically required by healthcare provider. During the initiation of therapy, hypotension may occur, particularly in patients with heart failure or post-MI patients. Use extreme caution with concurrent administration of potassium-sparing diuretics or potassium supplements, in patients with mild-to-moderate hepatic dysfunction (adjust dose), in those who may be sodium/water depleted (eg, on high-dose diuretics), and in the elderly. Avoid use in patients with CHF, unilateral renal artery stenosis, aortic/mitral valve stenosis, coronary artery disease, or hypertrophic cardiomyopathy, if possible. May be associated with deterioration of renal function and/or increases in serum creatinine, particularly in patients dependent on renin-angiotensin-aldosterone system.

Adverse Reactions (Reflective of adult population; not specific for elderly)
>10%:
Central nervous system: Dizziness (heart failure 17%)
Renal: Bun increased >50% (heart failure 17%)
1% to 10%:
Cardiovascular: Hypotension (1% to 7%), postural hypotension (2%), syncope (up to >1%)
Central nervous system: Fatigue (2% to 3%), headache (heart failure >1%)
Endocrine & metabolic: Serum potassium increased by >20% (4% to 10%), hyperkalemia (heart failure 2%)
Gastrointestinal: Diarrhea (heart failure 5%), abdominal pain (2%), nausea (>1%)
Hematologic: Neutropenia (2%)
Neuromuscular & skeletal: Arthralgia (3%), back pain (up to 3%)
Ocular: Blurred vision (heart failure >1%)
Otic: Vertigo (up to >1%)
Renal: Creatinine doubled (MI 4%), creatinine increased >50% (heart failure 4%), renal dysfunction (up to >1%)
Respiratory: Cough (1% to 3%)
Miscellaneous: Viral infection (3%)

Overdosage/Toxicology Only mild toxicity (hypotension, bradycardia, hyperkalemia) has been reported with large overdoses (up to 5 g of captopril and 300 mg of enalapril). No fatalities have been reported. Treatment is symptomatic (eg, fluids). Not removed by hemodialysis.

Drug Interactions Inhibits CYP2C9 (weak)
Eplerenone: May enhance the hyperkalemic effect of valsartan.
Lithium: Risk of toxicity may be increased by valsartan; monitor lithium levels.
NSAIDs: May decrease angiotensin II antagonist efficacy; effect has been seen with losartan, but may occur with other medications in this class; monitor blood pressure
Potassium salts: May increase the risk of hyperkalemia.
Potassium-sparing diuretics (amiloride, potassium, spironolactone, triamterene): Increased risk of hyperkalemia.
(Continued)

Valsartan *(Continued)*

Ethanol/Nutrition/Herb Interactions

Food: Decreases rate and extent of absorption by 50% and 40%, respectively.

Herb/Nutraceutical: Avoid dong quai if using for hypertension (has estrogenic activity). Avoid ephedra, yohimbe, ginseng (may worsen hypertension). Avoid garlic (may have increased antihypertensive effect).

Stability Store at controlled room temperature of 15°C to 30°C (59°F to 86°F). Protect from moisture.

Mechanism of Action Valsartan produces direct antagonism of the angiotensin II (AT2) receptors, unlike the ACE inhibitors. It displaces angiotensin II from the AT1 receptor and produces its blood pressure-lowering effects by antagonizing AT1-induced vasoconstriction, aldosterone release, catecholamine release, arginine vasopressin release, water intake, and hypertrophic responses. This action results in more efficient blockade of the cardiovascular effects of angiotensin II and fewer side effects than the ACE inhibitors.

Pharmacodynamics Onset of antihypertensive effect: 2 weeks (maximal: 4 weeks)

Pharmacokinetics

Distribution: V_d: 17 L (adults)

Protein binding: 95%, primarily albumin

Metabolism: To inactive metabolite

Bioavailability: 25% (range 10% to 35%)

Half-life: 6 hours

Time to peak, serum: 2-4 hours

Elimination: Feces (83%) and urine (13%) as unchanged drug

Dosage

Geriatrics & Adults:

Hypertension: Initial: 80 mg or 160 mg once daily (in patients who are not volume depleted); dose may be increased to achieve desired effect; maximum recommended dose: 320 mg/day

Heart failure: Initial: 40 mg twice daily; titrate dose to 80-160 mg twice daily, as tolerated; maximum daily dose: 320 mg

Left ventricular dysfunction after MI: Initial: 20 mg twice daily; titrate dose to target of 160 mg twice daily as tolerated; may initiate ≥12 hours following MI

Renal Impairment:

Cl_{cr} >10 mL/minute: No dosage adjustment necessary.

Dialysis: Not significantly removed.

Hepatic Impairment: In mild-to-moderate liver disease no adjustment is needed. Use caution in patients with liver disease. Patients with mild to moderate chronic disease have twice the exposure as healthy volunteers.

Administration Administer with or without food.

Monitoring Parameters Baseline and periodic electrolyte panels, renal function, BP; in CHF, serum potassium during dose escalation and periodically thereafter

Patient Information Do not stop taking this medication unless instructed by a physician; take a missed dose as soon as possible unless it is almost time for your next dose; call your physician immediately if you have symptoms of allergy or develop side effects including headache and dizziness. Avoid salt substitutes which contain potassium. May be taken with or without food.

Additional Information Increasing dose beyond 80 mg/day has less antihypertensive effect than the addition of a diuretic to the 80 mg/day dose. Valsartan may have an advantage over losartan due to minimal metabolism requirements and consequent use in mild to moderate hepatic impairment.

Special Geriatric Considerations No dosage adjustment is necessary when initiating angiotensin II receptor antagonists in the elderly. In clinical studies, no differences between younger adults and elderly were demonstrated. Many elderly may be volume depleted due to diuretic use and/or blunted thirst reflex resulting in inadequate fluid intake.

Dosage Forms Excipient information presented when available (limited, particularly for generics); consult specific product labeling.

Tablet:

Diovan®: 40 mg, 80 mg, 160 mg, 320 mg

Selected References

Cohn JN and Tognoni G, "A Randomized Trial of the Angiotensin-Receptor Blocker Valsartan in Chronic Heart Failure," *N Engl J Med*, 2001, 345(23):1667-75.

Munger MA and Furniss SM, "Angiotensin II Receptor Blockers: Novel Therapy for Heart Failure?" *Pharmacotherapy*, 1996, 16(2 Pt 2):59S-68S.

♦ **Valsartan and Amlodipine** *see* Amlodipine and Valsartan *on page 91*

Valsartan and Hydrochlorothiazide
(val SAR tan & hye droe klor oh THYE a zide)

Related Information
Hydrochlorothiazide *on page 756*
Valsartan *on page 1657*
Medication Safety Issues
Sound-alike/look-alike issues:
Diovan® may be confused with Darvon®, Dioval®, Zyban®
U.S. Brand Names Diovan HCT®
Canadian Brand Names Diovan HCT®
Index Terms Hydrochlorothiazide and Valsartan
Generic Available No
Pharmacologic Category Angiotensin II Receptor Blocker Combination; Antihypertensive Agent, Combination; Diuretic, Thiazide
Use Treatment of hypertension
Refer to individual agents.
Dosage
Geriatrics & Adults: Hypertension: Oral: Dose is individualized (combination substituted for individual components); dose may be titrated after 3-4 weeks of therapy.
Usual recommended starting dose of valsartan: 80 mg or 160 mg once daily (maximum: 320 mg/day) when used as monotherapy in patients who are not volume depleted
Usual recommended starting dose of hydrochlorothiazide: 12.5-25 mg once daily (maximum: 25 mg/day)
Renal Impairment: Cl_{cr} ≤30 mL/minute: Use of combination not recommended. Contraindicated in patients with anuria.
Hepatic Impairment: Use with caution.
Dosage Forms Excipient information presented when available (limited, particularly for generics); consult specific product labeling.
Tablet:
Diovan HCT® 80 mg/12.5 mg: Valsartan 80 mg and hydrochlorothiazide 12.5 mg
Diovan HCT® 160 mg/12.5 mg: Valsartan 160 mg and hydrochlorothiazide 12.5 mg
Diovan HCT® 160 mg/25 mg: Valsartan 160 mg and hydrochlorothiazide 25 mg
Diovan HCT® 320 mg/12.5 mg: Valsartan 320 mg and hydrochlorothiazide 12.5 mg
Diovan HCT® 320 mg/25 mg: Valsartan 320 mg and hydrochlorothiazide 25 mg

♦ **Valtrex®** *see Valacyclovir on page 1650*
♦ **Vancocin®** *see Vancomycin on page 1659*

Vancomycin (van koe MYE sin)

Related Information
Antibiotic Treatment of Adults With Infective Endocarditis *on page 1797*
Antimicrobial Activity Against Selected Organisms *on page 1728*
Prevention of Infective Endocarditis *on page 1803*
Recommendations for Preventing the Spread of Vancomycin Resistance *on page 1806*
Serum Drug Concentrations Commonly Monitored Guidelines *on page 1862*
Medication Safety Issues
Sound-alike/look-alike issues:
I.V. vancomycin may be confused with Invanz®
Vancomycin may be confused with vecuronium
U.S. Brand Names Vancocin®
Canadian Brand Names Vancocin®
Index Terms Vancomycin Hydrochloride
Generic Available Yes: Injection
Pharmacologic Category Antibiotic, Miscellaneous
Use Treatment of patients with the following infections or conditions: treatment of infections due to documented or suspected methicillin-resistant *S. aureus* or beta-lactam resistant coagulase negative *Staphylococcus*; treatment of serious or life-threatening infections (ie, endocarditis, meningitis) due to documented or suspected staphylococcal or streptococcal infections in patients who are allergic to penicillins and/or cephalosporins; empiric therapy of infections associated with central lines, VP shunts, vascular grafts, prosthetic heart valves; treatment of febrile granulocytopenic patient who has not responded after 48 hours to antibiotic treatment directed at gram-negative rod infections; used orally for staphylococcal enterocolitis or for antibiotic-associated pseudomembranous colitis produced by *C. difficile*
Contraindications Hypersensitivity to vancomycin or any component of the formulation; avoid in patients with previous severe hearing loss
(Continued)

Vancomycin *(Continued)*

Warnings/Precautions May cause nephrotoxicity; usual risk factors include pre-existing renal impairment, concomitant nephrotoxic medications, advanced age, and dehydration. Discontinue treatment if signs of nephrotoxicity occur; renal damage is usually reversible. May cause neurotoxicity; usual risk factors include pre-existing renal impairment, concomitant neuro-/nephrotoxic medications, advanced age, and dehydration. Ototoxicity is proportional to the amount of drug given and the duration of treatment. Tinnitus or vertigo may be indications of vestibular injury and impending bilateral irreversible damage. Discontinue treatment if signs of ototoxicity occur. Prolonged therapy (>1 week) or total doses exceeding 25 g may increase the risk of neutropenia; prompt reversal of neutropenia is expected after discontinuation of therapy. Prolonged use may result in fungal or bacterial superinfection, including *C. difficile*-associated diarrhea and pseudomembranous colitis. Use with caution in patients with renal impairment or those receiving other nephrotoxic or ototoxic drugs; dosage modification required in patients with impaired renal function (especially elderly). Rapid I.V. administration may result in hypotension, flushing, erythema, urticaria, and/or pruritus; rate of infusion should be ≥60 minutes.

Adverse Reactions (Reflective of adult population; not specific for elderly)

Oral:

>10%: Gastrointestinal: Bitter taste, nausea, vomiting

1% to 10%:

Central nervous system: Chills, drug fever

Hematologic: Eosinophilia

Parenteral:

>10%:

Cardiovascular: Hypotension accompanied by flushing

Dermatologic: Erythematous rash on face and upper body (red neck or red man syndrome - infusion rate related)

1% to 10%:

Central nervous system: Chills, drug fever

Dermatologic: Rash

Hematologic: Eosinophilia, reversible neutropenia

Overdosage/Toxicology Symptoms include ototoxicity and nephrotoxicity. There is no specific therapy for vancomycin overdose. Care is symptomatic and supportive. Peritoneal filtration and hemofiltration (not dialysis) have been shown to reduce the serum concentration of vancomycin. High flux dialysis may remove up to 25%.

Drug Interactions Increased toxicity: Anesthetic agents; other ototoxic or nephrotoxic agents

Stability Reconstituted 500 mg and 1 g vials are stable at either room temperature or under refrigeration for 14 days. **Note:** Vials contain no bacteriostatic agent. Solutions diluted for administration in either D_5W or NS are stable under refrigeration for 14 days or at room temperature for 7 days. Reconstitute vials with 20 mL of SWFI for each 1 g of vancomycin (10 mL/500 mg vial; 20 mL/1 g vial; 100 mL/5 g vial; 200 mL/10 g vial). The reconstituted solution must be further diluted with at least 100 mL of a compatible diluent per 500 mg of vancomycin prior to parenteral administration.

Intrathecal: Vancomycin is available as a powder for injection and may be diluted to 1-5 mg/mL concentration in preservative free 0.9% sodium chloride for administration into the CSF.

Mechanism of Action Inhibits bacterial cell wall synthesis by blocking glycopeptide polymerization through binding tightly to D-alanyl-D-alanine portion of cell wall precursor

Pharmacokinetics

Absorption:

Oral: Poor

I.M.: Erratic

Protein binding: 10%

Half-life: Biphasic: Terminal: Adults: 5-11 hours, half-life prolonged significantly with reduced renal function

Time to peak serum concentration: I.V.: Within 45-65 minutes

Elimination: As unchanged drug in urine (80% to 90%); oral doses are excreted primarily in feces

Geriatrics: Volume of distribution has been reported to be decreased 44% while total clearance decreased by 23% and the terminal half-life increased to 12 hours

Dosage

Geriatrics: Refer to adult dosing. Elderly patients may require greater dosage reduction than expected. Best to individualize therapy; dose (mg/kg/24 hours) = (0.227 x Cl_{cr}) + 5.67.

Adults:

Usual dosage range:

I.V.: 2-3 g/day (20-45 mg/kg/day) in divided doses every 6-12 hours; maximum 3 g/day; **Note:** Dose requires adjustment in renal impairment

Oral: 500-1000 mg/day in divided doses every 6 hours

Indication -specific dosing:

Catheter-related infections: Antibiotic lock technique: 2 mg/mL in SWFI/NS or D_5W; instill 3-5 mL into catheter port as a flush solution instead of heparin lock (**Note:** Do not mix with any other solutions.)

Colitis (*C. difficile*) (unlabeled use): Oral: 125-250 mg every 6 hours for 10 days

Endophthalmitis (unlabeled use): Intravitreal: Usual dose: 1 mg/0.1 mL NS instilled into vitreum; may repeat administration if necessary in 3-4 days, usually in combination with ceftazidime or an aminoglycoside

Note: Some clinicians have recommended using a lower dose of 0.2 mg/0.1 mL, based on concerns for retinotoxicity.

Hospital-acquired pneumonia (HAP): I.V.: 15 mg/kg/dose every 12 hours (American Thoracic Society [ATS] 2005 guidelines)

Infective endocarditis prophylaxis: I.V.:

Dental, oral, or upper respiratory tract surgery: 1 g 1 hour before surgery. **Note:** AHA guidelines now recommend prophylaxis only in patients undergoing invasive procedures and in whom underlying cardiac conditions may predispose to a higher risk of adverse outcomes should infection occur

GI/GU procedure: 1 g plus 1.5 mg/kg gentamicin 1 hour prior to surgery. **Note:** As of April 2007, routine prophylaxis no longer recommended by the AHA.

Meningitis (*Pneumococcus* or *Staphylococcus*):

I.V.: 30-45 mg/kg/day in divided doses every 8-12 hours **or** 500-750 mg every 6 hours (with third-generation cephalosporin for PCN-resistant *Streptococcus pneumoniae*); maximum dose: 2-3 g/day

Intrathecal: Up to 20 mg/day

Susceptible gram-positive infections: I.V.: 15-20 mg/kg/dose (usual: 750-1500 mg) every 12 hours

Renal Impairment: Vancomycin levels should be monitored in patients with any renal impairment:

Cl_{cr} >50 mL/minute: Start with 15-20 mg/kg/dose (usual: 750-1500 mg) every 12 hours

Cl_{cr} 20-49 mL/minute: Start with 15-20 mg/kg/dose (usual: 750-1500 mg) every 24 hours

Cl_{cr} <20 mL/minute: Will need longer intervals; determine by serum concentration monitoring

Dialysis: Variable, depending on method; poorly dialyzable by conventional hemodialysis (0% to 5%). Use of high-flux membranes and continuous renal replacement therapy (CRRT) increases vancomycin clearance, and generally requires replacement dosing.

Hemodialysis (HD): Following loading dose of 15-20 mg/kg, give 500 mg to 1 g after each dialysis session, depending on factors such as HD membrane type and flow rate; monitor levels closely.

Continuous ambulatory peritoneal dialysis (CAPD):

Administration via CAPD fluid: 15-30 mg/L (15-30 mcg/mL) of CAPD fluid

Systemic: 1 g loading dose, followed by 500 mg to 1 g every 48-72 hours with close monitoring of levels

Continuous renal replacement therapy (CRRT): Removal of vancomycin is highly dependent on the method of replacement, filter type, and flow rate. Appropriate dosing requires close monitoring of levels in relation to target trough. The following are general recommendations only, and require consideration of the aforementioned parameters.

CVVH: Following loading dose of 15-20 mg/kg, give 1 g every 48 hours

CVVHDF: Following loading dose of 15-20 mg/kg, give 1 g every 24 hours

Monitoring Parameters Peak and trough vancomycin serum concentrations, serum BUN and creatinine, hearing, culture and sensitivity results, I.V. site; signs of Red Man's syndrome

Reference Range

Therapeutic:

Depends on MIC of organism being treated, usually peak: 20-40 mcg/mL (SI: 14-27 μmol/L)

Trough: 5-10 mcg/mL (SI: 3.4-6.8 μmol/L)

Toxic: >80 mcg/mL (SI: >54 μmol/L)

Patient Information Report pain at infusion site, dizziness, fullness or ringing in ears with I.V. use; nausea or vomiting with oral use

(Continued)

Vancomycin *(Continued)*

Additional Information Vancomycin should not be used first line in *C. difficile*-induced diarrhea; to prevent resistance, it should be saved for patients who do not respond to metronidazole

Special Geriatric Considerations As a result of age-related changes in renal function and volume of distribution, accumulation and toxicity are a risk in the elderly. Careful monitoring and dosing adjustment is necessary.

Dosage Forms Excipient information presented when available (limited, particularly for generics); consult specific product labeling.

Capsule (Vancocin®): 125 mg, 250 mg

Infusion [premixed in iso-osmotic dextrose] (Vancocin®): 500 mg (100 mL); 1 g (200 mL)

Injection, powder for reconstitution: 500 mg, 1 g, 5 g, 10 g

Selected References

Cutler NR, Narang PK, Lesko LJ, et al, "Vancomycin Disposition: The Importance of Age," *Clin Pharmacol Ther*, 1984, 36(6):803-10.

"Recommendations for Preventing the Spread of Vancomycin Resistance. Recommendations of the Hospital Infection Control Practices Advisory Committee (HICPAC)," *MMWR*, 1995, 44(RR-12):1-13.

Rodvold KA, Blum RA, Fischer JH, et al, "Vancomycin Pharmacokinetics in Patients With Various Degrees of Renal Function," *Antimicrob Agents Chemother*, 1988, 32(6):848-52.

♦ **Vancomycin Hydrochloride** *see* Vancomycin *on page 1659*

♦ **Vandazole**™ *see* Metronidazole *on page 1031*

♦ **Vanos**™ *see* Fluocinonide *on page 641*

♦ **Vantin**® *see* Cefpodoxime *on page 265*

♦ **Vaprisol**® *see* Conivaptan *on page 364*

♦ **VAQTA**® *see* Hepatitis A Vaccine *on page 746*

Vardenafil *(var DEN a fil)*

Medication Safety Issues

Sound-alike/look-alike issues:

Levitra® may be confused with Lexiva®

U.S. Brand Names Levitra®

Canadian Brand Names Levitra®

Index Terms Vardenafil Hydrochloride

Generic Available No

Pharmacologic Category Phosphodiesterase-5 Enzyme Inhibitor

Use Treatment of erectile dysfunction

Contraindications Hypersensitivity to vardenafil or any component of the formulation; concurrent use of organic nitrates (nitroglycerin; scheduled dosing or as needed); concomitant use of alpha blockers

Warnings/Precautions There is a degree of cardiac risk associated with sexual activity; therefore, physicians may wish to consider the patient's cardiovascular status prior to initiating any treatment for erectile dysfunction. Use caution in patients with anatomical deformation of the penis (angulation, cavernosal fibrosis, or Peyronie's disease) and in patients who have conditions which may predispose them to priapism (sickle cell anemia, multiple myeloma, leukemia). Patients should be instructed to seek medical attention if erection persists >4 hours.

Not recommended for use in patients with congenital QT prolongation or those taking Class Ia or III antiarrhythmics. Concomitant use with alpha-blockers may cause hypotension; safety of this combination may be affected by other antihypertensives and intravascular volume depletion. Patients should be hemodynamically stable prior to initiating therapy. Use caution with alpha-blockers, effective CYP3A4 inhibitors, the elderly, or those with hepatic impairment (Child-Pugh class B); dosage adjustment is needed.

Rare cases of nonarteritic ischemic optic neuropathy (NAION) have been reported; risk may be increased with history of vision loss. Other risk factors for NAION include heart disease, diabetes, hypertension, smoking, age >50 years, or history of certain eye problems.

Safety and efficacy have not been studied in patients with the following conditions, therefore, use in these patients is not recommended at this time: Hypotension, uncontrolled hypertension, unstable angina, severe cardiac failure; a life-threatening arrhythmia, myocardial infarction, or stroke within the last 6 months; severe hepatic impairment (Child-Pugh class C); end-stage renal disease requiring dialysis; retinitis pigmentosa or other degenerative retinal disorders. The safety and efficacy of vardenafil with other treatments for erectile dysfunction have not been studied and are not recommended as combination therapy.

Adverse Reactions (Reflective of adult population; not specific for elderly)

>10%:
   Cardiovascular: Flushing (11%)
   Central nervous system: Headache (15%)
2% to 10%:
   Central nervous system: Dizziness (2%)
   Gastrointestinal: Dyspepsia (4%), nausea (2%)
   Neuromuscular & skeletal: CPK increased (2%)
   Respiratory: Rhinitis (9%), sinusitis (3%)
   Miscellaneous: Flu-like syndrome (3%)

Overdosage/Toxicology Doses of up to 120 mg caused back pain, myalgia, and/or abnormal vision in healthy volunteers. Treatment should be symptomatic and supportive.

Drug Interactions Substrate of CYP2C (minor), 3A5 (minor), 3A4 (major)
   Alpha-blockers: May lead to significant hypotension in some patients; initiate vardenafil at lowest possible dose if patient is stabilized on alpha-blocker. Initiate alpha-blocker at lowest possible dose and titrate cautiously in patients on a stable dose of vardenafil.
   Antifungal agents (imidazole): May increase the levels/effects of vardenafil. Vardenafil dose should be adjusted based on manufacturer's recommendations.
   CYP3A4 inhibitors: May increase the levels/effects of vardenafil. Example inhibitors include azole antifungals, clarithromycin, diclofenac, doxycycline, erythromycin, imatinib, isoniazid, nefazodone, nicardipine, propofol, protease inhibitors, quinidine, telithromycin, and verapamil.
   Macrolide antibiotics: May increase the levels/effects of vardenafil. Vardenafil dose should be adjusted based on manufacturer's recommendations.
   Nitroglycerin (or other nitrates): Concomitant use is contraindicated due to the potential for severe, potentially fatal, hypotensive responses.
   Protease inhibitors: May increase the levels/effects of vardenafil. Vardenafil dose should be adjusted based on manufacturer's recommendations.

Ethanol/Nutrition/Herb Interactions Food: High-fat meals decrease maximum serum concentration 18% to 50%. Serum concentrations/toxicity may be increased with grapefruit juice; avoid concurrent use.

Stability Store at controlled room temperature of 15°C to 30°C (59°F to 86°F).

Mechanism of Action Does not directly cause penile erections, but affects the response to sexual stimulation. The physiologic mechanism of erection of the penis involves release of nitric oxide (NO) in the corpus cavernosum during sexual stimulation. NO then activates the enzyme guanylate cyclase, which results in increased levels of cyclic guanosine monophosphate (cGMP), producing smooth muscle relaxation and inflow of blood to the corpus cavernosum. Vardenafil enhances the effect of NO by inhibiting phosphodiesterase type 5 (PDE-5), which is responsible for degradation of cGMP in the corpus cavernosum; when sexual stimulation causes local release of NO, inhibition of PDE-5 by vardenafil causes increased levels of cGMP in the corpus cavernosum, resulting in smooth muscle relaxation and inflow of blood to the corpus cavernosum; at recommended doses, it has no effect in the absence of sexual stimulation.

Pharmacokinetics

Absorption: Rapid
Distribution: V_d: 208 L; <0.01% found in semen 1.5 hours after dose
Metabolism: Hepatic
Bioavailability: 15%
   Geriatrics (≥65 years): 52%
   Hepatic impairment (Child-Pugh class B): 160%
Half-life: Terminal: Vardenafil and metabolite: 4-5 hours
Time to peak, plasma: 0.5-2 hours
Elimination: Feces (91% to 95% as metabolites); urine (2% to 6%)
Clearance: 56 L/hour

Dosage

Geriatrics: Erectile dysfunction: Elderly ≥65 years: Oral: Initial: 5 mg 60 minutes prior to sexual activity; to be given as one single dose and not given more than once daily.

Adults:

   Erectile dysfunction: Oral: 10 mg 60 minutes prior to sexual activity; dosing range: 5-20 mg; to be given as one single dose and not given more than once daily

   Dosing adjustment with concomitant medications:
      Alpha-blocker (dose should be stable at time of vardenafil initiation): Initial vardenafil dose: 5 mg/24 hours; if an alpha-blocker is added to vardenafil therapy, it should be initiated at the smallest possible dose, and titrated carefully.
      Atazanavir: Maximum vardenafil dose: 2.5 mg/24 hours
      Clarithromycin: Maximum vardenafil dose: 2.5 mg/24 hours
      Erythromycin: Maximum vardenafil dose: 5 mg/24 hours

(Continued)

Vardenafil *(Continued)*

Indinavir: Maximum vardenafil dose: 2.5 mg/24 hours
Itraconazole:
   200 mg/day: Maximum vardenafil dose: 5 mg/24 hours
   400 mg/day: Maximum vardenafil dose: 2.5 mg/24 hours
Ketoconazole:
   200 mg/day: Maximum vardenafil dose: 5 mg/24 hours
   400 mg/day: Maximum vardenafil dose: 2.5 mg/24 hours
Ritonavir: Maximum vardenafil dose: 2.5 mg/72 hours
Saquinavir: Maximum vardenafil dose: 2.5 mg/24 hours

Renal Impairment: Dose adjustment not needed for mild, moderate, or severe impairment; use has not been studied in patients on renal dialysis.

Hepatic Impairment: Child-Pugh class B: Initial: 5 mg 60 minutes prior to sexual activity (maximum dose: 10 mg); to be given as one single dose and not given more than once daily.

Administration Administer 60 minutes prior to sexual activity.

Monitoring Parameters Monitor for response and adverse reactions.

Patient Information Discuss with your physician the contraindications of vardenafil, particularly the use of nitrates. Report all adverse effects (eg, contact your physician and refrain from sexual activity). Do not take more than one dose per day. Take the dose about 60 minutes before sexual activity. Vardenafil has no effect without sexual stimulation. Do not increase the dose without speaking to your physician.

Special Geriatric Considerations In adults ≥65 years of age, vardenafil plasma concentrations were higher than younger males (mean C_{max} was 34% higher), therefore, initial dose should be lower than the usual adult dose. Since the elderly often have concomitant diseases, many of which may be contraindicated with the use of vardenafil, a thorough knowledge of disease and medications must be accessed.

Dosage Forms Excipient information presented when available (limited, particularly for generics); consult specific product labeling.
Tablet: 2.5 mg, 5 mg, 10 mg, 20 mg

♦ **Vardenafil Hydrochloride** *see* Vardenafil *on page 1662*

Varenicline *(var e NI kleen)*

U.S. Brand Names Chantix™
Canadian Brand Names Champix®
Index Terms Varenicline Tartrate
Generic Available No
Pharmacologic Category Partial Nicotine Agonist; Smoking Cessation Aid
Use Treatment to aid in smoking cessation
Contraindications Hypersensitivity to varenicline tartrate or any component of the formulation
Warnings/Precautions Use caution in renal dysfunction; dosage adjustment required. Safety and efficacy of varenicline with other smoking cessation therapies have not been established; increased adverse events when used concurrently with nicotine replacement therapy.

Adverse Reactions (Reflective of adult population; not specific for elderly)
>10%:
   Central nervous system: Insomnia (18% to 19%), headache (15% to 19%), abnormal dreams (9% to 13%)
   Gastrointestinal: Nausea (16% to 40%; dose related)
1% to 10%:
   Central nervous system: Somnolence (3%), nightmares (1% to 2%), lethargy (1% to 2%), malaise (≤7%)
   Dermatologic: Rash (≤3%)
   Gastrointestinal: Flatulence (6% to 9%), abdominal pain (6% to 7%), constipation (5% to 8%), dysgeusia (5% to 8%), xerostomia (5% to 6%), dyspepsia (5%), vomiting (1% to 5%), appetite increased (3% to 4%), anorexia (≤2%), gastroesophageal reflux (1%)
   Respiratory: Dyspnea (≤2%), rhinorrhea (≤1%)

Overdosage/Toxicology There is no experience with overdose. Treatment is symptom-directed and supportive. Varenicline is effectively removed by hemodialysis.

Drug Interactions Successful cessation of smoking may alter pharmacokinetic properties of other medications (eg, theophylline, warfarin, insulin).

Stability Store at controlled room temperature of 15°C to 30°C (59°F to 86°F).

Mechanism of Action Partial neuronal alpha$_4$ β_2 nicotinic receptor agonist; prevents nicotine stimulation of mesolimbic dopamine system associated with nicotine addiction. Also binds to 5 HT_3 receptor (significance not determined) with moderate affinity.

Varenicline stimulates dopamine activity but to a much smaller degree than nicotine does, resulting in decreased craving and withdrawal symptoms.

Pharmacokinetics
Absorption: Well absorbed; unaffected by food
Protein binding: ≤20%
Half-life elimination: 24 hours
Time to peak, plasma: 3-4 hours
Excretion: Primarily urine (92% as unchanged drug)

Dosage
Geriatrics & Adults: Smoking cessation: Oral:
Initial:
Days 1-3: 0.5 mg once daily
Days 4-7: 0.5 mg twice daily
Maintenance (week 2-12): 1 mg twice daily
Note: Start 1 week before target quit date. Patients who cannot tolerate adverse events may require temporary reduction in dose. If patient successfully quits smoking during the 12 weeks, may continue for another 12 weeks to help maintain success. If not successful in first 12 weeks, then stop medication and reassess factors contributing to failure.

Renal Impairment:
Cl_{cr} ≥30 mL/minute: No adjustment required
Cl_{cr} <30 mL/minute: Initiate: 0.5 mg once daily; maximum dose: 0.5 mg twice daily
Hemodialysis: Maximum dose: 0.5 mg once daily
Hepatic Impairment: Dosage adjustment not required

Administration Administer with food and glass of water.

Patient Information Inform prescriber of all prescription medications, OTC medications, or herbal products you are taking. Start medication 1 week prior to quit date designated. Take after eating with a full glass of water. You may experience nausea (small, frequent meals, frequent oral care, sucking lozenges, or chewing gum may help), vomiting, constipation (increasing exercise, fluids, fruit/fiber may help), headaches, problems sleeping, or unusual dreams. Report persistent symptoms to prescriber.

Additional Information In all studies, patients received an educational booklet on smoking cessation and received up to 10 minutes of counseling at each weekly visit. Dosing started 1 week before target quit date. Successful cessation of smoking may alter pharmacokinetic properties of other medications (eg, theophylline, warfarin, insulin).

Special Geriatric Considerations Dosage adjustment for renal function may be necessary. Although studies to date do not demonstrate any significant pharmacokinetic differences between elderly (65-75 years of age) and younger adults.

Dosage Forms Excipient information presented when available (limited, particularly for generics); consult specific product labeling.
Tablet, as tartrate:
Chantix™: 0.5 mg, 1 mg

♦ **Varenicline Tartrate** *see* Varenicline *on page 1664*
♦ **Varicella-Zoster (VZV) Vaccine (Zoster)** *see* Zoster Vaccine *on page 1713*
♦ **Vaseretic®** *see* Enalapril and Hydrochlorothiazide *on page 507*
♦ **Vasodilan® [DSC]** *see* Isoxsuprine *on page 844*

Vasopressin (vay soe PRES in)

Medication Safety Issues
Sound-alike/look-alike issues:
Pitressin® may be confused with Pitocin®
U.S. Brand Names Pitressin®
Canadian Brand Names Pressyn®; Pressyn® AR
Index Terms ADH; Antidiuretic Hormone; 8-Arginine Vasopressin
Generic Available Yes
Pharmacologic Category Antidiuretic Hormone Analog; Hormone, Posterior Pituitary
Use Treatment of diabetes insipidus; prevention and treatment of postoperative abdominal distention; differential diagnosis of diabetes insipidus
Unlabeled/Investigational Use Adjunct in the treatment of GI hemorrhage and esophageal varices; pulseless arrest (ventricular tachycardia [VT]/ventricular fibrillation [VF], asystole/pulseless electrical activity [PEA]); vasodilatory shock (septic shock)
Contraindications Hypersensitivity to vasopressin or any component of the formulation
Warnings/Precautions Use with caution in patients with seizure disorders, migraine, asthma, vascular disease, renal disease, cardiac disease; chronic nephritis with nitrogen retention. Goiter with cardiac complications, arteriosclerosis; I.V. infiltration may lead to severe vasoconstriction and localized tissue necrosis; also, gangrene of
(Continued)

Vasopressin *(Continued)*

extremities, tongue, and ischemic colitis. May cause water toxication; early signs include drowsiness, listlessness, and headache, these should be recognized to prevent coma and seizures. Elderly patients should be cautioned not to increase their fluid intake beyond that sufficient to satisfy their thirst in order to avoid water intoxication and hyponatremia; under experimental conditions, the elderly have shown to have a decreased responsiveness to vasopressin with respect to its effects on water homeostasis.

Adverse Reactions (Reflective of adult population; not specific for elderly)

Frequency not defined.

Cardiovascular: Arrhythmia, asystole (>0.4 units/minute), blood pressure increased, cardiac output decreased (>0.4 units/minute), chest pain, MI, vasoconstriction (with higher doses), venous thrombosis

Central nervous system: Pounding in the head, fever, vertigo

Dermatologic: Ischemic skin lesions, circumoral pallor, urticaria

Gastrointestinal: Abdominal cramps, flatulence, mesenteric ischemia, nausea, vomiting

Genitourinary: Uterine contraction

Neuromuscular & skeletal: Tremor

Respiratory: Bronchial constriction

Miscellaneous: Diaphoresis

Overdosage/Toxicology

Symptoms include drowsiness, weight gain, confusion, listlessness, and water intoxication. Water intoxication requires withdrawal of the drug. Severe intoxication may require osmotic diuresis and loop diuretics.

Drug Interactions

Decreased effect: Lithium, epinephrine, demeclocycline, heparin, and ethanol block antidiuretic activity to varying degrees.

Increased effect: Chlorpropamide, phenformin, urea, and fludrocortisone potentiate antidiuretic response.

Ethanol/Nutrition/Herb Interactions Ethanol: Avoid ethanol (due to effects on ADH).

Stability Store injection at room temperature; do not freeze. Protect from heat. Use only clear solutions.

Mechanism of Action Increases cyclic adenosine monophosphate (cAMP) which increases water permeability at the renal tubule resulting in decreased urine volume and increased osmolality; causes peristalsis by directly stimulating the smooth muscle in the GI tract; direct vasoconstrictor without inotropic or chronotropic effects

Pharmacodynamics

Nasal:

Onset of action: 1 hour

Duration: 3-8 hours

Parenteral: Duration:

Aqueous: 2-8 hours

Tannate: 24-72 hours

Pharmacokinetics Destroyed by trypsin in GI tract, must be administered parenterally or intranasally

Nasal:

Metabolism: In the liver and kidneys

Half-life: 15 minutes

Elimination: In urine

Parenteral:

Metabolism: Most of dose is metabolized by liver and kidney

Half-life: 10-20 minutes

Elimination: 5% of SubQ dose (aqueous) is excreted unchanged in urine after 4 hours

Dosage

Geriatrics & Adults:

Diabetes insipidus:

Note: Dosage is highly variable; titrated based on serum and urine sodium and osmolality in addition to fluid balance and urine output

I.M., SubQ: 5-10 units 2-4 times/day as needed (dosage range 5-60 units/day)

Continuous I.V. infusion: 0.5 milliunit/kg/hour (0.0005 unit/kg/hour); double dosage as needed every 30 minutes to a maximum of 0.01 unit/kg/hour

Intranasal: Administer on cotton pledget, as nasal spray, or by dropper

Abdominal distention: I.M.: 5 units stat, 10 units every 3-4 hours

GI hemorrhage (unlabeled use):

Continuous I.V. infusion: 0.5 milliunits/kg/hour (0.0005 unit/kg/hour); double dosage as needed every 30 minutes to a maximum of 10 milliunits/kg/hour

I.V.: Initial: 0.2-0.4 unit/minute, then titrate dose as needed; if bleeding stops, continue at same dose for 12 hours, taper off over 24-48 hours.

Pulseless arrest (unlabeled use) [ACLS protocol]: I.V; I.O.: 40 units; may give one dose to replace first or second dose of epinephrine. I.V./I.O. drug administration is preferred, but if no access, may give endotracheally at 2 to $2^1/_2$ times the I.V. dose. Mix with 5-10 mL of water or normal saline, and administer down the endotracheal tube.

Vasodilatory shock/septic shock (unlabeled use): I.V.: 0.01-0.04 units/minute for the treatment of septic shock. Doses >0.04 units/minute may have more cardiovascular side effects. Most case reports have used 0.04 units/minute continuous infusion as a fixed dose.

Hepatic Impairment: Some patients respond to much lower doses with cirrhosis.

Administration

I.V.: Use extreme caution to avoid extravasation because of risk of necrosis and gangrene. In treatment of varices, infusions are often supplemented with nitroglycerin infusions to minimize cardiac effects.

GI hemorrhage: Administration requires the use of an infusion pump and should be administered in a peripheral line.

Vasodilatory shock: Administration through a central catheter is recommended.

Infusion rates: 100 units in 500 mL D_5W rate

0.1 unit/minute: 30 mL/hour
0.2 unit/minute: 60 mL/hour
0.3 unit/minute: 90 mL/hour
0.4 unit/minute: 120 mL/hour
0.5 unit/minute: 150 mL/hour
0.6 unit/minute: 180 mL/hour

Intranasal (topical administration on nasal mucosa): Administer injectable vasopressin on cotton plugs, as nasal spray, or by dropper. Should not be inhaled.

Endotreacheal: If no I.V. /I.O. access may give endotracheally at 2 to $2^1/_2$ times the I.V. dose. Mix with 5-10 mL of water or normal saline, and administer down the endotracheal tube.

Monitoring Parameters EKG, serum and urine sodium, urine output, fluid input and output, urine specific gravity, urine and serum osmolality

Reference Range Plasma: 0-2 pg/mL (SI: 0-2 ng/L) if osmolality <285 mOsm/L; 2-12 pg/mL (SI: 2-12 ng/L) if osmolality >290 mOsm/L

Patient Information If nausea, abdominal cramping, or blanching of the skin occurs, take 1-2 glasses of water with each dose

Special Geriatric Considerations Elderly patients should be cautioned not to increase their fluid intake beyond that sufficient to satisfy their thirst in order to avoid water intoxication and hyponatremia. Under experimental conditions, the elderly have shown to have a decreased responsiveness to vasopressin with respect to its effects on water homeostasis.

Dosage Forms Excipient information presented when available (limited, particularly for generics); consult specific product labeling.

Injection, solution: 20 units/mL (0.5 mL, 1 mL, 10 mL)
Pitressin®: 20 units/mL (1 mL)

Selected References

"2005 American Heart Association Guidelines for Cardiopulmonary Resuscitation and Emergency Cardiovascular Care," *Circulation*, 2005, 112(24 Suppl): 1-211.

Dellinger RP, Carlet JM, Masur H, et al, "Surviving Sepsis Campagn Guidelines for Management of Severe Sepsis and Septic Shock," *Crit Care Med*, 2004, 32(3):858-73.

Lindeman RD, Lee TD Jr, Yiengst MJ, et al, "Influence of Age, Renal Disease, Hypertension, Diuretics, and Calcium on the Antidiuretic Responses to Suboptimal Infusions of Vasopressin," *J Lab Clin Med*, 1966, 68(2):206-23.

Miller JH and Shock NW, "Age Differences in the Renal Tubular Response to Antidiuretic Hormone," *J Gerontol*, 1953, 8:446-50.

♦ **Vasotec®** *see* Enalapril *on page 503*
♦ **Veg-Pancreatin 4X [OTC]** *see* Pancreatin *on page 1195*

Venlafaxine (ven la FAX een)

Related Information
Antidepressant Agents *on page 1742*
U.S. Brand Names Effexor®; Effexor® XR
Canadian Brand Names Effexor® XR; Novo-Venlafaxine XR
Generic Available Yes: Tablet
Pharmacologic Category Antidepressant, Serotonin/Norepinephrine Reuptake Inhibitor
Use Treatment of major depressive disorder; generalized anxiety disorder (GAD), social anxiety disorder (social phobia)
Unlabeled/Investigational Use Treatment of obsessive-compulsive disorder (OCD), chronic fatigue syndrome; hot flashes; neuropathic pain; panic disorder
Restrictions An FDA-approved medication guide concerning the use of antidepressants in children, adolescents, and young adults must be distributed when dispensing
(Continued)

Venlafaxine *(Continued)*

an outpatient prescription (new or refill) where this medication is to be used without direct supervision of a healthcare provider. Medication guides are available at http://www.fda.gov/cder/Offices/ODS/medication_guides.htm. Dispense to parents or guardians of children and adolescents receiving this medication.

Contraindications Hypersensitivity to venlafaxine or any component of the formulation; use of MAO inhibitors within 14 days; should not initiate MAO inhibitor within 7 days of discontinuing venlafaxine

Warnings/Precautions [U.S. Boxed Warning]: Antidepressants increase the risk of suicidal thinking and behavior in children, adolescents, and young adults (18-24 years of age) with major depressive disorder (MDD) and other psychiatric disorders; consider risk prior to prescribing. Short-term studies did not show an increased risk in patients >24 years of age and showed a decreased risk in patients ≥65 years. Closely monitor for clinical worsening, suicidality, or unusual changes in behavior; the patient's family or caregiver should be instructed to closely observe the patient and communicate condition with healthcare provider. A medication guide should be dispensed with each prescription.

The possibility of a suicide attempt is inherent in major depression and may persist until remission occurs. Monitor for worsening of depression or suicidality, especially during initiation of therapy (generally first 1-2 months) or with dose increases or decreases. Use caution in high-risk patients. Worsening depression and severe abrupt suicidality that are not part of the presenting symptoms may require discontinuation or modification of drug therapy. The patient's family or caregiver should be alerted to monitor patients for the emergence of suicidality and associated behaviors (such as agitation, irritability, hostility, impulsivity, and hypomania) and call healthcare provider.

May worsen psychosis in some patients or precipitate a shift to mania or hypomania in patients with bipolar disorder. Patients presenting with depressive symptoms should be screened for bipolar disorder. Monotherapy in patients with bipolar disorder should be avoided. **Venlafaxine is not FDA approved for the treatment of bipolar depression.**

The potential for severe reactions exists when used with MAO inhibitors, SSRIs/SNRIs or triptans (myoclonus, diaphoresis, hyperthermia, NMS features, seizures, and death). May cause sustained increase in blood pressure or tachycardia; dose related and increases are generally modest (12-15 mm Hg diastolic). Control pre-existing hypertension prior to initiation of venlafaxine. Use caution in patients with recent history of MI, unstable heart disease, or hyperthyroidism; may cause increase in anxiety, nervousness, insomnia; may cause weight loss (use with caution in patients where weight loss is undesirable); may cause increases in serum cholesterol. Use caution with hepatic or renal impairment. Venlafaxine has been associated with the development of SIADH and hyponatremia.

Interstitial lung disease and eosinophilic pneumonia have been rarely reported; may present as progressive dyspnea, cough, and/or chest pain. Prompt evaluation and possible discontinuation of therapy may be necessary. Venlafaxine may increase the risks associated with electroconvulsive therapy. Use cautiously in patients with a history of seizures. The risks of cognitive or motor impairment, as well as the potential for anticholinergic effects are very low. May cause or exacerbate sexual dysfunction. May impair platelet aggregation, resulting in bleeding.

Abrupt discontinuation or dosage reduction after extended (≥6 weeks) therapy may lead to agitation, dysphoria, nervousness, anxiety, and other symptoms. When discontinuing therapy, dosage should be tapered gradually over at least a 2-week period. If intolerable symptoms occur following a decrease in dosage or upon discontinuation of therapy, then resuming the previous dose with a more gradual taper should be considered. Use caution in patients with increased intraocular pressure or at risk of acute narrow-angle glaucoma.

Adverse Reactions (Reflective of adult population; not specific for elderly)
>10%:
    Central nervous system: Headache (25% to 34%), insomnia (15% to 23%), somnolence (12% to 23%), nervousness (6% to 21%), dizziness (11% to 20%)
    Gastrointestinal: Nausea (21% to 58%), xerostomia (12% to 22%), anorexia (8% to 20%), constipation (8% to 15%)
    Genitourinary: Abnormal ejaculation/orgasm (2% to 16%)
    Neuromuscular & skeletal: Weakness (8% to 17%)
    Miscellaneous: Diaphoresis (10% to 14%)
1% to 10%:
    Cardiovascular: Hypertension (dose related; 3% in patients receiving <100 mg/day, up to 13% in patients receiving >300 mg/day), vasodilation (3% to 4%), palpitation (3%), tachycardia (2%), chest pain (2%), postural hypotension (1%), edema
    Central nervous system: Abnormal dreams (3% to 7%), anxiety (5% to 6%), yawning (3% to 5%), agitation (2% to 4%), chills (3%), confusion (2%), abnormal thinking

(2%), depersonalization (1%), depression (1% to 3%), chills, fever, migraine, amnesia, hypoesthesia, trismus, vertigo

Dermatologic: Rash (3%), pruritus (1%), bruising

Endocrine & metabolic: Libido decreased (3% to 9%)

Gastrointestinal: Diarrhea (6% to 8%), vomiting (3% to 6%), dyspepsia (5%), abdominal pain (4%), flatulence (3% to 4%), taste perversion (2%), weight loss (1% to 4%), appetite increased, weight gain

Genitourinary: Impotence (4% to 10%), urinary frequency (3%), urination impaired (2%), urinary retention (1%), prostatic disorder

Neuromuscular & skeletal: Tremor (4% to 10%), hypertonia (3%), paresthesia (2% to 3%), twitching (1% to 2%), neck pain, arthralgia

Ocular: Abnormal or blurred vision (4% to 6%), mydriasis (2%

Otic: Tinnitus (2%)

Respiratory: Pharyngitis (7%), sinusitis (2%), cough increased, dyspnea

Miscellaneous: Infection (6%), flu-like syndrome (6%), trauma (2%)

Overdosage/Toxicology Symptoms include somnolence and occasionally tachycardia. Most overdoses resolve with only supportive treatment. Use of activated charcoal, inductions of emesis, or gastric lavage should be considered for acute ingestion. Forced diuresis, dialysis, and hemoperfusion are not effective due to the large volume of distribution.

Drug Interactions Substrate of CYP2C9 (minor), 2C19 (minor), 2D6 (major), 3A4 (major); **Inhibits** CYP2B6 (weak), 2D6 (weak), 3A4 (weak)

Buspirone: Concurrent use may result in serotonin syndrome; these combinations are best avoided.

Clozapine: Addition of venlafaxine has been associated with case reports of increased clozapine serum concentrations and seizures.

CNS depressants: May enhance the CNS depressant effects of venlafaxine; monitor.

CYP2D6 inhibitors: May increase the levels/effects of venlafaxine. Example inhibitors include chlorpromazine, delavirdine, fluoxetine, miconazole, paroxetine, pergolide, quinidine, quinine, ritonavir, and ropinirole.

CYP3A4 inducers: CYP3A4 inducers may decrease the levels/effects of venlafaxine. Example inducers include aminoglutethimide, carbamazepine, nafcillin, nevirapine, phenobarbital, phenytoin, and rifamycins.

CYP3A4 inhibitors: May increase the levels/effects of venlafaxine. Example inhibitors include azole antifungals, clarithromycin, diclofenac, doxycycline, erythromycin, imatinib, isoniazid, nefazodone, nicardipine, propofol, protease inhibitors, quinidine, telithromycin, and verapamil.

Haloperidol: Serum levels may be increased during concurrent administration; AUC may be increased by as much as 70%.

Indinavir: Serum levels may be reduced by venlafaxine (AUC reduced by 28%); clinical significance unknown.

Lithium: Concurrent use may increase risk of serotonin syndrome.

MAO inhibitors: Serotonin syndrome may result when venlafaxine is used in combination or within 2 weeks of an MAO inhibitor; these combinations should be avoided.

Meperidine: Concurrent use may increase risk of serotonin syndrome.

Mirtazapine: Concurrent use may increase risk of serotonin syndrome.

Nefazodone: Concurrent use may increase risk of serotonin syndrome; in addition, nefazodone may inhibit the metabolism of venlafaxine.

Selegiline: Concurrent use may predispose to serotonin syndrome; avoid concurrent use.

Serotonin agonists (eg, triptans): Concurrent use of venlafaxine with these agents may increase the risk of serotonin syndrome; monitor.

Serotonergic reuptake inhibitors (eg, SSRIs/SNRIs): Concurrent use of venlafaxine with these agents may increase the risk of serotonin syndrome; monitor.

Sibutramine: Concurrent use may increase risk of serotonin syndrome; avoid concomitant use.

Tramadol: Concurrent use may increase risk of serotonin syndrome.

Trazodone: Concurrent use may increase risk of serotonin syndrome.

Tricyclic antidepressants: Concurrent use may increase risk of serotonin syndrome.

Warfarin: Case reports of increased INR when venlafaxine was added to therapy.

Ethanol/Nutrition/Herb Interactions

Ethanol: Avoid ethanol (may increase CNS effects).

Herb/Nutraceutical: Avoid valerian, St John's wort, SAMe, kava kava, tryptophan (may increase risk of serotonin syndrome and/or excessive sedation).

Mechanism of Action Venlafaxine and its active metabolite, o-desmethylvenlafaxine (ODV), are potent inhibitors of neuronal serotonin and norepinephrine reuptake and weak inhibitors of dopamine reuptake. Venlafaxine and ODV have no significant activity for muscarinic cholinergic, H_1-histaminergic, or alpha$_2$-adrenergic receptors. Venlafaxine and ODV do not possess MAO-inhibitory activity.

Pharmacodynamics Onset of action: 1-3 weeks; 5-HT = NE

Pharmacokinetics

Absorption: 92% to 100%; not affected by food

(Continued)

Venlafaxine *(Continued)*

Distribution: V_d: 7.5 L/kg

Protein binding, plasma: 27% to 30%

Metabolism: Major active metabolite o-desmethylvenlafaxine (OVD); 2 less active metabolites; metabolic pathway (first-pass) are saturable

Peak concentration: 1.8-3 hours

Half-life (prolonged in renal and hepatic impairment):

Venlafaxine: 5 hours

OVD: 11 hours

Elimination: 1% to 10% excreted unchanged in urine; 30% OVD, 26% conjugated OVD, and 27% other metabolites

Not readily dialyzed

Dosage

Geriatrics: Refer to adult dosing. No specific recommendations for elderly, but may be best to start lower at 25-50 mg twice daily and increase as tolerated by 25 mg/dose. Extended-release formulation: 37.5 mg once daily, increase by 37.5 mg every 4-7 days as tolerated

Adults:

Depression:

Immediate-release tablets: 75 mg/day, administered in 2 or 3 divided doses, taken with food; dose may be increased in 75 mg/day increments at intervals of at least 4 days, up to 225-375 mg/day

Extended-release capsules: 75 mg once daily taken with food; for some new patients, it may be desirable to start at 37.5 mg/day for 4-7 days before increasing to 75 mg once daily; dose may be increased by up to 75 mg/day increments every 4 days as tolerated, up to a recommended maximum of 225 mg/day

GAD, social anxiety disorder: *Extended-release capsules:* 75 mg once daily taken with food; for some new patients, it may be desirable to start at 37.5 mg/day for 4-7 days before increasing to 75 mg once daily; dose may be increased by up to 75 mg/day increments every 4 days as tolerated, up to a maximum of 225 mg/day

Panic disorder: *Extended-release capsules:* 37.5 mg once daily for 1 week; may increase to 75 mg daily, with subsequent weekly increases of 75 mg/day up to a maximum of 225 mg/day.

Obsessive-compulsive disorder (unlabeled use): Titrate to usual dosage range of 150-300 mg/day; however, doses up to 375 mg daily have been used; response may be seen in 4 weeks

Neuropathic pain (unlabeled use): Dosages evaluated varied considerably based on etiology of chronic pain, but efficacy has been shown for many conditions in the range of 75-225 mg/day; onset of relief may occur in 1-2 weeks, or take up to 6 weeks for full benefit.

Hot flashes (unlabeled use): Doses of 37.5-75 mg/day have demonstrated significant improvement of vasomotor symptoms after 4-8 weeks of treatment; in one study, doses >75 mg/day offered no additional benefit; however, higher doses (225 mg/day) may be beneficial in patients with perimenopausal depression.

Attention-deficit disorder (unlabeled use): Initial: Doses vary between 18.75 to 75 mg/day; may increase after 4 weeks to 150 mg/day; if tolerated, doses up to 225 mg/day have been used

Note: When discontinuing this medication after more than 1 week of treatment, it is generally recommended that the dose be tapered. If venlafaxine is used for 6 weeks or longer, the dose should be tapered over 2 weeks when discontinuing its use.

Renal Impairment:

Cl_{cr} 10-70 mL/minute: Decrease dose by 25%.

Hemodialysis: Decrease total daily dose by 50% given after completion of dialysis.

Hepatic Impairment: Reduce total dosage by 50%.

Administration May be administered with food. Swallow extended release capsule whole; do not crush or chew. Alternatively, contents may be sprinkled on a spoonful of applesauce and swallowed immediately without chewing; followed with a glass of water to ensure complete swallowing of the pellets. If switching from a MAO inhibitor to venlafaxine, allow 2 weeks "washout" period before starting venlafaxine; allow 7 days "washout" if switching venlafaxine therapy to a MAO inhibitor.

Monitoring Parameters Blood pressure should be regularly monitored, especially in patients with a high baseline blood pressure; mental status for depression, suicidal ideation (especially at the beginning of therapy or when doses are increased or decreased), anxiety, social functioning, mania, panic attacks; cholesterol

Reference Range Not established

Test Interactions Increased thyroid, uric acid, glucose, potassium, AST, cholesterol (S)

Patient Information Use caution when driving or operating machinery; advise physician and pharmacist of any changes or additions in drug therapy; avoid alcohol; notify physician of rash or any other adverse event; may cause dry mouth, increased blood pressure

Special Geriatric Considerations Venlafaxine's low anticholinergic activity, minimal sedation, and hypotension properties makes this a valuable antidepressant in treating elderly with depression and GAD. No dose adjustment is necessary for age alone; adjust dose for renal function in the elderly.

Dosage Forms Excipient information presented when available (limited, particularly for generics); consult specific product labeling.
  Capsule, extended release:
    Effexor® XR: 37.5 mg, 75 mg, 150 mg
  Tablet: 25 mg, 37.5 mg, 50 mg, 75 mg, 100 mg
    Effexor®: 25 mg, 37.5 mg, 50 mg, 75 mg, 100 mg

♦ **Ventolin® HFA** *see* Albuterol *on page 40*
♦ **Veracolate [OTC]** *see* Bisacodyl *on page 173*
♦ **Veramyst™** *see* Fluticasone *on page 659*

Verapamil (ver AP a mil)

Related Information
  Calcium Channel Blockers *on page 1753*
Medication Safety Issues
  Sound-alike/look-alike issues:
    Verapamil may be confused with Verelan®
    Calan® may be confused with Colace®
    Covera-HS® may be confused with Provera®
    Isoptin® may be confused with Isopto® Tears
    Verelan® may be confused with verapamil, Virilon®, Voltaren®

  Significant differences exist between oral and I.V. dosing. Use caution when converting from one route of administration to another.

  International issues:
    Calan®: Brand name for vinpocetine in Japan
U.S. Brand Names Calan®; Calan® SR; Covera-HS®; Isoptin® SR; Verelan®; Verelan® PM
Canadian Brand Names Alti-Verapamil; Apo-Verap®; Apo-Verap® SR; Calan®; Chronovera®; Covera®; Covera-HS®; Gen-Verapamil; Gen-Verapamil SR; Isoptin® SR; Novo-Veramil SR; Nu-Verap; Riva-Verapamil SR; Verapamil Hydrochloride Injection, USP
Index Terms Iproveratril Hydrochloride; Verapamil Hydrochloride
Generic Available Yes: Excludes controlled onset products
Pharmacologic Category Antiarrhythmic Agent, Class IV; Calcium Channel Blocker
Use Treatment of angina (vasospastic, chronic stable, and unstable), hypertension
  I.V.: Treatment of supraventricular tachyarrhythmias (PSVT, atrial fibrillation, atrial flutter)
Unlabeled/Investigational Use Treatment of migraine, hypertrophic cardiomyopathy, bipolar disorder (manic manifestations)
Contraindications Hypersensitivity to verapamil or any component of the formulation; severe left ventricular dysfunction; hypotension (systolic pressure <90 mm Hg) or cardiogenic shock; sick sinus syndrome (except in patients with a functioning artificial pacemaker); second- or third-degree AV block (except in patients with a functioning artificial pacemaker); atrial flutter or fibrillation and an accessory bypass tract (WPW, Lown-Ganong-Levine syndrome)
Warnings/Precautions Use with caution in sick-sinus syndrome, severe left ventricular dysfunction, hepatic or renal impairment, and hypertrophic cardiomyopathy (especially obstructive). Abrupt withdrawal may cause increased duration and frequency of chest pain. Elderly may experience more constipation and hypotension. Monitor ECG and blood pressure closely in patients receiving I.V. therapy particularly in patients with supraventricular tachycardia. May prolong recovery from nondepolarizing neuromuscular-blocking agents.
Adverse Reactions (Reflective of adult population; not specific for elderly)
  >10%: Gastrointestinal: Gingival hyperplasia (19%)
  1% to 10%:
    Cardiovascular: Bradycardia (1.4% oral, 1.2% I.V.); first-, second-, or third-degree AV block (1.2% oral, unknown I.V.); CHF (1.8% oral); hypotension (2.5% oral, 3% I.V.); peripheral edema (1.9% oral); symptomatic hypotension (1.5% I.V.); severe tachycardia (1% I.V.)
    Central nervous system: Dizziness (3.3% oral, 1.2% I.V.), fatigue (1.7% oral), headache (2.2% oral, 1.2% I.V.)
(Continued)

Verapamil *(Continued)*

Dermatologic: Rash (1.2% oral)

Gastrointestinal: Constipation (12% up to 42% in clinical trials), nausea (2.7% oral, 0.9% I.V.)

Respiratory: Dyspnea (1.4% oral)

Overdosage/Toxicology Primary cardiac symptoms of calcium blocker overdose include hypotension and bradycardia. Hypotension is caused by peripheral vasodilation, myocardial depression, and bradycardia. Bradycardia results from sinus bradycardia, second- or third-degree atrioventricular block, or sinus arrest with junctional rhythm. Intraventricular conduction is usually not affected, so QRS duration is normal (verapamil prolongs the PR interval and bepridil prolongs the QT interval and may cause ventricular arrhythmias, including torsade de pointes).

The noncardiac symptoms include confusion, stupor, nausea, vomiting, metabolic acidosis and hyperglycemia.

Following initial gastric decontamination, if possible, repeated calcium administration may promptly reverse depressed cardiac contractility (but not sinus node depression or peripheral vasodilation). Glucagon, epinephrine, and inamrinone (amrinone) may treat refractory hypotension. Glucagon and epinephrine also increase the heart rate (outside the U.S., 4-aminopyridine may be available as an antidote). Dialysis and hemoperfusion are not effective in enhancing elimination, although repeat-dose activated charcoal may serve as an adjunct with sustained-release preparations.

In a few reported cases, overdose with calcium channel blockers has been associated with hypotension and bradycardia, initially refractory to atropine, but becoming more responsive to this agent when larger doses (approaching 1 g/hour for more than 24 hours) of calcium chloride were administered.

Drug Interactions Substrate of CYP1A2 (minor), 2B6 (minor), 2C9 (minor), 2C18 (minor), 2E1 (minor), 3A4 (major); **Inhibits** CYP1A2 (weak), 2C9 (weak), 2D6 (weak), 3A4 (moderate)

Alfentanil's plasma concentration is increased. Fentanyl and sufentanil may be affected similarly.

Amiodarone use may lead to bradycardia and decreased cardiac output. Monitor closely if using together.

Aspirin and concurrent verapamil use may increase bleeding times; monitor closely, especially if on other antiplatelet agents or anticoagulants.

Azole antifungals may inhibit the calcium channel blocker's metabolism; avoid this combination. Try an antifungal like terbinafine (if appropriate) or monitor closely for altered effect of the calcium channel blocker.

Barbiturates reduce the plasma concentration of verapamil. May require much higher dose of verapamil.

Beta-blockers may have increased pharmacodynamic interactions with verapamil (see Warnings/Precautions).

Buspirone's serum concentration may increase. May require dosage adjustment.

Calcium may reduce the calcium channel blocker's effects, particularly hypotension.

Carbamazepine's serum concentration is increased and toxicity may result; avoid this combination.

Cimetidine reduced verapamil's metabolism; consider an alternative H_2 antagonist.

Colchicine: Verapamil may increase colchicine toxicity (especially nephrotoxicity).

Cyclosporine's serum concentrations are increased by verapamil; avoid this combination. Use another calcium channel blocker or monitor cyclosporine trough levels and renal function closely.

CYP3A4 inducers: CYP3A4 inducers may decrease the levels/effects of verapamil. Example inducers include aminoglutethimide, carbamazepine, nafcillin, nevirapine, phenobarbital, phenytoin, and rifamycins.

CYP3A4 inhibitors: May increase the levels/effects of verapamil. Example inhibitors include azole antifungals, clarithromycin, diclofenac, doxycycline, erythromycin, imatinib, isoniazid, nefazodone, nicardipine, propofol, protease inhibitors, telithromycin, and quinidine.

CYP3A4 substrates: Verapamil may increase the levels/effects of CYP3A4 substrates. Example substrates include benzodiazepines, calcium channel blockers, cyclosporine, mirtazapine, nateglinide, nefazodone, sildenafil (and other PDE-5 inhibitors), tacrolimus, and venlafaxine. Selected benzodiazepines (midazolam and triazolam), cisapride, ergot alkaloids, selected HMG-CoA reductase inhibitors (lovastatin and simvastatin), and pimozide are generally contraindicated with strong CYP3A4 inhibitors.

Digoxin's serum concentration is increased; reduce digoxin's dose when adding verapamil.

Doxorubicin's clearance was reduced; monitor for altered doxorubicin's effect.

Erythromycin may increase verapamil's effects; monitor altered verapamil effect.

Ethanol's effects may be increased by verapamil; reduce ethanol consumption.

Flecainide may have additive negative effects on conduction and inotropy.

Grapefruit juice: Verapamil serum concentrations may be increased by grapefruit juice. Avoid concurrent use.

HMG-CoA reductase inhibitors (atorvastatin, cerivastatin, lovastatin, simvastatin): Serum concentration will likely be increased; consider pravastatin/fluvastatin or a dihydropyridine calcium channel blocker. If concurrent use with lovastatin is unavoidable, dose of lovastatin should not exceed 40 mg/day.

Lithium neurotoxicity may result when verapamil is added; monitor lithium levels.

Midazolam's plasma concentration is increased by verapamil; monitor for prolonged CNS depression.

Nafcillin decreases plasma concentration of verapamil; avoid this combination.

Nondepolarizing muscle relaxant: Neuromuscular blockade may be prolonged. Monitor closely.

Prazosin's serum concentration increases; monitor blood pressure.

Quinidine's serum concentration is increased; adjust quinidine's dose as necessary.

Rifampin increases the metabolism of calcium channel blockers; adjust the dose of the calcium channel blocker to maintain efficacy.

Risperidone: Verapamil may increase the levels and effects of risperidone.

Sildenafil, tadalafil, vardenafil: Blood pressure-lowering effects may be additive; use caution.

Tacrolimus's serum concentrations are increased by verapamil; avoid the combination. Use another calcium channel blocker or monitor tacrolimus trough levels and renal function closely.

Theophylline's serum concentration may be increased by verapamil. Those at increased risk include cigarette smokers.

Ethanol/Nutrition/Herb Interactions

Ethanol: Avoid or limit ethanol (may increase ethanol levels).

Food: Grapefruit juice may increase the serum concentration of verapamil; avoid concurrent use.

Herb/Nutraceutical: St John's wort may decrease levels. Avoid dong quai if using for hypertension (has estrogenic activity). Avoid ephedra, yohimbe, ginseng (may worsen arrhythmia or hypertension). Avoid garlic (may have increased antihypertensive effect).

Stability Store injection at room temperature; do not freeze. Protect from heat. Use only clear solutions. Physically compatible in solutions of pH of 3-6, but may precipitate in solutions having a pH ≥6. Protect I.V. solution from light.

Mechanism of Action Inhibits calcium ion from entering the "slow channels" or select voltage-sensitive areas of vascular smooth muscle and myocardium during depolarization; produces a relaxation of coronary vascular smooth muscle and coronary vasodilation; increases myocardial oxygen delivery in patients with vasospastic angina; slows automaticity and conduction of AV node.

Pharmacodynamics

Duration:
Oral: 6-8 hours; older adults have greater hypotensive effect than younger adults
I.V.: 10-20 minutes

Peak effect:
Oral (nonsustained tablets): 2 hours
I.V.: 1-5 minutes

Pharmacokinetics

Protein binding: 90%
Metabolism: Extensive in the liver; first-pass effect
Bioavailability: Oral: 20% to 30%
Half-life: Single dose: 2-8 hours, increased up to 12 hours with multiple dosing; increased half-life with hepatic cirrhosis
Elimination: 70% of dose excreted in urine (3% to 4% as unchanged drug) and 16% in feces

Dosage

Geriatrics:
Immediate release: Oral: 120-480 mg/24 hours divided 3-4 times/day
Sustained release: Oral: 120 mg/day; adjust dose after 24 hours by increases of 120 mg/day. When switching from immediate release forms, total daily dose may remain the same. Controlled onset: initiate therapy with 180 mg in the evening; titrate upward as needed to obtain desired response and avoiding adverse effects.

Adults:
Angina: Oral: Initial: 80-120 mg twice daily (elderly or small stature: 40 mg twice daily); range: 240-480 mg/day in 3-4 divided doses

Hypertension: Oral:
Immediate release: 80 mg 3 times/day; usual dose range (JNC 7): 80-320 mg/day in 2 divided doses
Sustained release: 240 mg/day; usual dose range (JNC 7): 120-360 mg/day in 1-2 divided doses; 120 mg/day in the elderly or small patients (no evidence of additional benefit in doses >360 mg/day).

(Continued)

Verapamil (Continued)

Extended release:

Covera-HS®: Usual dose range (JNC 7): 120-360 mg once daily (once-daily dosing is recommended at bedtime)

Verelan® PM: Usual dose range: 200-400 mg once daily at bedtime

Arrhythmia (SVT): I.V.: 2.5-5 mg (over 2 minutes); second dose of 5-10 mg (~0.15 mg/kg) may be given 15-30 minutes after the initial dose if patient tolerates, but does not respond to initial dose; maximum total dose: 20 mg

Renal Impairment: Cl_{cr} <10 mL/minute: Administer 50% to 75% of normal dose.

Hepatic Impairment: In cirrhosis, reduce dose to 20% to 50% of normal and monitor ECG.

Administration

Oral: Administer sustained release product with food or milk; sprinkling contents of capsules onto food does not affect absorption; should be dosed 1-2 times/day; **do not crush sustained release drug product.** Other oral formulations may be given with or without food.

I.V.: Rate of infusion: Over 2 minutes.

Monitoring Parameters Heart rate, blood pressure, signs and symptoms of congestive heart failure

Reference Range Therapeutic: 50-200 ng/mL (SI: 100-410 nmol/L) for parent; under normal conditions norverapamil concentration is the same as parent drug; Toxic: >90 mcg/mL

Patient Information Sustained release products should be taken with food and not crushed or chewed; limit caffeine intake; avoid alcohol; notify physician if angina pain is not reduced when taking this drug, irregular heartbeat, shortness of breath, swelling, dizziness, constipation, nausea, or hypotension occur; do not stop therapy without advice of physician

Additional Information Incidence of adverse reactions is most common with I.V. administration; discontinue disopyramide 48 hours before starting therapy, do not restart therapy until 24 hours after verapamil has been discontinued

Special Geriatric Considerations Elderly may experience a greater hypotensive response. Constipation may be more of a problem in the elderly. Calcium channel blockers are no more effective in the elderly than other therapies; however, they do not cause significant CNS effects which is an advantage over some antihypertensive agents. Generic verapamil products which are bioequivalent in young adults may not be bioequivalent in the elderly; use generics cautiously.

Dosage Forms Excipient information presented when available (limited, particularly for generics); consult specific product labeling.

Caplet, sustained release: 120 mg, 180 mg, 240 mg
Calan® SR: 120 mg, 180 mg, 240 mg
Capsule, extended release, controlled onset, as hydrochloride:
Verelan® PM: 100 mg, 200 mg, 300 mg
Capsule, sustained release, as hydrochloride: 120 mg, 180 mg, 240 mg, 360 mg
Verelan®: 120 mg, 180 mg, 240 mg, 360 mg
Injection, solution, as hydrochloride: 2.5 mg/mL (2 mL, 4 mL)
Tablet, as hydrochloride: 80 mg, 120 mg
Calan®: 40 mg, 80 mg, 120 mg
Tablet, extended release: 120 mg, 180 mg, 240 mg
Tablet, extended release, controlled onset, as hydrochloride:
Covera-HS®: 180 mg, 240 mg
Tablet, sustained release, as hydrochloride: 120 mg, 180 mg, 240 mg
Isoptin® SR: 120 mg, 180 mg, 240 mg

Selected References

Carter BL, Noyes MA, and Demmler RW, "Differences in Serum Concentrations of and Responses to Generic Verapamil in the Elderly," *Pharmacotherapy*, 1993, 13(4):359-68.

Chobanian AV, Bakris GL, Black HR, et al, "The Seventh Report of the Joint National Committee on Prevention, Detection, Evaluation, and Treatment of High Blood Pressure: The JNC 7 Report," *JAMA*, 2003, 289(19):2560-71.

♦ **Verapamil and Trandolapril** see Trandolapril and Verapamil on page 1611
♦ **Verapamil Hydrochloride** see Verapamil on page 1671
♦ **Verelan®** see Verapamil on page 1671
♦ **Verelan® PM** see Verapamil on page 1671
♦ **Versed** see Midazolam on page 1039

Verteporfin (ver te POR fin)

U.S. Brand Names Visudyne®
Canadian Brand Names Visudyne®
Generic Available No

Pharmacologic Category Ophthalmic Agent

Use Treatment of predominantly classic subfoveal choroidal neovascularization due to macular degeneration, presumed ocular histoplasmosis, or pathologic myopia

Unlabeled/Investigational Use Predominantly **occult** subfoveal choroidal neovascularization

Contraindications Hypersensitivity to verteporfin or any component of the formulation; porphyria

Warnings/Precautions Avoid exposing skin or eyes to direct sunlight or bright indoor light for 5 days following treatment. In case of emergency surgery within 48 hours of treatment, protect as much of the internal tissue as possible from intense light. Do not retreat patients who experience a decrease of vision ≥4 lines within 1 week of treatment unless vision recovers and the potential benefits and risks are carefully considered. Use of incompatible lasers (which do not provide the required light for photoactivation) can result in incomplete treatment, overtreatment, or damage to normal tissue.

Use in more than one eye has not been studied; however, it is recommended that if required, initial treatment should be applied to the more aggressive lesion first, followed by the second eye a week later (subsequent treatment may be concurrent). Standard precautions should be taken to avoid extravasation (eg free-flowing I.V. line, use of largest arm vein). Chest pain, vasovagal and hypersensitivity reactions have occurred rarely; observation of patient during infusion is suggested.

Use in patients with moderate-to-severe hepatic impairment, biliary obstruction, or under anesthesia has not been studied. Patients with dark irides, occult lesions, <50% classic choroidal neovascularization, or patients ≥75 years of age are less likely to benefit from therapy. Safety and efficacy of use for longer than 2 years has not been established.

Adverse Reactions (Reflective of adult population; not specific for elderly)

>10%:

Central nervous system: Headache

Local: Injection site reactions (including injection site extravasation, injection site rash)

Ocular: Blurred vision, visual acuity decreased, visual field defects, visual disturbances

1% to 10%:

Cardiovascular: Atrial fibrillation, hypertension, peripheral vascular disorder, varicose veins

Central nervous system: Fever, hypoesthesia, sleep disturbance, vertigo

Dermatologic: Eczema, photosensitivity

Gastrointestinal: Constipation, gastrointestinal cancers, nausea

Genitourinary: Prostatic disorder

Hematologic: Anemia, leukocytosis, leukopenia

Hepatic: Liver function tests increased

Neuromuscular & skeletal: Arthralgia, arthrosis, back pain (primarily during infusion), myasthenia, weakness

Ocular: Diplopia, lacrimation disorder

Treatment site: Blepharitis, cataracts, conjunctivitis/conjunctival injection, dry eyes, ocular itching, severe vision loss (1% to 4%, decrease in 4 lines or more within 7 days of treatment, partial recovery seen in many patients), subconjunctival, subretinal or vitreous hemorrhage.

Otic: Hearing loss

Renal: Albuminuria, creatinine increased

Respiratory: Cough, pharyngitis, pneumonia

Miscellaneous: Flu-like syndrome

Overdosage/Toxicology Nonperfusion of normal retinal vessels may result from overdose of drug and/or light in treated eye, and may lead to permanent vision loss. Prolongation of photosensitivity to light will also occur; extend light precautions proportional to overdose.

Drug Interactions Drug interaction studies have not been performed, however, the following are examples of medications that may influence the effect of verteporfin:

Increased efficacy: Calcium channel blockers, polymyxin B, and radiation therapy could enhance rate of uptake in vascular endothelium

Decreased efficacy: Thromboxane A2 inhibitors and other drugs that decrease clotting, vasoconstriction or platelet aggregation; beta-carotene, dimethyl sulfoxide, ethanol, formate, mannitol, and other drugs which decrease active oxygen molecules or scavenge radicals.

Griseofulvin, phenothiazines, sulfonamides, sulfonylureas, tetracyclines, thiazide diuretics, or other photosensitizing agents may increase photosensitivity.

Ethanol/Nutrition/Herb Interactions Ethanol: Ethanol may decrease efficacy of verteporfin.

Stability Store vial at 20°C to 25°C (68°F to 77°F). Each vial should be reconstituted with 7 mL of sterile water for injection, providing a total volume of 7.5 mL. Resulting
(Continued)

Verteporfin (Continued)

solution will be 2 mg/mL. Solution should be protected from light and used within 4 hours. Once reconstituted, verteporfin will be an opaque dark green solution. The total volume of solution needed to administer the dose should be withdrawn from the vial and further diluted in D_5W to a total volume of 30 mL. Infuse at 3 mL/minute over 10 minutes, using syringe pump and in-line filter.

Mechanism of Action Following intravenous administration, verteporfin is transported by lipoproteins to the neovascular endothelium in the affected eye(s), including choroidal neovasculature and the retina. Verteporfin then needs to be activated by nonthermal red light, which results in local damage to the endothelium, leading to temporary choroidal vessel occlusion.

Pharmacokinetics

Metabolism: Hepatic and by plasma esterases to diacid metabolite

Half-life elimination: Terminal: 5-6 hours, bi-exponential

Excretion: Feces

Dosage

Geriatrics: Refer to adult dosing. Patients ≥75 years were less likely to benefit from therapy in clinical trials.

Adults: Therapy is a two-step process; first the infusion of verteporfin, then the activation of verteporfin with a nonthermal diode laser (for light administration details, see Administration).

Subfoveal choroidal neovascularization: I.V.: 6 mg/m^2 body surface area

Note: Treatment in more than one eye: Patients who have lesions in both eyes should be evaluated and treatment should first be done to the more aggressive lesion. Following safe and acceptable treatment, the second eye can be treated one week later. Patients who have had previous verteporfin therapy, with an acceptable safety profile, may then have both eyes treated concurrently. Treat the more aggressive lesion followed immediately with the second eye. The light treatment to the second eye should begin no later than 20 minutes from the start of the infusion.

Hepatic Impairment: Half-life is increased by 20% with mild hepatic impairment. There are no clinical studies in patients with moderate-to-severe hepatic impairment.

Administration A free-flowing I.V. line should be established prior to starting infusion. Use of the largest arm vein, especially in the elderly, is suggested; avoid small veins in the back of the hand. Reconstituted solution should be given at 3 mL/minute over 10 minutes using a syringe pump and an in-line filter. If extravasation occurs, protect the site from light. Use of rubber gloves and eye protection is recommended. Skin and eye contact should be avoided and all materials should be disposed of properly.

Light administration: Following intravenous infusion, verteporfin must be light activated using a nonthermal diode laser. The system must provide a stable power output at a wavelength of 689±3 nm. Approved laser systems are listed in manufacturer's package insert. Light delivery should begin 15 minutes following the start of the 10-minute infusion. The light dose is J/cm^2 of neovascular lesion administered over 83 seconds at an intensity of 600 mW/cm^2. Instructions for determining lesion size and treatment spot size can also be found in the package insert.

Monitoring Parameters Intravenous site during infusion, to avoid extravasation; fluorescein angiography every 3 months to monitor choroidal neovascular leakage

Patient Information This medication can only be administered intravenously. Following administration, you will have a temporary increase in sensitivity to the sun. To prevent sunburn, avoid exposing unprotected skin, eyes, or other body parts to direct sunlight or bright indoor light for 5 days following treatment. Examples of bright indoor lights include tanning beds, bright halogen lights, or high powered lights, such as those used in a surgical operating rooms or dental offices. Wear protective clothing and dark sunglasses, UV sunscreens will **not** protect against this effect. Exposure to ambient indoor light is encouraged, and will help inactivate the medication. You may wish to wear a wristband as a reminder to avoid direct sunlight or bright indoor light during this time. Avoid alcohol. Avoid the use of other medications that may increase the risk of sunburn, such as griseofulvin, phenothiazines, sulfonamides, sulfonylureas, tetracyclines, and thiazide diuretics.

Additional Information Verteporfin also contains lactose, egg phosphatidylglycerol. Studies allowed treatment in only one eye per patient. Patients who have lesions in both eyes should be evaluated and treatment should first be done to the more aggressive lesion. Following safe and acceptable treatment, the second eye can be treated one week later. Patients who have had previous verteporfin therapy, with an acceptable safety profile, may then have both eyes treated concurrently. Treat the more aggressive lesion followed immediately with light application to the second eye. The light treatment to the second eye should begin no later than 20 minutes from the start of the infusion.

Dosage Forms Excipient information presented when available (limited, particularly for generics); consult specific product labeling.

Injection, powder for reconstitution: 15 mg [contains egg phosphatidylglycerol]

Vitamin E (VYE ta min ee)

Medication Safety Issues
Sound-alike/look-alike issues:
Aquasol E® may be confused with Anusol®

U.S. Brand Names Alph-E [OTC]; Alph-E-Mixed [OTC]; Aquasol E® [OTC]; Aquavit-E [OTC]; d-Alpha-Gems™ [OTC]; E-Gems® [OTC]; E-Gems Elite® [OTC]; E-Gems Plus® [OTC]; Ester-E™ [OTC]; Gamma E-Gems® [OTC]; Gamma-E Plus [OTC]; High Gamma Vitamin E Complete™ [OTC]; Key-E® [OTC]; Key-E® Kaps [OTC]

Index Terms *d*-Alpha Tocopherol; *dl*-Alpha Tocopherol

Generic Available Yes

Pharmacologic Category Vitamin, Fat Soluble

Use Prevention and treatment of hemolytic anemia secondary to vitamin E deficiency; dietary supplement

Unlabeled/Investigational Use Prevention and treatment of tardive dyskinesia, Alzheimer's disease

Contraindications Hypersensitivity to vitamin E or any component of the formulation; I.V. route

Warnings/Precautions May induce vitamin K deficiency.
(Continued)

Vitamin E *(Continued)*

Adverse Reactions (Reflective of adult population; not specific for elderly)
Frequency not defined.
Central nervous system: Fatigue, headache, weakness
Dermatologic: Contact dermatitis with topical preparation
Endocrine & metabolic: Gonadal dysfunction
Gastrointestinal: Diarrhea, intestinal cramps, nausea
Neuromuscular & skeletal: Weakness
Ocular: Blurred vision

Drug Interactions
Cholestyramine (and colestipol): May reduce absorption of vitamin E
Orlistat: May reduce absorption of vitamin E
Warfarin: Vitamin E may alter the effect of vitamin K actions on clotting factors resulting in an increase hypoprothrombinemic response to warfarin; monitor

Stability Protect from light.

Mechanism of Action
Prevents oxidation of vitamin A and C; protects polyunsaturated fatty acids in membranes from attack by free radicals and protects red blood cells against hemolysis

Pharmacokinetics
Absorption: Oral: Depends upon the presence of bile; absorption is reduced in conditions of malabsorption, and as dosage increases; water miscible preparations are better absorbed than oil preparations
Distribution: Distributes to all body tissues, especially adipose tissue, where it is stored
Metabolism: In the liver to glucuronides
Elimination: In feces and bile

Dosage
Geriatrics & Adults: One unit of vitamin E = 1 mg *dl*-alpha-tocopherol acetate. Oral:
Recommended daily allowance (RDA): 15 mg (22.5 units); upper limit of intake should not exceed 1000 mg/day
Vitamin E deficiency: 60-75 units/day
Prevention of vitamin E deficiency: Oral: 30 units/day
Cystic fibrosis: Oral: 100-400 units/day
Beta-thalassemia: Oral: 750 units/day
Sickle cell disease: Oral: 450 units/day
Alzheimer's disease: Oral: 1000 units twice daily
Tardive dyskinesia: Oral: 1600 units/day
Superficial dermatologic irritation: Topical: Apply a thin layer over affected area.

Reference Range
Therapeutic: 0.8-1.5 mg/dL (SI: 19-35 µmol/L), some method variation

Patient Information
Vitamin E toxicity appears as blurred vision, diarrhea, dizziness, flu-like symptoms, nausea, headache; swallow capsules whole, do not crush or chew

Additional Information
1 mg *dl*-alpha tocopherol acetate = 1 international unit

Special Geriatric Considerations
Elderly may have vitamin E prescribed for those with cardiovascular disease. Elderly should be advised not to take more than prescribed.

Dosage Forms
Excipient information presented when available (limited, particularly for generics); consult specific product labeling.
Capsule: 400 int. units, 1000 int. units
Key-E® Kaps: 200 int. units, 400 int. units
Capsule, softgel: 200 int. units, 400 int. units, 600 int. units, 1000 int. units
Alph-E: 200 int. units, 400 int. units
Alph-E-Mixed: 200 int. units [contains mixed tocopherols]; 400 int. units [contains mixed tocopherols], 1000 int. units [sugar free; contains mixed tocopherols]
Aqua Gem E®: 200 units, 400 units
d-Alpha-Gems™: 400 int. units [derived from soybean oil]
E-Gems®: 30 int. units, 100 int. units, 200 int. units, 400 int. units, 600 int. units, 800 int. units, 1000 int. units, 1200 int. units [derived from soybean oil]
E-Gems Plus®: 200 int. units, 400 int. units, 800 int. units [contains mixed tocopherols]
E-Gems Elite®: 400 int. units [contains mixed tocopherols]
Ester-E™: 400 int. units
Gamma E-Gems®: 90 int. units [also contains mixed tocopherols]
Gamma-E Plus: 200 int. units [contains soybean oil]
High Gamma Vitamin E Complete™: 200 int. units [contains soybean oil, mixed tocopherols]
Cream: 50 int. units/g (60 g), 100 int. units/g (60 g), 1000 int. units/120 g (120 g), 30,000 int. units/57 g (57 g)
Key-E®: 30 int. units/g (60 g, 120 g, 600 g)
Lip balm (E-Gem® Lip Care): 1000 int. units/tube [contains vitamin A and aloe]
Oil, oral/topical: 100 int. units/0.25 mL (60 mL, 75 mL); 1150 units/0.25 mL (30 mL, 60 mL, 120 mL); 28,000 int. units/30 mL (30 mL)

Alph-E: 28,000 int. units/30 mL (30 mL) [topical]
E-Gems®: 100 units/10 drops (15 mL, 60 mL)
Ointment, topical (Key-E®): 30 units/g (60 g, 120 g, 480 g)
Powder (Key-E®): 700 int. units per 1/4 teaspoon (15 g, 75 g, 1000 g) [derived from soybean oil]
Solution, oral drops: 15 int. units/0.3 mL (30 mL)
Aquasol E®: 15 int. units/0.3 mL (12 mL, 30 mL) [latex free]
Aquavit-E: 15 int. units/0.3 mL (30 mL) [butterscotch flavor]
Suppository, rectal/vaginal (Key-E®): 30 int. units (12s, 24s) [contains coconut oil]
Tablet: 100 int. units, 200 int. units, 400 int. units, 500 int. units
Key-E®: 200 int. units, 400 int. units

Selected References

Bieri JG, Corash L, and Hubbard VS, "Medical Uses of Vitamin E," *N Engl J Med*, 1983, 308(18):1063-71.
Hale TW, Rais-Bahrami K, Montgomery DL, et al, "Vitamin E Toxicity in Neonatal Piglets," *J Toxicol Clin Toxicol*, 1995, 33(2):123-30.
Hodis HN, Mack WJ, La Bree L, et al, "Serial Coronary Angiographic Evidence That Antioxidant Vitamin Intake Reduces Progression of Coronary Artery Atherosclerosis," *JAMA*, 1995, 273(23):1849-54.
Saperstein H, Rapaport M, and Rietschel RL, "Topical Vitamin E as a Cause of Erythema Multiforme-Like Eruption," *Arch Dermatol*, 1984, 120(7):906-8.

♦ **Vitamin K₁** see Phytonadione *on page 1257*

♦ **Vitrase®** see Hyaluronidase *on page 754*

♦ **Vitrasert®** see Ganciclovir *on page 697*

♦ **Vi Vaccine** see Typhoid Vaccine *on page 1646*

♦ **Vivactil®** see Protriptyline *on page 1343*

♦ **Viva-Drops® [OTC]** see Artificial Tears *on page 124*

♦ **Vivaglobin®** see Immune Globulin (Subcutaneous) *on page 796*

♦ **Vivelle®** see Estradiol *on page 549*

♦ **Vivelle-Dot®** see Estradiol *on page 549*

♦ **Vivotif®** see Typhoid Vaccine *on page 1646*

♦ **Voltaren®** see Diclofenac *on page 424*

♦ **Voltaren Ophthalmic®** see Diclofenac *on page 424*

♦ **Voltaren®-XR** see Diclofenac *on page 424*

Voriconazole (vor i KOE na zole)

U.S. Brand Names VFEND®
Canadian Brand Names VFEND®
Index Terms UK109496
Generic Available No
Pharmacologic Category Antifungal Agent, Oral; Antifungal Agent, Parenteral
Use Treatment of invasive aspergillosis; treatment of esophageal candidiasis; treatment of candidemia (in non-neutropenic patients); treatment of disseminated *Candida* infections of the skin and viscera; treatment of serious fungal infections caused by *Scedosporium apiospermum* and *Fusarium* spp (including *Fusarium solani*) in patients intolerant of, or refractory to, other therapy
Contraindications Hypersensitivity to voriconazole or any component of the formulation (cross-reaction with other azole antifungal agents may occur but has not been established; use caution); coadministration of CYP3A4 substrates which may lead to QT$_c$ prolongation (cisapride, pimozide, or quinidine); coadministration with barbiturates (long acting), carbamazepine, efavirenz (with standard [eg, not adjusted] voriconazole and efavirenz doses), ergot alkaloids, rifampin, rifabutin, ritonavir (≥800 mg/day), and sirolimus
Warnings/Precautions Visual changes are commonly associated with treatment. Patients should be warned to avoid tasks which depend on vision, including operating machinery or driving. Changes are reversible on discontinuation following brief exposure/treatment regimens (≤28 days).

Serious hepatic reactions (including hepatitis, cholestasis, and fulminant hepatic failure) have occurred during treatment, primarily in patients with serious concomitant medical conditions. However, hepatotoxicity has occurred in patients with no identifiable risk factors. Use caution in patients with pre-existing hepatic impairment (dose adjustment required).

Voriconazole tablets contain lactose; avoid administration in hereditary galactose intolerance, Lapp lactase deficiency, or glucose-galactose malabsorption. Suspension contains sucrose; use caution with fructose intolerance, sucrose-isomaltase deficiency, or glucose-galactose malabsorption. Avoid/limit use of intravenous formulation in patients with renal impairment; intravenous formulation contains excipient sulfobutyl ether beta-cyclodextrin (SBECD), which may accumulate in renal insufficiency. Infusion-related reactions may occur with intravenous dosing. Consider discontinuation of infusion if reaction is severe.
(Continued)

Voriconazole *(Continued)*

Use caution in patients with an increased risk of arrhythmia (concurrent QT_c-prolonging drugs, hypokalemia, cardiomyopathy, or prior cardiotoxic therapy). Correct electrolyte abnormalities before initiating therapy. Use caution in patients receiving concurrent non-nucleoside reverse transcriptase inhibitors (efavirenz is contraindicated).

Adverse Reactions (Reflective of adult population; not specific for elderly)

>10%: Ocular: Visual changes (dose dependent — photophobia, color changes, increased or decreased visual acuity, or blurred vision occur in ~21%)

2% to 10%:

Cardiovascular: Tachycardia (up to 2%), hyper-/hypotension (2%), vasodilation (2%)

Central nervous system: Fever (up to 6%), chills (up to 4%), headache (up to 3%), hallucinations (up to 3%)

Dermatologic: Rash (up to 7%)

Endocrine & metabolic: Hypokalemia (up to 2%)

Gastrointestinal: Nausea (1% to 5%), vomiting (1% to 4%), abdominal pain (2%)

Hepatic: Alkaline phosphatase increased (4% to 5%), AST increased (2% to 4%), ALT increased (2% to 3%), cholestatic jaundice (1% to 2%)

Ocular: Photophobia (2% to 3%)

Overdosage/Toxicology Visual changes may occur; one patient had photophobia for 10 minutes. Treatment is symptom-directed and supportive. Following intravenous overdose, toxicity from the vehicle, SBECD, may also occur. Both voriconazole and the intravenous vehicle may be eliminated via hemodialysis.

Drug Interactions Substrate of CYP2C9 (major), 2C19 (major), 3A4 (minor); **Inhibits** CYP2C9 (weak), 2C19 (weak), 3A4 (moderate)

Barbiturates (phenobarbital, secobarbital): May decrease the serum levels/effects of voriconazole; concurrent use is contraindicated.

Benzodiazepines (metabolized by oxidation): Alprazolam, diazepam, temazepam, triazolam, and midazolam serum concentrations/toxicity may be increased. Manufacturer suggests adjustment of benzodiazepine dose be considered.

Buspirone: Serum concentrations may be increased; monitor for sedation.

Busulfan: Serum concentrations may be increased; avoid concurrent use.

Calcium channel blockers: Serum levels may be increased (applies to those agents metabolized by CYP3A4, including felodipine, nifedipine, and verapamil).

Carbamazepine: May decrease the serum levels/effects of voriconazole; concurrent use is contraindicated.

Cisapride: Serum concentrations may be increased which may lead to malignant arrhythmias; concurrent use is contraindicated.

CYP2C9 inducers: May decrease the levels/effects of voriconazole. Example inducers include carbamazepine, phenobarbital, phenytoin, rifampin, rifapentine, and secobarbital.

CYP2C19 inducers: May decrease the levels/effects of voriconazole. Example inducers include aminoglutethimide, carbamazepine, phenytoin, and rifampin.

CYP3A4 substrates: Voriconazole may increase the levels/effects of CYP3A4 substrates. Example substrates include benzodiazepines, calcium channel blockers, cyclosporine, mirtazapine, nateglinide, nefazodone, sildenafil (and other PDE-5 inhibitors), tacrolimus, and venlafaxine. Selected benzodiazepines (midazolam and triazolam), cisapride, ergot alkaloids, selected HMG-CoA reductase inhibitors (lovastatin and simvastatin), and pimozide are generally contraindicated with strong CYP3A4 inhibitors.

Cyclosporine: Voriconazole increases the serum levels/effects of cyclosporine. Decrease cyclosporine dose and monitor. Readjust dose when voriconazole is discontinued.

Efavirenz: Serum levels/effects of voriconazole may be reduced, and efavirenz levels increased during therapy; concurrent use is contraindicated with standard doses of voriconazole. Adjusted doses of voriconazole and efavirenz may be used concurrently.

Ergot alkaloids: Serum levels may be increased by voriconazole, leading to ergot toxicity; concurrent use is contraindicated.

HMG-CoA reductase inhibitors (except pravastatin and fluvastatin): Serum levels/effects may be increased. The risk of myopathy/rhabdomyolysis may be increased. Switch to pravastatin/fluvastatin or monitor for development of myopathy. Manufacturer suggests that dosage adjustment of HMG-CoA reductase inhibitor may be necessary with concurrent use.

Methadone: Serum levels and duration/effects may be increased significantly; monitor and reduce methadone dose if necessary.

Omeprazole: Voriconazole may increase omeprazole serum levels. In patients taking ≥40 mg of omeprazole per day, dose of omeprazole should be reduced by half.

Oral (hormonal) contraceptives: May increase the levels/effects of voriconazole. Conversely, voriconazole may increase the levels/effects of ethinyl estradiol and norethindrone; monitor for adverse effects.

Phenytoin: Serum levels/effects of voriconazole may be decreased; adjust dose of voriconazole. Phenytoin levels may be increased; monitor phenytoin levels and adjust dose as needed.

Pimozide: Serum levels/toxicity may be increased; concurrent use is contraindicated.

QT_c-prolonging agents: Risk of arrhythmia (torsade de pointes) may be increased.

Quinidine: Serum levels may be increased; concurrent use is contraindicated.

Rifabutin: Rifabutin serum levels are increased by voriconazole; concurrent use is contraindicated.

Rifampin: Rifampin decreases voriconazole's serum concentration to levels which are no longer effective; concurrent use is contraindicated.

Ritonavir: Serum levels/effects of voriconazole are reduced; concurrent use of ritonavir ≥800 mg/day is contraindicated. Use caution with smaller doses (<800 mg/day) of ritonavir.

Sirolimus: Serum levels may be increased by voriconazole; concurrent use is contraindicated.

Tacrolimus: Serum levels may be increased by voriconazole. Reduce tacrolimus dose to $^1/_3$ of original dose and monitor. Readjust dose when voriconazole is discontinued.

Vinca alkaloids: Serum concentrations may be increased; consider reduced dosage of vinca alkaloid.

Warfarin: Anticoagulant effects may be increased; monitor INR.

Ethanol/Nutrition/Herb Interactions

Food: May decrease voriconazole absorption. Voriconazole should be taken 1 hour before or 1 hour after a meal.

Herb/Nutraceutical: St John's wort may decrease voriconazole levels.

Stability

Powder for injection: Store at 15°C to 30°C (59°F to 86°F). Reconstitute 200 mg vial with 19 mL of sterile water for injection (use of automated syringe is not recommended). Resultant solution (20 mL) has a concentration of 10 mg/mL. Prior to infusion, must dilute to 0.5-5 mg/mL with NS, LR, D_5WLR, D_5W$^1/_2$NS, D_5W, D_5W with KCl 20 mEq, $^1/_2$NS, or D_5WNS. Do not dilute with 4.2% sodium bicarbonate infusion. Reconstituted solutions are stable for up to 24 hours under refrigeration at 2°C to 8°C (36°F to 46°F).

Powder for oral suspension: Store at 2°C to 8°C (36°F to 46°F). Add 46 mL of water to the bottle to make 40 mg/mL suspension. Reconstituted oral suspension may be stored at 15°C to 30°C (59°F to 86°F). Discard after 14 days.

Tablets: Store at 15°C to 30°C (59°F to 86°F).

Mechanism of Action Interferes with fungal cytochrome P450 activity, decreasing ergosterol synthesis (principal sterol in fungal cell membrane) and inhibiting fungal cell membrane formation.

Pharmacokinetics

Absorption: Well absorbed after oral administration; administration of crushed tablets is considered bioequivalent to whole tablets

Distribution: V_d: 4.6 L/kg

Protein binding: 58%

Metabolism: Hepatic; saturable (may demonstrate nonlinearity)

Bioavailability: 96%

Half-life elimination: Variable, dose-dependent

Time to peak: Oral: 1-2 hours; 0.5 hours (crushed tablet)

Elimination: Urine (as inactive metabolites)

Dosage

Geriatrics & Adults:

Aspergillosis (invasive), scedosporiosis, fusariosis: I.V.: Initial: Loading dose: 6 mg/kg every 12 hours for 2 doses; followed by maintenance dose of 4 mg/kg every 12 hours

Candidemia and other deep tissue *Candida* infections: I.V.: Initial: Loading dose 6 mg/kg every 12 hours for 2 doses; followed by maintenance dose of 3-4 mg/kg every 12 hours

Endophthalmitis, fungal: I.V.: 6 mg/kg every 12 hours for 2 doses, then 200 mg orally twice daily

Esophageal candidiasis: Oral:

Patients <40 kg: 100 mg every 12 hours; maximum: 300 mg/day

Patients ≥40 kg: 200 mg every 12 hours; maximum: 600 mg/day

Note: Treatment should continue for a minimum of 14 days, and for at least 7 days following resolution of symptoms.

Conversion to oral dosing:

Patients <40 kg: 100 mg every 12 hours; increase to 150 mg every 12 hours in patients who fail to respond adequately

Patients ≥40 kg: 200 mg every 12 hours; increase to 300 mg every 12 hours in patients who fail to respond adequately

Dosage adjustment in patients unable to tolerate treatment:

I.V.: Dose may be reduced to 3 mg/kg every 12 hours

(Continued)

Voriconazole (Continued)

Oral: Dose may be reduced in 50 mg increments to a minimum dosage of 200 mg every 12 hours in patients weighing ≥40 kg (100 mg every 12 hours in patients <40 kg)

Dosage adjustment in patients receiving concomitant CYP450 enzyme inducers or substrates:

Cyclosporine: Reduce cyclosporine dose by $1/2$ and monitor closely.

Efavirenz: Oral: Increase maintenance dose of voriconazole to 400 mg every 12 hours and reduce efavirenz dose to 300 mg once daily

Phenytoin:

I.V.: Increase maintenance dosage to 5 mg/kg every 12 hours

Oral: Increase dose to 400 mg every 12 hours in patients ≥40 kg (200 mg every 12 hours in patients <40 kg)

Renal Impairment: In patients with Cl_{cr} <50 mL/minute, accumulation of the intravenous vehicle (SBECD) occurs. After initial loading dose, oral voriconazole should be administered to these patients, unless an assessment of the benefit:risk to the patient justifies the use of I.V. voriconazole. Monitor serum creatinine and change to oral voriconazole therapy when possible.

Hemodialysis: Oral dosage adjustment not required; for I.V. dosing, see dosage adjustment in renal impairment

Hepatic Impairment:

Mild-to-moderate hepatic dysfunction (Child-Pugh class A and B): Following standard loading dose, reduce maintenance dosage by 50%

Severe hepatic impairment: Should only be used if benefit outweighs risk; monitor closely for toxicity

Administration

Oral: Administer 1 hour before or 1 hour after a meal.

I.V.: Infuse over 1-2 hours (rate not to exceed 3 mg/kg/hour)

Monitoring Parameters Hepatic function, visual function, renal function

Dosage Forms Excipient information presented when available (limited, particularly for generics); consult specific product labeling.

Injection, powder for reconstitution: 200 mg [contains SBECD 3200 mg]

Powder for oral suspension: 200 mg/5 mL (70 mL) [contains sodium benzoate and sucrose; orange flavor]

Tablet: 50 mg, 200 mg [contains lactose]

Selected References

Breit SM, Hariprasad SM, Mieler WF, et al, "Management of Endogenous Fungal Endophthalmitis With Voriconazole and Caspofungin," Am J Ophthalmol, 2005, 139(1):135-40.

Dodds-Ashley ES, Zaas AK, Fang AF, et al, "Comparative Pharmacokinetics of Voriconazole Administered Orally as Either Crushed or Whole Tablets," Antimicrob Agents Chemother, 2006 [epub ahead of print]

Durand ML, Kim IK, D'Amico DJ, et al, "Successful Treatment of Fusarium Endophthalmitis with Voriconazole and Aspergillus Endophthalmitis With Voriconazole Plus Caspofungin," Am J Ophthalmol, 2005, 140(3):552-4.

Hariprasad SM, Mieler WF, Holz ER, et al, "Determination of Vitreous, Aqueous, and Plasma Concentration of Orally Administered Voriconazole in Humans," Arch Ophthalmol, 2004, 122(1):42-7.

♦ **VoSpire ER®** see Albuterol on page 40
♦ **Vytorin®** see Ezetimibe and Simvastatin on page 593
♦ **VZV Vaccine (Zoster)** see Zoster Vaccine on page 1713

Warfarin (WAR far in)

Related Information

Anticoagulants, Injectable on page 1741
Anticoagulant Therapy Guidelines on page 1813

Medication Safety Issues

Sound-alike/look-alike issues:

Coumadin® may be confused with Avandia®, Cardura®, Compazine®, Kemadrin®

High alert medication: The Institute for Safe Medication Practices (ISMP) includes this medication among its list of drugs which have a heightened risk of causing significant patient harm when used in error.

U.S. Brand Names Coumadin®; Jantoven™

Canadian Brand Names Apo-Warfarin®; Coumadin®; Gen-Warfarin; Novo-Warfarin; Taro-Warfarin

Index Terms Warfarin Sodium

Generic Available Yes: Tablet

Pharmacologic Category Anticoagulant, Coumarin Derivative

Use Prophylaxis and treatment of venous thrombosis, pulmonary embolism, and thromboembolic disorders; atrial fibrillation with risk of embolism; adjunct in the prophylaxis of systemic embolism after myocardial infarction; reduce risk of recurrent myocardial infarction

Unlabeled/Investigational Use Prevention of recurrent transient ischemic attacks

Restrictions An FDA-approved medication guide must be distributed when dispensing an outpatient prescription (new or refill) where this medication is to be used without direct supervision of a healthcare provider. Medication guides are available at http://www.fda.gov/cder/Offices/ODS/medication_guides.htm.

Contraindications Hypersensitivity to warfarin or any component of the formulation; hemorrhagic tendencies; hemophilia; thrombocytopenia purpura; leukemia; recent or potential surgery of the eye or CNS; major regional lumbar block anesthesia or surgery resulting in large, open surfaces; patients bleeding from the GI, respiratory, or GU tract; aneurysm; ascorbic acid deficiency; history of bleeding diathesis; prostatectomy; continuous tube drainage of the small intestine; polyarthritis; diverticulitis; emaciation; malnutrition; cerebrovascular hemorrhage; blood dyscrasias; severe uncontrolled or malignant hypertension; severe hepatic disease; pericarditis or pericardial effusion; subacute bacterial endocarditis; visceral carcinoma; following spinal puncture and other diagnostic or therapeutic procedures with potential for significant bleeding; history of warfarin-induced necrosis; an unreliable, noncompliant patient; alcoholism; patient who has a history of falls or is a significant fall risk; unsupervised senile or psychotic patient

Warnings/Precautions Use care in the selection of patients appropriate for this treatment. Ensure patient cooperation especially from the alcoholic, illicit drug user, demented, or psychotic patient. Use with caution in trauma, acute infection, moderate-severe renal insufficiency, prolonged dietary insufficiencies, moderate-severe hypertension, polycythemia vera, vasculitis, open wound, active TB, history of PUD, anaphylactic disorders, indwelling catheters, severe diabetes, thyroid disease, and menstruating and postpartum women. Use with caution in protein C deficiency. Use with caution in patients with heparin-induced thrombocytopenia and DVT. Warfarin monotherapy is contraindicated in the initial treatment of active HIT.

[U.S. Boxed Warning]: May cause major or fatal bleeding. Risk factors for bleeding include high intensity anticoagulation, age, variable INRs, history of GI bleeding, hypertension, cerebrovascular disease, serious heart disease, anemia, malignancy, trauma, renal insufficiency, drug-drug interactions, and long duration of therapy. Patient must be instructed to report bleeding, accidents, or falls. Patient must also report any new or discontinued medications, herbal or alternative products used, or significant changes in smoking or dietary habits. Necrosis or gangrene of the skin and other tissue can occur. "Purple toes syndrome" may rarely occur. Women may be at risk of developing ovarian hemorrhage at the time of ovulation. The elderly may be more sensitive to anticoagulant therapy.

Adverse Reactions (Reflective of adult population; not specific for elderly)
Bleeding is the major adverse effect of warfarin. Hemorrhage may occur at virtually any site. Risk is dependent on multiple variables, including the intensity of anticoagulation and patient susceptibility.

Cardiovascular: Angina, edema, hemorrhagic shock, hypotension, pallor, syncope, vasculitis

Central nervous system: Asthenia, dizziness, fever, headache, lethargy, malaise, pain, stroke

Dermatologic: Alopecia, bullous eruptions, dermatitis, rash, pruritus, urticaria

Gastrointestinal: Abdominal cramps, abdominal pain, anorexia, diarrhea, flatulence, gastrointestinal bleeding, mouth ulcers, nausea, taste disturbance, vomiting

Genitourinary: Hematuria, priapism

Hematologic: Agranulocytosis, anemia, hemorrhage, leukopenia, retroperitoneal hematoma, unrecognized bleeding sites (eg, colon cancer) may be uncovered by anticoagulation

Hepatic: Hepatic injury, hepatitis, jaundice, transaminases increased

Neuromuscular & skeletal: Osteoporosis (potential association with long-term use), paresthesia, weakness

Respiratory: Epistaxis, hemoptysis, pulmonary hemorrhage, tracheobronchial calcification

Miscellaneous: Hypersensitivity/allergic reactions

Skin necrosis/gangrene(<0.1%), due to paradoxical local thrombosis, is a known but rare risk of warfarin therapy. Its onset is usually within the first few days of therapy and is frequently localized to the limbs, breast, or penis. The risk of this effect is increased in patients with protein C or S deficiency.

"Purple toes syndrome," caused by cholesterol microembolization, also occurs rarely. Typically, this occurs after several weeks of therapy, and may present as a dark, purplish, mottled discoloration of the plantar and lateral surfaces. Other manifestations of cholesterol microembolization may include rash; livedo reticularis; gangrene; abrupt and intense pain in lower extremities; abdominal, flank, or back pain; hematuria, renal insufficiency; hypertension; cerebral ischemia; spinal cord infarction; or other symptoms of vascular compromise.

Overdosage/Toxicology See table. Symptoms include internal or external hemorrhage and hematuria. Avoid emesis and lavage to avoid possible trauma and incidental
(Continued)

Warfarin (Continued)

bleeding. When an overdose occurs, the drug should be immediately discontinued and vitamin K_1 (phytonadione) may be administered. When hemorrhage occurs, fresh frozen plasma transfusions have been used to help control bleeding by replacing clotting factors. In urgent bleeding, prothrombin complex concentrates may be needed. **Management of elevated INR:** See table.

Management of Elevated INR

INR	Symptom	Action
Above therapeutic range to <5	No significant bleeding	Lower or hold the next dose and monitor frequently; when INR approaches desired range, may resume dosing with a lower dose if INR was significantly above therapeutic range.
≥5 and <9	No significant bleeding	Omit the next 1or 2 doses; monitor INR and resume with a lower dose when the INR approaches the desired range. Alternatively, if there are other risk factors for bleeding, omit the next dose and give vitamin K_1 orally ≤5 mg; resume with a lower dose when the INR approaches the desired range. If rapid reversal is required for surgery, then given vitamin K_1 orally 2-4 mg and hold warfarin. Expect a response within 24 hours; another 1-2 mg may be given orally if needed.
≥9	No significant bleeding	Hold warfarin, give vitamin K_1 orally 5-10 mg, expect the INR to be reduced within 24-48 hours; monitor INR and administer additional vitamin K if necessary. Resume warfarin at lower doses when INR is in the desired range.
Any INR elevation	Serious bleeding	Hold warfarin, give vitamin K_1 (10 mg by slow I.V. infusion), and supplement with fresh plasma transfusion or prothrombin complex concentrate (Factor X complex); recombinant factor VIIa is an alternative to prothrombin complex concentrate. Vitamin K_1 injection can be repeated every 12 hours.
Any INR elevation	Life-threatening bleeding	Hold warfarin, give prothrombin complex concentrate, supplemented with vitamin K_1 (10 mg by slow I.V. infusion); repeat if necessary. Recombinant factor VIIa is an alternative to prothrombin complex concentrate.

Note: Use of high doses of vitamin K_1 (10.0-15.0) may cause resistance to warfarin for up to a week. Heparin or low molecular weight heparin can be given until the patient becomes responsive to warfarin.

Reference: Ansell J, Hirsh J, Poller L et al. "The Pharmacology and Management of the Vitamin K Antagonists," *Chest*, 2004, 126 (3 Suppl):204-33.

Drug Interactions **Substrate** of CYP1A2 (minor), 2C9 (major), 2C19 (minor), 3A4 (minor); **Inhibits** CYP2C9 (moderate), 2C19 (weak)

Acetaminophen: May enhance the anticoagulant effect of warfarin. Most likely to occur with daily acetaminophen doses >1.3 g for >1 week.

Allopurinol: May enhance the anticoagulant effect of warfarin. Reductions in warfarin will likely be required.

Aminoglutethimide: May increase the metabolism, via CYP isoenzymes, of warfarin. Monitor therapy for decreased warfarin effect.

Amiodarone: May enhance the anticoagulant effect of warfarin. An empiric warfarin dosage reduction of 30% to 50% at the initiation of warfarin may be considered.

Androgens: May enhance the anticoagulant effect of warfarin. Significant reductions in warfarin dosage may be needed during concomitant therapy.

Anticoagulants: May enhance the anticoagulant effect of warfarin.

Antifungal agents (imidazole): May decrease the metabolism, via CYP isoenzymes, of warfarin. Monitor for increased therapeutic/toxic effects of warfarin.

Antiplatelet agents: May enhance the anticoagulant effect of anticoagulants.

Antithyroid agents: May diminish the anticoagulant effects of warfarin. Monitor for decreased therapeutic effects.

Aprepitant: May decrease the serum concentration of warfarin. Monitor closely for 2 weeks following each course of aprepitant.

Azathioprine: May decrease the anticoagulant effect of warfarin. An adjustment in warfarin dose may be needed.

Barbiturates: May increase the metabolism, via CYP isoenzymes, of warfarin. Monitor for decreased therapeutic effect of warfarin. Anticoagulation dosage increase of 30% to 60% may be needed based upon monitored PT.

Bile acid sequestrants: May decrease absorption of warfarin. Separating the administration of doses by >2 hours may reduce the risk of interaction.

Bosentan: May increase metabolism, via CYP isoenzymes, of warfarin. Monitor for decreased effects.

Capecitabine: May decrease metabolism of warfarin. Monitor for evidence of excess anticoagulation.

Carbamazepine: May increase the metabolism, via CYP isoenzymes, of warfarin. Monitor for decreased therapeutic effects of warfarin.

Cephalosporins: May enhance the anticoagulant effect of warfarin. Monitor for increased evidence of bleeding, especially in cephalosporins that have NMTT side chain.

Cimetidine: May enhance the anticoagulant effect of warfarin. Monitor for increased therapeutic effects of warfarin.

Contraceptive, hormonal (estrogens): May diminish the anticoagulant effect of coumarin derivatives. In contrast, enhanced anticoagulant effects have also been noted with some products. Conversely, enhanced anticoagulant effect has also been reported. Avoid concomitant use. If combination therapy is necessary, monitor for changes in INR when contraceptive is added, discontinued, or when any change in dose of either agent occurs.

Contraceptives, hormonal (progestins): May diminish the anticoagulant effect of warfarin. Conversely, enhanced anticoagulant effect has also been reported. Avoid concomitant use. If combination therapy is necessary, monitor for changes in INR when contraceptive is added, discontinued, or when any change in dose of either agent occurs.

CYP2C9 inducers (strong): May increase the metabolism of warfarin. Examples of inducers include carbamazepine, fosphenytoin, phenobarbital, phenytoin, primidone, rifampin, rifapentine, and secobarbital. Monitor for decreased effect of warfarin.

CYP2C9 inhibitors may increase the levels/effects of warfarin. Example inhibitors include delavirdine, fluconazole, gemfibrozil, ketoconazole, nicardipine, NSAIDs, sulfonamides, and tolbutamide.

Dicloxacillin: May increase the metabolism, via CYP isoenzymes, of warfarin. Monitor for decreased therapeutic effects of warfarin.

Disulfiram: May increase the serum concentration of warfarin. Monitor for increased therapeutic effects of warfarin.

Drotrecogin Alfa: Warfarin may enhance the adverse/toxic effect of drotrecogin alfa. Monitor for increased risk of bleeding during concomitant therapy. If possible, avoid use of drotrecogin within 7 days of warfarin therapy, or if INR ≥3.

Etoposide: May enhance the anticoagulant effect of warfarin. Monitor for increased effects of warfarin.

Fibric acid derivatives: May enhance the anticoagulant effect of warfarin. Monitor for toxic effects of warfarin; may warrant a 25% to 33% reduction in the warfarin dosage.

Fluconazole: May decrease the metabolism, via CYP isoenzymes, of warfarin. Monitor for increased therapeutic/toxic effects of warfarin.

Fluorouracil: May enhance the anticoagulant effect of warfarin. Monitor for increased effects of warfarin.

Gefitinib: May enhance the anticoagulant effect of coumarin derivatives.

Glucagon: May enhance the anticoagulant effect of warfarin. Monitor for toxic effects of warfarin, especially if glucagon is administered in high doses.

Griseofulvin: May increase the metabolism, via CYP isoenzymes, of warfarin. Monitor for decreased therapeutic effects of warfarin.

HMG-CoA reductase inhibitors: May enhance the anticoagulant effect of warfarin. Monitor for increased effects of warfarin.

Ifosfamide: May enhance the anticoagulant effect of warfarin. Monitor for increased effects of warfarin.

Leflunomide: May enhance the anticoagulant effect of warfarin. Monitor for increased effects of warfarin.

Macrolide antibiotics: May decrease the metabolism, via CYP isoenzymes, of warfarin. Monitor for increased therapeutic effects of warfarin. CYP inhibitors (eg, clarithromycin, erythromycin, and troleandomycin) appear to pose the greatest risk. Azithromycin and telithromycin have also been implicated in a few cases.

Mefloquine: May enhance the anticoagulant effect of warfarin.

Mercaptopurine: May diminish the anticoagulant effect of warfarin. Monitor for decreased therapeutic effects of warfarin.

Metronidazole: May decrease the metabolism, via CYP isoenzymes, of warfarin. If concomitant therapy is necessary, consider an empiric reduction in warfarin dosage of approximately one-third. Monitor for increased therapeutic/toxic effects of warfarin.

(Continued)

Warfarin (Continued)

Mitotane: May diminish the anticoagulant effect of warfarin.

Nafcillin: May increase the metabolism of warfarin. Consider choosing an alternative antibiotic if available. Monitor for decreased therapeutic effects of warfarin if nafcillin is initiated. The effects on warfarin dosing may persist long after nafcillin is discontinued. Close monitoring is required even after nafcillin is discontinued.

NSAID (COX-2 inhibitor): May enhance the anticoagulant effect of coumarin derivatives.

NSAID (nonselective): May enhance the anticoagulant effect of warfarin. Monitor for increased signs and symptoms of bleeding.

Omega-3-acid ethyl esters: May enhance the anticoagulant effect of warfarin.

Orlistat: May enhance the anticoagulant effect of warfarin. Monitor for changes in effects of warfarin.

Phenytoin: May enhance the anticoagulant effect of warfarin. Warfarin may increase the serum concentration of phenytoin. Monitor for increased effects of warfarin and for increased serum concentrations/toxic effects of phenytoin.

Phytonadione: May antagonize the effects of warfarin. Monitor for decreased therapeutic effects of warfarin.

Propafenone: May increase the serum concentration of warfarin. Monitor for increased prothrombin times (PT)/therapeutic effects of warfarin.

Propoxyphene: May decrease the metabolism, via CYP isoenzymes, of warfarin. Monitor for increased prothrombin time/toxic effects of warfarin.

Proton pump inhibitors (omeprazole): May increase the serum concentration of warfarin. Monitor for increased effects of warfarin.

Quinidine: May enhance the anticoagulant effect of warfarin. Monitor for increased prothrombin times (PT)/therapeutic effects of warfarin.

Quinolone antibiotics: May enhance the anticoagulant effect of warfarin. Monitor for increased prothrombin time/toxic effects of warfarin.

Rifamycin derivatives: May increase the metabolism, via CYP isoenzymes, of warfarin. Monitor for decreased prothrombin times (PT)/therapeutic effects of warfarin.

Ropinirole: May enhance the anticoagulant effect of warfarin. Monitor for increased INR/effects of warfarin.

Salicylates: May enhance the anticoagulant effect of warfarin. Monitor for increased signs and symptoms of bleeding if used concomitantly.

Selective serotonin reuptake inhibitors (SSRIs): May enhance the anticoagulant effect of warfarin. Monitor for increased therapeutic/toxic effects of warfarin.

Sulfasalazine: May diminish the anticoagulant effect of warfarin. Monitor for decreased INR/effects of warfarin

Sulfinpyrazone: May decrease the metabolism, via CYP isoenzymes, of warfarin and may decrease the protein binding of warfarin. Monitor for increased prothrombin time (PT)/toxic effects of warfarin.

Sulfonamide derivatives: May enhance the anticoagulant effect of warfarin. Monitor for increased prothrombin time (PT)/toxic effects of warfarin.

Tetracycline derivatives: May enhance the anticoagulant effect of warfarin. Monitor for toxic effects of warfarin.

Thyroid products: May enhance the anticoagulant effect of warfarin. Monitor for increased hypoprothrombinemic effects of warfarin.

Tigecycline: May increase the serum concentration of warfarin. Monitor for increased effects of warfarin.

Tolterodine: May increase the effects of warfarin.

Treprostinil: May enhance the adverse/toxic effects of warfarin. Monitor for increased risk of bleeding when used concomitantly.

Tricyclic antidepressants: May enhance the anticoagulant effect of warfarin. Monitor for increased prothrombin times (PT)/toxic effects of warfarin.

Vitamin A: May enhance the anticoagulant effect of warfarin. Monitor for increased prothrombin time (PT)/effects of warfarin.

Vitamin E: May enhance the anticoagulant effect of warfarin. Monitor for increased prothrombin time (PT)/effects of warfarin. Likely only of significant concern with higher doses of vitamin E (eg, 1200 int. units/day).

Voriconazole: May increase the serum concentration of warfarin. Monitor for increased effects (eg, INR, bleeding) of warfarin.

Zafirlukast: May decrease the metabolism, via CYP isoenzymes, of warfarin. Monitor for increased prothrombin time (PT)/effects of warfarin.

Zileuton: May increase the serum concentration of warfarin. Monitor for increased effects of warfarin.

Ethanol/Nutrition/Herb Interactions

Ethanol: Avoid ethanol. Acute ethanol ingestion (binge drinking) decreases the metabolism of warfarin and increases PT/INR. Chronic daily ethanol use increases the metabolism of warfarin and decreases PT/INR.

Food: The anticoagulant effects of warfarin may be decreased if taken with foods rich in vitamin K. Vitamin E may increase warfarin effect. Cranberry juice may increase warfarin effect.

Herb/Nutraceutical: Cranberry, fenugreek, ginkgo biloba, glucosamine, may enhance bleeding or increase warfarin's effect. Ginseng (American), coenzyme Q_{10}, and St John's wort may decrease warfarin levels and effects. Avoid alfalfa, anise, bilberry, bladderwrack, bromelain, cat's claw, celery, coleus, cordyceps, dong quai, evening primrose oil, fenugreek, feverfew, garlic, ginger, ginkgo biloba, ginseng (American), ginseng (Panax), ginseng (Siberian), grapeseed, green tea, guggul, horse chestnut seed, horseradish, licorice, omega-3-acids, prickly ash, red clover, reishi, same (s-adenosylmethionine), sweet clover, turmeric, and white willow (all have additional antiplatelet activity).

Stability

Injection: Prior to reconstitution, store at 15°C to 30°C (59°F to 86°F). Following reconstitution with 2.7 mL of sterile water (yields 2 mg/mL solution), stable for 4 hours at 15°C to 30°C (59°F to 86°F). Protect from light.

Tablet: Store at 15°C to 30°C (59°F to 86°F). Protect from light.

Mechanism of Action
Interferes with hepatic synthesis of vitamin K-dependent coagulation factors (II, VII, IX, X)

Pharmacodynamics

Onset of action: Following rapid oral absorption, anticoagulation effects occur within 36-72 hours

Peak effect: Within 5-7 days; older adults are more sensitive to the effects of warfarin and usually respond to a lower mg/day dose

Pharmacokinetics

Absorption: Oral: Rapid, complete

Distribution: 0.14 L/kg

Protein binding: 99%

Metabolism: Hepatic, primarily via CYP2C9; minor pathways include CYP2C19, 1A2, and 3A4

Half-life elimination: 20-60 hours; Mean: 40 hours; highly variable among individuals

Clearance of R-warfarin may be reduced in older patients (>60 years of age)

Dosage

Geriatrics: Oral: Initial dose ≤5 mg. Usual maintenance dose: 2-5 mg/day. The elderly tend to require lower dosages to produce a therapeutic level of anticoagulation (due to changes in the pattern of warfarin metabolism).

Adults:

Prevention/treatment of thrombosis/embolism:

I.V. (administer as a slow bolus injection): 2-5 mg/day

Oral: Initial dosing must be individualized. Consider the patient (hepatic function, cardiac function, age, nutritional status, concurrent therapy, risk of bleeding) in addition to prior dose response (if available) and the clinical situation. Start 5-10 mg daily for 2 days. Adjust dose according to INR results; usual maintenance dose ranges from 2-10 mg daily (individual patients may require loading and maintenance doses outside these general guidelines).

Note: Lower starting doses may be required for patients with hepatic impairment, poor nutrition, CHF, elderly, high risk of bleeding, or patients who are debilitated. Higher initial doses may be reasonable in selected patients (ie, receiving enzyme-inducing agents and with low risk of bleeding).

Renal Impairment: No adjustment required, however, patients with renal failure have an increased risk of bleeding complications. Monitor closely.

Hepatic Impairment: Monitor effect at usual doses. The response to oral anticoagulants may be markedly enhanced in obstructive jaundice, hepatitis, and cirrhosis. INR should be closely monitored.

Administration

Oral: Administer with or without food. Take at the same time each day.

I.V.: Administer as a slow bolus injection over 1-2 minutes; avoid all I.M. injections

Monitoring Parameters
Prothrombin time (PT), PT ratio, international normalization ratio (INR); stool guaiac for blood; hemoglobin, hematocrit

Reference Range

INR = patient prothrombin time/mean normal prothrombin time

ISI = international sensitivity index

INR should be increased by 2-3.5 times depending upon indication. An INR >4 does not generally add additional therapeutic benefit and is associated with increased risk of bleeding.

Adult INR ranges based upon indication: See table on next page.

Warfarin levels are not used for monitoring degree of anticoagulation. They may be useful if a patient with unexplained coagulopathy is using the drug surreptitiously or if it is unclear whether clinical resistance is due to true drug resistance or lack of drug intake.

(Continued)

Warfarin *(Continued)*

INR Ranges (Adults) Based Upon Indication

Indication	Targeted INR	Targeted INR Range
Acute myocardial infarction (high risk)	2.5	2.0-3.0[1,2,3]
Atrial fibrillation	2.5	2.0-3.0
St Jude Medical bileaflet mechanical aortic valve	2.5	2.0-3.0
Bileaflet or tilting disk mechanical mitral valve	3	2.5-3.5
Caged ball or caged disk mechanical valve	3	2.5-3.5[1]
Mechanical prosthetic valve with systemic embolism despite adequate anticoagulation	3	2.5-3.5[1]
Carbomedics bileaflet/Medtronic Hall tilting disk mechanical aortic valve (NSR, NI LA size)	2.5	2.0-3.0
Mechanical valve and risk factors (atrial fibrillation, MI, left atrial enlargement, low EF, endocardial damage)	3	2.5-3.5[1]
Bioprosthetic mitral valve	2.5	2.0-3.0[2]
Bioprosthetic aortic valve	2.5	2.0-3.0[2] (or aspirin 81 mg/day)
Bioprosthetic mitral or aortic valve with atrial fibrillation	2.5	2.0-3.0
Rheumatic mitral valve disease and NSR (left atrial diameter >5.5 cm)	2.5	2.0-3.0
Venous thromboembolism	2.5	2.0-3.0
Lupus inhibitor (no other risk factors)	2.5	2.0-3.0
Lupus inhibitor and recurrent thromboembolism	3	2.5-3.5

[1]Combine with aspirin 81 mg/day

[2]Maintain anticoagulation for 3 months

[3]High-risk includes a large anterior MI, significant heart failure, intracardiac thrombus, thromboembolism

Normal prothrombin time (PT): 10.9-12.9 seconds. Healthy premature newborns have prolonged coagulation test screening results (eg, PT, aPTT, TT) which return to normal adult values at approximately 6 months of age. Healthy prematures, however, do not develop spontaneous hemorrhage or thrombotic complications because of a balance between procoagulants and inhibitors.

Patient Information It is imperative that you inform prescriber of all prescriptions, OTC medications, or herbal products you are taking. Do not take any new medication during therapy unless approved by prescriber. Take exactly as directed; if dose is missed, take as soon as possible. Do not double dose. Follow diet and activity as recommended by prescriber; check with prescriber before changing diet; carry Medi-Alert® ID identifying drug usage. Avoid alcohol. Do not make major changes in your dietary intake of vitamin K (green vegetables). You will have a tendency to bleed easily while taking this drug (use soft toothbrush, waxed dental floss, electric razor, and avoid scissors or sharp knives and other potentially harmful activities). May cause nausea, vomiting, disturbed taste (small frequent meals, frequent mouth care, sucking lozenges, or chewing gum may help). Report any unusual bleeding or bruising (eg, bleeding gums, nosebleed, blood in urine, dark stool, bloody emesis, heavier than usual menses, or menstrual irregularities); skin rash or irritation; unusual fever; persistent nausea or GI upset; pain in joints or back; swelling or pain at injection site; or unhealed wounds.

Special Geriatric Considerations Before committing an elderly patient to long-term anticoagulation therapy, the risk for bleeding complications secondary to falls, drug interactions, living situation, and cognitive status should be considered. A risk of bleeding complications has been associated with increased age.

Dosage Forms Excipient information presented when available (limited, particularly for generics); consult specific product labeling.

Injection, powder for reconstitution, as sodium:

Coumadin®: 5 mg

Tablet, as sodium: 1 mg, 2 mg, 2.5 mg, 3 mg, 4 mg, 5 mg, 6 mg, 7.5 mg, 10 mg

Coumadin®, Jantoven™: 1 mg, 2 mg, 2.5 mg, 3 mg, 4 mg, 5 mg, 6 mg, 7.5 mg, 10 mg

Selected References

Albers GW, Amarenco P, Easton JD, et al, "Antithrombotic and Thrombolytic Therapy for Ischemic Stroke: The Seventh ACCP Conference on Antithrombotic and Thrombolytic Therapy," *Chest*, 2004, 126(3 Suppl):483-512.

Ansell J, Hirsh J, Poller L, et al, "The Pharmacology and Management of the Vitamin K Antagonists: The Seventh ACCP Conference on Antithrombotic and Thrombolytic Therapy, " *Chest*, 2004, 126(3 Suppl):204-33.

Gurwitz JH, Avorn J, Ross-Degnan D, et al, "Aging and the Anticoagulant Response to Warfarin Therapy," *Ann Intern Med*, 1992, 116(11):901-4.

Harrington RA, Becker RC, Ezekowitz M, et al, "Antithrombotic Therapy for Coronary Artery Disease: The Seventh ACCP Conference on Antithrombotic and Thrombolytic Therapy," *Chest*, 2004, 126(3 Suppl):514-38

Redwood M, Taylor C, Bain BJ, et al, "The Association of Age With Dosage Requirement for Warfarin," *Age Ageing*, 1991, 20(3):217-20.

Salem DN, Stein PD, Al-Ahmad A, et al, "Antithrombotic Therapy in Valvular Heart Disease -- Native and Prosthetic: The Seventh ACCP Conference on Antithrombotic and Thrombolytic Therapy," *Chest*, 2004, 126(3 Suppl):457-82.

Shepherd AM, Hewick DS, Moreland TA, et al, "Age as a Determinant of Sensitivity to Warfarin," *Br J Clin Pharmacol*, 1977, 4(3):315-20.

- **Warfarin Sodium** *see* Warfarin *on page 1682*
- **Wart-Off® Maximum Strength [OTC]** *see* Salicylic Acid *on page 1441*
- **4-Way® 12 Hour [OTC]** *see* Oxymetazoline *on page 1184*
- **4 Way® Fast Acting [OTC]** *see* Phenylephrine *on page 1247*
- **4 Way® Menthol [OTC]** *see* Phenylephrine *on page 1247*
- **4 Way® No Drip [OTC]** *see* Phenylephrine *on page 1247*
- **4-Way® Saline Moisturizing Mist [OTC]** *see* Sodium Chloride *on page 1475*
- **WelChol®** *see* Colesevelam *on page 361*
- **Wellbutrin®** *see* BuPROPion *on page 198*
- **Wellbutrin XL™** *see* BuPROPion *on page 198*
- **Wellbutrin SR®** *see* BuPROPion *on page 198*
- **Westcort®** *see* Hydrocortisone *on page 762*
- **Westhroid®** *see* Thyroid *on page 1559*
- **White Mineral Oil** *see* Mineral Oil *on page 1045*
- **Wound Wash Saline™ [OTC]** *see* Sodium Chloride *on page 1475*
- **WR-139013** *see* Chlorambucil *on page 287*
- **Wycillin [DSC]** *see* Penicillin G Procaine *on page 1226*
- **Xalatan®** *see* Latanoprost *on page 878*
- **Xanax®** *see* Alprazolam *on page 54*
- **Xanax XR®** *see* Alprazolam *on page 54*
- **Xenaderm™** *see* Trypsin, Balsam Peru, and Castor Oil *on page 1642*
- **Xenical®** *see* Orlistat *on page 1163*
- **Xibrom™** *see* Bromfenac *on page 185*
- **Xifaxan™** *see* Rifaximin *on page 1409*
- **Xodol® 5/300** *see* Hydrocodone and Acetaminophen *on page 759*
- **Xodol® 7.5/300** *see* Hydrocodone and Acetaminophen *on page 759*
- **Xodol® 10/300** *see* Hydrocodone and Acetaminophen *on page 759*
- **Xolegel™** *see* Ketoconazole *on page 853*
- **Xopenex®** *see* Levalbuterol *on page 887*
- **Xopenex HFA™** *see* Levalbuterol *on page 887*
- **XPECT™ [OTC]** *see* Guaifenesin *on page 727*
- **Xylocaine®** *see* Lidocaine *on page 904*
- **Xylocaine® MPF** *see* Lidocaine *on page 904*
- **Xylocaine® Viscous** *see* Lidocaine *on page 904*

Xylometazoline (zye loe met AZ oh leen)

Medication Safety Issues
Sound-alike/look-alike issues:
Otrivin® may be confused with Lotrimin®
U.S. Brand Names Otrivin® [OTC] [DSC]; Otrivin® Pediatric [OTC] [DSC]
Canadian Brand Names Balminil
Index Terms Xylometazoline Hydrochloride
Generic Available No
Pharmacologic Category Imidazoline Derivative; Vasoconstrictor, Nasal
Use Symptomatic relief of nasal and nasopharyngeal mucosal congestion
Contraindications Known hypersensitivity to xylometazoline hydrochloride, narrow-angle glaucoma, patients receiving MAO inhibitors
Warnings/Precautions Excessive use may cause rebound congestion or chemical rhinitis; use with caution in patients with hypertension, diabetes, cardiovascular or coronary artery disease, hyperthyroidism, long-standing bronchial asthma
Adverse Reactions (Reflective of adult population; not specific for elderly)
Frequency not defined.
Cardiovascular: Palpitation
Central nervous system: Dizziness, drowsiness, headache, seizure
Ocular: Blurred vision, ocular irritation, photophobia
Miscellaneous: Diaphoresis
Drug Interactions No data reported
Mechanism of Action Stimulates alpha-adrenergic receptors in the arterioles of the conjunctiva and the nasal mucosa to produce vasoconstriction
Pharmacodynamics
Onset of action: Intranasal: Local vasoconstriction occurs within 5-10 minutes
(Continued)

Xylometazoline *(Continued)*

Duration: 5-6 hours

Dosage

Geriatrics & Adults: Nasal congestion: Nasal: Instill 2-3 drops or sprays (0.1%) in each nostril every 8-10 hours

Monitoring Parameters Blood pressure in hypertensive patients

Patient Information Do not exceed recommended dosage; do not use for more than 4 consecutive days; if symptoms persist, drug should be discontinued and a physician consulted; notify physician of insomnia, tremor, or irregular heartbeat; burning, stinging, or drying of the nasal mucosa may occur

Special Geriatric Considerations Evaluate the patient's ability to self-administer; use with caution in patients with cardiovascular disease.

Dosage Forms Excipient information presented when available (limited, particularly for generics); consult specific product labeling. [DSC] = Discontinued product

Solution, intranasal drops, as hydrochloride:

Otrivin® [DSC]: 0.1% (25 mL)

Otrivin® Pediatric [DSC]: 0.05% (25 mL)

Solution, intranasal spray, as hydrochloride (Otrivin® [DSC]): 0.1% (20 mL)

♦ **Xylometazoline Hydrochloride** *see* Xylometazoline *on page 1689*

Yellow Fever Vaccine *(YEL oh FEE ver vak SEEN)*

Related Information

Immunization Recommendations *on page 1787*

U.S. Brand Names YF-VAX®

Canadian Brand Names YF-VAX®

Generic Available No

Pharmacologic Category Vaccine

Use Induction of active immunity against yellow fever virus, primarily among persons traveling or living in areas where yellow fever infection exists

Contraindications Hypersensitivity to egg or chick embryo protein, or any component of the formulation; immunosuppressed patients

Warnings/Precautions Do not use in immunodeficient persons (including patients <24 months after hematopoietic stem cell transplant) or patients receiving immunosuppressants (eg, steroids, radiation). Patients who are immunosuppressed have a theoretical risk of encephalitis with yellow fever vaccine administration; consider delaying travel or obtaining a waiver letter. Patients on low-dose or short-term corticosteroids, or with asymptomatic HIV infection are not considered immunosuppressed and may receive the vaccine. Chicken embryos are used in the manufacture of this vaccine; have epinephrine available in persons with previous history of egg allergy if the vaccine must be used. The vial stopper contains latex.

Adverse Reactions (Reflective of adult population; not specific for elderly)

All serious adverse reactions must be reported to the U.S. Department of Health and Human Services (DHHS) Vaccine Adverse Event Reporting System (VAERS) 1-800-822-7967.

Frequency not defined (adverse reactions may be increased in patients <9 months or ≥65 years of age)

Central nervous system: Headache, myalgia, fever (incidence of these reactions have been reported to be as low as <5% and as high as 10% to 30% depending on the study)

Local: Injection site reactions (edema, hypersensitivity, mass, pain)

Neuromuscular & skeletal: Weakness

Miscellaneous: Hypersensitivity (immediate), vaccine-associated neurotropic disease (rare), viscerotropic disease (rare)

Drug Interactions Immunosuppressive agents: Decreased effect of live vaccines may occur. Use of yellow fever vaccine in immunosuppressed patients is contraindicated due to possible risk of encephalitis or other serious adverse reactions.

Stability Yellow fever vaccine is shipped with dry ice. Do not use vaccine unless shipping case contains some dry ice on arrival. Maintain vaccine continuously at a temperature between 0°C to 5°C (32°F to 41°F); do not freeze. Reconstitute only with diluent provided. Inject diluent slowly into vial and allow to stand for 1-2 minutes. Gently swirl until a uniform suspension forms; swirl well before withdrawing dose. Avoid vigorous shaking to prevent foaming of suspension. Vaccine must be used within 60 minutes of reconstitution. Keep suspension refrigerated until used.

Pharmacodynamics

Onset: Seroconversion: 10-14 days

Duration: ≥30 years

Dosage
Geriatrics: Refer to adult dosing. Monitor closely.

Adults: Immunization: SubQ: One dose (0.5 mL) ≥10 days before travel; Booster: Every 10 years

Administration For SubQ injection only. Do not administer I.M. or I.V.

Monitoring Parameters Monitor for adverse effects which may be seen 7-14 days after vaccination

Patient Information Immunity develops by the tenth day and **WHO** requires revaccination every 10 years to maintain travelers' vaccination certificates

Additional Information Federal law requires that the date of administration, the vaccine manufacturer, lot number of vaccine, and the administering person's name, title, and address be entered into the patient's permanent medical record. A desensitization procedure is available for persons with severe egg sensitivity. Consult manufacturer's labeling for details. Some countries require a valid international Certification of Vaccination showing receipt of vaccine. The WHO requires revaccination every 10 years to maintain traveler's vaccination certificate.

The following CDC agencies may be contacted if serologic testing is needed or for advice when administering yellow fever vaccine to patients with altered immune status:
Division of Vector-Borne Infectious Diseases: 970-221-6400
Division of Global Migration and Quarantine: 404-498-1600

Special Geriatric Considerations No special considerations except in patients with immunodeficient diseases.

Dosage Forms Excipient information presented when available (limited, particularly for generics); consult specific product labeling.

Injection, powder for reconstitution [17D-204 strain]: ≥4.74 Log_{10} plaque-forming units (PFU) per 0.5 mL dose [single-dose or 5-dose vial; produced in chicken embryos; packaged with diluent; vial stopper contains latex]

Selected References
Centers for Disease Control and Prevention, "General Recommendations on immunization. Recommendations of the Advisory Committee on Immunization Practices (ACIP) and the American Academy of Family Physicians (AAFP)," *MMWR*, 2002, 51(R-2):1-35.

Centers for Disease Control and Prevention, "Yellow Fever Vaccine. Recommendations of the Advisory Committee on Immunization Practices (ACIP)," *MMWR*, 2002, 51(R-2):1-11.

Centers for Disease Control and Prevention, "Guidelines for Preventing Opportunistic Infections Among Hematopoietic Stem Cell Transplant Recipients. Recommendations of CDC, the Infectious Disease Society of America, and the American Society of Blood and Marrow Transplantation," *MMWR*, 2004, 49(RR-10):89-90.

♦ **YF-VAX®** see Yellow Fever Vaccine on page 1690
♦ **YM087** see Conivaptan on page 364
♦ **Yodoxin®** see Iodoquinol on page 825
♦ **Zaditor® [OTC]** see Ketotifen on page 863

Zafirlukast (za FIR loo kast)

Related Information
Asthma on page 1767

Medication Safety Issues
Sound-alike/look-alike issues:
Accolate® may be confused with Accupril®, Accutane®, Aclovate®

U.S. Brand Names Accolate®

Canadian Brand Names Accolate®

Index Terms ICI-204,219

Generic Available No

Pharmacologic Category Leukotriene-Receptor Antagonist

Use Prophylaxis and chronic treatment of asthma

Contraindications Hypersensitivity to zafirlukast or any component of the formulation

Warnings/Precautions Zafirlukast is not FDA approved for use in the reversal of bronchospasm in acute asthma attacks, including status asthmaticus. Therapy with zafirlukast can be continued during acute exacerbations of asthma.

Hepatic adverse events (including hepatitis, hyperbilirubinemia, and hepatic failure) have been reported; female patients may be at greater risk. Discontinue immediately if liver dysfunction is suspected. Periodic testing of liver function may be considered. If hepatic dysfunction is suspected, liver function tests should be measured immediately. Do not resume or restart if hepatic function studies are consistent with dysfunction. Use caution in patients with alcoholic cirrhosis; clearance is reduced.

Rare cases of eosinophilic vasculitis (Churg-Strauss) have been reported in patients receiving zafirlukast. No causal relationship established. Monitor for eosinophilic vasculitis, rash, pulmonary symptoms, cardiac symptoms, or neuropathy.

Adverse Reactions (Reflective of adult population; not specific for elderly)
>10%: Central nervous system: Headache (13%)
(Continued)

Zafirlukast *(Continued)*

1% to 10%:

Central nervous system: Dizziness (2%), pain (2%), fever (2%)

Gastrointestinal: Nausea (3%), diarrhea (3%), abdominal pain (2%), vomiting (2%), dyspepsia (1%)

Hepatic: ALT increased (2%)

Neuromuscular & skeletal: Back pain (2%), myalgia (2%), weakness (2%)

Miscellaneous: Infection (4%)

Overdosage/Toxicology Ingestions of up to 200 mg have been reported. Rash and upset stomach were the predominant symptoms. Treatment should be symptomatic and supportive.

Drug Interactions Substrate of CYP2C9 (major); **Inhibits** CYP1A2 (weak), 2C8 (weak), 2C9 (moderate), 2C19 (weak), 2D6 (weak), 3A4 (weak)

Aspirin: Coadministration of zafirlukast with aspirin results in mean increased plasma levels of zafirlukast by 45%.

CYP2C9 inducers: May decrease the levels/effects of zafirlukast. Example inducers include carbamazepine, phenobarbital, phenytoin, rifampin, rifapentine, and secobarbital.

CYP2C9 substrates: Zafirlukast may increase the levels/effects of CYP2C9 substrates. Example substrates include bosentan, dapsone, fluoxetine, glimepiride, glipizide, losartan, montelukast, nateglinide, paclitaxel, phenytoin, warfarin, and zafirlukast.

Erythromycin: Coadministration of a single dose of zafirlukast with erythromycin to steady state results in decreased mean plasma levels of zafirlukast by 40% due to a decrease in zafirlukast bioavailability.

Theophylline: Coadministration of zafirlukast at steady state with a single dose of liquid theophylline preparations results in decreased mean plasma levels of zafirlukast by 30%, but no effects on plasma theophylline levels were observed. Cases of increased theophylline serum concentrations have been reported.

Warfarin: Coadministration of zafirlukast with warfarin results in a clinically-significant increase in prothrombin time (PT). Closely monitor prothrombin times of patients on oral warfarin anticoagulant therapy and zafirlukast, and adjust anticoagulant dose accordingly.

Ethanol/Nutrition/Herb Interactions Food: Decreases bioavailability of zafirlukast by 40%

Stability Store tablets at controlled room temperature (20°C to 25°C; 68°F to 77°F). Protect from light and moisture; dispense in original airtight container.

Mechanism of Action Zafirlukast is a selectively and competitive leukotriene-receptor antagonist (LTRA) of leukotriene D4 and E4 (LTD4 and LTE4), components of slow-reacting substance of anaphylaxis (SRSA). Cysteinyl leukotriene production and receptor occupation have been correlated with the pathophysiology of asthma, including airway edema, smooth muscle constriction, and altered cellular activity associated with the inflammatory process, which contribute to the signs and symptoms of asthma.

Pharmacokinetics

Absorption: Food reduces bioavailability by 40%

Protein binding: >99%, predominantly albumin

Metabolism: Extensive in the liver

Half-life: 10 hours

Time to peak serum concentration: 2-3 hours

Elimination: Urinary excretion (10%) and feces

Dosage

Geriatrics & Adults: Asthma: Oral: 20 mg twice daily

Renal Impairment:

Dosage adjustment not required.

Hepatic Impairment: Clearance of zafirlukast is reduced with a greater C_{max} and AUC of 50% to 60% in patients with alcoholic cirrhosis.

Administration Administer at least 1 hour before or 2 hours after a meal

Monitoring Parameters Monitor for improvements in air flow; monitor closely for sign/symptoms of hepatic injury; periodic monitoring of LFTs may be considered (not proved to prevent serious injury, but early detection may enhance recovery)

Patient Information Do not use to treat acute episodes of asthma. Do not increase or decrease the dose without consulting your physician.

Special Geriatric Considerations The mean dose (mg/kg) normalized AUC and C_{max} increase and plasma clearance decreases with increasing age. In patients >65 years of age, there is a two- to threefold greater C_{max} and AUC compared to younger adults. Some studies have demonstrated slightly higher adverse effect reports in elderly compared to younger adults: Headache (4.7%), diarrhea and nausea (1.8%), and pharyngitis (1.3%). No changes in dose recommended for elderly.

Dosage Forms Excipient information presented when available (limited, particularly for generics); consult specific product labeling.

Tablet: 10 mg, 20 mg

Zaleplon (ZAL e plon)

U.S. Brand Names Sonata®
Canadian Brand Names Sonata®; Starnoc®
Generic Available No
Pharmacologic Category Hypnotic, Nonbenzodiazepine
Use Short-term (7-10 days) treatment of insomnia (demonstrated to be effective for up to 5 weeks in controlled trial)
Restrictions C-IV
Contraindications Hypersensitivity to zaleplon or any component of the formulation
Warnings/Precautions Symptomatic treatment of insomnia should be initiated only after careful evaluation of potential causes of sleep disturbance. Failure of sleep disturbance to resolve after 7-10 days may indicate psychiatric and/or medical illness.

Use with caution in patients with depression, particularly if suicidal risk may be present. Use with caution in patients with a history of drug dependence. Abrupt discontinuance may lead to withdrawal symptoms. Hypnotics/sedatives have been associated with abnormal thinking and behavior changes including decreased inhibition, aggression, bizarre behavior, agitation, hallucinations, and depersonalization. These changes may occur unpredictably and may indicate previously unrecognized psychiatric disorders; evaluate appropriately. May impair physical and mental capabilities. Patients must be cautioned about performing tasks which require mental alertness (operating machinery or driving). Amnesia can occur. Use with caution in patients receiving other CNS depressants or psychoactive medications. Effects with other sedative drugs or ethanol may be potentiated. Postmarketing studies have indicated that the use of hypnotic/ sedative agents for sleep has been associated with hypersensitivity reactions including anaphylaxis as well as angioedema. An increased risk for hazardous sleep-related activities such as sleep-driving; cooking and eating food, and making phone calls while asleep have also been noted.

Use with caution in the elderly, those with compromised respiratory function, or renal and hepatic impairment. Because of the rapid onset of action, zaleplon should be administered immediately prior to bedtime or after the patient has gone to bed and is having difficulty falling asleep. Capsules contain tartrazine (FDC yellow #5); avoid in patients with sensitivity (caution in patients with asthma).

Adverse Reactions (Reflective of adult population; not specific for elderly)
1% to 10%:
    Cardiovascular: Chest pain, peripheral edema
    Central nervous system: Amnesia, anxiety, coordination impaired, depersonalization, depression, dizziness, fever, hallucination, hypoesthesia, lightheadedness, malaise, migraine, somnolence, vertigo
    Dermatologic: Photosensitivity reaction, pruritus, rash
    Gastrointestinal: Abdominal pain, anorexia, colitis, constipation, dyspepsia, nausea, xerostomia
    Genitourinary: Dysmenorrhea
    Neuromuscular & skeletal: Arthralgia, back pain, myalgia, paresthesia, tremor, weakness
    Ocular: Abnormal vision, eye pain
    Otic: Hyperacusis
    Miscellaneous: Parosmia
Overdosage/Toxicology Symptoms include CNS depression, ranging from drowsiness to coma. Mild overdose is associated with drowsiness, confusion, and lethargy. Serious cases may result in ataxia, respiratory depression, hypotension, hypotonia, coma, and rarely death. Treatment is supportive.
Drug Interactions Substrate of CYP3A4 (minor)
    Cimetidine: May increase zaleplon levels/effects; use 5 mg zaleplon as starting dose in patients receiving cimetidine.
    CNS depressants: Sedative effects may be additive with psychotropics; monitor for increased effect; includes anticonvulsants, antipsychotics, barbiturates, benzodiazepines, opioid analgesics, and other sedative agents.
    Flumazenil: May diminish the sedative effect of zaleplon.
    Rifamycin Derivatives: May decrease the levels/effects of zaleplon.
Ethanol/Nutrition/Herb Interactions
    Ethanol: Avoid ethanol (may increase CNS depression).
    Food: High fat meal prolonged absorption; delayed t_{max} by 2 hours, and reduced C_{max} by 35%.
    Herb/Nutraceutical: St John's wort may decrease zaleplon levels. Avoid valerian, St John's wort, kava kava, gotu kola (may increase CNS depression).
Stability Store at controlled room temperature of 20°C to 25°C (68°F to 77°F). Protect from light.
(Continued)

Zaleplon *(Continued)*

Mechanism of Action Zaleplon is unrelated to benzodiazepines, barbiturates, or other hypnotics. However, it interacts with the benzodiazepine GABA receptor complex. Nonclinical studies have shown that it binds selectively to the brain omega-1 receptor situated on the alpha subunit of the GABA-A receptor complex.

Pharmacodynamics
Peak effect: 1 hour
Duration: ~4 hours

Pharmacokinetics In older adults, no significant difference was seen in pharmacokinetics.
Absorption: Rapid
Bioavailability: 30%
Metabolism: Primarily metabolized by aldehyde oxidase and to a lesser extent inactive metabolites converted to glucuronides
Elimination: In urine, as metabolites.

Dosage
Geriatrics: Reduce dose to 5 mg at bedtime
Adults: Insomnia (short-term use): Oral: 10 mg at bedtime (range: 5-20 mg)
Renal Impairment: No adjustment for mild-to-moderate renal impairment; use in severe renal impairment has not been adequately studied.
Hepatic Impairment: Mild-to-moderate impairment: 5 mg; not recommended for use in patients with severe hepatic impairment.

Monitoring Parameters Mental status

Patient Information May cause drowsiness, dizziness, or lightheadedness. Avoid alcohol and other CNS depressants. Consult prescriber before taking any prescription or OTC medication. Do not operate machinery or drive while taking this medication. Dose should be taken immediately before bedtime or when you are in bed and cannot fall asleep.

Additional Information Prescription quantities should not exceed a 1-month supply. Zaleplon is primarily used to decrease sleep latency.

Special Geriatric Considerations In clinical trials, elderly responded to the 5 mg dose with decreased sleep latency. As with all hypnotics, assess underlying cause of insomnia.

Dosage Forms Excipient information presented when available (limited, particularly for generics); consult specific product labeling.
Capsule: 5 mg, 10 mg [contains tartrazine]

♦ **Zanaflex®** *see* Tizanidine *on page 1581*

Zanamivir *(za NA mi veer)*

U.S. Brand Names Relenza®
Canadian Brand Names Relenza®
Generic Available No
Pharmacologic Category Antiviral Agent; Neuraminidase Inhibitor

Use Treatment of uncomplicated acute illness due to influenza virus A and B; treatment should only be initiated in patients who have been symptomatic for no more than 2 days. Prophylaxis against influenza virus A and B

Unlabeled/Investigational Use Investigational: Prophylaxis against influenza A/B infections

Contraindications Hypersensitivity to zanamivir or any component of the formulation

Warnings/Precautions Patients must be instructed in the use of the delivery system. No data are available to support the use of this drug in patients who begin use for treatment after 48 hours of symptoms. Effectiveness has not been established in patients with significant underlying medical conditions or for prophylaxis of influenza in nursing home patients. Not recommended for use in patients with underlying respiratory disease, such as asthma or COPD, due to lack of efficacy and risk of serious adverse effects. Bronchospasm, decreased lung function, and other serious adverse reactions, including those with fatal outcomes, have been reported in patients with and without airway disease; discontinue with bronchospasm or signs of decreased lung function. For a patient with an underlying airway disease where a medical decision has been made to use zanamivir, a fast-acting bronchodilator should be made available, and used prior to each dose. Not a substitute for the flu vaccine. Consider primary or concomitant bacterial infections. Powder for oral inhalation contains lactose. Safety and efficacy of repeated courses or use with severe renal impairment have not been established.

Adverse Reactions (Reflective of adult population; not specific for elderly)
Most adverse reactions occurred at a frequency which was less than or equal to the control (lactose vehicle).

>10%:
  Central nervous system: Headache (prophylaxis 13% to 24%; treatment 2%)
  Gastrointestinal: Throat/tonsil discomfort/pain (prophylaxis 8% to 19%)
  Respiratory: Cough (prophylaxis 7% to 17%; treatment ≤2%), nasal signs and symptoms (prophylaxis 12%; treatment 2%)
  Miscellaneous: Viral infection (prophylaxis 3% to 13%)
1% to 10%:
  Central nervous system: Fever/chills (prophylaxis 5% to 9%; treatment <1.5%), fatigue (prophylaxis 5% to 8%; treatment <1.5%), malaise (prophylaxis 5% to 8%; treatment <1.5%), dizziness (treatment 1% to 2%)
  Dermatologic: Urticaria (treatment <1.5%)
  Gastrointestinal: Anorexia/appetite decreased (prophylaxis 2% to 4%), nausea (prophylaxis 1% to 2%; treatment ≤3%), diarrhea (prophylaxis 2% to 3%), vomiting (prophylaxis 1% to 2%; treatment 1% to 2%), abdominal pain (treatment <1.5%)
  Neuromuscular & skeletal: Muscle pain (prophylaxis 3% to 8%), musculoskeletal pain (prophylaxis 6%), arthralgia/articular rheumatism (prophylaxis 2%), arthralgia (treatment <1.5%), myalgia (treatment <1.5%)
  Respiratory: Infection (ear/nose/throat; prophylaxis 2%; treatment 2% to 5%), sinusitis (treatment 3%), bronchitis (treatment 2%), nasal inflammation (prophylaxis 1%)

Overdosage/Toxicology Information is limited, and symptoms appear similar to reported adverse events from clinical studies. Treatment should be symptom-directed and supportive

Drug Interactions Influenza virus vaccine: Zanamivir may diminish the therapeutic effect of live, attenuated influenza virus vaccine (FluMist™). The manufacturer of FluMist™ recommends that the administration of anti-influenza virus medications be avoided during the period beginning 48 hours prior to vaccine administration and ending 2 weeks after vaccine.

Stability Store at room temperature (25°C) 77°F. Do not puncture blister until taking a dose using the Diskhaler®.

Mechanism of Action Zanamivir inhibits influenza virus neuraminidase enzymes, potentially altering virus particle aggregation and release.

Pharmacokinetics
  Absorption: 4% to 17% of the inhaled dose
  Distribution: Plasma protein binding <10%
  Metabolism: None
  Half-life, serum: 2.5-5.1 hours
  Elimination: Urine (as unchanged drug); feces (unabsorbed drug)

Dosage
  Geriatrics & Adults: Influenza virus A and B:
    Prophylaxis: Oral inhalation:
      Household setting: Two inhalations (10 mg) once daily for 10 days. Begin within 1½ days following onset of signs or symptoms of index case.
      Community outbreak: Two inhalations (10 mg) once daily for 28 days. Begin within 5 days of outbreak.
    Treatment: Oral inhalation: Two inhalations (10 mg total) twice daily for 5 days. Doses on first day should be separated by at least 2 hours; on subsequent days, doses should be spaced by ~12 hours. Begin within 2 days of signs or symptoms.

Administration Inhalation: Must be used with Diskhaler® delivery device. Patients who are scheduled to use an inhaled bronchodilator should use their bronchodilator prior to zanamivir. With the exception of the initial dose when used for treatment, administer at the same time each day.

Patient Information This is **not** a substitute for the influenza vaccine. Use delivery device exactly as directed; complete full regimen, even if symptoms improve sooner. If you have asthma or COPD you may be at risk for bronchospasm; see prescriber for appropriate bronchodilator before using zanamivir. Stop using this medication and contact your physician if you experience shortness of breath, increased wheezing, or other signs of bronchospasm. You may experience dizziness or headache (use caution when driving or engaging in hazardous tasks until response to drug is known). Report unresolved diarrhea, vomiting, or nausea; acute fever or muscle pain; or other acute and persistent adverse effects.

Additional Information The majority of patients included in clinical trials were infected with influenza A; however, a number of patients with influenza B infections were also enrolled. Patients with lower temperature or less severe symptoms appeared to derive less benefit from therapy. No consistent treatment benefit was demonstrated in patients with chronic underlying medical conditions.

Special Geriatric Considerations A recent study demonstrated that most elderly were unable to use an inhaler device effectively.

Dosage Forms Excipient information presented when available (limited, particularly for generics); consult specific product labeling.
(Continued)

Zanamivir *(Continued)*

Powder for oral inhalation: 5 mg/blister (20s) [4 blisters per Rotadisk® foil pack, 5 Rotadisk® per package; packaged with Diskhaler® inhalation device; contains lactose]

Selected References

Centers for Disease Control, "Prevention and Control of Influenza. Recommendations of the Advisory Committee on Immunization Practices (ACIP)," *MMWR Recomm Rep,* 2005, 54(RR-8):1-40.

Diggory P, Fernandez C, Humphrey A, et al, "Comparison of Elderly People's Technique in Using Two Dry Powder Inhalers to Deliver Zanamivir: Randomised Controlled Trial," *BMJ,* 2001, 322(7286):577-9.

Ziconotide *(zi KOE no tide)*

Medication Safety Issues

High alert medication: The Institute for Safe Medication Practices (ISMP) includes this medication among its list of drugs which have a heightened risk of causing significant patient harm when used in error.

U.S. Brand Names Prialt®

Generic Available No

Pharmacologic Category Analgesic, Nonopioid; Calcium Channel Blocker, N-Type

Use Management of severe chronic pain in patients requiring intrathecal (I.T.) therapy and are intolerant or refractory to other therapies

Contraindications Hypersensitivity to ziconotide or any component of the formulation; history of psychosis; I.V. administration

I.T. administration is contraindicated in patients with infection at the injection site, uncontrolled bleeding, or spinal canal obstruction that impairs CSF circulation

Warnings/Precautions [U.S Boxed Warning]: Severe psychiatric symptoms and neurological impairment have been reported; interrupt or discontinue therapy if cognitive impairment, hallucinations, mood changes, or changes in consciousness occur. May cause or worsen depression and/or risk of suicide. Cognitive impairment may appear gradually during treatment and is generally reversible after discontinuation (may take up to 2 weeks for cognitive effects to reverse). Use caution in the elderly; may experience a higher incidence of confusion. Patients should be instructed to use caution in performing tasks which require alertness (eg, operating machinery or driving). May have additive effects with opiates or other CNS-depressant medications; may potentiate opioid-induced decreased GI motility; does not interact with opioid receptors or potentiate opiate-induced respiratory depression. Will not prevent or relieve symptoms associated with opiate withdrawal and opiates should not be abruptly discontinued. Unlike opioids, ziconotide therapy can be interrupted abruptly or discontinued without evidence of withdrawal.

Meningitis may occur with use of I.T. pumps; monitor for signs and symptoms of meningitis; treatment of meningitis may require removal of system and discontinuation of intrathecal therapy. Elevated serum creatine kinase can occur, particularly during the first 2 months of therapy; consider dose reduction or discontinuing if combined with new neuromuscular symptoms (myalgias, myasthenia, muscle cramps, weakness) or reduction in physical activity. Safety and efficacy have not been established with renal or hepatic dysfunction. Should not be used in combination with intrathecal opiates.

Adverse Reactions (Reflective of adult population; not specific for elderly)

>10%:

Central nervous system: Dizziness (46%), confusion (15% to 33%), memory impairment (7% to 22%), somnolence (17%), ataxia (14%), speech disorder (14%), headache (13%), aphasia (12%; including auditory and visual)

Gastrointestinal: Nausea (40%), diarrhea (18%), vomiting (16%)

Neuromuscular & skeletal: Creatine kinase increased (40%; ≥3 times ULN: 11%), weakness (18%), gait disturbances (14%)

Ocular: Blurred vision (12%)

2% to 10%:

Cardiovascular: Hypotension, peripheral edema, postural hypotension

Central nervous system: Abnormal thinking (8%), amnesia (8%), anxiety (8%), vertigo (7%), insomnia (6%), fever (5%), paranoid reaction (3%), delirium (2%), hostility (2%), stupor (2%), agitation, attention disturbance, balance impaired, burning sensation, coordination abnormal, depression, disorientation, fatigue, fever, hypoesthesia, irritability, lethargy, mental impairment, mood disorder, nervousness, pain, sedation

Dermatologic: Pruritus (7%)

Gastrointestinal: Anorexia (6%), taste perversion (5%), abdominal pain, appetite decreased, constipation, xerostomia

Genitourinary: Urinary retention (9%), dysuria, urinary hesitance

Neuromuscular & skeletal: Dysarthria (7%), paresthesia (7%), rigors (7%), tremor (7%), muscle spasm (6%), limb pain (5%), areflexia, muscle cramp, muscle weakness, myalgia

Ocular: Nystagmus (8%), diplopia, visual disturbance

Respiratory: Sinusitis (5%)

Miscellaneous: Diaphoresis (5%)

Overdosage/Toxicology Exaggerated pharmacological effects, including ataxia, confusion, dizziness, garbled speech, hypotension, nausea, nystagmus, sedation, spinal myoclonus, stupor, unresponsiveness, vomiting, and word-finding difficulty, are reported at doses >19.2 mcg/day. Respiratory depression was not observed. (Inadvertent intravenous or epidural administration may cause hypotension.) In case of overdose, ziconotide can be discontinued temporarily or withdrawn; additional treatment should be symptom-directed and supportive. Opioid antagonists are not effective. Most patients recover within 24 hours of discontinuing ziconotide therapy.

Drug Interactions CNS depressants: Ziconotide may enhance the adverse/toxic effects of other CNS depressants.

Ethanol/Nutrition/Herb Interactions Ethanol: Avoid ethanol (may increase CNS adverse effects).

Stability Prior to use, store vials at 2°C to 8°C (36°F to 46°F). Once diluted, may be stored at 2°C to 8°C (36°F to 46°F) for 24 hours; refrigerate during transit. Do not freeze. Protect from light.

Preservative free NS should be used when dilution is needed.

CADD-Micro® ambulatory infusion pump: Initial fill: Dilute to final concentration of 5 mcg/mL.

Medtronic SynchroMed® EL or SynchroMed® II infusion system: Prior to initial fill, rinse internal pump surfaces with 2 mL ziconotide (25 mcg/mL), repeat twice. Only the 25 mcg/mL concentration (undiluted) should be used for initial pump fill. When using the Medtronic SynchroMed® EL or SynchroMed® II Infusion System, solutions expire as follows:

25 mcg/mL: Undiluted:

Initial fill: Use within 14 days.

Refill: Use within 84 days.

100 mcg/mL:

Undiluted: Refill: Use within 84 days.

Diluted: Refill: Use within 40 days.

Mechanism of Action Ziconotide selectively binds to N-type voltage-sensitive calcium channels located on the nociceptive afferent nerves of the dorsal horn in the spinal cord. This binding is thought to block N-type calcium channels, leading to a blockade of excitatory neurotransmitter release and reducing sensitivity to painful stimuli.

Pharmacokinetics

Distribution: I.T.: V_d: ~140 mL

Protein binding: ~50%

Metabolism: Metabolized via endopeptidases and exopeptidases present on multiple organs including kidney, liver, lung; degraded to peptide fragments and free amino acids

Half-life elimination: I.V.: 1-1.6 hours (plasma); I.T.: 2.9-6.5 hours (CSF)

Excretion: I.V.: Urine (<1%)

(Continued)

Ziconotide *(Continued)*

Dosage

Geriatrics: Refer to adult dosing. Use with caution.

Adults: Chronic pain: I.T.: Initial dose: ≤2.4 mcg/day (0.1 mcg/hour)

Dose may be titrated by ≤2.4 mcg/day (0.1 mcg/hour) at intervals ≤2-3 times/week to a maximum dose of 19.2 mcg/day (0.8 mcg/hour) by day 21; average dose at day 21: 6.9 mcg/day (0.29 mcg/hour). A faster titration should be used only if the urgent need for analgesia outweighs the possible risk to patient safety.

Administration Not for I.V. administration. **For I.T. administration only** using Medtronic SynchroMed® EL, SynchroMed® II Infusion System, or CADD-Micro® ambulatory infusion pump.

Medtronic SynchroMed® EL or SynchroMed® II Infusion Systems:

Naive pump priming (first time use with ziconotide): Use 2 mL of undiluted ziconotide 25 mcg/mL solution to rinse the internal surfaces of the pump; repeat twice for a total of 3 rinses

Initial pump fill: Use only undiluted 25 mcg/mL solution and fill pump after priming. Following the initial fill only, adsorption on internal device surfaces will occur, requiring the use of the undiluted solution and refill within 14 days.

Pump refills: Contents should be emptied prior to refill. Subsequent pump refills should occur at least every 40 days if using diluted solution or at least every 84 days if using undiluted solution.

CADD-Micro® ambulatory infusion pump: Refer to manufacturers' manual for initial fill and refill instructions

Monitoring Parameters Monitor for psychiatric or neurological impairment; signs and symptoms of meningitis or other infection; serum CPK (every other week for first month then monthly); pain relief

Patient Information Avoid driving or operating machinery while on this medication. Avoid alcohol and other CNS depressants. Contact physician if you have new or worsening muscle pain, soreness, weakness, or darkened urine. Report nausea, vomiting, seizure, fever, headache, and/or stiff neck.

Special Geriatric Considerations Manufacturer reports that in all trials there was a higher incidence of confusion in the elderly compared to younger adults.

Dosage Forms Excipient information presented when available (limited, particularly for generics); consult specific product labeling.

Injection, solution, as acetate [preservative free]:

Prialt®: 25 mcg/mL (20 mL); 100 mcg/mL (1 mL, 2 mL, 5 mL)

Selected References

Staats PS, Yearwood T, Charapata SG, et al, "Intrathecal Ziconotide in the Treatment of Refractory Pain in Patients With Cancer or AIDS: A Randomized Controlled Trial," *JAMA*, 2004, 291(1):63-70.

Wermeling D, Drass M, Ellis D, et al, "Pharmacokinetics and Pharmacodynamics of Intrathecal Ziconotide in Chronic Pain Patients," *J Clin Pharmacol*, 2003, 43(6):624-36.

♦ Zilactin-L® [OTC] *see* Lidocaine *on page 904*

Zileuton *(zye LOO ton)*

Related Information

Asthma *on page 1767*

U.S. Brand Names Zyflo®; Zyflo CR™

Generic Available No

Pharmacologic Category 5-Lipoxygenase Inhibitor

Use Prophylaxis and chronic treatment of asthma in adults

Contraindications Hypersensitivity to zileuton or any component of the formulation; active liver disease or transaminase elevations greater than or equal to three times the upper limit of normal (≥3 times ULN)

Warnings/Precautions Not FDA approved for the reversal of bronchospasm in acute asthma attacks, including status asthmaticus; therapy may be continued during acute asthma exacerbations. Hepatic adverse effects have been reported; females >65 years and patients with pre-existing elevated transaminases may be at greater risk. Use caution with history of liver disease or alcoholic cirrhosis.

Adverse Reactions (Reflective of adult population; not specific for elderly)

>10%: Central nervous system: Headache (23% to 25%)

1% to 10%:

Central nervous system: Pain (8%)

Dermatologic: Rash

Gastrointestinal: Dyspepsia (8%), nausea (6%), abdominal pain (5%), diarrhea, vomiting

Hematologic: Leukopenia (1% to 3%)

Hepatic: ALT increased (2% to 3%)

Neuromuscular & skeletal: Asthenia (4%), myalgia (3%)

Respiratory: Pharyngitis, sinusitis, upper respiratory tract infection

Miscellaneous: Hypersensitivity reactions

Frequency not defined:
Cardiovascular: Chest pain
Central nervous system: Dizziness, fever, insomnia, malaise, nervousness, somno-
lence
Dermatologic: Pruritus
Gastrointestinal: Constipation, flatulence
Genitourinary: Urinary tract infection, vaginitis
Neuromuscular & skeletal: Arthralgia, hypertonia, neck pain/rigidity
Ocular: Conjunctivitis
Miscellaneous: Lymphadenopathy

Overdosage/Toxicology Symptoms of overdose in humans are limited. Oral minimum
lethal doses in mice and rats were 500-1000 and 300-1000 mg/kg, respectively
(providing >3 and 9 times the systemic exposure achieved at the maximum recommended human daily oral dose, respectively). No deaths occurred, but nephritis was
reported in dogs at an oral dose of 1000 mg/kg. Treat symptomatically. Institute
supportive measures as required. If indicated, achieve elimination of unabsorbed drug
by emesis or gastric lavage. Observe usual precautions to maintain the airway.
Zileuton is NOT removed by dialysis.

Drug Interactions Substrate (minor) of CYP1A2, 2C9, 3A4; **Inhibits** CYP1A2
(moderate)
CYP1A2 Substrates: Zileuton may increase the levels/effects of CYP1A2 substrates.
Example substrates include aminophylline, fluvoxamine, mexiletine, mirtazapine,
ropinirole, theophylline, and trifluoperazine.
Propranolol: Concomitant use results in a doubling of propranolol AUC and increased
beta-blocker activity. Monitor patient closely; reduce propranolol dose if necessary.
Theophylline: Concomitant use results in an approximate doubling of serum theophylline concentrations. Monitor concentrations closely; reduce theophylline dose.
Warfarin: Concomitant use results in a significant increase in prothrombin time. PT/INR
should be closely monitored; adjust warfarin dose.

Ethanol/Nutrition/Herb Interactions
Ethanol: Avoid ethanol (may increase CNS depression; may increase risk of hepatic
toxicity).
Food:
Zyflo CR™: Improved absorption when administered with food.
Zyflo®: Absorption not improved when taken with food.
Herb/Nutraceutical: St John's wort may decrease zileuton levels.

Stability Store tablets at 15°C to 30°C (59°F to 86°F). Protect from light.

Mechanism of Action Specific 5-lipoxygenase inhibitor which inhibits leukotriene
formation. Leukotrienes augment neutrophil and eosinophil migration, neutrophil and
monocyte aggregation, leukocyte adhesion, increased capillary permeability, and
smooth muscle contraction (which contribute to inflammation, edema, mucous secretion, and bronchoconstriction in the airway of the asthmatic.)

Pharmacokinetics
Absorption: Rapid
Distribution: 1.2 L/kg
Metabolism: Several metabolites in plasma and urine; metabolized by CYP1A2, 2C9,
and 3A4
Half-life elimination: 2.5 hours
Bioavailability: Unknown
Protein binding: 93%
Time to peak, serum: 1.7 hours
Excretion: Urine (~95% primarily as metabolites); feces (~2%)

Dosage
Geriatrics & Adults: Asthma: Oral:
Zyflo®: 600 mg 4 times/day
Zyflo CR™: 1200 mg twice daily
Renal Impairment: Adjustment not necessary in renal failure or with hemodialysis.
Hepatic Impairment: Contraindicated with hepatic dysfunction.

Administration May be administered without regard to meals (ie, with or without food)

Monitoring Parameters Evaluate hepatic transaminases at initiation of and during
therapy with zileuton. Monitor serum ALT before treatment begins, once-a-month for
the first 3 months, every 2-3 months for the remainder of the first year, and periodically
thereafter for patients receiving long-term zileuton therapy. If symptoms of liver
dysfunction (right upper quadrant pain, nausea, fatigue, lethargy, pruritus, jaundice or
"flu-like" symptoms) develop or transaminase elevations >5 times ULN occur, discontinue therapy and follow transaminase levels until normal.

Patient Information This medication is not for an acute asthmatic attack; in acute
attack, follow instructions of prescriber. Do not stop other asthma medication unless
advised by prescriber. Take with meals and at bedtime on a continuous bases; do not
discontinue even if feeling better (this medication may help reduce incidence of acute
(Continued)

Zileuton *(Continued)*

attacks). Avoid alcohol and other medications unless approved by your prescriber. You may experience mild headache (mild analgesic may help); fatigue or dizziness (use caution when driving); or nausea or heartburn (small frequent meals, frequent mouth care, sucking lozenges, or chewing gum may help). Report persistent headache, chest pain, rapid heartbeat, or palpitations; skin rash or itching; unusual bleeding (eg, tarry stools, easy bruising, or blood in stool, urine, or mouth); skin rash or irritation; muscle weakness or tremors; redness, irritation, or infections of the eye; flu-like symptoms; itching; jaundice or dark urine; or worsening of asthmatic condition.

Special Geriatric Considerations No differences in the pharmacokinetics found between younger adults and elderly; no dosage adjustments necessary. However, monitor liver effects closely as with any patient regardless of age.

Dosage Forms Excipient information presented when available (limited, particularly for generics); consult specific product labeling.

Tablet:
Zyflo®: 600 mg
Tablet, extended release:
Zyflo CR™: 600 mg

♦ **Zinacef**® *see* Cefuroxime *on page 275*
♦ **Zincate**® *see* Zinc Sulfate *on page 1700*

Zinc Sulfate *(zink SUL fate)*

Medication Safety Issues
Sound-alike/look-alike issues:
$ZnSO_4$ is an error-prone abbreviation (mistaken as morphine sulfate)

U.S. Brand Names Orazinc® [OTC]; Zincate®

Canadian Brand Names Anuzinc; Rivasol

Index Terms $ZnSO_4$ (error-prone abbreviation)

Generic Available Yes

Pharmacologic Category Trace Element

Use Zinc supplement (oral and parenteral); may improve wound healing in those who are deficient (pressure sores)

Contraindications Hypersensitivity to any component

Warnings/Precautions Do not use undiluted by direct injection into a peripheral vein because of potential for phlebitis, tissue irritation and potential to increase renal loss of minerals from a bolus injection

Adverse Reactions (Reflective of adult population; not specific for elderly)
Frequency not defined.
Central nervous system: Dizziness, restlessness
Gastrointestinal: Diarrhea, gastric ulcers, nausea, vomiting

Ethanol/Nutrition/Herb Interactions Food: Avoid foods high in calcium or phosphorus.

Stability Store oral liquid (injectable used orally) in refrigerator.

Pharmacokinetics
Absorption: Zinc and its salts are poorly absorbed from the gastrointestinal tract (20% to 30%)
Elimination: In feces with only traces appearing in urine

Dosage
Geriatrics & Adults:
Recommended Daily Allowance (RDA): Oral: 15 mg elemental zinc/day
Zinc deficiency: Oral: 110-220 mg zinc sulfate (25-50 mg elemental zinc)/dose 3 times/day
Parenteral TPN: I.V.:
Acute metabolic states: 4.5-6 mg/day
Metabolically stable: 2.5-4 mg/day
Stable with fluid loss from the small bowel: 12.2 mg zinc/L of TPN solution, or an additional 17.1 mg zinc (added to 1000 mL I.V. fluids) per kg of stool or ileostomy output

Monitoring Parameters Skin integrity

Reference Range Serum: 50-150 mcg/dL (<20 mcg/dL as solid test with dermatitis followed by alopecia)

Patient Information Take with food if GI upset occurs, but avoid foods high in calcium, phosphorous or phytate (high fiber foods)

Additional Information Zinc acetate can be used as an alternative to zinc sulfate in patients who cannot tolerate the gastrointestinal irritant effects of the sulfate salt

Special Geriatric Considerations May be useful to promote wound healing in patients with pressure sores.

Dosage Forms Excipient information presented when available (limited, particularly for generics); consult specific product labeling.

Capsule (Orazinc®, Zincate®): 220 mg [elemental zinc 50 mg]

Injection, solution [preservative free]: 1 mg elemental zinc/mL (10 mL); 5 mg elemental zinc/mL (5 mL)

Tablet (Orazinc®): 110 mg [elemental zinc 25 mg]

♦ **Ziox™** see Chlorophyllin, Papain, and Urea on page 293

♦ **Ziox 405™** see Chlorophyllin, Papain, and Urea on page 293

Ziprasidone (zi PRAS i done)

Related Information
Antipsychotic Agents on page 1747
Atypical Antipsychotics on page 1749

U.S. Brand Names Geodon®

Index Terms Zeldox; Ziprasidone Hydrochloride; Ziprasidone Mesylate

Generic Available No

Pharmacologic Category Antipsychotic Agent, Atypical

Use Treatment of schizophrenia; treatment of acute manic or mixed episodes associated with bipolar disorder with or without psychosis; acute agitation in patients with schizophrenia

Unlabeled/Investigational Use Treatment of Tourette's syndrome

Contraindications Hypersensitivity to ziprasidone or any component of the formulation; history (or current) prolonged QT; congenital long QT syndrome; recent myocardial infarction; history of arrhythmias; uncompensated heart failure; concurrent use of other QT_c-prolonging agents including amiodarone, arsenic trioxide, bretylium, chlorpromazine, cisapride, class Ia antiarrhythmics (quinidine, procainamide), dofetilide, dolasetron, droperidol, halofantrine, ibutilide, levomethadyl, mefloquine, mesoridazine, pentamidine, pimozide, probucol, some quinolone antibiotics (moxifloxacin, sparfloxacin, gatifloxacin), sotalol, tacrolimus, and thioridazine

Warnings/Precautions [U.S. Boxed Warning]: Patients with dementia-related behavioral disorders treated with atypical antipsychotics are at an increased risk of death compared to placebo. An increased incidence of cerebrovascular adverse events (including fatalities) has been reported in elderly patients with dementia-related psychosis. Risk may be increased by dehydration; use caution with concurrent diuretics. Ziprasidone is not approved for this indication.

May result in QT_c prolongation (dose related), which has been associated with the development of malignant ventricular arrhythmias (torsade de pointes). Note contraindications related to this effect. Avoid hypokalemia, hypomagnesemia. Use caution in patients with bradycardia. Discontinue in patients found to have persistent QT_c intervals >500 msec. Patients with symptoms of dizziness, palpitations, or syncope should receive further cardiac evaluation. May cause orthostatic hypotension.

May cause extrapyramidal symptoms. Impaired core body temperature regulation may occur; caution with strenuous exercise, heat exposure, dehydration, and concomitant medication possessing anticholinergic effects; not reported in premarketing trials of ziprasidone. Antipsychotic use may also be associated with neuroleptic malignant syndrome (NMS). Use with caution in patients at risk of seizures.

Atypical antipsychotics have been associated with development of hyperglycemia. There is limited documentation with ziprasidone and specific risk associated with this agent is not known. Use caution in patients with diabetes or other disorders of glucose regulation; monitor for worsening of glucose control.

Cognitive and/or motor impairment (sedation) is common with ziprasidone. Use with caution in disorders where CNS depression is a feature. Use with caution in Parkinson's disease. Antipsychotic use has been associated with esophageal dysmotility and aspiration; use with caution in patients at risk of pneumonia (ie, Alzheimer's disease). Caution in breast cancer or other prolactin-dependent tumors; elevates prolactin levels. Use caution in renal or hepatic impairment. Ziprasidone has been associated with a fairly high incidence of rash (5%). Significant weight gain has been observed with antipsychotic therapy; incidence varies with product. Monitor waist circumference and BMI.

The possibility of a suicide attempt is inherent in psychotic illness or bipolar disorder; use caution in high-risk patients during initiation of therapy. Prescriptions should be written for the smallest quantity consistent with good patient care.

Adverse Reactions (Reflective of adult population; not specific for elderly)
Note: Although minor QT_c prolongation (mean 10 msec at 160 mg/day) may occur more frequently (incidence not specified), clinically-relevant prolongation (>500 msec) was rare (0.06%) and less than placebo (0.23%).
(Continued)

Ziprasidone *(Continued)*

>10%:

Central nervous system: Extrapyramidal symptoms (2% to 31%), somnolence (8% to 31%), headache (3% to 18%), dizziness (3% to 16%)

Gastrointestinal: Nausea (4% to 12%)

1% to 10%:

Cardiovascular: Chest pain (5%), postural hypotension (5%), hypertension (2% to 3%), bradycardia (2%), tachycardia (2%), vasodilation (1%), facial edema, orthostatic hypotension

Central nervous system: Akathisia (2% to 10%), anxiety (2% to 5%), insomnia (3%), agitation (2%), speech disorder (2%), personality disorder (2%), psychosis (1%), akinesia, amnesia, ataxia, chills, confusion, coordination abnormal, delirium, dystonia, fever, hostility, hypothermia, oculogyric crisis, vertigo

Dermatologic: Rash (4%), fungal dermatitis (2%)

Endocrine & metabolic: Dysmenorrhea (2%)

Gastrointestinal: Weight gain (10%), constipation (2% to 9%), dyspepsia (1% to 8%), diarrhea (3% to 5%), vomiting (3% to 5%), salivation increased (4%), xerostomia (1% to 5%), tongue edema (3%), abdominal pain (2%), anorexia (2%), dysphagia (2%), rectal hemorrhage (2%), tooth disorder (1%), buccoglossal syndrome

Genitourinary: Priapism (1%)

Local: Injection site pain (7% to 9%)

Neuromuscular & skeletal: Weakness (2% to 6%), hypoesthesia (2%), myalgia (2%), paresthesia (2%), back pain (1%), cogwheel rigidity (1%), hypertonia (1%), abnormal gait, choreoathetosis, dysarthria, dyskinesia, hyper-/hypokinesia, hypotonia, neuropathy, tremor, twitching

Ocular: Vision abnormal (3% to 6%), diplopia

Respiratory: Infection (8%), rhinitis (1% to 4%), cough (3%), pharyngitis (3%), dyspnea (2%)

Miscellaneous: Diaphoresis (2%), furunculosis (2%), flu-like syndrome (1%), photosensitivity reaction, withdrawal syndrome

Overdosage/Toxicology Reported symptoms include somnolence, slurring of speech, and hypertension. Acute extrapyramidal symptoms may also occur. Treatment is symptom-directed and supportive. Not removed by dialysis.

Drug Interactions Substrate (minor) of CYP1A2, 3A4; **Inhibits** CYP2D6 (weak), 3A4 (weak)

Acetylcholinesterase inhibitors (central): May increase the risk of antipsychotic-related extrapyramidal symptoms; monitor.

Amphetamines: Efficacy may be diminished by antipsychotics. In addition, amphetamines may increase psychotic symptoms; avoid concurrent use.

Antihypertensives: Concurrent use of ziprasidone with an antihypertensive may produce additive hypotensive effects (particularly orthostasis).

Carbamazepine: May decrease serum concentrations of ziprasidone (AUC is decreased by 35%); other enzyme-inducing agents may share this potential.

CNS depressants: Sedative effects may be additive with ziprasidone; monitor for increased effect; includes barbiturates, benzodiazepines, opioid analgesics, ethanol, and other sedative agents.

Ketoconazole: May increase serum concentrations of ziprasidone (AUC is increased by 35% to 40%); other CYP3A4 inhibitors may share this potential. QT$_c$ prolongation was not demonstrated.

Levodopa: Ziprasidone may inhibit the antiparkinsonian effect of levodopa; avoid this combination.

Metoclopramide: May increase extrapyramidal symptoms (EPS) or risk.

Potassium- or magnesium-depleting agents: May increase the risk of serious arrhythmias with ziprasidone; includes many diuretics, aminoglycosides, cyclosporine, and amphotericin. Monitor serum potassium and magnesium levels closely.

QT$_c$-prolonging agents: May result in additive effects on cardiac conduction, potentially resulting in malignant or lethal arrhythmias; concurrent use is contraindicated. Includes amiodarone, arsenic trioxide, bretylium, chlorpromazine, cisapride, class Ia antiarrhythmics (quinidine, procainamide), dofetilide, dolasetron, droperidol, ibutilide, levomethadyl, mefloquine, mesoridazine, pentamidine, pimozide, probucol, some quinolone antibiotics (moxifloxacin), sotalol, tacrolimus, and thioridazine.

Ethanol/Nutrition/Herb Interactions

Ethanol: Avoid ethanol (may increase CNS depression).

Food: Administration with food increases serum levels twofold. Grapefruit juice may increase serum concentration of ziprasidone.

Herb/Nutraceutical: St John's wort may decrease serum levels of ziprasidone, due to a potential effect on CYP3A4. This has not been specifically studied. Avoid kava kava, chamomile (may increase CNS depression).

Stability

Capsule: Store at controlled room temperature of 15°C to 30°C (59°F to 86°F).

Vials for injection: Store at controlled room temperature of 15°C to 30°C (59°F to 86°F). Protect from light. Each vial should be reconstituted with 1.2 mL SWI. Shake vigorously. Will form a pale, pink solution containing 20 mg/mL ziprasidone. Following reconstitution, injection may be stored at room temperature up to 24 hours or up to 7 days if refrigerated. Protect from light.

Mechanism of Action Ziprasidone is a benzylisothiazolylpiperazine antipsychotic. The exact mechanism of action is unknown. However, *in vitro* radioligand studies show that ziprasidone has high affinity for D_2, D_3, $5-HT_{2A}$, $5-HT_{1A}$, $5-HT_{2C}$, $5-HT_{1D}$, and alpha$_1$-adrenergic; moderate affinity for histamine H_1 receptors; and no appreciable affinity for alpha$_2$-adrenergic receptors, beta-adrenergic, $5-HT_3$, $5-HT_4$, cholinergic, mu, sigma, or benzodiazepine receptors. Ziprasidone functions as an antagonist at the D_2, $5-HT_{2A}$, and $5-HT_{1D}$ receptors and as an agonist at the $5-HT_{1A}$ receptor. Ziprasidone moderately inhibits the reuptake of serotonin and norepinephrine.

Pharmacokinetics

Absorption: Well absorbed

Distribution: V_d: 1.5 L/kg

Protein binding: 99%, primarily to albumin and alpha-1-acid glycoprotein

Metabolism: Extensively hepatic, primarily via aldehyde oxidase

Bioavailability: Oral (with food): 60% (up to twofold increase with food); I.M.: 100%

Half-life: Oral: 7 hours; I.M.: 2-5 hours

Time to peak: Oral: 6-8 hours; I.M.: ≤60 minutes

Elimination: Feces (66%) and urine (20%) as metabolites; little as unchanged drug (1% urine, 4% feces)

Clearance: 7.5 mL/minute/kg

Dosage

Geriatrics: No dosage adjustment is recommended; consider initiating at a low end of the dosage range, with slower titration.

Adults:

Bipolar mania: Oral: Initial: 40 mg twice daily (with food)

Adjustment: May increase to 60 or 80 mg twice daily on second day of treatment; average dose 40-80 mg twice daily.

Schizophrenia: Oral: Initial: 20 mg twice daily (with food)

Adjustment: Increases (if indicated) should be made no more frequently than every 2 days; ordinarily patients should be observed for improvement over several weeks before adjusting the dose.

Maintenance: Range 20-100 mg twice daily; however, dosages >80 mg twice daily are generally not recommended.

Acute agitation (schizophrenia): I.M.: 10 mg every 2 hours **or** 20 mg every 4 hours (maximum: 40 mg/day). Oral therapy should replace I.M. administration as soon as possible.

Renal Impairment:

Oral: No dosage adjustment is recommended

I.M.: Cyclodextrin, an excipient in the I.M. formulation, is cleared by renal filtration; use with caution.

Ziprasidone is not removed by hemodialysis.

Hepatic Impairment: No adjustment necessary.

Administration Oral: Administer with food.

Monitoring Parameters Vital signs; serum potassium and magnesium; fasting lipid profile and fasting blood glucose/Hgb A_{1c} (prior to treatment, at 3 months, then annually); BMI, personal/family history of obesity, waist circumference; blood pressure; mental status, abnormal involuntary movement scale (AIMS), extrapyramidal symptoms. Weight should be assessed prior to treatment, at 4 weeks, 8 weeks, 12 weeks, and then at quarterly intervals. Consider titrating to a different antipsychotic agent for a weight gain ≥5% of the initial weight. The value of routine ECG screening or monitoring has not been established. Monitor orthostatic blood pressures 3-5 days after initiation of therapy or a dose increase.

Test Interactions Increased cholesterol, triglycerides, eosinophils

Patient Information Use this mediation exactly as directed; do not alter dosage or discontinue without consulting prescriber - may take 2-3 weeks to achieve desired results. Do not share this medication with anyone else. Avoid alcohol, caffeine, grapefruit or grapefruit juice, other prescription or OTC medication unless approved by prescriber. Maintain adequate hydration (2-3 L/day) unless instructed to restrict fluids. You may experience drowsiness, lightheadedness, impaired coordination, dizziness, or blurred vision (use caution when driving or engaging in tasks hazardous tasks until response to drug is known); dry mouth, nausea, or GI upset (small frequent meals, good mouth care, sucking lozenges or chewing gum may help); postural hypotension (rise slowly when changing position from lying or sitting to standing or when climbing stairs); urinary retention (void before taking medication); constipation (increased dietary fiber, fruit or fluids, and increased exercise may help). Report immediately persistent CNS effects (eg, trembling, altered gait or balance, excessive sedation, seizures, unusual muscle or skeletal movements, excessive anxiety, hallucinations, (Continued)

Ziprasidone (Continued)

nightmares, suicidal thoughts, or confusion); swelling or pain in breasts (male or female); altered menstrual pattern; sexual dysfunction; alteration in urinary pattern; vision changes; rash; difficulty breathing; or chest pain or palpitations.

Additional Information Blocks a number of CNS receptors, including dopamine, serotonin, alpha$_1$ adrenergic, and histamine receptors. Also inhibits reuptake of serotonin and epinephrine. Results in improvement in positive and negative symptoms of schizophrenia. The increased potential to prolong QT$_c$, as compared to other available antipsychotic agents, should be considered in the evaluation of available alternatives.

Special Geriatric Considerations Extrapyramidal syndrome symptoms occur less with this agent than phenothiazine and butyrophenone classes of antipsychotics.

Many elderly patients receive antipsychotic medications for inappropriate nonpsychotic behavior. Before initiating antipsychotic medication, the clinician should investigate any possible reversible cause; any stress or stress from any disease can cause acute "confusion" or worsening of baseline nonpsychotic behavior. Most commonly, acute changes in behavior are due to increases in drug dose or addition of a new drug to regimen, fluid electrolyte loss, infection, and changes in environment. Any changes in disease status and any organ system can result in behavior changes.

In the treatment of agitated, demented, elderly patients, authors of meta-analysis of controlled trials of the response to the traditional antipsychotics (phenothiazines, butyrophenones) in controlling agitation have concluded that the use of neuroleptics results in a response rate of 18%. Clearly, neuroleptic therapy for behavior control should be limited with frequent attempts to withdraw the agent given for behavior control. In light of significant risks and adverse effects in elderly population compared with limited data demonstrating efficacy in the treatment of dementia related psychosis, aggression, and agitation, an extensive risk:benefit analysis should be performed prior to use.

Since diabetes is prevalent in elderly, monitor closely when using this agent in this population.

Dosage Forms Excipient information presented when available (limited, particularly for generics); consult specific product labeling.
Capsule, as hydrochloride: 20 mg, 40 mg, 60 mg, 80 mg
Injection, powder for reconstitution, as mesylate: 20 mg

Selected References
American Diabetes Association; American Psychiatric Association; American Association of Clinical Endocrinologists; North American Association for the Study of Obesity, "Consensus Development Conference on Antipsychotic Drugs and Obesity and Diabetes," *Diabetes Care*, 2004, 27(2):596-601.
Schneider LS, Tariot PN, Dagerman KS, et al, "Effectiveness of Atypical Antipsychotic Drugs in Patients With Alzheimer's Disease," *N Engl J Med*, 2006, 355(15):1525-38.

Zoledronic Acid (zoe le DRON ik AS id)

U.S. Brand Names Reclast®; Zometa®
Canadian Brand Names Aclasta®; Zometa®
Index Terms CGP-42446; NSC-721517; Zoledronate
Generic Available No
Pharmacologic Category Antidote; Bisphosphonate Derivative
Use Treatment of hypercalcemia of malignancy, multiple myeloma, bone metastases of solid tumors, Paget's disease of bone
Unlabeled/Investigational Use Prevention of bone loss associated with aromatase inhibitor therapy in postmenopausal women with breast cancer; prevention of bone loss associated with androgen deprivation therapy in prostate cancer; treatment of postmenopausal osteoporosis
Contraindications Hypersensitivity to zoledronic acid, other bisphosphonates, or any component of the formulation

Warnings/Precautions Bisphosphonate therapy has been associated with osteonecrosis, primarily of the jaw; this has been observed mostly in cancer patients, but also in patients with postmenopausal osteoporosis and other diagnoses. Dental exams and preventative dentistry should be performed prior to placing patients with risk factors on chronic bisphosphonate therapy. Invasive dental procedures should be avoided during treatment.

Infrequently, severe (and occasionally debilitating) bone, joint, and/or muscle pain have been reported during bisphosphonate treatment. The onset of pain ranged from a single day to several months. Symptoms usually resolve upon discontinuation. Some patients experienced recurrence when rechallenged with same drug or another bisphosphonate; avoid use in patients with a history of these symptoms in association with bisphosphonate therapy.

May cause hypocalcemia in patients with Paget's disease, in whom the pretreatment rate of bone turnover may be greatly elevated. Hypocalcemia must be corrected before initiation of therapy. Ensure adequate calcium and vitamin D intake during therapy. Use caution in patients with disturbances of calcium and mineral metabolism (eg, hypoparathyroidism, thyroid surgery, malabsorption syndromes).

Adequate hydration is required during treatment (urine output ~2 L/day); avoid overhydration, especially in patients with heart failure.

Reclast®: Use is not recommended in patients with severe renal impairment (Cl_{cr} <35 mL/minute). When used in the treatment of Paget's disease significant renal deterioration has not been observed with the usual 5 mg dose administered over at least 15 minutes.

Zometa®: Use caution in renal dysfunction; dosage adjustment required. In cancer patients, renal toxicity has been reported with doses >4 mg or infusions administered over 15 minutes. Risk factors for renal deterioration include pre-existing renal insufficiency and repeated doses of zoledronic acid and other bisphosphonates. Dehydration and the use of other nephrotoxic drugs which may contribute to renal deterioration should be identified and managed. Use is not recommended in patients with severe renal impairment (serum creatinine >3 mg/dL) and bone metastases (limited data); use in patients with hypercalcemia of malignancy and severe renal impairment should only be done if the benefits outweigh the risks. Renal function should be assessed prior to treatment; if decreased after treatment, additional treatments should be withheld until renal function returns to within 10% of baseline. Diuretics should not be used before correcting hypovolemia. Renal deterioration, resulting in renal failure and dialysis has occurred in patients treated with zoledronic acid after single and multiple infusions at recommended doses of 4 mg over 15 minutes.

Use caution in patients with aspirin-sensitive asthma (may cause bronchoconstriction), hepatic dysfunction, and the elderly.

Adverse Reactions (Reflective of adult population; not specific for elderly)
Note: Percentages reported with Zometa®. In general, the rates of adverse reactions were decreased with Reclast® when used for Paget's disease of the bone.
>10%:
  Cardiovascular: Leg edema (5% to 21%), hypotension (11%)
  Central nervous system: Fatigue (39%), fever (32% to 44%), headache (5% to 19%), dizziness (18%), insomnia (15% to 16%), anxiety (11% to 14%), depression (14%), agitation (13%), confusion (7% to 13%), hypoesthesia (12%)
  Dermatologic: Alopecia (12%), dermatitis (11%)
  Endocrine & metabolic: Dehydration (5% to 14%), hypophosphatemia (12% to 13%), hypokalemia (12%), hypomagnesemia (11%)
  Gastrointestinal: Nausea (29% to 46%), constipation (27% to 31%), vomiting (14% to 32%), diarrhea (17% to 24%), anorexia (9% to 22%), abdominal pain (14% to 16%), weight loss (16%), appetite decreased (13%)
  Genitourinary: Urinary tract infection (12% to 14%)
  Hematologic: Anemia (22% to 33%), neutropenia (12%)
  Neuromuscular & skeletal: Bone pain (55%), weakness (5% to 24%), myalgia (23%), arthralgia (5% to 21%), back pain (15%), paresthesia (15%), limb pain (14%), skeletal pain (12%), rigors (11%)
  Renal: Renal deterioration (8% to 17%; up to 40% in patients with abnormal baseline creatinine)
  Respiratory: Dyspnea (22% to 27%), cough (12% to 22%)
  Miscellaneous: Cancer progression (16%), moniliasis (12%)
1% to 10%:
  Cardiovascular: Chest pain (5% to 10%)
  Central nervous system: Somnolence (5% to 10%)
  Endocrine & metabolic: Hypocalcemia (1% to 10%), hypermagnesemia (2%)
  Gastrointestinal: Dysphagia (5% to 10%), dyspepsia (10%), mucositis (5% to 10%), stomatitis (8%), sore throat (8%)
  Hematologic: Thrombocytopenia (5% to 10%), pancytopenia (5% to 10%), granulocytopenia (5% to 10%)
(Continued)

Zoledronic Acid *(Continued)*

Renal: Serum creatinine increased (grades 3/4: 2%)

Respiratory: Pleural effusion, upper respiratory tract infection (10%)

Miscellaneous: Metastases (5% to 10%), nonspecific infection (5% to 10%)

Overdosage/Toxicology Clinically-significant hypocalcemia, hypophosphatemia, and hypomagnesemia may occur. Doses >4 mg and infusion times <15 minutes are associated with a risk of renal toxicity. Treatment is symptom-directed and supportive.

Drug Interactions

Aminoglycosides: May lower serum calcium levels with prolonged administration. Concomitant use may have an additive hypocalcemic effect.

Nonsteroidal anti-inflammatory drugs (NSAIDs): May enhance the gastrointestinal adverse/toxic effects (increased incidence of GI ulcers) of bisphosphonate derivatives.

Phosphate supplements: Bisphosphonate derivatives may enhance the hypocalcemic effect of phosphate supplements.

Stability

Reclast®: Store at room temperature of 15°C to 30°C (59°F to 86°F). After opening, stable for 24 hours at 2°C to 8°C (36°F to 46°F).

Zometa®: Store vials at 15°C to 30°C (59°F to 86°F). Dilute solution for injection in 100 mL NS or D_5W prior to administration. Solutions for infusion may be stored for 24 hours at 15°C to 30°C (59°F to 86°F). Infusion of solution must be completed within 24 hours.

Mechanism of Action A bisphosphonate which inhibits bone resorption via actions on osteoclasts or on osteoclast precursors; inhibits osteoclastic activity and skeletal calcium release induced by tumors. Decreases serum calcium and phosphorus, and increases their elimination.

Pharmacokinetics

Distribution: Binds to bone

Protein binding: ~22%

Half-life: Triphasic; terminal half-life: 167 hours

Elimination: Urine (44% ± 18% as unchanged drug in 24 hours), feces (<3%)

Dosage

Geriatrics & Adults:

Hypercalcemia of malignancy (albumin-corrected serum calcium ≥12 mg/dL): I.V. (Zometa®): 4 mg (maximum) given as a single dose. Wait at least 7 days before considering retreatment. Dosage adjustment may be needed in patients with decreased renal function following treatment.

Multiple myeloma or metastatic bone lesions from solid tumors: I.V. (Zometa®): 4 mg every 3-4 weeks

Note: Patients should receive a daily calcium supplement and multivitamin containing vitamin D

Paget's disease (Reclast®, Aclasta® [not available in U.S.]): 5 mg infused over at least 15 minutes. **Note:** Data concerning retreatment is not available.

Postmenopausal osteoporosis (unlabeled use): 5 mg every 12 months

Prevention of aromatase inhibitor-induced bone loss in breast cancer (unlabeled use): 4 mg every 6 months

Prevention of androgen deprivation-induced bone loss in nonmetastatic prostate cancer (unlabeled use): 4 mg every 3-12 months

Renal Impairment:

Reclast®: Cl_{cr} <35 mL/minute: Not recommended

Zometa®: Multiple myeloma and bone metastases (at treatment initiation):

Cl_{cr} >60 mL/minute: 4 mg

Cl_{cr} 50-60 mL/minute: 3.5 mg

Cl_{cr} 40-49 mL/minute: 3.3 mg

Cl_{cr} 30-39 mL/minute: 3 mg

Cl_{cr} <30 mL/minute: Not recommended

Zometa®: Hypercalcemia of malignancy (at treatment initiation):

Mild-to-moderate impairment: No adjustment necessary

Severe impairment (serum creatinine >4.5 mg/dL): Evaluate risk versus benefit

Aclasta® [not available in U.S.]: Cl_{cr} >30 mL/minute: No adjustment recommended.

Renal toxicity (during treatment):

Hypercalcemia of malignancy: Evidence of renal deterioration: Evaluate risk versus benefit.

Multiple myeloma and bone metastases: Evidence of renal deterioration: Withhold dose until renal function returns to within 10% of baseline: renal deterioration defined as follows:

Normal baseline creatinine: Increase of 0.5 mg/dL

Abnormal baseline creatinine: Increase of 1 mg/dL

Reinitiate dose at the same dose administered prior to treatment interruption.

Hepatic Impairment: Specific guidelines are not available.

Administration Infuse over 15-30 minutes; do not infuse over <15 minutes. Infuse in a line separate from other medications. Patients should be appropriately hydrated prior to treatment.

Reclast®: If refrigerated, allow to reach room temperature prior to administration.

Monitoring Parameters Prior to initiation of therapy, dental exam and preventative dentistry for patients at risk for osteonecrosis

Reclast®: Alkaline phosphatase, serum creatinine, calcium and mineral levels

Zometa®: Serum creatinine prior to each dose; serum electrolytes, phosphate, magnesium, and hemoglobin/hematocrit should be evaluated regularly. Monitor serum calcium to assess response and avoid overtreatment.

Test Interactions Bisphosphonates may interfere with diagnostic imaging agents such as technetium-99m-diphosphonate in bone scans.

Patient Information This medication can only be administered intravenously. Avoid vitamins during infusion or for 2-3 hours after completion. You may experience some nausea or vomiting (small frequent meals, good mouth care, sucking lozenges, or chewing gum may help) or recurrent bone pain (consult prescriber for analgesic). Report unusual muscle twitching or spasms, severe diarrhea/constipation, acute bone pain, or other persistent adverse effects.

Additional Information Multiple myeloma or metastatic bone lesions from solid tumors: Take daily calcium supplement (500 mg) and daily multivitamin (with 400 int. units vitamin D).

Special Geriatric Considerations This drug requires adequate hydration and adjustments for creatinine clearance for its use. Elderly are often volume depleted secondary to drugs and a blunted thirst reflex. See disease related concerns in Dosage: Renal Impairment.

Dosage Forms Excipient information presented when available (limited, particularly for generics); consult specific product labeling. [CAN] = Canadian brand name

Infusion, solution [premixed]:
Aclasta® [CAN]: 5 mg (100 mL) [not available in U.S.]
Reclast®: 5 mg (100 mL)
Injection, solution:
Zometa®: 4 mg/5 mL (5 mL) [as monohydrate 4.264 mg]

Selected References

Body JJ, "Clinical Research Update: Zoledronate," *Cancer*, 1997, 80(Suppl):1699-701.

Brufsky A, Harker WG, Beck JT, et al, "Zoledronic Acid Inhibits Adjuvant Letrozole-Induced Bone Loss in Postmenopausal Women With Early Breast Cancer," *J Clin Oncol* 2007, 25(7):829-36.

Cheer SM and Noble S, "Zoledronic Acid," *Drugs*, 2001, 61(6):799-805.

Coleman RE and Seaman JJ, "The Role of Zoledronic Acid in Cancer: Clinical Studies in the Treatment and Prevention of Bone Metastases," *Semin Oncol*, 2001, 28(2 Suppl 6):11-6.

Gatti D and Adami S, "New Bisphosphonates in the Treatment of Bone Diseases," *Drugs Aging*, 1999, 15(4):285-96.

Lipton A, Small E, Saad F, et al, " The New Bisphosphonate, Zometa (Zoledronic Acid), Decreases Skeletal Complications in Both Osteolytic and Osteoblastic Lesions: A Comparison to Pamidronate," *Cancer Invest*, 2002, 20 Suppl 2:45-54.

Major PP and Coleman RE, "Zoledronic Acid in the Treatment of Hypercalcemia of Malignancy: Results of the International Clinical Development Program," *Semin Oncol*, 2001, 28(2 Suppl 6):17-24.

Reid IR, Miller P, Lyles K, et al, "Comparison of a Single Infusion of Zoledronic Acid With Risedronate for Paget's Disease," *N Engl J Med*, 2005, 353(9):898-908.

Zolmitriptan (zohl mi TRIP tan)

Medication Safety Issues
Sound-alike/look-alike issues:
Zolmitriptan may be confused with sumatriptan

U.S. Brand Names Zomig®; Zomig-ZMT™

Canadian Brand Names Zomig®; Zomig® Nasal Spray; Zomig® Rapimelt

Index Terms 311C90

Generic Available No

Pharmacologic Category Antimigraine Agent; Serotonin 5-HT$_{1B, 1D}$ Receptor Agonist

Use Acute treatment of migraine with or without aura

Contraindications Hypersensitivity to zolmitriptan or any component of the formulation; ischemic heart disease or Prinzmetal's angina; signs or symptoms of ischemic heart disease; uncontrolled hypertension; symptomatic Wolff-Parkinson-White syndrome or arrhythmias associated with other cardiac accessory conduction pathway disorders; use with ergotamine derivatives (within 24 hours of); use within 24 hours of another 5-HT$_1$ agonist; concurrent administration or within 2 weeks of discontinuing an MAO inhibitor; management of hemiplegic or basilar migraine

Warnings/Precautions Zolmitriptan is indicated only in patient populations with a clear diagnosis of migraine. Not for prophylactic treatment of migraine headaches. Cardiac events (coronary artery vasospasm, transient ischemia, myocardial infarction, ventricular tachycardia/fibrillation, cardiac arrest, and death) have been reported with 5-HT$_1$ agonist administration. Should not be given to patients who have risk factors for CAD (Continued)

Zolmitriptan *(Continued)*

(eg, hypertension, hypercholesterolemia, smoker, obesity, diabetes, strong family history of CAD, menopause, males >40 years of age) without adequate cardiac evaluation. Patients with suspected CAD should have cardiovascular evaluation to rule out CAD before considering zolmitriptan's use; if cardiovascular evaluation negative, first dose would be safest if given in the healthcare provider's office. Periodic evaluation of those without cardiovascular disease, but with continued risk factors should be done. Significant elevation in blood pressure, including hypertensive crisis, has also been reported on rare occasions in patients with and without a history of hypertension. Vasospasm-related reactions have been reported other than coronary artery vasospasm. Peripheral vascular ischemia and colonic ischemia with abdominal pain and bloody diarrhea have occurred. Use with caution in patients with hepatic impairment. Zomig-ZMT™ 2.5 mg tablet contains 2.81 mg phenylalanine.

Adverse Reactions (Reflective of adult population; not specific for elderly) Percentages noted from oral preparations.

1% to 10%:

Cardiovascular: Chest pain (2% to 4%), palpitation (up to 2%)

Central nervous system: Dizziness (6% to 10%), somnolence (5% to 8%), pain (2% to 3%), vertigo (≤2%)

Gastrointestinal: Nausea (4% to 9%), xerostomia (3% to 5%), dyspepsia (1% to 3%), dysphagia (≤2%)

Neuromuscular & skeletal: Paresthesia (5% to 9%), weakness (3% to 9%), warm/cold sensation (5% to 7%), hypoesthesia (1% to 2%), myalgia (1% to 2%), myasthenia (up to 2%)

Miscellaneous: Neck/throat/jaw pain (4% to 10%), diaphoresis (up to 3%), allergic reaction (up to 1%)

Overdosage/Toxicology Treatment is symptom-directed and supportive. It is not known if hemodialysis or peritoneal dialysis is effective.

Drug Interactions Substrate of CYP1A2 (minor)

Cimetidine: Zolmitriptan serum levels increased; avoid concurrent use.

Ergot-containing drugs (dihydroergotamine, methysergide): Concurrent use may lead to vasospastic reactions; separate use by at least 24 hours.

MAO inhibitors: Increase systemic exposure to zolmitriptan. Avoid concurrent use and use within 2 weeks of discontinuing a MAO inhibitor. Selegiline (selective MAO type B inhibitor) does not affect zolmitriptan levels.

Oral contraceptives: Zolmitriptan serum levels increased with concurrent use.

Propranolol: Increases zolmitriptan toxicity.

Serotonergic reuptake inhibitors (eg, SSRIs/SNRIs): Concurrent use of zolmitriptan with these agents may increase the risk of serotonin syndrome; monitor.

Serotonin agonists (eg, triptans): Concurrent use of zolmitriptan with these agents may increase the risk of serotonin syndrome; monitor.

Sibutramine: Concurrent use may lead to serotonin syndrome.

Ethanol/Nutrition/Herb Interactions Ethanol: Limit use (may have additive CNS toxicity).

Stability Store at 20°C to 25°C (68°F to 77°F). Protect from light and moisture.

Mechanism of Action Selective agonist for serotonin (5-HT$_{1B}$ and 5-HT$_{1D}$ receptors) in cranial arteries to cause vasoconstriction and reduce sterile inflammation associated with antidromic neuronal transmission correlating with relief of migraine

Pharmacodynamics Onset of action: Within 30 minutes to 1 hour

Pharmacokinetics

Absorption: Well absorbed

Distribution: V_d: 7 L/kg

Protein binding: 25%

Metabolism: Converted to an active N-desmethyl metabolite which is 2-6 times more potent than zolmitriptan

Bioavailability: 40%

Half-life: 2.8-3.7 hours

Time to peak serum concentrations: Tablet: 1.5 hours; orally-disintegrating tablet and nasal spray: 3 hours

Elimination: Urine (~60% to 65% of the total dose) and feces (30% to 40%)

Dosage

Geriatrics: Refer to adult dosing. No dosage adjustment needed, but elderly patients are more likely to have underlying cardiovascular disease and should have careful evaluation of cardiovascular system before prescribing.

Adults:

Migraine headache:

Oral:

Tablet: Initial: ≤2.5 mg at the onset of migraine headache; may break 2.5 mg tablet in half

Orally-disintegrating tablet: Initial: 2.5 mg at the onset of migraine headache

Nasal spray: Initial: 1 spray (5 mg) at the onset of migraine headache

Note: Use the lowest possible dose to minimize adverse events. If the headache returns, the dose may be repeated after 2 hours; do not exceed 10 mg within a 24-hour period. Controlled trials have not established the effectiveness of a second dose if the initial one was ineffective

Renal Impairment: No dosage adjustment recommended. There is a 25% reduction in zolmitriptan's clearance in patients with severe renal impairment (Cl_{cr} 5-25 mL/minute).

Hepatic Impairment: Administer with caution in patients with liver disease, generally using doses <2.5 mg. Patients with moderate-to-severe hepatic impairment may have decreased clearance of zolmitriptan, and significant elevation in blood pressure was observed in some patients.

Administration Administer as soon as migraine headache starts.

Tablets: May be broken

Orally-disintegrating tablets: Must be taken whole; do not break, crush or chew; place on tongue and allow to dissolve; administration with liquid is not required

Nasal spray: Blow nose gently prior to use. After removing protective cap, instill device into nostril. Block opposite nostril; breathe in gently through nose while pressing plunger of spray device. One dose (5 mg) is equal to 1 spray in 1 nostril.

Patient Information This drug is to be used to reduce your migraine, not to prevent or reduce number of attacks. Remove orally disintegrating tablet from blister package just before using. Place on tongue and allow to dissolve. Do not crush, break, or chew. Regular tablet may be broken in half for use. Do not remove protective cap from nasal spray until ready to use. Do not take within 24 hours of any other migraine medication without first consulting prescriber. Tell prescriber if you have ever had any heart problems (chest pain/pressure, angina, heart attack, high blood pressure, rapid heart-beats), high cholesterol, diabetes, or family history of heart disease. Tell prescriber if you are a smoker, have gone through menopause, or a male >40 years of age. If first dose brings relief, second dose may be taken anytime after 2 hours if migraine returns. If you have no relief with first dose, do not take a second dose without consulting prescriber. Do not exceed 10 mg in 24 hours. You may experience some dizziness or drowsiness; use caution when driving or engaging in tasks requiring alertness until response to drug is known. Frequent mouth care and sucking on lozenges may relieve dry mouth. Report immediately any chest pain, heart throbbing or tightness in throat; swelling of eyelids, face, or lips; skin rash or hives; easy bruising; blood in urine, stool, or vomitus; pain or itching with urination; or pain, warmth, or numbness in extremities.

Additional Information Not recommended if the patient has risk factors for heart disease (high blood pressure, high cholesterol, obesity, diabetes, smoking, strong family history of heart disease, postmenopausal woman, or a male >40 years of age).

This agent is intended to relieve migraine, but not to prevent or reduce the number of attacks. Use only to treat an actual migraine attack.

Special Geriatric Considerations No dosage adjustment needed, but elderly patients are more likely to have underlying cardiovascular disease and should have careful evaluation of the cardiovascular system before prescribing.

Dosage Forms Excipient information presented when available (limited, particularly for generics); consult specific product labeling.

Solution, nasal spray [single dose] (Zomig®): 5 mg/0.1 mL (0.1 mL)

Tablet (Zomig®): 2.5 mg, 5 mg

Tablet, orally disintegrating (Zomig-ZMT™): 2.5 mg [contains phenylalanine 2.81 mg/tablet; orange flavor]; 5 mg [contains phenylalanine 5.62 mg/tablet; orange flavor]

♦ **Zoloft®** see Sertraline on page 1457

Zolpidem (zole PI dem)

Medication Safety Issues
Sound-alike/look-alike issues:
Ambien® may be confused with Ambi 10®

U.S. Brand Names Ambien®; Ambien CR™

Index Terms Zolpidem Tartrate

Generic Available Yes: Excludes extended release

Pharmacologic Category Hypnotic, Nonbenzodiazepine

Use Short-term treatment of insomnia (sleep onset and/or sleep maintenance)

Restrictions C-IV

Contraindications Hypersensitivity to zolpidem or any component of the formulation

Warnings/Precautions Should be used only after evaluation of potential causes of sleep disturbance. Failure of sleep disturbance to resolve after 7-10 days may indicate psychiatric or medical illness. Hypnotics/sedatives have been associated with abnormal thinking and behavior changes including decreased inhibition, aggression, bizarre behavior, agitation, hallucinations, and depersonalization. These changes may occur unpredictably and may indicate previously unrecognized psychiatric disorders; evaluate appropriately. Sedative/hypnotics may produce withdrawal symptoms (Continued)

Zolpidem *(Continued)*

following abrupt discontinuation. Use with caution in patients with depression; worsening of depression, including suicidal ideation has been reported with the use of hypnotics. Intentional overdose may be an issue in this population. The minimum dose that will effectively treat the individual patient should be used. Prescriptions should be written for the smallest quantity consistent with good patient care. Causes CNS depression, which may impair physical and mental capabilities. Effects with other sedative drugs or ethanol may be potentiated. Use caution in the elderly; dose adjustment recommended. Closely monitor elderly or debilitated patients for impaired cognitive or motor performance. Avoid use in patients with sleep apnea or a history of sedative-hypnotic abuse. Postmarketing studies have indicated that the use of hypnotic/sedative agents for sleep has been associated with hypersensitivity reactions including anaphylaxis as well as angioedema. An increased risk for hazardous sleep-related activities such as sleep-driving; cooking and eating food, and making phone calls while asleep have also been noted. Discontinue treatment in patients who report a sleep-driving episode.

Use caution with respiratory disease. Use caution with hepatic impairment; dose adjustment required. Because of the rapid onset of action, administer immediately prior to bedtime or after the patient has gone to bed and is having difficulty falling asleep.

Adverse Reactions (Reflective of adult population; not specific for elderly)
Actual frequency may be dosage form, dose, and/or age dependent
>10%: Central nervous system: Dizziness, headache, somnolence
1% to 10%:
Cardiovascular: Blood pressure increased, chest discomfort/pain, palpitation
Central nervous system: Abnormal dreams, anxiety, apathy, amnesia, ataxia, attention disturbance, body temperature increased, confusion, depersonalization, depression, disinhibition, disorientation, drowsiness, drugged feeling, euphoria, fatigue, fever, hallucinations, hypoesthesia, insomnia, memory disorder, lethargy, lightheadedness, mood swings, sleep disorder, stress
Dermatologic: Rash, urticaria, wrinkling
Endocrine & metabolic: Menorrhagia
Gastrointestinal: Abdominal discomfort, abdominal pain, abdominal tenderness, appetite disorder, constipation, diarrhea, dyspepsia, flatulence, gastroenteritis, gastroesophageal reflux, hiccup, nausea, vomiting, xerostomia
Genitourinary: Urinary tract infection
Neuromuscular & skeletal: Arthralgia, back pain, balance disorder, myalgia, neck pain, paresthesia, psychomotor retardation, tremor, weakness
Ocular: Asthenopia, blurred vision, depth perception altered, diplopia, visual disturbance, red eye
Otic: Labyrinthitis, tinnitus, vertigo
Renal: Dysuria
Respiratory: Pharyngitis, sinusitis, upper respiratory tract infection, throat irritation
Miscellaneous: Allergy, binge eating, flu-like syndrome

Overdosage/Toxicology Symptoms include coma and hypotension. Treatment for overdose is supportive. Rarely is mechanical ventilation required. Flumazenil has been shown to selectively block binding to CNS receptors, resulting in reversal of CNS depression but not always respiratory depression. Hemodialysis is not likely to be of benefit.

Drug Interactions Substrate of CYP1A2 (minor), 2C9 (minor), 2C19 (minor), 2D6 (minor), 3A4 (major)
Antifungal agents (itraconazole and ketoconazole): Itraconazole and ketoconazole may decrease the metabolism of zolpidem; consider using lower dose of zolpidem; monitor closely.
Antipsychotics: Sedative effects may be additive with antipsychotics, including phenothiazines; monitor for increased effect.
CNS depressants: Sedative effects may be additive with other CNS depressants; monitor for increased effect; includes barbiturates, benzodiazepines, opioid analgesics, ethanol, and other sedative agents.
CYP3A4 inducers: CYP3A4 inducers may decrease the levels/effects of zolpidem. Example inducers include aminoglutethimide, carbamazepine, nafcillin, nevirapine, phenobarbital, phenytoin, and rifamycins.
CYP3A4 inhibitors: May increase the levels/effects of zolpidem. Example inhibitors include azole antifungals, clarithromycin, diclofenac, doxycycline, erythromycin, imatinib, isoniazid, nefazodone, nicardipine, propofol, protease inhibitors, quinidine, telithromycin, troleandomycin, and verapamil.
Rifamycin derivatives: May decrease levels/effects of zolpidem.

Ethanol/Nutrition/Herb Interactions
Ethanol: Avoid ethanol (may increase CNS depression).
Food: Maximum plasma concentration and bioavailability are decreased with food; time to peak plasma concentration is increased; half-life remains unchanged. Grapefruit juice may decrease the metabolism of zolpidem.

Herb/Nutraceutical: St John's wort may decrease zolpidem levels. Avoid valerian, St John's wort, kava kava, gotu kola (may increase CNS depression).

Mechanism of Action Structurally dissimilar to benzodiazepines. Selective hypnotic effects (with minor anxiolytic, myorelaxant, and anticonvulsant properties) mediated through selective affinity for the alpha-1 subunit of the omega-1 (benzodiazepine) receptor located on the $GABA_A$ receptor complex. Agonism at this site enhances GABA-ergic chloride conductance hyperpolarizing neuronal membranes thereby reducing the responsiveness to excitatory signals.

Pharmacodynamics
Onset of action: 30 minutes
Duration: 6-8 hours

Pharmacokinetics
Absorption: Rapid
Protein binding: 92%
Metabolism: Hepatic, primarily via CYP3A4 (~60%), to inactive metabolites
Half-life elimination: 2.5-2.8 hours (range 1.4-4.5 hours); Cirrhosis: Up to 9.9 hours
Time to peak, plasma: 2 hours; 4 hours with food
Excretion: As metabolites in urine, bile, feces

Dosage
Geriatrics:
Ambien®: 5 mg immediately before bedtime
Ambien CR™: 6.25 mg immediately before bedtime

Adults: Insomnia: Oral:
Ambien®: 10 mg immediately before bedtime; maximum dose: 10 mg
Ambien CR™: 12.5 mg immediately before bedtime

Renal Impairment: Dose adjustment not required; monitor closely.
Not dialyzable

Hepatic Impairment:
Ambien®: 5 mg
Ambien CR™: 6.25 mg

Administration Ingest immediately before bedtime due to rapid onset of action. Ambien CR™ tablets should not be divided, crushed, or chewed.

Monitoring Parameters Daytime alertness; respiratory and cardiac status; behavior profile

Reference Range 80-150 ng/mL

Patient Information Avoid alcohol and other CNS depressants while taking this medication; for fastest onset, take on an empty stomach; may cause daytime drowsiness

Additional Information Zolpidem causes less disturbances in sleep stages as compared to benzodiazepines; time spent in sleep stages 3 and 4 are maintained; zolpidem decreases sleep latency

Special Geriatric Considerations In doses >5 mg, there was subjective evidence of impaired sleep on the first post-treatment night. There have been few reports of increased hypotension and/or falls in the elderly with this drug. Can be considered a drug of choice in the elderly when a hypnotic is indicated. With Ambien CR™, the adverse event profile of 6.25 mg in elderly patients was similar to the 12.5 mg dose in younger adults. Until there is more experience with this dosage form, use with caution in the elderly.

Dosage Forms Excipient information presented when available (limited, particularly for generics); consult specific product labeling.
Tablet, as tartrate: 5 mg, 10 mg
Ambien®: 5 mg, 10 mg
Tablet, extended release, as tartrate:
Ambien CR™: 6.25 mg, 12.5 mg

Selected References
Holm KJ and Goa KL, "Zolpidem: An Update of Its Pharmacology, Therapeutic Efficacy and Tolerability in the Treatment of Insomnia," *Drugs*, 2000, 59(4):865-89.

Salva P and Costa J, "Clinical Pharmacokinetics and Pharmacodynamics of Zolpidem. Therapeutic Implications," *Clin Pharmacokinet*, 1995, 29(3):142-53.

Simcox DA, "Zolpidem-Associated Falls," *Consult Pharm*, 1995, 10:1378-80.

Zonisamide (zoe NIS a mide)

U.S. Brand Names Zonegran®
Canadian Brand Names Zonegran®
Generic Available Yes
Pharmacologic Category Anticonvulsant, Miscellaneous
Use Adjunct treatment of partial seizures in adults with epilepsy
Unlabeled/Investigational Use Treatment of bipolar disorder
Contraindications Hypersensitivity to zonisamide, sulfonamides, or any component of the formulation
Warnings/Precautions Rare, but potentially fatal sulfonamide reactions have occurred following the use of zonisamide. These reactions include Stevens-Johnson syndrome and toxic epidermal necrolysis, usually appearing within 2-16 weeks of drug initiation. Discontinue zonisamide if rash develops. Chemical similarities are present among sulfonamides, sulfonylureas, carbonic anhydrase inhibitors, thiazides, and loop diuretics (except ethacrynic acid). Use in patients with sulfonamide allergy is specifically contraindicated in product labeling, however, a risk of cross-reaction exists in patients with allergy to any of these compounds; avoid use when previous reaction has been severe.

Decreased sweating (oligohydrosis) and hyperthermia requiring hospitalization have been reported in children. Discontinue zonisamide in patients who develop acute renal failure or a significant sustained increase in creatinine/BUN concentration. Kidney stones have been reported. Use cautiously in patients with renal or hepatic dysfunction. Significant CNS effects include psychiatric symptoms, psychomotor slowing, and fatigue or somnolence. Fatigue and somnolence occur within the first month of treatment, most commonly at doses of 300-500 mg/day. Effects with other sedative drugs or ethanol may be potentiated. Abrupt withdrawal may precipitate seizures; discontinue or reduce doses gradually.

Adverse Reactions (Reflective of adult population; not specific for elderly)
Adjunctive Therapy: Frequencies noted in patients receiving other anticonvulsants:

>10%:
Central nervous system: Somnolence (17%), dizziness (13%)
Gastrointestinal: Anorexia (13%)
1% to 10%:
Central nervous system: Headache (10%), agitation/irritability (9%), fatigue (8%), tiredness (7%), ataxia (6%), confusion (6%), concentration decreased (6%), memory impairment (6%), depression (6%), insomnia (6%), speech disorders (5%), mental slowing (4%), anxiety (3%), nervousness (2%), schizophrenic/schizophreniform behavior (2%), difficulty in verbal expression (2%), status epilepticus (1%), tremor (1%), convulsion (1%), hyperesthesia (1%), incoordination (1%)
Dermatologic: Rash (3%), bruising (2%), pruritus (1%)
Gastrointestinal: Nausea (9%), abdominal pain (6%), diarrhea (5%), dyspepsia (3%), weight loss (3%), constipation (2%), dry mouth (2%), taste perversion (2%), vomiting (1%)
Neuromuscular & skeletal: Paresthesia (4%), weakness (1%), abnormal gait (1%)
Ocular: Diplopia (6%), nystagmus (4%), amblyopia (1%)
Otic: Tinnitus (1%)
Respiratory: Rhinitis (2%), pharyngitis (1%), increased cough (1%)
Miscellaneous: Flu-like syndrome (4%) accidental injury (1%)
Overdosage/Toxicology No specific antidotes are available, experience with doses >800 mg/day are limited. Emesis or gastric lavage, with airway protection, should be done following a recent overdose. General supportive care and close observation are indicated. Renal dialysis may not be effective due to low protein binding (40%).
Drug Interactions Substrate of CYP2C19 (minor), 3A4 (major)
CNS depressants: Sedative effects may be additive with other CNS depressants; monitor for increased effect; includes barbiturates, benzodiazepines, opioid analgesics, ethanol, and other sedative agents.
CYP3A4 inducers: CYP3A4 inducers may decrease the levels/effects of zonisamide. Example inducers include aminoglutethimide, carbamazepine, nafcillin, nevirapine, phenobarbital, phenytoin, and rifamycins.
CYP3A4 inhibitors: May increase the levels/effects of zonisamide. Example inhibitors include azole antifungals, clarithromycin, diclofenac, doxycycline, erythromycin, imatinib, isoniazid, nefazodone, nicardipine, propofol, protease inhibitors, quinidine, telithromycin, and verapamil.
Ethanol/Nutrition/Herb Interactions
Ethanol: Avoid ethanol (may increase CNS depression).
Food: Food delays time to maximum concentration, but does not affect bioavailability.
Stability Store at controlled room temperature 25°C (77°F). Protect from moisture and light.

Mechanism of Action The exact mechanism of action is not known. May stabilize neuronal membranes and suppress neuronal hypersynchronization through action at sodium and calcium channels. Does not affect GABA activity.

Pharmacokinetics

Distribution: V_d: 1.45 L/kg

Protein binding: 40%

Metabolism: Hepatic; forms N-acetyl zonisamide and 2-sulfamoylacetyl phenol (SMAP)

Half-life: 63 hours

Time to peak: 2-6 hours

Elimination: Urine, 62% (35% as parent drug, 65% as metabolites); feces, 3%

Dosage

Geriatrics: Data from clinical trials is insufficient for patients older than 65. Begin dosing at the low end of the dosing range.

Adults:

Adjunctive treatment of partial seizures: Oral: Initial: 100 mg/day. Dose may be increased to 200 mg/day after 2 weeks. Further dosage increases to 300 mg and 400 mg/day can then be made with a minimum of 2 weeks between adjustments, in order to reach steady state at each dosage level. Doses of up to 600 mg/day have been studied, however, there is no evidence of increased response with doses >400 mg/day.

Mania (unlabeled use): Oral: Initial: 100-200 mg/day; maximum: 600 mg/day (Kanba, 1994)

Renal Impairment: Slower titration and frequent monitoring are indicated in patients with renal or hepatic disease. There is insufficient experience regarding dosing/toxicity in patients with estimated GFR <50 mL/minute. Marked renal impairment (Cl_{cr} <20 mL/minute) was associated with a 35% increase in AUC.

Hepatic Impairment: Slower titration and frequent monitoring are indicated.

Administration Capsules should be swallowed whole. Dose may be administered once or twice daily. Doses of 300 mg/day and higher are associated with increased side effects. Steady-state levels are reached in 14 days.

Monitoring Parameters Serum creatinine and CNS side-effect potential

Patient Information May cause drowsiness, especially at higher doses. Do not drive a car or operate other complex machinery until effects on performance can be determined. Avoid alcohol and other CNS depressants. Contact healthcare provider immediately if seizures worsen or for any of the following symptoms: skin rash, sudden back pain, abdominal pain, blood in the urine, fever, sore throat, oral ulcers, or easy bruising. Swallow capsules whole, do not bite or break. It is important to drink 6-8 glasses of water each day while using this medication. Do not stop taking this or other seizure medications without talking to your healthcare professional first.

Special Geriatric Considerations Consider the CNS effects commonly experienced in the first month of therapy.

Dosage Forms Excipient information presented when available (limited, particularly for generics); consult specific product labeling.

Capsule: 25 mg, 50 mg, 100 mg

Zonegran®: 25 mg, 100 mg

♦ **ZORprin**® see Aspirin on page 127

♦ **Zostavax**® see Zoster Vaccine on page 1713

Zoster Vaccine (ZOS ter vak SEEN)

Medication Safety Issues

Both varicella vaccine and zoster vaccine are live, attenuated strains of varicella-zoster virus. Their indications, dosing, and composition are distinct. Varicella is indicated in children to prevent chickenpox, while zoster vaccine is indicated in older individuals to prevent reactivation of the virus which causes shingles. Zoster vaccine is **not** a substitute for varicella vaccine and should not be used in children.

U.S. Brand Names Zostavax®

Index Terms Shingles Vaccine; Varicella-Zoster (VZV) Vaccine (Zoster); VZV Vaccine (Zoster)

Generic Available No

Pharmacologic Category Vaccine

Use Prevention of herpes zoster (shingles) in patients ≥60 years of age

Contraindications Hypersensitivity to any component of the vaccine, including a history of anaphylactic/anaphylactoid reaction to gelatin or neomycin; individuals with blood dyscrasias, leukemia, lymphomas, or other malignant neoplasms affecting the bone marrow or lymphatic systems; primary and acquired immunodeficiency states; those receiving immunosuppressive therapy (including high-dose corticosteroids); active untreated tuberculosis

Warnings/Precautions Not for use in the treatment of active zoster outbreak or in the treatment of postherpetic neuropathy (PHN). Contact dermatitis to neomycin is not a

(Continued)

Zoster Vaccine *(Continued)*

contraindication to the vaccine. Avoid administration in patients with acute febrile illness; consider deferral of vaccination.

Immediate treatment for anaphylactoid reaction should be available during vaccine use; defer vaccination for at least 5 months following blood or plasma transfusions, immune globulin (IgG), or VZIG (avoid IgG or IVIG use for 2 months following vaccination); vaccinated individuals should not have close association with susceptible high-risk individuals (newborns, pregnant women, immunocompromised persons) for 6 weeks following vaccination.

Safety and efficacy in immunosuppressed patients or in patients receiving corticosteroid therapy (including inhaled steroids) have not been evaluated. Vaccination of immunosuppressed individuals may result in more severe manifestations of the attenuated virus (extensive rash or disseminated disease). Concurrent administration with antiviral medications with activity against VZV has not been evaluated. Use in patients with previous history of zoster has not been evaluated. Not for use in patients <60 years of age.

Adverse Reactions (Reflective of adult population; not specific for elderly)
All serious adverse reactions must be reported to the U.S. Department of Health and Human Services (DHHS) Vaccine Adverse Event Reporting System (VAERS) 1-800-822-7967.

>10%: Local: Injection site reaction (48%; includes erythema, tenderness, swelling, hematoma, pruritus, and/or warmth)

1% to 10%:
Central nervous system: Fever (2%), headache (1%)
Dermatologic: Skin disorder (1%)
Gastrointestinal: Diarrhea (2%)
Neuromuscular & skeletal: Weakness (1%)
Respiratory: Respiratory tract infection (2%), rhinitis (1%)
Miscellaneous: Flu-like syndrome (2%)

Drug Interactions

Corticosteroids: In patients receiving high doses of systemic corticosteroids for 14 days, wait at least 1 month between discontinuing steroid therapy and administering vaccine.

Immune globulin (including varicella zoster immune globulin): Do not administer together; vaccination should be deferred for at least 5 months following immune globulin administration. Immune globulins should not be given for at least 2 months following vaccination (unless benefits of use outweigh benefits of vaccination).

Immunosuppressant medications: The effect of the vaccine may be decreased and the risk of varicella disease in individuals who are receiving immunosuppressant drugs may be increased.

Influenza vaccine: Administration with trivalent inactivated influenza vaccine (TIV) did not decrease antibody response to either vaccine.

Stability During shipment, should be maintained at -15°C (5°F) or colder. Store powder in freezer at -15°C (5°F). Protect from light. Store diluent separately at room temperature or in refrigerator. Withdraw entire contents of the vial containing the provided diluent to reconstitute vaccine. Gently agitate to mix thoroughly. Withdraw entire contents of reconstituted vaccine vial for administration. Discard if reconstituted vaccine is not used within 30 minutes. Do not freeze reconstituted vaccine.

Mechanism of Action As a live, attenuated vaccine (Oka/Merck strain of varicella-zoster virus), zoster virus vaccine stimulates active immunity to disease caused by the varicella-zoster virus. Administration has been demonstrated to protect against the development of herpes zoster, with the highest efficacy in patients 60-69 years of age. It may also reduce the severity of complications, including postherpetic neuralgia, in patients who develop zoster following vaccination.

Pharmacokinetics

Onset of action: Seroconversion: ~6 weeks

Duration: Not established; protection has been demonstrated for at least 4 years

Dosage

Geriatrics & Adults: Shingles: Adults ≥60 years: SubQ: 0.65 mL administered as a single dose; there is no data to support readministration of the vaccine

Renal Impairment: No adjustment required.

Administration Do not administer I.V.; inject immediately after reconstitution. Inject SubQ into the outer aspect of the upper arm, if possible. Federal law requires that the date of administration, the vaccine manufacturer, lot number of vaccine, and the administering person's name, title and address be entered into the patient's permanent medical record.

Monitoring Parameters Fever, rash

Patient Information This vaccine is not a treatment for shingles, but may help prevent the occurrence of shingles or reduce the pain if shingles develops despite the vaccination. Avoid other vaccinations for 2 months following this vaccine unless approved by prescriber. Avoid close and/or prolonged contact with highly susceptible individuals (immunocompromised persons) for six weeks following vaccination; there is a rare risk of transmitting the vaccine virus to those who have not had chickenpox. Notify prescriber immediately of any acute reaction to vaccination (eg, difficulty breathing, chest pain, acute headache, rash or difficulty swallowing). May cause mild fever and some redness, pain, or swelling at injection site; consult prescriber if excessive or persisting.

Additional Information Federal law requires that the date of administration, the vaccine manufacturer, lot number of vaccine, and the administering person's name, title and address be entered into the patient's permanent medical record.

The varicella-zoster virus (VZV) is capable of causing two distinct manifestations of infection. Primary infection results in chickenpox (varicella). These infections tend to occur in young children or younger adults. Reactivation of latent infection (painful vesicular cutaneous eruption usually in a dermatomal pattern) occurs in older patients or in immunosuppressed populations. This is commonly referred to as shingles (herpes zoster). Although the vaccines are directed against the same causative organism, healthcare workers should be aware of differences in indications, dosing, populations, and composition of the vaccine. Neither vaccine is intended for administration during active outbreaks.

Special Geriatric Considerations This vaccine is intended for those >60 years of age. This live attenuated vaccine should be used with caution in patients with neoplastic disease or those who are immunosuppressed.

Dosage Forms Excipient information presented when available (limited, particularly for generics); consult specific product labeling.

Injection, powder for reconstitution [preservative free]

Zostavax®: 19,400 plaque-forming units (PFU) [contains gelatin, sucrose, and trace amounts of neomycin]

Selected References

Oxman MN, Levin MJ, Johnson GR, et al, "A Vaccine to Prevent Herpes Zoster and Postherpetic Neuralgia in Older Adults," *N Engl J Med*, 2005, 352(22):2271-84.

APPENDIX TABLE OF CONTENTS

APPENDIX TABLE OF CONTENTS *(Continued)*

ABBREVIATIONS, ACRONYMS, AND SYMBOLS

Abbreviation	Meaning
<	less than
>	greater than
≤	less than or equal to
≥	greater than or equal to
$\overline{aa}$, aa	of each
AA	Alcoholics Anonymous
ABG	arterial blood gases
ac	before meals or food
ACA	Adult Children of Alcoholics
ACLS	advanced cardiac life support
ad	to, up to
a.d.	right ear
ADHD	attention-deficit/hyperactivity disorder
ADLs	activities of daily living
ad lib	at pleasure
AIDS	acquired immune deficiency syndrome
AIMS	Abnormal Involuntary Movement Scale
a.l.	left ear
ALS	amyotrophic lateral sclerosis
AM	morning
AMA	against medical advice
amp	ampul
amt	amount
aq	water
aq. dest.	distilled water
ARC	AIDS-related complex
ARDS	adult respiratory distress syndrome
ARF	acute renal failure
a.s.	left ear
ASAP	as soon as possible
ASA-PS	American Society of Anesthesiologists - Physical Status P1: Normal, healthy patient P2: Patient having mild systemic disease P3: Patient having severe systemic disease P4: Patient having severe systemic disease which is a constant threat to life P5: Moribund patient; not expected to survive without the procedure P6: Patient declared brain-dead; organs being removed for donor purposes
a.u.	each ear
AUC	area under the curve
BDI	Beck Depression Inventory
bid	twice daily
BLS	basic life support
bm	bowel movement
BMI	body mass index
bp	blood pressure
BPH	benign prostatic hyperplasia
BPRS	Brief Psychiatric Rating Scale

ABBREVIATIONS, ACRONYMS, AND SYMBOLS *(Continued)*

Abbreviation	Meaning
BSA	body surface area
c	a gallon
c̄	with
CA	cancer
CABG	coronary artery bypass graft
CAD	coronary artery disease
cal	calorie
cap	capsule
CBT	cognitive behavioral therapy
cc	cubic centimeter
CCL	creatinine clearance
CF	cystic fibrosis
CGI	Clinical Global Impression
CIE	chemotherapy-induced emesis
cm	centimeter
CIV	continuous I.V. infusion
CNS	central nervous system
comp	compound
cont	continue
COPD	chronic obstructive pulmonary disease
CRF	chronic renal failure
CT	computed tomography
d	day
DBP	diastolic blood pressure
d/c	discontinue
dil	dilute
disp	dispense
div	divide
DOE	dyspnea on exertion
DSC	discontinued
DSM-IV	Diagnostic and Statistical Manual
DTs	delirium tremens
dtd	give of such a dose
DVT	deep vein thrombosis
Dx	diagnosis
ECG	electrocardiogram
ECT	electroconvulsive therapy
EEG	electroencephalogram
elix, el	elixir
emp	as directed
EPS	extrapyramidal side effects
ESRD	end stage renal disease
et	and
EtOH	alcohol
ex aq	in water
f, ft	make, let be made
FDA	Food and Drug Administration
FMS	fibromyalgia syndrome
g	gram
GA	Gamblers Anonymous

Abbreviation	Meaning
GAD	generalized anxiety disorder
GAF	Global Assessment of Functioning Scale
GABA	gamma-aminobutyric acid
GERD	gastroesophageal reflux disease
GFR	glomerular filtration rate
GITS	gastrointestinal therapeutic system
gr	grain
gtt	a drop
GVHD	graft versus host disease
h	hour
HAM-A	Hamilton Anxiety Scale
HAM-D	Hamilton Depression Scale
hs	at bedtime
HSV	herpes simplex virus
HTN	hypertension
IBD	inflammatory bowel disease
IBS	irritable bowel syndrome
ICH	intracranial hemorrhage
IHSS	idiopathic hypertrophic subaortic stenosis
I.M.	intramuscular
IOP	intraocular pressure
IU	international unit
I.V.	intravenous
kcal	kilocalorie
kg	kilogram
KIU	kallikrein inhibitor unit
L	liter
LAMM	L-α-acetyl methadol
liq	a liquor, solution
LVH	left ventricular hypertrophy
M.	mix; Molar
MADRS	Montgomery Asbery Depression Rating Scale
MAOIs	monamine oxidase inhibitors
mcg	microgram
MDEA	3,4-methylene-dioxy amphetamine
m. dict	as directed
MDMA	3,4-methylene-dioxy methamphetamine
mEq	milliequivalent
mg	milligram
mixt	a mixture
mL	milliliter
mm	millimeter
mM	millimolar
MMSE	mini mental status examination
MPPP	l-methyl-4-proprionoxy-4-phenyl pyridine
MR	mental retardation
MRI	magnetic resonance imaging
MS	multiple sclerosis
NF	National Formulary
NKA	no known allergies
NMS	neuroleptic malignant syndrome
no.	number

ABBREVIATIONS, ACRONYMS, AND SYMBOLS *(Continued)*

Abbreviation	Meaning
noc	in the night
non rep	do not repeat, no refills
NPO	nothing by mouth
NSAID	nonsteroidal anti-inflammatory drug
NV	nausea and vomiting
O, Oct	a pint
OA	osteoarthritis
OCD	obsessive-compulsive disorder
o.d.	right eye
o.l.	left eye
o.s.	left eye
o.u.	each eye
PANSS	Positive and Negative Symptom Scale
PAT	paroxysmal artrial tachycardia
pc, post cib	after meals
PCP	phencyclidine
PD	Parkinson's disease
PE	pulmonary embolus
per	through or by
PID	pelvic inflammatory disease
PM	afternoon or evening
P.O.	by mouth
PONV	postoperative nausea and vomiting
P.R.	rectally
prn	as needed
PSVT	paroxysmal superventricular tachycardia
PTA	prior to admission
PTSD	post-traumatic stress disorder
PUD	peptic ulcer disease
pulv	a powder
PVD	peripheral vascular disease
q	every
qad	every other day
qd	every day, daily
qh	every hour
qid	four times a day
qod	every other day
qs	a sufficient quantity
qs ad	a sufficient quantity to make
qty	quantity
qv	as much as you wish
RA	rheumatoid arthritis
REM	rapid eye movement
Rx	take, a recipe
rep	let it be repeated
s̄	without
sa	according to art
SAH	subarachnoid hemorrhage
sat	saturated
SBE	subacute bacterial endocarditis

Abbreviation	Meaning
SBP	systolic blood pressure
SIADH	syndrome of inappropriate antidiuretic hormone secretion
sig	label, or let it be printed
SL	sublingual
SLE	systemic lupus erythematosus
SOB	shortness of breath
sol	solution
solv	dissolve
$\overline{ss}$	one-half
sos	if there is need
SSKI	saturated solution of potassium iodide
SSRIs	selective serotonin reuptake inhibitors
stat	at once, immediately
STD	sexually transmitted disease
SubQ	subcutaneous
supp	suppository
SVT	supraventricular tachycardia
Sx	symptom
syr	syrup
tab	tablet
tal	such
TCA	tricyclic antidepressant
TD	tardive dyskinesia
tid	three times a day
TKO	to keep open
TPN	total parenteral nutrition
tr, tinct	tincture
trit	triturate
tsp	teaspoonful
Tx	treatment
ULN	upper limits of normal
ung	ointment
URI	upper respiratory infection
USAN	United States Adopted Names
USP	United States Pharmacopeia
UTI	urinary tract infection
u.d., ut dict	as directed
v.o.	verbal order
VTE	venous thromboembolism
VZV	varicella zoster virus
w.a.	while awake
x3	3 times
x4	4 times
YBOC	Yale Brown Obsessive-Compulsive Scale
YMRS	Young Mania Rating Scale

BODY SURFACE AREA (BSA)

$$\text{BSA (m}^2) = \frac{kg^{0.425} \times cm^{0.725} \times 71.84}{10,000}$$

or

$$\log \text{BSA (m}^2) = \frac{(\log kg \times 0.425) + (\log cm \times 0.725) + 1.8564}{10,000}$$

DuBois D and DuBois EF, "A Formula to Estimate the Approximate Surface Area if Height and Weight Be Known," *Arch Intern Med*, 1916, 17:863-71.

$$\text{BSA (m}^2) = \sqrt{\frac{\text{ht (in)} \times \text{wt (lb)}}{3131}} \quad \textit{or} \quad \text{BSA (m}^2) = \sqrt{\frac{\text{ht (cm)} \times \text{wt (kg)}}{3600}}$$

Lam TK and Leung DT, "More on Simplified Calculation of Body-Surface Area," *N Engl J Med*, 1988, 318(17):1130 (letter).

Mosteller RD, "Simplified Calculation of Body Surface Area," *N Engl J Med*, 1987, 317:1098 (letter).

BODY MASS INDEX (BMI)

$$\text{BMI} = \frac{\text{weight (kg)}}{[\text{height (m)}]^2}$$

CALCULATIONS

Ideal Body Weight

Adults (18 years and older) (IBW is in kg)

IBW (male) = 50 + (2.3 x height in inches over 5 feet)
IBW (female) = 45.5 + (2.3 x height in inches over 5 feet)

Lean Body Weight

Adults: Determination of lean body weight (LBW) in kg.

LBW = IBW + 0.4 (actual body weight - IBW)

Millimoles and Millequivalents

Definitions

mole	=	gram molecular weight of a substance (aka molar weight)
millimole (mM)	=	milligram molecular weight of a substance (a millimole is 1/1000 of a mole)
equivalent weight	=	gram weight of a substance which will combine with or replace 1 gram (1 mole) of hydrogen; an equivalent weight can be determined by dividing the molar weight of a substance by its ionic valence
milliequivalent (mEq)	=	milligram weight of a substance which will combine with or replace 1 milligram (1 millimole) of hydrogen (a milliequivalent is 1/1000 of an equivalent)

Calculations

moles	=	$\dfrac{\text{weight of a substance (grams)}}{\text{molecular weight of that substance (grams)}}$
millimoles	=	$\dfrac{\text{weight of a substance (milligrams)}}{\text{molecular weight of that substance (milligrams)}}$
equivalents	=	moles x valence of ion
milliequivalents	=	millimoles x valence of ion
moles	=	$\dfrac{\text{equivalents}}{\text{valence of ion}}$
millimoles	=	$\dfrac{\text{milliequivalents}}{\text{valence of ion}}$
millimoles	=	moles x 1000
milliequivalents	=	equivalents x 1000

Note: Use of equivalents and milliequivalents is valid only for those substances which have fixed ionic valences (eg, sodium, potassium, calcium, chlorine, magnesium bromine, etc). For substances with variable ionic valences (eg, phosphorous), a reliable equivalent value cannot be determined. In these instances, one should calculate millimoles (which are fixed and reliable) rather than milliequivalents.

CALCULATIONS (Continued)

Approximate Milliequivalents – Weights of Selected Ions

Salt	mEq/g Salt	Mg Salt/mEq
Calcium carbonate [$CaCO_3$]	20	50
Calcium chloride [$CaCl_2 \cdot 2H_2O$]	14	74
Calcium gluceptate [$Ca(C_7H_{13}O_8)_2$]	4	245
Calcium gluconate [$Ca(C_6H_{11}O_7)_2 \cdot H_2O$]	5	224
Calcium lactate [$Ca(C_3H_5O_3)_2 \cdot 5H_2O$]	7	154
Magnesium gluconate [$Mg(C_6H_{11}O_7)_2 \cdot H_2O$]	5	216
Magnesium oxide [MgO]	50	20
Magnesium sulfate [$MgSO_4$]	17	60
Magnesium sulfate [$MgSO_4 \cdot 7H_2O$]	8	123
Potassium acetate [$K(C_2H_3O_2)$]	10	98
Potassium chloride [KCl]	13	75
Potassium citrate [$K_3(C_6H_5O_7) \cdot H_2O$]	9	108
Potassium iodide [KI]	6	166
Sodium acetate [$Na(C_2H_3O_2)$]	12	82
Sodium acetate [$Na(C_2H_3O_2) \cdot 3H_2O$]	7	136
Sodium bicarbonate [$NaHCO_3$]	12	84
Sodium chloride [$NaCl$]	17	58
Sodium citrate [$Na_3(C_6H_5O_7) \cdot 2H_2O$]	10	98
Sodium iodine [NaI]	7	150
Sodium lactate [$Na(C_3H_5O_3)$]	9	112
Zinc sulfate [$ZnSO_4 \cdot 7H_2O$]	7	144

Valences and Approximate Weights of Selected Ions

Substance	Electrolyte	Valence	Ionic Wt
Calcium	Ca^{++}	2	40
Chloride	Cl^-	1	35.5
Magnesium	Mg^{++}	2	24
Phosphate	PO_4^{---}	3	95[1]
	HPO_4^{--}	2	96
	$H_2PO_4^-$	1	97
Potassium	K^+	1	39
Sodium	Na^+	1	23
Sulfate	SO_4^{--}	2	96[1]

[1]The atomic weight of phosphorus is 31, and of sulfur is 32.

CONVERSIONS

Apothecary-Metric Exact Equivalents

1 gram (g)	=	15.43 grains		0.1 mg	=	1/600 gr
1 milliliter (mL)	=	16.23 minims		0.12 mg	=	1/500 gr
1 grain (gr)	=	64.8 milligrams		0.15 mg	=	1/400 gr
1 fluid ounce (fl. oz)	=	29.57 mL		0.2 mg	=	1/300 gr
1 pint (pt)	=	473.2 mL		0.3 mg	=	1/200 gr
1 ounce (oz)	=	28.35 grams		0.4 mg	=	1/150 gr
1 pound (lb)	=	453.6 grams		0.5 mg	=	1/120 gr
1 kilogram (kg)	=	2.2 pounds		0.6 mg	=	1/100 gr
1 quart (qt)	=	946.4 mL		0.8 mg	=	1/80 gr
				1 mg	=	1/65 gr

Apothecary-Metric Approximate Equivalents[1]

Liquids			Solids		
1 teaspoonful	=	5 mL	1/4 grain	=	15 mg
1 tablespoonful	=	15 mL	1/2 grain	=	30 mg
			1 grain	=	60 mg
			1 1/2 grain	=	100 mg
			5 grains	=	300 mg
			10 grains	=	600 mg

[1]Use exact equivalents for compounding and calculations requiring a high degree of accuracy.

Pounds-Kilograms

1 pound = 0.45359 kilograms
1 kilogram = 2.2 pounds

Temperature

Celsius to Fahrenheit = (°C x 9/5) + 32 = °F
Fahrenheit to Celsius = (°F - 32) x 5/9 = °C

ANTIMICROBIAL ACTIVITY AGAINST SELECTED ORGANISMS

KEY TO TABLE

- **A** Recommended drug therapy
- **B** Alternate drug therapy
- **C** Organism is usually or always sensitive to this agent
- **D** Organism portrays variable sensitivity to this agent
- (Blank) This drug should not be used for this organism or insufficient data is available

GRAM-POSITIVE AEROBES

Class	Drug	Listeria monocytogenes	Corynebacterium jeikeium	Corynebacterium sp	Streptococcus, Viridans Group	Streptococcus pneumoniae	Streptococcus bovis (Group D)	Enterococcus sp	Streptococcus pyogenes (Group A)	Streptococcus agalactiae (Group B)	Staphylococcus epidermidis: Methicillin-Susceptible	Staphylococcus epidermidis: Methicillin-Resistant	Staphylococcus aureus: Methicillin-Susceptible	Staphylococcus aureus: Methicillin-Resistant
Penicillins	Amoxicillin				C	C	C		C	C				
	Ampicillin	A			C	C	C	A	C	C				
	Penicillin G	A	B	B	A	A	A	A	A	A				
	Penicillin V			C	C	C	C	C	C	C				
	Azlocillin													
	Mezlocillin				D	C	D	D	C	C				
	Piperacillin				D	C	D	C	C	C				
	Ticarcillin				D	C	D		C	C				
	Cloxacillin				D						D		A	A
	Dicloxacillin				D						D		A	A
	Methicillin				D						D		A	A
	Nafcillin				D						D		A	A
	Oxacillin				D						D		A	A
Penicillin-Related Antibiotics	Amoxicillin/Clavulanate	C			C	C	C	C	C	C	C		C	
	Ampicillin/Sulbactam	C			C	C	C	C	C	C	C		C	
	Ticarcillin/Clavulanate				C	C	C	D	C	C	C		C	
	Aztreonam													
	Imipenem/Cilastatin				C	C	C	D	C	C	C		C	
	Meropenem				C	C	C		C	C	C		C	
	Piperacillin/Tazobactam				C	C	C	C	C	C	C		C	
Other Antibiotics	Chloramphenicol	C				B		D						
	Clindamycin		D	D	C				C	C	B		B	
	Co-trimoxazole	B				C					B	C	B	C
	Daptomycin				C	C	D	C	C	C	C	C	C	C
	Linezolid				C	C		C	C	C	C	C	C	C
	Metronidazole													
	Quinupristin/Dalfopristin							D	C	C	C	C	C	C
	Rifampin			D							A	C	A	C
	Sulfonamides													
	Tetracyclines	C			C	C				C			A	D
	Tigecycline				C	C		C	C	C	C	C	C	C
	Vancomycin	D	A		B	B	B	B	B	B	A	B	A	B
UTI Agents	Indanyl Carbenicillin							D						
	Nitrofurantoin							D						

KEY TO TABLE

- **A** Recommended drug therapy
- **B** Alternate drug therapy
- **C** Organism is usually or always sensitive to this agent
- **D** Organism portrays variable sensitivity to this agent
- (Blank) This drug should not be used for this organism or insufficient data is available

GRAM-POSITIVE AEROBES

Class	Drug	Listeria monocytogenes	Corynebacterium jeikeium	Corynebacterium sp.	Streptococcus, Viridans Group	Streptococcus pneumoniae	Streptococcus bovis (Group D)	Enterococcus sp. (Group D)	Streptococcus agalactiae (Group B)	Streptococcus pyogenes (Group A)	Staphylococcus epidermidis: Methicillin-Resistant	Staphylococcus epidermidis: Methicillin-Susceptible	Staphylococcus aureus: Methicillin-Resistant	Staphylococcus aureus: Methicillin-Susceptible
1st Generation	Cefadroxil				B	B	C		B	B		B		B
1st Generation	Cefazolin				B	B	C		B	B		B		B
1st Generation	Cephalexin				B	B	C		B	B		B		B
1st Generation	Cephalothin				B	B	C		B	B		B		B
1st Generation	Cephapirin				B	B	C		B	B		B		B
2nd Generation and others	Cefaclor				C	C	C		C	C		D		D
2nd Generation and others	Cefamandole				C	C	C		C	C		C		C
2nd Generation and others	Cefmetazole				C	C	C		C	C		D		D
2nd Generation and others	Cefonicid				C	C	C		C	C		D		D
2nd Generation and others	Cefotetan				C	C	C		C	C		D		D
2nd Generation and others	Cefoxitin				C	C	C		C	C		D		D
2nd Generation and others	Cefpodoxime Proxetil				C	C	C		C	C		D		D
2nd Generation and others	Cefprozil				C	C	D		C	C				D
2nd Generation and others	Ceftibuten					D			C	C				
2nd Generation and others	Cefuroxime				C	C	C		C	C		D		D
2nd Generation and others	Cefuroxime Axetil				C	C			C	C		C		C
2nd Generation and others	Loracarbef				C	C	D		C	C		C		C
3rd Generation	Cefepime				C	C			C	C		C		C
3rd Generation	Cefixime				D	D			C	C				
3rd Generation	Cefoperazone				D	D	C		C	C		D		D
3rd Generation	Cefotaxime				D	D	C		C	C		D		D
3rd Generation	Ceftazidime				D		D		D	D				
3rd Generation	Ceftizoxime				D	D	C		C	C		D		D
3rd Generation	Ceftriaxone				C	C	C		C	C		D		D
Aminoglycosides	Amikacin	C	C				D	D						
Aminoglycosides	Gentamicin	A	B		A		D	A			A	D	A	D
Aminoglycosides	Netilmicin	C	C					C						
Aminoglycosides	Streptomycin						D	C						
Aminoglycosides	Tobramycin	C	C					D						D
Macrolides	Azithromycin	C			C	C			C	C				C
Macrolides	Clarithromycin	C			C	C			C	C				C
Macrolides	Dirithromycin	C			C	C			C	C				C
Macrolides	Erythromycin	C	C	A	C	B			B	B				C
Quinolones	Ciprofloxacin		D		D	D	D	D	D	D	D	D	D	D
Quinolones	Gatifloxacin				C	C	C	D	C	C		C		C
Quinolones	Levofloxacin				C	C	C	D	C	C	D	C	D	C
Quinolones	Moxifloxacin				C	C	C	D	C	C		C		C
Quinolones	Norfloxacin										D	D		
Quinolones	Ofloxacin		D			D	D	D	D	D	D	D	D	D

ANTIMICROBIAL ACTIVITY AGAINST SELECTED ORGANISMS (Continued)

KEY TO TABLE

- **A** — Recommended drug therapy
- **B** — Alternate drug therapy
- **C** — Organism is usually or always sensitive to this agent
- **D** — Organism portrays variable sensitivity to this agent
- (Blank) This drug should not be used for this organism or insufficient data is available

	GRAM-NEGATIVE AEROBES													
	Enteric bacilli											Cocci		
Drug	Yersinia enterocolitica	Shigella sp	Serratia sp	Salmonella sp	Providencia sp	Proteus sp	Proteus mirabilis	Klebsiella pneumoniae	Escherichia coli	Enterobacter sp[1]	Citrobacter sp[1]	Neisseria meningitidis	Neisseria gonorrhoeae	Moraxella (Branhamella) catarrhalis
Penicillin														
Amoxicillin				B			A		C			C	D	
Ampicillin		A		B			A		A			C	D	
Penicillin G												A	D	
Penicillin V													D	
Azlocillin														
Mezlocillin			A		B	B	C	B	C	A	A		D	
Piperacillin			A		B	B	C	B	C	A	A		D	
Ticarcillin			A		B	B	C	D	C	A	A		D	
Cloxacillin														
Dicloxacillin														
Methicillin														
Nafcillin														
Oxacillin														
Penicillin-Related Antibiotics														
Amoxicillin/Clavulanate				C			C	C	C			C	C	A
Ampicillin/Sulbactam		C		C			C	C	C			C	C	C
Ticarcillin/Clavulanate			A	C	C	B	C	B	C	A	A	C	C	C
Aztreonam			B	C	C	C	C	B	C	A	C		C	C
Imipenem/Cilastatin			B	C	B	B	B	B	C	B	B	D	C	C
Meropenem		C	B	C	B	B	B	B	C	B	B	C	C	C
Piperacillin/Tazobactam		C	A	C	B	B	B	B	C	A	A	C	C	C
Other Antibiotics														
Chloramphenicol	C			B						C		B		
Clindamycin														
Co-trimoxazole	C	A	C	B	A	C	B	C	A	C	C			A
Daptomycin														
Linezolid														
Metronidazole														
Quinupristin/Dalfopristin														
Rifampin												D		
Sulfonamides			C	C				C	C	C		D		
Tetracyclines	C	C						C	C		D	C	B	C
Tigecycline			C	C	C			C	C	C	C		C	
Vancomycin														
UTI Agents														
Indanyl Carbenicillin			C			C	C	C	C	C	C			
Nitrofurantoin								C	C	C	C			

[1] Citrobacter freundii, Citrobacter diversus, Enterobacter cloacae and Enterobacter aerogenes often have significantly different antibiotic sensitivity patterns. Speciation and susceptibility testing are particularly important.

KEY TO TABLE

A — Recommended drug therapy

B — Alternate drug therapy

C — Organism is usually or always sensitive to this agent

D — Organism portrays variable sensitivity to this agent

(Blank) This drug should not be used for this organism or insufficient data is available

GRAM-NEGATIVE AEROBES

	Enteric bacilli											Cocci		
Drug	*Yersinia enterocolitica*	*Shigella* sp.	*Serratia* sp.	*Salmonella* sp.	*Providencia* sp.	*Proteus* sp.	*Proteus mirabilis*	*Klebsiella pneumoniae*	*Escherichia coli*	*Enterobacter* sp.[1]	*Citrobacter* sp.[1]	*Neisseria meningitidis*	*Neisseria gonorrhoeae*	*Moraxella (Branhamella) catarrhalis*
1st Generation														
Cefadroxil							A	A	B					D
Cefazolin							A	A	B					D
Cephalexin							A	A	B					D
Cephalothin							A	A	B					D
Cephapirin							A	A	B					D
2nd Generation and others														
Cefaclor							C	A	B				C	B
Cefamandole						D	C	A	B				C	B
Cefmetazole	D	C	C		C	D	C	A	B				C	B
Cefonicid							C	A	B				C	B
Cefotetan	C	C	C		C	D	C	A	B				C	B
Cefoxitin				D	C	D	C	A	B				C	B
Cefpodoxime Proxetil							C	A	B				C	B
Cefprozil			C				C	D	B				C	B
Ceftibuten														
Cefuroxime	C	C				D	C	A	B				C	B
Cefuroxime Axetil							C	A	B			C	C	B
Loracarbef							C	C	B			C	C	B
3rd Generation														
Cefepime			C	C	C	C	C	C	C	B	B			C
Cefixime			C	C			C	C	A				C	B
Cefoperazone		B	A	A	A	A	C	A	A	B	B			B
Cefotaxime	A	B	A	A	A	A	C	A	A	B	B	B	C	B
Ceftazidime		B	A		A	A	C	A	A	B	B			B
Ceftizoxime	A	B	A	A	A	A	C	A	A	B	B	B		B
Ceftriaxone	A	B	A	A	A	A	C	A	A	B	B	B	C	B
Aminoglycosides														
Amikacin	A		C			C	C	C	C	C	C			
Gentamicin	A	D	C	D	D	C	C	C	C	C	C			
Netilmicin	A	D	C	D	D	C	C	C	C	C	C			
Streptomycin					D									
Tobramycin	A		C	D	D	C	C	C	C	C	C			
Macrolides														
Azithromycin													C	C
Clarithromycin													C	C
Dirithromycin														
Erythromycin													D	C
Quinolones														
Ciprofloxacin	C	B	C	B	C	C	C	C	C	B	B	C	A	C
Gatifloxacin								C	C	B	B			C
Levofloxacin	C	C	C	C	C	C	C	C	C	B	D	C	C	C
Moxifloxacin								C	C	B	B			C
Norfloxacin	C	C	C	C	C	C	C	C	C	B	B			C
Ofloxacin	C	C	C	C	C	C	C	C	C	B	B	C	A	C

[1] *Citrobacter freundii, Citrobacter diversus, Enterobacter cloacae* and *Enterobacter aerogenes* often have significantly different antibiotic sensitivity patterns. Speciation and susceptibility testing are particularly important

ANTIMICROBIAL ACTIVITY AGAINST SELECTED ORGANISMS (Continued)

KEY TO TABLE

- **A** Recommended drug therapy
- **B** Alternate drug therapy
- **C** Organism is usually or always sensitive to this agent
- **D** Organism portrays variable sensitivity to this agent
- (Blank) This drug should not be used for this organism or insufficient data is available

GRAM-NEGATIVE AEROBES — Other bacilli

Class	Drug	Vibrio cholerae	Stenotrophomonas maltophilia	Pseudomonas aeruginosa	Pasteurella multocida	Legionella pneumophila	Haemophilus influenzae	Haemophilus ducreyi	Gardnerella vaginalis	Francisella tularensis	Campylobacter jejuni	Brucella sp.	Bordetella pertussis	Alcaligenes	Acinetobacter sp.
Penicillin	Amoxicillin				C		B	C							
	Ampicillin				C		B	B		D					
	Penicillin G				A										
	Penicillin V				C										
	Azlocillin														
	Mezlocillin			A	C		D								A
	Piperacillin			A	C		D								A
	Ticarcillin			A	C		D								A
	Cloxacillin														
	Dicloxacillin														
	Methicillin														
	Nafcillin														
	Oxacillin														
Penicillin-Related Antibiotics	Amoxicillin/Clavulanate				B		B	B	C						C
	Ampicillin/Sulbactam				B		C	C	C						C
	Ticarcillin/Clavulanate		B	A	C		C								A
	Aztreonam			C			C								B
	Imipenem/Cilastatin			B			C								B
	Meropenem			B	C		C				C				B
	Piperacillin/Tazobactam			A	C		C								A
Other Antibiotics	Chloramphenicol		C		C		B			A	C	C			
	Clindamycin										C	C			
	Co-trimoxazole	A	A				A	B				B	A		
	Daptomycin														
	Linezolid			C											
	Metronidazole								A						
	Quinupristin/Dalfopristin														
	Rifampin					A	D			D		A			
	Sulfonamides				C			C				C			
	Tetracyclines	A			C		C	C			B	A	C		
	Tigecycline		C		C	C	C								C
	Vancomycin														
UTI Agents	Indanyl Carbenicillin			D											C
	Nitrofurantoin														

KEY TO TABLE

- **A** — Recommended drug therapy
- **B** — Alternate drug therapy
- **C** — Organism is usually or always sensitive to this agent
- **D** — Organism portrays variable sensitivity to this agent
- (Blank) This drug should not be used for this organism or insufficient data is available

GRAM-NEGATIVE AEROBES — Other bacilli

Class	Drug	Vibrio cholerae	Stenotrophomonas maltophilia	Pseudomonas aeruginosa	Pasteurella multocida	Legionella pneumophila	Haemophilus influenzae	Haemophilus ducreyi	Gardnerella vaginalis	Francisella tularensis	Campylobacter jejuni	Brucella sp.	Bordetella pertussis	Alcaligenes	Acinetobacter sp.
1st Generation	Cefadroxil						D								
1st Generation	Cefazolin						D								
1st Generation	Cephalexin						D								
1st Generation	Cephalothin						D								
1st Generation	Cephapirin						D								
2nd Generation and others	Cefaclor						B								
2nd Generation and others	Cefamandole				C		B								
2nd Generation and others	Cefmetazole				D		C								
2nd Generation and others	Cefonicid						C								
2nd Generation and others	Cefotetan				D		C								
2nd Generation and others	Cefoxitin				D		C		D						
2nd Generation and others	Cefpodoxime Proxetil						B								
2nd Generation and others	Cefprozil						B								
2nd Generation and others	Ceftibuten														
2nd Generation and others	Cefuroxime						B								
2nd Generation and others	Cefuroxime Axetil				D		B								
2nd Generation and others	Loracarbef						B								
3rd Generation	Cefepime			A			C								C
3rd Generation	Cefixime						A								D
3rd Generation	Cefoperazone		D	D	C		A	C							D
3rd Generation	Cefotaxime			D	C		C		C						A
3rd Generation	Ceftazidime		D	A			C		C						A
3rd Generation	Ceftizoxime			D			C		C						A
3rd Generation	Ceftriaxone			D	C		A	D							A
Aminoglycosides	Amikacin		C	A						C		C			C
Aminoglycosides	Gentamicin		C	A						C	A	C	C		C
Aminoglycosides	Netilmicin		C	A						C		C			C
Aminoglycosides	Streptomycin									A		C			
Aminoglycosides	Tobramycin		C	A						C		C			C
Macrolides	Azithromycin					D	B	C	C		C		C		
Macrolides	Clarithromycin					D	B	C			C		C		
Macrolides	Dirithromycin														
Macrolides	Erythromycin					D	A		C		C		A	A	
Quinolones	Ciprofloxacin	C	B	B	C	B	C	B	C	C	B	C			C
Quinolones	Gatifloxacin						C	C							
Quinolones	Levofloxacin			C			C	C							
Quinolones	Moxifloxacin							C							
Quinolones	Norfloxacin			C									B		D
Quinolones	Ofloxacin	C	B	D	C	C	C	C	C	C	C	B	C		C

ANTIMICROBIAL ACTIVITY AGAINST SELECTED ORGANISMS (Continued)

KEY TO TABLE

- **A** Recommended drug therapy
- **B** Alternate drug therapy
- **C** Organism is usually or always sensitive to this agent
- **D** Organism portrays variable sensitivity to this agent
- (Blank) This drug should not be used for this organism or insufficient data is available

		OTHERS									ANAEROBES			
Class	Drug	Treponema pallidum	Leptospira sp.	Borrelia burgdorferi (Lyme disease)	Rickettsia sp.	Mycoplasma pneumoniae	Ureaplasma urealyticum	Chlamydia trachomatis	Chlamydia psittaci	Chlamydia pneumoniae (TWAR)	Bacteroides sp. (Gram −)	Streptococcus, anaerobic (Gram +)	Clostridium difficile² (Gram +)	Clostridium perfringens (Gram +)
Penicillin	Amoxicillin			B								D	C	D
	Ampicillin			B								C	C	D
	Penicillin G	A	A	B								C	A	A
	Penicillin V	C	C	B								C	C	C
	Azlocillin													
	Mezlocillin											C	C	C
	Piperacillin											C	C	C
	Ticarcillin											C	C	C
	Cloxacillin													
	Dicloxacillin													
	Methicillin													
	Nafcillin													
	Oxacillin													
Penicillin-Related Antibiotics	Amoxicillin/Clavulanate										C	C		C
	Ampicillin/Sulbactam										C	C		C
	Ticarcillin/Clavulanate										C	C		C
	Aztreonam													
	Imipenem/Cilastatin										B	C		B
	Meropenem										B	C		B
	Piperacillin/Tazobactam										B	C		C
Other Antibiotics	Chloramphenicol				A						C	C	C	D
	Clindamycin										A	B		B
	Co-trimoxazole													
	Daptomycin													
	Linezolid													
	Metronidazole										A	D	A	A
	Quinupristin/Dalfopristin													
	Rifampin													
	Sulfonamides								D					
	Tetracyclines	B	B	A	A	A	A	A	B	B	D	C		C
	Tigecycline							C	C	C	C	C	C	C
	Vancomycin											B		B
UTI Agents	Indanyl Carbenicillin													
	Nitrofurantoin													

²Vancomycin is effective orally only.

KEY TO TABLE

- **A** Recommended drug therapy
- **B** Alternate drug therapy
- **C** Organism is usually or always sensitive to this agent
- **D** Organism portrays variable sensitivity to this agent
- (Blank) This drug should not be used for this organism or insufficient data is available

Class	Drug	Treponema pallidum	Leptospira sp.	Borrelia burgdorferi (Lyme disease)	Rickettsia sp.	Ureaplasma urealyticum	Mycoplasma pneumoniae	Chlamydia trachomatis	Chlamydia pneumoniae (TWAR)	Chlamydia psittaci	Bacteroides sp. (Anaerobe Gram −)	Streptococcus, anaerobic (Gram +)	Clostridium perfringens (Gram +)	Clostridium difficile 2 (Gram +)
1st Generation	Cefadroxil											B		
	Cefazolin											B		
	Cephalexin											B		
	Cephalothin											B		
	Cephapirin											B		
2nd Generation and others	Cefaclor													
	Cefamandole													
	Cefmetazole										C	C	C	
	Cefonicid													
	Cefotetan										B	C	C	
	Cefoxitin										B	C	C	
	Cefpodoxime Proxetil													
	Cefprozil													
	Ceftibuten													
	Cefuroxime											C	C	
	Cefuroxime Axetil													
	Loracarbef													
3rd Generation	Cefepime													
	Cefixime													
	Cefoperazone												D	
	Cefotaxime			C							D	C	C	
	Ceftazidime												D	
	Ceftizoxime			C							D	C	C	
	Ceftriaxone	C		A								C		
Aminoglycosides	Amikacin													
	Gentamicin													
	Netilmicin													
	Streptomycin													
	Tobramycin													
Macrolides	Azithromycin	D		C		B	C	C	C	C		D	D	
	Clarithromycin	D		D		B	C	C	C	C		D	D	
	Dirithromycin					C	C	C	C	C		D	D	
	Erythromycin	D		C		A	A	A	A	A		D	D	
Quinolones	Ciprofloxacin				D	D	D	D						
	Gatifloxacin						C					C		
	Levofloxacin						C	C	C					
	Moxifloxacin						C					C		
	Norfloxacin													
	Ofloxacin					D	D	D	C					

2 Vancomycin is effective orally only.

CREATININE CLEARANCE ESTIMATING METHODS IN PATIENTS WITH STABLE RENAL FUNCTION

These formulas provide an acceptable estimate of the patient's creatinine clearance **except** in the following instances.

- Patient's serum creatinine is changing rapidly (either increasing or decreasing).
- Patient is markedly emaciated.

In above situations, certain assumptions have to be made.

- In a patient with rapidly rising serum creatinine (ie, >0.5-0.7 mg/dL/day), it is best to assume that the patient's creatinine clearance is probably <10 mL/minute.
- In an emaciated patient, although their actual creatinine clearance is less than their calculated creatinine clearance (because of decreased creatinine production), it is not possible to easily predict how much less.

Adults (18 years and older)

Method 1: (Cockroft DW and Gault MH, *Nephron*, 1976, 16:31-41)

Estimated creatinine clearance (Cl_{cr}) (mL/min):

$$\text{Male} = \frac{(140 - age) \times BW\ (kg)}{72 \times S_{cr}}$$

$$\text{Female} = male \times 0.85$$

Note: Use of actual body weight (BW) in obese patients (and possibly patients with ascites) may significantly overestimate creatinine clearance. Some clinicians prefer to use an adjusted ideal body weight (IBW) in such cases [eg, IBW + 0.4(ABW-IBW)], especially when calculating dosages for aminoglycoside antibiotics.

Method 2: (Jelliffe RW, *Ann Intern Med*, 1973, 79:604)

Estimated creatinine clearance (Cl_{cr}) (mL/min/1.73 m^2):

$$\text{Male} = \frac{98 - 0.8\ (age - 20)}{S_{cr}}$$

$$\text{Female} = male \times 0.90$$

ANGIOTENSIN AGENTS

Comparison of Indications and Adult Dosages

Drug	Usual geriatric starting dose	Hypertension	CHF	Renal Dysfunction	Dialyzable	Strengths (mg)
			ACE Inhibitors			
Benazepril (Lotensin®)	5-10 mg/day	10-40 mg/day	Not FDA approved	Cl_{cr} <30 mL/min: 5 mg/day initially Maximum: 40 mg/day	Yes	Tablets 5, 10, 20, 40
Captopril (Capoten®)	12.5-25 mg tid	25-100 mg/day bid-tid	6.25-100 mg tid Maximum: 450 mg/day	Cl_{cr} 10-50 mL/min: 75% of usual dose Cl_{cr} <10 mL/min: 50% of usual dose	Yes	Tablets 12.5, 25, 50, 100
Enalapril (Vasotec®)	2.5-5 mg/day	2.5-40 mg/day qd-bid	2.5-20 mg bid Maximum: 20 mg/day	Cl_{cr} 30-80 mL/min: 5 mg/day initially Cl_{cr} <30 mL/min: 2.5 mg/day initially	Yes	Tablets 2.5, 5, 10, 20
Enalaprilat[1]	0.625-1.25 mg every 6 h over 5 min	0.625 mg, 1.25 mg, 2.5 mg q6h Maximum: 5 mg q6h	Not FDA approved	Cl_{cr} <30 mL/min: 0.625 mg q6h	Yes	1.25 mg/mL (1 mL, 2 mL vials)
Fosinopril (Monopril®)	5-10 mg/day	10-40 mg/day	10-40 mg/day	No dosage reduction necessary	Not well dialyzed	Tablets 10, 20, 40
Lisinopril (Prinivil®, Zestril®)	2.5-5 mg/day	10-40 mg/day Maximum: 40 mg/day	5-40 mg/day	Cl_{cr} 10-30 mL/min: 5 mg/day initially Cl_{cr} <10 mL/min: 2.5 mg/day initially	Yes	Tablets 2.5, 5, 10, 20, 30, 40
Moexipril (Univasc®)	3.75-7.5 mg/day	7.5-30 mg/day qd-bid Maximum: 30 mg/day	LV dysfunction (post-MI): 7.5-30 mg/day	Cl_{cr} <40 mL/min: 3.75 mg/day initially Maximum: 15 mg/day	Unknown	Tablets 7.5, 15
Perindopril (Aceon®)	2 mg/day	4-8 mg/day	4-8 mg/day Maximum: 16 mg/day	Cl_{cr} 30-60 mL/min: 2 mg/day Cl_{cr} 15-29 mL/min: 2 mg qod Cl_{cr} <15 mL/min: 2 mg on dialysis days	Yes	Tablets 2, 4, 8
Quinapril (Accupril®)	2.5-5 mg/day	10-40 mg/day qd-bid	5-20 mg bid	Cl_{cr} 30-60 mL/min: 5 mg/day initially Cl_{cr} <10-30 mL/min: 2.5 mg/day initially	Not well dialyzed	Tablets 5, 10, 20, 40
Ramipril (Altace®)	2.5-5 mg/day	2.5-20 mg/day qd-bid	2.5-10 mg/day	Cl_{cr} <40 mL/min: 25% of normal dose	Unknown	Capsules 1.25, 2.5, 5, 10
Trandolapril (Mavik®)	0.5-1 mg/day	1-4 mg/day Maximum: 8 mg/day qd-bid	LV dysfunction (post-MI): 1-4 mg/day	Cl_{cr} <30 mL/min: 0.5 mg/day initially	No	Tablets 1, 2, 4

ANGIOTENSIN AGENTS (Continued)

Comparison of Indications and Adult Dosages (continued)

Drug	Usual geriatric starting dose	Hypertension	CHF	Renal Dysfunction	Dialyzable	Strengths (mg)
Angiotensin II Receptor Blockers						
Candesartan (Atacand®)	No initial dosage adjustment necessary	8-32 mg/day	Target: 32 mg once daily	No dosage adjustment necessary	No	Tablets 4, 8, 16, 32
Eprosartan (Teveten®)	No initial dosage adjustment necessary	400-800 mg/day qd-bid	Not FDA approved	No dosage adjustment necessary	Unknown	Tablets 400, 600
Irbesartan (Avapro®)	No initial dosage adjustment necessary	150-300 mg/day	Not FDA approved	No dosage reduction necessary	No	Tablets 75, 150, 300
Losartan (Cozaar®)	No initial dosage adjustment necessary	25-100 mg qd or bid	Not FDA approved	No dosage adjustment necessary	No	Tablets 25, 50, 100
Olmesartan (Benicar®)	No initial dosage adjustment necessary; consider 5-10 mg/day	20-40 mg/day	Not FDA approved	No dosage adjustment necessary	Unknown	Tablets 5, 20, 40
Telmisartan (Micardis®)	No initial dosage adjustment necessary	20-80 mg/day	Not FDA approved	No dosage reduction necessary	No	Tablets 20, 40, 80
Valsartan (Diovan®)	No initial dosage adjustment necessary	80-320 mg/day	Target: 160 mg bid	Decrease dose only if Cl$_{cr}$ <10 mL/minute	No	Tablets 40, 80, 160, 320
Renin Inhibitors						
Aliskiren (Tekturna®)	No initial dosage adjustment necessary	150-300 mg once daily	Not FDA approved	No dosage adjustment necessary in mild-to-moderate impairment; not adequately studied in severe impairment	Unknown	Tablets 150, 300

Dosage is based on 70 kg adult with normal hepatic and renal function.
[1]Enalaprilat is the only available ACE inhibitor in a parenteral formulation.

ACE Inhibitors: Comparative Pharmacokinetics

Drug	Prodrug	Absorption (%)	Serum $t_{1/2}$ (h) Normal Renal Function	Serum Protein Binding (%)	Elimination	Onset of BP Lowering Action (h)	Peak BP Lowering Effects (h)	Duration of BP Lowering Effects (h)
Benazepril	Yes	37		~97	Renal (32%), biliary (~12%)	1	2-4	24
Benazeprilat			10-11 (effective)	~95%				
Captopril	No	60-75 (fasting)	1.9 (elimination)	25-30	Renal	0.25-0.5	1-1.5	~6
Enalapril	Yes	55-75	2 (elimination)	50-60	Renal (60%-80%), fecal	1	4-6	12-24
Enalaprilat			11 (effective)					
Fosinopril		36			Renal (~50%), biliary (~50%)	1		24
Fosinoprilat			12 (effective)	>99				
Moexipril	Yes		1	90	Fecal (53%), renal (8%)		1-2	>24
Moexiprilat			2-10	50				
Perindopril	Yes		1.5-3	60	Renal		3-7	
Perindoprilat			3-10 (effective)	10-20				
Quinapril	Yes	>60	0.8	97	Renal (~60%) as metabolite, fecal	1	2-4	24
Quinaprilat			2					
Ramipril	Yes	50-60	1-2	73	Renal (60%), fecal (40%)	1-2	3-6	24
Ramiprilat			13-17 (effective)	56				
Trandolapril	Yes		6	80	Renal (33%), fecal (66%)	1-2	6	≥24
Trandolaprilat			10	65-94				

ANGIOTENSIN AGENTS *(Continued)*

Angiotensin II Receptor Blockers and Renin Inhibitors: Comparative Pharmacokinetics

	Prodrug	Time to peak	Bioavail-ability	Food "area-under-the-curve"	Elimination half-life	Elimination altered in renal dysfunction	Precautions in severe renal dysfunction	Elimination altered in hepatic dysfunction	Precautions in hepatic dysfunction	Protein binding
Angiotensin II Receptor Blockers										
Candesartan (Atacand®)	Yes[1]	3-4 h	15%	No effect	9 h	Yes[2]	Yes	No	No	>99%
Eprosartan (Teveten®)	No	1-2 h	13%	No effect	5-9 h	No	Yes	No	Yes	98%
Irbesartan (Avapro®)	No	1.5-2 h	60%-80%	No effect	11-15 h	No	Yes	No	No	90%
Losartan (Cozaar®)	Yes[3]	1 h / 3-4 h[3]	33%	9%-10%	1.5-2 h / 6-9 h[3]	No	Yes	Yes	No	~99%
Olmesartan (Benicar®)	Yes	1-2 h	26%	No effect	13 h	Yes	Yes	Yes	No	99%
Telmisartan (Micardis®)	No	0.5-1 h	42%-58%	9.6%-20%	24 h	No	Yes	Yes	Yes	>99.5%
Valsartan (Diovan®)	No	2-4 h	25%	9%-40%	6 h	No	Yes	Yes	No	95%
Renin Inhibitors										
Aliskiren (Tekturna®)	No	1-3 h	~3%	85% (high-fat meal)	16-32 h	Yes[4]	Yes	No	No	?

[1] Candesartan cilexetil: Active metabolite candesartan.

[2] Dosage adjustments are not necessary.

[3] Losartan: Active metabolite E-3174.

[4] No initial dosage adjustment in mild-to-moderate impairment.

ANTICOAGULANTS, INJECTABLE

Name	Use	Limitation	Dose (SubQ unless otherwise noted)	Average MW (in daltons)
Low Molecular Weight Heparins				
Dalteparin (Fragmin®)	Prophylaxis	Abdominal surgery[1] Abdominal surgery[2]	2500 units/d 5000 units/d	4000-6000
		Hip surgery[1]	5000 units/d postoperatively	
	Treatment	DVT[3]	100 units/kg bid 200 units/kg qd	4000-6000
		Unstable[4] angina Non-Q-wave MI	120 units/kg (max: 10,000 units) q12h for 5-8 d	
Enoxaparin (Lovenox®)	Prophylaxis	Hip or knee replacement	30 mg twice daily[5]	3500-5500
		High-risk hip replacement or abdominal surgery	40 mg once daily	
	Treatment	DVT or PE	1 mg/kg q12h	
		Acute coronary	1 mg/kg q12h	
Tinzaparin (Innohep®)	Treatment	DVT or PE	175 anti-Xa int. units/kg/day	5500-7500
Heparin				
Heparin (Hep-Lock®)	Prophylaxis	Risk of thromboembolic disease	5000 units q8-12h	3000-30,000
	Treatment	Thrombosis or embolization	80 units/kg IVP then 20,000-40,000 units daily as continuous I.V. infusion	
	Treatment[3]	Unstable angina[3]	80 units/kg IVP then 20,000-40,000 units daily as continuous I.V. infusion	
Heparinoid				
Danaparoid	Prophylaxis	Hip replacement	750 units bid	6500
	Treatment[3]		2000 units q12h	
Selective Anti-Xa Inhibitor				
Fondaparinux[6] (Arixtra®)	Prophylaxis	Hip fracture Hip or knee replacement	2.5 mg once daily	1728
Coumarin Derivatives				
Warfarin (Coumadin®)	Prophylaxis	NS	Variable	NS
	Treatment		2-5 mg/d	

NS = not stated.

[1] Patients with low risk of DVT.

[2] Patients with high risk of DVT.

[3] Not FDA approved.

[4] Patients >60 years of age may require a lower dose of heparin.

[5] Patients weighing <100 lb or ≥65 years of age may receive 0.5 mg/kg/dose every 12 hours.

[6] Synthetic pentasaccharide.

ANTIDEPRESSANT AGENTS

Comparison of Usual Dosage, Mechanism of Action, and Adverse Effects

Drug	Initial Geriatric Dose (mg/d)	Usual Dosage (mg/d)	Dosage Forms	Therapeutic Drug Conc (ng/mL)	Sexual Dysfunction	Reuptake Inhibition		ACH	Adverse Effects				
						N	S		Drowsiness	Orthostatic Hypotension	Conduction Abnormalities	GI Distress	Weight Gain
Tricyclic Antidepressants & Related Compounds[1]													
Amitriptyline	10-25 mg at bedtime	100-300	T, I	100-250[2]	High	Moderate	High	4+	4+	3+	3+	1	4+
Amoxapine	25 mg twice daily	100-400	T	200-500	High	Moderate	Low[3]	2+	2+	2+	2+	0	2+
Clomipramine[4] (Anafranil)	25 mg at bedtime	100-250	C	80-100	Very high	Moderate	Very high	4+	4+	2+	3+	1+	4+
Desipramine (Norpramin)	10-25 mg at bedtime	100-300	T	125-160	High	High	Moderate	1+	2+	2+	2+	0	1+
Doxepin (Sinequan, Zonalon)	10-25 mg at bedtime	100-300	C, L	100-200[2]	High	Moderate	Low	3+	4+	2+	2+	0	4+
Imipramine (Tofranil, Tofranil-PM)	10-25 mg at bedtime	100-300	T, C	200-350[2]	High	Moderate	High	3+	3+	4+	3+	1+	4+
Maprotiline	25 mg at bedtime	100-225	T	200-300[2]	Moderate	Moderate	Low	2+	3+	2+	2+	0	2+
Nortriptyline (Pamelor)	10-25 mg at bedtime	50-150	C, L	50-150	High	Moderate	Low	2+	2+	1+	2+	0	1+
Protriptyline (Vivactil)	5-10 mg in morning	15-60	T	100-200	High	High	Low	2+	1+	2+	3+	1+	1+
Trimipramine (Surmontil)	25 mg at bedtime	100-300	C	180[2]	High	Low	Low	4+	4+	3+	3+	0	4+
Selective Serotonin Reuptake Inhibitors[5]													
Citalopram (Celexa)	20 mg in morning	20-60	T	—	Very high	Very low	Very high	0	0	0	0	3+[6]	1+
Escitalopram (Lexapro)	5-20 mg in morning	10-20	T	—	Very high	Very low	Very high	0	0	0	0	3+	1+
Fluoxetine (Prozac, Prozac Weekly, Sarafem)	10 mg in morning	20-80	C, L, T	—	Very high	Low	Very high	0	0	0	0	3+[6]	1+
Fluvoxamine[4]	50 mg at bedtime	100-300	T	—	Very high	Very low	Very high	0	0	0	0	3+[6]	1+

Comparison of Usual Dosage, Mechanism of Action, and Adverse Effects

Drug	Initial Geriatric Dose (mg)	Usual Dosage (mg/d)	Dosage Forms	Therapeutic Drug Conc (ng/mL)	Sexual Dysfunction	Reuptake Inhibition N	Reuptake Inhibition S	ACH	Drowsiness	Orthostatic Hypotension	Conduction Abnormalities	GI Distress	Weight Gain
Paroxetine (Paxil®, Paxil CR™)	10 mg in morning	20-50	T, L	—	Very high	Moderate	Very high	1+	1+	0	0	3+[6]	2+
Sertraline (Zoloft®)	25 mg in morning	50-200	T	—	Very high	Low	Very high	0	0	0	0	3+[6]	1+
Dopamine-Reuptake Blocking Compounds													
Bupropion (Wellbutrin®, Wellbutrin SR®, Wellbutrin XL™, Zyban®)	50-100	300-450[7]	T	50-100[2]	Low	Very low[8]	Very low[8]	0	0	0	1+/0	1+	0
Serotonin / Norepinephrine Reuptake Inhibitors[9]													
Duloxetine (Cymbalta®)	20 mg twice daily	40-60	C	—	High	NA	NA	1+	1+	0	1+	3+[6]	0
Venlafaxine (Effexor®, Effexor® XR)	25 mg 2-3 times/day IR, 37.5 mg daily XR	75-375	T	—	High	Low-high dose dependent	High	1+	1+	0	1+	3+[6]	0
5-HT$_2$ Receptor Antagonist Properties													
Nefazodone	50 mg twice daily	300-600	T	—	Low	Low	Low	1+	1+	2+	1+	1+	0
Trazodone (Desyrel®)	25 mg 2-3 times/day	150-600	T	800-1600	Low	Very low	Low	0	4+	3+	1+	1+	2+
Noradrenergic Antagonist													
Mirtazapine (Remeron®, Remeron® SolTab®)	7.5 mg at bedtime	15-45	T	—	Low	Very low	Very low	1+	3+	1+	1+	0	3+

ANTIDEPRESSANT AGENTS (Continued)

Comparison of Usual Dosage, Mechanism of Action, and Adverse Effects

Drug	Initial Geriatric Dose (mg/d)	Usual Dosage (mg/d)	Dosage Forms	Therapeutic Drug Conc (ng/mL)	Sexual Dysfunction	Reuptake Inhibition		Adverse Effects					
						N	S	ACH	Drowsiness	Orthostatic Hypotension	Conduction Abnormalities	GI Distress	Weight Gain
Monoamine Oxidase Inhibitors													
Isocarboxazid (Marplan®)	10 mg twice daily	10–30	T	—	Very high	—	—	2+	2+	2+	1+	1+	2+
Phenelzine (Nardil®)	7.5 mg	15–90	T	—	Very high	—	—	2+	2+	2+	0	1+	3+
Tranylcypromine (Parnate®)	10 mg twice daily	10–60	T	—	High	—	—	2+	1+	2+	1+	1+	2+

Key: N = norepinephrine; S = serotonin; ACH = anticholinergic effects (dry mouth, blurred vision, urinary retention, constipation); 0 - 4+ = absent or rare - relatively common. T = tablet, L = liquid, I = injectable, C = capsule, IR = immediate-release, SR = sustained-release.

[1]Important note: A 1-week supply taken all at once in a patient receiving the maximum dose can be fatal.

[2]Concentration represents a combination of parent drug and active metabolites.

[3]Also blocks dopamine receptors.

[4]Not approved by FDA for depression. Approved for OCD.

[5]Flat dose response curve, headache, nausea, and sexual dysfunction are common side effects for SSRIs.

[6]Nausea is usually mild and transient.

[7]Not to exceed 150 mg/dose to minimize seizure risk for IR and 200 mg/dose for SR.

[8]Norepinephrine and serotonin reuptake inhibition is minimal, but inhibits dopamine reuptake; metabolite inhibits norepinephrine reuptake.

[9]Do not use with sibutramine; relatively safe in overdose.

ANTIPARKINSONIAN AGENTS

Drugs Used for the Treatment of Parkinsonian Symptoms[1]

Drug	Mechanism	Initial Dose	Titration Schedule	Usual Daily Dosage	Recommended Dosing Schedule
		Dopaminergic Agents			
Amantadine (Symmetrel®)	NMDA receptor antagonist and inhibits neuronal reuptake of dopamine	100 mg every other day	100 mg/dose every week, up to 300 mg 3 times/d	100–200 mg	Twice daily
Apomorphine (Apokyn™)	D_2 receptors (caudate-putamen)	1–2 mg	Complex; based on tolerance and response to test dose(s)	Variable; <20 mg	Individualized; 3–5 times/d prn
Bromocriptine (Parlodel®)	Moderate affinity for D_2 and D_3 dopamine receptors	1.25 mg twice daily	2.5 mg every 2–4 wk	2.5–100 mg	3 times/d
Cabergoline (Dostinex®)[2]	Selective to D_2 dopamine receptors	0.5 mg once daily	0.25–0.5 mg/d every 4 wk	0.5–5 mg	Once daily
Entacapone (Comtan®)	COMT enzyme inhibitor	200 mg 3 times/d	Titrate down the doses of levodopa/carbidopa as required	600–1600 mg	3 times/d; up to 8 times/d
Levodopa/carbidopa (Sinemet® CR)	Converts to dopamine; binds to all CNS dopamine receptors	10–25/100 mg 2–4 times/d	0.5–1 tablet (10 or 25/100 mg) every 1–2 d	50/200 to 200/2000 mg (3–8 tablets)	3 times/d or twice daily (for controlled release)
Levodopa/carbidopa/ entacapone (Stalevo™)	Converts to dopamine; binds to all CNS dopamine receptors; COMT enzyme inhibitor	1 tablet 3–4 times/d (to replace previous dosing with individual agents)	As tolerated based on response and presence of dyskinesias	3–8 tablets per day	3–4 times/d
Pergolide (Permax®)	Low affinity for D_1 and maximal affinity for D_2 and D_3 dopamine receptors	0.05 mg/night	0.1–0.15 mg/d every 3 d for 12 d, then 0.25 mg/d every 3 d	0.05–5 mg	3 times/d
Pramipexole (Mirapex®)	High affinity for D_2 and D_3 dopamine receptors	0.125 mg 3 times/d	0.125 mg/dose every 5–7 d	1.5–4.5 mg	3 times/d
Rasagiline (Azilect®)	Inhibits MAO-B	0.5–1 mg once daily	≤1 mg daily	0.5–1 mg	Once daily
Ropinirole (Requip®)	High affinity for D_2 and D_3 dopamine receptors	0.25 mg 3 times/d	0.25 mg/dose weekly for 4 wk, then 1.5 mg/d every week up to 9 mg/d; 3 mg/d up to a max of 24 mg/d	0.75–24 mg	3 times/d

ANTIPARKINSONIAN AGENTS *(Continued)*

Drugs Used for the Treatment of Parkinsonian Symptoms[1] *(continued)*

Drug	Mechanism	Initial Dose	Titration Schedule	Usual Daily Dosage	Recommended Dosing Schedule
Rotigotine (Neupro®)	D_1, D_2, D_3 dopamine receptor agonist	2 mg/24 hours transdermal patch	Increase by 2 mg/24 hours weekly; maximum 6 mg/24 hours	2 mg/24 hours, 4 mg/24 hours, or 6 mg/24 hours	Once daily patch
Selegiline (Eldepryl®)	Inhibits MAO-B	5-10 mg twice daily	Titrate down the doses of levodopa/carbidopa as required	5-10 mg	Twice daily
Tolcapone (Tasmar®)	COMT enzyme inhibitor	100 mg 3 times/d	Titrate down the doses of levodopa/carbidopa as required	300-600 mg	3 times/d
Anticholinergic Agents					
Benztropine (Cogentin®)	Blocks cholinergic receptors, also has antihistamine effects	0.5-2 mg/d in 1-4 divided doses	0.5 mg/dose every 5-6 d	2-6 mg	1-2 times/d
Biperiden (Akineton®)	Blocks cholinergic receptors	2 mg 1-4 times/d	As tolerated	2-8 mg	1-4 times/d
Diphenhydramine (Benadryl®)	Blocks cholinergic receptors	12.5-25 mg 3-4 times/d	As tolerated	25-300 mg	3-4 times/d
Procyclidine (Kemadrin®)	Blocks cholinergic receptors	2.5 mg 3 times/d	Gradually as tolerated	7.5-20 mg	3 times/d
Trihexyphenidyl (Artane)	Blocks cholinergic receptors; also some direct effects	1-2 mg/d	2 mg/d at intervals of 3-5 d	5-15 mg	3-4 times/d

[1]The medications listed in the table represent treatment options for both idiopathic Parkinson's disease, as well as Parkinsonian symptoms resulting from other drug therapy.

[2]Cabergoline is not FDA approved for the treatment of Parkinson's disease.

ANTIPSYCHOTIC AGENTS

Antipsychotic Agent	Dosage Forms	I.M./P.O. Potency	Equiv. Dosages (approx) (mg)	Usual Adult Daily Maint. Dose (mg)	Sedation (Incidence)	Extrapyramidal Side Effects	Anticholinergic Side Effects	Orthostatic Hypotension	Comments
Aripiprazole (Abilify™)	Soln, tab		4	10-30	Low	Very low	Very low	Very low	Low weight gain; activating
Chlorpromazine (Thorazine® [DSC])	Conc, inj, supp, syr, tab	4:1	100	200-1000	High	Moderate	Moderate	Moderate / high	
Clozapine (Clozaril®)	Tab		100	75-900	High	Very low	High	High	~1% incidence of agranulocytosis; weekly-biweekly CBC required; potential for weight gain, lipid abnormalities, and diabetes
Fluphenazine (Permitil®, Prolixin®, Prolixin Decanoate®, Prolixin Enanthate®)	Conc, elix, inj, tab	2:1	2	0.5-20	Low	High	Low	Low	
Haloperidol (Haldol®, Haldol® Decanoate)	Conc, inj, tab	2:1	2	0.5-20	Low	High	Low	Low	
Loxapine (Loxitane®, Loxitane® C, Loxitane® I.M.)	Cap, conc, inj		10	25-250	Moderate	Moderate	Low	Low	
Mesoridazine (Serentil®)	Inj, liq, tab	3:1	50	30-400	High	Low	High	Moderate	Prolongs QTc; use only in treatment of refractory illness
Molindone (Moban®)	Conc, tab		15	15-225	Low	Moderate	Low	Low	May cause less weight gain
Olanzapine (Zyprexa®, Zyprexa® Zydis®)	Inj, tab, tab (oral-disintegrating)		4	5-20	Moderate / high	Low	Moderate	Moderate	Potential for weight gain, lipid abnormalities, diabetes
Perphenazine (Trilafon®)	Conc, inj, tab		10	16-64	Low	Moderate	Low	Low	
Pimozide (Orap®)	Tab		2	1-20	Moderate	High	Moderate	Low	Contraindicated with CYP3A inhibitors
Quetiapine (Seroquel®)	Tab		125	50-800	Moderate / high	Very low	Moderate	Moderate	Moderate weight gain; potential for lipid abnormalities; diabetes

ANTIPSYCHOTIC AGENTS *(Continued)*

Antipsychotic Agent	Dosage Forms	I.M./P.O. Potency	Equiv. Dosages (approx) (mg)	Usual Adult Daily Maint. Dose (mg)	Sedation (Incidence)	Extrapyramidal Side Effects	Anticholinergic Side Effects	Orthostatic Hypotension	Comments
Risperidone (Risperdal®)	Inj, soln, tab, tab (oral-disintegrating)		1	0.5-6	Low / moderate	Low	Very low	Moderate	Low to moderate weight gain; potential for diabetes
Thioridazine (Mellaril®)	Conc, tab		100	200-800	High	Low	High	Moderate / high	May cause irreversible retinitis pigmentosa at doses >800 mg/d; prolongs QTc; use only in treatment of refractory illness
Thiothixene (Navane®)	Cap, conc, powder for inj	4:1	4	5-40	Low	High	Low	Low / moderate	
Trifluoperazine (Stelazine® [DSC])	Conc, inj, tab		5	2-40	Low	High	Low	Low	
Ziprasidone (Geodon®)	Cap, powder for inj	2:1	40	40-160	Low / moderate	Low	Very low	Low / moderate	Low weight gain; contraindicated with QTc-prolonging agents

APPENDIX / COMPARATIVE DRUG CHARTS

ATYPICAL ANTIPSYCHOTICS

Drug	DR EPS	PROL	TD[1]	ACH	SZ	OH	LFTs	SED	WT GAIN	NMS	AGRAN	TX REFR	Lipid	DM	QTc
Aripiprazole (Abilify™)	No	No	Uncommon	Very low	Low	Low	Low	Low	Very low	?	?	Maybe	Very low	Very low	Low
Clozapine (Clozaril®)	No	No	Uncommon	High	DD	High	Low	High	High	Yes	Yes	Yes	High	High	Low
Risperidone (Risperdal®)	Yes	Yes	Uncommon	Very low	Low	Moderate	Low	Low	Low/Moderate	Yes	Yes[2]	Maybe	Low	Low/Moderate	Low
Olanzapine (Zyprexa®, Zyprexa® Zydis®)	Yes	Yes	Uncommon	Moderate	Low	Low/Moderate	Low/Moderate	Moderate	High	Yes	Yes[2]	Maybe	High	High	Low
Quetiapine (Seroquel®)	No	No	Uncommon	Moderate	Low	Moderate	Low/Moderate	Moderate	Moderate	Yes	Yes[2]	No	Moderate	Low/Moderate	Low
Ziprasidone (Geodon®)	Yes	Yes	Uncommon	Very low	Low	Low/Moderate	Low	Low	Very low	Yes	?	No	Very low	Very low	Moderate[3]

Note: Atypical antipsychotics are defined as 1) decrease or no EPS at doses producing antipsychotic effect; 2) minimum or no increase in prolactin; 3) decrease in both positive and negative symptoms of schizophrenia.

[1] Rate of TD ~⅕ that seen with conventional antipsychotics.

[2] Case reports.

[3] Dose related within 40-160 mg dosage range.

DR EPS = dose related extrapyramidal symptoms.

PROL = prolactin elevation (may cause amenorrhea, galactorrhea, gynecomastia, impotence).

TD = tardive dyskinesia.

ACH = anticholinergic side effects (dry mouth, blurred vision, constipation, urinary hesitancy).

SZ = seizures.

OH = orthostatic hypotension (blood pressure drops upon standing).

LFTs = increased liver function test results.

SED = sedation.

WT GAIN = weight gain.

NMS = neuroleptic malignant syndrome.

AGRAN = agranulocytosis (without white blood cells to fight infection).

TX REFR = efficacy in treatment refractory schizophrenia.

Lipid = lipid abnormalities; cholesterol and/or triglyceride elevations.

DM = diabetes (based on case reports).

QTc = QTc prolongation.

DD = dose dependent.

ANXIOLYTIC, SEDATIVE / HYPNOTIC, AND MISCELLANEOUS BENZODIAZEPINES

	Peak Blood Concentration (oral) (h)	Protein Binding %	Major Active Metabolite	Half-Life (parent) Adults (h)	Half-Life[1] (metabolite) Adults (h)	Adult Oral Dosage Range	Geriatric Oral Dosage Range
Anxiolytic							
Alprazolam (Alprazolam Intensol®, Xanax®)	1-2	80	No	12-15	—	0.75-4 mg/d	0.25-0.75 mg/d
Chlordiazepoxide (Librium®)	2-4	90-98	Yes	5-30	24-96	15-100 mg/d	10-20 mg/d[2]
Diazepam (Diastat® Rectal Delivery System, Diazepam Intensol®, Valium®)	0.5-2	98	Yes	20-80	50-100	4-40 mg/d	1-20 mg/d[2]
Lorazepam (Ativan®)[3]	1-6	88-92	No	10-20	—	2-4 mg/d	0.5-4 mg/d
Oxazepam (Serax®)	2-4	86-99	No	5-20	—	30-120 mg/d	20-45 mg/d
Sedative / Hypnotic							
Estazolam (ProSom®)	2	93	No	10-24	—	1-2 mg	0.5-1 mg
Flurazepam (Dalmane®)	0.5-2	97	Yes	Not significant	40-114	15-60 mg	15 mg[2]
Quazepam (Doral®)	2	95	Yes	25-41	28-114	7.5-15 mg	7.5 mg[2]
Temazepam (Restoril®)	2-3	96	No	10-40	—	15-30 mg	7.5-15 mg
Triazolam (Halcion®)	1	89-94	No	2.3	—	0.125-0.5 mg	0.0625-0.25 mg
Miscellaneous							
Clonazepam (Klonopin®)	1-2	86	No	18-50	—	1.5-20 mg/d	0.5-20 mg/d
Clorazepate (Tranxene®)	1-2	80-95	Yes	Not significant	50-100	15-60 mg/d	7.5-15 mg/d[2]
Midazolam	0.4-0.7[4]	95	No	2-5	—	NA	NA

[1]Significant metabolite.

[2]Not recommended for use in geriatric patients.

[3]Reliable bioavailability when given I.M.

[4]I.V. only.

NA = not available.

BETA-BLOCKERS

Agent	Adrenergic Receptor Blocking Activity	Lipid Solubility	Protein Bound (%)	Half-Life (h)	Bioavail-ability (%)	Primary (Secondary) Route of Elimination	Indications	Usual Dosage
Acebutolol (Sectral®)	beta$_1$	Low	15-25	3-4	40 7-fold[1]	Hepatic (renal)	Hypertension, arrhythmias	P.O.: 400-1200 mg/d
Atenolol (Tenormin®)	beta$_1$	Low	<5-10	6-9[2]	50-60 4-fold[1]	Renal (hepatic)	Hypertension, angina pectoris, acute MI	P.O.: 50-200 mg/d I.V.: 5 mg x 2 doses
Betaxolol (Kerlone®)	beta$_1$	Low	50-55	14-22	84-94	Hepatic (renal)	Hypertension	P.O.: 10-20 mg/d
Bisoprolol (Zebeta®)	beta$_1$	Low	26-33	9-12	80	Renal (hepatic)	Hypertension, heart failure	P.O.: 2.5-5 mg
Carteolol (Cartrol®)	beta$_1$ beta$_2$	Low	20-30	6	80-85	Renal	Hypertension	P.O.: 2.5-10 mg/d
Carvedilol (Coreg®)	beta$_1$ beta$_2$ alpha$_1$	ND	98	7-10	25-35	Bile into feces	Hypertension, heart failure (mild to severe)	P.O.: 6.25 mg twice daily
Esmolol (Brevibloc®)	beta$_1$	Low	55	0.15	NA 5-fold[1]	Red blood cell	Supraventricular tachycardia, sinus tachycardia	I.V. infusion: 25-300 mcg/Kg/min
Labetalol (Trandate®)	alpha$_1$ beta$_1$ beta$_2$	Moderate	50	5.5-8	18-30 10-fold[1]	Renal (hepatic)	Hypertension	P.O.: 200-2400 mg/d I.V.: 20-80 mg at 10-min intervals up to a maximum of 300 mg or continuous infusion of 2 mg/min
Metoprolol (Lopressor®, Toprol-XL®)	beta$_1$	Moderate	10-12	3-7	50 10-fold[1] (Toprol XL®: 77)	Hepatic/renal	Hypertension, angina pectoris, acute MI, heart failure (mild to moderate; XL formulation only)	P.O.: 100-450 mg/d I.V.: Post-MI 15 mg Angina: 15 mg then 2-5 mg/hour Arrhythmias: 0.2 mg/kg
Nadolol (Corgard®)	beta$_1$ beta$_2$	Low	25-30	20-24	30 5- to 8-fold[1]	Renal	Hypertension, angina pectoris	P.O.: 40-320 mg/d
Penbutolol (Levatol®)	beta$_1$ beta$_2$	High	80-98	5	≅100	Hepatic (renal)	Hypertension	P.O.: 20-80 mg/d
Pindolol	beta$_1$ beta$_2$	Moderate	57	3-4[2]	90 4-fold[1]	Hepatic (renal)	Hypertension	P.O.: 20-60 mg/d

BETA-BLOCKERS (Continued)

Agent	Adrenergic Receptor Blocking Activity	Lipid Solubility	Protein Bound (%)	Half-Life (h)	Bioavail-ability (%)	Primary (Secondary) Route of Elimination	Indications	Usual Dosage
Propranolol (Inderal®, various)	beta$_1$ beta$_2$	High	90	3-5[2]	30 20-fold[1]	Hepatic	Hypertension, angina pectoris, arrhythmias	P.O.: 40-480 mg/d I.V.: Reflex tachycardia 1-10 mg
Propranolol long-acting (Inderal-LA®)	beta$_1$ beta$_2$	High	90	9-18	20- to 30-fold[1]	Hepatic	Hypertrophic subaortic stenosis, prophylaxis (post-MI)	P.O.: 180-240 mg/d
Sotalol (Betapace®, Betapace AF®, Sorine®)	beta$_1$ beta$_2$	Low	0	12	90-100	Renal	Ventricular arrhythmias/ tachyarrhythmias	P.O.: 160-320 mg/d
Timolol (Blocadren®)	beta$_1$ beta$_2$	Low to moderate	<10	4	75 7-fold[1]	Hepatic (renal)	Hypertension, prophylaxis (post-MI)	P.O.: 20-60 mg/d P.O.: 20 mg/d

Dosage is based on 70 kg adult with normal hepatic and renal function.

Note: All beta$_1$-selective agents will inhibit beta$_2$ receptors at higher doses.

[1]Interpatient variations in plasma levels.

[2]Half-life increased to 16-27 hours in creatinine clearance of 15-35 mL/minute and >27 hours in creatinine clearance <15 mL/minute.

CALCIUM CHANNEL BLOCKERS

Comparative Pharmacokinetics

Agent	Bioavailability (%)	Protein Binding (%)	Onset of BP Effect (min)	Duration of BP Effect (h)	Half-Life (h)	Volume of Distribution	Route of Metabolism	Route of Excretion
Dihydropyridines								
Amlodipine (Norvasc®)	64-90	93-98	30-50	24	30-50	21 L/kg	Hepatic; inactive metabolites	Urine; 10% as parent
Felodipine (Plendil®)	20	>99	2-5 h	24	11-16	10 L/kg	Hepatic; CYP3A4 substrate (major); inactive metabolites; extensive first pass	Urine (70%; as metabolites); feces 10%
Isradipine (DynaCirc® [DSCI]) (immediate release)	15-24	95	20	>12	8	3 L/kg	Hepatic; CYP3A4 substrate (major); inactive metabolites; extensive first pass	Urine as metabolites
Nicardipine (Cardene®) (immediate release)	35	>95	30	≤8	2-4		Hepatic; CYP3A4 substrate (major); saturable first pass	Urine (60%; as metabolites); feces 35%
Nifedipine (Procardia®) (immediate release)	40-77	92-98	Within 20		2-5		Hepatic; CYP3A4 substrate (major); inactive metabolites	Urine as metabolites
Nimodipine (Nimotop®)	13	>95	ND	4-6	1-2		Hepatic; CYP3A4 substrate (major); metabolites inactive or less active than parent; extensive first pass	Urine (50%; as metabolites); feces 32%
Nisoldipine (Sular®)	5	>99	ND	6-12	7-12		Hepatic; CYP3A4 substrate (major); 1 active metabolite (10% of parent); extensive first pass	Urine as metabolites

CALCIUM CHANNEL BLOCKERS *(Continued)*

Comparative Pharmacokinetics

Agent	Bioavailability (%)	Protein Binding (%)	Onset of BP Effect (min)	Duration of BP Effect (h)	Half-Life (h)	Volume of Distribution	Route of Metabolism	Route of Excretion
Phenylalkylamines								
Verapamil (Calan®) (immediate release)	20-35	90	30	6-8	4.5-12		Hepatic; CYP3A4 substrate (major); 1 active metabolite (20% of parent); extensive first pass	Urine (70%; 3%-4% as unchanged drug); feces 16%
Benzothiazepines								
Diltiazem (Cardizem®) (immediate release)	~40	70-80	30-60	6-8	3-4.5	3-13 L/kg	Hepatic; CYP3A4 substrate (major); 1 major metabolite (20%-50% of parent); extensive first pass	Urine as metabolites

CORTICOSTEROIDS

Corticosteroids, Systemic Equivalencies

Glucocorticoid	Pregnancy Category	Approximate Equivalent Dose (mg)	Routes of Administration	Relative Anti-inflammatory Potency	Relative Mineralocorticoid Potency	Protein Binding (%)	Half-life Plasma (min)	Half-life Biologic (h)
Short-Acting								
Cortisone	D	25	P.O., I.M.	0.8	2	90	30	8-12
Hydrocortisone	C	20	I.M., I.V.	1	2	90	80-118	8-12
Intermediate-Acting								
Methylprednisolone[1]	—	4	P.O., I.M., I.V.	5	0	—	78-188	18-36
Prednisolone	B	5	P.O., I.M., I.V., intra-articular, intradermal, soft tissue injection	4	1	90-95	115-212	18-36
Prednisone	B	5	P.O.	4	1	70	60	18-36
Triamcinolone[1]	C	4	P.O., I.M., intra-articular, intradermal, intrasynovial, soft tissue injection	5	0	—	200+	18-36
Long-Acting								
Betamethasone	C	0.6-0.75	P.O., I.M., intra-articular, intradermal, intrasynovial, soft tissue injection	25	0	64	300+	36-54
Dexamethasone	C	0.75	P.O., I.M., I.V., intra-articular, intradermal, soft tissue injection	25-30	0	—	110-210	36-54
Mineralocorticoids								
Fludrocortisone	C	—	P.O.	10	125	42	210+	18-36

[1]May contain propylene glycol as an excipient in injectable forms.

CORTICOSTEROIDS *(Continued)*

GUIDELINES FOR SELECTION AND USE OF TOPICAL CORTICOSTEROIDS

The quantity prescribed and the frequency of refills should be monitored to reduce the risk of adrenal suppression. In general, short courses of high-potency agents are preferable to prolonged use of low potency. After control is achieved, control should be maintained with a low potency preparation.

1. Low-to-medium potency agents are usually effective for treating thin, acute, inflammatory skin lesions; whereas, high or super-potent agents are often required for treating chronic, hyperkeratotic, or lichenified lesions.

2. Since the stratum corneum is thin on the face and intertriginous areas, low-potency agents are preferred but a higher potency agent may be used for 2 weeks.

3. Because the palms and soles have a thick stratum corneum, high or super-potent agents are frequently required.

4. Low potency agents are preferred for the elderly. Elderly patients have thin, fragile skin.

5. The vehicle in which the topical corticosteroid is formulated influences the absorption and potency of the drug. Ointment bases are preferred for thick, lichenified lesions; they enhance penetration of the drug. Creams are preferred for acute and subacute dermatoses; they may be used on moist skin areas or intertriginous areas. Solutions, gels, and sprays are preferred for the scalp or for areas where a nonoil-based vehicle is needed.

6. In general, super-potent agents should not be used for longer than 2-3 weeks unless the lesion is limited to a small body area. Medium-to-high potency agents usually cause only rare adverse effects when treatment is limited to 3 months or less, and use on the face and intertriginous areas are avoided. If long-term treatment is needed, intermittent vs continued treatment is recommended.

7. Most preparations are applied once or twice daily. More frequent application may be necessary for the palms or soles because the preparation is easily removed by normal activity and penetration is poor due to a thick stratum corneum. Every-other-day or weekend-only application may be effective for treating some chronic conditions.

Corticosteroids, Topical

	Steroid	Vehicle
Very High Potency		
0.05%	Betamethasone dipropionate, augmented	Ointment, lotion
0.05%	Clobetasol propionate	Cream, foam, gel, lotion, ointment, shampoo, spray
0.05%	Diflorasone diacetate	Ointment
0.05%	Halobetasol propionate	Cream, ointment
High Potency		
0.1%	Amcinonide	Cream, ointment, lotion
0.05%	Betamethasone dipropionate, augmented	Cream
0.05%	Betamethasone dipropionate	Cream, ointment
0.1%	Betamethasone valerate	Ointment
0.05%	Desoximetasone	Gel
0.25%	Desoximetasone	Cream, ointment
0.05%	Diflorasone diacetate	Cream, ointment
0.05%	Fluocinonide	Cream, ointment, gel
0.1%	Halcinonide	Cream, ointment
0.5%	Triamcinolone acetonide	Cream

Corticosteroids, Topical *(continued)*

	Steroid	Vehicle
Intermediate Potency		
0.05%	Betamethasone dipropionate	Lotion
0.1%	Betamethasone valerate	Cream
0.1%	Clocortolone pivalate	Cream
0.05%	Desoximetasone	Cream
0.025%	Fluocinolone acetonide	Cream, ointment
0.05%	Flurandrenolide	Cream, ointment, lotion, tape
0.005%	Fluticasone propionate	Ointment
0.05%	Fluticasone propionate	Cream
0.1%	Hydrocortisone butyrate[1]	Ointment, solution
0.2%	Hydrocortisone valerate[1]	Cream, ointment
0.1%	Mometasone furoate[1]	Cream, ointment, lotion
0.1%	Prednicarbate	Cream, ointment
0.025%	Triamcinolone acetonide	Cream, ointment, lotion
0.1%	Triamcinolone acetonide	Cream, ointment, lotion
Low Potency		
0.05%	Alclometasone dipropionate[1]	Cream, ointment
0.05%	Desonide	Cream
0.01%	Fluocinolone acetonide	Cream, solution
0.5%	Hydrocortisone[1]	Cream, ointment, lotion
0.5%	Hydrocortisone acetate[1]	Cream, ointment
1%	Hydrocortisone acetate[1]	Cream, ointment
1%	Hydrocortisone	Cream, ointment, lotion, solution
2.5%	Hydrocortisone	Cream, ointment, lotion

[1]Not fluorinated.

GLAUCOMA DRUG THERAPY

Ophthalmic Agent (Brand)	Reduces Aqueous Humor Production	Increases Aqueous Humor Outflow	Average Duration of Action	Strengths Available
Cholinesterase Inhibitor[1]				
Echothiophate (Phospholine Iodide®)	No data	Significant	2 wk	0.125%
Direct-Acting Cholinergic Miotics				
Carbachol	Some activity	Significant	8 h	0.75% to 3%
Pilocarpine (various)	Some activity	Significant	5 h	0.5%, 1%, 2%, 3%, 4%
Sympathomimetics				
Apraclonidine (Iopidine®)	Moderate	Moderate	4 h	0.5%, 1%
Brimonidine (Alphagan®, Alphagan® P)	Moderate	Moderate	12 h	0.1%, 0.15%
Dipivefrin (Propine®)	Some activity	Moderate	12 h	0.1%
Epinephrine	Some activity	Moderate	18 h	0.25% to 2%
Beta-Blockers				
Betaxolol (Betoptic® S)	Significant	Some activity	12 h	0.5%
Carteolol	Yes	No	12 h	1%
Levobunolol (Betagan®)	Significant	Some activity	18 h	0.5%
Metipranolol (OptiPranolol®)	Significant	Some activity	18 h	0.3%
Timolol (Betimol®, Timoptic®)	Significant	Some activity	18 h	0.25%, 0.5%
Carbonic Anhydrase Inhibitors				
Acetazolamide (Diamox®)	Significant	No data	10 h	125 mg, 250 mg tab; 500 mg cap
Brinzolamide (Azopt®)	Yes	No data	8 h	1%
Dorzolamide (Trusopt®)	Yes	No	8 h	2%
Methazolamide	Significant	No data	14 h	25 mg, 50 mg
Prostaglandin Agonists				
Bimatoprost (Lumigan®)		Yes	≥24 h	0.03%
Latanoprost (Xalatan®)		Yes	≥24 h	0.005%
Travoprost (Travatan®)		Yes	20 h	0.004%

[1]All miotic drugs significantly affect accommodation.

HELICOBACTER PYLORI TREATMENT

Multiple Drug Regimens for the Treatment of *H. pylori* Infection

Drug	Dosages	Duration of Therapy
H$_2$-receptor antagonist[1]	Any one given at appropriate dose	4 weeks
plus		
Bismuth subsalicylate	525 mg 4 times/day	2 weeks
plus		
Metronidazole	250 mg 4 times/day	2 weeks
plus		
Tetracycline	500 mg 4 times/day	2 weeks
Proton pump inhibitor[1]	Esomeprazole 40 mg once daily	10 days
plus		
Clarithromycin	500 mg twice daily	10 days
plus		
Amoxicillin	1000 mg twice daily	10 days
Proton pump inhibitor[1]	Lansoprazole 30 mg twice daily or Omeprazole 20 mg twice daily	10-14 days
plus		
Clarithromycin	500 mg twice daily	10-14 days
plus		
Amoxicillin	1000 mg twice daily	10-14 days
Proton pump inhibitor[1]	Rabeprazole 20 mg twice daily	7 days
plus		
Clarithromycin	500 mg twice daily	7 days
plus		
Amoxicillin	1000 mg twice daily	7 days
Proton pump inhibitor	Lansoprazole 30 mg twice daily or Omeprazole 20 mg twice daily	2 weeks
plus		
Clarithromycin	500 mg twice daily	2 weeks
plus		
Metronidazole	500 mg twice daily	2 weeks
Proton pump inhibitor	Lansoprazole 30 mg once daily or Omeprazole 20 mg once daily	2 weeks
plus		
Bismuth	525 mg 4 times/day	2 weeks
plus		
Metronidazole	500 mg 3 times/day	2 weeks
plus		
Tetracycline	500 mg 4 times/day	2 weeks

[1]FDA-approved regimen.
Modified from Howden CS and Hunt RH, "Guidelines for the Management of *Helicobacter pylori* Infection," *AJG*, 1998, 93:2336.

INHALANT AGENTS

Medications Commonly Used for Asthma, Bronchospasm, and COPD

Agent	Indications	Onset	Duration	Frequency	Comments
Anticholinergics					
Ipratropium bromide (Atrovent®)	Bronchospasm associated with COPD	1-3 min	6 h	4 times/day	Additive bronchodilating effects used with α-, β$_2$-adrenergic agonists
Tiotropium (Spiriva®)	Bronchospasm associated with COPD			Daily	
Bronchodilators					
Albuterol (Proventil®, Proventil® HFA, Ventolin® HFA)	Prevention of exercise-induced bronchospasm; relief and prevention of bronchospasm	5 min	6-8 h	q4-6h	
Arformoterol (Brovana™)	Long-term maintenance treatment of bronchoconstriction in COPD	7-20 min		q12h	Not to be used for treatment of episodes of acute bronchospasm as rescue therapy
Epinephrine (various)	Treatment of bronchospasm	1-5 min	Individualize dosing		OTC; shorter-acting and less effective than prescription β-agonists
Formoterol (Foradil® Aerolizer™)	Long-term maintenance of asthma, prevention of bronchospasm; prevention of exercise-induced bronchospasm	Within 3 min	12 h	q12h	Not meant to relieve acute asthmatic symptoms
Ipratropium bromide and albuterol sulfate (Combivent®)	Patients with chronic obstructive pulmonary disease (COPD) on a regular aerosol bronchodilator who continue to have evidence of bronchospasm and who require a second bronchodilator	1-3 min		4 times/day	Additional doses may be administered; however, total doses should not exceed 12 in 24 hours
Levalbuterol (Xopenex®)	Bronchospasm with reversible obstructive airway disease	10-17 min	5-6 h	6-8 h intervals (nebulization); 4-6 h (inhaler)	
Metaproterenol sulfate (Alupent®)	Bronchial asthma and reversible bronchospasm; acute asthmatic attacks	5-30 min	4-6 h	q3-4h	Contraindicated in patients with arrhythmias; should not be used with other β-adrenergic aerosol inhalers because of additive effects
Pirbuterol acetate (Maxair™ Autohaler™)	Prevention and reversal of bronchospasm with reversible bronchospasm	Within 5 min	4-6 h	q4-6h	
Salmeterol (Serevent® Diskus®)	Long-term maintenance treatment of asthma and prevention of bronchospasm	20 min	12 h	q12h	Not meant to relieve acute asthmatic symptoms

Medications Commonly Used for Asthma, Bronchospasm, and COPD *(continued)*

Agent	Indications	Onset	Duration	Frequency	Comments
Corticosteroids[1]					
Beclomethasone dipropionate (various)	Bronchial asthma		6-8 h	Twice daily	Coughing and wheezing are more common
Budesonide (Pulmicort®)	Bronchial asthma		12 h	q12h	
Flunisolide (various)	Bronchial asthma		12 h	Twice daily	
Fluticasone (Flovent®)	Maintenance treatment of asthma as prophylactic therapy; also indicated for patients requiring oral corticosteroid therapy for asthma to assist in total discontinuation or reduction of total oral dose; **NOT** indicated for the relief of acute bronchospasm		–	Twice daily	May allow weaning from oral steroids in selected patients
Triamcinolone acetonide (Azmacort®)	Bronchial asthma		6-8 h	q6-8h	Asthma should be reasonably stable before Azmacort® treatment
Miscellaneous					
Cromolyn (Intal®)	Severe bronchial asthma; prevention of exercise-induced bronchospasm		6 h	4 times/day	Only useful in prophylaxis; has low toxicity and is as effective as theophylline in many patients
Nedocromil sodium (Tilade®)	Mild to moderate bronchial asthma		6 h	4 times/day	Must be taken regularly for benefit – even during symptom-free periods

[1]Not indicated for rapid relief of bronchospasm. Dysphonia and oral candidiasis can occur. Long-term use is associated with cataract formation.

LAXATIVES, CLASSIFICATION AND PROPERTIES

Laxative	Onset of Action	Site of Action	Mechanism of Action
Saline			
Magnesium citrate Magnesium hydroxide (Phillips'® Milk of Magnesia)	30 min to 3 h	Small and large intestine	Attract/retain water in intestinal lumen increasing intraluminal pressure; cholecystokinin release
Sodium phosphates (Fleet® Enema)	2-15 min	Colon	
Irritant / Stimulant			
Senna (Senokot®)	6-10 h	Colon	Direct action on intestinal mucosa; stimulate myenteric plexus; alter water and electrolyte secretion
Bisacodyl (Dulcolax®) tablets, suppositories	15 min to 1 h	Colon	
Castor oil	2-6 h	Small intestine	
Bulk-Producing			
Methylcellulose (Citrucel®) Psyllium (Metamucil®)	12-24 h (up to 72 h)	Small and large intestine	Holds water in stool; mechanical distention; malt soup extract reduces fecal pH
Lubricant			
Mineral oil	6-8 h	Colon	Lubricates intestine; retards colonic absorption of fecal water; softens stool
Surfactants / Stool Softener			
Docusate sodium (Colace®) Docusate calcium (Surfak®)	24-72 h	Small and large intestine	Detergent activity; facilitates admixture of fat and water to soften stool
Miscellaneous and Combination Laxatives			
Glycerin suppository	15-30 min	Colon	Local irritation; hyperosmotic action
Lactulose	24-48 h	Colon	Delivers osmotically active molecules to colon
Lubiprostone (Amitiza®)	24-48 h	Apical membrane of the GI epithelium	Activates intestinal chloride channels increasing intestinal fluid
Docusate/senna (Peri-Colace®)	8-12 h	Small and large intestine	Senna – mild irritant; docusate – stool softener
Polyethylene glycol 3350 (GlycoLax™, MiraLax™)	48 h	Small and large intestine	Nonabsorbable solution which acts as an osmotic agent
Sorbitol 70%	24-48 h	Colon	Delivers osmotically active molecules to colon

NARCOTIC / OPIOID ANALGESICS

Comparative Pharmacokinetics

Drug	Onset (min)	Peak (h)	Duration (h)	Half-Life (h)	Average Dosing Interval (h)	Equianalgesic Doses[1] (mg) I.M.	Equianalgesic Doses[1] (mg) Oral
Alfentanil	Immediate	ND	ND	1-2	—	ND	NA
Buprenorphine	15	1	4-8	2-3	—	0.4	—
Butorphanol	I.M.: 30-60; I.V.: 4-5	0.5-1	3-5	2.5-3.5	3 (3-6)	2	—
Codeine	P.O.: 30-60; I.M.: 10-30	0.5-1	4-6	3-4	3 (3-6)	120	200
Fentanyl	I.M.: 7-15 I.V.: Immediate	ND	1-2	1.5-6	1 (0.5-2)	0.1	NA
Hydrocodone	ND	ND	4-8	3.3-4.4	6 (4-8)	ND	ND
Hydromorphone	P.O.: 15-30	0.5-1	4-6	2-4	4 (3-6)	1.5	7.5
Levorphanol	P.O.: 10-60	0.5-1	4-8	12-16	6 (6-24)	2 (A) 1 (C)	4 (A) 1 (C)
Meperidine	P.O./I.M./SubQ: 10-15 I.V.: ≤5	0.5-1	2-4	3-4	3 (2-4)	75	300
Methadone	P.O.: 30-60; I.V.: 10-20	0.5-1	4-6 (A) >8 (C)	15-30	8 (6-12)	10 (A) 2-4 (C)	20 (A) 2-4 (C)
Morphine	P.O.: 15-60 I.V.: ≤5	P.O./I.M./SubQ: 0.5-1; I.V.: 0.3	3-6	2-4	4 (3-6)	10	60[2] (A) 30 (C)
Nalbuphine	I.M.: 30; I.V.: 1-3	1	3-6	5	—	10	—
Oxycodone	P.O.: 10-15	0.5-1	4-6	3-4	4 (3-6)	NA	20
Oxymorphone	5-15	0.5-1	3-6	2-3	3 (3-6)	1	10
Pentazocine	15-20	0.25-1	3-4	2-3	3 (3-6)	ND	130[3]-200[4]
Propoxyphene	P.O.: 30-60	2-2.5	4-6	3.5-15	6 (4-8)	ND	ND
Remifentanil	1-3	<0.3	0.1-0.2	0.15-0.3	—	ND	ND
Sufentanil	1.3-3	ND	ND	2.5-3	—	0.02	NA

ND = no data available. NA = not applicable. (A) = acute, (C) = chronic.

[1] Based on acute, short-term use. Chronic administration may alter pharmacokinetics and decrease the oral parenteral dose ratio. The morphine oral-parenteral ratio decreases to ~1.5-2.5:1 upon chronic dosing.

[2] Extensive survey data suggest that the relative potency of I.M.:P.O. morphine of 1:6 changes to 1:2-3 with chronic dosing.

[3] HCl salt.

[4] Napsylate salt.

Adapted from Principles of Analgesic Use in the Treatment of Acute Pain and Cancer Pain, 4th ed, Skokie, IL: The American Pain Society, 1999.

NARCOTIC / OPIOID ANALGESICS *(Continued)*

Comparative Pharmacology

Drug	Analgesic	Antitussive	Constipation	Respiratory Depression	Sedation	Emesis
Phenanthrenes						
Codeine	+	+++	+	+	+	+
Hydrocodone	+	+++		+		
Hydromorphone	++	+++	+	++	+	+
Levorphanol	++	++	++	++	++	+
Morphine	++	+++	++	++	++	++
Oxycodone	++	+++	++	++	++	++
Oxymorphone	++	+	++	+++		+++
Phenylpiperidines						
Alfentanil	++					
Fentanyl	++	+		+	+	+
Meperidine	++		+	++		
Remifentanil	++			++	+++	++
Sufentanil	+++					
Diphenylheptanes						
Methadone	++	++	++	++	+	+
Propoxyphene	+			+	+	+
Agonist / Antagonist						
Buprenorphine	++	N/A	+++	+++	++	++
Butorphanol	++	N/A	+++	+++	++	+
Nalbuphine	++	N/A	+++	+++	++	++
Pentazocine	++	N/A	+	++	++ or stimulation	++

SOME POTENTIAL PHOTOSENSITIZING AGENTS

Analgesics
Almotriptan
Nonsteroidal anti-inflammatory drugs[1]
    Celecoxib
    Diclofenac
    Flurbiprofen
    Ibuprofen
    Ketoprofen
    Meloxicam
    Nabumetone
    Naproxen
    Oxaprozin
    Piroxicam
    Tiaprofenic acid
Pentosan polysulfate sodium
Sulfasalazine
Sumatriptan
Zolmitriptan

Antineoplastics
Capecitabine
Dacarbazine
Dasatinib
Epirubicin
Floxuridine
Flucytosine
Fluorouracil
Flutamide
Imatinib
Leuprolide
Methotrexate
Porfimer
Thioguanine
UFT
Vinblastine

Antimicrobials
Amantadine
Atazanavir
Atovaquone and proguanil
Chloroquine
Dapsone
Demeclocycline[1]
Doxycycline[1]
Gentamicin
Griseofulvin
Interferon alpha-n3
Interferon beta-1b
Itraconazole
Kanamycin
Minocycline
Oxytetracycline
Pyrazinamide
Quinolones[1]
    Ciprofloxacin
    Gemifloxacin
    Levofloxacin
    Lomefloxacin
    Nalidixic acid
    Norfloxacin
    Ofloxacin
    Sparfloxacin

Sulfadiazine
Sulfadoxine and pyrimethamine
Sulfamethoxazole and trimethoprim
Sulfisoxazole
Tetracycline
Valacyclovir
Voriconazole

Cardiovascular Agents
Antilipemic agents
    Atorvastatin
    Fenofibrate
    Fluvastatin
    Gemfibrozil
    Lovastatin
    Pravastatin
    Simvastatin
ACE inhibitors
    Benazepril
    Enalapril
    Fosinopril
    Lisinopril
    Quinapril
    Ramipril
Beta-Blockers
    Carvedilol
    Metoprolol
    Sotalol
Calcium channel blockers
    Diltiazem
    Nifedipine
Diuretics
    Acetazolamide
    Furosemide
    Methazolamide
    Metolazone
    Thiazides[1]
        Chlorothiazide
        Chlorthalidone
        Hydrochlorothiazide
        Methyclothiazide
        Polythiazide
Miscellaneous cardiovascular agents
    Amiodarone[1]
    Losartan
    Quinidine[1]

CNS Agents
Antidepressants, tricyclic[1]
    Amitriptyline
    Amoxapine
    Clomipramine
    Desipramine
    Doxepin
    Imipramine
    Loxapine
    Maprotiline
    Nortriptyline
    Protriptyline
    Trimipramine

SOME POTENTIAL PHOTOSENSITIZING AGENTS *(Continued)*

Antidepressants, SSRI
  Fluoxetine
  Sertraline
Antidepressants, miscellaneous
  Bupropion
  Duloxetine
  Mirtazapine
  Nefazodone
Antihistamines
  Cetirizine
  Clemastine
  Cyproheptadine
  Diphenhydramine
  Loratadine
  Meclizine
Antipsychotic, miscellaneous
  Flupenthixol
  Haloperidol
  Molindone
  Quetiapine
  Risperidone
  Thiothixene
  Ziprasidone
  Zuclopenthixol
Antipsychotic, phenothiazine
  Chlorpromazine
  Fluphenazine
  Methotrimeprazine
  Perphenazine
  Pipotiazine
  Prochlorperazine
  Promethazine
  Trifluoperazine
Antiseizure agents
  Carbamazepine
  Felbamate
  Lamotrigine
  Oxcarbazepine
  Topiramate
  Valproic acid

Miscellaneous CNS agents
  Chlordiazepoxide
  Ropinirole
  Zaleplon

Hypoglycemic Agents
Chlorpropamide
Gliclazide
Glimepiride
Glipizide
Glyburide
Tolazamide
Tolbutamide

Skin Agents
Acitretin
Coal tar
Hexachlorophene
Silver sulfadiazine
Tretinoin
Triamcinolone

Miscellaneous Agents
Acamprosate
Alendronate
Anagrelide
Cevimeline
Cromolyn
Danazol
Droperidol
Glatiramer
Pilocarpine
Rabeprazole
Sildenafil
Tacrolimus
Thalidomide
Vardenafil
Verteporfin

[1]A 2004 NEJM paper identifies the marked drugs as being established as photosensitizing (Morison WL, "Clinical Practice. Photosensitivity," *N Engl J Med*, 2004, 350(11):1111-7). In light of sporadic and limited case reports, most other drugs labeled as photosensitizing are apparently only weakly and rarely so.

ASTHMA

MANAGEMENT OF ASTHMA IN ADULTS

Goals of Asthma Treatment

- Minimal or no chronic symptoms day or night
- Minimal or no exacerbations
- No limitations on activities; no school/work missed
- Minimal use of inhaled short-acting beta$_2$-agonist (<1 time/day, <1 canister/month)
- Minimal or no adverse effects from medications
- PEF >80% of personal best

All Patients

- Short-acting bronchodilator: **Inhaled beta$_2$-agonists** as needed for symptoms.
- Intensity of treatment will depend on severity of exacerbation; see "Management of Asthma Exacerbations".
- Use of short-acting inhaled beta$_2$-agonists on a daily basis, or increasing use, indicates the need to initiate or titrate long-term control therapy.

Education

- Teach self-management.
- Teach about controlling environmental factors (avoidance of allergens or other factors that contribute to asthma severity).
- Review administration technique and compliance with patient.
- May use a written action plan to help educate.

Stepwise Approach for Managing Asthma in Adults: Treatment[1]

Symptoms[2]	Lung Function[3]	Long-Term Control (Daily Medications)
STEP 4: Severe Persistent		
Day: Continual Night: Frequent	PEF/FEV$_1$ ≤60% PEF variability >30%	• **Preferred treatment:** – **High dose inhaled corticosteroid** **AND** – **Long-acting inhaled beta$_2$-agonist** AND, if needed – Long-term oral corticosteroids (2 mg/kg/day, generally do not exceed 60 mg/day). (Make repeated attempts to reduce systemic corticosteroids and maintain control with high-dose inhaled corticosteroids.)

ASTHMA *(Continued)*

Symptoms[2]	Lung Function[3]	Long-Term Control (Daily Medications)
STEP 3: Moderate Persistent		
Day: Every day Night: >1 night/week	PEF/FEV$_1$ >60% - <80% PEF variability >30%	• **Preferred treatment:** – **Low-medium dose inhaled corticosteroid** **AND** – **Long-acting inhaled beta$_2$-agonist** • Alternatives: – Increase inhaled corticosteroids within medium-dose range **OR** – Low-medium dose inhaled corticosteroids and either leukotriene receptor antagonist or theophylline
		If needed (especially with recurring severe exacerbations): • **Preferred treatment:** – Increase inhaled corticosteroids within medium-dose range, and add long-acting inhaled beta$_2$-agonist • Alternatives: – Increase inhaled corticosteroids in medium-dose range, and add either leukotriene receptor antagonist or theophylline
STEP 2: Mild Persistent		
Day: >2 days/week but <1 time/day Night: >2 nights/month	PEF/FEV$_1$ ≥80% PEF variability 20%-30%	• **Preferred treatment:** – **Low-dose inhaled corticosteroid** • Alternatives: Cromolyn, leukotriene receptor antagonist, nedocromil, or sustained release theophylline (serum concentration 5-15 mcg/mL)
STEP 1: Mild Intermittent		
Day: ≤2 days/week Night: ≤2 nights/month	PEF/FEV$_1$ ≥80% PEF variability <20%	No daily medication needed. A course of systemic corticosteroids is recommended for severe exacerbations.

[1]Classify severity. The presence of one of the features of severity is sufficient to place a patient in that category. An individual should be assigned to the most severe grade in which any feature occurs. The characteristics noted are general and may overlap because asthma is highly variable. Furthermore, an individual's classification may change over time.

[2]Patients at any level of severity can have mild, moderate, or severe exacerbations. Some patients with intermittent asthma experience severe and life-threatening exacerbations separated by long periods of normal lung function and no symptoms.

[3]PEF is % of personal best and FEV$_1$ is % predicted.

↓ **Step down**
Review treatment every 1-6 months; a gradual stepwise reduction in treatment may be possible.

↑**Step up**
If control is not maintained, consider step up. First, review patient medication technique, adherence, and environmental control.

Notes:

- **The stepwise approach presents general guidelines to assist clinical decision making; it is not intended to be a specific prescription. Asthma is highly variable; clinicians should tailor specific medication plans to the needs and circumstances of individual patients.**

- Gain control as quickly as possible; then decrease treatment to the least medication necessary to maintain control.

- A rescue course of systemic corticosteroids may be needed at any time and at any step.

- Some patients with intermittent asthma experience severe and life-threatening exacerbations separated by long periods of normal lung function and no symptoms. This may be especially common with exacerbations provoked by respiratory infections. A short course of systemic corticosteroids is recommended.

- At each step, patients should control their environment to avoid or control factors that make their asthma worse.

- Antibiotics are not recommended for treatment of acute asthma exacerbations except where there is evidence or suspicion of bacterial infection.

- Consultation with an asthma specialist is recommended for moderate or severe persistent asthma.

- Peak flow monitoring for patients with moderate-severe asthma should be considered.

ASTHMA *(Continued)*

Management of Asthma Exacerbations: Home Treatment[1]

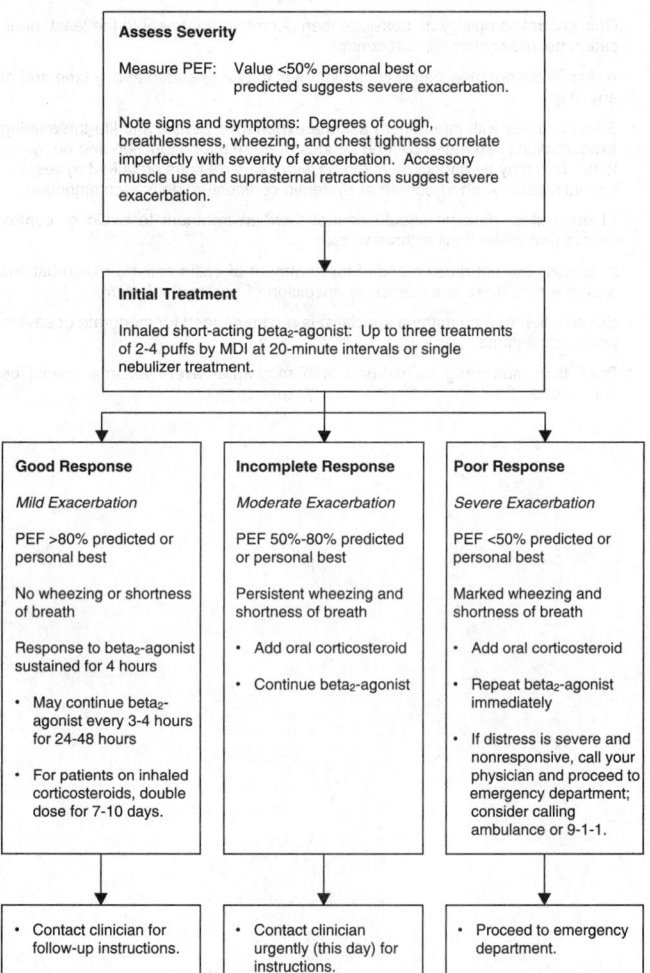

Assess Severity

Measure PEF: Value <50% personal best or predicted suggests severe exacerbation.

Note signs and symptoms: Degrees of cough, breathlessness, wheezing, and chest tightness correlate imperfectly with severity of exacerbation. Accessory muscle use and suprasternal retractions suggest severe exacerbation.

Initial Treatment

Inhaled short-acting beta$_2$-agonist: Up to three treatments of 2-4 puffs by MDI at 20-minute intervals or single nebulizer treatment.

Good Response

Mild Exacerbation

PEF >80% predicted or personal best

No wheezing or shortness of breath

Response to beta$_2$-agonist sustained for 4 hours

- May continue beta$_2$-agonist every 3-4 hours for 24-48 hours

- For patients on inhaled corticosteroids, double dose for 7-10 days.

- Contact clinician for follow-up instructions.

Incomplete Response

Moderate Exacerbation

PEF 50%-80% predicted or personal best

Persistent wheezing and shortness of breath

- Add oral corticosteroid

- Continue beta$_2$-agonist

- Contact clinician urgently (this day) for instructions.

Poor Response

Severe Exacerbation

PEF <50% predicted or personal best

Marked wheezing and shortness of breath

- Add oral corticosteroid

- Repeat beta$_2$-agonist immediately

- If distress is severe and nonresponsive, call your physician and proceed to emergency department; consider calling ambulance or 9-1-1.

- Proceed to emergency department.

[1]Patients at high risk of asthma-related death should receive immediate clinical attention after initial treatment. Additional therapy may be required.

Management of Asthma Exacerbations: Emergency Department and Hospital-Based Care

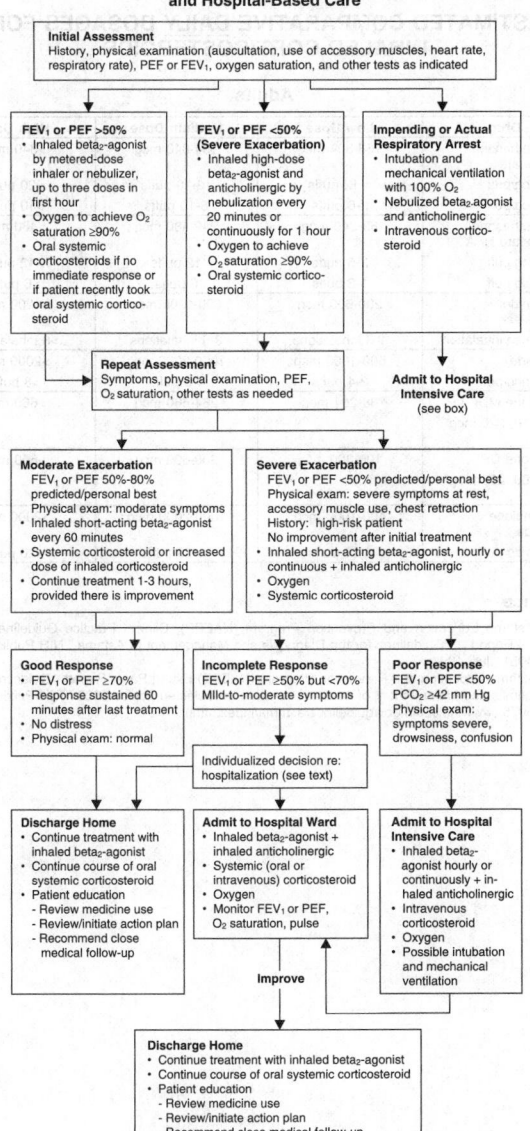

Initial Assessment
History, physical examination (auscultation, use of accessory muscles, heart rate, respiratory rate), PEF or FEV_1, oxygen saturation, and other tests as indicated

FEV_1 or PEF >50%
- Inhaled beta$_2$-agonist by metered-dose inhaler or nebulizer, up to three doses in first hour
- Oxygen to achieve O_2 saturation ≥90%
- Oral systemic corticosteroids if no immediate response or if patient recently took oral systemic corticosteroid

FEV_1 or PEF <50% (Severe Exacerbation)
- Inhaled high-dose beta$_2$-agonist and anticholinergic by nebulization every 20 minutes or continuously for 1 hour
- Oxygen to achieve O_2 saturation ≥90%
- Oral systemic corticosteroid

Impending or Actual Respiratory Arrest
- Intubation and mechanical ventilation with 100% O_2
- Nebulized beta$_2$-agonist and anticholinergic
- Intravenous corticosteroid

Repeat Assessment
Symptoms, physical examination, PEF, O_2 saturation, other tests as needed

Admit to Hospital Intensive Care
(see box)

Moderate Exacerbation
FEV_1 or PEF 50%-80% predicted/personal best
Physical exam: moderate symptoms
- Inhaled short-acting beta$_2$-agonist every 60 minutes
- Systemic corticosteroid or increased dose of inhaled corticosteroid
- Continue treatment 1-3 hours, provided there is improvement

Severe Exacerbation
FEV_1 or PEF <50% predicted/personal best
Physical exam: severe symptoms at rest, accessory muscle use, chest retraction
History: high-risk patient
No improvement after initial treatment
- Inhaled short-acting beta$_2$-agonist, hourly or continuous + inhaled anticholinergic
- Oxygen
- Systemic corticosteroid

Good Response
- FEV_1 or PEF ≥70%
- Response sustained 60 minutes after last treatment
- No distress
- Physical exam: normal

Incomplete Response
FEV_1 or PEF ≥50% but <70%
Mild-to-moderate symptoms

Poor Response
FEV_1 or PEF <50%
PCO_2 ≥42 mm Hg
Physical exam: symptoms severe, drowsiness, confusion

Individualized decision re: hospitalization (see text)

Discharge Home
- Continue treatment with inhaled beta$_2$-agonist
- Continue course of oral systemic corticosteroid
- Patient education
  - Review medicine use
  - Review/initiate action plan
  - Recommend close medical follow-up

Admit to Hospital Ward
- Inhaled beta$_2$-agonist + inhaled anticholinergic
- Systemic (oral or intravenous) corticosteroid
- Oxygen
- Monitor FEV_1 or PEF, O_2 saturation, pulse

Improve

Admit to Hospital Intensive Care
- Inhaled beta$_2$-agonist hourly or continuously + inhaled anticholinergic
- Intravenous corticosteroid
- Oxygen
- Possible intubation and mechanical ventilation

Discharge Home
- Continue treatment with inhaled beta$_2$-agonist
- Continue course of oral systemic corticosteroid
- Patient education
  - Review medicine use
  - Review/initiate action plan
  - Recommend close medical follow-up

ASTHMA *(Continued)*

ESTIMATED COMPARATIVE <u>DAILY</u> DOSAGES FOR INHALED CORTICOSTEROIDS

Adults

Drug	Low Dose	Medium Dose	High Dose
Beclomethasone dipropionate	168-504 mcg	504-840 mcg	>840 mcg
42 mcg/puff	4-12 puffs	12-20 puffs	>20 puffs
84 mcg/puff	2-6 puffs	6-10 puffs	>10 puffs
Beclomethasone dipropionate HFA	80-240 mcg	240-480 mcg	>480 mcg
40 mcg/puff	2-6 puffs	12 puffs	>12 puffs
80 mcg/puff	1-3 puffs	6 puffs	>6 puffs
Budesonide Turbuhaler®	200-600 mcg	600-1200 mcg	>1200 mcg
200 mcg/inhalation	1-3 inhalations	3-6 inhalations	>6 inhalations
Flunisolide	500-1000 mcg	1000-2000 mcg	>2000 mcg
250 mcg/puff	2-4 puffs	4-8 puffs	>8 puffs
Fluticasone MDI	88-264 mcg	264-660 mcg	>660 mcg
44, 110, 220 mcg/puff			
Fluticasone DPI	100-300 mcg	300-600 mcg	>600 mcg
50, 100, 250 mcg/dose			
Triamcinolone acetonide	400-1000 mcg	1000-2000 mcg	>2000 mcg
100 mcg/puff	4-10 puffs	10-20 puffs	>20 puffs

Reference

National Asthma Education and Prevention Program (NAEPP), Clinical Practice Guidelines, Expert Panel Report 2, "Guidelines for the Diagnosis and Management of Asthma," NIH Publication No. 97-4051, July 1997.

National Asthma Education and Prevention Program (NAEPP) Expert Panel Report, "Guidelines for the Diagnosis and Management of Asthma – Update on Selected Topics 2002," NIH Publication No. 02-5075 (www.nhlbi.nih.gov/guidelines/asthma/index.html)

HYPERLIPIDEMIA MANAGEMENT

MORTALITY

There is a strong link between serum cholesterol and cardiovascular mortality. This association becomes stronger in patients with established coronary artery disease. Lipid-lowering trials show that reductions in LDL cholesterol are followed by reductions in mortality. In general, each 1% fall in LDL cholesterol confers a 2% reduction in cardiovascular events. The aim of therapy for hyperlipidemia is to decrease cardiovascular morbidity and mortality by lowering cholesterol to a target level using safe and cost-effective treatment modalities. The target LDL cholesterol is determined by the number of patient risk factors (see the following Risk Factors and Goal LDL Cholesterol tables). The goal is achieved through diet, lifestyle modification, and drug therapy. The basis for these recommendations is provided by longitudinal interventional studies, demonstrating that lipid-lowering in patients with prior cardiovascular events (secondary prevention) and in patients with hyperlipidemia but no prior cardiac event (primary prevention) lowers the occurrence of future cardiovascular events, including stroke.

Major Risk Factors That Modify LDL Goals

Positive risk factors	Male ≥45 years
	Female ≥55 years
	Family history of premature coronary heart disease, defined as CHD in male first-degree relative <55 years; CHD in female first-degree relative <65 years
	Cigarette smoking
	Hypertension (blood pressure ≥140/90 mm Hg) or taking antihypertensive medication
	Low HDL (<40 mg/dL [1.03 mmol/L])
Negative risk factors	High HDL (≥60 mg/dL [1.6 mmol/L])[1]

[1]If HDL is ≥60 mg/dL, may subtract one positive risk factor.

Adult Treatment Panel (ATP) III LDL-C Goals and Cutpoints for Therapeutic Lifestyle Changes (TLC) and Drug Therapy in Different Risk Categories

Risk Category	LDL-C Goal	Initiate TLC	Consider Drug Therapy[1]
High risk: CHD[2] or CHD risk equivalents[3] (10-year risk >20%)	<100 mg/dL (optional goal: <70 mg/dL)[4]	≥100 mg/dL[5]	≥100 mg/dL[6] (<100 mg/dL: Consider drug options)[1]
Moderately high risk: 2+ risk factors[7] (10-year risk 10% to 20%)[8]	<130 mg/dL[9]	≥130 mg/dL[5]	≥130 mg/dL (100-120 mg/dL: Consider drug options)[10]
Moderate risk: 2+ risk factors[7] (10-year risk <10%)[8]	<130 mg/dL	≥130 mg/dL	≥160 mg/dL
Lower risk: 0-1 risk factor[11]	<160 mg/dL	≥160 mg/dL	≥190 mg/dL (160-189 mg/dL: LDL-lowering drug optional)

[1]When LDL-lowering drug therapy is employed, it is advised that intensity of therapy be sufficient to achieve at least a 30% to 40% reduction in LDL-C levels.

[2]CHD includes history of myocardial infarction, unstable angina, stable angina, coronary artery procedures (angioplasty or bypass surgery), or evidence of clinically significant myocardial ischemia.

[3]CHD risk equivalents include clinical manifestations of noncoronary forms of atherosclerotic disease (peripheral arterial disease, abdominal aortic aneurysm, and carotid artery disease [transient ischemic attacks or stroke of carotid origin or >50% obstruction of a carotid artery]), diabetes, and 2+ risk factors with 10-year risk for hard CHD >20%.

[4]Very high risk favors the optional LDL-C goal of <70 mg/dL, and in patients with high triglycerides, non-HDL-C <100 mg/dL.

[5]Any person at high risk or moderately high risk who has lifestyle-related risk factors (eg, obesity, physical inactivity, elevated triglyceride, low HDL-C, or metabolic syndrome) is a candidate for therapeutic lifestyle changes to modify these risk factors regardless of LDL-C level.

[6]If baseline LDL-C is <100 mg/dL, institution of an LDL-lowering drug is a therapeutic option on the basis of available clinical trial results. If a high-risk person has high triglycerides or low HDL-C, combining a fibrate or nicotinic acid with an LDL-lowering drug can be considered.

HYPERLIPIDEMIA MANAGEMENT *(Continued)*

[7]Risk factors include cigarette smoking, hypertension (BP ≥140/90 mm Hg or on antihypertensive medication), low HDL cholesterol (<40 mg/dL), family history of premature CHD (CHD in male first-degree relative <55 years of age; CHD in female first-degree relative <65 years of age), and age (men ≥45 years; women ≥55 years).

[8]Electronic 10-year risk calculators are available at www.nhlbi.nih.gov/guidelines/cholesterol.

[9]Optional LDL-C goal <100 mg/dL.

[10]For moderately high-risk persons, when LDL-C level is 100-129 mg/dL, at baseline or on lifestyle therapy, initiation of an LDL-lowering drug to achieve an LDL-C level <100 mg/dL is a therapeutic option on the basis of available clinical trial results.

[11]Almost all people with zero or 1 risk factor have a 10-year risk <10%, and 10-year risk assessment in people with zero or 1 risk factor thus not necessary.

Any person with elevated LDL cholesterol or other form of hyperlipidemia should undergo evaluation to rule out secondary dyslipidemia. Causes of secondary dyslipidemia include diabetes, hypothyroidism, obstructive liver disease, chronic renal failure, and drugs that increase LDL and decrease HDL (progestins, anabolic steroids, corticosteroids).

Elevated Serum Triglyceride Levels

Elevated serum triglyceride levels may be an independent risk factor for coronary heart disease. Factors that contribute to hypertriglyceridemia include obesity, inactivity, cigarette smoking, excess alcohol intake, high carbohydrate diets (>60% of energy intake), type 2 diabetes, chronic renal failure, nephrotic syndrome, certain medications (corticosteroids, estrogens, retinoids, higher doses of beta-blockers), and genetic disorders. Non-HDL cholesterol (total cholesterol minus HDL cholesterol) is a secondary focus for clinicians treating patients with high serum triglyceride levels (≥200 mg/dL). The goal for non-HDL cholesterol in patients with high serum triglyceride levels can be set 30 mg/dL higher than usual LDL cholesterol goals. Patients with serum triglyceride levels <200 mg/dL should aim for the target LDL cholesterol goal.

ATP classification of serum triglyceride levels:

- – Normal triglycerides: <150 mg/dL
- – Borderline-high: 150-199 mg/dL
- – High: 200-499 mg/dL
- – Very high: ≥500 mg/dL

NONDRUG THERAPY

Dietary therapy and lifestyle modifications should be individualized for each patient. A total lifestyle change is recommended for all patients. Dietary and lifestyle modifications should be tried for 3 months, if deemed appropriate. Nondrug and drug therapy should be initiated simultaneously in patients with highly elevated cholesterol (see LDL Cholesterol Goals and Cutpoints for Therapeutic Lifestyle Changes and Drug Therapy in Different Risk Categories table). Increasing physical activity and smoking cessation will aid in the treatment of hyperlipidemia and improve cardiovascular health.

Note: Refer to the National Cholesterol Education Program reference for details concerning the calculation of 10-year risk of CHD using Framingham risk scoring. Risk assessment tool is available on-line at http://hin.nhlbi.nih.gov/atpiii/calculator.asp?usertype=prof, last accessed March 14, 2002.

Total Lifestyle Change (TLC) Diet

	Recommended Intake
Total fat	25%-35% of total calories
Saturated fat[1]	<7% of total calories
Polyunsaturated fat	≤10% of total calories
Monounsaturated fat	≤20% of total calories
Carbohydrates[2]	50%-60% of total calories
Fiber	20-30 g/day
Protein	~15% of total calories
Cholesterol	<200 mg/day
Total calories[3]	Balance energy intake and expenditure to maintain desirable body weight/prevent weight gain

[1]*Trans* fatty acids (partially hydrogenated oils) intake should be kept low. These are found in potato chips, other snack foods, margarines and shortenings, and fast-foods.

[2]Complex carbohydrates including grains (especially whole grains, fruits, and vegetables).

[3]Daily energy expenditure should include at least moderate physical activity.

DRUG THERAPY

Drug therapy should be selected based on the patient's lipid profile, concomitant disease states, and the cost of therapy. The following table lists specific advantages and disadvantages for various classes of lipid-lowering medications. The expected reduction in lipids with therapy is listed in the Lipid-Lowering Agents table. Refer to individual drug monographs for detailed information.

Advantages and Disadvantages of Specific Lipid-Lowering Therapies

	Advantages	Disadvantages
Bile acid sequestrants	Good choice for ↑ LDL, especially when combined with a statin (↓ LDL ≤50%); low potential for systemic side effects; good choice for younger patients	May increase triglycerides; higher incidence of adverse effects; moderately expensive; drug interactions; inconvenient dosing
Niacin	Good choice for almost any lipid abnormality; inexpensive; greatest increase in HDL	High incidence of adverse effects; may adversely affect NIDDM and gout; sustained release niacin may decrease the incidence of flushing and circumvent the need for multiple daily dosing; sustained release niacin may not increase HDL cholesterol or decrease triglycerides as well as immediate release niacin
HMG-CoA reductase inhibitors	Produces greatest ↓ in LDL; generally well-tolerated; convenient once-daily dosing; proven decrease in mortality	Expensive
Gemfibrozil	Good choice in patients with ↑ triglycerides where niacin is contraindicated or not well-tolerated; gemfibrozil is well tolerated	Variable effects on LDL
Ezetimibe	Additional cholesterol-lowering effects when combined with HMG-CoA reductase inhibitors	Effects similar to bile acid sequestrants

HYPERLIPIDEMIA MANAGEMENT *(Continued)*

Lipid-Lowering Agents

Drug	Dose / Day	Effect on LDL (%)	Effect on HDL (%)	Effect on TG (%)
HMG-CoA Reductase Inhibitors				
Atorvastatin	10 mg 20 mg 40 mg 80 mg	-39 -43 -50 -60	+6 +9 +6 +5	-19 -26 -29 -37
Fluvastatin	20 mg 40 mg 80 mg	-22 -25 -36	+3 +4 +6	-12 -14 -18
Lovastatin	10 mg 20 mg 40 mg 80 mg	-21 -27 -31 -40	+5 +6 +5 +9.5	-10 -8 -8 -19
Pravastatin	10 mg 20 mg 40 mg 80 mg	-22 -32 -34 -37	+7 +2 +12 +3	-15 -11 -24 -19
Rosuvastatin	5 mg 10 mg 20 mg 40 mg	-45 -52 -55 -63	+13 +14 +8 +10	-35 -10 -23 -28
Simvastatin	5 mg 10 mg 20 mg 40 mg 80 mg	-26 -30 -38 -41 -47	+10 +12 +8 +13 +16	-12 -15 -19 -28 -33
Bile Acid Sequestrants				
Cholestyramine	4-24 g	-15 to -30	+3 to +5	+0 to +20
Colestipol	7-30 g	-15 to -30	+3 to +5	+0 to +20
Colesevelam	6 tablets 7 tablets	-15 -18	+3 +3	+10 +9
Fibric Acid Derivatives				
Fenofibrate	67-200 mg	-20 to -25	+1 to +34	-30 to -50
Gemfibrozil	600 mg twice daily	-5 to -10[1]	+10 to +20	-40 to -60
Niacin	1.5-6 g	-21 to -27	+10 to +35	-10 to -50
2-Azetidinone				
Ezetimibe	10 mg	-18	+1	-8
Omega-3-Acid Ethyl Esters	4 g	+44.5	+9.1	-44.9
Combination Products				
Ezetimibe and fenofibrate	10/160 mg	-20	+19	-44
Ezetimibe and simvastatin	10/10 mg 10/20 mg 10/40 mg 10/80 mg	-45 -52 -55 -60	+8 +10 +6 +6	-23 -24 -23 -31
Niacin and lovastatin	1000/20 mg 1000/40 mg 1500/40 mg 2000/40 mg	-30 -36 -37 -42	+20 +20 +27 +30	-32 -39 -44 -44

[1]May increase LDL in some patients.

Recommended Liver Function Monitoring for HMG-CoA Reductase Inhibitors

Agent	Initial and After Elevation in Dose	6 Weeks[1]	12 Weeks[1]	Periodically
Atorvastatin (Lipitor®)	x		x	x
Fluvastatin (Lescol®)	x		x	x
Lovastatin (Mevacor®)	x	x	x	x
Pravastatin (Pravachol®)	x			x
Simvastatin (Zocor®)	x			x

[1]After initiation of therapy or any elevation in dose.

Progression of Drug Therapy in Primary Prevention

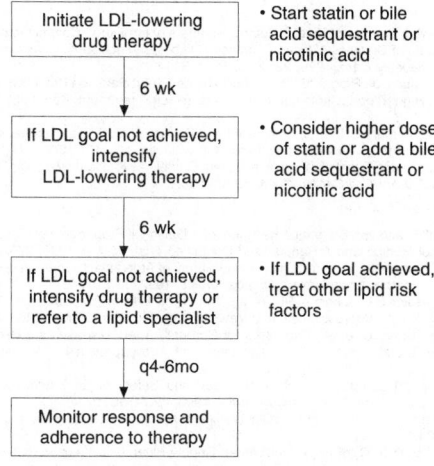

Initiate LDL-lowering drug therapy	• Start statin or bile acid sequestrant or nicotinic acid
↓ 6 wk	
If LDL goal not achieved, intensify LDL-lowering therapy	• Consider higher dose of statin or add a bile acid sequestrant or nicotinic acid
↓ 6 wk	
If LDL goal not achieved, intensify drug therapy or refer to a lipid specialist	• If LDL goal achieved, treat other lipid risk factors
↓ q4-6mo	
Monitor response and adherence to therapy	

DRUG SELECTION

Lipid Profile	Monotherapy	Combination Therapies
Increased LDL with normal HDL and triglycerides (TG)	Resin Niacin[1] Statin	Resin plus niacin[1] or statin Statin plus niacin[1,2]
Increased LDL and increased TG (200-499 mg/dL)[2]	Intensify LDL-lowering therapy	Statin plus niacin[1,3] Statin plus fibrate[3]
Increased LDL and increased TG (≥500 mg/dL)[2]	Consider combination therapy (niacin,[1] fibrates, statin)	
Increased TG	Niacin[1] Fibrates	Niacin[1] plus fibrates
Increased LDL and low HDL	Niacin[1] Statin	Statin plus niacin[1,2]

[1]Avoid in diabetics.

[2]Emphasize weight reduction and increased physical activity.

[3]Risk of myopathy with combination.

Resins = bile acid sequestrants; statins = HMG-CoA reductase inhibitors; fibrates = fibric acid derivatives (eg, gemfibrozil, fenofibrate).

COMBINATION DRUG THERAPY

If after at least 6 weeks of therapy at the maximum recommended or tolerated dose, the patient's LDL cholesterol is not at target, consider optimizing nondrug measures, prescribing a higher dose of current lipid-lowering drug, or adding another lipid-lowering medication to the current therapy. Successful drug combinations include statin and niacin, statin and bile acid sequestrant, or niacin and bile acid sequestrant. At maximum recommended doses, LDL cholesterol may be decreased by 50% to 60% with combination therapy. This is the same reduction achieved by atorvastatin 40 mg twice daily. If a bile acid sequestrant is used with other lipid-lowering agents, space doses 1 hour before or 4 hours after the bile acid sequestrant administration. Statins combined with either fenofibrate, clofibrate, gemfibrozil, or niacin increase the risk of rhabdomyolysis. In this situation, patient education (muscle pain/weakness) and careful follow-up are warranted.

HYPERLIPIDEMIA MANAGEMENT *(Continued)*

References

Guidelines

Gavin JR, Alberti KGMM, Davidson MB, et al, for the Members of the Expert Committee on the Diagnosis and Classification of Diabetes Mellitus, "American Diabetes Association: Clinical Practice Recommendations," *Diabetes Care*, 1999, 22(Suppl 1):S1-S114.

National Cholesterol Education Program, "Third Report of the Expert Panel on Detection, Evaluation, and Treatment of High Blood Cholesterol in Adults (Adult Treatment Panel III)," *JAMA*, 2001, 285:2486-97.

Grundy SM, Cleeman JI, Merz CN, et al, "Implications of Recent Clinical Trials for the National Cholesterol Education Program Adult Treatment Panel III Guidelines," *JACC*, 2004, 44(3):729.

Mosca L, Appel LJ, Benjamin EJ, et al, "Evidence-Based Guidelines for Cardiovascular Disease Prevention in Women," *J Am Coll Cardiol*, 2004, 43(5):900-21.

Others

Berthold HK, Sudhop T, and von Bergmann K, "Effect of a Garlic Oil Preparation on Serum Lipoproteins and Cholesterol Metabolism: A Randomized Controlled Trial," *JAMA*, 1998, 279:1900-2.

Bertolini S, Bon GB, Campbell LM, et al, "Efficacy and Safety of Atorvastatin Compared to Pravastatin in Patients With Hypercholesterolemia," *Atherosclerosis*, 1997, 130:191-7.

Blankenhorn DH, Nessim SA, Johnson RL, et al, "Beneficial Effects of Combined Colestipol-Niacin Therapy on Coronary Atherosclerosis and Venous Bypass Grafts," *JAMA*, 1987, 257:3233-40.

Brown G, Albers JJ, Fisher LD, et al, "Regression of Coronary Artery Disease as a Result of Intensive Lipid-Lowering Therapy in Men With High Levels of Apolipoprotein B," *N Engl J Med*, 1990, 323:1289-98.

Capuzzi DM, Guyton JR, Morgan JM, et al, "Efficacy and Safety of an Extended-Release Niacin (Niaspan®): A Long-Term Study," *Am J Cardiol*, 1998, 82:74U-81U.

Coronary Drug Project Research Program, "Clofibrate and Niacin in Coronary Heart Disease," *JAMA*, 1975, 231:360-81.

Dart A, Jerums G, Nicholson G, et al, "A Multicenter, Double-Blind, One-Year Study Comparing Safety and Efficacy of Atorvastatin Versus Simvastatin in Patients With Hypercholesterolemia," *Am J Cardiol*, 1997, 80:39-44.

Davidson MH, Dillon MA, Gordon B, et al, "Colesevelam Hydrochloride (Cholestagel): A New Potent Bile Acid Sequestrant Associated With a Low Incidence of Gastrointestinal Side Effects," *Arch Intern Med*, 1999, 159(16):1893-900.

Davidson M, McKenney J, Stein E, et al, "Comparison of One-Year Efficacy and Safety of Atorvastatin Versus Lovastatin in Primary Hypercholesterolemia," *Am J Cardiol*, 1997, 79:1475-81.

Frick MH, Heinonen OP, Huttunen JK, et al, "Helsinki Heart Study: Primary-Prevention Trial With Gemfibrozil in Middle-Aged Men With Dyslipidemia," *N Engl J Med*, 1987, 317:1237-45.

Garber AM, Browner WS, and Hulley SB, "Clinical Guideline, Part 2: Cholesterol Screening in Asymptomatic Adults, Revisited," *Ann Intern Med*, 1995, 124:518-31.

Johannesson M, Jonsson B, Kjekshus J, et al, "Cost-Effectiveness of Simvastatin Treatment to Lower Cholesterol Levels in Patients With Coronary Heart Disease. Scandinavian Simvastatin Survival Study Group," *N Engl N Med*, 1997, 336:332-6.

Jones P, Kafonek S, Laurora I, et al, "Comparative Dose Efficacy Study of Atorvastatin Versus Simvastatin, Pravastatin, Lovastatin, and Fluvastatin in Patients With Hypercholesterolemia," *Am J Cardiol*, 1998, 81:582-7.

Kasiske BL, Ma JZ, Kalil RS, et al, "Effects of Antihypertensive Therapy on Serum Lipids," *Ann Intern Med*, 1995, 133-41.

Lipid Research Clinics Program, "The Lipid Research Clinics Coronary Primary Prevention Trial Results: I. Reduction in Incidence of Coronary Heart Disease," *JAMA*, 1984, 251:351-64.

Mauro VF and Tuckerman CE, "Ezetimibe for Management of Hypercholesterolemia," *Ann Pharmacother*, 2003, 37(6):839-48.

Multiple Risk Factor Intervention Trial Research Group, "Multiple Risk Factor Intervention Trial: Risk Factor Changes and Mortality Results," *JAMA*, 1982, 248:1465-77.

Pitt B, Waters D, Brown WV, et al, "Aggressive Lipid-Lowering Therapy Compared With Angioplasty in Stable Coronary Artery Disease. Atorvastatin Versus Revascularization Treatment Investigators," *N Engl J Med*, 1999, 341(2):70-6.

Ross SD, Allen IE, Connelly JE, et al, "Clinical Outcomes in Statin Treatment Trials: A Meta-Analysis," *Arch Intern Med*, 1999, 159:1793-802.

Sacks FM, Pfeffer MA, Moye LA, et al, "The Effect of Pravastatin on Coronary Events After Myocardial Infarction in Patients With Average Cholesterol Levels," *N Engl J Med*, 1996, 335:1001-9.

Scandinavian Simvastatin Survival Study, "Randomized Trial of Cholesterol Lowering in 4444 Patients With Coronary Heart Disease: The Scandinavian Simvastatin Survival Study (4S)," *Lancet*, 1994, 344:1383-9.

Schrott HG, Bittner V, Vittinghoff E, et al, "Adherence to National Cholesterol Education Program Treatment Goals in Postmenopausal Women With Heart Disease. The Heart and Estrogen/Progestin Replacement Study (HERS)," *JAMA*, 1997, 277:1281-6.

Shepherd J, Cobbe SM, Ford I, et al, "Prevention of Coronary Heart Disease With Pravastatin in Men With Hypercholesterolemia, The West of Scotland Coronary Prevention Study Group," *N Engl J Med*, 1995, 333:1301-7.

Stein EA, Davidson MH, Dobs AS, et al, "Efficacy and Safety of Simvastatin 80 mg/day in Hypercholesterolemic Patients. The Expanded Dose Simvastatin U.S. Study Group," *Am J Cardiol*, 1998, 82:311-6.

OSTEOPOROSIS MANAGEMENT

PREVALENCE

Osteoporosis affects 25 million Americans of whom 80% are women. 27% of American women >80 years of age have osteopenia and 70% of American women >80 years of age have osteoporosis.

CONSEQUENCES

Osteoporosis results in 1.3 million bone fractures annually (low impact/nontraumatic) and pain, pulmonary insufficiency, decreased quality of life, and economic costs; >300,000 hip fractures with a 20% mortality rate and >700,000 vertebral fractures occur in women each year.

RISK FACTORS

- Advanced age
- Anorexia/hypogonadism, cancer, chronic renal disease, Cushing's disease, hyperparathyroidism, hyperprolactinemia, hyperthyroidism (current condition, history of, or use of excessive thyroid supplements), hypogonadism
- Caucasian or Asian race
- Early menopause
- Excessive alcohol intake
- Excessive exercise
- Family history
- Female gender
- Fracture in first degree relative
- History of low calcium intake
- Oophorectomy without hormone replacement
- Previous fracture as adult
- Recurrent falls
- Sedentary lifestyle
- Smoking
- Use of aluminum-containing antacids (excessive), anticonvulsants, ethanol, heparin or glucocorticoids (large doses or prolonged use), methotrexate, or cyclosporine
- Weight <127 lbs if female

DIAGNOSIS / MONITORING

- DXA bone density scan
- Osteomark® urine assay[1]
- History of fracture (low impact or nontraumatic)
- Compressed vertebrae
- Decreased height
- Hump-back appearance
- Excluded secondary causes

[1]Osteomark® urine assay measures bone breakdown fragments and may help assess therapy response earlier than DXA bone scan but diagnostic value is uncertain as Osteomark® does not reveal extent of bone loss. Bone markers may be tested to evaluate effectiveness of antiresorptive urine therapy.

PREVENTION

1. Adequate intake of dietary calcium (eg, dairy products)

2. Increased intake of vitamin D (eg, fortified dairy products, cod, fatty fish)

3. Weight-bearing exercise (eg, walking), as tolerated

4. Calcium supplement: 1000-1500 mg **elemental** calcium daily (divided in 500 mg increments); see table located at the end of this section. Do not administer orally with bran, foods high in oxalates, or whole grain cereals. Calcium carbonate is given with food to enhance bioavailability. Chewable and liquid products are available.

   Adults ≥51 years: Supplement 1200 mg **elemental** calcium.

   Women >65 years on estrogen replacement therapy: Supplement 1000 mg **elemental** calcium.

   Women >65 years not receiving estrogens and men >55 years: Supplement 1500 mg **elemental** calcium.

OSTEOPOROSIS MANAGEMENT *(Continued)*

- Contraindications: Hypercalcemia, renal calculi, ventricular fibrillation

- Side effects: Constipation, anorexia; to minimize constipation, add fiber supplement to diet and start with 500 mg/day for several months, then increase to 500 mg twice daily taken at different times than the fiber supplement

- Drug interactions: May potentiate digoxin toxicity, antagonize effects of calcium channel blockers (eg, verapamil), decrease potassium-binding ability of polystyrene sulfonate, and decrease absorption of tetracycline, atenolol, iron, quinolone antibiotics, alendronate, sodium fluoride, and zinc; high doses of calcium with thiazide diuretics may result in milk-alkali syndrome and hypercalcemia

5. Bisphosphonates: Alendronate 5 mg/day or 35 mg/week, ibandronate 2.5 mg/day or 150 mg/month, and risedronate 5 mg/day or 35 mg/week are approved for the prevention of osteoporosis in postmenopausal women. Risedronate 5 mg/day is also approved for the prevention of glucocorticoid-induced osteoporosis. Patients must be capable of following specific instructions related to drug administration (see Treatment for administration, side effects, and precautions).

6. Selective estrogen receptor modulators: SERMs are nonsteroidal modulators of estrogen-receptor mediated reactions. The key difference between these agents and estrogen replacement therapies is the potential to exert tissue-specific effects. Due to their chemical differences, these agents retain some of estrogen's beneficial effects on bone metabolism and lipid levels, but differ in their actions on breast and endometrial tissues, potentially limiting adverse effects related to nonspecific hormone stimulation. Among the SERMs, tamoxifen retains stimulatory effects in endometrial tissue, while raloxifene does not stimulate endometrial or breast tissue, limiting the potential for endometrial or breast cancer related to this agent. Raloxifene is the only SERM which has been approved by the FDA for osteoporosis prevention.

    Note: The effects on bone observed with SERMs appear to be less than that observed with estrogen replacement. In one study, the effect of raloxifene on hip bone mineral density was approximately half of that observed with conjugated estrogens. Raloxifene decreases total high-density lipoprotein cholesterol or triglyceride levels. Raloxifene has been shown to reduce the risk of breast cancer, not increase the risk of endometrial cancer, but increase the risk of DVT compared to placebo in postmenopausal women. Finally, SERMs do not block the vasomotor effects observed with menopause, which may limit compliance with therapy.

    Raloxifene: 60 mg/day; may be taken any time of the day without regard to meals but should be stopped 72 hours prior to or during prolonged immobilization due to risk of thromboembolic events (similar to reported risk of HRT).

    - Contraindications: Active thromboembolic disorder, prolonged immobilization (eg, postoperative recovery, prolonged bedrest)

    - Side effects: Hot flashes (vasomotor symptoms), increased risk of thromboembolism (DVT, PE) and superficial thrombophlebitis, flu-like symptoms (resolve with use), GI upset, vaginitis, UTI

    - Drug interactions: Ampicillin and cholestyramine decrease raloxifene absorption. Avoid ethanol.

7. Estrogens should not be considered first agents for preventing osteoporosis due to increased risk of breast cancer, heart disease, stroke, and deep-vein thrombosis (DVT) found in the Women's Health Initiative study. Estradiol, as well as various combination therapies, including ethinyl estradiol with norethindrone (femhrt®) and ethinyl with norgestimate (Ortho-Prefest®), have been approved for the prevention of osteoporosis.

8. Estrogen: 0.625 mg/day conjugated estrogen **or** its equivalent; initiate therapy slowly and monitor blood pressure in long-term use. In women with an intact uterus, administer with medroxyprogesterone acetate (MPA) 2.5-5 mg/day **or** another oral progesterone; unopposed estrogen can cause endometrial cancer.

    Note: Continuous therapy is preferred; especially useful if bone density is <80% of average and patient has symptoms of estrogen deficiency. Substantial evidence suggests that estrogen therapy increases bone mineralization; bone density increases over 1-2 years, then reaches a plateau. Therapy should be initiated after careful evaluation of risk:benefit ratio. Pretreatment mammogram and gynecological exam are advised along with routine breast exam due to possible increased risk of breast cancer with long-term use.

- Contraindications: Breast or estrogen-dependent cancer, undiagnosed abnormal genital bleeding, active thrombophlebitis, history of thromboembolism during previous estrogen therapy

  Note: It is important that patients on long-term estrogens avoid cigarette use. Conjugated estrogens (alone or in combination with a progestin) should not be used to prevent coronary heart disease. The HERS trial found that women with coronary disease derived no cardiovascular protection compared to those treated with placebo. In the Women's Health Initiative trial, a conjugated estrogen/progestin combination did not offer protection against heart disease. No cardiovascular benefits were seen, in fact, **more coronary heart disease was observed** in the treatment group.

- Side effects (more common/severe in women without estrogen for many years): Vaginal spotting/bleeding, nausea, vomiting, breast tenderness/enlargement, amenorrheic (with extended use), hypertension (less severe with lower doses), thromboembolic events (particularly in women who smoke). **Note:** If MPA is also used, it can increase vaginal bleeding, increase weight, edema, and mood changes.

- Drug interactions: May enhance the effects of hydrocortisone and prednisone; monitor for need to decrease corticosteroid dose. Anticoagulants: Increase potential for thromboembolic events with anticoagulants. CYP3A4 enzyme inducers (eg, carbamazepine, phenobarbital, rifampin) may decrease estrogen plasma concentrations; inhibitors (eg, clarithromycin, erythromycin, itraconazole, ketoconazole, ritonavir) may increase estrogen plasma concentrations. Avoid ethanol, grapefruit juice, St John's wort, black cohosh, dong quai, red clover, saw palmetto, and ginseng.

9. Vitamin D: 400-800 units/day (often satisfied by 1-2 multivitamins or fortified milk) in addition to calcium or a combined calcium and vitamin D supplement, **and/or** >15 minutes direct sunlight/day. Symptoms of deficiency include bone and tooth disorders, rickets, and osteomalacia.

   Note: Some older adults, especially those with significant renal or liver disease cannot metabolize (activate) vitamin D and require calcitriol or dosage adjustment per serum calcium level, the active form of vitamin D. Check 1,25 OH vitamin D level to confirm need for calcitriol. If required, administer 0.25 mcg calcitriol orally twice daily.

   - Contraindications: Hypercalcemia (weakness, headache, drowsiness, nausea, diarrhea), hypercalciuria, renal stones

   - Side effects: Hypercalcemia (uncommon); monitor 24-hour urine and serum calcium if using >1000 units/day. Overdose symptoms include excessive thirst, dehydration, anorexia, nausea, vomiting, headache, constipation, weakness, weight loss, hypercalcemia, kidney stones, arterial calcium deposits

   - Drug interactions: Drugs which can cause depletion of vitamin D include cholestyramine, anticonvulsants, corticosteroids, isoniazid, rifampin, H_2-receptor antagonists, and mineral oil. Vitamin A antagonizes some of the activity of vitamin D.

TREATMENT

1. Calcium, vitamin D, exercise, and estrogen: See table *on page 1783*.

2. Bisphosphonates: Administer ≥30 minutes before first food or drink (except water) with 6-8 ounces tap water (**not** mineral water) and remain upright (or raise head of bed to at least a 30° angle) to avoid ulcerative esophagitis.

   Note: Bisphosphonates may be useful even when the patient has severe osteoporosis (ie, ≥2.5 standard deviations below average young adult bone density, T-score, or history of low impact or nontraumatic fracture). Increasing bone density of hip and spine has been observed for at least 3 years (ie, no plateau as seen with estrogen). Therapy with calcium and vitamin D is advised (must be given at a different time of day than alendronate).

   Contraindications: Hypocalcemia (must be corrected prior to therapy), abnormalities of the esophagus which delay emptying (ie, stricture, achalasia), inability to stand or sit upright for at least 30 minutes

   - Alendronate (Fosamax®): Not recommended if Cl_{cr} <35 mL/minute.

     Osteoporosis **Males/postmenopausal females:** Treatment: 10 mg once daily **or** 70 mg once weekly.

OSTEOPOROSIS MANAGEMENT *(Continued)*

Glucocorticoid-induced osteoporosis: Treatment: 5 mg once daily; 10 mg once daily for postmenopausal women not receiving estrogen

Side effects: Hypocalcemia, hypophosphatemia, GI disturbances, musculoskeletal pain

Drug interactions: Increased GI effects with >10 mg alendronate and aspirin-containing products; wait at least 30 minutes after taking alendronate before taking any oral medications. Ranitidine can double the bioavailability of alendronate.

- Etidronate is not FDA-approved for postmenopausal osteoporosis and can decrease the quality of bone formation; **use alternative bisphosphonate**.

- Ibandronate (Boniva®): Not recommended if Cl_{cr} <30 mL/minute.

Osteoporosis: **Postmenopausal females:** 2.5 mg/day or 150 mg/month as a single monthly dose. Must be taken fasting with water and the patient must remain upright and fasting for **at least 60 minutes** after taking a dose.

Side effects: Gastrointestinal; back, joint, and muscle pain; osteonecrosis of the jaw

Drug interactions: Administer antacids and calcium supplements at a different time of the day so as not to interfere with absorption of ibandronate. Avoid ethanol.

- Risedronate (Actonel®): Not recommended if Cl_{cr} <30 mL/minute.

Osteoporosis: **Postmenopausal females:** 5 mg once daily **or** 35 mg once weekly

Glucocorticoid-induced osteoporosis: 5 mg once daily

Side effects: Flu-like symptoms

Drug interactions: Administer antacids and calcium supplements at a different time of the day so as not to interfere with absorption of risedronate. Avoid ethanol.

3. Calcitonin is indicated for the treatment of osteoporosis and may also be used as adjunctive therapy for hypercalcemia. Adequate dietary or supplemental calcium and vitamin D is essential. I.M. route is preferred if volume exceeds 2 mL. Administration in the evening may minimize flushing, nausea, and vomiting.

Hypercalcemia: Initial: 4 units/kg every 12 hours I.M., SubQ; may increase up to 8 units/kg every 12 hours (maximum every 6 hours)

Osteoporosis: **Postmenopausal females:** 100 units/day I.M., SubQ **or** 200 units/day (1 spray) intranasal; 1 spray (200 units) into 1 nostril daily (alternate right and left nostril daily); 5 days on and 2 days off is also effective but alternate day administration is not effective. If used only for pain, can decrease dose once pain is controlled.

- Contraindications: Hypersensitivity to salmon protein or gelatin diluent

- Side effects: Nasal dryness/irritation (periodically inspect), flushing, nausea, vomiting; SubQ 100 units/day: Many side effects including nausea, flushing, anorexia, and the discomfort/inconvenience of injection

4. Raloxifene: Refer to raloxifene information under "Prevention".

5. Teriparatide is indicated for the treatment of osteoporosis in postmenopausal women at high risk of fracture as well as the treatment of primary or hypogonadal osteoporosis in men at high risk of fracture.

- Dose: SubQ: 20 mcg once daily. **Note:** Initial administration should occur under circumstances in which the patient may sit or lie down, in the event of orthostasis.

- Contraindications: Should not be used in patients with a history of skeletal metastases, hyperparathyroidism, or pre-existing hypercalcemia. Metabolic bone disease other than osteoporosis should be excluded prior to initiating therapy.

- Warnings: Should be used with caution in patients with active or recent urolithiasis or in patients at risk of orthostasis patients as well as patients who may not tolerate transient hypotension. Due to concerns for a possible association between long term, high-dose use and osteosarcoma, teriparatide is not recommended for use longer than 2 years, and should be avoided in patients with an increased risk of osteosarcoma.

- Side effects: Transient hypercalcemia may be noted between 4 and 6 hours after a dose. Arthralgia, asthenia, and leg cramps may occur. May be associated with central nervous system effects such as dizziness, depression or vertigo. In addition, teriparatide use has been associated with gastrointestinal effects (nausea, dyspepsia) and rash.

6. Fall prevention: Minimize psychoactive and cardiovascular drugs, monitor BP for orthostasis, administer diuretics early in the day, and check environment for safety hazards.

Calcium Type	Elemental Calcium	Equivalent Elemental Calcium	Brand
Acetate	25%	667 mg = 169 mg	Phos-Lo® gelcaps and tablets
Carbonate	40%	364 mg = 145.6 mg	Florical® capsules and tablets
		400 mg = 160 mg	Mylanta® Children's chewable tablets
		420 mg = 168 mg	Chewable tablets: Alcalak, Amitone®, Titralac™
		500 mg = 200 mg	Chewable tablets: Cal-Gest, Chooz®, Tums®
		650 mg = 260 mg	Cal-Mint chewable tablets
		750 mg = 300 mg	Chewable tablets: Titralac™ Extra Strength, Tums® E-X, Tums® Extra Strength Sugar Free, Tums® Smooth Dissolve
		850 mg = 340 mg	Alka-Mints® chewable tablets
		1000 mg = 400 mg	Tums® Ultra chewable tablets
		1250 mg = 500 mg	Calci-Mix® capsules
			Chewable tablets: Calci-Chew®, Os-Cal® 500, Oysco 500, Oyst-Cal 500
		1250 mg/5 mL = 500 mg	Generic oral solution
		1500 mg = 600 mg	Chewable tablets: Calcarb 600, Caltrate® 600, Nephro-Calci®
Citrate	21%	950 mg = 200 mg	Citracal®
		2376 mg = 500 mg	Citracal® Liquitab effervescent tablets
Glubionate	6.5%	1.8 g = 115 g/5 mL	Various OTC and generic brands available
Gluconate	9%	500 mg = 45 mg	
Lactate	13%	325 mg = 42.25 mg	
Phosphate tribasic	39%	1565.2 mg = 600 mg	Posture®

References

Ashworth L, "Focus on Alendronate. A Nonhormonal Option for the Treatment of Osteoporosis in Postmenopausal Women," Formulary, 1996, 31:23-30.

Barrett-Connor E, Grady D, Sashegyi A, et al, "Raloxifene and Cardiovascular Events in Osteoporotic Postmenopausal Women: Four-Year Results From the MORE (Multiple Outcomes of Raloxifene Evaluation) Randomized Trial," JAMA, 2002, 287(7):847-57.

Grady D, Ettinger B, Moscarelli E, et al, "Safety and Adverse Effects Associated With Raloxifene: Multiple Outcomes of Raloxifene Evaluation," Obstet Gynecol, 2004, 104(4):837-44.

Hully S, Grady D, Bush T, et al, "Randomized Trial of Estrogen Plus Progestin for Secondary Prevention of Coronary Heart Disease in Postmenopausal Women. Heart and Estrogen/Progestin Replacement Study (HERS) Research Group," JAMA, 1998, 280(7):605-13.

Johnson SR, "Should Older Women Use Estrogen Replacement," J Am Geriatr Soc, 1996, 44:89-90.

Liberman UA, Weiss SR, and Brool J, "Effect of Oral Alendronate on Bone-Mineral Density and the Incidence of Fracture in Postmenopausal Osteoporosis," N Engl J Med, 1995, 333:1437-43.

"New Drugs for Osteoporosis," Med Lett Drugs Ther, 1996, 38:1-3.

NIH Concensus Development Panel on Optimal Calcium Intake, JAMA, 1994, 272:1942-8.

PCA Osteoporosis Prevention and Treatment Video-Teleconference (March 1, April 2 and 3, 1996).

"Writing Group for the Women's Health Initiative Investigators. Risks and Benefits of Estrogen Plus Progestin in Healthy Postmenopausal Women: Principle Results From the Women's Health Initiative Randomized Controlled Trial," JAMA, 2002, 288:321-33.

Multiple outcomes of raloxifene trial.

PARKINSON'S DISEASE MANAGEMENT

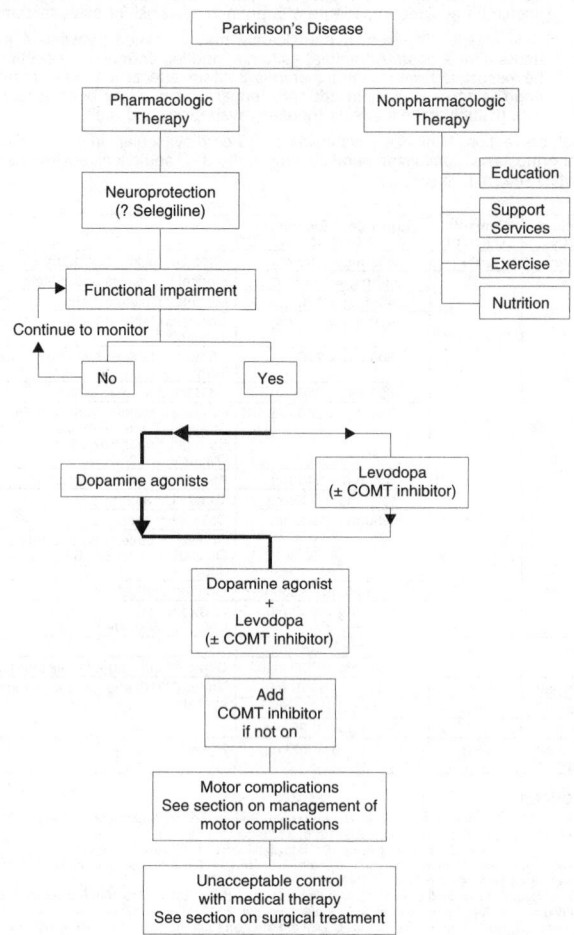

Recommendations for PD management are as follows:
- Ensure that correct diagnosis is made.
- Consider neuroprotective therapy as soon as diagnosis is made.
- Initiate symptomatic therapy with a dopamine agonist as appropriate.
- Supplement with levodopa when dopamine agonist monotherapy no longer provides satisfactory clinical control.
- Consider introducing supplemental levodopa therapy in combination with a COMT inhibitor to extend its elimination half-life.
- Consider surgical intervention when parkonsonism cannot be satisfactorily controlled with medical therapies.

Adapted from Olanow CW, Watts RL, and Koller WC, "An Algorithm (Decision Tree) for the Management of Parkinson's Disease (2001): Treatment Guidelines," *Neurology*, 2001, 56(11; Suppl 5):54.

TREATMENT OPTIONS FOR CONSTIPATION

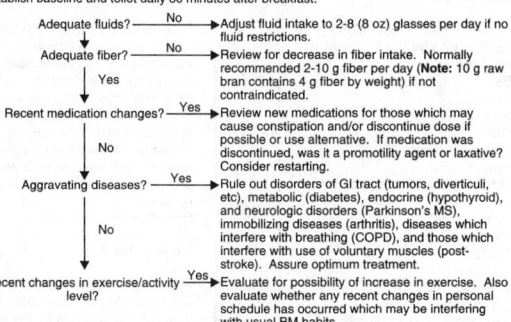

- Define constipation as no more than two bowel movements per week, or straining upon defecation 25% of the time or more. If possible, educate resident about this definition to develop cooperation.
- Verify constipation with digital exam and/or x-ray (radiography) if impaction is suspected. Establish baseline and toilet daily 30 minutes after breakfast.

Adequate fluids? — No → Adjust fluid intake to 2-8 (8 oz) glasses per day if no fluid restrictions.

Adequate fiber? — No → Review for decrease in fiber intake. Normally recommended 2-10 g fiber per day (**Note:** 10 g raw bran contains 4 g fiber by weight) if not contraindicated.

Yes

Recent medication changes? — Yes → Review new medications for those which may cause constipation and/or discontinue dose if possible or use alternative. If medication was discontinued, was it a promotility agent or laxative? Consider restarting.

No

Aggravating diseases? — Yes → Rule out disorders of GI tract (tumors, diverticuli, etc), metabolic (diabetes), endocrine (hypothyroid), and neurologic disorders (Parkinson's MS), immobilizing diseases (arthritis), diseases which interfere with breathing (COPD), and those which interfere with use of voluntary muscles (post-stroke). Assure optimum treatment.

No

Recent changes in exercise/activity level? — Yes → Evaluate for possibility of increase in exercise. Also evaluate whether any recent changes in personal schedule has occurred which may be interfering with usual BM habits.

Once constipation is identified and contributing factors are ruled out, determine if any signs or symptoms of fecal impaction are exhibited (distended abdomen, fever, vomiting, confusion).

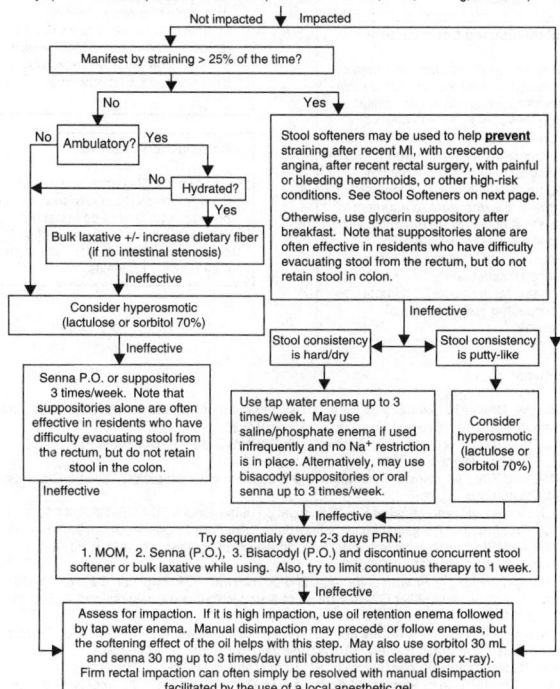

Not impacted | Impacted

Manifest by straining > 25% of the time?

No / Yes

Ambulatory? No / Yes

Hydrated? No / Yes

Bulk laxative +/- increase dietary fiber (if no intestinal stenosis)

Ineffective

Stool softeners may be used to help **prevent** straining after recent MI, with crescendo angina, after recent rectal surgery, with painful or bleeding hemorrhoids, or other high-risk conditions. See Stool Softeners on next page.

Otherwise, use glycerin suppository after breakfast. Note that suppositories alone are often effective in residents who have difficulty evacuating stool from the rectum, but do not retain stool in colon.

Ineffective

Consider hyperosmotic (lactulose or sorbitol 70%)

Ineffective

Stool consistency is hard/dry

Stool consistency is putty-like

Senna P.O. or suppositories 3 times/week. Note that suppositories alone are often effective in residents who have difficulty evacuating stool from the rectum, but do not retain stool in the colon.

Use tap water enema up to 3 times/week. May use saline/phosphate enema if used infrequently and no Na$^+$ restriction is in place. Alternatively, may use bisacodyl suppositories or oral senna up to 3 times/week.

Consider hyperosmotic (lactulose or sorbitol 70%)

Ineffective

Ineffective

Try sequentially every 2-3 days PRN:
1. MOM, 2. Senna (P.O.), 3. Bisacodyl (P.O.) and discontinue concurrent stool softener or bulk laxative while using. Also, try to limit continuous therapy to 1 week.

Ineffective

Assess for impaction. If it is high impaction, use oil retention enema followed by tap water enema. Manual disimpaction may precede or follow enemas, but the softening effect of the oil helps with this step. May also use sorbitol 30 mL and senna 30 mg up to 3 times/day until obstruction is cleared (per x-ray). Firm rectal impaction can often simply be resolved with manual disimpaction facilitated by the use of a local anesthetic gel.

TREATMENT OPTIONS FOR CONSTIPATION *(Continued)*

One should expect gradual rather than immediate results from a newly instituted laxative regimen. Additionally, nondrug interventions should be maintained during pharmacologic treatment of constipation as this is one of the cornerstones of long-term management.

Constipating Drugs

Aluminum (antacids, sucralfate)
Anticholinergics (antiparkinsons)
Antihistamines
CCBs
Levodopa
Opiates
MAOIs
Tricyclic antidepressants
Aluminum
Calcium (supplements & antacids)
Iron
Phenothiazines
Diuretics
Clonidine
Guanabenz
Guanfacine
Disopyramide
Irritant laxatives (with cathartic colon)
Vinca alkaloids
5-HT$_3$ antagonists
Anticonvulsants

Stool Softeners

Stool softeners have no laxative action and are not helpful in alleviating chronic constipation and may cause fecal incontinence. Short-term use is appropriate to minimize straining caused by hard stools following rectal surgery or recent MI or when defecation causes hemorrhoidal pain, rectal bleeding, crescendo angina, or other high risk condition.

Saline Laxatives

Regular use of saline laxatives is not recommended because their risks outweigh the benefits of the laxative. Saline laxatives are only indicated for acute bowel evacuation for diagnostic procedures.
Also, note that use of Milk of Magnesia in renally impaired residents can result in Mg^{++} toxicity (hypotension, muscle weakness, EKG changes, CNS changes).

Opioid-Induced Constipation

Stimulant laxatives such as senna or bisacodyl in combination with a stool softener such as docusate sodium often serve as an effective first-line regimen. Senna P.O. up to 4 tablets 2-3 times/day may be needed. Next, bisacodyl tablets P.O. at bedtime and up to 2-3 times/day if needed. If desired, use docusate to augment the effect of one or both medications, especially if stool is hard. If impaction can be ruled out, use bisocodyl suppository followed by fleet enema (if needed). If impaction is suspected, see last step of pathway.

Combination Laxatives

Use of products containing two or more laxatives is not advised because of a lack of documented therapeutic benefit over use of a single ingredient. Additionally, risks may outweigh benefits.

References

Bosshard W, Dreher R, Schnegg JF, et al, "The Treatment of Chronic Constipation in Elderly People: An Update," *Drugs Aging*, 2004, 21(14):911-30.

Burke C, "Avoiding Problems of GI Dysmotility in Patients Treated for Chronic Pain," *ASCP* 1995 Symposia Highlights, 7-8.

Floch MH and Wald A, "Clinical Evaluation and Treatment of Constipation," *Gastrolenterologist*, 1994, 2(1):50-60.

Harari D, Gurwitz JH, and Minaker KL, "Constipation in the Elderly," *JAGS*, 1993; 41:1130-40.

Hsieh C, "Treatment of Constipation in Older Adults," *Am Fam Physician*, 2005, 72(11):2277-84.

Izard MW and Ellison FS, "Treatment of Drug Induced Constipation with a Purified Senna Derivative," *Conn Med*, 1962; 26:589.

Lange RL and DiPiro JT, *Pharmacotherapy*, 2nd ed, Norwalk, CT: Appleton & Lange, 1993.

Maguire LC, Yon JL, and Miller E, "Prevention of Narcotic-Induced Constipation," *N Eng J Med*, 1981; 305:1651.

Ramkumar D and Rao SS, "Efficacy and Safety of Traditional Medical Therapies for Chronic Constipation: Systematic Review," *Am J Gastroenterol*, 2005, 100(4):936-71.

Tariq SH, "Constipation in Long-Term Care," *J Am Med Dir Assoc*, 2007, 8(4):209-18.

Wald A, "Is Chronic Use of Stimulant Laxatives Harmful to the Colon?" *J Clin Gastroenterol*, 2003, 36(5):386-9.

Wrenn K, "Fecal Impaction," *N Engl J Med*, 1989; 321:658-61.

IMMUNIZATION RECOMMENDATIONS

Recommended Adult Immunization Schedule, by Vaccine and Age Group
United States, October 2006 - September 2007

Vaccine	Age Group (years)		
	19-49	50-64	≥65
Tetanus, diphtheria, pertussis (Td/Tdap)[1]*	1-dose Td booster every 10 years		
	Substitute 1 dose of Tdap for Td		
Human papilloma-virus (HPV)[2]*	3 doses (females)		
Measles, mumps, rubella (MMR)[3]*	1 or 2 doses	1 dose	
Varicella[4]*	2 doses (0, 4-8 weeks)	2 doses (0, 4-8 weeks)	
Influenza[5]*	1 dose annually	1 dose annually	
Pneumococcal (polysaccharide)[6,7]	1-2 doses		1 dose
Hepatitis A[8]*	2 doses (0, 6-12 months, or 0, 6-18 months)		
Hepatitis B[9]*	3 doses (0, 1-2, 4-6 months)		
Meningococcal[10]	1 or more doses		

☐ For all persons in this category who meet the age requirements and who lack evidence of immunity (eg, lack documentation of vaccination or have no evidence of prior infection)

▨ Recommended if some other risk factor is present (eg, on the basis of medical, occupational, lifestyle, or other indications)

*Covered by the Vaccine Injury Compensation Program.
Note: These recommendations must be read along with the footnotes, which can be found following this schedule.

Recommended Adult Immunization Schedule, by Vaccine and Medical and Other Indications — United States, October 2006 - September 2007

Vaccine	Indication							
	Pregnancy	Congenital immunodeficiency, leukemia,[11] lymphoma, generalized malignancy, cerebrospinal fluid leaks, therapy with alkylating agents, antimetabolites, radiation, or high-dose, long-term corticosteroids	Diabetes, heart disease, chronic pulmonary disease, chronic alcoholism	Asplenia[11] (including elective splenectomy and terminal complement component deficiencies)	Chronic liver disease, recipients of clotting factor concentrates	Kidney failure, end-stage renal disease, recipients of hemodialysis	Human immuno-deficiency virus (HIV) infection[3,11]	Healthcare workers
Tetanus, diphtheria, pertussis (Td/Tdap)[1]*	1-dose Td booster every 10 years							
	Substitute 1 dose of Tdap for Td							
Human papilloma-virus (HPV)[2]*	3 doses for women ≤26 years of age (0, 2, 6 months)							
Measles, mumps, rubella (MMR)[3]*		1 or 2 doses						
Varicella[4]*		2 doses (0, 4-8 weeks)						2 doses
Influenza[5]*	1 dose annually		1 dose annually	1 dose annually				
Pneumococcal (polysaccharide)[6,7]	1-2 doses	1-2 doses						1-2 doses
Hepatitis A[8]*	2 doses (0, 6-12 months, or 0, 6-18 months)				2 doses (0, 6-12 months, or 0, 6-18 months)			
Hepatitis B[9]*	3 doses (0, 1-2, 4-6 months)				3 doses (0, 1-2, 4-6 months)			
Meningococcal[10]	1 dose			1 dose	1 dose			

☐ For all persons in this category who meet the age requirements and who lack evidence of immunity (eg, lack documentation of vaccination or have no evidence of prior infection)

▨ Recommended if some other risk factor is present (eg, on the basis of medical, occupational, lifestyle, or other indications)

■ Contraindicated

*Covered by the Vaccine Injury Compensation Program.
Note: These recommendations must be read along with the footnotes, which can be found following this schedule.

IMMUNIZATION RECOMMENDATIONS *(Continued)*

Footnotes to Recommended Adult Immunization Schedule

[1]**Tetanus, diphtheria, and acellular pertussis (Td/Tdap) vaccination.** Adults with uncertain histories of a complete primary vaccination series with diphtheria and tetanus toxoid-containing vaccines should begin or complete a primary vaccination series. A primary series for adults is 3 doses; administer the first 2 doses at least 4 weeks apart and the third dose 6-12 months after the second. Administer a booster dose to adults who have completed a primary series and if the last vaccination was received ≥10 years previously. Tdap or tetanus and diphtheria (Td) vaccine may be used; Tdap should replace a single dose of Td for adults aged <65 years who have not previously received a dose of Tdap (either in the primary series, as a booster or for wound management). Only one of two Tdap products (Adacel™ [sanofi pasteur, Swiftwater, Pennsylvania]) is licensed for use in adults. If the person is pregnant and received the last Td vaccination ≥10 years previously, administer Td during the second or third trimester; if the person received the last Td vaccination in <10 years, administer Tdap during the immediate postpartum period. A one-time administration of 1-dose of Tdap with an interval as short as 2 years from a previous Td vaccination is recommended for postpartum women, close contacts of infants aged <12 months, and all healthcare workers with direct patient contact. In certain situations, Td can be deferred during pregnancy and Tdap substituted in the immediate postpartum period, or Tdap can be given instead of Td to a pregnant woman after an informed discussion with the woman (see http://www.cdc.gov/nip/publications/acip-list.htm). Consult the ACIP statement for recommendations for administering Td as prophylaxis in wound management (http://www.cdc.gov/mmwr/preview/mmwrhtml/00041645.htm).

[2]**Human papillomavirus (HPV) vaccination.** HPV vaccination is recommended for all women aged ≤26 years who have not completed the vaccine series. Ideally, vaccine should be administered before potential exposure to HPV through sexual activity; however, women who are sexually active should still be vaccinated. Sexually active women who have not been infected with any of the HPV vaccine types receive the full benefit of the vaccination. Vaccination is less beneficial for women who have already been infected with one or more of the four HPV vaccine types. A complete series consists of 3 doses. The second dose should be administered 2 months after the first dose; the third dose should be administered 6 months after the first dose. Vaccination is not recommended during pregnancy. If a woman is found to be pregnant after initiating the vaccination series, the remainder of the 3-dose regimen should be delayed until after completion of the pregnancy.

[3]**Measles, mumps, rubella (MMR) vaccination.** *Measles component:* Adults born before 1957 can be considered immune to measles. Adults born during or after 1957 should receive ≥1 dose of MMR unless they have a medical contraindication, documentation of ≥1 dose, history of measles based on healthcare provider diagnosis, or laboratory evidence of immunity. A second dose of MMR is recommended for adults who 1) have been recently exposed to measles or in an outbreak setting; 2) have been previously vaccinated with killed measles vaccine; 3) have been vaccinated with an unknown type of measles vaccine during 1963-1967; 4) are students in postsecondary educational institutions; 5) work in a healthcare facility; or 6) plan to travel internationally. Withhold MMR or other measles-containing vaccines from HIV-infected persons with severe immunosuppression. *Mumps component:* Adults born before 1957 can generally be considered immune to mumps. Adults born during or after 1957 should receive 1 dose of MMR unless they have a medical contraindication, history of mumps based on healthcare provider diagnosis, or laboratory evidence of immunity. A second dose of MMR is recommended for adults who 1) are in an age group that is affected during a mumps outbreak; 2) are students in postsecondary educational institutions; 3) work in a healthcare facility; or 4) plan to travel internationally. For unvaccinated healthcare workers born before 1957 who do not have other evidence of mumps immunity, consider giving 1 dose on a routine basis and strongly consider giving a second dose during an outbreak. *Rubella component:* Administer 1 dose of MMR vaccine to women whose rubella vaccination history is unreliable or who lack laboratory evidence of immunity. For women of childbearing age, regardless of birth year, routinely determine rubella immunity and counsel women regarding congenital rubella syndrome. Do not vaccinate women who are pregnant or who might become pregnant within 4 weeks of receiving vaccine. Women who do not have evidence of immunity should receive MMR vaccine upon completion or termination of pregnancy and before discharge from the healthcare facility.

[4]**Varicella vaccination.** All adults without evidence of immunity to varicella should receive 2 doses of varicella vaccine. Special consideration should be given to those who 1) have close contact with persons at high risk for severe disease (eg, healthcare workers and family contacts of immunocompromised persons) or 2) are at high risk for exposure or transmission (eg, teachers of young children; child care employees; residents and staff members of institutional settings, including correctional institutions; college students; military personnel; adolescents and adults living in households with children; nonpregnant women of childbearing age; and international travelers). Evidence of immunity to varicella in adults includes any of the following: 1) documentation of 2 doses of varicella vaccine at least 4 weeks apart; 2) U.S.-born before 1980 (although for healthcare workers and pregnant women, birth before 1980 should not be considered evidence of immunity); 3) history of varicella based on diagnosis or verification of varicella by a healthcare provider (for a patient reporting a history of or presenting with an atypical case, a mild case, or both, healthcare providers should seek either an epidemiologic link with a typical varicella case or evidence of laboratory confirmation, if it was performed at the time of acute disease); 4) history of herpes zoster based on healthcare provider diagnosis; or 5) laboratory evidence of immunity or laboratory confirmation of disease. Do not vaccinate women who are pregnant or might become pregnant within 4 weeks of receiving the vaccine. Assess pregnant women for evidence of varicella immunity. Women who do not have evidence of immunity should receive dose 1 of varicella vaccine upon completion or termination of pregnancy and before discharge from the healthcare facility. Dose 2 should be administered 4-8 weeks after dose 1.

[5]**Influenza vaccination.** *Medical indications:* Chronic disorders of the cardiovascular or pulmonary systems, including asthma; chronic metabolic diseases, including diabetes mellitus, renal dysfunction, hemoglobinopathies, or immunosuppression (including immunosuppression caused by medications or HIV); any condition that compromises respiratory function or the handling of respiratory secretions or that can increase the risk of aspiration (eg, cognitive dysfunction, spinal cord injury, or seizure disorder or other neuromuscular disorder); and pregnancy during the influenza season. No data exist on the risk for severe or complicated influenza disease among persons with asplenia; however, influenza is a risk factor for secondary bacterial infections that can cause severe disease among persons with asplenia. *Occupational indications:* Healthcare workers and employees of long-term care and assisted living facilities. *Other indications:* Residents of nursing homes and other long-term care and assisted living facilities; persons likely to transmit influenza to persons at high risk (ie, in-home household contacts and caregivers of children aged 0-59 months, or persons of all ages with high-risk conditions); and anyone who would like to be vaccinated. Healthy, nonpregnant persons aged 5-49 years without high-risk medical conditions who are not contacts of severely immunocompromised persons in special care units can receive either intranasally administered influenza vaccine (fluMist®) or inactivated vaccine. Other persons should receive the inactivated vaccine.

[6]**Pneumococcal polysaccharide vaccination.** *Medical indications:* Chronic disorders of the pulmonary system (excluding asthma); cardiovascular diseases; diabetes mellitus; chronic liver diseases, including liver disease as a result of alcohol abuse (eg, cirrhosis); chronic renal failure or nephrotic syndrome; functional or anatomic asplenia (eg, sickle cell disease or splenectomy [if elective splenectomy is planned, vaccinate at least 2 weeks before surgery]); immunosuppressive conditions (eg, congenital immunodeficiency, HIV infection [vaccinate as close to diagnosis as possible when CD4 cell counts are highest], leukemia, lymphoma, multiple myeloma, Hodgkin disease, generalized malignancy, or organ or bone marrow transplantation); chemotherapy with alkylating agents, antimetabolites, or high-dose, long-term corticosteroids; and cochlear implants. *Other indications:* Alaska Natives and certain American Indian populations and residents of nursing homes or other long-term care facilities.

[7]**Revaccination with pneumococcal polysaccharide vaccine.** One-time revaccination after 5 years for persons with chronic renal failure or nephrotic syndrome; functional or anatomic asplenia (eg, sickle cell disease or splenectomy); immunosuppressive conditions (eg, congenital immunodeficiency, HIV infection, leukemia, lymphoma, multiple myeloma, Hodgkin disease, generalized malignancy, or organ or bone marrow transplantation); or chemotherapy with alkylating agents, antimetabolites, or high-dose, long-term corticosteroids. For persons aged ≥65 years, one-time revaccination if they were vaccinated ≥5 years previously and were aged <65 years at the time of primary vaccination.

[8]**Hepatitis A vaccination.** *Medical indications:* Persons with chronic liver disease and persons who receive clotting factor concentrates. *Behavioral indications:* Men who have sex with men and persons who use illegal drugs. *Occupational indications:* Persons working with hepatitis A virus (HAV)-infected primates or with HAV in a research laboratory setting. *Other indications:* Persons traveling to or working in countries that have high or intermediate endemicity of hepatitis A (a list of countries is available at http://www.cdc.gov/travel/diseases.htm) and any person who would like to obtain immunity. Current vaccines should be administered in a 2-dose schedule at either 0 and 6-12 months, or 0 and 6-18 months. If the combined hepatitis A and hepatitis B vaccine is used, administer 3 doses at 0, 1, and 6 months.

[9]**Hepatitis B vaccination.** *Medical indications:* Persons with end-stage renal disease, including patients receiving hemodialysis; persons seeking evaluation or treatment for a sexually transmitted disease (STD); persons with HIV infection; persons with chronic liver disease; and persons who receive clotting factor concentrates. *Occupational indications:* Healthcare workers and public-safety workers who are exposed to blood or other potentially infectious body fluids. *Behavioral indications:* Sexually active persons who are not in a long-term, mutually monogamous relationship (ie, persons with >1 sex partner during the previous 6 months); current or recent injection-drug users; and men who have sex with men. *Other indications:* Household contacts and sex partners of persons with chronic hepatitis B virus (HBV) infection; clients and staff members of institutions for persons with developmental disabilities; all clients of STD clinics; international travelers to countries with high or intermediate prevalence of chronic HBV infection (a list of countries is available at http://www.cdc.gov/travel/diseases.htm); and any adult seeking protection from HBV infection. Settings where hepatitis B vaccination is recommended for all adults: STD treatment facilities; HIV testing and treatment facilities; facilities providing drug-abuse treatment and prevention services; healthcare settings providing services for injection-drug users or men who have sex with men; correctional facilities; end-stage renal disease programs and facilities for chronic hemodialysis patients; and institutions and nonresidential daycare facilities for persons with developmental disabilities. *Special formulation indications:* For adult patients receiving hemodialysis and other immunocompromised adults, 1 dose of 40 mcg/mL (Recombivax HB®) or 2 doses of 20 mcg/mL (Engerix-B®).

[10]**Meningococcal vaccination.** *Medical indications:* Adults with anatomic or functional asplenia, or terminal complement component deficiencies. *Other indications:* First-year college students living in dormitories; microbiologists who are routinely exposed to isolates of *Neisseria meningitidis*; military recruits; and persons who travel to or live in countries in which meningococcal disease is hyperendemic or epidemic (eg, the "meningitis belt" of sub-Saharan Africa during the dry season [December-June]), particularly if their contact with local populations will be prolonged. Vaccination is required by the government of Saudi Arabia for all travelers to Mecca during the annual Hajj. Meningococcal conjugate vaccine is preferred for adults with any of the preceding indications who are aged ≤55 years, although meningococcal polysaccharide vaccine (MPSV4) is an acceptable alternative. Revaccination after 5 years might be indicated for adults previously vaccinated with MPSV4 who remain at high risk for infection (eg, persons residing in areas in which disease is epidemic).

[11]**Selected conditions for which *Haemophilus influenzae* type b (Hib) vaccine may be used.** Hib conjugate vaccines are licensed for children aged 6 weeks to 71 months. No efficacy data are available on which to base a recommendation concerning use of Hib vaccine for older children and

IMMUNIZATION RECOMMENDATIONS *(Continued)*

adults with the chronic conditions associated with an increased risk for Hib disease. However, studies suggest good immunogenicity in patients who have sickle cell disease, leukemia, or HIV infection or who have had splenectomies; administering vaccine to these patients is not contraindicated.

Adapted from "Centers for Disease Control and Prevention. Recommended Adult Immunization Schedule – United States, October 2006 - September 2007," *MMWR*, 2006, 55(40):Q1-4.

The Recommended Adult Immunization Schedule has been approved by the Advisory Committee on Immunization Practices (ACIP), the American College of Obstetricians and Gynecologists (ACOG), and the American Academy of Family Physicians (AAFP).

This schedule indicates the recommended age groups and medical indications for routine administration of currently licensed vaccines for persons ≥19 years of age, as of October 1, 2006. Licensed combination vaccines may be used whenever any components of the combination are indicated and when the vaccine's other components are not contraindicated. For detailed recommendations on **all** vaccines, including those used primarily for travelers or that are issued during the year, consult the manufacturers' package inserts and the complete statements from the Advisory Committee on Immunization Practices (http://www.cdc.gov/nip/publications/acip-list.htm).

Additional information about the vaccines in this schedule and contraindications for vaccination is also available at http://www.cdc.gov/nip or from the CDC-INFO Contact Center at 800-CDC-INFO (800-232-4636) in English and Spanish, 24 hours a day, 7 days a week.

Immunization in HIV-Infected Persons

Vaccination of immunocompromised patients depends on the characteristics of the vaccine and the patient. Vaccines are typically divided into two broad categories: those which contain live virus/bacteria or those which are derived from a component of the organism (or an inactivated organism). Live virus or live bacterial vaccines have been associated with severe complications in immunocompromised patients, and should generally be avoided [(except in selected circumstances (noted below)]. Inactivated, recombinant, subunit, polysaccharide, and conjugate vaccines and toxoids can be administered to all immunocompromised patients. However, it should be recognized that the response to these vaccines may be suboptimal. If indicated, all inactivated vaccines are recommended in usual doses and according to prescribed schedules. Pneumococcal, meningococcal, and Hib vaccines are recommended only for specific subpopulations, including functional or anatomic asplenia.

Special consideration must be given to immunization with measles and/or varicella vaccines. Persons with HIV are at a higher risk for severe complications from measles infection. In patients without severe immunocompromise, measles vaccination in HIV-infected persons has not been reported to cause severe and/or unusual adverse events. MMR vaccination is recommended for all HIV-infected persons who do not have evidence of severe immunocompromise (defined as a low age-specific total CD4+ T-lymphocyte count or a low CD4+ T-lymphocyte count as a percentage of total lymphocytes).

Varicella and/or herpes zoster infections are also associated with an increased risk of severe complications in children with HIV infection. Asymptomatic or mildly symptomatic HIV-infected children receiving varicella vaccination have demonstrated adequate response to the vaccine without evidence of severe and/or unusual events. However, experience has been limited. Varicella vaccine should be considered for children who are classified as CDC class N1, N2, A1, A2, B1, or B2 with age-specific CD4+ T-lymphocyte percentages >15%.

HIV-infected persons who are receiving IVIG may not respond to MMR or varicella vaccines (or an individual component) due to the presence of a passively acquired antibody. Measles vaccine should be considered approximately 2 weeks before the next scheduled dose of IVIG (unless otherwise contraindicated). Unless serologic testing confirms the production of specific antibodies, the vaccination should be repeated at the recommended interval. In patients receiving maintenance IVIG therapy, an additional dose of IVIG should be considered if the exposure to measles occurs ≥3 weeks following a standard dose. Persons with cellular immunodeficiency should not receive varicella vaccine; however, persons with humoral immunodeficiency should be vaccinated (including persons with dysgammaglobulinemia or hypogammaglobulinemia).

Summarized/adapted from Centers for Disease Control and Prevention, "General Recommendations on Immunization. Recommendations of the Advisory Committee on Immunization Practices (ACIP), *MMWR Recomm Rep*, 2006, 55(RR-15):1-56.

IMMUNIZATION RECOMMENDATIONS *(Continued)*

PREVENTION OF HEPATITIS A THROUGH ACTIVE OR PASSIVE IMMUNIZATION: RECOMMENDATIONS OF THE ADVISORY COMMITTEE ON IMMUNIZATION PRACTICES (ACIP)

PROPHYLAXIS AGAINST HEPATITIS A VIRUS INFECTION

Recommended Doses of Immune Globulin (IG) for Hepatitis A Pre-exposure and Postexposure Prophylaxis[1]

Setting	Duration of Coverage	IG Dose[2]
Pre-exposure	Short-term (1-2 months)	0.02 mL/kg
	Long-term (3-5 months)	0.06 mL/kg[3]
Postexposure	—	0.02 mL/kg

[1]Infants and pregnant women should receive a preparation that does not include thimerosal.

[2]IG should be administered by intramuscular injection into either the deltoid or gluteal muscle. For children <24 months of age, IG can be administered in the anterolateral thigh muscle.

[3]Repeat every 5 months if continued exposure to HAV occurs.

Recommended Dosages of Havrix®[1]

Vaccinee's Age (y)	Dose (EL.U.)[2]	Volume (mL)	No. Doses	Schedule (mo)[3]
2-18	720	0.5	2	0, 6-12
≥19	1440	1.0	2	0, 6-12

[1]Hepatitis A vaccine, inactivated, SmithKline Beecham Biologicals.

[2]Enzyme-linked immunosorbent assay (ELISA) units.

[3]0 months represents timing of the initial dose; subsequent numbers represent months after the initial dose.

Recommended Dosages of VAQTA®[1]

Vaccinee's Age (y)	Dose (units)	Volume (mL)	No. Doses	Schedule (mo)[2]
2-18	25	0.5	2	0, 6-18
≥19	50	1.0	2	0, 6

[1]Hepatitis A vaccine, inactivated, Merck & Company, Inc.

[2]0 months represents timing of the initial dose; subsequent numbers represent months after the initial dose.

Adapted from "Prevention of Hepatitis A Through Active or Passive Immunization: Recommendations of the Advisory Committee on Immunization Practices (ACIP)," *MMWR Recomm Rep*, 2006, 55(RR-07):1-23.

Recommended Dosages of Twinrix®[1]

Vaccinee's Age (y)	Dose (HepA / HepB)	Volume (mL)	No. Doses	Schedule (mo)[2]
≥18	720 EL.U./20 mcg	1	3	0, 1, 6

[1]Combined hepatitis A and hepatitis B vaccine manufactured by GlaxoSmithKline (Rixensart, Belgium).

[2]0 months represents timing of the initial dose; subsequent numbers represent months after the initial dose.

ADVERSE EVENTS AND VACCINATION

Reportable Events Following Vaccination[1]

Vaccine / Toxoid		Event	Onset Interval
Tetanus in any combination; DTaP, DTP, DTP-Hib, DT, Td, TT	A.	Anaphylaxis or anaphylactic shock	7 days
	B.	Brachial neuritis	28 days
	C.	Any sequela (including death) of above events	Not applicable
	D.	Events described in manufacturer's package insert as contraindications to additional doses of vaccine	See package insert
Pertussis in any combination; DTaP, DTP, DTP-Hib, P	A.	Anaphylaxis or anaphylactic shock	7 days
	B.	Encephalopathy (or encephalitis)	7 days
	C.	Any sequela (including death) of above events	Not applicable
	D.	Events described in manufacturer's package insert as contraindications to additional doses of vaccine	See package insert
Measles, mumps, and rubella in any combination; MMR, MR, M, R	A.	Anaphylaxis or anaphylactic shock	7 days
	B.	Encephalopathy (or encephalitis)	15 days
	C.	Any sequela (including death) of above events	Not applicable
	D.	Events described in manufacturer's package insert as contraindications to additional doses of vaccine	See package insert
Rubella in any combination; MMR, MR, R	A.	Chronic arthritis	42 days
	B.	Any sequela (including death) of above events	Not applicable
	C.	Events described in manufacturer's package insert as contraindications to additional doses of vaccine	See package insert
Measles in any combination; MMR, MR, M	A.	Thrombocytopenic purpura	7-30 days
	B.	Vaccine-strain measles viral infection in an immunodeficient recipient	6 months
	C.	Any sequela (including death) of above events	Not applicable
	D.	Events described in manufacturer's package insert as contraindications to additional doses of vaccine	See package insert
Inactivated polio (IPV)	A.	Anaphylaxis or anaphylactic shock	7 days
	B.	Any sequela (including death) of above events	Not applicable
	C.	Events described in manufacturer's package insert as contraindications to additional doses of vaccine	See package insert
Hepatitis B	A.	Anaphylaxis or anaphylactic shock	7 days
	B.	Any sequela (including death) of above events	Not applicable
	C.	Events described in manufacturer's package insert as contraindications to additional doses of vaccine	See package insert
Haemophilus influenzae type b (conjugate)	A.	Events described in manufacturer's package insert as contraindications to additional doses of vaccine	See package insert
Varicella	A.	Events described in manufacturer's package insert as contraindications to additional doses of vaccine	See package insert
Rotavirus	A.	Intussusception	30 days
	B.	Any sequela (including death) of above events	Not applicable
	C.	Events described in manufacturer's package insert as contraindications to additional doses of vaccine	See package insert
Pneumococcal conjugate	A.	Events described in manufacturer's package insert as contraindications to additional doses of vaccine	See package insert

[1]Effective date: July 1, 2005.
The Reportable Events Table (RET) reflects what is reportable by law (42 USC 300aa-25) to the Vaccine Adverse Event Reporting System (VAERS), including conditions found in the manufacturer's package insert. In addition, individuals are encouraged to report **any** clinically significant or unexpected events (even if you are not certain the vaccine caused the event) for **any** vaccine, whether or not it is listed on the RET. Manufacturers are also required by regulation (21CFR 600.80) to report to the VAERS program all adverse events made known to them for any vaccine.

Adapted from the website **http://www.vaers.org/reportable.htm**. For further information, contact VAERS at 1-800-822-7967.

AMINOGLYCOSIDE DOSING AND MONITORING

All aminoglycoside therapy should be individualized for specific patients in specific clinical situation. The following are guidelines for initiating therapy.

1. Loading dose based on estimated ideal body weight (IBW). **All patients require a loading dose independent of renal function.**

Agent	Dose
Gentamicin	2 mg/kg
Tobramycin	2 mg/kg
Amikacin	7.5 mg/kg

Significantly higher loading doses may be required in severely ill intensive care unit patients.

2. Initial maintenance doses as a percent of loading dose according to desired dosing interval and creatinine clearance (Cl_{cr}):

$$\text{Male } Cl_{cr} \text{ (mL/min)} = \frac{(140 - age) \times IBW}{72 \times \text{serum creatinine}}$$

$$\text{Female} = 0.85 \times Cl_{cr} \text{ males}$$

Cl_{cr}	Dosing Interval (h)		
(mL/min)	8	12	24
90	84%	—	—
80	80%	—	—
70	76%	88%	—
60	—	84%	—
50	—	79%	—
40	—	72%	92%
30	—	—	86%
25	—	—	81%
20	—	—	75%

Patients >65 years of age should not receive initial aminoglycoside maintenance dosing more often than every 12 hours.

3. Serum concentration monitoring

   a. Serum concentration monitoring is necessary for **safe** and **effective** therapy, particularly in patients with serious infections and those with risk factors for toxicity.

   b. Peak serum concentrations should be drawn 30 minutes after the completion of a 30-minute infusion. Trough serum concentrations should be drawn within 30 minutes prior to the administered dose.

   c. Serum concentrations should be drawn after 5 half-lives, usually around the third dose or thereafter.

4. Desired measured serum concentrations

	Peak (mcg/mL)	Trough (mcg/mL)
Gentamicin	6-10	0.5-2.0
Tobramycin	6-10	0.5-2.0
Amikacin	20-30	<5

5. For patients receiving hemodialysis:
    - administer the **same** loading dose
    - administer $2/3$ of the loading dose after each dialysis
    - **serum concentrations must be monitored**
    - watch for ototoxicity from accumulation of drug

6. For individual clinical situations the prescribing physician should feel free to consult Infectious Disease, the Pharmacology Service, or the Pharmacy.

"Once Daily" Aminoglycosides

High dose, "once daily" aminoglycoside therapy for treatment of gram-negative bacterial infections has been studied and remains controversial. The pharmacodynamics of aminoglycosides reveal dose-dependent killing which suggests an efficacy advantage of "high" peak serum concentrations. It is also suggested that allowing troughs to fall to unmeasurable levels decreases the risk of nephrotoxicity without detriment to efficacy. Because of a theoretical saturation of tubular cell uptake of aminoglycosides, decreasing the number of times the drug is administered in a particular time period may play a role in minimizing the risk of nephrotoxicity. Ototoxicity has not been sufficiently formally evaluated through audiometry or vestibular testing comparing "once daily" to standard therapy. Over 100 letters, commentaries, studies and reviews have been published on the topic of "once daily" aminoglycosides with varying dosing regimens, monitoring parameters, inclusion and exclusion criteria, and results (most of which have been favorable for the "once daily" regimens). The caveats of this simplified method of dosing are several, including assurance that creatinine clearances be calculated, that all patients are not candidates and should not be considered for this regimen, and that "once daily" is a semantic misnomer.

Because of the controversial nature of this method, it is beyond the scope of this book to present significant detail and dosing regimen recommendations. Considerable experience with two methods warrants mention. The Hartford Hospital has experience with over 2000 patients utilizing a 7 mg/kg dose, a dosing scheme for various creatinine clearance estimates, and a serum concentration monitoring nomogram.[1] Providence Medical Center utilizes a 5 mg/kg dosing regimen but only in patients with excellent renal function; serum concentrations are monitored 4-6 hours prior to the dose administered.[2] Two excellent reviews discuss the majority of studies and controversies regarding these dosing techniques.[3,4] An editorial accompanies one of the reviews and is worth examination.[5]

"Once daily" dosing may be a safe and effective method of providing aminoglycoside therapy to a large number of patients who require these efficacious yet toxic agents. As with any method of aminoglycoside administration, dosing must be individualized and the caveats of the method considered.

AMINOGLYCOSIDE DOSING AND MONITORING *(Continued)*

Footnotes

1. Nicolau DP, Freeman CD, Belliveau PP, et al, "Experience With a Once-Daily Aminoglycoside Program Administered to 2,184 Patients," *Antimicrob Agents Chemother*, 1995, 39:650-5.

2. Gilbert DN, "Once-Daily Aminoglycoside Therapy," *Antimicrob Agents Chemother*, 1991, 35:399-405.

3. Preston SL and Briceland LL, "Single Daily Dosing of Aminoglycosides," *Pharmacotherapy*, 1995, 15:297-316.

4. Bates RD and Nahata MC, "Once-Daily Administration of Aminoglycosides," *Ann Pharmacother*, 1994, 28:757-66.

5. Rotschafer JC and Rybak MJ, "Single Daily Dosing of Aminoglycosides: A Commentary," *Ann Pharmacother*, 1994, 28:797-801.

Aminoglycoside Penetration Into Various Tissues

Site	Extent of Distribution
Eye	Poor
CNS	Poor (<25%)
Pleural	Excellent
Bronchial secretions	Poor
Sputum	Fair (10%-50%)
Pulmonary tissue	Excellent
Ascitic fluid	Variable (43%-132%)
Peritoneal fluid	Poor
Bile	Variable (25%-90%)
Bile with obstruction	Poor
Synovial fluid	Excellent
Bone	Poor
Prostate	Poor
Urine	Excellent
Renal tissue	Excellent

Adapted from Neu HC, "Pharmacology of Aminoglycosides," *The Aminoglycosides*, Whelton E and Neu HC, eds, New York, NY: Marcel Dekker, Inc, 1981.

ANTIBIOTIC TREATMENT OF ADULTS WITH INFECTIVE ENDOCARDITIS

Table 1. Suggested Regimens for Therapy of Native Valve Endocarditis Due to Penicillin-Susceptible Viridans Streptococci and *Streptococcus bovis* (Minimum Inhibitory Concentration ≤0.12 mcg/mL)[1]

Antibiotic	Dosage and Route	Duration (wk)	Comments
Aqueous crystalline penicillin G sodium	12-18 million units/24 h I.V. either continuously or in 4-6 equally divided doses	4	Preferred in most patients older than 65 y and in those with impairment of the 8th cranial nerve or renal function
or			
Ceftriaxone sodium	2 g once daily I.V. or I.M.[2]	4	
Either penicillin or ceftriaxone regimen above with gentamicin sulfate[3]	3 mg/kg/24 h I.M./I.V. as single daily dose	2	When using combination therapy, both β-lactam and aminoglycoside regimen duration is 2 weeks; 2-week regimen not intended if known cardiac or extracardiac abscess, Cl$_{cr}$ <20 mL/min, 8th cranial nerve impairment or *Abiotrophia, Granulicatella,* or *Gemella* spp
Vancomycin hydrochloride[4]	30 mg/kg/24 h I.V. in 2 equally divided doses, not to exceed 2 g/24 h unless serum levels are monitored	4	Vancomycin therapy is recommended for patients allergic to β-lactams; peak serum concentrations of vancomycin should be obtained 1 h after completion of the infusion and should be in the range of 30-45 mcg/mL and trough of 10-15 mcg/mL for twice-daily dosing

[1]Dosages recommended are for patients with normal renal function. For nutritionally variant streptococci, see Table 3. I.V. indicates intravenous; I.M., intramuscular.

[2]Patients should be informed that I.M. injection of ceftriaxone is painful.

[3]Dosing of gentamicin on a mg/kg basis will produce higher serum concentrations in obese patients that in lean patients. Therefore, in obese patients, dosing should be based on ideal body weight. (Ideal body weight for men is 50 kg + 2.3 kg per inch over 5 feet, and ideal body weight for women is 45.5 kg + 2.3 kg per inch over 5 feet.) Relative contraindications to the use of gentamicin are age >65 years, renal impairment, or impairment of the eighth nerve. Other potentially nephrotoxic agents (eg, nonsteroidal anti-inflammatory drugs) should be used cautiously in patients receiving gentamicin.

[4]Vancomycin dosage should be reduced in patients with impaired renal function. Vancomycin given on a mg/kg basis will produce higher serum concentrations in obese patients than in lean patients. Therefore, in obese patients, dosing should be based on ideal body weight. Each dose of vancomycin should be infused over at least 1 hour to reduce the risk of the histamine-release "red man" syndrome.

ANTIBIOTIC TREATMENT OF ADULTS WITH INFECTIVE ENDOCARDITIS (Continued)

Table 2. Therapy for Native Valve Endocarditis Due to Strains of Viridans Streptococci and *Streptococcus bovis* Relatively Resistant to Penicillin G (Minimum Inhibitory Concentration >0.12 mcg/mL and ≤0.5 mcg/mL)[1]

Antibiotic	Dosage and Route	Duration (wk)	Comments
Aqueous crystalline penicillin G sodium	24 million units/24 h I.V. either continuously or in 4-6 equally divided doses	4	Cefazolin or other first-generation cephalosporins may be substituted for penicillin in patients whose penicillin hypersensitivity is not of the immediate type.
With gentamicin sulfate[2]	3 mg/kg/24 h I.M./I.V. as single daily dose	2	
Ceftriaxone sodium	2 g once daily I.V. or I.M.[2]	4	
With gentamicin sulfate[2]	3 mg/kg/24 h I.M./I.V. as single daily dose	2	
Vancomycin hydrochloride[3]	30 mg/kg/24 h I.V. in 2 equally divided doses, not to exceed 2 g/24 h unless serum levels are monitored	4	Vancomycin therapy is recommended for patients allergic to β-lactams.

[1]Dosages recommended are for patients with normal renal function. I.V. indicates intravenous; I.M., intramuscular.

[2]For specific dosing adjustment and issues concerning gentamicin (obese patients, relative contraindications), see Table 1 footnotes.

[3]For specific dosing adjustment and issues concerning vancomycin (obese patients, length of infusion), see Table 1 footnotes.

Table 3. Standard Therapy for Endocarditis Due to Enterococci[1]

Antibiotic	Dosage and Route	Duration (wk)	Comments
Aqueous crystalline penicillin G sodium	18-30 million units/24 h I.V. either continuously or in 6 equally divided doses	4-6	Native valve: 4-week therapy recommended for patients with symptoms ≤3 months in duration; 6-week therapy recommended for patients with symptoms >3 months in duration.
With gentamicin sulfate[2]	1 mg/kg I.M. or I.V. every 8 h	4-6	
Ampicillin sodium	12 g/24 h I.V. in 6 equally divided doses	4-6	Prosthetic valve or other prosthetic material: 6-week minimum therapy recommended
With gentamicin sulfate[2]	1 mg/kg I.M. or I.V. every 8 hours	4-6	Target gentamicin peak concentration of 3-4 mcg/mL and trough of <1 mcg/mL
Vancomycin hydrochloride[2,3]	30 mg/kg/24 h I.V. in 2 equally divided doses, not to exceed 2 g/24 h unless serum levels are monitored	6	Vancomycin therapy is recommended for patients allergic to β-lactams; cephalosporins are not acceptable alternatives for patients allergic to penicillin.
With gentamicin sulfate[2]	1 mg/kg I.M. or I.V. every 8 h	6	

[1]All enterococci causing endocarditis must be tested for antimicrobial susceptibility in order to select optimal therapy. This table is for endocarditis due to penicillin-, gentamicin-, and vancomycin-susceptible enterococci, viridans streptococci with a minimum inhibitory concentration of >0.5 mcg/mL, nutritionally variant viridans streptococci, or prosthetic valve endocarditis caused by viridans streptococci or *Streptococcus bovis*. If penicillin-resistant organisms, use vancomycin/gentamicin regimen above, or may use ampicillin/sulbactam (12 g/24 h in 4 divided doses) with gentamicin for 6 weeks. Antibiotic dosages are for patients with normal renal function. I.V. indicates intravenous; I.M., intramuscular.

[2]For specific dosing adjustment and issues concerning gentamicin (obese patients, relative contraindications), see Table 1 footnotes.

[3]For specific dosing adjustment and issues concerning vancomycin (obese patients, length of infusion), see Table 1 footnotes.

Table 4. Therapy for Native or Prosthetic Valve Endocarditis Due to Enterococci[1] Resistant to Vancomycin, Aminoglycosides, and Penicillin[2]

Antibiotic	Dosage and Route	Duration (wk)	Comments
E. faecium			
Linezolid	1200 mg/24 h P.O./I.V. in 2 divided doses	≥8	May cause severe, but reversible thrombocytopenia, particularly with extended therapy >2 weeks.
Quinupristin-dalfopristin	22.5 mg/kg/24 h I.V. in 3 divided doses	≥8	May cause severe myalgia; not effective against E. faecalis.
E. faecalis			
Imipenem/ cilastatin	2 g/24 h I.V. in 4 divided doses	≥8	Limited patient experience with these regimens.
With ampicillin sodium	12 g/24 h in 6 divided doses	≥8	
or			
Ceftriaxone sodium	2 g/24 h I.V./I.M.[3] once daily	≥8	Limited patient experience with these regimens.
With ampicillin sodium	12 g/24 h in 6 divided doses	≥8	

[1]Endocarditis caused by the organisms should be treated in consultation with an infectious disease specialist; bacteriologic cure with antimicrobial therapy alone may be <50% and valve replacement may be required.

[2]Dosages recommended are for patients with normal renal function. I.V. = intravenous; I.M. = intramuscular.

[3]Patients should be informed that I.M. injection of ceftriaxone is painful.

ANTIBIOTIC TREATMENT OF ADULTS WITH INFECTIVE ENDOCARDITIS *(Continued)*

Table 5. Therapy for Endocarditis Due to *Staphylococcus* in the Absence of Prosthetic Material[1]

Antibiotic	Dosage and Route	Duration	Comments
Methicillin-Susceptible Staphylococci			
Regimens for non-β-lactam-allergic patients			
Nafcillin sodium or oxacillin sodium	12 g/24 h I.V. in 4-6 divided doses	6 wk	Uncomplicated right side endocarditis may be treated for 2 weeks.
With optional addition of gentamicin sulfate[2]	3 mg/kg/24 h I.M./I.V. in 2-3 divided doses	3-5 d	Benefit of additional aminoglycosides has not been established.
Regimens for β-lactam-allergic patients (nonanaphylactic)			
Cefazolin (or other first-generation cephalosporins in equivalent dosages)	2 g I.V. every 8 h	6 wk	Cephalosporins should be avoided in patients with immediate-type hypersensitivity to penicillin; if penicillin-sensitive, vancomycin should be used.
With optional addition of gentamicin[2]	3 mg/kg/24 h I.M./I.V. in 2-3 divided doses	3-5 d	Benefit of additional aminoglycosides has not been established.
Methicillin-Resistant Staphylococci			
Vancomycin hydrochloride[3]	30 mg/kg/24 h I.V. in 2 equally divided doses; not to exceed 2 g/24 h unless serum levels are monitored	4-6 wk	Vancomycin therapy is recommended for patients allergic to β-lactams; peak serum concentrations of vancomycin should be obtained 1 h after completion of the infusion and should be in the range of 30-45 mcg/mL and trough of 10-15 mcg/mL for twice-daily dosing.

[1]For treatment of endocarditis due to penicillin-susceptible staphylococci (minimum inhibitory concentration ≤0.1 mcg/mL and non-beta-lactamase producing), aqueous crystalline penicillin G sodium 24 million units/24 h can be used instead of nafcillin or oxacillin. Shorter antibiotic courses have been effective in some drug addicts with right-sided endocarditis due to *Staphylococcus aureus*. I.V. indicates intravenous; I.M., intramuscular.

[2]For specific dosing adjustment and issues concerning gentamicin (obese patients, relative contraindications), see Table 1 footnotes.

[3]For specific dosing adjustment and issues concerning vancomycin (obese patients, length of infusion), see Table 1 footnotes.

Table 6. Treatment of Staphylococcal Endocarditis in the Presence of a Prosthetic Valve or Other Prosthetic Material[1]

Antibiotic	Dosage and Route	Duration (wk)	Comments
Methicillin-Susceptible Staphylococci			
Nafcillin sodium or oxacillin sodium[2]	12 g/24 h I.V. in 6 divided doses	≥6	First-generation cephalosporins or vancomycin should be used in patients allergic to β-lactam. Cephalosporins should be avoided in patients with immediate-type hypersensitivity to penicillin or with methicillin-resistant staphylococci.
With rifampin[3]	300 mg P.O./I.V. every 8 h	≥6	–
And with gentamicin sulfate[4,5]	3 mg/kg I.M./I.V. in 2-3 divided doses	2	Aminoglycoside should be administered in close proximity to vancomycin, nafcillin, or oxacillin.
Methicillin-Resistant Staphylococci			
Vancomycin hydrochloride[6]	30 mg/kg/24 h I.V. in 2 equally divided doses, not to exceed 2 g/24 h unless serum levels are monitored	≥6	–
With rifampin[3]	300 mg P.O./I.V. every 8 h	≥6	Rifampin increases the amount of warfarin sodium required for antithrombotic therapy.
And with gentamicin sulfate[4,5]	3 mg/kg I.M./I.V. in 2-3 divided doses	2	Aminoglycoside should be administered in close proximity to vancomycin, nafcillin, or oxacillin.

[1]Dosages recommended are for patients with normal renal function. I.V. indicates intravenous; I.M., intramuscular.

[2]May use aqueous penicillin G 24 million units/24 h in 4-6 divided doses if strain is penicillin susceptible (MIC ≤0.1 mcg/mL and non-beta-lactamase producing).

[3]Rifampin plays a unique role in the eradication of staphylococcal infection involving prosthetic material; combination therapy is essential to prevent emergence of rifampin resistance.

[4]For a specific dosing adjustment and issues concerning gentamicin (obese patients, relative contraindications), see Table 1 footnotes.

[5]Use during initial 2 weeks.

[6]For specific dosing adjustment and issues concerning vancomycin (obese patients, relative contraindications), see Table 1 footnotes.

ANTIBIOTIC TREATMENT OF ADULTS WITH INFECTIVE ENDOCARDITIS *(Continued)*

Table 7. Therapy for Native or Prosthetic Valve Endocarditis Due to HACEK Microorganisms (*Haemophilus parainfluenzae, Haemophilus aphrophilus, Actinobacillus actinomycetemcomitans, Cardiobacterium hominus, Eikenella corrodens,* and *Kingella kingae*)[1]

Antibiotic	Dosage and Route	Duration (wk)	Comments
Ceftriaxone sodium[2]	2 g once daily I.V. or I.M.[2]	4	Cefotaxime sodium or other third- or fourth-generation cephalosporins may be substituted.
Ampicillin/ sulbactam	12 g/24 h I.V. in 6 equally divided doses	4	
Ciprofloxacin	1000 mg/24 h orally or 800 mg/ 24 h I.V. in 2 divided doses	4	Use of fluoroquinolone recommended only if patient intolerant to ampicillin or cephalosporins; may substitute fluoroquinolone with equivalent coverage (eg, levofloxacin, moxifloxacin); if prosthetic material involved, treatment duration should be 6 weeks.

[1]Antibiotic dosages are for patients with normal renal function. I.V. indicates intravenous; I.M. intramuscular.

[2]Patients should be informed that I.M. injection of ceftriaxone is painful.

[3]Ampicillin should not be used if laboratory tests show β-lactamase production.

Reference

Baddour LM, Wilson WR, Bayer AS, et al, "Infective Endocarditis. Diagnosis, Antimicrobial Therapy, and Management of Complications. A Statement for Healthcare Professionals from the Committee on Rheumatic Fever, Endocarditis, and Kawasaki Disease, Council on Cardiovascular Disease in the Young, and the Councils on Clinical Cardiology, Stroke, and Cardiovascular Surgery and Anesthesia, American Heart Association," *Circulation*, 2005, 111(23):e394-434.

PREVENTION OF INFECTIVE ENDOCARDITIS

Recommendations by the American Heart Association
(*Circulation*, 2007, 115 [epub April 19, 2007])

Consensus Process – The recommendations were formulated by a writing group under the auspices of the American Heart Association (AHA), and included representation from the Infectious Diseases Society of America (IDSA), the American Academy of Pediatrics (AAP), and the American Dental Association (ADA). Additionally, input was received from both national and international experts on infective endocarditis (IE). These guidelines are based on expert interpretation and review of scientific literature from 1950 through 2006. The consensus statement was subsequently reviewed by outside experts not affiliated with the writing group and by the Science Advisory and Coordinating Committee of the American Heart Association. These guidelines are meant to aid practitioners but are not intended as the standard of care or as a substitute for clinical judgment.

Significant change from the previous 1997 guidelines – The previously published guidelines identified a broad range of cardiac conditions thought to predispose patients to a higher risk of IE. The document stratified these conditions into high-, moderate-, and low-risk categories, based on the likelihood of developing IE. The subsequent recommendations for prophylaxis were based on this classification, in conjunction with specification of numerous invasive procedures which were assumed to confer a higher risk of bacteremia, and therefore a higher risk of endocarditis. However, it is the consensus of the current writing group that existing data fail to show a clear link between many of these procedures, preexisting cardiovascular condition and IE. In the case of dental procedures, it was determined that the cumulative lifetime risk of developing bacteremia as a result of normal hygiene measures (eg, teeth brushing, flossing) vastly exceeded the risk associated with many of the procedures for which prophylaxis was previously recommended. Similarly, the writing group estimated that the absolute risk of developing IE as a result of dental procedures in patients with preexisting cardiac conditions was quite low, and there was little evidence to support the value of prophylactic antimicrobial efficacy in these cases.

In a major departure from the former recommendations, the current guidelines have been greatly simplified to place a much greater emphasis on a very limited number of underlying cardiac conditions (see below). These specific conditions have been associated with the highest risk of adverse outcomes due to IE. Patients should receive IE prophylaxis only if they are undergoing certain invasive procedures (see Table 1) and have one of the underlying cardiovascular conditions specified below.

Common situations for which routine prophylaxis was previously, but no longer recommended, include mitral valve prolapse, general dental cleanings and local anesthetic administration (noninfected tissue), and bronchoscopy (see Table 1).

Specific cardiac conditions for which IE antibiotic prophylaxis is recommended:

- Previous infective endocarditis

- Prosthetic cardiac valve

- Cardiac transplantation patients who develop valvulopathy

- Congenital heart disease (CHD), only under the following conditions:

    – Unrepaired cyanotic CHD, including palliative shunts and conduits

    – Completely repaired defects (with prosthetic materials/devices), regardless of method of repair, within the first 6 months after the procedure

    – Repaired CHD with residual defects at or adjacent to the site of repair

PREVENTION OF INFECTIVE ENDOCARDITIS *(Continued)*

Table 1. Guidance for Use of Prophylactic Antibiotic Therapy Based on Procedure or Condition[1]

Location of Procedure	Prophylaxis Recommended	Prophylaxis NOT Recommended
Dental	All invasive manipulations of the gingival or periapical region or perforation of oral mucosa	Anesthetic injections (through noninfected tissue), radiographs, placement of removable prosthodontic/orthodontic appliances or brackets, shedding of deciduous teeth, trauma-induced bleeding from lips, gums, or oral mucosa
Respiratory tract	Biopsy/incision of respiratory mucosa (eg, tonsillectomy/ adenoidectomy); drainage of abscess of empyema[2]	Bronchoscopy (unless incision of mucosa required)
Gastrointestinal (GI) or genitourinary (GU) tract	Established GI/GU infection or prevention of infectious sequelae[3]; elective cystoscopy or other urinary tract procedure with established enterococci infection/ colonization[3,4]	Routine diagnostic procedures, including esophagogastroduodenoscopy or colonoscopy; vaginal delivery and hysterectomy
Skin, skin structure, or musculoskeletal	Any surgical procedure involving infected tissue	Procedures conducted in noninfected tissue; tattoos and ear/ body piercing

[1]Patients should receive prophylactic antibiotic therapy if they meet the criteria for a specified procedure/condition in this table and they have a high-risk cardiovascular condition listed in the preceding text.

[2]If treating an infection of known staphylococcal origin, consider antistaphylococcal penicillin or cephalosporin, or vancomycin in beta-lactam-sensitive patients.

[3]Alternative agents with activity against enterococci to consider: Vancomycin (for beta-lactam-sensitive patients) or piperacillin.

[4]Eradication of enterococci from the urinary tract should be considered.

Table 2. Prophylactic Regimens for Oral / Dental, Respiratory Tract, Genitoruinary Tract, or Esophageal Procedures

Situation	Agent	Regimen to Be Given 30-60 Minutes Before Procedure[1]	
		Adults	Children
Standard general prophylaxis	Amoxicillin	2 g P.O.	50 mg/kg P.O.
Unable to take oral medications	Ampicillin **or**	2 g I.M./I.V.	50 mg/kg I.M./I.V.
	Cefazolin or ceftriaxone	1 g I.M./I.V.	50 mg/kg I.M./I.V.
Allergic to penicillin	Clindamycin **or**	600 mg P.O.	20 mg/kg P.O.
	Cephalexin[2] or other dose-equivalent first/ second generation cephalosporin **or**	2 g P.O	50 mg/kg P.O.
	Azithromycin or clarithromycin	500 mg P.O.	15 mg/kg P.O.
Allergic to penicillin and unable to take oral medications	Clindamycin **or**	600 mg I.V.	20 mg/kg I.V.
	Cefazolin or ceftriaxone[2]	1 g I.M./I.V.	50 mg/kg I.M./I.V.

[1]Total children's dose should not exceed adult dose.

[2]Cephalosporins should not be used in individuals with immediate-type hypersensitivity reaction (urticaria, angioedema, or anaphylaxis) to penicillins.

Reference:

Wilson W, Taubert KA, Gewitz M, et al, "Prevention of Infective Endocarditis. Guidelines From the American Heart Association. A Guideline From the American Heart Association Rheumatic Fever, Endocarditis, and Kawasaki Disease Committee, Council on Cardiovascular Disease in the Young, and the Council on Clinical Cardiology, Council on Cardiovascular Surgery and Anesthesia, and the Quality of Care and Outcomes Research Interdisciplinary Working Group," *Circulation*, 2007, 115 [epub April 19, 2007].

RECOMMENDATIONS FOR PREVENTING THE SPREAD OF VANCOMYCIN RESISTANCE

Recommendations of the Hospital Infection Control Practices Advisory Committee (HICPAC)

(*MMWR Morb Mortal Wkly Rep*, 1995, 44(RR-12))

Prudent Vancomycin Use

Vancomycin use has been reported consistently as a risk factor for infection and colonization with VRE and may increase the possibility of the emergence of vanco-mycin-resistant *S. aureus* (VRSA) and/or vancomycin-resistant *S. epidermidis* (VRSE). Therefore, all hospitals and other healthcare delivery services, even those at which VRE have never been detected, should a) develop a comprehensive, antimicrobial-utilization plan to provide education for their medical staff (including medical students who rotate their training in different departments of the healthcare facility), b) oversee surgical prophylaxis, and c) develop guidelines for the proper use of vancomycin (as applicable to the institution).

Guideline development should be part of the hospital's quality-improvement program and should involve participation from the hospital's pharmacy and therapeutics committee; hospital epidemiologist; and infection-control, infectious-disease, medical, and surgical staffs. The guidelines should include the following considerations:

1. Situations in which the use of vancomycin is appropriate or acceptable

    *   For treatment of serious infections caused by beta-lactam-resistant gram-positive microorganisms; vancomycin may be less rapidly bactericidal than are beta-lactam agents for beta-lactam-susceptible staphylococci

    *   For treatment of infections caused by gram-positive microorganisms in patients who have serious allergies to beta-lactam antimicrobials

    *   When antibiotic-associated colitis fails to respond to metronidazole therapy or is severe and potentially life-threatening

    *   Prophylaxis, as recommended by the American Heart Association, for endocarditis following certain procedures in patients at high risk for endocarditis

    *   Prophylaxis for major surgical procedures involving implantation of prosthetic materials or devices (eg, cardiac and vascular procedures and total hip replacement) at institutions that have a high rate of infections caused by MRSA or methicillin-resistant *S. epidermidis*. A single dose of vancomycin administered immediately before surgery is sufficient unless the procedure lasts >6 hours, in which case the dose should be repeated. Prophylaxis should be discontinued after a maximum of two doses.

2. Situations in which the use of vancomycin should be discouraged

    *   Routine surgical prophylaxis other than in a patient who has a life-threatening allergy to beta-lactam antibiotics

    *   Empiric antimicrobial therapy for a febrile neutropenic patient, unless initial evidence indicates that the patient has an infection caused by gram-positive microorganisms (eg, at an inflamed exit site of Hickman catheter) and the prevalence of infections caused by MRSA in the hospital is substantial

    *   Treatment in response to a single blood culture positive for coagu-lase-negative *Staphylococcus*, if other blood cultures taken during the same time frame are negative (ie, if contamination of the blood culture is likely). Because contamination of blood cultures with skin flora (eg, *S. epidermidis*) could result in inappropriate administration of vancomycin, phlebotomists and other personnel who obtain blood cultures should be trained to minimize microbial contamination of specimens.

- Continued empiric use for presumed infections in patients whose cultures are negative for beta-lactam-resistant gram-positive microorganisms
- Systemic or local (eg, antibiotic lock) prophylaxis for infection or colonization of indwelling central or peripheral intravascular catheters
- Selective decontamination of the digestive tract
- Eradication of MRSA colonization
- Primary treatment of antibiotic-associated colitis
- Routine prophylaxis for very low-birthweight infants (ie, infants who weigh <1500 g [3 lb 4 oz])
- Routine prophylaxis for patients on continuous ambulatory peritoneal dialysis or hemodialysis
- Treatment (chosen for dosing convenience) of infections caused by beta-lactam-sensitive gram-positive microorganisms in patients who have renal failure
- Use of vancomycin solution for topical application or irrigation

3. Enhancing compliance with recommendations
   - Although several techniques may be useful, further study is required to determine the most effective methods for influencing the prescribing practices of physicians
   - Key parameters of vancomycin use can be monitored through the hospital's quality assurance/improvement process or as part of the drug-utilization review of the Pharmacy and Therapeutics Committee and the medical staff

REFERENCE VALUES FOR ADULTS

CHEMISTRY

Test	Values	Remarks
Serum / Plasma		
Acetone	Negative	
Albumin	3.2-5 g/dL	
Alcohol, ethyl	Negative	
Aldolase	1.2-7.6 IU/L	
Ammonia	20-70 mcg/dL	Specimen to be placed on ice as soon as collected.
Amylase	30-110 units/L	
Bilirubin, direct	0-0.3 mg/dL	
Bilirubin, total	0.1-1.2 mg/dL	
Calcium	8.6-10.3 mg/dL	
Calcium, ionized	2.24-2.46 mEq/L	
Chloride	95-108 mEq/L	
Cholesterol, total	≤200 mg/dL	Fasted blood required – normal value affected by dietary habits. This reference range is for a general adult population.
HDL cholesterol	40-60 mg/dL	Fasted blood required – normal value affected by dietary habits.
LDL cholesterol	<160 mg/dL	If triglyceride is >400 mg/dL, LDL cannot be calculated accurately (Friedewald equation). Target LDL-C depends on patient's risk factors.
CO_2	23-30 mEq/L	
Creatine kinase (CK) isoenzymes		
CK-BB	0%	
CK-MB (cardiac)	0%-3.9%	
CK-MM (muscle)	96%-100%	
CK-MB levels must be both ≥4% and 10 IU/L to meet diagnostic criteria for CK-MB positive result consistent with myocardial injury.		
Creatine phosphokinase (CPK)	8-150 IU/L	
Creatinine	0.5-1.4 mg/dL	
Ferritin	13-300 ng/mL	
Folate	3.6-20 ng/dL	
GGT (gamma-glutamyltranspeptidase)		
male	11-63 IU/L	
female	8-35 IU/L	
GLDH	To be determined	
Glucose (preprandial)	<115 mg/dL	Goals different for diabetics.
Glucose, fasting	60-110 mg/dL	Goals different for diabetics.
Glucose, nonfasting (2-h postprandial)	<120 mg/dL	Goals different for diabetics.
Hemoglobin A_{1c}	<8	
Hemoglobin, plasma free	<2.5 mg/100 mL	
Hemoglobin, total glycosolated (Hb A_1)	4%-8%	
Iron	65-150 mcg/dL	
Iron binding capacity, total (TIBC)	250-420 mcg/dL	
Lactic acid	0.7-2.1 mEq/L	Specimen to be kept on ice and sent to lab as soon as possible.
Lactate dehydrogenase (LDH)	56-194 IU/L	

CHEMISTRY *(continued)*

Test	Values	Remarks
Lactate dehydrogenase (LDH) isoenzymes		
LD_1	20%-34%	
LD_2	29%-41%	
LD_3	15%-25%	
LD_4	1%-12%	
LD_5	1%-15%	
Flipped LD_1/LD_2 ratios (>1 may be consistent with myocardial injury) particularly when considered in combination with a recent CK-MB positive result.		
Lipase	23-208 units/L	
Magnesium	1.6-2.5 mg/dL	Increased by slight hemolysis.
Osmolality	289-308 mOsm/kg	
Phosphatase, alkaline		
adults 25-60 y	33-131 IU/L	
adults 61 y or older	51-153 IU/L	
infancy-adolescence	Values range up to 3-5 times higher than adults	
Phosphate, inorganic	2.8-4.2 mg/dL	
Potassium	3.5-5.2 mEq/L	Increased by slight hemolysis.
Prealbumin	>15 mg/dL	
Protein, total	6.5-7.9 g/dL	
SGOT (AST)	<35 IU/L (20-48)	
SGPT (ALT) (10-35)	<35 IU/L	
Sodium	134-149 mEq/L	
Thyroid stimulating hormone (TSH)		
adult ≤20 y	0.7-6.4 mIU/L	
21-54 y	0.4-4.2 mIU/L	
55-87 y	0.5-8.9 mIU/L	
Transferrin	>200 mg/dL	
Triglycerides	45-155 mg/dL	Fasted blood required.
Troponin I	<1.5 ng/mL	
Urea nitrogen (BUN)	7-20 mg/dL	
Uric acid		
male	2-8 mg/dL	
female	2-7.5 mg/dL	

Cerebrospinal Fluid

Test	Values	Remarks
Glucose	50-70 mg/dL	
Protein	15-45 mg/dL	CSF obtained by lumbar puncture.

Note: Bloody specimen gives erroneously high value due to contamination with blood proteins

Urine
(24-hour specimen is required for all these tests unless specified)

Test	Values	Remarks
Amylase	32-641 units/L	The value is in units/L and **not** calculated for total volume.
Amylase, fluid (random samples)		Interpretation of value left for physician, depends on the nature of fluid.
Calcium	Depends upon dietary intake	
Creatine		
male	150 mg/24 h	Higher value on children and during pregnancy.
female	250 mg/24 h	
Creatinine	1000-2000 mg/24 h	
Creatinine clearance (endogenous)		
male	85-125 mL/min	A blood sample must accompany urine specimen.
female	75-115 mL/min	
Glucose	1 g/24 h	
5-hydroxyindoleacetic acid	2-8 mg/24 h	

REFERENCE VALUES FOR ADULTS *(Continued)*

CHEMISTRY *(continued)*

Test	Values	Remarks
Iron	0.15 mg/24 h	Acid washed container required.
Magnesium	146-209 mg/24 h	
Osmolality	500-800 mOsm/kg	With normal fluid intake.
Oxalate	10-40 mg/24 h	
Phosphate	400-1300 mg/24 h	
Potassium	25-120 mEq/24 h	Varies with diet; the interpretation of urine electrolytes and osmolality should be left for the physician.
Sodium	40-220 mEq/24 h	
Porphobilinogen, qualitative	Negative	
Porphyrins, qualitative	Negative	
Proteins	0.05-0.1 g/24 h	
Salicylate	Negative	
Urea clearance	60-95 mL/min	A blood sample must accompany specimen.
Urea N	10-40 g/24 h	Dependent on protein intake.
Uric acid	250-750 mg/24 h	Dependent on diet and therapy.
Urobilinogen	0.5-3.5 mg/24 h	For qualitative determination on random urine, send sample to urinalysis section in Hematology Lab.
Xylose absorption test children	16%-33% of ingested xylose	
Feces		
Fat, 3-day collection	<5 g/d	Value depends on fat intake of 100 g/d for 3 days preceding and during collection.
Gastric Acidity		
Acidity, total, 12 h	10-60 mEq/L	Titrated at pH 7.

Blood Gases

	Arterial	Capillary	Venous
pH	7.35-7.45	7.35-7.45	7.32-7.42
pCO_2 (mm Hg)	35-45	35-45	38-52
pO_2 (mm Hg)	70-100	60-80	24-48
HCO_3 (mEq/L)	19-25	19-25	19-25
TCO_2 (mEq/L)	19-29	19-29	23-33
O_2 saturation (%)	90-95	90-95	40-70
Base excess (mEq/L)	-5 to +5	-5 to +5	-5 to +5

HEMATOLOGY

Complete Blood Count

Age	Hgb (g/dL)	Hct (%)	RBC (mill/mm^3)	RDW
0-3 d	15.0-20.0	45-61	4.0-5.9	<18
1-2 wk	12.5-18.5	39-57	3.6-5.5	<17
1-6 mo	10.0-13.0	29-42	3.1-4.3	<16.5
7 mo to 2 y	10.5-13.0	33-38	3.7-4.9	<16
2-5 y	11.5-13.0	34-39	3.9-5.0	<15
5-8 y	11.5-14.5	35-42	4.0-4.9	<15
13-18 y	12.0-15.2	36-47	4.5-5.1	<14.5
Adult male	13.5-16.5	41-50	4.5-5.5	<14.5
Adult female	12.0-15.0	36-44	4.0-4.9	<14.5

Age	MCV (fL)	MCH (pg)	MCHC (%)	Plts (x 10^3/mm^3)
0-3 d	95-115	31-37	29-37	250-450
1-2 wk	86-110	28-36	28-38	250-450
1-6 mo	74-96	25-35	30-36	300-700
7 mo to 2 y	70-84	23-30	31-37	250-600
2-5 y	75-87	24-30	31-37	250-550
5-8 y	77-95	25-33	31-37	250-550
13-18 y	78-96	25-35	31-37	150-450
Adult male	80-100	26-34	31-37	150-450
Adult female	80-100	26-34	31-37	150-450

REFERENCE VALUES FOR ADULTS *(Continued)*

WBC and Differential

Age	WBC (x 10^3/mm^3)	Segs	Bands	Lymphs	Monos
0-3 d	9.0-35.0	32-62	10-18	19-29	5-7
1-2 wk	5.0-20.0	14-34	6-14	36-45	6-10
1-6 mo	6.0-17.5	13-33	4-12	41-71	4-7
7 mo to 2 y	6.0-17.0	15-35	5-11	45-76	3-6
2-5 y	5.5-15.5	23-45	5-11	35-65	3-6
5-8 y	5.0-14.5	32-54	5-11	28-48	3-6
13-18 y	4.5-13.0	34-64	5-11	25-45	3-6
Adults	4.5-11.0	35-66	5-11	24-44	3-6

Age	Eosinophils	Basophils	Atypical Lymphs	No. of NRBCs
0-3 d	0-2	0-1	0-8	0-2
1-2 wk	0-2	0-1	0-8	0
1-6 mo	0-3	0-1	0-8	0
7 mo to 2 y	0-3	0-1	0-8	0
2-5 y	0-3	0-1	0-8	0
5-8 y	0-3	0-1	0-8	0
13-18 y	0-3	0-1	0-8	0
Adults	0-3	0-1	0-8	0

Segs = segmented neutrophils.
Bands = band neutrophils.
Lymphs = lymphocytes.
Monos = monocytes.

Erythrocyte Sedimentation Rates and Reticulocyte Counts

Sedimentation rate, Westergren	Children	0-20 mm/h
	Adult male	0-15 mm/h
	Adult female	0-20 mm/h
Sedimentation rate, Wintrobe	Children	0-13 mm/h
	Adult male	0-10 mm/h
	Adult female	0-15 mm/h
Reticulocyte count	Newborns	2%-6%
	1-6 mo	0%-2.8%
	Adults	0.5%-1.5%

ANTICOAGULANT THERAPY GUIDELINES

This information, for the use of heparin and warfarin in adults, was obtained from a review of current literature. This information is intended to optimize therapeutic anticoagulation by minimizing patient bleeding risks, decreasing the time required for titration to achieve a desired level of anticoagulation, and promoting efficient use of laboratory tests.

INITIATION OF I.V. HEPARIN THERAPY TREATMENT OF VENOUS THROMBOSIS AND PULMONARY EMBOLISM[1]

Monitoring	Dosing
Check baseline aPTT, PT/INR, CBC	Bolus 80 units/kg I.V. Initial drip 18 units/kg/hour I.V.
Check CBC with platelet count every 3 days, aPTT 6 hours post bolus and 6 hours after each dosing adjustment. When two consecutive aPTTs are therapeutic, monitor aPTT every 24 hours and readjust heparin drip as needed.	Refer to nomogram below

aPTT(s)[1]	Dosing
<35	80 units/kg bolus, increase drip 4 units/kg/hour
35-45	40 units/kg bolus, increase drip 2 units/kg/hour
46-70	No change
71-90	Reduce drip by 2 units/kg/hour
>90	Stop infusion 1 hour, reduce drip by 3 units/kg/hour

aPTT = activated partial thromboplastin time; PT/INR = prothrombin time/international normalized ratio; CBC = complete blood count and platelet count; s = seconds; kg = kilogram.

[1]It is recommended that each lab perform an *in vitro* heparin titration curve to establish the therapeutic range for a specific aPTT reagent which is equivalent to a heparin concentration of 0.3-0.4 International Units/mL. Thus, the therapeutic range will vary depending upon the aPTT reagent in use.

INITIATION OF ORAL ANTICOAGULATION WITH WARFARIN

Dosing of warfarin must be individualized according to patient response to the drug as indicated by the INR. Use of a large loading dose may increase the incidence of hemorrhagic and other complications, does not offer more rapid protection against thrombus formation, and is not recommended. Low initiation doses (eg, 2-5 mg/day) are recommended for elderly and/or debilitated patients and patients with potential for increased responsiveness to warfarin.

Step 1: Obtain baseline INR.

Begin therapy with warfarin with a dose of 2-5 mg per day with dosage adjustment based on results of INR determinations.

For patients on heparin: Since the anticoagulant effect of warfarin is delayed, heparin is preferred initially for rapid anticoagulation. Conversion to warfarin may begin concomitantly with unfractionated or low molecular weight heparin or may be delayed 3-6 days. When warfarin has produced two desired INR with at least 24 hours of separation, then the heparin may be discontinued.

Step 2: Day that the INR is stabilized in the therapeutic range: Check INR daily. Adjust warfarin dose based on the results of INR determinations.

Patients stabilized in the therapeutic range: Intervals between subsequent INR determinations should be based upon the physician's judgment of the patient's reliability and response to warfarin in order to maintain the individual within the therapeutic range. Acceptable intervals for INR determinations are normally within the range of 1-4 weeks after a stable dosage has been determined. Most patients are satisfactorily maintained on warfarin at a dose of 2-10 mg daily.

ANTICOAGULANT THERAPY GUIDELINES *(Continued)*

MONITORING INR (INTERNATIONAL NORMALIZED RATIO)

Because PT results are very dependent on the thromboplastin reagent used, a system of standardizing prothrombin time in oral anticoagulant therapy was introduced by the World Health Organization in 1983. It is based upon determination of an INR, which is equivalent to the PT ratio one would obtain if a sensitive reference thromboplastin were used for the PT.

- Thromboplastin sensitivity is determined by the manufacturer and is expressed as an International Sensitivity Index (ISI)

- The INR can be calculated as **INR = (Observed PT ratio)^{ISI}**

- Calculation of the INR from the PT ratio is usually performed by the laboratory

Reminder

- Be aware of potential drug interactions and other factors that may affect INR (refer to prescribing information for warfarin)

- Patient/staff education about warfarin is an important part of therapy. Effective therapeutic levels with minimal complications are in part dependent upon cooperative and well-instructed patients who communicate effectively with their physician. Various warfarin patient educational guides are available to health professionals on request.

DRUG INTERACTIONS WITH WARFARIN

Numerous factors, alone or in combination, including travel, changes in diet, environment, physical state, and medication may influence response of the patient to anticoagulants. It is generally good practice to monitor the patient's response with additional INR determinations in the period immediately after discharge from the hospital, and whenever other medications are initiated, discontinued, or taken irregularly. The factors on the following pages, alone or in combination, may be responsible for INCREASED INR response (other factors may also affect anticoagulant response).

Exogenous Factors

Potential drug interactions with warfarin are listed below by drug class. For specific drugs in these classes that have been reported to interact, see full prescribing information for warfarin.

Adrenergic stimulants, central
Alcohol abuse reduction preparations
Analgesics
Anesthetics, inhalation
Antiarrhythmics[1]
Antibiotics[1]
    Aminoglycosides (oral)
    Cephalosporins, parenteral
    Macrolides
    Metronidazole
    Miscellaneous
        Penicillins (intravenous high-dose)
    Quinolones (fluoroquinolones)
    Sulfonamides, long-acting
    Tetracyclines
Anticoagulants
Anticonvulsants[1]
Antidepressants[1]
Antimalarial agents
Antineoplastics[1]
Antiparasitic/antimicrobials
Antiplatelet drugs/effects
Antithyroid drugs[1]
Beta-adrenergic blockers
Bromelains
Cholelitholytic agents
Diabetes agents, oral
Diuretics[1]
Fungal medications, systemic[1]
Gastrointestinal, ulcerative colitis agents
Gout treatment agents
Hemorrheologic agents
Hepatotoxic drugs
Hyperglycemic agents
Hypertensive emergency agents
Hypnotics[1]
Hypolipidemics[1]
Monoamine oxidase inhibitors
Narcotics, prolonged
NSAIDs
Psychostimulants
Pyrazolones
Salicylates
Steroids, adrenocortical[1]
Steroids, anabolic (17-alkyl testosterone derivatives)
Thrombolytics
Thyroid drugs[1]
Tuberculosis agents[1]
Uricosuric agents
Vaccines
Vitamin E

Also: Other medications affecting blood elements which may modify hemostasis, dietary deficiencies, prolonged hot weather, unreliable INR determinations.

[1]Increased and decreased INR responses have been reported.

ANTICOAGULANT THERAPY GUIDELINES *(Continued)*

The following factors, alone or in combination, may be responsible for DECREASED INR response:

Exogenous Factors

Potential drug interactions with warfarin are listed below by drug class. For specific drugs in these classes that have been reported to interact, see full prescribing information for warfarin.

> Adrenal cortical steroid inhibitors
> Antacids
> Antianxiety agents
> Antiarrhythmics[1]
> Antibiotics[1]
> Anticonvulsants[1]
> Antidepressants[1]
> Antihistamines
> Antineoplastics[1]
> Antipsychotic medications
> Antithyroid drugs[1]
> Barbiturates
> Diuretics[1]
> Enteral nutritional supplements
> Fungal medications, systemic[1]
> Gastric acidity and peptic ulcer agents[1]
> Hypnotics[1]
> Hypolipidemics[1]
> Immunosuppressives
> Oral contraceptives, estrogen-containing
> Steroids, adrenocortical[1]
> Thyroid drugs[1]
> Tuberculosis agents[1]
> Vitamin K

Also: Diet high in vitamin K and unreliable INR determinations
[1]Increased and decreased INR responses have been reported.

Because a patient may be exposed to a combination of the above factors, the net effect of warfarin on INR response may be unpredictable. More frequent INR monitoring is therefore advisable. Medications of unknown interaction with coumarins are best regarded with caution. When these medications are started or stopped, more frequent INR monitoring is advisable.

It has been reported that concomitant administration of warfarin and ticlopidine may be associated with cholestatic hepatitis.

Effect on Other Drugs: Coumarins may also affect the action of other drugs. Hypoglycemic agents (chlorpropamide and tolbutamide) and anticonvulsants (phenytoin and phenobarbital) may accumulate in the body as a result of interference with either their metabolism or excretion.

THERAPY WITH WARFARIN

Warfarin is indicated for the prophylaxis and/or treatment of venous thrombosis and its extension, and pulmonary embolism.

Warfarin is indicated for the prophylaxis and/or treatment of the thromboembolic complications associated with atrial fibrillation and/or cardiac valve replacement.

Warfarin is indicated to reduce the risk of death, recurrent myocardial infarction, and thromboembolic events such as stroke or systemic embolization after myocardial infarction.

The benefits of oral anticoagulant therapy in reducing the occurrence of thromboembolic events in patients with atrial fibrillation has been confirmed by a number of major clinical trials. A pooled analysis of five major clinical trials demonstrated a 68% risk reduction of thromboembolic stroke in patients receiving warfarin (INR 2.0-3.0). The annual rate of major hemorrhage was 1.0% for the control group and 1.3% for the warfarin group.

Warfarin is contraindicated in:

- Patients where the risk of hemorrhage outweighs the potential clinical benefits of therapy
- Pregnancy
- Alcoholism/drug abuse
- Unsupervised dementia/psychosis

Thromboembolic Stroke Prevention in Patients With Atrial Fibrillation

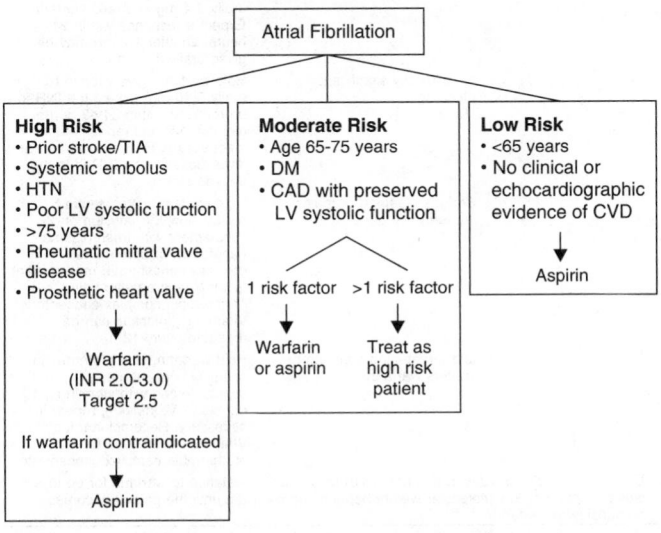

ANTICOAGULANT THERAPY GUIDELINES *(Continued)*

Seventh AACP Consensus Conference on Antithrombotic Therapy: Recommendations on Reversal of Elevated INR In Patients Taking Warfarin

INR	Symptoms	Recommendation
<5	No significant bleeding and rapid reversal not necessary	Lower or hold the next dose and monitor frequently; when INR approaches desired range, resume dosing with a lower dose.
>5 and <9	No significant bleeding	No other risk factors for bleeding, omit the next one or two doses, monitor INR and resume with a lower dose when the INR approaches the desired range.
		Alternatively, if there are other risk factors for bleeding, omit the next dose and give vitamin K_1 orally <5 mg; resume with a lower dose when the INR approaches the desired range.
		If rapid reversal is required for surgery, then given vitamin K_1 orally 2-4 mg and hold warfarin. Expect a response within 24 hours; another 1-2 mg may be given orally if needed.
>9	No clinically significant bleeding	Hold warfarin, give vitamin K_1 orally 5-10 mg, expect the INR to be reduced within 24-48 hours, monitor INR and repeat vitamin K if necessary. Resume warfarin at lower doses when INR is in the desired range.
	Serious bleeding or major warfarin overdose	Hold warfarin, give vitamin K_1 10 mg by slow I.V. infusion and supplement with fresh plasma transfusion or prothrombin complex concentrate; recombinant factor VIIa is an alternative to prothrombin complex concentrate. Vitamin K_1 injection can be repeated every 12 h.
	Life-threatening bleeding or serious warfarin	Hold warfarin, give prothrombin complex concentrate, supplemented with vitamin K_1 10 mg slow I.V. infusion; repeat if necessary. Recombinant factor VIIa is an alternative to prothrombin complex concentrate.

Use of high doses of vitamin K_1 (10.0-15.0) may cause resistance to warfarin for up to a week. Heparin or low molecular weight heparin can be given until the patient becomes responsive to warfarin.

Reference: Ansell J, Hirsh J, Poller L, et al, "The Pharmacology and Management of the Vitamin K Antagonists: The Seventh ACCP Conference on Antithrombotic and Thrombolytic Therapy," *Chest*, 2004, 126(3 Suppl):204S-233S.

References

Ansell J, Hirsh J, Poller L, et al, "The Pharmacology and Management of the Vitamin K Antagonists: The Seventh ACCP Conference on Antithrombotic and Thrombolytic Therapy," *Chest*, 2004, 126(3 Suppl):204S-233S.

Atrial Fibrillation Investigators, *Ann Intern Med*, 1994, 154:1449-57.

Connolly SJ, Laupacis A, Gent M, et al, "Canadian Atrial Fibrillation Anticoagulation (CAFA) Study," *J Am Coll Cardiol*, 1991, 18(2):349-55.

Coumadin® package insert.

Ezekowitz MD, Bridgers SL, James KE, et al, "Warfarin in the Prevention of Stroke Associated With Nonrheumatic Atrial Fibrillation. Veterans Affairs Stroke Prevention in Nonrheumatic Atrial Fibrillation Investigators," *N Engl J Med*, 1992, 327(20):1406-12.

Hirsh J and Raschke R, "Heparin and Low-Molecular-Weight Heparin: The Seventh ACCP Conference on Antithrombotic and Thrombolytic Therapy," *Chest*, 2004, 126(3 Suppl):188S-203S.

Petersen P, Boysen G, Godtfredsen J, et al, "Placebo-Controlled, Randomised Trial of Warfarin and Aspirin for Prevention of Thromboembolic Complications in Chronic Atrial Fibrillation. The Copenhagen AFASAK Study," *Lancet*, 1989, 1(8631):175-9.

Raschke RA, Reilly BM, Guidry JR, et al, "The Weight-Based Heparin Dosing Nomogram Compared With a 'Standard Care' Nomogram. A Randomized Controlled Trial," *Ann Intern Med*, 1993, 119(9):874-81.

"Stroke Prevention in Atrial Fibrillation Study. Final Results," *Circulation*, 1991, 84(2):527-39.

The American Geriatrics Society, Current Guidelines for Practice: Oral Anticoagulation for Older Adults, 2002, New York, NY.

"The Effect of Low-Dose Warfarin on the Risk of Stroke in Patients With Nonrheumatic Atrial Fibrillation. The Boston Area Anticoagulation Trial for Atrial Fibrillation Investigators," *N Engl J Med*, 1990, 323(22):1505-11.

"Warfarin Versus Aspirin for Prevention of Thromboembolism in Atrial Fibrillation: Stroke Prevention in Atrial Fibrillation II Study," *Lancet*, 1994, 343(8899):687-91.

CMS GUIDELINES FOR GRADUAL DOSE REDUCTION OF PSYCHOPHARMACOLOGICAL AGENTS IN NURSING FACILITY RESIDENTS

http://www.cms.hhs.gov/transmittals/downloads/R22SOMA.pdf
Section 483.25(l)

The following is an exerpt from Appendix PP of the Centers for Medicare and Medicaid Services (CMS) State Operations Manual concering gradual dose reduction in relation to specific classes of psychopharmacologic agents. The reader is refered to Table 1 (Medication Issues of Particular Relevance) in the above document, for further information regarding the use of psychopharmacological agents in nursing facilites.

CONSIDERATIONS SPECIFIC TO ANTIPSYCHOTICS

The regulation addressing the use of antipsychotic medications identifies the process of tapering as a "gradual dose reduction (GDR)" and requires a GDR, unless clinically contraindicated.

Within the first year in which a resident is admitted on an antipsychotic medication or after the facility has initiated an antipsychotic medication, the facility must attempt a GDR in two separate quarters (with at least one month between the attempts), unless clinically contraindicated. After the first year, a GDR must be attempted annually, unless clinically contraindicated.

For any individual who is receiving an antipsychotic medication to treat behavioral symptoms related to dementia, the GDR may be considered clinically contraindicated if:

- The resident's target symptoms returned or worsened after the most recent attempt at a GDR within the facility; and
- The physician has documented the clinical rationale for why any additional attempted dose reduction at that time would be likely to impair the resident's function or increase distressed behavior.

For any individual who is receiving an antipsychotic medication to treat a psychiatric disorder other than behavioral symptoms related to dementia (for example, schizophrenia, bipolar mania, or depression with psychotic features), the GDR may be considered contraindicated, if:

- The continued use is in accordance with relevant current standards of practice and the physician has documented the clinical rationale for why any attempted dose reduction would be likely to impair the resident's function or cause psychiatric instability by exacerbating an underlying psychiatric disorder; or
- The resident's target symptoms returned or worsened after the most recent attempt at a GDR within the facility and the physician has documented the clinical rationale for why any additional attempted dose reduction at that time would be likely to impair the resident's function or cause psychiatric instability by exacerbating an underlying medical or psychiatric disorder.

ATTEMPTED TAPERING RELATIVE TO CONTINUED INDICATION OR OPTIMAL DOSE

As noted, attempted tapering is one way to determine whether a specific medication is still indicated, and whether target symptoms and risks can be managed with a lesser dose of a medication. As noted, many medications in various categories can be tapered safely. The following examples of tapering relate to two common categories of concern: sedatives/hypnotics and psychopharmacologic medications (other than antipsychotic and sedatives/hypnotics medications).

TAPERING CONSIDERATIONS SPECIFIC TO SEDATIVES / HYPNOTICS

For as long as a resident remains on a sedative/hypnotic that is used routinely and beyond the manufacturer's recommendations for duration of use, the facility should attempt to taper the medication quarterly unless clinically contraindicated. Clinically contraindicated means:

- The continued use is in accordance with relevant current standards of practice and the physician has documented the clinical rationale for why any attempted dose reduction would be likely to impair the resident's function or cause psychiatric instability by exacerbating an underlying medical or psychiatric disorder; or
- The resident's target symptoms returned or worsened after the most recent attempt at tapering the dose within the facility and the physician has documented the clinical rationale for why any additional attempted dose reduction at that time would be likely to impair the resident's function or cause psychiatric instability by exacerbating an underlying medical or psychiatric disorder.

CONSIDERATIONS SPECIFIC TO PSYCHOPHARMACOLOGICAL MEDICATIONS (OTHER THAN ANTIPSYCHOTICS AND SEDATIVES / HYPNOTICS)

During the first year in which a resident is admitted on a psychopharmacological medication (other than an antipsychotic or a sedative/hypnotic), or after the facility has initiated such medication, the facility should attempt to taper the medication during at least two separate quarters (with at least one month between the attempts), unless clinically contraindicated. After the first year, a tapering should be attempted annually, unless clinically contraindicated. The tapering may be considered clinically contraindicated, if:

- The continued use is in accordance with relevant current standards of practice and the physician has documented the clinical rationale for why any attempted dose reduction would be likely to impair the resident's function or cause psychiatric instability by exacerbating an underlying medical or psychiatric disorder; or
- The resident's target symptoms returned or worsened after the most recent attempt at tapering the dose within the facility and the physician has documented the clinical rationale for why any additional attempted dose reduction at that time would be likely to impair the resident's function or cause psychiatric instability by exacerbating an underlying medical or psychiatric disorder.

PHARMACOTHERAPY OF URINARY INCONTINENCE

Incontinence Type	Drug Class	Drug Therapy	Adverse Effects and Precautions	Comments
Urge incontinence	Anticholinergic agents	Oxybutynin (2.5-5 mg 2-4 times/day, extended release 5-20 mg once daily, or transdermal 1 patch twice weekly delivering 3.9 mg/day), propantheline (7.5-30 mg at least 3 times/day), dicyclomine (10-20 mg twice daily), tolterodine (1-2 mg twice daily; extended release capsule: 2-4 mg once daily), trospium (20 mg once or twice daily), solifenacin (5-10 mg once daily), darifenacin (7.5-15 mg once daily)	Dry mouth, visual disturbances, constipation, dry skin, confusion	Anticholinergics are the first-line drug therapy. Propantheline and dicyclomine are not considered drugs of choice in older adults. Darifenacin and solifenacin may cause less anticholinergic side effects. Trospium may cause less CNS effects.
	Tricyclic antidepressants (TCAs)	Imipramine, desipramine, nortriptyline (25-100 mg/day)	Anticholinergic effects (as above), orthostatic hypotension, and cardiac dysrhythmia	TCAs are generally reserved for patients with an additional indication (eg, depression, neuralgia) at an initial dose of 10-25 mg 1-3 times/day.
Stress incontinence	Alpha-adrenergic agonists	Pseudoephedrine (15-60 mg 3 times/day)	Anxiety, insomnia, agitation, respiratory difficulty, sweating, cardiac dysrhythmia, hypertension, tremor; should not be used in obstructive syndromes and/or hypertension	Pseudoephedrine is the first-line drug therapy for women with no contraindication (notably hypertension).
Stress or combined urge/stress incontinence	Estrogen replacement agents	Conjugated estrogens (0.3-0.625 mg/day orally or 1 g vaginal cream at bedtime)	Should not be used if suspected or confirmed breast or endometrial cancer, active or past thromboembolism with past oral contraceptive, estrogen, or pregnancy; headache, spotting, edema, breast tenderness, possible depression\n\nGive progesterone with estrogen if uterus is present; pretreatment/periodic mammogram, gynecologic, breast exam advised	Estrogen (oral or vaginal) is an adjunctive therapy for postmenopausal women, as it augments alpha-agonists (eg, pseudoephedrine).\n\nProgestin (eg, medroxyprogesterone 2.5-10 mg/day) continuously or intermittently; combined oral or vaginal estrogen and pseudoephedrine in postmenopausal women, if single drug is inadequate; imipramine is an alternative therapy when first-line therapy is inadequate.
	Tricyclic antidepressants (TCAs)	Imipramine (10-25 mg 3 times/day)	May worsen cardiac conduction abnormalities, postural hypotension, anticholinergic effects	TCAs are generally reserved for patients with an additional indication (eg, depression, neuralgia) at an initial dose of 10-25 mg 1-3 times/day.

POTENTIALLY INAPPROPRIATE MEDICATIONS FOR GERIATRICS

Incontinence Type	Drug Class	Drug Therapy	Adverse Effects and Precautions	Comments
Overflow	Alpha-adrenergic antagonists	Terazosin (1 mg at bedtime with first dose in supine position and increase by 1 mg every 4 days to maximum 10 mg/day)	Postural hypotension, dizziness, vertigo, heart palpitations, edema, headache, anticholinergic effects	Possible benefit in men with obstructive symptoms of benign prostatic hyperplasia; monitor postural vital signs with first dose/each dose increase; may worsen female stress incontinence
		Doxazosin (1 mg at bedtime with first dose in supine position and increase by 1 mg every 7-14 days to maximum 8 mg/day)	Same as terazosin (may be smaller incidence of hypotension)	Same as terazosin
		Tamsulosin (0.4 mg-0.8 mg daily)	Postural hypotension, headache, dizziness	Less likelihood of postural hypotension than with terazosin or doxazosin
		Alfuzosin (10 mg daily)	Postural hypotension, headache, dizziness	Same as tamsulosin

Adapted from "Urinary Incontinence," *Clinical Practice Guideline*, 1996, American Medical Directors Association, reprinted with permission.

POTENTIALLY INAPPROPRIATE MEDICATIONS FOR GERIATRICS

Table 1. Critera Independent of Diagnoses or Conditions

Applicable Medication	Summary of Prescribing Concern	Severity
Amiodarone (Cordarone®)	Associated with QT interval problems and risk of provoking torsade de pointes. Lack of efficacy in older adults.	High
Amitriptyline (Elavil®), amitriptyline and chlordiazepoxide (Limbitrol®), and amitriptyline and perphenazine (Triavil®)	Because of its strong anticholinergic and sedation properties, amitriptyline is rarely the antidepressant of choice for elderly patients.	High
Amphetamines (excluding methylphenidate hydrochloride and anorexics)	CNS stimulant adverse effects.	High
Amphetamines and anorexic agents	These drugs have potential for causing dependence, hypertension, angina, and myocardial infarction.	High
Anticholinergics and antihistamines: Chlorpheniramine (Chlor-Trimeton®), diphenhydramine (Benadryl®), hydroxyzine (Vistaril®, Atarax®), cyproheptadine (Periactin), promethazine (Phenergan®), tripelennamine, dexchlorpheniramine (Polaramine®)	All nonprescription and many prescription antihistamines may have potent anticholinergic properties. Nonanticholinergic antihistamines are preferred in elderly patients when treating allergic reactions.	High
Barbiturates (all, except phenobarbital) except when used to control seizures	Are highly addictive and cause more adverse effects than most sedative or hypnotic drugs in elderly patients.	High
Benzodiazepines, long-acting: Chlordiazepoxide (Librium®), amitriptyline and chlordiazepoxide (Limbitrol®), clidinium and chlordiazepoxide (Librax®), diazepam (Valium®), quazepam (Doral®), halazepam (Paxipam®), and chlorazepate (Tranxene®)	These drugs have a long half-life in elderly patients (often several days), producing prolonged sedation and increasing the risk of falls and fractures. Short- and intermediate-acting benzodiazepines are preferred if a benzodiazepine is required.	High
Benzodiazepines, short-acting (doses greater than): Alprazolam (Xanax®) 2 mg; oxazepam (Serax®) 60 mg; lorazepam (Ativan®) 3 mg; temazepam (Restoril®) 15 mg; and triazolam (Halcion®) 0.25 mg	Because of increased sensitivity to benzodiazepines in elderly patients, smaller doses may be effective as well as safer. Total daily doses should rarely exceed the suggested maximums.	High
Chlorpropamide (Diabinese®)	It has prolonged half-life in elderly patients and could cause prolonged hypoglycemia. Additionally, it is the only oral hypoglycemic agent that causes SIADH.	High

Table 1. Critera Independent of Diagnoses or Conditions
(continued)

Applicable Medication	Summary of Prescribing Concern	Severity
Cimetidine (Tagamet®)	CNS adverse effects including confusion.	Low
Clonidine (Catapres®)	Potential for orthostatic hypotension and CNS adverse effects.	Low
Cyclandelate (Cyclospasmol®)	Lack of efficacy.	Low
Desiccated thyroid	Concerns about cardiac effects. Safer alternatives available.	High
Digoxin (Lanoxin®) (should not exceed >0.125 mg/day except when treating atrial arrhythmias)	Decreased renal clearance may lead to increased risk of toxic effects	Low
Diphenhydramine (Benadryl®)	May cause confusion and sedation. Should not be used as a hypnotic, and when used to treat emergency allergic reactions, it should be used in the smallest possible dose.	High
Dipyridamole, short-acting (Persantine®). Do not consider the long-acting dipyridamole (which has better properties than the short-acting in older adults) except with patients with artificial heart valves	May cause orthostatic hypotension.	Low
Disopyramide (Norpace®, Norpace® CR)	Of all antiarrhythmic drugs, this is the most potent negative inotrope and therefore may induce heart failure in elderly patients. It is also strongly anticholinergic. Other antiarrhythmic drugs should be used.	High
Doxazosin (Cardura®)	Potential for hypotension, dry mouth, and urinary problems.	Low
Doxepin (Sinequan®)	Because of its strong anticholinergic and sedating properties, doxepin is rarely the antidepressant of choice for elderly patients.	High
Ergot mesyloids (Hydergine®) and cyclandelate (Cyclospasmol®)	Have not been shown to be effective in the doses studied.	Low
Estrogens only (oral)	Evidence of the carcinogenic (breast and endometrial cancer) potential of these agents and lack of cardioprotective effect in older women.	Low
Ethacrynic acid (Edecrin®)	Potential for hypertension and fluid imbalances. Safer alternatives available.	Low
Ferrous sulfate >325 mg/day	Doses >325 mg/day do not dramatically increase the amount absorbed but greatly increase the incidence of constipation.	Low
Fluoxetine, daily (Prozac®)	Long half-life of drug and risk of producing excessive CNS stimulation, sleep disturbances, and increasing agitation. Safer alternatives exist.	High

POTENTIALLY INAPPROPRIATE MEDICATIONS FOR GERIATRICS *(Continued)*

Table 1. Critera Independent of Diagnoses or Conditions *(continued)*

Applicable Medication	Summary of Prescribing Concern	Severity
Flurazepam (Dalmane®)	This benzodiazepine hypnotic has an extremely long half-life in elderly patients (often days), producing prolonged sedation and increasing the incidence of falls and fracture. Medium- or short-acting benzodiazepines are preferable.	High
Gastrointestinal antispasmodic drugs: Dicyclomine (Bentyl®), hyoscyamine (Levsin® and Levsinex®), propantheline (Pro-Banthine), belladonna alkaloids (Donnatal® and others), and clidinium and chlordiazepoxide (Librax®)	GI antispasmodic drugs are highly anticholinergic and have uncertain effectiveness. These drugs should be avoided (especially for long-term use).	High
Guanadrel (Hylorel®)	May cause orthostatic hypotension.	High
Guanethidine (Ismelin®)	May cause orthostatic hypotension. Safer alternatives exist.	High
Indomethacin (Indocin® and Indocin® SR)	Of all available NSAIDs, this drug produces the most CNS adverse effects.	High
Isoxsuprine (Vasodilan®)	Lack of efficacy.	Low
Ketorolac (Toradol®)	Immediate and long-term use should be avoided in older persons, since a significant number have asymptomatic GI pathologic conditions.	High
Long-term use of full-dosage, longer half-life, non-COX-selective NSAIDs: Naproxen (Naprosyn®, Avaprox, and Aleve®), oxaprozin (Daypro®), and piroxicam (Feldene®)	Have the potential to produce GI bleeding, renal failure, high blood pressure, and heart failure.	High
Long-term use of stimulant laxatives: Bisacodyl (Dulcolax®), cascara sagrada, and Neoloid except in the presence of opiate analgesic use	May exacerbate bowel dysfunction.	High
Meperidine (Demerol®)	Not an effective oral analgesic in doses commonly used. May cause confusion and has many disadvantages to other narcotic drugs.	High
Meprobamate (Miltown®)	This is a highly addictive and sedating anxiolytic. Those using meprobamate for prolonged periods may become addicted and may need to be withdrawn slowly.	High
Mesoridazine (Serentil®)	CNS and extrapyramidal adverse effects.	High
Methyldopa (Aldomet®) and methyldopa and hydrochlorothiazide (Aldoril®)	May cause bradycardia and exacerbate depression in elderly patients.	High

Table 1. Critera Independent of Diagnoses or Conditions
(continued)

Applicable Medication	Summary of Prescribing Concern	Severity
Methyltestosterone (Android®, Testrad®, Virilon®)	Potential for prostatic hypertrophy and cardiac problems.	High
Mineral oil	Potential for aspiration and adverse effects. Safer alternatives available.	High
Muscle relaxants and antispasmodics: Methocarbamol (Robaxin®), carisoprodol (Soma®), chlorzoxazone (Paraflex®), metaxalone (Skelaxin®), cyclobenzaprine (Flexeril®), and oxybutynin (Ditropan®). Do not consider the extended-release Ditropan® XL.	Most muscle relaxants and antispasmodic drugs are poorly tolerated by elderly patients, since these cause anticholinergic adverse effects, sedation, and weakness. Additionally, their effectiveness at doses tolerated by elderly patients is questionable.	High
Nifedipine, short-acting (Adalat®, Procardia®)	Potential for hypotension and constipation.	High
Nitrofurantoin (Macrodantin®)	Potential for renal impairment. Safer alternatives available.	High
Orphenadrine (Norflex™)	Causes more sedation and anticholinergic adverse effects than safer alternatives.	High
Pentazocine (Talwin®)	Narcotic analgesic that causes more CNS adverse effects, including confusion and hallucinations, more commonly than other narcotic drugs. Additionally, it is a mixed agonist and antagonist.	High
Propoxyphene (Darvon®) and combination products (Darvon® with ASA, Darvon-N®, and Darvocet-N®)	Offers few analgesic advantages over acetaminophen, yet has the adverse effects of other narcotic drugs.	Low
Reserpine at doses >0.25 mg	May induce depression, impotence, sedation, and orthostatic hypotension.	Low
Thioridazine (Mellaril®)	Greater potential for CNS and extrapyramidal adverse effects.	High
Ticlopidine (Ticlid®)	Has been shown to be no better than aspirin in preventing clotting and may be considerably more toxic. Safer, more effective alternatives exist.	High
Trimethobenzamide (Tigan®)	One of the least effective antiemetic drugs, yet it can cause extrapyramidal adverse effects.	High

Adapted from Fick DM, Cooper JW, Wade WE, et al, "Updating the Beers Criteria for Potentially Inappropriate Medication Use in Older Adults: Results of a U.S. Consensus Panel of Experts," *Arch Intern Med*, 2003, 163(22):2716-24.

POTENTIALLY INAPPROPRIATE MEDICATIONS FOR GERIATRICS *(Continued)*

Table 2. Final Criteria Considering Diagnoses or Conditions

Disease or Condition	Drug	Concern	Severity
Anorexia and malnutrition	CNS stimulants: Dextroamphetamine and amphetamine (Adderall®), methylphenidate (Ritalin®), methamphetamine (Desoxyn®), pemolin, and fluoxetine (Prozac®)	Concern due to appetite suppressing effects	High
Arrhythmias	Tricyclic antidepressants (imipramine hydrochloride, doxepin hydrochloride, and amitriptyline hydrochloride)	Concern due to proarrhythmic effects and ability to produce QT interval changes.	High
Bladder outflow obstruction	Anticholinergics and antihistamines, gastrointestinal antispasmodics, muscle relaxants, oxybutynin (Ditropan®), flavoxate (Urispas®), anticholinergics, antidepressants, decongestants, and tolterodine (Detrol®)	May decrease urinary flow, leading to urinary retention.	High
Blood clotting disorders or receiving anticoagulant therapy	Aspirin, NSAIDs, dipyridamole (Persantine®), ticlopidine (Ticlid®), and clopidogrel (Plavix®)	May prolong clotting time and elevate INR values or inhibit platelet aggregation, resulting in an increased potential for bleeding.	High
Chronic constipation	Calcium channel blockers, anticholinergics, and tricyclic antidepressant (imipramine hydrochloride, doxepin hydrochloride, and amitriptyline hydrochloride)	May exacerbate constipation	Low
Cognitive impairment	Barbiturates, anticholinergics, antispasmodics, and muscle relaxants, CNS stimulants: Dextroamphetamine and amphetamine (Adderall®), methylphenidate (Ritalin®), methamphetamine (Desoxyn®), and pemolin	Concern due to CNS-altering effects	High
COPD	Benzodiazepines, long-acting: Chlordiazepoxide (Librium®), amitriptyline and chlordiazepoxide (Limbitrol®), clidinium and chlordiazepoxide (Librax®), diazepam (Valium®), quazepam (Doral®), and chlorazepate (Tranxene®). Beta-blockers: Propranolol	CNS adverse effects. May induce respiratory depression. May exacerbate or cause respiratory depression.	High
Depression	Long-term benzodiazepine use. Sympatholytic agents: Methyldopa (Aldomet), reserpine, and guanethidine (Ismelin)	May produce or exacerbate depression.	High
Gastric or duodenal ulcers	NSAIDs and aspirin (>325 mg) (coxibs excluded)	May exacerbate existing ulcers or produce new/ additional ulcers.	High

Table 2. Final Criteria Considering Diagnoses or Conditions
(continued)

Disease or Condition	Drug	Concern	Severity
Heart failure	Disopyramide (Norpace®), and high sodium content drugs (sodium and sodium salts [alginate bicarbonate, biphosphate, citrate, phosphate, salicylate, and sulfate])	Negative inotropic effect. Potential to promote fluid retention and exacerbation of heart failure.	High
Hypertension	Phenylpropanolamine hydrochloride (removed from the market in 2001), pseudoephedrine; diet pills, and amphetamines	May produce elevation of blood pressure secondary to sympathomimetic activity.	High
Insomnia	Decongestants, theophylline (Theodur), methylphenidate (Ritalin®), MAOIs, and amphetamines	Concern due to CNS stimulant effects	High
Obesity	Olanzapine (Zyprexa®)	May stimulate appetite and increase weight gain.	Low
Parkinson disease	Metoclopramide (Reglan®), conventional antipsychotics, and tacrine (Cognex®)	Concern due to their antidopaminergic/cholinergic effects	High
Seizures or epilepsy	Clozapine (Clozaril®), chlorpromazine (Thorazine®), thioridazine (Mellaril®), thiothixene (Navane®)	May lower seizure thresholds.	High
Seizure disorder	Bupropion (Wellbutrin®)	May lower seizure threshold.	High
SIADH/hyponatremia	SSRIs: Fluoxetine (Prozac®), citalopram (Celexa™), fluvoxamine (Luvox®), paroxetine (Paxil®), and sertraline (Zoloft®)	May exacerbate or cause SIADH.	Low
Stress incontinence	α-Blockers (doxazosin, prazosin, and terazosin), anticholinergic, tricyclic antidepressants (imipramine hydrochloride, doxepin hydrochloride, and amitriptyline hydrochloride), and long-acting benzodiazepines	May produce polyuria and worsening of incontinence	High
Syncope or falls	Short- to intermediate-acting benzodiazepine and tricyclic antidepressants (imipramine hydrochloride, doxepin hydrochloride, and amitriptyline hydrochloride)	May produce ataxia, impaired psychomotor function, syncope, and additional falls.	High

Adapted from Fick DM, Cooper JW, Wade WE, et al, "Updating the Beers Criteria for Potentially Inappropriate Medication Use in Older Adults: Results of a U.S. Consensus Panel of Experts," *Arch Intern Med*, 2003, 163(22):2716-24.

CYTOCHROME P450 ENZYMES: SUBSTRATES, INHIBITORS, AND INDUCERS

INTRODUCTION

Most drugs are eliminated from the body, at least in part, by being chemically altered to less lipid-soluble products (ie, metabolized), and thus are more likely to be excreted via the kidneys or the bile. Phase I metabolism includes drug hydrolysis, oxidation, and reduction, and results in drugs that are more polar in their chemical structure, while Phase II metabolism involves the attachment of an additional molecule onto the drug (or partially metabolized drug) in order to create an inactive and/or more water soluble compound. Phase II processes include (primarily) glucuronidation, sulfation, glutathione conjugation, acetylation, and methylation.

Virtually any of the Phase I and II enzymes can be inhibited by some xenobiotic or drug. Some of the Phase I and II enzymes can be induced. Inhibition of the activity of metabolic enzymes will result in increased concentrations of the substrate (drug), whereas induction of the activity of metabolic enzymes will result in decreased concentrations of the substrate. For example, the well-documented enzyme-inducing effects of phenobarbital may include a combination of Phase I and II enzymes. Phase II glucuronidation may be increased via induced UDP-glucuronosyltransferase (UGT) activity, whereas Phase I oxidation may be increased via induced cytochrome P450 (CYP) activity. However, for most drugs, the primary route of metabolism (and the primary focus of drug-drug interaction) is Phase I oxidation, and specifically, metabolism.

CYP enzymes may be responsible for the metabolism (at least partial metabolism) of approximately 75% of all drugs, with the CYP3A subfamily responsible for nearly half of this activity. Found throughout plant, animal, and bacterial species, CYP enzymes represent a superfamily of xenobiotic metabolizing proteins. There have been several hundred CYP enzymes identified in nature, each of which has been assigned to a family (1, 2, 3, etc), subfamily (A, B, C, etc), and given a specific enzyme number (1, 2, 3, etc) according to the similarity in amino acid sequence that it shares with other enzymes. Of these many enzymes, only a few are found in humans, and even fewer appear to be involved in the metabolism of xenobiotics (eg, drugs). The key human enzyme subfamilies include CYP1A, CYP2A, CYP2B, CYP2C, CYP2D, CYP2E, and CYP3A.

CYP enzymes are found in the endoplasmic reticulum of cells in a variety of human tissues (eg, skin, kidneys, brain, lungs), but their predominant sites of concentration and activity are the liver and intestine. Though the abundance of CYP enzymes throughout the body is relatively equally distributed among the various subfamilies, the relative contribution to drug metabolism is (in decreasing order of magnitude) CYP3A4 (nearly 50%), CYP2D6 (nearly 25%), CYP2C8/9 (nearly 15%), then CYP1A2, CYP2C19, CYP2A6, and CYP2E1. Owing to their potential for numerous drug-drug interactions, those drugs that are identified in preclinical studies as substrates of CYP3A enzymes are often given a lower priority for continued research and development in favor of drugs that appear to be less affected by (or less likely to affect) this enzyme subfamily.

Each enzyme subfamily possesses unique selectivity toward potential substrates. For example, CYP1A2 preferentially binds medium-sized, planar, lipophilic molecules, while CYP2D6 preferentially binds molecules that possess a basic nitrogen atom. Some CYP subfamilies exhibit polymorphism (ie, multiple allelic variants that manifest differing catalytic properties). The best described polymorphisms involve CYP2C9, CYP2C19, and CYP2D6. Individuals possessing "wild type" gene alleles exhibit normal functioning CYP capacity. Others, however, possess allelic variants that leave the person with a subnormal level of catalytic potential (so called "poor metabolizers"). Poor metabolizers would be more likely to experience toxicity from drugs metabolized by the affected enzymes (or less effects if the enzyme is responsible for converting a prodrug to it's active form as in the case of codeine). The percentage of people classified as poor metabolizers varies by enzyme and population group. As an example, approximately 7% of Caucasians and only about 1% of Orientals appear to be CYP2D6 poor metabolizers.

CYP enzymes can be both inhibited and induced by other drugs, leading to increased or decreased serum concentrations (along with the associated effects), respectively. Induction occurs when a drug causes an increase in the amount of smooth endoplasmic reticulum, secondary to increasing the amount of the affected CYP enzymes in the tissues. This "revving up" of the CYP enzyme system may take several days to reach peak activity, and likewise, may take several days, even months, to return to normal following discontinuation of the inducing agent.

CYP inhibition occurs via several potential mechanisms. Most commonly, a CYP inhibitor competitively (and reversibly) binds to the active site on the enzyme, thus preventing the substrate from binding to the same site, and preventing the substrate from being metabolized. The affinity of an inhibitor for an enzyme may be expressed by an inhibition constant (Ki) or IC50 (defined as the concentration of the inhibitor required to cause 50% inhibition under a given set of conditions). In addition to reversible competition for an enzyme site, drugs may inhibit enzyme activity by binding to sites on the enzyme other than that to which the substrate would bind, and thereby cause a change in the functionality or physical structure of the enzyme. A drug may also bind to the enzyme in an irreversible (ie, "suicide") fashion. In such a case, it is not the concentration of drug at the enzyme site that is important (constantly binding and releasing), but the number of molecules available for binding (once bound, always bound).

Although an inhibitor or inducer may be known to affect a variety of CYP subfamilies, it may only inhibit one or two in a clinically important fashion. Likewise, although a substrate is known to be at least partially metabolized by a variety of its CYP enzymes, only one or two enzymes may contribute significantly enough to its overall metabolism to warrant concern when used with potential inducers or inhibitors. Therefore, when attempting to predict the level of risk of using two drugs that may affect each other via altered CYP function, it is important to identify the relative effectiveness of the inhibiting/inducing drug on the CYP subfamilies that significantly contribute to the metabolism of the substrate. The contribution of a specific CYP pathway to substrate metabolism should be considered not only in light of other known CYP pathways, but also other nonoxidative pathways for substrate metabolism (eg, glucuronidation) and transporter proteins (eg, P-glycoprotein) that may affect the presentation of a substrate to a metabolic pathway.

HOW TO USE THE TABLES

The following CYP SUBSTRATES, INHIBITORS, and INDUCERS tables provide a clinically relevant perspective on drugs that are affected by, or affect, cytochrome P450 (CYP) enzymes. Not all human, drug-metabolizing CYP enzymes are specifically (or separately) included in the tables. Some enzymes have been excluded because they do not appear to significantly contribute to the metabolism of marketed drugs (eg, CYP2C18). In the case of CYP3A4, the industry routinely uses this single enzyme designation to represent all enzymes in the CYP3A subfamily. CYP3A7 is present in fetal livers. It is effectively absent from adult livers. CYP3A4 (adult) and CYP3A7 (fetal) appear to share similar properties in their respective hosts. The impact of CYP3A7 in fetal and neonatal drug interactions has not been investigated.

The **CYP Substrates table** contains a list of drugs reported to be metabolized, at least in part, by one or more CYP enzymes. An enzyme that appears to play a clinically significant (major) role in a drug's metabolism is indicated by "●", and an enzyme whose role appears to be clinically insignificant (minor) is indicated by "○". A clinically significant designation is the result of a two-phase review. The first phase considered the contribution of each CYP enzyme to the overall metabolism of the drug. The enzyme pathway was considered potentially clinically relevant if it was responsible for at least 30% of the metabolism of the drug. If so, the drug was subjected to a second phase. The second phase considered the clinical relevance of a substrate's concentration being increased twofold, or decreased by one-half (such as might be observed if combined with an effective CYP inhibitor or inducer, respectively). If either of these changes was considered to present a clinically significant concern, the CYP pathway for the drug was designated "major." If neither change would appear to present a clinically significant concern, or if the CYP enzyme was responsible for a smaller portion of the overall metabolism (ie, <30%), the pathway was designated "minor."

The **CYP Inhibitors table** contains a list of drugs that are reported to inhibit one or more CYP enzymes. Enzymes that are strongly inhibited by a drug are indicated by "●". Enzymes that are moderately inhibited are indicated by "◐". Enzymes that are weakly inhibited are indicated by "○". The designations are the result of a review of published clinical reports, available Ki data, and assessments published by other experts in the field. As it pertains to Ki values set in a ratio with achievable serum drug concentrations ([I]) under normal dosing conditions, the following parameters were employed: [I]/Ki ≥ 1 = strong; [I]/Ki 0.1-1 = moderate; [I]/Ki <0.1 = weak.

CYTOCHROME P450 ENZYMES: SUBSTRATES, INHIBITORS, AND INDUCERS *(Continued)*

The **CYP Inducers table** contains a list of drugs that are reported to induce one or more CYP enzymes. Enzymes that appear to be effectively induced by a drug are indicated by "●", and enzymes that do not appear to be effectively induced are indicated by "○". The designations are the result of a review of published clinical reports and assessments published by experts in the field.

In general, clinically significant interactions are more likely to occur between substrates and either inhibitors or inducers of the same enzyme(s), all of which have been indicated by "●". However, these assessments possess a degree of subjectivity, at times based on limited indications regarding the significance of CYP effects of particular agents. An attempt has been made to balance a conservative, clinically-sensitive presentation of the data with a desire to avoid the numbing effect of a "beware of everything" approach. Even so, other potential interactions (ie, those involving enzymes indicated by "○") may warrant consideration in some cases. It is important to note that information related to CYP metabolism of drugs is expanding at a rapid pace, and thus, the contents of this table should only be considered to represent a "snapshot" of the information available at the time of publication.

Selected Readings

Bjornsson TD, Callaghan JT, Einolf HJ, et al, "The Conduct of *in vitro* and *in vivo* Drug-Drug Interaction Studies: A PhRMA Perspective," *J Clin Pharmacol*, 2003, 43(5):443-69.

Drug-Drug Interactions, Rodrigues AD, ed, New York, NY: Marcel Dekker, Inc, 2002.

Levy RH, Thummel KE, Trager WF, et al, eds, *Metabolic Drug Interactions*, Philadelphia, PA: Lippincott Williams & Wilkins, 2000.

Michalets EL, "Update: Clinically Significant Cytochrome P-450 Drug Interactions," *Pharmacotherapy*, 1998, 18(1):84-112.

Thummel KE and Wilkinson GR, "*In vitro* and *in vivo* Drug Interactions Involving Human CYP3A," *Annu Rev Pharmacol Toxicol*, 1998, 38:389-430.

Zhang Y and Benet LZ, "The Gut as a Barrier to Drug Absorption: Combined Role of Cytochrome P450 3A and P-Glycoprotein," *Clin Pharmacokinet*, 2001, 40(3):159-68.

Selected Websites

http://www.gentest.com
http://www.imm.ki.se/CYPalleles
http://medicine.iupui.edu/flockhart
http://www.mhc.com/Cytochromes

CYP Substrates

● = major substrate
○ = minor substrate

Drug	1A2	2A6	2B6	2C8	2C9	2C19	2D6	2E1	3A4
Acenocoumarol	●				●	○			
Acetaminophen	○	○			○		○	○	○
Albendazole	○								○
Albuterol									●
Alfentanil									●
Almotriptan							○		○
Alosetron	○				●				○
Alprazolam									●
Aminophylline	●							○	○
Amiodarone	○			●		○	○		●
Amitriptyline	○		○		○	○	●		○
Amlodipine									●
Amoxapine							●		
Amphetamine							○		
Amprenavir					○				●
Aprepitant	○					○			●
Argatroban									○
Aripiprazole							●		●
Aspirin					○				
Atazanavir									●
Atomoxetine							○	●	
Atorvastatin									●
Azelastine	○						○	○	○
Azithromycin									○

CYP Substrates *(continued)*

Drug	1A2	2A6	2B6	2C8	2C9	2C19	2D6	2E1	3A4
Benzphetamine			○						●
Benztropine							○		
Betaxolol	●						●		
Bexarotene									○
Bezafibrate									○
Bisoprolol							○		●
Bortezomib	○				○	○	○		●
Bosentan					●				●
Brinzolamide									○
Bromazepam									●
Bromocriptine									●
Budesonide									●
Bupivacaine	○					○	○		○
Buprenorphine									●
BuPROPion	○	○	●		○		○	○	○
BusPIRone							○		●
Busulfan									●
Caffeine	●				○		○	○	○
Candesartan					○				
Capsaicin								○	
Captopril							●		
Carbamazepine				○					●
Carisoprodol						●			
Carteolol							○		
Carvedilol	○				●		●	○	○
Celecoxib					●				○
Cerivastatin									●
Cetirizine									○
Cevimeline							○		○
Chlordiazepoxide									●
Chloroquine							●		●
Chlorpheniramine							○		●
ChlorproMAZINE	○						●		○
ChlorproPAMIDE					○				
Chlorzoxazone	○	○					○	●	○
Cilostazol	○					●	○		●
Cinacalcet	○						○		○
Cisapride	○	○	○		○	○			●
Citalopram						●	○		●
Clarithromycin									●
Clobazam						●			●
Clofibrate									○
ClomiPRAMINE	●					●	●		○
Clonazepam									●
Clopidogrel	○								○
Clorazepate									●
Clozapine	●	○			○	○	○		○
Cocaine									●
Codeine[1]							●		○
Colchicine									●
Conivaptan									●
Cyclobenzaprine	●						○		○
Cyclophosphamide[2]		○	●		○	○			●
CycloSPORINE									●
Dacarbazine	●							●	
Dantrolene									●
Dapsone				○	●	○		○	●
Delavirdine							○		●
Desipramine	○						●		
Desogestrel						●			
Dexamethasone									○
Dexmedetomidine		●							
Dextroamphetamine							●		

CYTOCHROME P450 ENZYMES: SUBSTRATES, INHIBITORS, AND INDUCERS *(Continued)*

CYP Substrates *(continued)*

Drug	1A2	2A6	2B6	2C8	2C9	2C19	2D6	2E1	3A4
Dextromethorphan		O			O	O	●	O	O
Diazepam	O		O		O	●			●
Diclofenac	O		O	O	O		O		O
Digoxin									O
Dihydrocodeine[1]							●		
Dihydroergotamine									●
Diltiazem					O		O		●
Dirithromycin									O
Disopyramide									●
Disulfiram	O	O	O				O	O	
Docetaxel									●
Dofetilide									O
Dolasetron						O			O
Domperidone									O
Donepezil							O		O
Dorzolamide					O				O
Doxepin	●						●		●
DOXOrubicin							●		●
Doxycycline									●
Drospirenone									O
Duloxetine	●						●		
Dutasteride									O
Efavirenz			●						●
Eletriptan									●
Enalapril									●
Enflurane								●	
Eplerenone									●
Ergoloid mesylates									●
Ergonovine									●
Ergotamine									●
Erythromycin			O						●
Escitalopram						●			●
Esomeprazole						●			O
Estazolam									O
Estradiol	●	O	O		O	O	O	O	●
Estrogens, conjugated A/synthetic	●	O	O		O	O	O	O	●
Estrogens, conjugated equine	●	O	O		O	O	O	O	●
Estrogens, conjugated esterified	●		O		O		O		●
Estrone	●		O		O		O		●
Estropipate	●		O		O		O		●
Ethinyl estradiol					O				●
Ethosuximide									●
Etonogestrel									O
Etoposide	O							O	●
Exemestane									●
Felbamate								O	●
Felodipine									●
Fenofibrate									O
Fentanyl									●
Fexofenadine									O
Finasteride									O
Flecainide	O						●		
Fluoxetine	O		O		●	O	●	O	O
Fluphenazine							●		
Flurazepam									●
Flurbiprofen					O				
Flutamide	●								●
Fluticasone									●

CYP Substrates *(continued)*

Drug	1A2	2A6	2B6	2C8	2C9	2C19	2D6	2E1	3A4
Fluvastatin					○		○		○
Fluvoxamine	●						●		
Formoterol		○			○	○	○		
Fosamprenavir (as amprenavir)					○				●
Fosphenytoin (as phenytoin)					●	●			○
Frovatriptan	○								
Fulvestrant									○
Galantamine							○		○
Gefitinib									●
Gemfibrozil									○
Glimepiride					●				
GlipiZIDE					●				
Granisetron									○
Guanabenz	●								
Halazepam									○
Haloperidol	○						●		●
Halothane		○	○		○		○	●	○
Hydrocodone[1]							●		
Hydrocortisone									○
Ibuprofen					○	○			
Ifosfamide[3]		○	○	○	○	○			●
Imatinib	○				○	○	○		●
Imipramine	○		○			●	●		○
Imiquimod	○								○
Indinavir							○		●
Indomethacin					○	○			
Irbesartan					○				
Irinotecan			●						●
Isoflurane								●	
Isoniazid								●	
Isosorbide									●
Isosorbide dinitrate									●
Isosorbide mononitrate									●
Isradipine									●
Itraconazole									●
Ivermectin									○
Ketamine			●		●				●
Ketoconazole									●
Labetalol							●		
Lansoprazole					○	●			●
Letrozole		○							●
Levobupivacaine	○								○
Levonorgestrel									●
Lidocaine	○	○	○		○		●		●
Lomustine							●		
Lopinavir									○
Loratadine							○		○
Losartan					●				●
Lovastatin									●
Maprotiline							●		
MedroxyPROGESTERone									●
Mefenamic acid					○				
Mefloquine									●
Meloxicam					○				○
Mephobarbital			○		○	●			
Mestranol[4]					●				●
Methadone					○	○	○		●
Methamphetamine							●		
Methoxsalen		○							
Methsuximide						●			
Methylergonovine									●
Methylphenidate							●		

CYTOCHROME P450 ENZYMES: SUBSTRATES, INHIBITORS, AND INDUCERS *(Continued)*

CYP Substrates *(continued)*

Drug	1A2	2A6	2B6	2C8	2C9	2C19	2D6	2E1	3A4
MethylPREDNISolone									○
Metoclopramide	○						○		
Metoprolol						○	●		
Mexiletine	●						●		
Miconazole									●
Midazolam			○						●
Mifepristone									○
Miglustat									●
Mirtazapine	●				○		●		●
Moclobemide						●	●		
Modafinil									●
Mometasone furoate									○
Montelukast					●				●
Moricizine									●
Morphine sulfate							○		
Naproxen	○				○				
Nateglinide					●				●
Nefazodone							●		●
Nelfinavir					○	●	○		●
Nevirapine			○				○		●
NiCARdipine	○				○		○	○	●
Nicotine	○	○	○		○	○	○	○	○
NIFEdipine							○		●
Nilutamide						●			
Nimodipine									●
Nisoldipine									●
Norelgestromin									○
Norethindrone									●
Norgestrel									●
Nortriptyline	○					○	●		○
Olanzapine	○						○		
Omeprazole		○			○	●	○		○
Ondansetron	○				○		○	○	●
Orphenadrine	○		○				○		○
Oxybutynin									○
Oxycodone[1]							●		
Paclitaxel				●	●				●
Palonosetron	○						○		○
Pantoprazole						●			○
Paroxetine							●		
Pentamidine						●			
Pergolide									●
Perphenazine	○				○	○	●		○
Phencyclidine									●
Phenobarbital					○	●		○	
Phenytoin					●	●			○
Pimecrolimus									○
Pimozide	●								●
Pindolol							●		
Pioglitazone				●					○
Pipotiazine							●		●
Piroxicam					○				
Pravastatin									○
PrednisoLONE									○
PredniSONE									○
Primaquine									●
Procainamide							●		
Progesterone	○	○			○	●	○		●
Proguanil	○					○			○
Promethazine			●				●		

CYP Substrates *(continued)*

Drug	1A2	2A6	2B6	2C8	2C9	2C19	2D6	2E1	3A4
Propafenone	○						●		○
Propofol	○	○	●		●	○	○	○	○
Propranolol	●					○	●		○
Protriptyline							●		
Quazepam									○
Quetiapine							○		●
Quinidine					○			○	●
Quinine	○					○			○
Rabeprazole						●			●
Ranitidine	○					○	○		
Ranolazine							○		●
Repaglinide				●					●
Rifabutin									●
Riluzole	●								
Risperidone							●		○
Ritonavir	○		○				○		●
Rofecoxib					○				
Ropinirole	●								○
Ropivacaine	○		○				○		○
Rosiglitazone				●	○				
Rosuvastatin					○				○
Salmeterol									●
Saquinavir							○		●
Selegiline	○	○	●	○		○	○		○
Sertraline			○		○	●	●		○
Sevoflurane		○	○					●	○
Sibutramine									●
Sildenafil					○				●
Simvastatin									●
Sirolimus									●
Sorafenib									○
Spiramycin									●
Sufentanil									●
SulfaDIAZINE					●			○	○
Sulfamethoxazole					●				○
Sulfinpyrazone					●				○
SulfiSOXAZOLE					●				
Sunitinib									●
Tacrine	●								
Tacrolimus									●
Tamoxifen		○	○		●		●	○	●
Tamsulosin							●		●
Telithromycin	○								●
Temazepam			○		○	○			○
Teniposide									●
Terbinafine	○				○	○			○
Testosterone			○		○	○			○
Tetracycline									●
Theophylline	●				○		○	●	●
Thiabendazole	○								
Thioridazine						○	●		
Thiothixene	●								
Tiagabine									●
Ticlopidine									●
Timolol							●		
Tinidazole									○
Tiotropium							○		○
Tipranavir									●
TOLBUTamide					●	○			
Tolcapone		○							○
Tolterodine					○	○	●		●
Toremifene	○								●
Torsemide				○	●				

CYTOCHROME P450 ENZYMES: SUBSTRATES, INHIBITORS, AND INDUCERS (Continued)

CYP Substrates (continued)

Drug	1A2	2A6	2B6	2C8	2C9	2C19	2D6	2E1	3A4
Tramadol[1]			O				●		O
Trazodone							O		●
Tretinoin		O	O	●	O				
Triazolam									●
Trifluoperazine	●								
Trimethadione					O	O		●	O
Trimethoprim					●				●
Trimipramine						●	●		●
Troleandomycin									●
Valdecoxib					O				O
Valproic acid		O	O		O	O		O	
Vardenafil									●
Venlafaxine					O	O	●		●
Verapamil	O		O		O			O	●
VinBLAStine							O		●
VinCRIStine									●
Vinorelbine							O		●
Voriconazole					●	●			O
Warfarin	O				●	O			O
Yohimbine							O		
Zafirlukast					●				
Zaleplon									O
Zidovudine		O			O	O			O
Zileuton	O				O				O
Ziprasidone	O								O
Zolmitriptan	O								
Zolpidem	O				O	O	O		●
Zonisamide						O			●
Zopiclone					●				●
Zuclopenthixol							●		

[1]This opioid analgesic is bioactivated *in vivo* via CYP2D6. Inhibiting this enzyme would decrease the effects of the analgesic. The active metabolite might also affect, or be affected by, CYP enzymes.
[2]Cyclophosphamide is bioactivated *in vivo* to acrolein via CYP2B6 and 3A4. Inhibiting these enzymes would decrease the effects of cyclophosphamide.
[3]Ifosfamide is bioactivated *in vivo* to acrolein via CYP3A4. Inhibiting this enzyme would decrease the effects of ifosfamide.
[4]Mestranol is bioactivated *in vivo* to ethinyl estradiol via CYP2C8/9. See Ethinyl Estradiol for additional CYP information.

CYP Inhibitors

● = strong inhibitor
◐ = moderate inhibitor
○ = weak inhibitor

Drug	1A2	2A6	2B6	2C8	2C9	2C19	2D6	2E1	3A4
Acebutolol							○		
Acetaminophen									○
AcetaZOLAMIDE									○
Albendazole	○								
Alosetron	○							○	
Amiodarone	○	◐	○		◐	○	◐		◐
Amitriptyline	○				○	○	○	○	
Amlodipine	◐	○	○	○	○		○		○
Amphetamine							○		
Amprenavir						○			●
Anastrozole	○				○	○			○
Aprepitant					○	○			◐
Atazanavir	○			●	○				●
Atorvastatin									○
Azelastine			○		○	○	○		
Azithromycin									○
Bepridil							○		
Betamethasone									○
Betaxolol							○		
Biperiden							○		
Bortezomib	○				○	◐	○		○
Bromazepam								○	
Bromocriptine	○								○
Buprenorphine	○	○				○	○		
BuPROPion							○		
Caffeine	●								◐
Candesartan				○	○				
Celecoxib				◐			○		
Cerivastatin									○
Chloramphenicol					○				○
Chloroquine							◐		
Chlorpheniramine							○		
ChlorproMAZINE							●	○	
Chlorzoxazone								○	○
Cholecalciferol					○	○	○		
Cimetidine	◐				○	◐	◐	○	◐
Cinacalcet							○		
Ciprofloxacin	●								○
Cisapride							○		○
Citalopram	○		○			○	○		
Clarithromycin	○								●
Clemastine							○		○
Clofazimine									○
Clofibrate		○							
ClomiPRAMINE							◐		
Clopidogrel					○				
Clotrimazole	○	○	○	○	○	○	○	○	◐
Clozapine	○				○	○	◐	○	○
Cocaine							●		○
Codeine							○		
Conivaptan									●
Cyclophosphamide									○
CycloSPORINE					○				◐
Danazol									○
Delavirdine	○				●	●	●		●

CYTOCHROME P450 ENZYMES: SUBSTRATES, INHIBITORS, AND INDUCERS (Continued)

CYP Inhibitors (continued)

Drug	1A2	2A6	2B6	2C8	2C9	2C19	2D6	2E1	3A4
Desipramine		◐	◐				◐	○	◐
Dexmedetomidine	○				○		●		○
Dextromethorphan							○		
Diazepam						○			○
Diclofenac	◐				○			○	○
Dihydroergotamine									○
Diltiazem					○		○		◐
Dimethyl sulfoxide					○	○			
DiphenhydrAMINE							◐		
Disulfiram	○	○	○		○		○	●	○
Docetaxel									○
Dolasetron							○		
DOXOrubicin			◐				○		○
Doxycycline									◐
Drospirenone	○				○	○			◐
Duloxetine							◐		
Econazole								○	
Efavirenz					○	○			○
Enoxacin	●								●
Entacapone	○	○			○	○	○	○	
Eprosartan					○				
Ergotamine									○
Erythromycin	○								◐
Escitalopram							○		
Estradiol	○			○					
Estrogens, conjugated A/synthetic	○								
Estrogens, conjugated equine	○								
Ethinyl estradiol	○		○	○		○			○
Ethotoin						○			
Etoposide					○				○
Felbamate						○			
Felodipine				◐	○		○		○
Fenofibrate		○		◐	◐	○			
Fentanyl									○
Fexofenadine							○		
Flecainide							○		
Fluconazole	○				●	●			◐
Fluoxetine	◐		○		○	◐	●		○
Fluphenazine	○				○		○	○	
Flurazepam								○	
Flurbiprofen					●				
Flutamide	○								
Fluvastatin	○			○	◐		○		○
Fluvoxamine	●		○		○	●	○		○
Fosamprenavir (as amprenavir)						○			●
Gefitinib						○	○		
Gemfibrozil	◐			●	●	●			
Glyburide				○					○
Grapefruit juice									◐
Haloperidol							◐		◐
HydrALAZINE									○
HydrOXYzine							○		
Ibuprofen					●				
Ifosfamide									○
Imatinib					○		○		●

CYP Inhibitors *(continued)*

Drug	1A2	2A6	2B6	2C8	2C9	2C19	2D6	2E1	3A4
Imipramine	○					○	◐	○	
Indinavir					○	○	○		●
Indomethacin				●	○				
Interferon alfa-2a	○								
Interferon alfa-2b	○								
Interferon gamma-1b	○							○	
Irbesartan				◐	◐		○		○
Isoflurane			○						
Isoniazid	○	◐			○	●	◐	◐	●
Isradipine									○
Itraconazole									●
Ketoconazole	●	◐	○	○	●	◐	◐		●
Ketoprofen					○				
Labetalol							○		
Lansoprazole					○	◐	○		○
Leflunomide					○				
Letrozole		●				○			
Lidocaine	●						◐		◐
Lomefloxacin	○								
Lomustine							○		○
Loratadine					○	◐	○		
Losartan	○			◐	◐	○			○
Lovastatin					○		○		○
Mefenamic acid					●				
Mefloquine							○		○
Meloxicam					○				
Mephobarbital						○			
Mestranol	○		○			○			○
Methadone							◐		○
Methimazole	○	○	○		○		◐	○	○
Methotrimeprazine							○		
Methoxsalen	●	●			○	○	○	○	○
Methsuximide						○			
Methylphenidate							○		
MethylPREDNISolone				○					○
Metoclopramide							○		
Metoprolol							○		
Metronidazole					○				◐
Metyrapone		○							
Mexiletine	●								
Miconazole	◐	●	○		●	●	●	◐	●
Midazolam				○	○				○
Mifepristone							○		○
Mirtazapine	○								○
Mitoxantrone									○
Moclobemide	○					○	○		
Modafinil	○	○			○	●		○	○
Montelukast				○	○				
Nalidixic acid	○								
Nateglinide					○				
Nefazodone	○		○	○			○		●
Nelfinavir	○		○		○	○	○		●
Nevirapine	○						○		○
NiCARdipine					●	◐	◐		●
Nicotine		○						○	
NIFEdipine	◐				○		○		○
Nilutamide						○			
Nisoldipine	○								○
Nizatidine									○
Norfloxacin	●								◐

CYTOCHROME P450 ENZYMES: SUBSTRATES, INHIBITORS, AND INDUCERS *(Continued)*

CYP Inhibitors *(continued)*

Drug	1A2	2A6	2B6	2C8	2C9	2C19	2D6	2E1	3A4
Nortriptyline							○	○	
Ofloxacin	●								
Olanzapine	○				○	○	○		○
Omeprazole	○				◐	●	○		○
Ondansetron	○				○		○		
Orphenadrine	○	○	○		○	○	○	○	○
Oxcarbazepine						○			
Oxprenolol							○		
Oxybutynin				○			○		○
Pantoprazole					◐				
Paroxetine	○		◐		○	○	●		○
Peginterferon alfa-2a	○								
Peginterferon alfa-2b	○								
Pentamidine					○	○	○		○
Pentoxifylline	○								
Pergolide							●		○
Perphenazine	○						○		
Phencyclidine									○
Pilocarpine		○						○	○
Pimozide						○	○	○	○
Pindolol							○		
Pioglitazone				◐	○	○	◐		
Piroxicam					●				
Pravastatin					○		○		○
Praziquantel							○		
PrednisoLONE									○
Primaquine	●						○		○
Probenecid						○			
Progesterone					○	○			○
Promethazine							○		
Propafenone	○						○		
Propofol	◐				○	◐	○	○	●
Propoxyphene					○		○		○
Propranolol	○						○		
Pyrimethamine					◐		◐		
Quinidine					○		●		●
Quinine				◐	◐		●		○
Quinupristin									○
Rabeprazole					◐	◐	○		○
Ranitidine	○						○		
Ranolazine							○		○
Risperidone							○		○
Ritonavir					●	○	●	○	●
Rofecoxib	○								
Ropinirole	○						●		
Rosiglitazone				◐	○	○	○		
Saquinavir					○	○	○		◐
Selegiline	○	○			○	○	○	○	○
Sertraline	○		◐	○	○	◐	◐		◐
Sildenafil	○				○		○	○	○
Simvastatin				○	○		○		
Sirolimus									○
Sorafenib			○	○					
Sulconazole	○	○			○		○	○	○
SulfaDIAZINE					●				
Sulfamethoxazole					◐				
Sulfinpyrazone					◐				

CYP Inhibitors *(continued)*

Drug	1A2	2A6	2B6	2C8	2C9	2C19	2D6	2E1	3A4
SulfiSOXAZOLE					●				
Tacrine	○								
Tacrolimus									○
Tamoxifen			○	◐	○				○
Telithromycin							○		●
Telmisartan						○			
Teniposide					○				○
Tenofovir	○								
Terbinafine							●		
Testosterone									○
Tetracycline									◐
Theophylline	○								
Thiabendazole	●								
Thioridazine	○				○		◐	○	
Thiotepa			○						
Thiothixene							○		
Ticlopidine	○				○	●	◐	○	○
Timolol							○		
Tioconazole	○	○			○	○	○	○	
Tocainide	○								
TOLBUTamide				○	●				
Tolcapone					○				
Topiramate						○			
Torsemide						○			
Tranylcypromine	◐	●		○	○	◐	○	○	○
Trazodone							◐		○
Tretinoin					○				
Triazolam				○	○				
Trimethoprim				◐	◐				
Tripelennamine							◐		
Triprolidine							○		
Troleandomycin									◐
Valdecoxib					○	○	○		
Valproic acid					○	○	○		○
Valsartan					○				
Venlafaxine			○				○		○
Verapamil	○				○		○		◐
VinBLAStine									○
VinCRIStine									○
Vinorelbine							○		○
Voriconazole					○	○			◐
Warfarin					◐	○			
Yohimbine							○		
Zafirlukast	○			○	◐	○	○		○
Zileuton	◐								
Ziprasidone							○		○

CYTOCHROME P450 ENZYMES: SUBSTRATES, INHIBITORS, AND INDUCERS *(Continued)*

CYP Inducers

● = effectively induced
○ = not effectively induced

Drug	1A2	2A6	2B6	2C8	2C9	2C19	2D6	2E1	3A4
Aminoglutethimide	●					●			●
Amobarbital		●							
Aprepitant					○				○
Bexarotene									○
Bosentan					○				○
Calcitriol									○
Carbamazepine	●		●	●	●	●			●
Clofibrate			○					○	○
Colchicine				○	○			○	○
Cyclophosphamide			○	○	○				
Dexamethasone		○	○	○	○				○
Dicloxacillin									○
Efavirenz (in liver only)			○						○
Estradiol									○
Estrogens, conjugated A/synthetic									○
Estrogens, conjugated equine									○
Exemestane									○
Felbamate									○
Fosphenytoin (as phenytoin)			●	●	●	●			●
Griseofulvin	○				○	○			○
Hydrocortisone									○
Ifosfamide				○	○				
Insulin preparations	○								
Isoniazid (after D/C)								○	
Lansoprazole	○								
MedroxyPROGESTERone									○
Mephobarbital		○							
Metyrapone									○
Modafinil	○		○						○
Moricizine	○								○
Nafcillin									●
Nevirapine			●						●
Norethindrone						○			
Omeprazole	○								
Oxcarbazepine									●
Paclitaxel									○
Pantoprazole	○								○
Pentobarbital		●							●
Phenobarbital	●	●	●	●	●				●
Phenytoin			●	●	●	●			●
Pioglitazone									○
PredniSONE						○			○
Primaquine	○								
Primidone[1]	●		●	●	●				●
Rifabutin									●
Rifampin	●	●	●	●	●	●			●
Rifapentine				●	●				●
Ritonavir (long-term)	○			○	○				○
Rofecoxib									○
Secobarbital		●		●	●				
Sulfinpyrazone									○
Terbinafine									○
Topiramate									○
Tretinoin								○	
Troglitazone									○
Valproic acid		○							

[1]Primidone is partially metabolized to phenobarbital. See Phenobarbital for additional CYP information.

DEPRESSION SCALES

Short Form Geriatric Depression Scale*

NAME _____ AGE _____ SEX _____ DATE _____

WING _____ ROOM _____ PHYSICIAN _____

SCORING SYSTEM

Answers indicating depression are highlighted. Each BOLD-FACED answer counts one (1) point.

Score greater than 5 indicates probable depression

1.	Are you basically satisfied with your life?	YES / **NO**
2.	Have you dropped any of your activities and interests?	**YES** / NO
3.	Do you feel that your life is empty?	**YES** / NO
4.	Do you often get bored?	**YES** / NO
5.	Are you in good spirits most of the time?	YES / **NO**
6.	Are you afraid that something bad is going to happen to you?	**YES** / NO
7.	Do you feel happy most of the time?	YES / **NO**
8.	Do you often feel helpless?	**YES** / NO
9.	Do you prefer to stay in your room/facility, rather than going out and doing new things?	**YES** / NO
10.	Do you feel you have more problems with memory than most?	**YES** / NO
11.	Do you think it is wonderful to be alive?	YES / **NO**
12.	Do you feel worthless the way you are now?	**YES** / NO
13.	Do you feel full of energy?	YES / **NO**
14.	Do you feel that your situation is hopeless?	**YES** / NO
15.	Do you think that most people are better off than you?	**YES** / NO

SCORE

NOTES / CURRENT MEDICATIONS:

ASSESSOR:

*This scale may be used when evaluating residents who do not have limited cognition.

DEPRESSION SCALES *(Continued)*

Cornell Scale for Depression in Dementia*

NAME _____ AGE _____ SEX _____ DATE _____

WING _____ ROOM _____ PHYSICIAN _____

Ratings should be based on symptoms and signs occurring during the week before interview. No score should be given if symptoms result from physical disability or illness.

SCORING SYSTEM

a = Unable to evaluate   0 = Absent

1 = Mild to Intermittent   2 = Severe

Score greater than 12 = Probable Depression

A. MOOD-RELATED SIGNS   a   0   1   2
1. Anxiety; anxious expression, rumination, worrying
2. Sadness; sad expression, sad voice, tearfulness
3. Lack of reaction to pleasant events
4. Irritability; annoyed, short tempered

B. BEHAVIORAL DISTURBANCE   a   0   1   2
5. Agitation; restlessness, hand wringing, hair pulling
6. Retardation; slow movements, slow speech, slow reactions
7. Multiple physical complaints *(score 0 if gastrointestinal symptoms only)*
8. Loss of interest; less involved in usual activities *(score only if change occurred acutely, i.e., in less than one month)*

C. PHYSICAL SIGNS   a   0   1   2
9. Appetite loss; eating less than usual
10. Weight loss (score 2 if greater than 5 pounds in one month)
11. Lack of energy; fatigues easily, unable to sustain activities

D. CYCLIC FUNCTIONS   a   0   1   2
12. Diurnal variation of mood; symptoms worse in the morning
13. Difficulty falling asleep; later than usual for this individual
14. Multiple awakening during sleep
15. Early morning awaking; earlier than usual for this individual

E. IDEATIONAL DISTURBANCE   a   0   1   2
16. Suicidal; feels life is not worth living
17. Poor self-esteem; self-blame, self-depreciation, feelings of failure
18. Pessimism; anticipation of the worst
19. Mood congruent delusions; delusions of poverty, illness, or loss

NOTES / CURRENT MEDICATIONS: SCORE

ASSESSOR:

*This scale may be used to evaluate residents with limited cognition.

DISCOLORATION OF FECES
DUE TO DRUGS

Black
Acetazolamide
Alcohols
Alkalies
Aluminum hydroxide
Aminophylline
Aminosalicylic acid
Amphetamine
Amphotericin
Antacids
Anticoagulants
Aspirin
Betamethasone
Bismuth
Charcoal
Chloramphenicol
Chlorpropamide
Clindamycin
Corticosteroids
Cortisone
Cyclophosphamide
Cytarabine
Digitalis
Ethacrynic acid
Ferrous salts
Floxuridine
Fluorides
Fluorouracil
Halothane
Heparin
Hydralazine
Hydrocortisone
Ibuprofen
Indomethacin
Iodine drugs
Iron salts
Levarterenol
Levodopa
Manganese
Melphalan
Methylprednisolone
Methotrexate

Methylene blue
Oxyphenbutazone
Phenacetin
Phenolphthalein
Phenylbutazone
Phenylephrine
Phosphorous
Potassium salts
Prednisolone
Procarbazine
Pyrvinium
Reserpine
Salicylates
Sulfonamides
Tetracycline
Theophylline
Thiotepa
Triamcinolone
Warfarin

Blue
Chloramphenicol
Methylene blue

Dark Brown
Dexamethasone

Gray
Colchicine

Green
Indomethacin
Iron
Medroxyprogesterone

Greenish Gray
Oral antibiotics
Oxyphenbutazone
Phenylbutazone

Light Brown
Anticoagulants

Orange-Red
Phenazopyridine
Rifampin

Pink
Anticoagulants
Aspirin
Heparin
Oxyphenbutazone
Phenylbutazone
Salicylates

Red
Anticoagulants
Aspirin
Heparin
Oxyphenbutazone
Phenolphthalein
Phenylbutazone
Pyrvinium
Salicylates
Tetracycline syrup

Red-Brown
Oxyphenbutazone
Phenylbutazone
Rifampin

Tarry
Ergot preparations
Ibuprofen
Salicylates
Warfarin

White / Speckling
Aluminum hydroxide
Antibiotics (oral)
Indocyanine green

Yellow
Senna

Yellow-Green
Senna

Adapted from Drugdex® — Drug Consults, Micromedex, Vol 62, Denver, CO: Rocky Mountain Drug Consultation Center, 1998.

DISCOLORATION OF URINE DUE TO DRUGS

Black
Cascara
Cotrimoxazole
Ferrous salts
Iron dextran
Levodopa
Methocarbamol
Methyldopa
Naphthalene
Pamaquine
Phenacetin
Phenols
Quinine
Sulfonamides

Blue
Anthraquinone
DeWitt's pills
Indigo blue
Indigo carmine
Methocarbamol
Methylene blue
Mitoxantrone
Nitrofurans
Resorcinol
Triamterene

Blue-Green
Amitriptyline
Anthraquinone
DeWitt's pills
Doan's® pills
Indigo blue
Indigo carmine
Magnesium salicylate
Methylene blue
Resorcinol

Brown
Anthraquinone dyes
Cascara
Chloroquine
Hydroquinone
Levodopa
Methocarbamol
Methyldopa
Metronidazole
Nitrofurans
Nitrofurantoin
Pamaquine
Phenacetin
Phenols
Primaquine
Quinine
Rifabutin
Rifampin
Senna
Sodium diatrizoate
Sulfonamides

Brown-Black
Isosorbide mono- or
  dinitrate
Methyldopa
Metronidazole
Nitrates
Nitrofurans
Phenacetin
Povidone iodine
Quinine
Senna

Dark
p-Aminosalicylic acid
Cascara
Levodopa
Metronidazole
Nitrites
Phenacetin
Phenol
Primaquine
Quinine
Resorcinol
Riboflavin
Senna

Green
Amitriptyline
Anthraquinone
DeWitt's pills
Indigo blue
Indigo carmine
Indomethacin
Methocarbamol
Methylene blue
Nitrofurans
Phenols
Propofol
Resorcinol
Suprofen

Green-Yellow
DeWitt's pills
Methylene blue

Milky
Phosphates

Orange
Chlorzoxazone
Dihydroergotamine
  mesylate
Heparin sodium
Phenazopyridine
Phenindione
Rifabutin
Rifampin
Sulfasalazine
Warfarin

Orange-Red-Brown
Chlorzoxazone
Doxidan
Phenazopyridine
Rifampin
Warfarin

Orange-Yellow
Fluorescein sodium
Rifampin
Sulfasalazine

Pink
Aminopyrine
Anthraquinone dyes
Aspirin
Cascara
Danthron
Deferoxamine
Methyldopa
Phenazopyridone
Phenolphthalein
Phenothiazines
Phenytoin
Salicylates
Senna

Purple
Phenolphthalein

Red
Anthraquinone
Cascara
Chlorpromazine
Daunorubicin
Deferoxamine
Dihydroergotamine
  mesylate
Dimethyl sulfoxide
DMSO
Doxorubicin
Heparin
Ibuprofen
Methyldopa
Oxyphenbutazone
Phenacetin
Phenazopyridine
Phenolphthalein
Phenothiazines
Phensuximide
Phenylbutazone
Phenytoin
Rifampin
Senna

Red-Brown
Cascara
Deferoxamine
Methyldopa
Oxyphenbutazone
Pamaquine
Phenacetin
Phenazopyridine
Phenolphthalein
Phenothiazines
Phenylbutazone
Phenytoin
Quinine
Senna

Red-Purple
Chlorzoxazone
Ibuprofen
Phenacetin
Senna

Rust
Cascara
Chloroquine
Metronidazole
Nitrofurantoin
Pamaquine
Phenacetin
Quinacrine
Riboflavin
Senna
Sulfonamides

Yellow
Nitrofurantoin
Phenacetin
Quinacrine
Riboflavin
Sulfasalazine

Yellow-Brown
Aminosalicylate acid
Bismuth
Cascara
Chloroquine
DeWitt's pills
Methylene blue
Metronidazole
Nitrofurantoin
Pamaquine
Primaquine
Quinacrine
Senna
Sulfonamides

Yellow-Pink
Cascara
Senna

Adapted from Drugdex® — Drug Consults, Micromedex, Vol 62, Denver, CO: Rocky Mountain Drug Consultation Center, 1998.

FEVER DUE TO DRUGS

Most Common

Atropine	Cephalosporins	Procainamide
Amphotericin B	Interferon	Quinidine
Asparaginase	Methyldopa	Salicylates (high doses)
Barbiturates	Penicillins	Streptomycin
Bleomycin	Phenytoin	Sulfonamides

Less Common

Allopurinol	Hydralazine	Nitrofurantoin
Antihistamines	Hydroxyurea	Pentazocine
Azathioprine	Imipenem	Procarbazine
Carbamazepine	Iodides	Propylthiouracil
Cimetidine	Isoniazid	Rifampin
Cisplatin	Mercaptopurine	Streptokinase
Colistimethate	Metoclopramide	Triamterene
Diazoxide	Nifedipine	Vancomycin
Folic acid	NSAIDs	

References

Cunha BA, "Antibiotic Side Effects," *Med Clin North Am*, 2001, 85(1):149-85.

Mackowiak PA and LeMaistre CF, "Drug Fever: A Critical Appraisal of Conventional Concepts. An Analysis of 51 Episodes in Two Dallas Hospitals and 97 Episodes Reported in the English Literature," *Ann Intern Med*, 1987, 106(5):728-33.

Tabor PA, "Drug-Induced Fever," Table 2, "Drugs Implicated in Causing a Fever," *Drug Intell Clin Pharm*, 1986, 20(6):416.

LIQUID COMPATIBILITY OF ANTIPSYCHOTICS AND MOOD STABILIZERS

Drug	Water	Saline	Milk	Coffee	Tea	Apple Juice	Grape Juice	Grapefruit Juice	Orange Juice	Prune Juice	Cola	7-Up / Sprite
Carbamazepine[1]	C	C	C	C	C		C	C	C	C	C	C
Lithium	C	C	C	C		X	X				X	X
Valproate	C	C	C	U	U			C	C	U	U	C
Chlorpromazine[1]	C	C	C	X	X	X	X	C	C	C	X	X
Fluphenazine	C	C	C	X	X	X		X	C	C	C	
Haloperidol	C	X	X	C	X	C	X	C	C		C	C
Loxapine	C			C				C	C		C	
Mesoridazine	C		C	C					C			
Risperidone	C	C	C	C	X	X			C		X	C
Thioridazine	C	C	X	X	X	X	X	C	C	X	X	
Thiothixene	C		C	X	X	X		C	C	C	X	C
Trifluoperazine	C		C	U	C	X	X	C	C	C	C	C

C = compatible; X = incompatible; U = conflicting data; blank = no data.

[1]Carbamazepine is not compatible with chlorpromazine.

ORAL MEDICATIONS THAT SHOULD NOT BE CRUSHED

There are a variety of reasons for crushing tablets or capsule contents prior to administering to the patient. Patients may have nasogastric tubes which do not permit the administration of tablets or capsules; an oral solution for a particular medication may not be available from the manufacturer or readily prepared by pharmacy; patients may have difficulty swallowing capsules or tablets; or mixing of powdered medication with food or drink may make the drug more palatable.

Generally, medications which should not be crushed fall into one of the following categories.

- **Extended-Release Products**. The formulation of some tablets is specialized as to allow the medication within it to be slowly released into the body. This is sometimes accomplished by centering the drug within the core of the tablet, with a subsequent shedding of multiple layers around the core. Wax melts in the GI tract. Slow-K® is an example of this. Capsules may contain beads which have multiple layers which are slowly dissolved with time.

    Common Abbreviations for Extended-Release Products

CD	Controlled dose
CR	Controlled release
CRT	Controlled-release tablet
LA	Long-acting
SR	Sustained release
TR	Timed release
TD	Time delay
SA	Sustained action
XL	Extended release
XR	Extended release

- **Medications Which Are Irritating to the Stomach**. Tablets which are irritating to the stomach may be enteric-coated which delays release of the drug until the time when it reaches the small intestine. Enteric-coated aspirin is an example of this.

- **Foul-Tasting Medication**. Some drugs are quite unpleasant to taste so the manufacturer coats the tablet in a sugar coating to increase its palatability. By crushing the tablet, this sugar coating is lost and the patient tastes the unpleasant tasting medication.

- **Sublingual Medication**. Medication intended for use under the tongue should not be crushed. While it appears to be obvious, it is not always easy to determine if a medication is to be used sublingually. Sublingual medications should indicate on the package that they are intended for sublingual use.

- **Effervescent Tablets**. These are tablets which, when dropped into a liquid, quickly dissolve to yield a solution. Many effervescent tablets, when crushed, lose their ability to quickly dissolve.

Recommendations

1. It is not advisable to crush certain medications.

2. Consult individual monographs prior to crushing capsule or tablet.

3. If crushing a tablet or capsule is contraindicated, consult with your pharmacist to determine whether an oral solution exists or can be compounded.

Drug Product	Dosage Form	Dosage Reasons / Comments
Accuhist®	Tablet	Slow release[8]
Accutane®	Capsule	Mucous membrane irritant
Aciphex™	Tablet	Slow release
Adalat® CC	Tablet	Slow release
Adderall XR™	Capsule	Slow release[1]
Advicor®	Tablet	Slow release
Afeditab™ CR	Tablet	Slow release
Aggrenox®	Capsule	Slow release **Note:** Capsule may be opened; contents include an aspirin tablet that may be chewed and dipyridamole pellets that may be sprinkled on applesauce
Alavert™ Allergy Sinus 12 Hour	Tablet	Slow release
Allegra-D®	Tablet	Slow release
Altocor™	Tablet	Slow release
Arthritis Bayer® Time Release	Capsule	Slow release
Arthrotec®	Tablet	Enteric-coated
A.S.A.® Enseals®	Tablet	Enteric-coated
Asacol®	Tablet	Slow release
Ascriptin® A/D	Tablet	Enteric-coated
Ascriptin® Extra Strength	Tablet	Enteric-coated
Augmentin XR™	Tablet	Slow release[2, 8]
Avinza™	Capsule	Slow release[1] (not pudding)
Avodart™	Capsule	Teratogenic potential[9]
Azulfidine® EN-tabs®	Tablet	Enteric-coated
Bayer® Aspirin EC	Caplet	Enteric-coated
Bayer® Aspirin, Low Adult 81 mg	Tablet	Enteric-coated
Bayer® Aspirin, Regular Strength 325 mg	Caplet	Enteric-coated
Biaxin® XL	Tablet	Slow release
Biltricide®	Tablet	Taste[8]
Bisacodyl	Tablet	Enteric-coated[3]
Bontril® Slow-Release	Capsule	Slow release
Calan® SR	Tablet	Slow release[8]
Carbatrol®	Capsule	Slow release[1]
Cardene® SR	Capsule	Slow release
Cardizem®	Tablet	Slow release
Cardizem® CD	Capsule	Slow release[1]
Cardizem® LA	Tablet	Slow release
Cardizem® SR	Capsule	Slow release[1]
Carter's Little Pills®	Tablet	Enteric-coated
Cartia® XT	Capsule	Slow release
Ceclor® CD	Tablet	Slow release
Ceftin®	Tablet	Taste[2] **Note:** Use suspension for children
CellCept®	Capsule, tablet	Teratogenic potential[9]
Charcoal Plus®	Tablet	Enteric-coated
Chloral Hydrate	Capsule	**Note:** Product is in liquid form within a special capsule[2]
Chlor-Trimeton® 12-Hour	Tablet	Slow release[2]
Cipro™	Tablet	Taste[5]
Cipro® XR	Tablet	Slow release
Claritin-D® 12-Hour	Tablet	Slow release
Claritin-D® 24-Hour	Tablet	Slow release
Colace®	Capsule	Taste[5]
Colestid®	Tablet	Slow release
Comhist® LA	Capsule	Slow release[1]

ORAL MEDICATIONS THAT SHOULD NOT BE CRUSHED
(Continued)

Drug Product	Dosage Form	Dosage Reasons / Comments
Commit™	Lozenge	**Note:** Integrity compromised by chewing or crushing
Compazine® Spansule®	Capsule	Slow release[2]
Concerta®	Tablet	Slow release
Contac® 12-Hour	Tablet	Slow release
Cotazym-S®	Capsule	Enteric-coated[1]
Covera-HS™	Tablet	Slow release
Creon® 5, 10, 20	Capsule	Slow release[1]
Crixivan®	Capsule	Taste **Note:** Capsule may be opened and mixed with fruit puree (eg, banana)
Cymbalta®	Capsule	Enteric-coated
Cytovene®	Capsule	Skin irritant
Cytoxan®	Tablet	**Note:** Drug may be crushed, but maker recommends using injection
Dallergy®	Capsule	Slow release
Dallergy-JR®	Capsule	Slow release
Deconamine® SR	Capsule	Slow release[2]
Defen L.A.®	Tablet	Slow release[8]
Depakene®	Capsule	Slow release mucous membrane irritant[2]
Depakote®	Tablet	Slow release
Depakote® ER	Tablet	Slow release
Desoxyn®	Tablet	Slow release
Desyrel®	Tablet	Taste[5]
Detrol® LA	Capsule	Slow release
Dexedrine® Spansule®	Capsule	Slow release
Diamox® Sequels®	Capsule	Slow release
Dilacor® XR	Capsule	Slow release
Dilatrate-SR®	Capsule	Slow release
Diltia XT®	Capsule	Slow release
Ditropan® XL	Tablet	Slow release
Dolobid®	Tablet	Irritant
Donnatal® Extentab®	Tablet	Slow release[2]
Drisdol®	Capsule	Liquid filled[4]
Drixoral®	Tablet	Slow release[2]
Drixoral® Plus	Tablet	Slow release
Drixoral® Sinus	Tablet	Slow release
Dulcolax®	Capsule	Liquid-filled
Dulcolax®	Tablet	Enteric-coated[3]
Duratuss® G	Tablet	Slow release[9]
Duratuss® GP	Tablet	Slow release[8]
Dynabac®	Tablet	Enteric-coated
DynaCirc® CR	Tablet	Slow release
Easprin®	Tablet	Enteric-coated
EC-Naprosyn®	Tablet	Enteric-coated
Ecotrin® Adult Low Strength	Tablet	Enteric-coated
Ecotrin® Maximum Strength	Tablet	Enteric-coated
Ecotrin® Regular Strength	Tablet	Enteric-coated
E.E.S.® 400	Tablet	Enteric-coated[2]
Effexor® XR	Capsule	Slow release
Efidac/24® Pseudoephedrine	Tablet	Slow release
Efidac® 24	Tablet	Slow release

Drug Product	Dosage Form	Dosage Reasons / Comments
E-Mycin®	Tablet	Enteric-coated
Entex® LA	Capsule	Slow release[2]
Entex® PSE	Capsule	Slow release
Entocort™ EC	Capsule	Enteric-coated[1]
Ergomar®	Tablet	Sublingual form[7]
Eryc®	Capsule	Enteric-coated[1]
Ery-Tab®	Tablet	Enteric-coated
Erythrocin Stearate	Tablet	Enteric-coated
Erythromycin Base	Tablet	Enteric-coated
Eskalith CR®	Tablet	Slow release
Evista®	Tablet	Taste; teratogenic potential[9]
Extendryl JR	Capsule	Slow release[2]
Extendryl SR	Capsule	Slow release[2]
Feldene®	Capsule	Mucous membrane irritant
Feosol®	Tablet	Enteric-coated[2]
Feratab®	Tablet	Enteric-coated[2]
Fergon®	Tablet	Enteric-coated
Fero-Grad 500®	Tablet	Slow release
Ferro-Sequels®	Tablet	Slow release
Flagyl ER®	Tablet	Slow release
Flomax®	Capsule	Enteric-coated[1]
Fosamax®	Tablet	Mucous membrane irritant
Fumatinic®	Capsule	Slow release
Geocillin®	Tablet	Taste
Gleevec®	Tablet	Taste[8] Note: May be dissolved in mineral oil or apple juice
Glucophage® XR	Tablet	Slow release
Glucotrol® XL	Tablet	Slow release
Gris-PEG®	Tablet	Note: Crushing may result in precipitation of larger particles.
Guaifed®	Capsule	Slow release
Guaifed®-PD	Capsule	Slow release
Guaifenex® DM	Tablet	Slow release[8]
Guaifenex® LA	Tablet	Slow release[8]
Guaifenex® PSE	Tablet	Slow release[8]
Guaimax-D®	Tablet	Slow release
Hista-Vent® DA	Tablet	Slow release[8]
Humibid® DM	Tablet	Slow release
Humibid® LA	Tablet	Slow release
Iberet® Filmtab	Tablet	Slow release[2]
Iberet®-500	Tablet	Slow release[2]
Iberet-Folic-500®	Tablet	Slow release
ICAPS® Time Release	Tablet	Slow release
Imdur™	Tablet	Slow release[8]
Inderal® LA	Capsule	Slow release
Inderide® LA	Capsule	Slow release
Indocin® SR	Capsule	Slow release[1,2]
InnoPran XL™	Capsule	Slow release
Ionamin®	Capsule	Slow release
Isoptin® SR	Tablet	Slow release
Isordil® Sublingual	Tablet	Sublingual form[7]
Isosorbide Dinitrate Sublingual	Tablet	Sublingual form[7]
Isosorbide SR	Tablet	Slow release
K+ 8®	Tablet	Slow release[2]
K+ 10®	Tablet	Slow release[2]
Kadian®	Capsule	Slow release[1] Note: Do not give via N/G tubes

ORAL MEDICATIONS THAT SHOULD NOT BE CRUSHED
(Continued)

Drug Product	Dosage Form	Dosage Reasons / Comments
Kaon-Cl®	Tablet	Slow release[2]
K-Dur®	Tablet	Slow release
Klor-Con®	Tablet	Slow release[2]
Klor-Con® M	Tablet	Slow release[2]
Klotrix®	Tablet	Slow release[2]
K-Lyte®	Tablet	Effervescent tablet[6]
K-Lyte/Cl®	Tablet	Effervescent tablet[6]
K-Lyte DS®	Tablet	Effervescent tablet[6]
K-Tab®	Tablet	Slow release[2]
Lescol® XL	Tablet	Slow release
Levbid®	Tablet	Slow release[8]
Levsinex® Timecaps®	Capsule	Slow release
Lexxel®	Tablet	Slow release
Lipram 4500	Capsule	Enteric-coated[1]
Lipram-CR	Capsule	Enteric-coated[1]
Lipram-PN	Capsule	Enteric-coated[1]
Lipram-UL	Capsule	Enteric-coated[1]
Lipram (all products)	Capsule	Slow release[1]
Liquibid-PD	Tablet	Slow release[8]
Lithobid®	Tablet	Slow release
Lodine® XL	Tablet	Slow release
Lodrane® LD	Capsule	Slow release[1]
Mag-Tab® SR	Tablet	Slow release
Maxifed®	Tablet	Slow release
Maxifed® DM	Tablet	Slow release
Maxifed-G®	Tablet	Slow release
Mestinon® Timespan®	Tablet	Slow release[2]
Metadate® CD	Capsule	Slow release[1]
Metadate™ ER	Tablet	Slow release
Methylin™ ER	Tablet	Slow release
Micro-K®	Capsule	Slow release
Motrin®	Tablet	Taste[5]
MS Contin®	Tablet	Slow release[2]
Mucinex®	Tablet	Slow release
Myfortic®	Tablet	Slow release
Naprelan®	Tablet	Slow release
Nasatab® LA	Tablet	Slow release[8]
Nexium®	Capsule	Slow release[1]
Niaspan®	Tablet	Slow release
Nicotinic Acid	Capsule, tablet	Slow release
Nifediac™ CC	Tablet	Slow release
Nitrostat®	Tablet	Sublingual route[7]
Norflex™	Tablet	Slow release
Norpace® CR	Capsule	Slow release form within a special capsule
Oramorph SR®	Tablet	Slow release[2]
Oruvail®	Capsule	Slow release
OxyContin®	Tablet	Slow release
Palgic®-D	Tablet	Slow release[8]
Pancrease®	Capsule	Enteric-coated[1]
Pancrease® MT	Capsule	Enteric-coated[1]
Pancrecarb MS®	Capsule	Enteric-coated[1]
PanMist®-DM	Tablet	Slow release[8]
PanMist®-Jr	Tablet	Slow release[8]

Drug Product	Dosage Form	Dosage Reasons / Comments
PanMist®-LA	Tablet	Slow release[8]
Pannaz®	Tablet	Slow release[8]
Papaverine Sustained Action	Capsule	Slow release
Paxil CR™	Tablet	Slow release
Pentasa®	Capsule	Slow release
Perdiem® Fiber Therapy	Granules	Wax coated
PhenaVent™ D	Tablet	Slow release
Plendil®	Tablet	Slow release
Prelu-2®	Capsule	Slow release
Prevacid®	Capsule	Slow release
Prevacid®	Suspension	Slow release **Note:** Contains enteric-coated granules
Prilosec®	Capsule	Slow release
Procainamide HCl SR	Tablet	Slow release
Procanbid®	Tablet	Slow release
Procardia®	Capsule	Delays absorption[2, 5]
Procardia XL®	Tablet	Slow release **Note:** AUC is unaffected.
Profen II®	Tablet	Slow release[8]
Profen II DM®	Tablet	Slow release[8]
Profen Forte™ DM	Tablet	Slow release
Pronestyl®-SR	Tablet	Slow release
Propecia®	Tablet	**Note:** Women who are, or may become, pregnant, should not handle crushed or broken tablets
Proscar®	Tablet	**Note:** Women who are, or may become, pregnant, should not handle crushed or broken tablets
Protonix®	Tablet	Slow release
Quibron-T/SR®	Tablet	Slow release[2]
Rescon-Jr	Tablet	Slow release
Respa-DM®	Tablet	Slow release[8]
Respaire®-120 SR	Capsule	Slow release
Ritalin-SR®	Tablet	Slow release
Rondec-TR®	Tablet	Slow release[2]
Rythmol® SR	Capsule	Slow release
Sinemet® CR	Tablet	Slow release
SINUvent® PE	Tablet	Slow release[8]
Slo-Niacin®	Tablet	Slow release[8]
Slow-Mag®	Tablet	Slow release
Somnote™	Capsule	Liquid filled
Sudafed® 12-Hour	Capsule	Slow release[2]
Sular®	Tablet	Slow release
Symax SR	Tablet	Slow release
Taztia XT™	Capsule	Slow release
Tegretol®-XR	Tablet	Slow release
Temodar®	Capsule	**Note:** If capsules are accidentally opened or damaged, rigorous precautions should be taken to avoid inhalation or contact of contents with the skin or mucous membranes[9]
Tessalon®	Capsule	Slow release
Theo-24®	Tablet	Slow release[2]
Theochron®	Tablet	Slow release
Tiazac®	Capsule	Slow release
Topamax®	Capsule	Taste[1]
Topamax®	Tablet	Taste
Touro™ CC	Tablet	Slow release

ORAL MEDICATIONS THAT SHOULD NOT BE CRUSHED
(Continued)

Drug Product	Dosage Form	Dosage Reasons / Comments
Touro EX®	Tablet	Slow release
Touro LA®	Tablet	Slow release
Trental®	Tablet	Slow release
TripTone®	Tablet	Slow release
Tylenol® Arthritis Pain	Tablet	Slow release
Tylenol® 8 Hour	Tablet	Slow release
Ultrase®	Capsule	Enteric-coated[1]
Ultrase® MT	Capsule	Enteric-coated[1]
Uniphyl®	Tablet	Slow release
Urocit®-K	Tablet	Wax-coated
Verelan®	Capsule	Slow release[1]
Videx® EC	Capsule	Slow release
Voltaren®-XR	Tablet	Slow release
VoSpire ER™	Tablet	Slow release
Wellbutrin SR®	Tablet	Slow release
Wellbutrin XL™	Tablet	Slow release
Xanax XR®	Tablet	Slow release
Z-Cof LA	Tablet	Slow release[8]
Zephrex LA®	Tablet	Slow release
ZORprin®	Tablet	Slow release
Zyban®	Tablet	Slow release

[1]Capsule may be opened and the contents taken without crushing or chewing; soft food such as applesauce or pudding may facilitate administration; contents may generally be administered via nasogastric tube using an appropriate fluid, provided entire contents are washed down the tube.

[2]Liquid dosage forms of the product are available; however, dose, frequency of administration, and manufacturers may differ from that of the solid dosage form.

[3]Antacids and/or milk may prematurely dissolve the coating of the tablet.

[4]Capsule may be opened and the liquid contents removed for administration.

[5]The taste of this product in a liquid form would likely be unacceptable to the patient; administration via nasogastric tube should be acceptable.

[6]Effervescent tablets must be dissolved in the amount of diluent recommended by the manufacturer.

[7]Tablets are made to disintegrate under the tongue.

[8]Tablet is scored and may be broken in half without affecting release characteristics.

[9]Skin contact may enhance tumor production; avoid direct contact.

Adapted from Mitchell JF, "Oral Dosage Forms That Should Not Be Crushed-2004," available at www.hospitalpharmacyjournal.com.

PRESSURE ULCER TREATMENT

Specific Treatment Options by Category	Description by Category	Advantages by Category	Disadvantages by Category
Surgical Debridement Indicated when there is evidence of cellulitis or sepsis	Surgical excision of eschar by physician; may require concomitant treatment with systemic antimicrobials.	Repaid removal of necrotic tissue. Large wounds may be partially debrided reducing risk to resident.	May require hospitalization for procedure. Caution must be used with those who are immunosuppressed, debilitated, or have bleeding disorders. May leave some necrotic debris in place.
Autolytic Debriders Absorption, hydrocolloid, and transparent dressings Indicated in wounds with minimal exudate. Do not use in presence of infection.	Use of occlusive dressings or dressings which impart moisture to soften and liquefy necrotic tissue.	Selective form of debridement (does not harm healing tissue). Effective alternative for debridement of small wounds. Readily available.	May lead to infection in large necrotic wounds. Not indicated for clinically infected wounds due to increased bacterial growth beneath dressing.
Enzymatic Debriders Uses topical agents such as collagenase, papain, fibrinolysin, and deoxyribonuclease; promotes growth of granulation tissue. Indicated in patients in long-term care or who cannot tolerate surgery. Accuzyme® Biozyme-C® Elase® Elase-Chloromycetin® Ethezyme™ Granulex Panafil® Panafil ® SE Santyl®	Enzyme topically applied to necrotic surface; usually covered with wet gauze and/or transparent dressing; applying a protectant (ie, moisture barrier cream) to surrounding tissue may be indicated; often requires concomitant treatment with topical or systemic antimicrobials; discontinue when wound is red and granulating or if it bleeds easily when cleansed.	Less traumatic than surgical debriding. Ease of application. Cost-effective debridement therapy.	Cross-hatching recommended if thick eschar is present. Some detergents and antiseptics may inactivate certain products. Effect on viable tissue varies by product. Takes longer than surgical debridement. May need barrier cream around wound to protect healthy skin. Requires secondary dressing.
Mechanical Debriders Wet-to-dry gauze dressings, hydrotherapy, wound irrigation and scrubbing the wound with gauze. Best for wounds with thick exudate, slough on loose necrotic tissue.	Removal of eschar using mechanical forces that pull off necrotic tissue; discontinue when wound is red and granulating or if it bleeds easily when cleansed.	Promotes softening and loosening of eschar. Potentially less traumatic than surgical debridement. Economical. Readily available.	Generally not as effective in severely necrotic wounds. Must monitor for signs of injury to healthy tissue.
Cleansing Solutions Acetic acid Hydrogen peroxide Lactated Ringer's Normal saline Shur-Clens®	Cleansing solution that also hydrates; some products are bactericidal.	Cleanses wound. Maintains moist environment.	Can disturb granulation tissue. Can be cytotoxic if not diluted or used too vigorously.

PRESSURE ULCER TREATMENT *(Continued)*

Specific Treatment Options by Category	Description by Category	Advantages by Category	Disadvantages by Category
Topical Antibiotics Betadine® Gentamicin Mupirocin Neosporin® Silvadene®	Antimicrobial solutions, ointments and creams; indicated for prophylaxis or for treatment of an infected wound.	Easy to apply. Water miscible creams easy to remove. Helps control bacterial growth until necrotic tissue can be debrided.	May have cytotoxic effects which may delay wound healing. Ointments are difficult to remove. Allergic reactions may occur. Bacteria may become resistant with prolonged use.
Absorption Dressings Bard® dressings Debrisan® DuoDERM® FlexiGel Strands® Intrasite® Iodoflex® Iodosorb® Sorbsan®	Includes granules, flakes, paste, and pads; placed directly into wound bed to absorb exudate; provides minor debriding action by retaining wound debris.	Absorbs wound exudate while maintaining wound moisture. Cleanses wound bed. Reduces wound odor.	Some dressings require irrigation to remove from wound. May increase time for dressing changes. May impair granulation and epithelialization by drying wound bed, if exudate is minimal. Permeable to fluids and bacteria. Contraindicated with tunneling. May sting upon application. Requires secondary dressing.
Gauze Dressings	Fine mesh gauze dressing used as vehicle for soaks, lubricants, or antimicrobials.	Economical. Readily available. Effective delivery of solution if kept moist. Cost-effective filler for large wounds.	May cause bleeding, pain, and remove healthy granulation tissue if allowed to dry. Requires increased nursing time to keep dressing moist.
Hydrocolloid Dressings DuoDERM® Ultec®	Dressing that reacts with exudate to form a gel; creates a physical barrier and maintains a moist/acidic environment.	Totally occlusive; protects wound from physical injury and contamination. Maintains moist environment. Easy removal without adhesion to wound surface. May remain on wound for up to 5 days. Waterproof dressing allows resident to shower.	Difficult to observe wound. May promote development of infection in deep wounds. May accumulate excess fluid and macerate tissue. Dressing may soften, and wrinkles may increase pressure on wound base.
Nonadherent Dressings Adaptic® Exu-Dry® Telfa® Vaseline® Gauze	Nonocclusive, absorbent dressing; may be used with topical medications.	Easy to use. Inexpensive. Nontraumatic.	Nonocclusive. Does not physically protect wound site from injury. Less absorptive than plain gauze. Need secondary dressing.
Transparent Dressings Acu-Derm® Bioclusive® Blisterfilm® Op-Site® Tegaderm® Uniflex®	Adhesive, transparent, thin film-type semipermeable dressing; semipermeable membrane allows moisture and oxygen exchange.	A barrier to contamination that also keeps wound moist. Allows for easy visual inspection. Good adhesive properties. Waterproof dressing allows resident to shower. Reduces pain. Time saving.	May lead to tissue maceration in extremely moist wounds. Some products are difficult to apply, and wrinkling may occur. May promote infection if necrotic tissue is present. Potential for adhesive injury. Expensive.

Specific Treatment Options by Category	Description by Category	Advantages by Category	Disadvantages by Category
Hydrogels Carrington® Wound Gel Elastogel® Intrasite® Gel Vigilon®	Topicals with absorptive and moisturizing properties.	Nonadherent. May cool and/or soothe wound. Easy to apply. Conforms to wound bed.	Usually requires protective outer dressing. May require multiple daily dressing changes. May macerate surrounding tissue.
Pain Pain may be present in pressure ulcers and does not respond well to oral drugs at doses low enough to avoid side effects	Extemporaneous preparation may be helpful topically. 1 mL injectable morphine sulfate in 8 g of Intrasite® gel applied topically once daily; cover with Tegaderm® dressing.		

References

Agency for Health Care Policy and Research, "Pressure Ulcers in Adults: Prediction and Prevention," Clinical Practice Guideline Number 3, AHCPR Publication No. 92-0050, May 1992.

Agency for Health Care Policy and Research, "Treatment of Pressure Ulcers," Clinical Practice Guideline Number 15, AHCPR Publication No. 95-0652, December 1994.

Flock P, "Pilot Study to Determine the Effectiveness of Diamorphine Gel to Control Pressure Ulcer Pain," *J Pain Symptom Manage*, 2003, 25(6):547-54.

Goode PS and Thomas DR, "Pressure Ulcers. Local Wound Care," *Clin Geriatr Med*, 1997, 13(3):543-52.

Lee LK and Ambrus JL, "Collagenase Therapy for Decubitus Ulcers," *Geriatrics*, 1975, 30(5):91-3, 97-8.

Lyder CH, "Pressure Ulcer Prevention and Management," *JAMA*, 2003, 289(2):223-6.

Pullen R, Popp R, Volkers P, et al, "Prospective Randomized Double-Blind Study of the Wound-Debriding Effects of Collagenase and Fibrinolysin/Deoxyribonuclease in Pressure Ulcers," *Age Ageing*, 2002, 31(2):126-30.

Rao DB, Sane PG, and Georgiev EL, "Collagenase in the Treatment of Dermal and Decubitus Ulcers," *J Am Geriatr Soc*, 1975, 23(1):22-30.

Zeppetella G, Paul J, and Ribeiro MD, "Analgesic Efficacy of Morphine Applied Topically to Painful Ulcers," *J Pain Symptom Manage*, 2003, 25(6):555-8.

SERUM DRUG CONCENTRATIONS COMMONLY MONITORED GUIDELINES

Drug	When to Sample	Therapeutic Concentration[1]	Usual Half-Life	Steady State (Ideal Sampling Time)	Potentially Toxic Concentration[1]
Antibiotics					
Gentamicin Tobramycin	30 min after 30 min infusion Trough: <0.5 h before next dose	Peak: 4-10 mcg/mL Trough: <2.0 mcg/mL	2 h	15 h	Peak: >12 mcg/mL Trough: >2 mcg/mL
Amikacin		Peak: 20-35 mcg/mL Trough: <8 mcg/mL	2 h	15 h	Peak: >35 mcg/mL Trough: >8 mcg/mL
Vancomycin	Peak: 1 h after 1 h infusion Trough: <0.5 h before next dose	Peak: 30-40 mcg/mL Trough: 5-10 mcg/mL	6-8 h	24 h	Peak: >80 mcg/mL Trough: >13 mcg/mL
Anticonvulsants					
Ethosuximide	Trough: Just before next oral dose	40-100 mcg/mL	30-60 h	10-13 d	>100 mcg/mL
Lamotrigine	Prior to dose	0.25-29 mcg/mL	25-33 h		
Gabapentin			5-6 h		
Phenobarbital	Trough: Just before next dose	15-40 mcg/mL	40-120 h	20 d	>40 mcg/mL
Phenytoin Free phenytoin	Trough: Just before next dose Draw at same time as total serum concentration	10-20 mcg/mL 1-2 mcg/mL	Concentration dependent	5-14 d	>20 mcg/mL
Primidone	Trough: Just before next dose (**Note:** Primidone is metabolized to phenobarb, order levels separately)	5-12 mcg/mL	10-12 h	5 d	>12 mcg/mL
Bronchodilators					
Aminophylline (I.V.)	18-24 h after starting or changing a maintenance dose given as a constant infusion	10-20 mcg/mL	Nonsmoking adults: 8 h Smoking adults: 4 h	2 d	>20 mcg/mL
Theophylline (P.O.)	Peak: Not recommended Trough: Just before next dose	10-20 mcg/mL	4-8 h	2 d	>20 mcg/mL
Cardiovascular Agents					
Digitoxin	Peak: Not necessary Trough: Prior to dose	20-35 ng/mL	7-8 days	5 wk	>45 ng/mL
Digoxin	Trough: Just before next dose (serum concentration drawn earlier than 6 h after a dose will be artificially elevated)	0.5-2 ng/mL	36 h	5 d	>2 ng/mL
Lidocaine	Steady-state concentrations are usually achieved after 6-12 h	1.2-5.0 mcg/mL	1.5 h	5-10 h	>6 mcg/mL

Drug	When to Sample	Therapeutic Concentration[1]	Usual Half-Life	Steady State (Ideal Sampling Time)	Potentially Toxic Concentration[1]
Procainamide	Trough: Just before next oral dose I.V.: 6-12 h after infusion started Combined procainamide plus NAPA	4-10 mcg/mL NAPA: 6-10 h, 5-30 mcg/mL	Procain: 2.7-5 h >30 (NAPA + procain)	20 h	>10 mcg/mL
Quinidine	Trough: Just before next oral dose	2-5 mcg/mL	6 h	24 h	>10 mcg/mL
Psychotropic Agents					
Amitriptyline plus nortriptyline	12 hours after the last dose	100-250 ng/mL	Amitriptyline: 9-25 h Nortriptyline: 28-31 h	4-8 d	>500 ng/mL
Carbamazepine	12 hours after the last dose	4-12 mcg/mL 4-8 mcg/mL in combination with other anticonvulsants	15-20 h	7-12 d	>12 mcg/mL
Desipramine	12 hours after the last dose	125-160 ng/mL	12-54 h	3-11 d	>300 ng/mL
Imipramine plus desipramine	12 hours after the last dose	150-300 ng/mL	9-24 h	2-5 d	>500 ng/mL
Lithium	12 hours after the last dose	0.6-1.2 mEq/mL	18-20 h	2-7 d	>3 mEq/mL
Nortriptyline	12 hours after the last dose	50-150 ng/mL	28-31 h	4-19 d	>500 ng/mL
Valproic acid	12 hours after the last dose	50-100 mcg/mL	5-20 h	4 d	>150 mcg/mL
Other Agents					
Cyclosporine	Trough: Just before next dose or 12-18 h after oral dose	Months post-transplant: Plasma: 50-150 ng/mL Whole blood: 150-450 ng/mL	17-40 h	Variable 5 half-lives	>400 ng/mL
Salicylates	Peak: 2 h after oral ingestion Trough: Just before next oral dose	150-400 mcg/mL	3-15 h	15-75 h	>400 mcg/mL

[1]Due to methodology differences, reference ranges may vary from laboratory to laboratory; check with the laboratory service used for their appropriate levels.

PHARMACOLOGIC CATEGORY INDEX

Acetylcholinesterase Inhibitor

Acetylcholinesterase Inhibitor (Central)

Acne Products

Adrenergic Agonist Agent

Alkalinizing Agent

Alkalinizing Agent, Oral

Alpha$_1$ Agonist

Alpha$_1$ Blocker

Alpha$_1$ Blocker, Ophthalmic

Alpha$_2$-Adrenergic Agonist

Alpha$_2$ Agonist, Ophthalmic

Alpha-Adrenergic Inhibitor

Alpha/Beta Agonist

5 Alpha-Reductase Inhibitor

Amebicide

Aminoquinoline (Antimalarial)

5-Aminosalicylic Acid Derivative

Ammonium Detoxicant

Amylinomimetic

Vasodilator *(Continued)*

Vasopressin Analog, Synthetic

Vasopressin Antagonist

Vitamin D Analog

Vitamin, Fat Soluble

Vitamin, Water Soluble

Xanthine Oxidase Inhibitor

Other Products Offered by Lexi-Comp®

Anesthesiology & Critical Care Drug Handbook

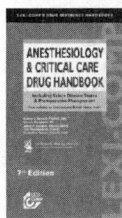

Designed for anesthesiologists, critical care practitioners, and all healthcare professionals involved in the care of surgical or ICU patients.

Includes: Comprehensive drug information to ensure the appropriate clinical management of patients; Intensivist and Anesthesiologist perspective; Over 2000 medications most commonly used in the preoperative and critical care setting; and Special Topics/Issues section with frequently encountered patient conditions

Clinician's Guide to Diagnosis

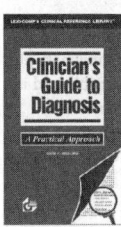

A reference with a practical approach to commonly-encountered symptoms, designed to follow the logical thought process of a seasoned clinician.

Includes: Evidence-based, easy-to-find answers to the questions that commonly arise in the symptom evaluation process; Over 35 algorithms that provide parallel references to the information in each chapter

Clinician's Guide to Internal Medicine

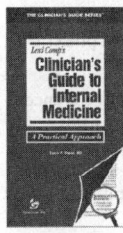

Quick access to essential information covering diagnosis, treatment, and management of commonly-encountered patient conditions in Internal Medicine.

Includes: Practical approaches ideal for point-of-care use; Algorithms to establish a diagnosis and select the appropriate therapy; and Tables to summarize diagnostic and therapeutic strategies

Clinician's Guide to Laboratory Medicine

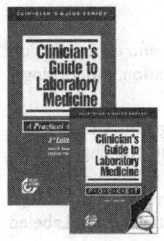

A resource providing a logical step-by-step process from an abnormal lab test to diagnosis. This two-book set provides you with a full size guide and a portable pocket version for convenient referencing.

Includes: 137 chapters; 700 charts, tables, and algorithms; and sections such as neurology, infectious diseases, and obstetrics/gynecology

Other Products Offered by Lexi-Comp®

Drug Information Handbook

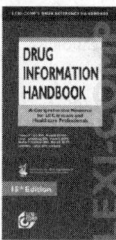

This easy-to-use drug reference is for the pharmacist, physician, or other healthcare professional requiring fast access to comprehensive drug information.

Over 1400 drug monographs are detailed with up to 33 fields of information per monograph. A valuable appendix includes hundreds of charts and reviews of special topics such as guidelines for treatment and therapy recommendations. A pharmacologic category index is also provided.

Published in cooperation with APhA.

Drug Information Handbook with International Trade Names Index

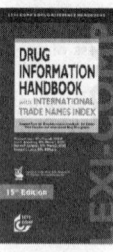

Drug Information Handbook with International Trade Names Index includes the same content of our *Drug Information Handbook*, plus International drug monographs for use worldwide! Published in cooperation with APhA, this easy-to-use drug reference is compiled especially for the pharmacist, physician, or other healthcare professional seeking quick access to comprehensive drug information.

Drug Information Handbook for Advanced Practice Nursing

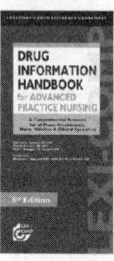

Designed to assist the Advanced Practice Nurse with prescribing, monitoring, and educating patients.

Includes: Over 4800 generic and brand names, cross-referenced by page number; Drug names and important Nursing fields highlighted in RED; Labeled and investigational indications; Adult, Geriatric, and Pediatric dosing; and Up to 58 fields including critical information on Patient Education and Physical Assessment

Drug Information Handbook for Nursing

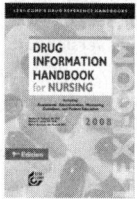

Designed for registered professional nurses and upper-division nursing students requiring dosing, administration, monitoring, and patient education information.

Includes: Over 4800 generic and brand drug names cross-referenced by page number; Drug names and Nursing fields in RED; Fields of information include: Nursing Actions: Physical Assessment, and Patient Education; and Administration: I.V. Detail, Storage, Reconstitution, and Compatibility; and Labeled and investigational indications

To order call Customer Service at 1-866-397-3433 or go to www.lexi.com.
Outside of the U.S. call: 330-650-6506 or www.lexi.com

Other Products Offered by Lexi-Comp®

Drug Information Handbook for Oncology

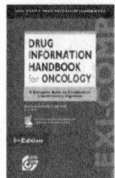

Designed for oncology professionals requiring information on combination chemotherapy regimens and dosing protocols.

Includes: Monographs containing warnings, adverse reaction profiles, drug interactions, dosing for specific indications, vesicant, emetic potential, combination regimens, and more; Where applicable, a special Combination Chemotherapy field that will link you to specific oncology monographs; Special Topics such as Cancer Treatment Related Complications, Bone Marrow Transplantation, and Drug Development

Drug Information Handbook for Perioperative Nursing

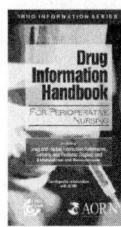

Designed especially for perioperative nurses, Registered Nurses practicing in operative and interventional procedure settings, and upper-division nursing students seeking a distinctive reference for dosing, administration, monitoring, and patient education criteria for perioperative patient care environments.

Includes: Up to 40 fields per monograph including Medication Safety data; Adult, Pediatric, and Geriatric Dosing guidelines; and information on each phase of the perioperative encounter, with emphasis on special situations central to perioperative patient care

Drug Information Handbook for Psychiatry

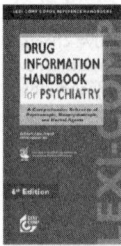

Designed for any healthcare professional requiring quick access to comprehensive drug information as it relates to mental health issues.

Includes: Detailed drug monographs for psychotropic, nonpsychotropic, and herbal medications; Special fields such as Mental Health Comment (useful clinical pearls), Medication Safety Issues, Effects on Mental Status, and Effects on Psychiatric Treatment

Laboratory Test Handbook

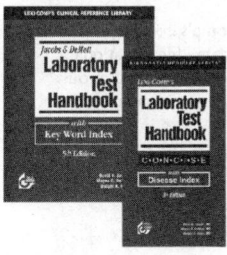

An invaluable source of information for anyone interested in diagnostic laboratory testing. Includes: 960 tests; Up to 25 fields per test; Extensive cross-referencing; Over 12,000 references; and Key Word Index: test result, disease, organ system and syndrome.

Clinicians, nurse practitioners, residents, nurses, and students will appreciate the Concise version of the *Laboratory Test Handbook* for its convenience as a quick reference. This abridged version includes 876 tests.

To order call Customer Service at 1-866-397-3433 or go to www.lexi.com.
Outside of the U.S. call: 330-650-6506 or www.lexi.com

Other Products Offered by Lexi-Comp®

Pediatric Dosage Handbook

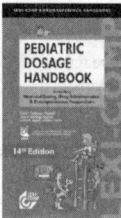

This book is designed for any healthcare professional requiring quick access to comprehensive pediatric drug information. Each monograph contains multiple field of content, including usual dosage by age group, indication and route of administration. Drug interactions, adverse reactions, extemporaneous preparations, pharmacodynamics/pharma-cokinetics data, and medication safety issue are covered.

Pediatric Dosage Handbook with International Trade Names Index also available.

Pharmacogenomics Handbook

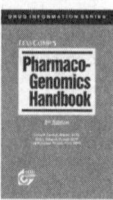

Ideal for any healthcare professional or student wishing to gain insight into the emerging field of pharmacogenomics.

Includes: Information concerning key genetic variations that may influence drug disposition and/or sensitivity; brief introductions to fundamental concepts in genetics and genomics. A foundation for all clinicians who will be called on to integrate rapidly-expanding genomic knowledge into the management of drug therapy.

Pharmacology Companion Guide

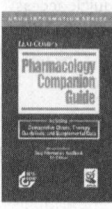

This guide supplies the best of Lexi-Comp's comparative charts, therapy guidelines, and supplemental data. Ideal for healthcare providers who require a quick reference to all the key appendix information found in our popular *Drug Information Handbook* or as a companion to our PDA software.

Includes: Abbreviations and measurements; ACLS Algorithms; Cytochrome P450 and Drug Interactions; and Laboratory Values

Pediatric Pharmacology Companion Guide

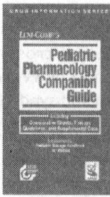

This guide supplies the best of Lexi-Comp's comparative charts, therapy guidelines, and supplemental data. Ideal as a quick reference to all the key appendix information found in our popular *Pediatric Dosage Handbook* or as a companion to our PDA software.

Includes: Apgar Scoring System; CPR Pediatric Drug Dosages; Immunization Guidelines; and Pediatric ALS Algorithms

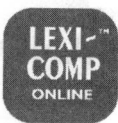
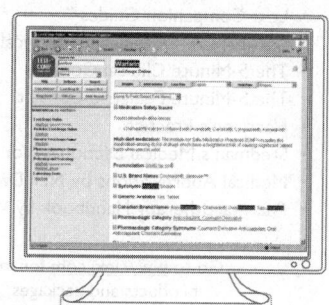

Ot[h]   ®

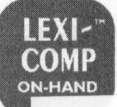

Lexi-Comp ON-HAND

Available for Palm OS® , Pocket PC, and

At Lexi-[Comp]... [commun]ally [d]rug information [at] ... [care]. Our [content is not subject to] third party recommendations or suggestions, but is based on the contributions of our respected authors, internal clinical team, and the thousands of professionals within the healthcare industry who constantly review and validate our data.

With Lexi-Comp® ON-HAND, you can be confident you are accessing the most up-to-date information on the latest warnings and new drug information. All updates are included with your annual subscription.

Lexi-Comp ON-HAND databases include:

- Lexi-Drugs®
- Pediatric Lexi-Drugs®
- Lexi-Interact™
- Lexi-Natural Products™
- Lexi-Poisoning & Toxicolog[y]
- Lexi-Infectious Diseases™
- Lexi-Lab & Diagnostic Proc[edures]
- Nursing Lexi-Drugs®
- Perioperative Nursing Lexi[-Drugs]
- Dental Lexi-Drugs®
- Lexi-Pharmacogenomics™
- Lexi-PALS™ (Patient Advisory Leaflets)
- Lexi-Drug ID™
- Lexi-CALC™
- Lexi-I.V. Compatibility™
- Lexi-Companion Guides™
- Lexi-NBCA™ (Nuclear, Biological, & Chemical Agent) Exposures
- The 5-Minute Clinical Consult
- The 5-Minute Pediatric Consult
- Harrison's Practice
- Stedman's Medical Dictionary for the Health Professions and Nursing
- Medical Abbreviations by Neil Davis
- Pharmacotherapy Handbook by Wells

Erythromycin   Jump
Pharmacologic Category
Antibiotic, Macrolide; Antibiotic,
Ophthalmic; Antibiotic, Topical;
Topical Skin Product; Topical Skin
Product, Acne

Use
Systemic: Treatment of susceptible
bacterial infections including S.
pyogenes, some S. pneumoniae,
some S. aureus, M. pneumoniae,

Go to www.lexi.com for more information on Lexi-Comp's products and packages. See opposite page for clinical areas covered by the LEXI-COMP® Knowledge Solution™.